DERMATOLOGY IN GENERAL MEDICINE

EDITORS

Thomas B. Fitzpatrick, M.D., Ph.D., D.Sc. (Hon)

Edward C. Wigglesworth Professor of Dermatology, Emeritus
Chairman Emeritus, Department of Dermatology
Harvard Medical School
Chief Emeritus, Dermatology Service
Massachusetts General Hospital
Boston, Massachusetts

Arthur Z. Eisen, M.D.

Winfred A. and Emma R. Showman Professor of Medicine
Chairman, Division of Dermatology
Washington University School of Medicine
Dermatologist-in-Chief
Barnes Hospital
St. Louis, Missouri

Klaus Wolff, M.D.

Professor and Chairman, Department of Dermatology
University of Vienna Medical School
Head, Division of General Dermatology
Vienna General Hospital
Vienna, Austria

Irwin M. Freedberg, M.D.

George Miller MacKee Professor and Chairman
Ronald O. Perelman Department of Dermatology
New York University Medical Center
New York, New York

K. Frank Austen, M.D.

Theodore B. Bayles Professor of Medicine
Harvard Medical School
Chairman, Department of Rheumatology and Immunology
Brigham and Women's Hospital
Boston, Massachusetts

COLOR ILLUSTRATION EDITOR

Richard Allen Johnson, M.D.C.M.

Harvard Medical School
New England Deaconess Hospital
Boston, Massachusetts

Fourth Edition

DERMATOLOGY IN GENERAL MEDICINE

VOLUME II

EDITORS

Thomas B. Fitzpatrick, M.D.

Arthur Z. Eisen, M.D.

Klaus Wolff, M.D.

Irwin M. Freedberg, M.D.

K. Frank Austen, M.D.

McGraw-Hill, Inc.

HEALTH PROFESSIONS DIVISION

*New York St. Louis San Francisco Auckland Bogotá Caracas Lisbon
London Madrid Mexico Milan Montreal New Delhi Paris
San Juan Singapore Sydney Tokyo Toronto*

Dermatology in General Medicine
Fourth Edition

1234567890 KGPKGP 9876543

Set Volume: ISBN 0-07-909350-7
  Volume I: ISBN 0-07-021207-4
  Volume II: ISBN 0-07-021208-2

This book was set in Times Roman by York Graphic Services, Inc.
The editors were J. Dereck Jeffers and Mariapaz Ramos Englis;
the production supervisor was Roger Kasunic. Index was
prepared by Irving Conde Tullar. Text and cover were
designed by Marsha Cohen/Parallelogram.
Arcata Graphics/Kingsport was printer and binder.

INTERNATIONAL EDITION
Copyright 1993

Exclusive rights by McGraw-Hill, Inc., for manufacture and export.
This book cannot be re-exported from the country to which it is
consigned by McGraw-Hill.
When ordering this title, use:
        Set: ISBN 0-07-112952-9
   Volume I: ISBN 0-07-112659-7
  Volume II: ISBN 0-07-112660-0

Library of Congress Cataloging in Publication Data

Dermatology in general medicine/editors. Thomas B. Fitzpatrick
. . . [et al.]. —4th ed.

   p. cm.
   includes bibliographical references and index.
   ISBN 0-07-909350-7 (set) ISBN 0-07-021207-4 (v.1).
   ISBN 0-07-021208-2 (v.2) 1. Dermatology. 2. Cutaneous
manifestations of general diseases. 1. Fitzpatrick. Thomas B.
(Thomas Bernhard), date. . . . [DNLM: 1. Skin Diseases. 2. Skin
Manifestations. WR 100 D4383 1993]
RL 71.D46   1993
616.5—dc20
DNLM/DLC
for Library of Congress   92-48388
                                                   CIP

NOTICE

Medicine is an ever-changing science. As new research and clinical experience broaden our knowledge, changes in treatment and drug therapy are required. The editors and the publisher of this work have checked with sources believed to be reliable in their efforts to provide information that is complete and generally in accord with the standards accepted at the time of publication. However, in view of the possibility of human error or changes in medical sciences, neither the editors nor the publisher nor any other party who has been involved in the preparation or publication of this work warrants that the information contained herein is in every respect accurate or complete, and they are not responsible for any errors or omissions or for the results obtained from use of such information. Readers are encouraged to confirm the information contained herein with other sources. For example and in particular, readers are advised to check the product information sheet included in the package of each drug they plan to administer to be certain that the information contained in this book is accurate and that changes have not been made in the recommended dose or in the contraindications for administration. This recommendation is of particular importance in connection with new or infrequently used drugs.

The color photographs herein are from the collections of the Departments of Dermatology at the University Medical Center, Leiden; the University of Vienna Medical School, Vienna; and Harvard Medical School, Massachusetts General Hospital, Boston; and submitted by the individual authors.

The following companies are gratefully acknowledged for making educational grants that helped make possible the publication of this edition:

Neutrogena Dermatologics
Ortho Pharmaceutical Corporation
Roche Dermatologics
Schering Corporation
Stiefel Laboratories, Inc.

CONTENTS

PART THREE Disorders Presenting in the Skin and Mucous Membranes

PART FOUR   Dermatology and Internal Medicine

PART FIVE   Diseases due to Microbial Agents

CONTRIBUTORS

A. Bernard Ackerman, M.D. Professor of Dermatology and Dermatopathology, Director of Dermatopathology, New York University Medical Center, New York, New York [98, 107, 110, 118]

Cheryl D. Ackerman, M.D. Pittsburgh, Pennsylvania [118]

Raymond D. Adams, M.A., M.D., M.A.(Hon.), D.Sc.(Hon.), M.D.(Hon.) Bullard Professor of Neuropathy (Emeritus), Harvard Medical School, Massachusetts General Hospital, Boston, Massachusetts [184]

Robert M. Adams, M.D. Clinical Professor of Dermatology, Stanford University School of Medicine, Stanford, California [141]

Rhoda Alani, M.D. Resident in Dermatology, Harvard Medical School, Boston, Massachusetts [204]

Steffen Albrecht, M.D., F.R.C.P.C. Neuropathology Fellow, Department of Pathology, Baylor College of Medicine, Houston, Texas [103]

Elaine L. Alexander, M.D., Ph.D. Assistant Professor, The Johns Hopkins Medical Institutions, Division of Molecular and Clinical Rheumatology, Department of Medicine, The Johns Hopkins University, Baltimore, Maryland [181]

Carl H. Anders, M.D. Assistant Clinical Professor of Pathology and Laboratory Medicine, University of California at Los Angeles, Los Angeles, California [110]

Paul J. Anderson, M.D., Ph.D. Assistant Professor of Medicine, Harvard Medical School; Division of Tumor Immunology, Dana-Farber Cancer Institute; Department of Rheumatology and Immunology, Brigham and Women's Hospital, Boston, Massachusetts [34]

R. Rox Anderson, M.D. Associate Professor of Dermatology, Harvard Medical School, Assistant in Dermatology, Massachusetts General Hospital, Boston, Massachusetts [140]

Elliot J. Androphy, M.D. Department of Dermatology, Tufts University School of Medicine, New England Medical Center, Boston, Massachusetts [212]

Kenneth A. Arndt, M.D. Professor of Dermatology, Harvard Medical School; Dermatologist-in-Chief, Beth Israel Hospital, Boston, Massachusetts [68, 86, 87, 88, 229]

Eva Åsbrink, M.D., Ph.D. Associate Professor of Dermatology, Department of Dermatology, Karolinska Institutet, Stockholm, Sweden [193]

Dalal Assaad, M.D., F.R.C.P. Consultant Dermatologist and Dermatopathologist, Sunnybrook Medical Centre; Assistant Professor, University of Toronto, Toronto, Canada [97]

K. Frank Austen, M.D. Theodore B. Bayles Professor of Medicine, Harvard Medical School; Chairman, Department of Rheumatology and Immunology, Brigham and Women's Hospital, Boston, Massachusetts [1]

Howard P. Baden, M.D. Professor of Dermatology, Department of Dermatology, Harvard Medical School; Massachusetts General Hospital, Boston, Massachusetts [20, 42, 43, 44, 62]

Ann Sullivan Baker, M.D. Assistant Professor of Medicine, Harvard Medical School; Associate Physician, Infectious Disease Unit, Massachusetts General Hospital, Boston, Massachusetts [226]

Raymond L. Barnhill, M.D. Associate Professor of Pathology, Harvard Medical School; Associate Pathologist, Massachusetts General Hospital, Boston, Massachusetts [82]

Eugene A. Bauer, M.D. Professor and Chairman, Department of Dermatology, Stanford University Medical Center, Stanford, California [60]

Donald V. Belsito, M.D. Associate Professor, Ronald O. Perelman Department of Dermatology and Department of Pathology, New York University Medical Center, New York, New York [119, 121, 122]

Jeffrey D. Bernhard, M.D. Professor of Medicine, Director, Division of Dermatology, Director of Phototherapy Center, Department of Medicine; Associate Dean for Admissions, University of Massachusetts Medical Center, Worcester, Massachusetts [4]

Arthur P. Bertolino, M.D., Ph.D. Associate Clinical Professor of Dermatology, Ronald O. Perelman Department of Dermatology, New York University Medical Center, New York, New York [19, 61]

David R. Bickers, M.D. Professor and Chairman, Department of Dermatology, Case Western Reserve University; Director, Department of Dermatology, University Hospitals of Cleveland and Veterans Administration Hospital, Cleveland, Ohio [150]

Alf Bjornberg, M.D. Department of Dermatology, University of Lund, Lund, Sweden [83]

Kerry L. Blacker, M.D. Assistant Clinical Professor, Department of Dermatology, University of California, San Francisco, San Francisco, California [142]

Edward E. Bondi, M.D. Associate Professor of Dermatology, Department of Dermatology, University of Pennsylvania School of Medicine, Philadelphia, Pennsylvania [108]

Conrado C. Bondoc, M.D. Associate Professor of Surgery, Harvard Medical School; Associate Visiting Surgeon, Massachusetts General Hospital and Shriners Burns Institute, Boston, Massachusetts [126]

Kathryn E. Bowers, M.D. Clinical Instructor, Harvard Medical School; Staff Dermatologist, Beth Israel Hospital, Boston, Massachusetts [205]

Irwin M. Braverman, M.D. Professor, Department of Dermatology, Yale University School of Medicine, New Haven, Connecticut [28]

Stephen Michael Breathnach, M.A., M.D., Ph.D.,

Numbers in brackets refer to chapters written or cowritten by the contributors.

xix

M.R.C.P., Senior Lecturer and Consultant, Dermatologist, Institute of Dermatology and St. John's Dermatology Centre, St. Thomas' Hospital, London, England   [149]

Robert A. Briggaman, M.D. Professor of Dermatology and Chairman, Department of Dermatology, University of North Carolina School of Medicine, Chapel Hill, North Carolina [55, 60]

Walter H. C. Burgdorf, M.D. Professor and Chairman, Department of Dermatology, The University of New Mexico School of Medicine, Albuquerque, New Mexico   [91, 94, 100, 101]

Robert E. Burgeson, Ph.D. Research Director, Portland Research Unit, Shriners Hospital for Crippled Children, Portland, Oregon   [23]

John F. Burke, M.D. Helen Andrus Benedict Professor of Surgery, Harvard Medical School; Chief of Trauma Services, Massachusetts General Hospital, Boston, Massachusetts   [126]

Stephen A. Cannistra, M.D. Assistant Professor of Medicine, Harvard Medical School; Program Director, Gynecologic Oncology, Dana-Farber Cancer Institute, Boston, Massachusetts [35]

Ruggero Caputo, M.D. Professor of Dermatology, 1° Dermatology Clinic, University of Milan, Milan, Italy   [102]

D. Martin Carter, M.D., Ph.D. Professor and Senior Physician, Laboratory for Investigative Dermatology, The Rockefeller University; Professor of Medicine and Co-Chief, Division of Dermatology, Cornell University Medical Center, New York, New York   [75]

Emily Christian, M.D. Associate Professor in Physical Therapy, University of Alabama, Birmingham, Alabama   [29]

Angela M. Christiano, M.D. Research Assistant Professor, Department of Dermatology, Thomas Jefferson University, Philadelphia, Pennsylvania   [24]

Enno Christophers, M.D. Professor and Chairman, Department of Dermatology and Venereology, University of Kiel, Germany   [39, 59]

Richard A. F. Clark, M.D. Professor and Chair, Department of Dermatology, State University of New York at Stony Brook, Stony Brook, New York   [38]

Jay D. Coffman, M.D. Professor of Medicine, Boston University School of Medicine; Chief, Peripheral Vascular Section, University Hospital, Boston, Massachusetts   [167]

Louis Z. Cooper, M.D. Director of Pediatrics, St. Luke's/Roosevelt Hospital Center, New York, New York   [199]

Lynn A. Cornelius, M.D. Assistant Professor of Medicine (Dermatology), Division of Dermatology, Washington University School of Medicine, St. Louis, Missouri   [162]

Roger C. Cornell, M.D. Senior Consultant in Dermatology, Scripps Clinic and Research Foundation; Clinical Professor of Dermatology, Department of Medicine, University of California at San Diego, La Jolla, California   [230]

Thomas G. Cropley, M.D. Assistant Professor of Medicine, Division of Dermatology, University of Massachusetts Medical Center, Worcester, Massachusetts   [5]

Clyde S. Crumpacker, M.D. Associate Professor of Medicine, Harvard Medical School; Infectious Disease Unit, Beth Israel Hospital, Boston, Massachusetts   [203]

Mark V. Dahl, M.D. Professor of Dermatology, Department of Dermatology, University of Minnesota, Minneapolis, Minnesota   [95]

Robert J. Desnick, Ph.D., M.D. Professor of Pediatrics and Genetics, Chief, Medical and Molecular Genetics, The Mount Sinai Medical Center, New York, New York   [153]

John J. DiGiovanna, M.D. Investigator, Dermatology Branch, National Cancer Institute, National Institutes of Health, Bethesda, Maryland   [236]

Andrzej A. Dlugosz, M.D. Biotechnology Fellow, Laboratory of Cellular Carcinogenesis and Tumor Promotion, Division of Cancer Etiology, National Cancer Institute, National Institutes of Health, Bethesda, Maryland   [70]

Jeffrey S. Dover, M.D., F.R.C.P.C. Assistant Professor of Dermatology, Harvard Medical School; Chief, Division of Dermatology, New England Deaconess Hospital, Boston, Massachusetts   [129, 215]

Robin Dover, B.Sc. Ph.D. Histopathology Unit, Imperial Cancer Research Fund, Royal College of Surgeons, London, England   [11]

Donald T. Downing, Ph.D. Professor, Department of Dermatology, University of Iowa College of Medicine, Iowa City, Iowa   [14]

Louis Dubertret, M.D. Chef de Service, Clinique des Maladies Cutanées, Hôpital Saint-Louis, Paris, France   [96]

Richard L. Edelson, M.D. Professor of Dermatology and Chairman, Department of Dermatology, Yale University School of Medicine, New Haven, Connecticut   [105]

Alfred R. Eichmann, M.D. Associate Professor of Dermatology, Städtische Poliklinik für Haut und Geschlechtskrankheiten, Zürich, Switzerland   [217, 220, 224]

Arthur Z. Eisen, M.D. Winfred A. and Emma R. Showman Professor of Medicine; Chairman, Division of Dermatology, Washington University School of Medicine; Dermatologist-in-Chief, Barnes Hospital, St. Louis, Missouri   [1, 22, 173]

Peter M. Elias, M.D. Clinical Professor of Dermatology, University of California School of Medicine; Chief, Dermatology Service, Veterans Administration Medical Center, San Francisco, California   [16, 49, 50, 51]

Christine M. Eng, M.D. Assistant Professor of Pediatrics and Genetics, The Mount Sinai Medical Center, New York, New York   [153]

Edgar G. Engleman, M.D. Professor of Pathology and Medicine, Stanford University School of Medicine, Stanford, California   [32]

Ervin H. Epstein, Jr., M.D. Clinical Professor of Dermatology and Research Dermatologist, Department of Dermatology, University of California at San Francisco, San Francisco, California [7, 109]

Fuad S. Farah, M.D. Professor of Medicine and Chief, Section of Dermatology, State University of New York Upstate Medical Center, Syracuse, New York   [225]

Evan R. Farmer, M.D. Professor of Dermatology, The Johns Hopkins University School of Medicine, Baltimore, Maryland [117]

David S. Feingold, M.D. Professor and Chairman, Department of Dermatology, Tufts University School of Medicine, New England Medical Center, Boston, Massachusetts   [223]

Jessica Fewkes, M.D. Assistant Professor of Dermatology, Harvard Medical School; Associate Dermatologist, Massachusetts General Hospital, Boston, Massachusetts   [238]

Thomas B. Fitzpatrick, M.D., Ph.D., D.Sc.(Hon.) Edward C. Wigglesworth Professor of Dermatology, Emeritus; Chairman Emeritus, Department of Dermatology, Harvard Medical School; Chief Emeritus, Dermatology Service, Massachusetts

General Hospital; Consultant in Dermatology, Brigham and Women's Hospital and The Children's Hospital, Boston, Massachusetts   [1, 4, 5, 18, 80, 82, 137, 139, 240]

Raul Fleischmajer, M.D. Professor and Chairman, Department of Dermatology, The Mount Sinai Medical Center, New York, New York   [177]

Shoshana Frankenburg, Ph.D. Research Associate, Department of Dermatology, The Hebrew University of Jerusalem, Jerusalem, Israel   [225]

Andrew G. Franks, Jr., M.D., F.A.C.P. Associate Clinical Professor of Dermatology, New York University School of Medicine; Associate Rheumatologist, Hospital for Joint Disease, New York University Medical Center, New York, New York   [166]

Irwin M. Freedberg, M.D. George Miller MacKee Professor and Chairman, Ronald O. Perelman Department of Dermatology, New York University Medical Center, New York, New York   [1, 13, 19, 41, 61, 152, 189]

Ruth K. Freinkel, M.D. Professor of Dermatology and Cell Biology, Department of Dermatology, Northwestern University, Chicago, Illinois   [169]

Peter O. Fritsch, M.D. Professor and Chairman, Department of Dermatology, University of Innsbruck, Innsbruck, Austria   [49, 50, 51, 175]

Lynn From, M.D., F.R.C.P.C. Associate Professor, Department of Pathology; University of Toronto, Pathologist-in-Chief, Women's College Hospital, Toronto, Ontario, Canada   [97, 103]

Vincent A. Fulginiti, M.D. Dean, College of Medicine, Tulane University, New Orleans, Louisiana   [209]

Helmut Gadner, M.D. Professor of Pediatrics and Director, St. Anna Children's Hospital, Vienna, Austria   [160]

George T. Gallagher, D.M.D., D.M.Sc. Associate Professor of Oral Pathology, Department of Oral Medicine and Oral Pathology, Harvard School of Dental Medicine, Boston, Massachusetts   [111]

W. Ray Gammon, M.D. Professor of Dermatology, University of North Carolina at Chapel Hill; North Carolina Memorial Hospital, Chapel Hill, North Carolina   [55]

Richard W. Gange, M.D.* Assistant Professor of Dermatology, Harvard Medical School; Assistant in Dermatology, Massachusetts General Hospital, Boston, Massachusetts   [133]

Paul A. Gatenby, M.B.B.S., Ph.D. Associate Professor, Department of Medicine, University of Sydney; Department of Clinical Immunology, Royal Prince Alfred Hospital, Sydney, Australia   [32]

Raif S. Geha, M.D. Professor of Pediatrics, Harvard Medical School; Chief, Division of Immunology, Children's Hospital, Boston, Massachusetts   [120]

Stephen E. Gellis, M.D. Assistant Professor of Dermatology (Pediatrics), Harvard Medical School; Clinical Director of Dermatology, Children's Hospital, Boston, Massachusetts   [198]

Feroze N. Ghadially, M.B., B.S.(Bom), M.B., B.S.(Lond), M.D., Ph.D., D.Sc.(Lond), Hon. D.Sc.(Guelph), F.R.C. Path., F.R.C.P.(C), F.R.S.A. Izaak Walton Killam Laureate of the Canada Council; Professor Emeritus of the University of Saskatchewan; Adjunct Professor of the University of Ottawa;

Pathologist, Ottawa Civic Hospital; Consultant, Canadian Reference Centre for Cancer Pathology, Ottawa, Ontario, Canada   [76]

Ruby Ghadially, M.B., Ch.B.(Sheffield), F.R.C.P.(C) Department of Dermatology, University of California, San Francisco, San Francisco, California   [76]

Irma Gigli, M.D. Professor of Medicine and Chief, Division of Dermatology, University of California, San Diego, School of Medicine, San Diego, California   [36, 115]

Barbara Gilchrest, M.D. Chairman, Department of Dermatology, Boston University School of Medicine, Boston, Massachusetts   [10]

Gerald J. Gleich, M.D. Professor of Medicine and Immunology, Mayo Medical School; Consultant, Department of Immunology and Division of Allergic Diseases and Internal Medicine, Mayo Clinic and Mayo Foundation; Rochester, Minnesota   [90]

Sergij Goerdt, M.D. Münster, Germany   [27]

Gregory I. Goldberg, Ph.D. Associate Professor of Biochemistry and Molecular Biophysics in Medicine (Dermatology), Washington University School of Medicine, St. Louis, Missouri   [22]

Lowell A. Goldsmith, M.D. Chairman, Department of Dermatology, University of Rochester Medical Center, Rochester, New York   [7, 147, 148]

Sanford M. Goldstein, M.D. Assistant Clinical Professor, Department of Dermatology, University of California, San Francisco, San Francisco, California   [26]

Robert W. Goltz, M.B., M.D. Adjunct Professor of Medicine, University of California, San Diego; Chief, Dermatology, La Jolla Veterans Administration Hospital, La Jolla, California   [100]

Robin A.C. Graham-Brown, B.Sc., M.B., F.R.C.P. Consultant Dermatologist, The Leicester Royal Infirmary, Leicester, England   [163]

Richard D. Granstein, M.D. Associate Professor of Dermatology, Harvard Medical School; Associate Dermatologist, Massachusetts General Hospital, Boston, Massachusetts   [132]

Ellen M. Gravallese, M.D. Assistant Professor of Medicine, Harvard Medical School; Associate Rheumatologist and Immunologist, Associate Pathologist, Brigham and Women's Hospital; Department of Cancer Biology, Harvard School of Public Health, Boston, Massachusetts   [174]

Malcolm W. Greaves, M.D. Professor and Chairman, Institute of Dermatology, St. Thomas' Hospital, London, England   [31]

Joop M. Grevelink, M.D. Instructor in Dermatology, Harvard Medical School; Assistant Dermatologist, Massachusetts General Hospital; Director, MGH Dermatology Laser Center, Boston, Massachusetts   [140]

Nicole Grois, M.D. St. Anna Children's Hospital, Vienna, Austria   [160]

F. Carl Grumet, M.D. Professor of Pathology, Director of Tranfusion Service and Histocompatibility Laboratories, Stanford University Medical Center, Stanford University School of Medicine, Palo Alto, California   [32]

Roy M. Gulick, M.D. Instructor of Medicine, Harvard Medical School; Beth Israel Hospital, Boston, Massachusetts   [203]

B. Hanchard, M.D. Professor of Pathology, Department of Pathology, University of the West Indies, Kingston, Jamaica   [214]

*Deceased

Leonard C. Harber, M.D. Rhodebeck Professor of Dermatology, Columbia University, College of Physicians and Surgeons of New York; Attending Physician, The Presbyterian Hospital, New York, New York   [136]

Ken Hashimoto, M.D. Professor and Chairman, Department of Dermatology, Wayne State University School of Medicine, Detroit, Michigan   [78]

Conrad Hauser, M.D. Associate Professor of Dermatology, Clinique de Dermatologie, Hôpital Cantonal Universitaire, Geneva, Switzerland   [12]

John L. M. Hawk, M.D., F.R.C.P. Consultant Dermatologist, St. Thomas Hospital, London, England   [133, 135]

Harley A. Haynes, M.D. Associate Professor of Dermatology, Department of Dermatology, Harvard Medical School; Director, Dermatology Division, Brigham and Women's Hospital; Chief, Dermatology, West Roxbury Veterans Administration Hospital, Boston, Massachusetts   [183]

Peter W. Heald, M.D. Associate Professor of Dermatology, Department of Dermatology, Yale University School of Medicine, New Haven, Connecticut   [105]

Peter J. Heenan, M.B., F.R.C.Path., F.R.C.P.A. Hospital and University Pathology Services, The Queen Elizabeth II Medical Centre, Nedlands, Australia   [45]

Helmut Hintner, M.D. Professor of Dermatology, Head, Division of Dermatology, Landes-Krankenhaus Salzburg, Salzburg, Austria   [49]

Vincent C.Y. Ho., M.D., F.R.C.P.C. Assistant Professor, Division of Dermatology, University of British Columbia, Vancouver, British Columbia, Canada   [77]

Karen Holbrook, Ph.D. Professor of Anatomy, Department of Biological Structure, University of Washington School of Medicine, Seattle, Washington   [8]

Karl Holubar, M.D. Professor of Dermatology and the History of Medicine, Chairman, Institute for the History of Medicine, Vienna, Austria   [179]

Herbert Hönigsmann, M.D. Professor of Dermatology, Head, Division of Special and Environmental Dermatology, Department of Dermatology, University of Vienna Medical School, Vienna, Austria   [58, 89, 139]

Antoinette F. Hood, M.D. Professor of Dermatology, The Johns Hopkins University School of Medicine, Baltimore, Maryland   [117, 143, 200]

Yoshiaki Hori, M.D., Ph.D., Professor and Chairman, Department of Dermatology, Yamanashi Medical College, Yamanashi, Japan   [80]

Anders Hovmark, M.D. Associate Professor of Dermatology, Department of Dermatology, Karolinska Institutet, Stockholm, Sweden   [193]

George J. Hruza, M.D. Assistant Professor of Dermatology (Medicine), Otolaryngology, and Plastic Surgery, Washington University School of Medicine, St. Louis, Missouri   [238]

Chung-Hong Hu, M.D. President, Taipei Medical College, Taiwan, and Clinical Professor of Dermatology, Stanford University School of Medicine, Stanford, California   [84]

Ronald D. Hunt, D.V.M. Professor of Comparative Pathology, Harvard Medical School; Director, New England Regional Primate Research Center, Southborough, Massachusetts   [208]

Harry J. Hurley, Jr., M.D. Clinical Professor of Dermatology, University of Pennsylvania, Philadelphia, Pennsylvania   [67]

Stephania Jablonska, M.D. Professor, Department of Derma-

tology, Warsaw Academy of Medicine, Warsaw, Poland   [213]

Simon M. Jackson, M.D. Dermatology Service, Veterans Administration Medical Center, San Francisco, California   [16]

Robert J. Jacob, M.D. Orthopaedic Surgeon, Louisville, Kentucky   [210]

Jean-Claude Jamoulle, Ph.D. Laboratoire Algovital, Cannes, France   [228]

Brian V. Jegasothy, M.D. Professor and Chairman, Department of Dermatology, University of Pittsburgh Medical Center, Pittsburgh, Pennsylvania   [118]

Kowichi Jimbow, M.D. Division of Dermatology, Heritage Medical Research Centre, University of Alberta, Edmonton, Alberta, Canada   [18]

Olle Johansson, M.D. Associate Professor, Department of Histology and Neurobiology, Experimental Dermatology Unit, Karolinska Institute, Stockholm, Sweden   [29]

Richard Allen Johnson, M.D.C.M. Instructor in Dermatology, Harvard Medical School; Clinical Associate in Dermatology, Massachusetts General Hospital; Dermatologist, New England Deaconess Hospital, Boston, Massachusetts   [112, 202, 205, 207, 215]

Joseph L. Jorizzo, M.D. Professor and Chairman, Department of Dermatology, Bowman Gray School of Medicine, Winston-Salem, North Carolina   [165, 185]

Stephen I. Katz, M.D., Ph.D. Marion B. Sulzberger Professor of Dermatology, Uniformed Services University of the Health Sciences; Chief, Dermatology Branch, National Cancer Institute, National Institutes of Health, Bethesda, Maryland   [54, 56, 92, 176, 233]

Robert O. Kenet, M.D., Ph.D. Visiting Instructor in Medicine, Cornell University Medical College, New York, New York   [82]

Helmut Kerl, M.D. Professor and Chairman, Department of Dermatology, University of Graz, Graz, Austria   [79, 107]

Rebecca E.I. Kerr, M.B., Ch.B., F.R.C.P., Consultant in Dermatology, The Royal Infimary; Honorary Clinical Lecturer, The University of Glasgow, Glasgow, Scotland   [65]

Abdul-Ghani Kibbi, M.D. Department of Dermatology, American University of Beirut, Beirut, Lebanon   [6]

Lloyd E. King, Jr., M.D., Ph.D. Professor of Medicine, Vanderbilt University; Chief of Dermatology, Vanderbilt University and Veterans Administration Medical Centers, Nashville, Tennessee   [227]

Sidney N. Klaus, M.D. Professor and Chairman, Department of Dermatology, Hebrew University, Jerusalem, Israel   [225]

Lynn M. Klein, M.D. Resident in Dermatology, Ronald O. Perelman Department of Dermatology, New York University Medical Center, New York, New York   [19]

Albert M. Kligman, M.D., Ph.D. Professor of Dermatology, Emeritus, Duhring Laboratories, Department of Dermatology, University of Pennsylvania, Philadelphia, Pennsylvania   [240]

Lorraine H. Kligman, Ph.D. Associate Research Professor, Department of Dermatology, University of Pennsylvania, Philadelphia, Pennsylvania   [240]

Amy D. Klion, M.D. Medical Staff Fellow, Laboratory of Parasitic Diseases, National Institute of Allergy and Infectious Diseases, National Institutes of Health, Bethesda, Maryland   [225]

George S. Kobayashi, Ph.D. Professor, Departments of Internal Medicine and Microbiology and Immunology, Washington University School of Medicine, St. Louis, Missouri [194, 195]

Caroline S. Koblenzer, M.D. Associate Clinical Professor of Dermatology and Dermatology-in-Psychiatry, University of Pennsylvania, Philadelphia, Pennsylvania [3]

Irene E. Kochevar, Ph.D. Associate Professor, Harvard Medical School; Wellman Laboratories of Photomedicine, Massachusetts General Hospital, Boston, Massachusetts [131]

Howard K. Koh, M.D. Associate Professor of Dermatology, Boston University School of Medicine, Boston, Massachusetts [82]

Sophia N. Kotliar, M.D. Resident in Pathology, Northwestern Memorial Hospital, Northwestern University Medical School, Chicago, Illinois [155]

Kenneth H. Kraemer, M.D. Research Scientist, Laboratory of Molecular Carcinogenesis, National Cancer Institute, National Institutes of Health, Bethesda, Maryland [69, 158]

Margaret L. Kripke, Ph.D. Professor and Chairman, Vivian L. Smith Chair in Immunology, Department of Immunology, The University of Texas, M.D. Anderson Cancer Center, Houston, Texas [72]

Thomas S. Kupper, M.D. Thomas B. Fitzpatrick Associate Professor of Dermatology, Harvard Medical School; Director of Dermatological Research, Brigham and Women's Hospital, Boston, Massachusetts [9]

Joseph C. Kvedar, M.D. Department of Dermatology, Harvard Medical School; Massachusetts General Hospital, Boston, Massachusetts [20, 62]

Alfred T. Lane, M.D. Associate Professor of Dermatology and Pediatrics, Stanford University School of Medicine, Stanford, California [239]

Charles M. Lapiere, M.D., Ph.D. Department of Dermatology, University of Liège, Liège, Belgium [154]

Olle Larkö, M.D. Associate Professor, Department of Dermatology and Venereology, University of Gothenburg, Göteborg, Sweden [138]

Thomas J. Lawley, M.D. Professor and Chairman, Department of Dermatology, Emory University School of Medicine, Atlanta, Georgia [33, 162, 168]

Gerald S. Lazarus, M.D. Hartzell Professor and Chairman, Department of Dermatology, University of Pennsylvania School of Medicine; Chief, Department of Dermatology, Hospital of the University of Pennsylvania, Philadelphia, Pennsylvania [108, 232]

Ullin W. Leavell, Jr. M.D. Dermatology Associates of Kentucky, Lexington, Kentucky [210]

Kristin M. Leiferman, M.D. Associate Professor of Dermatology, Mayo Medical School; Consultant, Department of Dermatology, Mayo Clinic, Rochester, Minnesota [90]

Walter F. Lever, M.D.* Professor Emeritus of Dermatology, Tufts University School of Medicine, Boston, Massachusetts [57, 78]

Paul C. Levins, M.D. Resident, Department of Dermatology, Harvard Medical School, Boston, Massachusetts [140]

S. William Levy, M.D. Clinical Professor of Dermatology,

University of California, San Francisco Medical Center, San Francisco, California [128]

William H. Leyva, M.D. Clinical Assistant Professor, Departments of Medicine (Dermatology) and Pathology, University of Kentucky College of Medicine, Lexington, Kentucky [227]

Donald Y.M. Leung, M.D., Ph.D. Professor of Pediatrics, University of Colorado Health Sciences; Head, Division of Pediatric Allergy–Immunology, National Jewish Center for Immunology and Respiratory Medicine, Denver, Colorado [120, 216]

Henry W. Lim, M.D. Associate Professor of Dermatology, New York University School of Medicine; Chief, Dermatology Service, New York Veterans Administration Medical Center, New York, New York [150]

Andrew N. Lin, M.D. Assistant Professor and Associate Physician, Laboratory for Investigative Dermatology, The Rockefeller University; Adjunct Assistant Professor (Medicine), Cornell University Medical Center, New York, New York [75]

Douglas R. Lowy, M.D. Chief, Laboratory of Cellular Oncology, National Cancer Institute, National Institutes of Health, Bethesda, Maryland [71, 211, 212]

Anne W. Lucky, M.D. Adjunct Associate Professor of Dermatology and Pediatrics, University of Cincinnati College of Medicine; Director, Pediatric Dermatology Clinic, Children's Hospital Medical Center, Cincinnati, Ohio [216]

Anton Luger, M.D. Professor of Dermatology, Ludwig Boltzmann Institut für Dermato-Venerologische Serodiagnostik, Krankenhaus der Stadt Wien-Lainz, Vienna, Austria [218, 219]

Nancy B. Lyon, M.D., Ph.D. Resident, Department of Dermatology, Harvard Medical School, Boston, Massachusetts [240]

Frederick D. Malkinson, M.D. Chairman, Department of Dermatology, Rush–Presbyterian–St. Luke's Medical Center, Chicago, Illinois [127]

Janet M. Marks, M.D. Dermatologist, Royal Victoria Infirmary, Newcastle-upon-Tyne, England [164]

Ann G. Martin, M.D. Assistant Professor of Medicine (Dermatology), Division of Dermatology, Washington University School of Medicine, St. Louis, Missouri [194, 195]

José M. Mascaro, M.D. Professor and Chairman, Department of Dermatology, Hospital Clinic, Barcelona, Spain [85]

A. Colin McDougall, M.D., F.R.C.P. Honorary Consultant, Department of Dermatology, The Slade Hospital, Headington, Oxfordshire, England [192]

Marilynne McKay, M.D. Associate Professor of Dermatology, Emory University School of Medicine, Atlanta, Georgia [113]

Donald S. McLaren, M.D., Ph.D., F.R.C.P. Associate Professor and Head, Nutritional Blindness Prevention Programme, International Centre for Eye Health, Institute of Ophthalmology, University of London, London, England [145]

David I. McLean, M.D., F.R.C.P. Associate Professor and Head, Division of Dermatology, Department of Medicine, University of British Columbia; British Columbia Cancer Agency and Vancouver General Hospital, Vancouver, British Columbia, Canada [77, 183]

Paula V. Mendenhall, Pharm.D. Director, Global Manufacturing Planning, Syntex Corporation, Palo Alto, California [229]

Dean D. Metcalfe, M.D. Head, Mast Cell Physiology Section,

*Deceased

Laboratory of Clinical Investigation, National Institute of Allergy and Infectious Diseases, National Institutes of Health, Bethesda, Maryland   [161]

Martin C. Mihm, Jr., M.D.   Professor of Pathology, Harvard Medical School; Chief, Dermatopathology, Massachusetts General Hospital and Harvard Medical School, Boston, Massachusetts   [6, 82, 200]

Sharon Milgram, M.D.   Department of Neuroscience, The Johns Hopkins University School of Medicine, Baltimore, Maryland   [29]

John A. Mills, M.D.   Associate Professor of Medicine, Harvard Medical School; Physician, Massachusetts General Hospital, Boston, Massachusetts   [172]

David B. Mosher, M.D.   Clinical Instructor in Dermatology, Department of Dermatology, Harvard Medical School; Clinical Associate, Massachusetts General Hospital, Boston, Massachusetts   [80]

Janet A. Moy, M.D.   Assistant Professor, Ronald O. Perelman Department of Dermatology, New York University Medical Center, New York, New York   [144]

Kenneth H. Neldner, M.D.   Professor and Chairman, Department of Dermatology, Texas Tech University Health Sciences Center, Lubbock, Texas   [146]

James Niederman, M.D.   Department of Epidemiology and Public Health, Yale University School of Medicine, New Haven, Connecticut   [206]

W.C. Noble, Ph.D., D.Sc., F.R.C.Path., F.I.Biol.   Professor of Microbiology, Institute of Dermatology, St. Thomas Hospital, London, England   [17]

Paul G. Norris, M.A., M.R.C.P.   Consultant Dermatologist, Addenbrooke's Hospital, Cambridge, England   [133, 135]

Thomas B. Nutman, M.D.   Senior Investigator, Laboratory of Parasitic Disease, National Institute of Allergy and Infectious Disease, National Institutes of Health, Bethesda, Maryland   [225]

Jean-Paul Ortonne, M.D.   Professor of Dermatology, Nice University School of Medicine; Chief, Department of Dermatology, Hôpital Pasteur, Nice, France   [80]

Michael N. Oxman, M.D.   Professor of Medicine and Pathology, University of California at San Diego; Chief of Infectious Diseases and Clinical Virology Sections, Veterans Administration Medical Center, San Diego, California   [204]

Elizabeth Heller Page, M.D.   Sunnybrook Hospital, University of Toronto Clinic, Toronto, Ontario, Canada   [125]

Amy S. Paller, M.D.   Associate Professor of Pediatrics and Dermatology, Division of Immunology/Rheumatology, Northwestern University School of Medicine; Head, Division of Dermatology, The Children's Hospital, Chicago, Illinois   [156]

John A. Parrish, M.D.   Edward C. Wigglesworth Professor and Chairman, Department of Dermatology, Harvard Medical School; Professor, Division of Health Sciences Technology, Massachusetts Institute of Technology; Chief, Dermatology Service, Massachusetts General Hospital; Director, Wellman Laboratories of Photomedicine; Director, Massachusetts General Hospital–Harvard Cutaneous Biology Research Center, Boston, Massachusetts   [130, 131, 138]

Robert H. Parrott, M.D.   Department of Pediatrics, George Washington University School of Medicine, Washington, D.C.   [201]

Madhu A. Pathak, B.Sc.(Hon.), M.S.(Tech.), M.S., Ph.D.   Senior Associate in Dermatology, Department of Dermatology, Harvard Medical School, Massachusetts General Hospital, Boston, Massachusetts   [131, 137, 139, 150]

Barry S. Paul, M.D.   Clinical Instructor in Dermatology, Harvard Medical School, Boston, Massachusetts   [138]

Monica Peacocke, M.D.   Assistant Professor, Department of Dermatology, Tufts University School of Medicine, New England Medical Center, Boston, Massachusetts   [223]

Gary L. Peck, M.D.   Professor of Dermatology, University of Maryland School of Medicine, Baltimore, Maryland   [236]

Alice P. Pentland, M.D.   Associate Professor in Medicine, Molecular Biology and Pharmacology, Division of Dermatology, Washington University School of Medicine, St. Louis, Missouri   [37]

John H. Perrin, Ph.D.   Professor of Medicinal Chemistry, Department of Medicinal Chemistry, College of Pharmacy, University of Florida, Gainesville, Florida   [229]

Scott B. Phillips, M.D.   Chief, Dermatology Clinical Investigations Unit, Massachusetts General Hospital, Harvard Medical School, Boston, Massachusetts   [42, 44]

Stephanie H. Pincus, M.D.   Professor and Chairman, Department of Dermatology, State University of New York at Buffalo, Buffalo, New York   [113]

Sheldon R. Pinnell, M.D.   Chairman, Department of Dermatology, Duke University Medical Center, Durham, North Carolina   [157]

Gerd Plewig, M.D.   Professor and Chairman, Department of Dermatology, Ludwig Maximilian-University, Munich, Germany   [64, 123]

Jordan S. Pober, M.D., Ph.D.   Professor of Pathology, Immunobiology and Biology, Yale University School of Medicine; Director, Molecular Cardiobiology, Boyer Center for Molecular Medicine, New Haven, Connecticut   [27]

Machiel K. Polano, M.D.   Emeritus Professor and Chairman, Department of Dermatology, University Hospital, Lieden, The Netherlands   [152]

Walter C. Quevedo, Jr., Ph.D.   Professor of Biology and Medicine, Brown University, Providence, Rhode Island   [18]

Christopher J. Quirk, M.B., F.A.C.D.   Department of Dermatology, Fremantle Hospital, Fremantle, Australia   [45]

Rhonda Rand, M.D.   Dermatologist, Beverly Hills, California   [68]

Klemens Rappersberger, M.D.   Associate Professor of Dermatology, Division of General Dermatology, Department of Dermatology, University of Vienna Medical School, Vienna, Austria   [99]

Marvin S. Reitz, Jr., M.D.   Laboratory of Tumor Cell Biology, National Cancer Institute, National Institutes of Health, Bethesda, Maryland   [214]

Arthur R. Rhodes, M.D., M.P.H.   Professor of Dermatology, University of Pittsburgh School of Medicine, Pittsburgh, Pennsylvania   [81, 120]

Johannes Ring, M.D., Ph.D.   University of Hamburg, Arzil. Direktor der Universitats-Hautklinik und Poliklinik, Hamburg, Germany   [120]

Douglas J. Ringler, V.M.D.   Associate Professor of Comparative Pathology, Harvard Medical School; Chairman, Division of

Comparative Pathology, New England Regional Primate Research Center, Southborough, Massachusetts [208]

Fred S. Rosen, M.D. James L. Gamble Professor of Pediatrics, Harvard Medical School; President, Center for Blood Research, Boston, Massachusetts [115]

Tamzin A. Rosenwasser, M.D. Fellow in Dermatology, Washington University School of Medicine, St. Louis, Missouri [173]

Sanford I. Roth, M.D. Professor of Pathology, Northwestern University Medical School; Attending Pathologist, Northwestern Memorial Hospital, Chicago, Illinois [155]

Richard B. Rothenberg, M.D. Assistant Director of Science, National Center for Chronic Disease Prevention and Health Promotion, Centers for Disease Control, Atlanta, Georgia [221, 222]

Naomi F. Rothfield, M.D. Professor of Medicine and Chief, Division of Rheumatic Diseases, University of Connecticut Health Center, Farmington, Connecticut [171]

Neville R. Rowell, M.D., F.R.C.P. Emeritus Professor of Dermatology, Department of Dermatology, The General Infirmary at Leeds, University of Leeds, Leeds, England [178]

Eric H. Rubin, M.D. Instructor in Medicine, Harvard Medical School, Dana-Farber Cancer Institute, Boston, Massachusetts [35]

Jorge L. Sanchez, M.D. Department of Dermatology, University of Puerto Rico, Puerto Rico [98]

Miguel R. Sanchez, M.D. Assistant Professor of Dermatology, Ronald O. Perelman Department of Dermatology, New York University Medical Center, New York, New York [218, 219]

Imrich Sarkany, M.D. Honorary Consultant Dermatologist, Royal Free Hospital, London, England [163]

Kenzo Sato, M.D., Ph.D. Professor of Dermatology, The University of Iowa College of Medicine, Iowa City, Iowa [15, 66]

Hans Schaefer, Ph.D. Professor of Biochemistry and Director, Centre International de Recherches Dermatologiques Galderma, Valbonne, France [228]

William Schaffner, M.D. Professor and Chairman, Department of Preventive Medicine, Chief, Division of Infectious Diseases, Department of Medicine, Vanderbilt University School of Medicine, Nashville, Tennessee [197]

Mark Jordan Scharf, M.D. Assistant Professor, Division of Dermatology, University of Massachusetts Medical Center, Worcester, Massachusetts [226]

Gundula Schaumburg-Lever, M.D. Associate Professor of Dermatology; Head, Dermatopathology Laboratory, Department of Dermatology, University of Tübingen, Germany [57]

Robert J. Scheuplein, Ph.D. Deputy Director for Toxicological Sciences, Food and Drug Administration, Center for Food Safety and Applied Nutrition, Washington, D.C. [30]

Lynda C. Schneider, M.D. Assistant Professor of Pediatrics, Harvard Medical School; Director, Allergy Program, Children's Hospital, Boston, Massachusetts [120]

Urs W. Schnyder, M.D. Professor and Chairman Emeritus, Department of Dermatology, University Hospital of Zurich, Zurich, Switzerland [46]

Robert A. Schwartz, M.D., M.P.H., F.A.C.P. Professor and Chairman, Division of Dermatology, UMDNJ Medical School,

Newark, New Jersey [73, 74]

J. Edwin Seegmiller, M.D. Head, Division of Arthritis, University of California, San Diego, La Jolla, California [151]

H. Jean Shadomy, M.A., Ph.D. Professor of Microbiology and Immunology, Medicine, Pathology, and Biology, Virginia Commonwealth University–Medical College of Virginia, Richmond, Virginia [196]

Om P. Sharma, M.D. Professor of Medicine and Director, Sarcoidosis Clinic, Pulmonary and Critical Care Medicine, University of Southern California School of Medicine, Los Angeles, California [182]

Neil H. Shear, M.D. Sunnybrook Health Science Centre A3, Toronto, Ontario, Canada [125]

Elizabeth F. Sherertz, M.D. Professor, Department of Dermatology; Director of Occupational and Contact Dermatitis, Bowman Gray School of Medicine, Winston-Salem, North Carolina [165]

M. Priscilla Short, M.D. Assistant Professor (Neurology), Harvard Medical School; Assistant Neurologist, Massachusetts General Hospital, Boston, Massachusetts [184]

Jerome L. Shupack, M.D. Professor of Clinical Dermatology, Ronald O. Perelman Department of Dermatology, New York University Medical Center, New York, New York [235]

Jeremiah E. Silbert, M.D. Director, Connective Tissue Research Laboratory, Bedford, Massachusetts [25]

Meredith A. Simon, D.V.M. New England Regional Primate Research Center, Southborough, Massachusetts [208]

Mihael Skerlev, M.D. Department of Dermatology and Venerology, Medical School of Zagreb University and KBC Salata, Zagreb, Yugoslavia [207]

Kenneth B. Sloan, Ph.D. Associate Professor, Department of Medicinal Chemistry, University of Florida, Gainesville, Florida [229]

Arthur J. Sober, M.D. Associate Professor of Dermatology, Harvard Medical School; Associate Dermatologist, Massachusetts General Hospital, Boston, Massachusetts [82]

Nicholas A. Soter, M.D. Professor of Dermatology, Ronald O. Perelman Department of Dermatology, New York University School of Medicine; Medical Director, Charles C. Harris Skin and Cancer Pavillion; Attending Physician, Tisch Hospital, The University Hospital of New York University, New York, New York [114, 116, 121, 237]

H. Peter Soyer, M.D. Associate Professor, Department of Dermatology, University of Graz, Graz, Austria [79]

John R. Stanley, M.D. Senior Investigator, Dermatology Branch, National Cancer Institute, National Institutes of Health, Bethesda, Maryland [52, 53]

Robert S. Stern, M.D. Associate Professor of Dermatology, Harvard Medical School; Dermatologist, Beth Israel Hospital, Boston, Massachusetts [2, 142]

Wolfram Sterry, M.D. Professor and Chairman, Department of Dermatology, University of Ulm, Ulm, Germany [39, 106]

Mary Ellen Stewart, Ph.D. Associate Research Scientist, Department of Dermatology, University of Iowa College of Medicine, Iowa City, Iowa [14]

Matthew J. Stiller, M.D. Assistant Professor of Dermatology, Ronald O. Perelman Department of Dermatology, New York University Medical Center, New York, New York [235]

Georg Stingl, M.D. Professor of Dermatology, Head, Division of Immunology, Allergy and Infectious Diseases, Department of Dermatology, University of Vienna Medical School, Vienna, Austria   [12, 93, 99]

Howard L. Stoll, Jr., M.D.   Clinical Associate Professor, Dermatology, Roswell Park Memorial Institute and State University of New York at Buffalo School of Medicine, Buffalo, New York   [73, 74]

Richard B. Stoughton, M.D.*   Emeritus Professor of Dermatology, Department of Medicine, University of California, San Diego, La Jolla, California   [230]

John S. Strauss, M.D.   Professor and Head, Department of Dermatology, The University of Iowa Hospitals and Clinics, Iowa City, Iowa   [14, 63]

Gunnar Swanbeck, M.D.   Professor and Chairman, Department of Dermatology, University of Gothenberg, Göteborg, Sweden   [138, 234]

Morton N. Swartz, M.D., F.A.C.P.   Professor of Medicine, Harvard Medical School; Chief, Infectious Disease Unit, Massachusetts General Hospital, Boston, Massachusetts   [187, 188]

George Szabó, Ph.D., M.Sc.   Senior Associate in Anatomy (Ret.), Harvard Medical School; Visiting Research Professor, Department of Oral Pathology, Tufts University School of Dental Medicine, Boston, Massachusetts   [18]

Gert Tappeiner, M.D.   Associate Professor, Department of Dermatology, Division of General Dermatology, University of Vienna Medical School, Vienna, Austria   [191]

Francisco A. Tausk, M.D.   Professor, Department of Neuroscience, The Johns Hopkins University School of Medicine, Baltimore, Maryland   [29]

Thomas F. Tedder, Ph.D.   Assistant Professor of Pathology, Harvard Medical School; Division of Tumor Immunology, Dana Farber Cancer Institute, Boston, Massachusetts   [34]

John Thomson, M.D., F.R.C.P., D.Obst., R.C.O.G.   Honorary Clinical Lecturer, The University of Glasgow, Consultant in Dermatology, The Royal Infirmary; Glasgow, Scotland   [65]

Arthur K.F. Tong, M.B., B.S.(Lond)   Dermatologist, Quincy Hospital, Quincy, and New England Memorial Hospital, Stoneham, Massachusetts   [231]

Erwin Tschachler, M.D.   Associate Professor of Dermatology, Department of Dermatology, Division of Immunology, Allergy and Infectious Diseases, University of Vienna, Vienna, Austria   [214]

Jouni Uitto, M.D., Ph.D.   Professor of Dermatology and Biochemistry and Molecular Biology, Chairman, Department of Dermatology, Jefferson Medical College, Thomas Jefferson University, Philadelphia, Pennsylvania   [21, 23]

Marian I. Ulrich, M.D.   Section of Immunology, Instituto de Biomedicina, Caracas, Venezuela   [192]

John P. Utz, M.D.   Professor of Medicine, Georgetown University School of Medicine, Washington, D.C.   [196]

Christopher F.H. Vickers, M.D., F.R.C.P.   Professor of Dermatology, University of Liverpool; Royal Liverpool Hospital and Alder Hey Children's Hospital, Liverpool, England   [231]

Guy F. Webster, M.D., Ph.D.   Assistant Professor of Dermatology, Director of Center for Cutaneous Pharmacology, Thomas Jefferson University, Jefferson Medical College, Philadelphia, Pennsylvania   [235]

Arnold N. Weinberg, M.D.   Professor of Medicine, Harvard Medical School; Physician, Infectious Disease Unit, Massachusetts General Hospital, Boston, Massachusetts   [186, 187, 188, 190]

Richard J. Wenstrup, M.D.   Department of Pediatrics, Duke University Medical Center, Durham, North Carolina   [157]

Victoria P. Werth, M.D.   Assistant Professor of Dermatology, University of Pennsylvania School of Medicine; Chief of Dermatology, Department of Veterans Affairs Medical Center, Philadelphia, Pennsylvania   [232]

Philip W. Wertz, Ph.D.   Associate Professor Dows Institute for Dental Research, University of Iowa College of Dentistry, Iowa City, Iowa   [14]

William Weston, M.D.   Professor and Chairman, Department of Dermatology; Professor of Pediatrics, University of Colorado Medical Center, Denver, Colorado   [239]

Jonathan K. Wilkin, M.D.   Professor, Departments of Pharmacology and Medicine; Director, Division of Dermatology, Ohio State University College of Medicine, Columbus, Ohio   [170]

John D. Wilkinson, M.D.   Department of Dermatology, Wycombe General Hospital, High Wycombe, England   [124]

David C. Wilson, M.D.   Assistant Professor (Medicine), Division of Dermatology, The Vanderbilt Clinic, Nashville, Tennessee   [227]

Robert Winchester, M.D.   Department of Pediatrics, Director, Division of Autoimmune and Molecular Diseases, Columbia University, College of Physicians and Surgeons, New York, New York   [40, 180]

Bruce U. Wintroub, M.D.   Professor and Chairman, Department of Dermatology, University of California, San Francisco; Associate Dean, University of California, San Francisco/Mount Zion School of Medicine, San Francisco, California   [26, 142]

Karen Wiss, M.D.   Assistant Professor of Medicine and Pediatrics; Director of Pediatric Dermatology, Dermatology Department, University of Massachusetts Medical Center, Worcester, Massachusetts   [202]

Klaus Wolff, M.D.   Professor and Chairman, Department of Dermatology; Head, Division of General Dermatology, University of Vienna Medical School, Vienna General Hospital, Vienna, Austria   [1, 6, 8, 58, 89, 93, 99, 139, 191]

Elisabeth Ch. Wolff-Schreiner, M.D.   Associate Professor of Dermatology, Department of Dermatology, Division of General Dermatology, University of Vienna Medical School, Vienna, Austria   [47, 48, 104]

David T. Woodley, M.D.   Professor and Chairman, Department of Dermatology, Northwestern University School of Medicine, Chicago, Illinois   [55]

Nicholas A. Wright, M.D.   Professor and Director of Histopathology, University of London Royal Postgraduate Medical School, Hammersmith Hospital, London, England   [11]

Kim B. Yancey, M.D.   Associate Professor Department of Dermatology, The Uniformed Services University of the Health Sciences, Bethesda, Maryland   [168]

Benjamin K. Yokel, M.D.   Former Chief Resident in Dermatology, The Johns Hopkins University School of Medicine, Baltimore, Maryland   [143]

Antony R. Young, Ph.D.   Department of Photobiology, St.

*Deceased

John's Institute of Dermatology, United Medical and Dental Schools of Guy's and St. Thomas Hospitals, University of London, England   [134]

Stuart H. Yuspa, M.D.   Chief, Laboratory of Cellular Carcinogenesis and Tumor Promotion, Division of Cancer Etiology, National Cancer Institute, National Institutes of Health, Bethesda, Maryland   [70]

Dorothea Zucker-Franklin, M.D.   Professor of Medicine, Department of Medicine, New York University Medical Center, New York, New York   [159]

PREFACE

"To furnish the means of acquiring knowledge is . . . the greatest benefit that can be conferred upon mankind . . . "

Report on the establishment of the
Smithsonian Institution (c. 1846)

The publication of the Fourth Edition of *Dermatology in General Medicine* is a special event for us. The book was conceived in 1965 at a time when there was a pressing need for a modern textbook of dermatology, and this was one of the reasons we undertook the task of writing a new comprehensive textbook of dermatology. Another reason for taking on this new venture was that a new generation of dermatologists had new ideas and had accelerated research on the biology of the skin and on the pathophysiology of skin diseases and their views and concepts of the biology and diseases of the skin had not yet been incorporated into a modern text. In the First Edition we presented our view of dermatology:

Dermatology can be considered relevant and important in general medicine because:

1. *The skin exhibits important clues to diseases in other systems, and these can often be specifically identified by the skin biopsy. Thus, the skin can contribute to the solution of puzzling diagnostic problems in general medicine. The physician must be capable of identifying the changes in the skin that are incidental findings during a general physical examination but cannot be disregarded. The physician cannot know what to overlook unless he is familiar with the spectrum of lesions commonly encountered during the examination of the skin.*

2. *The skin can be an important cause of disability and discomfort. The general physician does not always appreciate the significance of skin lesions and therefore does not refer patients with dermatologic disorders to the dermatologist for appropriate therapy. Too often, dermatologic disease is treated incorrectly for months, the physician's approach to therapy being oral antimycotics and topical and systemic corticosteroids. The postponement of effective treatment not uncommonly leads to an irreversible dissemination of the disorder, prolongs the discomfort, and aids and abets disfigurement.*

3. *The skin can be used to ascertain the fundamental mechanisms of disease, inasmuch as it is the most accessible solid tissue. The one-gene-one-enzyme concept was initiated by Sir Archibald Garrod's study of, among other diseases, albinism.*

This book attempts to place dermatology in the continuum of general medicine and to acquaint the general physician with the vast array of cutaneous lesions that indicate pathology in other organ systems.

For the First Edition of *Dermatology in General Medicine,* we were fortunate to have had as collaborating editors the dermatopathologist, Dr. Wallace H. Clark, Jr., the immunologist, Dr. John H. Vaughan, and the dermatologists, Dr. Eugene J. Van Scott and Dr. Kenneth A. Arndt.

From all indications *Dermatology in General Medicine* in these two decades has had a salutary effect on the practice of dermatology and is generally regarded throughout the world as an authoritative textbook of dermatology and of dermatologic manifestations of multisystem diseases—a treasury of information, which contains a large collection of photographs of clinical disorders, in color for the first time in this Fourth Edition. Most of the excellent photomicrographs taken by Dr. Wallace H. Clark, Jr., for the First Edition are still included.

Increasingly, clinicians and scientists have had their eyes opened regarding the depth and breadth of dermatology. The presentation of the skin manifestations of multisystem diseases has made this book popular with internists (especially rheumatologists, endocrinologists, infectious disease physicians, and gastroenterologists), primary care physicians, pediatricians, and plastic surgeons. For the scientist, for the physician interested in research, and for the inquiring clinician, there are comprehensive chapters on the biology and pathophysiology of skin. Some chapters are virtual monographs, e.g., neurocutaneous diseases, melanocytic nevi, biology and disorders of melanin pigmentation, skin manifestations of AIDS, *inter alia.*

For this Fourth Edition, there have been extensive revisions and additions to existing chapters with 100 new authors. A number of new chapters have been added, including:

In Part I—*Introduction:* Dermatologic Diagnosis by Recognition of Clinical Morphologic Patterns and Syndromes.

In Part II—*Biology and Pathophysiology of Skin:* Genetics in Relation to the Skin; The Epidermis: An Immunologic Microenvironment; Skin as an Organ of Protection; Ecology and Host Resistance in Relation to Skin Disease; The Cellular and Molecular Biology of the Human Mast Cell; Endothelium: Differentiation and Activation; Cutaneous Microvasculature; Neurobiology of the Skin; and Arachidonic Acid Metabolism.

In Part III—*Disorders Presenting in the Skin and Mucous Membranes:* Carcinogenesis: Ultraviolet Radiation; Cutaneous Neuroendocrine Carcinoma: Merkel Cell; Cutaneous Manifestations in the Immunosuppressed Host; Skin Problems in Amputees; Sports Dermatology; Mucocutaneous Complications of Antineoplastic Therapy; and Cutaneous Manifestations of Drug Abuse.

In Part IV—*Dermatology and Internal Medicine:* Genetic Immunodeficiency Diseases; Cryoglobulinemia and Cryofibrinogenemia.

In Part V—*Diseases due to Microbial Agents:* Lyme Borreliosis.

In Part VII—*Pediatric and Geriatric Dermatology:* Geriatric Dermatology.

To assure high quality of the clinical color photographs for this edition, we have been fortunate to have the discriminatory guidance of Dr. Richard Allen Johnson as the Color Illustration Editor, who, with the assistance of the Editors, selected the clinical color photographs. The authors have a special word of appreciation for the skillful collaboration of Patricia K. Novak, who has been an important editorial colleague for all four of the editions of this book; the editors also acknowledge the help of Arlene Stolper Simon in this and previous editions. McGraw-Hill, Inc., has been very patient and cooperative in producing this complex text and we acknowledge the cooperation of J. Dereck Jeffers, Mariapaz Ramos Englis, Roger Kasunic, and Mark Elszy.

The Editors

DERMATOLOGY IN GENERAL MEDICINE

PART FOUR

Dermatology and Internal Medicine

Cutaneous Lesions in Nutritional, Metabolic, and Heritable Disorders

CHAPTER 145

Donald S. McLaren

Nutrients are chemical substances that must be ingested in appropriate amounts if health is to be maintained. About 50 nutrients are known for humans, disorders involving about half of which are associated with characteristic clinical manifestations. The skin and its appendages are affected in many instances. Most of these clinical states result from nutrient deficiency, whether primary due to inadequate dietary intake or secondary to problems in utilization, but not uncommonly toxicity from excessive intake may also induce disease. Although diseases such as pellagra, scurvy, and kwashiorkor have skin lesions prominent among their symptomatology, it is important to appreciate that they, like all nutritional disorders, are generalized conditions affecting many systems. Furthermore, an inadequate diet tends to lead to multiple deficiencies. The accessibility of the skin and its appendages and mucous membranes to examination makes them especially valuable in clinical diagnosis.

Energy and Protein

Experimental Starvation in Adults

The most thorough study of the effects of inanition on the skin of human volunteers was made as part of the monumental Minnesota experiment.[1] The skin of the subjects, after 23 weeks on a diet providing only 1570 kcal, was thinner than normal, dry, inelastic, pallid, and grayish in color. It was described as being cold and "dead" to the touch with a tendency to cyanosis in cold weather. All these signs were very suggestive of those commonly seen in old age. Less regular in occurrence was the rough gooseflesh appearance similar to the follicular hyperkeratosis associated by some workers with vitamin A deficiency (see "Vitamin A Deficiency" below). A patchy, dirty brownish pigmentation situated anywhere on the body, but most commonly on the face, was found to some degree but never sufficiently marked to resemble the skin changes of pellagra (see below). The hair was dry, dull, and "staring," with a tendency to cease growing and to fall out very easily, very much as described in protein-energy malnutrition in children (see "Kwashiorkor" below).

Cutaneous Changes in Nutritional Disorders

Privation Starvation in Adults

In times of famine and war many abnormal appearances of the skin have been described, in addition to the obvious loss of subcutaneous fat, which most noticeably affects normally prominent depots of fat (e.g., buttocks) and muscle masses (thighs, back) that waste, causing bones to protrude. Some of these changes may be attributed to starvation in terms of calories, but others are undoubtedly more closely related to the breakdown of sanitary and medical facilities at such times. Pallor of the skin is often more than can be explained by anemia, and the skin is abnormally cold as a result of vasoconstriction. In victims of famine and prisoners of war, the skin has frequently been described as dry, rough, scaly, thin, and inelastic—resembling the skin of old age. A similar appearance is found in anorexia nervosa and, indeed, in any prolonged wasting disease, whatever the cause. In undernourished, dark-skinned people fine, mosaic-like fissuring of the skin is extremely common, as are burnished, hyperpigmented lesions over the shins and dorsa of the feet. These appearances are probably related to repeated minor trauma in individuals with chronic marginal undernutrition resulting from habitually consuming a diet low in most essential nutrients.

Follicular hyperkeratosis and folliculosis have been reputed to be associated with undernutrition. The former is recognized clinically as small, hard, elevated nodules around the hair follicles, giving the skin a "nutmeg grater" texture. The follicles may be filled with keratotic plugs. Exactly what is meant by *folliculosis* in nutrition survey reports is far from clear. It usually seems to mean a relative prominence of the hair follicle due to thinning of the epidermal, dermal, and subcutaneous layers of the skin; it is also called *follicular pouting* and *permanent gooseflesh*. The clinical significance of these appearances is unclear (see "Vitamin A Deficiency" below).

Pigmentary changes in the skin are characteristic in semistarvation. Their color is usually brownish, darker than ordinary suntan, and they usually manifest around the mouth and eyes and on the malar prominences. Less commonly, the hands, arms, and trunk are involved. The changes are not like those seen in pellagra.

Changes in the hair have also been reported to occur frequently in semistarvation. It is thin, grows slowly, falls out prematurely, and rapidly becomes gray. The nails grow slowly and may be fissured. Some have reported a pronounced development of downy hair (lanugo) all over the body, especially on the face and nape of the neck in children, as well as in patients with anorexia nervosa.

Starvation in Children (Marasmus)

Total inanition in the child, with intake of all nutrients greatly reduced but especially protein and energy, soon leads to suppression of growth, negative nitrogen balance due to catabolism of tissue protein for energy, and the state of *marasmus* (Greek, "wasting"). This is one form of what is now termed *protein-energy malnutrition* of early childhood (see also "Kwashiorkor" below). It is widely prevalent throughout the developing regions of the world and is to a large extent responsible for the high mortality in infancy and early childhood. The disturbed nutrition is usually secondary to weaning problems resulting from ignorance, poor hygiene, and economic and cultural factors.[2]

In contrast to kwashiorkor, there is classically no clinical edema or dermatosis in marasmus. As in the undernourished, the skin is dry, wrinkled, and loose, due to marked loss of subcutaneous fat. The "monkey facies" with loss of the buccal fat pads is characteristic (Fig. 145-1). Emaciation may be extreme (Fig. 145-2). There is some evidence to suggest that pitting edema is seen only if the subcutaneous fat is largely preserved, as in kwashiorkor.

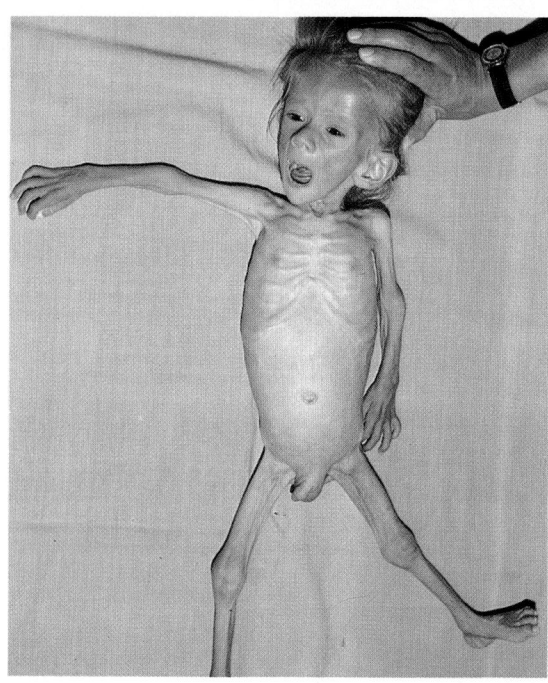

FIGURE 145-2 Marasmus. General appearance with advanced disease.

Kwashiorkor

This form of protein-energy malnutrition results from a diet quantitatively and qualitatively poor in protein and essential amino acids but with an adequate and often excessive intake of energy from starch or sugar. Characteristically, the weanling child is affected; in addition to the dermatosis and hair changes to be described below, there are typically retarded growth, hypoalbuminemia, edema, moon face, fatty liver, and psychomotor changes. Much less commonly, a similar clinical picture has been reported in school-age children and young adults, and several cases are on record following extensive intestinal surgical treatment resulting in a secondary type of protein malnutrition.

The skin lesions are not invariably present in kwashiorkor, but when present they are diagnostic and characteristic. They are more frequent and severe in dark-skinned races; the basic change is depigmentation. The first sign is circumoral pallor; pallor is also marked on the legs. The skin is stretched with edema, and the pallor may be due as much to thinning and distention of the skin as to actual loss of pigment. Localized losses of pigment may follow abrasions, wounds, ulceration, or other injuries (Fig. 145-3).

The characteristic dermatosis in white-skinned infants starts with erythema. At first the skin blanches on pressure, but this is rapidly followed by small, dusky, purple patches that do not blanch. On dark skins, purple areas darken within a few hours of appearing. They have a burnished surface and feel almost waxy to the touch. They have an absolutely sharp edge and appear raised above the surrounding skin, as if small particles of enamel paint had been applied. They are most common in areas subject to pressure, especially if combined with moisture resulting from sweat or any other secretions or discharge. The diaper area is affected early, as also are the trochanters, knees, ankles, elbows, and areas of pressure on the trunk. The dermatosis seldom appears on areas exposed to sunlight and, in contrast to pellagra, it spares the feet and dorsa of the hands.

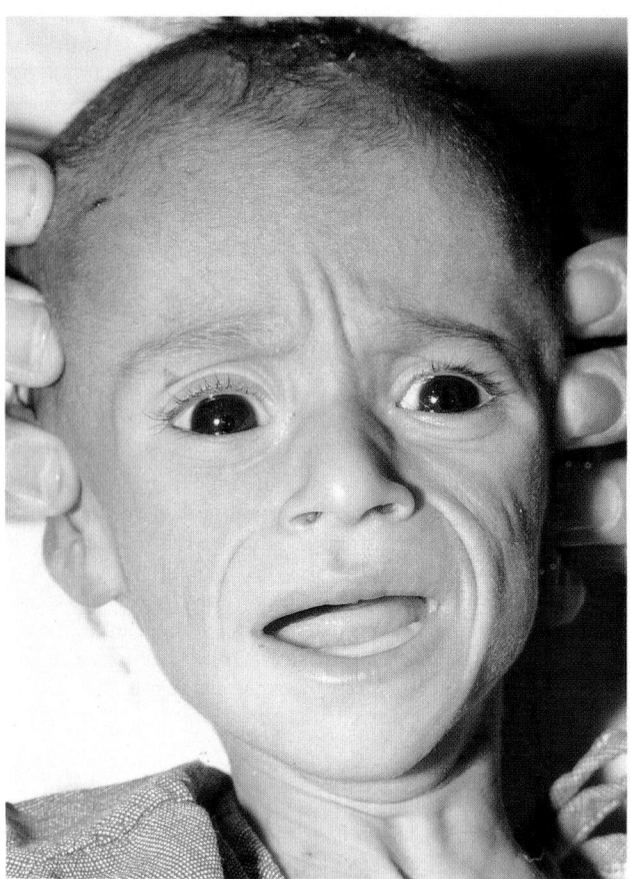

FIGURE 145-1 Marasmus. "Monkey facies" in an Arab infant with wrinkled skin and loss of subcutaneous fat.

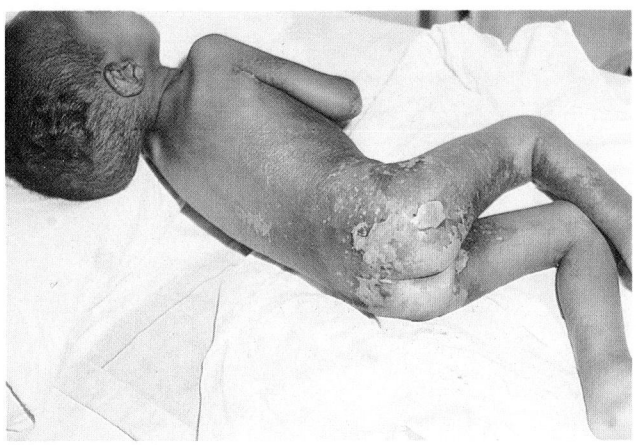

FIGURE 145-3 Kwashiorkor. "Flaky paint" dermatosis.

Whereas in mild cases patients show only a superficial desquamation, in severe cases there are large areas of erosion in which much skin is lost. This characteristic dermatosis was given the descriptive names of "enamel paint," "flaky paint," and "crazy paving" dermatosis. Advanced cases may also show linear fissuring in the flexures around the pinna, on the back of the knee, in front of the elbow, in the axilla, between the toes, at the edge of the foreskin, and in the center of the lips. All these lesions appear to be precipitated by intermittent tension, and those occurring at the corners of the mouth should be distinguished from the angular stomatitis of riboflavin deficiency, in which there is usually a heaped-up, sodden appearance (Fig. 145-4, see also Fig. 145-13). It has been observed that the skin changes of kwashiorkor bear a remarkable resemblance to those of acrodermatitis enteropathica (see Chap. 146). A well-controlled clinical trial to determine the relationship between kwashiorkor and zinc deficiency has not been carried out. Patients show multiple nutritional deficiencies, including that of zinc, and response of the skin and other abnormalities to a complete diet is dramatic.

One of the milder skin changes in kwashiorkor, and the most commonly observed sign involving the skin in fair-skinned children, is a dry, fine desquamation with cracking along the natural

lines to give "mosaic skin" or "cracked skin." The shins, outer sides of the thighs, and back of the trunk are among the other areas commonly affected. In fair Arab children, the changes are especially prone to affect the forehead with some hyperpigmentation (Fig. 145-5).

Occasionally on the dorsum of the foot, on the buttocks, or on sites not obviously related to pressure, a large bulla may form and break, leaving a shallow depression.

In advanced kwashiorkor the skin is very easily damaged. Bony points on the pelvis and over the elbows and knees are easily rubbed raw. Special care has to be taken in nursing these cases, most especially if metabolic experiments are being carried out that necessitate keeping the child on a special bed for continuous collection of stools and urine.

True pellagrous skin changes can occur in children with evidence of kwashiorkor. This is especially apt to arise when children are weaned onto a diet containing much maize flour, as in south and central Africa.

The nails are often thin and soft in kwashiorkor, and this may be particularly obvious when healthy new nails start to grow, forming a mass at the nail base that is completely separated from the old nail.

The hair in kwashiorkor shows depigmentation, is sparse, thin in texture, and comes out easily. None of these changes is specific to kwashiorkor; in malnourished Arab children they are seen about as frequently accompanying marasmus. Kwashiorkor may be diagnosed without the presence of hair changes, although this is rather unusual. Hair that is normally black becomes brown or reddish, and brown hair turns blond. Somehow the idea has spread that kwashiorkor means "red boy," red referring to the hair change. The word *kwashiorkor*, however (taken from the Ga language of Ghana), means "the sickness of the weanling," an apt description of the pathogenesis of the condition. There are many causes of bleaching

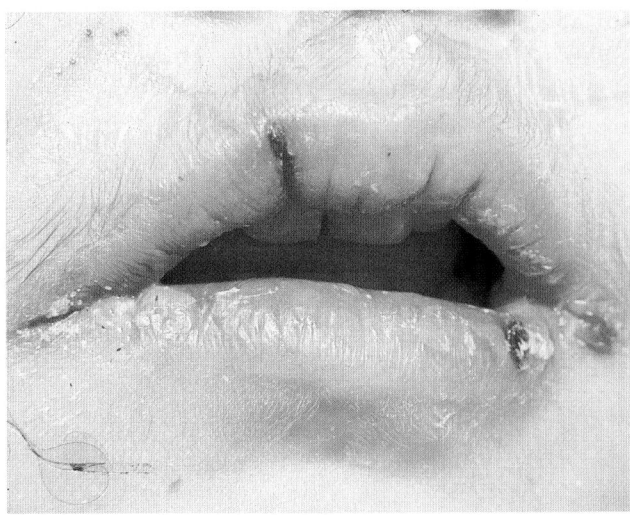

FIGURE 145-4 Kwashiorkor. Fissuring of lips in a child (compare with riboflavin in Fig. 145-13).

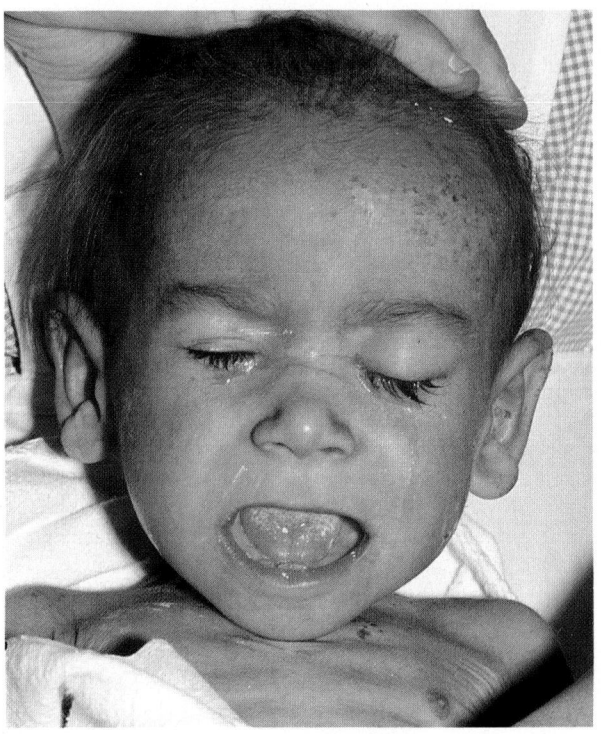

FIGURE 145-5 Kwashiorkor. Scaly hyperpigmented dermatosis of the forehead in an Arab child.

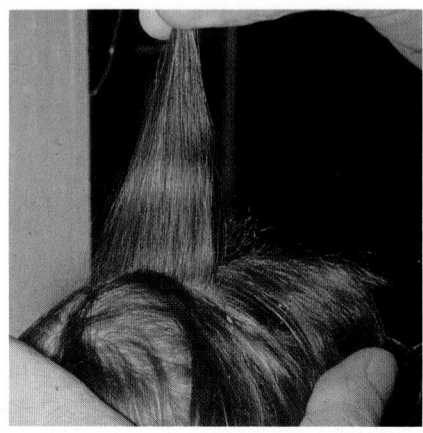

a

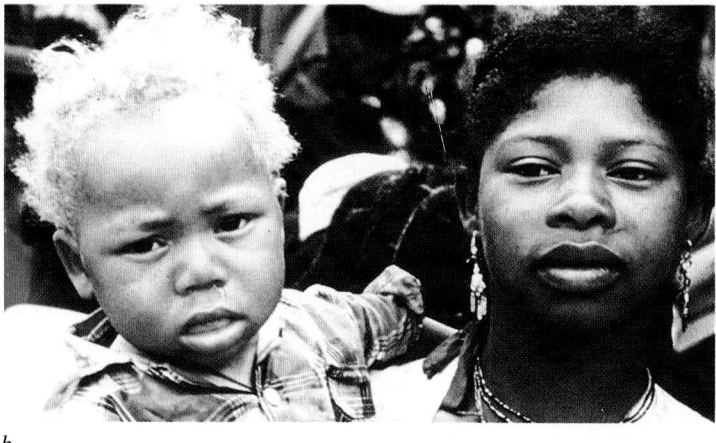

b

FIGURE 145-6   Kwashiorkor. (*a*) Flag sign in a Salvadoran child. (*b*) Hypomelanization of the hair and skin.

of the hair other than malnutrition—such as sunlight and oxidizing agents—and care must be taken in interpretation. Especially striking is the flag sign (*signe de la bandera*) affecting long and normally dark hair. The hair grown during periods of inadequate nutrition is pale, so that alternating bands of dark and pale hair can be seen along a single strand, recording alternating periods of adequate and inadequate nutrition (Fig. 145-6).

The other changes undergone by the hair are more constant and more reliable than the alterations in color described above. The growth of hair is sparse and it comes out easily. There may be recession from the temporal region and loss from the back of the head, probably due to pressure when the child lies down. Loss of hair may be extreme in advanced cases. The texture of the hair becomes softer and finer than normal for a child of that age and culture. It tends to be unruly and to resemble the ''staring'' coat of some animals described in nutritional deficiency. The eyelashes may undergo the same change, having a so-called ''broomstick'' appearance.

In health, most of the scalp hairs are in the anagen, or active, growth phase and few in the telogen, or resting, phase. In early protein-energy malnutrition this is reversed, and analysis of the hair cycle has been advocated as a diagnostic procedure.[3]

Cancrum Oris (Noma, Necrotizing Ulcerative Gingivitis)

The cause of this destructive lesion (Fig. 145-7), usually involving the face in the region of the mouth, is not clear. Malnutrition in the form of kwashiorkor or marasmus is almost always present, but it is sometimes difficult to decide whether the nutritional deficiency is primary or whether it is secondary to the obvious interference with normal feeding. Likewise, the role played by the constantly present Vincent's organisms is obscure.

Infants and preschool children are most commonly affected. Cancrum oris is reported not infrequently from all parts of Africa, some areas in southeast Asia, and tropical America, especially in relation to famine. It used to occur in Europe following measles, typhus, or typhoid fever.

Most cases probably start as an area of ulcerative gingivitis with a tender, firm swelling of the upper gum and underlying bone and some swelling of the overlying part of the face. Very soon the teeth loosen, and inflammation spreads into the underlying bone

with osteitis and a sequestrum. The cheek usually ulcerates, producing a cavity leading directly into the mouth. Occasionally the process originates in the nose, vulva, or elsewhere.

Without treatment there is rapid progress of the disease, frequently leading to death. Broad-spectrum antibiotics halt the progression of the disease, although massive residual defects continue to present extremely difficult cosmetic surgery problems, particularly in relation to the relatively primitive medical facilities available where the disease occurs. A full diet is of great value, especially one rich in protein, high in energy value, and providing all vitamins and essential elements. Feeding difficulties can now be overcome if total parenteral nutrition is available.

Tropical Ulcer (Tropical Sloughing Phagedena)

This chronic condition, chiefly affecting the lower limbs above the malleoli, shares with cancrum oris the frequent background of general malnutrition of the patient and the occurrence of Vincent's

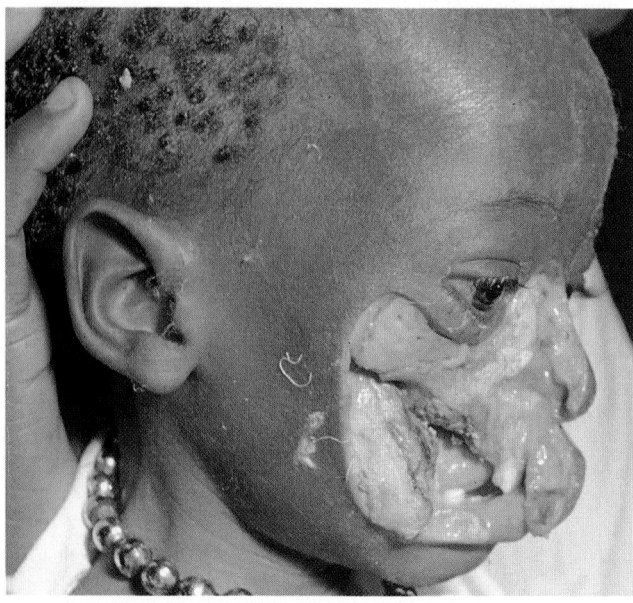

FIGURE 145-7   Cancrum oris (noma). Massive destruction of the face in a Tanzanian child.

organisms in the lesions. A recent survey[4] of 170 patients in Zambia, Gambia, South India, and Papua New Guinea found that children and teenagers were most commonly affected. There was no correlation between the development of an ulcer and nutritional status found in this survey. Nevertheless, a good diet, rest, and antibiotics give good results and healing is usually complete within six months.

The disease starts with the formation of a larger or smaller blister with serosanguinolent contents. When the bulla ruptures, an ash-gray moist slough is exposed. The sloughing process extends rapidly, until the skin and subcutaneous fascia over quite a large area may be converted into a yellowish, moist, foul-smelling ulcer. In extensive cases, muscles, tendons, nerves, vessels, and even the periosteum may have shared in the gangrenous process. Even after healing, deformity may ensue from ankylosis, and a contracting cicatrix may strangulate a vital part, necessitating amputation. Smaller healed tropical ulcers leave behind tissue-paper-like scars with pigmented edges. These are prone to break down.

Obesity

Skin disorders tend to be common in the obese. Excessive fat folds lead to intertrigo from friction between skin surfaces and to maceration of the skin from accumulated moisture in the folds. Infection frequently supervenes, particularly with staphylococci, dermatophytes, and yeast. The obese become overheated easily and sweat more profusely because of the thick layers of subcutaneous fat; areas of inflammation and skin rashes are thus exaggerated. Many obese patients have either a diabetic tendency or frank diabetes with all the accompanying dermatoses. It is important in all these circumstances that due attention be paid during treatment to measures aimed at correction of the underlying obesity; otherwise, local treatment of the skin lesions will remain purely palliative.

Vitamins

Vitamin A (Retinol)

This fat-soluble vitamin is found only in the animal kingdom. Many plants contain one or more of the several provitamin carotenoids of which beta-carotene is the most active. Vitamin A, as the aldehyde (retinal), has a well-defined role in night vision, and the earliest clinical manifestation of vitamin A deficiency is impairment of dark adaptation. In animals, deficiency of vitamin A has been shown to have profound effects, including cessation of growth, death, congenital malformations, and severe damage especially to epithelial tissues. In both humans and animals, severe deficiency produces destructive eye lesions affecting the conjunctiva (xerosis conjunctivae, Bitot's spots) and cornea (xerosis corneae and keratomalacia). Recent work suggests that even subclinical deficiency of vitamin A is associated with increased morbidity from infections and mortality in young children.[5]

Vitamin A Deficiency There is general agreement that severely malnourished patients with the pathognomonic ocular lesions of vitamin A deficiency may also show changes in the skin attributable to the same cause. The skin over large areas of the body is dry, wrinkled, and covered with fine scales. These changes were described in China more than 50 years ago,[6] together with deep, excavated lesions, which were termed *dermomalacia*. Marked changes

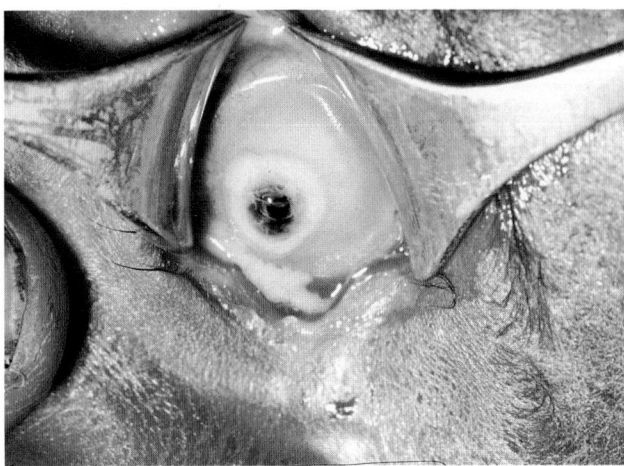

FIGURE 145-8 Vitamin A deficiency, advanced keratomalacia. 5-month old Arab child. Note hyperkeratosis of facial skin. Serum vitamin A level was 2 μg/dL (normal, 20 to 50 μg).

of this type are extremely uncommon, even in children with bilateral keratomalacia (Figs. 145-8 and 145-9).

Histologically, those skin lesions that can confidently be attributed to vitamin A deficiency represent primary hyperkeratinization and hyperplasia of the epidermis, including the lining of the hair follicles and sebaceous glands. Most characteristically in the conjunctiva and cornea, vitamin A deficiency causes metaplasia, but in the skin there is an accentuation of a process of progressive keratinization normally inherent here.

In infants and very young children, before the pilosebaceous follicle has fully matured, simple xerosis, or xeroderma, is usually the characteristic feature. The stratum corneum is usually several times its normal thickness, and there is blockage of sweat ducts and hyperkeratinization of the follicle lining.

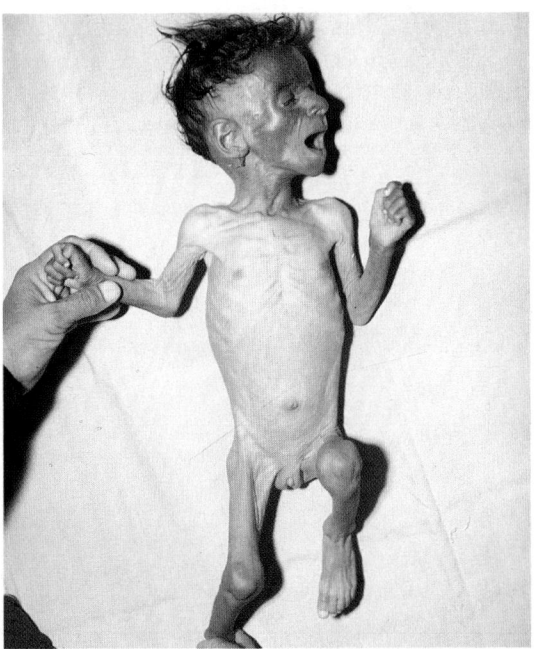

FIGURE 145-9 Vitamin A deficiency. General appearance in the same patient as Fig. 145-8.

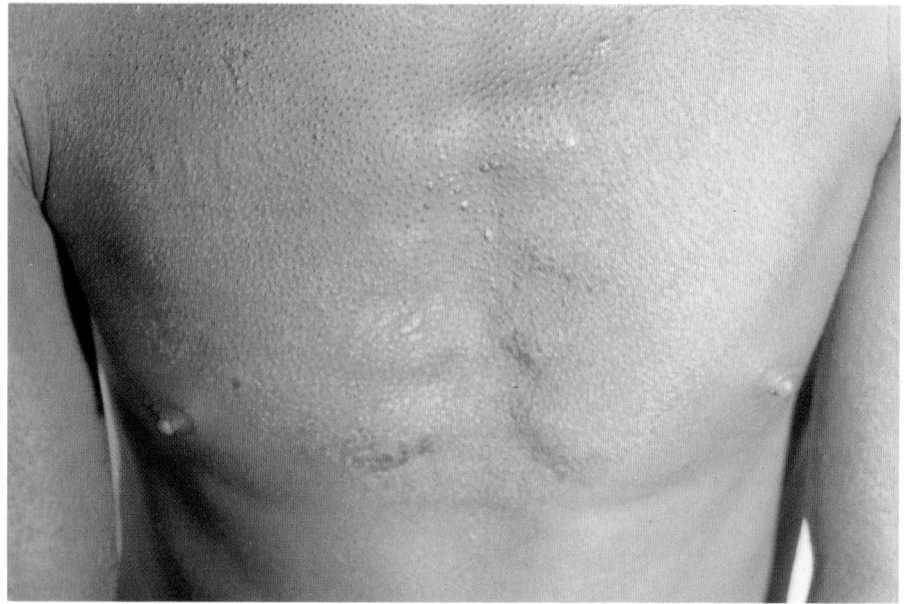

FIGURE 145-10 Vitamin A deficiency. Typical perifollicular hyperkeratosis of the chest in a Tanzanian adult male.

Adults, especially those who have exhibited the advanced ocular manifestations, have shown grosser changes. The stratum corneum forms a broad network of horny plates, with abundant desquamation of fine scales. The stratum lucidum and stratum granulosum remain unchanged. The basal layers are unaltered except for increased melanin deposition. Sebaceous glands are reduced in number, sweat gland ducts are occluded by keratinous material, and although the glands are normal in appearance, they are probably hypofunctional. Except for perifollicular infiltration, the dermis is normal.

It is significant that the follicular reaction is minimal in those cases with marked hyperkeratosis and pathognomonic eye lesions; this is in contrast to the pronounced reaction in the very common follicular hyperkeratosis usually accompanied by generalized hyperkeratosis or eye changes.

It is a follicular eruption (Figs. 145-10 and 145-11), termed *follicular hyperkeratosis* by Frazier and Hu,[6] that has proved to be so controversial. It is interesting to note that Pillat, the ophthalmologist, made no reference to such a finding, although he was working in the same hospital and the 14 cases that Frazier and Hu reported were drawn from a group of 209 soldiers with ocular lesions seen by Pillat. The follicular changes were described as occurring on a background of generally dry and rough skin. Spinous papules

appeared at the tips of the hair follicles. First affected were the anterolateral aspects of the thighs and the posterolateral parts of the upper forearms. The eruptions slowly spread to the extensor surface of upper and lower limbs, the shoulders, the lower part of the abdomen, and, to a lesser extent, the chest, back, and buttocks. Each papule had a keratotic plug at its apex, projecting as a hard spinous process. The eruption was usually abundant and symmetric. With a generally good diet and cod liver oil (up to 30 mL daily) the skin lesions improved slowly, but even after 2 months the skin had not regained its normal appearance.

Subsequently, under the name of *phrynoderma,* or "toad skin," such follicular changes, frequently of a much milder nature and more limited distribution, have been attributed to nutritional deficiency. Not only deficiency of vitamin A, but deficiency of linoleic acid or vitamins of the B complex have all been implicated.

The evidence from deprivation experiments in humans does not support the contention that follicular hyperkeratosis can be associated specifically with vitamin A deficiency. In the Sheffield experiment,[7] 20 men and 3 women received a diet deficient in vitamin A and carotene for periods ranging from 6½ to 25 months. With regard to the minimal skin changes observed, it was concluded that the enlargement and hyperkeratosis of the hair follicles that occurred among both the supplemented and the deprived group

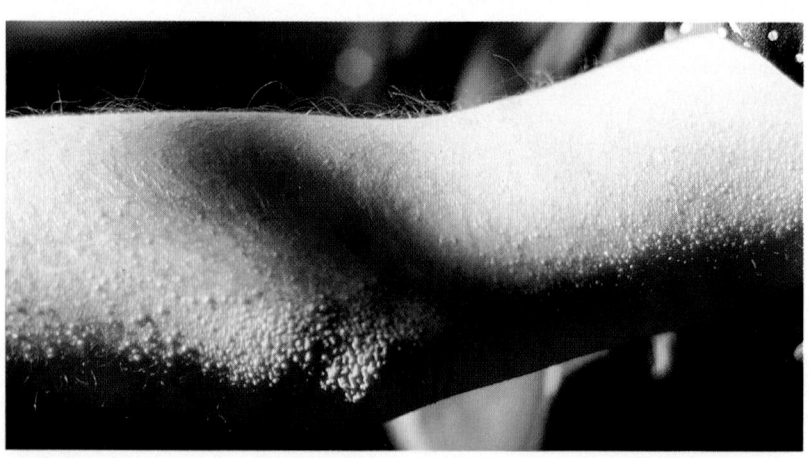

FIGURE 145-11 Vitamin A deficiency. Marked perifollicular hyperkeratosis on the arm in an undernourished Iranian child.

fluctuated in both extent and size of the eruption independently of the state of vitamin A nutrition.

In view of the lack of proof of nutritional deficiency as the cause of hyperfollicular keratosis, it is especially important to explore the possibility of other diagnoses. The distribution of the lesions and infrequency of pustulation should rule out acne vulgaris; the rarity of the eruption in postpubertal females and in adolescent children seems incompatible with keratosis pilaris, and the relatively rare Darier's disease may be excluded by the absence of familial tendency and the demonstration of dyskeratotic changes in the skin specimen.

Massive oral vitamin A therapy has been advocated for many skin conditions of unknown cause, including some mentioned above, that pose problems of differential diagnosis. Other conditions that have been treated with vitamin A include pityriasis rubra pilaris, keratosis palmaris et plantaris, ichthyosis, and pachyonychia. In none of these conditions has a deficiency of vitamin A been demonstrated.

Various synthetic vitamin A derivatives, known as retinoids, are effective in a variety of dermatologic diseases in which keratinization is disturbed (see Chap. 236).[8] Prolonged use and high dosage of these compounds has led to toxic reactions, including severe fetal abnormalities in offspring of women who have become pregnant while receiving the drugs.[9]

Vitamin A Toxicity (Hypervitaminosis A)   The skin is frequently involved in both acute and chronic forms of vitamin A toxicity. Desquamation over large areas of the body, accompanied by severe headache and vomiting, has occurred in arctic explorers after a single meal of the liver of polar bear, bearded seal, or sledge dogs previously fed on the livers of these animals. Chronic poisoning results from injudicious therapeutic use of the vitamin or its derivatives. The bizarre symptomatology includes coarsening of the skin with pruritus and loss of hair. Frequently the true diagnosis is made only when it occurs to someone to have the serum level of vitamin A checked by the laboratory. The unfortunate patients have been labeled as having brain tumors, psychoneurosis, generalized infectious arthritis, Addison's disease, hepatitis, or dermatomyositis before the true nature of the process has been determined.

Both acute and chronic manifestations of hypervitaminosis A must be watched for in young children; increasing numbers of such cases are being reported in the literature. Central nervous system and bone changes are especially common, but pruritus and desquamation are not infrequent.

Withdrawal of vitamin A brings about gradual improvement over several weeks, and, in spite of the alarming manifestations of vitamin A poisoning, no fatalities have been reported to date.

Carotenoderma   The time taken to produce clinically appreciable pigmentation depends to some extent on dietary consumption of carotenoids. In one instance 1.8 kg of carrots were consumed weekly for 7 months. Children develop carotenoderma more readily than adults. An infant showed the characteristic yellowish skin pigmentation after only 2 months on the breast milk of its carotenemic mother, while another, born pigmented to such a mother, remained yellow until weaned. Appropriate laboratory tests, including determination of total serum carotenoids (usual range for healthy adults: 40 to 150 μg/dL), will differentiate hypercarotenosis from such conditions as hemolytic anemia, pernicious anemia, or obstructive jaundice. It is especially likely to occur during wartime, with rationing of meat, butter, and cheese, and with increased consumption of fresh green leafy vegetables—rich

sources of beta-carotene. It is endemic in parts of the world such as central and west Africa where red palm oil is used for cooking.

Excess carotene is, in part, excreted in sweat and reabsorbed by the horny layer of the skin. Carotenoderma is said to develop more readily in those who sweat profusely. Deposition occurs first and predominantly in the nasolabial folds and over the forehead, where sebaceous glands abound, and on the palms and soles where the horny layer of the skin is thickest. It has to be borne in mind that some carotene is present in all normal skin. Carotene is found to a lesser degree on the upper eyelids, inner canthi, ears, and anterior folds of the axillae, and over areas subject to pressure, e.g., the elbows, knees, and malleoli. This uneven distribution helps to distinguish carotenoderma from jaundice.

Carotenoderma is usually not noticeable until the serum level is three or four times normal. The color of the skin is canary yellow, ochre, or golden. It never has the bronze, orange, saffron, or green tint of jaundice. Mucous membranes, including the sclerae, are not stained by carotene. Subconjunctival or submucosal fat, if present, may be stained and lead to confusion. Other points of differentiation from jaundice are that hypercarotenosis does not cause itching and does not significantly change the color of urine or stools, although plasma is bright yellow. As far as is known, hypercarotenosis in all its forms appears to be harmless. If of dietary origin, it slowly disappears when the intake is reduced to normal levels.

In diabetes mellitus there is frequently a raised serum carotene level, but carotenoderma develops in only about 10 percent of cases. In this disease it is probably due to a high dietary consumption, but there may possibly be impaired conversion of carotene to vitamin A. Some patients with hypothyroidism also have carotenoderma and this may be related to the known function of thyroid hormone in facilitating carotene conversion. Hypercarotenemia has been consistently reported in anorexia nervosa. It occasionally results in carotenoderma and is of obscure origin.

Vitamins of the B Complex

Niacin (Pellagra)   The amide of niacin is an important constituent of coenzyme I (oxidized form of nicotinamide-adenine dinucleotide, NAD) and coenzyme II (reduced form of nicotinamide-adenine dinucleotide, NADP) that either donate or accept hydrogen ions in vital oxidation-reduction reactions. The essential amino acid, tryptophan, can be converted in the body to niacin, about 60 mg of tryptophan being the dietary equivalent of 1 mg of niacin. The cause of pellagra is still not entirely clear. It may arise from a diet deficient in niacin or tryptophan, or more commonly both, and amino acid imbalance may also play a part. A predominantly maize diet is usually implicated, but only if the maize is steamed or cooked. In parts of Latin America maize flour is lime-treated and made into tortillas; this process releases niacin from an insoluble form called niacytin and usually prevents the occurrence of pellagra. Besides the dermatosis, there are important gastrointestinal and nervous system changes.

The dermatosis is usually preceded by prodromal symptoms, especially of the digestive system. The skin changes are characteristic and pathognomonic, and their distribution is determined especially by exposure to the sun and by localized pressure. The diagnosis of pellagra is difficult in the absence of the dermatosis, which begins as erythema on the dorsa of the hands, with pruritus and burning. It is characteristically symmetric with slight edema of the skin. In some patients, several days after the onset of the erythema, blisters appear; these run together to form bullae and then break. In others, dry brown scales form. On the face, the scales are thicker, larger, and frequently become pustular.

In the second stage, the dermatosis becomes hard, rough, cracked, blackish, and brittle. The epidermis of the fingers thickens, and the articular folds disappear. Painful fissures develop in the palms and on the digits. The skin may look like that of a goose; hence the term *goose skin*. When the deficiency state is far advanced, the skin becomes progressively harder, drier, more cracked, and covered with scales and blackish crusts that are due to hemorrhages.

The usual sites are the face, neck, and dorsal surfaces of the hands, arms, and feet. The changes are rarely seen elsewhere. The dorsa of the hands are the most frequent site; here the lesions may extend up the arm to form the "glove" or "gauntlet" of pellagra (Fig. 145-12a). The symmetry and clear line of demarcation from normal skin are especially striking. On the feet the lesions usually do not rise proximally to the malleoli, which are included; the heels remain free. Distally, the eruption ends at the toes or on the backs of the great toes. The front and back of the leg may be involved to form a "boot."

On the face the symmetry of the lesions is striking. They tend to spread from the sides to the rest of the nose, the forehead, cheeks, chin, lips, and, more rarely, eyelids and ears. The "butterfly" appearance, common to lupus erythematosus, is frequent. On the forehead there is always a narrow border of normal skin between the erythema and the hair. The face is often only slightly affected. The facial lesions never appear independently of lesions on the hands and elsewhere.

Casal's "necklace" extends as a fairly broad band, or collar, entirely around the neck (Fig. 145-12b). If the band is incomplete, the lesions are striking in their symmetry. The upper border reaches from somewhat below the hairline to the larynx anteriorly. The lower border begins under the vertebral prominences and extends to the edge of the manubrium. In many instances the necklace has an anterior continuation, or broad "cravat," extending from the manubrium over the sternum to the level of the nipples, ending in a point or square. Men, women, and children have the necklace, and it is always accompanied by the characteristic dermatosis elsewhere.

Other sites occasionally affected are the shoulders, elbows, forearms, and knees. The so-called pellagrous vulvitis, vaginitis, and lesions of the perianal region and scrotum are dealt with as part of the "oro-oculo-genital" syndrome [see "Riboflavin (Oro-Oculo-Genital Syndrome)" below].

Healing usually takes place centrifugally with the line of demarcation remaining actively inflamed after the center of the lesion has desquamated. Specific therapy consists of the oral administration of 100 to 300 mg of niacinamide daily in divided doses. The amide is preferable since it does not precipitate the vasomotor disturbances resulting from administration of niacin in large doses. A similar dose is given subcutaneously when diarrhea or a noncooperative patient makes oral administration ineffective or difficult. Multivitamins (especially other vitamins of the B complex) and a high-quality protein diet (about 100 g per day) should be given.

Riboflavin (Oro-Oculo-Genital Syndrome)   This vitamin has coenzyme function in the chain of reversible oxidation-reduction reactions on which tissue respiration depends. A variety of lesions has been produced by animal experimental deficiency, but in humans the changes appear mainly in the skin and mucous membranes.

For many years a syndrome resembling pellagra but without the typical dermatosis had been known, going by the rather confusing name of *pellagra sine pellagra*. Sebrell and Butler[10] studied a group of patients on a diet low in riboflavin and nicotinic acid and showed that the manifestations of pellagra sine pellagra were due to riboflavin deficiency. The changes commenced with pallor of the

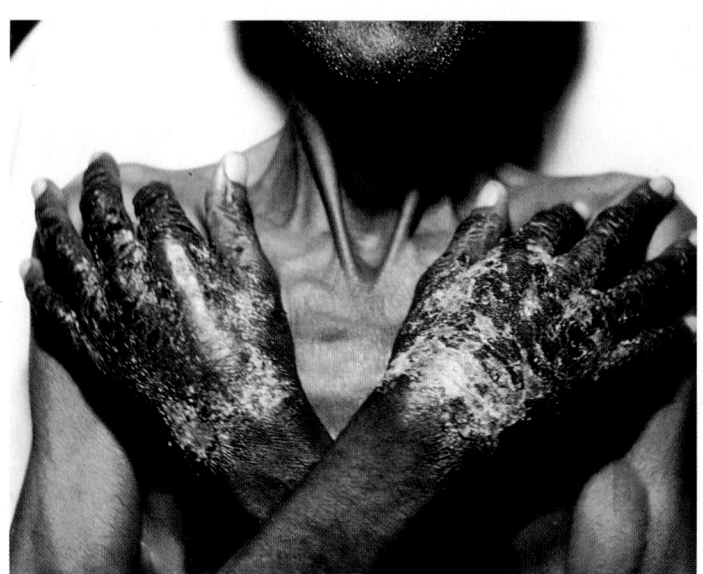

a

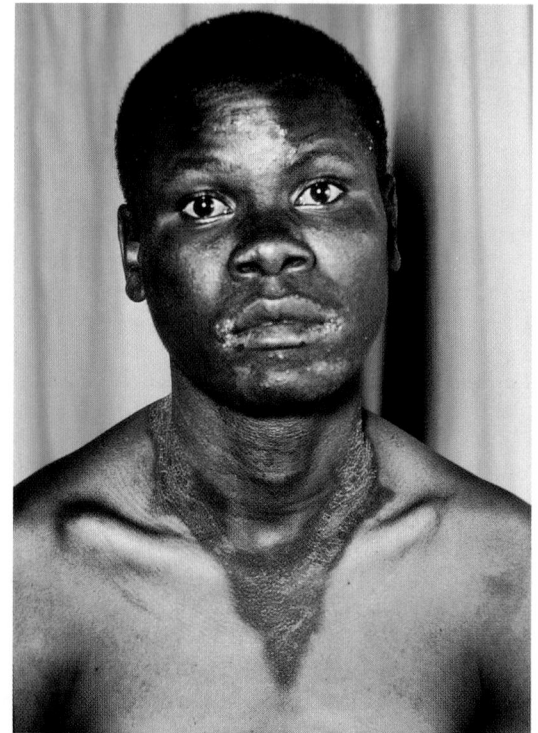

b

FIGURE 145-12 Pellagra. Acute dermatosis: (*a*) "Glove" or "gauntlet" exudative and crusted lesions on the hands. (*b*) Casal's "necklace" on the neck with facial involvement.

mucosa in the angles of the mouth. This was soon followed by maceration and superficial linear fissures (Fig. 145-13). These fissures remained moist and became crusted. The skin of the nasolabial folds, on the alae nasi, in the vestibule of the nose, and sometimes on the ears and at the inner and outer canthi of the eyelids became rather greasy and scaly (Fig. 145-14).

In addition to these changes, other alterations of the skin and mucous membranes have been associated with human riboflavin deficiency, but it needs to be emphasized that none is pathognomonic. These changes include (1) soggy, white, angular lesions of the mouth, usually termed *perlèche* (French, *perlècher,* "to lick thoroughly with the tongue"), often associated with moniliasis; (2) involvement of the vermilion border of the lips including vertical fissuring, usually termed *cheilosis* (Greek, *cheilos,* "lip"); (3) a glossitis in which the tongue frequently has a magenta color; (4) rarely corneal vascularization; and (5) lesions of the scrotum and vulva.

The dermatosis affecting the genital area has frequently been reported to be the earliest manifestation of riboflavin deficiency and also one of the most common. It may begin either as a patchy redness associated with scaling of the superficial epithelium or as a fine, powdery desquamation without any color change. In chronic cases lichenification is a feature, and far-advanced lesions are raw and extend up the shaft of the penis or onto the inner aspects of the thighs. The response to treatment (5 mg of riboflavin daily) is usually quite dramatic.

Sideropenic anemia with epithelial lesions (Plummer-Vinson syndrome), which has a little understood relationship to postcricoid carcinoma, may be accompanied by evidence of riboflavin deficiency as well as deficiency of iron and other vitamins of the B complex.

Pyridoxine (Vitamin B₆) Pyridoxine acts mainly as a coenzyme in the decarboxylation and transamination of a number of amino acids. It also plays a role in the conversion of linoleic to arachidonic acid and in adrenocortical function. It is now well established that occasional cases of both microcytic hypochromic and megalo-

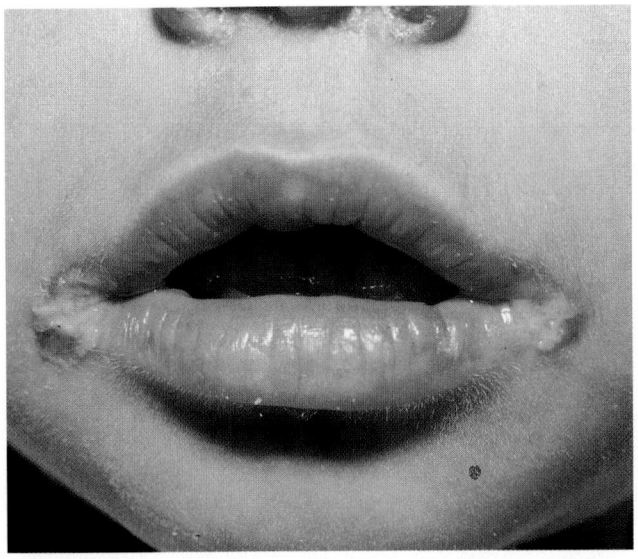

FIGURE 145-13 Riboflavin deficiency. Angular stomatitis with maceration in an Arab child. Riboflavin excretion in the urine was diminished.

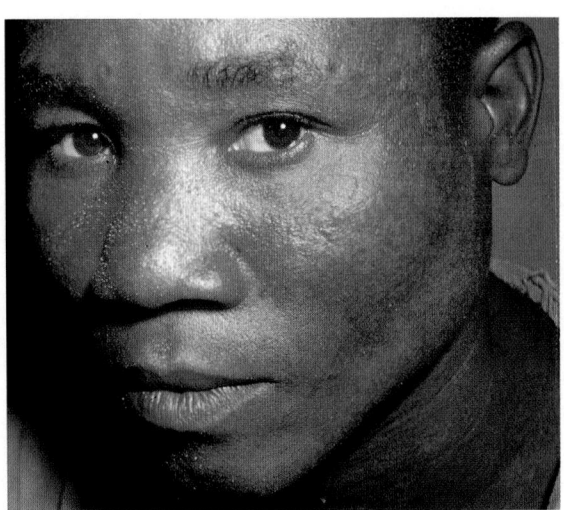

FIGURE 145-14 Riboflavin deficiency. Early nasolabial seborrhea in an African boy.

blastic types of anemia may respond to pyridoxine therapy. In pyridoxine dependency, in which there is no deficiency of the coenzyme form of the vitamin but a defect in the apoenzyme itself, reversal of the clinical and biochemical changes is obtained only with massive doses of pyridoxine. One form of dependency is familial xanthurenic aciduria with urticaria as the main feature.

Adults may live on a pyridoxine-deficient diet for up to 2 months and remain symptom-free. However, Vilter and his associates[11] described symptoms of pyridoxine deficiency after prolonged administration of an antimetabolite, desoxypyridoxine. The symptoms included seborrhea-like changes around the eyes, nose, and mouth and cheilosis. No response occurred to thiamin, riboflavin, or niacinamide, but the process cleared completely with pyridoxine. During the test period, there was increased excretion of xanthurenic acid.

Drugs that may impair pyridoxine metabolism include isoniazid, hydralazine, DL-penicillamine, and oral contraceptives.

Vitamin B₁₂ (Cobalamin) This vitamin, together with folic acid, is involved in the synthesis of deoxyribonucleic acid (DNA). There are several reports of patients with vitamin B₁₂ deficiency having symmetric hyperpigmentation of the extremities over the palms and dorsal aspects of the hands and around the wrists and forearms, and also involving the lower limbs with a similar distribution. In one case, epidermal cells in areas of pigmentation had abnormally large nuclei. Lesions have responded to treatment with vitamin B₁₂.

Biotin This substance is a growth factor for yeast and also the curative factor for raw egg-white injury which results from avidin antagonism of biotin. A generalized exfoliative dermatitis results.

A similar, milder condition has been produced experimentally in human volunteers fed a diet with minimal biotin and containing large amounts of raw egg-white. A prompt response occurred with 75 to 300 μg biotin per day. Several patients receiving prolonged total parenteral nutrition without added biotin have developed scaling eczematoid lesions of the arms, legs, and feet; nasal and genital excoriations; cheilosis; waxy pallor of the face; alopecia; lethargy; and hypotonia; all of which responded to added biotin.[12]

Pantothenic Acid This is a component of coenzyme A and is involved in the process of acetylation. No deficiency symptoms

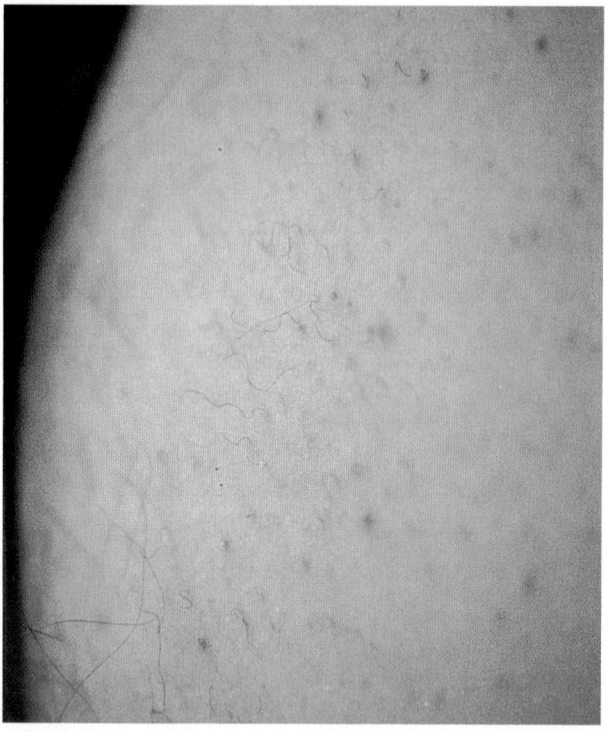

a

have resulted during controlled human experiments in which volunteers were fed deficient diets. These results fail to substantiate frequent claims that have been made for the efficacy of pantothenic acid in the treatment of the "burning feet" syndrome.

Vitamin C (Scurvy)

In the deficiency state, collagen formation is impaired as a result of failure in hydroxylation of protocollagen proline and lysine. Clinically, changes have been described in bones, mucous membranes, skin (Fig. 145-15), and blood.

In human deprivation experiments,[13,14] the first changes noted were enlargement and keratosis of the hair follicles, chiefly on the outer aspect of the upper arm. The follicles became plugged by horny material in which the hair was coiled or looped, the so-called swan neck deformity. The number of enlarged follicles increased over ensuing weeks and months; the main areas affected were the upper arms, back, buttocks, backs of thighs, calves, and shins. A few weeks later the enlarged follicles turned red, due to congestion and proliferation of blood vessels around the hair follicles. The color deepened to dark purple over another week or two when the follicles became hemorrhagic; there was no bleaching on compression. Follicles on the legs showed the greatest tendency to become hemorrhagic. If acne had been present in a mild form at the start of

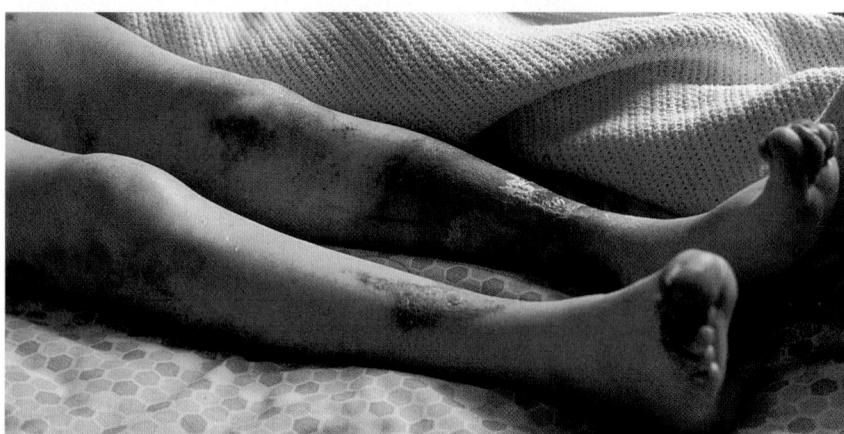

b

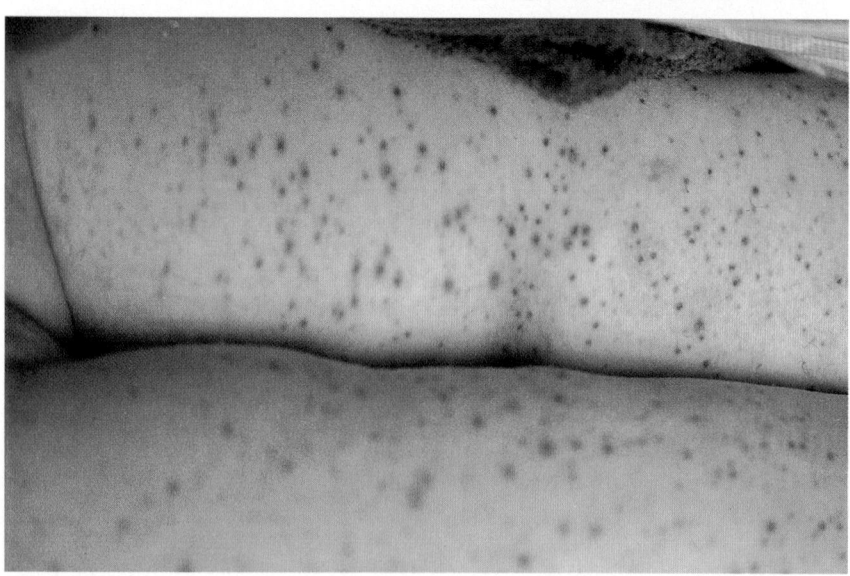

c

FIGURE 145-15 Vitamin C deficiency (scurvy). 61-year-old male in Edinburgh, Scotland. (*a*) "Swan neck" deformity of the hairs. (*b*) Ecchymoses over the legs, especially around a varicose ulcer on the left. (*c*) Numerous perifollicular petechial hemorrhages over the backs of the thighs.

the experiment, the lesions increased in size and became hemorrhagic.

Gum changes were most marked in those volunteers who showed evidence of gingivitis and periodontal disease at the start of the experiment. The earliest signs, after about 6 months of deprivation, were reddening, swelling, and tiny hemorrhages in the tips of the interdental papillae. Grosser changes observed in a few subjects consisted of a purplish, swollen, and spongy appearance of the gums, part of the tissue becoming necrotic with some bleeding. Aphthous ulcers, tenderness and pain, nontypical hemorrhages into the gums, and small extravasations without swelling in places other than the interdental papillae were all observed just as frequently in the supplemented group as in those not supplemented, and were therefore not related to the diet. Gum changes did not occur in edentulous subjects.

During the later stages of experimental deficiency, scars, where experimental wounds had been excised, became red and livid as a result of hemorrhages into the scar tissue and surrounding skin. New wounds made at the stage of profound scurvy failed to heal at the normal rate.

Scorbutic patients respond dramatically to the administration of vitamin C. Infants should receive 150 to 300 mg of vitamin C daily by mouth, in divided doses, for 10 days, followed by 150 mg daily for a month. Thereafter, a daily intake of 30 to 60 mg should be ensured in the form of fresh citrus fruits and juices. Adults should receive up to 800 mg daily in divided doses, for 1 week, and half this amount daily thereafter until complete recovery.

Vitamin K

Vitamin K is necessary for the synthesis in the liver of clotting factors II (prothrombin), VII (proconvertin), IX (Christmas factor), and X (Stuart-Power factor). Hypothrombinemia and deficiency of the other clotting factors in vitamin K deficiency may cause bleeding to occur almost anywhere in the body, including the skin. Ecchymoses may appear, associated with mild trauma, and massive hemorrhage may occur beneath the skin within muscles, particularly of the extremities. In hemorrhagic disease of the newborn, areas of predilection are the umbilicus, skin, nose and mouth, intestine, and brain. Differentiation has to be made from scurvy, hemophilia, and thrombocytopenia, but the clinical features are different, as are results of tests of clotting time, plasma prothrombin, bleeding time, and capillary fragility.

Intramuscular phytonadione (vitamin K_1) is curative, 10 mg in adults, 2 mg in young children, and 1 mg in newborns who should receive it routinely.

Essential Fatty Acids

On a fat-free diet rats failed to thrive and developed a scaly dermatosis. Certain polyunsaturated fatty acids (linoleic, linolenic, and arachidonic) are curative. Arachidonic acid is synthesized in the body from linoleic acid, which is an essential dietary nutrient. It has recently become evident that linoleic acid deficiency causes skin lesions; linolenic acid deficiency may lead to neurologic damage.

Linoleic acid deficiency caused growth failure and a dry, scaly skin in young children fed a deficient diet. Prolonged total parenteral nutrition, with concentrated glucose as the sole source of energy, has also resulted in deficiency, evidenced first by an abnormal plasma fatty acid pattern (a ratio of 20:3 ω 9 to 20:4 of 0.4 or over is diagnostic) and later by skin changes similar to those produced in experimental animals. These changes can be prevented by infusing at least 500 mL of 10 percent fat emulsion twice a week.[15]

Essential Elements

Iron

Chronic iron deficiency causes spoon-shaped deformity (koilonychia) of fingernails and toenails. Iron overload results in bronzing of the skin (see "Hemochromatosis" in Chap. 66) and is a major factor in porphyria cutanea tarda (see Chap. 150).

Zinc

Acrodermatitis enteropathica is an autosomal recessive condition due to impaired absorption of zinc (see Chap. 146). Deficiency has frequently been reported in patients receiving prolonged total parenteral nutrition[16] when zinc is not added to the nutrients. Clinical signs have included eczematous lesions of the face, mouth, and genitalia.

Copper

Menkes' kinky (steely) hair disease is an X-linked recessive disorder caused by defective copper absorption (see Chap. 61). Infants on an exclusively milk diet or prolonged total parenteral nutrition have developed a copper-responsive syndrome consisting of anemia, bone changes, psychomotor retardation, and depigmentation of hair and skin with distended blood vessels due to defective elastin formation.[17]

Selenium

Several patients on prolonged parenteral nutrition in the United States developed a syndrome that included a white appearance of the fingernail beds and dyschromotrichia that were reversed by selenium.[18] Acute poisoning with selenium is often fatal, and skin changes include alopecia, paronychia, and red pigmentation of nails, hair, and teeth.[19]

Manganese

A report exists of a single case of manganese deficiency, occurring in a volunteer who inadvertently received a deficient diet, developed transient dermatitis, changes in hair color, and slow growth of hair.[20]

References

1. Keys A et al: *The Biology of Human Starvation,* 2 vols. Minneapolis, Univ of Minnesota Press, 1950
2. McLaren DS: Skin in protein calorie malnutrition. *Arch Dermatol* **123**:1674, 1987

3. Bradfield RB: Hair tissue as a medium for the differential diagnosis of protein calorie malnutrition. *J Pediatr* **84**:294, 1974

4. Robinson DC et al: The clinical and epidemiologic features of tropical ulcer (tropical phagedinic ulcer). *Int J Dermatol* **27**:49, 1988

5. Sommer A et al: Impact of vitamin A supplementation on childhood morality: A randomized controlled community trial. *Lancet* **1**:1169, 1986

6. Frazier CN, Hu CK: Nature and distribution according to age of cutaneous manifestations of vitamin A deficiency. *Arch Dermatol Syphilol* **33**:825, 1936

7. Hume EM, Krebs HA (Comps): *Vitamin A Requirements of Human Adults: Experimental Study of Vitamin A Deprivation in Man. Report of Vitamin A Subcommittee of Accessory Food Factors Committee.* Medical Research Council Special Report Series, no. 264. London, Her Majesty's Stationery Office, 1949

8. Olsen TG: Therapy of acne. *Med Clin North Am* **66**:851, 1982

9. Lammer EJ et al: Retinoic acid embryopathy. *N Engl J Med* **313**:837, 1985

10. Sebrell WH, Butler RE: Riboflavin deficiency in man: Preliminary note. *Public Health Rep* **53**:2282, 1938

11. Vilter RW et al: Effect of vitamin B_6 deficiency induced by desoxypyridoxine in human beings. *J Lab Clin Med* **42**:335, 1953

12. Innis SM, Allardyce DB: Possible biotin deficiency in adults receiving long-term parenteral nutrition. *Am J Clin Nutr* **37**:185, 1983

13. Bartley W et al: *Vitamin C Requirements of Human Adults. Report by Vitamin C Subcommittee of Accessory Food Factors Committee and A.E. Barnes, and Others.* Medical Research Council Special Report Series, no 280. London, Her Majesty's Stationery Office, 1953

14. Hodges RE et al: Clinical manifestations of ascorbic acid deficiency in man. *Am J Clin Nutr* **24**:432, 1971

15. Fleming CR et al: Essential fatty acid deficiency in adults receiving total parenteral nutrition. *Am J Clin Nutr* **29**:976, 1976

16. Younoszai HD: Clinical zinc deficiency in total parenteral nutrition: Zinc supplementation. *J Parenter Enteral Nutr* **7**:72, 1983

17. Bennani-Smires C et al: Infantile nutritional copper deficiency. *Am J Dis Child* **134**:1155, 1980

18. Brown MR et al: Proximal muscle weakness and selenium deficiency associated with long term parenteral nutrition. *Am J Clin Nutr* **43**:549, 1986

19. Ruta DA, Haider S: Attempted murder by selenium poisoning. *Br Med J* **299**:316, 1989

20. Doisy EA: Human manganese deficiency, in *Trace Substances in Environmental Health,* VI, edited by DD Hemphill. Minneapolis, Univ of Minnesota Press, 1972, p 193

CHAPTER 146

Kenneth H. Neldner

Acrodermatitis Enteropathica and Other Zinc-Deficiency Disorders

Acrodermatitis Enteropathica

Acrodermatitis enteropathica (AE) is a rare, inherited disorder, transmitted as an autosomal recessive trait. Prior to the discovery that the disorder was caused by an inability to absorb sufficient zinc from the diet, the disease was usually fatal in infancy or early childhood. It is now rapidly and dramatically cured by simple dietary supplementation with zinc salts.

The clinical syndrome is characterized by a phenotypic triad of acral dermatitis, alopecia, and diarrhea. The distribution of the rash (face, hands, feet, anogenital area) has become recognized as a virtually pathognomonic cutaneous marker for zinc deficiency, whether secondary to hereditary AE or to any of the numerous nonhereditary causes for zinc deficiency, which produce an identical clinical picture to that of classic hereditary AE.

Historical Aspects

Acrodermatitis enteropathica was originally described by Danbolt and Closs[1] in 1943. In 1953 Dillaha et al.[2] reported modest therapeutic success with oral diiodohydroxyquin which was effective in controlling some aspects of AE, at least to a degree that would allow the children to survive, though with varying degrees of morbidity. While studying a patient with AE and associated lactose intolerance in 1973, Moynahan and Barnes[3] made the observation during various dietary manipulations that alterations in zinc concentrations affected the well-being of the patient, leading to the discovery that AE was a disease of zinc deficiency.

Epidemiology

Hereditary acrodermatitis enteropathica has worldwide distribution with no apparent predilection for race or gender. Because of the early interest in the disease throughout Europe, particularly northern Europe, there are seemingly larger numbers of cases reported from these geographic areas.

The ease of diagnosis and treatment of AE has now relegated it to the status of a relatively minor and seemingly insignificant disease. It remains, however, one of the more intriguing disorders known to medical science because seldom in human physiology have so many physical (and emotional) signs and symptoms been attributable to a deficiency of one single element, all of which are dramatically reversed by simple dietary supplementation with zinc. The opportunities for research are legion, yet the disease is seldom studied, perhaps due in part to the fact that it is now so easily treated that cases are seldom referred to academic centers.

Etiology

After AE was discovered to be a disorder of zinc deficiency, the one missing link in its pathogenesis was to determine the mechanism by which zinc is absorbed from the diet, a process that is not totally lacking in hereditary AE because the patients can absorb a small amount of zinc from an average diet. A simple increase in dietary zinc will rapidly raise plasma levels to normal and cure the disease. The fact that zinc in human milk is much more available biologically to infants with AE than zinc from bovine milk, with essentially equal zinc concentration, has led to much interest and speculation. The two milks have been compared in an effort to find a basic transport mechanism for zinc such as a possible species-specific zinc-binding ligand (ZBL) for humans that might be abnormal or deficient in AE. Thus far, the search has shown the process to be complex and controversial.

Eckert et al.[4] found the zinc in human milk to be associated with a low molecular weight ligand ($\sim$10,000) and the zinc of bovine milk was contained in higher molecular weight fractions. Hurley et al.[5] and Casey et al.[6] have found a similarly sized zinc ligand in human duodenal-pancreatic secretions adding to the impression that the size of the ZBL was critical. Casey and coworkers also found that the low molecular weight ligand of duodenal-pancreatic secretions of patients with AE contained much less zinc than similar secretions from normal controls, suggesting that the ZBL in the duodenum of patients with AE was in some way less efficient.

Cousins and Smith[8] found only 10 percent of the zinc in fat-free human milk to be associated with a low molecular weight ZBL ($<$2000). When additional zinc was added in vitro almost all of it became associated with this fraction, suggesting that the overall concentration of zinc in milk determined how much of it appeared in which fraction. They postulated that the difference in total protein of human milk (5.3 mg/mL) compared to bovine milk (29.0 mg/mL) also influenced the bioavailability of zinc in some unknown way.

Lönnerdal et al.[9] and Menard and Cousins[10] found intestinal zinc to be complexed with citrate (molecular weight 600 to 650), which they believe to be a major intestinal ZBL. However, Oestreicher and Cousins[11] have reported that the addition of citrate to milk does not enhance absorption of zinc in the rat.

To further complicate the picture, other ZBLs have been reported to exist. Song[12] has proposed that prostaglandin E_2 has a role in zinc absorption from the gut. Evans and Johnson[13] proposed that picolinic acid, present in milk and duodenal contents, has a high affinity for zinc. On the other hand, Rebello et al.[14] found the intestinal concentration of picolinic acid to be so low that a significant role in zinc absorption was questioned.

Other factors, such as the overall state of total-body zinc nutriture of the host, will influence zinc absorption, i.e., the zinc-depleted individual will absorb zinc much more avidly than one in a zinc adequate or excess state. Poorly understood interactions with other trace elements, particularly copper, lead, iron, cadmium, and chelating drugs, are known to alter absorption.[15] Once zinc is ab-

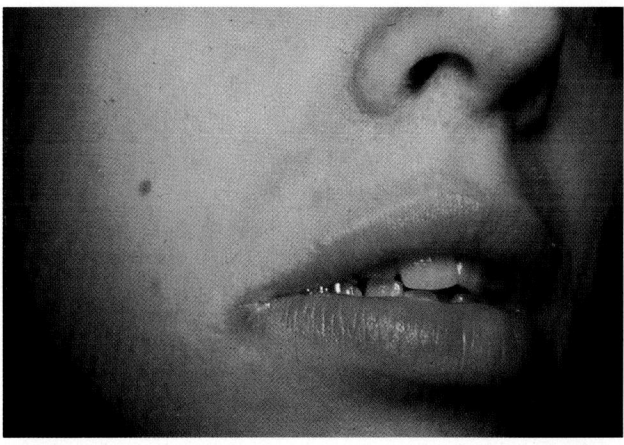

a

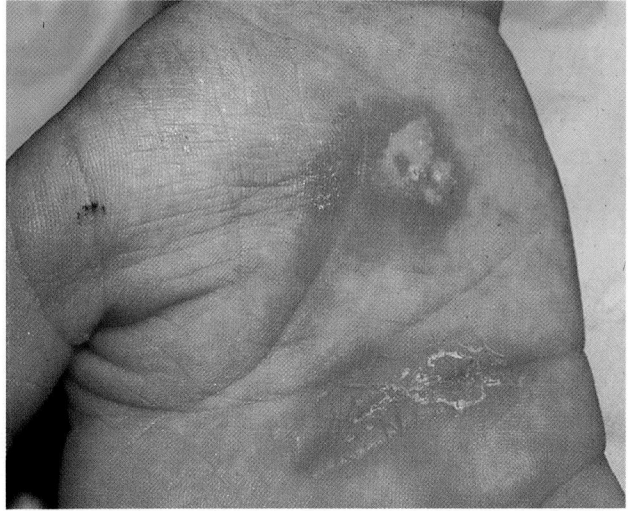

b

FIGURE 146-2 Acrodermatitis enteropathica in older individuals showing typical lesions. (*a*) Facial and (*b*) palmar.

sorbed by the intestinal villous brush border, another complex series of homeostatic events involving metallothioneins regulates the transport of zinc into the circulation and then on to the liver and kidneys, where a final poorly understood homeostatic surveillance system operates to regulate how much zinc will be preserved and how much excreted. These mechanisms appear to function normally in AE. The defect, therefore, is believed to be somewhere in the early stages of zinc absorption where the bioavailability of the chemical form and the structure in which dietary zinc is presented to the intestinal mucosal brush border in some way causes malabsorption.

Clinical Manifestations

Hereditary Zinc Deficiency   Classic hereditary AE usually begins within days to a few weeks after birth in infants bottle-fed with bovine milk or soon after weaning from the breast in older infants. Acral dermatitis begins slowly with dry, scaly, eczematous plaques on the face, scalp, and anogenital areas (Figs. 146-1 and 146-2). Perlèche is a common early sign and it has also been called a sign

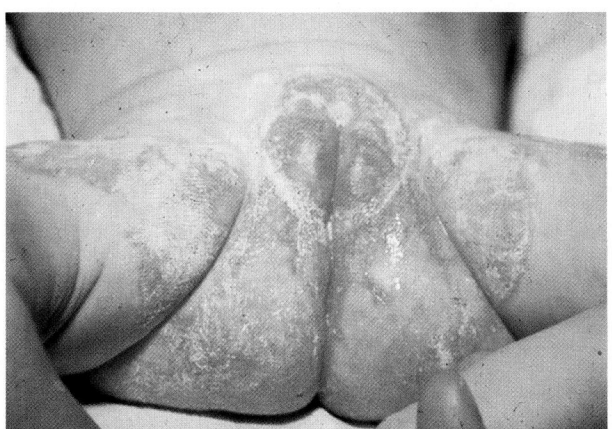

FIGURE 146-1 Acrodermatitis enteropathica. Erosive, eczematous, and secondarily infected lesions: genital area.

heralding relapse.[16] All lesions become progressively worse as vesicobullous, pustular, and erosive lesions develop. Superficial oral aphthous-like lesions may appear. The hands and feet are soon involved, commonly with paronychia and a brightly erythematous dermatitis of the palmar and finger creases plus annular lesions with collarette scaling. As the dermatitis worsens, secondary infections with bacteria and *Candida albicans* are common aggravating factors. Alopecia gradually worsens with time. Diarrhea is the most variable manifestation and may be only intermittent or totally absent. If diarrhea is severe and persistent, the clinical course will be further complicated by the loss of fluids, electrolytes, and other nutrients.

Within a few weeks, growth failure becomes measurable and becomes more apparent as the child approaches adolescence, when hypogonadism in males also becomes obvious. Emotional and mental disturbances are common manifestations of zinc deficiency, although difficult to evaluate. They are often best appreciated at the time when zinc supplementation is instituted, resulting in other rapid improvement in mood, disposition, and overall mental status within 24 to 48 h.

Photophobia develops gradually and is believed to be due to malfunction of retinal binding protein, known to be zinc-dependent. Other manifestations include anorexia, hypogeusia, hyosmia, and anemia. A "zebra striped" light and dark banding of hair may be seen with polarized light microscopy.[17]

Prior to the use of zinc in AE, fertility was low in those who reached reproductive age, and congenital malformations were common, particularly neural tube defects. The disease was often fatal during infancy. In those with milder cases who survived and those who received larger amounts of dietary zinc for unrelated reasons, the manifestations were less severe but usually resulted in growth retardation and dwarfism, delayed puberty, hypogonadism in male adolescents, continuing skin problems (dry skin and/or acral dermatitis of varying degrees), frequent infections, delayed wound healing, and mental disturbances.[18] There are rare reports of spontaneous remission occurring in adolescence.[19]

In recent years a number of infants with presumed hereditary AE have been reported who had all the typical findings of AE as outlined above, but who were found subsequently to have hypozincemia as a result of a very low concentration of zinc in their mother's milk.[20] In these infants, zinc supplementation cured the problem dramatically. As soon as the infants were weaned, they no longer required supplemental zinc, indicating that they suffered from simple acute dietary zinc deficiency and did not possess the hereditary defect in zinc absorption. No specific genetic reasons were found for the low maternal milk zinc levels. The mothers most likely became marginally zinc deficient due to the increased demands for zinc during pregnancy and lactation.

A possible role for biotin in AE has been proposed, particularly in premature infants with zinc deficiency who responded better to a combination of zinc and biotin than to zinc alone.[21] There has been no evidence found for a biotinidase deficiency in these infants. Such a deficiency has been described recently in rare premature infants with a dermatitis that resembled AE to some extent but was found solely related to a defect in biotin metabolism.[22]

Nonhereditary Acquired Zinc Deficiency As more is learned of the biochemical role of zinc in a vast array of physiologic functions, the subject of AE and zinc deficiency can no longer be viewed as a simple genetically determined event. Based on the knowledge gained from hereditary AE, it is now possible to recognize a similar pattern of signs and symptoms in patients with zinc deficiency from many other causes. In fact, the term *acrodermatitis*

enteropathica is now being used in a generic sense to include all patients with acral dermatitis due to zinc deficiency. This anatomic distribution is now recognized as the sine qua non and hallmark of zinc deficiency, whether on a hereditary or nonhereditary basis (Fig. 146-3).

A list of disorders and postsurgical states that are now recognized to be causes for zinc deficiency is presented in Table 146-1. The most common are those involving the gastrointestinal tract, such as chronic inflammatory bowel disease with diarrhea and/or malabsorption, steatorrhea, pancreatic insufficiency, and cirrhosis or surgically induced conditions such as total or partial gastrectomies and bowel resections, with or without blind-loop syndromes. Any catabolic chronic disease is also likely to induce zinc deficiency. Alcoholics are particularly prone to zinc deficiency.[23] The clinical expression will depend on the severity and duration of the deficiency and the age of the patient. As expected, there is almost total overlap with hereditary AE. The potential manifestations are summarized in Table 146-2.

Marginal Zinc Deficiency

A new area of interest lies not at the severe end of the spectrum, but rather at the other end, i.e., individuals whose dietary zinc intake is marginal, but still adequate to prevent overt clinical manifestations. There is a growing body of evidence to suggest that such individu-

TABLE 146-1
Conditions and Disorders that May Cause Zinc Deficiency

Disorder	Etiology
Gastrointestinal	
Mucosal diseases	Diarrhea
Malabsorption syndromes	Diarrhea
Pancreatic disorders	Reduced zinc ligands
Cirrhosis	Increased urinary loss
Postgastrectomy syndrome	Diarrhea
Blind-loop syndromes	Diarrhea
Dietary factors	
High dietary phytate	Chelation
Alcoholism	Increased urinary loss
Total parenteral nutrition	Lack of zinc supplementation
Faddish weight-reduction diets	Inadequate dietary zinc
Bulimia	Inadequate dietary zinc
Anorexia nervosa	Inadequate dietary zinc
Trauma	
Burns	Exudation, catabolism
Postsurgical procedure	Catabolism, anorexia
Malignancy	
All types	Catabolism, anorexia
Renal disorders	
Renal tubular disease	Failure to absorb zinc
Nephrotic syndrome	Proteinuria
Dialysis	Loss of zinc in dialyzate
Infection	
Parasitic	Chronic blood loss
Bacterial, viral	Redistribution, urinary loss
Miscellaneous	
Antimetabolite drug therapy	Catabolism
Chelation drug therapy	Chelation-urinary loss
Diabetes mellitus	Urinary loss
Hemolytic anemias	Urinary loss of erythrocyte zinc
Collagen-vascular diseases	Catabolism
Pregnancy/lactation	Increased fetal requirements

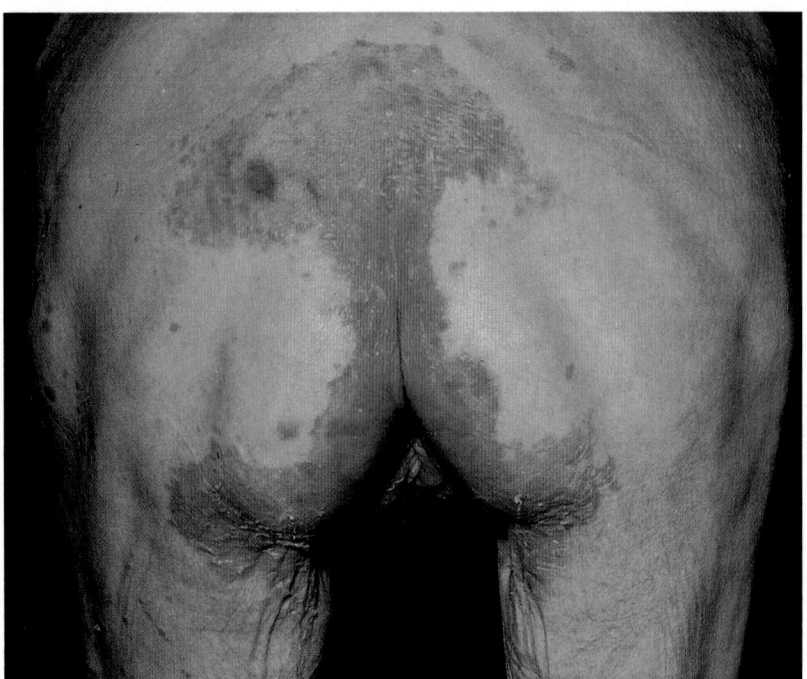

a

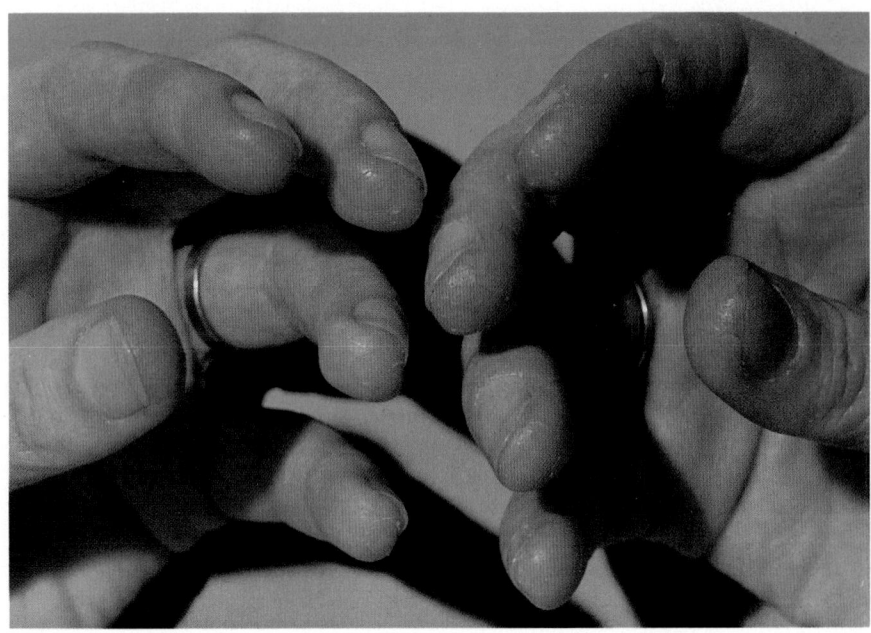

FIGURE 146-3   Zinc deficiency.
(*a*) There are plaques of dry, scaly,
eczematous skin around the buttocks.
The lesions often become secondarily
infected with *Candida albicans*
(*b*) Hands. The fingers are enlarged,
there are paronychia and bright erythema
on the terminal phalanges.   *b*

als are at significant long-term risk for a number of as yet ill-defined systemic and cutaneous disorders. In order to demonstrate more clearly the effects of this level of deficiency, animal studies are essential because it is almost impossible to maintain humans on a constant level of any nutrient for long periods and continue to monitor a broad range of possible physiologic consequences. Several pieces of evidence to support the contention that marginal zinc deficiency may be a silent and unrecognized partner in the pathogenesis of diverse and seemingly unrelated skin and systemic diseases are summarized in Table 146-3.

Numerous human and animal studies have demonstrated T-cell and immune effects at all levels of zinc deprivation, including marginal levels, if extended over long periods of time.[24–27] The possibility for cause or aggravation of diseases of diverse nature seems very likely although difficult to prove. As immune function declines, an increased susceptibility to infection soon follows.[28] This is well demonstrated in the more severe forms of animal and human zinc deficiency. Marginal zinc deficiency in infants and children has been shown to cause failure to thrive across a broad range of anthropometric parameters.[29]

In both AE and an animal model of AE (Danish black pied Friesian breed of cattle), thymic atrophy is one consequence. As a result, thymocytes and cellular immune functions, particularly a wide range of T-cell functions, are depressed. This aspect of zinc deficiency has been reviewed by Good et al.[30] Neutrophils, peripheral blood monocytes, tissue macrophages, and mast cells are

TABLE 146-2

Clinical Manifestations of Moderate to Severe Zinc Deficiency Observed in Nonhereditary Acquired Conditions

Rough dry skin
Progressively severe, patterned acral dermatitis (the diagnostic hallmark)
Perlèche (angular stomatitis)
Seborrheic dermatitis-like eruption
Alopecia
Diarrhea (variable)
Hypogeusia
Anorexia
Mental disturbances
Delayed wound healing
Growth retardation (children and adolescents)
Delayed puberty
Hypogonadism in developing males
Defective embryogenesis (neural tube defects)

known to require optimal concentrations of zinc for normal function.[31] Zinc also plays an important, although not completely understood, role in essential fatty acid metabolism.[32,33] Recent reviews of the biochemistry and physiology of zinc metabolism have been written by Prasad[34,35] and Forbes.[36]

Wound healing requires many nutrients, one of which is zinc. Patients with low plasma zinc levels and poor wound healing decrease their healing time following zinc supplementation. However, there is believed to be no pharmacologic effect from high doses of oral zinc if zinc status is otherwise normal. A determination of the plasma zinc level is therefore indicated in patients with leg ulcers or other slow-healing wounds or infections.

A proven role for zinc in the treatment of other dermatologic disorders has been somewhat controversial. Claims for efficacy in acne have been made and disputed.[37,38] A recent study found epidermal zinc to be low in dermatitis herpetiformis, acne, psoriasis, and Darier's disease, but plasma levels were low only in dermatitis herpetiformis.[39] Bruske et al.[40] found low serum levels in patients with vitiligo. Others found low serum and epidermal zinc in atopic eczema, but dietary zinc supplementation had no readily apparent efficacy, indicating that if zinc does play a role, it is probably not primary, but one that could conceivably facilitate healing once the primary damage has been done.[41] It should be recalled that the topical use of zinc (calamine, zinc oxide) is one of the oldest dermatologic medications known, being recorded in a 2000 B.C. Ebers papyrus.

Superoxide dismutase (SOD) is an important free radical scavenger and a zinc-copper-manganese metalloenzyme. Low SOD concentrations have been reported in the skin in severe zinc deficiency but have not been studied in marginally deficient humans or animals. Free radical scavengers as a group (SOD, selenium, vitamin E, vitamin C, catalases) protect against oxidative damage to all cell membranes, DNA macromolecules, and other vital cellular components. Free radicals are also potent carcinogens. The impor-

TABLE 146-3

Potential Long-Term Effects of Low-Grade, Marginal Zinc Deficiency

Abnormal lymphocyte function
Increased susceptibility to infection
Delayed wound healing
Aggravation of other dermatologic disorders
Impaired free radical scavenging

tant role of zinc and other trace elements and vitamins in disease prevention has been thoroughly reviewed recently.[42]

Biochemistry of Zinc Metabolism

Even though zinc has been known to be required for normal growth and development in the rat since 1934, it was not established as an essential human nutrient by the National Research Council until 1974, when a recommended dietary allowance (RDA) was set at 15 mg per day.

The adult body contains 2 to 3 g of zinc, which is about half the iron content and some 10 to 20 times more than other trace elements such as copper, magnesium, and nickel. The zinc cation exists almost totally in the Zn^{2+} oxidation state and does not readily undergo further oxidation or reduction, providing a stability that is believed to be significant in zinc biochemistry, such as hydrolysis and transfer or addition to double bonds.

The average diet in the United States provides approximately 12 to 15 mg of elemental zinc per day. Body stores and homeostatic mechanisms combine to ensure adequate supplies during times of reduced intake; however, during periods of dietary deprivation, the body will soon fall into a negative metabolic balance. In the rat, a negative balance develops within a few days after being fed a zinc-deficient diet, causing a rapid reduction in DNA synthesis.[43] Normally, about 30 percent of the daily intake is absorbed, although this figure is variable. Specific mechanisms of absorption have been discussed under "Etiology." The intravascular transport of zinc is primarily as a loosely bound complex with albumin (60 to 70 percent) and lesser amounts are more tightly bound to α_2-macroglobulin (10 to 20 percent), transferrin (1 to 5 percent), amino acid chelates (5 to 10 percent), and IgG (<1 percent).

All body tissues contain zinc. Muscle, bone, and the prostate gland have the richest stores. In the skin, zinc is concentrated in the epidermis, which contains up to five or six times greater concentration than the dermis.[44,45] Zinc also concentrates in hair, but changes in host zinc nutriture will be reflected in hair zinc concentration only after prolonged periods of deprivation (or excess), so its quantitation is unreliable for assessment of short-term or recent events.

The principal biochemical function of zinc is through its incorporation into a wide range of enzymes. Since zinc was discovered in 1940 to be present in carbonic anhydrase, the list of zinc metalloenzymes has grown to over 200, if those from nonhuman species are included.[46] All six classes of enzymes contain zinc metalloenzymes, the largest number being found in the hydrolases (class III). There are two basic types of zinc-activated enzymes; one is a metal-enzyme complex that readily dissociates but requires the presence of zinc for continued activity, and the other is one in which zinc is firmly bound to the active site so that it will not dissociate during isolation of the enzyme.

Laboratory Diagnosis of Zinc Deficiency

The laboratory verification of zinc deficiency is the same for hereditary deficiency (AE) or any of the acquired forms. Plasma or serum zinc levels are currently the easiest, best, and most commonly used method for assessing zinc status. However, it is well recognized that blood levels fluctuate rapidly following infection, injury, burns, or any sudden stressful stimuli, resulting in redistribution of zinc from the blood to other body compartments. Blood levels during such events may, therefore, not correctly reflect total zinc nutriture. Normal plasma levels are 70 to 110 μ/dL. (Serum levels are 80 to 120 $\mu g/dL$.) Urinary zinc excretion is highly variable under normal circumstances but it gradually decreases as zinc deficiency progresses. The normal urinary excretion ranges from 200 to 500 $\mu g/24$ h. Hair zinc concentration is commonly measured but again reflects only the long-term zinc status. Its use and interpretation will therefore depend upon the clinical situation and type of information desired. Serum alkaline phosphatase activity is a moderately sensitive indicator of zinc status, although not a particularly early marker of deficiency. Its activity remains near normal until profound and prolonged deficiency exists. Leukocyte zinc has been shown to be quite sensitive to early minor changes in total-body zinc nutriture but it has the disadvantage of being a difficult and expensive assay.[47]

It should also be emphasized that specimen collections and laboratory technique are important. Contamination with environmental zinc in collecting tubes or containers plus laboratory contamination in the handling and transfer of specimens and in the preparation of laboratory chemicals and solutions is a constant threat. Spurious laboratory results will, therefore, almost always be on the side of higher than actual values, which may lead to a missed diagnosis of impending or borderline zinc deficiency. The time between collection of blood and separation of serum and plasma also effects zinc concentration, with increases in the plasma up to 6 percent during the first 2 h if not separated.[48]

Treatment of Zinc Deficiency

The treatment of zinc deficiency is essentially that of dietary or intravenous supplementation with zinc salts, no matter what the etiology. In most instances, dietary supplementation with two to three times the RDA in doses of 30 to 55 mg of elemental Zn^{2+} daily will be adequate to restore a normal zinc status within days to a few weeks, depending on the degree of depletion. In all circumstances, a rapid clinical response will occur with dramatic reversal of many manifestations within hours to days.[18] Severe infected and erosive skin lesions will heal within 1 to 2 weeks without additional topical therapy. Diarrhea, if present, often stops within 24 h. Rapid improvement in mental disturbances is usually detectable within 24 to 48 h. In children, a surge of total-body and hair growth can be detected within 3 to 4 weeks after commencing zinc therapy.

Any of the zinc compounds available appear to work well (zinc sulfate, zinc acetate, zinc gluconate, zinc chloride, amino acid chelates). However, $ZnSO_4$ has been recommended more for oral supplementation and $ZnCl_2$ for intravenous use. Dosage prescribed must be based on the amount of elemental zinc present in the preparation, which varies from one compound to another. For example, a standard capsule of 220 mg of $ZnSO_4 \cdot 7H_2O$ contains approximately 55 mg Zn^{2+} which is an adequate daily dose for most deficient individuals.

High pharmacologic doses of oral zinc have been recommended by some investigators for the therapy of sickle cell anemia, acne, delayed wound healing, and leg ulcers. All of these conditions will improve with zinc therapy if a preceding zinc deficiency existed. However, in general, proof is lacking for a pharmacologic effect over and above that of restoration of a normal zinc nutritional status. Furthermore, the threat of zinc toxicity must be guarded against if prolonged high doses are ingested.[49]

Zinc Toxicity

Most heavy metals, including zinc, become toxic if taken to excess. Moderate overdose is eliminated through homeostatic mechanisms involving decreased absorption and/or increased urinary and biliary excretions. However, plasma levels of 150 to 300 $\mu g/dL$ (normal, 70 to 110 $\mu g/dL$) are easily achieved by persons ingesting zinc supplements of 50 to 100 mg Zn^{2+} daily. Such doses usually produce no immediately apparent adverse effects, although the long-term safety of such a dose is unknown.

$ZnSO_4$, is listed in the *U.S. Pharmacopeia* as an emetic. Not surprisingly its most common adverse effect is gastric irritation with nausea, vomiting, and mild gastric hemorrhage.

Acute and fatal zinc toxicity has been reported following large accidental oral and intravenous overdose.[50] Chronic toxicity among zinc smelter workers is known as "metal fume fever" and causes fevers, chills, gastroenteritis, and pulmonary symptoms.[51] Rats and mice fed moderate overdose for long periods have shown reduced growth rates, anemia, declining rates of reproduction, and hypertrophy of the adrenal cortex and pancreatic islets.[52] The finding that moderate to high (160 mg Zn^{2+} daily) overdose was atherogenic in humans was reported by Hooper et al.,[53] but it has been found more recently that lower doses of zinc have no effect on high-density lipoprotein cholesterol.[54]

A reciprocal interaction with copper is well recognized.[55] Patients receiving prolonged oral zinc supplementation are prone to develop hypocupremia as a consequence of long-standing hyperzincemia. One adverse effect of hypocupremia is a refractory microcytic anemia that will not respond to iron therapy until the serum copper level is normalized.[56] Neutropenia and hypoceruloplasminemia also occur with hypocupremia.

It is recommended that patients on long-term zinc therapy should be monitored periodically with the following tests: plasma zinc concentrations taken as a fasting a.m. specimen to regulate dosage, complete hemogram with erythrocyte indices, leukocyte differential count, serum copper level, and a stool examination for occult blood.

References

1. Danbolt N, Closs K: Acrodermatitis enteropathica. *Acta Derm Venereol (Stockh)* **23**:172, 1943
2. Dillaha CJ et al: Acrodermatitis enteropathica: Review of the literature and a report of a case successfully treated with Diodiquin. *JAMA* **152**:509, 1953
3. Moynahan EJ, Barnes PM: Zinc deficiency and a synthetic diet for lactose intolerance. *Lancet* **1**:676, 1973
4. Eckert CD et al: Zinc binding: A difference between human and bovine milk. *Science* **195**:789, 1977
5. Hurley LS et al: Zinc binding ligands in milk and intestine: A role in neonatal nutrition. *Proc Natl Acad Sci USA* **74**:3547, 1977
6. Casey CE et al: Zinc binding in human duodenal secretions. *Lancet* **2**:423, 1978
7. Casey CE et al: Zinc binding in human duodenal secretions. *J Pediatr* **95**:1008, 1979
8. Cousins RJ, Smith KT: Zinc-binding properties of bovine and human milk in vitro: Influence of changes in zinc content. *Am J Clin Nutr* **33**:1083, 1980
9. Lönnerdal B et al: Isolation of a low molecular weight zinc binding ligand from human milk. *J Inorg Biochem* **12**:71, 1980
10. Menard MD, Cousins RJ: Effect of citrate, glutathione and picolinate

on zinc transport by brush border membrane vesicles from rat intestine. *J Nutr* **113**:1653, 1983

11. Oestreicher P, Cousins RJ: Influence of intraluminal constituents on zinc absorption by isolated, vascularly profused rat intestine. *J Nutr* **112**:1978, 1982

12. Song MK: Evidence for an important role of prostaglandin E$_2$ and F$_2$ in the regulation of zinc transport in the rat. *J Nutr* **109**:2152, 1979

13. Evans GW, Johnson PE: Characterization and quantitation of a zinc binding ligand from human milk. *Pediatr Res* **14**:870, 1980

14. Rebello T et al: Picolinic acid in milk, pancreatic juice and intestine: Inadequate for role in zinc absorption. *Am J Clin Nutr* **35**:1, 1982

15. Solomons NW: Competitive mineral-mineral interaction in the intestine: Implications for zinc absorption in humans, in *Nutritional Bioavailability of Zinc,* edited by GE Inglett. Washington, DC, ACS Symposium Series, 1983, p 247

16. Mostafa WZ, Al-Zayer AA: Acrodermatitis enteropathica in Saudi Arabia. *Int J Dermatol* **29**:134, 1990

17. Traupe H et al: Polarizing microscopy of hair in AE. *Pediatr Dermatol* **3**:300, 1986

18. Neldner KH, Hambridge KM: Zinc therapy of acrodermatitis enteropathica. *N Engl J Med* **292**:879, 1975

19. Van Wouwe JP: Clinical and laboratory diagnoses of AE. *Eur J Pediatr* **149**:2, 1989

20. Lee MG et al: Transient symptomatic zinc deficiency in a full term breast fed infant. *J Am Acad Dermatol* **23**:375, 1990

21. Lagier P et al: Zinc and biotin deficiency during prolonged parenteral nutrition in the infant. *Press Med* **31**:1795, 1987

22. Nyhan WL: Inborn errors of biotin metabolism. *Arch Dermatol* **123**:1696, 1987

23. Gaveau D et al: Cutaneous manifestations of zinc deficiency in ethylic cirrhosis. *Ann Dermatol Venereol* **114**:39, 1987

24. Fraber PJ et al: Zinc deficiency and immune function. *Arch Dermatol* **123**:1699, 1987

25. Anttila PH et al: Abnormal immune response during hypozincemia in AE. *Acta Paediatr Scand* **75**:988, 1986

26. Fraber PJ et al: Interrelationships between zinc and immune function. *Fed Proc* **45**:1475, 1986

27. Couvreur Y et al: Zinc deficiency and lymphocyte subpopulations, a study by flow cytometry. *J Parenter Enterol Nutr* **10**:239, 1986

28. David TJ et al: Low serum zinc in children with atopic eczema. *Br J Dermatol* **111**:597, 1984

29. Walravens PA et al: Zinc supplementation in infants with a nutritional pattern of failure to thrive: A double blind controlled study. *Pediatrics* **83**:532, 1989

30. Good RA et al: Zinc and immunity, in *Clinical, Biochemical, and Nutritional Aspects of Trace Elements,* edited by AS Prasad. New York, Alan R Liss, 1982, p 189

31. Beisel WR: The role of zinc in neutrophil function, in *Clinical, Biochemical and Nutritional Aspects of Trace Elements,* edited by AS Prasad. New York, Alan R Liss, 1982, p 203

32. Neldner KH et al: Acrodermatitis enteropathica. *Arch Dermatol* **110**:711, 1974

33. Walldius G et al: The effects of diet and zinc treatment of the fatty acid compositions of serum lipids and adipose tissue and/or serum lipoproteins in two adolescent patients with AE. *Am J Clin Nutr* **38**:512, 1983

34. Prasad AS: Chemical biochemistry and nutritional spectrum of zinc deficiency in human subjects: An update. *Nutr Rev* **41**:197, 1983

35. Prasad AS: Clinical endocrinologic and biochemical effects of zinc deficiency. *Spec Top Endocrinol Metab* **7**:45, 1985

36. Forbes RM: Use of laboratory animals to define physiological functions and bioavailability of zinc. *Fed Proc* **43**:2835, 1984

37. Michaëlsson G et al: A double-blind study of the effect of zinc and oxytetracycline in acne vulgaris. *Br J Dermatol* **97**:561, 1977

38. Orris L et al: Oral zinc therapy of acne. *Arch Dermatol* **114**:1018, 1977

39. Michaëlsson G, Ljunghall K: Patients with acne, psoriasis, dermatitis herpetiformis, and Darier's disease have low epidermal zinc concentrations. *Acta Derm Venereol (Stockh)* **70**:304, 1990

40. Brüske K, Salfeld K: Zinc and its status in some dermatologic diseases—a statistical assessment. *Z Hautkr* **62**(suppl):125, 1987

41. David TJ et al: Low serum zinc in children with atopic eczema. *Br J Dermatol* **111**:597, 1984

42. Slater TF, Block G eds: Antioxidant vitamins and beta-carotene in disease prevention. *Am J Clin Nutr* **53**(suppl):1895, 1991

43. Prasad AS, Oberleas D: Thymidine kinase activity and incorporation of thymidine in DNA in zinc deficient tissues. *J Lab Clin Med* **83**:634, 1974

44. Michaëlsson G et al: Zinc in epidermis and dermis of normal subjects. *Acta Derm Venereol (Stockh)* **60**:295, 1980

45. Molokhia M, Portnoy B: Neutron activation and analysis of trace elements in skin: III. Zinc in normal skin. *Br J Dermatol* **81**:759, 1969

46. Vallee BL, Galdes A: The metallobiochemistry of zinc enzymes. *Adv Enzymol* **56**:284, 1984

47. Prasad AS et al: Experimental zinc deficiency in humans. *Ann Intern Med* **89**:483, 1978

48. English JL, Hambidge KM: Plasma and serum zinc concentration effect of time between collection and separation. *Clin Chim Acta* **175**:211, 1988

49. Prasad AS et al: Hypocupremia induced by zinc therapy in adults. *JAMA* **240**:2166, 1978

50. Brocks A et al: Acute intravenous zinc poisoning. *Br Med J* **28**:1390, 1977

51. Papp JP: Metal fume fever. *Postgrad Med* **43**:160, 1968

52. Aughey E et al: The effect of oral zinc supplementation in the mouse. *J Comp Pathol* **87**:1, 1977

53. Hooper PL et al: Zinc lowers high-density lipoprotein-cholesterol levels. *JAMA* **244**:1960, 1980

54. Crounse SF et al: Zinc ingestion and lipoprotein values in sedentary and endurance trained men. *JAMA* **252**:785, 1984

55. Kirchgessner M et al: Interactions of essential metals in human psychology, in *Clinical, Biochemical and Nutritional Aspects of Trace Elements,* edited by AS Prasad. New York, Alan R Liss, 1982, p 477

56. Solomons NW et al: Studies on the bioavailability of zinc in humans: Mechanism of the intestinal interaction of non-heme iron and zinc. *J Nutr* **113**:337, 1983

CHAPTER 147

Lowell A. Goldsmith

Cutaneous Changes in Errors of Amino Acid Metabolism: Tyrosinemia II, Phenylketonuria, and Argininosuccinic Aciduria

This chapter concerns skin disorders in which an abnormality of amino acid metabolism causes specific cutaneous syndromes. The general aspects of amino acid metabolism are reviewed elsewhere.[1–3] Table 147-1 summarizes the cutaneous manifestations in disorders of amino acid metabolism.

Tyrosinemia Type II

Definition

Tyrosinemia type II (Richner-Hanhart syndrome) is a distinctive clinical syndrome involving the eyes, skin, and central nervous system. Tyrosine is elevated because of a deficiency of hepatic tyrosine aminotransferase.

General Features of the Patients

Less than 100 patients with this clinical syndrome have been reported. All had tyrosinemia, phenolicaciduria, and inflammatory skin and eye lesions.[4] The sexes are affected equally; the disease is worldwide in distribution. There is often consanguinity, which is strongly suggestive of autosomal recessive inheritance.[4]

Dermatologic Features Patients have hyperkeratotic skin lesions limited to the palms and soles.[5–8] Lesions usually begin during the first year of life; in one patient, the first lesions appeared at age 6.[9] The skin lesions are painful, nonpruritic, and are frequently associated with hyperhidrosis (Fig. 147-1). The pain can be intense enough to cause patients to crawl rather than apply pressure to the

lesions. Bullous lesions may occur and rapidly progress to erosions; these then become crusted and hyperkeratotic. Lesions are often linear. The fingertips and hypothenar eminences are commonly involved. One patient had hyperkeratotic subungual lesions; one patient may have been hyperpigmented.

Ophthalmologic Features Eye lesions occur weeks to months before the skin lesions. Eye symptoms start as early as 2 weeks of age and as late as 8 years. Tearing, redness, pain, and photophobia are early signs; late signs include corneal clouding and central or paracentral opacities which initially are intraepithelial and can progress to superficial or deep dendritic ulcers (Fig. 147-2). Neovascularization is prominent. The eye disease may lead to scarring, nystagmus, and exodeviation. One patient had a persistent conjunctival plaque.[9] Topical therapy is ineffective, and herpes simplex and bacterial cultures are consistently negative.

Neurologic Features Mental retardation of varying degrees is reported, as is normal mental development.

Other Organ System Involvement Renal and liver function tests have been uniformly normal. One of the patients has multiple congenital anomalies, including microcephaly, cleft lip and palate, inguinal hernias, talipes equinovarus, and the absence of one kidney.[10] This patient (see below) has chromosomal deletions which may explain these other defects.

Laboratory Findings

Amino Acid Abnormalities The blood and urine tyrosine levels of the affected patients are markedly elevated. Other amino acids have

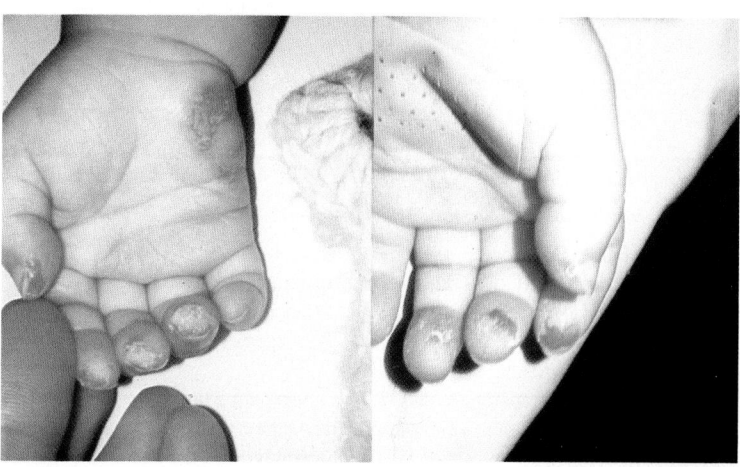

FIGURE 147-1 Hyperkeratotic and erosive lesions in a patient with tyrosinemia II.

TABLE 147-1
Inherited Disorders of Amino Acid and Organic Acid Metabolism with Skin Manifestations

Disease	Skin manifestation	Enzyme deficiency/ pathophysiology (mode of inheritance)
Alkaptonuria	Ochronosis Black cerumen, eccrine and apocrine secretions	Homogentisic acid oxidase (AR)*
Argininosuccinic aciduria	Trichorrhexis nodosa Rough skin	Argininosuccinase (AR)
Aspartylglycosaminuria	Thick skin Coarsening of facies Sagging skin folds Increased acne Photosensitivity	Aspartylglycosaminidase (AR)
Biotinidase deficiency	Erythematous rash Alopecia Oral candidiasis Seborrheic dermatitis Glossitis	Biotinidase (AR)
Citrullinemia	Light, short hair with interrupted cuticle	Argininosuccinate synthetase (AR)
Hartnup disease	Pellagra-like lesions Photosensitivity	Defect of neutral amino (AR) acid transport in renal and intestinal brush border; increased excretion of tryptophan metabolites
Histidinemia	Light-colored hair and eyes	Histidinase (AR) Decreased epidermal urocanic acid
Holocarboxylase synthetase deficiency	Skin rash Alopecia	Holocarboxylase synthetase (AR)
Homocystinuria	Fine, sparse friable hair Thin skin Livedo reticularis Malar flush Vascular occlusions Marfanoid habitus	Cystathionine β-synthetase (AR)
Hydroxykynureninuria	Chronic stomatitis Ulcerated gums, gingivitis Photosensitivity	Kynureninase (AR)
Hyperprolinuria I	Ichthyosis	? Proline dehydrogenase deficiency (AR)
Iminodipeptiduria (Prolidase deficiency)	Chronic skin ulcers Recurrent infections	Prolidase (AR)
Isovaleric acidemia	Odor of sweaty feet, alopecia	Isovaleryl-CoA dehydrogenase (?)*
Methionine malabsorption syndrome	White hair Dried celery or oast house odor Edema	Defective methionine transport (?)
Phenylketonuria	Hypopigmentation Atopic dermatitis Scleroderma	Phenylalanine hydroxylase (AR) Dihydropteridine reductase Defective dihydrobiopterin synthesis
Tyrosinemia II	Painful, acral erosions Hyperkeratosis Corneal/conjunctival plaques and erosions	Tyrosine aminotransferase (AR)
Tryptophanuria with dwarfism	Photosensitivity	One patient (?)
Xanthurenic aciduria	Urticaria Dermatitis	Kynureninase (AD)*

*AR: Autosomal recessive; AD: Autosomal dominant; ?: Unknown or unclear inheritance

not been increased. Urinary tyrosine metabolites are elevated; these include p-hydroxyphenylpyruvic acid, p-hydroxyphenyllatic acid, p-hydroxyphenylacetic acid, tyrosine, and N-acetyltyrosine (Fig. 147-3). All of the metabolic effects are consequences of the deficiency of hepatic tyrosine aminotransferase.

Tyrosine aminotransferase (TAT) is a pyridoxal phosphate-dependent cytoplasmic enzyme which transaminates tyrosine, forming p-hydroxyphenylpyruvate (PHPPA). The liver is the rich-est source of TAT; this specific TAT is not present in skin. The liver biopsy shows little or no soluble TAT, although there is normal or slightly increased mitochondrial tyrosine (aspartate) transaminase activity.[8,11] In mitochondria, aspartate aminotransferase uses tyrosine as a substrate and is responsible for the production of increased amounts of PHPPA from the increased amounts of tyrosine available in tyrosinemia II. Since mitochondria do not have PHPPA oxidase activity, PHPPA and its metabolic products increase and

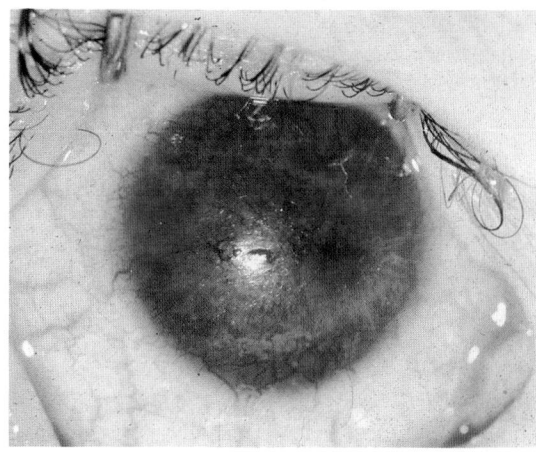

a

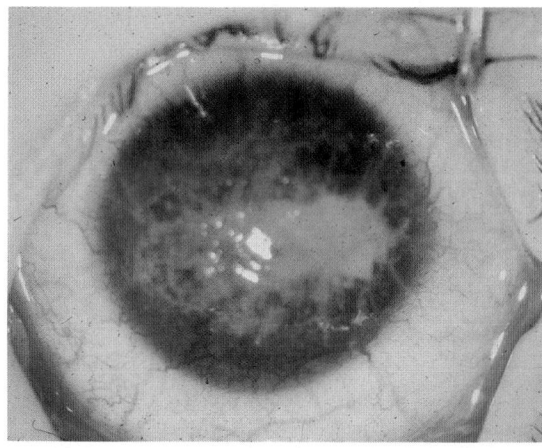

b

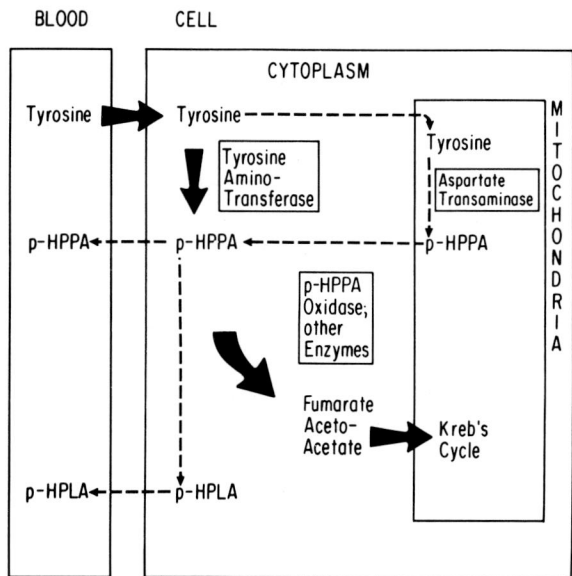

c

FIGURE 147-2 Corneal changes in tyrosinemia II. Cornea before treatment, left eye (*a*) corneal opacity and neovascularization are prominent. The right eye (*b*) has even more extensive involvement. After 6 weeks of therapy, there is marked clearing of the lesions (*c*).

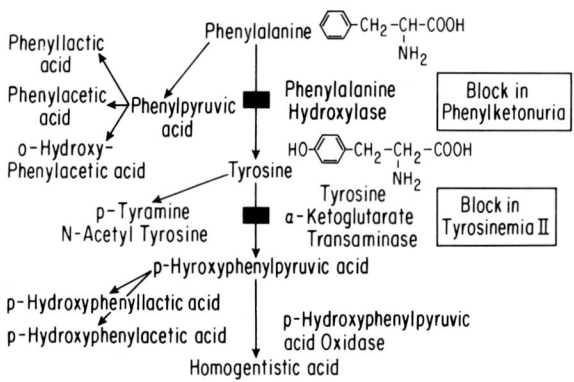

FIGURE 147-3 Metabolic scheme of phenylalanine, tyrosine, and their derivatives.

appear in the urine.[11] This creates the unusual situation in which metabolites are increased both proximally and distally to the defective enzyme (Fig. 147-4).

Histopathology Routine histopathology is not diagnostic; it shows hyperkeratosis, parakeratosis, and acanthosis. In one patient, the biopsy was interpreted as showing epidermolytic hyperkeratosis[5]; however, review of the published biopsy does not support that specific diagnosis.

In one patient, the palmar papules showed parakeratosis with homogeneous, refractile, eosinophilic inclusions 2 to 3 μm in diameter in the stratum corneum and stratum spinosum.[9] Electron microscopy in one case suggested that the 2- to 3-μm inclusions were lipid-like granules. Discrete 100-Å filaments and myelin-like figures were intermixed with lipid-like droplets.[9] These electron microscopy results were interpreted as showing possibly lysosomal activation. Extensive electron microscopy studies in three patients showed increases in tonofibrils and keratohyalin and very tightly packed microtubular and microfibrillar masses.[12]

FIGURE 147-4 Tyrosine metabolism in normal subjects and in tyrosinemia II. The hepatic metabolism is depicted with the normal metabolic pathways in bold arrows. The pathway in disease is in broken arrows.

The conjunctival plaques of one patient showed eosinophilic inclusions in the superficial epithelial cells and a plasma cell infiltrate. Electron microscopy revealed aggregated clumps of chromatin, and increased numbers of fibrils, forming bundles.[13] The superficial epithelial cells contained membrane-bound, alcian-blue-positive inclusion bodies, 0.5 to 1.0 μm in diameter. Endothelial cells of the vessels contained similar inclusions and whorled membranous substances. In fibroblasts, dark bodies consisting of fine, needlelike crystals were found. A second conjunctival biopsy, 2 years after the initial biopsy, revealed no infiltration, but persistence of the inclusions in the epithelium and fibrocytes was seen.[13]

Genetics   Tyrosine aminotransferase maps to chromosome 16, the 16q22-q24 region. Detailed studies of the Oregon patient show her to be a double heterozygote with a contiguous deletion syndrome.[14] On her maternal 16q she has a deletion of at least 11 of 12 TAT exons and a small de novo deletion in q22.1::q22.3. Her other somatic defects which have not been part of the tyrosinemia syndrome may be related to the deletions. Restriction fragment polymorphisms for the TAT gene will begin to allow prenatal diagnosis in families known to be carrying the trait.[15]

Pathophysiology of the Skin and Eye Lesions in Tyrosinemia II
Rats fed a 12 percent protein diet with 0.5 to 2.0 percent tyrosine developed a syndrome resembling tyrosinemia II, with weight loss, a shortened life span, keratitis, conjunctivitis, alopecia, cheilitis, and inflammatory toe changes.[16] The high tyrosine syndrome in rats was ameliorated by increasing the protein content of the diet or by adding threonine or thiouracil.[17] Inducers of tyrosine aminotransferase, e.g., glucagon, phenobarbital, corticosteroids, and catatoxic steroids devoid of glucocorticoid activity (e.g., pregnenolone-16-α-carbonitrile, or progesterone), prevented the syndrome.[18]

The affected animals had photophobia, corneal erosions, exudate, and panblepharitis. Microscopically, the initial lesion was epithelial edema associated with disorganization of the basal cells and polymorphonuclear leukocyte (PMNL) infiltration.[19] The PMNL invaded the epithelium stroma and the anterior chamber. After one week, the cornea was opaque, thickened, and vascularized. By 2 to 3 weeks, the cornea was ulcerated.

The eyes contained birefringent crystals limited to the areas of corneal damage. The crystals were long (10 to 25 μm), slender (0.5 to 1.1 μm), and appeared to be membrane-bound; the crystals passed from cell to cell and penetrated nuclei. Multinucleate cells, vacuoles, autophagic vacuoles, and multivesicular bodies were present, which suggested lysosomal activation by the tyrosine crystals.

In unpublished studies, skin lesions in the rats were limited to the bottoms of the feet and the nail beds. The histologic changes were limited to the volar surfaces of the feet and the nail beds. Initially, there was dyskeratosis followed by local areas of intense PMNL infiltration, erosions, crusting, and hyperkeratosis. Subcorneal collections of PMNL were seen first focally and then diffusely. By days 5 to 7, there were extravasated erythrocytes, basal cell vesiculation, subepidermal vesiculation, and necrotic epidermis. Biopsies of epidermis from the tail and back, even after epidermal cell division was stimulated, showed no evidence of inflammation.

There are ranch mink and dogs with the clinical metabolic features of tyrosinemia.[20,21] The reason for the localization of the lesions to the eyes and volar skin in human, mink, and canine tyrosinemia II and in experimental tyrosinemia is unknown. Studies of the rat cornea showed that inflammation was limited to the location of crystal deposition, suggesting the importance of tyrosine crystals as a factor in the initiation of inflammation.[22] Electron microscopic studies of both human and rat tissues showed evidence of lysosomal activation and cytoskeletal disorganization.

In vitro studies showed that tyrosine crystals can cause release of lysosomal enzymes and as yet uncharacterized heat-labile chemotactic factors.[23,24] The model of tyrosine crystals as lysosome labilizers is unique in that the tyrosine crystals are not phagocytosed into the cell but form within the cell and possibly within lysosomes. Within the cells, the initially soluble tyrosine, either because of changes in pH, ionic strength, carrier proteins, or other protective factors, crystallizes and then interacts with lysosomes and other membrane-bound structures. It is hypothesized that by this mechanism tyrosine crystals induce lysosomal rupture with subsequent release of proteolytic enzymes and chemotactic factors, which in turn initiate PMNL infiltration and grossly visible inflammation.

Treatment

With a low-tyrosine, low-phenylalanine diet (Mead Johnson), there is a rapid decrease in tyrosine to normal levels (Fig. 147-5). Skin and eye lesions resolved within days in all individuals treated with the diet.[7] Normal growth and development took place in a patient when kept on the diet for 30 months starting at the age of 14 months. In this patient, 6 weeks after diet therapy was begun, the corneas were much clearer and less injected (Fig. 147-2c) and the patient had vision sufficient to follow colored objects during play. At age 6 years, examination showed only remnants of vessels, and vision was normal except for myopia. Other patients have had slower resolution of symptoms. A 55-year-old man with tyrosinemia II had diffuse plantar hyperkeratosis (Fig. 147-6) which responded to a low-tyrosine, low-phenylalanine diet.[8]

Two adults have responded objectively to an aromatic retinoid (Ro 10-9359) (1.0 mg/kg per day). Interestingly, there was resolution without decrease in plasma tyrosine.[25] In none of the patients studied has there been response to cortisone acetate, ascorbic acid, pyridoxine, or folic acid, which are cofactors or known inducers of TAT and PHPPA oxidase.

Since the consequences of tyrosinemia II are serious, and a safe treatment is available, a patient presenting with any atypical bullous or hyperkeratotic disease on the palms and soles in the first months of life should be screened for tyrosine and its metabolites; simple screening tests (nitrosonaphthol in the presence of nitric acid and sodium nitrite) are available in most hospital laboratories.[1] Amino acid analysis by ion-exchange chromatography is necessary to confirm the diagnosis and follow the response to diet therapy.

Differential Diagnosis

Clinical Disorders of Tyrosine Metabolism   The disorders of tyrosine metabolism have a bewildering set of names. Tyrosinemia II (Richner-Hanhart syndrome) is distinct from the others; none of the others has any skin manifestations. These diseases are more completely reviewed elsewhere.[4]

Neonatal tyrosinemia is a common transient condition with decreased amounts of PHPPA oxidase apoenzyme and a relative deficiency of ascorbic acid contributing to the tyrosinemia,

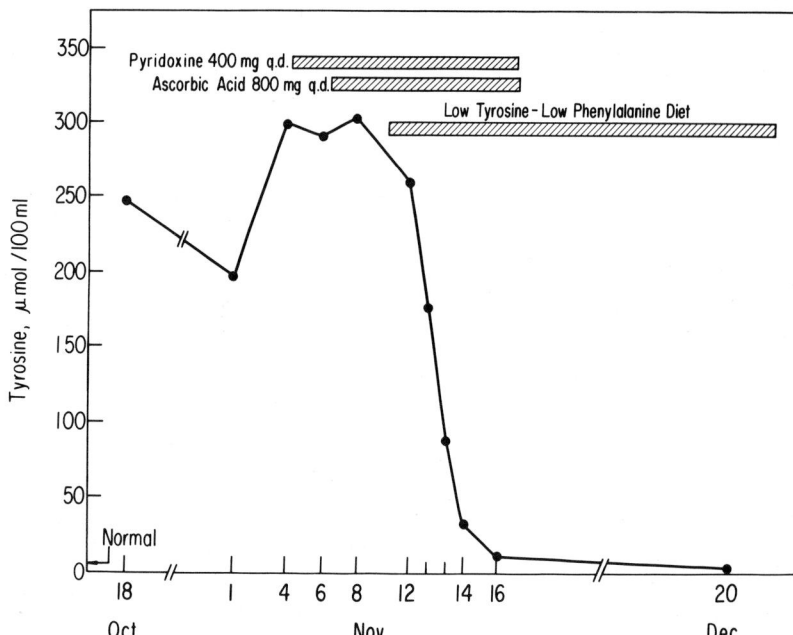

FIGURE 147-5 The response of elevated plasma tyrosine to a low-tyrosine, low-phenylalanine diet and failure of response to various cofactors in a patient with tyrosinemia II.

tyrosinuria, and increased excretion of tyrosine metabolites. Treatment is with ascorbic acid supplementation and a low-protein diet.

Hereditary tyrosinemia (tyrosinosis, tyrosinemia type I) is an autosomal recessive, severe liver and renal disease. In the first six months of life, there are fever, edema, vomiting, a peculiar odor, hematuria, diarrhea, jaundice, hepatosplenomegaly, and the Fanconi syndrome. The basic biochemical defect is fumarylacetoacetate deficiency with resulting increases in succinylacetone. Tyrosinemia, tyrosinuria, increased plasma PHPPA, hypermethioninemia, increased δ-aminolevulinic acid, increased catecholamines, and the renal findings of the Fanconi syndrome are present. Succinylacetone inhibits δ-aminolevulinic acid dehydratase and probably other enzymes, leading to the multiplicity of metabolic defects.

Some other patients with disorders of tyrosine metabolism have had similar metabolic profiles to those seen in tyrosinemia II but have not had the complete clinical syndrome.[4]

Classical Richner-Hanhart Syndrome The Richner-Hanhart syndrome classically consists of keratosis palmoplantaris, persistent dendritic lesions of the cornea with unaffected corneal sensitivity, photophobia, tearing, profound mental retardation, and autosomal recessive inheritance. In a review of the classical syndrome, 14 cases from 10 families are discussed.[26] All had corneal disease, 12 had keratosis palmoplantaris, and 8 were retarded. Consanguinity was common. Although none of the 14 patients had the extensive eye lesions of the patient in Fig. 147-2, it is suspected most of these patients had tyrosinemia II.

An autosomal dominant syndrome of volar keratosis and keratitis which is clinically similar to tyrosinemia was described in one family by Zmegac and Sarajlic.[27] The lesions were more extensive than those in the classical Richner-Hanhart syndrome but were similar to those seen in patients with tyrosinemia II. The keratitis of the Spanglang-Tappeiner syndrome, which is associated with palmar

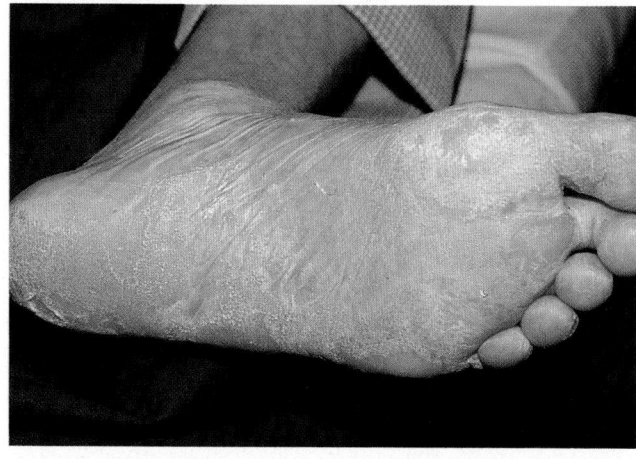

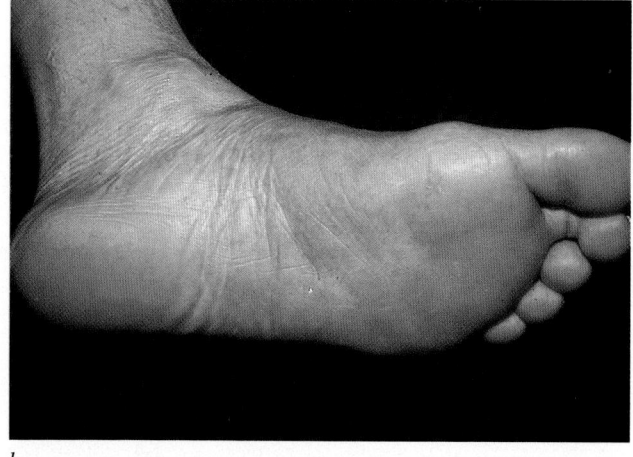

a   *b*

FIGURE 147-6 Diffuse plantar hyperkeratosis in an adult with tyrosinemia (*a*). The hyperkeratosis cleared on a low-tyrosine, low-phenylalanine diet without topical treatment (*b*).

and plantar keratosis, appears to be related to lipid infiltration of the cornea.[28]

Phenylketonuria

Definition

Phenylketonuria (PKU) is an autosomal recessive disease caused by a deficiency of hepatic phenylalanine hydroxylase or cofactors for phenylalanine hydroxylase. The increased levels of phenylalanine are associated with mental retardation, seizures, decreased pigmentation of the skin, hair and eyes, and eczematous dermatitis.

Clinical Features

This common metabolic defect occurs in 1 of 10,000 births and can be detected by screening procedures in neonatal life. One percent of institutionalized retarded patients have PKU. Mental retardation, athetosis, restlessness, increased tendon reflexes and muscle tone, hyperkinesis, tremors, and seizures accompany the untreated disease. The general features of the disease, its detailed genetics, biochemistry, heterozygote detection, prenatal diagnosis, and treatment are reviewed elsewhere.[29,30] Although there is a detailed understanding of the genetic abnormalities at the PKU locus and other related loci there has been little research into the skin manifestations associated with PKU.

Patients with phenylketonuria have an increased incidence of eczematous dermatitis, pigment dilution of hair and skin color, and occasionally sclerodermatous skin changes. Other changes reported included a decreased number of pigmented nevi, and an increased incidence of keratosis pilaris.[31] Skin phenylalanine levels are higher in PKU skin than in normal skin.[32]

Fleisher and Zeligman and Braun-Falco and Geissler found an increased incidence of atopic dermatitis in PKU.[31,33] In the former study, atopic dermatitis was present in 3 of 23 patients; in the latter, it was present in 15 of 25 patients. A potential mechanism suggested for the increased incidence of atopic disease is an increased tendency to vasoconstriction in PKU.[34] Dramatic clearing of eczema with a low-phenylalanine diet has been reported in some patients. It is possible that an inborn tendency to eczematous dermatitis has been nonspecifically triggered in these patients, although normal patients with eczema have no abnormality of phenylalanine metabolism detectable after a phenylalanine load.[35] Patients with PKU often have a lighter hair and eye color than their siblings.[36] The color changes may be especially striking in the rare black or Japanese patient with PKU whose eye or hair color may be very different from that of other members of the ethnic group. With a low-phenylalanine diet, or with aging alone, hair color darkens. When tyrosine is added to the diet of patients with PKU, hair darkens; if tyrosine is removed, the hair will lighten and banded hair is produced. The increased levels of phenylalanine and its oxidation products (phenylpyruvic acid, o-hydroxyphenylacetic acid, phenylacetic acid) inhibit the enzyme, tyrosinase, and therefore reduce melanization.[37]

The sclerodermatous changes in PKU are very striking and have been reviewed by Jablonska and Stachow.[38] Nine patients with PKU have had the onset of indurated areas of skin during the first year of life, most prominently on the thighs and associated with contractures. Acral areas of the body were least affected in contradistinction to systemic sclerosis. Biopsy showed increased fibroblasts and histiocytes, and atrophy of skin appendages. The elastic fibers were scanty and fragmented and were thus different from those found in true scleroderma. With dietary control, the sclerodermatous lesions cleared. The lesions may be due to alterations in tryptophan metabolism which occur in patients with phenylketonuria; tryptophan absorption is decreased in the presence of high blood levels of phenylalanine.[39] Tryptophan and scleroderma-like skin lesions are associated in the eosinophilia-myalgia syndrome.[40] In two sibs with phenylketonuria one had atrophoderma of Pasini and Perini and the other localized scleroderma.[41] In experimental phenylketonuria, there is an abnormal tubulin due to a decreased posttranslational addition of tyrosine to tubulin's α-chain.[42] This may explain some of the tissue effects in PKU.

Diagnosis

Phenylalanine can be quantitated by ion exchange chromatography. Increased levels of its metabolites in the urine are detected by a screening test in which $FeCl_3$ forms a bluish green (olive-green) color in the presence of phenylpyruvic acid. The chemical determination distinguishes PKU from the various forms of oculocutaneous albinism and Chédiak-Higashi disease, which are also associated with pigment dilution.

Treatment

A low-phenylalanine diet results in increased pigmentation and, often, clearing of the eczema. Over-rigorous control of diet can lead to protein deficiency and an eczematous dermatitis.

Argininosuccinic Aciduria (ASA)

Definition and Clinical Features

Argininosuccinic aciduria is characterized by hepatomegaly, mental retardation, seizures, episodic lethargy and ataxia, autosomal recessive inheritance, and friable, brittle hair with the morphology of trichorrhexis nodosa. The deficiency of an essential cytosolic enzyme in the urea cycle, argininosuccinase (argininosuccinate lyase), causes citrullinemia and an increase in blood ammonia. Argininosuccinate is increased in the blood and spinal fluid and is excreted in large amounts (2 to 9 g a day) in the urine.

The detailed clinical and biochemical features of the disease and the principles of therapy have been reviewed.[43] The disease presents in the neonatal period as failure to thrive and ammonia intoxication, or, in the second year of age, with psychomotor retardation, seizures, and ataxia. The hair abnormality is more characteristic of the late onset disease. Weaning and a change to a diet with higher protein content can be precipitating factors in clinical disease. Essential to current therapeutic regimens are diets providing adequate energy, protein and arginine.[44]

The molecular pathology of the nucleic acids in this disease has been clarified, but the detailed pathophysiology of the hair defect remains to be studied.[44] Argininosuccinase cDNA has been cloned, sequenced, mapped to chromosome 7 and is about 60 percent homologous to the δ-crystallins of the lens. Although there are at least 12 different mutant alleles, they all belong to one complementation group. Defining the molecular pathology allows prenatal diagnosis, so therapy can be instituted expeditiously.

Hair Defects

Clinical and Morphologic   About half of the reported patients have had abnormally friable hair with visible trichorrhexis nodosa; the other half have grossly normal hair.[43,45] Brushing and combing accentuate breaking (i.e., "brittle" hair).[45] No definite correlation can be made between liver ASase level, argininosuccinic acid levels, arginine levels, and the degree of hair abnormalities; some patients with severe ASA have had seemingly normal hair. Some patients' hair has improved with diet or without specific therapy.[46,47] One patient of Hartlage et al. had trichorrhexis nodosa at birth and improvement in her hair with the addition of increased amounts of arginine to the diet.[48] Eyelashes, eyebrows, and general body hair, as well as the nails, may be involved.[45,49]

There is variation in diameter within the same hair and torsion, grooving, and irregular contours of the intrafollicular portions of growing hairs.[45] With polarizing microscopy, there is no uniform cortical or medullary structure and no correlation of the lesion to polarized or nonpolarized regions.[45] Stains of the hair with acridine orange and subsequent fluorescent microscopy show red fluorescence instead of the green fluorescence seen in ordinary, mechanically induced trichorrhexis nodosa.[49]

Molecular Nature of Hair Defect   During stress-strain testing in air, ASA hair broke prematurely at the end of the Hookean portion of the stress-strain curve, and Young's modulus of elasticity was less than 50 percent of normal.[50] In two patients, there was no argininosuccinic acid in the hair, and the only abnormality in amino acid content was a decreased serine level.[51] In another patient the amino acid content was normal except for a cystine value one-half that of normal.[50]

The basic nature of the hair defect is not known. Are the brittle hair and the trichorrhexis nodosa a consequence of the deficiency of a product from the urea cycle, e.g., arginine, or is the hair defect related to an excess of one of the products which are increased due to argininosuccinate lyase deficiency? The administration of argininosuccinic acid to adult rats did not cause any specific effects, although there are no data on whether the argininosuccinic acid was absorbed from the gut.[47]

Increasing arginine in the diet aids hair growth and structure in this disease, suggesting that the decrease in arginine may be related to the defective hair. Since the urea cycle is depressed in ASA, the arginine required for protein synthesis would come predominantly from dietary sources. Hair protein is rich in arginine (up to 10 percent of the amino acid residues are arginine) and, furthermore, the citrulline present in certain specialized proteins in the medulla and internal root sheath is derived from arginine.[52] Increased ammonia levels also might inhibit ϵ-(γ-glutamyl) lysine bond formation, which is important for stabilization of the internal root sheath and medulla. The fumarate derived from ASA is important for the Krebs tricarboxylic acid cycle, and this cycle might be altered in ASA with consequent abnormalities of hair metabolism and growth.

Other Disorders of the Urea Cycle[43,44]

In citrullinemia, a rare recessive disease due to the absence of argininosuccinic acid synthetase, there are somatic and mental retardation and increased levels of blood, urine, and cerebral spinal fluid citrulline, low to normal values of plasma arginine, and increased blood ammonia.[43] Hair from a patient with citrullinemia was lightly pigmented, grew only to a length of 6 cm, and showed irregular areas of dystrophy and interruption of the cuticle.[53] The hair of an adult with the syndrome was said to be normal. More clinical details on the hair of these and similar patients and further studies of their hair would be of interest.

Deficiency of the cytosolic enzyme argininosuccinic acid synthetase is associated with trichorrhexis nodosa.[44] Its overall clinical presentation is almost identical to that of argininosuccinic aciduria, although the plasma citrulline levels are usually higher (>1 mM) in the former disease. Enzymatic and genetic analysis confirm the diagnosis.[44]

In lysinuric protein intolerance, which is due to defective transport, the skin may be hyperelastic, joints hypermobile, and the hair sparse and brittle.[43] One-half of the patients have been from Finland. Mice with deficiency in the X-linked urea cycle enzyme, ornithine carbamyl transferase, have sparse hair, but hair defects are not described in humans with the mutation.

Diagnosis

Retardation, ammonia intolerance, and abnormal hair will suggest these syndromes. The diagnosis is confirmed by high-voltage electrophoresis or ion-exchange chromatography of the urine, blood, or spinal fluid. Only a tiny percentage of the cases of trichorrhexis nodosa and brittle hair are due to ASA.

Microargininosuccinic Aciduria

In true ASA, urinary ASA ranges between 2 and 9 g per day. In contradistinction, there have been instances of normal individuals excreting a few milligrams of argininosuccinic acid a day, and some of these patients have had monilethrix, trichorrhexis nodosa, or pili torti.[54–56] In some of these cases ASA was not correctly identified, or there may have been dietary sources.[56] In any case, it is difficult to make a cause-and-effect relationship between these trivial levels of ASA and the associated hair defects.

References

1. Scriver CR et al: *Amino Acid Metabolism and Its Disorders.* Philadelphia, Saunders, 1973
2. Nyhan WL: *Heritable Disorders of Amino Acid Metabolism: Patterns of Clinical Expression and Genetic Variation.* New York, Wiley, 1974
3. Scriver CR et al (eds): *The Metabolic Basis of Inherited Disease,* 6th ed. New York, McGraw-Hill, 1989
4. Goldsmith LA, LaBerge C: Tyrosinemia and related disorders, in *The Metabolic Basis of Inherited Disease,* 6th ed., edited by CR Scriver et al. New York, McGraw-Hill, 1989, p 547
5. Zaleski WA et al: Skin lesions in tyrosinosis: Response to dietary treatment. *Br J Dermatol* **88**:335, 1973
6. Billson FA, Danks DM: Corneal and skin change in tyrosinemia. *Aust J Ophthalmol* **3**:112, 1975
7. Goldsmith LA, Reed J: Tyrosine-induced eye and skin lesions. A treatable genetic disease. *JAMA* **236**:382, 1976
8. Goldsmith LA et al: Hepatic enzymes of tyrosine metabolism in tyrosinemia II. *J Invest Dermatol* **73**:530, 1979
9. Goldsmith LA et al: Tyrosinemia with plantar and palmar keratosis and keratitis. *J Pediatr* **83**:798, 1973
10. Burns RP: Soluble tyrosine aminotransferase deficiency: An unusual cause of corneal ulcers. *Am J Ophthalmol* **73**:400, 1972

11. Fellman JH et al: Soluble and mitochondrial forms of tyrosine aminotransferase. Relationship to human tyrosinemia. *Biochemistry* **8**:615, 1969

12. Bohnert A, Anton-Lamprecht I: Richner-Hanhart's syndrome: Ultrastructural abnormalities of epidermal keratinization indicating a causal relationship to high intracellular tyrosine levels. *J Invest Dermatol* **79**:68, 1982

13. Bienfang DC et al: The Richner-Hanhart syndrome. Report of a case with associated tyrosinemia. *Arch Ophthalmol* **94**:1133, 1976

14. Natt E et al: Inherited and de novo deletion of the tyrosine aminotransferase gene locus at 16q22.1-q22.3 in a patient with tyrosinemia type II. *Hum Genet* **77**:352, 1987

15. Westphal EM et al: The human tyrosine aminotransferase gene: Characterization of restriction fragment length polymorphisms and haplotype analysis in a family with tyrosinemia type II. *Hum Genet* **79**:260, 1988

16. Schweizer W: Studies on the effect of L-tyrosine on the white rat. *J Physiol (Lond)* **106**:167, 1947

17. Alam SQ et al: Effect of threonine on the toxicity of excess tyrosine and cataract formation in the rat. *J Nutr* **89**:91, 1966

18. Selye H: Steroids influencing the toxicity of L-tyrosine. *J Nutr* **101**:515, 1971

19. Beard ME et al: Histopathology of keratopathy in the tyrosine-fed rat. *Invest Ophthalmol* **13**:1037, 1974

20. Goldsmith LA et al: Tyrosine aminotransferase deficiency in mink (*Mustela vison*): A model for human tyrosinemia II. *Biochem Genet* **19**:687, 1981

21. Jezyk PF et al: Screening for inborn errors of metabolism in dogs and cats, in *Animal Models of Inherited Metabolic Diseases,* edited by RJ Desnick. New York, Alan R. Liss, 1983, p 93

22. Gipson IK et al: Crystals in corneal epithelial lesions of tyrosine fed rats. *Invest Ophthalmol* **14**:937, 1975

23. Goldsmith LA: Hemolysis and lysosomal activation by solid-state tyrosine. *Biochem Biophys Res Commun* **64**:558, 1975

24. Lohr KM et al: Corneal organ cultures in tyrosinemia release chemotactic factors. *J Lab Clin Med* **105**:573, 1985

25. Hunziker N et al: Richner-Hanhart syndrome (RHS)—tyrosinemia type II and oral aromatic retinoid (Ro 10-9359). Report of two cases, in *Retinoids. Advances in Basic Research and Therapy,* edited by CE Orfanos et al. New York, Springer-Verlag, 1981, p 453

26. Franceschetti AT et al: Die cornea beim Richner-Hanhart Syndrom. *Ber Dtsch Ophthalmol Ges* **71**:109, 1971

27. Zmegac ZJ, Sarajlic MV: A rare form of an inheritable palmar and plantar keratosis. *Dermatologica* **130**:40, 1964

28. Geeraets WJ: *Ocular Syndromes,* 3d ed. Philadelphia, Lea & Febiger, 1976

29. Tourian A, Sidbury JB: Phenylketonuria and hyperphenylalaninemia, in *The Metabolic Basis of Inherited Disease,* 5th ed, edited by JB Stanbury et al. New York, McGraw-Hill, 1982, p 270

30. Scriver CR et al: The Hyperphenylalaninemias, in *The Metabolic Basis of Inherited Disease,* 6th ed, edited by CR Scriver et al. New York, McGraw-Hill, 1989, p 495

31. Braun-Falco O, Geissler H: Hauterscheinungen bei Phenylketonurie. *Med Welt* **37**:1941, 1964

32. Fisch RO et al: Studies of phenylketonuria with dermatitis. *J Am Acad Dermatol* **4**:284, 1981

33. Fleisher TL, Zeligman I: Cutaneous findings in phenylketonuria. *Arch Dermatol* **81**:898, 1960

34. Solomon LM, Desai K: Phenylketonuria. *Cutis* **4**:1233, 1968

35. Vickers CFH: Eczema and phenylketonuria. *Trans St Johns Hosp Dermatol Soc* **50**:56, 1964

36. Berg JM, Stern J: Iris color in phenylketonuria. *Ann Hum Genet* **22**:370, 1958

37. Miyamoto M, Fitzpatrick TB: Competitive inhibition of mammalian tyrosinase by phenylalanine and in relationship to hair pigmentation in phenylketonuria. *Nature* **179**:199, 1957

38. Jablonska S, Stachow A: Scleroderma-like lesions in phenylketonuria (PKU), in *Scleroderma and Pseudoscleroderma,* 2d ed, edited by S Jablonska. Warsaw, Polish Medical Publishers, 1975, p 489

39. Yarbro MT, Anderson JA: Tryptophan metabolism in phenylketonuria. *J Pediatr* **68**:895, 1966

40. Belongia AE et al: An investigation of the cause of the eosinophilia-myalgia syndrome associated with tryptophan use. *N Engl J Med* **323**:357, 1990

41. Lasser AE et al: Phenylketonuria and scleroderma. *Arch Dermatol* **114**:1215, 1978

42. Rodriguez JA, Borisy GG: Experimental phenylketonuria: Replacement of carboxyl terminal tyrosine by phenylalanine in infant rat brain tubulin. *Science* **206**:463, 1979

43. Walser M: Urea cycle disorders and other hereditary hyperammonemic syndromes, in *The Metabolic Basis of Inherited Disease,* 5th ed, edited by JB Stanbury et al. New York, McGraw-Hill, 1983, p 402

44. Brusilow SW, Horwich AL: Urea cycle enzymes, in *The Metabolic Basis of Inherited Disease,* 6th ed, edited by CR Scriver et al. New York, McGraw-Hill, 1989, p 629

45. Rauschkolb EW et al: Hair fragility—an important clue to aminoacidopathy in mental retardation. *Cutis* **4**:1315, 1968

46. Coryell ME et al: A familial study of a human enzyme defect, argininosuccinic aciduria. *Biochem Biophys Res Commun* **14**:307, 1964

47. Westall RG: Treatment of argininosuccinic aciduria. *Am J Dis Child* **113**:160, 1967

48. Hartlage RL et al: Argininosuccinic aciduria: Perinatal diagnosis and early dietary management. *J Pediatr* **85**:86, 1974

49. Levin B et al: Argininosuccinic aciduria. An inborn error of amino acid metabolism. *Arch Dis Child* **36**:622, 1961

50. Potter JL et al: Argininosuccinic-aciduria—the hair abnormality. *Am J Dis Child* **127**:724, 1974

51. Van Sande M: Hair amino acids: Normal values and results in metabolic errors. *Arch Dis Child* **45**:678, 1970

52. Rogers GE, Harding HWJ: Molecular mechanisms in the formation of hair, in *Biology and Disease of the Hair,* edited by T Kobori, W Montagna. Baltimore, University Park Press, 1976, p 411

53. Porter PS: The genetics of human hair growth. *Birth Defects* **7**:69, 1971

54. Grosfeld JCM et al: Argininosuccinic aciduria in monilethrix. *Lancet* **2**:789, 1964

55. Winther A, Bundgaard L: Argininosuccinic aciduria in hereditary hair diseases. *Acta Derm Venereol (Stockh)* **48**:567, 1968

56. Efron ML, Hoefnagel D: Argininosuccinic acid in monilethrix. *Lancet* **1**:321, 1966

CHAPTER 148

Lowell A. Goldsmith

Cutaneous Changes in Errors of Amino Acid Metabolism: Alkaptonuria

Definition

Alkaptonuria is a rare autosomal recessive disorder caused by deficiency of homogentisic acid oxidase, the sole catabolic enzyme for homogentisic acid (HGA). Excessive HGA is excreted in the urine, which often turns dark, and HGA accumulates in connective tissues, including the dermis.

Historical Aspects[1]

In 1859, Boedeker originally used the term *alcapton* to denote a urinary substance with great avidity for oxygen at an alkaline pH; later, he spelled the word *alkapton*. In 1866, Virchow saw the diffuse bluish-black pigmentation of connective tissue, in a presumably alkaptonuric individual, and called the condition *ochronosis* because of the ochre (yellow) hue seen microscopically. The prediction of Garrod, set forth in 1908, that alkaptonuria was caused by a specific enzyme deficiency was fully confirmed 50 years later when La Du and associates demonstrated the absence of hepatic HGA oxidase in an alkaptonuric patient.

Epidemiology

Alkaptonuria is inherited as an autosomal recessive trait; those pedigrees which support a dominant mode of transmission and contain a high degree of consanguinity, when subjected to careful scrutiny, and are actually "pseudodominants." In populations, alkaptonuria is rare (1:250,000), but clusters of high incidence are found in certain groups with significant inbreeding, e.g., in Slovakia and Santo Domingo. In Slovakian newborns the incidence is 1:25,000.[2] Disease distribution is worldwide, and there is an approximately equal incidence in the sexes.

Etiology and Pathogenesis[3]

The biochemical pathway by which phenylalanine and tyrosine normally undergo oxidative degradation to acetoacetic acid is shown in Fig. 148-1. HGA (2,5-dihydroxyphenylacetic acid), the last molecule in the sequence to contain an intact aromatic ring, is cleaved to maleylacetoacetic acid. The enzyme catalyzing ring cleavage, HGA oxidase, is normally present in the soluble fraction of liver and kidney cells, but not in other cells. It is highly specific for HGA. Atmospheric oxygen, ferrous ion, and sulfhydryl groups are required for enzymatic function. Quinones inhibit the enzyme. HGA oxidase activity is totally absent in both liver and kidney tissue from alkaptonuric subjects. Whether there is inactive enzy-

matic protein is unknown, and the detailed molecular pathobiology of the disease is not understood. In patients with alkaptonuria, HGA undergoes renal excretion or is transformed to ochronotic pigment within connective tissue. HGA may not be present in the first days of life due to the absence of enzymatic activity of other enzymes in the pathway of tyrosine catabolism.

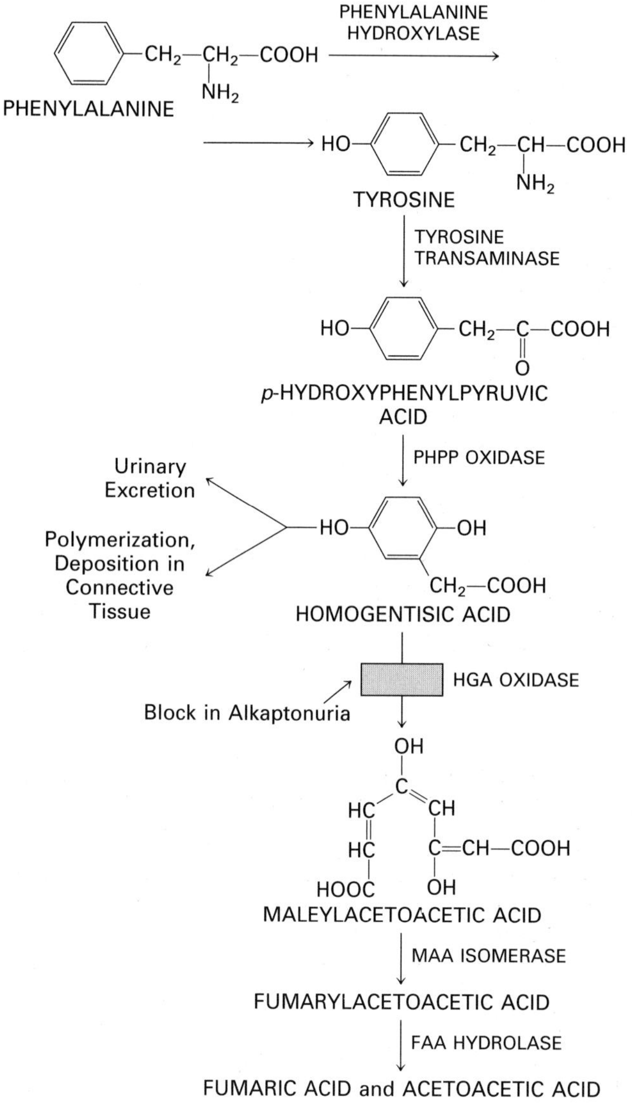

FIGURE 148-1 Metabolic pathway of phenylalanine and tyrosine degradation.

The renal clearance of HGA is extremely high (up to 400 to 500 mL/min) in both normal and alkaptonuric subjects, indicating active tubular secretion of HGA.[3] This explains how with relatively low fasting plasma concentrations of HGA (in the range of 3 mg/dL), excretion may be up to 4 to 8 g/day in alkaptonuria. Drugs which inhibit this secretion may be an important factor in ochronosis. Once excreted, HGA (which is itself colorless in solution) gradually oxidizes to dark products. Oxidation occurs by degrees when the urine is exposed to air, but it can be markedly hastened by alkalinization. Urinary pH is the major variable causing the darkening of the urine, and some patients with acidic urine may *never* have spontaneously black urine. Urinary HGA varies at least tenfold in concentration. A diet high in protein or tyrosine increases the amount of HGA excreted in disease.

The precise manner by which HGA accumulation in tissues leads to ochronosis is only partially understood. A presumed HGA polymer has never been characterized. When HGA is injected into guinea pigs, it has a high predilection to localize in skin and cartilage; benzoquinoneacetic acid (BQA), the highly reactive quinone of HGA, binds irreversibly to connective tissue. Homogentisic acid polyphenol oxidase, a copper-containing enzyme in human, guinea pig, and rabbit skin and cartilage, catalyzes the oxidation of HGA into ochronotic pigment. In the presence of increased HGA, this enzyme may form BQA, which can then be polymerized by the same polyphenol oxidase.[4]

The demonstration of experimental ochronosis by prolonged feeding of high tyrosine diets to rats may be of particular value in delineating the precise interaction between HGA and its products and connective tissue.[5] In this animal model, joint capsules, sternum, and trachea were affected, and there was increased nonsulfated acid mucopolysaccharides and decreased sulfated mucopolysaccharides. HGA and BQA were in the subcutaneous tissue. Alkaptonuria also has been produced in experimental animals by L-phenylalanine feeding, diets deficient in sulfur amino acids or tryptophan and the iron chelator, α,α'-dipyridyl. In patients with tyrosinemia II there is no evidence of increased HGA or of dermal pigmentation (see Chap. 147).

Homogentisic acid inhibits the enzyme lysyl hydroxylase in chick embryo calvaria, suggesting that a reduction of the structural integrity of collagen consequent to deficient hydroxylysine-derived cross-linkages may be responsible for cartilaginous degeneration in alkaptonuria.[6] The plasma level of HGA, approximately 0.1 mM, would cause 30 percent inhibition of lysyl hydroxylase. Milch has shown that autooxidized polymers of HGA combine with collagen chains to form significant cross-linking in vitro.[7]

Clinical Manifestations[1,2]

Although many classic descriptions of the clinical presentation of alkaptonuria cite dark urine as the initial manifestation, this is not always the case. The urine is most apt to discolor rapidly at a pH above 7.0 and when reducing substances such as ascorbic acid, which normally protect HGA from oxidation, are not present in sufficient quantity.

An early diagnosis of alkaptonuria is frequently made when: (1) it is specifically sought because of family history; (2) discoloration of diapers occurs after cleansing in (alkaline) soap; (3) the urinary pH favors the polymerization of HGA; or (4) testing for urinary glucose with Benedict's solution yields an orange precipitate (indicating a reducing substance) accompanied by a dark super-

natant. A positive Benedict's reaction and a negative glucose analysis with a glucose oxidase test reagent strongly suggest the diagnosis.

Although the diagnosis of alkaptonuria may be made during childhood, individuals rarely develop pathologically significant changes in connective tissue until they reach their third or fourth decade. If coincidental renal disease prevents effective HGA excretion, the development of ochronosis may be accelerated and diffuse hyperpigmentation results.[8,9]

Dark brown or black cerumen may be present in the first decade even in those less than 5 years of age.[2] Axillary skin pigmentation (greenish blue, blue, greenish yellow, or brown) may be present late in the first decade and may be accompanied by underwear staining. The pigmentation is in the pattern of glandular orifices.

A grayish-blue tinge overlying ear cartilage occurs relatively early in the course of ochronosis. Later in the disease, structural changes result in loss of transillumination, stiffening, irregular contours, and eventually, in the third decade, calcification of the pinnae. The tympanic membrane may be blue. Tinnitus and variable degrees of deafness have been ascribed to ochronotic degeneration of the tympanic membrane and underlying ossicles. Laryngeal and tracheal cartilage become heavily pigmented but do not cause symptoms.

The visible changes that occur with the passage of time are due primarily to the formation of ochronotic pigment granules in the dermis and sweat follicles, and, most importantly, to the transmission of ochronotic discoloration through thin areas of skin overlying pigmented cartilage and tendon. The latter type, which is fairly uniform in ochronosis, is most apparent at the nose tip, ear (Fig. 148-2), costochondral junctions, and extensor tendons of the hands. Intrinsic pigmentation of the skin is typically less prominent but may occur in a butterfly pattern on the nose and cheeks (Fig. 148-3). Rarely, bluish-gray fingernails and intensely dark nevi have been reported.[1]

Ochronotic pigment sometimes accumulates in the outer ocular tissues: sclerae (Figs. 148-4 and 148-5), corneas, conjunctivae, and tarsal plates. Scleral discoloration is generally restricted to that portion of the globe exposed by the palpebral fissure. The scleral pigmentation is usually triangular in shape, with the base of the triangle facing the cornea at the site of recti muscle insertion.[3] Tiny "oil droplets" of ochronotic pigment appear at the inner and outer poles of the corneas in advanced ochronosis.

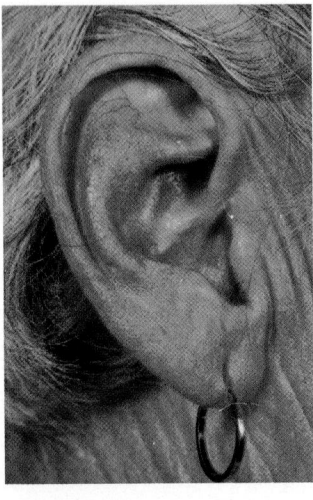

FIGURE 148-2 Ochronotic discoloration seen through the thin area of skin overlying the pigmented cartilage of the ear.

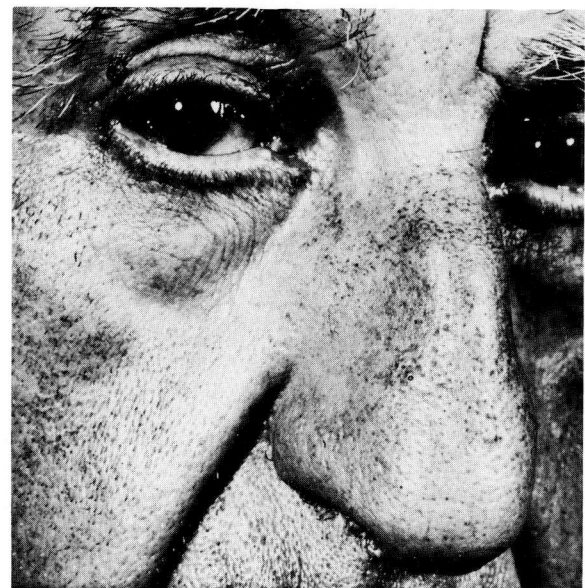

FIGURE 148-3 Punctate, blue dermal pigmentation in alkaptonuric ochronosis in a butterfly distribution on the nose and cheeks.

Insidious progression of ochronotic arthropathy, which generally begins in the third and fourth decades in males and about 10 years later in females, is the most disabling manifestation of alkaptonuria. The disease is more severe in males. Bouts of acute inflammation may occur. Hip, knee, and shoulder limitation are early signs. Lumbar pain, lordosis, kyphosis, and sciatica are common. X-rays show a characteristic appearance of early calcification of the intervertebral disc and later narrowing of the intervertebral spaces, with eventual disc collapse and progressive loss of height (Fig. 148-6). In addition to the spine, ochronotic arthropathy typically involves larger joints, such as the shoulders, knees, and hips. The hands and feet are generally spared. Pseudogout may coexist with ochronosis.[10]

There is some suggestion of an increased incidence of cardiovascular disease in ochronosis, but accelerated arteriosclerosis has

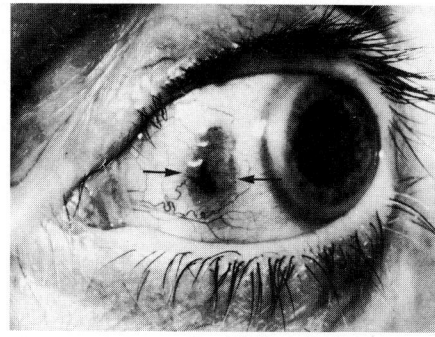

FIGURE 148-4 Ochronosis (alkaptonuria) has pathognomonic ocular signs. The first sign to appear is that of grayish black scleral pigmentation anterior to the tendon insertions of the horizontal recti muscles (arrows). At times pigmentation of the elastic tissue in pinguecula may be stained a dark brown or black and usually has the configuration of small, dark rings. In advanced cases of ochronosis, Bowman's membrane, adjacent to the limbus, may have areas of black pigmentation.

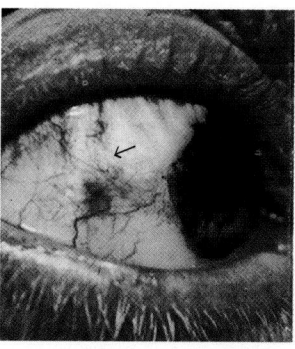

FIGURE 148-5 Ochronotic scleral pigmentation.

not been clearly documented. At postmortem examination, pigmentation is commonly observed in the heart valves, annuli, and in arteriosclerotic plaques. A case of aortic valve stenosis has been attributed to the deposition of ochronotic pigment.[11]

Prostatic symptoms in older males frequently are due to the formation of soft pigmented calculi in the alkaline secretions of the ducts and sinuses of that gland. Porous black renal stones containing calcium, phosphate, and oxalate have also been reported.

Laboratory Findings

Aside from the excretion of HGA, alkaptonuric patients show no abnormalities discernible on routine clinical laboratory tests. Normal individuals do not excrete HGA; therefore, darkening of the urine upon addition of sodium hydroxide is presumptive evidence of alkaptonuria.

Other tests based on the reducing properties of HGA include the black reaction after treatment with $FeCl_3$, and blackening of photographic emulsion paper upon application of a drop of alkaptonuric urine followed by a drop of sodium hydroxide (Fig. 148-7). A screening test with sodium hydroxide-impregnated filter paper is sensitive and useful for field studies.[2] Specific identification and quantitation of urinary (as well as blood) HGA can be achieved by the use of a direct spectrophotometric method employing HGA oxidase.

With the development of ochronotic arthropathy, x-rays of the spine show characteristic disc calcification which rarely occurs in other forms of spondylitis. Periostitis, ligament calcification, and sacroiliac sclerosis are not features of ochronotic spondylitis.

Pathology

Yellow to light brown (ochre) color pigment granules, which gave the original designation of ochronosis, are present as free bodies and in dermal macrophages.[12] Irregular masses may be over 100 μm in diameter. The pigment is not bleached by 10% H_2O_2 after 72 h.[12]

Electron microscopic studies show smaller-sized homogeneous bodies fusing to form larger non-membrane-bound structures.[12] Although the original pigment is brown, Tyndall scattering of light makes involved skin appear blue.

The tendency of connective tissue, in particular, cartilage, to gradually darken over the years constitutes the cardinal pathologic finding in alkaptonuria. Intervertebral discs are pigmented ("jet black") and darken when examined. Articular cartilage, when

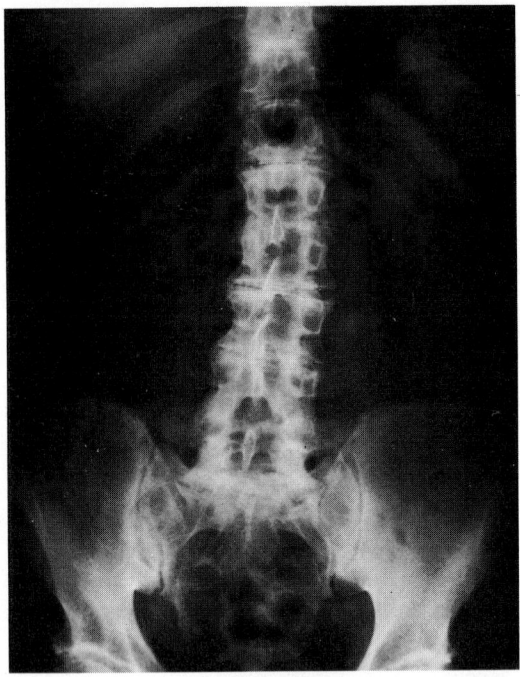

a

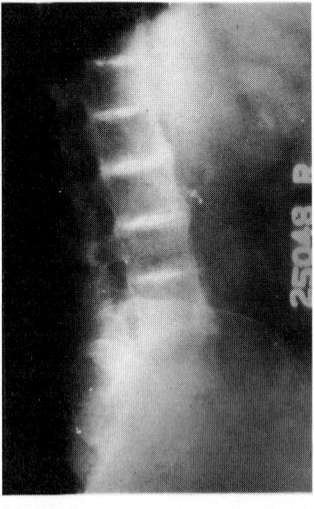

b

FIGURE 148-6 Roentgenographic findings in ochronosis. (*a*) Calcification of the intervertebral discs and disc collapse. (*b*) Marked intervertebral disc calcification.

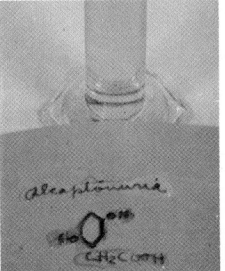

FIGURE 148-7 Urine from the patient with alkaptonuria. The urine itself was used to write on the photographic paper, then alkali was added. The homogentisic acid in the urine acted as a photographic developer.

made. Other causes of dark urine—melaninuria, porphyria, myoglobinuria, bilirubinuria, hematuria, etc.—ought not to be confused with alkaptonuria. An ochronotic-like pigmentation of skin and cartilage has been iatrogenically produced by quinacrine administration over a period of months and at the site of quinine injections.[15] Pigmentation due to antimalarial treatment is usually much more pronounced on mucosal surfaces and will fluoresce with a Wood's lamp.

Ochronotic pigmentation has also resulted from chronic application of carbolic acid to cutaneous ulcers, a form of therapy rarely used today. In a patient described by Osler and Garrod, the blue color was present on the sclera, the conchar concavity of the antihelix, and the extensor tendons of the hands.[16] The pigmentation on the eyes and ears regressed during hospitalization and upon discontinuation of carbolic acid. The light-related distribution of pigmentation was noted by the authors.

It is possible that the *reversible* ochronotic pigmentation caused by prolonged carbolic acid treatment is due to HGA polyphenol oxidase polymerizing the carbolic acid to an HGA-polymer-*like* substance which differs from the polymer found in the genetic disease by its reversibility.

Exogenous ochronosis has been reported in a number of South Africans who used 2% or stronger hydroquinone bleaching creams for a prolonged period.[17,18] Forty-two percent of women and fifteen percent of men who used hydroquinones had exogenous ochronosis.[18] A similar condition is seen in American blacks.[19] The dermal material was autofluorescent, electron dense, and was phagocytosed, although another study emphasized the elastotic nature of the dermal fibers in the abnormal skin.[20] The precise etiology of the pigmentation remains to be determined. An occupationally induced blue-black dermal pigmentation resembling ochronosis has been described in a tiler who handled glues, varnishes, dyes, diluents, and stain removers.[21] Ochronotic arthropathy does not occur in these exogenous forms of hyperpigmentation.

heavily pigmented, displays the degenerative changes of fibrillation, fissuring, fragmentation, and erosion to bare bone.[13] Phagocytosis of collagen fibrils is found in synovial macrophages.[14]

Diagnosis and Differential Diagnosis

The diagnosis of alkaptonuria may be made on the basis of typical urinary discoloration or may await the onset of ochronosis in adulthood. Inasmuch as the disease behaves in a quite stereotypical manner with few confusing variants in its mode of presentation, it has been concluded that the diagnosis need only be thought of to be

Treatment

It is disappointing that despite advances in our biochemical understanding of alkaptonuria and the disposition of accumulated HGA to form ochronotic pigment in connective tissue, this information has yet to be translated into a successful therapeutic program for managing the disease. The treatment of ochronotic arthropathy centers about the proper balance of rest, physiotherapy, and analgesia. Prosthetic joint replacement is apt to be of considerable benefit for patients with advanced degenerative joint changes. Exogenous cutaneous ochronosis induced by hydroquinone has been treated with the carbon dioxide laser.[22]

Course and Prognosis

The ultimate course in adults with alkaptonuria is that of increasing pigmentation and skeletal incapacity. Little can be done to interrupt this progression; however, the disease is not incompatible with a normal life span, and the oldest patient on record lived to 99 years of age.

References

1. O'Brien WM et al: Biochemical, pathologic and clinical aspects of alcaptonuria, ochronosis and ochronotic arthropathy. *Am J Med* **34**:813, 1963
2. Srsen S: Alkaptonuria. *Johns Hopkins Med J* **145**:217, 1979
3. LaDu BN: Alcaptonuria, in *The Metabolic Basis of Inherited Disease,* 6th ed, edited by CS Scriver et al. New York, McGraw-Hill, 1989, p 775
4. Zannoni VG et al: Oxidation of homogentisic acid to ochronotic pigment in connective tissue. *Biochim Biophys Acta* **177**:94, 1969
5. Blivaiss BB et al: Experimental ochronosis: induction in rats by long-term feeding with L-tyrosine. *Arch Pathol* **82**:45, 1966
6. Murray JC et al: *In vitro* inhibition of chick embryo lysyl hydroxylase by homogentisic acid. A proposed connective tissue defect in alkaptonuria. *J Clin Invest* **59**:1071, 1977
7. Milch RA: Studies of alcaptonuria: mechanisms of swelling of homogentisic acid-collagen preparations. *Arthritis Rheum* **4**:253, 1961
8. Wyre CHW: Alkaptonuria with extensive ochronsis. *Arch Derm* **115**:461, 1979
9. Abreo K et al: Clinicopathologic conference: A fifty year old man with skin pigmentation, arthritis, chronic renal failure and methemoglobinemia. *Am J Med Genet* **14**:97, 1983
10. Rynes RI et al: Pseudogout in ochronosis. *Arthritis Rheum* **18**:21, 1975
11. Gould L et al: Cardiac manifestations of ochronosis. *J Thorac Cardiovasc Surg* **72**:788, 1976
12. Attwood HD et al: A histologic, histochemical and ultrastructural study of dermal ochronosis. *Pathology* **3**:115, 1971
13. O'Brien WM et al: Studies on the pathogenesis of ochronotic arthropathy. *Arthritis Rheum* **4**:137, 1961
14. Gaines JJ et al: An ultrastructural and light microscopy study of the synovium in ochronotic arthropathy. *Hum Pathol* **18**:1160, 1987
15. Bruce S et al: Exogenous ochronosis resulting from quinine injections. *J Am Acad Dermatol* **15**:357, 1986
16. Reid E et al: On ochronosis: Report of a Case, the clinical features, the urine. *Q J Med* **1**:199, 1908
17. Findlay GH et al: Exogenous ochronosis and pigmented colloid milium from hydroquinone bleaching creams. *Br J Dermatol* **93**:613, 1975
18. Hardwick N et al: Exogenous ochronosis: an epidemiological study. *Br J Dermatol* **120**:229, 1989
19. Hoshaw RA et al: Ochronosis-like pigmentation from hydroquinone bleaching creams in American Blacks. *Arch Dermatol* **121**:105, 1985
20. Tidman MJ et al: Hydroquinone-induced ochronosis—light and electron-microscopic features. *Clin Exper Dermatol* **II**:224, 1986
21. Dupre A et al: Idiopathic pigmentation of the hands: professional exogenous ochronosis? New entity? *Arch Dermatol Res* **266**:1, 1979
22. Diven DG et al: Hydroquinone-induced localized exogenous ochronosis treated with dermabrasion and CO$_2$ laser. *J Dermatol Surg Oncol* **16**:1018, 1990

CHAPTER 149

Stephen Michael Breathnach

Amyloidosis of the Skin

The generic term *amyloidosis* signifies the abnormal extracellular tissue deposition of one of a family of biochemically unrelated proteins that share certain characteristic staining properties, including apple green briefringence of Congo red–stained preparations viewed under polarized light, and a fibrillar ultrastructure.[1–5] Paired, 7.5- to 10-nm, rigid, linear, nonbranching, aggregated, hollow fibrils of indefinite length, arranged in a loose meshwork, constitute the bulk of amyloid deposits, regardless of clinicopathologic type or the tissue involved. Amyloid fibrils have been shown by x-ray diffraction crystallography and infrared spectroscopy to have, at least in part,[3] a beta-pleated sheet configuration, which probably accounts for their ability to bind Congo red.[6]

Classification of Amyloidosis

Amyloid deposition may occur throughout many organs of the body (systemic amyloidosis) or may be restricted to a single tissue site (organ-limited or localized amyloidosis) (Table 149-1). In both cases it is usually associated with considerable tissue dysfunction. Interest in amyloidosis has increased tremendously with the realization that it is involved in the pathology of aging and of neurodegenerative diseases, including Alzheimer's disease and strokes.[7–9] Systemic types of amyloidosis include those associated with plasma cell dyscrasia, either overt as in multiple myeloma or occult as in "primary" systemic amyloidosis,[10] and amyloidosis secondary to a variety of chronic diseases. The latter include acute recurrent and chronic infections, rheumatoid arthritis, juvenile chronic arthritis, ankylosing spondylitis, Reiter's syndrome, Behçet's syndrome, Sjögren's syndrome, systemic lupus erythematosus (very rarely), inflammatory bowel disease, Hodgkin's disease, and some solid nonlymphoid tumors.[1,2,4,11–14] Secondary systemic amyloidosis has been reported as a complication of a number of dermatoses,[1,14,15] such as recurrent venous ulceration, generalized psoriasis and psoriatic arthritis,[16] lepromatous leprosy, hidradenitis suppurativa, chronically infected burns, chronic skin infection in drug addicts,[17] nodular nonsuppurative panniculitis,[18] ulcerated or metastatic basal cell carcinoma,[19] acne conglobata,[20] epidermolysis bullosa of dystrophic[21] and acquired types, and X-linked anhidrotic ectodermal dysplasia.

The systemic amyloidoses associated with subunit proteins derived from immunoglobulins (either primary or myeloma-associated) are known as AL amyloidoses. Those associated with inflammatory disease are known as AA amyloidoses, while the hereditary syndromes derived from prealbumin are known as AH amyloidoses.

TABLE 149-1

Classification of Amyloid and Biochemical Nature of Fibril Proteins

Clinical syndrome	Fibril proteins and precursors
I Systemic amyloidosis	
A Associated with immunocyte dyscrasia	
1 Primary systemic (occult dyscrasia)	AL fibrils derived from monoclonal immunoglobulin light chains
2 Myeloma-associated	
B Associated with chronic active diseases (secondary or reactive systemic amyloidosis)	AA fibrils derived from serum amyloid A protein (SAA)
C Hereditary syndromes	
1 Predominantly neuropathic forms (autosomal dominant)	
a Type I (Portuguese, Japanese, Swedish, Jewish kindreds)	Prealbumin fibrils
b Type II (Swiss, German kindreds; Indiana-Maryland type)	Prealbumin fibrils
c Type III (Scottish, Irish, English kindreds; Iowa type)	? Apolipoprotein A1 fibrils
d Type IV (Finnish kindreds)	Gelsolin (actin modulating protein)
2 Predominantly nephropathic forms	
a Familial Mediterranean fever (autosomal recessive)	AA fibrils from SAA
b Ostertag type (autosomal dominant)	Unknown
c Muckle-Wells' type	Unknown
3 Predominantly cardiomyopathic forms	
a Danish type	Prealbumin fibrils
b Appalachian type	Prealbumin fibrils
c Cardiomyopathy with persistent atrial standstill	Unknown
D Senile systemic amyloidosis (formerly senile cardiac amyloidosis)	Prealbumin ASc_1 fibrils from plasma prealbumin
II Localized (organ-limited) amyloidosis	
A Hereditary syndromes	
1 Hereditary cerebral hemorrhage with amyloidosis	
a Icelandic type	Cystatin C (γ trace) fibrils
b Dutch type	β-protein fibrils
B Periarticular, bony, and renal amyloid in chronic hemodialysis patients	β-2 microglobulin derived from high plasma levels
C Cerebral amyloid angiopathy and cortical plaques in Alzheimer's disease, senile dementia, Down's syndrome	β-protein fibrils, transmembrane precursor encoded on chromosome 21
D Senile amyloidosis (heart, joints, seminal vesicles)	Atrial natriuretic peptide-related fibrils in isolated atrial amyloid; otherwise unknown
E Ocular deposits (corneal, conjunctival)	Unknown
F Endocrine amyloidosis (APUD organs, APUDomas)	
1 Elderly non-insulin-dependent diabetics, benign insulinomas of the pancreas, normal aged pancreas	Islet amyloid polypeptide fibrils (homology with calcitonin gene-related peptides)
2 Medullary carcinoma of the thyroid	Precalcitonin-related fibrils
G Nodular (skin, lung, genitourinary tract)	AL fibrils derived from monoclonal immunoglobulin light chains
H Primary localized cutaneous (Macular amyloidosis and lichen amyloidosus)	? Keratin-derived
I Secondary localized cutaneous (Microscopic deposits secondary to a variety of cutaneous lesions)	? Keratin-derived

SOURCE: Derived from references 1–4.

Clinically evident involvement of the skin is frequent in primary systemic and myeloma-associated systemic amyloidosis, but occurs only rarely, if at all, in secondary systemic amyloidosis.[14] Although there is a degree of overlap, primary and myeloma-associated systemic amyloidosis typically involve the tongue, heart, gastrointestinal tract, skeletal and smooth muscle, carpal ligaments, nerves, and skin, whereas secondary systemic amyloidosis affects the liver, spleen, kidneys, and adrenals.[1,12,22] Skin manifestations are associated with a number of systemic heredofamilial syndromes of amyloid deposition, including familial Mediterranean fever,[23] the Muckle-Wells' syndrome,[24] and heredofamilial amyloid polyneuropathy.[25] Localized cutaneous amyloidosis may be of primary (nodular, and macular amyloid and lichen amyloidosus) or secondary type (Table 149-1).[26–28]

Etiology and Pathogenesis

Amyloid material may accumulate as a result of a variety of different pathogenic mechanisms, and the biochemical composition of amyloid fibrils varies according to the clinicopathologic type of amyloidosis.[1–5] The various known amyloid fibril proteins are listed in Table 149-1. Only those relevant to cutaneous disease will be discussed further.

Systemic Amyloidosis

Amyloid deposition in primary and myeloma-associated systemic amyloidosis occurs as a result of plasma cell dyscrasia, and the fibrils are composed of immunoglobulin light chain material (protein AL),[1–4] either intact light chains, light chain fragments (particularly the variable aminoterminal region), or both.[29,30] Abnormal light chain material is almost always present in the serum or urine, even in so-called primary systemic amyloidosis, and can be demonstrated on tissue culture of bone marrow cells from affected patients.[31,32] Patients who have apparent nonsecretory myeloma may have low absolute rates of monoclonal immunoglobulin synthesis, and the protein products may have high tissue affinity.[31] Proteolytic digestion of only a proportion of Bence Jones proteins results in amyloid fibril formation,[33] which may account for the fact that amyloidosis develops in only about 15 percent of patients with myelomatosis. Amyloidogenic immunoglobulin AL monoclonal proteins appear to be preferentially of lambda type, of lower molecular weight, and of lower isoelectric point.[31,34]

In secondary systemic amyloidosis and familial Mediterranean fever, the fibrils are composed of a nonimmunoglobulin protein, designated *protein AA*.[1–4,35] A precursor of protein AA, known as serum amyloid A protein (protein SAA), is present in the serum of normal individuals as an apolipoprotein of high-density lipoprotein (HDL$_3$) and behaves as an acute-phase reactant. A number of types of familial amyloidosis, which may manifest initially with progressive neuropathy, cardiomyopathy, or renal involvement, are related to a variant of transthyretin (prealbumin) inherited as a dominant trait, produced by a point mutation leading to an amino acid substitution in the transthyretin gene.[1–4,36,37] However, in senile systemic amyloidosis the amino acid primary structure of the transerythrithin, of which the fibrils are composed, is normal, so that factors other than the primary structure of the protein must be involved in the amyloid deposition.[9]

Localized Cutaneous Amyloidosis

Secondary Localized Cutaneous Amyloidosis Deposition of clinically insignificant microscopic amounts of amyloid in relation to a variety of cutaneous lesions is the most common type of localized cutaneous amyloidosis. Reported predisposing conditions include intradermal nevi, sweat gland tumors, pilomatrixoma, dermatofibroma, seborrheic keratosis, solar elastosis, photosensitive annular elastolytic giant cell granuloma, actinic keratosis, porokeratosis of Mibelli, Bowen's disease, and basal cell carcinoma,[26,27,38–42] as well as following PUVA therapy.[43]

Primary Localized Cutaneous Amyloidosis (PLCA) PLCA comprises macular, papular (lichen amyloidosus), and the rare nodular (tumefactive) forms.[26–28] Nodular PLCA may be regarded as akin to extramedullary plasmacytoma, because the fibrils are of immunoglobulin AL type and are thought to arise as a result of local aberrant light chain material production by clonally expanded plasma cells.[44–46] Fibrils in lichen amyloidosus and macular amyloidosis do not bind antibodies to protein AA or prealbumin,[47] and although immunoglobulins, κ and λ light chains, and complement are frequently observed in deposits of macular and papular PLCA,[48,49] they are not thought to be integral constituents of the fibrils as they are readily eluted.[48,50] Instead, the concept has arisen of focal epidermal damage and filamentous degeneration of keratinocytes, followed by apoptosis and conversion of filamentous masses (colloid bodies) into amyloid material in the papillary dermis.[51,52] In support of this theory is the fact that dermal amyloid deposits in these forms of PLCA cross-react immunohistochemically with keratin.[53,54] However, the tertiary structure of epidermal keratin is of alpha helical type, rather than the beta-pleated sheet configuration typical of amyloid. Furthermore, the pathogenesis cannot be this simple because colloid (keratin) bodies produced in other dermatoses, such as lichen planus, are not transformed into amyloid. One theory proposes that in lichen amyloidosus specific immunologic tolerance to the presence of colloid bodies in the papillary dermis favors their transformation into amyloid by macrophages or fibroblasts,[39] whereas in lichen planus a brisk inflammatory response ensures their removal.

Nonfibrillar Amyloid Proteins

In addition to the fibrillar component, amyloid deposits invariably contain up to 14 percent by dry weight of a protein termed *amyloid P (plasma) component* (AP),[55,56] which is derived from and identical to serum amyloid P component (SAP), a protein present in the blood of all normal individuals. AP is also constantly associated with the microfibrillar sheath of elastic fibers throughout the body in normal adults.[57] The role of AP in the pathogenesis of amyloidosis is unknown, but there has been speculation that it may be involved in the deposition and maintenance of amyloid deposits. In this regard, it is of interest that AP is absent from nonamyloidotic monoclonal immunoglobulin deposits. AP shows calcium-dependent binding to isolated amyloid fibrils in vitro, which may account for the frequent observation of amyloid deposition in the vicinity of elastic fibers.[56,58] Amyloid deposits also always contain glycosaminoglycans.[59]

Clinical Manifestations

Primary and Myeloma-Associated Systemic Amyloidosis

The field has been extensively reviewed.[1,2,10,12,60–62] These conditions are very rare below the age of 40 years, the mean age of onset being about 65 years; there is a slight male preponderance. Diagnosis is often delayed because of nonspecific presenting symptoms; these include fatigue, weight loss, paresthesias, hoarseness, edema, dyspnea, and syncope secondary to orthostatic hypotension. The classic presentation with symptoms of carpal tunnel syndrome, macroglossia (which occurs in about 10 percent of cases and may result in painful dysphagia), specific mucocutaneous lesions, hepatomegaly, and edema should always alert the clinician to the presence of an underlying plasma cell dyscrasia.

Noncutaneous Changes Hepatomegaly occurs in about 50 percent of patients at presentation, but splenomegaly occurs in less than 10 percent. Pitting edema is common and may be the result of the nephrotic syndrome or of congestive cardiac failure, both of which occur in about 30 percent of cases; rarely, it may be a complication of protein-losing enteropathy from amyloid involvement of the small bowel. Ascites may develop. Angina, infarction, arrhythmias, or orthostatic hypotension may develop as a consequence of cardiac infiltration. Congestive cardiac failure or arrhythmias account for death in about 40 percent of cases of AL-type systemic amyloidosis. Pulmonary involvement is common but usually asymptomatic. Amyloid infiltration of blood vessels may lead to claudication of the legs or jaw, and gastrointestinal tract involvement may simulate inflammatory bowel disease with hemorrhage; malabsorption is found in 5 percent of cases. The carpal tunnel syndrome has been reported in up to 25 percent of patients with primary systemic amyloidosis.[10] Peripheral neuropathy,[63] initially of the lower extremities, tends to pursue a chronic course and may be accompanied by superimposed autonomic neuropathy, leading to orthostatic hypotension, diarrhea, loss of bladder control, or impotence. Muscle weakness may be caused by neuropathy or by direct infiltration of muscle or its vascular supply, and infiltration between muscle fibers leading to pseudohypertrophy is recognized.

Lymphadenopathy, which occurs in about 10 percent of patients, or Sjögren's syndrome[64] may occasionally be presenting

TABLE 149-2
Cutaneous Lesions in Primary and Myeloma-Associated Systemic Amyloidosis

Common	Less common
Petechiae, purpura, ecchymoses	Pigmentary changes
Waxy, translucent or purpuric papules	Scleroderma-like infiltration
Nodules	Bullous lesions
Plaques	Alopecia
Tumefactive lesions	Cord-like blood vessel thickening
	Nail dystrophy
	Amyloid elastosis
	Cutis laxa

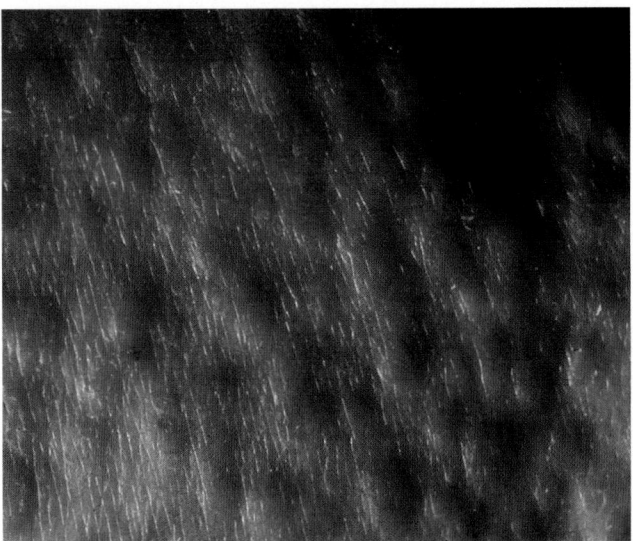

FIGURE 149-2 Papular lesions of cutaneous amyloidosis. (*Courtesy of Klaus Wolff, M.D.*)

features. Amyloid deposition in joints may mimic rheumatoid arthritis, and deposition around the shoulders may cause extensive soft tissue enlargement (the shoulder-pad sign).[65] Among the hematologic complications of systemic amyloidosis are isolated factor X deficiency,[66] disseminated intravascular coagulation, and fibrinolysis with severe bleeding.

Mucocutaneous Findings Clinically evident mucocutaneous involvement occurs in up to 40 percent of cases (Table 149-2).[13,26,60,62] The surface of the tongue may be smooth and dry, or studded with waxy papules, nodules, plaques, or bullae; there may be fissuring, ulceration, hemorrhage, and tooth indentations on the lateral border.

The most common skin signs consist of petechiae, purpura, and ecchymoses occurring spontaneously or after minor trauma. These are the result of amyloid infiltration of blood vessel walls. Purpuric lesions are especially found in flexural regions, such as the eyelids (Fig. 149-1), nasolabial folds, neck, axillae, umbilicus, and anogenital area, as well as in the mouth. Eyelid purpura following pinching (pinch purpura) and periorbital purpura following

coughing, vomiting, the Valsalva maneuver, forced expiration during spirometric testing, or proctoscopy (postproctoscopic palpebral purpura) are very characteristic. Targetlike lesions may develop as transient purpuric halos around Campbell de Morgan spots.[67] Pigmentary changes include jaundice due to hepatic disease, cardiac failure, or severe hemorrhage, pallor due to anemia, and hyperpigmentation due to hemorrhage.

Waxy, smooth, shiny, papules (Fig. 149-2), nodules, and plaques, which may be skin- or amber-colored with a hemorrhagic appearance, are the most characteristic skin lesions. Translucent lesions may resemble vesicles. Flexural areas are sites of predilection, including the eyelids, retroauricular region, neck, axillae, umbilicus and inguinal and anogenital regions. Lesions may also be found on the central face, lips, tongue, and buccal mucosa. Nodules, which occur at any site, may resemble condylomata lata on perianal and vulval skin and, when widespread, may appear like xanthomata.[68] Plaques may be isolated or coalesce to produce large tumefactive lesions. Diffuse amyloid infiltration may produce a sclerodermatous appearance of the face, hands, and feet.[69] Alternatively, a myxedema-like appearance may develop; scalp lesions may resemble cutis verticis gyrata or lead to patchy or universal alopecia.[70]

Signs that occur rarely include bullae of the skin or mucous membranes as a result of shearing within dermal amyloid deposits.[71,72] Extensive amyloid infiltration may lead to cordlike thickening of superficial blood vessels.[73,74] Dystrophic nail changes, including brittleness, crumbling, subungual striations, and partial or complete anonychia, may be a presenting sign.[75,76] Amyloid elastosis is an unusual, recently recognized syndrome in which papulonodular cutaneous lesions are associated with widespread amyloid infiltration of visceral and cutaneous blood vessels, particularly in relation to elastic fibers.[58,77] Acquired cutis laxa has also been described.[78,79]

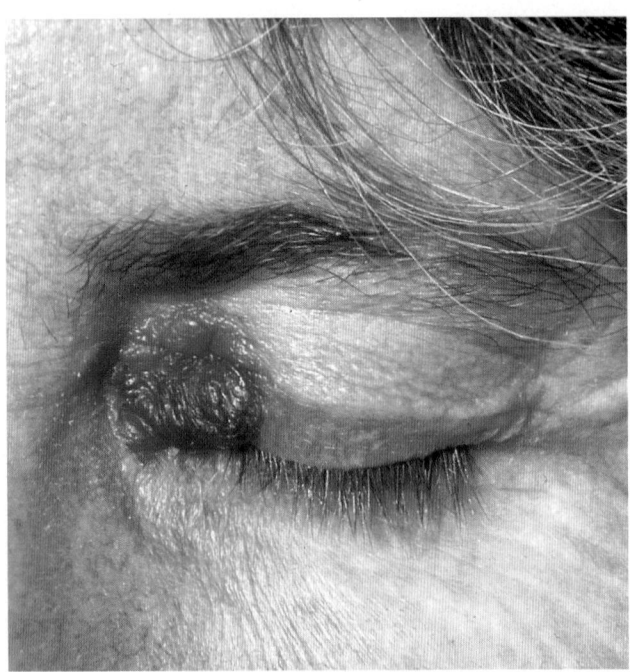

FIGURE 149-1 Amyloidosis of the eyelid with purpura. (*Courtesy of Klaus Wolff, M.D.*)

Heredofamilial Amyloidosis[1]

Familial Mediterranean fever, inherited as an autosomal recessive trait, may involve erysipelas-like lesions on the lower legs, urticaria, Henoch-Schönlein purpura, and vasculitic nodules. Associated features are intermittent fevers and a tendency to peritonitis, pleurisy, synovitis, and renal amyloidosis.[23] The Muckle-Wells' syndrome, inherited as an autosomal dominant trait, is characterized by periodic attacks of urticaria, fever, and limb pains, associated with progressive perceptive nerve deafness and renal amyloidosis.[24] Trophic skin changes may develop in heredofamilial amyloid polyneuropathy.[25] The Finnish type of heredofamilial neuropathic amyloidosis, characterized by cranial neuropathy and corneal lattice dystrophy, may be associated with cutis laxa.[80]

Localized Cutaneous Amyloidosis

Nodular Localized Cutaneous Amyloidosis[81–83]   This presents clinically with single or, more commonly, multiple lesions on the limbs (Fig. 149-3), face, trunk, or genitalia. These appear indistinguishable from those associated with plasma cell dyscrasia–related systemic amyloidosis and vary in size from a few millimeters to several centimeters. Japanese reports suggest an association with Sjögren's syndrome.[46] The condition may follow a prolonged benign course over many years; however, some patients later develop paraproteinemia and overt systemic amyloidosis.[27,28]

Macular Amyloidosis and Lichen Amyloidosus (PLCA)[26–28,62] Macular amyloidosis, which tends to persist unchanged for many years, is a pruritic eruption of small brownish macules distributed typically in a rippled, symmetric fashion on the upper back (Fig. 149-4), limbs, and occasionally chest and buttocks. Lichen amyloidosus is a persistent, pruritic eruption of multiple discrete hyperkeratotic papules, which may coalesce to form plaques, distributed principally on the shins. These may be spread to the calves, ankles, dorsa of the feet, and thighs, and the extensor aspects of the arms and abdominal or chest wall may also be involved.[84] Because macular amyloidosis and lichen amyloidosus may coexist in an affected individual (biphasic amyloidosis), they are regarded as variants of a single pathologic process.[85]

Lichen amyloidosus is more common among the Chinese,[84] and macular amyloidosis is more common among Central and

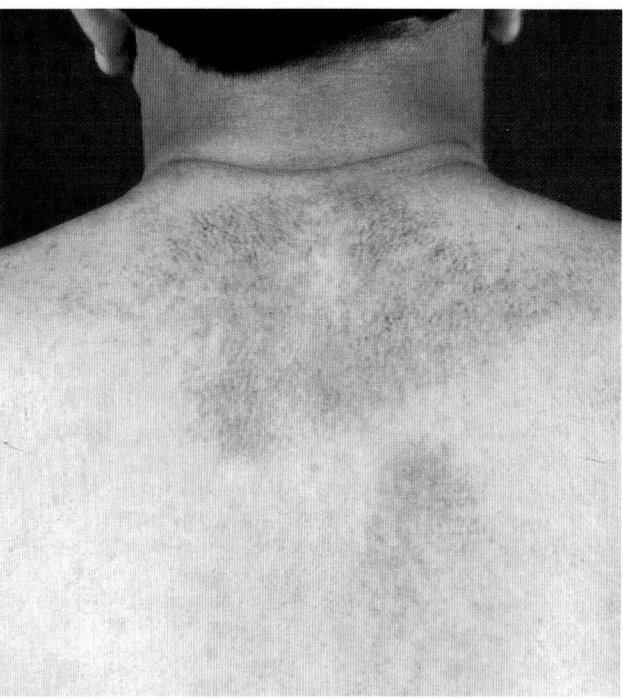

FIGURE 149-4   Macular amyloidosis of the upper back. (*Courtesy of Klaus Wolff, M.D.*)

South Americans,[86] Middle Easterners,[87] and Asians. This apparent racial incidence may, in the case of the Japanese, be contributed to by a habit of rubbing the skin vigorously with a nylon towel or brush ("friction amyloidosis").[88,89] The importance of genetic factors in the development of PLCA is emphasized by the occurrence of familial cases.[90–93] PLCA has occasionally been reported to be associated with connective tissue diseases (including systemic sclerosis, primary biliary cirrhosis, and systemic lupus erythematosus)[28] and in a few kindreds with pachonychia congenita[94] or multiple endocrine neoplasia type 2a.[95]

Unusual variants of PLCA include macular forms, simulating nevoid hyperpigmentation[96] or causing periocular hyperpigmentation,[97] and a poikiloderma-like form.[98] Primary cutaneous amyloidosis of the auricular concha (small papules are grouped on the concha of the ear) is also believed to be a variant of PLCA and may coexist with lichen amyloidosus.[99,100]

Anosacral Cutaneous Amyloidosis   This is a rare syndrome described in elderly Japanese males, in which pigmented macules and glossy hyperkeratotic lesions radiate out from the anus.[101] It has been attributed to the aging process.

Laboratory and Special Examination

Primary and Myeloma-Associated Systemic Amyloidosis[1,2,10,12,61]

Anemia is not a prominent feature, the leukocyte and differential counts are usually within normal limits, and the erthrocyte sedimentation rate is usually less than 50 mm/h (Westergren). Thrombocytosis > 500,000/mm^2 occurs in up to 10 percent of patients. Hepatic function abnormalities are usually minor apart from hypoalbuminemia, but the serum creatinine is raised in 50 percent, and

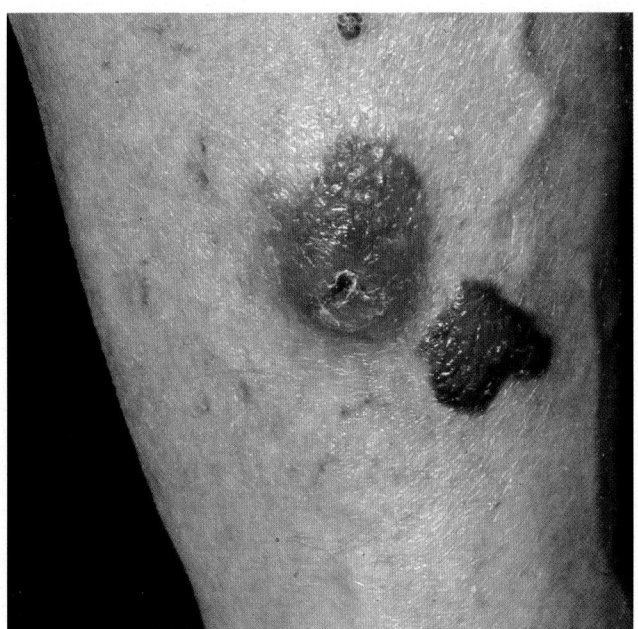

FIGURE 149-3   Nodular amyloidosis of the leg. (*Courtesy of Klaus Wolff, M.D.*)

proteinuria is present in about 80 percent of patients; hypercalcemia occurs in a third of myeloma patients but is rare in primary cases.

Immunoglobulin estimation reveals reduced IgG levels in half the primary and two-thirds of the myeloma-associated cases. Serum protein electrophoresis shows a spike pattern in slightly less than half the primary and two-thirds of the myeloma patients. However, the spike is usually of modest size and may be missed; monoclonal light chains rarely produce a recognizable band. Immunoelectrophoresis of serum reveals a monoclonal protein in two-thirds of patients with AL amyloidosis; only 45 percent have a monoclonal heavy chain, whereas 20 percent have free monoclonal light chains (Bence Jones proteinemia).[1] The ratio of λ light chains to κ light chains is 3:1 in patients with AL amyloidosis, in contrast to uncomplicated multiple myeloma patients, in whom the ratio is 1:2.

The heat test for Bence Jones protein is usually negative.[1] Immunoelectrophoresis of concentrated urine reveals a monoclonal light chain in about two-thirds of cases (λ to κ ratio 2:1). When screening of both serum and urine is performed, the frequency of patients with an identifiable monoclonal protein rises to about 86 percent.[1,10] Nevertheless, in some patients with the clinical features of AL amyloidosis, it is not possible to demonstrate a paraprotein, even after follow-up for as long as 24 years.[102]

Histopathology

Systemic Amyloidosis

In primary and myeloma-associated systemic amyloidosis,[13,26,103,104] papular lesions contain amorphous, often fissured, faintly eosinophilic masses in the papillary dermis, and there is associated thinning or obliteration of the rete ridges. There may be diffuse amyloid deposition in the reticular dermis and subcutis in nodular lesions and plaques. There is usually little in the way of any associated inflammatory infiltrate. Amyloid infiltration of blood vessel walls, pilosebaceous units, arrector pili muscles, the lamina propria of sweat glands and ducts, and around individual fat cells in the subcutis as "amyloid rings" is characteristic. Amyloid deposits in the nail fold and bed of dystrophic nails have been reported.[75]

In secondary systemic amyloidosis, amyloid deposits may be found deep in the dermis in small blood vessels and around adnexal structures, as well as surrounding individual cells in the subcuticular fat.[105] In the Swedish type of heredofamilial amyloid polyneuropathy, amyloid deposits are found in the dermis and subcutis associated with arrector pili muscles, sweat glands, and nerves in clinically normal skin.[106]

Localized Cutaneous Amyloidosis[26,27]

Nodular PLCA The histopathology resembles that of primary systemic amyloidosis with the single exception that in nodular PLCA there is usually a marked infiltrate of plasma cells.[103,107]

Lichen Amyloidosus and Macular PLCA Amyloid deposits are usually confined to the papillary dermis and do not involve blood vessels or adnexal structures. Early lesions contain small, multifaceted, amorphous globules within the papillae, which are easily missed without the use of special stains. Later lesions show globules that coalesce, expand the papillae, and displace the rete ridges laterally. In lichen amyloidosus the deposits are slightly larger and

are accompanied by irregular acanthosis and hyperkeratosis of the overlying epidermis.

Use of Special Stains[26,62,108]

The special stains for amyloid include the triphenyl-methane dyes, methyl and cresyl violet, for the demonstration of metachromasia; the PAS method; the substantive cotton dyes, Congo red and Sirius red, with or without fluorescence or polarized light microscopy; and fluorescence with thiazole dyes, such as thioflavine T. Alternative cotton dyes, including Pagoda red, RIT scarlet No. 5, and RIT cardinal red no. 9, may be used; fluorescence methods using an optical brightener for cellulose (Phorwhite BBU) and immunohistochemical staining with anti-SAP have also been advocated. Unfortunately, methyl violet and Congo red staining may be equivocal and inadequate for detecting small deposits of amyloid; false-positive results occur in colloid milium and lipoid proteinosis. False-positive staining with thioflavine T is seen with stromal hyaline deposits, collagen fibers, and colloid bodies in lichen planus; anti-SAP also stains colloid bodies and elastotic elastic fibers. Thus, none of the existing stains is absolutely reliable, and ultrastructural examination may sometimes be necessary.

AL-type amyloid, unlike AA-type amyloid, retains its affinity for Congo red and its typical polarization characteristics after exposure to potassium permanganate.[109] Immunohistochemical staining with specific antisera is used to differentiate between the various types of fibril protein in amyloid deposits.[110]

Diagnosis

The diagnosis of cutaneous amyloidosis depends on the histochemical, immunohistochemical, or ultrastructural demonstration of amyloid material in a skin biopsy specimen. Biopsy of even clinically normal forearm skin has been reported positive in up to 50 percent of patients with primary and myeloma-associated disease.[60]

Other Diagnostic Procedures in Systemic Amyloidosis[1,2,12,61]

Fine-needle biopsy of subcutaneous fat of clinically normal abdominal skin has become established as a simple, minimally invasive diagnostic test with a 60 to 85 percent positive yield in AL-type and AA-type systemic amyloidosis, as well as in heredofamilial amyloidosis.[2,111] In AL- and AA-type amyloidosis, rectal biopsy is positive in up to 80 percent of patients, but the specimen must contain submucosal tissue; jejunal biopsy is positive in about two-thirds of patients, but gingival biopsy in only 19 percent.[112] Gastric biopsy may produce a higher yield than rectal biopsy in AL-type amyloidosis.[113] Ninety-six percent of hepatic and 90 percent of renal and of splenic percutaneous needle biopsies are positive.[114] Bone marrow aspiration may be positive in up to 45 percent of patients. Electrocardiography, echocardiography,[115] angiocardiography, technetium scanning, and endomyocardial biopsy are useful in the diagnosis of amyloid heart disease. Sural nerve biopsy in patients with peripheral neuropathy, synovial fluid analysis in patients with arthropathy,[116] and examination of tissue removed at carpal tunnel decompression may be helpful. Scanning with ^{123}I-labeled serum amyloid P component enables specific localization and imaging of amyloid deposits in vivo.[117]

Distinction between Primary and Myeloma-Associated Amyloidosis

Differentiation between the two ends of the spectrum of AL-type amyloidosis is of prognostic significance but is by no means clear-cut.[10] In one series, over half of myeloma patients had more than 15 percent plasma cells in the marrow (mean 23 percent plasma cells) compared with none of the primary patients (mean 4 percent plasma cells).[12] Similarly, 50 percent of myeloma patients show radiologic evidence of bone involvement, compared with only 6 percent of primary patients. In general, myeloma is not present if a patient has no lytic bone lesions, hypercalcemia, or anemia; has only a small serum or urine monoclonal component; and has fewer than 25 percent bone marrow plasma cells.[10]

Treatment

Systemic Amyloidosis[1,2]

Assessment of response to therapy is hindered by the lack of reliable methods for the quantification of the extent of amyloid in individual patients and by the fact that apparent spontaneous clinical remissions of amyloid nephropathy may occur despite histologic evidence of progressive amyloid infiltration.[1]

Reactive AA-type (Secondary) Amyloidosis Resolution or remission has followed therapy of underlying disease, including nephrectomy for hypernephroma, antibiotic treatment of chronic infection, and etretinate and PUVA therapy for psoriasis.[1,16,62] Colchicine prevents the development of amyloidosis and deterioration of renal function in patients with familial Mediterranean fever.[118] Dimethyl sulfoxide (DMSO) may improve renal function and is relatively nontoxic,[119] but its use is limited because of the associated offensive breath odor. Cytotoxic therapy has prolonged survival in patients with underlying rheumatic diseases.[120]

AL-Type (Primary) Amyloidosis The effect of combined melphalan and prednisone therapy seems in general not to be significantly different from that of placebo on the survival of patients with primary systemic amyloid.[121] Nonetheless, there have been occasional responses,[1,2,66,122] especially in a subset of patients with a κ type monoclonal protein and without cardiac amyloidosis.[123] Thus, despite the relatively high risk of development of leukemia or a dysmyelopoietic syndrome, it has been recommended that all patients should receive a trial of chemotherapy.[124] Colchicine improved survival in one series[125] but not in another trial.[126] Neither DMSO nor vitamin E[127] appear to be beneficial in terms of prolonged survival, although DMSO cleared skin lesions in one patient.[128]

Diuretics are the mainstay of therapy for congestive cardiac failure, because digoxin may result in arrhythmias and calcium channel-blocking agents are contraindicated.[129] Cardiac transplantation has been used for intractable cases.[130] Renal failure may be treated with regular dialysis; hemodialysis membranes are nearly impermeable to the immunoglobulin light chain precursors of protein AL, so that peritoneal dialysis may be preferable.[131] Renal amyloidosis is not an absolute contraindication to transplantation, although amyloid may reaccumulate in the transplanted kidney; patients with AA-type amyloidosis seem to survive longer than those with AL-type amyloidosis.[132]

Localized Cutaneous Amyloidosis Deposits of nodular PLCA may be excised surgically or treated with the carbon dioxide laser, but tend to recur.[133] Macular and papular (lichen amyloidosus) forms of PLCA unfortunately respond poorly to topical steroids combined with systemic antihistamines to alleviate pruritus. Dermabrasion has been advocated for lichen amyloidosus.[134] There have been anecdotal reports of response to topical DMSO therapy in some patients,[135,136] but not in others.[137,138] Etretinate therapy may also be beneficial in a proportion of patients[139,140] but not in all.[141]

Prognosis

The prognosis of systemic amyloidosis, especially of the primary and myeloma-associated variants, remains poor as there is no very effective therapy; cardiac and renal failure are the major causes of death.[1,2] In most reported series the median survival of patients with primary systemic amyloidosis without myeloma is from 12 to 20 months, compared with only 5 months for patients with myeloma-associated amyloidosis.[1,10,12,61,125,142] The overall 5-year survival for primary systemic amyloidosis is about 20 percent.[10] Prognosis depends on response to therapy and the extent of disease; the median survival of patients with primary amyloidosis with response to chemotherapy was 28 months, compared to 7.5 months in nonresponders.[61,142] Patients presenting with amyloid neuropathy without associated cardiac, renal, or hepatic involvement have a significantly better prognosis (median survival 40 to 50 months; 5-year survival 31.6 percent), whereas congestive heart failure indicates a very poor prognosis (median survival 7.7 months, 5-year survival 2.4 percent).[10,63]

References

1. Kyle RA, Gertz MA: Systemic amyloidosis. *Crit Rev Oncol Hematol* **10**:49, 1990
2. Stone MJ: Amyloidosis: A final common pathway for protein deposition in tissues. *Blood* **75**:531, 1990
3. Pepys MB: Amyloidosis: Some recent developments. *Q J Med* **67**(252):283, 1988
4. Hawkins PN: Amyloidosis. *Blood Rev* **2**:270, 1988
5. Glenner GG: Amyloid deposits and amyloidosis. The β-fibrilloses. *N Engl J Med* **302**:1283, 1980
6. Klunk WE et al: Quantitative evaluation of Congo Red binding to amyloid-like proteins with a beta-pleated sheet conformation. *J Histochem Cytochem* **37**:1273, 1989
7. Selkoe DJ: Aging, amyloid and Alzheimer's disease. *N Engl J Med* **320**:1484, 1989
8. Vinters HV: Amyloid and the central nervous system: The neurobiology, genetics and immunocytochemistry of a process important in neurodegenerative diseases and stroke. *Monogr Pathol* **32**:55, 1990
9. Westermark P et al: Fibril in senile systemic amyloidosis is derived from normal transthyretin. *Proc Natl Acad Sci USA* **87**:2843, 1990
10. Gertz MA, Kyle RA: Primary systemic amyloidosis—a diagnostic primer. *Mayo Clin Proc* **64**:1505, 1989
11. Dhillon V et al: Amyloidosis in the rheumatic diseases. *Ann Rheum Dis* **48**:696, 1989
12. Kyle RA, Bayrd ED: Amyloidosis: Review of 236 cases. *Medicine* **54**:271, 1975
13. Brownstein MH, Helwig EB: The cutaneous amyloidoses: II. Systemic forms. *Arch Dermatol* **102**:20, 1970

14. Brownstein MH, Helwig EB: Secondary systemic amyloidosis: Analysis of underlying disorders. *South Med J* **64**:491, 1971

15. Brownstein MH, Helwig EB: Systemic amyloidosis complicating dermatoses. *Arch Dermatol* **102**:1, 1970

16. af Ekenstam E et al: Response of secondary amyloidosis in psoriasis to treatment with etretinate and ultraviolet light. *Br Med J* **293**:733, 1986

17. Neugarten J et al: Amyloidosis in subcutaneous heroin abusers ("skin popper's amyloidosis"). *Am J Med* **81**:635, 1986

18. Pallares R et al: Amyloidosis (AA type) associated with nodular nonsuppurative panniculitis. *Ann Intern Med* **99**:488, 1983

19. Beck HI et al: Giant basal cell carcinoma with metastasis and secondary amyloidosis: Report of case. *Acta Derm Venereol (Stockh)* **63**:564, 1983

20. Pérez-Villa F et al: Renal amyloidosis secondary to acne conglobata. *Int J Dermatol* **28**:132, 1989

21. Yi S et al: Complicating systemic amyloidosis in dystrophic epidermolysis bullosa, recessive type. *Pathology* **20**:184, 1988

22. Isobe T, Osserman EF: Patterns of amyloidosis and their association with plasma cell dyscrasia, monoclonal immunoglobulins and Bence Jones proteins. *N Engl J Med* **290**:473, 1974

23. Sohar E et al: Familial Mediterranean fever: A survey of 470 cases and a review of the literature. *Am J Med* **43**:227, 1967

24. Muckle TJ: The Muckle-Wells' syndrome. *Br J Dermatol* **100**:87, 1979

25. Rubinow A, Cohen AS: Skin involvement in familial amyloidotic polyneuropathy. *Neurology* **31**:1341, 1981

26. Wong C-K, Breathnach SM (eds): Cutaneous amyloidosis. *Clin Dermatol* **8(2)**, 1990

27. Brownstein MH, Helwig EB. The cutaneous amyloidoses: I. Localized forms. *Arch Dermatol* **102**:8, 1970

28. Black MM: Primary localized amyloidosis of the skin: Clinical variants, histochemistry and ultrastructure, in *Amyloidosis*, edited by O Wegelius et al. London, Academic, 1976, p 479

29. Glenner GG et al: Amyloid fibril proteins: Proof of homology with immunoglobulin light chains by sequence analyses. *Science* **172**:1150, 1971

30. Terry WD et al: Structural identity of Bence Jones and amyloid fibril proteins in a patient with plasma cell dyscrasia and amyloidosis. *J Clin Invest* **52**:1276, 1973

31. Buxbaum JN et al: Monoclonal immunoglobulin deposition disease; light chain and light and heavy chain deposition diseases and their relation to light chain amyloidosis. Clinical features, immunopathology, and molecular analysis. *Ann Intern Med* **112**:455, 1990

32. Buxbaum J: Aberrant immunoglobulin synthesis in light chain amyloidosis. Free light chain and light chain fragment production by human bone marrow cells in short-term tissue culture. *J Clin Invest* **78**:798, 1986

33. Glenner GG et al: Creation of "amyloid" fibrils from Bence Jones proteins in vitro. *Science* **174**:712, 1971

34. Bellotti V et al: Relevance of class, molecular weight and isoelectric point in predicting human light chain amyloidogenicity. *Br J Haematol* **74**:65, 1990

35. Husby G et al: Serum amyloid A (SAA)—the precursor of protein AA in secondary amyloidosis. *Adv Exp Med Biol* **243**:185, 1988

36. Varga J, Wohlgethan JR: The clinical and biochemical spectrum of hereditary amyloidoses. *Semin Arthr Rheum* **18**:14, 1988

37. Sakaki Y et al: Human transthyretin (prealbumin) gene and molecular genetics of familial amyloidotic polyneuropathy. *Mol Biol Med* **6**:161, 1989

38. Malak JA, Smith EW: Secondary localized cutaneous amyloidosis. *Arch Dermatol* **86**:465, 1962

39. Runne U, Orfanos CE: Amyloid production by dermal fibroblasts. Electron microscopic studies on the origin of amyloid in various dermatoses and skin tumors. *Br J Dermatol* **97**:155, 1977

40. Hashimoto K, Brownstein MH: Localized amyloidosis in basal cell epitheliomas. *Acta Derm Venereol (Stockh)* **53**:331, 1973

41. MacDonald DM, Black MM: Secondary localized cutaneous amyloidosis in melanocytic naevi. *Br J Dermatol* **103**:553, 1980

42. Lee Y-S et al: Photosensitive annular elastolytic giant cell granuloma with cutaneous amyloidosis. *Am J Dermatopathol* **11**:443, 1989

43. Hashimoto K, Kumakiri M: Colloid-amyloid bodies in PUVA-treated human psoriatic patients. *J Invest Dermatol* **72**:70, 1979

44. Husby G et al: Characterization of an amyloid fibril protein from localized amyloidosis of the skin as lambda immunoglobulin light chains of variable subgroup I (A lambda I). *Clin Exp Immunol* **45**:90, 1981

45. Sletten K et al: Amino acid sequences in amyloid proteins of κ III immunoglobulin light-chain origin. *Scand J Immunol* **18**:557, 1983

46. Kitajima Y et al: Partial amino acid sequence of an amyloid fibril protein from nodular primary cutaneous amyloidosis showing homology to λ immunoglobulin light chain of variable subgroup III (A λ III). *J Invest Dermatol* **95**:301, 1990

47. Breathnach SM et al: Primary localized cutaneous amyloidosis: Dermal amyloid deposits do not bind antibodies to amyloid A protein, prealbumin or fibronectin. *Br J Dermatol* **107**:453, 1982

48. MacDonald DM et al: Localized cutaneous amyloidosis: A clinical review of 100 cases including immunofluorescent studies, in *Amyloid and Amyloidosis*, edited by GG Glenner et al. Amsterdam, Excerpta Medica, 1980, p 239

49. Habermann MC, Montenegro MR: Primary cutaneous amyloidosis: Clinical, laboratorial and histopathological study of 25 cases: Identification of gammaglobulins and C3 in the lesions by immunofluorescence. *Dermatologica* **160**:240, 1980

50. Ito K, Hashimoto K: Antikeratin autoantibodies in the amyloid deposits of lichen amyloidosus and macular amyloidosis. *Arch Dermatol Res* **281**:377, 1989

51. Kumakiri M, Hashimoto K: Histogenesis of primary localized cutaneous amyloidosis: Sequential change of epidermal keratinocytes to amyloid via filamentous degeneration. *J Invest Dermatol* **73**:150, 1979

52. Kumakiri M et al: Presence of basal lamina-like substance with anchoring fibrils within the amyloid deposits of primary localized cutaneous amyloidosis. *J Invest Dermatol* **81**:153, 1983

53. Kobayashi H, Hashimoto K: Amyloidogenesis in organ-limited cutaneous amyloidosis: An antigenic identity between epidermal keratin and skin amyloid. *J Invest Dermatol* **80**:66, 1983

54. Yoneda K et al: Immunohistochemical staining properties of amyloids with anti-keratin antibodies using formalin-fixed, paraffin-embedded sections. *J Cutan Pathol* **16**:133, 1989

55. Pepys MB et al: Biology of serum amyloid P component. *Ann N Y Acad Sci* **389**:286, 1982

56. Breathnach SM, Hintner H: Amyloid P-component and the skin. *Clin Dermatol* **8(2)**:46, 1990

57. Breathnach SM et al: Amyloid P component is located in elastic fibre microfibrils in normal human tissue. *Nature* **293**:652, 1981

58. Sepp N et al: Amyloid elastosis: Analysis of the role of amyloid P component. *J Am Acad Dermatol* **22**:27, 1990

59. Snow AD et al: Sulfated glycosaminoglycans: A common constituent of all amyloids? *Lab Invest* **56**:120, 1987

60. Rubinow A, Cohen AS: Skin involvement in generalized amyloidosis: A study of clinically involved and uninvolved skin in 50 patients with primary and secondary amyloidosis. *Ann Intern Med* **88**:781, 1978

61. Kyle RA, Greipp PR: Amyloidosis (AL): Clinical and laboratory features in 229 cases. *Mayo Clin Proc* **58**:665, 1983

62. Breathnach SM: Amyloid and amyloidosis. *J Am Acad Dermatol* **18**:1, 1988

63. Duston MA et al: Peripheral neuropathy as an early marker of AL amyloidosis. *Arch Intern Med* **149**:358, 1989

64. Gogel HK et al: Primary amyloidosis presenting as Sjögren's syndrome. *Arch Intern Med* **143**:2325, 1983

65. Katz GA et al: The shoulder-pad sign—a diagnostic feature of amyloid arthropathy. *N Engl J Med* **288**:354, 1973

66. Camoriano JK et al: Resolution of acquired factor X deficiency and amyloidosis with melphalan and prednisone therapy. *N Engl J Med* **316**:1133, 1987

67. Brear SG et al: Target-like skin lesions in primary amyloidosis. *Br J Dermatol* **112**:209, 1985

68. Chapman RS et al: Xanthoma-like skin lesions as a presenting feature in primary systemic amyloidosis. *Br J Clin Pract* **27**:271, 1973

69. Leach WB et al: Primary systemic amyloidosis presenting as scleroderma. *Can Med Assoc J* **83**:263, 1960

70. Wheeler GE, Barrows GH: Alopecia universalis. A manifestation of occult amyloidosis and multiple myeloma. *Arch Dermatol* **117**:815, 1981

71. Breathnach SM: Bullous amyloidosis, in *Management of Blistering Diseases,* edited by F Wojnorowska, RA Briggaman. Oxford, Chapman and Hall, 1990, p 289

72. Johnson TM et al: Bullous amyloidosis. *Cutis* **43**:346, 1989

73. Breathnach SM, Wells GC: Amyloid vascular disease: Cord-like thickening of mucocutaneous arteries, intermittent claudication and angina in a case with underlying myelomatosis. *Br J Dermatol* **102**:591, 1980

74. Henry RB III et al: Vascular amyloid in a patient with multiple myeloma. *J Am Acad Dermatol* **15**:379, 1986

75. Breathnach SM et al: Systemic amyloidosis with an underlying lymphoproliferative disorder. Report of a case in which nail involvement was a presenting feature. *Clin Exp Dermatol* **4**:495, 1979

76. Pineda MS et al: Nail alterations in systemic amyloidosis: Report of one case. *J Am Acad Dermatol* **18**:1357, 1988

77. Winkelmann RK et al: Amyloid elastosis: A new cutaneous and systemic pattern of amyloidosis. *Arch Dermatol* **121**:498, 1985

78. Newton JA et al: Cutis laxa associated with amyloidosis. *Clin Exp Dermatol* **11**:87, 1986

79. Yoneda K et al: Elastolytic cutaneous lesions in myeloma-associated amyloidosis. *Arch Dermatol* **126**:657, 1990

80. Boysen G et al: Familial amyloidosis with cranial neuropathy and corneal lattice dystrophy. *J Neurol Neurosurg Psych* **42**:1020, 1979

81. Northcutt AD, Vanover MJ: Nodular cutaneous amyloidosis involving the vulva. Case report and literature review. *Arch Dermatol* **121**:518, 1985

82. Clement MI et al: Nodular localized primary cutaneous amyloidosis. *Clin Exp Dermatol* **12**:460, 1987

83. Ann C-C et al: Nodular amyloidosis. *Clin Exp Dermatol* **13**:20, 1988

84. Wong C-K: Lichen amyloidosus: A relatively common skin disorder in Taiwan. *Arch Dermatol* **110**:438, 1974

85. Piamphongsant T, Kullavanijaya P: Diffuse biphasic amyloidosis. *Dermatologica* **153**:243, 1979

86. Wolf M, Tolmach JA: Macular amyloidosus. *Arch Dermatol* **99**:373, 1969

87. Kurban AK et al: Primary localized macular cutaneous amyloidosis: Histochemistry and electron microscopy. *Br J Dermatol* **85**:52, 1971

88. Hashimoto K et al: Nylon brush macular amyloidosis. *Arch Dermatol* **123**:633, 1987

89. Wong C-K et al: Friction amyloidosis. *Int J Dermatol* **27**:302, 1988

90. De Pietro WP: Primary familial cutaneous amyloidosis: A study of HLA antigens in a Puerto Rican family. *Arch Dermatol* **117**:639, 1981

91. Sagher F, Shanon J: Amyloidosis cutis: Familial occurrence in three generations. *Arch Dermatol* **87**:171, 1963

92. Rajagopalan K, Tay CH: Familial lichen amyloidosis. Report of 19 cases in 4 generations of a Chinese family in Malaysia. *Br J Dermatol* **87**:123, 1972

93. Newton JA et al: Familial primary cutaneous amyloidosis. *Br J Dermatol* **112**:201, 1985

94. Tidman MJ et al: Pachonychia congenita with cutaneous amyloidosis and hyperpigmentation—a distinct variant. *J Am Acad Dermatol* **16**:935, 1987

95. Gagel RF et al: Multiple endocrine neoplasia type 2a associated with cutaneous lichen amyloidosis. *Ann Intern Med* **111**:802, 1989

96. Black MM, Maibach HI: Macular amyloidosis simulating naevoid hyperpigmentation. *Br J Dermatol* **90**:461, 1974

97. Van den Bergh WHHW, Starink TM: Macular amyloidosis, presenting as periocular hyperpigmentation. *Clin Exp Dermatol* **8**:195, 1983

98. Ogino A, Tanaka S: Poikiloderma-like cutaneous amyloidosis. Report a case and review of the literature. *Dermatologica* **155**:301, 1977

99. Hicks BC et al: Primary cutaneous amyloidosis of the auricular concha. *J Am Acad Dermatol* **18**:19, 1988

100. Bakos L et al: Primary amyloidosis of the concha. *J Am Acad Dermatol* **20**:525, 1989

101. Ive FA, Wilkinson DS: Diseases of the umbilical, perianal and genital regions: Anosacral cutaneous amyloidosis, in *Textbook of Dermatology,* 4th ed, edited by A Rook et al. Oxford, Blackwell, 1986, p 2173

102. Crow KD: Primary amyloidosis. *Br J Dermatol* **97**(suppl 15):58, 1977

103. Lever WF, Schaumburg-Lever G: Metabolic diseases: Amyloidosis, in *Histopathology of the Skin,* 7th ed. Philadelphia, Lippincott, 1990, p 452

104. Westermark P: Amyloidosis of the skin: A comparison between localized and systemic amyloidosis. *Acta Derm Venereol (Stockh)* **59**:341, 1979

105. Westermark P: Occurrence of amyloid deposits in the skin in secondary systemic amyloidosis. *Acta Pathol Microbiol Immunol Scand Sect A* **80**:718, 1972

106. Shirahama T et al: Ultrastructure of skin biopsies from patients with heredo-familial amyloid polyneuropathy, in *Amyloid and Amyloidosis,* edited by GG Glenner et al. Amsterdam, Excerpta Medica, 1980, p 132

107. Masuda C et al: Histopathological and immunohistochemical study of amyloidosis cutis nodularis atrophicans—comparison with systemic amyloidosis. *Br J Dermatol* **199**:33, 1988

108. Elghetany MT et al: Methods for staining amyloid in tissues: A review. *Stain Technol* **63**:201, 1988

109. Wright JR et al: Potassium permanganate reaction in amyloidosis: A histologic method to assist in differentiating forms of this disease. *Lab Invest* **36**:274, 1977

110. Fujihara S et al: Identification and classification of amyloid in formalin-fixed, paraffin-embedded tissue sections by the unlabelled immunoperoxidase method. *Lab Invest* **43**:358, 1980

111. Duston MA et al: Sensitivity, specificity, and predictive value of abdominal fat aspiration for the diagnosis of amyloidosis. *Arthr Rheum* **32**:82, 1989

112. Blum A, Sohar E: The diagnosis of amyloidosis. Ancillary procedures. *Lancet* **1**:721, 1962

113. Yamada M et al: Gastrointestinal amyloid deposition in AL (primary or myeloma-associated) and AA (secondary) amyloidosis: Diagnostic value of gastric biopsy. *Hum Pathol* **16**:1206, 1985

114. Pasternak A: Fine needle aspiration biopsy of the spleen in the diagnosis of systemic amyloidosis, in *Amyloidosis,* edited by O Wegelius et al. London, Academic, 1976, p 393

115. von Kemp K et al: Echocardiography and magnetic resonance imaging in cardiac amyloidosis. *Acta Cardiol* **44**:29, 1989

116. Lakhanpal S et al: Synovial fluid analysis for diagnosis of amyloid arthropathy. *Arthr Rheum* **30**:419, 1987

117. Hawkins PN et al: Diagnostic radionuclide imaging of amyloid: Biological targeting by circulating human serum amyloid P component. *Lancet* **1**:1413, 1988

118. Zemer D et al: Colchicine in the prevention and treatment of the amyloidosis of familial Mediterranean fever. *N Engl J Med* **314**:1001, 1986

119. Scheinberg MA et al: DMSO and colchicine therapy in amyloid disease. *Ann Rheum Dis* **43**:421, 1984

120. Berglund K et al: Alkylating cytostatic treatment in renal amyloidosis secondary to rheumatic disease. *Ann Rheum Dis* **46**:757, 1987

121. Kyle RA, Greipp PR: Primary systemic amyloidosis: Comparison of melphalan and prednisone versus placebo. *Blood* **52**:818, 1978

122. Benson MD: Treatment of AL amyloidosis with melphalan, prednisone and colchicine. *Arthr Rheum* **29**:683, 1986

123. Fielder K, Durie BGM: Primary amyloidosis associated with multiple myeloma. Predictors of successful therapy. *Am J Med* **80**:413, 1986

124. Gertz MA, Kyle RA: Acute leukemia and cytogenetic abnormalities complicating melphalan treatment of primary systemic amyloidosis. *Arch Intern Med* **150**:629, 1990

125. Cohen AS et al: Survival of patients with primary (AL) amyloidosis: Colchicine-treated cases from 1976 to 1983 compared with cases seen in previous years (1961 to 1973). *Am J Med* **82**:1182, 1987

126. Kyle RA et al: Primary systemic amyloidosis. Comparison of melphalan/prednisone versus colchicine. *Am J Med* **79**:708, 1985

127. Gertz MA, Kyle RA: Phase II trial of α-tocopherol (vitamin E) in the treatment of primary systemic amyloidosis. *Am J Hematol* **34**:55, 1990

128. Wang W-J et al: Response of systemic amyloidosis to dimethyl sulfoxide. *J Am Acad Dermatol* **15**:402, 1986

129. Gertz MA et al: Worsening of congestive heart failure in amyloid heart disease treated by calcium channel-blocking agents. *Am J Cardiol* **55**:1645, 1985

130. Conner R et al: Heart transplantation for cardiac amyloidosis: Successful one-year outcome despite recurrence of the disease. *J Heart Transplant* **7**:165, 1988

131. Browning MJ et al: Continuous ambulatory peritoneal dialysis in systemic amyloidosis and end-stage renal disease. *J R Soc Med* **77**:189, 1984

132. Pasternack A et al: Renal transplantation in 45 patients with amyloidosis. *Transplantation* **42**:598, 1986

133. Truhan AP et al: Nodular primary localized cutaneous amyloidosis: Immunohistochemical evaluation and treatment with the carbon dioxide laser. *J Am Acad Dermatol* **14**:1058, 1986

134. Wong CK, Li WM: Dermabrasion for lichen amyloidosus. Report of a long-term study. *Arch Dermatol* **118**:302, 1982

135. Monfrecola G et al: Lichen amyloidosus: A new therapeutic approach. *Acta Derm Venereol (Stockh)* **65**:453, 1985

136. Pravata G et al: Unusual localization of lichen amyloidosus. Topical treatment with dimethylsulfoxide. *Acta Derm Venereol (Stockh)* **69**:259, 1989

137. Bonnetblanc JM et al: Dimethyl sulphoxide and macular amyloidosus. *Acta Derm Venereol (Stockh)* **60**:91, 1980

138. Lim KB et al: Lack of effect of dimethyl sulphoxide (DMSO) on amyloid deposits in lichen amyloidosis. *Br J Dermatol* **119**:409, 1989

139. Helander I, Hopsu-Havu VK: Treatment of lichen amyloidosus by etretinate. *Clin Exp Dermatol* **11**:574, 1986

140. Marschalkó M et al: Etretinate for the treatment of lichen amyloidosis. *Arch Dermatol* **124**:657, 1988

141. Aram H: Failure of etretinate (RO 10-9359) in lichen amyloidosus. *Int J Dermatol* **25**:206, 1986

142. Kyle RA et al: Primary systemic amyloidosis: Multivariate analysis for prognostic factors in 168 cases. *Blood* **68**:220, 1986

CHAPTER 150

David R. Bickers, Madhu A. Pathak, and

Henry W. Lim

The Porphyrias

The porphyrias are among the most intriguing diseases of humans. Widely variable, even bizarre in their clinical manifestations, these disorders of porphyrin or porphyrin-precursor metabolism result from aberrations in the control of the porphyrin-heme biosynthetic pathway. Heme, the end product of the pathway, is a tetrapyrrole in which protoporphyrin (PROTO) is chelated with ferrous iron. Because of its special ability to bind and release oxygen, heme functions in numerous metabolic pathways of living organisms. Heme is the prosthetic group for a number of important cellular proteins, including hemoglobin, myoglobin, catalases, peroxidases, and cytochromes P_{450}, P_{448}, a_3, etc.; without this iron-chelated tetrapyrrole, most essential biochemical pathways in the body could not function. Heme is essential for oxygen binding and transport (as hemoglobin and myoglobin), for electron transport (as cytochromes), and for mixed-function oxidases such as cytochrome P_{450}, etc. Chlorophyll, a magnesium-chelated porphyrin, is another important tetrapyrrole and is critical for photosynthesis, the specialized energy-storing system found in plants in which the conversion of light energy into stabilized chemical energy is achieved with a sequence of oxidation-reduction reactions. The corrin ring, a cobalt-chelated tetrapyrrole, is a major constituent of vitamin B_{12}, the lack of which results in pernicious anemia. Porphyrins, therefore, are ubiquitous and essential biochemical constituents of living beings. The biologic importance of the porphyrins and their iron complexes in metabolism lies in their capacity to act as mediators of oxidation reactions, either as oxidative components in the metabolism of steroids, drugs, and environmental chemicals or as a means of exchanging gases, such as oxygen and carbon dioxide, between the environment and the tissues of the body.

Daily synthesis of porphyrins and heme in humans occurs in amounts sufficient to provide for the body's metabolic requirements. The control of heme synthesis is so precise that, under normal circumstances, microgram quantities or less of pathway intermediates are present in plasma, red blood cells (RBC), urine, and stool (see Table 150-1).

Porphyria results from either inherited or acquired enzymatic abnormalities in heme synthesis. There are eight enzymes contributing to excessive accumulation of heme pathway intermediates in the body. Most of the human porphyrias appear to be characterized by deficient activity of specific enzymes, as shown in Table 150-2; each of these enzymes will be discussed separately. The different porphyrias arising from such derangements of normal heme synthesis manifest patterns of accumulation and excretion of specific porphyrins and/or their precursors.[1] In general, the major porphyrin or porphyrin precursor excreted in a given porphyria is the oxidized substrate for the specific deficient or defective enzyme. The different porphyrias arising from such derangements of normal heme synthesis are also characterized by accumulation and excretion of specific intermediate porphyrins and/or their precursors (Table 150-3). These intermediates, when present in excess amounts,

TABLE 150-1
Normal Values of Porphyrins and Porphyrin Precursors in Humans

Porphyrins or precursors	Urine (μg/24 h)	RBC (μg/100 mL packed cells)	Plasma (μg/100 mL)	Feces (μg/g dry wt)
δ-Aminolevulinic acid (ALA)	<4000	—	15–23	—
Porphobilinogen (PBG)	<1500	—	—	—
Uroporphyrin (URO)	<40	0–2.0	0–2	10–50
Coproporphyrin (COPRO)	<280	0–2.0	0–1	10–50
Protoporphyrin(PROTO)	Absent	<90	0–2	0–20
X-porphyrin	Absent	Absent	Absent	Trace
Isocoproporphyrin(ISOCOPRO)	Absent	Absent	Absent	—
	(nmol/day)	(nmol/dL)	(nmol/dL)	(nmol/g dry weight)
δ-Aminolevulinic acid (ALA)	8.8×10^3	—	$1.1–1.8 \times 10^2$	—
Porphobilinogen (PGB)	4.6×10^4	—	—	—
Uroporphyrin (URO)	<40	—	24	—
Coproporphyrin (COPRO)	<280	—	46	—
Protoporphyrin (PROTO)	0	285	0.5	134

exert toxic effects that are likely responsible for the expression of clinical porphyria.

The porphyrias are of particular dermatologic interest because several of them have distinct cutaneous manifestations that may permit diagnosis from clinical signs alone. Furthermore, simple laboratory procedures, easily performed in a physician's office, can confirm a clinically suspected diagnosis in many instances and can also help to initiate appropriate therapeutic measures for the amelioration of the biochemical derangements and the clinical symptoms of these diseases.

Historical Aspects

One of the first known reported cases of cutaneous porphyria was that of Schultz,[2] who described a 33-year-old man with marked cutaneous photosensitivity and splenomegaly that he called pemphigus leprosus, a bullous disease. The excreted urine was red. Spectroscopic studies by Schultz and subsequently by Baumstark[3] identified abnormal urinary pigments, which were named urorubrohematin and urofuscohematin. This abnormal pigment was most likely uroporphyrin (URO), and this patient probably had porphyria, but of what type is disputed.[4] Anderson[5] reported two brothers with a scarring photosensitivity that he called hydroa aestivale. Beginning in childhood, this disease was said to be associated with "hematoporphyrin" in the urine. Anderson implied that the abnormal urinary pigment was related to the skin disease.

Detailed studies by Günther in 1911 led to the first classification of the porphyrias.[6] Günther felt that the dark pigment in the urine of patients with porphyria was the synthetic porphyrin, hematoporphyrin, but subsequent studies by Fischer proved that this pigment was a natural porphyrin, which he named URO as it was isolated from the urine of a patient with congenital porphyria.[7] The detailed study of Mathias Petry, the celebrated but unfortunate patient with congenital erythropoietic porphyria (EP), added greatly to modern knowledge of porphyria and of the cutaneous photosensitivity associated with it.[8] This is an excellent example of the interaction of basic science and clinical medicine leading to important new knowledge about the metabolic basis of a human disease.

Other types of porphyrias known as acute intermittent porphyria (AIP) and porphyria cutanea tarda (PCT) were first defined in Sweden by Waldenström in 1937.[9] The former, with abdominal and neurologic symptoms, was found to be very common in the northernmost provinces of Sweden, around Lapland, and to be comparatively rare in South Africa. Subsequently, Brunsting,[10] Waldenström,[11] and Schmid[12] further characterized PCT in various human populations and showed that environmental factors such as drugs and chemicals (xenobiotics) could influence the clinical expression of this disease. Barnes,[13] Dean,[14] and Dean and Barnes[15] described a type of porphyria occurring predominantly in South Africans and characterized by cutaneous manifestations identical to those of PCT and acute attacks identical to those of AIP. Defined as variegate porphyria (VP), this disease is now known to occur throughout the world.[16,17]

Another porphyria of bone marrow origin, erythropoietic protoporphyria (EPP), was described in 1961 by Magnus et al. in England,[18] and an extremely rare disorder, erythropoietic coproporphyria, was identified in Germany by Heilmeyer and Clotten in 1964.[19] In 1955, Berger and Goldberg in Scotland first described hereditary coproporphyria (HCP).[20] In 1969, hepatoerythropoietic porphyria (HEP) was described by Pinõl-Aguadé,[21] as was a type of porphyria associated with sideroblastic anemia.[22] Doss et al.[23] described hereditary aminolevulinic acid (ALA) dehydratase deficiency porphyria in 1979. In 1990, Poh-Fitzpatrick et al.[24] described a porphyria associated with Alagille syndrome, a familial form of cholestatic liver disease.

Porphyrin-Heme Biosynthesis

Most mammalian cells, including those in the epidermis and dermis, can synthesize the heme required for formation of essential heme-proteins; however, the major sites of heme synthesis in the body are the bone marrow and the liver.

Heme is the prosthetic group for a number of hemoproteins, including hemoglobin, myoglobin, mitochondrial cytochromes, microsomal cytochromes (including cytochrome P_{450}), catalase, peroxidase, tryptophan pyrrolase, prostaglandin endoperoxide syn-

TABLE 150-2
Enzyme Activities in Various Porphyrias

Enzyme	Tissue	Disease displaying enzymatic defect
δ-Aminolevulinic acid (ALA) synthase	Liver, kidney, fibroblasts, and lymphocytes	Increased activity in AIP, HCP, VP
δ-Aminolevulinic acid (ALA) dehydratase	Erythrocytes, liver, and kidney	Decreased in lead intoxication; decreased in a rare type of acute hepatic porphyria
Porphobilinogen (PBG) deaminase	Erythrocytes, liver, fibroblast, lymphocytes, and amnion cells	Decreased in AIP
Uroporphyrinogen III (UROGEN III) cosynthase	Erythrocytes and fibroblasts	Decreased in congenital EP
Uroporphyrinogen (UROGEN) decarboxylase	Erythrocytes and liver	Decreased in PCT (sporadic and familial) and HEP
Coproporphyrinogen (COPROGEN) oxidase	Fibroblasts, lymphocytes and liver	Decreased in HCP
Protoporphyrinogen (PROTOGEN) oxidase	Liver and fibroblasts	Decreased in VP
Ferrochelatase	Bone marrow, fibroblasts	Decreased in EPP, lead poisoning and ? in VP

NOTE: AIP, acute intermittent porphyria; EP, erythropoietic porphyria; EPP, erythropoietic protoporphyria; HCP, hereditary coproporphyria; HEP, hepatoerythropoietic porphyria; PCT, porphyria cutanea tarda; VP, variegate porphyria.

TABLE 150-3
Biochemical Features of the Porphyrias

Type of porphyria	Blood				Stool			Urine				
	RBC URO	RBC COPRO	RBC PROTO	Plasma	URO	COPRO	PROTO	Color	ALA	PBG	URO	COPRO
Erythropoietic												
Erythropoietic porphyria (EP)	++++	+++	+++	↑URO & COPRO	+	+++	+	Pink to red	N	N	++++*	++*
Erythropoietic protoporphyria (EPP)	N	N to +	++++	↑PROTO	N	++	++ to ++++	N	N	N	N	N
Hepatic												
Acute intermittent porphyria (AIP)												
Latent	N	N	N	N	N to +	N to +	N to +	Red to purple	+ to +++	+ to +++	N	N to +
Acute	N	N	N	N	N to +	N to +	N to +	Red to purple	++ to ++++	++ to ++++	+++	++
Porphyria variegata (VP)												
Latent	N	N	N	?N	N	+++	++++	N	N	N	N	N
Acute	N	N	N	?N	++	++	+++	Pink to red	++ to +++	++ to +++	+++	+++
Porphyria cutanea tarda (PCT)	N	N	N	↑URO	++	+++	+ ISOCOPRO	Pink to red	N	N	++++	++
Hereditary coproporphyria (HCP)												
Latent	N	N	N	?N	++	++++	N to +	N	N to +	N to +	N	N
Acute	N	N	N	?N	+	+++	N to +	Red	++ to N	++ to N	++	++++
Hepatoerythropoietic porphyria (HEP)	N	+/−	++++	↑URO	N	ISOCOPRO	N	Pink to red			+++	ISOCOPRO
ALA dehydratase deficiency porphyria	N	N	++	↑ALA ↑COPRO ↑PROTO	N	+	+	?	+++	N	+	++

NOTE: N, normal; +, above normal; ++, moderately increased; +++ and ++++, greatly increased; URO, uroporphyrin; COPRO, coproporphyrin; PROTO, protoporphyrin; ISOCOPRO, isocoproporphyrin. Findings of major diagnostic importance are boxed.
*Type I isomers.

thase, and the soluble form of guanylate cyclase. The two body organs that produce the vast majority of heme in humans are the liver and the bone marrow. Approximately 85 percent of heme synthesis occurs in bone marrow where it is utilized for the production of hemoglobin. Most remaining heme synthesis occurs in the liver for making cytochrome P_{450}, catalase, and various mitochondrial cytochromes. Heme is a critical cellular constituent essential for a variety of metabolic processes, primarily because of its unique ability to take up and release oxygen and to facilitate electron transport. Heme synthesis is regulated by the interplay of a number of factors and is directly dependent upon its concentration within cells and upon the requirements of the cell for production of the various hemoproteins described above. Many of these have rapid turnover times (minutes to hours), thereby necessitating continuously high rates of hepatic heme synthesis (e.g., cytochrome P_{450}, an important membrane-bound enzyme in the liver involved in the detoxification and metabolism of drugs, has a half-life of 90 to 180 min). This regulation (and indeed the ability to synthesize heme at all) is dependent upon a series of eight intracellular enzymes, whose sequential catalytic activity contributes to heme synthesis. The first (ALA synthase) and the last three enzymes involved in heme synthesis (COPROGEN oxidase, PROTOGEN oxidase, and ferrochelatase) are localized in mitochondria, and the remaining intermediate enzymes (ALA dehydratase, PBG deaminase, UROGEN III cosynthase, and UROGEN decarboxylase) are localized in the cytosol. Heme breakdown is catalyzed by the microsomal enzymes

NADPH–cytochrome C reductase, heme oxygenase, and biliverdin reductase, which convert the cyclic tetrapyrrole to bile pigments. cDNAs for six of the eight enzymes in the heme synthesis pathway and two of the three enzymes in the heme catabolic pathway have been cloned and defined in mammalian cells.[1] Abnormal control of heme synthesis may result from partial defects in enzymes of the pathway, and this may occur as the result of inherited and/or environmental factors. One result of such abnormal control is the accumulation in the body of one or more heme pathway intermediates, such as the porphyrins or their precursors, which are associated with the clinical disorders that are collectively referred to as the porphyrias. Studies by Schmid and coworkers first clearly proved that the porphyrias reflect derangements in heme synthesis in the liver or the bone marrow.[25] Although a diagnosis of porphyria can often be made from a careful history and physical examination, the definitive diagnosis rests upon measurements of porphyrin and/or porphyrin excretion or the activity of one or another of the enzymes in the heme pathway (Table 150-3). Each porphyria demonstrates a unique pattern of porphyrin or porphyrin-precursor accumulation in blood or excretion in urine and/or feces. To fully comprehend the meaning as well as the importance of these measurements, it is necessary to have a clear understanding of current concepts regarding the regulation of heme synthesis. The steps involved in the biosynthesis of porphyrins and heme synthesis and its regulation are outlined in Figs. 150-1 to 150-4 and have recently been summarized with extensive references to the details of the individual steps.[26]

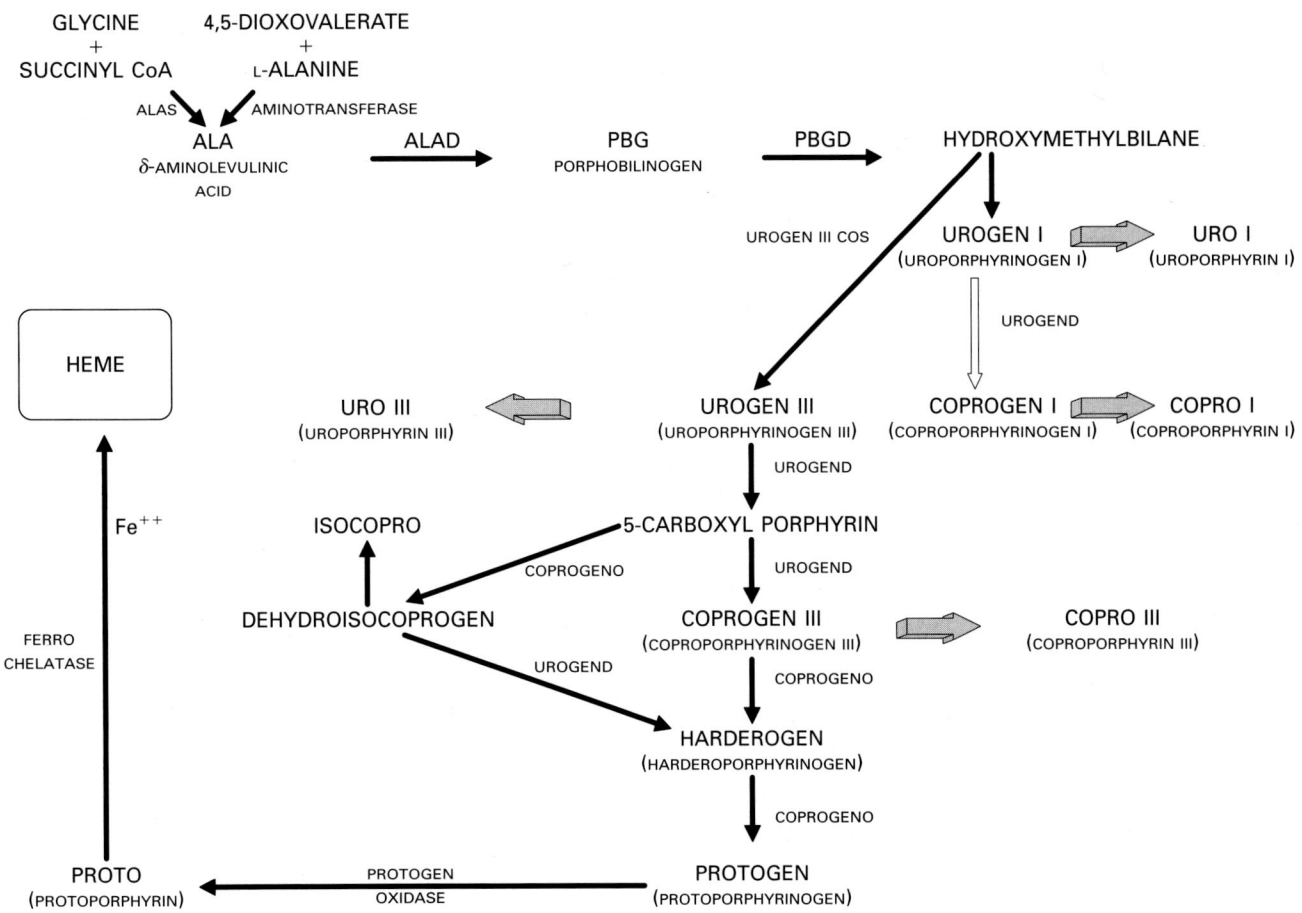

FIGURE 150-1 The porphyrin-heme biosynthetic pathway (see also legend for Fig. 150-2).

Delta-Aminolevulinic Acid (ALA) Synthase
(Fig. 150-2)

Heme synthesis begins in the mitochondrion of the cell where succinate and glycine (single molecules of glycine and succinyl CoA) are conjugated to form a five-carbon aminoketone delta-aminolevulinic acid (ALA). The reaction requires pyridoxal 5′-phosphate as a cofactor. ALA synthase is the mitochondrial enzyme that catalyzes the formation of ALA and is a homodimer of two identical catalytically active subunits of molecular mass 55 kDa, linked to catalytically inactive substrates of higher molecular mass.[27]

The major significance of this enzyme is its regulatory role in controlling the rate of heme synthesis in the liver. The putative pool of hepatocellular free heme is thought to regulate heme synthesis by directly influencing the activity of mitochondrial ALA synthase in two ways: (1) by inhibiting ALA synthase activity or (2) by controlling its rate of synthesis. ALA synthase activity is increased in the liver of patients with those hepatic porphyrias in which acute attacks characterized by a neurologic–visceral symptom complex occur. This increase in ALA synthase is a major marker for AIP, VP, and HCP. It is also an inducible enzyme in the liver, and factors that lead to further increases in activity of ALA synthase are accompanied by exacerbation of the clinical manifestations of these types of porphyria. Conversely, factors that reduce ALA synthase

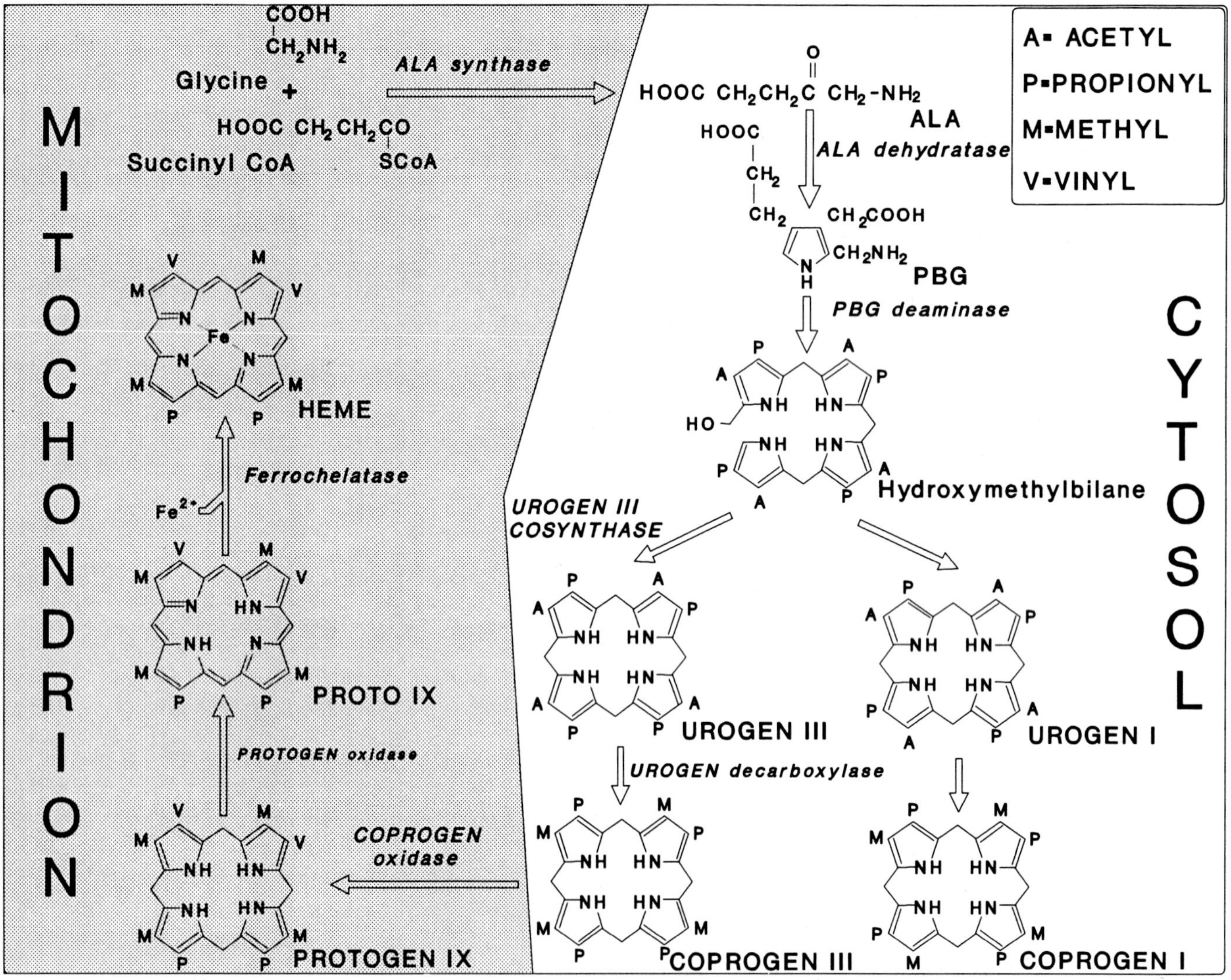

FIGURE 150-2 Major steps in the porphyrin-heme biosynthetic pathway: (*1*) Delta-aminolevulinic acid (ALA) synthase can be formed from glycine and succinyl CoA, which is the primary source in mammalian systems and is catalyzed by the mitochondrial enzyme δ-aminolevulinic acid synthase (ALAS). Two molecules of aminolevulinic acid form the monopyrrole porphobilinogen (PBG). (*2*) Four molecules of PBG are converted by PBG deaminase to a linear tetrapyrrole, hydroxymethylbilane, which can cyclize spontaneously to form uroporphyrinogen (UROGEN) I. (*3*) The four acetyl groups of UROGEN I are sequentially decarboxylated by UROGEN decarboxylase to form coproporphyrinogen (COPROGEN) I.

(*4*) Hydroxymethylbilane can also be converted to UROGEN III by the enzyme UROGEN III cosynthase. In this reaction one of the monopyrrole rings is "flipped over," thereby altering the sequence of the side chains. (*5*) The acetyl groups of UROGEN III are sequentially decarboxylated by UROGEN decarboxylase to form coproporphyrinogen III. (*6*) Coproporphyrinogen III is converted to protoporphyrinogen (PROTOGEN) IX by the enzyme COPROGEN oxidase, which oxidatively decarboxylates each of the propionyl groups. (*7*) PROTOGEN IX is converted to protoporphyrin (PROTO) IX by PROTOGEN oxidase. PROTO IX is converted to heme by ferrochelatase, which catalyzes the insertion of ferrous iron into the molecule.

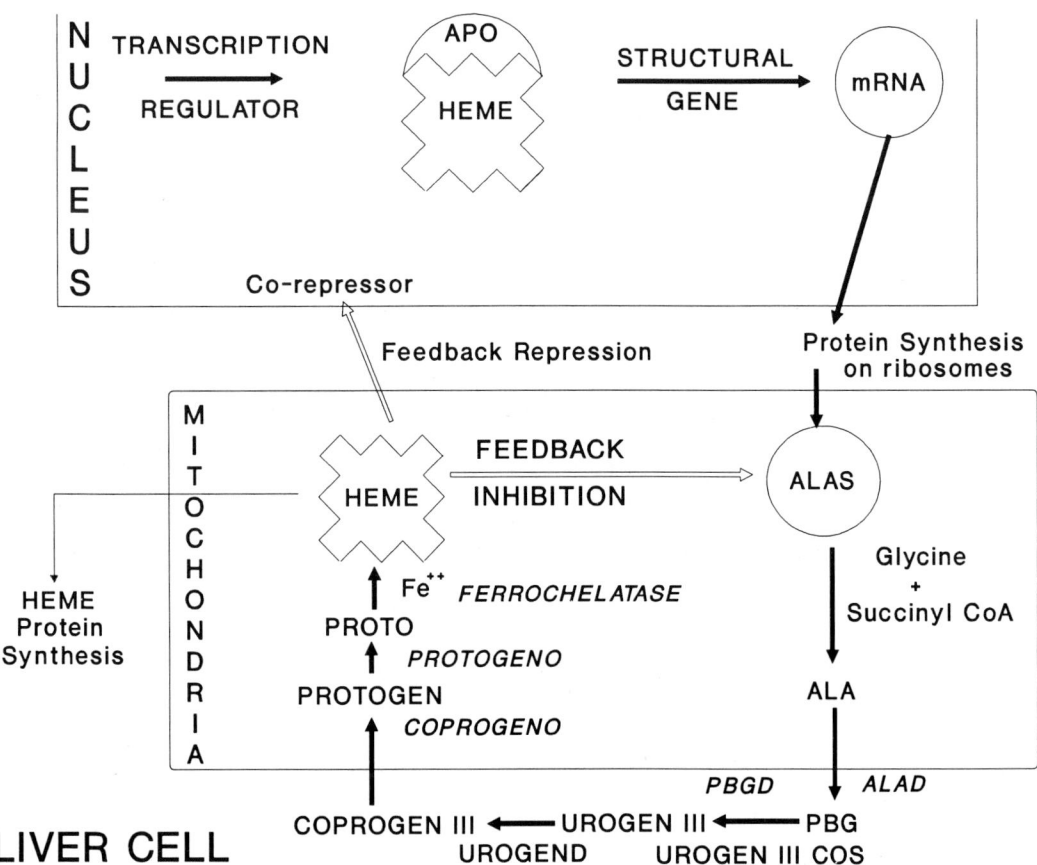

FIGURE 150-3 Heme is capable of regulating its synthesis by either directly inhibiting or repressing the synthesis of its rate-limiting enzyme, ALA synthase. The repression may result from the binding of heme, as a co-repressor, to an apo-repressor protein (APO) which, when combined with heme, becomes a functional unit which blocks transcription of ALA synthase mRNA.

activity are often useful therapeutically in those porphyrias characterized by elevated activity of the enzyme. The importance of ALA synthase for the regulation of heme synthesis will be discussed later in the chapter. ALA synthase in the erythroid compartment behaves in a rather different manner in that it is not inducible by xenobiotics that augment the synthesis of the hepatic enzyme. Immunochemical differences exist between the hepatic and erythroid enzyme in various animal species.[28]

Using chicken ALA synthase cDNA clones isolated from both liver and erythroid cells, Riddle et al.[27] have shown that at least two separate genes encode ALA synthase mRNAs found in these tissues and that the erythroid gene product is expressed exclusively in erythroid cells, whereas the hepatic form is expressed ubiquitously.

It should be pointed out that there is some evidence to suggest that a second mitochondrial enzyme in mammalian liver, known as L-alanine-4,5-dioxovalerate (DOVA) aminotransferase, can catalyze a transamination between L-alanine and DOVA, yielding ALA (Fig. 150-2) and pyruvate.[29] The importance of this reaction for production of tetrapyrroles in certain plants is well known but its role in human heme synthesis remains to be defined.

Delta-Aminolevulinic Acid (ALA) Dehydratase

In the next reaction, two molecules of ALA are combined in the presence of an enzyme known as ALA dehydratase to form the monopyrrole porphobilinogen (PBG) (Fig. 150-2). ALA dehydratase is present in the cytoplasm of the cell. Its activity is 50 to 100-fold higher than ALA synthase so that virtually all of the ALA synthesized is converted to PBG.[26] No tissue-specific enzymes have been identified for ALA dehydratase, but polymorphic charge isozymes are known to occur in human populations.[30]

Liver cDNA–expression libraries have been employed to isolate cDNA clones that encode for the rat and human enzyme.[1,31,32] ALA dehydratase from human liver was shown to be encoded by an open reading frame of 990 bp that possessed a high degree of homology with the enzyme in rats.[31,32] The ALA dehydratase from rat liver and the mouse erythroid compartment are also highly homologous.[33] Genetic variation in the level of ALA dehydratase may be due to differences in copy number of the gene.

Porphobilinogen (PBG) Deaminase

This, the third enzyme in the pathway, combines four molecules of the monopyrrole PBG to form the linear tetrapyrrole, hydroxymethylbilane (Fig. 150-2), which cyclizes spontaneously to form the initial porphyrinogen, or tetrapyrrole, known as uroporphyrinogen I (UROGEN I) (Fig. 150-2). Depending on the manner in which the PBG molecules are arranged, several different isomers of the tetrapyrroles are possible. The sole difference between type I and type III porphyrinogens is that one of the four pyrrole rings is "flipped over." Only two of them (labeled I and III) are known to occur in the mammalian heme synthetic pathway. PBG deaminase has been purified from human RBC and shown to have a molecular mass of approximately 36 to 40 kDa and a pH optimum of 8.2.[34]

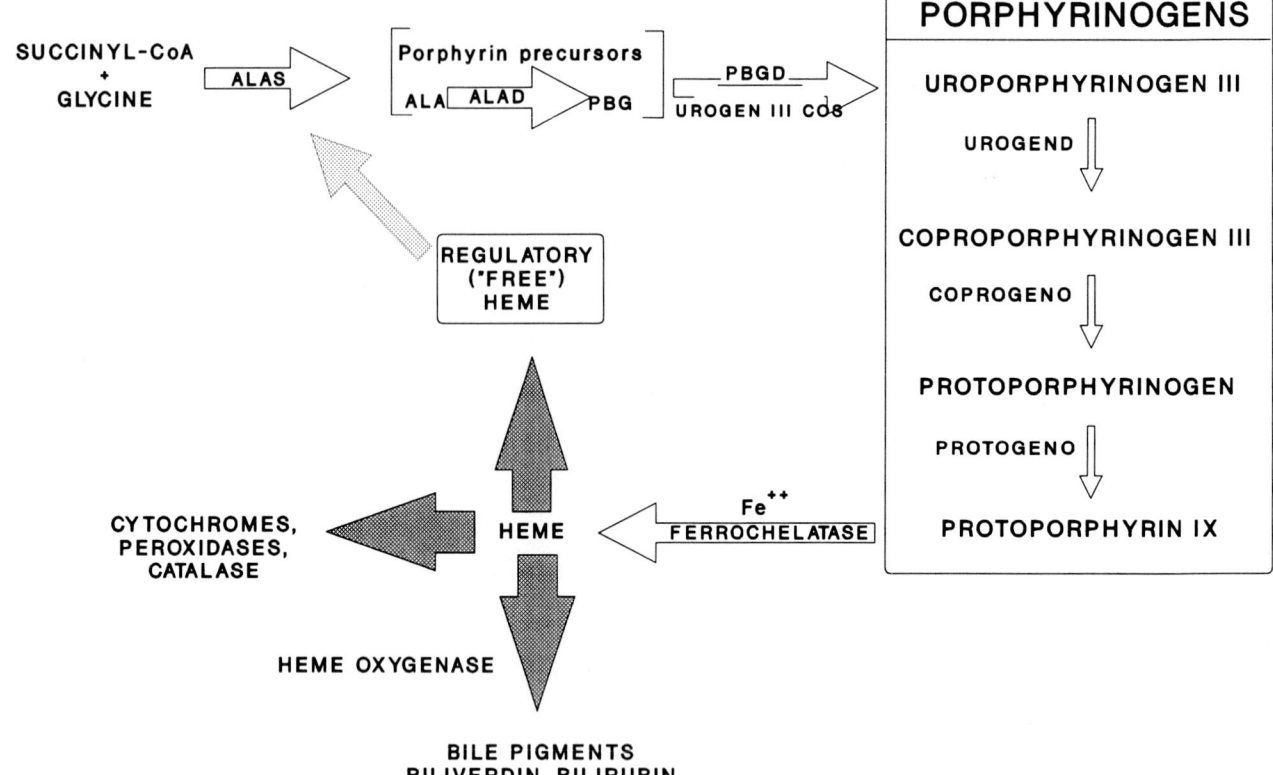

FIGURE 150-4 A regulatory pool of "free" heme unbound to apo-proteins may be the critical determinant for regulation of synthesis of ALA synthase activity.

The PBG deaminase gene has been cloned and characterized.[35] It is split into 15 exons spread over 10 kb of DNA. The two isoforms of the enzyme are encoded by two distinct mRNAs that arise from two overlapping transcription units, the first of which (upstream) is active in all tissues and its promoter has some features of a housekeeping promoter, whereas the second, located 3 kb downstream, is active only in erythroid cells and displays structural homology with beta globin gene promoters.

PBG deaminase is present in the lowest concentration of any enzyme in the heme pathway except for ALA synthase. This suggests that factors (genetic or acquired) that influence PBG deaminase activity may have important regulatory influences on the rate of heme synthesis. Consequently, if excessive PBG is formed because of increased ALA synthase activity, as is often seen in the acute hepatic porphyrias, there may be only partial conversion of this monopyrrole to UROGEN I. These factors account for the elevated urinary PBG characteristic of attacks of the acute hepatic porphyrias. PBG deaminase activity is known to be reduced by about 50 percent in the tissue of patients with AIP and is currently thought to be the primary enzymatic abnormality in this autosomal dominant disorder.[36]

ALA and PBG, the two aliphatic nonporphyrin precursors of heme, are excreted primarily in the urine; normally this amounts to less than 4000 and 1500 μg of each, respectively, per 24 h (Table 150-1). However, in some types of porphyria (AIP and VP), there may be a 10- to 100-fold increase in urinary excretion of ALA and PBG, which can be detected using relatively simple diagnostic tests. For example, PBG reacts with Ehrlich's reagent, which contains p-dimethylaminobenzaldehyde in hydrochloric acid, to give a positive red-color reaction (Watson-Schwartz test) during attacks of AIP and VP.[37] The cherry-red chromogen is not extracted into chlo-

roform or butanol and remains in the aqueous phase when PBG is elevated. The Hoesch test is a simpler modification of the Watson-Schwartz test that has found increasing application.[38]

Uroporphyrinogen (UROGEN) III Cosynthase

The fourth enzyme in the heme pathway is UROGEN III cosynthase, which catalyzes the formation of uroporphyrinogen III from hydroxymethylbilane or from PBG if PBG deaminase is also present. By simple inversion of one PBG molecule during synthesis of UROGEN I, the III isomer is formed (Fig. 150-2). This apparently minor structural alteration is of considerable biologic importance as only the III isomer can proceed to the formation of heme. Heme is a type III porphyrin, and no type I heme has been identified in nature, thus making production of the I isomer an essentially "dead end" pathway. The formation of UROGEN III is catalyzed by the cytoplasmic enzyme UROGEN III cosynthase, which is closely linked to PBG deaminase. This enzyme has been purified from human erythrocytes and has a molecular mass of approximately 30 kDa; it is thermolabile, exhibits maximum catalytic activity at pH 7.4,[39] and is inhibited by heavy metals such as zinc, cadmium, and copper.[40]

The human gene for UROGEN III cosynthase has also been cloned and sequenced and encodes a protein of 265 amino acids with a predicted mass of about 28.6 kDa.[41] In most tissues, UROGEN III cosynthase is present in considerable excess as compared to PBG deaminase, thus assuring maximum conversion of the I to the III isomer. The only difference between the I and III isomers of each of the porphyrinogens is the reversal of the side chains on the "D" ring of the tetrapyrrole molecule.

Uroporphyrinogen (UROGEN) Decarboxylase

UROGEN I and III each contain eight carboxyl groups as side chains, four of which are acetate ($-CH_2COOH$) and four of which are propionate ($-CH_2-CH_2-COOH$) moieties (Fig. 150-2). The soluble cytosolic enzyme UROGEN decarboxylase catalyzes the sequential decarboxylation of the four carboxyl groups of the acetic acid side chains to methyl groups to form coproporphyrinogen (acetate groups to methyl groups) (Fig. 150-2). Decarboxylation first occurs on ring D, then the enzyme turns around to decarboxylate rings A, B, and C in a clockwise fashion. This converts the original 8-carboxyl porphyrinogen (UROGEN I or III) first to 7-carboxyl, then to 6-carboxyl, and 5-carboxyl porphyrinogen. The 5-carboxyl porphyrinogen can then undergo decarboxylation of its last acetyl group to form the 4-carboxyl porphyrinogen that is known as coproporphyrinogen (COPROGEN I or III) (Fig. 150-2). These intermediates are also referred to as hepta-, hexa-, penta-, and tetracarboxylate porphyrinogens. As discussed above, COPROGEN I cannot be further metabolized to heme. The purified human enzyme from erythrocytes has a molecular mass of about 41 kDa and its activity is inhibited by metals such as copper, mercury, and lead. The human cDNA for UROGEN decarboxylase has been isolated, and the deduced sequence was found to be equivalent to 367 amino acids, consistent with the molecular mass and the amino acid composition of the purified protein.[1,42] The gene is approximately 3 kb in length and includes 10 exons.

UROGEN decarboxylase activity is reduced in the liver of patients with PCT and HEP.[43] Approximately 20 percent of patients with PCT have a 50 percent decrease in UROGEN decarboxylase concentration in all tissues; this form of PCT is inherited as an autosomal dominant trait with low penetrance (type II PCT).[44] In type I PCT, also known as the sporadic form, the enzyme deficiency is limited to the liver. A form of type II PCT in which the activity and concentration of erythrocyte enzyme is normal suggests that an autosomal gene, not necessarily at the UROGEN decarboxylase locus, could influence the expression of type II PCT.[45] Normal amounts of mRNA for the enzyme are present in type II PCT, and a splice site mutation has been found in one pedigree with type II (familial) PCT that causes a deletion of exon 6 from the mRNA.[46] The resulting protein is shorter than the normal protein, missing the amino acids encoded by exon 6, and this aberrant protein lacks catalytic activity and is rapidly degraded.

In HEP, UROGEN decarboxylase activity is usually 5 to 10 percent of normal, and the disease occurs as a result of inherited mutant alleles from each parent.[47] One mutation that has been identified in some, but not all, families with HEP is a 281 (Gly → Glu) shift.[48]

Coproporphyrinogen (COPROGEN) Oxidase

This is a mitochondrial enzyme located at the outer surface of the inner membrane. COPROGEN III has four carboxyl groups, each of which is part of a propionate side chain. COPROGEN oxidase, a mitochondrial enzyme of molecular mass 72 kDa, catalyzes the sequential oxidative removal of the carboxyl group from two of the propionate groups, forming first 3-carboxyl porphyrinogen, or harderoporphyrinogen (HARDEROGEN), and then 2-carboxyl-porphyrinogen, or protoporphyrinogen (PROTOGEN)[49] (Fig. 150-2). The activity of this enzyme is reduced in patients with HCP.

A unique modification of normal heme synthesis also occurs in PCT. No additional enzymes or enzymatic reactions are involved, but there is a reversal in the sequence of action of the enzymes UROGEN decarboxylase and COPROGEN oxidase. As shown in Fig. 150-1, UROGEN decarboxylase normally acts on 5-carboxylporphyrinogen to decarboxylate the final remaining acetate group, forming a tetracarboxyl porphyrinogen known as COPROGEN III. This is subsequently converted to PROTOGEN by COPROGEN oxidase (Fig. 150-1 and 150-2). However, in PCT where UROGEN decarboxylase is deficient, COPROGEN oxidase may first oxidatively decarboxylate a propionate group on 5-carboxylporphyrinogen to form dehydroisocoproporphyrinogen (Fig. 150-1). The acetyl group on dehydroisocoproporphyrinogen can be decarboxylated by UROGEN decarboxylase to form HARDEROGEN, resulting in diversion back into the normal heme synthesis pathway (Fig. 150-1). Alternatively, dehydroisocoproporphyrinogen can undergo hydration to isocoproporphyrinogen (Fig. 150-1). These steps rarely, if ever, occur during the normal process of heme synthesis but become important in certain of the porphyrias such as PCT, where they provide one explanation for the increased isocoproporphyrin (ISOCOPRO) characteristically found in the feces of patients with this diease.

Protoporphyrinogen (PROTOGEN) Oxidase

The oxidation of PROTOGEN to PROTO is catalyzed by the enzyme PROTOGEN oxidase, an integral protein of the inner mitochondrial membrane (Fig. 150-2). This reaction can also occur nonenzymatically, but the enzyme appears to be necessary for heme synthesis to proceed at a normal rate.[50] There is experimental evidence to indicate that PROTOGEN oxidase activity is reduced in patients with VP.[51] PROTOGEN oxidase isolated from rat liver mitochondria has been shown to have a molecular mass of 35 kDa and requires molecular oxygen to catalyze the oxidation of PROTOGEN to PROTO.

Ferrochelatase

The final step in the formation of heme, the incorporation of ferrous iron (Fe^{2+}) into PROTO, is catalyzed by the enzyme ferrochelatase at the matrix face of the inner mitochondrial membrane (Fig. 150-2). This enzyme is also referred to as heme synthase or proto-heme-ferro-lyase. Unlike other enzymes in the heme biosynthesis pathway, which require reduced forms of the porphyrins (porphyrinogens) as substrates, ferrochelatase can utilize oxidized PROTO. This lysine-rich enzyme has a molecular mass of 63 kDa and a pH optimum of 7.8. Ferrochelatase activity has been shown to be reduced in various tissues of patients with EPP.[52]

Murine ferrochelatase has been cloned, and two mRNA transcripts have been identified in multiple tissues.[53] The enzyme appears to be identical in both erythroid and hepatic cells. The protein has 367 amino acid residues and a molecular mass of about 41.7 kDa. The cDNA for human ferrochelatase has also been cloned, sequenced, and shown to have 88 percent identity to the mouse enzyme.[54]

The end product of the pathway, ferrous-PROTO (FePROTO) or heme, diffuses out of the mitochondrion into the cytoplasm, where it is available to function as a prosthetic group by combining with appropriate apoproteins.

It is important to emphasize that porphyrinogens (reduced porphyrins) are the true intermediates in heme synthesis. The irreversibly oxidized porphyrins, with the exception of PROTO, do not function as substrates for the enzymes of the pathway. Free porphyrins are not known to contribute any useful biologic function. These porphyrins exhibit an absorption spectrum with a major peak in the 400-nm region, the so-called Soret band, and smaller absorption peaks between 500 and 640 nm. These oxidized porphyrins induce photodynamic effects in skin tissue and subcellular elements when exposed to ultraviolet and short visible light (360 to 420 nm) or red wavelengths (640 to 700 nm). Thus, porphyrins are actually heme pathway by-products, which are of special interest to dermatologists because of their unique photosensitizing properties.

Pathophysiology of Cutaneous Lesions in Porphyrias

One of the most common cutaneous manifestations of the porphyrias is photosensitivity; it is observed in patients with several of these disorders (EP, EPP, PCT, VP, HCP, and HEP) in whom plasma and tissue porphyrins are increased. Patients with AIP, in whom only nonphotosensitizing porphyrin precursors (ALA, PBG) are formed in substantially increased amounts, do not have photosensitivity. In addition, none of the four patients reported with ALA dehydratase–deficiency porphyria have exhibited photosensitivity.

Patients with the erythropoietic types of porphyria frequently complain of a burning sensation and pruritus following exposure to sunlight. A "primary" effect of sun exposure on cutaneous photosensitivity in EPP has been described in which threshold exposure on one day that evokes barely any symptoms, or none, will augment the reaction caused by additional sunlight on the following day.[55] The cause of this is unknown, but the phenomenon suggests that the repair of porphyrin photosensitization skin damage may be prolonged. These subjective symptoms are notably absent in patients with PCT. Although much has been learned about the pathophysiology of photosensitivity and sclerodermoid skin changes in the porphyrias, the causes of the pigmentary alterations and hypertrichosis seen in some of these patients remain to be elucidated.

Porphyrins have certain unique photobiologic and spectroscopic properties. The metal-chelated porphyrins (e.g., heme or FePROTO) show no fluorescence. Porphyrins that are chelated to other paramagnetic metals, such as Mn^{2+}, Co^{2+}, or Zn^{2+} (e.g., chlorophyll, ZnPROTO), also do not fluoresce. This is the reason that patients with lead intoxication, in which ZnPROTO is elevated, do not have photosensitivity.[56] However, metal-free porphyrins (e.g., URO, COPRO, PROTO) in acidic solutions show a major absorption peak in the 400- to 410-nm region (Soret band); they also exhibit four additional absorption bands with decreasing intensity between 500 and 700 nm. Exposure of porphyrins to the Soret band spectra results in two major fluorescence emission peaks at the 600- to 610-nm and 640- to 660-nm regions.[56]

The first experimental evidence for the photosensitizing property of porphyrins in human skin was provided by the heroic self-experiment of Meyer-Betz, reported in 1913.[57] After injecting himself intravenously with 200 mg of hematoporphyrin and exposing his skin to sunlight, he observed marked erythema and edema in light-exposed body areas, especially on his face and hands. With the increasing use of hematoporphyrin derivative (HPD) and other porphyrins for photodynamic therapy of human malignancy, porphyrin-induced photosensitivity is reported to be occurring with increasing frequency.[58]

Although there is no single clearly defined pathway that can currently explain the photosensitization evoked by porphyrins and light, there are a number of potential cellular and soluble factors that could be responsible. Among them, reactive oxygen species, certain cells (erythrocytes, mast cells, polymorphonuclear cells, and fibroblasts), and soluble mediators (the complement system, factor XII-dependent pathways, and the eicosanoids) will be discussed (Table 150-4). It is likely that interactions among these factors will prove to be responsible for the pathogenesis of the cutaneous lesions in the porphyrias.

Reactive Oxygen Species

Porphyrins such as URO, COPRO, and PROTO absorb light intensely in their Soret bands. Absorption of this radiant energy results in the generation of "excited" state molecules (Fig. 150-5). The initial excited state molecule generated is one which has an extremely short half-life of less than 0.01 μs. Singlet excited state porphyrins may spontaneously convert to a triplet state molecule, another excited state molecule that has a lower energy level but a longer half-life (in the order of microseconds to milliseconds). Because of their long half-life, porphyrin molecules in their triplet state are more likely to react with biologic molecules and are likely candidates to mediate most porphyrin-associated photobiologic reactions. Excited state porphyrin molecules subsequently return to their normal ground states by releasing their absorbed energy in the form of light (fluorescence is emitted by singlet state molecules and phosphorescence by triplet states), heat, or by transferring energy to cell constituents (cell membranes, organelles, proteins, DNA) (Fig. 150-6).

Excited porphyrins in their singlet and triplet states can also transfer their absorbed energy to oxygen molecules, thereby creating reactive "excited" oxygen states.[59] Cellular and tissue damage induced by photoactivated porphyrins is believed to occur primarily as a result of the formation of reactive singlet oxygen ($^1O_2$), as illustrated in Figs. 150-5 and 150-7.[60,61] Various forms of reactive oxygen species capable of causing tissue damage are known to exist, including singlet oxygen ($^1O_2$) and superoxide anion (O_2^-). In some cases the sensitized porphyrin may react with oxygen to yield hydrogen peroxide (H_2O_2) or with water to form hydroxyl radicals ($\cdot OH$)'. Those processes in which activated oxygen species play a role in photosensitization are referred to as photodynamic reactions.[62] Most of the porphyrin-mediated cutaneous photosensitization reactions are essentially photodynamic and can be minimized or prevented if reactive oxygen is eliminated from the reaction system through inactivation processes known as quenching or scavenging.

Although these concepts regarding excited porphyrins and reactive oxygen species are valid in simple systems, their applicability to complex tissues such as the skin remains to be established. Several hypotheses have been advanced regarding the mechanism of porphyrin-induced photosensitivity. One hypothesis involves the transfer of energy from excited species of oxygen to water or to lipids, creating hydrogen and/or lipid peroxides. These peroxides,

TABLE 150-4

Factors Contributing to the Development of Cutaneous Lesions in Porphyrias

Sunlight, especially blue and red light (380–760 nm)
Reactive oxygen species ($^1O_2$, O_2^-, H_2O_2, $\cdot OH$)
Cells
    Erythrocytes
    Mast cells
    Polymorphonuclear leukocytes
    Fibroblasts
Soluble mediators
    The complement system
    Factor XII-dependent pathways
    The eicosanoids

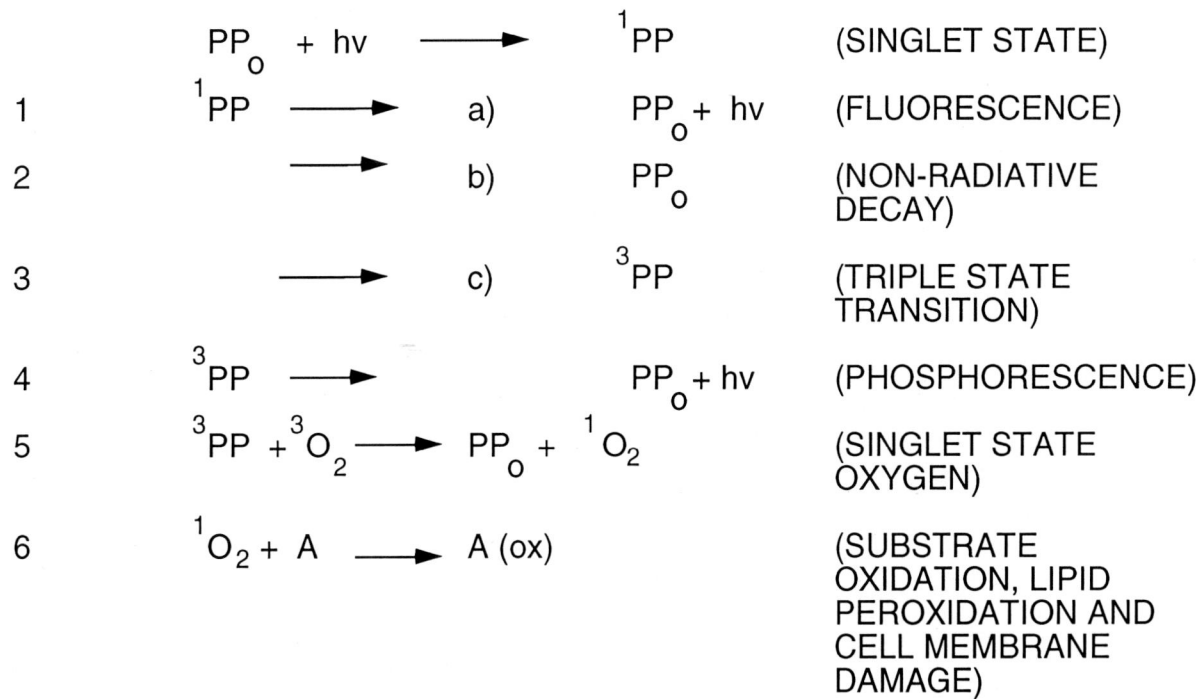

$$PP_O + hv \longrightarrow {}^1PP \quad \text{(SINGLET STATE)}$$

1   $${}^1PP \longrightarrow \text{a)} \quad PP_O + hv \quad \text{(FLUORESCENCE)}$$

2   $$\longrightarrow \text{b)} \quad PP_O \quad \text{(NON-RADIATIVE DECAY)}$$

3   $$\longrightarrow \text{c)} \quad {}^3PP \quad \text{(TRIPLE STATE TRANSITION)}$$

4   $${}^3PP \longrightarrow \quad PP_O + hv \quad \text{(PHOSPHORESCENCE)}$$

5   $${}^3PP + {}^3O_2 \longrightarrow PP_O + {}^1O_2 \quad \text{(SINGLET STATE OXYGEN)}$$

6   $${}^1O_2 + A \longrightarrow A \,(ox) \quad \text{(SUBSTRATE OXIDATION, LIPID PEROXIDATION AND CELL MEMBRANE DAMAGE)}$$

FIGURE 150-5 Photoexcited porphyrins release energy in a variety of ways when returning to their ground state, and these may contribute to damaging reactions in biologic systems.

in turn, can evoke damage in lipid-rich cellular membranes (Fig. 150-7). Evidence for this type of reaction has come from the demonstration of porphyrin-UV–induced cross-linkage of proteins within RBC membranes[63] and destruction of fibroblast membrane sulfhydryl groups.[64] If such damage occurs in plasma membranes in cells in or adjacent to the skin, it could result in tissue destruction and possibly explain the photosensitivity seen in the cutaneous por-

phyrias. Goldstein and Harber showed that photoexcitation of PROTO-enriched RBC resulted in the formation of hydrogen peroxide and lipid peroxides, each of which would be highly destructive to lipid-rich membranous structures.[65] There is evidence in RBC of peroxidation of cholesterol groups in the cell membrane resulting in hemolysis following exposure to UV radiation and PROTO.[66]

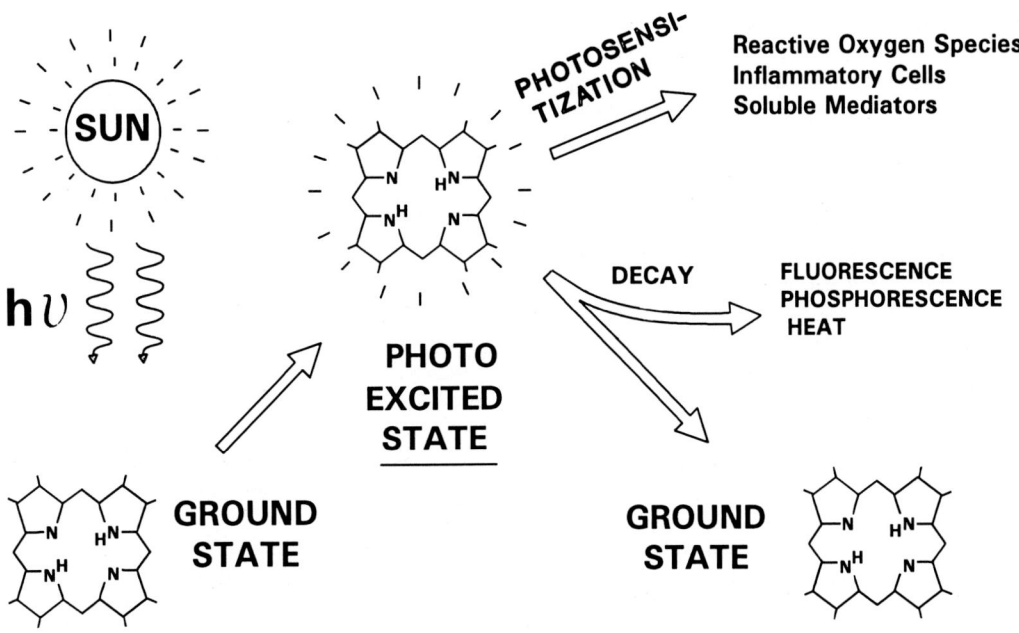

FIGURE 150-6 Porphyrins in ground state upon absorption of radiant energy (hv) undergo transition to photoexcited states. The photoexcited porphyrins react with molecular oxygen, inflammatory cells, and release soluble mediators; these in turn may contribute to damaging reactions in biologic systems such as skin.

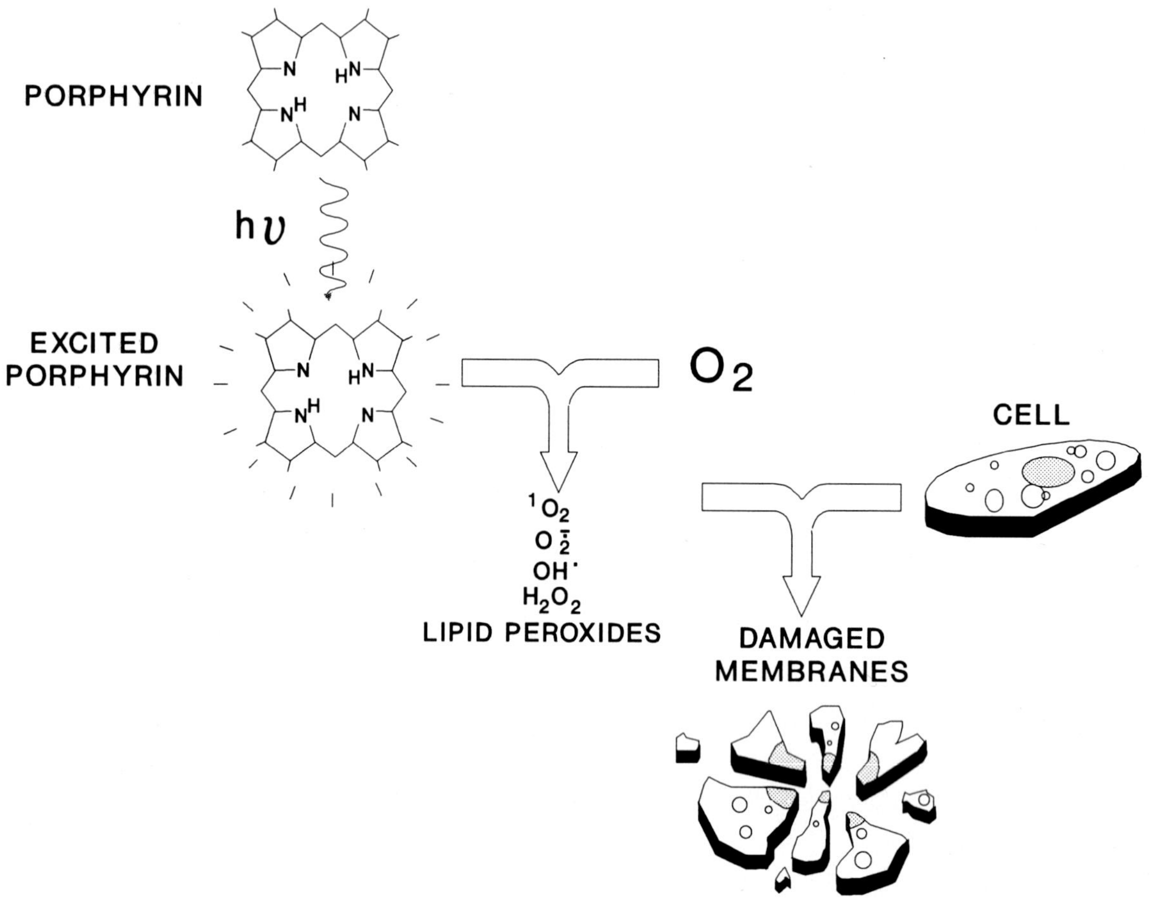

FIGURE 150-7 Photoexcited porphyrins in their triplet state transfer the absorbed energy to oxygen (O_2) molecules, thereby producing reactive oxygen species ($^1O_2$, O_2^-, $\cdot OH$, and lipid peroxides). These reactive oxygen species interact with cell membranes to cause tissue damage.

Several other studies have also supported the participation of reactive oxygen species in porphyrin-induced phototoxicity. The release of inflammatory mediators from mast cells induced by photoexcited PROTO can be suppressed by catalase, which inactivates hydrogen peroxide by converting it to water and oxygen.[67] Singlet oxygen has been shown to mediate porphyrin-induced photodamage to hepatic and epidermal microsomal cytochrome P_{450}.[68] Porphyrin and radiation-induced damage of lysosomal and mitochondrial membranes have also been reported.[69,70] DNA exposed to visible light and hematoporphyrin manifests selective degradation of the guanine moiety.[71] In vivo, beta-carotene, a scavenger of singlet oxygen, has been shown to be effective in diminishing the severity of cutaneous photosensitivity in patients with EPP.[72] In a murine model, it was demonstrated that xanthine oxidase–generated superoxide anions also play a significant role in the development of the phototoxicity induced by HPD.[73]

Erythrocytes

Erythrocytes have been used extensively in the study of porphyrin-membrane interactions. Photoexcited PROTO elicits peroxidation of cholesterol groups in cell membranes, whereas URO or COPRO has shown no such effect. This differential effect, also observed in studies using mast cells, polymorphonuclear leukocytes, and fibroblasts, most likely relates to variations in lipid-water partitioning of the different porphyrins, which may relate to their polarity. The lipophilic PROTO, a 2-carboxyl porphyrin, is more damaging to membranes as compared to the more water-soluble COPRO and URO.[74,75]

Mast Cells

Mast cell degranulation occurs in the exposed skin of patients with EPP.[76] Irradiation of PROTO-treated mast cells in vitro induces release of mast cell–derived mediators, although exposure to lower doses of PROTO and radiation results in inhibition of secretagogue-induced histamine release from these cells.[67,77] In contrast, no mediator release is detectable when cells are radiated in the presence of URO.[67] These findings may help to explain the differences in the clinical presentation of patients with EPP and PCT. The elevated PROTO in patients with EPP may induce the release of mast cell mediators in vivo following sun exposure, resulting in painful, pruritic erythema and edema. The absence of these changes in patients with PCT may be explained by the apparent inability of photoexcited URO to damage cutaneous mast cells.

Studies conducted in animal models have further confirmed the participation of mast cells in porphyrin-induced phototoxicity. It has been shown that phototoxicity is associated with elevated serum histamine levels and dermal mast cell degranulation,[78] and that the phototoxic response can be suppressed by pretreatment with antihistamines (H_1 blockers) and by intradermal injection of a mast cell secretagogue (compound 48/80).[79]

Polymorphonuclear Cells

Exposure of human polymorphonuclear leukocytes (PML) to PROTO and radiation in vitro results in membrane damage, whereas photo-excited URO induces no such alterations.[80] These results are strikingly similar to those obtained in studies with mast cells (see above). In an animal model, the porphyrin-induced phototoxic response was associated with dermal PML infiltrate,[78,81] and the phototoxicity was markedly suppressed in leukopenic animals.[79] These results appear to suggest that PML may be necessary but not sufficient for the complete manifestation of phototoxicity induced by porphyrins.

Fibroblasts

Differential phototoxic effects of various porphyrins have also been verified in studies using dermal fibroblasts. An increase in collagen biosynthesis is observed following incubation of fibroblasts with URO.[82] This effect is independent of irradiation and may partly explain the sclerodermoid changes observed in patients with PCT, which can occur in sun-exposed and in sun-protected areas. In contrast, PROTO induces photolysis of fibroblasts in vitro.[83,84]

The Complement System

The participation of the complement system in porphyrin-induced phototoxicity was initially suggested by immunofluorescent studies identifying selected complement components localized within vessel walls at the dermal-epidermal junction in patients with cutaneous porphyria.[85,86] In addition to endothelial cell damage, histologic changes consistent with those mediated by complement activation products, i.e., mast cell degranulation and infiltration of PML, are observed during the acute phase of photosensitivity in the skin of patients with EPP.[76] In vitro irradiation of sera obtained from patients with EPP and PCT results in complement activation.[87] In animal models, porphyrin-induced phototoxicity is associated with complement activation and is suppressed in complement-depleted animals as well as in animals congenitally deficient in the fifth component of complement.[88,89] Generation of complement-derived chemotactic activity is also seen following exposure of the skin of patients with EPP and PCT to Soret band radiation.[90]

Factor XII-Dependent Pathways of Coagulation

Activation of Hageman factor-dependent pathways in the presence of PROTO has been demonstrated in vitro.[91] In contrast, neither URO nor COPRO induces such activation. Whether this activation, which is independent of irradiation, contributes to the pathogenesis of porphyrin-induced phototoxicity remains to be determined.

The Eicosanoids

Porphyrins and radiation have been reported to affect eicosanoid metabolism. Incubation of mouse peritoneal macrophages or radiation-induced fibrosarcoma tumor cells in vitro with hematoporphyrin derivative PHOTOFRIN II, followed by 630-nm radiation, re-

sults in dose-dependent generation of prostaglandin E_2 (PGE_2).[92] In a protoporphyric mouse model, the ability of epidermal eicosanoid-metabolizing enzymes to generate eicosanoids is markedly suppressed following irradiation, a suppression secondary to photooxidative injury to enzymes during the phototoxic response.[93]

Summary

Cutaneous phototoxicity in porphyrias is directly related to the interaction of porphyrins with light of the Soret and other bands, resulting in the generation of reactive oxygen species; this in turn can induce lipid peroxidation and cell membrane alterations. Release of mediators and enzymes from cells such as mast cells and PML contributes to the inflammatory response; the latter is modulated by the effects of porphyrins on the complement system, factor XII-dependent pathways, and the eicosanoids. Variations in solubility influenced by the lipid-water partitioning of porphyrins may account for the unique phototoxic manifestations observed in various types of porphyria.

Classification of the Porphyrias

At present, most classifications of the porphyrias are based on the primary site of expression of the specific enzymatic defect and the abnormal porphyrin profile of patients with these disorders.

The porphyrias have been classified by Günther,[6] Waldenström,[9,11] Watson et al.,[75] and Schmid et al.[25] The classification used here (Table 150-5) is an extension of that originally proposed by Watson et al.[75]

Erythropoietic Porphyria (EP) (Table 150-6)

Synonyms for EP include Günther's disease, congenital hematoporphyria, and erythropoietic uroporphyria.

Historic Aspects

This disease was originally named hematoporphyria congenita by Günther in 1911, and the first published case of porphyria was probably of this type.[2]

TABLE 150-5
Classification of Human Porphyria

Tissue origin	Type	Inheritance
Erythropoietic	Erythropoietic porphyria (EP)	Autosomal recessive
	Erythropoietic protoporphyria (EPP)	Autosomal dominant
	Erythropoietic coproporphyria (ECP)	Autosomal dominant
Hepatic	Acute intermittent porphyria (AIP)	Autosomal dominant
	Variegate porphyria (VP)	Autosomal dominant
	Hereditary coproporphyria (HCP)	Autosomal dominant
	Porphyria cutanea tarda (PCT)	Variable, autosomal dominant
	ALA dehydratase porphyria	Autosomal recessive
Hepatoerythropoietic	Hepatoerythropoietic porphyria (HEP)	Autosomal recessive

TABLE 150-6
Erythropoietic Porphyria

Synonyms	Günther's disease, congenital hematoporphyria, erythropoietic uroporphyria
Inheritance	Autosomal recessive
Age of onset	Usually infancy or first decade
Incidence	Very rare ($<$200 reported cases)
Photosensitivity	Marked, early in childhood
Skin reactions	Early: Vesicles, bullae, erosions, hypertrichosis of lanugo hair and thickened brows and eyelashes, hypermelanosis, skin photosensitivity
	Late: Scarring with atrophy, mutilating deformities of hands, ears, face, and nose, cicatrizing alopecia, sclerodermoid changes
Clinical findings	Hemolytic anemia, erythrodontia, splenomegaly, skin photosensitivity, pink-red urine, fluorescent red blood cells and normoblasts, scleral ulceration of the eyes
Biochemical defects	Excretory: Mainly elevated URO I and COPRO I in urine and COPRO I in feces; URO $>$ COPRO
	RBC and plasma: Increased URO I and PROTO
	Enzymatic: UROGEN III cosynthase deficiency primarily in bone marrow
	? Increased PBG deaminase activity
	? Decreased UROGEN decarboxylase in some cases
Management	Hemolysis may improve after splenectomy; avoidance of sunlight and treatment of secondary skin infections

Between 1911 and 1936, Günther and Fischer performed a most detailed study of a patient with porphyria named Mathias Petry. In this study, an excessive excretion of a new type of porphyrin was identified, and because the porphyrin was in highest concentration in the urine, Fischer named it URO.[7] This was the first definite evidence that the type of porphyrin observed in excess in human porphyria was not hematoporphyrin. An excellent review of EP has been published by Ippen and Fuchs.[94]

Etiology

The etiology of EP remains unknown, although most clinical evidence suggests that EP is due to presumably decreased activity of UROGEN III cosynthase, inherited as an autosomal recessive trait.[95]

Genetics

The UROGEN III cosynthase gene has been cloned and its nucleotide sequence determined.[41] Two distinct point mutations have been identified in codons 73 and 53 of the gene.[96]

Epidemiology

EP has been observed to occur in countries around the world. Fewer than 200 cases had been reported until 1992. Nearly all begin in childhood and only a few in adult life.[97,98] EP also occurs in a number of mammals, including swine, cattle, and cats,[99] and these animal models have greatly aided research in this disease.

Clinical Manifestations

The disease usually presents itself in the first few months of life with moderate to severe cutaneous photosensitivity associated with pinkish red urine.[94,100] EP causes the most mutilating skin lesions of any of the porphyrias. The photosensitivity is due to the excessive URO I and COPRO I in RBC, plasma, and skin, which may result in photolysis of porphyrin-rich cells.

The skin manifestations include skin fragility and vesicles and bullae, which may contain pink fluorescent fluid. Secondary infec-

tion, delayed healing, and scar formation may occur. This may lead to loss of acral tissue, such as the tips of the ears, the nose, and fingers (Fig. 150-8a, -8b), and facial mutilation. Hirsutism, with long, dark, lanugo-like hair, may occur and is particularly evident in light-exposed areas such as the face, neck, and extremities. The scalp may develop a cicatrizing alopecia. Other chronic findings include eye changes (photophobia, keratoconjunctivitis, ectropion, symblepharon, and even loss of vision) and irregular hyper- and hypopigmentation of the skin. Erythrodontia (red-stained teeth) is a common finding in both deciduous and permanent teeth and is virtually pathognomonic of EP. The urine also fluoresces reddish pink.

In addition, splenomegaly, porphyrin-rich gallstones, and fluorescent bone marrow normoblasts are often observed. Hemolytic anemia associated with shortened erythrocyte lifespan (36 vs. 120 days) is seen. Whether the hemolytic anemia is due to "photohemolysis" of circulating porphyrin-laden erythrocytes or to an associated intracorpuscular red cell defect is unresolved.[101]

Laboratory Findings

The primary defect in EP involves a decreased activity of UROGEN III cosynthase that results in accumulation and increased excretion of predominantly type I porphyrins. The pink to burgundy red color of the urine from excess URO I is often visible on inspection (Fig. 150-8c). Marrow normoblasts exhibit relatively stable fluorescence and contain markedly elevated URO I, COPRO I, and PROTO. Urinary excretion of ALA and PBG is normal. COPRO I may be present in large amounts in the feces. Typical biochemical findings of EP are summarized in Tables 150-3 and 150-6.

Histopathology

The bullous lesion of EP is subepidermal with minimal degrees of inflammation. Thickening of collagen bundles may be seen in areas of scarring. Perivascular deposits of porphyrin can be found when the unstained sections of skin or liver are viewed with a fluorescence microscope.

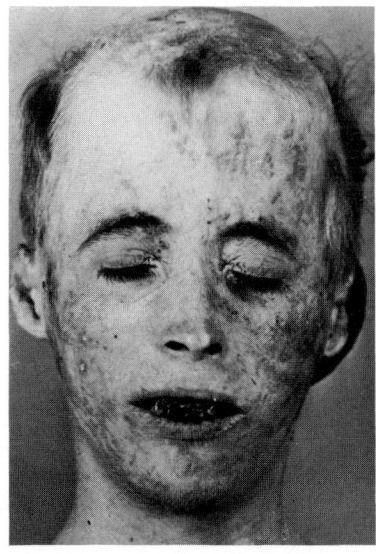
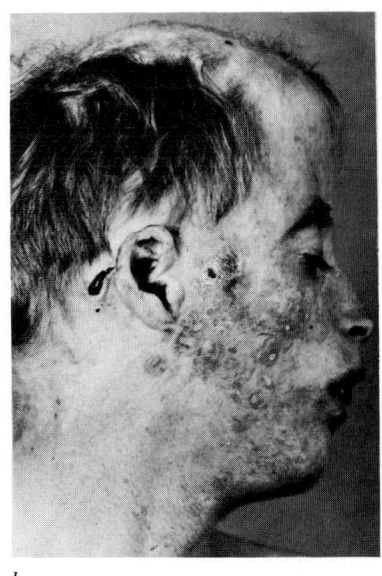
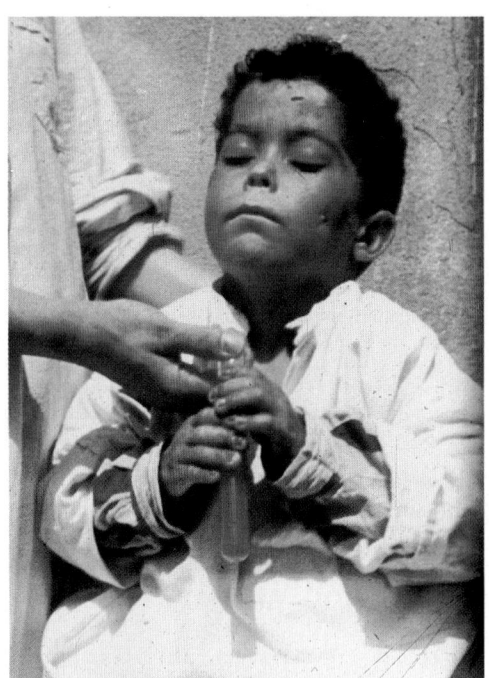

a   *b*

c

FIGURE 150-8 Two cases of congenital erythropoietic porphyria (Gunther's disease). (*a* and *b*) Severe scarring, damage of the ear and nose cartilage, hair loss, and discolored teeth. (*Courtesy of A. Wiskemann, M.D., and J. Kimmig, M.D.*) (*c*) Burgundy red urine of a patient with congenital porphyria.

Differential Diagnosis

The diagnosis of EP can usually be made from the early onset of severe cutaneous photosensitivity associated with red fluorescent urine and erythrodontia. Distinguishing EP from other congenital types of photodermatoses is important. Cutaneous findings in patients with xeroderma pigmentosum, epidermolysis bullosa, hydroa vacciniforme, and bullous pemphigoid may mimic those in patients with EP, but the porphyrin profiles of the former conditions are completely normal. Patients with hepatic porphyrias such as PCT and VP can be differentiated from patients with EP by the normal PROTO content of their erythrocytes. The cutaneous manifestations of HEP may be strikingly similar to those of EP, and measurement of the enzymes UROGEN III cosynthase (decreased in EP) and UROGEN decarboxylase (decreased in HEP) will distinguish the two. A recent report has pointed out the dual occurrence of HCP and EP in a single patient who inherited the HCP trait from her mother and the EP trait from both of her parents.[102]

Treatment

The treatment of EP is essentially preventive and symptomatic and includes avoidance of sun exposure, surveillance of the anemia, and treatment of recurrent skin infections. Protection from sunlight is absolutely essential and this alone may be of substantial benefit. Patients should be instructed to wear broad-brimmed hats and other photoprotective clothing. Topical sunscreens are relatively little used as the only ones effective at wavelengths greater than 400 nm are light opaque (SPF > 30) and contain zinc oxide or titanium dioxide, which are cosmetically unacceptable to many patients. The efficacy of oral administration of beta-carotene (120 to 180 mg daily) in EP is not proved, although there are reports that it may improve light tolerance (DJ Cripps, personal communication). Splenectomy because of intractable hemolytic anemia has occa-

sionally resulted in marked improvement both in the anemia and in cutaneous photosensitivity. Suppression of erythropoiesis by transfusion of packed erythrocytes causes a marked decrease in porphyrin production and excretion[103]; however, iron overload is a drawback. Intravenous hematin to repress porphyrin biosynthesis has been used successfully in one patient.[104] Oral treatment of a single patient with activated charcoal (60 g three times a day) for 9 months was found to lower the porphyrin levels in plasma and skin and there was complete remission of photosensitivity during the treatment period.[105] Charcoal interferes with the enterohepatic recirculation of the porphyrin and thereby enhances porphyrin clearance from the body. However, chronic use of charcoal was shown to decrease vitamin B_{12}, vitamin D, and folic acid, which returned to normal with supplementation.

Erythropoietic Protoporphyria (EPP)
(Table 150-7)

Synonyms for EPP include erythrohepatic porphyria and protoporphyria.

Historical Aspects

Although the disorder was first reported by Kosenow and Treibs[106] and Langhof et al.,[107] it was first clearly defined and named by Magnus et al.[18] who, in 1961, showed a relationship between the protoporphyrinemia and the cutaneous photosensitivity in the Soret band manifested in the form of solar urticaria. This disease escaped detection for many years for at least two reasons: (1) objective clinical signs of skin photosensitivity associated with EPP are much milder than those of EP, and (2) excessive porphyrins are almost never found in the urine of patients with EPP due to the virtual insolubility of PROTO in water.

TABLE 150-7
Erythropoietic Protoporphyria

Synonyms	Erythrohepatic protoporphyria, protoporphyria
Inheritance	Autosomal dominant, variable penetrance
Age of onset	Early childhood (1–4 years)
Photosensitivity	Mild to severe, onset immediate (in minutes)
Skin reactions	Early: Edematous plaques, erythema, urticaria (occasional), purpura, rare bullae on the nose and hands
	Late: Shallow waxy scars over nose and dorsa of hands; aged knuckles; skin thickening of exposed areas; erosions, crusts, and diffuse infiltration and wrinkling of the face
Differential diagnosis	Congenital EP, lipoid proteinosis, exaggerated sunburn
Clinical findings	Pruritus, burning, and stinging of skin during sun exposure; erythema and edema 12–24 h after exposure; waxy thickening of the knuckles and nose with fine linear scarring; nails may show onycholysis; gallstones may be present; cholelithiasis, terminal hepatic failure in a small percentage of patients; anemia uncommon
Biochemical defects	Excretory: Urine—normal porphyrins; feces—elevated PROTO
	RBC and plasma: Increased PROTO; RBC show orange-red fluorescence
	Enzymatic: Ferrochelatase deficiency in skin fibroblasts, liver, and bone marrow.
Management	Beta-carotene (60–180 mg/day) to ameliorate photosensitivity; oral PUVA phototherapy when combined with beta-carotene may also improve sun tolerance

Etiology

The specific enzyme defect in EPP is ferrochelatase, which has been shown to be decreased in RBC, mitogen-stimulated lymphocytes, and cultured skin fibroblasts of patients and unaffected carriers of EPP.[52,108] Because the activity of ferrochelatase in cultured skin fibroblasts of EPP patients is only 10 to 25 percent of normal,[109] questions have been raised about the dominant inheritance of the disease.

Genetics

Murine and human cDNAs for ferrochelatase have been cloned recently and should provide the basis for future studies to identify the molecular defect in EPP.[53] Norris et al.,[110] using a new assay for ferrochelatase, studied 9 families including 14 patients with EPP. Two distinct inheritance patterns were identified: the first was autosomal dominant and the second was autosomal recessive. In some families studied, both parents had normal enzyme activity and the inheritance could not be determined. Deyback et al.[111] have reported a single patient with EPP with homozygous deficiency of the enzyme whose parents both manifest evidence of partially decreased ferrochelatase activity. This genetic heterogeneity requires further research to clarify the inheritance of EPP, which was initially believed to be a simple autosomal dominant trait.[112]

Epidemiology

Although the exact incidence of EPP is unknown, it has been reported with increasing frequency since 1961, indicating that it is one of the more common types of cutaneous porphyria. Studies from one laboratory performing diagnostic tests for RBC porphyrins in patients with suspected cutaneous photosensitivity indicated that 8 percent of such samples demonstrate elevated RBC PROTO levels diagnostic of EPP. The disease has been reported from many countries around the world, and possibly no ethnic group is spared.[113]

Clinical Manifestations

The disease begins early in life and is characterized by cutaneous photosensitivity and by elevated PROTO in RBC, feces, and plasma; there is no excess porphyrin excretion in the urine except when hepatic failure occurs as a terminal event. The acute episodes of cutaneous photosensitivity include burning, stinging (smarting), and pruritus in light-exposed skin, particularly of the nose, cheeks, and dorsal aspects of the hands. These are followed by erythema, edema (Fig. 150-9), urticarial lesions, and rarely purpura. Photosensitivity may occur within minutes of sun exposure; it often starts early in the spring, continues through the summer, and diminishes in the winter. The skin lesions may resolve slowly, leaving small, atrophic, waxy or pitted scars (Fig. 150-10a, -10b). There may be some pursing of perioral skin (pseudorhagades). The skin of the knuckles and fingers, particularly over the metacarpophalangeal and interphalangeal joints, often appears thickened, wrinkled, and waxy, suggesting a premature aging (so-called old knuckles, in a child). This subtle change is pathognomonic, particularly in children. Superficial scarring on the bridge of the nose and small circular shallow scars may be seen on the face. Vesicular or bullous lesions rarely occur in EPP in temperate climates, although they have occurred in patients exposed to tropical sunlight. The porphyrin abnormality persists throughout life, although some patients seem to be less symptomatic as they get older.

Controversy has existed concerning the tissue origin of the excessive PROTO. Some have shown that RBC PROTO levels

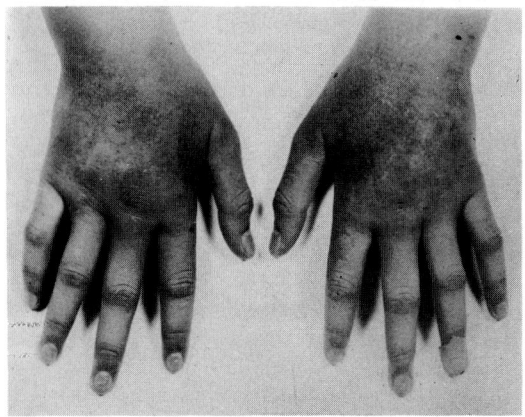

FIGURE 150-9   A case of erythropoietic protoporphyria showing swelling and purpura on dorsa of hands resulting from exposure to solar radiation. (*Courtesy of E. Gasser-Wolff, M.D.: Helv Paediatr Acta 20:598, 1965.*)

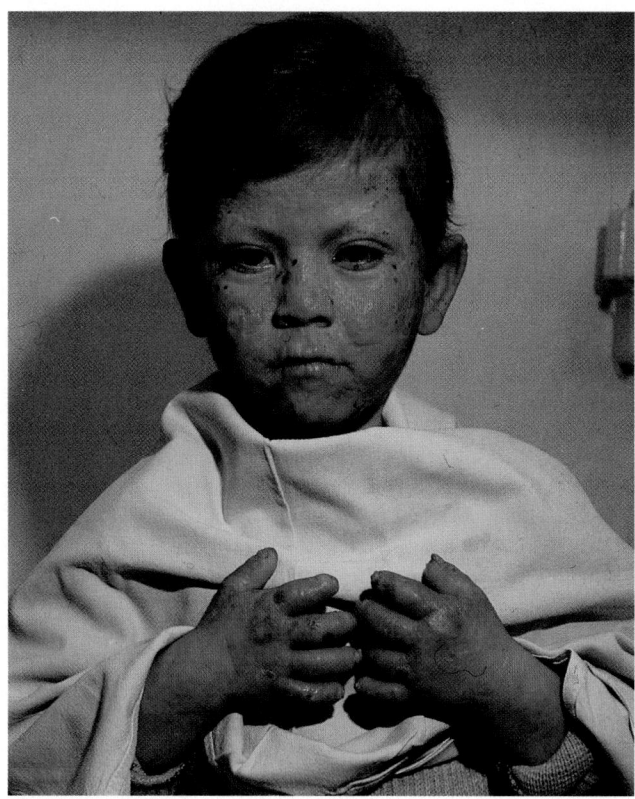

a

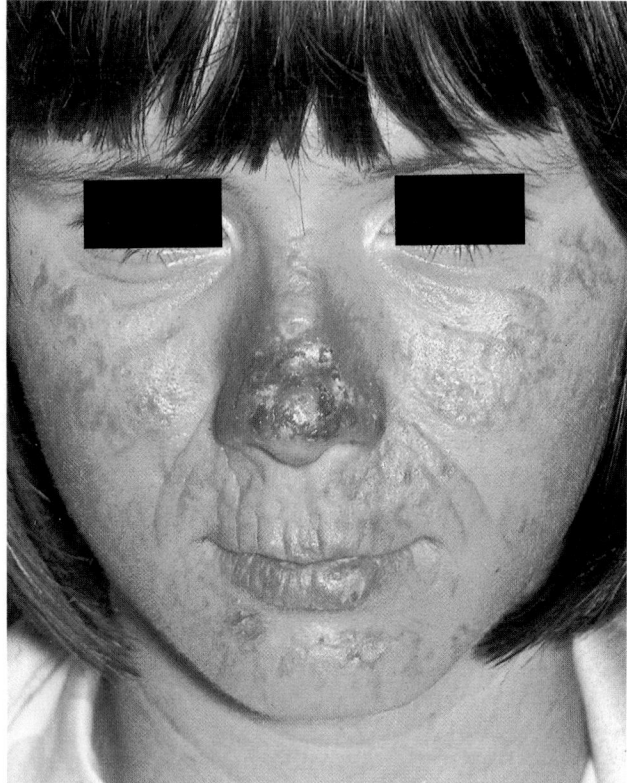

b

FIGURE 150-10 (*a*) A case of erythropoietic protoporphyria showing atrophic waxy scars, mutilations, and crusted lesions on face and hands. The hands also show severe edema. The mutilating skin lesions are the result of severe photosensitivity due to excessive protoporphyrin. (*Courtesy of A. Kurban, M.D., American University of Beirut.*) (*b*) A 15-year-old patient

with erythropoietic protoporphyria with severe sensitivity to sunlight. The nose, lower lip, and chin show erythematous, in part erosive, and crusted lesions. Nose and cheeks show erythematous lesions, a few small slightly depressed scars, and peculiar waxy thickening of skin. Linear scars are seen between the nose and mouth.

alone are sufficient to explain the increased levels of PROTO,[114,115] whereas others have suggested that hepatic PROTO production contributes to the excessively high levels of circulating PROTO.[116]

Associated findings are few in most patients with EPP. There is no erythrodontia, hypertrichosis, milia, sclerodermoid change, or hyperpigmentation. Hemolytic anemia is decidedly uncommon, although about 11 percent of patients with EPP have a mild anemia of unknown cause.[113]

Gallstones have been reported in some patients with EPP at a relatively early age; in one series, 12 percent of patients had chole-lithiasis, of whom three underwent cholecystectomy.[117] Careful study of all gallstones obtained at surgery from two EPP patients showed that they contained large amounts of PROTO (Pathak and Bickers, unpublished observations).

Light microscopy of liver biopsies has revealed slight portal and periportal fibrosis and deposition of brown pigment, which may occlude bile canaliculi and ducts; it is also present in hepato-cytes, in Kupffer cells, and in periportal macrophages. The pig-ment is birefringent on polarization microscopy.[118] Hepatocytes may also contain cytoplasmic or mitochondrial inclusions, which at the ultrastructural level appear as needlelike crystals, probably due to precipitated PROTO[119] (Fig. 150-11).

Terminal hepatic failure has been reported in a small percent-age of patients with EPP.[120,121] All these individuals were jaun-diced, had hepatic cirrhosis, and died in hepatic coma or as a con-sequence of portal hypertension. Risk factors for this type of

hepatic failure remain unknown, but it is likely that the deposits of crystalline PROTO lead to hepatocyte injury. Experimental studies have shown that perfusion of rat liver with PROTO induces a dose-dependent cholestasis that could contribute to the hepatotoxic effect of PROTO.[122]

Laboratory Findings

The diagnosis of EPP is made by detecting elevated levels of free PROTO in the RBC and/or feces (see Tables 150-3 and 150-7). In addition, there may be increased plasma PROTO, increased fecal COPRO, and occasionally slightly increased RBC COPRO. In in-complete expression of EPP, only the fecal PROTO may be ele-vated. Examination of a blood smear under a fluorescent micro-scope reveals red-fluorescing RBC (5 to 30 percent). This fluorescence is often transient and quite light sensitive, and the procedure should be carried out in subdued light or preferably in the dark. Poh-Fitzpatrick et al.[123] have devised a rapid quantitative microfluorometric assay for free erythrocyte and plasma PROTO that is useful as a screening test for suspected EPP. Finger-prick samples of blood collected on filter paper are used for this test. In one series of 32 patients with EPP, the RBC PROTO levels ranged from 131 to 1617 μg/dL of RBC (normal < 90 μg/dL of RBC).[112,124]

The photosensitizing activity of porphyrins is most probably related to the light absorption and emission characteristics of these

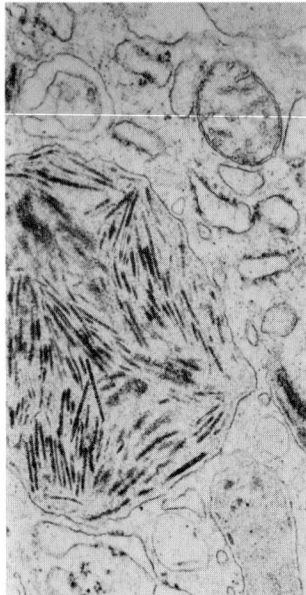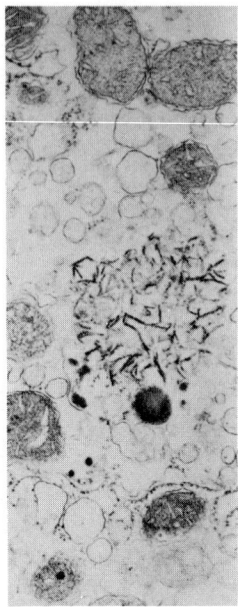

FIGURE 150-11 Electron micrographs of a percutaneous liver biopsy specimen obtained from a patient with erythropoietic protoporphyria. Numerous rod-shaped crystals and electron-dense clumps of pigment are seen in the hepatocytes and Kupffer cells. When viewed under the microscope, these dense clumps of pigment exhibit an orange-red fluorescence and striking birefringence. (*Courtesy of K. Wolff, M.D., and H. Hönigsmann, M.D., University of Vienna.*)

tetrapyrroles (see Table 150-8). There is good evidence to suggest that unchelated (metal-free) PROTO is responsible for the skin photosensitivity reactions in EPP. Evidence for this has come from studies designed to explain the perplexing observation that in lead poisoning and in iron-deficiency anemia, conditions in which RBC PROTO levels are similar to those found in EPP, cutaneous photosensitivity does not occur. Studies by Piomelli et al.[114] and Lamola et al.[125] suggest that in these nonphotosensitizing disorders the excessive PROTO is probably chelated with zinc and bound to globin chains in the RBC, which renders it incapable of diffusing into the plasma and then into cutaneous tissue. This explains why plasma PROTO is not elevated in these nonphotosensitizing disorders. In EPP, however, the majority of the excessive PROTO is probably unchelated or free. Free PROTO can diffuse out of the RBC and is detectable in the plasma of patients with EPP who manifest cutaneous photosensitivity.[101] In one study, a patient with sideroblastic anemia had marked increases in free PROTO, both in the RBC and in the plasma, but had no cutaneous photosensitivity.[126] Because

ferrochelatase activity was normal in this patient, it is possible that the excessive free PROTO was either chelated with zinc or readily converted to heme in the skin, thereby precluding cutaneous accumulation of PROTO and associated photosensitivity. It has also been suggested that the absence of hemolytic anemia in EPP is due to the unique capacity of PROTO to move out of the RBC and to bind to albumin in the plasma.[127] The porphyrin does not remain within the lipid-rich red cell membrane sufficiently long for light exposure to cause damage, and serum albumin has a potent inhibitory effect on photohemolysis in EPP.

Histopathology

Immediately following irradiation, endothelial cell damage, mast cell degranulation, and polymorphonuclear cells are seen in the dermis.[76] In sun-exposed areas, there is often marked eosinophilic homogenization and thickening of vessels in the papillary dermis due to the accumulation of an amorphous, homogeneous, slightly basophilic (hyaline-like) substance in and around the vessel walls.[112] The perivascular deposits of concentric eosinophilic layers of hyaline-like material stain strongly positive with periodic acid–Schiff (PAS) and are diastase positive (see Fig. 150-12). Histochemical studies suggest that this material may be a neutral glycoprotein with smaller amounts of acid mucopolysaccharide and lipids.[128] The histologic findings are similar to those of lipoid proteinosis (hyalinosis cutis et mucosae).[129] Electron microscopic studies in EPP show that the amorphous material consists of a multilayered, partially fragmented basement membrane and finely fibrillar material of moderate density that permeates and surrounds the vessel walls.[130] Other studies have shown that type IV collagen and laminin as well as amyloid P and fibronectin are deposited in the walls of dermal blood vessels.[131]

Differential Diagnosis

EPP must be differentiated from other causes of photosensitivity, primarily hydroa aestivale, polymorphous light eruption (PMLE), idiopathic solar urticaria, and other types of porphyria. Contact dermatitis and angioedema should also be considered. In PMLE, the lesions are characteristically papules, plaques, and papulovesicles. A family history of photosensitivity is less common. Burning and smarting of the skin during or soon after sun exposure is unusual in PMLE, whereas it is a common occurrence in EPP. Porphyrin profile and skin biopsy with PAS staining may also be helpful in differentiating between PMLE and EPP. Idiopathic solar urticaria can be easily differentiated from EPP; it is not associated with elevated RBC or fecal PROTO. Contact dermatitis may in-

TABLE 150-8
Fluorescence Characteristics of Porphyrin-Containing Plasma Diluted with 1:10 Phosphate Buffered Solution

Type	Excitation, nm	Emission, nm	Fluorescent porphyrins
Erythropoietic porphyria (EP)	398	619	URO I, COPRO I
Erythropoietic protoporphyria (EPP)	409	634	PROTO
Porphyria cutanea tarda (PCT)	398	619	URO I, III, COPRO III
Variegate porphyria (VP)	405	626	COPRO III, PROTO
Acute intermittent porphyria (AIP)	398	619	URO III
Hereditary coproporphyria (HCP)	398	619	COPRO III
Hepatoerythropoietic porphyria (HEP)	398	619	URO I

SOURCE: Modified from Poh-Fitzpatrick.[243]

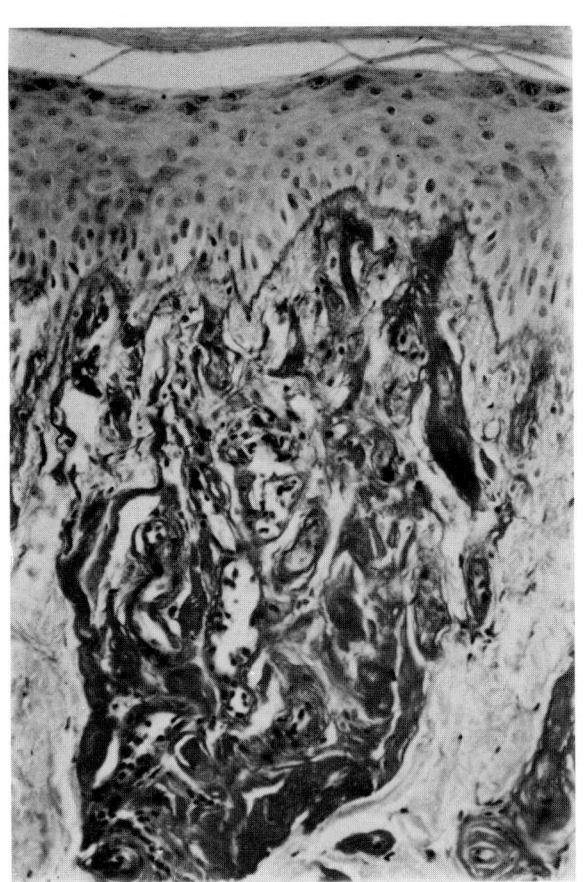

a

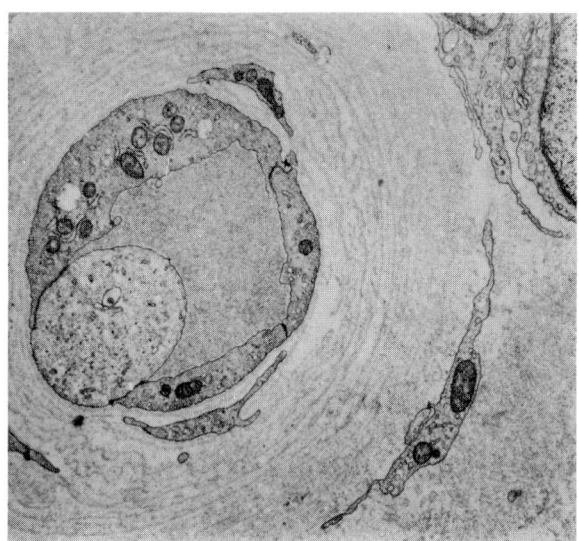

c

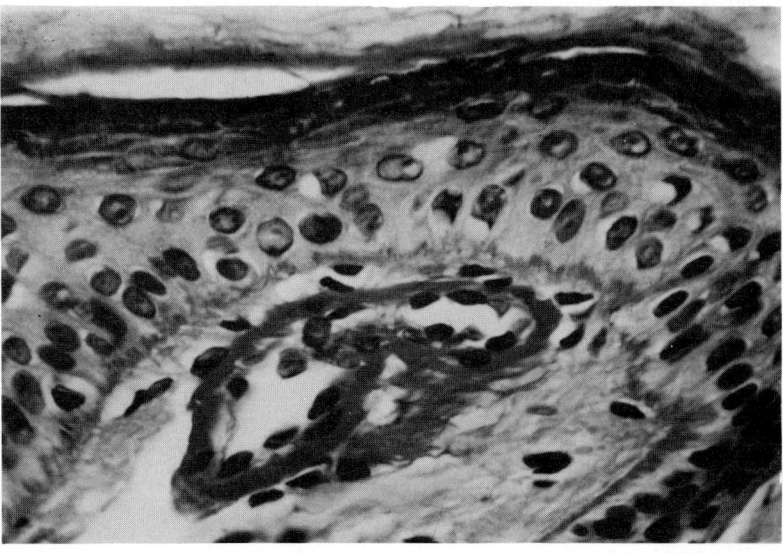

b

FIGURE 150-12 (*a*) A biopsy of light-exposed skin from a patient with erythropoietic protoporphyria. There is marked thickening of the blood vessel walls of the upper dermis. The capillaries in the upper dermis are surrounded by a hyaline-like material. (*b*) PAS stain of biopsy from light-exposed skin from a patient with erythropoietic protoporphyria, showing PAS-positive carbohydrate protein complex with lipid also present. These histologic features were not unlike those found in lipoid proteinosis. (*c*) Electron micrograph of biopsy of chronically exposed skin from a patient with erythropoietic protoporphyria. Multiple concentric basal laminae surrounding dermal blood vessels and finely fibrillar material admixed with amorphous masses within perivascular tissue are shown. (*Courtesy of K. Wolff, M.D., and H. Hönigsmann, M.D., University of Vienna.*)

volve non-light-exposed areas such as the skin folds and the submental areas. Patch testing with a suspected allergen and negative porphyrin values help to differentiate this condition. The lesions of angioedema may occur anywhere on the body, including the mucous membranes. Because discomfort is often disproportionate to visible lesions, EPP has been confused with psychoneurosis or even malingering. This problem in differential diagnosis is readily solved by porphyrin determinations. Erythropoietic coproporphyria (ECP), an extremely rare condition, should also be considered in the differential diagnosis.[19] Clinically, it resembles EPP and could only be diagnosed by chromatographic study of RBC porphyrins.

Treatment

The treatment of photosensitivity in EPP has been aided by the use of orally administered beta-carotene (Solatene). Topical sunscreens, antimalarial drugs, cholestyramine, and vitamins E and C have all been suggested but have not been shown to be effective.[112] As reported by Mathews-Roth et al.,[132] beta-carotene (60 to 180 mg per day by mouth) has been found helpful in preventing or minimizing the symptoms of skin photosensitivity reactions of EPP. Eighty-four percent of 133 patients claimed to triple their tolerance to sunlight after an adequate course of beta-carotene exceeding 2 months. The therapeutic effectiveness of the drug has been confirmed by several groups of investigators.[133] These results are, however, based on limited controlled laboratory testing and uncontrolled clinical impressions; the one controlled trial failed to confirm the therapeutic effectiveness of beta-carotene.[134] To achieve optimal photoprotection, serum carotene levels should be maintained at a minimum of 600 μg/dL. In adult patients, this can usually be achieved by oral administration of 2 to 6 capsules of 30 mg each per day, which will produce serum carotene levels of 600 to 800 μg/dL after 4 to 6 weeks of therapy. Children under 12 years of age may receive 30 to 90 mg daily. Maximum effectiveness may not occur until 1 to 2 months after initiating therapy; hence patients should receive therapy in early spring through the fall season (February to October in the northern hemisphere). The drug is remarkably well tolerated at these doses, and there are no known toxic systemic effects of beta-carotene. Occasionally diarrhea occurs in a small number of patients. Orange or rusty discoloration of stools is common and is not an indication for discontinuing treatment. The only other side effect of note is the visible yellowing of the skin that occurs as a result of carotenoderma and this is more noticeable on the palms and soles. Topical application of beta-carotene in cream form (1 to 5%) to light-exposed skin areas of EPP patients is totally ineffective; the photolability of carotenoid pigments results in rapid destruction of the applied beta-carotene (Pathak, unpublished observations). Oral PUVA photochemotherapy combined with beta-carotene may be helpful in some patients.

The mechanism of the photoprotective effect of beta-carotene is not precisely known. Beta-carotene does not function as a sunscreen; it does, however, appear to be capable of quenching excited singlet oxygen and of trapping free radicals formed by the interaction of light with PROTO and molecular oxygen.[135]

Uncontrolled studies have shown some clinical and biochemical improvement using the anionic binding resin cholestyramine and the antioxidant vitamin E.[121] Hematin infusions have been used to decrease the production of heme temporarily and are associated with a decrease in fecal and plasma PROTO in some patients.[115] The use of RBC exchange with autologous washed cells has also been explored for its ability to induce clinical and biochemical remission of EPP. Bechtel et al. showed that transfusion therapy in

one patient with EPP resulted in a marked decrease in photosensitivity associated with a decline in free erythrocyte PROTO levels.[136] Hypertransfusion therapy to suppress erythropoiesis, however, cannot be recommended. The potential hazards of transfusion, particularly in terms of infectious diseases, are a contraindication.

Management of the hepatic failure is particularly difficult. Orally administered bile salts have been used in an effort to diminish the enterohepatic circulation of the excessive PROTO[137] and to enhance the capacity of the liver to clear excess PROTO. Another approach was reported using large amounts of orally administered iron in a patient with EPP who manifested incipient hepatic failure as well as elevated erythrocyte and plasma PROTO levels and concomitant iron deficiency anemia.[138] Oral iron therapy exacerbated the disease in another patient.[139] Liver transplantation has also been used successfully in a small number of patients.[140]

Erythropoietic Coproporphyria (ECP)

There are only three known cases of this entity that have been published. Heilmeyer and Clotten have described the disorder in some detail.[19] Elevated PROTO and COPRO were found in the RBC of one patient. Topi et al.[141] described two brothers with cutaneous photosensitivity similar to that of EPP but with elevated RBC PROTO and COPRO III in both. Very little is known about this disease.

Porphyria Cutanea Tarda (PCT)
(Table 150-9)

Synonyms for PCT include type I, symptomatic porphyria, acquired hepatic porphyria, and chemical porphyria.

Historical Aspects

PCT was originally classified by Günther as hematoporphyria chronica. He described it as a syndrome of skin lesions and darkly colored urine occurring later in life than either congenital or acute porphyria without acute attacks of abdominal pain or neurologic dysfunction.[6] Waldenström[9,11] first named the disease PCT and observed that Swedish patients with acute attacks of porphyria (AIP) never developed cutaneous porphyria. He suggested that these two disorders were completely distinct, PCT being primarily acquired and AIP familial.

Following Waldenström's description of PCT in 1937, scattered case reports appeared in the literature. Early experience with this disorder in the United States was carefully described by Brunsting and his coworkers at the Mayo Clinic.[10,142] Later, patients with a comparable clinical picture were described in South Africa.[143] Finally, and even more confusing, it became clear that there were a small number of patients in the United States and a larger number in South Africa who manifested both the cutaneous changes of PCT as well as intermittent attacks of AIP. In South Africa, this was called VP, whereas initially in the United States it was known as mixed porphyria.[144] There is general agreement now on the use of the term VP to describe this disorder in the United States.[16,17]

TABLE 150-9
Porphyria Cutanea Tarda

Synonyms	Symptomatic porphyria, acquired hepatic porphyria, chemical porphyria
Inheritance	Mixed or variable autosomal dominant in some patients
Types	Acquired or type I; inherited (familial types II and III)
Age of onset	Usually in third or fourth decade; rare before puberty; prevalence: most common porphyria
Photosensitivity	Moderate to severe; bullae on dorsa of hands and feet
Skin reactions	Vesicular, bullous and ulcerative lesions, primarily on light-exposed skin; increased skin fragility to mechanical trauma; hyperpigmentation and sclerodermoid plaques; scarring alopecia, milia on fingers and hands, hypertrichosis and periorbital violaceous suffusion, dystrophic calcification and photoonycholysis
Clinical findings	Diabetes mellitus in about 25 percent of patients; rare hepatic tumor; increased liver iron stores; increased serum iron; pink fluorescence in urine with Wood's lamp; unlike VP, acute attacks are absent in PCT
Biochemical defects	Excretory: Increased urinary URO (I > III) and 7-carboxyl porphyrins (III > I); increased COPRO in urine; increased ISOCOPRO in feces
	RBC: Normal porphyrins
	Plasma: Increased 8- and 7-carboxyl porphyrins
	Enzymatic: Deficiency of UROGEN decarboxylase in liver (type I) and RBC (type II) and their families
Differential diagnosis	Pseudo PCT, VP, epidermolysis bullosa acquisita
Treatment or management	Stop ethanol or estrogens and other precipitating chemicals or drugs; phlebotomy (500 mL weekly or biweekly) until Hb is 10–11 g/dL and serum Fe is reduced to 50–60 μg/dL
	Alternative therapy: chloroquine 125 mg twice weekly

Etiology

Complete understanding of the etiology of PCT has been hampered by clinical evidence suggesting that there are several distinct forms of the disease. Thus, many patients who, in retrospect, clearly had VP were often initially classified as having PCT if the cutaneous manifestations of their disease predominated.[145] The additional knowledge that exposure to toxic environmental chemicals such as hexachlorobenzene (HCB) or chlorinated phenols induced a PCT-like syndrome, despite no clear evidence of genetic susceptibility, also made classification of PCT difficult.

Most classifications of PCT separate the disorder into at least two broad categories, both associated with decreased UROGEN decarboxylase activity: (1) PCT-symptomatic, or sporadic (also referred to as acquired or type I), (2) PCT-hereditary, or type II. In symptomatic (sporadic) PCT, the enzyme is deficient only in the liver, which could be explained either by a different gene defect restricted to the liver or by exposure to chemicals that selectively inhibit the hepatic but not the RBC enzyme[146] (Table 150-10). Some of these substances (e.g., alcohol and estrogen) may provoke porphyria only in selected individuals, and others (e.g., HCB) in practically all exposed individuals.

In hereditary (type II) PCT, UROGEN decarboxylase is decreased approximately 50 percent in all tissues, including RBC and cultured skin fibroblasts.[43,44,147] The defect is inherited in an autosomal dominant fashion. The enzyme defect is cross-reactive immunologic material (CRIM)-negative. Elder et al.[44] have employed an immunochemical assay to measure UROGEN decarboxylase in a large number of unrelated patients with PCT. Decreased enzyme concentration appears to follow a bimodal distribution, suggesting two overlapping groups of patients: a large group (>80 percent) with normal UROGEN decarboxylase concentration, and a small group (<20 percent) in whom the amount of detectable enzyme was about half normal. Some patients with type II PCT were found to have UROGEN decarboxylase activity at the lower end of the normal range. Penetrance of type II PCT is relatively low, so that the majority of individuals with the inherited enzyme defect do not manifest the disease.

On the other hand, it is important to emphasize that not every patient with a positive family history of PCT will have type II disease. Roberts et al.[148] showed that several patients with one or more relatives with clearcut PCT had normal UROGEN decarboxylase concentrations and yet were clinically and biochemically indistinguishable from individuals with type I PCT. These patients could either have inherited some form of UROGEN decarboxylase that is immunochemically indistinguishable from the normal enzyme but which is uniquely susceptible to inhibition in the liver, or they may have a second inherited enzyme deficiency unrelated to UROGEN decarboxylase. These possibilities require further investigation. This latter category of PCT has been designated as type III by some investigators.[149]

It is also unclear from some of the early studies whether patients who were reported as having hereditary PCT actually had VP, an autosomal dominant disorder. Studies by Watson et al. in the United States[150] and by Day et al. in South Africa[151] have shown that PCT and VP may occur in different members of the same family, so-called dual porphyria. Another form of dual porphyria in which PCT and AIP co-exist has been described.[152]

The most frequently incriminated agents that contribute to the development of PCT (type I, acquired, or sporadic) are alcohol, estrogens, iron, polychlorinated hydrocarbons, HCB, and hemodialysis in patients with renal failure. Some of these precipitating factors are discussed briefly below:

Alcohol Heavy alcohol intake has long been recognized to exacerbate PCT. Ethanol has been shown to induce hepatic ALA synthase

TABLE 150-10
Drugs and Chemicals Associated with the Clinical Expression of Porphyria Cutanea Tarda

Ethyl alcohol	Iron
Estrogenic hormones	Tetrachlorodibenzo[*p*]-dioxin
Hexachlorobenzene	
Chlorinated phenols	Polychlorinated biphenyls (PCB)
	Herbicides 2,4-dichloro- and trichloro-phenoxy acetic acid

in patients with PCT.[153] Erythrocyte UROGEN decarboxylase activity is diminished in healthy subjects following acute ethanol ingestion and in chronic alcoholics.[154] Ethanol can also inhibit the activity of other enzymes in the heme pathway, including ferrochelatase and ALA dehydratase. Chronic alcoholism leads to suppression of erythropoiesis[155] and increased absorption of dietary iron, although whether the increased iron absorption of alcoholism contributes to the pathogenesis of the disease and to the characteristic hepatic siderosis of PCT is unknown. The fact that ALA synthase is increased in cirrhotic liver of individuals without porphyria raises questions concerning the relevance of alcohol effects on ALA synthase in the clinical expression of PCT.[156]

Estrogens   The widespread use of estrogens as contraceptive agents or as hormone supplements for postmenopausal replacement therapy in females and as adjunctive hormonal therapy in males with prostatic carcinoma has been associated with PCT.[157] The mechanism of the estrogen effect on the expression of PCT is not established. Diethylstilbesterol, an estrogen, induces hepatic ALA synthase,[158] but this would not explain the distinctive porphyrin excretion pattern found in PCT. The vast majority of patients receiving estrogens do not manifest the biochemical abnormalities associated with PCT.

Hexachlorobenzene   This fungicide caused an "epidemic" of a PCT-like syndrome in southeastern Turkey in the 1950s.[159] It was added as a preservative to wheat intended for planting but, because of a famine, several thousand individuals of diverse ethnic origin, mostly children, ingested the seed wheat and subsequently developed typical PCT. Over 4000 cases of this syndrome were reported from 1956 to 1961. The porphyrin excretion pattern and the cutaneous findings in these patients were similar to those seen in PCT evoked by ethanol or estrogens. The outbreak of PCT in Turkey caused by ingestion of HCB indicated that the disease can be acquired in nongenetically predisposed individuals.

Twenty-five years after onset, the most common clinical findings in these HCB-poisoned individuals were those of chronic porphyria, including sclerodermoid scarring (84 percent), hyperpigmentation (78 percent), hirsutism (49 percent), thyromegaly, and increased skin fragility (38 percent).[160] A painless arthritis was seen in two out of three affected individuals, and a variety of neurologic signs and symptoms were seen in the majority. Stool and urine porphyrins remained elevated in many patients.

Studies have shown that the chronic administration of HCB to experimental animals produces excessive porphyrin accumulation in the liver in a pattern quite similar to that seen in PCT in humans.[161] These data are consistent with the hypothesis that chlorinated hydrocarbons, such as HCB, or their metabolites inhibit hepatic UROGEN decarboxylase, leading to excessive hepatic storage of URO and other acetate substituted porphyrins.[162,163] Experimental studies have also shown that HCB can inactivate UROGEN decarboxylase by abolishing catalytic activity without changing the amount of immunoreactive enzyme protein.[164] Additional studies on the porphyrinogenic effects of HCB, dioxin, and PCB suggest that metabolic activation of the compounds mediated by cytochrome P_{450} is associated with a decrease in UROGEN decarboxylase activity.[162,163] Chemical porphyria, similar to PCT, is caused by other chlorinated hydrocarbons such as the polychlorinated biphenyls and 2,3,7,8-tetrachlorodibenzo-*p*-dioxin (TCDD), a by-product in the synthesis of the herbicide 2,4,5-trichlorophenoxyacetic acid.[165]

Tetrachlorodibenzo-p-dioxin (TCDD)   TCDD is a toxic environmental pollutant chemical. Among its numerous effects are chloracne, liver damage, and hepatic porphyria in experimental animals and perhaps also in humans.[166,167] It has been shown that the hepatic porphyrinogenic effect of TCDD can be abolished in mice by first depleting them of iron.[167] Furthermore, it is known that highly inbred mouse strains vary in their susceptibility to induction of hepatic porphyria by TCDD, indicating that the porphyrogenic effect of this hydrocarbon is modulated by as yet undefined genetic factors.[168]

Iron   Serum iron and ferritin concentrations are elevated or in the upper range of normal in PCT, suggesting a possible role of iron in the pathogenesis of the disease.[169] Hepatic iron overload accompanies clinical PCT in practically all cases, and elevation of plasma iron is found in one-third to one-half of patients.[157] In PCT, the quantity of iron that can be mobilized by phlebotomy indicates that total iron stores are approximately twice normal.[170] Ferrokinetic studies in patients with PCT are said to be normal.[171] The long remissions that follow repeated phlebotomy and the apparent ineffectiveness of this treatment if supplemental iron is administered concomitantly suggest that iron plays a role in the excessive hepatic porphyrin production of PCT. PCT is particularly common where alcoholism and iron overload occur together.

The role of iron in the pathogenesis of PCT is undoubtedly a complex one, and several hypotheses have been proposed to explain it. Some believe that iron is capable of directly inhibiting UROGEN decarboxylase.[170] However, studies with purified UROGEN decarboxylase prepared from human erythrocytes have shown that the purified enzyme is not inhibited by Fe^{2+} or Fe^{3+}.[172] Chronic iron overload can produce peroxidative damage to lipid-rich mitochondrial and microsomal membranes in the liver of experimental animals, but the relationship of this toxic effect to changes in hepatic heme synthesis has not been clearly defined.[173]

Iron may have a permissive effect on the inhibition by chlorinated phenols of UROGEN decarboxylase,[167,168] and it can also enhance the induction response of hepatic ALA synthase to drugs.[174] Although such an iron-augmented increase in ALA synthase activity could lead to enhanced porphyrinogenesis, this alone would not explain the porphyrin excretion pattern seen in PCT. Kushner et al. have shown that addition of ferrous iron to liver in vitro causes a marked increase in porphyrin synthesis and inhibits UROGEN III cosynthase activity.[175] This latter effect would explain the URO isomer I excess characteristic of PCT. The multiple effects of iron on heme synthesis have been summarized recently.[169]

From these known effects of alcohol, estrogens, chlorinated hydrocarbons, and iron on the heme pathway, it is clear that each of these could contribute to the excessive hepatic porphyrinogenesis characteristic of PCT. How the putative effects of alcohol, estrogens, and iron contribute to the hepatic UROGEN decarboxylase activity and associated porphyrin metabolism remains unclear. The clinical expression of PCT is therefore dependent upon the interaction of a number of factors, both genetic and environmental. However, it is important to note that the ingestion of drugs usually associated with inducing attacks of the acute hepatic porphyrias (see Table 150-11) has not been reported to exacerbate PCT.

Genetics

UROGEN decarboxylase is the fifth enzyme in the heme pathway, and the cDNA and gene for the human enzyme have been isolated

TABLE 150-11

Examples of Drugs Potentially Hazardous in Patients with the Acute Hepatic Porphyrias

Amidopyrine	Hydralazine
Aminoglutethimide	Isopropylmeprobamate
Aminopyrine	Mephenytoin
Amphetamines	Meprobamate
Antipyrine	Methyldopa
Barbiturates	Methylprylon
Bemegride	N-butylscopolammonium bromide
Carbamazepine	Nalidixic acid
Carbromal	Nikethamide
Chloromethazone	Nitrazepam
Chloropropamide	Nortriptyline
Chloroquine	Novobiocin
Danazol	Pargyline
Dapsone	Pentazocine
Diclophenac	Pentylenetetrazole
Diethylpropione	Phenoxybenzamine
Diphenylhydantoin	Phenylbutazone
Dramamine	Primadone
Enflurane	Pyrazinamide
Ergot preparation	Rifampin
Erythromycin	Sedormid
Ethclorvynol	Succinimides
Ethinamate	Sulfonamides
Ethosuximide	Sulfonethylmethane
Ethyl alcohol	Sulfonylureas
Fentanyl	Synthetic estrogens, progestins
Furosemide	Theophylline
Furoxene	Tolazamide
Glutethimide	Tolbutamide
Griseofulvin	Trimethadione
Halothane	Valproic acid
Heavy metals	

and sequenced. The human enzyme is a single polypeptide of 367 amino acids with a molecular mass of about 40.8 kDa. In one family with PCT, a specific mutation resulting in UROGEN decarboxylase deficiency was shown to be a glycine → valine substitu-

tion at amino acid 281.[176] This resulted in a marked decrease in the half-life of the enzyme from more than 100 h to around 4 h. The same mutation could not be identified in several other families, suggesting that there is genetic heterogeneity in PCT.

Epidemiology

PCT occurs throughout the world,[177] and it is the most common of all the porphyrias. The disease most often begins in middle-aged individuals but can develop earlier. Prior to the widespread use of oral contraceptives, PCT developed predominantly in males. Brunsting's experience at the Mayo Clinic clearly illustrates this point because of 34 patients, 26 were male and more than 90 percent consumed moderate to heavy amounts of alcohol.[10]

In contrast, the experience of Grossman et al. indicates that the sex incidence is approximately equal[157]; in this series, 21 patients were male and 19 were female. The rising incidence of PCT in females is probably due to the widespread ingestion of estrogens in oral contraceptives or in hormone supplements.[178] It should be noted that males treated with estrogens, for example as adjunctive therapy for carcinoma of the prostate, have also developed PCT.

Clinical Manifestations

Vesicles and bullae occur predominantly in areas subject to repeated trauma (see Figs. 150-13 to 150-15). There is an increased skin fragility, usually on the dorsa of the hands but occasionally on the feet as well (Fig. 150-15). The traumatized skin becomes crusted and, as the lesions resolve, areas of scarring may ensue. Numerous small milia can develop, particularly on the fingers and hands. These are pearly white to yellow, spherical subepidermal inclusions 1 to 5 mm in diameter and characteristically they are present in each of the hepatic porphyrias with cutaneous photosensitivity (PCT and VP) (Figs. 150-14, -15). Although the cutaneous

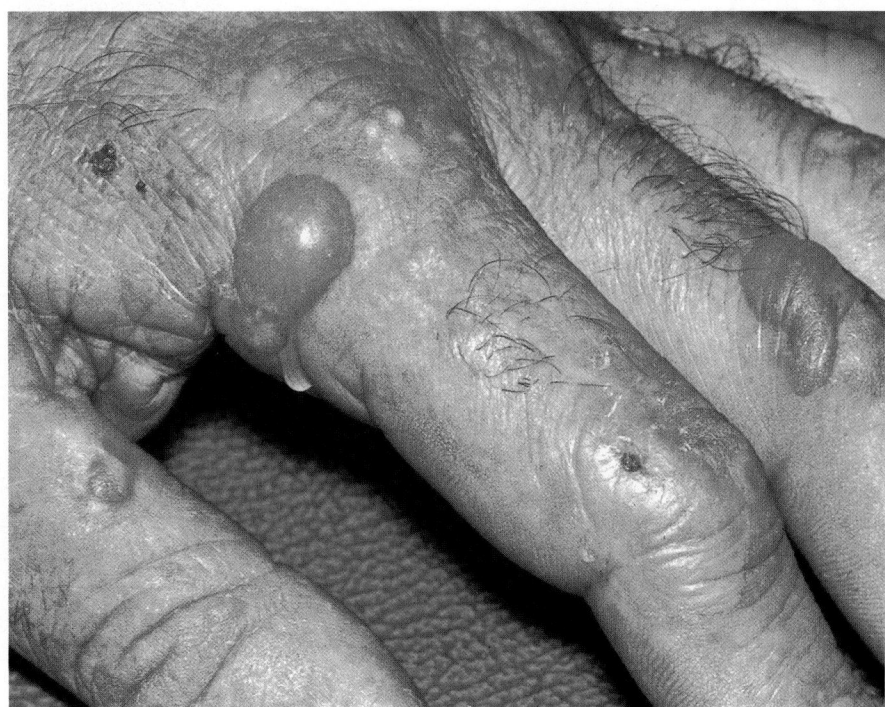

FIGURE 150-13 A case of porphyria cutanea tarda showing bullae filled with clear fluid. Elsewhere are remnants of blisters, and on the second metacarpophalangeal joint are small white papules of hard consistency (milia). On the index finger there is a pink atrophic scar.

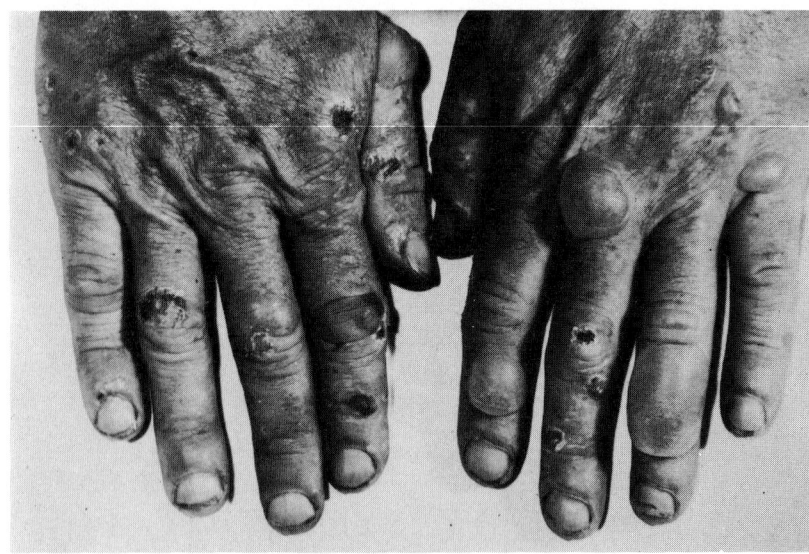

FIGURE 150-14 A case of porphyria cutanea tarda showing bullae and erosions on the hands. (*Courtesy of A. Wiskemann, M.D., and J. Kimmig, M.D., University Skin Clinic, Hamburg.*)

lesions are primarily seen on the light-exposed areas, patients are often unaware that sunlight plays a role in producing their lesions because the acute photosensitivity, so characteristic of the erythropoietic porphyrias, is rare in PCT (Fig. 150-16). However, most patients do recognize that their skin condition worsens in the spring and summer and seems to improve in the fall and winter. Porphyrin excretion in PCT appears to increase in summer months and decrease in winter months.[179] It remains unknown whether increased duration of sun exposure and photocatalyzed oxidation of porphyrin precursors account for this seasonal variation in porphyrin excretion and clinical expression of the disease.

Other skin changes seen in PCT include hyperpigmentation and hypopigmentation that may be mottled, resembling chloasma (Fig. 150-17). There may be an associated purplish red ("heliotrope") suffusion of the central part of the face, particularly involv-

ing the periorbital areas, which may bear a striking resemblance to the plethora seen in polycythemia rubra vera (see Fig. 150-17). This is not seen in the porphyrias of bone marrow origin.

Hypertrichosis (nonvirilizing) is a useful diagnostic sign that often brings the female patient to the dermatologist (Fig. 150-18). Facial hypertrichosis develops gradually and is more apparent in

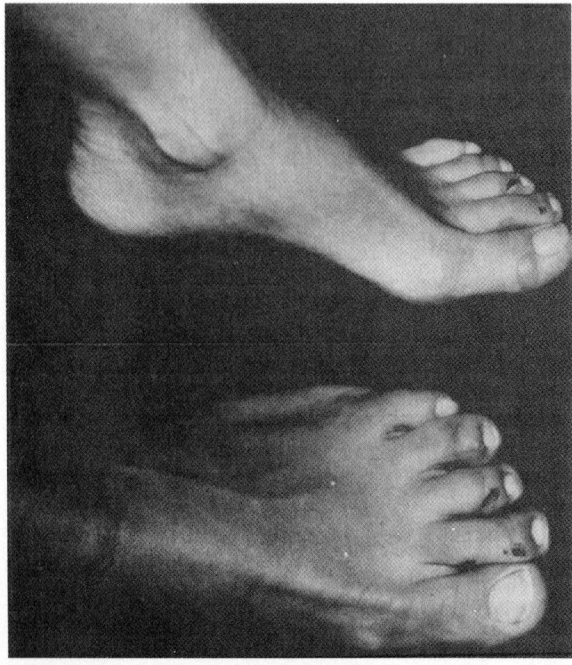

FIGURE 150-15 A bullous eruption with erosions on the feet in a patient with porphyria cutanea tarda.

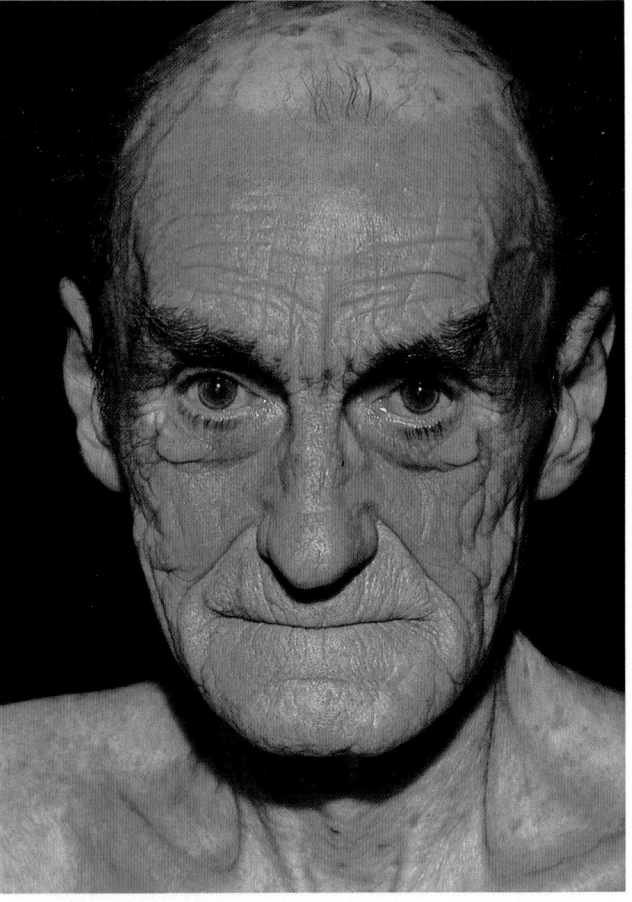

FIGURE 150-16 Porphyria cutanea tarda. Purple-red suffusion ("heliotrope") of central facial skin, most pronounced in the periorbital areas; hypermelanosis in sun-exposed areas.

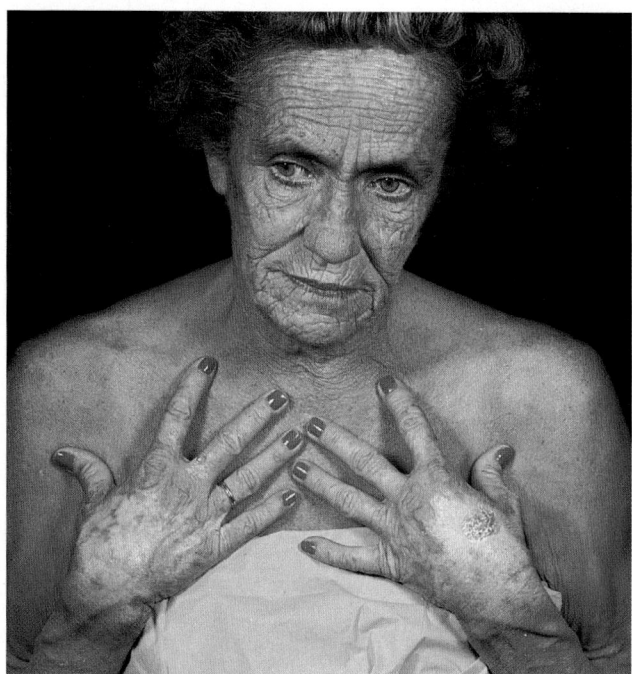

FIGURE 150-17 Porphyria cutanea tarda. The patient exhibits marked "wrinkling" of the face and depigmented scars on the dorsa of the hands.

females. The hair may vary in texture between fine and coarse and in color between light and dark. These hairs are particularly prominent along the temples and the cheeks but may occasionally involve the trunk and extremities in severe cases. Such hair may continue to grow, darken, and thicken, particularly on the cheeks, the forehead between the eyes, and at the hairline of the scalp. Males may complain that shaving is more difficult and that the growth pattern of their beard has changed. Hypertrichosis may be the presenting symptom in women, and a particularly severe form of hypertrichosis may occur in younger children with PCT. In the reports of HCB poisoning in Turkey, some of the children were described as "monkey-like" because of marked hypertrichosis.[180] The mechanism of this phenomenon is unknown; androgen levels are reported to be normal. It is possible that surface receptors or growth factors for hair bulb keratinocytes are activated by the dual action of light and porphyrins. The hypertrichosis of PCT usually improves slowly following appropriate treatment with phlebotomies.

Sclerodermoid plaques (Fig. 150-18) may develop on both light-exposed and light-protected body areas. These are usually scattered, waxy yellow to white, indurated plaques that closely resemble, both clinically and histopathologically, morphea or scleroderma. There is some evidence to indicate that PCT may occur concomitantly with true scleroderma but this seems to be quite rare. As discussed earlier, URO I stimulates collagen synthesis in human skin fibroblasts.[82] In some patients, calcification has developed in these sclerodermoid plaques, necessitating excision and grafting.

PCT-like syndromes are occasionally seen in association with other conditions, including hepatic tumors,[181] hepatitis,[182] and lupus erythematosus.[183] Subepidermal bullous dermatoses mimicking PCT clinically and histologically have been described (see "Pseudoporphyria" below). A number of cases have occurred in patients with renal failure undergoing hemodialysis.[184] Associations with sarcoidosis[185] and Sjögren's syndrome[186] have also been reported.

PCT and Human Immunodeficiency Virus (HIV)/AIDS

In 1987, the first reported association between PCT and HIV was described in which three men with cutaneous symptoms and biochemical signs of PCT developed AIDS.[187] Since then, additional HIV infected patients have been reported with PCT.[188] In many patients the signs and symptoms of PCT preceded the diagnosis of HIV infection, whereas in others they followed the diagnosis. The risk factors for HIV infection include homosexuality, transfusion, and intravenous drug abuse. Although the pathophysiology of this association is not understood, it has been suggested that the virus may lead to impairment of hepatic function, resulting in the clinical manifestations of PCT.[187]

Pseudoporphyria

This term is used to describe patients who clinically exhibit cutaneous manifestations of PCT without the characteristic abnormal porphyrin profile. This disorder may develop in association with ingestion of certain drugs such as furosemide,[189] nalidixic acid,[190] tetracycline,[191] naproxen,[192] and pyridoxine.[193] In the drug-induced type of pseudoporphyria, the blistering process is subepidermal with little or no dermal inflammation. Staining with PAS reveals little or no deposition around upper dermal blood vessels and capillary walls. Indirect immunofluorescence studies conducted on split skin reveal no dermal deposition of fluorescent material in pseudoporphyria.[192] Direct immunofluorescence studies have shown patchy granular deposition of IgG and C3 at the basement membrane zone in pseudoporphyria, PCT, and in epidermolysis bullosa acquisita (EBA).

In unpublished observations involving a few recent cases of pseudoporphyria, homogeneous diffuse staining to all classes of immunoglobulins and albumin was also observed in the membrane propria of eccrine ducts, the perineurium, and around deeper vessels. Whether this is characteristic for pseudoporphyria or can be observed in PCT remains to be established.

A bullous dermatosis that is morphologically and histologically indistinguishable from PCT has also been observed in patients with chronic renal failure receiving maintenance hemodialysis. Initially, porphyrin levels in urine, stool, and plasma were found to be in the normal range.[194] Although it was believed that no porphyrin abnormalities occurred in these patients, subsequent studies revealed that true PCT with excess porphyrins can develop in some dialyzed patients.[184] An additional subset of patients undergoing long-term hemodialysis may exhibit increased plasma porphyrin levels, even though there is no clinical evidence of porphyria. This appears to be related to binding of porphyrins to nondialyzable plasma proteins.

Laboratory Findings

Virtually all patients with PCT have excessive total body iron stores manifested as increased serum iron, ferritin, and/or hepatocellular iron. Occasionally, there is mild erythrocytosis and cryoglobulinemia.[195] An abnormal glucose tolerance test occurs in 25 percent of patients.

Patients with PCT excrete increased amounts of porphyrins in the urine, which may exhibit characteristic pink-red fluorescence when examined with a Wood's lamp. The porphyrin excretion pattern of PCT (see Table 150-9) has three main features: (1) increased urinary excretion of URO and of other acetate-substituted porphyrins, (2) a distinctive pattern of excretion of isomer series I and III

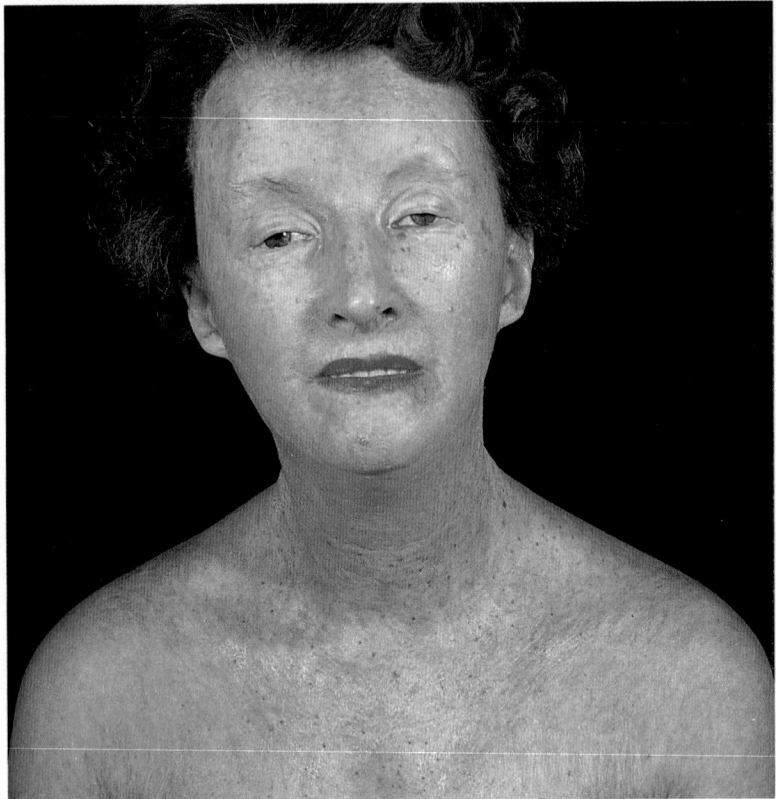

a

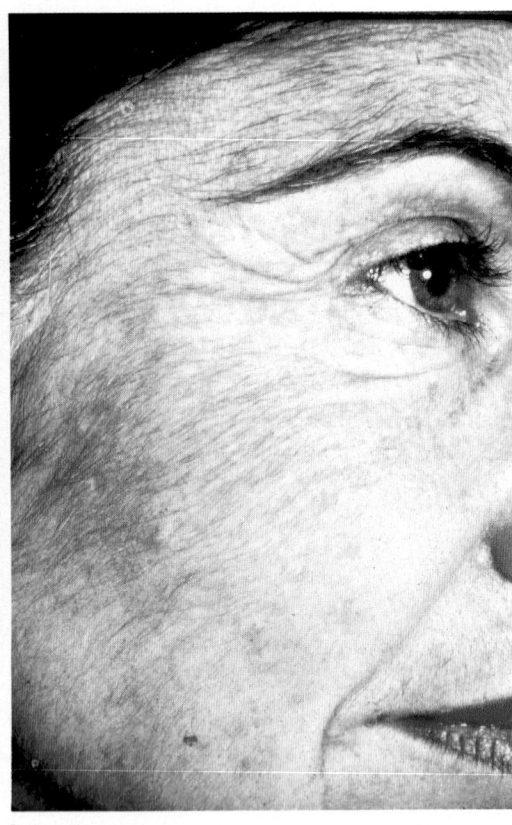

b

FIGURE 150-18 Porphyria cutanea tarda. (*a*) Well-demarcated, shiny, sclerodermoid plaques on the chest. (*b*) Facial hypertrichosis in a female patient with porphyria cutanea tarda who received estrogen therapy. Thick black hair growth is seen on the cheeks and in the periorbital region. This growth of hair often extends to the forehead. (*Reproduced with permission of Yearbook of Dermatology, Chicago, Year Book, 1975 and Professor L. C. Harber.*)

porphyrins, and (3) increased excretion of fecal ISOCOPRO.[196,197] PCT patients excrete greatly increased amounts of urinary 8-carboxyl URO and also porphyrins with 7-, 6-, and 5-carboxyl groups; 4-carboxyl porphyrin (COPRO) is also increased but to a lesser extent than URO and rarely surpasses 600 μg per 24 h (see Table 150-3). In PCT, the hepatic UROGEN decarboxylase deficiency results in the accumulation of 5-carboxylporphyrinogen III (Figs. 150-1 and 150-2). This can be utilized as a substrate by the enzyme COPROGEN oxidase and it forms dehydroisocoproporphyrinogen, which in turn is oxidized to ISOCOPRO, resulting in the characteristic elevation of this compound in the feces of these patients.

The 8-carboxyl URO and 7-carboxyl porphyrins are the predominant urinary porphyrins in PCT (>90 percent of total porphyrins). The urinary porphyrin excretion pattern is a mixture of type I and type III isomers. URO is about 60 percent type I isomer and 40 percent type III; the 7- and 6-carboxyl porphyrins are >90 percent type III and <10 percent type I isomer; the 5- and 4-carboxyl porphyrins are about 50 percent each isomer. This distinctive isomer pattern is found consistently in patients with PCT.[197]

In general, only trace amounts of URO are present in the stools of normal individuals. The porphyrin content of stool is increased in PCT and consists primarily of ISOCOPRO (type III), 7-carboxyl porphyrin, and lesser amounts of URO and COPRO. The total daily 24-h fecal porphyrin excretion may exceed total urinary porphyrin excretion.

The ratio of URO to COPRO in the urine is often helpful in differentiating PCT and VP. Thus, in PCT, the URO:COPRO ratio is usually >3:1, whereas in VP the ratio is usually <1:1. Occasionally, 24-h urine porphyrins will be normal or only slightly increased in a patient with the cutaneous findings of PCT. This should alert the physician to evaluate stool porphyrins as these are elevated in patients with VP (see "Variegate Porphyria" below).

The constellation of clinical and laboratory findings, including examination of the urine with a readily available Wood's lamp, often suffices to make the tentative diagnosis of PCT. Suspected PCT can frequently be confirmed by acidifying a random urine sample with a few drops of 10% hydrochloric acid or acetic acid and looking for orange-red fluorescence. The sensitivity of the screening test can be enhanced by addition of a small amount of talcum powder to a 5-mL sample of urine, shaking, centrifuging, and examining the talc pellet for fluorescence. If in doubt, this test can be modified as follows[198]: To 5 mL of urine (freshly voided or 24-h specimen), add 5 to 10 drops (0.5 mL) glacial acetic acid and 2.5 mL ethyl acetate. Shake and allow to settle. Examine the upper aqueous layer with a Wood's lamp for characteristic red-pink porphyrin fluorescence.

It should be emphasized that patients who appear clinically to have PCT may have a negative urine fluorescent screening test for porphyrins. In such patients, it is absolutely essential to perform quantitative 24-h urine URO and COPRO determinations and stool PROTO and COPRO determinations, which often permit differentiation of PCT from VP. However, some patients with VP will have normal fecal porphyrin excretion, and recent studies indicate that bile porphyrin measurements may be helpful in evaluating such patients.[199]

Biochemical tests for liver function may be performed to identify liver disease. Elevated serum transaminases and γ-glutamyl-transpeptidase levels may occur. Serum iron and ferritin concentrations may be elevated. The measurement of erythrocyte UROGEN decarboxylase is useful for detection of mutant-gene carriers in pedigrees having a proband with familial PCT.[200]

Histopathology

The characteristic histopathologic finding in PCT is a subepidermal bulla (Figs. 150-19 and 150-20). Bullae characteristically show a corrugated, undulating base that has been termed *festooned*.[201] There is little or no inflammatory infiltrate. PAS stain reveals a mild degree of thickening of the papillary vessel wall, not nearly so marked as that seen in patients with EPP. Reticulin staining demonstrates slight proliferation of fibers along the basement membrane. Direct immunofluorescence studies reveal deposition of C3 and IgG in a granular pattern at the dermal-epidermal junction and in and around vessel walls in affected individuals.[86] These changes are most apparent in sun-exposed areas of patients with active disease and high urinary porphyrin excretion, and they decrease substantially in patients after appropriate treatment. It is also possible that the deposition of immunoglobulins and complement is a nonspecific result of injury to the cutaneous tissue. The locus of damage to the upper dermal vessels and the dermal-epidermal junction suggests that damage to these areas evoked by porphyrin photosensitivity may be responsible for the unique skin fragility seen in PCT. Several studies have shown increased porphyrin concentrations in the skin of patients with PCT.[202,203] With rare exception, blisters have not been induced by phototesting; however, Rimington et al.,[204] using a monochromator, have been able to produce both erythema and delayed edema in the skin of patients with PCT.

Differential Diagnosis

Other dermatoses that can be confused with PCT include VP, HEP, HCP, pseudoporphyria, scleroderma, and the acquired type of epidermolysis bullosa. Each of these can be differentiated on histopathologic grounds, by immunofluorescence tests, or by appropri-

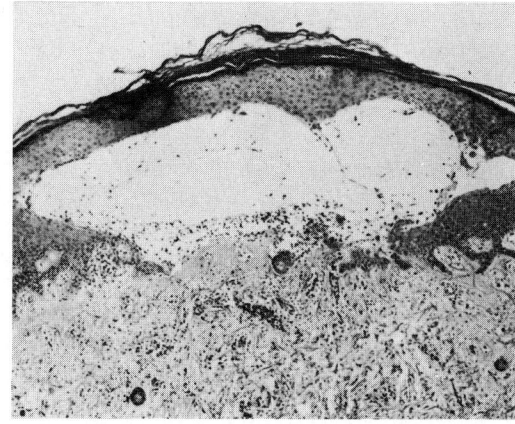

FIGURE 150-19 Porphyria cutanea tarda: subepidermal vesiculation in an early lesion. The subepidermal vesiculation of porphyria may occur with only a sparse, inflammatory cell infiltrate. ×40. (*Courtesy of W. H. Clark, Jr., M.D., University of Pennsylvania.*)

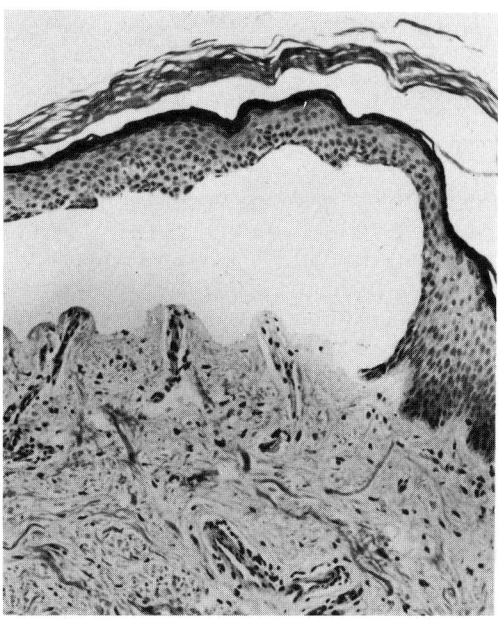

FIGURE 150-20 Porphyria cutanea tarda: subepidermal vesiculation in a late lesion. There is virtually no inflammatory response, but the form of the dermal papillae is partially preserved. ×100. (*Courtesy of W. H. Clark, Jr., M.D., University of Pennsylvania.*)

ate porphyrin studies. Careful evaluation of urine, stool, plasma, or bile porphyrins will almost always permit confirmation of the diagnosis of PCT. It should be emphasized that patients with PCT are not prone to the acute life-threatening attacks characteristic of the acute hepatic porphyrias. A very limited number of drugs and chemicals, particularly alcohol, estrogens, and selected halogenated hydrocarbons, seem capable of eliciting the disease in susceptible individuals (Table 150-11). Drugs such as barbiturates, which are contraindicated in AIP, have been administered to PCT patients without untoward effect. Nonsteroidal anti-inflammatory drugs such as naproxen, antibiotics such as the tetracyclines and nalidixic acid, and a variety of other agents may rarely produce clinical signs closely resembling PCT (see ''Pseudoporphyria'' above). VP has skin lesions identical to PCT. However, in VP, stool PROTO and COPRO excretion is usually increased (PROTO > COPRO), and urinary porphyrin levels are only moderately increased (COPRO > URO).[199,200] In PCT, stool ISOCOPRO is elevated, and total urinary porphyrin (URO > COPRO) is much higher than that observed in VP.

Treatment

Initially, a careful history should be taken in an effort to identify an environmental toxin, e.g., alcohol, estrogen, or chlorinated hydrocarbon, that may have triggered the disease. These should be strictly avoided if possible; often this alone can lead to gradual improvement. However, in most patients with PCT, more aggressive treatment is usually appropriate to accelerate the rate of clinical and biochemical improvement, and this currently consists of either repeated phlebotomy[205,206] or orally administered antimalarials, either chloroquine or hydroxychloroquine,[207,208] or a combination of both.[209] Other forms of treatment that have been described include administration of iron chelators,[210,211] oral administration of cholestyramine,[212] and, more recently, the combination of genetically engineered erythropoietin combined with phlebotomy in one patient with concomitant anemia secondary to chronic renal failure.[213]

Phlebotomy Phlebotomy is the treatment of choice for PCT. Numerous reports have emphasized the safety and efficacy of this form of therapy,[205,214] which was introduced by Ippen in 1961. Phlebotomy is effective because it depletes the excessive hepatic iron stores characteristic of PCT. Biochemical remission of PCT has occurred in patients treated with phlebotomy who had iron overload as well as in patients with quantitatively normal iron stores. Replenishment of iron following phlebotomy-induced remission of PCT may result in biochemical and clinical exacerbation of the disease.[169] Abstinence from the porphyrinogenic agent alone, especially alcohol, may induce a clinical and biochemical remission, although this may take months to years.

There are several interesting hypotheses concerning the mechanism whereby phlebotomy-induced depletion of excess iron leads to improvement in PCT and these include the following:

1. *Iron effect on ALA synthase.* Iron can enhance the induction response of ALA synthase to drugs and the hepatic porphyrinogenic response to HCB in experimental animals, and its depletion could render ALA synthase less inducible and thereby diminish hepatic porphyrinogenesis.[169]
2. *Iron depletion effects on other heme pathway enzymes.* The studies of Kushner et al.,[170,175] showing that ferrous iron inhibits UROGEN decarboxylase and increases the rate of hepatic porphyrin synthesis from ALA or PBG, suggest that removal of iron can allow UROGEN decarboxylase activity to return to normal and/or reduce excessive porphyrinogenesis.
3. *Iron effects on hepatic lipid peroxidation.* Iron depletion could reverse this response of the liver to iron overload.[173]
4. *Iron effects on oxidation of URO.* Removal of iron could result in a diminished capacity of the ferrous metal to irreversibly oxidize the UROGEN substrate to nonmetabolizable porphyrins.[215]

Phlebotomy can be carried out as an ambulatory procedure. The total amount of blood removed has varied widely, usually ranging from 1500 to 12,000 mL. It is most convenient to use plastic blood-drawing bags available in any blood bank. Approximately 500 mL of blood is removed at weekly or biweekly intervals until the hemoglobin decreases to approximately 10g/dL or until the serum iron drops to 50 to 60 μg/dL. Patients are strongly encouraged to discontinue or decrease exposure to porphyrinogenic agents as this usually hastens clinical and biochemical remission.

It is particularly important to reassure the patient that clinical improvement may not become apparent for variable intervals after beginning the phlebotomies. Porphyrin excretion continues to fall long after phlebotomies are discontinued. Ramsay et al.[214] have shown that in more than 90 percent of patients treated with regular phlebotomy, urinary URO excretion reached normal levels (<100 μg per 24 h) after 5 to 12 months. Blistering is the first sign to disappear, followed by improvement in skin fragility and in hypertrichosis over a period of 3 to 18 months. Even sclerodermoid changes can resolve slowly, although this may take several years. There is little or no published information on long-term follow-up of treatment, but most relapsed patients have again responded to repeated courses of phlebotomies.[206] The length of remission induced by phlebotomy varies widely and ranges from 6 months to more than 10 years. At least 10 to 20 percent of patients will relapse within 1 year.

Phlebotomy is a safe, effective, and relatively simple form of therapy with minimum associated morbidity. A few patients may complain of mild to moderate fatigue and weakness during the treatment period, but this usually resolves as the hemoglobin returns to normal. Phlebotomy remains the treatment of choice for uncomplicated PCT.

Antimalarials In some patients, phlebotomy is not recommended or is contraindicated owing to the presence of anemia or cardiopulmonary disorders or HIV infection. In such cases low-dose antimalarial therapy may be useful. The antimalarial aminoquinolines, chloroquine (Aralen) and hydroxychloroquine (Plaquenil), have been recommended for treating PCT.[207,208] In 1957, London[216] first suggested that chloroquine was useful in treating PCT. The cutaneous signs of the disease cleared within 1 year in one patient who received 500 mg daily for several months. However, such doses will trigger severe hepatotoxicity in many PCT patients and this is no longer an acceptable approach. Experience with low doses has proven that such a toxic response is not necessary for therapeutic benefit.[208,209] The clinical and biochemical remission of PCT obtained with chloroquine appears to be identical in all respects to that evoked by phlebotomy. However, it has been reported that rapid relapse occurred in several patients treated with hydroxychloroquine.[217] There is a marked increase in urinary URO excretion in patients receiving higher doses of the antimalarial. The effect of chloroquine seems to be due to rapid removal of a drug-porphyrin complex from the liver.[218] Taljaard et al.,[219] however, feel that chloroquine chelates to iron in the hepatocyte and that the bound iron is then excreted.

Low-dose (125 mg twice weekly) chloroquine therapy has been shown to be effective in PCT. The concept of using low-dose chloroquine therapy to reduce the severity of the hepatotoxic effect in PCT was first suggested by Saltzer et al.[220] Remission of the disease was obtained in a single patient who received 50 mg of chloroquine twice weekly for 7 months. Taljaard et al.[219] extended these studies and reported good results in seven of eight PCT patients treated with chloroquine sulfate (330 mg base) twice weekly for several months. Kordac et al.[208] have reported the successful use of low-dose chloroquine (125 mg twice weekly for 8 to 18 months) in more than 100 patients with PCT. Complete clinical and biochemical remission occurred in all patients. Furthermore, the majority of these patients remained in remission for at least 4 years.

The authors suggest the following regimen for chloroquine administration in PCT. After obtaining baseline urinary porphyrin values and liver function tests, a single "test dose" of chloroquine base of 125 mg is administered. Liver function tests are repeated in 1 week, and if there are no abnormalities, the drug is then administered in doses of 125 mg twice weekly. Liver function tests and urinary porphyrins are monitored bi-monthly, and the medication continued until urinary URO is <100 μg per 24 h. This usually requires 6 to 12 months of treatment. Studies comparing the therapeutic efficacy of phlebotomy with that of low-dose chloroquine have verified the efficacy of each.[221,222]

Swanbeck and Wennersten[209] suggest that the combination of phlebotomy and chloroquine treatment may reduce the severity of the hepatotoxic response to chloroquine and also induce remission of the disease. Patients are treated with a series of one to four phlebotomies prior to starting chloroquine (250 mg daily for 7 days). The procedure is repeated when signs of biochemical or clinical relapse develop, which may occur in 1 to 2 years.

It should be emphasized that despite the tendency of the antimalarials to evoke hepatotoxic responses in patients with PCT, there is no evidence to suggest that the changes in hepatocellular pathology characteristic of PCT worsen as a result of treatment with these drugs.[223] The antimalarials may cause retinopathy, and the low-dose regimen helps to minimize the risk of this complication. Pretreatment and semiannual ophthalmologic examinations should be obtained on patients treated with these drugs.

Acute Intermittent Porphyria (AIP)
(Table 150-12)

Synonyms include Swedish porphyria and pyrroloporphyria.

Historical Aspects

The disease has been known since the late nineteenth century. The first detailed clinical description of AIP was that of Waldenström[9] who described a total of 179 cases in Sweden. Of these, 103 were said to have acute porphyria characterized by periodic attacks of abdominal pain with constipation, nervous and mental symptoms, and paralysis. This was accompanied by increased urinary excretion of PBG. Several excellent reviews have summarized the clinical and biochemical features of AIP.[26,224,225] The disease may affect the peripheral, autonomic, or central nervous systems with neuropathic symptoms and dysfunction.

Several groups showed that increased hepatic ALA synthase activity occurred in AIP.[36,225] It is now clear that the enzyme PBG deaminase, which converts PBG to UROGEN I, is deficient in various tissues of affected individuals and latent carriers of the disease. This helps to explain the excessive ALA and PBG excretion of AIP. PBG deaminase activity in AIP is approximately 50 percent of that in unaffected normal individuals, consistent with an autosomal dominant mode of inheritance. The decreased PBG deaminase may lead to a partial block in heme synthesis, which in turn decreases the regulatory heme pool and leads to derepression of the synthesis of mRNA for ALA synthase.

A most important concept is that, although AIP appears to be inherited as an autosomal dominant trait, most latent carriers of the PBG deaminase defect never express the clinical phenotype.[200] The gene defect alone seems to be inconsequential unless the individual is exposed to precipitating factors, among which are drugs (see Table 150-11).[226,227]

Genetics

AIP has been thoroughly studied from the perspective of genetics using the techniques of molecular biology. The disease manifests considerable genetic pleomorphism that relates to varying mutations of PBG deaminase.[200] Grandchamp et al.[228] have shown tissue-specific expression of PBG deaminase in AIP. An additional peptide of 17 amino acid residues at the NH_2 terminus of the nonerythropoietic isoform accounts for its increased molecular mass. Furthermore, the smaller erythroid form is limited to that compartment.

Three intragenic restriction fragment length polymorphisms (RFLPs) have been identified in AIP and can be used for linkage analysis and presymptomatic carrier detection.[229] The polymerase chain reaction (PCR) has been used to amplify a 3.3-kb genomic fragment of the human PBG deaminase gene in which these restriction sites are located.[230] The technique was shown to be capable of detecting asymptomatic carriers of the defective enzyme.

Epidemiology

AIP is an autosomal dominant disease which is rarely, if ever, manifested before puberty. Most published series emphasize the female predominance of affected patients, ranging from ratios of 1.5:1 to 2.0:1.[26] The incidence in the human population is approximately 1.5:100,000 in most areas of the world. However, in Scandinavia, particularly Lapland, Waldenström[9] has shown that the incidence is much higher (1:1000).

Clinical Manifestations (see Table 150-12)

All of the clinical signs and symptoms of AIP may be related to the effects of porphyrin precursors on the autonomic nervous system.[2] The acute attack is characterized by abdominal pain and neurologic and psychiatric symptoms and is often precipitated by ingestion of drugs such as those listed in Table 150-11. Acute attacks of AIP are accompanied by seizures, especially in patients with hyponatremia resulting from vomiting and inappropriate fluid therapy.

There are no cutaneous lesions related to photosensitivity in AIP. This is logical as the abnormal excretion pattern of the disease consists mostly of the porphyrin precursors ALA and PBG, which are not photosensitizers.

TABLE 150-12
Acute Intermittent Porphyria

Synonym	Swedish porphyria
Inheritance	Autosomal dominant
Age of onset	10 to 40; extremely rare prior to puberty
Incidence	1.5:100,000; more common in Scandinavia and Lapland
Photosensitivity	Absent
Skin reactions	None
Clinical findings	Acute attacks with a neurovisceral symptom complex; this includes abdominal pain, constipation, nausea, vomiting, abdominal distension, muscle weakness occasionally leading to paralysis and death; motor neuropathy; bizarre, neurotic or psychotic behavior; acute attacks often precipitated by drugs, hormones (progesterone, estrogen), and nutritional factors, including starvation
Biochemical defects	Excretory: Elevated ALA and PBG in the urine during and between attacks; stool porphyrins are normal Erythrocytes: Normal porphyrins Enzymatic: 50% PBG deaminase deficiency in liver, RBC, lymphocytes, and skin fibroblasts; increased hepatic ALA synthase; hormones, drugs, and nutritional factors may increase ALA synthase; decreased hepatic sex steroid 5-α-reductase
Management	High carbohydrate diet, intravenous glucose, or hematin, and avoidance of drugs known to exacerbate porphyria

These patients usually have abdominal pain (80 to 90 percent) during an acute attack (between attacks patients are often completely symptom free). The pain may be diffuse or localized and is often intermittent and spastic. Vomiting and constipation are frequently associated. Mild fever and leukocytosis may occur, making differential diagnosis extremely difficult. This is one reason many patients with AIP undergo repeated exploratory laparotomies before the diagnosis is finally established.

Peripheral neuropathy is a major part of the clinical syndrome in many patients. This may vary from localized pain and weakness to complete generalized flaccid paralysis. Patients may succumb to the disease, usually due to respiratory failure, or may improve slowly, although residual muscle weakness may persist for extended periods in some cases.

Laboratory Findings

The primary biochemical abnormality in AIP is PBG deaminase deficiency, which causes excessive urinary excretion of ALA and PBG. Urinary porphyrins may also be elevated (Table 150-3). Urinary excretion of ALA and PBG as high as 100 mg/24 h may occur during an acute attack. During clinical remission of the disease, urinary excretion of ALA and PBG decreases but usually remains above normal values. This is in contrast to patients with VP who often exhibit normal urinary excretion of ALA and PBG between acute attacks.

Two rapid screening tests are available to test freshly voided urine for increased PBG. The first is simply to expose the urine to bright sunlight for several hours. Darkening to a deep red color suggests that PBG is present but does not prove it. (Porphobilin, another dark pigment, can also be photocatalytically formed in urine.) The second rapid screening test, known as the Hoesch test, is also a simple procedure for detecting excessive urinary PBG.[231] To 2 mL of Ehrlich's reagent (3 g of p-dimethylaminobenzaldehyde dissolved in 125 mL of acetic acid and 24 mL of perchloric acid) 2 drops of fresh urine are added. A uniform cherry-red color of the sample indicates a positive reaction. This test is based upon the formation of a chromogen by PBG and Ehrlich's aldehyde reagent that produces a red pigment with strong absorbance at 552 nm. The well-known Watson-Schwartz test is based on this same principle, although a number of refinements have helped to enhance its accuracy.[232] In patients with suspected AIP, quantitative 24-h measurement of urinary ALA and PBG is essential.

Histopathology

Histopathologic findings of skin are unremarkable.

Differential Diagnosis

The clinical manifestations of AIP are so variable and resemble so many different diseases that Waldenström has used the term *little imitator* to describe it.[9,11] Several excellent reviews have summarized the differential clinical features of AIP.[26]

Treatment

Although there is still no specific treatment for AIP, several therapeutic modalities have been used, including glucose loading, hematin infusion, and administration of a gonadotropin-releasing hormone analogue.[233–235] Avoidance of precipitating factors such as drugs (Table 150-11), sex steroid hormones, starvation, etc., are important preventive measures. AIP patients should be provided with medical warning bracelets and with lists of drugs to avoid. A list of drugs thought to be safe for AIP patients is provided in Table 150-13.

Variegate Porphyria (VP) (Table 150-14)

Synonyms include South African porphyria, PCT hereditaria, mixed porphyria, and protocoproporphyria.

Historical Aspects

This disease has been a source of confusion among the human porphyrias. In 1957, Waldenström revised his original 1937 classification of the porphyrias and described two different types of PCT: PCT symptomatica and PCT hereditaria (protocoproporphyria).[11] PCT symptomatica was said to be the typical PCT with onset of cutaneous lesions in middle age or later, occurring predominantly in males who ingested moderate to heavy quantities of ethanol. PCT hereditaria was said to occur in individuals at a much younger age (15 to 30 years). Large amounts of PROTO and COPRO were excreted in the stool, and these patients had acute attacks indistinguishable from those of AIP. Waldenström suggested that this disease be named protocoproporphyria to separate it from PCT in which fecal porphyrins were usually elevated to a lesser extent.

Barnes[13,236] had described a similar disorder in South Africa. However, not being a physician, he found it difficult to pursue detailed clinical studies. Soon thereafter Geoffrey Dean migrated to South Africa and in collaboration with Barnes began a careful evaluation of families affected with this type of porphyria.[14,15,237] Because it presents in a variety of forms, Dean and Barnes proposed the name porphyria variegata to describe the porphyria commonly seen in the South African white population. Dean has summarized this entire adventure in a fascinating book.[238] These patients manifest intermittent attacks typical of AIP, usually following ingestion of barbiturates or sulfonamides. These attacks, predominantly af-

TABLE 150-13

Drugs Considered to be Safe (or Probably Safe) in Patients with the Acute Hepatic Porphyrias

Acetaminophen	Insulin
Adrenaline	Labetalol
Amitryptyline	Lithium
Aspirin	Mandelate
Atropine	Methenamide
Bromide	Naproxen
Cephalosporins	Narcotic analgesics
Chloralhydrates	Neostigmine
Chloramphenicol	Nitrofurantoin
Chlordiazepoxide	Nitrous oxide
Colchicine	Oxazepam
Digoxin	Penicillin and derivatives
Diphenhydramine	Phenothiazines
EDTA	Propranolol
Ether	Prostigmine
Glucocorticoids	Rauwolfia alkaloids
Guanethidine	Streptomycin
Heparin	Succinylcholine
Hyocine	Tetracycline
Hypocine	Thiouracil
Ibuprofin	Thyroxine
Indomethacin	

TABLE 150-14
Variegate Porphyria

Synonyms	Mixed porphyria; South African genetic porphyria; protocoproporphyria hereditaria; PCT hereditaria
Inheritance	Autosomal dominant
Age of onset	Usually between ages 15 to 30
Incidence	Common in South Africa (3/1000); relatively rare elsewhere
Photosensitivity	Similar to PCT (see Table 150-9)
Skin lesions	Similar to PCT (see Table 150-9)
Clinical findings	Neurovisceral symptomatology similar to AIP; acute attacks similar to AIP precipitated by barbiturates, dapsone, and drugs (estrogens); history of acute episodes of abdominal pain, nausea, vomiting, behavioral disturbances, paralysis, and seizures
Biochemical defects	Excretory: Increased PROTO, COPRO, and X-porphyrins (ether-acetic acid insoluble) in feces; PROTO > COPRO III; increased ALA and PBG in urine during acute attacks; normal between attacks
	Enzymatic: Decreased PROTOGEN oxidase in fibroblasts, some evidence for decreased ferrochelatase; increased hepatic ALA synthase
Management	Avoidance of precipitating factors (drugs); treatment for neurovisceral symptoms similar to AIP, photoprotection for photosensitivity

fecting females, are identical to those described in Waldenström's patients with AIP, and most, if not all, such acute attacks could be avoided by eliminating exposure to inducing drugs. Furthermore, Dean was able to obtain detailed histories and family trees from the patients and subsequently saw numerous family members, predominantly males, with a clinical picture practically identical to that of PCT, hence the name VP. The disease has now been recognized worldwide.[16,17]

Etiology

Dowdle et al.[225] have shown that hepatic ALA synthase is elevated in the liver of patients with VP just as in those with AIP. This is a nonspecific finding as it occurs in each of the acute hepatic porphyrias. A 50 percent decrease in PROTOGEN oxidase activity is now recognized as the primary enzyme defect in VP.[51] The enzyme acts specifically on PROTOGEN IX, the penultimate step in heme synthesis, and cannot catalyze the oxidation of COPROGEN I or III or UROGEN I.

Genetics

The gene for PROTOGEN oxidase has not yet been cloned. Homozygous cases of VP have been described.[239]

Epidemiology

This form of porphyria is quite common among the white and so-called Cape-coloured South Africans because of the "founder" effect. A high proportion of the present white population is descended from a pair of early Dutch settlers who emigrated to South Africa from Holland in 1680.[14,15] The disease is inherited as an autosomal dominant trait, and the incidence in South Africa is the highest in the world, approximately 1:300 individuals in the white population.

The cutaneous manifestations of PCT and VP are for the most part indistinguishable. Among the native black population of South Africa, typical PCT without associated acute attacks also occurs.[143] There is apparently no family history, and porphyrin excretion patterns are as for PCT, not VP. Excessive intake of home-brewed spirits (Kaffir beer) and dietary overload of iron from cooking ves-

sels are considered important factors in the development of this disease. Thus VP occurring in the descendants of the Dutch immigrants of South Africa is quite distinct from the PCT seen in the native black population. Finally, Dean has pointed out that the so-called Cape-coloured, who are descendants of white European and Indian immigrants who intermarried with black natives, may have VP and PCT in the same family.[238] Factors that precipitate or lead to activation of AIP also appear to induce VP (various drugs, starvation, etc.). All patients with suspected PCT should be screened for VP because VP has a life-threatening potential, and death can follow the ingestion of these drugs.

Clinical Manifestations

The clinical manifestations of VP include those of AIP and PCT, either or both of which may occur in the same individual. In general, females have more frequent acute attacks typical of AIP and males are more likely to have the cutaneous lesions of PCT. Two major differences between VP and PCT are: (1) the skin reactions which usually develop at an earlier age (second and third decades) as compared to PCT (fourth and fifth decades) and (2) the neurovisceral symptomatology. The clinical features of VP are: (1) positive personal or family history of chronic skin involvement with or without attacks of abdominal pain, constipation, vomiting, muscle weakness, and neuropsychiatric manifestations of stupor and coma; and (2) photocutaneous lesions associated with minor mechanical trauma. The skin lesions of VP are indistinguishable from those of PCT. These include bullae, erosions, or ulcers following minor trauma of light-exposed skin (Fig. 150-21). Hyperpigmentation, milia, hypertrichosis, and increased skin fragility are also seen. They appear to be more common in the hot climate of South Africa and are less frequently seen in cold climates. Blisters are often blood-tinged, heal slowly, and form milia with some scarring. Occasionally the patient gives a history of acute sun sensitivity occurring during or soon after a period of exposure; this may include burning, erythema, and edema. In its chronic state, the skin changes include crusting, depigmented scarring, and hypertrichosis (Fig. 150-22). The skin manifestations do not correlate with the acute attacks in most patients. These clinical and biochemical features are usually seen after puberty, except in the homozygous patients who may develop signs and symptoms at or shortly after birth.[239]

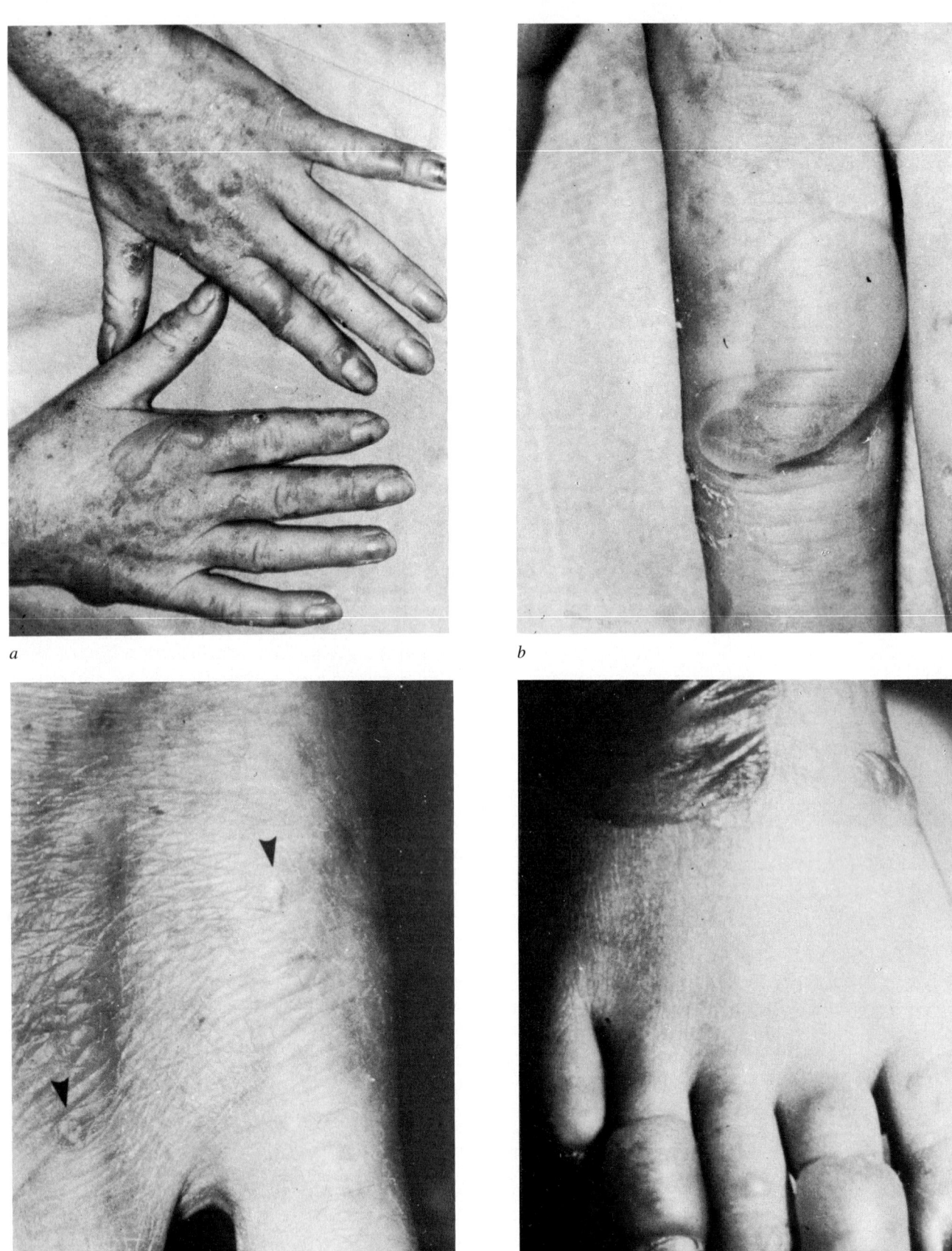

a

b

c

d

FIGURE 150-21 A case of variegate porphyria. (*a*) Blisters, crusted erosions, and pigmentary changes over the dorsa of the hands and fingers. (*b*) Close-up view of index finger shows an intact blister with milia and pigmentary changes. (*c*) Healing phase shows milia (arrows) and pigmentary changes. (*d*) Large bullae of dorsum of foot and toes. *Note:* Patients with porphyria cutanea tarda have indistinguishable cutaneous findings.

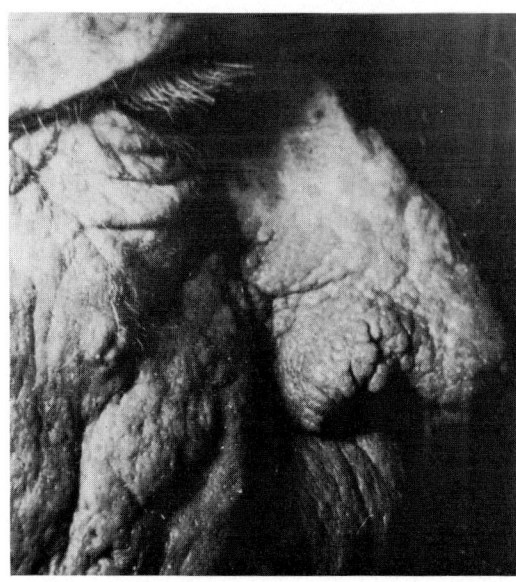

a

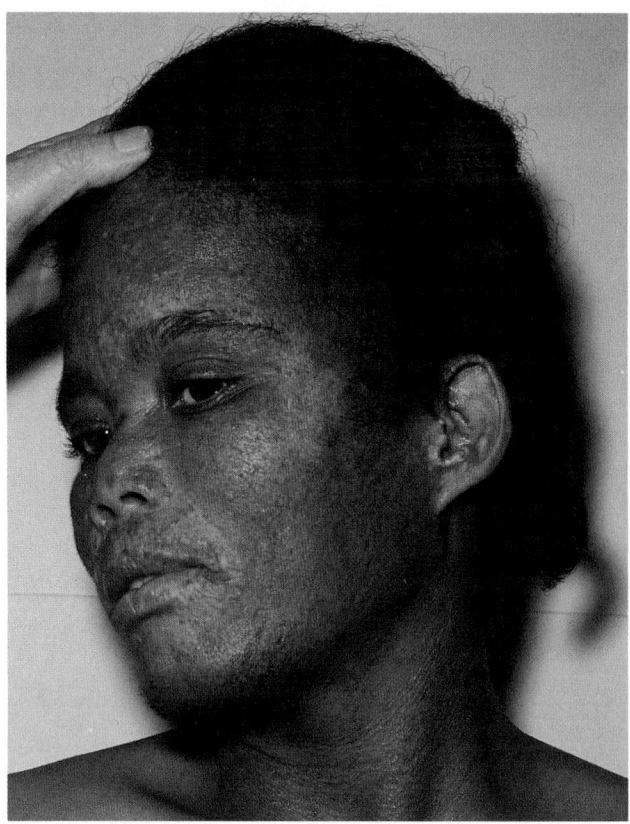

b

FIGURE 150-22   Variegate porphyria. (*a*) A peculiar leathery thickening of skin of the face of a patient chronically exposed to strong sunlight. A similar appearance has been noted in South African patients with erythropoietic protoporphyria. (*Courtesy of G. H. Findlay, M.D., F. P. Scott, M.D., and D. J. Cripps, M.D.; Br J Dermatol 78:69, 1966.*) (*b*) A South African pigmented patient showing less severe photodamage; the melanin appears to be photoprotective.

Laboratory Findings

Urinary ALA and PBG are elevated during acute attacks of VP (when the Watson-Schwartz test may be positive) but characteristically fall to normal levels between attacks (see Table 150-3), whereas in AIP patients, the urinary ALA and PBG are elevated, both during and between attacks. Another distinguishing feature of the two disorders is the stool porphyrin excretion. Asymptomatic patients with VP usually, but not always, have marked elevations of stool PROTO and COPRO between attacks.[200] These may fluctuate somewhat during acute attacks. PROTO typically exceeds COPRO. In AIP, fecal porphyrins are not elevated between attacks and usually increase only slightly during attacks. Rimington et al.[240] have suggested that a markedly hydrophilic, ether-acetic acid–insoluble porphyrin-peptide conjugate is present in the stool of patients with VP. The name X-porphyrin was given to this peculiar porphyrin, as it could only be extracted from stool with a mixture of urea and the detergent, Triton-X. Elder et al.[241] have questioned the usefulness of measuring the X-porphyrin as it was also detected in the stools of patients with active PCT; the levels overlapped considerably with those found in patients with VP.

Eales et al.[242] have suggested that certain patterns of fecal and urinary porphyrin excretion may help in distinguishing VP from PCT, e.g., urinary URO is only moderately elevated in VP and is usually less than COPRO. This is in marked contrast to active PCT where the reverse is seen, i.e., urinary URO is much higher than COPRO. Again in VP, fecal porphyrins exceed 500 μg/g dry weight in 92 percent of patients, whereas in PCT this amount of stool porphyrin is excreted by only 1 percent of patients. Furthermore, the ratio of stool PROTO to COPRO in VP usually exceeds 1.5:1, whereas in PCT the ratio is almost always <1:1 due to the increased ISOCOPRO content characteristic of this disease. Stool porphyrin excretion patterns consistent with both VP and PCT have been found in different members of single families.[150,151] These types of findings have led to the suggestion that measurement of bile porphyrins may be decisive in confirming a diagnosis of VP when excretory porphyrin patterns are ambiguous.[199]

Poh-Fitzpatrick has shown that saline-diluted plasma specimens from patients with VP have characteristic fluorescence emission spectra (626-nm emission peak) that can be used to differentiate this disease from other forms of acute porphyria, PCT, EPP, and lead poisoning (Table 150-8).[243]

Histopathology

The skin lesions of VP are subepidermal bullae indistinguishable from those of PCT.

Differential Diagnosis

The differential diagnosis of VP should be considered from two perspectives. Acute attacks of abdominal pain and neurologic signs and symptoms are identical to those described for AIP. Fecal and biliary PROTO and COPRO determinations and plasma fluorescence spectra are decisive in making the diagnosis. The skin lesions of VP are identical to those of PCT, and, as such, the differential diagnosis includes the bullous diseases as well as other photosensitivity disorders. In HCP there may be identical acute attacks, but markedly elevated fecal COPRO III is diagnostic for this disease. HEP must also be considered, but this usually begins in childhood and is characterized by markedly deficient erythrocyte UROGEN decarboxylase and elevated erythrocyte PROTO as well as increased stool ISOCOPRO. The presence of skin lesions rules out AIP. The determination of urinary ALA and PBG concentrations may help to rule out PCT and HEP. Screening of family members by measuring fecal porphyrins may also be helpful in differentiating VP and PCT.

Treatment

Preventive treatment of VP is identical to that described in AIP, i.e., avoidance of inducing drugs (see Table 150-11). Glucose loading and hematin infusions have also been used with ill-defined success. Phlebotomy and the antimalarials are not effective.[244,245]

Hereditary Coproporphyria (HCP)
(Table 150-15)

Idiopathic coproporphyria is a synonym for HCP.

Historical Aspects

This rare disorder was first described by Watson et al.[246] in two completely asymptomatic individuals who excreted large amounts of COPRO III in the feces and to a lesser extent in the urine. The condition was named HCP by Berger and Goldberg,[20] who described similar findings in a 10-year-old Swiss boy and three relatives. These individuals were also completely asymptomatic.

In 1967, Goldberg et al.[247] reported 10 cases of HCP and reviewed 20 more in the literature. They found that HCP was associated with acute attacks similar in many ways to those seen in AIP and VP, although severe neurologic sequelae seemed to occur less often. In addition, most acute attacks of HCP seemed to be precipitated by ingestion of drugs responsible for the exacerbation of AIP. During acute attacks, urinary ALA and PBG are elevated just as in AIP and VP; however, a marked elevation of fecal COPRO is diagnostic of HCP.

Cutaneous photosensitivity has been reported in some patients; many of them have associated hepatocellular dysfunction and jaundice. Brodie et al.[248] reviewed the known cases of HCP and found that 20 percent had suffered cutaneous photosensitivity reactions of

an unspecified type and 35 percent acute attacks similar to those of AIP or VP.

Etiology

The etiology of HCP is unknown. There is deficiency of COPROGEN oxidase activity in cultured skin fibroblasts, in RBC, and in leukocytes of affected individuals.[249,250] Enzyme activity is approximately 50 percent of that of normal individuals or patients with other forms of porphyria. Hepatic ALA synthase is reported to be elevated in this disease.[251]

Epidemiology

The disease appears to occur worldwide and, like AIP, to have a female preponderance and probably also an autosomal dominant transmittance. Less than 200 cases have been reported. A patient with HCP who developed AIDS has been reported.[252]

An extremely rare form of porphyria known as harderoporphyria appears to be a variant of HCP in which COPROGEN oxidase activity is very low (10 percent of control values).[253] This disease has been identified in three siblings, and it is said that these patients may be homozygous for a gene that causes HCP in some families.

Clinical Manifestations

The acute attacks are similar to those of AIP, and neurovisceral symptomatology predominates in HCP. This includes abdominal pain, vomiting, constipation, neuropathies, and psychiatric symptoms. The oral hypoglycemic agent glipizide has been reported to exacerbate a coproporphyria-like syndrome that was reversible following discontinuation of the drug.[254] Cutaneous photosensitivity occurs in 20 percent of cases.[255] In general, it appears that this disorder is not associated with acute attacks as severe as those of AIP or VP.

Laboratory Findings

HCP is characterized by increased excretion of COPRO III in urine and feces. Markedly elevated fecal COPRO, more than 90 percent of which is the III isomer, is present at all times in these patients. In

TABLE 150-15
Hereditary Coproporphyria (HCP)

Synonym	Idiopathic coproporphyria
Inheritance	Autosomal dominant
Age of onset	Any age
Incidence	Rare (less than 50 cases reported)
Photosensitivity	Occurs infrequently
Skin reactions	Usually blistering
Clinical findings	Neurovisceral symptomatology similar to but milder than that of AIP; acute attacks precipitated by barbiturates and other drugs
Biochemical defects	Excretory: Marked elevation of fecal and urinary COPRO III during and between attacks; fecal PROTO may be modestly elevated; ALA and PBG elevated during acute attacks
	Enzymatic: COPROGEN oxidase deficiency in lymphocytes and fibroblasts; increased hepatic ALA synthase
Management	Similar to AIP or VP (avoidance of precipitating factors)

addition, the feces also contain increased amounts of hepta-, hexa-, and pentacarboxylic porphyrins. Urinary COPRO III is also raised, as are ALA and PBG, during attacks. The latter usually fall to near normal levels in remission.

Histopathology

No histology has yet been reported.

Differential Diagnosis

Acute attacks are similar to those of AIP. The differential diagnosis rests on stool porphyrin determinations and measurement of COPROGEN oxidase in fibroblasts or leukocytes. The skin lesions are said to resemble PCT, although no definitive evidence for this has been reported. Fecal predominance of COPRO III is more suggestive of HCP than VP, in which PROTO and COPRO are usually increased.

Treatment

Avoidance of inducing drugs, glucose loading, and hematin infusions may be helpful.

Hepatoerythropoietic Porphyria (HEP)
(Table 150-16)

HEP is also known as hepatoerythrocytic porphyria.

Historical Aspects

In 1969, Pinõl Aguadé et al. first reported the occurrence of a new and at first biochemically unclassifiable type of porphyria in Spain.[21] Since that time, less than 30 cases of a similar nature have been reported.[256–258] The skin manifestations resemble both PCT and EP and are characterized by severe photosensitivity, bullae, erosions, and mutilating scarring deformities that often begin in early childhood.

Etiology

The cause of HEP is unknown, but the available evidence indicates that this disease is a homozygous form of type II PCT and is inherited as an autosomal recessive trait. The primary enzyme defect is a profound deficiency of UROGEN decarboxylase activity.[44] Measurement of the enzyme in hemolyzed whole blood or skin fibroblasts from three unrelated patients with the disease showed that it was 7 to 8 percent of normal levels. The father of one HEP patient was heterozygous for the same enzyme defect, suggesting that patients with HEP are homozygous for the gene that causes PCT. There is no evidence, as yet, to show that clinical expression of HEP is related to exposure to environmental drugs or chemicals, as is true for PCT. Toback et al.[258] reported clinical, biochemical, and enzymatic studies in a three-generation family lineage in which a second-generation 31-year-old male was shown to have HEP. Both of the proband's parents and each of his three children had a moderate deficiency of UROGEN decarboxylase.

Epidemiology

Patients with HEP have been reported in Europe and America.

Genetics

deVerneuil et al.[47,48] cloned and sequenced a cDNA for UROGEN decarboxylase from a patient with HEP and identified a mutation consisting of a single base substitution, (281, Gly → Glu) that was present in some but not all families with the disease. In a further study, UROGEN decarboxylase cDNA was cloned from another patient, and comparison of the mutant and wild type sequences showed a single base difference within the coding sequence leading to replacement of glutamic acid by a lysine at codon 167 of the mutant protein.[259] This was not detected in six unrelated patients with type II PCT, indicating heterogeneity in the mutations responsible for PCT and HEP phenotypes.

Clinical Manifestations

This disease is usually manifest in early childhood with dark urine being the most frequently observed sign. Severe cutaneous photosensitivity includes blistering and pruritus. The photosensitivity

TABLE 150-16
Hepatoerythropoietic Porphyria (HEP)

Synonym	Hepatoerythrocytic porphyria
Inheritance	Autosomal recessive
Age of onset	Early infancy, before age 2
Incidence	Extremely rare (<20 cases)
Photosensitivity	Marked
Skin reactions	Early: Subepidermal vesicles, bullae, erosions, scarring, mutilation, hypertrichosis
	Late: Scleroderma-like scarring, hyperpigmentation, mutilating scarring deformities of acral areas such as hands, ears, face, and nose; cicatrizing alopecia
Clinical findings	Moderate normochromic anemia; ? hemolytic anemia; erythrodontia; pink urine; serum Fe normal
Biochemical defects	Excretory: Elevated URO (I–III) and 7-carboxyl porphyrin (III) in urine; elevated URO, COPRO, and ISOCOPRO in feces
	RBC: Elevated PROTO, usually Zn PROTO
	Enzymatic: Markedly decreased RBC UROGEN decarboxylase
Management	Avoidance of sun; phlebotomy not indicated, oral charcoal therapy may be attempted

seems to diminish with age and is followed by hypertrichosis, hyperpigmentation, and scleroderma-like scarring similar to that seen in Günther's disease. Ocular manifestations include ectropion associated with cutaneous sclerosis and scleromalacia perforans. Splenomegaly has occurred in a small percentage of affected individuals, particularly after the age of 10, and hemolytic anemia has been documented as well. In some patients, liver function tests have been abnormal, but serum iron and iron binding are normal. In summary, the clinical manifestations of HEP resemble a combination of EP and PCT.

Laboratory Findings

Elevated urinary URO (I and III) and 7-carboxyl porphyrins (>90 percent III), elevated fecal COPRO and ISOCOPRO, and elevated RBC PROTO (zinc-chelated) have been observed in all patients. These findings suggest that there is abnormal porphyrin synthesis in both the liver and the bone marrow. In contrast to PCT patients, serum iron concentrations are usually normal in HEP.

Histopathology

Skin biopsies have shown subepidermal bullae similar to PCT. PAS-positive material in and around dermal capillaries has been observed.

Differential Diagnosis

The differential diagnosis is that of childhood porphyria and includes EP, PCT, and EPP. EP manifests erythrodontia and mutilating scarring, whereas EPP often presents with acute photosensitivity. Unlike EP, in which increased RBC URO is a characteristic finding, in HEP there is elevated RBC PROTO of the zinc-chelated type. The urinary porphyrin pattern is similar to that found in PCT with high URO (URO:COPRO ratio > 5:1). The elevated PROTO in RBC helps to distinguish HEP from PCT. Urinary porphyrin analysis can differentiate HEP and EPP because urinary porphyrins are normal in EPP.

Treatment

There is no known treatment aside from careful photoprotection.

ALA Dehydratase Deficiency Porphyria
(Table 150-17)

This is a rare type of acute hepatic porphyria, and only a few patients have been reported.[23,260] Clinically, these patients have symptoms similar to AIP, and no skin lesions have been noted. Stress and ethanol ingestion have been reported to precipitate attacks. The patients have erythrocyte ALA dehydratase activity which is <5 percent of normal. Although it has been suggested that ALA dehydratase deficiency porphyria may represent a homozygous ALA dehydratase defect, recent cloning of a mutant ALA dehydratase cDNA in a patient showed that the patient was doubly heterozygous for two independent mutant alleles of ALA dehydratase.[261]

TABLE 150-17
ALA Dehydratase Deficiency Porphyria

Inheritance	Autosomal recessive
Age of onset	Any age
Incidence	Extremely rare; <10 cases
Photosensitivity	None
Clinical findings	Symptoms similar to AIP
Biochemical findings	Excretory: Elevated ALA, COPRO, and URO in urine, COPRO and PROTO in feces. RBC: Elevated PROTO Enzymatic: Markedly decreased ALA dehydratase activity
Management	Symptomatic; avoidance of known stimulating factors for acute hepatic porphyria

In the few patients studied, the urinary porphyrin profile revealed elevated ALA, COPRO, and, to a lesser extent, URO. Fecal porphyrins revealed mildly elevated COPRO and PROTO in one patient, elevated COPRO in another, and a normal profile in two others. Erythrocyte PROTO was elevated in all patients. Increases of plasma ALA, COPRO, and PROTO have been reported.[260] The reason for the elevated porphyrins in these patients is not understood.

Abnormal Porphyrin Profile and Sideroblastic Anemia

Some cases of sideroblastic anemia may be associated with an abnormal porphyrin profile.[22,262,263] Clinically, these patients may have photosensitivity most consistent with the features of EPP and they subsequently develop sideroblastic anemia; in some, the two conditions may develop within a few months of each other. All patients have elevated PROTO in RBC and/or plasma; many also have elevated stool PROTO levels. Urinary COPRO and URO are also elevated. The activities of ferrochelatase and, less frequently, of ALA synthase may be decreased. Chromosomal abnormalities, which include deletions in chromosomes 18 and 20, have been described.

References

1. Sassa S: Regulation of the genes for heme pathway enzymes in erythroid and nonerythroid cells. *Int J Cell Cloning* **8**:10, 1990
2. Schultz JH: *Ein Fall von Pemphigus leprosus complicirt durch Lepra visceralis.* Greifswald, Kunike, 1874
3. Baumstark F: Zwei pathologische Harnfarbstoffe. *Arch Dtsch Ges Physiol* **9**:568, 1874
4. Taddeini L, Watson CJ: The clinical porphyrias. *Semin Hematol* **5**:335, 1968
5. Anderson TM: Hydroa aestivale in two brothers, complicated with the presence of haematoporphyrin in the urine. *Br J Dermatol* **10**:1, 1898
6. Günther J: Die Hamatoporphyrie. *Dtsch Arch Klin Med* **105**:89, 1911
7. Fischer H: Über das Urinporphyrin. *Z Physiol Chem* **95**:34, 1915
8. Fischer H et al: Zur Kenntnis der naturlichen. Porphyrine: Chemische Befund bei einem Fall von Porphyrinurie (Petry). *Z Physiol Chem* **150**:44, 1925
9. Waldenström J: Studien über Porphyrie. *Acta Med Scand* (suppl) **82**:1, 1937

10. Brunsting LA: Observations on porphyria cutanea tarda. *Arch Dermatol Syphilol* **70**:551, 1954

11. Waldenström J: The porphyrias as inborn errors of metabolism. *Am J Med* **22**:758, 1957

12. Schmid R: Cutaneous porphyria in Turkey. *N Engl J Med* **263**:397, 1960

13. Barnes HD: A note on porphyrinuria with a resumé of eleven South African cases. *Clin Proc* **4**:269, 1945

14. Dean G: Porphyria. *Br Med J* **2**:1291, 1953

15. Dean G, Barnes HD: Porphyria in Sweden and South Africa. *S Afr Med J* **33**:246, 1959

16. Fromke VL et al: Porphyria variegata. Study of a large kindred in the United States. *Am J Med* **65**:80, 1978

17. Mustajoki P: Variegate porphyria. *Ann Intern Med* **89**:238, 1978

18. Magnus IA et al: Erythropoietic protoporphyria: A new porphyria syndrome with solar urticaria due to protoporphyrinaemia. *Lancet* **2**:448, 1961

19. Heilmeyer L, Clotten R: Congenital erythropoietic coproporphyria. *German Med Monthly* **9**:353, 1964

20. Berger H, Goldberg A: Hereditary coproporphyria. *Br Med J* **2**:85, 1955

21. Pinõl-Aguadé J et al: A case of biochemically unclassifiable hepatic porphyria. *Br J Dermatol* **81**:270, 1969

22. Rothstein G et al: Sideroblastic anemia with dermal photosensitivity and greatly increased protoporphyrin. *New Engl J Med* **280**:587, 1969

23. Doss M et al: New type of hepatic porphyria with porphobilinogen synthase defect and intermittent acute manifestation. *Klin Wochenschr* **57**:1123, 1979

24. Poh-Fitzpatrick MB et al: Cutaneous photosensitivity and coproporphyrin abnormalities in Alagille syndrome. *Gastroenterol* **99**:831, 1990

25. Schmid R et al: Porphyrin content of bone marrow and liver in the various forms of porphyria. *Arch Intern Med* **93**:167, 1954

26. Kappas A et al: The porphyrias, in *The Metabolic Basis of Inherited Disease,* 6th ed, edited by CR Scriver et al. New York, McGraw-Hill, 1989, 1305

27. Riddle RD et al: Expression of δ-aminolevulinate synthase in avian cells: Separate genes encode erythroid specific and nonspecific isozymes. *Proc Natl Acad Sci USA* **86**:792, 1989

28. Yamamoto M et al: An immunochemical study of δ-aminolevulinate synthase and δ-aminolevulinate dehydratase in liver and erythroid cells of rat. *Arch Biochem Biophys* **245**:76, 1986

29. Morton KA et al: Biosynthesis of delta-aminolevulinic acid and heme from 4,5-dioxovalerate in the rat. *J Clin Invest* **71**:1744, 1983

30. Ben Ezzer J et al: Genetic polymorphism of delta-aminolevulinate dehydrase in several population groups in Israel. *Hum Genet* **37**:229, 1987

31. Wetmur JG et al: Molecular cloning of a cDNA for human δ-aminolevulinate dehydratase. *Gene* **43**:123, 1986

32. Bishop TR et al: Isolation of a rat liver δ-aminolevulinate dehydrase (ALAD) cDNA clone: Evidence for unequal ALAD gene dosage among inbred mouse strains. *Proc Natl Acad Sci USA* **83**:5568, 1986

33. Bishop T et al: Cloning and sequence of mouse erythroid δ-aminolevulinate dehydratase cDNA. *Nucleic Acids Res* **17**:1775, 1989

34. Anderson PM, Desnick RJ: Purification and properties of uroporphyrinogen I synthase from human erythrocytes. Identification of stable enzyme-substrate intermediates. *J Biol Chem* **255**:1993, 1980

35. Chretien S et al: Alternative transcription and splicing of the human porphobilinogen deaminase gene result either in tissue-specific or in housekeeping expression. *Proc Natl Acad Sci USA* **85**:6, 1988

36. Strand LJ et al: Heme biosynthesis in intermittent acute porphyria: Decreased hepatic conversion of porphobilinogen to porphyrins and increased delta-aminolevulinic acid synthetase activity. *Proc Natl Acad Sci USA* **67**:1315, 1970

37. Watson CJ, Schwartz S: A simple test for urinary porphobilinogen. *Proc Soc Exp Biol Med* **47**:393, 1941

38. Lamon J et al: The Hoesch test: Bedside screening for urinary uroporphyrinogen in patients with suspected porphyria. *Clin Chem* **20**:1438–1440, 1974

39. Tsai SF et al: Purification and properties of uroporphyrinogen III synthase from human erythrocytes. *J Biol Chem* **262**:1268, 1987

40. Clement RP et al: Rat hepatic uroporphyrinogen III cosynthase: Purification, properties and inhibition of metal ions. *Arch Biochem Biophys* **214**:657, 1982

41. Tsai S-F et al: Human uroporphyrinogen III synthase: Molecular cloning, nucleotide sequence and expression of a full-length cDNA. *Proc Natl Acad Sci, USA* **85**:7049, 1988

42. Romeo P-H et al: Molecular cloning and nucleotide sequence of a complete human uroporphyrinogen decarboxylase cDNA. *J Biol Chem.* **261**:9825, 1986

43. Kushner JP et al: An inherited enzymatic defect in porphyria cutanea tarda: Decreased uroporphyrinogen decarboxylase activity. *J Clin Invest* **58**:1089, 1976

44. Elder GH et al: Genetics and pathogenesis of human uroporphyrinogen decarboxylase defects. *Clin Biochem* **22**:163, 1989

45. Held JL et al: Erythrocyte uroporphyrinogen decarboxylase activity in porphyria cutanea tarda: A study of 40 consecutive patients. *J Invest Dermatol* **93**:332, 1990

46. Garey JR et al: Uroporphyrinogen decarboxylase: A splice site mutation causes the deletion of exon 6 in multiple families with porphyria cutanea tarda. *J Clin Invest* **86**:1416, 1990

47. deVerneuil H et al: Uroporphyrinogen decarboxylase structural mutant (gly^{281} → glu) in a case of porphyria. *Science* **234**:732, 1986

48. deVerneuil H et al: Prevalence of the 281 (Gly → Glu) mutation in hepatoerythropoietic porphyria and porphyria cutanea tarda. *Hum Genet* **78**:101, 1988

49. Yoshinaga T, Sano S: Coproporphyrinogen oxidase. I. Purification, properties and activation by phospholipids. *J Biol Chem* **255**:4722, 1980

50. Poulson R: The enzymic conversion of protoporphyrinogen IX to protoporphyrin IX in mammalian mitochondria. *J Biol Chem* **251**:3730, 1976

51. Brenner DA, Bloomer JR: The enzymatic defect in variegate porphyria. Studies with human cultured skin fibroblasts. *N Engl J Med* **302**:765, 1980

52. Bonkowsky HL et al: Heme synthetase activity in human protoporphyria: Demonstration of the defect in liver and cultured skin fibroblasts. *J Clin Invest* **56**:1139, 1975

53. Taketani S et al: Molecular cloning, sequencing and expression of mouse ferrochelatase. *J Biol Chem* **265**:19377, 1990

54. Nakahashi Y et al: The molecular defect of ferrochelatase in a patient with erythropoietic protoporphyria. *Proc Natl Acad Sci USA* **89**:281, 1992

55. Poh-Fitzpatrick MB: The "primary phenomenon" for acute phototoxicity in erythropoietic protoporphyria? *J Am Acad Dermatol* **21**:311, 1989

56. Lamola AA et al: Erythropoietic protoporphyria and lead intoxication: The molecular basis for difference in cutaneous photosensitivity. *J Clin Invest* **56**:1528, 1975

57. Meyer-Betz F: Untersuchungen über die biologische (photodynamische) Wirkung des Hamatoporphyrins und andere derivate des Blut und Gallenfarbstoffes. *Dtsch Arch Klin Med* **112**:476, 1913

58. Harty JI et al: Complications of whole bladder dihematoporphyrin ether photodynamic therapy. *J Urol* **141**:1341, 1989

59. Bodaness RS, Chan PC: Singlet oxygen as a mediator in the hematoporphyrin-catalyzed photooxidation of NADPH to NADP+ in deuterium oxide. *J Biol Chem* **252**:8554, 1977

60. Kessel D, Rossi E: Determinants of porphyrin-induced photo-oxidation characterized by fluorescence and absorption spectra. *Photochem Photobiol* **35**:37, 1982

61. Bickers DR et al: Hematoporphyrin photosensitization of epidermal microsomes results in destruction of cytochrome P-450 and in decreased monooxygenase activities and heme content. *Biochem Bio-*

phys Res Commun **108**:1032, 1982

62. Blum HF: *Photodynamic Action and Diseases Caused by Light.* Princeton, Reinhold, 1941

63. Girotti AW: Protoporphyrin-sensitized photodamage in isolated membranes of human erythrocytes. *Biochemistry* **18**:4403, 1979

64. Schothorst AA et al: Photochemical damage to skin fibroblasts caused by protoporphyrin and violet light. *Arch Dermatol Res* **268**:31, 1980

65. Goldstein BD, Harber LC: Erythropoietic protoporphyria: Lipid peroxidation and red cell membrane damage associated with photohemolysis. *J Clin Invest* **51**:892, 1972

66. Lamola AA et al: Cholesterol hydroperoxide formation in red cell membranes and photohemolysis in erythropoietic protoporphyria. *Science* **179**:1131, 1973

67. Lim HW et al: Differential effects of protoporphyrin and uroporphyrin on murine mast cells. *J Invest Dermatol* **88**:281, 1987

68. Dixit R et al: Destruction of cytochrome P-450 by reactive oxygen species generated during photosensitization of hematoporphyrin derivative. *Photochem Photobiol* **37**:173, 1983

69. Sandberg S, Romslo I: Phototoxicity of protoporphyrin as related to its subcellular localization in mice livers after short-term feeding with griseofulvin. *Biochem J* **198**:67, 1981

70. Coppola A et al: Ultrastructural changes in lymphoma cells treated with hematoporphyrin and light. *Am J Pathol* **99**:175, 1980

71. Canti G et al: Hematoporphyrin-treated murine lymphocytes: In vitro inhibition of DNA synthesis and light-mediated inactivation of cells responsible for GVHR. *Photochem Photobiol* **34**:589, 1981

72. Mathews-Roth MM et al: Beta-carotene as an oral photoprotective agent in erythropoietic protoporphyria. *JAMA* **228**:1004, 1974

73. Athar M et al: A novel mechanism for the generation of superoxide anions in hematoporphyrin derivative–mediated cutaneous photosensitization. Activation of the xanthine oxidase pathway. *J Clin Invest* **83**:1137, 1989

74. Emiliani C, Delmelle M: The lipid solubility of porphyrins modulates their phototoxicity in membrane models. *Photochem Photobiol* **37**:487, 1983

75. Watson CJ et al: The manifestations of the different forms of porphyria in relation to chemical findings. *Trans Assoc Am Physicians* **64**:345, 1951

76. Schnait FG et al: Erythropoietic protoporphyria—submicroscopic events during the acute photosensitivity flare. *Br J Dermatol* **92**:545, 1975

77. Yen A et al: Dual effects of protoporphyrin and long wave ultraviolet light on histamine release from rat peritoneal and cutaneous mast cells. *J Immunol* **144**:4327, 1990

78. He D et al: The late phase of hematoporphyrin derivative–induced phototoxicity in mice: Release of histamine and histologic changes. *Photochem Photobiol* **50**:91, 1989

79. Lim HW et al: Delayed phase of hematoporphyrin-induced phototoxicity: Modulation by complement, leukocytes and antihistamines. *J Invest Dermatol* **84**:114, 1985

80. Sandberg S et al: Porphyrin-induced photodamage to isolated human neutrophils. *Photochem Photobiol* **34**:471, 1981

81. Baart De La Faille H et al: Experimental protoporphyria in hairless mice, in *Photodermatitis*, in *Inflammation: Mechanisms and Treatment*, edited by DA Willoughby, JP Girouds. Baltimore, University Park Press, 1980, p 603

82. Varigos G et al: Uroporphyrin I stimulation of collagen biosynthesis in human skin fibroblasts. A unique dark effect of porphyrin. *J Clin Invest* **69**:129, 1982

83. Latham PS, Bloomer JR: Protoporphyrin-induced photodamage: Studies using cultured skin fibroblasts. *Photochem Photobiol* **37**:553, 1983

84. Wakulchik SD et al: Photolysis of protoporphyrin-treated human fibroblasts *in vitro*. Studies on the mechanism. *J Lab Clin Med* **96**:158, 1980

85. Cormane RH et al: Histopathology of the skin in acquired and hereditary porphyria cutanea tarda. *Br J Dermatol* **85**:531, 1971

86. Epstein JH et al: Cutaneous changes in the porphyrias. *Arch Dermatol* **107**:689, 1973

87. Lim HW et al: Generation of chemotactic activity in serum from patients with erythropoietic protoporphyria and porphyria cutanea tarda. *N Engl J Med* **304**:212, 1981

88. Lim HW, Gigli I: Role of complement in porphyrin-induced photosensitivity. *J Invest Dermatol* **76**:4, 1981

89. Torinuki W et al: Activation of the alternative complement pathway by 405-nm light in serum from porphyric rat. *Acta Derm Venereol (Stockh)* **64**:367, 1984

90. Lim HW et al: Activation of the complement system in patients with porphyrias after irradiation *in vivo*. *J Clin Invest* **74**:1976, 1984

91. Becker CG et al: Activation of factor XII-dependent pathways in human plasma by hematin and protoporphyrin. *J Clin Invest* **76**:413, 1985

92. Henderson BW, Donovan JM: Release of prostaglandin E2 from cells by photodynamic treatment in vitro. *Cancer Res* **49**:6896, 1989

93. He D, Lim HW: Irradiation of protoporphyric mice induces down regulation of epidermal eicosanoid metabolism. *J Invest Dermatol* **97**:488, 1991

94. Ippen H, Fuchs T: Congenital porphyria. *Clin Haematol* **9**:323, 1980

95. Romeo G et al: Uroporphyrinogen III cosynthetase activity in an asymptomatic carrier of congenital erythropoietic porphyria. *Biochem Genet* **4**:719, 1970

96. Deybach J-C et al: Point mutations in the uroporphyrinogen III synthase gene in congenital erythropoietic porphyria (Günther's disease). *Blood* **75**:1763, 1990

97. Magnus IA: The cutaneous porphyrias. *Semin Hematol* **5**:380, 1968

98. Horiguchi Y et al: Late onset erythropoietic porphyria. *Br J Dermatol* **121**:255, 1989

99. Watson CJ et al: Some studies of the comparative biology of human and bovine erythropoietic porphyria. *Arch Intern Med* **103**:436, 1959

100. Nordmann Y, Deybach JC: Congenital erythropoietic porphyria. *Semin Liver Dis* **2**:154, 1982

101. Poh-Fitzpatrick MB: Erythropoietic porphyrias: Current mechanistic, diagnostic and therapeutic considerations. *Semin Haematol* **14**:211, 1977

102. Nordmann Y et al: Coexistent hereditary coproporphyria and congenital erythropoietic porphyria (Günther disease). *J Inherit Metab Dis* **13**:687, 1990

103. Piomelli S et al: Complete suppression of the symptoms of congenital erythropoietic porphyria by long term treatment with high level transfusions. *N Engl J Med* **314**:1019, 1986

104. Watson CJ, Bossenmaier I: Repression by hematin of porphyrin biosynthesis in erythrocyte precursors in congenital erythropoietic porphyria. *Proc Natl Acad Sci USA* **71**:278, 1974

105. Pimstone NR et al: Therapeutic efficacy of oral charcoal in congenital erythropoietic porphyria. *N Engl J Med* **316**:390, 1987

106. Kosenow W, Treibs A: Lichtüberemfindlichkeit und porphyrinamine. *Z Kinderheilkd* **73**:82, 1953

107. Langhof H et al: Untersuchungen zur Familieren Protoporphyrinamischen Lichturticaria. *Arch Klin Exp Dermatol* **212**:506, 1961

108. Bloomer JR: Characterization of deficient heme synthase activity in protoporphyria with cultured skin fibroblasts. *J Clin Invest* **65**:321, 1980

109. Sassa S et al: Studies in porphyria. Functional evidence for a partial deficiency of ferrochelatase activity in mitogen-stimulated lymphocytes from patients with erythropoietic protoporphyria. *J Clin Invest* **69**:809, 1982

110. Norris PG et al: Genetic heterogeneity in erythropoietic protoporphyria: A study of the enzymatic defect in nine affected families. *J Invest Dermatol* **95**:260, 1990

111. Deybach JC et al: Ferrochelatase in erythropoietic protoporphyria: The first case of a homozygous form of the enzyme deficiency, in *Porphyrins and Porphyrias*, edited by Y Nordmann. Paris, Colloque, INSERM, John Libbey EURO text, vol. 134, 1986, p 163

112. DeLeo VA et al: Erythropoietic protoporphyria. *Am J Med* **60**:8, 1976

113. Schmidt H et al: Erythropoietic protoporphyria: A clinical study based on 29 cases in 14 families. *Arch Dermatol* **110**:58, 1974

114. Piomelli S et al: Erythropoietic protoporphyria and lead intoxication: The molecular basis for difference in cutaneous photosensitivity. I. Different rates of disappearance of protoporphyrin from the erythrocytes, both in vivo and in vitro. *J Clin Invest* **56**:1519, 1975

115. Lamon JM et al: Hepatic protoporphyrin production in human protoporphyria. Effects of intravenous hematin and analysis of erythrocyte protoporphyrin distribution. *Gastroenterology* **79**:115, 1980

116. Scholnick P et al: Erythropoietic protoporphyria: Evidence for multiple sites of excess protoporphyrin formation. *J Clin Invest* **50**:203, 1971

117. Cripps DJ, Scheuer PJ: Hepatobiliary changes in erythropoietic protoporphyria. *Arch Pathol* **80**:500, 1965

118. Klatskin G, Bloomer JR: Birefringence of hepatic pigment deposits in erythropoietic protoporphyria: Specificity and sensitivity of polarization microscopy in the identification of hepatic protoporphyrin deposits. *Gastroenterology* **67**:295, 1974

119. Wolff K et al: Liver inclusions in erythropoietic protoporphyria. *Eur J Clin Invest* **5**:21, 1975

120. Scott AJ et al: Erythropoietic protoporphyria with features of a sideroblastic anemia terminating in liver failure. *Am J Med* **54**:251, 1973

121. Romslo I et al: Erythropoietic protoporphyria terminating in liver failure. *Arch Dermatol* **118**:668, 1982

122. Avner DL et al: Protoporphyrin-induced cholestasis in the isolated in situ perfused rat liver. *J Clin Invest* **67**:385, 1981

123. Poh-Fitzpatrick MB et al: Rapid quantitative assay for erythrocyte porphyrins. *Arch Dermatol* **110**:225, 1974

124. Poh-Fitzpatrick MB, Lamola AA: Direct spectrofluorometry of diluted erythrocytes and plasma: A rapid diagnostic method in primary and secondary porphyrinemias. *J Lab Clin Med* **87**:362, 1976

125. Lamola AA et al: Erythropoietic protoporphyria and Pb intoxication: The molecular basis for difference in cutaneous photosensitivity. II. Differential binding of erythrocyte protoporphyrin to hemoglobin. *J Clin Invest* **56**:1528, 1975

126. Romslo I et al: Sideroblastic anemia with markedly increased free erythrocyte protoporphyrin without dermal photosensitivity. *Blood* **59**:628, 1982

127. Sandberg S, Brun A: Light-induced protoporphyrin release from erythrocytes in erythropoietic protoporphyria. *J Clin Invest* **70**:693, 1982

128. Peterka EA et al: Erythropoietic protoporphyria. II. Histological and histochemical studies of cutaneous lesions. *Arch Dermatol* **92**:357, 1965

129. Cripps DJ et al: Four cases of erythropoietic protoporphyria presenting as light-sensitive lipoid proteinosis. *Proc R Soc Med* **57**:1095, 1964

130. Ryan EA, Madill GT: Electron microscopy of the skin in erythropoietic protoporphyria. *Br J Dermatol* **80**:561, 1968

131. Breathnach SM et al: Immunohistochemical studies of amyloid P component and fibronectin in erythropoietic protoporphyria. *Br J Dermatol* **108**:267, 1983

132. Mathews-Roth MM et al: Beta-carotene therapy for erythropoietic protoporphyria and other diseases. *Arch Dermatol* **113**:1229, 1977

133. Krook G, Haeger-Aronsen B: Beta-carotene in the treatment of erythropoietic protoporphyria. A short review. *Acta Dermatol Venereol* **100**(suppl): 125, 1982

134. Corbett NF et al: The long term treatment with beta-carotene in erythropoietic protoporphyria: A controlled trial. *Br J Dermatol* **97**:653, 1977

135. Carraro C, Pathak MA: Studies on the nature of in vitro and in vivo photosensitization reactions by psoralens and porphyrins. *J Invest Derm* **90**:267, 1988

136. Bechtel MA et al: Transfusion therapy in a patient with erythropoietic protoporphyria. *Arch Dermatol* **47**:99, 1981

137. McCullough AJ et al: Fecal protoporphyrin excretion in erythropoietic protoporphyria: Effect of cholestyramine and bile acid feeding. *Gastroenterology* **94**:177, 1988

138. Gordeuk VR et al: Iron therapy for hepatic dysfunction in erythropoietic protoporphyria. *Ann Intern Med* **105**:27, 1986

139. Milligan A et al: Erythropoietic protoporphyria exacerbated by iron therapy. *Br J Dermatol* **119**:63, 1988

140. Polson RJ et al: The effect of liver transplantation in a 13-year-old boy with erythropoietic protoporphyria. *Transplantation* **46**:386, 1988

141. Topi G et al: Coproporphirie erithropoetique congenitales observée chez un frère et une soeur. *Ann Dermatol Venereol* **104**:68, 1977

142. Brunsting LA, Mason HL: Porphyria with cutaneous manifestations. *Arch Dermatol Syphilol* **60**:66, 1949

143. Eales L: Cutaneous porphyria: Observations on 111 cases in three racial groups. *S Afr J Lab Clin Med* **6**:63, 1960

144. Watson CJ: The problem of porphyria: Some facts and questions. *N Engl J Med* **263**:1205, 1960

145. Holti G et al: Investigation of porphyria cutanea tarda. *Q J Med* **27**:1, 1958

146. Elder GH et al: Decreased activity of hepatic uroporphyrinogen decarboxylase in sporadic porphyria cutanea tarda. *N Engl J Med* **299**:274, 1978

147. Benedetto AV et al: Porphyria cutanea tarda in three generations of a single family. *N Engl J Med* **298**:358, 1978

148. Roberts AG et al: Heterogeneity of familial porphyria cutanea tarda. *J Med Genet* **25**:669, 1988

149. Held JL et al: Erythrocyte uroporphyrinogen decarboxylase activity in porphyria cutanea tarda: A study of 40 consecutive patients. *J Invest Dermatol* **93**:332, 1989

150. Watson CJ et al: Porphyria variegata and porphyria cutanea tarda in siblings: Chemical and genetic aspects. *Proc Natl Acad Sci USA* **72**:5126, 1975

151. Day RS et al: Coexistent variegate porphyria and porphyria cutanea tarda. *N Engl J Med* **307**:36, 1982

152. Doss MO: New form of dual porphyria: Coexistent acute intermittent porphyria and porphyria cutanea tarda. *Eur J Clin Invest* **19**:20, 1989

153. Shanley BC et al: Effect of ethanol on liver and aminolaevulinate synthetase activity and urinary porphyrin excretion in symptomatic porphyria *Br J Haematol* **17**:389, 1969

154. McColl KEL et al: Abnormal haem biosynthesis in chronic alcoholics. *Eur J Clin Invest* **11**:461, 1981

155. Hourihane DO, Weir DG: Suppression of erythropoiesis by alcohol. *Br Med J* **1**:86, 1970

156. Kodama T et al: Changes in aminolevulinate synthase and aminolevulinate dehydratase activity and cirrhotic liver. *Gastroenterology* **84**:236, 1983

157. Grossman ME et al: Porphyria cutanea tarda. Clinical features and laboratory findings in 40 patients. *Am J Med* **67**:277, 1979

158. Levere RD: Stilbesterol-induced porphyria: Increased in hepatic delta-aminolevulinic acid synthetase. *Blood* **28**:569, 1966

159. Ochner RK, Schmid R: Acquired porphyria in man and rat due to hexachlorobenzene intoxication. *Nature* **189**:499, 1961

160. Cripps DJ et al: Porphyria turcica. Twenty years after hexachlorobenzene intoxication. *Arch Dermatol* **116**:46, 1980

161. Courtney KD: Hexachlorobenzene (HCB): A review. *Environ Res* **20**:225, 1979

162. Elder GH et al: The effect of the porphyrinogenic compound, hexachlorobenzene, on the activity of hepatic uroporphyrinogen decarbosylase in the rat. *Clin Sci Mol Med* **51**:71, 1976

163. Sinclair PR et al: Chlorinated biphenyls induce cytochrome P450IA2 and uroporphyrin accumulation in cultures of mouse hepatocytes. *Arch Biochem Biophys* **281**:225, 1990

164. Elder GH, Sheppard DM: Immunoreactive uroporphyrinogen decarboxylase is unchanged in porphyria caused by TCDD and hexachlorobenzene. *Biochem Biophys Res Commun* **109**:113, 1982

165. Poland AP, Glover E: 2,3,7,8-Tetrachlorodibenzo-*p*-dioxin: A potent inducer of delta-aminolevulinic acid synthetase. *Science* **179**:476, 1973

166. Schwartz BA et al: Toxicology of chlorinated dibenzo(p)dioxins. *Env Health Perspec* **5**:87, 1973

167. Sweeney GD et al: Iron deficiency prevents liver toxicity of 2,3,7,8-tetrachlorodibenzo-p-dioxin. *Science* **204**:332, 1979

168. Jones KG, Sweeney GD: Dependence of the porphyrogenic effect of 2,3,7,8-tetrachlorodibenzo(p)dioxin upon inheritance of aryl hydrocarbon hydroxylase responsiveness. *Toxicol App Pharmacol* **53**:42, 1980

169. Bonkovsky HL: Iron and the liver. *Am J Med Sci* **301**:32, 1991

170. Kushner JP et al: The role of iron in the pathogenesis of porphyria cutanea tarda. II. Inhibition of uroporphyrinogen decarboxylase. *J Clin Invest* **56**:661, 1975

171. Blekkenhorst GH et al: Iron and porphyria cutanea tarda: Activation of uroporphyrinogen decarboxylase by ferrous iron. *S Afr Med J* **56**:918, 1979

172. deVerneuil H et al: Purification and properties of uroporphyrinogen decarboxylase from human erythrocytes. A single enzyme catalyzing the four sequential decarboxylations of uroporphyrinogens I and III. *J Biol Chem* **258**:2454, 1983

173. Feldman ES, Bacon BR: Hepatic mitochondrial oxidative metabolism and lipid peroxidation in experimental hexachlorobenzene-induced porphyria with dietary carbonyl iron overload. *Hepatology* **9**:686, 1989

174. Bonkovsky HL: Mechanism of iron potentiation of hepatic uroporphyria: Studies in cultured chick embryo liver cells. *Hepatology* **10**:354, 1989

175. Kushner JP et al: The role of iron in the pathogenesis of porphyria cutanea tarda: An in vitro model. *J Clin Invest* **51**:3044, 1972

176. Garey JR et al: A point mutation in the coding region of uroporphyrinogen decarboxylase associated with familial porphyria cutanea tarda. *Blood* **73**:892, 1989

177. Elder GH: The cutaneous porphyrias. *Semin Dermatol* **9**:63, 1990

178. Enriquez de Salamanca R et al: Patterns of porphyrin excretion in female estrogen-induced porphyria cutanea tarda. *Arch Dermatol Res* **274**:179, 1982

179. Burnett JW, Pathak MA: Effect of light upon porphyrin metabolism of rats. *Arch Dermatol* **89**:257, 1964

180. Cam C, Nigogosyan G: Acquired toxic porphyria cutanea tarda due to hexachlorobenzene. *JAMA* **183**:88, 1963

181. Solis JA et al: Association of porphyria cutanea tarda and primary liver cancer. *J Dermatol* **9**:131, 1982

182. Burnett JW et al: Haemophilia, hepatitis and porphyria. *Br J Dermatol* **97**:353, 1977

183. Clemmensen O, Thomsen K: Porphyria cutanea tarda and systemic lupus erythematosus *Arch Dermatol* **118**:160, 1982

184. Poh-Fitzpatrick MB et al: Porphyria cutanea tarda in two patients treated with hemodialysis for chronic renal failure. *N Engl J Med* **299**:292, 1978

185. Mann RJ, Harman RR: Porphyria cutanea tarda and sarcoidosis. *Clin Exp Dermatol* **7**:619, 1982

186. Ramasamy R, Kubik MM: Porphyria cutanea tarda in association with Sjögren's syndrome. *Practitioner* **226**:1297, 1982

187. Wissel PS et al: Porphyria cutanea tarda associated with the acquired immune deficiency syndrome. *Am J Hematol* **25**:107, 1987

188. Cohen PR: Porphyria cutanea tarda in human immunodeficiency virus-infected patients. *JAMA* **264**:1315, 1990

189. Burry JN, Lawrence JR: Phototoxic blisters from high furosemide dosage. *Br J Dermatol* **94**:495, 1976

190. Ramsay CA, Obreshkova E: Photosensitivity from nalidixic acid. *Br J Dermatol* **91**:523, 1974

191. Epstein JH et al: Porphyria-like cutaneous changes induced by tetracycline hydrochloride photosensitization. *Arch Dermatol* **112**:661, 1976

192. Suarez SM et al: Bullous photosensitivity to naproxen: "Pseudoporphyria." *Arthritis Rheum* **33**:903, 1990

193. Baer RL, Stillman MA: Cutaneous skin changes probably due to pyridoxine abuse. *J Am Acad Dermatol* **10**:527, 1984

194. Goldman CI, Taylor J: Porphyria cutanea tarda and bullous dermatoses associated with chronic renal failure. A review. *Cleve Clin Q* **50**:151, 1983

195. Biro I et al: Cryoglobulinemia and porphyria hepatica chronica (porphyria cutanea tarda). *Acta Derm Venereol (Stockh)* **44**:226, 1964

196. Elder GH: Porphyrin metabolism in porphyria cutanea tarda. *Semin Hematol* **14**:227, 1977

197. Elder GH et al: Laboratory investigation of the porphyrias. *Ann Clin Biochem* **27**:395, 1990

198. Cripps DJ, Peters HA: Fluorescing erythrocytes and porphyrin screening tests on urine, blood and stool. *Arch Dermatol* **96**:712, 1967

199. Logan GM et al: Bile porphyrin analysis in the evaluation of variegate porphyria. *N Engl J Med* **324**:1408, 1991

200. Kushner JP: Laboratory diagnosis of the porphyrias. *N Engl J Med* **324**:1432, 1991

201. Wolff K et al: Microscopic and fine structural aspects of porphyrias. *Acta Derm Venereol (Stockh)* **100**(Suppl): 17, 1982

202. Pathak MA, Burnett JW: The porphyrin content of skin. *J Invest Dermatol* **43**:119, 1964

203. Molina L et al: Skin porphyrin assay in porphyria. *Clin Chim Acta* **83**:55, 1978

204. Rimington C et al: Porphyria and photosensitivity. *Q J Med* **36**:29, 1967

205. Ippen H: Allgemeinsymptome der spaten Hautporphyrie (Porphyria cutanea tarda) als Hisweise fur deren Behandlung. *Dtsch Med Wochenschr* **86**:127, 1961

206. Lundvall O: Phlebotomy treatment of porphyria cutanea tarda. *Acta Derm Venereol (Stockh)* **100**(suppl): 107, 1982

207. Vogler WR et al: Biochemical effects of chloroquine therapy in porphyria cutanea tarda. *Am J Med* **49**:316, 1970

208. Kordac V et al: Chloroquine in the treatment of porphyria cutanea tarda. *N Engl J Med* **296**:949, 1977

209. Swanbeck G, Wennersten G: Treatment of porphyria cutanea tarda with chloroquine and phlebotomy. *Br J Dermatol* **97**:77, 1977

210. Rocchi E et al: Iron removal therapy in porphyria cutanea tarda—phlebotomy versus slow subcutaneous desferrioxamine infusion. *Br J Dermatol* **114**:621, 1986

211. Praga M et al: Treatment of hemodialysis-related porphyria cutanea tarda with desferroxamine. *N Engl J Med* **316**:547, 1987

212. Stathers GM: Porphyrin-binding effect of chloestyramine. *Lancet* **2**:780, 1966

213. Anderson KE et al: Erythropoietin for the treatment of porphyria cutanea tarda in a patient on long-term hemodialysis. *N Engl J Med* **322**:315, 1990

214. Ramsay CA et al: The treatment of porphyria cutanea tarda by venesection. *Q J Med* **43**:1, 1974

215. Mukerji SK, Pimstone NR: Free radical mechanism of oxidation of uroporphyrinogen in the presence of ferrous iron. *Arch Biochem Biophys* **281**:177, 1990

216. London ID: Porphyria cutanea tarda: Report of a case successfully treated with chloroquine. *Arch Dermatol* **75**:801, 1957

217. Malkinson FD, Levitt L: Hydroxychloroquine treatment of porphyria cutanea tarda. *Arch Dermatol* **116**:1147, 1980

218. Scholnick PL et al: The molecular basis of the action of chloroquine in porphyria cutanea tarda. *J Invest Dermatol* **61**:226, 1973

219. Taljaard JJF et al: Studies on low-dose chloroquine therapy and the action of chloroquine in symptomatic porphyria. *Br J Dermatol* **87**:261, 1972

220. Saltzer EI et al: Porphyria cutanea tarda: Remission following chloroquine administration without adverse effects. *Arch Dermatol* **98**:496, 1968

221. Malina L, Chlumsky J: A comparative study of the results of phlebotomy therapy and low-dose chloroquine treatment in porphyria cutanea tarda. *Acta Derm Venereol (Stockh)* **61**:346, 1981

222. Cainelli T et al: Hydroxychloroquine versus phlebotomy in the treatment of porphyria cutanea tarda. *Br J Dermatol* **108**:593, 1983

223. Chlumska A et al: Liver changes in porphyria cutanea tarda patients treated with chloroquine. *Br J Dermatol* **102**:261, 1980

224. Mustajoki P: Acute intermittent porphyria. *Semin Dermatol* **5**:155, 1986

225. Dowdle EB et al: Delta-aminolevulinic acid synthetase activity in normal and porphyric human liver. *S Afr Med J* **41**:1093, 1967

226. DeMatteis F: Disturbances of liver porphyrin metabolism caused by drugs. *Pharmacol Rev* **17**:523, 1967

227. McColl KEL, Moore MR: The acute porphyrias—an example of pharmacogenetic disease. *Scott Med J* **26**:32, 1981

228. Grandchamp B et al: Tissue specific expression of porphobilinogen deaminase. Two isozymes from a single gene. *Eur J Biochem* **1621**:105, 1987

229. Kauppinen R et al: RFLP analysis of three different types of acute intermittent porphyria. *Hum Genet* **85**:160, 1990

230. Lee J-S et al: Haplotyping of the human porphobilinogen deaminase gene in acute intermittent porphyria by polymerase chain reaction. *Hum Genet* **84**:241, 1990

231. Hoesch K: Über die Auswertung der Urobilinogenurie und die ''umgekehrte'' Urobilinogenurie. *Dtsch Med Wochenschr* **72**:704, 1947

232. Tiepermann RV, Doss M: Simple diagnostic test for urinary porphobilinogen and porphyrins, in *Porphyrins in Human Diseases*, First International Porphyrin Meeting, Freiburg, edited by M Doss, P Nawrocki. Basel, Karger, 1976, p 249

233. Mustajoki P et al: Heme in the treatment of porphyrias and hematological disorders. *Semin Hematol* **26**:1, 1989

234. Herrick AL et al: Controlled trial of haem arginate in acute hepatic porphyria. *Lancet* **1**:1295, 1989

235. Anderson KE et al: Gonadotropin releasing hormone analogue prevents cyclical attacks of porphyria. *Arch Intern Med* **150**:1469, 1990

236. Barnes HD: Further South African cases of porphyrinuria. *S Afr J Clin Sci* **2**:117, 1951

237. Dean G, Barnes HD: The inheritance of porphyria. *Br Med J* **2**:89, 1955

238. Dean G: *The Porphyrias*. Philadelphia, Lippincott, 1963

239. Kordac V et al: Homozygous variegate porphyria. *Lancet* **1**:851, 1984

240. Rimington C et al: The excretion of porphyrin-peptide conjugates in porphyria variegata. *Clin Sci* **35**:211, 1968

241. Elder GH et al: Faecal ''X'' porphyrin in the hepatic porphyrias. *Enzyme* **17**:29, 1974

242. Eales L et al: The place of screening tests and quantitative investigations in the diagnosis of the porphyrias, with particular reference to variegate and symptomatic porphyria. *S Afr Med J* **40**:63, 1966

243. Poh-Fitzpatrick MB: A plasma porphyrin fluorescence marker for variegate porphyria. *Arch Dermatol* **116**:543, 1980

244. Cramers M, Jepsen LV: Porphyria variegata: Failure of chloroquine treatment. *Acta Derm Venereol* **60**:89, 1980

245. Perrot H et al: La porphyrie variegata (à propos de 4 cas). *Lyon Med* **235**:905, 1976

246. Watson CJ et al: Studies of coproporphyrin III. Idiopathic coproporphyrinuria, a hitherto unrecognized form characterized by lack of symptoms in spite of the excretion of large amounts of coproporphyrin. *J Clin Invest* **28**:465, 1949

247. Goldberg A et al: Hereditary coproporphyria. *Lancet* **1**:632, 1967

248. Brodie NJ et al: Hereditary coproporphyria. *Q J Med* **46**:229, 1977

249. Grandchamp B, Nordmann Y: Decreased lymphocyte and coproporphyrinogen oxidase activity in hereditary coproporphyria. *Biochem Biophys Res Commun* **74**:1089, 1977

250. Elder GH et al: The primary enzyme defect in hereditary coproporphyria. *Lancet* **2**:1217, 1976

251. McIntyre N et al: Hepatic delta-aminolevulinic acid synthetase in an attack of hereditary coproporphyria and during remission. *Lancet* **1**:560, 1971

252. Herrero C et al: Acquired immunodeficiency syndrome in a patient affected by hereditary coproporphyria: Safety of zodovudine treatment. *Arch Dermatol* **126**:122, 1990

253. Nordmann Y et al: Harderoporphyria: A variant hereditary coproporphyria. *J Clin Invest* **72**:1139, 1983

254. Moder KG: A coproporphyria-like syndrome induced by glipizide. *Mayo Clin Proc* **66**:312, 1991

255. Hunter JAA et al: Hereditary coproporphyria: Photosensitivity, jaundice and neuropsychiatric manifestations associated with pregnancy. *Br J Dermatol* **84**:301, 1971

256. Pinõl-Aguadé J et al: Hepato-erythrocytic porphyria: A new type of porphyria. *Ann Dermatol Syphiligr (Paris)* **102**:129, 1975

257. Lim HW, Poh-Fitzpatrick MB: Hepatoerythropoietic porphyria: A variant of childhood-onset porphyria cutanea tarda. *J Am Acad Dermatol* **11**:1103, 1984

258. Toback AG et al: Hepatoerythropoietic porphyria: Clinical, biochemical, and enzymatic studies in a three generation family lineage. *N Engl J Med* **316**:646, 1987

259. Romana M et al: Identification of a new mutation responsible for hepatoerythropoietic porphyria. *Eur J Clin Invest* **21**:225, 1991

260. Thunell S et al: Aminolevulinate dehydratase porphyria: A clinical and biochemical study. *J Clin Chem Clin Biochem* **25**:5, 1987

261. Ishida N et al: Message amplification phenotyping of an inherited δ-aminolevulinate dehydratase deficiency in a family with acute hepatic porphyria. *Biochem Biophys Res Commun* **172**:237, 1990

262. Sato Y et al: A case of sideroblastic anemia with dermal photosensitivity and increased erythrocyte protoporphyrin. *Jpn J Clin Hematol* **22**:1971, 1981

263. Lim HW et al: Photosensitivity, abnormal porphyrin profile, and sideroblastic anemia—a case report and review of the literature. *J Am Acad Dermatol* **27**:287, 1992

CHAPTER 151

J. Edwin Seegmiller

Skin Manifestations of Gout

The sudden onset of a severe monarticular arthritis usually involving a peripheral joint constitutes the typical clinical presentation of acute gouty arthritis. It is seen predominantly in males during mature years who often give a family history of the same disease. These clinical features are preceded by many years of hyperuricemia, which leads to deposition of needle-shaped crystals of monosodium urate from the supersaturated serum in and about the joints.[1-3] Phagocytosis of the deposited crystals by polymorphonuclear leukocytes leads to an acute inflammatory response with swelling, redness, and acute tenderness similar to that generated by invading microorganisms, thus accounting for the frequent confusion of the acute attack of gout with an acute septic process. Larger aggregates of the crystals give rise to the characteristic tophi found in the subcutaneous tissue most often on the ear or overlying joints, tendons or cartilage as a later manifestation of the gout. If the disease is untreated, the tophi will show a progressive enlargement over the years, and when they are near the surface of the skin, they show a characteristic mottled, salmon-pink color. Large tophi may spontaneously drain a clear, amber fluid containing white flecks of crystals of monosodium urate. Microscopic examination of this draining fluid, of material removed from the tophus with a needle, or of joint fluid aspirated from an acutely inflamed joint reveals needle-shaped crystals, negatively birefringent under cross-polarizing filters, which are diagnostic of gout. These same deposits are frequently found in the kidney of gout patients and are associated with a progressive renal damage, while precipitation of free uric acid in the urinary tract can form renal calculi in a significant portion of gouty patients. Many relatives of gouty patients, who may never develop the disease, nevertheless show asymptomatic hyperuricemia sometimes associated with renal calculi.

A wide range of other diseases are found in association with hyperuricemia and gout. Included are psoriasis,[4] proliferative disorders of the hemopoietic system, hypertension, obesity, primary or secondary renal damage, myocardial infarction, hyper- or hypoparathyroidism, and myxedema. Hyperuricemia and gout can result from thiazides and other diuretics, from excessive alcohol ingestion, and they can be a late effect of lead poisoning. In addition, hyperuricemia accompanies Down syndrome (mongolism), type I glycogen storage disease (absence of glucose-6-phosphatase), hereditary nephritis, pituitrin-resistant diabetes insipidus, and an X-linked neurologic disorder with compulsive automutilation (Lesch-Nyhan syndrome).[2] The latter is caused by a severe X-linked genetic deficiency of the enzyme hypoxanthine-guanine phosphoribosyltransferase. Another X-linked form of gout, which is associated with deafness in some families, results from a threefold increase in phosphoribosylpyrophosphate synthetase activity.[5,6] A start has been made in identifying genetic deficiencies of specific enzymes of purine metabolism associated with gouty arthritis from purine overproduction[7]; however, these are very rare defects. Only recently has a start been made in identifying hereditary defects in metabolism responsible for the much more common dominantly-inherited familial gout. Oberhaensli et al,[8] using noninvasive ^{31}P magnetic resonance spectroscopy, detected an abnormal response to ingested fructose by heterozygotes for hereditary fruc-

tose intolerance (aldolase B deficiency). Three of the nine heterozygotes had clinical gout.[8] Subsequently, the same technology revealed a similar pattern in two of eleven patients with a family history of gout.[9]

Historical Aspects

Gout has been on the forefront in the historical development of many medical concepts. The unusual clinical features permitted it to be distinguished from other ailments by Hippocrates at a very early stage in medical history and the specific treatment of the acute attack with the drug colchicine was introduced in the fifth century. Sydenham's description in 1563 of his own personal experience with the disease remains a classic of descriptive medicine. The early interest of the chemists in the disease, and, more recently, the biochemists, has resulted in substantial advances in our scientific understanding of gout throughout the years. Scheele in 1776 first isolated uric acid from a urinary concretion and some 20 years later Wallaston isolated the same substance from a gouty tophus which he reportedly removed from his own ear. The demonstration of hyperuricemia in gout by Garrod in 1848 provided the first use of an abnormality in a chemical component of serum as an aid to the diagnosis of a metabolic disease. It also provided the first application of chemical principles to the understanding of the pathology of the disease.[1]

No disease has enjoyed a more royal patronage than gout. The list of gouty personages of fame is astonishingly long and, through their vicissitudes, gout has changed the course of history. A less admirable image has been the popular association of gout with luxurious living and excessive indulgence in natural appetites, giving rise to the moralistic view that gout is nature's retribution for intemperate living and quite impossible to treat medically. This view is being dispelled to some extent by the identification of both specific hereditary and environmental factors that can contribute to the development of hyperuricemia and gout. Furthermore the introduction of new drugs and the more effective use of colchicine have now minimized the disability and deformity heretofore produced by this ancient malady.[10]

Epidemiology

Gouty arthritis accounts for 5 percent of the patients seen with arthritis at major clinics. It has been found in all races but appears in unusually high incidence among Filipinos who have emigrated to the United States or Hawaii and certain people of the South Pacific islands, where it is frequently associated with obesity. Gout is primarily a disease of males (95 percent of cases) and usually appears between the third and sixth decades of life. When it does appear in women it is usually after the menopause. The fact that the mean serum urate of women is lower than that of men by about 1 mg/dL until after the menopause provides the most reasonable explanation for this sex difference in incidence of the disease. The frequency of hyperuricemia and gout is increasing in the more affluent countries of the world. A low but statistically significant, positive correlation between serum urate concentration and intelligence as well as academic and professional achievement has been reported.

Etiology and Pathogenesis

The principal clinical features of gouty arthritis can be related to the limited solubility of uric acid and its monosodium salt in body fluids. The crystals of monosodium urate monohydrate deposited in and about the joints can produce an inflammatory reaction. A vicious cycle of inflammatory reactions leading to more crystal deposition and additional inflammatory reaction directed toward such crystals has been proposed to account for the acute attack of gouty arthritis (Fig. 151-1). Colchicine presumably interrupts the cycle through a metabolic effect on leukocytes. At the more acid pH of the urinary tract, crystals of free uric acid are precipitated and give rise to kidney stones in 20 to 40 percent of gouty patients.

The demonstration by Simkin[11] that urate moves from a traumatic effusion of a joint at a rate roughly half that of water, provides a mechanism for concentrating urate transiently within the joint cavity, particularly if the joint had been previously injured. The possibility of such an injury in the form of preexisting osteoarthritis setting the stage for a traumatic effusion of the first metatarsophalangeal joint by reason of the high weight-bearing stresses to which it is subject in normal walking provides an ingenious explanation for the predilection of gouty arthritis to attack the first meta-

tarsophalangeal joint. Presumably the onset of the attack during the early morning hours reflects crystal formation during the partial resolution of the traumatic effusion which would attend the elevation of the feet to the horizontal position during nocturnal slumber.

The hyperuricemia of gout results from a variety of biochemical and physiologic abnormalities, as shown in Fig. 151-2. In some patients the diminished renal excretion of uric acid accounts for the hyperuricemia, while in others an excessive production of uric acid from increased purine biosynthesis is found either as a primary metabolic abnormality or secondary to the turnover of tissue nucleic acids in a myeloproliferative disease. In still other gouty patients both excessive synthesis of uric acid and decreased renal excretion of uric acid are found. Patients with gout are therefore a very heterogeneous group; a variety of specific underlying disorders of physiology or metabolism rather than a uniform defect in a single enzyme accounts for their hyperuricemia.

As noted above, several types of specific enzyme defects associated with purine overproduction have been identified among patients with severe gout. Two of these are X-linked disorders. One is a deficiency in an enzyme of purine metabolism, hypoxanthine-guanine phosphoribosyltransferase (HPRT), and is associated with the most severe degree of excessive production of uric acid yet found and with a wide range of clinical expression.[12] Patients with virtually complete deficiency of HPRT show a severe and incapacitating neurologic disease often classed as cerebral palsy, consisting of choreoathetosis, spasticity, and some degree of mental retardation with a dramatic, compulsive self-mutilation (the Lesch-Nyhan syndrome). Other patients with as little as 1 percent of normal HPRT activity in the erythrocytes have no neurologic disease and present with a high incidence of uric acid renal calculi and severe gouty arthritis in adolescence or early adult life. Patients in families

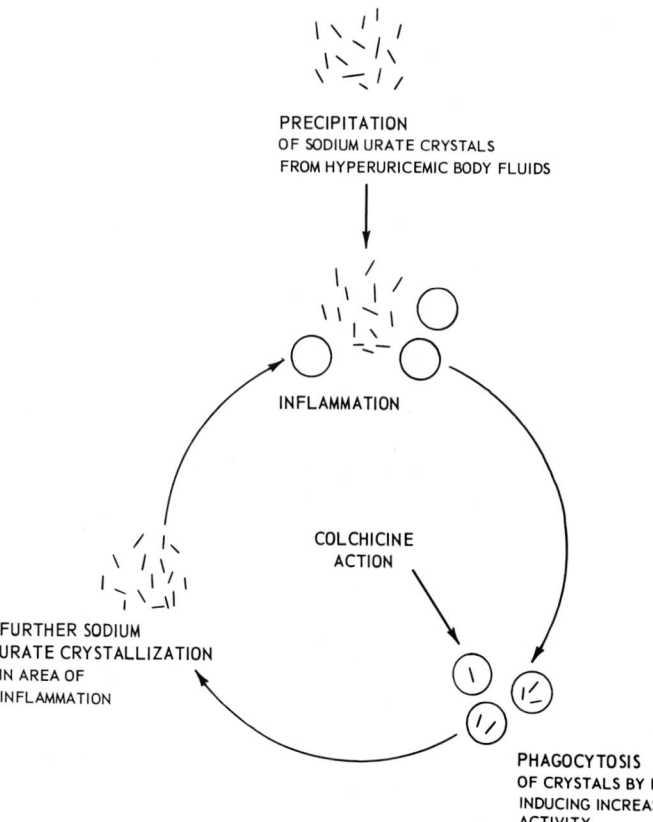

PRECIPITATION
OF SODIUM URATE CRYSTALS
FROM HYPERURICEMIC BODY FLUIDS

INFLAMMATION

COLCHICINE
ACTION

FURTHER SODIUM
URATE CRYSTALLIZATION
IN AREA OF
INFLAMMATION

PHAGOCYTOSIS
OF CRYSTALS BY LEUKOCYTES
INDUCING INCREASED METABOLIC
ACTIVITY

FIGURE 151-1 A possible mechanism of acute gouty arthritis. *(From Seegmiller JE, Howell RR: Arthritis Rheum 5:616, 1962. Reproduced with permission of the publisher.)*

NORMAL

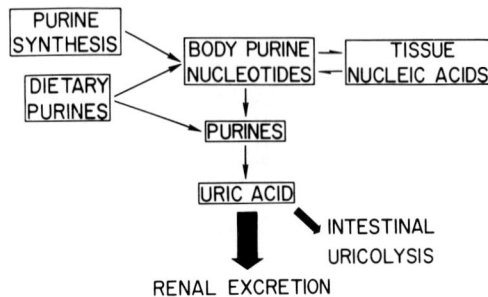

PRIMARY GOUT
With overproduction of uric acid

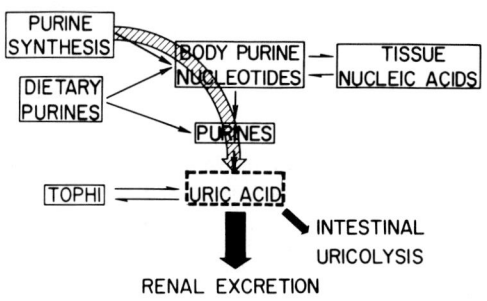

SECONDARY GOUT
Associated with myeloproliferative disease

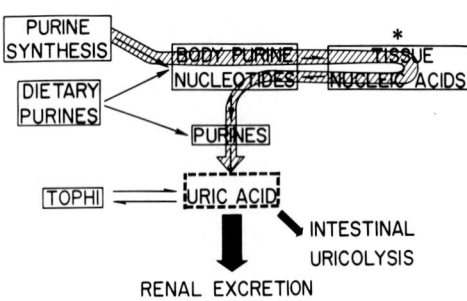

PRIMARY GOUT
With diminished renal excretion of uric acid

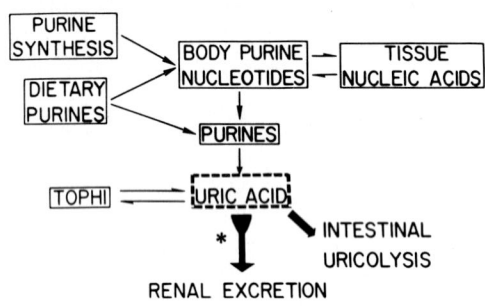

FIGURE 151-2 Origin and disposition of uric acid in normal man and causes of hyperuricemia in gout. *(From Seegmiller JE et al: N Engl J Med 268:712, 764, 821, 1963. Reproduced with permission of the publisher.)*

having lesser amounts of HPRT enzyme manifest, in addition, a variety of mild neurologic disorders.

The second X-linked disorder associated with gout and overproduction of purine consists of a high specific activity (2 to 3 times normal) of the enzyme phosphoribosylpyrophosphate synthetase. Two families have been found in whom this enzyme defect is associated with deafness.[5,6] Cells of patients with both of these disorders show a high intracellular concentration of the substrate for the presumed rate-limiting reaction of purine synthesis, phosphoribosylpyrophosphate.

Severe gouty arthritis is also a major clinical problem of patients with type I glycogen storage disease (glucose-6-phosphatase deficiency) who live to adult life. They show not only a renal retention of uric acid associated with a profound lactic acidemia and ketonemia but also an excessive rate of purine synthesis. Some evidence has been presented in support of the view that the overproduction of purines results from an intermittent glucogen-mediated increase in glycogen breakdown which induces a secondary depletion of ATP and inorganic phosphate within the cells, thus leading to an excessive rate of purine synthesis. Both the lactic acidemia and excessive rate of purine synthesis can be alleviated by continuous feedings by a nasal gastric tube, suggesting that they are a direct consequence in these patients of hypoglycemia.[13] A similar depletion of ATP and of inorganic phosphate with an accompanying hyperuricemia induced by fructose consumption in heterozygotes for hereditary fructose intolerance has been proposed to account for the concurrence of these disorders in a significant portion of the patients with familial gout.[8,9]

Not all patients with essential hyperuricemia develop gout, but the chance of developing gouty arthritis seems to be increased by the degree of hyperuricemia and the duration of exposure to hyperuricemia.

Clinical Manifestations

History

Acute Gout A typical patient with gout is an adult male, usually in his thirties or forties, who gives a history of the sudden onset over a few hours of an excruciating, throbbing pain, usually in a single peripheral joint, frequently the first metatarsophalangeal joint, which appears warm, red, and so exquisitely tender that even the touch of a bedsheet may be intolerable to the patient. The patient is incapacitated and unable to use the limb. Frequently the overlying warmth and redness is interpreted as a cellulitis from an infectious process or as a sprain developing after minimal trauma. If undiagnosed and untreated, the acute attack will gradually subside over a period of days to weeks with complete recovery of normal function lasting months to years.

Tophaceous Gout If untreated, the natural history is one of recurrent acute attacks in different joints over the years at progressively more frequent intervals. Eventually full recovery between attacks does not occur, thereby merging into the stage of chronic tophaceous gout. At this stage the cumulative tophaceous deposits erode into bone and cartilage, causing structural damage that is only partially reversible. Impairment of renal function by the disease can lead to a progressive decrease in ability to excrete uric acid, thereby accelerating the pathologic process.

Cutaneous Findings

The area involved by the acute attack shows the classic signs of an acute inflammatory process consisting of warmth, tenderness, swelling, as well as varying degrees of redness (Fig. 151-3). As the acute attack diminishes, the involved area often assumes a violaceous hue and the skin may show desquamation.

The tophaceous deposit is a highly specific lesion of gout which should not be confused with the deposits of xanthoma tuberosum, rheumatoid nodules, or Darwinian tubercles of the ear. Subcutaneous lesions have a characteristic salmon-pink color and are seen most commonly on the helix of the ear (Fig. 151-4*a*), over the bursa of the elbow Fig. 151-4*b*, and about the digits of the hands and feet (Fig. 151-4*c*, *d*). When very large, they usually drain a chalky white material consisting of crystals of monosodium urate. In gout associated with psoriasis, the excessive uric acid synthesis is a consequence of the more rapid turnover of nucleic acid associated with proliferation of the epidermal cells and is diminished when the proliferation process is brought under control.[4]

Other Physical Findings

A fever and systemic symptoms not infrequently accompany the acute attack. Although the acute attack of gout does not produce permanent joint damage, the bony erosions from tophaceous deposits are readily demonstrable by x-ray as characteristic punched-out lesions in subchondral areas of the bone of peripheral joints, most commonly the first metatarsophalangeal joint. Gout patients have a high incidence of renal calculi that may produce symptoms. The physical findings characteristic of any one of the variety of underlying diseases associated with hyperuricemia listed above may also be found.

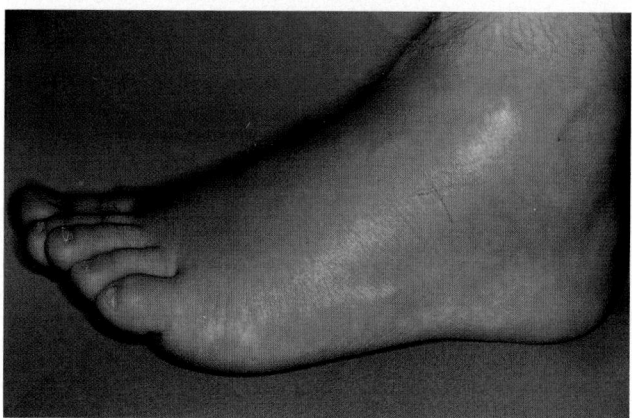

FIGURE 151-3 Acute gout. This middle-aged male experienced sudden onset of excruciating, throbbing pain in the foot. Clinically, the involved area was red, hot, and exquisitely tender. The first episode of acute gout is often confused with bacterial cellulitis.

Laboratory Findings

Hyperuricemia (a serum urate above 7.0 mg/dL) is found in virtually all gouty patients, although an occasional patient may show a serum urate value in the high normal range, particularly during the acute attack. As methodology has improved, the number of instances of gouty arthritis with normal serum urate has diminished. Leukocytosis and an increased sedimentation rate accompany the generalized inflammatory reaction. In advanced stages of renal damage the serum creatinine is first elevated, followed by an increase in uric acid content. Laboratory tests also may show evidence of polycythemia, hemolytic anemia, other hematologic disorders, abnormalities of calcium metabolism, or hypothyroidism among gouty patients.

Pathology

The characteristic lesion of gout is the deposit of crystals of needle-shaped monosodium urate and the accompanying inflammatory reaction of the surrounding tissue. However, tissue deposits of urate crystals almost invariably are dissolved away during formalin fixation and aqueous staining routinely used in preparation of histologic specimens. Fixation in absolute ethanol or freezing is required for preservation of crystals in histologic materials. Crystals are brilliantly anisotropic when viewed microscopically with polarized light, and in the staining technique of DeGalantha the urate crystals appear brownish black. Deposits of elongated urate crystals in the interstices of the renal pyramids are seen in many of the patients with long-standing gout. These deposits are accompanied by evidence of chronic pyelonephritis which does not need to be bacterial in origin. A high incidence of arteriolar nephrosclerosis and chronic glomerulonephritis also has been found.

Diagnosis and Differential Diagnosis

In most patients the clinical features of the acute attack are sufficiently characteristic to permit a presumptive diagnosis if the possibility of gout is but considered. The subsequent demonstration of hyperuricemia and the clinical response of the arthritis to colchicine within 24 to 48 h of treatment provides confirmation of the diagnosis. A positive diagnosis can be established by demonstration of urate crystals in the material removed with a needle or expressed from a subcutaneous tophus or in fluid aspirated from a synovial effusion. Monosodium urate crystals have a needle-like shape and are intensely birefringent, so are readily detected through polarizing filters attached to an ordinary light microscope. The acute attack of gout is often confused with severe cellulitis or septic arthritis; however, regional lymphadenopathy is seldom seen in acute gout and a septic process is often surrounded by doughlike, pitting edema. Synovial fluid examination and culture provide a definitive answer. Biopsy of the subcutaneous nodule with fixation in alcohol provides histologic distinction between the gouty tophus and the rheumatoid nodule of rheumatoid arthritis. Chondrocalcinosis (pseudogout) also shows birefringent crystals (calcium pyrophosphate) in the synovial fluid, but the calcium deposited in the knee or wrist joint serves to distinguish it from gout by x-ray. Other types of arthritis to be considered include osteoarthritis, Reiter's syndrome, and palindromic rheumatism.

Treatment

Acute Gouty Arthritis

The affected joints should be kept at complete rest. A narcotic is often required for analgesia. As early as possible in the attack, one of the drugs discussed below should be administered to control the inflammation. Treatment with drugs that lower serum urate should not be started until the acute attack is well under control because of their tendency to cause an exacerbation of the acute attack.

Colchicine (0.5 mg) is given hourly until relief is obtained or until nausea, vomiting, or diarrhea occur, at which time the drug is discontinued. Because of its specific effect on acute gouty arthritis, colchicine remains the drug of choice for the presenting attack, particularly if the diagnosis is in doubt. It is helpful in aborting an incipient attack and less effective if given late in the course of an

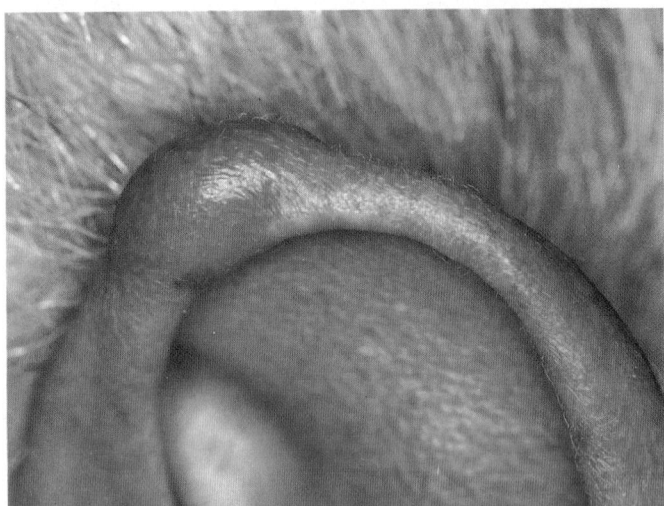

a

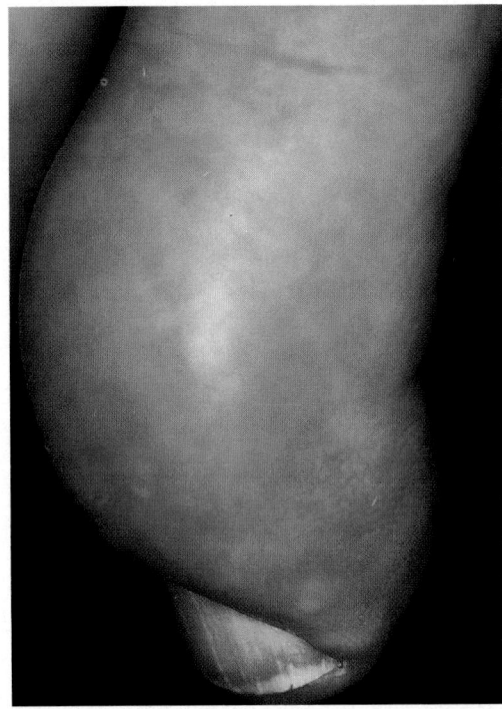

c

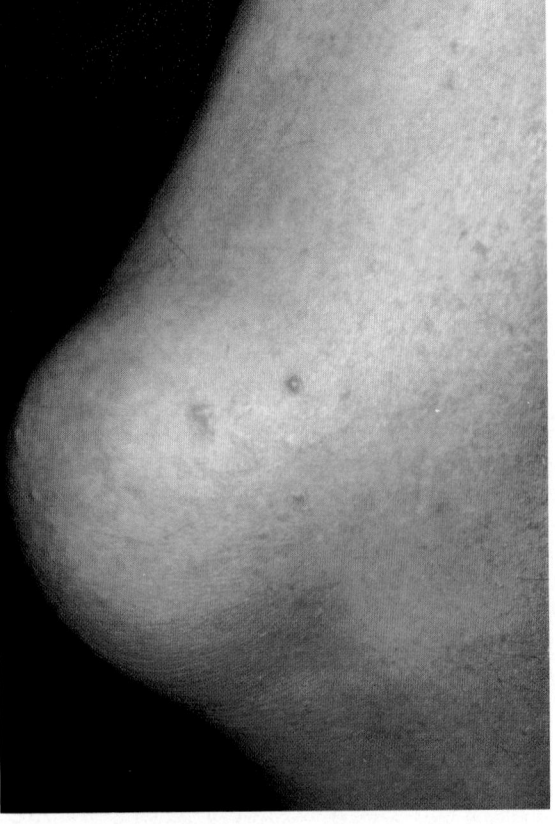

b

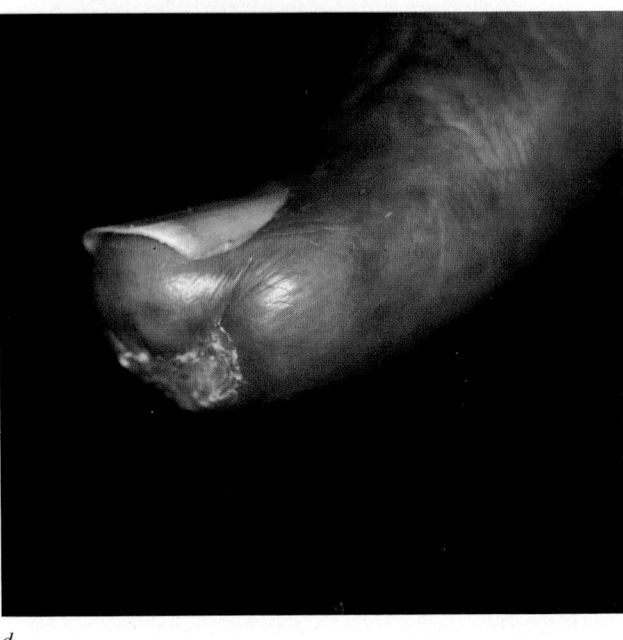

d

FIGURE 151-4 Tophaceous gout. Deposits of uric acid are seen in the (*a*) helix of the ear, (*b*) olecranon bursa of the elbow, (*c*) dorsum of the finger, (*d*) tip of the finger, and (*e*) around multiple joints on the dorsum of the hands and wrists.

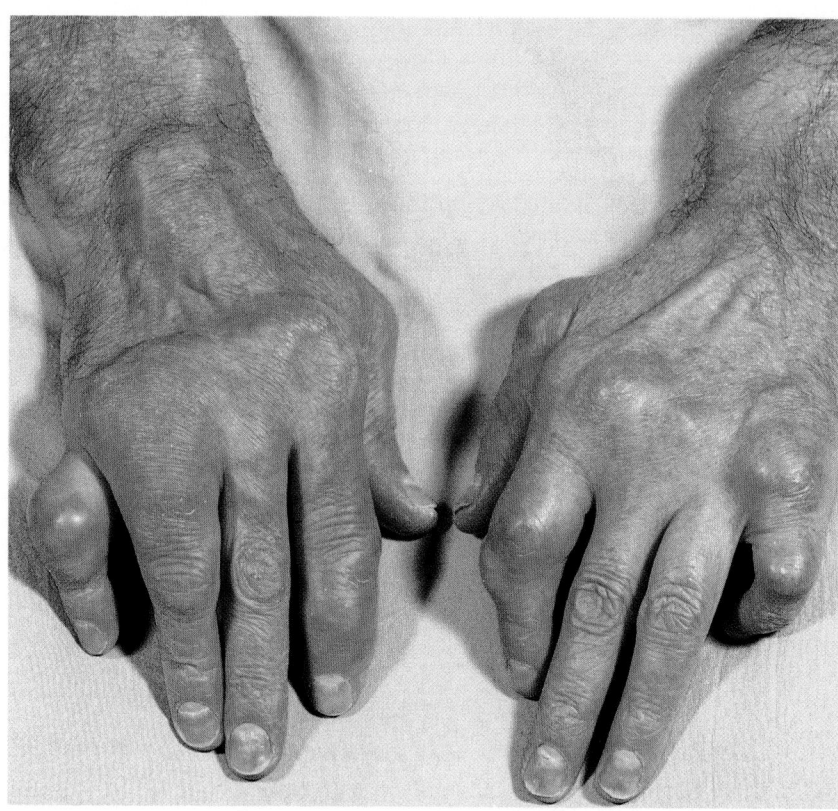

FIGURE 151-4 *(continued)*   e

attack. Administration of 2.0 mg diluted in 20 mL of saline by the intravenous route is very effective, particularly for a patient with peptic ulcer or before or after surgery since this route avoids the gastrointestinal side effects that often accompany oral colchicine. No more than 5 mg in divided doses should be given by the intravenous route over a 48-h period and even this dose should be given only to patients with normal renal function. It is best delivered into the tubing of a running intravenous system in order to avoid the painful consequences of extravasation.

Adrenocorticotropic hormine (ACTH) in long-acting repository gel form at a dosage of 50 to 100 units administered intramuscularly provides effective control of even very severe attacks. Colchicine (0.5 mg, 2 to 3 times daily) should be given concurrently to prevent a ''rebound'' attack.

Alternative methods of terminating the acute attack of gouty arthritis include phenylbutazone or oxyphenbutazone given orally at a dose of 0.4 g followed by 0.1 to 0.2 g at 4 and 8 h, and by 0.1 g four times daily for the second and third day. The drug is then stopped.

Indomethacin at a dose of 50 mg three times daily for 2 to 3 days is also effective but sometimes produces the side effect of headache. Other newer anti-inflammatory drugs have also been found to be effective in terminating acute attacks of gouty arthritis.

Preventive Therapy

Colchicine, 0.5 mg taken 2 to 4 times daily depending on tolerance to gastrointestinal side effects, is very effective in preventing acute attacks. However, it does nothing to prevent the more serious joint destruction by tophaceous deposits. This aspect of the disease, as well as the progressive renal damage, presumably can be arrested by lowering the serum urate concentration to the normal unsaturated range (below 7.0 mg/dL) by the use of one of a number of drugs. The serum urate should be determined every few weeks as a guide to the proper dose of medication during the period when therapy is initiated. Prophylactic daily colchicine is especially important during the initiation and the first 3 to 4 months of therapy with drugs used to lower the serum urate content in order to suppress the tendency of gout patients to develop acute attacks during this time. Patients should always be warned that they are at greater risk for developing an acute attack during this period and should be advised to take an extra tablet of colchicine at the appearance of the very first symptom suggestive of an impending acute attack.

Since therapy with a drug for lowering the serum urate is a commitment to lifelong medication, the proper drug for each particular patient's need should be selected. This can be determined most readily by assessing the 24-h urinary excretion of uric acid while the patient is maintained on a diet virtually free of purine compounds. For this purpose meat, fish, fowl, the high-purine vegetables (peas, beans, and other leguminous plants), as well as all fermented or alcohol-containing beverages and caffeine-containing drinks are eliminated from the diet for a 6-day period. Twenty-four-hour urines are then collected over the last 3 days of the diet, each in a separate bottle containing 3 mL of toluene as preservative, and the urine is stored at room temperature until analysis to minimize the deposition of crystalline uric acid that tends to occur at lower temperatures. Uricosuric drugs, as well as drugs that cause urate retention such as salicylate and most antihypertensive drugs except the spironolactones are also eliminated during the evaluation period on the diet. The drug acetaminophen (Tylenol) should be used in place of aspirin or other salicylate-containing medication for mild analgesia by all gout patients.

The purine-free diet and urine collection are most conveniently instituted immediately after the patient presents with his acute attack of gout. At this time he is well motivated to follow a diet virtually free of purines. In addition, time must be allowed for resolving the acute attack of gout before instituting any therapy with uricosuric drugs, otherwise the acute attack may not be as promptly resolved.

The 24-h urines are analyzed for uric acid and creatinine; the latter compound provides an index of complete 24-h collection. Excretion of quantities of uric acid greater than 600 mg for 24 h is indicative of purine overproduction and is indication for beginning the xanthine oxidase inhibitor allopurinol (Zyloprim), which blocks uric acid production by specifically reducing purine overproduction. Other indications for allopurinol are a uric acid/creatinine ratio of the morning urine above 0.7, a history of renal calculi composed of uric acid, or the presence of impaired renal function. It is effective in preventing uric acid stone formation as well as dissolving calculi already formed. It can be used in combination with uricosuric drugs, if necessary, but such combined therapy is seldom required.

Allopurinol has a prolonged therapeutic action and is available in 0.1- and 0.3-g tablets. The usual dosage is 0.1 to 0.4 g daily and is particularly useful for patients resistant or intolerant to uricosuric drugs. In addition, it is specifically indicated for patients who are producing excessive quantities of uric acid in the 24-h urine as stated above.

Excretion of quantities of uric acid less than 600 mg per 24 h in the absence of evidence of renal impairment indicates a normal production of uric acid and a probable specifically diminished renal clearance of uric acid as the basis for hyperuricemia. Therefore, a uricosuric drug provides the specific correction to normalize this aberration of renal physiology.

Probenecid acts to increase the renal excretion of uric acid. It is begun at a low dose of 0.25 g twice daily and gradually increased over a week's time to the usual maintenance dose of 0.5 g 2 to 3 times daily. It may be increased to as high as 3.0 g daily if necessary to produce a normal serum urate concentration.

Sulfinpyrazone provides a much greater uricosuric action and is often required in the presence of renal impairment. It is begun at a dose of 50 mg twice daily and increased over a week to 0.1 g 3 to 4 times daily. Up to 0.8 g per day can be administered if necessary. The serum urate should initially be evaluated at monthly intervals and the dose of allopurinol or uricosuric drug increased as needed to bring the serum urate to the unsaturated range of 6 mg/dL or less.

Adjuncts to Treatment

A high fluid intake of at least 3 L per day will be of value in preventing uric acid precipitation in the urinary tract. Since low-calorie diets can exacerbate hyperuricemia and provoke acute attacks of gout, any weight reduction is best deferred until the serum urate concentration has been brought under control and the disease is quiescent. Avoidance of high-purine foods may be helpful until the serum urate has been brought under control, then a regular diet is advised.

Prognosis

As a result of improvement in therapy over the past three decades almost all patients with gouty arthritis can now look forward to a full and productive life without serious disability from their arthritis or uric acid stones of the urinary tract. This can be achieved by early diagnosis, continuous medical supervision, and institution of a preventive program of management which includes assessment of serum urate concentration taken before the morning medications at 6-month intervals with appropriate adjustment of drug dosage to assure the maintenance of serum urate concentrations well within the normal range of less than 7.0 mg/dL.

Whether the recent demonstrations of an aberration of fructose metabolism in at least some patients with hereditary gout can lead to a beneficial effect from restriction of dietary fructose in these patients remains to be demonstrated clinically. Restriction of fructose could account for the beneficial effect of the diet reported by Stirpe et al. in some gout patients.[14]

References

1. Garrod AB: *The Nature and Treatment of Gout and Rheumatic Gout.* London, Walton and Maberly, 1859
2. Seegmiller JE: Diseases of purine and pyrimidine metabolism, in *Metabolic Control and Disease,* 8th ed, edited by PK Bondy, LE Rosenberg. Philadelphia, Saunders, 1980, p 777
3. Wyngaarden JB, Kelley WN: *Gout and Hyperuricemia.* New York, Grune & Stratton, 1976
4. Eisen AZ, Seegmiller JE: Uric acid metabolism in psoriasis. *J Clin Invest* **40**:1486, 1961
5. Becker MA et al: Variant human phosphoribosylpyrophosphate synthetase altered in regulatory and catalytic functions. *J Clin Invest* **65**:109, 1980
6. Simmonds HA et al: Evidence of a new syndrome involving hereditary uric acid overproduction, neurological complications and deafness. *Adv Exp Med Biol* **165 (pt A)**:97, 1984
7. Seegmiller JE: Disorders of purine and pyrimidine metabolism, in *The Principles and Practice of Medical Genetics,* edited by A Emery, D Rimoin. New York, Churchill Livingstone, 1984, p 97
8. Oberhaensli RD et al: Study of hereditary fructose intolerance by use of ^{31}P magnetic resonance spectroscopy. *Lancet* **2**:931, 1987
9. Seegmiller JE et al: Fructose-induced aberration of metabolism in familial gout identified by ^{31}P magnetic resonance spectroscopy. *Proc Natl Acad Sci* **87**:8326, 1990
10. Talbott JR, Yu T-F: *Gout and Uric Acid Metabolism.* New York, Stratton Intercontinental Medical Book Corp, 1976
11. Simkin PA: The pathogenesis of podagra. *Ann Intern Med* **86**:230, 1977
12. Seegmiller JE: Inherited deficiency of hypoxanthine-guanine phosphoribosyltransferase in X-linked uric aciduria (the Lesch-Nyhan syndrome and its variants), in *Advances in Human Genetics,* edited by H Harris, K Hirschhorn. New York, Plenum, vol 6, p 75
13. Greene HL et al: ATP depletion. A possible role in hyperuricemia in glycogen storage disease Type I. *J Clin Invest* **62**:321, 1978
14. Stirpe F et al: Fructose-induced hyperuricemia. *Lancet* **2**:1310, 1970

CHAPTER 152

Machiel K. Polano

Xanthomatoses and Dyslipoproteinemias

Xanthomas are tumors or infiltrations of the skin, varying from yellow (Greek *xanthos*) to brown or red-purple in color.[1] When they arise in tendons, the overlying skin retains its normal color or is somewhat yellow. When xanthomas are flat, they are traditionally called xanthelasma (*èlasma,* "plaque"). Histologically, xanthomas are composed of fibroblasts, histiocytes, macrophages, and, often, Touton giant-cells, all laden with lipids; the lipids are seen as vacuoles in hematoxylin-eosin (H&E)-stained sections and react positively with Sudan III and oil red O. Other inflammatory cells may also be present (see Figs. 152-1, 152-2, and 152-3).

Classification of xanthomas

Xanthomas arise in a broad spectrum of conditions, the most important of which are those arising in association with specific defects in lipoprotein metabolism (dyslipoproteinemias). They also occur in normolipoproteinemic patients. This leads to the following classification:

1. *Normolipemic xanthomas*
   a. Xanthomas associated with reticuloses such as xanthoma disseminatum, Hand-Schüller-Christian disease, Abt-Letterer-Siwe disease (see Chap. 160)
   b. Juvenile xanthogranuloma, also known as nevoxanthoendothelioma (see Chap. 160) (Fig. 152-4)

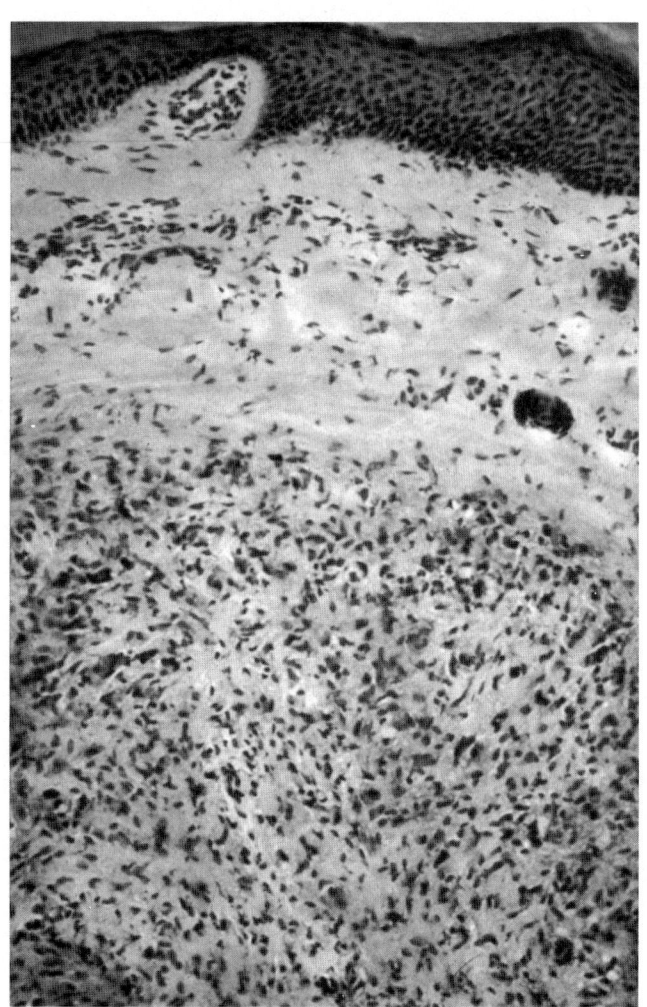

FIGURE 152-1 Histology of xanthoma tendinosum stained with hematoxylin and eosin. Low magnification.

Based on the chapter in previous editions by H. Bryan Brewer, Jr., and Donald S. Frederickson

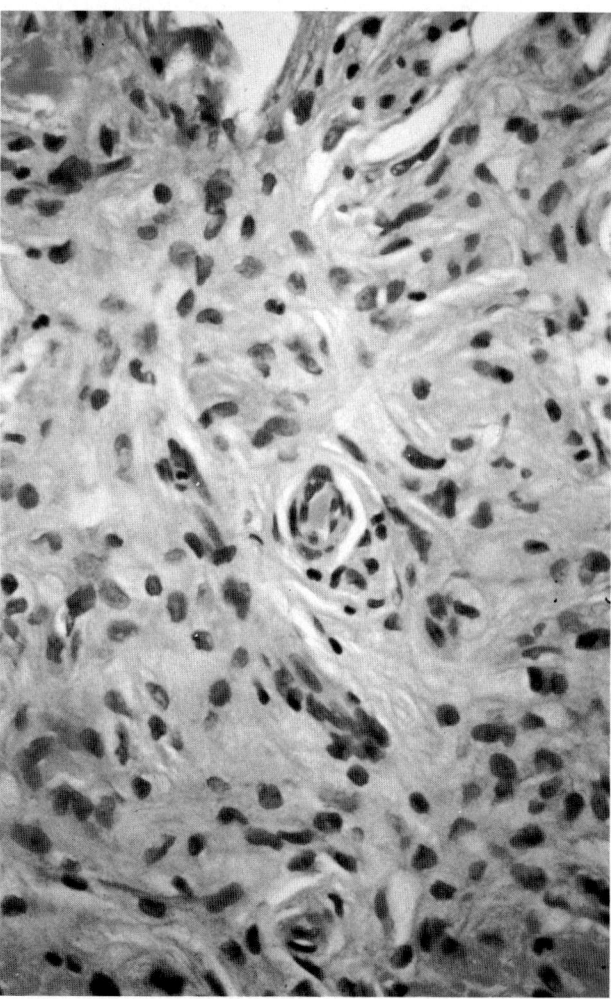

FIGURE 152-2 Higher magnification of section of xanthoma tendinosum showing foam cells and fibroblasts.

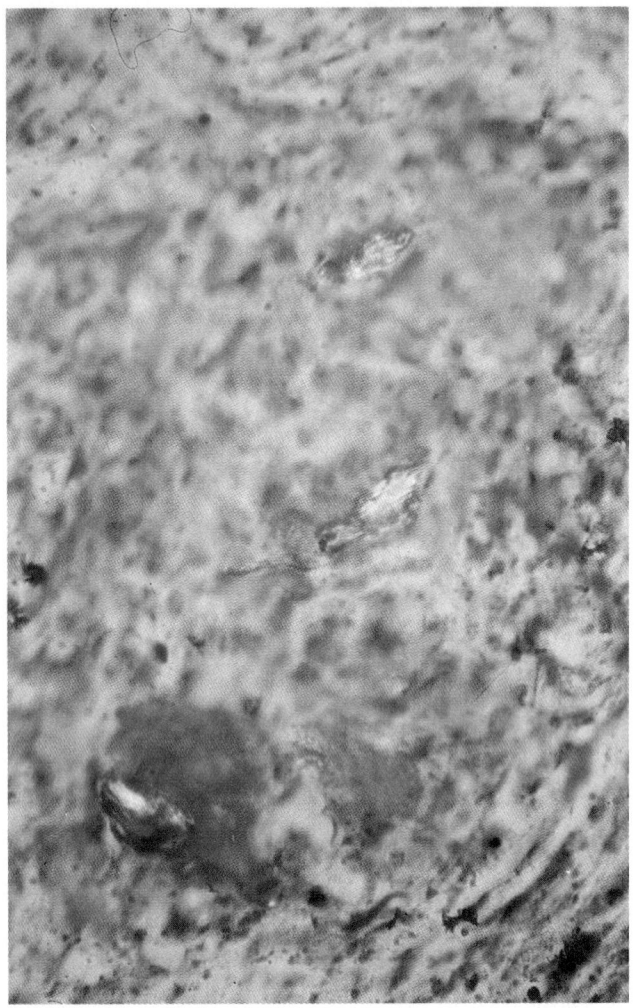

FIGURE 152-3 Section of eruptive xanthoma stained with oil red 0.

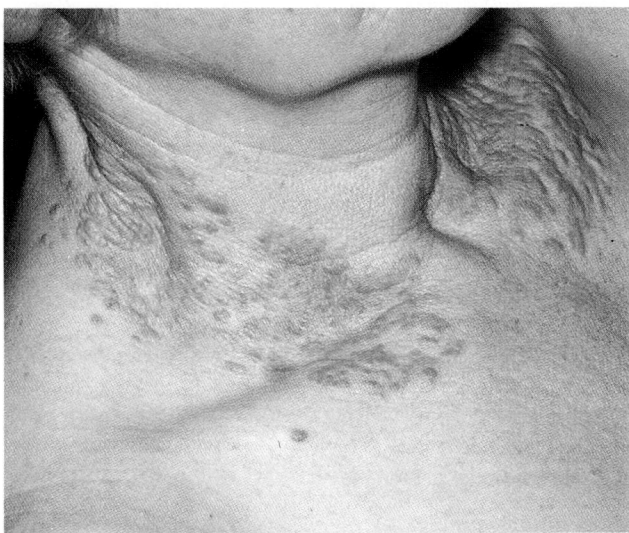

FIGURE 152-5 Disseminated flat xanthoma (xanthoma planum) on the neck.

   c. Xanthoma planum disseminatum (Winkelman-Altman) (Figs. 152-5 and 152-6)

   d. Xanthelasma palpebrarum. In the literature these are often referred to simply as xanthelasma. Although palpebral xanthelasma occur regularly in dyslipoproteinemic patients, in the majority of cases no systemic cause can be found (Fig. 152-7).

   e. Xanthomas arising secondarily in lymphedema or associated with various skin tumors, such as histiocytoma

 2. *Dyslipoidemic xanthomas*[2,3]

   a. Primary dyslipoidemic xanthomas, which are a symptom, in most cases, of a genetically caused dyslipoproteinemia.

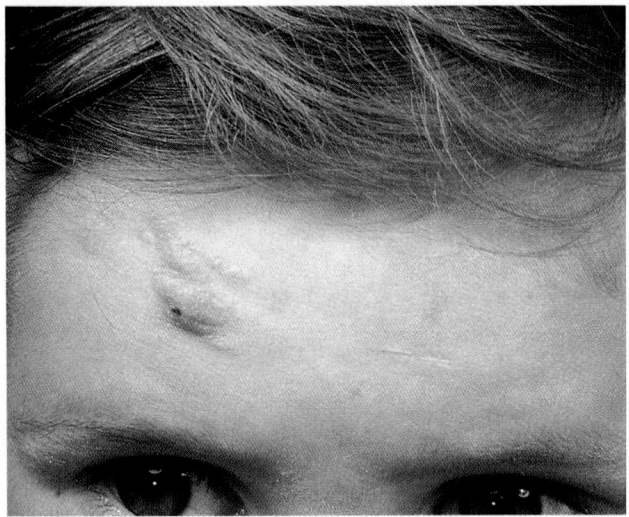

FIGURE 152-4 Juvenile xanthogranuloma, also known as nevoxanthoendothelioma.

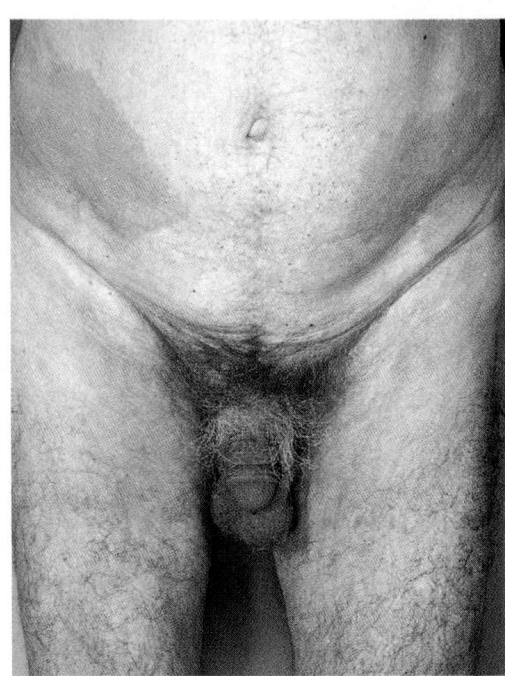

FIGURE 152-6 Disseminated flat xanthoma in the "bathing trunk" area.

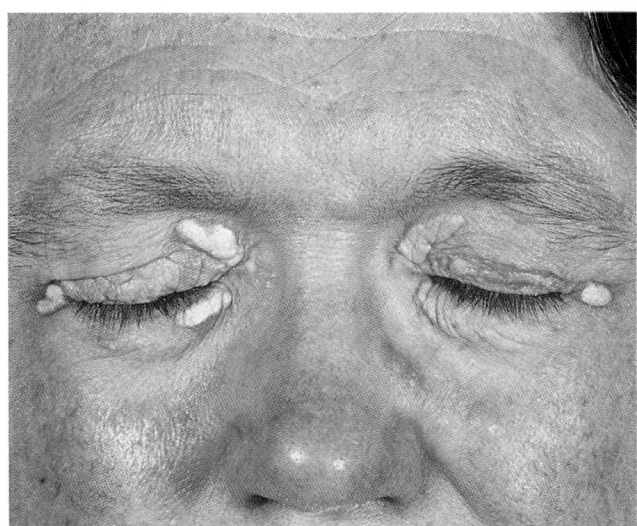

FIGURE 152-7 Palpebral xanthelasma in a patient with familial hypercholesterolemia. A similar clinical picture may be seen in normolipemic patients.

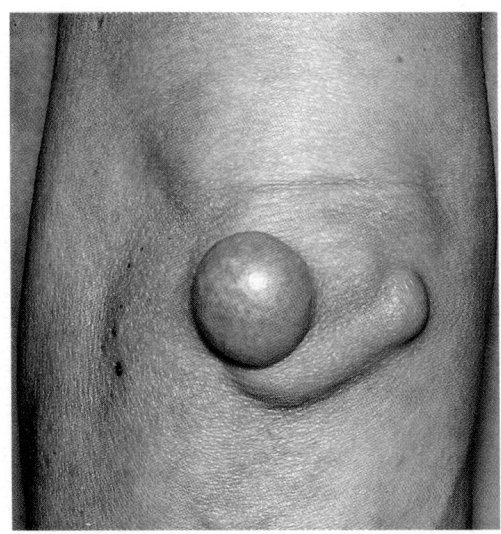

FIGURE 152-8 Tuberous and tendon xanthomas in a patient with familial hypercholesterolemia.

In addition to xanthomas, the process is associated with signs and symptoms in other organ systems, most significantly in the cardiovascular system.

    b. Classified as secondary lipoproteinemia with xanthomatosis are those cases in which the hyperlipoproteinemia is secondary to another metabolic disease, such as diabetes, hypothyroidism, or primary biliary cirrhosis.

The following cutaneous lesions may be distinguished in primary hyperlipoproteinemia:

1. *Xanthelasma palpebrarum.* Yellow plaques on the eyelids predominantly the nasal side (Fig. 152-7).
2. *Xanthoma tendinosum.* Subcutaneous tumors of varying dimension, especially in the Achilles tendons and extensor tendons of the hands. The overlying skin color is normal. Related to the tendinous xanthomas are subperiostal xanthomas below the knees (Figs. 152-8 and 152-9).
3. *Xanthoma papuloeruptivum.* Small, yellow-brown, sometimes red papules, which seem to spring up in crops. They have a predilection for the buttocks and thighs, but also occur on the arms, elbows, and palms (Figs. 152-10, 152-11, and 152-12).
4. *Xanthoma tuberoeruptivum.* Tumors in most cases on the elbows, originating from a coalescence of papules (Fig. 152-13).
5. *Xanthoma tuberosum.* Tumors with a smooth surface on the buttocks, elbows, and knees (Figs. 152-14, 152-15, and 152-16).
6. *Xanthoma and xanthochromia striata palmaris.* Yellow discoloration and linear infiltration of the creases of the palms, often combined with papular xanthomas of the palms. The striate discolorations and xanthomas of the palms regularly occur together. The term planar xanthoma is best avoided as it causes confusion with the diffuse plane xanthomas that occur in normolipemic patients (Figs. 152-17 and 152-18).

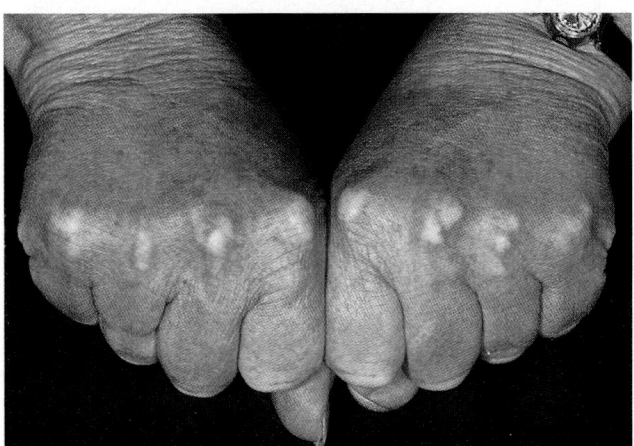

FIGURE 152-9 Tendon xanthomas of the hands in a patient with hypercholesterolemia.

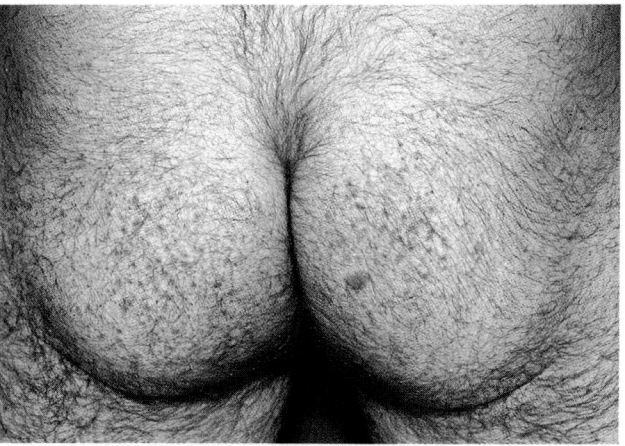

FIGURE 152-10 Eruptive xanthomas of the buttocks in a patient with hyperchylomicronemia.

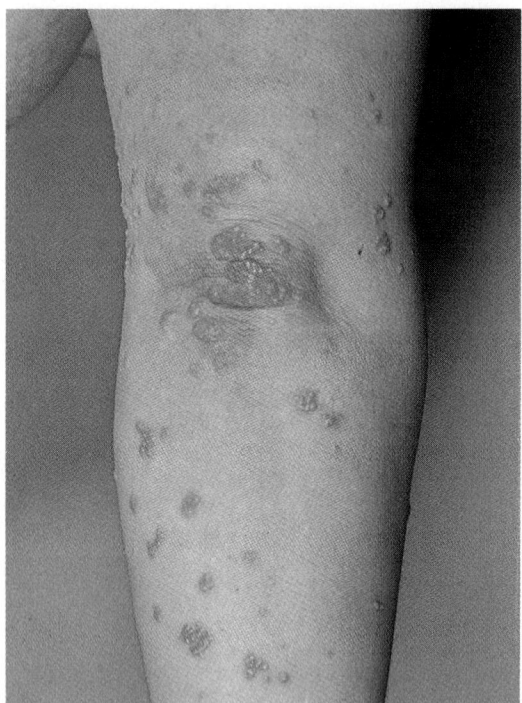

FIGURE 152-11 Eruptive and tuberoeruptive xanthomas of the arm in a patient with hyperchylomicronemia and hyper-VLDL-emia (type V).

7. *Xanthoma intertriginosum.* This term has been introduced recently for xanthomas in the fingerwebs and the anal cleft (Figs. 152-19 and 152-20).

Histologic Examination

Examination of the histopathology and histochemistry of xanthomas seems to offer the possibility of extrapolation of observations made in the skin to the vascular problems associated with the process. Xanthomas are characterized by foam cells, and Braun-Falco and Eckert[4] distinguish small clusters of cells that show birefringence due to cholesterol in polarized light (type I) from large perivascular cells with foamy cytoplasm (type II). In one study, histochemical investigation of 27 xanthomas indicated that eruptive xanthomas contained relatively more free fatty acids and triglycerides and less cholesterol esters than tuberous and tendinous xanthomas. The triglycerides in the xanthomas contained more oleic acid and less linoleic acid than the plasma.[5] Comparison of regressing with nonregressing xanthomas showed that the former have a relatively lower cholesterol ester and a higher phospholipid content. This difference influences the physical properties of the lipid mixtures.[6]

Lipoprotein Metabolism

Large quantities of poorly soluble lipids are transported in extracellular fluids, including plasma, as lipoproteins, which are particles composed of several lipids (including cholesterol, triglycerides, and phospholipids), and proteins called *apolipoproteins*. Abnor-

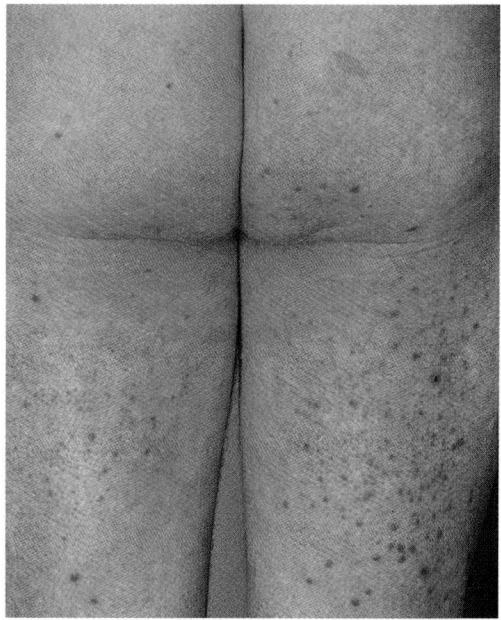

FIGURE 152-12 Eruptive xanthomas in a patient with familial dysbetalipoproteinemia.

malities of lipid transport often present clinically as abnormal plasma concentrations of cholesterol or triglycerides (dyslipidemia means hyper- or hypolipidemia). Such abnormalities are best understood by their translation into dyslipoproteinemias and by quantitating the concentrations and composition of the plasma lipoproteins in which lipids are transported. A frequent clinical expression of hyperlipoproteinemias is the occurrence of the xanthomas discussed above, in which there are deposits of lipoprotein components in various parts of the skin. Frequently primary-care physicians and dermatologists are the first called upon to interpret such

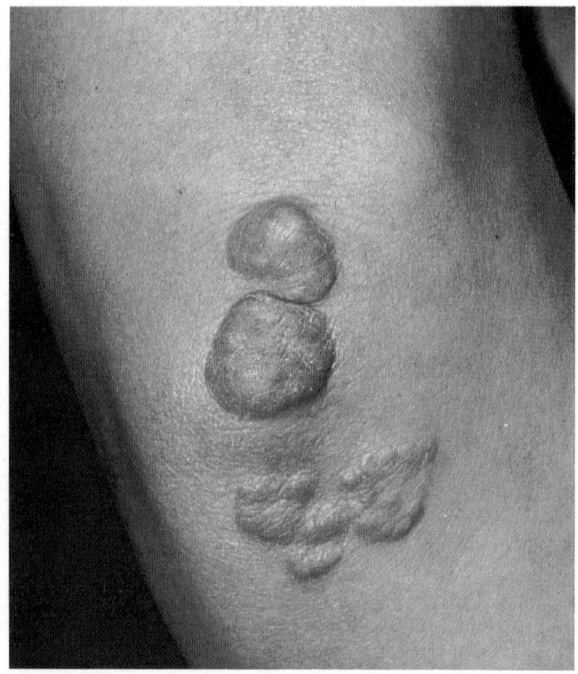

FIGURE 152-13 Tuberoeruptive xanthomas in a patient with familial dysbetalipoproteinemia.

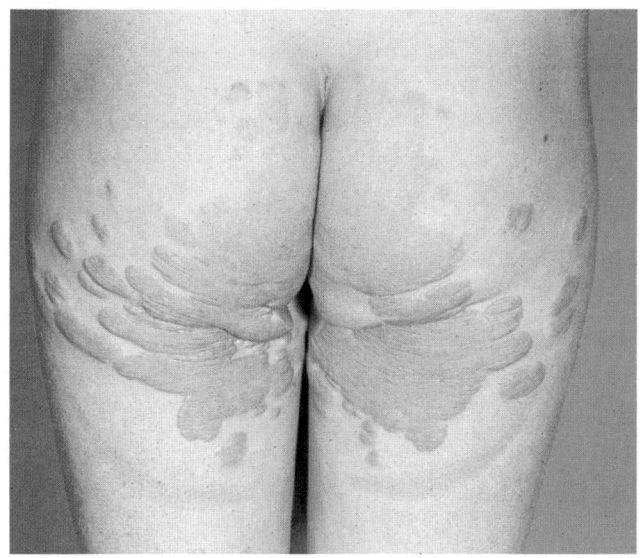

FIGURE 152-14 Flat and fibrous xanthomas of the buttocks in association with homozygous familial hypercholesterolemias.

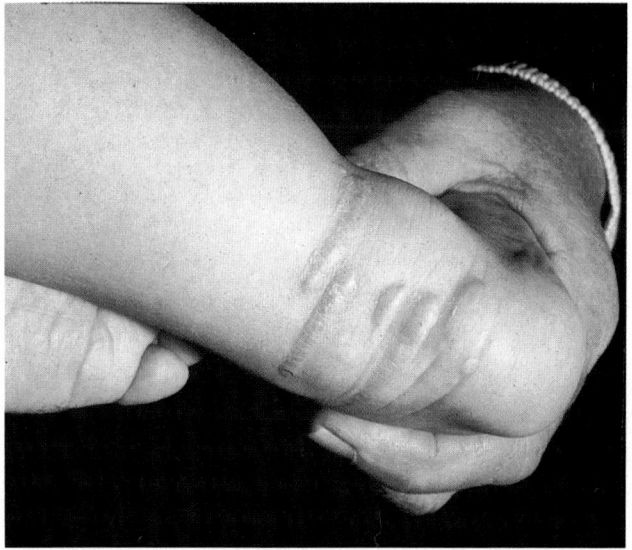

FIGURE 152-15 Tuberous xanthomas on the Achilles tendon region in a patient with familial hypercholesterolemia.

lesions. The diseases represented are diverse, numerous, and of considerable importance, especially because of their relationship to cardiovascular disease. Moreover, by early interpretation of the signs and symptoms and by institution of appropriate treatment, later severe complications may be prevented.

Knowledge of the chemistry of lipoproteins is growing steadily. The minimum required for proper understanding of the basis for dyslipidemia, dyslipoproteinemia, and xanthomatosis is presented here. Normal values for plasma concentrations of cholesterol and triglycerides and several fractions are given in Table 152-1.

Classification of Lipoproteins

In clinical medicine as well as in research laboratories, lipoproteins are usually classified on the basis of either their electrophoretic mobility or their hydrated density. Plasma lipoproteins can be sepa-

rated by electrophoresis into those that remain at the origin and those that migrate into the beta (β lipoproteins), pre-β lipoproteins, or alpha$_1$ (α lipoproteins) globulin zones. In addition, five major classes of lipoproteins are separable by preparative ultracentrifugation: chylomicrons, very low density lipoproteins (VLDL), intermediate-density lipoproteins (IDL), low-density lipoproteins (LDL), and high-density lipoproteins (HDL). The lipoproteins that remain at the origin on electrophoresis are chylomicrons, those of the pre-β mobility are VLDL, those of β mobility are LDL, and those of α mobility are HDL.

Apolipoproteins[7]

Thirteen major human plasma apolipoproteins have been identified and characterized (Table 152-2). The major apolipoproteins associated with LDL is apoB, and the two principal apolipoproteins of HDL are apoA-I and apoA-II. C-I, C-II, C-III. E_2, E_3, and E_4 are

TABLE 152-1
Normal Plasma Lipid and Lipoprotein Levels

Age	Cholesterol		Triglycerides		VLDL		LDL		HDL	
Male										
0–19	155	(120–195)	65	(55–115)	10	(1–20)	95	(65–130)	50	(35–70)
20–29	170	(125–225)	100	(45–185)	15	(2–30)	110	(70–155)	45	(30–65)
30–39	200	(145–265)	130	(50–285)	25	(4–50)	130	(80–190)	45	(30–65)
40–49	210	(155–270)	150	(55–300)	25	(5–55)	140	(95–195)	45	(30–65)
50–59	215	(155–275)	145	(60–290)	25	(5–55)	145	(90–200)	45	(30–70)
60+	215	(160–280)	135	(65–245)	20	(2–40)	145	(90–200)	50	(30–75)
Female										
0–19	160	(125–205)	70	(35–125)	10	(2–15)	100	(65–140)	50	(35–70)
20–29	175	(125–235)	90	(40–165)	15	(2–30)	110	(65–160)	55	(35–80)
30–39	185	(135–240)	90	(40–185)	15	(2–30)	115	(75–165)	55	(35–80)
40–49	200	(150–265)	105	(45–210)	15	(3–40)	130	(80–180)	60	(35–90)
50–59	225	(165–290)	125	(55–250)	20	(2–45)	75	(90–205)	60	(40–90)
60+	230	(170–290)	130	(60–270)	15	(1–45)	150	(95–220)	65	(35–95)

Values are adopted from Lipid Research Clinics Study and expressed as mg/dL. Values are mean with 5 and 95 percentile limits in parentheses; VLDL, LDL, and HDL values are expressed in terms of cholesterol content (*Lipid Research Clinics Population Studies Data Book, vol 1. DHHS, NIH Publication No. 80-1527, 1980*).

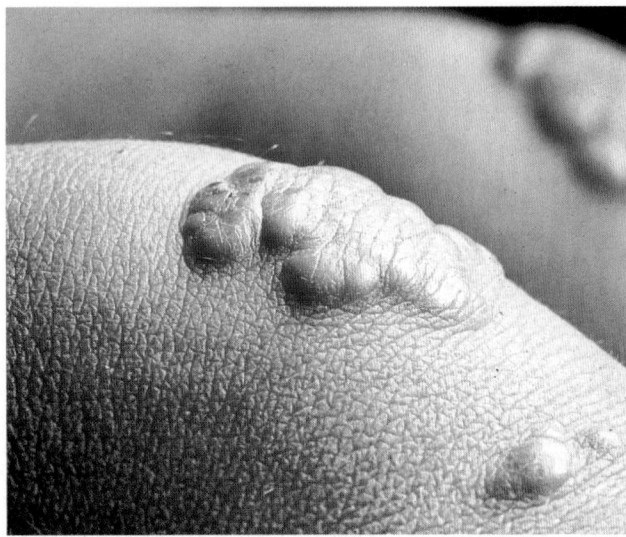

FIGURE 152-16 Tuberous xanthomas of the knees in a patient with homozygous familial hypercholesterolemia.

TABLE 152-2
Major Human Plasma Apolipoproteins

Apolipo-protein	Major density class	Approximate molecular weight	Major site of synthesis in humans
A-I	HDL	28,000	Liver-intestine
A-II	HDL	18,000	Liver-intestine
A-IV	Chylomicrons	45,000	Intestine
B-100	VLDL-IDL-LDL	375,000	Liver
B-48	Chylomicrons-VLDL-IDL	180,000	Intestine
C-I	Chylomicrons-VLDL-HDL	6,500	Liver
C-II	Chylomicrons-VLDL-HDL	10,000	Liver
C-III$_{0-2}$	Chylomicrons-VLDL-HDL	10,000	Liver
D	HDL	20,000	?
E$_{2-4}$	Chylomicrons-VLDL-HDL	40,000	Liver
F	HDL	30,000	?
G	VHDL	75,000	?
H	Chylomicrons	45,000	?

the apolipoproteins found associated with VLDL and chylomicrons, as noted in Table 152-2. In addition to serving as structural constituents of the lipoproteins, the functions of the apolipoproteins include: (1) participating as cofactors or activators of enzymes involved in lipoprotein-lipid metabolism; (2) interacting with a specific receptor site on cells and thereby directing lipoprotein catabolism; and (3) facilitating exchange of lipids (cholesteryl esters, triglycerides, and phospholipids) between various lipoprotein particles. The physiologic functions of a number of different apolipoproteins are summarized in Table 152-3.

The Apolipoprotein B Cascades[8]   A conceptual overview of the known features of lipoprotein metabolism is shown schematically in Fig. 152-21. The metabolic relationships of the principal lipoprotein classes containing apoB may be considered to consist of two major "cascades." The first apoB cascade involves the stepwise metabolism of chylomicrons secreted by the intestine. The major function of these triglyceride-rich lipoproteins is to transport dietary lipids from the intestine to the liver. The chylomicrons se-

creted by the intestine contain a form of apoB synthesized by the intestine, designated as apoB-48. Shortly after secretion, the triglyceride-rich chylomicrons rapidly acquire other apolipoproteins, particularly apoC-II and apoE transferred from HDL. ApoC-II is a cofactor required for optimal activity of lipoprotein lipase (Table 152-3), an enzyme attached to the capillary endothelium that catalyzes, under influence of heparin, the hydrolysis of triglycerides to

TABLE 152-3
Physiologic Functions of Human Plasma Apolipoproteins

Physiologic function	Apolipoprotein
Cofactor for enzyme	
Lipoprotein lipase	apoC-II
Lecithin cholesterol acyltransferase (LCAT)	apoA-I
Ligand on lipoprotein particle for interaction with receptor sites on cells	
Chylomicron remnant	apoE
LDL	apoB-100
HDL	apoA-I and apoE
Structural protein on lipoprotein particle	
Intestinal chylomicron	apoB-48
Hepatogenous VLDL	apoB-100
HDL	apoA-I

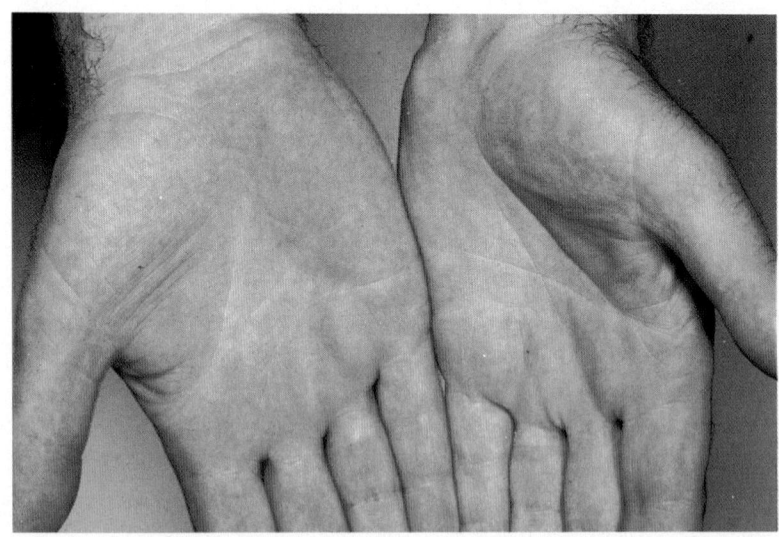

FIGURE 152-17 Xanthochromia of the palms in a patient with familial dyslipoproteinemia.

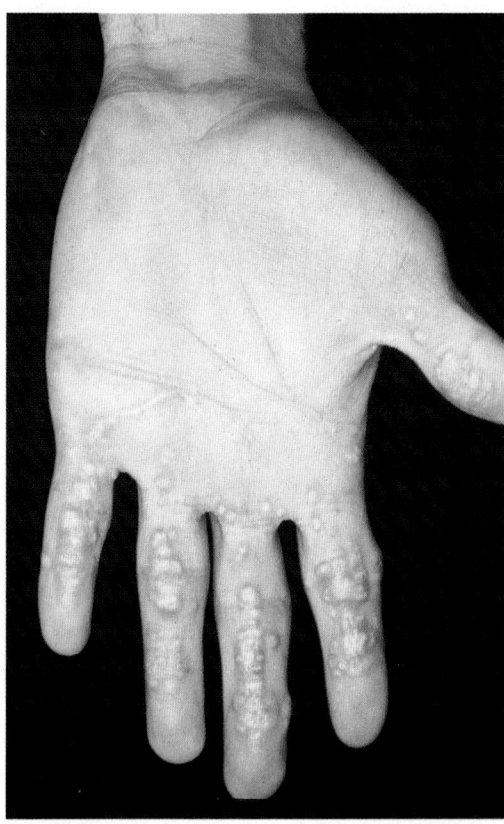

FIGURE 152-18 Xanthochromia of the palm associated with papular xanthomas in a patient with familial dyslipoproteinemia.

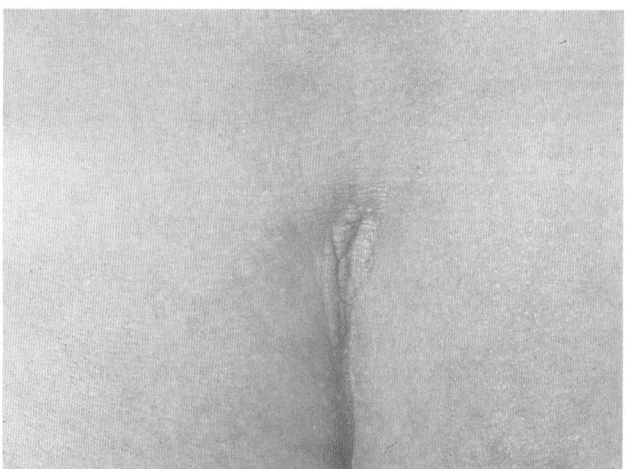

FIGURE 152-19 Intertriginous xanthomas of the gluteal cleft in a patient with homozygous familial hypercholesterolemia.

free fatty acids and monoglycerides. After entering the plasma, the triglycerides on chylomicrons rapidly undergo hydrolysis by lipoprotein lipase, and the chylomicrons are sequentially reduced to "remnants," first having the density of VLDL and then of IDL. The chylomicron remnants are then removed from the plasma by binding to receptors in the liver having an affinity for apoE. The remnants are then taken up by endocytosis, and their constituents are catabolized by the hepatocytes (Fig. 152-21).

The second apoB cascade involves hydrolysis of triglyceride-rich VLDL secreted by the liver. These lipoprotein particles contain apoB-100, a larger molecular weight form of apoB also secreted by the liver. The triglycerides on VLDL also undergo hydrolysis by lipoprotein lipase and are serially converted to lipoproteins with the density of IDL and, finally, LDL. During the conversion of IDL to LDL, apoC-II and apoE dissociate from IDL and reassociate with HDL. The resulting LDL contains apoB-100 almost exclusively (Fig. 152-21). A second lipolytic enzyme, hepatic lipase, appears to be involved in the conversion of IDL to LDL; this enzyme may function both as a triglyceride hydrolase and as a phospholipase.

LDL containing apoB-100 interacts with receptors on the membrane of cells in the liver and on adrenal and smooth muscle cells and fibroblasts. This receptor has a high affinity for apolipoproteins B and E. Following interaction with LDL, the receptor and lipoproteins undergo endocytosis, and the components of LDL are catabolized (Fig. 152-21).

Recently plasma apolipoprotein(a) [Lp(a)] has been described.[9] It contains apoB-100 and a high molecular weight protein that is specific for Lp(a). The Lp(a) content of the plasma varies widely between normal individuals; there is no clear cutoff value

for "normal." It is clear, however, that the high Lp(a) values enhance the risk for arteriosclerotic disease and may also cause the development of characteristic subcutaneous xanthomas similar to the xanthomas caused by familial hypercholesterolemia.

High Density Lipoproteins

HDL arise in plasma by several pathways, including direct synthesis and secretion by the intestine and liver. The HDL particles in plasma also acquire lipids and apolipoproteins arising from the catabolism of triglyceride-rich apoB containing lipoproteins. It is thought that HDL function partly as a "reservoir" for apolipoproteins (e.g., apoC-II and apoE) during lipoprotein metabolism. HDL may also interact with specific receptors to initiate the transport of excess cholesterol from cells back to the liver. This process is often termed *reverse cholesterol transport* or *scavenger activity*. It begins with the removal from cells of cholesterol largely as unesterified sterol, which is subsequently esterified in the plasma by the enzyme lecithin cholesteryl acyltransferase (LCAT). The choles-

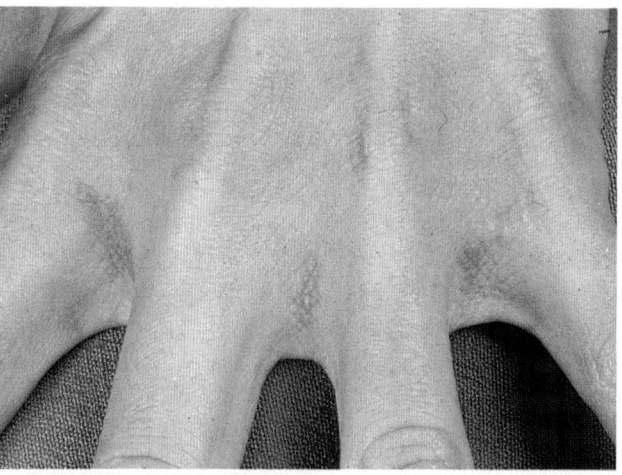

FIGURE 152-20 Intertriginous xanthomas of the hands in a patient with homozygous familial hypercholesterolemia.

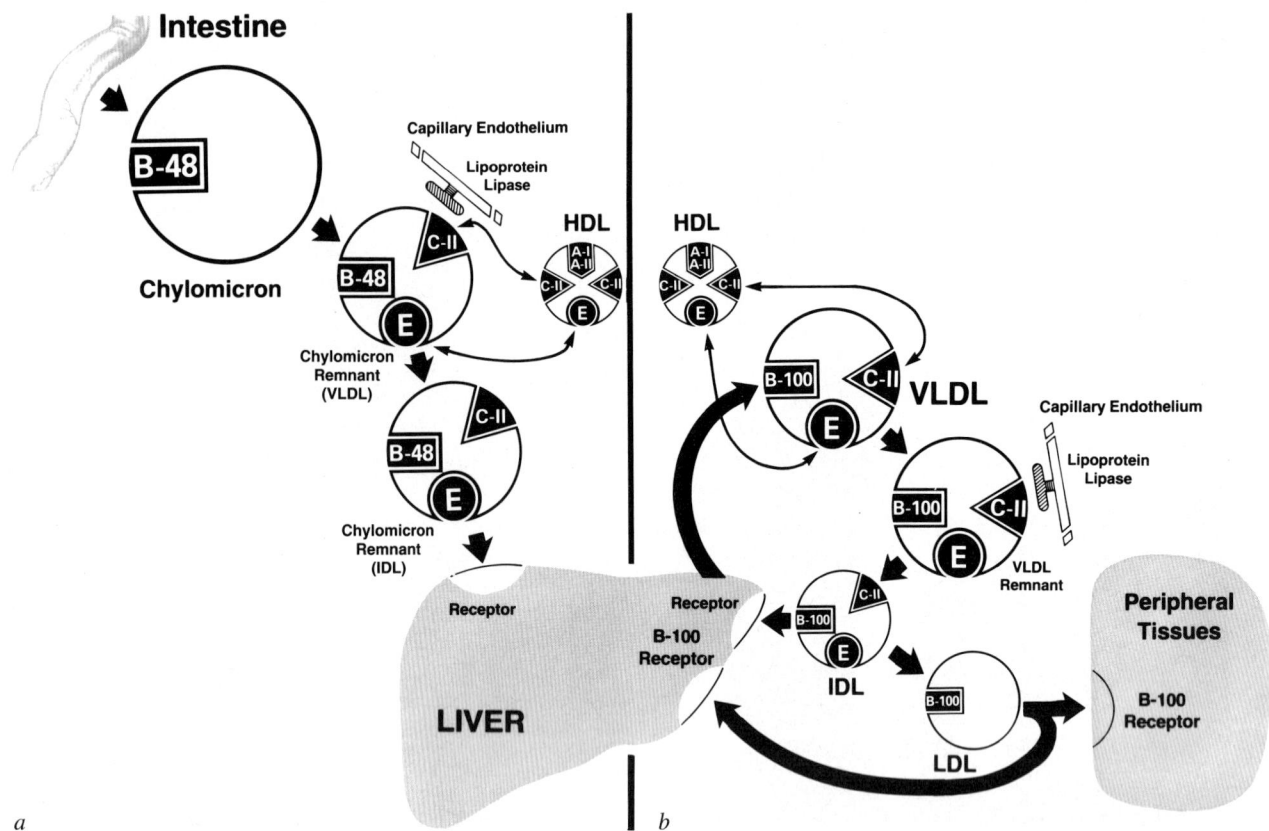

a   *b*

FIGURE 152-21 Schematic overview of human lipoprotein metabolism. The metabolism of the principal lipoprotein classes containing apoB may be conceptualized as consisting of two major cascades. (*a*) The *first apoB cascade* involves chylomicrons containing apoB-48 secreted by the intestine. The triglycerides on the chylomicrons undergo lipolysis by the enzyme lipoprotein lipase and chylomicron remnants are formed with densities initially of VLDL and finally of IDL. (*b*) The *second apoB cascade* involves triglyceride-rich VLDL containing apoB-100 secreted by the liver. The triglycerides on VLDL are hydrolyzed and VLDL undergoes serial conversion to IDL and then LDL. During metabolism some of the VLDL remnants are taken up by the liver. Shortly after secretion, triglyceride-rich particles from both the liver and intestines acquire apoC-II and apoE from HDL. ApoC-II is a cofactor for lipoprotein lipase, and apoE facilitates the receptor-mediated endocytosis and catabolism of remnants by the liver. ApoB-100, the predominant apolipoprotein on LDL, interacts with a high-affinity receptor on peripheral cells and hepatocytes, culminating in LDL endocytosis and catabolism of LDL. (See text for further details.)

teryl esters are transferred to the core of the lipoprotein particles and they exchange between different lipoprotein particles, such as HDL and VLDL. The esterification of cholesterol in plasma, the exchange of cholesteryl esters between lipoproteins, and the HDL-facilitated movement of intracellular cholesterol into plasma are important elements in cholesterol metabolism that are related to the development of atherosclerosis. During this process the disc-shaped HDL becomes spherical (HDL$_2$) and further transforms into HDL$_3$.

Dyslipoproteinemia

Specific defects in lipoprotein metabolism usually involve either abnormal increases (hyperlipoproteinemia) or decreases (hypo-lipoproteinemia) in the concentrations of specific classes of plasma lipoproteins. Sometimes, in addition, abnormal plasma lipoproteins are present. Certain dyslipoproteinemias may be associated with distinct clinical syndromes. History, physical examination, and laboratory evaluation all contribute to establishing the diagnosis.

Lipoprotein Patterns

Until 1950 it was only possible to estimate the lipid content of the plasma (cholesterol content, phospholipid content, and triglyceride content), and even today estimation of the lipid content is the first and often the only examination that is made. Since the work of Gofman et al.,[10] we have been able to distinguish several lipoprotein classes, each with a specific content of lipids. They may be. estimated following paper or gel electrophoresis or by preparative ultracentrifugation as described above. Table 152-4 summarizes the lipid content of the various lipoprotein classes.

The classification of lipoprotein disturbances by Fredrickson et al., which was adopted by the World Health Organization in 1970,[11,12] has been very important. Since then it has become clear that the patterns that they described do not distinguish specific diseases but may be the symptoms of various monogenetic, polygenetic, or other metabolic diseases. However, this classification scheme still remains important for our study of dys-lipoproteinoses. The lipoprotein patterns can be separated into the five types noted in Table 152-5.

TABLE 152-4
Composition of the Various Lipoproteins

	Chylo-microns	Pre-beta VLDL	Beta LDL	Alpha HDL
Density	< 0.98	0.98–1.006	1.006–1.063	>1.063
SF value*	400	20–400	0–20	—
Total sterol, %	2.8	17–20	39–58	20–26
Triglycerides, %	88	49–56	7–16	13–20
Phospholipids, %	8	12–20	24–32	44–17
Proteins, %	2	8–10	20–25	48–54

*SF: flotation after analytical ultracentrifugation.

Hypolipoproteinemia is also separable into syndromes expressed as reductions in HDL or in apoB-containing lipoproteins (i.e., chylomicrons, VLDL, IDL, and LDL). Sometimes concentrations of both are affected. Initial classification helps to sharpen differential diagnosis, including separation of primary (genetic) defects from dyslipoproteinemias secondary to other disorders; to anticipate the clinical course, including complications; and to select the most effective therapy. Consideration of lipoproteins, rather than lipids, also provides a more flexible basis for adjusting to the rapidly expanding knowledge about these disorders.

Hyperlipoproteinemias[13]

Chylomicronemia (Type I and Type V Hyperlipoproteinemia) (Fig. 152-22)

CLINICAL SYNDROME. Plasma triglyceride concentrations are labile depending primarily upon the time relationship of sampling to the intake of fat. In general, fasting plasma triglyceride concen-

trations >300 mg/dL are abnormal (Table 152-1). Chylomicrons are normally present in plasma only a few hours after consumption of a fatty meal. At plasma concentrations of triglycerides >1500 mg/dL, there is usually a distinct accumulation of chylomicrons, visible as a definite creamy layer on top of plasma left overnight in a refrigerator at 4°C. If the infranatant is cloudy, significant elevations of VLDL or IDL are also present.

The *chylomicronemia syndrome* may be present at triglyceride concentrations of >1500 to 2000 mg/dL. The clinical manifestations are eruptive xanthomas, lipemia retinalis, and, sometimes, pancreatitis. Additional symptoms may include dry eyes and dry mouth, numbness or tingling in the extremities, abdominal pains, depression, memory loss, and emotional lability. Hepatosplenomegaly may be present. The majority of the symptoms are ameliorated with a reduction in plasma triglycerides. A history of prior exploratory surgery because of abdominal pain is not unusual, and patients may ultimately develop chronic pancreatitis.

Patients classified as having type I hyperlipoproteinemia or exogenous hypertriglyceridemia have elevated triglycerides appearing primarily in chylomicrons. In those classified as having type V hyperlipoproteinemia or mixed endogenous/exogenous hypertriglyceridemia, the elevated triglycerides are found in both chylomicrons and VLDL. Patients having either type have elevations of apoB-48 and apoB-100 in triglyceride-rich lipoproteins, indicating increased liver and intestinal lipoprotein production.

In the past, the xanthomas occurring in patients with lipemic plasma were designated as *xanthoma diabeticorum*. Currently, diabetic patients with eruptive xanthoma and the chylomicronemia syndrome combined with elevated VLDL levels are considered as having type V hyperlipoproteinemia.

The type of defect in patients with severe hypertriglyceridemia is actually suggested by the age of onset of the chylomicronemia syndrome. Patients with signs and symptoms before puberty nearly always have genetic defects in triglyceride metabolism involving lipoprotein lipase activity (Fig. 152-22). Such primary deficiency

TABLE 152-5
Abnormal Lipoprotein Patterns in Familial Hyperlipoproteinemia

Type	Definitive lipoprotein abnormalities	Appearance of plasma*	Usual changes in lipid concentrations[†]
I	1. Chylomicrons present and markedly increased 2. VLDL, LDL, HDL normal or decreased	Cream layer on top, clear below	C normal,[‡] TG ++ (C/TG < 0.2)
II	1. LDL ++ 2. VLDL normal (type IIa); or VLDL + (type IIb)	Usually clear, may be slightly turbid	C ++, TG normal or + (C/TG usually >1.5)
III	1. Presence of beta VLDL ("floating beta," LDL of abnormal lipid composition)	Usually turbid, often with faint cream layer	C +, TG + (C/TG variable, often = 1)
IV	1. VLDL ++ 2. Chylomicrons absent 3. LDL not increased	Usually turbid; no cream layer	C + or normal, TG ++ (C/TG variable)
V	1. Chylomicrons present 2. VLDL ++	Cream layer on top, turbid below	C +, TG ++ (C/TG usually >0.15 and <0.6)

* After standing at 4°C for ≥18 h.
[†] C, cholesterol; TG, triglycerides.
[‡] ++, increased: implies in excess of whatever cut-off limit is used.

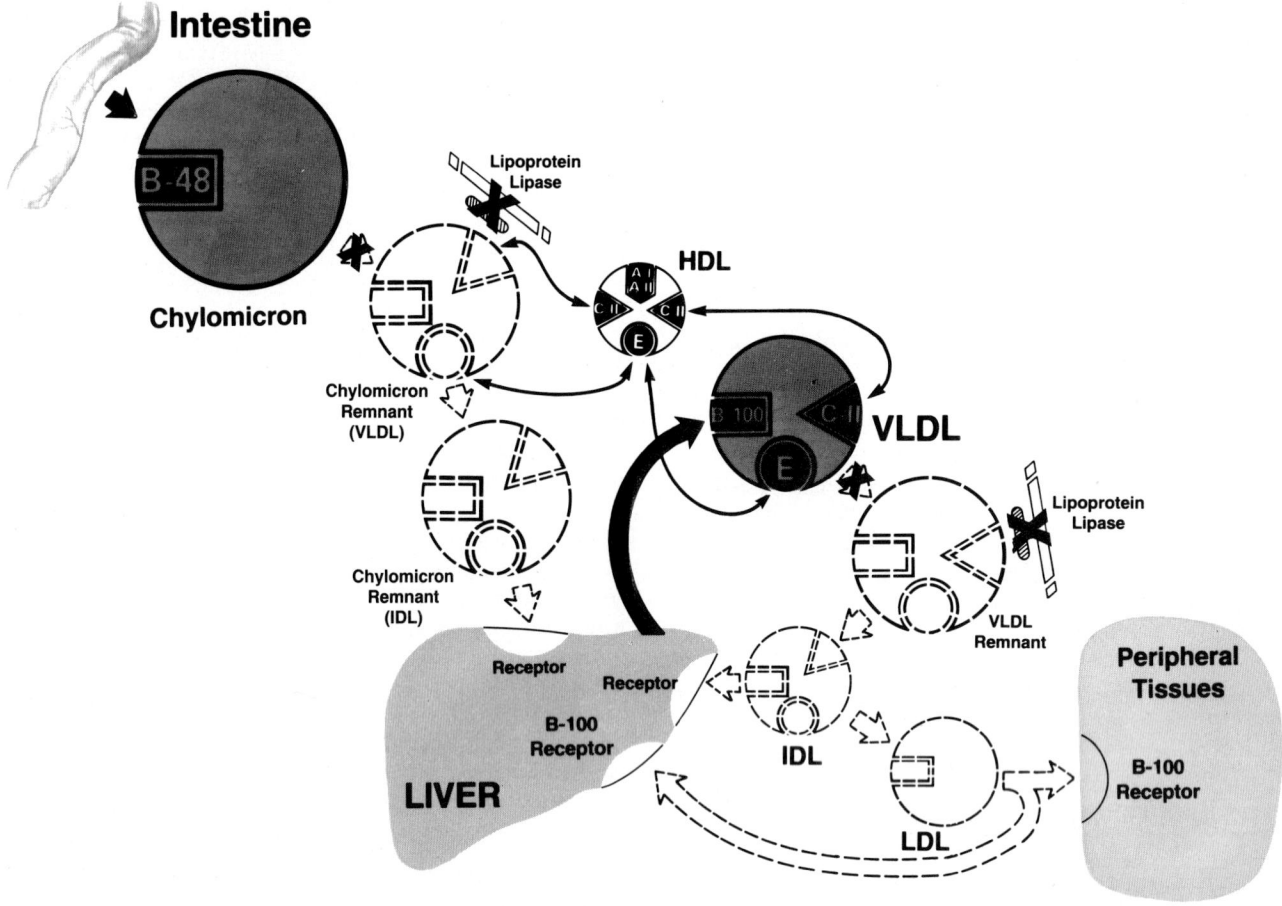

FIGURE 152-22 Schematic view of the block in lipoprotein metabolism in patients with the chylomicronemia syndrome and the type I phenotype. Molecular defects underlying this syndrome include primarily a deficiency of lipoprotein activity and a deficiency of the cofactor for lipoprotein lipase, apoC-II.

of lipoprotein lipase activity results in defective lipolysis of chylomicrons and hepatogenous VLDL, with accumulation of very large triglyceride-rich lipoprotein particles in plasma—the classic type I phenotype.

A deficiency of apoC-II has been recognized as another possible cause of severe hypertriglyceridemia and the type I phenotype. These patients have a severe reduction in lipoprotein lipase activity secondary to an absence of normal amounts of the apoC-II cofactor. The clinical manifestations of apoC-II deficiency appear before puberty. However, the signs and symptoms tend to be less dramatic than in familial lipoprotein lipase deficiency.

As a third cause of chylomicronemia, a very rare familial lipoprotein lipase inhibitor has been identified. The differentiation of whether the hyperlipidemia is secondary to chronic pancreatitis or vice versa may sometimes be academic with respect to the clinical care of the patient.

GENETIC ASPECTS.[14] The locus for the gene coding for lipoprotein lipase is situated on chromosome 8 at band 22. Recently a number of mutations have been described in the gene including duplications, deletions, and insertions. The gene for the apoC-II gene is on chromosome 19. It has four exons and three introns and spans 3320 nucleotides. The nature of the mutation in the apoC-II gene in the group of patients with chylomicronemia is still under investigation. When C-II is deficient, lipoprotein lipase cannot recognize the VLDL remnants or hydrolyze the triglyceride component.

PHYSICAL EXAMINATION. The characteristic skin lesions accompanying the chylomicronemia syndrome are eruptive xanthomas (Figs. 152-10 and 152-11). These are usually asymptomatic, discrete papules 5 to 6 mm in size, with a yellow center and red halo. During resolution, the inflammatory character of the lesions resolves, and the papules become waxy yellow in appearance. The lesions result from the phagocytosis of triglyceride-rich lipoproteins by macrophages in the skin. Eruptive xanthomas may appear suddenly in showers and disappear with a decline in the acute transient elevations in plasma triglycerides. Eruptive xanthomas have a predilection to form on pressure points on the extensor surfaces of the elbows, back, buttocks (Figs. 152-10 and 152-11), and knees. Occasionally, eruptive xanthomas may become confluent and merge into tuberoeruptive xanthomas.

Lipemia retinalis can be detected in the fundus of the eye when triglyceride levels reach 3000 to 4000 mg/dL (Fig. 152-23). The retinal arterioles and venules appear pale pink due to light scattering by the large chylomicron particles. Vision is not affected. Hepatosplenomegaly, associated with abdominal pain and tenderness, is a frequent physical manifestation of the hyperchylomicronemia syndrome. The hepatosplenomegaly is secondary to lipid accumulation in the parenchymal and reticuloendothelial tissues. Acute right and left upper quadrant pain may develop with rapid elevations in plasma triglycerides, often mimicking an acute abdominal emergency. With reduction in plasma triglycerides, hepatospleno-

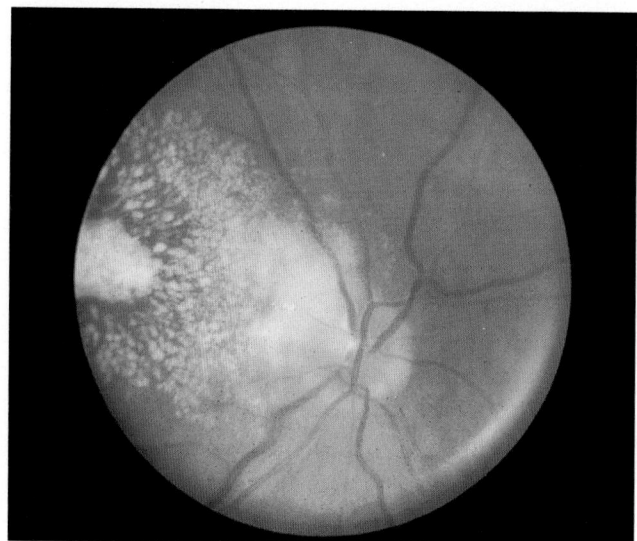

FIGURE 152-23 Lipemia retinalis in type V hyperlipidemia.

megaly may decrease and the symptoms abate. Abdominal pain in patients with the hyperchylomicronemia syndrome is frequently due to acute pancreatitis, which may have a fatal outcome. Chronic pancreatitis is a frequent and important sequela of the syndrome.

Neuropsychiatric symptoms are frequently present in patients with severe elevations in plasma triglycerides, especially with primary type V hyperlipoproteinemia. The symptoms are often bizarre, follow no neurologic patterns, and include paresthesias, dysthesias, acute memory loss, personality changes, depression, and mild dementia. Physical findings are not consistent with any specific neurologic syndrome. The severity of the symptoms appears to be correlated with the elevation of the plasma triglycerides.

THERAPY.   Patients with severe chylomicronemia with or without VLDL elevations respond to dietary restriction of fats. However, selected patients with type V hyperlipoproteinemia may require drug therapy with norethindrone acetate, nicotinic acid, or gemfibrozil. The hyperlipoproteinemia in patients whose clinical course is complicated by an additional disease (e.g., diabetes, hypothyroidism) can be markedly improved by treatment of the acquired disease.

Familial Dysbetalipoproteinemia[11] (Type III Hyperlipoproteinemia) (Fig. 152-24)

CLINICAL SYNDROME.   Patients with delayed removal of lipoprotein remnants often develop hyperlipidemia and clinical symptomatology in the fourth and fifth decades. This dyslipoproteinemia has been designated as *type III hyperlipoproteinemia* and is of particular importance due to the increased incidence of premature cardiovascular disease. Untreated patients have virtually pathognomonic yellow lines or infiltrations in the palmar creases of their hands and palmar xanthomas (xanthoma striata palmaris) (Figs. 152-17 and 152-18). They also have tuberoeruptive xanthomas on the elbows, knees, and buttocks (Fig. 152-12). Plasma concentrations of both triglycerides and cholesterol are elevated (frequently about equally). The principal elevation of the plasma lipoproteins involves IDL. These lipoproteins are cholesterol rich, migrate as an extra beta band on high-resolution agarose gel electrophoresis of plasma, and migrate in the beta position on lipoprotein electrophor-

esis following separation by ultracentrifugation of the plasma lipoproteins at a density <1.006 g/mL. These beta-migrating lipoproteins have been designated as floating beta lipoproteins. An additional important diagnostic feature of this dyslipoproteinemia is a VLDL-cholesterol to plasma triglyceride ratio >0.3. In addition, the ratio of cholesterol to triglycerides in VLDL is >0.5 in the syndrome.[15]

APOLIPOPROTEIN E.   A key role in the metabolism and cellular uptake of triglyceride-rich lipoproteins is played by apoE. Population and structural analyses have indicated that apoE is controlled at a single genetic locus with an unusual degree of polymorphism. There are three common apoE alleles in the general population, which have been designated E^2, E^3, and E^4. The three E apolipoproteins encoded by these three alleles are separable by isoelectrofocusing and are called apoE$_2$, apoE$_3$, and apoE$_4$. Six major apoE phenotypes are present in the population, including homozygotes for apolipoprotein E$_2$, E$_3$, and E$_4$ as well as heterozygotes for apolipoproteins E$_{2/3}$, E$_{2/4}$, and E$_{3/4}$.

Epidemiologic studies have established the frequency of the E alleles and lipoprotein profiles in the general and hyperlipidemic population. The predominant E isoprotein in the normolipidemic population is apoE$_3$. An increased frequency of the E^2 allele (apoE$_2$ phenotype) or E^0 allele (apoE absence) has been observed in patients with type III hyperlipoproteinemia. In early adult life, nearly all patients with the apoE$_{2/2}$ phenotype are normolipidemic and, in fact, may be hypolipidemic. Patients with the apoE$_{2/2}$ phenotype and no hyperlipidemia are categorized as normolipidemic E^2 homozygotes, or patients with dysbetalipoproteinemia. They also have an elevated synthesis and plasma level of apoE.

In the fourth and fifth decades, some patients either lacking apoE (E^0) or with the apoE$_{2/2}$ phenotype develop hyperlipidemia and have a lipoprotein pattern characteristic of type III. Genetic and kindred studies in hyperlipidemic patients have suggested that the apoE$_{2/2}$ phenotype is a necessary, but not sufficient, factor for dyslipoproteinemia and xanthomas of the xanthoma striata palmaris type. Other factors such as obesity, age, body mass, gender, and hormonal levels are required for the patient to become hyperlipidemic and to develop the clinical signs of type III hyperlipoproteinemia.

Recent genetic investigations into the apoE defects using molecular biologic techniques have detected at least 24 different isoforms of apoE, often named after the place where the isoform was initially described. Thus, marked differences in the apoE alleles exist in various populations. Still, the vast majority of patients with familial dysbetalipoproteinemia are homozygous for the apoE$_2$/E$_2$ phenotype. The rarer isoforms, such as E$_1$ Harrisburg, E$_2$ Christchurch, and E$_3$ Leiden, may be dominantly expressed.

To illustrate the way various apoE isoforms have been detected, the apoE$_3$ Leiden isoform will be described.[16–18] This variant was found originally in five probands without apparent family relation. Further genealogic studies showed that these patients had a common ancestor in the seventeenth century, and that in this pedigree 37 additional heterozygous apoE$_3$ Leiden subjects could be traced. All presented with more or less severe familial dysbetalipoproteinemia, and the expression of the genetic defect was almost exclusively dependent on age. The apoE$_3$ Leiden allele can be differentiated from the apoE$_4$ allele by the inclusion of 21 nucleotides in exon 4 coding for seven additional amino acids. This mutation causes the E isoform coded by this allele to focus at the E$_3$ position in isoelectric focusing. The E$_3$ Leiden consequently can be described as E$_3$. The location of the mutation in the apoE just outside the putative receptor domain for the hepatocyte affects the

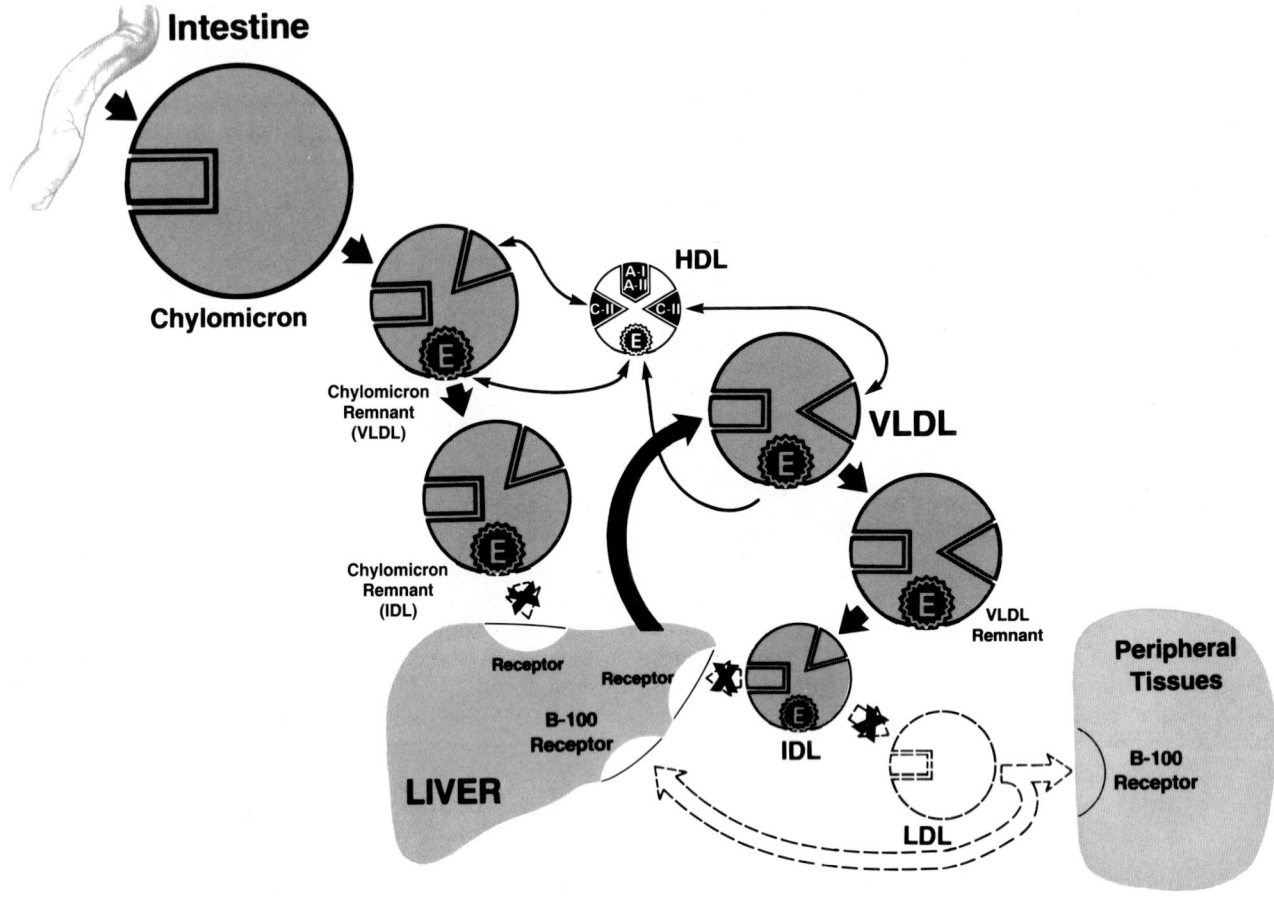

FIGURE 152-24 Schematic model of the defect in lipoprotein metabolism in patients with type III hyperlipoproteinemia. The block is characterized by a defect in removal of remnants of both the chylomicron and hepatogenous VLDL cascades due to a defect in the apoE-mediated uptake of lipoprotein remnants. These patients may be missing apoE (E° allele) or more commonly have an abnormal apoE (apoE$_2$, E^2 allele) resulting in the accumulation of lipoproteins and hyperlipidemia.

conformation of the receptor-binding in the liver irreversibly and causes dominant familial dysbetalipoproteinemia without the necessity of other factors.

The lipoproteins that accumulate in type III hyperlipoproteinemia contain both apoB-48 and apoB-100, indicating that there is defective metabolism of lipoproteins of both intestinal (chylomicron) and liver (VLDL) origin (Fig. 152-24). The delay in catabolism of these lipoproteins is due to the absence of apoE or the presence of apoE$_2$, which results in defective binding to the hepatic apoE receptor. Remnants, therefore, persist in the circulation for an abnormally long time and are susceptible to uptake by macrophages. Lipid accumulation in the macrophages underlies the development of xanthomas and deposits such as those that occur in endothelium. Presumably, this is also the basis for the increased incidence of coronary and peripheral arterial disease in patients with type III hyperlipoproteinemia.

PHYSICAL EXAMINATION.   As described above, one of the fascinating features of type III hyperlipoproteinemia is the appearance of xanthoma striata palmaris that are nearly pathognomonic of the disorder (Fig. 152-18). They are frequently accompanied by tuberoeruptive lesions over the elbows, knees, and buttocks (Fig. 152-13). The patients rarely also develop Achilles tendon xanthomas.

Other physical findings in patients with type III hyperlipoproteinemia relate to the increased frequency of atherosclerosis observed in these patients, including evidence of both cardiac as well as peripheral vascular disease. The atherosclerotic lesions in patients with type III hyperlipoproteinemia are similar to those observed in the absence of hyperlipidemia or in other hyperlipidemic phenotypes. Since the syndrome first presents with xanthomas, treatment is possible before cardiovascular symptoms develop.

THERAPY.   Before the institution of therapy for type III hyperlipoproteinemia, aggravating factors should be excluded, including diabetes mellitus or other diseases that mimic or exaggerate the abnormal lipoprotein patterns (systemic lupus erythematosus, paraproteinemias, and especially hypothyroidism). Modification of diet and caloric restriction are very effective in lowering plasma lipids in patients with the uncomplicated phenotype. Additional lowering may be achieved by drug therapy with nicotinic acid or gemfibrozil. Clofibrate is less appropriate, as more side effects have been described. Alcohol intake should be sharply limited as it often exaggerates the hyperlipidemia. Effective control of type III hyperlipoproteinemia with diet and/or drug therapy leads to rapid resolution of xanthomas and presumably cardiovascular lesions.

Elevated LDL Levels (Type II Hyperlipoproteinemias)
(Fig. 152-25)

Elevated LDL levels are found in distinctive monogenetic and polygenetic diseases. The following syndromes must be distinguished:

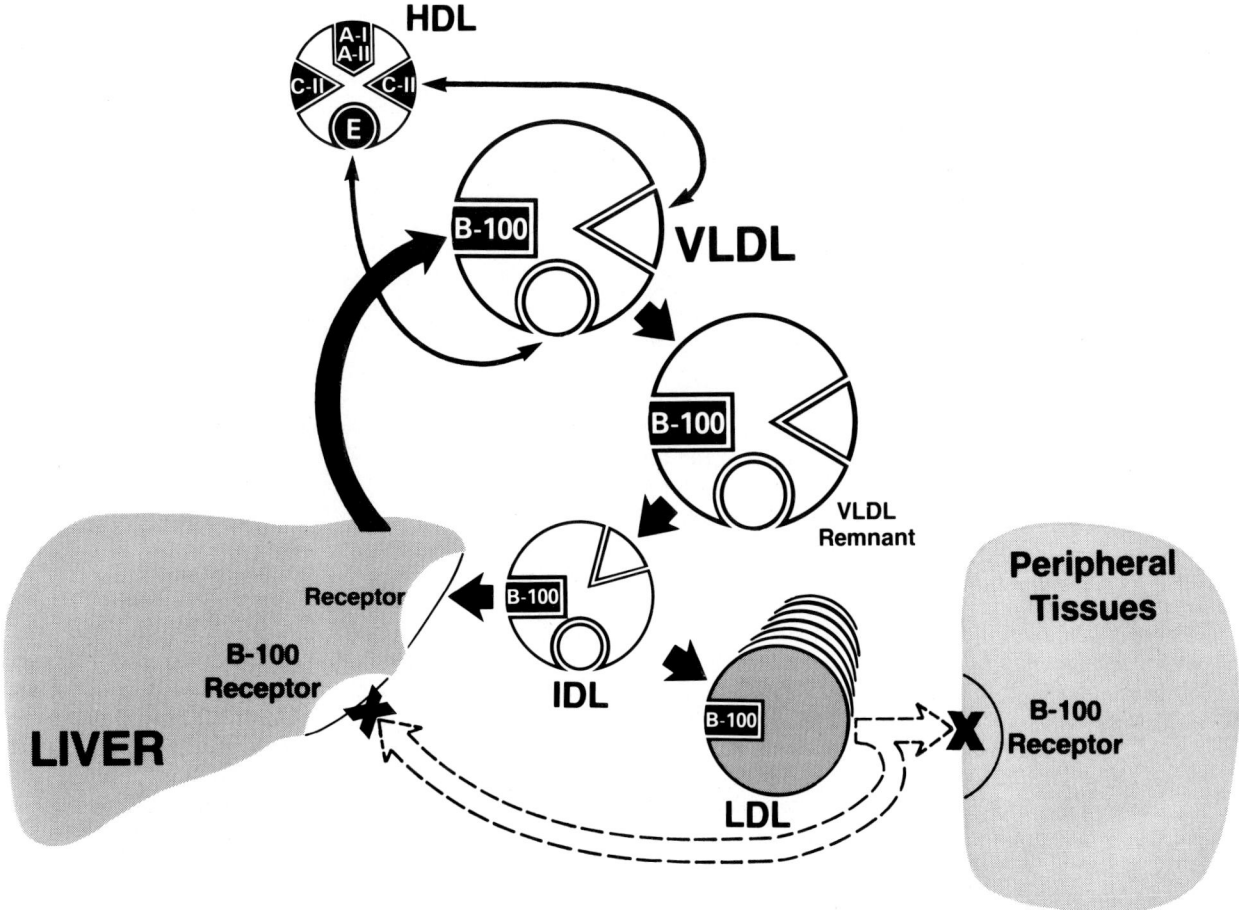

FIGURE 152-25 Schematic view of the defect in familial hypercholesterolemia characterized by tendon xanthomas and hyperbetalipoproteinemia observed in patients with hypercholesterolemia and the type II phenotype. The molecular defect in famial hypercholesterolemia is a defect in the LDL receptor process on both liver and peripheral cells.

1. Familial hypercholesterolemia (FH)[19]
2. Familial combined hyperlipidemia (FCH)
3. Polygenetic (''common'') hypercholesterolemia

Familial Hypercholesterolemia One of the most important dyslipoproteinemias, FH is a relatively common codominant disease with a gene frequency of approximately 1:500 in the general population. Heterozygotes for FH have elevated plasma cholesterol and LDL levels from birth. By adult years the heterozygous patient's plasma cholesterol is usually in the 300 to 400 mg/dL range. Clinical manifestations typically do not develop until the third and fourth decades. At this time xanthomas appear, most characteristically in the Achilles tendons and extensor tendons of the hands (Fig. 152-9) and occasionally in tendons about the knee and elbow (Fig. 152-8). Arcus juvenilis and xanthelasma palpebrarum (Fig. 152-7) may also be present.

In male heterozygous FH patients, there is a tendency to develop coronary artery disease several decades earlier than other 30- to 60-year-old males. Premature occurrence of coronary artery disease also occurs in female heterozygotes but lags about 10 years behind male heterozygotes.

Homozygotes for FH have markedly elevated cholesterol and LDL at birth, and during the first few years of life plasma cholesterol levels range from 700 to 1200 mg/dL. In the early years, a unique yellowish xanthoma may develop in the interdigital webs of the hands and in the cleft between the buttocks and at pressure points or sites of trauma, particularly over the knees, elbows, and buttocks (Figs. 152-14, 152-15, and 152-16). Large xanthomas, particularly in the Achilles tendons but also over the elbows, ankles, and hands, are characteristic of homozygous FH, as are arcus juvenilis and xanthelasma palpebrarum. Of paramount clinical importance in homozygous patients is the very early development of severe coronary artery disease; myocardial infarction can occur in the first and second decades of life, and life expectancy rarely extends beyond the third decade.

The molecular defect in FH is now well understood and has been extensively studied in fibroblasts and the liver. Circulating LDL normally binds to a high-affinity receptor on cellular membranes, initiating a receptor-mediated endocytosis. In FH, one of numerous primary defects in the structure and function of the LDL receptor results in defective cellular uptake of LDL (Fig. 152-25). The resulting deficiency of LDL uptake results in a marked increase in circulating plasma LDL and a reduction in the uptake of LDL by high-affinity processes. The steady-state level of LDL in these patients is above the LDL level of normal subjects.

Our understanding of the underlying molecular defect in FH started with the discovery of pits coated with a fuzzy coat on the surface of cultivated fibroblasts by Anderson et al.,[20] using ferritin-conjugated LDL. This was confirmed by Vermeer et al.,[21] using anti-apoB serum and the immunoperoxidase technique. In fibroblasts from homozygous FH patients, no LDL-reactive material was found. In heterozygotes, half of the reactive material was present. Further investigations[22,23] showed that the coated pits normally present a receptor for LDL. After LDL is bound to the receptor by a high-affinity process, it transforms into a coated vesicle, which fuses with other coated vesicles into an endosome. Lysosomal enzymes break up the endosome; the receptor migrates back to the coated pit; and the cholesterol is internalized in the cytoplasm where it reduces the intracellular synthesis of cholesterol by downregulating 3-hydroxyl, 3-methylglutaryl CoA reductase (HMG CoA-reductase), the main enzyme regulating intracellular cholesterol synthesis. Due to the genetic defect in FH patients, the production of the receptor is severely inhibited. In the heterozygote, half the normal quantity of the receptor is present. Initially, it was presumed that in the homozygote no LDL receptor would be produced. Recent investigations have shown that there are mutations in which partial production of the LDL receptor is possible.[24]

The LDL receptor gene locus is situated on the distal part of the arm of chromosome 19. It spans 45 kb, comprising 18 exons and 17 introns. Several classes of mutations of the gene may be distinguished:

1. *Class I:* These so-called null alleles make up 50 percent of the homozygous patients. In this class different point mutations, deletions, and mutations in the promotor region are found; no LDL receptor protein is synthesized.
2. *Class 2:* These are the mutations that result in a defective LDL receptor, since proteins are synthesized which fail to migrate from the endoplasmic reticulum to the Golgi apparatus.
3. *Class 3:* Receptors are formed with proteins that are not able to bind LDL.
4. *Class 4:* Apparently normal LDL receptors are formed but they do not cluster in coated pits and are not able to internalize LDL.

This classification of homozygotes is important from the perspective of therapy. In cases of the null allele, no effect of statine therapy may be expected, whereas in the other classes, therapy with statines may be tried.

PHYSICAL EXAMINATION. Heterozygotes as well as homozygotes for FH have tendon xanthomas located in the Achilles tendons and the tendons of the dorsa of the hands. In homozygotes, the characteristic and usually earliest physical manifestation of hypercholesterolemia is the appearance of intertriginous xanthomas in the webs of the hands and tuberous xanthomas on the elbows, knees, and buttocks (Figs. 152-19 and 152-20). These xanthomas do not appear in the heterozygous adult with FH. Palpebral xanthelasmas often accompany type II hyperlipoproteinemia; however, these lesions are not diagnostic of hyperlipoproteinemia and may be seen in normal subjects.

Histologically, tendon xanthomas contain macrophages so laden with lipid droplets that they form foam cells, which are interspersed among the fibrous stroma. The cytoplasmic lipid droplets predominantly contain cholesteryl esters, which are birefringent and positive for the oil red O stain. Arcus juvenilis, a grayish white ring in the cornea, is due to the accumulation of lipid droplets. Superficially, the arcus appears to extend not quite to the limbus, leaving a clear margin of iris. By slit-lamp examination, however, the lipid droplets extend diagonally through the entire thickness of the cornea. Arcus in children is practically always a sign of hyperbetalipoproteinemia. In older subjects its diagnostic value gradually diminishes with age. In blacks, arcus is commonly observed without hyperlipidemia.

THERAPY. The treatment of adults with FH begins with a low-fat, low-cholesterol diet (less than 300 mg/day) with a polyunsaturated:saturated fat ratio of 1.0 to 1.5. Diet, however, is insufficient to reduce the cholesterol adequately. Niacin is of moderate benefit, and a major advance is the introduction of the cholesterol-binding resin, cholestyramine, and the MHG CoA-reductase inhibitors,[25] the statins.

In the gut, the resin absorbs cholesterol that was excreted with the bile and prevents it from being reabsorbed. In this way the enterohepatic cholesterol cycle is interrupted. The other drugs stimulate the production of LDL receptors by inhibiting intracellular cholesterol production. Although cholestyramine administration may be offensive to patients due to its taste, the combined treatments leads to superior results compared to monotherapy with a statin.

In patients with homozygous FH and residual LDL receptor activity, the same therapy as in heterozygotes may be tried. In the case of null alleles, more-drastic measures must be advised because of the severity of the disease. A low-fat, low-cholesterol diet should be used with combination drug therapy. Occasionally, good results have been reported from partial ileal bypass, portocaval shunt, plasmapheresis, and liver transplantation.

Familial Combined Hyperlipidemia One of the most common monogenetic disorders in humans is FCH. The gene frequency, assuming a single defect, has been estimated to be as high as 1:300. The clinical manifestations of FCH generally appear in the fourth and fifth decades. The characteristic feature of FCH is paradoxically the variability of the plasma lipoprotein phenotype in the proband and the affected relatives. The most frequent lipoprotein patterns observed are types IIa, IIb, III, and IV. The molecular defect in FCH is unknown, and the diagnosis is presumptive and established only by analysis of the pattern of dyslipoproteinemia in the propositus and family members. No homozygotes for FCH have been identified, although a number of genetic compounds, i.e., one gene for FCH and the other for some other form of hyperlipoproteinemia, have been suspected. Available data suggest that at least a subset of patients with FCH have increased synthesis of LDL and an increased ratio of apoB-100 to cholesterol in plasma LDL. A receptor-mediated defect in LDL catabolism, such as that present in FH, has not been shown. The largest proportion of patients with FCH have no xanthomas, although tendon xanthomas, arcus juvenilis, and xanthelasma may be observed. The most frequent, as well as significant, clinical manifestation of FCH is the development of premature cardiovascular disease.

Therapy is dependent upon the type of lipoprotein pattern. In the majority of patients presenting with lipoprotein patterns IIa or IIb without xanthomata, the pattern is due to undefined genetic and environmental factors. Because these patients present no xanthomas or other dermatologic disease, they are not discussed further.

Elevation of Plasma VLDL without Elevated Chylomicrons (Hyper-VLDL-emia, Hyperlipemia, Type IV)

In 1950, Thanhauser[26] separated hyperlipemia from hypercholesterolemia. This hypertriglyceridemia later proved to be due to elevated VLDL levels in the plasma. Due to the cholesterol content of the VLDL, the cholesterol level in these patients can also be elevated while the LDL is normal. These patients must be distinguished from those with chylomicronemia (types I and V) and familial dysbetalipoproteinemia (FD) (type III), who also present with elevated VLDL.

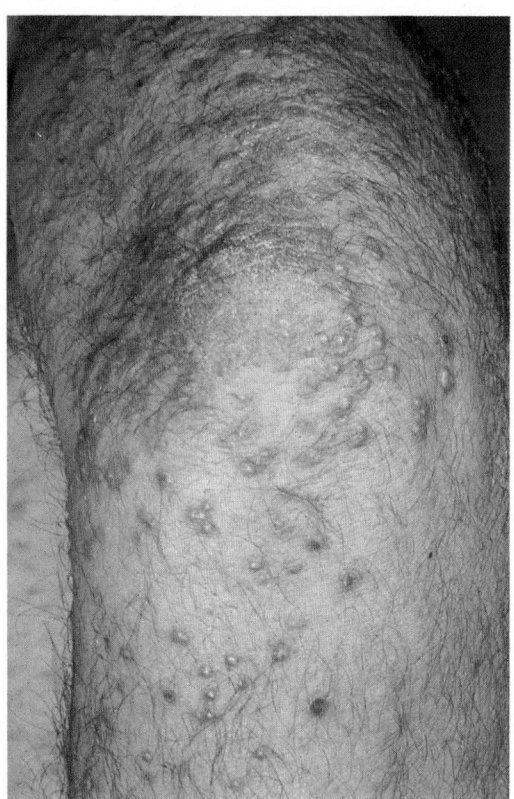

FIGURE 152-26   Papular eruptive xanthomas in hyper-VLDL-emia (type IV disease).

The frequency of xanthomata (Fig. 152-26) in this group is largely dependent upon the origin of patients who are studied. In our series[27] we found, among 74 patients with xanthoma and hyperlipoproteinemia, 7 with type IV pattern in the blood. Other authors have found xanthomas only rarely in hyper VLDL lipoproteinemias.

The typical type IV patient is obese and sensitive to carbohydrates. Oral contraceptives and alcohol excess cause exacerbation of their condition and may cause the appearance of eruptive xanthomas. When the serum triglyceride content rises above 2000 mg/dL, abdominal pain due to pancreatitis may occur. The frequency of cardiovascular complications is not absolutely clear. Such problems certainly occur but they are less frequent than in FH or FD. The pathogenesis of hyper VLDLemia has not been clarified.

THERAPY.   A low-calorie, low-carbohydrate diet with avoidance of alcohol generally gives excellent results. The xanthomata disappear, and the lipoprotein levels become normal. In case diet is not sufficient, pharmacologic agents are to be recommended.

Xanthomata in Secondary Dyslipoproteinemia

In addition to primary dyslipoproteinemias, other metabolic diseases may cause dyslipoproteinemia that results in xanthomatosis. Included among these processes are eruptive xanthomas in diabetic hyperlipemia, various types of xanthomas in primary biliary cirrhosis, diffuse plane xanthomas in multiple myeloma,[28] and hyperlipoproteinemia in hypothyroidism. Treatment must be directed against the primary disease.

References

1. Parker F: Xanthomas and hyperlipidemia. *J Am Acad Dermatol* **13**:1, 1985
2. Vermeer BJ et al: Xanthomatosis and other clinical findings in patients with elevated levels of very low density lipoproteins. *Br J Dermatol* **106**:657, 1979
3. Seymour CA: Xanthoma and abnormalities of lipid metabolism and storage, in *Textbook of Dermatology,* 5th ed, edited by RH Champion et al. Oxford, Blackwell, 1992, p 2314
4. Braun-Falco O, Eckert F: Macroscopic and microscopic structure of xanthomatous eruptions, in *Metabolic Disorders and Nutrition Correlated with Skin,* edited by BJ Vermeer et al. *Curr Probl Dermatol* **20**:54, 1991
5. Baes H et al: Lipid composition of various types of xanthoma. *J Invest Dermatol* **51**:286, 1968
6. Vermeer BJ et al: The lipid composition and localization of free and esterified cholesterol in different types of xanthoma. *J Invest Dermatol* **78**:305, 1982
7. Havel RJ, Kane JP: Structure and metabolism of plasma lipoproteins, in *The Metabolic Basis of Inherited Diseases,* 6th ed, edited by CR Scriver et al. New York, McGraw-Hill, 1989, p 1129
8. Kane JP, Havel RJ: Disorders of the biogenesis and secretion of lipoproteins containing the B apolipoproteins, in *The Metabolic Basis of Inherited Diseases,* 6th ed, edited by CR Scriver et al. New York, McGraw-Hill, 1989, p 1139
9. Boerwinkle E et al: Apolipoprotein(a) gene accounts for greater than 90% of the variation in plasma lipoprotein(a) concentrations. *J Clin Invest* **90**:52, 1992
10. Gofman JW et al: Ultracentrifugal studies on lipoproteins of human serum. *J Biol Chem* **179**:973, 1949
11. Mahley RW, Rall SC Jr: Type III hyperlipoproteinemia, in *The Metabolic Basis of Inherited Diseases,* 6th ed, edited by CR Scriver et al. New York, McGraw-Hill, 1989, p 1195
12. Fredrickson DS et al: Fat transport in lipoproteins: An integrated approach to mechanism and disorders. *N Engl J Med* **267**:34, 1967
13. Brunzell JB: Familial lipoprotein lipase deficiency and other causes of the chylomicronemia syndrome, in *The Metabolic Basis of Inherited Diseases,* 6th ed, edited by CR Scriver et al. New York, McGraw-Hill, 1989, p 1165
14. Langlois S et al: A major insertion accounts for a significant proportion of mutations underlying lipoprotein lipase deficiency. *Proc Natl Acad Sci USA* **86**:948, 1989
15. Hazzard WR et al: Abnormal lipid composition of very low density lipoproteins in diagnosis of broad-beta disease (type 3 hyperlipoproteinemia). *Metabolism* **21**:1009, 1972
16. Vermeer BR et al: Familial dysbetalipoproteinemia: A genetically heterogeneous disease caused by mutations of the ligand apolipoprotein E. *J Invest Dermatol* **98**:58s, 1992
17. Smit M et al: Apoprotein E polymorphism in the Netherlands and its effect on plasma lipid and apolipoprotein levels. *Hum Genet* **80**:287, 1988
18. de Knijff P et al: Familial dysbetalipoproteinemia associated with apolipoprotein E₃-Leiden in an extended multigeneration pedigree. *J Clin Invest* **88**:643, 1991
19. Goldstein JL, Brown MS: Familial hypercholesterolemia, in *The Metabolic Basis of Inherited Diseases,* 6th ed, edited by CR Scriver et al. New York, McGraw-Hill, 1989, p 1215
20. Anderson RGW et al: Localization of low density lipoprotein receptors on plasma membrane of normal human fibroblasts and their absence in cells from a familial hypercholesterolemia homozygote. *Proc Natl Acad Sci USA* **73**:2434, 1976
21. Vermeer BJ et al: Binding of unmodified low density lipoproteins to human fibroblasts. An investigation by immunoelectron microscopy. *Biochim Biophys Acta* **553**:169, 1979
22. Goldstein JL et al: Binding site on macrophages that mediates uptake and degradation of acetylated low density lipoprotein provoking massive cholesterol deposition. *Proc Natl Acad Sci USA* **76**:333, 1979

23. Goldstein JL, Brown MS: Lipoprotein receptors, genetic defense against atherosclerosis. *Clin Res* **30**:417, 1982

24. Kastelein JJP, Ten Cate JW: The low density lipoprotein receptor. *Ned Tijdschr* **135**:646, 1990

25. Mol MJ et al: Effects of synvinolin on plasma lipids in familial hypercholesterolemia. *Lancet* **2**:936, 1986

26. Thanhauser SJ: Lipidoses, in *Diseases of the Intracellular Lipid Metabolism,* 3d ed. New York, Grune & Stratton, 1958

27. Hessel LW et al: Primary hyperlipoproteinemia in xanthomatosis. *Clin Chim Acta* **69**:405, 1976

28. Marien KJ, Smeenk G: Plane xanthomata associated with multiple myeloma and hyperlipoproteinemia. *Br J Dermatol* **93**:407, 1975

CHAPTER 153

Robert J. Desnick and Christine M. Eng

Fabry Disease: α-Galactosidase A Deficiency (Angiokeratoma Corporis Diffusum Universale)

Fabry disease, an inborn error of glycosphingolipid metabolism, results from the defective activity of the lysosomal enzyme, α-galactosidase A. The enzymatic defect, transmitted by an X-linked recessive gene, leads to the progressive deposition of neutral glycosphingolipids with terminal α-galactosyl moieties in most visceral tissues and fluids of the body (Fig. 153-1). The predominant glycosphingolipid accumulated in this disorder is globotriaosylceramide. The birefringent glycosphingolipid deposits are primarily found in the lysosomes of the vascular endothelium; progressive endothelial accumulation results in ischemia and infarction and leads to the major clinical manifestations of the disease. These glycosphingolipids also accumulate in perithelial and smooth muscle cells of the cardiovascular-renal system and, to a lesser extent, in reticuloendothelial, myocardial, and connective tissue cells of the cornea, kidney, and other tissues, and in ganglion and perineural cells of the autonomic nervous system.

Clinically, hemizygous males have a characteristic skin lesion, which led to the descriptive name of *angiokeratoma corporis diffusum universale.* They also have acroparesthesias, episodic crises of excruciating pain, corneal and lenticular opacities, hypohidrosis, and cardiac and renal dysfunction. Death usually occurs in adult life from renal, cardiac, and/or cerebral complications of their vascular disease. Heterozygous females are usually asymptomatic and are most likely to show the corneal opacities.

Historical Aspects

In 1898, two dermatologists, Anderson[1] in England and Fabry[2] in Germany, independently described the first patients with angiokeratoma corporis diffusum. Anderson designated his case as one of angiokeratoma. His original patient was a 39-year-old male who had proteinuria, finger deformities, varicose veins, and lymphedema. Because of the proteinuria, Anderson suspected that the disease was a generalized disorder and astutely suggested that abnormal vessels might be present in the kidneys as well as in the skin. He also correctly noted that "the vascular lesion was not a new formation, as implied by the suffix 'oma', but an ectasia of cutaneous capillaries."[1] Fabry originally made the diagnosis of purpura nodularis in a 13-year-old male whom he followed over the next 30 years (Fig. 153-2). He documented the presence of albuminemia,

further described the cutaneous lesions, noting the presence of small vessel aneurysms,[3] and subsequently classified his case to be one of *angiokeratoma corporis diffusum,* a designation that has persisted.

Several individuals made early contributions to the clinical description of the disease. Steiner and Voerner[4] and Gunther[5] described a hemizygous male with anhidrosis and intermittent acroparesthesias that were aggravated by hot or cold weather. Examination of a skin biopsy showed atrophy of the sweat glands and aneurysmal dilatation of the capillaries. Weicksel[6] first described the characteristic corneal opacities and the vascular abnormalities in the retina and conjunctiva. In 1947, Pompen and coworkers[7] reported the first postmortem findings in two affected brothers who died from renal failure. The most significant observation was the presence of abnormal vacuoles in blood vessels throughout their bodies. From these findings, they suggested that the disease was a

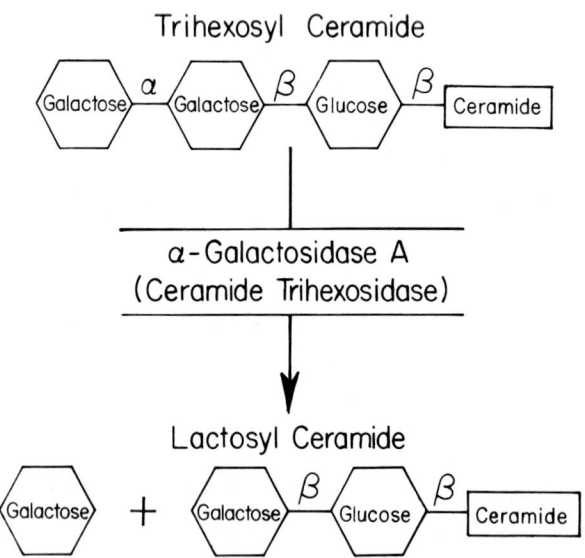

FIGURE 153-1 The metabolic defect in Fabry disease. Defective α-galactosidase A activity results in the accumulation of its major glycosphingolipid substrate, trihexosyl ceramide, which is also termed *globotriaosylceramide.*

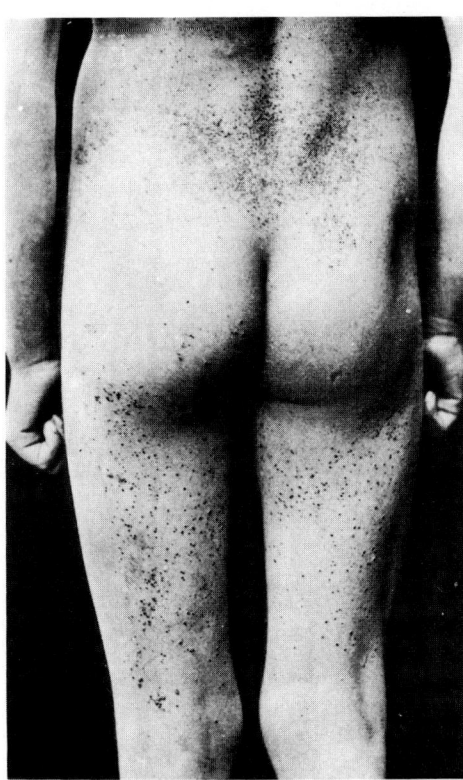

FIGURE 153-2   Distribution of angiokeratoma in the 30-year-old patient originally described by Fabry.[2]

generalized storage disorder. Subsequently, Scriba definitively established the lipid nature of the storage material[8] and Hornbostel and Scriba were the first to confirm the diagnosis histologically in a living patient by demonstrating the refractile lipid deposits in vessels of a skin biopsy specimen.[9] Although the familial occurrence of the disease was recognized earlier,[10] it was not until 1965 that Opitz et al.[11] documented the X-linked recessive inheritance of the disorder by pedigree analysis.

In 1963, Sweeley and Klionsky[12] isolated and characterized the two major accumulated neutral glycosphingolipids—globotriaosylceramide (Gal-Gal-Glc-Cer) and galabiosylceramide (Gal-Gal-Cer)—from the kidney of a Fabry hemizygote obtained at autopsy. On the basis of these findings, they classified Fabry disease as a sphingolipidosis. Subsequent chemical analyses of various Fabry tissues and fluids[13–16] have demonstrated the marked accumulation of Gal-Gal-Glc-Cer and, to a lesser extent, Gal-Gal-Cer. In addition, the accumulation of blood group B substances, glycosphingolipids with terminal α-galactosyl moieties, have been reported in affected individuals with B or AB blood types.[17]

In 1967, Brady et al.[18] demonstrated that the enzymatic defect was the defective activity of ceramide trihexosidase, a lysosomal galactosyl hydrolase required for the catabolism of Gal-Gal-Glc-Cer (Fig. 153-1). Kint,[19] using synthetic substrates, characterized the defective enzymatic activity as an α-galactosyl hydrolase (designated α-galactosidase A). Shortly thereafter, workers in several laboratories independently demonstrated that the accumulated glycosphingolipid substances, including blood group B substances, all had α-linked terminal galactosyl residues. The elucidation of the specific enzymatic defect permitted the enzymatic diagnosis of affected hemizygous males, identification of

heterozygous carrier females,[20,21] and the prenatal diagnosis of hemizygous fetuses.[22,23] In addition, pilot trials of α-galactosidase A replacement for the experimental treatment of patients with this lysosomal storage disease have been reported.[24–26] The recent molecular cloning of the full-length cDNA and entire gene encoding human α-galactosidase A[27,28] has facilitated the characterization of the various mutations causing the disease, improved the accuracy of carrier diagnosis, and stimulated efforts to treat the disease using the recombinant enzyme.

Various designations have been used to identify this disorder. In keeping with the terminology applied to other lipidoses and for the benefit of information retrieval, it would seem advisable to retain the commonly used eponym and to append the specific enzymatic defect. Thus, an appropriate designation is *Fabry disease: α-galactosidase A deficiency*. Comprehensive reviews on the clinical, pathologic, biochemical, and genetic aspects of the disease are available.[29–32]

Clinical Manifestations

The Hemizygote

The clinical manifestations of Fabry disease predominantly result from the progressive deposition of Gal-Gal-Glc-Cer in the vascular endothelium (Table 153-1). Onset of the disease usually occurs during childhood or adolescence. Early manifestations include periodic crises of severe pain in the extremities (acroparesthesias), the appearance of vascular cutaneous lesions (angiokeratoma), hypohidrosis, and the characteristic corneal and lenticular opacities.

Pain   The single most debilitating symptom of Fabry disease is the pain, of which two types have been described: episodic crises and constant discomfort.[10,33] The painful crises most often begin in childhood or in early adolescence and signal clinical onset of the disease. Lasting from minutes to several days, these "Fabry crises" consist of agonizing, burning pain initially in the palms and soles. Often the pain will radiate to the proximal extremities and other parts of the body. Attacks of abdominal or flank pain may simulate appendicitis or renal colic. The painful crises are usually triggered by exercise, fatigue, emotional stress, or rapid climatic changes in temperature and humidity. With increasing age, the periodic crises usually decrease in frequency and severity; however, in some patients, they may occur more frequently and the pain can be so excruciating that the patient may contemplate suicide. Because the pain is usually associated with a low-grade fever and an elevated erythrocyte sedimentation rate, these symptoms have fre-

TABLE 153-1
Major Clinical Manifestations in Hemizygotes with Fabry Disease*

Vascular glycolipid deposition	Manifestation
Skin	Angiokeratoma
Peripheral nerves	Excruciating pain; acroparesthesias
Heart	Ischemia and infarctions
Brain	TIAs[†] and strokes
Kidney	Renal failure

*Average age at death, 41 years.
[†]TIA, transient ischemic attack.

quently led to the misdiagnosis of rheumatic fever, neurosis, or erythromelalgia.[33]

In addition to these intermittent crises, most patients complain of a nagging, constant discomfort in their hands and feet, characterized by burning, tingling paresthesias.[33] These acroparesthesias may occur daily, usually during late afternoon, and may represent an attenuated form of the excruciating episodic crises. Although pain is a hallmark of the disease, it should be noted that about 10 to 20 percent of older patients deny any history of Fabry crises or acroparesthesias.

Skin Lesion Angiectases may be one of the earliest manifestations and may lead to diagnosis in childhood. There is a progressive increase in the number and size of these cutaneous vascular lesions with age. Classically, the angiokeratomas develop slowly as clusters of individual, punctate, dark red to blue-black angiectases in the superficial layers of the skin (Figs. 153-3, 153-4). The lesions may be flat or slightly raised and do not blanch with pressure. There is slight hyperkeratosis notable in larger lesions. The clusters of lesions are most dense between the umbilicus and the knees and have a tendency toward bilateral symmetry. The hips, back, thighs, buttocks, penis, and scrotum are most commonly involved, but there is a wide variation in the pattern of distribution and density of the lesions. Involvement of the oral mucosa and conjunctiva is common, and other mucosal areas may also be involved. Variants without the characteristic skin lesions have been reported.[34-37] Although the angiectases may not be detected readily in some patients, careful examination of the skin, especially the scrotum and umbilicus, may reveal the presence of isolated lesions. In addition to these vascular lesions, anhidrosis or, more commonly, hypohidrosis is an early and almost constant finding.

Cardiac, Cerebral, and Renal Vascular Manifestations With increasing age, the major morbid symptoms of the disease result from the progressive infiltration of glycosphingolipid in the vascular system. Cardiac disease occurs in most hemizygous males; common clinical manifestations include anginal chest pain, myocardial ischemia and infarction, congestive heart failure, and cardiac enlargement.[38,39] These findings may be accentuated by systemic hypertension related to vascular involvement of renal parenchymal vessels. Mitral insufficiency is the most frequent valvular lesion.

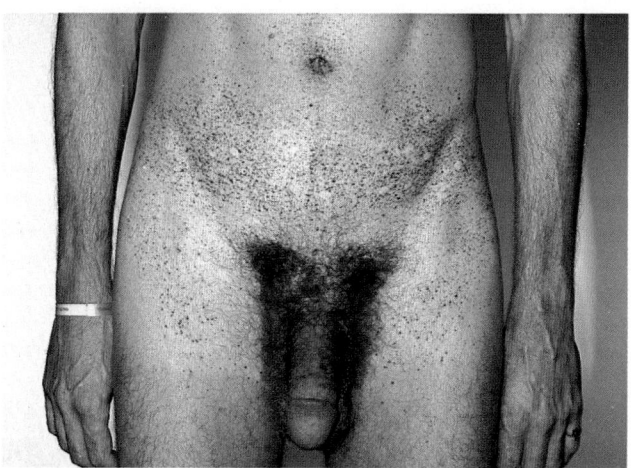

FIGURE 153-4 Angiokeratoma in a 28-year-old hemizygote with Fabry disease are seen in the "swim-suit" distribution.

Involvement of the myocardium and possibly the conduction system results in electrocardiographic abnormalities, which may show left ventricular hypertrophy, ST segment changes, and T wave inversion; other abnormalities including arrhythmias and an abbreviated PR interval have been reported.[40] Electrocardiographic patterns consistent with myocardial infarction have been seen. However, several cases with electrocardiographic changes indicating infarction had no evidence of myocardial necrosis at postmortem examination; the electrocardiographic changes were probably related to glycosphingolipid deposition in the myocardium.[39] Echocardiographic studies reveal an increased incidence of mitral valve prolapse and an increased thickness of the interventricular septum and the left ventricular posterior wall, particularly in affected older males.[41,42] In addition, hypertrophic obstructive cardiomegaly has been reported.[43]

Cerebrovascular manifestations result primarily from multifocal small-vessel involvement and may include thromboses, basilar artery ischemia and aneurysm, seizures, hemiplegia, hemianesthesia, aphasia, labyrinthine disorders, or frank cerebral hemorrhage. Personality changes and psychotic behavior may become manifest with increasing age. A transient state of disorientation and confusion may occur in association with electrolyte imbalance secondary to renal disease. Severe neurologic signs may be present without evidence of major thrombosis or hypertension and are presumably due to multifocal small-vessel occlusive disease.

Progressive glycosphingolipid deposition in the kidney results in proteinuria and other signs of renal impairment, with gradual deterioration of renal function and development of azotemia in middle age. During childhood and adolescence, protein, casts, red cells, and desquamated kidney and urinary tract cells may appear in the urine. Birefringent lipid globules with characteristic "Maltese crosses" can be observed free in the urine and within desquamated urinary sediment cells by polarization microscopy (Fig. 153-5). With age, progressive renal impairment is evidenced by significant proteinuria, isosthenuria (specific gravities of 1.008 to 1.012), and alterations of other renal tubular functions including tubular reabsorption, secretion, and excretion.[44] Polyuria and a syndrome similar to vasopressin-resistant diabetes insipidus occasionally develop. Gradual deterioration of renal function and the development of azotemia usually occur in the third to fourth decades of life, although renal failure has been reported in the second decade. Death most

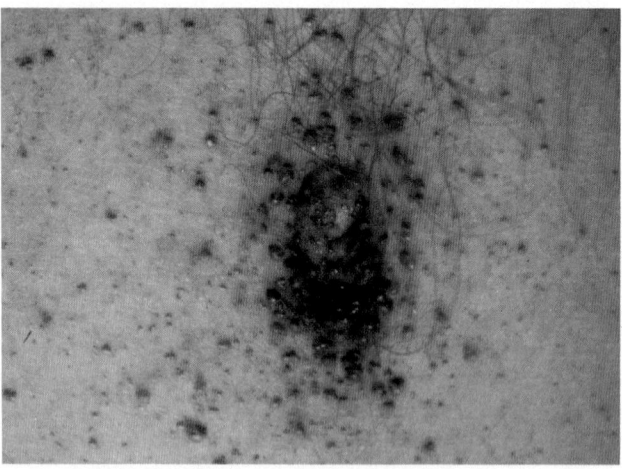

FIGURE 153-3 Clusters of dark red angiokeratomas in a hemizygote with Fabry disease.

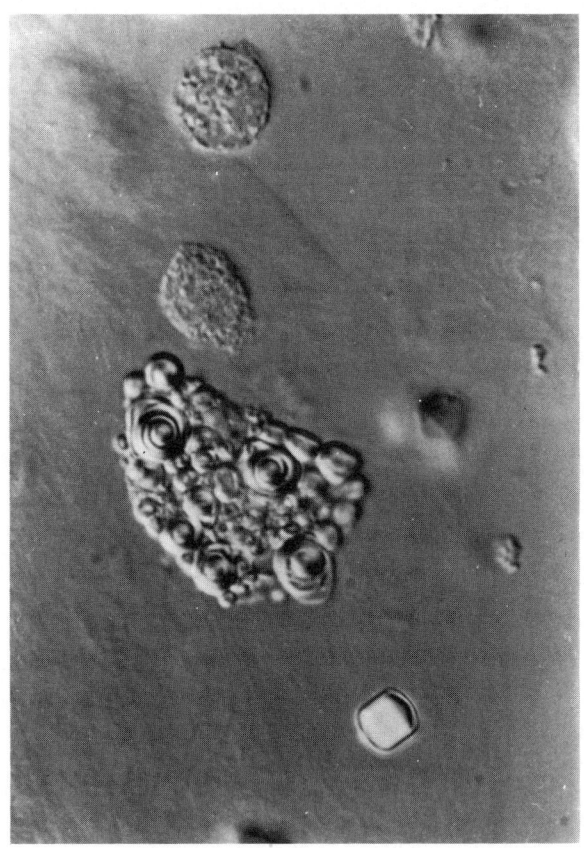

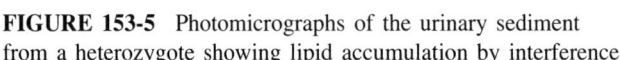

a

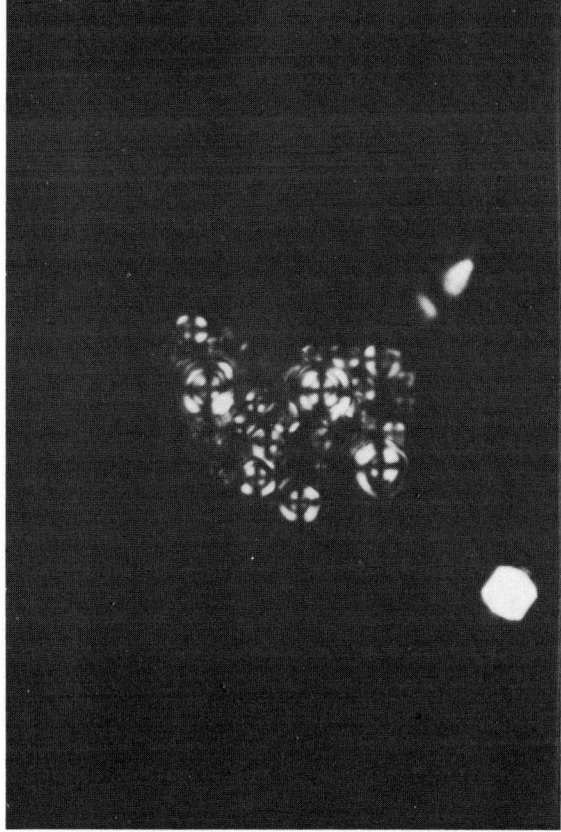

b

FIGURE 153-5 Photomicrographs of the urinary sediment from a heterozygote showing lipid accumulation by interference- microscopy (*a*) and polarization light microscopy (*b*). Note that Maltese crosses are observed under polarization. ×1000.

often results from uremia unless chronic hemodialysis or renal transplantation is undertaken. The mean age at death of 104 hemizygous males who were not treated for uremia was 41 years,[45] but occasionally an affected individual has survived into his early sixties.

Ocular Features   Ocular involvement is most prominent in the cornea, lens, conjunctiva, and retina.[46–48] A characteristic corneal opacity, observed only by slit-lamp microscopy, is found in males with the disease and in most heterozygous females (Fig. 153-6). The earliest lesion is a diffuse haziness in the subepithelial layer. In more advanced cases, the opacities appear as whorled streaks extending from a central vortex to the periphery of the cornea. Typically, the whorl-like opacities are inferior and cream-colored; however, they range from white to golden brown and may be very faint. An identical familial corneal dystrophy, termed *cornea verticullata,* was described by Gruber[49] in 1946; subsequent investigation of these patients revealed that they were hemizygotes and heterozygotes for Fabry disease.[48] An indistinguishable, drug-induced phenocopy of the Fabry corneal dystrophy occurs in patients on long-term chloroquine or amiodarone therapy (see "Genetics"). Interestingly, a report has suggested that the corneal lesions regress in patients who wear contact lenses.[50]

Two specific types of lenticular changes have been described. A granular anterior capsular or subcapsular deposit has been observed in about one-third of hemizygous males, but rarely in heterozygous females. Typically, these lenticular opacities are bilateral

and inferior in position. They frequently appear in a "propeller-like" distribution, i.e., wedge-shaped with their bases near the lenticular equator and aligned radially with the apices toward the center of the anterior capsule. A second, and possibly unique, lenticular opacity has been observed in both hemizygous and heterozygous individuals.[46,47] It may be the first ocular manifestation to appear. The opacity is posterior, linear, and appears as a whitish, almost translucent, spokelike deposit of fine granular material on or near the posterior cortex. This unusual opacity has been termed the *Fabry cataract*[46] and is best seen by retroillumination.

Conjunctival and retinal vascular lesions are common and represent part of the diffuse systemic vascular involvement. These vascular lesions occur early in life in normotensive individuals and are characterized by mild to marked tortuosity of the conjunctival and retinal vessels. There is an aneurysmal dilation of thin-walled venules as well as angulation and segmental, sausage-like dilatation of veins typically seen on the inferior bulbar conjunctiva. As the disease progresses, retinal changes associated with the development of hypertension and uremia may be superimposed. Vision is not impaired by the vascular lesions in the conjunctiva and retina or by the corneal dystrophy. However, acute visual loss has occurred in hemizygotes as a result of unilateral total central retinal artery occlusion.[46]

Other ocular findings have included lid edema in the absence of renal insufficiency, myelinated nerve fibers radiating from the optic disc, mild optic atrophy, papilledema, peripapillary edema, nystagmus, and internuclear ophthalmoplegia.[46–48]

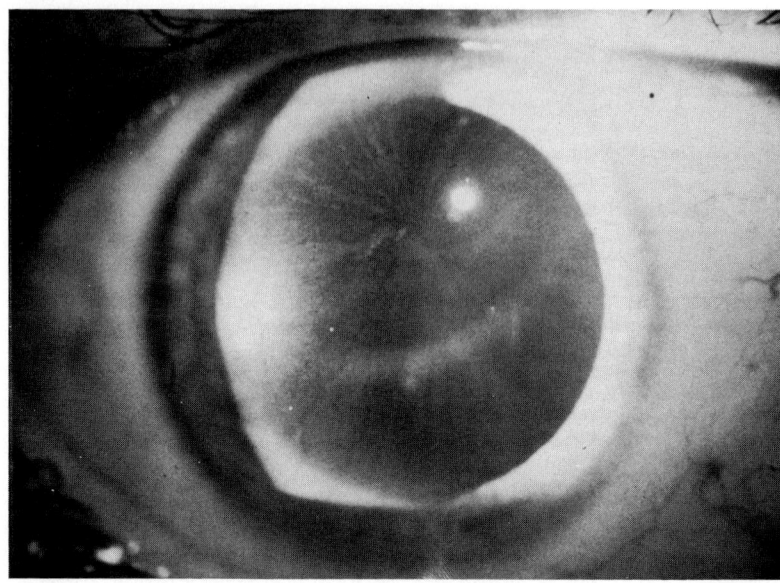

FIGURE 153-6 Corneal opacity in a heterozygote observed by slit-lamp microscopy. The corneal involvement results from subepithelial glycosphingolipid deposition.

Other Clinical Features Because of the widespread visceral distribution of the glycosphingolipid deposits, signs and symptoms of this disorder arise in many other organs and systems. Several patients have had chronic bronchitis, wheezing respiration, or dyspnea with alveolar capillary block. Pulmonary function studies in older hemizygotes may show significant airflow obstruction, reduced diffusing capacity, and a reduction in the $Vmax_{25}$ values. Roentgenographic studies may reveal hyperinflation and/or bullous disease. Smokers have greater airflow obstruction than expected from smoking alone. In general, hemizygotes do not manifest significant clinical or functional pulmonary involvement on a primary basis.[51] Presumably the reported findings of pneumothorax, pleural effusions, and pulmonary edema were secondary to primary cardiac, vascular, and/or renal insufficiency. However, primary pulmonary involvement has been reported in the absence of cardiac or renal disease.[52]

Lymphedema of the legs may be present in adulthood without hypoproteinemia, varices, or any clinically manifest vascular disease. This symptom presumably reflects the progressive glycosphingolipid deposition in the lymphatic vessels and lymph nodes. Many patients have varicose leg veins and hemorrhoids. Priapism has also been reported.

Episodic diarrhea and, to a lesser extent, nausea, vomiting, and flank pain, are the most common gastrointestinal complaints[53]; these symptoms may be related to deposition of glycosphingolipid in intestinal small vessels and in the autonomic ganglia of the bowel.[54] Perforation of the small bowel has been described. Although intestinal malabsorption has been reported, it is not a recognized feature of the disease. Radiologic studies reveal thickened, edematous folds and mild dilatation of the small bowel, a granular-appearing ileum, and the loss of haustral markings throughout the colon, particularly in the distal segments.[53] The symptomatology and pathophysiology of the gastrointestinal involvement have been reviewed.[53–55]

Anemia is probably due to decreased red blood cell survival. A decreased serum iron concentration, normal red blood cell fragility, and an elevated reticulocyte count have been reported.[29] Lipid-laden, foamy-appearing macrophages are present in the bone marrow. The spleen is not enlarged.

Many patients have evidence of musculoskeletal involvement. A characteristic permanent deformity arises from changes in the distal interphalangeal joints of the fingers, causing limited extension of the terminal joints.[10] Avascular necrosis of the head of the femur or talus, multiple small infarct-like opacities in the femoral heads, and involvement of the metacarpals, metatarsals, and temporal mandibular joint have been described.

Many hemizygous males appear to have retarded growth or delayed puberty and sparse, fine facial and body hair. In some kindreds, an acromegalic-like appearance has been reported. Affected individuals may complain of fatigue and weakness and may be incapacitated for prolonged periods of time.

The Heterozygote

The clinical course and prognosis of heterozygotes and hemizygotes differ significantly. Heterozygotes experience little difficulty in adult life when affected males already have severe renal and/or cardiac involvement. Although most biochemically documented heterozygotes are asymptomatic throughout a normal life span, with increasing age many manifest minor symptoms of the disease (Table 153-2). Some heterozygotes will develop cardiac involvement with advanced age.[56] However, a few heterozygotes have been reported in which the expression was comparable to that observed in severely affected males.[38,57] In contrast, obligate heterozygotes (daughters of affected males) without clinical or biochemical evidence of the disease have also been described,[58] further documenting the extensive variability of heterozygote expression in this disease. Of more than 150 heterozygotes reported in the literature, corneal involvement is the most frequent and often the singular manifestation[46]; frequently, the corneal dystrophy is more prominent than in affected males in the same family due to lyonization. However, biochemically documented and/or obligate heterozygous females without corneal opacities have been described.[10,47,58]

The skin lesions are much less prominent in affected females than in males; often they are not clinically manifest. The lesions may occur in the characteristic distribution; isolated lesions may

TABLE 153-2
Clinical Manifestations in Heterozygotes for Fabry Disease

Manifestation	Estimated incidence, %*	Remarks
Corneal dystrophy	~80	Useful for heterozygote identification
Angiokeratoma	~30	Single or isolated lesions
Acroparesthesias	<10	Infrequent; hands and feet
Hypohidrosis	<1	Rare variants†
Cardiac involvement	<1	Rare variants†
CNS involvement	<1	Rare variants†
Renal failure	<1	Rare variants†

*Based on review of over 122 heterozygous females, 1–85 years old, evaluated at our center.
†Rare variants with 0–5% α-galactosidase A activity.

occasionally be seen on the breasts, lips, and trunk. The lesions have been detected in heterozygotes during childhood. Skin biopsies of clinically uninvolved skin from obligate heterozygotes obtained in the first decade of life contain deposits of glycosphingolipid in the vascular endothelial and smooth muscle cells.

Other manifestations may include intermittent pain in the extremities, edema (particularly of the ankles), vascular lesions in the conjunctiva and retina, and cardiovascular changes such as hypertension, electrocardiographic abnormalities, and left ventricular hypertrophy.[10,35,44] Basilar artery aneurysms have also been reported. Urologic symptoms in heterozygotes include hyposthenuria; the occurrence of erythrocytes, leukocytes, and granular and hyaline casts in the urinary sediment; proteinuria; and other signs of renal impairment. Mucosal lesions, hypohidrosis, and diarrhea have been recorded less frequently. Heterozygotes may develop a distal interphalangeal joint arthritis of the finger.

Pathology

Morphologically, Fabry disease is characterized by widespread tissue deposits of crystalline glycosphingolipid that show birefringence with typical Maltese crosses under polarization microscopy

(Fig. 153-5). The glycosphingolipid is deposited in all areas of the body, occurring predominantly in the lysosomes of endothelial, perithelial, and smooth muscle cells of blood vessels (Fig. 153-7) and, to a lesser degree, in histiocytic and reticular cells of connective tissue. Lipid deposits are also prominent in epithelial cells of the cornea and glomeruli and tubules of the kidney, in muscle fibers of the heart, and in ganglion cells of the autonomic system.

Pathology of the Skin

The skin lesions are telangiectases or small superficial angiomas (Fig. 153-8). After a silent period, cumulative vascular damage leads eventually to clinically apparent and progressive angiectases. This sequence is suggested by the biopsy finding of lipid deposits in areas of clinically normal skin[59,60] or in patients with no skin lesions,[61] and by recognition of patients who have visceral lesions but whose skin lesions either were of minimal consequence or were delayed. The pathologic involvement was observed in the vascular endothelium and perithelium of clinically normal skin from a 1-year-old hemizygote.[60]

Capillaries, venules, and arterioles contain pathologic lipid storage in the endothelium, perithelium, and smooth muscle (Fig. 153-7). There is marked dilatation of the capillaries of the dermal papillae. Deeper vessels show less dilatation and aneurysm formation. Lipid stores have been noted in arrectores pilorum muscles, sweat gland epithelium, and perineural cells.[59-63] Similar findings have been observed in gingival tissues. Atrophic or scarce sweat and sebaceous glands have been reported.

The fully developed classic lesions are usually located in the upper dermis, where they may produce elevation, flattening, or hypertrophy of the epithelium. The larger lesions may have a slight to moderate keratosis, hence the term *angiokeratoma*. As in all forms of angiokeratomas, the hypertrophy and hyperkeratosis may be secondary to pressure on the epithelium by the underlying dilated vessel.

Pathology of the Kidney

The earliest lesions are due to the accumulation of glycosphingolipid in endothelial and epithelial cells of the glomerulus and of

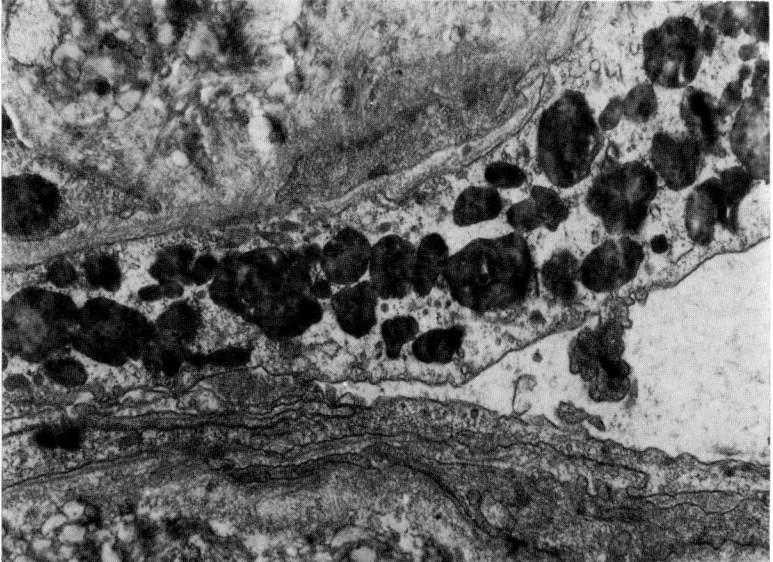

FIGURE 153-7 Electron micrograph of a section of an arteriole from the jejunum of a hemizygote showing the marked accumulation of concentric lamellar inclusions in the lysosomes of the vascular endothelium. The progressive lysosomal deposition of the glycosphingolipid substrate leads to the narrowing and eventual occlusion of the vascular lumen. ×25,000. (*Courtesy of J. G. White, M.D., University of Minnesota.*)

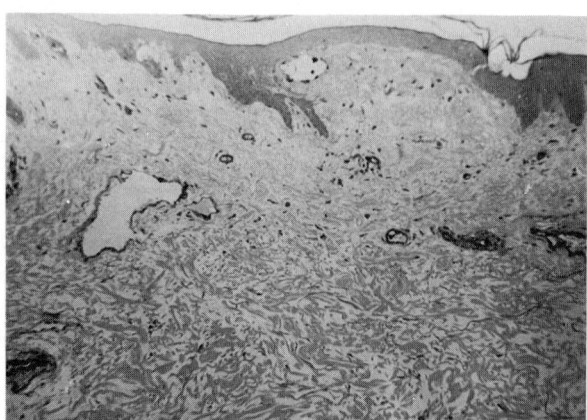

FIGURE 153-8 Telangiectatic vessels in the dermis that are typical of the changes seen in the skin.

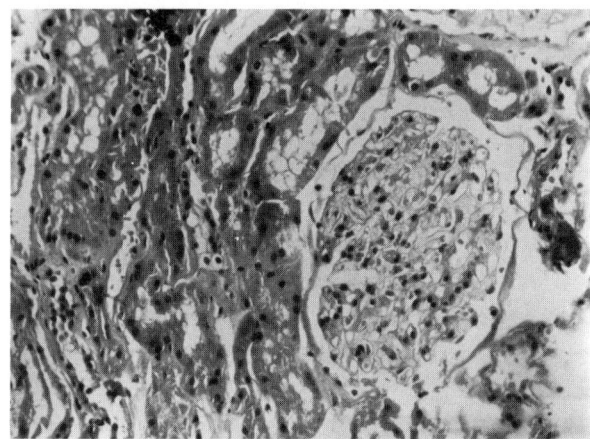

FIGURE 153-9 Photomicrograph of glomerulus and renal tubules from a 35-year-old hemizygote. The epithelial cells of the parietal and visceral layers of Bowman's capsule show multiple vacuoles from which the stored glycosphingolipids were extracted during fixation and staining (Zenker's fixation, paraffin embedding, hematoxylin and eosin). ×225.

Bowman's space and in the epithelium of the loops of Henle and of distal tubules (Fig. 153-9). In later stages and, to a lesser degree, proximal tubules, interstitial histiocytes, and fibrocytes may show lipid accumulation. Lipid-laden distal tubular epithelial cells desquamate and may be detected in the urinary sediment (Fig. 153-5).

Concurrently, renal blood vessels are involved progressively and often extensively. An early finding is the presence of arterial fibrinoid deposits, which may result from the necrosis of severely involved muscular cells. Other histologic changes in the kidney are the sequelae of nonspecific, end-stage renal disease with evidence of severe arteriolar sclerosis, glomerular atrophy and fibrosis, pseudotubular proliferation of residual glomerular epithelium, tubular atrophy, and diffuse interstitial fibrosis. Kidney size increases during the third decade of life, followed by a decrease in the fourth and fifth decades. The renal involvement has been the subject of comprehensive reviews.[43,62,64,65]

Pathology of the Nervous System

Vascular involvement is also prominent in the nervous system[66–73] and presumably accounts for the observation of minor electroencephalographic and electromyographic abnormalities in these patients. In addition, vascular ischemia and lipid deposition in the perineurium may cause the peripheral nerve conduction abnormalities of slowed conduction velocities and distal latency, respectively. In both heterozygotes and affected males, glycosphingolipid deposition in nervous tissue appears to be limited to perineural sheath cells of peripheral nerves, neurons of the peripheral and central autonomic nervous system, and certain primary neurons of somatic afferent pathways.[8,67–71,74] Lipid deposition was observed in Schwann cells by some investigators but not by others.[70,71] Qualitative[67–70] and quantitative[68] studies of peripheral sensory neurons in sural nerves and spinal ganglia have shown preferential loss of small myelinated and unmyelinated fibers as well as small cell bodies of spinal ganglia.[69,75,76]

Brainstem centers that are involved include the nuclei gracilis and cuneatus, the dorsal autonomic vagal nuclei, salivary nuclei, nucleus ambiguus, thalamus, reticular substance, mesencephalic nucleus of the fifth nerve, and the substantia nigra.[69,70] Hemisphere involvement has been noted in the amygdaloid, hypothalamic, and hippocampal nuclei. Recent studies have revealed abnormal lipid deposits in the fifth and sixth cortical layers of the inferior temporal

gyrus, the Edinger-Westphal nucleus, the parasympathetic cell column, and the midline nucleus.[70] Lipid storage in neuronal cells of the anterior and posterior lobes of the pituitary has been described. Detailed reviews of the neurologic findings are available.[70,74]

Pathology of the Eye

Histologically, abnormal glycosphingolipid deposits are found in endothelial, perivascular, and smooth muscle cells of all ocular and orbital vessels, in smooth muscle of the iris and ciliary body, in perineural cells, and in connective tissue of the lens and cornea.[77,78] Inclusions have been localized in the epithelium of the conjunctiva, cornea, and lens, and, by electron microscopy, in the basal layer of conjunctival epithelial cells as well as in the surface epithelium. There may be hyperplasia and edema of corneal epithelial cells. Bowman's membrane appears normal and no deposits are observed in the stroma or endothelium by light or electron microscopy. It has been suggested that the whorl-like corneal dystrophic pattern may result from the formation of a series of subepithelial ridges or from the reduplication of the basement membrane.[76,77]

Pathology of the Heart

The progressive deposition of glycosphingolipid in myocardial cells and valvular fibroblasts appears to be a primary cause of cardiac disease in affected males and some heterozygotes.[16,38,39] Gross cardiomegaly involving all chambers has been observed. Most commonly, the left atrium and ventricle are enlarged, and the ventricular walls and septum are markedly thickened; right atrial and ventricular dilatation and enlargement are variable findings. Within the myocardial cells there is extensive glycosphingolipid deposition around the nucleus and between myofibrils. The vessels show marked hypertrophy of the endothelial cells and smooth muscle cells secondary to lipid deposition.

Mitral and tricuspid valves have numerous lipid-laden cells embedded in fibrous tissue.[16] The most common valvular defect is thickening and interchordal hooding of the leaflets of the mitral valve, with normal chordae tendineae and either normal or thickened and shortened papillary muscles. The tricuspid valve may be similarly involved; the aortic and pulmonary valves are usually normal. Clinical and pathologic features of cardiac involvement in both affected males and heterozygotes have been reviewed.[16,38,39]

Histochemistry and Ultrastructure

The accumulated glycosphingolipids are birefringent and show a Maltese cross configuration in polarized light (Fig. 153-5). They can be stained in frozen sections with lipid-soluble dyes and may be removed from tissues by the process of dehydration and embedding in paraffin. If lipid-solubilizing procedures are used, empty vacuoles are observed by light microscopy. Most of the lipid crystals are retained through alcohol dehydration but are lost on exposure to xylene or pyridine. Exposure of formalin-fixed tissue to 3% potassium chromate for 1 week helps to preserve the lipid; improved fixation of the lipid deposits can be achieved with 1% calcium formol. A comparison of various fixation and embedding techniques to preserve the storage material has been reported.[79] A modified PAS stain specific for neutral glycosphingolipids[80] and a positive test for sphingosine[81] have served to confirm the chemical identification of the accumulated glycosphingolipids. Peroxidase- or fluorescent-labeled *Banderiaea simplicifolia* lectin, which is specific for α-D-galactosyl residues, and anti-globotriaosylceramide antibodies also have been used to stain the glycosphingolipid substrates selectively.[79,82,83]

The ultrastructural characteristics of the lesions and of the lipid inclusions in various tissues from affected males have been described extensively.[84–86] At high resolution, a typical pattern of concentric or lamellar inclusions with alternating light- and dark-staining bands is observed (Fig. 153-10). The periodicity of these bands has been reported variably as 40 to 50 Å, 50 to 60 Å, 60 to 65 Å, or as great as 98 Å. The electron-dense component is 20 to 30 Å in thickness. These inclusions have coarser periods of 150 to 200 Å.

The Metabolic Defect in Fabry Disease

The Enzymatic Defect

The primary metabolic defect in Fabry disease is the defective activity of the lysosomal enzyme, α-galactosidase A,[18,19] in the tissues and fluids of affected individuals. The deficient activity in affected hemizygotes and heterozygotes has been demonstrated with the radiolabeled natural substrate, globotriaosylceramide,[18] and with synthetic chromogenic or fluorogenic substrates.[19–21] Studies with the synthetic substrates have revealed that affected hemizygotes have residual α-galactosidase activity that is approximately 10 to 25 percent of that observed in material from normal subjects. The residual activity was determined to be due to the presence of another enzyme, α-N-acetylgalactosaminidase (previously designated α-galactosidase B) on the basis of differential physical, kinetic, and immunologic properties.[20,21,87–91]

The inability to detect α-galactosidase A activity in affected hemizygotes is consistent with the accumulation of glycosphingolipid substrates with terminal α-galactosyl moieties. The intermediate levels of α-galactosidase A activity in most heterozygous females are associated with a less severe accumulation of

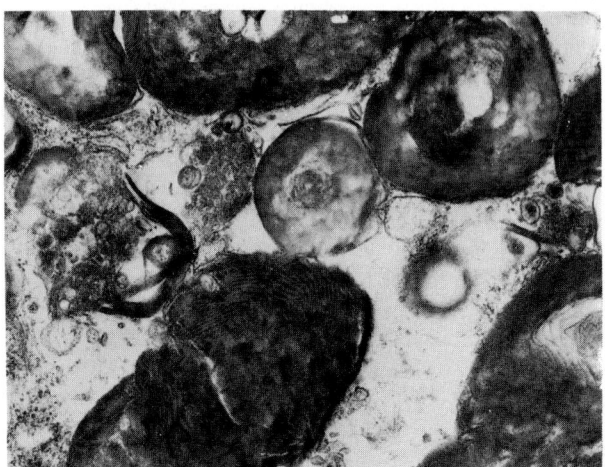

FIGURE 153-10 Electron photomicrograph of a section of the mitral valve from a hemizygote with Fabry disease, showing the concentric lamellar inclusions in lysosomes of fibrocytes. $\times$ 65,000. (*Courtesy of H. L. Sharp, M.D.*)

globotriaosylceramide in plasma, urinary sediment, and cultured skin fibroblasts, as shown in Table 153-3. In addition, the observed transmission of the defective α-galactosidase A activity in families with Fabry disease is consistent with the inheritance of a mutant gene for this catalytic gene product on the X chromosome (see "Molecular Genetics of α-Galactosidase A").

α-Galactosidase A isolated from normal tissues and fluids is a relatively heat-labile glycoprotein that catalyzes the hydrolysis of substrates possessing α-galactosyl residues, including various synthetic water-soluble substrates and naturally occurring glycosphingolipids and glycoproteins. Maximal activity of α-galactosidase A is obtained at about pH 4.5 with 4-methylumbelliferyl-α-galactoside. The Michaelis constant (K_m) of the reaction with this substrate is about 2.5 mmol.[20,89,92–94] The highest specific activities obtained to date were reported with human liver,[93] spleen, and placenta.[92] In addition, heat-stable sphingolipid activator protein-1 (Saposin B) has been identified that enhances α-galactosidase activity in vitro.[95] The molecular mass of native α-galactosidase A from human tissues is approximately 101 kDa[92–94,96] Polyacrylamide gel electrophoresis in the presence of sodium dodecylsulfate (SDS) has consistently shown a diffuse band of subunits with a

TABLE 153-3

Mean Concentration of Globotriaosylceramide and Galabiosylceramide in Various Sources from Normal Individuals and Hemizygotes and Heterozygotes with Fabry Disease[13,14,158]

Glycosphingolipid source	Normal	Heterozygotes	Hemizygotes
Globotriaosylceramide			
Plasma	2.1*	4.5	7.6
Urinary sediment	26.1*	405	1570
Cultured fibroblasts	660*	2260	2430
Galabiosylceramide			
Plasma	nd†	nd	nd
Urinary sediment	trace	183	247
Cultured fibroblasts	nd	nd	nd

*Concentrations expressed as nmol/mL plasma, nmol/24-h urine, nmol/g dry weight cultured fibroblasts.

†nd, not detectable.

molecular mass of about 49 kDa,[27,92–94,97] indicating that the enzyme probably has a homodimeric structure. Biosynthetic studies have shown that the enzyme is synthesized as a 58-kDa precursor, which is processed to a mature 49-kDa enzyme in cultured Chang liver cells and human fibroblasts.[97,98]

α-Galactosidase A is a glycoprotein containing three asparagine-linked complex oligosaccharide chains. Multiple forms are observed upon isoelectric focusing of purified preparations from plasma and various tissues due to differential processing of their oligosaccharide chains. The isoelectric points of the tissue forms of α-galactosidase A range from 4.4 to as high as 5.1,[92] whereas the plasma form has a pI of 4.2.[94] It has been suggested that the plasma enzyme form may contain 10 to 12 sialic acid residues, whereas the placental form of α-galactosidase A has only 1 or 2 residues.[92] This property is of considerable importance in connection with the circulatory half-life of enzyme administered intravenously to patients with Fabry disease,[26] and may also be a factor determining which organs acquire enzyme activity after infusion.

The more heat-stable form of α-galactosidase activity in human tissues, called α-galactosidase B, has been purified to apparent homogeneity from human liver and placenta. Kinetic studies of α-galactosidase B indicate that it probably functions in vivo as an α-N-acetylgalactosaminidase rather than as an α-galactosidase. Based on biochemical and immunologic studies, it has been concluded that α-galactosidase B is probably identical to the α-N-acetylgalactosaminidases isolated independently from various sources by monitoring activity with p-nitrophenyl-α-N-acetylgalactosaminide.

The Nature of Accumulated Glycosphingolipids

The deficient activity of α-galactosidase A in patients with Fabry disease leads to the progressive accumulation of glycosphingolipids with terminal α-galactosyl residues in the lysosomes of most nonneural tissues and in body fluids. These substances are structurally and metabolically members of a family of glycosphingolipids that are widely distributed in human tissues as normal constituents of plasma membranes and possibly of subcellular membranes as well. The lipoidal moiety of glycosphingolipids is a hydrophobic structure called *ceramide,* which consists of a mixture of 4-sphingenine long-chain aliphatic amines joined in amide linkages with various fatty acids. Carbohydrate groups are attached by a glycosidic linkage between the reducing end of the carbohydrate and the terminal hydroxyl group of the ceramide:

$$\text{Carbohydrate}\cdots\text{O}-\underset{\underset{\displaystyle \underset{\text{CO(CH}_2)_{22}\text{CH}_3}{\text{CO(CH}_2)_{22}\text{CH}_3}}{\overset{|}{\underset{\displaystyle \overset{|}{\text{NH}}}{\text{CH}}}}{\text{CH}_2}\overset{\overset{\displaystyle \text{HO}}{|}}{\text{CH}}\overset{\overset{\displaystyle \text{H}}{|}}{\text{CH}}\text{C}{=}\text{C(CH}_2)_{12}\text{CH}_3$$

Ceramide

The glycosphingolipids involved in Fabry disease are of the type called neutral glycosphingolipids, as contrasted with the gangliosides, which contain one or more acidic sialic acid groups, and the sulfoglycosphingolipids, which contain a sulfate monoester group on the carbohydrate moiety.

In living organisms, the glycosphingolipids are localized in the membranes of cells and in transport complexes such as lipoproteins. During their synthesis, and when exchanged from one membrane to another, they may be attached to cytosolic exchange proteins.[99] Glycosphingolipids of the plasma membrane are believed

to be associated primarily with the outer half of the bilayer in such a way that the carbohydrate residues extend from the surface of the cell into the extracellular environment.

In Fabry disease there is widespread accumulation of the glycosphingolipid, globotriaosylceramide [Gal(α1 → 4)Gal(β1 → 4)Glc(β1 → 1′)Cer], particularly in the lysosomes of vascular endothelial cells as well as in epithelial and perithelial cells of most organs. Chemical analyses have shown that the accumulated glycosphingolipids isolated from tissues of patients with Fabry disease are identical with those of normal tissues. The positions of glycosidic linkages, the anomeric configurations of these linkages, and the fatty acid compositions of globotriaosylceramide from normal and Fabry tissue have been rigorously established.[29] The complete structure of this glycosphingolipid, shown in Fig. 153-11a has been chemically synthesized.[100] It is notable that globotriaosylceramide is a cell-specific marker for Burkitt lymphoma.[101]

A second neutral glycosphingolipid, galabiosylceramide [Gal(α1 → 4)Gal(β1 → 1′)Cer], also occurs in abnormally high concentrations in the kidneys, pancreas, and urinary sediment of patients with Fabry disease.[12,14,15] Some of this glycosphingolipid may also occur abnormally in other tissues, such as lung and the right-sided heart structures.[16] The chemical structure of the carbohydrate moiety of galabiosylceramide obtained from Fabry kidney has been established.[29] The complete structure is shown in Fig. 153-11b.

Other accumulated glycosphingolipids were identified in patients who had blood group B activity. Certain tissues from such patients contained abnormal quantities of two neutral glycosphingolipids that inhibit blood group B–specific hemagglutination (IV^2-α-fucosyl-IV^3-α-galactosyllactotetraosylceramide and IV^2-α-fucosyl-IV^3-α-galactosylneolactotetraosylceramide).[17] These substances have been shown to occur on the membranes of human erythrocytes that express the blood group B antigens.[17] The structures of the glycosphingolipids from Fabry tissues were established by biochemical, enzymatic, and immunologic properties to be identical to the H$_1$ and H$_2$ glycosphingolipids of human erythrocytes.[17] The complete structures of these blood group B–active glycosphingolipids are shown in Fig. 153-11c, -11d.

Abnormal Distribution in Tissues

The distribution of glycosphingolipids in the organs and tissues of patients with Fabry disease has been investigated.[12,15] Increased concentrations of globotriaosylceramide were found in all sources analyzed except erythrocytes,[13,15] which indicates that most tissues are involved in the catabolism of these glycosphingolipids. In one affected male, the magnitude of glycosphingolipid accumulation was 30- to 300-fold higher than normal levels.[15] The greatest levels of accumulation were observed in kidney, lymph nodes, vessels, prostate, and autonomic ganglia. Globotriaosylceramide accumulation in various tissues was compared in hemizygotes and heterozygotes.[102] Hemizygotes had markedly increased levels in the kidney, whereas a heterozygote had the highest accumulation in the heart. Accumulation of galabiosylceramide has been reported to occur only in the kidney, pancreas, heart, lungs, and urinary sediment.[12,14–16] Table 153-3 indicates the average levels of globotriaosylceramide and galabiosylceramide in plasma, urinary sediment, and cultured skin fibroblasts from hemizygotes, heterozygotes, and normal subjects. The two blood group B–active neutral glycosphingolipids have only been found to accumulate in Fabry patients who have blood group B specificity.[17]

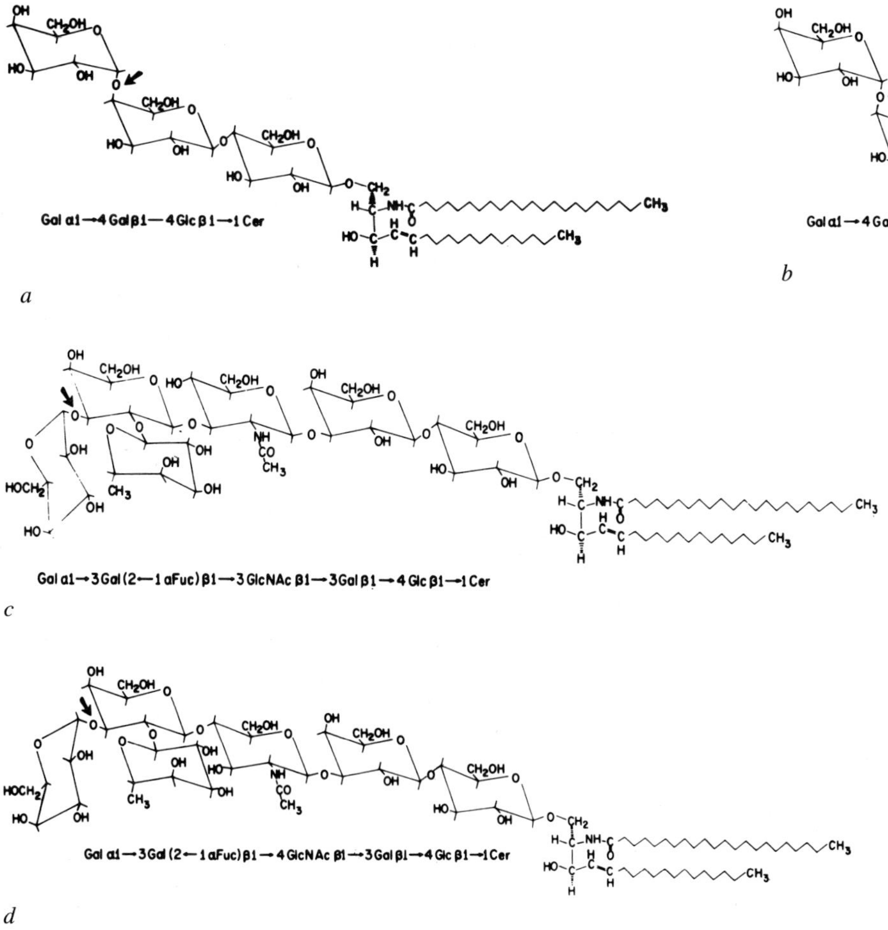

a

Gal α1→4 Gal β1→4 Glc β1→1 Cer

b

Gal α1→4 Gal β1→1 Cer

c

Gal α1→3 Gal (2←1 αFuc) β1→3 GlcNAc β1→3 Gal β1→4 Glc β1→1 Cer

d

Gal α1→3 Gal (2←1 αFuc) β1→4 GlcNAc β1→3 Gal β1→4 Glc β1→1 Cer

FIGURE 153-11 Complete chemical structures of the neutral glycosphingolipids that accumulate in Fabry disease.
(*a*) Globotriaosylceramide, Gal-Gal-Glc-Cer, the major accumulated substrate. (*b*) Galabiosylceramide, Gal-Gal-Cer. (*c* and *d*) The blood group B antigenic glycosphingolipids that accumulate in blood group B and AB patients. The arrows indicate the α-galactosyl bonds, which are normally cleaved by α-galactosidase A.

The Molecular Genetics of α-Galactosidase A

Our understanding of human α-galactosidase A and Fabry disease has been advanced dramatically by the recent isolation of the cDNA and genomic sequences encoding this lysosomal enzyme.[27,28,103,104] The full-length cDNA sequence provided the primary structure of the enzyme, and the subsequent isolation of the chromosomal gene allowed characterization of its structural organization and regulatory elements. Initial analyses of the mutations in unrelated Fabry families have identified a variety of molecular lesions underlying the genetic heterogeneity of this disease. More accurate carrier diagnosis has become possible by identification of the specific lesions in families and by analysis of locus-specific or linked restriction fragment length polymorphisms (RFLPs). Expression of full-length cDNA and genomic sequences together with site-specific mutagenesis should provide information on the structure and function of the enzyme, as well as provide large amounts of recombinant enzyme for therapeutic replacement trials.

Gene Assignment

Somatic cell hybridization studies of human-hamster hybrid fibroblasts initially localized the α-galactosidase A gene to a region on the long arm of the X chromosome, Xq21 → q22, using a series of somatic cell hybrids made from a human cell line with an X,2,15 translocation, 46X,t(X;2;15)(q22;p12;p12).[105] More recently, this

localization was further refined to the region Xq21.33 → Xq22 by in situ hybridization using radiolabeled α-galactosidase A cDNA as a probe,[103] and by close linkage to several RFLPs[106–109] that map to this region (e.g., DXS17, DXS87, and DXS287).

Characterization of the Full-length α-Galactosidase A cDNA

The pcDAG126 full-length cDNA insert encoding α-galactosidase A contains 60 base pairs (bp) of 5′ untranslated sequence and a 1287-bp open reading frame that encodes a 31-amino acid signal peptide and the 398 residues of the mature enzyme subunit. The predicted signal peptide is consistent in size with that estimated from maturation studies in which human α-galactosidase A synthesized as an ~50.5-kDa precursor glycoprotein and then proteolytically cleaved to a mature ~46-kDa lysosomal glycoprotein.[98]

Searches of amino acid sequence databases have revealed remarkable amino acid homology with human α-*N*-acetylgalactosaminidase (also known as α-galactosidase B).[110] Overall amino acid identity between the two lysosomal enzymes is 46 percent. A few other sequences have very limited similarity to human α-galactosidase A.[103] The predicted amino acid sequences of the yeast α-galactosidase A cDNA and the *melA* gene of *Escherichia coli* have a few short regions of homology with the human enzyme.[111] The only other lysosomal enzyme with any homology to α-galactosidase A is human α-fucosidase,[112] in which there is a nucleotide region, spanning bp 31 to 178, with 52 percent homology to α-galactosidase A, bp 34 to 168, when four gaps totaling 18 bases are introduced.

The α-Galactosidase A Gene

Genomic clones containing the entire α-galactosidase A gene and about 20 kb of flanking sequence have been isolated and characterized.[104] The gene is approximately 12 kb and contains seven exons (Fig. 153-12). The exons range in length from 92 to 291 bp, while the introns vary from 200 bp to 3.7 kb. All intron-exon splice junctions follow the "GT/AG" rule[113] and are consistent with the consensus sequences for splice junctions of RNA polymerase II–transcribed genes.[114] Exon 1 contains the entire 5' untranslated region, the sequence encoding the signal peptide, and the first 33 residues of the mature enzyme subunit. There are 12 Alu-repetitive sequences in or immediately adjacent to the gene (Fig. 153-12); thus, the gene has an Alu element per kilobase. The gene contains several possible regulatory elements in the 5' flanking region, including a TAATAA sequence, five CCAAT box sequences, and two GC box consensus sequences for the promoter-binding transcription factor Sp1.[104]

The Molecular Pathology of Fabry Disease

The availability of the full-length cDNA and genomic sequences for α-galactosidase A has facilitated investigation of the lesions causing Fabry disease. Southern hybridization analyses have identified gene rearrangements,[115,116] Northern hybridization analyses and ribonuclease A studies[116–119] have detected abnormalities in RNA processing and/or stability, and the amplification and sequencing techniques have identified specific point mutations in the α-galactosidase A gene.[116,118,120–122] Continued characterization of these lesions should provide insight into the frequency and nature of the mutations causing this disease. In addition, the identification of the mutation in a given Fabry family permits the precise diagnosis of other family members, including accurate carrier detection.

Gene Rearrangements

Southern hybridization analyses of genomic DNAs from over 200 unrelated Fabry hemizygotes identified six gene rearrangements, including a partial duplication and five partial gene deletions.[115,116,118] The breakpoints of the five partial gene deletions and one partial gene duplication were subsequently determined.[123]

Only one deletion resulted from an Alu-Alu recombination. The remaining five involved illegitimate recombinational events between short direct repeats of 2 to 6 bp at the deletion or duplication breakpoints. Recently, two additional α-galactosidase A gene rearrangements were described in unrelated Japanese hemizygotes, both involving short direct repeats.[124,125] These findings suggest that slipped mispairing or intrachromosomal exchanges involving short direct repeats are responsible for the generation of most of these α-galactosidase A gene rearrangements.

Transcript Abnormalities and Splice Site Alterations

Northern hybridization and ribonuclease A studies have been performed to assess the quality and quantity of the α-galactosidase A mRNA in affected hemizygotes from unrelated families. An interesting mRNA abnormality was observed in a family of Japanese ancestry. Affected males had a shorter 1.2-kb message, whereas heterozygotes had the short 1.2-kb mRNA as well as the normal 1.4-kb transcript. Ribonuclease A protection studies permitted the localization of the lesion, and subsequent sequencing demonstrated the deletion of the 198-bp exon 6 from the mature transcript. The exon 6 deletion was the result of a G to T single bp substitution occurring at the 5' splice site of intron 6. This G to T transversion altered the invariant GT consensus 5' splice site (Fig. 153-13), resulting in abnormal splicing of the α-galactosidase A pre-mRNA.[119]

Point Mutations

The ability to use the polymerase chain reaction to amplify the coding region or to use various mutation detection techniques has led to the identification of a variety of point mutations causing Fabry disease. As shown in Fig. 153-13, four missense and one nonsense mutations have been identified in classically affected hemizygotes and variants with milder disease phenotypes. These include point mutations resulting in P40S (the normal proline replaced by a serine at position 40)[122] and T44X.[120] Several mutations have been identified in atypical variants with milder disease phenotypes. An A356T mutation[116] that obliterated an MspI site was identified in a mildly affected Fabry patient with residual enzymatic activity. In addition, there were several atypical variants whose primary manifestations were cardiovascular. An atypical variant with late-onset cardiac involvement had a R301Q mutation that resulted in about 5 percent residual α-galactosidase A activity.[120] His cardiac manifestations included electrocardiographic abnormalities consistent with hypertrophy of the left ventricle and both ventricular septa. Biopsy of the left ventricular endocardium

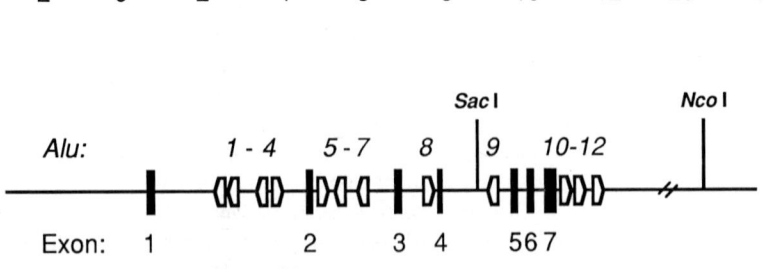

FIGURE 153-12 Schematic of the α-galactosidase A gene. Exons 1–7 are shown by bold rectangles. The positions and orientations of the 12 Alu-repetitive elements are indicated. The nucleotide coordinates for the α-galactosidase A gene (top) are as reported for the entire 12,436-bp sequence.[28] The position of the SacI and NcoI RFLPs in intron 4 and about 10-kb downstream from exon 7, respectively, are shown.

FIGURE 153-13 Mutations in the α-galactosidase A gene. Four missense mutations (P40S, M296V, R301Q, and R356W)[116,120–122] and one exon 1 nonsense mutation (T44X)[120] have been identified in classic and variant patients. In addition, a G → T transversion at the 5′ donor splice site of intron 6 results in the elimination of exon 6 from the processed mRNA.[119]

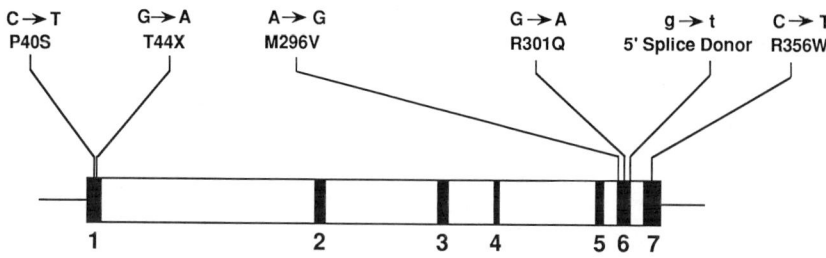

revealed vacuolar degeneration of myocardial cells and the typical lamellar inclusion bodies in lysosomes. Another interesting variant was a 56-year-old male who presented with cardiac symptoms and was diagnosed by pathology characteristic of Fabry disease on an endocardial biopsy. He had no history of acroparesthesias, corneal involvement, or hypohidrosis. In addition, ultrastructural examination revealed the absence of lysosomal glycosphingolipid accumulation in endothelial cells of endomyocardium, liver, skeletal muscle, rectum, and skin. These findings were associated with about 5 to 10 percent of normal α-galactosidase A activity in various sources. This variant, with manifestations limited to the myocardium, had a missense mutation, M296V.[121] It is notable that both variants with cardiac disease had mutations that cause amino acid substitutions within 6 residues of each other.

Pathophysiology

The pattern of glycosphingolipid deposition in Fabry disease, particularly its predilection for vascular endothelial and smooth muscle cells, is uniquely different from that seen in other glycosphingolipidoses.[126] However, the origin of the accumulated glycosphingolipid substrates has not been fully clarified. Certainly there is a significant contribution from the endogenous synthesis and subsequent lysosomal accumulation of terminal α-galactosyl-containing glycosphingolipids following autophagy of cellular membranous material with these lipid substrates. Endogenous metabolism is presumably the major source of substrate accumulation in avascular sites, such as cornea, and in neural cells, which are presumably protected from the increased circulating levels of Gal-Gal-Glc-Cer by the blood-brain barrier. In addition, the turnover of Gal-Gal-Glc-Cer and particularly its precursor, globotriaosylceramide (globoside), which are present in higher concentrations in normal renal tissue than in any other tissue, are presumably responsible for the endogenous renal deposition of the Fabry substrate.

The unique cellular and tissue distribution of accumulated Gal-Gal-Glc-Cer, particularly in the vascular endothelium (Fig. 153-7) and smooth muscle, suggests that a significant intracellular contribution may be derived by the endocytosis or diffusion of Gal-Gal-Glc-Cer from the circulation where the concentration is three- to tenfold higher than that of normal individuals. In Fabry hemizygotes and normal individuals, the circulating Gal-Gal-Glc-Cer is primarily transported in the low density (LDL) and high density (HDL) lipoprotein fractions.[29,127–129] In plasma from hemizygotes, the accumulated Gal-Gal-Glc-Cer is distributed in the LDL and HDL fractions in proportions similar to those in normal plasma, approximately 60 and 30 percent, respectively. The finding that little, if any, substrate deposition occurs in Fabry hepatocytes (in contrast to the accumulation in Kupffer cells[79,130]) supports the contention that Gal-Gal-Glc-Cer synthesized by the

hepatocyte is associated with lipoprotein and secreted as a complex.[131] In support of this concept is the fact that patients with hypercholesterolemia have proportional plasma elevations of both LDL and neutral glycosphingolipids, including Gal-Gal-Glc-Cer.[127] The circulating Gal-Gal-Glc-Cer then presumably gains access to vascular endothelial and smooth muscle cells throughout the body by the high-affinity lipoprotein receptor–mediated uptake pathway.[132–134] Deposits in other tissues may also be derived to a lesser extent from receptor-independent diffusion or by nonabsorptive endocytosis of globoside- or Gal-Gal-Glc-Cer-lipoprotein complexes from the plasma. Since lysosomes in all cells are deficient in the α-galactosidase A activity needed to degrade the accumulated glycosphingolipids, they accumulate within extended multivesicular bodies, or, in more advanced stages, as free intracytoplasmic masses, which may lead to cellular dysfunction or degeneration.

In addition to hepatocyte biosynthesis, glycosphingolipids are synthesized in the bone marrow, where they become incorporated into the membranes of the formed blood elements.[13,135,136] It has been postulated that erythrocyte globoside (Gal-Nac-Gal-Gal-Glc-Cer), the predominant glycosphingolipid of erythrocytes and the catabolic precursor of Gal-Gal-Glc-Cer (Fig. 153-11), may be another major metabolic source of the circulating pathogenic lipid. Globoside is presumably released into the circulation from senescent erythrocytes[135] and is subsequently catabolized (presumably in the spleen) to Gal-Gal-Glc-Cer. In Fabry disease, the Gal-Gal-Glc-Cer cannot be metabolized and may be partly released into the circulation where it can be incorporated into both HDL and LDL fractions[131] and/or rapidly cleared by the liver, as has been shown for intravenously administered neutral glycosphingolipids.[137] Thus, the turnover of erythrocyte and other membrane glycosphingolipids may contribute significantly to the substrate load in Fabry disease. In addition, a minor amount of Gal-Gal-Glc-Cer may be "excreted" into the circulation from the secondary lysosomes of various cell types throughout the body. Because the glycosphingolipid cannot be catabolized in the circulation, it would slowly accumulate at a rate reflecting the turnover of various cells, the contribution from exocytosis, lipoprotein uptake, and/or diffusion.

The metabolism of at least two related compounds is also abnormal, as demonstrated by the accumulation of galabiosylceramide, Gal-Gal-Cer, and the blood group B antigenic substances. Hemizygous and heterozygous individuals who are blood group type B or AB appear to be more severely affected, presumably due to the additional accumulation of B-specific glycosphingolipids.[31] Thus, the total amount of glycosphingolipid stored in a given tissue depends on time, the rate of accumulation from intracellular and circulatory sources, the possibilities for excretion, the individual's ABO blood type, and the presence or absence of residual α-galactosidase A activity (see "Genetic Variants").

The pattern of glycosphingolipid accumulation, predominantly in the cardiovascular-renal system, best correlates pathophysiologically with the major clinical manifestations of the disease as selectively described below.

Pathophysiology of the Vasculature

Narrowing, dilatation, motor unresponsiveness, and instability of blood vessels are major features of the altered physiology in Fabry disease. The swollen vascular endothelial cells, often accompanied by endothelial proliferation, encroach upon the lumen (Fig. 153-7), causing a focal increase of intraluminal pressure, dilatation, and angiectases as well as peripheral ischemia or frank infarction.[138] Such changes are frequently the precursors of thromboses and infarcts of the brain and other tissues. Muscle and peripheral nerve ischemia may contribute to the pain or fatigue.[7,139]

There may be progressive aneurysmal dilatation of the weakened vascular wall. This process is apparent in the progressive dilatation and microaneurysm formation of the retinal and conjunctival vessels and in the transition from normality to telangiectasia and frank angiokeratoma in the skin.

Observed alterations of vasomotor control may reflect either the vascular lesions themselves or the extensive glycosphingolipid deposits in autonomic ganglia and perineural sheath cells.[73,140,141] Both hemizygotes and heterozygotes with Fabry disease demonstrate an impaired ability for vasoconstriction, and the more severely involved hemizygotes show, in addition, an inability of vasodilatation. Such a combined vascular and neural lesion may also explain the clinically observed temperature intolerance.[142]

Pathophysiology of the Nervous System

The involvement of peripheral and central autonomic nerve cells may be responsible for the paresthesias, pain, hypohidrosis, such gastrointestinal symptoms as nausea and diarrhea, and a variety of vague neurologic signs and symptoms. Fukuhara et al.[139] found marked degeneration of the secretory cells and myoepithelial cells of sweat glands by electron microscopy and proposed that the hypohidrosis was due to local lipid deposition rather than autonomic nervous system involvement. The episodic fevers may be related to lesions of the hypothalamus.[74] The observations of a selective decrease in the number of unmyelinated and small myelinated fibers in peripheral nerves[67,70,71,75,140,143,144] have led to the suggestion that the selective damage to these fibers may account for the pain production and hypohidrosis in this disorder. Studies of autonomic function revealed sympathetic and parasympathetic dysfunction, particularly in distal cutaneous responses.[73,140] Alternatively, it has been suggested that the lipid deposition in the vasa nervorum may lead to the acroparesthesias, rather than involvement of the autonomic nervous system.[139,140,143]

Pathophysiology of the Kidney

The observed abnormalities in renal function have their basis in lesions of the nephron and of the renal vasculature, and possibly in disorders of the posterior pituitary and hypothalamus. Early glycosphingolipid deposits antedate clinical signs and symptoms. During this early period, the lesions of the renal vasculature are less prominent than those of the nephron, and renal architecture is maintained. The observed mild proteinuria may be explained by altera-

tion of the glomerular epithelial cells and their foot processes[64] or by increased desquamation of lipid-laden tubular epithelial cells.[82]

Loss of renal concentrating ability with polyuria and polydypsia may occur well in advance of a significant decrease in glomerular filtration or evidence of renal failure.[44] The defect in concentrating ability may be due to decreased water permeability of the distal tubules and collecting ducts secondary to lipid deposition. The diabetes insipidus-like syndrome, which is not related to faulty electrolyte transfer in distal tubules, may result from tubular insensitivity to antidiuretic hormone or to combined dysfunction of the renal tubular cells and lesions of the glycosphingolipid-laden supraoptic nucleus and antidiuretic center of the hypothalamus. The later and more severe renal changes are the result of vascular lesions and of hypertension.

Pathophysiology of the Heart

The progressive deposition of glycosphingolipids in the myocardial cells, the valvular fibroblasts, and the coronary vessels is the primary cause of cardiac disease in hemizygotes and some heterozygotes.[16,38,39] The frequent findings of left ventricular hypertrophy and mitral insufficiency are presumably related to the fact that the left ventricular myocardium and the mitral valve are the sites of the most marked lipid deposition in the heart.[16] The abnormally short PR interval and the finding of cardiomyopathy on electrocardiography may be related to lipid deposition in the myocardium and/or conduction system.[40] The marked deposition of Gal-Gal-Glc-Cer in the coronary arteries leads to myocardial ischemia and frank infarction.[16,38,39]

Other Involvement

Pulmonary symptoms have been attributed to involvement of lung vasculature or bronchial and mucous gland epithelium.[51] The airflow obstruction may be due to the loss of elastic recoil secondary to lipid deposition in lung parenchyma. The lymphedema presumably results from lymphatic obstruction or venous insufficiency secondary to lipid-laden endothelial cells.

Reports of growth retardation, delayed puberty, abnormal beard, or impaired fertility associated with a decrease of gonadotropins may correlate with observations of testicular atrophy[145] or with glycosphingolipid storage in anterior and posterior lobes of the pituitary gland[79] or in the interstitial cells of the testis. No explanations have been offered for the frequently observed acromegalic-like appearance.

Genetics

Mode of Inheritance

Fabry disease is transmitted by an X-linked recessive gene, located at Xq21.33 → q22 (see "The Molecular Genetics of α-Galactosidase A"), which normally encodes the gene product, α-galactosidase A. The frequency of Fabry disease has not been determined; the disease is rare, and it is estimated that the incidence is about 1:40,000. Of the over 400 described cases of affected hemizygous males, most are Caucasian; however, African American, Latin American, Native American, Egyptian, and Asian cases have been observed. The Fabry gene is highly penetrant in the hemizygote. Clinical onset is variable, occurring usually during childhood, but may be delayed until the second or third decade. Both intrafamilial and interfamilial variations in the clinical expression have been reported, the intrafamilial being less than the interfamilial variation.

Expressivity in the heterozygote is variable. Approximately 30 percent of the heterozygotes have a few, isolated skin lesions, a smaller percentage have the characteristic intermittent pain in the extremities, and about 80 percent have whorl-like corneal dystrophy. Proven heterozygotes may be completely asymptomatic throughout a normal life span. Obligate heterozygotes without any clinical manifestations and with normal levels of leukocyte α-galactosidase A and urinary sediment glycosphingolipids have been reported.[58,146] In contrast, complete clinical and biochemical expression of the disease, as severe as in affected hemizygotes, has been documented in several heterozygotes.[38,146] The markedly variable expression of the Fabry gene in heterozygous females is anticipated for X-linked enzymatic deficiencies by the random X-inactivation hypothesis.[147] At the cellular level, this hypothesis predicts that heterozygotes for X-linked enzymatic defects will have two populations of cells, one with mutant and the other with normal enzymatic activity. Two such populations have been isolated from individual cultured skin fibroblasts from obligate heterozygotes, one with normal and the other with defective α-galactosidase A activities.[148] Ultrastructural examination of renal tissue from heterozygotes has also demonstrated two populations of glomerular, interstitial, and vascular cells: one normal, the other in which glycosphingolipid deposition was observed.

Genetic Variants

Although most affected hemizygotes present with the classic clinical features and disease progression, rare variants have been described with milder disease manifestations.[36,116,121,149–151] In contrast to the typical patients who have nondetectable α-galactosidase A activity, biochemical investigation of these variants has revealed the presence of residual α-galactosidase A activity. The occurrence of the residual activity in the variants is consistent with less substrate accumulation and attenuation or absence of the characteristic clinical manifestations. For example, variants in their midfifties with disease manifestations limited to the myocardium and 5 percent residual activity have been recently described.[120,121] In addition, Bach et al.[150] described a 51-year-old asymptomatic male who had 10 percent of normal α-galactosidase A activity and normal levels of globotriaosylceramide in his urinary sediment. Further enzymatic studies revealed that the residual enzymatic activity had a K_m value which was fourfold higher than normal and an increased stability. Kobayashi et al.[151] studied a 26-year-old Japanese variant who had a history of acroparesthesias but no angiokeratomas, keratopathy, or hypohidrosis. Although the level of α-galactosidase A activity in this variant was typical of classical hemizygotes, loading studies indicated that his cultured skin fibroblasts were able to hydrolyze some of the exogenously supplied substrate.

Phenocopies

A phenocopy is a phenotypic mimic or simulation of a specific genetic trait. Since a phenocopy is usually the result of environ-

mental factors, it is not inherited. There are two such phenocopies for Fabry disease, one that mimics the characteristic corneal opacity and another that causes renal functional and ultrastructural changes resembling those in affected hemizygotes. Since the diagnosis of Fabry disease is often suspected from an eye examination or renal evaluation for proteinuria, these phenocopies have significant diagnostic import.

The whorl-like keratopathy of Fabry disease is readily distinguishable from the corneal opacities of other lysosomal storage diseases but is clinically and ultrastructurally identical to the corneal dystrophy associated with long-term chloroquine therapy.[152,153] Chloroquine has been shown to rapidly concentrate in lysosomes, increase the intralysosomal pH, decrease the activity of specific lysosomal hydrolases, alter the rate of proteolysis, and cause the formation of lysosomal inclusions. Based on these findings, it has been proposed that the chloroquine-induced keratopathy results from the pH inactivation of lysosomal α-galactosidase A and the subsequent accumulation of Gal-Gal-Glc-Cer.[136] In support of this concept is the finding that corneal α-galactosidase A is more sensitive to increasing pH in vitro than other lysosomal hydrolases.[154] Similar studies have shown that chloroquine inactivated the α-galactosidase A activity in cultured human skin fibroblasts.[155] These findings demonstrate the likely mechanism responsible for the phenocopy and represent the first biochemical elucidation of a human phenocopy. More recently, amidarone has also been shown to cause a phenocopy of the Fabry keratopathy; although presumed to act like chloroquine, the mechanism underlying the amidarone-induced pathology has not been characterized.[156]

Another tissue-specific phenocopy of Fabry disease occurs in individuals who are environmentally exposed to silica dust. The pulmonary complications of silicolipoproteinosis have been described, but the renal manifestations of proteinuria and lipiduria have received little attention. Ultrastructural examination of renal tissue from these individuals has revealed the typical electron-dense lamellar inclusions in the lysosomes of glomerular epithelial and endothelial cells and proximal and distal tubular cells observed in Fabry disease.[157] The levels of α-galactosidase A and urinary sediment glycosphingolipids were normal in one such patient.[157] Although the mechanism responsible for the silica-induced phenocopy is unknown, the finding of such lesions in biopsied renal tissue should include silicosis as well as Fabry disease in the differential diagnosis.

Genetic Counseling

Genetic counseling should be made available to all families in which the diagnosis of Fabry disease is made. Inheritance of the Fabry gene from affected males and heterozygotes should be considered, since both genotypes transmit the gene. All sons of affected males will be unaffected, but all daughters will be obligate carriers of the gene. Heterozygous females have a 50 percent chance of transmitting the gene to sons who will have the disease and a 50 percent chance of transmitting the gene to daughters who will be carriers. On the average, half the sons of heterozygous females will have the disease and half the daughters will be carriers. All possible carriers among close female relatives should be examined clinically and biochemically for heterozygote identification. Fabry disease has been detected antenatally from cultured fetal cells and amniotic fluid obtained by amniocentesis as well as from chorionic villus samples (see "Prenatal Diagnosis").

Diagnosis

Clinical Evaluation

The clinical diagnosis in affected males is most readily made from the history and by observation of the characteristic skin lesions and corneal dystrophy. The most common childhood symptom before the appearance of the cutaneous lesions is recurrent fever in association with pain of the hands and feet. The disorder has often been misdiagnosed as rheumatic fever, neurosis, erythromelalgia, or collagen vascular disease. Differential diagnosis of the cutaneous lesions must exclude the angiokeratoma of Fordyce,[158,159] angiokeratoma of Mibelli,[160] and angiokeratoma circumscriptum,[161,162] none of which have the typical histologic or ultrastructural pathology of the Fabry lesion (Fig. 153-8). The angiokeratoma of Fordyce are similar in appearance to those of Fabry disease, but are limited to the scrotum and usually appear after age 30. The angiokeratoma of Mibelli are warty lesions on the exterior surfaces of extremities in young adults that are associated with chilblains. Angiokeratoma circumscriptum or naeviformis can occur anywhere on the body, are clinically and histologically similar to those of Fordyce, and are not associated with chilblains.

Angiokeratoma reportedly similar to or indistinguishable from the clinical appearance and distribution of the cutaneous lesions in Fabry disease have been described in patients with other lysosomal storage diseases, including fucosidosis,[163] sialidosis (α-neuraminidase deficiency with or without β-galactosidase deficiency),[164] adult-type β-galactosidase deficiency,[165] aspartylglucosaminuria,[166] a lysosomal disorder that presents with mental retardation and some features of the mucopolysaccharidoses,[167] and an adult-onset variant of α-N-acetylgalactosaminidase deficiency.[168] Ultrastructural examination of these lesions reveals lysosomal substrate deposition that differs in the fine structural appearance of the respective storage material. In addition, patients with classically appearing angiokeratoma but no other clinical symptoms or morphologic evidence of lysosomal storage have been described[169,170]; these patients have normal levels of α-galactosidase A and other lysosomal hydrolase activities. Clinical and pathologic details of the differential diagnosis of the skin lesion are available in reviews.[59,171-174]

Presumptive diagnosis of hemizygotes can be made by a careful ophthalmologic examination, demonstration of the birefringent inclusions in the urinary sediment, or by skin or bone marrow biopsy. The observation of the characteristic corneal dystrophy by slit-lamp examination should aid in the diagnosis. Biopsied skin will reveal the refractile lipid inclusions (Maltese crosses) in blood vessels.[60] Lipid-containing macrophages may also be observed in bone marrow aspirates. Women suspected of being heterozygous carriers of the Fabry gene should be carefully examined for evidence of the characteristic corneal opacity by slit-lamp microscopy and for isolated skin lesions, particularly on the breasts, back, trunk, and posterolateral thighs. Detection may also be accomplished by the histologic finding of lipid-laden cells in biopsied skin, tissues, or in the urinary sediment.

Biochemical Confirmation

All suspect hemizygotes should be confirmed biochemically by the demonstration of deficient α-galactosidase A activities in plasma or serum, leukocytes, tears, biopsied tissues, or cultured skin fibroblasts.[20,21,86,87,175,176] Alternatively, multiprocedural glycosphingolipid analyses can be accomplished to demonstrate the increased levels of Gal-Gal-Glc-Cer in urinary sediment, plasma, or cultured skin fibroblasts[13,14,177] (Table 153-3).

Suspect heterozygotes should be identified biochemically by their intermediate levels of α-galactosidase A activity in the above sources (Fig. 153-14). Although many obligate heterozygous females can be detected by low or intermediate levels of α-galactosidase A activity in various sources, the biochemical identification of female carriers of the Fabry gene is problematic due to random X-chromosomal inactivation.[147] Thus, heterozygotes can express levels of enzymatic activity ranging from essentially zero to normal, consistent with reports of obligate heterozygotes with normal α-galactosidase A activity and no keratopathy.[178-180] If borderline levels of enzymatic activity are obtained, then heterozygotes can be identified by the demonstration of both normal and mutant cell populations by α-galactosidase A assays of single hair roots[181-184] or by cloning[148] or cell sorting[185] of individual fibroblasts. Such studies are laborious, procedurally difficult, and extremely time-consuming; require special expertise to perform; and may be difficult to interpret.[146] In addition, the diagnosis may be made by the demonstration of increased concentrations of Gal-Gal-Glc-Cer and Gal-Gal-Cer in urinary sediment.

Molecular Diagnosis of Heterozygotes

For families in which a specific α-galactosidase A gene lesion has been identified, heterozygote detection is specific. However, in the many Fabry families in which a gene lesion has not been identified, the use of RFLPs in or near the α-galactosidase A locus, or closely linked to it, would be useful. To date, two RFLPs in and near the α-galactosidase A gene have been recognized. A SacI RFLP was found within intron 4 of the gene and an NcoI RFLP about 10 kb downstream of the gene (Fig. 153-12); these RFLPs are informative in about 10 and 15 percent of families, respectively.[186] Other closely linked RFLPs have been identified proximal (e.g., DXS1 and DXS3), near (e.g., DXS17, DXS87, and DXS88), and distal (e.g., DXS11) to the locus for α-galactosidase A.[106-108,187-189] Studies of the segregation of DXS17 and DXS87 in Fabry families have indicated the usefulness of these probes for heterozygote detection,[106,107] as they were informative in about 50 percent of the 60 families evaluated.[108] Based on the Lod scores and recombination fractions for these families, it is estimated that these probes were about 1 to 2 centimorgans from the α-galactosidase A locus, indicating their usefulness in informative families.[37,108,190]

Prenatal Diagnosis

Prenatal diagnosis of Fabry disease can be accomplished by the assay of α-galactosidase A activity in chorionic villi obtained at 9 to 10 weeks of pregnancy[191] or in cultured amniotic cells obtained by amniocentesis at approximately 15 weeks of pregnancy.[22,23,192,193] The prenatal diagnosis of an affected hemizygous male fetus minimally requires the demonstration of deficient α-galactosidase A activity and an XY karyotype.

Biochemical and ultrastructural studies of tissues from fetuses with Fabry disease have been reported.[22,191,193] Consistent with the prenatal diagnosis, the α-galactosidase A activity was defective in all tissues studied; increased concentrations of globotriaosylceramide were found in all tissues analyzed with the exception of neural tissues.[192] Histologic and light microscopic examination of

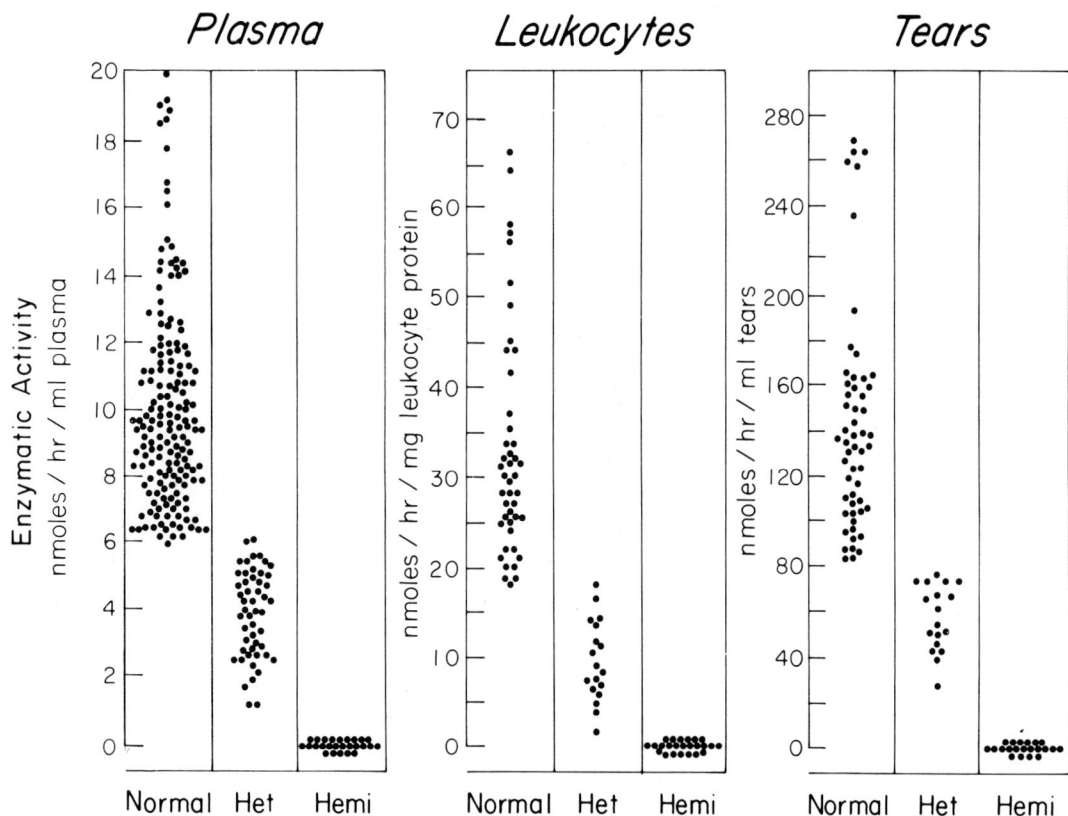

FIGURE 153-14 Levels of α-galactosidase A activity in plasma (or serum), isolated leukocytes, and tears from normal individuals and heterozygotes (Het) and hemizygotes (Hemi) with Fabry disease.

various tissues were unremarkable, but ultrastructural examination revealed electron-dense concentric lamellar inclusions in the lysosomes of vascular endothelium, myocardial cells, renal tubules, and epithelial and endothelial cells of renal glomeruli.[192,193]

Treatment

Medical Management

In Fabry disease, the chronicity of the clinical events causes severe debilitation and incapacity that extends over years. The single most debilitating and morbid aspect of Fabry disease is the excruciating pain. The pathophysiologic events that cause the incapacitating episodes of pain or the chronic burning acroparesthesias have not been clarified. Numerous drugs have been tried for the relief of these agonizing pains.[10] The α-adrenergic blocking agent, phenooxybenzamine, which increases peripheral vascular flow, has been administered for pain relief, although this drug provided relief in a hemizygote on several occasions, priapism and epistasis were early complications in two other hemizygotes.[194] With the exception of centrally acting narcotic analgesics, which have been only partially effective, conventional analgesic agents have not been successful. However, prophylactic administration of low-maintenance dosages of diphenylhydantoin have been found to provide relief from the periodic crises of excruciating pain and constant discomfort in hemizygotes and heterozygotes.[33] Carbamazepine also provides pain relief.[195] The combination of diphenylhydantoin and carbamazepine significantly reduced the pain in an affected hemizy-

gote,[196] and subsequent reports have further documented the effectiveness of diphenylhydantoin and/or carbamazepine in the prevention and amelioration of these debilitating pains.[197]

Care of patients with regard to cardiac, pulmonary, and central nervous system manifestations remains nonspecific and symptomatic. Obstructive lung disease has been documented in older hemizygotes and heterozygotes, with more severe impairment in smokers; therefore, patients should be discouraged from smoking. Since renal insufficiency is the most frequent late complication in patients with this disease, chronic hemodialysis and/or renal transplantation have become life-saving procedures. In addition to treatment of the renal failure, kidney transplantation has been undertaken to determine if the allograft could provide normal α-galactosidase A for substrate metabolism.[56,198] Hypothetically, the normal kidney might metabolize the accumulated substrate by uptake and catabolism within the allograft and/or by the release of the active enzyme into the circulation for uptake and metabolism in other tissues, such as the vascular endothelium. Although biochemical and/or clinical improvement has been reported in several recipients,[56,198–202] no biochemical effect could be demonstrated in other recipients.[203–206] Patients with successful engraftment who survived for more than 10 years have expired from cardiac disease complications[207,208] or from sepsis.[209] Thus, the use of renal allografts to alter the rate of progressive substrate accumulation remains unclear, and further studies are required to determine the long-term biochemical effects of this strategy. In view of these results, renal transplantation should be undertaken only in patients with clinically significant renal failure.

At present, the most practical and effective therapy is preventive. Screening of all suspect heterozygotes, genetic counseling, and prenatal diagnostic studies should be made available to all at-risk families (see "Genetics"). Family and vocational counseling should be provided, especially to families with affected children. Often, parents, teachers, and/or physicians misinterpret the excruciating pain experienced during childhood as psychosomatic, especially in the absence of any objective physical or laboratory findings. Since physical exertion, emotional stresses, and fatigue, as well as rapid changes in the environmental temperature and humidity, can trigger these painful episodes, appropriate arrangements must be made with physical education teachers and other individuals to minimize or eliminate stressful activities. In addition, young hemizygotes should be allowed to pursue selected activities and be permitted to stop these activities at their own discretion. Within this perspective, reasonable occupational and vocational objectives should be pursued. Vocational counseling should discourage occupations that require significant manual dexterity, physical exertion, emotional stress, or exposure to rapid changes in temperature or humidity.

Enzyme Replacement and Substrate Depletion Strategies

Attempts to replace the defective α-galactosidase A activity with normal enzyme have been undertaken in vitro and in vivo. Studies using partially purified α-galactosidase A from fig[210] and human sources (references 211, 212, and DL Johnson and RJ Desnick, unpublished results) supplied in the media of cultured skin fibroblasts from Fabry hemizygotes demonstrated the ability of the exogenous enzyme to gain access to and catabolize the accumulated substrate, Gal-Gal-Glc-Cer. These in vitro studies indicated the feasibility of enzyme replacement and, in particular, demonstrated that low levels (~5 percent) of exogenous enzyme, particularly the high-uptake form,[211] were capable of effecting normalization of substrate metabolism.

Several in vivo exploratory studies of enzyme replacement have been undertaken to determine the effectiveness and whether such endeavors can decrease the circulating accumulated substrate concentration. Normal plasma containing active enzyme has been administered to hemizygotes with Fabry disease.[24] Although active enzyme and decreased levels of Gal-Gal-Glc-Cer were demonstrated in the recipients' plasma, the major limitation was the short half-life ($t_{1/2}$ ~95 min) of the infused enzymatic activity. Brady and coworkers[25] partially purified a tissue form of α-galactosidase A from human placenta and administered single intravenous doses to two patients (6000 and 11,000 units, respectively). The exogenous activity was rapidly cleared from the recipients' circulation with half-lives of 10 and 12 min, respectively. The plasma substrate was decreased about 50 percent at 45 min, with a return to the preinfusion level by 48 h. In addition, the administered activity was detected in percutaneously biopsied liver at 1 h.[25]

Subsequently, a clinical trial of enzyme replacement was performed involving multiple injections of purified splenic and plasma forms of α-galactosidase A into two brothers with Fabry disease.[26] This trial confirmed the previously observed differences in clearance rates of enzyme from the circulation and demonstrated for the first time the differential substrate depletion and reaccumulation kinetics for enzyme purified from tissue versus plasma sources.[211] The differential plasma clearance of these enzyme forms was presumably related to differences in the posttranslational modifications of these glycoproteins. The splenic form, which was rapidly cleared from the circulation ($t_{1/2}$ ~10 min), contained few sialic acid residues. The plasma form, however, was highly sialylated and was retained in the circulation ($t_{1/2}$ ~70 min).[26] These results are in accordance with the Ashwell model for the prolonged retention of sialylated glycoproteins in the circulation and the rapid clearance of desialylated glycoproteins.[213]

A marked difference in the clearance of circulating substrate was observed after the administration of these isozymes.[26,214,215] α-Galactosidase A isolated from human spleen effected a rapid decrease in the plasma concentration of accumulated substrate. The level of the circulating substrate decreased to approximately 50 percent of the preinfusion values 15 min after injection, followed by a rapid return to preinfusion levels by 2 to 3 h. In contrast, the administration of α-galactosidase A from human plasma resulted in prolonged depletion of the circulating substrate. At 2 h after injection, the levels of Gal-Gal-Glc-Cer were decreased by 50 to 70 percent of the preinfusion values. Significantly, low levels were retained up to 12 to 24 h, and the substrate levels slowly returned to preinfusion levels after 36 to 72 h. When the total amount of substrate cleared with time was calculated by integrating the mean concentrations of Gal-Gal-Glc-Cer, the plasma enzyme appeared to have cleared about 25 times more substrate over time than the splenic form. When two doses were administered on subsequent days, the plasma substrate level was reduced into the normal range.[214] In addition, these clinical trials demonstrated that multiple doses of either partially purified enzyme, administered over a 117-day period, did not elicit an immune response in the recipients. Although these studies demonstrated the feasibility of enzyme therapy for Fabry disease, the current limitation of this approach is the unavailability of the purified human enzyme. Efforts are underway to use genetic engineering techniques to produce large amounts of recombinant α-galactosidase A for future trials of replacement therapy.

Fetal liver has been transplanted in three hemizygotes with Fabry disease in an attempt to replace the deficient enzyme.[216] The rise and subsequent fall in the levels of serum α-fetoprotein evidenced the initial survival and subsequent maturation (or possible loss) of the fetal cells. Following transplantation, the α-galactosidase A levels in sera and leukocytes were unchanged, and the substrate levels in urine and sera were slightly decreased. There have been no further reports concerning fetal liver transplantation effectiveness.

Another approach that has been employed to deplete the accumulated circulating substrate is chronic plasmapheresis.[217] Three plasmaphereses, performed at 2-day intervals, resulted in a 70 percent reduction of the level of circulating Gal-Gal-Glc-Cer to a value within the normal range. A total of 23 mg of substrate was removed. The plasma substrate levels slowly returned to preplasmapheresis levels in 5 days. Similar results have been observed with chronic plasmapheresis performed over a 6-month period (DF Bishop and RJ Desnick, unpublished data). Clearly, this approach will remove quantities of circulating substrate, but it entails a significant effort for limited effectiveness. Another therapeutic attempt to decrease the plasma substrate levels involved chronic phlebotomies that were performed in an attempt to remove senescent erythrocytes, a source of the accumulated glycosphingolipid.[218] However, following chronic blood depletion for almost 6 months, the levels of plasma Gal-Gal-Glc-Cer unexpectedly increased, indicating that this approach was not therapeutic. Reviews of the various approaches for the treatment of enzyme deficiency diseases are now available.[214,219,220]

References

1. Anderson W: A case of angiokeratoma. *Br J Dermatol* **10**:113, 1898
2. Fabry J: Ein Beitrag zur Kenntnis der Purpura haemorrhagica nodularis (Purpura papulosa hemorrhagica Hebrae). *Arch Dermatol Syphilol* **43**:187, 1898
3. Fabry J: Weiterer Beitrag zur Klinik des Angiokeratoma naeviforme (Naevus angiokeratosus). *Dermatol Wochenschr* **90**:339, 1930
4. Steiner L, Voerner H: Angiomatosis miliaris: eine ideipathische Gefasserkrankung. *Dtsch Arch Klin Med* **96**:105, 1909
5. Gunther H: Anhidrosis and Diabetes insipidus. *Z Klin Med* **78**:53, 1913
6. Weicksel J: Angiomatosis, bzw. Angiokeratosis universalis (eine sehr selthene Haut und Gafasskrankheit). *Dtsch Med Wochenschr* **51**:898, 1925
7. Pompen AWM et al: Angiokeratoma corporis diffusum (universale) Fabry, as a sign of an unknown internal disease: Two autopsy reports. *Acta Med Scand* **128**:234, 1947
8. Scriba K: Zur Pathogenese des Angiokeratoma corporis diffusum Fabry mit kardio-vasorenalem Symptomenkomplex. *Verh Dtsch Ges Pathol* **34**:221, 1950
9. Hornbostel H, Scriba K: Zur Diagnostik des Angiokeratoma Fabry mit kardio-vasorenalem Symptomenkomplex als Phosphatid-speicherungskrankheit durch Probeexcision der Haut. *Klin Wochenschr* **31**:68, 1953
10. Wise D et al: Angiokeratoma corporis diffusum: A clinical study of eight affected families. *Q J Med* **31**:177, 1962
11. Opitz JM et al: The genetics of angiokeratoma corporis diffusum (Fabry's disease) and its linkage with Xg(a) locus. *Am J Hum Genet* **17**:325, 1965
12. Sweeley CC, Klionsky B: Fabry's disease: Classification as a sphingolipidosis and partial characterization of a novel glycolipid. *J Biol Chem* **238**:3148, 1963
13. Vance DE et al: Concentrations of glycosyl ceramides in plasma and red cells in Fabry's disease: A glycolipid lipidosis. *J Lipid Res* **10**:188, 1969
14. Desnick RJ et al: Diagnosis of glycosphingolipidoses by urinary sediment analysis. *N Engl J Med* **284**:739, 1971
15. Schibanoff JM et al: Tissue distribution of glycosphingolipids in a case of Fabry's disease. *J Lipid Res* **10**:515, 1969
16. Desnick RJ et al: Cardiac valvular anomalies in Fabry's disease: Clinical, morphologic and biochemical studies. *Circulation* **54**:818, 1976
17. Wherret JR, Hakomori S: Characterization of a blood group B glycolipid, accumulating in the pancreas of a patient with Fabry's disease. *J Biol Chem* **218**:3046, 1973
18. Brady RO et al: Enzymatic defect in Fabry's disease: Ceramide trihexosidase deficiency. *N Engl J Med* **276**:1163, 1967
19. Kint JA: Fabry's diseae, α-galactosidase deficiency. *Science* **167**:1268, 1970
20. Desnick RJ et al: Fabry's disease. Enzymatic diagnosis of hemizygotes and heterozygotes. *J Lab Clin Med* **81**:157, 1973
21. Johnson DL et al: Fabry disease: Diagnosis of hemizygotes and heterozygotes by α-galactosidase A activity in tears. *Clin Chim Acta* **63**:81, 1975
22. Brady RO et al: Fabry's disease: Antenatal diagnosis. *Science* **172**:172, 1971
23. Desnick RJ, Sweeley CC: Prenatal detection of Fabry's disease, in *Antenatal Diagnosis,* edited by A Dorfman. Chicago, University of Chicago Press, 1971, p 185
24. Mapes CA et al: Enzyme replacement in Fabry's disease, an inborn error of metabolism. *Science* **1969**:987, 1980
25. Brady RO et al: Replacement therapy for inherited enzyme deficiency: Use of purified ceramidetrihexosidase in Fabry's disease. *N Engl J Med* **289**:9, 1973
26. Desnick RJ et al: Enzyme therapy XII: Enzyme therapy in Fabry's disease: Differential enzyme and substrate clearance kinetics of plasma and splenic α-galactosidase isozymes. *Proc Natl Acad Sci USA* **76**:5326, 1979
27. Calhoun DH et al: Fabry disease: Isolation of a cDNA clone encoding human α-galactosidase A. *Proc Natl Acad Sci USA* **82**:7364, 1985
28. Kornreich R et al: Nucleotide sequence of the human α-galactosidase A gene. *Nucleic Acids Res* **17**:3301, 1989
29. Desnick RJ et al: Fabry disease: α-galactosidase deficiency; Schindler disease: α-N-acetylgalactosaminidase deficiency, in *The Metabolic Basis of Inherited Disease,* 6th ed, edited by CR Scriver et al. New York, McGraw-Hill, 1989, p 1751
30. Kahlke W: Angiokeratoma corporis diffusum (Fabry's disease), in *Lipids and Lipidoses,* edited by G Schettler. Berlin, Springer, 1967, p 332
31. Kint JA, Carton D: Fabry's disease, in *Lysosomes and Storage Diseases,* edited by HG Hers, F Van Hoof. New York, Academic, 1973, p 347
32. Dean K, Sweeley C: Fabry disease, in *Practical Enzymology of the Sphingolipidoses,* edited by RH Glew, SP Peters. New York, Alan R Liss, 1977, p 173
33. Lockman LA et al: Relief of pain of Fabry's disease by diphenylhydantoin. *Neurology* **23**:871, 1973
34. Urbain G et al: Fabry's disease without skin lesions. *Lancet* **1**:1111, 1967
35. Wallace RD, Cooper WJ: Angiokeratoma corporis diffusum universale (Fabry). *Am J Med* **39**:656, 1965
36. Clarke JTR et al: Ceramide trihexosidosis (Fabry's disease) without skin lesions. *N Engl J Med* **284**:233, 1971
37. Ainsworth SK, Smith RM: A case study of Fabry's disease occurring in a Black kindred without peripheral neuropathy or skin lesions. *Lab Invest* **38**:373, 1978
38. Ferrans VJ et al: The heart of Fabry's disease: A histochemical and electron microscopic study. *Am J Cardiol* **24**:95, 1969
39. Becker AE et al: Cardiac manifestations of Fabry's disease. Report of a case with mitral insufficiency and electrocardiographic evidence of myocardial infarction. *Am J Cardiol* **36**:829, 1975
40. Mehta J et al: Electrocardiographic and vectocardiographic abnormalities in Fabry's disease. *Am Heart J* **93**:699, 1977
41. Bass JL et al: The M-mode echocardiogram in Fabry's disease. *Am Heart J* **100**:807, 1980
42. Goldman M et al: Echocardiographic abnormality and disease severity in Fabry disease. *Am J Coll Cardiol* **7**:1157, 1986
43. Colucci WS et al: Hypertrophic obstructive cardiomyopathy due to Fabry's disease. *New Engl J Med* **2**:926, 1982
44. Pabico RC et al: Renal pathologic lesions and functional alterations in a man with Fabry's disease. *Am J Med* **55**:415, 1973
45. Colombi A et al: Angiokeratoma corporis diffusum—Fabry's disease. *Helv Med Acta* **34**:67, 1967
46. Sher NA et al: The ocular manifestations in Fabry's disease. *Arch Ophthalmol* **97**:671, 1979
47. Spaeth GL, Frost P: Fabry's disease: Its ocular manifestations. *Arch Ophthalmol* **74**:760, 1965
48. Franceschetti ATh: La cornea verticillata (Gruber) et ses relations avec la maladie de Fabry (Angiokeratoma corporis diffusum). *Ophthalmologica* **156**:232, 1968
49. Gruber H: Cornea verticillata. *Ophthalmologica* **111**:120, 1946
50. Terlinde R et al: Ruckbildung der cornea verticillata bei Morbus Fabry durch kontaktlinsen-erste beobachtungen. *Contactologia* **4**:20, 1982
51. Bartimmon EE et al: Pulmonary involvement in Fabry's disease: A reappraisal. Follow up of a San Diego kindred and review of the literature. *Am J Med* **53**:755, 1972
52. Kariman K et al: Pulmonary involvement in Fabry's disease. *Am J Med* **64**:911, 1978
53. Rowe JW et al: Intestinal manifestations of Fabry's disease. *Ann Intern Med* **81**:628, 1974

54. Sheth KJ et al: Gastrointestinal structure and function in Fabry's disease. *Am J Gastroenterol* **76**:246, 1981

55. O'Brien BD et al: Pathophysiologic and ultrastructural basis for intestinal symptoms in Fabry's disease. *Gastroenterology* **82**:957, 1982

56. Broadbent JC et al: Fabry cardiomyopathy in the female confirmed by endomyocardial biopsy. *Mayo Clin Proc* **56**:623, 1981

57. Desnick RJ et al: Correction of enzymatic deficiencies by renal transplantation: Fabry's disease. *Surgery* **72**:203, 1972

58. Avila JL et al: Fabry's disease: Normal α-galactosidase activity and urinary-sediment glycosphingolipid levels in two obligate heterozygotes. *Br J Dermatol* **89**:149, 1973

59. Sagebiel RW, Parker F: Cutaneous lesions of Fabry's disease: Glycolipid lipidosis—light and electron microscopic findings. *J Invest Dermatol* **50**:208, 1968

60. Breathnach SM et al: Anderson-Fabry disease: Characteristic ultrastructural features in cutaneous blood vessels in a 1 year old boy. *Br J Dermatol* **103**:81, 1980

61. Tarnowski WM, Hashimoto K: New light microscopic skin findings in Fabry's disease. *Acta Dermatol Venereol* **49**:386, 1969

62. Morel-Maroger L et al: Des rapports avec l'angiokeratose de Fabry et la cytodystrophie renale familiale. *Bull Soc Med Hosp Paris* **117**:49, 1966

63. Hashimoto K et al: Angiokeratoma corporis diffusum (Fabry): Histochemical and electron microscopic studies of the skin. *J Invest Dermatol* **44**:119, 1965

64. McNary W, Lowenstein LM: A morphological study of the renal lesion in angiokeratoma corporis diffusum universale (Fabry's disease). *J Urol* **93**:641, 1965

65. Burkholder PM et al: Clinicopathologic, enzymatic and genetic features in a case of Fabry's disease. *Arch Pathol Lab Med* **104**:17, 1980

66. Grunnet ML, Spilsbury PR: The central nervous system in Fabry's disease. *Arch Neurol* **28**:231, 1973

67. Kocen RS, Thomas PK: Peripheral nerve involvement in Fabry's disease. *Arch Neurol* **22**:81, 1970

68. Kahn P: Anderson-Fabry disease: A histopathological study of three cases with observations on the mechanism of production of pain. *J Neurol Neurosurg Psychiatry* **36**:1053, 1973

69. Ohnishi A, Dyck PJ: Loss of small peripheral sensory neurons in Fabry disease. Histologic and morphometric evaluation of cutaneous nerves, spinal ganglia, and posterior columns. *Arch Neurol* **31**:120, 1974

70. Sung JH et al: Neuropathology of Fabry's disease. *Proceedings of the VIIth International Congress of Neuropathology,* ICS no 362. Excerpta Medica Cong Ser, vol 1, 1975, p 267

71. Sung JH: Autonomic neurons affected by lipid storage in the spinal cord of Fabry's disease: Distribution of autonomic neurons in the sacral cord. *J Neuropathol Exp Neurol* **38**:87, 1979

72. Cable WJ et al: Fabry disease: Significance of ultrastructural localization of lipid inclusions in dermal nerves. *Neurology* **32**:347, 1982

73. Cable WJ et al: Fabry disease: Impaired autonomic function. *Neurology* **32**:347, 1982

74. Rahman AN, Lindenberg R: The neuropathology of hereditary dystopic lipidosis. *Arch Neurol* **9**:373, 1963

75. Gemignani F et al: Pathological study of the sural nerve in Fabry's disease. *Eur Neurol* **23**:173, 1984

76. Hozumi I et al: Accumulation of glycosphingolipids in spinal and sympathetic ganglia of a symptomatic heterozygote of Fabry's disease. *J Neurosci* **90**:273, 1989

77. Witschel H, Mathyl J: Morphological elements of the specific ocular changes in Morbus Fabry. *Klin Monatsbl Augenheilkd* **154**:599, 1969

78. Font RF, Fine BS: Ocular pathology in Fabry's disease. Histochemical and electron microscopic observations. *Am J Ophthalmol* **73**:419, 1972

79. Farragina T et al: Light and electron microscopic histochemistry of Fabry disease. *Am J Pathol* **103**:247, 1981

80. Lehner T, Adams CWM: Lipid histochemistry of Fabry's disease. *J Pathol Bacteriol* **95**:411, 1968

81. Van Mullem PJ, Ruiter M: Histochemical studies on lipid metabolism in so-called Fabry's disease (angiokeratoma corporis diffusum). *Arch Klin Exp Derm* **232**:148, 1968

82. Chatterjee S et al: Immunohistochemical localization of glycosphingolipid in urinary renal tubular cells in Fabry's disease. *Am J Clin Pathol* **82**:24, 1984

83. Robinson D, Khalfan HA: Fabry's disease. Identification of carrier status by fluorescent/electron binding. *Biochem Soc Trans* **12**:1063, 1984

84. Van Mullem PJ, Ruiter M: Fine structure of the skin in angiokeratoma corporis diffusum (Fabry's disease). *J Pathol* **101**:221, 1970

85. Hashimoto K et al: Angiokeratoma corporis diffusum (Fabry disease). *Arch Dermatol* **112**:1416, 1976

86. Nakamura T et al: Angiokeratoma corporis diffusum (Fabry disease): Ultrastructural studies of the skin. *Acta Dermatol Venereol (Stockh)* **61**:37, 1981

87. Beutler E, Kuhl W: Biochemical and electrophoretic studies of α-galactosidase in normal man, in patients with Fabry's disease, and in *Equidae*. *Am J Hum Genet* **24**:237, 1972

88. Wood S, Nadler HL: Fabry's disease: Absence of an α-galactosidase isozyme. *Am J Hum Genet* **24**:250, 1972

89. Beutler E, Kuhl W: Purification and properties of human α-galactosidases. *J Biol Chem* **247**:7195, 1972

90. Dean KJ et al: The identification of α-galactosidase B from human liver as an α-N-acetylgalactosaminidase. *Biochem Biophys Res Commun* **77**:1411, 1977

91. Schram AW et al: The identity of α-galactosidase B from human liver. *Biochim Biophys Acta* **482**:138, 1977

92. Bishop EF, Desnick RJ: Affinity purification of α-galactosidase A from human spleen, placenta and plasma with elimination of pyrogen contamination. *J Biol Chem* **256**:1307, 1981

93. Dean KJ, Sweeley CC: Studies on human liver α-galactosidases. I. Purification of α-galactosidase A and its enzymatic properties with glycolipid and oligosaccharide substrates. *J Biol Chem* **254**:9994, 1979

94. Bishop DF, Sweeley CC: Plasma α-galactosidase A. Properties and comparisons with tissue α-galactosidases. *Biochim Biophys Acta* **525**:399, 1978

95. Gartner S et al: Activator protein for the degradation of globotriaosylceramide by human α-galactosidase. *J Biol Chem* **258**:12378, 1983

96. Kusiak JW et al: Purification and properties of the two major isozymes of α-galactosidase from human placenta. *J Biol Chem* **253**:184, 1978

97. LeDonne NC et al: Biosynthesis of α-galactosidase A in cultured Chang liver cells. *Arch Biochem Biophys* **224**:186, 1983

98. Lemansky P et al: Synthesis and processing of α-galactosidase A in human fibroblasts. Evidence for different mutations in Fabry disease. *J Biol Chem* **262**:2062, 1987

99. Crain RC, Zilversmit DB: Net transfer of phospholipid by the nonspecific phospholipid transfer proteins from bovine liver. *Biochim Biophys Acta* **620**:37, 1980

100. Shapiro D, Archer AJ: Total synthesis of ceramide trihexoside accumulating with Fabry's disease. *Chem Phys Lipids* **197**:206, 1978

101. Nudelman E et al: A glycolipid antigen associated with Burkitt lymphoma defined by a monoclonal antibody. *Science* **220**:509, 1983

102. Hozumi et al: Biochemical and clinical analysis of accumulated glycolipids in symptomatic heterozygotes of angiokeratoma corporis diffusum (Fabry's disease) in comparison with hemizygotes. *J Lipid Res* **31**:335, 1990

103. Bishop EF et al: Human α-galactosidase A: Nucleotide sequence of a cDNA clone encoding the mature enzyme. *Proc Natl Acad Sci USA* **83**:4859, 1986

104. Bishop EF et al: Structural organization of the α-galactosidase A gene: Further evidence for the absence of a 3′ untranslated region. *Proc Natl Acad Sci USA* **85**:3903, 1988

105. Fox MF et al: Regional localization of α-galactosidase (GLA) to Xpter → q22, hexosaminidase B (HEXB) to 5q13 → qter, and arylsulfatase B (ARSB) to 5pter → q13. *Cytogenet Cell Genet* **38**:45, 1984

106. Morgan SH et al: Anderson-Fabry disease—family linkage studies using two polymorphic X-linked DNA probes. *Pediatr Nephrol* **1**:536, 1987

107. MacDermot KD et al: Anderson Fabry disease. Close linkage with highly polymorphic DNA markers DXS17, DXS87 and DXS88. *Hum Genet* **77**:263, 1987

108. Desnick RJ et al: Fabry disease. Molecular diagnosis of hemizygotes and heterozygotes. *Enzyme* **38**:54, 1987

109. Yang HM et al: Subregional localization of anonymous Xq DNA probe by deletion mapping. *Cytogenet Cell Genet* **46**:722, 1988

110. Wang AE, Desnick RJ: Structural organization and complete sequence of the human α-N-acetylgalactosaminidase gene: Homology with the α-galactosidase A gene provides evidence for evolution from a common ancestral gene. *Genomics* **10**:133, 1991

111. Liljestrom PL, Liljestrom P: Nucleotide sequence of the *mel*A gene, coding for α-galactosidase in *Escherichia coli*. K-12. *Nucleic Acids Res* **15**:2213, 1987

112. Fukushima H et al: Molecular cloning of a cDNA for human α-L-fucosidase. *Proc Natl Acad Sci USA* **82**:1262, 1985

113. Breathnach R, Chambon P: Organization and expression of eukaryotic split genes coding for proteins. *Annu Rev Biochem* **50**:349, 1981

114. Mount SM: A catalogue of splice junction sequences. *Nucleic Acids Res* **10**:459, 1982

115. Bernstein HS et al: Fabry disease: Analysis of mutations in the human α-galactosidase A gene. *Am J Hum Genet* **39**:A188, 1986

116. Bernstein HS et al: Fabry disease: Gene rearrangements and a coding region point mutation in the α-galactosidase A gene. *J Clin Invest* **83**:1390, 1989

117. Prywes R, Roder RG: Inducible binding of a factor to the c-*fos* enchancer. *Cell* **47**:777, 1986

118. Desnick RJ et al: Fabry disease: Molecular genetics of α-galactosidase deficiency. *Clin Res* **36**:612A, 1988

119. Sakuraba H et al: Invariant exon skipping in the human α-galactosidase A pre-mRNA: A g^{+1} to t substitution in a 5′ splice site causing Fabry disease. *Genomics* **12**:643, 1992

120. Sakuraba H et al: Identification of point mutations in the α-galactosidase A gene in classical and atypical hemizygotes with Fabry disease. *Am J Hum Genet* **47**:784, 1990

121. von Scheidt W et al: An atypical variant of Fabry's disease with manifestations confined to the myocardium. *N Engl J Med* **324**:395, 1991

122. Koide T et al: A case of Fabry's disease in a patient with no α-galactosidase A activity caused by a single amino acid substitution of Pro-40 by Ser. *FEBS Lett* **259**:353, 1990

123. Kornreich R et al: α-Galactosidase A gene rearrangements causing Fabry disease. Identification of short direct repeats at breakpoints in an *Alu* rich gene. *J Biol Chem* **265**:9319, 1990

124. Ishii S et al: Fabry disease: Detection of 13 bp deletion in α-galactosidase A gene and its application to gene diagnosis of heterozygotes. *Ann Neurol* **29**:560, 1990

125. Fukuhara Y et al: Partial deletion of human α-galactosidase A gene in Fabry disease: Direct repeat sequences as a possible cause of slipped mispairing. *Biochem Biophys Res Commun* **170**:296, 1990

126. Johnson DL, Desnick RJ: Molecular pathology of Fabry's disease: Physical and kinetic properties of α-galactosidase A in cultured human endothelial cells. *Biochim Biophys Acta* **538**:195, 1978

127. Dawson G et al: Distribution of glycosphingolipids in the serum lipoproteins of normal human subjects and patients with hypo- and hyperlipidemias. *J Lipid Res* **17**:125, 1976

128. Clarke JTR et al: Neutral glycosphingolipids of serum lipoproteins in Fabry's disease. *Biochim Biophys Acta* **431**:317, 1976

129. Van den Bergh FAJTM, Tager JM: Localization of neutral glycosphingolipids in human plasma. *Biochim Biophys Acta* **441**:391, 1976

130. Meuweissen SGM et al: Ultrastructural and biochemical liver analyses in Fabry's disease. *Hepatology* **2**:263, 1982

131. Clarke JTR, Stoltz JM: Uptake of radiolabeled galactosyl-(α1 → 4)-galactosyl-(β1 → 4)-glucosylceramide by human lipoproteins in vitro. *Biochim Biophys Acta* **441**:165, 1976

132. Stein O, Stein Y: High density lipoproteins reduce the uptake of low density lipoproteins by human endothelial cells in culture. *Biochim Biophys Acta* **431**:363, 1976

133. Goldstein JL, Brown MS: The low density lipoprotein pathway and its relation to atherosclerosis. *Annu Rev Biochem* **46**:897, 1977

134. Voldavsky I et al: Role of contact inhibition in the regulation of receptor-mediated uptake of low density lipoprotein in cultured vascular endothelial cells. *Proc Natl Acad Sci USA* **75**:356, 1979

135. Dawson G, Sweeley CC: *In vivo* studies on glycosphingolipid metabolism in porcine blood. *J Biol Chem* **245**:410, 1970

136. Tao RVP: Biochemistry and metabolism of mammalian blood glycosphingolipids. Ph.D. Thesis, Michigan State University, 1973

137. Barkai A, DeCesare JL: Influence of sialic acid groups on retention of glycosphingolipids in blood plasma. *Biochim Biophys Acta* **398**:287, 1975

138. Nakamura T et al: Angiokeratoma corporis diffusum (Fabry disease): Ultrastructural studies of the skin. *Acta Derm Venereol (Stockh)* **61**:37, 1981

139. Fukuhara N et al: Fabry's disease on the mechanism of the peripheral nerve involvement. *Acta Neuropathol* **33**:9, 1975

140. Dvorak AM et al: Diagnostic electron microscopy. II. Fabry's disease: Use of biopsies from uninvolved skin. Acute and chronic changes involving the microvasculature and small unmyelinated nerves. *Pathol Annu* **16**:139, 1981

141. Seino Y et al: Peripheral hemodynamics in patients with Fabry's disease. *Am Heart J* **105**:783, 1983

142. Morgan, SH et al: The neurological complications of Anderson-Fabry disease (α-galactosidase A deficiency)—investigation of symptomatic and presymptomatic patients. *Q J Med* **277**:491, 1990

143. Sheth KJ, Swick HM: Peripheral nerve conduction in Fabry disease. *Ann Neurol* **7**:319, 1980

144. Pelissier JF et al: Morphological and biochemical changes in muscle and peripheral nerve in Fabry's disease. *Muscle Nerve* **4**:381, 1981

145. Vogelberg KH et al: Lipoidchemische Untersuchungen beim Angiokeratoma corporis diffusum (Fabry-syndrome). *Klin Wochenschr* **47**:916, 1969

146. Rjetra PJGM et al: The use of biochemical parameters for the detection of carriers of Fabry's disease. *J Mol Med* **1**:237, 1976

147. Lyon M: Gene action in the X-chromosome of the mouse (*Mus musculus L*) *Nature* **190**:372, 1961

148. Romeo G, Migeon BR: Genetic inactivation of the α-galactosidase locus in carriers of Fabry's disease. *Science* **170**:180, 1970

149. Bishop DF et al: Fabry disease: An asymptomatic hemizygote with significant residual α-galactosidase A activity. *Am J Hum Genet* **33**:71A, 1981

150. Bach G et al: Pseudodeficiency of α-galactosidase A. *Clin Genet* **21**:59, 1982

151. Kobayashi T et al: Fabry's disease with partially deficient hydrolysis of ceramide trihexoside. *J Neurol Sci* **67**:179, 1985

152. Francois J, de Becker L: Les manifestations oculaires de l'intoxication chloroquine. *Ann Oculist* **198**:513, 1965

153. Desnick RJ et al: Fabry keratopathy: Molecular pathology of the chloroquine-induced phenocopy. *Am J Hum Genet* **26**:26a, 1974

154. Whitley CB: Studies of heritable and induced lysosomopathies. Ph.D. Thesis, University of Minnesota, 1977

155. De Groot PG et al: Inactivation by chloroquine of α-galactosidase in cultured human skin fibroblasts. *Exp Cell Res* **136**:327, 1981

156. Whitley CB et al: Amiodarone phenocopy of Fabry's keratopathy. *JAMA* **249**:2177, 1983

157. Banks DE et al: Silicon nephropathy mimicking Fabry's disease. *Am J Nephr* **3**:279, 1983

158. Imperial R, Heliwig EB: Angiokeratoma of the scrotum (Fordyce type). *J Urol* **98**:379, 1967

159. Fordyce JA: Angiokeratoma of the scrotum. *J Cutan Genitourin Dis* **14**:81, 1896

160. Traub EF, Tolmach JA: Angiokeratoma. Comprehensive study of the literature and report of a case. *Arch Dermatol Syphilol* **24**:39, 1931

161. Dammert K: Angiokeratosis naeviformis—a form of naevus telangiectatieus lateralis (naevus flammeus). *Dermatologica* **130**:17, 1965

162. Goldman L et al: Thrombotic angiokeratoma circumscriptum simulating melanoma. *Arch Dermatol* **117**:138, 1981

163. Epinette WW et al: Angiokeratoma corporis diffusum with α-L-fucosidase deficiency. *Arch Dermatol* **107**:755, 1973

164. Miyatake T et al: Adult type neuronal storage disease with neuraminidase deficiency. *Ann Neurol* **6**:232, 1978

165. Wenger DA et al: Adult G_{M1} gangliosidosis: Clinical and biochemical studies on two patients and comparison to other patients called variant or adult G_{M1} gangliosidosis. *Clin Genet* **17**:323, 1980

166. Gehler J et al: Clinical and biochemical delineation of aspartylglycosaminuria as observed in two members of an Italian family. *Helv Paediatr Acta* **36**:179, 1981

167. McCallum DI et al: Angiokeratoma corporis diffusum with features of a mucopolysaccharidosis. *J Med Genet* **17**:21, 1980

168. Kanzaki T et al: Lysosomal α-N-acetylgalactosaminidase deficiency, the enzymatic defect in angiokeratoma corporis diffusum with glycopeptiduria. *J Clin Invest* **88**:707, 1991

169. Holmes RC et al: Angiokeratoma corporis diffusum in a patient with normal enzyme activities. *J Am Acad Dermatol* **10**:384, 1984

170. Crovato F, Rebora A: Angiokeratoma corporis diffusum and normal enzyme activities. *J Am Acad Dermatol* **12**:885, 1985

171. Frost P et al: Fabry's disease: Glycolipid lipidosis. Skin manifestations. *Arch Intern Med* **117**:440, 1966

172. Imperial R, Heliwig EB: Angiokeratoma: A clinicopathological study. *Arch Dermatol* **95**:166, 1967

173. Van Mullem PJ, Ruiter M: Electron microscopic study of the skin in angiokeratoma corporis diffusum. *Arch Klin Exp Dermatol* **226**:453, 1966

174. Elleder M et al: An atypical ultrastructural pattern in Fabry's disease: A study on its nature and incidence in seven cases. *Ultrastruct Pathol* **14**:467, 1990

175. Ho MW et al: Fabry's disease: Evidence for a physically altered α-galactosidase. *Am J Hum Genet* **24**:256, 1972

176. Mayes JS et al: Differential assay for lysosomal α-galactosidase in human tissues and its application to Fabry's disease. *Clin Chim Acta* **112**:247, 1981

177. Dawson G et al: Glycosphingolipids in cultured human fibroblasts. II. Characterization and metabolism in fibroblasts from patients with inborn errors of glycosphingolipid and mucopolysaccharide metabolism. *J Biol Chem* **247**:5951, 1972

178. Spaeth GL, Frost P: Fabry's disease: Its ocular manifestations. *Arch Ophthalmol* **74**:760, 1965

179. Avila JL et al: Fabry's disease: Normal α-galactosidase activity and urinary-sediment glycosphingolipid levels in two obligate heterozygotes. *Br J Dermatol* **89**:149, 1973

180. Francois J: Heterozygotes for sex-linked traits and Mary Lyon's inactivation theory. XIV. Fabry's dystopic lipidosis, in *Proceedings of the III International Congress of Human Genetics*. Baltimore, Johns Hopkins Press, 1967, p 423

181. Grimm T et al: Fabry's disease: Heterozygote detection by hair root analysis. *Hum Genet* **32**:329, 1976

182. Spence MW et al: Heterozygote detection in angiokeratoma corporis diffusum (Anderson-Fabry disease). *J Med Genet* **14**:91, 1977

183. Vermorken AJM et al: Fabry's disease: Biochemical and histochemical studies on hair roots for carrier detection. *Br J Dermatol* **98**:191, 1978

184. Beaudet AL, Caskey CT: Detection of Fabry's disease heterozygotes by hair root analysis. *Clin Genet* **13**:251, 1978

185. Jongkind JF et al: Detection of Fabry's disease heterozygotes by enzyme analysis in single fibroblasts after cell sorting. *Cell Genet* **23**:243, 1985

186. Desnick RJ et al: Fabry disease: Molecular diagnosis of hemizygotes and heterozygotes. *Enzyme* **38**:54, 1987

187. Davies KE: Molecular genetics of the human X chromosome. *J Med Genet* **22**:243, 1985

188. Drayna D, White R: Genetic linkage map of the human X-chromosome. *Science* **230**:753, 1985

189. Williard HF et al: Report of the committee on human gene mapping by recombinant DNA techniques, in *Human Gene Mapping 8. Cytogenet Cell Genet* **40**:360, 1985

190. Bagdale JD et al: Fabry's disease: A correlative clinical, morphologic and biochemical study. *Lab Invest* **18**:681, 1968

191. Kleijer WJ et al: Prenatal diagnosis of Fabry's disease by direct analysis of chorionic villi. *Prenatal Diagn* **7**:283, 1987

192. Malouf M et al: Ultrastructural changes in antenatal Fabry's disease. *Am J Pathol* **82**:132, 1976

193. Desnick RJ et al: Prenatal diagnosis of glycosphingolipidoses: Sandhoff's and Fabry's diseases. *J Pediatr* **83**:149, 1973

194. Funderburk SJ et al: Priapism after phenoxybenzamine in a patient with Fabry's disease. *N Engl J Med* **290**:630, 1974

195. Lenoir G et al: La maladie de Fabry. Traitement du syndrome acrodyniforme par la carbamazepine. *Arch Fr Pediatr* **34**:704, 1977

196. Atzpodien W et al: Angiokeratoma corporis diffusum (Morbus Fabry). Biochemische diagnostik im Blutplasma. *Dtsch Med Wochenschr* **100**:423, 1975

197. Dupperrat B et al: Maladie de Fabry. Angiokeratomes presents a la naissance. Action de la diphenylhydantoine sur les crises douloureuses. *Ann Dermatol Syphiligre* **102**:392, 1975

198. Philippart M et al: Reversal of an inborn sphingolipidosis (Fabry's disease) by kidney transplantation. *Ann Intern Med* **77**:195, 1972

199. Desnick RJ et al: Fabry disease: Correction of the enzymatic deficiency by renal transplantation, in *Enzyme Therapy in Genetic Diseases*, edited by RJ Desnick et al. Baltimore, Williams & Wilkins, 1973, p 188

200. Jacky E: Fabrysche Erkrankung (Angiokeratoma corporis diffusum universale): gunstiger Verlauf nach Nierentransplantation. *Schweiz Med Wochenschr* **106**:703, 1976

201. Buhler FR et al: Kidney transplantation in Fabry's disease. *Br Med J* **3**:28, 1973

202. Clement M et al: Renal transplantation in Anderson-Fabry disease. *J R Soc Med* **75**:557, 1982

203. Clarke JTR et al: Enzyme replacement therapy by renal allotransplantation in Fabry's disease. *N Engl J Med* **287**:1215, 1972

204. Spense MW et al: Failure to correct the metabolic defect by renal allotransplantation in Fabry's disease. *Ann Intern Med* **84**:13, 1976

205. Grunfeld JP et al: Le transplantation renale chez les sujets atteints de maladie de Fabry. *Nouv Presse Med* **4**:2081, 1975

206. Van den Bergh FAJTM et al: Therapeutic implications of renal transplantation in a patient with Fabry's disease. *Acta Med Scand* **200**:249, 1976

207. Bannwart F: Morbus Fabry. Licht- und elektronenmikroskopischer Herzbefund 12 Jahre nach erfolgreicher Nierentransplantation. *Schweiz Med Wochenschr* **112**:1742, 1982

208. Kramer W et al: Progressive cardiac involvement by Fabry's disease despite successful renal allotransplantation. *Int J Cardiol* **7**:72, 1984

209. Mosnier JF et al: Recurrence of Fabry's disease in a renal allograft eleven years after successful renal transplantation. *Transplantation* **51**:759, 1991

210. Dawson G et al: Correction of the enzymatic defect in cultured fibroblasts from patients with Fabry's disease: Treatment with purified α-galactosidase from Ficin. *Pediatr Res* **7**:684, 1973

211. Mayes JS et al: Endocytosis of lysosomal α-galactosidase A by cultured fibroblasts from patients with Fabry disease. *Am J Hum Genet* **34**:602, 1982

212. Hasholt L, Sorensen, SA: A microtechnique for quantitative measurements of acid hydrolases in fibroblasts. Its application in diagnosis of Fabry disease and enzyme replacement studies. *Clin Chim Acta* **142**:257, 1984

213. Ashwell G, Morell AG: The role of surface carbohydrates in the

hepatic recognition and transport of circulating glycoproteins. *Adv Enzymol* **41**:99, 1974

214. Desnick RJ et al: Enzyme therapy XVII: Metabolic and immunologic evaluation of α-galactosidase A replacement in Fabry disease, in *Enzyme Therapy in Genetic Diseases: 2*, edited by RJ Desnick. New York, Alan R Liss, 1980. p 393

215. Bishop DF et al: Enzyme therapy XX: Further evidence for the differential *in vivo* fate of human splenic and plasma forms of α-galactosidase A in Fabry disease. Recovery of exogenous activity from hepatic tissue, in *Lysosomes and Lysosomal Storage Diseases,* edited by JW Callahan, JA Lowden. New York, Raven, 1981, p 381

216. Touraine JL et al: Maladie de Fabry: Deux maladies ameliores par la greffe de cellules de foie foetal. *Nouv Presse Med* **8**:1499, 1979

217. Pyeritz RE et al: Plasma exchange removes glycosphingolipid in Fabry disease. *Am J Med Genet* **7**:301, 1980

218. Beutler E et al: The effect of phlebotomy as a treatment of Fabry disease. *Biochem Med* **30**:363, 1983

219. Desnick RJ, Grabowski, GA: Advances in the treatment of inherited metabolic diseases. *Adv Hum Genet* **11**:281, 1981

220. Desnick RJ (editor): *Treatment of Genetic Diseases*. New York, Churchill Livingstone, 1991

CHAPTER 154

Lipoid Proteinosis

Ch. M. Lapiere

Lipoid proteinosis, also called *hyalinosis cutis et mucosae* and *Urbach-Wiethe disease,* is an uncommon, recessively inherited disorder characterized by noninflammatory persistent papules on the skin and mucous membranes. The papules are produced by the accumulation of a basement membrane-like material in various connective tissues. The pathogenesis of the disease is not yet clear. Therapy is mainly symptomatic. For a complete review, see ref. 1.

History

In 1929, two Viennese, E. Urbach and C. Wiethe, a dermatologist and an otorhinolaryngologist, described an entity that they called *lipoidosis cutis et mucosae*[2] on the basis of histologic investigations demonstrating the deposition, in skin and mucous membranes, of a lipoid material associated with protein. The initial name was later modified to *lipoid proteinosis* to avoid confusion with other lipoidoses. At the present time, the most common names given to this syndrome are *lipoid proteinosis or hyalinosis cutis et mucosae*. It may be referred to as Urbach-Wiethe disease eponymously.

Genetics

Parental consanguinity, affected siblings, and equal numbers of male and female patients suggest autosomal recessive transmission. Most of the reported patients have a European background and more than half of them belong to or are related to the Germanic linguistic group. Interesting studies performed in the Afrikaaner population of South Africa suggest that most of the reported cases in that country derive from descendants of a brother and a sister who emigrated to South Africa from Germany in the middle of the seventeenth century.

Clinical Presentation

The first clinical sign is often hoarseness, caused by infiltration of the laryngeal mucosa, that has developed by birth or develops in early childhood. Skin lesions usually appear shortly afterward or simultaneously. The development of the clinical signs may be precipitated by an intercurrent disease as benign as, for example, vaccination.

Location of Lesions

Papular, nodular, or diffuse yellow waxy infiltrates are located on the face, the axillae, and the scrotum. Skin lesions resembling pitted acne scars may be located not only on the face but also in non-acneogenic regions. Other lesions of the face resemble solar elastosis because of the deposition of yellow material inducing a marked thickening of the skin with deep wrinkles (Fig. 154-1). The classic and most easily recognizable sign, although not always present, is the beaded arrangement of waxy papules along the eyelids (Fig. 154-1). Lesions on the scalp may occur and cause alopecia. Lesions on non-sun-exposed skin can be present, as well as alterations of the mucous membranes. The tongue is often firm and its mobility may be limited (Fig. 154-2). The tonsils and other areas

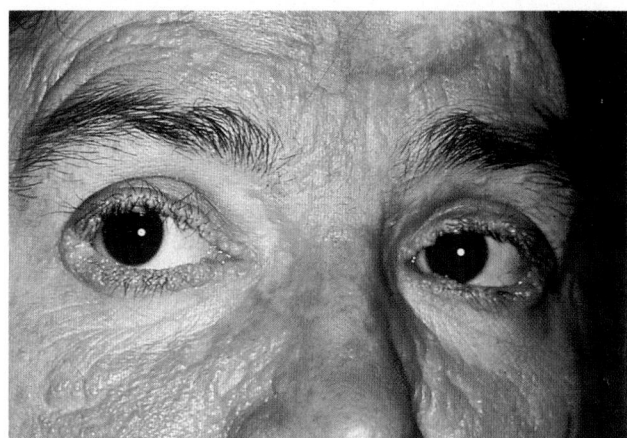

FIGURE 154-1 Lipoid proteinosis. Note the beaded arrangement of waxy papules along the margin of both eyelids and the pseudo solar elastosis of the cheeks and forehead. *(Courtesy of O. Braun-Falco, Munich.)*

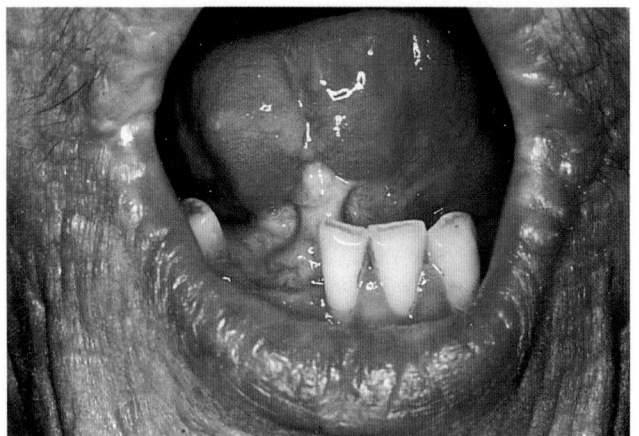

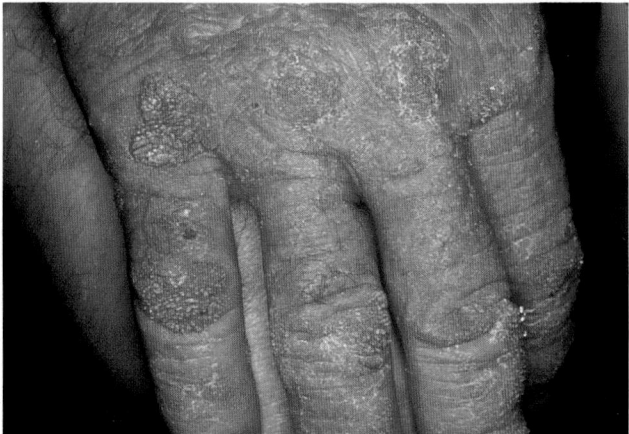

a

FIGURE 154-2 Discoloration of the lips in lipoid proteinosis. Limitation of mobility of the tongue is related to infiltration of the frenulum. *(Courtesy of O. Braun-Falco, Munich.)*

in the oral cavity may be infiltrated. A yellow discoloration of the lips is characteristic (Fig. 154-2). The skin lesions may be traumatized and present in the form of an oozing infiltrate leading to hyperkeratosis. Hyperkeratosis is also observed on the palm and dorsum of the hands (Fig. 154-3*a*, -3*b*), elbows, knees (Fig. 154-4), and buttocks, possibly related to frequent trauma in these locations.

Involvement of Other Organs

Recurrent parotitis is related to occlusion of the salivary canal. The teeth are abnormal in almost 30 percent of patients: patients will lack permanent upper lateral incisors. Except for lesions in the oropharyngeal cavity, alterations of the digestive tract are uncommon and reported only as autopsy findings in a few patients. The respiratory tract may be involved by infiltration of the vocal cords and obstruction.

A bilateral intracranial sickle-shaped sub-cellar calcification has been observed in 50 percent of the patients but not all of them present with epilepsy or any other signs of cerebral dysfunction. Abnormalities of the peripheral nervous system are uncommon; four South African patients had peripheral nervous system lesions that may have been due to congenital analgesia.

Infiltration of the eyelids induces malfunction of the eyelashes, causing corneal ulceration. Alopecia of the eyelashes and eyebrows is observed. Focal degeneration of the macula has been found in a third of the examined patients.

Cardiac, endocrine, and urogenital disorders have been seen but are not clearly a part of the spectrum of this disease.

Deposition of hyaline material around the blood vessels is seen by microscopy to be present in internal organs. It indicates that the defect is a generalized disease. These changes appear to be asymptomatic.

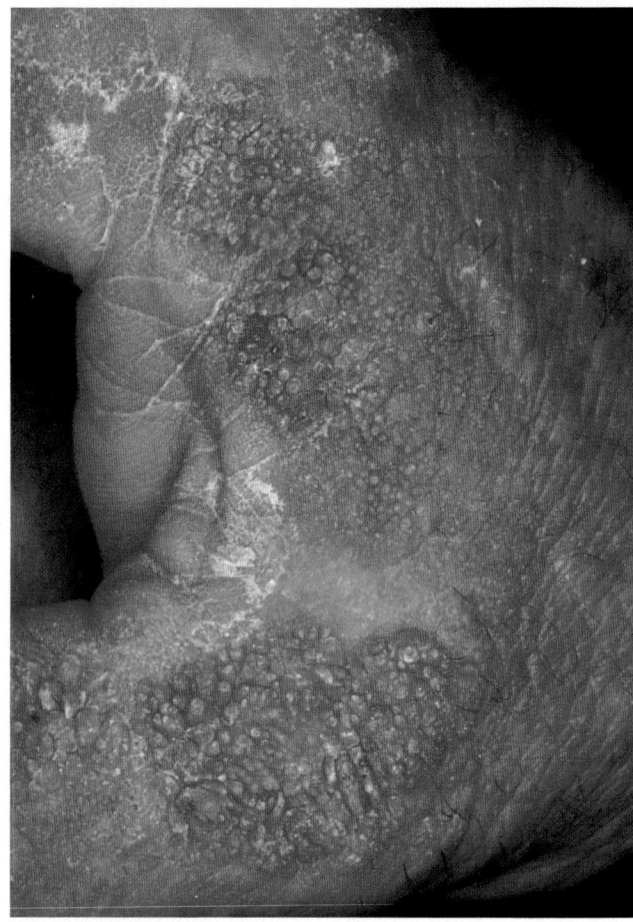

b

FIGURE 154-3 Hyperkeratotic papular lesions on dorsum of hands (*a*), interdigital web, and the sides of the fingers (*b*) in lipoid proteinosis.

Clinical Course and Prognosis

Except for the risk of respiratory obstruction in infancy, the disease is compatible with a normal life span. Lesions of the upper respiratory tract may cause problems in patients with tracheotomy or disease of the trachea. Quality of life is seriously impaired by the disfiguring lesions and the permanent hoarseness.

Laboratory Findings

No laboratory finding is typical of lipoid proteinosis. In some patients, abnormal glucose metabolism has been reported. Porphyrins, liver function, protein electrophoresis, lipids, and lipoproteins are normal in the classic form of the disease. There may be signs of

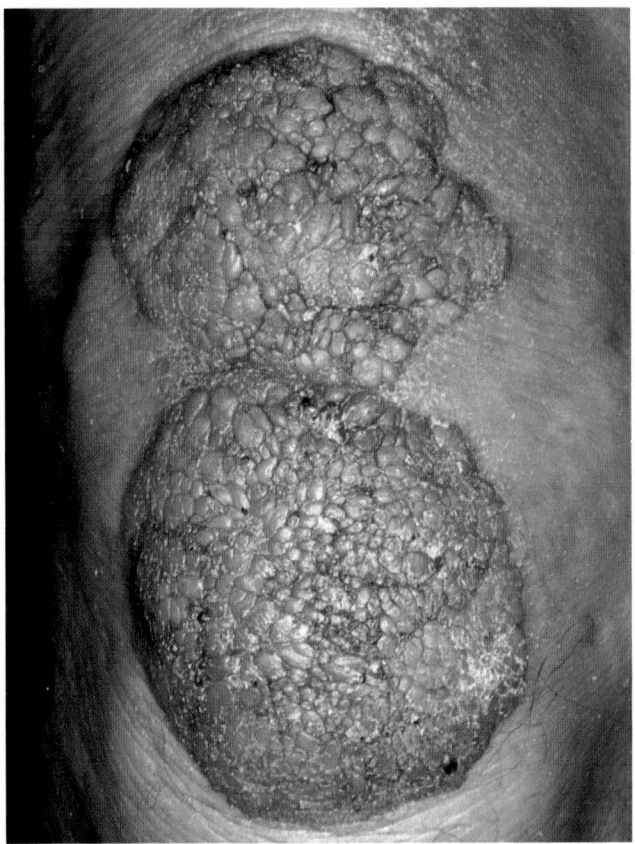

FIGURE 154-4   Verrucous nodular lesion on the knee in lipoid proteinosis.

chronic or acute inflammation (increased alpha$_2$ or gamma globulins). Elevated serum calcium has been reported rarely.

Differential Diagnosis

Lipoid proteinosis has to be differentiated from other diseases related to the deposition of amorphous material in the dermis. The differential diagnosis applies at both clinical and histopathologic levels.

Porphyria, mainly erythropoietic protoporphyria, shows deposition of a PAS-positive material around the blood vessels, mainly in sun-exposed areas. Light sensitivity is not a feature of lipoid proteinosis, and the observation of lesions in nonexposed sites aids the diagnosis. The site of the biopsy should be provided to the pathologist for differential diagnosis.

Lipid deposition in the various forms of xanthomatosis is rarely a problem of differential diagnosis. Furthermore, xanthoma cells never occur in lipoid proteinosis.

Amyloidosis may resemble lipoid proteinosis. Its development is often more progressive and accompanied by involvement of the kidneys, heart, etc. Amyloid deposition may occur in the skin of lipoid proteinosis patients. The clinical presentation of diabetic microangiopathy is often different from that of lipoid proteinosis but the pathologic picture may be confusing.

A recent report of acquired hyalinosis cutis et mucosae in a patient with monoclonal immunoglobulinopathy requires attention.[3] This form of the syndrome can be differentiated by immunoelectrophoresis of the plasma proteins.

Morphologic Findings

The main manifestations of the disease are related to the deposition of an amorphous or laminated material in the connective tissues. The location and the immunohistochemical nature of the deposit support its relation to components of the basement membrane zone. It displays a PAS-positive reaction that resists digestion by enzymes and contains collagen type IV and laminin. The deposition of this material is progressive and often located next to cells that are known to synthesize a basement membrane.[4]

Little is known about the initial stage of the disease. Most often biopsy specimens are collected from obvious lesions and show deposition of the amorphous eosinophilic material initially around walls of the small and medium size blood vessels in the papillary dermis, which shows a pronounced "onion-skin" proliferation of the adventitia. The hyaline material is also found around the smooth muscle cells of the arrectores pilorum and ultimately involves the surrounding dermis of the sweat glands. The myoepithelial cells may also be involved in the development of these lesions. The amount of amorphous material increases with time to progressively encase the adnexae, filling up the dermis and pushing aside most of the normal collagen bundles (Fig. 154-5).

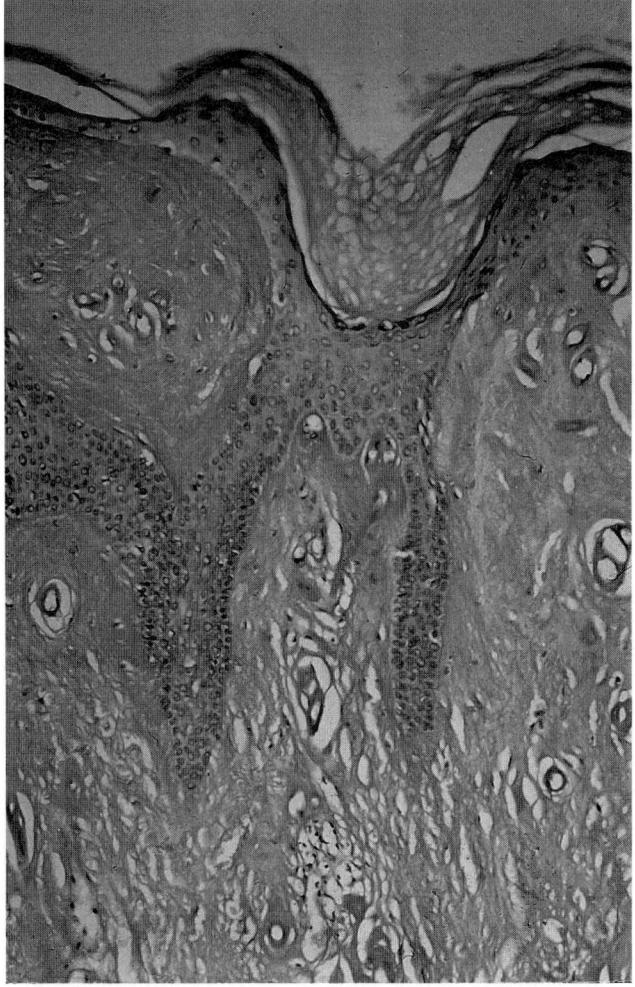

FIGURE 154-5   Extensive deposition of a PAS-positive material in the papillary dermis of a pitted acne scar lesion in lipoid proteinosis.

By electron microscopy, the deposit appears to be composed of small granules and short filaments of low electron density, 3 to 5 nm in diameter. Electron-dense bodies (mineralized) are located around the sweat glands.

The deposit in lipoid proteinosis is mainly composed of non-collagen protein, although the concentric layers of basement membrane-like material contain collagen types III and IV and laminin, as shown by immuno-detection. A portion of this material, solubilized by reduction and injected to produce antibodies in rabbits, induced antibodies that recognize antigens also detectable in normal skin.[5] This indicates that the disease might be related to the overproduction and/or the lack of degradation of a normal component of the human skin.

The lipid nature of the deposit remains controversial. Solubilization in various solvents gave nonreproducible information. It stains with lipophilic agents, suggesting that unsaturated hydrophobic lipids might be present.

The pathogenesis of the disease is still uncertain. Observations by Bauer et al.[6] of accumulations of cytoplasmic inclusions and vacuoles in culture of cells derived from lipoid proteinosis-afflicted skin suggest that the defect might be a storage disease. This intracellular material is rich in hexuronic acids and is sulphated. It has a lower than normal degradation rate, suggesting defective hydrolytic activity, as found in some mucolipidoses. In vitro, the fibroblasts collected from the affected skin also display an increased biosynthetic activity for collagen type IV (basement membrane collagen) and laminin.[7]

Therapy

There is presently no effective therapy. Topical corticosteroids have been extensively used with beneficial effect.

Plastic surgery to remove lesions has been used in some patients. Dermabrasion has also been used. The use of these therapies is questionable because trauma has seemed to increase deposition of the pathologic material. Some beneficial effect has, however, been reported.

Recently, treatment by oral dimethyl sulfoxide has been claimed to be successful.[8]

References

1. Hofer PA: Urbach-Wiethe disease (lipoglucoproteinosis: lipoid proteinosis; hyalinosis cutis et mucosae). A review. *Acta Dermatol Venereol (Stockh)* **53**(71): 1973
2. Urbach E, Wiethe C: Lipoidosis cutis et mucosae. *Virchows Arch Path Anat* **273**:285, 1929
3. Von der Helm D et al: Acquired hyalinosis cutis et mucosae in plasmacytoma with monoclonal IgG-lambda gammapathy. *Hautarzt* **40**(3):153, 1989
4. Pierard GE et al: A clinicopathologic study of six cases of lipoid proteinosis. *Am J Dermatopathol* **10**(4):300, 1989
5. Fleischmajer R et al: Ultrastructure and composition of connective tissue in hyalinosis cutis et mucosae skin. *J Invest Dermatol* **82**:252, 1984
6. Bauer EA et al: Lipoid proteinosis: In vivo and in vitro evidence for a lysosomal storage disease. *J Invest Dermatol* **76**:119, 1981
7. Olsen DR et al: Expression of basement membrane zone genes coding for type IV procollagen and laminin by human skin fibroblasts in vitro: Elevated alpha I (IV) collagen mRNA levels in lipoid proteinosis. *J Invest Dermatol* **90**:734, 1988
8. Wong CK, Lin CS: Remarkable response of lipoid proteinosis to oral dimethyl sulfoxide. *Br J Dermatol* **119**:541, 1988

<hr>

CHAPTER 155

Sophia N. Kotliar and Sanford I. Roth

Cutaneous Mineralization and Ossification

Mineralization (calcification)* in biology is defined as the deposition of insoluble crystalline or amorphous salts in tissue. In the context of this chapter, it will be used to define the condition where salts are deposited in the absence of bone formation. Ossification is the formation of true bone tissue, either mineralized or non-mineralized. Cutaneous mineralization and ossification occur as primary or secondary phenomena. Primary (idiopathic) mineralization and ossification occur without preceding local or systemic alterations. Secondary mineralization may result from local or systemic changes in calcium or phosphorus metabolism, whereas

Mineralization is a universal term, whereas the more commonly applied term is *calcification*. As both a cation, usually calcium, and an anion, typically phosphate or carbonate, are deposited, many use the terms interchangeably. Because we feel that the general term is more correct, we will use *mineralization* exclusively.

secondary ossification is almost always associated with local abnormalities in the skin or a preexisting secondary mineralization. When secondary mineralization or ossification occur as a result of a systemic abnormality of metabolism, it is often accompanied by similar findings in other organs. The term *ectopic* is redundant, as by definition deposition of mineral or bone within the skin is a localization "away from the normal site." The adjective *dystrophy* is used when the mineralization is associated with local phenomena, whereas *metastatic* refers to an association with systemic abnormalities. Primary mineralization is rare when compared to the incidence of primary ossification. Both primary mineralization and ossification are less frequent than their secondary counterparts.

In this chapter we will outline the physiology of ossification and mineralization and discuss some of the specific lesions associated with secondary mineralization and/or ossification. Mineralization that occurs in the context of abnormalities of anion metabolism (other than carbonate and phosphate), such as gout, is discussed in Chap. 151.

Bone Formation

Normal bone formation is a highly regulated process that begins with the deposition of an organized collagen matrix by specialized mesenchymal cells, the osteoblasts.[1] The osteoblasts are derived from undifferentiated mesenchymal cells, referred to as osteoprogenitor cells. In the embryo, ossification begins either de novo, in fibrous connective tissue (membrane bone), or by replacement of a preformed, cartilaginous anlage (enchondral bone). In children, bone growth proceeds by the formation of new membranous bone around the diaphysial bone of the primary center of ossification, or by replacement of the cartilage anlage at the epiphysial growth plate. In adults, bone remodeling occurs by osteoclastic resorption of old bone and replacement with new bone. The organization of the bone matrix depends largely upon the rate of bone formation. Rapidly forming bone lays down a meshwork or feltlike pattern of collagen fibers (woven bone), whereas more slowly forming bone lays down parallel lamellae of collagen fibers (lamellar bone). The cortex of tubular bones is composed of compact sheets of lamellar bone. Medullary bone (trabecular bone) is composed of trabeculae of lamellar bone. During the deposition of the bone matrix, the osteoblasts become trapped within the matrix and further mature to the terminally differentiated osteocytes. Bone remodeling is continuous throughout life. Compact lamellar bone is remodeled by osteoclastic resorption, with tunneling of vascular-filled cavities (Haversian canals). Concentric lamellae of new bone fill these cavities forming the Haversian systems.

Collagenous proteins account for 85 to 90 percent of the total protein in the organic matrix of bone, whereas the remaining 10 to 15 percent of the proteins are noncollagenous.[2] More than 200 different proteins have been identified in bone, and although many are identical to serum proteins, several are unique to bone. The exact role of these proteins is currently the subject of intense research, but already over 60 have been shown to affect bone formation, growth, or resorption. The collagen matrix of bone and skin are very similar, both consisting of a mixture of primarily type I collagen, lesser amounts of type III collagen, and still smaller amounts of type V collagen. All of these molecules are composed of triple helices organized in very similar structures. In skin, type III collagen fibers form a surface layer over the more common type I collagen fibers.

The tropocollagen of type I is encoded by two genes, $\alpha1(I)$ (COL1A1) and $\alpha2(I)$ (COL1A2). Type I tropocollagen is composed of three polypeptides, two of one type and one of a second type, in 2:1 ratio $[\alpha1(I)]_2\alpha2(I)$. Each polypeptide chain is approximately 1000 amino acids long. The central portion is an alpha helix and contains 338 contiguous repeating triplet sequences. Three molecules fold together in the central area to form a triple helical structure with short terminal nonhelical segments (forming a total molecular length of approximately 300 nm). The structure for the type I fiber, as first deduced by Hodge and Petruska,[3] is a linear array of triple helical tropocollagen with a quarter-length lateral stagger, which allows for overlap regions and gap, or "hole," regions. A detailed review of the collagens is beyond the scope of this chapter, but one has recently been published by van der Rest and Garrone.[4] As well, the subject is treated in Chap. 21 of this book.

Glimcher[5,6] has recently presented a detailed analysis of the mineralization of bone, which we have summarized. Prior to depo-

sition of mineral in bone, the collagen fibers have a characteristic histologic appearance, known as *osteoid* (nonmineralized bone). The differences in the type I collagen of bone and other tissues are probably related to posttranslational modifications of the type I collagen, as well as to interactions with other collagenous and noncollagenous molecules. Phosphorylation of the collagen and the interaction with phosphoproteins may also play a key role in the initiation of mineralization in bone. It is clear that this process in normal bone is closely regulated and requires cells, the osteoblasts and osteocytes.

Mineralization of bone is dependent on a number of intra- and extracellular factors, including pH, hormones (parathyroid, estrogens, etc.), vitamins (D), paracrine factors, and local ion concentrations. Osteoblasts are also required. Shortly after bone formation begins, mineralization is initiated with the deposition of mineral salts either in or near the gap regions of the collagen fibers. There is much dispute over the exact nature of the initial deposits.[7,8] Whether crystal formation is preceded by deposition of amorphous calcium phosphate is still open to dispute. Glimcher[5] has proposed that the initial solid deposits in bone are poorly crystalline type B (carbonate) apatite, with ~5 percent carbonate and 5 to 10 percent phosphate. However, shortly after the initial deposits, identifiable hydroxyapatite crystals are recognizable. Although it may be artifact, it is apparent that the earliest ultrastructurally recognized mineral forms are crystals. The mineral crystals of bone are the smallest crystals recognizable in biology. By transmission electron microscopy, they appear as tablets of book-shaped crystals having a mean maximum dimension of about 5 to 10 nm × 40 to 50 nm × 1.5 to 3.5 nm.

The initial phases of mineralization in lamellar bone are relatively rapid, with 65 to 75 percent occurring within days; full mineralization of lamellar bone may require weeks to months. In fully mineralized lamellar bone the hydroxyapatite is deposited within and on the surface of the collagen fibers. In fully mineralized woven bone, in addition to crystals within the collagen fibers, hydroxyapatite is present in clusters without apparent association with the collagen fibers.

Calcium and phosphate ions exist in the extracellular fluid and serum in a metastable concentration, that is, their concentrations exceed the solubility product constant. The mechanisms for maintaining the metastable state are not entirely clear, but under normal conditions in most tissues the phase transformation to the solid state does not occur. The calcium ions are known to be complexed with albumin and other compounds in both serum and extracellular spaces. In the mineralizing tissues (bone, dentin, enamel), the posttranslationally modified proteins may serve as a nidus for precipitation of the salts. We know that reconstituted collagen from any source under the proper conditions may mineralize in vitro, even in the absence of cells. However, in tissue, cells (osteoblasts) are necessary for mineralization. Ions such as pyrophosphate, phosphorylation of the collagen, proteoglycans, other substances produced by the osteoblasts, and local pH may also play a role in the control of this process.

Though there are posttranslational differences in the type I collagen from bone and other tissues such as skin, there is no full understanding as to why one mineralizes and the other does not under normal circumstances.[5] It has been shown that activation and regulation of the type I collagen genes are coordinated. Both genes are active in numerous tissues, and are nonhousekeeping single-copy genes. Numerous recent studies have indicated differences in the regulation of these genes between osteoblasts and fibroblasts. Some of these differences include a higher rate of basal collagen synthesis in the osteoblasts; production of almost exclusively type I collagen in osteoblasts; and regulation of collagen synthesis by vitamin D, parathyroid hormone, insulin, and other hormones in osteoblasts but not in fibroblasts. Pavlin et al.[9] recently demonstrated a differential response to the internal regulatory sequences in the COL1A1 gene between osteoblasts and fibroblasts. Their studies suggest that in the 5' flanking promotor there is a sequence that is preferentially active in osteoblastic cells.

In woven bone and cartilage, initiation occurs within so-called matrix vesicles that form by budding from chondrocyte and osteoblast cell surface membranes,[10,11] although some controversy still exists as to the exact relationship of the matrix vesicles and collagen fibers in bone. The matrix vesicles present a sequestered microenvironment where calcium ions are concentrated by the calcium affinity of acidic phospholipids, and inorganic phosphate accumulates as a result of membrane-bound phosphatases. Once these matrix vesicles form mineral, further mineralization proceeds. Ectopic crystals and those formed in matrix vesicles are needle-shaped, and the accumulation of crystals is in a disordered starburst pattern. Some workers claim that the matrix vesicles serve as a transport mechanism for the bone crystals from the initiation site to the collagen fibers.[10,11]

Extraosseous Ossification

Bone formation was induced experimentally by the insertion of urinary bladder epithelium in the fascial sheath of the rectus muscle by Huggins.[12] Subsequently, other types of epithelial cells have been shown to be capable of inducing extraosseous ossification. Later studies have demonstrated that acellular, defatted bone and tooth matrix were capable of inducing cartilage and enchondral bone formation. Subsequent to these initial observations, other workers discovered that bone morphogenic proteins (BMPs) were responsible for these phenomena.[13,14] The BMPs are polypeptides (BMP-1, BMP-2A, BMP-2B, and BMP-3 having been most extensively studied) that induce cartilage formation and, in some cases, subsequent enchondral bone formation (BMP-2A) when injected into the soft tissues or skin. BMP-2A and BMP-3 are members of the transforming growth factor β supergene family.[14,15] The role of these polypeptides in normal bone formation is as yet unproven, although Tabas et al.[15] have demonstrated chromosomal association with human and rat disorders of bone formation.

Cutaneous Ossification

Cutaneous ossification is relatively rare in normal dermatopathology practice. Burgdorf and Nasemann[16] found cutaneous ossification in only 35 cases out of 20,000 consecutive biopsies (0.175 percent). Out of the 467 cases of cutaneous ossification reported and reviewed by Roth et al.,[17] there were 59 (12.6 percent) in which no preexisting lesion could be identified (Table 155-1). These cases were classified as primary cutaneous ossification. The remainder were secondary lesions associated with preexisting neoplasia, with neoplastic-like lesions (197, 42.2 percent), or with nonneoplastic lesions (211, 45.2 percent). In neither primary nor secondary ossification is the etiology or pathogenesis clear. Localized lesions of primary cutaneous ossification are often referred to as "osteoma cutis."

TABLE 155-1

Previously Reported Cases of Secondary Ossification Associated with Neoplasms

	Roth *et al.*[17]* No (%)	Burgdorf & Nasemann[16] No (%)
Nevi		
Without inflammation	29 (17)	3 (14)
With inflammation	6 (4)	
Basal cell carcinoma	10 (6)	2 (10)
Chondroid syringoma	13 (8)	
Pilomatrixoma†	98 (59)	7 (33)
Miscellaneous tumors		
Hemangioma	3 (2)	
Dermatofibroma	1(0.6)	
Extra-abdominal desmoid	1(0.6)	
Neurilemmoma	1(0.6)	
Chondroma	1(0.6)	
Senile keratosis	1(0.6)	
Epidermal cyst	2 (1)	2 (10)
Pilar cyst		3 (14)
Trichoepithelioma	1(0.6)	
Fibrohistiocytic lesions		4 (19)
Atypical fibroxanthoma‡(32)		
Neurofibroma‡(33)		
Malignant melanoma‡(34,35)		
Total Cases	167(100)	21(100)
No demonstrable associated or preexisting lesion ("Primary cutaneous ossification")	59	10

*Including cases from the literature.

†It should be noted that in the series by Roth et al.,[17] the number of pilomatrixomas previously reported should have been 94, plus 4 unreported tumors making a total of 98.

‡Cases reported subsequent to the previous two series.

Primary Ossification (Osteoma Cutis)   Lever and Schaumburg-Lever[18] classified primary ossification into four groups: (1) widespread osteomas present since birth or early life without Albright's hereditary osteodystrophy; (2) single, large, plaquelike osteomas present since birth; (3) single small osteomas arising in later life and in various locations, with or without epidermal elimination (we have separated these latter two groups); and (4) multiple miliary osteomas of the face in women.

Neonatal, Tumorlike, Multiple, Widespread Osteomas with or without Myositis Ossificans   Involvement of both males and females has been reported.[19–21] In one case[19] of a 33-year-old woman and her 7-year-old daughter, the mother had a localized lesion of the foot and the daughter had multiple lesions over the face. The histopathology showed cancellous lamellar bone, at different depths in the dermis and subcutaneous tissue, extending into the fascia in one case. In another case,[21] the patient subsequently developed myositis ossificans.

Neonatal, Plaquelike, Single Osteomas   The first case of this condition was described in 1892 by Sherwell[22] and in 1894 by Coleman[23] as cited by Combes and Vanina.[24] In the series reported by Roth et al.,[17] there were four cases of this syndrome. The patients ranged in age from 15 months to 5 years. Combes and Vanina[24] reported a case that began in the neonatal period. Burgdorf and Nasemann's series also includes a case.[16] The bone consisted of a plate of cancellous, membranous, woven, and lamellar bone at the dermal-subcutaneous junction. The bony spicules extended into both the dermis and subcutaneous tissue. In the latter case they followed the fibrous septa of the adipose tissue. In the dermis the spicules surrounded the dermal appendages, without apparent deformation of these structures. The bone was largely limited to the lower third of the dermis and resembled that seen in armadillo skin. Osteoblasts and osteocytes appeared normal. Foci of osteoclastic resorption with Howship's lacunae were seen along the bony spicules. Fatty and hemopoietic marrow were present. Subsequently, similar cases have been reported with the ossification extending into the muscle fascia but not into the muscle itself. In all of the reported cases, all aspects of calcium metabolism that were studied have been normal. In all forms of primary ossification, the appendages are spared, and the bone surrounds them.

Late Onset, Single Osteomas with Epidermal Elimination

Duperrat and Vanbremeersch[25] were the first to describe this condition, and a subsequent case has been reported by Delacrétaz and Koenig.[26] The bone is in the upper portion of the reticular and papillary dermis, often adjacent to the epidermis. There is overlying ulceration and crust.

Late Onset, Single Osteomas without Epidermal Elimination

In the series by Roth et al.,[17] 21 of 120 (17.5 percent) cases fell into this group. There were no identifiable other preexisting or associated lesions. The ossification was generally localized to the dermis and occasionally had an overlying area of ulceration (Fig. 155-1). The plaques of bone were most frequently on the scalp or extremities. The bone was woven or lamellar, membranous without cartilage, with focal areas of rimming osteoblasts (including osteoclasts), and marrow, either fatty or hemopoietic. Additional cases were described by Burgdorf and Nasemann,[16] and Vončina.[27]

Late Onset, Multiple Miliary Osteomas of the Face and Scalp

This condition consists of multiple small 0.1- to 0.4-cm papular

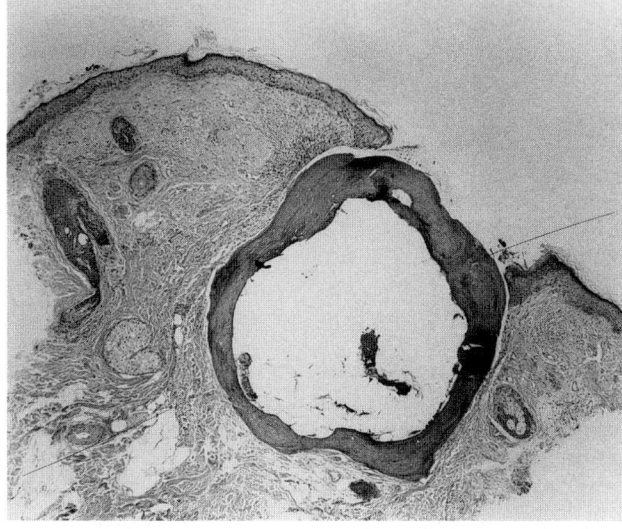

FIGURE 155-1 Solitary osteoma cutis. The lamellar bone exhibits a central marrow space that is occupied primarily with fat. There is an overlying ulceration. The adjacent skin and subcutaneous tissue are within normal limits. ×34.

lesions over the face, from the scalp line to the chin. It was first mentioned in the literature by Wilckens in 1858, and subsequently by Virchow in 1864, as cited by Hopkins[28] in his report of a similar case in 1928. The specimens reported by Wilckens and Virchow both consisted of multiple small spherules of bone without overlying skin. The bone consisted of compact lamellar bone with Haversian systems and a marrow cavity. All of the patients so far described have been adult women.[18,29,30] Although most have had accompanying acne or acneform lesions for long periods, the case reported by Helm et al.[31] was in a 67-year-old woman who had no previous acneform lesions. In the latter case, true hemopoietic marrow was also found.

Secondary Cutaneous Ossification

Cutaneous ossification occurs in association with a wide variety of conditions, including neoplasms, inflammatory processes, scarring, metabolic conditions, and preexisting cutaneous mineralization. Both membranous bone formation and enchondral ossification are seen: some lesions contain only one form and others contain both types. In the literature, the disease is somewhat more frequent in women than men.

Neoplasms   The most common cutaneous neoplasm with ossification is the pilomatrixoma (calcifying epithelioma of Malherbe). When reviewing the cases at the Armed Forces Institute of Pathology, Roth et al.[17] found that 42 of 162 cases of neoplasms with ossification were pilomatrixomas, and 94 (including 38 of the 42 AFIP cases) of 315 cases in the literature were pilomatrixomas (Table 155-1). The mineralization and ossification are an integral part of this tumor. Approximately 15 to 20 percent of the tumors show ossification, and 75 percent show mineralization. The mineralization is usually intracellular, with the calcium salts deposited within the cytoplasm of the ghost cells. It may be visible as hematoxylin-stained granules on ordinary stains or made more apparent by staining with the von Kossa stain. Some tumors contain large areas of amorphous calcium salts, replacing the tumor cells. Areas of mineralization may be seen in the connective tissue adjacent to viable tumor cells, although it is not clear whether or not these represent areas where the tumor cells have been replaced. A foreign-body giant cell reaction can be seen in the region of the mineralization. The pathogenesis of the mineralization in association with this tumor is not clear.

When ossification is present in a pilomatrixoma, it occurs within the connective tissue adjacent to the dermis. The bone occurs as spicules of woven or lamellar cancellous bone. Although there are osteocytes present, surface osteoblasts are not common. Fatty or, rarely, hemopoietic marrow may be present, though uncommon.

Ossification is associated with a wide variety of other neoplasms (Table 155-1). In the vast majority of these tumors, the ossification is in the connective tissue adjacent to the tumors. It is rarely associated with necrosis or ossification of the tumor itself. The bone varies from small, highly calcified spherules of lamellar bone to spicules and sheets of lamellar and woven bone. Central areas of fatty and hemopoietic marrow are seen within the spherules or spicules. The amount of surrounding osteoblastic activity is highly variable. Osteocytes are characteristic of the type of bone (lamellar or woven). Osteoclasts and Howship's lacunae are occasionally present.

TABLE 155-2
Previously Reported Cases of Secondary Ossification Associated with Nonneoplastic Conditions

	Roth et al.[17] No. (%)	Burgdorf & Nasemann[16] No. (%)
Cicatrices		
Abdominal	93 (44)	
Extraabdominal	2 (1)	
Suspected	7 (3)	
Chronic venous insufficiency	71 (33)	
Inflammatory Conditions		
Trauma	18 (8.4)	2 (50)
Pyogenic granuloma	1 (0.5)	1 (25)
Injection site	1 (0.5)	
Folliculitis	1 (0.5)	
Callus	1 (0.5)	
Scleroderma	1 (0.5)	
Dermatomyositis	1 (0.5)	
Calcinosis cutis	3 (1)	
Sebaceous gland hyperplasia		1 (25)
Miscellaneous or undetermined(36)	13 (6)	
Molluscum contagiosum*(37)		
Morphea, linear*(38,39)		
Total Cases	213 (100)	4 (100)

*Cases reported subsequent to the previous two series.

Nonneoplastic Conditions   Many nonneoplastic conditions (Table 155-2) are associated with cutaneous ossification (Fig. 155-2). The histology of the bone in these conditions is essentially identical to that secondary to neoplasms. The etiology and pathogenesis of the process is still not clear.

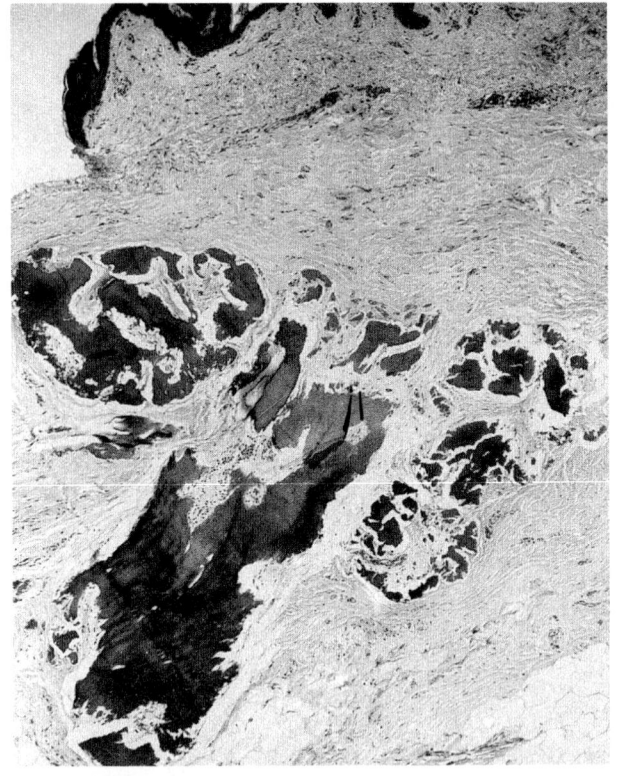

FIGURE 155-2 Ossification in a cutaneous scar. ×55.

Pseudohypoparathyroidism (Albright's Hereditary Osteodystrophy) and Pseudopseudohypoparathyroidism   Pseudohypoparathyroidism is a group of hereditary diseases in which the patients have the metabolic signs of hypoparathyroidism, hypocalcemia, and hyperphosphatemia but are unresponsive to parathyroid hormone. It is thought to be due to defects either in the parathyroid hormone receptor and/or in the postreceptor cascade of the kidneys and the bone. The patients have a characteristic appearance: round facies, short stature, brachydactyly, and other abnormalities of bone structure. Pseudopseudohypoparathyroidism is a disease in which the patients have an appearance and bony abnormalities similar to those with pseudohypoparathyroidism, except that their calcium metabolism is normal. The mode of inheritance of these diseases is not clear, although it is thought to be X-linked. The structural defects and the metabolic defects are separately inherited, as pseudohypoparathyroidism and pseudopseudohypoparathyroidism may be seen in the same family. In addition to ectopic mineralization, including cutaneous mineralization, the patients have foci of cutaneous ossification. Though ectopic mineralization is seen in true hypoparathyroidism, true ossification is rarely seen. Ectopic bone is rarely seen in pseudopseudohypoparathyroidism.

The histopathology of the cutaneous bone reveals spicules of woven and lamellar bone in the deep dermis and subcutaneous tissue. Osteoblasts, osteocytes, and osteoclasts are present. The spicules may partially or completely surround areas of fatty and, rarely, hemopoietic marrow.

Cutaneous Mineralization

Extraosseous mineralization occurs secondarily to local alterations in the tissue, such as necrosis of the collagen or abnormalities of the elastic tissue (dystrophic). Systemic alterations in calcium and phosphorus metabolism may also result in extraosseous depositions of mineral in various sites, including the skin and subcutaneous tissues (metastatic). Pathologic mineralization is characterized by abnormal deposits of calcium salts with small amounts of other mineral salts, including iron and magnesium salts, at sites not normally mineralized. It differs from ossification in that the mineral salts are not organized by osteoblasts. It occurs as a two-stage process, involving initiation of a calcium phosphate nidus and proceeding through crystal propagation. Initiation of mineralization in metastatic and dystrophic mineralization is somewhat different from that seen in bone.

The pathogenesis of cutaneous mineralization has not been entirely elucidated. However, the most commonly accepted theory is based on experimental studies on calciphylaxis by Selye et al.[40] In their experimental studies, sensitization of the tissue occurs by exposure to parathyroid hormone and is followed by exposure to a microenvironment having an elevated calcium-phosphate product (in the range of 70 mg/dL or higher) thereby causing precipitation.[40] Similar findings have been proposed for cutaneous mineralization, though the sensitizing agent may be different.

In metastatic and dystrophic mineralization, the mitochondria serve as the initiating vesicles. Mitochondria possess a great affinity for calcium and inorganic phosphate and thus have the ability to concentrate calcium and phosphate to the concentration required for mineral formation. However, under normal physiologic conditions, mitochondrial mineralization is amorphous and temporary and serves as an intracellular repository for calcium when there are transient physiologic increases in cytosolic calcium levels. If excessive cytosolic levels of calcium are attained, secondary to very high extracellular calcium levels or due to failure of the cell membrane calcium pumps, the intracellular concentrations of calcium and phosphate exceed the solubility product. The mitochondrial sequestration of calcium phosphate continues until mitochondrial respiration is impeded, the cell pH falls, and cell death ensues. The first mineral formed within the mitochondria is probably amorphous and exhibits little or no crystallinity by x-ray diffraction studies. However, it is rapidly converted to crystalline hydroxyapatite. Once initiation occurs, mineralization propagates. Crystal formation is dependent on many factors, including calcium and phosphate concentrations in the extracellular and intracellular fluid, the presence of mineral inhibitors [such as pyrophosphate, adenosine triphosphate (ATP), and anionic proteins], collagen, and pH. Mineralization and crystal deposition are thus not only a sign of cell death; they may be the cause of cell death and organ dysfunction in calcific disease.[41] Induction of abnormal mineralization may occur as a result of a systemic process having elevated concentrations of calcium and/or of inorganic phosphate.

Mineralization may also occur as a result of a local phenomenon in which tissue damage and necrosis occur, producing a series of events not well understood. Some investigators suggest that dystrophic mineralization occurs secondarily to cell membrane damage causing calcium influx and mitochondrial mineral formation. However, others suggest that the process is entirely extracellular and that decreases in pH and loss of inhibitors (as occur in tissue necrosis) may be the initiating events in the precipitation of calcium and phosphorus. Ultrastructurally, nucleation of mineralization in many cases appears to be related to collagen and elastic fibers.[42,43]

Histologically, end stages of metastatic and dystrophic mineralization have similar appearances: the amorphous calcium salt deposits stain deep blue with hematoxylin and eosin and black with the von Kossa stain. The calcium may be present as fine granules or large deposits. The large deposits tend to evoke a foreign-body giant cell reaction.

Metastatic Mineralization

Metastatic mineralization is associated with increased concentrations of calcium and/or inorganic phosphate. It is usually a generalized phenomenon occurring throughout the body but it primarily affects the interstitial tissue of the blood vessels, kidney, lungs, and gastric mucosa. The skin is occasionally involved. Although metastatic mineralization is more common in the deep organs, this discussion will be limited to cutaneous mineralization. A wide variety of conditions may cause metastatic mineralization, including primary hyperparathyroidism, secondary hyperparathyroidism associated with renal failure, solid neoplasms, hematologic malignancies, vitamin D intoxication, sarcoid and other granulomatous diseases, idiopathic hypercalcemia of infancy, milk-alkali syndrome, and tumoral calcinosis. Although metastatic mineralization occurs in a wide variety of conditions (Table 155-3), only the more common will be discussed.

Renal Failure and Secondary Hyperparathyroidism   Renal failure is associated with decreased filtration of serum phosphorus and impaired renal production of 1,25(OH)$_2$ vitamin D. In the absence of 1,25(OH)$_2$ vitamin D, calcium absorption from the gastro-

intestinal tract is decreased, as is renal tubular reabsorption of calcium, leading to a depression of serum calcium. Hypocalcemia then results in elevated parathyroid hormone production and induces secondary hyperparathyroidism. The elevated parathyroid hormone causes skeletal resorption, mobilizing calcium and phosphorus. Thus, serum calcium levels tend to normalize. Phosphorus levels, however, remain markedly elevated. Since the solubility product may be exceeded because of elevations of either ion, mineralization of skin and subcutaneous tissue occur. The areas of mineralization are generally localized to the periarticular subcutaneous tissue. The size and number of these mineralized sites appear to correlate with the degree of hyperphosphatemia. The mineralization tends to disappear if phosphate levels are reduced by dialysis.

Another syndrome associated with chronic renal failure is systemic calciphylaxis of Selye.[40] This is a rare disease in which hyperphosphatemia and hyperparathyroidism are common findings but hypercalcemia is an inconstant finding. It is a process of abnormal calcium deposition in various organs that presents with two different pathologic pictures: (1) diffuse mineralization of the medial layer of the small and intermediate vessels with subsequent ischemia and necrosis of the skin of the distal extremities; and (2) soft tissue mineralization resulting from the deposition of calcium in the connective tissue of various organs, most commonly the lungs, kidneys, stomach, heart, and skin. Parathyroidectomy may be curative. However, some patients, despite all therapeutic intervention, develop gangrene.

Milk-Alkali Syndrome   Milk-alkali syndrome is due to an excessive ingestion of calcium and absorbable antacids, such as calcium carbonate, resulting in hypercalcemia, alkalosis, and renal failure. Phosphorus levels are normal. Acute manifestations are weakness, myalgia, irritability, and apathy. Chronic cases, referred to as Burnett's syndrome, present with severe hypercalcemia, irreversible renal failure, and phosphate retention, accompanied by ectopic mineralization: nephrocalcinosis, renal calculi, and subcutaneous mineralization that tends to occur around joints.

Vitamin D Intoxication   Vitamin D intoxication as a consequence to chronic ingestion of large doses of vitamin D (usually at least 50 to 100 times the normal physiologic requirement or doses in excess of 50,000 to 100,000 units/day) will produce hypercalcemia, and renal function may become impaired. Subcutaneous mineralization may also occur. However, it appears that some degree of hyperphosphatemia may be necessary to propagate mineralization. The mineralization occurs in periarticular tissue and joints.

Primary Hyperparathyroidism   Rare cases of primary hyperparathyroidism with cutaneous mineralization have been reported.

Malignancies   Metastatic mineralization has been described in patients with malignancies, especially lymphomas and carcinomas of the lung. Leukemia also has been associated with metastatic mineralization. It has been shown that many of these neoplasms produce a parathyroid hormone-like (or related) protein that produces hypercalcemia and hypophosphatemia. The hypercalcemias of lymphomas and leukemias, such as that associated with human T-cell leukemia virus 1 (HTLV-1) (almost universally associated with hypercalcemia), are felt to be the result of production of various lymphokines by the tumor cells.

Tumoral Calcinosis   Tumoral calcinosis, formerly classified as a dystrophic mineralization, has been reclassified as metastatic cal-

TABLE 155-3
Cutaneous Mineralization

I Dystrophic mineralization	**II** Metastatic mineralization
A Localized	**A** Hypercalcemia
1 Degenerative	**1** Destructive bone disease
a Parasitic infections[44]	**a** Metastatic carcinoma
b Hemiplegia[45]	**b** Lymphoma[78]
2 Inflammatory/trauma	**c** Multiple myeloma[79]
a Acne	**d** Leukemia[80]
b Foreign body granuloma	**e** Paget's disease
c Postinfection	**2** Milk-alkali syndrome[81]
(**1**) Herpes[46]	**3** Primary and secondary hyperparathyroidism[82,83]
(**2**) Cytomegalovirus[47]	**4** Sarcoid[84]
d Scars	**5** Vitamin D intoxication[85]
(**1**) Burns[48,49]	**6** Calciphylaxis of Selye[86–88]
(**2**) Trauma[50,51]	**7** Idiopathic hypercalcemia of infancy[89]
(**3**) Surgical	**B** Normocalcemic/hypocalcemic
(**4**) Post EEG[52,53]	**1** Hyperphosphatemic
(**5**) Neonatal heel sticks[54]	**a** Chronic renal failure and uremia[90–92]
e Keloid[55]	**b** Tumoral calcinosis[93–95]
f Hematoma	**c** Primary hypoparathyroidism
g Venous stasis ulcers	**d** Pseudohypoparathyroidism[96]
h Post calcium chloride, calcium gluconate extravasation[56,57]	**e** Rothmund-Thomson syndrome[97,98]
i Phlebitis[58,59]	**2** Normophophosphatemic
3 Neoplastic	**a** Primary hyperoxaluria[99]
a Benign	**III** Idiopathic mineralization
(**1**) Angioma	**A** Localized
(**2**) Pilomatrixoma[60]	**1** Idiopathic calcinosis of the penis[100]
(**3**) Epidermal cyst	**2** Subepidermal calcified nodule[101]
(**4**) Lipoma	**3** Idiopathic scrotal calcinosis[102–104]
(**5**) Syringoma[61]	**4** Idiopathic vulvar calcinosis[105]
b Malignant	**5** Mineralization of the breast[106,107]
(**1**) Basal cell carcinoma	**B** Generalized
(**2**) Sclerosing adnexal carcinoma, low grade (microcystic adnexal carcinoma)	**1** Pseudopseudohypoparathyroidism
(**3**) Liposarcoma	
B Generalized	
1 Acquired	
a Scleroderma/CREST syndrome[62–64]	
b Dermatomyositis[65,66]	
c Systemic lupus erythematosus[67–69]	
d Discoid lupus erythematosus[70]	
e Porphyria cutanea tarda[71–73]	
f Thibierge-Weissenbach syndrome[74]	
g Werner's syndrome	
h Subcutaneous fat necrosis of the newborn[75,76]	
2 Inheritable	
a Ehlers-Danlos syndrome	
b Pseudoxanthoma elasticum[77]	

cification. Calcium levels are normal; however, mild hyperphosphatemia is present. Patients are young, with a male predominance, and present with calcific masses periarticular to larger joints, primarily the hips and elbows. Urinary calcium excretion is decreased and urinary hydroxyproline is increased, possibly related to increased collagen breakdown.

Miscellaneous Conditions Various other conditions have been associated with metastatic cutaneous mineralization, including Paget's disease of bone, sarcoid, idiopathic hypercalcemia of infancy, pseudohypoparathyroidism, primary hypoparathyroidism, and Rothmund-Thomson syndrome. In these conditions either calcium or phosphate levels are elevated.

Dystrophic Mineralization

Dystrophic mineralization is the more common form of cutaneous mineralization and occurs as calcium salts are deposited in previ-

ously damaged or degenerating tissue. It tends to occur without evidence of systemic metabolic abnormalities, and calcium and inorganic phosphate ion concentrations in the extracellular fluid are normal. Dystrophic mineralization occurs secondarily to tissue injury (Fig. 155-3) and is classically associated with focal areas of devitalized tissue or tissue necrosis. This focal necrosis serves as the initiator of mineralization. Serum calcium and inorganic phosphate concentrations are normal in these processes. Multiple other systemic processes that have normal serum calcium and phosphate levels also produce dystrophic mineralization; however the mineralization is widespread throughout the body. Examples of conditions with dystrophic mineralization include trauma, chronic inflammation, and prolonged venous stasis. A wide variety of lesions may feature mineralization (Table 155-3), including benign and malignant tumors, either in the associated stroma or in necrotic or keratinized tumor cells. The ghost cells of pilomatrixoma are often the nidus for mineralization (Fig. 155-4). Other diseases associated with mineralization include Ehlers-Danlos syndrome, pseudoxan-

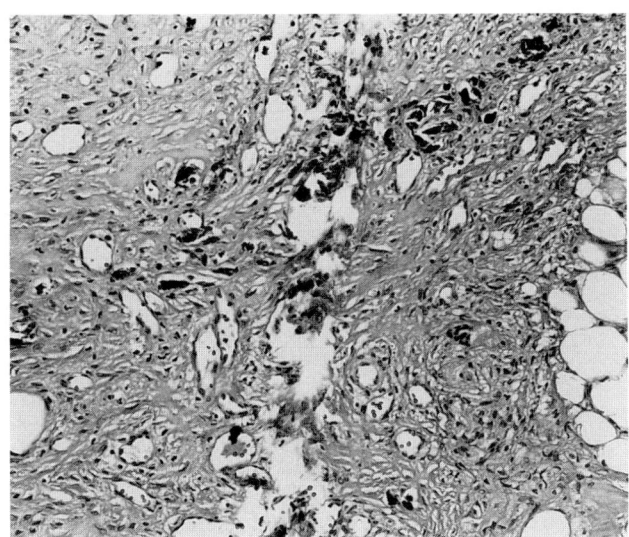

FIGURE 155-3 Mineralization of the deep dermis associated with an overlying wound. ×123.

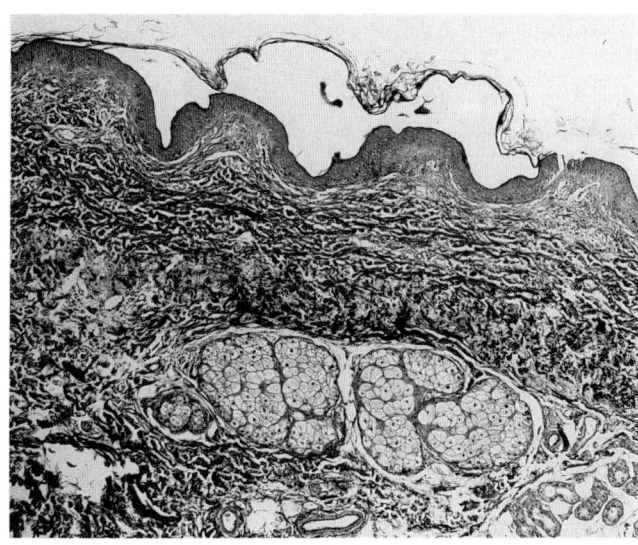

FIGURE 155-5 Pseudoxanthoma elasticum exhibits swollen and irregular elastic fibers staining faintly basophilic secondary to calcium imbibition. ×106.

thoma elasticum (Fig. 155-5), Werner's syndrome, porphyria cutanea tarda, scleroderma/CREST syndrome (Calcinosis cutis, Raynaud's phenomenon, Esophageal dysfunction, Sclerodactyly, and Telangiectasia), systemic lupus erythematosus, and dermatomyositis. The generalized dystrophic mineralization that occurs in these disorders may present as numerous large deposits of calcium (calcinosis universalis) or as a few localized deposits (calcinosis cir-

cumscripta). Calcinosis universalis occurs primarily in patients with dermatomyositis, but has been seen in patients with systemic scleroderma. The deposits of calcium salts are found in the skin and subcutaneous tissue and often in muscles and tendons. In dermatomyositis, these dystrophic nodules gradually resolve if the patient survives. Calcinosis circumscripta occurs over extensor surfaces such as the elbows in patients with systemic scleroderma.

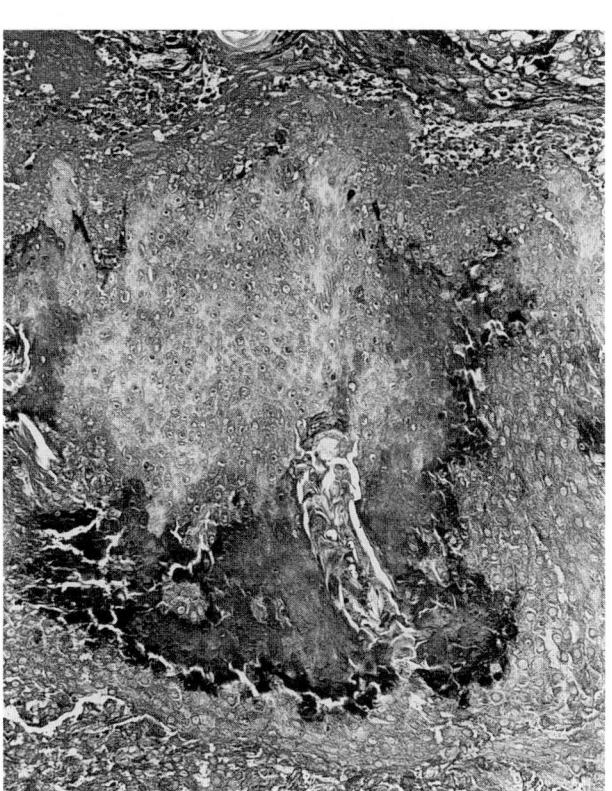

FIGURE 155-4 A pilomatrixoma exhibiting the characteristic appearance of ghost cells, basophilic cells, and areas of mineralization surrounding the tumor. ×160.

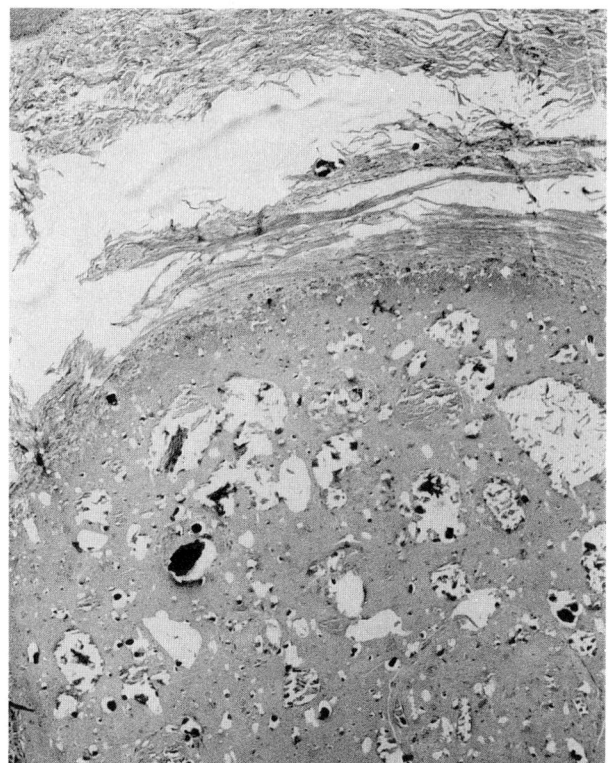

FIGURE 155-6 Idiopathic scrotal calcinosis exhibits a well-demarcated border with fairly homogeneous eosinophilic material with discrete areas of mineralization. ×55.

Primary (Idiopathic) Mineralization

A number of cutaneous sites have been reported to develop cutaneous mineralization. These cases have been reported to have normal calcium and phosphorus levels and do not have associated pathologic processes. In scrotal calcinosis, it has been suggested that the mineralization occurs in eccrine glands. However, this has not been clearly documented. The pathogenesis of mineralization of the dermis of the scrotum (Fig. 155-6), penis, vulva, and breast have not been elucidated to this date. A study of the dermal mineralization in superficial dystrophic calcification revealed a "flowerlike" arrangement of the apatite crystals around the collagen bundles.[42] The initial mineralization of the elastic fibers has been linked to the microfibrils, in contrast to the pseudoxanthoma elasticum where the central core of the elastic fiber is mineralized.[108]

References

1. Gurley AM, Roth SI: Bone, in *Histology for Pathologists*, edited by SS Sternberg. New York, Raven, 1992, p 61

2. Veis A, Sabsay B: The collagen of mineralized matrices, in *Bone and Mineral Research/5*, edited by WA Peck. Amsterdam, Elsevier, 1987, p 1

3. Hodge AJ, Petruska JA: Recent studies with the electron microscope on ordered aggregates of the tropocollagen molecule, in *Aspects of Protein Synthesis*, edited by GN Gamachandran. New York, Academic, 1963, p 289

4. van der Rest M, Garrone R: Collagen family of proteins. *FASEB J* **5**:2814, 1991

5. Glimcher MJ: Mechanism of calcification: Role of collagen fibrils and collagen-phosphoprotein complexes *in vitro* and *in vivo*. *Anat Rec* **224**:139, 1989

6. Glimcher MJ: The nature of the mineral component of bone and the mechanism of calcification, in *Disorders of Bone and Mineral Metabolism*, edited by FL Coe, MJ Favus. New York, Raven, 1992, p 265

7. Posner AS: Bone mineral and the mineralization process, in *Bone and Mineral Research/5*, edited by WA Peck. Amsterdam, Elsevier, 1987, p 65

8. Posner AS: The mineral of bone. *Clin Orthoped Rel Res* **200**:87, 1985

9. Pavlin D et al: Differential utilization of regulatory domains within the α1(I) collagen promoter in osseous and fibroblastic cells. *J Cell Biol* **116**:227, 1992

10. Anderson HC: Mechanism of mineral formation in bone, in *Pathology Reviews* edited by E Rubin, I Damjanov. Clifton, NJ, Humana, 1990, p 13

11. Marks SC Jr, Popoff SN: Bone cell biology: The regulation of development, structure, and function in the skeleton. *Am J Anat* **183**:1, 1988

12. Huggins CB: The formation of bone under the influence of epithelium of the urinary bladder. *Arch Surg* **22**:377, 1931

13. Urist MR et al: Bone cell differentiation and growth factors. *Science* **220**:680, 1983

14. Massagu EJ: The transforming growth factor-beta family. *Annu Rev Cell Biol* **6**:507, 1990

15. Tabas JA et al: Bone morphogenic protein: Chromosomal localization for BMP1, BMP2A, and BMP3. *Genomics* **9**:283, 1991

16. Burgdorf W, Nasemann T: Cutaneous osteomas: A clinical and histopathologic review. *Arch Dermatol Res* **260**:121, 1977

17. Roth SI et al: Cutaneous ossification. Report of 120 cases and review of the literature. *Arch Pathol* **76**:44, 1963

18. Lever WF, Schaumburg-Lever G: *Histopathology of the Skin*, 7th ed. Philadelphia; Lippincott, 1990, p 731

19. Maclean GD et al: Connective tissue ossification presenting in the skin. *Arch Dermatol* **94**:168, 1966

20. O'Donnell TF Jr, Geller SA: Primary osteoma cutis. *Arch Dermatol* **104**:325, 1971

21. Vero F et al: Disseminated congenital osteoma of the skin with subsequent development of myositis ossificans. *JAMA* **129**:728, 1945

22. Sherwell J: Case for diagnosis. *J Cut Genito-Urin Dis* **10**:119, 1892

23. Coleman W: Osteosis of the skin of the foot. *J Cut Genito-Urin Dis* **12**:185, 1894

24. Combes FC, Vanina R: Osteosis cutis. *AMA Arch Dermatol* **69**:613, 1954

25. Duperrat B, Vanbremeersch F: Ostéome perforant verruciforme post-traumatique. *Ann Dermatol Syphiligr* **90**:37, 1963

26. Delacrétaz J, Koenig R: Ostéome perforant. Dans le cadre d'une ostéomatose régionale acquise. *Dermatologica* **156**:251, 1978

27. Vončina D: Osteoma cutis. *Dermatologica* **148**:257, 1974

28. Hopkins JG: Multiple miliary osteomas of the skin, report of a case. *Arch Dermatol Syphilol* **18**:706, 1928

29. Costello MJ: Metaplasia of bone, report of a case. *Arch Dermatol Syphilol* **56**:536, 1947

30. Rossman RE, Freeman RG: Osteoma cutis, a stage of preosseous calcification. *Arch Dermatol* **89**:68, 1964

31. Helm F et al: Multiple miliary osteomas of the skin. Report of a case. *Arch Dermatol* **96**:681, 1967

32. Chen KTK: Atypical fibroxanthoma of the skin with osteoid production. *Arch Dermatol* **116**:113, 1980

33. Kapoor R et al: Solitary neurofibroma of the foot—an unusual case with extensive calcification and ossification. *Australasia Radiol* **30**:150, 1986

34. Urmacher C: Unusual stromal pattern in truly recurrent and satellite metastatic lesion of malignant melanoma. *Am J Dermatopathol* **6**(suppl 1):331, 1984

35. Moreno A et al: Osteoid and bone formation in desmoplastic malignant melanoma. *J Cutan Pathol* **13**:128, 1984

36. Matsumoto K et al: Osteoma cutis associated with disordered ossification of the clavicle. A case report. *Clin Orthoped* **246**:106, 1989

37. Naert F, Lachapelle JM: Multiple lesions of molluscum contagiosum with metaplastic ossification. *Am J Dermatopathol* **22**:238, 1989

38. Handfield-Jones SE et al: Ossification in linear morphoea with hemifacial atrophy—treatment by surgical excision. *Clin Exp Dermatol* **13**:385, 1988

39. Monroe AB et al: Platelike cutaneous osteoma. *J Am Acad Dermatol* **16**:481, 1987

40. Selye H et al: Sensitization to calciphylaxis by endogenous parathyroid hormone. *Endocrinology* **71**:554, 1962

41. Anderson HC: Calcific diseases. A concept. *Arch Pathol Lab Med* **107**:341, 1983

42. Fartasch M et al: Mineralization of collagen and elastic fibers in superficial dystrophic cutaneous calcification: An ultrastructural study. *Dermatologica* **181**:187, 1990

43. Paegle RD: Ultrastructure of mineral deposits in calcinosis cutis. A case study. *Arch Pathol* **82**:474, 1966

44. Pastel A, Grupper C: [Subcutaneous calcification, generalized calcinosis in nodular chains. Cysticercosis.] *Bull Soc Fr Dermatol Syphiligr* **76**:28, 1969

45. Rosin AJ: Ectopic calcification around joints of paralyzed limbs in hemiplegia, diffuse brain damage and other neurologic diseases. *Ann Rheum Dis* **34**:499, 1975

46. Beers BB et al: Dystrophic calcinosis cutis secondary to intrauterine herpes simplex. *Pediatr Dermatol* **3**:208, 1986

47. Grattan CE et al: Metastatic calcification and cytomegalovirus infection. *Br J Dermatol* **119**:785, 1988

48. Heim M et al: Calcinosis cutis—a rare late complication of burns. *Burns Incl Therm Inj* **12**:502, 1986

49. Coskey RJ, Mehregan AH: Calcinosis cutis in a burn scar. *J Am Acad Dermatol* **11**:666, 1984

50. Pitt AE et al: Self-healing dystrophic calcinosis following trauma with transepidermal elimination. *Cutis* **45**:28, 1990

51. Ellis IO et al: Plumber's knee: Calcinosis cutis after repeated minor trauma in a plumber. *Br Med J* **288**:1723, 1984

52. Mancuso G et al: Cutaneous necrosis and calcinosis following electroencephalography. *Dermatologica* **181**:324, 1990

53. Wiley HE 3d, Eaglstein WE: Calcinosis cutis in children following electroencephalography. *JAMA* **242**:455, 1979

54. Leung A: Calcification following heel sticks. *J Pediatr* **106**:168, 1985

55. Redmond WJ, Baker SR: Keloidal calcification. *Arch Dermatol* **119**:270, 1983

56. Goldminz D et al: Calcinosis cutis following extravasation of calcium chloride. *Arch Dermatol* **124**:922, 1988

57. Hironaga M et al: Cutaneous calcinosis in a neonate following extravasation of calcium gluconate. *J Am Acad Dermatol* **6**:392, 1982

58. Bosch RJ et al: [Post-phlebitis cutaneous calcinosis. Histochemical study.] *Med Cutan Ibero Lat Am* **13**:77, 1985

59. Miura T et al: Calcinosis cutis developing after phlebitis. *Dermatologica* **146**:292, 1973

60. Solanki P et al: Pilomatrixoma. Cytologic features with differential diagnostic considerations. *Arch Pathol Lab Med* **111**:294, 1987

61. Maroon M et al: Calcinosis cutis associated with syringomas: A transepidermal elimination disorder in a patient with Down syndrome. *J Am Acad Dermatol* **23**:372, 1990

62. Nielsen AO et al: Calcinosis in generalized scleroderma. *Acta Dermatol Venereol (Stockh)* **60**:301, 1980

63. Muller SA et al: Calcinosis cutis: Its relationship to scleroderma. *Arch Dermatol* **80**:15, 1959

64. Velayos EE et al: The 'CREST' syndrome. Comparison with systemic sclerosis (scleroderma). *Arch Intern Med* **139**:1240, 1979

65. Magid D et al: Dermatomyositis with calcinosis cutis. Case report 317. *Skeletal Radiol* **14**:126, 1985

66. Wang WJ et al: Calcinosis cutis in juvenile dermatomyositis: Remarkable response to aluminum hydroxide therapy. *Arch Dermatol* **124**:1721, 1988

67. Rothe MJ et al: Extensive calcinosis cutis with systemic lupus erythematosus. *Arch Dermatol* **126**:1060, 1990

68. Nomura M et al: Large subcutaneous calcification in systemic lupus erythematosus. *Arch Dermatol* **126**:1057, 1990

69. Kabir DI, Malkinson FD: Lupus erythematosus and calcinosis cutis. *Arch Dermatol* **100**:17, 1969

70. Johansson E et al: Diffuse soft tissue calcifications (calcinosis cutis) in a patient with discoid lupus erythematosus. *Clin Exp Dermatol* **13**:193, 1988

71. Strumia R et al: Cutaneous calcinosis with transepithelial elimination in porphyria cutanea tarda. Chemico-structural characterization. *G Ital Dermatol Venereol* **125**:201, 1990

72. Wilson PR: Porphyria cutanea tarda with cutaneous "scleroderma" and calcification. *Australas J Dermatol* **30**:93, 1989

73. Gianadda B et al: [Calcifications in porphyria cutanea tarda sclerodermiforme.] *Ann Dermatol Venereol* **109**:75, 1982

74. Legros R et al: [Physiochemical analysis of subcutaneous calcifications in a case of Thibierge-Weissenbach syndrome.] *Ann Dermatol Venereol* **113**:535, 1986

75. Noojin RO et al: Subcutaneous fat necrosis of newborn: Certain etiologic considerations. *J Invest Dermatol* **12**:331, 1949

76. Harrison GA, McNee JW: Sclerema neonatorum, with special reference to chemistry of subcutaneous tissues, with histological report. *Arch Dis Child* **1**:63, 1926

77. Goodman RM et al: Pseudoxanthoma elasticum: A clinical and histopathological study. *Medicine* **42**:297, 1963

78. Panicek DM et al: Calcification in untreated mediastinal lymphoma. *Radiology* **166**:735, 1988

79. Raper RF, Ibels LS: Osteosclerotic myeloma complicated by diffuse arteritis, vascular calcification and extensive cutaneous necrosis. *Nephron* **39**:389, 1985

80. Abe M et al: Hypercalcemia and metastatic calcification in adult T-cell leukemia—pathogenesis of hypercalcemia. *Fukushima J Med Sci* **31**:85, 1985

81. Werner P et al: Reversible metastatic calcification associated with excessive milk and alkali intake. *Am J Med* **14**:108, 1953

82. Yoong AK, Smallman LA: Cutaneous gangrene, metastatic and secondary hyperparathyroidism. *Histopathology* **18**:92, 1991

83. Khafif RA et al: Acute hyperparathyroidism with systemic calcinosis. Report of a case. *Arch Intern Med* **149**:681, 1989

84. Kroll JJ et al: Subcutaneous sarcoidosis with calcification. *Arch Dermatol* **106**:894, 1972

85. Wilson CW et al: Vitamin D poisoning with metastatic calcification. *Am J Med* **14**:116, 1953

86. Khafif RA et al: Calciphylaxis and systemic calcinosis. Collective review. (Published erratum appears in *Arch Intern Med* **150**:2592, 1990.) *Arch Intern Med* **150**:967, 1990

87. Adrogue HJ et al: Systemic calciphylaxis revisited. *Am J Nephrol* **1**:177, 1981

88. Asmundsson P et al: A case of calciphylaxis. Case report. *Scand J Urol Nephrol* **22**:155, 1988

89. McAleer JK, Mercer RD: Subcutaneous fat necrosis with calcification and hypercalcemia in an infant. Report of a case. *Cleve Clin Quart* **31**:179, 1964

90. Reginato AJ et al: Arthropathy and cutaneous calcinosis in hemodialysis oxalosis. *Arthritis Rheum* **29**:1387, 1986

91. Parfitt AM: Soft-tissue calcification in uremia. *Arch Intern Med* **124**:544, 1969

92. Katz AI et al: Secondary hyperparathyroidism and renal osteodystrophy in chronic renal failure. Analysis of 195 patients, with observations on the effects of chronic dialysis, kidney transplantation and subtotal parathyroidectomy. *Medicine* **48**:333, 1969

93. Frame B et al: Massive osteolysis and tumoral calcinosis. *Am J Med* **50**:408, 1971

94. Prasad VL et al: Tumoral calcinosis. *World J Surg* **13**:803, 1989

95. Pursley TV et al: Cutaneous manifestations of tumoral calcinosis. *Arch Dermatol* **115**:1100, 1979

96. Hewitt M, Chambers TL: Early presentation of pseudohypoparathyroidism. *J R Soc Med* **81**:666, 1988

97. Aydemir EH et al: Rothmund-Thomson syndrome with calcinosis universalis. *Int J Dermatol* **27**:591, 1988

98. Anonymous: Rothmund-Thomson syndrome with calcinosis cutis. *Br J Dermatol* **81**:79, 1969

99. Smeenk G, Vink R: Calcinosis cutis metastatica in a patient with primary hyperoxaluria. *Dermatologica* **134**:356, 1967

100. Hutchinson IF et al: Idiopathic calcinosis cutis of the penis. *Br J Dermatol* **102**:341, 1980

101. Shmunes E, Wood MG: Subepidermal calcified nodules. *Arch Dermatol* **105**:593, 1972

102. Dare AJ, Axelsen RA: Scrotal calcinosis: Origin from dystrophic calcification of eccrine duct milia. *J Cutan Pathol* **15**:142, 1988

103. Nakamura S et al: Idiopathic calcinosis of the scrotum. *J Dermatol* **12**:369, 1985

104. Zamora S et al: Calcific dystrophy of scrotal skin. *Br J Urol* **54**:198, 1982

105. Balfour PJ, Vincenti AC: Idiopathic vulvar calcinosis. *Histopathology* **18**:183, 1991

106. Berkowitz JE et al: Dermal breast calcifications: Localization with template-guided placement of skin marker. *Radiology* **163**:282, 1987

107. Kopans DB et al: Dermal deposits mistaken for breast calcifications. *Radiology* **149**:592, 1983

108. Renie WA et al: Pseudoxanthoma elasticum: High calcium intake in early life correlates with severity. *Am J Med Genetics* **19**:235, 1984

CHAPTER 156

Amy S. Paller

Genetic Immunodeficiency Diseases

Immunodeficiency disorders may be associated with a variety of cutaneous abnormalities, and recognition of these clinical features may allow an early diagnosis of primary immunodeficiency. Cutaneous abnormalities may include cutaneous infections, atopic- or seborrheic-like dermatitis, macular erythemas, alopecia, poor wound healing, purpura, petechiae, telangiectasias, pigmentary dilution, cutaneous granulomas, angioedema, and lupus-like changes (Table 156-1). Other clinical consequences of impaired immunocompetence often include failure to thrive, visceral infection, autoimmune disorders, allergic reactions, and neoplasia.

The classification of genetic immunodeficiency disorders includes: (1) disorders of lymphocytes, including antibody deficiency disorders, severe combined immunodeficiency, partial combined immunodeficiency, and predominantly T-cell defects; (2) disorders of phagocytic cells; and (3) disorders of complement proteins. The characteristic clinical signs of each group suggest proper classification, and laboratory tests may be employed to confirm the diagnosis. In the past decade, great advances have been made in prenatal diagnosis of immunodeficiency, specifically in diagnosis of carriers of X-linked disorders[1] by analysis of X-chromosomal inactivation and in gene localization.

Signs of Immunodeficiency

In general, immunodeficiency should be suspected when patients have recurrent infections of increased duration and severity, particularly with unusual organisms. Incomplete clearing of infections or poor response to antibiotics may be associated. Affected infants often grow poorly (failure to thrive). The most common noncutaneous abnormalities are infections, diarrhea, vomiting, hepatosplenomegaly, arthritis, adenopathy or lack of nodes where they would be expected, and hematologic abnormalities. The clinical characteristics of each group of immunodeficiency disorders are outlined in Table 156-2.

Antibody Deficiency Disorders

X-Linked Hypogammaglobulinemia

X-linked hypogammaglobulinemia (XLH) is characterized by recurrent pyogenic infections that often begin 5 to 6 months after birth with the disappearance of maternal immunoglobulins.[2] Recurrent otitis, sinusitis, bronchitis, and pneumonitis are the earliest infectious manifestations and are usually caused by pneumococci, streptococci, or *Haemophilus*. Untreated pulmonary infections may lead to chronic progressive bronchiectasis. Other common bacterial infections include conjunctivitis, osteomyelitis, septic arthritis, and meningitis. Protracted diarrhea may be due to infection, particularly with *Giardia, Salmonella, Campylobacter,* or cryptosporidial organisms.

Skin infections, especially furunculosis and impetigo, occur in 28 percent of patients and often surround body orifices. An atopic-like eczematous eruption that fails to improve with immunoglobulin therapy has been described in many affected children. Pyoderma gangrenosum and cutaneous granulomas have been reported.

TABLE 156-1
Cutaneous Manifestations of Immunodeficiency Disorders

Atopic-like dermatitis
  X-linked hypogammaglobulinemia
  IgA deficiency
  IgM deficiency
  Elevated IgM with hypogammaglobulinemia
  Common variable immunodeficiency
  Wiskott-Aldrich syndrome
  Hyperimmunoglobulinemia E syndrome
  Chronic granulomatous disease
Seborrheic-like dermatitis
  Severe combined immunodeficiency
  Ataxia-telangiectasia
  Leiner's disease
Cutaneous abscesses
  Hyperimmunoglobulinemia E syndrome
  Chronic granulomatous disease
  Leukocyte adhesion deficiency
Petechiae and/or purpura
  Wiskott-Aldrich syndrome
  Chédiak-Higashi syndrome
  Griscelli syndrome
Mucocutaneous telangiectases
  Ataxia-telangiectasia
Pigmentary dilution
  Chédiak-Higashi syndrome
  Griscelli syndrome
Graft-versus-host disease
  Severe combined immunodeficiency
  Di George syndrome
  Nezelof syndrome
Cutaneous granulomas
  Chronic granulomatous disease
  Ataxia-telangiectasia
  X-linked hypogammaglobulinemia
  Common variable immunodeficiency
  Severe combined immunodeficiency
Pyoderma gangrenosum-like ulcerations
  X-linked hypogammaglobulinemia
  IgA deficiency
  Leukocyte adhesion deficiency
  Chronic granulomatous disease
  Hyperimmunoglobulinemia E syndrome
  Chédiak-Higashi syndrome
Cutaneous candidal infections
  Severe combined immunodeficiency
  Di George syndrome
  Nezelof syndrome
  Chronic mucocutaneous candidiasis
Angioedema
  Hereditary angioedema
Lupus-like cutaneous changes
  IgA deficiency
  Elevated IgM with hypogammaglobulinemia
  Carriers of chronic granulomatous disease
  Deficiency of early complement components

TABLE 156-2

Classification of Genetic Immunodeficiency Disorders by Clinical Characteristics

Features of antibody deficiency disorders
  Recurrent infections with pathogenic extracellular encapsulated bacteria
  Chronic sinopulmonary infections
  Normal handling of fungal and viral infections, except enterovirus infections
  Minimal growth retardation
  Paucity of palpable lymphoid tissue (XLH)
  Compatible with survival for many years except if persistent enteroviral infections, malignancy, or autoimmune disease
Features of cellular (T-lymphocyte) immunodeficiency
  Recurrent infections with low-grade or opportunistic infections, particularly with fungi, *Pneumocystis carinii,* and viruses
  Growth retardation, wasting, diarrhea
  Susceptible to graft-versus-host disease, fatal infections from live vaccines
  High incidence of malignancy
  Shortened life span
Features of neutrophil disorders
  Recurrent skin and pulmonary infections
  Lymphadenopathy, hepatosplenomegaly
  Ulcerative stomatitis
Features of complement deficiency disorders
  Autoimmune disorders (early components)
  Bacterial infections, especially neisserial (alternative, late components)
  Angioedema (C1 esterase inhibitor deficiency)

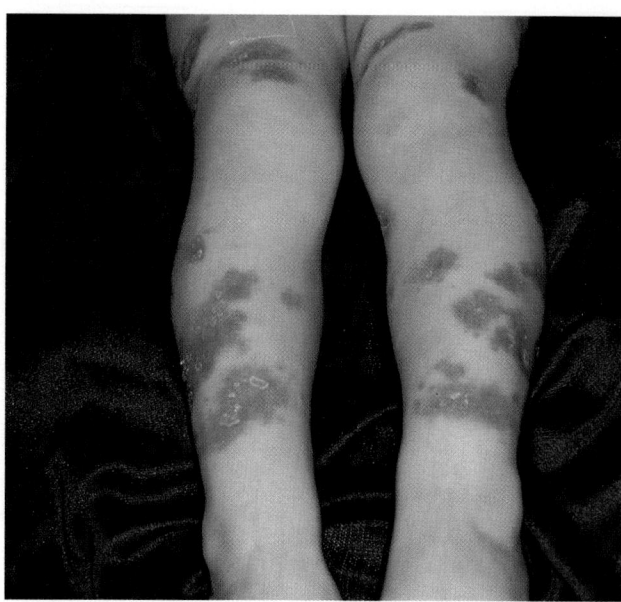

FIGURE 156-1 Noncaseating granulomas on the legs of a child with common variable immunodeficiency. Cultures and special stains showed no organisms.

Childhood exanthematous disorders are handled appropriately, but the infections may recur owing to a failure to develop specific antibodies. Three virus groups cause problems: enterovirus, hepatitis B virus, and rotavirus. Patients have developed paralysis following administration of polio vaccine. A rheumatoid-like arthritis, characterized by chronic inflammation and swelling of the large joints, may develop in as many as one-third to one-half of boys with XLH.[2,3] Disseminated echovirus infection has caused meningoencephalitis and a dermatomyositis-like disorder with brawny edema, induration of the muscles with accompanying weakness, muscle contractures, and poikiloderma in more than 35 patients.[2,4]

The underlying defect in XLH is a failure of maturation of the pre-B cell to a differentiating B cell; B-cell precursors are found in the bone marrow in normal numbers. Serum concentrations of IgG, IgA, and IgM are far below the 95 percent confidence limits for appropriate controls (usually less than 100 mg/dL total immunoglobulin).[5] Cell-mediated immunity is normal. Early intravenous immunoglobulin replacement markedly reduces the risk of infections, although it may not be helpful in diminishing the risk and morbidity of chronic enterovirus infection or of lymphoreticular malignancy (as high as 6 percent).[5]

The gene for XLH has been localized to Xq21.3-Xq22,[6] allowing prenatal diagnosis of the disorder by DNA analysis. Carrier detection is possible by analyzing the patterns of X-chromosome inactivation, with selective inactivation of the abnormal X chromosome in B lymphocytes from female carriers.[7]

Common Variable Immunodeficiency

Common variable immunodeficiency (CVID) usually presents in young adults but occasionally occurs during childhood. Patients have infections similar to those in patients with X-linked hypogammaglobulinemia particularly sinopulmonary infections, but are less

susceptible to enteroviral infections. Many patients with CVID have malabsorption syndromes, and noncaseating granulomas of skin (Fig. 156-1), lungs, liver, and spleen have been reported in a number of patients with CVID. Lymphoid tissues are often enlarged, and splenomegaly with hypersplenism is found in 25 percent of patients. Autoimmune disorders are especially frequent (22 percent), particularly autoimmune thrombocytopenia, autoimmune hemolytic anemia, rheumatoid arthritis, sicca syndrome, and pernicious anemia. Alopecia areata and lupus have also been described. In 11 percent of patients, other family members are also immunodeficient (hypogammaglobulinemia, IgA deficiency).[8] The incidence of lymphoreticular malignancy is markedly increased, particularly in the fifth and sixth decades of life.

Immunoglobulin levels may be as low as or lower than in X-linked hypogammaglobulinemia. It is believed that this is due to intrinsic abnormalities in B cells. The numbers of circulating T and B lymphocytes are usually normal. Approximately one-half of patients have T-cell dysfunction as well, with the incidence increasing with advancing age (Fig. 156-2). Recently, molecular genetic studies have suggested that both CVID and IgA deficiency are linked to the same susceptibility gene on chromosome 6 in the class III MHC region.[9]

Selective Immunoglobulin Disorders

IgA deficiency occurs in approximately 1 per 600 persons, most of whom are healthy. However, affected patients tend to have an increased incidence of upper respiratory tract infections (especially viral), allergies and atopic dermatitis, chronic gastroenteritis, and autoimmune disorders with circulating autoimmune antibodies.[10] Approximately one-third of patients with IgA deficiency have IgE anti-IgA antibody, and risk transfusion reactions if immunoglobulin is given.

Selective IgM deficiency is associated with an increased risk of pneumococcal and neisserial infections, warts, and eczema. Pa-

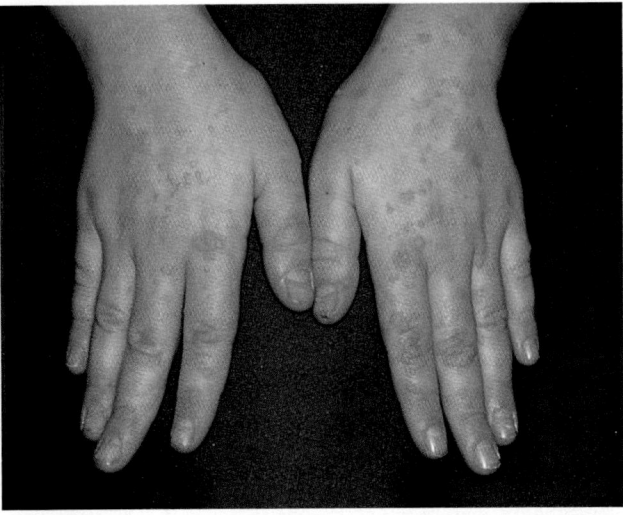

FIGURE 156-2 Flat warts on the hands of a girl with CVID. The warts were widespread, including face, trunk, and extremities, and did not respond to therapy during a 3-year treatment period.

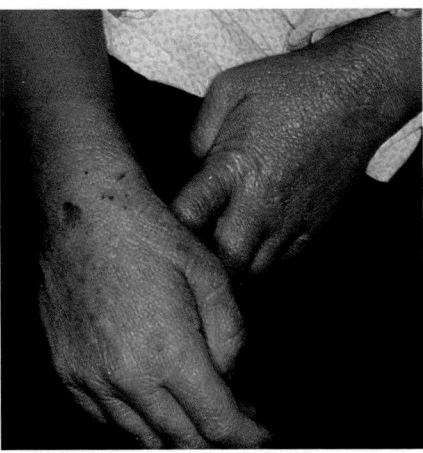

FIGURE 156-3 Severe atopic dermatitis in a patient with the Wiskott-Aldrich syndrome. Note the serosanguineous crust.

tients with hypogammaglobulinemia associated with elevated IgM levels have recurrent respiratory tract infections, eczematous dermatitis, and autoimmune disorders[11]; most cases are X-linked (gene probably at Xq24-27), but an autosomal variety may occur in female patients.

X-Linked Lymphoproliferative Disease (Duncan's)

X-linked lymphoproliferative (XLP) disease, or Duncan's disease, is characterized by an abnormal immune response to Epstein-Barr virus (EBV) infection.[12] Prior to EBV infection, patients with XLP have normal immunologic responses. With EBV infection, patients respond abnormally to the antigen and fail to develop EBV-specific serologic responses. The majority of patients die early because of severe hepatitis, liver necrosis, and hepatic failure. Patients who survive the acute EBV infection (25 percent) develop acquired agammaglobulinemia and chronic infectious mononucleosis, progressing to malignant lymphoma and marked T-lymphocyte depletion of lymph nodes, thymus, and spleen. The locus for X-linked lymphoproliferative disease has been mapped to the Xq26 region.[13]

Combined Antibody and T-Cell Deficiency

Wiskott-Aldrich Syndrome

The Wiskott-Aldrich syndrome (WAS) is an X-linked recessive disorder characterized by hemorrhage due to thrombocytopenia and platelet dysfunction, recurrent pyogenic infections, and recalcitrant dermatitis.[14] WAS usually manifests initially during the first weeks or months of life with bleeding, especially with bloody diarrhea. Epistaxis, hematemesis, hematuria, mucocutaneous petechiae, and intracranial hemorrhage may also occur. Recurrent bacterial infections begin in infancy as placentally transmitted maternal antibody levels diminish. These infections include furunculosis, conjunctivitis, otitis media and externa, pansinusitis, pneumonia, meningitis,

and septicemia. Infections with encapsulated bacteria such as pneumococcus, *Haemophilus influenzae,* and *Neiserria meningitidis* predominate. With advancing age, T-cell function progressively deteriorates, and patients become increasingly susceptible to infections due to herpes and other viruses and to *Pneumocystis carinii.*

The atopic dermatitis of patients with WAS usually develops during the first few months of life and may be quite severe. The face, scalp, and flexural areas are the most severely involved, although patients commonly have widespread involvement with progressive lichenification. The rash is often more exfoliative than that of atopic dermatitis in normal individuals, and excoriated areas frequently have serosanguineous crust (Fig. 156-3). Secondary bacterial infection of eczematous lesions is common, as are eczema herpeticum (Fig. 156-4) and molluscum.

Hepatosplenomegaly is common, and lymphadenopathy, transient arthritis with joint effusions, nephropathy, and nodular vasculitis with arteritis are occasionally present. IgE-mediated allergic

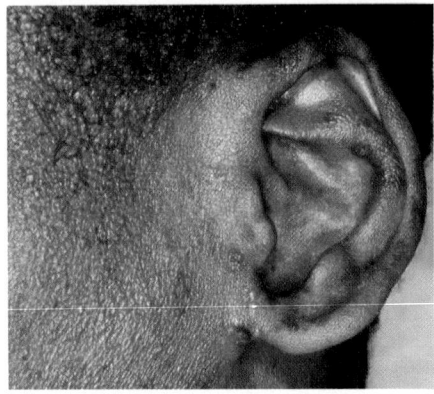

FIGURE 156-4 Herpetic infection with pustules on the ear of a patient with the Wiskott-Aldrich syndrome. The patient was blind in his left eye owing to previous ocular involvement with herpes simplex. Following the pictured infection, the patient was administered prophylactic oral acyclovir and had no subsequent herpetic infections during 5 years of follow-up. (*From Paller AS: Hereditary immunodeficiency disorders, in Genetic Disorders of the Skin, edited by JC Alper. Chicago, Mosby Year Book, 1991, Chap 7, pp 105–123.*)

problems such as urticaria, food allergies, and asthma are seen in addition to the atopic dermatitis.

The thrombocytopenia of WAS is persistent, and platelet counts may range from 1 to 80 platelets per mL. The platelets are small, and platelet aggregation is defective.[15] Patients may also have Coombs-positive hemolytic anemia, leukopenia, lymphopenia, and eosinophilia. Levels of IgM and sometimes IgG are low, and isohemagglutinins are absent. IgA, IgE, and IgD levels are usually elevated. Delayed hypersensitivity skin test reactivity is diminished, and patients fail to respond to polysaccharide antigens. The number of T lymphocytes and the response in vitro to mitogens may be normal in early life but often decreases with advancing age.

Many patients with WAS die during infancy, usually as a result of severe infections, especially of the respiratory and central nervous systems, or as a result of severe hemorrhage, especially intracranial. Twenty percent of patients with WAS develop lymphoreticular malignancies, especially non-Hodgkin's lymphoma[16] with a predominance of extranodal and brain involvement. Ten percent of patients die from these malignancies, usually as adolescents or young adults.

Appropriate antibiotics and transfusions of platelets and plasma decrease the risk of fatal infections and hemorrhage. Intravenous infusions of gammaglobulin are also useful in some patients. Splenectomy has been advocated to ameliorate the bleeding abnormality in patients with recurrent severe hemorrhage. Bone marrow transplantation is the treatment of choice for patients with recurrent problems. Full engraftment results in normal platelet numbers and functions, immunologic status, and clearance of the dermatitis (T-lymphocyte engraftment).[17] Topical corticosteroid preparations and systemic gammaglobulin may improve the dermatitis, and chronic administration of oral acyclovir is appropriate for patients with recurrent eczema herpeticum.

A lymphocyte and platelet surface glycoprotein (sialophorin, leukosialin, CD43), a component of the T-lymphocyte activation pathway, is deficient or defective in WAS patients.[18] Sialophorin is not the primary genetic defect, however, because the WAS locus lies at the pericentric region of the X chromosome[19] and CD43 has been localized to chromosome 16.[20]

Female carriers for WAS may be detected by the selective inactivation of the abnormal X chromosome in T and B cells and in platelets.[1] Studies of maternal X-chromosome inactivation have also been used to diagnose two boys with atypical WAS.[21] Prenatal diagnosis has been achieved in the first trimester by DNA markers.[22]

Ataxia-Telangiectasia

Ataxia-telangiectasia (AT) is an autosomal recessive disorder characterized by ataxia, oculocutaneous telangiectases, sinopulmonary infections, immunodeficiency, and the development of lymphoreticular malignancies.[23] The characteristic oculocutaneous telangiectases usually appear at 3 to 6 years of age near the ocular canthi and progress across the bulbar conjunctivae (Fig. 156-5). Cutaneous telangiectases may subsequently develop on the malar prominences, ears, eyelids, anterior chest, and popliteal and antecubital fossae. The telangiectases may be subtle and resemble fine petechiae, especially in the flexural areas. The development of telangiectases may be related to sun exposure, because ocular but not cutaneous telangiectases develop in affected black children.[23]

Progeric changes of the skin and hair occur in 90 percent of patients.[23] During adolescence, the facial skin may become pro-

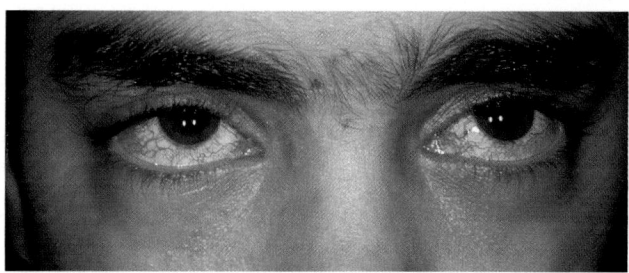

FIGURE 156-5 Bulbar conjunctival telangiectases in a patient with ataxia-telangiectasia. (*From Paller AS: Hereditary immunodeficiency disorders, in Genetic Disorders of the Skin, edited by JC Alper. Chicago, Mosby Year Book, 1991, Chap 7, pp 105–123.*)

gressively more atrophic and sclerotic, causing the face to appear masklike. Occasionally the ears, arms, and hands also become sclerodermatous. The hair may be diffusely gray by adolescence, and subcutaneous fat is generally lost in childhood.

Patients with AT often develop recurrent severe impetigo. Seborrheic dermatitis occurs in many patients, and the associated blepharitis may lead to a diagnosis of blepharoconjunctivitis rather than ocular telangiectasia. Mottled hyper- and hypopigmentation frequently occur and, together with the telangiectases and atrophy, can resemble the poikiloderma of radiodermatitis, actinic damage, or scleroderma.[24] Other pigmentary changes include café au lait spots that may be found in a dermatomal distribution,[24] multiple ephilides, and vitiligo. Hirsutism of the arms and legs, alopecia areata, multiple warts, atopic dermatitis, keratosis pilaris, nummular eczema, and acanthosis nigricans have all been described in association with AT.[24] Recently, nine patients with AT and noninfectious cutaneous granulomas have been described.[25,26]

Usually, the progressive cerebellar ataxia first becomes apparent during infancy as swaying of the head and trunk and the apraxia of eye movements. In childhood, dysarthric speech, drooling, choreoathetosis, and myoclonic jerks become prominent. Patients usually require a wheelchair by teenage years. Recurrent bacterial and viral sinopulmonary infections occur in up to 80 percent of patients; these are the most common cause of death, which is usually from bronchiectasis and respiratory failure. Patients with AT may also have growth retardation (approximately three-quarters) and endocrine disorders, especially ovarian agenesis or testicular hypoplasia and insulin-resistant diabetes. Malignant lymphoreticular neoplasms develop in 10 to 15 percent of patients, usually by adolescence.

Patients with AT tend to have both humoral and cellular immunologic abnormalities. Serum IgA and IgE are absent or deficient in the majority of patients. Circulating anti-IgA antibodies are common in patients with IgA deficiency. Defective cell-mediated immunity is found in 70 percent of patients. Virtually all patients have elevated levels of alpha fetoprotein, and many have detectable carcinoembryonic antigen. Other laboratory abnormalities in patients with AT are elevated hepatic transaminases, in 40 to 50 percent, and glucose intolerance.

Spontaneous chromosomal abnormalities (fragments, breaks, gaps, and translocations) occur 2 to 18 times more frequently in patients with AT than in normal individuals. Rearrangements of chromosomes 7 and 14, and especially 14:14 translocations, seem to predict the development of lymphoreticular malignancy. DNA isolated from fibroblasts of patients is extremely sensitive to ionizing radiation and to radiomimetic agents such as bleomycin. Heterozygotes for the AT gene (1 percent of the U.S. population) are at high risk for neoplasia, especially female breast cancer.[27]

The gene for AT has been localized to chromosome 11q22-23.[28] Prenatal diagnosis has been achieved by measurement of amniotic alpha fetoprotein levels, by increased spontaneous breakage of chromosomes of fetal amniocytes, and by the presence of a clastogenic factor in the amniotic fluid.[29]

The therapy for AT is supportive and includes administration of antibiotics for infection, physiotherapy for pulmonary bronchiectasis, physical therapy to prevent contractures in patients with neurologic dysfunction, and sunscreens and sun avoidance to diminish actinic-like changes. Lymphoreticular malignancies are the second most common cause of death, leading to the demise of 15 percent of patients with AT. Radiation and radiomimetic chemotherapeutic agents, especially bleomycin, may lead to extensive tissue necrosis. The administration of small doses of other chemotherapeutic drugs and low-dose, fractionated radiation is the least harmful means of managing these malignancies. Death usually occurs by late childhood or early adolescence; however, the oldest surviving patient died at the age of 50 years.

Severe Combined Immunodeficiency

Severe combined immunodeficiency (SCID) includes a group of heterogeneous disorders characterized by similar clinical manifestations and immunologic deficiencies of both humoral and cell-mediated immunity. Most patients with SCID are boys with an X-linked recessive inheritance pattern, but autosomal recessive and sporadic modes have been described. The overall incidence of SCID is from 1 in 100,000 to 1 in 500,000 live births.

Infants with SCID usually fail to gain weight by 3 to 6 months of age, following the onset of recurrent infections. Persistent mucocutaneous candidiasis is often present at the time of diagnosis, and systemic candidal infections occasionally occur. Patients with SCID may also have chronic diarrhea and malabsorption caused by viral infections. *P. carinii* pneumonia is often a presenting feature. Although bacterial infections usually respond to systemic antibiotics, viral infections tend to be fatal. Infants with SCID lack palpable lymphoid tissue, despite recurrent infections.

In addition to cutaneous bacterial and candidal infections, the most common cutaneous eruptions are morbilliform or resemble seborrheic dermatitis. In some infants with SCID, biopsy sections show graft-versus-host disease (GVHD). GVHD may result from the in utero exposure to maternal lymphocytes or from transfusion with nonirradiated blood products, or it may follow bone marrow transplantation.

All patients with SCID have abnormalities of both cell-mediated and humoral immunity, although the extent of deficiency is variable. Although the classification of SCID is rudimentary to date, subgroups have been defined on the basis of morphologic features, biochemical abnormalities, and cellular immunologic alterations. Two of the better defined subsets of severe combined immunodeficiency disease are: (1) adenosine deaminase (ADA) deficiency, and (2) bare lymphocyte syndrome.

Twenty percent of all patients with SCID and 50 percent of those with autosomal inheritance have a deficiency of ADA, an enzyme of the purine salvage pathway.[30,31] The lymphocyte defect is due to the toxic effects of accumulated deoxyadenosine and adenosine. Some patients have chondroosseous dysplasia. The gene has been mapped to chromosome 20q13.

Patients with bare lymphocyte syndrome, the autosomal recessive form of SCID, have poor expression of HLA antigens and beta$_2$ microglobulin on the surface of lymphocytes.[32]

One newly described form of SCID is deficiency of CD4 (inducer) T lymphocytes, which results in functional dysglobulinemia despite normal B-cell numbers. Interleukin 2 (IL-2) secretion and receptor expression are markedly reduced.[33] A specific defect in the production of IL-2 with CD4 + T cells present has also been found recently in some patients with SCID.[34,35] Administration of intravenous IL-2 causes clinical and immune function improvement.[36] In another newly described form of SCID, patients have features of graft-versus-host disease and a novel T-lymphocyte population.[37]

SCID must be differentiated from acquired immunodeficiency syndrome (AIDS). In addition to the lack of HIV antigen and anti-HIV antibodies in patients with SCID, other features help to differentiate the disorders. Despite the lymphopenia of SCID, the inverted CD4/CD8 ratio of AIDS is not found. Most patients with SCID have low levels of immunoglobulins, in contrast to the hypergammaglobulinemia of infants with AIDS.[38]

In families with a previously affected sibling of a known phenotype, prenatal detection of SCID is possible by fluorescence-activated cell sorting of fetal blood with monoclonal antibodies or by analysis of enzyme levels in cultured amniocytes.[39,40] Carrier mothers of boys with X-linked SCID may be detected by the selective inactivation of the abnormal X chromosome in T and B cells; these techniques may determine X linkage of the disorder in "sporadic" male cases.[41]

The definitive treatment of choice for SCID is bone marrow transplantation. Affected children rarely survive beyond 2 years without transplantation. Removal of postthymic cells from parental marrow may diminish the risk of GVHD in patients with SCID without an HLA-identical donor.[38]

T-Lymphocyte Disorders

Chronic Mucocutaneous Candidiasis

Patients with chronic mucocutaneous candidiasis (CMCC) have recurrent mucocutaneous candidal infections that vary from mild scaling plaques with some dystrophic nails and recurrent thrush (Fig. 156-6) to severe generalized granulomatous plaques. Associ-

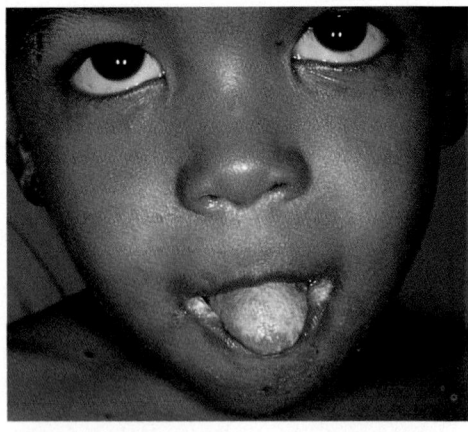

FIGURE 156-6 Recurrent thrush and candidal cheilitis in a patient with chronic mucocutaneous candidiasis.

ations with other immunodeficiencies, endocrinopathies, abnormalities of iron metabolism, and a variety of other conditions have been described.[42] CMCC may be sporadic, or inherited in an autosomal dominant or autosomal recessive pattern.

CMCC has been classified into four major variants. The most severe and typical form is early onset CMCC with moderate to severe candidiasis and usually keratotic candidal granulomas (Fig. 156-7) with extensive skin and scalp involvement, in addition to oral infection. Endocrinopathy may be associated. A second form has mild to moderate candidiasis and usually no associated endocrinopathy. *Candida*-endocrinopathy syndrome is associated with endocrinopathies that may present years after the chronic candidal infections are noted. Autoantibodies are frequently found. Hypoparathyroidism (70 percent) and hypoadrenalism (37 percent) are the most common associated endocrine disorders, but hypothyroidism, diabetes, pernicious anemia, and chronic active hepatitis may also occur. Late onset CMCC is the mildest form and may be limited to paronychia or buccal mucosal involvement. CMCC may also be a feature of patients with other primary problems, such as multiple carboxylase deficiency, a condition that is responsive to biotin,[43] and in association with ectodermal dysplasia.[44]

Visceral infections with *Candida* are rarely associated except in patients with other immunodeficiencies, but a variety of infections due to other organisms, particularly bacteria and dermatophytes, may occur.[45] A variety of T-lymphocyte abnormalities have been described, although many patients have abnormal immunologic responses only to candidal organisms. Skin tests to candidal antigens are usually negative, and lymphocytes do not respond in vitro to candidal antigens although the response to phytohemagglutinin is generally normal.

Lesions often respond to the intermittent administration of ketoconazole,[46] but patients are refractory to topical agents that are effective in normal individuals. Amphotericin B and flucytosine may be effective as well, but they are associated with a greater risk of side effects.

Di George Syndrome

Di George syndome (congenital thymic aplasia) results from developmental defects of the third and fourth pharyngeal pouches. Although most patients have T-cell defects, some have only mild T-cell abnormalities, whereas others have SCID with B-cell immu-

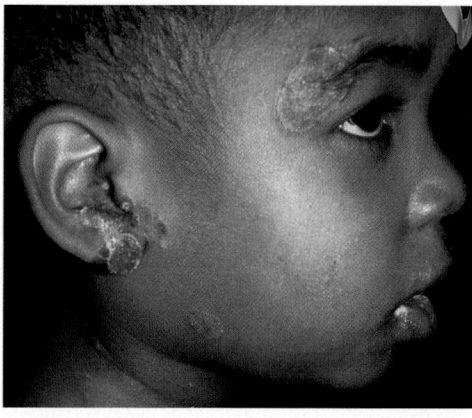

FIGURE 156-7 Cutaneous candidal infections with a hyperkeratotic candidal granuloma. The child responded to oral ketoconazole, but not to topical agents.

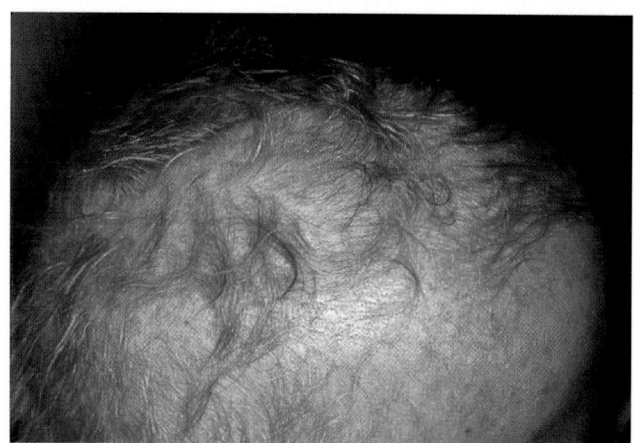

FIGURE 156-8 Sparse hypopigmented hair in a patient with the cartilage-hair hypoplasia syndrome. (*From Brennan and Pearson,[51] with permission.*)

nodeficiency as well,[47] presumably due to the effect of T cells on B-cell function. The thymic shadow is absent or reduced at birth. Infants often have neonatal tetany with hypocalcemia due to the aplastic parathyroid glands. The cardiac anomalies are most commonly truncus arteriosus, septal defects, and abnormal aortic arch vessels. Characteristic facial features of Di George syndrome include a short philtrum, low-set malformed ears, and hypertelorism.

Many patients have recurrent mucocutaneous candidal infections as neonates, as well as increased susceptibility to viral infections, *P. carinii,* and other fungal infections. Graft-versus-host disease may develop in infants that are given nonirradiated blood products. Although most cases are sporadic, many families with an autosomal dominant form of inheritance have been described.[48] Di George syndrome is often associated with loss of a portion of the proximal long arm of chromosome 22,[49] and monosomy 22q11 and 10p13 have been noted in approximately 18 percent of patients. Bone marrow transplantation has corrected the immune defect in three patients with complete Di George syndrome.

Cartilage-Hair Hypoplasia Syndrome

Cartilage-hair hypoplasia syndrome is an autosomal recessive disorder that is most common in Amish individuals. Patients have fine, sparse, hypopigmented hair (Fig. 156-8) and metaphyseal dysostosis that results in short-limbed dwarfism. Most patients have defective cell-mediated immunity, and patients may be particularly susceptible to severe disseminated varicella.[50] A subset of patients who have additional defective humoral immunity has been described. Patients may have soft, doughy skin with degenerated elastic tissue.[51]

Nezelof Syndrome

Most patients with Nezelof syndrome present later in infancy or childhood with infections similar to those of patients with SCID. Gram-negative sepsis and pneumonia are common, as are candidal infections of the mouth, perianal area, skin (Fig. 156-9), esophagus, and gastrointestinal tract that do not respond to topical therapy. Severe viral and *P. carinii* infections may also occur. Patients characteristically have lymphopenia, but other leukocyte counts are

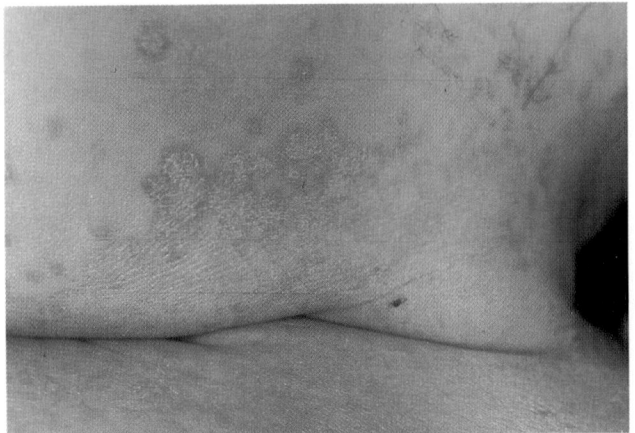

FIGURE 156-9 Cutaneous candidal infection in an infant with Nezelof syndrome.

normal. T cells are deficient, but immunoglobulin levels are normal or near-normal. Despite the presence of immunoglobulin, antibody production is suboptimal or absent. A subgroup of patients with Nezelof syndrome have purine nucleoside phosphorylase (PNP) deficiency, an autosomal recessive disorder that is due to absence of an enzyme of the purine salvage pathway.[52] Between 10 and 15 percent of children with ADA deficiency have a less severe form of Nezelof syndrome, with the onset of T-cell immunodeficiency after 6 months of age and normal immunoglobulin levels.[52]

Disorders of Phagocytic Cells

Chronic Granulomatous Disease

Chronic granulomatous disease (CGD) is a heterogeneous group of X-linked and autosomal recessive disorders characterized by severe recurrent infections due to an inability of phagocytic leukocytes to kill intracellular organisms by generation of oxidative metabolites. Most patients with the disorder are male. The recurrent infections of patients of CGD usually begin during the first year of life.[53] Pyodermas with associated regional lymphadenopathy and dermatitis, especially periorificial, may occur during infancy. Staphylococcal abscesses are common, particularly of the perianal area. Cutaneous granulomas occur less frequently than cutaneous infections and are nodular and often necrotic. The granulomas can occlude vital structures, especially of the gastrointestinal and genitourinary systems. Intraoral ulcerations resembling aphthous stomatitis, chronic gingivitis, perioral ulcers, scalp folliculitis, and seborrheic dermatitis have also been described in many patients.

The lymph nodes, lungs, liver, spleen, and gastrointestinal tract are the most frequent areas of noncutaneous involvement. Suppurative lymphadenitis with abscess and fistula formation usually affects cervical nodes. Pneumonia occurs in almost all affected children and may lead to abscess formation, cavitation, and empyema. Hepatosplenomegaly has been reported in 80 to 90 percent of patients; more than 30 percent of patients develop hepatic abscesses, and hepatic granuloma formation is common.

Normal bactericidal activity after phagocytosis requires the nicotinamide adenine dinucleotide (NADPH) oxidase system, which consists of NADPH, a flavoprotein, and an unusual phagocyte cytochrome b_{558}. Patients with CGD have deficient killing

because this membrane-associated NADPH oxidase system fails to produce superoxide and other toxic oxygen metabolites. In most patients with the X-linked form of CGD, b_{558} is not detectable.[54] Some patients with X-linked CGD also have deficient flavoprotein. In a variant form of X-linked CGD, cytochrome b_{558} is present but dysfunctional.[55] Most patients with autosomal recessive CGD have normal cytochrome b_{558}[56] but are deficient in 47-kDa and 67-kDa NADPH oxidase cytosolic factors.[57]

The types of microbial organisms that cause infections in patients with CGD are usually catalase-positive and require intracellular killing; such organisms include *Staphylococcus aureus, Salmonella,* and *Aspergillus.* Long-term prophylactic trimethoprim-sulfamethoxazole therapy decreases the incidence of bacterial infection without increasing the incidence of fungal infection.[58,59] The intensive humoral and granulomatous responses can be explained as compensatory reactions. The screening test for CGD is the nitroblue tetrazolium (NBT) reduction assay. Quantitative NBT tests and chemiluminescence assays may also be performed. Patients frequently have leukocytosis, anemia, elevated sedimentation rate, and hypergammaglobulinemia, but immune function is otherwise normal.

Heterozygous carriers for X-linked cytochrome b_{558}-negative CGD do not have the increased risk of infections but may have discoid or systemic lupus erythematosus, severe aphthous stomatitis,[60] or granulomatous cheilitis.[61] The histopathology of the discoid lupus in not typical, and immunofluorescence examination is negative.[62]

Therapy of CGD includes antimicrobial agents for infections and debridement and drainage of abscesses. Leukocyte transfusions have been used for rapidly progressive life-threatening infections. Bone marrow transplantation has been performed in some patients with CGD.[63,64] Gamma-interferon induces the mRNA that codes for the defective cytochrome b and it has been shown to increase the functional cytochrome b, superoxide generation, and bactericidal activity.[65-67] Patients with X-linked CGD and ``variant'' CGD showed clinical improvement after administration of gamma-interferon. Systemic corticosteroids have been helpful for patients with obstructive visceral granulomas.[68] Prenatal diagnosis has been performed by the NBT slide test.[69] The defective gene in CGD has been localized to Xp21.

Hyperimmunoglobulinemia E Syndrome

The hyperimmunoglobulinemia E (HIE) syndrome is characterized by (1) markedly increased levels of IgE, (2) recurrent cutaneous and systemic pyogenic infections, (3) atopic-like dermatitis, (4) peripheral eosinophilia, and (5) defective neutrophil chemotaxis.[70,71] Buckley's syndrome and Job's syndrome are subsets of the HIE syndrome. The disorder is usually sporadic, but familial cases that have been described suggest an autosomal dominant trait with incomplete penetrance.

The dermatitis of HIE syndrome begins in infancy and resembles atopic dermatitis, but intertriginous, retroauricular, and hairline areas are also frequently involved. Most patients develop extensive lichenification (Fig. 156-10), and many patients have other manifestations of atopy. Patients develop progressive coarsening of facial features (Fig. 156-11). Skin infections include impetigo, furunculosis, paronychia, cellulitis, and characteristic abscesses (``cold'' abscesses) (Fig. 156-11) that do not demonstrate the anticipated degree of erythema, warmth, and purulence. The abscesses most commonly occur on the head and neck and in intertriginous

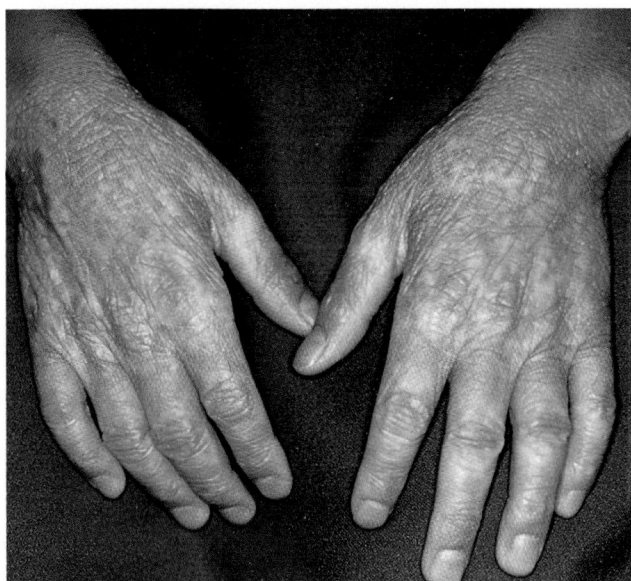

FIGURE 156-10 Extensive lichenification in a patient with hyperimmunoglobulinemia E syndrome and severe atopic dermatitis.

areas. Pulmonary bacterial pneumonia, abscesses, and empyema are the most frequent systemic infections and may result in pneumatoceles that become the nidus for further bacterial and fungal infections. The most common infecting organisms are *Staph. aureus* and *H. influenza*.

Elevated serum IgE levels (>2000 IU) are characteristic and may be related to defective T-suppressor-cell function. The most common functional defect in host resistance is defective neutrophil chemotaxis, particularly during severe infections.

Antistaphylococcal antibiotics are effective for most cutaneous infections in patients with HIE. Ascorbic acid[72] and cimetidine[73] have decreased the number of infections and the chemotactic defect in some patients. Isotretinoin has been reported to eliminate the recurrent staphylococcal abscesses in an isolated patient, without any change in immunologic status.[74] The cutaneous and pulmonary abscesses often require incision and drainage and may require

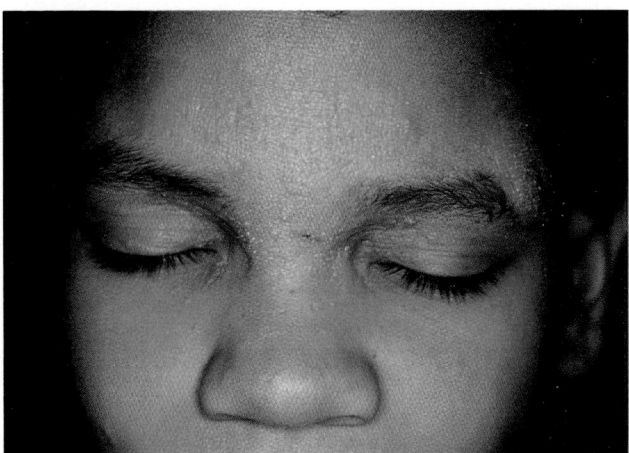

FIGURE 156-11 Coarse facial features and ''cold'' abscess and furuncle in a patient with hyperimmunoglobulinemia E syndrome.

surgical removal. Recently, gamma-interferon has been shown to decrease IgE levels without altering IgG and IgM levels in two patients with HIE.[75]

Leukocyte Adhesion Deficiency

Leukocyte adhesion deficiency is a rare, autosomal recessive disorder that affects the adherence of neutrophils, lymphocytes, and monocytes.[76,77] Patients have frequent skin infections, mucositis, and otitis. The skin infections often present as necrotic abscesses that resemble pyoderma gangrenosum, but the inflammatory response and production of purulent material are impaired. Patients may have delayed separation of the umbilical cord. Cellulitis of the face and perirectal area is common. Gingivitis with periodontitis results in loss of teeth. Life-threatening severe bacterial or fungal infections may occur. Poor wound healing leads to paper-thin or dysplastic cutaneous scars.

Adherence of leukocytes relates in part to a group of cell surface glycoproteins (integrins) that share a common 95-kDa beta subunit (CD18) that is encoded on the distal portion of the long arm of chromosome 21. The beta subunit is linked to three distinct alpha chains to form three different surface glycoproteins. These glycoproteins, the iC3b receptor (CR3), LFA-1, and p150,95, are absent or deficient in affected patients. As a result, neutrophil and monocyte chemotaxis and phagocytosis are impaired. The severity of clinical involvement is proportional to the degree of glycoprotein deficiency. Death usually occurs by 2 years of age unless successful bone marrow transplantation is performed.

Chédiak-Higashi Syndrome

This rare, autosomal recessive disorder is characterized by incomplete oculocutaneous albinism and severe recurrent infections.[78] Parental consanguinity is often reported. Pigmentary dilution is present in 75 percent of patients. Ocular hypopigmentation may cause photophobia, and strabismus and nystagmus are common. The skin is typically fair, but slate-colored areas of pigmentation may be present. The hair frequently has a silvery sheen (Fig. 156-12a). Infections most commonly involve the skin, lungs, and respiratory tract and are usually due to *Staph. aureus, Streptococcus pyogenes,* and *Pneumococcus.* Deep ulcerations resembling pyoderma gangrenosum have also been described. Seizures and progressive neurologic deterioration, with muscle weakness and cranial and peripheral neuropathy, have occurred in some patients in early childhood.

An ''accelerated phase,'' which resembles lymphoma, occurs by late childhood and is characterized by widespread visceral infiltration by atypical lymphoid and histiocytic cells. This lymphoma-like stage is precipitated by viruses, particularly by EBV infection.[79,80] Hepatosplenomegaly, lymphadenopathy, pancytopenia, jaundice, a leukemia-like gingivitis, and pseudomembraneous sloughing of the buccal mucosa are associated.[81] The thrombocytopenia and depletion of coagulation factors lead to petechiae, bruising, and gingival bleeding. The mean age of death for patients with Chédiak-Higashi syndrome is 6 years, usually from overwhelming infection or hemorrhage during the lymphoma-like ''accelerated phase.''

Giant granules are typically found in circulating neutrophils, melanocytes, renal tubular cells, and neurons. Hair shafts have clumped pigment granules (Fig. 156-12b). The granules are

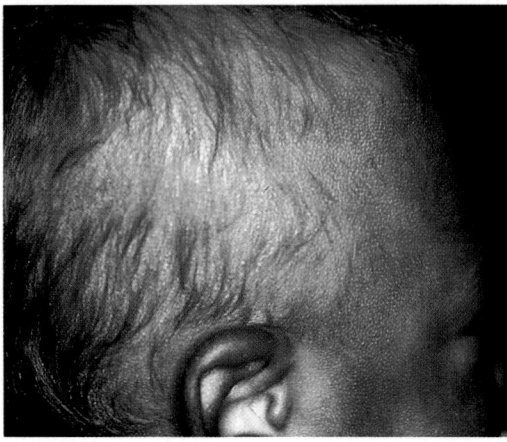

a

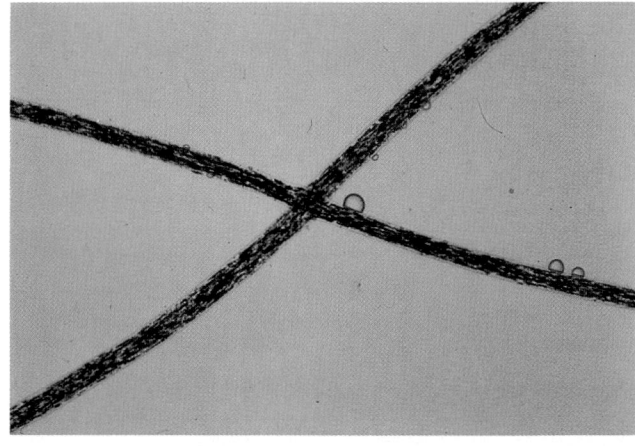

b

FIGURE 156-12 Chédiak-Higashi Syndrome. (*a*) Silvery sheen to hair in a black infant; patient had darkly pigmented eyes and skin. (*b*) Clumped pigment granules in hairs. (×100, original magnification.)

thought to result from markedly delayed discharge of lysosomal and peroxidative enzymes from cells, perhaps because of associated microtubular anomalies. Diminished chemotaxis of neutrophils and decreased antibody-dependent cellular cytotoxicity and natural killer cell function are often associated.

The treatment of choice for patients with Chédiak-Higashi syndrome is bone marrow transplantation, which corrects the immunologic status but does not affect pigment dilution.[82] Acyclovir,[83] high-dose intravenous gammaglobulin,[84] and vincristine and prednisone have been used to control the accelerated phase. Ascorbic acid corrects the microtubular defects in vitro, but has no clinical ameliorative effect.[85] Interferon has been demonstrated by some authors to partially restore natural killer cell function.

Griscelli Syndrome

As in Chédiak-Higashi syndrome, patients with Griscelli syndrome have pigmentary dilution with silver-gray hair, recurrent systemic and cutaneous pyogenic infections, and cutaneous abscesses. Early hepatosplenomegaly, progressive neurologic deterioration, lymphohistiocytosis, and neutropenia and thrombocytopenia may occur.[86] Large clumps of pigment are seen in the hair shaft, and melanosomes accumulate in melanocytes. Patients with Griscelli syndrome also have hypogammaglobulinemia and defective cell-mediated immunity. Polymorphonuclear leukocytes do not show giant granules. Griscelli syndrome has been uniformly fatal but can now be reversed by successful bone marrow transplantation.[87]

Complement Deficiency Disorders (See also Chaps. 36 and 115)

Except for autosomal dominant hereditary angioedema, complement deficiencies are inherited as autosomal recessive disorders.[88,89] Although many patients with complement component deficiencies are clinically normal, patients with deficiences of the early components of the classical complement pathway (C1, C4, C2) may demonstrate lupus-like disorders, and patients with defi-

ciencies of later components and components of the alternate pathway may have recurrent infections (Table 156-3).

The most common deficiency of complement protein is of C2. Autoimmune disorders occur in 10 percent of patients who are heterozygous (incidence 1:100) and in almost 50 percent of patients who are homozygous (1:10,000) for deficiency of C2. The most common abnormality in affected patients is a photosensitivity-like rash (Fig. 156-13), which often resembles subacute lupus erythematosus but may resemble discoid lupus plaques or the malar erythema of SLE. Lupus-like alopecia is often described. Unexplained fevers, arthritis, and arthralgias are found in 80 percent of patients, whereas 50 percent of patients have leukopenia and oral ulcerations. Other features of SLE are found less frequently. Renal disease, if present, is usually mild. Although lupus-like manifestations are most commonly described, patients may have other autoimmune disorders, such as dermatomyositis, juvenile rheumatoid arthritis, vasculitis, and cold urticaria.

Elevated anti-Ro (SSA) antibody titers are found in 75 percent of patients with SLE and C2 deficiency, and rheumatoid factor is positive in 40 percent of patients. In contrast to SLE, antinuclear

TABLE 156-3
Complement Deficiency Disorders

C1q	SLE, infections, glomerulonephriris
C1r	SLE, infections, glomerulonephritis
C1s	SLE
C1INH	Herediary angioedema
C4	SLE with palmoplantar keratoderma, glomerulonephritis, HSP, urticaria
C2	SLE, DLE, infections, HSP
C3	Gram-positive infections, SLE, vasculitis
Properdin	Neisserial infections
C3b INA	Infections, aquagenic urticaria
C5	Neisserial infections
C6	Neisserial infections
C7	Neisserial infections, SLE, scleroderma
C8	Neisserial infections, SLE
C9	Neisserial infections

NOTE: DLE, discoid lupus erythematosus; HSP, Henoch-Schöenlein purpura; INA inactivator; INH, inhibitor; SLE, systemic lupus erythematosus.
SOURCE: Modified from Paller AS: *Adv Dermatol* **6**:212, 1991, by permission of Mosby Year Book.

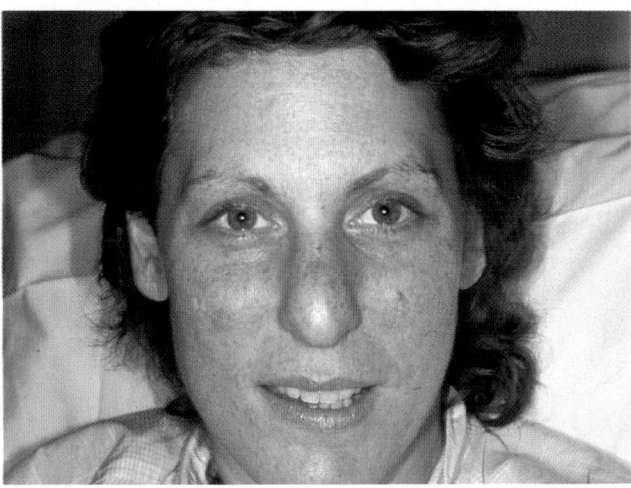

FIGURE 156-13   Malar erythema in a patient with C2 deficiency. The patient was ANA-negative but had high titers of anti-Ro antibodies.

antibodies and anti-DNA antibodies are often of low titer or absent, and the lupus band test is usually negative. CH_{50} is markedly decreased or zero. Radioimmunodiffusion assays may be used to demonstrate the selective deficiency of C2.

Hereditary Angioedema

Hereditary angioedema (HAE) (formerly called hereditary angioneurotic edema) is an autosomal dominant disorder characterized by nonpruritic edema of the face, extremities, and respiratory and gastrointestinal tracts without associated typical urticaria.[90] Episodes of angioedema usually begin in early childhood and become more severe with advancing age. Many patients cite trauma as an eliciting factor. A prodrome of localized tingling of the skin, hoarseness, altered taste, abdominal pain, and difficulty in swallowing may be reported. The angioedema typically increases progressively for several hours and then persists for 2 to 3 days. Laryngeal obstruction occurs most frequently in adults, and up to 25 percent of patients die from airway compromise. Patients with HAE may also demonstrate manifestations of autoimmune disorders, especially systemic or discoid lupus erythematosus.[91]

Levels of C4 and C2 are low during attacks of angioedema, and C4 tends to be depressed between episodes as well. CH_{50} is often normal. C1 esterase inhibitor (C1̄INH) level is diminished (85 percent of patients) or dysfunctional (15 percent). The drug of choice for patients with HAE is danazol, which stimulates the synthesis of functional C1̄INH. Antifibrinolytics and fresh frozen plasma have been used for more acute situations.

Leiner's Disease

Leiner's disease is characterized by severe seborrheic dermatitis, diarrhea, failure to thrive, and recurrent gram-negative and candidal infections during infancy. Although originally reported as a disorder due to defective yeast opsonization from dysfunctional C5,[92] it is now clear that so-called Leiner's syndrome describes a constellation of clinical findings that may be manifestations of a variety of immunodeficiency disorders, including defective

yeast opsonization,[92] C3 deficiency,[93] severe combined immunodeficiency, hypogammaglobulinemia, and hyperimmunoglobulinemia E.[94]

References

1. Winkelstein JA, Fearon E: Carrier detection of the X-linked primary immunodeficiency diseases using X-chromosome inactivation analysis. *J Allergy Clin Immunol* **85**:1090, 1990

2. Lederman HM, Winkelstein JA: X-linked agammaglobulinemia: An analysis of 96 patients. *Medicine (Baltimore)* **64**:145, 1985

3. Ackerson BK et al: Echovirus 11 arthritis in a patient with X-linked agammaglobulinemia. *Pediatr Infect Dis J* **6**:485, 1987

4. Bardelas JA et al: Fatal ECHO 24 infection in a patient with hypogammaglobulinemia: Relationship to dermatomyositis-like syndrome. *J Pediatr* **90**:396, 1977

5. Buckley RH: Immunodeficiency. *J Allergy Clin Immunol* **72**:627, 1983

6. Kwan S-P et al: Mapping of the X-linked agammaglobulinemia locus by use of restriction fragment-length polymorphism. *J Clin Invest* **77**:649, 1986

7. Fearon ER et al: Carrier detection in X-linked agammaglobulinemia by analysis of X-chromosome inactivation. *N Engl J Med* **316**:427, 1987

8. Cunningham-Rundles C: Clinical and immunologic analyses of 103 patients with common variable immunodeficiency. *J Clin Immunol* **9**:22, 1989

9. Schaffer FM et al: Individuals with IgA deficiency and common variable immunodeficiency share complex polymorphisms of major histocompatibility complex class III genes. *Proc Natl Acad Sci USA* **86**:8015, 1989

10. Sennhauser FH et al: Anti-IgA antibodies in IgA deficient children. *J Clin Immunol* **8**:356, 1988

11. Mayer L et al: Evidence for a defect in "switch" T cells in patients with immunodeficiency and hyperimmunoglobulinemia M. *N Engl J Med* **314**:409, 1986

12. Saemundsen AK et al: Documentation of Epstein-Barr virus (EBV) infection in immunodeficient patients with life-threatening lymphoproliferative diseases by EBV complementary RNA/DNA and viral DNA/DNA hybridization. *Cancer Res* **41**:4237, 1981

13. Sanger WG et al: Partial Xq25 deletion in a family with the X-linked lymphoproliferative disease (XLP). *Cancer Genet Cytogenet* **47**:163, 1990

14. Perry GS III et al: The Wiskott-Aldrich syndrome in the United States and Canada (1892–1979). *J Pediatr* **97**:72, 1980

15. Corash L et al: Platelet-associated immunoglobulin, platelet size, and the effect of splenectomy in the Wiskott-Aldrich syndrome. *Blood* **65**:1439, 1985

16. Cotelingam JD et al: Malignant lymphoma in patients with the Wiskott-Aldrich syndrome. *Cancer Invest* **3**:515, 1985

17. Parkman R et al: Complete correction of the Wiskott-Aldrich syndrome by allogeneic bone marrow transplantation. *N Engl J Med* **298**:921, 1978

18. Mentzer SJ et al: Sialophorin, a surface sialoglycoprotein defective in Wiskott-Aldrich syndrome, is involved in human T lymphocyte proliferation. *J Exp Med* **165**:1383, 1987

19. Peacocke M, Siminovitch KA: Linkage of the Wiskott-Aldrich syndrome with polymorphic DNA sequences from the human X chromosome. *Proc Natl Acad Sci USA* **84**:3430, 1987

20. Pallant A et al: Characterization of cDNAs encoding human leukosialin and localization of the leukosialin gene to chromosome 16. *Proc Natl Acad Sci USA* **86**:1328, 1989

21. Puck JM et al: Atypical presentation of Wiskott-Aldrich syndrome: Diagnosis in two unrelated males based on studies of maternal T cell X chromosome inactivation. *Blood* **75**:2369, 1990

22. Schwartz M et al: First-trimester diagnosis of Wiskott-Aldrich syn-

drome by DNA markers. *Lancet* **2**:1405, 1989

23. Boder E: Ataxia-telangiectasia: An overview, in *Ataxia-Telangiectasia: Genetics, Neuropathology, and Immunology of a Degenerative Disease of Childhood,* edited by RA Gatti, M Smith. New York, Alan R Liss, 1985, p 1

24. Cohen LE et al: Common and uncommon cutaneous findings in patients with ataxia-telangiectasia. *J Am Acad Dermatol* **10**:431, 1984

25. Fleck RM et al: Ataxia-telangiectasia associated with sarcoidosis. *Pediatr Dermatol* **3**:339, 1986

26. Paller AS et al: Granulomatous lesions in patients with ataxia-telangiectasia. *J Pediatr* **119**:917, 1991

27. Swift M: Genetic aspects of ataxia-telangiectasia. *Immunodeficiency Rev* **2**:67, 1981

28. Gatti RA et al: Localization of an ataxia-telangiectasia to chromosome 11q22-23. *Nature* **336**:577, 1988

29. Schwartz S et al: Tests appropriate for the prenatal diagnosis of ataxia-telangiectasia. *Prenatal Diagnosis* **5**:9, 1985

30. Hirschhorn R: Genetic deficiencies of adenosine deaminase and purine nucleoside phosphorylase: Overview, genetic heterogeneity and therapy. *Birth Defects* **19**:73, 1983

31. Carson DA, Carrera CJ: Immunodeficiency secondary to adenosine deaminase deficiency and purine nucleoside phosphorylation deficiency. *Semin Hematol* **27**:260, 1990

32. Touraine J-L, Betuel H: The bare lymphocyte syndrome: Immunodeficiency resulting from the lack of expression of HLA antigens. *Birth Defects* **19**:83, 1983

33. Sleasman JW et al: Combined immunodeficiency due to the selective absence of CD4 inducer T lymphocytes. *Clin Immunol Immunopathol* **55**:401, 1990

34. Weinberg K, Parkman R: Severe combined immunodeficiency due to a specific defect in the production of interleukin 2. *N Engl J Med* **322**:1718, 1990

35. DiSanto JP et al: Absence of interleukin 2 production in a severe combined immunodeficiency disease syndrome with T cells. *J Exp Med* **171**:1697, 1990

36. Pahwa R et al: Recombinant interleukin 2 therapy in severe combined immunodeficiency disease. *Proc Natl Acad Sci USA* **86**:5069, 1989

37. Wirt DP et al: Novel T-lymphocyte population in combined immunodeficiency with features of graft-versus-host disease. *N Engl J Med* **321**:370, 1989

38. Buckley RH: Advances in the diagnosis and treatment of primary immunodeficiency diseases. *Arch Intern Med* **146**:377, 1986

39. Linch DC et al: Prenatal diagnosis for severe combined immunodeficiency. *Birth Defects* **19**:121, 1983

40. Durandy A, Griscelli C: Prenatal diagnosis of severe combined immunodeficiency and X-linked agammaglobulinemia. *Birth Defects* **19**:125, 1983

41. Conley ME et al: X-linked severe combined immunodeficiency. Diagnosis in males with sporadic severe combined immunodeficiency and clarification of clinical findings. *J Clin Invest* **85**:1548, 1990

42. Dwyer JM: Chronic mucocutaneous candidiasis. *Annu Rev Med* **32**:491, 1981

43. Ahonen P et al: Clinical variation of autoimmune polyendocrinopathy-candidiasis-ectodermal dystrophy (APECED) in a series of 68 patients. *N Engl J Med* **322**:1829, 1990

44. Williams ML et al: Alopecia and periorificial dermatitis in biotin-responsive multiple carboxylase deficiency. *J Am Acad Dermatol* **9**:97, 1983

45. Herrod HG: Chronic mucocutaneous candidiasis in childhood and complications of non-*Candida* infection: A report of the Pediatric Immunodeficiency Collaborative Study Group. *J Pediatr* **116**:377, 1990

46. Horsburgh C, Kirkpatrick C: Long-term therapy of chronic mucocutaneous candidiasis with ketoconazole: Experiences with twenty-one patients. *Am J Med* **74**(suppl):23, 1983

47. Muller W et al: The Di George sequence. II. Immunologic findings in partial and complete forms of the disorder. *Eur J Pediatr* **149**:96, 1989

48. Stevens CA et al: Di George anomaly and velocardiofacial syndrome. *Pediatrics* **85**:526, 1990

49. Fibison WJ: Molecular studies of Di George syndrome. *Am J Hum Genet* **46**:888, 1990

50. Polmar SH, Pierce GF: Cartilage hair hypoplasia: Immunological aspects and their clinical implications. *Clin Immunol Immunopathol* **40**:87, 1986

51. Brennan T, Pearson R: Abnormal elastic tissue in cartilage hair hypoplasia. *Arch Dermatol* **124**:1411, 1988

52. Edwards NL: Immunodeficiencies associated with errors in purine metabolism. *Med Clin North Am* **69**:505, 1985

53. Babior BM, Woodman RC: Chronic granulomatous disease. *Semin Hematol* **27**:247, 1990

54. Segal AW et al: Absence of cytochrome b245 in chronic granulomatous disease. *N Engl J Med* **308**:245, 1983

55. Dinauer MC et al: A missense mutation in the neutrophil cytochrome b heavy chain in cytochrome-positive X-linked chronic granulomatous disease. *J Clin Invest* **84**:2012, 1989

56. Weening R et al: Cytochrome b deficiency in an autosomal form of chronic granulomatous disease. *J Clin Invest* **75**:915, 1985

57. Clark RA et al: Genetic variants of chronic granulomatous disease: Prevalence of deficiencies of two cytosolic components of the NADPH oxidase system. *N Engl J Med* **321**:647, 1989

58. Margolis DM et al: Trimethoprim-sulfamethoxazole prophylaxis in the management of chronic granulomatous disease. *J Infect Dis* **162**:723, 1990

59. Mouy R et al: Incidence, severity, and prevention of infections in chronic granulomatous disease. *J Pediatr* **114**:555, 1989

60. Brandrup F et al: Discoid lupus erythematosus-like lesions and stomatitis in female carriers of X-linked chronic granulomatous disease. *Br J Dermatol* **104**:495, 1981

61. Dusi S et al: Chronic granulomatous disease in an adult female with granulomatous cheilitis. Evidence for an X-linked pattern of inheritance with extreme lyonization. *Acta Haematol* **84**:49, 1990

62. Sillevis Smitt JH et al: Discoid lupus erythematosus-like lesions in carriers of X-linked chronic granulomatous disease. *Br J Dermatol* **122**:643, 1990

63. Kamani N et al: Bone marrow transplantation in chronic granulomatous disease. *J Pediatr* **105**:42, 1984

64. DiBartolomeo P et al: Reconstitution of normal neutrophil function in chronic granulomatous disease by bone marrow transplantation. *Bone Marrow Transplant* **4**:695, 1989

65. Ezekowitz R, Newburger P: New perspectives in chronic granulomatous disease. *J Clin Immunol* **8**:419, 1988

66. Gallin JI, Malech HL: Update on chronic granulomatous diseases of childhood: Immunotherapy and potential for gene therapy. *JAMA* **263**:1533, 1990

67. Ezekowitz R et al: Partial correction of the phagocyte defect in patients with X-linked chronic granulomatous disease by subcutaneous interferon gamma. *N Engl J Med* **319**:146, 1988

68. Chin TW et al: Corticosteroids in treatment of obstructive lesions of chronic granulomatous disease. *J Pediatr* **111**:349, 1989

69. Newberger PE et al: Prenatal diagnosis of chronic granulomatous disease. *N Engl J Med* **300**:178, 1979

70. Hill H: The syndrome of hyperimmunoglobulinemia-E in recurrent infections. *Am J Dis Child* **136**:767, 1982

71. Donabedian H. Gallin J: Hyperimmunoglobulin-E recurrent-infection (Job's) syndrome: Review of the NIH experience in the literature. *Medicine (Baltimore)* **62**:195, 1983

72. Guarda R et al: Hyperimmunoglobulinemia E syndrome (Buckley's syndrome). Clinical case associated with mucopolysacchariduria with good therapeutic response to ascorbic acid. *Rev Med Chil* **113**:442, 1985

73. Simon G et al: Cimetidine in the treatment of hyperimmunoglobulinemia E with impaired chemotaxis. *J Infect Dis* **147**:1121, 1983

74. Shuttleworth D et al: Hyperimmunoglobulin E syndrome: Treatment with isotretinoin. *Br J Dermatol* **119**:93, 1988

75. King CL et al: Regulation of immunoglobulin production in hyperimmunoglobulin E recurrent-infection syndrome by interferon gamma. *Proc Natl Acad Sci USA* **86**:10085, 1989

76. Malech H. Gallin J: Neutrophils in human diseases. *N Engl J Med* **317**:687, 1987

77. Kishimoto TK et al: The leukocyte integrins. *Adv Immunol* **46**:149, 1989

78. Blume RS, Wolff SM: The Chédiak-Higashi syndrome: Studies in four patients and a review of the literature. *Medicine (Baltimore)* **51**:247, 1972

79. Merino F et al: Chronic active Epstein-Barr virus infection in patients with Chédiak-Higashi syndrome. *J Clin Immunol* **6**:299, 1986

80. Kinugawa N: Epstein-Barr virus infection in Chédiak-Higashi syndrome mimicking acute lymphocytic leukemia. *Am J Pediatr Hematol Oncol* **12**:192, 1990

81. Rubin CM et al: The accelerated phase of Chédiak-Higashi syndrome: An expression of the virus-associated hemophagocytic syndrome? *Cancer* **56**:524, 1985

82. Griscelli C, Virelizier J-L: Bone marrow transplantation in a patient with Chédiak-Higashi syndrome. *Birth Defects* **19**:333, 1983

83. Conley M, Henle W: Acyclovir in accelerated phase of Chédiak-Higashi syndrome. *Lancet* **1**:212, 1987

84. Kinugawa N, Ohtani T: Beneficial effects of high-dose intravenous gammaglobulin on the accelerated phase of Chédiak-Higashi syndrome. *Helv Pediatr Acta* **40**:169, 1985

85. Boxer LA et al: Correction of leukocyte function in Chédiak-Higashi syndrome by ascorbate. *N Engl J Med* **295**:1041, 1976

86. Griscelli C et al: A syndrome associating partial albinism and immunodeficiency. *Am J Med* **65**:691, 1978

87. Schneider LC et al: Bone marrow transplantation (BMT) for the syndrome of pigmentary dilution and lymphohistiocytosis (Griscelli's syndrome). *J Clin Immunol* **10**:146, 1990

88. Guenther LC: Inherited disorders of complement deficiencies. *J Am Acad Dermatol* **9**:815, 1983

89. Schur PH: Inherited complement component abnormalities. *Annu Rev Med* **37**:333, 1986

90. Frank MM et al: Hereditary angioedema: The clinical syndrome and its management. *Ann Intern Med* **84**:580, 1976

91. Massa MC, Connolly SM: An association between C1 esterase inhibitor deficiency and lupus erythematosus. *J Am Acad Dermatol* **7**:255, 1982

92. Miller ME, Koblenzer PJ: Leiner's disease and deficiency of C5. *J Pediatr* **80**:879, 1972

93. Sonea MJ et al: Leiner's disease associated with diminished third component of complement. *Pediatr Dermatol* **4**:105, 1987

94. Glover M et al: Syndrome of erythroderma, failure to thrive and diarrhea in infancy. A manifestation of immunodeficiency. *Pediatrics* **81**:66, 1988

CHAPTER 157

Richard J. Wenstrup and Sheldon R. Pinnell

Heritable Disorders of Connective Tissue with Skin Changes

Heritable disorders of connective tissue are generalized defects that are due to mutations in the genes for components of connective tissues or in enzymes modifying them. They involve many tissues, reflecting organ distribution of those components. Virtually all are inherited in a simple mendelian manner.[1,2]

Marfan Syndrome

Patients with Marfan syndrome may have major abnormalities in primarily three organ systems[3]: the eye, especially dislocation of the lenses; the skeletal system, especially excessive length of extremities, loose-jointedness, kyphoscoliosis, and anterior chest deformity; and the cardiovascular system, especially aortic aneurysm and mitral valve redundancy. Skin manifestations consist of striae distensae, a common finding, and elastosis perforans serpignosa, a rare finding.

Clinical Manifestations

Skeletal (Figs. 157-1 and 157-2) The skeletal features, particularly the long, narrow extremities, figured prominently in Marfan's initial description in 1896 of the syndrome that bears his name. Some have suggested that Marfan's original patient in fact had congenital contractural arachnodactyly rather than the disorder now defined as Marfan syndrome. Patients with the Marfan syndrome are usually taller than unaffected same-sex siblings. There is skeletal disproportion, with the most consistent and reliable measure being an abnormally low ratio of upper segment to lower segment. The segments are measured below and above the top of the pubic symphysis. In practice, two measurements are made with the patient standing: height and lower segment (top of the pubic symphysis to the floor). In adult Caucasians the mean ratio is about 0.92, and in adult American blacks it is about 0.87. The excessive length of the extremities is responsible for the abnormally low upper-segment-to-lower-segment ratio (US/LS) in Marfan syndrome. Shortening of the trunk by kyphoscoliosis exaggerates the low US/LS. When kyphoscoliosis is more than minimal, the US/LS should not be used. Another abnormal measurement includes the comparison of the arm span (fingertip to fingertip) with height; the arm span is usually longer by several centimeters.

The ribs appear to undergo the same excessive longitudinal growth as do the bones of the extremities. Depression of the sternum (pectus excavatum) or projection (pectus carinatum) or an asymmetric deformity of the anterior chest results.

Joint hyperextensibility is often striking in patients with Marfan syndrome but is not found in all patients. Flat-footedness, hyperextensibility at the knees (genu recurvatum) and elbows, and occasional dislocation of joints are manifestations of the loose-jointedness. Because of joint hyperextensibility and long, narrow extremities, the patient is often able to touch his or her umbilicus with the right hand passed around the back and approaching the umbilicus from the left. A relatively narrow palm of the hand with a long thumb and hyperextensibility is the basis of Steinberg's sign:

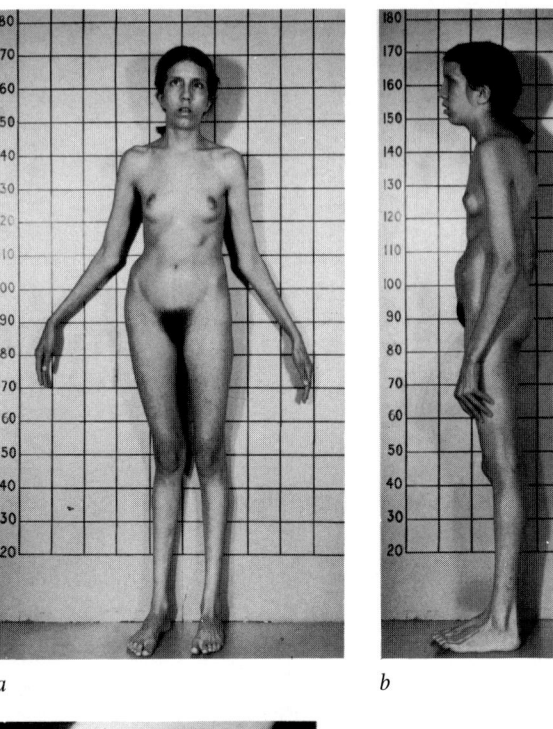

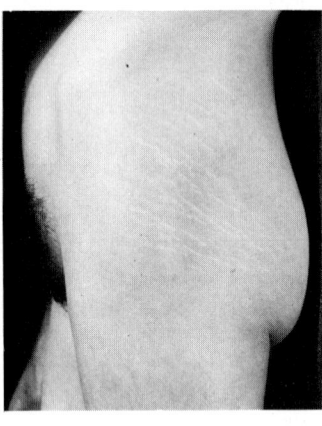

a   *b*

c

Cardiovascular The most common serious cardiovascular feature of Marfan syndrome is a weakness of the aortic media which leads to diffuse aneurysm. Aneurysm may develop in the first year of life or not until the fifth or sixth decades. The ascending aorta is the most severely affected region of the aorta, although the defect is clearly generalized, because the ascending aorta is exposed to more pulsatile fatigue in the aorta. Although the ascending aorta shows the main change, abdominal aneurysm without notable thoracic involvement has occurred in a few patients.

Echocardiography of the proximal aorta is a very sensitive noninvasive diagnostic procedure for aortic root involvement. It must be performed on any patient in whom the diagnosis of the Marfan syndrome is considered, and patients with documented aortic dilation should be monitored yearly for progression. The mitral valve may be redundant, resulting in regurgitation. Echocardiography can also determine whether prolapse of the mitral valve is pres-

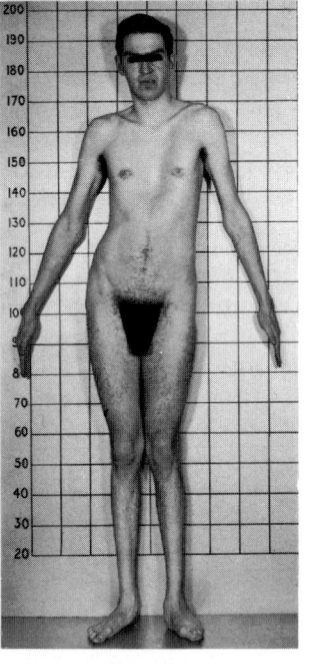

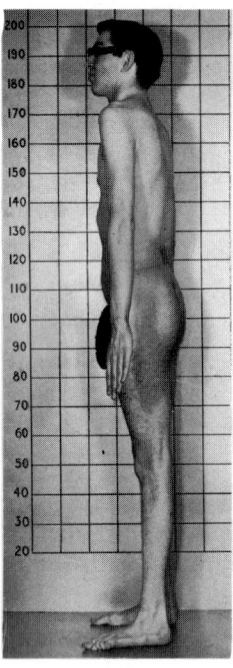

a   *b*

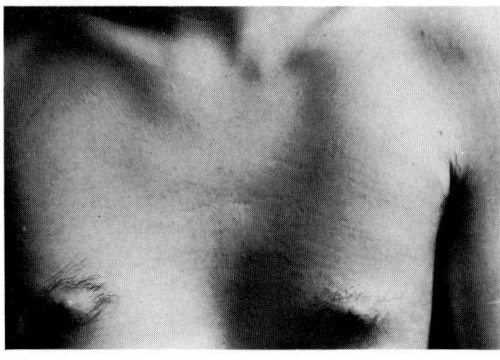

c

FIGURE 157-1 Marfan syndrome, (*a*) Frontal and (*b*) lateral views of a 15-year-old girl with Marfan syndrome. Note the tall stature, arachnodactyly, kyphoscoliosis, round shoulders, and strabismus. (*c*) Striae distensae over the hips in the same patient.

The thumb propped across the palm extends well beyond the ulnar margin of the hand.

Ocular Virtually all patients with Marfan syndrome have myopia. The orbit is abnormally long. In addition, about 70 percent of patients have ectopia lentis.[3] The lens is usually displaced upward. With significant dilation, the margin of the lens may be visible in the lower part of the pupil. Dislocation of the lens into the anterior chamber or trapping of the lens in the pupil sometimes occurs, and acute glaucoma may result. Detection of mild ectopia lentis requires full dilation of the pupils and slit-lamp examination for redundancy of the suspensory ligament of the lens. Therefore, clinical exclusion of ectopia lentis in an individual suspected of having Marfan syndrome must include a slit-lamp exam after dilation of the pupils. Detachment of the retina is also an ocular component of Marfan syndrome.

FIGURE 157-2 Marfan syndrome. (*a*) Frontal and (*b*) lateral views of a 20-year-old boy with Marfan syndrome. Note the tall stature, depressed sternum, scoliosis, and arachnodactyly. The father and a younger brother were also affected. This patient falls among the approximately 30 percent who do not have ectopia lentis. His brother, however, did have ectopia lentis. (*c*) Striae distensae over the pectoral and deltoid areas.

ent, whether mitral regurgitation is present, and whether mitral valve regurgitation is hemodynamically significant.

Other Features   A high-arched palate, crowding of the anterior teeth, and inguinal hernia are both common manifestations of the syndrome. Pulmonary manifestations include cystic changes, emphysema, and spontaneous pneumothorax. The skeletal musculature is often underdeveloped and hypotonic.

Skin Changes   Although often not a conspicuous feature of Marfan syndrome, two types of change have been observed. Most patients show striae distensae, particularly in the pectoral and deltoid areas and over the thighs. Elastosis perforans serpignosa has been described in some Marfan variants.[4]

Genetic Defect

Marfan syndrome was recently shown to be caused by heterozygous mutations in the gene for fibrillin, a connective tissue protein found to coassociate with elastin in tissues. Approximately 80 percent of patients with Marfan syndrome have a positive family history; in the rest the syndrome results from de novo mutations in the sperm or ova of the parents. Thereafter, the syndrome is inherited as an autosomal dominant condition. The clinical severity of Marfan syndrome differs considerably between and within families. The interfamilial heterogeneity is doubtless due to different kinds of mutation at the fibrillin locus on chromosome 15. Differences within families are probably due to extragenetic influences and/or to differences at other loci that code for extracellular matrix proteins.

After fibrillin was discovered in 1986,[5] it was found to be abundant in tissues prominently affected with the Marfan syndrome—the ascending aorta, suspensory ligament of the lens, periosteum, and skin. There was dramatically decreased binding of fluorescent antibodies to fibrillin in skin and dermal fibroblast matrix in patients with Marfan syndrome,[6] and the decreased antifibrillin staining cosegregated with the Marfan clinical phenotype in several Marfan families.[7] At approximately the same time, family linkage studies by several investigators mapped Marfan syndrome to the long arm of chromosome 15, which was also found to be the chromosomal locus of a fibrillin gene.[8] Restriction fragment length polymorphisms within the fibrillin gene itself have been tightly linked to Marfan syndrome in several large families, with no recombinants; this finding confirms the genetic cause of the disorder to be mutation within the fibrillin gene.

Homocystinuria

Homocystinuria is the most common disorder due to inherited defects in the metabolism of methionine. The major form of the disease discussed here is characterized by deficiency in the enzyme β cystathionine synthase and is autosomal recessive in inheritance. The major clinical manifestations include dolichostenomelia, ectopia lentis, and chest and spinal deformity; the latter two make it superficially similar to Marfan syndrome. Generalized osteoporosis, arteriovenous thrombosis, and mental retardation are prominent features that allow relatively easy discrimination from Marfan syndrome. The cutaneous manifestations include malar flush, thin hair and skin, and cutis reticulata.

Clinical Manifestations

Vascular   The most serious and life-threatening complication of β cystathionine synthase deficiency is arterial and venous thrombosis. Acute occlusion of the coronary arteries can cause myocardial infarction, renal occlusion can cause severe hypertension, occlusion of carotid or cerebral arteries can cause stroke, and blindness can be caused by ophthalmic artery occlusion. Venous thromboses may cause renal vein thrombosis or portal vein thrombosis and pulmonary embolism. These manifestations are usually seen in the homozygous state with the full-blown clinical syndrome. However, recent data suggest that heterozygotes for a mutation at the β cystathionine synthase locus may be at increased risk for myocardial infarction. The vascular complications of homocystinuria are the cause of increased mortality in these patients. At least 20 percent of patients die prematurely from thrombotic complications.

Ocular   Most patients with homocystinuria have ectopia lentis in the first decade of life. Ectopia lentis is progressive in β cystathionine synthase deficiency; it is stable in Marfan syndrome. Rupture of the sclera and retinal detachment have also been reported. Nearly all patients have significant myopia.

Skeletal   Patients with homocystinuria have the same asthenic habitus as those seen with Marfan syndrome and have a high incidence of scoliosis, thoracic asymmetry, and pectus excavatum. However, joint hyperextensibility is not a feature of this disorder; more characteristic is mild joint limitation. There is an increased incidence of pathologic fractures in patients with homocystinuria because of generalized osteopenia.

Other Features   Mental retardation is a common but variable feature of β cystathionine synthase deficiency. In addition, a recent survey reported that slightly over half of the patients with documented β cystathionine synthase deficiency had psychiatric disorders such as depression, chronic behavioral disorders, obsessive-compulsive disorder, and other personality disorders.[9]

Cutaneous Features   A prominent malar flush has been reported in many patients, which is most easily seen after vigorous exercise or after cold exposure. Hair is thinned. The dermis is usually thin and dermis reticularis is commonly seen on the extremities. In patients with deep venous thromboses, collateral venous channels are rarely visible through the skin.

Metabolic Defect

β Cystathionine synthase catalyzes the condensation of homocystine and serine; in its absence, homocysteine is converted to homocystine which is greatly increased in blood and appears in urine. Some homocystine is converted back to methionine which is also elevated in blood and urine. Cystine, which normally is supplied to the body by metabolism of methionine, becomes an essential amino acid in patients with β cystathionine synthase deficiency.

There has been considerable controversy over the mechanisms by which β cystathionine synthase and elevated homocystine cause the clotting abnormality and the connective tissue findings characteristic of homocystinuria. With regard to the clotting abnormality, experimental work suggests that elevated homocystine alters the aggregation of platelets, is toxic to endothelial surfaces, or alters the activity of soluble factors that regulate thrombosis, such as antithrombin III, but no widely accepted general explanation has taken hold.

With regard to the connective tissue findings of ectopia lentis, osteoporosis, and the vertebral and thoracic abnormalities, there is good evidence that elevated homocystine inhibits cross-linking of collagen. Harris and Sjoerdsma[10] demonstrated a decrease of cross-linking of collagen in skin from two patients with homocystinuria. Specifically, they found an excess of monomeric collagen relative to the amount of dimerized collagen chains in reducing gels. The mechanism for decreased cross-linking in vivo is unknown. It might be in the earliest step in cross-linking, which is catalyzed by lysyl oxidase, or in later steps, which serve to mature the cross-links. The biologic basis for mental retardation and psychiatric disturbance in patients with homocystinuria is also unknown.

Genetics

The great majority of patients with homocystinuria have primary deficiency of β cystathionine synthase (reviewed by Mudd et al.[11]) A minority have acquired (dietary) deficiency of cobalamin or heritable disorders that prevent conversion of dietary cobalamin to its biologically active forms; rarely, some have defects that cause decreased availability of 5-methyltetrahydrofolate, which is also required in the metabolism of methionine.

The clinical syndrome of homocystinuria due to β cystathionine synthase deficiency is inherited as an autosomal recessive trait, based on segregation analysis of a number of families, on the increased incidence of homocystinuria in consanguineous matings, and in the finding of intermediate decreases of β cystathionine synthase activity in liver biopsy specimens from parents of some patients. Recently the gene for β cystathionine synthase has been isolated and has been located on the long arm of chromosome 21 (21q22.3). Molecular analysis of the β cystathionine synthase locus in patients should provide an explanation for clinical heterogeneity in this condition. It is expected that several different disease alleles

exist. One subtype is clinically milder, with few or no central nervous system (CNS) or psychiatric complications, and usually with residual β cystathionine synthase activity. These patients respond to administration of vitamin B_6 (pyridoxine) in doses of about 100 mg per day by clearing homocystine from the urine. Pyridoxine-unresponsive patients usually have no β cystathionine synthase activity and more severe clinical findings. If heterozygosity for a β cystathionine synthase gene mutation does predispose to increased risk for myocardial infarction, then that risk would be dominantly inherited.

Osteogenesis Imperfecta

Osteogenesis imperfecta (OI) is a generalized connective tissue disorder in which the primary clinical manifestation is osseous fragility.[12,13] There is an extremely wide range of clinical severity, from mild osseous fragility in childhood with no bony deformities, to a severe deforming disorder that is lethal in the perinatal period. The wide range of severity in OI is reflected in Table 157-1, adapted from that of Sillence and colleagues.[12]

Nearly all cases of OI are due to heterozygosity for different kinds of mutations in the proα1(I) and proα2(I) genes of type I collagen (reviewed by Byers[1,14] and Prockop[15]).

Clinical Description

Skeleton An increased incidence of fractures defines the clinical syndrome. Fractures are always present in utero in OI types II and III and also may occur in the milder forms. Skeletal deformity is a hallmark of all but the mildest forms of osteogenesis imperfecta; OI type II is so severe that it is readily detected by the beginning of the second trimester of pregnancy. Deformity of long bones at birth does not necessarily result from in utero fractures, but may be the

TABLE 157-1
Clinical Subtypes and Associated Defects in Osteogenesis Imperfecta (OI)

OI type	Clinical features	Inheritance	Biochemical defects
I	Normal stature; little or no deformity; blue scleras; hearing loss in about 50% of individuals; dentinogenesis imperfecta rare and may distinguish a subset	AD	Decreased production of type I procollagen; Substitution for residue other than glycine in triple helix of α1(I)
II	Lethal in the perinatal period; minimal calvarial mineralization; beaded ribs, compressed femurs, marked long bone deformity, platyspondylisis	AD (new mutation) AR (rare)	Rearrangements in the COL1A1 and COL1A2 genes; substitutions for glycyl residues in the triple-helical domain of the α1(I) or α2(I) chain; Small deletion in α2(I) on the background of a null allele
III	Progressively deforming bones, usually with moderate deformity at birth; scleras variable in hue, often lighten with age; dentinogenesis common; hearing loss common; stature very short	AR (rare) AD	Frameshift mutation that prevents incorporation of proα2(I) into molecules (noncollagenous defects); Point mutations in the α1(I) or α2(I) chain
IV	Normal scleras; mild to moderate bone deformity and variable short stature; dentinogenesis common; hearing loss occurs in some	AD	Point mutations in the α2(I) chain; rarely, point mutations in the α1(I) chain; small deletions in the α2(I) chain

Note: AD = autosomal dominant, AR = autosomal recessive.
Source: Sillence et al.[12]

result of molding under the strain of normal muscle tone in the fetus. "Codfish vertebrae" (hollowing out of vertebral bodies by pressure from expansile intervertebral disks) or flat vertebrae are observed in some patients, particularly older patients in whom senile or postmenopausal changes exaggerate the change, or in younger patients who are immobilized after fractures or osteotomies.

Fracture frequency usually decreases after puberty, but there is a second fracture peak in late adulthood. Patients with more severe OI phenotypes also have dentinogenesis imperfecta, which presents as graying, opalescent teeth that are prone to erosion.

Other Connective Tissue   Because type I collagen is found in nearly all tissues, it is not surprising that clinical problems stemming from dysfunction of other connective tissues are increased in OI. Joint laxity and occasional joint dislocation are relatively common in milder forms of OI. Tendon rupture and, rarely, rupture of blood vessels are probably increased in patients with OI compared with the general population.

Hearing   Deafness develops in many patients with OI by the third decade of life. There appears to be a mixture of otosclerosis and sensorineural deafness involved in OI hearing loss.

Skin   Patients with OI, particularly OI type I, have thin skin with wider scars than normal after incisions. This same subset of patients also has increased bruisability after mild trauma, probably because of abnormal collagen fibril structure in the walls of small blood vessels or in the supporting connective tissues.

Basic Defect

There are two general classes of type I collagen mutations distinguished by their biochemical effects on cultured dermal fibroblasts. One class of mutations, almost always associated with mild OI (type I, Table 157-1), results in loss of expression of one proα1(I) allele and half-normal production of type I collagen from cultured dermal fibroblasts[16-18] (Fig. 157-3). A second class of mutations, usually associated with more severe OI (types II, III, and IV), results in type I collagen molecules with an altered triple helical structure.[18] Some of these structural mutations are deletions or insertions of peptidyl material, but the great majority are single amino acid substitutions for glycine residues in α1(I) or α2(I) chains that disrupt the Gly-X-Y repeat structure of the triple helical domain.

Biochemical studies of abnormal type I collagen molecules synthesized by OI fibroblasts have consistently shown that molecules have increased posttranslational modifications—primarily lysyl hydroxylation and glycosylation—that are limited to the portion of the molecule that is amino-terminal to the site of a glycine substitution (reviewed by Byers[1]). Molecules assemble and wind from the carboxyl to the amino-terminal end, but winding is slowed through the region of the substitution. Unwound chains are either further modified before molecular assembly, or else the final conformation of the helix amino-terminal to the mutation is altered sufficiently to allow posttranslational modifications after the helix is formed. These biochemical features form the basis of current methods of biochemical screening for this form of OI. In addition, abnormal molecules are secreted more slowly from cultured fibroblasts and have decreased thermal stability.

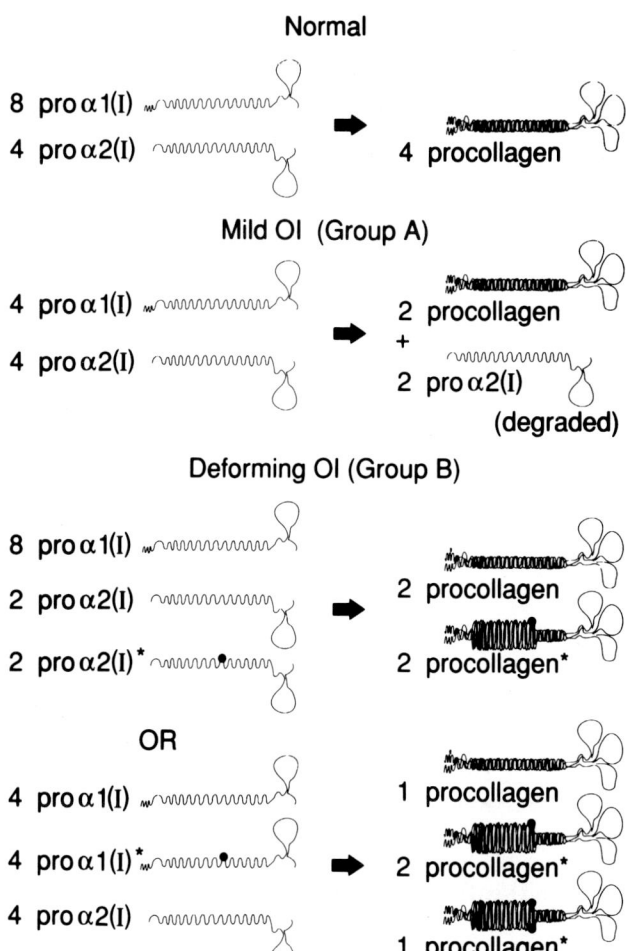

FIGURE 157-3   Stoichiometric relationship of normal and abnormal α chains of type I collagen resulting from dominant mutations that produce the observed biochemical phenotypes of OI. Mild OI is caused by 50 percent reduction of proα1(I) chains. More severe OI is caused by production of molecules that contain mutant chains (the site of mutation is indicated by the black dot in the triple-helical domain). Proα chains in these molecules undergo increased posttranslational modification amino-terminal to the site of the mutation, may be inefficiently secreted with increased degradation within cells, and result in defective collagen fibrillogenesis. The broadened area of the triple helix depicts overmodification.

Genetics

There is convincing evidence from family linkage studies and from biochemical and molecular characterizations of OI cell strains, that almost all patients with OI are heterozygous for mutations in the genes for the proα1(I) and proα2(I) chains of type I collagen that lie in chromosomes 17 and 7, respectively. Although earlier clinical genetic studies of OI suggested that the most severe forms (types II and III) were autosomal recessive because of recurrences in the offspring of clinically unaffected parents, there is clear evidence that these recurrences are in most cases caused by germline mosaicism for a type I collagen mutation. A relatively minor subset of OI types II and III may be caused by an autosomal recessive mutation at a different locus.

TABLE 157-2
Ehlers-Danlos Syndromes (EDS): Clinical, Genetic, and Biochemical Characteristics

Type	Clinical features	Inheritance	Biochemical defects
I Gravis	Soft, hyperextensible skin; easy bruising; thin, atrophic scars; hypermobile joints; varicose veins; prematurity of affected newborns	AD	Not known
II Mitis	Similar to EDS type I but less severe	AD	Not known
III Familial hypermobility	Soft skin; large and small joint hypermobility	AD	Not known
IV Arterial	Thin, translucent skin with visible veins; easy bruising; absence of skin and joint extensibility; arterial, bowel, and uterine rupture	AD	Abnormal type III collagen synthesis, secretion, or structure: deletions and point mutations in the gene
		(AR)	Not known
V X-linked	Similar to EDS type II	XLR	Not known
VI	Soft muscle hypotonia; scoliosis; joint laxity; hyperextensible skin	AR	Lysyl hydroxylase deficiency
VII Arthro-chalasis multiplex congenita	Congenital hip dislocation, severe joint hypermobility; soft skin with normal scarring	AD	Deletion of exons from type I collagen genes that encode the amino-terminal propeptide cleavage sites
VII Perio-dontal	Generalized periodontitis; soft hyperextensible skin	AD	Not known
IX	Soft, extensible, lax skin; bladder diverticulae and rupture; short arms, limited pronation and supination; broad clavicles; occipital horns	XLR	Abnormal copper utilization with defect in lysyl oxidase
X	Similar to EDS type II, with abnormal clotting studies	AR	Possible defect in fibronectin

Note: AD = autosomal dominant, AR = autosomal recessive, XLR = X-linked recessive.

Ehlers-Danlos Syndromes

The Ehlers-Danlos syndromes (EDS) are a genetically, biochemically, and clinically distinct group of inherited disorders with common characteristics of joint laxity, skin hyperextensibility, and skin fragility.[1,19,20] Ten distinct subtypes have been described (Table 157-2), but many individuals with these clinical features do not fit into a distinct subtype.

Clinical Description

EDS Type I Ehlers-Danlos syndrome type I, the *gravis* form, is characterized by joint laxity, hyperextensibility of skin, poor wound healing, and autosomal dominant inheritance (Figs. 157-4 to 157-6). The skin is soft and velvety and can be stretched easily. The dermis is fragile and is easily bruised. Scars after trauma or surgical procedures are thinned and atrophic and may stretch considerably after healing, having a characteristic "cigarette paper" appearance. About half of affected individuals with EDS I are delivered prematurely as infants because of premature rupture of fetal membranes, presumably due to abnormalities in structure of fetal tissues. A significant number of individuals with EDS type I have cardiac defects, most commonly mitral valve prolapse. A few EDS type I patients have dilation and occasionally rupture of the ascending aorta or proximal pulmonary artery. Musculoskeletal features seen in EDS type I include joint hyperextensibility in all patients and a fairly high frequency of scoliosis and pes planus (flat feet). The joint hypermobility can be associated with the onset of osteoarthritis in the third or fourth decade.

EDS Type II Ehlers-Danlos type II is clinically similar to EDS type I, except that the skin is less fragile and there is normal or near-normal scar formation. Ultrastructural findings shown thickened collagen fibrils in skin, similar to findings in the dermis in patients with EDS type I.

EDS Type III Ehlers-Danlos type III, also known as the familial benign hypermobility syndrome, is characterized primarily by hyperextensibility of large and small joints and autosomal dominant inheritance. Individuals with EDS type III are at risk for premature onset of osteoarthritis in the third or fourth decade. There are no known abnormalities in collagen associated with EDS type III.

EDS Type IV Ehlers-Danlos type IV is a condition characterized by thin, translucent skin with easy bruisability but normal scar formation. Affected individuals are at high risk for life-threatening rupture of the large intestine, uterus, or medium-sized arteries. The most common sites of arterial rupture are the mesenchymal arteries in the abdomen, the splenic artery, renal arteries, and the descending aorta. There may also be an increased incidence of stroke in patients with EDS type IV. Another life-threatening complication is uterine rupture in the peripartum period.[21] EDS type IV is clinically distinct from other EDS subtypes in that there is no skin hyperextensibility or abnormal scarring, and joint hyperextensibility is not as prominent a finding as in other forms of EDS.

Although EDS type IV was initially thought to be autosomal recessive in inheritance, most EDS type IV individuals have family histories compatible with autosomal dominant inheritance, and linkage analysis has documented dominant inheritance in several EDS type IV families.

EDS Type V EDS type V is a rare X-linked disorder characterized by mild skin hyperelasticity, mildly abnormal scarring, and joint hyperextensibility. Female carriers are asymptomatic. There are only a few well-documented families with EDS type V in the litera-

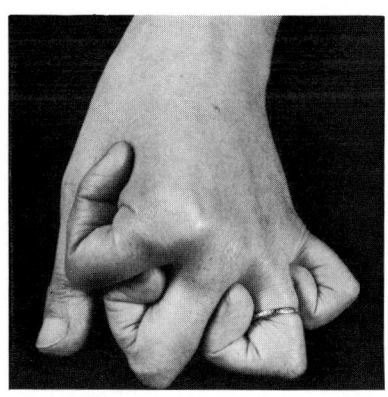
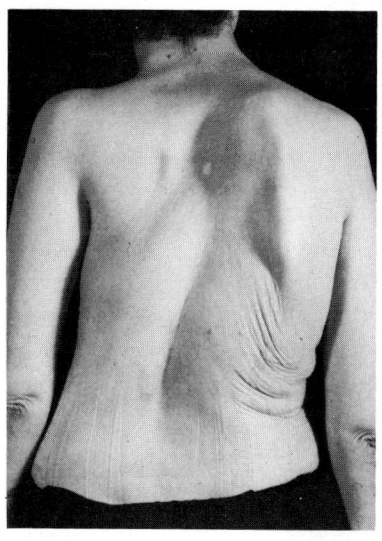
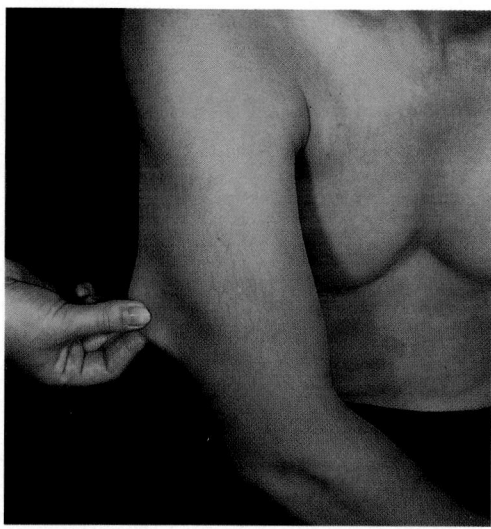

a   *b*   *c*

FIGURE 157-4 The Ehlers-Danlos syndrome in a 37-year-old woman. (*a*) Loose-jointedness is demonstrated. (*b*) Note the severe scoliosis as well as the loose, puckered skin over the elbows. (*c*) Loose skin is demonstrated over the elbow. The patient is blind from retinal detachment, as is a brother with the Ehlers-Danlos syndrome.

ture. This rare disorder clinically resembles EDS type II except that the latter disorder has autosomal dominant inheritance. Thus, in clinical situations in which diagnosis of EDS types V and II are both possible, the much more common EDS type II should be considered unless family history clearly suggests X-linked inheritance.

EDS Type VI A recent review of the clinical findings in 10 patients with documented lysyl hydroxylase deficiency indicates that the cardinal features of lysyl hydroxylase deficiency are neonatal onset of joint laxity, kyphoscoliosis, and hypotonia.[22] Ocular fragility, which was observed in the original reports of lysyl hydroxylase deficiency, was found in only a minority of patients. Skin fragility, easy bruisability, and dermal hyperextensibility occurred to some extent in most patients. Three of ten individuals in the study with EDS type VI suffered a potentially catastrophic arterial rupture.

EDS Type VII Ehlers-Danlos type VII (arthrochalasia multiplex) is characterized by extreme joint laxity, multiple joint dislocations, and congenital hip dislocations that are difficult to repair surgically.

EDS Type VIII Ehlers-Danlos type VIII is a rare autosomal dominant condition characterized by soft, hyperextensible skin, abnormal scarring, easy bruising, hyperextensible joints, and generalized periodontitis. It resembles the *gravis* form of EDS type I but can be clinically distinguished from the latter disorder by the periodontitis and by the characteristic purplish discoloration of scars on the shins. The molecular basis of EDS type VIII is unknown.

EDS Type IX Ehlers-Danlos type IX is a rare disorder characterized by lax, extremely soft skin at birth, and later development of skeletal deformities such as occipital horns, short humeri, and short, broad clavicles. Inheritance is X-linked recessive. Affected males may also have bladder diverticuli which can result in hydronephrosis, and a chronic diarrhea of unknown etiology. Intellect is usually unaffected.

EDS Type X Arneson and coworkers[23] reported a single family in which two siblings of unaffected parents had joint hyperextensibility, mitral valve prolapse, easy bruisability, and poor wound healing. Clotting studies performed to evaluate excessive bleeding at incision sites were normal except for a striking defect in the platelet adhesion that is normally observed in response to exposure of platelets to collagen. Addition of purified fibronectin to the patients' plasma improved platelet adhesiveness. The authors suggested that this disorder may be due to a defect in fibronectin.

Basic Defect

Many abnormalities in collagen synthesis result in the EDS. Histology of skin from patients with EDS reveals reduced collagen content and disorganization of fiber bundles.[24] Two patients with EDS have been reported to have deficient synthesis of the $\alpha 2(I)$ collagen chain.[25-27] They apparently make and use collagen composed of three $\alpha 1(I)$ chains rather than the normal two $\alpha 1(I)$ and one $\alpha 2(I)$ chains. Type IV EDS results from defects in synthesis, structure, or secretion of type III collagen.[28,29] Collagen fibers are small and irregular in skin and blood vessels.[30,31] Several mutations have been described in the triple helical region of the type III collagen molecule. These include multiexon deletions,[32,33] single point mutations,[34,35] and splicing defects.[36–39] A low serum level of the aminopropeptide of type III procollagen confirms the diagnosis.[40]

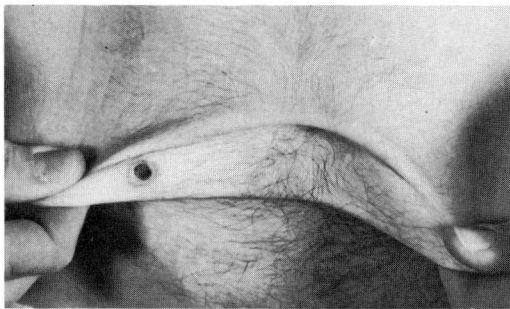

FIGURE 157-5 Abnormally stretchable skin of a patient with Ehlers-Danlos syndrome.

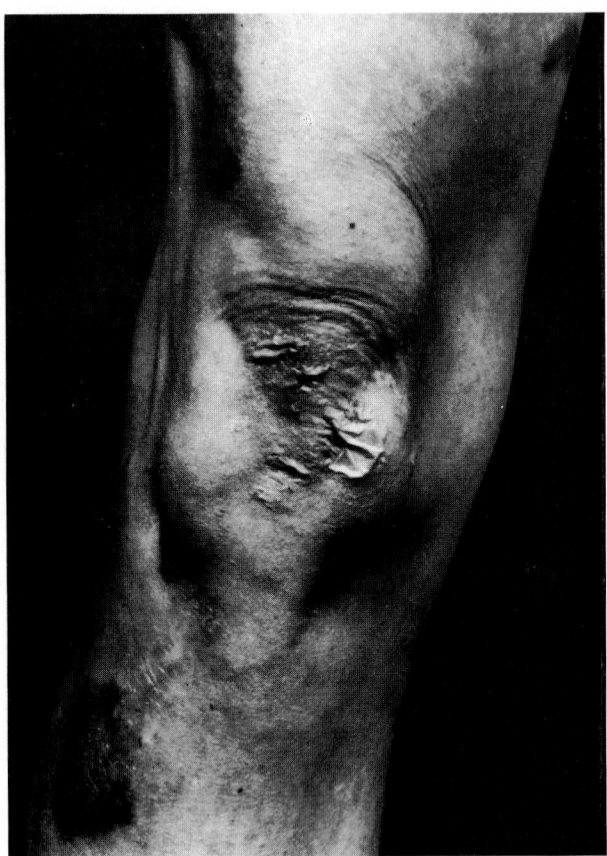

FIGURE 157-6 Atrophic scarring and a pseudotumor in a patient with the Ehlers-Danlos syndrome.

In type VI EDS, collagen is hydroxylysine-deficient because of a deficiency of lysyl hydroxylase.[41,42] Although hydroxylysine-deficient collagen is efficiently secreted, it is not capable of normal cross-linking[43]; hydroxylysine is essential for collagen cross-linking. A mutant lysyl hydroxylase has been found to have abnormal thermal stability and altered affinity for its cofactor, ascorbic acid.[44] A second mutant enzyme had normal thermal and kinetic behavior.[45]

In type VII EDS, conversion of type I procollagen to collagen is abnormal; the result is persistence of the aminoterminal propeptide. The incompletely cleaved procollagen is unable to participate in normal fibrillogenesis and collagen cross-linking. The disorder may result from mutations deleting the cleavage site in either $pro\alpha1(I)$ or $pro\alpha2(I)$ collagen[46] or from abnormal procollagen N-proteinase activity.[47] Defects resulting from a mutant cleavage enzyme have been difficult to confirm because of difficulty in detecting the enzyme in cells and tissue.

In type IX EDS, an abnormality in copper metabolism causes deficient lysyl oxidase activity.[48,49] This copper-dependent enzyme is necessary for collagen cross-linking. Lysyl oxidase deficiency has also been described in some patients with type V EDS,[50] but is normal in others.[51] In type X EDS, abnormal platelet aggregation appears to be associated with a fibronectin abnormality.[23]

Pseudoxanthoma Elasticum

Pseudoxanthoma elasticum is a genetic disorder of connective tissue characterized by progressive mineralization of elastic fibers.[52]

The disorder consists of characteristic skin lesions involving flexural sites, ocular involvement (angioid streaks and retinal hemorrhage), and cardiovascular manifestations (gastrointestinal hemorrhage, hypertension and occlusive vascular disease). The disease may be inherited as an autosomal dominant or autosomal recessive trait and has a prevalence estimated at 1 in 100,000.[52] The cause of the disorder is unknown. Progressive calcification and fragmentation of elastic fibers in skin, in Bruch's membrane in the eye, and in blood vessels appear to be responsible for the clinical manifestations of the disorder.

Clinical Manifestations

Skin Yellowish papules giving a "plucked chicken" appearance in flexural skin occur at an average age of 13.5 years.[53] Commonly affected areas include antecubital, popliteal, inguinal, neck, axillae, and periumbilical areas, as well as oral, vaginal, and rectal mucosa (Fig. 157-7). Involvement may be progressive and involve the entire skin. In time, the skin may become lax and hang in folds, particularly in the neck, axillae, and groin. Plastic surgery can ordinarily be undertaken without complication, although calcium-containing material may be extruded.[54] Diagnosis can be made by biopsy of affected skin. The characteristic histology consists of fragmentation and calcification of elastic fibers in the middle and lower third of the dermis (Fig. 157-8). Although normal elastic fibers do not stain with hematoxylin/eosin, altered elastic fibers in pseudoxanthoma elasticum stain blue because of their calcium content. Elastosis perforans serpiginosa may coexist in patients with pseudoxanthoma elasticum.[53]

Eye Angioid streaks, the characteristic ocular lesion of pseudoxanthoma elasticum, are red to brown curvilinear bands radiating from the optic disk. Although they are irregular and generally wider, they are often mistaken for blood vessels. They occur commonly in patients with pseudoxanthoma elasticum (85%), but may be found in those with other conditions, including Paget's disease of bone and sickle-cell disease.[56] Angioid streaks apparently result from breaks in Bruch's membrane associated with faulty elastic fibers in its outer portion, the lamina elasticum. Fibrovascular ingrowth may result in retinal hemorrhage, detachment, and severe visual loss. Because laser repair may be sight-sparing, early diagnosis and regular examination are critically important. Other ocular lesions include a characteristic yellowish mottling of the posterior pole called "leopard spotting" and a reticular pigmentary pattern in the retina.[57]

Vascular Disease Calcification of the elastic media of blood vessels with subsequent intimal proliferation leads to serious complications in this disorder. Claudication is the most common problem; pulses in adults are often obliterated. Angina pectoris or abdominal angina may become incapacitating. Hypertension is prevalent in adults[52] and appears to be associated with renal artery involvement. It may occur early in the disease.

Gastrointestinal hemorrhage, apparently due to fragile submucosal vessels, may occur early and often is the presenting sign. Bleeding may also occur in the urinary tract. For unknown reasons, cerebrovascular disease appears to be less common than expected.

Other Despite an abundance of elastic tissue, lungs are not prominently affected in pseudoxanthoma elasticum.[52] Pregnancy is surprisingly uncomplicated; hemorrhage is generally not a problem.[58] The rate of first trimester miscarriage may be increased.[58]

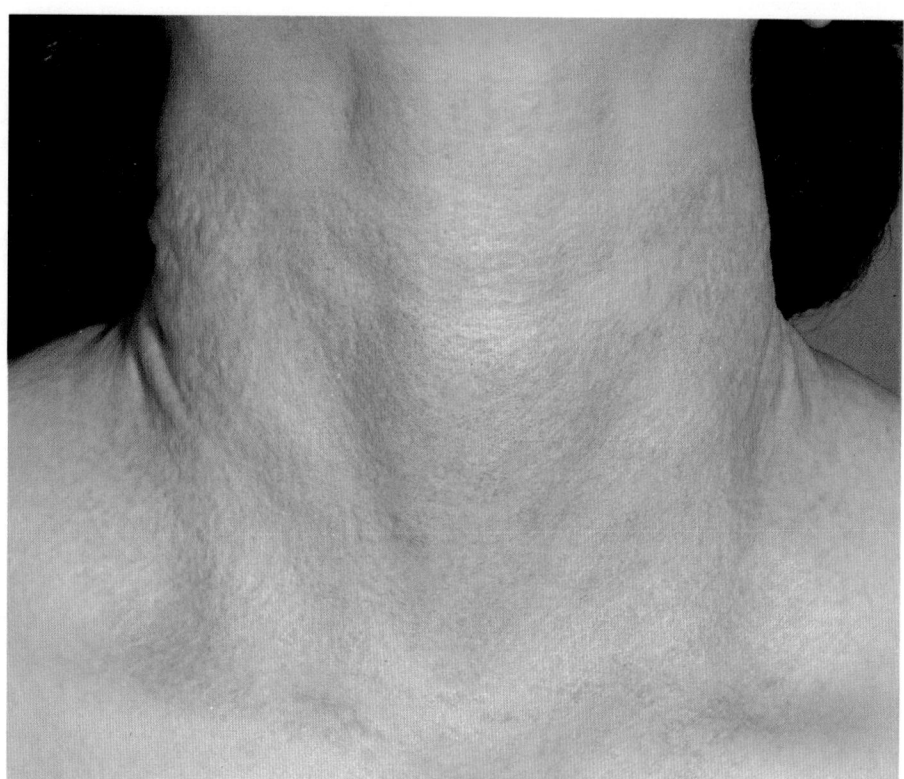

FIGURE 157-7 Pseudoxanthoma elasticum. Papules on the neck. There is a distinct yellowish hue. Loose, thickened skin with a pebbled appearance on the neck.

Basic Defect

Although the basic defect in pseudoxanthoma elasticum is un-known, there is a progressive calcification of elastin with fragmentation of elastic fibers in the area of calcification.[59] In dermal blood vessels, abnormal elastin in the internal elastic lamina may be detected in the absence of mineralization.[60] Abnormal amounts of proteoglycans have been detected in skin and urine of patients with pseudoxanthoma elasticum.[61] Abnormal proteolytic[62] and elastolytic[63] activity have been reported in dermal fibroblasts from patients with the disorder. Skin changes consistent with pseudoxanthoma elasticum have been reported in patients with cystinuria who are taking D-penicillamine.[64] Penicillamine can inhibit intermolecular cross linking of collagen and elastin. The severity of pseudoxanthoma elasticum may be influenced by calcium ingestion.[52,65]

Genetics

Two autosomal dominant and three autosomal recessive forms of pseudoxanthoma elasticum have been reported (Table 157-3).[66-69]

Most patients appear to inherit their disorder as an autosomal recessive trait, although new dominant mutations cannot be excluded. The least common form of the disorder involves skin only and presents with generalized skin sagging clinically similar to cutis laxa.[70]

Cutis Laxa (Dermatochalasis, Generalized Elastolysis)

Cutis laxa is a rare group of disorders in which the skin hangs loosely in folds, causing a prematurely aged appearance. The disorder may be inherited (autosomal dominant, autosomal recessive, or X-linked recessive) or acquired.

Clinical Manifestations

Skin In cutis laxa, the skin gives the appearance of being too large for the rest of the body. It tends to sag in areas where the skin is

TABLE 157-3
Pseudoxanthoma Elasticum

Clinical characteristics		AD1 (N = 12)	AD2 (N = 52)	AR1 (N = 54)	AR2 (N = 3)	AR3 (N = 39)
Skin	Classic flexural	100%	24%	77%	—	100%
	Generalized	—	—	100%	—	—
Cardiovascular system	Hypertension	75%	7.8%	19.7%	—	41%
	Angina/claudication	56%	—	—	—	20.5%
Opthalmic manifestations	Angioid streaks	34%	47%	47%	—	76.9%
	Retinal deterioration	75%	7.8	35%	—	51.3%
Marfanoid features	High arched palate, loose jointedness, blue scleras	—	50%	10%	—	—

Note: AD = autosomal dominant, AR = autosomal recessive.
Source: Adapted from Viljoen et al.[58]

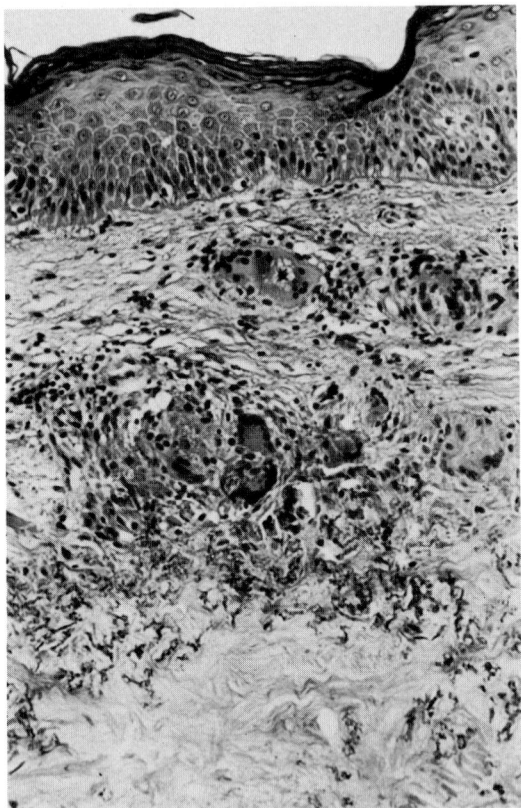

FIGURE 157-8 Pseudoxanthoma elasticum. The pathology affects the connective tissue of most of the reticular dermis. Even in routine hematoxylin and eosin preparations one may see the tightly, but irregularly coiled, basophilic elastic fibers. The collagen associated with the fibrils is also abnormal; the broad collagen bundles so characteristic of the reticular dermis are replaced by irregular and rather confluent collagen fibrils. ×160. (*Micrograph by Wallace H. Clark, Jr., M.D.*)

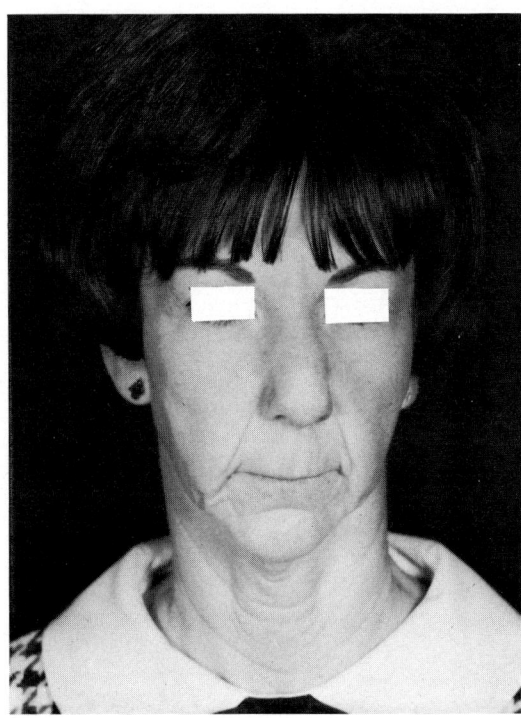

FIGURE 157-9 Cutis laxa in a 15-year-old girl. The skin hangs in loose folds, giving the appearance of premature aging. (*Courtesy of Peter Beighton, M.D.*)

normally loose, e.g., around the face and eyes (Fig. 157-9). Sagging jowls may result in a "bloodhound" look. The skin may be excessively wrinkled and appear prematurely aged. At birth, the skin may be noticeably soft, loose, and hyperextensible; in contrast to the skin of EDS, it returns slowly to its normal position after being stretched. Skin fragility, easy bruisability, joint hypermobility, and poor wound healing are not usually associated with cutis laxa. Cosmetic surgery can ordinarily be undertaken without complication.

Other Features Beighton[71] pointed out characteristic facial features including a hooked nose, inverted nostrils, and a long upper lip. The cry of an affected infant may be hoarse, and a low-pitched voice is often associated with redundancy of the vocal chords. Hernias (inguinal, umbilical, and obturator) as well as diverticula of the gastrointestinal and genitourinary tracts are common.[72] Angiographic studies in patients with cutis laxa have revealed tortuous blood vessels with a peculiar corkscrew appearance.[73] Aortic dilation and peripheral pulmonary artery stenosis have been described. The most severe manifestation of cutis laxa is progressive emphysema which may lead to early death from cor pulmonale. One form of cutis laxa is associated with growth retardation and congenital hip dislocation.[74–77]

Basic Defect

Elastic fibers are fragmented and diminished in number in the skin of patients with cutis laxa.[78,79] In addition, collagen fiber morphology may be defective.[80] In skin fibroblasts from some patients with cutis laxa, levels of elastin production as well as mRNA for elastin may be diminished.[81,82] Structural mutations in elastin have not yet been identified. In one patient markedly elevated serum elastolytic activity was reported.[83] An X-linked form of cutis laxa associated with diminished lysyl oxidase activity and abnormal copper metabolism has been reclassified as type IX EDS.[84,85]

Genetics

Autosomal dominant, autosomal recessive, and X-linked recessive forms of cutis laxa are recognized. The dominant form of cutis laxa is basically a cosmetic problem and the prognosis is good. Onset may be delayed and appear to be an acquired defect. One autosomal recessive form of cutis laxa is associated with severe cardiorespiratory complications and early death.[71] Another less severe form is characterized by growth retardation and ligamentous laxity.[74–77] X-linked cutis laxa (type IX EDS) is characterized by mild joint laxity, bladder diverticula, hernias, and cranial occipital exostoses or horns.[85] Acquired forms of cutis laxa have been reported, often following an ill-defined febrile illness.[86–89]

Cutis laxa may occur in offspring of mothers taking penicillamine for cystinuria.[90] Penicillamine is known to interfere with cross-linking of collagen and elastin. Other inherited disorders with cutis laxa as an associated feature include De Barsy syndrome, Patterson syndrome (McKusick 16917), "wrinkly skin" syndrome, geroderma osteodysplastica, pseudoxanthoma elasticum, and SCARF syndrome.[91] Cutis laxa may also be associated with amyloidosis and plasma cell dyscrasia.[92]

Genetic Mucopolysaccharidoses

The mucopolysaccharide storage diseases[93] or mucopolysaccharidoses are hereditary disorders characterized by the progressive accumulation of mucopolysaccharides (glycosaminoglycans) in various tissues. Each of those outlined in Table 157-4 is caused by deficiency of a specific lysosomal enzyme normally involved in the degradation of one or more species of mucopolysaccharide. Ten enzymatically distinct types of mucopolysaccharidosis have been identified and most appear to have allelic variants. In most of these conditions the skin is diffusely thickened and hirsute. Pebbly lesions overlie the inferior end of the scapulae in Hunter's syndrome (MPS II).

Pathophysiology

Lysosomes are the disposal and reclamation systems of the cell. The mucopolysaccharidoses (and some other conditions discussed in this book such as Fabry's disease) fulfill the criteria for lysosomal storage disease as defined by Hers.[94]

1. As seen by electron microscopy, the cellular inclusions are bound by single membranes and stain positively for acid phosphatase.
2. The disorders are progressive.
3. Multiple organs are affected.
4. The stored material is biochemically heterogeneous, e.g., both dermatan sulfate and heparin sulfate in MPS I and II.

Mucopolysaccharides consist of a protein core to which is attached multiple side chains made up of alternating uronic acid and hexosamine residues, some of which are sulfated. The side chains are digested by enzymes that work sequentially. Thus, even though different enzymes are deficient in Hurler (MPS I) and Hunter (MPS II) syndromes, the same two mucopolysaccharides appear in excess in the urine because each of the two enzymes is involved at a distinct and different point in the degradation of these mucopolysaccharides.

Neufeld and her colleagues performed the now famous complementation experiments (reviewed by Newton et al.[93]), with cells of patients with different forms of mucopolysaccharidosis. Cocultivation of fibroblasts from different mucopolysaccharidoses led to mutual cross-correction of the abnormal intracellular retention of ^{35}S mucopolysaccharides. Surprisingly, Hurler and Scheie syndromes, previously considered separate entities called MPS I and V, respectively, were found not to cross-correct, indicating that they have the same defect; phenotypically indistinguishable cases

TABLE 157-4
Classification of the Mucopolysaccharidoses

Number	Eponym	Clinical manifestations	Enzyme deficiency	Glycosaminoglycan affected
MPS I H	Hurler	Corneal clouding, dysostosis multiplex, organomegaly, heart disease, mental retardation, death in childhood	α-L-iduronidase	Dermatan sulfate, heparan sulfate
MPS I S	Scheie	Corneal clouding, stiff joints, normal intelligence and life span	α-L-iduronidase	Dermatan sulfate, heparan sulfate
MPS I H/S	Hurler-Scheie	Phenotype intermediate between I H and I S	α-L-iduronidase	Dermatan sulfate, heparan sulfate
MPS II (severe)	Hunter (severe)	Dysostosis multiplex, organomegaly, no corneal clouding, mental retardation, death before 15 years	Iduronate sulfatase	Dermatan sulfate, heparan sulfate
MPS II (mild)	Hunter (mild)	Normal intelligence, short stature survival from 20s to 60s	Iduronate sulfatase	Dermatan sulfate, heparan sulfate
MPS III A	Sanfilippo A	Profound mental deterioration, hyperactivity, relatively mild somatic manifestations	Heparan N-sulfatase	Heparan sulfate
MPS III B	Sanfilippo B	Phenotype similar to III A	α-N-acetylglucosaminidase	Heparan sulfate
MPS III C	Sanfilippo C	Phenotype similar to III A	Acetyl-CoA:α-glucosaminide acetyl transferase	Heparan sulfate
MPS III D	Sanifilippo D	Phenotype similar to III A	N-acetylglucosamine 6-sulfatase	Heparan sulfate
MPS IV A	Morquio A	Distinctive skeletal abnormalities, corneal clouding, odontoid hypoplasia; milder forms known to exist	Galactose 6-sulfatase	Keratan sulfate, chondroitin 6-sulfate
MPS IV B	Morquio B	Spectrum of severity as in IV A	β-Galactosidase	Keratan sulfate
MPS VI	Maroteaux-Lamy	Dysostosis multiplex, corneal clouding, normal intelligence; survival to teens in severe form; milder forms known to exist	N-acetylgalactosamine 4-sulfatase (arylsulfatase B)	Dermatan sulfate
MPS VII	Sly	Dysostosis multiplex, hepatosplenomegaly; wide spectrum of severity	β-Glucuronidase	Dermatan sulfate, heparan sulfate, chondroitin 4- and 6-sulfates

of Sanfilippo syndrome (MPS III) were found to be of several different types, on the basis of mutual cross-correction.

Several classes of mucopolysaccharidoses are now identified through demonstration of deficiency of ten specific lysosomal enzymes (Table 157-4). α-Iduronidase is the enzyme deficiency in the MPS I group of conditions and includes Hurler and Scheie syndromes which are thought to be allelic, i.e., due to homozygosity for different mutant genes at the same locus. Several of the other forms of MPS also have alleles that result in severe and mild forms. In the case of the MPS I class, genetic compounds are suspected, i.e., patients who have a Hurler gene on one chromosome and a Scheie gene on the other; cases of an intermediate phenotype that may represent the genetic compound at the α-L-iduronidase locus have been identified.

Clinical Manifestations

Table 157-4 summarizes the clinical manifestations for each of the mucopolysaccharidoses. Clinical manifestations are primarily in the eye, heart, brain, bony skeleton, skin, and other systems.

Eye Corneal clouding occurs in all forms except MPS II and III and is only minor in MPS IV. A pigmentary retinal degeneration develops in the Scheie (MPS I S) and Hunter (MPS II) syndromes, and glaucoma is a complication particularly of MPS I S. Chronic papilledema is a feature of Hunter syndrome (MPS II.)

Heart A pseudoatherosclerosis develops from intimal deposition of mucopolysaccharides, and coronary insufficiency (angina pectoris) may occur in children with Hurler syndrome (MPS I H). The major cardiac problems, other than cor pulmonale, are valvular and occur in most of the polysaccharidoses. Aortic valve disease is a feature, for example, of Scheie syndrome (MPS I S), and patients with the mild variety of MPS VI have required valve replacement. Patients with MPS IV have had aortic regurgitation.

Brain Progressive deterioration of intellect is a cardinal feature of (MPS I H) and Sanfilippo syndromes. In Scheie's (MPS I S) and Maroteaux-Lamy syndromes (MPS VI) intellect is normal or near normal. In the mild form of Hunter syndrome (MPS II), intellectual capacity is normal in some areas such as computational function, but abnormal in other areas such as verbal performance; in the severe form of MPS II, intellectual function is progressively and severely reduced.

Hydrocephalus is frequent in MPS I and severe MPS II. Arachnoid cysts erode in the area of the sella turcica. In the case of the Hurler-Scheie compound syndrome, erosion into the nasal cavity with chronic spinal fluid rhinorrhea has been noted.

Skeleton The changes in the bony skeleton are generically referred to as dysostosis multiplex. The skeletal x-rays of most patients with the mucopolysaccharidoses have similar features with varying degrees of severity.

Skin The only truly distinctive skin change of the mucopolysaccharidoses is the "pebbling" over the inferior angle of the scapulae in MPS II (Hunter syndrome). In addition, a generalized thickening of the skin is found in most of the conditions. Generalized hirsutism is also a striking feature of most, perhaps all, of the mucopolysaccharidoses. Meyer et al.[95] showed that rabbits injected with mucopolysaccharides grew hair in shaved areas more rapidly than did untreated rabbits.

Genetics

All the mucopolysaccharidoses are recessive and all except MPS II are autosomal recessive. Hunter syndrome is classically X-linked recessive. Multiple allelic forms of individual mucopolysaccharidoses with different phenotypes (the Hurler-Scheie phenomenon) have been identified, as well as the same phenotype resulting from different enzyme deficiencies (Sanfilippo syndrome).

References

1. Byers PH: Disorders of collagen biosynthesis and structure, in *The Metabolic Basis of Inherited Diseases*, 6th ed., edited by CR Scriver, et al., New York, McGraw-Hill, 1989, p 2805
2. McKusick VA: *Heritable Disorders of Connective Tissue*, 4th ed. St. Louis, Mosby, 1972, p 292
3. Pyeritz RE: Marfan Syndrome, in *Principles and Practice of Medical Genetics*, edited by AEH Emery, DL Rimion, Edinburgh, Churchill Livingstone, 1983, p 820
4. Haber J: Miescher's elastoma (elastoma intrapapillare perforans verruciforme). *Br J Dermatol* 71:85, 1959
5. Sakai LY et al: Fibrillin, a new 350-kD glycoprotein, is a component of extracellular microfibrils. *J Cell Biol* 103:2499, 1986
6. Hollister DW et al: Immunohistologic abnormalities of the microfibrillar-fiber system in the Marfan syndrome. *N Engl J Med* 323:152, 1990
7. Kaimulainen K et al: Location on chromosome 15 of the gene defect causing Marfan syndrome. *N Engl J Med* 323:935, 1990
8. Lee B et al: Linkage of Marfan syndrome and a phenotypically related disorder to two different fibrillin genes. *Nature* 352:330, 1991
9. Abbot MH et al: Psychiatric manifestations of homocystinuria due to cystathionine beta-synthase deficiency: Prevalence, natural history, and relationship to neurologic impairment and vitamin B_6 responsiveness. *Am J Med Genet* 26:959, 1990
10. Harris ED Jr, Sjoerdsma A: Effect of penicillamine on human collagen and its possible application to treatment of scleroderma. *Lancet* 2:996, 1966
11. Mudd SH et al: Disorders of transsulfuration, in *The Metabolic Basis of Inherited Diseases*, 6th ed., edited by CR Scriver et al., New York, McGraw-Hill, 1989, p 693
12. Sillence DO et al: Genetic heterogeneity in osteogenesis imperfecta. *J Med Genet* 16:101, 1979
13. Smith R: *The Brittle Bone Syndrome: Osteogenesis Imperfecta*. London, Butterworths, 1983
14. Byers PH: *Trends Genet* 6:293, 1990
15. Prockop DJ: Mutations that alter the primary structure of type I collagen. *J Biol Chem* 265:15349, 1990
16. Rowe DW et al: Diminished type I collagen synthesis and reduced $\alpha 1$(I) collagen messenger RNA in cultured fibroblasts from patients with dominantly inherited (type I) osteogenesis imperfecta. *J Clin Invest* 76:504, 1985
17. Willing MC et al: Frameshift mutation near the 3' end of the COLA1A gene of the type I collagen predicts an elongated proα1(I) chain and results in osteogenesis imperfecta. *J Clin Invest* 85:282, 1990
18. Wenstrup RJ et al: Distinct biochemical phenotypes predict clinical severity in nonlethal variants of osteogenesis imperfecta. *Am J Hum Genet* 46:975, 1990
19. Beighton P. *The Ehlers-Danlos Syndrome*. London, Heinemann, 1970
20. McKusick VA. *Heritable Disorders of Connective Tissue*. St. Louis, Mosby, 1972
21. Rudd NL et al: Pregnancy complications in type IV Ehlers-Danlos syndrome. *Lancet* 1:50, 1983
22. Wenstrup RJ et al: Ehlers-Danlos syndrome type VI: Clinical manifes-

tations of lysyl hydroxylase deficiency. *J Pediatrics* **151**:145, 1989

23. Arneson MA et al: A new form of Ehlers-Danlos syndrome: Fibronectin corrects defective platelet function. *JAMA* **244**:144, 1980

24. Junqueira LCU, Roscoe JT: Reduced collagen content and fibre bundle disorganization in skin biopsies of patients with Ehlers-Danlos syndrome. *Histochemistry* **17**:1197, 1985

25. Sasaki T et al: Ehlers-Danlos syndrome: A variant characterized by the deficiency of proα2 chain of type I procollagen. *Arch Dermatol* **123**:76, 1987

26. Hata R et al: Existence of malfunctioning proα2(I) genes in a patient with a proα2(I)-chain-defective variant of Ehlers-Danlos syndrome. *J Biochem* **174**:231, 1988

27. Kojima T et al: Case report and study of collagen metabolism in Ehlers-Danlos syndrome type II. *J Dermatol* **15**:155, 1988

28. Superti-Furga A et al: Molecular defects of type III procollagen in Ehlers-Danlos syndrome type IV. *Hum Genet* **82**:104, 1989

29. Anonymous: Type III collagen deficiency. *Lancet* **2**:197, 1989

30. Vitellaro-Zuccarello L et al: Ultrastructural study of the dermis in a case of type IV Ehlers-Danlos syndrome. *J Submicrosc Cytol* **17**:695, 1985

31. Crowther MA et al: Vascular collagen fibril morphology in type IV Ehlers-Danlos syndrome. *Connective Tissue Res* **25**:209, 1991

32. Vissing H et al: Multiexon deletion in the procollagen III gene is associated with mild Ehlers-Danlos syndrome type IV. *J Biol Chem* **266**:5244, 1991

33. Superti-Furga A et al: Ehlers-Danlos syndrome type IV: A multi-exon deletion in one of the two COL3A1 alleles affecting structure, stability, and processing of type III procollagen. *J Biol Chem* **263**:6226, 1988

34. Tromp G et al: A single base mutation that substitutes serine for glycine 790 of the α1(III) chain of type III procollagen exposes an arginine and causes Ehlers-Danlos syndrome IV. *J Biol Chem* **264**:1349, 1989

35. Tromp G et al: Single base mutation in the type III procollagen gene that conveys the codon for glycine 883 to aspartate in a mild variant of Ehlers-Danlos syndrome IV. *J Biol Chem* **264**:19313, 1989

36. Lee B et al: G to T transposition at position +5 of a splice donor site causes skipping of the preceding exon in the type III procollagen transcripts of a patient with Ehlers-Danlos syndrome type IV. *J Biol Chem* **266**:5256, 1991

37. Kuivaniemi H et al: Identical G^{+1} to A mutations in three different introns of the type III procollagen gene (COL3A1) produce different patterns of RNA splicing in three variants of Ehlers-Danlos syndrome IV. *J Biol Chem* **265**:12067, 1990

38. Kontusaari S et al: Inheritance of an RNA splicing mutation ($G^{+1\ IVS20}$) in the type III procollagen gene (COL3AI) in a family having aortic aneurysms and easy bruisability: Phenotypic overlap between familial arterial aneurysms and Ehlers-Danlos syndrome type IV. *Am J Hum Genet* **47**:112, 1990

39. Cole WG et al: A base substitution at a splice site in the COL3AI gene causes exon skipping and generates abnormal type III procollagen in a patient with Ehlers-Danlos syndrome type IV. *J Biol Chem* **265**:17070, 1990

40. Steinmann B et al: Ehlers-Danlos syndrome type IV: A subset of patients distinguished by low serum levels of the amino-terminal propeptide of type III procollagen. *Am J Med Genet* **34**:68, 1989

41. Pinnel SR et al: A heritable disorder of connective tissue: Hydroxylysine-deficient collagen disease. *N Engl J Med* **286**:1013, 1972

42. Krane SM et al: Lysyl-protocollagen hydroxylase deficiency in fibroblasts from siblings with hydroxylysine-deficient collagen. *Proc Natl Acad Sci USA* **69**:2899, 1972

43. Eyre DR, Glimcher MJ: Reducible crosslinks in hydroxylysine-deficient collagens of a heritable disorder of connective tissue. *Proc Natl Acad Sci USA* **69**:2594, 1972

44. Quinn KS, Krane SM: Abnormal properties of collagen lysyl hydroxylase from skin fibroblasts of siblings with hydroxylysine-deficient collagen. *J Clin Invest* **57**:83, 1976

45. Miller RL et al: Ascorbate action on normal and mutant human lysyl

hydroxylases from cultered dermal fibroblasts. *J Invest Dermatol* **72**:241, 1979

46. Vasan NS et al: A mutation in the proα2(I) gene (COL1A2) for type I procollagen in Ehlers-Danlos syndrome type VII: Evidence suggesting that skipping of exon 6 in RNA splicing may be a common cause of the phenotype. *Am J Hum Genet* **48**:305, 1991

47. Lichtenstein JR et al: Defect in conversion of procollagen to collagen in a form of the Ehlers-Danlos syndrome. *Science* **182**:298, 1973

48. Byers PH et al: X-linked cutis laxa. Defective cross-link formation in collagen due to decreased lysyl oxidase activity. *N Engl J Med* **303**:61, 1980

49. Peltonen L et al: Alterations in copper and collagen metabolism in the Menkes syndrome and a new subtype of the Ehlers-Danlos syndrome. *Biochemistry* **22**:6156, 1983

50. Di Ferrante N et al: Lysyl oxidase deficiency in Ehlers-Danlos syndrome type V. *Connective Tissue Res* **33**:49, 1975

51. Siegel RC et al: Cross-linking of collagen in the X-linked Ehlers-Danlos type V. *Biochem Biophys Res Commun* **88**:281, 1979

52. Neldner KH: Pseudoxanthoma elasticum. *Clin Dermatol* **6**:1, 1988

53. Neldner KH: Pseudoxanthoma elasticum. *Int J Dermatol* **27**:98, 1988

54. Viljoen DL et al: Plastic surgery in pseudoxanthoma elasticum: Experience in nine patients. *Plastic Reconstruct Surg* **85**:233, 1990

55. Smith EW et al: Reactive perforating elastosis: features of certain genetic disorders. *Bull Johns Hopkins Hosp* **111**:235, 1962

56. Connor PJ et al: Pseudoxanthoma elasticum and angioid streaks: A review of 106 cases. *Am J Med* **30**:537, 1961

57. McDonald HR et al: Reticular-like pigmentary patterns in pseudoxanthoma elasticum. *Opthalmology* **95**:306, 1988

58. Viljoen DL et al: The obstetric and gynaecological implications of pseudoxanthoma elasticum. *Br J Obstet Gynecol* **94**:884, 1987

59. Tsuji T: Three-dimensional architecture of altered dermal elastic fibers in pseudoxanthoma elasticum: Scanning electron microscopic studies. *J Invest Dermatol* **82**:518, 1984

60. Walker EA et al: The mineralization of elastic fibers and alterations of extracellular matrix in pseudoxanthoma elasticum. *Arch Dermatol* **125**:70, 1989

61. Longas MO et al: Glycosaminoglycans of skin and urine in pseudoxanthoma elasticum: Evidence for chondroitin 6-sulfate alteration. *Clin Chim Acta* **155**:227, 1986

62. Gordon SG et al: Cysteine protease characteristics of the proteoglycanase activity from normal and pseudoxanthoma elasticum (PXE) fibroblasts. *J Lab Clin Med* **102**:400, 1983

63. Schwartz E et al: Elastase-like protease and elastolytic activities expressed in cultured dermal fibroblasts derived from lesional skin of patients with pseudoxanthoma elasticum, actinic elastosis, and cutis laxa. *Clin Chim Acta* **176**:219, 1988

64. Meyrick Thomas RH et al: Elastosis perforans serpiginosa and pseudoxanthoma elasticum-like skin change to D-penicillamine. *Clin Exp Dermatol* **10**:386, 1985

65. Renie WA et al: Pseudoxanthoma elasticum: High calcium intake in early life correlates with severity. *Am J Med Genet* **19**:235, 1984

66. Pope FM: Autosomal dominant pseudoxanthoma elasticum. *J Med Genet* **11**:152, 1974

67. Pope FM: Two types of autosomal recessive pseudoxanthoma elasticum. *Arch Dermatol* **110**:209, 1974

68. Viljoen DL et al: Heterogeneity of pseudoxanthoma elasticum: Delineation of a new form? *Clin Genet* **32**:100, 1987

69. De Paepe A et al: Pseudoxanthoma elasticum: Similar autosomal recessive subtype in Belgian and Afrikaner families. *Am J Med Genet* **38**:16, 1991

70. Rongioletti F et al: Generalized pseudoxanthoma elasticum with deficiency of vitamin K-dependent clotting factors. *J Am Acad Dermatol* **21**:1150, 1989

71. Beighton P: The dominant and recessive forms of cutis laxa. *J Med Genet* **9**:216, 1972

72. Gorlin RJ, Cohen MM: Craniofacial manifestations of Ehlers-Danlos syndromes, cutis laxa syndromes, and cutis laxa-like syndromes. *Birth Defects* **25**:39, 1990

73. Meine F et al: Radiographic findings in congenital cutis laxa. *Radiology* **113**:687, 1974

74. Sakati NO et al: Syndrome of cutis laxa, ligamentous laxity, and delayed development. *Pediatrics* **72**:850, 1983

75. Rogers JG, Danks DM: Cutis laxa with delayed development. *Aust Paediatr J* **21**:281, 1985

76. Patton MA et al: Congenital cutis laxa with retardation of growth and development. *J Med Genet* **24**:556, 1987

77. Ogur G et al: Syndrome of congenital cutis laxa with ligamentous laxity and delayed development: Report of a brother and sister from Turkey. *Am J Med Genet* **37**:6, 1990

78. Hashimoto K, Kanzaki T: Cutis laxa: Ultrastructural and biochemical studies. *Arch Dermatol* **111**:861, 1975

79. Oku T et al: Congenital cutis laxa. *Dermatologica* **179**:79, 1989

80. Marchase P et al: A familial cutis laxa syndrome with ultrastructural abnormalities of collagen and elastin. *J Invest Dermatol* **75**:399, 1980

81. Olsen DR et al: Cutis laxa: Reduced elastin gene expression in skin fibroblast cultures as determined by hybridizations with a homologous cDNA and an exon 1-specific oligonucleotide. *J Biol Chem* **263**:6464, 1988

82. Sephel GC et al: Heterogeneity of elastin expression in cutis laxa fibroblast stains. *J Invest Dermatol* **93**:147, 1989

83. Anderson LL et al: Characterization and partial purification of a neutral protease from the serum of a patient with autosomal recessive pulmonary emphysema and cutis laxa. *J Lab Clin Med* **105**:537, 1985

84. Byers PH et al: X-linked cutis laxa. Defective cross-link formation in collagen due to decreased lysyl oxidase activity. *N Engl J Med* **303**:61, 1980

85. Kaitila II et al: A skeletal and connective tissue disorder associated with lysyl oxidase deficiency and abnormal copper metabolism, in *Skeletal Dysplasias*, edited by CJ Papadatos, CS Bartsocas. New York, Alan R. Liss, 1982, p 307

86. Reed WB et al: Acquired cutis laxa. Primary generalized elastolysis. *Arch Dermatol* **103**:661, 1971

87. Verhagen AR, Woerderman MJ: Post-inflammatory elastolysis and cutis laxa. *Br J Dermatol* **92**:183, 1975

88. Lewis PG et al: Postinflammatory elastolysis and cutis laxa. *J Am Acad Dermatol* **22**:40, 1990

89. Koch SE, Williams ML: Acquired cutis laxa: Case report and review of disorders of elastolysis. *Ped Dermatol* **2**:282, 1985

90. Rosa FW: Teratogen update: Penicillamine. *Teratology* **33**:127, 1986

91. Koppe R et al: Ambiguous genitalia associated with skeletal abnormalities, cutis laxa, craniostenosis, psychomotor retardation, and facial abnormalities (SCARF syndrome). *Am J Med Genet* **34**:305, 1989

92. Newton JA et al: Cutis laxa associated with amyloidosis. *Clin Exp Derm* **2**:87, 1986

93. Neufeld EF, Muenzer J: The mucopolysaccharidoses, in *The Metabolic Basis of Inherited Diseases*, 6th ed., edited by CR Scriver et al. New York, McGraw-Hill, 1989, p 1565

94. Hers H: Inborn lysosomal disease. *Gastroenterology* **48**:625, 1965

95. Meyer K et al: Effect of acid mucopolysaccharides on hair growth in rabbit. *Proc Soc Exp Biol Med* **108**:59, 1961

CHAPTER 158

Kenneth H. Kraemer

Heritable Diseases with Increased Sensitivity to Cellular Injury

A group of heritable diseases with differing clinical features share the common characteristics of in vitro or in vivo cellular hypersensitivity to damage by some physical or chemical agents (Table 158-1). Diseases with autosomal recessive, X-linked, and autosomal dominant inheritance fall in this group. These diseases include xeroderma pigmentosum, Cockayne syndrome, trichothiodystrophy, Bloom syndrome, Fanconi anemia, dyskeratosis congenita, basal cell nevus syndrome, ataxia-telangiectasia, and familial dysplastic nevus syndrome. Clinical abnormalities involve cutaneous, ocular, nervous, immune, hemopoietic, skeletal, or gastrointestinal systems. Some are associated with an increased incidence of neoplasia. Several have progressive degeneration of previously normal bodily functions.

The cellular hypersensitivity is often useful diagnostically. Furthermore, it may suggest pathogenic mechanisms and measures for therapeutic or prophylactic intervention. The molecular basis of the cellular hypersensitivity is just beginning to be understood in some of these disorders.

In this chapter, clinical features and laboratory abnormalities of seven of the heritable diseases with cellular hypersensitivity listed in Table 158-1 will be presented (ataxia-telangiectasia and familial dysplastic nevus syndrome are reviewed in Chaps. 184 and 81. The diseases will be discussed in terms of the systems affected, the cellular hypersensitivity, and the relevance of the cellular abnormality to the clinical symptoms. The major tests used to measure cellular hypersensitivity and to assess DNA repair are described in Chap. 69.

Xeroderma Pigmentosum

Xeroderma pigmentosum (XP) serves as the prototype heritable disease with increased sensitivity to cellular injury.[1-4] It is an autosomal recessive disease with sun sensitivity, photophobia, early onset of freckling, and subsequent neoplastic changes on sun-exposed surfaces. There is cellular hypersensitivity to ultraviolet (UV) radiation and to certain chemicals in association with abnormal DNA repair. Some patients have progressive neurologic degeneration.[3,5]

Frequency

Xeroderma pigmentosum occurs with an estimated frequency of 1:1,000,000 in the United States. It is more common in Japan.[1,4] Patients have been reported worldwide in all races including whites, Asians,[4] blacks, and Native Americans.[3] Consanguinity is common.

TABLE 158-1
Heritable Diseases with Cellular Hypersensitivity

Disease	Clinical abnormalities					Cellular abnormalities	
	Cutaneous	Ocular	Nervous	Hemo-poietic	Neoplasia*	Type*	Mechanism
Autosomal recessive							
Xeroderma pigmentosum	Sun sensitivity, atrophy, frecking	Photophobia, UV conjuncti-vitis, UV keratitis	Deafness, progressive mental deterioration	Normal	BCC, SCC, melanoma	UV-induced cell killing, mutagenesis, chromosome breakage, SCE	Abnormal DNA repair
Ataxia-telangiectasia	Telangiec-tasia, x-ray sensitivity	Conjunctival telangiec-tasia, oculomotor dyspraxia	Progressive ataxia	Humoral and cellular immune defects	Lympho-reticular, GI	Spontaneous chromosome breakage, x-ray-induced cell killing and chromosome breakage	Abnormal DNA repair?
Cockayne syndrome	Sun sensitivity	Retinal pigmentation	Progressive mental deterioration	Normal	None	UV-induced cell killing, SCE	Abnormal DNA repair
Trichothio-dystrophy	Sun sensitivity	Normal	Mental retardation	Normal	None	UV-induced cell killing	Abnormal DNA repair
Bloom syndrome	Telangiec-tasia, sun sensitivity	Normal	Normal	Defective immunity	Leukemia, GI	Spontaneous chromosome breakage	Abnormal DNA ligase?
Fanconi anemia	Hyperpig-mentation	Normal	Normal	Anemia	Leukemia, liver	Spontaneous chromosome breakage, diepoxybutane-induced chromosome breakage	Abnormal DNA cross-link repair
X-linked							
Dyskeratosis congenita	Poikeloderma, nail dystrophy	Stenosis of lacrimal duct	Normal	Anemia	GI	Psoralen-induced SCE	?
Autosomal dominant							
Basal cell nevus syndrome	Palmar pits, x-ray sensitivity	Cataract, coloboma	Mental retardation (some patients)	Normal	BCC, medullo-blastoma, ovarian tumors	UVB-induced cell killing (some patients)	?
Familial dysplastic nevus syndrome	Dysplastic nevi	Normal	Normal	Normal	Cutaneous melanoma	UV-induced cell killing, mutagenesis (some patients)	?

*BCC, basal cell carcinoma; SCC, squamous cell carcinoma; SCE, sister chromatid exchange; GI, gastrointestinal.

Clinical Features

Skin Approximately half of the XP patients have a history of acute sunburn reaction on minimal UV exposure. The other patients apparently tan normally without excessive burning. In all patients numerous freckle-like hyperpigmented macules appear (Fig. 158-1). The median age of onset of the cutaneous symptoms is between 1 and 2 years (Fig. 158-2).[3] These abnormalities are strikingly limited to sun-exposed areas (Fig. 158-1e). Continued sun exposure causes the patient's skin to become dry and parchment-like with increased pigmentation, hence the name *xeroderma pigmentosum* ("pigmented dry skin") (Fig. 158-1a). Premalignant actinic kera-

toses develop at an early age (Fig. 158-1b). The appearance of sun-exposed skin in children with XP is similar to that occurring in farmers and sailors after many years of extreme sun exposure.

Cancer Xeroderma pigmentosum patients under 20 years of age have a greater than 1000-fold increased risk of cutaneous basal cell or squamous cell carcinoma or melanoma.[3] The median age of onset of nonmelanoma skin cancer reported in XP patients was 8 years, in comparison to 60 years in the general population (Fig. 158-2).[3] Multiple primary cutaneous neoplasms, including melanomas, commonly occur.

Review of the world literature has revealed a substantial number of cases of oral cavity neoplasms, particularly squamous cell carcinoma of the tip of the tongue (a presumed sun-exposed location).[3,6] Brain (sarcoma and medulloblastoma), central nervous system (astrocytoma of the spinal cord),[7] lung, uterine, breast, pancreatic, gastric, renal,[8] and testicular tumors and leukemias have been reported in a few patients.[3] Overall, these reports suggest an approximate ten- to twentyfold increase in internal neoplasms in xeroderma pigmentosum.[3]

Eyes Ocular abnormalities are almost as common as the cutaneous abnormalities and are an important feature of XP[3] (Fig. 158-1*c*). The posterior portion of the eye (retina) is shielded from UV radia-

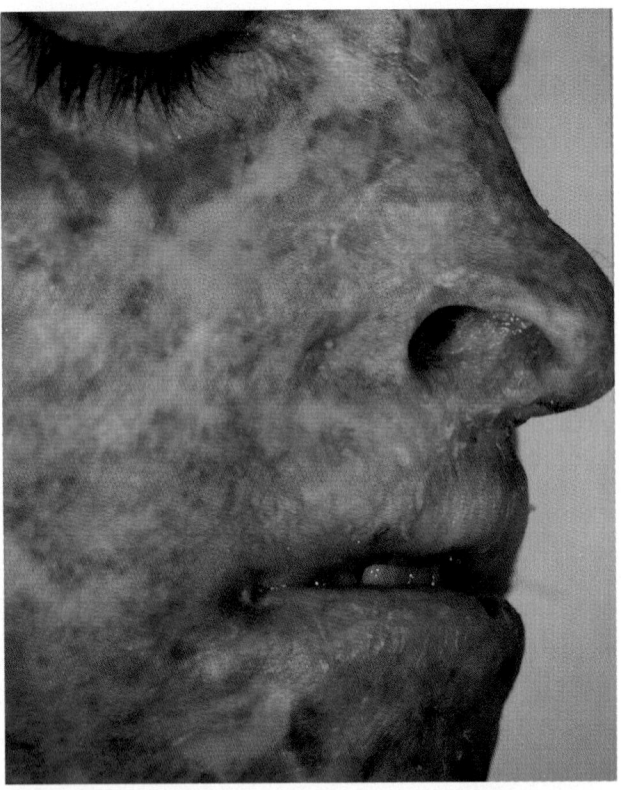

a

tion by the anterior portion (lids, cornea, and conjunctiva). Clinical findings are strikingly limited to these anterior, UV-exposed structures. Photophobia is often present and may be associated with prominent conjunctival injection. Continued UV exposure of the eye may result in severe keratitis, leading to corneal opacification and vascularization. The lids develop increased pigmentation and loss of lashes. Atrophy of the skin of the lids results in ectropion, entropion, or, in severe cases, complete loss of the lids. Benign conjunctival inflammatory masses or papillomas of the lids may be present. Epithelioma, squamous cell carcinoma, and melanoma of UV-exposed portions of the eye are common.[3,9]

Nervous System Neurologic abnormalities have been reported in approximately 30 percent of patients[1,3,5]; their onset may be early in infancy or, in some patients, delayed until the second decade. The neurologic abnormalities may be mild (e.g., isolated hyporeflexia) or severe, with progressive mental retardation, sensorineural deafness, spasticity, or seizures[1,3,5,10] (Fig. 158-1*d*). The most severe form, known as the DeSanctis-Cacchione syndrome, involves the cutaneous and ocular manifestations of classic XP plus additional neurologic and somatic abnormalities, including microcephaly, progressive mental deterioration, low intelligence, hyporeflexia or areflexia, choreoathetosis, ataxia, spasticity, Achilles tendon shortening with eventual quadraparesis, markedly retarded growth, and immature sexual development.[1,3,5] The complete DeSanctis-Cacchione syndrome has been recognized in very few patients; however, many XP patients have one or more of its neurologic features. In clinical practice, deep tendon reflex testing and routine audiometry can usually serve as a screen for the presence of XP-associated neurologic abnormalities.

The predominant neuropathologic abnormality found at autopsy in patients with neurologic symptoms was loss (or absence) of neurons, particularly in the cerebrum and cerebellum.[1,5,11] There is evidence for a primary axonal degeneration in these patients.[1,5,12]

Laboratory Abnormalities

There have been no consistent routine clinical laboratory abnormalities in patients with XP. Tests of cellular hypersensitivity to UV

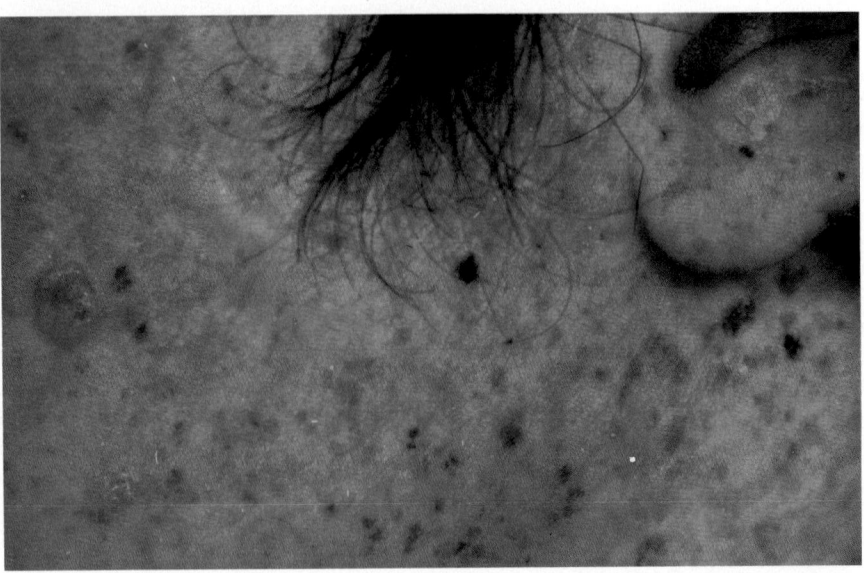

FIGURE 158-1 Xeroderma pigmentosum. (*a*) Pigmentary changes, atrophy, dryness, and cheilitis in a 16-year-old patient. (*b*) Cheek of a 14-year-old patient with pigmented macules of varying size and intensity, actinic keratosis, basal cell carcinoma, and a surgical scar. (*c*) Corneal clouding, prominent conjunctival blood vasculature, and loss of lashes. (*d*) A 26-year-old patient with deafness and mental retardation. (*e*) A myriad of pigmented macules of varying size and intensity and scattered achromic areas on the back of a 14-year-old patient, with marked sparing of sun-protected buttocks.

b

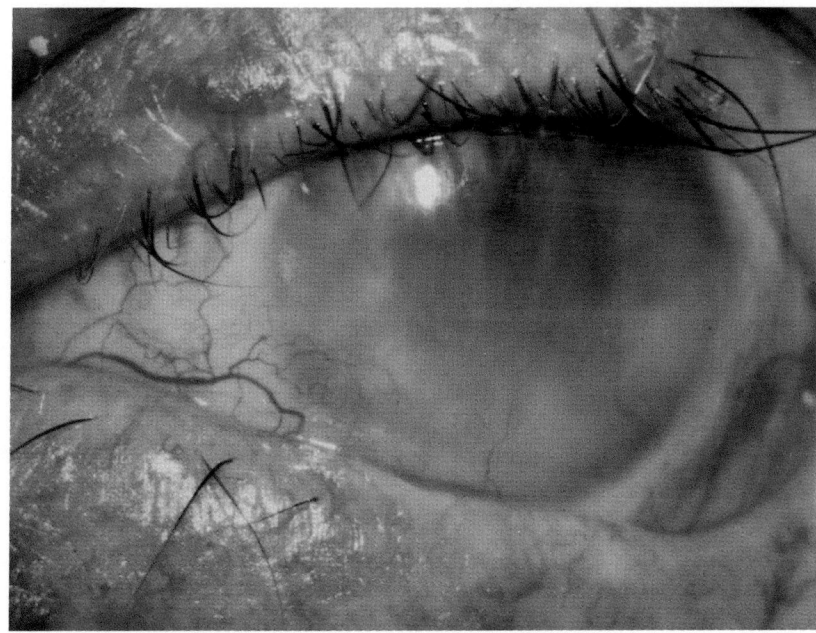

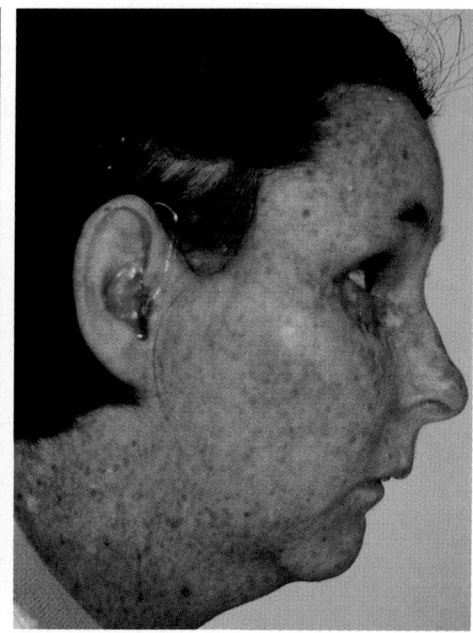

c   *d*

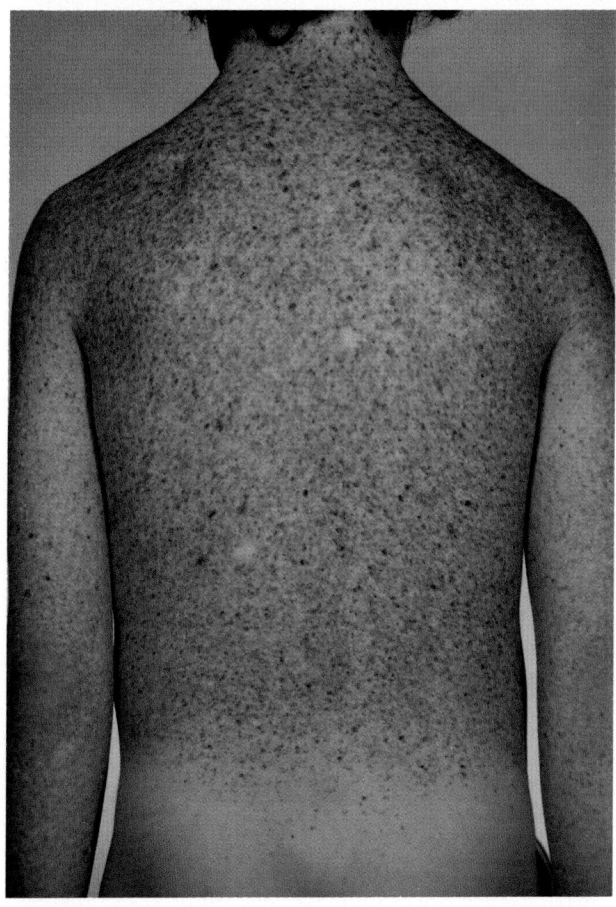

e

FIGURE 158-1 *(continued)*

damage, however, have shown uniformly abnormal results[1,2,13–15] (see also Chap. 69).

Cellular Hypersensitivity Cultured cells from XP patients generally grow normally when not exposed to damaging agents. How-

ever, the population growth rate (see Fig. 69-1) or single cell colony-forming ability (see Fig. 69-2) is reduced to a greater extent than normal following exposure to UV radiation. A range of post-UV colony-forming abilities has been found with fibroblasts from patients, some having extremely low post-UV colony-forming ability and others having nearly normal survival.[16]

Xeroderma pigmentosum fibroblasts are deficient in their ability to repair some UV-damaged viruses or plasmids to a functionally active state[1,2,17–19] (see Figs. 69-3, 69-4, and 69-5). These *host-cell reactivation* assays have detected an abnormality in every form of XP tested.

Ultraviolet-irradiated xeroderma pigmentosum fibroblasts produce more mutations per survivor than normal fibroblasts.[1,2] Xeroderma pigmentosum cells also introduce more mutations into UV-damaged plasmids than do normal cells[19] (see Fig. 69-5*b*). If prevented from dividing for an interval after irradiation, normal cells repair the damage induced with resultant increased survival and fewer mutants per survivor. This phenomenon has been called *potentially lethal damage recovery*. Xeroderma pigmentosum fibroblasts exhibit diminished or absent recovery from potentially lethal damage after UV irradiation, thereby indicating a defect in cellular recovery mechanisms.[2]

Chromosome Abnormalities Xeroderma pigmentosum cells are generally found to have a normal karyotype without excessive chromosome breakage or increased sister chromatid exchanges (see Fig. 69-7). Following exposure to UV radiation, however, an abnormally large increase in chromosome breakage and in sister chromatid exchanges have been observed.[1,2,20] The extent of this induced abnormality varies in different patients.

DNA Repair In 1968, the hypersensitivity of cultured XP cells to UV damage was reported by Cleaver[13] to be the result of defective DNA repair. He found defective UV-induced repair replication, indicating a defect in the nucleotide excision repair system (see Fig. 69-10). In 1970, Epstein et al.[21] demonstrated that the DNA repair defect was also present in vivo by measurements of unscheduled DNA synthesis in the skin of patients. The fact that most XP cells have a normal response to treatment with x-rays was interpreted as

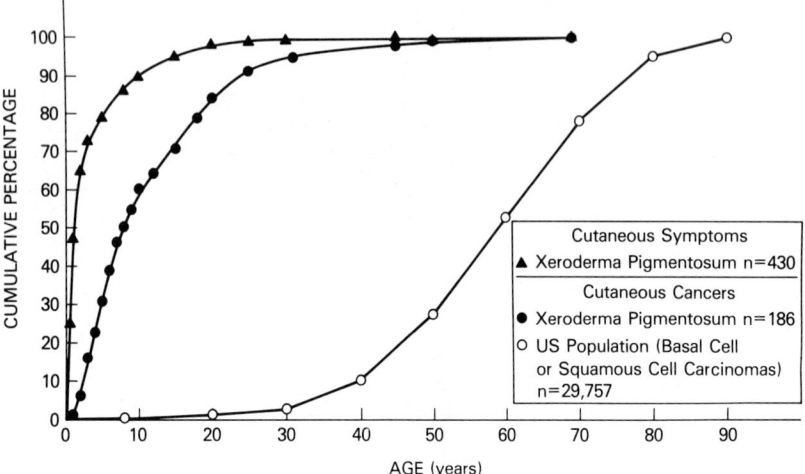

FIGURE 158-2 Xeroderma pigmentosum. Age at onset of clinical symptoms and skin cancers. Age at onset of cutaneous symptoms (generally sun sensitivity or pigmentation) was reported for 430 patients. Age at first skin cancer was reported for 186 patients and is compared with the age distribution for 29,757 patients with basal cell carcinoma or squamous cell carcinoma in the U.S. general population. (*From Kraemer et al.[3]*)

indicating that the UV DNA excision repair defect was at the level of endonuclease function. The repair system is probably more complex than indicated in Fig. 69-9. The defective genes for several forms of XP have been cloned[22–25] and their functions are being investigated.

Complementation Groups   In 1972, investigators in the Netherlands, by using cell fusion techniques (see Fig. 69-11), demonstrated genetic heterogeneity among the XP DNA repair defects.[26] They fused cultured fibroblasts from two different patients, then measured UV-induced unscheduled DNA synthesis. The unfused cells had the typical low level of UV-induced unscheduled DNA synthesis seen in most XP fibroblasts. Fusion of cells from certain pairs of patients resulted in the presence of fused cells with nearly normal levels of unscheduled DNA synthesis (see Fig. 69-12). In these heterokaryons each cell provides components that the other was lacking, resulting in enhanced DNA repair. These "complementing cells" thus have different DNA repair defects. Fibroblasts from patients with the same DNA repair defect do not correct each other when fused and are said to be in the same complementation group. In 1975, Kraemer et al.[27] reported that the first five comple-

mentation groups discovered had characteristic residual rates of UV-induced unscheduled DNA synthesis. They were named A through E in order of increasing DNA repair activity. Groups F and G were discovered more recently.[2] Their rates of unscheduled DNA synthesis overlap with groups C and A, respectively. Thus, assignment of cells to complementation groups must be based on fusion studies, not on the rate of DNA repair. Up to 1992, seven such DNA excision repair–deficient complementation groups have been identified (Table 158-2).

In 1971, Burk et al.[28] reported a patient with clinically severe XP who had normal unscheduled DNA synthesis in his fibroblasts, lymphocytes, and even his tumor cells.[1] This patient subsequently was termed an XP *variant*. Studies of cellular hypersensitivity revealed a slightly increased sensitivity to UV-induced inhibition of cell growth and colony-forming ability, to adenovirus host-cell reactivation,[17] and to UV-induced mutations in vitro. DNA repair studies revealed the presence of a defect in a second DNA repair system, that of postreplication repair (see Fig. 69-9).[2,15,29] Cells from this patient had a delayed rate of increase of the molecular weight of newly replicating DNA following UV irradiation. Furthermore, these cells were especially sensitive to inhibition of this

TABLE 158-2
Xeroderma Pigmentosum: Characteristics of DNA Repair Complementation Groups

Complementation group	Skin cancer	Neurologic abnormalities*	Number of patients, location†	DNA repair, % of normal	Gene cloned (chromosome location)
A	Yes	Severe or mild	63, Japan	<2	Yes (chr 9)
B	Yes	XP/CS	3, US, Europe	3–7	Yes (chr 2)
C	Yes	No	62, US, Europe, Egypt	10–25	No
D	Yes	Moderate	28, US, Europe	25–50	Yes (chr 19)
	No	TTD	6, US, Europe		
	Yes	XP/CS	1, France		
E	Yes	No	20, Europe, Japan	40–50	No
F	Yes	No	16, Japan, Europe	10–20	No (chr 15)
G	Yes	Yes	3, Europe, Japan	<5	No
	No	XP/CS	1, US		
Variant	Yes	No	54, US, Europe, Japan	100	No

*XP/CS, patients with XP–Cockayne syndrome complex; TTD, patients with trichothiodystrophy (without XP.)
†source: References 1, 2, 3, 4, and 85 and personal communications.

process by caffeine. Xeroderma pigmentosum variant patients have also been identified in Japan[4] and Europe.[30]

Prenatal Diagnosis This has been accomplished by measuring UV-induced unscheduled DNA synthesis in cultured amniotic fluid cells[31] (see Fig. 69-10).

Drug and Chemical Hypersensitivity Hypersensitivity responses to a number of DNA-damaging agents other than UV radiation have been found with XP cells (Table 158-3).[2,14,32,33] These agents include drugs (psoralens, chlorpromazine), cancer chemotherapeutic agents [platinum, bis(chloroethyl)nitrosourea (BCNU)], and chemical carcinogens (benzo[a]pyrene derivatives). Presumably, these agents induce DNA damage of which repair involves portions of the DNA repair pathways that are defective in patients with XP.

Treatment

Management of patients with XP is based on early diagnosis, lifelong protection from UV radiation exposure, and early detection and treatment of neoplasms. Diagnosis rests on clinical features and is confirmed by laboratory tests of cellular hypersensitivity.

Sun Protection Patients should be educated to protect all body surfaces from UV radiation by wearing protective clothing,[34] UV-absorbing glasses, and long hair-styles. They should adopt a lifestyle to minimize UV exposure and use sunscreens with high sun protective factor (SPF) ratings (minimum SPF 15) daily. Patients should be examined frequently by a family member who has been instructed in recognition of cutaneous neoplasms. A set of color photographs of the entire skin surface with close-ups of lesions (including a ruler) are often extremely useful to both the patient and the physician in detecting new lesions. Patients should be examined by a physician at frequent intervals, (about every 3 to 6 months depending on severity of skin disease). Premalignant lesions such as actinic keratoses may be treated by freezing with liquid nitrogen or with topical 5-fluorouracil. Larger areas have been treated with therapeutic dermatome shaving or dermabrasion to remove the more damaged superficial epidermal layers and permit repopulation by relatively UV-shielded cells from the follicles and glands.

Since cells from XP patients are also hypersensitive to environmental mutagens, such as benzo[a]pyrene found in cigarette smoke (Table 158-3), prudence dictates that patients should be protected against these agents. A patient who smoked cigarettes for

TABLE 158-3
Xeroderma Pigmentosum: DNA-Damaging Agents Inducing Cellular Hypersensitivity

Drugs
    Psoralens plus long-wavelength UV radiation (PUVA)
    Chlorpromazine
    Nitrofurantoin
    Mitomycin C
    Anthramycin
    Platinum
    Bis(chloroethyl)nitrosourea (BCNU)
Carcinogens
    Aflatoxin
    Benzo[a]pyrene
    Nitroquinoline oxide derivatives (4NQO)
    Acetoaminofluorene derivatives (AAF)
    Phenanthrene derivatives

more than 10 years died of bronchogenic carcinoma of the lungs at age 35.[3]

Cancers Cutaneous neoplasms are treated in the same manner as in patients who do not have XP. This involves electrodesiccation and curettage, surgical excision, or micrographic surgery. Because multiple surgical procedures are often necessary, removal of undamaged skin should be minimized. Extremely severe cases have been treated by excision of large portions of facial surface and grafting with uninvolved skin.[35]

Most XP patients are not abnormally sensitive to therapeutic x-rays. However, because cultured cells from a few patients were found to be hypersensitive to x-rays, when x-ray therapy is indicated, an initial small dose is advisable to test for clinical hypersensitivity.

High-dose oral isotretinoin has been shown to be effective in preventing new neoplasms in patients with multiple skin cancers.[7] Because of its toxicity (hepatic, hyperlipidemic, teratogenic, calcification of ligaments and tendons, premature closure of the epiphyses), oral isotretinoin should be reserved for XP patients who have had multiple skin cancers.

Eyes The eyes should be protected by wearing UV-absorbing glasses with side shields. Methylcellulose eye drops or soft contact lenses have been used to keep the cornea moist and to protect against mechanical trauma in patients with deformed eyelids. Corneal transplantation has restored vision in patients with severe keratitis with corneal opacity. Neoplasms of the lids, conjunctiva, and cornea are usually treated surgically.

Clinical-Laboratory Correlations

Patients with XP are hypersensitive to UV radiation and so are their cultured cells. Cutaneous and ocular abnormalities are strikingly limited to UV-exposed areas and usually spare such UV-shielded locations as the axillae, buttocks, and retina.

Complementation Groups At least eight different molecular defects are associated with the clinical abnormalities recognized as XP, as indicated by the existence of seven DNA excision repair-deficient complementation groups [A–G] and the variant form (Table 158-2).

Complementation group A contains patients with the most severe neurologic and somatic abnormalities (the DeSanctis-Cacchione syndrome) as well as patients with minimal or no neurologic abnormalities.[1,2,4] This form is seen in the United States, Europe, and the Middle East; it is the most common form of XP in Japan.[4] The gene for this form of XP (XPAC) was cloned in 1990 by Tanaka and coworkers.[22,23] The gene is located on human chromosome 9[22,36] and codes for a 273-amino acid protein that may have a DNA binding region (zinc finger).[22] Patients with group A XP have been found to have single base substitution mutations in this gene.[23]

Complementation group B is composed of one patient who had the cutaneous abnormalities characteristic of XP (including neoplasms) in conjunction with neurologic and ocular abnormalities typical of Cockayne's syndrome.[1,37] The defective gene in complementation group B (ERCC-3) was identified in 1990 by Weeda et al.[24] This gene, on human chromosome 2, also corrects a DNA repair defect in hamster cells. It codes for a protein of 782 amino acids that has sequence similarity to a DNA helicase. The patient with complementation group B had a single base substitution mutation within this gene.

Patients in complementation group C, with rare exceptions, have XP with skin and ocular involvement but without neurologic abnormalities.[1,2,30] This is the most common group in the United States, Europe, and Egypt but has rarely been found in Japan.

Patients in complementation group D may have late onset of neurologic abnormalities in their second decade of life or no neurologic abnormalities.[1,2,30] A patient with clinical symptoms of both XP and Cockayne syndrome, whose cells were previously assigned to complementation group H, was recently reassigned to complementation group D.[38] In addition, cells from patients with a photosensitive form of trichothiodystrophy (without XP) were also assigned to XP complementation group D.[39–41] The gene responsible for this defect may also be involved in a DNA repair defect in UV-sensitive cultured hamster cells (ERCC-2).[25]

Complementation group E at present has been found in one kindred in Europe and several in Japan.[2,30,42] These patients had relatively mild cutaneous abnormalities without neurologic involvement. Cells from some, but not all, of the group E patients lack a DNA damage-binding protein.[43]

Complementation group F patients have been found mainly in Japan.[2,4,44,45] These patients have mild clinical symptoms without neurologic abnormalities or skin cancer. The residual rate of DNA repair, however, is very low (only 10 to 20 percent of normal). Human chromosome 15 appears to contain a gene that partially corrects the defect in group F cells.[46]

Two patients in complementation group G have been identified in Europe. Both had neurologic abnormalities without skin cancer. Fibroblasts from one of the patients were found to be hypersensitive to killing by x-rays as well as by UV radiation.[2] Another patient in complementation group G, seen at the National Institutes of Health, had clinical features of both XP and severe Cockayne syndrome and died at age 6 years weighing only 15 pounds.

Xeroderma pigmentosum variant cells have normal DNA nucleotide excision repair and thus do not fall in any of the complementation groups of cells with defective DNA excision repair.[1,2] There is, however, defective postreplication repair[1,2,29] (see Fig. 69-9). Xeroderma pigmentosum variants have been identified in the United States,[1,2] Europe,[30] and Japan.[4] Very few of the variant patients have neurologic abnormalities. The cutaneous and ocular abnormalities have been severe in some patients and mild in others. A family with four affected individuals was described in Germany[47]; they had extensive sun exposure and the late onset of cutaneous cancers and had originally been thought to represent a separate disorder (pigmented xerodermoid).[47] Subsequent laboratory studies showed the findings typical of XP variants.

Environmental-Genetic Interaction The cutaneous and ocular changes in XP patients are consistent with the notion that repeated insults by environmental agents, particularly UV radiation, produce repeated bouts of DNA damage. Because of defective DNA repair, this damage results in cell death, diminished cell growth, or somatic cell mutations. Through mechanisms that are not completely understood, these cellular alterations lead to atrophy, hyper- and hypopigmentation, and telangiectasia, as well as a 1000-fold increase in malignant neoplasms. Thus, XP provides strong support for the somatic mutation theory of carcinogenesis. In addition, rigorous protection from UV radiation from early infancy in a few patients has been shown to prevent most of the serious cutaneous and ocular abnormalities.

The neurologic abnormalities in some XP patients demonstrate the clinical features of progressive degeneration.[1,2,5] Severely affected patients lose their ability to walk and talk. Histologically, the picture is of a primary neuronal degeneration with loss (or absence) of neurons but without evidence of vascular abnormality, deposition of abnormal material, or inflammatory reaction. It has been hypothesized,[1] in analogy to the cutaneous degenerative changes, that the neurologic degeneration is a manifestation of unrepaired DNA damage. Since mature neurons do not divide, unrepaired DNA damage would lead to cell death without replacement by other neurons. This process would lead to progressive loss of neurologic function. The specific cause of such damage, whether by exogenous or endogenous agents, and the explanation of why some neurons are more severely affected than others is not known. The severity of the neurologic symptoms in XP patients with associated neurologic disease has been shown to correlate with the UV sensitivity of their skin fibroblasts.[2,5]

Heterozygotes Xeroderma pigmentosum heterozygotes (parents and some other relatives) are carriers of the gene for XP but are clinically normal. There is limited epidemiologic evidence to indicate that these people have an increased risk of developing skin cancer.[48] Most tests of cell function or DNA repair yield normal responses with cells from XP heterozygotes. A nonspecific test of hypersensitivity to x-ray-induced chromosome breakage has been reported to be abnormal with cells from obligate heterozygotes for XP.[49] Cloning of the defective genes in different XP complementation groups should provide a direct assay for detection of XP heterozygotes.[23]

Registry In order to gather information on clinical abnormalities in XP and to provide information to physicians, a registry has been established. Patients with XP should be reported to the registry, from which additional clinical information is available:

Xeroderma Pigmentosum Registry
c/o Department of Pathology
Medical Science Building, Room C520
UMDNJ—New Jersey Medical School
185 South Orange Avenue
Newark, NJ 07103

Cockayne Syndrome

Cockayne syndrome is a very rare autosomal recessive degenerative disease with cutaneous, ocular, neurologic, and somatic abnormalities[37,50–54] (Table 158-1). A review published in 1987 described 129 cases reported in the literature.[50]

Clinical Features

In 1936, Cockayne described a syndrome characterized by cachectic dwarfism, deafness, and pigmentary retinal degeneration with a characteristic "salt and pepper" appearance of the retina. The skin had photosensitivity[54] without the excessive pigmentary abnormalities seen in XP. There was marked loss of subcutaneous fat resulting in a "wizened" appearance, with typical "bird-headed" facies and prominent "Mickey Mouse" ears. Other ocular findings included cataracts and optic atrophy. Neurologic abnormalities, in addition to deafness, include peripheral neuropathy, normal pressure hydrocephalus, and microcephaly. Birth weight and early development are usually normal. The disease onset is usually in the second year of life, with slowly progressive neurologic degeneration. Intellectual deterioration may be nonuniform with some functions preserved better than others. A severe infantile form has been described[51] as well as a milder form with late onset.[52,53]

Cockayne syndrome is not associated with an increased incidence of neoplasia.

Laboratory Abnormalities

Clinical laboratory testing often shows sensorineural deafness, neuropathic electromyogram, and slow motor nerve conduction velocity.[37] The electroencephalogram may be abnormal. X-ray examination may show a thickened skull and microcephaly.[55] Computed tomography (CT) may be diagnostically useful in the detection of normal pressure hydrocephalus[37] and calcification of the basal ganglia (Fig. 158-3). Magnetic resonance imaging (MRI) of the brain shows atrophy and hypomyelination of the cerebrum and cerebellum. Bone age is usually normal. Height and weight are usually well below the third percentile for age.

Cellular Hypersensitivity   As with XP, cultured cells (fibroblasts or lymphocytes) from Cockayne syndrome patients are hypersensitive to UV-induced inhibition of growth and colony-forming ability.[2,56–58]

Host-cell reactivation of UV-damaged adenovirus[17] or plasmids is reduced, although generally to a lesser extent than in XP. The mutant frequency was elevated in circulating lymphocytes from two Cockayne syndrome donors.[54]

Chromosome Abnormalities   Chromosome karyotype and sister chromatid exchange frequency is usually normal in untreated cells.

One patient had a deletion of a portion of chromosome 10, suggesting that a gene for Cockayne syndrome is located there.[52] Ultraviolet treatment of Cockayne syndrome cells results in a greater than normal increase in sister chromatid exchanges[20,58] (see Fig. 69-7 for explanation of this assay). These cellular abnormalities are similar to those of XP.

Cockayne syndrome cells do not have the same DNA repair defects as XP cells. The uusual tests of DNA excision repair are normal. In 1990, Venema et al.[59] reported that normal cells repair the DNA of UV-damaged active genes at a faster rate than inactive genes, and this preferential repair is absent in Cockayne syndrome cells. There is also evidence that Cockayne syndrome cells are unable to repair photoproducts of the cyclobutane dimer type in UV-treated plasmids but are able to repair nondimer photoproducts.[60]

Cockayne syndrome cells have a prolonged decrease in the rate of RNA synthesis following UV irradiation.[61] This test has been used to demonstrate three different complementation groups (A, B, and C) in Cockayne syndrome,[62,63] presumably reflecting three different molecular defects. According to recent reports, the gene for Cockayne syndrome complementation group B may be ERCC-6, a human gene on chromosome 10 that was originally identified because it corrects a DNA repair defect in hamster cells.

Prenatal Diagnosis   In Cockayne syndrome patients, this has been performed[64] based on the delay in recovery of post-UV RNA synthesis and the increased killing by UV.

Clinical-Laboratory Correlation

Cockayne syndrome, like XP, is a disease of progressive neurologic degeneration. Pathologically, Cockayne syndrome shows de-

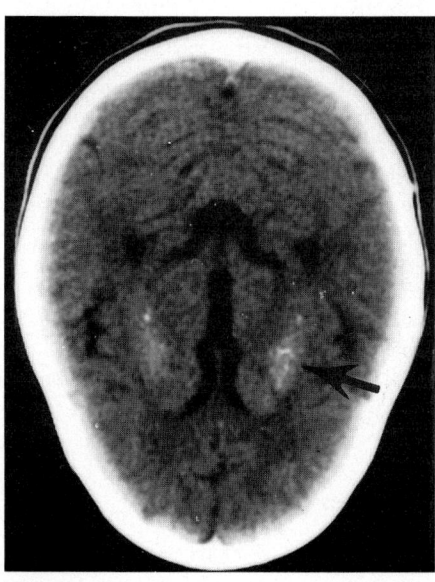

a

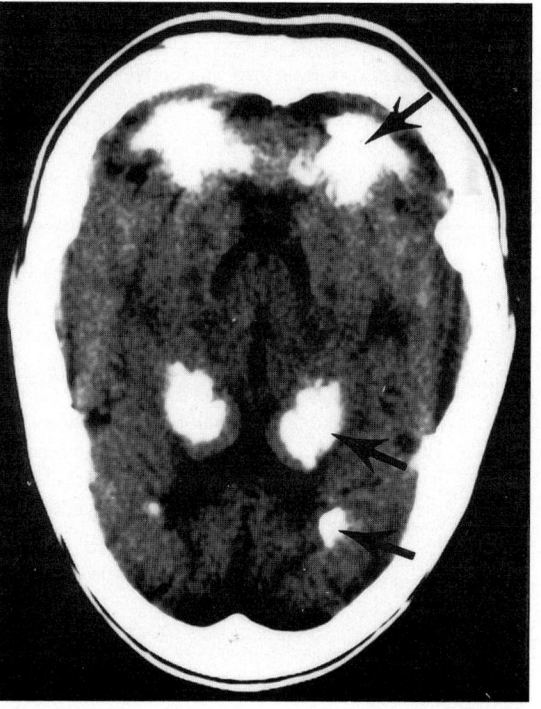

b

FIGURE 158-3   Cockayne syndrome. Calcification of brain visualized on CT scan. (*a*) A 2-year-old patient with bilateral calcification of basal ganglia (arrow). (*b*) A 15-year-old patient with extensive calcification involving basal ganglia, cerebellum, and cerebral hemispheres (arrows).

myelinization of neurons, whereas XP shows primary axonal degeneration. These findings are consistent with the theory that the myelin-producing cells or neurons (respectively) are damaged repeatedly but do not recover fully and so die.[1,5,37] Because mature neurons cannot divide, the dead neurons are not replaced, resulting in progressive loss of neurologic functioning. As in XP, the cause of this damage and the reason for the precise anatomic location of the damage is not known.

Despite similar UV hypersensitivity to cell killing in Cockayne syndrome as in XP, patients with Cockayne syndrome do not have an increased frequency of cutaneous (or internal) neoplasia. In the literature, the Cockayne syndrome patients with multiple skin cancers also had XP.[1,37,38] Thus cellular UV hypersensitivity does not necessarily result in increased neoplasia. The neoplastic process may be more closely related to the defect in DNA repair present in XP but absent in Cockayne syndrome.

Cockayne Syndrome–Xeroderma Pigmentosum Complex

A few patients with Cockayne syndrome have also been found to have clinical features of XP. These include freckling on sun exposed skin and cutaneous neoplasms. Cells from these patients have reduced DNA excision repair, characteristic of XP. Clinically, these patients may be distinguished from XP patients with neurologic abnormalities by the presence of the Cockayne syndrome features of pigmentary retinal degeneration, calcification of the basal ganglia, normal pressure hydrocephalus, and hyperreflexia. Cells from patients with this complex have been found to be in three different XP complementation groups [B, D (formerly H), and G], implying that several different genes are implicated in this disorder (Table 158-2). The gene[24] that corrects the defect in the one patient in XP complementation group B (XP11BE, whose cells are also in Cockayne syndrome complementation group C) is ERCC-3, a human gene on chromosome 2 that also corrects a DNA repair defect in hamster cells.

Trichothiodystrophy

Patients with trichothiodystrophy,[41,65–67] also called Tay syndrome[68] or IBIDS syndrome, have *i*chthyosis, sulfur-deficient *b*rittle hair, *i*ntellectual impairment, *d*ecreased fertility, and *s*hort stature. Some patients are also sun sensitive (Table 158-1). Trichothiodystrophy is not associated with cancer. It is an autosomal recessive disease, and a small number of affected families have been described in Italy[69] and elsewhere. Trichothiodystrophy may be part of a group of similar rare disorders variously known as Amish brittle hair syndrome,[70] Sabinas brittle hair syndrome,[71] or Pollitt syndrome[72]; they all have low cystine content of hair and additionally may have brittle nails, cataracts, hypogonadism, microcephaly, or ataxia.

Laboratory Abnormalities

Fibroblasts from some trichothiodystrophy patients with sun sensitivity have been found to have similar abnormalities to patients with XP.[39–41,69,73] The cells are hypersensitive to killing by UV radiation and have reduced unscheduled DNA synthesis. Fusion studies have revealed them to be in XP complementation group D.[39–41] Fibroblasts from trichothiodystrophy patients without sun sensitivity have normal UV survival and normal unscheduled DNA synthesis.[40,73]

Bloom Syndrome

Bloom syndrome is an autosomal recessive disease characterized by sun sensitivity, facial telangiectasia, short stature, and immunodeficiency[74–82] (Table 158-1). Patients have an increased frequency of various internal neoplasms, including acute leukemia and carcinomas of skin, breast, and gastrointestinal tract. Less than 200 patients have been reported.[78] Bloom syndrome is most frequent among Ashkenazi Jews in whom the carrier rate has been estimated as 1:120.[75] Fourteen patients have been reported from Japan.[79]

Clinical Features

Facial erythema and telangiectasia superficially resembling lupus erythematosus are often present within the first few weeks after birth in the malar area, nose, and around the ears.[74,78,80,82] Sun exposure accentuates these abnormalities and may induce bullae, bleeding, and crusting of the lips and eyelids. The telangiectatic lesions often involve the ears and dorsa of the hands but characteristically spare the trunk, buttocks, and lower extremities. The intensity of the facial lesions may vary from minimal telangiectasia around the lips to severe erythema of the malar area, cheeks, and nose (Fig. 158-4). Café au lait spots are common, at times accompanied by adjacent depigmented areas.

Affected children are generally born at full term but are of low birth weight, averaging approximately 2000 g. Patients are well proportioned but small. Adult height is usually under 150 cm. Patients have a long, narrow head, with a characteristic facies consisting of a narrow prominent nose, relatively hypoplastic malar areas, and a receding chin. Major skeletal abnormalities are unusual. Neurologic abnormalities are uncommon and intelligence is generally normal.

Bloom syndrome patients are predisposed to multiple severe infections of the respiratory or gastrointestinal tracts. There is a tendency for the frequency of infections to decrease with advancing age. There is immune dysfunction,[76,80] and diabetes is common.

Sexual development generally appears to be normal, but male infertility due to defective sperm is the rule.[77]

Approximately 20 percent of Bloom syndrome patients develop neoplasms; half occur before age 20 years.[75,78] Bloom syndrome patients have been estimated to have a 150- to 300-fold increased frequency of development of lymphatic and nonlymphatic leukemia, lymphosarcoma, lymphoma, and carcinoma of the oral cavity and digestive system.

Laboratory Studies

Laboratory studies of immunity have shown diminished immunoglobulin levels, reduced cellular proliferative response to mitogens, and decreased proliferation in the mixed leukocyte reaction.[76,80]

Studies of gonadal function in males revealed azoospermia, and a high follicle-stimulating hormone response to luteinizing hormone–releasing hormone.[77] The studies indicated that primary

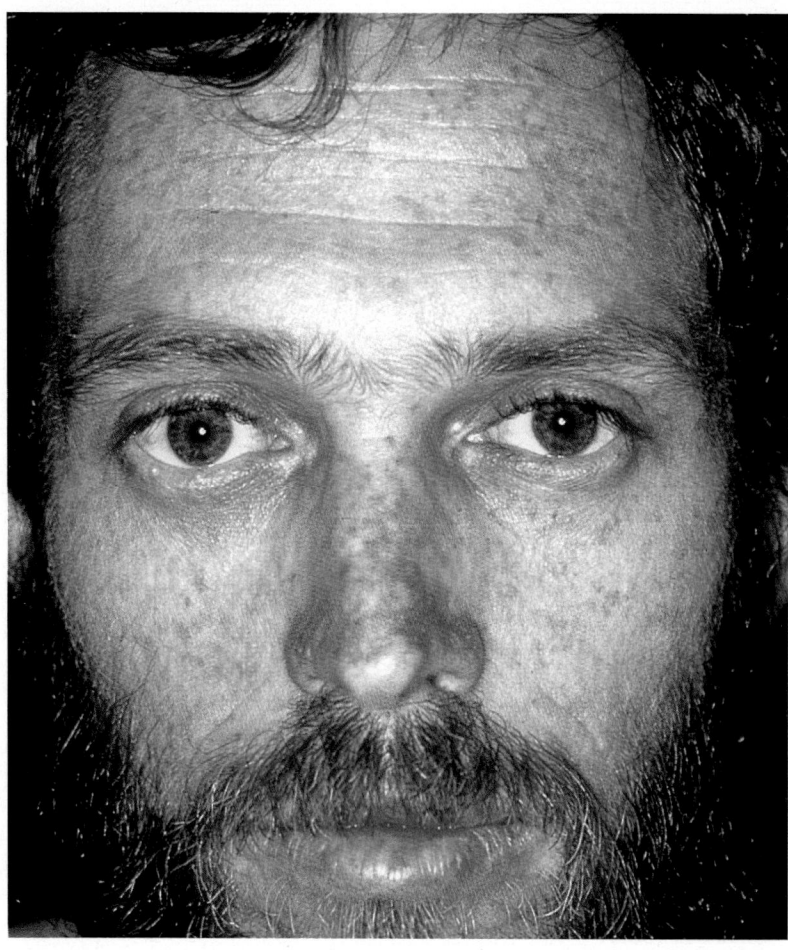

FIGURE 158-4 Bloom syndrome. Prominent telangiectasia in malar distribution.

hypogonadism mainly affected the tubular element of the testis. There was relative sparing of the androgen-secreting Leydig cells resulting in normal secondary sexual development.

Chromosome Abnormalities Bloom syndrome cells have a characteristic elevated frequency of chromosome abnormalities, accompanied by a markedly elevated rate of spontaneous sister chromatid exchanges (see Figs. 69-7 and 69-8) and spontaneous hypermutability of circulating blood cells.[83–87] The chromosome abnormalities include a high frequency of chromosomal breakage and rearrangements, including isochromatid gaps and breaks, transverse breakage at centromeres, dicentric chromosomes, and acentric fragments. The most characteristic of these aberrations, the quadriradial configuration was found in 0.5 to 14.0 percent of all dividing phytohemagglutinin-stimulated lymphocytes from Bloom syndrome patients (see Fig. 69-6).[83] Quadriradials are believed to be the result of a rearrangement before the onset of mitosis, resulting from the exchange of chromatid segments of two homologous chromosomes. The quadriradial is almost never found in cells from normal individuals. Increased sister chromatid exchanges and the presence of quadriradials are considered essential for the diagnosis of Bloom syndrome.

The carcinogens, 4-nitroquinoline-*N*-oxide, *N*-methyl-*N'*-nitro-*N*-nitrosoguanidine, aflatoxin, and methylnitrosourea, induce a greater increase in sister chromatid exchanges in Bloom syndrome lymphocytes than in lymphocytes from normal persons.[88–90] Bloom syndrome cells show an abnormally large increase in chro-

mosome aberrations when treated with x-rays in the G2 phase of the cell cycle.[91]

Fusion (see Fig. 69-11) of Bloom syndrome fibroblasts with rodent cells, or with normal human fibroblasts, results in a normal rate of sister chromatid exchanges in the fused cells.[92,93] This result implies that the defect in Bloom syndrome cells is the consequence of the loss of a normal function rather than the acquisition of a new abnormal function. There is apparently only one complementation group, despite the different ethnic backgrounds of these patients.[94]

Cell Killing There are a few reports of cellular hypersensitivity to agents such as UVB, but this has not been a consistent finding. Cells from three Japanese Bloom syndrome patients were hypersensitive to killing by mitomycin C[95] and to *N*-ethyl-*N*-nitrosourea.[89]

Bloom syndrome fibroblasts were reported to have an 8- to 10-fold increase in the spontaneous mutation rate and a 50- to 100-fold increase in frequency of in vivo mutations at the glycophorin A (MN blood group) locus.[87]

The molecular basis for these abnormalities remains elusive. The rate of DNA chain elongation was found to be significantly slower than with normal fibroblasts.[96] Two laboratories independently reported decreased DNA ligase I activity (an enzyme involved in DNA replication).[97–99] Bloom syndrome cells show diminished ability to ligate plasmids that have been linearized by a restriction enzyme.[100] There have not yet been any published reports of abnormalities in a cloned DNA ligase gene in Bloom syndrome cells. Abnormal antibody reactivity of a uracil DNA glycosylase was reported from one laboratory.[101]

Clinical-Laboratory Correlation

The clinical diagnosis of Bloom syndrome is confirmed by the findings of increased sister chromatid exchange and increased chromosome breakage, including the presence of quadriradials.

    The high frequency of neoplasia in Bloom syndrome may be related to the chromosome breakage or the immune deficiency, as in ataxia-telangiectasia. The observation of an increased spontaneous mutation rate in cultured cells suggests that somatic mutations may play a role in the neoplasia. Homologous chromosome exchange (as in quadriradials) or genetic recombination[102] may be a mechanism whereby heterozygous (recessive) traits become homozygous within somatic cells and thereby result in mutation or neoplasia.

Fanconi Anemia

Fanconi anemia is an autosomal recessive disease with progressive loss of all formed elements of the blood (pancytopenia) (Table 158-1). Patients may also have malformations of the heart, kidney, or limbs.[103–112] Internal neoplasms such as leukemia occur at increased frequency. Blood cells show increased spontaneous chromosome breakage. Approximately 300 patients have been identified in the United States.[109]

Clinical Features

Cutaneous abnormalities have been present in almost 80 percent of the patients. Hyperpigmentation develops from birth or early childhood. The hyperpigmentation is diffuse and accentuated over the neck, joints, and trunk. Café au lait spots and achromic lesions are also present. Following repeated blood transfusions, hyperpigmentation due to iron overloading may be present.

    Hemopoietic manifestations usually have their onset before age 10 years. These consist of a hypocellular bone marrow with progressive decrease in the number of circulating platelets, granulocytes, and erythrocytes. Of 129 patients with Fanconi anemia, 66 percent had skeletal malformations.[104] These included aplasia or hypoplasia of the thumb, metacarpals, or radius; less frequently, hip dislocation or scoliosis have been reported. About 60 percent of patients have short stature and most have low birth weight. Malformations of other organ systems have also been observed: 28 percent of patients have renal deformities including renal aplasia and horseshoe kidney; 21 percent have ocular abnormalities including strabismus and microphthalmia; 20 percent of patients have hypogonadism. Central nervous system abnormalities (hyperreflexia and mild mental retardation) have been observed in fewer than 20 percent of patients. Deafness due to deformities of the ear anatomy is present in fewer than 10 percent of patients. Heart defects (patent ductus arteriosus, aortic stenosis, auricular septum defect) have been observed in 8 patients.

    Patients with Fanconi anemia have a high incidence of neoplasia, particularly nonlymphatic leukemia.[106] In recent years hepatomas have been noted with increasing frequency; there is some suspicion that these may be a late effect of the anabolic steroids used to treat the anemia.[107]

The course is often progressively downhill with death from infection, hemorrhage, or neoplasia.

Laboratory Abnormalities

Clinical laboratory abnormalities reflect the bone marrow failure. There is a hypocellular marrow with thrombocytoplasia, leukopenia, and anemia.

Chromosome Abnormalities   Fanconi anemia is associated with a high frequency of spontaneous chromosomal abnormalities.[109,113,114] These include gaps, breaks, and translocations. With Fanconi anemia cells the chromosomal abnormalities are increased to a greater extent than with normal cells following treatment with diepoxybutane, mitomycin C, psoralen plus UVA, or isonicotinic acid hydrazide (INH).[109,114–118]

    The baseline frequency of sister chromatid exchanges is normal (see Fig. 69-7 for explanation of this assay). However, following treatment with psoralen plus UVA, the increase in sister chromatid exchanges in Fanconi anemia lymphocytes is less than in normal fibroblasts.

Cell Killing   Colony-forming ability of cultured fibroblasts is hypersensitive to inhibition by treatment with agents that form crosslinks in DNA.[118,119] These include mitomycin C, busulfan, nitrogen mustard, and psoralen plus UVA. Colony-forming ability has a normal response to killing by UV radiation. 8-Methoxypsoralen hypersensitivity has been used as the basis of a complementation assay defining two complementation groups (A and B).[120] One is associated with increased sensitivity to the effects of DNA cross-linking agents, whereas the other is not. There is an apparent rodent cell homologue to Fanconi anemia.[121] A gene for Fanconi anemia was located on chromosome 20q.[122]

    The mechanism of the cellular hypersensitivity to DNA cross-linking agents is thought to involve defective DNA repair.[118,119] A detailed understanding of this defect has not yet been attained. Some Fanconi anemia fibroblasts have been reported to have defective removal of an x-ray-induced thymidine analogue, thymine glycol.

Heterozygotes   Cells from heterozygous carriers of Fanconi anemia have an abnormal chromosomal response to damage from diepoxybutane[113] or from nitrogen mustard,[116] intermediate between homozygotes and normal persons.

Prenatal Diagnosis   The chromosomal aberrations induced by diepoxybutane have been used successfully as a test for prenatal diagnosis of Fanconi anemia.[109,114] Many more chromosome aberrations are induced by diepoxybutane in cultured amniotic fluid cells from fetuses with Fanconi anemia than from normal fetuses.

Clinical-Laboratory Correlation

Fanconi anemia is a progressive, degenerative disease with major involvement of the hematologic system. There is a high frequency of spontaneous chromosomal breakage in association with a high rate of neoplasia, particularly nonlymphatic leukemia. Immunodeficiency is not prominent. Cells are hypersensitive to killing and to induction of chromosome aberrations by DNA cross-linking agents. At present, incorporating these diverse observations into a unitary theory involves considerable speculation. The progressive nature of the disease is similar to XP and ataxia-telangiectasia and suggests the presence of accumulated cellular damage. "Spontaneous" chromosomal breakage may be a manifestation of this damage. Fanconi anemia shows more chromosome aberrations than Bloom syndrome but in Bloom syndrome most aberrations are between homologous chromosomes, whereas in Fanconi anemia they are between nonhomologous chromosomes. The neoplasia may be related to the chromosome breakage. However, when considering two diseases with spontaneous chromosome breakage (Fanconi anemia and ataxia-telangiectasia), lymphoid leukemia is absent in Fanconi anemia and predominant in ataxia-telangiectasia. In contrast, nonlymphoid leukemia predominates in Fanconi anemia and is absent in ataxia-telangiectasia. Thus other modifying factors, perhaps the immune defects in ataxia-telangiectasia, may be at work.

The postulated damage may be caused by agents similar to the DNA cross-linking agents to which the Fanconi anemia cells are hypersensitive.

Clinical symptoms in Fanconi anemia have been observed to vary from mild to severe but to be similar in multiple affected children within a family. Similarly, cells from different patients have shown different degrees of sensitivity to x-radiation damage and repair. This suggests that genetic heterogeneity may exist within Fanconi's anemia.

Registry In order to gather information on clinical abnormalities in Fanconi anemia and to provide information to physicians, a registry has been established. Patients with Fanconi anemia may be reported to:

Fanconi Anemia Registry
c/o Dr. Arleen D. Auerbach
Laboratory for Investigative Dermatology
The Rockefeller University
1230 York Avenue
New York, NY 10021

Dyskeratosis Congenita

Dyskeratosis congenita, the Zinsser-Engman-Cole syndrome, is an X-linked multisystem disease with cutaneous, mucosal, ocular, gastrointestinal, and hematologic abnormalities and an increased incidence of cancer (Table 158-1). More than 100 cases have been recorded in the literature, including some female cases.[123–126] Patients have been reported from the United States, Europe, Japan,[127] China, and India.

Clinical Features

The most common features are hyperpigmentation, dystrophic nails, and leukoplakia.[123] During the first decade of life, patients develop reticulated poikiloderma of sun-exposed areas, with hyperpigmentation and occasionally bullae. Nail dystrophy is present in virtually all patients beginning at approximately age 2 to 5 years. The nails initially split easily, then develop longitudinal ridging with irregular free edges. Eventually the nails become smaller resulting in only rudiments remaining. The fingernails are usually involved before the toenails. Other skin abnormalities include atrophic, wrinkled skin over the dorsum of hands and feet and hy-

perhidrosis and hyperkeratosis of palms and soles with disappearance of dermal ridges (absence of fingerprints).

Leukoplakia may be present in any mucosal site. The oral mucosa is the most frequent but leukoplakia has also been found in the urethra, glans penis, vagina, and rectum. Mucosal surfaces such as the esophagus, urethra, and lacrimal duct may become constricted and stenotic, resulting in dysphagia, dysuria, and epiphora. Multiple dental caries and early loss of teeth are common. Approximately half of patients have subnormal intelligence. Patients may have multiple infections.

There is an increased incidence of neoplasia, particularly squamous cell carcinoma of the mouth, rectum, cervix, vagina, esophagus, and skin. A large British kindred had Hodgkin's disease and adenocarcinoma of the pancreas.[124] Several patients had multiple primary neoplasms, and most neoplasms occurred in the third or fourth decade. None of the patients had leukemia.

Half of the patients develop anemia secondary to bone marrow failure in the second or third decade. Leukopenia and thrombocytopenia may also be present, resulting in a hematologic picture similar to Fanconi anemia.

Laboratory Studies

Immune function has been studied in only a small number of patients. Defects in immunoglobulin levels and in cell-mediated immunity were found in some patients.[127]

There have been several reports of intracranial calcifications, especially of the basal ganglia.[125,128]

Chromosomes are usually normal in untreated cells. There is a report of one patient with elevated spontaneous sister chromatid exchanges.[129] Peripheral blood lymphocytes showed abnormally large numbers of chromosome breaks following treatment with either bleomycin or x-irradiation during the G2 phase of the cell cycle.[130,131] (See Chap. 69 for a discussion of these assays.)

Treatment of peripheral blood leukocytes from two patients with psoralens plus UV radiation in vitro induced abnormally large increases in sister chromatid exchanges.[132] Cultured fibroblasts from two patients had increased sensitivity to killing by mitomycin C.[133]

Clinical-Laboratory Correlation

A gene for dyskeratosis has been assigned to the q28 region of the X chromosome by linkage analysis.[134] There is also evidence for an autosomal form.[126]

Dyskeratosis congenita, like Fanconi anemia, is associated with anemia and increased incidence of neoplasia.[111] However, patients with dyskeratosis congenita do not have the developmental malformations or spontaneous chromosomal breakage seen in Fanconi anemia. In both disorders there is a suggestion of an abnormal chromosomal response to the DNA cross-linking induced by psoralens. In dyskeratosis congenita, abnormally large increases in numbers of sister chromatid exchanges were induced in lymphocytes,[132] whereas in Fanconi anemia there was an abnormally small increase.

As in ataxia-telangiectasia, dyskeratosis congenita has increased neoplasia and immune deficiency. However, the types of neoplasia most commonly seen in ataxia-telangiectasia, lymphoma and leukemia, have not been reported in dyskeratosis congenita. The mechanism and the extent of cellular abnormalities in dyskeratosis congenita are presently not understood.

Basal Cell Nevus Syndrome

Basal cell nevus syndrome (nevoid basal cell carcinoma syndrome, fifth phacomatosis, Gorlin syndrome, Gorlin-Goltz syndrome) is a progressive degenerative multisystem disorder characterized by early onset of mandibular cysts and basal cell carcinomas.[135–138] Inheritance is autosomal dominant with variable penetrance (Table 158-1).

There may be a high spontaneous mutation rate. The frequency of the basal cell nevus syndrome is not known, but the disease is not rare. Basal cell nevus syndrome has been estimated to be present in 22 percent of basal cell carcinoma patients younger than 19 years and in 2 percent of basal cell carcinoma patients younger than 45 years.[136]

Clinical Features

The early features of the basal cell nevus syndrome do not usually involve the skin (Table 158-4). Patients may be born with congenital blindness (due to coloboma, cataracts, or glaucoma) or hydrocephalus. Multiple cysts of the mandible or maxilla with keratinized lining (odontogenic keratocysts) may occur early in the

TABLE 158-4
Basal Cell Nevus Syndrome: Clinical Features

Cutaneous abnormalities
  Multiple basal cell carcinomas
  Pits in palms and soles
  Benign lesions: milia, cysts, lipomas, fibromas
Characteristic facies
  Broad nasal root
  Frontal and biparietal bossing
  Hypertelorism
  Lateral displacement of inner canthi
Osseous abnormalities
  Oral: jaw cysts (odontogenic keratocysts), defective
    dentition, ameloblastoma
  Ribs: bifid, splayed, fused, missing, pectus
    excavatum
  Vertebrae: spina bifida occulta, kyphoscoliosis
  Short fourth metacarpals (brachymetacarpalism)
  Pseudocystic lytic lesions of bones (hamartomas)
Ocular abnormalities
  Hypertelorism
  Dystopia canthorum
  Strabismus
  Congenital blindness: cataracts, coloboma, glaucoma
Neurologic abnormalities
  Calcification of the dura: lamellar calcification
    of falx cerebri, tentorium cerebelli
  Calcified sellae turcica: bridged sella, fused
    clinoids
  Congenital hydrocephalus
  Mental retardation
Endocrine abnormalities
  Male hypogonadism: absent or undescended testes
  Female: ovarian fibromas, calcified ovarian cysts
Internal neoplasms
  Medulloblastoma
  Meningioma
  Ovarian fibrosarcoma
  Cardiac fibroma
  Fetal rhabdomyoma
  Ameloblastoma of jaw cyst
  Squamous cell carcinoma of jaw cyst
  Seminoma

disease. Patients have a characteristic facies with broad nasal root, frontal bossing, well-developed supraorbital ridges, hypertelorism, and mild mandibular prognathism. There may be lateral displacement of the inner canthi (dystopia canthorum).

The most common cutaneous abnormality is the presence of multiple basal cell carcinomas. These usually have their onset between puberty and 35 years of age.[136] They occur predominantly in sites exposed to sunlight but are also present in shielded sites. Patients may have from a few to dozens or hundreds of basal cell carcinomas.

The term *nevus*, in basal cell nevus syndrome, is an old medical term referring to any circumscribed lesion believed to arise under genetic influence. It referred to vascular or nonvascular growths and not just nevus cell nevi or "moles," as in the terminology of today. The *nevi* in the basal cell nevus syndrome are true basal cell carcinomas. They may be flesh-colored or reddish brown with a pearly appearance. Most lesions remain relatively stable for many years. A few may become locally invasive, showing increasing size, ulceration, and bleeding.

More than 50 percent of patients have minute pits (epidermal defects in keratin production) of the palms and soles.[136] These are more common in adults than children. There may be only a few to hundreds of these pits. They are more numerous on the lateral surfaces of the palms and soles. Other cutaneous lesions include milia, multiple cysts, lipomas, and fibromas or desmoids.

The keratocysts of the jaws develop progressively during the second or third decade.[136] More than 80 percent of patients have radiographically visible cysts by age 40 years. The odontogenic keratocysts are lined with squamous epithelium. They have extensive keratinization and walls of connective tissue. They may range in size from a few millimeters to several centimeters in diameter. Recurrences after surgery are common. Teeth may be carious, misshapen, or in abnormal locations. Ameloblastomas, an oral analogue of the basal cell carcinoma, and squamous cell carcinoma may rarely occur.

Brachymetacarpalism (Albright's sign) consists of a short fourth metacarpal.[139] It is easily seen by examining the knuckles on the dorsum of a clenched fist and verified by hand x-ray (Fig. 158-5a). In addition to its presence in the basal cell nevus syndrome, Albright's sign is seen in pseudohypoparathyroidism, Turner's syndrome, pseudopseudohypoparathyroidism, and in about 10 percent of the normal population.[136] Rib or vertebral abnormalities are common. Lamellar calcification of the falx is often a valuable diagnostic sign (Fig. 158-5b).[140]

Mental retardation is present in a minority of patients. The electroencephalogram may show nonspecific abnormalities. Congenital abnormalities include agenesis of the corpus callosum and congenital hydrocephalus.

Other abnormalities in some patients include male hypogonadism with absent or undescended testes, infantile external genitalia, female pubic hair pattern, and scanty facial hair. Ovarian fibromas and pelvic calcification may be present. Lymphatic mesenteric cysts may necessitate laparotomy.[135] Some patients have been reported with kidney malformations (horseshoe kidney, L-shaped kidney, unilateral renal agenesis).[136]

Patients with the basal cell nevus syndrome are subject to internal neoplasms in addition to cutaneous basal cell carcinomas. These include ameloblastomas of the oral cavity, fibrosarcomas of the jaw, ovarian fibromas,[141] teratomas, cystadenomas, and cardiac tumors.[142] Meningioma and craniopharyngioma have been reported.[136] Medulloblastoma of the brain is present in increased frequency, estimated at 2 to 3 percent,[143] including development

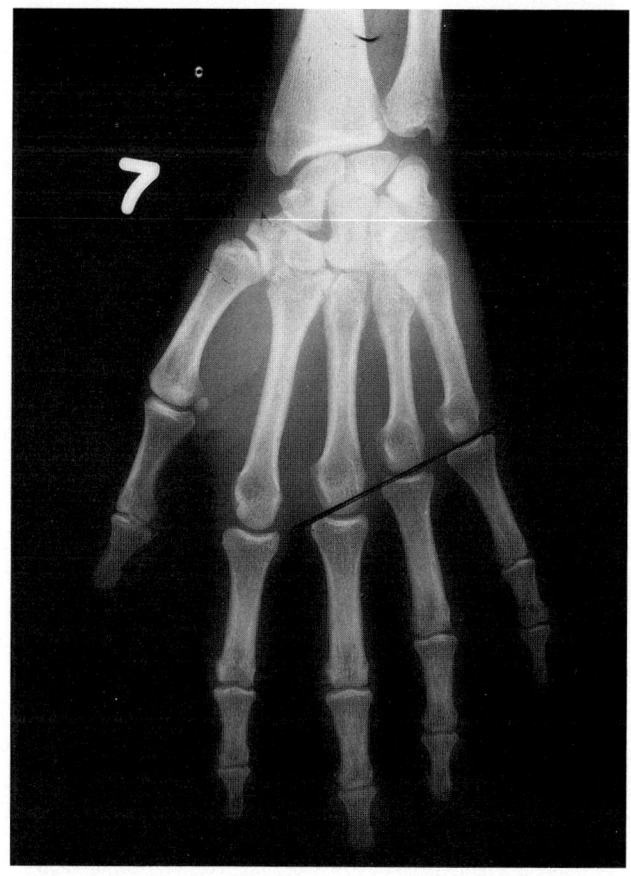

a

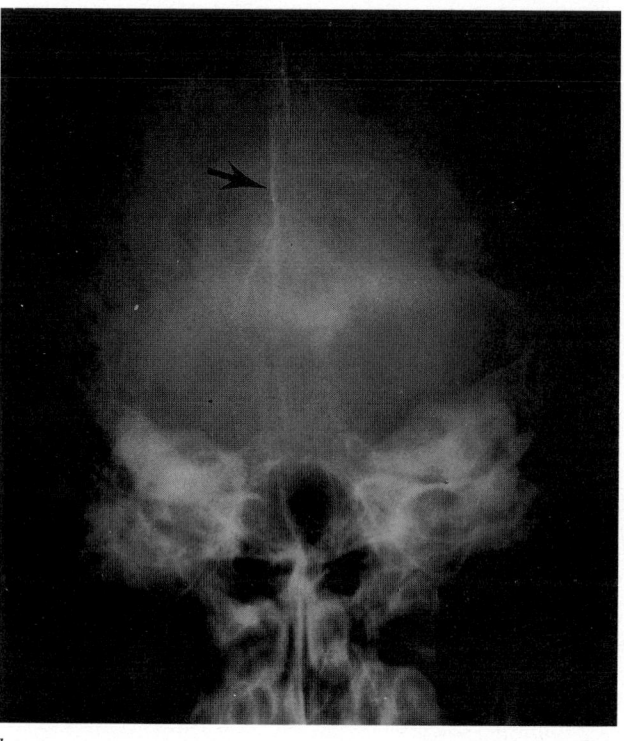

b

FIGURE 158-5 Basal cell nevus syndrome. (*a*) Short fourth metacarpal (Albright's sign). A line drawn through the distal ends of the fifth and fourth metacarpals intersects the third metacarpal proximal to its end. (*b*) Lamellar calcification of the falx (arrow).

within the first 2 years of life.[136] Treatment of the medulloblastoma with standard dosage of radiotherapy has resulted in a remarkable phenomenon: numerous basal cell carcinomas appeared in the irradiated skin within 4 years.[144] A similar induction of numerous large basal cell carcinomas followed treatment of cutaneous basal cell carcinomas with radiation (Fig. 158-6).

Laboratory Abnormalities

Most standard clinical laboratory tests are normal in patients with basal cell nevus syndrome. Chromosome abnormalities have been found in a small number of patients.[145] However, normal rates of chromosome breakage and baseline sister chromatid exchanges were found in 20 patients and 15 unaffected relatives.[146]

X-Ray Hypersensitivity   The clinical observation of the induction of numerous basal cell carcinomas in skin in the field of radiotherapy for treatment of central nervous system neoplasms prompted the study of x-ray sensitivity of cultured cells from patients with basal cell nevus syndrome. Studies of dermal fibroblasts have shown normal survival response following x-ray.[147,148] There was defective repair of potentially lethal damage following x-radiation in one patient, who also had an increased level of mutated circulating T cells.[148] One laboratory reported increased sensitivity to killing of fibroblasts by UVB but not by UVC radiation.[149] (See Chap. 69 for a discussion of these assays.)

Treatment

Because patients may have large numbers of basal cell carcinomas they should be followed regularly for evidence of invasive growth. Lesions showing signs of aggression should be surgically removed by excision, micrographic surgery, or similar techniques. Large numbers of smaller tumors have been treated by cryotherapy or by electrodesiccation and curettage. However, it is often impossible to remove all tumors and most have a clinically benign course. Oral retinoids (isotretinoin or etretinate) in high doses have been reported to be useful in preventing new tumors in isolated cases,[150–152] but no controlled series has been presented. Radiotherapy is not indicated for treatment of skin cancers because of the marked sensitivity to induction of basal cell carcinomas (Fig. 158-6). The jaw cysts can be treated surgically but have a high rate of recurrence.

Clinical-Laboratory Correlations

There is striking induction of basal cell carcinomas by x-ray. However, a corresponding cellular radiohypersensitivity has not been

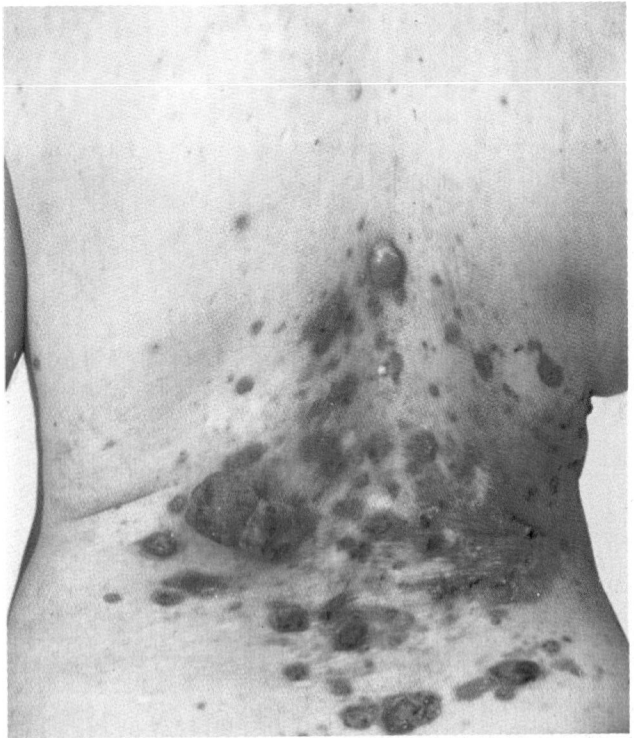

FIGURE 158-6 Basal cell nevus syndrome. Multiple, large, fungating basal cell carcinomas arising in a portion of the lower back treated years earlier with superficial x-ray for therapy of basal cell carcinomas.

demonstrated. Perhaps the defect is limited to the epidermal basal cells and not found in the dermal fibroblasts that are usually cultured.

Patients with basal cell nevus syndrome have features of progressive degeneration, with occurrence of multiple jaw cysts and basal cell carcinomas. This progressive deterioration may be an example of the two-hit hypothesis of Knudson (originally proposed to explain neoplasia in retinoblastoma).[153] The first hit represents the inherited gene defect and the second would be due to environmental DNA damage, presumably caused by x-radiation or UVB. In this regard, Shimada et al.[154] reported that the life span of cultured dermal fibroblasts from a basal cell nevus syndrome patient was substantially extended by introduction of a single oncogene (v-myc) that did not extend the life span of normal control cells.

Conclusion

Increased sensitivity to some physical and chemical agents has been recognized in a small number of heritable diseases in recent years (Table 158-1). Clinical hypersensitivity to sunlight or to radiotherapy has been shown to be manifested by a corresponding cellular hypersensitivity in XP, Cockayne syndrome, trichothiodystrophy, and ataxia-telangiectasia (see Chap. 184).

In XP, Cockayne syndrome, and in some patients with trichothiodystrophy, the cellular hypersensitivity has been shown to be related to defective DNA repair.

Spontaneous chromosomal breakage is a feature of Bloom syndrome, Fanconi anemia, and ataxia-telangiectasia. As with

most of these disorders, the molecular mechanisms involved in these chromosomal abnormalities is just beginning to be understood.

Recognition of the hypersensitivity in these disorders has significance for diagnosis of several of these disorders (see Chap. 69 for a discussion of these diagnostic tests). Diagnosis of Bloom syndrome, Fanconi anemia, XP, and Cockayne syndrome may be facilitated by examining chromosomal abnormalities or DNA repair. Prenatal diagnosis has been accomplished in XP, Cockayne syndrome, and Fanconi anemia on the basis of cellular hypersensitivity to UV radiation[31,64] and to diepoxybutane.[109]

Although these heritable diseases are rare, carriers of the affected genes can be calculated to comprise several percent of the general population. These individuals are usually free of clinical symptoms. However, epidemiologic studies have suggested that they may have an increased risk of neoplasia. In particular, heterozygous carriers of ataxia-telangiectasia may have a fivefold increased risk of dying from ovarian, stomach, or biliary tract cancer below age 45.[155] Since they may comprise 1 percent of the general population, they may thus represent 5 percent of the persons dying from these cancers below age 45 years. There is a similar suggestion that persons heterozygous for XP have an increased risk of developing skin cancer.[47] Many of these individuals may be at an increased risk from exposure to environmental agents. There are thus implications for cancer control, preventive medicine, and occupational medicine. At present, however, there is no laboratory test that can reliably detect the asymptomatic carriers of most of these disorders. However, as the defective genes are identified, molecular biologic techniques should permit carrier identification.

There is a tantalizing link between these cellular abnormalities and certain common clinical problems such as neoplasia, neurologic degeneration, and immune deficiency. Progressive cutaneous, neoplastic, or neurologic degeneration (as in XP, ataxia-telangiectasia, Cockayne syndrome, dyskeratosis congenita, or basal cell nevus syndrome) may be the result of impaired survival of cells subjected to damage by exogenous or endogenous physical or chemical agents. Immune deficiency is seen in ataxia-telangiectasia, Bloom syndrome, and dyskeratosis congenita. The immune deficiency may be related to in utero damage, to defective DNA processing at a crucial stage of embryonic development, or to other, not presently identified, defects. A better understanding of the relationship between these clinical abnormalities and the cellular defects in these patients will undoubtedly provide insights into disease processes in normal individuals.

References

*1. Robbins JH et al: Xeroderma pigmentosum: An inherited disease with sun sensitivity, multiple cutaneous neoplasms, and abnormal DNA repair. *Ann Intern Med* **80**:221, 1974

*2. Cleaver J, Kraemer KH: Xeroderma pigmentosum, in *The Metabolic Basis of Inherited Disease,* 6th ed, edited by CR Scriver et al. New York, McGraw-Hill, 1989, p 2949

*3. Kraemer KH et al: Xeroderma pigmentosum: Cutaneous, ocular and neurologic abnormalities in 830 published cases. *Arch Dermatol* **123**:241, 1987

*4. Takebe H et al: Genetics and skin cancer of xeroderma pigmentosum in Japan. *Jpn J Cancer Res* **78**:1135, 1987

*Indicates general references

5. Robbins JH et al: Neurological disease in xeroderma pigmentosum: Documentation of a late onset type of the juvenile onset form. *Brain* **114**:1335, 1991

6. Keukens F et al: Xeroderma pigmentosum: Squamous cell carcinoma of the tongue. *Acta Derm Venereol (Stockh)* **69**:530, 1989

7. Kraemer KH et al: Prevention of skin cancer with oral 13-*cis* retinoic acid in xeroderma pigmentosum. *N Engl J Med* **318**:1633, 1988

8. Tomas M et al: Renal leiomyosarcoma associated with xeroderma pigmentosum. *Arch Esp Urol* **42**:484, 1989

9. Johnson MW et al: Malignant melanoma of the iris in xeroderma pigmentosum. *Arch Ophthalmol* **107**:402, 1989

10. Mimaki T et al: Neurological manifestations in xeroderma pigmentosum. *Ann Neurol* **20**:70, 1986

11. Mimaki T et al: EEG and CT abnormalities in xeroderma pigmentosum. *Acta Neurol Scand* **80**:136, 1989

12. Kanda T et al: Peripheral neuropathy in xeroderma pigmentosum. *Brain* **113** (part 4):1025, 1990

13. Cleaver JE: Defective repair replication of DNA in xeroderma pigmentosum. *Nature* **218**:652, 1968

14. Thielmann HW et al: Clinical symptoms and DNA repair characteristics of xeroderma pigmentosum patients from Germany. *Cancer Res* **51**:3456, 1991

*15. Friedberg EC, Hanawalt PC (editors): *DNA Repair: A Laboratory Manual of Research Procedures*. New York, Marcel Dekker, 1981

16. Andrews AD et al: Xeroderma pigmentosum neurological abnormalities correlate with colony forming ability after ultraviolet radiation. *Proc Natl Acad Sci USA* **75**:1984, 1978

*17. Day RS: Human adenoviruses as DNA repair probes, in *DNA Repair Processes*, edited by WW Nichols, DG Murphy. Miami, Symposium Specialists, 1977, p 119

18. Protić-Sabljić M, Kraemer KH: One pyrimidine dimer inactivates expression of a transfected gene in xeroderma pigmentosum cells. *Proc Natl Acad Sci USA* **82**:6622, 1985

19. Bredberg A et al: Restricted ultraviolet mutational spectrum in a shuttle vector propagated in xeroderma pigmentosum cells. *Proc Natl Acad Sci USA* **83**:8273, 1986

20. Chang WS et al: Ultraviolet light-induced sister chromatid exchanges in xeroderma pigmentosum and in Cockayne's syndrome lymphocyte cell lines. *Cancer Res* **38**:1601, 1978

21. Epstein JH et al: Defect in DNA synthesis in skin of patients with xeroderma pigmentosum demonstrated in vivo. *Science* **168**:1477, 1970

22. Tanaka K et al: Analysis of a human DNA excision repair gene involved in group A xeroderma pigmentosum and containing a zinc-finger domain. *Nature* **348**:73, 1990

23. Satokata I et al: Characterization of a splicing mutation in group A xeroderma pigmentosum. *Proc Natl Acad Sci USA* **87**:9908, 1990

24. Weeda G et al: A presumed DNA helicase encoded by ERCC-3 is involved in the human repair disorders xeroderma pigmentosum and Cockayne's syndrome. *Cell* **62**:777, 1990

25. Flejter WL et al: Correction of xeroderma pigmentosum complementation group D mutant cell phenotypes by chromosome and gene transfer: Involvement of the human ERCC2 DNA repair gene. *Proc Natl Acad Sci USA* **89**:261, 1992

26. De Weerd-Kastelein EA et al: Genetic heterogeneity of xeroderma pigmentosum demonstrated by somatic cell hybridization. *Nature* **238**:80, 1972

27. Kraemer KH et al: Genetic heterogeneity in xeroderma pigmentosum: Complementation groups and their relationship to DNA repair rates. *Proc Natl Acad Sci USA* **72**:59, 1975

28. Burk PG et al: Ultraviolet stimulated thymidine incorporation in xeroderma pigmentosum lymphocytes. *J Lab Clin Med* **77**:759, 1971

29. Boyer JC et al: Defective postreplication repair in xeroderma pigmentosum variant fibroblasts. *Cancer Res* **50**:2593, 1990

30. Jung EG et al: Heterogeneity of xeroderma pigmentosum (XP); variability and stability within and between the complementation groups C, D, E, I and variants. *Photodermatol* **3**:125, 1986

31. Ramsay CA et al: Prenatal diagnosis of xeroderma pigmentosum: Report of the first successful case. *Lancet* **2**:1109, 1974

32. Hansson J, Wood RD: Repair synthesis by human cell extracts in DNA damaged by *cis*- and *trans*-diamminedichloroplatinum(II). *Nucleic Acids Res* **17**:8073, 1989

33. Dijt FJ et al: Formation and repair of cisplatin-induced adducts to DNA in cultured normal and repair-deficient human fibroblasts. *Cancer Res* **48**:6058, 1988

34. Bech-Thomsen N et al: Xeroderma pigmentosum lesions related to ultraviolet transmittance by clothes. *J Am Acad Dermatol* **24**:365, 1991

35. Ashall G et al: Facial resurfacing in xeroderma pigmentosum: Are we spoiling the ship for a ha'p'orth of tar? *Br J Plast Surg* **40**:610, 1987

36. Henning KA et al: Gene complementing xeroderma pigmentosum group A cells maps to distal human chromosome 9q. *Somat Cell Mol Genet* **16**:395, 1990

37. Brumback RA et al: Normal pressure hydrocephalus: Recognition and relationship to neurological abnormalities in Cockayne's syndrome. *Arch Neurol* **35**:337, 1978

38. Moshell AN et al: A new patient with both xeroderma pigmentosum and Cockayne syndrome establishes the new xeroderma pigmentosum complementation group H. in *Cellular Responses to DNA Damage*, edited by E Friedberg, B Bridges. New York, Alan R. Liss, 1983, p 209

39. Stefanini M et al: Xeroderma pigmentosum (complementation group D) mutation is present in patients affected by trichothiodystrophy with photosensitivity. *Hum Genet* **74**:107, 1986

40. Lehmann AR et al: Trichothiodystrophy, a human DNA repair disorder with heterogeneity in the cellular response to ultraviolet light. *Cancer Res* **48**(21):6090, 1988

41. Rebora A, Crovato F: PIBI(D)S syndrome: Trichothiodystrophy with xeroderma pigmentosum (group D) mutation. *J Am Acad Dermatol* **16**:940, 1987

42. Kondo S et al: Assignment of three patients with xeroderma pigmentosum to complementation group E and their characteristics. *J Invest Dermatol* **90**:152, 1988

43. Chu G, Chang E: Xeroderma pigmentosum group E cells lack a nuclear factor that binds to damaged DNA. *Science* **242**:564, 1988

44. Yamamura K et al: Clinical and photobiological characteristics of xeroderma pigmentosum complementation group F: A review of cases from Japan. *Br J Dermatol* **121**:471, 1989

45. Kondo S et al: Late onset of skin cancers in 2 xeroderma pigmentosum group F siblings and a review of 30 Japanese xeroderma pigmentosum patients in groups D, E and F. *Photodermatol* **6**:89, 1989

46. Saxon PJ et al: Human chromosome 15 confers partial complementation of phenotypes of xeroderma pigmentosum group F cells. *Am J Hum Genet* **44**:474, 1989

47. Hofmann H et al: Pigmented xerodermoid: First report of a family. *Bull Cancer* **65**:347, 1978

48. Swift M, Chase C: Cancer in families with xeroderma pigmentosum. *J Natl Cancer Inst* **62**:1415, 1979

49. Parshad R et al: Carrier detection in xeroderma pigmentosum. *J Clin Invest* **85**:135, 1990

*50. Cantani A et al: Rare syndromes. I. Cockayne syndrome: A review of the 129 cases so far reported in the literature. *Riv Eur Sci Med Farmacol* **9**:9, 1987

51. Jaeken J et al: Clinical and biochemical studies in three patients with severe early infantile Cockayne syndrome. *Hum Genet* **83**:339, 1989

52. Fryns JP et al: Apparent late-onset Cockayne syndrome and interstitial deletion of the long arm of chromosome 10 (del(10) (q11.23q21.2)). *Am J Med Genet* **40**:343, 1991

53. Kennedy RM et al: Cockayne syndrome: An atypical case. *Neurology* **30**:1268, 1980

54. Norris PG et al: Abnormal erythemal response and elevated T lymphocyte HRPT mutant frequency in Cockayne's syndrome. *Br J Dermatol* **124**:453, 1991

55. Riggs W, Seibert J: Cockayne's syndrome: Roentgen findings. *Am J Roentgenol* **116**:623, 1972

56. Andrews AD et al: Cockayne's syndrome fibroblasts have increased sensitivity to ultraviolet light but normal rates of unscheduled DNA synthesis. *J Invest Dermatol* **70**:237, 1978

57. Wade MH, Chu EHY: Effects of DNA damaging agents on cultured fibroblasts derived from patients with Cockayne's syndrome. *Mutat Res* **59**:49, 1979

58. Marshall RR et al: Increased sensitivity of cell strains from Cockayne's syndrome to sister chromatid exchange induction and cell killing by UV light. *Mutat Res* **69**:107, 1980

59. Venema J et al: The genetic defect in Cockayne syndrome is associated with a defect in repair of UV-induced DNA damage in transcriptionally active DNA. *Proc Natl Acad Sci USA* **87**:4707, 1990

60. Barrett SF et al: Defective repair of cyclobutane pyrimidine dimers with normal repair of other DNA photoproducts in a transcriptionally active gene transfected into Cockayne syndrome cells. *Mutat Res* **255**:281, 1991

61. Lehmann AR et al: Abnormal kinetics of DNA synthesis in ultraviolet light-irradiated cells from patients with Cockayne's syndrome. *Cancer Res* **39**:4237, 1979

62. Tanaka K et al: Genetic complementation groups in Cockayne syndrome. *Somat Cell Genet* **7**:445, 1981

63. Lehmann AR: Three complementation groups in Cockayne syndrome. *Mutat Res* **106**:347, 1982

64. Lehmann AR et al: Prenatal diagnosis of Cockayne's syndrome. *Lancet* **1**:486, 1985

65. Price VH et al: Trichothiodystrophy. *Arch Dermatol* **116**:1375, 1980

66. Przedborski S et al: Trichothiodystrophy, mental retardation, short stature, ataxia, and gonadal dysfunction in three Moroccan siblings. *Am J Med Genet* **35**:566, 1990

*67. Itin PH, Pittelkow MR: Trichothiodystrophy: Review of sulfur-deficient brittle hair syndromes and association with the ectodermal dysplasias. *J Am Acad Dermatol* **22**:705, 1990

68. Tay CH: Ichthyosiform erythroderma, hair shaft abnormalities, and mental and growth retardation: A new recessive disorder. *Arch Dermatol* **104**:4, 1971

69. Nuzzo F et al: Search for consanguinity within and among families of patients with trichothiodystrophy associated with xeroderma pigmentosum. *J Med Genet* **27**:21, 1990

70. Jackson CE et al: 'Brittle' hair with short stature, intellectual impairment, and decreased fertility: An autosomal recessive syndrome in an Amish kindred. *Pediatrics* **54**:201, 1974

71. Howell RR et al: The Sabinas brittle hair syndrome. *Am J Hum Genet* **33**:957, 1981

72. Pollitt RJ, Stonier PD: Proteins of normal hair and of cystine-deficient hair from mentally retarded siblings. *Biochem J* **122**:433, 1971

73. Broughton BC et al: Relationship between pyrimidine dimers, 6–4 photoproducts, repair synthesis and cell survival: Studies using cells from patients with trichothiodystrophy. *Mutat Res* **235**:33, 1990

74. Bloom D: Congenital telangiectatic erythema resembling lupus erythematosus in dwarfs. *Am J Dis Child* **88**:754, 1954

75. German J et al: Bloom's syndrome. VII. Progress report for 1978. *Clin Genet* **15**:361, 1979

76. Weemaes CMR et al: Immune responses in four patients with Bloom syndrome. *Clin Immunol Immunopathol* **12**:12, 1979

77. Kauli R et al: Gonadal function in Bloom's syndrome. *Clin Endinocrinol* **6**:285, 1977

*78. German J, Passarge E: Bloom's syndrome. XII. Report from the Registry for 1987. *Clin Genet* **35**:57, 1989

79. German J, Takebe H: Bloom's syndrome. XIV. The disorder in Japan. *Clin Genet* **35**:93, 1989

80. Van Kerckhove CW et al: Bloom's syndrome. Clinical features and immunologic abnormalities of four patients. *Am J Dis Child* **142**:1089, 1988

81. Cairney AE et al: Wilms tumor in three patients with Bloom syndrome. *J Pediatr* **111**:414, 1987

*82. Gretzula JC et al: Bloom's syndrome. *J Am Acad Dermatol* **17**:479, 1987

83. Chaganti RSK et al: A manyfold increase in sister chromatid ex-

changes in Bloom's syndrome lymphocytes. *Proc Natl Acad Sci USA* **71**:4508, 1974

84. Kuhn EM, Therman E: Cytogenetics of Bloom's syndrome. *Cancer Genet Cytogenet* **22**:1, 1986

85. Rosin MP, German J: Evidence for chromosome instability in vivo in Bloom syndrome: Increased numbers of micronuclei in exfoliated cells. *Hum Genet* **71**:187, 1985

86. Vijayalaxmi et al: Bloom's syndrome: Evidence for an increased mutation frequency in vivo. *Science* **221**:851, 1983

87. Langlois RG et al: Evidence for increased in vivo mutation and somatic recombination in Bloom's syndrome. *Proc Natl Acad Sci USA* **86**:670, 1989

88. Shiraishi Y: Bloom syndrome B-lymphoblastoid cells are hypersensitive towards carcinogen and tumor promoter-induced chromosomal alterations and growth in agar. *EMBO J* **4**:2553, 1985

89. Kurihara T et al: Hypersensitivity of Bloom's syndrome fibroblasts to *N*-ethyl-*N*-nitrosourea. *Mutat Res* **184**:147, 1987

90. Shiraishi Y: Hypersensitive character of Bloom syndrome B-lymphoblastoid cell lines usable for sensitive carcinogen detection. *Mutat Res* **175**:179, 1986

91. Aurias A et al: Radiation sensitivity of Bloom's syndrome lymphocytes during S and G2 phases. *Cancer Genet Cytogenet* **16**:131, 1985

92. Alhadeff B et al: High rate of sister chromatid exchanges of Bloom's syndrome is corrected in rodent human somatic cell hybrids. *Cytogenet Cell Genet* **27**:8, 1980

93. Shiraishi Y: Effects of cell fusion and deoxynucleosides on sister-chromatid exchanges in B-lymphoblastoid cell lines from 5 Bloom syndrome patients. *Mutat Res* **199**:75, 1988

94. Weksberg R et al: Bloom syndrome: A single complementation group defines patients of diverse ethnic origin. *Am J Hum Genet* **42**:816, 1988

95. Hook GJ et al: Sensitivity of Bloom syndrome fibroblasts to mitomycin C. *Mutat Res* **131**:223, 1984

96. Hand R, German J: Bloom's syndrome: DNA replication in cultured fibroblasts and lymphocytes. *Hum Genet* **38**:297, 1977

97. Willis AE, Lindahl T: DNA ligase I deficiency in Bloom's syndrome. *Nature* **325**:355, 1987

98. Chan JY et al: Altered DNA ligase I activity in Bloom's syndrome cells. *Nature* **325**:357, 1987

99. Willis AE et al: Structural alterations of DNA ligase I in Bloom syndrome. *Proc Natl Acad Sci USA* **84**:8016, 1987

100. Rünger TM, Kraemer KH: Error-prone *in vivo* end joining of linear plasmid DNA by Bloom's syndrome cells. *EMBO J* **8**:1419, 1989

101. Seal G et al: Immunological alteration of the Bloom's syndrome uracil DNA glycosylase in Epstein-Barr virus-transformed human lymphoblastoid cells. *Mutat Res* **243**:241, 1990

102. Bubley GJ, Schnipper LE: Effects of Bloom's syndrome fibroblasts on genetic recombination and mutagenesis of herpes simplex virus type 1. *Somat Cell Mol Genet* **13**:111, 1987

103. Nilsson LR: Chronic pancytopenia with multiple congenital abnormalities (Fanconi's anemia). *Acta Pediatrica* **49**:518, 1960

*104. Gmyrek D, Syllm-Rapoport I: Fanconi's anemia: Analysis of 129 described cases. *Z Kinderheilkd* **91**:294, 1964

105. Schroeder TM et al: Formal genetics of Fanconi's anemia. *Hum Genet* **32**:257, 1976

*106. Auerbach AD, Allen RG: Leukemia and preleukemia in Fanconi anemia patients. A review of the literature and report of the International Fanconi Anemia Registry. *Cancer Genet Cytogenet* **51**:1, 1991

107. Linares M et al: Hepatocellular carcinoma and squamous cell carcinoma in a patient with Fanconi's anemia. *Ann Hematol* **63**:54, 1991

108. Macdougall LG et al: Fanconi anemia in black African children. *Am J Med Genet* **36**:408, 1990

*109. Auerbach AD et al: International Fanconi Anemia Registry: Relation of clinical symptoms to diepoxybutane sensitivity. *Blood* **73**:391, 1989

110. Shahidi NT: Fanconi anemia, dyskeratosis congenita, and WT syn-

drome. *Am J Med Genet* **3**(suppl):263, 1987

*111. Fujiwara Y et al: Heritable disorders of DNA repair: Xeroderma pigmentosum and Fanconi's anemia. *Curr Probl Dermatol* **17**:182, 1987

112. Abbondanzo SL et al: Hepatocellular carcinoma in an 11-year-old girl with Fanconi's anemia. Report of a case and review of the literature. *Am J Pediatr Hematol Oncol* **8**:334, 1986

113. Auerbach AD, Wolman SR: Carcinogen-induced chromosome breakage in chromosome instability syndromes. *Cancer Genet Cytogenet* **1**:21, 1979

114. Auerbach AD et al: Prenatal identification of potential donors for umbilical cord blood transplantation for Fanconi anemia. *Transfusion* **30**:682, 1990

115. Sasaki M, Tonomura A: A high susceptibility of Fanconi's anemia to chromosome breakage by DNA cross-linking agents. *Cancer Res* **33**:1829, 1973

116. Berger R et al: Sister chromatid exchanges induced by nitrogen mustard in Fanconi's anemia: Application to the detection of heterozygotes and interpretation of the results. *Cancer Genet Cytogenet* **2**:259, 1980

117. Schroeder TM, Stahl-Mauge C: Mutagenic effects of isonicotinic acid hydrazide in Fanconi's anemia. *Hum Genet* **52**:309, 1979

118. Matsumoto A et al: Repair analysis of mitomycin C-induced DNA crosslinking in ribosomal RNA genes in lymphoblastoid cells from Fanconi's anemia patients. *Mutat Res* **217**:185, 1989

119. Fujiwara Y et al: Cross-link repair in human cells and its possible defect in Fanconi's anemia cells. *J Mol Biol* **113**:635, 1977

120. Diatloff-Zito C et al: Partial complementation of the Fanconi anemia defect upon transfection by heterologous DNA. Phenotypic dissociation of chromosomal and cellular hypersensitivity to DNA crosslinking agents. *Hum Genet* **86**:151, 1990

121. Arwert F et al: The Chinese hamster cell mutant V-H4 is homologous to Fanconi anemia (complementation group A). *Cytogenet Cell Genet* **56**:23, 1991

122. Mann WR et al: Fanconi anemia: Evidence for linkage heterogeneity on chromosome 20q. *Genomics* **9**:329, 1991

*123. Sirnavin C, Trowbridge AA: Dyskeratosis congenita: Clinical features and genetic aspects. Report of a family and review of the literature. *J Med Genet* **12**:339, 1975

124. Connor JM, Teague RH: Dyskeratosis congenita. Report of a large kindred. *Br J Dermatol* **105**:321, 1981

125. Kelly TE, Stelling CB: Dyskeratosis congenita: Radiologic features. *Pediatr Radiol* **12**:31, 1982

126. Pai GS et al: Etiologic heterogeneity in dyskeratosis congenita. *Am J Med Genet* **32**:63, 1989

127. Kawaguchi K et al: Dyskeratosis congenita (Zinsser-Cole-Engman syndrome). An autopsy case presenting with rectal carcinoma, noncirrhotic portal hypertension, and *Pneumocystis carinii* pneumonia. *Virchows Arch* **417**:247, 1990

128. Mills SE et al: Intracranial calcifications and dyskeratosis congenita. *Arch Dermatol* **115**:1437, 1979

129. Burgdorf W et al: Sister chromatid exchange in dyskeratosis congenita. *J Med Genet* **14**:256, 1977

130. Pai GS et al: Bleomycin hypersensitivity in dyskeratosis congenita fibroblasts, lymphocytes, and transformed lymphoblasts. *Cytogenet Cell Genet* **52**:186, 1989

131. DeBauche DM et al: Enhanced G2 chromatid radiosensitivity in dyskeratosis congenita fibroblasts. *Am J Hum Genet* **46**:350, 1990

132. Carter DM et al: Psoralen-DNA cross-linking photoadducts in dyskeratosis congenita: Delay in excision and promotion of sister chromatid exchange. *J Invest Dermatol* **73**:97, 1979

133. Nagasawa H, Little JB: Suppression of cytotoxic effect of mitomycin-C by superoxide dismutase in Fanconi's anemia and dyskeratosis congenita fibroblasts. *Carcinogenesis* **4**:795, 1983

134. Connor JM et al: Assignment of the gene for dyskeratosis congenita to Xq28. *Hum Genet* **72**:348, 1986

*135. Berlin NI et al: Basal cell nevus syndrome. *Ann Intern Med* **64**:403, 1966

*136. Gorlin RJ: Nevoid basal-cell carcinoma syndrome. *Medicine (Baltimore)* **66**:98, 1987

137. Woolgar JA et al: The basal cell naevus syndrome. *Br J Hosp Med* **38**:344, 1987

138. Pratt MD, Jackson R: Nevoid basal cell carcinoma syndrome. A 15-year follow-up of cases in Ottawa and the Ottawa Valley. *J Am Acad Dermatol* **16**:964, 1987

139. Slater S: An evaluation of the metacarpal sign (short fourth metacarpal). *Pediatrics* **46**:468, 1970

140. Dunnick NR et al: Nevoid basal cell carcinoma syndrome: Radiographic manifestations including cystlike lesions of the phalanges. *Radiology* **127**:331, 1978

141. Johnson AD et al: Nevoid basal cell carcinoma syndrome: Bilateral ovarian fibromas in a 3½-year-old girl. *J Am Acad Dermatol* **14**:371, 1986

142. Cotton JL et al: Cardiac tumors and the nevoid basal cell carcinoma syndrome. *Pediatrics* **87**:725, 1991

143. Evans DG et al: The incidence of Gorlin syndrome in 173 consecutive cases of medulloblastoma. *Br J Cancer* **64**:959, 1991

144. Strong LC: Theories of pathogenesis: Mutation and cancer, in *Genetics of Cancer,* edited by JJ Mulvihill et al. New York, Raven, 1977, p 401

145. Happle R, Hoehn H: Cytogenetic studies on cultured fibroblast-like cells derived from basal cell carcinoma tissue. *Clin Genet* **4**:17, 1973

146. Bale AE et al: Sister chromatid exchange and chromosome fragility in the nevoid basal cell carcinoma syndrome. *Cancer Genet Cytogenet* **42**:273, 1989

147. Little JB et al: Radiation sensitivity of cell strains from families with genetic disorders predisposing to radiation-induced cancer. *Cancer Res* **49**:4705, 1989

148. Newton JA et al: Radiobiological studies in the naevoid basal cell carcinoma syndrome. *Br J Dermatol* **23**:573, 1990

149. Applegate LA et al: Hypersensitivity of skin fibroblasts from basal cell nevus syndrome patients to killing by ultraviolet B but not by ultraviolet C radiation. *Cancer Res* **50**:637, 1990

150. Cristofolini M et al: Aromatic retinoid in the chemoprevention of the progression of nevoid basal-cell carcinoma syndrome. *J Dermatol Surg Oncol* **10**:778, 1984

151. Peck GL: Long-term retinoid therapy is needed for maintenance of cancer chemopreventive effect. *Dermatologica* **175**(suppl 1):138, 1987

152. Goldberg LH et al: Effectiveness of isotretinoin in preventing the appearance of basal cell carcinomas in basal cell nevus syndrome. *J Am Acad Dermatol* **21**:144, 1989

153. Knudson AG et al: Mutation and childhood cancer: A probabilistic model for the incidence of retinoblastoma. *Proc Natl Acad Sci USA* **72**:5116, 1975

154. Shimada T et al: Lifespan extension of basal cell nevus syndrome fibroblasts by transfection with mouse pro or v-myc genes. *Int J Cancer* **39**:649, 1987

155. Swift M et al: Breast and other cancers in families with ataxia-telangiectasia. *N Engl J Med* **316**:1289, 1987

Cutaneous Manifestations
of Hematologic Disorders

CHAPTER 159

Dorothea Zucker-Franklin

Cutaneous Manifestations
of Hematologic Diseases

The skin may provide many clues leading to the diagnosis of hematologic disease, but in the final analysis cutaneous manifestations can be expressed only in a limited number of ways. These consist of: (1) extravasation of whole blood; (2) infiltration by migrating blood cells (i.e., devoid of platelets and erythrocytes); (3) changes in color or pigmentation; and (4) ulceration, which, when located in specific areas, suggests ischemia or infection attributable to underlying hematologic disease. Although there will be some overlap, and some of the conditions are discussed in greater detail elsewhere in this volume, it will be useful to base our discussion in this chapter on the order described above.

Blood Extravasation

Bleeding into the skin, as manifested by petechiae or ecchymoses requiring hematologic evaluation, is due either to a disorder in hemostasis or to an impairment of coagulation, but rarely to both. Vasculitis as is seen in connective tissue disorders or infections, telangiectasia, vitamin C deficiency, senile purpura due to fragility of vessels or skin (Fig. 159-1), and traumatic, factitial (self-induced, Fig 159-2) or other exogenously inflicted lesions are not within the purvue of hematology, although they must be included in the list of differential diagnoses.

Disorders of Hemostasis

Bleeding into the skin, as manifested by purpura, easy or spontaneous bruising, is usually due to impaired primary hemostasis. Primary hemostasis is mediated by platelets, their interaction with injured or pathologically altered vessel walls, and with each other. A defect in primary hemostasis can be due to an abnormal number of platelets in the circulation or to their abnormal function. The "secondary stage" of hemostasis depends on the formation of a fibrin clot, which stabilizes the so-called platelet plug. Disorders in coagulation or its physiologic sequel, fibrinolysis, lead to frank bleeding, which is less likely to have cutaneous manifestations. Therefore, defects in primary hemostasis are of greater concern to

the dermatologist, and the coagulopathies involving congenital or acquired defects in clotting factors will not be considered here.

Thrombocytopenia The normal platelet count ranges from 200 to 400×10^9/L, but skin manifestations (e.g., spontaneous purpura or ecchymoses) usually do not occur unless the count falls below $50,000/\mu$L. Platelet counts below $70,000/\mu$L, when obtained by

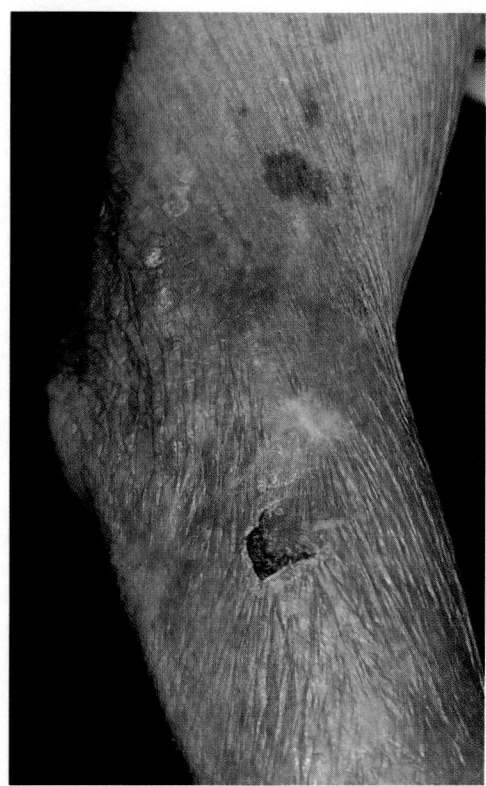

FIGURE 159-1 Senile purpura (Bateman's purpura). Advanced dermatoheliosis is seen on the arms of this 70-year-old male associated with purpura and tears that follow minimal trauma to the skin.

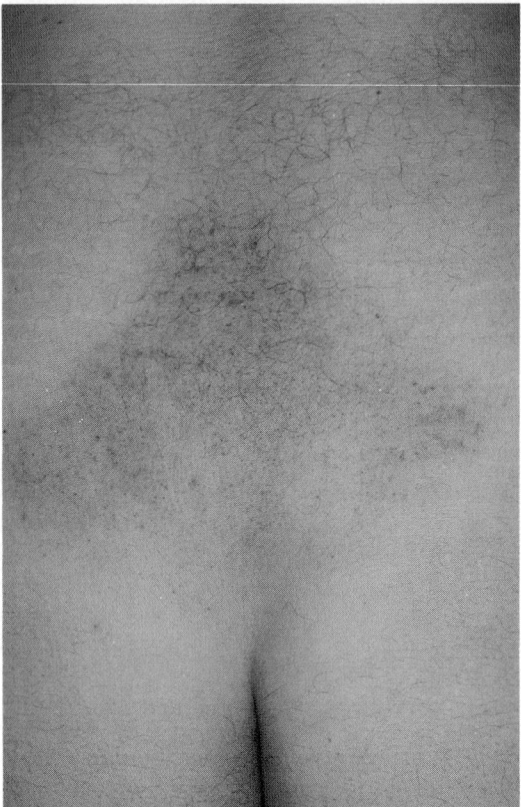

FIGURE 159-2 Traumatic ecchymosis. This large area of ecchymosis was noted on the lower back of a patient who had pressed the skin to the back of the bathtub and then pulled away, resulting in a suction cuplike effect on the cutaneous tissue, which caused hemorrhage.

machine, may be inaccurate and should be confirmed by inspection of a routine blood smear to detect such artifacts as platelet clumps, giant platelets, or platelet satellitism. The latter condition refers to a phenomenon in which platelets adhere to leukocytes in vitro (Fig. 159-3) and thereby cause pseudothrombocytopenia.[1] Platelet aggregates or very large platelets are gated with lymphocytes in automated particle counters. If thrombocytopenia has been confirmed, it is necessary to determine by bone marrow examination whether this condition is due to underproduction of platelets or their accelerated destruction in the peripheral blood.

THROMBOCYTOPENIA DUE TO PLATELET DESTRUCTION. Since platelets are derived from megakaryocytes (Fig. 159-4), a normal or increased number of megakaryocytes suggests that there is accelerated destruction of platelets in the periphery. This holds true for the vast majority of patients whose thrombocytopenia is due to a shortened platelet life span caused by immune mechanisms. The antibodies directed against platelets usually belong to the IgG class of immunoglobulins[2] but may also be of the IgM or IgA class.[3] They can be demonstrated in the serum as well as associated with platelets.[4] Although immune thrombocytopenia may be a chronic accompaniment of many conditions [e.g., connective tissue diseases such as systemic lupus erythematosus, chronic lymphocytic leukemia, and, more recently, the acquired immunodeficiency syndrome (AIDS)], in most instances no underlying disease is evident. The condition is then referred to as idiopathic thrombocytopenic purpura (ITP) (Fig. 159-5). ITP is most prevalent in individuals

between the ages of 20 and 40 and is arbitrarily considered chronic when it lasts for more than 6 months. The sensitized platelets are removed by the spleen, but splenic enlargment is rare. Platelet transfusions are to no avail since the transfused platelets, like the patient's own platelets, are subject to sensitization by the circulating antibody. Apart from splenectomy, which may prolong platelet life span, immunosuppression with steroids or other agents is often efficacious. The administration of intravenous immunoglobulin has also proved to be beneficial, although it is usually not curative.[5,6] The effectiveness of immunoglobulin is partially explained by its ability to bind to the Fc receptors on macrophages, thereby producing a blockade of the reticuloendothelial system. Because platelets also express Fc receptors for immunoglobulin, which bind all subclasses of IgG without regard to specificity, aggregated IgG and immune complexes also react with them and cause their removal by the reticuloendothelial system. This may be one of the reasons why ITP has been found to be an almost invariable hematologic abnormality in patients with AIDS and the AIDS-related syndrome[7] (see also "Underproduction of Platelets," below). The autoimmune thrombocytopenia just described is usually accompanied by subclinical hemolysis.[8] ITP associated with frank hemolytic anemia is referred to as Evans' syndrome.[9] The acute form of ITP is usually seen in children, often following exanthems. It may be severe but is almost always reversible.

Sensitization of circulating platelets may also be caused by drugs, the classic ones being sulfonamides, quinine, and quinidine.

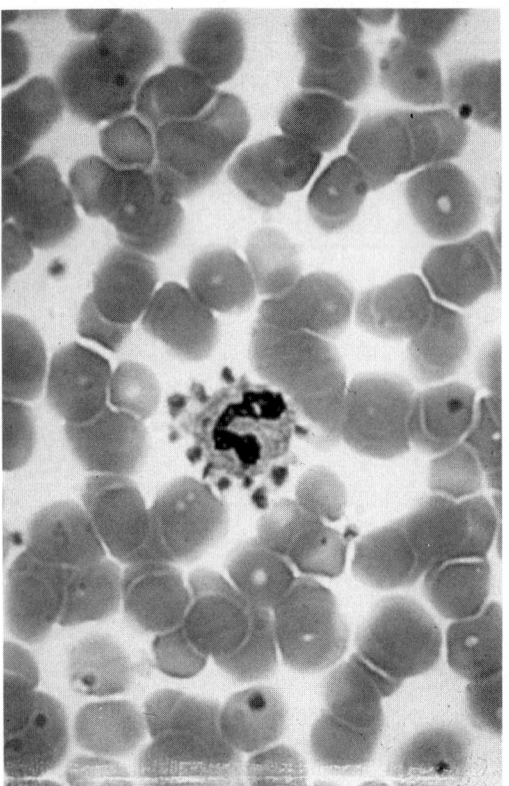

FIGURE 159-3 Platelet satellitism in a specimen anticoagulated with EDTA. In this in vitro phenomenon, platelets rosette around leukocytes. Although the phenomenon may have no clinical significance, it may be responsible for spurious thrombocytopenia, particularly when platelet levels are established by electronic counting.

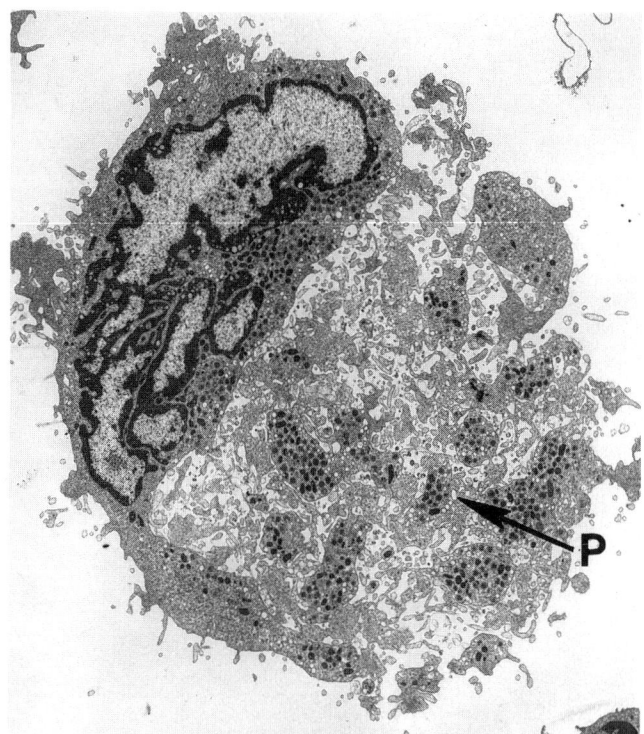

FIGURE 159-4 Megakaryocyte illustrating the process of thrombocytopoiesis (i.e., platelet release) which occurs by random fragmentation of the cytoplasm in which platelet fields are preformed. *P* indicates demarcated platelet field within megakaryocyte cytoplasm. Magnification ×3000.

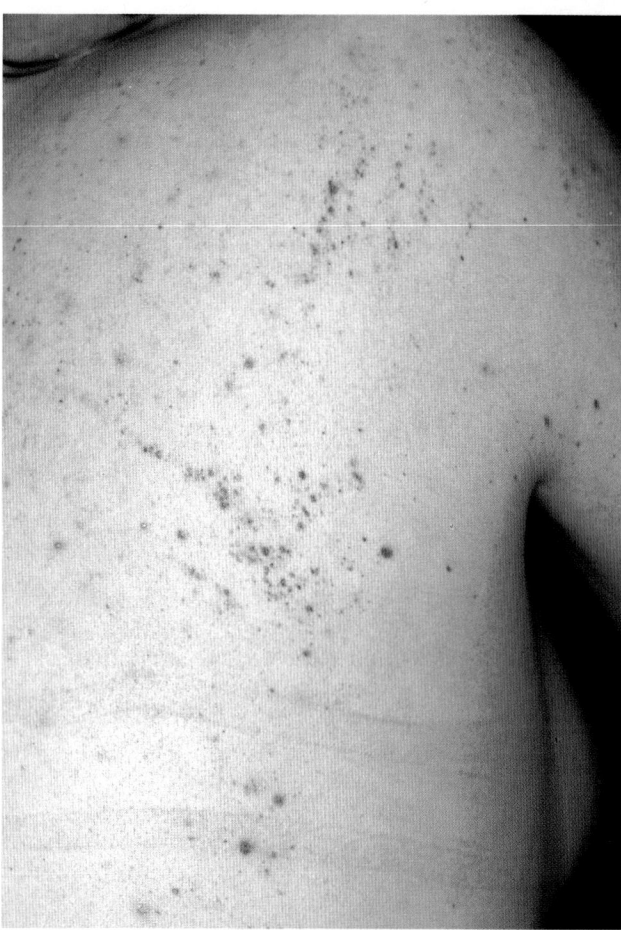

FIGURE 159-5 Idiopathic thrombocytopenic purpura. Numerous dermal hemorrhages, manifested by nonblanching pinpoint-to-pinhead, dusky-red petechiae are seen on the back of this young woman who presented with petechiae.

These agents were believed to bind like haptens to plasma protein carriers. The antibody was thought to be directed against the hapten-protein complex and bind to platelets as "innocent bystanders."[10] Although this is a classic theory, there is more recent evidence showing that antibodies responsible for drug-induced thrombocytopenia bind to platelets by their Fab regions.[11,12] In some instances, the target glycoproteins of the platelet membrane have been identified.[13] More than 50 different medications have been reported to be responsible for this kind of immune destruction of platelets, and the list is still growing. Other mechanisms (e.g., direct injury to the platelet membrane) occur with some drugs and toxins. Thrombocytopenia due to medications or other ingested substances may develop shortly after the drug is taken or may occur in a patient who has taken the same medication with impunity for long periods of time. Patients should always be questioned about the consumption of soft drinks or mixers that may contain quinine. An otherwise healthy individual may develop purpura due to thrombocytopenia precipitated by acute sensitization in this fashion.[14] In any case, the thrombocytopenia should resolve within a week after drug administration has been discontinued. A rare but fulminant development of immune thrombocytopenia is post-transfusion purpura, which appears 1 to 2 weeks after transfusion in an individual who has been sensitized by an uncomplicated pregnancy or prior transfusion. As a rule, the platelets of such patients lack the Pl^{A1} antigen, which is present in 97 percent of the general population. Sensitization is caused by fetal platelets bearing this antigen or by transfusion with Pl^{A1}-positive platelets. The reaction is so severe that frank hemorrhage may overshadow cutaneous manifestation.[15]

Nonimmunologic Causes for Increased Platelet Destruction Increased platelet destruction may be attributable to mechanical injury, such as increased blood turbulence caused by vascular grafts, intravascular calcification, or prosthetic heart valves. The remaining causes for thrombocytopenia in the face of a normal bone marrow are due to excessive platelet consumption, usually resulting from the involvement of the platelets in some form of intravascular coagulation. A dramatic example of such a state is thrombotic thrombocytopenic purpura (TTP, Moschcowitz syndrome),[16] a fulminant multisystem syndrome which, in addition to purpura, presents with Coombs'-negative hemolytic anemia, fever, renal failure, and fluctuating neurologic manifestations.[17] Such patients rarely consult a dermatologist. A skin or mucosal biopsy is often requested as it may show the pathologic hallmark of TTP. The "hyalin" microthrombi which occlude the microvasculature are composed of degranulated platelets and endothelial cell debris, PAS-positive amorphous material, and variable amounts of fibrin. The development of TTP may be triggered by diverse stimuli, such as viremia, bacteremia, pregnancy, oral contraceptives, and a variety of connective tissue disorders. The hemolytic uremic syndrome (HUS) is a related condition which primarily affects arterioles and the renal glomerular capillaries. For the sake of completion, disseminated intravascular coagulation (DIC) must be included as a mechanism for thrombocytopenia. However, DIC refers to a syn-

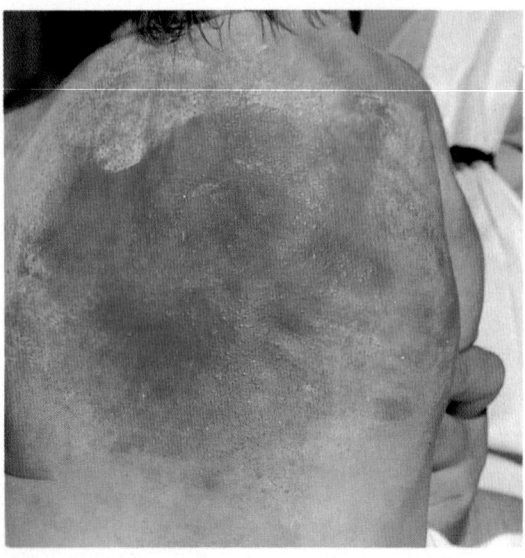

a

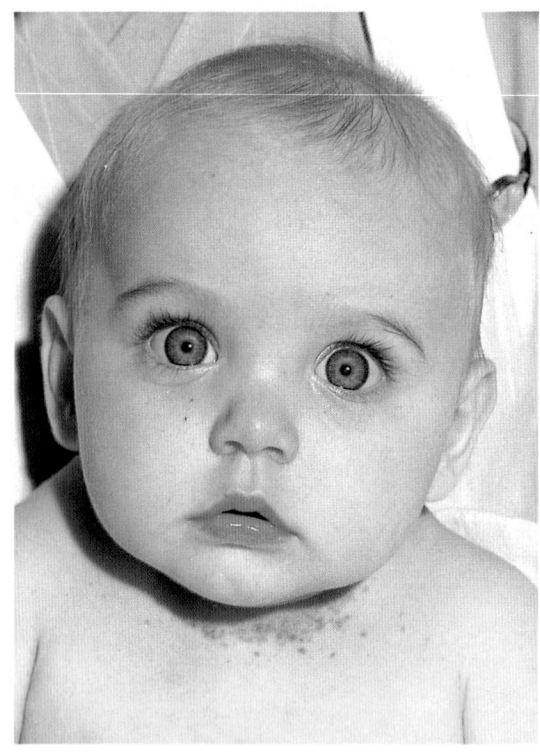

b

FIGURE 159-6 Thrombocytopenic purpura: Kasabach-Merritt syndrome. (*a*) Posterior view of the infant shows a large cavernous hemangioma in which platelets were sequestered and destroyed, resulting in thrombocytopenia. (*b*) The anterior neck of the infant shows numerous nonblanching petechiae.

drome which not only involves platelets but also implies consumption of fibrinogen and the activation of numerous clotting factors. As a result, there is widespread deposition of fibrin in small blood vessels and activation of the fibrinolytic system. Such intravascular coagulation may cause paradoxical bleeding. The coagulation factors consumed are those involved in normal coagulation (i.e., fibrinogen, prothrombin, and factors V, VIII, and XIII). The generation of plasma thrombin results in platelet aggregation, degranulation, and removal by the reticuloendothelial system. DIC is not a single disease but accompanies conditions that are associated with vascular lesions, tissue destruction associated with sepsis, neoplasia, massive trauma, abruptio placentae, snake poisons, and many other factors which initiate the coagulation cascade.

Local consumption coagulopathy may also cause thrombocytopenia. This occurs with vascular malformations, such as the Kasabach-Merritt syndrome (Fig. 159-6). In this syndrome giant hemangiomas, often located in the liver, lung, or other viscera, produce sufficient blood turbulence to activate coagulation factors and platelets. The consumption of fibrinogen, factor V, and factor VIII is similar to that found in DIC. Because of their massive sequestration, autologous platelets labeled with indium-III can be used to localize such hemangiomas radiographically.[18] In rare instances, Kaposi's sarcoma, which is discussed in detail elsewhere in this volume (Chap. 99), may cause thrombocytopenia by the same mechanism. It should be realized that thrombocytopenia may be only "relative." This is seen with splenomegaly of almost any cause. In health, approximately 30 percent of available platelets are stored in the spleen. Splenic enlargement may increase this number to more than 80 percent. Thrombocytopenia caused by this mechanism rarely results in purpura.

THROMBOCYTOPENIA DUE TO PLATELET UNDERPRODUCTION. The reason for thrombocytopenia due to defective platelet production is usually evident on bone marrow examination. Megakaryocytes are decreased or abnormal. This is seen in viral infections and even after inoculation with live measles vaccine. Vacuolation, nu-

clear degeneration, and a reduced number of megakaryocytes have been described in parvovirus, mumps, varicella, Epstein-Barr virus, rubella, and cytomegalovirus infection. In patients with AIDS, the finding of proviral sequences of the human immune deficiency virus (HIV-1)[19] and aberrant megakaryocyte morphology[20] suggests that underproduction of platelets is, at least in part, responsible for thrombocytopenia. Marrow replacement by leukemic cells or infiltration by tumor cells which originate in extramedullary sites may affect the number of megakaryocytes.

A congenital disorder associated with underproduction of platelets is the Wiskott-Aldrich syndrome. This X-linked condition affects males and is characterized by obstinate eczema, thrombocytopenia, and susceptibility to infection because of impairment in the cellular as well as humoral immune response. Both platelets and megakaryocytes have deranged ultrastructure and are half the normal size.[21,22] Also, patients usually have a Coombs' positive hemolytic anemia and a leukocyte chemotactic defect. Splenectomy results in improvement of platelet number and function but does not alleviate eczema and the impaired immune response. Transplantation with normal hematopoietic and lymphopoietic stem cells is the only treatment that may prove curative. Thrombocytopenia manifested by purpura is not infrequently the first sign of the myelodysplastic (preleukemic) syndrome. In addition, there are numerous exogenous agents that can cause generalized marrow aplasia. Substances that have a relatively specific effect on platelet production include thiazide diuretics, alcohol, and estrogens. Nutritional deficiencies, such as iron, vitamin B_{12}, and folic acid, affect platelet production as well. These may present with purpura as a first sign before more widespread symptoms become evident.

Defects of Platelet Function

Purpura and/or ecchymosis in the face of a normal platelet count makes investigation of platelet function mandatory. A prolonged bleeding time is an invariable accompaniment. Bleeding time is tested by placing a blood pressure cuff around the patient's upper arm at a pressure of 40 mmHg. Superficial incisions are made 5 cm distal to the antecubital fossa, a stopwatch is started, and the blood is blotted at 30-s intervals. Bleeding should not exceed 7 min. Although the test is simple, it should be performed by an expert, as falsely shortened bleeding times may be recorded when platelet abnormalities are subtle. Because aspirin and preparations containing aspirin prolong the bleeding time, any patient with purpura should be questioned about the ingestion of aspirin. When a bleeding time test is to be performed, the patient should be instructed to omit ingestion of such agents for at least 1 week.

Congenital Platelet Disorders

Glanzmann Thrombasthenia   *Glanzmann thrombasthenia* is a relatively rare disorder which is inherited in an autosomal recessive manner. Therefore, a family history of consanguinity is important. Clinical symptoms, which typically consist of mucocutaneous bleeding, epistaxis, petechiae, purpura, and menorrhagia, are due to the inability of platelets to aggregate in response to adenosine diphosphate (ADP) or other platelet agonists. Quantitative and/or qualitative defects in the glycoprotein IIb/IIIa complex of the platelet membrane are responsible for this defect.[23,24] These membrane proteins serve as receptors for fibrinogen, fibronectin, vitronectin, and von Willebrand factor (see below). The deficiency prevents normal interaction of activated platelets with each other and the subendothelium. Clot retraction is impaired. Since the degree of this abnormality varies from mild to severe, a patient with a very mild form may consult a dermatologist. The only available treatment, necessary when bleeding is severe, is transfusion with normal platelets, which should be HLA-matched to prevent alloimmunization.

Bernard-Soulier Syndrome   *Bernard-Soulier syndrome* is an extremely rare condition which is inherited as an autosomal recessive disorder and which usually becomes manifest in infancy. The platelet membranes lack glycoprotein Ib, which serves as the major receptor for von Willebrand factor (see below). Antibodies raised against GPIb disrupt adhesion of normal platelets.[25] Platelets thus affected also appear to be much larger in size than their normal counterparts.

von Willebrand Disease   von Willebrand disease is the most common congenital platelet anomaly associated with a prolonged bleeding time. Its prevalence has been estimated to range from 3 to 4 per 100,000. The most common form is transmitted as an autosomal dominant trait with variable penetrance. The pathophysiology of the disease is as complex as its inheritance and goes beyond what can be discussed in this space. Briefly, von Willebrand factor (vWF) is synthesized in megakaryocytes and endothelial cells. In platelets, it is stored in the α-granules, and it circulates in plasma with a molecular weight ranging from 500,000 to 20 million. The larger multimers are hemostatically more competent. Thrombin, ADP, collagen, and other agonists induce the expression of vWF on the platelet surface. Platelet vWF is more effective in supporting adherence to collagen than plasma vWF. To diagnose this condition, coagulation as well as platelet tests are necessary. Among these are an activated thromboplastin time, factor VIII coagulant activity, ristocetin cofactor activity, ristocetin-induced platelet aggregation, and vWF antigen. One or more of these tests may be abnormal. Addition of the antibiotic ristocetin to platelet-rich

plasma causes normal platelets to aggregate. This test is abnormal in 70 percent of patients with vWF deficiency and is a good screening test.

Impaired Platelet Function due to Pathology of Granules   A normal platelet count with a prolonged bleeding time may be attributable to a reduction in platelet granules or their impaired secretion. The platelet α-granules contain fibrinogen, fibronectin, vWF, thrombospondin, platelet factor 4, and β-thromboglobulin. These substances are released when platelets are activated. In the gray platelet syndrome, or α-storage pool disease, such granules are decreased in number or absent. Hence, the platelets appear gray on routine blood smears. Dense granule deficiency, or δ-storage pool disease, refers to a condition in which platelets lack granules that contain adenine nucleotides and serotonin. The condition may coexist with other clinical aberrations. Of particular interest to dermatologists is the Hermansky-Pudlak syndrome in which δ-storage pool disease of platelets is associated with oculocutaneous tyrosine-positive albinism and the accumulation of pigment-laden macrophages in many organs. The ability of platelets to aggregate is defective, and their response to a low concentration of collagen is diminished.[26,27]

Impaired Platelet Function due to Extrinsic Factors

A host of acquired systemic conditions, such as uremia, myeloproliferative diseases, and the dysproteinemias, may affect platelet function adversely. In most of these conditions, cutaneous manifestations are not primary. Multiple myeloma and its variants, particularly the macroglobulinemias, are noteworthy in this regard. The exact relationship between the type and level of the paraprotein and the platelet dysfunction is somewhat vague.[28] However, sometimes the paraprotein may have a sensitizing effect on platelets.[29,30] In some patients, the degree of platelet destruction and thrombocytopenia may mimic ITP. In others, the platelet count is not decreased but the paraprotein may react with specific platelet membrane proteins, resulting in abnormalities that resemble conditions like von Willebrand disease.

Benign hypergammaglobulinemic purpura refers to a condition involving primarily the lower extremities. The patient may experience local tenderness, burning, itching, transient petechiae, and urticarial eruptions, which may become confluent. As the urticaria subsides, petechiae and purpuric lesions remain. Although this condition may accompany diverse systemic diseases, a dermatologist may be consulted because of the predominant skin manifestations. The circulating protein is usually polyclonal, and the causes are so varied that the number of papers on the subject appears to exceed the occurrences of the syndrome.

Circulating cryoproteins are also associated with purpura. Cryoglobulinemia of the "essential" or primary type is almost always associated with it. Exposure to cold results in the precipitation of a complex of IgG and immunoglobulins having anti-IgG activity which may cause Raynaud's phenomenon, livedo reticularis, and plasma hyperviscosity. Three main types of cryoglobulins are recognized. Type I cryoglobulins are monoclonal and comprise 5 to 10 percent of the total number. Type II consist of mixed immunoglobulin complexes, usually monoclonal IgM with antibody specificity for polyclonal IgG. A large percentage of these have χ light chains. No underlying disease may be found. Type III cryoglobulins are polyclonal mixed and contain, in addition to immune complexes, some non-immunoglobulin substances, such as complement, polynucleotides, and viral antigens. In addition to the platelet malfunction and/or thrombocytopenia, impaired blood flow due to cryoprecipitates in capillaries of the skin accounts for the purpura. Ulceration of the skin may also ensue. Several good reviews of this subject are available,[31,32] including Chap. 162.

Thrombocythemia

Bleeding into the skin is also a frequent accompaniment of thrombocythemia, which should be considered when platelet counts over 600,000/μL are sustained for a prolonged time. In benign reactive thrombocytosis, which is common in such conditions as iron deficiency, acute bleeding, chronic inflammation, and after splenectomy, the underlying problem is usually obvious and the platelet count rarely exceeds 1000×10^9/μL. In contrast, primary or essential thrombocythemia is a clonal disorder originating from a single abnormal multipotential stem cell.[33] Megakaryocyte colony-forming units are both increased in number and able to grow autonomously (i.e., without the addition of growth factors). Marrow karyotypes in these patients are usually normal. Clinically, this disease is distinct from polycythemia vera (PV), a disease in which the thrombocythemia is accompanied by an elevated hematocrit, an expanded red cell volume, and leukocytosis. Pruritus is common in PV but not in essential thrombocythemia. The thrombocythemia associated with other myeloproliferative diseases is easily recognized as part of a larger complex affecting many cell lineages. In all these conditions platelet function may be impaired.

Finally, the Gardner-Diamond syndrome (painful bruising), a rare disorder of uncertain etiology, should be mentioned in a section on purpura.[34] There is local itching, burning, or pain before the lesions appear. The extremities, particularly the hands, are most frequently involved. The presence of erythema may differentiate the lesions from simple bruises. Autoerythocyte sensitivity and autosensitization to DNA have been substantiated in some cases. However, because most patients have associated psychiatric disorders, the term *psychogenic purpura* has been suggested.[35]

Infiltration of the Skin by Leukocytes

A normal response of the skin to trauma or infection calls for the diapedesis and migration of white blood cells to the site. Leukocytes (neutrophils, eosinophils, basophils, and monocytes) become involved in all cutaneous infections. Each type of cell provides a specific function and is attracted to the site by chemotactic factors for which the cell in question has receptors. Therefore, one cell type may dominate another depending on the stimulus. Infiltration of the skin with eosinophils, mast cells, and basophils, as is seen in urticaria pigmentosa (Chap. 161), or with normal or neoplastic mononuclear cells, as is seen in mycosis fungoides (Chap. 105), is discussed elsewhere in this volume. The present discussion is limited to neutrophils.

Localized bacterial infections that elicit leukocyte infiltrates (e.g., furuncles, carbuncles, or cellulitis) are usually not indicative of blood disease. In contrast, recurrent, chronic neutrophilic dermatosis (Sweet's syndrome) is a febrile illness involving erythematous, eczematous patches on the arms, face, and legs which progress to brown painful plaques that may ulcerate. The histopathology of the skin is that of a dense leukocytic infiltrate, and there is blood neutrophilia.[36] At least 10 percent of the patients will develop mye-

logenous leukemia or another hemopoietic stem cell disease. Therefore, it may be prudent to look for karyotypic abnormalities in the bone marrow cells of afflicted patients, even when only marrow hyperplasia is reported. Leukemic infiltrates of the skin in patients with frank leukemia are not unusual (Fig. 159-7). Sweet's syndrome was first reported as a unique form of infective dermatitis occuring primarily in Jamaican children. Recently, the development of this condition has also been attributed to immunosuppression caused by infection with HTLV-I.[37]

As mentioned, in the healthy individual, infiltration of the skin with leukocytes is a physiologic, if not always a desirable, response. However, neutropenia, as well as defects in neutrophil function, permit invasion of the skin and mucous membranes with microorganisms that are not usually considered pathogenic (e.g., staphylococci or gram-negative bacteria present in the environment).

The lower limit of a normal neutrophil count is 1800/μL, but even 1000/μL poses no threat. Counts of 500/μL or less are invariably associated with fever, erythema without pus, and painful ulcers. The causes for neutropenia are numerous and include insults to the bone marrow by drugs, toxins, and neoplastic infiltrates as well as destruction of the cells in the circulation by immune mechanisms or sequestration by the spleen. Congenital and cyclic neutropenias are well-established syndromes with similar skin manifestations.[38,39] Recently, it has been possible to alleviate these conditions by the administration of hematopoietic growth factors, such as granulocyte/macrophage colony-stimulating factor (GM-CSF). In the face of a normal white blood cell count, difficulty in handling invasive microorganisms may also be due to functional impairment of the cells. The function of neutrophils depends on their ability to adhere, to respond to chemotactic stimuli, to phagocytose, and to kill ingested pathogens. Defects in each of these processes have been identified.[40,41]

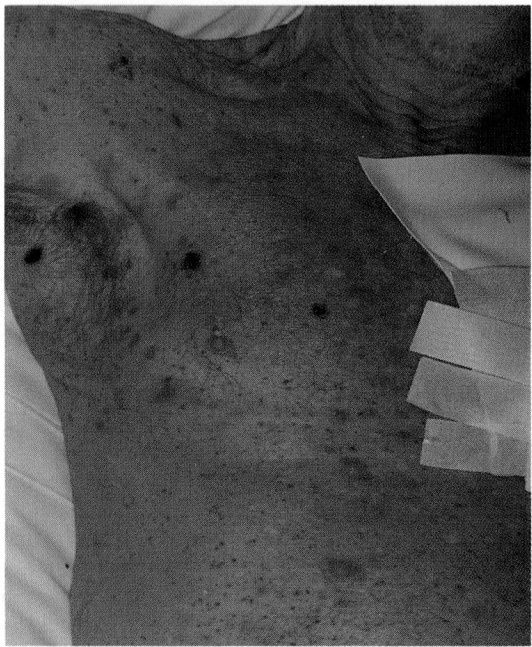

FIGURE 159-7 Leukemia cutis. Slightly hemorrhagic papules are seen on the chest of a 70-year-old male with acute myelogenous leukemia.

Pathology Related to Defects in Granules

Chronic Granulomatous Disease of Childhood (CGD)   Leukocytes of patients with CGD ingest bacteria normally but fail to kill them. The defect in bactericidal function is due to the inability of the cells to generate hydrogen peroxide and free oxygen radicals.[42] Because the usual mode of inheritance is X-linked, males are more often affected than females.[43] Overall, the male-to-female ratio is 6:1. CGD has been reviewed repeatedly (see Refs. 44,45). Patients develop infections at multiple sites, including lymph nodes, liver, lung, and bone. Skin lesions are eczematous and purulent but gradually become granulomatous as infections smolder. The diagnosis is accomplished by means of the nitroblue tetrazolium (NBT) dye test, in which the diseased leukocytes are unable to reduce the colorless NBT dye to blue-black.

There are various forms of CGD. The major classification criteria depend on the cytochrome-b spectrum measured on extracts of disrupted neutrophils. Type I is X-linked, cytochrome-b negative, and accounts for 66 percent of patients; Type II is autosomal recessive, cytochrome-b positive, and accounts for 30 percent; and Type III is autosomal recessive, cytochrome-b negative, and accounts for most of the remainder. Catalase-positive microbes, such as *S. aureus*, can multiply intracellularly. In contrast, organisms that generate their own hydrogen peroxide, such as pneumococci and streptococci, are readily killed by CGD leukocytes. Patients suffer the sequelae of severe chronic infection, but the attack rate and severity of the disease is exceedingly variable. Treatment is largely supportive and includes the use of prophylactic antibiotics. Recently, bone marrow transplantation and treatment with interferon-γ[46] have been advocated.

Chédiak-Higashi Syndrome[47–50]   This autosomal recessive disease is now recognized as a generalized defect in the function of cytoplasmic granules. Although the increased susceptibility to infection of afflicted patients is, to a large extent, attributable to the inability of leukocyte lysosomes to fuse with phagocytic vacuoles, practically all granulated cells are involved.[49] Pathologic aggregation of melanosomes results in albinism of hair, skin, and ocular fundi. Thus, the dermatologist confronted by a patient with partial or complete albinism or photosensitivity should be aware of the syndrome. The diagnosis is established by the presence in all blood cells of large inclusions, which can be seen on routine Wright-stained smears. It is believed that the membranes of Chédiak-Higashi cells are more fluid than those of normal cells. During neutrophil development, there is fusion of the primary granules with each other, as well as with secondary granules and the membranes of other organelles. This fusion gives rise to huge secondary lysosomes that contain a reduced content of hydrolytic enzymes. Granulocyte precursors may also die in the bone marrow, resulting in neutropenia. The granules of platelets are affected as well. Thus, despite normal platelet counts, there is inadequate hemostasis because the platelet storage granules are not properly released. The prognosis is poor. Many affected individuals die in childhood and those who survive may have a rapid, downhill course.

Myeloperoxidase Deficiency   This condition is inherited as an autosomal recessive trait that affects neutrophils but not eosinophils. Although the enzyme potentiates microbicidal effectiveness, the functional impairment is not severe. The patients rarely have pyogenic infections, but persistent lesions caused by fungi may occur.[51]

Membrane and Cytoskeletal Dysfunction of Neutrophils

Leukocyte adherence deficiency is a congenital disorder manifested by cutaneous infection, lack of pus formation despite blood neutrophilia, and impaired wound healing. In this syndrome the leukocytes lack a family of related surface glycoproteins designated CD11/CD18.[52,53] These proteins mediate migration, adhesion, phagocytosis, complement, and antibody-dependent phagocytosis. The neutrophils of these patients are unable to adhere firmly to surfaces and to respond to chemotactic signals. They fail to recognize microorganisms coated with opsonic complement fragments, like C3bi. Despite elevated blood neutrophil levels, there is a paucity of cells at inflammatory sites. The severity of the disease correlates with the degree of glycoprotein deficiency. Bone marrow transplantation is the only available treatment that can prevent a fatal outcome in severe cases. Patients with leukocyte adhesion deficiency have normal polymerizable actin.[52] In contrast, a syndrome that is clinically similar to the one seen in patients who lack CD11/CD18 may also result from a failure of actin to polymerize into filaments.[54] Such a defect interferes with normal motility of the cells as well.

Defects Extrinsic to Neutrophils

Inasmuch as directed migration of neutrophils to inflammatory sites depends on chemotaxis, and phagocytosis depends on the presence of various opsonins, many extracellular factors orchestrate the cell's function. The most profound disturbances arise from abnormalities in the complement system, particularly C3. C3 deficiency is inherited as an autosomal recessive trait. Heterozygotes have half the normal level of C3. Pyogenic infections may also result from a deficiency in C3b inactivator, a protein inhibitor of the alternative complement pathway. Its absence leads to hypercatabolism of C3 and factor B. The subject is discussed in greater detail elsewhere in this text (Chaps. 36 and 115).

In addition, impaired neutrophil motility with pyogenic cutaneous manifestations is seen in the hyperimmunoglobulin E syndrome.[55] To date, it has not been possible to show a relationship between the serum IgE level and the degree of neutrophil dysfunction.[56]

Finally, neutrophil function may be affected by numerous diseases and metabolic states as well as by ingested and medically administered agents. Prominent among the latter are glucocorticoids, especially in very high doses over long periods. Steroids inhibit neutrophil locomotion, chemotaxis, phagocytosis, and degranulation.[57,58] However, their administration on alternate days may avoid this problem.[59]

Change in Color and Pigmentation of the Skin

With the exception of the variety of colors associated with extravasated blood or with frank jaundice due to hemolytic anemia, changes in skin pigmentation are usually not due to primary hematologic disease. However, the astute dermatologist may observe a number of lesions that are related to blood diseases. Ecchymoses may be red, purple, yellowish, or green depending on the size of the hemorrhage and its age. The brown pigmentation resulting from repeated petechiae due to platelet disorders or dysproteinemias is often found in areas of high venous pressure, such as the lower legs. It will not blanch on digital pressure. Chronic stasis with extravasation of blood cells results in permanent hyperpigmentation due not only to the deposition of hemosiderin, but also to the increased deposition of melanin. These lesions are referred to by various eponyms, such as the pigmentary dermatosis of Schamberg (Fig. 159-8),[60] purpura annularis telangiectodes (Majocchi disease),[61,62] and the pigmented purpuric lichenoid dermatitis of Gougerot and Blum.[63] These lesions are not related to any blood dyscrasias.

Anemia

Pallor of the skin is associated with severe anemia of any cause. The palmar creases are useful to assess the degree of anemia. In the fully open hand, the palmar creases appear pink unless the hemoglobin level is less than 7 g/dL. If such a low level of hemoglobin is due to chronic iron deficiency, there should be other skin manifestations, such as dryness, coarseness, brittle hair and nails, and a smooth tongue. When anemia is associated with some degree of hemolysis (as in vitamin B_{12} or folate acid deficiency), the skin may have a lemon-yellow hue. It is not unusual to see blotchy hyper- or hypopigmentation in full-blown pernicious anemia. This may be irreversible even after the anemia has been treated with parenteral administration of vitamin B_{12}. Pernicious anemia is recognized as an autoimmune disease in which atrophy of the gastric mucosa is prominent. The elaboration of intrinsic factor is impeded by humoral as well as cellular immune mechanisms. Intrinsic factor is necessary for the absorption of cobalamin. Autoantibodies against gastric parietal cells are found in 90 percent of patients with pernicious anemia. The literature on various aspects of this subject is vast. Therefore, the interested reader is referred to reviews (see Refs. 64, 65). Not infrequently, the disease is associated with autoimmune thyroiditis, hypoparathyroidism, and Addison disease.[66] Patients with pernicious anemia also have a higher than expected incidence of antibodies directed against other epithelia, and it is therefore not surprising that components of the integument may be targets. Vitiligo has been reported in as many as 10 percent of the patients.[67] Folate deficiency, which also results in megaloblastic anemia, is usually due to malnutrition, as seen in alcoholics, food faddists, and the elderly. It is associated with atrophy of the filiform papillae of the tongue and cheilosis.

Cyanosis

A grayish-blue color of the skin (i.e., cyanosis) connotes an excess of reduced hemogloblin. In the absence of cardiopulmonary disease, this may be due to the presence of methemoglobin or sulfhemoglobin. To be grossly visible the minimum of methemoglobin must be 1.5 to 2.0 g/dL and the concentration of sulfhemoglobin 0.5 g/dL. Methemoglobin is a form of hemoglobin in which ferrous ions have been oxidized to the ferric state. Such hemoglobin is less able to carry oxygen. There are three types of methemoglobinemia. The hereditary type, which is transmitted as an autosomal recessive trait, is due to a deficiency in NADH-diaphorase, an enzyme that catalyzes a step in methemoglobin reduction.[68] The second type is due to toxic drugs or chemicals that oxidize hemoglobin in excess of the amount that can be reduced by available reducing enzymes.[69,70] The rate of hemoglobin oxidation

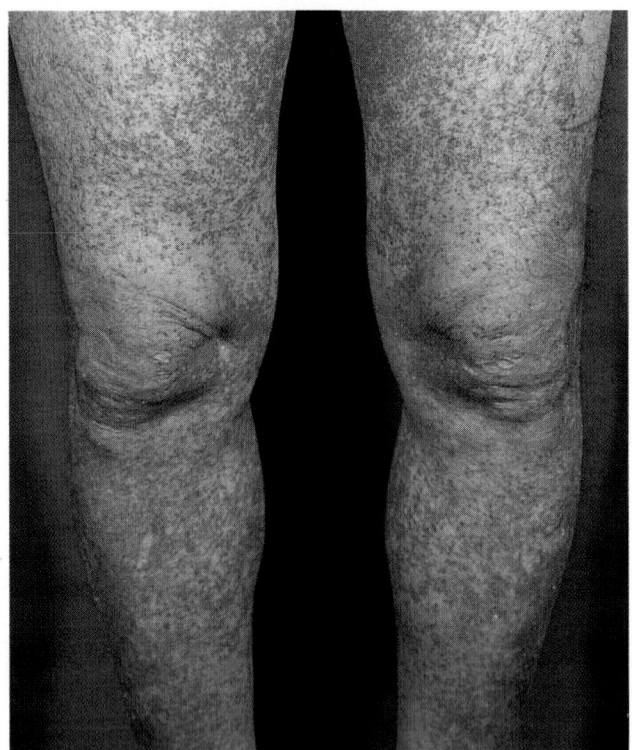

a

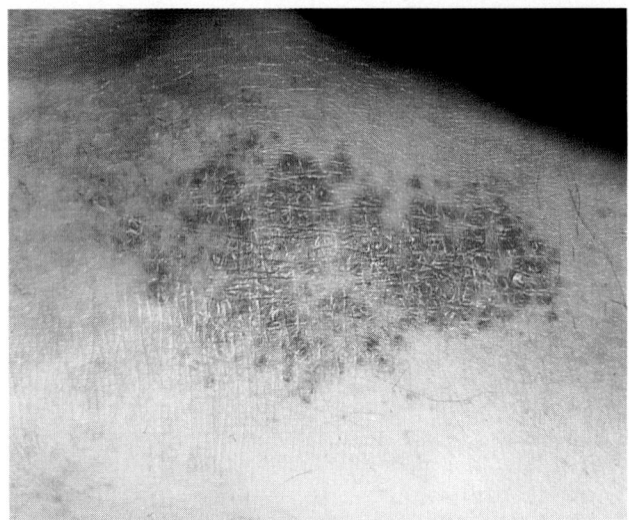

b

FIGURE 159-8 Progressive pigmentary purpura (Schamberg's disease). (*a*) Innumerable small ''cayenne pepper'' colored, nonpalpable, fresh dermal hemorrhages are seen on the legs; older hemorrhages have more of a tan color. (*b*) Close-up.

is accelerated by many drugs, including sulfonamides, dapsone, analine derivatives, nitrates, nitroglycerin,[71,72] and local anesthetics. Patients with hereditary NADH-diaphorase deficiency may be particularly sensitive to such drugs. Administration of reducing agents, such as ascorbic acid or methylene blue, may be helpful. The third type of methemoglobinemia is known as hemoglobin M disease.[73] The hemoglobin M diseases are due to inherited abnormalities in the structure of the globin portion of hemoglobin. They are often transmitted as autosomal dominant traits. Therefore most patients affected with cyanosis due to hemoglobin M will have an affected parent. The hemoglobin M disorders rarely produce health problems. Their effect is mainly cosmetic. To date, more than 20 hemoglobinopathies that result in the formation of methemoglobin with an abnormal oxygen affinity have been described.[74] Some patients may have hemolytic anemia apart from cyanosis. Sulfhemoglobinemia may also cause the skin to have a bluish tinge. It appears to be a benign disorder which often recurs repeatedly in the same person after exposure to certain drugs. Unlike methemoglobin, which can be reduced, the formation of sulfhemoglobin is not reversible and persists for the life span of the erythrocytes carrying the pigment. The differential diagnosis of these forms of hemoglobinemia depends largely on spectrophotometric and electrophoretic analyses.

A ruddy cyanosis or acrocyanosis is seen in conditions associated with abnormally high levels of hemoglobin. This may be secondary or compensatory in situations with a decreased availability of oxygen, or it may be primary as is the case in polycythemia vera. Polycythemia vera is a hemopoietic stem cell disorder which involves all hemopoietic cell lines, even though erythroid proliferation usually appears dominant. Because cutaneous findings such as plethora, ecchymoses, and intense pruritus occur in about 15 percent of patients,[75] such individuals may consult a dermatologist before the diagnosis of the blood disease is made. The pruritus may be sudden in onset after a warm bath or shower and is often of limited duration.[76] It is attributed to the release from mast cells or basophils of secretory products, which are always elevated in this disorder.[77] The triad of increased total red cell volume with a normal plasma volume, a normal arterial oxygen saturation, and splenomegaly establish the diagnosis. In the absence of splenomegaly, two of the following additional findings should be present to make the diagnosis definitive: (1) a platelet count over 400×10^9/L; (2) a leukocytosis of 12×10^9/L; (3) an elevated leukocyte alkaline phosphatase score; and (4) an elevated serum B_{12} level or unbound B_{12} binding capacity. Phlebotomy is the treatment of choice for relief of symptoms of hypervolemia and hyperviscosity, but it does not relieve pruritus or thrombocytosis. Myelosuppressive therapy or radioactive phosphorus (^{32}P) is indicated to reduce the incidence of thrombosis. However, since the survival of patients with polycythemia vera is often 10 years or more, the development of acute leukemia or other neoplasms may emerge in the course of such treatments. This is seen in about 35 percent of patients and is believed to be, in part, attributable to the use of alkylating agents or ^{32}P.[78]

Ulceration

By far the most common ulcerations are self-inflicted excoriations as a response to intense pruritus accompanying such hematologic disorders as Hodgkin disease, polycythemia vera, or cutaneous lymphomas. Spontaneously appearing ulcers or scars from healed ulcers are found over the internal or external maleoli in up to 75 percent of patients with sickle cell disease (Fig. 159-9) who live in tropical areas.[79] However, leg ulcers are also seen in other hemolytic anemias such as thalassemia[80] and congenital spherocytosis.[81] Although this manifestation is attributable to ischemia, its pathogenesis is not entirely clear since ulcerative lesions are seen even when the anemia is relatively mild or when it has been alleviated by

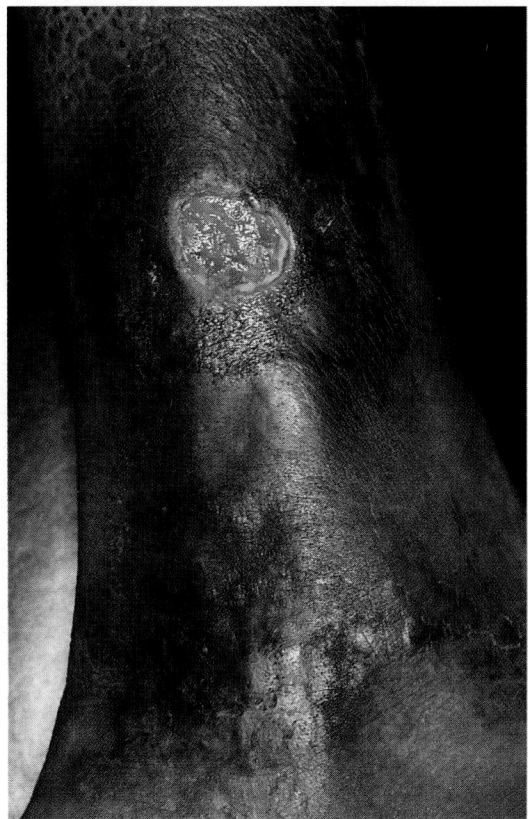

FIGURE 159-9   Sickle cell disease with ulceration. This 34-year-old male with sickle cell disease experienced the formation of an ulcer on the leg, just proximal to the ankle while hiking at an elevation of 4000 meters.

splenectomy. The spontaneous ulcerations associated with cutaneous T cell lymphomas are addressed elsewhere in this volume (see Chap. 105).

References

1. Kjeldsberg CR, Swanson J: Platelet satellitism. *Blood* **43**:831, 1974
2. Rosse WF et al: Subclasses of IgG antibodies in immune thrombocytopenic purpura (ITP). *Br J Haematol* **46**:109, 1970
3. Panzer S et al: Platelet-associated immunoglobulins IgG, IgM, IgA and complement C_3 in immune and non-immune thrombocytopenic disorders. *Am J Hematol* **23**:89, 1986
4. McMillan R et al: Platelet-associated and plasma anti-glycoprotein autoantibodies in chronic ITP. *Blood* **70**:1040, 1987
5. Bussel JB et al: Intravenous gammaglobulin treatment of chronic idiopathic thrombocytopenic purpura. *Blood* **62**:480, 1983
6. Bussel JB, Pham LC: Intravenous treatment with gammaglobulin in adults with immune thrombocytopenic purpura: Review of the literature. *Vox Sang* **52**:206, 1987
7. Walsh CM et al: On the mechanism of thrombocytopenic purpura in sexually active homosexual men. *N Engl J Med* **311**:635, 1984
8. Zucker-Franklin D, Karpatkin S: Red cell and platelet fragmentation in idiopathic autoimmune thrombocytopenic purpura. *N Engl J Med* **297**:517, 1977
9. Evans RS et al: Primary thrombocytopenic purpura and acquired hemolytic anemia; evidence for common etiology. *Arch Intern Med* **87**:48, 1951

10. Shulman NR: Immunoreactions involving platelets. IV. Studies on the pathogenesis of thrombocytopenia in drug purpura using test doses of quinidine in sensitized individuals; their implications in idiopathic thrombocytopenic purpura. *J Exp Med* **107**:711, 1958

11. Christie DJ et al: Fab-mediated binding of drug-dependent antibodies to platelets in quinidine and quinine-induced thrombocytopenia. *J Clin Invest* **75**:310, 1985

12. Smith ME et al: Binding of quinine- and quinidine-dependent drug antibodies to platelets is mediated by the Fab domain of the immunoglobulin G and is not Fc dependent. *J Clin Invest* **79**:912, 1987

13. Christie DJ et al: Quinine- and quinidine-platelet antibodies can react with GPIIb/IIIa. *Br J Haematol* **67**:213, 1987

14. Belkin GA: Cocktail purpura. An unusual case of quinine sensitivity. *Ann Intern Med* **66**:583, 1967

15. Mueller-Eckhardt C et al: Post-transfusion thrombocytopenic purpura: Immunological and clinical studies in two cases and review of the literature. *Blut* **40**:249, 1980

16. Moschcowitz E: An acute febrile pleiochromic anemia with hyaline thrombosis of terminal arterioles and capillaries—an undescribed disease. *Arch Intern Med* **36**:89, 1925

17. Amorosi EL, Ultmann JE: Thrombotic thrombocytopenic purpura: Report of 16 cases and review of literature. *Medicine (Baltimore)* **45**:139, 1966

18. Warrell RP, Jr et al: Intratumoral consumption of indium-III labeled platelets in a patient with hemangiomatosis and intravascular coagulation (Kasabach-Merritt syndrome). *Cancer* **52**:2256, 1983

19. Zucker-Franklin D, Cao Y: Megakaryocytes of human immunodeficiency virus-infected individuals express viral RNA. *Proc Natl Acad Sci* **86**:5595, 1989

20. Zucker-Franklin D et al: Structural changes in the megakaryocytes of patients infected with the human immune deficiency virus (HIV-I). *Am J Pathol* **134**:1295, 1989

21. Grottum KA et al: Wiskott-Aldrich syndrome: Qualitative platelet defects and short platelet survival. *Br J Haematol* **17**:373, 1969

22. Corash L et al: Platelet-associated immunoglobulin, platelet size, and the effect of splenectomy in the Wiskott-Aldrich syndrome. *Blood* **65**:1439, 1985

23. Phillips DR, Agin PP: Platelet membrane defects in Glanzmann's thrombasthenia. Evidence for decreased amounts of two major glycoproteins. *J Clin Invest* **60**:535, 1977

24. George JN et al: Molecular defects in interactions of platelets with the vessel wall. *N Eng J Med* **311**:1084, 1984

25. McMichael AJ et al: Monoclonal antibody to human glycoprotein. I. Effects on human platelet function. *Br J Haematol* **49**:501, 1981

26. Hermansky F, Pudlak P: Albinism associated with hemorrhagic diathesis and unusual pigmented reticular cells in the bone marrow: Report of two cases with histochemical studies. *Blood* **14**:162, 1959

27. DePinho RA, Kaplan KL: The Hermansky-Pudlak syndrome. Report of three cases and review of pathophysiology and management considerations. *Medicine (Baltimore)* **64**:192, 1985

28. Furie B: Acquired coagulation disorders and dysproteinemias in hemostasis and thrombosis, in *Basic Principles and Clinical Practice,* 2d ed, edited by R Coleman et al. Philadelphia, Lippincott, 1987, p 841

29. Varticovski L et al: Anti-platelet and anti-DNA in a Waldenstrom macroglobulinemia and ITP. *Am J Hematol* **24**:351, 1987

30. Richards F et al: Correlation between serum IgG, platelet membrane IgG, and platelet function in hypergammaglobulinaemic states. *Br J Haematol* **41**:585, 1979

31. Meltzer M et al: Cryoglobulinemia—a clinical and laboratory study. *Am J Med* **40**:828, 837, 1966

32. Gorevic PD et al: Mixed cryoglobulinemia: Clinical aspects and long term follow-up of 40 patients. *Am J Med* **69**:287, 1980

33. Fialkow PJ et al: Evidence that essential thrombocythemia is a clonal disorder with origin in a multipotent stem cell. *Blood* **58**:916, 1981

34. Gardner FH, Diamond LK: Auto-erythrocyte sensitization; a form of purpura producing painful bruising following autosensitization to red blood cells in certain women. *Blood* **10**:675, 1955

35. Ratnoff OD: The psychogenic purpuras, a review of autoerythrocyte sensitization, autosensitization to DNA, hysterical and factitial bleeding, and religious stigmata. *Semin Hematol* **17**:192, 1980

36. Sweet RD: Acute neutrophilic dermatosis. *Br J Dermatol* **100**:93, 1979

37. Le Grenade L: Affective dermatitis of Jamaican children: A marker for HTLV-1 infection. *Lancet* **336**:1345, 1990

38. Kostmann R: Infantile genetic agranulocytosis. A review with presentation of 10 new cases. *Acta Paediatr Scand* **64**:362, 1975

39. Lange RD: Cyclic hematopoiesis: Human cyclic neutropenia. *Exp Hematol* **11**:435, 1983

40. Baehner RL: Disorders of leukocytes leading to recurrent infection. *Pediatr Clin North Am* **19**:935, 1972

41. Gallin JI et al: Disorders of phagocyte chemotaxis. *Ann Intern Med* **92**:520, 1980

42. Quie PG et al: In vitro bactericidal capacity of human polymorphonuclear leukocytes: Diminished activity in chronic granulomatous disease of childhood. *J Clin Invest* **46**:668, 1967

43. Holmes B et al: Chronic granulomatous disease in females. *N Engl J Med* **283**:217, 1970

44. Tauber AI et al: Chronic granulomatous disease: A syndrome of phagocyte oxidase deficiencies. *Medicine* **62**:286, 1983

45. Boxer LA, Morganroth ML: Neutrophil function disorders. *Dis Mon* **33**:681, 1987

46. Ezekowitz RA et al: Recombinant interferon gamma augments phagocyte superoxide production in X-chronic granulomatous disease gene expression in X-linked variant chronic granulomatous disease. *J Clin Invest* **80**:1009, 1987

47. Chédiak M: Nouvelle anomalie leucocytaire de caractère constitutional familial. *Rev Hematol* **7**:362, 1952

48. Higashi O: Congenital gigantism of peroxidase granules: First case ever reported of qualitative abnormality of peroxydase. *Tohoku J Exp Med* **59**:315, 1954

49. Blume RS, Wolff SM: The Chédiak-Higashi syndrome: Studies in four patients and a review of the literature. *Medicine (Baltimore)* **51**:247, 1972

50. Root RK et al: Abnormal bactericidal, metabolic and lysosomal functions of Chédiak-Higashi Syndrome leukocytes. *J Clin Invest* **51**:649, 1972

51. Lehrer RI, Cline MJ: Leukocyte myeloperoxidase deficiency and disseminated candidiasis: The role of myeloperoxidase in resistance to *Candida* infection. *J Clin Invest* **48**:1478, 1969

52. Howard T et al: Actin polymerization in C_3 receptor (CR3 or CDW 18 glycoprotein complex) deficient neutrophils. *Clin Res* **35**:477A, 1987

53. Anderson DC, Springer TA: Leukocyte adhesion deficiency; An inherited defect in Mac-1, LFA-1 and p150, 95 glycoproteins. *Ann Rev Med* **38**:175, 1987

54. Boxer LA et al: Neutrophil actin dysfunction and abnormal neutrophil behavior. *N Engl J Med* **291**:1093, 1974

55. Donabedian H, Gallin JI: The hyperimmunoglobulin E recurrent-infection (Job's) syndrome. A review of the NIH experience and the literature. *Medicine (Baltimore)* **62**:195, 1983

56. Leung DY, Geha RS: Clinical and immunologic aspects of the hyperimmunoglobulin E syndrome. *Hematol Oncol Clin North Am* **2**:81, 1988

57. Hammerschmitt DE et al: Corticosteroids inhibit complement-induced granulocyte aggregation. A possible mechanism for their efficacy in shock states. *J Clin Invest* **63**:798, 1979

58. Oseas RS et al: Mechanism of dexamethasone inhibition of chemotactic factor induced granulocyte aggregation. *Blood* **59**:265, 1982

59. Dale DC et al: Alternate-day prednisone. Leukocyte kinetics and susceptibility to infections. *N Engl J Med* **291**:1154, 1974

60. Templetoin HJ: Progressive pigmentary dermatosis (Schamberg); with review of the literature, report of two cases and comparison with angioma serpiginosum and purpura annularis telangiectodes. *Arch Dermatol & Syph* **16**:141, 1927

61. Randall SJ et al: Pigmented purpuric eruptions. *Arch Dermatol* **64**:177, 1951

62. Nichamin SJ, Brough AJ: Chronic progressive pigmentary purpura. Purpura annularis telangiectodes of Majocchi-Schamberg. *Am J Dis Child* **116**:429, 1968

63. Gougerot J, Blum P: Purpura angioscleureux prurigeneux avec éléments lichénoides (presentation de malade). *Bull Soc Fr Dermatol Syphilol* **32**:161, 1925

64. Irvin WJ: Immunologic aspects of pernicious anemia. *N Engl J Med* **273**:432, 1968

65. Doniach D et al: Autoimmunity in pernicious anemia and atrophic gastritis. *Ann NY Acad Sci* **124**:644, 1965

66. Logue G, Rosse W: Immunologic mechanisms in autoimmune hemolytic disease. *Semin Hematol* **13**:277, 1976

67. Howitz J, Schwartz M: Vitiligo, achlorhydria and pernicious anemia. *Lancet* **1**:1331, 1971

68. Gibson QH: The reduction of methemoglobin in red blood cells and studies on the cause of idiopathic methemoglobinemia. *Biochem J* **42**:13, 1948

69. Bodansky O: Methemoglobinemia and methemoglobin-producing compounds. *Pharmacol Rev* **3**:144, 1951

70. Kiese M: The biochemical production of ferrihemoglobin-forming derivatives from aromatic amines, and mechanisms of ferrihemoglobin formation. *Pharmacol Rev* **18**:1091, 1966

71. Damergis JA et al: Methemoglobinemia after sulfamethoxazole and trimethoprim. *JAMA* **249**:590, 1983

72. Gibson GR et al: Methemoglobinemia produced by high-dose intravenous nitroglycerin. *Ann Intern Med* **96**:615, 1982

73. Bonaventura J, Riggs A: Hemoglobin kansas, a human hemoglobin with a neutral amino acid substitution and an abnormal oxygen equilibrium. *J Biol Chem* **243**:980, 1968

74. Beutler E: Hemoglobinopathies producing cyanosis, in *Hematology,* 4th ed. Edited by WJ Williams et al. NY, McGraw-Hill, 1957, p 746

75. Winklemann RK, Muller SA: Pruritus. *Annu Rev Med* **15**:53, 1964

76. Greaves MW et al: Aquagenic pruritus. *Br Med J* **11**:2008, 1981

77. Gilbert HS et al: A study of histamine in myeloproliferative disease. *Blood* **28**:795, 1966

78. Berk PD et al: Therapeutic recommendations in polycythemia vera based on Polythemia Vera Study Group protocols. *Semin Hematol* **23**:132, 1986

79. Serjeant GR et al: Leg ulceration in sickle cell anemia. *Arch Intern Med* **133**:690, 1974

80. Samitz MH et al: Leg ulcers in Mediterranean anemia. *Arch Dermatol* **90**:567, 1964

81. Beinhauer LG, Gruhn JG: Dermatologic aspects of congenital spherocytic anemia. *Arch Dermatol* **75**:642, 1957

CHAPTER 160

Helmut Gadner and Nicole Grois

The Histiocytosis Syndromes

Introduction

The histiocytosis syndromes comprise a group of rare diseases whose etiology and pathogenesis are poorly understood. They embrace a number of clinical entities displaying a spectrum of highly variable clinical features and are characterized by the infiltration and accumulation of cells of the monocyte/macrophage lineage.

The origin of these cells from hematopoietic precursor cells in the bone marrow, their circulation in the peripheral blood after maturation, and seeding in almost every organ forming "resident" macrophages (e.g., Kupffer cells in the liver, Langerhans cells in the skin) explain why these diseases develop such diverse clinical phenotypes. Macrophages are intimately involved in the presentation of antigens to T-lymphocytes and possess a large repertoire of secretory products which may eventually be responsible for some of the variable clinical features and signs.[1] However, to date it has not been clarified whether the various disease entities are based on different maturational stages of the cells involved or result from defective macrophage/T-cell interactions or a cytokine dysequilibrium.

Because of the fundamental lack of knowledge regarding the underlying pathogenetic processes there is confusion about the terminology and nomenclature relating to these disorders, and this has impeded clinicians in developing appropriate diagnostic programs, effective treatment regimens, and more precise criteria for the prediction of prognosis.[2]

In an attempt to overcome these problems the Writing Group of the Histiocyte Society has proposed a state of the art classification of histiocytosis syndromes[3] with the aim of establishing specific criteria required for definite diagnosis. According to this rec-

ommendation histiocytosis syndromes are grouped into three classes, as shown in Table 160-1.

Class I disease, termed *Langerhans cell histiocytosis* (previously called *histiocytosis X*), is defined by the identification of lesional cells as Langerhans cells.

The lesional cells in *class II* disorders are benign mononuclear cells which lack the characteristics of Langerhans cells. The following diseases are included in this category: hemophagocytic lymphohistiocytosis, infection-associated hemophagocytic syndrome, sinus histiocytosis with massive lymphadenopathy, xanthogranuloma, reticulohistiocytoma and other unclassified disorders (see also Chap. 102).

Class III embraces truly malignant histiocytic disorders characterized by the presence of histiocytes with malignant features. This disease group comprises: acute monocytic leukemia (FAB M5), malignant histiocytosis, and histiocytic lymphoma (histiocytic sarcoma).

Apart from these three categories of disorders a variety of diseases show histiocytic infiltrations in the skin and other organs.[1] These diseases may be reactive syndromes due to bacterial, fungal, parasitic, or viral infections. Thus, tuberculosis, toxoplasmosis, rubella syndrome, and congenital cytomegaly may simulate a histiocytic disorder. An accumulation of normal histiocytes that mimics a reactive syndrome may even result from stimuli by inert agents, such as beryllium or zirconium. The well-known lipid storage diseases like Gaucher disease, Nieman-Pick disease, gangliosidosis type 1, Fabry disease, and lipogranulomatosis (Farbers disease), and sarcoidosis can also imitate a histiocytosis syndrome.

The proliferation of normal histiocytes found in various humoral and cell-mediated immunodeficiencies and in graft-versus-

TABLE 160-1
Classification of Histiocytosis Syndromes

	Class I	Class II	Class III
Disease	Langerhans cell histiocytosis	Histiocytosis of mononuclear phagocytes	Malignant histiocytic disorders
Cell type	Langerhans cell	Mononuclear phagocyte	Malignant cells of the monocyte/macrophage system
Cellular features, morphology	CD1 positivity Birbeck granules	Normal histiocytes (not Langerhans cells)	Typical malignant features

SOURCE: According to the Writing Group of the Histiocyte Society, modified.[3]

host disease may also be difficult to distinguish from a true histiocytic disorder, unless an adequate diagnostic program is used.[4]

Class I Disease

Langerhans Cell Histiocytosis

Definition and Historical Aspects Langerhans cell histiocytosis (LCH) is a new term for a disease, described under a variety of names, such as Hand-Schüller-Christian syndrome, Abt-Letterer-Siwe disease, eosinophilic granuloma, pure cutaneous histiocytosis, type II histiocytosis, self-healing histiocytosis, nonlipid reticuloendotheliosis, Hashimoto-Pritzker syndrome, Langerhans cell granulomatosis, and histiocytosis X.[3] The disease is considered a reactive, proliferative process characterized by the accumulation of histiocytes along with infiltrates consisting of lymphocytes, eosinophils, and fibroblasts. Many tissues and organs may be involved presenting either as isolated lesions or as multisystem disease. The lesional histiocytes are recognized as dendritic cells which share numerous characteristics of epidermal Langerhans cells. This has led to the term *Langerhans cell histiocytosis,* which has replaced the previous designation *histiocytosis X.*

It was the merit of Lichtenstein[5] in 1953 to propose a single term for three previously described and well-known clinical conditions: eosinophilic granuloma, Hand-Schüller-Christian syndrome, and Abt-Letterer-Siwe disease. He felt that these three syndromes represent the same basic disease but vary in degree, stage of involvement, and localization. Since no causative agent for the disease was known, the "X" was used to emphasize the obscure etiology. However, this unitary hypothesis was never universally accepted, especially by clinicians who observed too many different clinical pictures, until the lesional cell was identified as the Langerhans cell.

Epidemiology The occurrence of the disease is universal with no specific epidemiologic aspect. However, repeated cases in certain kindreds have been reported. The disease affects predominantly infants and young children but may persist until adulthood. Infrequently onset may occur in adulthood. The incidence is about 0.2 to 1.0/100,000 children per year. Males outnumber females by a ratio of about 2:1.[6] The acute disseminated form occurs particularly in children under the age of 2 years (60–70 percent; congenital, 10 percent). The chronic disseminated form shows a frequency peak between the ages of 2 and 10 years; and more than 40 percent of the localized form occurs between the ages of 5 and 15 years.[7]

Etiology and Pathogenesis The exact etiology of Langerhans cell histiocytosis is unknown, and the pathogenesis is not understood. Currently, the disease is widely accepted to be a reactive process rather than a malignancy. This theory is supported by the analysis of the DNA-content of lesional cells, showing that the cells of the patients investigated so far had an entirely normal DNA-content[8] and by the fact that spontaneous remissions occur. It has been postulated that either an atypical immunologic response or autoimmunity may be involved in the disease. The disorder may be triggered by a defect in intercellular communication (e.g., T-cell/macrophage interaction) and/or by a dysequilibrium of cytokines.[9–11] There is also some evidence that in adults with pulmonary disease cigarette smoking plays a key role in the development of the disease.

Clinical Manifestation The clinical picture is highly variable, ranging from single or multiple lesions in one organ, e.g., bone, skin, or lymph nodes, to multiple organ involvement (called multisystem disease). Signs and symptoms at presentation depend on the localization and extent of the disease and comprise localized or generalized pain, skin rash, and general symptoms, which are prominent in disseminated disease, e.g., fever, irritability, or failure to thrive. The time from onset to diagnosis is between 1 and 3 months in the majority of patients.[12]

The organ most frequently involved is the skeleton (82 percent) (Table 160-2). Lesions described as eosinophilic granuloma may present as monostotic (Fig. 160-1) or poliostotic manifestations. Predominantly affected are the skull (Fig. 160-1), especially the calvarial region, followed by lesions in the mastoid, mandible, or periorbital area. Involvement of the mandible and maxillary bone leads to loss of teeth.

Purulent chronic otitis media may indicate a granuloma in the petrous bone. Lesions are also detected quite frequently in the pelvic bones, in ribs or vertebrae, as well as in long bones.

The majority of patients with disseminated disease also show bone lesions (74 percent) (Tables 160-2 and 3). Other organ manifestations include soft tissue, skin, liver, spleen, lungs, bone marrow, lymph nodes, and central nervous system. The frequency of the various organ manifestations is shown in Table 160-3.

Diabetes insipidus resulting from involvement of the hypothalamic/pituitary region may be the first and only symptom in patients with monostotic or with disseminated disease. It can precede the diagnosis of LCH for years or develop during the course of the disease. The triad of exophthalmus, multiple skull lesions, and diabetes insipidus represents a rare form of multisystem disease with a rather chronic course previously known as *Hand-Schüller-Christian syndrome.*

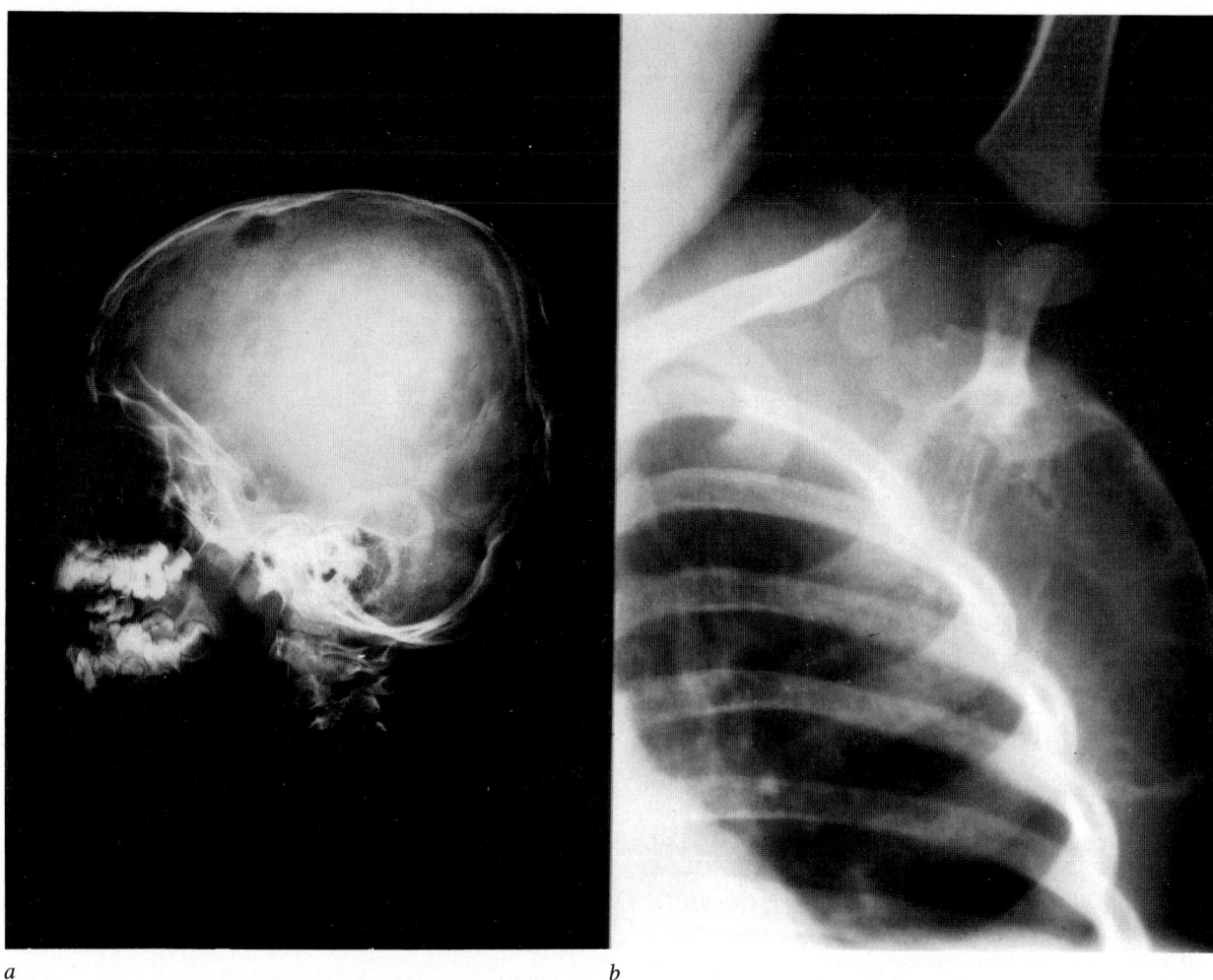

FIGURE 160-1 Langerhans cell histiocytosis. Typical lytic bone lesion, characterized by well-defined margins without evidence of reactive osteogenesis. (*a*) Isolated eosinophilic granuloma of the skull in a 6-year-old child. (*b*) Scapula involvement in a 2-year-old boy with bone distension and a huge contiguous soft tissue mass.

TABLE 160-2
Distribution of Bone Lesions, n = 163 (82%)

Site	Unifocal, n = 77; (n%)	Multifocal, n = 28; (n%)	Multisystem disease n = 78; (n%)	Total n = 163; (n%)
Skull	31 (40,3)	15 (53,6)	37 (47,4)	84 (51,5)
Calvarial	24 (31,2)	13 (46,4)	36 (46,1)	73 (44,7)
Mastoid	4	4	2	10 (6,1)
Basis	2	2	3	7 (4,2)
Mandible	3	4	5	12 (7,3)
Maxilla	1	2	5	8 (4,9)
Orbita	3	2	8	13 (7,9)
Thorax	3	9 (32,1)	16 (20,5)	28 (17.1)
Ribs	3	2	12 (15,3)	17 (10,4)
Clavicle	1	5	2	8 (4,9)
Scapula	0	4	5	9 (5,5)
Vertebrae	9 (11,5)	11 (35,7)	7	27 (16,5)
Pelvis	10 (13,0)	8	14 (17,9)	32 (19,3)
Ileum	5	7	7	19 (11,6)
Ischium	2	1	5	8 (4,9)
Long bone	19 (24,7)	27 (96,4)	29 (37,1)	75 (46,0)

SOURCE: Data from DAL-HX 83 Study.[12]

TABLE 160-3

Distribution of Organ Involvement in Multisystem Disease

Organ	Group B (n = 57)	Group C (n = 21)	Total [n = 78, (%)]
Bone	47	11	58 (74,4)
Skin	23	18	41 (52,6)
Soft tissue (ST)	31	2	33 (42,3)
ST contiguous to bone lesion	25	—	25 (32,0)
ST contiguous to lymph node lesion	2	—	2 (2,6)
Mediastinal mass	2	1	25 (32,0)
Hepatomegaly	9	16	25 (32,0)
Lymph node	13	10	23 (29,5)
Splenomegaly	4	14	18 (23,1)
Lungs	4	9	13 (16,6)
Bone marrow	2	9	11 (14,1)
Gingiva	7	3	10 (12,8)
Gastrointestinal tract	4	5	9 (11,5)
Anus	3	2	5 (6,4)

Group B: pts. with soft tissue with/without bone involvement.
Group C: pts. with multisystem disease with organ dysfunction (liver, lungs, hematopoietic system).
SOURCE: Data from DAL-HX 83 Study.[12]

Abt-Letterer-Siwe disease is usually seen in children less than 1 year old. It is characterized by typical cutaneous lesions and multisystem disease, often associated with organ dysfunction. Criteria defining organ dysfunction are shown in Table 160-4.[13]

DERMATOLOGIC MANIFESTATIONS. Skin involvement is reported in roughly 30 to 40 percent of the patients. A wide range of clinical presentations with heterogenous cutaneous eruptions and a variable clinical course are recognized (Fig. 160-2).

Isolated cutaneous lesions may manifest in early or later infancy and may resolve spontaneously or persist for several months to years.[14] Areas of predilection are the trunk, abdomen, and scalp. Classic lesions are multiple erythematous papules covered by a scale; they may have a greasy-seborrheic, hemorrhagic, vesicular-pustular, or crusted appearance (Fig. 160-2a, b, d) and may ulcerate (Fig. 160-2c). In chronic disease the color of the papules may be yellowish and xanthomatous.

Especially in the intertriginous regions, e.g., groin, perianal area, axilla, and skin folds on the neck or behind the ears, the

TABLE 160-4

Dysfunction Criteria in Langerhans Cell Histiocytosis

1. *Liver dysfunction*
   Hypoproteinemia (total protein < 5.5 g/dL) and/or hypoalbuminemia <1.5 g/L
   Edema
   Ascites
   Hyperbilirubinemia (>1.5 g/dL, not due to hemolysis)
2. *Pulmonary dysfunction*
   Tachypnea and/or dyspnea, cyanosis, cough
   Pneumothorax
   Pleural effusion
3. *Hematopoietic system dysfunction*
   Anemia (Hb <10 g/dL, not due to iron deficiency or infection)
   Leukopenia (<4.0 × 10⁹/L)
   Granulocytopenia (<1.5 × 10⁹/L)
   Thrombocytopenia (<100 × 10⁹/L)

SOURCE: According to Lahey,[13] modified.

eruptions tend to become erosive and to ulcerate, forming confluent ulcers and granulomas (Fig. 160-3). In the ear canal lesions usually present as pruritic, wet, exudative, and crusted eruptions, usually with bacterial superinfection, mimicking otitis externa.

Rarely, LCH may manifest as a solitary cutaneous or subcutaneous nodule covered by intact skin. In the genital and perianal region such nodules may break down, evolving into punched out ulcers with little tendency to heal (Fig. 160-3).

Cutaneous lesions may be the only manifestation of LCH or may accompany involvement of other organs. Cutaneous lesions may also antedate multisystem disease, which develops within a year or later. In this case the disease rarely goes into remission without therapy. Although LCH is predominantly a disease of infants and children, the described cutaneous lesions may also occur in adults. This is particularly true for the genital ulcers and the widespread granulomatous and ulcerating lesions in the intertriginous regions.

Localized or disseminated lesions also occur on the *mucous membranes,* usually on the buccal mucosa, palate, and gingiva, but also in the gastrointestinal, urogenital, and vaginal tract, presenting as whitish granulomatous plaques that transform into ulcers with a tendency to bleeding. Gingival ulcers are punched out and are often accompanied by the loss of one or more teeth.

Congenital self-healing reticulohistiocytosis (Hashimoto-Pritzker syndrome) presumably represents a special form of purely cutaneous LCH, first described in 1973.[15] This clinical entity is characterized by the congenital or perinatal occurrence of numerous firm nodules of a brownish-red to dark-blue color scattered over the trunk, face, and scalp. Mucous membranes are always spared. There is no other organ involvement and hematologic abnormalities like neutropenia and lymphocytosis are rarely found. Typically the lesions resolve spontaneously without any treatment within a few months, leaving a residual hyperpigmentation. Morphologically, ultrastructurally, and immunophenotypically lesional cells resemble Langerhans cells.

Laboratory and Special Examinations There exist general guidelines for the evaluation of patients with LCH.[16] The aim of the adoption of a standardized diagnostic approach is a uniform classification according to the extent of the disease; this also facilitates cooperation and communication with respect to treatment and basic research. Recommended studies are divided into two categories:

1. Baseline evaluations to be performed uniformly in every newly diagnosed patient (Table 160-5), and
2. Investigations required upon specific indication (Table 160-6).

Pathology On the cellular level LCH lesions appear to be reactive rather than inflammatory or malignant. Granulomas show a clear predilection for the clinical sites of manifestation, e.g., bone, skin, thymus, pituitary, lung, liver, spleen, lymph node, and bone marrow. The lesions consist of an aggregation of Langerhans cells with an admixture of other cell types and exhibit a proliferative and locally destructive behavior (Fig. 160-4a). The Langerhans cells are about twice the size of other lesional cells, they have a homogeneous pink cytoplasm in hematoxylin-eosin stained section, and exhibit lobulated, "coffee bean"-like nuclei.[1,17] In the skin there is marked epidermotropism of these cells (Fig. 160-4a). Regular components of the infiltrate are eosinophils, neutrophils, phagocytic macrophages, and a variable number of lymphocytes.

Lesions initially have a high cellular content, which decreases with time. Simultaneously, the number of phagocytic

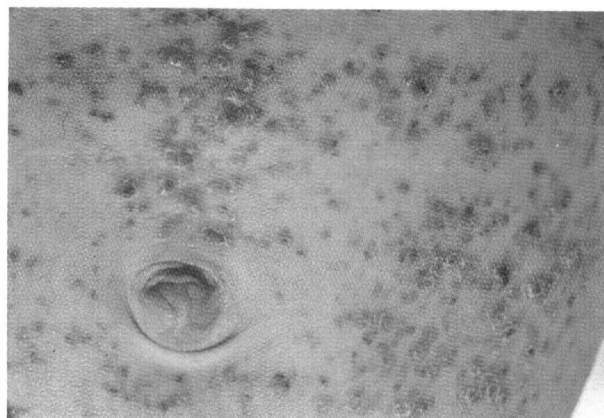

a

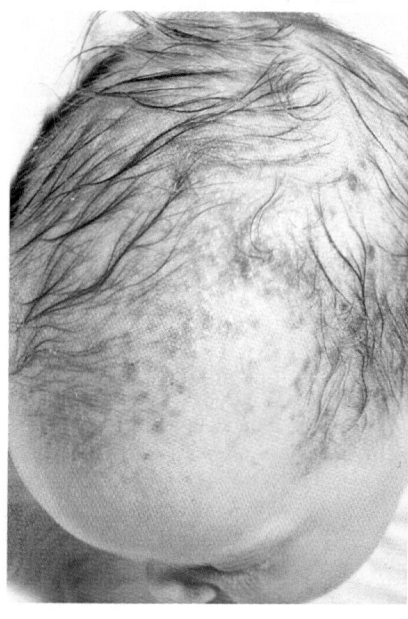

b

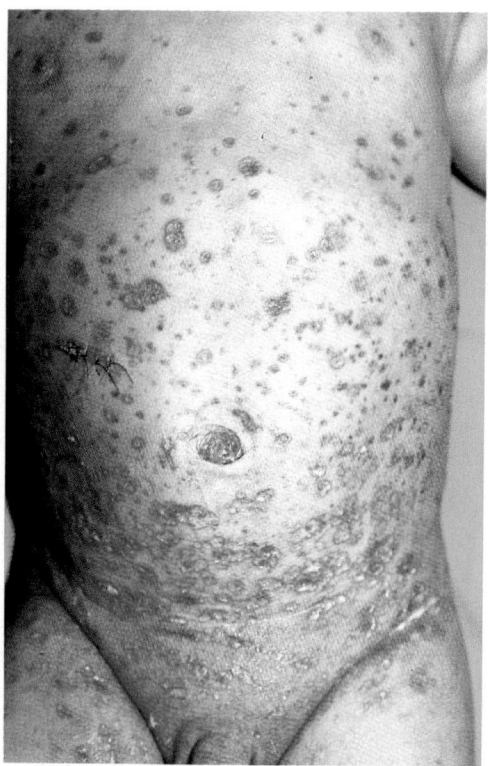

c

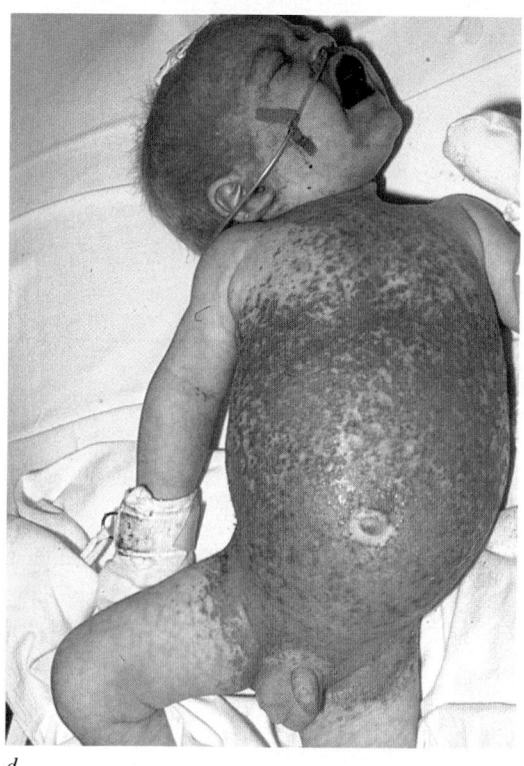

d

FIGURE 160-2   Langerhans cell histiocytosis. Classic skin
lesions. (*a*) Abdominal area of an infant with multiple
erythematous papules covered by a scale and/or crust.
(*b*) Seborrheic papules on the scalp mimicking seborrhoic
dermatitis. (*c*) Infant with multiple ulcerated skin lesions on the
trunk. (*d*) A severe case of Abt-Letterer-Siwe disease with
confluent, erosive, and crusted lesions forming ulcers in the
groins; distension of the abdomen reflects marked
hepatosplenomegaly. [*Parts (a), (b), (c) courtesy of Klaus
Wolff, M.D.*]

macrophages and fibroblasts increases, resulting in a xanthomatous
and fibrotic pattern. Multinucleated giant cells resembling osteoclasts are frequently seen in lesions in bone, lymph nodes, and
thymus. There is no evidence that they are produced by fusion of
Langerhans cells.

There is no correlation between the histopathologic picture
and the aggressiveness or the extent of the disease. However, the
sites of manifestation and the duration of the disease clearly influence the character of the pathologic lesion. Under favorable circumstances the process can heal with a fibrotic repair or eventually

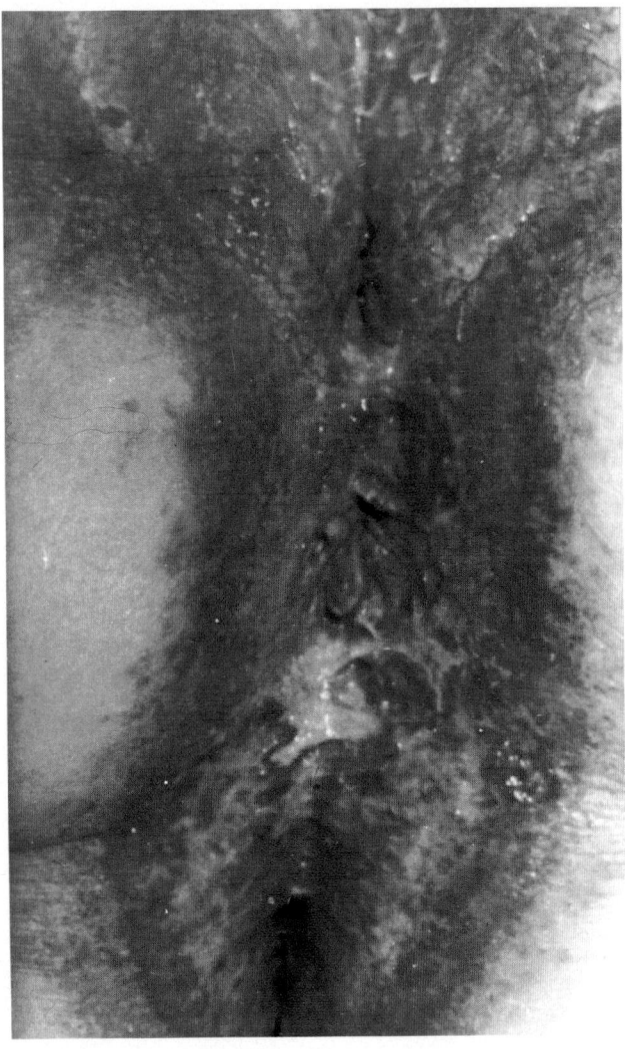

a

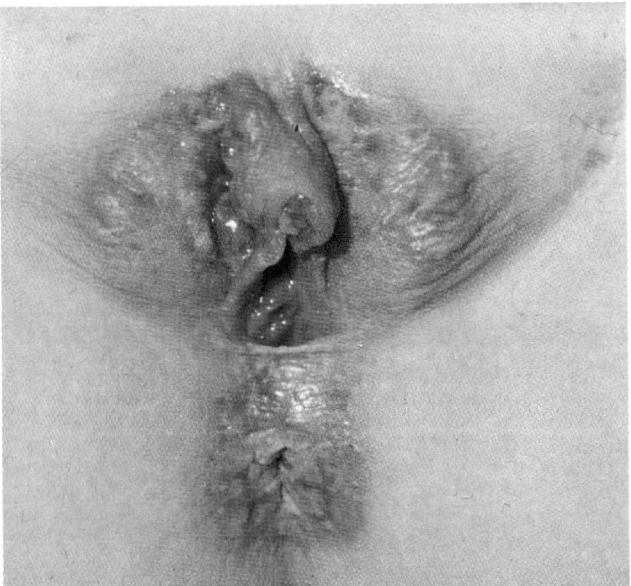

b

FIGURE 160-3 Langerhans cell histiocytosis. (*a*) Acute pruritic, exudative, and ulcerative lesions in the anogenital region of a 65-year-old woman. (*b*) Chronic ulcerated lesions in a female infant with subcutaneous nodules. (*Courtesy of Klaus Wolff, M.D.*)

TABLE 160-5
Baseline Diagnostic Evaluations

Clinical
Complete history: fever, pain, irritability, failure to thrive, loss of appetite, diarrhea, polydipsia, polyuria, activity level
Complete physical examination: measurement of temperature, height, weight, head circumference, skin and skalp rashes, purpura, bleeding, aural discharge, orbital abnormalities, lymphadenopathies, gum and palatal lesions, dentition, soft tissue swelling, dyspnea, tachypnea, intercostal retractions, liver and spleen size, ascites, edema, jaundice, neurologic examination, papilledema, cranial nerve abnormalities, cerebellar dysfunction

Laboratory and Radiographic
Hemoglobin and/or hematocrit
White blood count and differential
Platelet count
Liver function tests (SGOT, SGPT, alkaline phosphatase, bilirubin, total protein, albumin)
Coagulation studies (PT, PTT, fibrinogen)
Immunoglobulins
Chest radiograph, PA and lateral
Skeletal radiograph survey (radionuclide bone scan is not as sensitive as the skeletal radiograph survey in most patients)
Urine osmolality (measurement after overnight water deprivation)

SOURCE: The Histiocyte Society.[16]

with a total involution.

Immunohistochemically the lesional cells are identified by the demonstration of important markers, such as alpha-D-mannosidase, S-100 protein, and peanut agglutinin, as well as the finding of Birbeck granules by electron microscopy[3] (Table 160-7). The proliferating cells in LCH share numerous immunophenotypic features with the normal Langerhans cell of the skin. The most important is the presence of CD1 antigenic determinants on the cell surface (Fig. 160-4*b*).

Depending on the state of activation and/or differentiation, the marker expression may vary substantially. This heterogeneity, however, does not correlate with the clinical course and the prognosis of the disease.[18]

Diagnosis and Differential Diagnosis In order to achieve a high level of diagnostic confidence the Histiocyte Society has proposed three terms which reflect different levels of diagnostic accuracy.

1. *Definitive diagnosis* requires the detection of *Birbeck granules* in lesional cells by electron microscopy or the demonstration of CD1 positivity on the cell surface.
2. The term *diagnosis* is justified by typical characteristics on light microscopy and the additional presence of two or more of the following features: positive stain for ATP-ase, S-100 protein, alpha-D-mannosidase, or peanut lectin.
3. If the biopsy material is examined exclusively by conventional staining only a *presumptive diagnosis* is accepted.[16]

From a clinical point of view the typical multisystem disease with skin manifestations (Abt-Letterer-Siwe syndrome) and the chronic form of Hand-Schüller-Christian disease are rather easy to diagnose. More problems may arise in the evaluation of isolated

TABLE 160-6
Investigations Required upon Specific Indication

Test	Indication
Bone marrow aspirate and trephine biopsy	Anemia, leukopenia, or thrombocytopenia
Pulmonary function tests	Abnormal chest radiograph, tachypnea, intercostal retractions
Lung biopsy, preceded by bronchoalveolar lavage, when available; when diagnostic, obviates lung biopsy	Patients with abnormal chest radiograph in whom chemotherapy is being considered, to exclude opportunistic infection
Small bowel series and biopsy	Unexplained chronic diarrhea or failure to thrive, evidence of malabsorption
Liver biopsy	Liver dysfunction, including hypoproteinemia not due to protein-losing enteropathy, to differentiate active LCH of the liver from cirrhosis
CT of brain/hypothalamic-pituitary axis, with IV contrast enhancement (MRI preferable if available)	Hormonal, visual, or neurologic abnormalities
Panoramic dental radiography of mandible and maxilla; oral surgery consultation	Oral involvement
Endocrine evaluation	Short stature, growth failure, diabetes insipidus, hypothalamic syndromes, galactorrhea, precocious or delayed puberty; CT or MRI abnormality of hypothalamus/pituitary
Otolaryngology consultation and audiogram	Aural discharge, deafness

SOURCE: The Histiocyte Society.[16]

skin disease or atypical involvement. In this situation a physician should carefully rule out other possibilities, such as seborrheic or atopic dermatitis, juvenile xanthogranuloma, xanthoma disseminatum, or unusual infections. In localized skin disease, especially when solitary nodes are present, the distinction from malignant lymphoma, malignant histiocytosis, or a metastatic solid tumor may be difficult. In multisystem disease without prominent skin lesions the disease may mimic familial hemophagocytic lymphohistiocytosis or a virus-associated hemophagocytic syndrome. Localized bone lesions have to be distinguished from osteomyelitis or other bone tumors. (For other "nonhistiocytosis X" histiocytic syndromes see Chap. 102)

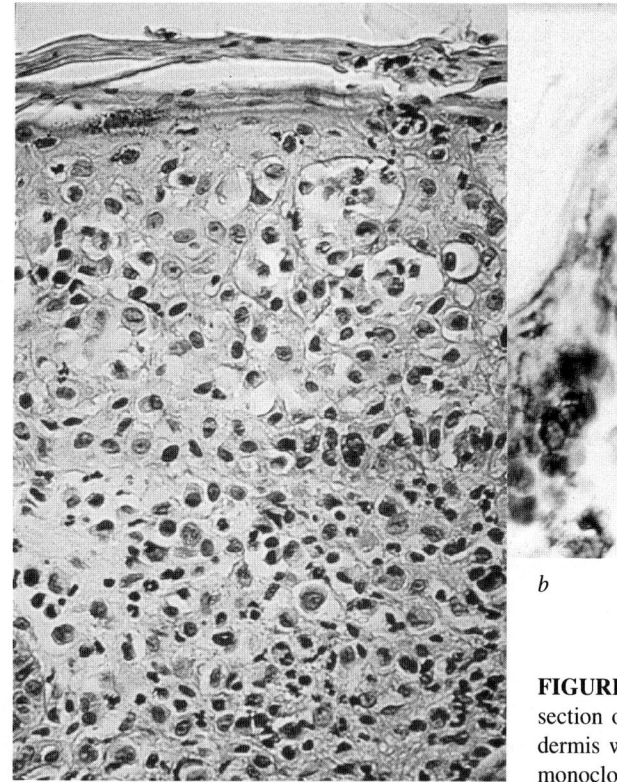

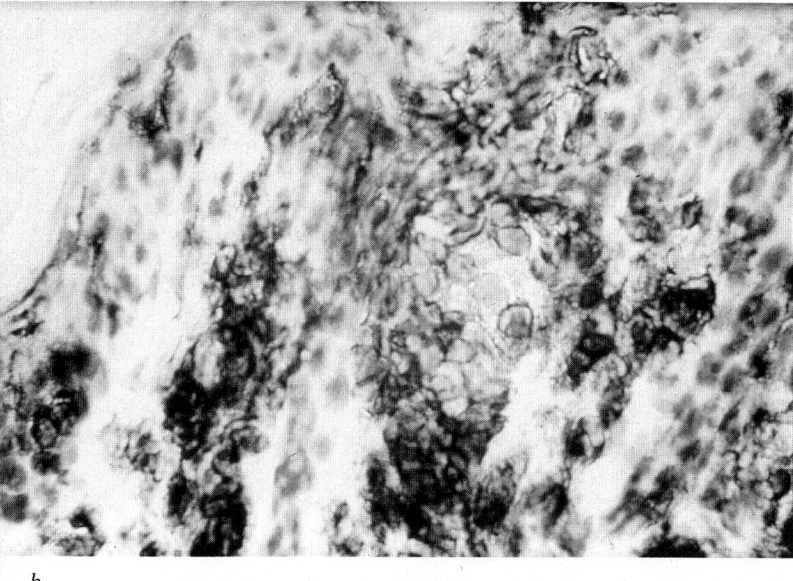

FIGURE 160-4 Langerhans cell histiocytosis. (*a*) Hematoxylin-eosin stained section of a skin biopsy showing clusters of Langerhans cells in the papillary dermis with exocytosis into the epidermis. (*b*) Similar section stained with a monoclonal antibody to the CD1 antigenic determinant. (*Courtesy of Klaus Wolff, M.D.*)

TABLE 160-7
Specific Features of Histiocytes

	Normal and pathologic Langerhans cell	Paracortical interdigitating cell	Ordinary histiocyte
Nonspecific esterase	−	−	+
Alpha$_1$-antichemotrypsin	−	−	+
Alpha-D-Mannosidase	+	+	−
S-100 protein	+	+	−
CD1	+	+	−
CDw14	+	+	+
Birbeck granules	+	−	−

S-100 = a neuroprotein; CD1 = antigenic determinant on surface of thymocytes, intertigitating cells, normal and pathologic Langerhans cells; CDw14 = antigen found on monocytes, macrophages, and dendritic cells.
SOURCE: Modified according to the Writing Group of the Histiocyte Society.[3]

Staging

Since treatment depends on the extent of the disease, an adequate staging procedure is important. Many attempts have been made to establish a generally accepted staging of the disease according to clinical or histologic criteria. None has proved satisfactory, but young age, extent of disease, and presence of organ dysfunction seem to be variables which appear most important for prognosis.[12,13,19,20]

The International LCH Study of the Histiocyte Society proposes the stratification into *single system disease* and *multisystem disease*. Single system disease is divided into single site and multiple site disease (Table 160-8).

Treatment

As there is no specific treatment established for LCH, several therapeutic approaches are used.[2]

Local treatment such as intralesional injection of corticosteroids (50–150 mg depot-methylprednisolone),[21] surgical excision (curettage), or radiation treatment may achieve very good results in monostotic bone involvement. Surgical excision is the treatment of choice for isolated lymph node infiltration or isolated skin lesions.

The handling of patients with skin disease may be crucial. Disseminated skin lesions may be controlled by PUVA photochemotherapy or topical nitrogen mustard.[22] Mild skin lesions may respond to topical corticosteroids.

Systemic chemotherapy may be indicated when local treatment is not successful in localized disease and in case of multisystem disease. Systemic treatment with steroids and cytotoxic drugs, either alone or in combination, has been shown to be effective in controlling symptoms in most patients. More aggressive therapy is considered to be of no advantage and even hazardous. In poliostotic manifestation, mild systemic treatment with steroids and/or vinblastine is recommended.

Common therapy regimens for multisystem disease include prednisone, vinblastine, 6-mercaptopurine, or methotrexate given as single agents or in combination for 3 to 6 months.[2,7,22] Recently the epipodophyllotoxin etoposide (VP 16) has shown promising effects in the prevention and treatment of diabetes insipidus.[23] Cyclophosphamide, chlorambucil, and anthracyclines, (all used at one time), should be avoided in the initial treatment and given with great caution in nonresponding patients as salvage therapy because of their potential carcinogenic properties. Children under 2 years of age with multisystem disease and organ dysfunction especially need systemic control of their disease using a nonaggressive regimen. Drug dosages are summarized in Table 160-9.

Radiotherapy should be reserved for bony lesions which are unusually large and painful or are in crucial weight-bearing locations. Another indication may be the extension of disease from a vertebral lesion to the spinal chord. The dose employed should be 6 to 8 Gy and should not exceed 10 Gy. Limited data in adults, however, suggest that higher doses of radiotherapy are required for control of the disease. There is no agreement concerning the role of radiotherapy in management of diabetes insipidus.[24]

Only preliminary data exist on the efficacy of alternative treatment approaches. There is no convincing evidence that thymic hormones or thymic factors are superior to chemotherapy[25] in controlling the disease in unselected patients. A few reports concern the use of alpha-interferon[26] in chronic recurrent disease, especially with poliostotic lesions, and of cyclosporine in acute disseminated disease.[27] In only a few cases with chronic recurrent disease allogeneic bone marrow transplantation has been performed with success.[28] More extensive trials are required to confirm these preliminary observations.

TABLE 160-8
Stratification of Langerhans Cell Histiocytosis According to the Extent of Disease

Single system disease	
Single site:	monostotic bone disease
	isolated skin disease
	solitary lymph node involvement
Multiple site:	polyostotic bone disease
	multiple lymph node involvement
Multisystem disease	
Multiple organ involvement: with/without organ dysfunction	

SOURCE: Proposal of the International LCH Study Group, by permission of the Histiocyte Society.

TABLE 160-9
Drug Dosages in Common Treatment Protocols

Drug	Dose	Frequency
Prednisone	40–60 mg/m² p.o. or i.v.	Daily for 28 days
High dose methyl-prednisolone	30 mg/kg i.v. (20′ infusion)	3 days in a row every three weeks
Vinblastine	6 mg/m² i.v.	Weekly
VP-16 (etoposide)	150–200 mg/m² i.v.	Daily for 3 days every 3 weeks
6-Mercaptopurine	50–80 mg/m² p.o.	Daily
Methotrexate	20–30 mg/m² p.o.	Weekly

Course and Prognosis

The course of the disease may be acute, subacute, or chronic as well as progressive, stable, or sometimes spontaneously regressing. The progress is unpredictable in the single patient.[2,22]

The prognosis of *localized disease*, usually confined to bone, is considered to be excellent, occasionally even without any treatment in monostotic as well as in polyostotic disease. In the case of solitary lymph node involvement the cure rate is also nearly 100 percent after surgical excision.

Similarly good results are to be expected in isolated skin disease, where surgical excision of single lesions or PUVA photochemotherapy induces remissions, and spontaneous regression may occur. On the other hand, skin manifestations in disseminated disease signal a rather poor prognosis. A poor outcome is signaled not by the skin manifestations per se but by their combination with other organ involvement, especially with organ dysfunction in infants.[12]

In *disseminated disease* the prognosis depends on age, extent of the disease, number of involved organs, and the presence of dysfunction of liver, lungs, and/or hemopoietic system.[2,12,14] Children under 2 years of age as well as patients older than 60 years have a bad prognosis, with a mortality rate of up to 50 percent or more.[29] If the disease progresses for years with recurrences and remissions the chance of sequelae is high.

Late defects may be observed in up to 50 percent of the survivors.[30] The most important are orthopedic disabilities, hearing impairment, and diabetes insipidus, followed by neuroendocrinologic, neuropsychologic, and neurologic defects. Diabetes insipidus may develop in up to 50 percent.[31,32] Other sequelae include retardation of growth, chronic pulmonary dysfunction, and liver cirrhosis. These sequelae emphasize the importance of early treatment.[12]

Class II Diseases

Hemophagocytic Lymphohistiocytosis

Definition and Historical Aspects A variety of names have been used for this disease, such as familial histiocytic reticulosis, congenital hemophagocytic reticulosis, familial erythrophagocytic lymphohistiocytosis, and familial erythrophagocytic reticulosis, as originally described by Farquhar and Claireaux in 1952.[33]

Epidemiology This is a rare, usually familial, disorder affecting infants and very young children. The pattern of inheritance appears to be autosomal recessive, but sporadic cases may occur.

Etiology and Pathogenesis The etiology and pathogenesis are unknown. Defects of both cellular and humoral immunity have been reported but are considered secondary phenomena. It has been speculated that the disease results from a T-cell defect (impairment of T-cell function, reduction of natural killer cells) causing an immunodeficiency, which is followed by compensatory macrophage activation with hemophagocytosis.[34,35]

Clinical Manifestations The clinical picture is characterized by severe deterioration of the patient's general condition, fever, anorexia, vomiting, and irritability. Marked hepatosplenomegaly and pancytopenia with bleeding diathesis are already evident early in the disease. Meningeal involvement with lymphohistiocytic pleocytosis and increased protein levels in the cerebrospinal fluid frequently causes neurologic symptoms. Lymph node enlargement and, usually, maculopapular noncharacteristic and transient skin rashes are rare. Bone involvement is not seen.[36]

Laboratory Findings Typical laboratory findings in hemophagocytic histiocytosis are hypertriglyceridemia (probably secondary) and hypofibrinogenemia and other signs of liver dysfunction. Hyponatremia is frequently found. A high serum ferritin and elevated soluble interleukin-2 receptor levels may reflect disease activity.[37,38]

Pathology Histopathologically there is a diffuse tissue infiltration by benign lymphocytes and histiocytes displaying a varying degree of hemophagocytosis. The disease principally affects the spleen, liver, bone marrow, lymph nodes, and meninges.[39]

Diagnosis In the early stages the diagnosis may be difficult, since bone marrow examination may fail to demonstrate hemophagocytosis by histiocytes. Splenic biopsy is considered superior to liver biopsy in yielding a diagnosis. In case of severe coagulopathy, biopsy should be performed with caution.

Treatment Treatment with corticosteroids, chemotherapy, splenectomy, and exchange transfusion have been used successfully to induce temporary remissions. Among the cytostatic drugs, etoposide (VP16) in combination with corticosteroids seems to be most promising in achieving remission and prolonging survival (over many years in some cases).[40] Concomitant treatment of the central nervous system (intrathecal methotrexate or irradiation) is important.[41] Cyclosporine and marrow transplantation are other options.[42]

Course and Prognosis The course of the disease in untreated cases is rapidly fatal, due to infections, hepatic failure, bleeding, or cerebral dysfunction.

Infection-Associated Hemophagocytic Syndrome

Definition and Historical Aspects This nonhereditary disease first described by Risdall et al. in 1979[43] probably presents the most frequent condition associated with hemophagocytic lymphohistiocytosis. It occurs in older children and adults. Males are more often affected.

Etiology and Pathogenesis The pathophysiologic mechanism of this condition remains unclear. There are, however, many suggestions of an underlying immune dysfunction mainly due to T-cell defects, namely a decreased response to mitogens, reduced natural killer cell activity, and an impaired T-cytotoxic response to Epstein-Barr virus infection.[4] T lymphocytes secreting excessive amounts of macrophage activating cytokines (e.g., interleukin 2, tumor necrosis factor, gamma-interferon, prostaglandin E_2) have been demonstrated.[37,38,44]

The majority of the cases reported so far were associated with proven viral infections, mainly Epstein-Barr virus, CMV, herpes simplex, and varicella virus, as well as adenovirus or rubella virus. However, bacterial infections, such as tuberculosis, brucella, salmonella, and *E. coli,* and protozoal infections, such as leishmania, have also been described.[1] The identification of the causative pathogen is essential for diagnosis and treatment.

Immunologically compromised patients and patients with the Chédiak-Higashi, Griscelli, or X-linked lymphoproliferative syndromes may develop a fatal form of the disease.[4,45,46] In patients with the X-linked lymphoproliferative syndrome a genetic susceptibility to Epstein-Barr virus is a well-established etiologic factor.[47]

Clinical Manifestations The clinical picture is very similar to that seen in familial hemophagocytic lymphohistiocytosis; it is characterized by fever, failure to thrive, abdominal pain, pancytopenia, petechiae, hepatosplenomegaly with liver function abnormalities, and coagulation abnormalities. In addition, pulmonary involvement and, frequently, central nervous system signs and symptoms as well as skin rashes usually due to viral infection may occur.[2]

Pathology The most important pathologic feature of the disease is the detection of histiocytic hyperplasia with hemophagocytosis in bone marrow, liver, spleen, or lymph nodes. The histiocytic cells appear benign without Langerhans cell features and reflect a reactive process.[1,3]

Treatment and Prognosis Therapy is frustratingly ineffective. Most patients die from coagulopathy or secondary infections. Antimicrobial or antiviral treatment of the underlying infection should be administered. Currently, the use of the chemotherapeutic agent etoposide has shown promising results which are superior to those obtained with other cytostatic drugs. Concomitant administration of prednisone or exchange transfusions may be effective. In some cases the use of cyclosporine has shown to be clearly beneficial.[42] So far, it is not clear if prostaglandin synthesis inhibition by indomethacin combined with etoposide may be another effective therapeutic alternative.[48] The disease is usually self-limiting but often rapidly fatal. The mortality rate is considered to be about 30 to 40 percent.

Class III Diseases

Malignant Histiocytosis

Definition and Historical Aspects Malignant histiocytosis is characterized by adenopathy, hepatosplenomegaly with jaundice, anemia, leukopenia, wasting, and fever. It was first described in 1939 by Scott and Robb-Smith who used the name *histiocytic medullary reticulosis.*[49] The term *malignant histiocytosis* was introduced by Rappaport in 1966.[50]

Since then various cases with similar clinical presentations have been reported under different names, such as *histiocytic reticulosis, malignant reticulosis,* and *histiocytic leukemia.* The histologic distinction of malignant histiocytosis from other lymphoreticular malignancies turned out to be very difficult, leading to confusion in the literature.[51] Since modern diagnostic techniques have become available, true malignant histiocytosis is only rarely diagnosed. The majority of the previously assigned clinical syndromes (more than 90 percent of the cases) are now regarded as large cell anaplastic lymphoma or Ki 1 lymphoma[52,53] (see also Chap. 106).

Epidemiology Malignant histiocytosis is a non-hereditary malignant disease with a male preponderance. There is a wide age distribution with a peak incidence between 30 and 45 years. Occasionally the disease has been observed in children and very rarely in infants.[54–57]

Etiology and Pathogenesis The etiology of the disease is unknown. The higher incidence in certain areas of Asia and Africa has led to the speculation that an oncogenic virus transmitted by an arthropod vector in a susceptible population plays a causative role.[1]

Chromosomal aberrations have been reported in malignant histiocytosis and in Ki 1 lymphoma. Recently, cytogenetic studies have shown a reciprocal translocation between chromosome 2 and 5, involving bands 2p 23 and 5q 35. The breakpoint at the q35 region on chromosome 5 is close to the position of fms protooncogen, suggesting that an abnormality of this gene may be the causative factor in this disease.[58]

Clinical Manifestations Clinical features include fever and general symptoms, such as wasting, weakness, anorexia, weight loss, sweats, pains, chills, and nausea, in the majority of cases. Localized or generalized lymph node enlargement, predominantly in the cervical, axillary and hilar, mediastinal as well as abdominal region, is the most common physical finding and often the initial symptom. Other important features are splenomegaly, hepatomegaly with jaundice (which is often a terminal event), pulmonary involvement (including pleural effusion), and central nervous system manifestations.[54–57]

Cutaneous and subcutaneous nodules, often located on the trunk, especially in the abdominal wall (Fig. 160-5*a*), transient maculopapular, micronodular, or erythematous rashes (Fig. 160-5*b*) are frequently seen. In pediatric patients cutaneous lesions are more frequent (54 percent) than in adults (20 percent).[55] Rarely, subcutaneous nodules or a soft tissue mass are the only clinical manifestation.

Bone lesions (lytic or sclerotic) are also very rarely observed.[59] In a high percentage of cases—more often in disseminated, widespread disease—a typical bone marrow infiltration is found.

Limited and generalized disease are distinguished according to the extent of the disease at the time of diagnosis, and the Ann Arbor and Murphy classifications of Hodgkin's and non-Hodgkin's lymphoma are used for staging.[60,61] Roughly 70 to 80 percent of cases show stage III or IV disease at diagnosis.

Laboratory and Special Examinations Typically, anemia, thrombocytopenia, and leukopenia are present (sometimes also leukocytosis) and reflect bone marrow infiltration by the malignant histiocytes. In some cases circulating atypical histiomonocytes are detected in the peripheral blood.

The erythrocyte sedimentation rate is usually raised. In widespread disease and also late in the course, liver dysfunction is present (hyperbilirubinemia, elevated transaminases, hypercholesterinemia, hypertriglyceridemia, coagulopathy, elevation of lactate dehydrogenase). Occasionally there is a positive Coombs' test and elevated lysozyme levels in the serum or urine. A high level of serum ferritin may be a nonspecific marker of disease activity.[37]

Pathology Histologically the disease is characterized by a destructive local or systemic infiltration by malignant cells of proven mononuclear/phagocytic origin (Fig. 160-6), usually ordinary histio-

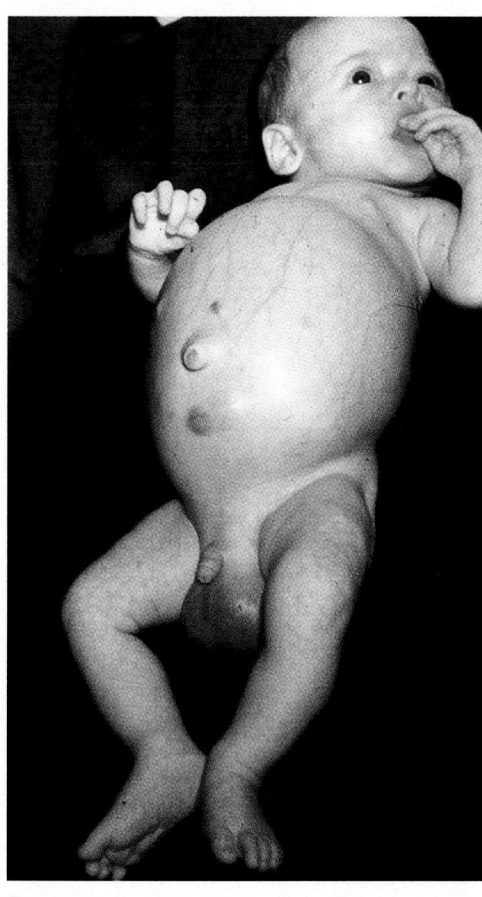

a

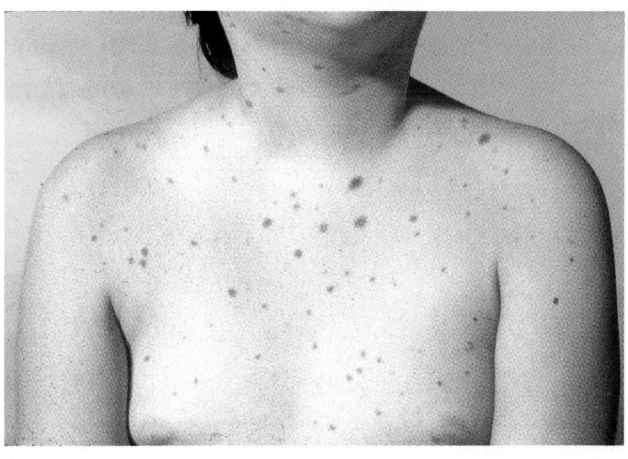

b

FIGURE 160-5 Generalized "true" malignant histiocytosis. (*a*) Infant with massive hepatosplenomegaly and ascites and scrotal edema presenting with typical cutaneous and subcutaneous bluish nodules. (*b*) Large cell anaplastic (Ki1-positive) lymphoma in a 13-year-old girl presenting with multiple disseminated maculopapular, micronodular, and erythematous skin lesions. [*Part (b) Courtesy of J. Ritter, M.D.*]

cytes, rarely interdigitating dendritic cells, and most rarely Langerhans cells.[51]

The sites of predilection are lymph nodes, splenic red pulp, hepatic sinusoids, bone marrow, lung, skin, bone, and various other tissues.[1,51,56]

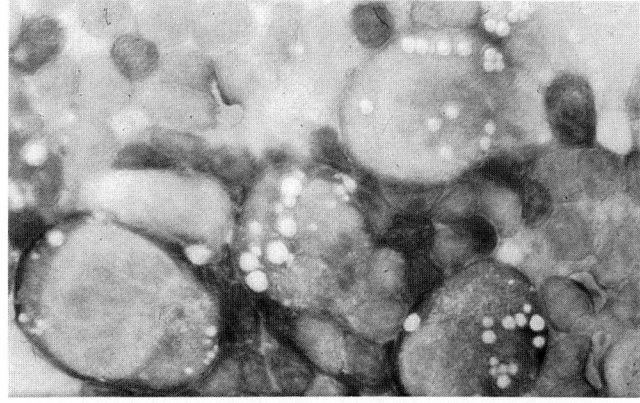

FIGURE 160-6 Malignant histiocytosis. Hematoxylin-eosin stain of a lymph node infiltrated with tumor cells which resemble immature histiocytes with oval irregular nuclei with small nucleoli and abundant vacuolated cytoplasm. In the center of the picture there is a multinucleated giant cell. (*Courtesy of J. Ritter, M.D.*)

Hemophagocytosis, especially erythrophagocytosis, and lysozyme positivity can often be observed in tumor cells.

Intracellular ferritin has been found in tumor cells, suggesting that ferritin may represent a tumor-associated antigen which probably plays a regulatory role for tumor cell differentiation.[62]

Large cell anaplastic lymphoma (i.e., Ki1 lymphoma) and true malignant histiocytosis share clinicopathologic similarities and overlapping immunologic features (Table 160-10)[51-53] (see also Chap. 106).

Characteristic for large cell anaplastic lymphoma (Ki1 lymphoma) is the expression of cell-surface–associated CD 30 antigen (Ki 1 antigen). Most of these cells display T-lymphoid markers and some B-lymphoid markers, suggesting the presence of a T-lineage–associated hematolymphoid neoplasm.[63] These findings are also supported by gene rearrangement studies and investigations showing the expression of other markers such as epithelial membrane antigens and interleukin-2 receptors[64] (Table 160-10). The diagnosis of "true" malignant histiocytosis is based on the demonstration of at least two histiocytic markers with a negative reaction to pan B/T antigens[53] (Table 160-10).

Diagnosis and Differential Diagnosis To avoid further confusion in the nomenclature, the diagnosis has to be confirmed by applying all modern immunohistochemical, cytogenetical, and molecular biologic techniques according to a uniform and generally accepted program.

The diagnosis of malignant histiocytosis demands bone marrow aspiration and bone marrow biopsy in case of bone marrow

TABLE 160-10

Phenotypical Characteristics of LCH, Malignant Histiocytosis, and Large Cell Anaplastic Lymphoma

Langerhans cell histiocytosis		Malignant histiocytosis		Large cell anaplastic lymphoma	
CD45 (LCA)	+	CD45 (LCA)	+/(−)	CD45 (LCA)	+/−
CD1 (OKT6)	+	CD14 (LEU-M3)	+/−	CD30	+/(−)
CD4 (LEU-3a)	+	CD68 (KI-M6)	+/−	CD25 (IL2R)	+/−
S-100 protein	+	KI-M8	+/−	B/T marker	+/−
		M-CSF (CSF-1)	+		
		ANAE	+		
Birbeck granula	+	Lysotyme	+/−		
		pan B/T marker	−		
		t(2;5) (p23;q35)	+/−	t(2;5) (p23;q35)	+/−

For the diagnosis of MH: Tumor cells have to be positive for at least two histiocytic markers with negative reactions for pan B/T markers.

For the diagnosis of LCAL: The morphology is decisive.

SOURCE: According to Bucsky and Fellner.[53]

involvement but preferably biopsy of lymph nodes and other involved organs. Radiographic and sonographic findings are important to detect the involvement of intrathoracal and abdominal lymph nodes and other organs. Lymphangiography is no longer the method of choice since CT and MRI as well as ultrasound are available.

A number of infectious and reactive processes may simulate the clinicopathologic features of malignant histiocytosis as a result of the activation of benign or malignant macrophages. Misdiagnoses include hemophagocytic syndromes such as familial or sporadic hemophagocytic lymphohistiocytosis, virus-associated hemophagocytic syndrome, bacterial infection (typhoid fever, miliary tuberculosis), systemic leishmaniasis, disseminated Langerhans cell histiocytosis, massive lymph adenopathy with sinus histiocytosis, malignant metastatic carcinoma, Hodgkin's disease, and histiocytic lymphoma.[1]

Treatment and Prognosis Without treatment the disease usually is progressive and generally fatal. Children seem to have a better prognosis than adults.[65] Large cell anaplastic lymphoma may occasionally present as localized disease of lymph nodes or skin (stage I or II) and take a benign course. Even spontaneous and transient regressions have been reported. In some cases splenectomy is followed by remission lasting for some months.[66]

In the face of early reports indicating a very poor prognosis with a median survival of 6 months, chemotherapy has proved to be the treatment of choice in malignant histiocytosis. In the majority of patients a rapid remission is obtained, but early relapse occurs frequently. With combination-chemotherapy regimens (usually vincristine, prednisone, cyclophosphamide, and adriamycin), the beneficial effect of cytotoxic treatment has been clearly documented by the 18 to 75 percent disease-free survival rates.[55,57,65,66]

The inclusion of adriamycin in the therapy programs was of major importance for the improvement of the treatment results. Etoposide has recently also shown promising effects. In pediatric practice polychemotherapy protocols used in non-Hodgkin's lymphoma have demonstrated excellent results.[67] The advantage of additional irradiation and of a central nervous system prophylaxis remains unclear and does not appear to be essential for cure. The same is true for splenectomy. Other treatment modalities, such as bone marrow transplantation, should be considered as a therapeutic option in individual cases.

Monocytic Leukemia

Definition Monocytic leukemia is a variant of acute nonlymphocytic leukemia classifed as M5 according to the FAB scheme.[68] The lesional cell is the monocyte, present in the peripheral blood and bone marrow.

Morphologically the disease is grouped into two subtypes:

1. In the poorly differentiated subtype M5a, more common in children, the large leukemic cells display abundant relatively agranular cytoplasm with characteristic basophilic color and occasional vacuoles. Due to the immaturity of these cells the disease is termed *acute monoblastic leukemia*.

2. In contrast, in the subtype M5b, more often seen in adults, the pathologic monocytes may have characteristically twisted, indented, and folded nuclei with more mature features. This differentiated form is considered compatible with the term *acute monocytic leukemia*.

Epidemiology and Pathogenesis The disease mostly affects adults. In children, the disease is rare and accounts for 20 to 25 percent of acute nonlymphocytic leukemias. Congenital forms have also been described.[69]

Clinical Manifestations The typical clinical features of leukemia are present along with gum hypertrophy (Fig. 160-7c), lymphadenopathy, and hepatosplenomegaly.

The prominent extramedullary involvement may be associated with a high number of leukocytes in the peripheral blood at diagnosis, causing a high risk of early death due to leukostasis and hemorrhage. Disseminated intravascular coagulation may occur at presentation or develop after initiation of chemotherapy.[70] Central nervous system involvement is frequently seen at diagnosis or during the course of disease.

Leukemia cutis is defined as localized or disseminated skin infiltration by leukemic cells. The lesions are usually small (2 to 5 mm), raised, pinkish, nontender, painless, and not pruritic, and are located on the trunk and extremities[71] (Fig. 160-7a). They may also involve the face and other areas (Fig. 160-7b). These cutaneous manifestations present as papules, nodules, plaques, and ulceronecrotic lesions and are clearly distinguishable from petechiae resulting from capillary hemorrhage in a thrombocytopenic patient.

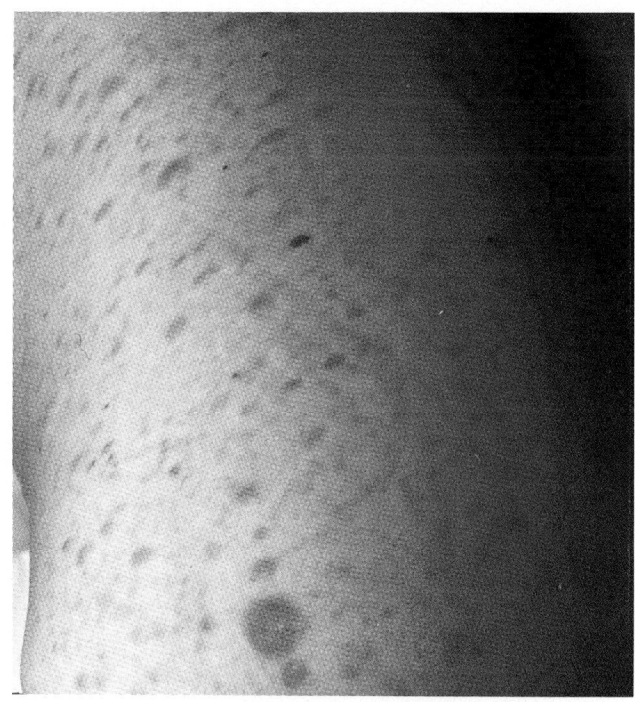

a

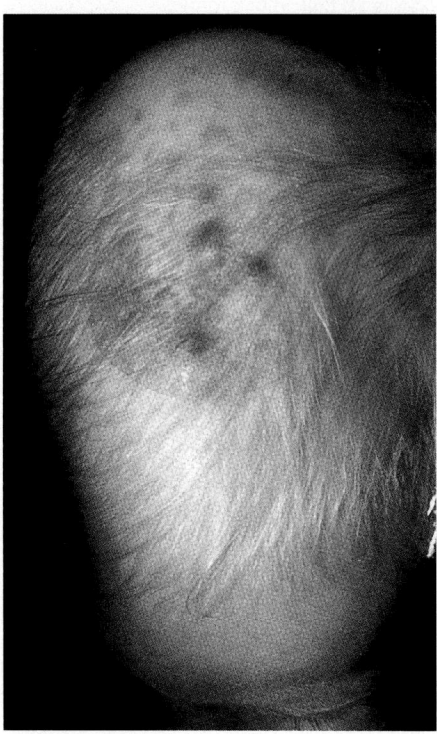

b

Special Examinations Characteristic of the FAB-M5 leukemias is the presence of an elevated lysozyme level in serum and urine. Cytochemically the pathologic monocyte may be peroxidase- (or Sudan black-) positive and PAS-positive. Positive staining for non-specific esterase is inhibited by sodium fluoride.

Pathology Histologically a perivascular, interstitial or diffuse in-filtration by leukemic cells with monocytic (or myelomonocytic)

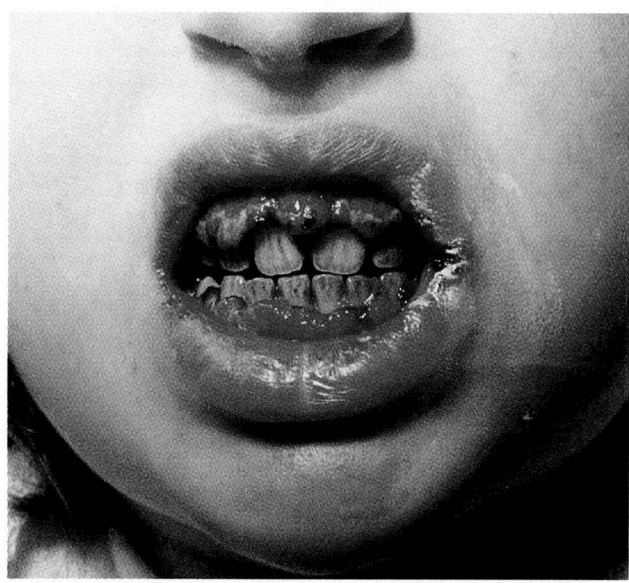

c

FIGURE 160-7 Monocytic/monoblastic leukemia. (*a*) Pinkish, partially hemorrhagic nontender nodules and papules on the trunk. (*b*) Scalp lesions in a 2-year-old boy with chronic myelomonocytic leukemia. (*c*) A teenage girl with acute monoblastic leukemia presenting with typical gum hyperplasia. [*Part (a) courtesy of D. Lutz, M.D.*]

features is seen. The subcutaneous tissue often is involved and a thin grenz zone is seen between the epidermis and the leukemic lesions. The diagnosis can be confirmed by touch preparations in addition to the peripheral blood and bone marrow smears.[1]

Treatment and Prognosis The treatment follows protocols for sys-temic leukemia, including central nervous system prophylaxis. The principles of modern therapy are based on intermittent application of intensive sequential combination chemotherapy.[69] An alternative is allogeneic bone marrow transplantation, if an appropriate mar-row donor is available.

The prognosis for monocytic leukemia is unfavourable in comparison to most of the other morphologic subtypes of acute nonlymphocytic leukemia. Skin involvement is considered a poor prognostic parameter.[72] It rarely is the only sign of the leukemic process and usually reflects progression of the disease or signals an imminent hematologic recurrence.

References

1. Groopman JE, Golde DW: The histiocytic disorders: A pathophysio-logic analysis. *Ann Intern Med* **94**:95, 1981

2. Ladisch S: Histiocytosis, in *Hematology and Oncology,* Butter-worth's International Medical Reviews, Pediatrics 1, edited by MLN Willoughby and SE Siegal. Butterworth Scientific, London, 1983, p 95

3. Writing Group of the Histiocyte Society: Histiocytosis syndromes in children. *Lancet* **24**:208, 1987

4. Nesbit ME et al: The immune system and the histiocytosis syndromes. *Am J Pediatr Hematol* **3**:141, 1981

5. Lichtenstein L: Histiocytosis X—integration of eosinophilic granu-loma of bone, "Letterer-Siwe disease," and "Schüller-Christian dis-

ease'' as related manifestations of a single nosologic entity. *Arch Pathol Lab Med* **56**:84, 1953

6. Slater JM, Swarm OJ: Eosinophilic granuloma of bone. *Med Pediatr Oncol* **8**:151, 1980

7. Gadner H et al: Histiocytoses: Diagnosis and treatment. *Monogr Paediatr* **18**:368, 1986

8. McLelland J et al: A flow cytometric study of Langerhans cell histiocytosis. *Br J Dermatol* **120**:485, 1989

9. Barbey S et al: Histiocytosis X Langerhans cells react with antiinterleukin-2 receptor monoclonal antibody. *Pediatr Pathol* **7**:569, 1987

10. Larrick WJ et al: Activated Langerhans cells release tumor necrosis factor. *J Leukocyte Biol* **45**:429, 1989

11. Neumann Ch et al: Interferon gamma is a marker for histiocytosis X cells in the skin. *J Invest Dermatol* **91**:280, 1988

12. Gadner H et al: Langerhans cell histiocytosis in Kindesalter-Ergebnisse der DAL-HX 83 Studie. Klin Pädiat **199**:173, 1987

13. Lahey ME: Histiocytosis X—an analysis of prognostic factors. *J Pediatr* **87**:184, 1975

14. Lee CW et al: Recurrent cutaneous Langerhans cell histiocytosis in infancy. *Br J Dermatol* **119**:259, 1988

15. Hashimoto K et al: Congenital self-healing reticulohistiocytosis. Report of the seventh case with histochemical and ultrastructural studies. *J Am Acad Dermatol* **11**:447, 1984

16. Clinical Writing Group of the Histiocyte Society: Histiocytosis syndromes in children: II. Approach to the clinical and laboratory evaluation of children with Langerhans cell histiocytosis. *Med Pediatr Oncol* **17**:492, 1989

17. Favara BE, Jaffe R: Pathology of Langerhans cell histiocytosis. *Hematol Oncol Clin North Am* **1**:75, 1987

18. Groh V, et al: The phenotypic spectrum of histiocytosis X cells. *J Invest Dermatol* **90**:441, 1988

19. Broadbent V: Favourable prognostic features in histiocytosis X: Bone involvement and absence of skin disease. *Arch Dis Child* **61**:1219, 1986

20. Lahey ME: Prognosis in reticuloendotheliosis in children. *J Pediatr* **60**:664, 1962

21. Cohen M et al: Direct injection of methyl sodium succinate in the treatment of solitary eosinophilic granuloma of the bone. *Radiology* **136**:289, 1980

22. McLelland J et al: Current controversies. *Hematol Oncol Clin North Am* **1**:147, 1987

23. Broadbent V et al: Etoposide (VP16) in the treatment of multisystem Langerhans cell histiocytosis (histiocytosis X). *Med Pediatr Oncol* **17**:97, 1989

24. Selch MT, Parker RG: Radiation therapy in the management of Langerhans cell histiocytosis. *Med Pediatr Oncol* **18**:97, 1990

25. Osband ME et al: Histiocytosis-X. Demonstration of abnormal immunity, T-cell histamine H2-receptor deficiency, and successful treatment with thymic extract. *N Engl J Med* **304**:146, 1981

26. Jakobson AM et al: Treatment of Langerhans cell histiocytosis with alpha-interferon. *Lancet* **2**:1520, 1987

27. Mahmoud H et al: Cyclosporine therapy for advanced Langerhans cell histiocytosis. *Blood* **77**:721, 1991

28. Stoll M et al: Allogeneic bone marrow transplantation for Langerhans' cell histiocytosis. *Cancer* **66**:284, 1990

29. Novice F et al: Letterer-Siwe disease in adults. *Cancer* **63**:166, 1989

30. Komp DM: Long-term sequelae of histiocytosis X. *Am J Pediatr Hematol Oncol* **3**:165, 1981

31. Dunger DB et al: The frequency and natural history of diabetes insipidus in children with Langerhans-cell histiocytosis. *N Engl J Med* **321**:1157, 1989

32. Avery ME et al: The course and prognosis of reticuloendotheliosis. *Am J Med* **22**:636, 1957

33. Farquhar JW, Claireaux AF: Familial hemophagocytic reticulosis. *Arch Dis Child* **27**:519, 1952

34. Aricò M et al: Natural cytotoxicity impairment in familial hemophagocytic lymphohistiocytosis. *Arch Dis Child* **63**:292, 1988

35. Hansmann ML et al: Familial hemophagocytic lymphohistiocytosis

macrophages showing immunohistochemical properties of activated macrophages and T-accessory cells. *Pediatr Hematol Oncol* **6**:237, 1989

36. Janka GE: Familial hemophagocytic lymphohistiocytosis. *Eur J Pediatr* **140**:221, 1983

37. Esumi N et al: Hyperferritinemia in malignant histiocytosis, virus-associated hemophagocytic syndrome, and familial erythrophagocytic lymphohistiocytosis. *Acta Paediatr Scand* **78**:268, 1989

38. Komp DM et al: Elevated soluble interleukin-2 receptor in childhood hemophagocytic histiocytic syndromes. *Blood* **73**:2128, 1989

39. Landing BH: Lymphohistiocytosis in childhood. *Perspect Pediatr Pathol* **9**:48, 1987

40. Ware R et al: Familial erythrophagocytic lymphohistiocytosis: Late relapse despite continuous high-dose VP-16 chemotherapy. *Med Pediatr Oncol* **18**:27, 1990

41. Howells DW et al: Central nervous system involvement in the erythrophagocytic disorders of infancy: The role of cerebrospinal fluid neopterins in their differential diagnosis and clinical management. *Pediatr Res* **28**:116, 1990

42. Oyama Y et al: Haemophagocytic syndrome treated with cyclosporin A: A T cell disorder? *Br J Hematol* **73**:276, 1989

43. Risdall RJ et al: Virus-associated hemophagocytic syndrome. A benign histiocytic proliferation distinct from malignant histiocytosis. *Cancer* **44**:993, 1979

44. Maury CPJ, Pettersson T: Detection of circulating tumour necrosis factor in systemic histiocytosis. *Br J Hematol* **71**:293, 1989

45. Wilson ER et al: Fatal Epstein Barr virus associated hemophagocytic syndrome. *J Pediatr* **98**:260, 1981

46. Blanche S et al: Epstein-Barr virus-associated hemophagocytic syndrome: Clinical presentation and treatment. *Pediatr Hematol Oncol* **6**:233, 1989

47. Purtilo DT et al: X-linked lymphoproliferative syndrome provides clues to the pathogenesis of Epstein-Barr virus-induced lymphomagenesis, in *Unusual Occurrences as Clues to Cancer Etiology,* edited by RW Miller et al. Japan Sci Soc Press, Tokyo/Taylor & Francis Ltd, 1988, p 149

48. Brown RE et al: Endoperoxidation, hyperprostaglandinemia and hyperlipidemia in a case of erythrophagocytic lymphohistiocytosis: Reversal with VP-16 and indomethacin. *Cancer* **60**:2388, 1987

49. Scott RD, Robb-Smith AHT: Histiocytic medullary reticulosis. *Lancet* **2**:194, 1939

50. Rappaport H: Tumors of the hematopoietic system; in *Atlas of Tumor Pathology*. Armed Forces Institute of Pathology, Washington, DC, 1966, p 49

51. Wilson MS et al: Malignant histiocytosis. A reassessment of cases previously reported in 1975 based on paraffin section immunophenotyping studies. *Cancer* **66**:530, 1990

52. Schnitzer B et al: Ki-1 lymphomas in children. *Cancer* **61**:1213, 1988

53. Bucsky P et al: Zur Frage der Definition der malignem Histiozytose und des großelligen anaplastischen (Ki-1) Lymphoms im Kindesalter. *Klin Pädiat* **201**:233, 1989

54. Warnke RA et al: Malignant histiocytosis (histiocytic medullary reticulosis). 1. Clinicopathologic study of 29 cases. *Cancer* **35**:215, 1975.

55. Zucker JM et al: Malignant histiocytosis in childhood. Clinical study and therapeutic results in 22 cases. *Cancer* **45**:2821, 1980

56. Byrne GE, Rappaport H: Malignant histiocytosis. *GANN Monogr Cancer Res* **15**:145, 1973

57. Rilke F et al: Malignant histiocytosis: A clinicopathologic study of 18 consecutive cases. *Tumori* **64**:211, 1978

58. Morgan R et al: Lack of involvement of the c-fms and N-myc genes by chromosomal translocation t(2;5) (p23;q35) common to malignancies with features of so-called malignant histiocyosis. *Blood* **73**:2155, 1989

59. Vanel D et al: Radiological findings in 23 pediatric cases of malignant histiocytosis (MH). *Eur J Radiol* **3**:60, 1983

60. Carbone PP et al: Report of the Committee on Hodgkin's Disease Staging Classification. *Cancer Res* **31**:1960, 1971

61. Murphy S: Childhood non-Hodgkin's lymphoma. *N Engl J Med*

299:1446, 1978

62. Ya-You J et al: An immunocytochemical study on the distribution of ferritin and other markers in 36 cases of malignant histiocytosis. *Cancer* **64**:1281, 1989

63. Weiss LM et al: Sinusoidal hematolymphoid malignancy ("malignant histiocytosis") presenting as atypical sinusoidal proliferation. A study of nine cases. *Cancer* **58**:1681, 1986

64. Delsol G et al: Coexpression of epithelial membrane antigen (EMA), Ki-1, and interleukin-2 receptor by anaplastic large cell lymphomas. Diagnostic value in so-called malignant histiocytosis. *Am J Pathol* **130**:59, 1988

65. Brugieres L et al: Malignant histiocytosis: Therapeutic results in 27 children treated with a single polychemotherapy regimen. *Med Pediatr Oncol* **17**:193, 1989

66. Huhn D et al: Malignant histiocytosis: Clinical findings and therapy. *Klin Wochenschr* **58**:31, 1980

67. Heitger A et al: Das großzellige anaplastische Lymphom im Kindesalter—Klinische Erfahrungen bei einer histologisch neu definierten Entität. *Klin Pädiatr* **201**:237, 1989

68. Bennet JM et al: Proposed revised criteria for the classification of acute myeloid leukemia: A report of the French-American-British Cooperative Group. *Ann Intern Med* **103**:626, 1985

69. Creutzig U et al: *Acute Myelogenous Leukemia in Childhood. Implications of Therapy Studies for Future Risk-Adapted Treatment Strategies.* Springer Verlag, Berlin, 1990

70. Andoh K et al: Tissue factor activity in leukemic cells. *Cancer* **59**:748, 1987

71. Haubenstock A et al: Isolated leukemia cutis—A case report. *Am J Hematol* **24**:437, 1987

72. Shaikh BS et al: Histologically proven leukemia cutis carries a poor prognosis in acute nonlymphocytic leukemia. *Cutis* **39**:57, 1987

CHAPTER 161

Dean D. Metcalfe

The Mastocytosis Syndrome

Mastocytosis is a condition characterized by mast cell hyperplasia in the bone marrow, liver, spleen, lymph nodes, gastrointestinal tract, and skin. Clinically, the disease is often accompanied by evidence of mast cell activation which includes pruritus, flushing, urtication, abdominal pain, nausea, vomiting, diarrhea, bone pain, vascular instability, headache, and neuropsychiatric difficulties. Mastocytosis can occur at any age and demonstrates a slight male-to-female predominance (1.5:1.0). The prevalence of the disease is unknown and familial occurrence appears unusual.

Mastocytosis is divided into distinct clinicopathologic entities on the basis of clinical presentation, pathologic findings, and prognosis. A recent consensus revised classification for mastocytosis is shown in Table 161-1.[1] Patients in the indolent category have a good prognosis, while patients in the other three groups do poorly. Indolent mastocytosis is delineated on the basis of the presence of syncope, cutaneous disease, ulcer disease, malabsorption, bone marrow involvement, skeletal disease, hepatosplenomegaly, and lymphadenopathy. In most cases patients with indolent disease gradually accrue more mast cells as symptoms progress but can be managed successfully for decades using medications that provide symptomatic relief.

The second most common form of mastocytosis is that associated with a hematologic disorder. In this group, examination of the bone marrow and peripheral blood reveals the hematologic abnormality. The prognosis in these patients is determined by the course of the associated hematologic disorder.

Patients in the third category have an aggressive form of mastocytosis; these individuals have poor prognostic features but do not have a distinctive hematologic disorder or mast cell leukemia. There exists a subset of patients with aggressive mastocytosis who have a distinct syndrome termed *lymphadenopathic mastocytosis with eosinophilia* because of the pronounced eosinophilia, hepatosplenomegaly, and lymphadenopathy. Patients with aggressive disease rapidly increase mast cell numbers and are difficult to manage medically. Prognosis is less favorable compared with patients with indolent mastocytosis.

The fourth category of mast cell disease is mast cell leukemia; it is the rarest form and has the most fulminant behavior. The peripheral blood smear shows numerous immature mast cells. Mast cell leukemia is distinguished from the other categories by its unique pathologic and clinical picture.

Etiology and Pathogenesis

Human mast cells originate from pluripotent (CD34+) bone marrow cells and are circulated through the blood stream and lymphatics to specific sites within the body where they mature into fully granulated cells.[2] The targeting of mast cells to defined locations appears to be determined by the sequential expression of cell surface adhesion molecules including a laminin-binding protein.[3] Thus mast cells are often identified in proximity to basement membrane, nerves, and glandular structures rich in laminin. The skin and gastrointestinal tract, which interface the external environment,

TABLE 161-1
Consensus Revised Classification

I. Indolent
A. Syncope
B. Cutaneous disease
C. Ulcer disease
D. Malabsorption
E. Bone marrow mast cell aggregates
F. Skeletal disease
G. Hepatosplenomegaly
H. Lymphadenopathy
II. Hematologic disorder
A. Myeloproliferative
B. Myelodysplastic
III. Aggressive
Lymphadenopathic mastocytosis and eosinophilia
IV. Mastocytic leukemia

TABLE 161-2
Mast Cell Mediators and Their Contribution to Pathogenesis

Mediators	Effects
Granule-associated	
Histamine	Pruritus, urticaria, increased vasopermeability, gastric hypersecretion, bronchoconstriction
Heparin	Local anticoagulation, osteoporosis
Tryptase, chymotryptic proteases	Bone lesions
Lipid-derived	
Sulfidopeptide leukotrienes	Increased vasopermeability, bronchoconstriction, vasoconstriction (LTC_4); increased vasopermeability, bronchoconstriction, vasodilation (LTD_4 and LTE_4)
Prostaglandin D_2	Vasodilation, bronchoconstriction
Platelet-activating factor	Increased vasopermeability, vasodilation, bronchoconstriction
Cytokines	
Proinflammatory factor	Fibrosis (TGF-β); activation of vascular endothelial cells, cachexia (TNF-α)
Growth enhancing	Mast cell growth factors (IL-3, stem cell factor); eosinophilia (IL-5)

are particularly rich in mast cells. Mast cells at these sites are believed to contribute to host defense against parasites.[4]

The regulation of mast cell number and mast cell differentiation is under the control of factors produced both in the hematopoietic marrow and by cells in the tissues in which mast cells finally reside. For example, early mast cell differentiation depends on the colony stimulating factor interleukin 3 (IL-3)[5] and is inhibited by granulocyte/macrophage colony-stimulating factor (GM-CSF).[6] Final maturation and granule composition may depend on the production of specific mast cell growth factors including stem cell factor produced by fibroblasts and stromal cells.[7]

The pathogenesis of mastocytosis is largely the result of the increased production of mast cell mediators, which have effects both at the site of their production or remote from their origin, irrespective of the etiology of the increased burden of mast cells or the category of disease. Mast cell mediators are of three categories; all may circulate through the blood stream and lymphatics to produce biologic effects observed in patients with mastocytosis (Table 161-2).

Clinical Features

The four categories of mastocytosis share clinical features that are due to the excess production of mast cell-dependent mediators, although some aspects of disease may predominate in a specific category. The skin, gastrointestinal tract, lymph nodes, liver, spleen, bone marrow, and skeletal system contribute the most significant management problems. The respiratory tract and endocrine systems are seldom if ever involved. Also patients with mastocytosis do not suffer from recurrent bacterial, fungal, or viral infections even though mast cells release mediators such as histamine that can inhibit immune responses in vitro.

Urticaria pigmentosa is the most common skin manifestation of mastocytosis in both children (Fig. 161-1) and adults (Fig. 161-4). It is seen in over 90 percent of patients with indolent mastocytosis, and in less than 50 percent of patients with mastocytosis with an associated hematologic disorder or those with lymphadenopathic mastocytosis with eosinophilia. The lesions of urticaria pigmentosa appear as small, yellow-tan to reddish-brown macules or slightly raised papules scattered over the body. The palms, soles, face, and scalp may be free of lesions. Mild trauma, including scratching or rubbing of the lesions, usually causes urtication and erythema around the macules; this is known as Darier's sign. Urticaria pigmentosa is associated with a variable amount of pruritus, which may be exacerbated by changes in climatic temperature, skin friction, ingestion of hot beverages or spicy foods, ethanol, and certain drugs. The diagnosis is confirmed by characteristic skin histopathology.[8]

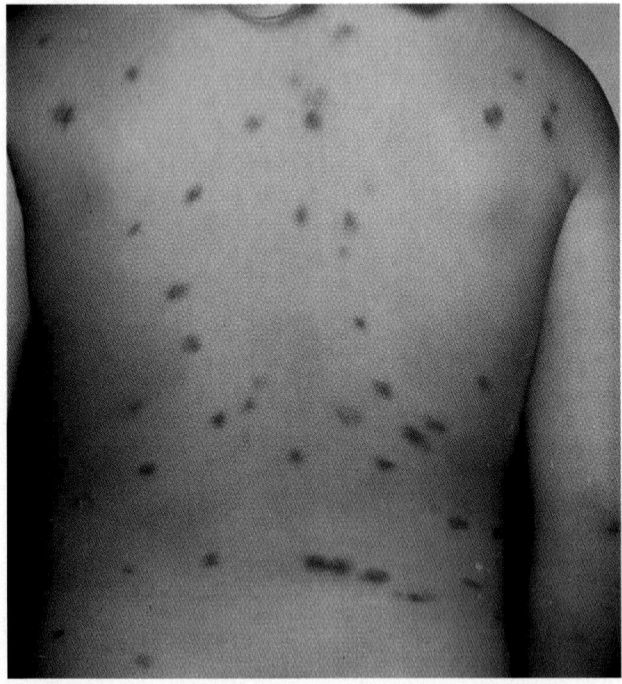

FIGURE 161-1 Urticaria pigmentosa in a child with cutaneous disease only.

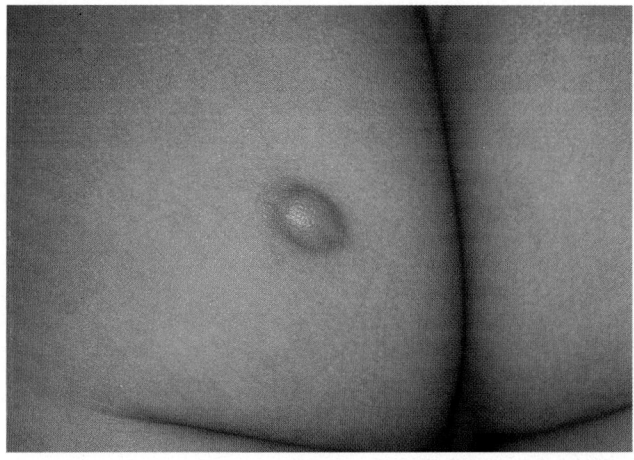

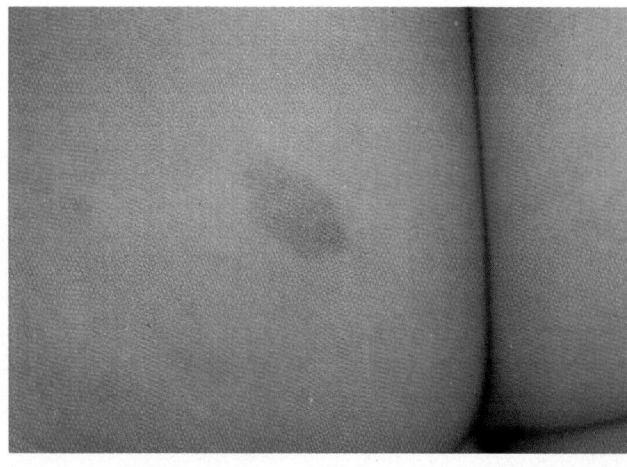

a   *b*

FIGURE 161-2 Solitary mastocytoma. (*a*) A tan macule is seen on the buttocks of an 18-month-old child. (*b*) After

the child's diaper was changed, the lesion became an urticarial plaque.

Diffuse cutaneous mastocytosis consists of a diffuse mast cell infiltration of the skin without discrete lesions. It usually occurs before the age of 3 years. The entire cutaneous integument is involved. The skin is normal to yellow-brown in color and is diffusely thickened.[9]

Solitary lesions called mastocytomas (Fig. 161-2) do occur but are quite rare. Their onset is generally before 6 months of age. In most cases such lesions spontaneously involute.

Young children with urticaria pigmentosa or diffuse cutaneous mastocytosis may have bullous eruptions with hemorrhage (Fig. 161-3).[9,10] Eruptions of blisters may be seen spontaneously or in association with infection or immunization. Blisters may occur at birth and thus are in the differential diagnosis of neonatal disorders with blisters.

Telangiectasia macularis eruptiva perstans is observed in less than 1 percent of cases of mastocytosis (Fig. 161-4). It appears as tan to brown macules and patchy erythema. Telangiectasias are observed. This form of cutaneous disease in mastocytosis is observed exclusively in adults.[11] A rare type of erythrodermic cutaneous mastocytosis has also been described.[12]

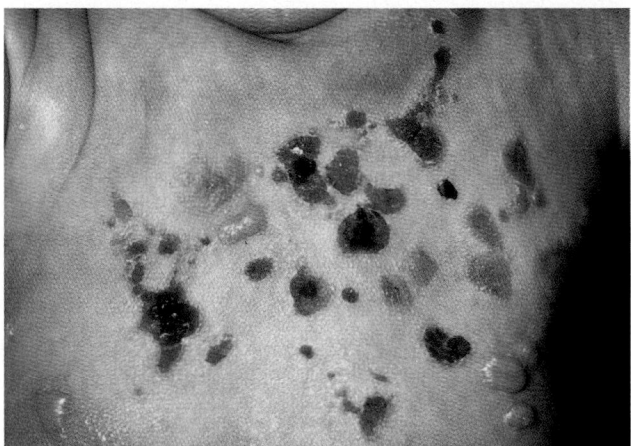

FIGURE 161-3 Bullous eruption on the back of a child with diffuse cutaneous mastocytosis and indolent mastocytosis.

Patients with mastocytosis often develop gastrointestinal disease. Gastric hypersecretion due to elevated plasma histamine with resultant gastritis and peptic ulcer disease is the most common problem.[13] Diarrhea and abdominal pain are also common and are followed by the onset of malabsorption in approximately one in three patients. Roentgenographic abnormalities fall into three major categories: peptic ulcers; abnormal mucosal patterns such as mucosal edema, multiple nodular lesions, coarsened mucosal folds, or multiple polyps; and motility disturbances. Histologic sections of jejunal biopsies have shown moderate blunting of the villi; however significant mast cell hyperplasia is uncommon.

Significant hepatic disease in indolent systemic mastocytosis is relatively infrequent, and liver function tests are often normal. The most common chemical abnormality is an elevated alkaline phosphatase, which must be distinguished from bone-derived alkaline phosphatase (which may also be elevated). Serious manifestations of hepatic and splenic involvement, including portal hypertension and ascites associated with liver fibrosis,[14] are more common in patients who have mastocytosis with an associated hematologic disorder or in those with aggressive mastocytosis.

Splenic involvement is frequently observed in patients with mastocytosis; it was found in 28 (48 percent) of one group of 58 patients.[15] The authors of this study reviewed the pathologic features of 16 spleens. All but one of the spleens showed a paratrabecular distribution of mast cell infiltrates: 10 (64 percent) perifollicular, two (14 percent) follicular, and one (7 percent) diffuse. Various degrees of trabecular fibrosis were present in biopsies examined, as were eosinophilic infiltrates. Seventy-one percent of biopsies showed extramedullary hematopoiesis. Markedly increased splenic weights (greater than 700 g) generally occurred in patients who fit into unfavorable categories of mastocytosis, i.e., aggressive mastocytosis or mastocytosis with an associated hematologic disorder.

Bone marrow lesions consist of focal and paratrabecular aggregates of spindle-shaped mast cells, often mixed with eosinophils, lymphocytes, and occasional plasma cells, histiocytes, and fibroblasts (Fig. 161-5).[16–20] These lesions are rarely seen in children.[21] Anemia, leukopenia, thrombocytopenia, and eosinophilia may occur in association with systemic disease.[20] Bone marrow infiltration with mast cells may induce bone changes that cause

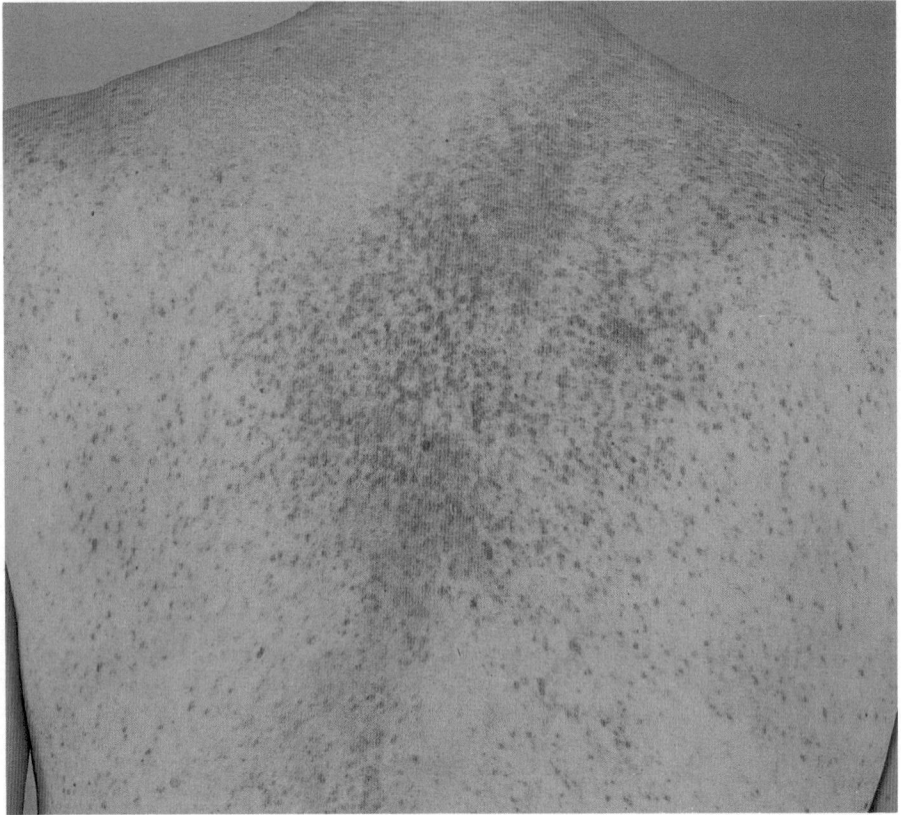

a

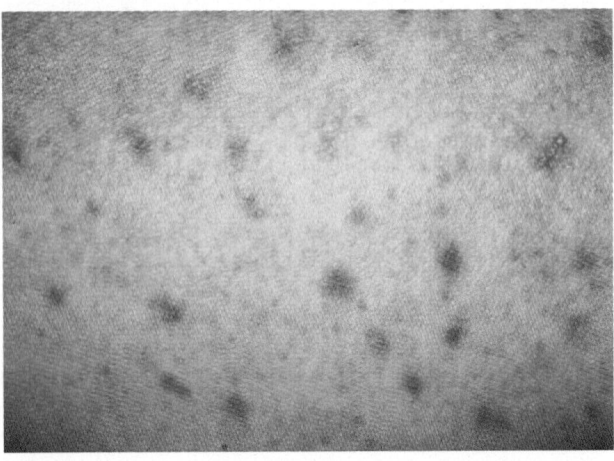

b

FIGURE 161-4 Urticaria pigmentosa in an adult with indolent systemic mastocytosis. (*a*) Hundreds of lentigo-like macules are seen on the back of this adult. If vigorously rubbed, these lesions will show urtication and become erythematous, raised, and pruritic. (*b*) Close-up.

radiographically detectable lesions in up to 70 percent of patients. The proximal long bones are most often affected, followed by the pelvis, ribs, and skull. Skeletal scintigraphy (bone scan) is more sensitive than a radiographic survey in detecting and locating active lesions.[22] Bone pain affects 19 to 28 percent of patients. In patients with severe or advanced disease, pathologic fractures may occur.

Patients in every category of mastocytosis sometimes experience flushing or vascular collapse.[20] In occasional patients, such reactions may be provoked by alcohol, aspirin, exercise, or infections.

Neuropsychiatric abnormalities have been reported.[23,24] Problems include decreased attention span, memory impairment, and irritability. Depression as a consequence of chronic disease or possibly mediated by mast cell products is a possibility.

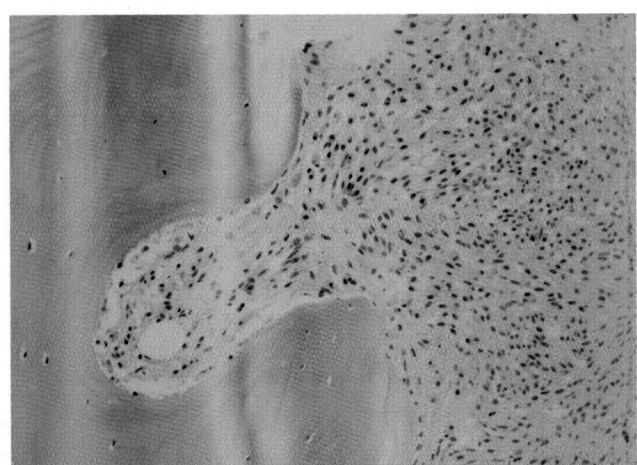

FIGURE 161-5 Bone marrow biopsy shows a characteristic lesion of systemic mastocytosis with paratrabecular infiltrates of mast cells and bony erosion. Mast cells are spindle-shaped, resembling fibroblasts or histiocytes.

Diagnosis

The diagnosis of mastocytosis is suspected on clinical grounds and confirmed by histology. Supporting evidence is derived from biochemical and radiographic data (Table 161-3).[1,17,20,25] Mast cells may be overlooked on histologic sections depending on the fixation and/or stain employed. The most useful stains for mast cells include metachromatic stains, such as toluidine blue and Giemsa, enzymatic stains, such as chloroacetate esterase and aminocaproate esterase, and avidin, which binds to heparin.[24] These procedures highlight the granules in the cytoplasm of the mast cell, thereby facilitating identification. In trephine core bone marrow biopsies, decalcification interferes with subsequent attempts to visualize mast cells granules, making their identification more difficult.

Fortunately most patients with mastocytosis have either urticaria pigmentosa or diffuse cutaneous mastocytosis, which can be recognized on physical examination. These diagnoses should be confirmed by skin biopsy. Blind skin biopsies must be interpreted with caution because other skin conditions including eczema and chronic urticaria are associated with a two- to fourfold increase in dermal mast cells as noted below.

In patients with urticaria pigmentosa, mast cells are found in increased numbers in the dermal papillae, particularly near blood vessels.[8,26–28] Mast cells may distribute in a bandlike infiltrate of the papillary dermis (Fig. 161-6) or appear as nodular infiltrates from the papillary dermis to subcutaneous tissues. Analysis of the relationship between mast cells and blood vessels has suggested that mast cells in patients with mastocytosis first increase around blood vessels and later appear in tissues distant from vessels. Mast cells may also be found in increased numbers in skin between lesions of urticaria pigmentosa. The greatest increases in mast cell number do occur beneath urticaria pigmentosa macules and papules where, on average, there is a fifteen- to twentyfold increase in mast cells. However, in occasional patients only a two- to fourfold increase in mast cells is found beneath these lesions. Two- to fourfold increases in mast cell number have also been documented in patients with recurrent episodes of flushing or anaphylaxis,[8] or in other skin involved in scleroderma,[29] chronic urticaria,[30] and prolonged antigenic contact.[31] These observations document the need to correlate the gross skin examination with skin mast cell numbers and to avoid diagnosis of urticaria pigmentosa relying solely on small increases in dermal mast cells. Cutaneous responses to intradermal histamine are unchanged in patients with urticaria pigmentosa.[32]

In patients with diffuse cutaneous mastocytosis, prominent bandlike infiltrates are observed, which may be indistinguishable from some lesions of urticaria pigmentosa or from tissue obtained from mastocytomas. Cutaneous mast cell hyperplasia in patients with telangiectasia macularis eruptiva perstans is observed around the capillary-venules of the superficial plexus.

TABLE 161-3
Consensus Diagnostic Workup for Mastocytosis Suspected on Clinical Grounds

Routine studies
  Skin examination—gross and microscopic
  Bone marrow biopsy and aspiration
  24-h urine for mediators
Additional studies
  Bone scan/skeletal survey
  GI workup—upper GI series, small bowel x-ray,
    CT scan, endoscopy
  EEG, neuropsychiatric workup

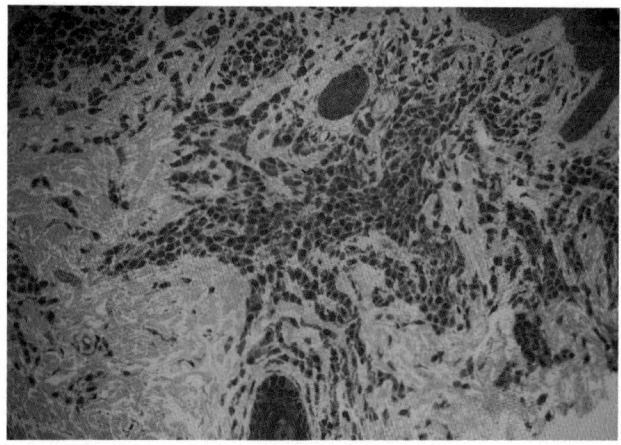

FIGURE 161-6 Mast cell hyperplasia in the dermis of a patient with systemic mastocytosis.

Dermal mast cells in patients with mastocytosis have been examined by both light and electron microscopy. When mast cells were examined for tryptase and chymase using specific antibodies to these proteases, only tryptase-positive, chymase-positive mast cells (MC_{TC}) were identified.[33] Because MC_{TC} are by far the predominant mast cell type in skin, while tryptase-positive, chymase-negative mast cells (MC_T) predominate in alveolar walls and in the gastrointestinal mucosa, the exclusive presence of MC_{TC} in dermal lesions of mastocytosis supports the concept that the mast cell hyperplasia observed is not clonal in nature. Upon electron microscopy and morphometric analysis, lesional mast cells from adults with systemic mastocytosis had a larger mean cytoplasmic area, nuclear size, and granule diameter than mast cells from normal individuals.[28] Bilobed or highly identical nuclei were more numerous.

Mastocytosis should be suspected in patients without skin lesions if they have one or more of the following: unexplained ulcer disease or malabsorption, radiographic or ^{99m}Tc bone scan abnormalities, hepatomegaly, splenomegaly, lymphadenopathy, peripheral blood abnormalities, or unexplained flushing or anaphylaxis. Elevated levels of plasma[34,35] or urinary histamine or histamine metabolites,[36] prostaglandin D_2 (PGD_2) metabolites in the urine,[37] or plasma mast cell tryptase[38] are not diagnostic but do raise the index of suspicion of mastocytosis. However, reliable tests for these substances are not generally available except in research laboratories.

In the absence of skin lesions, patients suspected of having mastocytosis should have a bone marrow biopsy and aspirate for diagnosis and categorization of the type of mastocytosis. Patients with urticaria pigmentosa or diffuse cutaneous mastocytosis should also have this procedure, particularly if they have peripheral blood abnormalities, hepatomegaly, splenomegaly, or lymphadenopathy, to determine if they have an associated hematologic disorder. Other tissue specimens, such as lymph nodes, spleen, liver, and gastrointestinal mucosa define the extent of mast cell involvement but are usually obtained only as dictated by necessity. For example, gastrointestinal biopsies are obtained only if a gastrointestinal workup is indicated, and lymph nodes are biopsied only if lymphoma is considered.

Patients suspected of having mastocytosis should have 24-h urine 5-hydroxyindoleacetic acid (5-HIAA) and urinary metanephrines measured to help eliminate the possibility of a carcinoid tumor or pheochromocytoma. That patients with mastocytosis do not excrete increased amounts of 5-HIAA suggests that serotonin, present in the mast cells of some species, is not synthesized by human mast cells. Idiopathic anaphylaxis and flushing must also be ruled out. Patients with these disorders do not have histologic evidence of significant mast cell proliferation and should have normal plasma histamine levels between episodes of anaphylaxis.[35]

Treatment

The primary objective of treatment in all categories of mastocytosis is to control mast cell mediator-induced signs and symptoms such as vascular collapse, gastric hypersecretion, gastrointestinal cramping, and pruritus. H_1 receptor antagonists such as hydroxyzine and doxepin are helpful in reducing pruritus, flushing, and tachycardia. If insufficient relief occurs, the addition of an H_2 antagonist such as ranitidine or cimetidine may be beneficial. However many patients continue to complain of bone pain, headaches, and flushing, resulting in part from the inability to block the effects of high levels of histamine with histamine antagonists and the presence of other mast cell mediators.

Disodium cromoglycate (cromolyn sodium) is known to inhibit degranulation of mast cells and may have some efficacy in the treatment of mastocytosis, particularly in relieving gastrointestinal complaints.[23,39,40] Cromolyn sodium does not lower plasma or urinary histamine levels in patients with mastocytosis.[39] Ketotifen, an antihistamine with mast cell-stabilizing properties, helps by relieving the pruritus and whealing associated with mastocytosis.[41] However, in a double-blind placebo-controlled trial of ketotifen vs. hydroxyzine in the treatment of pediatric mastocytosis, it was concluded that ketotifen offered no advantage over hydroxyzine, which was equally as effective at relieving symptoms.[42] Neither ketotifen nor hydroxyzine lowered plasma or urinary histamine levels.

Epinephrine is used to treat episodes of vascular collapse.[43] Patients should be prepared to self-administer this drug. If subcutaneous epinephrine is insufficient, intensive therapy for vascular collapse should be instituted. Patients with recurrent episodes of vascular collapse may be placed on H_1 and H_2 antihistamines to lessen the severity of attacks. Episodes of vascular collapse may be spontaneous but have also been observed after stings from insects.

Methoxsalen with long-wave ultraviolet radiation (PUVA) has been shown to relieve pruritus and whealing after 1 to 2 months of treatment.[44-48] Improvement is associated with a temporary decrease in dermal mast cells. Pruritus recurs within 3 to 6 months after stopping treatment. Photochemotherapy should be used only in instances of extensive cutaneous disease unresponsive to other forms of therapy. Some patients report a diminution in the number or intensity of cutaneous lesions after exposure to natural sunlight.

Topical corticosteroids, such as 0.05 percent betamethasone diproprionate ointment under plastic-film occlusion for 8 h per day over 8 to 12 weeks, can be used to treat extensive urticaria pigmentosa or diffuse cutaneous mastocytosis. Mast cell numbers decrease as the lesions clear. These lesions eventually recur after discontinuation of therapy,[48,49] although the treatment may lead to improvement in the cutaneous lesions for up to 1 year.

Treatment of gastrointestinal disease is directed as controlling peptic symptoms, diarrhea, and malabsorption.[9] Gastric acid hypersecretion leading to peptic symptoms and ulcerations is controlled with H_2 antagonists. Diarrhea is difficult to manage, and H_2 antagonists are generally not effective. Anticholinergics may give partial relief. In patients with severe malabsorption, systemic corticosteroids have been effective. Ascites is also difficult to control. Portal hypertension in one patient was successfully managed with a portacaval shunt.[50] Another patient with an exudative ascites was treated successfully with systemic corticosteroid therapy.[51]

Patients with mastocytosis and an associated hematologic disorder are managed as dictated by the specific hematologic abnormality. In patients with mast cell leukemia, chemotherapy has not yet been shown to produce remission or to prolong survival.[19] Chemotherapy has no place in the treatment of indolent mastocytosis.[25] A recent study suggested that splenectomy may improve survival in patients with forms of mastocytosis that have a poor prognosis.[52]

Prognosis

Prognosis must be addressed separately for each category of mastocytosis. One study[20] found seven variables that were strongly associated with poor survival: constitutional symptoms, anemia, thrombocytopenia, abnormal liver function tests, a lobated mast cell nucleus, a low percentage of fat cells in the bone marrow biopsy, and an associated hematologic disorder. Other poor prognostic variables include absence of urticaria pigmentosa, male sex, absence of skin and bone symptoms, hepatomegaly, splenomegaly, and normal bone x-ray findings.

As a group, patients with indolent mastocytosis and skin involvement alone have the best prognosis. Among children with isolated urticaria pigmentosa, at least 50 percent of cases resolve by adulthood.[53,54] Adults with urticaria pigmentosa usually progress gradually to systemic disease, and rarely may develop hematologic disease. Diffuse cutaneous mastocytosis is usually associated with indolent systemic disease. Patients with mastocytosis with an associated hematologic disorder have a variable course dependent on the prognosis of their hematologic disorder. With mast cell leukemia, mean survival is less than 6 months. Survival with lymphadenopathic mastocytosis with eosinophilia is 1 to 2 years without therapy. The prognosis appears to improve with aggressive symptomatic management.

References

1. Metcalfe DD: Conclusions. *J Invest Dermatol* **96**:64S, 1991
2. Kirshenbaum AS et al: Demonstration of the origin of human mast cells from CD 34+ bone marrow progenitor cells. *J Immunol* **146**:1410, 1991
3. Thompson HL et al: Laminin promotes mast cell attachment. *J Immunol* **143**:2323, 1989
4. Nutman T: The role of mast cells in the host defense against parasites, in *The Mast Cell in Health and Disease,* edited by M Kaliner, D Metcalfe. New York, Marcel Dekker, 1992, in press
5. Ihle JN et al: Biological properties of homogeneous interleukin 3. I. Demonstration of WEHI-3 growth-factor activity, mast cell growth-factor activity, P cell-stimulating factor activity and histamine-producing factor activity. *J Immunol* **131**:282, 1983
6. Bressler RB et al: Inhibition of the growth of interleukin-3 dependent mast cells from murine bone marrow by recombinant granulocyte-macrophage stimulating factor. *J Immunol* **143**:135, 1989
7. Zsebo KM et al: Stem cell factor is encoded at the S1 locus of the mouse and is the ligand for the C-Kit tyrosine kinase receptor. *Cell* **63**:213, 1990

8. Garriga MM et al: A survey of the number and distribution of mast cells in the skin of patients with mast cell disorders. *J Allergy Clin Immunol* **82**:425, 1988

9. Orkine M et al: Bullous mastocytosis. *Arch Dermatol* **101**:547, 1970

10. Golitz LE et al: Bullous mastocytosis: Diffuse cutaneous mastocytosis with extensive blisters mimicking scalded skin syndrome or erythema multiforme. *Pediatr Dermatol* **1**:288, 1984

11. Soter N: The skin in mastocytosis. *J Invest Dermatol* **96**:32S, 1991

12. Hissard R et al: Etude d'un cas de mastocytose. *Ann Med (Paris)* **52**:583, 1951

13. Cherner JA et al: Gastrointestinal dysfunction in systemic mastocytosis: A prospective study. *Gastroenterology* **95**:657, 1988

14. Horny H-P et al: Liver findings in generalized mastocytosis: A clinicopathologic study. *Cancer* **63**:532, 1989.

15. Travis WD, Li C-Y: Pathology of the lymph node and spleen in systemic mast cell disease. *Modern Pathol* **1**:4, 1988

16. Webb TA et al: Systemic mast cell disease: A clinical and hematopathologic study of 26 cases. *Cancer* **49**:927, 1982

17. Horny H-P et al: Bone marrow findings in systemic mastocytosis. *Hum Pathol* **16**:808, 1985

18. Travis WD et al: Significance of systemic mast cell disease with associated hematologic disorders. *Cancer* **62**:954, 1988

19. Travis WD et al: Mast cell leukemia: Report of a case and review of the literature. *Mayo Clin Proc* **61**:957, 1986

20. Travis WD et al: Systemic mast cell disease: Analysis of 58 cases and literature review. *Medicine* **67**:345, 1988

21. Kettelhut BV et al: Hematopathology of the bone marrow in pediatric cutaneous mastocytosis: A study of seventeen patients. *Am J Clin Pathol* **91**:558, 1989

22. Rosenbaum RC et al: Patterns of skeletal scintigraphy and their relationship to plasma and urinary histamine levels in systemic mastocytosis. *J Nucl Med* **25**:859, 1984

23. Soter NA et al: Oral disodium cromoglycate in the treatment of systemic mastocytosis. *N Engl J Med* **301**:465, 1979

24. Rogers MO et al: Mixed organic brain syndrome as a manifestation of systemic mastocytosis. *Psychosomatic Med* **48**:437, 1986

25. Friedman BS, Metcalfe DD: Mastocytosis, in *Biochemistry of the Acute Allergic Reactions, Fifth International Symposium,* edited by AI Tauber et al. New York, Alan R. Liss, 1989, pp 163–173

26. Kasper CS, Tharp MD: Quantification of cutaneous mast cells using morphometric counting and a conjugated avidin stain. *J Am Acad Dermatol* **16**:326, 1987

27. Mihm MC et al: Mast cell infiltrates of the skin and the mastocytosis syndrome. *Hum Pathol* **4**:231, 1973

28. Tharp MD et al: Ultrastructural morphometric analysis of lesional skin: Mast cells from patients with systemic and nonsystemic mastocytosis. *J Am Acad Dermatol* **18**:298, 1988

29. Nishioka K et al: Mast cell numbers in scleroderma. *Arch Dermatol* **123**:205, 1987

30. Elias J et al: Studies of the cellular infiltrate of chronic idiopathic urticaria: Prominence of T-lymphocytes, monocytes, and mast cells. *J Allergy Clin Immunol* **78**:914, 1986

31. Mitchell EB et al: Increase in skin mast cells following chronic house dust mite exposure. *Br J Dermatol* **114**:65, 1986

32. Keffer JM et al: Analysis of the wheal and flare reactions that follow the intradermal injection of histamine and morphine in adults with recurrent unexplained anaphylaxis and systemic mastocytosis. *J Allergy Clin Immunol* **83**:595, 1989

33. Irani A-M et al: Mast cells in cutaneous mastocytosis: Accumulation of the MC$_{TC}$ type. *Clin Exp Allergy* **20**:53, 1990

34. Kettelhut BV, Metcalfe DD: Plasma histamine in the evaluation of pediatric mastocytosis. *J Pediatr* **111**:419, 1987

35. Friedman BS et al: Analysis of plasma histamine levels in patients with mast cell disorders. *Am J Med* **87**:649, 1989

36. Keyzer JJ et al: Improved diagnosis of mastocytosis by measurement of urinary histamine metabolites. *N Engl J Med* **309**:1603, 1983

37. Roberts LJ II et al: Increased production of prostaglandin D$_2$ in patients with systemic mastocytosis. *N Engl J Med* **303**:1400, 1980

38. Schwartz LB et al: Tryptase levels as an indicator of mast cell activation in systemic anaphylaxis and mastocytosis. *N Engl J Med* **316**:1622, 1987

39. Frieri M et al: Comparison of the therapeutic efficacy of cromolyn sodium with that of combined chlorpheniramine and cimetidine in systemic mastocytosis: Results of a double-blind clinical trial. *Am J Med* **78**:9, 1985

40. Horan RF et al: Cromolyn sodium in the management of systemic mastocytosis. *J Allergy Clin Immunol* **85**:852, 1990

41. Czarnetski BM: A double blind cross-over study of the effect of ketotifen in urticaria pigmentosa. *Dermatologica* **166**:44, 1983

42. Kettelhut BV et al: A double blind placebo controlled trial of ketotifen versus hydroxyzine in the treatment of pediatric mastocytosis. *J Allergy Clin Immunol* **83**:866, 1989

43. Turk J et al: Intervention with epinephrine in hypotension associated with mastocytosis. *J Allergy Clin Immunol* **71**:189, 1983

44. Christophers E et al: PUVA-treatment of urticaria pigmentosa. *Br J Dermatol* **98**:701, 1978

45. Granerus G et al: Decreased urinary histamine metabolite after successful PUVA treatment of urticaria pigmentosa. *J Invest Dermatol* **76**:1, 1981

46. Vella-Briffa D et al: Photochemotherapy (PUVA) in the treatment of urticaria pigmentosa. *Br J Dermatol* **109**:67, 1983

47. Czarnetski PM et al: Phototherapy of urticaria pigmentosa: Clinical response and changes of cutaneous reactivity, histamine, and chemotactic leukotrienes. *Arch Dermatol Res* **277**:105, 1985

48. Laoker RM, Schechter NM: Cutaneous mast cell depletion results from topical corticosteroids usage. *J Immunol* **135**:2368, 1985

49. Barton J et al: Treatment of urticaria pigmentosa with corticosteroids. *Arch Dermatol* **121**:1516, 1985

50. Bonnet P et al: Intractable ascites in systemic mastocytosis treated by portal diversion. *Digestive Dis Sci* **32**:209, 1987

51. Reisberg IR, Oyakawa S: Mastocytosis and malabsorption, myelofibrosis and massive ascites. *Am J Gastroenterology* **82**:54, 1987

52. Friedman B et al: Splenectomy in the management of systemic mast cell disease. *Surgery* **107**:94 1990

53. Sondergaard J, Asbo-Hansen E: Mastocytosis in childhood, in *Pediatric Dermatology,* edited by R Happle et al. Berlin, Springer-Verlag, 1987, pp 148–154

54. Kettelhut BV, Metcalfe DD: Pediatric mastocytosis *J Invest Dermatol* **96**:15S, 1991

CHAPTER 162

Lynn A. Cornelius and Thomas J. Lawley

Cryoglobulinemia and Cryofibrinogenemia

Definition

Cryoglobulins are circulating immunoglobulins complexed with other immunoglobulins or proteins that reversibly precipitate in the cold. The symptoms of type I cryoglobulinemia are caused by vascular occlusion resulting from protein precipitation; mixed cryoglobulinemia (type II or III) is an immune complex disease (see below).

History

The existence of cryoproteinemia as a clinical entity was first noted by Wintrobe and Buell in 1933.[1] The immunoglobulin composition of these cryoproteins was recognized by Waldenstrom in 1943.[2] Four years later, Lerner and Watson[3] performed the first large-scale examination of pathologic sera for cryoglobulins and found them in 11 percent.

Classification

The classification of cryoglobulinemia consists of three distinct groups initially described by Brouet et al[4] based on immunoglobulin type. Type I cryoglobulins consist of a single monoclonal immunoglobulin, usually an IgG or an IgM. Patients with type I cryoglobulinemia usually have an underlying B-cell malignancy such as multiple myeloma or a B-cell lymphoma. Type II and type III cryoglobulins consist of rheumatoid factors (usually IgM) complexed with IgG and thus constitute immune complexes. Type II cryoglobulins are single monoclonal immunoglobulins that cryoprecipitate with polyclonal immunoglobulins (usually IgG). Type III cryoglobulins are polyclonal immunoglobulins that form cryoprecipitates with polyclonal IgG or a nonimmunoglobulin serum component. Type I, II, and III cryoglobulins may be associated with various disease states (Table 162-1); these associations will be further addressed.

TABLE 162-1
Selected Diseases Associated with Cryoglobulins

Cryoglobulin	Disease state
Type I	Multiple myeloma, chronic lymphocytic leukemia, Waldenström's macroglobulinemia
Type II	Multiple myeloma, Waldenström's macroglobulinemia, chronic lymphocytic leukemia, rheumatoid arthritis, Sjögren's syndrome
Type III	Systemic lupus erythematosus, rheumatoid arthritis, Sjögren's syndrome, infectious mononucleosis, cytomegalovirus infections, biliary cirrhosis

Isolation Techniques

The isolation and characterization of cyoglobulins is described in detail by Gorevic.[5] In brief, cryoproteins are isolated from blood that has clotted at 37°C. The serum is separated and then maintained at 4°C. Most type I cryoprecipitates will be evident within 24 h, whereas mixed type III cryoglobulins may require several days of incubation for precipitation. Therefore it is important to hold serum for approximately 1 week before final determination is made of the presence of a cryoprecipitate. The reversibility of the formation of the cryoprecipitate is confirmed through rewarming to 37°C. The precipitate is purified by repeated washing and low-speed cold centrifugation. Of note is that cryoglobulins may become associated with serum lipids and remain suspended during centrifugation, thereby obscuring the formation of a visible precipitate.[6]

The concentration of cryoglobulins may be expressed as a percentage of the volume of the total collected serum, milligrams per milliliter, or a cryocrit. Type I cryoglobulins are typically present in concentrations greater than 5 mg/mL. In contrast, type III cryoglobulins are usually present in lesser amounts, i.e., cryocrits less than 1 percent.[7] Alternatively quantitation may be accomplished by determining the protein concentration of the dissolved cryoprecipitate. A method for rapid cryoglobulin screening has been described[8]; this method uses centrifugation, incubation of paired serum samples at 37°C and 4°C for 1 h, and comparison of optical densities via spectrophotometry of the sera held at the two temperatures. Symptom severity is generally thought to reflect cryoprotein concentration in the serum as well as the temperature at which cryoprecipitation takes place; some reports, however, have described dramatic clinical symptoms at relatively low cryoglobulin concentrations.[9] The components of the cryoglobulin are identified by use of specific antibodies against suspected protein such as immunoglobulin or complement components.

Cryoglobulin Characteristics

Type I Monoclonal Cryoglobulins

Type I cryoglobulins are monoclonal immunoglobulins, typically IgM or IgG, although IgA and Bence Jones proteins have been identified. In a review of 86 patients with cryoglobulinemia, Brouet et al[4] reported that 25 percent of patients had only monoclonal cryoglobulins. Further characterization of these cryoglobulins revealed a predominance of IgM immunoglobulin. IgG and IgM light chain types did not differ significantly from normal serum immunoglobulin types. Amino acid abnormalities as well as changes in the composition of carbohydrate side chains have been noted in monoclonal as well as in mixed cryoglobulins.[10] The carbohydrate abnormalities have been hypothesized to contribute to the decreased solubility of the immunoglobulins.[11] However such abnormalities are not invariably found, and the precipitation of cryoglobulins most likely results from varied interactions of the constituent molecules at decreased temperatures.[12] The large molecular size of IgM monoclonal cryoglobulins may predispose these immunoglobulins to precipitation; it has been postulated that cryoprecipitation is an extension of the normal solubility.[13] In some monoclonal IgG cryoprecipitates, the cryoprecipitate determinant seems to reside in the variable region of the immunoglobulin since the activity may be retained in the F(ab')2 fragment.[5]

Some idiotypic relatedness may exist among monoclonal IgG cryoglobulins; one study's finding of cross-reactivity among 5 of 15 IgG cryoglobulins suggested similar variable region structures and, possibly, antigenic specificities.[14] Complement components are not routinely found as components of type I cryoglobulins.

Mixed Cryoglobulins

Type II cryoglobulins consist of two immunoglobulin components, one of which is monoclonal. The most common composition is that of a monoclonal IgM rheumatoid factor complexed with a polyclonal IgG. Although the serum concentration of type II cryoglobulin is often very high, a typical monoclonal spike is not always apparent on immunoelectrophoresis. IgG monoclonal rheumatoid factors are identified in about 10 percent of cases of type II cryoglobulinemia, but IgA monoclonal rheumatoid factors are rare. Some evidence suggests that there is an increased prevalence of kappa light chains in the monoclonal IgM and that in some instances the monoclonal IgM has restricted specificity for IgG. Exceptions to this restricted specificity occur.

The most common type (approximately 50 percent) of cryoglobulins identified are type III mixed cryoglobulins. These cryoglobulins usually occur in low concentration and consist of polyclonal immunoglobulin complexes or polyclonal immunoglobulin-nonimmunoglobulin cryoprecipitates. These cryoglobulins are found in association with diseases that may involve the formation of immune complexes. Again, IgM-IgG cryoglobulins are most frequent.[4] The finding of complement system components in these cryoprecipitates, in particular C1q,[15] provides substantial evidence for the immune complex nature of this phenomenon. Indeed, these cryoglobulins activate complement in vitro, and patients with type III cryoglobulinemia often have decreased serum complement levels. Various antigens, both autologous and exogenous, have been found associated with polyclonal immunoglobulins in this disease. Polyclonal IgG-antilipoprotein autoantibodies,[16] IgM anti-hepatitis A virus,[17] and antifibronectin antibodies[18] have been described. DNA has been identified in the cryoglobulins of patients with systemic lupus erythematosus (SLE).[19] However DNA and anti-DNA antibodies have also been found in cryoglobulins in patients with glomerulonephritis, who did not necessarily have SLE.[20]

Pathophysiology

Type I cryoglobulins demonstrate a self-association of monoclonal immunoglobulins at temperatures ranging from 0 to 30°C or more. Monoclonal cryoglobulins are present in substantial amounts, often ranging from 1 to 30 mg/mL.[4] They may precipitate as a gel, a flocculent precipitate, or in some instances as crystals. The specific physical forces involved in causing precipitates of type I cryoglobulins seem to include temperature-induced conformational changes, deficient carbohydrate side chains, and nucleation reactions.[5] In some instances type I cryoglobulins, even when present in large amounts, may not result in signs or symptoms of disease. Clinical manifestations of type I disease usually consist of occlusive peripheral vascular phenomena such as Raynaud's phenomenon, cutaneous ulcers, or gangrene. Renal disease and peripheral neuropathy are much less common (see "Clinical Features" below).

Types II and III cryoglobulins tend to be present in relatively small amounts. These monoclonal (type II) or polyclonal (type III) rheumatoid factor-IgG complexes usually occur with a concomitant disease process such as connective tissue disease, infection, hepatic disease, or lymphoproliferative disease. The exception is the occurrence of type III cryoglobulins in so-called essential mixed cryoglobulinemia. These cryoglobulins function as immune complexes and in many instances are effective activators of complement. Therefore analysis of types II and III cryoglobulins often reveals the presence of C1q in addition to other immunoglobulins. Patients with mixed cryoglobulinemia not only have immune complexes composed of cryoprecipitable material, but may also have distinctive circulating immune complexes that are noncryoprecipitable and predominately composed of IgG.[21] These latter immune complexes may contribute to the presentation of the disease in these patients.

Earlier work on the complement system in cryoglobulinemia revealed decreased levels of "whole complement" (CH50), C1, C4, and C2.[22] Normal levels of C3 and elevated levels of later components were sometimes found, leading to the hypothesis of hyposynthesis and/or hypercatabolism of the early complement components in this disease.[23,24] However a number of other clinical studies have identified patients with mixed cryoglobulinemia who do evidence depressed levels of C3, along with decreases in CH50, C2, and C4.[25]

The actual deposition of immunoglobulins and complement in involved tissues has been evaluated. The immunoglobulins in the serum cryoprecipitate of patients with mixed cryoglobulinemia have been identified, along with complement, in involved renal vessels; the histologically normal vasculature evidenced immunoglobulin deposition without complement.[26] In a long-term follow-up of 40 patients with mixed cryoglobulinemia, Gorevic et al[25] performed immunofluorescence studies of the skin in 16 cases. In 50 percent of the patients, immune reactants and complement were present in the vessel walls; the uninvolved skin of five patients did not reveal immunoglobulin or complement. The absence of immune reactants and/or the lack of complement deposition in uninvolved tissue is notable in these reports. Studies such as these have been cited as evidence for the pathogenic role of immune complex deposition in cryoglobulinemia. However immunofluorescence may in fact be negative.[5]

Clinical Features

The classical presentation of a patient with cryoglobulinemia is the appearance of purpura. Cold sensitivity is not an invariable feature of cryoglobulinemia. Patients may also evidence serum cryoprecipitates in the absence of clinical symptoms. Some patients with type I cryoglobulins may present solely with cutaneous lesions and ultimately may develop significant vascular compromise with subsequent visceral injury.[4]

The usual organ systems affected in cryoglobulinemia are the skin, kidneys, liver, and musculoskeletal and nervous systems. In general, type I cryoglobulins are typically associated with acrocyanosis, retinal hemorrhage, Raynaud's phenomenon, and arterial thrombosis.[5] Types II and III cryoglobulins are associated with arthritis or arthralgias and vascular purpura.[5] Renal and neurologic symptoms may be found in patients with types II and III cryoglobulins.[4] In a series of 40 patients with mixed cryoglobulins, Gorevic et al[25] reported that 100 percent had recurrent palpable purpura, 73 percent had polyarthralgias, and 55 percent had renal disease.

Cutaneous Features

Purpura is considered to be a cutaneous hallmark of cryoglobulinemia. It is usually located distally, most typically on the lower extremities. Showers of these lesions may occur spontaneously, may be provoked by cold exposure, or may be induced by long periods of standing or sitting.[4] Noninflammatory purpura, with histologic evidence of an amorphous eosinophilic precipitate within the vasculature, is characteristically seen in type I cryoglobulinemia,[27] but may also occur in types II and III.[28] Leukocytoclastic vasculitis, presenting clinically as palpable purpura, is characteristic of the mixed cryoglobulinemias. The lesions are intermittent in nature (typically lasting 3 to 10 days) and usually are nonpruritic.[25] As mentioned before, immunofluorescence findings are variable.

Synovitis, serositis, digital ulcerations, and gangrene have been described in cryoglobulinemia. Urticaria may occasionally occur in association with cryoglobulinemia, and cold urticaria has also been found.[29,30] Raynaud's phenomenon and ulcerations of the lower extremities have been reported.[25]

Renal Disease

Reports indicate that 30 to 60 percent of patients with essential mixed cryoglobulinemia have, or will develop, renal involvement.[5] In one large series,[31] pathologic evaluation revealed predominantly a membranoproliferative glomerulonephritis. The initial clinical presentation may include diastolic hypertension, edema, or frank renal failure. Laboratory findings may include proteinuria, hematuria, pyuria, and red cell casts.[25] Immunofluorescence is characteristically positive and reflects the immunoglobulin and/or complement components identified in the isolated cryoglobulin.

Other

Neurologic symptoms may occur in a small percentage of patients and typically consist of a peripheral sensorimotor polyneuropathy, which may present as paresthesias or foot drop.[25] Articular manifestations, more common in types II and III cryoglobulinemias, rarely involve a distinct arthritis,[5] although arthralgias are reported.[32] Hepatic involvement consists of hepatomegaly and splenomegaly, while the most common liver function abnormality is elevation of alkaline phosphatase.[25] As previously described, serologic studies for hepatitis may be positive. Other manifestations of vascular occlusive phenomena or immune complex disease may affect the eye and gastrointestinal system.

Associated Diseases

Lymphoproliferative and autoimmune disorders are the most frequently associated diseases. Lymphoproliferative diseases are associated with types I or II cryoglobulins and autoimmune disorders with type III. Lymphoproliferative diseases include macroglobulinemia and lymphomas. Autoimmune disorders most typically include rheumatoid arthritis, SLE, and Sjögren's syndrome. Epidermolysis bullosa acquisita has also been described in association with mixed cryoglobulins.[33]

Essential mixed cryoglobulinemia describes the presence of cryoglobulins and the concomitant manifestation of symptoms without an identifiable connective tissue, neoplastic, or infectious process. Levo et al[34] recognized the high frequency of liver involvement in these patients and identified hepatitis B surface antigen, hepatitis B surface antibody, or Dane particles associated with most of their sera or cryoprecipitates. These researchers postulated that most of these cases resulted from hepatitis B virus or other viral infections. This association is presently well recognized. However there remains a cohort of patients for whom the designation *essential cryoglobulinemia* continues to be appropriate.

Treatment

Treatment in cryoglobulinemia is based on the severity of disease presentation. Mild cutaneous symptoms may not require therapeutic intervention. Dermatologic and articular manifestations may be improved by nonsteroidal antiinflammatory agents. More severe visceral involvement, particularly renal disease, may require corticosteroid therapy in conjunction with cytotoxic agents. Melphalan, chlorambucil, or cyclophosphamide may benefit some patients.[5] Plasmapheresis has also been employed in patients with rapidly progressive disease refractory to conventional therapy. Unfortunately a postpheresis rebound in disease activity may occur. Plasma exchange is usually instituted together with immunosuppressive or cytotoxic agents in an attempt at better disease control as well as avoidance of rebound. High-dose intravenous gamma globulin therapy has been described as beneficial in one patient with essential mixed cryoglobulinemia and leukocytoclastic vasculitis.[35]

Cryofibrinogenemia

Cryofibrinogens are cryoproteins in anticoagulated blood or plasma that reversibly precipitate in the cold and are composed of fibrinogen. In the evaluation of cryofibrinogens, it is imperative that blood collection be performed in citrate, oxalate, or ethylenediaminetetraacetic acid. Heparin may produce false-positive precipitates (heparin-precipitable fraction) through the formation of heparin-fibronectin cryoprecipitable complexes, the formation of which may be enhanced by the presence of fibrinogen.[5]

Many earlier investigators found evidence of cryofibrinogens in a small percentage of normal subjects. Some reports describe cryofibrinogen complexes composed of fibrin, fibrinogen, and fibrin split products together with albumin, fibronectin, and von Willebrand factor.[36] Taken together, these reports may, in fact, reflect the formation of cryoprecipitates composed of these plasma proteins upon freeze-thawing of normal plasma.[5] Cutaneous manifestations of cryofibrinogenemia may include purpura, ecchymosis, gangrene, and ulcerations.[37] Associated disease states most commonly include malignancies and thromboembolic diseases. Diabetes and hyperglycemia have been described, as have pregnancy, oral contraceptive agents, and pseudotumor cerebri.[38] The treatment of cryofibrinogenemia is that of the underlying disease or associated condition.

References

1. Wintrobe NM, Buell MV: Hyperproteinemia associated with multiple myeloma: With report of a case in which an extraordinary hyperproteinemia was associated with thrombosis of the retinal veins and symptoms suggesting Raynaud's disease. *Bull Johns Hopkins Hosp* **52**:156, 1933

2. Waldenstrom J: Klinska metoder for pavisande an hyperproteinam: Oc deras praktiska for diagnostiken. *Nord Med* **20**:2288, 1943

3. Lerner AB, Watson CJ: Studies of cryoglobulins. II. The spontaneous precipitation of protein from serum at 5°C in various disease states. *Am J Med Sci* **214**:416, 1947

4. Brouet JC et al: Biological and clinical significance of cryoglobulinemia: Report of 86 cases. *Am J Med* **57**:775, 1974

5. Gorevic PD: Cryopathies: Cryoglobulins and cryofibrinogenemia, in *Immunological Diseases,* edited by M Samter et al. Boston/Toronto: Little, Brown, 1978, p 1687

6. Winfield JB: Cryoglobulinemia. *Hum Pathol* **14**:350, 1983

7. Lospalluto J et al: Cryoglobulinemia based on interaction between a macroglobulin and 7S gammaglobulin. *Am J Med* **32**:142, 1962

8. Kalovidouris AE, Johnson L: Rapid cryoglobulin screening: An aid to the clinician. *Ann Rheum Dis* **37**:444, 1978

9. Letendre L, Kyle RA: Monoclonal cryoglobulinemia with high thermal insolubility. *Mayo Clin Proc* **57**:629, 1982

10. Zinneman HH, Caperton E: Cryoglobulinemia in a patient with Sjögren's syndrome, and factors of cryoprecipitation. *J Lab Clin Med* **89**:483, 1977

11. Levo Y: Nature of cryoglobulinaemia. *Lancet* **1**:285, 1980

12. Litman G et al: Molecular basis for the temperature-dependent insolubility of cryoglobulins. IX. Physicochemical characterization of an IgG1 K monoclonal cryoglobulin exhibiting marginal low temperature-dependent insolubility. *Mol Immunol* **17**:337, 1980

13. Middaugh CR et al: Physicochemical characterization of six monoclonal cryoimmunoglobulins: Possible basis for cold dependent insolubility. *Proc Natl Acad Sci USA* **75**:3440, 1978

14. Abraham GN et al: Idiopathic relatedness of human monoclonal IgG cryoglobulins. *Immunology* **48**:315, 1983

15. Stastny P, Ziff M: Cold-insoluble complexes and complement levels in systemic lupus erythematosus. *N Engl J Med* **280**:1376, 1969

16. Kodama H: Determination of cryoglobulins as lipoprotein-autoantibody immune complexes and antigenic determinants against an-

tilipoprotein autoantibody. *Clin Exp Immunol* **28**:437, 1977

17. Ilan Y et al: Vasculitis and cryoglobulinemia associated with persisting cholestatic hepatitis A virus infection. *Am J Gastroenterol* **85**:586, 1990

18. Beaulieu AD et al: The influence of fibronectin on cryoprecipitate formation in rheumatoid arthritis and systemic lupus erythematosus. *Arthritis Rheum* **24**:1383, 1981

19. Winfield JB et al: Specific concentration of polynucleotide complexes in the serum cryoprecipitates of patients with SLE. *J Clin Invest* **56**:563, 1975

20. Roberts JL, Lewis EJ: Immunochemical demonstration of cryoprecipitable anti-native DNA antibody in the serum of patients with glomerulonephritis. *J Immunol* **124**:127, 1980

21. Lawley TJ et al: Multiple types of immune complexes in patients with mixed cryoglobulinemia. *J Invest Dermatol* **75**:297, 1980

22. Linscott WD, Kane JP: The complement system in cryoglobulinaemia: Interaction with immunoglobulins and lipoproteins. *Clin Exp Immunol* **21**:510, 1975

23. Tarantino A et al: Serum complement pattern in essential cryoglobulinaemia. *Clin Exp Immunol* **32**:77, 1978

24. Haydey RP et al: A newly described control mechanism of complement activation in patients with mixed cryoglobulinemia (cryoglobulins and complement). *J Invest Dermatol* **74**:328, 1980

25. Gorevic PD et al: Mixed cryoglobulinemia: Clinical aspects and long term follow-up of 40 patients. *Am J Med* **69**:287, 1980

26. Feiner HD: Relationship of tissue deposits of cryoglobulin to clinical features of mixed cryoglobulinemia. *Hum Pathol* **14**:710, 1983

27. Lever WF, Schaumburg-Lever G: *Histopathology of the Skin,* 7th ed. Philadelphia: JP Lippincott, 1990, p 191

28. Cattaneo R et al: The cryoglobulinemic vasculitis. *Ricera Clinica Laboratorio* **16**:327, 1986

29. Costanzi JJ et al: Activation of complement by a monoclonal cryoglobulin associated with cold urticaria. *J Lab Clin Med* **74**:902, 1969

30. Rawnsley HM, Shelley WB: Cold urticaria with cryoglobulinemia. *Arch Dermatol* **98**:12, 1968

31. Tarantino A et al: Renal disease in essential mixed cryoglobulinemia. *Q J Med* **197**:1, 1981

32. Weinberger A et al: Articular manifestations of essential cryoglobulinemia. *Semin Arthritis Rheum* **10**:224, 1981

33. Krivo JM, Miller F: Immunopathology of epidermolisis bullosa acquisita. *Arch Dermatol* **114**:1218, 1978

34. Levo YL et al: Association between hepatitis B virus and essential mixed cryoglobulinemia. *N Engl J Med* **296**:1501, 1977

35. Boom BW et al: Severe leukocytoclastic vasculitis of the skin in a patient with essential mixed cryoglobulinemia treated with high-dose γ-globulin intravenously. *Arch Dermatol* **124**:1550, 1988

36. Ireland TA et al: Cutaneous lesions in cryofibrinogenemia. *Clin Lab Obstet* **105**:67, 1984

37. Martin S: Cryofibrinogenemia, monoclonal gammopathy, and purpura. *Arch Dermatol* **115**:208, 1979

38. Smith SB, Arkin C: Cryofibrinogenemia: Incidence, clinical correlations and a review of the literature. *Am J Clin Pathol* **58**:524, 1972

Cutaneous Manifestations of Gastrointestinal and Renal Disorders

CHAPTER 163

Imrich Sarkany and Robin A.C. Graham-Brown

An association between the skin and the liver has been recognized for centuries (Fig. 163-1). It has been taken over by folklore, which in the Middle Ages labeled females with various vascular skin blemishes as witches, still accepts a "bottlenose" as a sign of an alcoholic with liver trouble, and describes a variety of pigmented skin lesions as "liver spots." Even the term *spider* is said to have originated in the New York underworld where barmaids spotted "spiders" as evidence of advanced liver disease in their customers.

The alterations of nails and hair and the vascular, pigmentary, and allergic changes found in the skin of patients with hepatobiliary disease may also occur in its absence or in association with physiologic states. For example, spider nevi may be seen in normal children and in pregnant women. There may be no visible skin changes in patients with severe or advanced liver disease, and dramatic cu-

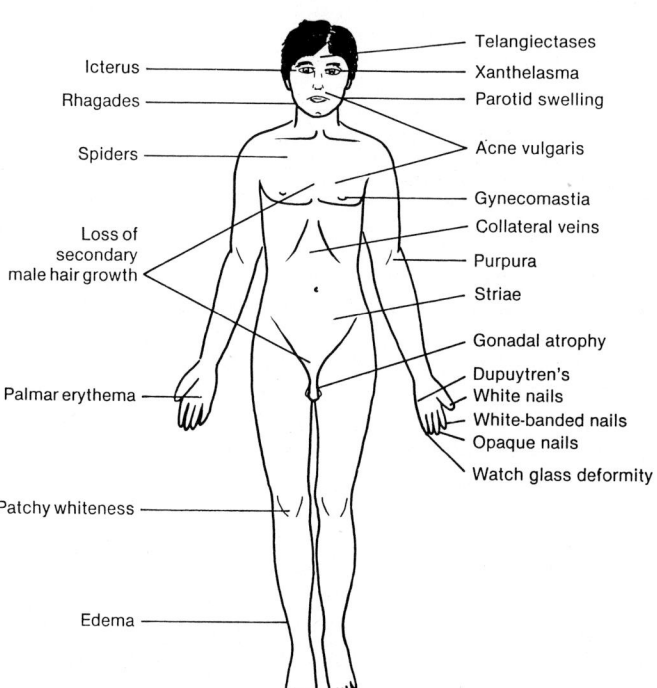

FIGURE 163-1 The main skin changes in liver disease.

Labels:
Icterus
Rhagades
Spiders
Loss of secondary male hair growth
Palmar erythema
Patchy whiteness
Edema
Telangiectases
Xanthelasma
Parotid swelling
Acne vulgaris
Gynecomastia
Collateral veins
Purpura
Striae
Gonadal atrophy
Dupuytren's
White nails
White-banded nails
Opaque nails
Watch glass deformity

The Hepatobiliary System and the Skin

taneous manifestations may be seen in those with minimal hepatic dysfunction. Severe itching may antedate other features of biliary cirrhosis by months or years.

Hyperestrogenism in male alcoholics, even in the absence of cirrhosis, may manifest itself with gynecomastia, vascular spiders, and changes in body hair and fat distribution.[1]

Several types of interaction between the skin and the hepatobiliary system are encountered in clinical practice:

1. Liver disease may cause skin changes: Primary disorders of hepatic functions may induce changes in the skin and its appendages. Jaundice, itching, pigmentary abnormalities, and alterations in nails and hair fall into this category. These are the cutaneous changes best recognized by physicians as contributing to an early diagnosis of hepatobiliary disease.
2. The skin and the liver may be involved by the same pathologic process, or by exposure to exogenous chemicals, as in patients with vinyl chloride disease. Damage to the liver, skin, adnexa, and other organs may also be part of an inherited disorder, such as argininosuccinic aciduria or tuberous sclerosis.
3. Skin disease may cause liver abnormalities. Disturbances of hepatic function due to skin disease have been documented.
4. The liver may be damaged by the drugs used to treat skin disease. Methotrexate is the best known example of this association.

Skin Lesions due to Hepatobiliary Disease

When skin lesions occur in association with liver disease, they are generally not specific to a particular hepatic pathology, but the most florid cutaneous lesions are generally seen in patients with chronic active hepatitis and in alcoholics.

Jaundice

Jaundice, or icterus, is the generalized yellow or ocher coloration of the skin, mucous membranes, and other body tissues imparted by the bile pigment bilirubin. Both jaundice and pigmentation are most prominent in disease states that produce extrahepatic biliary obstruction, and in primary biliary cirrhosis. Clinically detectable jaundice is always indicative of disease and must be distinguished from olive or sallow skin complexions, carotenemia, the yellowish skin pigmentation produced by quinacrine and busulfan, and lycopenemia due to ingestion of tomato juice.

Pathogenesis Jaundiced skin, varying in hue from faint golden to dark greenish yellow, results from increased local cellular or connective tissue binding of the tetrapyrrole bilirubin (or its metabolites). The tissue pigment, which has a special affinity for elastin, is derived from the perfusing blood and lymph, circulating almost exclusively as a tightly bound complex with serum albumin (2 moles of bilirubin per mole of protein). The elevated serum bilirubin level results, in turn, from an imbalance between overall pigment production and excretion.

Tissue-serum equilibration is slow and the intensity of clinical icterus often fails to reflect the concurrent serum bilirubin level. Hyperbilirubinemia may therefore antedate the onset of detectable jaundice by 1 or more days and, conversely, scleral and cutaneous icterus may persist despite falling or normal serum bilirubin levels. Local changes in vascular permeability may "sequester" bile pigment or impair its equilibration with the general circulation—hence the occasional finding of jaundice of different intensity in areas of edema. The correlation between cutaneous staining and serum pigment levels is especially poor in newborn infants. A further discrepancy between tissue and serum pigment levels in infants may result from the administration of drugs such as sulfisoxazole and salicylates, which apparently uncouple protein-bound bilirubin and favor its passage into body tissues.[2]

Clinically detectable jaundice appears when sufficient bilirubin has become tissue-bound, generally implying in adults that total serum levels have exceeded 2.5 to 3.0 mg/dL (normally less than 1.5 mg/dL) over a period of days. Jaundice is often not obvious in newborn infants until serum levels reach 6.0 to 8.0 mg/dL (1 mg = 17 μmol/L).

Etiology Between 80 and 90 percent of bilirubin entering the circulation of normal adults is derived from degradation of red cell hemoglobin within the reticuloendothelial system; the remainder arises from red cell precursors in the marrow and from nonhemoglobin heme compounds in the liver. This newly formed pigment is albumin-bound, unconjugated, and reacts only slightly (and "indirectly") with the standard diazo reagent. In the normal adult liver, which has a metabolic reserve of fivefold increases in pigment production without the development of jaundice, unconjugated and albumin-free pigment is coupled by microsomal enzymes with glucuronic acid, transported to bile canaliculi, and excreted actively as the water-soluble diglucuronide that reacts "directly" with the diazo reagent.[3]

No current etiologic classification of jaundice is complete or physiologically sound, but a functional approach based on conjugated and total serum bilirubin concentrations has some merit (Table 163-1). Thus most types of clinical jaundice are caused predominantly either by overproduction or by underconjugation of bilirubin (with less than 15 percent conjugated, or "direct-reacting," pigment in the serum) or by liver cell damage and impaired excretion (with greater than 15 percent conjugated pigment in the serum).

Clinical Features Jaundice is a cardinal sign of disease and requires careful evaluation. Its onset, evolution, and implications

TABLE 163-1
Functional Classification of Jaundice

Unconjugated ("indirect") hyperbilirubinemia
  Newborn and infant
    "Physiologic"—functional hepatic immaturity
    Hemolysis—Rh, ABO, sepsis, drug factors
    Prematurity
    Transient familial hyperbilirubinemia—maternal steroid
      inhibitors
    Crigler-Najjar syndrome—glucuronyl transferase deficiency
      (hereditary)
  Adult
    Excess bilirubin production
      Hemolysis
        Congenital
        Acquired
      Dyserythropoietic—"shunt" hyperbilirubinemia
    Deficient conjugation
      Familial
        Constitutional hepatic dysfunction (Gilbert's
          syndrome)
        Crigler-Najjar syndrome type II
      Acquired
        Posthepatic
        Associated disease—cardiac, enteric, metabolic
        Drug-induced
  Diagnostic features
    Serum-conjugated bilirubin less than 15% of total
    Absence of bilirubinuria
    Low to normal urine urobilinogen
    Absence of other liver function disturbances
    Normal morphologic features of liver

Conjugated ("direct-reacting") hyperbilirubinemia
  Hepatic cell damage
    Acute—viral, toxic, anoxic, metabolic
    Chronic—cirrhosis, metabolic
  Impaired bile excretion
    Extrahepatic obstruction
    Intrahepatic cholestasis—atresias, viral, drugs,
      hormones, pregnancy, benign recurrent cholestasis
    Familial (defect confined to bilirubin excretion)
      Dubin-Johnson syndrome—excretory defect and cell pigment
      Rotor's syndrome—excretory defect and no pigment
  Diagnostic features
    Serum-conjugated bilirubin more than 15% of total
    Bilirubinuria common
    Urine urobilinogen often elevated
    Other liver functions often abnormal in hepatic cell
      damage and impaired bile excretion
    Characteristic morphologic abnormalities of liver

depend on the underlying disease process. Hyperbilirubinemia and cutaneous icterus themselves produce neither symptoms nor harmful effects in adults.

Slight jaundice is frequently unremarked by patients and family: poor lightening, dark skin coloration, and subtle progression often combine to delay the clinical diagnosis for days or weeks. Careful inspection of peripheral ocular sclerae in natural or bluish light is the best clinical method for detecting minimal jaundice; the high elastic tissue content of sclerae apparently accounts for this preferential staining. Prolonged and deep jaundice may assume a greenish-tan quality, the result perhaps of melanosis and partial oxidation of bilirubin to biliverdin.

The intensity of jaundice and levels of serum bilirubin in patients with biliary atresia, acquired bile duct obstruction, or defective bilirubin conjugation tend to stabilize despite continued pigment production: The fate or disposition of the excess pigment is still uncertain. Some degradation of bilirubin has been shown to occur with exposure to ultraviolet radiation. This phenomenon is the basis for phototherapy of babies to prevent kernicterus in severe neonatal jaundice: The colorless breakdown products are probably excreted in the urine. The urine becomes dark yellow and then tea-colored as conjugated serum bilirubin exceeds an inconstant "threshold" value of 0.4 to 0.6 mg/dL. Bilirubinemia is not a feature of unconjugated hyperbilirubinemic states. Since most of the brown color of normal feces is produced by urobilins derived from degradation of bilirubin in the intestine, the jaundice of impaired pigment excretion or bile obstruction is associated with "clay-colored" stools.

Diagnosis   The precise diagnosis of jaundice requires a methodical consideration of all the factors that may be responsible (Table 163-1). Careful history and clinical examination should indicate the underlying disease in 60 to 70 percent of cases; a selected group of liver function tests should afford a diagnosis in another 10 to 15 percent; special procedures may be required to establish a definitive diagnosis in the remainder.

Treatment and Course   Jaundice in patients with acute hepatitis resolves spontaneously. A small percentage of patients with acute hepatitis, predominantly those with hepatitis type A, may enter a cholestatic phase with jaundice and severe itching. These patients may be "whitewashed" by a short course of systemic corticosteroids. The jaundice of chronic liver disease may improve when the underlying liver involvement improves. Patients with chronic active hepatitis often lose their jaundice to a large extent after successful therapy with corticosteroids and patients with primary biliary cirrhosis may also show lessening of jaundice after treatment with penicillamine. The jaundice of biliary obstruction resolves when the obstruction is relieved. In addition to phototherapy in babies, help may be offered to patients with Gilbert's and the Crigler-Najjar syndromes, in which benign unconjugated hyperbilirubinemia is found in association with otherwise normal liver function. Microsomal enzyme inducers, such as phenobarbital, result in a lowering of bilirubinemia.

Melanosis and Other Pigmentary Changes

Apart from jaundice there are other color changes that have diagnostic value in chronic liver disease. These changes may be diffuse or circumscribed. A *diffuse* muddy gray color in patients with long-standing cirrhosis is essentially due to epidermal melanin, especially in the basal layer. There may be a yellowish tinge in the presence of jaundice and the deposition of hemosiderin in the skin.

Melanin pigmentation of the skin in patients with primary biliary cirrhosis initially involves exposed areas but gradually becomes generalized. It is a common feature of this disease and may be an early presenting sign which may become clinically obtrusive.[4] Pigmentation as impressive as that seen in primary biliary cirrhosis rarely occurs in other forms of chronic liver disease and is generally not a feature of secondary biliary cirrhosis.

Blotchy, *circumscribed* areas of dirty brown pigmentation in an irregular distribution are also occasionally seen. Accentuation of normal freckling and of areolar pigmentation may appear. Localized linear pigmentation may be found in the creases of the fingers and palms. Circumscribed pigmentation may occur in perioral and periorbital areas, resembling chloasma; such pigmentation has been described by older English-speaking clinicians as *chloasma*

hepaticum, while the French call it *masque biliaire*.[5] Facial chloasma in a man or a nonpregnant woman should alert the clinician to the possibility of liver disease.

Patchy depigmentation[6] refers to white pea-sized flecks—guttate hypomelanosis on the skin of the buttocks, back, thighs, and forearms which is sometimes seen in cirrhosis and may be associated with spiders. These paler patches may be uniformly depigmented, or there may be a central spider. These pale flecks may be analogous to the white flecks seen in individuals with spiders, including pregnant women, who may develop white patches around vascular spiders due to a vasoconstrictor response to cold.

Hemochromatosis is an inherited condition in which excess iron is deposited in the liver, pancreas, heart, and joints. Skin pigmentation is so striking that its alternative name is "bronzed diabetes." The metallic gray or bronze-brown color of hemochromatosis is usually generalized,[7] and buccal mucosal and conjunctival pigmentation may also be present in 20 percent of cases.

Etiology and Pathogenesis   The etiology and pathogenesis of hyperpigmentation in chronic liver disease are obscure. The slow progression of generalized brownish pigmentation, related to advancing liver disease, suggests a humoral mechanism, perhaps comparable to that seen with excessive adrenocorticotropic hormone (ACTH) or melanocyte-stimulating hormone (MSH),[8] but MSH levels are not raised.

A different mechanism for pigmentation in primary biliary cirrhosis was suggested by Burton and Kirby,[9] who showed that bile salts caused itching when applied to blister bases in normal subjects. They postulated that cytotoxic properties of bile salts caused the release of proteolytic enzymes, which are known to be potent pruritogens, and activate epidermal tyrosinases, possibly by splitting a small blocking peptide from the inactive precursor, prototyrosinase, and so producing pigmentation. They suggested that the continued release of low concentrations of proteolytic enzymes in the skin could account for both the pigmentation and the pruritus of patients with chronic obstructive jaundice. However, in a recent study, a decrease in serum bile acid concentrations achieved by percutaneous transhepatic biliary drainage had little or no effect on pruritus and it was concluded that bile acids had no causative role in the pruritus of cholestatic liver disease.[10]

A histologic and ultrastructural study of cutaneous pigmentation in primary biliary cirrhosis[11] has claimed that the pigmentation was due to excess melanin, widely dispersed throughout the epidermis, often accumulating into giant compound melanosomes and frequently spilling over into the dermis. No deposits of stainable iron were observed. Similar changes were seen in one patient with alcoholic cirrhosis and skin pigmentation. Compared with skin from matched sites in control patients with alcoholic cirrhosis and no pigmentation, the melanocyte/keratinocyte ratio was not significantly higher in patients with primary biliary cirrhosis. However, in the latter patients, melanosomes persisted to unusually high levels in the epidermis and were packaged in larger membrane-bound clusters than in controls. It was not clear whether the excess melanin resulted from increased melanogenesis or defective melanin degradation. No hormonal (β-MSH and ACTH) or chemical (bile salt irritation) stimuli were shown to increase melanogenesis.

In hemochromatosis, faulty intestinal absorption of iron and a failure of the mucosal block results in increased absorption of iron. Skin darkening is generalized but is most marked over sun-exposed skin and in traumatized areas. The mucosal surfaces of the mouth and eyes are occasionally affected. Cutaneous pigmentation is not caused by the presence of hemosiderin in the skin, but is produced by melanin, although iron, melanin, and lipofuscin are all demonstrable histochemically.

Hemosiderin granules are inconstantly seen in macrophages within the dermis and its appendages, perhaps contributing to the slate-gray quality of hemochromatotic skin.[12] Others[7] have stressed the high incidence of ichthyosis-like states and koilonychia, and the presence of siderosis in eccrine sweat glands has been claimed to be of diagnostic help. After phlebotomy, histologic siderosis and clinical skin pigmentation decreased, whereas melanosis remained histologically unchanged. Hepatic iron stores and markers of iron overload in alcoholics and in patients with idiopathic hemochromatosis have also been investigated,[13] and liver iron concentration remains the best way of assessing iron stores in these two groups of patients. Liver iron concentrations were elevated in approximately one-third of alcoholics, irrespective of liver damage, but there was no overlap with values found in patients with idiopathic hemochromatosis.

Good evidence that increased pigmentation in hemochromatosis is caused by melanin and not iron is provided by a patient with both vitiligo and hemochromatosis who was reported by Perdrup and Poulsen.[14] They showed that, although histochemically there was iron in the white area of vitiligo as well as in the remainder of the skin, the vitiliginous areas remained completely white because of the absence of melanin. The remainder of the skin showed the expected hyperpigmentation due to excess melanin.

Other cutaneous pigmentary changes associated with liver disease may be due to derangement of porphyrin or cholesterol metabolism. In porphyria cutanea tarda, the light-exposed parts of the body are subject to blister formation, bruising, and excoriations. The healed sites show residual pigmentation which is usually accompanied by various degrees of general melanin hyperpigmentation on the face and hands. The yellow and orange lesions of xanthomatosis and xanthelasma are common in biliary cirrhosis, especially in the primary form. These changes are also frequently seen in the absence of liver disease. While pigmentation is usually seen late in the course of liver disease, its late occurrence is not invariable. The main exceptions are primary biliary cirrhosis and hemochromatosis, in which pigmentation occurs early.

Diagnosis and Management of Pigmentation In the differential diagnosis of generalized pigmentation related to hepatobiliary disease, certain endocrinopathies and chronic debilitating diseases should be considered. Primary adrenal insufficiency (Addison's disease) and certain pituitary tumors may produce pigmentary changes of the skin and mucous membranes. Similarly, chronic diseases, such as lymphoma, tuberculosis, and malabsorption syndromes, may produce pigmentation and hepatic dysfunction. Liver biopsy may be essential in making the definitive diagnosis. A good example of the need for liver biopsy is iron-storage disease, in which liver specimens stained for hemosiderin are much more certain indicators of iron storage than preparations of skin, marrow, or urinary sediment.[13]

Once the liver is chronically damaged, as in cirrhosis, it never regains its normal structure.[15] However the liver cells retain such enormous regenerative capacity that functional compensation may be attained. Bed rest in acute cases, control of alcoholism, improved nutrition, selective use of corticosteroids, and surgical correction of mechanical biliary obstruction may arrest or reverse the secondary cutaneous pigmentary changes.

Vascular Changes

Patients with chronic liver disease often have telangiectatic changes, mainly over the areas of the body exposed to light: the face, neck, forearms, and hands. They resemble the vascular changes not infrequently seen in sailors and farmers whose skin is damaged by the sun and wind. Numerous tiny telangiectases sometimes give the impression of a diffuse, almost exanthematic redness.[16] They are known as "dollar paper markings" since they resemble the small threads in paper money held up against the light. They fade on pressure with a glass slide and rarely pulsate. Minimal dilatation of venules is the most likely cause of these diffuse vascular changes.

Spider Nevus The vascular spider, arterial spider, or spider angioma is the most representative and classical vascular lesion of chronic liver disease, although it may also be seen in alcoholics without liver involvement. It derives its name from its resemblance to a spider because it consists of a central arteriole represented by a red point from which numerous small twisted vessels radiate (Fig. 163-2). The arterial spider is bright red and ranges in size from a pinhead to 2 cm. When sufficiently large it can be seen or felt to pulsate, especially when pressed with a glass slide. Pressure on the central arteriole with the head of a pin or a matchstick causes blanching of the whole lesion, including its branches, as would be expected from an arterial structure. Because the spider contains red arterial blood, it is not demonstrable by infrared photography.[15]

Spider nevi are most common on the face, necklace area, forearms, hands, and upper part of the chest (Fig. 163-2), i.e., mainly over the region drained by the superior vena cava. Only rarely are they found in the mucous membranes of the nose, mouth, and pharynx. They fade after death.[16,17] Spider nevi may be seen in 10 percent of the normal general population and not infrequently in children of all ages. They may appear in large numbers during pregnancy and generally disappear rapidly after parturition, although some lesions may persist. With or without palmar erythema, they may also be seen in patients with thyrotoxicosis, in

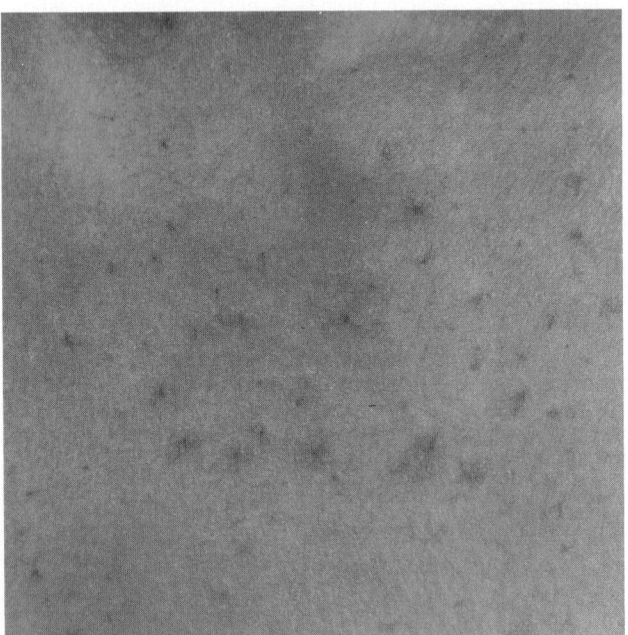

FIGURE 163-2 Spider nevi in a patient with cirrhosis. (*Courtesy of Klaus Wolff, M.D.*)

those with rheumatoid arthritis who are receiving estrogen therapy, and in women after taking an oral contraceptive. A familial incidence of spider nevi has also been reported.

Regression of spiders in patients with liver disease is possible with improvement of the underlying condition. Persistence of the lesions is more likely. However, spiders are functionally reversible. It is not clear whether the central artery is obliterated when they disappear or whether it persists morphologically but simply fails to fill because the filling pressure in it is no longer sufficient. It has also been suggested that the rarely encountered association of unilateral nevoid telangiectasia and liver disease could be manifestations of a disease involving skin and liver vessels, as in hereditary hemorrhagic telangiectasia.[18]

The selective distribution of vascular spiders is not understood. Traditionally, vascular spiders and palmar erythema[15] have been attributed to estrogen excess, particularly since they are also found during pregnancy when circulating estrogens are increased. Estrogens have an enlarging, dilating effect on the spiral arterioles of the endometrium; this mechanism may explain the similar cutaneous spiders in men[19] receiving estrogen therapy for prostatic cancer, although such occurrences are exceptional. However there are many difficulties in explaining the precise pathogenesis of vascular spiders in patients with chronic liver disease.

The blood pressure in these small arteries has been measured at 50 to 70 mmHg: The temperature is 2 to 3°C higher than that of the surrounding skin. Morphologic studies with the help of reconstruction methods[20] have demonstrated that spiders represent an arterial end organ with five separate parts: (1) a cutaneous arterial net, (2) a central spider arteriole, (3) a subepidermal ampulla, (4) a star-shaped arrangement of efferent spider vessels, and (5) capillaries. Martini and Staubesand[21] have demonstrated that the central spider vessel comes from the subcutis, winds up to the epidermis, and there branches out as an end artery. The efferent branches of the dilated arteriole show no evidence of a transition into veins. The spider is not, therefore, an arteriovenous anastomotic structure. The structure of the wall of the central artery is striking in that its media is considerably thicker on one side than the other. The muscular component of the vessel wall disappears as it approaches the surface; it gradually resembles a vein, and just below the epidermis gives the impression of a dilated vascular bed formed by a thin endothelial tube.

More recently, Pirovino and colleagues have examined the relationship of vascular spiders to sex hormone levels and to capillary circulation in the nail fold.[22] Several structural and functional capillary microscopic parameters differed significantly between patients with cirrhosis and control subjects. However, nothing separated patients with cirrhosis with spiders from those without. In addition, serum estradiol and total testosterone were comparable in patients with cirrhosis and control subjects. Free serum testosterone was reduced in male patients with cirrhosis, particularly in those with spider nevi. The estradiol/free testosterone ratio was highest in male patients with spiders. Cirrhosis was associated with structural and functional effects in cutaneous capillaries, whether or not spiders were present.

Palmar Erythema   Palmar erythema or "liver palm" occurs in two clinical forms. In the first variety (Fig. 163-3), there is an exaggeration of normal mottling, the hands are warm and bright red, especially on the palm itself, on the dorsa of the hands, and on fingers and the bases of nails. The second type of palmar erythema is characterized by well-demarcated redness of the hypothenar eminence which gradually spreads to other parts of the hand.[23] The

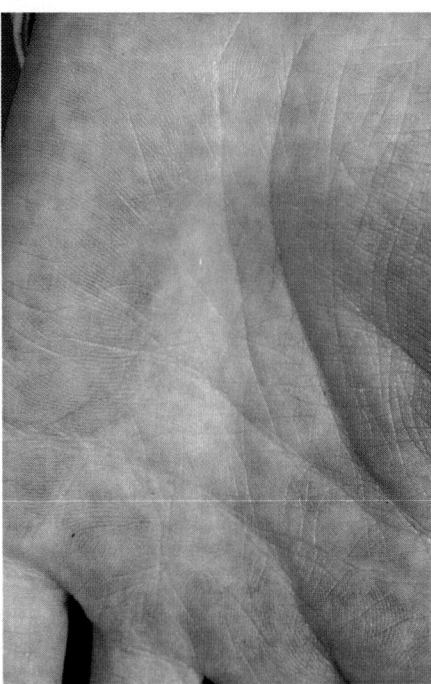

FIGURE 163-3   Palmar erythema or "liver palms" showing the characteristic blotchy redness.

soles of the feet may show similar changes. The mottling blanches on pressure and, when a glass slide is pressed on the palm, it flushes synchronously with the pulse rate.[15] Patients may complain of throbbing or tingling palms. "Liver palms" occur not only in liver disease, but also during pregnancy and in a number of chronic diseases such as chronic polyarthritis, chronic lung disease, subacute bacterial endocarditis, chronic febrile diseases, leukemia, and thyrotoxicosis.

It has been suggested that palmar erythema in liver disease and pregnancy is due to hyperestrogenism, and palmar erythema has also been ascribed to the ingestion of those oral contraceptives with a higher estrogen content. The high incidence of palmar erythema in patients with an alcoholic fatty liver has been blamed on direct effects of ethanol on the vasculature.[24] In a number of individuals, the characteristic mottling and blotchy redness are of no clinical significance and palmar flushing may be familial.

Other Vascular Changes   Corkscrew scleral vessels, i.e., tortuous small arteries that traverse the margins of the ocular sclerae, have been described in many patients with chronic liver disease and have been thought to indicate increased local cutaneous arterial perfusion and vasodilatation (W.A. Tisdale and R.C. Williams, unpublished observations, 1960). The pathogenesis of all the vascular changes in cirrhosis is not understood, but it has been claimed that cardiac output is frequently increased, total peripheral resistance may be decreased, and arteriovenous shunting may occur within the lungs, liver, and extremities.[25] The various vascular phenomena such as spiders and palmar erythema could be explained by actual structural arteriovenous shunts or functional alterations.

In portal hypertension, whether associated with cirrhosis or noncirrhotic liver disease or with portal vein block, portal systemic collateral vessels may develop and may be an important clue to the existence of portal hypertension. Often the umbilical vein is dilated and visible in the epigastrium, an occurrence more common than the often quoted *caput medusae*.

Purpuric lesions ranging from pinpoint size to large ecchymoses may occur with acquired clotting defects of liver disease. They occur mainly on the lower limbs, may be transient and recurrent, and are sometimes accompanied by follicular hyperkeratosis, although they are usually not associated with vitamin C deficiency. Bruising is common at the sites of venipuncture.

Hormone-Induced Changes of the Skin

Hormonal disturbances have been claimed to be responsible for a variety of skin and hair changes in patients with cirrhosis. There is occasionally a decrease in the rate of growth of facial hair in men, but loss of forearm, axillary, and pubic hair may occur in both men and women. Pectoral alopecia and female pubic hair distribution may be seen in men, as may loss of libido and potency, testicular atrophy, and oligospermia. Striae distensae occur in both men and women in association with chronic liver disease (Fig. 163-4) on the abdomen and on the thighs. They arise in the absence of ascites or systemic corticosteroid therapy but may accompany either. They are particularly associated with chronic active hepatitis of the lupoid type. Dupuytren's contracture and swelling of the parotid gland, as well as gynecomastia, are more frequently seen in chronic cirrhosis than in otherwise healthy individuals. It has been generally assumed that gynecomastia and many other changes are due to hyperestrogenism due to a failure of the liver to inactivate estrogens in chronic liver disease. Martini[6] has pointed out that many of these so-called hormonal changes, including gynecomastia, Dupuytren's contracture, and parotid swelling, occur more commonly in patients with cirrhosis who are alcoholics, and has suggested that they might be the result of dietary deficiencies. In chronic alcoholics, there are other "pseudoendocrine" effects even in the absence of liver disease.[26] These effects include facial mooning, truncal obesity, and proximal muscle wasting, all features reminiscent of Cushing's syndrome. This "pseudo-Cushing's syndrome" reverts to normal when alcohol is discontinued.

The precise abnormality responsible for gynecomastia is unknown. A number of different hormonal disturbances have been invoked, including increased secretion of estrogen, increased conversion of androgen to estrogen, altered binding of androgen by globulins, decreased estrogen metabolism, increased production of growth hormone and other pituitary hormones, and altered local tissue response. Some of these concepts are more plausible than others. For example, the suggestion that gynecomastia may be due to an increased concentration of sex hormone-binding globulin found in chronic liver disease is worthy of consideration. Since testosterone is more tightly bound to sex hormone-binding globulin than estradiol, an increase in the concentration of sex hormone-binding globulin causes a greater increase in the binding of testosterone than of estradiol and increases the ratio of free estradiol to free testosterone in the plasma. This increased ratio may lead to the development of secondary sexual characteristics. Shuster and Marks[27] have investigated estrogen metabolism in patients with erythroderma showing evidence of gynecomastia. They found hyperestrogenism and increased urinary estrogen excretion in a number of these cases. They postulated that the skin disease itself might lead to hyperestrogenism resulting occasionally in gynecomastia.

An exuberant growth of condylomata acuminata of the vulva and vagina has been described in women with cirrhosis[28] and has been linked to the occasional appearance of large moist warts in pregnancy, presumably as a result of increased urinary estrogens.

Chemically Induced Changes of the Skin

Porphyria cutanea tarda and erythropoietic protoporphyria are dealt with in Chap. 150. Liver disease is frequently associated with the former and the liver is the source of fecal protoporphyrin in the latter. In porphyria cutanea tarda, fragility of the skin and bulla formation in sun-exposed areas are often accompanied by purpuric and ecchymotic lesions, scarring, hyperpigmentation, and a sclerodermoid quality of the skin. Hypertrichosis, particularly over the malar and periorbital regions, may be present. In erythropoietic protoporphyria, the most striking skin changes are small atrophic scars on the nose, the malar eminences, the pinnae, and occasionally the dorsa of the fingers.

A wide range of xanthomatous lesions may be seen in patients with biliary cirrhosis and other hyperlipemic states. These lesions are described in detail in Chap. 152.

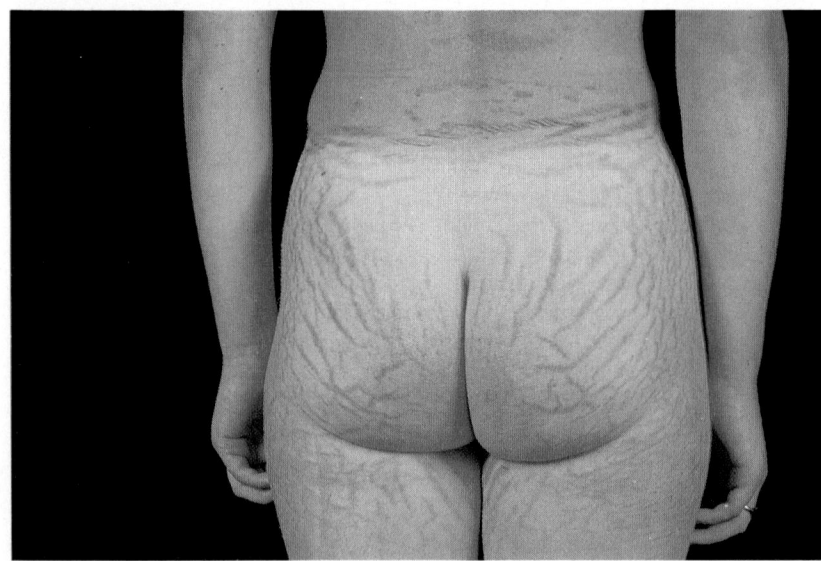

FIGURE 163-4 Widespread stretch marks in a 16-year-old boy with chronic active hepatitis.

Immunologic Manifestations of Liver Disease

Abnormal immunologic mechanisms have been implicated in some forms of hepatitis and cirrhosis, especially chronic active hepatitis and primary biliary cirrhosis. While these liver diseases may show evidence of nonspecific cutaneous involvement encountered in other forms of hepatic dysfunction, they may, more interestingly, be accompanied by skin changes that form part of a multisystem autoimmune process.

In a study of the premonitory phase of hepatitis B in 100 patients over a period of 2 weeks before the onset of the disease, Veyre and Brette[29] found that 33 percent of the patients developed urticaria and, to a lesser extent, various erythemas and purpura. They considered that these changes were due to immune disturbances resembling serum sickness (see below).

Exacerbation of chronic urticaria following ingestion of aspirin is well recognized.[30,31] In a few patients with chronic urticaria aspirin reactivity is complicated by jaundice and liver histology shows changes of atypical portal cirrhosis.[32] It is possible that this is another allergic cutaneous manifestation of liver disease.

One patient with localized scleroderma and chronic active hepatitis and several patients with scleroderma in association with primary biliary cirrhosis have been seen by these authors. Scleroderma and primary biliary cirrhosis have also been noted together by others.[33–36] Reynolds et al[37] found six cases of systemic sclerosis among 41 patients with primary biliary cirrhosis. Recently the syndrome of primary biliary cirrhosis and limited scleroderma has been expanded to include a serologic marker—the anticentromere antibody—and keratoconjunctivitis sicca.[38] The acronym *PACK* (*P*rimary biliary cirrhosis, *A*nticentromere antibody, *C*REST syndrome, and *K*eratoconjunctivitis sicca) has been suggested for this entity.

Chronic Active Hepatitis and the Skin   Read et al[39] found that in about one-quarter of their series of 81 patients with chronic active hepatitis, there were cutaneous striae even before corticosteroid therapy (Fig. 163-4) and a number of skin eruptions including acne, "erythematous" rashes, lupus erythematosus-type changes, localized scleroderma, purpura, and splinter hemorrhages under the nails and at the nail bases. An allergic capillaritis of the skin in patients with juvenile cirrhosis (chronic active hepatitis) was described by Sarkany.[40] The skin changes are clinically characteristic: The chronic skin eruption is mainly on the trunk and less marked on the limbs (Fig. 163-5); it may persist for years but fluctuates with the severity of the disease and with response to therapy; there are active inflammatory papules with a central pustular element, later forming a crust and leading to atrophy and formation of a characteristically depressed scar. Eventually the pink color fades and a persistent, pale, depressed, circular or oval lesion remains which resembles a postvaccination scar. In fresh cases only the inflammatory papule with pus or a crust in the center may be present, while later all elements or only the residual scars may be seen. Systemic corticosteroids have a suppressive effect and the skin changes may not necessarily correspond to the severity of the liver disease.

Histopathologically the epithelium contains a crater in which there is a parakeratotic plug. In the subbasal region there are patchy quantities of fibrin and a dermal infiltrate consisting of lymphocytes, histiocytes, and eosinophils. Many capillaries show edema and cuffing with a paraaminosalicylic acid (PAS)-positive fibrin-like material. There appears to be increased permeability of small

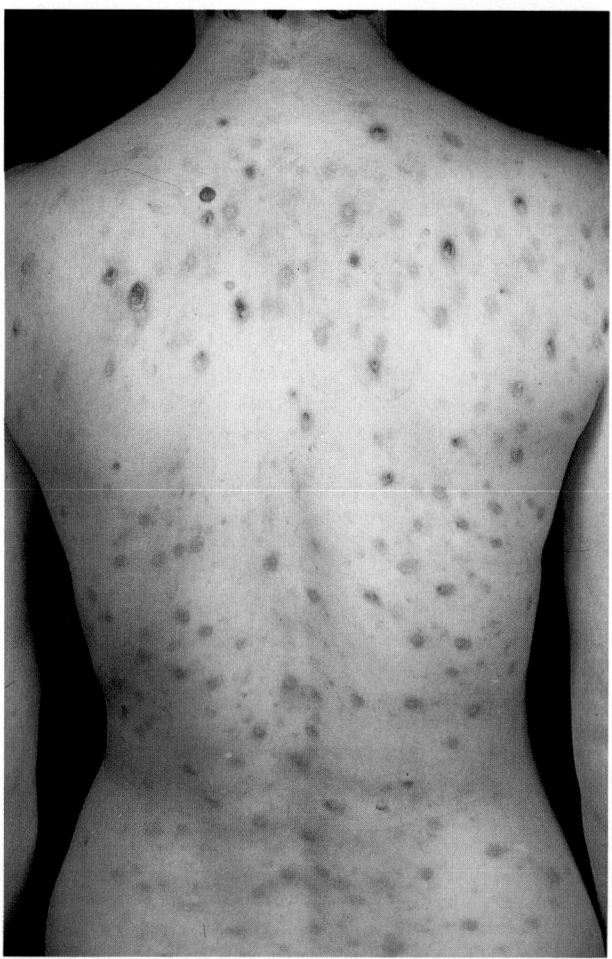

FIGURE 163-5   Eruption of red papules with central crusts and depressed scars caused by allergic capillaritis in a patient with chronic active hepatitis.

vessels associated with endothelial swelling, permeation of plasma, fibrin formation, and resulting hyalinosis. The microscopic changes are characteristic of an allergic response.

Chronic active hepatitis, when not associated with the hepatitis B virus, is also known as juvenile cirrhosis, lupoid hepatitis, and plasma cell hepatitis.[41–43] Although originally thought to occur in nonalcoholic young women, it is now known to affect all age groups. Jaundice and fever may be accompanied by other immunologic disorders, in particular ulcerative colitis, rheumatoid arthritis, glomerulonephritis, or Hashimoto's disease. The number of diseases associated with chronic active hepatitis continues to increase: Pyoderma gangrenosum has been added in relatively recent years.[44–46] Raised serum transaminases and IgG levels, and antinuclear factors, smooth muscle antibodies, and other antibodies are found.[47] Liver histology shows cell damage with rosette formation and hepatic fibrosis leading to postnecrotic cirrhosis with infiltration by lymphocytes and plasma cells. The allergic capillaritis of the skin fits into this overall picture of a liver disease associated with wide-ranging autoimmune phenomena. Exactly similar clinical and histologic findings have been reported from other centers.[48]

In a wider range of cases of acute and chronic hepatitis,[49] less uniform clinical and histologic skin reaction patterns were found.

These patterns included urticarial, macular, and papular rashes and raised purpuric lesions. Corresponding histologic features were various degrees of cutaneous vasculitis, some with a primarily lymphocytic venulitis with focal necrosis, while the purpuric lesions were represented by neutrophilic necrotizing vasculitis involving small vessels. The finding of vascular deposits of immunoglobulins, complement, and fibrin in skin, as well as hypocomplementemia in these patients, suggested that the cutaneous changes resulted from immune complex-mediated vascular injury.

Cutaneous Manifestations and Primary Biliary Cirrhosis The diagnosis of primary biliary cirrhosis is based on a typical clinical picture, liver function tests suggesting cholestasis, antimitochondrial antibodies, and characteristic histology. Various cutaneous changes may be seen, including the nonspecific skin changes usually associated with liver disease. In addition, cutaneous capillaritis, scleroderma and systemic sclerosis (see above), and lichen planus are all seen in patients with this form of cirrhosis.

An IgM-associated membranous glomerulonephritis has been reported in association with primary biliary cirrhosis and cutaneous capillaritis.[50] Capillaritis associated with IgM and C3 in skin lesions might indicate that immunologic events contributed to the production of the itchy papules and vesicles. Furthermore the deposition of circulating immune complexes, including both IgG and IgM, might account for both renal and cutaneous lesions.

Another skin disease that has been reported in association with primary biliary cirrhosis is lichen planus. A group of five patients with lichen planus and primary biliary cirrhosis was reported by the authors,[51] who suggested that this coexistence was more than coincidental and most likely due to the fact that both conditions involve altered immune function. An earlier report[52] had claimed an association between erosive lichen planus and cirrhosis, but the documentation of the liver disease was not sufficiently precise. Of more interest was a report from the Mayo Clinic, in which a larger number of patients with primary biliary cirrhosis appeared to develop lichen planus after the administration of penicillamine, although in some the skin lesions developed in the absence of the drug.[53]

Immunopathologic mechanisms play an important role in both lichen planus and primary biliary cirrhosis, and the evidence for this association has been reviewed.[51] It has also been pointed out that primary biliary cirrhosis shares features with chronic graft-versus-host disease.[54] Similar changes are seen in the liver, and damage to the lacrimal and salivary glands in both gives rise to the sicca syndrome.[54] Lichen planus is the skin disease that most resembles the cutaneous features of graft-versus-host reactions, and the appearance of lichen planus in patients with primary biliary cirrhosis provides an additional link and suggests common pathogenetic mechanisms.[51]

One other immunopathologic link between primary biliary cirrhosis and the skin is provided by cutaneous immunofluorescence.[55–57] IgM has been demonstrated at the basement membrane zone and around blood vessels; C3, fibrin, IgA, and IgG have also been seen but less frequently. Such positivity is not related to high IgM levels and is not a washout effect.[58] The pattern of immune deposition is similar or identical to that seen in lupus erythematosus. This is an important finding because it represents an additional accessible immunologic marker and diagnostic aid in primary biliary cirrhosis. Some authors have claimed that penicillamine therapy can alter or abolish the immunofluorescence,[55] but we have not found this effect.[57] Positive cutaneous immunofluorescence is not unique in liver disease, because IgA deposits in the skin in

alcoholic liver disease have been shown to correlate with characteristic deposition of IgA in the liver.[59]

Nail Changes in Liver Disease

Although a variety of changes have been described, the nails of many patients with liver disease are normal and nail abnormalities are a less constant physical sign that spiders or liver palms. However, in cirrhotic patients, clubbing, white nails, watchglass deformity, flat nails, white bands, striations, and brittleness may be found.

While *clubbing* of the fingers is primarily a sign of lung and heart disease, it is also quite common in all forms of cirrhosis, especially primary biliary cirrhosis. The incidence of clubbing even in cardiothoracic disease is not known, and quoted figures vary from 10 to 80 percent. In one large series 60 percent of patients with subacute bacterial endocarditis were said to develop clubbing, but no precise figures were given for extrapulmonary disease, especially cirrhosis and ulcerative colitis.[60] However, in a group of 106 patients with primary biliary cirrhosis and chronic active hepatitis, clubbing was present in 18 cases (16 percent) (M.J. Whelton, personal communication). In a study of 35 cases of chronic active hepatitis, Cook[61] found five patients with clubbing (14 percent), while two had opaque white nails. Martini[62] noted an association between the incidence of clubbing and palmar erythema. Cirrhosis and lung disease share an increased blood flow,[63] but the exact pathogenesis of clubbing is not understood. Bean[23] believes that it may be the result of the same forces that operate in liver disease.

The anatomic basis of clubbing is an increased thickness of the nail bed due to edema, cellular infiltration, increased vascularity, or a combination of all or some of these factors. These changes are largely responsible for the characteristic shape of the clubbed digit, but other vascular and tissue changes may be contributory factors.[60] Most of the changes of clubbing are probably the result of an increase in connective tissue between the nail and bone, although the increased peripheral blood flow, which is variable, is probably an essential requirement, if not a primary cause, for all clubbing. It has been suggested that there are, in fact, two types of clubbing: one, principally associated with lung disease, that is characterized mainly by an increase in the amount of connective tissue; and a second variety due mainly to increased blood flow in the distal portion of the finger. The importance of the vascular element is demonstrated by the findings of Mendlowitz,[64–66] who examined patients with clubbing and found that the blood flow of the distal portion of the fingers in patients with clubbing was greater than normal digits and that the gradient of pressure, diminishing toward the periphery of the finger, was lost. In all cases of clubbing there was a marked increase in blood pressure in the digital arteries compared with controls. It has also been shown that when clubbing disappears, a reduction in blood flow follows. It must be concluded, therefore, that the rise in peripheral blood flow is one of the factors in the formation of clubbing.

The development of clubbing in association with lung or heart disease has also been blamed on the action of reduced ferritin due to inadequate oxidation. Reduced ferritin levels dilate the arteriovenous anastomoses in the finger tips by antagonizing the vasoconstrictor effect of circulating adrenaline. The demonstration of portopulmonary anastomoses bypassing the pulmonary capillary bed in postmortem studies of patients with cirrhosis has been taken as evidence of a right-to-left shunt in cases of clubbing associated with cirrhosis.[67] But there was no such correlation, nor were portopulmonary anastomoses demonstrated in life, in a group of patients with cirrhosis.[68] Reid[69] postulated, nevertheless, that cyanosis and finger clubbing in patients with hepatic cirrhosis were due to arteriovenous pleural shunts or pleural spider nevi. The (convex) *watchglass deformity* of the nail has been considered to be simply a milder form of clubbing.

White nails may be seen occasionally in normal individuals and in a variety of diseases, especially in patients with cryoglobulinemia, Raynaud's syndrome, and systemic scleroderma. However, intensely white nails are characteristic of cirrhosis (Figs. 163-6 and 163-7). Terry[70] reported white nails in 82 of 100 patients with cirrhosis. The white color was not within the nail plate but was due to opacification of the nail bed since the whiteness did not move with nail growth nor did it alter when blood was forced into the subungual tissue by compression of digital vessels. In severe cases all fingernails may be affected and show a ground-glass opacity of almost the entire nail bed (Fig. 163-7). There may be a zone of normal pink at the distal edge of the nail (Fig. 163-6). The white nail is probably due to overgrowth of connective tissue between the nail and the bone which reduces the amount of blood in the subcapillary plexus. Watchglass deformity may accompany white nails (Figs. 163-6 and 163-7). In one patient with alcoholic liver disease, all the fingernails showed multiple transverse white bands that later disappeared and turned into typical white nails.[71] The changes were located in the nail bed and were thought to be due to vascular effects. *Opaque nails*[72] and thinned nail folds with a wide cuticle[73] have also been reported in patients with alcoholic liver disease.

Flat or spoon nails[74] are less common in patients with liver disease. They are either flat or concave, pale in color, and frequently show longitudinal ridging. In idiopathic hemochromatosis, koilonychia[7] was said to be the most common of the nail abnormalities but was not related to anemia. A deficit of sulfhydrated amino acids metabolized by the liver has been suggested with vitamin C deficiency as a possible cofactor. Faulty iron metabolism has been incriminated in the development of koilonychia in other forms of liver disease. *Brittle nails* have also been blamed on liver disease, often without adequate documentation.

Azure lunules, a bluish color of the lunular portion of nails, occur in hepatolenticular degeneration (Wilson's disease).[75] One of the authors has seen azure lunules and corneal changes resembling Kayser-Fleischer rings in a patient with argyria,[76] a finding subsequently also described by Whelton and Pope.[77] The characteristic

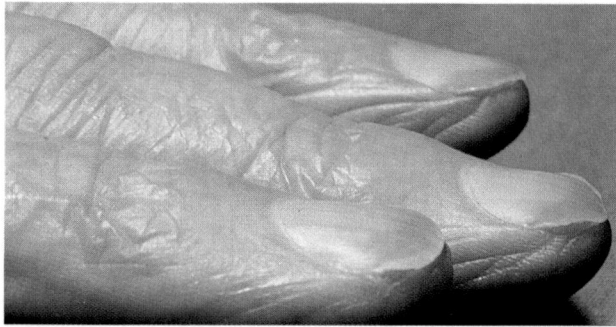

FIGURE 163-6   Flat white nails with slight convex watchglass deformity showing a distal pink band in a patient with liver disease.

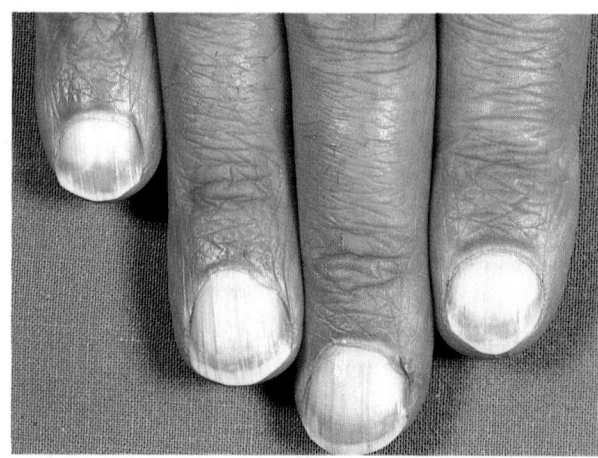

FIGURE 163-7   Terry's white nails in a patient with cirrhosis.

nail changes of lichen planus, including longitudinal ridging, pterygium formation, and permanent nail loss, have been reported in primary biliary cirrhosis.[78]

Itching

Pruritus is one of the most common and distressing symptoms associated with diseases of the hepatobiliary tract. It may be mild and transient or so severe and prolonged that it dominates the clinical picture of the disease. The exact incidence of pruritus in liver disease is not known, but Wüst[79] found evidence of intensive pruritus in 40 percent of a series of 1000 patients with liver disease. Now more sophisticated methods of measurement of itch with sensitive limb movement meters exist.[80]

In hepatitis, itching may affect selectively the lower limbs and is frequently missed as an early sign of the disease, but occasionally pruritus occurs in the later icteric phase of the illness. It may be transient or last 4 to 6 weeks. Itching was found in 40 percent of adults with viral hepatitis but only in 3 percent of children.[79] Although usually most marked on the extremities, severe pruritus may affect the trunk, but the neck and face are rarely, and the genitalia hardly ever, involved. Pruritus may be debilitating in patients with primary biliary cirrhosis, mechanical biliary obstruction, or other causes of cholestasis. Drugs may also induce cholestasis, e.g., erythromycin, oral contraceptives, phenothiazines, chlorpropamide, paraaminosalicylic acid, and nitrofurantoin. Pruritus is the presenting symptom in over 50 percent of cases of primary biliary cirrhosis and may precede jaundice by months or even years. As parenchymal destruction of cirrhosis increases and hepatocellular failure supervenes, itching may subside spontaneously.

Pathogenesis of Pruritus (see also Chap. 31)   The physiologic basis of pruritus is not completely known. While there are no specific receptors for itch, there is a rich cutaneous nerve network in the papillary dermis that subserves this sensation. The itch stimulus is carried by slow-conducting C fibers to the spinal cord and from there in the anterolateral spinothalamic tracts to the thalamus and the posterior central gyrus. Mechanical, electrical, and thermal stimuli can cause itching by their effects on the skin; irritant and allergic processes in the skin may cause histamine release which may cause itching, but proteolytic enzymes and prostaglandins have also been shown to be involved in the chemical mediation of pruritus.

The mechanism of itching in jaundice is still not known. The association of itching with the absence of bile from the feces, whether as a result of cholestasis or hepatitis, suggests that pruritus is due to some substance normally excreted in the bile. Perhaps bile salts irritate cutaneous sensory nerves. Bile acids have been identified in the skin of patients with pruritus, but no direct relationship has been found between itching and the concentration of any particular conjugated or free bile acid. A great overlap of values of bile acid levels has been shown in patients with cholestasis with and without pruritus. Moreover, when pruritus stops in terminal liver failure, serum bile acids may still be elevated. Thus there is strong evidence against a direct, causative role for retained bile acids in the pruritus of cholestasis.[81] However the relief of itching by the bile salt-chelating resin cholestyramine suggests that bile salts are implicated, and the disappearance of pruritus when liver cells fail certainly indicates that whatever is responsible is manufactured by the liver.

One reason for the poor correlation between serum bile salt concentration and pruritus may be the variation in bile salt composition. The pruritic effect of purified bile salts has been tested by applying them to blister bases.[82] All salts tested were pruritogens, but the dihydroxy salts (especially unconjugated chenodeoxycholate) were more potent than the trihydroxy salts. Plasma bile salt levels, especially fasting conjugated-cholate measurements, have been claimed to be a useful screening test for identifying possible hepatobiliary disease.[83]

Chemical mediators of itching may act by directly depolarizing cutaneous nerves or by releasing endogenous pruritogens such as histamine or proteolytic enzymes. Although bile salts liberate small amounts of histamine on perfusion of animal skin[84] and blood histamine levels increase in experimental obstructive jaundice,[85] the poor correlation between pruritus and plasma histamine in liver disease[86] and the poor therapeutic response to antihistamines suggest that histamine is not the major mediator of pruritus in liver disease.[82]

Clinical Features   In liver disease, itching implies cholestasis or mechanical biliary obstruction. Pruritus is significant in primary biliary cirrhosis, cholestatic hepatitis, benign recurrent cholestasis, cholestasis of pregnancy or induced by oral contraceptives, and sclerosing cholangitis. Itching in hepatobiliary disease may be transient or continuous and may or may not be accompanied by jaundice. It is usually generalized. There may be no visible skin change, but more often there are scratch marks and excoriations. Macular, papular, or urticarial lesions may be present, and in long-standing cases lichenified plaques or the nodules of prurigo are found. Histologically these changes are nonspecific. In the differential diagnosis, a whole range of systemic diseases and skin conditions must be considered. Itching of pregnancy has been found to be associated with cholestasis with or without jaundice and has tended to recur in subsequent pregnancies in half the cases. An increased prevalence of cholelithiasis was discovered in these patients.[87] Itching may occur in other systemic disorders, such as Hodgkin's disease, but the pruritus in thyrotoxicosis may cause particular difficulties in diagnosis, because the latter's cutaneous manifestations of hyperpigmentation, onycholysis, and palmar erythema may have some resemblance to those seen in liver disease.[88]

Management   The itching of acute viral hepatitis and mild drug-induced cholestasis requires only sympathetic understanding and reassurance, mild sedation, and local applications such as calamine lotion with 1% phenol or 0.25% menthol or both. Persistent and troublesome itching of primary biliary cirrhosis may require more effective topical antipruritics such as Eurax cream or lotion (crotamiton 10%), topical corticosteroids, or systemic phenothiazines. More effective is the basic anion-exchange resin cholestyramine, which sequesters bile acids within the intestine and lowers levels in serum (and tissue). In many patients up to 6 sachets per day are used, starting one-half hour before and giving more one-half hour after the meal, when serum bile acids are at their lowest and the largest amounts reach the intestine.

Patients taking cholestyramine to control their itching have been found to have low vitamin C concentrations. Although there may be a causal relationship, patients with cirrhosis are, in any case, well known to have deficiencies of many water- and fat-soluble vitamins.[89] Cholestyramine is known to bind to vitamin C and precipitate it out of the diet,[90] and it binds to many other drugs as well. For this reason, any other medication should be given between and as far apart as possible from administrations of cholestyramine. An alternative to cholestyramine is colestipol.

Itching due to mechanical obstruction of bile requires surgical correction. Plasmapheresis has also been tried in the treatment of cholestatic pruritus, with variable results. The improvement in a proportion of patients was said to be dramatic and surprisingly long-lasting. Serum bile acids fell in the patients in whom the pruritus improved, but not in a patient who responded less favorably.[91,92] Rifampicin has also been found to reduce pruritus in primary biliary cirrhosis in a double-blind, crossover trial.[93] It has been compared to phenobarbital in another study, and found to be superior.[94] The mechanism of action remains unknown. A combination of phototherapy and cholestyramine seemed to work in a patient when the drug alone had failed.[95]

Disorders in which both Skin and Liver May Be Involved

There are many systemic diseases that involve both the skin and the liver, but in which the changes are not dependent on one another, do not always both occur, or may appear separated by an interval of months or years. A list of some of the more important is given in Table 163-2.

Argininosuccinic aciduria (see Chap. 147) is a rare autosomal recessive disorder characterized by ataxia, seizures, severe mental retardation, hepatomegaly and liver dysfunction, and brittle hair.

TABLE 163-2
Disorders in which both Skin and Liver May Be Involved

Arginosuccinic aciduria	Neurofibromatosis
Ataxia telangiectasia	Pityriasis rotunda with hepatoma
Dermatomyositis	Porphyrias
Drug reactions	Porphyria cutanea tarda
Eruptive neonatal angiomatosis	Variegate porphyria
Graft-versus-host disease	Erythropoietic (erythrohepatic)
Hereditary hemorrhagic	porphyria
telangiectasia (Osler-Weber-	Hereditary coproporphyria
Rendu disease)	Sarcoidosis
Histiocytoses	Syphilis
Immunodeficiency states	Systemic lupus erythematosus
Mastocytosis	Tuberous sclerosis
Mucocutaneous lymph node	Vinyl chloride disease
syndrome (Kawasaki disease)	

The hair shaft abnormality is found, on microscopy, to be trichorrhexis nodosa. Blood, urine, and CSF levels of argininosuccinic acid are raised and ammonia may also be present.

Ataxia telangiectasia (see Chap. 184) is another recessive disorder. Cutaneous and ocular telangiectases are associated with cerebellar ataxia and immunologic defects. There has also been a report of posthepatitis B cirrhosis in a patient with this disorder.[96] Many patients develop neoplasms, predominantly hematologic, but there has been a report of a hepatoma in one patient.[97] It is of interest, therefore, but alpha-fetoprotein levels are often raised in ataxia telangiectasia.

Dermatomyositis is not associated with any specific hepatic changes, but in older patients it may be the presenting sign of an underlying cancer, often with hepatic secondaries. It is important to note, however, that raised aminotransferases in dermatomyositis may not arise from the liver, but from damaged muscle.

Drug-induced hepatitic lesions may be characterized by cholestasis and the associated skin component by erythema. Cholestatic jaundice possibly associated with a generalized hypersensitivity reaction has resulted from erythromycin estolate, but other forms of erythromycin do not cause hepatitis. Intrahepatic cholestasis and cutaneous bullae have been reported together during glyburide therapy.[98] Interestingly, a bullous eruption has also been seen with chronic active hepatitis and glomerulonephritis.[99] Drugs frequently used in the management of liver disease may also produce cutaneous side effects. Vitamin K_1 (phytonadione) is used widely and erythematous, tender, indurated plaques may occur at the site of intramuscular injections.[100] Localized sclerodermatous changes may develop subsequently.[101]

Eruptive neonatal angiomatosis is a very rare condition in which multiple angiomata may occur anywhere on the skin surface during the first few weeks of life. Vascular lesions may also occur in internal organs, including the liver. Both liver and skin may be prominently involved in both acute and chronic phases of *graft-versus-host reactions,* the cutaneous features of which are discussed in Chap. 117. Although these features are most commonly seen in patients receiving bone marrow transplants, similar states have been described in association with disseminated cancers.[102]

Laparoscopic examination of patients with *hereditary hemorrhagic telangiectasia* has revealed small vascular lesions on the surface of the liver.[103] Arteriovenous fistulae and cirrhosis have also been described. Both skin and liver may be involved in several of the *histiocytoses,* including histiocytosis X (Langerhans cell histiocytosis), malignant histiocytosis, and cytophagic histiocytic panniculitis. There are several congenital disorders in which *immunodeficiency* results in multiple infections of skin and liver, or in which there are significant cutaneous markers. Examples include ataxia telangiectasia (see above), Chédiak-Higashi syndrome, in which fair skin and gray hair are seen, and chronic granulomatous disease. Acquired immunodeficiency states, including AIDS, may result in cutaneous and hepatic infections. Kaposi's sarcoma in AIDS patients frequently affects both skin and liver.

Hepatomegaly is a relatively common accompaniment to the cutaneous changes of *mastocytosis.* Ten to fifteen percent of children with *mucocutaneous lymph node syndrome* (Kawasaki disease) develop upper abdominal pain associated with hepatobiliary changes, usually nonspecific elevation of liver enzymes, due to vasculitic changes or bile duct inflammation. However, in up to 5 percent of cases, hydrops of the gallbladder develops.[104] Extrahepatic biliary obstruction due to neural masses has been reported in patients with *neurofibromatosis,* and there are also reports of hepatoma,[105] polycystic liver disease,[106] and unexplained pruritus and

cholestasis[107] in patients with this disorder. The *porphyrias* are covered in detail in Chap. 150.

Sarcoidosis may cause many different skin changes, and sarcoidal infiltration of the liver may accompany many of them. Cutaneous sarcoid-like granulomata have rarely been seen in patients with primary biliary cirrhosis, and it should be noted that hepatic granulomata may also occur in tuberculosis, glandular fever, syphilis, and as a result of the administration of several drugs (phenylbutazone, sulfonamides, and allopurinol).

In *syphilis* a cutaneous chancre may antedate hepatitis by months and hepatic gummata by years. However true syphilitic hepatitis in the secondary stage has been well documented,[108] presenting with pruritus and cholestatic jaundice. Liver biopsy showed centrilobular cholestasis with liver cell swelling and pleomorphism. Rapid disappearance of symptoms and signs followed treatment with penicillin.

In a retrospective study of 238 patients with *systemic lupus erythematosus* (SLE),[109] 43 patients were found to have liver disease, including cirrhosis, chronic active hepatitis, and fatty change. In one patient a granulomatous hepatitis appeared and subsided simultaneously with an exacerbation of the SLE.[110] Autopsy in some patients with SLE has revealed multiple nodular hyperplasia without cirrhosis, which has been interpreted as a regenerative-hyperplastic process.[111] Hepatic lesions are well described in *tuberous sclerosis.* These are usually hamartomatous malformations involving fat, smooth muscle, and blood vessels, but portal fibrosis may occur. There is one report of clumps of large, abnormal hepatocytes.[112]

Liver function abnormalities are common in patients with *vinyl chloride disease,* and there may be hepatosplenomegaly and frank cirrhosis. Additionally, angiosarcomata of the liver may develop.[113]

The association of hepatocellular carcinoma in 10 South African blacks with *pityriasis rotunda* has been reported. The curious circular and arcuate scaly hyperpigmented lesions typical of this rare dermatosis affected mainly the trunk, lower back, and buttocks.[114]

Hepatitis and the Skin

Viral hepatitis may be due to three different viruses: type A, type B, and type non-A non-B.

Hepatitis B infection is a serious worldwide problem, accounting for an enormous burden of morbidity, mortality, and economic consequences, whether due to its acute effects or to its chronic sequelae, including primary hepatoma.[115] It has been estimated that there may be 200 million carriers in the world at large. The complete virus is known as a Dane particle[116] and carries several specific, identifiable antigens that are clinically important. First there is a surface antigen, HBsAg, which is useful in identifying the carrier state. Within the particle is the core antigen (HBcAg), which indicates recent infection. Finally there is HBeAg, a subunit of the viral core, the detection of which indicates a high degree of infectivity. It is now possible to treat some patients with active hepatitis B infection, and one of the major indications is the presence of HBe antigenemia with progressive liver damage.[117] Agents that have been used include vidarabine, alpha-interferons, and combinations of alpha- and gamma-interferons, acyclovir, and corticosteroids.[118]

Hepatitis B has a marked tendency to induce a chronic infective state, 10 percent of infected subjects becoming carriers. Furthermore, 90 percent of infants born of mothers infected with the virus will develop an ongoing infection.[119] This prevalence has significant implications for health professionals, and the risk of infection to dermatologists has been extensively studied. After a letter by Pegum[120] reported an increased incidence of hepatitis B virus in dermatologists who operated without gloves, a survey was conducted among members of the Australasian College of Dermatologists. This survey revealed that, of 67 individuals tested, only two had anti-HBs and anti-HBc, indicating past infection. Only one had HBsAg and HBeAg and was therefore a carrier.[121] These results were well within the expected prevalence in the Australian population, and were lower than would be expected from a random sample of health workers routinely exposed to blood and its products.

In the United States, an editorial in the *Journal of the American Academy of Dermatology*[122] reviewed the risks of acquiring hepatitis. A survey of 593 American dermatologists showed that glove wearing did not correlate with hepatitis B serologic positivity, although evidence of previous infection was found in 15.4 percent, a rate indicating that dermatologists were an at-risk population compared with professionals in many other branches of medicine.[123] Not unexpectedly there was a correlation between positivity and a history of blood transfusion, tattooing, or homosexuality.

In Germany, the steps that should be taken if a dermatologist or other personnel should experience a needle prick or other injury during blood-contaminated procedures have been specified.[124] The patient's serum should be screened rapidly for hepatitis B antigen and, if positive, individuals other than those known to be immune should be given hyperimmune globulin immediately. This should be followed by the administration of vaccine: an initial injection, followed by boosters at 1 month and 6 months. Immunity should last for about 5 years. The first vaccine was produced by using plasma from known hepatitis B carriers and separating the outer surface (HBsAg) from the infectious core.[125,126]

AIDS has never been transmitted by the hepatitis vaccine in spite of its source (homosexual men) and the vaccine is therefore considered entirely safe.[116] A genetically engineered vaccine has now also been used successfully. Health care workers, including dermatologists exposed to hemophilia or cancer patients or those with hepatic or renal disease, together with surgeons, dentists, and physicians treating homosexuals, should be offered vaccination. Immunization should also be made available to infants of infected mothers, homosexuals, and intravenous drug abusers in an attempt to reduce the medical and economic burden of this preventable, but incurable, disease.[127]

Skin Manifestations of Hepatitis B

Circulating immune complexes contribute to the pathogenesis of the extrahepatic manifestations of hepatitis B infection and there are four well-documented cutaneous associations: a serum sickness-like syndrome; essential mixed cryoglobulinemia; polyarteritis nodosa; and papular acrodermatitis of childhood (Gianotti-Crosti syndrome).

A *serum sickness-like syndrome* occurs in about 20 to 30 percent of patients with hepatitis B infection. Urticaria may be the predominant, or sole, feature, but polyarthralgia, a true arthritis, proteinuria, and hematuria may also occur. The skin changes may become vasculitic. This phase usually lasts from 1 to 6 weeks before jaundice appears.[128] The skin lesions are associated with the perivascular deposition of immune complexes containing HBsAg,

IgM or IgG, and C3.[128–130] That this is a true serum sickness is suggested by the appearance of HBsAg, then anti-HBs in association with depressed complement levels and evidence of immune complex deposition. It seems likely that these immune complexes are involved directly in the pathologic damage to vessels.[130–132]

Another immune complex-mediated disease that may occur in patients with prolonged hepatitis B exposure is *essential mixed cryoglobulinemia*. Patients develop purpura, acropathy, and weakness, and renal involvement is common.[133,134] Histopathologically there is a necrotizing vasculitis. Cryoglobulins are present and show a mixed pattern, with IgG and IgM in near equal amounts.[131] Anti-HBs has been found more commonly than HBsAg in these patients (in contrast to the findings in polyarteritis nodosa; see below), suggesting that excess antibody production with minimal antigenemia is responsible.

Polyarteritis nodosa has been well documented in association with hepatitis B infection.[135,136] Indeed it has been suggested that 50 percent of all cases of polyarteritis nodosa should suggest the presence of HBsAg, although hepatic dysfunction is usually mild and often results only in elevation of enzymes. The disease may present soon after an attack of hepatitis B, but there may be a delay of years.[137] Electron microscopy has shown the virion of the hepatitis B virus in the serum of these patients, and circulating immune complexes containing HBsAg and immunoglobulin have been demonstrated. A leukocytoclastic vasculitis may develop and, if so, immunofluorescence for HBsAg in the dermal vessels is often positive.[137–139]

Papular acrodermatitis of childhood (Gianotti-Crosti syndrome) affects children aged 2 to 6 years and is characterized by the appearance of a papular eruption on the face and limbs. This eruption usually lasts 2 to 3 weeks and is accompanied by lymphadenopathy and acute hepatitis, which is anicteric and lasts for about 2 months.[140] Histologically the nodes show a reactive reticulohistiocytic lymphadenitis. These features are associated with HBs antigenemia of the ''ayw'' subtype,[141] which persists for months or years in more than one-third of patients and is accompanied by continuously elevated liver enzymes. Anti-HBs is not detected in the dermatitic phase of the illness but becomes positive about 6 to 12 months later. All children who ultimately become HBsAg negative develop these antibodies, suggesting that they may play an important role in recovery.[141]

Skin Changes in Hepatitis A and in Non-A Non-B Hepatitis

Hepatitis A is spread largely by the oral-fecal route and is most common in young adults who have visited countries with poor standards of hygiene. An early phase has been documented in which a discrete, transient, maculopapular, urticarial, or petechial rash has developed, together with joint symptoms.[142] Non-A non-B hepatitis accounts for most cases of posttransfusion hepatitis, but also occurs sporadically, and epidemically in India. A relapsing papulovesicular rash on the trunk, extremities, and occasionally the face has been reported in about one-third of patients.[143]

The Effects of Skin Disease on the Liver

A number of metabolic and other disturbances occur as a consequence of skin disease, and some of them reflect abnormalities of hepatic function.

Extensive Loss of Skin

Large areas of skin may be lost after thermal burns, but also in severe pemphigus, staphylococcal scalded skin syndrome, and toxic epidermal necrolysis. It has been known for many years from autopsy specimens that degenerative changes appear in the liver of severely burned patients. Liver enzyme abnormalities are common and a rise in transaminases often occurs early during acute shock immediately after a bad burn.[144] These early changes appear to be nonspecific and have no prognostic value. A much more significant finding is cholestatic jaundice, which generally occurs in the more severely affected patients in whom complications such as pneumonia or septicemia have arisen. This jaundice is preceded by a gradual rise in the alkaline phosphatase, and liver biopsies confirm cholestasis together with nonspecific inflammatory changes. The mortality among patients with this type of jaundice remains very high.[145]

Exfoliative Dermatitis

The systemic effects of exfoliative dermatitis are considerable.[27] There is a high cardiac output due to increased blood flow, the metabolic rate is increased, and there are several hematologic abnormalities, including leukocytosis and anemia. Many patients develop high-output cardiac failure and dehydration and are prone to infections, especially pneumonia. Patients with exfoliative dermatitis may develop hypoalbuminemia, gynecomastia, and hepatomegaly—features suggestive of hepatic dysfunction. For many years it was thought that these changes were due to actual hepatic complications, but it now seems more likely that they are due to a combination of excessive protein loss from shed scale[146,147] and hemodilution, the latter probably being the more important.[148] Certainly the protein abnormalities disappear very rapidly once the skin disease is treated.[149] Similarly the apparent folic acid deficiency in patients with exfoliative dermatitis, which in theory could be attributed to liver dysfunction, has been shown to be a true deficiency.[150,151] The hepatomegaly seen in exfoliative dermatitis is probably largely due to congestion: Liver enzymes are generally normal, and, when liver biopsies have been performed, the liver architecture is unaffected in most instances.

Psoriasis

Features suggesting hepatic dysfunction, similar to the changes described above in exfoliative dermatitis, may occur in severe, widespread psoriasis. Some patients with generalized pustular psoriasis develop jaundice, which has been attributed to a combination of oligemia, general toxicity, and drugs.[152] However, abnormalities in liver architecture have been described in several patients with uncomplicated plaque psoriasis.[153] The most common finding is a fatty change, but focal necrosis, periportal inflammation, and fibrosis have also been found. There has been controversy over what these changes represent. Most authors consider it highly unlikely that they are due solely to psoriasis,[153] and it has been proposed that they arise from other factors, such as alcohol ingestion.[154] There has been debate about whether psoriatics have an increased alcohol intake compared with controls, because early studies failed to demonstrate a direct relationship between psoriasis and alcohol consumption.[153]

However a French study of 1987 patients admitted to the hospital found that psoriasis was significantly more common in those whose daily alcohol consumption exceeded 50 g, although they were unable to demonstrate a link with histologic evidence of alcoholic liver disease.[155] In another report, alcoholism was found more often in patients with psoriasis than in patients with other skin diseases.[156] More evidence comes from Monk and Neill,[157] who found that males with very bad psoriasis had a significantly higher alcohol intake. In addition, men with bad psoriasis frequently had serious alcohol-related medical and social problems. It remains unclear whether alcohol has a direct pharmacologic role in determining the severity of a patient's psoriasis, or whether severe psoriasis leads to excessive drinking, which would tend to reduce patient compliance with treatment and follow-up, establishing a vicious circle of poor disease control and increased alcohol abuse.

Systemic Sclerosis and Morphea

Three to four percent of patients with primary biliary cirrhosis develop systemic sclerosis, usually in a slowly progressive form.[38] There are also reports of morphea in patients with primary biliary cirrhosis. Apart from these associations, the liver in patients with scleroderma is usually normal, although mild fibrosis around bile ducts and portal tracts has been found in some patients. There have also been reports of ascites without evidence of hepatic disease in systemic sclerosis.

Dermatitis Herpetiformis

Abnormalities of liver function tests have been found in a significant proportion of patients with dermatitis herpetiformis.[158] These abnormalities were not due to concomitant autoimmune liver disease, which was specifically excluded, but patients on a gluten-free diet generally had a lower incidence of abnormalities than those on a normal diet.

Lichen Planus

Two centers specializing in the treatment of liver disease have independently reported lichen planus in patients with primary biliary cirrhosis,[51,53] and the relationship has been thoroughly reviewed by Sarkany.[159] We have already pointed out that lichenoid changes are a common accompaniment of chronic graft-versus-host disease, that primary biliary cirrhosis has many other features of graft-versus-host reactions, and that it seems likely that common pathogenetic mechanisms probably play a role in lichen planus, primary biliary cirrhosis, and chronic graft-versus-host disease.[51]

There have, however, also been claims that there is an equally striking association between lichen planus and chronic active hepatitis.[160–163] In direct contrast to these reports are studies[164–166] that have failed to demonstrate any association between otherwise uncomplicated oral or cutaneous lichen planus and autoimmune liver disease. It is not clear why there should be such disparity between findings. One explanation is that many of the positive reports have been uncontrolled, have not clearly defined the liver disease, or have been retrospective reviews. It is notable that all three of the negative reports to date have been careful, prospective studies. Another possibility is that racial factors may be important, because many of the positive studies have been from Italy, whereas the negative findings have been predominantly among Northern Europeans. The only definitively confirmed association between lichen planus and liver disease appears to be the tendency for patients with primary biliary cirrhosis to develop lichen planus lesions, particularly after the use of penicillamine.

Cancers of the Skin

It is important to remember that some skin cancers are capable of producing hepatic metastases, especially melanoma and Kaposi's sarcoma.

Hepatotoxic Effects of Drugs Used in the Treatment of Skin Disease

Several drugs used frequently in managing patients with skin disease, and some hardly used for anything else, and are known to be hepatotoxic. Table 163-3 lists some of the most important.

Danazol, the drug of choice for hereditary angioedema, may rarely cause cholestatic jaundice. More importantly, however, it may exacerbate preexisting liver dysfunction and porphyrias. It should only be used with caution in patients with a history of liver injury. *Azathioprine* is a widely used immunosuppressive agent in dermatologic practice. Marginal elevation of hepatic enzymes is very common in patients receiving azathioprine, and occasionally cholestasis may occur. Serious hepatic damage is, however, rare. Both *griseofulvin* and the antiandrogen *cyproterone acetate* are contraindicated in patients with preexisting liver disease. Liver tumors have been reported in laboratory animals fed cyproterone, and griseofulvin may exacerbate porphyrias. Hepatitis has been reported in patients receiving *ketoconazole*,[167] and some patients have died. This problem has limited the drug's usefulness, but newer and safer agents are now available for systemic treatment of fungal diseases.

Psoralens have been reported to cause hepatitis[168] and are also said to reduce antipyrine clearance,[169] suggesting a possible interaction with other drugs metabolized in the liver. The *retinoids*, etretinate and isotretinoin, are both capable of inducing liver enzyme abnormalities,[170,171] and hepatitis may rarely occur among patients receiving these agents. Liver enzyme abnormalities seem to be a particular problem with etretinate if it is given with methotrexate, a combination that is no longer recommended.[172] *Stanozolol* is an androgenic agent that induces fibrinolysis and is used to treat venous disease, Raynaud's phenomenon, and Behçet's syndrome. Raised transaminases are common when stanozolol is given but usually return to normal when it is stopped. Stanozolol, like danazol, may exacerbate the porphyrias.

The problem of *methotrexate* hepatoxicity is probably the most important of all, because methotrexate is so effective as an antipsoriatic drug. It has been known for years that it is hepatotoxic,[153] causing a variety of histologic changes: small areas of necrosis in early stages, followed by stellate periportal fibrosis, with portal-portal and portal-central vein bridging, leading ultimately to full-blown cirrhosis. Patients with diabetes, obese individuals, and those who consume high levels of alcohol seem to be at an increased risk, as do the elderly and those receiving high doses of the drug.[153] However there does not appear to be a relationship between the pharmacokinetics of methotrexate and ensuing fibrosis.[173] Nor does the patient's HLA status help.[174]

Clearly, once patients are on methotrexate, it is important to monitor hepatic function carefully, but it is accepted that conventional blood liver function tests have no value in assessing methotrexate-induced liver damage[153] and clinicians have had to resort to liver biopsies. Attempts have been made to find other screening methods, including bile salt concentrations,[175] isotope and ultrasound scans,[176,177] antipyrine and indocyanine green clearance tests,[178] and, most recently, serum aminoterminal propeptide of type III procollagen levels.[179] However, none of these tests has yet established itself as a safe way of monitoring liver damage in methotrexate-treated patients with psoriasis, and liver biopsy remains the only proven method until further research confirms that noninvasive tests can safely replace it.

TABLE 163-3
Potentially Hepatotoxic Drugs Used in the Treatment of Skin Disease

Azathioprine	Methotrexate
Cyproterone acetate	Psoralens
Danazol	Retinoids
Griseofulvin	Stanozolol
Ketoconazole	

References

1. Morgan MY: Sex and alcohol. *Br Med Bull* **38**:43, 1982
2. Diamond I, Schmid R: Experimental bilirubin encephalopathy: The mode of entry of bilirubin-^{14}C into the central nervous system. *J Clin Invest* **45**:678, 1966
3. Arias IM: Hepatic aspects of bilirubin metabolism. *Annu Rev Med* **17**:257, 1966
4. Schaffner F: Primary biliary cirrhosis. *Clin Gastroenterol* **4**:351, 1975
5. Bohnstedt RM: Haut und Leber, in *Leber, Haut und Skelett*, edited by L Wannagat. Stuttgart, George Thieme, 1964
6. Martini GA: Leber und Haut, in *Leber, Haut und Skelett*, edited by L Wannagat. Stuttgart, George Thieme, 1964
7. Chevrant-Breton J et al: Cutaneous manifestations of idiopathic hemochromatosis. *Arch Dermatol* **113**:161, 1977
8. Lerner AB, McGuire JS: Melanocyte-stimulating hormone and adrenocorticotrophic hormone. *N Engl J Med* **270**:539, 1964
9. Burton JL, Kirby J: Pigmentation and biliary cirrhosis. *Lancet* **1**:458, 1975
10. Bartholomew TC et al: Bile acid profiles of human serum and skin interstitial fluid and their relationship to pruritus studied by gas chromatography-mass spectrometry. *Clin Sci* **63**:65, 1982
11. Mills PR et al: Melanin pigmentation of the skin in primary biliary cirrhosis. *J Cutan Pathol* **8**:404, 1981
12. Finch SC, Finch CA: Idiopathic hemochromatosis, an iron storage disease. A. Iron metabolism in hemochromatosis. *Medicine (Baltimore)* **34**:381, 1955
13. Chapman RW et al: Hepatic iron stores and markers of iron overload in alcoholics and patients with idiopathic hemochromatosis. *Dig Dis Sci* **27**:909, 1982
14. Perdrup A, Poulsen H: Hemochromatosis and vitiligo. *Arch Dermatol* **90**:34, 1964
15. Sherlock S: *Diseases of the Liver and Biliary System*, 6th ed. Oxford, Blackwell, 1981
16. Bean WB: The cutaneous arterial spider: A survey. *Medicine (Baltimore)* **24**:243, 1945
17. Bean WB: The arterial spider and similar lesions of the skin and mucous membrane. *Circulation* **8**:117, 1953
18. Capron JP et al: Unilateral nevoid telangiectasia and chronic liver disease. *Am J Gastroenterol* **76**:47, 1981
19. Bean WB: *Vascular Spiders and Related Lesions of the Skin*. Oxford, Blackwell, 1959

20. Schirren C: Hautveränderungen beie inneren Erkrankungen, in *Handbuch der Haut- und Geschlechtskrankheiten,* edited by HA Gottron. Berlin, Springer-Verlag, 1967, p 569

21. Martini GA, Staubesand J: Zur Morphologie der Gefässpinnen (''vascular spiders'') in der Haut Leberkranker. *Virchows Arch [Pathol Anat]* **324**:147, 1953

22. Pirovino M et al: Cutaneous spider nevi in liver cirrhosis: Capillary, microscopical and hormonal investigations. *Klin Wochenschr* **66**:289, 1988

23. Bean WB: *Vascular Spiders.* Oxford, Blackwell, 1958

24. Tarao K et al: The incidence of palmar erythema in patients with alcoholic fatty liver. *Jap J Gastroenterol* **83**:2365, 1986

25. Kontos HA et al: General and regional circulatory alterations in cirrhosis of the liver. *Am J Med* **37**:526, 1964

26. Morgan MY: Alcohol and the endocrine system. *Br Med Bull* **38**:35, 1982

27. Shuster S, Marks J: *Systemic Effects of Skin Disease.* London, Heinemann, 1970

28. Blank H: Common viral diseases of the skin. *Med Clin North Am* **43**:1401, 1959

29. Veyre B, Brette R: L'hépatite B à la phase prémonitoire. *Nouv Presse Med* **4**:1349, 1975

30. Calnan CD: Release of histamine in urticaria pigmentosa. *Lancet* **1**:996, 1957

31. Warin RP: The effect of aspirin in chronic urticaria. *Br J Dermatol* **72**:350, 1960

32. Moore-Robinson M, Warin RP: Effect of salicylates in urticaria. *Br Med J* **4**:262, 1967

33. Murray-Lyon IM et al: Scleroderma and primary biliary cirrhosis. *Br Med J* **3**:258, 1970

34. Rau R et al: Liver involvement in scleroderma. *Schweiz Med Wochenschr* **104**:1877, 1974

35. McCoy DG: Spontaneous rupture of the liver in a case of scleroderma. *J Irish Med Assoc* **60**:474, 1967

36. De Graaf P et al: Princire biliaire cirrose met sclerodermie en hypothyreidie. *Tijdschr Gastroenterol* **18**:151, 1975

37. Reynolds TB et al: Primary biliary cirrhosis with scleroderma, Raynaud's phenomenon and telangiectasis. New syndrome. *Am J Med* **50**:302, 1971

38. Powell FC et al: Primary biliary cirrhosis and the CREST syndrome—new terminology? *Q J Med* **62**:75, 1987

39. Read AE et al: Active ''juvenile'' cirrhosis considered as part of a systemic disease and the effect of corticosteroid therapy. *Gut* **4**:378, 1963

40. Sarkany I: Juvenile cirrhosis and allergic capillaritis of the skin. A hepato-cutaneous syndrome. *Lancet* **2**:666, 1966

41. Mackay IR et al: Lupoid hepatitis and the hepatic lesions of systemic lupus erythematosus. *Lancet* **1**:65, 1959

42. Good RA: Plasma-cell hepatitis, and extreme hypergammaglobulinaemia in adolescent females. *Am J Dis Child* **92**:508, 1956

43. Page AR, Good RA: Plasma-cell hepatitis, with special attention to steroid therapy. *Am J Dis Child* **99**:288, 1960

44. Byrne JPH et al: Pyoderma gangrenosum associated with active chronic hepatitis. *Arch Dermatol* **112**:1297, 1976

45. Norris DA et al: Pyoderma gangrenosum. Abnormal monocyte function corrected in vitro with hydrocortisone. *Arch Dermatol* **114**:906, 1978

46. Burns DA, Sarkany I: Active chronic hepatitis and pyoderma gangrenosum: Report of a case. *Clin Exp Dermatol* **4**:465, 1979

47. Bouchier IAD et al: Serological abnormalities in patients with liver disease. *Br Med J* **1**:592, 1964

48. Kurwa A (for Waddington E): Hepato-cutaneous syndrome (juvenile cirrhosis, allergic capillaritis of the skin, proctocolitis and arthritis). *Br J Dermatol* **80**:839, 1968

49. Popp JW et al: Cutaneous vasculitis associated with acute and chronic hepatitis. *Arch Intern Med* **141**:623, 1981

50. Rai GS et al: Primary biliary cirrhosis, cutaneous capillaritis, and IgM-associated membranous glomerulonephritis. *Br Med J* **1**:817, 1977

51. Graham-Brown RAC et al: Lichen planus and primary biliary cirrhosis. *Br J Dermatol* **106**:699, 1982

52. Rebora A et al: Erosive lichen planus and cirrhotic hepatitis. *Ital Gen Rev Dermatol* **15**:123, 1978

53. Seehafer JR et al: Lichen planus-like lesions caused by penicillamine in primary biliary cirrhosis. *Arch Dermatol* **117**:140, 1981

54. Epstein O et al: Primary biliary cirrhosis is a dry gland syndrome with features of chronic graft-versus-host disease. *Lancet* **1**:1166, 1980

55. Randle HW et al: Cutaneous immunofluorescence in primary biliary cirrhosis. *JAMA* **246**:1679, 1981

56. Hendricks AA et al: Cutaneous immunoglobulin deposition in primary biliary cirrhosis. *Arch Dermatol* **118**:634, 1982

57. Graham-Brown RAC, Sarkany I: Positive cutaneous immunofluorescence in primary biliary cirrhosis. Personal observations, 1983

58. Lindgren S et al: IgM deposition in skin biopsies from patients with primary biliary cirrhosis. *Acta Med Scand* **210**:317, 1981

59. Swerdlow MA et al: IgA deposits in skin in alcoholic liver disease. *Arch Dermatol* **118**:950, 1982

60. Ginsburg J: Clubbing of the fingers, in *Handbook of Physiology—Circulation III,* edited by NF Hamilton, P Dow. Waverly Press, Baltimore, 1965, p 2377

61. Cook GC: Active chronic hepatitis and its response to corticosteroid therapy. MD thesis. University of London, 1965

62. Martini GA: Über Gefässveränderungen der Haut bei Leberkranken. *Z Klin Med* **153**:470, 1955

63. Martini GA, Hagemann JE: Über Fingernagelveränderungen bei Lebercirrhose als Folge veränderter peripherer Durchblutung. *Klin Wochenschr* **34**:25, 1956

64. Mendlowitz M: Some observations on clubbed fingers. *Clin Sci* **3**:387, 1938

65. Mendlowitz M: Measurements of blood flow and blood pressure in clubbed fingers. *J Clin Invest* **20**:113, 1941

66. Mendlowitz M: *Digital Circulation.* New York, Grune & Stratton, 1954

67. Calabresi P, Abelmann WH: Porto-caval and porto-pulmonary anastomoses in Laennec's cirrhosis and in heart failure. *J Clin Invest* **36**:1257, 1957

68. Shaldon S et al: The demonstration of porto-pulmonary anastomoses in portal cirrhosis with the use of radioactive krypton (Kr^{35}). *N Engl J Med* **265**:410, 1961

69. Reid L: Cyanosis and finger clubbing in liver disease explained? *Med Trib Int* Ed (Gr Br) **2**(2):25, 1967

70. Terry RB: White nails in hepatic cirrhosis. *Lancet* **1**:757, 1954

71. Jenssen O: White fingernails preceded by multiple transverse white bands. *Acta Derm Venereol (Stockh)* **61**:261, 1981

72. Lewin K: The finger nail in general disease. A macroscopic and microscopic study of 87 consecutive autopsies. *Br J Dermatol* **77**:431, 1965

73. Young AW: Cutaneous stigmata of alcoholism. *Alcohol Health Res World,* Summer 1974, p 24

74. Kleeberg J: Flat finger-nails in cirrhosis of the liver. *Lancet* **2**:248, 1951

75. Bearn AG, McKusick VA: Azure lunulae: An unusual change in the fingernails in two patients with hepatolenticular degeneration (Wilson's disease). *JAMA* **166**:904, 1958

76. Sarkany I: The skin lesions associated with liver disease. *Prog Dermatol* **4**:1, 1969

77. Whelton MJ, Pope FM: Azure lunules in argyria. *Arch Intern Med* **121**:267, 1968

78. Sowden JM et al: Isolated lichen planus of the nails associated with primary biliary cirrhosis. *Br J Dermatol* **121**:659, 1989

79. Wüst H: Zur Klinik und Therapie des Pruritus bei Lebererkrankungen, in *Leber, Haut und Skelett,* edited by L Wannagat. Stuttgart, George Thieme, 1964

80. Summerfield JA, Welch ME: The measurement of itch with sensitive

limb movement meters. *Br J Dermatol* **102**:275, 1981

81. Freedman MR et al: Pruritus in cholestasis: No direct causative role for bile acid retention. *Am J Med* **70**:1011, 1981

82. Kirby J et al: Pruritic effect of bile salts. *Br Med J* **4**:693, 1974

83. Lawrence CM et al: Plasma bile salt levels in patients presenting with generalised pruritus: An improved indicator of occult liver disease. *Ann Clin Biochem* **22**:232, 1985

84. Schachter M: The release of histamine by pethidine, atropine, quinine and other drugs. *Br J Pharmacol* **7**:646, 1952

85. Anrep GV, Barsoum GS: Blood histamine in experimental obstruction of the common bile duct. *J Physiol (Lond)* **120**:427, 1953

86. Mitchell RG et al: Histamine metabolism in diseases of the liver. *J Clin Invest* **33**:1199, 1954

87. Furhoff A-K: Itching in pregnancy: A 15-year follow-up study. *Acta Med Scand* **196**:403, 1974

88. Barnes HM: Pruritus and thyrotoxicosis. *Trans St Johns Hosp Dermatol Soc* **60**:59, 1974

89. Leading article: Liver disease and vitamin C. *Br Med J* **1**:735, 1977

90. Beattie AD, Sherlock S: Ascorbic acid deficiency in liver disease. *Gut* **17**:571, 1976

91. Garden JM et al: Pruritus in hepatic cholestasis. *Arch Dermatol* **121**:1415, 1985

92. Lauterburg BH et al: Treatment of pruritus of cholestasis by plasma perfusion through USP-charcoal-coated glass beads. *Lancet* **2**:53, 1980

93. Ghent CN, Carruthers SG: Treatment of pruritus in primary biliary cirrhosis with rifampicin. *Gastroenterol* **94**:488, 1988

94. Bachs L et al: Comparison of rifampicin with phenobarbitone for treatment of pruritus in biliary cirrhosis. *Lancet* **1**:574, 1989

95. Cerio R et al: A combination of phototherapy and cholestyramine for the relief of pruritus in primary biliary cirrhosis. *Br J Dermatol* **116**:265, 1987

96. Casaril M et al: Atassia teleangiectasia. *Minn Med* **73**:2183, 1982

97. Weinstein S et al: Ataxia telangiectasia with hepatocellular carcinoma in a 15-year-old girl and studies of her kindred. *Arch Pathol Lab Med* **109**:1000, 1985

98. Wongpaitoon V et al: Intrahepatic cholestasis and cutaneous bullae associated with glibenclamide therapy. *Postgrad Med J* **57**:244, 1981

99. Breathnach SM et al: A severe bullous eruption occurring in a patient with chronic active hepatitis and glomerulonephritis. *Arch Dermatol* **116**:1061, 1980

100. Barnes HM, Sarkany I: Adverse skin reaction from vitamin K_1. *Br J Dermatol* **95**:653, 1976

101. Brunskill N et al: Pseudosclerodermatous reaction to phytomenadione (Texier's syndrome). *Clin Exp Dermatol* **13**:276, 1988

102. Graham-Brown RAC et al: A graft-versus-host-disease-like eruption with carcinomatosis. *Br J Dermatol* **116**:249, 1987

103. Solis-Herruzo JA et al: Laparascopic findings in hereditary haemorrhagic telangiectasia (Osler-Weber-Rendu disease). *Endoscopy* **16**:137, 1984

104. Melish M et al: Kawasaki syndrome: An update. *Hosp Practice* **17**(3):99, 1982

105. Ettinger LJ, Freeman AI: Hepatoma in a child with neurofibromatosis. *Am J Dis Child* **133**:528, 1979

106. Varma SC et al: Association of von Recklighausen's neurofibromatosis with adult polycystic disease of kidneys and liver. *Postgrad Med J* **58**:117, 1982

107. Monk BE et al: Neurofibromatosis, generalized pruritus and cholestatic liver function—Report of two cases. *Clin Exp Dermatol* **10**:590, 1985

108. Sarkany I: Pruritus and cholestatic jaundice due to secondary syphilis. *Proc R Soc Med* **66**:237, 1973

109. Runyon BA et al: The spectrum of liver disease in systemic lupus erythematosus. *Am J Med* **69**:187, 1980

110. Feurle GE et al: Granulomatous hepatitis in systemic lupus erythematosus. Report of a case. *Endoscopy* **14**:153, 1982

111. Kuramochi S et al: Systemic lupus erythematosus associated with multiple nodular hyperplasia of the liver. *Acta Pathol Jpn* **32**:547, 1982

112. Grasso S et al: Unusual liver lesion in tuberous sclerosis. *Arch Pathol Lab Med* **106**:49, 1982

113. Walker A: Occupational acro-osteolysis (two cases). *Proc R Soc Med* **68**:343, 1975

114. Di Bisceglie AM et al: Pityriasis rotunda. *Arch Dermatol* **122**:802, 1986

115. Rogers RB et al: Hepatitis and the skin. *J Am Acad Dermatol* **7**:552, 1981

116. Sherlock S: Virus hepatitis. The Harveian Oration. Royal College of Physicians, London, 1981

117. Sherlock S, Thomas HC: Treatment of chronic hepatitis due to hepatitis B virus. *Lancet* **2**:1343, 1985

118. Alexander G, Williams R: Antiviral treatment in chronic infection with hepatitis B virus. *Br Med J* **292**:915, 1986

119. Thomas HC, Scully LJ: Antiviral therapy in hepatitis B infection. *Br Med Bull* **41**:374, 1985

120. Pegum JS: Wound suturing without gloves. *Lancet* **2**:269, 1982

121. Armati RP, McCullagh RB: Hepatitis in dermatologists. *Med J Aust* **142**:78, 1983

122. Graham-Smith JR, Chalker DK Jr: Editorial. *J Am Acad Dermatol* **8**:252, 1983

123. Leydon JJ et al: Serologic survey for markers of hepatitis B infection in dermatologists *J Am Acad Dermatol* **12**:676, 1985

124. Steigleder GK: Was tun, wenn sich ein Artz oder einer seiner Mitarbeiter bei einer Massnahme beim Patienten mit dem gebrauchten Instrument verletz? *Zeitsch Haut Krankheiten* **58**:355, 1983

125. Hilleman MR et al: Purified and inactivated human hepatitis B vaccine: Progress report. *Am J Med Sci* **270**:401, 1975

126. Maupas P et al: Efficacy of hepatitis B vaccine in prevention of early HBsAg carrier state in children: Controlled trial in an endemic area (Senegal). *Lancet* **1**:289, 1981

127. Finch RG: Time for action on hepatitis B immunisation. *Br Med J* **294**:197, 1987

128. Dienstag LJ et al: Urticaria associated with acute viral hepatitis type B. Studies of pathogenesis. *Ann Intern Med* **89**:34, 1978

129. Popp JW et al: Cutaneous vasculitis associated with acute and chronic hepatitis. *Arch Intern Med* **141**:623, 1981

130. Neumann HAM et al: Hepatitis B surface antigen deposition in the blood vessel walls of urticarial lesions in acute hepatitis B. *Br J Dermatol* **104**:383, 1981

131. McElgunn PSJ: Dermatologic manifestations of hepatitis B virus infection. *J Am Acad Dermatol* **8**:539, 1983

132. Conn DL et al: Immunologic mechanisms in systemic vasculitis. *Mayo Clin Proc* **51**:511, 1976

133. Levo Y et al: Association between hepatitis B virus and essential mixed cryoglobulinemia. *N Engl J Med* **296**:1501, 1977

134. Heim LR: Cryoglobulins: Characterizations and classification. *Cutis* **23**:259, 1979

135. Gocke DJ et al: Association between polyarteritis nodosa and Australia antigen. *Lancet* **2**:1149, 1970

136. Trepo CG et al: The role of circulating hepatitis B antigen/antibody immune complexes in the pathogenesis of vascular and hepatic manifestations in polyarteritis nodosa. *J Clin Pathol* **27**:863, 1974

137. Cohen RO et al: Clinical features, prognosis and response to treatment in polyarteritis. *Mayo Clin Proc* **55**:146, 1980

138. Duffy J et al: Polyarthritis, polyarteritis and hepatitis B. *Medicine (Baltimore)* **55**:19, 1976

139. Sams WM Jr: Necrotizing vasculitis. *J Am Acad Dermatol* **3**:1, 1980

140. Gianotti F: Papular acrodermatitis of childhood. An Australia antigen disease. *Arch Dis Child* **48**:794, 1973

141. Colombo M et al: Immune response to hepatitis B virus in children with papular acro-dermatitis. *Gastroenterology* **73**:1103, 1977

142. Doutre MS, Beylot C: Les signes cutanes lies aux virus de l'hepatite. *Ann Dermatol Venereol* **110**:647, 1983

143. Lier H et al: Cutaneous papulo-vesicular eruptions in non-A, non-B hepatitis. *Hepatogastroenterology* **32**:11, 1985

144. Czaja AJ et al: Acute liver disease after cutaneous thermal injury. *J Trauma* **15**:887, 1975

145. Pruitt BA: Other complications of burn injury, in *Burns: A Team Approach,* edited by CP Artz et al. Philadelphia, Saunders, 1979, p 523

146. Pegum JS: Exfoliative dermatitis associated with liver changes and hypoproteinemia. *Guy's Hosp Reports* **100**:304, 1951

147. Tickner A, Basit A: Serum proteins and liver function in exfoliative dermatitis. *Br J Dermatol* **72**:138, 1960

148. Shuster S, Wilkinson P: Protein metabolism in exfoliative dermatitis and erythroderma. *Br J Dermatol* **75**:344, 1963

149. Bauer F: Generalized exfoliative dermatitis and liver function. *Aust J Dermatol* **2**:69, 1953

150. Knowles JP et al: Folic-acid deficiency in patients with skin disease. *Lancet* **1**:1138, 1963

151. Knowles JP et al: Folic-acid metabolism in liver disease. *Clin Sci* **24**:39, 1963

152. Ryan TJ, Baker H: Systemic corticosteroids and folic acid antagonists in the treatment of generalized pustular psoriasis. *Br J Dermatol* **81**:134, 1969

153. Zachariae H: Psoriasis and the liver, in *Psoriasis,* edited by HH Roegnigk, HI Maibach. New York, Marcel Dekker, 1985, p 45

154. Berge G et al: Liver biopsy in psoriasis. *Br J Dermatol* **82**:250, 1970

155. Chaput JC et al: Psoriasis, alcohol and liver disease. *Br Med J* **291**:25, 1985

156. Morse RM et al: Alcoholism and psoriasis. *Alcohol Clin Exp Res* **9**:396, 1985

157. Monk BE, Neill SM: Alcohol consumption and psoriasis. *Dermatologica* **173**:57, 1986

158. Wojnarowska F, Fry L: Hepatic injury in patients with dermatitis herpetiformis. *Acta Dermatovenereol* **61**:165, 1981

159. Sarkany I: The skin-liver connection. The Prosser-White Oration 1987. *Clin Exp Dermatol* **13**:151, 1988

160. Rebora A: Lichen planus and the liver. *Lancet* **2**:805, 1981

161. Rebora A et al: Chronic active hepatitis and lichen planus. *Acta Dermatovenereol* **62**:351, 1982

162. Rebora A, Rongioletti F: Lichen planus and chronic active hepatitis. *J Am Acad Dermatol* **10**:840, 1984

163. Korkij W et al: Liver abnormalities in patients with lichen planus. *J Am Acad Dermatol* **11**:609, 1984

164. Mobacken H et al: Lichen planus and the liver. *Acta Dermatovenereol* **64**:570, 1984

165. Shuttleworth D et al: The autoimmune background in lichen planus. *Br J Dermatol* **115**:199, 1986

166. McDonagh AJG et al: Lichen planus is not commonly a skin marker of primary biliary cirrhosis. *Dermatologica* **180**:111, 1990

167. Heiberg JK et al: Toxic hepatitis during ketoconazole treatment. *Br Med J* **183**:825, 1981

168. Pariser DM, Wyles RJ: Toxic hepatitis from oral methoxalen photochemotherapy (PUVA). *J Am Acad Dermatol* **3**:248, 1980

169. Chretien P et al: Effects of oral methoxypsoralen photochemotherapy (PUVA) on liver function and antipyrin kinetics. *Int J Clin Pharm Res* **3**:343, 1983

170. Orfanos CE: Laboratory investigations in psoriasis under oral retinoid treatment. *Dermatologica* **159**:62, 1979

171. Marsden JR et al: Effects of isotretinoin on serum lipids and lipoproteins, liver and thyroid function. *Clin Chim Acta* **143**:243, 1984

172. Zachariae H et al: Methotrexate and etretinate as concurrent therapies in the treatment of psoriasis. *Arch Dermatol* **120**:155, 1983

173. Jones SK et al: Methotrexate pharmacokinetics in psoriatic patients developing hepatic fibrosis. *Arch Dermatol* **122**:666, 1986

174. Pestana A et al: Predictive value of HLA antigen for methotrexate-induced liver damage in patients with psoriasis. *J Am Acad Dermatol* **12**:26, 1985

175. Lawrence CM et al: Assessment of liver function using fasting bile salt concentrations in psoriasis prior to and during methotrexate therapy. *Clin Chim Acta* **129**:341, 1983

176. Geronemus RG et al: Liver biopsies vs. liver scans in methotrexate-treated patients with psoriasis. *Arch Dermatol* **118**:649, 1982

177. Coulson IH et al: A comparison of liver ultrasound with liver biopsy histology in psoriatics receiving long-term methotrexate therapy. *Br J Dermatol* **116**:491, 1987

178. Birnie GG et al: Hepatic metabolic function in patients receiving long-term methotrexate therapy: Comparison with topically treated psoriatics, patient controls and cirrhotics. *Hepatogastroenterology* **32**:163, 1985

179. Zachariae H et al: Serum aminoterminal propeptide of type III procollagen: A non-invasive test for liver fibrogenesis in methotrexate-treated psoriatics. *Acta Dermatovenereol* **69**:241, 1989

CHAPTER 164

Janet M. Marks

The Skin and Disorders of the Alimentary Tract

Diseases of the skin and alimentary tract frequently occur together and, just as examination of the whole patient should be part of a full dermatologic assessment, it is important to examine the skin of everyone who presents with a gastrointestinal problem. Because of the skin's unique position, any abnormal signs are easily seen there. In a gastrointestinal emergency such as bleeding or acute abdominal pain, skin signs may even influence the decision on whether surgical intervention is necessary. In less urgent situations skin signs also help; they may predate any other signs of illness including those of malignant disease, although the practical usefulness of early skin signs is often reduced in such patients because the malignancy may already have spread.

This chapter deals with changes in the skin that are associated with diseases of the pharynx, esophagus, stomach, pancreas, and intestines and their main presenting signs and symptoms (Table 164-1). Investigation and treatment of the gastrointestinal aspects of combined disease may well need the expertise of gastroenterologists for such specialized procedures as endoscopy and laser surgery, which are beyond the scope of this book. In other situations

TABLE 164-1

Gastrointestinal Signs and Symptoms in Dermatologic Disease

Dysphagia
Gastrointestinal bleeding
Abdominal pain
Diarrhea and malabsorption

the dermatologist will be the expert, especially when mucosal disease is an extension of skin disease and responds to the same or similar treatment.

Dysphagia

There are four main categories of disease in which skin signs may be associated with difficulty in swallowing: rashes that extend to the pharynx and esophagus, oro-oculogenital syndromes, carcinoma of the esophagus, and collagen vascular diseases (Table 164-2).

Rashes that Extend to the Pharynx and Esophagus

Infections   Infections of the skin and mouth are discussed fully elsewhere (see Chaps. 186 to 193, 198 to 216). Symptoms caused by extension of infections to the esophagus, for example by *Candida albicans* or herpes simplex, are rare except in immunocompromised patients (see Chaps. 195, 203). Dysphagia is one of the most common gastrointestinal symptoms of acquired immunodeficiency syndrome (AIDS). *Candida albicans* is the most frequent pathogen, although opportunistic viruses can also be responsible.[1] Ulcerative hairy leukoplakia, well recognized in the mouth in patients with AIDS, has also been described in the esophagus as a rare cause of dysphagia[2] (see Chap. 215).

Blistering Diseases   The blistering diseases may be congenital or acquired.

CONGENITAL EPIDERMOLYSIS BULLOSA   Serious esophageal involvement with blisters, erosions, and later sometimes strictures occurs in the severe forms of this disease, particularly the recessive generalized dystrophic and recessive letalis forms. Now that prenatal diagnosis is possible and some pregnancies with an affected fetus are terminated, fewer cases can be expected. Early treatment is a matter of debate, particularly if it involves high-dosage corticosteroids, a regimen no longer advocated as much as it once was.[3] Reconstructive surgery for the hands and esophagus can be successful if the early years are survived. Phenytoin has been used in the recessive dystrophic form for its effect on collagenase, and although there are reports of improvement of the skin in such cases,[4] its effect on esophageal lesions is not known.

ACQUIRED "IMMUNOLOGIC" BLISTERING DISEASES   The lesions of pemphigus, bullous pemphigoid, acquired epidermolysis bullosa, and dermatitis herpetiformis may occur on mucosae (Fig. 164-1), but it is in mucous membrane pemphigoid (MMP) that dysphagia is most troublesome and most long lasting. Here blistering may be followed by scarring and esophageal stenosis. In one clinical study of 81 patients with MMP, 35 patients had lesions in the pharynx and 6 in the esophagus; 2 needed dilatation of their esophageal stricture.[5]

Papulosquamous Conditions   Lichen planus can cause symptoms when it involves the esophagus and, considering the frequency with which oral lesions occur, it is surprising that the esophagus has been investigated so little. One endoscopic study of 19 patients with lichen planus, all of whom had mouth lesions, showed that 5 had visible changes with papules in 4 and severe ulceration in 1; the histologic changes were consistent with lichen planus.[6] Isolated cases of esophageal involvement in Darier's disease and acanthosis nigricans have been reported.

Oro-Ocular-Genito-Cutaneous Syndromes

In Stevens-Johnson syndrome and Behçet's disease, dysphagia may result from ulceration of buccal, pharyngeal, and less often esophageal mucosae. In Stevens-Johnson syndrome there is usually crusting and ulceration of the lips. In Behçet's disease the ulcers probably represent one extreme end of the spectrum of aphthous ulceration; intestinal involvement, probably of a arteritic nature, sometimes coexists and can cause confusion in distinguishing Crohn's disease with mouth ulceration from Behçet's disease.

Carcinoma of the Esophagus

In the Plummer-Vinson (Paterson-Kelly) syndrome, a postcricoid web is associated with koilonychia, angular stomatitis, and a sore tongue. The common cause is iron deficiency with or without anemia. About 5 to 10 percent of patients with a postcricoid web develop carcinoma at the site. Patients with celiac disease have an increased risk of developing gastrointestinal malignancies includ-

TABLE 164-2
Skin Abnormalities that Occur with Dysphagia

Rashes that extend to the esophagus
  Infections
  Blistering diseases, congenital and acquired
  Papulosquamous diseases (lichen planus, Darier's disease, acanthosis nigricans)
Oro-oculogenital syndromes
  Stevens-Johnson syndrome
  Behçet's disease
Carcinoma of the esophagus
  Iron deficiency
  Dermatitis herpetiformis
  Tylosis
  Inorganic arsenic ingestion
Collagen vascular diseases
  Systemic sclerosis
  Dermatomyositis

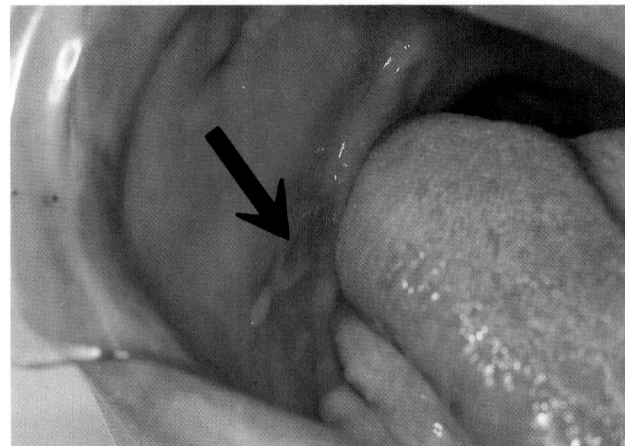

FIGURE 164-1   Ulceration of the mouth in a patient with mucous membrane pemphigoid.

ing carcinoma of the esophagus.[7] It might be expected therefore that dermatitis herpetiformis with its strong association with celiac disease would carry a similar risk. The syndrome of tylosis and carcinoma of the esophagus, although much quoted, is exceedingly rare. Two families have been described[8] in whom both tylosis and carcinoma were inherited as dominant traits. The cancer occurred only in those with skin lesions, which usually appeared first and so acted as a useful marker for special follow-up. Eventually 95 percent of those with tylosis developed cancer. Finally treatments used for dermatologic conditions, particularly medicinal inorganic arsenic,[9] can increase the risk of malignancy. Useful dermatologic markers are skin cancers and palmoplantar keratoses.

Collagen Vascular Diseases

Vasculitic ulcers in the mouth and pharynx occur, though relatively infrequently, in systemic lupus erythematosus (SLE) and probably in other diseases of this group as well. Dysphagia also occurs, particularly in systemic sclerosis and dermatomyositis, as a result of changes in various components of the esophageal and pharyngeal wall.

Systemic Sclerosis   The esophagus is probably the internal organ most often involved in systemic sclerosis. Symptoms, especially dysphagia and heartburn, occur frequently, and radiologic or manometric abnormalities can be detected in up to 70 percent of cases of systemic sclerosis.[10] The basis of the esophageal abnormalities that result in decreased peristalsis, dilatation, and stricture formation is thought to be fibrosis similar to that in the skin, although muscle and nerve may be affected as well. Abnormalities at the gastroesophageal junction lead to acid regurgitation and peptic ulceration with all its complications and are another cause of dysphagia. Blocking gastric acid secretion with H_2 blockers such as ranitidine or by the proton pump inhibitor omeprazole may relieve symptoms and limit mucosal damage. Esophageal dilatation and other surgical procedures are necessary in some patients.

Dermatomyositis   In this collagen vascular disease and occasionally in others, the muscles of swallowing can be affected in a fashion similar to the proximal skeletal muscles. Regardless of whether there is an underlying neoplasm, a myopathy, especially when it involves muscles of swallowing, is an indication for urgent treatment with adequate doses of systemic corticosteroids and possibly azathioprine as well.

Gastrointestinal Bleeding

Gastrointestinal bleeding (Table 164-3) may present as hematemesis, melena, or passing of fresh blood in the stools according to the level of the gastrointestinal tract at which the bleeding occurs. The skin may give diagnostic clues in cases of congenital malformation of blood vessels common to the skin and gastrointestinal tract, genetic defects of collagen and elastic tissue, and Kaposi's sarcoma. Vasculitis, ulcerative colitis, Crohn's disease, polyposis, and cancers may also produce bleeding. They may also present as abdominal pain or disturbances of bowel habit and will be dealt with later. Finally drugs used in dermatology can produce gastrointestinal hemorrhage.

TABLE 164-3
Skin Abnormalities in Patients with Gastrointestinal Bleeding

Congenital malformations of blood vessels
    Hereditary hemorrhagic telangiectasia
    Blue rubber bleb nevi
Inherited defects of connective tissue
    Ehlers-Danlos syndrome
    Pseudoxanthoma elasticum
Kaposi's sarcoma
Drugs used to treat skin disease
Vasculitis
Polyposis
Ulcerative colitis and Crohn's disease
Gastrointestinal tumors

Vascular Abnormalities

Hereditary Hemorrhagic Telangiectasia   The vascular dilatations that characterize this condition occur particularly on skin and on oral, nasal, and gastrointestinal mucosa and may bleed at any of these sites. They have to be differentiated from other telangiectases, including those of systemic sclerosis, that do not bleed. Although the condition is inherited as an autosomal dominant trait, lesions may not be apparent until young adult life. Treatment with large doses of estrogens reduces bleeding at some sites,[11] perhaps by increasing keratinization of the mucosa, but this process is unlikely to be relevant to most cases of gastrointestinal bleeding. When bleeding is severe, inhibition of fibrinolysis, e.g., by ϵ-aminocaproic acid, is a suggested method of treatment. However, as with estrogens, there are no controlled trials to support its usefulness.

Blue Rubber Bleb Nevus Syndrome   This condition[12] is another that is associated with gastrointestinal bleeding and is also inherited as an autosomal dominant trait. The cavernous hemangiomata are venous in origin; in the skin they look and feel as their name suggests, and in the bowel they project as submucous tumors into the lumen particularly of the small intestine.

Inherited Defects of Connective Tissue

Ehlers-Danlos Syndrome   At least nine types of this disease are now known. They probably represent defects in the different enzymes concerned with collagen formation and degradation, although the precise abnormality has not been defined in all cases. Rupture of vessels in the gastrointestinal tract and elsewhere occurs mainly in Ehlers-Danlos syndrome type IV, in which the variety of collagen (type III) found in the skin, gastrointestinal tract, and blood vessels is defective.[13] Diverticula and hiatus and inguinal hernias occur in addition to bleeding and perforation in the gastrointestinal tract (see Chap. 157).

Pseudoxanthoma Elasticum   The defect of this condition is in elastic fibers. The disease will probably turn out to be a series of enzyme defects, as with the Ehlers-Danlos syndrome; four types have been described.[14] Gastrointestinal bleeding and signs of blockage of major arteries are clinical features (see Chap. 157).

Kaposi's Sarcoma

This tumor of the vascular endothelium and pericapillary cells presents clinically with vascular macules, papules, and nodules in skin and mucosae. When it involves other organs, the gastrointestinal tract is a common site. Spread of lesions is thought not to be from metastases but to represent a field change in the vascular endothelium. Although such an aggressive form of Kaposi's sarcoma has long been known in Africans, much of the present interest is in its appearance in large numbers of patients with AIDS. Gut involvement may be asymptomatic, but severe bleeding is a possible complication[1] (see Chap. 99).

Drugs Used in Dermatology

Gastrointestinal bleeding in a patient with a dermatologic disease may be the result of therapy; systemic corticosteroids and methotrexate are two important culprits. Bleeding from the gastrointestinal tract is among the most important causes of morbidity and mortality with these drugs.

Abdominal Pain

Rare instances in which skin signs help in the diagnosis of abdominal pain include herpes zoster, urticaria and angioedema, porphyria, Anderson-Fabry disease, and pancreatitis. Vasculitis, polyposis, inflammatory bowel disease, and cancers have several possible gastrointestinal presentations including abdominal pain and will also be discussed (Table 164-4).

Herpes Zoster

Involvement of the sensory roots of T_6-L_1 may produce abdominal pain; the most difficult time to diagnose this condition is before the

TABLE 164-4
Skin Abnormalities in Patients with Abdominal Pain

Herpes zoster
Angioedema
Porphyria
Anderson-Fabry disease
Vasculitis
　Henoch-Schönlein disease
　Collagen vascular diseases
　Malignant atrophic papulosis
Polyposis
　Gardner's syndrome
　Peutz-Jeghers syndrome
　Canada-Cronkhite syndrome
　Neurofibromatosis
　Ulcerative colitis
Inflammatory bowel disease: ulcerative colitis and Crohn's disease
Pancreatitis
Gastrointestinal tumors
　Signs of wasting
　Metastases
　Dermatomyositis
　Acanthosis nigricans
　Hypertrichosis lanuginosa
　Carcinoma of esophagus, stomach, small bowel, large bowel, and
　　pancreas

spots appear. Grouped blisters, usually unilateral and involving the distribution of one or more of the above dorsal roots, are fairly characteristic. It is easy to confirm the diagnosis by appropriate virologic techniques. Especially in immunocompromised patients, there may be a chickenpox-like spread outside the main area. The pain of postherpetic neuralgia may persist long after the skin lesions have healed, but there are usually scars to help with the diagnosis. Occasionally blisters of herpes zoster in the distribution of S_2, S_3, and S_4 (perineum and adjacent areas) are associated with perineal pain and, if motor fibers are involved, with disturbance of defecation[15] (see Chap. 204).

Angioedema

Acute attacks of urticaria and angioedema of the skin, when accompanied by edema of the bowel, may present as abdominal pain. This gut edema is probably more common in familial hereditary angioedema than in other forms. Though rare, it is a very important diagnosis to make because of the fatalities that occur from laryngeal edema, and unnecessary operation is particularly undesirable. Clues are a family history with an autosomal dominant inheritance, subcutaneous and other mucosal edema often without urticaria, and low levels of C1 esterase inhibitor in the blood (see Chap. 115).

Porphyria Variegata

Acute intermittent porphyria most often poses problems in the diagnosis of abdominal pain, but in patients with acute intermittent porphyria there are *no* abnormalities in the skin. The skin signs of porphyria are most common in porphyria cutanea tarda, in which abdominal symptoms do not occur. It is in the rare porphyria variegata that skin involvement and attacks of abdominal pain coexist. The skin on the backs of the hands and forearms and other light-exposed areas breaks down on minimal trauma, and blisters, when chronic, result in scarring and milia formation. Acute attacks may be precipitated by ingestion of one of a large number of drugs, e.g., estrogen and griseofulvin,[16] and all patients and physicians should be aware of the list of forbidden drugs (see Chap. 150). The urine may turn red on standing. The diagnosis is made by biochemical estimation of porphyrins in urine and particularly feces. Simple "screening" tests on urine are not sufficient to rule out the diagnosis, especially between attacks (see Chap. 150).

Anderson-Fabry Disease (Angiokeratoma Corporis Diffusum)

In this rare disease, which is inherited as a sex-linked recessive trait, there is a deficiency of the lysosomal enzyme α-galactosidase. Internal signs and symptoms are many and varied depending on the site of deposition of uncleaved glycosphingolipid. Unexplained pains at various sites are one form of presentation, and the diagnosis is easily missed if the skin signs are not elicited.[17] These angiokeratomata may not appear until adolescence and even then can be very unimpressive. Diagnosis based on enzyme assay is possible in prenatal cases as well as in established cases, and female carriers can usually be identified. It is important therefore that affected families and individuals are singled out for testing with the help of their skin signs. Treatment with renal transplant has been exceptionally successful, but characterization of the α-galactosidase gene offers the possibility in the future of treatment by enzyme replacement (see Chap. 153).

Vasculitis

There are many cases of acute vasculitis of mesenteric vessels in which similar disease affects the skin. Skin signs are also associated with chronic mesenteric vessel obstruction.

Anaphylactoid Purpura (Henoch-Schönlein Disease) This leukocytoclastic vasculitis with deposits of IgA in the skin is manifested as palpable purpura, especially on the legs and buttocks. It is accompanied by joint swelling, hematuria, and abdominal colic with blood in the stools. Bleeding from the gut, abdominal pain, and, in children, intussusception occur. Skin biopsy can be helpful in diagnosis.

Collagen Vascular Diseases Acute involvement of different sized vessels in the small and large intestines occurs in this group of diseases; occasionally such an episode causes death. The skin signs of small-vessel disease are likely to be present as well. Chronic obliteration of small intestinal vessels in these diseases can result in malabsorption.[18]

Malignant Atrophic Papulosis It is difficult to know whether this subacute vasculitis of skin, brain, and gut vessels[19] is a separate disease entity or if it is a variety of one of the more common vascular diseases, but the histologic finding of endarteritis with thrombosis is said to be diagnostic. The scars in the skin take on a porcelain-like appearance and the patient usually dies from vascular disease or perforation of the bowel. Although a bad prognosis is the rule, skin lesions can be present for years with apparent fitness in other respects.[20]

Polyposis

True polyps are adenomatous tumors and are rare except in the colon and rectum. Polypoid lesions which are hamartomatous or inflammatory occur in all parts of the gut.[21] All may have dermatologic associations.

Gardner's Syndrome In Gardner's syndrome[22] adenomatous polyps with a high risk of malignancy occur particularly in the colon; they are associated with multiple epidermoid cysts, fibromas, and lipomas as well as osteomas of the facial bones. The syndrome is inherited as an autosomal dominant trait. The skin lesions occur early in life and are an important marker of the polyposis, so regular colonoscopy can be done in patients at risk to detect and deal with malignant changes early. Epidermoid cysts and polyposis coli also occur separately in families, and the relationship to Gardner's syndrome is still not worked out. Establishing that relationship should be possible soon, however, with improved techniques and gene localization in Gardner's syndrome.

Peutz-Jeghers Syndrome (see Chap. 80) In this syndrome[23] the polyps are hamartomatous and occur mainly in the small intestine. The risk of malignancy was overstressed in the past mainly because of misinterpretation of the hamartomatous histology. Nevertheless, true malignant change with metastasis does occur in these polyps, and there is also an increased risk of malignancy in general in these

patients.[24] The skin changes are small dark freckles around the mouth, on the lips, and on the distal parts of the fingers and toes; patchy pigmentation occurs inside the mouth. With increasing age the characteristic freckles tend to disappear, leaving the mouth pigmentation which may be indistinguishable from that due to racial factors or Addison's disease. The syndrome is inherited as an autosomal dominant trait, but some members of the family seem to have either the skin signs or the intestinal changes but not both. As with Gardner's syndrome, the relationship of these groups should soon be known.

Canada-Cronkhite Syndrome In this rare acquired disease with alopecia and abnormal nails, inflammatory polyps are present in the stomach as well as the bowel. A protein-losing enteropathy is part of the syndrome, but the hair and nail changes precede the bowel trouble and so do not seem to be the result of the lack of protein. The alopecia is patchy and the nail changes are characteristic but not diagnostic.[25] It has been suggested that the inverted triangle of normal nail with surrounding dystrophy is due to growth of the ventral nail.

Neurofibromatosis Twenty-five percent of patients with neurofibromatosis are said to have gastrointestinal involvement, usually in the form of tumors which can be polypoid.[26] Most of these tumors are neurofibromas, but leiomyomas and rarely other tumors including malignant ones also occur. Gastrointestinal neurofibromatosis is a feature of von Recklinghausen neurofibromatosis (NF1) and consequently skin lesions are usually found (see Chap. 184).

Ulcerative Colitis Inflammatory polyposis occurs in this condition and is important in relation to malignancy.

Inflammatory Bowel Disease: Ulcerative Colitis and Crohn's Disease

Abdominal pain occurs in both of these inflammatory bowel diseases, although they may also present with gastrointestinal bleeding or diarrhea; ulcerative colitis also predisposes to carcinoma of the colon. The skin complications of the two diseases are similar, although some occur with different frequencies; in particular granulomata are much more common in Crohn's disease (Table 164-5).

Pyoderma Gangrenosum (see Chap. 93) Although it is generally agreed that this skin condition has a significant association with inflammatory bowel disease, it also occurs in rheumatoid disease, myeloma, and leukemias and in a number of patients who are otherwise well. Figures about associated diseases vary partly as a result of the referral pattern of patients studied and partly because of different diagnostic criteria.[27] One study found that half the patients with pyoderma gangrenosum had ulcerative colitis but less than 10 percent of patients with ulcerative colitis had pyoderma

TABLE 164-5
Skin Lesions in Ulcerative Colitis and Crohn's Disease

Pyoderma gangrenosum
Granulomata
Erythema nodosum
Aphthous ulcers
Malnutrition
Erythemas, lichen planus, vascular thrombosis
Rashes at ileostomy and colostomy sites

gangrenosum. Another retrospective study found about one-third of 86 patients with pyoderma gangrenosum had inflammatory bowel disease, with ulcerative colitis and Crohn's disease featured almost equally.[28] Investigation of the bowel is worthwhile even in the absence of symptoms because relevant disease has been found in pyoderma gangrenosum in the absence of symptoms. The pathogenesis of the disease is not understood: There are no specific bacteriologic, histologic, or immunologic findings. Vasculitis is present in a number of cases but by no means all. The ulcers usually heal with treatment of the bowel but this is not always so.

Granulomata These nodules occur in the mouth in patients with Crohn's disease, where they may coalesce to give a cobblestone appearance to the mucosa. Alternatively they can cause a diffuse granulomatous thickening of the lips. Not all granulomatous cheilitis is due to Crohn's disease, though this type of lip involvement may predate bowel disease by several years. Granulomata also occur round the anus and vulva, at colostomy and ileostomy sites, and in association with scars, sinuses, and fistulas. So-called metastatic granulomas occur at sites remote from the bowel.[29]

Erythema Nodosum Ulcerative colitis and Crohn's disease are relatively uncommon causes of this rash. When they occur, skin lesions are usually associated with an exacerbation of the bowel disease.

Aphthous Ulcers These lesions are reported to occur in 8 percent of patients with ulcerative colitis[30] and 6 percent of patients with Crohn's disease.[31] They may be the presenting feature of either of these conditions or of celiac disease, so investigation of the bowel should be considered in patients with intractable mouth ulcers. Bowel studies are, however, not necessary or rewarding in patients with aphthous ulcers in general.

Malnutrition Various signs of specific and nonspecific deficiencies can arise from inflammatory bowel disease or its treatment with elemental diets, which are described below.

Miscellaneous Skin Conditions Annular erythemas, vascular thromboses, erythema multiforme, lichen planus, and rosacea have been described in association with inflammatory bowel disease. It is not always clear that they are caused by the bowel condition, especially in cases in which drugs that might be responsible have been given.

Rashes at Colostomy and Ileostomy Sites These rashes are most common in patients with inflammatory bowel disease but are not confined to patients with these diseases: They are seen regardless of the primary disease for which the operation was done, if conditions are adverse. They are worst in those with ileostomies in which gut enzymes digest the skin and in those who also have ureters transplanted into the bowel. The following factors are important.

SITING AND FASHIONING OF STOMA It is important that stomas are correctly sited and fashioned so that bowel contents are directed away from the skin into the colostomy or ileostomy bag. Resiting and refashioning by a surgeon may be necessary.

FLUIDITY OF BOWEL CONTENTS (see above) It may be possible to improve fluidity by drugs and dietary manipulation.

ILL-FITTING APPLIANCE It is important that appliances do not leak and that adhesives are satisfactory; otherwise the skin will suffer. It may be possible to protect the skin to some extent with a silicone barrier cream or aluminum paint, as long as they do not interfere with adhesion.

INFECTION The skin at the site may become infected by *C. albicans* or bacteria from the gut. Systemic treatment to clear the infection is preferable to topical applications which may sensitize the skin.

KOEBNER'S PHENOMENON These lesions may occur in psoriatic individuals and are best treated with topical cortiosteroid, e.g., clobetasol. If the cream base is used and allowed to sink into the skin, it does not interfere with adhesion.

CONTACT ECZEMA Contact eczema may be irritant or allergic.[32] There are many potential allergens including the rubber or plastic of the bag, adhesives, deodorants, substances used to clean the skin, and medicaments applied. Patch testing must be tailored to individual patients and their appliances. The variety of appliances is now legion, so if a contact allergen is identified it should be possible to find an appliance that does not contain it. In some cases of weeping eczema it may be necessary to admit the patient to the hospital and manage the condition without an appliance while the skin heals, although the advantage of this measure is likely to be outweighed by the disadvantage of more soiling of the skin. Drying agents like silver nitrate may help the skin, but usually a topical corticosteroid cream is satisfactory.

PATIENT ATTITUDE AND SUPPORT Overall management of difficult cases depends on close cooperation between the surgeon, physician, dermatologist, stoma nurse, and not least the patient. A number of ileostomy and colostomy "clubs" exist for patient self-help.

Acute and Chronic Pancreatitis

If these diseases give rise to diagnostic problems when they present with abdominal pain, skin signs may be helpful.

Acute Pancreatitis Bruising of the skin around the umbilicus (Cullen's sign) or in the flanks (Grey Turner's sign) is a well-known feature of acute pancreatitis, though it occurs only in a small proportion of cases.

Chronic Pancreatitis Fat necrosis, resulting in tender, subcutaneous nodules that may ulcerate is a skin sign of chronic pancreatitis. The fat necrosis is probably due to liberation of pancreatic enzymes into the circulation (see Chap. 108).

Gastrointestinal Cancer and Other Malignancies

When these cancers present as pain it may be from ulceration, perforation, colic, or spread to involve nerves. Many skin changes, some organ-specific or tumor-specific and some not, occur in association.

Signs of Weight Loss or Cachexia These signs include dry skin (acquired ichthyosis) with cracking and eczematization of the cracks (eczema craquelé), poor hair and nails, and hyperpigmentation. They are not specific to malignancy and occur also in patients with malabsorption syndromes (see below).

Metastases Any tumor may metastasize to the skin where it usually appears as one or more vascular lumps or hard nodules. The scalp is a common site. Metastases at the umbilicus (Sister Joseph nodules) occur particularly with carcinoma of the stomach, colon, and ovary (Fig. 164-2). A number of skin tumors metastasize to the gut. Malignant melanoma does so in as many as 60 percent accord-

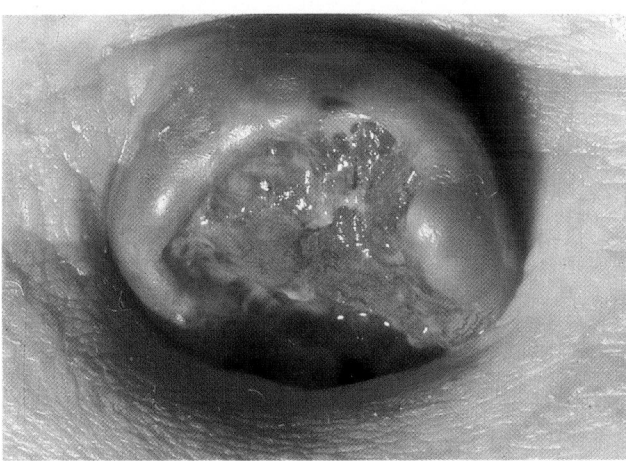

FIGURE 164-2 Umbilical metastasis (Sister Joseph nodule) from intraabdominal adenocarcinoma.

ing to one postmortem series. Metastases do not always produce symptoms but they may be massive and cause bleeding, anemia, ulceration, and malabsorption as well as pain.[33]

Dermatomyositis (see Chap. 172)   This collagen vascular disease, when it occurs in adults, may be due to underlying malignant disease; 15 to 34 percent of cases are said to show such an association.[34] The acceptance of different criteria for diagnosis as well as the degree of investigation to which patients have been subjected in searching for cancer are partly responsible for the variation in different series. The associated tumors are the ones most prevalent in a particular population. Gastric and colonic cancers are less frequent than bronchogenic and breast cancers in Europe and North America; in the Chinese, in whom nasopharyngeal carcinoma is a common tumor, this type of cancer is also most often associated with dermatomyositis. There is no doubt that the rash and myopathy can regress after removal of the tumor and, since dermatomyositis may be a relatively early sign of internal malignancy, its recognition is potentially life saving. Overall, however, investigation of patients with dermatomyositis for malignancy gives a poor return in finding cancers not detectable clinically or by the simplest of tests, and this low diagnostic yield should temper the vigor of investigation of an individual case.[35]

Acanthosis Nigricans (see also Chaps. 169, 183)   This generic term encompasses a number of separate disorders, including genetodevelopmental or nevoid disorders, those due to friction or maceration, as in obesity, and epidermotropic disorders, as in acromegaly. In this chapter only the form seen in malignancy is relevant (Fig. 164-3), and it seems likely that eventually a circulating epidermotropic factor will be found. In this context it is interesting that in two-thirds of patients with acanthosis nigricans and cancer the tumor is gastric, and that urogastrone which is a potent physiologic inhibitor of gastric secretion is similar in structure to human epidermal growth factor. It is rare for a tumor not to be found in this type of acanthosis nigricans, and the rash may regress if the tumor, usually an adenocarcinoma of the stomach or bowel, is removed. However recognition of the disorder is more important diagnostically than therapeutically, since the tumor is already well established in 80 to 90 percent of patients at the time of diagnosis of the rash.

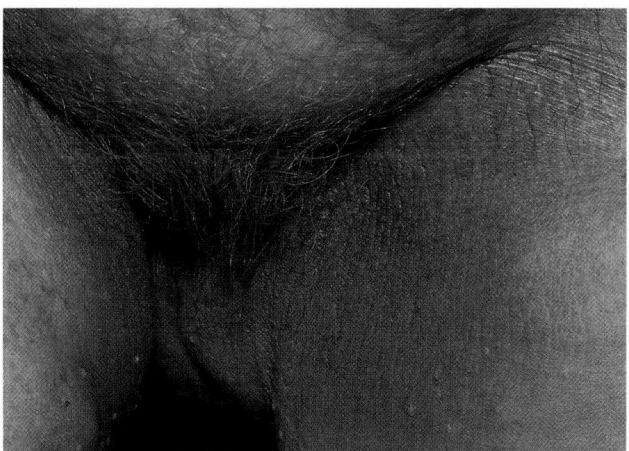

a

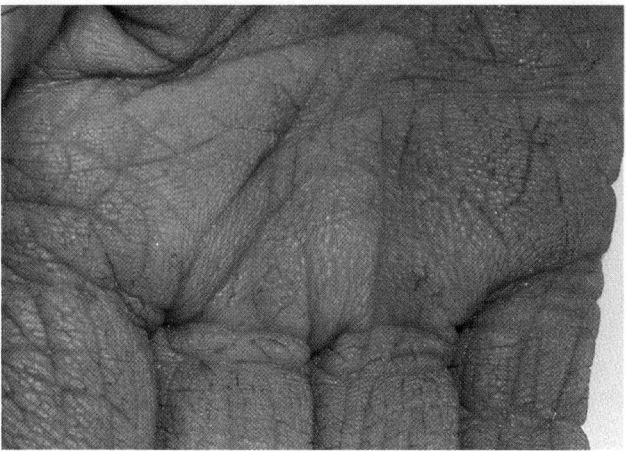

b

FIGURE 164-3 Patient with acanthosis nigricans due to adenocarcinoma of jejunum. (*a*) Rash in groins. (*b*) ''Tripe hands.''

Hypertrichosis Lanuginosa   This excessive growth of lanugo hair (Fig. 164-4), which may cover the whole body, is a rare complication of malignant disease, including gastrointestinal cancer. The mechanism of its production is not understood, but inappropriate cortisol production may be to blame.

Nonspecific Rashes   Urticarias, erythemas, and vasculitis are among the nonspecific rashes that occur occasionally, apparently as a result of malignant disease, though much more often the same rashes have a less sinister cause. A suggested special relationship of pemphigoid to neoplasia remains unproved.

Signs of Special Gastrointestinal Tumors

CARCINOMA OF THE ESOPHAGUS   These signs are discussed above in the section on dysphagia.

CARCINOMA OF THE STOMACH   Vitiligo is a rare presenting sign of carcinoma of the stomach. The association is through atrophic gastritis and pernicious anemia, which themselves have an association with vitiligo. A similar comparatively increased chance of developing carcinoma of the stomach might be expected in patients with alopecia areata, dermatitis herpetiformis, and lichen

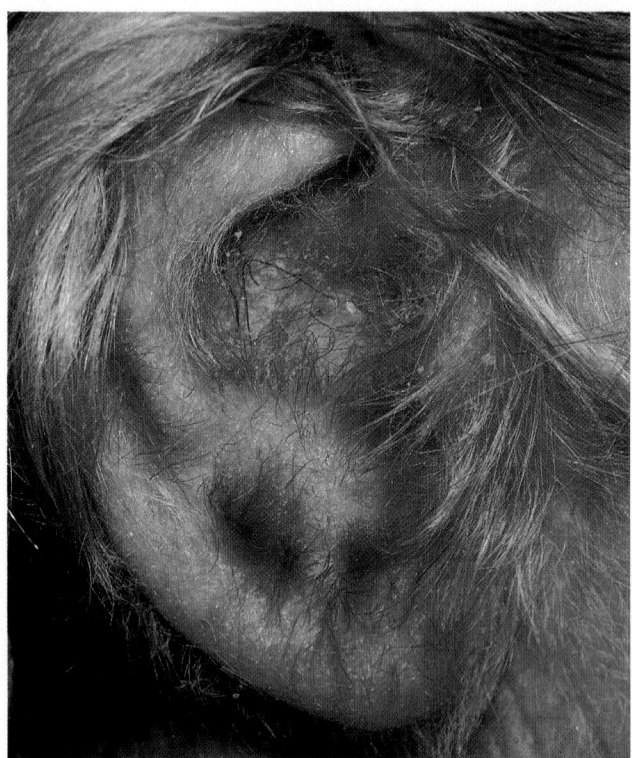

FIGURE 164-4 Hypertrichosis lanuginosa in a patient with metastatic adenocarcinoma.

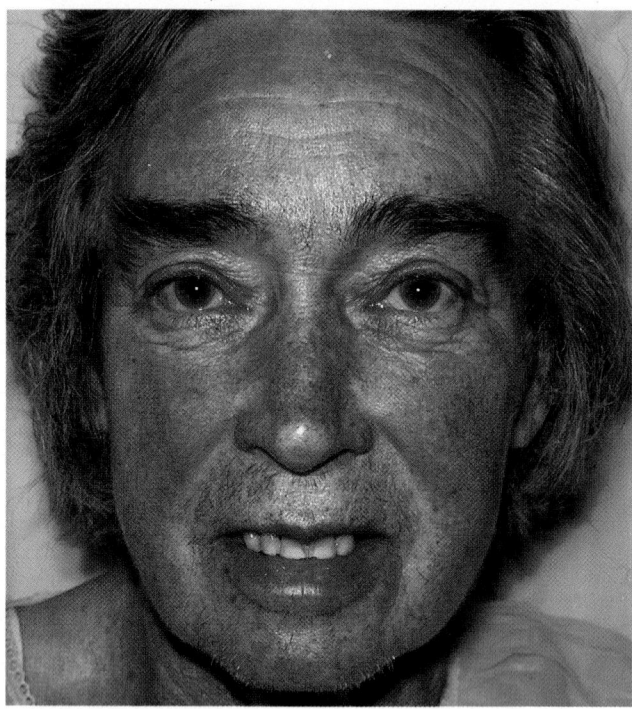

FIGURE 164-5 Facial rash in a patient with liver metastases from a carcinoid tumor of the small bowel.

sclerosus, who also have an increased incidence of parietal cell antibodies.

SMALL BOWEL TUMORS *Carcinoid syndrome* (see also Chap. 170) Carcinoid tumors produce a number of vasoactive substances including 5-hydroxytryptamine (5HT), histamine, prostaglandins, bradykinin, and tachykinins. It was initially thought that 5HT was the cause of the carcinoid flush (Fig. 164-5), but 5HT alone does not produce the full symptomatology. Bradykinin, subsequently blamed, has not been shown to be responsible either. The most common carcinoid tumors, those of the appendix and small bowel, do not produce flushing because the vasoactive substances do not reach the systemic circulation. Thus this type of symptom usually indicates metastasis to the liver or a primary tumor at a different site, e.g., lung or ovary. Diagnosis by measuring hydroxyindoleacetic acid (HIAA), a breakdown product of 5HT, in the urine is unsatisfactory for reasons stated above and because even if it is present in attacks it may be absent in between. Unsuccessful attempts have been made to correlate the different types of carcinoid flush—bright red, cyanotic, edematous, diffuse, less widespread, intermittent and permanent—with different mediators, and treatment with a number of antagonists has as a rule been unsatisfactory.[36]

Mastocytosis (see Chap. 161) Most mast cell infiltrates are benign. Troublesome effects of benign and malignant tumors are due to the histamine they produce. Urticaria pigmentosa may involve organs other than the skin; the rarer diffuse mast cell infiltration of the skin is usually accompanied by widespread infiltration of internal tissues. The small bowel and pancreas are among the organs affected, and malabsorption can result. Celiac disease has been described in patients with mastocytosis[37] and is another cause of malabsorption in these patients. Osteomalacia can occur as a consequence, and it may be difficult to differentiate from the osteo-

porosis that sometimes results from the liberation of heparin-like substances from the mast cells. Not all the gastrointestinal effects of mastocytosis are due to infiltration by mast cells, because the liberation of large amounts of pharmacologically active substances from the skin lesions, e.g., during bathing, can lead to diarrhea and abdominal pain.

Lymphoma (also see below) The occurrence of malignant disease with dermatitis herpetiformis has been mentioned above. When a lymphoma occurs in a patient with celiac disease, with or without dermatitis herpetiformis, it can be difficult to diagnose early because the clinical signs are often vague and nonspecific. "Ulcers, nodules and skin rashes" have been described as arising at the onset of the lymphoma in one series of cases.[38]

Patients with lymphomas, including those of the bowel, are prone to skin complications of immunosuppression due either to the disease or its treatment. There is increased susceptibility to infection with viruses, bacteria, fungi, and protozoa, including those that are not normally pathogenic. Herpes simplex and herpes zoster may occur and tend to be widely disseminated, and *C. albicans* infection may become systemic or accompanied by granuloma formation.

CARCINOMA OF THE LARGE BOWEL Skin signs occur in conjunction with the potentially malignant forms of polyposis and in conjunction with ulcerative colitis, which should be regarded as a premalignant condition. Paget's disease in the perianal skin is, like mammary Paget's disease, associated with an underlying carcinoma. This tumor is not always in adjacent tissue, but most commonly does arise in rectal mucosa, apocrine glands, or cloacal remnants. A rare presentation in the last case is chronic anal fistula.

CARCINOMA OF THE PANCREAS *Carcinoma of exocrine cells* Migratory superficial thrombophlebitis occurs in association with neoplasia, particularly carcinoma of the pancreas.

Glucagonoma (see also Chap. 183) This neoplasm is one of the APUD (*A*mine *P*recursor *U*ptake and *D*ecarboxylation) cell tumors. They produce excessive amounts of regulatory gastrointestinal peptide hormones such as glucagon, pancreatic polypeptide, vasoactive intestinal peptide (VIP), gastrin, and insulin. Some produce a single peptide and others several different ones. Those that produce glucagon usually arise in the islet cells of the pancreas, though not invariably so. The tumors may be benign or malignant, but in the case of glucagonoma they are usually malignant.

The distinctive necrolytic migratory erythematous rash associated with glucagonoma[39] is occasionally seen also with tumors that produce other peptides and rarely in patients who apparently have no tumor at all.[40,41]

The rash is most commonly seen around orifices (Fig. 164-6a), in flexures (Fig. 164-6b), and on the fingers. It starts as erythematous papules which coalesce and spread outward; then vesicles appear in the center of the lesions and proceed through crusting to postinflammatory pigmentation. The eventual appearance is a geographic circinate pattern (Fig. 164-6b). Histologic examination shows superficial necrolysis with separation of the outer layers of the epidermis and infiltration with lymphocytes and histiocytes. Patients with glucagonoma are usually ill with weight loss, diarrhea, malabsorption, sore mouth, diabetes, psychiatric disturbance, anemia, hypoaminoacidemia, and hypozincemia. In a few, however, the rash is a relatively early sign of the tumor and is particularly important to diagnose in those with benign or slow-growing tumors.

Diagnosis is by detection of excess glucagon in the blood by radioimmunoassay using antibodies directed especially against the C-terminal of the glucagon amino acid sequence. Fresh frozen plasma from a fasting patient is required, and the specimen must be transported in a tube containing the enzyme inhibitor aprotinin (Trasylol) to one of the limited number of laboratories that perform the assay. If specimens of tumor are available, immunochemical stains specific to the peptide will settle the matter. The tumor may be localized by ultrasound, isotope scan, or CT scan.

If the tumor can be removed, the rash will disappear. If removal is not possible a specific peptide antagonist, streptozotocin, has been given with good results. Another form of treatment involves somatostatin, a peptide that inhibits the release of a number of gastrointestinal peptides. Symptomatic treatment of the rash with topical corticosteroids and antiyeast preparations may help, as may potassium permanganate baths.

The mechanism that produces the rash is not known. It does not appear to be the direct result of glucagon, although a rash has been described in a patient who was given glucagon as treatment for acute pancreatitis. The similarity of the rash to that of zinc deficiency, essential fatty acid (EFA) deficiency, or hypoaminoacidemia has led to theories that these deficiencies are to blame, but correcting them does not usually improve the rash. VIP, which is closely related to glucagon, has a number of actions on the skin, producing erythema, edema, and increased sweat, but the relation of this and other peptides produced in the skin to the rash of glucagonoma is not known.

Diarrhea and Malabsorption

Some of the skin associations of gastrointestinal diseases that produce diarrhea have already been mentioned and include angioedema, carcinoid, mastocytosis, glucagonoma, pancreatitis, bowel cancers, ulcerative colitis, and Crohn's disease. When the diarrhea is due to steatorrhea, there are additional possibilities. Many skin

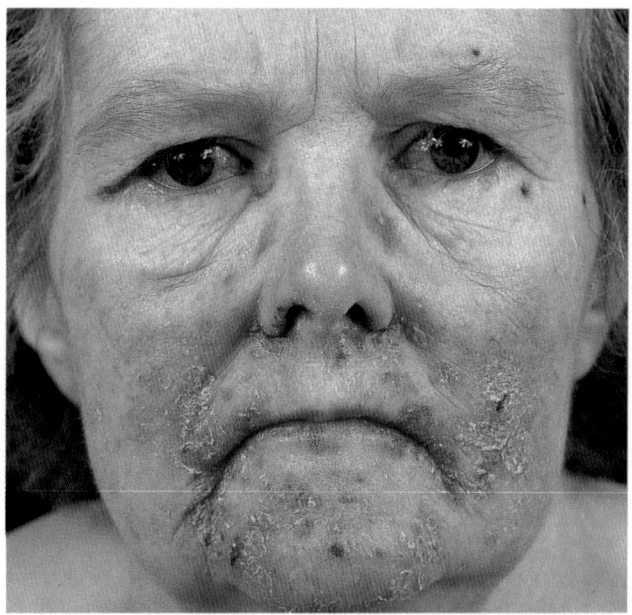

a

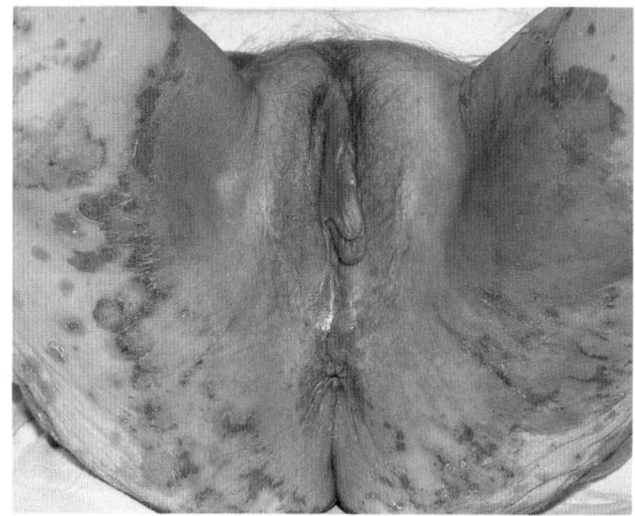

b

FIGURE 164-6 The glucagonoma syndrome. Papulovesicular lesions (*a*) with erosions, crusting and fissures around the orifices and (*b*) appearing as geographic, circinate "necrolytic migratory erythema" in the groin. (*Fig. 6a courtesy of Klaus Wolff, M.D.*).

changes occur in association with malabsorption, some as a result of it, some due to a disease process that affects the bowel as well as the skin, and some because of a genetic susceptibility to two different diseases. In addition, skin disease can actually cause malabsorption.[42]

Skin Changes due to Malabsorption

Some skin changes due to malabsorption (Table 164-6) are quite specific, e.g., the rash of zinc deficiency, while others are nonspecific, e.g., those that occur as a result of wasting or of illness in general.

TABLE 164-6
Malabsorption and Skin Disease

Skin changes due to malabsorption
   Nonspecific
      Acquired ichthyosis and itch
      Hair and nail changes
      Hyperpigmentation
      Skin texture and elasticity
      Eczematous and psoriatic rashes
      Jejunoileal and jejunocolic anastomoses
   Specific nutrients
      Zinc
      Essential fatty acids
      Vitamins
Malabsorption due to skin disease
   Dermatogenic enteropathy
Collagen vascular disease
Dermatitis herpetiformis and celiac disease

Nonspecific Cutaneous Effects Nonspecific effects do not depend on the nature of the underlying disease. Although they are most common in patients who have lost weight, for example, from malabsorption or malignant disease, they are not necessarily confined to this group. Usually by the time the skin is involved it is apparent that the patient is systemically ill, but this sequence is not invariable; for instance, patients with malignant lymphoma may have pruritus long before they have clinical evidence of underlying disease.

ACQUIRED ICHTHYOSIS AND ITCH The skin of sick people often feels dry; this dryness is one of the main causes of the itch about which they may complain. The skin resembles that seen in dominantly inherited ichthyosis of mild degree. It is not known whether a genetic predisposition is necessary for the development of the acquired form, but the frequency with which it occurs makes this doubtful. The cracks in the skin often become eczematized and the resulting clinical picture, on the shins particularly, is described as crazy-paving eczema. The presence of this sign not only in patients with malabsorption but also in those with cancer, chronic renal disease, and chronic hepatic disease as well, led to the postulation that malabsorption was the common factor and that this in turn was due to flattening of the intestinal mucosa such as has been described in malignant disease. The possibility has not been investigated systematically, but villous atrophy has been found with acquired ichthyosis due to lymphoma.[42] More likely is the possibility of EFA deficiency or a comparable defect due either to malabsorption or to abnormal metabolism within the skin. Although some studies show a decrease in plasma linoleic acid in wasting disease, they do not show an increase in plasma 5,8,11-eicosatrienoic acid, which is thought to be the metabolic marker of severe EFA deficiency (see below).

The dryness that has been described in association with malabsorption is a major factor in the production of itch in patients with lymphoma and other malignant disease, although some of these patients itch without any visible abnormality of their skin. The mechanism is not understood. It is still not known, for instance, whether unconjugated bile salts like chenodeoxycholate, which are important in the itch of biliary obstruction, are important here too. The investigation for systemic disease in a patient who is apparently well and yet suffers from pruritus is an exercise of few returns. Most people itch because of a common skin disease. Hypoferremia is a rare cause of itch. It is related to decreased iron concentration itself rather than to any accompanying anemia, be-

cause it disappears within hours of intravenous administration of iron. A group of male patients with itch and hypoferremia who subsequently developed lymphoma has been described,[43] so further investigation may be worthwhile in a patient with unexplained itch in these circumstances.

HAIR AND NAILS Hair and nails are frequently abnormal in poorly nourished people. Deficiencies of specific nutrients such as protein, iron, zinc, and folic acid may be found, but in most cases the mechanism is not known and is likely to be multifactorial. Changes in hair and nails in malnourished patients whose main dietary deficiency is protein have been studied in those with kwashiorkor.[44] These changes include reduction in both linear growth and diameter of the shaft, making the hair liable to break; there is also an increase in the percentage of hairs in telogen at any one time. Thus the clinical picture is that of chronic telogen effluvium.

Nails are generally poor and brittle in these patients and there may be episodic slowing of growth resulting in horizontal ridges (Beau's lines). When koilonychia occurs in malnourished patients, it usually indicates iron deficiency with or without anemia. The transverse white bands that appear in the nails of patients with hypoalbuminemia remain unexplained.

SKIN COLOR One of the most interesting skin changes associated with malabsorption as well as with malignant disease is hyperpigmentation due to melanin. This discoloring may be gross and indistinguishable from that of Addison's disease with hyperpigmentation in the palmar creases and buccal mucosa. It is not due to an increase in circulating melanocyte-stimulating hormone peptide.

SKIN TEXTURE AND ELASTICITY In the course of wasting diseases the skin becomes thinner from loss of collagen. This thinning occurs in patients with anorexia nervosa and after experimental dietary deprivation in the rat. The effect may be exaggerated clinically by loss of subcutaneous fat. The skin is also less elastic and does not spring back normally after stretching.

ECZEMATOUS AND PSORIASIFORM RASHES DUE TO MALABSORPTION These rashes occur in association with malabsorption regardless of its cause, although they have been observed most often in patients with celiac disease and tropical sprue.[45–47] A number of specific deficiencies including EFA deficiency have been postulated as causes, but they have not been substantiated in the group as a whole. Treatment of the malabsorption is always effective in curing the rash. Although atypicality of the eczematous and psoriasiform rashes has been stressed in the past, there do not seem to be any special diagnostic features in the rashes now occasionally associated with malabsorption. Associated acquired ichthyosis and hyperpigmentation were other points stressed, but neither is confined to patients wasting from malabsorption. Furthermore, hyperpigmentation is common in extensive rashes and in these patients it is not related to the presence or absence of malabsorption.

In the absence of clear indications, investigation of the bowel in such cases is not necessary: No cases of celiac disease were found by small-intestinal mucosal biopsy of 100 unselected consecutive patients with eczema and psoriasis (personal observation). This result is of course in direct contrast to findings in patients with dermatitis herpetiformis, in which biopsy uncovers many previously unsuspected cases of celiac disease.

JEJUNOILEAL AND JEJUNOCOLIC ANASTOMOSES The increase in the number of patients with obesity treated by these bypass operations has led to the recognition of certain metabolic consequences, most of which are of unknown etiology. Apart from dryness of the skin and hair loss, which are presumably due to malabsorption, inflammatory and vasculitic skin lesions occur together with fever, leukocytosis, and arthralgia.[48]

Cutaneous Effects of Malabsorption of Specific Nutrients

ZINC DEFICIENCY AND ACRODERMATITIS ENTEROPATHICA (also see Chap. 146) Zinc deficiency can occur from malabsorption due to celiac disease and inflammatory bowel disease; it is relatively common when elemental feeds are deficient in zinc. Although there are reasons for believing deranged zinc metabolism, due to malabsorption or not, may have adverse effects on the skin, it has been difficult to prove that common skin conditions are particularly associated with zinc deficiency. Low plasma zinc concentrations have been found in patients with psoriasis and leg ulcers as well as in those with many other unrelated diseases.[49] This association does not mean that there is a deficiency in the body as a whole or that zinc is helpful in therapy. Dynamic studies of zinc metabolism using Zn-65 have been few and show there is a wide variation of absorption and reexcretion into the bowel and no evidence of overall zinc deficiency in patients with stasis leg ulcers.[50]

Acrodermatitis enteropathica usually presents at the time of weaning. The rash is the same as that of zinc deficiency of other causes with blistering on the hands and feet and around the mouth and anus; alopecia and "failure to thrive" are other features. Absorption of zinc is impaired,[51] although the mechanism is still not understood. Moynahan[53] suggested that dietary zinc is chelated in the bowel by an abnormal small-molecular-weight ligand which may be in the mucosa or in pancreatic secretions. Large doses of oral zinc result in sufficient absorption to overcome the defect, as does breast milk in which the zinc is bound to another ligand. Zinc deficiency is thought to be associated with abnormalities of essential fatty acid metabolism and there are certain similarities between the rashes of zinc deficiency and EFA deficiency.

ESSENTIAL FATTY ACID DEFICIENCY The appearance of a scaly rash in experimental animals with EFA deficiency is well known, and a dry skin with cracking of the horny layer has been reported in children fed diets low in linoleic acid. Adults receiving parenteral nutrition had similar skin problems until the cause was recognized and rectified. Other information comes from patients who have scaly skin as a result of malabsorption from small gut resection.[53] They have low levels of linoleic acid and an abnormal metabolite 5,8,11-eicosatrienoic acid in the plasma. Clinically their skin is improved by topical linoleic acid such as that found in sunflower seed oil. In other wasting conditions, including celiac disease, levels of plasma linoleic acid are again low but the abnormal metabolite is not found; it is not certain how specific this finding is to EFA deficiency but it seems reasonable to treat patients with a scaly skin that may be due to this condition with sunflower seed oil.

How the scaliness of EFA deficiency is brought about is not clear. Barrier function is impaired and there is an increase in transepidermal water loss. It is difficult to explain why the horny layer cracks as if it were poorly hydrated, yet percutaneous water movement is increased. As in other scaly dermatoses, there is an increase in total lipid synthesis in the skin with as yet incompletely defined qualitative changes in the different lipid classes. EFA deficiency impairs prostaglandin synthesis and topical prostaglandin (PGE_2) improves the skin changes in animals. The role claimed for EFA deficiency in scaly, inflammatory dermatoses like eczema and psoriasis will not be discussed here.

MALABSORPTION OF VITAMINS AND OTHER NUTRIENTS The rashes due to deficiency of vitamins A, B, C, and K, usually in combination, occur in severe small-bowel abnormalities. In addition malabsorption of vitamin K occurs in obstructive jaundice. Deficiency of vitamin A, whether due to malabsorption or not, is no longer thought to be a causal factor in pityriasis rubra pilaris and other scaly dermatoses, as was once suggested. The mechanism of action of the vitamin A-related aromatic retinoids in some of these conditions is not thought to involve the bowel.

Folate, iron, and zinc deficiency may contribute to the poor hair growth of malnutrition. Malabsorption of protein, or protein-losing enteropathy, leads to edema of the skin as in kwashiorkor. In this condition, however, there are many deficiencies in addition to that of protein and it is difficult to attribute the physical signs to a specific one. There has been a suggestion that an aflatoxin from fungi growing on cereals in humid climates may be as important as malnutrition.

Malabsorption due to Skin Disease

Dermatogenic Enteropathy[54] A large proportion of patients with extensive skin disease get mild malabsorption as a result: In one study of 30 patients with erythroderma, steatorrhea was found in 22. Malabsorption of fat has been most studied in patients with eczema and psoriasis, in whom steatorrhea is proportional to the extent of the skin disease and responds rapidly to topical treatment of the rash. Dermatogenic enteropathy is not related to gluten sensitivity or celiac disease, and structural changes, if they occur at all, are minimal.[55] The mechanism of its production is unknown, but it is one of the systemic effects of skin disease; similar malabsorption appears to occur in other chronic diseases.

Symptoms of dermatogenic enteropathy are rare, and their importance lies in the confusion that can occur if they are not recognized for what they are in a patient with a rash and malabsorption. If in doubt, a small intestinal biopsy can be done, and a flat biopsy will exclude a dermatogenic cause and point to celiac disease. Treatment of dermatogenic enteropathy, other than by clearing the rash, is not necessary; in particular, a gluten-free diet should not be given.

Malabsorption in Collagen Vascular Diseases

This malabsorption can occur as a result of poor peristalsis from changes in the small intestinal wall in patients with systemic sclerosis, or by chronic obliteration of mesenteric vessels in those with polyarteritis and other forms of vasculitis.[18] The small intestinal changes in patients with systemic sclerosis are structurally similar to those that occur in the esophagus and the large bowel; in the latter case they are accompanied by saccules or wide-mouthed diverticula found on barium enema examination in a large proportion of patients.[56] The structural changes in the small bowel wall that interfere with peristalsis result in malabsorption by allowing bacterial colonization higher up the bowel than is usual and produce, in effect, a blind loop syndrome. There is also some evidence of a primary enterocyte defect that may contribute to the malabsorption.[57] Clinical symptoms and signs of diarrhea and steatorrhea are severe in some cases but can be improved at least for a time by broad-spectrum antibiotics such as lincomycin.

Dermatitis Herpetiformis (See also Chap. 56)

Dermatitis herpetiformis is perhaps the most important and interesting skin disease associated with malabsorption. When malabsorption occurs it is due to celiac disease. Diagnosis of dermatitis herpetiformis thus has gastrointestinal implications, and it is important that it should not be made without its specific features, i.e., diagnosis usually requires the opinion of a dermatologist to whom the specific physical signs and histologic and immunologic features are well known. Although an itchy rash predominantly affecting extensor surfaces with grouped papules and small tense blisters is usual, atypical forms occur, including large blister forms: The exacerbation of the rash by iodides, its response to treatment with sulfones and sulfonamides, and the histologic finding of papillary-tip microabscesses in recent (nonblistered) lesions all help in diagnosis but are not totally specific. The finding of granular or fibrillary IgA deposits in clinically uninvolved skin is likewise not completely specific[58]: It is nevertheless the most valuable single criterion in reliable hands, but even this finding should not be the sole criterion for diagnosis, and it is inadvisable for nondermatologists to label a rash dermatitis herpetiformis from the immunofluorescence findings alone.[59] When facilities are not available, or their quality is in doubt, the author has shown that a combination of clinical and histologic features and response to treatment is as good as the results of immunofluorescence. In linear IgA disease celiac disease occurs but probably less often and the different frequencies of the HLA types, DQW1 and 2, suggest that linear IgA disease is different from classical dermatitis herpetiformis.[60] It must be remembered however that numbers in this relatively rare group are still small.

Celiac Disease in Dermatitis Herpetiformis Although there was initially some difficulty in accepting that the enteropathy of dermatitis herpetiformis was celiac disease,[61] this is no longer the case. Doubt arose mainly because of the mildness of the enteropathy in dermatitis herpetiformis compared with that of celiac disease as it usually presents to the gastroenterologist. Severe celiac disease does occur in patients with dermatitis herpetiformis but is rare, most cases being mild, subclinical, or latent. Celiac disease can usefully be considered as the proverbial iceberg with a submerged zone of subclinical disease of unknown, but probably considerable, dimension. Thus it can be expected that much of the celiac disease discovered will indeed be subclinical if the cases selected for small intestinal mucosal biopsy are those that present to the dermatologist with what we now know is a marker of celiac disease. The structural abnormalities are, as in celiac disease, sometimes patchy, worse in the proximal small bowel, and responsive to withdrawal gluten.

Diagnosis and Incidence of Celiac Disease in Dermatitis Herpetiformis Although the exact incidence of this condition is not known, it is unlikely to be high because 10 to 20 percent of patients have rashes and only a proportion of these are dermatitis herpetiformis. By contrast, the proportion of patients with dermatitis herpetiformis who have celiac disease is high. The precise number depends on the criteria used for diagnosing celiac disease. Only 33 percent of the author's series[58] have clinical or biochemical evidence of celiac disease, but 58 percent have structural abnormalities on stereomicroscopic or histologic examination.

Attempts have been made to extend the diagnostic criteria of celiac disease, and, if we take a raised interepithelial lymphocyte count in the small bowel even in the absence of other abnormalities as indicating celiac disease,[62] the incidence in our patients with dermatitis herpetiformis becomes 81 percent. Whatever criteria are used for diagnosis, the percentage of patients with dermatitis herpetiformis in whom celiac disease can be demonstrated still falls short of 100 percent. This shortfall may well change with new techniques.

Relationship of Dermatitis Herpetiformis and Celiac Disease The nature of this relationship remains unknown. In particular the presence of clinical celiac disease is obviously not necessary for the development of dermatitis herpetiformis, and malabsorption cannot be the cause of the rash. Likewise the role of gluten, which is generally thought to be important in the production of the rash, is not known. Although the gut almost always responds to gluten withdrawal, the response of the skin is less clear and its time course is remarkably prolonged. Moreover, the responses of skin and gut can occur independently of one another.[63] Patients with dermatitis herpetiformis and celiac disease have a significant increase in the incidence of HLA B8, DR3, and DQW2. This increase occurs even in the patients with dermatitis herpetiformis who apparently do not have celiac disease and suggests a genetic association. Although the consensus view is that the rash as well as the bowel defect is caused by gluten sensitivity, the evidence that gluten alone is responsible is still not entirely convincing.

Treatment of Dermatitis Herpetiformis with a Gluten-free Diet There are several reasons for wanting to treat dermatitis herpetiformis with a gluten-free diet. Obviously patients with clinical and biochemical evidence of celiac disease should be treated this way. It is more difficult to advise people with dermatitis herpetiformis who have only structural changes in the small bowel mucosa or no detectable changes at all. When malignant disease, especially lymphoma of the gastrointestinal tract, has been reported in patients with dermatitis herpetiformis, it has usually been in conjunction with celiac disease.[64] In this disease it seems likely that control of the disease with a gluten-free diet protects against malignancy; ideally patients with dermatitis herpetiformis should be placed on a gluten-free diet for this reason, although the small numbers of patients make it difficult to know if it prevents lymphomas.

Quite apart from prescribing a gluten-free diet for the bowel in patients with dermatitis herpetiformis, there is the question of prescribing it for the skin. A number of patients develop dermatitis herpetiformis when they are on a gluten-free diet for celiac disease and when their enteropathy is, as a result, well controlled. Nevertheless the general view is that a strict gluten-free diet enables the rash to be controlled without dapsone, or with a much reduced dose of dapsone, in a significant proportion of patients, although this control may take months or years. Those intolerant of dapsone are candidates for dietary management, if diet is effective. Otherwise patients may prefer dapsone to the inconvenience of a lifelong dietary restriction.

References

1. Gazzard BG: HIV disease and the gastroenterologist. *Gut* **29**:1497, 1988
2. Kitchen V et al: Ulcerating pharyngo-oesophageal leukoplakia, in *Advanced HIV Disease*. Montreal, 5th International Conference on AIDS, **244**:262, 1989
3. Moynahan E: The treatment and management of epidermolysis bullosa. *Clin Exp Dermatol* **7**:665, 1982
4. Cooper T, Bauer E: Therapeutic efficacy of phenytoin in recessive dystrophic epidermolysis bullosa. *Arch Dermatol* **120**:490, 1984
5. Hardy KM et al: Benign mucous membrane pemphigoid. *Arch Dermatol* **104**:467, 1971
6. Dickens C et al: The oesophagus in lichen planus: Endoscopic studies. *Br Med J* **300**:84, 1990

7. Holmes GKT et al: Malignancy in coeliac disease—effect of a gluten free diet. *Gut* **30**:333, 1989

8. Howel-Evans W et al: Carcinoma of the oesophagus with keratosis palmaris et plantaris (tylosis). *Q J Med* **27**:413, 1958

9. Robson AO, Jelliffe AM: Medicinal arsenic poisoning and lung cancer. *Br Med J* **2**:207, 1963

10. Weihrauch TR, Korling GW: Manometric assessment of oesophageal involvement in progressive systemic sclerosis, morphoea and Raynaud's disease. *Br J Dermatol* **107**:325, 1982

11. Harrison DF: Familial haemorrhagic telangiectasia: 20 cases treated with systemic oestrogen. *Q J Med* **33**:25, 1964

12. Bean WB: *Vascular Spiders and Related Lesions of the Skin.* Springfield, Charles C Thomas, 1958

13. Pope FM et al: Patients with Ehlers-Danlos syndrome type IV lack type III collagen. *Proc Natl Acad Sci USA* **72**:1314, 1975

14. Pope FM: Autosomal dominant pseudoxanthoma elasticum. *J Med Genet* **11**:152, 1974

15. Jellinek EH, Tulloch WS: Herpes zoster with dysfunction of bladder and anus. *Lancet* **2**:1219, 1976

16. Moore MR et al: Drugs and the acute porphyrias. *Trends Pharmacol Sci* **2**:330, 1981

17. Morgan SH, Crawford M d'A: Anderson-Fabry disease. A commonly missed diagnosis. *Br Med J* **297**:872, 1988

18. Carron DB, Douglas AP: Steatorrhoea in vascular insufficiency of the small intestine. *Q J Med* **34**:331, 1963

19. Degos R et al: Dermatite papulosquameuse atrophiante. *Bull Soc Fr Dermatol Syphiligr* **52**:60, 1942

20. Hall-Smith P: Malignant atrophic papulosis (Degos' disease). *Br J Dermatol* **81**:817, 1969

21. Bussey H, Morson B: Familial polyposis coli, in *Gastrointestinal Tract Cancer,* edited by M Lipkin, R Good. New York, Plenum, 1978, p 275

22. Gardner EJ: A genetic and clinical study of intestinal polyposis, a predisposing factor for carcinoma of the colon and rectum. *Am J Hum Genet* **3**:167, 1951

23. Jeghers H et al: Generalised intestinal polyposis and melanin spots of the oral mucosa, lips and digits. *N Engl J Med* **241**:993, 1961

24. Spigelman AD et al: Cancer and the Peutz-Jeghers syndrome. *Gut* **30**:1588, 1989

25. Cunliffe W, Anderson J: Case of Cronkhite-Canada syndrome with associated jejunal diverticulosis. *Br Med J* **4**:601, 1967

26. Davis GB, Berk RN: Intestinal neurofibromas in von Recklinhausen's disease. *Am J Gastroenterol* **60**:410, 1973

27. Hickman JG, Lazarus GS: Pyoderma gangrenosum: A reappraisal of associated systemic diseases. *Br J Dermatol* **102**:235, 1980

28. Powell FC et al: Pyoderma gangrenosum: A review of 86 patients. *Q J Med* **55**:173, 1985

29. McCallum DI, Kinmont PDL: Dermatological manifestations of Crohn's disease. *Br J Dermatol* **80**:1, 1968

30. Edwards FC, Truelove SC: The course and prognosis of ulcerative colitis. *Gut* **5**:1, 1964

31. Croft CB, Wilkinson AR: Ulceration of mouth, pharynx and larynx in Crohn's disease of the intestine. *Br J Surg* **59**:249, 1972

32. Cronin E: In *Contact Dermatitis.* Edinburgh, Churchill Livingstone, 1980, p 886

33. Silverman JM, Hamlin JA: Large melanoma metastases to the gastrointestinal tract. *Gut* **30**:1783, 1989

34. Rowell NR: The connective tissue diseases, in *Textbook of Dermatology,* 5th ed, edited by A Rook et al. Oxford, Blackwell, 1992, p 2163

35. Cox NH et al: Dermatomyositis and malignancy in an audit of the value of extensive investigation. *Br Med J* **121**:47, 1989

36. Graham-Smith DD: The carcinoid syndrome. *Gut* **28**:1413, 1987

37. Scott BB et al: Involvement of the small intestine in systemic mast cell disease. *Gut* **16**:918, 1975

38. Austad WI et al: Steatorrhoea and malignant lymphoma. *Am J Dig Dis* **12**:475, 1967

39. Mallinson et al: A glucagonoma syndrome. *Lancet* **2**:1, 1974

40. Choksi VA et al: An unusual skin rash associated with a pancreatic polypeptide producing tumour of the pancreas. *Ann Intern Med* **108**:64, 1988

41. Thivolet J: Necrolytic migratory erythema without glucagonoma. *Arch Dermatol* **117**:4, 1981

42. Shuster S: The gut and the skin, in *Third Symposium of Advanced Medicine. Proceedings of a Conference Held at Royal College of Physicians, London,* edited by AM Dawson. London, Pitman Medical, 1967, p 349

43. Vickers CFH: Nutrition and the Skin, in *Tenth Symposium on Advanced Medicine.* London, Pitman Medical, 1974

44. Sims RT: Hair as an indicator of incipient and developed malnutrition and response to therapy—principles and practice, in *An Introduction to the Biology of the Skin,* edited by RH Champion et al. Oxford, Blackwell, 1970, p 387

45. Cook WT et al: Symptoms, signs and diagnostic features of idiopathic steatorrhoea. *Q J Med* **22**:57, 1953

46. Badenoch J: Steatorrhoea in the adult. *Br Med J* **2**:879, 1960

47. Wells GC: Skin disorders and malabsorption. *Br Med J* **2**:937, 1962

48. Kennedy C: The spectrum of inflammatory skin disease following jejuno-ileal bypass for morbid obesity. *Br J Dermatol* **105**:425, 1981

49. Greaves MW, Boyd TRC: Plasma-zinc concentrations in patients with psoriasis, other dermatoses and venous leg ulceration. *Lancet* **2**:1019, 1967

50. Hawkins T et al: Whole body monitoring and other studies of zinc 65 metabolism in patients with dermatological disease. *Clin Exp Dermatol* **1**:243, 1976

51. Lombeck et al: Akrodermatitis enteropathica eine Zinkstoffwechselstorung mit Zinkmalapsorption. *Z Kinderheilkd* **120**:181, 1975

52. Moynahan EJ: Acrodermatitis enteropathica: A lethal inherited human zinc deficiency. *Lancet* **2**:399, 1974

53. Prottey C et al: Correction of the cutaneous manifestations of essential fatty acid deficiency in man by application of sunflower seed oil to the skin. *J Invest Dermatol* **64**:918, 1975

54. Shuster S, Marks J: Dermatogenic enteropathy—a new cause for steatorrhoea. *Lancet* **1**:1367, 1965

55. Marks J, Shuster S: Small intestinal mucosal abnormalities in various skin diseases—fact or fancy. *Gut* **11**:281, 1970

56. Harper R, Jackson DC: Progressive systemic sclerosis. *Br J Radiol* **38**:825, 1965

57. Hendel L et al: Enterocyte function in progressive systemic sclerosis. *Gut* **28**:435, 1987

58. Marks J: Dogma and dermatitis herpetiformis. *J Clin Exp Dermatol* **2**:189, 1977

59. Karlsson I et al: Absence of cutaneous IgA in coeliac disease without dermatitis herpetiformis. *Br J Dermatol* **99**:621, 1978

60. Sachs J et al: A comparative serological and molecular study of linear IgA disease and dermatitis herpetiformis. *Br J Dermatol* **118**:759, 1988

61. Weinstein WM et al: What is coeliac sprue, in *Coeliac Disease. Proceedings of an International Conference Held at the Royal Postgraduate Medical School, London,* edited by CC Booth, RH Dowling. Edinburgh, Churchill Livingstone, 1970, p 232

62. Fry L et al: Lymphocytic infiltration of epithelium in diagnosis of gluten-sensitive enteropathy. *Br Med J* **3**:371, 1972

63. Fry L et al: Long-term follow up of dermatitis herpetiformis with and without gluten withdrawal. *Br J Dermatol* **107**:631, 1982

64. Leonard JN et al: Increased incidence of malignancy in dermatitis herpetiformis. *Br Med J* **286**:16, 1983

CHAPTER 165

Joseph L. Jorizzo and Elizabeth F. Sherertz

A number of diseases are characterized by distinctive cutaneous and renal manifestations. These diseases are covered extensively elsewhere in this volume and a partial list is outlined in Table 165-1. Occasionally skin biopsy may be helpful in establishing a diagnosis of renal disease such as IgA nephropathy.[1,2] The remainder of this discussion will be devoted to a review of cutaneous changes related to chronic renal failure, changes seen in patients on dialysis, and changes seen in patients who have undergone renal transplantation. These subjects have also been reviewed recently.[3,4]

Cutaneous Changes Related to Chronic Renal Failure

The sequelae of chronic renal failure are complex and involve multiple systems. Careful examination of the skin, hair, nails, and mucous membranes reveals many abnormalities in these patients and may be an important component of the first impression made by these patients.

Changes in skin color may be striking. Pallor is usually present and results from anemia. A sallow, yellowish cast to the skin is caused by urochrome deposition in skin.[5] Hyperpigmentation often occurs and may be accentuated in a photodistribution. This hyperpigmentation may be related to abnormal excretion of β-MSH with associated increases in skin pigmentation.[6]

TABLE 165-1

Some Examples of Diseases with Prominent Cutaneous and Renal Manifestations

Immunologic/rheumatologic diseases
  Poststreptococcal glomerulonephritis
  Systemic lupus erythematosus
  Scleroderma
  Necrotizing vasculitis
    Small-vessel necrotizing venulitis
    Larger vessel
      Polyarteritis nodosa
      Wegener's granulomatosis
Hematologic/oncologic diseases
  Thrombotic thrombocytopenic purpura
  Dysproteinemia
  Leukemia/lymphoma
  Solid tumors
Genetic/metabolic diseases
  Diabetes mellitus
  Gout
  Tuberous sclerosis
  Neurofibromatosis
  Nail patella syndrome
  Angiokeratoma corporis diffusum universale (Fabry's disease)
Other diseases
  Familial Mediterranean fever
  Amyloidosis
  Sarcoidosis

Cutaneous Changes in Renal Disorders

Extensive ecchymoses are a sequela of hemostatic abnormalities. Dry skin and poor skin turgor are related to the dehydration that accompanies chronic renal failure.

Calcinosis cutis can occur in this setting due to secondary hyperparathyroidism.[7] Hard papules, nodules, or plaques which may manifest chalky discharge are typical. Calcium deposits in blood vessels may result in cutaneous ulceration. A distinctive necrotizing panniculitis has also been described in this setting.[8] Primary oxalosis resulting in renal failure has been associated with livedo reticularis in which oxalate crystals may be found on biopsy.[9]

"Half-and-half" nails have been described in patients with chronic renal failure and consist of a proximal white half of the nail due to edema of the nail bed and a distinct normal distal portion (Fig. 165-1). This abnormality does not correlate with the severity of the uremia.[10] Uremic frost is a classic manifestation of chronic renal failure. This finding was not uncommon when described in 1865 as white deposits on the skin of the face and neck in patients dying of uremia. The presumed mechanism was deposition of crystallized urea from sweat. This finding is rare today.

Cutaneous Changes Particularly Prevalent in Patients on Dialysis

Pruritus

Generalized pruritus without a primary cutaneous eruption can be a sign of underlying internal disease in as many as 50 percent of patients who present with this cutaneous sign. Uremia is detected in a percentage of these patients (2 of 44 patients in a recent series).[11] Conversely 70 to 90 percent of patients with chronic renal failure are affected by "prolonged bothersome itch."[12,13] Dialysis appears to be an important trigger of pruritus. The pruritus is often intermittent, occurring in intense paroxysms. In one study 37 percent of 237 dialysis patients experienced pruritus at a given point in time.[12]

The pathogenesis of uremic pruritus remains unclear. Pruritus is not a feature of acute renal failure. Subtotal parathyroidectomy has been associated with relief of pruritus in patients with secondary hyperparathyroidism due to chronic renal failure. A direct role for parathyroid hormone in causing uremic pruritus has been questioned because of the failure of intradermal injections of parathyroid hormone analogs to cause pruritus, and because of negative immunohistochemical studies for parathyroid hormone in skin biopsy specimens.[14] Parathyroid hormones have been postulated to cause mast cell proliferation in skin, and histamine has been postulated to cause uremic pruritus.[15] Other studies have shown increased mast cells in the skin of pruritic patients on dialysis, but no relationship to parathyroid levels.[16] Whether mast cell numbers might be increased or decreased in uremic patients is controversial. A recent study showed no difference in cutaneous mast cell numbers in uremic patients with or without pruritus.[17]

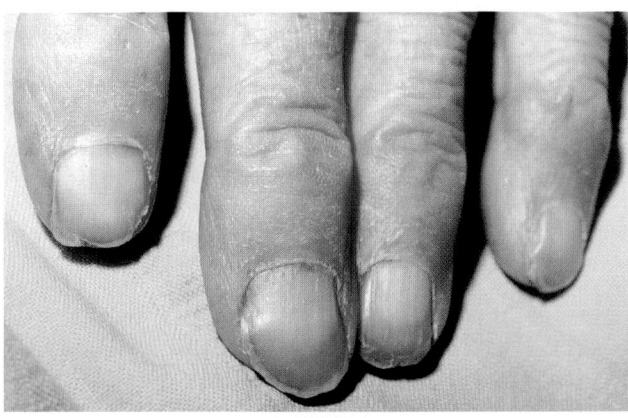

FIGURE 165-1 Half-and-half nails in a patient with chronic renal failure.

Xerosis may also contribute to pruritus in these patients.[18] Atrophy of sweat glands and sebaceous glands is seen histologically in these patients and may contribute to the xerosis. However recent studies have also questioned whether insufficient hydration even exists in the epidermis of uremic patients on dialysis.[19] A dialysis-resistant, transplant-responsive microangiopathy occurs in skin of patients in renal failure but it is still unclear how this may contribute to pruritus.[20]

Hyperphosphatemia is associated with uremic pruritus, and a lowering of serum phosphorus levels is often associated with control of pruritus. The mechanism by which ultraviolet B ameliorates uremic pruritus may involve a decrease in skin phosphorus content, possibly via an effect on vitamin D.[21] It is also possible that ultraviolet B has direct effects on mast cells or other inflammatory cells. Levels of vitamin A may be increased in the epidermis of patients with uremia. The epidermal retinol content may be reduced after ultraviolet B therapy.[22] Recent immunohistochemical studies have shown neuron-specific enolase immunoreactive nerve fibers sprouting through the epidermis in dialysis patients but not in control subjects, raising the question of whether abnormal patterns of cutaneous innervation may occur in dialysis patients and account for their pruritus.[23] No significant difference exists in the distribu-

tion of neurochemical markers, such as neuropeptides, in uremic patients versus control subjects.[24]

In summary, despite ongoing investigation, the cause of uremic pruritus remains undefined. A multifactorial etiology is likely.

Treatment for uremic pruritus can be difficult. Ultraviolet B therapy has become a mainstay of therapy. Treatment of half of the body produces generalized improvement, implying a systemic effect.[25] Other described systemic therapies including lidocaine, mexiletine, activated oral charcoal, and oral cholestyramine are impractical, are associated with complications such as binding of therapeutic drugs, or have other unacceptable side effects.[13] Topical antipruritic agents including pramoxine, emollients, and carefully administered antihistamines with central nervous system effects are somewhat useful as therapeutic adjuncts.[26] It is important to rule out other causes of pruritus in uremic patients, such as scabies.[27]

Bullous Disease

A bullous dermatosis resembling porphyria cutanea tarda has been well described in patients undergoing chronic hemodialysis. Bullae favor sun-exposed skin and heal with scarring and milia formation (Fig. 165-2). The other cutaneous signs of porphyria cutanea tarda, such as hirsutism, are absent. Histopathologically the bullae are indistinguishable from lesions of porphyria cutanea tarda.[28] A similar process occurs in patients taking furosemide or nalidixic acid, and many of these patients had renal failure.[29] The absence of urine output has complicated the evaluation of patients with chronic renal failure for true porphyria which, not surprisingly, can also occur in this setting.[30] Most patients with the bullous dermatosis of hemodialysis have normal uroporphyinogen decarboxylase activity and normal fecal and plasma porphyrin studies.[31] Further assessment of porphyrin metabolism abnormalities is warranted in these patients.

Perforating Disease

As many as 10 percent of patients on dialysis develop various perforating disorders described as Kyrle's disease,[32] perforating follic-

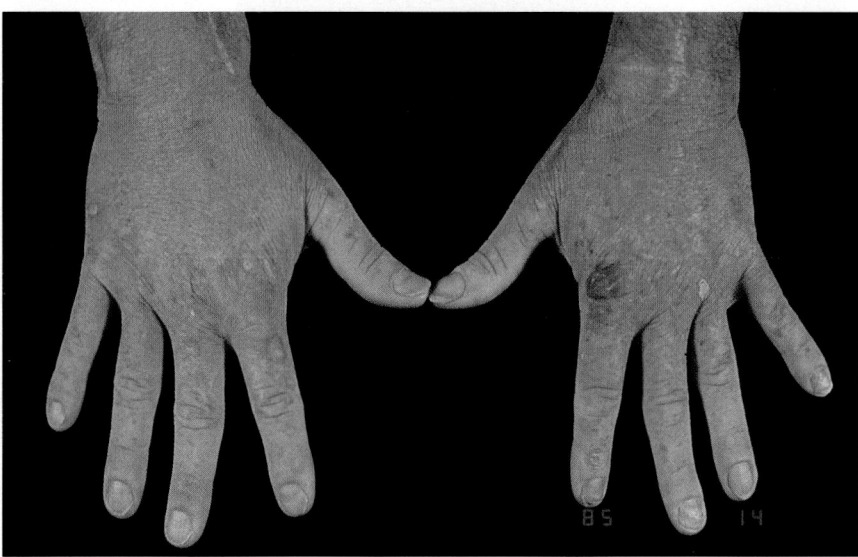

FIGURE 165-2 Bullous dermatosis in a patient undergoing chronic hemodialysis.

ulitis,[33] or reactive perforating collagenosis.[34] Clinical and histologic similarities among these cases of perforating diseases associated with uremia are striking, and an argument has been made to unify them as acquired perforating disease of chronic renal failure[35] (see Chap. 48). Diabetes mellitus is a frequent finding in these patients and a recent patient had acquired immunodeficiency syndrome and end-stage renal disease.[36] The mechanism of connective tissue alteration in these disorders is unknown. Trauma such as from scratching may play a role.

Various therapies have been described for perforating disorders, including keratolytics, topical 5-fluorouracil, topical corticosteroids, and topical retinoic acid.[35] Aggressive control of uremic pruritus with ultraviolet B and control of the serum phosphorus level is also beneficial.

Other Skin Disease

Contact dermatitis to dialysis tubing, nickel (needles), and topical medicaments may occur in patients on dialysis. A benign vascular proliferation called acroangiodermatitis or pseudo-Kaposi's sarcoma can occur over arteriovenous fistula sites (Fig. 165-3) and may resolve only with thrombosis or removal of the fistula.[37] Increased carriage of *Staphylococcus aureus* has been found in patients undergoing peritoneal dialysis and hemodialysis and may predispose patients to folliculitis, furunculosis, or catheter site infections. "Dialysis acne" has been noted in patients receiving hemodialysis and has been associated with testosterone therapy given to stimulate hematopoiesis.[38] Infectious eccrine hidradenitis may occur in patients on dialysis and present as crops of violaceous papules or pustules.[39]

Cutaneous Changes in Renal Transplant Patients

Patients with renal and other transplants have a host of cutaneous problems including reactions to medications, infections occurring

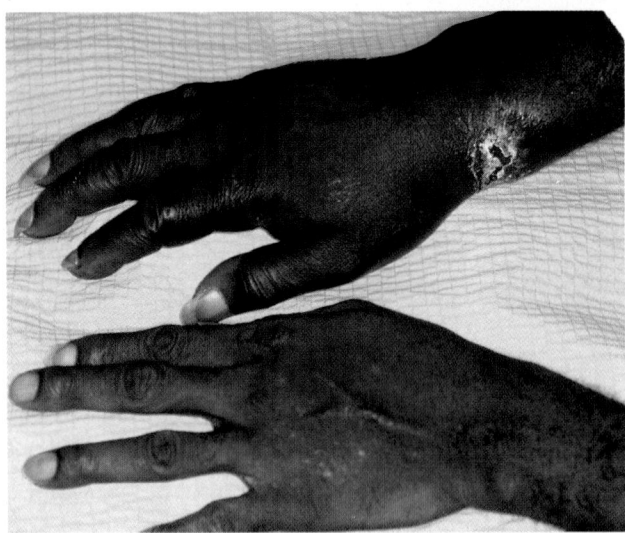

FIGURE 165-3 Acroangiodermatitis (pseudo-Kaposi's sarcoma) due to vascular proliferation distal to the site of an arteriovenous fistula.

in the setting of the iatrogenic immunosuppression required in these patients, and neoplasms occurring in the setting of immunosuppression. A review of the direct cutaneous sequelae of systemic corticosteroids is beyond the scope of this review, as is a review of the sequelae of other therapy, but they are described elsewhere.[4]

Cutaneous infections are well described in renal transplant patients. Human papilloma virus infections are particularly problematic.[40] Widespread infections with molluscum contagiosum, dermatophytes, *Candida,* and tinea versicolor are common in these patients as well. Septic vasculitis or other cutaneous manifestations of disseminated infection with unusual bacteria, virus, acid-fast organisms, and fungi are unfortunately not rare in this patient population. Systemic infections with *Pneumocystis carinii, Candida, Aspergillus, Nocardia,* and cytomegalovirus may be associated with significant morbidity in these patients.

Squamous cell carcinomas and keratoacanthomas may occur with increased frequency, possibly as a result of reduced immune surveillance.[41] Basal cell carcinomas may also occur with increased frequency. The incidence of Kaposi's sarcoma also appears to be increased. The dermatologist should be involved in the pretransplantation evaluation of renal patients to treat warts and actinic keratoses, to educate patients about sun protection, and to establish cutaneous surveillance as part of the follow-up.

References

1. Zawada GT, Ramirez G: The skin in IgA nephropathies. *Cutis* **36**:341, 1985
2. Hene RJ et al: The relevance of IgA deposits in vessel walls of clinically normal skin. *Arch Intern Med* **146**:745, 1986
3. Gupta AK et al: Cutaneous associations of chronic renal failure and dialysis. *Int J Dermatol* **25**:498, 1986
4. Abel EA: Cutaneous manifestations of immunosuppression in organ transplant recipients. *J Am Acad Dermatol* **21**:161, 1989
5. Kopple JD, Massry SG: Uremic toxins: What are they? How are they identified? *Semin Nephrol* **3**:263, 1983
6. Smith AG: Role of the kidney in regulating plasma immunoreactive beta-melanocyte stimulating hormone. *Br Med J* **1**:874, 1976
7. Kolton B, Pedersen J: Calcinosis cutis and renal failure. *Arch Dermatol* **110**:256, 1974
8. Mehregan DA, Winkelmann RK: Cutaneous gangrene, vascular calcification, and hyperparathyroidism. *Mayo Clin Proc* **64**:211, 1989
9. Greer KE et al: Primary oxalosis with livedo reticularis. *Arch Dermatol* **116**:213, 1980
10. Leyden JJ, Wood MG: The half and half nail of uraemic onychodystrophy. *Arch Dermatol* **105**:591, 1972
11. Kantor GR, Lookingbill DP: Generalized pruritus and systemic disease. *J Am Acad Dermatol* **9**:375, 1983
12. Gilchrest BA et al: Clinical failures of pruritus among patients undergoing maintenance hemodialysis. *Arch Dermatol* **118**:154, 1982
13. Denman ST: A review of pruritus. *J Am Acad Dermatol* **14**:375, 1986
14. Stahle-Backdahl M et al: Experimental and immunochemical studies on the possible role of parathyroid hormone in uremic pruritus. *Ann Intern Med* **225**:411, 1989
15. Gilchrest BA: Pruritus: Pathogenesis, therapy, and significance in systemic disease states. *Arch Intern Med* **142**:101, 1982
16. Matsumoto M et al: Pruritus and mast cell proliferation of the skin in end stage renal failure. *Clin Nephrol* **23**:285, 1985
17. Klein LR et al: Cutaneous mast cell quantity in pruritic and non-pruritic hemodialysis patients. *Int J Dermatol* **27**:557, 1988
18. Young AW et al: Dermatologic evaluation of pruritus in patients on hemodialysis. *NY State J Med* **73**:2370, 1973
19. Stahle-Backdahl M: Stratum corneum hydration in patients undergo-

ing maintenance hemodialysis. *Acta Derm Venereol (Stockh)* **68**:531, 1988

20. Gilchrest BA et al: Clinical and histological cutaneous findings in uremia: Evidence from a dialysis-resistant, transplant-responsive microangiopathy. *Lancet* **2**:1271, 1980.

21. Blackley JD et al: Uremic pruritus and skin ion content. *Am J Kidney Dis* **5**:236, 1985

22. Berne B et al: UV treatment of uraemic pruritus reduces the vitamin A content of skin. *Eur J Clin Invest* **14**:203, 1984

23. Stahle-Backdahl M: Uremic pruritus: Clinical and experimental studies. *Acta Derm Venerol (Stockh)* (suppl) **145**:1, 1989

24. Johansson O et al: Immunohistochemical screening for neurochemical markers in uremic patients on maintenance hemodialysis. *Skin Pharmacol* **1**:265, 1988

25. Gilchrest BA et al: Ultraviolet phototherapy of uremic pruritus: Long-term results and possible mechanisms of action. *Ann Intern Med* **91**:17, 1979

26. Jorizzo JL et al: Prurigo: A clinical review. *J Am Acad Dermatol* **4**:723, 1981

27. Lempert KD: Pseudouremic pruritus: A scabies epidemic in a dialysis unit. *Am J Kidney Dis* **5**:117, 1985

28. Gilchrest BA et al: Bullous dermatosis of hemodialysis. *Ann Intern Med* **83**:480, 1975

29. Kennedy AC, Lyell A: Acquired epidermolysis bullosa due to a high dose furosemide. *Br Med J* **1**:1509, 1976

30. Poh-Fitzpatrick MB, Masuillo AS et al: Porphyria cutanea tarda associated with chronic renal disease and hemodialysis. *Arch Dermatol* **116**:191, 1980

31. Matarredona J et al: Bullous dermatosis of hemodialysis. *J Dermatol* **12**:410, 1985

32. Hood AF et al: Kyrle's disease in patients with chronic renal failure. *Arch Dermatol* **118**:85, 1982

33. Hurwitz RM et al: Perforating folliculitis in association with hemodialysis. *Am J Dermatol* **4**:101, 1982

34. Cochran RJ et al: Reactive perforating collagenosis of diabetes mellitus and renal failure. *Cutis* **31**:55, 1983

35. Patterson JW: The perforating disorders. *J Am Acad Dermatol* **10**:561, 1984

36. Bank DE et al: Reactive perforating collagenosis in a setting of double disaster: Acquired immunodeficiency syndrome and end-stage renal disease. *J Am Acad Dermatol* **21**:371, 1989

37. Goldblum OM et al: Pseudo-Kaposi's sarcoma of the hand associated with an acquired, iatrogenic arteriovenous fistula. *Arch Dermatol* **121**:1038, 1985

38. Fuchs E et al: Dialysis acne. *J Am Acad Dermatol* **23**:125, 1990

39. Moreno A et al: Infectious eccrine hidradenitis in a patient undergoing hemodialysis. *Arch Dermatol* **121**:1106, 1985

40. Rudlinger R et al: Human papilloma virus infections in a group of renal transplant recipients. *Br J Dermatol* **115**:681, 1986

41. Gupta AK et al: Cutaneous malignant neoplasms in patients with renal transplants. *Arch Dermatol* **122**:1288, 1986

Cutaneous Manifestations of Disorders of the Cardiovascular and Pulmonary Systems

CHAPTER 166

Andrew G. Franks, Jr.

Cutaneous Aspects of Cardiopulmonary Disease

Descriptions of abnormalities of the skin in association with diseases of the heart and lungs are among those first recorded in medical antiquity. While many are familiar and easily recognizable by the physician, others are unique and may remain a diagnostic challenge (Table 166-1). The primary objective of this chapter is to present the cutaneous manifestations of selected cardiopulmonary diseases; however, in addition, interesting associations between the skin, heart, and lung are also included.

A number of situations in which the skin and the cardiopulmonary system are both involved are described elsewhere in this volume. These conditions include pruritus associated with cardiac failure or pulmonary insufficiency (see Chap. 31), pigmentary changes associated with hemochromatosis or endocrine abnormalities (see Chaps. 163 and 169), the hyperlipidemias (see Chap. 152), mucocutaneous lymph node syndrome (see Chap. 216), lipoid proteinosis (see Chap. 154), and amyloidosis (see Chap. 149).

Alterations in Skin Quality

The skin may be warm in patients with erythroderma or exfoliative dermatitis due to shunting or increased metabolism with or without high-output congestive failure. Hyperthyroidism with increased cardiac output and vasodilation may lead to increased skin temperature. Conversely the temperature may be reduced in patients with hypothyroidism and low-output congestive failure secondary to atherosclerotic disease or myocardial infarction.

Systemic amyloidosis may cause waxy induration of the skin and when stroked it may become hemorrhagic (''pinch purpura''). Cardiac conduction disturbances, myocardial disease, and orthostatic hypotension are common.

Hyperelastic velvety skin that rebounds to the original position after being stretched, ''cigarette-paper'' scars, and hyperextensible joints are characteristic of the Ehlers-Danlos syndrome (see Chap. 157). Mitral and tricuspid prolapse, dilatation of the aorta and pulmonary artery, arterial rupture, a variety of congenital heart diseases, and panacinar emphysema may accompany this syndrome.[1]

A progressive looseness of the skin with pendulous folds and droopy eyelids can be a clue to cutis laxa (see Chap. 157). This condition may be associated with generalized hyperelastosis that may cause aortic dilatation and rupture, congestive heart failure, or pulmonale with pulmonary artery stenosis and progressive emphysema.[2]

The skin of patients with pseudoxanthoma elasticum is thick, lax, and yellowish, especially over the axillae, antecubital area, and neck (Fig. 166-1). The skin around the mouth may sag. Yellow patches may occur on mucous membranes, especially the labia. The arteries may be calcified, and the aortic and mitral valves thickened. Angina pectoris and claudication are frequent symptoms.[3]

TABLE 166-1
Diseases with Heart and Skin Involvement

Joint and connective tissue diseases	Nevoid or genetic disorders
Rheumatoid arthritis	Progressive lentigines
Systemic lupus erythematous	(Moynahan syndrome)
Reiter's syndrome	Watson syndrome
Behçet's syndrome	Neurofibromatosis
Systemic scleroderma	Tuberous sclerosis
Dermatomyositis	LEOPARD syndrome
Rheumatic fever	LAMB syndrome
Ehlers-Danlos syndrome	NAME syndrome
Cutis laxa	Danoff syndrome
Marfan's syndrome	Infectious diseases
Periarteritis nodosa	Varicella
Multicentric reticulohistiocytosis	Gonococcemia
Metabolic diseases	Subacute and acute bacterial
Hemochromatosis	endocarditis
Amyloidosis	Chagas' disease
Fabry's disease	Diphtheria
Carcinoid tumors	Miscellaneous (protozoal,
Myxedema	viral, rickettsial, and
Hyperlipidemias	bacterial infections)
Hyperthyroidism	Diseases of uncertain etiology
	Sarcoidosis
	Whipple's disease
	Mucocutaneous lymph node
	syndrome
	Degos' disease

Source: Modified and reprinted with permission from *Dermatologic Capsule & Comment,* edited by TB Fitzpatrick. September 1987, p 9.

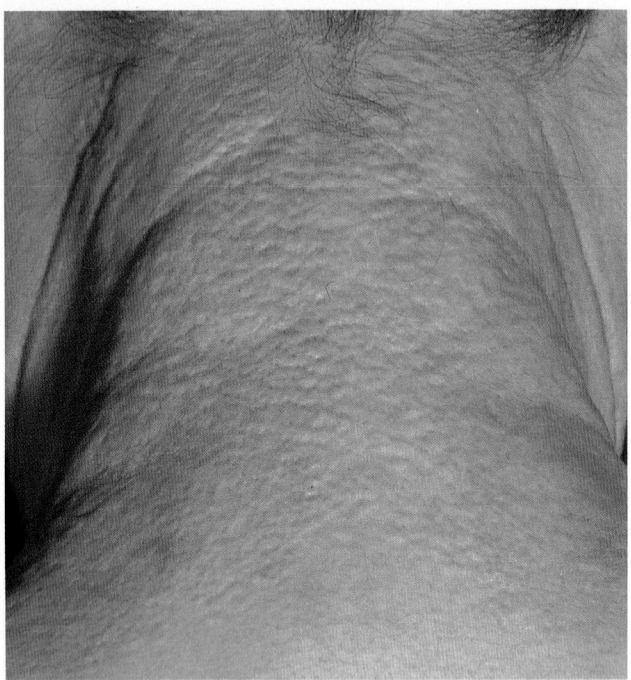

FIGURE 166-1 Pseudoxanthoma elasticum. Thickened, pebbly, yellowish lesions on the neck. *(Courtesy of Klaus Wolff, M.D.)*

In Werner's syndrome (progeria) the skin appears atrophic and tight; there is marked loss of subcutis, with ulcerations of the legs and severe coronary atherosclerosis; death by myocardial infarction is frequent at an early age.[4]

Changes in Skin Color

Changes in skin color are due to a number of variables including hemoglobin, melanin, carotene, vasoactivity, metals, and miscellaneous other phenomena.

Cyanosis

An increase in the absolute amount of desaturated (reduced) hemoglobin results in a purplish or bluish discoloration of the skin. By definition, cyanosis is divided into "central" and "peripheral" types, the latter being the more common. Conceptually the terms refer to the level of arterial oxygen saturation, and not to the anatomic source of the cyanosis. Thus central cyanosis occurs in states that produce low arterial oxygen saturation, such as congenital heart disease with intracardiac or intrapulmonary right-to-left shunting as well as most severe pulmonary diseases. Peripheral cyanosis occurs in states that have normal arterial oxygen saturation but reduced blood flow, such as low-output cardiac failure of any etiology, and local vasospastic phenomena. Pulmonary embolism may result in a combination of central cyanosis due to intrapulmonary shunting and peripheral cyanosis due to low cardiac output.

Central cyanosis is usually present on the warm areas of the skin such as the tongue, oral mucosae, and conjunctivae. Peripheral cyanosis is usually seen on the cool areas such as the nose, lips,

earlobes, and fingertips. However this distinction is not absolute since both central and peripheral cyanosis may affect any of the aforementioned areas of the body. Detection of cyanosis may be difficult, even to the experienced observer. Although the tongue is probably the area where it is most easily detected, a number of false-positive evaluations may occur. Therefore examination of the fingertips and conjunctivae, while less sensitive, may reflect the underlying condition more clearly. In the anemic patient, detection of cyanosis may be impossible since the absolute amount of reduced hemoglobin is not increased. To avoid confusion with staining of the skin, either topically or from systemic deposits of heavy metals or other chemicals, it is important to note that cyanosis fades when pressure is applied since the color is within the blood vessels.[5]

Cyanosis that is more intense in the fingers than in the toes suggests complete transportation of the great vessels, with either a preductal coarctation or complete interruption of the aortic arch, pulmonary hypertension, and a reversed shunt through a patent ductus arteriosus. If the cyanosis is slightly more on the right hand, coarctation of the aorta is more likely. Equal cyanosis of both hands suggests complete aortic interruption.[6]

Cyanosis and clubbing of the toes associated with cyanosis in the left hand and a normal right hand suggest pulmonary hypertension with a reversed shunt through a patent ductus arteriosus bringing saturated blood to the left arm and both legs.[7]

Redness/Flushing

Redness of the skin may be due to an increase in the amount of saturated hemoglobin, an increase in the diameter or actual number of skin capillaries, or a combination of these factors.

Erythroderma or exfoliative dermatitis with intense redness may be associated with so much capillary dilatation that high-output cardiac failure occurs, especially in compromised patients.[8]

Polycythemia may produce the characteristic "ruddy" complexion, but may also cause a peculiar coloration termed *erythremia,* which is a combination of redness and cyanosis. The tongues, lips, nose, earlobes, conjunctivae, and fingertips especially demonstrate this coloration. Erythremia results when increased amounts of saturated hemoglobin produce the redness and when increased amounts of desaturated hemoglobin produce cyanosis because of the inability of the body to oxygenate fully the increased absolute amounts of hemoglobin. The absence of nail clubbing may help differentiate patients with polycythemia vera from those patients with cardiopulmonary disease who develop secondary polycythemia. In addition, the hypervolemic state of polycythemia vera is associated with increased stroke volume and may lead to high-output cardiac failure, while pulmonary infarction may result from venous thrombosis and embolization caused by hyperviscosity.[9]

Paroxysmal intense flushing of the face, neck, chest, and abdomen, often with telangiectases of the face and neck, may occur in patients with carcinoid tumors that have metastasized to the liver and thereby produce increased amounts of serotonin (see Chap. 170). Serotonin and histamine are responsible for the bronchospasm seen in this syndrome. Fibrosis of the right side of the heart may lead to a combination of stenosis and regurgitation at the tricuspid valve and pulmonary stenosis. If cyanosis occurs, the combination of flushing and cyanosis may produce the reddish, cyanotic erythremia seen in some patients with polycythemia. Occasionally patients in whom this syndrome develops have a patent ductus arteriosus or foramen ovale, and metastases occur in the lung. In this setting, left-sided cardiac lesions may also occur.[10]

Systemic mastocytosis may produce flushing as a result of vasodilatation and may be associated with telangiectasia (see Chap. 161). Histamine release from degranulated mast cells is the pathogenetic mechanism. Cardiopulmonary alterations include hypotension and bronchospasm.[11]

Pheochromocytomas may cause flushing of the face and forehead as well as redness and cyanosis of the hands (see Chap. 170). Generalized, extreme flushing, mimicking carcinoid, may occur in Sipple's syndrome, in which levels of prostaglandin, serotonin, and catecholamine are increased.[12]

Edema of the face, arms, and hands associated with redness and/or cyanosis may indicate obstruction of the superior vena cava due to mediastinal disease.

Erythromelalgia (Labile Hyperthermia)   Atherosclerosis, hypertension, and polycythemia may produce this peculiar pattern of erythema on the hands and feet, or it may be idiopathic. During the episodes, and especially when exposed to heat, patients complain of pain, warmth, and swelling of the areas, which sometimes extend to the elbows and knees. The pulse is either normal or slightly increased in intensity.[13]

Palmar Erythema   Palmar erythema may occur in many healthy women, but recent onset or increased intensity of this condition raise the possibility of liver involvement (see Chap. 163). Palmar erythema may be associated with high-output cardiac failure. The erythema primarily involves the hypothenar eminence but may also affect the thenar eminence and the fingertips. Other factors, including pregnancy and hyperthyroidism, may cause this condition.[5]

Jaundice

Hyperbilirubinemia and jaundice may occur in patients in heart failure as a result of raised intrahepatic pressure due to passive congestion. Hemorrhagic pulmonary infarction with destruction of red cells and hemoglobin may also produce jaundice, especially in patients with passive congestion of the liver. Constrictive pericarditis and tricuspid valvular disease may produce jaundice secondary to cardiac cirrhosis. Under fluorescent light, jaundice may be difficult to assess.[4]

Alterations in Sweating

Sweating may be prominent in a number of cardiopulmonary states such as acute myocardial infarction, cardiogenic shock, left ventricular failure, massive pulmonary emboli, and pulmonary edema. Pallor and clamminess or coldness of the extremities and exposed surfaces are also often found. When associated with hypertension, excessive sweating may suggest pheochromocytoma. There may also be additional features such as flushing, most prominent in those patients with Sipple's syndrome in whom prostaglandin and serotonin production by the tumor may simulate carcinoid. Myocardial infarction may occur or cardiac failure may develop due to a metabolic cardiomyopathy. Neurofibromatosis and café au lait macules have been found in as many as 10 percent of patients, especially those with bilateral pheochromocytoma.[12]

The sodium and chloride content of sweat is increased in patients with cystic fibrosis and may lead to an increase in skin wrinkling after immersion, as when bathing.[14]

Alterations of Nails, Hands, and Arms

Nail Clubbing

Nail clubbing and osteoarthropathy are distinct entities that may be associated with significant cardiopulmonary abnormalities (Fig. 166-2).

Clinically, nail clubbing has various manifestations. Beaking or distal curvature of the nail may occur. There may be loss of the normal 15° angle between the nail and cuticle (unguophalangeal angle). Sponginess or "floating" of the nail when pressure is applied is also characteristic. Finally the size of the terminal tuft may increase. This change may be quantified by measuring the depth of the finger at the base of the nail and dividing by the depth of the finger at the distal interphalangeal (DIP) joints. The ratio should normally be less than 1.0.

Clubbing most commonly occurs in patients with bronchogenic carcinoma, suppurative lung disease, endocarditis, and congenital heart disease, but it may be idiopathic or familial.[4]

Quincke Pulse

Flushing of the nail beds synchronous with the heartbeat is one sign of aortic regurgitation called Quincke pulsation.[7]

In addition, the fingernail beds may be used to evaluate the microcirculation. Capillary "fill" is estimated by pressing down on the nail bed until blanching occurs. Following release, there should be immediate filling and a pink appearance. However perfusion of the skin may not reflect perfusion of internal organs.

Hypertrophic Osteoarthropathy

Hypertrophic osteoarthropathy often has clubbing as a feature, but in addition there is an associated arthralgia and/or arthritis of the fingers, wrists, knees, and ankles, as well as painful periostitis revealed as subperiosteal new bone formation on x-ray. Suffusion of the digits may be prominent, with pitting edema. Shiny skin with increased sweating and paronychial thickening are sometimes noted.

Although hypertrophic osteoarthropathy is most often associated with malignant tumors of the chest, there are numerous other disorders that produce this syndrome. In addition, some cases are primary or idiopathic. Pachydermoperiostosis, a primary form, is frequently familial. Its onset is around puberty and it has a number of cutaneous manifestations. Distinctive thickening and furrowing of the skin of the scalp, forehead, and cheeks may create a leonine facies. Other features include excessive sweating, especially of the hands and feet, severe seborrhea of the scalp and face, and dermatitis of the hands and feet.[15] Familial clubbing alone may also be found and may represent a partial expression of this syndrome. Thyroid acropachy may mimic osteoarthropathy but is most often painless.

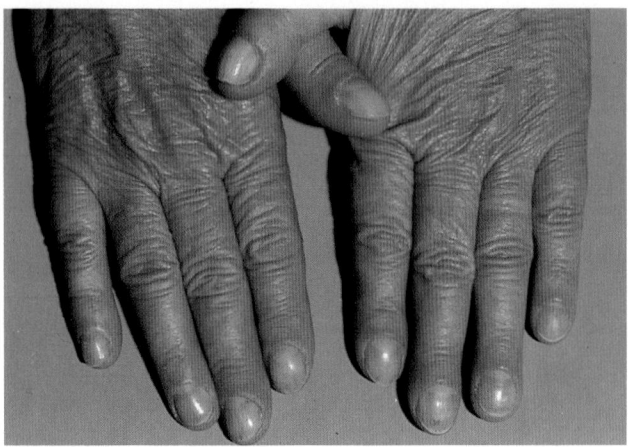

FIGURE 166-2 Clubbing of fingernails. *(Courtesy of Klaus Wolff, M.D.)*

Shoulder-Hand Syndrome

The shoulder-hand syndrome is a painful periarthritis or adhesive capsulitis of the shoulder (''frozen shoulder''), usually on the left side, associated with erythema, sweating, shiny induration, edema, tenderness, pain, and immobility of the ipsilateral hand. Neurotrophic ulcerations of the fingers and thickening of the palmar aponeurosis with nodules and/or Dupuytren's contracture may be late sequelae. This syndrome was observed in up to 15 percent of patients with myocardial infarction in the past when bed rest was prolonged, but it is now uncommon. Other predisposing conditions include arterial embolization, cerebrovascular accidents, and protective disuse of the arms for any reason.[16]

The Heart and the Skin

Coronary Heart Disease

Familial Hyperlipidemia The risk of coronary artery disease (CAD) may increase with elevation of plasma cholesterol and triglyceride concentrations.[17,18] Familial hyperlipidemias comprise a group of metabolic disorders with elevated plasma cholesterol and/or triglyceride, and some may be associated with a high incidence of CAD. Xanthomatosis may be present in patients with these disorders, and they have been associated for many years with a high incidence of CAD.[19] As noted previously, the lipidoses are discussed in Chap. 152.

Earlobe Crease A number of reports relate coronary artery disease to the presence of a diagonally positioned skin crease along the earlobe.[20–23] These creases may be unilateral or bilateral. It is not known whether such creases are congenital or acquired, nor is the mechanism of their formation understood.

Their association with other risk factors including hyperlipidemia has not been evaluated. However their presence suggests an increased risk for CAD based on clinical,[24] angiographic,[25] and postmortem[26] studies.

Cholesterol Emboli (See Chap. 167) In patients with advanced atherosclerosis of the abdominal aorta, cholesterol crystals may microembolize to the lower extremities, particularly after invasive vascular procedures or surgery. The pulses may remain normal.[27,28] In addition to complaints of pain in the legs, buttocks, and low back, as well as myalgia, restless legs, or abdominal symptoms, both renal insufficiency and various skin lesions frequently develop.[29] Livedo reticularis affecting the lower abdomen and back, buttocks, legs, and feet may occur.[30] Ulcerations on the legs and feet, surrounded by an erythematous or violaceous halo and a small scab, may be present.[31] Cyanosis and digital gangrene may simulate necrotizing vasculitis.[32,33]

Indurated plaques and nodules have been noted as well,[34] and their association with livedo reticularis and ulceration may mimic polyarteritis nodosa.[35] These plaques and nodules are firm, violaceous, painful, and necrotic in the center. They are most prominent on the thighs and calves. Superficial skin biopsy is often nondiagnostic; deep skin and muscle biopsy revealing the intraarteriolar site of pathology is more useful.[36,37] The characteristic findings are arterioles occluded by multinucleated foreign-body giant cells and fibrosis surrounding biconvex, needle-shaped clefts corresponding to the cholesterol crystal microemboli.[38]

Postbypass Skin Changes Coronary artery bypass surgery is commonly performed using the superficial veins of the legs as donor-graft sites. A dermatitis has been reported to occur along the saphenous vein graft scars on the medial aspect of the legs.[39,40] Patients with this problem have no history of venous stasis, thrombophlebitis, ankle edema, or skin disease. Examination generally reveals a reddish-brown, slightly scaling, and fissured dermatitis along the distal part of a well-healed saphenous vein graft scar. Each case developed 2 to 6 months after surgery and the patients returned to full activity. The cause is unclear but may be related to the high incidence of postoperative thrombophlebitis[41] and resultant stasis dermatitis. The dermatitis responds to topical corticosteroids.

Recurrence is usual and most patients have required continued treatment. Interestingly, one patient[39] had two episodes of secondary infection with coagulase-positive *Staphylococcus aureus* at the vein graft site which antibiotics cleared. In one large series of over 2000 patients undergoing coronary revascularization with saphenous vein, 1 percent had leg wound complications at the vein graft site within the immediate postoperative period. Most had either *S. aureus* or mixed gram-negative infections, primarily in the thigh area.[42]

In another group of patients, recurrent cellulitis develops in the healed vein graft many months after surgery. These patients present with fever and chills; erythema may extend along the entire vein graft site, accompanied by pain and tenderness. Swelling may be significant, and often the patients are initially considered to have thrombophlebitis. Although cultures are not always positive, beta-hemolytic streptococcus was isolated in a number of cases. Treatment with intravenous antibiotics followed by oral antibiotics cleared the infection, but recurrence was not unusual.[43]

The presence of an associated tinea pedis in patients with this complication was reported[44] as well. The authors recommend that all patients considered for vein graft surgery be examined carefully for evidence of tinea infections of the feet, which, if found, should be treated vigorously with antifungal medication prior to surgery. Vein graft dermatitis with the subsequent secondary infection may also play a role in the development of cellulitis.

Cardiomyopathy

Cutaneous abnormalities may aid in the diagnosis and subsequent treatment of some kinds of cardiomyopathy. These disorders of the myocardium affect ventricular function and may produce cardiac failure. A useful classification divides cardiomyopathies into dilated, nondilated, and hypertrophic types. It has recently been stressed that each type of cardiomyopathy has a distinct differential diagnosis and that little etiologic overlap occurs.[45]

Thus a specific cutaneous finding in conjunction with the appropriate studies to determine the type of cardiomyopathy may be very important in making the correct diagnosis. Either radionuclide ventriculography or two-dimensional echocardiography estimates ventricular volume and left ventricular ejection fraction. These measurements are utilized to distinguish among the three types of cardiomyopathy. Tables 166-2 and 166-3 list the causes of cardiomyopathy according to type.

Myxoma

Atrial myxomas, the most common primary tumors of the heart, are benign hamartomatous intracardiac tumors that may produce a wide variety of clinical symptoms and signs and may simulate a number of disease states.

The cardiopulmonary findings reviewed in one series of 24 cases[46] included in order of frequency: congestive heart failure (54 percent), mitral murmur (38 percent), chest pain (29 percent), pulmonary edema (25 percent), and embolic phenomena (21 percent).

Additionally, valvular insufficiency, constrictive pericarditis, conduction blocks, arrhythmias, and intracardiac shunts may occur. Variable murmurs may be an important clue.

Pulmonary emboli and pulmonary hypertension may also occur, in addition to other systemic findings, including fever, cachexia and malaise, arthralgias, arthritis, clubbing, hypergammaglobulinemia, anemia or polycythemia, thrombocytosis or thrombocytopenia, and leukocytosis.[46]

The cutaneous manifestations of atrial myxomas may be dramatic. In addition to biphasic digital color changes on cold exposure,[47] various cutaneous lesions have been described which simulate collagen vascular disease or vasculitis: tender, violaceous, nonblanching, annular, and serpiginous lesions of the digital pads, as well as splinter hemorrhages presenting as a systemic vasculitis[48] or infective endocarditis. Others have reported characteristic pruritic, erythematous papules as well as cyanosis and ecchymosis of the extremities.[49] A reddish-violet malar flush along with macular erythema and cyanosis of digits simulated acute rheumatic fever in one patient.[50]

Another patient with arthritis and nonblanching erythema was thought to have rheumatoid arthritis.[51] The diagnosis may be made by biopsy of the skin and subcutaneous tissue in an area of embolic infarct. Myxomatous emboli with large pale-staining cytoplasms and stellate nuclei may be found among occluded blood vessels.[46]

Before the introduction of the echocardiogram in 1960, over 80 percent of patients were undiagnosed at postmortem. The diagnosis may now be made earlier and more frequently during routine echocardiography, allowing successful surgical intervention.

Recently various associations of atrial myxoma with mucocutaneous pigmented lobules, including lentigines (Fig. 166-3), nevomelanocytic nevi and blue nevi, as well as dermal myxomatous nodules, have been described[52,53] (Table 166-4).

TABLE 166-2
Causes of Cardiomyopathy by Type

Dilated
  Coronary artery disease with multiple infarcts*
  Alcoholic*
  Peripartum
  Valvular*
  Infectious acute inflammatory myocarditis*
  Chagas' disease*
  Sarcoid*
  Doxorubin toxicity
  Uremia*
  Hemochromatosis*
  Pheochromocytoma*
  Hypocalcemia
  Diabetes mellitus*
  Nutritional (? selenium)
  Idiopathic
Nondilated
  Amyloid heart disease*
  Endomyocardial diseases
    Löffler's disease*
    Pseudoxanthoma elasticum*
    Endomyocardial fibrosis (Davies' disease)
  Neoplastic*
    Melanoma*
  Ventricular thrombosis
    Polycythemia vera*
    Mitral valve prosthesis
  Idiopathic
Hypertrophic
  Genetic form (? autosomal dominant)
  Acquired or secondary forms
    Neurofibromatosis*
    Lentiginosis*
    Hyperthyroidism*
    Hypothyroidism*
    Noonan's syndrome
    Hypertension
    Valvular or subvalvular obstruction of left ventricular
      outlet tract
    Pompe's disease
    Friedreich's ataxia
    In infants of diabetic mothers

*May have significant cutaneous features.
Source: Modified from Johnson and Palacios.[45]

Leopard Syndrome

Multiple lentigines syndrome, an autosomal dominant disorder, has been associated with numerous abnormalities of variable clinical expression including disturbances of the heart.[54,55] Each letter of the mnemonic "leopard" represents a feature of the syndrome: L, lentigines, multiple; E, electrocardiogram conduction defects; O, ocular telorism; P, pulmonary stenosis; A, abnormalities of genitalia; R, retardation of growth; D, deafness, sensorineural[55] (see Chap. 80).

Other malformations and related disorders have also been reported.[56] Multiple lentigines which are usually present at birth are the most characteristic feature of the syndrome. They vary in size, shape, and shades of brown to black. While the entire body, including the palms and soles may be covered, the oral mucosa and lips are spared.[55,56]

The abnormal pigmentation may also be found in the iris and retina.[57] There is a tendency for the lentigines to increase in number and size with age, especially around puberty, but they are not af-

TABLE 166-3
Infectious Causes of Acute Dilated Cardiomyopathy*

Coxsackie virus B	Cytomegalovirus
Coxsackie virus A	Mumps
Echo virus	Psittacosis
Poliovirus	*Cryptococcus neoformans*
Arbovirus (dengue, chikungunya fever)	*Candida albicans*
Toxoplasma gondii	*Trichinella spiralis*
Trypanosoma cruzi	*Schistosoma mansoni*
Mycoplasma pneumoniae	*Corynebacterium diphtheriae*
Varicella	*Neisseria meningitidis*
Variola	*Leptospira*
Influenza	Polymicrobial bacterial
Rabies	myocarditis

*Most have cutaneous features.
Source: Modified from Johnson and Palacios.[45]

TABLE 166-4
Clinical Findings Associated with Atrial Myxoma

LEOPARD syndrome*†	NAME syndrome‡
Lentiginosis	Nevi
Electrocardiographic	Atrial
abnormalities	Myxoid neurofibrotoma
Ocular hypertelorism	Ephelides
Pulmonic stenosis	Danoff syndrome§
Abnormal genitalia	Adrenocortical micronodular
Retardation	dysplasia
Deafness	Lentigines
LAMB syndrome‡	Atrial myxoma
Lentigines	Spindle cell tumors
Atrial myxoma	
Mucocutaneous myxomas	
Blue nevi	

*Skeletal deformities can occur frequently.
†Autosomal dominant inheritance.
‡Inheritance pattern not determined.
§Possible autosomal dominant inheritance
Source: Reprinted with permission from *Dermatologic Capsule & Comment,* Fitzpatrick TB (ed), September 1987, p 10.

fected by sun exposure because they appear in areas not normally exposed to sunlight.[55,56,58]

Giant melanosomes were found in dermal melanophages, melanocytes, and keratinocytes in all epidermal layers in a patient with multiple lentigines syndrome.[59]

The disorder may arise in the neuroectoderm.[58] Involvement of the neural crest in the development of the inner ear and the sympathetic nervous system may explain some features of the system.[56]

The types of cardiac involvement include electrocardiogram conduction disturbances and anatomic malformation. Axis deviation,[56] prolonged P-R intervals,[60] left anterior hemiblock,[56] bundle branch block,[61] and complete heart block[57] have been reported.

Hypertrophic cardiomyopathy appears to be the most common anatomic abnormality.[58,62] Subaortic stenosis is the most common valvular lesion.[58] Although earlier reports suggested that pulmonary stenosis was frequent,[55] some of the clinical and physiological

features pf hypertrophic cardiomyopathy mimic pulmonary stenosis and were clarified only after catheterization[62] or echocardiography.[63]

Because the clinical expression of the conduction disturbances and the anatomic malformation vary in onset and severity, frequent cardiac evaluation should be performed.

Subacute Bacterial Endocarditis

The cutaneous manifestations of bacterial endocarditis are important clues to the diagnosis, although less frequently than in the preantibiotic era. They include Osler's nodes, Janeway lesions, subungual splinter hemorrhages, cutaneous purpura and petechiae, and conjunctival petechiae (Roth's spots).

Petechiae are the most common mucocutaneous manifestation of bacterial endocarditis, their incidence varying from 20 to 40 percent of patients with both acute and subacute bacterial endocarditis.[64,65] Small, red, or violaceous macules that do not blanch subsequently become brownish and fade. Purpuric lesions, both flat and elevated, have also been associated with subacute endocarditis without evidence of platelet dysfunction and may represent a leukocytoclastic vasculitis.[66,67] The petechiae may be observed on the skin, especially on the heels, shoulders, and legs, but the conjunctiva and oral mucosa must also be evaluated.[68]

Osler's nodes and Janeway lesions may both present as erythematous or hemorrhagic macules, papules, or nodules (Fig. 166-4). However, while Osler's nodes are exquisitely painful, tender, and located distally on the digital tufts, Janeway lesions are nontender and located proximally on the palms and soles.[69,70] Osler's original description in 1885 did not specify the tenderness of these lesions,[71] but his later report[72] did emphasize the findings noted above.

Histologically Osler's nodes are a perivasculitis or necrotizing vasculitis without microabscess formation or other evidence of infection or emboli.[73–76] However Osler himself considered them septic emboli.[71] Cultures have generally been negative, although more recent reports have reemphasized the possibility of septic microemboli with microabscess formation.[77] Janeway lesions have also been described histologically as a vasculitis with microabscess

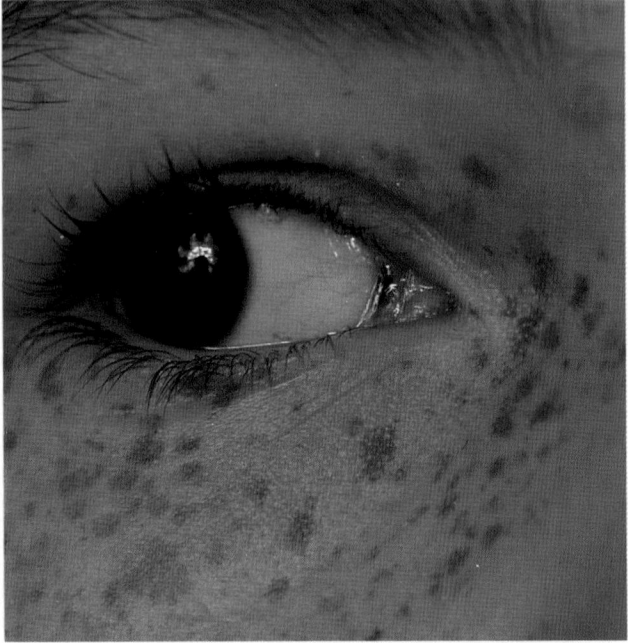

FIGURE 166-3 Lentiginous lesions in the atrial myxoma syndrome complex. This child has the LAMB syndrome (see Table 166-4). *(Courtesy of Klaus Wolff, M.D.)*

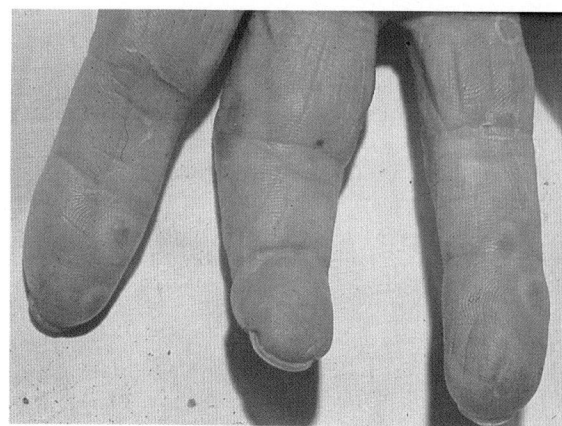

FIGURE 166-4 Osler nodules. *(Courtesy of Klaus Wolff, M.D.)*

formation.[78] The cutaneous and conjunctival petechiae are histologically similar.[79]

Current theories regard the pathogenesis of both Osler's nodes and Janeway lesions as immunologic or allergic due to immune complex deposition.[80,81] Some reports dispute this concept, suggesting that the initial event is a septic microembolism that subsequently causes the endothelial swelling and perivasculitis seen in older lesions.[77] Thus organisms may be occasionally cultured initially, but later the lesions become sterile.

That infected arterial catheters may precipitate clinical lesions comparable to Osler's nodes, Janeway lesions, and splinter hemorrhages supports the concept that these lesions are infectious in etiology.[82-84] Osler's nodes and Janeway lesions have been found in patients with other conditions, particularly systemic lupus erythematosus, gonococcemia, hemolytic anemia, and typhoid fever.[85-87]

An unusual presentation of endocarditis caused by *Erysipelothrix rhusiopathiae,* with bullae of the hand initially mimicking herpes zoster, has been noted.[88] This organism, while rare, is sometimes seen in butchers and fish handlers and is responsible for erysipeloid. In contrast to this "cutaneous only" form (see Chap. 190), the systemic infection may lead to endocarditis. Early diagnosis of the offending organism may be made by the history of exposure to meats and fish and the bullous eruption on the violaceous base. Of importance, the bullae that are subepidermal are usually sterile. Diagnosis can be made by culturing the tissue.[89] *E. rhusiopathiae* is a slender, curved, nonmotile, non-spore-forming gram-positive bacillus. It is a facultative anaerobe that produces alpha hemolysis on sheep blood sugar.

The Lungs and the Skin

Yellow Nail Syndrome

Yellow nails with primary lymphedema were described in 1964.[90] Separately, primary lymphedema and pleural effusion were reported.[91] The triad of yellow nails, primary lymphedema, and pleural effusion was then recognized,[92] followed by a number of reports with partial or complete features.

The characteristics of nails include thickening, transverse ridging, diminished growth, increased curvature with a "hump," and onycholysis. The lunulae and cuticles may be absent. The color may vary from pale yellow to green[93,94] (Fig. 166-5). The nail changes are secondary to congenitally hypoplastic lymphatics.[95]

The lymphedema in this disorder is also due to congenitally hypoplastic lymphatics.[90] It is characteristically slowly progressive and somewhat asymmetric, with induration and hyperkeratosis extending to the thighs. Periodic lymphangitis is frequent and may contribute to the swelling.[92]

Respiratory findings include sinusitis, bronchiectasis, and pleural effusions. Symptoms vary from mild to severe, and some patients require repeated thoracentesis, treatment for pneumonia secondary to bronchiectasis, and drainage of the sinusitis. Patients may have a productive or nonproductive cough, dyspnea, frequent upper respiratory infections, and pneumonia. Chest x-rays may be normal but generally reveal evidence of fibrosis and/or effusion at the bases.[95]

Pulmonary features and lymphedema may not occur until late in the course; therefore follow-up of patients who present with this type of nail dystrophy is recommended.[95] Finally a number of patients have developed lymphomas or sarcomas with metastases.[95]

Pulmonary Arteriovenous Fistulas

Pulmonary arteriovenous fistulas are congenital abnormalities of capillary development that may not become clinically apparent until late adolescence.[96] Osler-Rendu-Weber disease (hereditary hemorrhagic telangiectasia), an autosomal dominant trait, may be present in one-third to one-half of such patients.[97] It is characterized clinically by punctate, linear, or spider-like telangiectasias of the skin, especially the upper body, oral and nasal mucous membranes, and nail beds (Fig. 166-6). The radiating arms about an elevated punctum are the most characteristic feature, especially on the lips and tongue. They are distinguished from true spider telangiectasis in that they do not pulsate.[98]

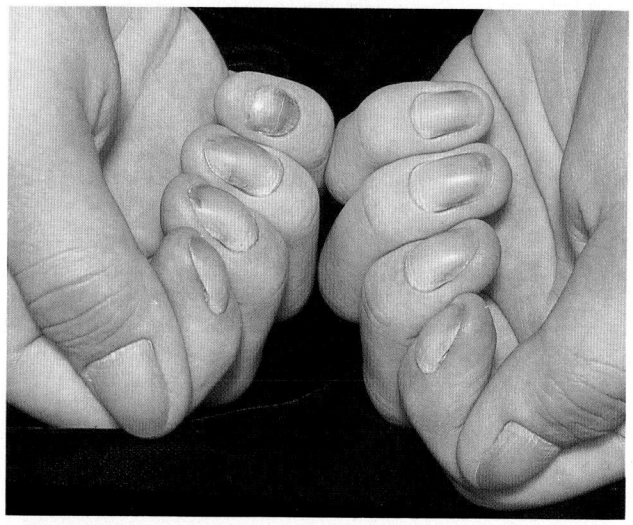

FIGURE 166-5 Yellow nail syndrome. There is thickening, increased curvature, and yellowish discoloration of all fingernails. This patient had lymphedema of the extremities and bronchiectasis with multiple recurrent respiratory infections. *(Courtesy of Klaus Wolff, M.D.)*

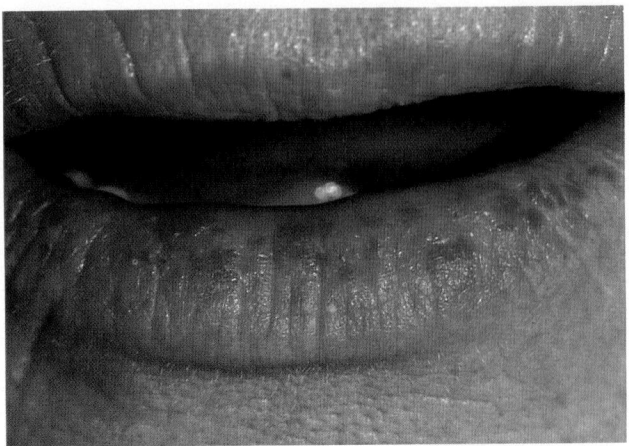

FIGURE 166-6 Osler-Rendu-Weber disease. Note the punctate and splinter-like telangiectasia on the lips. *(Courtesy of Klaus Wolff, M.D.)*

Recurrent epistaxis is the most frequent presenting symptom and may begin in early childhood or adolescence. Other organ systems besides the lungs may be involved, including the liver, gastrointestinal and genitourinary tracts, and central nervous system, and recurrent hemorrhage may result. Bleeding may be enhanced by an associated von Willebrand's disease.[99]

The pulmonary findings in those patients with an arteriovenous fistula of the lungs include dyspnea, hemoptysis, cyanosis, clubbing, polycythemia, and pulmonary bruits accentuated by inspiration. Chest x-rays reveal nodular "coinlike" lesions, sometimes initially considered to be metastatic disease.

Asthma-Eczema Complex (Atopy) (See Chap. 120)

The association of atopic (infantile) eczema, asthma, and hay fever is well known. Although infants with eczema are at increased risk of asthma and hay fever, there appears to be a difference in prevalence of each component. Different hereditary patterns probably exist, with some patients developing only one or two components of the atopic diathesis. The early onset of eczema, its severity, and its duration past the age of 2 years all appear to favor the later development of asthma and/or hay fever.

Mediators of the atopic inflammatory response may be released by sensitized IgE-mast cell complexes present along the tracheobronchial tree. Dust, pollen, and dander may initiate this response.

Although asthma may be divided into extrinsic and intrinsic types, most patients have overlapping clinical features. The extrinsic group has known external allergies (to dust, pollen, and dander), a higher prevalence of associated eczema and hay fever, and a higher prevalence of positive atopic family history.[100]

Cutaneous Findings in Chronic Pulmonary Diseases

Chronic obstructive pulmonary disease (COPD) is actually a group of disorders including chronic bronchitis, bronchiectasis, emphysema, and asthma. The incidence and mortality of COPD have increased recently and approach that of heart disease in the United States. Smoking habits as well as increased longevity of the popu-

lation may be responsible, in part, for this increase. Genetic, infectious, occupational, and environmental factors also contribute.

Two basic types of COPD have been described: type A, or emphysematous, and type B, or bronchial. Clinically both may present with dyspnea, cough, wheezing, and recurrent respiratory infections. Type A patients have been termed "pink puffers" since they usually hyperventilate and maintain arterial oxygen tension. Type B patients have been termed "blue bloaters" since they frequently are hypoxic with cyanosis and associated right congestive heart failure. These patients, especially if young, should be evaluated for the possibility of cystic fibrosis.

Cigarette stains on the fingertips may be helpful in determining the cause of COPD when the patient's history is unclear.[101]

Cystic Fibrosis

Cystic fibrosis is an autosomal recessive disorder of the exocrine glands that subsequently involves the tracheobronchial tree, pancreas, and gastrointestinal tract. The basic alteration of mucus is unknown, but viscid mucous plugs may cause fecal impaction, intussusception, and rectal prolapse in infancy. Pancreatic insufficiency may subsequently predominate but it is the pulmonary disease that is the most significant feature. Progressive lung disease with chronic bronchitis, emphysema, and cor pulmonale from cystic fibrosis is a leading cause of death among patients with genetic disorders in the United States. As patients live longer with appropriate antibiotic care and tracheobronchial toilet, other features such as cirrhosis, hemoptysis, and pneumothorax have been noted.[102]

The cutaneous features of this disorder result from increased amounts of electrolyte in the sweat, which leads to excessive skin wrinkling when the palms and soles are immersed in water. Although this feature is not always present, it may be a valuable clue to the disease. Parents are often aware of, but not disturbed by, the wrinkling.[103]

Larva Migrans and Pulmonary Involvement (See Chap. 225)

Cutaneous larva migrans or creeping eruption may occasionally cause minimal respiratory symptoms and be associated with transient pulmonary infiltrates and a peripheral eosinophilia (Löffler's syndrome). The skin lesions are initially nonspecific and highly pruritic, and subsequently progress to erythematous, serpiginous, tunnel-like tracks. Older lesions are frequently excoriated and crusted.

Visceral larva migrans or toxocariaris may lead to granulomatous involvement of the liver, lungs, heart, muscle, brain, and eyes. Marked eosinophilia, hyperglobulinemia, pneumonitis with wheezing, recurrent bronchitis, fever, and tender hepatomegaly frequently occur. Skin lesions may present as patchy urticaria or erythematous papular eruptions.[104]

Fat Embolism Syndrome

Petechiae, respiratory insufficiency, and cerebral dysfunction after long bone fracture are termed the fat embolism syndrome. Petechiae alone after fractures should suggest this syndrome. Histologically fat globules are present within the dermal and pulmonary vessels. Additional factors such as hyperglycemia, diabetes, or elevated beta-lipoproteins may play a contributing role.

The petechiae are most commonly on the neck, axillae, shoulder, chest, and conjunctivae, and often appear before other manifestations. They begin about the second or third day after injury, appear in crops, and are almost never found on the face or posterior aspects of the body. When widespread, they tend to herald more significant cerebral and pulmonary dysfunction. In addition, cyanosis may be prominent.[105]

The respiratory involvement may begin with dyspnea, tachypnea, or hemoptysis. Tachycardia, fever, and pulmonary edema may occur. X-rays may show patchy densities or linear streaks progressing to the bilateral opacities characteristic of the adult respiratory distress syndrome.[106]

Cerebral dysfunction includes restlessness, irritability, delirium, and coma. Additional features include jaundice, renal involvement, anemia, thrombocytopenia, and elevated sedimentation rate.

Selected Diseases Affecting the Cardiopulmonary System

Lipoid Proteinosis (Hyalinosis Cutis et Mucosae) (See Chap. 154)

Affected individuals are homozygous for a mutant recessive autosomal gene[107] but have normal chromosome findings.[108] The disease is worldwide in distribution. Deposition of the amorphous "hyalin," while primarily affecting the mucous membranes and skin, has also been found in other organ systems, including the respiratory tract and heart.[109]

Oropharyngeal and laryngeal mucous membranes are usually affected early in the course of the disease, during infancy or childhood. The tongue enlarges and acquires a firm consistency and a smooth, glistening surface (Fig. 166-7a). Hoarseness due to laryngeal infiltration is often the initial finding and may be present at birth.[110] Laryngeal and tracheal infiltration may progress to obstruction and cause respiratory insufficiency requiring tracheostomy.[111] The trachea and main-stem bronchus may be thickened and studded with wartlike hyaline projections.[110] An increased risk of aspiration pneumonia has been reported,[112] as well as repeated upper respiratory infections.[113] Cardiovascular involvement is rare, but conduction defects and arrhythmias have been reported.[110]

The skin abnormalities usually appear in childhood shortly after the onset of mucous membrane changes. These consist of waxy, translucent induration, followed by papules, nodules, and plaques, characteristically on the face (Fig. 166-7b), which are easily traumatized.[114] A beadlike pattern on the palpebral margins and angles of the mouth is common.[115]

Additional cutaneous manifestations include pitted acne-like scarring, alopecia, hyperkeratosis particularly over elbows, knees, and knuckles, and onychodystrophy.[110]

Multicentric Reticulohistiocytosis (See Chap. 179)

Multicentric reticulohistiocytosis (MRH) is an uncommon disorder presenting with characteristic mucocutaneous lesions and a deforming arthritis[116,117] in association with systemic symptoms such as fever, malaise, weight loss, and myopathy.[118–120] The cardiopul-

monary complications include pulmonary infiltrates,[121] pleural effusions,[119,122] pericarditis,[116] cardiomegaly,[116] congestive heart failure,[116] angina pectoris,[116] myocardial infarction,[123] and pulmonary infarction.[123]

The eruption is composed of yellow to brown, firm papules and nodules especially localized about the hands and face. The dorsum of the hand is more commonly involved than the palm. The paronychial zone and lateral aspects of the digits, with accentuation about the finger joints, are also typically affected.[118] Involvement of the scalp, ears, and nose may coalesce, resulting in a leonine appearance.[124] The mucous membranes are also involved and infiltration of the lips, gingiva, tongue, and pharynx are reported.[118] Histologically these lesions are composed of histiocytic, multinucleated giant cells that are both PAS-positive and sudanophilic.[121] The PAS-positive material is thought to represent a mucoprotein or glycoprotein and the sudanophilic material may represent a combination of triglycerides, cholesterol, neutral fat, phospholipids, and glycolipids.[125]

The arthritis is frequently inflammatory[117] and, when associated with the nail dystrophy that occurs in the disease,[126] it may mimic psoriatic arthritis. There is early involvement of the distal interphalangeal (DIP) joints. Rheumatoid arthritis may be considered, but MRH patients are seronegative.[126]

An association of MRH with malignancy has been recorded in a few reports,[118,121,127] suggesting the need for complete evaluation of these patients.[127]

Sarcoidosis (See Chap. 182)

Sarcoidosis is a multisystem granulomatous disease with unknown cause and widespread manifestations.[128] Cardiac involvement consisting of myocardial or conduction system granulomata may be occult, but it may be clinically evident in about 20 percent of the patients.[129] Ventricular arrhythmias and conduction disturbances are responsible for the palpitations, presyncope, and syncope reported.[130] Congestive heart failure and chest pain occur less frequently and may be due to cardiomyopathy or cor pulmonale.[131] Additionally, prolapsed mitral valves, papillary muscle dysfunction, and aneurysm formation may be found rarely.[132] The prognosis for patients with cardiac involvement is unfavorable.[130]

Sarcoidosis affecting the pulmonary system may be suggested by lupus pernio[133] with involvement of the hilar nodes, bronchi, and/or alveoli resulting in obstructive and/or restrictive dysfunction. Respiratory failure is often the most difficult clinical problem, characterized by shortness of breath, dyspnea, and hypoxemia.[134]

The cutaneous features of sarcoidosis may not be clinically apparent at the time of cardiac involvement but occur in about 30 percent of patients.[128] Lesions are found especially about the eyes, nose, nasolabial folds, and mouth (lupus pernio).

The quality of clinical lesions varies considerably, but such features as a distinctive red color, translucency, and central atrophy with ringed borders should suggest the diagnosis. Flat-topped papules with or without scale are also common.[128] These lesions histologically reveal a granulomatous pattern with epithelioid tubercles and giant cells. Additionally erythema nodosum and erythema multiforme may occur as nonspecific reactive phenomena.[134] Although sarcoid lesions generally are not pruritic and do not ulcerate, exceptions have been documented.[135,136]

While there are at least two forms of sarcoidosis, acute (transient) and chronic (persistent), no definite correlation between skin and internal involvement has been made. However those patients

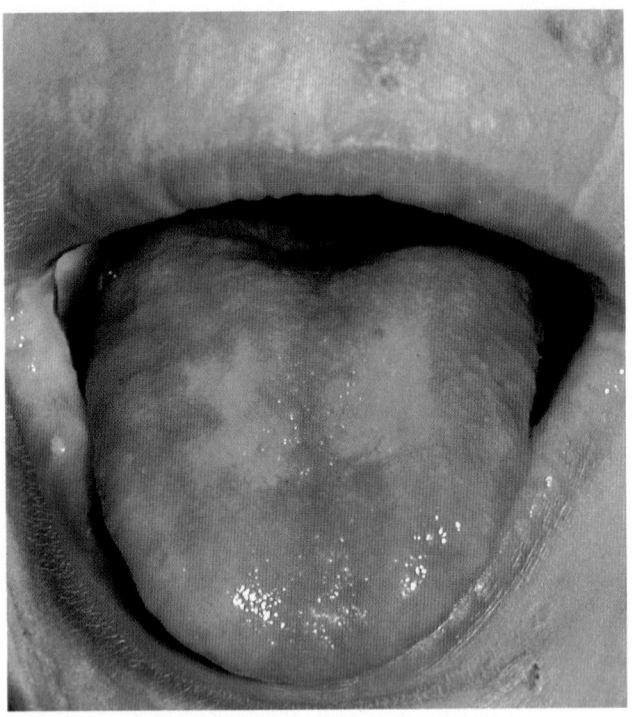

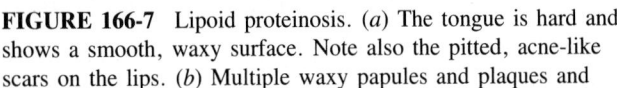

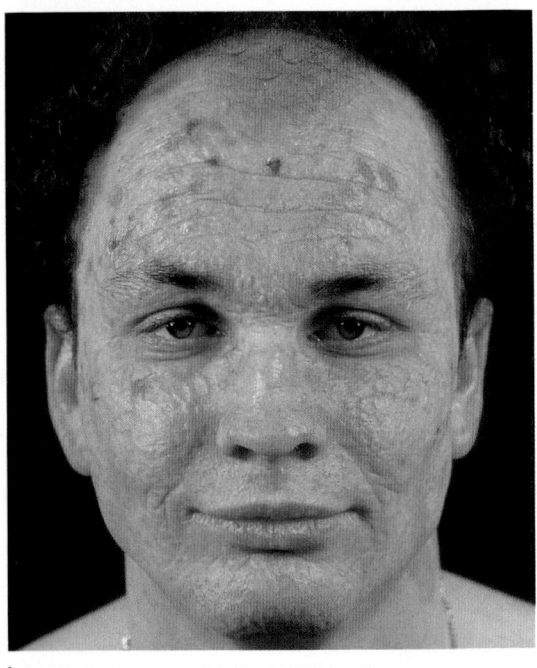

a

b

FIGURE 166-7 Lipoid proteinosis. (*a*) The tongue is hard and shows a smooth, waxy surface. Note also the pitted, acne-like scars on the lips. (*b*) Multiple waxy papules and plaques and pitted, acne-like scarring in the face. Note also the alopecia in this 20-year-old man. (*Courtesy of Klaus Wolff, M.D.*)

who present abruptly with hilar adenopathy and nonspecific skin involvement, such as erythema nodosum (Löfgren's syndrome), appear to respond to corticosteroid therapy and have fewer recurrences and a more favorable prognosis.[134]

Amyloidosis (See Chap. 149)

Involvement of the heart may be associated with all three systemic forms of amyloidosis but appears to be clinically predominant in the primary myeloma-associated types.[137] Senile amyloidosis may also affect the heart but is often asymptomatic.[138] Clinical findings include dizziness, palpitations, syncope, orthostatic hypotension, and congestive heart failure. Chest x-ray may reveal cardiomegaly. ECGs may show low-voltage, abnormal Q waves, conduction defects, and arrhythmias.[139] Echocardiography may reveal a restrictive cardiomyopathy with enlargement of the left ventricular wall and obstruction of the outflow tract. Pathologically, infiltration of the endocardium, myocardium, pericardium, valves, and coronary vessels may occur.[139]

Upper and lower respiratory tract involvement also occurs in all systemic forms of amyloidosis, but it is clinically predominant in primary and myeloma-associated types. Macroglossia may impede respiration, especially when complicated by bleeding. The larynx and trachea may become infiltrated, causing hoarseness, cough, and respiratory stridor. Bronchial and lung parenchymal involvement may cause asthma-like symptoms, hemoptysis, and severe pulmonary disease.[140] Chest x-rays may reveal interstitial type involvement and occasionally amyloid nodules may mimic a malignant tumor.[141] Pulmonary function studies may reveal obstructive or restrictive dysfunction depending on the location of the amyloid deposition.[140]

Cutaneous involvement occurs most often in the primary and myeloma-associated types and therefore serves as a marker for cardiopulmonary involvement.[142] Translucent papules and plaques may be found on the eyelids, nasolabial folds, mouth, neck, and upper trunk. A sclerodermoid appearance may occur with extensive involvement, especially with the myeloma-associated type.[142]

Areas of petechiae, purpura, and hemorrhage (pinch purpura) occur readily due to early involvement of dermal blood vessels. Pinch purpura may occur in areas of previously involved skin or in areas that appear clinically normal, and this distribution suggests the high incidence of dermal blood vessel involvement. Therefore a skin biopsy of clinically normal skin in a patient suspected of having amyloidosis may demonstrate deposition within the vessels in as many as 50 percent of patients.[142,143]

Lymphomatoid Granulomatosis (See Chap. 106)

This infiltrative systemic disease affects the skin, lungs, central nervous system, kidneys, and other organs in a characteristic histologic pattern.[116] Pulmonary involvement may begin with transient alveolar or interstitial infiltrates and effusions on chest x-ray, which subsequently may progress to nodular, masslike densities. These lesions may cavitate and be responsible for profuse hemoptysis.[144] Although many patients remain asymptomatic, cough, dyspnea, and chest pain may occur.[145] Cardiac involvement is uncommon but when present may involve the coronary vessels with subsequent myocardial ischemia.[146]

Skin lesions are found in up to half of all patients and are varied in appearance, often not suggestive of vasculitis. Erythematous papules, nodules, and plaques are found and sometimes ulcerate. These lesions usually reveal the characteristic histologic pattern of lymphoreticular cells surrounding and infiltrating blood vessels.[147]

Collagen Vascular Diseases

The cardiopulmonary complications of the various collagen vascular diseases may sometimes be associated with a specific cutaneous sign or constellation of features.

Rheumatoid Arthritis (See Chap. 178)

Extraarticular manifestations of rheumatoid arthritis, especially in the pulmonary system, appear to correlate with subcutaneous nodules and vasculitic skin lesions. The nodules may become necrobiotic and ulcerate, causing pain, secondary infection, and poor healing. The vasculitic lesions include palpable purpura, splinter hemorrhages, digital pitting, ulceration, or gangrene, sometimes in association with Raynaud's phenomenon, and pyoderma gangrenosum.[148-150]

In addition, laboratory evidence of high-titer rheumatoid factor, hypocomplementemia, cryoimmunoglobulinemia, and hypereosinophilia may be associated with the extraarticular manifestations including cardiopulmonary disease.[144,151-153] These manifestations occur more commonly in men with long-standing disease, but they may not necessarily correlate with arthritis activity at the time.[154] The pulmonary disease consists of pleural effusions, localized or diffuse parenchymal infiltrates, or rarely, lung nodules. Complaints include dypsnea, cough, pleuritic chest pain, and hemoptysis. Cardiac involvement may not be clinically apparent, although autopsy studies have revealed a high incidence of cardiac lesions related to granuloma or vasculitis.[155]

Systemic Lupus Erythematosus (See Chap. 171)

Cutaneous manifestations of systemic lupus erythematosus (SLE) appear in over 75 percent of patients during the course of their disease. While the extent of the cutaneous features in SLE may not correlate with the severity of visceral disease, the trend toward serologic and clinical subsets has suggested certain associations.

Photosensitive dermatitis, discoid-type lesions, Raynaud's phenomenon, and polyarthritis are associated with an increased incidence of serositis, including pleurisy, pericarditis, and noninfectious peritonitis.[156] The incidence of significant serositis may be higher in patients with drug-induced SLE syndromes, particularly when induced by procainamide.[157]

Pleuropulmonary Disease in SLE   Pleuritis may be present during the course of the disease in about half of patients with SLE. Chest pain may become subacute or chronic because of adhesions and may be confused with costochondritis. Pleural effusions with or without a friction rub may also occur.[156] Parenchymal lung involvement in SLE is usually due to secondary factors such as infections or pulmonary emboli.[158] Primary lung involvement in SLE may be classified as follows: (1) diffuse interstitial pneumonitis, (2) acute pneumonitis, (3) intrapulmonary hemorrhage, (4) diaphragm dysfunction with decreased lung volume (shrinking lung syndrome), (5) pulmonary hypertension with cor pulmonale, and (5) fibrosing alveolitis.[159-164]

Respiratory difficulty may also be due to acute epiglottitis, necrotic and ulcerative laryngitis, and tracheobronchitis.[165]

Cardiac involvement in patients with SLE is frequently subclinical.[156] Pericarditis may be more common in patients with drug-induced syndromes or those with photosensitive discoid lesions.[156] Chest pain may be present, especially when associated with effusion. A friction rub may be heard. The ECG changes primarily are T-wave abnormalities.[166]

Myocarditis is often undiagnosed and may be associated with prolonged P-R intervals, heart block, and arryhthmias.[167] Since the introduction of corticosteroid therapy, an increased incidence of atherosclerotic-related myocardial infarction has been reported.[167]

Valvular heart disease in patients with SLE is most often of the Libman-Sacks type, frequently is associated with antiphospholipid antibodies, and is manifested by systolic murmurs which may occur in almost one-half of all patients. These murmurs are rarely clinically significant.[167] Although diastolic murmurs may occur due to noninfectious mitral stenosis or aortic insufficiency, the onset of a new diastolic murmur should provoke a search for subacute bacterial endocarditis (SBE).[168] The cutaneous clues of SBE, such as splinter hemorrhages, Osler's nodes, Janeway lesions, and Roth's spots, should be searched for, although they may occur in SLE without infection. It appears that SLE, as well as other cutaneous vascular diseases, may be associated with complete heart block in newborn infants. In SLE this may be due to placental transfer of maternal antibodies, especially anti-Ro antibody.[169] The newborn infants of patients with SLE may also have distinctive evanescent cutaneous eruptions including prominent telangiectasia and periorbital erythema.[170]

Systemic Sclerosis (See Chap. 173)

Microvascular abnormalities are among the earliest pathologic changes seen in patients with systemic sclerosis, a finding supporting the concept of a primary vascular defect in the disease.[171] Characteristically the vascular lesions are characterized by intimal proliferation with loose connective tissue at the internal elastic membrane, medial thinning, and adventitial fibrosis.[172]

Many of the cutaneous features of this disorder are directly attributable to vascular abnormalities. Vasospastic episodes (Raynaud's) are often the first cutaneous findings. Telangiectases, also found early in the disease, are typically polygonal and sharply defined, commonly appearing as "mats" about the malar area of the face and upper trunk. Nail fold capillary changes also occur early in the disease as dilated and distorted capillary loops alternating with avascular areas on wide-field capillary microscopy.[173] Skin involvement generally follows three stages: edematous, fibrotic, and atrophic.

Pulmonary Abnormalities   Dypsnea on exertion, occurring in about half the patients, is usually the most common symptom. Chronic, nonproductive cough and pleuritic chest pain may also occur. Examination may reveal dry rales, especially at the bases, as well as diminished breath sounds and pleural rubs. Chest x-ray may show a diffuse reticulonodular interstitial pattern, cystic changes, calcification, pleural effusion, or scarring. Pulmonary function tests reveal diminished diffusing capacity, decreased volume, and decreased compliance characteristic of restrictive disease.[174]

Abnormalities of the respiratory system may not be due only to parenchymal lung disease. For example, pulmonary hypertension with cor pulmonale and congestive heart failure may develop independently of parenchymal disease. Biopsies of the lung show the typical changes described earlier around the small pulmonary arteries and arterioles.[175] Esophageal dysmotility may cause aspiration pneumonia and acute respiratory insufficiency.[144] Finally, abrupt changes in respiratory function suggest the possibility of a bronchoalveolar carcinoma in association with long-standing pulmonary fibrosis.[174]

Cardiovascular Disease in Systemic Sclerosis   Acute or chronic pericarditis is an important feature of the disease and, when associated with congestive heart failure, may be a marker for incipient renal failure. Pericardial effusions may be occult, and constrictive pericarditis and tamponade may occur.[176]

Transient vasospasm may involve the coronary vessels and cause myocardial ischemia with angina. Additionally, small-vessel involvement of the myocardium may lead to fibrosis (scleroderma heart).[177]

Fibrosis of the conduction system may cause arrhythmias and sudden death. Right ventricular hypertrophy due to cor pulmonale with congestive heart failure and pulmonary hypertension is observed.[178] The presence of the CREST variant may be associated with biliary cirrhosis and may not imply diminished cardiopulmonary or renal involvement in all cases as originally described.

In 1976 an attempt to correlate nail fold capillary abnormalities with visceral manifestations was reported.[173] The increased tortuosity of capillaries and areas of avascularity suggest an increased probability of cardiopulmonary and renal disease.[173]

Relapsing Polychondritis (See Chap. 176)

Relapsing polychondritis is characterized by inflammation and destruction of cartilage and connective tissues including those of the cardiopulmonary system. The pathogenesis is unknown, although it appears to be an autoimmune process frequently associated with other immunologic disorders such as SLE and rheumatoid arthritis.[179]

Auricular chondritis with pain, swelling, and redness of the pinna but complete sparing of the lobes is characteristic. Nasal chondritis may be associated with rhinorrhea and epistaxis and progress to "saddle-nose" deformity. Ocular involvement includes episcleritis and iritis. Various skeletal complaints including arthralgias, polyarthritis, costochondritis, and manubriosternal arthritis may be found.[180] Vasculitis involving multiple-size vessels may occur and simulate giant cell arteritis or polyarteritis nodosa. Cutaneous involvement includes dermal vasculitis sometimes associated with panniculitis. Additional cutaneous manifestations include postinflammatory hyperpigmentation, alopecia, nail dystrophy, and subcutaneous fat necrosis.[181]

Respiratory tract involvement may begin with hoarseness or tenderness of the anterior trachea. Degeneration of the laryngeal, tracheal, and/or bronchial rings may lead to progressive insufficiency or sudden collapse requiring emergency tracheostomy. Adequate ventilatory support may not be possible if advanced scarring and deformity are present.[180]

Cardiac involvement includes degeneration of the aortic ring with valvular insufficiency and aneurysmal dilatation. "Floppy" mitral valve syndrome also occurs. Pericardial and myocardial abnormalities have been reported.[182]

References

1. Di Mario C et al: Coronary aneurysms in a case of Ehlers-Danlos syndrome. *Jpn Heart J* **29**:421, 1988
2. Merten DF, Rooney R: Progressive pulmonary emphysema associated with congenital generalized elastosis (cutis laxa). *Pediatr Radiol* **113**:691, 1974
3. Slade AK et al: Pseudoxanthoma elasticum presenting with myocardial infarction. *Br Heart J* **63**:372, 1990
4. Silverman ME, Hurst JW: Inspection of the patient, in *The Heart, Arteries and Veins,* 5th ed. New York, McGraw-Hill, 1982, p 165
5. DeGowin EL, DeGowin RL: *Bedside Diagnostic Examination,* 4th ed. New York, Macmillan, 1981
6. Chesler E et al: Anatomic basis for delivery of right ventricular blood into localized segments of the systemic arterial system. *Am J Cardiol* **21**:72, 1968
7. Silverman ME, Hurst JW: The hand and the heart. *Am J Cardiol* **22**:718, 1968
8. Hecht HH: On cardiocutaneous syndromes. *Trans Assoc Am Physicians* **80**:91, 1967
9. Cobb LA et al: Circulatory effects of chronic hypervolemia in polycythemia vera. *J Clin Invest* **39**:1722, 1960
10. Engelman K: The carcinoid syndrome, in *Textbook of Medicine,* 16th ed, edited by JB Wyngaarden, LH Smith JR. Philadelphia, Saunders, 1982, p 1312
11. Schosser RH et al: Mastocytosis, in *Cutaneous Aspects of Internal Disease,* edited by JP Callen. Chicago, Year Book, 1981, p 539
12. Gifford FW et al: Clinical features, diagnosis and treatment of pheochromocytoma. *Mayo Clin Proc* **39**:281, 1964
13. Babb RR et al: Erythermalgia: Review of 51 cases. *Circulation* **29**:136, 1964
14. Johns MK: Skin wrinkling in cystic fibrosis. *Med Biol Illus* **25**:205, 1975
15. Altman RD, Tenenbaum J: Hypertrophic osteoarthropathy, in *Textbook of Rheumatology,* edited by WN Kelley et al. Philadelphia, Saunders, 1981, p 1647
16. Steinbrocker O: The shoulder-hand syndrome: Present perspective. *Arch Phys Med Rehabil* **49**:388, 1968
17. Kannel WB et al: Serum cholesterol, lipoprotein, and the risk of coronary heart disease. The Framingham study, *Ann Intern Med* **74**:1, 1971
18. Carlson LA, Bottiger LE: Ischaemic heart disease in relation to fasting values of plasma triglycerides and cholesterol. Stockholm prospective study. *Lancet* **1**:865, 1972
19. Muller C: Angina pectoris in hereditary xanthomatosis. *Arch Intern Med* **64**:674, 1939
20. Frank ST: Aural sign of coronary artery disease (letter). *N Engl J Med* **289**:327, 1973
21. Lichstein E et al: Diagonal ear-lobe crease: Incidence and significance as a coronary risk factor (abstr). *Clin Res* **21**:949, 1973
22. Lichstein E et al: Diagonal ear-lobe crease: Prevalence and implications as a coronary risk factor. *N Engl J Med* **290**:615, 1974
23. Christiansen J et al: Diagonal ear-lobe crease in coronary heart disease (letter). *N Engl J Med* **293**:308, 1975
24. Wyre H: The diagonal ear-lobe crease: A cutaneous manifestation of coronary artery disease. *Cutis* **23**:328, 1979
25. Sternlieb JJ et al: The ear crease sign in coronary artery disease (abstr). *Circulation* **50**:152, 1974
26. Cumberland GD et al: Ear-lobe creases and coronary atherosclerosis. *Am J Forensic Med Pathol* **8**:9, 1987
27. Fisher ER et al: Disseminated atheromatous emboli. *Am J Med* **29**:176, 1960
28. Carvajal JA et al: Atheroembolism: An etiologic factor in renal insufficiency, gastrointestinal, and peripheral vascular diseases. *Arch Intern Med* **119**:593, 1967
29. Rosman HS et al: Cholesterol embolization: Clinical findings and implications. *J Am Coll Cardiol* **15**:1296, 1990

30. Moldveen-Geronimus M, Merriam JC: Cholesterol embolization. From pathological curiosity to clinical entity. *Circulation* **35**:946, 1967

31. Stewart WM et al: Les manifestations cutanées des embolies de cristaux de cholesterol. *Ann Dermatol Venereol (Paris)* **104**:5, 1977

32. Crane C: Atherothrombotic embolism to lower extremities in arteriosclerosis. *Arch Surg* **94**:96, 1967

33. Calhoun P: Cholesterol emboli causing gangrene of the extremities. *Arch Dermatol* **111**:1373, 1975

34. Fischer DA, Kistner RL: Athero-thrombotic emboli in the lower extremities. *Arch Dermatol* **104**:533, 1971

35. Deschamps P et al: Livedo reticularis and nodules due to cholesterol embolism in the lower extremities. *Br J Dermatol* **97**:93, 1977

36. Maurizi CP et al: Atheromatous emboli. A postmortem study with special references to the lower extremities. *Arch Pathol* **86**:528, 1968

37. Anderson WR, Richard AM: Evaluation of lower extremity muscle biopsies in the diagnosis of atheroembolism. *Arch Pathol* **86**:535, 1968

38. Anderson WR: Necrotizing angiitis associated with embolization of cholesterol. *Am J Clin Pathol* **43**:65, 1965

39. Carr RD, Rau RC: Dermatitis at vein graft site in coronary artery bypass patients. *Arch Dermatol* **117**:814, 1981

40. Bart RS: Dermatitis at vein graft site (letter). *Arch Dermatol* **119**:97, 1983

41. Timmis GC: *Cardiovascular Review: 1980.* Baltimore, Williams & Wilkins, 1980, p 220

42. Giacomo A et al: Leg wound complications associated with coronary revascularization. *J Thorac Cardiovasc Surg* **81**:403, 1981

43. Baddour LM, Bisno AL: Recurrent cellulitis after saphenous venectomy for coronary bypass surgery. *Ann Intern Med* **97**:493, 1982

44. Greenberg J et al: Vein-donor cellulitis after coronary artery bypass surgery. *Ann Intern Med* **97**:565, 1982

45. Johnson RA, Palacios I: Dilated cardiomyopathies of the adult. *N Engl J Med* **307**:1051, 1119, 1982

46. Bullkley BH, Hutchins GM: Atrial myxomas: A fifty year review. *Am Heart J* **97**:639, 1979

47. Kounis NG: Left atrial myxoma presenting with intermittent claudication and Raynaud's phenomenon: Echocardiographic patterns of tumor size. *Br J Med* **56**:356, 1977

48. Byrd WE et al: Left atrial myxomas presenting as a systemic vasculitis. *Arthritis Rheum* **23**:240, 1980

49. Feldman AR et al: Cutaneous manifestations of atrial myxoma. *J Am Acad Dermatol* **21**: 1080, 1989

50. McWhirter WR, Tetteh-Lartey EV: A case of atrial myxoma. *Br Heart J* **36**:839, 1974

51. Currey HLF et al: Right atrial myxoma mimicking a rheumatic disorder. *Br Med J* **1**:547, 1967

52. Atherton DJ et al: A syndrome of various pigmented lesions, myxoid neurofibromata and atrial myxoma: The NAME syndrome. *Br J Dermatol* **103**:421, 1980

53. Rhodes AR et al: Mucocutaneous lentigines, cardiomucocutaneous myxomas, and multiple blue nevi: The "LAMB" syndrome. *J Am Acad Dermatol* **10**:72, 1984

54. Moynahan EJ: Multiple symmetrical moles with psychic and somatic infantilism and genital hypoplasia. *Proc R Soc Med* **55**:959, 1962

55. Gorlin RJ et al: Multiple lentigines syndrome. *Am J Dis Child* **117**:652, 1969

56. Norlund JJ et al: The multiple lentigines syndrome. *Arch Dermatol* **107**:259, 1973

57. Smith RF et al: Generalized lentigo: Electrocardiographic abnormalities, conduction disorders and arrhythmia in three cases. *Am J Cardiol* **25**:501, 1970

58. Polani PE, Moynahan EJ: Progressive cardiomyopathic lentiginosis. *Q J Med* **41**:205, 1972

59. Weiss LW, Zelickson AS: Giant melanosomes in multiple lentigines syndrome. *Arch Dermatol* **113**:491, 1977

60. Matthews NL: Lentigo and electrocardiographic changes. *N Engl J Med* **278**:780, 1968

61. Walther RJ et al: Electrocardiographic abnormalities in a family with generalized lentigo. *N Engl J Med* **275**:1220, 1966

62. Somerville J, Bonham-Carter RE: The heart in lentiginosis. *Br Heart J* **34**:58, 1972

63. Hopkins BC et al: Familial hypertrophic cardiomyopathy and lentiginosis. *Aust NZ J Med* **5**:359, 1975

64. Pankey GA: Subacute bacterial endocarditis at the University of Minnesota Hospital, 1939 through 1959. *Ann Intern Med* **55**:550, 1961

65. Pankey GA: Acute bacterial endocarditis at the University of Minnesota Hospital, 1939 through 1959. *Am Heart J* **64**:583, 1962

66. Horwitz LD, Silber R: Subacute bacterial endocarditis presenting as purpura. *Arch Intern Med* **120**:483, 1967

67. Rubenfeld S, Kyung-What M: Leukocytoclastic angiitis in subacute bacterial endocarditis. *Arch Dermatol* **113**:1073, 1977

68. Myall RW et al: Mucosal and dermal lesions seen in bacterial endocarditis. *J Am Dent Assoc* **78**:120, 1969

69. Libman E: The clinical features of subacute streptococcal (and influenzal) endocarditis in the bacterial stage. *Med Clin North Am* **2**:117, 1918

70. Janeway E: Certain clinical observations upon heart disease. *Med News* **75**:257, 1899

71. Osler W: Gulstonian lectures on malignant endocarditis. *Lancet* **1**:415, 459, 505, 1885

72. Osler W: Chronic infectious endocarditis. *Q J Med* **2**:219, 1909

73. Merklen P, Wolf M: Participation des endothéliites arteriocapillaries au syndrome de l'endocardite maligne lente. *Presse Med* **36**:97, 1928

74. Lian C et al: Histopathologie de nodule d'Osler, étude sur l'endothéliite de l'endocardite maligne à évolution lente. *Presse Med* **37**:497, 1929

75. Von Gemmengen GR, Winkelmann RK: Osler's nodes of subacute bacterial endocarditis. *Arch Dermatol* **95**:91, 1967

76. Cornil L et al: Contribution a l'étude histologique du nodule d'Osler. *Ann Anat Pathol* **13**:675, 1936

77. Alpert JS et al: Pathogenesis of Osler's nodes. *Ann Intern Med* **85**:471, 1976

78. Kerr A: *Subacute Bacterial Endocarditis.* Springfield, IL, Charles C. Thomas, 1956, p 101

79. Kennedy JE, Wise GN: Clinicopathologic correlation of retinal lesions, subacute bacterial endocarditis. *Arch Ophthalmol* **74**:658, 1965

80. Weinstein L: "Modern" infective endocarditis. *JAMA* **223**:260, 1975

81. Weinstein L, Schlesinger JJ: Pathoanatomic, pathophysiologic and clinical correlation in endocarditis. *N Engl J Med* **291**:832, 1122, 1974

82. Michaelson ED, Walsh RE: Osler's node—a complication of prolonged arterial cannulation. *N Engl J Med* **283**:472, 1970

83. Matthews J, Gibbons RB: Embolization complicating radial artery puncture. *Ann Intern Med* **75**:87, 1971

84. Fanning L, Aronson M: Osler node, Janeway lesions and splinter hemorrhages: Occurrence with an infected arterial catheter. *Arch Dermatol* **113**:648, 1977

85. Rudusky BM: Recurrent Osler's nodes in systemic lupus erythematosus. *Angiology* **20**:33, 1969

86. Keil H: The rheumatic subcutaneous nodules and simulating lesions. *Medicine (Baltimore)* **17**:261, 1938

87. Howard EJ: Osler's nodes. *Am Heart J* **59**:633, 1960

88. Park CH et al: Erysipelothrix endocarditis with cutaneous lesion. *South Med J* **69**:1101, 1976

89. Grieco MH, Sheldon C: *Erysipelothrix rhusiopathiae. Ann NY Acad Sci* **174**:523, 1970

90. Samman PD, White WF: The "yellow nail" syndrome. *Br J Dermatol* **76**:153, 1964

91. Hurwitz PA, Pinals DJ: Pleural effusion in chronic hereditary lymphedema (Nonne, Milroy, Meige's disease): Report of two cases.

Radiology **82**:246, 1964

92. Emerson PA: Yellow nails, lymphoedema, and pleural effusions. *Thorax* **21**:247, 1966

93. Runyon BA: Pleural-fluid kinetics in a patient with lymphedema, pleural effusions and yellow nails. *Am Rev Respir Dis* **119**:821, 1979

94. DeCoste SD et al: Yellow nail syndrome. *J Am Acad Dermatol* **22**:608, 1990

95. Hiller E et al: Pulmonary manifestations of the yellow nail syndrome. *Chest* **61**:452, 1972

96. Shumacker HB Jr, Waldhausen JA: Pulmonary arteriovenous fistulas in children. *Ann Surg* **158**:713, 1963

97. Dines DE et al: Pulmonary arteriovenous fistulas. *Mayo Clin Proc* **58**:176, 1983

98. Harrison DF: Familial haemorrhagic telangiectasia. *Q J Med* **33**:25, 1964

99. Conlon CL et al: Telangiectasia and von Willebrand's disease in two families. *Ann Intern Med* **89**:921, 1978

100. Meijer A: Asthma predictors in infantile atopic dermatitis. *J Asthma Res* **12**:181, 1975

101. Burrows B: Chronic airway diseases, in *Textbook of Medicine,* 16th ed, edited by JB Wyngaarden, LH Smith Jr. Philadelphia, Saunders, 1982, p 363

102. Di Sant'Agnese PA, Davis PB: Cystic fibrosis in adults. *Am J Med* **66**:121, 1979

103. Johns MK: Skin wrinkling in cystic fibrosis. *Med Biol Illus* **25**:205, 1975

104. Katz R et al: The natural course of creeping eruption and treatment with thiabendazole. *Arch Dermatol* **91**:420, 1965

105. Tachakra SS: Distribution of skin petechiae in fat embolism rash. *Lancet* **1**(7954):284, 1976

106. Cole WG, Oakes BW: Skin petechiae and fat embolism. *Aust NZ J Surg* **42**:401, 1973

107. Gordon H et al: Lipoid proteinosis in an inbred Namaqualand community. *Lancet* **1**:1032, 1969

108. Burnett JW, Marcy SM: Lipoid proteinosis. *Am J Dis Child* **105**:81, 1963

109. Caplan RM: Visceral involvement in lipoid proteinosis. *Arch Dermatol* **95**:149, 1967

110. Hofer PA: Urbach-Wiethe disease: A review. *Acta Derm Venerol (Stockh)* **53**(suppl 71):1, 1973

111. Caplan RM: Lipoid proteinosis: A review including some new observations. *Univ Mich Med Bull* **28**:365, 1962

112. Weidner WA et al: Roentgenographic findings in lipoid proteinosis: A case report. *Am J Roentgenol* **110**:457, 1970

113. Sanderson KV: Lipoid proteinosis. *Proc R Soc Med* **63**:888, 1970

114. Heyl T: Lipoid proteinosis. I. The clinical picture. *Br J Dermatol* **75**:465, 1963

115. Jensen AD et al: Lipoid proteinosis. *Arch Ophthalmol* **88**:273, 1972

116. Warin RP et al: Reticulohistiocytosis (lipoid dermato-arthritis). *Br Med J* **1**:1387, 1957

117. Bortz AI, Vincent M: Lipoid dermato-arthritis and arthritis mutilans. *Am J Med* **30**:951, 1961

118. Barrow MV, Holubar K: Multicentric reticulohistiocytosis: A review of thirty-three patients. *Medicine (Baltimore)* **48**:287, 1969

119. Ehrlich GE et al: Multicentric reticulohistiocytosis (lipoid dermato-arthritis): A multisystem disorder. *Am J Med* **52**:830, 1972

120. Anderson TE et al: Myositis and myotonia in a case of multicentric reticulohistiocytosis. *Br J Dermatol* **80**:39, 1968

121. Orkin M et al: A study of multicentric reticulohistiocytosis. *Arch Dermatol* **89**:640, 1964

122. Flam M et al: Multicentric reticulohistiocytosis: Report of a case with atypical features and electron microscopic study of skin lesions. *Am J Med* **52**:841, 1972

123. Fast A: Cardiopulmonary complications in multicentric reticulohistiocytosis. *Arch Dermatol* **112**:1139, 1976

124. Braverman IM: In *Skin Signs of Systemic Disease,* 2d ed. Philadephia, Saunders, 1981, p 208

125. Barrow MV et al: Identification of tissue lipids in lipoid der-

matoarthritis (multicentric reticulohistiocytosis). *Am J Clin Pathol* **47**:312, 1967

126. Barrow MV: The nails in multicentric reticulohistiocytosis. *Arch Dermatol* **95**:200, 1967

127. Catterall MD, White JE: Multicentric reticulohistiocytosis and malignant disease. *Br J Dermatol* **98**:221, 1978

128. James DG et al: A worldwide review of sarcoidosis. *Ann NY Acad Sci* **278**:321, 1976

129. Matsui Y et al: Clinicopathological study on fatal myocardial sarcoidosis. *Ann NY Acad Sci* **278**:455, 1976

130. Stein E et al: Clinical course of cardiac sarcoidosis. *Ann NY Acad Sci* **278**:470, 1976

131. Lorell B et al: Cardiac sarcoidosis. *Am J Cardiol* **42**:143 1978

132. Roberts WC et al: Sarcoidosis of the heart. *Am J Med* **63**:86, 1977

133. Jorizzo JL et al: Sarcoidosis of the upper respiratory tract in patients with nasal rim lesions. *J Am Dermatol* **22**:439, 1990

134. Jones Williams W, Davies BH: *Eighth International Conference on Sarcoidosis and Other Granulomatous Disease.* Cardiff, Wales, Alpha Omega Publishing, 1984

135. Fong YW, Sharma OP: Pruritic maculopapular skin lesions in sarcoidosis. *Arch Dermatol* **111**:362, 1975

136. Schiffner V, Sharma OP: Ulcerative sarcoidosis. *Arch Dermatol* **113**:676, 1977

137. Meaney E et al: Cardiac amyloidosis, constrictive pericarditis and restrictive cardiomyopathy. *Am J Cardiol* **38**:347, 1976

138. Westermark P et al: Senile cardiac amyloidosis: Evidence of two different amyloid substances in the aging heart. *Scand J Immunol* **10**:303, 1979

139. Kyle RA, Bayrd ED: Amyloidosis: Review of 236 cases. *Medicine (Baltimore)* **54**:271, 1975

140. Celli BR et al: Patterns of pulmonary involvement in systemic amyloidosis. *Chest* **74**:543, 1978

141. Brauner GJ et al: Acquired bullous disease of the skin and solitary amyloidoma of the lung. *Am J Med* **57**:978, 1974

142. Rubinow A, Cohen AS: Skin involvement in generalized amyloidosis. *Ann Intern Med* **88**:781, 1978

143. Brownstein MH, Helwig EB: The cutaneous amyloidoses. II. Systemic forms. *Arch Dermatol* **102**:20, 1970

144. Hunninghake GW, Fauci AS: Pulmonary involvement in the collagen vascular diseases. *Am Rev Respir Dis* **119**:471, 1979

145. Liebow AA et al: Lymphomatoid granulomatosis. *Hum Pathol* **3**:457, 1972

146. Israel HL et al: Wegener's granulomatosis, lymphomatoid granulomatosis and benign lymphocytic angiitis and granulomatosis of the lung: Recognition and treatment. *Ann Intern Med* **87**:691, 1977

147. Minars N et al: Lymphomatoid granulomatosis of the skin. *Arch Dermatol* **111**:493, 1975

148. Gordon DA et al: The extra-articular features of rheumatoid arthritis: A systemic analysis of 127 cases. *Am J Med* **54**:445, 1973

149. Gardner DL et al: Pulmonary hypertension in rheumatoid arthritis: Report of a case with intimal sclerosis of the pulmonary and digital arteries. *Scott Med J* **2**:183, 1957

150. Stolman LP et al: Pyoderma gangrenosum and rheumatoid arthritis. *Arch Dermatol* **111**:1020, 1975

151. Mongan ES et al: A study of the relation of seronegative and seropositive rheumatoid arthritis to each other and to necrotizing vasculitis. *Am J Med* **47**:23, 1969

152. Winchester RJ et al: Observations on the eosinophilia of certain patients with rheumatoid arthritis. *Arthritis Rheum* **14**:650, 1971

153. Weisman M, Zvaifler N: Cryoimmunoglobulinemia in rheumatoid arthritis. *J Clin Invest* **56**:725, 1975

154. Hurd ER: Extraarticular manifestations of rheumatoid arthritis. *Semin Rheum Dis* **8**:151, 1979

155. Bonfiglio T, Atwater E: Heart disease in patients with seropositive rheumatoid arthritis: A controlled autopsy study and review. *Arch Intern Med* **127**:714, 1969

156. Fries JF, Holman HR: *Systemic Lupus Erythematosis: A Clinical Analysis.* Philadelphia, Saunders, 1975, p 64

157. Byrd RB, Schanger B: Pulmonary sequelae in procaine amide induced lupus-like syndrome. *Dis Chest* **55**:170, 1969

158. Dubois EL, Tuffanelli DL: Clinical manifestations of systemic lupus erythematosus. *JAMA* **190**:104, 1964

159. Eisenberg H et al: Diffuse interstitial lung disease in systemic lupus erythematosus. *Ann Intern Med* **79**:37, 1973

160. Simonson JS et al: Pulmonary hypertension in systemic lupus erythematosus. *J Rheumatol* **16**:918, 1989

161. Eagen JW et al: Pulmonary hemorrhage in systemic lupus erythematosus. *Medicine (Baltimore)* **57**:545, 1978

162. Gibson GJ et al: Diaphragm function and lung involvement in systemic lupus erythematosus. *Am J Med* **63**:926, 1977

163. Perez HD, Kramer N: Pulmonary hypertension in systemic lupus erythematosus: Report of four cases and review of the literature. *Semin Arthritis Rheum* **11**:177, 1981

164. Sperryn PN: Systemic lupus erythematosus with fibrosing alveolitis. *Proc R Soc Med* **64**:58, 1971

165. Toomey JM et al: Acute epiglottis due to systemic lupus erythematosus. *Laryngoscope* **84**:522, 1974

166. Ropes MW: *Systemic Lupus Erythematosus.* Cambridge, MA, Harvard Univ Press, 1976

167. Bulkley BH, Roberts WC: The heart in systemic lupus erythematosus and the changes induced in it by corticosteroid therapy. A study of 36 necropsy patients. *Am J Med* **58**:243, 1975

168. Dubois EL: *Lupus Erythematosus: A Review of the Current Studies of Discoid and Systemic Lupus Erythematosus,* 2d ed. Los Angeles, Univ of Southern California Press, 1976

169. McCue CM et al: Congenital heart blocks in newborns of mothers with connective tissue disease. *Circulation* **56**:82, 1977

170. McCune AB et al: Maternal and fetal outcome in neonatal lupus erythematosus. *Ann Intern Med* **106**:518, 1987

171. Campbell PM, LeRoy ED: Pathogenesis of systemic sclerosis: A vascular hypothesis. *Semin Arthritis Rheum* **4**:351, 1975

172. D'Angelo WA et al: Pathologic observations in systemic sclerosis (scleroderma): A study of 58 autopsy cases and 58 matched controls. *Am J Med* **46**:428, 1969

173. Maricq HR et al: Skin capillary abnormalities as indicators of organ involvement in scleroderma (systemic sclerosis), Raynaud's syndrome and dermatomyositis. *Am J Med* **61**:862, 1976

174. Peters-Golden M et al: Clinical and demographic predictors of loss of pulmonary function in systemic sclerosis. *Medicine* **63**:221, 1984

175. Hurwitz AL et al: Esophageal dysfunction and Raynaud's phenomenon in patients with scleroderma. *Am J Dig Dis* **21**:601, 1976

176. McWhorter JE, LeRoy EC: Pericardial disease in scleroderma (systemic sclerosis). *Am J Med* **57**:566, 1974

177. Gupta MF et al: Scleroderma heart disease with skin flow velocity in coronary arteries. *Chest* **67**:116, 1975

178. Bulkely BH et al: Myocardial lesions of progressive systemic sclerosis: A cause of cardiac dysfunction. *Circulation* **53**:483, 1976

179. Arkin CR, Masi AT: Relapsing polychondritis: Review of current status and case report. *Semin Arthritis Rheum* **5**:41, 1975

180. Herman VH: Polychondritis, in *Textbook of Rheumatology,* edited by WN Kelley et al. Philadelphia, Saunders, 1981, p 1500

181. Bergfeld WF: Relapsing polychondritis with positive direct immunofluorescence. *Arch Dermatol* **114**:127, 1978

182. Cipriano PR et al: Multiple aortic aneurysms in relapsing polychondritis. *Am J Cardiol* **37**:1097, 1976

CHAPTER 167

Jay D. Coffman

Cutaneous Changes in Peripheral Vascular Disease

Physiology of the Cutaneous Circulation

Central Control of Cutaneous Blood Flow

The central nervous system regulates blood flow through the sympathetic nervous system. The primary centers regulating and integrating cutaneous blood flow are the hypothalamus, medulla oblongata, and spinal cord. The hypothalamus regulates blood flow through the arteriovenous (A-V) anastomoses to control body temperature and has been referred to as the "heat loss center." It controls the vasoconstrictor fibers in association with the vasomotor center. Emotional cutaneous vascular responses also occur here. The hypothalamus integrates messages from higher cortical centers to coordinate its function. The medulla oblongata contains the vasodepressor and pressor vasomotor centers which are influenced by the hypothalamus, baroreceptors, chemoreceptors, and somatic afferent nerves. The vasomotor centers are believed to be the primary controlling factor of cutaneous and muscle vasoconstrictor tone. The vasodilator and vasoconstrictor areas may act as an integrated unit and are primarily involved in vascular reflexes arising from the baroreceptors in the carotid sinus and aorta. From the medulla ob-

longata, nerves run in the intermediolateral cell columns of the spinal cord to the sympathetic ganglia and hence to the peripheral sympathetic nerves. There are also spinal vasomotor reflexes which are elicited by stimulation of the peripheral receptors. The efferent limbs are the cutaneous sympathetic vasoconstrictor fibers. These reflexes are segmentally or regionally arranged in the spinal cord.

Digital Blood Flow

The digits contain a dual circulation that consists of the capillaries and the A-V anastomoses. Finger blood can vary from less than 1 to 180 mL/min per 100 mL of tissue.[1] The capillaries supply the nutritional blood flow for the digits. In normal subjects, the capillary blood flow is therefore preserved during reflex sympathetic vasoconstriction of body cooling.[2] The capillary flow may be 100 percent of the total finger blood flow during body cooling when the A-V shunts are closed but only 10 to 20 percent in a warm environment when the shunts are open.

Arteriovenous Anastomoses   The A-V anastomoses are coiled blood vessels with thick muscular walls and many nerve endings. They directly connect the arterial with the venous circulation and bypass the capillary beds. These shunts are most numerous in the nail bed but also are present in the digital tips and palmar surfaces.[3] They have also been found in the palm of the hand and sole of the foot, and in the ear. Their main function is to control body temperature but they may also maintain the temperature of the digits.

Digital blood flow is decreased by activation of the sympathetic nerves and increased by withdrawal of their activity. In contrast to other cutaneous vascular beds, a neurogenic vasodilatory mechanism has not been demonstrated.[4] Reflex sympathetic vasoconstriction results in digital vasoconstriction which is absent in sympathectomized limbs; digital nerve block also results in a very large digital blood flow. Body warming elicits a reflex vasodilation in the hand or foot which has been shown to be due to a release of vasoconstrictor tone. The reflex may originate either in cutaneous receptors or by central nervous system stimulation.

Local Cooling and Cold Vasodilatation   Local cooling reduces finger blood flow, but not as much as reflex sympathetic vasoconstriction does.[5] The mechanism of the local cooling vasoconstriction is unknown but may be due to an increased sensitivity of α_2-adrenoceptors at low temperatures.[6]

If a finger is cooled for 15 minutes at less than 10°C, blood flow almost ceases but then vasodilatation occurs and the temperature of the finger rises to about 28°C. The temperature of the finger then fluctuates as periods of vasoconstriction alternate with periods of vasodilatation (the hunting reaction). The mechanism of the cold vasodilatation is unknown but it occurs only in areas containing A-V anastomoses.[3] It is not an axon reflex. Atropine and antihistamines do not affect it[7] and it occurs in the absence of a sympathetic innervation. It is a very valuable mechanism to warm the cold-exposed parts sufficiently to preserve movement and sensation. Young adults and men have the greatest cold vasodilatation response while blacks have a lesser response and Japanese a greater vasodilatation than Caucasians.[8-10] Thus the reaction may determine the sensitivity of a group or race to cold.

Digital Vasoconstriction and Vasodilator Receptors   In vitro and in vivo methods have shown that α_1- and α_2-adrenoceptors are present in hand arteries and veins and digital blood vessels.[11,12] Proximal digital artery strips are more sensitive to α_1- than α_2-adrenoceptor antagonists but distal arteries need both adrenoceptor antagonists to prevent their contraction in response to norepinephrine.[13] In vivo studies in man indicate that α_2-adrenoceptors are more important than α_1-adrenoceptors during reflex sympathetic vasoconstriction and that α_2-adrenoceptors predominantly affect A-V anastomoses in the finger.[12]

In vitro and in vivo studies have also demonstrated the presence of S_2-serotonergic receptors in human hand arteries and veins and in digital blood vessels.[11,14] Intraarterial serotonin decreases finger blood flow which is antagonized by ketanserin, an S_2-serotonergic antagonist.[14] Serotonin decreases both capillary and A-V shunt flow. During reflex sympathetic vasoconstriction produced by body cooling, S_2 blockade increases finger blood flow which indicates that serotonin may be an important mechanism of vasoconstriction in the digits.

Histamine and cholinergic agents increase finger blood flow and the responses are inhibited by appropriate antagonists.[15,16] If the digital vascular bed is vasoconstricted by norepinephrine or angiotensin, isoproterenol increases finger blood flow.[17] However, isoproterenol does not increase finger blood flow during reflex sympathetic vasoconstriction. The β-adrenergic vasodilator mechanism has been shown to affect only A-V shunts. The physiologic importance of the β-adrenoceptors, and of histaminergic and cholinergic receptors, remains to be determined.

Forehead Cutaneous Blood Flow

Forehead vasculature is relatively nonreactive to various stimuli. The blood flow is very large, approximately 28.4 mL/min per 100 mL of tissue, and exceeds that of the calf, forearm, or trunk skin.[18] During cold exposure, vasoconstriction is absent and loss of body heat continues. Head gear must be used to prevent heat loss in cold climates. Despite blanching of the forehead skin during intravenous epinephrine infusion and flushing afterward, forehead blood flow does not change. These findings confirm that skin color is often not related to skin blood flow but reflects changes in the dermal venous plexuses.[19] Some pharmacologic agents, such as nicotinic acid and papaverine, do increase skin temperature of the forehead. The reason for the large forehead blood flow is unknown; it has been postulated that it is necessary to keep the brain temperature normal.[20]

Cutaneous Blood Flow of the Forearm

The cutaneous blood flow of the forearm varies from almost 0 to 70.5 mL/min per 100 mL of tissue.[21] In contrast to the digits, the skin of the forearm has both a sympathetic vasoconstrictor and vasodilator innervation. Skin blood flow and temperature decrease in response to cooling or baroreceptor stimulation. These responses occur via α-adrenoceptors, especially the α_1-adrenoceptors.[22] During body cooling, a longitudinal temperature gradient from the warmer trunk to the cooler distal extremities is maintained by the sympathetic nervous system.

During body heating, an increase in forearm skin blood flow surpasses that expected from the release of sympathetic vasoconstrictor tone.[23] This vasodilatory response is absent in areas devoid of sweat glands. Bradykinin has been implicated in this reaction.[24] During activation of the sweat glands, a proteolytic enzyme is released into the tissues where it acts on bradykininogen to produce the potent vasodilator, bradykinin. A local sympathetic venoarteriolar reflex also controls forearm and calf skin blood flow and is activated by increased venous pressure in the limbs.

Age- and Sex-Related Changes

In males skin blood flow in the deltoid region, anterior chest, and dorsum of the hands and feet decreases with age.[25] Skin blood flow decreases by 30 to 40 percent from 20 to 70 years of age. Females in general have lower skin blood flow than males, but only after menarche and before menopause.[26] During the menstrual cycle, finger blood flow decreases during the luteal phase compared with flow during the preovulatory phase.[27]

Obstructive Arterial Diseases

Arteriosclerosis Obliterans

Arteriosclerosis obliterans is characterized by muscle pain or fatigue on exercise, or by pain, ulcers, or gangrene of the distal lower extremities during rest due to stenosis or obstruction of large arteries by atheroma and thrombosis.

Epidemiology Intermittent claudication due to arteriosclerosis obliterans affects about 1 percent of the population over 35 years of age. It occurs predominantly in males. Most patients have superficial femoral artery disease and develop symptoms in the seventh decade, but symptoms from aortoiliac disease usually occur a decade earlier.[28]

Etiology and Pathogenesis Arteriosclerosis is similar to vascular disease that occurs in other areas of the body. Arteriosclerosis obliterans develops in patients who smoke at twice the frequency that it does in nonsmokers.[29] About 50 percent of patients have hyperlipoproteinemia. It is very common in patients with hypertension. Arteriosclerosis develops in patients with diabetes mellitus at an earlier age than in those without diabetes, and they have more severe and progressive disease. The distribution of the disease is different in that diabetics have less aortoiliac arteriosclerosis and more disease of the vessels between the knees and the ankles than nondiabetics; superficial femoral artery disease is similar in both populations.[30]

The cause of atheromas is not known, but progressive build-up of cholesterol plaques narrows the vessel lumen and finally occlusion may occur by thrombosis. Since the disease progresses slowly, collateral blood vessels develop to supply the extremity distal to the stenosis or obstruction. Therefore the blood supply to the limb is usually adequate at rest, but the blood pressure distal to the lesions is decreased because of the high resistance of the collateral vessels.[30] During exercise, the diseased segment of the artery limits the needed increase in blood flow. The perfusion pressure distal to the lesion falls further on muscle vasodilation during exercise, and then muscle contraction may actually stop blood flow. Pain or severe fatigue occurs but the exact metabolites producing the symptoms are unknown. With rest, an adequate blood flow returns and symptoms disappear usually within 5 min. In patients with inadequate collateral blood supply, usually due to occlusion of both the superficial and deep femoral arteries or to occlusion of all three calf blood vessels, rest pain, ulceration, or gangrene occurs because of deficient oxygenation and nutrition of the distal tissue.

Clinical Manifestations HISTORY. The patient complains of pain, fatigue, or tiredness in the muscles distal to the diseased arterial segment when walking (intermittent claudication).[30] The calf muscles, which do the most work during walking, are most commonly symptomatic with disease at any vascular level. The distance covered before symptoms appear is quite constant for each patient, except that shorter distances can be covered when walking on inclines or carrying heavy bundles. The symptoms are usually relieved within 5 min by rest, even while standing. Patients with inadequate collateral circulation complain of coldness, hyperesthesia, rest pain, discolored toes, or skin breakdown. Rest pain may be so severe that the patient cannot sleep or sleeps with the leg in a dependent position. Such patients then may develop edema of the lower parts of the extremity.

SYSTEM REVIEW. The patient may complain of ischemic cardiac or cerebrovascular symptoms due to similar disease of the arterial supply to the heart or brain. Nearly all patients are smokers. Diabetes and hypertension are common concomitant diseases.

PHYSICAL EXAMINATION. The limbs in patients with only intermittent claudication may appear normal, although there may be hair loss, coldness, and thickened or malformed toe nails. In patients with aortoiliac disease, there may be global atrophy of the lower limbs. Pulses will be decreased or absent distal to the diseased arterial segment, and there may be bruits over the distal vessels. A diastolic component to the bruit indicates a very limited collateral blood flow because the pressure distal to the obstruction is so low that flow continues throughout the cardiac cycle. In patients with severe ischemia, the skin is apt to be atrophic, dry, and shiny. In patients with rest pain, the foot is usually bright red and cold in dependency. Rest pain occurs in the foot; the muscles rarely have symptoms during rest. Ulcerations usually start at the tips of the toes and are extremely painful, except when a diabetic neuropathy is present. Ulcers occasionally start on the lower calves (Fig. 167-1). The ulcers have a sloughing gray or black base. Skin of the heels may be cracked. When gangrene occurs, usually one or more toes become black, dry, and mummified.

Laboratory and Special Examinations The collateral circulation to limbs affected by arteriosclerosis obliterans can be evaluated by simple tests.[30] With the patient supine, elevation of the limb at a 45° angle for 2 min should not produce pallor. The collateral circulation is not adequate if the toes and feet become pale. If the patient then assumes a sitting position with the legs dependent, the times for filling of the foot veins and flushing of the feet can be measured. The veins should fill within 20 s and the feet flush immediately in a warm environment. When these times exceed 30 s, the collateral circulation is inadequate and the patient must be observed frequently for the development of rest pain, ulcers, or gangrene. Venous filling times cannot be used to evaluate collateral circulation in patients with varicose veins.

An objective test to document the disease is the measurement of ankle systolic blood pressures. Ankle systolic pressure in the supine position should be equal to or greater than brachial artery systolic pressure. An ankle-to-arm systolic pressure index is usually calculated; values greater than 0.95 are considered normal while values less than 0.5 indicate severe disease. If the index is 0.95 or greater and the patient's symptoms are typical for the disease, the ankle pressures should be measured before and after exercise of the limb. In normal subjects, the ankle pressure may fall slightly for 30 s after exercise but then usually rises higher than the preexercise level. In patients with diseased arteries, the systolic ankle pressure falls after exercise and may not return to preexercise levels for several minutes. In patients with diabetes mellitus or renal disease, the arteries may have medial calcification which pre-

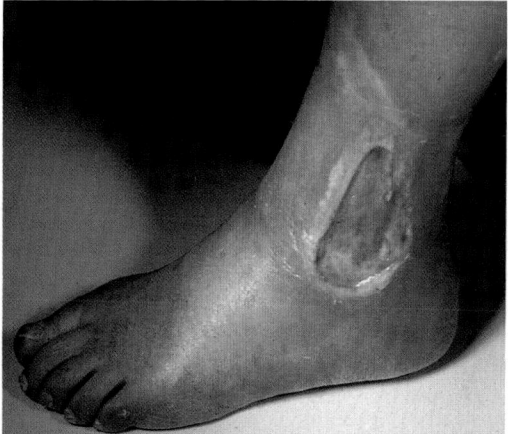

FIGURE 167-1 An ischemic ulcer in a patient with arteriosclerosis obliterans. The location on the lateral aspect of the ankle is typical. The base of the ulcer shows fibrous tissue with scant granulation tissue and the outline of tendons. The distal foot and toes are cyanotic from ischemia.

vents compression by a pressure cuff. In these patients, plethysmography or oscillometry is usually helpful and shows decreased arterial pulsations in the limb compared with the opposite extremity.

Arteriography can be used to demonstrate the location and extent of disease in the arteries but supplies no hemodynamic information. It is usually used only before vascular surgery and not as a diagnostic test.

Pathology   There is a focal accumulation of lipids, mucopolysaccharides, blood and blood products, fibrous tissue, and calcium deposits in the intima of arteries. Localized areas of thickening of the intima by fibroblastic proliferation and phagocytes laden with lipid material are seen. The media is atrophic and is characterized by thin strands of smooth muscle, disrupted elastic lamella, collagen tissue, and calcium deposits. Enlarging plaques encroach on the lumen despite dilation of the artery, and the plaques may ulcerate. Hemorrhages occur in the arterial wall. Thrombi may form and occlude the narrowed arterial lumen.

Diagnosis and Differential Diagnosis   The diagnosis of arteriosclerosis obliterans can usually be made on the basis of the typical history of intermittent claudication and by palpation of all pulses in the limbs. In questionable cases, ankle systolic blood pressures should be measured at rest and, if needed, after exercise.

In patients with diabetes mellitus, ulcers may develop on the heel, toes, or anterior calf when the pulse is normal. These painless ulcers are due to repetitive trauma not noticed by the patient because of peripheral neuropathy (Fig. 167-2). Other causes of neuropathy also lead to neurotropic ulcers. Surrounding callus formation is typical of these ulcers.

Thromboangiitis obliterans also causes intermittent claudication, ulcers, and gangrene. It occurs in a younger age group than arteriosclerosis obliterans and is often associated with superficial thrombophlebitis and vasospasm. It affects medium and smaller arteries and the upper extremities more commonly than arteriosclerosis obliterans. Neurogenic claudication is often a difficult differential diagnosis and is due to compression or intermittent ischemia of the lower spinal cord or corda equina on exercise. Etiologic factors are prolapsed intervertebral disks and stenosis or hypertrophic bony ridging of the spinal canal. In contrast to arteriosclerosis obliterans, leg pain may occur in the erect position without exercise, neurologic signs may be present before or after exercise, and peripheral pulses are normal.

Other rare causes of intermittent claudication are adventitial cysts of the popliteal artery, compression of the popliteal artery by abnormal insertion of calf muscles, deep venous obstruction of the iliofemoral region, and abnormalities of muscle phosphorylases (McArdle's syndrome). Patients with these entities usually have normal pulses and a history not compatible with arteriosclerosis obliterans.

Treatment   For patients with intermittent claudication and an adequate collateral circulation, an exercise regime is the treatment of choice.[31] The patient is instructed to exercise to tolerable pain, rest, and then exercise again for 30 to 60 min daily beyond his or her normal activity. The exercise must be performed in one session; any type of exercise is beneficial as long as it is in the upright position. In several studies, about 80 percent of patients have increased their walking distance. Patients must also quit smoking because smokers have a greater rate of amputation[28] and vascular graft occlusion than nonsmokers. Patients should also be instructed

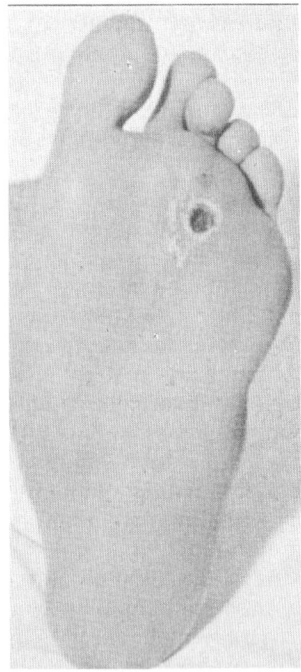

FIGURE 167-2   A neurotropic ulcer over the metatarsal heads in a patient with diabetes mellitus and neuropathy. The ulcer is deep, surrounded by callus, and painless.

to keep their feet warm, clean, and dry; extremes of temperature should be avoided because ischemic tissue is more susceptible to burning at lower temperatures and to frostbite than normal tissues. Cuts or severe bruises of the limbs or feet should be reported to a physician immediately.

Vasodilator drugs have not been shown to be of value in treatment.[32] Pentoxifylline, an agent that has hemorrheologic effects, has improved treadmill walking distance in some studies.[33] Antiplatelet drugs, such as ticlopidine[34] and aspirin with dipyridamole, may have a beneficial effect in patients with intermittent claudication. Concomitant diseases including polycythemia, hypertension, diabetes, and hyperlipoproteinemias should be treated.

Surgical or angioplasty procedures are usually reserved for patients with intermittent claudication that interferes with employment, ischemic symptoms at rest, or ulcers and gangrene. Sympathectomy is not valuable in treating intermittent claudication but may allow small ulcers or areas of gangrene to heal.

In patients with rest pain, ulcers, or gangrene who cannot undergo revascularization, treatment is difficult. A period of rest with the legs dependent may help some patients but amputation is a frequent outcome. Parenterally administered prostacyclin and prostaglandin E_1 have been the subject of favorable reports, but neither has been adequately evaluated or is available in the United States.

Prevention   Measures that may help prevent arteriosclerosis obliterans are targeted at its risk factors.[32] It is very important not to smoke tobacco. Hypertension and diabetes mellitus should be controlled. Hyperlipoproteinemias should be treated. Although control of hypertension prevents strokes, it is not known if careful control of hypertension or diabetes prevents large-vessel disease. Evidence is accumulating that control of hypercholesterolemia prevents progression of atherosclerotic complications.

Course and Prognosis   In most studies, 60 to 90 percent of patients with intermittent claudication due to arteriosclerosis obliterans remained stable over a period of 5 to 9 years. In one study, 93 percent of the patients with superficial femoral artery disease without diabetes had unchanged or improved symptoms over 9 years.[35] Patients with diabetes mellitus, however, have progressive disease, and their amputation rate is fourfold greater than that of patients without diabetes. About 30 to 50 percent of patients with intermittent claudication have coronary artery or cerebrovascular disease.[36] Mortality in these patients is much greater than in the normal population and is mainly due to myocardial infarction and stroke.

Arterial Emboli

Emboli to the peripheral vasculature originate from thrombi in the heart or proximal blood vessels and cause symptoms and signs of acute ischemia.

Epidemiology   The epidemiology of arterial emboli is that of the underlying disease.

Etiology and Pathogenesis   The greatest incidence of arterial emboli results from mural thrombi in patients with myocardial infarction and from atrial thrombi in patients with atrial fibrillation and mitral valve disease. Emboli are also common in patients with atrial fibrillation without valvular disease,[37] and in patients with prosthetic heart valves, chronic congestive heart failure, cardiomyopathy, endocarditis, and the sick sinus syndrome. Paradoxical emboli originate from deep venous thromboses; the embolus travels to the right side of the heart and then to the left side via the foramen ovale to reach peripheral arteries. Emboli may also originate from thrombi in aneurysms in any proximal blood vessel.

Emboli usually lodge at the bifurcation of arteries; the most common sites are the superficial-deep femoral artery junction, the aortoiliac junction, and the popliteal artery above its trifurcation.

Symptoms and signs are due to the abrupt interruption of the arterial supply to an extremity without collateral blood vessels. A collateral blood supply opens almost immediately in an otherwise normal extremity, which prevents cell death and gangrene in most patients. Lactic acid and other metabolites of ischemia form in the tissues and probably cause the symptoms. If the embolus disintegrates or is removed, tissue swelling occurs because of leaky capillaries.

Clinical Manifestations   HISTORY.   Approximately 50 percent of patients have a sudden onset of pain in an extremity.[38] The other patients have a more insidious onset of pain over several hours. Characteristically, the pain intensifies with time. Most patients also complain of paresthesias or numbness. Twenty percent of patients have muscle weakness or paralysis.

SYSTEM REVIEW.   A history of the underlying heart disease may be found.

PHYSICAL EXAMINATION.   Distal to an embolus, pulses are absent. Coldness and paleness of the extremity are usually well demarcated at a distance below the embolus site. Occasionally the embolus site can be palpated as a localized area of tenderness. An important clinical sign is collapsed veins in the extremity due to slow to absent blood flow. If the patient is seen later in the course of the illness, the limb pallor is replaced by a blotchy cyanosis and muscles may be tender. Edema occurs as collateral circulation develops. Without adequate development of collateral blood flow, the skin of the toes, foot, and lower limb may develop blebs and dry gangrene.

Laboratory and Special Examinations   Doppler measurement of ankle systolic pressure is very low, or arterial sounds over the pedal arteries are absent or nonpulsatile. Plethysmography or oscillometry shows no arterial pulsations in the limb distal to the embolus. Arteriography shows the embolus as a segmental occlusion with sharp borders; the proximal and distal arteries are normal.

Pathology   The pathologic picture is the same as that of the thrombus from which the embolus originated. The embolus lodges in the vessel and there may be clotting of blood distally. Some emboli fragment, and the fragments may become emboli in distal vessels. If not removed or fragmented, the embolus organizes and becomes bound down to the arterial wall. In some patients, the occluded vessel may recanalize.

Diagnosis and Differential Diagnosis   The clinical picture of severe pain that develops over a short period with a cold, pale, pulseless extremity in a patient with a known source for an embolus confirms the diagnosis. Usually no special tests are needed. The differential diagnosis of an acute thrombosis of a previously diseased artery may be difficult. The clinical picture is the same. Acute thrombosis should be suspected when there is a history of intermittent claudication, when the opposite limb is pulseless, and when a source for an embolus is lacking. In acute thrombosis of a stenosed artery, collateral blood vessels may be already developed, and symptoms may abate quickly compared with arterial emboli. In difficult cases, arteriography may be necessary to differentiate the two conditions. Arteriography will show arteriosclerosis of the vasculature proximal and distal to the occlusion to rule out an embolus.

Treatment   Anticoagulation with heparin should be started immediately to prevent thrombus formation proximal and distal to the embolus but also to prevent recurrent embolization. Thrombolytic agents can be used before anticoagulation and are successful without complications in about one-third of patients.[39] The affected extremity should be dependent; the body and limb should be kept warm but heat should not be applied directly to the ischemic limb for fear of burns. Adequate analgesia must be given for the intense pain.

If conservative therapy is not effective in improving the color and temperature of the extremity and pain in 2 to 4 h, or if paralysis occurs, embolectomy by Fogarty catheter or a direct surgical approach is indicated. Patients with aortoiliac emboli usually require embolectomy because progression to gangrene is more common than in patients with more distal emboli. The best results from embolectomy are within 12 h of the embolic event but success is possible even after 48 h. After a surgical approach, anticoagulation must be continued indefinitely to prevent recurrent embolization. After embolectomy, the limb may become edematous, tender, and warm, signs that sometimes lead to a mistaken diagnosis of thrombophlebitis.

Prevention   The incidence of arterial emboli from heart disease can be markedly decreased by chronic anticoagulation with warfarin.[40] Emboli from aneurysms can be prevented by surgical correction of the aneurysm.

Course and Prognosis   After either medical or surgical treatment, muscle fibrosis with tendon shortening or intermittent claudication is not uncommon.[38] The overall prognosis depends on the patient's underlying disease and the incidence of recurrent emboli. The mortality in most studies exceeds 20 percent because of the underlying disease.[41] The prognosis for the affected limb depends on the size of the vessel with the embolus, the age of the patient, and the rapidity of treatment. Emboli to large vessels in an elderly patient lead to more amputations than smaller vessel emboli in younger patients.

Atheromatous Embolism

Atheromatous embolism is the embolization of small pieces of atheromatous debris from arteries to the extremities or body organs. This disease has also been called the trash foot syndrome.

Epidemiology   In 100 consecutive autopsies of patients predominantly greater than 50 years old, 4 percent revealed atherosclerotic emboli.[42] In another autopsy series, only 0.79 percent of 2126 patients over 60 years of age had such emboli, but many cases may have been missed.[43] Usually patients are men over 50 years of age.

Etiology and Pathogenesis   Instigating causes are often absent, but coughing or straining has been postulated as the factor that breaks loose the emboli. Catheterization of blood vessels and intravenous streptokinase therapy have been associated with embolization.[44] Coumarin derivatives have also been blamed, but it is more likely that they aggravate the lesions and prevent healing.[45] The emboli usually originate in the aorta or proximal blood vessels that are severely involved with atherosclerotic lesions. An aneurysm can also be the source. The lining of the atherosclerotic vessels is usually irregularly ulcerated and shaggy. Soft atheromas erode into the vessel lumen and release cholesterol crystals and amorphous atheromatous material. Fibrinoplatelet emboli may also be involved in some cases.[46] The clinical picture is caused by ischemia of the skin and muscle due to the emboli, although all organs of the body may be involved.

Clinical Manifestations   HISTORY.   Patients present with unilateral or bilateral discolored or ulcerated painful toes.[44] They may complain of painful and tender calf muscles and a rash on the lower calf or foot.

SYSTEM REVIEW.   Some patients have a history of intermittent claudication. If the entire aorta is involved, transient ischemic attacks or strokes, renal failure, hemorrhagic pancreatitis, and gastrointestinal ulcerations and bleeding may occur. In these patients, almost all organs except the lung contain cholesterol crystals.[47]

PHYSICAL EXAMINATION.   Physical examination reveals tender, blue toes, and there may be ecchymoses of the sole and lateral aspects of the feet. In some patients, the entire extremities and trunk of the body may show ecchymotic lesions and petechiae in a reticular pattern (Fig. 167-3). Ulcers or gangrene may be present. Normally perfused tissue surrounds the ischemic areas. The calf muscles are often tender. Livedo reticularis and petechiae may be present on the calf and foot. The upper extremities are involved in patients with disease of the aortic arch (Fig. 167-4). Occasionally there are elevated nodular lesions of skin.[48] Pedal and proximal pulses are usually normal, but there may be systolic bruits over the aorta or common femoral arteries. Fever may be present.

Laboratory and Specific Examinations   Eosinophilia is common and has been described in up to 80 percent of patients with renal atheromatous emboli.[49] The sedimentation rate is often elevated. In patients with multisystem involvement there may be elevated renal function tests, increased amylase levels, blood in the urine or stool,

and anemia. Angiography demonstrates diffuse atherosclerotic involvement of the vessels proximal to the lesions.

Pathology   Skin or muscle biopsies may reveal the characteristic elongated, needle-shaped clefts of cholesterol crystals in small arterial vessels.[50] There may be inflammatory infiltrates, intimal thickening, and perivascular fibrosis. Giant cells may also be present.

Diagnosis and Differential Diagnosis   The diagnosis of atheromatous emboli is suggested by the blue or ulcerated painful toes, livedo reticularis, petechiae, tender calf muscles, and elevated skin plaques in the presence of normal pulses. A definite diagnosis can often be made by skin, muscle, or renal biopsies.[50] Occasionally cholesterol emboli may be visualized in the retinal arterioles.

In the differential diagnosis of the blue toe syndrome, several other entities must be considered (Table 167-1). Biopsy of skin or muscle showing cholesterol crystals usually rules out other causes. Without visualization of cholesterol emboli, the pathologic picture resembles that of polyarteritis nodosa; angiography helps in such cases. Small emboli from the heart due to endocarditis, intracardiac thrombi, or arrhythmias are common but can be differentiated from atheromatous emboli by the clinical picture.

Treatment   Atheromatous emboli can be stopped by surgical bypass or endarterectomy to remove or exclude the source. However, many of these patients have contraindications to major surgery. In these patients, therapeutic doses of subcutaneous heparin or aspirin and dipyridamole can be tried but should be continued for at least 1 year if successful.[46,51,52] Warfarin should usually be avoided, especially in patients with toe ulcers. Many patients do not respond to any therapy except surgery.

Prevention   One modality of prevention is to avoid catheterization of severely atherosclerotic blood vessels.

Course and Prognosis   The syndrome usually subsides and lesions heal after successful surgical or medical treatment. Sometimes the emboli cease spontaneously. When surgery cannot be performed and emboli continue, amputations may be necessary. Patients with malignant multisystem disease usually die within a year if treatment is unsuccessful.[53]

Thromboangiitis Obliterans

Thromboangiitis obliterans is an inflammatory occlusive disease affecting medium and small arteries and veins. In 1908 Buerger described in detail a group of patients and so his name is attached to the disease, although the disease was recognized previously.[54]

Epidemiology   The prevalence of the disease is greatest in eastern Europe, the Mediterranean area, and Asia. Many more males are afflicted than females, although the incidence among females has increased in recent years.[55] Patients are usually between the age of 20 and 40 years.

Etiology and Pathogenesis   The etiology of thromboangiitis obliterans remains unknown. Almost all patients who develop this disease are smokers, and the syndrome sometimes abates when patients stop smoking. However, patients do not have an increased sensitivity to subcutaneous injections of nicotine or tobacco extracts or altered blood flow responses to smoking. An increased

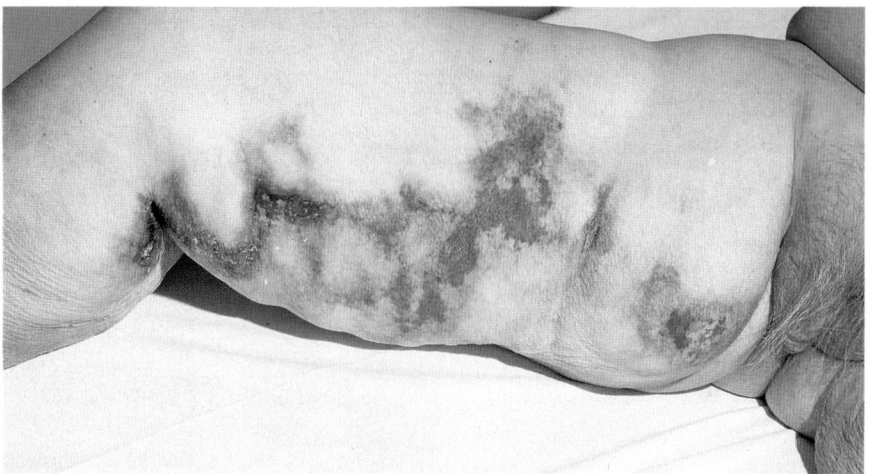

a

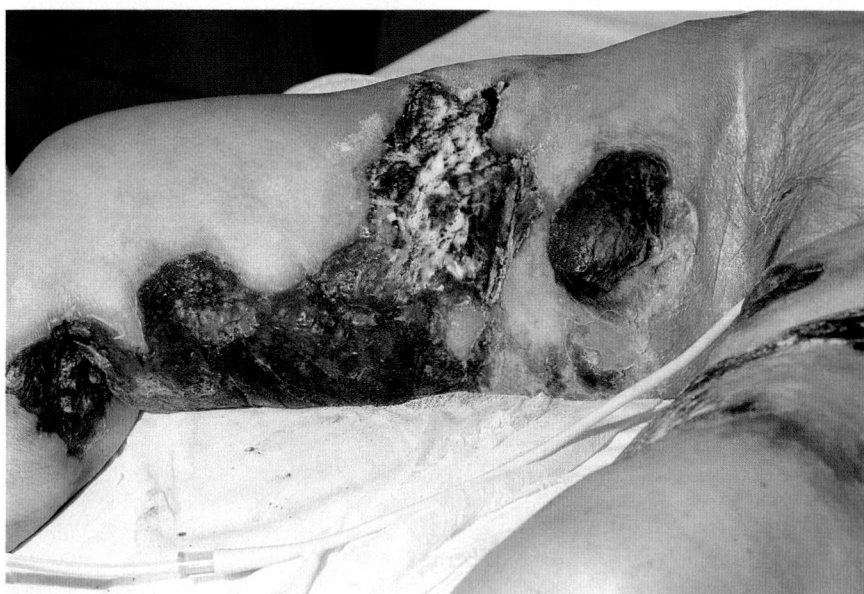

FIGURE 167-3 Multiple atheromatous emboli to the lower body and limbs in a patient with extensive atheromatous disease of the aorta. (*a*) Livedoid vascular pattern with early infarcts. (*b*) Within several days the initial lesion has become much more extensive. (*Courtesy of Klaus Wolff, M.D.*)

b

frequency of HLA-A9 and HLA-B5 or HLA-B8 has been reported but not found by all investigators.[56–58] One study has shown a cell-mediated sensitivity to types I and III collagen and low titers of anticollagen antibody in this disease but not in arteriosclerosis obliterans.[59] The significance of this finding is unknown. It may be that the disease is a vasculitis induced by several different causes. For some reason, the prevalence of the disease has declined sharply in the United States. The pathogenesis of thromboangiitis obliterans involves the production of tissue ischemia and all its manifestations by an inflammatory reaction of medium and small arteries of the extremities, and by obstruction by thrombi.

Veins may also be involved. Occasionally cardiac, intestinal, and cerebral vessels are involved.

Clinical Manifestations   HISTORY.   The most common initial complaints are claudication of the foot or lower calf, digital cyanosis or gangrene, or rest pain. Patients may present with ulcers of the toes or fingers because, although the lower extremities are affected

most often, more than one-third of patients have upper extremity involvement. Ulcerations or gangrenous areas are characteristically extremely painful. Vasospasm or migratory superficial thrombophlebitis may occur in 40 percent of patients.

SYSTEM REVIEW.   Almost all patients are tobacco smokers.

PHYSICAL EXAMINATION.   Physical exam may reveal cyanotic, ulcerated, or gangrenous, very painful digits. The dorsalis pedis and posterior tibial pulses may be absent. In the upper extremity, the ulnar pulse is often absent. During episodes of thrombophlebitis, small indurated red, tender nodules are found; they follow the course of superficial veins and are common on the thigh or calf. Typical changes of Raynaud's phenomenon with well-demarcated pallor or cyanosis of the digits may be seen on exposure to cold; one or more extremities may be involved.

Laboratory and Special Examinations   There are no specific blood studies. Arteriography shows segmental occlusions of medium and small blood vessels with normal vessel walls between

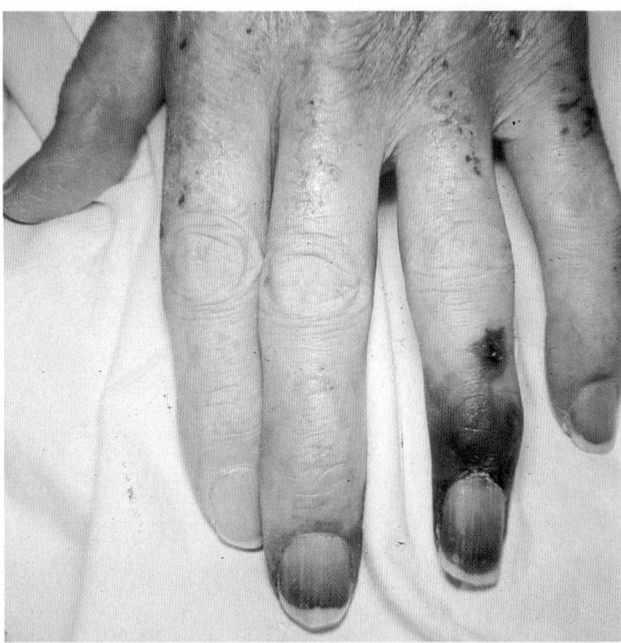

FIGURE 167-4 Atheromatous emboli to the fingers in an elderly patient with extensive atheromatous disease of the aorta. There is gangrene of the third and fourth distal fingers and ecchymotic discrete areas proximally. Radial and ulnar pulses were normal.

diseased areas, no arteriosclerosis of proximal vessels, and a corkscrew configuration of collateral vessels originating from occluded vessels.[60]

Pathology In the acute stage, there is a panvasculitis of arteries and veins. The diagnostic finding is arterial thrombi with foci of microabscesses and giant cells. In the chronic stage, only fibrotic obliteration of the arteries is seen; the diagnosis can only be surmised since arteriosclerosis is absent.

Diagnosis and Differential Diagnosis The diagnosis should be considered in young male smokers presenting with symptoms and signs of distal extremity ischemia, migratory thrombophlebitis, and Raynaud's phenomenon. Arteriography may suggest the diagnosis but only a biopsy of an artery during the active phase of the disease showing the characteristic pathologic picture is diagnostic.

Arteriosclerosis obliterans occurs in an older age group, larger vessels are involved, Raynaud's phenomenon is infrequent, and the upper extremities are rarely involved. In patients with diabetes mellitus, the arteriosclerosis may affect medium-size vessels, but the

TABLE 167-1
Differential Diagnosis of the Blue Toe Syndrome

Polycythemia
Thrombocytosis
Emboli from the heart
Atheromatous emboli
Connective tissue diseases
Primary Raynaud's disease
Circulating anticoagulants
Polyarteritis
Vasculitis
Malignancy with or without cryoglobulins or macroglobulins

blood sugar is normal in patients with thromboangiitis obliterans. Raynaud's phenomenon associated with scleroderma may present with a similar picture, but systemic symptoms, proximal skin changes, and antinuclear antibodies will help in the diagnosis.

Treatment There is no specific treatment. Patients must give up smoking and in some the disease will abate. Otherwise treatment of the disease is the same as for arteriosclerosis obliterans or Raynaud's phenomenon. Corticosteroids have not been beneficial. Sympathectomy may be valuable in patients with a prominent vasospastic component.

Prevention The only preventive measure is never to smoke.

Course and Prognosis The course of the disease is marked by exacerbations and remissions, but finally the disease usually becomes quiescent after many years. Cessation of tobacco smoking sometimes hastens disappearance of the disease. Amputations of digits or even extremities may be necessary, especially in patients who continue to smoke.[61] Patients often have a normal life expectancy.

Erythromelalgia (Erythermalgia)

Erythromelalgia is characterized by paroxysmal attacks of burning pain and redness of one or more extremities brought on by dependency or increased temperature in the presence of normal pulses. The syndrome was described by Mitchell in 1878[62] and better defined as an entity by Smith and Allen in 1938.[63]

Epidemiology

Primary erythromelalgia occurs more in males than females and at all ages.[64] Secondary erythromelalgia has an equal sex distribution and occurs mostly after the third decade. Familial cases have been described sometimes associated with nephritis.[65] One epidemic of the syndrome occurred in China and was thought to be caused by pox virus.[66]

Etiology and Pathogenesis

The etiology of primary erythromelalgia is unknown. Attacks can be produced during occlusion of the circulation to the extremity, which argues against a vascular cause. Abnormalities of prostaglandin metabolism have been postulated because intradermal injection of prostaglandins produces abnormal bullous reactions and increased amounts of prostaglandin-like substance have been found in skin perfusates of patients.[67] This mechanism could account for the marked relief of the syndrome by cyclooxygenase inhibitors in some patients.

In secondary erythromelalgia due to thrombocythemia or polycythemia vera, a qualitative abnormality of platelets has been blamed.[68] Since all diseases with increased platelets do not develop into this syndrome, it is unlikely to be only a quantitative effect. Secondary erythromelalgia is also seen in patients with hypertension, myeloproliferative diseases, lupus erythematosus, and vasculitis. It has been reported during treatment with nifedipine.[69]

Clinical Manifestations

History Patients complain of paroxysmal attacks of localized pain, heat, and redness in the hands, feet, and sometimes more proximally in the extremities. The pain is described as burning, sharp, stabbing, or stinging. Attacks are produced by exposure to heat, dependency of the extremity, or exercise and are relieved by cooling or elevation of the extremity. In the primary syndrome and familial cases, the legs are often affected symmetrically whereas all four extremities are usually involved in secondary erythromelalgia.[64] In the secondary cases, symptoms of the underlying disease may also be present.

Physical Examination Examination during attacks reveals warm, red, extremely sensitive extremities with normal pulses. Between attacks, the extremities appear normal.

Laboratory and Special Examinations

In primary erythromelalgia, all laboratory studies are normal. To rule out secondary causes, platelets and white blood cells must be measured. Antinuclear antibodies should be determined if lupus erythematosus is suspected.

Pathology

Pathologic exams of patients with primary erythromelalgia have not been reported. In the secondary syndrome due to thrombocytosis or polycythemia, fibromuscular dysplasia, internal elastic membrane splitting, and thrombotic occlusions of the arterioles have been described.[68]

Diagnosis and Differential Diagnosis

Criteria for the diagnosis of erythromelalgia include attacks of burning pain in feet or hands; initiation or aggravation of the attacks by standing, exercising, or exposure to heat; relief by elevation or cooling; painful areas that are red, congested, and warm; and refractoriness to treatment.[70] Often attacks can be produced by immersion of the extremity in water at 32 to 36°C. During attacks the skin temperature usually exceeds 31°C. A dramatic relief of attacks by aspirin is also diagnostic but does not occur in all patients.

The differential diagnosis includes the rubor of severe ischemic vascular disease due to arteriosclerosis obliterans or thromboangiitis obliterans. However pulses are absent and the extremity pales upon elevation in these diseases. Arthritis, gout, neuromas, fasciitis, and neuropathies must be considered. Raynaud's phenomenon may have a red, reactive, hyperemic phase with throbbing pain, but this phase is preceded by pallor or cyanotic attacks. Some patients who present with an erythromelalgia syndrome later develop Raynaud's phenomenon. A syndrome called palmar-plantar erythrodysesthesia with painful, red areas has also been described during chemotherapy, but a rash and bullae are usually present.[71]

Treatment

Acute attacks are often relieved by cooling or elevation of the extremity, but otherwise treatment of primary erythromelalgia has been unsatisfactory. Therefore a plethora of drugs including vaso-dilator and vasoconstrictor agents, steroids, antihistamines, β-adrenoceptor blocking agents, and aspirin has been recommended. Desensitization to heat and sympathectomy have also been tried but are not usually successful. In the secondary syndrome due to thrombocytosis or polycythemia vera, complete relief occurs upon treatment with the cyclooxygenase inhibitors, aspirin or indomethacin.[68] The syndrome usually remits with treatment of the thrombocythemia.

Prevention

Attacks may be prevented by avoiding exposure to heat or prolonged dependency of the involved limb.

Prognosis

Patients with the primary disease often learn how to avoid attacks and live with the symptoms. However some patients become totally disabled by the pain and have to live a sedentary existence. In thrombocytosis and polycythemia, acrocyanosis and necrosis of fingers and toes has been described, but these changes may be caused by platelet thrombi rather than by the erythromelalgia.

Vasospastic Diseases and Diseases due to Cold Exposure

Raynaud's Disease and Phenomenon

Raynaud's phenomenon is the occurrence of episodic attacks of well-demarcated blanching or cyanosis of one or more digits on exposure to cold. Maurice Raynaud described the condition in 1888.[72] In 1901 Hutchinson described multiple etiologies for digital vasospastic attacks and suggested the term Raynaud's phenomenon.[73]

Epidemiology Primary Raynaud's disease usually occurs in patients 15 to 40 years of age but may occur in young children and patients over 50 years of age.[74] There is a 4:1 female/male predominance.[75] Some studies have found an equal distribution among men and women and among blacks and whites.[76] Prevalence studies are few and estimate that Raynaud's phenomenon occurs in 4.6 to 30 percent of randomized questioned populations.[76–78] Although cold is usually required to produce the attacks, geographic studies have not been reported.

Etiology and Pathogenesis The pathogenesis of Raynaud's phenomenon or episodic vasospastic attacks is unknown. Normal circulatory control mechanisms have been studied in patients to determine if abnormalities exist. The following are some of the most important findings reported:

1. Ischemic attacks can be produced in single fingers by local cooling and in sympathetically denervated or blocked fingers.[79]
2. Local cooling of the hand augments the reflex sympathetic vasoconstriction induced by cooling of the nape of the neck in patients with Raynaud's disease but not in normal subjects.[80]

Sensitization of α-adrenoceptors by cold exposure was hypothesized.

3. Plasma levels of catecholamines are not increased in the venous drainage of the hands of patients with Raynaud's disease.[81]

4. Systolic pressures at the brachial, proximal digit, and distal fingertip in a cool environment are significantly lower in patients with Raynaud's disease than in normal subjects.[5]

5. In most patients with Raynaud's phenomenon, there is an abrupt loss of distal systolic pressure after release of arterial occlusion of single fingers at 14 to 18°C, which does not occur in normal individuals.[82]

6. During body cooling to induce reflex digital vasoconstriction, capillary blood flow significantly decreases in patients with Raynaud's disease and phenomenon compared with normal subjects.[83] The reduced capillary blood flow is reversed by warming the body.

The first three findings support the theory that there may be a local fault in which the blood vessels are abnormally sensitive to cold, rather than the alternate theory of overactivity of the sympathetic nervous system. The local cold sensitivity would lead to an increased vasoconstrictor response to normal stimuli in Raynaud's disease. The second point indicates that that response may be at the receptor level. Increased levels of α_2-adrenoceptors of platelets have been found in patients with primary Raynaud's disease compared with normal subjects and patients with secondary Raynaud's phenomenon.[84] Also patients with primary Raynaud's disease have an increased digital vasoconstrictor response to an intraarterial α_2-adrenoceptor and not to α_1-adrenoceptor agonists.[85]

Concerning the fourth point, the intravascular pressure not only provides the potential energy for blood to flow, it also maintains the patency of blood vessels. In many of the secondary causes of Raynaud's phenomenon, there are vascular obstructions that would produce a low distal blood pressure. Under these circumstances, a normal sympathetic vasoconstrictor stimulus could lead to vessel closure and an ischemic attack. In Raynaud's disease, digital arteries often appear normal on arteriograms; however, if the digital systolic pressures are lower than normal, the same sequence of events could occur. This phenomenon would explain the finding described in point 5.

The decreased capillary flow in a cool environment (point 6), often to extremely low levels, helps explain the pathogenesis of ischemic attacks, because the capillaries provide nutritional blood flow. The sympathetic nervous system can be implicated since the decreased capillary flow during body cooling is partially reversible upon body warming.

Serotonin has also been incriminated as important in the induction of ischemic attacks in Raynaud's disease because a serotonin inhibitor reduced the intensity and duration of the response of patients to immersion of their hands in cold water.[86] Patients also have an increased sensitivity to intraarterial infusions of serotonin.[85] However, ketanserin, an S_2-serotonergic antagonist, relieves vasospastic attacks but does not prevent their induction.[87]

Measurements of blood viscosity by several investigators have yielded inconsistent results.[88–90] They may be raised in patients with systemic sclerosis or Raynaud's phenomenon. Consistent abnormalities in plasma fibrinogen, cold agglutinins, or cryoglobulins have not been demonstrated in Raynaud's disease but are important in certain secondary cases. Thus aberrations in hemorrheology in the idiopathic disease have not been documented. Platelets may be involved in the pathogenesis of the phenomenon; plasma β-thromboglobulin has been reported to be increased in patients.[91] Serial plasmapheresis has been used to treat severe Raynaud's disease; thus the hemorrheology theory is left open for further investigation.

In summary, a combination of factors may lead to digital artery closure on cold exposure. These factors include vasoconstriction due to reflex sympathetic activity and local cold, low systemic blood pressure, external pressure on the digit, increased sensitivity of certain receptors to cold, and release of vasoactive agents from platelets.

The connective tissue diseases are the most common causes of secondary Raynaud's phenomenon (Table 167-2). Among patients with scleroderma, 80 to 90 percent manifest Raynaud's phenomenon and/or persistent vasospasm. It is the presenting symptom in about one-third of patients and may be the only manifestation of the disease for years. Raynaud's phenomenon occurs in 10 to 35 percent of patients with systemic lupus erythematosus and in about 30 percent with dermatomyositis. It is also sometimes present in patients with rheumatoid arthritis or the vasculitides. In patients with rheumatoid arthritis, cold hands with mottled red and white areas are more common. Arteriograms of patients with connective tissue diseases usually show digital and sometimes ulnar or radial artery obstructions.

Raynaud's phenomenon may be occupational in origin and is especially common in people who use vibratory tools to cut stone or wood. Approximately 30 percent of chain saw users in forestry develop the phenomenon, and it is clearly related to the duration of the exposure.[92] Traumatic vasospastic disease also occurs among various other manual workers such as pianists, typists, riveters, and butchers. Arteriograms have shown digital, radial, ulnar, or palmar arch thromboses in these workers.

Any neurologic condition that produces permanent disuse of a limb can produce a sympathetic nervous system disturbance to that limb. This disturbance is usually manifested by persistent vasospasm with coldness, paleness or cyanosis, and even ulcerations, but Raynaud's phenomenon may occur. Nerve root pressure or nerve entrapment may produce Raynaud's phenomenon. It is often present in patients with the carpal tunnel syndrome and then may involve only the first, index, and middle fingers; the thenar muscles may atrophy. Tapping the median nerve at the wrist may produce shooting pain in the distribution of the median nerve (Tinel's sign). Demonstration of a prolonged conduction time in the median nerve is the definitive diagnostic test. Raynaud's phenomenon may occur secondary to neurovascular compression at the thoracic outlet. Such compression may be due to cervical ribs; abnormalities of the scalenus anticus muscle; bony abnormalities of the cervical vertebrae, clavicle, or first rib; or shoulder compression syndromes (the costoclavicular or hyperabduction syndrome). To confirm the diagnosis, assumption of postures to exaggerate the abnormality must reproduce the symptoms or produce a pale hand from which radial pulse disappears. Loss of the pulse is not diagnostic nor are nerve conduction studies.

Several drugs have been implicated as causing Raynaud's phenomenon. Propranolol, one of the most widely used β-adrenoceptor blockers for cardiovascular diseases and migraine headaches, is probably the most frequent offender.[93] The exact mechanism is not known, but cardioselective β-adrenoceptor blocking drugs have not been shown to be free of this side effect. Ergot preparations and methysergide used to treat migraine headaches also cause the phenomenon. Ergotamine is a powerful α-adrenoceptor vasoconstrictor agonist and may produce gangrene of the fingers.[94] Methysergide, a serotonin antagonist and agonist,

TABLE 167-2
Causes of Raynaud's Phenomenon

Connective tissue disease
  Scleroderma
  Systemic lupus erythematosus
  Dermatomyositis and polymyositis
  Mixed connective tissue disease
  Rheumatoid arthritis
  Polyarteritis and vasculitis
  Sjögren syndrome
Obstructive arterial disease
  Arteriosclerosis obliterans
  Thromboangiitis obliterans
  Arterial embolism
Neurogenic disorders
  Thoracic outlet syndrome
  Carpal tunnel syndrome
  Reflex sympathetic dystrophy
  Hemiplegia
  Poliomyelitis
  Multiple sclerosis
  Syringomyelia
Drugs
  Beta-adrenergic blockers
  Ergot preparations
  Methysergide
  Bleomycin and vinblastine
  Clonidine
  Bromocriptine
  Cyclosporine
Trauma
  Vibratory tools
  Hypothenar hammer syndrome
  Pianists, typists
  Meat cutters
Hematologic causes
  Cryoproteins
  Cold agglutinins
  Macroglobulins
  Polycythemia
Miscellaneous
  Hypothyroidism
  Vinyl chloride disease
  Neoplasms
  Vasculitis and hepatitis B
    antigenemia
  Arteriovenous fistula
  Intraarterial injections

produces peripheral vascular symptoms or signs in about 7 percent of patients.[95] It potentiates the effect of catecholamines on blood vessels but may also cause a sensitivity reaction because vasospasm may follow administration of small doses. Industrial exposure to vinyl chloride polymerization processes may produce acroosteolysis of the distal phalanges of the fingers in a small percentage of workers, and Raynaud's phenomenon may also occur. Arteriograms in these patients show digital artery obstructions.[96] The chemotherapeutic agents bleomycin and vinblastine also may cause the phenomenon.[97] The abuse of methylamphetamine has been followed by vasospasm. Intraarterial use of many medications may lead to vasospasm and gangrene of the fingers.

Patients with cold-precipitable plasma proteins, macroglobulins, and polycythemia can exhibit Raynaud's phenomenon, probably as a result of rheologic disturbances or actual occlusion of small vessels. Cold agglutinins may occasionally cause the syndrome because of blockage of the vessels by agglutinated erythrocytes; an associated vasospastic condition has not been found.[98] Similarly, cryoglobulins can induce ischemic episodes in digits. These epi-

sodes are usually associated with monoclonal gammopathies, particularly macroglobulinemia, or polyclonal gammopathies, such as rheumatoid arthritis. Cryoglobulins are most commonly seen in patients with multiple myeloma but they also occur in those with leukemia, lymphoblastoma, or rarely as an idiopathic condition.

The most common hormonal disturbance causing Raynaud's phenomenon is hypothyroidism; the condition usually remits with thyroid replacement. Manifestations of peripheral vasospasm may also be seen in patients with pheochromocytoma or carcinoid tumors.

Clinical Manifestations HISTORY. Patients complain of episodic attacks of well-demarcated, white or blue digits on exposure to cold and sometimes induced by emotional stimuli (Fig. 167-5). During the attacks, one or more fingers or toes may be numb and may be described as "dead." The thumbs are often spared. On rewarming, the digits may become bright red and throbbing pain may occur. When pain is a prominent symptom in the ischemic phase, a secondary cause should be suspected. Attacks may last minutes to hours. Patients may experience one or more attacks per cold season or multiple attacks throughout the year. The fingers are the digits most commonly involved, but vasospastic attacks may occur in the toes in 40 percent of patients.

SYSTEM REVIEW. In patients with primary disease, systemic symptoms are lacking, although migraine headaches and variant angina pectoris may be more common.[99] Patients with secondary Raynaud's phenomenon may have other symptoms of their underlying disease.

PHYSICAL EXAMINATION. Examination usually shows no abnormalities in patients with primary disease, and vasospastic attacks are difficult to induce in the office. If an attack is witnessed, there is well-demarcated blanching or cyanosis of the digits extending from the tip to varying levels of the digit. The digits distal to the line of ischemia are cold while the proximal skin is pink and warmer. The hands and feet are not involved except in some secondary etiologies. On rewarming, blanched digits may become cyanotic because of the slow blood flow, and then bright red because of reactive hyperemia. The digits appear normal between attacks but may be cool and moist with excess perspiration. The radial and ulnar pulses are normal. Patients may show the nail change known as pterygium, that is, widening of the cuticle to several millimeters and thinning of the proximal skin fold which merges with the cuticle. Other signs are trophic changes including tense and atrophic skin, deformity of the nails, and shortening and contracture of the digits (sclerodactyly). Gangrene is rare and affects only the tips of fingers. Patients with secondary Raynaud's phenomenon may show other manifestations of their underlying disease; persistent ischemic discoloration of digits suggests a secondary cause.

Laboratory and Special Examinations The results of blood and urine studies are normal in patients with primary Raynaud's disease. The effect of local cooling with an ischemic stimulus has been used as a diagnostic test for Raynaud's phenomenon but does not differentiate primary from secondary disease.[100] Compared with normal subjects, patients with Raynaud's phenomenon have a greater reduction in finger systolic pressure upon cooling and many have a loss of pressure or digital artery closure.

Nailfold capillary microscopy may be valuable in diagnosing secondary causes of Raynaud's phenomenon but is not helpful in diagnosing primary disease. Patients with scleroderma, mixed connective tissue disease, and dermatomyositis may have enlarged,

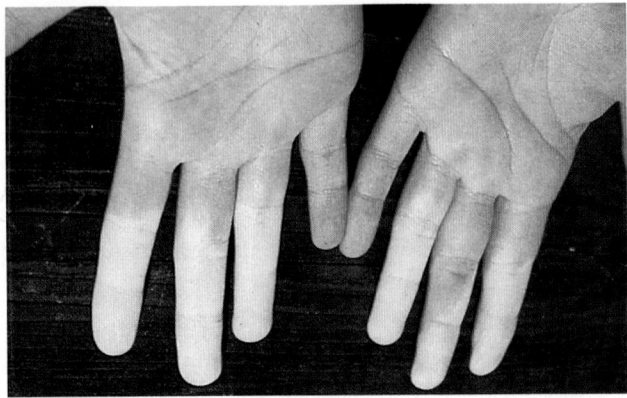

a

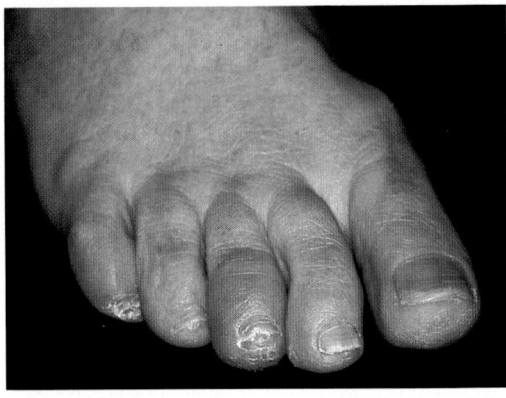

b

FIGURE 167-5 (*a*) A vasospastic attack in a young woman with Raynaud's phenomenon. Well-demarcated blanching of the fingers on exposure to cold is present. Ulnar and radial pulses were normal. The hand is not involved. The attacks were episodic. (*b*) Chilblains are, at times, confused with vasospasm; however, the extremities are cold and red but never white.

deformed capillary loops surrounded by avascular areas.[101] Abnormal capillary loops and a prominent subpapillary venous plexus occur in patients with lupus erythematosus, while bushy capillary formations are most prominent in those with mixed connective tissue disease.

Pathology   Histologic examination of digital arteries has been done in few patients with mild primary Raynaud's disease and results have been normal.[102] Patients with more severe disease show evidence of intimal hyperplasia, narrowing or total occlusion of arteries, or thrombi.

Diagnosis and Differential Diagnosis   The diagnosis is usually made from the history of typical episodic attacks of well-demarcated white or blue discoloration of the digits on cold exposure.[103] Attacks are very difficult to induce in patients with the idiopathic disease despite immersion of the hands in ice water during total body cooling. Patients with enough symptoms to seek a physician's advice should have a complete workup to exclude secondary causes. The history will elicit symptoms of connective tissue disease (arthralgias, arthritis, dysphagia, heartburn, facial rash from the sun, persistent tans), a drug-related etiology, symptoms of the obstructive arterial diseases (intermittent claudication, migratory thrombophlebitis), and exposure to vibratory tools or continuous finger trauma.

   Physical examination should pay attention to all pulses, blood pressure in both arms, telangiectasis, subcutaneous nodules, swollen or deformed joints, skin texture, discoloration of the eyelids, bruits in the neck, thyroid size, relaxation time of reflexes, neurologic deficits, and organomegaly. The thoracic outlet maneuvers should be performed and Tinel's sign sought. Blood analyses for anemia, polycythemia, leukopenia, sedimentation rate, serum protein electrophoresis, antinuclear antibodies, rheumatoid factor, cryoglobulins, and cold agglutinins are necessary. A urinalysis should be done especially to look for proteinuria and red blood cell casts. A chest film will rule out cervical ribs. The results of the history, examination, and tests should all be normal before a patient is reassured that the benign, idiopathic disease is probably the diagnosis. The effect of local cooling on finger systolic blood pressure can be used as a diagnostic test but does not differentiate primary from secondary Raynaud's phenomenon.[100]

In 1932 Allen and Brown[104] proposed the following criteria for the diagnosis of primary Raynaud's disease to exclude patients with connective tissue diseases:

1. Vasospastic attacks precipitated by exposure to cold or emotional stimuli.
2. Bilateral involvement of extremities.
3. Absence of gangrene or, if present, limited to the skin of the fingertips.
4. No evidence of an underlying disease that could be responsible for vasospastic attacks.
5. History of symptoms for at least 2 years.

   These criteria are very helpful but fail to exclude some patients with connective tissue diseases, especially scleroderma.

   The main differential diagnoses are chilblains (perniosis) (Fig. 166-5*b*), cold digits, and acrocyanosis. Many patients complain of cold, sometimes painful digits but color changes are absent. This condition may be one extreme of the spectrum of normal sympathetic nerve activity. In patients with acrocyanosis, the hands and feet are involved (whereas only the digits are in Raynaud's phenomenon), the color change is persistent and not episodic, a pallor phase is absent, and there is no predilection for males or females.

Treatment   Most patients with Raynaud's disease respond to reassurance that they have a benign disease and to instructions to wear loose-fitting, warm clothes covering as much of the body as possible to prevent reflex sympathetic vasoconstriction and to avoid cold, especially with pressure on the digits.[103] Tobacco smoking should be discouraged because nicotine induces cutaneous vasoconstriction; smokers are more numerous among patients with Raynaud's disease[78] and traumatic vasospastic disease[92] than among those without these conditions. The underlying cause must be treated in patients with secondary Raynaud's phenomenon. In those with obstructive arterial disease, the large-vessel involvement must be corrected. In patients with traumatic vasospastic disease, avoidance of the instigating cause will ameliorate, but not always completely cure, the symptoms. Drug-induced ischemic attacks usually respond to withdrawal of the offending agent, but in acute episodes of severe vasoconstriction, intravenous or intraarterial nitroprusside may be needed. Shoulder buildup exercises are often successful in patients with thoracic outlet syndromes and should be tried for several months before surgery is considered. Hematologic abnormalities often respond to treatment of the underlying disease. Vasospastic symptoms in patients with connective tissue diseases usually must be treated symptomatically or with drugs.

Drug therapy can be used in the more severe cases of the disease or phenomenon but is only successful in about 50 percent of patients.[103] The calcium channel blocking agent nifedipine has had the most success. Several studies have shown that nifedipine decreases the frequency, duration, and severity of attacks in about two-thirds of patients with primary or secondary Raynaud's phenomenon.[105,106] Diltiazem but not verapamil may also be beneficial.[107,108] Both reserpine and guanethidine increase capillary blood flow during cold exposure in patients and have the advantage of once-a-day administration.[83] Painful ulcerations or gangrene have been reported to respond to intraarterial reserpine, but a controlled study found no benefit compared with saline injections.[109] Prazosin, an α_1-adrenoceptor agonist, produces a moderate benefit.[110] Other sympatholytic drugs including methyldopa, phenoxybenzamine, and tolazoline have also been recommended. Nitrates or their ointments have their proponents but are usually used in combination with other agents. Parenteral prostaglandins have been reported to be beneficial but oral preparations are not available.[111] Oral forms of other direct-acting agents such as niacin and papaverine are not useful, nor are the drugs that are principally muscle vasodilators, nylidrin and isoxsuprine.[112]

Stanozolol, a fibrinolytic agent, has been shown to increase hand blood flow in patients but evidently does not act by decreasing blood viscosity.[88] Serial plasmapheresis has been reported to ameliorate symptoms of the disease in more severely afflicted patients; its mode of action is undetermined.[91] Either biofeedback or Pavlovian conditioning[113] may provide some benefit to patients, but the former requires a time commitment by the patient. Upper extremity sympathectomy has no value in controlling the disease or the phenomenon; its benefit lasts only 6 months to 2 years. Lumbar sympathectomy does produce lasting relief for Raynaud's phenomenon of the lower extremity but may be accompanied by increased sympathetic activity in the upper limbs.

Prevention   Moving to a warmer climate alleviates symptoms in about 50 percent of patients.[74] Some of the secondary causes can be prevented. Measures have been instituted to decrease the vibration of tools and to shorten hours for workers to prevent traumatic vasospastic disease. Vasoconstrictor drugs must be used with care to prevent overdoses. Mechanics and meat cutters should be warned not to use the hand as a hammer.

Course and Prognosis   Among patients with primary Raynaud's disease, approximately 38 percent of patients have no change in symptoms over time, 36 percent improve, 16 percent develop more severe attacks, and in 10 percent the syndrome disappears.[74] Sclerodactyly develops in 3.3 percent. Less than 1 percent have digital amputations although digital trophic changes occur in 13 percent. Although trophic changes of the fingers may develop in many patients, the prognosis is fairly good.[114] Unfortunately scleroderma is difficult to diagnose and some patients develop manifestations of this disease many years after the onset of Raynaud's phenomenon.

Acrocyanosis

Acrocyanosis is a persistent, symmetric blue discoloration of the digits, hands, or feet on cold exposure while pulses are normal. In 1896 Crocq described patients whose hands and feet slowly became blue on exposure to cool or cold environments.[115]

Epidemiology   The age range is 20 to 45 years.[116] Acrocyanosis is not more frequent in either men or women. The incidence is unknown and no geographic information is available.

Etiology and Pathogenesis   The etiology is unknown. Inactivity[116] and emotional problems[115] have been blamed. It has been postulated that vasoconstriction of the small cutaneous arteries and arterioles leads to decreased blood flow while secondary dilatation of the capillaries and subpapillary venous plexus enhances the cyanosis.[117] Skin blood flow is markedly reduced and capillary pressure is probably low. Sympathetic nerve blocks relieve the cyanosis. Because the vasoconstriction is reversible, gross structural changes of the vasculature are unlikely.[118,119] One study found heightened arteriolar tone at average room temperature.[120] During sleep, the cyanosis may disappear and may not be induced by local cooling,[121] a finding suggesting an abnormal vasomotor response of central origin.

Clinical Manifestations   HISTORY.   Patients complain of persistently blue or reddish discoloration of the digits, hands, and feet of both upper and lower extremities which extends sometimes as far proximally as the wrists or ankles. The involved parts feel cool and sweat excessively; puffiness and numbness but not pain may be complaints.

SYSTEM REVIEW.   Patients have no complaints except for the symptoms in the extremities.

PHYSICAL EXAMINATION.   Examination of the patient shows only cyanotic digits, hands, and feet in a cool or cold environment and usually excess sweating of the extremities. The pulses are normal. Cyanosis is usually relieved by warming the affected parts. The nose, cheeks, chin, and pinna may rarely manifest cyanosis. Trophic changes except digital swelling do not occur.

Laboratory and Special Examinations   The results of blood and urine examinations are normal.

Pathology   Pathologic studies are rare; minimal hypertrophy of the medial coats of cutaneous arterioles has been described.[116] Capillary dilatation and abnormalities have been reported by microscopy of the nail beds.[122]

Diagnosis and Differential Diagnosis   The diagnosis is based on the persistent, symmetric bluish discoloration of the digits, hands, or feet accompanied by increased sweating and a normal history and physical examination. If generalized cyanosis is a consideration, arterial oxygen saturation should be measured. The lack of episodic, well-demarcated color changes rules against Raynaud's phenomenon.

A more severe disease termed "remittent necrotizing acrocyanosis" usually appears suddenly in late adult life without regard for seasons and lasts weeks to months.[123] In addition to the color changes, ulcers and gangrene of the fingers often occur. It is distinguished from benign acrocyanosis by the presence of pain. Biopsies have shown occlusion of small arteries and arterioles by cellular proliferation or hyaline thrombi. The cause is unknown but it is probably different from the symmetric cyanosis and gangrene seen rarely in acute infections.

Treatment   Treatment is usually unnecessary because acrocyanosis is mainly a cosmetic problem. It does respond to drugs that interfere with sympathetic nerve activity such as reserpine.

Prevention   Keeping the extremities and body warm may decrease sympathetic nerve activity and attenuate the discoloration.

Course and Prognosis   The syndrome usually persists but the prognosis is very good because trophic digital changes do not occur.

Livedo Reticularis

Livedo reticularis is characterized by a reddish blue mottling of the skin in a ''fishnet'' reticular pattern. Livedo reticularis with ulceration was originally described by Milian in 1929 as *atrophie blanche en plaque;* he considered it a manifestation of syphilis.[124]

Epidemiology   All types of livedo reticularis occur most commonly in young women less than 40 years of age.

Etiology and Pathogenesis   Livedo reticularis has been called by many names including idiopathic livedo reticularis, cutis marmorata, livedo annularis, livedo racemosa, sympathetic livedo reticularis, and asphyxia reticularis. Livedo reticularis with ulceration is also known as livedo or livedoid vasculitis and atrophie blanche. A variety of names always reflects an unknown etiology.

Secondary livedo reticularis usually accompanies vasospastic conditions such as primary and secondary Raynaud's phenomenon, acrocyanosis, and vasculitis. It is often a manifestation of an underlying disease and may be a clue to its diagnosis. It has been reported in association with connective tissue diseases especially lupus erythematosus, obstructive arterial diseases, endocrine disorders, neurogenic diseases, drug reactions, hyperviscosity states, hypertension, and lymphomas. It has been shown to be induced by amantadine, a drug used for Parkinson's disease and influenza. It is an important diagnostic manifestation in atheromatous embolization. Livedo reticularis with cerebrovascular lesions has been described (Sneddon's syndrome),[125] this manifestation may be part of a syndrome with arterial and venous thromboses, spontaneous abortions, and anticardiolipin antibodies (Fig. 167-6).[126]

Livedo reticularis with ulceration may result from a localized vasculitis.[127] Immunofluorescence studies have shown immunoglobulin M deposits. Complement factors, fibrin, and sometimes IgA have also been found in the vessel walls, which suggests an immune complex pathogenesis. Other investigators believe that this disease may be caused by blood or tissue abnormalities that induce thromboses of arterioles.[128] A defect in the fibrinolytic system may be present. Abnormalities of platelet adhesiveness have also been reported.[129,130]

Amantadine causes livedo reticularis and is known to release norepinephrine from central and peripheral nerve terminals and to enhance the action of norepinephrine and dopamine on several peripheral tissues.[131] These actions, combined with amantadine's ability to inhibit uptake of dopamine and norepinephrine in neurons, could lead to arteriolar constriction.

Vasospasm or obstruction of the small perpendicular arterioles in the dermis is the probable cause of the fishnet appearance of the skin. The red to blue periphery of each web of the net would be due to deoxygenated blood in surrounding horizontally arranged venous plexuses.[132] Elevation of the extremity therefore decreases the intensity of the color changes by emptying the veins. The reversibility of the color pattern with warming, the frequent association with vasospastic diseases of the digits, and the beneficial response to sympathetic blocking agents suggest increased sympathetic nerve activity as the cause of benign livedo reticularis.

Clinical Manifestations   HISTORY.   Patients with benign livedo reticularis have no complaints except for the cosmetic appearance

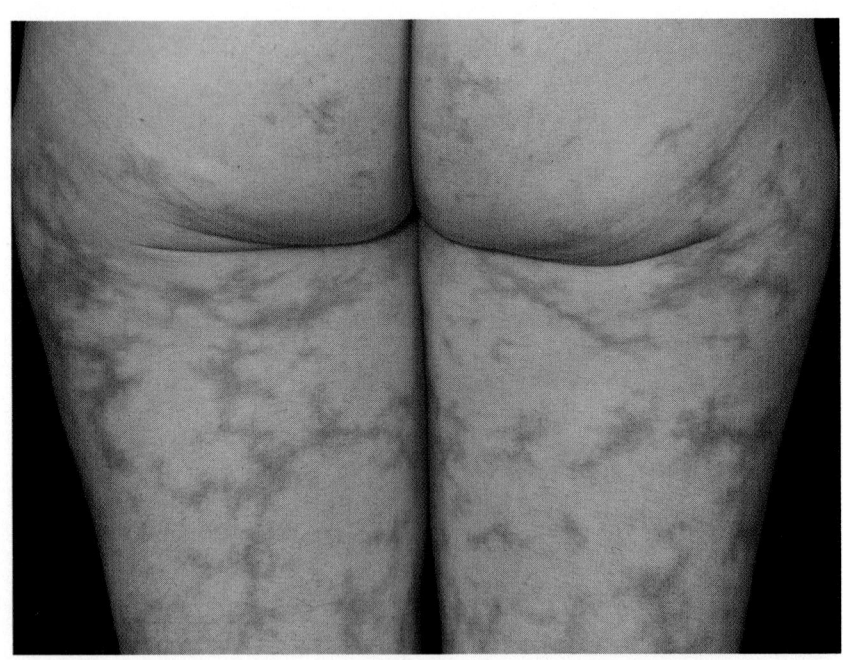

FIGURE 167-6   Livedo reticularis of the buttocks and thighs in a woman who had a cerebrovascular thrombosis. This is an example of Sneddon's syndrome. (*Courtesy of Klaus Wolff, M.D.*)

of the cutaneous fishnet. Numbness and pain are rare but a subjective feeling of coldness is common. Patients with secondary livedo reticularis may complain of symptoms of their underlying disease. Persistence of the fishnet pattern during warming and purpuric macular lesions or skin nodules that ulcerate are the complaints in patients with livedo reticularis with ulceration. Most patients only have the painful ulcers in the winter while others have them in the summer also.

SYSTEM REVIEW.   There are no systemic complaints in patients with benign or ulcerating disease. In patients with secondary livedo reticularis, there may be symptoms of venous or arterial thrombosis, lupus erythematosus, atherosclerotic emboli, or cerebrovascular disease.

PHYSICAL EXAMINATION.   In the benign form, a fishnet pattern affects mainly the extremities, and the webs are rose, violet, red, or blue. Between the webs, the skin appears pale. The colors are aggravated by exposure to cold and may disappear on warming. The examination is normal except for the skin. In patients with livedo reticularis with ulceration, purpuric lesions, cutaneous nodules, or ulcers may be found (Fig. 167-7). The ulcers are usually covered with eschars and surrounded by red inflammation. They are very tender. About 50 percent of patients have edema of the legs which often occurs before the ulcerations. Healed ulcers leave a smooth ivory-white plaque of atrophic skin surrounded by hyperpigmented borders and telangiectatic blood vessels (atrophie blanche) (Fig. 167-7b). Most ulcers are found on the lower part of the legs, ankles, and dorsum of the feet (Fig. 167-7a).

Patients with secondary livedo reticularis may have other manifestations of their underlying disease. They may have the benign or ulcerated form, but patients with Sneddon's syndrome (livedo reticularis and cerebrovascular lesions) need not necessarily have ulceration or atrophie blanche (Fig. 167-6).

Laboratory and Special Examinations   In patients with livedo reticularis with or without ulceration, no specific blood or urine tests are abnormal.[127]

Pathology   In benign livedo reticularis and that due to drug therapy, biopsies have shown nonspecific changes or increased numbers of dilated capillaries.[133,134] A segmental hyalinizing vasculitis of the middle dermal vessels has been described in the ulcerative disease.[127,133] The vessel walls are thickened with or without lymphocytic cuffing; hyaline degeneration and areas of focal arteriolar thromboses are present. Hemorrhages and new blood vessel proliferation may be seen. In Sneddon's syndrome, there is also a noninflammatory hyalinization and thickening of vessel walls and vascular occlusions which are seen only in biopsies from the center of the mesh of the fishnet pattern.

Diagnosis and Differential Diagnosis   Diagnosis of the benign form is easily made from the typical fishnet pattern on the skin. In patients with ulcers, other causes of lower extremity ulcers must be ruled out. Secondary causes must be sought before the diagnosis is considered benign or ulcerated livedo reticularis. Livedo reticularis with ulceration is therefore a diagnosis by exclusion of underlying diseases.

Treatment   The benign type of livedo reticularis needs no treatment. The skin discoloration can be covered with cosmetics or, as a last resort, sympatholytic agents can be tried for patients bothered by the social stigma.

In livedo reticularis due to secondary causes, the underlying disease should be treated. Patients with anticardiolipin antibodies and thromboses should be treated with anticoagulants. Treatment of livedo reticularis with ulceration has been unsuccessful. Saline soaks and analgesic ointments are helpful. Antiplatelet agents[129,130] and agents that induce fibrinolysis[135] are the most recently recommended therapies. Dextran infusions, nicotinic acid, pentoxifylline, nifedipine, heparin, corticosteroids, cytoxan, methotrexate, radiotherapy, sympathetic blocking agents, and other therapies have all been reported to benefit some patients. Since the disease is rare, there are no large controlled studies of treatment modalities.

Prevention   Only measures to keep the body and extremities warm may help prevent livedo reticularis.

Course and Prognosis   The benign condition has an excellent prognosis. In livedo reticularis with ulceration, the painful ulcers are often recurrent and may be disabling. The lower limbs and feet become scarred; amputations have been necessary for deep ulcers and severe pain.[133]

Reflex Sympathetic Dystrophy

Reflex sympathetic dystrophy or causalgia is a syndrome of persistent pain and swelling of an extremity usually following minor or major injuries, certain illnesses, or surgical procedures. Mitchell made the classic descriptions of reflex sympathetic dystrophy in 1864 and 1872.[136,137]

Epidemiology   The syndrome is seen most commonly in adults in the fifth to seventh decade, but there are several reports of the disease in children. The syndrome has been reported in 2 to 14 percent of patients with nerve injuries[138] and in 22 percent of patients with myocardial infarction.[139] In the latter patients, it is referred to as the shoulder-hand syndrome.

Etiology and Pathogenesis   Reflex sympathetic dystrophy usually follows fractures, compression injuries, gun shot wounds, or surgical procedures but can occur with minor blunt trauma or sprains.[140] The shoulder-hand syndrome is seen in patients after myocardial infarctions, strokes, or prolonged immobilization of an extremity. The pathogenesis is unknown but the condition has been postulated to be due to injured sensory fibers transmitting constant signals to the spinal cord which results in stimulation of sympathetic centers.[141] A decrease followed by an increase in sympathetic activity would then occur. There are definite signs of disturbed sympathetic activity in the affected limb. Others consider that there is a central nervous system component because patients sometimes have bilateral abnormalities.[142] Most evidence points to an increase in blood flow to the bones in the affected extremity leading to osteoporosis.

Clinical Manifestations   HISTORY.   There is a history of major or minor trauma, or prolonged immobilization of a limb. Occasionally, no inciting event can be discerned. Patients complain of severe, unrelenting pain and sensitivity of the afflicted limb. The extremity may feel hot or cold. Increased sweating, pale or bluish discolorations, and cold sensitivity are other possible signs. Vasospastic attacks of white or blue digits may also be experienced and suggest a diagnosis of Raynaud's phenomenon.

PHYSICAL EXAMINATION.   At first, the affected part may be warm, dry, swollen, and extremely sensitive to even light touch.

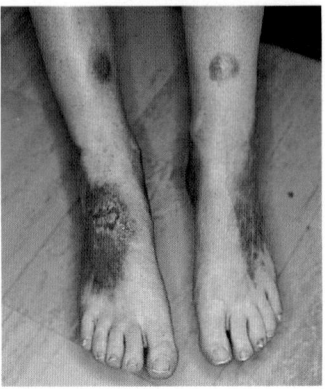

a

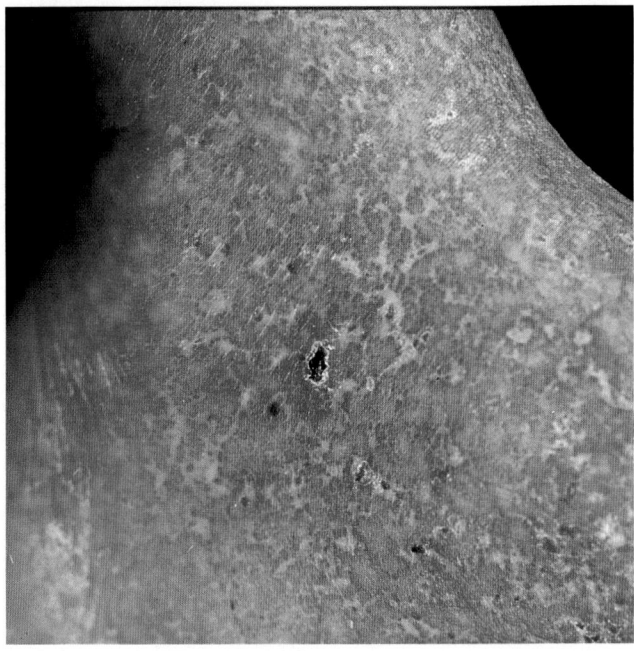

b

FIGURE 167-7 (*a*) Recurrent irregular, extremely painful ulcers of the feet and lower legs in a 32-year-old woman with livedo reticularis with ulceration. Pigmented areas of healed ulcers are present. Ulcerations had been recurrent since age 16 with no relation to seasons. Pedal pulses were normal. (*b*) Close-up of atrophie blanche with irregular porcelain-white atrophic scars, ulceration, and crusting in a similar patient. (*Courtesy of Klaus Wolff, M.D.*)

This initial presentation is followed by a cold, pale, and swollen phase with hyperhidrosis. The patient usually is very protective of the involved limb and withdraws it from examination because of severe sensitivity. Part or all of a hand or foot or extremity may be involved. Some investigators report bilateral signs in many patients.[142] Pulses are normal.

Laboratory and Special Examinations Blood and urine studies are usually normal although an increased sedimentation rate may be found. X-ray of the involved part may show patchy demineralization of bone (Sudeck's atrophy), which does not correlate with the duration of the syndrome.[143] Radionuclide studies may show an asymmetric increase of the isotope in the affected extremity compared with the nonaffected extremity.[143] However isotope localization may also be decreased in children.[144] There is no test that is positive in all patients.

Pathology Skin, subcutaneous tissue, and muscle show nonspecific changes. Affected bone has increased vascularity and prominent osteoclastic activity. Synovial biopsies show proliferation and disarray of synovial lining cells, an increased number of small blood vessels, and some lymphocytic infiltration.[142]

Diagnosis The diagnosis is based on the presence of persistent pain and tenderness in an extremity with signs of vasomotor instability such as increased warmth or coldness, pallor or cyanosis, increased or decreased sweating, and swelling in comparison with the contralateral extremity. It is helpful but not necessary to have a history of trauma or immobilization, an x-ray showing patchy osteoporosis, or a positive radionuclide bone scan.

Treatment As soon as this entity is recognized, it is most important to institute a physical therapy program for the affected extremity. If there is no improvement, other treatment modalities should be tried. Treatments that have been reported effective include chemical sympathetic nerve blockade, pharmacologic (regional intravenous reserpine or guanethidine) or surgical sympathectomy, phenoxybenzamine, ketanserin, calcitonin, vasodilator agents (ni-

fedipine, naftidrofuryl hydrogen oxalate), intravenous droperidol, systemic corticosteroids, transcutaneous nerve stimulation, and casting of the involved extremity. As with any disease for which multiple therapies are recommended, patients often do not respond to some or any treatments. Early in the course, ganglionic blockade or surgical sympathectomy has the most success, but most treatments are ineffective after the syndrome has been present more than a few months.

Course and Prognosis Many patients respond to physical therapy with or without sympathetic nerve blocks or sympathectomy to relieve pain if treated early, but recovery to a normal status usually takes 1 to 2 years. The extremity atrophies in other patients and continues to be extremely painful, cold, and swollen. The pain is difficult to relieve and may require narcotics. These patients often have a psychiatric problem, but it is difficult to ascertain whether it preceded the condition or was the natural outcome of this disabling, painful illness.

Frostbite

Frostbite is due to freezing of tissues and the resulting tissue injury.

Epidemiology Frostbite may occur in any area where the temperature reaches 0°C although higher temperatures coupled with strong winds can also freeze tissue. It is especially a danger to mountain climbers.

Etiology and Pathogenesis Tissue damage results from intense vasoconstriction and ice crystal formation. The circulation stops in the frozen area. Crystal formation leads to cellular dehydration and hyperviscosity. Injury appears to affect mainly the endothelial cells of arterioles.[145] After thawing, intravascular platelet aggregation and swelling of the interstitium occur, and much later leukocytes appear and red blood cells extravasate.

High winds and cold are more dangerous than cold alone. Wet skin is also more conducive to frostbite because water in the corneum triggers crystallization not only in the corneum but also in underlying tissue.[146] The pathogenesis is similar to immersion foot, which is due to prolonged exposure of the extremities to wetness plus cold. Immersion foot at warm temperatures shows only hyperhydration of the plantar stratum corneum.

Clinical Manifestations HISTORY.   Patients relate exposure to extreme cold, cold with wetness, or a high wind chill factor. The frozen part may have become numb and stiff with a white or waxy, hard appearance. On rewarming, burning pain, paresthesias, and flushing of the skin are common complaints.

PHYSICAL EXAMINATION.   Before rewarming, the damaged area will be pale, indurated, and less sensitive.[147] The nose, ear lobes, cheeks, fingers, or toes are most frequently affected. After rewarming, the part is reddened, swollen, and painful. Blisters, sometimes hemorrhagic, may form early or in several days. Joint contractures may develop early. In severe cases, there is no recovery of tissue color on rewarming and dry gangrene develops. Autoamputation of the mummified areas often takes place after several weeks.

Pathology   There is morphologic injury to the endothelial cells during freezing of the skin. After thawing there is intravascular platelet aggregation and interstitial swelling followed by red blood cell extravasation and leukocyte invasion. Subcutaneous edema forms and may result in vesicles and bullae. A hyperemic zone separates injured from normal tissue. Thrombosis occurs mostly in arterioles. These changes either revert toward normal or go on to necrosis and gangrene. Depending on the depth of freezing, muscle, nerve, and bone destruction can be seen in addition to cutaneous necrosis.

Diagnosis and Differential Diagnosis   The diagnosis is made from the history of cold exposure with or without high wind and wetness and from the clinical picture. There is little reason to differentiate the condition from cold immersion foot since the prognosis and treatment are similar.

Treatment   Frostbite is usually classified as only superficial or deep since the extent of tissue damage is difficult to determine in the early phases.[147] Management should be conservative until the full depth of tissue damage is known. Conservation prevents unnecessary removal of viable tissue. If superficial frostbite occurs, quick rewarming by placing the affected part in the axilla or against a companion's warm body may help. The hands or feet should not be rubbed together or with snow. Rewarming the affected parts in a water bath at 40 to 42°C (104 to 108°F) is the only effective treatment. It takes about 30 min until the entire part becomes flushed; rewarming may be painful. Dependency of the limb should be avoided to prevent edema. Weight bearing should be avoided. The areas of frostbite should only be cleaned gently and blisters should be left intact. Most authorities recommend avoiding debridement until all healing has occurred, which may take months. Early surgical or medical sympathectomy may be beneficial.[148,149]

Prevention   To prevent frostbite not only the hands and feet but also the head and body must be kept warm. Multiple layers of clothing that trap air should be worn. Tight or wet clothing causes a greater risk. Exposed persons should observe each other for signs of frostbite on exposed areas.

Course and Prognosis   Depending on the depth of frostbite, tissue may be lost eventually by amputation. Sequelae of healed frostbite include hyperhidrosis, paresthesias, cold sensitivity, Raynaud's phenomenon, and pain with use.

Diseases of the Veins

Thrombophlebitis

Thrombophlebitis or deep venous thrombosis is caused by thrombotic obstruction of veins with or without an inflammatory response to the thrombus.

Etiology and Pathogenesis   Deep venous thrombosis results from slow blood flow, hypercoagulability, or changes in the venous walls. The most common causes are shown in Table 167-3. Some malignancies such as those of the lung, pancreas, and stomach are associated with thrombophlebitis, and it may be of the migratory variety. Oral contraceptives significantly reduce activated factor X inhibitory activity and induce venous thrombosis. In recent years, coagulation factor deficiencies predisposing to thrombophlebitis have been discovered. These are often hereditary deficiencies and include antithrombin III, proteins C and S, and fibrinolytic factor deficiencies.[150,151] Actual deficiencies in these factors may occur or there may be abnormal inactive molecular forms. Thrombophlebitis and arterial thrombi may occur in patients with antiphospholipid antibodies and are most common in patients with lupus erythematosus.

Superficial thrombophlebitis is usually due to infections or trauma to superficial veins from needles or catheters. A migratory variety is seen in patients with thromboangiitis obliterans and malignancies. Mondor's disease is an inflamed subcutaneous vein from the breast to the axillary region that has no special associations.[152]

The thrombus originates in an area of low or no venous flow, and the extrinsic pathway for blood coagulation is probably the most important factor.[153] Occlusion of a vein by a thrombus blocks venous return and leads to increased venous pressure and edema in the distal limb. An inflammatory response to the thrombus causes pain and tenderness. Prominent collateral veins appear early to bypass the obstruction and relieve the edema; recanalization may

TABLE 167-3

Predisposing Factors in Deep Venous Thrombosis

Common factors	Less common factors
Major surgery	Sickle cell anemia
Fractures	Homocystinuria
Congestive heart failure	Protein C or S deficiency
Acute myocardial infarction	Antithrombin III deficiency
Stroke	Antiphospholipid antibodies
Pregnancy and postpartum	Ulcerative colitis
Spinal cord injuries	
Shock	
Oral contraceptives	
Malignancies	
Venous varicosities	
Previous history of venous thrombosis	
Severe pulmonary insufficiency	
Prolonged immobilization	

occur in several weeks. If the venous pressure is too high, arterial inflow may rarely be compromised and ischemia of the distal limb occurs. The thrombus within the vein often has a free-floating tail which may break off to produce a pulmonary embolus. The free-floating tail is bound down to the vein wall in about 10 days. Organization of the thrombus in the vein destroys the venous valves and leads to the postphlebitic syndrome.

Clinical Manifestations HISTORY. Patients may complain of pain or aching in the involved limb, have no symptoms, or notice limb swelling. Some patients have the symptoms of pulmonary emboli without symptoms of the extremities.

SYSTEM REVIEW. Patients may have a history of malignancy, oral contraceptive use, a recent long trip with prolonged immobility, or a family history of thrombophlebitis.

PHYSICAL EXAMINATION. The clinical picture varies widely from subtle signs of swelling to a tensely swollen, warm, tender limb with prominent, distended collateral veins. Swelling may first be detected by noting increased turgor of the muscles or by carefully measuring limb circumference compared with the opposite limb. Pitting edema may occur. A tender cord may be felt where the vein is thrombosed.

In patients with iliofemoral thrombophlebitis, the limb is swollen from the foot to the inguinal region, tenderness is not present in the limb because the thrombus is proximal, and collateral veins may form from the thigh to the abdominal wall (Fig. 167-8). The limb may be very pale (phlegmasia alba dolens) or may be cyanotic with cold digits if the arterial inflow is compromised (phlegmasia coerulea dolens). In patients with thrombosis of calf veins, the calf and foot are swollen and warm; there is deep tenderness with or without a palpable cord. Resistance to dorsiflexion of the foot may be increased (Homans' sign). Subclavian venous thrombosis causes swelling of an upper limb with fullness of the supraclavicular area and collateral veins to the anterior chest wall and around the shoulder.

Thrombosis of the superior vena cava causes swelling of both upper limbs and face including the eyelids. Thrombophlebitis of a superficial vein or varicosity is evidenced by painful induration of the vein with redness and increased heat. Migratory cases have successive areas of superficial veins involved over a variable period. Mondor's disease is manifested by a tender cord from the breast to the axillary region; during healing the venous cord shortens and puckers the skin.[152]

Laboratory and Special Examinations There are a variety of tests to detect venous obstruction including doppler examination, impedance plethysmography, and rheoplethysmography.[154] These tests have a high sensitivity and specificity but only for proximal venous thrombosis and not for calf disease. Venous imaging by B-mode duplex ultrasound scanning is an extremely valuable test that can diagnose proximal venous thrombi by indirect means or actual visualization of the thrombi.[155] It is replacing other tests including the definitive venogram. For thrombophlebitis of the calf veins, the localization in the leg of intravenously administered I^{125} fibrinogen is the only definitive test besides venography. White blood cell counts and sedimentation rates are usually normal but may be high in patients with extensive or inflammatory thrombophlebitis.

Pathology The thrombus is composed of fibrin, red blood cells, and platelets. Both white thrombi (platelet aggregates) and red thrombi (fibrin and red blood cells) have been described in the

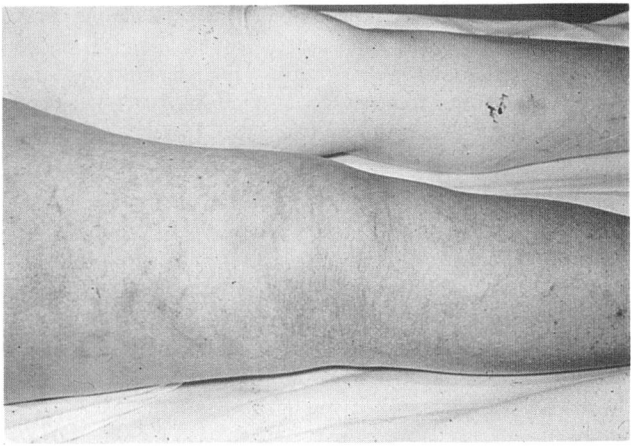

FIGURE 167-8 Acute iliofemoral deep venous thrombosis in a woman postpartum. The thigh and calf are very swollen compared with the opposite limb and have a blotchy cyanotic discoloration.

initial deposits. The thrombus propagates proximally and consists predominantly then of fibrin interspersed with red cells. The reaction of the underlying vein wall may show minimal to marked inflammatory changes with infiltration of white blood cells and loss of endothelium. Leukocytes, lymphocytes, phagocytes, and edema may be seen in the vein wall. Fibroblasts predominate in the later stages to form scar tissue. The thrombus may also undergo the same process and thereby adhere to the vein wall. Some thrombi recanalize. The venous valves within the area of the thrombus are permanently damaged as the thrombus adheres to the vein wall.

Diagnosis and Differential Diagnosis Thrombophlebitis is difficult to diagnose clinically. The symptoms and signs are nonspecific; studies have shown that the clinical diagnosis is incorrect in about 50 percent of patients.[156] Definitive tests by doppler examination, plethysmography, or preferably venous scanning are necessary to make the diagnosis. A venogram is necessary only when these tests give indeterminate results. Although a cause is often not found for a painful or swollen extremity, patients with these problems have a benign prognosis if noninvasive tests do not detect deep venous thrombosis.[157] Superficial thrombophlebitis can be diagnosed by the characteristic clinical picture although lymphangiitis and cellulitis must be considered; the former is usually signaled by red streaking up the limb and tender lymph nodes proximally while the latter is marked by a more diffuse involvement of the extremity.

The most common differential diagnoses of thrombophlebitis include rupture of the plantar muscle which produces an ecchymotic area in the dependent ankle area and sometimes a tender knot over the muscle. Ruptured synovial membrane of the knee joint can imitate thrombophlebitis; knee joint fluid, inflammation, or arthritis are clues to the diagnosis but an arthrogram may be needed.

Treatment The treatment for deep venous thrombosis is anticoagulation.[153] Heparin is given by intravenous infusion at a dosage of approximately 1000 U/h after a loading dose of 5000 U. The aim is to keep the partial thromboplastin time (PTT) at 1.5 to 2 times normal, but it is very important to reach this level within the first day.[158] Warfarin can be started orally at the same time at a dosage of 10 mg daily to prolong the prothrombin time to 1.33 to 1.5 times normal.[159] Warfarin should overlap heparin for 5 days until all necessary blood factors are depressed by the warfarin. Patients are then usually treated with warfarin for 3 months which is when thrombophlebitis or pulmonary emboli are most likely to recur.

Fibrinolytic agents have been used in patients with acute deep venous thrombosis but have not been very successful; their failure may be due to patients' presenting late in the course of the disease.[160] These agents should be given a trial in patients with iliofemoral or subclavian venous thrombosis when possible.

Ambulation is usually allowed when symptoms and signs subside, but elastic stockings with 30 mmHg pressure should be worn for 3 months. In patients in whom anticoagulation is contraindicated, who hemorrhage during anticoagulation, or who have pulmonary emboli while adequately anticoagulated, the therapy of choice is insertion of an inferior vena cava filter.

When gangrene of the toes is impending in patients with iliofemoral venous thrombosis, surgical removal of the thrombus often alleviates the condition even though there is rethrombosis of the vein. Septic thrombophlebitis is treated by removal of catheters and appropriate antibiotic therapy. However, removal of the affected area of the vein may be required in resistant cases.

Prevention Minidose heparin (5000 U subcutaneously every 12 h) is effective prophylaxis against deep venous thrombosis for surgical patients and patients with myocardial infarctions, strokes, or congestive heart failure.[161] For surgery, the heparin must be started preoperatively since the disease starts on the operating table. Minidose heparin does not protect patients undergoing orthopedic procedures or patients with fractures. Warfarin, pneumatic intermittent compression boots, or daily dextran infusions can be used in these patients. Early ambulation after surgery and elastic stockings are also excellent preventive measures in combination with the above methods.

Course and Prognosis Most cases of thrombophlebitis subside within 10 days but many patients have persistent limb swelling, especially with iliofemoral and subclavian venous thrombosis. The postphlebitic syndrome may develop in some patients within 2 years while it may not occur for 20 years in others.

Varicose Veins

Varicose veins are dilated, distended, tortuous veins with incompetent valves.

Epidemiology Varicose veins are more common in women than men and usually appear during the child-bearing years. They are more common in countries whose inhabitants eat a low-fiber diet than in African countries where the diet is high in fiber.[162]

Etiology and Prognosis A hereditary influence in some patients with varicose veins is suggested by the occurrence of the disorder in several members of the same family and the appearance of varices during adolescence. Because varicosities, hemorrhoids, and diverticula of the colon are infrequent in populations subsisting on a high-fiber diet, constipation, and hence increased intraabdominal pressure, have been incriminated for all three entities.[162] Pregnancy is one of the prime causes of varicose veins because of venous relaxation due to increased hormones, expansion of blood volume, and increased venous pressure especially in the limb whose iliac vein is compressed by the enlarged uterus. Increased venous pres-

sure in the limbs during pregnancy is also caused by the arteriovenous fistula-like nature of the placenta which allows a high pressure flow into the uterine and iliac veins.[163] Thrombophlebitis leads to the formation of varicosities by destroying venous valves. Arteriovenous communications also cause varices.

The first abnormality inducing varicosities is a weakening of the commissures of the valves upon dilatation.[164] The dilatation leads to incompetence of the valves and increased venous pressure distally. The increased venous pressure creates a vicious cycle by causing further dilatation of the vein and valves. The increased venous pressure is also transmitted to the capillaries and the result is leakage of fluid into the subcutaneous tissues and muscles.

Clinical Manifestations HISTORY. Most patients have no symptoms but seek medical advice because of the cosmetic appearance. Some patients do complain of fatigue or aching in the calves or swelling of the ankles at the end of the day. The swelling disappears with bed rest overnight. Rarely patients with very large varicosities complain of lightheadedness or blurry vision caused by venous pooling on standing.

SYSTEM REVIEW. Many patients have a history of constipation, hemorrhoids, and pregnancies. In some patients a history of thrombophlebitis precedes the onset of the varicosities.

PHYSICAL EXAMINATION. Varicose veins can be seen as dilated, tortuous, sacculated superficial veins (Fig. 167-9). They are often thick-walled. The greater saphenous vein is most commonly involved but varicosities may be found anywhere on the legs and

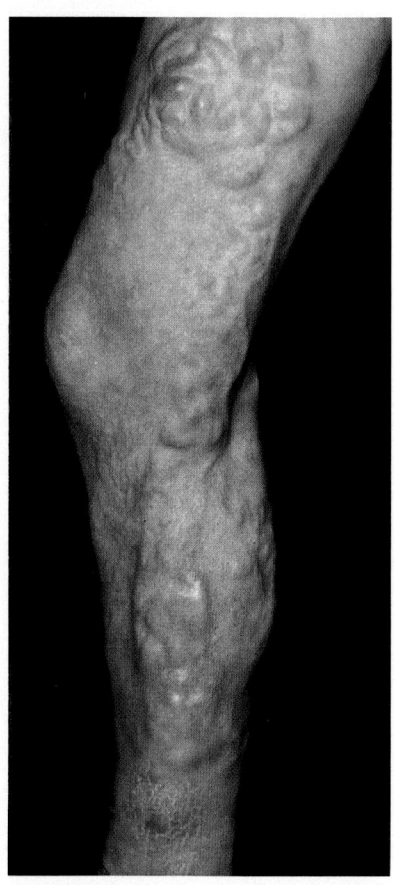

FIGURE 167-9 Extensive superficial varicose veins of the thigh and calf. (*Courtesy of Klaus Wolff, M.D.*)

feet without involvement of the saphenous veins. There may be pitting edema at the ankle area or increased turgor of the calf muscles. In patients with very large varicosities, systemic blood pressure may fall when they stand. Many patients have prominent, multiple, fine cutaneous veins on the thighs which are not varicose veins; they usually appear after age 20 in women and increase in number.

Laboratory and Special Examinations   The incompetent valves of varicose veins can be demonstrated by applying a tourniquet on an elevated extremity so that the superficial veins are empty (Fig. 167-10). When the patient assumes an erect posture, release of the tourniquet allows rapid filling of a varicose vein if the valves are incompetent. Venography is seldom necessary but will show the dilated, tortuous veins and incompetent valves.

Pathology   The pathology is variable: Some varicose veins appear normal but dilated so that the venous valves no longer are in opposition; others have damaged, deformed valves and fibrotic vein walls.[165]

Diagnosis and Differential Diagnosis   The diagnosis of varicose veins rests primarily on seeing and palpating the varices. The tourniquet test described above delineates the incompetent valves.

Treatment   Symptoms caused by varicose veins respond to heavy-gauge elastic stockings (30 mmHg or more.)[166] They will prevent further enlargement of veins and edema but will not reverse the size of varicosities. Patients often say their legs feel better with the elastic support even if they denied previous symptoms. Stockings must be put on within 30 min after arising and worn to bedtime. Panty girdles or garters should never be worn.

Ligation and stripping of veins is usually reserved for patients with very large and symptomatic varicosities. The operation has markedly decreased in popularity since the veins may be needed in the future for arterial bypass. Small- to medium-sized varicosities can be injected with a sclerosing solution (0.5 to 1 mL of sodium

tetradecyl sulfate, Sotradecol). This solution causes inflammation and then fibrosis of the vein. It is often very successful for cosmetic purposes but may leave discoloration where the fibrosed vein lies.

Prevention   Many varicose veins would be prevented if women wore elastic support hose during pregnancy. Chronic constipation should always be avoided.

Course and Prognosis   Without adequate external support, varicose veins continue to enlarge in most but not all patients. New varicose veins usually appear in a 10-year period after stripping or sclerosing injections. Some patients develop a postphlebitic syndrome.

Postphlebitic Syndrome

The postphlebitic syndrome is characterized by edema, stasis pigmentation, and ulcers of the lower extremities due to venous stasis.

Epidemiology   Studies are lacking on the epidemiology but it is more common in females than males. Whites and blacks appear to be equally affected.

Etiology and Pathogenesis   The postphlebitic syndrome may occur soon after an episode of deep venous thrombosis or up to 20 years later.[167,168] It has been a common belief that most patients have had thrombophlebitis, although many do not give a history of the disease. It can occur in patients with superficial varicosities or incompetent deep veins; the perforating veins may also have defective valves.

Valve destruction due to thrombophlebitis is the main factor in causing increased venous pressure in the leg. The edema is due to leakage of fluid from the capillaries. Stasis pigmentation results from escape of red blood cells into the tissues, which results in an inflammatory reaction to the deposited hemoglobin. The exact mechanism of spontaneous ulcer formation is unknown. A reason-

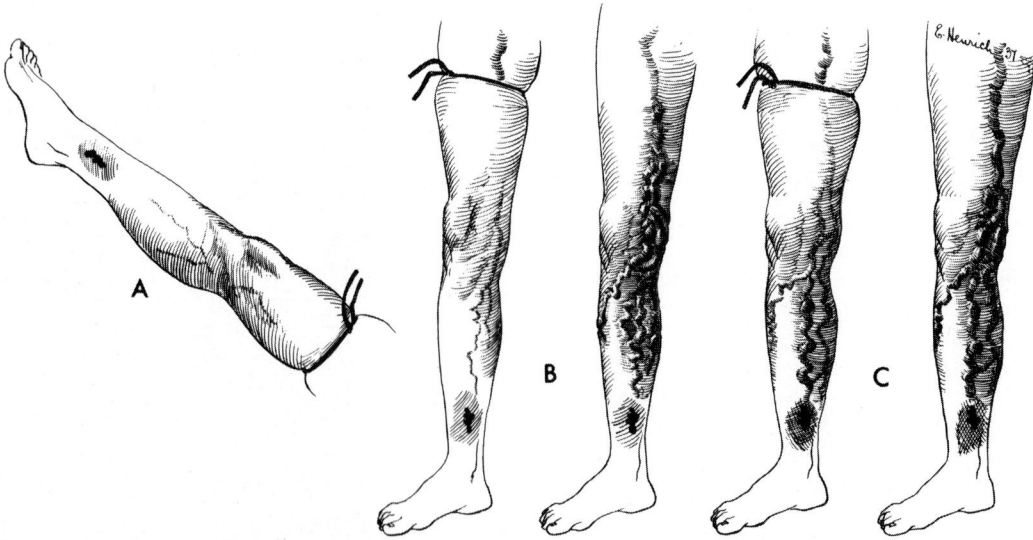

FIGURE 167-10   Varicose veins. Demonstration of venous reflux by the Trendelenburg test. (*a*) Elevation of the leg empties the varices. (*b*) While the patient is standing, varices remain empty until the tourniquet is removed, showing reflux from the saphenous vein. (*c*) Reflux takes place via communicating veins before removal of the tourniquet, with additional reflux from the saphenous vein when the tourniquet is removed.

able explanation is that there is ischemia in the area in the erect state because high venous pressure prevents capillary blood flow. Venous blood drawn from the ulcer area is often "black" from desaturation. Marked fibrosis in the subcutaneous tissue may develop, and channels can be palpated where veins course in the fibrotic tissue.

Clinical Manifestations HISTORY. Patients complain of swelling of the limb, discoloration of the calf and ankle area, and ulcers or breakdown of skin. Since the ulcers are often painless, patients may not see a physician for several weeks to months after the beginning of an ulcer. Patients may or may not have a history of thrombophlebitis. Some patients present with fever, chills, and redness of the involved extremity due to cellulitis.

SYSTEM REVIEW. No systemic symptoms are present unless infection occurs.

PHYSICAL EXAMINATION. Pitting edema of the extremity is usually present but varicose veins are not always apparent. There is brownish to dark pigmentation and often extensive scaling of the skin, especially on the medial side of the ankle and lower calf. Although cellulitis may occur, the leg may also be red, warm, and tender from an inflammatory reaction to the pigment in the dermis. Small erosions to very large but usually not deep ulcers may develop (Fig. 167-11). The ulcers usually have a red base of granulation tissue. They also occur on the medial ankle or lower calf in the majority of cases. Sometimes a fluctuant area denoting an incompetent perforating vein can be palpated at the base or near an ulcer, or a varicosity can be traced draining the ulcer area. The subcutaneous tissue may be indurated and retraction of the lower third of the leg may occur with pitting edema above it. One or both legs may be involved with the signs of the postphlebitic syndrome.

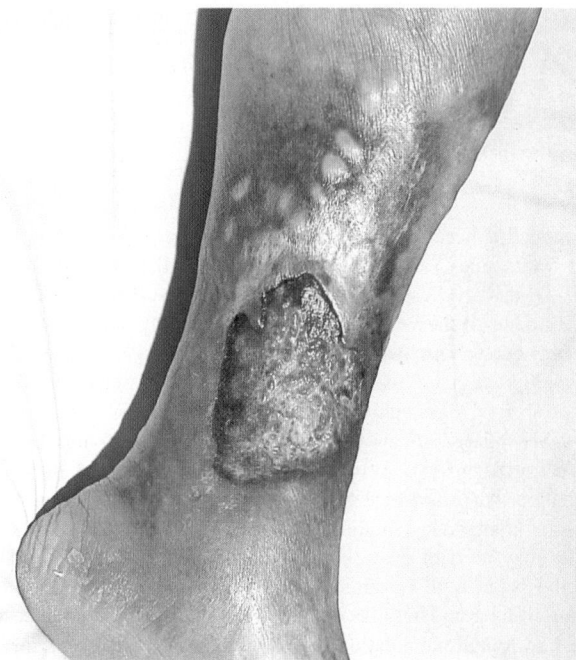

FIGURE 167-11 A large venous ulcer in a patient with the postphlebitic syndrome. This painless ulcer is shallow and has good granulation tissue. Surrounding tissue shows typical stasis pigmentation as well as subcutaneous tissue fibrosis and contraction.

Laboratory and Special Examinations Incompetence of the superficial or deep venous systems can be determined by tourniquet tests, doppler or plethysmographic examinations, or ascending and descending venography. Besides the tourniquet test described in the preceding section on varicose veins, incompetent perforators can be detected by applying two tourniquets at various levels of an extremity with the veins empty (Fig. 167-10). Then, when the patient assumes the standing position, the segment of the superficial vein between the two tourniquets will fill when the underlying perforator has an incompetent valve.

Pathology In the area of postphlebitic changes there may be edema, inflammation, fibrosis, hemosiderin deposits, and tissue breakdown of the skin and subcutaneous tissues. In late cases, venous walls are thickened, and endothelial proliferation and fragmentation of the walls of venules and arterioles of the skin may be seen.

Diagnosis and Differential Diagnosis The characteristic picture of edema, stasis pigmentation, and ulcers is diagnostic of the postphlebitic syndrome. The differential diagnosis includes lymphedema, in which there is no stasis pigmentation or ulcers. Other causes of ulcers discussed below are usually painful, whereas venous ulcers are painless or only tender. Demonstration of superficial or deep venous valvular incompetence by plethysmography, doppler examination, or venography may be needed when varicosities are absent.

Treatment The treatment of the postphlebitic syndrome is elastic compression to prevent venous stasis. Ace bandages or elastic stockings (30 mmHg or more compression) must be worn throughout the day whenever sitting or standing.[169] It also helps to sleep with the foot of the bed elevated 18 cm so that the patient starts the day with as little tissue fluid as possible. Itching or inflammation of stasis dermatitis usually yields to corticosteroids applied in cream or ointment. Insertion of segments of arm veins with competent valves in the popliteal area has been performed to treat the postphlebitic syndrome[170]; only about 50 percent remain patent and some patients appear to benefit.

Prevention Elastic stockings with suitable venous compression prevent progression of venous insufficiency to the postphlebitic syndrome. Similarly, elastic compression may prevent recurrence of venous ulcers late in the disease.

Course and Prognosis Without treatment, stasis dermatitis usually progresses to venous ulceration. Recurrent ulcers and episodes of cellulitis then follow. With adequate elastic compression and sometimes surgical procedures to decrease venous pressure in the area, the course will stabilize. However, the prognosis depends on a great effort and on the cooperation of the patient.

Lymphedema

Lymphedema is the occurrence of chronically swollen extremities due to inadequate drainage of interstitial tissue fluid by the lymphatic vessels.

Epidemiology

The prevalence of primary lymphedema is less than 1 in 6000.[171] One male is affected for every three females. Secondary lymphedema is more common in countries with warm climates because of the greater prevalence of filariasis there.

Etiology and Pathogenesis

Primary lymphedema is most often seen in girls and women and appears between ages 10 and 25 years.[172] It may be congenital, appear at puberty (praecox), or occur after age 35 (tardum) (Table 167-4). Milroy's disease is both familial and congenital. Other lymphatic defects causing chylous pleural effusions or ascites, malabsorption, yellow fingernails and toenails, or intrahepatic cholestasis may rarely accompany primary lymphedema.[173] A genetic defect causing distichiasis and lymphedema has been described but affects males more than females.[174]

Secondary lymphedema is caused by obstruction of lymphatic flow by surgical removal or radiation fibrosis of lymph nodes, infiltration by malignancies of lymph vessels or nodes, or destruction of lymphatics by recurrent infections or filariasis.

The pathogenesis of lymphedema is the accumulation of tissue fluid due to a failure of lymphatic drainage.

Clinical Manifestations

History Patients often do not notice the swelling of the limb because the onset is very gradual and the edema is painless. The swelling may also disappear overnight which leads to delay in seeking medical advice.

System Review Unless other systems are involved, the system review is normal in patients with primary lymphedema. In patients with pleural effusions, cough and shortness of breath may develop. The abdomen may swell with ascites. Intestinal lymphangiectasis may produce pale-colored stools and diarrhea. Patients with secondary lymphedema have symptoms of the underlying disease.

TABLE 167-4
Classification of Lymphedema

Primary
  Congenital
  Familial (Milroy's disease)
  Idiopathic
    Praecox
    Tardum
    Variant with yellow nails and pleural effusions
Secondary
  Infection
    Bacterial
    Filariasis
    Viral (cat-scratch fever)
  Radical lymph node excision or surgical scarring
  Malignant infiltration
  Fibrosis
    Radiation therapy
    Stasis
    Localized myxedema
    Panniculitis
    Idiopathic or pharmacologic retroperitoneal fibrosis

Physical Examination There is soft, pitting edema of the distal extremity at the onset of lymphedema. In the later stages, the swelling becomes indurated and nonpitting (Fig. 167-12a). The skin may thicken and resist wrinkling; hair follicles are prominent. Some patients proceed to develop disfigured extremities with thick folds of skin and hyperkeratosis (Fig. 167-12b). Patients may present with cellulitis of the involved extremity because lymphedematous limbs are susceptible to infection.

In primary lymphedema the lower extremities are involved most often and bilateral swelling occurs in about 50 percent of patients. In secondary lymphedema usually only one extremity is involved. Discoloration of nails, distichiasis, jaundice, and signs of pleural effusion or ascites may occur rarely in patients with primary lymphedema.

Laboratory and Special Examinations

Invasive diagnostic tests are not usually necessary. The results of blood and urine studies are normal in primary lymphedema and in most cases of secondary lymphedema. Lymphoscintigraphy with radioisotopic preparations is useful in differentiating lymphedema from other causes of extremity edema.[175] Lymphangiography should usually be avoided because it is painful and involves an incision with the chance of infection.

Pathology

The pathologic picture as determined by lymphangiography varies from aplasia or hypoplasia to varicosities of the lymphatic channels.[172] Primary lymphedema with distichiasis is associated with bilateral hyperplasia of the lymphatic vessels.[174] In secondary cases, there may be neoplastic involvement of lymph nodes or fibrosis of lymph nodes and lymph vessels.

Diagnosis and Differential Diagnosis

The diagnosis of lymphedema can usually be made by physical examination because the patient has a swollen, painless limb without varicosities, stasis pigmentation, or collateral veins (Table 167-5). Invasive tests are not necessary in most patients. Noninvasive studies of the venous system or venography may be indicated to rule out venous disease. Lymphoscintigraphy and rarely lymphangiography are used to distinguish the lipomatous nodular masses of lipodystrophy (see Chap. 109).

Secondary lymphedema should be considered in most patients before a diagnosis of primary lymphedema is made. A history of radiation or radium treatment, surgery of lymph nodes, or symptoms of malignancy should be ascertained. Patients from endemic areas may need blood tests or biopsies to detect filariasis. Males should be carefully examined for prostate cancer which is often signaled by a unilateral swollen limb due to lymph node invasion. An ultrasound examination of the abdomen is usually performed especially in females to rule out tumors or enlarged lymph nodes. Occasionally, women complain of swollen legs but no edema or other pathology can be found in the large legs. This configuration of the legs is usually familial. Clues to the absence of pathology are symmetric measurements of the ankles, calves, and thighs; small ankles in comparison to the calves and thighs; and lack of edema.

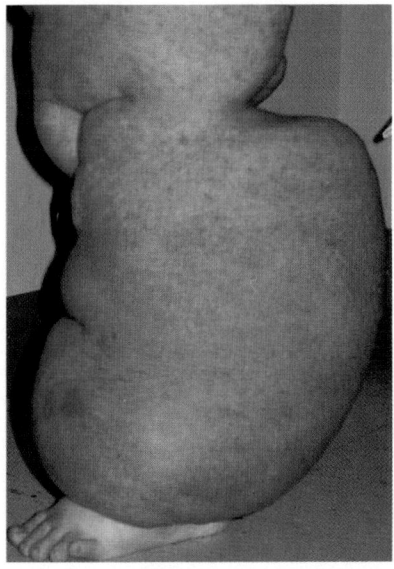

a

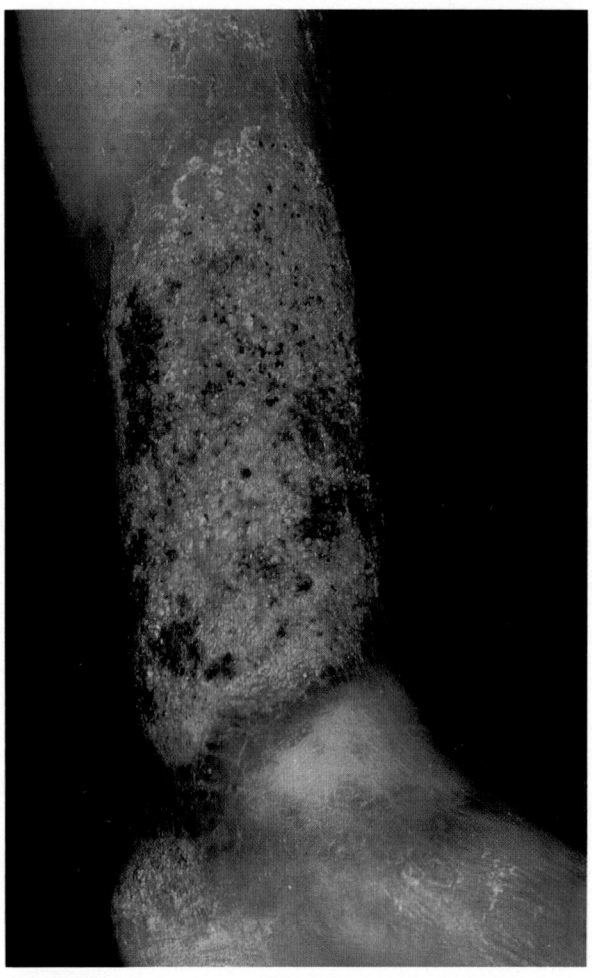

b

FIGURE 167-12   Lymphedema. (*a*) A 47-year-old male with extreme painless swelling which began at birth. (*b*) Elephantiasis nostras verucosa; edema has been replaced by fibrosis, hyperkeratosis, and hyperpigmentation.

Treatment

It is important to minimize edema of the extremities to prevent subcutaneous fibrosis, skin thickening, and recurrent episodes of cellulitis. Elastic garments with at least 30 mmHg of pressure but sometimes as much as 60 mmHg must be worn from morning to bedtime. These elastic garments should have graded pressure from the distal to the proximal extremity. The patient should also sleep with the foot of the bed elevated 18 cm to promote drainage of tissue fluid overnight. A low-sodium diet and occasional but not continuous use of diuretics may be helpful. In patients with edema resistant to conservative measures, a sequential pneumatic compression device may be used.[176] However, these machines must be used for at least 4 h on the extremity each night, are uncomfortable, and only move the fluid more proximally in some patients.

For very large, incapacitating limbs or for lymphangiosarcoma, various surgical procedures have been performed including removal of the subcutaneous tissue[177] and lymphovenous anastomoses.[178] Removal of the subcutaneous tissue leaves a very scarred but more usable limb. Lymphovenous anastomosis is less successful in primary than secondary lymphedema. Lymphatic grafts are also being used with some benefit.[179]

Prevention

Lymphedema cannot be prevented. Some patients have recurrent episodes of cellulitis and lymphangiitis in the involved limb. Each attack destroys more lymphatic vessels and aggravates the lymphedema. These patients should be treated with antibiotic prophylaxis, usually with penicillin.[180] The acute attacks produce a red, warm extremity with increased swelling; red streaks may be seen on the proximal extremity extending from the inflamed area, and regional lymph nodes may be enlarged and tender. Fever and leukocytosis may accompany the infection. The most common offending organisms are the coagulase-positive *Staphylococcus* and the hemolytic *Streptococcus*. Even when organisms cannot be cultured, therapy should be directed to these bacteria.

Course and Prognosis

Primary lymphedema usually progresses to a chronically swollen limb. Some patients with primary lymphedema and many patients with secondary lymphedema remain stable. Malignant degeneration of the lymphatic vessels—called lymphangiosarcoma—develops in 1 percent of cases and is more common in patients with secondary lymphedema due to mastectomy (see Chap. 98). The edema sometimes abates in patients with lymphedema associated with Turner's syndrome.

TABLE 167-5
Differential Diagnosis of Lymphedema

Postphlebitic syndrome
Edema of inactivity (old age)
Hereditary "piano legs"
Edema of constitutional disease
Lipodystrophy
Idiopathic or cyclic edema
Arthritis and synovitis
Panniculitis
Localized myxedema

Differential Diagnosis and Treatment of Ulcers

Differential Diagnosis

Table 167-6 lists the common and some uncommon etiologies and characteristics of extremity ulcers. The most common ulcer is due to venous stasis. Arterial ulcers due to large-vessel disease are next in frequency and then the neurotropic ulcers of diabetic neuropathy. History and physical examination help in the differential diagnosis of most ulcers. Normal pulses are usually present in the limbs except in patients with ulcers due to large-vessel arterial disease. Pain is characteristically absent to mild in patients with venous, neurotropic, and neoplastic ulcers. An ulcer with a red granulating base is usually venous (Fig. 167-11). Excess callus formation around a painless ulcer on pressure points suggests a neuropathic ulcer (Fig. 167-2). Very painful, often serpiginous ulcers occur on the feet and legs of patients with vasculitis, connective tissue diseases, and livedo reticularis with ulceration (Fig. 167-7a). Most secondary causes of Raynaud's phenomenon may lead to digital ulcers. Ulcers may also occur over subcutaneous calcifications of patients with scleroderma and will not usually heal until the calcium is extruded. These ulcerations usually occur on the digits, wrists, elbows, knees, or ankles.

A painful ulceration may occur on the posterolateral aspect of the calf in patients with hypertension.[181] These lesions may start as purplish blebs and then ulcerate with a black eschar which is surrounded by purpura (Fig. 167-13). The etiology is unknown but biopsy of surrounding tissue shows thrombosis and hyalinization of arterioles. A variety of infections may cause ulcerations and diagnosis is usually difficult without a culture or biopsy. Ulceration of the nonischemic lesion of necrobiosis lipoidica in patients with diabetes mellitus is uncommon. Malignancies of the skin must always be considered in patients with indolent, nonhealing ulcers.

Treatment

VENOUS ULCERS Venous ulcers should be treated twice a day with bandages soaked with warm 0.9% sodium chloride solution for 20 to 30 min. After the area is patted dry, zinc oxide ointment or gauze impregnated with Vaseline should be applied, gauze pads added, and the limb wrapped with elastic bandages from the foot to above the ulcer. Additional compression of the ulcer-bearing area or an obvious perforating vein is often necessary. Sponge rubber pieces can be cut to fit the area and applied under the elastic bandage. If there is inflammation around the ulcer, corticosteroid creams are useful. Systemic antibiotics may be needed for obviously infected ulcers or for a surrounding cellulitis. Fibrin-covering material may have to be debrided weekly.

Patients can remain ambulatory during treatment but should sleep with the leg elevated 18 cm above heart level. Rest periods of 30 to 60 min with leg elevation above heart level twice a day should be recommended. Edema of the limb slows the healing process. Small to moderate-size ulcers heal with this regime, but large ulcers often need skin grafts. Rarely the entire fibrosed area must be excised surgically followed by ligation of the perforating veins and skin grafting. Sometimes injections of sclerosing solutions or surgi-

TABLE 167-6
Differential Diagnosis of Ulcers

Type	Cause	Location	Pain	Characteristics
Venous	Postphlebitic syndrome Arteriovenous shunts	Medial lower leg-ankle	Absent to mild	Red base of granulation tissue; surrounding pigmentation, induration, edema; warm foot
Arterial				
Large vessel	Arteriosclerosis obliterans Thromboangiitis obliterans	Usually toes or foot	Severe	Black or gray base, shallow, irregular; no granulation tissue; cold foot with dependent rubor
Small vessel	Raynaud's phenomenon Vasculitis Atherosclerotic emboli	Toes, fingers, or lower legs	Severe	Irregular, inflamed edges, whitish base
Neurotropic	Diabetes mellitus and other neuropathies; spinal cord lesions	Over metatarsal arch, heel, toes	None	Often deep and infected; surrounded by thick callus
Hypertensive	Hypertension	Lateral or posterior calf	Severe	Black to white base surrounded by purpura
Infectious	Bacterial, fungal, syphilis, tuberculosis	Arms or legs	Absent to moderate	Purulent, erythematous margins, raised edges, linear; may be multinodular in lymphatic distribution
Hematologic	Sickle cell anemia Thalassemia	Lower legs	Moderate	Often punched-out with sharp edges and deep; white base; can also resemble small-vessel arterial ulcers
Neoplastic	Cancer Sarcoma	No predilection	Usually not painful	Raised edges above skin level; nonhealing
Pyoderma gangrenosum	Ulcerative colitis and unknown etiologies	Calves and thighs	Often severe	Black base with rolled edges of violaceous red color; often purulent; very painful

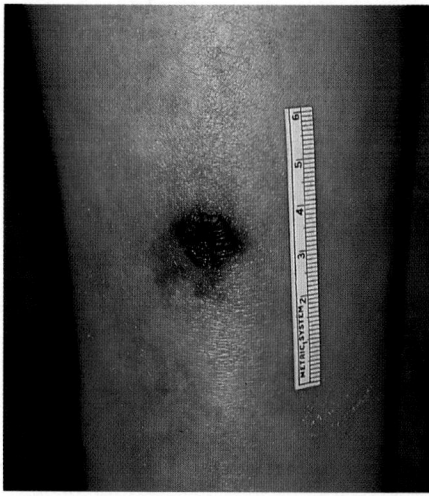

FIGURE 167-13 A hypertensive ulcer in a 56-year-old woman. The usual location is the lateral aspect of the calf. The base has a black eschar with surrounding ecchymotic tissue. Pain was extreme. All pulses in the extremity were normal.

cal ligation of incompetent superficial veins or perforators that feed the ulcer area will suffice.

ARTERIAL ULCERS Arterial ulcers should be treated twice a day with bandages soaked with warm 0.9% saline solution for 20 to 30 min. If debridement is necessary, the saline-soaked bandages should be allowed to dry overnight. Removal of the dry bandage cleanses the ulcer of dead tissue. Enzymatic debriding agents often cause inflammatory reactions and should not be used. Patients should sleep with the limb dependent by elevating the head of the bed 18 cm. Ulcers should be cultured and appropriate systemic antibiotics used when indicated. Elastic bandages should never be applied to an ischemic limb. The lesion should be protected from trauma by a loose wrapping bandage. Pain medications may be needed but care must be exercised to prevent addiction to narcotics. When good granulation tissue covers the whole base of the ulcer, skin grafting can be considered.

GANGRENE Dry gangrene of the digits or lower limbs should be allowed to demarcate by itself. Soaking or ointments are unnecessary. The edges of the gangrenous areas should be kept open if possible and observed frequently for infection. Pain medication is usually necessary for 2 to 3 months in patients with digital gangrene. It often takes several months to heal digital ulcers or gangrene, or ulcers of livedo reticularis, sickle cell disease, hypertension, or vasculitis. Conservatism and patience will save many digits. Infected (wet) gangrenous areas must be debrided and appropriate antibiotics administered. Amputation may be necessary.

References

1. Greenfield ADM, Shepherd JT: A quantitative study of the response to cold of the circulation through the fingers of normal subjects. *Clin Sci* **9**:323, 1950
2. Coffman JD: Total and nutritional blood flow in the finger. *Clin Sci* **42**:243, 1972
3. Grant RT, Bland EF: Observations on arteriovenous anastomoses in human skin and in the bird's foot with special reference to the reaction to cold. *Heart* **15**:385, 1931
4. Sarnoff SJ, Simeone FA: Vasodilator fibers in the human skin. *J Clin Invest* **26**:453, 1947
5. Cohen RA, Coffman JD: Reduced fingertip arterial pressures in Raynaud's disease. *J Vasc Med Biol* **1**:21, 1989
6. Flavahan NA et al: The effect of cooling on alpha$_1$- and alpha$_2$-adrenergic responses in canine saphenous and femoral veins. *J Pharmacol Exp Ther* **238**:139, 1986
7. Whittow GC: Effect of antihistamine substances on cold vasodilatation in the finger. *Nature* **176**:511, 1955
8. Hirai K et al: Differences in the vascular hunting reaction between Caucasians and Japanese. *Angiology* **21**:502, 1970
9. Iampietro PF et al: Response of Negro and white males to cold. *J Appl Physiol* **19**:798, 1959
10. Yoshimura H, Iida T: Studies on the reactivity of skin vessels to extreme cold. *Jpn J Physiol* **1**:147, 1950; **2**:177, 1952; **2**:310, 1952
11. Arneklo-Nobin B, Owman C: Adrenergic and serotonergic mechanisms in human hand arteries and veins studied by fluorescence histochemistry and in vitro pharmacology. *Blood Vessels* **22**:2, 1985
12. Coffman JD, Cohen RA: Role of alpha-adrenoceptor subtypes mediating sympathetic vasoconstriction in human digits. *Eur J Clin Invest* **18**:309, 1988
13. Flavahan NA et al: Human postjunctional alpha-1 and alpha-2 adrenoceptors: Differential distribution in arteries of the limbs. *J Pharmacol Exp Ther* **241**:341, 1987
14. Coffman JD, Cohen RA: Serotonergic vasoconstriction in human fingers during reflex sympathetic response to cooling. *Am J Physiol* **254**:H889, 1988
15. Coffman JD et al: The effect of histamine on human fingertip circulation. *Clin Sci* **66**:343, 1984
16. Coffman JD, Cohen RA: A cholinergic vasodilator mechanism in the human finger. *Am J Physiol* **252**:H594, 1987
17. Cohen RA, Coffman JD: β-adrenergic vasodilator mechanism in the finger. *Circ Res* **49**:1196, 1981
18. Coffman JD: Forehead blood flow measured by radioisotope disappearance rates. *Am J Physiol* **217**:1134, 1969
19. Wetzel NC, Zotterman Y: On differences in the vascular coloration of various regions of the normal human skin. *Heart* **13**:357, 1926
20. Froese G, Burton AC: Heat losses from the human head. *J Appl Physiol* **10**:235, 1957
21. Cooper KE et al: The blood flow in skin and muscle of the human forearm. *J Physiol* **128**:258, 1955
22. Jie K et al: Identification of vascular postsynaptic α_1- and α_2-adrenoceptors in man. *Circ Res* **54**:447, 1984
23. Edholm OG et al: The effect of body heating on the circulation in skin and muscle. *J Physiol* **134**:612, 1956
24. Fox RH, Hilton SM: Bradykinin formation in human skin as a factor in heat vasodilatation. *J Physiol* **142**:219, 1958
25. Tsuchida Y: Age-related changes in skin blood flow at four anatomic sites of the body in males studied by Xenon-133. *Plast Reconstr Surg* **85**:556, 1990
26. Bollinger A, Schlumpf M: Finger blood flow in healthy subjects of different age and sex and in patients with primary Raynaud's disease. *Acta Chir Scand* **465**(suppl): 42, 1975
27. Bartelink ML et al: Changes in skin blood flow during the menstrual cycle: The influence of the menstrual cycle on the peripheral circulation in healthy female volunteers. *Clin Sci* **78**:527, 1990
28. Juergens JL et al: Arteriosclerosis obliterans: Review of 520 cases with special reference to pathogenic and prognostic factors. *Circulation* **21**:188, 1960
29. Kannel WB, Shurtleff D: Cigarettes and the development of intermittent claudication. *Geriatrics* **28**:61, 1973
30. Coffman JD: Intermittent claudication and rest pain: Physiological concepts and therapeutic approaches. *Prog Cardiovasc Dis* **22**:53, 1979
31. Ekroth R et al: Physical training of patients with intermittent claudication. *Surgery* **84**:640, 1978
32. Coffman JD: Principles of conservative treatment of occlusive arterial disease, in *Clinical Vascular Disease*, edited by JA Spittell Jr. Philadelphia, F.A. Davis, 1983, p 1

33. Porter JM et al: Pentoxifylline efficacy in the treatment of intermittent claudication: Multicenter controlled double-blind trial with objective assessment of chronic occlusive arterial disease patients. *Am Heart J* **104**:66, 1982

34. Balsano F et al: Ticlopidine in the treatment of intermittent claudication: A 21-month double blind trial. *J Lab Clin Med* **114**:84, 1989

35. Schadt DT et al: Chronic atherosclerotic occlusion of the femoral artery. *JAMA* **175**:937, 1961

36. Coffman JD: Intermittent claudication: Not so benign. *Am Heart J* **112**:1127, 1986

37. Hinton RC et al: Influence of etiology of atrial fibrillation on incidence of systemic embolism. *Am J Cardiol* **40**:509, 1977

38. Jacobs AL: *Arterial Embolism in the Limbs*. Edinburgh, E. & S. Livingston, 1959

39. Amery A et al: Outcome of recent thromboembolic occlusions of limb arteries treated with streptokinase. *Br Med J* **4**:639, 1970

40. Szekely P: Systemic embolism and anticoagulant prophylaxis in rheumatic heart disease. *Br Med J* **1**:1209, 1964

41. Freund U et al: Mortality rate following lower limb arterial embolectomy: Causative factors. *Surgery* **77**:201, 1975

42. Maurizi CP et al: Atheromatous emboli. *Arch Pathol* **86**:528, 1968

43. Kealy WF: Atheroembolism. *Circulation* **30**:611, 1978

44. Coffman JD: Clincal forum: Atheroembolism after cardiac surgery. *J Vasc Med Biol* **1**:37, 1989

45. Feder W, Auerbach R: ''Purple toes'': An uncommon sequela of oral coumarin drug therapy. *Ann Intern Med* **55**:911, 1961

46. Brewer ML et al: Blue toe syndrome: Treatment with anticoagulants and delayed percutaneous transluminal angioplasty. *Radiology* **166**:31, 1988

47. Eliot RS et al: Atheromatous embolism. *Circulation* **30**:611, 1964

48. Deschamps P et al: Livedo reticularis and nodules due to cholesterol embolism in the lower extremities. *Br J Dermatol* **97**:93, 1977

49. Kasinath BS et al: Eosinophilia in the diagnosis of atheroembolic renal disease. *Am J Nephrol* **7**:173, 1987

50. Anderson WR, Richards AM: Evaluation of lower extremity muscle biopsies in the diagnosis of atheroembolism. *Arch Pathol* **86**:535, 1968

51. Comerford JA et al: Digital ischaemia and palpable pedal pulses. *Br J Surg* **74**:493, 1987

52. Morris-Jones W et al: Gangrene of the toes with palpable pulses: Response to platelet suppressive therapy. *Ann Surg* **193**:462, 1981

53. Kaufman JL et al: Disseminated atheroembolism from extensive degenerative atherosclerosis of the aorta. *Surgery* **102**:63, 1987

54. Buerger L: Thrombo-angiitis obliterans: A study of vascular lesions leading to presenile spontaneous gangrene. *Am J Med Sci* **136**:567, 1908

55. Lie JT: Thromboangiitis obliterans (Buerger's disease) in women. *Medicine* **66**:65, 1987

56. McLaughlin GA et al: Association of HLA-A9 and HLA-B5 with Buerger's disease. *Br Med J* **2**:1165, 1976

57. Mills JL et al: Buerger's disease in the modern era. *Am J Surg* **154**:123, 1987

58. Ohtawa T et al: HLA antigens in thromboangiitis obliterans. *JAMA* **230**:1128, 1974

59. Adar R et al: Cellular sensitivity to collagen in thromboangiitis obliterans. *N Engl J Med* **308**:1113, 1983

60. Suzuki S et al: Buerger's disease (thromboangiitis obliterans): An analysis of the arteriograms of 119 cases. *Clin Radiol* **33**:235, 1982

61. Olin JW et al: The changing spectrum of thromboangiitis obliterans (Buerger's disease). *Circulation* **80**(suppl II):226, 1989

62. Mitchell SW: On a rare vaso-motor neurosis of the extremities and on the maladies with which it is confounded. *Am J Med Sci* **76**:2, 1878

63. Smith LA, Allen EV: Erythermalgia (erythromelalgia) of the extremities: A syndrome characterized by redness, heat, pain. *Am Heart J* **16**:175, 1938

64. Babb RR et al: Erythermalgia: Review of 51 cases. *Circulation* **29**:136, 1964

65. Cohen IJK, Samorodin CS: Familial erythromelalgia. *Arch Dermatol* **118**:963, 1982

66. Zheng ZM et al: Pox viruses isolated from epidemic erythromelalgia in China. *Lancet* **1**:296, 1988

67. Jorgensen HP, Sondergaard J: Pathogenesis of erythromelalgia. *Arch Dermatol* **114**:112, 1978

68. Michiels JJ et al: Erythromelalgia caused by platelet-mediated arteriolar inflammation and thrombosis in thrombocythemia. *Ann Intern Med* **102**:466, 1985

69. Fisher JR et al: Nifedipine and erythromelalgia (letter). *Ann Intern Med* **98**:671, 1983

70. Brown GE: Erythromelalgia and other disturbances of the extremities accompanied by vasodilation and burning. *Am J Med Sci* **183**:468, 1932

71. Baer MR et al: Palmar-plantar erythrodysesthesia and cytarabine. *Ann Intern Med* **102**:556, 1985

72. Raynaud M: *On Local Aphyxia and Symmetrical Gangrene of the Extremities*. Translated by T. Barlow. London, The Syndenham Society, 1888, p 99

73. Hutchinson J: Raynaud's phenomenon. *Med Press Circ* **23**:403, 1901

74. Gifford RW, Hines EA: Raynaud's disease among women and girls. *Circulation* **16**:1012, 1957

75. Hines EA Jr, Christensen NA: Raynaud's disease affecting men. *JAMA* **129**:1, 1945

76. Maricq HR et al: Prevalence of Raynaud's phenomenon in the general population. *J Chronic Dis* **39**:423, 1986

77. Lewis T, Pickering GW: Observations upon maladies in which the blood supply to digits ceases intermittently or permanently and upon bilateral gangrene of digits: Observations relevant to so-called Raynaud's disease. *Clin Sci* **1**:327, 1934

78. Olsen N, Nielsen SL: Prevalence of primary Raynaud's phenomenon in young females. *Scand J Clin Lab Invest* **37**:761, 1978

79. Lewis T: Experiments relating to the peripheral mechanism involved in spasmodic arrest of the circulation on the fingers: A variety of Raynaud's disease. *Heart* **15**:7, 1929

80. Jamieson GG et al: Cold hypersensitivity in Raynaud's phenomenon. *Circulation* **44**:254, 1971

81. Kontos HA, Wasserman JA: Effect of reserpine in Raynaud's phenomenon. *Circulation* **39**:259, 1969

82. Krahenbuhl B et al: Closure of digital arteries in high vascular tone states as demonstrated by measurement of systolic blood pressure in the fingers. *Scand J Clin Lab Invest* **37**:71, 1977

83. Coffman JD, Cohen AS: Total and capillary fingertip blood flow in Raynaud's phenomenon. *N Engl J Med* **285**:259, 1971

84. Edward JM et al: α_2-Adrenergic receptor levels in obstructive and spastic Raynaud's syndrome. *J Vasc Surg* **5**:38, 1987

85. Coffman JD, Cohen RA: α_2-Adrenergic and 5HT-2 receptor hypersensitivity in Raynaud's phenomenon. *J Vasc Med Biol* **2**:100, 1990

86. Halperin A et al: Raynaud's disease, Raynaud's phenomenon and serotonin. *Angiology* **11**:151, 1960

87. Seibold JR, Terregino CA: Selective antagonism of S_2-serotonergic receptors relieves but does not prevent cold-induced vasoconstriction in primary Raynaud's phenomenon. *J Rheumatol* **13**:337, 1986

88. Ayres ML et al: Blood viscosity, Raynaud's phenomenon and the effect of fibrinolytic enhancement. *Br J Surg* **68**:51, 1981

89. Jahnsen T et al: Blood viscosity and local response to cold in primary Raynaud's phenomenon. *Lancet* **2**:1001, 1977

90. Pringle R et al: Blood viscosity in Raynaud's phenomenon. *Lancet* **1**:1086, 1965

91. Zahavi J et al: Plasma exchange and platelet function in Raynaud's phenomenon. *Thromb Res* **19**:85, 1980

92. Theriault G et al: Raynaud's phenomenon in forestry workers in Quebec. *Can Med Assoc J* **126**:1404, 1982

93. Marshall AJ et al: Raynaud's phenomenon as a side effect of beta-blockers in hypertension. *Br Med J* **1**:1498, 1976

94. Cranley JJ et al: Impending gangrene of four extremities secondary to ergotism. *N Engl J Med* **269**:727, 1963

95. Graham JR: Methysergide for prevention of headache. *N Engl J Med* **270**:67, 1964

96. Falappa P et al: Angiographic study of digital arteries in workers exposed to vinyl chloride. *Br J Indust Med* **39**:169, 1982

97. Teutsch C et al: Raynaud's phenomenon as a side effect of chemotherapy with vinblastine and bleomycin for testicular carcinoma. *Cancer Treatment Res* **61**:925, 1977

98. Marshall RJ et al: Vascular responses in patients with high serum titres of cold aggutinins. *Clin Sci* **12**:255, 1953

99. Miller D et al: Is variant angina the coronary manifestation of a generalized vasospastic disorder? *N Engl J Med* **304**:763, 1981

100. Nielsen SL: Raynaud's phenomenon and finger systolic pressure during cooling. *Scand J Clin Lab Invest* **38**:765, 1978

101. Maricq HR et al: Diagnostic potential of in vivo capillary microscopy in scleroderma and related disorders. *Arthritis Rheum* **23**:183, 1980

102. Lewis T: The pathological changes in the arteries supplying the fingers in warm-handed people and in cases of so-called Raynaud's disease. *Clin Sci* **3**:287, 1938

103. Coffman JD: *Raynaud's Phenomenon.* New York, Oxford University Press, 1989

104. Allen EV, Brown GE: Raynaud's disease: A critical review of minimal prerequisites for diagnosis. *Am J Med Sci* **183**:187, 1932

105. Rodeheffer RJ et al: Controlled double-blind trial of nifedipine in the treatment of Raynaud's phenomenon. *N Engl J Med* **308**:880, 1983

106. Smith CD, McKendry RJR: Controlled trial of nifedipine in the treatment of Raynaud's phenomenon. *Lancet* **2**:1299, 1982

107. Kahan A et al: A randomized double blind trial of diltiazem in the treatment of Raynaud's phenomenon. *Ann Rheum Dis* **44**:30, 1985

108. Kinney EL et al: The treatment of severe Raynaud's phenomenon with verapamil. *J Clin Pharmacol* **22**:74, 1982

109. McFadyen IJ et al: Intra-arterial reserpine administration in Raynaud's syndrome. *Arch Intern Med* **132**:526, 1973

110. Wollersheim H et al: Double-blind, placebo-controlled study of prazosin in Raynaud's phenomenon. *Clin Pharmacol Ther* **40**:219, 1986

111. Clifford PC et al: Treatment of vasospastic disease with prostaglandin E$_1$. *Br Med J* **281**:1031, 1980

112. Coffman JD: Vasodilator drugs in peripheral vascular disease. *N Engl J Med* **300**:713, 1979

113. Jobe JB et al: Induced vasodilation as treatment for Raynaud's disease. *Ann Intern Med* **97**:706, 1982

114. Farmer RG et al: Raynaud's disease with sclerodactylia. *Circulation* **23**:13, 1961

115. Crocq C: De l'acrocyanosis. *Semin Med* **16**:297, 1896

116. Stern ES: The aetiology and pathology of acrocyanosis. *Br J Dermatol Syphilol* **49**:100, 1937

117. Lewis T, Landis EM: Observations upon vascular mechanisms in acrocyanosis. *Heart* **15**:29, 1930

118. Peacock JH: Vasodilatation in the human hand: Observations on primary Raynaud's disease and acrocyanosis of the upper extremities. *Clin Sci* **17**:575, 1957

119. Peacock JH: A comparative study of the digital cutaneous temperatures and hand blood flows in the normal hand, primary Raynaud's disease and primary acrocyanosis. *Clin Sci* **18**:25, 1959

120. Larsson Y: The vasoconstrictor tone of the cutaneous arterioles in acroasphyxia, hypertension, and in the cold pressor test. *Acta Med Scand* **130**(suppl 206):146, 1948

121. Day R, Klingman W: Effect of sleep on skin temperature reactions in case of acrocyanosis. *J Clin Invest* **18**:271, 1939

122. Jacobs MJHM et al: Nomenclature of Raynaud's phenomenon: A capillary microscopic and hemorrheologic study. *Surgery* **101**:136, 1987

123. Edwards EA: Remittent necrotizing acrocyanosis. *JAMA* **161**:1530, 1956

124. Milian G: Les atrophies cutanées syphilitiques. *Bull Soc Fr Dermatol Syphig* **36**:865, 1929

125. Sneddon IB: Cerebrovascular lesions and livedo reticularis. *Br J Dermatol* **77**:180, 1965

126. Weinstein C et al: Livedo reticularis associated with increased titers of anticardiolipin antibodies in systemic lupus erythematosus. *Arch Dermatol* **123**:596, 1987

127. Winkelmann RK et al: Clinical studies of livedoid vasculitis (segmental hyalinizing vasculitis). *Mayo Clin Proc* **49**:746, 1974

128. Cunliffe WJ, Menon IS: The association between cutaneous vasculitis and decreased blood fibrinolytic activity. *Br J Dermatol* **84**:99, 1971

129. Drucker CR, Duncan WC: Antiplatelet therapy in atrophie blanche and livedo vasculitis. *J Am Acad Dermatol* **7**:359, 1982

130. Yamamoto M et al: Antithrombic treatment in livedo vasculitis. *J Am Acad Dermatol* **18**:57, 1988

131. Heimans RLH et al: Some actions of amantadine on peripheral tissues. *J Pharm Pharmacol* **24**:869, 1972

132. William CM, Goodman H: Livedo reticularis. *JAMA* **85**:955, 1925

133. Barker NW et al: Livedo reticularis: A peripheral arteriolar disease. *Am Heart J* **21**:592, 1941

134. Pearce LA et al: Amantadine hydrochloride: Alteration in peripheral circulation. *Neurology* **24**:46, 1974

135. Milstone LM et al: Classification and therapy of atrophie blanche. *Arch Dermatol* **119**:963, 1983

136. Mitchell SW et al: *Gunshot Wounds and Other Injuries of Nerves.* Philadelphia, Lippincott, 1864

137. Mitchell SW: *Injuries of Nerves and Their Consequences.* Philadelphia, Lippincott, 1872

138. Richards RL: Causalgia. *Arch Neurol* **16**:339, 1967

139. Johnson AC: Disabling changes in the hands resembling sclerodactylia following myocardial infarction. *Ann Intern Med* **19**:433, 1943

140. Homans J: Minor causalgia: A hyperesthetic neurovascular syndrome. *N Engl J Med* **222**:870, 1940

141. Drucker WR et al: Pathogenesis of post-traumatic sympathetic dystrophy. *Am J Surg* **97**:454, 1959

142. Kozin F et al: The reflex sympathetic dystrophy syndrome. *Am J Med* **60**:321, 1976

143. Kozin F et al: Bone scintigraphy in reflex sympathetic dystrophy syndrome. *Radiology* **138**:437, 1981

144. Laxer RM: Technetium 99m-methylene diphosphonate bone scans in children with reflex neurovascular dystrophy. *J Pediatrics* **106**:437, 1985

145. Marzella L et al: Morphologic characterization of acute injury to vascular endothelium of skin after frostbite. *Plast Reconstr Surg* **83**:67, 1989

146. Molnar GW et al: Effect of skin wetting on finger cooling and freezing. *J Appl Physiol* **35**:205, 1973

147. Washburn B: Frostbite. *N Engl J Med* **266**:974, 1962

148. Porter JM et al: Intra-arterial sympathetic blockade in the treatment of clinical frostbite. *Am J Surg* **132**:625, 1976

149. Golding MR et al: The role of sympathectomy in frostbite with a review of 68 cases. *Surgery* **57**:774, 1965

150. Comp PC et al: Familial protein S deficiency is associated with recurrent thrombosis. *J Clin Invest* **74**:2082, 1984

151. Clouse LH, Comp PC: The regulation of hemostasis: The protein C system. *N Engl J Med* **314**:1298, 1986

152. Abramson DJ: Mondor's disease and string phlebitis. *JAMA* **196**:1087, 1966

153. Coffman JD: Deep venous thrombosis and pulmonary emboli: Etiology, medical treatment and prophylaxis. *J Thorac Imag* **4**:4, 1989

154. Hull R et al: Replacement of venography in suspected venous thrombosis by impedance plethysmography and ^{125}I fibrinogen leg scanning. *Ann Intern Med* **94**:12, 1981

155. Lensing AWA et al: Detection of deep vein thrombosis by real-time B-mode ultrasonography. *N Engl J Med* **320**:342, 1989

156. Barnes RW et al: The fallibility of the clinical diagnosis of venous thrombosis. *JAMA* **234**:605, 1975

157. Huisman MV et al: Serial impedance plethysmography for suspected deep venous thrombosis in outpatients. *N Engl J Med* **314**:823, 1986

158. Hull RD et al: Continuous intravenous heparin compared with inter-

mittent subcutaneous heparin in the initial treatment of proximal vein thrombosis. *N Engl J Med* **315**:1109, 1986

159. Hull R et al: Different intensities of oral anticoagulation therapy in the treatment of proximal vein thrombosis. *N Engl J Med* **307**:1676, 1982

160. Samama MM: Deep vein thrombosis of inferior limbs: Are thrombolytic agents superior to heparin? *Semin Thromb Hemost* **13**:178, 1987

161. Clagett GP, Reisch JS: Prevention of venous thromboembolism in general surgical patients. *Ann Surg* **208**:227, 1988

162. Burkitt DP: Varicose veins: Facts and fantasy. *Arch Surg* **111**:1327, 1976

163. Burwell CS: The placenta as a modified arteriovenous fistula, considered in relation to the circulatory adjustments to pregnancy. *Am J Med Sci* **195**:1, 1938

164. Edwards EA, Edwards JE: The effect of thrombophlebitis on the venous valve. *Surg Gynecol Obstet* **65**:310, 1937

165. Leu HJ et al: Morphological alterations of non-varicose and varicose veins. *Basic Res Cardiol* **74**:435, 1979

166. Tolins SH: Treatment of varicose veins: An update. *Am J Surg* **145**:248, 1983

167. Jacobs P: Pathogenesis of the postphlebitic syndrome. *Ann Rev Med* **34**:91, 1983

168. McEnroe CS et al: Correlation of clinical findings with venous hemodynamics in 386 patients with chronic venous insufficiency. *Am J Surg* **156**:148, 1988

169. O'Donnell TF et al: Effect of elastic compression on venous hemodynamics in postphlebitic limbs. *JAMA* **242**:2766, 1979

170. Taheri SA et al: Status of vein valve transplant after 12 months. *Arch Surg* **117**:1313, 1982

171. Dale RF: The inheritance of primary lymphoedema. *J Med Genetics* **22**:274, 1985

172. Kinmonth JB: *The Lymphatics: Diseases, Lymphography, and Surgery*. Baltimore, Williams & Wilkins, 1972

173. Dilley JJ et al: Primary lymphedema associated with yellow nails and pleural effusions. *JAMA* **204**:607, 1968

174. Dale RF: Primary lymphoedema when found with distichiasis is of the type defined as bilateral hyperplasia by lymphography. *J Med Genet* **24**:170, 1987

175. Weissleder R, Thrall JH: The lymphatic system: Diagnostic imaging studies. *Radiology* **172**:315, 1989

176. Richmand DM et al: Sequential pneumatic compression for lymphedema. *Arch Surg* **120**:1116, 1985

177. Servelle M: Surgical treatment of lymphedema: A report of 652 cases. *Surgery* **101**:485, 1987

178. Gloviczki P et al: Microsurgical lymphovenous anastomosis for treatment of lymphedema: A critical review. *J Vasc Surg* **7**:647, 1988

179. Baumeister RG, Siuda S: Treatment of lymphedemas by microsurgical lymphatic grafting: What is proved? *Plast Reconstr Surg* **85**:64, 1990

180. Babb RR et al: Prophylaxis of recurrent lymphangiitis complicating lymphedema. *JAMA* **195**:871, 1966

181. Schnier BR et al: Hypertensive ischemic ulcer: A review of 40 cases. *Am J Cardiol* **17**:560, 1966

Cutaneous Manifestations of Alterations and Disorders of the Endocrine System

CHAPTER 168

Thomas J. Lawley and Kim B. Yancey

Skin Changes and Diseases in Pregnancy

Cutaneous changes and eruptions during pregnancy are exceedingly common and in some cases a cause for substantial anxiety on the part of the prospective mother. These alterations may range from normal cutaneous changes that occur in almost all pregnancies, to common skin diseases that are not associated with pregnancy, to eruptions that appear to be specifically associated with pregnancy. Likewise the concerns of the patient may range from cosmetic appearance, to the chance of recurrence of the particular problem in a subsequent pregnancy, to its potential effects on the fetus in terms of morbidity and mortality. In this chapter the cutaneous changes that are specifically associated with pregnancy will be discussed.

Cutaneous Changes Commonly Associated with Pregnancy

While the influences that the individual hormones have on the skin are incompletely understood, it is thought that they are responsible, either primarily or secondarily, for many of the cutaneous changes that are normally seen during pregnancy.

Pigmentation The nipples, areolae, and external genitalia become hyperpigmented during pregnancy. The linea alba becomes the pigmented linea nigra. Occasionally hyperpigmentation is noted in the axillae and the proximal medial portions of the thighs. The most noticeable pigmentary change during pregnancy is the development of a masklike hyperpigmentation of the face, known as chloasma or melasma, in over 50 percent of women[3] (Fig. 168-1). This tendency is exacerbated by sun exposure in susceptible individuals and may also be exacerbated by birth control pills in nonpregnant women. Additionally, preexisting nevi or ephelides frequently darken during pregnancy. The degree of hyperpigmentation tends to be related to the skin type of the individual, with lightly complected individuals developing less intense pigmentation. In all of these instances there is usually partial, and at times complete, regression of the hyperpigmentation occuring gradually following termination of pregnancy. The physiology of the hyperpigmentation appears to be related to the increased production of estrogens and perhaps to increased levels of progesterone or melanocyte-stimulating hormone.

Hair Mild to moderate hirsutism is frequently seen during pregnancy. The hirsutism tends to resolve shortly after delivery or in some instances in the third trimester. After delivery, the resulting telogen effluvium may be severe, resulting in significant hair loss from 1 to 5 months post partum. In these instances regrowth, usually within 1 year, is the rule.

Connective Tissue The most common change in connective tissue is the development of striae distensae over the abdomen, hips, but-

Hormonal Changes

Pregnancy is a time of significant and complex physiologic changes. Some of these changes are due to the de novo production of a variety of protein and steroid hormones by the fetoplacental unit as well as by the increased activity of the maternal pituitary, thyroid, and adrenal glands. The currently recognized hormones produced by the placenta include the protein hormones human chorionic gonadotropin (HCG), human placental lactogen (HPL) or human somatomammotropin, human chorionic thyrotropin, and human chorionic corticotropin, as well as the steroid hormones progesterone and estrogen.[1,2] A description of the chemistry, function, and metabolism of these hormones is beyond the scope of this chapter, but it should be kept in mind that the production and the serum levels of these hormones are dynamic. For instance, HCG levels peak between the 10th and 12th weeks of gestation although they remain elevated throughout pregnancy. The levels of progesterone and estrogen rise throughout the first and second trimesters of pregnancy and plateau during the third trimester. The levels of these hormones are of diagnostic significance in certain obstetric conditions and complications, but their exact impact on cutaneous physiology as well as their influence on the immunology of the skin and the inflammatory response are essentially unknown.

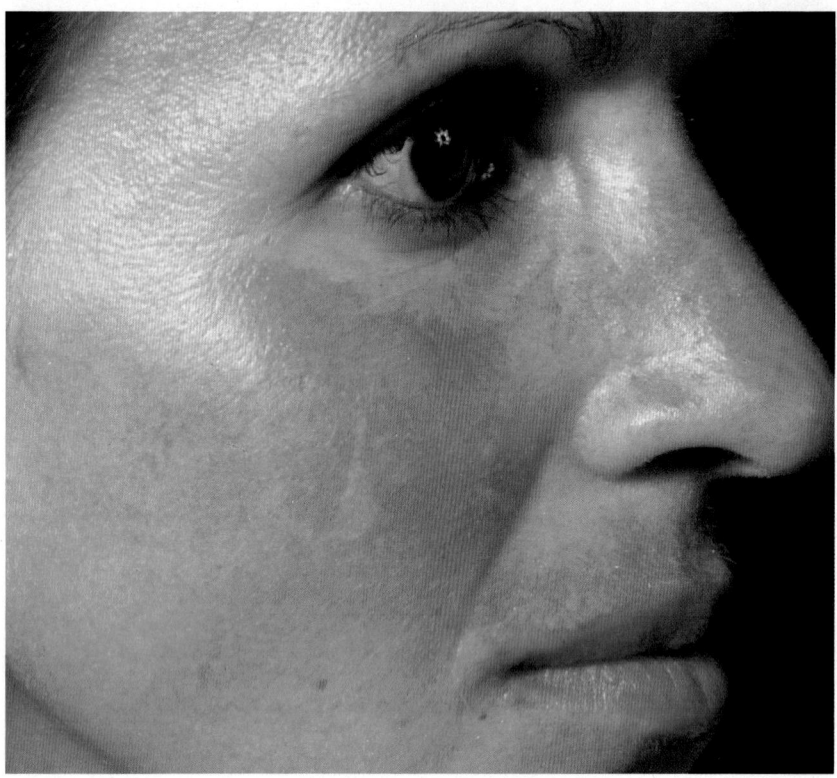

FIGURE 168-1   Melasma. (*Courtesy of Klaus Wolff, M.D.*)

tocks, and sometimes the breasts (Fig. 168-2). Striae distenae occur in up to 90 percent of pregnant women.[4] The exact cause of striae is unknown, although a combination of increased adrenal cortical activity associated with increased lateral stress on the connective tissue due to increased size of the various portions of the body are thought to be important. Striae distensae initially appear as pink to purple atrophic bands (Fig. 168-2) sometimes associated with mild pruritus. Following delivery they become pale and less apparent. There is no known effective treatment that will resolve striae distensae. Skin tags, sometimes known as molluscum fibrosum gravidarum, often appear on the lateral portions of the neck and axillae during pregnancy and may persist following delivery.

Vascular   Hyperemia is physiologic during pregnancy. This combined with a tendency toward vascular proliferation results in a number of common cutaneous changes during pregnancy. Up to two-thirds of women will develop palmar erythema and/or spider angiomas during pregnancy.[5] Vascular distention resulting in part from increased intraabdominal pressure is thought to be responsible for the edema and venous varicosities that commonly occur on the legs and feet. Hemorrhoids also occur for the same reasons. Vascular tumors such as glomus tumors or hemangiomas may appear or enlarge during pregnancy. The pregnancy tumor of the gingiva is a pyogenic granuloma that may appear in the second or third trimester and resolves shortly after delivery.

Well-Defined Dermatoses Associated with Pregnancy

A variety of cutaneous diseases have been reported to be associated with pregnancy (Table 168-1). Most of these "diseases" are poorly characterized both clinically and pathophysiologically. In a number

of instances their very existence as disease entities is in doubt. Even with diseases that are reasonably well-defined clinically, there is some dispute with regard to nomenclature. The section that follows is an attempt to describe the best known and most common of these diseases.

Herpes Gestationis (See also Chap. 54)

Herpes gestationis is an extremely pruritic, recurrent, bullous dermatosis of pregnancy and the immediate postpartum period. Its name is a total misnomer as it is not related to any viral infectious agent. Pemphigoid gestationis has been suggested as an alternative name for this disease. Herpes gestationis is immunologically mediated.

History   Milton first used the term *herpes gestationis* in 1872.[6] In 1973 Provost and Tomasi demonstrated that herpes gestationis is a distinct, immunologically mediated disease.[7]

Clinical Manifestations   Herpes gestationis is an extremely pruritic eruption that may occur at any time during pregnancy or immediately post partum. The primary lesions of herpes gestationis are small papulovesicles that are often grouped and frequently occur on a background of erythema and/or urticarial plaques (Fig. 168-3). These lesions often develop into frank vesicles and in some instances into bullae. As these lesions are extremely itchy, it is also common to see numerous crusts and excoriations. The eruption may be widespread, but the most frequent areas of initial involvement are the abdomen, particularly the umbilicus as well as the periumbilical area, and the extremities. The eruption frequently spreads to involve palms, soles, chest, and back. Mucous membrane lesions are rare.

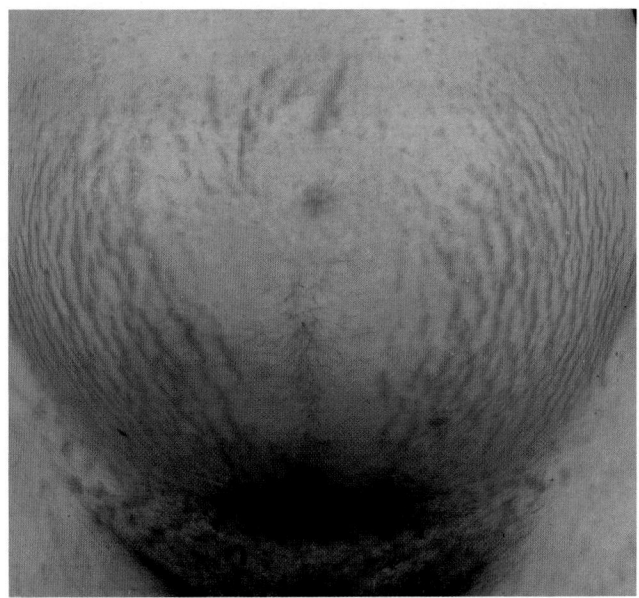

FIGURE 168-2   Striae distensae. (*Courtesy of Klaus Wolff, M.D.*)

TABLE 168-1
Dermatoses of Pregnancy

Well-defined eruptions
   Herpes gestationis (pemphigoid gestationis)
   Pruritic urticarial papules and plaques of pregnancy (PUPPP)
   Recurrent cholestasis of pregnancy
   Impetigo herpetiformis

Poorly defined eruptions
   Prurigo gestationis (Besnier)
   Papular dermatitis of pregnancy (Spangler)
   Follicular eruption of pregnancy
   Autoimmune progesterone dermatitis

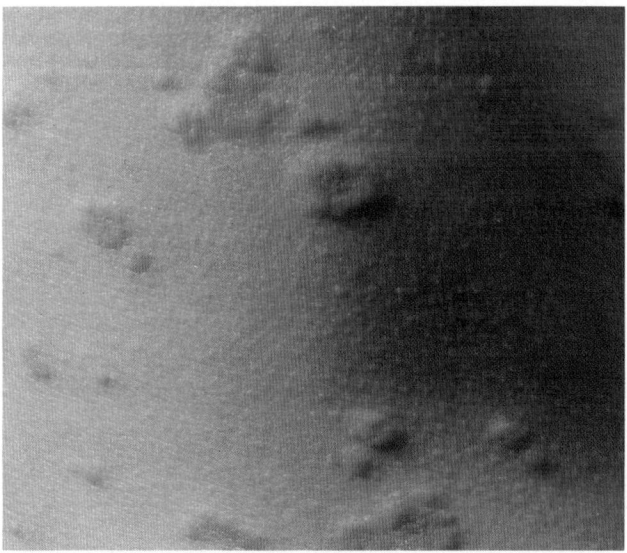

a

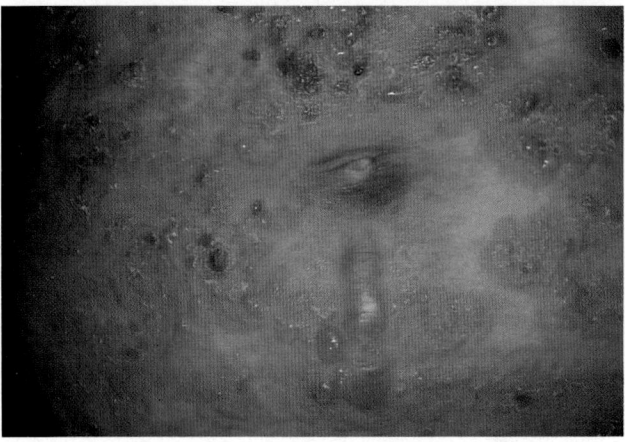

b

FIGURE 168-3   Herpes gestationis. (*a*) Primary lesions are papular and urticarial lesions. (*b*) Grouped vesicles, bullae, and urticarial plaques in a circinate configuration.

The eruption may begin at any time during pregnancy. In a survey of 41 immunologically proven cases of herpes gestationis, 8 cases began in the first trimester, 15 cases in the second trimester, 12 in the third trimester, and 6 cases began immediately post partum.[8] Flares of controlled disease are also especially prone to occur at or near the time of delivery. In the same survey cited above,[8] 46 percent of patients had an exacerbation of disease shortly after delivery. Therefore 61 percent of patients in this study flared or developed herpes gestationis in the postpartum period.

Histopathology   An early lesion of herpes gestationis is characterized by edema of the dermal papillae with an infiltrate of eosinophils, lymphocytes, and a few neutrophils (Fig. 168-4). The epidermis may show spongiosis and focal necrosis of basal cells over the tips of the dermal papillae. There is also a superficial and mid-dermal perivascular infiltrate of eosinophils, lymphocytes, and histiocytes. The accumulation of edema may result in the formation of teardrop-shaped vesiculobullae in dermal papillae of older lesions. It is often not possible to distinguish herpes gestationis completely from other subepidermal bullous skin diseases by histopathologic studies alone.

Immunopathology   DIRECT IMMUNOFLUORESCENCE.   Direct immunofluorescence microscopy of perilesional or normal skin of herpes gestationis patients reveals the presence of the third component of complement (C3) deposited along the basement membrane zone in a linear band (Fig. 168-5). The diagnosis of herpes gestationis should not be made without this finding. Deposits of IgG are found in the same area in 40 to 50 percent of patients.[8] Other immunoreactants occasionally found at the basement membrane zone in herpes gestationis patients are IgM, IgA, Clq, C4, C5, and factor B. C3 deposits have persisted for more than 1 year after the cutaneous lesions have resolved. C3 deposits have also been found in the skin of infants of affected mothers.

INDIRECT IMMUNOFLUORESCENCE.   Circulating IgG anti-basement membrane zone antibodies are demonstrable in only 25 percent of herpes gestationis patients using conventional indirect immunofluorescence microscopy techniques. The use of a complement-binding technique will demonstrate the presence of "HG factor" in about 75 percent of patients. It has been clearly shown that the HG factor is an IgG_1 anti-basement membrane zone antibody that is present in low titer yet avidly fixes complement.[9,10] The latter explains why C3 deposits are more readily detected in situ than IgG deposits as two IgG molecules activating complement

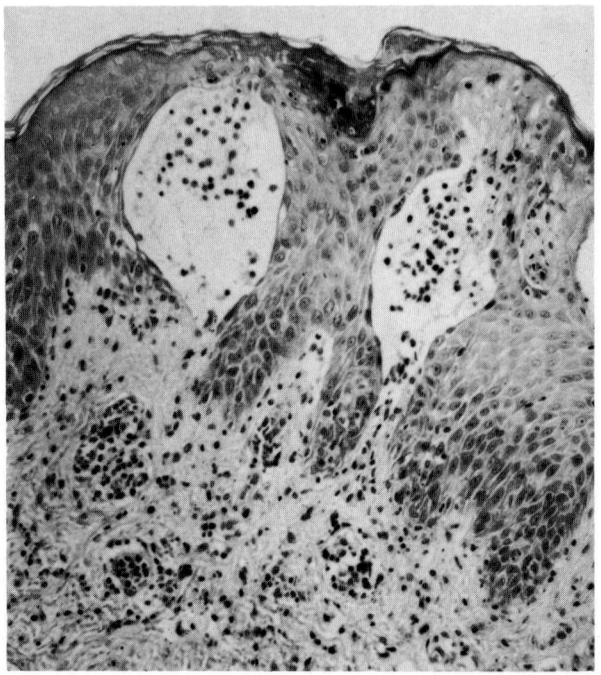

FIGURE 168-4 Biopsy of an early lesion of herpes gestationis showing microvesicle formation. The inflammatory infiltrate consists of lymphocytes and eosinophils with an admixture of polymorphonuclear neutrophils.

result in the deposition of 500 to 1000 C3 molecules at the site of activation, in this case the basement membrane zone. HG factor has also been detected in the cord blood of some infants born to affected mothers.

IMMUNOELECTRON MICROSCOPY. The deposits of C3 at the basement membrane zone have been shown to be located in the lamina lucida.[11,12] Immunoreactants may also be deposited along the dermal side of the basal cell plasma membrane.[11]

IMMUNOCHEMICAL STUDIES. Sera from a number of herpes gestationis patients bind a 180-kDa protein in extracts of human epidermal cells.[13] This same antigen is present in extracts of human amnion and is also recognized by a number of patients with bullous pemphigoid.[14] Recently, a human epidermal cDNA corresponding to this 180-kDa protein has been isolated.[15] Moreover, antisera

raised against a fusion protein encoded by this cDNA react with the 180-kDa epidermal antigen by immunoblot and bind basal keratinocyte hemidesmosomes by immunoelectron microscopy.[15] These findings provide some degree of unity between herpes gestationis and bullous pemphigoid patients in that an antigen recognized by their circulating autoantibodies is apparently identical.

IMMUNOGENETIC STUDIES. Patients with herpes gestationis demonstrate an increased incidence of HLA-B8, HLA-DR3, and the HLA-DR3, -DR4 paired haplotype.[16]

Course As mentioned above, herpes gestationis may begin at any time during pregnancy but tends to remit spontaneously within a few weeks of delivery. There is a tendency for it to recur in subsequent pregnancies and it usually begins earlier in the subsequent pregnancy than it did in the first. Exacerbation of the disease may be induced by birth control pills in patients with a prior history of herpes gestationis.

One study has indicated an increased incidence of fetal morbidity and mortality in herpes gestationis,[8] but another large study did not confirm this.[17] Other data suggest an increased incidence in small-for-gestational-age infants in herpes gestationis patients.

Treatment The treatment of patients with herpes gestationis is aimed at relief of symptoms and amelioration of maternal cutaneous disease. Systemic corticosteroids are the most frequently used treatment and are usually quite effective in doses of 20 to 40 mg per day of prednisone. The corticosteroid should be tapered as tolerated by the patient. In some instances it can be stopped even before delivery. In view of the frequency of postpartum disease exacerbations, the physician must be prepared to quickly reinstitute or increase therapy at the time of delivery. In very mild cases of herpes gestationis, vigorous use of topical corticosteroids will sometimes suffice. Infants born of mothers treated with prolonged courses of high-dose systemic corticosteroids should be monitored for adrenal insufficiency. It is not known whether maternal therapy decreases the risk of fetal morbidity or mortality.

Pruritic Urticarial Papules and Plaques of Pregnancy

Pruritic urticarial papules and plaques of pregnancy (PUPPP) is a common, intensely pruritic dermatosis that usually occurs late in the third trimester of pregnancy. It typically affects primigravidas.

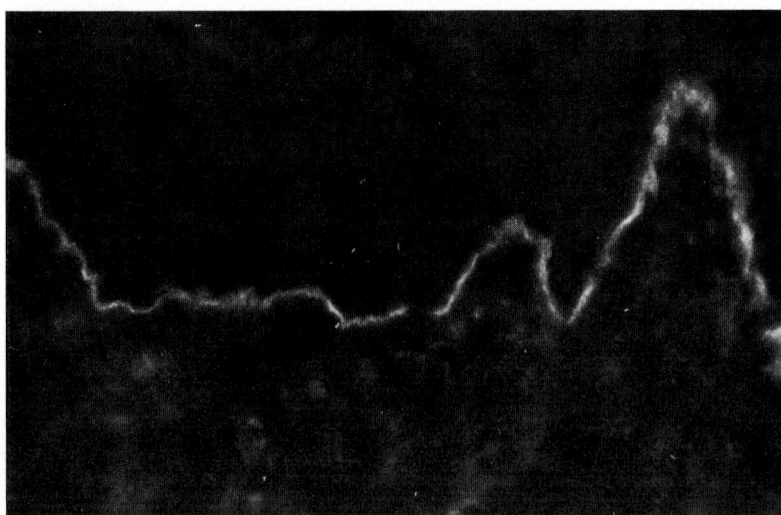

FIGURE 168-5 Direct immunofluorescence microscopy of perilesional skin from a patient with herpes gestationis. C3 deposits are present in the basement membrane zone.

History   The eruption was first described in detail and named by Lawley et al. in 1979.[18] Previously Nurse[19] and Bourne[20] reported similar eruptions that probably represented PUPPP. Nurse termed these eruptions *prurigo of pregnancy—late type,* and Bourne used the term *toxemic rash of pregnancy.* Subsequently Holmes et al. have used the name *polymorphous eruption of pregnancy* to describe a somewhat similar group of patients.[17]

Clinical Features   PUPPP is characterized by the onset of tiny (1 to 2 mm) erythematous papules on the abdomen, most often in the latter part of the third trimester of pregnancy.[18,21–24] The papules frequently begin in the striae distensae (Fig. 168-6*a*) but soon coalesce to form large erythematous plaques centered around the umbilicus. The lesions are extraordinarily itchy, and patients frequently are unable to sleep at night. Curiously, despite the intense pruritus, excoriations are extremely unusual. The urticarial papules and plaques spread over the course of a few days to involve the buttocks and thighs (Fig. 168-6*b*). The morphology of the lesions as well as their anatomic progression is in general rather uniform from patient to patient. In some instances lesions will also occur on the arms, forearms, and legs. Lesions on or above the breasts are rare, and lack of involvement of the face is a consistent feature. Close observation of the primary erythematous papules often reveals a surrounding narrow pale halo. Occasionally some papules are so edematous as to appear as papulovesicles.

   Almost all reported cases have begun in the third trimester and most after the 35th week. The onset of PUPPP in the immediate postpartum period is rare. Although this eruption can occur in any pregnancy, it is most frequently seen in primigravidas. In the experience at the National Institutes of Health with 25 patients, 19 (76 percent) were primigravidas.[21] All of these patients had their onset of disease in the third trimester except one, who developed lesions in the immediate postpartum period. The average time of onset was the 36th week of gestation, and the most frequent week of onset was the 39th. In all 25 patients, lesions began on the abdomen, and nearly one-half specifically indicated onset in their periumbilical striae distensae. A recent study found an increased maternal weight gain, increased neonatal birth weight, and an increased incidence of twinning in 30 PUPPP patients, and the authors theorized that abdominal distention or a reaction to it may play a role in the development of this disorder.[25]

Histopathology and Immunofluorescence   The histopathologic findings in PUPPP are not specific. Biopsy of skin reveals a superficial and often mid-dermal perivascular lymphohistiocytic infiltrate associated, in some cases, with a variable number of eosinophils and edema of the papillary dermis. Epidermal changes may include mild focal spongiosis and parakeratosis.

   Direct immunofluorescence microscopy of lesional or perilesional skin is routinely negative.

Course   The natural history of PUPPP appears to be spontaneous resolution of most cases within a few days after delivery. Unlike herpes gestationis, postpartum onset or exacerbation of PUPPP is exceptional. There does not appear to be a tendency for it to recur in subsequent pregnancies, although a few cases have been reported. Moreover, there does not appear to be an increased incidence of fetal morbidity or mortality associated with it.[21,22] There is report of an infant being born with lesions. In our series of PUPPP patients, follow-up revealed that eight patients had subsequent pregnancies and that none was complicated by PUPPP.[21]

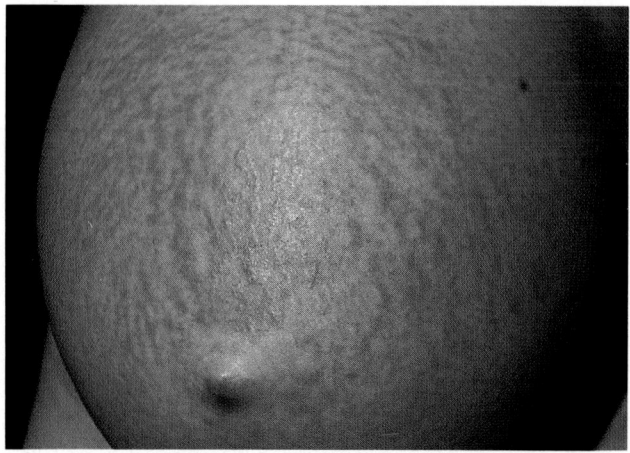

a

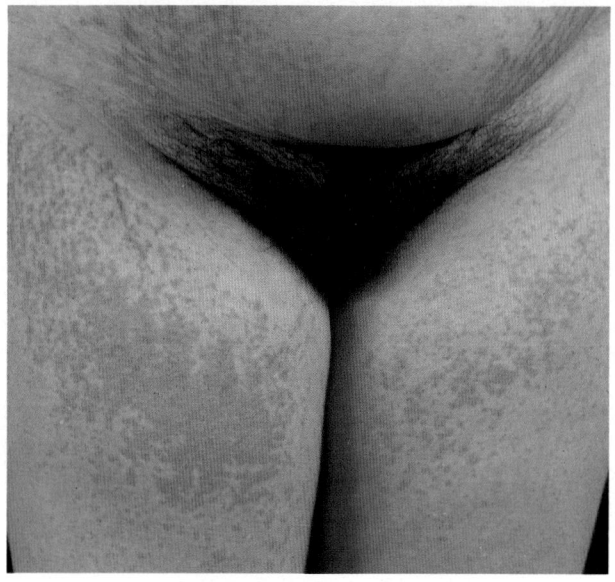

b

FIGURE 168-6   Pruritic urticarial papules and plaques of pregnancy. (*a*) The earliest lesions are tiny erythematous papules frequently localized to the striae distensae. (*b*) They then coalesce to form erythematous plaques and spread to involve buttocks and thighs. (*Courtesy of Klaus Wolff, M.D.*)

Differential Diagnosis   In most instances the diagnosis of PUPPP is not difficult. The classic presentation is a primigravida late in the third trimester with an extraordinarily pruritic eruption of papules and plaques that began in the striae distensae on the abdomen and spread to involve the buttocks and thighs, sparing the upper chest and face. Herpes gestationis must be considered as a diagnostic possibility in some instances, although usually prominent vesicular and/or bullous lesions are found in these patients. Direct immunofluorescence microscopy of perilesional skin should be performed if herpes gestationis is considered.

   It must also be kept in mind that all of the eruptions that occur in nonpregnant individuals may also occur in pregnancy and should not be confused with those dermatoses that are apparently pregnancy-specific. Thus erythema multiforme, drug eruptions, contact dermatitis, and insect bites can at times be confused with pregnancy-related dermatoses.

Treatment Intense (five to six times per day) therapy with potent topical corticosteroids seems to provide symptomatic relief in almost all cases. New lesions will usually stop appearing within 2 to 3 days, and most patients can then begin to taper the frequency of applications. In many instances patients will be able to stop all therapy prior to delivery. Brief tapering courses of systemic corticosteroids will also provide relief. H₁ antihistamines do not appear to be effective.

Recurrent Cholestasis of Pregnancy (Prurigo Gravidarum)

Recurrent cholestasis of pregnancy, also known as *prurigo gravidarum* or *benign recurrent intrahepatic cholestasis,* is a hepatic condition usually occurring late in pregnancy and first manifested by severe generalized pruritus followed by the appearance of clinical jaundice. It is thought to be hormonally induced in susceptible individuals. Its incidence has been estimated at 0.02 to 2.4 percent of pregnancies.[26]

History Recurrent cholestasis of pregnancy was first separated from other causes of jaundice in pregnancy by Svanborg and Ohlsson.[27]

Clinical Features Recurrent cholestasis of pregnancy has no primary cutaneous lesions although secondary excoriations may occur. The first symptom of recurrent cholestasis of pregnancy is pruritus. The severity may vary from moderate to severe, and in the early stages the pruritus may manifest itself only at night. Although often localized at first, the pruritus tends to become generalized.[28] The pruritus may precede the onset of clinical jaundice by up to 4 weeks although, rarely, it can be much longer. Patients may also complain of fatigue and anorexia and, in some instances, may develop nausea and vomiting. Most cases occur during the third trimester, although the onset has been reported as early as the first trimester. In fully developed cases numerous excoriations may be seen in conjunction with icterus. Patients may complain of right quadrant fullness or tenderness as well as dark urine and light-colored stools.

Course The pruritus associated with recurrent cholestasis of pregnancy usually remits within a few days after delivery. There is a tendency for this disorder to recur in subsequent pregnancies, and there have been reports of several members of families being affected, suggesting a genetic predisposition in some instances.[29] There have also been documented instances where patients who had developed recurrent cholestasis of pregnancy also developed cholestatic jaundice while taking synthetic estrogens and progestational agents for contraception.[29] It is not entirely clear whether estrogen or progesterone is the primary inciting agent and it may be that they work synergistically. Also the precise pathophysiology of the cholestasis is unknown. Finally, there have been patients who have been diagnosed as having recurrent cholestasis of pregnancy who did not develop clinical jaundice.

There appears to be an increased incidence of prematurity and low birth weights in the offspring of patients with recurrent cholestasis of pregnancy. In addition, postpartum hemorrhage is also more likely in these women. The incidence of untoward events seems to be highest in patients with both jaundice and pruritus.[30]

Treatment Attempts should be made to control pruritus with bland emollients and topical antipruritic regimens. In many instances these will provide adequate relief to the patient. The addition of antihistamines is at times of some benefit. Therapy with cholestyramine may occasionally be effective.[31]

Impetigo Herpetiformis

Impetigo herpetiformis is a form of pustular psoriasis that occurs during pregnancy and may be life threatening (see also Chap. 39). It is exceedingly rare and only approximately 100 cases have been reported.[32]

History This disorder was first reported in 1872 by Hebra in five pregnant women, four of whom died.[33]

Clinical Manifestations Impetigo herpetiformis tends to occur in the third trimester of pregnancy, although cases have been reported as early as the first trimester. Many of the affected women have had no personal or family history of psoriasis. Cases recurring in subsequent pregnancies have been reported.

The earliest lesions are erythematous patches occurring in the groin, axillae, and anterior as well as posterior neck.[34] At their margins these erythematous patches are studded with tiny superficial pustules (Fig. 168-7). The lesions expand by peripheral extension, with new pustules occurring at the leading edges while the old pustules at the interior of the expanding lesions break down, resulting in crusting or in some cases impetiginization. Pruritus is unusual in impetigo herpetiformis. Large areas of the body may be affected eventually, and in flexural areas the lesions may become vegetative. In some cases mucous membranes may be affected and subungual pustules can cause onycholysis.

Most patients also have constitutional signs and symptoms, the most common being fever and chills accompanied at times by nausea, vomiting, and diarrhea. In the past, delirium, convulsions, and tetany secondary to hypocalcemia were often reported, but these complications as well as bacterial sepsis are infrequently seen in the modern era.

Histology The histopathology of impetigo herpetiformis is the same as that of pustular psoriasis. The characteristic finding in an early lesion is the presence of collections of polymorphonuclear

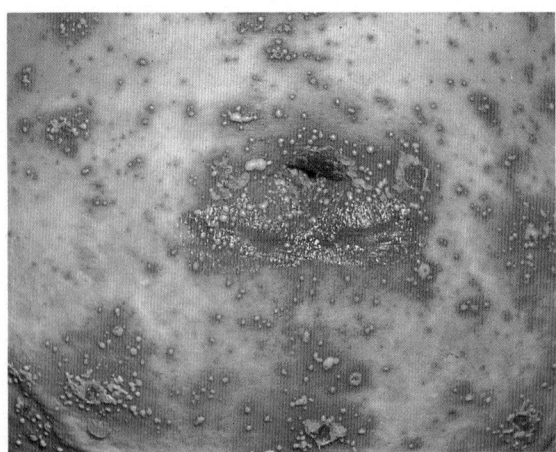

FIGURE 168-7 Impetigo herpetiformis. This is pustular psoriasis occurring in pregnancy. Erythematous patches that are studded with tiny superficial pustules. (*Courtesy of Klaus Wolff, M.D.*)

neutrophils in spongiotic foci in the epidermis, known as spongiform pustules of Kogoj. In mature lesions, the spongiform pustules become quite large and may assume a subcorneal location. Parakeratosis and elongation of rete ridges are also often found.

Laboratory Results   Elevated white blood cell counts and sedimentation rates are quite common in impetigo herpetiformis. When these occur in the presence of fever, infection must be ruled out. The unopened pustules are sterile, but the skin may become secondarily infected. Decreased serum calcium and decreased serum albumin are sometimes found.

Course   The disease tends to remit promptly after delivery but may recur in subsequent pregnancies.[35] There may be an increased risk of fetal morbidity and mortality associated with placental insufficiency.

Treatment   Systemic corticosteroids appear to be the treatment of choice in impetigo herpetiformis, with prednisone in doses of up to 60 mg per day being necessary at times to control the eruption.[35–38] Once under control, the prednisone can be tapered judiciously, but there is a risk of sudden exacerbation of disease if tapered too rapidly.

Patients should be monitored for systemic and cutaneous infections and treated with appropriate antibiotics when indicated. Serum calcium and albumin levels should also be followed, and replacement therapy undertaken if levels become too low.

Poorly Defined Eruptions Associated with Pregnancy

Prurigo Gestationis (Besnier)

Prurigo gestationis is a pruritic dermatosis that may occur any time in the fourth to ninth month of gestation but has peak incidence between the 20th and 34th weeks of pregnancy. It is characterized by the occurrence of small papules, most of which are excoriated, on the proximal limbs and upper trunk. In some instances the limb lesions tend to be distributed on extensor surfaces. Although Costello estimated a 2 percent incidence of prurigo gestationis in otherwise normal pregnancies, this is clearly a large overestimation.[39] Nurse[19] has suggested an incidence of 0.5 percent, but this also is probably much too high as 25 percent of Nurse's series of patients probably had PUPPP.

The eruption tends to resolve quickly after delivery, although postinflammatory hyperpigmentation may persist for some time. Therapy with topical corticosteroids is apparently helpful. It is uncommon for prurigo gestationis to recur in subsequent pregnancies, and there is no known increased incidence of fetal morbidity or mortality associated with this disease.

Papular Dermatitis of Pregnancy

Papular dermatitis of pregnancy is a rare, controversial eruption described by Spangler et al. in 1962.[40] The very existence of this disease is in doubt owing to the paucity of subsequent reports of well-described cases. Spangler estimated the incidence to be 1 case in 2400 pregnancies, but this is surely a vast overestimation.

Clinical Manifestations   As described by Spangler, papular dermatitis of pregnancy is a pruritic eruption that may begin at any time during pregnancy. It is characterized by the appearance of small erythematous papules, usually 3 to 5 mm in diameter, that are often surmounted by a 1- to 2-mm central papule or central crust. Spangler indicated that the lesions were excoriated so rapidly that it was extremely rare to find an intact papule. The distribution of the lesions was generalized with no predilection for any area.

Histology   Spangler did not report biopsies of any of his cases. A biopsy of an unexcoriated papule in a case reported by Michaud et al. showed hyperkeratosis, spongiosis, exocytosis, elongation of the rete ridges, and a perivascular infiltrate of lymphocytes in the papillary dermis.[41] Direct immunofluorescence testing of skin for deposits of IgG, IgA, IgM, and C3 was negative.

Laboratory Results   Patients with papular dermatitis of pregnancy have markedly elevated levels of urinary chorionic gonadotropin. Some patients also have low levels of urinary estriol[42] and plasma hydrocortisone. The half-life of plasma hydrocortisone is also decreased for the group as a whole.

Treatment   Therapy with systemic corticosteroids is reported to be effective in controlling the eruption.[4,26] At times doses of up to 100 mg of prednisone per day are necessary.

Diethylstilbestrol, once recommended by Spangler and Emerson,[42] should not be used due to the increased risk of vaginal carcinoma in offspring born to mothers treated with this agent. Spangler himself later withdrew this therapeutic recommendation.[43]

Course   The disease has been reported to recur in subsequent pregnancies. Spangler reported a 27 percent incidence of fetal death in untreated cases, whereas there was no fetal loss in treated cases. A recent careful reevaluation of these data has demonstrated a 12 percent incidence of fetal loss in patients with papular dermatitis of pregnancy.[3] The previously reported higher incidence was caused by the inclusion of fetal wastage in pregnancies in which there was no cutaneous eruption. Several of these mothers would almost surely be classified as habitual aborters today.

Miscellaneous Disorders

Six patients with an eruption termed *pruritic folliculitis of pregnancy* were described by Zoberman and Farmer.[44] The onset of their eruption ranged from the fourth to the ninth month of gestation and their lesions consisted of 3- to 5-mm excoriated, erythematous papules. The lesions were generalized in five patients and confined to the extremities and abdomen in one. The striking feature of the histopathology of five of these cases was the presence of folliculitis, with the hair follicles showing intraluminal pustule formation. The skin biopsy of one patient did not reveal folliculitis but only a mild perivascular infiltrate in the upper dermis and parakeratosis at the edges of the acrotrichium. Direct immunofluorescence microscopy was negative in all four patients tested. Two patients reported similar eruptions in previous pregnancies. All of the offspring born of these pregnancies were healthy. Of the five patients available for follow-up, two had the eruption resolve at delivery, two had it resolve one month after delivery, and in one patient it resolved spontaneously within a week of onset.

An eruption termed *autoimmune progesterone dermatitis of pregnancy* has been reported in one patient.[45] The eruption was characterized by the appearance of papules and pustules on the extensor surfaces of the thighs, arms, forearms, hands, and buttocks. The eruption began early in pregnancy and the patient experienced a spontaneous abortion in the third month. The patient reported a similar eruption associated with a previous pregnancy that also terminated in a spontaneous abortion in the second month. The eruption was exacerbated by an oral contraceptive. Intradermal skin tests with aqueous progesterone produced delayed hypersensitivity reactions whose histology was similar to that found in naturally occurring lesions. However, the patient did not develop an exacerbation of her skin lesions premenstrually, a time during which progesterone levels are elevated. The exact relation of progesterone to this eruption as well as the existence of autosensitivity to progesterone is unclear.

References

1. Jaffe RB: Endocrine physiology of normal pregnancy, in *Obstetrics and Gynecology,* edited by DN Danforth. Philadelphia, Harper & Row, 1982, p 342

2. Osathanondoh R, Tulchinsky D: Placental polypeptide hormones, in *Maternal-Fetal Endocrinology,* edited by D Tulchinsky, KJ Ryan. Philadelphia, Saunders, 1980, p 17

3. Winton GB, Lewis CW: Dermatoses of pregnancy. *J Am Acad Dermatol* **6**:977, 1982

4. Scoggins RB: Skin changes and diseases in pregnancy, in *Dermatology in General Medicine,* 2d ed, edited by TB Fitzpatrick et al. New York, McGraw-Hill, 1979, p 1363

5. Demis DJ: Skin conditions during pregnancy, in *Clinical Dermatology,* edited by DJ Demis et al. Hagerstown, MD, Harper & Row, 1980, p 1

6. Milton JL: *The Pathology and Treatment of Diseases of the Skin.* London, Robert Hardwicke, 1872, p 205

7. Provost TT, Tomasi TB, Jr: Evidence for complement activation via the alternate pathway in skin diseases: Herpes gestationis, systemic lupus erythematosus and bullous pemphigoid. *J Clin Invest* **53**:1779, 1973

8. Lawley TJ et al: Fetal and maternal risk factors in herpes gestationis. *Arch Dermatol* **114**:552, 1978

9. Jordon RE et al: The immunopathology of herpes gestationis: Immunofluorescent studies and characterization of "HG factor." *J Clin Invest* **57**:1426, 1976

10. Katz SI et al: Herpes gestationis: Immunopathology and characterization of the HG factor. *J Clin Invest* **57**:1434, 1976

11. Yaoita H et al: Herpes gestationis: Ultrastructure and ultrastructural localization of in vivo-bound complement: Modified tissue preparation and processing for horseradish peroxidase staining of skin. *J Invest Dermatol* **66**:383, 1976

12. Honigsmann H et al: Herpes gestationis: Fine structural pattern of immunoglobulin deposits in the skin in vivo. *J Invest Dermatol* **66**:389, 1976

13. Morrison LH et al: Herpes gestationis autoantibodies recognize a 180-kDa human epidermal antigen. *J Clin Invest* **81**:2023, 1988

14. Roth J et al: Herpes gestationis and bullous pemphigoid autoantibodies detect a 180-kDa antigen in human amnion. *Clin Res* **36**:690, 1988

15. Diaz LA et al: Isolation of a human epidermal cDNA corresponding to the 180-kDa autoantigen recognized by bullous pemphigoid and herpes gestationis sera. *J Clin Invest* **86**:1088, 1990

16. Shornick JK: Herpes gestationis. *J Am Acad Dermatol* **17**:539, 1987

17. Holmes RC et al: A comparative study of toxic erythema of pregnancy and herpes gestationis. *Br J Dermatol* **106**:499, 1982

18. Lawley TJ et al: Pruritic uritcarial papules and plaques of pregnancy. *JAMA* **241**:1696, 1979

19. Nurse DS: Prurigo of pregnancy. *Australas J Dermatol* **9**:258, 1968

20. Bourne G: Toxemic rash of pregnancy. *Proc R Soc Med* **55**:462, 1962

21. Yancey KB et al: Pruritic urticarial papules and plaques of pregnancy (PUPPP): Clinical experience in 25 patients. *J Am Acad Dermatol* **10**:473, 1984

22. Ulhin SR: Pruritic urticarial papules and plaques of pregnancy. *Arch Dermatol* **117**:238, 1981

23. Ahmed AR, Kaplan R: Pruritic urticarial papules and plaques of pregnancy. *J Am Acad Dermatol* **4**:679, 1981

24. Callen JP, Hanno R: Pruritic urticarial papules and plaques of pregnancy (PUPPP). A clinicopathologic study. *J Am Acad Dermatol* **5**:401, 1981

25. Cohen LM et al: Pruritic urticarial papules and plaques of pregnancy and its relationship to maternal-fetal weight gain and twin pregnancy. *Arch Dermatol* **125**:1534, 1989

26. Sasseville D et al: Dermatoses of pregnancy. *Int J Dermatol* **20**:223, 1981

27. Svanborg A, Ohlsson S: Recurrent jaundice of pregnancy. *Am J Med* **27**:40, 1939

28. Holzbach RT: Jaundice in pregnancy. *Am J Med* **61**:367, 1976

29. DePagter AGF et al: Familial benign recurrent intrahepatic cholestasis. *Gastroenterology* **71**:202, 1976

30. Johnston WG, Baskett TF: Obstetric cholestasis: A 14-year review. *Am J Obstet Gynecol* **133**:299, 1979

31. Laatikainen T: Effect of cholestyramine and phenobarbital on pruritus and serum bile levels in cholestasis of pregnancy. *Am J Obstet Gynecol* **132**:501, 1978

32. Braverman IM: Pregnancy and the menstrual cycle, in *Skin Signs of Systemic Disease.* Philadelphia, Saunders, 1981, p 761

33. Hebra F von: On some affections of the skin occurring in pregnant and puerperal women. *Wien Med Wochenschr* **48**:1197, 1872. Abstracted in *Lancet* **1**:399, 1872

34. Baker H, Ryan TJ: Generalized pustular psoriasis: A clinical and epidemiological study of 104 cases. *Br J Dermatol* **80**:771, 1968

35. Beveridge GW et al: Impetigo herpetiformis in two successive pregnancies. *Br J Dermatol* **78**:106, 1966

36. Sauer G: Impetigo herpetiformis. *Arch Dermatol* **83**:119, 1961

37. Oosterling RJ et al: Impetigo herpetiformis or generalized pustular psoriasis. *Arch Dermatol* **114**:1527, 1978

38. Oumeish OY et al: Some aspects of impetigo herpetiformis. *Arch Dermatol* **118**:103, 1982

39. Costello MJ: Eruptions of pregnancy. *NY State J Med* **41**:849, 1941

40. Spangler AS et al: Papular dermatitis of pregnancy. *JAMA* **181**:577, 1962

41. Michaud RM et al: Papular dermatitis of pregnancy. *Arch Dermatol* **118**:1003, 1982

42. Spangler AS, Emerson K: Estrogen levels and estrogen therapy in papular dermatitis of pregnancy. *Am J Obstet Gynecol* **110**:534, 1971

43. Spangler AS: Letter to the editor. *Am J Obstet Gynecol* **113**:570, 1972

44. Zoberman E, Farmer E: Pruritic folliculitis of pregnancy. *Arch Dermatol* **112**:1534, 1976

45. Bierman SM: Autoimmune progesterone dermatitis. *Arch Dermatol* **107**:896, 1973

CHAPTER 169

Ruth K. Freinkel

Cutaneous Manifestations of Endocrine Diseases

General Considerations

Hormones regulate physiologic processes by modification of existing activities rather than by initiation of reactions de novo. Thus, in the skin as elsewhere, excesses or deficiencies of hormones generally result in quantitative rather than qualitative changes in cutaneous function and morphology. However, the expression of altered hormonal balance is determined to some extent by intrinsic properties of skin in various areas. The capacity of cutaneous structures to respond, local hemodynamics, and extrinsic factors such as light and trauma will influence the distribution as well as quantity of hormonally induced changes in the skin.

The expression of endocrine disorders in the skin may reflect both alterations in total body economy and direct actions on cutaneous structures. For example, abnormalities in fluid and electrolyte balance resulting from endocrine abnormalities produce changes in skin turgor. As a major site for dissipation and conservation of heat, the skin may reflect derangements in thermogenesis in endocrine disease; skin temperature, vascular dilatation, and sweating reflect such changes.

Intermediary metabolism is controlled by balanced actions of hormones. Control is exerted by both direct effects on cells and indirect effects via circulating fuels and other regulatory substances. Expression of hormonal effects at the cellular level is a function of circulating levels of hormones and the ability of the tissue to respond. Excessive amounts of hormones accentuate activity of a cutaneous structure to the degree that it can respond. Hormone deficiency may result in diminished function of a responsive structure or be expressed by effects of unbalanced or excessive activity of other hormones (e.g., excess ACTH in adrenal insufficiency).

For certain hormones the skin displays the responsiveness of a specific target tissue (e.g., sex hormones); other hormones have global effects on tissues that are expressed also in skin (e.g., thyroid hormone); still other hormones have little or no discernible effects on the skin (e.g., adrenal mineralocorticoids). Because cell turnover, synthesis of structural proteins, lipids, and mucopolysaccharides, and a vast network of blood vessels are affected by hormones, the skin affords a sensitive barometer of endocrine disease. In subsequent sections, the effects of various endocrinopathies on the skin will be considered in detail. In keeping with the concept that hormones regulate rather than initiate functions, the discussion will be formulated in terms of *too little* and *too much* of given hormones.

Finally, not all of the cutaneous manifestation of endocrine disorders can be attributed to direct effects of hormones on the skin itself. Thus, vitiligo in Addison's disease and pretibial myxedema in Graves' disease appear to reflect underlying pathologic processes that also initiate the endocrinopathy.

Thyroid Hormone

Effects of Thyroid Hormone on the Skin

Thyroid hormones act on fundamental mechanisms of energy metabolism, fuel metabolism, and biosynthetic and degradative processes at the cellular level. They appear to have diverse primary sites of action at the level of cell membranes, mitochondria, and gene transcription that enhance substrate availability and oxidative metabolism and regulate functional properties,[1] including those of keratinocytes and fibroblasts.[2,3]

Available data suggest that thyroid hormone plays a pivotal role in embryonic development of mammalian skin as well as in maintenance of normal cutaneous function in adult skin. Ablation of the thyroid gland of sheep in utero retards formation of hair follicles and other adnexal structures as well as development of the dermis and epidermis.[4] Extrapolation from experiments in amphibian skin suggests that the effects of thyroid hormone on fetal development involve stimulation of mitotic activity as well as differentiation. Oxygen consumption,[5] epidermal mitotic activity, and protein synthesis[6] are increased by thyroid hormone. Thyroid hormone appears to be necessary for both the initiation and maintenance of hair growth[7] and for normal secretion of sebum.[8]

Thyroid hormones affect production of collagen and mucopolysaccharides by dermal fibroblasts. Acid-soluble collagen is increased, insoluble collagen is decreased, and accumulation of glycosaminoglycans is retarded by thyroid hormone.

Lack of thyroid hormone is expressed by changes in all of the above functions in the skin. However, excess amounts of thyroid hormone do not correlate with abnormal acceleration of these functions.

Thyroid hormones also appear to affect pigmentation, and both hyper- and hypopigmentation are seen in hyperthyroidism.

Some of the effects of thyroid hormones on the skin are mediated indirectly by generalized effects on heat production and cardiovascular dynamics. Excessive sweating and increased cutaneous blood flow result from hyperthyroidism. To what extent these changes impinge on local cutaneous metabolism cannot be assessed.

Finally, it should be pointed out that some of the cutaneous changes in thyroid disease cannot be attributed directly to the effects of thyroid hormones. Altered activity in neurotransmitters may be responsible for actions that appear to result from altered levels of thyroid hormones. The autoimmune states that underlie Graves' disease and Hashimoto's thyroiditis appear to be responsible for some of the more striking cutaneous changes.

Cutaneous Manifestations of Too Much Thyroid Hormone

Thyrotoxicosis is the syndrome that results from excessive amounts of thyroid hormone. It may be due to Graves' disease, toxic nodular goiter, administration of excessive amounts of thyroid hormone, or as a transient phase in subacute thyroiditis.

The skin is above all warm, moist, and smooth. The warmth, which is due to peripheral vasodilatation and increased blood flow, is often accompanied by a persistent flush of the face, redness of the elbows, and palmar erythema. There is excessive sweating generally, but this is particularly pronounced on the palms and soles where eccrine glands are under sympathetic control. Other evidence of vasomotor instability is seen in evanescent blushing over the head and neck.

The epidermis is thin but not atrophic, and the stratum corneum is well hydrated. Altered texture of the hair and diffuse alopecia are commonly observed. Nails exhibit a characteristic onycholysis in which the free edge of the nail curves upward (Plummer's nail).

Other cutaneous manifestations may include generalized pruritus, chronic urticaria, and alopecia areata.[9] Hyperpigmentation of a diffuse or patchy nature is not uncommon and generally occurs on the face. Vitiligo occurs in approximately 7 percent of patients with Graves' disease but is not abnormally more frequent in other forms of hyperthyroidism.[10] It may antedate the endocrine disorders and is not improved by treatment of the thyrotoxicosis.

Graves' Disease   Graves' disease is an autoimmune disorder manifesting goiter and thyrotoxicosis, infiltrative ophthalmopathy, acropachy, and an infiltrative dermopathy (pretibial myxedema) (Fig. 169-1). Although these features can occur independently of each other, pretibial myxedema usually occurs in the presence of ophthalmopathy. Correction of the thyrotoxicosis has no effect on the skin lesions, which are found in about 5 percent of patients with Graves' disease. Indeed half of the cases of pretibial myxedema occur after the patient has been rendered euthyroid. The clinical picture may not be pathognomonic, as similar lesions have been reported in patients with primary hypothyroidism and Hashimoto's thyroiditis.[11]

The lesions occur most frequently on the anterior tibia and dorsa of the feet and are morphologically varied. They are usually bilateral but not symmetric. The lesions commonly consist of pink, flesh-colored, or purplish nodules (Fig. 169-2). A diffuse brawny edema may be present without nodules. Less common is an elephantiasis nostras variant in which the extremity becomes enlarged and covered with verrucous nodules. Thickening of the skin of the extensor surface of the forearm (preradial myxedema) has been reported.[12] The dermal changes are like those of myxedema proper. Excessive amounts of hyaluronic acid and chondroitin are present in lesions as well as in clinically normal skin.[13]

The pathogenic mechanisms are not clear. Circulating factors in the sera of affected patients have been shown to stimulate synthesis of mucopolysaccharides in dermal fibroblasts.[14] It has been speculated that antithyroid immunoglobulins bind to dermal sites and stimulate production of the carbohydrates.

Treatment of pretibial myxedema is not very successful. Systemic or intralesional corticosteroids or topical application of potent steroids under occlusion may afford some relief.

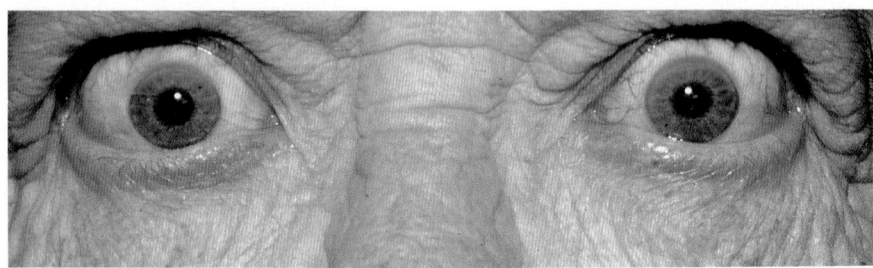

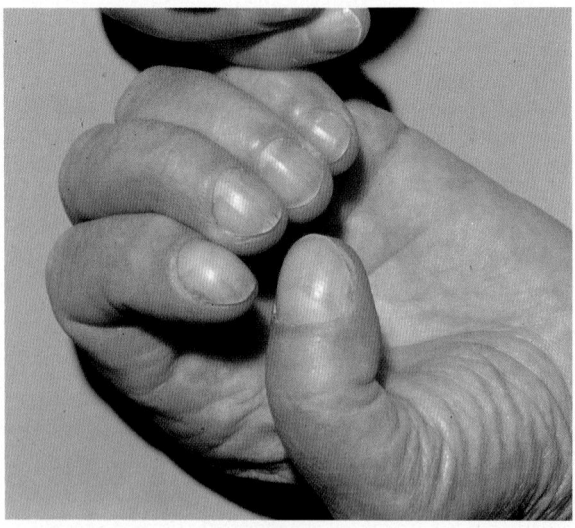
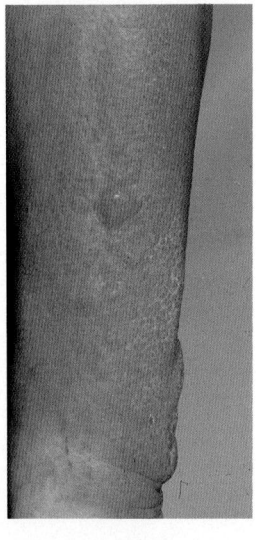

FIGURE 169-1 Hyperthyroidism. This composite illustrates the proptosis, the acropathy, and the pink or skin-colored papules, plaques, and nodules of pretibial myxedema.

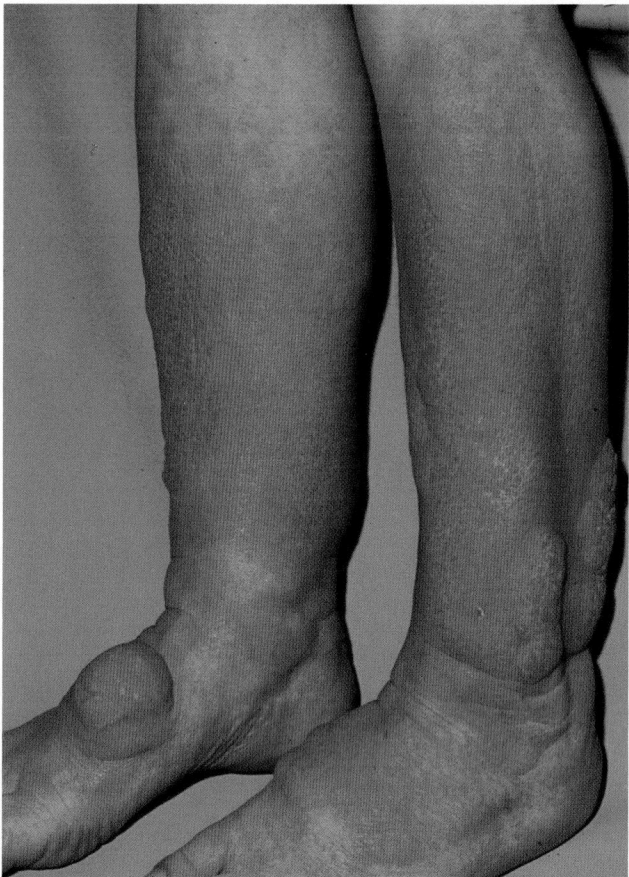

FIGURE 169-2 Hyperthyroidism with pretibial myxedema. Note infiltrated plaques that also extend to the calf and are partially hyperkeratotic. There is also an isolated nobule on the dorsum of the right foot.

Cutaneous Manifestations of Too Little Thyroid Hormone

Thyroid deficiency occurs when there is decreased production of thyroid hormone due to loss of functioning thyroid tissue, inadequate stimulation of the thyroid gland due to failure of the pituitary or hypothalamus, or absolute or relative impairment in biosynthesis of thyroid hormone due to either extrinsic or intrinsic factors. The resultant endocrine disorder derives its name, myxedema, from its most prominent manifestation in the skin.

In hypothyroidism, the skin is cold, xerotic, and pale. The coldness is due to reduced core temperature and cutaneous vasoconstriction. The latter is also in part responsible for the pallor. Xerosis is due to a change in skin texture and poor hydration of the stratum corneum. The epidermis is thin and hyperkeratotic, and there is follicular plugging. Because the changes are generalized, they can be differentiated from similar alterations in the skin of atopic individuals and in keratosis pilaris, where the findings are more prominent on the extremities. Fine wrinkling imparts a parchment-like quality to the skin, especially in hypothyroidism secondary to pituitary failure.

A yellowish discoloration of the skin is sometimes present and is accentuated on the palms and soles and nasolabial folds. This is due to the accumulation of carotene in stratum corneum, secondary to carotenemia. Elevated blood levels of carotene have been attrib-uted to a hepatic defect in the conversion of β carotene to vitamin A.

The hair is dry, coarse, and brittle and grows slowly. There is both patchy and diffuse loss of scalp hair, a very characteristic loss of the outer third of the eyebrow, and diminished body hair. Massive telogen effluvium may occur when there is abrupt onset of hypothyroidism, and the percentage of scalp hairs in telogen is generally increased in hypothyroid states. The chronology of the reversal of these changes when thyroid hormone is administered suggests that hair loss is due to both premature anagen arrest and failure in initiation of anagen.[15] Hypothyroid patients, especially children, frequently develop long, lanugo-type hair on the back, shoulders, and extremities.

Diminished sebum secretion contributes to the coarse appearance of the hair. Nails grow slowly and tend to be brittle.

The most striking change in the skin is due to dermal accumulation of mucopolysaccharides (myxedema). Although these accumulations are more striking in acral parts, the distribution of myxedema is not affected by a dependent position. Generally myxedema is diffuse, but focal mucinous papules, responsive to L-thyroxine, have been described.

The facial changes are especially characteristic (Fig. 169-3). The nose is broadened and lips are thickened. The tongue is large, smooth, and clumsy. There may be sticky secretions on the eyelids, which show fine wrinkling and a flaccid and translucent puffiness. Drooping of the upper lid may occur in the absence of edema due to decreased sympathetic stimulation of the superior palpebral muscle. At rest, the face lacks expressiveness, and changing emotions are registered slowly because of the concomitant lethargy. This facies is almost pathognomonic, although it may be simulated in untreated pernicious anemia and the nephrotic syndrome.

The hypothyroid skin heals slowly, and this tendency is proportional to the degree of hormone deficiency.

The mucopolysaccharides that accumulate in the dermis are hyaluronic acid and chondroitin sulfate. They appear first in the papillary dermis and are most prominent around hair follicles and vessels. They separate the collagen bundles and there may be some secondary degeneration of collagen.

All of the changes are reversible by judicious use of thyroid hormone. Mobilization of myxedematous deposits is one of the earliest indications of the action of thyroid hormone replacement and is characterized by a rise in serum sodium and a fall in hematocrit,[16] due to the conjoint release of water and electrolytes bound to the hydrophilic mucopolysaccharides.

The mechanism that causes myxedema is not clear. There is evidence in animals and tissue culture supporting actions of thyroid hormone on both restraint of synthesis and catabolism of mucopolysaccharides. Crude thyrotropic hormone has been reported to cause dermal accumulation of mucopolysaccharides,[17] suggesting a role for pituitary factors, which are elevated in primary thyroid failure. However, while myxedema is less prominent in hypothyroidism secondary to pituitary failure, it need not be absent. Thus, it is likely that lack of thyroid hormone is the primary factor in causing myxedema, but that interactions with pituitary and/or other hormones may play a facilitating role.

Parathyroid Hormone

Effects of Parathyroid Hormone on the Skin

Parathyroid hormone regulates the flux of calcium between extra- and intracellular compartments in responsive tissues (i.e., kidney

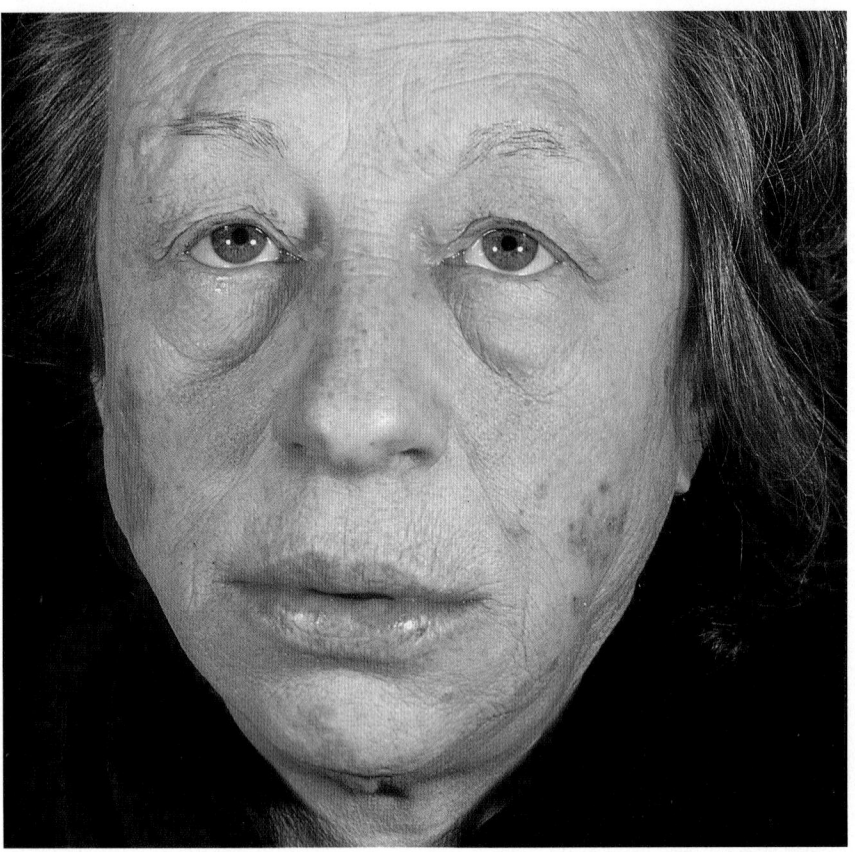

FIGURE 169-3 Hypothyroidism. This patient has many of the typical features of hypothyroidism: a cold, dry, pale skin; absence of hair in the lateral third of the eyebrows; and a puffiness of the face and lips due to the accumulation of water and mucopolysaccharides in the dermis. The hair is dry, coarse, and brittle. The nose is broadened, the tongue is large, smooth, red, and clumsy, and there is drooping of the eyelids. The face lacks expression and is the most pathognomonic of any of the features.

and bone) and the metabolism of vitamin D. A role for this hormone in the skin has not been established. However, receptors for parathyroid hormone have been identified in dermal fibroblasts, and the hormone affects collagen synthesis in dermal fibroblasts in vitro. The possible role of parathyroid hormone in the skin is clouded by the presence of a parathyroid-like protein in keratinocytes that stimulates adenylcyclase and acts on dermal fibroblasts at concentrations that are lower than those of parathyroid hormone.[18]

Hypercalcemia may result in calcium deposits in the skin, irrespective of its cause. Moreover, clinical experience suggests[19] that abnormalities of calcium and phosphate per se produce profound changes in the skin, attesting to the importance of these ions in normal skin physiology.

Cutaneous Manifestation of Excessive Parathyroid Hormone

Primary hyperparathyroidism is not associated with any cutaneous manifestation except, rarely, pruritus and deposition of calcium. Because of this, intractable pruritus in renal disease has been attributed to the presence of secondary hyperparathyroidism. An increased amount of calcium has been reported in the skin of such patients, and some, but not all, have experienced relief of itching after parathyroidectomy.[20] However, it should be noted that such patients are usually being treated with chronic dialysis, and that itching is frequently intensified by the treatment. Furthermore itching in uremic patients may be alleviated by irradiation of the skin with UVB. Thus, the mechanism of pruritus in chronic renal disease and in hyperparathyroidism has not been elucidated.

Cutaneous Manifestation of Too Little Parathyroid Hormone

Primary failure of the parathyroid glands may occur as an isolated phenomenon or as part of an autoimmune syndrome of multiple endocrine failure. In the latter case, it may be associated with Hashimoto's thyroiditis, Addison's disease, ovarian failure, or pernicious anemia; alopecia areata and vitiligo may be present in this syndrome. The least common cause of hypoparathyroidism is peripheral refractoriness to parathyroid hormone (pseudohypoparathyroidism). The most common cause is ablation of the parathyroids as a complication of thyroidectomy.

In all types of hypoparathyroidism the skin is dry, scaly, hyperkeratotic, and puffy. Nails become opaque and brittle and develop transverse ridges. Hair may be coarse and sparse. Eczematous dermatitis and hyperkeratotic and maculopapular eruptions have been reported. Since these changes are reversed when calcium levels are normalized, they appear to relate directly to the lack of calcium rather than to the level of parathyroid hormone.

Primary hypoparathyroidism is frequently associated with chronic mucocutaneous candidiasis.[21] The infection commonly involves the nails and oral mucosa, but there may be vulvovaginitis and candidal intertrigo. Candidiasis may present on glabrous skin as an annular or scaling eruption resembling a dermatophytosis.

These infections are not altered by regulation of blood calcium and phosphorous levels and are attended by defects in cellular immune mechanisms. They may antedate the onset of hypoparathyroidism by years. The presence of autoantibodies to parathyroid tissue in 30 percent of cases as well as autoantibodies to melanocytes[22] and other endocrine tissues has suggested that the fungal infections are related to the disturbance of immune function that underlies the endocrinopathy.[23]

Glucocorticoids

Effects of Glucocorticoids on the Skin

The effects of glucocorticoids on the skin are best appreciated by observation of the changes produced by excess hormone. Although endogenous hypercortisolism is uncommon, the iatrogenic disease has become all too familiar due to the common use of synthetic corticosteroids in nonendocrine disorders. These will be discussed in detail elsewhere but do not differ qualitatively from those produced by endogenous hormone. (See Chaps. 230 and 232).

The actions of corticosteroids on the skin has been extensively studied both in vivo and in vitro. Cortisol decreases the mass of dermal connective tissue due to direct effects on dermal fibroblasts. The hormone decreases synthesis as well as accumulation of glycosaminoglycans and alters their composition[24,25] possibly via receptor-mediated mechanisms. Corticosteroid increases collagen cross-linking, decreases activity of collagenase,[26,27] but probably does not affect the relative proportions of types I and III collagen. Although corticosteroid inhibits production of collagen,[28] dermal atrophy may also reflect diminished numbers of dermal fibroblasts.[29]

Corticosteroid appears to regulate diurnal variations in mitotic activity of the epidermis.[30] Mitotic peaks correlate inversely with serum cortisol levels,[31] and these effects may be mediated via adenylcyclase. Differentiation of epidermal cells is accelerated by the hormone in vitro.[32,33]

Corticosteroid retards growth of hair in experimental animals, possibly due to effects on initiation of anagen[34] and mitotic activity. However, excess endogenous corticosteroid produces hypertrichosis, whereas deficiency of the hormone causes loss of axillary hair, suggesting that the hormone plays a physiologic role in maintaining hair growth, at least in some sites. There is little clear evidence of an effect on sebaceous glands; however, follicular hyperkeratosis is frequently observed and plays a role in steroid-induced acne.

Corticosteroids profoundly affect the immune system and inflammatory reactions. While the immunosuppressive actions are the basis of the use of corticosteroids as anti-inflammatory agents, steroid-induced immunomodulation may play a role under physiologic conditions and in some of the manifestations of endogenous hypercortisolism. Among the effects are constraints on the production of interleukins, the actions of growth factors such as epidermal growth factor and platelet-derived growth factor, and synthesis of prostanoids due to inhibition of phospholipase A.[35] Anti-inflammatory effects are also abetted by stabilization of lysosomes, with resulting inhibition of release of proteases and other mediators.[36]

The skin is a major site for degradation and interconversion of glucocorticoids and other steroid hormones, as has been established by numerous studies. In particular, interconversion of cortisone and cortisol[37,38] is relevant to the effects of hormone excess. Cortisol has much greater effects on the skin and inflammatory reactions than cortisone. Exquisite regulation of interconversion of these two endogenous hormones, which has been shown in such physiologic events as wound healing, may provide control of proliferative events.[39]

Despite all of the above, it is not clear what role glucocorticoids play in maintenance of normal structure and function of the adult skin. In contrast to the effects of hormone excess, its lack seems to result in no clinically discernible changes in cutaneous integrity. However, the protean nature of glucocorticoid effects on the skin suggest that they play a regulatory role here as elsewhere. Indeed, high-affinity receptors for these hormones have been demonstrated in dermal fibroblasts as well as in keratinocytes. Perhaps the absence of gross structural and functional changes in the presence of too little glucocorticoid attests to the ability of the skin to function without fine tuning of such varied activities as mitotic division and collagen synthesis.

Effects of ACTH on the Skin

Effects of glucocorticoids on the skin cannot be discussed without mentioning the extraadrenal actions of pituitary corticotropin. Although corticosteroids do not directly affect pigmentation, corticotropin and its structurally related pituitary peptides MSH-α and -β stimulate melanogenesis. These hormones belong to a series of peptides that arises from the prohormone, pro-opiomelanocortin, that also includes the endorphins. In addition to effects on melanocytes, ACTH may also directly influence sebum secretion via lipotropic effects.[40]

Cutaneous Manifestations of Too Much Glucocorticoid

Hypercortisolism can arise from (1) functioning tumors of the adrenal cortex (Cushing's syndrome), (2) inappropriate secretion of ACTH by the pituitary (Cushing's disease), or (3) production of ACTH by nonpituitary neoplasia (ectopic ACTH syndrome). In all three types the effects of excess glucocorticoids may be mixed, but in varying degrees, with those of excess mineralocorticoids and androgenic steroids.

The skin becomes generally atrophic. The epidermis is thin and shiny and may show slight scaling. The dermis is also thin and loose, especially where subcutaneous fat is diminished. The skin becomes friable and easily damaged. Wound healing is markedly impaired; even slight injuries may fail to heal and become ulcerated and secondarily infected. Patients are prone to develop dermatophytosis as well as tinea versicolor.

There is increased vascular fragility, and patients often display petechiae and ecchymoses from slight trauma, especially in dependent parts. Decreased vascular tone is evident in purplish mottling of the lower extremities (cutis marmorata).

Among the characteristic lesions of glucocorticoid excess are the broad, purple striae that usually appear in areas of stretched skin on the trunk as well as elsewhere. They differ from the commonly found striae of adolescence, pregnancy, and obesity only with respect to their inordinate depth and breadth and intense color. The color fades when the disease is arrested, but the atrophy remains. The lesions represent another index of the loss of integrity of the dermal connective tissue and the failure of normal regenerative powers.

Hyperpigmentation is unusual in Cushing's syndrome but may occur in Cushing's disease in which production of ACTH (and related peptides) is increased; it has also been reported with ectopic ACTH production. Acanthosis nigricans occurs but is usually mild.

Plethora is common and accompanied by telangiectasia on the face (Fig. 169-4). This is usually attributed to associated polycy-

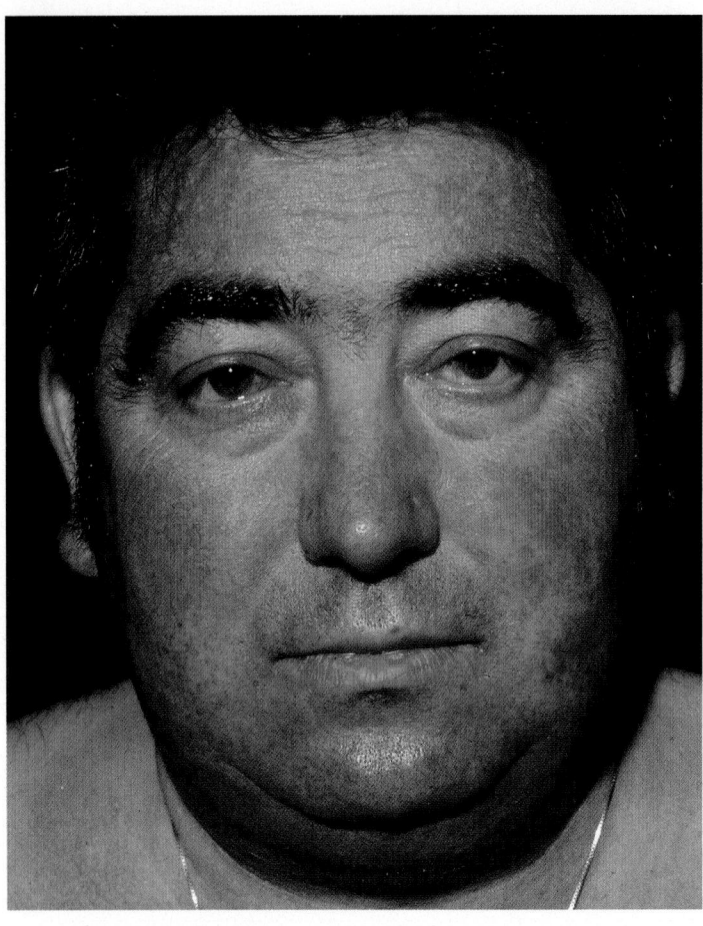

FIGURE 169-4 Hypercortisolism (Cushing's disease). Plethoric moon facies.

themia, although it occurs in the absence of increased red cell mass (personal observation).

Hypertrichosis and acne are common. The excess hair is usually found on the face on the upper lip, chin, and lateral cheeks. Pure hypercortisolism (as seen in iatrogenic Cushing's syndrome), does not induce true beard growth; rather the hair tends to be more lanugo-like. Intense hirsutism, involving body hair as well and accompanied by male-pattern alopecia, is sufficiently unusual in bilateral adrenal hyperplasia to justify suspicion of an adrenal tumor producing androgenic steroids.

One of the striking features of excess glucocorticoids is the change in appearance and body habitus. Excessive deposits of fat over the clavicles and back of the neck (buffalo hump) and abdomen are accompanied by loss of subcutaneous fat over the extremities. In addition, there is deposition of fat in the cheeks, giving the face a rounded appearance (moon facies). The central obesity may be associated with muscle wasting. Reduced height and kyphosis as a result of osteoporosis and compression fractures of the vertebrae may add to the altered appearance.

Cutaneous Effects of Too Little Glucocorticoid

Deficiency of glucocorticoids (i.e., Addison's disease) can occur when the adrenal cortex is (1) atrophic, either idiopathically or secondary to destructive disease (e.g., tuberculosis) or surgical ablation; or (2) inadequately stimulated by ACTH or when glucocorticoid synthesis is thwarted by abnormality in the biosynthetic sequence (e.g., adrenogenital syndrome). Although the clinical

manifestations of these disorders vary to some extent with causative factors, glucocorticoid deficiency is common to all. Except in adrenogenital syndrome, there is also a lack of adrenal androgens. This produces clinical stigmata of androgen deficiency only when gonadal function is also diminished (e.g., after menopause).

Although large amounts of glucocorticoids have a marked effect on the skin, their absence causes surprisingly little change. Unless the patient is severely debilitated, texture of the skin appears normal. Loss of body hair, however, is common and is most striking in the axilla. Since replacement with cortisone may partly restore axillary hair, some of the effect may be ascribable to glucocorticoid per se. Except for fibrosis and calcification of the pinna, mesenchymal changes are not apparent in the dermis.

The most striking cutaneous change of chronic adrenal insufficiency is hyperpigmentation, which occurs almost uniformly. In 20 to 40 percent of cases it is the first sign of the disease.[41] Hyperpigmentation that results from excess ACTH is one of the chief differentiating features between adrenal insufficiency due to pituitary disease and that due to primary adrenal failure.

The hyperpigmentation is generalized and represents an accentuation of normal pigment distribution. It is often noted as the persistence of a tan acquired in the summer, and it is always darker in sun-exposed areas (Fig. 169-5a). Darkening also occurs in areas of trauma, recent scars, and points of pressure and friction (elbows, knees, skin folds, and palmar creases) (Fig. 169-5b). Skin in sexual areas (nipples, areola, axilla, perineum, and genitalia) becomes darker. In parous females the linea alba darkens. Hair may darken and longitudinal pigmented bands appear on the nails. Pigmentation appears on mucosal surfaces, especially the buccal mucosa,

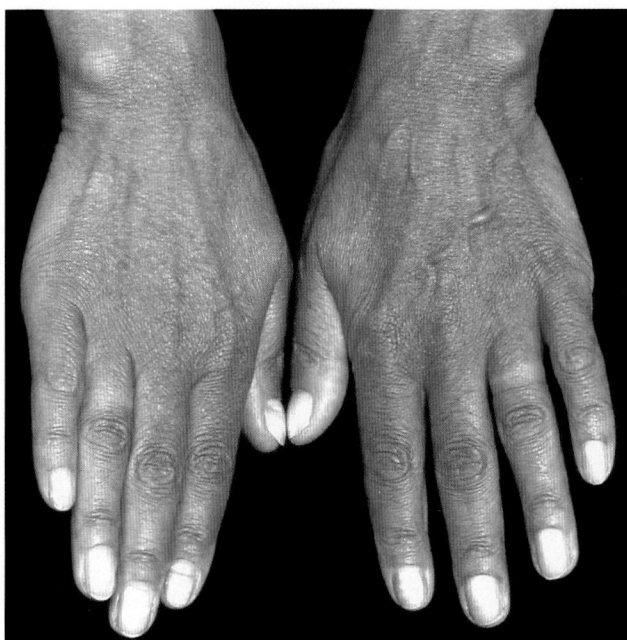

a

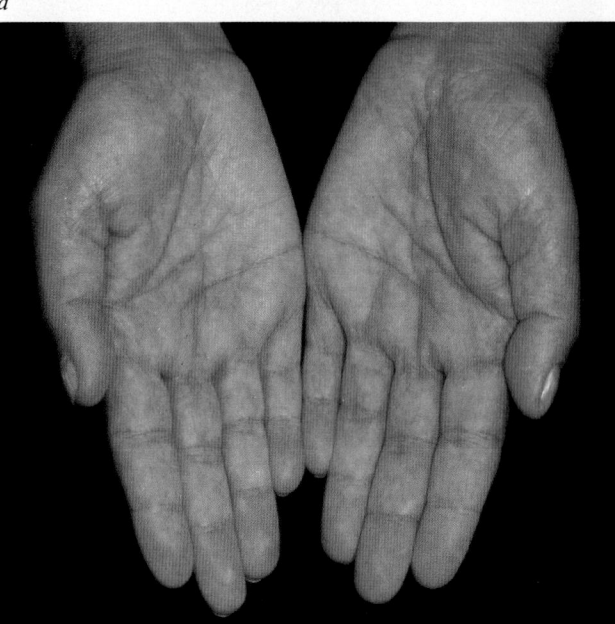

b

FIGURE 169-5 Addison's disease. Hyperpigmentation of the hands: (*a*) dorsa; (*b*) palmar creases. (*Courtesy of Klaus Wolff, M.D.*)

gums, and tongue. Such pigmentation is normally present in non-Caucasians and may darken. From the above description it is obvious that the hyperpigmentation is relative and can be evaluated only in terms of the patient's previous skin color (see also Chap. 80). Replacement therapy produces a gradual diminution of the color. In the treated Addisonian patient, waxing and waning of the intensity of pigmentation may be one of the most sensitive indices of changing requirements for maintenance doses of corticosteroids.

Other pigmentary changes are also observed. An early and sometimes prominent change is darkening of pigmented nevi and the appearance of lentigo-like lesions. Vitiligo is associated with primary adrenal failure in as many as 15 percent of cases and may

precede clinical manifestations of adrenal cortical insufficiency. Some studies have suggested that vitiligo associated with Addison's disease is limited to patients with multiglandular deficiency syndromes,[42] as is the association with mucocutaneous candidiasis.

One of the more unusual variants of hyperpigmentation due to pituitary stimulation occurs after bilateral adrenalectomy for adrenal hyperplasia. This syndrome (Nelson's syndrome, Fig. 169-6) is characterized by intense hyperpigmentation as well as amenorrhea and signs of an expanding pituitary lesion (see also Chap. 80).[43] The pituitary adenomas in this condition produce extremely high levels of ACTH/MSH. Because the neoplasms are not usually observed prior to adrenalectomy, some theories ascribe their development to loss of feedback to the pituitary that follows the loss of glucocorticoids after adrenalectomy.

Sex Hormones

Effect of Sex Hormones on the Skin

Androgenic hormones have trophic actions on the skin as a whole, but certain parts of the skin such as sexual zones are particularly sensitive. Moreover, hair follicles and sebaceous glands appear to be particularly responsive. Under the influence of androgenic hormones, mitotic activity, cell turnover time, and thickness of epidermis are increased. Growth of sebaceous glands is enhanced, and measurements of sebum production are sensitive indices of androgenicity.[44] Hair growth is markedly affected by androgens, as is detailed in Chap. 61. Pigmentation is increased by androgens not only in sexual skin but generally. This effect appears to be due, at least in part, to direct effects on the synthesis of melanin[45] and on packaging of melanosomes.[46] Androgens also cause thickening of the dermis with increase in skin collagen content.[47]

The nature of the effects appears to be identical for all androgenic hormones, irrespective of their source (adrenal or gonadal). Of circulating hormones, testosterone is the most potent. However, other androgens have trophic effects on cutaneous structures and may be quantitatively more important, either because they are more abundant in the circulation (as may be the case for adrenal androgens in women) or because of target tissue sensitivity.

A detailed review of the mechanism of action of androgens and other steroid hormones is beyond the scope of this chapter. Briefly, testosterone and other sex steroids circulate in association with transport proteins (sex hormone–binding globulin) and enter the cell in free form. Within cells, testosterone may be converted into dihydrotestosterone (DHT) by 5α-reductase. Conversions of other androgens by reductases, dehydrogenases, and isomerases produce intermediates that may be converted to DHT. For cutaneous structures, androgen responsiveness appears to depend more upon the availability of DHT rather than testosterone itself.

DHT and other active androgenic steroids are bound to specific high-affinity receptor proteins in the cytosol and translocated into the nucleus. The receptor-hormone complex bound to nuclear proteins initiates protein synthesis and sets the anabolic machinery into motion. Thus anabolic effects of androgenic hormones are determined by conversion to DHT, specificity and prevalence of receptors, and nuclear binding sites. As the skin itself is an important site for metabolism of sex steroids, adrenal and ovarian androgens, such as androstenedione and dehydroepiandrosterone, may be a more important source of androgenic stimulation in the female than

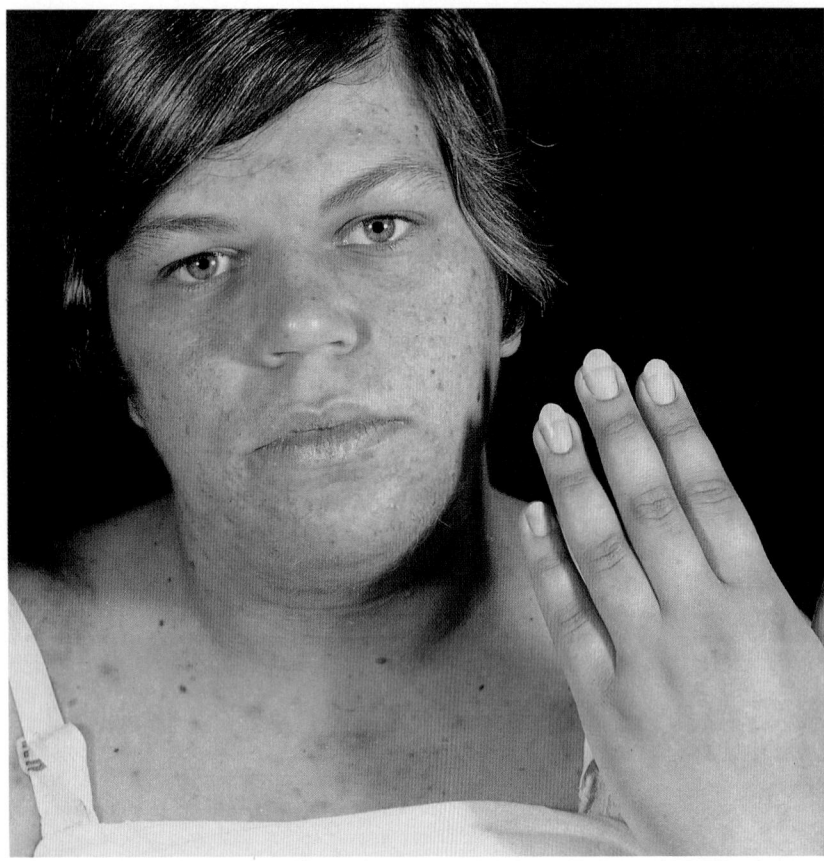

FIGURE 169-6 Pituitary adenema with Nelson's syndrome. This patient is a skin phototype II who became markedly hyperpigmented as the result of a functioning tumor of the pituitary. The patient had a chromophobe adenoma that excreted large amounts of ACTH and associated peptides.

the limited amounts of circulating testosterone.[48] A considerable body of evidence suggests that there are marked differences in the sensitivity of various portions of the skin to androgenic stimulation. These differences may reside in differences in the activity and distribution of androgen-metabolizing enzymes, such as hydroxy steroid dehydrogenases and isomerases as well as α-reductases,[49] and in intracellular androgen-binding proteins.[50]

Studies in animals have suggested that anterior pituitary hormones may facilitate the effects of testosterone. Although the mechanisms remain controversial, such studies have shown that pituitary hormones facilitate the uptake and/or conversion of testosterone to DHT.[40,51]

Estrogens likewise have significant effects on skin, mainly in the sexual zones. They may accelerate the rate of maturation of epidermal cells[52] even as they induce cornification of vaginal mucosa. It has been demonstrated that there are increases in both mitotic division and thickness of the epidermis in estrogen-treated women after castration[53] and alterations in collagen formation in the skin.[54,55]

For the most part, however, the effect of estrogens on skin under physiologic conditions remains poorly defined. The suppression of sebaceous glands by pharmacologic amounts of estrogen is a well-known phenomenon that can be only partially explained by suppression of the pituitary-ovarian axis and reduced production of ovarian androgen. Some direct effect on the target tissue must be invoked to explain the increased response of sebaceous glands to dosages of estrogen in excess of those required for suppression of ovarian function. Presence of high-affinity estrogen receptors in the skin suggests a role for direct effects of these hormones.

Cutaneous Manifestations of Diseases Characterized by Too Much Sex Hormone

Too Much Androgen The clinical manifestations of androgen excess are recognized as virilization when they occur in the adult female and as precocious puberty when present in preadolescent children. Although cutaneous changes are similar for various endocrine disorders in which virilization occurs, diagnostic differentiation can be made on the basis of additional features.

In virilizing syndromes, the skin becomes thickened and coarse. Pores on the face enlarge, and there is excessive oiliness. Typical acne vulgaris may develop. In children, the straight hairline is molded to conform to the adult configuration (calvities frontalis adolescentium); androgenetic alopecia may develop (see Chap. 61). Growth of body hair is accelerated so that coarse hair appears on the extremities, on the anterior chest, and in the beard area. Pubic and axillary hair develops in children. The genitalia show masculinization; the clitoris enlarges in women, and in prepubertal males there is penile hypertrophy and increasing folding of the scrotal skin. If virilization occurs during fetal life in females, pseudohermaphroditism may result. Hyperpigmentation of the perineum, external genitalia, axillae, aureolae, and nipples is present.

The skin changes are accompanied by effects on musculature and distribution of body fat characteristic of the male. In children, excess androgens initially accelerate growth of the long bones but also cause premature closure of the epiphyses, resulting in short stature.

The adrenogenital syndrome is one of the more common of the hereditary disorders characterized by virilization. The biochemical lesion is a defect in the synthesis of glucocorticoids and mineralo-corticoids, most commonly due to defective hydroxylation of carbon-21 or -11 of the steroid nucleus. Pituitary secretion of ACTH is then not restrained by negative feedback because of the relative absence of hydroxylated steroids. As a result the adrenal cortex is driven to secrete increased amounts of androgenic steroids. The resulting disorder is a combination of adrenal glucocorticoid and mineralocorticoid deficiency in the face of virilization. Moreover, the increased availability of ACTH may effect generalized hyperpigmentation (as in Addison's disease). Partial deficiencies of 3β-hydroxylase steroid dehydrogenase, as well as 11- or 21-hydroxylases, have also been recognized to underlie hirsutism and recalcitrant acne in postadolescent women.[56] A number of syndromes have been described in which hirsutism, androgenetic alopecia, and acne occur and for which the pathogenesis is not clearly established (see Chap. 63). Elevated levels of free testosterone, dehydroepiandrosterone, and urinary ketosteroids may be present even without polycystic ovaries in such patients. Such rather milder signs of hyperandrogenization should provoke an investigation of androgenic hormone levels.

Too Much Estrogen   Excess estrogens may result from estrogen-producing tumors of the ovary or testes or rarely from hypothalamic disorders. It results in precocious puberty in the female. In males, gynecomastia may be the only manifestation. However, testicular atrophy may follow, with diminished androgen-dependent functions.

The widespread use of oral contraceptive agents containing combinations of synthetic estrogens and progestins has introduced a spectrum of cutaneous changes due to prolonged exposure to sex hormones.[57] Many of these are similar to the cutaneous changes encountered in pregnancy (see Chap. 168). Vaginal candidiasis is common, 5 percent of patients develop melasma, and hair loss during or after withdrawal of these drugs may occur. Telangiectasia, spider angioma, and palmar erythema may appear. Some agents ameliorate acne whereas others make it worse, depending on the androgenicity of the progestin and the quantity of estrogen. Other cutaneous disorders are occasionally precipitated or worsened by oral contraceptive agents; these include erythema nodosum, porphyria cutanea tarda, herpes gestationis, and systemic lupus erythematosus.

Cutaneous Manifestations of Too Little Sex Hormone

Absolute or relative lack of sex hormone may result from (1) congenital disorders in which gonads fail to develop; (2) end organ unresponsiveness in the target tissue due to defects in metabolism or receptors of sex hormones; (3) destruction of gonads by disease or castration; (4) suppression of gonadal function by hormone administration; or (5) pituitary disturbance resulting in lack of gonadotrophic hormones.

It should be noted, however, that while gonadal testosterone is the prime source of androgens in the male, adrenal androgens may provide some androgenicity for the skin in the male and a major source for androgens in females. Skin changes due to lack of gonadal hormones are therefore not as complete as they might be if there were only a single source for androgenization. Moreover, peripheral metabolism of steroid hormones may provide some minimal sources in the absence of gonadal function.

The skin changes that result from lack of androgens depend in large measure upon the age and sex of the patients. If males are deprived of testosterone before puberty, the fully developed picture of eunuchoidism or infantilism results; the skin remains thin and fine, and sebaceous glands, apocrine glands, and sexual hair remain dormant. Facial pores are small, and there is neither oiliness nor acne. As time goes on, the skin around the eyes and lips develops the fine wrinkling characteristic of aging. The hairline remains straight over the forehead and low over the temples. Beard, axillary, and pubic hair do not develop and neither does androgenetic alopecia. Pallor of the skin is an outstanding feature. There is not only less pigment in sexual zones but generally. Reduced cutaneous blood flow may contribute to the pallor.

The penis remains small, and scrotal skin does not develop deep furrows. Delayed somatic maturation is evident in poor muscular development and and excessive subcutaneous fat in the pectoral and girdle regions. Delayed closure of the epiphyses results in prolonged growth of the long bones so that normal height may be achieved by virtue of disproportionate length of the extremities.

The picture is modified if hypoandrogenicity develops after puberty. Although initiation of growth of body hair and beard requires androgens, maintenance of some growth usually persists. Thus in the postpubertal male castrate, axillary and pubic hair usually remains although it may be sparse and slow growing. Terminal hair on the body and beard shows even less change. Regular shaving of the beard may still be necessary but at longer intervals.

Because sebaceous glands require constant androgenization, sebum secretion is markedly reduced. Although the texture of the skin is less coarse and may be finely wrinkled, it does not revert to a prepubertal state. Replacement therapy with androgens will reverse all these changes.

Pituitary Hormones

The adenohypophysis and neurohypophysis are the source of a number of hormones, some of which regulate activity of endocrine glands: ACTH, gonadotropins, and thyrotropin (TSH). They also include somatotropin (growth hormone, GH), prolactin, MSH, and lipotropin that do not seem to stimulate endocrine glands but to act on other tissues. Peptides that are indistinguishable from their pituitary counterparts may be produced ectopically by solid tumors. To what extent ectopic production of pituitary-like tropic hormones may occur under other physiologic or pathologic conditions is not known; however it has recently been shown that keratinocytes produce ACTH and MSH.[58]

The implications of disordered adenohypophoseal function for the skin must be formulated in terms of direct actions mediated via target gland hormones stimulated by tropic pituitary hormones. The latter introduce multiple potentialities so that alterations of the skin in pituitary disorders usually present a composite of endocrine effects. For example, hyperandrogenicity is often seen in women with excess prolactin. The prolactin inhibits gonadotropin and may precipitate the development of polycystic ovary disease, with increased levels of adrenal androgens resulting in hirsutism and acne.

Direct effects of pituitary hormones on the skin have not been convincingly demonstrated in humans with the exception of MSH and ACTH. However, numerous studies in animals have suggested that somatotropin (GH), prolactin, and TSH, as well as ACTH and MSH may facilitate response of sebaceous glands to androgenic stimulation, suggesting that pituitary peptides have subtle effects directly on the skin.

The next two sections deal with two disorders of pituitary function that are well-defined and illustrate the complexity of composite endocrine effects on the skin, that is, too much GH (acromegaly) and too little of all anterior pituitary hormones (panhypopituitarism).

Cutaneous Manifestations of Too Much Growth Hormone: Acromegaly

Excessive GH elaboration is commonly associated with eosinophilic adenomas of the pituitary. Although elaboration of other hormones such as gonadotropins may be compromised, the preponderant changes in the skin and the rest of the body are those due to excessive amounts of GH. The cutaneous changes are most pronounced in the dermis, with a hyperplasia due to increased amounts of glycosaminoglycans[59] and an attendant retention of water. Whether collagen is also increased remains controversial.

These effects, like those on skeletal tissue, are mediated by growth factors, collectively known as *somatomedins,* which have now been identified to be the circulating insulin-like growth factor(s) (IGF). Of the two major IGF responsible for growth and insulin-like effects, IGF-1 is more responsive to stimulation by GH than IGF-2. Although circulating somatomedin is made primarily in the liver, many other tissues, such as fibroblasts, produce somatomedin-like peptides under control of GH (and other growth factors) that act via autocrine and paracrine mechanisms. It is possible that acanthosis nigricans, a frequent feature of acromegaly, may result from circulating or even locally produced IGF.

In acromegaly there is also hyperplasia of the epidermis and dermal appendages. Whether this is an effect on epidermal cells per se or secondary to alterations of the connective tissue is not yet clear. For example, in certain nonendocrine conditions characterized by similar mesenchymal hyperplasia, changes in the epidermis

and its appendages are quite analogous to those in acromegaly, for example, pachydermaperiostosis.

GH may also exert effects on pilosebaceous structures by potentiating the effectiveness of androgens. Such actions have been demonstrated in animals; data in humans are not definitive. Thus, isolated deficiency of GH in sexual ateliotic dwarfs may not be associated with significant depression of sebaceous gland activity,[44] but pilosebaceous functions are usually sustained in acromegaly even after hypogonadism develops.

Although the most striking clinical expression of acromegaly is due to effects on bone and cartilage, there are usually prominent changes in the skin (Fig. 169-7). Clinically, the effect on the integument can be described as "too much skin." The skin is thickened and has a doughy feel; this is most marked over the face and on the extremities, where skeletal changes are also most prominent. Furrowing and accentuation of folds contributes to the coarsening of the facial features. Deepening of creases on the forehead and nasolabial folds gives the patients a scowling, somber expression. In some cases, overgrowth of the dermis results in bizarre ridging of the skin of the scalp (cutis vertices gyrata). Eyelids become thick and edematous. The lower lip is enlarged and protruding and there is macroglossia. The nose becomes elongated, and the exuberant hypertrophy of soft tissue usually exceeds the cartilaginous overgrowth. Increased soft tissue in the alae nasi gives the nose an unmistakable triangular configuration. Similar changes occur on the hands and feet. Folds of skin over bony prominences on the hands are accentuated. The pads of the digits become fleshy, and fingers assume a blunted shape. The heel pads on the feet are predictably thickened. Indeed, measurement of heel pad thickness has been used to assess clinical status in acromegaly,[60] although such measurements do not always show regression in treated acromegalics. The overgrowth of fibrous tissue leads to production of small sessile or pedunculated fibromas that are found in 20 to 30 percent of patients.[61]

There is thickening of the epidermis with accentuation of markings and enlarged pores. Nails become thick and hard. Exces-

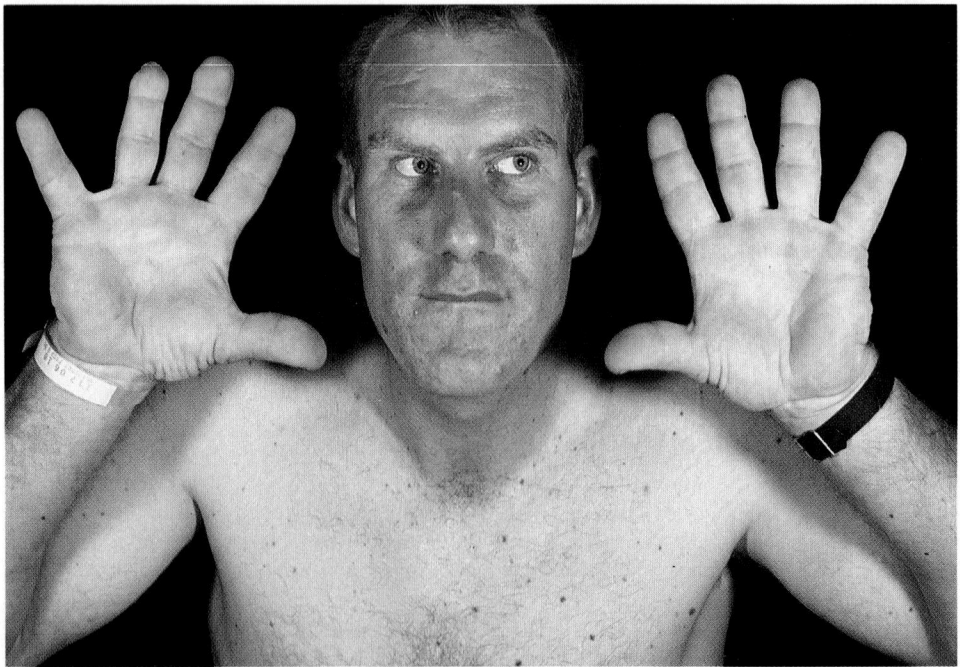

FIGURE 169-7 Acromegaly. Coarse facies with enlargement of the nose, chin, hands, and fingers.

sive eccrine and apocrine sweating occurs in the majority of patients and may be implicated in the heightened incidence of abscesses in the axillae and intergluteal cleft. Although breast tissue often becomes atrophic in women, along with other stigmata of hypogonadism, galactorrhea may occur.

Hypertrichosis occurs in about half of the patients. However, it differs from that in virilizing syndromes in that it does not affect the beard area. The skin is said to be oily, but acne is not a common feature.

Hyperpigmentation has been observed in about 40 percent of patients. The increase in color is generalized but not marked.

As activity of the disease diminishes, skin changes become stationary and may even regress. Occasionally in the late stages of the disease a predominating hypogonadism may contribute to regression of changes, especially in hair growth.

Acanthosis nigricans is associated with acromegaly in at least 10 percent of patients.[62]

Effects of Too Little of All Pituitary Hormones: Panhypopituitarism

A variety of conditions may compromise the anterior pituitary and thereby the elaboration of all pituitary hormones. Acute infarction may occur as in postpartum hemorrhage (Sheehan's syndrome). Slower failure may be due to destruction of the gland by chronic infection (syphilis and tuberculosis), granulomatous inflammation (sarcoid), neoplastic invasion (histiocytosis X, metastatic cancer), or by tumors arising within the pituitary (chromophobe adenomas) or contiguous structures (craniopharyngioma).

The alterations of the skin in panhypopituitarism depend on how much pituitary tissue has been destroyed and the effects of integrated deprivation of those hormones that have been considered singly in earlier portions of the chapter. Individual hormonal deficits may not be as pronounced as in primary failure of the target glands as some autonomous function of target glands may persist in the absence of tropic stimulation. Moreover, the effects of the lack of one hormone may be modified by the lack of others. For example, although the patient with panhypopituitarism may have severe hypothyroidism, myxedema is often mild. This may be due to the lack of other hormones that stimulate synthesis of mucopolysaccharides.

Pallor of the skin with a yellowish tinge is a prominent feature. Melanin content is apparently diminished, especially in the sexual areas. There may be increased sensitivity to sunlight and less pigmentation of traumatized and inflamed skin. Lack of the normal pink color of the cheeks, earlobes, and palms contributes to the pallor, but mucous membranes retain their normal hue unless the patient is anemic. The texture of the skin is dry but smoother and softer than in primary hypothyroidism. The face may be puffy. The facies tend to be less expressive because of a diminution in skin folds. Thinness of the skin and subcutaneous tissues results in fine wrinkling around the eyes and mouth making the patient look older.

Loss of body hair occurs in all patients early in the course. Axillary hair is affected first, and a reduced need for axillary shaving may be an initial symptom. Pubic hair loss takes longer to develop and is less consistent. Beard growth slows but is not altogether lost in adult males. Scalp hair tends to be fine and dry and there may be generalized thinning. Sebaceous secretions and sweating also decrease.

Diabetes Mellitus

Diabetes mellitus is a metabolic disorder characterized by disturbances in traffic of fuels, primarily as affected by insulin. The abnormalities arise from heterogeneous mechanisms that fall into two major groups: insulin-dependent diabetes mellitus (IDDM), also known as type 1, and non-insulin-dependent diabetes mellitus (NIDDM), also known as type 2. IDDM, which frequently but not always begins in younger life, is characterized by absolute deficiency in pancreatic and circulating insulin. Patients commonly (60 to 90 percent) have circulating antibodies to pancreatic islet cells and distinctive patterns of major histocompatibility antigens. NIDDM occurs in older populations, is often linked to obesity, and frequently has a hereditary pattern. Pancreatic and circulating insulin are not lacking but are insufficient to meet the needs of peripheral tissues.

Disposition of ingested nutrients and recall of endogenous fuels are faulty in all types of diabetes. The common denominator is insufficient action of insulin on peripheral tissues. Whereas this is due to lack of pancreatic insulin in IDDM, in NIDDM the problem is one of relative insufficiency despite the presence of insulin stores in the pancreas and even high levels of circulating insulin. Sluggish release of insulin from the pancreas in response to glucose challenge, peripheral resistance to insulin action at the level of tissue receptors,[63,64] and abnormal insulin[65] are among the pathogenic mechanisms operative in NIDDM.

The acute derangements resulting in hyperglycemia, hyperlipidemia, symptomatic diabetes, and ketoacidosis are usually correctable by appropriate therapy. However, all forms of diabetes are associated in the long term with multiple degenerative disorders affecting the cardiovascular system, nervous system, eyes, and skin. Effects on large and small blood vessels (macro- and microangiopathy) are the cardinal pathologic factors, although direct effects of the metabolic derangements on certain tissues may play a significant role. It is generally accepted that the changes are all due to chronic metabolic derangements that are not entirely regulated by available hypoglycemic strategies. Although there is some evidence that prolonged "tight" control may lessen degenerative complications or even induce regression of vascular changes (e.g., thickened capillary basement membranes[66,67]), definitive studies are not yet available, and practical long-term therapeutic regimens have not been developed to meet such ends.

The skin shares both in the effects of acute metabolic derangements and in the chronic degenerative complications of diabetes. This is not surprising as the skin is an actively metabolizing tissue depending on insulin and circulating fuels for metabolic and biosynthetic activity.

Insulin affects the utilization of glucose in skin,[68] even though it is not required to facilitate the entry of glucose into epidermal cells.[69] Increase in apparent intracellular content of glucose in diabetic skin suggests that insulin regulates glucose disposition in cutaneous cells.[70]

Insulin profoundly affects various cutaneous compartments. It is required for growth and differentiation of keratinocytes in culture systems. Healing of experimental wounds, which involves both dermis and epidermis, is delayed in diabetic animals until they are treated with insulin. However, the most pronounced effects of insulin may be on the dermal fibroblasts. In experimental diabetes there is less soluble dermal collagen and it is more cross-linked.[71] These changes parallel the findings in dermal collagen of diabetics, which shows a decrease in acid-soluble collagen and more glycosylation than in age-matched controls.[72] Dermal fibroblasts from diabetic mice produce more fibronectin than do control cells.[73]

Consideration of the cutaneous manifestations of diabetes may be divided into those that accompany acute metabolic derangements and those that correlate with the presence of chronic degenerative complications. In addition, there are dermatologic disorders that occur more frequently in diabetics but that do not correlate with either acute metabolic derangements or degenerative changes.

Cutaneous Manifestations Correlated with Gross Metabolic Derangements

Certain cutaneous disorders occur in diabetic patients specifically in relation to hyperglycemia and hyperlipidemia and are reversible when these abnormalities are corrected.

Infections   Poorly controlled diabetes may be associated with bacterial and fungal infections of the skin. The infections most frequently encountered are staphylococcal pyodermas, candidiasis, erythrasma, and epidermophytosis. Although the prevalence of the latter two appears to be increased in diabetics, such a correlation has not been established for staphylococcal and candidal infections. Moreover, it is not clear whether the diabetic host is more susceptible to infection or less able to deal with it once the infection is established.

Abnormalities in leukocyte function, including diminished chemotaxis, phagocytosis, and killing of organisms, have been demonstrated in diabetics who are hyperglycemic.[74] These effects may be due in part to the hyperosmolality of hyperglycemic serum.[75] Such effects may also include the consequences of insulin lack on insulin-dependent action of cytokines such as interleukins.[76] The diminished leukocyte response may also be due to the inability of leukocytes to migrate through thickened capillary walls as well as to the diminished diffusion of nutrients to sustain extravascular inflammatory cells. Furthermore, repair of minor trauma may be affected both by delayed wound healing and compromised dermal vasculature, thereby providing access for pathogenic organisms.

Vulvovaginitis due to *Candida albicans* is a common complication of poorly controlled diabetes. Involvement of other intertriginous skin and nails is frequently seen together with the vaginal infection. The candidiasis responds readily to control of hyperglycemia and does not occur more frequently in aglycosuric diabetics than in the normal population. Although generalized pruritus is not a feature of diabetes,[77] vulvar itching with candidiasis should alert the clinician to the possible presence of diabetes unless other obvious precipitating causes can be invoked.

Pyodermas, especially furunculosis, were formerly a more serious complication of diabetes. The availability of antibiotics and better control of diabetes has lessened both the morbidity and incidence of septic skin infections in the diabetic population. Nonetheless, pyogenic infections do occur more frequently in poorly controlled patients; conversely, control of well-regulated diabetes can be interrupted by intercurrent pyogenic infection.

Infections of the lower extremities constitute a particular hazard for the diabetic patient. The presence of atherosclerosis and peripheral neuropathy leads to ulceration and gangrene as well as poor wound healing. The damaged and devitalized skin provides a fertile breeding ground for secondary infections. Moreover, the

increased incidence of epidermophytosis of the feet provides portals of entry for pathogenic organisms.

Prevention of such infections requires meticulous care of the feet. Such care should be incorporated into every diabetic regimen and includes the regular services of a podiatrist and twice-daily foot washing with tepid water followed by thorough drying and use of emollients. Prompt attention to foot wounds, blisters, minor infections, and epidermophytosis is indicated.

Xanthomatosis (See also Chap. 152)   Hyperlipidemia involving triglycerides and cholesterol more than phospholipids is common in diabetics, even in those with rather mild elevations of blood glucose. Xanthomas, secondary to the chylomicronemia, are characteristically multiple and tend to occur rapidly in crops. Small reddish-yellow nodules up to 0.5 cm in diameter present in clusters primarily on extensor surfaces and buttocks. They may be pruritic initially and are much smaller and more inflammatory than the tendon and tuberous xanthomas associated with hypercholesterolemia. They are clinically indistinguishable from xanthomas secondary to other states associated with chylomicronemia.

The lesions are laden with neutral lipid-rich histiocytes. Ultrastructural studies have demonstrated that chylomicrons migrate through the dermal capillary walls and are phagocytosed by tissue macrophages and perithelial cells. In freshly erupted xanthomas, the lipid composition of the lesion reflects that of plasma chylomicrons, containing about 45 percent triglycerides. Resolving or evolving lesions gradually lose triglycerides and become relatively richer in cholesterol.[78] Rapid regression occurs when diabetes is brought under control.

Xanthelasma occurs in most hyperlipidemic states, including diabetes, but may occur without demonstrable abnormality of plasma lipids; it does not usually regress when therapy for diabetes is instituted. Hyperlipidemia is sometimes accompanied by yellowish discoloration of the palms, soles, and nasolabial folds due to deposition of carotene.

Cutaneous Manifestations of Diabetes Correlated with Chronic Degenerative Complications

It is now generally accepted that microangiopathy characteristic of diabetes occurs in the dermal vasculature as well as in other small blood vessels and may result in decreased cutaneous blood flow. Reduplication and thickening of basement membranes have been shown in diabetic skin.[79] Veil cells are seen more frequently surrounding cutaneous vessels.[80] It has been postulated that these cells produce excessive amounts of basement membrane-like material accounting for vascular thickening. In addition to changes in blood vessels, there are changes in dermal connective tissue and in cutaneous innervation. Thus, the cutaneous manifestations that appear to correlate with multisystem degenerative complications are probably attributable to biochemical and anatomic disturbances within the skin itself.

Diabetic Dermopathy   These lesions were first described as atrophic circumscribed brownish lesions of the lower extremities.[81] The presence of small blood vessel changes led to the term *diabetic dermopathy*,[82] although the pathogenic significance of vascular changes in relation to the lesions remains to be established. The lesions are asymptomatic, irregularly shaped patches occurring primarily over the anterior lower legs; their surfaces are depressed and they have a light brown color (Fig. 169-8). Lesions appear in crops

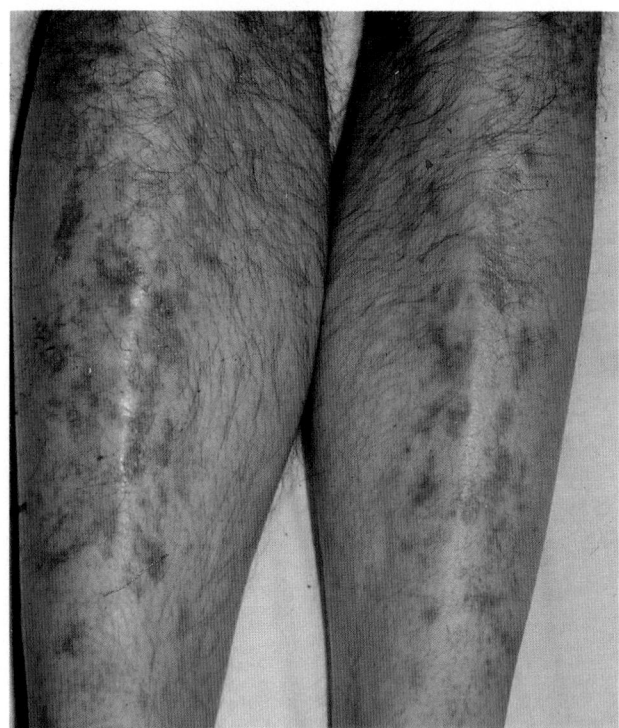

FIGURE 169-8   Diabetes mellitus with diabetic dermopathy. Hyperpigmented scars are seen on the anterior lower leg at sites of trauma. The absence of hair on the lower legs is associated with peripheral vascular disease.

and gradually resolve over 12 to 18 months; however, the constant appearance of new lesions gives the impression of a stationary course. Although the initial report[81] did not note antecedent cutaneous changes, other authors[82–84] have noted the presence of red patches, sometimes with scaling and erosion, prior to the development of the pigmented atrophic patches. Despite their resemblance to scars, recall of antecedent trauma is seldom elicited.

Histologically, dermal arterioles and capillaries display intimal thickening and deposition of PAS-positive fibrillar material in vessel walls. Capillary basement membranes are thickened with focal deposition of PAS-positive material. Hemosiderin and extravasated red cells are often present, and accumulation of leukocytes around vessels has been described.

Although these lesions are not clinically distinguishable from posttraumatic scarring on the legs of older patients with compromised circulation, they appear more frequently and in greater numbers in diabetics. They are more common in men than women (2:1) and are often accompanied by evidence of significant microangiopathy elsewhere.

Erythema and Necrosis   Reddening of the face (rubeosis faciei) and of the extremities has been described in long-standing diabetes. Erysipelas-like areas on the lower legs and feet, which may or may not eventuate in frank necrosis, and destructive lesions of underlying bone have also been described.[85] These painless areas are often edematous and do not differ clinically from the erythema that accompanies gangrene of the toes and feet due to arterial insufficiency. Cardiac failure, unilateral edema from venous occlusion, and arterial insufficiency have been cited as precipitating factors.

Bullous Lesions   Although the appearance of bullae in diabetics was noted earlier, the first carefully studied series of 15 patients was presented in 1963.[86] In this and subsequent reports, the bullae appeared spontaneously, usually on the extremities, especially the feet (Fig. 169-9). Generally the bullae heal in several weeks without significant scarring, although they may recur. The bullae are subepidermal, and ultrastructural studies have demonstrated the plane of separation to be in the basement membrane zone above the basal lamina.[87] In some cases distribution of the lesions in light-exposed areas suggests porphyria cutanea tarda, but abnormalities of porphyrin metabolism have not been found. Neither trauma nor immunologic mechanisms have been implicated.

The cause of this rare manifestation of diabetes is unknown. At least 75 percent of patients have significant diabetic retinopathy, and in one series of three patients dermopathy and cutaneous angiopathy were present.[83] The localization of the plane of separation suggests that weakness in the basement membrane zone is an underlying factor. That this may be the case is suggested by reports of a reduced threshold to formation of suction blisters on the forearms of insulin-dependent diabetics.[88]

Thickened Skin, Stiff Joints, and Scleredema Adultorum   As many as one-third of diabetics (both IDDM and NIDDM) have tight, thickened, and waxy skin over the dorsa of the hands.[89] An associated change is the presence of multiple, minute, flesh-colored papules (pebbles) on the dorsum of the fingers, knuckle pads, and periungual areas.[90] A possibly related connective tissue change is limited mobility of joints, especially of the proximal interphalangeal joints of patients with IDDM.[91] The contractures can be demonstrated by an inability to approximate the palmar surfaces of the fingers when the palms are pressed together.[92] The changes are strongly correlated with an increased risk for microangiopathy.

Scleredema adultorum, a well-defined entity (see Chap. 177), has only been recognized as a cutaneous manifestation of diabetes in the past few decades. It consists of induration of the skin beginning on the posterior and lateral neck. The painless swelling may gradually spread to the face, shoulders, anterior neck, and upper torso; it may eventually involve the abdomen, arms, and hands. The hard skin does not pit on pressure. Demarcation from normal skin may be sharp or poorly defined.

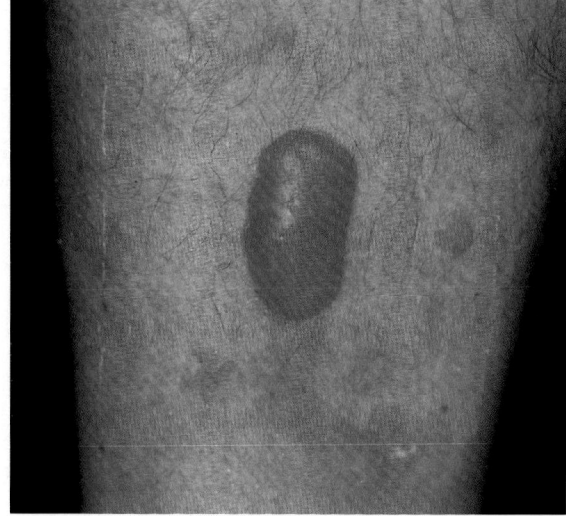

FIGURE 169-9   Diabetes mellitus with bullous dermatosis. Two intact bullae are seen on the anterior lower leg.

Histologically there are thickened collagen bundles and deposition of glycosaminoglycans, chiefly hyaluronic acid in the dermis.

In contrast to the identical changes occurring after infection (especially streptococcal), scleredema associated with diabetes may not remit even after long periods of time. Diabetic scleredema occurs mainly in obese diabetics with evidence of vascular complications.[93,94]

Although the underlying mechanisms for these various connective tissue abnormalities remain to be elucidated, it may be postulated that they represent the clinical manifestations of altered metabolism of collagen and mucopolysaccharide due to insulin deprivation.

Cutaneous Neuropathy   Autonomic disturbances may accompany the sensory neuropathy that is a common degenerative complication (Fig. 169-10). This may manifest as anhydrosis, either confined to extremities or generalized.[95] Involved areas of skin show abnormalities in autonomic fibers adjacent to eccrine sweat glands.[96]

Cutaneous Disorders That Are More Common in Diabetes Without Regard to Metabolic Derangements or Degenerative Changes

Certain skin disorders are more frequently associated with diabetes. Although the literature abounds with reports of well-defined cutaneous diseases occurring more frequently in diabetics, only a few of these associations have withstood careful scrutiny.

Necrobiosis Lipoidica Diabeticorum   This very distinctive skin disease is perhaps the best example of such an association, occurring in about 0.3 percent of diabetics. These relatively asymptomatic lesions, which are three times more common in women than in men, are characteristically found on the anterior and lateral surfaces of the lower legs. They may also be present on the face, arms, and trunk. There may be one or several lesions, either unilaterally or bilaterally. The lesion begins as a small, dusky-red elevated nodule with a sharply circumscribed border. It slowly enlarges, becoming a plaque irregular in outline, flattened, and eventually depressed as the dermis becomes more atrophic (Fig. 169-11). The color becomes more brownish yellow except for the border, which may remain red. Coalescing or enlarging lesions may in time encompass the entire anterior tibial area. The epidermis is smooth or slightly scaly and atrophic. Delicate vessels can be seen through the surface (Fig. 169-11). The lesions may be anesthetic due to destruction of cutaneous nerves.[97] The lesions of necrobiosis lipoidica diabeticorum (NLD) are extremely chronic and indolent; shallow, often painful ulcers frequently appear in long-standing lesions. In the early stages, NLD may resemble granuloma annulare or sarcoid (Fig. 169-11), but the well-developed plaque is characteristic and easily recognized.

The primary pathologic changes are in the lower dermis, where collagen is markedly altered with focal areas of loss of normal structure, swelling, basophilia, and distortion of the bundles (necrobiosis). Cross-striations and diameters of collagen fibers are irregular. Although the amount of collagen is actually decreased, the relative proportions of types I and III are preserved. Fibroblasts cultured from lesional skin have been reported to make less collagen.[98] There is also loss and fragmentation of elastic fibers.

In these areas, there are aggregations of inflammatory cells including epithelioid cells, histiocytes, and multinucleated giant

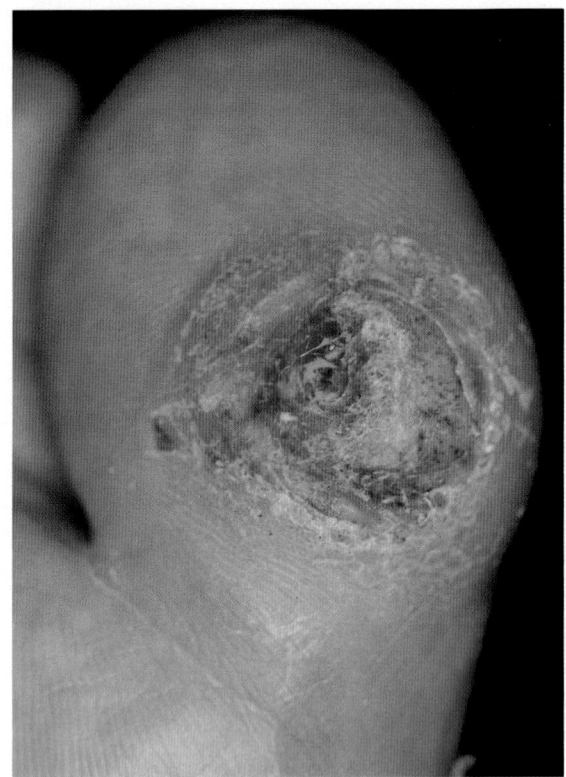

FIGURE 169-10   Diabetes mellitus with neuropathy and neuropathic ulcer. A large ulcer is present on the plantar aspect of the great toe, surrounded by a ring of callus and associated with diminished sensation. Osteomyelitis of the underlying bone is common.

cells, sometimes containing asteroid bodies. The late appearance of foam cells accounts for the designation *lipoidica*. The vasculature is always involved, with endothelial proliferation and occlusion of the lumina of arterioles and venules. Capillary walls are thickened with focal deposits of PAS-positive material that may also be present in the lumen.

The precise correlation between NLD and diabetes remains somewhat controversial. The disease was first described in patients with well-established diabetes but subsequently reported in patients without evident diabetes. In a study of 171 patients,[99] the majority had diabetes when NLD developed; in most of the rest diabetes developed later, or there were other stigmata such as a close relative with the disease or abnormal cortisone-glucose tolerance tests. Only about 10 percent of patients with NLD do not fall into any of these categories. The induction of abnormal carbohydrate tolerance with glucocorticoids has been demonstrated in the majority of patients with NLD and without evident diabetes.[100] Although NLD has not usually been linked to degenerative complications, a more recent study of a small number of patients suggests a greater prevalence of IDDM, limited joint mobility, and microvascular disease than had previously been reported.[98]

Thus, despite the lack of full concordance, NLD seems to be a valid marker for diabetes. However, the nature of the association and the pathogenesis remain unclear. Because NLD occurs in both IDDM and NIDDM, its pathogenesis cannot be related to genetic factors, underlying autoimmune disease, or other causes of diabetes. It can be reasonably assumed that the granulomatous response is secondary to alterations in dermal collagen. The controversy

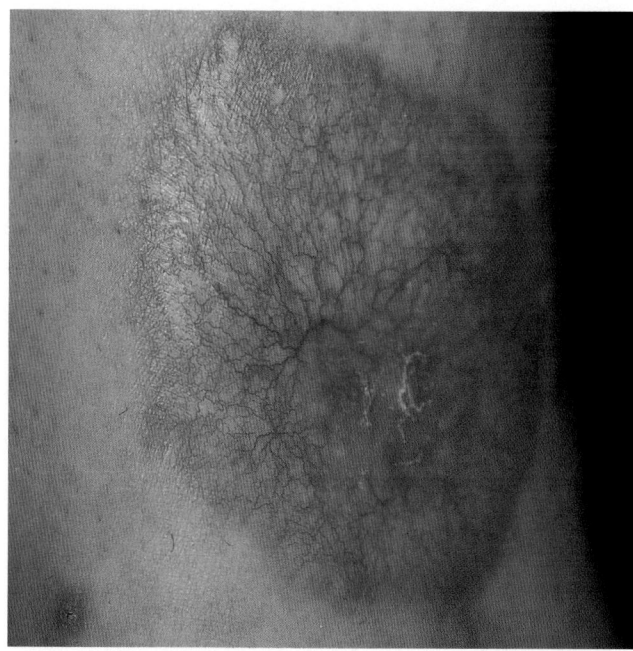

a

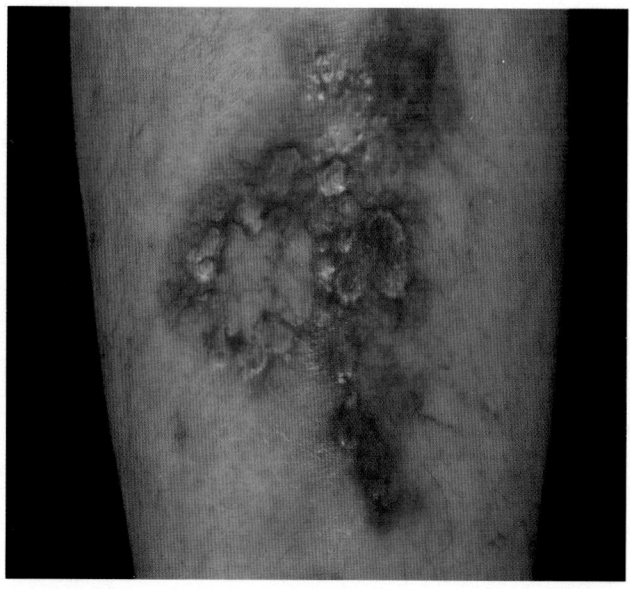

c

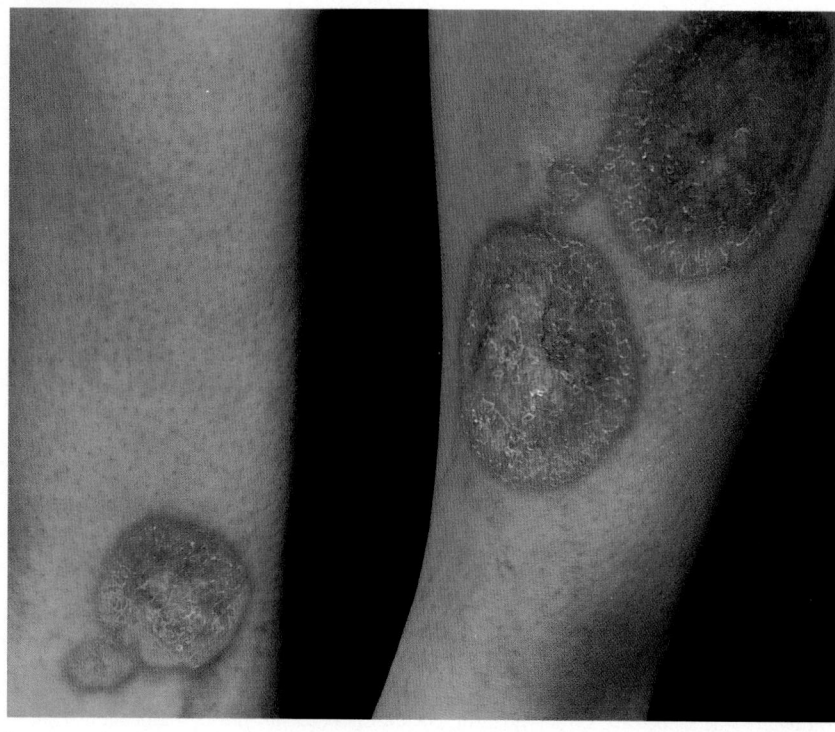

b

FIGURE 169-11 Diabetes mellitus with necrobiosis lipoidica diabeticorum (NLD). (*a*) A single orange plaque with atrophy of the overlying epidermis and arborizing telangiectasis is seen on the lower leg of a juvenile diabetic; the crust marks the spot of early ulceration. (*b*) Older lesions with striking central atrophy involving both the epidermis and dermis. (*c*) NLD of longstanding with sharply demarcated atrophic areas, sites of healed ulcerations. (*Courtesy of Klaus Wolff, M.D.*)

concerns the nature of the degenerative change in collagen. It is not clear whether this is secondary to an underlying vascular disease or develops independently. The latter would ascribe the changes in dermal collagen and vasculature to some primary disorder of connective tissue (as yet unknown). On the other hand, the invariable presence of arteriolar changes deep into and within the areas of collagen degeneration suggests an interrelation between the two components of NLD. It has been hypothesized that increased platelet aggregation may be a trigger factor in the vascular changes.

Immunoglobulins, complement (C3 and C4), and fibrinogen are present in blood vessels in lesional and, in some cases, non-

lesional skin.[101,102] These findings are in concordance with the presence of inflammatory changes in adjacent clinically normal skin.[103] Whether or not an immune process is a factor in the pathogenesis of NLD has not been resolved.

Treatment of NLD is not very satisfactory. Progression of lesions does not correlate with normalization of hyperglycemia. Local therapy with topical applications of steroids under occlusion or by intralesional injection may afford some improvement of active lesions. There have been some enthusiastic reports on the use of aspirin and dipyrimidole, but these have not been confirmed in a rigorous double-blind trial.[104] In rebuttal it has been pointed out that the dose of aspirin is a critical factor in achieving an optimal effect on platelet aggregation, and that favorable effects were obtained with very small doses of aspirin: 3.5 mg/kg every 48 to 72 h.[105] Among other agents that have been reported to be helpful are clofazimine[106] and nicotinamide.[107]

Granuloma Annulare (See Chap. 95)   Similarity between the pathologic changes of NLD and granuloma annulare and sporadic reports of diabetes in patients with granuloma annulare has led to a search for the presence of an abnormal carbohydrate metabolism in the latter disease. Although there is little evidence to support association of overt diabetes with granuloma annulare, abnormal carbohydrate metabolism after cortisone administration has been reported by some authors. Others have failed to confirm such findings in patients with typical disease[108] or have not convincingly confirmed such an association in patients with generalized or atypical granuloma annulare.[109]

Vitiligo (See Chap. 80)   Vitiligo occurs with greater than expected incidence (4.8 percent) in patients with NIDDM.[110] It may precede the onset of clinically evident diabetes. Vitiligo has also been reported in association with IDDM; in one series, four out of five children also had autoantibodies to adrenal, thyroid, or gastric parietal cells.[111] Such autoantibodies have not been reported in patients with NIDDM and vitiligo in the absence of other endocrine disease. The association of the pigment disorder and diabetes per se thus requires further clarification.

Acanthosis Nigricans (See also Chaps. 164, 183)   This disorder is characterized by velvety papillomatous hyperplasia of the epidermis with intense hyperpigmentation most prominently displayed in axillary, inguinal, and inframammary folds and increases of the neck (Fig. 169-12). In more severe forms it may be more generalized and accompanied by verrucous patches on knuckles and other extensor surfaces, hyperkeratosis of the palms and soles, and other hyperplastic lesions. Acanthosis nigricans is associated with two types of disorders. The severer form is usually found in patients with advanced malignant disease (Chap. 183). The more limited form is more frequently found in association with a variety of endocrinopathies,[62,112] including acromegaly, Cushing's syndrome, polycystic ovary disease (Fig. 169-12), and diabetes. Mild forms also occur in obesity without evident endocrine disorder.

It appears likely that a common pathogenetic mechanism accounts for acanthosis nigricans linked to endocrinopathy. Studies of patients with a variety of endocrine diseases and acanthosis nigricans suggest that insulin resistance is a common denominator even in the absence of overt diabetes. It was first shown to be associated with insulin resistance in patients with the rare syndrome of lipoatrophic diabetes.[113] Subsequently, acanthosis nigricans has been associated with all three types of insulin resistance: type A, in which insulin resistance is due to receptor defects; type B, in which insulin resistance is conferred by effects of circulating antireceptor antibodies; and type C, in which postreceptor defects inhibit insulin action.

The mechanism for pathogenesis in insulin-resistant states has been proposed to involve the action of insulin on the IGF receptor. Hyperinsulinemia, induced by insulin resistance, provides excess insulin that may then compete for IGF receptors on keratinocytes and thus stimulate growth.[114] The fact that hypercortisolism induces insulin resistance may explain acanthosis nigricans in cushingoid states and is probably relevant in other endocrinopathies.

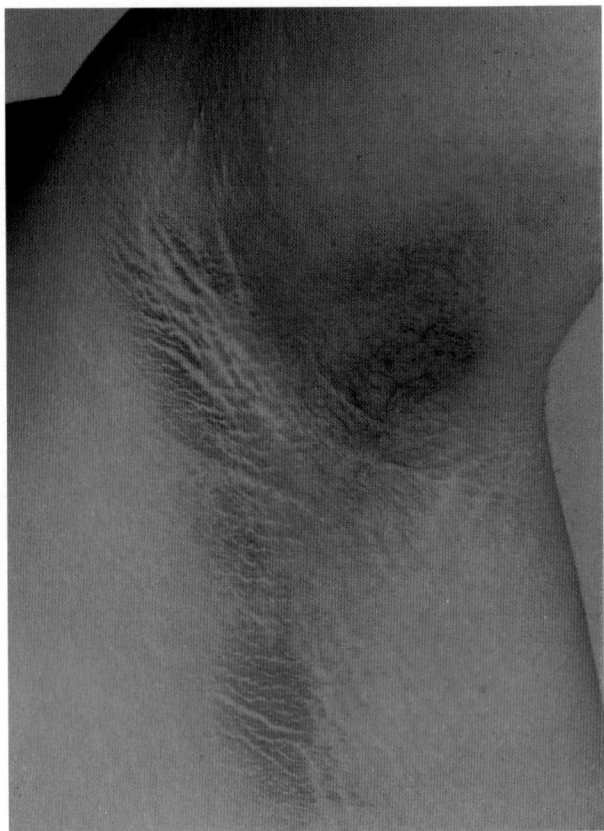

FIGURE 169-12   Diabetes mellitus with acanthosis nigricans. Velvety, papillomatous hyperplasia of the skin with hyperpigmentation is seen in the axilla of the patient with insulin-resistant diabetes mellitus. (*Courtesy of Klaus Wolff, M.D.*)

Kyrle's Disease/Reactive Perforating Collagenosis (See Chap. 48) This uncommon skin disease is characterized by hyperkeratotic follicular and perifollicular papules. The pathologic process involves transepidermal elimination of dermal material that may represent altered collagen. The perforating disease occurs in diabetics with renal failure but is also associated with renal failure without diabetes.[115,116]

Glucagonoma Syndrome (See also Chaps. 164, 183)

An unusual and striking cutaneous disease is found in patients with glucagon-secreting islet cell tumors. Although there is hyperglycemia as a consequence of excess glucagon secretion, the cutaneous findings are not a manifestation of diabetes.

The glucagonoma syndrome was first recognized as such by Mallinson et al.,[117] although there was an undiagnosed dermatitis in the first confirmed case of glucagonoma reported in 1966.[118] Although the eruption may begin as a recalcitrant nonspecific eczematous dermatitis, the typical pattern[119] consists of migrating marginated areas of erythema with blisters that heal with hyperpigmentation. The eruption waxes and wanes, involving different areas especially on the lower abdomen, buttock, perineum, and legs. A beefy red tongue, angular cheilitis, and nail dystrophy may be present.[120] The somewhat diverse clinical features may also suggest various bullous dermatoses, pustular psoriasis, or acrodermatitis enteropathica. Histologically there is necrosis and cleft formation in the upper epidermis. This picture, now known as *necrolytic migratory erythema*, is considered to be characteristic of an underlying glucagonoma.

However, the relationship of the cutaneous lesions and the tumor are still obscure. About 75 percent of the associated tumors are malignant, and widespread metastases are often present when the tumor is diagnosed.[120] Regression of the cutaneous lesions follows removal of the tumor. Somatostatin, which depresses glucagon levels, may also suppress the skin lesions.[121] Because skin lesions do not accompany many of the tumors, despite elevated levels of circulating glucagon, it is not yet clear what role the hormone plays. Possibly some other factor secreted by the tumor is responsible. In this regard a report of necrolytic migratory erythema in two patients with normal glucagon levels and without a pancreatic tumor is of interest.[122]

References

1. Ingbar SH: The thyroid gland, in *Williams' Textbook of Endocrinology*, 7th ed, edited by JD Wilson, DW Foster. Philadelphia, Saunders, 1985, p 743
2. Holt PJ: In vitro responses of epidermis to triiodothyronine. *J Invest Dermatol* 71:202, 1978
3. Smith TJ et al: The effect of thyroid hormone in glycosaminoglycans accumulation in human skin fibroblasts. *Endocrinol* 108:2397, 1981
4. Chapman RE et al: The effects of fetal thyroidectomy and thyroxin: A demonstration on the development of skin and wool follicles of sheep fetuses. *J Anat* 117:419, 1974
5. Freinkel RK: Effect of thyroxine administration on the metabolism of guinea pig skin. *J Invest Dermatol* 38:31, 1962
6. Holt PJA, Marks R: The epidermal response to change in thyroid states. *J Invest Dermatol* 68:229, 1977
7. Ebling FJ: Hormonal control and methods of measuring sebaceous secretions. *J Invest Dermatol* 62:161, 1974
8. Goolamali AK et al: Thyroid disease and sebaceous gland function. *Br Med J* 1:432, 1976
9. Barrow MV, Bird ED: Pruritus in hyperthyroidism. *Arch Dermatol* 93:237, 1966
10. Ochi Y, deGroot LJ: Vitiligo in Graves' disease. *Ann Intern Med* 71:935, 1969
11. Lynch PJ et al: Pretibial myxedema and nonthyrotoxic thyroid disease. *Arch Dermatol* 107:107, 1973
12. Wortsman J et al: Preradial myxedema in thyroid states. *Arch Dermatol* 117:635, 1981
13. Bierewaltes WH, Bollet AJ: Mucopolysaccharide content of skin in patients with pretibial myxedema. *J Clin Invest* 38:945, 1959
14. Cheung HS et al: Stimulation of fibroblast biosynthetic activity by serum of patients with pretibial myxedema. *J Invest Dermatol* 71:12, 1978
15. Freinkel RK, Freinkel N: Hair growth and alopecia in hypothyroidism. *Arch Dermatol* 106:349, 1972
16. Ingbar SH, Freinkel N: Hypothyroidism. *Dis Mon*, September, 1958
17. Dyrbe MO et al: Effect of thyroxine, thyrotrophic and somatotrophic hormones on skin of dwarf mice. *Proc Soc Exp Biol Med* 102:417, 1959
18. Wu TL et al: Skin-derived fibroblasts respond to human parathyroid hormone like adenylcyclase-stimulating protein. *J Clin Endocrinol Metab* 651:105, 1987
19. Hirano K et al: Cutaneous manifestations in idiopathic hypoparathyroidism. *Arch Dermatol* 109:242, 1975
20. Kleeman CR et al: The disappearance of intractable pruritus after parathyroidectomy in uremic patients with secondary hyperparathyroidism. *Trans Assoc Am Physicians* 81:203, 1968
21. Sutphin A et al: Five cases (three in siblings) of idiopathic hypoparathyroidism associated with moniliasis. *J Clin Endocrinol* 3:625, 1943
22. Hertz KC et al: Autoimmune vitiligo: Detection of antibodies to melanin producing cells. *N Engl J Med* 297:634, 1977
23. Blizzard RM, Gibbs JH: Candidiasis: Studies pertaining to its association with endocrinopathies and pernicious anemia. *Pediatrics* 42:231, 1968
24. Dorfman A, Schiller S: Effect of hormones on the metabolism of acid mucopolysaccharide of connective tissue. *Recent Prog Horm Res* 14:427, 1958
25. Sarnstrand B et al: Effect of glucocorticoids on glycosaminoglycans metabolism in cultured skin fibroblasts. *J Invest Dermatol* 79:412, 1982
26. Oxlund H et al: Changes in the mechanical properties, thermal stability, reducible cross-links and glycosyl-lysines in rat skin induced by corticosteroid treatment. *Acta Endocrinol* 101:312, 1982
27. Koob TJ et al: Hormonal interactions in mammalian collagenase regulation. Comparative studies in human skin and rat uterus. *Biochim Biophys Acta* 629:13, 1980
28. Asboe-Hansen G, Blumenkrantz N: Cortisol effects on collagen biosynthesis in embryonic explants and in vitro hydroxylation of procollagen. *Acta Endocrinol* 83:665, 1976
29. Booth BA et al: Steroid induced dermal atrophy: Effects of glucocorticoids on collagen metabolism in human skin fibroblast cultures. *Int J Dermatol* 21:333, 1982
30. Fisher LB, Maibach HI: Effect of corticosteroids on human epidermal mitotic activity. *Arch Dermatol* 103:39, 1971
31. Schell H et al: Evidence of diurnal variation of human epidermal cell proliferation. *Arch Dermatol Res* 271:41, 1980
32. Sugimoto M, Endo H: Effect of hydrocortisone on keratinization of chick embryonic skin cultured in chemically defined medium. *Nature* 222:1270, 1969
33. Laurence EB, Christophers E: Selective action of hydrocortisone on post mitotic epidermal cells in vivo. *J Invest Dermatol* 66:222, 1976
34. Morril SD, Hermann F: Influence of systemically administered cortisone on hair growth in mice. *J Invest Dermatol* 47:243, 1961
35. Galey CI et al: Activation of phospholipase A₂ and C in murine keratinocytes by phorbol ester 12-O-tetradecanophorbol-13-acetate. *Clin Res* 31:567A, 1983
36. Weissmann G, Thomas L: The effect of corticosteroids upon connective tissue and lysosomes. *Recent Prog Horm Res* 20:215, 1964
37. Hsia SL, Hao YL: Transformation of cortisone to cortisol in human skin. *Steroids* 10:489, 1967
38. Malkinson FD et al: In vitro studies of adrenal steroid metabolism in the skin. *J Invest Dermatol* 32:101, 1959
39. Nabors CJ, Berliner DL: Corticosteroid metabolism during wound healing. *J Invest Dermatol* 52:465, 1969
40. Shuster S, Thody AJ: The control and measurement of sebum secretion. *J Invest Dermatol* 62:172, 1974
41. Soffer LJ et al: *The Human Adrenal Gland*. Philadelphia, Lea & Febiger, 1961
42. McGregor BC et al: Vitiligo and multiglandular insufficiencies. *JAMA* 219:724, 1972
43. Nelson DH et al: ACTH-producing pituitary tumors following adrenalectomy for Cushing's syndrome. *Ann Intern Med* 52:561, 1960
44. Pochi PE, Strauss JS: Endocrinological control of the development and activity of the human sebaceous gland. *J Invest Dermatol* 62:191, 1974
45. Wilson MJ, Spaziane E: The melanogenic response to testosterone in scrotal epidermis: Effects on tyrosinase activity and protein synthesis. *Acta Endocrinol* 81:435, 1970
46. Glimcher ME et al: Ultrastructure of normals and castrates and the effects of testosterone and ultra violet (UVLB) irradiation on scrotal skin of rats. *J Exp Zool* 207:249, 1979

47. Black MM et al: Osteoporosis, skin collagen and androgens. *Br Med J* **4**:773, 1970

48. Hodgins MB, Hay JB: Steroid metabolism in human skin: Its relation to sebaceous gland growth and acne vulgaris. *Biochem Soc Trans* **4**:605, 1976

49. Hay JB, Hodgins MB: Distribution of androgen metabolizing enzymes in isolated tissues of human forehead and axillary skin. *J Endocrinol* **79**:29, 1978

50. Sawaya ME et al: Increased androgen binding capacity in scalp of male pattern baldness. *J Invest Dermatol* **92**:91, 1989

51. Ebling FJ: Hormonal control and methods of measuring sebaceous secretions. *J Invest Dermatol* **62**:161, 1974

52. Ebling FJ: Endocrine factors affecting cell replacement and cell loss in the epidermis and sebaceous glands of the female albino rat. *J Endocrinol* **12**:38, 1955

53. Puonnen R: Effect of castration and peroral estrogen treatment on the skin. *Acta Obstet Gynecol Scand* **21**(suppl):3, 1972

54. Smith QT, Allison DJ: Changes of collagen content in skin, femur, and uterus of 17β estradiol benzoate treated rats. *Endocrinol* **79**:486, 1966

55. Yang SL et al: The effect of estrogens on collagen synthesis at the site of a skin graft. *Am J Obstet Gynecol* **116**:694, 1973

56. Rose LI et al: Adrenocortical hydroxylase deficiencies in acne vulgaris. *J Invest Dermatol* **66**:324, 1976

57. Jelineck JE: Cutaneous side effects of oral contraceptives. *Arch Dermatol* **101**:181, 1970

58. Köck A et al: MSHα and ACTH production by human keratinocytes: A link between the neuronal and the immune system (abstr) *J Invest Dermatol* **95**:543A, 1990

59. Matsuoka LY et al: Histochemical characterization of cutaneous involvement of acromegaly. *Arch Intern Med* **142**:1820, 1982

60. Gouding GAW et al: Heel pad thickness: Determination by high resolution ultrasound. *J Ultrasound Med* **4**:173, 1985

61. Davidoff LM: Studies in acromegaly. III. The anamnesis and symptomatology in one hundred cases. *Endocrinology* **10**:461, 1926

62. Brown J, Winkelmann RK: Acanthosis nigricans: A study of 90 cases. *Medicine* **47**:33, 1968

63. Reaven GM: Insulin resistance in noninsulin dependent diabetes mellitus. Does it exist and can it be measured? *Am J Med* **74** (suppl 1A):3, 1983

64. Flier JS et al: Antibodies that impair insulin receptor binding in an unusual diabetic syndrome with severe insulin resistance. *Science* **190**:63, 1975

65. Shoelson S et al: Three mutant insulins in man. *Nature* **302**:1, 1983

66. Raskin PR et al: The effect of diabetic control on the width of skeletal muscle capillary basement membrane in patients with Type I diabetes mellitus. *N Engl J Med* **309**:1546, 1983

67. Camerini-Davlos RA et al: Drug induced reversal of early diabetic microangiopathy. *N Engl J Med* **309**:1551, 1983

68. Hsia SL: *Essays in Biochemistry,* vol 7, *Potentials in Exploring the Biochemistry of Human Skin.* New York, Academic, 1971, p 1

69. Halprin KM, Ohkawara A: Glucose entry into human epidermis. *J Invest Dermatol* **49**:561, 1967

70. Peterka ES, Fusaro RM: Cutaneous carbohydrate studies. IV. The skin glucose content of fasting diabetics with and without infection. *J Invest Dermatol* **46**:459, 1966

71. Chang KJ et al: Increased cross linkages in experimental diabetes. *Diabetes* **29**:778, 1980

72. Schnider SL, Kohn RR: Effects of age and diabetes mellitus on the solubility and nonenzymatic glycosylation of human skin collagen. *J Clin Invest* **67**:1630, 1981

73. Phan Than L et al: Increased biosynthesis and processing of fibronectin in fibroblasts from diabetic mice. *Proc Natl Acad Sci USA* **84**:1911, 1987

74. Sabin JA: Bacterial infections in diabetes mellitus. *Br J Dermatol* **91**:481, 1974

75. Drachman RH et al: Studies on the effect of experimental nonketotic diabetes mellitus on antibacterial defense. *J Exp Med* **124**:227, 1966

76. Lang CH et al: IL-1 induced increases in glucose utilization are insulin mediated. *Life Sci* **45**:2127, 1989

77. Neilly JB et al: Pruritus in diabetes mellitus: Investigation of prevalence and correlation with diabetes control. *Diabetes Care* **9**:273, 1986

78. Parker F, Short JM: Xanthomatosis associated with hyperlipoproteinemia. *J Invest Dermatol* **55**:71, 1970

79. Braverman I: Ultrastructural features of aging in the skin of normal adults and juvenile diabetes. *Clin Res* **28**:247A, 1980

80. Braverman IM, Fonfuko E: Studies in cutaneous aging. II. The microvasculature. *J Invest Dermatol* **78**:444, 1982

81. Melin H: An atrophic circumscribed skin lesion in the lower extremities of diabetics. *Acta Med Scand* **423**(suppl):1, 1964

82. Binkley GW: Dermopathy in the diabetic syndrome. *Arch Dermatol* **92**:625, 1965

83. Kurwa A et al: Concurrence of bullous and atrophic skin lesions in diabetes mellitus. *Arch Dermatol* **103**:607, 1971

84. Bauer M, Levan NE: Diabetic dermangiopathy. *Br J Dermatol* **83**:528, 1970

85. Lithner F: Lesions of the legs in diabetics. *Acta Med Scand* **589**(suppl):1, 1976

86. Rocca FF, Pereyra E: Phlyctenar lesions in the feet of diabetic patients. *Diabetes* **12**:220, 1963

87. Bernstein JE et al: Bullous eruptions of diabetes mellitus. *Arch Dermatol* **115**:324, 1979

88. Bernstein JE et al: Reduced threshhold to suction-induced blister formation in insulin dependent diabetics. *J Am Acad Dermatol* **8**:790, 1983

89. Clark CV et al: Decreased skin wrinkling in diabetes mellitus. *Diabetes Care* **7**:224, 1984

90. Huntley AC: Finger pebbles: A common finding in diabetes mellitus. *J Am Acad Dermatol* **14**:612, 1984

91. Grgic A et al: Joint contracture: A common manifestation of childhood diabetes. *J Pediatr* **88**:584, 1975

92. Rosenblum AL et al: Limited joint mobility in childhood diabetes indicates increased risk for microvascular disease. *N Engl J Med* **23**:1919, 1981

93. Fleischmajor R, Lara JV: Scleredema adultorum: A histochemical and biochemical study. *Arch Dermatol* **92**:643, 1965

94. Cohen BA et al: Scleredema adultorum of Buschke and diabetes mellitus. *Arch Dermatol* **101**:27, 1970

95. Goodman JI: Diabetic anhydrosis. *Am J Med* **41**:831, 1966

96. Faerman I et al: Autonomic neuropathy in the skin: A histological study of the sympathetic nerve fibers in diabetic anhidrosis. *Diabetologica* **22**:96, 1982

97. Mann JR, Harman RRM: Cutaneous anesthesia in necrobiosis lipoidica diabeticorum. *Br J Dermatol* **110**:323, 1984

98. Oikarinen A et al: Necrobiosis lipoidica: Ultrastructural and biochemical demonstration of a collagen defect. *J Invest Dermatol* **88**:227, 1987

99. Muller SA, Winkelmann RK: Necrobiosis lipoidica diabeticorum, a clinical and pathological investigation of 171 cases. *Arch Dermatol* **93**:272, 1966

100. Narva WM et al: Necrobiosis lipoidica diabeticorum with apparently normal diabetic tolerance. *Arch Intern Med* **115**:718, 1965

101. Ullman S, Dahl MV: Necrobiosis lipoidica, an immunofluorescence study. *Arch Dermatol* **113**:1671, 1977

102. Quimby SR et al: Cutaneous immunopathology of necrobiosis lipoidica diabeticorum. *Arch Dermatol* **124**:1364, 1983

103. Boulton AJM et al: Necrobiosis lipoidica diabeticorum: A clinicopathological study. *J Am Acad Dermatol* **18**:530, 1988

104. Statham B et al: A randomized double blind comparison of an aspirin-dipyridamole combination versus a placebo in the treatment of necrobiosis lipoidica. *Acta Derm Venereol* **61**:270, 1981

105. Karkavitsas K et al: Aspirin in the management of necrobiosis lipoidica. *Acta Derm Venereol* **62**:183, 1982

106. Mensing H: Clofazimine, therapeutic alternative in necrobiosis lipoidica diabeticorum and granuloma annulare. *Hautarzt* **40**:99, 1989

107. Handfield-Jones S et al: High dose nicotinamide in the treatment of necrobiosis lipoidica diabeticorum. *Br J Dermatol* **118**:693, 1987

108. Williamson DM, Dykes RW: Carbohydrate metabolism in granuloma annulare. *J Invest Dermatol* **58**:400, 1972

109. Haim S et al: Generalized granuloma annulare: Relationship to diabetes mellitus as revealed in 8 cases. *Br J Dermatol* **83**:302, 1970

110. Dawber RPR: Vitiligo in mature-onset diabetes. *Br J Dermatol* **80**:275, 1968

111. Macaron C et al: Vitiligo and juvenile diabetes mellitus. *Arch Dermatol* **113**:1515, 1977

112. Matsuoka LY et al: Spectrum of endocrine abnormalities associated with acanthosis nigricans. *Am J Med* **83**:719, 1985

113. Kahn CR et al: Syndromes of insulin resistance and acanthosis nigricans. *N Engl J Med* **294**:739, 1976

114. Geffner ME, Golde DW: Selected insulin action on skin, ovary, heart in insulin resistant states. *Diabetes Care* **11**:500, 1988

115. Poliak SC et al: Reactive perforating collagenosis is associated with diabetes mellitus. *N Engl J Med* **306**:81, 1982

116. Zarate AR et al: Hyperkeratosis penetrans (HKP), a rare dermatological disease with high incidence in patients on hemodialysis. *Proceedings of the Dialysis Transplant Forum* 1978, p 99

117. Mallinson CN et al: A glucagonoma syndrome. *Lancet* **2**:1, 1974

118. McGavran MH et al: A glucagon-secreting α cell carcinoma of the pancreas. *N Engl J Med* **274**:1408, 1966

119. Binnick GN et al: The glucagonoma syndrome. *Arch Dermatol* **113**:749, 1977

120. Rappesberger K et al: Das Glukagonom-Syndrom. *Hautarzt* **38**:589, 1987

121. Sohier J et al: Rapid improvement of skin lesions in glucagonomas with intravenous somatostatin infusions. *Lancet* **1**:40, 1980

122. Goodenberger DM et al: Necrolytic migratory erythema without glucagonoma. *Arch Dermatol* **115**:1429, 1979

CHAPTER 170

J.K. Wilkin

Skin Changes in the Flushing Disorders and the Carcinoid Syndrome

Flushing Disorders

Flushing is a transient reddening of the face and frequently other areas, including the neck, upper chest, and epigastric areas. The erythema is easily extinguished with direct pressure, and the redness subsides between flushing episodes. The latter feature excludes patients with a "red face," for example, due to drug photosensitivity, in whom the erythema is much longer-lived (fixed) and not subject to transient, pronounced changes in intensity.

Despite the limited distribution of the erythema, flushing is the visible sign of a generalized increase in cutaneous blood flow.[1] The greater visibility of the superficial cutaneous vasculature and the greater capacity of these vessels for erythrocytes provide for this limited distribution of observed erythema. This also explains the limited flush distribution seen after obviously systemic stimuli.

Pathophysiology: Two Basic Mechanisms

Because flushing is a phenomenon of transient vasodilation, the mechanisms of vasodilation provide a physiologic scheme for classifying flushing reactions.[2] There is a dual control of vascular smooth muscle by autonomic nerves and by circulating vasoactive agents. Autonomic nerves also control the eccrine sweat glands, so that whenever vasodilation is mediated by autonomic nerves, it is accompanied by eccrine sweating.

Accordingly, two mechanisms of flushing can be distinguished at the bedside or in the office: neural-mediated flushing, which includes eccrine sweating ("wet flush"), and flushing from agents that act directly on vascular smooth muscle ("dry flush"). An important caveat to the clinician is that the presence or absence of eccrine sweating is specifically associated contemporaneously with the actual flushing, that is, the transient reddening. It is not rare for a patient with carcinoid syndrome to have a flushing reaction of such intensity that it is *followed* by coexisting pallor and diaphoresis. The "wet pallor" does not invalidate the clinical usefulness of the preceding dry flush.

Consequences: The Cutaneous Stigmata

In susceptible persons, frequent, intense flushing leads to a cluster of physical signs, called *rosacea*. Rosacea is characterized by erythema or cyanosis in the flush distribution, telangiectasia, papules, pustules, and eventually connective tissue hypertrophy, including rhinophyma. Frequent, intense flushing may lead to loss of vascular tone, resulting in the permanent background erythema. That the venules in the superficial plexus are involved, and not the superficial collecting veins, is compatible with infrared studies of rosacea.[3] Thus, the shunting of a considerable volume of blood during a flushing reaction directly into the venules of the subpapillary plexus, leading to loss of tone, may represent a significant step in the pathogenesis of the erythematotelangiectatic component of rosacea.

Various observations support the view that flushing is an important factor in the pathogenesis of rosacea.[4] There is a correlation between the severity of ocular rosacea (which is largely vascular) and the tendency to strong flushing. Patients with severe flushing due to carcinoid develop all of the various rosacea stigmata, including ocular rosacea, facial telangiectasia, and severe connective tissue hypertrophy. Patients with severe flushing due to mastocytosis can similarly develop rosacea in less than a year after the onset of flushing episodes. Mild rosacea is more common in women and usually appears after age 35 when the frequency of hot flashes and flushing increases. Flushing is typically the earliest component of rosacea to be apparent. Rosacea is exacerbated during vasodilator therapy accompanied by flushing. Finally, extrafacial rosacea may occur in extrafacial areas of flushing.

The pathophysiologic mechanism by which flushing leads to rosacea probably involves edema formation.[4] This edema is usually subclinical or only barely perceptible, although the frequent occurrence of overt facial edema in the course of rosacea has been documented. It follows a severe flushing episode and may last only a day initially. Over time it can become more persistent. Rosacea stigmata are typically in those areas of the face overlying relatively inactive musculature, where the edema fluid tends to persist. Rosacea responds to massage therapy, thereby supporting the pathologic role for edema.

Evaluation of the Patient with a Flushing Disorder

It is important to consider the clinical characteristics of the patient with flushing before embarking on an expensive laboratory evaluation. Four key elements of information must be obtained: provocative and palliative factors, morphology, associated features, and temporal characteristics.

Provocative and palliative factors should be sought first. This information may permit a more focused differential diagnosis, for example, alcohol-related, drug-related, or eating-related flushing (Table 170-1).

Morphology of the flushing reaction may suggest not only the cause of the flushing but also, in the case of carcinoidosis, the anatomic origin of the disorder. Important points to consider include: one basic feature that comes and goes versus discrete phases or stages; patchy versus confluent; bright pink to cyanotic; pallor, preceding or following; and dry skin versus perspiration.

Associated findings, when present, aid in the differential diagnosis. Bronchospasm, abdominal cramps, diarrhea, headaches, urticaria, and pruritus can provide important clues.

Temporal characteristics include the timing of the specific features during each flushing reaction and the frequency of the flushing reactions. Since this is often the weakest part of the patient's account, a 2-week diary will provide data of better quality. The patient should record qualitative and quantitative aspects of the flushing reaction and list all occupational exposures, physical exercise, and exogenous agents, especially food, beverages, and drugs. In a patient with caffeine-withdrawal flushing, it was the absence of an exogenous agent at the critical time in a 2-week diary that led to the diagnosis.[5] The 2-week diary should be considered whenever the cause of the flushing is not immediately obvious.

When the diagnosis remains obscure after evaluation of the 2-week diary, the patient is given an exclusion diet listing foods high in histamine, foods and drugs that affect urinary 5-hydroxyindoleacetic acid (5-HIAA) tests, and foods and beverages that cause flushing. If the flushing reactions completely disappear, restoring the excluded items individually can identify the causative agent. If the flushing reactions continue unchanged, then histamine and urinary 5-HIAA may be assayed.

Occasionally, the exclusion diet will eliminate nonspecific factors that lower the threshold for flushing, perhaps by additive effects. Careful attention must be directed to a variety of such nonspecific factors, which must be avoided as much as possible. Examples are legion: menopause exacerbates flushing in the dumping syndrome; warming augments gustatory flushing; and alcohol can enhance a menopausal flush.

Hyperthermic Flushing

Hyperthermic stress can be exogenous, such as a hot day, or endogenous, for example, resulting from exercise. In many patients heat can cause flushing or overheating can lower the threshold to flushing from other causes, such as menopausal flushing. Although hyperthermia is usually considered in the context of the total body thermal economy, the actual physiologic thermostat resides in the anterior hypothalamus. Thus, the ingestion of hot beverages and the resultant increased heat in the oral cavity may cause flushing by a countercurrent heat-exchange mechanism.[6]

Menopausal (Climacteric) Flushing

Although the name suggests the cessation of menses, some women develop menopausal-like symptoms in their middle thirties while still having cyclic menses. They have flushing just before or during their periods each month, when the estrogen levels are lowest. Hot beverages, physical exertion, and emotional upsets can provoke menopausal flushing. Although natural climacteric flushing is extremely rare in men, surgical climacteric flushing in men is not uncommon after orchiectomy.[7] Pharmacologic menopause with flushing can be induced by a variety of drugs: 4-hydroxyandrostenedione, danazol, tamoxifen, clomiphene citrate, decapeptyl, and leuprolide.

Surgical menopause with flushing can occur any time after puberty when there is surgical loss of ovarian function. Bilateral tubal ligation can also compromise the vascular supply to the ovaries, possibly resulting in menopausal symptoms.

Several characteristics of climacteric flushing suggest the clinical diagnosis. First, drenching perspiration, which is often the most distressing component of the climacteric flush, implicates a neural-mediated mechanism. Second, waking episodes at night accompanied by flushing and sweating are typical. Third, the prodromal sensation of overheating before the onset of flushing and sweating suggests a dysfunction in the thermoregulatory mechanism. Several lines of recent evidence indicate that the site of dysfunction lies in the central catecholaminergic system.[4]

Most women choose hormonal replacement therapy for menopausal flushing. However, nonhormonal alternatives exist, such as clonidine hydrochloride. The smallest dosage form of clonidine hydrochloride marketed in the United States is the 0.1-mg tablet. The patient should be instructed to crush one tablet daily. Half the powder is taken in the morning and the other half in the evening before bed. This regimen of 0.05 mg twice daily is sufficient for many patients.[8] Some patients may require 0.1 mg twice daily.

Emotional Flushing

Some people with fair skin and a readily visible superficial cutaneous vasculature of the face are extremely troubled by blushing. It is critical to discern at the outset whether the blushing is simply intense and the emotional dynamics are normal or whether there is a significant emotional disturbance that is accompanied by frequent blushing.

Therapies for flushing attending normal emotional responses include biofeedback, hypnosis, paradoxical intention, and nadolol. Nadolol is a nonselective beta blocker that can attenuate the vascular response to anxiety in most patients at a dose of 40 to 80 mg daily. The long plasma half-life (14 to 24 h) permits a once-daily dose. Nadolol is a convenient therapy for patients with rosacea who have flushing associated with anxiety or who otherwise describe emotional flushing.[9]

Rosacea Flushing

Although the term *rosacea flushing* has been used, there is no evidence to date that suggests that flushing in rosacea is qualitatively

TABLE 170-1
Differential Diagnosis of Flushing Reactions

I Flushing reactions related to alcohol
    Increased susceptibility in mongoloid populations
    Occupational ''degreasers'' flush occurs in workmen drinking beer
    after exposure to industrial solvents.
        Trichloroethylene vapor
        N,N-dimethylformamide
        N-butyraldoxime
        Carbon disulfide
        Xylene
    Fermented alcoholic beverages (beer, sherry) may contain tyramine
    or histamine, which induce flushing.
    Drugs
        Disulfiram
        Chlorpropamide
        Calcium carbamide
        Phentolamine
        Griseofulvin
        Metronidazole
        Ketoconazole
        Chloramphenicol
        Quinacrine
        Beta-lactams with methyltetrazolethiol side chain (cephalosporin
        antibiotics)
            Cefamandole
            Cefoperazone
            Moxalactam
    Eating *Coprinus* mushrooms
    Carcinoid flushing
    Mastocytosis flushing

II Flushing related to food additives
    Monosodium glutamate (MSG) putatively provokes flushing, but
    this is not verified.
    Sodium nitrite in cured meats (frankfurters, bacon, salami, ham)
    may cause headache and flushing.
    Sulfites (potassium metabisulfite) may cause wheezing and flushing.

III Flushing associated with eating
    Hot beverages cause flushing through countercurrent heat exchange
    into blood vessels leading to the anterior hypothalamus.
    Auriculotemporal flushing, especially after cheese, chocolate, lemon,
    highly spiced foods.
    Gustatory flushing, especially after chewing a chili pepper.
    Dumping syndrome, especially after a meal or ingestion of hot liquids
    or hypertonic glucose.
    Spoiled scombroid (tuna, mackerel, skipjack, and bonito) and
    nonscombroid (mahi-mahi, bluefish, amberjack, herring, sardines,
    and anchovies) fishes and cheeses. Histamine is the probable toxin.

IV Neurologic flushing
    Anxiety
    Simple blushing
    Brain tumors
    Spinal cord lesions (autonomic hyperreflexia)
    Migraine headaches
    Parkinson's disease
    Climacteric (menopausal) flushing: ''hot flashes''
    Cholinergic erythema

V Flushing due to drugs
    All vasodilators (e.g., nitroglycerin, prostaglandins, synthetic
    calcitonin-gene-related peptide)
    All calcium channel blockers
        Nifedipine
        Verapamil
        Diltiazem
    Nicotinic acid (not nicotinamide)
    Morphine and other opiates
    Amyl nitrite and butyl nitrite (recreational drugs)
    Cholinergic drugs, e.g., metrifonate, an anthelminthic
    Bromocriptine used in Parkinson's disease
    Thyrotropin-releasing hormone (TRH)
    Tamoxifen
    Cyproterone acetate
    Oral triamcinolone used with psoriatic arthritis
    Cyclosporine
    Rifampin

VI Flushing due to systemic diseases
    Carcinoid syndrome
    Mastocytosis
    Basophilic chronic granulocytic leukemia
    Pheochromocytoma
    Medullary carcinoma of thyroid
    Pancreatic tumors (e.g., VIPoma)
    Renal cell carcinoma
    Horseshoe kidneys (Rovsing's syndrome)

different from flushing in the general population. However, quantitative differences based on such factors as the reactivity of the vasculature, the visibility of the vasculature, and the enhanced release of endogenous mediators are quite likely.[4]

Monosodium Glutamate Flushing

Monosodium glutamate (MSG) is widely regarded as a cause of flushing in the ''Chinese restaurant syndrome.'' However, a true MSG-induced flushing reaction must be extremely rare, if it occurs at all.[10] Patients should be encouraged to look beyond MSG at other dietary agents, such as red pepper (capsaicin), other spices, nitrites and sulfites (additives in many foods), thermally hot food and beverages, and alcohol.

Pheochromocytoma

Flushing is so rare in patients diagnosed as having pheochromocytoma that its presence casts doubt on the diagnosis.[11] If flushing occurs at all, it is seen after a paroxysm of hypertension, tachycardia, palpitations, chest pain, severe throbbing headaches, and excessive perspiration. Pallor is present during the attack, and mild flushing may occur after the attack as a rebound from the facial cutaneous vasoconstriction.

Mastocytosis (See Chap. 161)

Carcinoid Syndrome

Pathology

Although malignant carcinoid neoplasms are not rare, the carcinoid syndrome is. Less than 4 percent of 3718 patients with abdominal carcinoid tumors had the carcinoid syndrome.[12] The lack of neuroendocrine product-related symptomatology in most patients may be related to the detoxifying effect of the liver or to low levels of bioactive hormone produced by the tumors. The presence of the carcinoid syndrome implies either hepatic metastases, extraabdominal carcinoid tumor, or large or multiple primary intraabdominal lesions with sufficient biomass to produce more hormone than the liver can degrade.

Carcinoid tumors, which are derived from enterochromaffin (Kulchitsky) cells, produce a variety of humoral agents, even within a single tumor. Carcinoid tumors develop different histologic patterns and biochemical characteristics according to primary growth sites and embryonic derivation.[13,14] The appendix is the most common site, and the ileum is the second most common site. Ileal tumors are the most common source of the classic carcinoid syndrome, and the ileum is the most frequent origin for metastasizing carcinoid. Other sites for carcinoid tumors include the rectum, duodenum, stomach, colon, biliary tract, and pancreas. Less than 10 percent of carcinoid tumors originate outside the gastrointestinal tract, in sites such as ovary, testis, skin, and bronchus.[15]

The carcinoid syndrome and tumors have important characteristics that correlate with the site of origin.[13,14] Most important is the comparison between those tumors that originate in the embryologic foregut (bronchus, stomach, pancreas) and the carcinoids of the midgut (small intestine to midcolon). Although tumors from both sites produce serotonin, foregut carcinoid tumors also produce histamine, which may explain the associations of peptic ulcer disease with foregut rather than midgut carcinoid tumors. Furthermore, the flushing reaction associated with foregut tumors as compared with midgut tumors is brighter (salmon pink to red), more persistent, and more intense; shows a geographic pattern; and has prominent associated findings, including lacrimation, sweating (with pallor), vomiting, and asthma. Bronchial carcinoids show a closer relationship to foregut tumors and have a similar associated type of flushing, which is also of considerable intensity. Midgut tumors are associated with a cyanotic flush, giving an appearance of mixed cyanosis, erythema, and pallor. This flush occurs more frequently and is regarded as the classic pattern for carcinoid syndrome. Hypotension and bronchoconstriction are more common with the flushing reactions associated with midgut tumors. Hindgut (descending colon and rectal) tumors do not lead to flushing or other manifestations of carcinoid syndrome.

Clinical Manifestations

Cutaneous findings are multiple, and many can be grouped according to probable pathogenesis. Thus, pellagra-like lesions result from the excessive utilization of tryptophan by the carcinoid tumor, leaving little for the daily niacin requirement. These lesions include hyperkeratosis; xerosis; scaling of the legs, forearms, and trunk; angular cheilitis; and glossitis.

Severe carcinoid flushing can explain the rosacea stigmata, including ocular rosacea, scleral reddening, facial telangiectasia and cyanosis, and severe frontophyma, rhinophyma, and zygophyma.[4,15] The flushing, found in nearly all patients with carcinoid syndrome, can be especially intense, with facial edema occurring during the attacks.

Additional skin manifestations associated with carcinoid syndrome include yellow-brown or brown-gray patches on the forehead, back, and wrists; pruritus; pruritus with pressure-induced "orange blotches"[16]; scleroderma-like changes[17,18]; acropachyderma and pachyperiostitis[19]; cutaneous metastatic nodules[19]; erythematous, telangiectatic, atrophic patches with central ulcera-

tion[20]; pyoderma gangrenosum[21]; erythema annulare centrifugum and white banding of the toe nails[22]; blisters that heal leaving white scarlike lesions and white macular lesions surrounded by an erythematous halo[23]; and reddish cyanotic, hyperkeratotic papules.[24]

Gastrointestinal manifestations may precede or coexist with the carcinoid syndrome. Chronic watery diarrhea occurs in 85 percent of patients.[25] Abdominal pain, constipation, nausea, vomiting, malabsorption, anorexia, weight loss, small bowel obstruction, and rectal bleeding may also precede the full carcinoid syndrome.

Respiratory manifestations include wheezing, stridor, dyspnea, coughing, and bronchospasm.[25] Additional findings include arthritis, psychiatric symptoms, osteoblastic bone lesions associated with bronchial carcinoid metastases, acromegaly, neurofibromatosis, Cushing's disease, and a unique retinal lesion consisting of very small, punched-out areas of postischemic changes in the peripheral retina.[15]

Fibrotic reactions are curious manifestations occurring in collagenous and elastic tissues. Endocardial fibrosis with valve damage is classically on the ventricular surface of the tricuspid valve and the pulmonary arterial surface of the pulmonic valve, producing valvular stenosis followed by insufficiency.[25] Hypotensive episodes, edema of the lower limbs, murmurs, and congestive heart failure can occur. Less commonly, the fibrotic valvular damage is left-sided due to either bronchial carcinoids or the combination of hepatic metastases with an atrial septal defect.[26]

The fibrotic reactions to surgery, fibrosis of the bladder, and fibrosis of the peritoneum may be of the same nature as the valvular lesions, that is, young fibrous tissue hyperproliferation that is purely collagenous and not elastic. A distinctly different type of reaction is the elastic vascular sclerosis of mesenteric blood vessels. This unique process, which occurs only with ileal carcinoid tumors, can lead to ischemic ileal necrosis. Serotonin may have a direct role in the fibrotic processes.[15]

Diagnosis and Serotonin Metabolism

The essential diagnostic criterion of carcinoid syndrome is biochemical evidence of serotonin overproduction.[7] This is usually established by an elevated output of urinary 5-HIAA, which is normally 2 to 10 mg per day. In carcinoid syndrome it is often over 40 mg per day. Various foods and drugs can affect the urinary excretion of 5-HIAA (Table 170-2), and specimens for determination of urinary 5-HIAA excretion should be collected during the third day of an exclusion diet. It cannot be overemphasized that a qualitative (screening, or "spot") test for urinary 5-HIAA is of value only when positive. If carcinoid tumor is suspected clinically and the qualitative test is negative, a quantitative assay should be performed on a sample from a 24-h urine collection. Excretion fluctuates, so that repeated measurements may be necessary. Occasional patients are reported with carcinoid syndrome and normal 5-HIAA excretion.[27] These patients have hyperserotoninemia, and they lack the metabolic machinery to convert serotonin to 5-HIAA.

Provocative tests, which should be performed in an appropriate clinical setting, can also be valuable. Epinephrine, 5 μg, or calcium gluconate, 10 to 15 mg/kg, administered intravenously over 4 h, may produce a flush mimicking a spontaneous attack.[28] Selective abdominal vein catheterization with blood sampling for serotonin determination in a platelet-poor plasma fraction can both determine whether carcinoid tumor is present and identify the site in cases in which urine 5-HIAA levels and liver scintiscan are negative and angiograms are inconclusive.[29] Recently, a radiolabeled

TABLE 170-2

Foods and Drugs That Affect Urinary Excretion of 5-Hydroxyindoleacetic Acid

Foods	
Avocados	Red plums
Bananas	Tomatoes
Eggplant	Walnuts
Pineapples	

Drugs	
ACTH	Mephenesin
Acetaminophen	Methamphetamine
Acetanilid	Methenamine
Bromocriptine	Methocarbamol
Caffeine	Methyldopa
Chlorpromazine	Methysergide
Fluorouracil	Monoamine oxidase inhibitors
Guaifenesin	Phenacetin
Glyceryl guaiacolate	Phenmetrazine
Heparin	Phenothiazines
Imipramine	Promethazine
Isoniazid	Reserpine
Lugol's solution	Somatostatin analogues (e.g., octreotide)
Melphalan	

TABLE 170-3

Factors That Precipitate Flushing in the Carcinoid Syndrome

Foods and beverages
    Hot (thermal) food/beverages
    Spicy food
    Chocolate
    Cheeses
    Tomatoes
    Avocados
    Red plums
    Walnuts
    Eggplant
    Ingestion of any food
    Alcohol
Emotional stress
Valsalva maneuver
    Straining during defecation
    Vigorous coughing
Sudden, direct pressure on a large carcinoid tumor
    Physical examination
    Intraoperative manipulation
Spontaneous

octreotide scanning technique has been shown to be a rapid and safe procedure for the visualization of primary tumors or metastases in patients with carcinoid tumors.[30] A positive scan can also predict the ability of octreotide therapy to control symptoms of hormonal hypersecretion.

It is important to remember that the tissue diagnosis of carcinoid tumor in a patient with flushing does not unequivocally establish the diagnosis of carcinoid syndrome.[7]

Management and Prognosis

Even though carcinoid syndrome may appear relatively homogeneous clinically, biochemical and pharmacologic heterogeneity is present. Serotonin may affect the qualitative nature of the flush, that is, the cyanotic aspect, but it is not the mediator of the flushing reaction. In fact, the hypersecretion of serotonin and the flushing reaction can be pharmacologically dissociated.[4] Corticosteroids and bromocriptine have been effective in patients with bronchial carcinoid tumors.[31,32] Serotonin antagonists and depleters, such as methysergide and parachlorophenylalanine, respectively, may effectively control the diarrhea but have no effect on the flushing.[33-35] Another serotonin antagonist, ketanserin, has been successful perioperatively in a patient with the carcinoid syndrome undergoing hepatic artery embolization.[36] Cyproheptadine, which is a serotonin antagonist among other properties, has been helpful in controlling flushing.[33] Antihistamines may be especially useful in patients with foregut carcinoid tumors that produce histamine. Clonidine controls carcinoid flushing in some patients in whom the release of catecholamines, which act on the tumor cells, may be an important factor.[37,38] Thus, the pharmacologic basis for management of carcinoid flushing reactions is complex.

Importantly, somatostatin is a potent antagonist of the flushing reaction associated with both gastric and ileal carcinoid tumors.[39-41] Since somatostatin is effective in midgut carcinoid flushing, where histamine is without a major role, it is likely that somatostatin does more than simply inhibit the release of histamine. However, clinical use of somatostatin is limited because of its short half-life and intravenous delivery.

The somatostatin analogue octreotide has pharmacologic effects similar to those of somatostatin but a much longer half-life, making subcutaneous therapy possible. Octreotide not only controls the flushing and diarrhea of carcinoid syndrome but also may suppress cancerous cell growth.[42] Octreotide must be given by subcutaneous injection at least once a day and usually twice a day. Octreotide has also been used intravenously with success to treat carcinoid crisis during anesthesia.[43]

In addition to the specific pharmacologic agents used to control flushing, the dermatologist should determine that the patient is receiving an adequate niacin supplement (as nicotinamide, not nicotinic acid, since the latter causes flushing). Patients should avoid foods, agents, and activities that precipitate symptoms (Table 170-3).

At present, antitumor drugs and subtotal tumor resection lead to variable results in the patient with carcinoid syndrome. Only total surgical removal can offer cure, and this is unfortunately seldom feasible.

References

1. Wilkin JK: Why is flushing limited to a mostly facial cutaneous distribution? *J Am Acad Dermatol* **19**:309, 1988
2. Burnstock G, Iwayama T: Fine-structural identification of autonomic nerves and their relation to smooth muscle. *Prog Brain Res* **34**:389, 1971
3. Wilkin JK, Josephs JA: Infrared photographic studies of rosacea. *Arch Dermatol* **116**:678, 1980
4. Wilkin JK: Flushing reactions, in *Recent Advances in Dermatology*, No. 6, edited by AJ Rook, HI Maibach. New York, Churchill Livingstone, 1983, p 157
5. Wilkin JK: The caffeine withdrawal flush: Report of a case of "weekend flushing." *Military Med* **151**:123, 1986
6. Wilkin JK: Oral thermal-induced flushing in erythematotelangiectatic rosacea. *J Invest Dermatol* **76**:15, 1981
7. Wilkin JK: Climacteric flushing in a patient with carcinoid tumour. *Br J Dermatol* **112**:357, 1985
8. Edington RF et al: Clonidine (Dixarit) for menopausal flushing. *Can Med Assoc J* **123**:23, 1980

9. Wilkin JK: Effect of nadolol on flushing reactions in rosacea. *J Am Acad Dermatol* **20**:202, 1989

10. Wilkin JK, Fortner G: Does monosodium glutamate cause flushing? *J Am Acad Dermatol* **15**:225, 1986

11. Bravo EL, Gifford RW: Pheochromocytoma: Diagnosis, localization and management. *N Engl J Med* **311**:1298, 1984

12. Wilson H: Carcinoid syndrome. *Curr Probl Surg* (11):36, 1970

13. Williams ED, Sandler M: The classification of carcinoid tumors. *Lancet* **1**:238, 1963

14. Soga J, Tazawa K: Pathologic analysis of carcinoids. *Cancer* **28**:990, 1971

15. Wilkin JK, Demis DJ: Carcinoidosis (carcinoid syndrome), in *Clinical Dermatology,* edited by DJ Demis, RL Dobson, JS McGuire. Philadelphia, Harper & Row, 1985, 4-12, p 1

16. Mengel C: Cutaneous manifestations of malignant carcinoid syndrome. *Ann Intern Med* **58**:989, 1963

17. Zarafonetis C, Lorber S: Association of functioning carcinoid syndrome and scleroderma. *Am J Med Sci* **236**:1, 1958

18. Fries JF et al: Scleroderma-like lesions and the carcinoid syndrome. *Arch Intern Med* **131**:550, 1973

19. Walker J: Metastasizing argentaffinomas from dermatologists point of view. *S Afr Med J* **31**:1271, 1957

20. Bean SF, Fusaro RM: An unusual manifestation of the carcinoid syndrome. *Arch Dermatol* **98**:268, 1968

21. Lee SS et al: Pyoderma gangrenosum with carcinoid tumor. *Cutis* **18**:791, 1976

22. Everall JD et al: Unusual cutaneous associations of a malignant carcinoid tumour of the bronchus: Erythema annulare centrifugum and white banding of the toe nails. *Br J Dermatol* **93**:341, 1975

23. Smith AS, Greaves MW: Blood prostaglandin activity associated with noradrenaline-produced flush in the carcinoid syndrome. *Br J Dermatol* **90**:547, 1974

24. Lachapelle J-M et al: Syndrome carcinoide: Manifestations cutanées chroniques florides. *Ann Dermatol Venereol* **104**:66, 1977

25. Beaton H, Dineen P: Gastrointestinal carcinoids and the malignant carcinoid syndrome. *Surg Gynecol Obstet* **152**:268, 1981

26. Waldenstrom J, Ljungberg E: Studies on the functional circulatory influence from metastasizing carcinoid tumours and their possible relation to enteramine production. *Acta Med Scand* **152**:293, 1955

27. Davis RB, Rosenberg JC: Carcinoid syndrome associated with hyperserotoninemia and normal 5-hydroxyindoleacetic acid excretion. *Am J Med* **30**:167, 1961

28. Kaplan EL et al: A new provocative test for the diagnosis of the carcinoid syndrome. *Am J Surg* **123**:173, 1972

29. Nobin A et al: Selective mesenteric vein catheterization and plasma serotonin determination in patients with carcinoid tumors. *World J Surg* **7**:223, 1983

30. Lamberts SWJ et al: Somatostatin-receptor imaging in the localization of endocrine tumors. *N Engl J Med* **323**:1246, 1990

31. Reith PR et al: Prolonged suppression of a corticotropin-producing bronchial carcinoid by oral bromocriptine. *Arch Intern Med* **147**:989, 1987

32. Sebastian A et al: The spectrum produced by malignant carcinoid tumor. *Calif Med* **106**:64, 1967

33. Brown H et al: Functioning carcinoid tumors, in *Cancer of the Gastrointestinal Tract*. Chicago, Year Book, 1967, p 155

34. Satterlee WG, Serpick A, Bianchine JR: The carcinoid syndrome: Chronic treatment with parachlorophenylalanine. *Ann Intern Med* **72**:919, 1970

35. Engelman K et al: Inhibition of serotonin synthesis by para-chlorophenylalanine in patients with the carcinoid syndrome. *N Engl J Med* **277**:1103, 1967

36. Houghton K, Carter JA: Peri-operative management of carcinoid syndrome using ketanserin. *Anaesthesia* **41**:596, 1986

37. Wilkin JK, Rountree CB: Blockade of carcinoid flush with cimetidine and clonidine. *Arch Dermatol* **118**:109, 1982

38. Metz SA et al: Suppression of plasma catecholamines and flushing by clonidine in man. *J Clin Endocrinol Metab* **46**:83, 1978

39. Roberts LJ et al: Carcinoid: Provocation by pentagastrin and inhibition by somatostatin. *Gastroenterology* **84**:272, 1983

40. Thulin L et al: Efficacy of somatostatin in a patient with carcinoid syndrome. *Lancet* **2**:43, 1978

41. Quatrini M et al: Effects of somatostatin infusion in four patients with malignant carcinoid syndrome. *Am J Gastroenterol* **78**:149, 1983

42. Maton PN: Use in patients with gut neuroendocrine tumors, p 41, in Gordon P, moderator: Somatostatin and somatostatin analogue (SMS 201-995) in treatment of hormone-secreting tumors of the pituitary and gastrointestinal tract and non-neoplastic diseases of the gut. *Ann Intern Med* **110**:35, 1989

43. Marsh HM et al: Carcinoid crisis during anesthesia: Successful treatment with a somatostatin analogue. *Anesthesiology* **66**:89, 1987

SECTION 29

Cutaneous Manifestations
of Multisystem Diseases

CHAPTER 171

Naomi F. Rothfield

Lupus Erythematosus

Chronic Discoid Lupus Erythematosus

Chronic discoid lupus erythematosus (CDLE) is a skin disease characterized by the presence of well-defined, raised, erythematous lesions that spread slowly with an irregular outline while the centers of the lesions heal with scaling, atrophy, and scarring. The lesions are located most often on the face, ears, and scalp. A number of clinical varieties of the disease are described below.

Although the lesions, which may be of varying sizes, are generally located above the neck, some patients have more extensive lesions on the neck, back and shoulders, forearms, and even the legs. On the basis of clinical experience, patients have been separated into those having the localized form, in which there are no lesions or virtually no lesions below the neck, and those with widespread lesions, which may affect extensive areas of the body. Some believe that patients with widespread lesions are more likely to develop systemic disease.

In order to avoid confusion with systemic and generalized lupus erythematosus, the term *widespread* is recommended for the description of CDLE involving many areas as opposed to the term *localized,* which is used when the disease is restricted to the face and scalp. The terms *generalized* or *disseminated,* when used to describe widespread CDLE, lead to confusion with the systemic (or acute, generalized) variety, in which constitutional symptoms, multiple-system involvement, and laboratory abnormalities are the main findings and in which skin manifestations may or may not be present. In contrast with systemic lupus erythematosus (SLE), the skin lesions are the principal, and generally single, finding of CDLE, both in the localized and widespread forms.

Historical Aspects

The erythematous and atrophic nature of the skin disease caused Cazenave to classify it in 1851 as a variety of lupus and to give it its name. Since then it has been divorced from a tuberculous cause, but the descriptive name *lupus* (meaning to have the appearance of something that has been gnawed at by a wolf) has remained. Kaposi, in 1872, separated the chronic discoid form from the acute systemic form.

Epidemiology

CDLE is not a rare disease but its prevalance is unknown. Although CDLE can be found occasionally in infants as well as in older persons, most cases are found in adults between the ages of 25 and 45.[1] Women are affected twice as often as men, and the disease occurs in all races.

Etiology and Pathogenesis

The cause of CDLE is unknown. There are few reports of CDLE in relatives of patients with the disease. A number of individuals with a hereditary deficiency of the second complement component (C2) have lesions of discoid lupus as their only clinical abnormality.[2]

Various factors induce the appearance of lesions of CDLE in predisposed individuals. Approximately 40 percent of the patients with CDLE suffer exacerbation of the disease during summer.[1] The lesions of a few patients also become worse under the influence of cold and wind. Other forms of trauma, such as thermal burns and direct physical force (contusion), have been implicated in causing the lesions of CDLE at the site of the trauma. Occasionally seen is the aberrant localization of lesions of CDLE, for example, on the buttock (due to a burn) or on the thigh (due to a contusion), in patients who previously had a few lesions normally distributed on the face and scalp.

A number of female patients with CDLE have noted exacerbation of their lesions during the premenstrual and menstrual period. This phenomenon also occurs in other dermatologic diseases and probably is a nonspecific increase in responsiveness of the skin due to changes in hormone levels.

The demonstration of immunoglobulins and complement proteins in the dermal-epidermal junction of lesions from patients with CDLE has led to renewed interest in the immunologic abnormalities of these patients. The absence of significant titers of antinuclear antibodies, the lack of antibodies to native DNA, and the normal serum levels of complement proteins suggest that the pathogenesis of CDLE differs from that of SLE (see below).

Clinical Manifestations

CDLE generally starts with one or more raised, sharply limited papules on the butterfly area of the face or on the scalp, forehead (Fig. 171-1), or ears, although any site may be affected.[3] The papule may be slightly pruritic or asymptomatic. It enlarges slowly and eventually presents the typical clinical form described below. Occasionally the eruption is much more widespread at onset and consists of several erythematous, rather rapidly enlarging, slightly elevated lesions that may be mistaken for a form of tinea. The mature

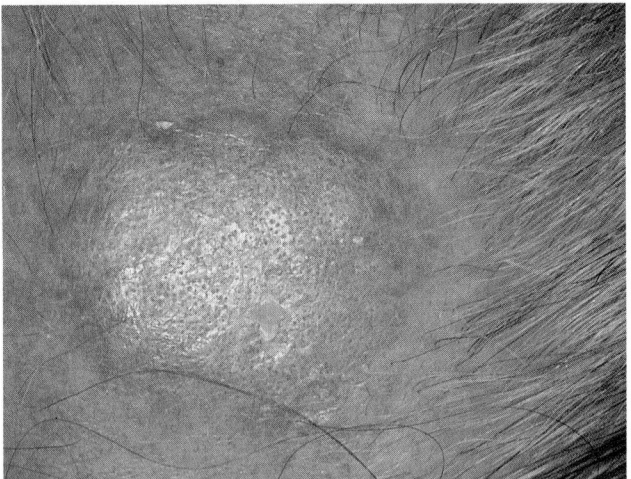

FIGURE 171-1 Lupus erythematosus, chronic discoid (CDLE). Typical early erythematous plaque on the forehead showing hyperkeratosis and accentuation of hair follicle infundibulum in a 60-year-old male with a 25-year history of CDLE. The lesion had been present for 3 months; no atrophy was present at this stage.

lesions generally consist of sharply outlined papules and plaques with bright erythema, edema, and some elevation when the process is beginning, and eventually showing central atrophy and depression (Fig. 171-2). As the plaque enlarges, the center fades and becomes atrophic, while the edges retain their edematous and erythematous appearance. The outline of the lesion is irregular. Active areas often show telangiectasia, and as the acute stage subsides, there is development of follicular scales with follicular plugging. Eventually, atrophy develops from the center of the lesions outward (Fig. 171-3a, b).

Thus, the three events—erythema, hyperkeratosis, and atrophy—follow each other. The lesions are usually concentric, with erythema at the periphery and atrophy at the center. However, most often one of the processes is much more marked than the others; after the process has burned itself out, only a white atrophic plaque remains, generally with loss of pigment and occasionally also with small areas of hyperpigmentation. Leukoderma may be extensive in the affected skin of black patients.

Areas most commonly affected are the malar areas, the nose, the scalp, and the external ears. However, any area of the head may be involved, including the oral mucosa, particularly the palate (Figs. 171-3c, 171-4), which may show a fairly sharply outlined erythematous patch with dilation of the blood vessels. The edges of the eyelids or the lips may also be involved and are at times the only areas affected, leading to some diagnostic difficulties. Lesions on the lip frequently have characteristic silvery white scales at the margin. Intraoral discoid lupus may be painful and may be confused both clinically and histologically with lichen planus. Immunohistology will help confirm discoid lesions. The palms and soles are rarely involved. When they are, there is marked hyperkeratosis of up to 1-in. thickness and immobility of the fingers. When the disease is widespread, it may involve the upper chest, the back, the arms, and much more rarely the lower extremities, with papules and plaques having the characteristic appearance.

The hypertrophic form of CDLE occurs in about 2 percent of patients who usually also have typical discoid lesions elsewhere. This form consists of raised, indurated, hyperkeratotic lesions,

generally on the face or on the extensor surfaces of the upper extremities or palms and soles. As the lesions mature they form nodules, and squamous cell carcinomas have been reported to arise in these lesions. The hypertrophic form may be confused with hypertrophic psoriasis or with hypertrophic lichen planus.

The profundus form (Kaposi-Irgang) may be associated with CDLE. This form presents with deep cutaneous nodules often associated with the usual discoid variety (Fig. 171-5).[4] A panniculitis involves the subdermal fat, with typical lesions of discoid lupus overlying the nodules or with normal-appearing epidermis. Lesions are most commonly present on the arms, buttocks, thighs, and breasts. These movable nodules are also found on the forehead, cheeks, chin, and eyelids. Histologically, the lesions are characterized by the presence of hyaline necrosis of fat with lymphocytic aggregates or lymphoid nodules in the fat. Calcification is common. Direct immunofluorescence may be helpful in the diagnosis. The lesions eventually heal with deep atrophy of the involved areas.

Laboratory Findings

A search for abnormal laboratory values in patients with CDLE is generally unrewarding, even when patients and controls are carefully selected. Antinuclear antibodies are rarely positive. Significant levels of antibodies to native DNA are not found, and the levels of C3 and C4 are not depressed. There is a higher than normal prevalence of genetic C2 deficiency in patients with CDLE, which may account for multiple cases with or without additional cases of SLE in the same family.[2,5]

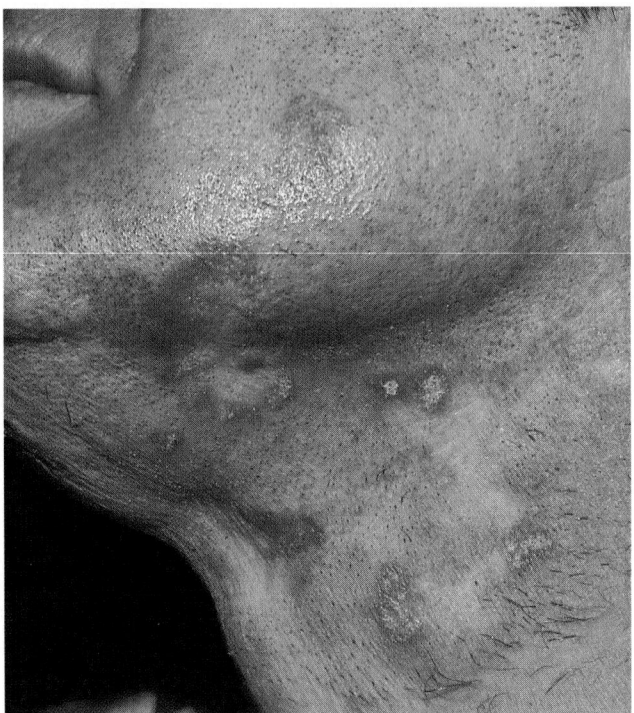

FIGURE 171-2 CDLE. Round-to-ovoid, slightly indurated, red-violaceous patches, fairly sharply demarcated, on the neck and face. Most patches show a slight follicular keratotic scaling, and some show central atrophy. Hypopigmentation and scarring mark the sites of lesions that have resolved.

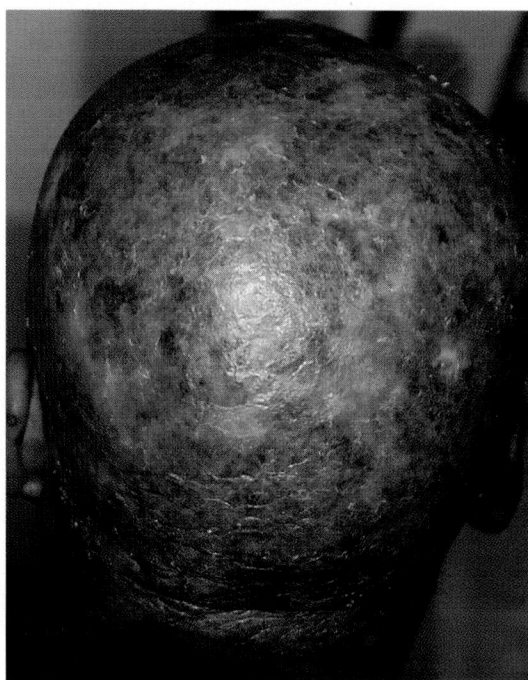

a

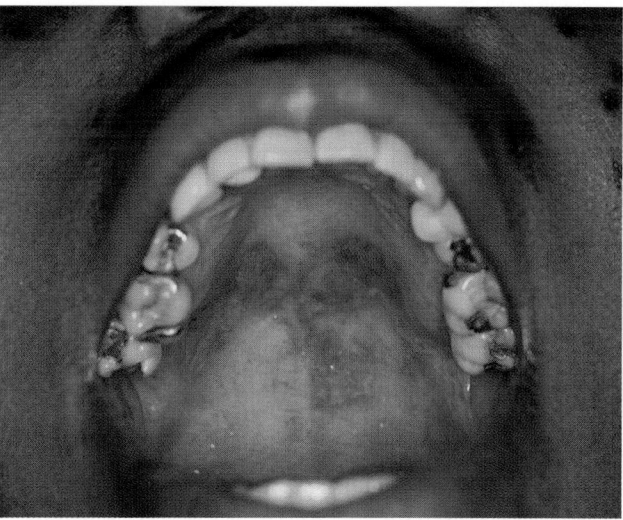

c

FIGURE 171-3 CDLE in a 45-year-old African-American female with a 20-year history of untreated CDLE. (*a*) Confluent lesions of the scalp have resulted in extensive scarring alopecia. (*b*) Characteristic involvement of the ear shows lesions with atrophy and postinflammatory hyperpigmentation, as well as inflammatory red plaques on the scalp with postinflammatory hypopigmentation. (*c*) Plaques of CDLE on the mucosa of the hard and soft palate showing similar morphology to cutaneous lesions.

layer damage. The basal margin is preserved, but the basal cells show some disorganization with liquefaction degeneration (Fig. 171-6). Basal cells show poor cohesion with vacuolization and irregularity of size. The upper dermis is edematous and the small blood vessels are dilated. The inflammatory round cell infiltrate of

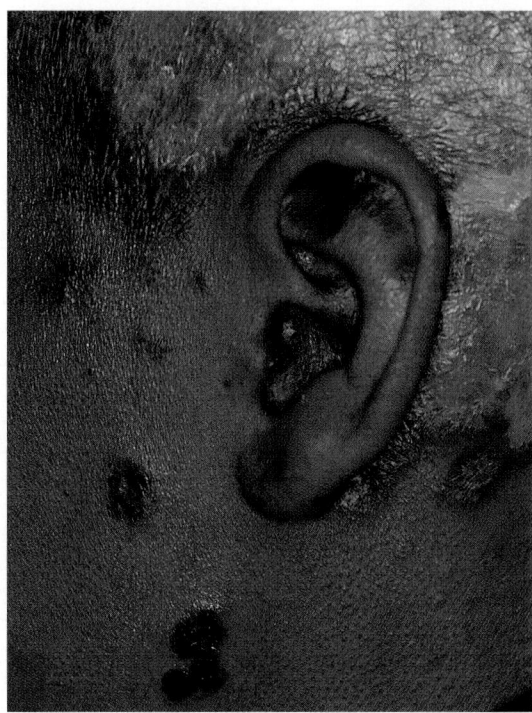

b

Histopathology

As would be expected, the appearance of CDLE varies according to the type of clinical lesion from which the biopsy is taken and reflects the visible skin alterations. The epidermis may be hyperkeratotic or atrophic, depending on the stage of the disease. When there is a hyperkeratosis, it is primarily follicular with formation of horny plugs dilating the follicular orifices. The epidermis itself is generally thin. The most characteristic feature is the evidence of basal

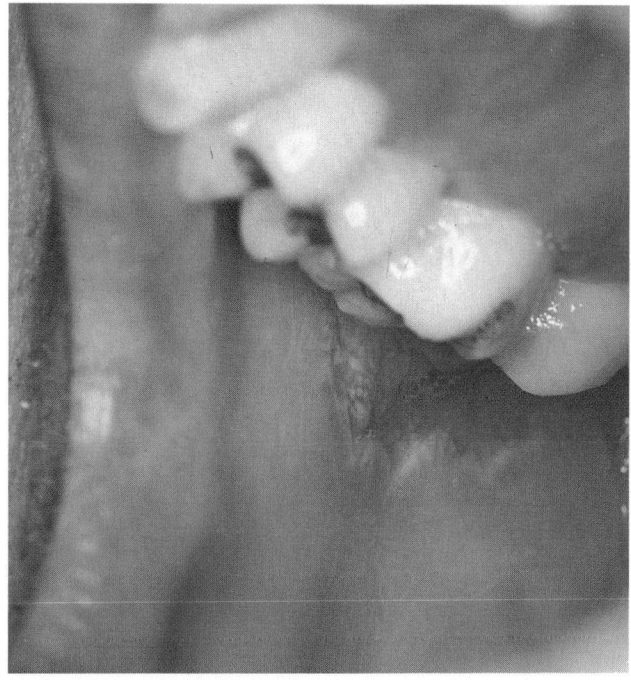

FIGURE 171-4 CDLE. Closeup of a plaque of CDLE on the buccal mucosa.

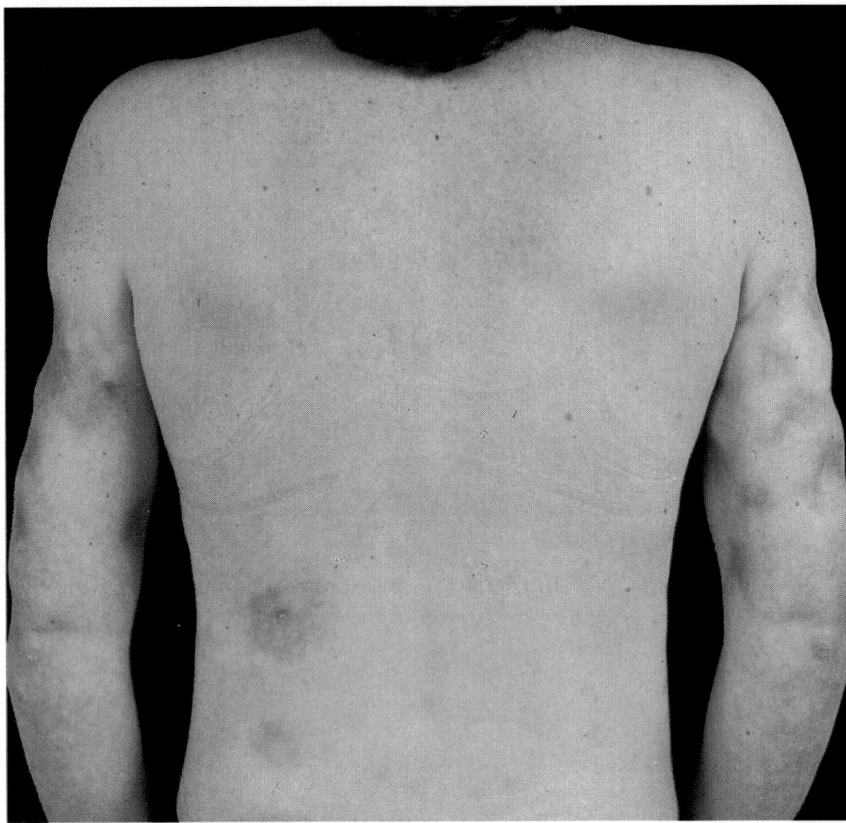

FIGURE 171-5 CDLE. Chronic panniculitis has resulted in large, sunken areas of overlying skin; erythema and atrophy of skin are seen.

lymphocytes and histiocytes is patchy and is localized around the hair follicle and the sebaceous glands and vessels. Eventually, the appendages atrophy and disappear. Staining with PAS reveals the subepidermal, thickened basement zone.

In electron microscopic studies, early lesions of CDLE reveal minimal, nonspecific changes. Chronic lesions show disintegration and necrosis of basal cell cytoplasm and lamination or multiplication of the basal lamina at the dermal-epidermal junction and around blood vessels.

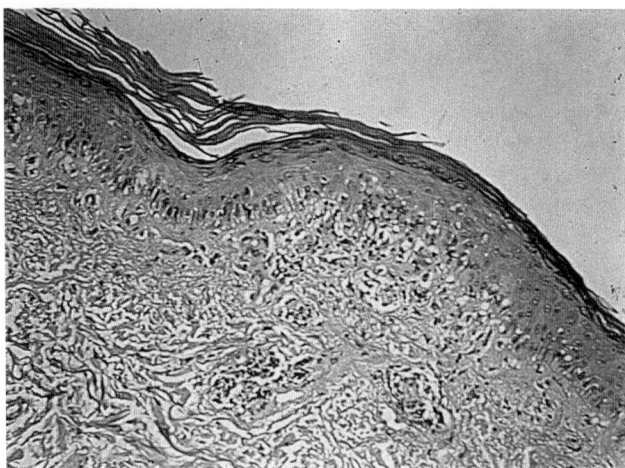

FIGURE 171-6 CDLE. Histology of lesion showing marked basal cell layer damage with vacuolization and irregularity of basal cell size. Some hyperkeratosis is evident.

Immunohistology

Biopsy specimens of lesions from patients with CDLE usually contain deposits of immunoglobulins and proteins of the classical and alternative complement pathways. With direct immunofluorescence, a narrow region of the dermal-epidermal junction is specifically stained by fluorescein isothiocyanate–conjugated immunoglobulins when the specimen is viewed under UV light (Fig. 171-7). The deposits appear in a granular, globular, or dense pattern at the dermal-epidermal junction. IgM is usually demonstrated, IgG is much less common, and complement proteins are rare. Biopsies from lesions are usually positive if the lesions are at least 6 weeks old and have remained active. Ultrastructural studies with horseradish peroxidase–conjugated antibodies have revealed that the reactive zone in CDLE is similar to that found in SLE lesions, i.e., deposits at the dermal-epidermal junction occupy the uppermost layers of the dermis immediately beneath the basal cells.

Diagnosis and Differential Diagnosis

Most cases of CDLE do not present great difficulty in diagnosis. However, some of the lesions may at times be confused with various diseases and require histopathologic and immunopathologic examination in order to rule out or to confirm the diagnosis. The histologic picture is usually clear-cut enough to allow a definite diagnosis. The following diseases commonly may be confused with CDLE.

Chronic Polymorphous Light Eruptions   The plaquelike polymorphous light eruptions (PLE) may very closely resemble and, in

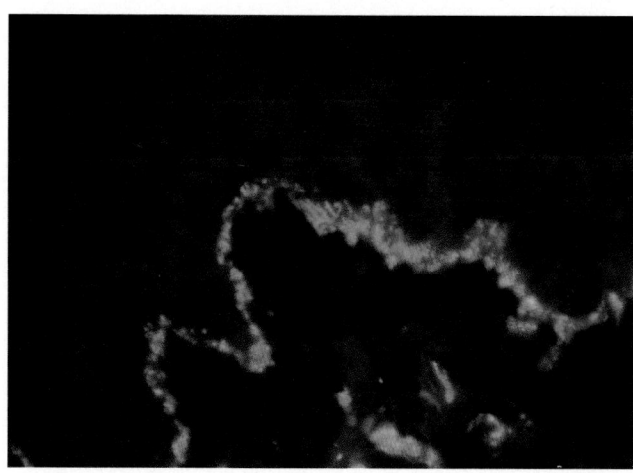

FIGURE 171-7   CDLE. Direct immunofluorescence of lesional skin biopsy showing a distinct granular fluorescence in the dermal-epidermal junction with fluorescein isothiocyanate conjugated goat anti-IgG.

fact, be indistinguishable clinically as well as histologically from early CDLE of the photosensitive variety. The lesions occur on the light-exposed areas of the body, including the butterfly area of the face, during the late spring or early summer after exposure to the sun, as does CDLE in many instances. The early histologic picture is quite similar. However, immunopathologic studies are negative in chronic PLE and are positive in about 90 percent of active CDLE lesions. Phototests with proper wavelength light will reproduce the disease on uninvolved skin of patients with PLE, whereas only one-third of CDLE patients will respond. The presence of lesions in the scalp or on areas protected from sunlight rules out the possibility that the eruption is due to light sensitivity. In addition, the development of adherent scales and of atrophy in the areas of the lesions suggest the diagnosis of CDLE. These characteristics do not occur in chronic PLE.

Seborrheic Dermatitis and Psoriasis   Seborrheic dermatitis or early psoriasis of the sun-sensitive type may also be distributed over the malar and butterfly areas of the face. These diseases can be confused with CDLE of the superficial, erythematous form; however, the biopsy is generally fairly conclusive in these cases. Immunopathology studies are negative in psoriasis and in seborrheic dermatitis. It is important to consider psoriasis in the differential diagnosis, as this disease may be considerably aggravated if antimalarial drugs are administered systemically.

Tinea   Isolated plaques of tinea due to *Trichophyton rubrum* may at times simulate the appearance of fairly typical CDLE when the lesions occur on the bearded area of the face. The raised, erythematous border and the central scaling with apparent atrophy may be present. Examination of the scrapings is helpful in these cases; biopsy will also rule out CDLE.

Sarcoidosis   Certain cases of sarcoid involving the skin present with raised erythematous lesions with advancing edges on the face, ears, scalp, arms, and upper trunk. Clinically, the picture may be very similar to certain forms of CDLE in its early active stages. These sarcoidal lesions do not progress to scarring. Histopathologic examination establishes the correct diagnosis.

Basal Cell Epithelioma (Superficial Type) and Rosacea   Superficial basal cell epithelioma may also simulate an isolated lesion of CDLE. There is an advancing raised border with telangiectasia and a central scaling with atrophy quite similar to that found in the more torpid lesions of CDLE. Here again, the biopsy is diagnostic. Rosacea may be difficult to distinguish from CDLE. However, erythematous papules containing tiny pustules at their apex are frequent in rosacea and absent in CDLE, and the characteristic atrophy seen in CDLE does not occur in rosacea. Immunoglobulins may be found in the dermal-epidermal junction in lesions of rosacea.

Scalp Lesions that may Resemble CDLE   Lichen planopilaris (lichen planus of the scalp), pseudopelade of Brocq, and tinea tonsurans may all resemble CDLE. Burnt-out lichen planopilaris may be quite similar to burnt-out CDLE, and in this case a biopsy may not be helpful because of the lack of active specific inflammatory infiltrate in the scarred, atrophic areas of either disease. Pseudopelade generally presents a more scattered and patchy appearance then the well-defined plaques of CDLE. Tinea tonsurans can be differentiated by using suitable laboratory examinations for fungi.

Lymphocytic Infiltration of the Skin (Jessner-Kanof)   This peculiar dermatosis affects primarily the face, although occasionally it is found on other parts of the body. It is generally confused clinically with the early stages of CDLE. Lesions are discoid, slightly elevated, and reddish, starting as small papules and expanding peripherally with occasional clearing in the center. There is no follicular hyperkeratosis, and the lesions regress without scarring. This is a relatively rare disease, and the diagnosis may be doubtful until a biopsy has been done.

Treatment

Patients with a history of aggravation of CDLE by physical trauma, cold, and sunlight should have adequate protection. Sunscreens are appropriate in winter as well as during warmer weather as wind and winter sun may be very harmful. Patients should always wear wide-brimmed hats when out of doors. Long sleeves and high-necked garmets should be worn by patients with lesions below the face. A preparation containing an opaque sunscreen is useful for protection of the lips.

Intralesional and Topical Treatment   Active lesions must be treated aggressively because they can lead to scarring. Short-term treatment for 1 to 2 weeks is helpful at the time of institution of antimalarial therapy. Any of the commonly used topical corticosteroids (classes 3, 4, 5) can be used on lesions, including those on the face. Intralesional steroids are very useful in patients with a few plaques. Intralesional triamcinolone acetonide diluted to a concentration of 3 to 4 mg/mL is most often used.

Systemic Therapy   Antimalarial agents are the drug of choice and are effective in most patients with CDLE.[6] Chloroquine and hydroxychloroquine (Plaquenil) are the drugs most commonly used. Chloroquine (250 mg) and hydroxychloroquine (200 mg) are given once or twice daily for 3 to 4 weeks and then the dose is reduced to once daily. A response is seen after 4 to 8 weeks. The drug may be slowly discontinued after lesions respond, but it is not uncommon for new lesions to appear or for old lesions to become active again 3 to 6 months after discontinuation. Quinacrine (100 mg) may be tried in patients who do not respond to either chloroquine or hydroxychloroquine, or quinacrine may be added to the regimen. All of the antimalarials cause ocular damage, including retinopathy.[7,8] The author followed a patient who took 100 mg of quinacrine daily for 18 years before she developed retinopathy. Other ocular abnormalities include effects on extraocular muscles leading to trouble in focusing, halos around lights (due to reversible corneal deposits), pigmentation of the skin, and myopathy. Patients should be examined by an ophthalmologist before therapy and every 4 to 6 months thereafter.

    Thalidomide has been used successfully to treat CDLE in Europe, but relapses occurred within a year in 70 percent of patients and significant polyneuritis occurred in 25 percent of patients.[6,9] Dapsone has been used in a dose of 100 mg per day with good results, but relapses within 3 months and significant side effects have lessened the enthusiasm for this agent.[6] Retinoids have been used for those patients who failed to improve with corticosteroids, thalidomide, and antimalarials.[6] Retinoids are very effective, especially in hyperkeratotic discoid lesions. Adverse reactions are common, and extreme caution must be used in women of child-bearing age because the drugs are teratogens. Azathioprine is occasionally used to treat very refractory lesions and hyperkeratotic lesions of the soles and palms.

Prognosis

Most patients with CDLE do extremely well. Progression to systemic disease is rare (from 1 to 5 percent). There are no laboratory markers to indicate which patients will progress. Patients should be reassured that they have a local and self-limited disease.

Systemic Lupus Erythematosus (SLE)

SLE is a systemic disease affecting multiple organ systems that is characterized by the presence of antibodies to nuclear antigens.

Historical Aspects

The term *lupus* was used during the early nineteenth century to characterize a destructive disease consisting of spreading ulcerations of the face. Kaposi distinguished the acute from the chronic variety in 1872, and in 1903 Osler described the systemic form of the disease without the skin lesions. The pathology of the disease was defined by Libman and Sacks, Gross, and Baehr. In 1948 the LE cell was described by Hargraves and associates, and in 1958 Friou and associates described a method to detect antinuclear antibodies using fluorescent antihuman globulin.

Epidemiology

SLE is the most common connective tissue disease. The prevalence has been reported as 50.8 per 100,000 of individuals over age 17. The prevalence in white females age 18 to 65 is about 1/1000 and in black females is 1/250.[10] In this age range, the disease is nearly 10 times more frequent in females than in males. Among children and the elderly, the disease is only twice as frequent in females than in males.

Etiology and Pathogenesis

Genetic   About 10 percent of patients with SLE have a first-degree relative with the disease. Multiple HLA associations have been reported, particularly for B8, DR2, DR3, DRw52, DQw1, and DQw2. The null gene for C4 occurs more often in patients with SLE and in their families.

Environmental   Drugs such as hydralazine, procainamide, isoniazid, methyldopa, sulfonamides, phenytoin, and penicillamine have been implicated as causing a lupus-like illness. Oral contraceptives have been suggested to induce the disease. The role of infectious agents is still to be defined. Toxins, food substances, and other environmental factors have not been implicated. Significant sunlight exposure clearly precedes the onset of SLE in about one-third of patients, particularly in New England and New York.

Pathogenesis   The immune system is clearly abnormal in patients with SLE. T cells do not control the activity of B cells, which are producing large numbers of autoantibodies. Some of the autoantibodies, e.g., anti-DNA, participate directly in the renal disease by forming immune complexes in the glomeruli. Other autoantibodies form complexes with their antigen and lead to vasculitis. Immunoglobulins and complement are found in skin lesions and also in normal skin. However, in the skin lesions the later complement proteins are also found.

    At the present time, SLE is thought to be a disorder in which genetic defects are present but not yet delineated. These defects lead to defective homeostasis between B and T cells so that when the individual is challenged by ultraviolet light, by infection, or by an unknown stimulus, the B cells become hyperactive, leading to a variety of autoantibodies.

Clinical Manifestations

History   Because SLE is a multisystem disease, a complete review of systems must be obtained and should include questions relating to the presence of the clinical manifestations listed in Table 171-1. One of the most outstanding complaints of untreated patients with SLE is fatigue. Not infrequently, this is misdiagnosed as psychoneurosis, and the patient is dismissed from the physician's care. The fatigue is a very real part of the clinical manifestations of SLE. Frequently, the first manifestations of SLE are misdiagnosed as an infectious process, and the patient may receive antibiotics. The appearance of a diffuse erythematous maculopapular eruption may then be mistaken for an allergic reaction to the antibiotic. It is extremely important to determine whether the patient has a history of a disorder that can be considered a manifestation of SLE, such as idiopathic thrombocytopenic purpura, rheumatoid arthritis, Sjögren's syndrome, chronic hepatitis, pleuritis, or convulsions. It is important to determine whether the patient has taken hydralazine, procainamide, penicillin, anticonvulsants, sulfonamides, or birth control pills. The family history is important in ascertaining whether there is a history of SLE or CDLE in a first-degree relative (in about 10 percent of patients) or whether there is a history of hemolytic anemia, thrombocytopenia, chronic spontaneous miscarriages, or clotting abnormalities (suggestive of the anticardiolipin antibody syndrome).

Cutaneous Lesions   Some type of cutaneous involvement is present in about 85 percent of patients. An erythematous rash of a

TABLE 171-1
The 1982 Revised Criteria for Classification of Systemic Lupus Erythematosus*

Criterion	Definition
1. Malar rash	Fixed erythema, flat or raised, over the malar eminences, tending to spare the nasolabial folds
2. Discoid rash	Erythematous raised patches with adherent keratotic scaling and follicular plugging; atrophic scarring may occur in older lesions
3. Photosensitivity	Skin rash as a result of unusual reaction to sunlight, by patient history or physician observation
4. Oral ulcers	Oral or nasopharyngeal ulceration, usually painless, observed by a physician
5. Arthritis	Nonerosive arthritis involving two or more peripheral joints, characterized by tenderness, swelling, or effusion
6. Serositis	*a.* Pleuritis—convincing history of pleuritic pain or rub heard by a physician or evidence of pleural effusion *or* *b.* Pericarditis—documented by ECG or rub or evidence of pericardial effusion
7. Renal disorder	*a.* Persistent proteinuria— > 0.5 g/day or greater than 3+ if quantitation not performed *or* *b.* Cellular casts—may be red cell, hemoglobin, granular, tubular, or mixed
8. Neurologic disorder	*a.* Seizures—in the absence of offending drugs or known metabolic derangements, e.g., uremia, ketoacidosis, or electrolyte imbalance *or* *b.* Psychosis—in the absence of offending drugs or known metabolic derangements, e.g., uremia, ketoacidosis, or electrolyte imbalance
9. Hematologic disorder	*a.* Hemolytic anemia—with reticulocytosis *or* *b.* Leukopenia— < 4000/μL total on two or more occasions *or* *c.* Lymphopenia— < 1500/μL on two or more occasions *or* *d.* Thrombocytopenia— < 100,000/μL in the absence of offending drugs
10. Immunologic disorder	*a.* Positive LE cell preparation *or* *b.* Anti-DNA—antibody to native DNA in abnormal titer *or* *c.* Anti-Sm—presence of antibody to Sm nuclear antigen *or* *d.* False-positive serologies for syphilis—known to be positive for at least 6 months and confirmed by *Treponema pallidum* immobilization or fluorescent treponemal antibody absorption test
11. Antinuclear antibody	An abnormal titer of antinuclear antibody by immunofluorescence of an equivalent assay at any point in time and in the absence of drugs known to be associated with "drug-induced lupus" syndrome

*The proposed classification is based on 11 criteria. For the purpose of identifying patients in clinical studies, a person shall be said to have SLE if any 4 or more of the 11 criteria are present, serially or simultaneously, during any interval of observation.
SOURCE: Reprinted from *Arthritis Rheumatism,* copyright 1982. Used by permission of the American College of Rheumatology.[22]

variety of types is the most frequent cutaneous manifestation. The typical erythematous blush in the butterfly area (Fig. 171-8) was present at the time of diagnosis in 52 percent of the author's first 356 patients with SLE. Only 16 of the 356 patients developed a blush for the first time later in the course of the disease. The blush is a very slightly edematous lesion located on both cheeks and across the bridge of the nose. It is commonly the first manifestation of the disease, preceding by weeks or months the onset of multisystem disease, and occurs very frequently after sun exposure. At the onset the patient may mistake this butterfly blush for a sunburn and seek medical advice only after the lesion has persisted for a few weeks or after new areas of erythema have appeared elsewhere. This "butterfly blush" is particularly obvious in fair-skinned individuals and may be transiently observed in some patients after very brief exposure to sun. The lesion heals well and without scarring or pigmentation.

The second most common erythematous rash in patients with SLE is a maculopapular rash, which may resemble a drug eruption and which frequently occurs after sun exposure. These lesions are often pruritic and may be located any place on the body, although sites of predilection are above the waistline. Scattered macular lesions are occasionally also located on the palms and fingers (Fig. 171-9) and, rarely, on the soles of the feet. In most instances, the maculopapular eruption also heals without scarring or hyperpig-

mentation. However, the lesions may persist and become crusted, and eventually some superficial atrophy may develop.

CDLE lesions occur in patients with SLE. In the author's first series of 356 patients with SLE, CDLE patients were present in 19 percent. Among these patients, 39 percent had had the CDLE lesions for 2 to 35 years prior to the onset of multiple system disease, 53 percent had CDLE lesions develop within 6 months of the diagnosis of SLE, and only 8 percent developed CDLE lesions after the diagnosis of SLE had been made. The patients with SLE and CDLE lesions did not differ from the rest of the patients with SLE except for a significantly higher incidence of Raynaud's phenomenon and photosensitive rashes. No difference was noted in the incidence of severe renal disease.

Widespread, nonscarring photosensitive erythematous lesions that are either annular or papular have been termed *subacute cutaneous lupus erythematosus.*[11] These lesions were thought to be histologically distinguishable from the lesions of CDLE but recent studies have shown that the histologic differentiation of discoid and subacute lupus cannot be made on the basis of the histologic features.[12,13] The main distinguishing feature of the subacute lesion is the lack of thick adherent scales and the lack of atrophic scarring and follicular involvement. Patients with so-called subacute lesions nearly always meet the American Rheumatism Association's Criteria for the Classification of SLE (Table 171-1). In many of the

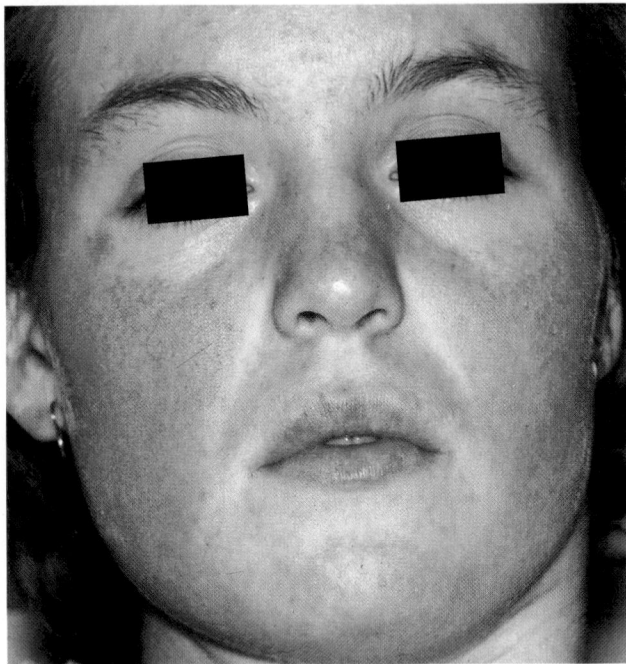

FIGURE 171-8 Lupus erythematosus, systemic (SLE). Erythematous, slightly edematous, sharply demarcated erythema are seen on the cheeks in a "butterfly" pattern.

The locations of the rash in patients with SLE vary greatly, although most patients have facial involvement. Twenty percent of patients have no facial rash of any type but do have skin lesions on other areas. Discoid lesions commonly involve the scalp; less frequently, the maculopapular erythematous lesions are present in the scalp. In both instances, patchy alopecia may occur. The CDLE lesions result in scarring, and therefore these areas of alopecia are permanent. The erythematous scaly lesions of SLE usually heal without scarring, and the hair most often regrows in the previously involved areas. Diffuse alopecia was present during an exacerbation of the disease in 60 percent of the author's patients. With therapy, there is a regrowth of hair, and during periods of clinical remission the patients do not complain of falling hair. The onset of diffuse alopecia is, in some patients, the first manifestation of an impending flare-up of the disease and can be used as a criterion of disease activity in these patients during regulation of therapy. Patients who have lost most of their hair at the time of the first severe illness should be reassured that, as they improve, their hair will grow back. Patchy alopecia is less common and also occurs during periods of clinical disease activity. The new hair growing in as the patient improves on therapy gives the patient's hair a stubbly look. As the patient continues to be free of clinical or serologic evidence of active disease, the new hair grows longer.

A common location of lesions of vasculitis with ulceration is on the extensor surface of the forearms. Less commonly, lesions are noted on the dorsa of the hands, on the palms, on or near the small joints of the fingers, and on the fingertips. Periungual erythema (Fig. 171-9b) has been noted in 10 percent of the author's patients and palmar erythema in 10 percent. Atrophie blanche lesions closely resembling lesions found in malignant atrophic papulosis (Degos' disease) occasionally occur. The patients usually have erythematous papular or infiltrated lesions that gradually develop porcelain-white centers with telangiectasia of their margins and may be found in areas of livedo reticularis. Small splinter hemorrhages are ocasionally observed.

author's patients with SLE, lesions typical of discoid and subacute forms are found. The patients with either subacute or discoid lesions are usually very sun-sensitive and have anti-Ro antibodies (see below). The subacute rash is also seen in infants with the congenital lupus syndrome associated with anti-Ro antibodies. In addition, many of the patients with SLE and C2 or C4 deficiency have lesions of either discoid lupus or subacute lupus.

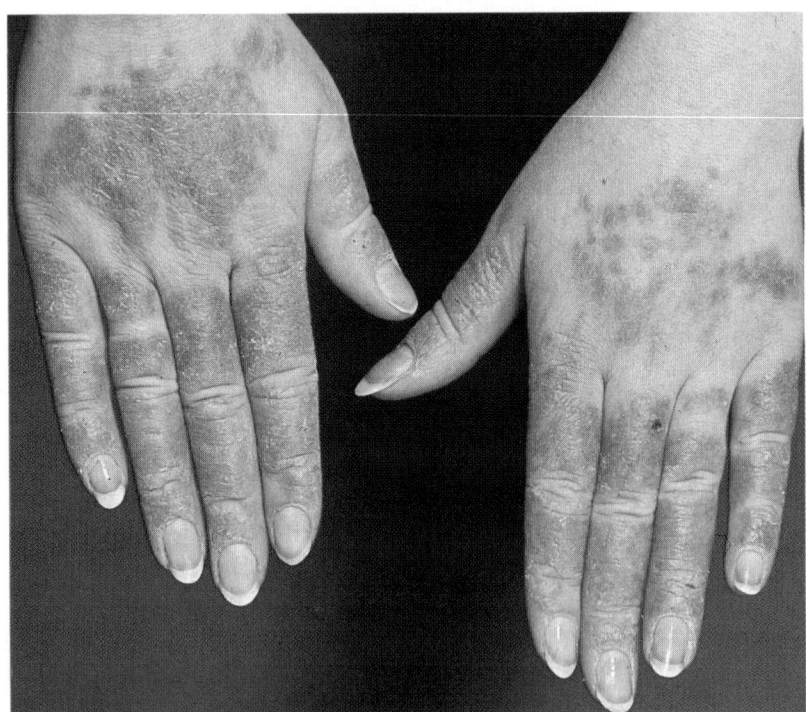

a

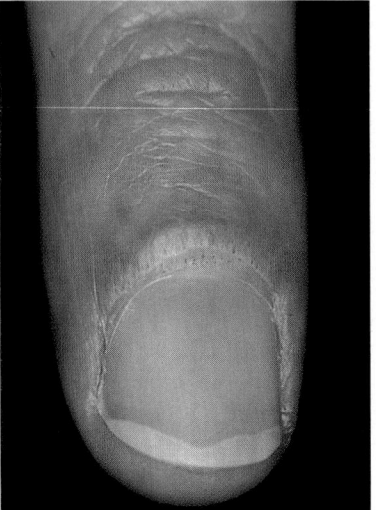

b

FIGURE 171-9 SLE. (*a*) Red-to-violaceous, well-demarcated plaques on the dorsa of the fingers and hands with periungual erythema sparing the knuckles. (*b*) Closeup of periungual erythema and telangiectasia.

Livedo reticularis is not uncommon in patients with SLE, especially in those with active disease. It is especially common on the lower extremities, around the elbows, knees, and ankles and is present when the skin is warm. Fixed livedo reticularis of the upper extremities and of the trunk is due to vasculitis and is usually seen in patients with severe active disease; it may be associated with antiphospholipid antibodies, false-positive tests for syphilis, and/or the lupus anticoagulant. Purple discoloration of the toes when these are in a dependent position is also common. Livedo reticularis may precede severe cyanosis and gangrene in some patients. Mucosal ulcers, appearing very much like aphthous stomatitis, are common (36 percent of the author's patients). The lesions are usually present on the palate, but the vaginal, laryngeal, and nasal mucosa are occasionally involved. These mucosal ulcers are seen most commonly in patients with SLE who have severe skin lesions. Mucosal ulcers are usually asymptomatic and superficial and disappear within a few days of increased corticosteroid therapy. They are frequently the first clinical finding of a flare-up of the disease.

Nasal septal ulcerations may rarely occur, especially during disease activity, and may lead to septal perforation.[14] Although septal ulcers are asymptomatic, patients with perforations complain of epistaxis and nasal obstruction due to secretions or crusts. Perforations characteristically involve the anteroinferior part of the cartilaginous septum. The nasal mucosal margin becomes erythematous and edematous at times of disease activity and returns to normal when disease activity is controlled by increasing the dose of corticosteroids. Leg ulcers are usually located near the malleoli, are punched-out, and are exquisitely tender. The ulcerations may be the first manifestation of SLE, preceding multisystem disease by many years. They heal very slowly and may require skin grafting. Bullous lesions are infrequently seen and their presence should not rule out the diagnosis of SLE. In patients with thrombocytopenia, the bullae may be hemorrhagic. Periorbital edema occurs in some patients with an acute onset of lupus nephritis and may recur in these patients with the recurrence of hematuria. Urticaria and erythema multiforme are uncommon and may be related to increased clinical activity of the disease. Ecchymoses and petechiae may be observed in association with thrombocytopenia. In addition, many patients with SLE with no demonstrable hematologic abnormality complain of easy bruisability prior to the onset of multisystem disease. The most common cause of ecchymoses in patients with SLE is long-term steroid therapy.

Gangrene of the extremities due to arteritis of medium-sized arteries occurs rarely. Gangrene may be preceded by severe Raynaud's phenomenon or livedo reticularis.

Lupus profundus (panniculitis) (Fig. 171-5) is occasionally noted in patients with SLE who may also have lesions of CDLE. Soft-tissue calcification is noted rarely in SLE and occurs without myositis.[15] These patients have no abnormalities of calcium and phosphorus metabolism or of the serum alkaline phosphatase. Rheumatoid nodules are present in about 6 percent of patients with SLE and are usually associated with a nonerosive deforming arthritis.

General Manifestations   Fever, fatigue, weight loss, and generalized malaise are very common manifestations of SLE. At the time of diagnosis 68 percent of our patients had loss of weight, 83 percent had fever, and moderate to severe fatigue was present in 76 percent. Fever may be low-grade or spiking. It is important to remember that fever may represent the presence of infection in a patient with SLE and that infection should therefore always be ruled out.

Joint Manifestations   Joint involvement is the most common manifestation of SLE, occurring in 95 percent of patients. Arthritis with pain on motion, tenderness, or effusion is present in about 80 percent and arthralgia is present in an additional 15 percent of patients. The proximal interphalangeal, knee, wrist and metacarpophalangeal joints are most often involved. The joint involvement is usually strikingly symmetric. Morning stiffness was present in 50 percent of our patients. Deforming arthritis occurs in 15 percent of patients with SLE who have typical swan neck deformities and ulnar deviation of fingers. These deformities, unlike those in rheumatoid arthritis, reveal no bony erosions. Synovial fluid is usually clear with good viscosity and a low white blood cell count with predominance of mononuclear cells. Tendinitis is occasionally present, and tendon rupture occasionally occurs. Aseptic necrosis of the femoral head, knee, or wrist may occur late in the disease in corticosteroid-treated patients.

Myalgia and Myositis   At the time of diagnosis, myalgia was present in one-third of our patients. Pain and tenderness of muscles was much less common, and muscle weakness was rare. In patients with SLE treated with corticosteroids for more than a few months in moderate to high doses (40 to 60 mg per day), weakness of the proximal muscles may occur due to the therapy. Chloroquine myopathy has also been described.[16]

Renal Disease   Clinically evident kidney involvement occurs in approximately 55 to 60 percent of patients with SLE. The overall prognosis depends on the type and severity of the renal lesions. Patients with normal kidneys on renal biopsy [World Health Organization (WHO) class I] have no clinical evidence of renal disease. Patients with mesangial hypercellularity and immune deposits confined to the mesangium (WHO class II) usually have only mild proteinuria and have an excellent outcome as long as they are adequately treated and their systemic disease does not become active. Patients with focal proliferative lupus nephritis (WHO class III) usually have proteinuria and hematuria and occasionally may present with the nephrotic syndrome. These patients respond promptly to high doses of corticosteroids, and the renal disease does not progress unless future disease activity occurs. Patients with diffuse proliferative nephritis (WHO class IV) usually have significant proteinuria, hematuria, and may have red cell casts.[17,18] Renal insufficiency, severe nephrotic syndrome, and hypertension may be present. This type of renal disease is present in only about 20 percent of patients. At the present time, these patients have a good 5-year survival without dialysis, which is probably due to the more aggressive treatment used and to the use of serologic tests such as complement levels and antibodies to native DNA in monitoring the disease activity. Mild focal lupus nephritis is the most common form of renal disease and has an excellent prognosis.[17,18] The least common form of lupus nephritis is membranous nephritis (WHO class V), which is characterized by significant proteinuria, nephrotic syndrome, and, in some patients, hematuria. In patients with lupus nephritis, hypertension is a poor prognostic sign and should be treated aggressively. In addition to the WHO Classification, the biopsy is graded as to activity and sclerosis.[18] The possibility of eventual dialysis is significantly greater if the sclerotic index is high.

Cardiopulmonary Manifestations   The most common symptom is pleuritic chest pain, which is present in about 40 percent of patients. Pleural effusions are found somewhat less often and are usually exudates. Pulmonary infiltrates due to lupus pneumonitis occur in only 10 percent of patients, and the major manifestation is dyspnea. Rarely pulmonary hemorrhage may occur. It is very important to rule out infectious causes for any pulmonary infiltrate in a patient with SLE, and such patients should be aggressively studied and treated for infectious pneumonitis until this is done.

The most common cardiac manifestation is pericarditis, which occurs in about 25 percent of patients. Tachycardia, an enlarging heart, congestive heart failure, arrhythmias, and conduction defects are noted in an occasional patient. Coronary arteritis may lead to myocardial infarction in an occasional patient. More frequently, coronary artery disease is noted late in the course of the disease in patients treated with corticosteroids and is due to atherosclerosis of coronary arteries. Valvular involvement with dysfunction is rare. Subacute and acute bacterial endocarditis may be superimposed on a valve damaged by Libman-Sacks endocarditis.

Nervous System Manifestations   Peripheral neuropathy occurs in about 14 percent of patients and usually produces a mixed sensorimotor disturbance similar to mononeuritis multiplex. Guillain-Barré syndrome occasionally may also be present. Transverse myelitis occurs in less than 4 percent of patients. Movement disorders such as chorea or choreoathetosis are rarely observed but may be the first manifestation of disease. Grand mal seizures are noted in about 15 percent of patients early in the disease. Other types of seizure disorders, including Jacksonian seizures, psychomotor epilepsy, petit mal, and temporal lobe epilepsy, are rare.

Organic brain syndromes are characterized by impairment of orientation, perception, memory, and intellectual function.[19] This type of psychosis is found early in the course of the disease and is very rare later in the course if the patient remains in remission after the initial treatment. The 5-year survival was not influenced by the presence of organic brain syndrome at the time of diagnosis in our series of patients studied in New York at the Bellevue Hospital.[20] Severe headaches may occur in patients with SLE and may be associated with organic brain syndrome or seizures. In addition, these headaches, which are usually clinically indistinguishable from classic migraine headaches, may appear in patients with brain infarcts demonstrated by computed tomography (CT scan) or in patients with abnormal signals on magnetic resonance imaging (MRI). Arteritis of the cerebral arteries has been found in a small number of patients with severe headaches or evidence of cerebral vascular accidents who have been studied by arteriography.

Cerebrospinal fluid abnormalities occurred in 32 percent of the neuropsychiatric episodes in 37 patients reported by Feinglass et al.[19] Protein elevations occurred in one-half of the fluids, and increased numbers of white blood cells were occasionally noted. The electroencephalogram is usually abnormal in patients with organic brain syndrome or seizure disorders but may also be abnormal in patients without central nervous system manifestations. CT and MRI are reported abnormal in some patients with central nervous system disease but may eventually return to normal after treatment. Although cerebral atrophy is frequently reported, this finding may be nonspecific and should not be interpreted as evidence of central nervous system disease due to SLE.

Psychological abnormalities are very common in patients with SLE, especially in recently diagnosed individuals. Disfigurement due to the disease (skin lesions, alopecia) and due to the corticosteroid therapy leads to significant reactive depression in many patients. Unless the physician provides adequate psychological support and uses allied health professionals such as nurses or support groups, patients may be confused and noncompliant. Patients who are depressed and/or anxious should be encouraged to verbalize and

to seek additional help from a psychologist or psychiatrist, if necessary. The psychological abnormalities must be distinguished from organic brain syndrome and should not be considered as manifestations of the disease requiring increases in corticosteroid therapy.

Gastrointestinal Manifestations   Gastrointestinal manifestations such as nausea, vomiting, or anorexia are present in about 20 percent of patients at the time of diagnosis or during periods of disease activity. Abdominal pain is uncommon, occurring in only 10 percent, but is a very important symptom. Crampy abdominal pain associated with localizing signs and rebound tenderness should be viewed as a surgical emergency. Perforation of the large or small bowel or infarction without perforation is due to mesenteric arteritis. Such patients have other evidence of disease activity and should have the earliest surgical intervention possible since only those who have received surgery early have survived. Other abdominal pain may be due to non-SLE causes such as rupture of an ovarian cyst, tubal-ovarian abscess, or appendicitis. Early diagnosis and surgical intervention are crucial in these patients.

Ascites is rarely present in patients with SLE, but may be massive when it does occur. Dysphagia may be present and is usually associated with Raynaud's phenomenon. Hepatomegaly occurs in about 30 percent of patients, and liver enzyme abnormalities may also occur. Biopsy-proved chronic active hepatitis may be associated with active SLE. Splenomegaly is present in 20 percent of patients and is usually not associated with hemolytic anemia.

Lymphadenopathy   Enlarged lymph nodes are present in about one-half of patients during disease activity. These nodes may be moderately enlarged in children and may be associated with hepatosplenomegaly, suggesting a diagnosis of lymphoma.

Ocular Manifestations   Conjunctivitis and episcleritis occur in about 15 percent of patients and are usually associated with extensive cutaneous lesions. Occlusion of the central retinal artery may occur, as well as blindness from retinal arteritis. Recently, an association between thrombosis of retinal vessels and the presence of the antiphospholipid antibody has been recognized. Cytoid bodies are present in about 8 percent of patients. These are hard white lesions adjacent to retinal vessels, which appear during disease activity and are due to retinal artery vasculitis. Keratoconjunctivitis sicca may occur in patients with SLE.

Parotid Gland Manifestations   Acute enlargement of one or both parotid glands occurs occasionally in patients with SLE. The swelling may be painful and usually returns to normal as the systemic disease is controlled. This enlargement may be associated with the presence of Sjögren's syndrome.

Menstrual Abnormalities and Pregnancy   Some patients report that they have an increase in SLE symptoms, such as joint pain or rashes, immediately prior to their menstrual periods. Pregnancy is associated with flare of the disease if the disease is active at the time of conception. Thus, pregnancy should be avoided for the first few years of the disease or until it is well controlled with low doses of corticosteroids. Postpartum flare of the disease can be controlled by increasing corticosteroid doses during labor.

Hematologic Abnormalities   One or more hematologic abnormalities are present in nearly all patients with SLE who have clinical evidence of active disease. Most common is a mild to moderate normocytic normochromic anemia, which occurs in one-half of patients. Hemolytic anemia with reticulocytosis occurs in only 10 percent of patients. Leukopenia with white blood cell counts <4000/μL was present in only 17 percent of our 356 patients. Most patients with active disease have an absolute lymphophenia. Mild thrombocytopenia is present in one-third of patients with SLE, but significant thrombocytopenia (<100,000 platelets/μL) occurs less frequently.

Laboratory Findings in Systemic Lupus Erythematosus

A broad spectrum of autoantibodies may be found in patients with SLE. Antinuclear antibodies (ANA) are usually detected for screening purposes by the indirect fluorescence antibody technique. ANA are positive in nearly all patients with SLE who have clinical evidence of active disease. Occasionally, a patient who has been in corticosteroid-induced prolonged remission is found to have exceedingly low levels of ANA that are in the normal range. ANA are found in many other diseases, and the diagnosis of SLE should never be made in a patient with a positive ANA and the absence of multisystem disease. Anti-DNA antibodies are much more specific and, depending on the laboratory, may be found in significant levels only in patients with SLE. These antibodies usually become lower in titer when the disease is less active and disappear in remission. The anti-DNA antibodies are present in only 70 percent of patients with active disease.[21] Anti-single stranded DNA antibodies are not specific for SLE and are not a useful clinical test. Anti-Sm, an acidic nuclear protein, is very specific for patients with SLE and may be present in patients for years whether or not the disease is active. Unfortunately, anti-Sm is present in only about 20 percent of patients with SLE. Anti-RNP is not specific for SLE. Anti-Ro and anti-La are also not specific for SLE but are also found in Sjögren's syndrome. Anti-Ro is important because it has been identified in all of the mothers who have a baby born with congenital heart block.

The lupus anticoagulant can be identified by the presence of a slight prolongation of the thromboplastin time and a more marked prolongation of the partial thromboplastin time. This prolongation of the partial thromboplastin time cannot be corrected by the addition of equal volumes of normal plasma to the patient's plasma at varying dilutions. This in vitro clotting abnormality is due to an antibody to phospholipid and may be detected by an antiphospholipid antibody test using enzyme-limited immunosorbent assay or by the presence of a false-positive test for syphilis. The lupus anticoagulant is associated with increased arterial and venous clotting and is usually found in patients with SLE who present with stroke, thrombophlebitis, and renal vein or mesenteric artery thrombosis. The lupus anticoagulant usually disappears with corticosteroid therapy. The lupus anticoagulant is frequently noted in patients with a false-positive test for syphilis. IgG anticardiolipin antibodies may be associated with arterial or venous thrombosis, chorea, and livedo reticularis.

Polyclonal hypergammaglobulinemia is common in patients with SLE as is an increased erythrocyte sedimentation rate. Serum complement levels are generally decreased in active SLE, especially in those patients with active nephritis. The first complement component to decrease is generally C4, followed by C3, C1q, and the total hemolytic complement activity (CH50). The C4 level usually remains depressed longest. Low complement levels are generally thought to result from complement consumption with fixation by antigen-antibody complexes. However, there is evidence that in some patients with SLE the major determinant of a low C3 level is its decreased synthesis.

Pathology and Immunopathology

The pathologic findings in patients with SLE who have died untreated may reveal no features typical of SLE. The characteristic histologic changes of SLE are hematoxylin bodies, which are LE bodies or masses of bluish dense homogeneous material. They are identical to the inclusion body of the LE cell and may be seen in many tissues. These are specific for SLE. Verrucous endocarditis of Libman-Sack, present in nearly all autopsied patients, are microscopic or macroscopic vegetations. The characteristic onionskin appearance found in the spleen is present in 15 percent of cases and is due to concentric periarterial fibrosis, which may be the end stage of an earlier focal arteritis. Changes in lymph nodes, muscles, pericardium, pleura, and synovium are mild and nonspecific. Characteristically, vasculitis of small vessels is present in many organs.

Skin histology varies with the clinical lesion. In the acute SLE rash there are distinct characteristics: thinning of the epidermis, liquefaction degeneration of the basal layer with disruption of the dermal-epidermal junction, edema of the upper dermis, scattered infiltrate of lymphocytes in the dermis, and fibrinoid degeneration of the connective tissue with fibrinoid clumps, which stain with alcian blue because the clumps contain mucopolysaccharides. Many skin lesions in SLE are not specific for the disease and display nonspecific vasculitis.

Examination of the normal-appearing skin by direct immunofluorescence can also be useful in the diagnosis of patients with SLE. The presence of subepidermal immunoglobulin and complement protein deposits in uninvolved skin of patients with cutaneous LE is evidence for systemic disease. The presence of IgM alone at the dermal-epidermal junction of normal skin suggests benign, nonaggressive disease and is not diagnostic of SLE.

Diagnosis and Differential Diagnosis

The diagnosis of SLE is based on the presence of multisystem disease in addition to the presence of antinuclear antibodies. The Revised Criteria for the Classification of SLE proposed by the American Rheumatism Association[22] are shown in Table 171-1. These criteria are not to be used in individual patients except as guidelines. Only about 50 percent of SLE patients meet these criteria at the time a diagnosis of SLE is made.[23] A low serum complement level is present in about 70 percent of patients with SLE and when both low C3 and high anti-double stranded DNA antibodies are present the diagnosis of SLE is almost certain.[21] Some patients with other diseases may meet the criteria, e.g., patients with early forms of scleroderma. Alopecia and Raynaud's phenomenon are not included in the Revised Criteria but are very important manifestations to consider in the diagnosis of patients with multisystem disease. Some of the conditions that may be confused with SLE include subacute bacterial endocarditis, gonococcal or meningococcal septicemia with arthritis and skin lesions, drug reactions, lymphoma and leukemia, thrombotic thrombocytopenic purpura, sarcoidosis, secondary syphilis, bacterial septicemia, and leprosy.

Treatment

The basis of treatment is the use of corticosteroids, which should be given in a dose adequate to control the multisystem disease and to return the anti-DNA antibodies and complement levels to normal. Depending on the activity and severity of the disease, the dose of corticosteroids may vary from 10 mg to 1 g intravenously per day. Cyclophosphamide is used in patients with severe vasculitis and in patients with diffuse proliferative lupus nephritis. In patients with repeated flares of the disease at moderately high doses of corticosteroids, azathioprine may be useful in order to allow the patient to be maintained on a lower corticosteroid dose. Antimalarials are very useful in patients with skin abnormalities, alopecia, or mucosal ulcers and may allow a lower dose of maintenance corticosteroids to be taken. Other therapies are experimental and space does not allow discussion of their use.

Course and Prognosis

Survival studies show significant improvement over the past decade with most series showing a 5-year survival of about 95 percent. Most patients require constant medical management to keep their disease under control on the lowest possible corticosteroid dose. Pregnancy, infection, and surgery may all precipitate an excerbation, but most exacerbations occur without a demonstrable cause. If the patient is under good medical care and is compliant, minor flares can easily be managed by an immediate, small increase of corticosteroids. Major exacerbations late in the course are unusual. Isolated thrombocytopenia may occur as an isolated event 10 to 15 years after the disease has been adequately treated. In general, patients with SLE, even those with renal disease, do well and live normal productive lives.

References

1. Rothfield NF et al: Chronic discoid lupus erythematosus: A study of 65 patients and 65 controls. *N Engl J Med* **269**:1155, 1963
2. Agnello V: Complement deficiency states. *Medicine* **57**:1, 1978
3. Hymes SR, Jordon RE: Chronic cutaneous lupus erythematosus. *Med Clin North Am* **73**:1055, 1989
4. Peters MS, Su WPD: Lupus erythematosus panniculitis. *Med Clin North Am* **73**:1113, 1989
5. Belin DC et al: Familial discoid lupus erythematosus associated with familial heterozygote C2 deficiency. *Arthritis Rheum* **23**:898, 1980
6. Lo JS et al: Treatment of discoid lupus erythematosus. *Int J Dermatol* **28**:497, 1989
7. Henkind P, Rothfield NF: Ocular abnormalities in patients treated with synthetic antimalarial drugs. *N Engl J Med* **269**:433, 1963
8. Meislin AG, Rothfield NF: Systemic lupus erythematosus in childhood. *Pediatrics* **42**:37, 1968
9. Knop J et al: Thalidomide in the treatment of sixty cases of chronic discoid lupus erythematosus. *Br J Dermatol* **109**:461, 1983
10. Fessel WJ: Systemic lupus erythematosus in the community. *Arch Intern Med* **134**:1027, 1974
11. Sontheimer RD et al: Subacute cutaneous lupus erythematosus. A cutaneous marker for a distinct lupus erythematosus subset. *Arch Dermatol* **115**:1409, 1979
12. Bangert JL et al: Subacute cutaneous lupus erythematosus and discoid lupus erythematosus. *Arch Dermatol* **120**:332, 1984
13. Jerdan MS et al: Histopathologic comparison of the subsets of lupus erythematosus. *Arch Dermatol* **126**:52, 1990
14. Synder GG III et al: Nasal septal perforation in systemic lupus erythematosus: *Arch Otology* **99**:456, 1974
15. Rothe MJ et al: Extensive calcinosis cutis with systemic lupus erythematosus. *Arch Dermatol* **126**:1060, 1990
16. Itobashi HH, Kokman E: Chloroquine neuromyopathy. A reversible granulovacuolar myopathy. *Arch Pathol* **93**:209, 1972
17. Baldwin DS et al: The clinical course of the proliferative and membranous forms of lupus nephritis. *Ann Intern Med* **75**:929, 1970
18. Morel-Maroger L et al: The course of lupus nephritis: Contribution of serial renal biopsies. *Adv Nephrol* **6**:79, 1976
19. Feinglass EJ et al: Neuropsychiatric manifestations of systemic lupus erythematosus: Diagnosis, clinical spectrum, and relationship to other features of the disease. *Medicine (Baltimore)* **55**:323, 1976
20. Urman JD, Rothfield NF: Corticosteroid treatment in systemic lupus erythematosus: Survival studies. *JAMA* **238**:2272, 1977
21. Weinstein A et al: Antibodies to native DNA and serum complement (C3) levels. *Am J Med* **74**:206, 1983
22. Tan EM et al: Revised criteria for the classification of systemic lupus erythematosus. *Arthritis Rheum* **25**:1271, 1982
23. Levin RE et al: A comparison of the sensitivity of the 1971 and 1982 American Rheumatism Association criteria for the classification of systemic lupus erythematosus. *Arthritis Rheum* **27**:530, 1984

CHAPTER 172

John A. Mills   # Dermatomyositis

Dermatomyositis and polymyositis are the most common idiopathic inflammatory myopathies, a group of diseases that also includes juvenile dermatomyositis, inclusion body myopathy, and giant cell myositis. Myositis is also a variable component of other connective tissue diseases such as systemic lupus erythematosus, scleroderma, and Sjögren's syndrome. When myopathy is associated with clinical features of another connective tissue disease, precise classification is often difficult.

Myopathies caused by infection, drugs, or toxins should be distinguished from the idiopathic inflammatory myopathies. The syndrome of acute rhabdomyolysis, which is usually a consequence of severe metabolic stress in individuals with a latent abnormality of muscle metabolism, is also a distinct disorder. However, patients who are ultimately diagnosed as having an inflammatory myopathy may sometimes present with rhabdomyolysis.

Dermatomyositis and polymyositis have been considered to be essentially the same disease except for the presence or absence of a rash. Their relationship is being reexamined in the light of recent serologic studies, although they are still commonly considered together in most medical literature.

There is no completely satisfactory classification of the idiopathic inflammatory myopathies.[1] On the basis of histology, inclusion body myopathy, giant cell myositis, and juvenile dermatomyositis can be distinguished from the other disorders. The histology of adult dermatomyositis, polymyositis, and myositis in patients with other connective tissue diseases is indistinguishable at the present time.

Historical Aspects

The first detailed description of dermatomyositis was that of Wagner in 1863.[2] No extensive clinical experience was reported in the English literature until that of O'Leary and Waisman from the Mayo Clinic in 1940.[3] Studies of two large patient series appeared in 1957 and 1958.[4,5] These, together with an analysis of 153 cases by Carl Pearson's group in 1977,[6] form the basis of much of our current clinical information.

The dermatologic manifestations were probably first described in detail by Unverrecht in 1887,[7] but they were not clearly distinguished from those of systemic lupus erythematosus until Kiel reported his meticulous observations in 1942.[8]

The recognition that dermatomyositis and polymyositis may affect other organ systems including the heart, lungs, and gastrointestinal tract is comparatively recent. The vascular pathology of juvenile dermatomyositis was first recognized in 1953 by Wedgewood et al.,[9] although that form of the disease occurs occasionally in adults as well.

Epidemiology

Both dermatomyositis and polymyositis may occur at any age. There is a peak in childhood and another in the age range from 45 to 65 years. The latter peak includes those with dermatomyositis and polymyositis associated with malignant disease.

The age-adjusted incidence of dermatomyositis and polymyositis combined varies in different studies from 1 to 10 per 10^6 population per year with a prevalence of about 10 cases per 10^6 population.[10] There appears to be little difference in the prevalence among different ethnic groups, at least in North America.

Several demographic studies have suggested that more cases begin in the spring than at other times of the year. That seems to be true for juvenile dermatomyositis and for a group of patients who have in their serum the Jo 1 antibody.[1] In juvenile dermatomyositis there is evidence for an association with coxsackievirus B infection, which is also more common in the spring.

Etiology

The etiology of dermatomyositis and polymyositis remains unknown. An autoimmune pathogenesis is implicated by the sharing of clinical, pathologic, and serologic features of the idiopathic myopathies with other connective tissue diseases. As is the case for many connective tissue diseases, there is an overrepresentation of the HLA-DR3 phenotype in both Caucasians and blacks with idiopathic inflammatory myopathies. The association is particularly strong in patients with the anti-Jo 1 antibody.[11]

A viral etiology for inflammatory myopathies has been suspected for many years. Viral infections often precede attacks of rhabdomyolysis. Both intact virus and viral genome have been identified in muscle from patients with myositis temporally associated with influenza-, echo-, and coxsackievirus infections.[12] Echovirus infection can induce a diffuse myositis in children with X-linked agammaglobulinemia.[13]

The discovery that a number of the myositis-associated antibodies such as Jo 1 and PL 12 appear to be directed against tRNA synthetases has increased interest in the possible role of picornavirus in the etiology of inflammatory myopathies. That group of viruses has surface proteins similar to aminoacyl tRNA synthetases. Thus, the presence of antibody to tRNA synthetase might be a consequence of infection with a picornavirus. In a study of adult dermatomyositis, in situ hybridization with RNA probes for a murine picornavirus revealed evidence of infection in the muscle of three of five cases studied.[14] A recent study has failed to find any of 7 frequently indicted virus genomes in muscle biopsies from 44 patients with idiopathic inflammatory myopathy.[15] Myositis occurs in patients with AIDS[16] and in some seems to be precipitated by treatment with zidovudine (AZT). Details of the pathogenesis are not yet known.

A role for immune complex in the pathogenesis of dermatomyositis, particularly in children but also in some adults, has been established by demonstrating the presence of the membrane attack complex of serum complement in the blood vessels of biopsy specimens from muscle.[17] A fundamental difference between dermatomyositis and polymyositis was identified when none of the biopsies from the fourteen patients with polymyositis showed immune complex deposition. However, the pathogenic importance of complement activation by immune complex is challenged by the fact that dermatomyositis can occur in patients with hereditary complement deficiency.[18]

Drugs are a common cause of diffuse myopathy.[19] However, only a few have been shown to produce a true myositis, and none has been implicated as a cause of dermatomyositis. Various studies of immunologic mechanisms by which myositis could be induced have yielded conflicting results. The evidence for a humoral pathogenesis, at least with respect to juvenile dermatomyositis and some cases of the adult syndrome, has been summarized above. The predominantly lymphocytic cellular infiltrate in involved muscle has stimulated numerous studies of cell-mediated immunity as a pathogenic mechanism.[20] Mononuclear cells from the peripheral blood of patients with myositis have been reported to be cytotoxic to cultured human or animal myocytes.[21] There is controversy concerning the phenotype of the inflammatory cells found in muscle biopsies. In dermatomyositis, especially in children, most of the lymphocytes are B cells and T cells of the CD4 phenotype, whereas in polymyositis, CD8-bearing T cells seems to predominate.[22] This finding further distinguishes the two disorders.

Finally, the possible association of dermatomyositis with malignant tumors in adults has provoked speculation about the role of tumor immunity in the pathogenesis of such cases.[23] Some patients exhibit delayed skin sensitivity to extracts of their tumors; the significance of this observation is uncertain.

Clinical Manifestations

Progressive weakness is the major clinical manifestation of both dermatomyositis and polymyositis. Usually, muscles of the trunk and limb girdles are affected more than peripheral ones. Difficulty in rising from low chairs, climbing stairs, or holding the arms above the head are common symptoms. In the case of young children, impaired mobility is observed by the parents, while older children may notice decreased athletic ability. Half of the patients complain of myalgia or have some muscle tenderness. However, in contrast to infectious myositis, pain is rarely a prominent symptom of the idiopathic myopathies. The weakness is constant and is usually progressive. Those characteristics help to differentiate myositis from myasthenia, most metabolic myopathies, and also psychogenic weakness.

Muscle weakness, which is almost always bilateral and symmetric, is best evaluated by testing muscle groups such as the abductors or adductors of the arms, flexors, or extensors of the thigh, or neck flexors. Except in rare cases, hand grips and ankle flexors will be appreciably stronger. Patients should be observed for the presence of a Trendelenburg gait or an exaggerated lumbar lordosis. Muscle atrophy is rarely seen when the patient presents to a physician, although the muscles may feel flabby. However, patients whose disease has progressed slowly over relatively long periods may show muscle atrophy out of proportion to weakness. When patients are first seen, it may be difficult to detect weakness on testing in a third of the cases in spite of clearly described symptoms. The facial and bulbar muscles are usually spared, but may be affected, particularly in cases associated with a malignancy or with myasthenia.

Dermatomyositis has cutaneous manifestations that are essentially pathognomonic and without which the diagnosis cannot be made with confidence. The skin lesions are almost always present at the time the patient presents with weakness. Occasionally, they precede the myositis, and a few cases with only skin involvement have been reported.[24]

The most specific skin manifestation is a maculopapular erythema on bony prominences such as the knuckles, elbows, and knees that appears in about 70 percent of cases. The first lesions are small and discrete but may enlarge and coalesce, forming red to purple plaques with telangiectasia, scale, and sometimes small eschars (Fig. 172-1). Over time, the involved areas become atrophic and depigmented. The papular lesions were described by Gottron and are named after him[25]; the more polymorphic, erythematous, or atrophic plaques are referred to as Gottron's sign.

A blotchy erythema, especially on sun-exposed skin, occurs in about a third of patients (Fig. 172-2). More chronic macular erythema and poikilodermatous lesions may also develop on the trunk and proximal parts of the limbs.[26]

A distinctive, but often more subtle, sign is an erythematous blush on the eyelids and around the eyes. It has a lavender shade similar to the flower of the valerian, from which comes the term heliotrope erythema (Fig. 172-3). The intensity of the periorbital blush may vary considerably from hour to hour. This skin manifestation may be the only one in children and some adults. It is present in about 60 percent of cases.

Nail margin telangiectasia, often with a few thrombosed vessels and cuticular hypertrophy, may be observed in cases of myositis, including connective tissue overlap syndromes, as well as in patients with polymyositis or dermatomyositis[27] (Fig. 172-4).

Various other skin rashes have been reported in association with polymyositis, including dermatitis herpetiformis[28] and lichen planus (Fig. 172-5). Patients with connective tissue overlap syndromes may have lupus-like or sclerodermatous skin involvement.

Calcinosis universalis is a distressing late complication of juvenile dermatomyositis.[29] The calcium is deposited diffusely in fascial planes of skin and muscle (Fig. 172-6). Subcutaneous calcium deposits over extensor surfaces frequently lead to chronic ulcers.

Arthralgia is an early symptom of dermatomyositis in about one-third of cases. The severity of the arthritis seems to diminish as weakness becomes more prominent, except in patients with connective tissue overlap syndromes in whom arthritis may be chronic.[30] Other manifestations of overlap syndromes are Raynaud's phenomenon and the sicca syndrome.

Although there is little smooth muscle pathology in these disorders, lower esophageal dysfunction has been documented by barium swallow in up to 30 percent of patients.[31] Less commonly, but especially when myositis is associated with a malignancy, oropharyngeal weakness may develop.

The myocardium is affected in patients with dermatomyositis with a frequency that varies in different series depending on the care with which cardiac features have been sought.[32] Electrocardiographic abnormalities are detected in about 40 percent of patients with idiopathic inflammatory myopathies. Clinically significant arrhythmias are infrequent but may be life-threatening when present.

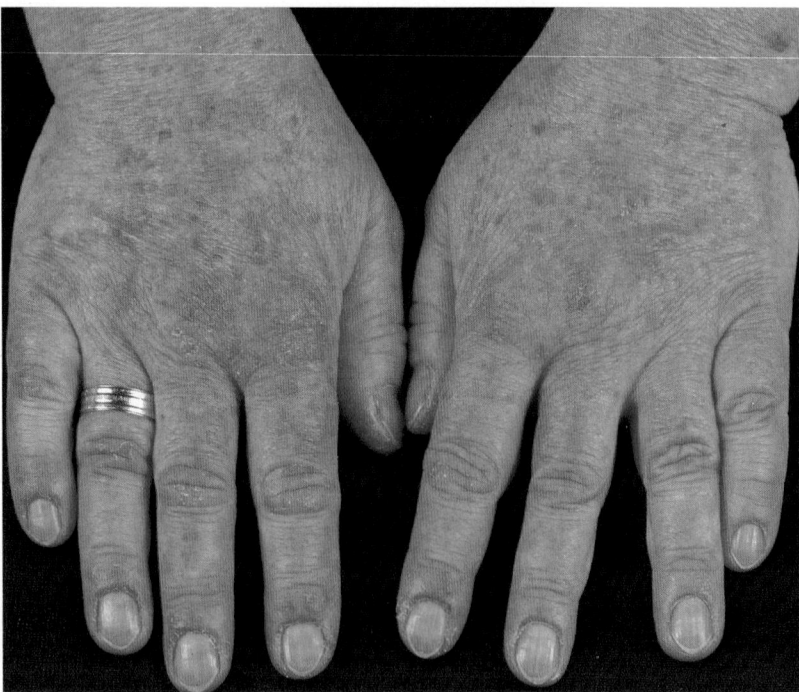

FIGURE 172-1 Dermatomyositis. In this patient can be seen a vivid red color of the nail fold which is produced by multiple telangiectases. Also on the knuckles there are plaques and papules, which tend to be over bony prominences; these are called *Gottron's papules* but are not specific for dermatomyositis.

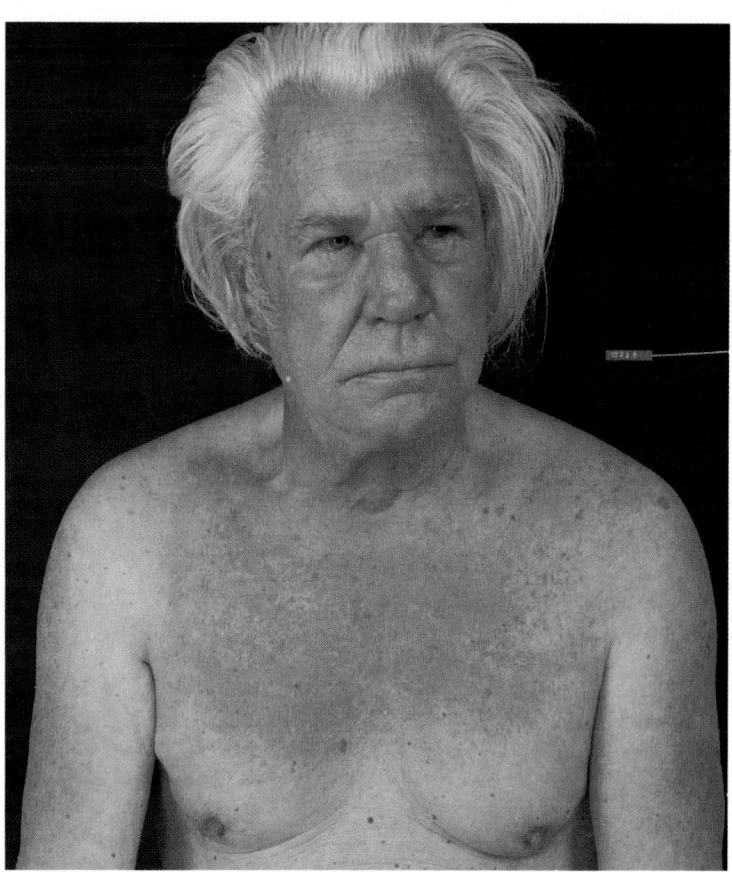

FIGURE 172-2 Dermatomyositis. The fiery erythema on the upper chest and neck is composed of numerous telangiectases. There is also considerable edema of the eyelids and a heliotrope color of the upper eyelids.

Another serious complication of dermatomyositis and polymyositis is progressive pulmonary fibrosis, which affects about 10 percent of patients. It is especially common in patients with connective tissue overlap syndromes and in association with the presence of the anti-Jo 1 or anti-PL 12 antibodies.[33] Symptoms are progressive dyspnea and nonproductive cough. Additionally, life-threatening hypoxemia can occur insidiously in patients with severe myositis of the respiratory muscles. These respiratory complications together with cardiomyopathy are responsible for most deaths of patients with idiopathic inflammatory myopathies.[34]

Laboratory Findings and Special Examinations

Abnormal laboratory tests associated with the primary myopathies include elevations of the serum muscle enzymes, an abnormal electromyogram, and pathologic changes in affected muscles. Any one of these laboratory abnormalities may be absent in up to one-third of cases, either because of sampling errors or because of timing of the examination.[6] The serum level of creatine phosphokinase (CPK) is the most reliable indicator of disease activity. The CPK is mostly of the MM isotype, although in patients with chronic disease up to 20 percent may be of the MB isotype. In some cases, either before or after treatment, the degree of CPK elevation seems not to reflect disease activity. The serum aldolase level is usually less sensitive than that of the CPK, although it is more specific than SGOT or LDH, the levels of which are also raised in most patients.

The electromyogram is usually abnormal when affected muscles are tested. Diagnostically helpful findings include increased electrical activity in response to needle insertion, fibrillation potentials, positive sharp waves, and the dominance of relatively low voltage, short-duration action potentials.[35] Early recruitment and a normal interference pattern are present, except when patients are tested late in the course of the disease. At that time, hypertrophy of

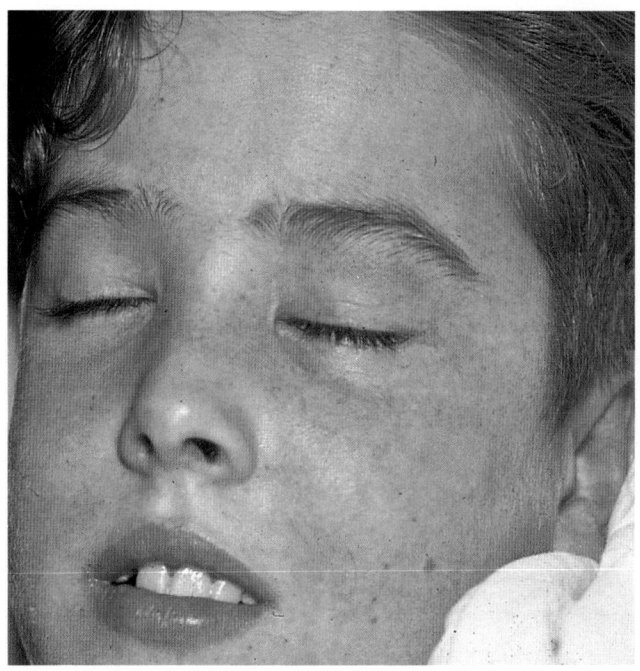

FIGURE 172-3 "Heliotrope" periorbital erythema.

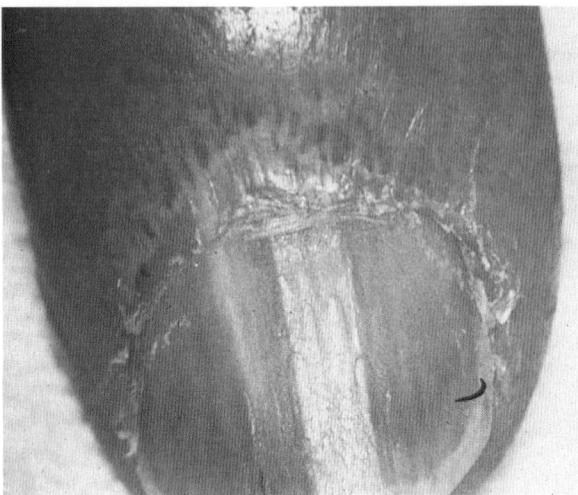

FIGURE 172-4 Dermatomyositis. Telangiectatic and thrombosed nail margin capillaries with cuticular hypertrophy.

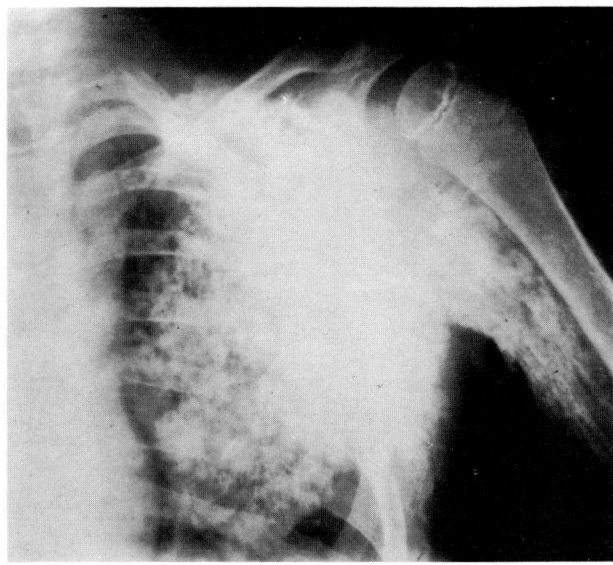

FIGURE 172-6 Calcinosis universalis. Calcification of subcutaneous tissue and pectoralis fascia in a child with dermatomyositis.

remaining fibers, muscle regeneration, or reenervation of segmentally denervated fibers may produce neuropathic features as well.[36] The presence of neuropathic findings early in the clinical course strongly suggests a carcinoma-associated myopathy.

Muscle biopsies are subject to sampling error unless relatively large specimens are obtained. When the disease is active, biopsies are usually abnormal, but the changes may not be very specific. A biopsy helps to rule out inclusion body myositis and myopathy caused by parasites, toxoplasmosis, or sarcoidosis. Muscle pathology is described in more detail in the next section.

An increasing variety of autoantibodies has been identified in the serum of patients with idiopathic inflammatory myopathy. Of special interest are the antibodies directed against tRNA synthe-

tases. These seem to correlate with the presence of extramuscular disease manifestations.[11]

Patients who have features of one of the connective tissue overlap syndromes frequently have antibodies characteristic of those diseases, such as anti-DNA, anti-RNP, or anti-Ro.[1] A few have rheumatoid factor, which may lead to misdiagnosis in patients who present with polyarthritis.

An ECG and chest x-ray should be performed to rule out cardiac or pulmonary complications. Tests of ventilation must be followed in any patient suspected of having significant respiratory muscle involvement, accompanied by blood gas determination as appropriate.

Patients who are over age 50 at onset should be evaluated for the presence of a malignant tumor. Inasmuch as the great majority are common tumors, a chest x-ray, gastrointestinal evaluation, and careful breast and genitourinary examinations are sufficient unless symptoms point elsewhere.

Pathology

The muscle pathology of the idiopathic inflammatory myopathies is being reevaluated in light of the serologic abnormalities described in the preceding section. Three basic pathologic processes are usually present, although to variable degrees. These are segmental muscle fiber necrosis, interstitial inflammation, and a vasculopathy. The extent to which any one of these features is seen varies with the individual case and with the number of biopsies obtained.

In most adults with dermatomyositis, the prominent histologic abnormality is a segmental fiber necrosis with a variable inflammatory infiltrate consisting of lymphocytes and macrophages.[37] Lymphocytes predominate in the early histology. The inflammatory infiltrate may be diffusely distributed in the interstitium or focally around small blood vessels. Biopsies obtained some time after disease onset show myocyte regeneration characterized by activated sarcolemmal nuclei with displacement of the nuclei into myofibers that take a basophilic stain. The morphologic features of inclusion

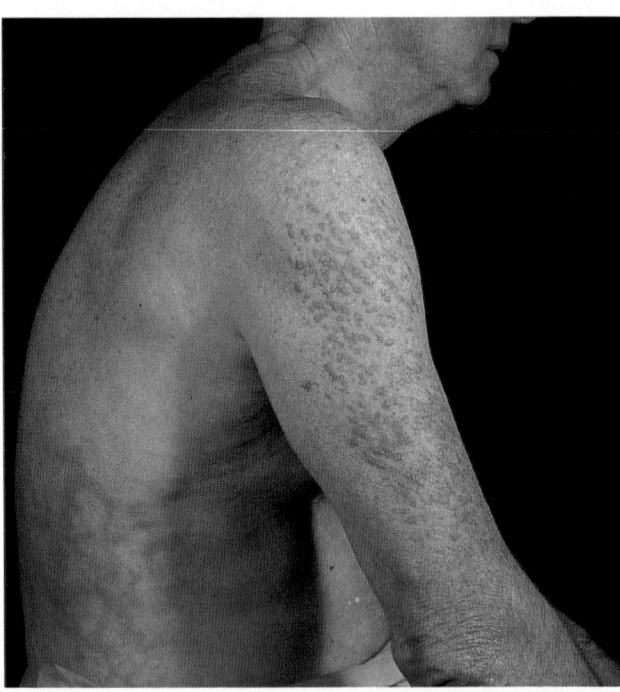

FIGURE 172-5 Lichen planus-like skin lesions in a patient with dermatomyositis.

body myositis are most easily identified in sections stained by the modified trichrome method.

Children and some adults with dermatomyositis show vascular pathology characterized by a perivascular lymphocytic infiltrate, an obliterative endarteropathy, and perifascicular myofiber atrophy.[9] There may be little fiber necrosis or other inflammatory infiltrate. This pattern of muscle pathology is also found in some patients with overlap syndromes. In patients with vasculopathy, immune complex, including the terminal complement components, can be identified in the vessel walls.[17]

The dermatopathology of dermatomyositis is characterized by focal vacuolar degeneration of the basal epithelial cells, basement membrane degeneration, and epidermal atrophy.[38] Although microvascular dilatation is prominent, the inflammatory component is usually sparse and localized around the superficial blood vessels. Areas of mucinous change in the dermis are common in both clinically involved and uninvolved skin. In areas of more severe inflammation there may be a subepidermal fibrinoid deposition. Although these pathologic changes are similar to those of SLE, immune complex is not found at the epidermal basement membrane. In more chronic lesions, the morphologic features of poikiloderma are usually present as well.

The lung pathology takes several forms.[39] Bronchiolitis obliterans is the most frequent finding, but in some instances the features are those of "usual interstitial pneumonitis." Vasculopathy, including vasculitis, and endothelial proliferation may be present in patients with features of other connective tissue diseases, such as the CREST syndrome.

The cardiac pathology is also relatively nonspecific, consisting of microfocal myofiber degeneration with interstitial fibrosis, but with little inflammatory infiltrate.[40]

Treatment

The primary treatment for dermatomyositis is prednisone or methylprednisolone in a single morning dose of 1 mg per kilogram body weight.[41] More frequent dosing is rarely necessary. Patients should avoid strenuous exertion for the first few weeks until serum levels of muscle enzymes begin to fall. The value of bed rest has not been tested in a controlled manner, but rest may be desirable for patients with very active disease.[42]

The serum CPK usually begins to fall 2 to 3 weeks after treatment is started, although an initial decrease may occur in the first few days with bed rest alone. Even in steroid-responsive patients it can take 6 to 10 weeks of treatment for a 50 percent drop in the serum CPK to occur. At that point, it is advisable to start a slow taper of prednisone, making decrements of about 15 percent of the dose at 2-week intervals. From 3 to 6 months of therapy may be required to obtain a full remission. Once the dose has been reduced to 30 mg/day, further tapering to an alternate day schedule may be possible with a concomitant reduction of steroid side effects.[41]

The return of strength usually lags some weeks behind the fall in serum enzymes. It is important to manage the prednisone dose by the level of serum enzymes rather than by strength measurements because of the risk that the supervention of steroid myopathy may confuse the clinical evaluation. Because of their greater propensity to produce myopathy, the more potent fluorinated glucocorticoids should not be used to treat myositis.

In 10 to 15 percent of cases, muscle enzymes do not return completely to normal levels but remain in the range of two to five times normal in spite of a continued gain of muscle strength. In that circumstance, a repeat muscle biopsy is warranted after 6 months of therapy. If no evidence of myositis is present, tapering of the prednisone dose should continue.

A considerable number of patients, up to 30 percent in some series, either fail to regain strength, have persistently high serum muscle enzyme levels, or relapse as the prednisone dose is reduced. Inclusion body myositis is particularly resistant to treatment. Numerous other drugs have been used to treat such patients. Although it is likely that the idiopathic inflammatory myopathies are heterogeneous and thus might respond selectively to different drugs, that has not been evident to date. There are few prospective comparative trials of other therapy. High-dose bolus or "pulse" methylprednisolone has been recommended for juvenile dermatomyositis.[43] In the case of adults with glucocorticoid-resistant disease, most authorities favor intravenous methotrexate in a dose of 40 to 50 mg once weekly for 6 to 10 weeks.[44] When methotrexate is ineffective, patients are frequently treated with cytotoxic drugs. Azathioprine is one of the few drugs that has been tested in a comparative fashion. About 50 percent of patients whose disease is not adequately controlled by prednisone have been reported to improve when azathioprine is added.[45] Doses are in the range of 2 to 3 mg/kg per day. Treatment with cytotoxic drugs should be undertaken only by those who have previous experience with such therapy. Cyclophosphamide, orally or intravenously, seems to be less effective than either methotrexate or azathioprine.[46]

Plasmapheresis[47] and cyclosporine[48] have also been used to treat prednisone-resistant cases. Cyclosporine itself may cause a myopathy.[49] Both successes and failures have been reported. Recently, intravenous gamma globulin infusions have produced encouraging results in children and that therapy is undergoing evaluation in adults.[50]

During the acute phase of the disease, severely weak patients should have respiratory dynamics monitored closely. The appearance of pulmonary fibrosis or congestive failure portends a poor prognosis. No effective therapy for these complications has been found, although there are a few case reports of benefit after treatment with high-dose methylprednisolone, plasmapheresis, or cyclophosphamide.[51] Overwhelming infection is a common cause of death in such patients.

The skin rash of dermatomyositis usually improves with glucocorticoid therapy. Topical treatment is of little value, but hydroxychloroquine may be efficacious in resistant cases.[52]

No treatment is available for calcinosis universalis that develops in some children during recovery from dermatomyositis. Surgical excision of the calcified tissue has been helpful when used selectively to treat specific functional problems. Colchicine, 0.6 mg once or twice daily, may be useful to treat the chronic ulcers associated with subcutaneous calcium deposits.

Physical therapy to restore muscle strength and function is important once the myositis has been adequately controlled. That point is usually indicated by a substantial fall in the level of serum CPK and the beginning of a return of muscle strength. It is not known whether physical therapy started earlier is detrimental, but higher levels of physical activity early in the disease are frequently accompanied by a rise of serum CPK. This rise may reflect further muscle damage and, at the least, confuses the evaluation of the response to treatment.[53] Isotonic exercise may be preferable to isometric and especially to eccentric contraction, because of the possibility that the latter might cause additional ischemic muscle injury. Exercise does not stimulate muscle repair, but restores strength through hypertrophy of the remaining undamaged fibers.

Differential Diagnosis

Diagnosis is not difficult when the typical rash of dermatomyositis occurs in a patient with symmetric, predominantly proximal muscle weakness. Because of the similarity of their cutaneous manifestations, systemic lupus erythematosus or overlap connective tissue syndromes with prominent myositis are the principal alternative diagnoses.

When a rash is not present or is not characteristic, the differential diagnosis of polymyositis is much more extensive. It includes infectious and metabolic myopathies, drug-induced myolysis, muscular dystrophy (particularly the limb girdle type), and other neuromuscular disorders. Levels of serum CPK or aldolase more than ten times greater than normal are rarely seen in myopathies other than dermatomyositis and polymyositis, except in rhabdomyolysis secondary to trauma or metabolic disorders.

Patients with dermatomyositis do not always have serum enzyme levels that are greatly elevated, and the values may not parallel the severity of muscle weakness. Furthermore, it may be difficult to detect muscle weakness by objective testing in up to 30 percent of cases. In the absence of a rash, the family history may suggest a diagnosis of muscular dystrophy or a metabolic myopathy. Pain and fever are rarely prominent in patients with dermatomyositis or polymyositis. When present, they implicate infectious myopathies such as trichinosis or viral myositis.

When the presence of myositis is uncertain or when a neuropathy is suspected, an electromyogram (EMG) should be the next diagnostic step. The detection of atypical myopathic, short-duration, low-amplitude action potentials with a normal interference pattern helps to exclude most metabolic myopathies and neuromuscular diseases. Clinically affected muscles should be examined by EMG. Even so, the focal nature of the process may result in a falsely negative or indeterminate electromyographic study. A muscle biopsy should be performed when the EMG is not indicative of a myositis or when other causes of myositis, such as trichinosis, toxoplasmosis, or inclusion body myositis, are suspected. It is important not to biopsy the muscles examined by EMG so as to avoid needle artifacts. Muscle biopsy is also subject to sampling errors, and at least 2 to 3 cm^3 should be obtained from a clinically affected muscle and examined in both longitudinal and transverse sections. Chronic myositis has been described in patients infected with *Borrelia bergdorferi*.[54] In the appropriate circumstances a test for Lyme disease should be performed.

Assays for the autoantibodies that have been detected in the various forms of idiopathic myositis, such as Jo 1, PL 12, or Ku, are still not routinely available. Because of a low sensitivity they are of little primary diagnostic value but may call attention to the presence of other disease manifestations with which they are associated.

Prevention

The etiology of this group of diseases is unknown. No preventive measures have been identified. The rash of dermatomyositis can frequently be induced with light. Patients with dermatomyositis should avoid unnecessary sun exposure.

Course

The natural history of dermatomyositis is not known precisely. Clinical observation before the advent of glucocorticoid therapy indicated that most patients eventually succumbed to their disease,[3] although its course was extremely variable. Death was often caused by infection secondary to general debility. However, in about one-third of cases remissions, some permanent, were documented. At the present time, with optimum treatment about 85 percent of patients can be expected to survive, although almost one-half are left with some weakness and about 20 percent are substantially disabled.[34] The prognosis is worse when other organ systems such as the lungs and heart are affected. In that regard, the presence of the anti Jo 1 or PL 12 antibodies may be of prognostic significance. The recovery from juvenile dermatomyositis is complicated by calcinosis universalis in about 50 percent of cases. This process may advance for several years after clinical recovery from the myositis and result in severe disability. It has been suggested that intensive treatment early in the course of the disease may reduce the risk or severity of calcinosis.[43]

Pregnancy in patients with polymyositis or dermatomyositis is usually well tolerated, although an exacerbation of the disease is common, and glucocorticoid therapy is necessary in most instances. The prognosis for the fetus is much less satisfactory. Only 55 percent of pregnancies were successfully completed in one study. Spontaneous abortion occurred in 33 percent. Inasmuch as prednisone does not cross the placenta, it is not clear that glucocorticoid is the responsible factor.[55]

References

1. Plotz PH: Current concepts in the idiopathic inflammatory myopathies: Polymyositis, dermatomyositis, and related disorders. *Ann Intern Med* **111**:143, 1989
2. Wagner E: Fall einer seltenen Muskelkrankheit. *Arch Heilkd* **4**:282, 1863
3. O'Leary PA, Waisman M: Dermatomyositis: A study of 40 cases. *Arch Derm Syphilol* **41**:1001, 1940
4. Everett MA, Curtis AC: Dermatomyositis. *Arch Intern Med* **100**:70, 1957
5. Walton JN, Adams RD: *Polymyositis*. Edinburgh, Livingston, 1958
6. Bohan A et al: A computer assisted analysis of 153 patients with polymyositis and dermatomyositis. *Medicine* **56**:255, 1977
7. Unverrecht H: Polymyositis acuta progressiva. *Z Clin Med* **12**:553, 1887
8. Keil H: The manifestations in the skin and mucous membranes in dermatomyositis with special reference to the differential diagnosis from systemic lupus erythematosus. *Ann Intern Med* **16**:828, 1942
9. Wedgewood RJ et al: Dermatomyositis. Report of 26 cases in children with discussion of endocrine therapy in 13. *Pediatrics* **12**:447, 1953
10. Cronin ME, Plotz PH: Idiopathic inflammatory myopathies. *Rheum Dis Clin North Am* **16**:655, 1990
11. Goldstein R et al: HLA-D region genes associated with autoantibody responses to histidyl-transfer t-RNA synthetase (Jo 1) and other translation-related factors in myositis. *Arthritis Rheum* **33**:1240, 1990
12. Bowles NE: Dermatomyositis, polymyositis, and coxsackie B virus infections. *Lancet* **1**:1004, 1987
13. Crennen IM et al: Echovirus polymyositis in patients with hypogammaglobulinemia; failure of high dose intravenous gamma globulin therapy and review of the literature. *Am J Med* **81**:35, 1986
14. Rosenberg NL et al: Evidence for a novel picornavirus in human dermatomyositis. *Ann Neurol* **26**:204, 1989
15. Leff RL et al: Viruses in idiopathic inflammatory myopathies: Absence of candidate viral genomes in muscle. *Lancet* **339**:1192, 1992
16. Simpson DM, Bender AN: Human immunodeficiency virus-associated myopathy: Analysis of 11 patients. *Ann Neurol* **24**:79, 1988
17. Kissel JT et al: Microvascular deposition of complement membrane attack complex in dermatomyositis. *N Engl J Med* **314**:329, 1988

18. Leddy J et al: Hereditary complement (C2) deficiency with dermatomyositis. *Am J Med* **58**:83, 1975

19. Strongwater SL: Overview and clinical manifestations of inflammatory myositis, polymyositis, and dermatomyositis. *Mt Sinai J Med* **55**:435, 1988

20. Ytterberg S: Cellular immunity in polymyositis/dermatomyositis. *Mt Sinai J Med* **55**:494, 1988

21. Hayashi Y et al: Muscle regeneration and cell mediated cytotoxicity in the autologous muscle culture of dermatomyositis. *Acta Derm Venereol (Stockh)* **70**:53, 1990

22. Engel AG, Arahata K: Mononuclear cells in myopathies, quantitation of functionally distinct subsets, recognition of antigen-specific cell mediated cytotoxicity in some diseases and implications for the pathogenesis of the different inflammatory myopathies. *Hum Pathol* **17**:704, 1986

23. Lakhanpal S et al: Polymyositis-dermatomyositis and malignant lesions: Does an association exist? *Mayo Clinc Proc* **61**:645, 1986

24. Krain LS: Dermatomyositis in six patients without initial muscle involvement. *Arch Derm* **111**:241, 1975

25. Gottron H: Hautveranuderungen bei dermatomyositis, in *VIII Congres International de Dermatologie et de Syphilologie,* edited by S Lomholt. Compts Rendus de Seances, Copenhagen, 1930, p 826

26. Callen JP: Dermatomyositis. *Dis Month* **33**:242, 1987

27. Maricq HR et al: Skin capillary abnormalities as indicators of organ development in scleroderma, Raynaud's syndrome, and dermatomyositis. *Am J Med* **61**:862, 1976

28. Kalovidouris AE et al: Polymyositis/dermatomyositis associated with dermatitis herpetiformis. *Arthritis Rheum* **32**:1178, 1989

29. Bowyer SK et al: Childhood dermatomyositis: Factors predicting functional outcome and development of dystrophic calcification. *J Pediatr* **103**:882, 1983

30. Oddis CV et al: A subluxing arthropathy associated with the anti Jo 1 antibody in polymyositis/dermatomyositis. *Arthritis Rheum* **33**:1640, 1990

31. Horowitz M et al: Abnormalities of gastric and esophageal emptying in polymyositis and dermatomyositis. *Gastroenterology* **90**:434, 1986

32. Askari AD: The heart in polymyositis and dermatomyositis. *Mt Sinai J Med* **55**:479, 1988

33. Targoff IN, Arnett FC: Clinical manifestations in patients with antibody to P1-12 antigen. *Am J Med* **88**:241, 1990

34. Hochberg MC et al: Adult onset polymyositis/dermatomyositis. An analysis of clinical and laboratory features and survival in 76 patients with a review of the literature. *Semin Arthritis Rheum* **15**:168, 1986

35. Warmolts JR: Electrodiagnosis in neuromuscular disorders. *Ann Intern Med* **99**:599, 1981

36. Bromberg MB, Albers JW: Electromyography in idiopathic myositis. *Mt Sinai J Med* **55**:459, 1988

37. DiGirolami U, Smith TW: Muscle pathology—a teaching monograph. *Am J Pathol* **107**:231, 1982

38. Janis JF, Winklemann RK: Histopathology of the skin in dermatomyositis. *Arch Dermatol* **97**:640, 1968

39. Tazelaar HD: Interstitial lung disease in polymyositis and dermatomyositis. Clinical features and prognosis as correlated with histologic findings. *Am Rev Respir Dis* **141**:727, 1990

40. Haupt HM, Hutchins GM: The heart and cardiac conduction system in polymyositis-dermatomyositis. A clinicopathologic study of 16 autopsied patients. *Am J Cardiol* **50**:998, 1982

41. Henriksson KG, Sandstedt P: Polymyositis, treatment and prognosis. A study of 107 patients. *Acta Neurol Scand* **65**:280, 1982

42. Round JM et al: Cellular infiltrates in human skeletal muscle: Exercise-induced damage as a model for inflammatory muscle disease? *J Neurol Sci* **82**:1, 1987

43. Laxer RM et al: Intravenous pulse methylprednisolone treatment of juvenile dermatomyositis. *Arthritis Rheum* **30**:328, 1987

44. Metzger AL et al: Polymyositis and dermatomyositis: Combined methotrexate and corticosteroid therapy. *Ann Intern Med* **81**:182, 1974

45. Bunch TW: Prednisone and azathioprine for polymyositis. *Arthritis Rheum* **24**:45, 1981

46. Cronin ME et al: The failure of intravenous cyclophosphamide therapy in refractory idiopathic inflammatory myopathy. *J Rheumatol* **16**:1225, 1989

47. Dau PC: Plasmapheresis in idiopathic inflammatory myopathy, experience with 35 patients. *Arch Neurol* **38**:544, 1981

48. Jones DW: Cyclosporine treatment for intractable polymyositis. *Arthritis Rheum* **30**:959, 1987

49. Goy JJ et al: Myopathy as a possible side-effect of cyclosporine. *Lancet* **1**:1446, 1989

50. Chervin P et al: Intravenous immunoglobulin for polymyositis and dermatomyositis. *Lancet* **336**:116, 1990

51. Al-Janadi M et al: Cyclophosphamide treatment of interstitial pulmonary fibrosis in polymyositis/dermatomyositis. *J Rheumatol* **16**:1592, 1989

52. Woo TY et al: Cutaneous lesions of dermatomyositis are improved by hydroxychloroquine. *J Am Acad Dermatol* **10**:592, 1984

53. Ramirez G et al: Adult onset polymyositis-dermatomyositis. Description of 25 patients with emphasis on treatment. *Semin Arthritis Rheum* **20**:114, 1990

54. Schoener J et al: Myositis during *Borrelia burgdorferi* infection. *J Neurol Neursurg Psychiatry* **52**:1002, 1989

55. Mintz G: Dermatomyositis. *Rheum Dis Clin North Am* **15**:375, 1989

CHAPTER 173

Tamzin A. Rosenwasser and Arthur Z. Eisen

Scleroderma is a chronic disease of unknown cause that affects the microvasculature and loose connective tissue and is characterized by fibrosis and obliteration of vessels in the skin, lungs, gastrointestinal tract, kidneys, and heart. It may occur in a localized form or as a systemic disease, systemic sclerosis (systemic scleroderma, SSc), which is often progressive and fatal. SSc is characterized clinically by induration and thickening of the skin. The fibrous deposition and vascular obliteration seen in the skin also occur in certain internal organs.

Classification

Several clinical forms of localized scleroderma are recognized, including morphea, generalized morphea, and linear scleroderma. Localized scleroderma is not a life-threatening disease but can cause disfigurement. The most common type is morphea, in which the lesions are usually single or few in number. In the generalized form of morphea, symmetric and bilateral lesions occur. The absence of Raynaud's phenomenon, acrosclerosis, and organ involvement differentiates generalized morphea from systemic scleroderma. A guttate variant of morphea has been described, but it may be a variant of lichen sclerosus et atrophicus. In linear scleroderma the lesions are arranged in a bandlike linear distribution and may involve the deeper layers of the skin and underlying structures. Deformities, such as hemiatrophy, may be associated with linear scleroderma.

It has been proposed[1] that SSc be divided into two distinct subsets: limited SSc (lSSc) and diffuse SSc (dSSc). Sixty percent of patients with SSc are in the lSSc group, which includes individuals with the CREST syndrome, so-called for its features of calcinosis cutis, Raynaud's phenomenon, esophageal dysfunction, sclerodactyly, and telangiectasia. Patients with lSSc typically are women who are older than patients with dSSc, with a long history (10 to 15 years) of Raynaud's phenomenon; skin involvement limited to the digits or hands, face, feet, and forearms; nail fold capillary dilatation; and early onset of facial and digital telangiectasias. In addition, they have a high incidence of anticentromere antibodies (70 to 80 percent). Systemic involvement (notably pulmonary hypertension) may not appear for years (often decades), and many patients outlive their disease and die of other causes. (Miners, users of vibrating machines, and those exposed to chemicals or plastics may develop a seronegative form of lSSc.)

In contrast, the typical patient with dSSc is well until the abrupt onset of swelling (nonpitting) of the hands and feet associated with Raynaud's phenomenon and hidebound changes in the skin, often sparing only the back and buttocks. Polyarticular symmetric synovitis, tenosynovitis, and tendon friction rubs are often present. Nail fold capillary dilatation and destruction are common, and there is an early onset of internal organ involvement. Anticentromere antibodies are uncommon, but Scl-70 (antitopoisomerase 1) antibodies are present in approximately 30 percent of the patients. In some patients, skin involvement rapidly progresses initially and

Scleroderma

then subsides slowly over years.[1] Cases have been reported[2] of patients with dSSc who do not develop extensive or severe internal organ involvement. These patients form a subset whose disease is termed *chronic dSSc*.

Epidemiology

Localized scleroderma is relatively uncommon. Women are affected about three times as often as men. From reported cases, the disease appears much more common in whites than in blacks. In a large series,[3] 75 percent of patients with morphea had their onset between ages 20 and 50. In linear scleroderma, the age of onset is earlier, with a significant number occurring in the first two decades of life.

Systemic scleroderma is four times more common in women than in men, and evidence is growing that SSc may be more frequent among black than white women.[4,5] The disease incidence increases with age in white females but remains stable among black females throughout adulthood. It may occur at any age but is relatively uncommon in childhood. Most patients suffer their onset between ages 30 and 50.

The average annual incidence is estimated at 2.7 new cases of SSc per million population.[4] In a random sample of approximately 7000 subjects from the general population of South Carolina,[2] the estimated prevalence of SSc was between 1.4 to 5.4 times greater than the highest previously reported incidence rate. The reason for this finding is not known. In a large combined study of 309 patients from two different geographic areas of the country, the 7-year survival after entry into the study was 35 percent.[6] A significantly decreased survival rate was found in older patients. Females had a significantly better survival rate than males, and the mortality from scleroderma for black females was significantly greater than for white females. In a study of 177 patients,[1] the 10-year survival was 71 percent in patients with sclerodactyly only, 58 percent in patients with skin stiffness proximal to the metacarpophalangeal joint but sparing the trunk, and only 21 percent in those with diffuse skin stiffness including the trunk. Anticentromere antibody correlated strongly with patients having sclerodactyly only and may be a marker for milder disease. The classification of SSc into the lSSc and dSSc subsets is important prognostically as it has been estimated that the survival rates for 1, 6, and 12 years of patients with dSSc are only 80 percent, 30 percent, and 15 percent, respectively, whereas those of patients with lSSc are 98 percent, 80 percent, and 50 percent, respectively.[2]

Scleroderma-like Disorders

SSc is more common in underground coal and gold miners.[7] In male patients with silicosis who are over 40 years of age, the likelihood of developing SSc is approximately 190 times greater than in males not exposed to silica and is 50 times greater than in males without silicosis but exposed to silica dust.[8] Silica exposure itself seems to be a principal factor in the cause of the disease.

An unusual form of scleroderma characterized by Raynaud's phenomenon, morphea-like skin changes, capillary abnormalities of the nail fold (similar to those seen in SSc), osteolysis of the distal phalanges, and hepatic and pulmonary fibrosis has been reported in workers exposed to polyvinyl chloride.[9] The relationship of this disorder to SSc remains unclear. Bleomycin also produces pulmonary fibrosis, Raynaud's phenomenon, and cutaneous changes indistinguishable from those of SSc.[10] The development of these changes appears to be dose-dependent and is reversible upon discontinuation of the drug. Other agents connected with sclerodermatous disease include epoxy resins, metaphenylenediamine, pentazocine, and denatured rapeseed oil. Systemic scleroderma has been reported after augmentation mammoplasty with silicone gel implants (for review see reference 11). The disease may develop many years after surgery and may be related to the leakage of silicone from the implants, which triggers a persistent inflammatory reaction with resultant fibrosis. Removal of the silicone implant may cause the disease to remit and should be tried, especially if the patient develops hypertension.[12] Scleroderma-like skin changes may be associated with scleromyxedema, porphyria cutanea tarda, and graft-versus-host disease. Similar skin changes, primarily in the legs, have been described in the carcinoid syndrome, but these entities, though related, are clearly separable from scleroderma diseases per se. Familial cases of SSc have been reported, but a clear-cut genetic predisposition for the disease has not been established.

Clinical Manifestations

Localized morphea is characterized by circumscribed sclerotic plaques with ivory-colored centers and, if the disease is in an active state, violaceous borders (Fig. 173-1). The lesion often begins as a reddened area that may show some nonpitting edema. The center gradually becomes white or yellowed. Often there is a diminished sweat response and an absence of hair in the lesion. The plaques, whether slightly elevated or depressed, are indurated but not bound to the deeper structures. Most commonly, the lesions are single or few in number, but they may be multiple. They range in size from 1

to 30 cm.[3] Uncommonly, localized morphea may occur after radiation therapy at the site of treatment. Its development is not related to dosage or to the severity of the acute reaction. Whether it results from the well-recognized fibroblastic response to irradiation is unknown.

Generalized morphea, a severe form of the local disease, differs from it in that involvement of the skin is widespread, with multiple indurated plaques and hyperpigmentation, and there is often muscle atrophy. The plaques may be larger, but in the early stages are often indistinguishable from lesions of localized morphea. They involve the upper trunk, abdomen, buttocks, and legs. Generalized morphea is not associated with systemic disease.

Antinuclear antibodies, elevated immunoglobulins, and rheumatoid factor have been reported in all forms of localized scleroderma,[10,11] but the overall incidence is uncertain. The prognosis is good; the disease often becomes inactive in 3 to 5 years.[3] Slight atrophy, often with hyperpigmentation, may be the only persisting sequel of either form of morphea; disability from muscle atrophy may also be a sequel of severe cases of morphea.

Guttate morphea may be a variant of localized morphea or of lichen sclerosis et atrophicus. Morphea and lichen sclerosis et atrophicus can occur simultaneously in the same patient. The coexistence of these two disorders in ten patients has been reported, with the same lesion frequently showing histologic evidence of both diseases.[13] Guttate morphea is characterized by multiple small chalk-white lesions, which lack the firm character of morphea, involving primarily the neck and upper trunk.

Linear scleroderma is a form of the disease that occurs as a linear band, usually with a single unilateral lesion. The lower extremities are most often involved, followed by upper extremities, frontal areas of the head, and anterior thorax.[3] If the upper and lower extremities are involved, the lesions are homolateral. Calcinosis within a linear lesion occurs rarely. Frontal or frontal parietal linear scleroderma is called *coup de sabre,* and is characterized by atrophy and a furrow in the skin (Fig. 173-2). The depression may be extensive, causing facial hemiatrophy, sometimes with atrophy of the tongue on the same side. Linear frontal lesions and active morphea plaques may coexist on the same side of the face. An important distinction between linear scleroderma and morphea is that linear scleroderma involves not only superficial but also deeper layers of the skin, with fixation to underlying structures. Because

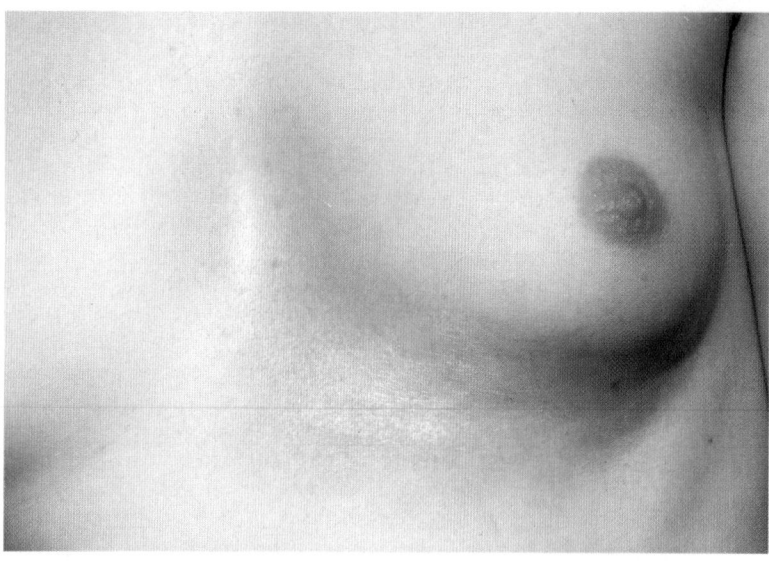

FIGURE 173-1 Morphea. There is an indurated, poorly defined plaque under the left breast. The lesion is multicolored with a central, yellow, ''carnauba-wax'' area surrounded by a lilac border.

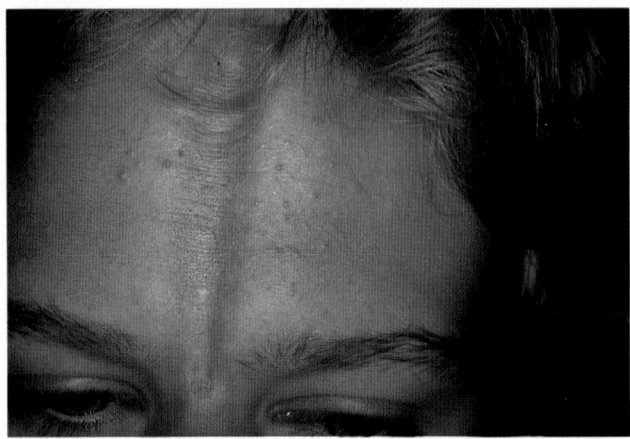

FIGURE 173-2 *Coup de sabre.* Linear, atrophic depression involving the forehead.

linear scleroderma occurs most often during the first two decades of life, it may cause severe deformities, such as hemiatrophy of an extremity or a side of the face, or contractures. Linear scleroderma may also be associated with anomalies of the vertebral column, the most common being spina bifida occulta.[1,14] *Melorheostosis,* an unusual linear, dense, cortical hyperostosis often affecting an involved limb, but occasionally widespread, may rarely occur.[15]

Although there are several reports [16,17] that the tick-borne spirochete *Borrelia burgdorferi,* which is responsible for Lyme disease, plays a role in the pathogenesis of morphea, these studies have not been confirmed. In addition, there is no evidence that the antibiotic therapy used successfully in treating Lyme disease is effective in treating morphea. The coexistence of morphea and acrodermatitis chronica atrophicans (a disorder in which *B. burgdorferi* may well be the causative agent) does occur[18] but may be coincidental. Further studies will be required to either confirm or dispel a link between morphea and the spirochete causing Lyme disease.

Eosinophilia has been reported to occur in localized scleroderma. In one such study[19] eosinophilia (>400 cells/μL) was most common in generalized morphea and linear scleroderma and uncommon in morphea. Eosinophilia signified active disease. Antinuclear antibodies are commonly present in localized scleroderma and are found in 50 percent of cases when HEp-2 cells are used as the substrate.[20] The incidence of antinuclear antibodies is greatest in linear scleroderma, being present in at least 67 percent of the patients examined in one study.[21] Antibodies to single-stranded DNA (ssDNA) have been reported in 59 percent of cases, with the highest levels in patients with generalized morphea,[20] especially those with clinically active disease.

The *Parry-Romberg syndrome* (facial hemiatrophy) may be a form of linear scleroderma, but this has not been established (see Chap. 184). This syndrome is characterized by hyperpigmentation followed by atrophy of the dermis, subcutaneous fat, muscle, and sometimes the underlying bone. The atrophy is usually deeper than that seen in *coup de sabre,* but the skin is less often bound down. It may be impossible to distinguish the two disorders. Whether scleroderma-like hemiatrophy of the face, which spreads to the homolateral or contralateral side of the body, forms a variant of the Parry-Romberg syndrome has not been established. A case has been reported[22] of progressive facial hemiatrophy with a positive ANA, rheumatoid factor, and elevated gamma globulins, findings which may be associated with linear scleroderma.

In *systemic scleroderma* the clinical manifestations depend on the sites involved. The initial complaints are usually related either to Raynaud's phenomenon or to chronic, usually nonpitting, edema of the hands and fingers. As many as one-third of patients first have pain and stiffness of the fingers and knees. In some cases, the first manifestation is active polyarthritis, often migratory. In other cases, severe erosive digital osteoarthritis (related to the CREST syndrome, particularly in females) occurs first. Flexion contractures and sclerodactyly are present, and on x-ray, digital tuft resorption, subcutaneous calcification, joint space narrowing and focal erosions of the periarticular bone are seen. Usually, skin changes precede visceral involvement by several years, but occasionally this order is reversed.[23]

The disease then extends to involve the upper extremities (Fig. 173-3), trunk, face, and finally the lower extremities, which may sometimes be spared. In the early stages, the peculiar, painless, slightly pitting edema often lasts several months before tightening of the skin occurs. Isolated periorbital edema may occur in the early edematous phase in patients with few other manifestations of SSc. Often the skin feels indurated and stiff, and as it progresses to the atrophic state, it becomes tense, smooth, hardened, and eventually firmly bound to the underlying structures (Fig. 173-4). The skin of the face becomes masklike and expressionless, with loss of the normal facial lines and then thinning of the lips and constriction of the opening of the mouth (microstomia). Radial furrowing around the mouth is seen (Fig. 173-5). Uncommonly, the mucous membranes are involved, with painful induration of the gums and tongue. A prominent feature is tightening of the skin over the nose, giving it a small sharp appearance. The neck sign, ridging and tightening of the skin of the neck on extending the head, is commonly seen. Matlike telangiectases may develop (Fig. 173-5), especially about the face and upper trunk. There may be thinning or complete loss of hair and anhidrosis in the affected areas. Generalized hyperpigmentation, like that of Addison's disease but with no evidence of adrenal insufficiency or elevated plasma MSH-β, can occur and may antedate the sclerosis. Focal hyper- or hypopigmentation may represent a postinflammatory response in the areas of sclerosis.

Sclerodactyly causes the fingers to become tapered, with marked skin atrophy. As in systemic lupus erythematosus (SLE) and dermatomyositis, periungual telangiectasia is seen. In as many as 75 percent of cases of SSc, enlarged, dilated nail fold capillaries forming "giant" or sausage-shaped loops can be seen by capillary microscopy of the nail folds (done with an ophthalmoscope),[24] and this examination can be useful in confirming the diagnosis.[25] The pattern in scleroderma can be distinguished from the changes in SLE but not from those seen in dermatomyositis. Capillary microscopy may be of prognostic value in Raynaud's disease, because if nail fold capillary changes are present, the patient is more likely to develop SSc later. Another common problem is recurrent painful ulceration of the fingertips (Fig. 173-6). Slow-healing ulcers over the knuckles may also occur. These ulcers may heal with stellate scarring, become chronic, or, rarely, become gangrenous. Flexion contractures of the stiff fingers trouble many patients. Resorption of bone may cause dissolution of terminal phalanges, and cutaneous calcification develops in some cases, especially around fingertips and bony prominences but also in any area involved with scleroderma. These calcifications may ulcerate, extrude calcified material, and reepithelialize very slowly.

Dental x-rays of patients with SSc often show widening of the periodontal membrane and loss of the lamina dura. Bone absorption at the angle of the mandible may occur, perhaps secondary to tightness of facial skin and atrophy of the underlying muscles.

Systemic involvement manifests itself in many ways. Esophageal dysfunction is the most common internal manifestation (over

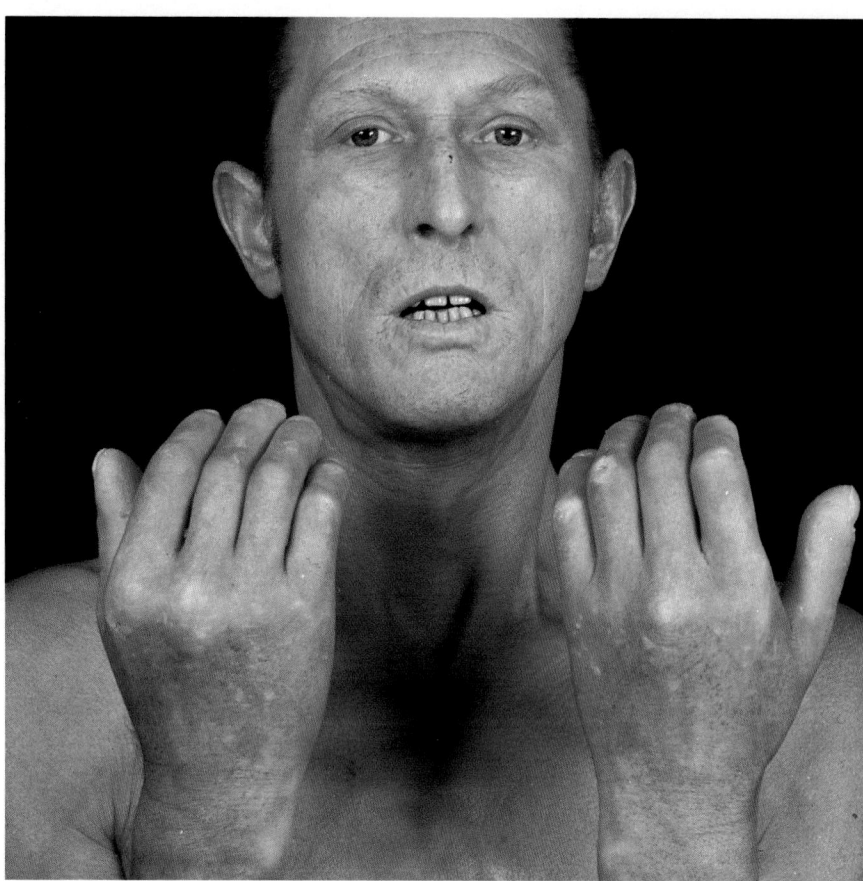

FIGURE 173-3 Scleroderma. The connective tissue changes in the face result in loss of the normal facial lines producing a masklike appearance, a thinning of the lips, and a perioral furrowing (rhagades). The hands exhibit a sclerodactylia with tapering of the fingers and a waxy, shiny, atrophic skin. There are flexion contractures and ulceration of the skin overlying the bony prominences on the right hand.

90 percent). Dysphagia is due to diminished peristalsis, especially in the distal two-thirds of the esophagus, easily seen on radiologic or manometric study. Heartburn from reflex esophagitis due to a loss of tone in the lower esophageal sphincter occurs commonly, but hemorrhage is rare. Dysphagia may occur long before skin involvement,[26] thereby giving rise to the idea of systemic sclerosis sine scleroderma. Abnormal esophageal motility has also been reported in Raynaud's phenomenon, dermatomyositis, and lupus erythematosus. In SSc the small intestine may be involved, producing symptoms of constipation, diarrhea, bloating, and sometimes malabsorption. Common findings on x-ray include delayed transit with prolonged retention of barium and distension of the small bowel, all secondary to atonia.

Another important feature of SSc is pulmonary involvement with fibrosis. Patients complain of exertional dyspnea, and small

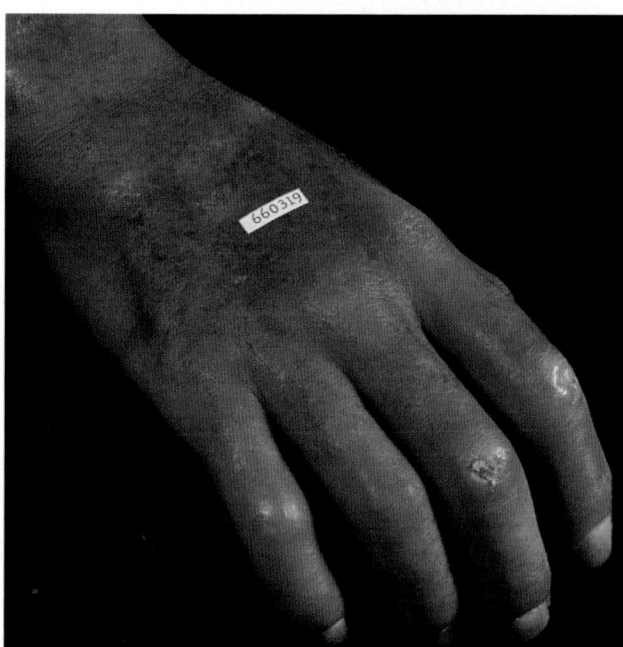

FIGURE 173-4 Scleroderma. Skin is atrophic and appears tense and smooth and has become firmly bound to the underlying structures.

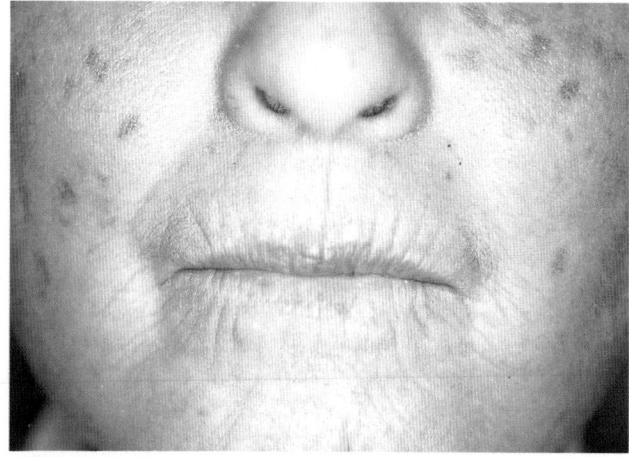

FIGURE 173-5 Radial furrowing around the mouth and matlike telangiectasis are prominent on the cheeks in a patient with scleroderma.

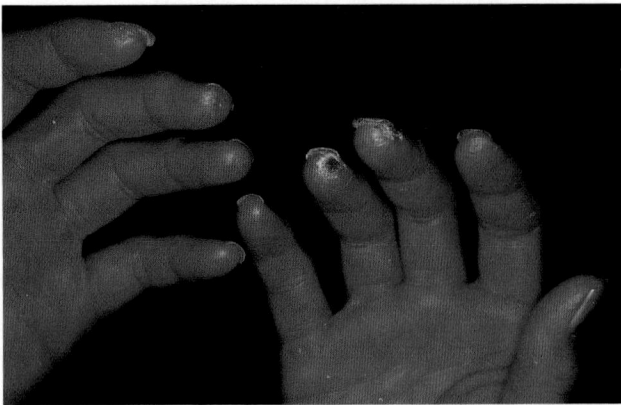

FIGURE 173-6 Ulceration of the fingertips in a patient with Raynaud's phenomenon and scleroderma.

airway disease is an early sensitive indicator of pulmonary involvement that often precedes measurable impairment of gas diffusion.[27] Alveolitis, which can be detected by bronchoalveolar lavage, occurs frequently in SSc, and patients with persistent alveolitis show progressive reduction in pulmonary function over time.[28] Early treatment with prednisone and cyclophosphamide may result in significant clinical improvement. Early pulmonary involvement, functionally characterized by a lowered diffusing capacity of the alveolocapillary membrane, correlates with morphologic changes of the nail fold capillaries.[29] Cardiac involvement in SSc may cause conduction defects, heart failure, or pericarditis; the latter is often associated with effusion and sometimes with tamponade. The overall prevalence of myocardial fibrosis in SSc in approximately 50 to 70 percent. Myocardial fibrosis is associated with microvascular coronary vasospasm, which has been linked to a myocardial Raynaud's phenomenon.[30]

Renal involvement occurs in about 45 percent. Some patients have slowly progressive uremia, but for most the renal failure is abrupt and associated with a malignant form of hypertension. There has been some suggestion that the acute renal failure and hypertension were induced by corticosteroids, but these findings have clearly occurred in patients who had never received corticosteroids.[23]

CREST Syndrome

A clinical variant of scleroderma is the CREST syndrome. The telangiectasias are most evident on the skin of the face (Fig. 173-5), upper trunk, and hands, but they also occur on the lips and oral mucosa and throughout the entire gastrointestinal tract. Gastrointestinal bleeding from the lesions occurs uncommonly. The CREST syndrome is a more slowly progressive form of the disease; it develops later in life than dSSc and so has a more favorable prognosis. It is not entirely a benign syndrome because the esophageal dysfunction is identical to that of the more severe forms of the disease, and occasionally pulmonary hypertension and biliary cirrhosis occur. Anticentromere antibodies have been identified in 50 to 96 percent of patients with CREST syndrome, but in only 12 to 25 percent of patients with dSSc.[31,32] Anticentromere antibodies have prognostic value since they may appear before the development of the full CREST syndrome and are associated with less systemic involvement. Antitopoisomerase I antibodies are more

frequently associated with dSSc (approximately 30 percent), and patients having these antibodies appear to have a less favorable prognosis than patients with anticentromere antibodies.[32]

Three patients with a high titer of IgG antibody to a 34-kDa protein, fibrillarin, associated with U3-RNP, were characterized by diffuse skin involvement, widespread telangiectasia and internal (gastrointestinal, lung, renal) manifestations, lack of anticentromere antibodies, and a progressive course.[33] Patients with SSc need to be studied to determine if these characteristics define a subset.

Patients with combined features of scleroderma, lupus erythematosus, and myositis have been grouped under the heading of *mixed connective tissue disease* (MCTD). The patients have high titers of antibody to a ribonucleoprotein, the extractable nuclear antigen.[34] Patients with SSc have not been found to have this antibody.

Eosinophilic Fasciitis and Eosinophilia-Myalgia Syndrome

Other syndromes that cause scleroderma-like skin changes, such as eosinophilic fasciitis (Shulman's syndrome) and the eosinophilia-myalgia syndrome are discussed in Chap. 90.

Toxic Oil Syndrome

The toxic oil syndrome occurred in epidemic form in Spain in 1981 and affected approximately 25,000 people.[35-39] It resulted from the consumption of denatured rapeseed oil sold as olive oil for cooking. To date, ingestion of the denatured rapeseed oil has caused approximately 600 deaths and has left 300 individuals disabled by a chronic multisystem disease. This syndrome has the features of a toxic allergic reaction, with an acute phase associated with a morbilliform-type eruption, pruritus, fever, interstitial pneumonitis, myalgia, and liver function abnormalities. Serum IgE levels were elevated in 37 to 50 percent of the cases. Approximately 5 percent of those affected presented with seizures and encephalopathy. Several months after onset, a chronic phase begins which is characterized by severe neuromuscular abnormalities, generalized edema, scleroderma-like skin lesions, joint contractures, Sjögren-like syndrome, and pulmonary hypertension. The histopathology of the skin lesions is similar to that described in another disease, the eosinophilia-myalgia syndrome[40] (see Chap. 90). In both phases the primary injury is vascular, with evidence of perivascular inflammation, intimal proliferation, reduplication of the basal lamina, endothelial damage, and luminal obliteration.[39] Immunofluorescence with antiprocollagen and antifibronectin antibodies and electron microscopy confirmed the vascular damage.

The exact cause of the syndrome remains obscure, but it appears that the ingestion of aniline-degraded reprocessed rapeseed oil leads to a chronic autoimmune disease. An oil of comparable chemical composition to case-related oils has been produced, and an in vitro toxicologic assay with mouse neuroblastoma and rat liver epithelial cells has been developed.[41] Extracts from aniline-treated rapeseed oil and several high-performance liquid chromatography fractions were toxic to these cells when compared to appropriate controls. It appears that at least some of the puzzling aspects of this syndrome may soon be solved.

Cutaneous Histopathology

The features of morphea or SSc seen in any histologic section of a skin biopsy depend on the stage of the disease and the biopsy site (Figs. 173-7 to 173-9). In morphea, specimens from the peripheral violaceous border show many inflammatory cells among collagen bundles of the lower two-thirds of the reticular dermis and the fibrous trabeculae of the subcutaneous tissue, and among the fat cells of the subcutaneous tissue. Usually lymphocytes and histiocytes predominate; but there may be large numbers of plasma cells, and occasionally there are mast cells. Formation of typical lymphoid follicles with germinal centers may be seen. Mononuclear cell infiltrates are much less common in SSc than in localized scleroderma and are often less severe.

Associated with the inflammatory infiltrate are collagen changes, which first occur in the lower third of the dermis and in the fibrous trabeculae of the subcutaneous tissues. Later in the disease the changes extend to the upper portion of the dermis and consist of a markedly increased eosinophilia of collagen, broadening of collagen bundles, and decreased space between collagen bundles. Biopsies from the central region of well-developed lesions of morphea may show only collagen changes but no inflammation. In these later stages of morphea the pathology is similar to that of SSc. The collagen bundle pattern is altered so that most bundles appear to parallel the dermal-epidermal junction. The inflammatory stage is followed by the replacement of the subcutaneous tissue by hyalinized connective tissue. On electron microscopy, the fibrous trabeculae of the subcutaneous tissue are increased in thickness by deposition of immature collagen fibrils smaller in diameter than normal, suggesting increased collagen synthesis.

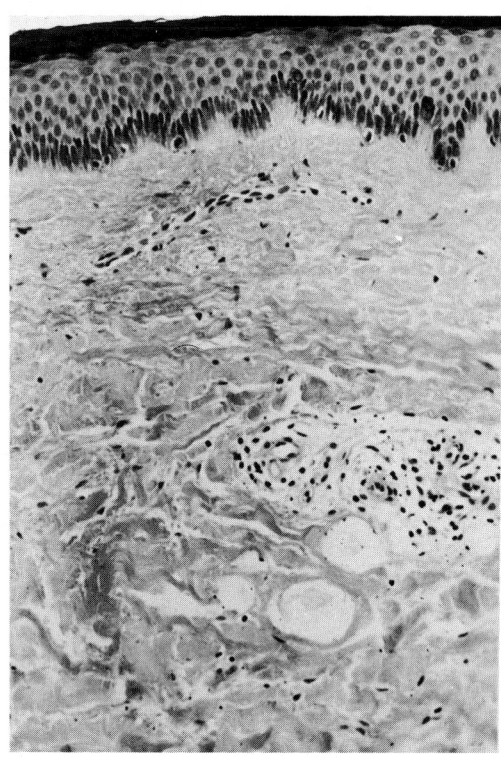

FIGURE 173-8 Scleroderma. The collagen bundle pattern of the reticular dermis is virtually obliterated, and one cannot distinguish between papillary and reticular dermis. ×160. (*Micrograph by Wallace H. Clark, Jr., M.D.*)

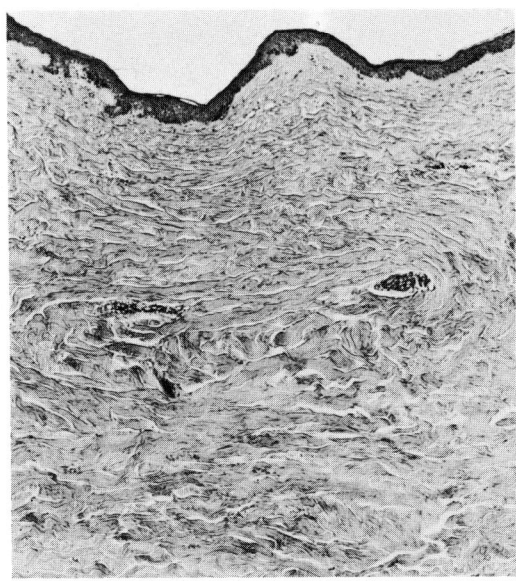

FIGURE 173-7 Scleroderma. The changes of generalized scleroderma and localized scleroderma (morphea) overlap; the former, however, is dominated by dense, acellular sclerosis, and the latter shows varying degrees of inflammation with some extension into the subcutis. Figs. 173-7 and 173-8 show the pathologic changes of scleroderma and Fig. 173-9 shows the pathologic changes of morphea. In this photomicrograph one sees broad collagen bundles which tend to parallel each other, diminished interbundle spaces, and few cells of any kind. ×40. (*Micrograph by Wallace H. Clark, Jr., M.D.*)

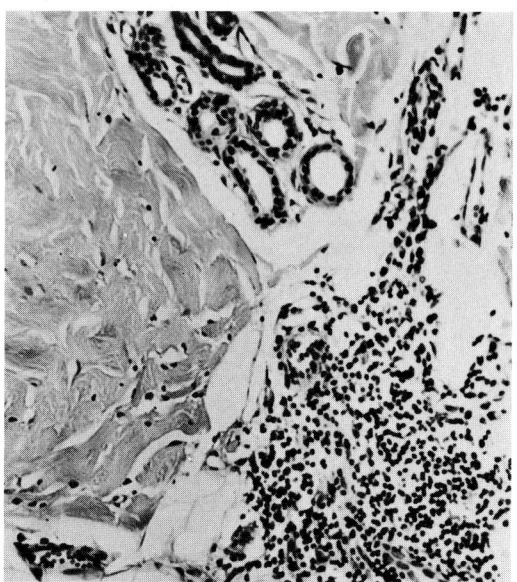

FIGURE 173-9 Morphea. The connective tissue changes in morphea seem to extend from the lower reticular dermis outward and are usually indistinguishable from the changes of generalized scleroderma. Biopsies taken from the margins of morphea lesions, however, frequently show extensive inflammation; such inflammation may be patchy, as one sees here, or it may involve the reticular dermis rather diffusely, presenting some difficulty in histologic diagnosis. ×40. (*Micrograph by Wallace H. Clark, Jr., M.D.*)

A form of localized scleroderma termed *morphea profunda*, presenting with either solitary or generalized lesions, has also been described.[42] The lesions are associated with a subcutaneous, dense, mononuclear cell infiltrate with abundant plasma cells and with extensive sclerosis and hyalinization of the connective tissue and occasional involvement of the underlying fascia. Lymphoid aggregates with germinal center formation have been described in some of the solitary lesions.

The pathology of SSc is similar to that of morphea. The lower two-thirds of the dermis and the subcutaneous fibrous trabeculae sclerose. Panniculitis may also be a prominent feature in the early stages. Subcutaneous fat is replaced by hyalinized connective tissue and this process is particularly evident around eccrine sweat glands. The collagen bundles appear pale, homogeneous, and swollen, but the collagen bundle swelling, increased eosinophilia, and inflammation are not as prominent as in morphea. The glycosaminoglycans of ground substance also may be markedly increased. In the late stages of SSc, secondary changes, such as absence of pilosebaceous units, eccrine ducts, and glands, and effacement of the rete ridges of the epidermis may be evident. These abnormalities indicate that the disease process is advanced. Electron microscopy has revealed randomly arranged "immature" collagen fibrils, from 100 to 400 Å in diameter, in contrast to mature collagen fibrils from 700 to 800 Å. Whether the immature fibrils represent newly synthesized collagen remains speculative.

Vessels of all sizes may be involved in SSc, and vascular involvement is an important, although inconsistent, feature. In the early stages, there may be only dilatation of capillaries and lymphatics. Then intimal proliferation and complete occlusion of the vessel may occur. These changes may also be seen in muscle capillaries. Occlusive vascular changes are not found in morphea, but the precise implications of the difference are unclear. Possibly they are somehow related to the spontaneous involution of morphea. In morphea, skeletal muscle fibers underlying affected skin may be structurally damaged in the absence of changes in muscle capillaries.

Pathogenesis

The cause of scleroderma is still unknown. Among the questions yet to be answered are the following: What is the precipitating cause of scleroderma? How does this cause relate to the toxic compounds and physical agents that also cause scleroderma or similar conditions? What cellular events occur in the primary response to the etiologic agents, and what chain of inter- and intracellular events then ensues? How does a person's immunologic make-up influence the outcome of an encounter with whatever causes scleroderma? Are the autoantibodies pathogenic or epiphenomena, and what provokes them to appear? What causes fibrosis, and what makes it advance or regress?

We believe that in scleroderma endothelium suffers some basic insult, and one end result is tissue ischemia. There is a loss of capillaries, with an earlier stage of capillary abnormality visible on nail fold capillaroscopy, and faulty vascular function, as seen in Raynaud's phenomenon, which is a prominent, but not invariant feature of scleroderma. Histologically, the endothelial cells are swollen, with gaps between the cells, and there exist surrounding cellular infiltrates, particularly of T cells, but also of lymphocytes and monocytes. Serum of patients with SSc appears to contain a factor cytotoxic for endothelial cells. Penning et al.[43] found that when sera from 39 patients with SSc were co-cultured with normal human monocytes, 23 percent were highly cytotoxic for endothelial cells in vitro. The cytotoxic factor was present in the IgG fraction. Kahaleh and LeRoy[44] had previously identified a cytotoxic activity in serum from patients with SSc that could be inhibited by protease inhibitors, and their findings have been confirmed and extended by others.[45] The damaged endothelium may also be activated endothelium; as Pober et al. point out,[46] the above histology characterizes endothelium activated to a state of increased synthesis, secretion, and immune participation. Serum from patients with SSc contains laminin fragments, type IV collagen, and dimeric nonfunctional von Willebrand factor,[47,48] all considered to be indices of endothelial damage. Damaged endothelium induces a procoagulant state,[49] which may contribute to the pathology of this disease. Small vessels show intimal proliferation and basal lamina reduplication; some of these changes may reflect activation or damaged endothelium attempting to regenerate, but eventually the vessels are obliterated. Deguchi et al.[50] showed that fibroblasts from seven patients with SSc had a fibronectin gene mutation adjacent to the cell attachment site, causing an Ala to Gly substitution. Perhaps this factor plays some role in the disease by causing aberrant cell interaction.

The primary etiologic agent(s) of SSc precipitate pathogenic events that involve circulating cells of the immune system as well as endothelial cells and fibroblasts. As yet, we do not know what sequence of events ensues from the encounter of a patient with the causative agent(s) of SSc, but it seems likely that the factors that mediate tissue damage, including the damage to endothelium, are produced by macrophages, T cells, mast cells, endothelial cells themselves, or, most probably, a combination of them. These cells all communicate with one another and with fibroblasts.

Several cytokines and growth factors have been studied in SSc. They include interleukin 2 (IL-2),[51,52] soluble IL-2 receptor,[53] IL-1α and -1β, tumor necrosis factor (TNF) from monocytes,[54] platelet-derived growth factor (PDGF),[55] and β-thromboglobulin.[56] IL-1α, IL-1β, and TNF activate cultured endothelial cells to produce procoagulant and proinflammatory molecules,[46,57] including ELAM-1, IL-1, and class I MHC antigens. Interferon-γ, not yet well studied in SSc, can cause endothelium to express class II MHC molecules, which bind foreign antigens and present them to helper T cells.[58] IL-1α, IL-1β, and TNF also stimulate fibroblast growth.[54] T cells activated by a mitogen, antigen, or cytokine make IL-2, which can bind to receptors on other T cells and cause them to proliferate. Kahaleh and Leroy[51] examined the effect of sera from patients with SSc in supporting growth of an IL-2-dependent cytotoxic T-cell line and found a significant mitogenic effect in sera from 41 of 47 patients with SSc, 9 of 20 with rheumatoid arthritis, and 0 of 14 normal controls. There were also higher serum levels of IL-2 in patients with SSc compared to normals, and incubation experiments with IL-2 alone or with SSc versus normal sera suggested an IL-2 inhibitor present in normal serum is absent in SSc serum. IL-2 causes natural killer cells to stick to human endothelial cells,[59] possibly killing them, and causes pulmonary edema and vasoconstriction,[60] as does IL-1β.[61] The killer cells activated by IL-2 contain serine esterases, which may be implicated in the cytotoxicity of sera from patients with SSc.[62] Guinan et al.[63] found endothelial cells to be capable of boosting IL-2 levels; they propose that this contributes to a unique ability of endothelial cells to boost T-cell responses to limiting quantities of antigen. Antigens are detected in the body by virtue of their interactions with receptors on cells of the immune system. A class of T cells expressing receptors encoded by gamma and delta genes binds soluble antigens and MHC class I or II molecules. Kratz et al.[64] analyzed the restriction fragment length polymorphisms (RFLP) of the gamma T-cell receptor gene; they found that 41.0 percent of patients with SSc have an 11.3-kb allele of the Pvu 2 RFLP, whereas only 21.7 percent of the controls have it. This Pvu 2 site is near the polymorphic C gamma 2 gene. Perhaps T-cell receptors expressing certain alleles of this gene interact with antigen in such a way as to predispose toward abnormal function of the immune response. There may also be other such idiosyncrasies in the antigen receptor system. Although we do not know what this evidence means, it does provide an idea of how the immune mechanism might interact with an antigen in a dysfunctional way.

Mast cells have been investigated in scleroderma because they are associated with some conditions in which fibrosis is common. For example, in chronic graft-versus-host (GVH) disease of mice, in which there is cutaneous fibrosis similar to that in SSc, mast cells seemed to disappear from the skin; actually they could be demonstrated to be present, but were degranulated, and their synthetic apparatus indicated active synthesis. In scleroderma, mast cells are increased in affected skin only in early disease,[65] and in skin not yet affected, there were increased numbers of total and degranulated mast cells; 10 of the 11 patients had fibrosis of that skin within 1.5 years of the biopsy.[66]

Mast cells may need to be stimulated by mediators from mononuclear cells to cause fibrosis. Several investigators have shown that histamine mediates fibrosis, and elevated histamine levels have been found in patients with SSc.[67] Heparin also may stimulate fibroblasts in vitro. TNF is an effector in acute GVH disease[68] and increases the production of plasminogen activator inhibitor in human endothelial cells in vitro and in rats in vivo.[69] It mediates release of PDGF from endothelial cells in culture,[70] and PDGF itself has been shown histologically to be deposited in endothelium in association with mononuclear cell infiltrates.

Chromosome breaking (clastogenic) activity has been identified in plasma ultrafiltrates of patients with SSc.[71] The clastogenic fractions were shown to be compatible with inosine diphosphate and inosine triphosphate, and these nucleotides, when added to other normal cells, also doubled the incidence of chromosomal damage. Superoxide dismutase protected chromosomes from damage by ITP. The authors of this study speculate that ischemia causes depletion of ATP, and the ITP is produced under those conditions. This area of research may turn out to be very fruitful, especially if it converges with the research on the various cytokines and growth factors that may be active mediators of the disease.

Collagen overproduction in SSc seems to be a reactive, rather than a constitutive reaction[66]; presumably some factor(s) drive normal (or formerly normal) fibroblasts to make too much collagen. A subset of the fibroblast population may be particularly susceptible to the effects of such triggering factors.[72] Although the mechanism is unknown, there is evidence that collagen genes are turned on. Cells from sclerodermatous areas produce increased amounts of collagen types I and III without a change in collagenase synthesis.[73] Analysis of fibroblast cell lines from patients with progressive morphea revealed an increase in collagen synthesis and $pro\alpha1$ collagen mRNAs in affected skin.[74] However, this could be due to increased stability of the mRNA, as well as to increased transcription. A deeper understanding of the pathogenesis of SSc may come when we know more about regulatory sequences in the 5′ region of the collagen genes: what factors turn them on and off, how cytokines modulate their expression, and which sequences are important for interaction with cis- and trans-acting factors.

Transforming growth factor β (TGF-β) transcriptionally activates the mouse $\alpha2(I)$ and $\alpha1(III)$ collagen promoters in NIH 3T3 fibroblasts and ROS 17/2 cells through its effect on their nuclear factor 1 binding sites.[75] TGF-β also increases steady-state amounts of type I and type III collagen (known to be increased in SSc skin) and fibronectin in normal human dermal fibroblasts, and the stimulation continues for at least 72 h after removal of TGF-β.[76] $TGF-\beta_2$ mRNA (but not $TGF-\beta_1$) and $pro\alpha1(I)$ collagen are co-localized in the inflammatory infiltrate that surrounds the dermal blood vessels in the inflammatory stage of SSc but not in the fibrotic stage of the disease.[77] Neither gene was expressed in the dermis of patients with SLE or dermatomyositis. This finding suggests that $TGF-\beta_2$, produced by perivascular inflammatory cells, results in an increased gene expression of type I collagen in closely approximated fibroblasts, thus playing a major role in mediating the fibrotic process in SSc. The production of IL-1α, IL-1β, and TNF in vitro by monocytes of patients with SSc is significantly greater than that by monocytes from normal individuals.[54] Because these cytokines stimulate fibroblast growth, their overproduction by monocytes from patients with SSc may be important in pathogenesis. When the transcription rate of the type I collagen gene in fibroblasts from affected skin and unaffected skin of three patients with localized scleroderma was measured, from 3 to almost 5 times as much $pro\alpha2(I)$ collagen mRNA was found in the affected skin as in the unaffected.[78] The highly suggestive evidence about the damage to endothelium, presumptively mediated by cells or products of cells of the immune system, brings us to the question of what triggers the activities of those cells. Autoantibodies in patients with autoimmune diseases cross-react with a retroviral gag protein.[79] Maul et al.[80] have cloned DNA topoisomerase 1 (an antigen to which antibodies are found in dSSc), sequenced it, and found the smallest peptide recognized by dSSc serum. An 11-amino acid–long piece has six sequential amino acids identical to a sequence in the p30 gag protein of some mammalian retroviruses. Furthermore, the 70-kDa RNP epitope of MCTD is separated by only one amino acid from the 6-amino acid match of topoisomerase 1 with the same p30 gag protein. The authors discuss the idea that autoantibodies are epiphenomena representing fingerprints of a virus that has caused disease by transforming T cells or target cells such as fibroblasts or endothelial cells. This field of inquiry and the hypothesis developed by those working in it provide a plausible theoretical framework for further study.

Animal models for scleroderma include an induced rat disease[81] and a genetic disease of mice.[82] The autosomal dominant tight-skin mouse mutant[82] shows connective tissue changes but no vascular changes. The mice do have abundant mast cells with prominent degranulation in their skin. Most important is the finding[83] that oral disodium cromoglycate and ketotifen, both inhibitors of mast cell degranulation, decrease mast cell degranulation and fibrosis in the tight-skin mouse.

Course

In patients with morphea or linear scleroderma, the disease may last from a few months to many years. In approximately one-half of the cases, the lesions disappear or soften, leaving areas of hyperpigmentation or depigmentation. In some, the disease may involute completely. In the *coup de sabre* type of scleroderma, the lesions remain unchanged or become more extensive. It is unlikely that true localized scleroderma progresses into systemic scleroderma, although such a progression has been reported in 6 of 106 cases (5.7 percent) in patients with generalized disease,[84] and three cases have been reported in which localized scleroderma with hemiatrophy was associated with SLE, SSc, or a rheumatoid arthritis-like picture.[85]

In SSc, evidence of visceral involvement develops in most of the patients if they are followed long enough. In some cases, the disease may progress rapidly, and the severity of vital organ involvement determines the outcome. The prognosis is particularly poor in those with cardiopulmonary involvement, in those who develop hypertension and renal insufficiency, and in those who are 45 years or older at the time the initial diagnosis is made. Current therapy has increased the 1-year survival rate in scleroderma renal crisis from less than 25 percent to greater than 75 percent, but there is a small group of patients with rapidly progressive dSSc who develop multiorgan failure despite intensive treatment.[86] In about half the patients the disease reaches a plateau or shows signs of regression and may result in only a moderate degree of disability.

Management

The treatment of localized scleroderma remains unsatisfactory. The use of topical corticosteroids and the intralesional injection of steroids into plaques of morphea have been unrewarding. Patients with limited involvement may require no treatment, since in most cases the lesions resolve spontaneously. Antimalarials, phenytoin, colchicine, and systemic corticosteroids have been used in generalized morphea but provide little proven benefit. Of 11 patients with severe localized scleroderma treated with D-penicillamine, six improved after 3 to 6 months of therapy, with skin softening, resumed growth of affected limbs, and cessation of appearance of new lesions.[87] The mean length of treatment was 21 months (range 15 to 53), with a mean daily dose ranging from 2.0 to 5.0 mg/kg. Careful monitoring for renal and hematologic toxicity is essential. Physiotherapy or surgery to prevent contractures may be necessary in linear scleroderma.

Many agents have been tried in the therapy of SSc and found wanting. They include antimalarials, bismuth, relaxin, EDTA, aminocaproic acid, dimethylsulfoxide, *p*-aminobenzoate, colchicine, and immunosuppressive drugs. Systemic corticosteroids may be of some benefit for limited periods early in the disease or for specific inflammatory lesions (myositis, alveolitis, myocarditis) but do not alter the overall course of the disease. Among the agents currently being studied in the hope of finding something capable of at least modifying the course or severity of the disease are recombinant interferon-γ, recombinant tissue plasminogen activator (rtPA), fish oil, and factor XIII.

Several studies of SSc fibroblasts in vitro show that interferons may influence their collagen overproduction toward normal levels. In one study with SSc fibroblasts, collagen production was halved with low doses of interferon-γ and reduced about 60 to 85 percent with higher doses, and a coordinate reduction occurred in the types I and III collagen mRNAs compared with untreated cells.[88] In another study of confluent cultures of normal and SSc fibroblasts, the SSc fibroblasts produced 69 percent more collagen.[89] Interferon-α_2, -β, and -γ all inhibited collagen production in both normal and SSc fibroblasts, but collagen synthesis in the normal cells returned

to baseline after two to three passages, whereas in the SSc fibroblasts collagen production remained reduced for 31 days (18 cell divisions); the degree of collagen reduction in SSc fibroblasts resulted in near-normal collagen production. After 31 days, re-treatment with the interferons again inhibited growth and collagen production in normal fibroblasts, but did not inhibit collagen production any further in SSc fibroblasts; this result was interpreted to mean that the fibroblasts had not been completely restored to normalcy. Such studies have not yet been carried out in patients. Fritzler and Hart[90] describe a patient with a 15-year history of the CREST form of lSSc who had an acute myocardial infarction, was treated with rtPA and heparin, and had swift and significant improvement of skin tightness, ulcers, and Raynaud's phenomenon. Because the improvement followed so suddenly and closely after the rtPA, the report suggests a new modality to study.

It is possible that eicosapentaenoic acid, derived from fish oil, will benefit patients with Raynaud's phenomenon. Although we do not know which of the effects of fish oil may be responsible, DiGiacomo et al.[91] found that patients with primary Raynaud's phenomenon have a longer time before cold induces vasospasm, and 5 of 11 lost inducibility of Raynaud's after cold exposure. Patients also had increased digital systolic blood pressure.

Rook et al.[92] exposed peripheral blood leukocytes of patients with SSc to UVA light after giving the patients 8-methoxypsoralen by mouth, and compared the results to the effect of treatment with D-penicillamine. In a blind test, examiners assessed the results in 22 patients treated with phototherapy and 21 treated with D-penicillamine. Seventy-seven percent had an improved skin score on phototherapy compared to 33 percent on D-penicillamine. Disease progression occurred in 3 of 22 on phototherapy, but in 10 of 21 on D-penicillamine. Histology showed a decrease in deep dermal collagen, and pulmonary function tests were unchanged. Although these results suggest a possible ameliorative treatment for patients with SSc, it is important to realize that the measurements were subjective and that untreated and sham photopheresis controls were not used.

It has been suggested that penicillamine, which is a lathyrogen in animals and can produce an increase in soluble collagen in sclerodermatous skin, may be effective in treating SSc. The results of a retrospective analysis[93] of 73 patients with SSc treated with high-dose penicillamine, 500 to 1500 mg (median 750 mg) daily for an average of 24 months, are encouraging. Significant improvement was not noted in the treated patients until 19 to 42 months after the initiation of therapy. An impressive reduction in skin thickness and in the rate of new visceral organ involvement, especially for the kidney, was found in the treated group. In addition, patients treated with penicillamine had a 5-year cumulative survival rate of 88 percent compared with a 5-year survival rate of 66 percent for the comparison group. These changes were not found in patients treated with colchicine or immunosuppressive agents. Fibroblast cultures from forearm skin biopsies of three patients obtained before and after they had shown a marked decrease in skin thickness during a year or more of penicillamine therapy were examined for glycosaminoglycan and collagen production.[94] No differences were observed in the synthesis of these connective tissue components. These findings indicate that, although penicillamine has a clinical effect on the connective tissue, the fibroblasts from the thinned skin retain their potential for increased collagen and glycosaminoglycan synthesis. In a prospective trial of D-penicillamine in 69 patients with recent onset of rapidly progressive dSSc,[95] there were two nonresponders and nine unable to receive a full trial; the 58 remaining patients had marked regression of sclerosis. D-penicillamine prevents formation of stable collagen cross-links, making the newly formed collagen more vulnerable to degradation. It would not be expected to reverse the basic defect. Of 21 patients whose sclerosis decreased to less than 10 percent of body surface, 15 remained stable after D-penicillamine was stopped.

Gruber and Kaufman[96] treated two patients with ketotifen (an inhibitor of mast cell degranulation), 3 mg orally twice a day, and observed dramatic normalization of early severe SSc in both.

Malabsorption has been successfully treated in some patients by means of long-term, broad-spectrum antibiotics, because bacterial overgrowth occurring in the atonic loops of the bowel plays a major factor in malabsorption. Scleroderma renal crisis is the most acute life-threatening problem that occurs in dSSc. Recent studies indicate that use of the angiotensin-converting enzyme (ACE) inhibitor captopril markedly improves survival and may permit discontinuation of dialysis in some patients.[86] The authors advocate that all SSc patients with new onset hypertension, with or without evidence of renal involvement, should be treated and maintained on an ACE inhibitor.

Patients with Raynaud's phenomenon should be carefully instructed to protect their hands from thermal, chemical, and mechanical trauma. Application of emollients to the hands may be helpful in preventing drying and fissuring of the skin. The calcium-channel blockers nifedipine and verapamil[97,98] have been used to treat Raynaud's phenomenon. Although there is variability in the response to therapy, and some patients fail to respond, at least with nifedipine, 66 percent of the patients treated showed subjective symptomatic improvement in double-blind controlled clinical trials. Intraarterial reserpine is no longer recommended. Serotonin has been implicated in the pathogenesis of the vasospasm associated with Raynaud's phenomenon. Ketanserin, a selective antagonist of 5-hydroxytryptamine receptors (5-HT$_2$) blocks the vasoconstriction and platelet aggregation induced by serotonin, significantly decreases the frequency of vasospastic episodes, and improves the subjective symptoms of patients with either primary or secondary Raynaud's phenomenon.[99] Further studies will be required to establish the efficacy of this drug in SSc. Sympathectomy is ineffective in the management of Raynaud's phenomenon secondary to scleroderma and should not be recommended.

Cyclosporine has been used in one patient with generalized morphea, resulting in a marked, long-term improvement in the skin, and in four patients with SSc.[100] Improvement, as indicated by partial regression of cutaneous fibrosis and the healing of fingertip and leg ulcers, occurred in three of the four patients with SSc treated with cyclosporine. The fourth patient developed acute renal failure and arterial hypertension. Because this patient refused a kidney biopsy, it was not possible to determine whether the findings were secondary to the rapidly progressing disease or due to cyclosporine nephrotoxicity. Until further studies are undertaken, the risk of renal compromise secondary to cyclosporine makes this drug unsuitable for general use in the treatment of SSc.

References

1. Barnett AJ et al: A survival study of patients with scleroderma diagnosed over 30 years (1953–1983): The value of a simple cutaneous classification in the early stages of the disease. *J Rheumatol* **15**:276, 1988

2. Leroy EC et al: Scleroderma (systemic sclerosis): Classification, subsets and pathogenesis. *J Rheumatol* **15**:202, 1988

3. Christianson HB et al: Localized scleroderma: A clinical study of two hundred thirty-five cases. Arch Dermatol **74**:629, 1956

4. Medsger TA Jr, Masi AT: Epidemiology of systemic sclerosis (scleroderma). *Ann Intern Med* **74**:714, 1971

5. Maricq HR: Prevalence of scleroderma spectrum disorders in the general population of South Carolina. *Arthritis Rheum* **32**:998, 1989

6. Medsger TA et al: Survival with systemic sclerosis (scleroderma). *Ann Intern Med* **75**:369, 1971

7. Rodnan GP et al: The association of progressive systemic sclerosis (scleroderma) with coal miners' pneumoconiosis and other forms of silicosis. *Ann Intern Med* **66**:323, 1967

8. Haustein U-F: Silica-induced scleroderma. *J Am Acad Dermatol* **22**:444, 1990

9. Veltman G et al: Clinical manifestations and course of vinylchloride disease. *Ann N Y Acad Sci* **245**:6, 1975

10. Finch WR et al: Bleomycin-induced scleroderma. *J Rheumatol* **7**:651, 1980

11. Varga J et al: Systemic sclerosis after augmentation mammoplasty with silicone implants. *Ann Intern Med* **111**:377, 1989

12. Gutierrez FJ, Espinoza LR: Progressive systemic sclerosis complicated by severe hypertension: Reversal after silicone implant removal. *Am J Med* **89**:390, 1990

13. Uitto J et al: Morphea and lichen sclerosis et atrophicus. *J Am Acad Dermatol* **3**:271, 1980

14. Rubin L: Linear scleroderma: Association with abnormalities of spine and nervous system. *Arch Dermatol Syphilol* **58**:1, 1948

15. Soffa DJ et al: Melorheostosis with linear sclerodermatous changes. *Diagn Radiol* **114**:577, 1975

16. Aberer E: Is localized scleroderma a *Borrelia* infection? *Lancet* **2**:278, 1985

17. Aberer E et al: Evidence for spirochetal origin of circumscribed scleroderma (morphea). *Acta Derm Venereol* **67**:225, 1987

18. Coulson IH et al: Acrodermatitis chronica atrophicans with coexisting morphea. *Br J Dermatol* **121**:263, 1989

19. Falanga V, Medsger TA: Frequency, levels, and significance of blood eosinophilia in systemic sclerosis, localized scleroderma, and eosinophilic fasciitis. *J Am Acad Dermatol* **17**:648, 1987

20. Falanga V, Medsger TA: Antinuclear and anti-single-stranded DNA antibodies in morphea and generalized morphea. *Arch Dermatol* **123**:350, 1987

21. Takehara K et al: Antinuclear antibodies in localized scleroderma. *Arthritis Rheum* **26**:612, 1983

22. Hickman JW, Shiels WS: Progressive facial hemiatrophy. *Arch Intern Med* **113**:716, 1964

23. Rodnan GP: Progressive systemic sclerosis (scleroderma), in *Arthritis and Allied Conditions,* edited by DJ McCarty. Philadelphia, Lea & Febiger, 1979, p 762

24. Minkin W, Rabban NB: Office nail fold capillary microscopy using ophthalmoscope. *J Am Acad Dermatol* **7**:190, 1982

25. Maricq HR et al: Predictive value of capillary microscopy in patients with Raynaud's phenomenon. *Arthritis Rheum* **23**:716, 1980

26. Rodnan GP et al: Progressive systemic sclerosis sine scleroderma. *JAMA* **180**:665, 1962

27. Guttadauria M et al: Pulmonary function in scleroderma. *Arthritis Rheum* **20**:1071, 1977

28. Silver RM et al: Evaluation and management of scleroderma lung disease using bronchoalveolar lavage. *Am J Med* **88**:470, 1990

29. Groen H et al: Pulmonary diffusing capacity disturbances are related to nail fold capillary changes in patients with Raynaud's phenomenon with and without an underlying connective tissue disease. *Am J Med* **89**:34, 1990

30. Follansbee WP et al: A controlled clinicopathologic study of myocardial fibrosis in systemic sclerosis (scleroderma). *J Rheumatol* **17**:656, 1990

31. Moroi Y et al: Antibody to centromere (kinetocore) in scleroderma sera. *Proc Natl Acad Sci USA* **77**:1627, 1980

32. Weiner ES et al: Clinical association of anticentromere antibodies and antibodies to topoisomerase 1: A study of 355 patients. *Arthritis*

Rheum **31**:378, 1988

33. Kurzhals G et al: Clinical association of autoantibodies to fibrillarin with diffuse scleroderma and disseminated telangiectasia. *J Am Acad Dermatol* **23**:832, 1990

34. Sharp GC et al: Mixed connective tissue disease: An apparently distinct rheumatic disease syndrome associated with a specific antibody to an extractable nuclear antigen (ENA). *Am J Med* **52**:148, 1972

35. Tabuenca JM: Toxic-allergic syndrome caused by ingestion of rapeseed oil denatured with aniline. *Lancet* **2**:567, 1981

36. Rigau-Perez JG et al: Epidemiologic investigation of an oil-associated pneumonic paralytic eosinophilic syndrome in Spain. *Am J Epidemiol* **119**:250, 1984

37. Kilbourne EM et al: Clinical epidemiology of toxic-oil syndrome: Manifestations of a new illness. *N Engl J Med* **309**:1408, 1983

38. Castroviejo-Pascual I: A multisystem disease caused by adulterated rapeseed oil. *Brain Dev* **10**:84, 1988

39. Phelps RG et al: Clinical pathologic and immunopathologic manifestations of the toxic oil syndrome, analysis of fourteen cases. *J Am Acad Dermatol* **18**:313, 1988

40. Varga J et al: Development of diffuse fasciitis with eosinophilia during L-tryptophan treatment: Demonstration of elevated type I collagen gene expression in affected tissues. *Ann Intern Med* **112**:344, 1990

41. Slack PT et al: Toxic oil disaster. *Nature* **345**:583, 1990

42. Whittaker SJ et al: Solitary morphoea profunda. *Br J Dermatol* **120**:431, 1989

43. Penning CA et al: Antibody-dependent cellular cytotoxicity of human vascular endothelium in systemic sclerosis. *Clin Exp Immunol* **57**:548, 1984

44. Kahaleh MB, LeRoy EC: Endothelial injury in scleroderma. A protease mechanism. *J Lab Clin Med* **101**:553, 1983

45. Meyer O et al: Vascular endothelial cell injury in progressive systemic sclerosis and other connective tissue diseases. *Clin Exp Rheumatol* **1**:29, 1983

46. Pober JS et al: Cytokine-mediated activation of vascular endothelium. Physiology and pathology. *Am J Pathol* **133**:426, 1988

47. Kahaleh MB et al: Increased factor VIII/von Willebrand factor antigen and von Willebrand factor activity in scleroderma and Raynaud's phenomenon. *Ann Intern Med* **94**:482, 1981

48. Gerstmeier H et al: Levels of type IV collagen and laminin fragments in serum from patients with progressive systemic sclerosis. *J Rheumatol* **15**:969, 1988

49. Stern D et al: An endothelial cell-dependent pathway of coagulation. *Proc Natl Acad Sci USA* **82**:2523, 1985

50. Deguchi Y et al: Mutant fibronectin gene in skin fibroblasts of sclerotic lesions from patients with progressive systemic sclerosis. *Arthritis Rheum* **32**:247, 1989

51. Kahaleh MB, LeRoy EC: Interleukin-2 in scleroderma: Correlation of serum level with extent of skin involvement and disease duration. *Ann Intern Med* **110**:446, 1989

52. Umehara H et al: Enhanced production of interleukin-2 in patients with progressive systemic sclerosis: Hyperactivity of CD-4 positive T cells? *Arthritis Rheum* **31**:401, 1988

53. Clements PJ et al: Elevated serum levels of soluble interleukin 2 receptor, interleukin 2 and neopterin in diffuse and limited scleroderma: Effect of chlorambucil. *J Rheumatol* **17**:908, 1990

54. Umehara H et al: Enhanced production of interleukin-1 and tumor necrosis factor α by cultured peripheral blood monocytes from patients with scleroderma. *Arthritis Rheum* **33**:893, 1990

55. Gay S et al: Immunohistologic demonstration of platelet-derived growth factor (PDGF) and cis-oncogene expression in scleroderma. *J Invest Dermatol* **92**:301, 1989

56. Kahaleh MB et al: Elevated levels of circulating platelet aggregates and beta-thromboglobulin in scleroderma. *Ann Intern Med* **96**:610, 1982

57. Cotran RS, Pober JS: Endothelial activation: Its role in inflammatory and immune reactions, in *Endothelial Cell Biology*, edited by N Simionescu, M Simionescu. New York, Plenum, 1988, p 335

58. Pober JS et al: Ia expression by vascular endothelium is inducible by activated T cells and by human δ-interferon. *J Exp Med* **157**:1339, 1983

59. Aronson FR et al: IL-2 rapidly induces natural killer cell adhesion to human endothelial cells. A potential mechanism for endothelial injury. *J Immunol* **141**:158, 1988

60. Ferro TJ et al: IL-2 induces pulmonary edema and vasoconstriction independent of circulating lymphocytes. *J Immunol* **142**:1916, 1989

61. Goldblum SE et al: Provocation of pulmonary vascular endothelial injury in rabbits by human recombinant interleukin-1 beta. *Infect Immunol* **56**:2255, 1988

62. Hameed A et al: Characterization of three serine esterases isolated from human IL-2 activated killer cells. *J Immunol* **141**:3142, 1988

63. Guinan EC et al: Vascular endothelial cells enhance T cell responses by markedly augmenting IL-2 concentrations. *Cell Immunol* **118**:166, 1989

64. Kratz LE et al: Association of scleroderma with a T cell antigen receptor δ gene restriction fragment length polymorphism. *Arthritis Rheum* **33**:569, 1990

65. Hawkins RA et al: Increased dermal mast cell populations in progressive systemic sclerosis: A link in chronic fibrosis. *Ann Intern Med* **102**:182, 1985

66. Claman HN: Mast cells and fibrosis: The relevance to scleroderma. *Rheum Dis Clin North Am* **16**:141, 1990

67. Falanga V et al: Elevated plasma histamine levels in systemic sclerosis (scleroderma). *Arch Dermatol* **126**:336, 1990

68. Piguet P-F et al: Tumor necrosis factor/cachectin is an effector of skin and gut lesions of the acute phase of graft-vs-host disease. *J Exp Med* **166**:1280, 1987

69. van Hinsbergh VW et al: Tumor necrosis factor increases the production of plasminogen activator inhibitor in human endothelial cells in vitro and in rats in vivo. *Blood* **72**:1467, 1988

70. Hajjar KA et al: Tumor necrosis factor mediated release of platelet derived growth factor from cultured endothelial cells. *J Exp Med* **166**:235, 1987

71. Auclair C et al: Clastogenic inosine nucleotide as components of the chromosome breakage factor in scleroderma patients. *Arch Biochem Biophys* **278**:238, 1990

72. Kahari V-M et al: Identification of fibroblasts responsible for increased collagen production in localized scleroderma by in situ hybridization. *J Invest Dermatol* **90**:664, 1988

73. Uitto J et al: Scleroderma: Increased biosynthesis of triple helical type I and type III procollagen with unaltered expression of collagenase by skin fibroblasts in culture. *J Clin Invest* **64**:921, 1979

74. Vuorio T et al: Activation of type 1 collagen genes in cultured scleroderma fibroblasts. *J Cell Biochem* **28**:105, 1985

75. Rossi P et al: A nuclear factor 1 binding site mediates the transcriptional activation of a type 1 collagen promoter by transforming growth factor β. *Cell* **52**:405, 1988

76. Varga J et al: Transforming growth factor β (TGF β) causes a persistent increase in steady-state amounts of type I and type III collagen and fibronectin mRNA's in normal human dermal fibroblasts. *Biochem J* **247**:597, 1987

77. Kulozik M et al: Co-localization of transforming growth factor β2 with α1(1) procollagen mRNA in tissue sections of patients with systemic sclerosis. *J Clin Invest* **86**:917, 1990

78. Kahari V-M et al: Elevated pro α 2(I) collagen mRNA levels in cultured scleroderma fibroblasts result from an increased transcription rate of the corresponding gene. *FEBS Lett* **215**:331, 1987

79. Query CC, Keene JD: A human autoimmune protein associated with U1 RNA contains a region of homology that is cross-reactive with retroviral p30 gag antigen. *Cell* **51**:211, 1987

80. Maul GG et al: Determination of an epitope of the diffuse systemic sclerosis marker antigen DNA topoisomerase I: Sequence similarity with retroviral p30[gag] protein suggests a possible cause for autoimmunity in systemic sclerosis. *Proc Natl Acad Sci USA* **86**:8492, 1989

81. Bos GMJ et al: Chronic cyclosporine-induced autoimmune disease in the rat: A new experimental model for scleroderma. *J Invest Der-*

matol **93**:610, 1989

82. Menton DN et al: The structure and tensile properties of the skin of tight-skin (Tsk) mutant mice. *J Invest Dermatol* **70**:4, 1978

83. Walker M et al: Ketotifen prevents skin fibrosis in the tight skin mouse. *J Rheumatol* **17**:57, 1990

84. Curtis AC, Jansen TG: The prognosis of localized scleroderma. *Arch Dermatol* **78**:749, 1958

85. Tuffanelli DL et al: Linear scleroderma with hemiatrophy: Report of three cases associated with collagen-vascular disease. *Dermatologica* **132**:51, 1966

86. Steen VD et al: Outcome of renal crisis in systemic sclerosis in relation to availability of angiotensin converting enzyme (ACE) inhibitors. *Ann Intern Med* **113**:352, 1990

87. Falanga V, Medsger TA: D-penicillamine in the treatment of localized scleroderma. *Arch Dermatol* **126**:609, 1990

88. Rosenbloom J et al: Inhibition of excessive scleroderma fibroblast collagen production by recombinant γ-interferon. Association with a coordinate decrease in types I and III procollagen messenger RNA levels. *Arthritis Rheum* **29**:851, 1986

89. Duncan MR, Berman B: Persistence of a reduced-collagen-producing phenotype in cultured scleroderma fibroblasts after short-term exposure to interferons. *J Clin Invest* **79**:1318, 1987

90. Fritzler MJ, Hart DA: Prolonged improvements of Raynaud's phenomenon and scleroderma after recombinant tissue plasminogen activator therapy. *Arthritis Rheum* **33**:274, 1990

91. DiGiacomo RA et al: Fish oil dietary supplementation in patients with Raynaud's phenomenon: A double-blind controlled prospective study. *Am J Med* **86**:158, 1989

92. Rook AH et al: Effective treatment of progressive systemic sclerosis with extracorporeal photochemotherapy. *Clin Res* **38**:420A, 1990

93. Steen VD et al: D-penicillamine therapy in progressive systemic sclerosis (scleroderma). A retrospective study. *Ann Intern Med* **97**:652, 1982

94. Shapiro LS et al: D-penicillamine treatment of progressive systemic sclerosis (scleroderma). A comparison of clinical and in vitro effects. *J Rheumatol* **10**:316, 1983

95. Jimenez SA, Sigal H: A fifteen-year prospective study of treatment of rapidly progressive systemic sclerosis (PSS) with D-penicillamine (D-PEN). *Arthritis Rheum* **32**:S34, 1989

96. Gruber BL, Kaufman LD: Ketotifen induced remission in progressive early diffuse scleroderma. Evidence for the role of mast cells in disease and pathogenesis. *Am J Med* **89**:392, 1990

97. Rodheffer RJ et al: Controlled double-blind trial of nifedipine in the treatment of Raynaud's phenomenon. *N Engl J Med* **308**:880, 1983

98. Thomas RH et al: Nifedipine in the treatment of Raynaud's phenomenon in patients with systemic sclerosis. *Br J Dermatol* **117**:237, 1987

99. Coffman JD et al: International study of ketanserin in Raynaud's phenomenon. *Am J Med* **87**:264, 1989

100. Worle B et al: Cyclosporin in localized systemic scleroderma. A clinical study. *Dermatologica* **181**:215, 1990

CHAPTER 174

Ellen M. Gravallese

Systemic Vasculitis

The clinical syndromes that fall in the category designated *systemic vasculitis* are defined histologically by the presence of an inflammatory cell infiltrate in blood vessel walls, usually with vessel wall necrosis. Fibrinoid necrosis, or fibrin-like deposits in necrotic vessel walls, is often seen. Although this histologic definition is straightforward, the spectrum of diseases encompassed in this category is wide. Clinical manifestations are variable depending on the size and site of the vessels involved and the extent of end organ damage caused by vascular compromise.[1] This chapter covers the clinical syndromes in which vasculitis is the primary process or is a prominent component, but does not include cutaneous necrotizing venulitis or the giant cell arteritides, which are covered in separate chapters.

A number of clinicopathologic schemes for the classification of vasculitic syndromes have been proposed since the original description of necrotizing vasculitis by Kussmaul and Maier.[2] At the time of this description, all vasculitides were considered to be polyarteritis nodosa. Subsequently, Zeek described four vasculitic syndromes[3,4] that were distinct from polyarteritis nodosa. Since that time, new classification schemes have been set forth,[5–8] based on size of the vessels involved, association with known diseases or etiologic factors, and clinicopathologic correlations. A modification of one classification scheme[9] originally proposed by Fauci et al.[5] is summarized in Table 174-1. The classification of the vasculitic syndromes has become increasingly important as effective therapeutic regimens for disease entities such as Wegener's granulomatosis have been described.[10,11] However, certain patients continue to defy classification, and overlap among described syndromes exists.[12–14] Classification would ideally be based on pathogenetic mechanisms. However, many of the vasculitic syndromes remain idiopathic, and in cases where an etiologic agent has been identified, such as in the case of hepatitis B antigen-associated vasculitis, several different clinical syndromes may result.[15–18]

Cutaneous manifestations of systemic vasculitis are common, and a wide range of lesions is seen. When skin is involved with a vasculitic process, it must be determined whether the vasculitis is isolated to the skin or is more diffuse. For example, skin lesions in polyarteritis nodosa may be the primary disease manifestation or may be part of a picture of systemic involvement.[19–21] Involvement of a spectrum of cutaneous vessels has been described in both Wegener's granulomatosis[10] and in allergic angiitis and granulomatosis.[22] Biopsy often allows identification of the size of the vessels involved as well as of the histologic process.

Polyarteritis Nodosa

Since the time of Zeek's classification of vasculitic syndromes,[3,4] polyarteritis nodosa has been considered a distinct clinical entity. However, some authors[5,9] include allergic angiitis and granulomatosis in the polyarteritis nodosa group, which also includes an overlap syndrome with features of both entities.[14] The idiopathic form of polyarteritis nodosa is discussed, although a similar vasculitic syndrome has been noted in association with viral infections, including hepatitis B[23,24] and human immunodeficiency virus[25,26];

intravenous use of amphetamines[27]; serous otitis media[28]; hairy cell leukemia[29]; hyposensitization therapy[30]; and collagen-vascular diseases including rheumatoid arthritis.[31] Predominantly small- and medium-sized arteries are affected.[3,4,32] Clinical symptoms reflect the location of the affected vessels and the extent of organ system damage secondary to vessel destruction and thrombosis. Limited vessel involvement has been described.[20,33–35] If untreated, less than 15 percent of patients with systemic disease survive for 5 years.[36] With therapy, the 5-year survival of patients with systemic disease approaches 60 percent.[37,38]

Clinical Manifestations

Polyarteritis nodosa typically affects patients in middle age, with a male predominance. Constitutional symptoms such as malaise, weakness, fever, and weight loss are common.[39] Renal complications occur in about 70 percent of patients, and clinical signs include proteinuria, urinary sediment abnormalities, and hypertension.[38,40] The two forms of renal disease are vasculitis of small- and medium-sized renal arteries and necrotizing glomerulonephritis, often with crescent formation.[40] The term *microscopic polyarteritis* has been suggested to describe a subgroup of patients with small-vessel vasculitis and focal segmental necrotizing glomerulonephritis[40,41]; polyarteritis nodosa limited to the kidneys has also been described.[33,34]

Peripheral neuropathy occurs in about 60 percent of patients and may result in motor and sensory deficits in a pattern of mononeuritis multiplex or polyneuropathy.[36,38] The central nervous system is less commonly involved, but changes in mental status, seizures, and cerebral vascular accident may occur.[42] Myalgias and arthralgias are common, and frank arthritis may appear early in the disease.[38] Abdominal pain is the most common symptom of gastrointestinal tract involvement[37]; hemorrhage, infarction, and perforation may occur in the gallbladder and in the small and large bowel. Coronary arteritis, myocardial infarction, and congestive heart failure are also described.[43] Pulmonary manifestations are rare in classic polyarteritis nodosa.

The incidence of skin involvement approaches 50 percent of cases[37,39] and is partly dependent on how polyarteritis nodosa is defined. Cutaneous and subcutaneous nodules occur over affected vessels, most commonly in the lower extremities (Fig. 174-1*a*). They tend to appear in crops and clusters, are sometimes painful,

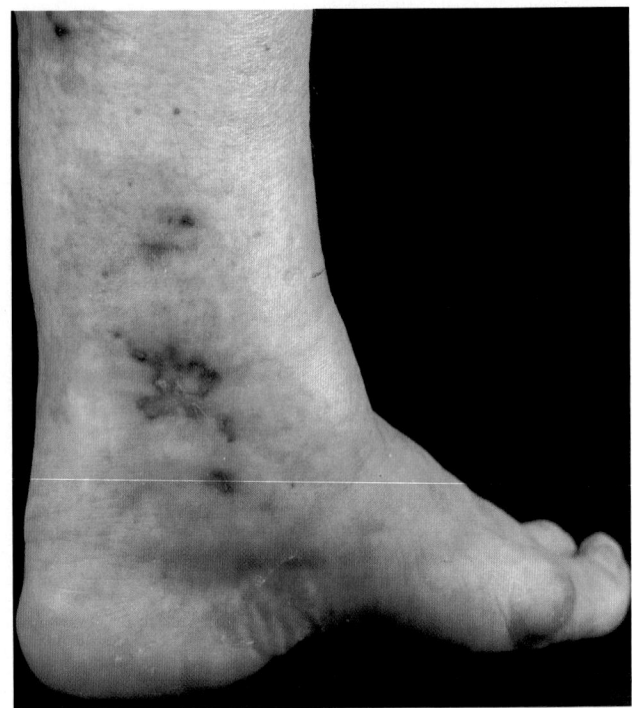

a

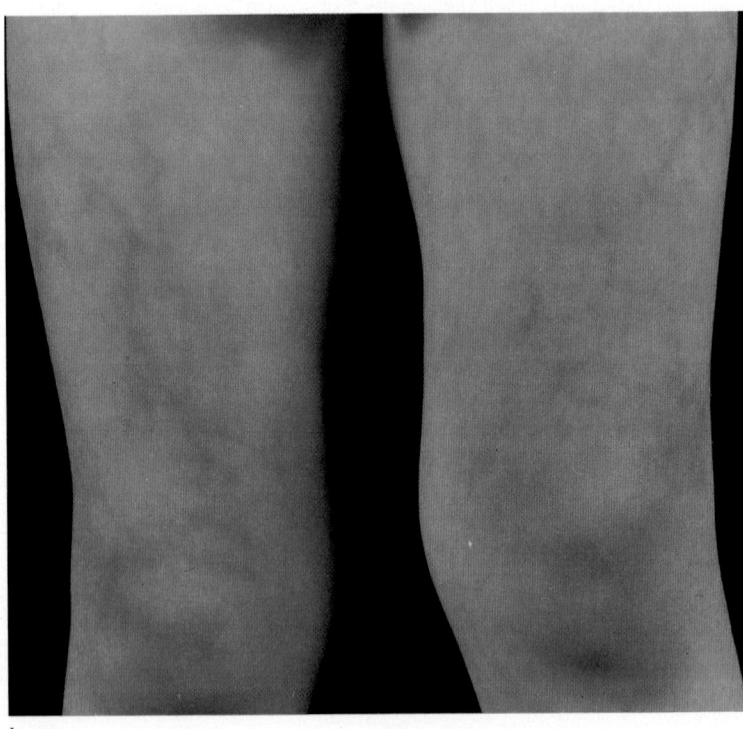

FIGURE 174-1 Polyarteritis nodosa. (*a*) There are nodular ulcerations occurring on the medial aspect of the lower leg. Scarring is present in the site of the previous lesions. (*b*) This is a livedo pattern. On biopsy, lesions were polyarteritis nodosa.

b

and persist for days to months. Although characteristic, they are seen in less than 20 percent of patients.[44] In the acute stage of disease, urticarial lesions and subcutaneous hemorrhage are described.[37,44] Other cutaneous manifestations include ulcers, livedo reticularis (Fig. 174-1b),[21] maculopapular eruptions, nail fold and digital pulp infarcts, and a nonspecific erythematous rash.[45] Although palpable purpura is described, some authors would not include such cases in the category of classic polyarteritis nodosa, but rather in an overlap category.

Cutaneous polyarteritis nodosa[19,20,46] has been described as a distinct clinical entity with a benign prognosis, although its existence has been challenged.[21] Fever, arthralgia, myalgia, and localized neuropathy may accompany cutaneous lesions, but visceral involvement is felt not to occur. The most common presentation is that of painful cutaneous nodules, typically located asymmetrically on the lower legs. Livedo reticularis (Fig. 174-1b) and ulceration may result. Excisional biopsy specimens of affected skin reveal a necrotizing vasculitis of small- or medium-sized arteries, and direct immunofluorescence is positive for immunoglobulin and/or complement in the vessel wall in the majority of cases. Cutaneous involvement in classic systemic polyarteritis appears to confer a more favorable prognosis.[21,37]

Pathology

Classic polyarteritis nodosa is a disease of small- and medium-sized arteries, with a predilection for sites of vessel bifurcation. Extension to arterioles is unusual but does occur.[4] Focal involvement of vessels is characteristic, and within vessels, segmental inflammation may be seen.[4,32] The inflammatory infiltrate is panmural and pleomorphic, and acute lesions include infiltration of polymorphonuclear leukocytes and fibrinoid necrosis of the vessel wall (Fig. 174-2). Resultant weakening of the vessel wall may lead to the formation of aneurysms, and vessel thrombosis is common. Rarely, the infiltrate may be granulomatous.[32] Vessels heal with proliferation and fibrosis, and lesions at different stages of activity are commonly seen.[5] Biopsy of clinically affected organs gives the highes diagnostic yield.

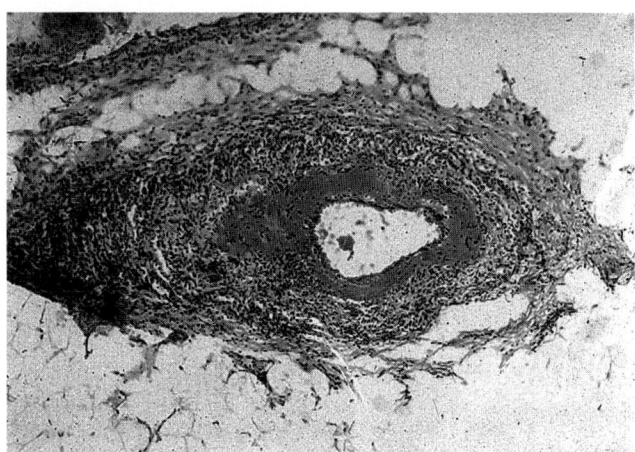

FIGURE 174-2 Artery from a patient with polyarteritis nodosa, demonstrating fibrinoid necrosis, pleomorphic panmural infiltrate, and disruption of the internal elastic lamina. H&E, ×100.

Laboratory Features

Nonspecific laboratory features include an elevated erythrocyte sedimentation rate, anemia, leukocytosis, elevated liver function tests, and abnormalities of renal function and urinary sediment. Antinuclear antibodies, rheumatoid factor, and eosinophilia may also be present.[37,38] Circulating immune complexes are described,[47] and, less commonly, hypocomplementemia is seen.[48] Visceral angiography of the hepatic, renal, celiac, and mesenteric circulations is helpful in the diagnosis of polyarteritis nodosa if characteristic aneurysms are demonstrated (Fig. 174-3). However, similar aneurysms can be seen in several other diseases including Wegener's granulomatosis[49] and systemic lupus erythematosus.[50]

Wegener's Granulomatosis

In 1936, Wegener defined the clinical features of the disease now known as Wegener's granulomatosis.[51] This idiopathic disease is

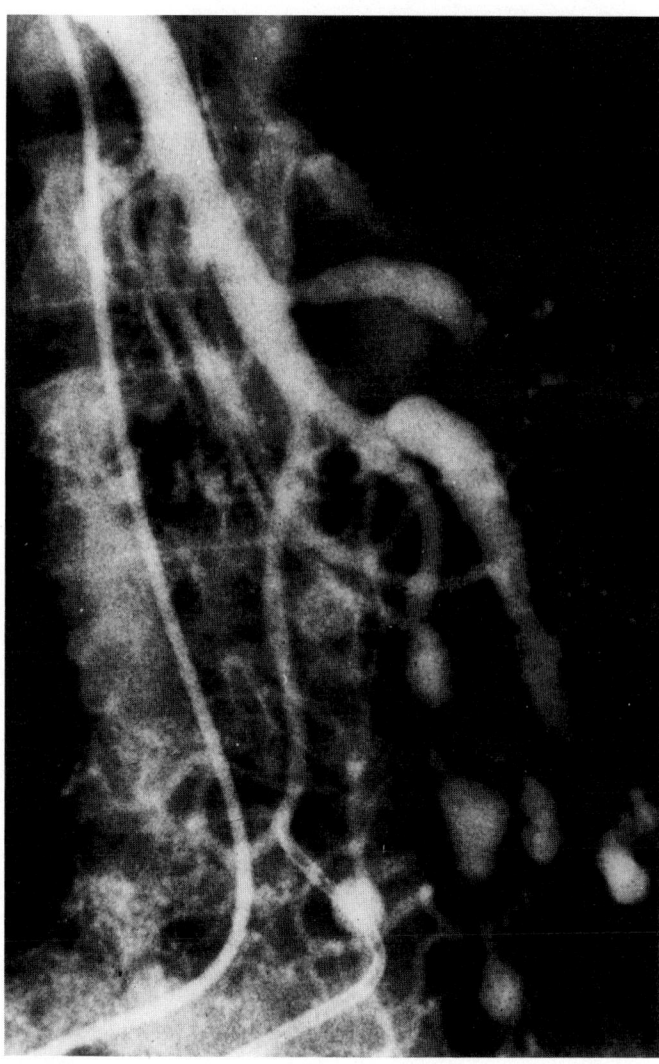

FIGURE 174-3 Selective abdominal arteriogram in polyarteritis nodosa. Small saccular aneurysms are present in the branches of the superior mesenteric artery. (*Reprinted from the Revised Clinical Slide Collection on the Rheumatic Diseases, copyright 1981. Used by permission of the American College of Rheumatology.*)

characterized by necrotizing granulomatous inflammation and vasculitis affecting predominantly small arteries and veins.[10,11] The disease is probably a continuum; it may present with limited organ involvement, which remains limited for variable periods of time.[52–54] In its generalized form there is involvement of the upper and lower respiratory tract, kidney, and often other organs including skin. Protracted mucosal and skin involvement have been described, with an average of 6.5 years from onset of symptoms to diagnosis.[55] If left untreated, the generalized form of the disease is usually fatal, with more than 90 percent of patients dying within 2 years of disease onset.[56] With the advent of cytotoxic therapy, more than 90 percent of patients can have long-term remissions.[10,11]

Clinical Manifestations

Wegener's granulomatosis can occur in any age group; it has been reported in children as young as 3 months of age.[52] However, it occurs most commonly in men, aged 40 to 50,[57] with a male:female ratio of about 3:2.[10] The initial clinical presentations vary, but patients typically present with upper airway disease and nonspecific complaints including fever, malaise, arthralgia, and weight loss. In one large series,[11] sinusitis was the presenting symptom in 67 percent of the patients, with 71 percent of patients having pulmonary infiltrates at presentation. Renal failure was present at presentation in only 11 percent of patients in this series.

Necrotizing granulomas involving the paranasal sinuses are common and can lead to pansinusitis with secondary bacterial infection.[10] Other symptoms include serous otitis media, hearing loss, persistent rhinorrhea and congestion, and nasal mucosal ulcerations.[10] Granulomatous involvement of the nasal septum with dissolution of cartilage leads to the typical saddle nose deformity. Pulmonary involvement may be asymptomatic with single or multiple pulmonary nodules, typically with cavitation. Pulmonary symptoms may include cough, sputum production, chest pain, dyspnea, and hemoptysis.[11,58] Pleural effusions are also seen.[11] Massive pulmonary hemorrhage can occur and may rarely precede other symptoms.[59,60]

Renal disease is present in about 80 to 85 percent of cases.[11,61] The most common histologic finding in the kidney is focal segmental glomerulonephritis, and crescent formation may occur. Immune complex deposition may be seen.[11,62,63] Although vasculitis and granuloma formation can be seen on renal biopsy, granulomatous changes were seen in only 3 of 18 renal biopsies in one series[64]; therefore, renal biopsy is not the diagnostic procedure of choice. A granulomatous reaction around inflamed glomeruli has been described,[65] as has interstitial nephritis.[61] Crescentic glomerulonephritis can precede classic Wegener's granulomatosis by as long as 6 to 7 years.[66]

Cutaneous manifestations are common in Wegener's granulomatosis, reported in 40 to 50 percent of cases,[67–69] and may be part of the initial presentation.[10,68] Rarely, cutaneous manifestations may precede other disease manifestations by many months.[68,70] Papular or plaquelike and ulcerative lesions (Fig. 174-4) are most commonly seen[10,68]; but vesicles, urticarial lesions, purpura, subcutaneous nodules, petechiae,[69,71] and panniculitis[69] have also been described. Purpuric and hemorrhagic lesions show necrotizing vasculitis on biopsy.[10] Biopsies of skin lesions performed in one clinical series revealed a spectrum of lesions including vasculitis, granulomatous vasculitis, necrotizing granuloma, granulomatous inflammation, and chronic inflammation.[10] Although granuloma-

tous inflammation and necrotizing granuloma are suggestive of the diagnosis, only one of eight patients who underwent biopsy in this series had the necrotizing granulomatous vasculitis typical of Wegener's granulomatosis. Fienberg reported three cases with prolonged mucosal and skin involvement.[55]

Ocular manifestations occur in about 30 to 50 percent of cases[72–74]; they include corneal and scleral ulcerations, uveitis, keratitis, proptosis, conjunctivitis, orbital pseudotumor,[75] and vasculitis of the retinal, ciliary, and optic vessels. Arthralgias and, less commonly, true arthritis do occur.[10] Cardiac involvement includes pericarditis, coronary arteritis, myocardial infarction, pancarditis, and granulomatous valvulitis.[10,76,77] The nervous system is affected in 25 to 54 percent of patients,[61,78] with polyneuritis or mononeuritis multiplex being the most common presentation.[78]

Pathology

Histologic documentation is necessary for the definitive diagnosis of Wegener's granulomatosis. The classic generalized form of the disease encompasses the triad of necrotizing granulomas of the upper and/or lower respiratory tract, necrotizing granulomatous vasculitis, most commonly involving small arteries and veins, and glomerulonephritis, usually focal segmental. However, all three criteria may not be present simultaneously.[32,79] Due to their necrotic nature, biopsy of upper airway lesions is diagnostic in only half of the cases.[11] Pulmonary lesions are best demonstrated on open lung biopsy[11] and include single or confluent necrotizing granulomas with a geographic pattern of parenchymal necrosis and giant cells in variable numbers. Necrotizing or granulomatous vasculitis is also typically seen, although parenchymal necrosis and vasculitis appear to be distinct processes.[80] Acute, chronic, and healed lesions may all be present at the same time. Necrosis appears to be the first pathologic lesion. Subsequently recruitment of monocytes and histiocytes, which define the granulomatous response, occurs.[55,80] Rarely, an eosinophilic infiltrate may be seen, requiring differentiation of Wegener's granulomatosis from Churg-Strauss syndrome.[81]

Laboratory Features

Most of the laboratory features seen in Wegener's granulomatosis are nonspecific and include an elevated sedimentation rate, normochromic normocytic anemia, thrombocytosis, and, occasionally, leukocytosis.[11] It has been proposed that the level of C-reactive protein, an acute phase reactant, is useful in following disease activity.[82] Low titer rheumatoid factor and circulating immune complexes may be present.[11] Chest radiograph, serum blood urea nitrogen, creatinine, and urinary sediment should be obtained to detect pulmonary and renal disease.

A recently described laboratory feature of Wegener's granulomatosis is the antineutrophil cytoplasmic autoantibody (ANCA). First described in 1982 by Davies et al.,[83] ANCA was not clearly associated with Wegener's granulomatosis until 1985 when IgG autoantibodies against cytoplasmic components of polymorphonuclear granulocytes and monocytes were found in 25 of 27 patients with active Wegener's granulomatosis.[84] In this study, a strong correlation between antibody positivity and disease activity was noted. It is now clear that when alcohol-fixed neutrophils are used as substrates, two patterns of ANCA positivity exist. One is a pattern of perinuclear staining (P-ANCA), which is associated with

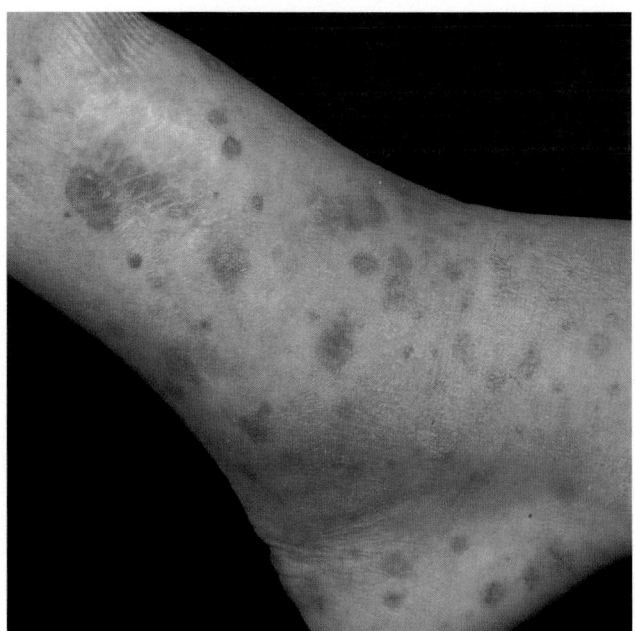

a

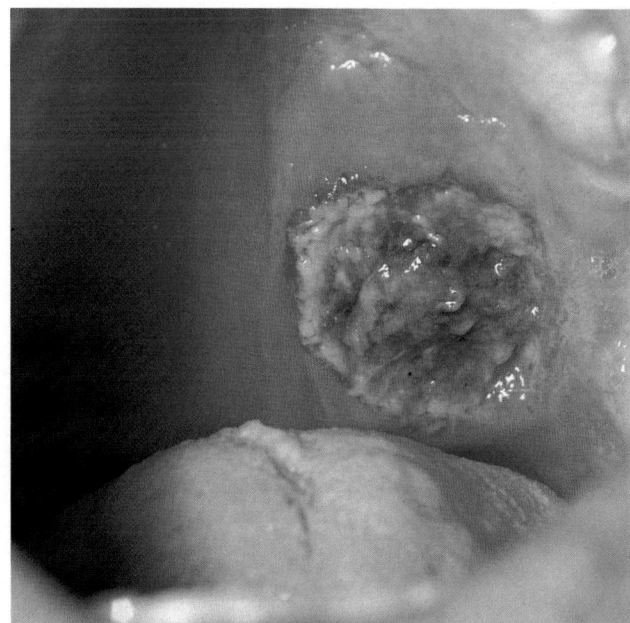

c

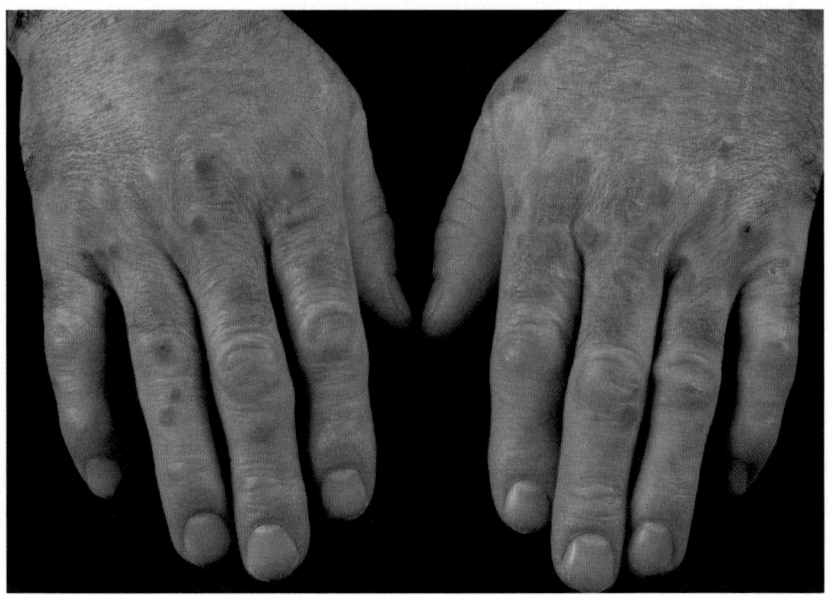

b

FIGURE 174-4 Wegener's granulomatosis. (*a*) Typical areas of palpable purpura are seen on the lower leg and foot. (*b*) Erythematous, purpuric, nonblanching nodules on the dorsa of the fingers and hands. (*c*) There is a very large ulcer on the palate covered by a sphacelus (a dense, necrotic membrane).

antibodies against antigens, including myeloperoxidase, in the primary granules of neutrophils.[85] The second is a true cytoplasmic staining (C-ANCA); one antigen involved in this pattern is a neutrophil serine protease.[85,86] C-ANCA positivity has been reported to have a sensitivity of 96 percent in patients with generalized active Wegener's granulomatosis; sensitivity falls to 41 percent in patients with generalized disease that is in remission. Positivity was seen less commonly in patients with active localized disease.[87] Although C-ANCA positivity correlates well with disease activity in Wegener's granulomatosis, it is not seen uniquely in this disease and has been described in nonimmune complex necrotizing crescentic glomerulonephritis and in other vasculitic syndromes.[86,87] ANCA positivity thus remains a useful tool in the diagnosis of

Wegener's granulomatosis, but histopathologic criteria are still required. The possible role of these antibodies in the pathogenesis of vasculitis is discussed below.

Allergic Angiitis and Granulomatosis (Churg-Strauss Syndrome)

Allergic angiitis and granulomatosis was first described in 1951 by Churg and Strauss[22] as a clinical entity distinct from polyarteritis nodosa. The original description included 13 patients with asthma, peripheral eosinophilia, and necrotizing vasculitis. Subsequently, among 111 autopsy cases of polyarteritis nodosa, 32 had features of the syndrome described by Churg and Strauss.[88] Although several authors still consider this entity to be a subgroup of polyarteritis nodosa (Table 174-1), distinguishing features include a history of asthma or allergic phenomena, pulmonary disease, peripheral and tissue eosinophilia, granulomatous lesions, vasculitis of capillaries and veins as well as of small- and medium-sized arteries, and rarity of renal failure.[89] Cutaneous manifestations are more common than in polyarteritis nodosa and are present in more than 60 percent of cases.[90] In the pre-corticosteroid era, the disease was usually fatal, but with corticosteroid therapy prognosis is favorable.[89]

Clinical Manifestations

Although generally considered rare, allergic angiitis and granulomatosis is probably underreported as a distinct clinical entity. The mean age of onset is 40 to 50 years, with a roughly equal incidence in males and females.[91] Adult-onset asthma or allergic symptoms such as rhinitis usually precede vasculitic manifestations by months to decades[91] and may be absent when vasculitic manifestations appear.[90] However, the onset of asthma can coincide with that of vasculitis.[90] Peripheral eosinophilia can be as high as 81 percent of the peripheral leukocyte count,[90] and eosinophilic tissue infiltrates can occur in the absence of peripheral eosinophilia.[91] A correlation between eosinophilia and asthma in patients with vasculitis has been reported.[36] Pulmonary involvement is seen in most patients and manifests as diffuse, patchy, nodular, or transient[90,91] infiltrates on a chest radiograph. Pulmonary lesions usually do not cavitate,[91] in contrast to those in Wegener's granulomatosis. Pleural effusions have been reported.[91]

Multiple organ systems can be involved in the vasculitic phase of disease. Peripheral neuropathy presenting most typically as mononeuritis multiplex occurs in more than 60 percent of cases.[89,90] The gastrointestinal tract is commonly affected, with granulomas of the stomach, liver, and bowel, as well as mucosal ulcerations, pseudopolyps, and bowel perforation secondary to

TABLE 174-1
The Clinical Spectrum of Vasculitis

Polyarteritis nodosa group
    Classic polyarteritis nodosa
    Allergic angiitis and granulomatosis (Churg-Strauss disease)
    Overlap syndrome
Hypersensitivity vasculitis
    Henoch-Schönlein purpura
    Serum sickness and serum sickness-like reactions
    Vasculitis associated with infectious diseases
    Vasculitis associated with neoplasms
    Vasculitis associated with connective tissue diseases
    Vasculitis associated with other underlying diseases
    Congenital deficiencies of the complement system
    Erythema elevatum diutinum
Wegener's granulomatosis
Giant cell arteritides
    Cranial or temporal arteritis
    Takayasu's arteritis
Other vasculitic syndromes
    Lymphomatoid granulomatosis
    Mucocutaneous lymph node syndrome (Kawasaki's disease)
    Behçet's disease
    Vasculitis isolated to the central nervous system
    Thromboangiitis obliterans (Buerger's disease)
    Miscellaneous vasculitides

SOURCE: Data from Wolff,[9] p 2026

necrotizing vasculitis.[90,91] Cardiac lesions include pericarditis,[92] cardiac granulomas and fibrosis, eosinophilic infiltrates, and coronary artery vasculitis[91]; cardiac complications accounted for 48 percent of deaths in one series.[91] Although hypertension is common, renal disease is generally less severe than in Wegener's granulomatosis and polyarteritis nodosa, and renal failure is uncommon.[91] Granulomatous lesions of the lower urinary tract and prostate have been described,[90] and arthralgia or arthritis can also occur.[90,91]

Skin is among the most common sites of involvement in the vasculitic phase. Purpura of the extremities is the most common cutaneous lesion.[91] Biopsy reveals vasculitis, usually of venules. Tender subcutaneous nodules on the extremities and scalp are also a common but not pathognomonic feature.[91,93,94] Biopsy of these lesions shows the characteristic granulomas originally described by Churg and Strauss,[22] and subsequently described in other conditions including Wegener's granulomatosis, other connective tissue diseases, lymphoproliferative diseases, and infection.[69,93] Other cutaneous manifestations include maculopapular lesions, vesicles, livedo reticularis, and hemorrhagic lesions sometimes accompanied by necrosis or urticaria.[94,95]

Pathology

The vasculitis in allergic angiitis and granulomatosis may be indistinguishable from that seen in polyarteritis nodosa, may have a prominent eosinophilic infiltrate, or may be granulomatous. Small- and medium-sized arteries as well as veins and venules may be affected, including pulmonary and systemic vessels.[96] The granulomas classically have an eosinophilic core of necrotic collagen surrounded by histiocytes, lymphocytes, and often giant cells.[22] Eosinophilic tissue infiltrate is often seen. Several authors have stressed that granulomas, vasculitis, and eosinophilic tissue infiltrates need not be present simultaneously.[89,91,96]

Laboratory Features

Apart from the eosinophil count, laboratory studies are not particularly useful in the diagnosis of allergic angiitis and granulomatosis. An elevated erythrocyte sedimentation rate is often present and a fall may reflect response to treatment.[91] Normochromic normocytic anemia and leukocytosis are common.[90] Although immune complexes have been demonstrated in tissues in this disease,[91] they are not usually present. Elevated serum IgE levels may be present in the vasculitic phase.[91]

Kawasaki Syndrome (Mucocutaneous Lymph Node Syndrome)

The mucocutaneous lymph node syndrome was described first in the Japanese literature by Kawasaki[97] and later in the English literature.[98,99] It is thus also known by the eponym "Kawasaki syndrome." This syndrome is a systemic vasculitis of childhood that is self-limited, with a propensity for coronary artery involvement. More than half of the cases occur in children under 2 years of age.[98] Adult cases are rare but have been reported.[100] Its relationship to infantile polyarteritis nodosa remains controversial.[101–103] Originally the syndrome was thought to be a benign process, but a fatality rate of 0.5 to 2.8 percent is reported, mainly due to coronary artery vasculitis.[98,104,105]

Clinical Manifestations

The diagnosis of Kawasaki syndrome is made on the basis of a constellation of clinical findings. Fever, often 40°C or greater, unresponsive to antibiotic therapy, is the principal finding and usually precedes other signs. Bilateral nonpurulent conjunctival injection is seen within 1 to 5 days. Changes in the mucous membranes include reddening and fissuring of the lips, prominent erythematous papillae of the tongue ("strawberry tongue"), and injection of the oral and pharyngeal mucosae.[98,99]

Cutaneous manifestations begin with reddening of the palms and soles, usually in the third to fifth day, which may spread to the trunk.[98] This is followed by an indurative edema and subsequent desquamation beginning usually on the tips of the fingers and toes and around the nails.[105] A polymorphous rash may also be present, most commonly maculopapular or morbilliform, but also scarlatiniform or macular. It may resemble erythema multiforme or rarely may be urticarial or vesicular.[105] Nonsuppurative cervical adenopathy is the least frequent of the principal signs.[99] Associated features include pyuria, arthralgia or arthritis, central nervous system involvement, and gastrointestinal manifestations.[99]

Cardiovascular involvement is the most important prognostic feature, and ectasia or aneurysms of the coronary arteries occur in 15 to 20 percent of cases.[104,106] These can lead to thrombosis with myocardial infarction or to rupture.[107] Other cardiac manifestations include pericarditis; myocarditis, often with subsequent congestive heart failure; arrhythmias and sudden death; electrocardiographic abnormalities; and, rarely, valvulitis.[104]

Pathology

Although coronary arteries are most commonly affected by vasculitis, vessels of all sizes from capillaries and venules to large arteries may be involved.[107,108] Pathologic studies of both cardiac[107] and cutaneous[109] lesions suggest that the pathologic changes begin in the microvasculature. Acute perivasculitis is seen in the early stages. During the stage of arterial involvement, a panvasculitis involving adventitia, media, and intima exists with an infiltration of many cell types, including neutrophils, lymphocytes, plasma cells, monocytes, and fibroblasts.[107] The vasculitis resembles polyarteritis nodosa except that fibrinoid necrosis of the media appears to be uncommon.[107]

Laboratory Features

Laboratory features are generally nonspecific. Leukocytosis with a shift to the left, thrombocytosis, and an elevated erythrocyte sedimentation rate are commonly seen.[98,99] A mild normochromic normocytic anemia is also frequent.[104] Two-dimensional echocardiography has proven useful in detecting coronary artery aneurysms.[110] Immune complexes have been noted, but their role in pathogenesis is unclear.[111] An increase in the ratio of helper T cells to suppressor/cytotoxic T cells has also been reported,[112] as has an expansion of the B-cell compartment.[113] The role of endothelial cell antigens in pathogenesis is discussed below.

Thromboangiitis Obliterans (Buerger's Disease)

Thromboangiitis obliterans is an uncommon inflammatory vascular syndrome occurring almost exclusively in tobacco smokers, with a marked predominance in males, particularly of Oriental descent. Symptoms usually occur between 20 and 40 years of age.[114,115] Clinical symptoms may be abrupt or gradual in onset, and cutaneous manifestations include recurrent episodes of cold, painful extremities with ulceration and gangrene. Aside from the discontinuation of tobacco, therapeutic options are limited,[116] and amputation is often required.

Small- and medium-sized arteries and veins are affected, most commonly in the extremities, although visceral[117] and cerebral[118] vessels also have been involved. Acute lesions are diagnostic, with histologic findings including panmural inflammation of the vessel wall, associated with thrombosis of the vessel lumen with microabscess formation and multinucleated giant cells. As lesions heal, they become less distinctive and may eventually be difficult to distinguish from arteriosclerosis or organized thrombus.[115,119]

Primary Angiitis of the Central Nervous System

This rare form of vasculitis involves vessels of the central nervous system and, as such, has no cutaneous manifestations. It occurs over a wide range of ages and usually presents with unexplained headache and subsequent neurologic deterioration.[120,121] The mortality rate is high. Small intracranial arteries, arterioles, and veins are typically affected with a segmental, granulomatous vasculitis, although polyarteritis-like vasculitis may be seen.[122] Similarity to the vascular syndrome in varicella zoster infection[123] has led to the implication of an infectious etiology in this disease.

Miscellaneous Vasculitic Syndromes

Vasculitic syndromes that are beyond the scope of this review but should be mentioned include Cogan's syndrome,[124] Behçet's disease[125,126] (Chap. 185), erythema elevatum diutinum (Chap. 92), and isolated retinal vasculitis.

Pathogenesis

In systemic vasculitis, inflammation of the blood vessel wall and endothelial cell damage lead to narrowing of the vessel lumen. There is often accompanying thrombosis and subsequent ischemic organ damage. The pathogenetic mechanisms leading to the inflammation and destruction of the vessel wall are poorly understood. Three possible mechanisms have been proposed: deposition of immune complexes into the vessel wall, the production of specific antibody directed against a component of the blood vessel wall or against other antigens, and direct interactions between components of the blood vessel wall and activated T lymphocytes.[127] The most widely accepted pathogenetic mechanism is that of passive deposition of immune complexes in the vessel wall.[5] However, this mechanism is best established for certain of the vasculitides within the hypersensitivity group (Table 174-1) and is less clearly involved in the vasculitic syndromes discussed in this chapter. Evidence for both of the second two mechanisms is now beginning to emerge.

Experimental studies in animals support the hypothesis that immune complex deposition can mediate vascular damage. In animal models of acute serum sickness, circulating immune complexes are formed from antibody reacting with free antigen.[128,129] Factors that influence subsequent deposition of preformed immune complexes in vessel walls include vascular permeability, size and composition of the immune complex, and hydrodynamic factors, among others.[128] Antibody may also react with localized tissue antigen, as in the Arthus reaction.[130] Once deposited in the vessel wall, immune complexes activate the complement cascade, leading to the release of chemotactic factors and the recruitment of polymorphonuclear leukocytes. Release of proteolytic enzymes and toxic hydroxyl radicals then promotes vessel wall destruction. The presence of hypocomplementemia[48,131] and immune complexes in the serum and tissues of patients with active vasculitis would support this proposed pathogenetic mechanism. However, in the "primary" systemic vasculitides other than polyarteritis nodosa, further evidence is largely indirect.

Although classic polyarteritis nodosa remains idiopathic, some knowledge of pathogenetic mechanisms can be gained by examining the polyarteritis nodosa-like vasculitis associated with known diseases. For example, a role for immune complexes has been demonstrated in polyarteritis nodosa associated with hepatitis B viral infection, in which hepatitis B surface antigen–antibody complexes have been demonstrated in the serum of patients with active vasculitis,[132] and hepatitis B antigen, immunoglobulin, and complement have been demonstrated by immunofluorescence in blood vessel walls and in fibrinoid lesions.[133,134] However, the majority of patients with polyarteritis nodosa do not show evidence of hepatitis B infection.

The polyarteritis nodosa-like vasculitis seen in association with hairy cell leukemia may provide an example of the second proposed pathogenetic mechanism for vessel wall damage, that of antibody-mediated vasculitis. It is postulated that vessel wall destruction in this setting is due to the production of recently described antibodies that cross-react with leukemic cells and with endothelial cells.[135] Because endothelial cells are in direct contact with the bloodstream, several other studies have focused on potential mechanisms for endothelial cell damage in vasculitis. Circulating cytotoxic antibodies that react with endothelial cells have been described in a spectrum of vasculitic syndromes.[136] In this regard, studies on Kawasaki syndrome have elucidated a possible mechanism of endothelial cell damage and subsequent vasculitis. Patients with Kawasaki syndrome produce elevated levels of interleukin 1 (IL-1)[137] and tumor necrosis factor (TNF).[138] Both cytokines induce the expression of endothelial surface antigens.[139] In addition, antibodies in the sera of acutely ill patients with Kawasaki syndrome caused complement-mediated lysis of IL-1 or TNF-stimulated cultured endothelial cells.[140]

It is thus postulated that cytokine production in Kawasaki syndrome induces expression of novel endothelial cell antigens, and that antibodies directed against these antigens are then produced, with subsequent formation of antigen-antibody complexes and endothelial cell lysis. Such endothelial damage may be an early event in the pathogenesis of vessel wall destruction. The primary cytokine-inducing event remains unclear, although several infectious agents have been implicated, including rickettsia-like organisms.[141] Antecedent respiratory illness has been associated with outbreaks in the United States.[142]

Although the pathogenetic role of the recently described C-ANCA autoantibodies in patients with Wegener's granulomatosis remains hypothetical, this may provide an additional example of blood vessel wall damage mediated by antibody. Etiologic infectious agents and environmental antigens have been sought in Wegener's granulomatosis, but none has been identified. The disease has been presumed to be immune-mediated because of the inflammation and granuloma formation, the deposits of immune complexes seen in some patients,[10,143] and the dramatic response to immunosuppressive therapy.[11] Indirect evidence for the pathogenetic role of the C-ANCA autoantibody includes the correlation between ANCA positivity and activity of disease and the low frequency of C-ANCA positivity in nonvasculitic syndromes.[87] ANCA antibodies can enter neutrophils,[84] and one target antigen has been demonstrated on the plasma membrane of neutrophils.[144] Preliminary evidence suggests that IgG from ANCA-positive serum causes degranulation of neutrophils in vitro.[86] In addition, intravascular lysis of leukocytes has been described in early tissue injury in Wegener's granulomatosis.[145] Thus, these autoantibodies may cause neutrophil activation, leading to release of proteolytic enzymes with subsequent tissue and vessel damage.

Beyond the possible pathogenetic role of the ANCA antibodies, their presence in the spectrum of diseases including Wegener's granulomatosis, crescentic glomerulonephritis without pulmonary involvement, and microscopic polyarteritis nodosa suggests that these diseases may be related and have a similar pathogenesis. This is of particular interest in view of the reported cases of isolated crescentic glomerulonephritis that eventually evolve into generalized Wegener's granulomatosis.[66]

Although definitive evidence for cell-mediated immune mechanisms in the human vasculitic syndromes is lacking, the role of blood vessel wall components, including endothelial cells and vascular smooth muscle cells, in the initiation of nonimmune complex-mediated vasculitis has begun to be investigated experimentally. Human vascular endothelial cells can act as antigen-presenting cells,[146] thus supporting the notion that endothelial cell–T cell interactions may be initiated at the site of vessel wall damage. One experimental study in BALB/c mice has demonstrated the induction of vasculitis in lung, brain, and other organs by the transfer of syngeneic lymphocytes that were previously activated by cultured endothelial cells from outbred mice.[147] A role for vascular smooth muscle cells in the recruitment of lymphocytes in vasculitis in the autoimmune MRL/1pr mouse has also been proposed.[148] These mice have high levels of circulating immune complexes, which have been implicated in vessel wall damage as well, underscoring the concept that different pathogenetic mechanisms may be acting in concert to produce vessel wall damage.

The pathogenetic mechanisms involved in the development of granulomas and granulomatous vasculitis in Wegener's granulomatosis and in allergic angiitis and granulomatosis remain unclear. Immunohistochemical studies in Wegener's granulomatosis have demonstrated that the cells infiltrating pulmonary vessels are predominantly T cells and monocytes,[149] supporting an underlying cellular immune mechanism. Cellular mechanisms have also been postulated in granuloma formation, with sensitized T lymphocytes releasing lymphokines, leading to recruitment of macrophages and giant cell formation.[5,89] Immune complexes may also play a role, as it has been shown that insoluble immune complexes can induce granuloma formation.[150] Little has been added in recent years to an understanding of the specific pathogenetic mechanisms involved in allergic angiitis and granulomatosis, although eosinophils may play a central role; eosinophil cationic proteins, which are toxic to tissues, have been demonstrated in the granulomas of patients with this disease.[151]

Therapy

When the diagnosis of cutaneous vasculitis is made on skin biopsy, a history, physical examination, and laboratory studies should be performed to establish or exclude the presence of systemic vasculitis. Cutaneous polyarteritis nodosa usually has a benign, though recurrent, course, and therapy includes meticulous local care of ulcerated lesions. In some patients, corticosteroid therapy may be required.[46] Corticosteroid therapy has been widely used in systemic polyarteritis nodosa and has been reported to be of benefit in inducing remission and improving 5-year survival.[36,38] Therapy with cytotoxic agents including cyclophosphamide[152,153] and azathioprine[154] has contributed significantly to remission in severe cases of arteritis of the polyarteritis nodosa group. When added to corticosteroid therapy, cytotoxic agents in one retrospective study allowed for a 5-year survival rate of 80 percent as compared to 53 percent in patients treated with corticosteroids alone.[154] Allergic angiitis and granulomatosis may be more responsive to steroids alone than classic polyarteritis nodosa.[54] Monoclonal antibody therapy for systemic vasculitis with antibodies directed toward lymphocyte and monocyte surface markers is currently being evaluated.[155]

Although corticosteroids alone were once advocated in Wegener's granulomatosis,[156] the addition of cytotoxic agents has vastly improved survival in this disease.[10,157] In one prospective study, complete remissions were achieved in 93 percent of patients with a regimen of cyclophosphamide and prednisone,[11] and it is generally agreed that cyclophosphamide is the cytotoxic agent of choice. The use of trimethoprim-sulfamethoxazole has been advocated by some authors[158] for limited forms of disease, but this remains controversial.[159]

Intravenous gamma globulin therapy in Kawasaki syndrome[160] was originally proposed on the hypothesis that circulating immune complexes were important in disease pathogenesis and that such therapy might block tissue deposition of immune complexes. Whether or not this is its mechanism of action, intravenous gamma globulin is highly effective in suppressing inflammation and preventing coronary artery aneurysm formation.[161] Steroids are no longer recommended, as studies have revealed an increased incidence of aneurysms in steroid-treated patients.[162] Salicylate therapy is advocated,[104] although recommended dosages and treatment duration vary.*

References

1. Lie JT: Diagnostic histopathology of major systemic and pulmonary vasculitic syndromes. *Rheum Dis Clin North Am* **16**:269, 1990
2. Kussmaul A, Maier R: Über eine bisher nicht beschreibene eigenthümliche Arterienerkrankung (Periarteritis nodosa), die mit Morbus Brightii und rapid fortschreitender allgemeiner Muskellähmung einhergeht. *Dtsch Arch Klin Med* **1**:484, 1866
3. Zeek PM: Periarteritis nodosa: A critical review. *Am J Clin Pathol* **22**:777, 1952
4. Zeek PM: Periarteritis nodosa and other forms of necrotizing angiitis. *N Engl J Med* **248**:764, 1953
5. Fauci AS et al: The spectrum of vasculitis: Clinical, pathologic, immunologic, and therapeutic considerations. *Ann Intern Med* **89**:660, 1978
6. McCluskey RT, Fienberg R: Vasculitis in primary vasculitides, granulomatoses and connective tissue diseases. *Hum Pathol* **14**:305, 1983
7. Alarcón-Segovia D: Classification of the necrotizing vasculitides in man. *Clin Rheum Dis* **6**:223, 1980
8. Hunder GG et al: The American College of Rheumatology 1990 criteria for the classification of vasculitis. *Arthritis Rheum* **33**:1065, 1990
9. Wolff SM: The vasculitic syndromes, in *Cecil Textbook of Medicine,* 18th ed, edited by JB Wyngaarden, LH Smith, Philadelphia, Saunders, 1988, p 2025
10. Fauci AS, Wolff SM: Wegener's granulomatosis: Studies in eighteen patients and a review of the literature. *Medicine (Baltimore)* **52**:535, 1973
11. Fauci AS et al: Wegener's granulomatosis: Prospective clinical and therapeutic experience with 85 patients for 21 years. *Ann Intern Med* **98**:76, 1983
12. DeShazo RD et al: Systemic vasculitis with coexistent large and small vessel involvement. A classification dilemma. *JAMA* **238**:1940, 1977
13. Yousem SA, Hochholzer L: Overlap syndromes: Wegener's granulomatosis and Churg-Strauss syndrome. *Semin Respir Med* **10**:162, 1989
14. Leavitt RY, Fauci AS: Polyangiitis overlap syndrome. Classification and prospective clinical experience. *Am J Med* **81**:79, 1986
15. Sergent JS: Vasculitides associated with viral infections. *Clin Rheum Dis* **6**:339, 1980
16. Kohler PF et al: Chronic membranous glomerulonephritis caused by hepatitis B antigen-antibody immune complexes. *Ann Intern Med* **81**:448, 1974
17. Levo Y et al: Association between hepatitis B virus and essential mixed cryoglobulinemia. *N Engl J Med* **296**:1501, 1977
18. Gorevic PD et al: Mixed cryoglobulinemia: Clinical aspects and long-term follow-up of 40 patients. *Am J Med* **69**:287, 1980
19. Borrie P: Cutaneous polyarteritis nodosa. *Br J Dermatol* **87**:87, 1972
20. Diaz-Perez JL, Winkelmann RK: Cutaneous periarteritis nodosa. *Arch Dermatol* **110**:407, 1974
21. Meyrick Thomas RH, Black MM: The wide clinical spectrum of polyarteritis nodosa with cutaneous involvement. *Clin Exp Dermatol* **8**:47, 1983
22. Churg J, Strauss L: Allergic granulomatosis, allergic angiitis and periarteritis nodosa. *Am J Pathol* **27**:277, 1951
23. Sergent JS et al: Vasculitis with hepatitis B antigenemia: Long-term observations in nine patients. *Medicine (Baltimore)* **55**:1, 1976
24. Duffy J et al: Polyarthritis, polyarteritis, and hepatitis B. *Medicine (Baltimore)* **55**:19, 1976
25. Berg RA et al: Vasculitis in a suspected AIDS patient. *South Med J* **79**:914, 1986
26. Calabrese LH et al: Systemic vasculitis in association with human immunodeficiency virus infection. *Arthritis Rheum* **32**:569, 1989
27. Citron BP et al: Necrotizing angiitis associated with drug abuse. *N Engl J Med* **283**:1003, 1970
28. Sergent JS, Christian CL: Necrotizing vasculitis after acute serous otitis media. *Ann Intern Med* **81**:195, 1974
29. Elkon KB et al: Hairy-cell leukaemia with polyarteritis nodosa. *Lancet* **2**:280, 1979
30. Phanuphak P, Kohler PF: Onset of polyarteritis nodosa during allergic hyposensitization treatment. *Am J Med* **68**:479, 1980

*None of these drugs has been specifically approved for these purposes by the Food and Drug Administration at the time of publication.

31. Ball J: Rheumatoid arthritis and polyarteritis nodosa. *Ann Rheum Dis* **13**:277, 1954

32. Lie JT: Illustrated histopathologic classification criteria for selected vasculitic syndromes. *Arthritis Rheum* **33**:1074, 1990

33. Chen KTK: Renal-limited polyarteritis nodosa. *Hum Pathol* **18**:1074, 1987

34. Croker BP et al: Clinical and pathologic features of polyarteritis nodosa and its renal-limited variant: Primary crescentic and necrotizing glomerulonephritis. *Hum Pathol* **18**:38, 1987

35. Fayemi AO et al: Necrotizing vasculitis of the gallbladder and the appendix. *Am J Gastroenterol* **67**:608, 1977

36. Frohnert PP, Sheps SG: Long-term follow-up study of periarteritis nodosa. *Am J Med* **43**:8, 1967

37. Sack M et al: Prognostic factors in polyarteritis. *J Rheumatol* **2**:411, 1975

38. Cohen RD et al: Clinical features, prognosis and response to treatment in polyarteritis. *Mayo Clin Proc* **55**:146, 1980

39. Fauci AS: Vasculitis. *J Allergy Clin Immunol* **72**:211, 1983

40. Davson J et al: The kidney in periarteritis nodosa. *Q J Med* **17**:175, 1948

41. Savage COS et al: Microscopic polyarteritis: Presentation, pathology and prognosis. *Q J Med* **56**:467, 1985

42. Ford RG, Siekert RG: Central nervous system manifestations of periarteritis nodosa. *Neurology* **15**:114, 1965

43. Holsinger DR et al: The heart in periarteritis nodosa. *Circulation* **25**:610, 1962

44. Lyell A, Church R: The cutaneous manifestations of polyarteritis nodosa. *Br J Dermatol* **66**:335, 1954

45. Travers RL et al: Polyarteritis nodosa: A clinical and angiographic analysis of 17 cases. *Sem Arthritis Rheum* **8**:184, 1979

46. Diaz-Perez JL, Winkelmann RK: Cutaneous periarteritis nodosa: A study of 33 cases, in *Vasculitis,* edited by K Wolff, RK Winkelmann. Philadelphia, Saunders, 1980, p 273

47. Leib ES et al: Correlation of disease activity in systemic necrotizing vasculitis with immune complexes. *J Rheumatol* **8**:258, 1981

48. Conn DL et al: Immunologic mechanisms in systemic vasculitis. *Mayo Clin Proc* **51**:511, 1976

49. Baker SB, Robinson DR: Unusual renal manifestations of Wegener's granulomatosis. Report of two cases. *Am J Med* **64**:883, 1978

50. Longstreth PL et al: Renal microaneurysms in a patient with systemic lupus erythematosus. *Radiology* **113**:65, 1974

51. Wegener F: Über generalisierte, septische Gefässerkrankungen. *Verh Dtsch Ges Pathol* **29**:202, 1936

52. Carrington CB, Liebow AA: Limited forms of angiitis and granulomatosis of Wegener's type. *Am J Med* **41**:497, 1966

53. Cassan SM et al: The concept of limited forms of Wegener's granulomatosis. *Am J Med* **49**:366, 1970

54. Specks U, DeRemee RA: Granulomatous vasculitis. Wegener's granulomatosis and Churg-Strauss syndrome. *Rheum Dis Clin North Am* **16**:377, 1990

55. Fienberg R: The protracted superficial phenomenon in pathergic (Wegener's) granulomatosis. *Hum Pathol* **12**:458, 1981

56. Walton EW. Giant-cell granuloma of the respiratory tract (Wegener's granulomatosis). *Br Med J* **2**:265, 1958

57. Fahey JL et al: Wegener's granulomatosis. *Am J Med* **17**:168, 1954

58. DeRemee RA et al: Wegener's granulomatosis. Anatomic correlates, a proposed classification. *Mayo Clin Proc* **51**:777, 1976

59. Haworth SJ et al: Pulmonary haemorrhage complicating Wegener's granulomatosis and microscopic polyarteritis. *Br Med J* **290**:1775, 1985

60. Myers JL, Katzenstein A-LA: Wegener's granulomatosis presenting with massive pulmonary hemorrhage and capillaritis. *Am J Surg Pathol* **11**:895, 1987

61. Wolff SM et al: Wegener's granulomatosis. *Ann Intern Med* **81**:513, 1974

62. Pinching AJ et al: Wegener's granulomatosis. Observations on 18 patients with severe renal disease. *Q J Med* **208**:435, 1983

63. Weiss MA, Crissman JD: Renal biopsy findings in Wegener's granulomatosis: Segmental necrotizing glomerulonephritis with glomerular thrombosis. *Hum Pathol* **15**:943, 1984

64. Appel GB et al: Wegener's granulomatosis—clinical-pathologic correlations and long-term course. *Am J Kidney Dis* **1**:27, 1981

65. Heptinstall RH: Polyarteritis (periarteritis) nodosa, other forms of vasculitis and rheumatoid arthritis, in *Pathology of the Kidney,* vol 2. Boston, Little Brown, 1983, p 793

66. Woodworth TG et al: Severe glomerulonephritis with late emergence of classic Wegener's granulomatosis. Report of 4 cases and review of the literature. *Medicine* (Baltimore) **66**:181, 1987

67. DeOreo GA: Wegener's granulomatosis. *Arch Dermatol* **81**:169, 1960

68. Reed WB et al: The cutaneous manifestations in Wegener's granulomatosis. *Acta Derm Venereol* **43**:250, 1963

69. Hu C-H et al: Cutaneous manifestations of Wegener granulomatosis. *Arch Dermatol* **113**:175, 1977

70. Edwards MB et al: Wegener's granulomatosis: A case with primary mucocutaneous lesions. *Oral Surg* **46**:53, 1978

71. Cupps TR, Fauci AS: Wegener's granulomatosis. *Int J Dermatol* **19**:76, 1980

72. Bullen CL et al: Ocular complications of Wegener's granulomatosis. *Ophthalmology* **90**:279, 1983

73. DeRemee RA et al: Extrapulmonary manifestations of Wegener's granulomatosis and other respiratory vasculitides. *Semin Respir Med* **9**:403, 1988

74. Haynes BF et al: The ocular manifestations of Wegener's granulomatosis: Fifteen years experience and review of the literature. *Am J Med* **63**:131, 1977

75. Cassan SM et al: Pseudotumor of the orbit and limited Wegener's granulomatosis. *Ann Intern Med* **72**:687, 1970

76. Gatenby PA et al: Myocardial infarction in Wegener's granulomatosis. *Aust NZ J Med* **6**:336, 1976

77. Gerbracht DD et al: Reversible valvulitis in Wegener's granulomatosis. *Chest* **92**:182, 1987

78. Drachman DA: Neurological complications of Wegener's granulomatosis. *Arch Neurol* **8**:145, 1963

79. Lie JT: Classification of pulmonary angiitis and granulomatosis: Histopathologic perspectives. *Semin Respir Med* **10**:111, 1989

80. Fienberg R: A morphologic and immunohistologic study of the evolution of the necrotizing palisading granuloma of pathergic (Wegener's) granulomatosis. *Semin Respir Med* **10**:126, 1989

81. Yousem SA, Lombard CM: The eosinophilic variant of Wegener's granulomatosis. *Hum Pathol* **19**:682, 1988

82. Hind CRK et al: Objective monitoring of activity in Wegener's granulomatosis by measurement of serum C-reactive protein concentration. *Clin Nephrol* **21**:341, 1984

83. Davies DJ et al: Segmental necrotizing glomerulonephritis with antineutrophil antibody: Possible arbovirus aetiology? *Br Med J* **285**:606, 1982

84. Van der Woude FJ et al: Autoantibodies against neutrophils and monocytes: Tool for diagnosis and marker of disease activity in Wegener's granulomatosis. *Lancet* **1**:425, 1985

85. Falk RJ, Jennette JC: Anti-neutrophil cytoplasmic autoantibodies with specificity for myeloperoxidase in patients with systemic vasculitis and idiopathic necrotizing and crescentic glomerulonephritis. *N Engl J Med* **318**:1651, 1988

86. Jennette JC et al: Anti-neutrophil cytoplasmic autoantibody-associated glomerulonephritis and vasculitis. *Am J Pathol* **135**:921, 1989

87. Nölle B et al: Anticytoplasmic autoantibodies: Their immunodiagnostic value in Wegener granulomatosis. *Ann Intern Med* **111**:28, 1989

88. Rose GA, Spencer H: Polyarteritis nodosa. *Q J Med* **26**:43, 1957

89. Leavitt RY, Fauci AS: Pulmonary vasculitis. *Am Rev Respir Dis* **134**:149, 1986

90. Chumbly LC et al: Allergic granulomatosis and angiitis (Churg-Strauss syndrome). Report and analysis of 30 cases. *Mayo Clin Proc* **52**:477, 1977

91. Lanham JG et al: Systemic vasculitis with asthma and eosinophilia:

A clinical approach to the Churg-Strauss syndrome. *Medicine (Baltimore)* **63**:65, 1984

92. Sokolov RA et al: Allergic granulomatosis. *Am J Med* **32**:131, 1962

93. Finan MC, Winkelmann RK: The cutaneous extravascular necrotizing granuloma (Churg-Strauss granuloma) and systemic disease: A review of 27 cases. *Medicine (Baltimore)* **62**:142, 1983

94. Crotty CP et al: Cutaneous clinicopathologic correlation of allergic granulomatosis. *J Am Acad Dermatol* **5**:571, 1981

95. Strauss L et al: Cutaneous lesions of allergic granulomatosis. A histopathologic study. *J Invest Dermatol* **17**:349, 1951

96. Lie JT: The classification of vasculitis and a reappraisal of allergic granulomatosis and angiitis (Churg-Strauss syndrome). *Mt Sinai J Med* **53**:429, 1986

97. Kawasaki T: Acute febrile mucocutaneous syndrome with lymphoid involvement with specific desquamation of the fingers and toes in children. *Jpn J Allergy* **16**:178, 1967

98. Kawasaki T et al: A new infantile acute febrile mucocutaneous lymph node syndrome (MLNS) prevailing in Japan. *Pediatrics* **54**:271, 1974

99. Melish ME et al: Mucocutaneous lymph node syndrome in the United States. *Am J Dis Child* **130**:599, 1976

100. Butler DF et al: Adult Kawasaki syndrome. *Arch Dermatol* **123**:1356, 1987

101. Tanaka N et al: Kawasaki disease: Relationship with infantile periarteritis nodosa. *Arch Pathol Lab Med* **100**:81, 1976

102. Landing BH, Larson EJ: Are infantile periarteritis nodosa with coronary artery involvement and fatal mucocutaneous lymph node syndrome the same? Comparison of 20 patients from North America with patients from Hawaii and Japan. *Pediatrics* **59**:651, 1977

103. Ettlinger RE et al: Polyarteritis nodosa in childhood: A clinical pathologic study. *Arthritis Rheum* **22**:820, 1979

104. Wortmann DW, Nelson AM: Kawasaki syndrome. *Rheum Dis Clin North Am* **16**:363, 1990

105. Morens DM et al: National surveillance of Kawasaki disease. *Pediatrics* **65**:21, 1980

106. Kato H et al: Fate of coronary aneurysms in Kawasaki disease: Serial coronary angiography and long-term follow-up study. *Am J Cardiol* **49**:1758, 1982

107. Fujiwara H, Hamashima Y: Pathology of the heart in Kawasaki disease. *Pediatrics* **61**:100, 1978

108. Yanagisawa M et al: Myocardial infarction due to coronary thromboarteritis, following acute febrile mucocutaneous lymph node syndrome (MLNS) in an infant. *Pediatrics* **54**:277, 1974

109. Hirose S, Hamashima Y: Morphologic observations on the vasculitis in the mucocutaneous lymph node syndrome. *Eur J Pediatr* **129**:17, 1978

110. Capannari TE et al: Sensitivity, specificity and predictive value of two-dimensional echocardiography in detecting coronary artery aneurysms in patients with Kawasaki disease. *J Am Coll Cardiol* **7**:355, 1986

111. Mason WH et al: Circulating immune complexes in Kawasaki syndrome. *Pediatr Infect Dis* **4**:48, 1985

112. Leung DYM et al: Immunoregulatory T cell abnormalities in mucocutaneous lymph node syndrome. *J Immunol* **130**:2002, 1983

113. Barron K et al: Abnormalities of immunoregulation in Kawasaki syndrome. *J Rheumatol* **15**:1243, 1988

114. McKusick VA et al: Buerger's disease: A distinct clinical and pathologic entity. *JAMA* **181**:5, 1962

115. McKusick VA, Harris WS: The Buerger syndrome in the Orient. *Bull Johns Hopkins Hosp* **109**:241, 1961

116. Shionoya S et al: Diagnosis, pathology and treatment of Buerger's disease. *Surgery* **75**:695, 1974

117. Deitch EA, Sikkema WW: Intestinal manifestation of Buerger's disease: Case report and literature review. *Am Surg* **47**:326, 1981

118. Drake ME Jr: Winiwarter-Buerger disease ("thromboangiitis obliterans") with cerebral involvement. *JAMA* **248**:1870, 1982

119. Lie JT: Thromboangiitis obliterans (Buerger's disease) revisited. *Pathol Ann* **23** (part 2):257, 1988

120. Calabrese LH, Mallek JA: Primary angiitis of the central nervous system. Report of 8 new cases, review of the literature, and proposal for diagnostic criteria. *Medicine (Baltimore)* **67**:20, 1987

121. Cupps TR et al: Isolated angiitis of the central nervous system: Prospective diagnostic and therapeutic experience. *Am J Med* **74**:97, 1983

122. Lie JT: The classification and diagnosis of vasculitis in large and medium-sized blood vessels. *Pathol Ann* **22** (part 1):125, 1987

123. Blue MC, Rosenblum WI: Granulomatous angiitis of the brain with herpes zoster and varicella encephalitis. *Arch Pathol Lab Med* **107**:126, 1983

124. Cheson BD et al: Cogan's syndrome: A systemic vasculitis. *Am J Med* **60**:549, 1976

125. O'Duffy JD et al: Behçet's disease: Report of 10 cases, 3 with new manifestations. *Ann Intern Med* **75**:561, 1971

126. Chajek T, Fainaru M: Behçet's disease: Report of 41 cases and a review of the literature. *Medicine (Baltimore)* **54**:179, 1975

127. Moore PM: Immune mechanisms in the primary and secondary vasculitides. *J Neurol Sci* **93**:129, 1989

128. Cochrane CG, Koffler D: Immune complex disease in experimental animals and man, in *Advances in Immunology,* vol 16, edited by FJ Dixon, HG Kunkel. New York, Academic, 1973, p 185

129. Dixon FJ et al: Pathogenesis of serum sickness. *Arch Pathol Lab Med* **65**:18, 1958

130. Cochrane CG et al: The role of polymorphonuclear leukocytes in the initiation and cessation of the Arthus vasculitis. *J Exp Med* **110**:481, 1959

131. Soter NA et al: The complement system in necrotizing angiitis of the skin. Analysis of complement component activities in serum of patients with concomitant collagen-vascular diseases. *J Invest Dermatol* **63**:219, 1974

132. Trepo CG et al: The role of circulating hepatitis B antigen-antibody immune complexes in the pathogenesis of vascular and hepatic manifestations in polyarteritis nodosa. *J Clin Pathol* **27**:863, 1974

133. Gocke DJ et al: Association between polyarteritis and Australia antigen. *Lancet* **2**:1149, 1970

134. Nowoslawski A et al: Tissue localization of Australia antigen immune complexes in acute and chronic hepatitis and liver cirrhosis. *Am J Pathol* **68**:31, 1972

135. Posnett DN et al: A membrane antigen (HC1) selectively present on hairy cell leukemia cells, endothelial cells and epidermal basal cells. *J Immunol* **132**:2700, 1984

136. Brasile L et al: Identification of an autoantibody to vascular endothelial cell-specific antigens in patients with systemic vasculitis. *Am J Med* **87**:74, 1989

137. Maury CPJ et al: Circulating interleukin-1β in patients with Kawasaki disease. *N Engl J Med* **319**:1670, 1988

138. Furukawa S et al: Peripheral blood monocyte/macrophages and serum tumor necrosis factor in Kawasaki disease. *Clin Immunol Immunopathol* **48**:247, 1988

139. Pober JS et al: Two distinct monokines, interleukin 1 and tumor necrosis factor, each independently induce biosynthesis and transient expression of the same antigen on the surface of cultured human vascular endothelial cells. *J Immunol* **136**:1680, 1986

140. Leung DYM et al: Two monokines, interleukin 1 and tumor necrosis factor, render cultured vascular endothelial cells susceptible to lysis by antibodies circulating during Kawasaki syndrome. *J Exp Med* **164**:1958, 1986

141. Carter RF et al: Rickettsia-like bodies and splenitis in Kawasaki disease. *Lancet* **2**:1254, 1976

142. Bell DM et al: Kawasaki syndrome: Description of two outbreaks in the United States. *N Engl J Med* **304**:1568, 1981

143. Ronco P et al: Immunopathological studies of polyarteritis nodosa and Wegener's granulomatosis: A report of 43 patients with 51 renal biopsies. *Q J Med* **206**:212, 1983

144. Csernok E et al: Ultrastructural localization of proteinase 3, the target antigen of anticytoplasmic antibodies circulating in Wegener's granulomatosis. *Am J Pathol* **137**:1113, 1990

145. Donald KJ et al: An ultrastructural study of the pathogenesis of tissue injury in limited Wegener's granulomatosis. *Pathology* **8**:161, 1976

146. Hirschberg H et al: Antigen-presenting properties of human vascular endothelial cells. *J Exp Med* **152**:249s, 1980

147. Hart MN et al: Experimental autoimmune type of vasculitis resulting from activation of mouse lymphocytes to cultured endothelium. *Lab Invest* **48**:419, 1983

148. Mayer CF, Reinisch CL: The role of vascular smooth muscle cells in experimental autoimmune vasculitis. I. The initiation of delayed type hypersensitivity angiitis. *Am J Pathol* **117**:380, 1984

149. Gephardt GN et al: Pulmonary vasculitis (Wegener's granulomatosis): Immunohistochemical study of T and B cell markers. *Am J Med* **74**:700, 1983

150. Spector WG, Heesom N: The production of granulomata by antigen-antibody complexes. *J Pathol* **98**:31, 1969

151. Tai P-C et al: Deposition of eosinophil cationic protein in granulomas in allergic granulomatosis and vasculitis: The Churg-Strauss syndrome. *Br Med J* **289**:400, 1984

152. Fauci AS et al: Cyclophosphamide-induced remissions in advanced polyarteritis nodosa. *Am J Med* **64**:890, 1978

153. Fauci AS et al: Cyclophosphamide therapy of severe systemic necrotizing vasculitis. *N Engl J Med* **301**:235, 1979

154. Leib ES et al: Immunosuppressive and corticosteroid therapy of polyarteritis nodosa. *Am J Med* **67**:941, 1979

155. Mathieson PW et al: Monoclonal-antibody therapy in systemic vasculitis. *N Engl J Med* **323**:250, 1990

156. Fred HL et al: A patient with Wegener's granulomatosis exhibiting unusual clinical and morphologic features. *Am J Med* **37**:311, 1964

157. Hollander D, Manning RT: The use of alkylating agents in the treatment of Wegener's granulomatosis. *Ann Intern Med* **67**:393, 1967

158. DeRemee RA: The treatment of Wegener's granulomatosis with trimethoprim/sulfamethoxazole: Illusion or vision? Current controversies in rheumatology. *Arthritis Rheum* **31**:1068, 1988

159. Leavitt RY et al: Response: The role of trimethoprim/sulfamethoxazole in the treatment of Wegener's granulomatosis. *Arthritis Rheum* **31**:1073, 1988

160. Furusho K et al: High-dose intravenous gammaglobulin for Kawasaki disease. *Lancet* **2**:1055, 1984

161. Newburger JW et al: The treatment of Kawasaki syndrome with intravenous gamma globulin. *N Engl J Med* **315**:341, 1986

162. Kato H et al: Kawasaki disease: Effect of treatment on coronary artery involvement. *Pediatrics* **63**:175, 1979

CHAPTER 175

Peter O. Fritsch

Giant Cell Arteritis

Giant cell arteritis (GCA) is a histopathologic term applied to a specific type of granulomatous vasculitis of medium-sized and large arteries, characterized by destruction of the tunica media, intramural giant cell-rich granulomas, intima cell proliferation, and vascular occlusion. GCA is the pathologic substrate of temporal arteritis (TA), polymyalgia rheumatica (PMR), and Takayasu's arteritis. Takayasu's arteritis is set apart by distinct clinical differences (see below), but PMR and TA share many general features in common and are presently regarded as clinically different but overlapping manifestations of the same disease process.[1-3] PMR is a generalized "rheumatic" disease without skin symptoms, primarily affecting the muscles of the shoulder and limb girdles; TA is a seemingly localized affliction of branches of the carotid artery, notably the superficial temporal artery, which may be accompanied by skin symptoms.

Temporal Arteritis and Polymyalgia Rheumatica

Historical Aspects

Temporal arteritis was first observed by Hutchinson in 1890[4] and described in detail by Horton and coworkers in 1932.[5] Bruce[6] is credited with having first mentioned PMR as "senile rheumatic gout" in 1888. In 1957, Barber[7] recognized this condition as a separate clinical entity distinct from rheumatoid arthritis and coined the term polymyalgia rheumatica. The connection of PMR with GCA was proposed in 1966 by Dixon et al.[8] and others ("polymyalgia arteritica").

Epidemiology

Polymyalgia rheumatica and temporal arteritis are fairly common conditions of old age, although the incidence reported varies greatly due to uncertainties of case definition (1 to 20 per 100,000 per year).[1,9] Rarely developing before 50 years of age, they steadily become more frequent thereafter and may affect approximately 0.5 percent of the population over 70 years of age. Peak incidence occurs in the seventh and eighth decades; there may be a higher prevalence in females (2:1) and in populations of northern latitudes.[1] PMR and TA occur in all racial groups[10] and are weakly associated with HLA-DR3 and HLA-DR4.[1] PMR is two to four times as common as TA. Biopsies of clinically unaffected temporal arteries in patients with PMR reveal GCA in up to 50 percent, but the transition from PMR to TA probably occurs in only approximately 15 percent. An incidence of 1.7 percent of GCA was found by Ostberg in nonselected autopsy material.[11]

Etiology and Pathogenesis

The cause of PMR and TA is unknown. Their association with bacterial and viral infection,[1,2] malignant tumors and monoclonal gammopathy,[3] and hormonal disturbances[12] has been anecdotally reported. Actinic and infrared damage[13] have been hypothesized to be a trigger of a generalized autoimmune reaction against elastic fibers. In a case control study, Machado et al.[14] observed a significant correlation with smoking and a less strong association with atherosclerotic vascular disease.

PMR and TA are no longer regarded as immune complex vasculitis,[1,15,16] although immunoglobulins and complement are occasionally found in the vascular lesions (which are notably devoid of leukocytes). The inflammatory infiltrate, as typically found in granulomas, contains mostly CD4+ lymphocytes and HLA-DR+ macrophages (along with interdigitating reticulum cells) and CD8+ lymphocytes more peripherally[15,16]; B and K cells are notably absent. Some CD4+ lymphocytes express interleukin 2 receptors, which they lose shortly after initiation of corticosteroid treatment.[16] Together with the absence of significant necrosis and the presence of multinucleated giant cells, this situation suggests a granulomatous cellular immune reaction directed against an inert and poorly digestible antigenic determinant of the vessel wall. Stimulation of peripheral lymphocytes of patients with PMR by arterial antigens has been shown in vitro.[15] Elastic fiber material, possibly chemically altered by aging processes or actinic damage, would be a likely candidate.[16] Alternatively, degenerate smooth muscle cells may become targets of macrophage cytotoxicity.[15]

Clinical Features

Polymyalgia Rheumatica PMR may develop insidiously or rapidly, within several days or a few weeks. Nonspecific systemic signs such as low-grade fever, malaise, fatigue, anorexia, weight loss, and depression accompany the characteristic symptoms of symmetric myalgias and rigidity, predominantly of the muscles of the neck, shoulders, and hips. The myalgias of PMR typically inhibit actions that involve these muscle groups (like combing the hair and getting out of bed or up from a chair) and tend to worsen in the second half of the night.[1,2] Myalgias may mimic muscle weakness, although physical examination usually reveals neither muscle tenderness nor reduction of strength. Mild and transient arthralgias of the large joints may occur, but synovitis is absent.[17] Electromyography is normal,[1,2]

Temporal Arteritis TA may exhibit a plethora of mostly nonspecific clinical symptoms, the most striking and consistent being severe and bilateral headache and scalp tenderness. Three clusters of symptoms may be distinguished: the PMR complex, symptoms arising from involvement of one or several cranial arteries, and symptoms from extracranial artery involvement. Typically, TA evolves according to a three-stage course.[18]

The *prodromal stage* may take from a few weeks to several years and is characterized by the clinical symptoms of PMR. While PMR persists, headaches of gradually increasing intensity develop.

The *acute stage* is characterized by severe, usually bilateral headache, which may be diffuse or localized to the temporofrontal, -parietal, or -occipital regions. Pains are described as superficial, burning, at times with a lancinating quality. The scalp areas affected are tender, edematous, and inflamed. The superficial temporal arteries are prominent, meandering, infiltrated, tender, and show focal nodular thickening; their pulses are weak or absent (Fig. 175-1).

At this stage, symptoms of involvement of other cranial arteries may become manifest. Activity-dependent pain of facial muscles (masseter, pharynx, tongue) that subsides after rest is a pathognomonic sign of TA (jaw claudication). In approximately 50 percent, the retinal and/or other arteries supplying the eye are involved, leading to ophthalmologic symptoms of different kinds and intensity: transitory impairment of vision, blurring and amblyopia, diplopia, ptosis, ischemic optic neuritis, and sudden transitory (amaurosis fugax) or, more often, permanent blindness and ophthalmoplegia.[19] Eye involvement is usually bilateral. Involvement of other cranial arteries may lead to deafness, nausea, disturbances of

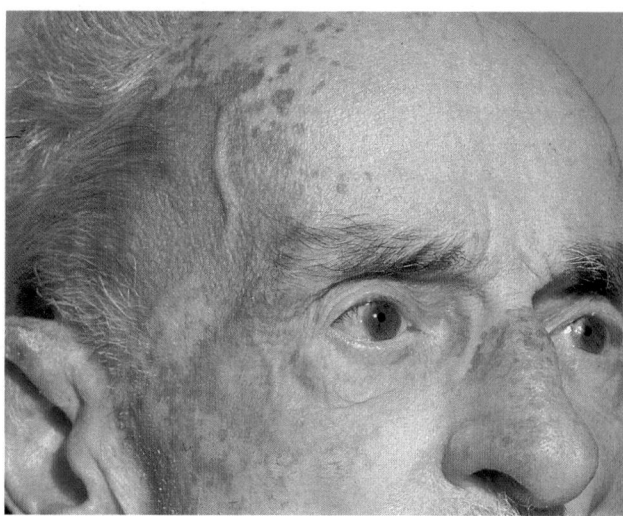

FIGURE 175-1 Giant cell arteritis. There is an obvious involvement of the superficial temporal arteries which are swollen and tortuous.

speech,[20] subarachnoid hemorrhage, psychoses, and dementia.[21] As a rare complication, cerebral artery involvement may result in lethal ischemic stroke.

Although rare, sudden and complete occlusion of the affected vessels may lead to acute gangrene[18,22] (Fig. 175-2*a*). This serious complication most often arises in the scalp regions supplied by the superficial temporal arteries. Accompanied by a paroxysmal worsening of the headache, it begins as a bandlike ischemic lesion along the afflicted artery, rapidly enlarges, and acquires bizarre irregular outlines. Initially, the necrosis is dry but may soon become bullous-hemorrhagic and transform into deep ulcers, which may extend down to the calvaria and even lead to bone perforation. Again, involvement is usually bilateral, with a narrow band of uninvolved skin often remaining in the sagittal region. Necrosis of the tongue is another rare but typical complication.

Involvement of extracranial arteries is relatively frequent (up to 15 percent); the resulting clinical symptoms are either absent or mild. The aorta and the large arteries of the aortic arch (particularly the subclavian artery) are most frequently involved.[23] Hemorrhage from an aortic aneurysm is a rare but fatal complication; of a less dramatic nature are the aortic arch syndrome and angina pectoris- and claudicatio intermittens-like disturbances. In the latter case, weak or absent pulses and bruits may be detected over affected arteries.

If untreated, the disease activity tends to decrease over several weeks or months, leading to the *chronic stage*. Headache and systemic signs gradually diminish and finally disappear; myalgias persist the longest. The inflamed temporal arteries transform into pulseless, wirelike fibrotic strands. Even the large and deep ulcers of the scalp, if present, tend to heal spontaneously, over a period of several months (Fig. 175-2*b*).

Unusual clinical features of TA may comprise isolated involvement of arteries of internal organ systems, e.g., the digestive tract, the central and peripheral nervous systems, the heart, and the joints.[1]

Laboratory Examinations

No specific laboratory tests are available for the diagnosis of PMR and TA. Except for a markedly increased erythrocyte sedimentation

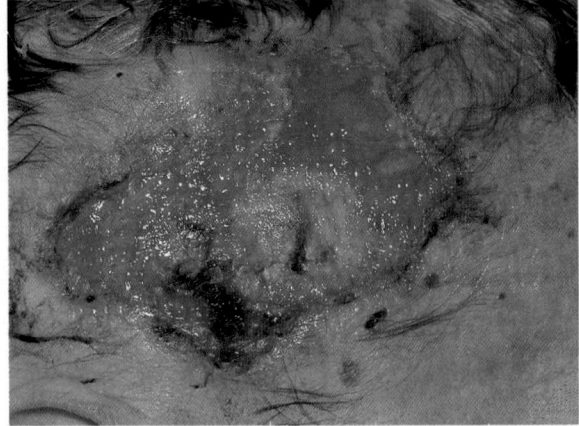

a

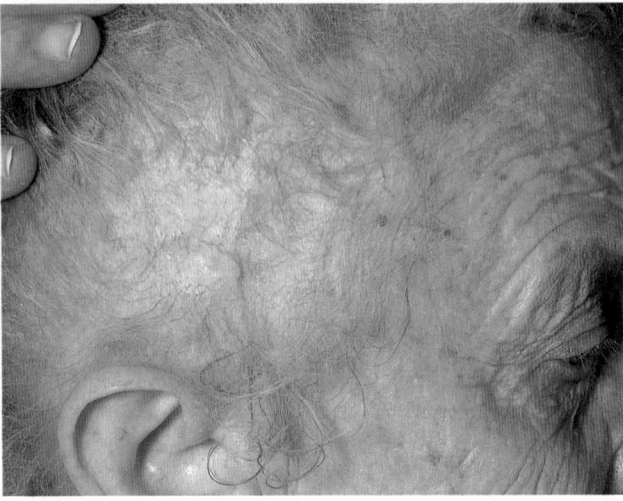

b

FIGURE 175-2 (*a*) Temporoparietal scalp gangrene in an 89-year-old female with temporal arteritis (acute stage) (*b*) Spontaneous healing with scarring 3 months after initiation of systemic corticosteroid treatment.

rate (ESR) (>80 mm/h) and the presence of acute-phase reactants in most patients in the active phase, laboratory results as a rule prove noncontributory. Recently, a constant and significant depletion of peripheral CD8+ lymphocytes has been reported,[24] even in those few cases with low acute-phase response.[25] Occasionally, low serum calcium, anemia, leukocytosis, thrombocytosis, elevated transaminases and immunoglobulins, and immune complexes may be present.

Histopathology

The characteristic arterial lesions are focal and thus can often be detected only in multiple biopsies and/or serial sections. The earliest changes are fibrinoid degeneration and, although usually not very conspicuous, necrosis of the smooth muscle cells of the tunica media; these are followed by mononuclear cell infiltrates and granuloma formation with a variable number of foreign body type multinuclear giant cells (Fig. 175-3*a*). The granuloma centers around the lamina elastica interna, which is split up and partially destroyed (Fig. 175-3*b*). Concentric or eccentric subendothelial proliferation

results in narrowing or occlusion of the vascular lumen. Older lesions display calcium deposits and fibrosis. In all stages thrombi may be found, which are probably responsible for sudden vascular occlusion. Immunoglobulin and complement deposits have been reported but are not a regular finding.

Diagnosis and Differential Diagnosis

The diagnosis of PMR is a diagnosis of exclusion. Tentative clinical diagnosis rests on the following criteria [modified from reference 26]: over 50 years of age, a history of proximal muscle myalgia for more than 4 weeks, ESR elevation greater than 50 mm/h, and responsiveness to low-dose corticosteroid treatment. PMR must be distinguished by clinical and laboratory criteria from rheumatoid arthritis, dermatomyositis, fibromyositis, degenerative disorders of the spine and joints, infectious myositis, and malignant neoplasms with paraneoplastic syndrome. Biopsies of the temporal artery are not routinely performed but are recommended if corticosteroid treatment proves ineffective in cases of suspected PMR.[1,2]

The diagnosis of TA rests on the demonstration of GCA in biopsies of the superficial temporal artery (only exceptionally of muscle arteries). In contrast to PMR, histologic proof should be sought in all suspected cases of TA (including those without obvious involvement of the temporal artery). Successful biopsy requires incision at the correct anatomic site[27] and excision of a sufficiently large artery specimen (>2 cm) because of the focal distribution of vascular lesions. If properly performed, the sensitivity of this procedure is estimated at over 90 percent.[1] Complications (e.g., scalp gangrene)[28] resulting from biopsies of the superficial temporal artery are very rare inasmuch as compensatory circuits are already formed in most cases. As an exception, however, blinding and fatal ischemic stroke have been reported in cases where the artery was part of a more complex compensatory circuit involving ocular and cerebral arteries. Therefore, before biopsy Doppler sonography has been recommended.[29] As an alternative of comparable sensitivity, pneumoplethysmography of the eye has been reported.[30] Doppler ultrasound investigation and arteriography are useful for the diagnosis of GCA of extracranial arteries. In the clinical differential diagnosis of TA, glaucoma, neuralgia of the trigeminal nerve, migraine, cerebral tumors, and, if scalp gangrene is present, cellulitis, deep trichomycosis, extensive basal cell carcinomas, angiosarcoma, and other tumors must be considered.

Therapy

Both PMR and TA are exquisitely sensitive to systemic corticosteroids. In view of the advanced age of the patients, carefully controlled administration is necessary.[2,31,32]

PMR, as a rule, responds within several days to low-dose prednisone therapy (10 to 40 mg/day), administered in divided doses initially and slowly tapered to maintenance doses (4 to 10 mg/day) according to clinical improvement and normalization of the ESR. Withdrawal of steroids may be tried after several months, but continued administration is often required for 1 to 2 years or indefinitely. After discontinuation of steroids, careful, frequent observation of the patient is necessary in view of the risk for the development of TA. Nonsteroidal antiphlogistic drugs act more slowly and less effectively.

TA requires rapid institution of steroids in much higher doses to relieve pain quickly and prevent irreversible complications

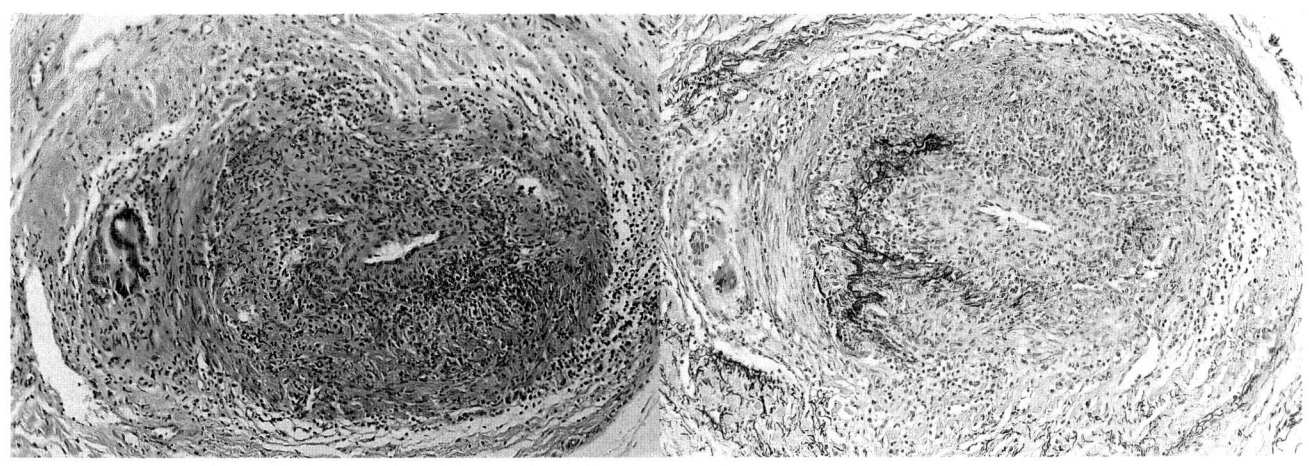

a   *b*

FIGURE 175-3 Histopathology of temporal arteritis. Intramural lymphohistiocytic granuloma with giant cells, intima proliferation, subtotal occlusion of vascular lumen, and splitting up and destruction of lamina elastica interna. ×25, HE (*a*) and elastica stain (*b*).

(blindness). The initial dose of prednisone may range from 40 to 100 mg/day in divided doses, followed by slow tapering to maintenance doses (10 mg/day or less). The clinical response is dramatic in most instances. Myalgias and headache subside within days to weeks, and claudicatio intermittens and pulselessness usually take several weeks. The ESR normalizes within several weeks, whereas depletion of peripheral CD8+ lymphocytes reportedly takes 2 years to gradually revert to normal.[24] The rapid onset of treatment is particularly important in case of ophthalmologic complications or acute gangrene, since irreversible damage may otherwise result; high-dose steroid treatment may reverse blindness if initiated within 24 h. Later, success is unlikely.[1] Systemic steroids should be continued for at least 6 months up to 2 years; some patients require treatment for 4 to 5 years.[32] No reliable criteria are available to determine the optimal time of steroid withdrawal; reversal of CD8+ lymphocytes to normal has been suggested.[29] Relapses not infrequently occur when attempts are made to taper the dose and within the first year after steroid withdrawal, but become less likely at later stages. Regular observation is nevertheless warranted for several years. Nonsteroidal anti-inflammatory drugs have little or no effect. Immunosuppressive drugs may help to spare steroids, but controlled trials of their use in TA are not available.

Prognosis

PMR and TA are regarded by many as principally self-limited conditions; spontaneous resolution occurs after an average of 5 to 7 years, although often with functional deficits in TA. There are no data on the mortality of untreated TA but it appears to be low. A fatal outcome can result from cerebrovascular ischemia or aorta and large vessel involvement or from overwhelming infection in the acute stage. In patients treated for TA, life expectancy is equal to that of the general population.[33]

Takayasu's Arteritis

Takayasu's arteritis is a chronic, progressive GCA predominantly affecting the aorta, its large branches, and the pulmonary arteries. Originally described in Japan,[34] it appears to have its highest incidence in Southeast Asia (ranging from 1/1000 to 1/5000 females per year.)[35] Recently, cases were reported from Africa and South America.[36] In Western countries, the incidence appears to be low even though cases may go undiagnosed. Takayasu's arteritis has a strong prevalence in females (8:1) and presents between the second and fourth decades in most patients.[36] It has been tentatively linked to infection (syphilis, tuberculosis)[37] and autoimmune diseases (SLE, rheumatoid arthritis) but is now regarded as part of the spectrum of GCA.[38] The histopathology of Takayasu's arteritis resembles that of TA, although the process appears to begin at the adventitia-media boundary.[36] In Japanese patients, an association with the HLA-Bw52 haplotype and certain C4 haplotypes has been found.[39]

Clinical Features

Takayasu's arteritis follows a two-stage course. The early, preocclusive phase is characterized by nonspecific general symptoms such as fever, malaise, weight loss, dyspnea, myalgias, and arthralgias. Months to years later, vascular occlusion leads to protean clinical pictures depending on the location of arterial stenosis or dilatation/aneurysm formation. Lupi-Herrera and associates[37] have identified four main patterns of arterial involvement: the aortic arch and its branches only (type I), the abdominal aorta only (type II), a combination of both (type III), and any of the above plus pulmonary artery involvement (type IV). Hypertension due to renal artery involvement is a frequent finding, as are pulselessness (subclavian artery involvement), vascular bruits, and retinal vascular malformations.[34]

Dermatologic Signs

The skin is usually uninvolved in Takayasu's arteritis. In the acute phase, Raynaud's syndrome, a malar flush, and erythema nodosum-like lesions may be observed.[40] Rarely, ulcerative lesions due to cutaneous granulomatous vasculitis, occasionally resembling erythema induratum, may be present.

Laboratory Data

As in other manifestations of GCA, laboratory findings are nonspecific. The ESR is typically elevated; leukocytosis, anemia, fibrinogenemia, and acute-phase proteins may be present as well as occasional immune complexes. Antistreptolysin titers and tuberculin tests often prove positive.[36]

Diagnosis

In the absence of histopathologic proof, diagnosis depends on circumstantial evidence: age (below 40 years), absence of vascular risk factors (smoking, diabetes, hyperlipidemia, oral contraceptives), elevated ESR, and arterial criteria (aortic stenosis or aneurysm, stenosis or occlusion of subclavian and/or carotid arteries, arterial parietal thickening).

Therapy and Prognosis

Corticosteroids are the treatment of choice in the early phase of Takayasu's arteritis. However, the response to corticosteroids is less complete and striking than in the other forms of GCA; long-term therapy (2 years and more) is often necessary.[36] In the later stages of Takayasu's arteritis, corticosteroids are of little effect, and vascular reconstructive surgery may be warranted. Antibiotics, anticoagulants, and antiaggregant drugs have been tried, but their value remains to be demonstrated. Supportive therapy for heart and/or kidney failure is required. Mortality rates reported are highly discrepant, ranging from 75 percent within 2 years[41] to 14 percent in 19 years.[37] The main causes of death are heart and renal failure and myocardial infarction.[36]

References

1. Allen BA, Studenski SA: Polymyalgia rheumatica and temporal arteritis. *Med Clin North Am* **70**:369, 1986
2. Hart FD: Polymyalgia rheumatica. Its correct diagnosis and treatment. *Drugs* **33**:280, 1987
3. Case records of the Massachusetts General Hospital, Case 23-1990: Polymyalgia rheumatica–giant cell arteritis syndrome. *N Engl J Med* **322**:1656, 1990
4. Hutchinson J: Diseases of the arteries. 1. On a peculiar form of thrombotic arteritis of the aged which is sometimes productive of gangrene. *Arch Surg* **1**:323, 1890
5. Horton BT et al: An undescribed form of arteritis of the temporal vessels. *Proc Mayo Clin* **8**:700, 1932
6. Bruce W: Senile rheumatic gout. *Br Med J* **2**:811, 1888
7. Barber HS: Myalgic syndrome with constitutional effects: Polymyalgia rheumatica. *Ann Rheum Dis* **16**:230, 1957
8. Dixon AJ et al: Polymyalgia rheumatica and temporal arteritis. *Ann Rheum Dis* **25**:203, 1966
9. Nordborg E, Bengtsson BA: Epidemiology of biopsy-proven giant cell arteritis (GCA). *J Intern Med* **227**:233, 1990
10. Gonzalez EB et al: Giant-cell arteritis in the Southern United States. An 11-year retrospective study from the Texas gulf coast. *Arch Intern Med* **149**:1561, 1989
11. Ostberg G: Prospective study of aortic and of aortic-temporal artery changes, respectively. *Acta Pathol Microbiol Scand* **237**:38, 1973
12. Wiseman P et al: Hypothyroidism in polymyalgia rheumatica and giant cell arteritis. *Br Med J* **298**:647, 1989
13. O'Brien JP: A new risk factor in vascular disease. Excessive solar and other actinic radiation in giant-cell arteritis and atherosclerosis. *Int J Dermatol* **26**:345, 1987
14. Machado EBV et al: A population-based case-control study of temporal arteritis: Evidence for an association between temporal arteritis and degenerative vascular disease? *Int J Epidemiol* **18**:836, 1989
15. Shiki H et al: Temporal arteritis: Cell composition and the possible pathogenetic role of cell-mediated immunity. *Hum Pathol* **20**:1057, 1989
16. Cid MC et al: Immunohistochemical analysis of lymphoid and macrophage cell subsets and their immunologic activation markers in temporal arteritis. *Arthritis Rheum* **32**:884, 1989
17. Kyle V et al: Rarity of synovitis in polymyalgia rheumatica. *Ann Rheum Dis* **49**:155, 1990
18. Fritsch P et al: Temporal arteritis, in *Vasculitis. Major Problems in Dermatology,* vol 10, edited by K Wolff and RK Winkelmann. London, Lloyd Luke, 1980, p 285
19. Mehler MF, Rabinowich L: The clinical neuro-ophthalmologic spectrum of temporal arteritis. *Am J Med* **85**:839, 1988
20. Nelson DA: Speech pathology in giant cell arteritis. Review and case report. *Ann Otol Rhinol Laryngol* **98**:859, 1989
21. Pascuzzi RM et al: Mental status abnormalities in temporal arteritis: A treatable cause of dementia in the elderly. *Arthritis Rheum* **32**:1308, 1989
22. Hitch JH: Dermatologic manifestations of giant-cell (temporal, cranial) arteritis. *Arch Dermatol* **101**:409, 1970
23. Ninet JP et al: Subclavian and axillary involvement in temporal arteritis and polymyalgia rheumatica. *Am J Med* **88**:13, 1990
24. Dasgupta B et al: Selective depletion and activation of CD8+ lymphocytes from peripheral blood of patients with polymyalgia rheumatica and giant cell arteritis. *Ann Rheum Dis* **48**:307, 1989
25. Elling H et al: CD8+ lymphocyte subset in polymyalgia rheumatica and arteritis temporalis. Inverse relationship between the acute hepatic phase reactants and the CD8+ T-cell subset. *Clin Exp Rheumatol* **7**:627, 1989
26. Bird HA et al: An evaluation of criteria for polymyalgia rheumatica. *Ann Rheum Dis* **38**:434, 1979
27. Daumann C et al: Der Verlauf der Arteria temporalis superficialis. Anatomische Studien als Voraussetzung für eine Arterien-Biopsie. *Klin Monatsbl Augenheilkd* **194**:37, 1989
28. Foged EK: Chronische Ulceration nach Biopsie der Arteria temporalis. *Hautarzt* **32**:647, 1981
29. Vollrath-Junger C, Gloor B: Warum eine Dopplersonographie vor jeder Biopsie der A. temporalis? *Klin Monatsbl Augenheilkd* **195**:169, 1989
30. Bosley TM et al: Ocular pneumoplethysmography can help in the diagnosis of giant-cell arteritis. *Arch Ophthalmol* **107**:379, 1989
31. Kyle V, Hazleman BL: Treatment of polymyalgia rheumatica and giant cell arteritis. I. Steroid regimens in the first two months. II. Relation between steroid dose and steroid associated side effects. *Ann Rheum Dis* **48**:658, 1989.
32. Kyle V, Hazleman BL: Stopping steroids in polymyalgia rheumatica and giant cell arteritis. Treatment usually lasts for two to five years. *Br Med J* **300**:344, 1990
33. Nordborg E, Bengtsson B-Å: Death rates and causes of death in 284 consecutive patients with giant cell arteritis confirmed by biopsy. *Br Med J* **299**:549, 1989
34. Takayasu M: Case with unusual changes of the central vessels in the retina. *Acta Soc Ophthalmol Jpn* **12**:544, 1908
35. Wong VCW et al: Pregnancy and Takayasu's arteritis. *Am J Med* **75**:597, 1983
36. Van der Heijden JTM et al: Takayasu's arteritis. Case report and review of the literature. *Neth J Med* **27**:74, 1984
37. Lupi-Herrera E et al: Takayasu's arteritis. Clinical study of 107 cases. *Am Heart J* **93**:94, 1977

38. Cairns SA, Oleesky S: Takayasu's disease and giant cell arteritis—a single disease? *Br Med J* **11**:127, 1977
39. Numano F et al: Hereditary factors in Takayasu disease. *Exp Clin Immunogenet* **6**:236, 1989
40. Francès C et al: Cutaneous manifestations of Takayasu arteritis. *Der-*

matologica **181**:266, 1990
41. Fraga A et al: Takayasu's arteritis: Frequency of systemic manifestations (study of 22 patients) and favorable response to maintenance steroid therapy with adrenocorticosteroids (12 patients). *Arthritis Rheum* **15**:617, 1972

CHAPTER 176

Stephen I. Katz

Relapsing Polychondritis

Relapsing polychondritis is a rare disease manifested by recurring episodes of inflammation in cartilagenous tissues throughout the body.

Historical Aspects

The disease was first described by Jaksch-Wartenhorst in 1921[1] and given the name polychondropathia in 1923.[2] In 1960, Pearson et al.[3] suggested the name *relapsing polychondritis* to emphasize its episodic nature, which leads to degeneration and replacement of cartilagenous structures by fibrous tissue. In 1976, McAdam et al. reviewed 159 reported cases of relapsing polychondritis, including 23 patients whom they had seen over the 15-year period of 1960 to 1975.[4] They also empirically defined diagnostic criteria that included the most common clinical features.

Etiology and Pathogenesis

Considerable evidence suggests that relapsing polychondritis is an autoimmune disease mediated by immunity to type II collagen. In humans, type II collagen is restricted to cartilage and constitutes more than 50 percent of the proteins of cartilage.

The concurrence of relapsing polychondritis with various rheumatic and autoimmune diseases initially led to the suggestion that an immunologic dysfunction might play a role in the pathogenesis of relapsing polychondritis.[4] Indeed, several investigators had reported abnormal cellular and humoral immunologic phenomena in relapsing polychondritis.[5-10] However, most of the reported findings lacked specificity for relapsing polychondritis, and the antigens used were not well characterized. Foidart et al.[11] detected antibodies to type II collagen in the sera of 6 of 23 patients with relapsing polychondritis. All patients in whom antibodies were detected had active disease. Subsequently, Terato et al.,[12] using an enzyme-linked immunosorbent assay (ELISA), found antibodies to type II collagen in the sera of 50 percent of patients with relapsing polychondritis but in only 15 percent of patients with rheumatoid arthritis and 4 percent of normal individuals.

The demonstration of antibodies to type II collagen in sera of patients with relapsing polychondritis raises the question of whether these antibodies are functionally active in vivo or whether they simply represent an epiphenomenon secondary to injury to cartilage and consequent exposure to the relevant antigens. That the antibodies are directed mainly against native rather than denatured

collagen would favor the former possibility.[11] Also, the epitope specificity of the antibodies is different in patients with rheumatoid arthritis and those with relapsing polychondritis.[12] The clinical manifestations may then be influenced by this specificity. Experimentally induced autoimmunity to type II collagen in rats[13,14] results in acute arthritis, suggesting that immune responses to type II collagen may play a role in inciting an inflammatory reaction in cartilage. Moreover, some rats sensitized with type II collagen also develop inflammatory ear lesions characterized by an intense, destructive chondritis, which resembles relapsing polychondritis histologically.[15] The observation that relapsing polychondritis may be transferred from an afflicted mother to her newborn child and that the child may then recover completely from the disease[16] also suggests an important role for antibodies in the pathogenesis of relapsing polychondritis. Finally, the finding in vivo of deposits of immunoglobulin and complement in inflamed cartilage in two patients with relapsing polychondritis[17] supports the likelihood that immunity to type II collagen plays a role in the pathogenesis of relapsing polychondritis.

Clinical Manifestations

The most frequent presenting manifestations are auricular chondritis and arthritis.[4,18] The chondritis is characterized by the sudden onset of redness, warmth, swelling, and tenderness limited to the cartilagenous portion of the external ears. Often only one ear is involved initially, and the ear lobe is typically uninvolved. The acute inflammation usually subsides spontaneously in 1 to 2 weeks. It is characterized by recurrences that appear after highly variable periods—from weeks to months. Eventually 85 to 90 percent of patients with relapsing polychondritis will develop auricular chondritis.[4,18] Nasal chondritis follows the same pattern as the auricular chondritis and eventually occurs in 54 to 70 percent of patients. The recurrent episodes of chondritis usually result in the destruction of normal cartilagenous structures and their fibrotic replacement. Clinically this process results in floppy or cauliflower ears and nasal deformities (Figs. 176-1 and 176-2).

Arthritis, which may involve only one or many small or large joints, is the second most frequent presenting sign and is eventually manifested in 52 to 80 percent of patients. At its onset, the arthritis is often migratory and is frequently associated with effusions, but it may be monoarticular and difficult to distinguish from gouty or infectious arthritis.

Other organ system involvement includes the eyes, where the inflammation may involve almost every part of the eye and adnexal

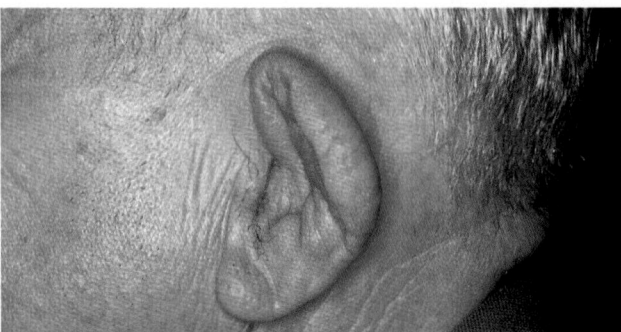

FIGURE 176-1 Relapsing polychondritis. Cartilagenous portion of ear is deformed and fibrotic.

structures,[4,19] manifesting as conjunctivitis, episcleritis, keratitis, and iritis (Fig. 176-3); the respiratory tract, where symptoms may include hoarseness, aphonia, and dyspnea; the inner ear, where symptoms may include nausea, vomiting, tinnitus, and deafness as a result of audiovestibular damage; and, less frequently, the cardiovascular system. Approximately 30 percent of patients have an associated rheumatic or autoimmune disease, and 5 to 14 percent of patients also have leukocytoclastic vasculitis.[4,18]

Laboratory Findings

The only laboratory finding that is consistently abnormal is an elevated erythrocyte sedimentation rate. The white blood count is elevated and/or the hemoglobin or hematocrit is decreased in more than half of patients.[4] Indirect immunofluorescence and ELISA studies have detected circulating antibodies to type II collagen in one-third to one-half of patients.[11]

Pathology

Relapsing polychondritis is characterized by a loss of the normal basophilia of cartilage with a perichondrial inflammatory infiltrate (Fig. 176-4). The earliest of the inflammatory cells are thought by some to be neutrophils and by others to be mononuclear cells. The end stage of the disease is characterized by the fibrotic replacement of cartilage.

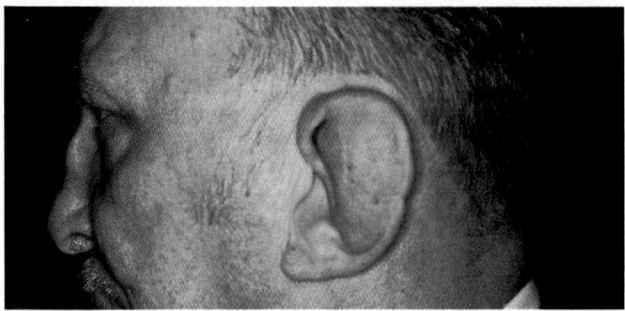

FIGURE 176-2 Relapsing polychondritis. "Cauliflower" ear and nasal deformity.

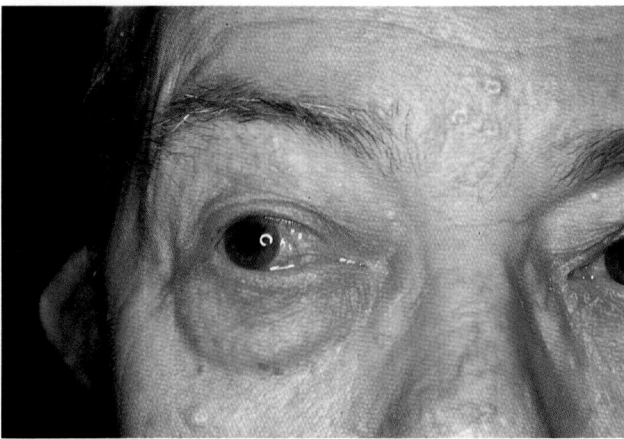

FIGURE 176-3 Relapsing polychondritis. Acute episcleritis.

Diagnosis

McAdam et al.[4] suggested that the diagnosis of relapsing polychondritis can be made when three of the following criteria are present along with histologic confirmation of the chondritis:

1. Bilateral auricular chondritis
2. Nonerosive seronegative inflammatory polyarthritis
3. Nasal chondritis
4. Ocular inflammation
5. Respiratory chondritis
6. Audiovestibular damage

Ordinarily, relapsing polychondritis presents little problem in diagnosis. However, there are patients who have only auricular and nasal chondritis and none of the other manifestations of relapsing polychondritis. If the histology shows perichondrial inflammation and the loss of the normal cartilagenous basophilia and if other conditions are excluded, a diagnosis of relapsing polychondritis should be made.

Concurrent rheumatalogic diseases may, at times, obscure the diagnosis of relapsing polychondritis. Cellulitis of the ear or nose may be confused on rare occasion with relapsing polychondritis; however, sparing of the ear lobe favors the diagnosis of relapsing polychondritis.

Treatment

Because of the highly variable course of relapsing polychondritis, individualized therapy is the key to optimum management. Systemic corticosteroids are helpful in controlling the acute inflammation. Seventy-five percent of patients in McAdam's series required chronic corticosteroid therapy; the average dose of prednisone was 25 mg/day.[4] Immunosuppressive therapy may also be efficacious in severe progressive disease.[4] Dapsone has also been reported to be an effective treatment[20,21]; however, our experience and that of others[18] with dapsone in relapsing polychondritis have been disappointing. The frequent spontaneous remissions that occur during

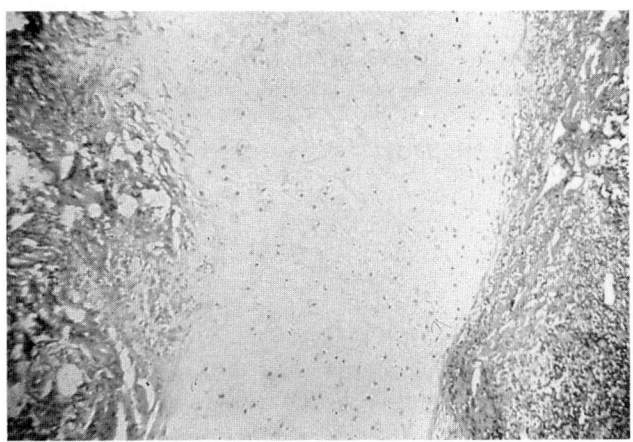

FIGURE 176-4 Relapsing polychondritis. Histopathology showing loss of basophilic staining of cartilage and perichondrial inflammatory infiltrate.

the acute episodes have made evaluation of most treatments difficult. The more chronic manifestations of relapsing polychondritis can be managed with indomethacin in some patients.

Course and Prognosis

The course of relapsing polychondritis is unpredictable. The acute chondritis in most patients lasts for 1 to 4 weeks, but in a few it may be more prolonged. Some patients have a relatively mild course with few episodes of chondritis. Other patients may have multiple episodes of chondritis. The degree of tissue destruction and fibrosis is difficult to predict early in the course of the disease. About one-third of the patients die as a result of relapsing polychondritis. The most frequent causes of death are airway collapse or obstruction, cardiovascular complications including systemic vasculitis and ruptured aneurysms, and infections (probably secondary to corticosteroid-induced immunosuppression).[4,18]

References

1. Jaksch-Wartenhorst R: Arztliche vortragsabende. *Prag Med Klin* **17**:342, 1921
2. Jaksch-Wartenhorst R: Polychondropathia. *Wien Arch Inn Med* **6**:93, 1923
3. Pearson CM et al: Relapsing polychondritis. *N Engl J Med* **263**:51, 1960
4. McAdam LP et al: Relapsing polychondritis. Prospective study of 23 patients and a review of the literature. *Medicine* **55**:193, 1976
5. Herman JH, Dennis MV: Immunopathologic studies in relapsing polychondritis. *J Clin Invest* **52**:549, 1973
6. Rajapakse DA, Bywaters EGL: Cell-mediated immunity to cartilage proteoglycan in relapsing polychondritis. *Clin Exp Immunol* **16**:497, 1974
7. Dolan DL et al: Relapsing polychondritis. *Am J Med* **41**:285, 1966
8. Hundeiker M et al: Infiltrat und Knorpelzerstorung bei polychondritis (Histochemische und immunofluoreszenz-histologische Befunde). *Z Haut Geschl Kr* **45**:437, 1970
9. Hughes RAC et al: Relapsing polychondritis. *Q J Med* **41**:363, 1972
10. Rogers PH et al: Relapsing polychondritis with insulin resistance and antibodies to cartilage. *Am J Med* **55**:243, 1973
11. Foidart JM et al: Antibodies to type II collagen in relapsing polychondritis. *N Engl J Med* **299**:1203, 1978
12. Terato K et al: Specificity of antibodies to type II collagen in rheumatoid arthritis. *Arthritis Rheum* **33**:1493, 1990
13. Trentham DE et al: Autoimmunity to type II collagen: An experimental model of arthritis. *J Exp Med* **146**:857, 1977
14. Trentham DE et al: Humoral and cellular sensitivity to collagen in type II collagen-induced arthritis in rats. *J Exp Med* **154**:535, 1981
15. Cremer MA et al: Auricular chondritis in rats: An experimental model of relapsing polychondritis induced with type II collagen. *J Exp Med* **154**:535, 1981
16. Arundell FW, Haserick JR: Familial chronic atrophic polychondritis. *Arch Dermatol* **82**:439, 1960
17. Valenzuela R et al: Relapsing polychondritis: Value of immunomicroscopic examination of ear biopsy. *Hum Pathol* **11**:19, 1980
18. Michet CJ et al: Relapsing polychondritis—survival and predictive role of early disease manifestations. *Ann Intern Med* **104**:74, 1986
19. Isaak BL et al: Ocular and systemic findings in relapsing polychondritis. *Ophthalmology* **93**:681, 1986
20. Barranco VP et al: Treatment of relapsing polychondritis with dapsone. *Arch Dermatol* **112**:1286, 1976
21. Martin J et al: Relapsing polychondritis treated with dapsone. *Arch Dermatol* **112**:1272, 1976

CHAPTER 177

Raul Fleischmajer

Scleredema and Papular Mucinosis

Scleredema

Scleredema is a connective tissue disease that was recognized as a distinct entity by Buschke in 1902. The disease affects all races and appears to be more prevalent among females. In a review of 209 cases by Greenberg et al.,[1] 29 percent were children under 10 years, 22 percent were between 10 and 20 years old, and 49 percent were adults.

Pathogenesis

The cause of scleredema is unknown. Streptococcal hypersensitivity, injury of lymph channels, alterations of pituitary function, and peripheral nerve abnormalities have been proposed as hypotheses; but none has been substantiated. The dermis is markedly increased in thickness, although it appears that this finding is due in part to the replacement of the subcutaneous tissue by connective tissue (Fig. 177-1). Chemical analysis of the dermis reveals an increase in hydroxyproline and hexosamines proportional to the increase in skin thickness. Fractionation of acid mucopolysaccharides shows a normal distribution of hyaluronic acid and dermatan sulfate. The water content of the skin is normal.[2] Using electron microscopy, Teller and Vester[3] noted clumping of collagen fibrils, increase in ground substance, and collagen fibrils with reduced diameter. The urinary excretion of hydroxyproline and hydroxylysine appears

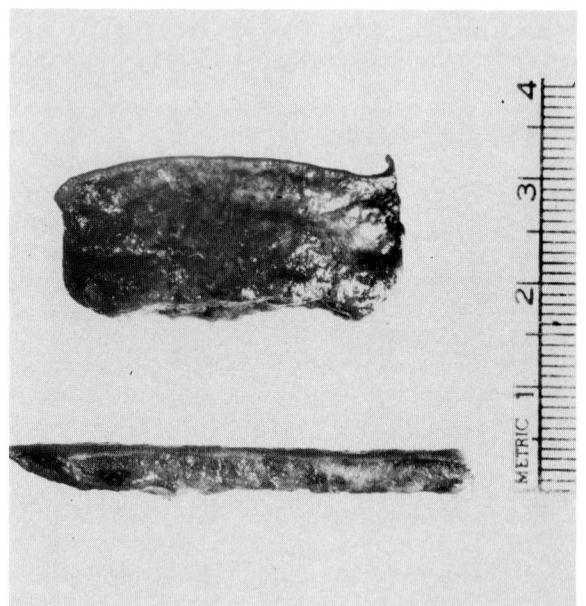

FIGURE 177-1 Scleredema skin from the back (top) and normal control. Note the marked increase in thickness. (*From Fleischmajer et al.*[2])

normal.[4] Scleredema has been found in association with a monoclonal gammopathy. Serum immunoglobulins are usually of the IgG type, although IgA and IgM have also been reported. The chains are either of the kappa or lambda type.[5,6] The association of multiple myeloma and scleredema has been documented in one case.[6] There is some evidence that the serum of scleredema patients may contain a factor that stimulates collagen synthesis.[6]

Clinical Manifestations

Skin involvement may be preceded by a prodrome of low-grade fever, malaise, myalgia, and arthralgia. A few days to 6 weeks before the onset, 65 percent of patients develop an infection, usually of streptococcal origin.[1] Influenza, scarlet fever, measles, mumps, tonsillitis, pharyngitis, otitis, furuncles, erysipelas, and impetigo have all been observed.

The onset is frequently sudden and consists of marked, nonpitting, symmetric induration of the skin, usually affecting the posterior and lateral aspects of the neck and then spreading to the face, shoulders, arms, and thorax (Fig. 177-2). The buttocks, legs, and abdomen are less frequently involved, and hands and feet are affected in about 10 percent of the cases. The disease usually reaches maximal involvement in about 1 to 2 weeks, although it may continue spreading for 2 to 3 additional months.

The induration is of wooden-like consistency, waxy white or shiny in appearance, and rather diffuse so that there is no sharp line of demarcation between involved and noninvolved areas as in localized scleroderma. Folding of the skin is almost impossible, and the normal markings are lost. When the face is involved, there is lack of expression and often difficulty in opening the mouth. Curtis and Shulak[7] described a transient, erythematous, macular or papular eruption during the early stage of the disease. Pain is absent, although paresthesias may occur. Heart abnormalities occur; in children the most common are diastolic gallop without evidence of cardiac failure, a nonspecific S-T depression, and T-wave inversion, usually reverting to normal in 3 to 9 months. Carditis secondary to rheumatic fever has also been noted.[4]

A syndrome has been recognized consisting of scleredema of long duration, obesity, maturity onset, latent or overt diabetes, and a high incidence of cardiovascular disease.[2,8] Diabetic retinopathy is not uncommon.[2,9] Most patients are quite resistant to antidiabetic therapy, including insulin, chlorpropamide, and phenformin. Furthermore, antidiabetic therapy has no effect on the evolution of the scleredema.

Laboratory Findings

Most laboratory tests are usually normal except for an increase in ASO titer in some patients.[2] A glucose tolerance test should be performed to rule out diabetes mellitus.[2,8] Hyperinsulinism may be present.

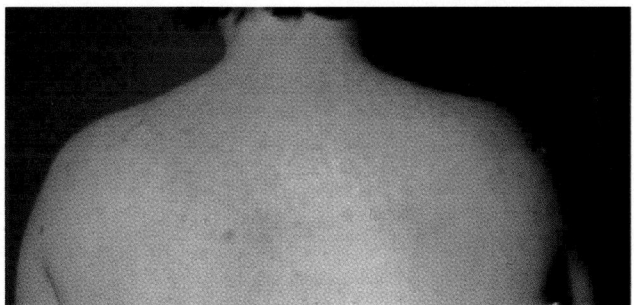

FIGURE 177-2   Scleredema of 41-year duration affecting the neck and back.

Pathology

The epidermis and its appendages are normal. The dermis reveals collagen bundles separated by large interfascicular spaces. The papillary layer is prominent and slightly edematous. In the upper dermis, there may be mild perivascular or scattered infiltrates consisting mostly of lymphocytes and histiocytic type cells (Fig. 177-3). An increase in mast cells has also been noted.[7,10] The secretory coils of the eccrine sweat glands are found in the upper third or mid-dermis. The subcutaneous tissue is reduced, probably due to its replacement by connective tissue.[2] The ground substance reveals an increase in metachromatic material with toluidine blue,[10] and this material also stains positive with alcian blue at pH 2.5. The alcian blue at pH 0.5, which stains sulfated acid mucopolysaccharides, is negative.[11] Hyaluronidase digestion completely removes the alcian blue–positive material, suggesting an increase in hyaluronic acid. However, this increase is only temporary and is not seen in all patients.

Differential Diagnosis

Scleredema has to be differentiated from the early edematous stage of systemic scleroderma. In systemic scleroderma, Raynaud's phenomenon, predilection for hands, abnormal pigmentation, telengiectasia, ischemia, and atrophic skin changes usually occur; these findings are not seen in scleredema. Scleredema should also be differentiated from trichinosis, dermatomyositis, scleromyxedema, myxedema, progeria, sclerema neonatorum, edema neonatorum, primary systemic amyloidosis, and edema from cardiac or renal origin.

Treatment

There is no effective treatment.

Course and Prognosis

Prognosis is usually good, and in most patients the disease undergoes spontaneous resolution in 6 months to 2 years. However, Curtis and Shulak[7] noted that 25 percent of patients showed no tendency toward resolution. The disease persists indefinitely in those patients with associated diabetes mellitus. In the Fleischmajer et al.[2] series, duration ranged from 2 to 41 years.

Papular Mucinosis

Papular mucinosis, or lichen myxedematosus, is a rare disease characterized by a papular-lichenoid eruption, mucin deposition, and a paraproteinemia. A clinical variant of papular mucinosis is

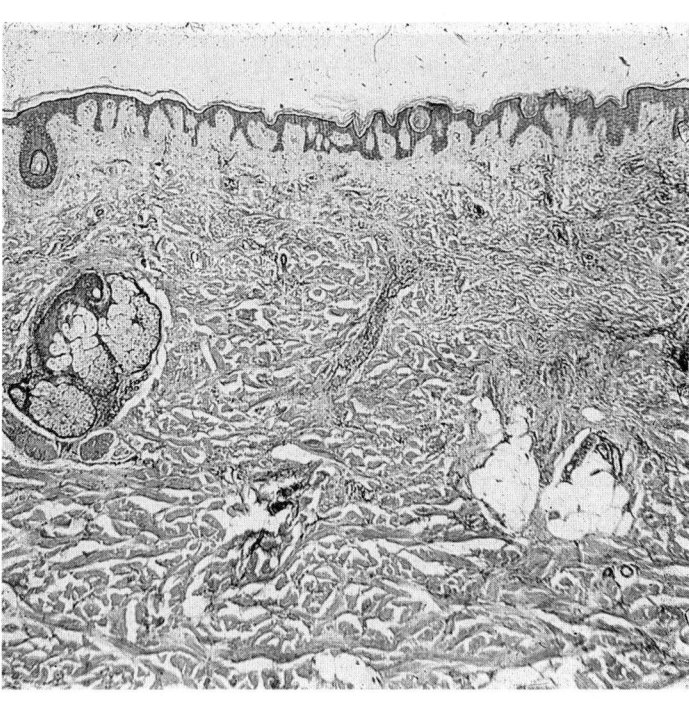

FIGURE 177-3   Scleredema. Edematous papillary layer, mild perivascular cellular infiltrates and collagen bundles separated by large interfascicular spaces. H&E, ×18.

scleromyxedema, in which the disease is more generalized and is accompanied by erythema and sclerosis.[12]

Pathogenesis

The pathogenesis of papular mucinosis remains unknown. This disease is frequently associated with a paraproteinemia that consists of a myeloma-like, homogeneous serum globulin of the IgG type, with predominantly lambda light chains, although kappa light chains have also been noted.[13,14] Less commonly, paraproteins of the IgM and IgA types have been identified. The paraprotein in papular mucinosis is a 7S, papain-sensitive globulin, which is strongly basic due to its high content in lysine.[15] It has a molecular mass of about 110 kDa (normal IgG is 160 kDa), thus suggesting that this IgG globulin is incomplete by missing a significant antigenic portion of the Fc fragment.[16] The initial suggestion that papular mucinosis represents a plasma cell dyscrasia has never been substantiated. Its association with multiple myeloma is rare, if it occurs at all. Furthermore, the paraprotein in multiple myeloma is usually a monoclonal IgG with kappa light chains. It has been shown that serum from papular mucinosis patients can stimulate DNA synthesis and proliferation of normal human fibroblasts in vitro.[17] However, removal of the paraprotein from culture media did not decrease fibroblast mitosis, thus suggesting that another serum factor may be responsible for this proliferative effect.

Clinical Manifestations

The disease affects adults from 30 to 70 years of age, has no sex predilection, and usually runs a chronic course. The primary lesion is a dome-shaped papule, skin color or erythematous, 2 to 4 mm in diameter; the lesions may be densely grouped in a lichenoid fashion or may show a linear arrangement. The areas most frequently affected are the dorsa of the hands and fingers, axillary folds, and external surfaces of the arms and legs. Coalescence of papules on the face, particularly in the glabella area, results in longitudinal folding, giving the appearance of leonine facies (Fig. 177-4). The lesions are usually asymptomatic, although mild pruritus may be present. In scleromyxedema, large parts of the body may be involved; the skin shows erythematous, scleroderma-like induration accompanied by reduced mobility of lips, arms, hands, and legs. Other skin lesions include urticaria, nodules, and cysts.[18] Although the disease primarily affects the skin, systemic manifestations have been described, such as severe proximal myopathy, inflammatory polyarthritis,[19,20] central nervous system symptoms resembling acute organic brain syndrome,[21] esophageal aperistalsis, and hoarseness.[22,23]

Laboratory Findings

The paraproteinemia is present in most patients, particularly in those with the clinical form of scleromyxedema. Immunofluorescence microscopy of the skin lesions occasionally shows deposits of IgG, with or without IgM, in the papillary and upper reticular dermis.[14,16] However, others have failed to reproduce these findings.[24] Other inconsistent findings refer to elevated sedimentation rate, leukocytosis with eosinophilia, albuminuria, and plasma cell aggregates in the bone marrow.

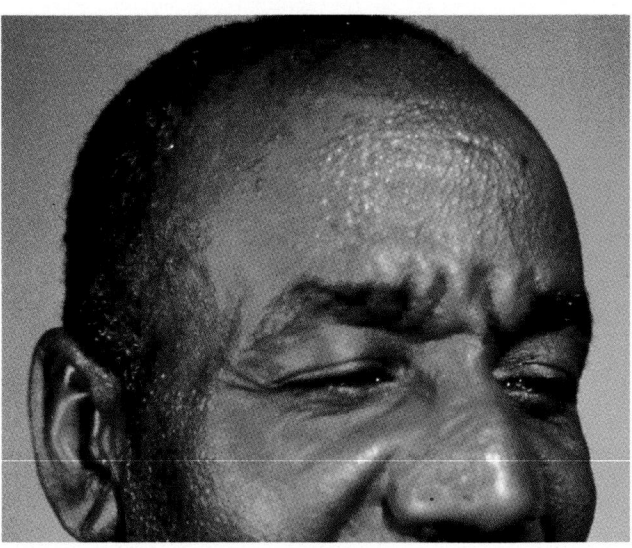

FIGURE 177-4 Papular mucinosis. Note discrete papules on the forehead and longitudinal folding of the glabella. (*Courtesy of L. Shapiro, M.D.*)

Pathology

The most striking changes are in the upper dermis, which shows a horizontal band of mucinous material between collagen bundles. This material is a glycosaminoglycan that stains with alcian blue at pH 2.5 and is susceptible to hyaluronidase digestion (Fig. 177-5). The epidermis may appear thinner due to pressure from the mucinous deposits. There is an increase in fibroblasts, which appear plump and stellate, and dermal fibrosis. Cellular infiltrates may be present around the small blood vessels and appendages and consist mostly of lymphocytes with some histiocytic types and polymorphonuclear cells.[25] An increase in plasma cells has also been noted.[24] Electron microscopy reveals fibroblasts with long cytoplasmic processes and dilated rough endoplasmic reticulum. In addition, there are numerous thin collagen fibrils, suggestive of young collagen.[26] Muscle biopsies reveal an atypical necrotizing myopathy with fiber necrosis, severe type II fiber atrophy, and vacuolization.[20] Mucin deposits have also been reported in the adventitia of blood vessels in kidney, heart, adrenal glands, pancreas, and kidney papillae. However, internal involvement in papular mucinosis still remains controversial.[24] Papular mucinosis has to be differentiated histologically from follicular mucinosis, amyloidosis, hyalinosis cutis et mucosae, scleredema, scleroderma, cutaneous focal mucinosis, pretibial myxedema, and colloid degeneration.

Diagnosis and Differential Diagnosis

Diagnosis is based on the presence of papular lesions, the demonstration of mucin in the dermis, and the presence of paraproteinemia. Clinically, papular mucinosis should be differentiated from scleredema, scleroderma, amyloidosis, disseminated granuloma annulare, malignant lymphomas, and dermatomyositis. The more localized forms should be differentiated from colloid degeneration, lichen planus, morbus moniliformis, and epithelioma adenoides cysticum.

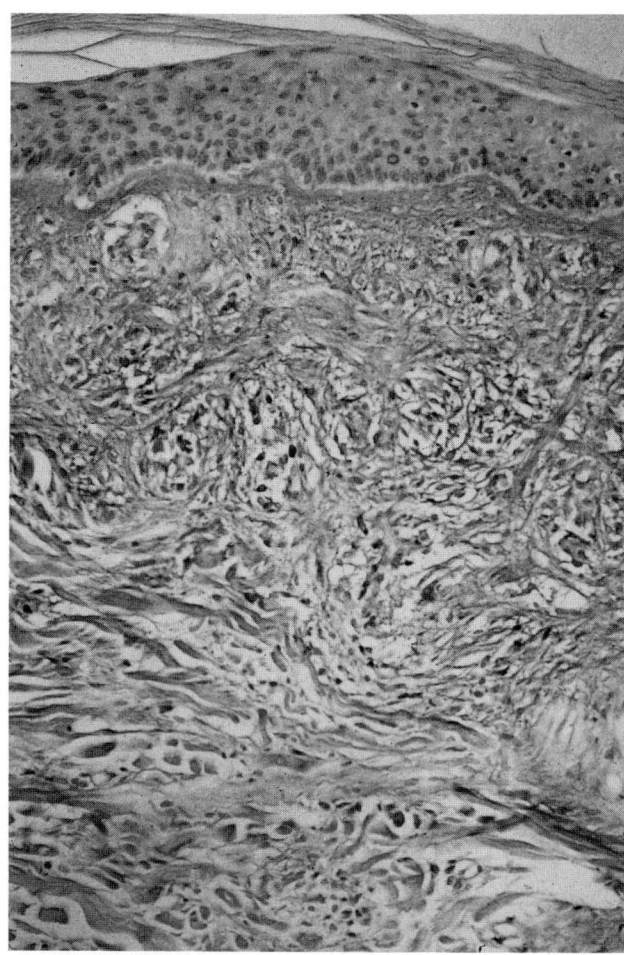

FIGURE 177-5 Scleromyxedema. Mucin and numerous plump fibroblasts in the upper dermis. Alcian blue, pH 2.5. (*Courtesy of L. Shapiro, M.D.*)

Treatment

The treatment of papular mucinosis remains unsatisfactory. Topical therapy is of no help. Complete clearance of lesions was reported with melphalan (1 to 10 mg per day) and cyclophosphamide (200 mg per day), alone or in combination with prednisone.[27–30] However, because side effects can be severe, these drugs should be restricted to patients with widespread disease.

Course and Prognosis

The disease runs a chronic course and usually has no tendency toward spontaneous resolution. The prognosis for long-term survival is good. Reported causes of death appear to be unrelated to the disease and included tuberculosis, pneumonia, and vascular thrombosis.

References

1. Greenberg LM et al: Scleredema adultorum in children. *Pediatrics* **32**:1044, 1963

2. Fleischmajer R et al: Scleredema and diabetes mellitus. *Arch Dermatol* **101**:21, 1970

3. Teller H, Vester G: Elektronenmikroskopische Untersuchungsergebnisse an der Interzellularsubstanz des Coriums beim Skleroedema adultorum Buschke. *Z Haut Geschlechskr* **23**:142, 1957

4. Yogman M, Echeverria P: Scleredema and carditis: Report of a case and review of the literature. *Pediatrics* **54**:108, 1974

5. Kovary PM et al: Monoclonal gammopathy in scleredema: Observations of three cases. *Arch Dermatol* **117**:536, 1981

6. Ohta A et al: Paraproteinemia in patients with scleredema: Clinical findings and serum effects on skin fibroblasts in vitro. *J Am Acad Dermatol* **16**:96, 1987

7. Curtis AC, Shulak BM: Scleredema adultorum. *Arch Dermatol* **92**:526, 1965

8. Cohn BA et al: Scleredema adultorum of Buschke and diabetes mellitus. *Arch Dermatol* **101**:27, 1970

9. Breinin GM: Scleredema adultorum: Ocular manifestations. *Arch Ophthalmol* **50**:155, 1953

10. Braun-Falco O: Neueres zur Hispathalogie des Scleroedema adultorum (Buschke). *Dermatol Wochenschr* **125**:409, 1952

11. Fleischmajer R, Lara JV: Scleredema: A histochemical and biochemical study. *Arch Dermatol* **92**:643, 1965

12. Gottron HA: Skleromyxodem (Eine eigenartige Erscheinungsform von Myxothesaurodermie). *Arch Dermatol Syphilol* **199**:71, 1954

13. Osserman EF, Takatsuki K: Role of an abnormal myeloma-type, serum gamma globulin in the pathogenesis of the skin lesions of papular mucinosis (lichen myxedematosus). *J Clin Invest* **42**:962, 1963

14. McCarthy JT et al: An abnormal serum globulin in lichen myxedematosus. *Arch Dermatol* **89**:446, 1964

15. Lawrence DA et al: Immunochemical analysis of the basic immunoglobulin in papular mucinosis. *Immunochemistry* **9**:41, 1972

16. Kitamura W et al: Immunochemical analysis of the monoclonal paraprotein in scleromyxedema. *J Invest Dermatol* **70**:305, 1978

17. Harper RA, Rispler J: Lichen myxedematosus serum stimulates human skin fibroblast proliferation. *Science* **188**:545, 1978

18. Wright RC et al: Scleromyxedema. *Arch Dermatol* **112**:63, 1976

19. McAdam LP et al: Papular mucinosis with myopathy, arthritis and eosinophilia: A histopathologic study. *Arthritis Rheum* **20**:989, 1977

20. Verity MA et al: Scleromyxedema myopathy: Histochemical and electron microscopic observations. *Am J Clin Pathol* **69**:446, 1978

21. Ochitill HN, Amberson J: Acute cerebral symptomatology: A rare presentation of scleromyxedema. *J Clin Psychiatry* **39**:471, 1978

22. Braverman IM: *Skin Signs of Systemic Disease,* 2d ed. Philadelphia, Saunders, 1981, p 233

23. Alligood TR et al: Scleromyxedema associated with esophageal aperistalsis and dermal eosinophilia. *Cutis* **28**:60, 1981

24. Farmer ER et al: Papular mucinosis: A clinicopathologic study of four patients. *Arch Dermatol* **118**:9, 1982

25. Perry HO et al: Further observations on lichen myxedematosus. *Ann Intern Med* **53**:955, 1960

26. Lever WF, Schaumburg-Lever G: Lichen myxedematosus, in *Histopathology of the Skin,* 5th ed. Philadelphia, Lippincott, 1975, p 405

27. Feldman et al: Scleromyxedema: A dramatic response to melphalan. *Arch Dermatol* **99**:51, 1969

28. Harris RB et al: Treatment of scleromyxedema with melphalan. *Arch Dermatol* **115**:295, 1979

29. Jessen RT et al: Lichen myxedematosus: Treatment with cyclophosphamide. *Int J Dermatol* **17**:833, 1978

30. Howsden SM et al: Lichen myxedematosus: A dermal infiltrative disorder responsive to cyclophosphamide therapy. *Arch Dermatol* **111**:1325, 1975

CHAPTER 178

Neville R. Rowell

Skin Manifestations of Rheumatic Diseases

Dermatologists are frequently asked to diagnose and manage patients with rheumatic diseases, although many may already be under the care of a general physician or rheumatologist. Histologic, immunohistologic, immunologic, and other investigations of such patients often require multidepartmental cooperation. This chapter deals with disorders in which joint involvement is a prominent feature and excludes the so-called connective tissue diseases, such as discoid and systemic lupus erythematosus, morphea, systemic sclerosis, Sjögren's syndrome, and dermatomyositis, which are dealt with elsewhere.

Rheumatoid Arthritis

In the United Kingdom rheumatoid arthritis affects 0.5 percent of adult males and 1.8 percent of adult females. The prevalence increases with age so that by 64 years of age 2 percent of males and 5 percent of females are affected. The onset is sudden (20 percent) or insidious. A symmetric polyarthritis affects the proximal interphalangeal and metacarpophalangeal joints, the wrists, ankles, knees, and cervical spine. Patients complain of stiffness, particularly in the early morning; the joints are painful, warm, and tender. Fever, weight loss, anemia, and lassitude are prominent when the disease is active. The severity of the joint disease determines the extraarticular manifestations. These include pleurisy, pleural effusions, pericarditis, and nonspecific valvulitis.

The eyes may be involved. Episcleritis is nonspecific and normally mild. Scleritis implies deep inflammation of the sclera and may be painful. The inflammation can be diffuse, nodular, or necrotizing; the latter may lead to perforation (scleromalacia perforans) (Fig. 178-1) and loss of the eye. Healing of scleritis leads to a translucent scar through which the blue-black choroid can be seen. Other complications of scleritis are uveitis, glaucoma, and cataracts. Keratolysis of the cornea and corneal perforation may be the result of vasculitis of the circumcorneal vessels. Treatment is with corticosteroid drops or systemic steroids.

Rheumatoid Nodules

Discrete nontender subcutaneous swellings occur in 20 percent of patients (Fig. 178-2). They are larger and more constant than those seen in rheumatic fever and usually occur in patients with severe disease and positive tests for rheumatoid and antinuclear factors. However, they can occur in mild disease and in anarthritic rheumatoid disease.[1] A variant called *rheumatoid nodulosis* has been described[2] in which nodules occur in palindromic rheumatism with little signs of synovitis. Nodules may precede joint changes by many years. The size is variable but may be up to several centimeters in diameter. They are subcutaneous or dermal and occur particularly at sites of repeated minor trauma. Common sites include the ulnar border of the forearms, and to a lesser extent the back of the hands, knees, heels, scapulae, sacrum, buttocks, and ears. They may be missed over the sacrum in immobile patients. Ulceration occurs with trauma, and secondary infection results in staphylococcal septicemia and septic arthritis. The underlying bone may be eroded.[3] Variants include violaceous papules, sometimes with centripetal scaling.

Histology of a rheumatoid nodule shows abundant fibrous tissue with areas of fibrinoid necrosis surrounded by a palisade of

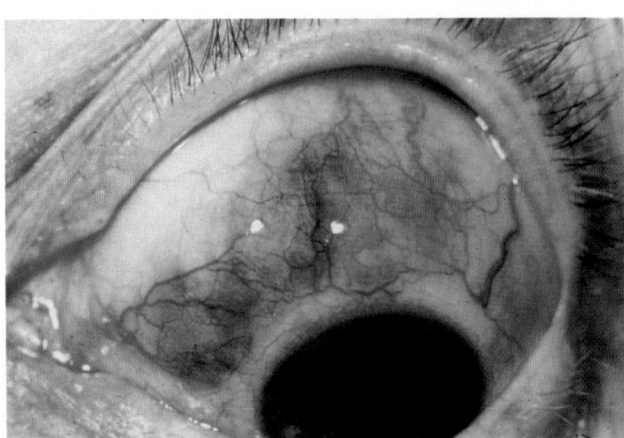

FIGURE 178-1 Scleromalacia in rheumatoid arthritis.

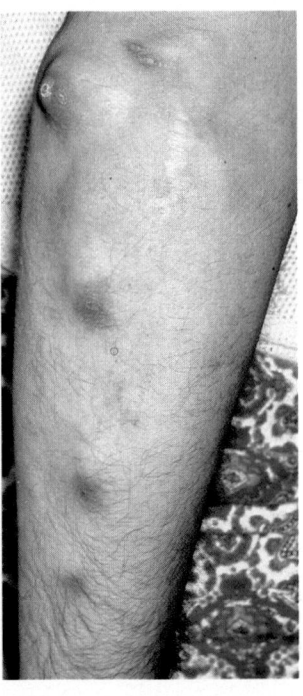

FIGURE 178-2 Rheumatoid nodules on the back of the forearm.

fibroblasts and histiocytes. Outside this is a band of lymphocytes and plasma cells. Reticulum fibers as seen in young granulation tissue, nuclear debris, and amorphous material occur in the necrotic areas. The histology of granuloma annulare shows similar changes. The appearances are different from those of the nodules of rheumatic fever, in which there is more fibrinoid material and edema of the collagen. Fibrosis is minimal or absent, and cellular infiltration with lymphocytes, histiocytes, and fibroblasts is not a prominent feature. Nodules persist and, apart from superficial ulceration, seldom cause trouble. Treatment is ineffective and removal is rarely required.

Linear Subcutaneous Bands

Vertical, firm, nontender, elongated subcutaneous bands 3.5 mm in width may occur rarely on the trunk and thighs of patients with rheumatoid arthritis and nodules.[4] They occur particularly in the anterior and posterior folds of the axilla, are more visible when the arms are raised, and may extend downwards as far as the iliac crest. Histology shows features similar to rheumatoid nodules.

Vascular Lesions

Erythema of the peripheral margins of the palms is common and is similar to that seen in liver disease, systemic lupus erythematosus, and pregnancy. Raynaud's phenomenon is uncommon.[5]

Patients with vasculitis usually have high titers of rheumatoid and antinuclear factors.[6] Subcutaneous nodules, pulmonary involvement, and episcleritis are frequent. Vasculitis occurs more frequently in females than males. Characteristic digital lesions (Fig. 178-3) around the nails and in the pulp of the fingers occurred in 34 percent of males and 18 percent of females in one series.[7] Lesions result from small infarcts and last only a few days. They are usually painless and may be missed unless the area is examined with a magnifying glass in a good light. Initially red, they fade to a brown stain, sometimes with scaling, and usually disappear completely, although scarring and grooving of the nail may occur. The digital lesions resemble those due to trauma, such as encountered by tailors using needles and woodworkers hitting their fingers with hammers.[7] Small nodules also occur in the pulps of the fingers. Vasculitis, however, may be more dramatic, with gangrene of the fingers and toes that may extend to involve most of the hand or foot. Purpuric and necrotic areas can occur elsewhere on the skin. They are usually painless and do not result from trauma. Lesions

vary from petechiae to necrotic areas with scabbing several centimeters in diameter. They heal slowly and may result in scarring. Bullae of fingers and toes can spread widely. Livedo reticularis, pyoderma gangrenosum, and delayed pressure urticaria are other cutaneous manifestations.

Vasculitis in rheumatoid disease is frequently widespread throughout the body. In the gastrointestinal tract[8] it leads to abdominal pain, multiple ischemic ulcerations, gangrene of the bowel, intraperitoneal hemorrhages, and splenic infarction. Occlusion of the vasa nervosum gives rise to sensory and motor neuropathy.[9] Arteritis may also involve the heart and lungs, but the kidneys are usually spared.

Leg Ulcers

Although it might be expected that ulceration of the legs in rheumatoid arthritis[10] is commonly associated with arteritis, this has not been our experience. Gravitational factors are much more frequent and are exaggerated by immobility, dependency, and difficulty in walking. This is another reason for keeping such patients mobile. Gravitational ulcers resemble those seen in patients without rheumatoid arthritis and usually occur in shiny, brawny, hairless skin. Arteritic ulcers are most frequent in females with rheumatoid nodules and positive tests for rheumatoid and antinuclear factors. Although rheumatoid arthritis can occur with systemic lupus erythematosus, diagnosis of the latter should not depend on the presence of antinuclear factor alone, as this can occur in rheumatoid disease. Arteritic ulcers are usually deep, punched out, and very slow to heal. They sometimes start as breaking-down purpura or subcutaneous nodules. The surrounding skin is usually of normal color and not fibrosed.

Local treatment is as for gravitational ulceration with supporting bandages, but arteritic ulcers may require systemic steroids. There is no evidence that steroids induce or enhance ulceration. Many patients with arteritic ulceration have never had steroids. Dapsone, 100 mg daily, alone or with colchicine, has healed arteritic leg ulceration in some patients.[11]

Transparent Skin and Osteoporosis

Transparent skin is seen frequently in patients with rheumatoid arthritis and is closely associated with osteoporosis.[12] It is not related to corticosteroid therapy. Transparent skin is best seen on the back of the hands, usually of women over 60 years of age. The degree increases with age. The skin is loose and inelastic, the surface is smooth, and pigment is lacking. The details of even small veins can be seen easily. There is an increased tendency to so-called senile purpura. Histology shows no characteristic features.

Pseudoscleroderma and Cold Flexed Fingers

Sclerotic changes resembling those seen in systemic sclerosis may occur in the hands of patients with rheumatoid arthritis. Joint pain, tenderness, and swelling also occur in systemic sclerosis, and thus the distinction between the two diseases may not be easy in the absence of other manifestations. Moreover, rheumatoid arthritis and systemic sclerosis can occur in the same patient.[13]

Patients whose hands can be described by the term *cold flexed fingers*[14] have hands that are cool and are held in semiflexion but

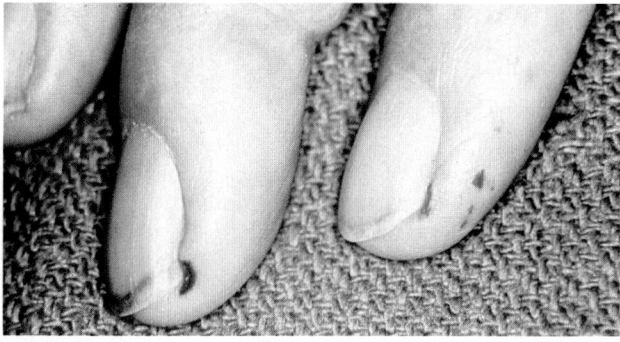

FIGURE 178-3 Characteristic small digital infarcts in rheumatoid arthritis.

are without other features at presentation. These patients can eventually progress to having either rheumatoid arthritis or systemic sclerosis.

Pustular Panniculitis

Multiple red subcutaneous nodules that ulcerate and discharge purulent material have been described.[15] Histologic examination shows fat necrosis and neutrophilic dust in the subcutaneous tissue with surrounding fibrosis. This type of panniculitis may respond to dapsone and tetracycline.

Rheumatoid Neutrophilic Dermatitis

This rare entity[16] occurs in patients with severe rheumatoid arthritis as symmetric erythematous papules or nodules up to 8 mm diameter and as plaques on the extensor aspects of the joints, particularly of the hands and arms. Crusting is frequent. Individual lesions may last from 1 to 3 weeks and resolve without scarring or ulceration, whereas others may ulcerate. Histologically, there is a dense neutrophilic infiltrate throughout the entire dermis. Sometimes there are small abscesses in the dermal papillae. Vasculitis is absent, although vascular dilatation may be seen. The differential diagnosis includes erythema elevatum diutinum in which there is a leukocytoclastic vasculitis, rheumatoid nodules, Sweet's syndrome, pyoderma gangrenosum, and the intestinal bypass arthritis-dermatitis syndrome.

Other Cutaneous Features

A rash like that of Still's disease (see below) occurred in 7 of 500 adults with rheumatoid arthritis in one series.[17] Steroid-induced skin manifestations are common in patients with rheumatoid arthritis. Many have been treated with oral corticosteroids for long periods and have experienced the usual side effects, including the purple discoloration similar to so-called senile purpura on the forearms and elsewhere. This discoloration is due to extravasation of blood from vessels that are unsupported as a result of decreased dermal collagen. The dose of steroids should be kept as low as possible. It has been claimed[18] that the addition of azathioprine may allow a reduction of the steroid dose by up to one-third. Rashes due to therapy with other drugs such as penicillamine, gold, and chloroquine are also encountered.

Pressure sores may be a problem. They usually result from immobility in a bed or chair, but bed sores can start as breaking-down rheumatoid nodules. A vivid yellow color of the skin has been reported[19] and is due to inspissated sweat. It is removed by vigorous washing.

Felty's Syndrome

Felty's syndrome is a combination of rheumatoid arthritis, splenomegaly, and leukopenia. There is also a normocytic normochromic anemia, thrombocytopenia, lymphadenopathy, and loss of weight. The total white count is usually less than 2500/μL with fluctuating neutropenia. Patients have severe erosive arthritis with positive tests for rheumatoid and antinuclear factors. The cutaneous features include recurrent infections, pigmentation, and ulceration of the

skin. Ulceration of the perianal area may resemble that in Crohn's disease and may be difficult to heal.

The pathogenesis is not clear. Neutropenia is associated with splenomegaly and may be due to depression of granulopoiesis or destruction of the white cells. Some patients improve after splenectomy.

Association of Rheumatoid Arthritis with Other Diseases

Both classic rheumatoid arthritis and rheumatoid-like changes in the hands can occur with other connective tissue diseases, such as systemic lupus erythematosus, Sjögren's syndrome, systemic sclerosis, and dermatomyositis. Rheumatoid arthritis has also been reported to occur with scleredema of Buschke.[20] Rheumatoid arthritis may be distinguished from systemic lupus erythematosus by virtue of the fact that immunoglobulin and complement are not found at the dermal-epidermal junction in patients with rheumatoid arthritis,[21] even in those with a high level of antinuclear factor.

Many other diseases have been reported in patients with rheumatoid arthritis,[22] but some of these associations may be coincidental. They include pemphigus vulgaris and foliaceus, pemphigoid, dermatitis herpetiformis, acquired epidermolysis bullosa, subcorneal pustular dermatosis, and the yellow nail syndrome.

Still's Disease (Juvenile Chronic Arthritis)

Still's disease affects children up to the age of 16 years. By definition it lasts more than 3 months and involves four or more joints. In 10 percent of those affected, the disease resembles adult rheumatoid arthritis, and these patients have a poor prognosis. The remaining 90 percent fall into three main subtypes. In the first or *systemic type*, fever, worse in the afternoon, is usually associated with a macular rash, lymphadenopathy, splenomegaly, hepatosplenomegaly, pleurisy, and pericarditis. The arthritis is relatively mild. The second or *polyarticular type* affects young girls, and any joint may be involved. Systemic features are minimal. In the third or *pauciarticular type*, the male/female sex ratio is equal. The arthritis affects less than five joints, usually ankles, knees, or elbows. Patients with onset before 8 years are usually girls, and chronic iridocyclitis is a prominent feature. Rheumatoid factor is usually absent, but tests for antinuclear factor are positive. The late-onset patients with pauciarticular arthritis are usually boys, and the large joints of their lower limbs and spine are typically affected. The disease is associated with HLA-B27 and is the equivalent of juvenile ankylosing spondylitis.

The Rash of Still's Disease

Surprisingly, the rash of Still's disease[17] was not recognized by Still in his original description of the disease.[23] The rash occurs in about 25 percent of patients, particularly in boys. The incidence decreases with age. The rash (Fig. 178-4) consists of small, nonitching, salmon-pink, erythematous macules or papules, 3 mm or less in diameter, on the trunk, limbs, and face. The margin is irregular, and there may be central and surrounding pallor. The lesions are smaller than the erythema marginatum of rheumatic fever and do spread. The rash tends to occur at midday and in the

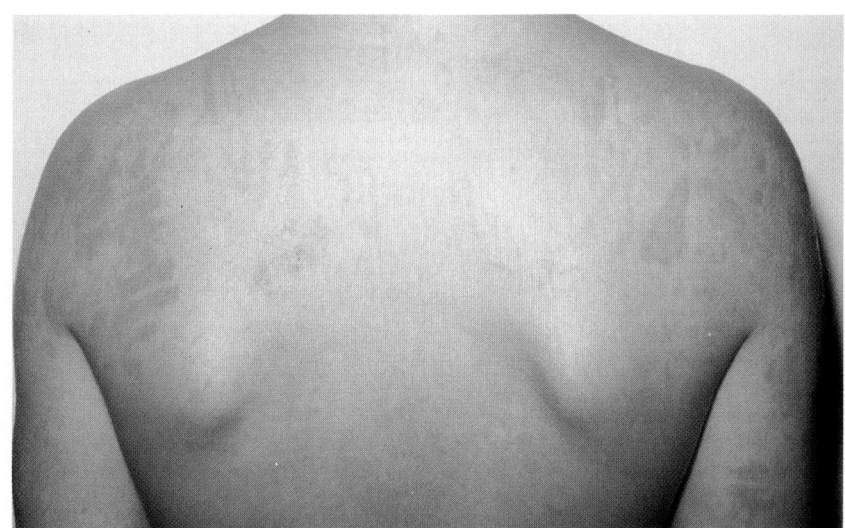

FIGURE 178-4 Transitory rash of Still's disease.

evening, associated with increased temperature of the environment and with fever. It is usually accompanied by splenomegaly, lymphadenopathy, and a raised erythrocyte sedimentation rate. The rash and fever accompany or follow arthritis but occasionally may precede other manifestations by up to 9 years. The duration of the rash is variable, and it may occur intermittently over many years. It has no relation to prognosis.[24] The rash, fever, and arthritis may continue for years[25]; there may be residual ankylosis in the carpus, tarsus, and neck as well as distal interphalangeal joint involvement and occasional destructive lesions.

Subcutaneous Nodules

Occasionally nodules occur in Still's disease. Histologically they resemble the nodules of rheumatic fever rather than those of rheumatoid arthritis.[26]

Acute Rheumatism (Rheumatic Fever)

Acute rheumatism occurs predominantly in childhood. The triad consists of fever, arthritis, and carditis. The condition is attributed to an abnormal immune response to infection with group A beta-hemolytic streptococci. There has been a marked decline in rheumatic fever in the western world during this century, but the disease is still important in developing countries. The incidence is less than 5 per 100,000 in the west compared with 100 to 1000 per 100,000 in developing countries, where carditis is severe and may affect up to 50 percent of patients. The condition occurs between the ages of 6 and 15 and is rare under 4 years of age.

There is usually a history of a sore throat 1 to 3 weeks before the onset, which may be sudden or gradual. Arthritis moves from joint to joint. Carditis can occur without other factors. Chorea is now rare (less than 0.5 percent). The average duration of the disease is 10 to 15 weeks. There is no specific diagnostic test. Treatment consists of rest, aspirin for the pain, and prednisone if carditis is aggressive. However, the overall value of prednisone is disputed. Early treatment of sore throats is the best preventive measure; once the disease has developed, patients should have prophylactic penicillin for at least 10 years and longer if there is established heart disease.

Erythema Marginatum

This finding is specific for rheumatic fever, occurring in about 25 percent of patients.[27] Characteristically it consists of rapidly spreading erythematous rings (Fig. 178-5). The margins are raised (erythema marginatum) or flat (erythema annulare or circinatum). Lesions start as macular areas of erythema that spread at the rate of 2 to 10 mm in 12 h, leaving a pale or slightly pigmented inactive center. They are usually circular but can be polycyclic or irregular. They occur on the trunk, especially in the axillae, and on the limbs. Occasionally the back of the hands and the face may be involved. Itching, urticaria, and purpura occur infrequently. Livedo reticularis has been reported.[28] The rash must be distinguished from the rash of Still's disease, which does not spread, familial annular erythema, neonatal lupus erythematosus, urticaria (sometimes penicillin-induced), erythema multiforme, and the rash of infectious mononucleosis. The rash usually precedes joint involvement, but the rash and carditis can occur without arthritis.

Histologically, there is a perivascular cellular infiltrate with many necrotic polymorphonuclear leukocytes similar to the appearances of Henoch-Schönlein purpura, although extravasated erythrocytes are common in the latter. There may be collections of neutrophils in the dermal papillae. Direct immunofluorescence for immunoglobulins and complement is negative. Biopsy may be helpful in the early stages before the development of arthritis and carditis.[29] The rash may last only a few hours but can recur over weeks or months. It is unaffected by treatment.

Erythema Papulatum

Very rarely, papules a few millimeters in diameter occur on the flexor aspects of the elbows and knees and last for 6 to 8 days.[30] They may resemble the lesions of granuloma annulare. Histologically, there is parakeratosis, edema of the basal layer with a focal perivascular lymphocytic infiltrate quite distinct from that seen in erythema marginatum.

Subcutaneous Nodules

Multiple subcutaneous nodules 2 to 5 mm in diameter occur in 34 percent of patients, mainly over bony prominences such as the

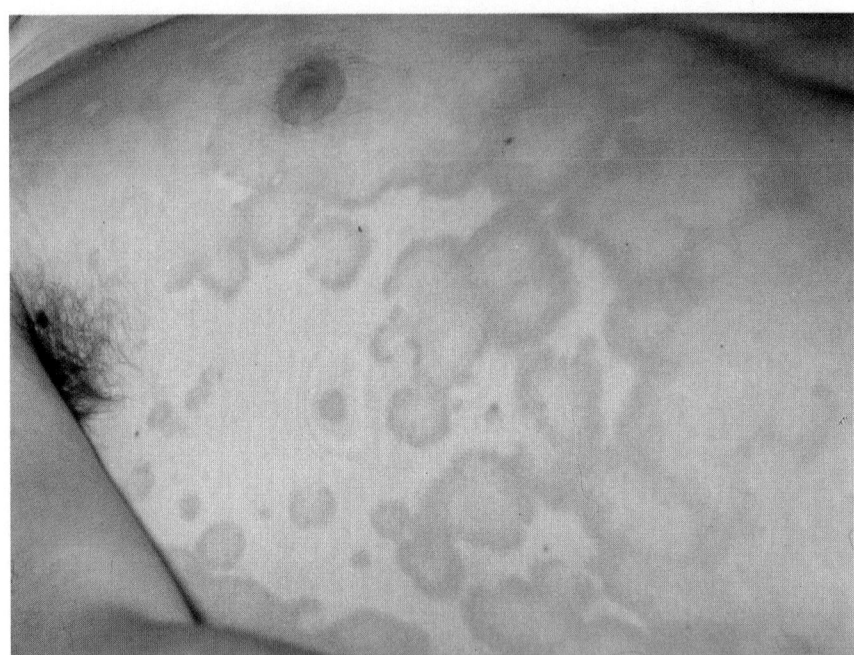

FIGURE 178-5 Erythema marginatum in rheumatic fever.

knuckles, olecranon processes, humoral epicondyles, and occiput.[31] They are sometimes better seen on the feet. They may develop later in the disease when the erythrocyte sedimentation rate has returned to normal. Carditis is frequent.

Histologically there is a lattice-like formation of fibrinoid separating thick-walled vessels. Lymphocytes are infrequent, and palisading by fibroblasts is less prominent than in rheumatoid arthritis.

Other Disorders with Skin Manifestations and Arthritis

Many viral infections,[32] including adenovirus and cocksackie virus, occur with a rash, lymphadenopathy, and arthritis. Arthritis also occurs with rubella,[33] either naturally acquired or after vaccination. Arthritis is also a feature of psoriasis (Chap. 39) and Lyme disease (Chap. 193).

Familial diseases with rash and arthritis include familial cold urticaria,[34] Muckle-Wells syndrome,[35] hereditary inflammatory vasculitis with nodules,[36] erythrokeratoderma with deafness,[37] recurrent rash with episcleritis and rheumatism,[38] and familial arthropathy with rash, uveitis, and mental retardation.[39]

References

1. Bagraturi L: Prognosis in the anarthritic rheumatoid syndrome. *Br Med J* **1**:513, 1963
2. Ginsberg MH et al: Rheumatoid nodulosis: An unusual variant of rheumatoid disease. *Arthritis Rheum* **18**:49, 1975
3. Dorfman HD et al: Bone erosion in relation to subcutaneous rheumatoid nodules. *Arthritis Rheum* **13**:69, 1970
4. Dykman CJ et al: Linear subcutaneous bands in rheumatoid arthritis. *Ann Intern Med* **63**:134, 1965
5. Carroll GJ et al: The prevalence of Raynaud's syndrome in rheumatoid arthritis. *Ann Rheum Dis* **40**:567, 1981
6. Bywaters EGL, Scott JT: The natural history of vascular lesions in rheumatoid arthritis. *J Chronic Dis* **16**:905, 1963
7. Goulding JR et al: Arteritis of rheumatoid arthritis. *Br J Dermatol* **77**:207, 1965
8. Lindsay MK et al: Acute abdomen in rheumatoid arthritis due to necrotizing arteritis. *Br Med J* **2**:592, 1973
9. Pallis CA, Scott JT: Peripheral neuropathy in rheumatoid arthritis. *Br Med J* **1**:1141, 1965
10. Wilkinson M, Kirk J: Leg ulcers complicating rheumatoid arthritis. *Scot Med J* **10**:175, 1965
11. Bernard P et al: Dapsone and rheumatoid vasculitis leg ulcerations. *J Am Acad Dermatol* **18**:140, 1988
12. McConkey B, Fraser GM: Transparent skin and osteoporosis. *Ann Rheum Dis* **24**:219, 1965
13. Baron M et al: The coexistence of rheumatoid arthritis and scleroderma. *J Rheumatol* **9**:947, 1982
14. Rowell NR: Cold flexed fingers, in *Textbook of Dermatology*, 4th ed, edited by A Rook et al. Oxford, Blackwell, 1986, p 1368
15. Newton J, Wojnarowska FT: Pustular panniculitis in rheumatoid arthritis. *Br J Dermatol* **119**:97, 1988
16. Sanchez JL, Cruz A: Rheumatoid neutrophilic dermatitis. *J Am Acad Dermatol* **22**:922, 1990
17. Isdale IC, Bywaters EGL: The rash of rheumatoid arthritis and Still's disease. *Q J Med* **25**:377, 1956
18. Mason M et al: Azathioprine in rheumatoid arthritis: *Br Med J* **1**:420, 1969
19. Spender JK: On some of the rarer complications of rheumatoid arthritis. *Br Med J* **1**:905, 1892
20. Miyagawa S et al: Scleredema of Buschke associated with rheumatoid arthritis and Sjögren's syndrome. *Br J Dermatol* **121**:517, 1989
21. Tuffanelli DL: Cutaneous immunopathology: Recent observations. *J Invest Dermatol* **65**:153, 1975
22. Jorizzo JL, Daniels JC: Dermatologic conditions reported in patients with rheumatoid arthritis. *J Am Acad Dermatol* **8**:439, 1983
23. Still GF: On a form of chronic joint disease in children. *Med-Chir Tr (London)* **80**:47, 1897
24. Calabro JJ, Marchesano JM: Juvenile rheumatoid arthritis. *N Engl J*

Med 277:696, 1967

25. Elkon K et al: Adult-onset Still's disease: Twenty year follow-up and further studies of patients with active disease. *Q J Med* 25:377, 1956
26. Bywaters EGL et al: Subcutaneous nodules of Still's disease. *Ann Rheum Dis* 17:278, 1958
27. Hill AGS: Skin manifestations in rheumatic disorders. *Trans St John's Hosp Dermatol Soc* 50:105, 1965
28. Haber H: Zur Atiologie der livedo racemosa. *Arch Dermatol Syphilol* 163:1, 1931
29. Troyer C: Erythema marginatum in rheumatic fever: Early diagnosis by skin biopsy. *J Am Acad Dermatol* 8:724, 1983
30. Gadrat J: Erythema papulaux rhumatismal: Lesions dermiques du type Aschoff-Klinge. *Bull Soc Fr Dermatol Syphiligr* 44:1782, 1937
31. Bywaters EGL, Thomas GT: Bed rest, salicylates and steroid in rheumatic fever. *Br Med J* 1:1628, 1961
32. Malawista SE, Steere AC: Viral arthritis, in *Textbook of Rheumatol-ogy*, edited by WN Kelley et al. Philadelphia, Saunders, 1981, p 1586
33. Chambers RJ, Bywaters EGL: Rubella synovitis. *Ann Rheum Dis* 22:263, 1963
34. Kile RL, Rusk HA: Case of cold urticaria with an unusual family history. *JAMA* 114:1067, 1940
35. Muckle TJ, Wells M: Urticaria, deafness, amyloidosis: A new heredo-familial syndrome. *Q J Med* 31:235, 1962
36. Reed WB et al: Hereditary inflammatory vasculitis with persistent nodules. *Br J Dermatol* 87:299, 1972
37. Beare JM et al: Atypical erythrokeratoderma with deafness, physical retardation and peripheral neuropathy. *Br J Dermatol* 87:309, 1972
38. Jones BR, Champion RH: Still's disease: Rash in mother and daughter. *Br J Dermatol* 88:35, 1975
39. Ansell BM et al: Familial arthropathy with rash, uveitis and mental retardation. *Proc R Soc Med* 68:584, 1975

CHAPTER 179

Karl Holubar

Multicentric Reticulohistiocytosis

Multicentric reticulohistiocytosis (MR) is a systemic granulomatous disease of unknown cause. The disease is rare and is characterized by a distinct histopathology. Skin, mucosa, synovia, bone, and internal organs may be involved. Cutaneous nodules and destructive arthritis are the most prominent clinical features. A paraneoplastic character of MR is discussed.

Historical Aspects

In 1952, Caro and Senear[1] first studied sections of a patient with these features and called the syndrome *reticulohistiocytic granuloma*, a term reemphasized by Ackerman in 1978.[2] Goltz and Laymon in 1954 created the term *multicentric reticulohistiocytosis*,[3] which most authors now use,[4-7] because of the multifocal origin and the systemic nature of the process. At least a dozen synonyms appear in the literature,[4-7] including lipoid dermatoarthritis, giant cell (reticulo)histiocytosis, (giant cell) reticulohistiocytoma, and nondiabetic cutaneous xanthomatosis. By the early 1950s the entity of MR was established (see reference 5 for additional references).

Epidemiology

Two comprehensive reviews are available,[5,6] and about 100 cases have been reported, but many others may have gone undiagnosed. There appears to be no geographic area of prevalence. Caucasians predominate, but this finding may merely reflect the higher number of reports from North America and Europe; patients of African, South American, Japanese, and American-Indian ancestry have also been reported.[5,6,8] In two studies a greater number of women were found to be affected[5,9]; in a third study an equal distribution was found between the sexes.[6] The mean age of onset was 43 years.[5] After an average of 8 years the disease burns out and becomes inactive. Recently, adolescent patients have also been identified.

Etiology and Pathogenesis

The etiology of MR remains obscure, and its pathogenesis can only be speculated upon.[5,6] The hallmark of the disease is a granulomatous, proliferative process of histiocytes, some of which are multinucleated and laden with lipids. The stimulus is not known and no specific metabolic defect has been found; there is no evidence of an infective agent and there are no convincing data on a compromise of the immune status of the host. There is little if any evidence[10] to permit the categorization of MR with disorders of deranged lipid metabolism.

Clinical Manifestations

Skin and joint symptoms dominate the clinical picture. Almost two-thirds of patients note arthritis first; one-fifth note skin nodules first; and in another fifth skin and joint changes appear simultaneously. About half of the patients develop mucous membrane manifestations.[5]

Skin Changes

The face (particularly the nose and paranasal areas), hands (particularly the nail folds, Fig. 179-1), ears, forearms, scalp (especially behind the ears), neck, and trunk are involved in decreasing order of frequency. The hemispherical, nontender nodular lesions have a reddish brown hue; they vary in size from a few millimeters to

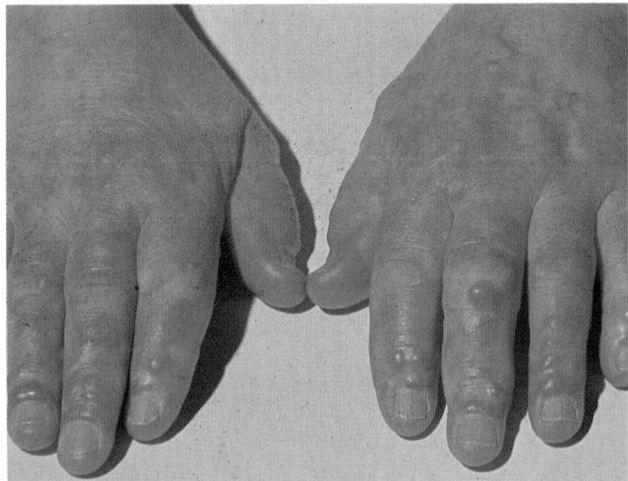

FIGURE 179-1 Hands of a patient with active skin lesions of multicentric reticulohistiocytosis. Note periungual array of some of the nodules. (*From Barrow and Holubar,[5] with permission of Hautarzt.*)

conglomerate nodules measuring several centimeters. Ulceration does not normally occur. Erythema may precede the formation of nodules. Pruritus may be a prominent symptom.

Articular Changes

There is symmetric involvement of the interphalangeal joints, knees, shoulders, wrists, hips, ankles, feet, elbows, and vertebral joints, in decreasing order of frequency. The arthritis is destructive (arthritis mutilans); bone and cartilage are destroyed and severe deformation ensues. The disease progresses rapidly in the beginning, tapers, and finally burns out. There is a marked discrepancy between the severity of the radiographic findings and the underlying bone destruction, and the relatively mild clinical symptoms. In far-advanced cases the fingers are considerably shortened but can be pulled out to their full length, leading to such designations as *la main en lorgnette*, opera-glass hand, telescope fingers, and concertina-hand. There is no periostal reaction or osteoporosis.

Mucosal Changes

Roughly half the patients have mucosal lesions[5]; the lips, buccal mucosa, tongue,[11] gingiva, nasal septum, and larynx[8,12] are involved. Physically, the nodules mimic those in the skin (Fig. 179-2).

Other Clinical Manifestations

These include xanthelasmata; lesions along tendon sheaths; lesions in the myocardium and the lungs[13]; adenopathy; pathologic fractures; hypertension; and hyperextensible joints. In a number of cases a definitive diagnosis of MR could not be substantiated; and the association of unusual findings may have been fortuitous, as in one patient with carpal tunnel syndrome, Dupuytren's contracture, and pleural effusion[7]; two patients with cardiopulmonary complications[13,14]; one patient with splenomegaly and pancytopenia[15]; one

patient with a gamma heavy-chain paraprotein[16]; and one patient with involvement of the salivary glands and pericardial effusion.[17] Gold et al.[18] alluded to a possible relationship between MR and tuberculosis. Chevrant-Breton[6] in her review quoted reports on ocular, neurologic, and (terminal) hematologic changes.

Laboratory Findings

A recent report[19] cites an association of MR with type IV hyperlipidemia; another[10] considers MR "another lipid disorder with normolipidemic xanthomatosis." These are chance findings. Otherwise, only nonspecific laboratory findings have become known in individual cases: anemia, elevated sedimentation rate, leukocytosis, eosinophilia, hypo- and hypercholesterolemia, hypergammaglobulinemia, and the presence of cold agglutinins and cryoglobulins.

Pathology

Skin and Mucous Membranes

The histopathology of skin lesions is fairly uniform.[5,6,20–24] The nodules are nonencapsulated, moderately well circumscribed, and occupy the entire dermis or parts of it. Frequently there is a narrow zone of noninfiltrated connective tissue between the infiltrates and the slightly atrophic epidermis. Lesions consist of histiocytic cells, irregular in size and shape (Fig. 179-3a). Many have transformed into multinucleated giant cells, generally up to 250 μm in diameter, but occasionally larger (Fig. 179-3b). They contain up to 20 or more aggregated nuclei with a distinct nuclear membrane and prominent nucleoli. The cytoplasm is slightly eosinophilic, has a granular appearance ("ground-glass cytoplasm"), and may be foamy or show tiny vacuoles. There are no Tuton type giant cells.

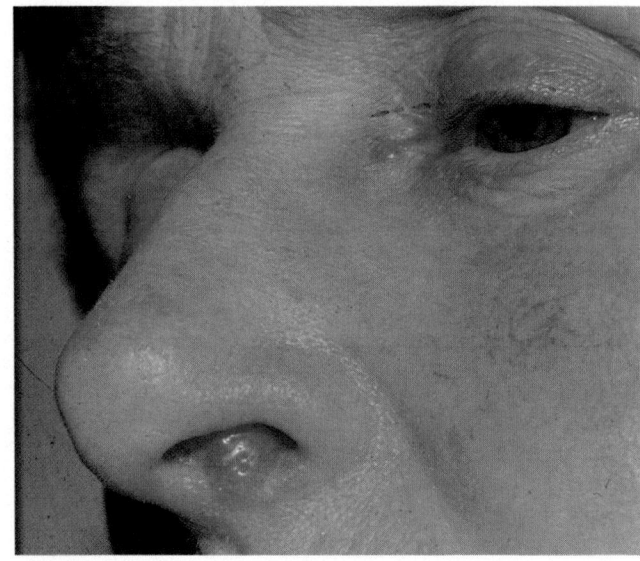

FIGURE 179-2 Multicentric reticulohistiocytosis. Mucocutaneous nodular infiltrate on nasal mucosa and adjoining skin.

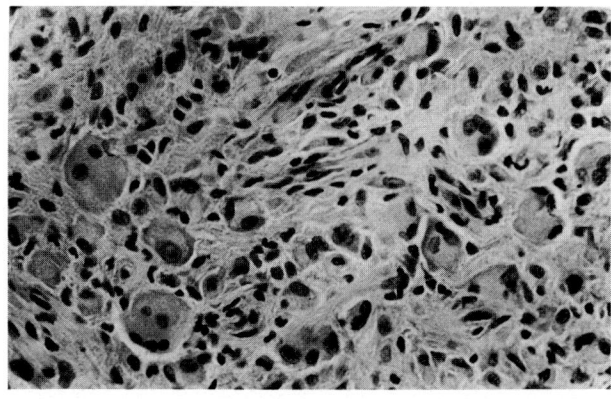

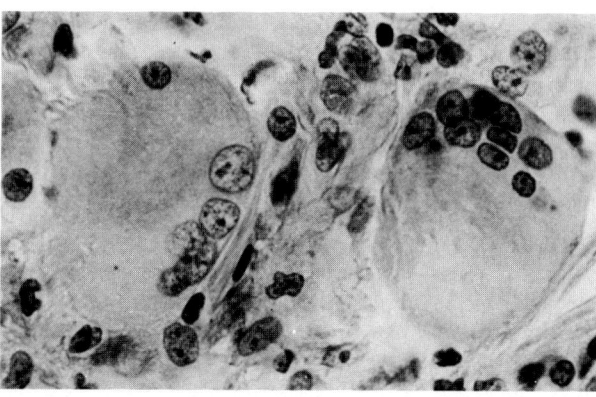

a

b

FIGURE 179-3 Microphotograph of a lesion of the patient shown in Fig. 179-1. Note histiocytic infiltrate *(a)* and multinucleated giant cells with aggregated nuclei and "ground glass" cytoplasm *(b)*. ×100 *(a)*, ×250 *(b)*. *(From Holubar and Mach,[4] with permission of Hautarzt.)*

MR nodules contain lymphocytes, which are more numerous in early lesions, and plasma cells, eosinophils, mast cells, and occasionally, extravasated erythrocytes. With increasing age of the lesions, lymphocytes and giant cells decrease in number, fibroblasts appear, and fibrosis ensues. Lesions are well vascularized and capillaries show endothelial hypertrophy. In places, histiocytes and giant cells show a perivascular arrangement. Elastic fibers are fragmented, clumped, and thickened, particularly in early lesions.

Histochemical Investigations

The cytoplasm of histiocytes and giant cells is PAS-positive, and hyaluronidase- and diastase-resistant, suggesting the presence of glycoproteins; it contains phospholipids, neutral fats, and iron.[5] Biochemical studies have failed to reveal an isolated enzyme defect responsible for lipid accumulation.[5]

Electron Microscopy

There are no Langerhans cell granules in the histiocytic cells. Both histiocytes and giant cells show lobulated nuclei with indented contours and margination of nuclear chromatin, an enlarged Golgi apparatus, and hyperplastic endoplasmic reticulum with dilated cysternae. Lipid-laden vacuoles are present and numerous small, electron-dense, ovoid or rod-shaped cytoplasmic granules, up to 250 nm in size, have been described. These are positive for acid phosphatase, as are autophagic vacuoles.[20,22] Complex interdigitation of membranes of adjacent histiocytic cells has been described as a characteristic feature. In addition, collagen phagocytosis has been observed.[25] The histiocytes of MR have been characterized by their iron uptake, positivity of acid phosphatase, unspecific esterase, and lysozyme.[5,6,20,22,25,26]

The histopathology of synovial lesions is identical to that of skin lesions; the number of giant cells and histochemical reactions are variable.

Lesions in Other Tissues

The morphology and localization of cutaneous nodules, the typical articular symptoms, and radiographic findings (symmetric involve-

ment of distal interphalangeal joints) are highly suggestive of MR. Histopathologic examination of a nodule permits the diagnosis. Various disorders have to be differentiated from MR[5,6]: rheumatoid arthritis, the various types of xanthomas, Farber's disseminated lipogranulomatosis, lepromatous leprosy, lipoid proteinosis, sarcoidosis, histiocytosis X, juvenile and adult xanthogranuloma, solitary reticulohistiocytoma, generalized eruptive histiocytoma, congenital reticulohistiocytoma of Hashimoto and Pritzker,[27] and Zayid and Farraj's familial histiocytic dermatoarthritis.[28] MR is not familial or congenital. Many of these diagnoses will be ruled out by the absence of one of the typical features of MR, such as acral or facial nodules, mutilating arthritis, characteristic histopathology, and the history of the patient.

Associated Conditions

Concomitant diseases have been mentioned[5]: thyroid disorders; tuberculosis; diabetes; hemoblastoses; cancer of the colon, breast, bronchus, cervix, ovary, and stomach; and mesothelioma of the pleura.[29] An association with sarcoma and lymphoma has also been reported. The tumors may progress and MR may remit; in contrast, MR may progress despite removal of the tumor. Many investigators therefore remain skeptical with regard to the alleged paraneoplastic nature of MR.[6] Recently, Green et al.[30] reported on OKT3 and OKT4 T-cell markers in histiocytes of MR; Amor et al.[12] speculated on histiocyte pathology in MR that might lead to a compromise of the immune status of the host and favor development of neoplasms. A careful tumor search is warranted in MR.

Treatment

Gianotti and Caputo[31] state that, "Treatment is usually not helpful." Corticosteroids (also as pulse therapy[32]), ACTH, antimalarials, salicylates, indomethacin, pyrazolone, clofibrate, and various antimitotic compounds such as penicillamine[11,33] and topical nitrogen mustard[34] have been used, but no controlled studies have been performed. Antimitotic agents such as nitrogen mustard, chlorambucil, vinca alkaloids, and cyclophosphamide appear to be a rational choice for therapy, but the possibility that MR is a paraneoplastic condition must be kept in mind. Surgical measures have also been used.[33]

Course and Prognosis

Skin nodules and arthritis do not necessarily run parallel. Articular changes may wax and wane and finally evolve into mutilating arthritis, whereas skin nodules may not appear at all or may erupt in successive crops with new infiltrates being superimposed on older, regressing ones. The course of MR is capricious, and prediction is difficult; about half the patients will eventually suffer from prominent destructive arthritis. As a rule, the disease burns out after 5 to 8 years,[5,6] leaving the patient with severe articular deformations and disfigurement of the hands, face, and scalp.

ACKNOWLEDGMENT

Supported in part by Schering AG Berlin, Germany.

References

1. Caro MR, Senear FE: Reticulohistiocytoma of the skin. *Arch Dermatol* **65**:701, 1952
2. Ackerman AB: *Histologic Diagnosis of Inflammatory Skin Diseases*. Philadelphia, Lea & Febiger, 1978, p 472
3. Goltz RW, Laymon CW: Multicentric reticulohistiocytosis. *Arch Dermatol* **69**:717, 1954
4. Holubar K, Mach K: Histiocytosis giganto-cellularis. *Hautarzt* **17**:440, 1966
5. Barrow MV, Holubar K: Multicentric reticulohistiocytosis. *Medicine (Baltimore)* **48**:287, 1969
6. Chevrant-Breton J: La réticulo-histiocytose multicentrique. Revue de la littérature récente (depuis 1969). *Ann Dermatol Venereol* **104**:745, 1977
7. Flam M et al: Multicentric reticulohistiocytosis. *Medicine (Baltimore)* **52**:841, 1972
8. Bechelli LM et al: Réticulo-histiocytose multicentrique. *Méd Hyg* **45**:856, 1987
9. Catteral MD, White JE: Multicentric reticulohistiocytosis and malignant disease. *Br J Dermatol* **98**:221, 1978
10. Kesäniemi YA et al: Multicentric reticulohistiocytosis, another lipid disorder with normolipidemic xanthomatosis? *Atherosclerosis* **68**:179, 1987
11. Zagala A et al: Réticulohistiocytose multicentrique. *Rev Rhum Mal Osteoartic* **54**:145, 1987
12. Amor B et al: Réticulo-histiocytose multicentrique. *Rev Rhum Mal Osteoartic* **54**:113, 1987
13. Fast A: Cardiopulmonary complications in multicentric reticulohistiocytosis. *Arch Dermatol* **112**:1139, 1976
14. Jessop S, Gordon W: Multicentric reticulohistiocytosis. *S Afr Med J* **49**:2191, 1975
15. Piett J-C et al: Réticulohistiocytome multicentrique avec splénomegalie et pancytopénie. *Ann Dermatol Venereol* **109**:801, 1982
16. Randall JRS et al: Atypical multicentric reticulohistiocytosis with paraproteinemia. *Arch Dermatol* **113**:1576, 1977
17. Furey N et al: Multicentric reticulohistiocytosis with salivary gland involvement and pericardial effusion. *J Am Acad Dermatol* **8**:679, 1983
18. Gold KD et al: Relationship between multicentric reticulohistiocytosis and tuberculosis. *JAMA* **237**:2213, 1977
19. Gharpuray MB et al: Multicentric reticulohistiocytosis. *Int J Dermatol Venerol Leprol* **55**:253, 1989
20. Coode PE et al: Multicentric reticulohistiocytosis: Report of two cases with ultrastructure, tissue culture and immunology studies. *Clin Exp Dermatol* **5**:281, 1980
21. Burgdorf WHC et al: Immunohistochemical identification of lysozyme in cutaneous lesions of alleged histiocytic nature. *Am J Clin Pathol* **75**:162, 1981
22. Tani M et al: Multicentric reticulohistiocytosis. *Arch Dermatol* **117**:495, 1981
23. Krmpotic L et al: Multizentrische Reticulohistiozytose. *Hautarzt* **31**:384, 1980
24. Ackerman AB et al: *Differential Diagnosis in Dermatopathology*. Philadelphia, Lea & Febiger, 1982, p 166
25. Caputo R et al: Collagen phagocytosis in multicentric reticulohistiocytosis. *J Invest Dermatol* **76**:342, 1981
26. Brégon C et al: Réticulohistiocytose multicentrique. *Rev Rhum Mal Osteoartic* **49**:59, 1982
27. Hashimoto K, Pritzker MS: Electron microscopic study of reticulohistiocytoma. *Arch Dermatol* **107**:263, 1973
28. Zayid I, Farraj S: Familial histiocytic dermatoarthritis. A new syndrome. *Am J Med* **54**:793, 1973
29. Coupe MO et al: Multicentric reticulohistiocytosis. *Br J Dermatol* **116**:245, 1987
30. Green CA et al: A case of multicentric reticulohistiocytosis: Uncommon clinical signs and a report of T-cell marker characteristics. *Br J Dermatol* **115**:623, 1986
31. Gianotti F, Caputo R: Histiocytic syndromes: A review. *J Am Acad Dermatol* **13**:383, 1985
32. Pandhi RK et al: Multicentric reticulohistiocytosis: Response to dexamethasone pulse therapy. *Arch Dermatol* **126**:251, 1990
33. Chevrant-Breton J, Mosser J: La réticulo-histiocytose multicentrique. *Méd Hyg* **43**:922, 1985
34. Brandt F et al: Topical nitrogen mustard therapy in multicentric reticulohistiocytosis. *J Am Acad Dermatol* **6**:260, 1982

CHAPTER 180

Robert Winchester

Reiter's Syndrome

Reiter's syndrome is a genetically determined and often protracted host response to specific antecedent enteric or genitourinary infection. In its characteristic form Reiter's syndrome is manifest as an abruptly appearing reactive asymmetric inflammation of the synovium and periarticular tissues accompanied by mucocutaneous, ophthalmic, and genitourinary involvement. The disorder is recognized by a set of clinical manifestations that are usually highly distinctive: acute oligoarthritis, primarily involving knee and ankle; enthesopathy, especially of the Achilles tendon; dactylitis; urethritis, cervicitis; mouth ulcers; conjunctivitis; balanitis; keratodermia blennorrhagicum; and onychodystrophy. Because there is no specific diagnostic test, diagnosis is sometimes complicated by forme fruste expression of the features of the illness or by a protracted evolution of the full illness in time. The nomenclature of Reiter's syndrome has been complicated by the artificial subdivision of the illness into complete and incomplete forms, designations that refer to the number of characteristic features that are present. Similarly, the term *reactive arthritis* should be thought of as essentially synonymous with Reiter's syndrome, although in its original usage reactive arthritis referred primarily to the development of arthritis induced by an enteric infection in the absence of mucocutaneous manifestations.

Reiter's syndrome is a member of a family of diseases termed the *seronegative spondyloarthropathies* that have in common varying degrees of arthrocutaneous and sometimes ocular manifestations (Table 180-1). They exhibit familial clustering, an inherited predisposition associated with the presence of certain major histocompatibility gene complex (MHC) class I alleles, such as HLA-B27, and are frequently precipitated by infection with certain microorganisms. In addition to psoriatic arthritis and Reiter's syndrome, which often have striking cutaneous involvement, the spondyloarthropathy group includes other entities that less frequently affect the skin. These spondyloarthropathies usually exhibit a tendency to involve periarticular structures, notably tendons and ligaments and their insertions, leading to tendinitis, dactylitis, and fasciitis. This process is designated *enthesopathy*. Nail involvement is often prominent. The mechanism of disease of the spondyloarthropathies appears to involve an as yet imprecisely characterized immune reaction that is clearly distinguished from the immune reaction of rheumatoid arthritis by the absence of immunoreactants

such as rheumatoid factor, and by the occurrence of these disorders with undiminished, and often enhanced, intensity in the setting of the frank immunosuppression of advanced HIV infection. Reiter's syndrome and pustular psoriasis with arthritis are increasingly being seen as related entities, a finding reemphasized by the arthrocutaneous syndromes of HIV infection.

Historical Aspects

The earliest mentions of the characteristic triad of arthritis, conjunctivitis, and urethritis following enteric or venereal infections were in 1776 by Stoll[1] and in 1818 by Brodie.[2] The distinction of this triad from the similar findings in gonococcal infection was difficult. Indeed, the term *keratodermia blennorrhagicum* was introduced at the end of the last century to refer to a supposed complication of gonococcal infection.[3] Reiter's syndrome was independently described by Reiter and by Feissinger and Leroy in the setting of the appalling sanitary conditions of the Balkan and Western fronts in World War I that led to epidemics of dysentery.[4] Again in a military context, the distinctive epidemiology of Reiter's syndrome was documented by the epidemiologic study of more than 150,000 Finns who developed shigellosis in 1944, of whom Reiter's syndrome was found in 344, and of 602 similarly infected sailors on the cruiser *Little Rock,* of whom Reiter's syndrome developed in 9. Complete and still unsurpassed clinical descriptions of Reiter's syndrome were the culmination of the period of the clinical definition of the illness.[5-7] More recently, at a clinical level, the understanding of the importance of ligament and tendon insertional inflammation, or enthesopathy, as a general manifestation of Reiter's syndrome was advanced by the work of Ball.[8]

The fundamental observation in 1973 by Brewerton et al.,[9] that susceptibility to Reiter's syndrome was strongly associated with the MHC class I specificity HLA-B27, ushered in the intense period of current interest in this disease and made Reiter's syndrome the first instance of a human immune response to a bacterial infection that was genetically regulated by allelic forms of MHC molecules. This observation pointed to the role of the human MHC as the site of immune response genes.[9] The role of HLA-B27 in

TABLE 180-1
The Spondyloarthropathies

Disease	HLA marker of susceptibility	Mucocutaneous involvement
Reiter's syndrome	HLA-B27, HLA-B7	Marked
Psoriatic arthritis	HLA-Cw6,-Bw13 etc., HLA-B27	Marked
Ankylosing spondylitis	HLA-B27	No
Enteric arthritis (ulcerative colitis, Crohn's disease)	HLA-B27 (axial disease)	Occasional
Behçet's syndrome?	HLA-B5	Marked
Whipple's disease?	HLA-B27	No

Reiter's syndrome was confirmed by returning to the survivors of the two epidemiologic studies and identifying this HLA specificity in approximately 80 percent of the 50 Finns and 5 sailors with Reiter's syndrome who were available for study; the expected low levels were found in the unaffected controls. Further understanding of the pathogenesis of Reiter's syndrome was provided by the recognition that adjuvant arthritis was an experimental model of the illness; accordingly, interest has focused on the role of heat-shock proteins as inciting elements of an untoward immune response that could underlie this disorder.[10] The recognition that Reiter's syndrome can occur in persons with advanced AIDS emphasized that the CD4 T-cell lineage was not involved in its pathogenesis. Attention was therefore directed to the role of the residual T cells of the CD8 lineage, introducing the notion of a CD8 T cell-driven disease process.[11,12]

Epidemiology

There are two epidemiologically distinct forms of Reiter's syndrome. One, the venereal or endemic form, follows a sexually transmitted route and is initiated by urethritis. The other is the epidemic or postdysenteric form that follows enteric infection. The analysis of Reiter's syndrome is made difficult by the fact that both urethritis and bowel inflammation can be components of the Reiter's syndrome reaction as well as antecedent inducing factors associated with a predisposing infection. The sex ratio is approximately equal in the postdysenteric form[13] but is greatly male-biased in the clinically equivalent form that follows urethritis, perhaps because nonspecific urethritis is much more common among men. Reiter's syndrome develops in from 1 to 3 percent of individuals with nonspecific urethritis.[14–16] Since epidemic enteric infections are relatively uncommon in the United States, Reiter's syndrome is largely a disease of males, and male predominance ranges from 85 to 88 percent.[17,18] The most frequent age of onset is in the early twenties,[17] but Reiter's syndrome has been recognized from childhood into the sixth decade.[17,19]

In general, Reiter's syndrome is more prevalent among Caucasians, perhaps because the frequency of HLA-B27 is relatively high among this ethnic group.[20] In addition, other incompletely defined genetic factors appear to be involved. HLA-B27 is the major determinant of susceptibility to both Reiter's syndrome and ankylosing spondylitis. However, in some families with HLA-B27 there is a strong concentration of Reiter's syndrome without ankylosing spondylitis, whereas in others the opposite is the case.[21,22] A similar divergence between Reiter's syndrome and ankylosing spondylitis is evident among certain groups of American Indians and Inupiat Eskimos in whom HLA-B27 is prevalent. For example, the Haida and Pima have a high frequency of ankylosing spondylitis, and the Navaho and Inupiat have a high frequency of Reiter's syndrome.[23–26]

As would be anticipated in a disorder with an infectious etiology, characteristic modes of transmission, a genetic susceptibility associated with an allele that has a complex distribution, and no specific diagnostic test to identify atypical clinical presentations, it is difficult to arrive at a reliable estimate of the prevalence or incidence of Reiter's syndrome. In the rural midwestern United States, the annual age-adjusted incidence[27] is reported to be 3.5 per 100,000. This figure varies greatly according to socioeconomic status, life-style, and various other factors. Reiter's syndrome is considered to be the most common cause of arthritis in young males.[28,29]

Etiology and Pathogenesis

Infectious Etiology

The postdysenteric form of Reiter's syndrome is initiated by infection with a specific set of gram-negative enteric organisms that are designated as *arthritogenic*. These include *Salmonella enteritidis, typhimurium,* and *heidelberg; Shigella flexneri,* types 1b and 2a, and *dysenteriae,* but not *sonnei; Yersini enterocolitica* and *pseudotuberculosis;* and *Campylobacter fetus* and *Clostridium difficile.*[30–37] Among the *Salmonella* and *Shigella* infections that result in Reiter's syndrome there is a very close connection between the ability to induce Reiter's syndrome and the presence of a distinctive plasmid.[38] In contrast, the infectious etiology of the endemic or venereal form of Reiter's syndrome has been more difficult to define. *Chlamydia trachomatis* has been implicated as a possible agent. This agent can be cultured from over one-third of men with nonspecific urethritis regardless of whether or not they develop Reiter's syndrome. *C. trachomatis* infection has been associated with a spectrum of spondyloarthropathy-like illnesses of which only a small proportion meet criteria for Reiter's syndrome.[39] Additional support for the specific role of *C. trachomatis* infection of the joint tissues has been brought forward with the identification of elementary bodies of the organism in the synovial membrane[40] and the finding of a high frequency of serologic reactivity to the 57-kDa heat-shock protein of *C. trachomatis* in both non-HIV- and HIV-associated forms of Reiter's syndrome[41] (Y. Molad, personal communication). In an animal model of Reiter's syndrome, the recombinant form of the 57-kDa chlamydial heat-shock protein has been shown to induce the Reiter's syndrome-like eye lesions.[10]

In contrast to the clear epidemiologic implication of microorganisms, in individual cases it is often difficult to establish a role of a specific microorganism because the clinical response of Reiter's syndrome follows the apparent inciting infection by 1 to 4 weeks, and therefore cultures are usually negative. For this reason primary emphasis has been placed on analyzing the serologic and cellular responses to microorganisms present in the blood and joint fluids of the patient with Reiter's syndrome. In infection with *Yersinia,* elevated titers of IgA antibodies correlate with the development of Reiter's syndrome, and these antibodies are primarily directed to lipopolysaccharide components of the organism.[42,43] Similar antibodies are found in instances of Reiter's syndrome incited by other microorganisms.[44] Paradoxically, the cellular response to microbial antigens in the blood of those who develop Reiter's syndrome is lower than in others who are similarly infected but who do not develop Reiter's syndrome; however, there is a much greater response in the lymphocytes of the joint fluid compared to those in the blood of those who develop the disease.[45,46] These findings again raise the question of whether microbial antigens persist, possibly because the cellular component of the immune response in susceptible individuals is incapable of effectively eliminating them. Such strain-related persistence is associated with the development of *Yersinia*-induced reactive arthritis in a rat model,[47] and there is increasing evidence for the demonstration of *Yersinia, Chlamydia,* and *Salmonella* antigens in the tissue of affected persons.[48–51]

Genetic Factors

There is a clear-cut familial aggregation of Reiter's syndrome; it is found in one out of ten blood relatives of the proband. As discussed previously, the inheritance of either Reiter's syndrome or ankylosing spondylitis, or both, is a characteristic of each family.[52–54] In each family either Reiter's syndrome or ankylosing spondylitis, or both, segregate with the HLA-B27 haplotype.

In the Caucasian population at large, cross-sectional studies demonstrate a close association between HLA-B27 and Reiter's syndrome; this HLA specificity is found in 80 percent of 906 patients and 9 percent of 13,477 ethnically matched controls.[20] The relative risk is 37, showing that the presence of HLA-B27 marks the potential for an untoward immune response. Furthermore, of the 20 percent of HLA-B27-negative patients with Reiter's syndrome, many have one of a group of HLA class I specificities termed *HLA-B27 cross-reacting antigens* (CREGs) because they share structural and antigenic similarities with HLA-B27.[55] The CREGs include HLA-B7, HLA-Bw22, HLA-Bw40, and HLA-Bw42. In a study by Inman,[56] HLA-B27 accounted for only 5 of 25 persons developing postenteric Reiter's syndrome, whereas CREG specificities were present in the remainder; the role of the latter HLA alleles is therefore emphasized.[56] Among non-Caucasians the association with HLA-B27 is less encompassing. From 14 to 37 percent of non-Caucasian patients with Reiter's syndrome have HLA-B27, whereas the frequency of the HLA specificity in healthy controls is only 2 percent or less. However, the intensity of the association with HLA-B27 determined by the relative risk is not decreased.[57] When Reiter's syndrome occurs in individuals infected with HIV, the same genetic predisposition is found that is primarily defined by the presence of HLA-B27.[58] In general, the intensity of the association between Reiter's syndrome and HLA-B27 is appreciably less than that observed between the same specificity and ankylosing spondylitis, where the relative risk is over 90 and susceptibility is not associated with CREG specificities.[20] Therefore, ankylosing spondylitis may be related more directly to a particular structure in the HLA-B27 molecule itself, while Reiter's syndrome is most probably developed in response to a shared determinant encoded by HLA-B27 and several evolutionarily related alleles of the CREG group (Fig. 180-1). Six alleles found at differ-

ent frequencies in various ethnic groups encode the HLA-B27 specificity[59,60] (Fig. 180-2). Recent evidence indicates that all but one of these alleles are associated with reactive arthritis or ankylosing spondylitis.[61] The B*2703 allele is found primarily in black Africans.

An important question that is not yet completely answered is the following: In a setting of infection by an arthritogenic organism, what is the risk of an HLA-B27-positive or a CREG-positive person for developing Reiter's syndrome? In effect this question asks what the penetrance is of the trait of developing Reiter's syndrome in this situation, given the presence of HLA-B27. In the instance of the epidemic on the cruiser *Little Rock,* depending on the assumptions made about HLA gene frequency in the crew, from 10 to 20 percent of genetically susceptible individuals developed Reiter's syndrome.[31] The risk of developing Reiter's syndrome in an HLA-B27-positive person has been calculated to be as high as 20 percent,[62] but in other epidemics such as that among the Finns the risk is as much as an order of magnitude lower.[19]

The fact that HLA-B27 is independently associated with other diseases in the spondyloarthropathy family, such as anterior uveitis or ankylosing spondylitis, complicates the analysis of certain of the manifestations of Reiter's syndrome. Because the percentage of patients with Reiter's syndrome that exhibit these findings is small, they might not be specific parts of the Reiter's syndrome symptom complex but rather could be attributed directly to the effects of the presence of HLA-B27.

Immunologic Mechanisms

Three experimental models are particularly relevant to the pathogenesis of Reiter's syndrome. Adjuvant arthritis in rats resulting from the administration of inactivated *Mycobacterium tuberculosis* is a strain-specific response characterized by tendinitis, keratodermia blennorrhagicum, urethritis, and ophthalmitis, which resem-

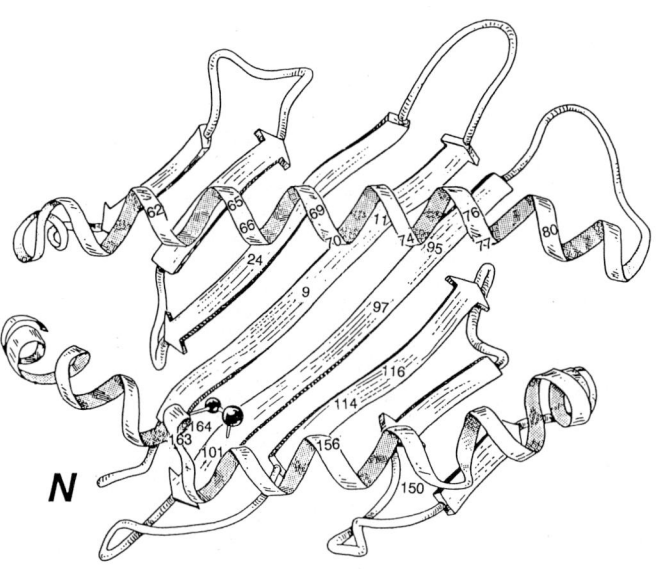

a

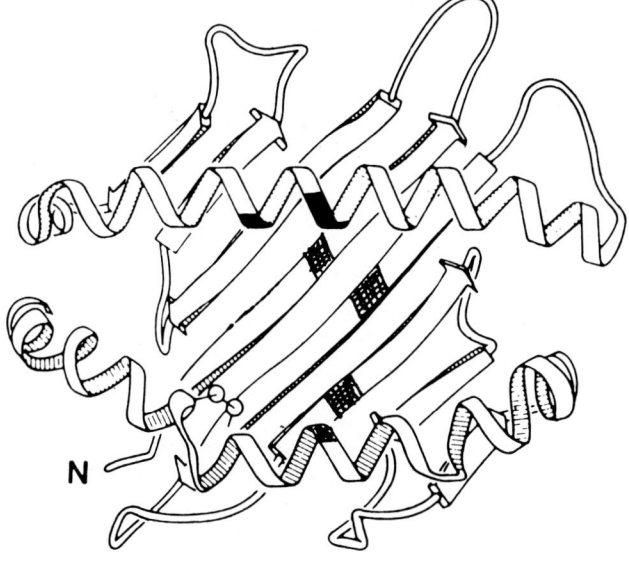

b

FIGURE 180-1 (*a*) The conformation of the MHC class I molecule as described by Bjorkman et al.[127] from the perspective of a T-cell receptor looking down at the antigen-binding portion of the molecule. The polypeptide backbone of the class I molecule consists of two α helices that form the walls of the antigen-presenting cleft and the eight strands of antiparallel β-pleated sheet that form the base. (*b*) The dark areas indicate the location of the amino acid substitutions that define the HLA-B27 specificities (see Fig. 180-2).

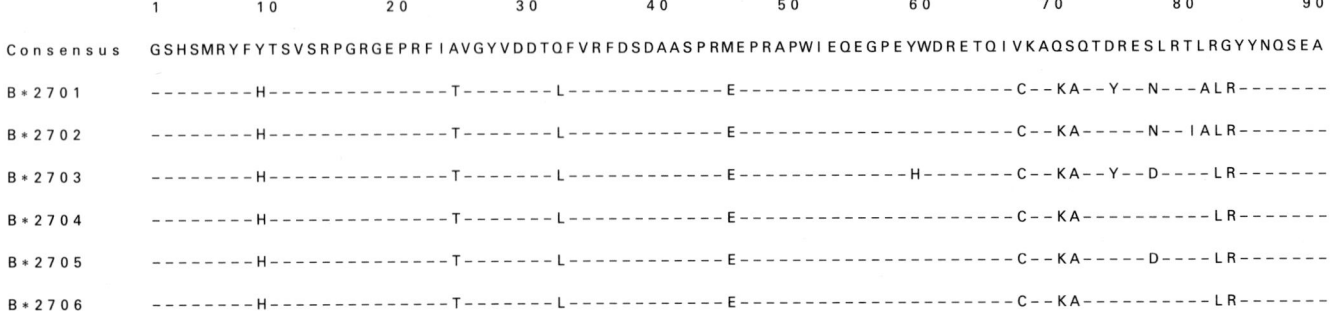

FIGURE 180-2 Amino acid sequences of alleles encoding the HLA-B27 specificity. This illustrates the amino acid substitutions that distinguish the 6 HLA alleles that each bear the HLA-B27 specificity, compared with the class I consensus sequence. The B*2703 allele is reported to confer a much lower risk of ankylosing spondylitis and reactive arthritis[61] than the other five allelic products. This difference is primarily based on the nonconservative replacement of tyrosine (Y) by a positively charged histidine (H) residue at position 59 in the B*2703 allele.

bles Reiter's syndrome.[18,63] Similarly, the 57-kDa heat-shock protein of *Chlamydia* induces experimental eye inflammation that mimics the reactive inflammation induced by the whole organism and in turn that in Reiter's syndrome.[10] The expression of the HLA-B27 molecule in mice at levels from five to ten times those of the mouse MHC molecules resulted in phenotypically normal animals which, however, had enhanced susceptibility to *Yersinia* infection.[64] Taken together with the previous information, this finding suggests the paradigm that Reiter's syndrome is a specific immunologic reaction to a microorganism antigen presented by MHC molecules to T cells. The expression of this molecule at five to ten times still higher levels in rats resulted in an extensive arthrocutaneous reaction with many features resembling psoriasis and psoriatic arthritis.[65]

Of the two T-cell lineages CD4 and CD8, the possibility that CD4 lineage T cells play an important role in the pathogenesis of Reiter's syndrome was eliminated by the observation that Reiter's syndrome can occur in persons with advanced HIV infection at a time when there is no effective CD4 T cell helper function.[11] Because the CD8 T-cell arm is relatively intact and CD8 T cells recognize antigen presented in the context of MHC class I molecules such as HLA-B27, the immunologic drive in Reiter's syndrome may be mediated through CD8 cells.[58] This conclusion would fit with the fact that susceptibility is associated with certain class I alleles such as HLA-B27.[66] Consistent with this possibility is the absence of autoantibodies such as antinuclear antibodies and rheumatoid factors, whose presence might be expected if this mechanism were CD4 T-cell driven. These autoantibodies are present in diseases such as systemic lupus erythematosus (SLE) and rheumatoid arthritis, which ameliorate with progression of the CD4 immune deficiency and appear to be CD4 T cell-driven.[67] Therefore, a CD8 or equivalent immune response initiated by some antigenic determinant and dependent on the presence of HLA-B27 molecule likely underlies Reiter's syndrome.

The nature of the immune response remains unknown. It could develop through one of at least two quite dissimilar mechanisms. One possibility is that the HLA-B27 molecule and its CREG species induce a highly specific immunologic tolerance to the arthritogenic organisms through a process of deleting specific T-cell clones during the formation of the T-cell repertoire, thereby creating a "hole" in the T-cell repertoire. These clones would be necessary for the normal elimination of the organism, which does not occur in the HLA-B27-positive person. In this model of microbial persistence, the resulting sustained immune response to the organism would be incapable of eliminating the organism, similar to the situation in leprosy, but would be of sufficient intensity to give rise to the clinical disease. The pathogenic immune response would be both induced and sustained by the persisting foreign microorganism or equivalent foreign antigens in the environment. The clear identification of chlamydial or yersinial antigens in the synovial tissues in patients during the first month of illness supports this hypothesis.[40]

A variant of this mechanism involves nonantigen-specific stimulation of T lymphocytes by bacterial superantigens. Superantigens are molecules encoded either by a microorganism such as certain heat-shock proteins or by endogenous genes such as the integrated murine mouse mammary tumor retrovirus. They bind to particular Vβ gene segment products that comprise a portion of the TCR β chain and interact with MHC molecules. The interactions are nonclonal, are nonantigen specific, and are not restricted by specific MHC types. This mechanism would involve sustained drive of particular T-cell clones or possibly an initial phase of superantigen-driven T-cell proliferation, followed by a phase in which a particular T-cell clone, perhaps positively selected by the HLA-B27 molecule early in ontogeny, becomes stimulated by a self antigen.[68] Whereas the first model relies on selective microbial persistence in HLA-B27-positive individuals because of a defect in the ability to eliminate the viable microorganism, a second, related, model postulates the persistence of residual microorganismal antigens. Genetically responsive individuals defined by HLA-B27 would then mount an immune response to the antigen. Similarly, a superantigen mechanism could operate as described for the first model.

A third "autoimmune" model postulates that upon stimulation by arthritogenic microorganisms, the immune system loses tolerance for self molecules through mimicry of specific self antigens by molecules of the microorganism. This loss of tolerance most likely would arise through an induced response to minor antigenic determinants on self molecules for which tolerance does not exist and which are usually not seen as antigenic. This process is termed *mimicry*. The resulting pathogenic immune response, occurring most probably at the CD8 T-cell level, is essentially autoimmune in character with its persistent driving element a component of self. It differs from the other two mechanisms in that microbial antigens only induce the abnormality but play no part in its sustained presence.

Mimicry at the level of antibody recognition can be divided into two types, linear and interrupted. Three examples of linear mimicry between HLA-B27 molecules and those of *Klebsiella* nitrogenase reductase, the *Shigella flexneri*-pHS-2 plasmid-encoded protein, and the *Yersinia enteritidis* plasmid-encoded protein respectively involve 6, 5, and 4 amino acid residues shared with the MHC class I allelic product.[37,69]

A significant problem with the notion of a linear epitope is that the secondary structure of proteins results in conformations such as the α helix or the β-pleated sheet, in which amino acids are displayed on different faces of the molecule, making recognition by a known receptor unlikely. In the instance of discontinuous epitopes recognized by monoclonal antibodies to cross-reacting epitopes shared by HLA-B27 and molecules of the microorganism, one such conformation has been identified on *Yersinia* outer membrane protein A.[70] There is no sequence homology between these two structures. In support of some type of mimetic mechanism is the identification of what might be termed *autoantibodies* that react with synthetic peptides representing short stretches of the HLA-B27 molecule but that do not react with the intact molecule.[71,72] Evidence against a mimetic model between HLA-B27 and microbes has been provided by the finding that B lymphocytes from patients with Reiter's syndrome synthesize very few or no antibodies that react with candidate Enterobacteriaceae antigens and HLA-B27.[73] In the case of T cells, it is likely that the antigenic structure would be linear because of the requirement for presentation of small fragments of peptide by MHC molecules. In any event, it is difficult to conceive how a response to HLA-B27 molecules, which are found on essentially all nucleated cells, could account for the selective clinical findings of Reiter's syndrome. Although the first two mechanisms are more plausible given the current state of understanding, our knowledge is still insufficient to distinguish which of these is the most likely possibility, or whether other mechanisms may operate.

Pathology

Skin

Histologically the appearance of established keratodermia blennorrhagicum is indistinguishable from that of pustular psoriasis, with hyperkeratosis and parakeratosis, elongation and hypertrophy of the rete pegs, general epidermal hyperplasia, and extensive neutrophilic infiltration with formation of microabscesses and spongiform pustules. The initial lesion is a vesicular, pustular, or erythematous macule. Balanitis in circumcised individuals has a similar histologic appearance, whereas the moist lesion of uncircumcised males and the mouth ulcers are otherwise similar but are not keratinized.[14,15,74] Differentiation from psoriasis may be helped by the presence of a greatly thickened horny layer in Reiter's syndrome.

Musculoskeletal System

The characteristic lesions of the entheses have not been studied in great detail but apparently contain small numbers of lymphocytes and proliferating fibroblasts. The appearance of the synovium is typical of any nonspecific chronic synovitis but with rather more marked vascular involvement and fibroblast proliferation. Edema, vascular congestion, increased surface fibrin, lining cell proliferation, infiltration with neutrophils and lymphocytes, and consider-

able fibroblast proliferation are found. Occlusion by platelet and fibrin thrombi, simulating that caused by endotoxins, is common.[25,40] The inciting antigen may be demonstrable.

Systemic

Sixty-seven percent of patients with Reiter's syndrome are reported to have either acute ileocolitis or evidence of Crohn's disease upon biopsy, with most having no gastrointestinal symptoms.[75] Five percent of patients have granulomatous lesions found at the aortic root and annulus that may cause abnormalities in conduction, including complete heart block and frank aortic regurgitation. Secondary amyloidosis with AA protein deposition is a rare complication usually found after a long course of the illness.[76,77] Nephropathy characterized by casts and proteinuria but not distinguishable from analgesic nephropathy has been reported.[78]

Clinical Manifestations

Natural History

The chronologic evolution of Reiter's syndrome is a distinctive feature that often provides the clue to diagnosis. The enteric or genitourinary infection that initiates Reiter's syndrome is followed by a characteristic latent period of 1 week to 1 month, during which the initial symptoms attributable to the infection subside. Urethritis and conjunctivitis are usually the first manifestations of Reiter's syndrome; they are followed within several days by the often abrupt and diagnostically characteristic onset of arthritis. The mucocutaneous involvement occurs independently, sometimes at or preceding the phase of urethritis and conjunctivitis and sometimes developing after the onset of arthritis. During the acute phase of Reiter's syndrome, constitutional symptoms and signs are prominent, including fever, fatigue, malaise, and weight loss that can be profound. Occasionally, the manifestations of the syndrome evolve over a protracted period.[18]

Skin Disease

Circinate balanitis is the most common cutaneous finding, being reported in an average of 36 percent of patients with Reiter's syndrome.[9,18,79–82] The lesion is initially vesicular with little or no surrounding erythema and evolves differently according to whether or not the male is circumcised. Irregular moist superficial ulcers form in the uncircumcised male and may coalesce to give a circinate distribution (Fig. 180-3). These ulcers may occasionally become secondarily infected. In the circumcised male the lesions evolve to form hard crusts and plaques. Painless mucosal ulcers of varying size on the tongue, palate, buccal mucosa, and lips are usually transient and cause little or no morbidity. This stomatitis is found in an average of 17 percent of patients.[9,18,79–82]

The initial lesions of keratodermia blennorrhagicum are small vesicles or erythematous macules that may coalesce and are usually surrounded by an erythematous base. The vesicle wall becomes progressively thickened, forming a small papule, nodule, or even a horny excrescence (Fig. 180-4). The appearance of the lesions varies from a scaling plaquelike process that resembles pustular psoriasis

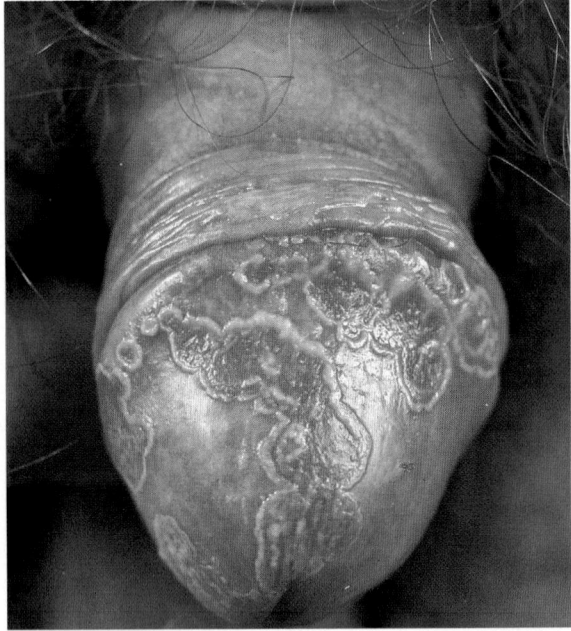

FIGURE 180-3 Reiter's syndrome, balanitis circinata. Illustrated in this patient is circinate balanitis with moist, well-demarcated erosions with slightly raised border.

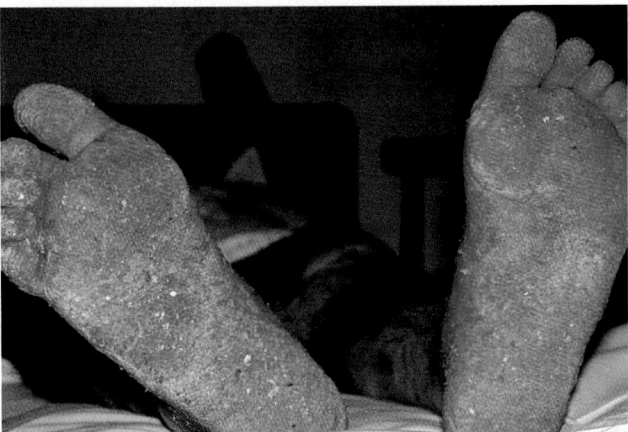

FIGURE 180-5 Severe keratodermia blennorrhagicum with marked dyskeratotic change in an HIV-positive person. The margins of the dyskeratotic process are intensely inflamed.

to combinations of crusting, exudation, and erosion associated with erythema. Lesions of keratodermia blennorrhagicum are found in an average of 15 percent of patients.[9,18,79,81,82] Keratodermia blennorrhagicum is most commonly found on the soles, toes, and palms where the lesions are often densely scattered. More isolated lesions occur on the glans penis, scrotum, trunk, limbs, and scalp. In severe cases, notably those associated with HIV infection, the keratodermia blennorrhagicum may be distributed over the entire body, with an intensification on the digits in a pattern that resembles the lesions of pustular psoriasis and in the groin in the pattern of inverse psoriasis or sebopsoriasis. The soles may exhibit unusually marked keratotic changes (Fig. 180-5). The keratodermia blennorrhagicum lesions may last for weeks to months, disappear, and then

recur.[14,15,83] In patients with HIV infection, the initial Reiter's syndrome-like illness may gradually assume the chronic features of pustular psoriatic arthritis.

Joint Disease

The foot, ankle, and knee are the principal sites of musculoskeletal involvement. Joint disease includes both enthesopathy, mainly of the plantar fascia and Achilles tendon, and arthritis of the subtalar, ankle, and knee joints. The arthritis is generally abrupt in onset and may be florid, particularly in the knee joint where massive effusion may lead to rupture of the popliteal Baker's cyst and the syndrome of pseudothrombophlebitis. The joint inflammation occasionally subsides and does not recur; more commonly it remains as a chronic problem, manifesting itself as either sustained or recrudescent arthritis. The small or large joints of the upper limbs may be involved, but only in association with predominant arthritis of the large joints of the legs. In the instances of Reiter's syndrome associated with HIV infection, the course of the joint disease is some-

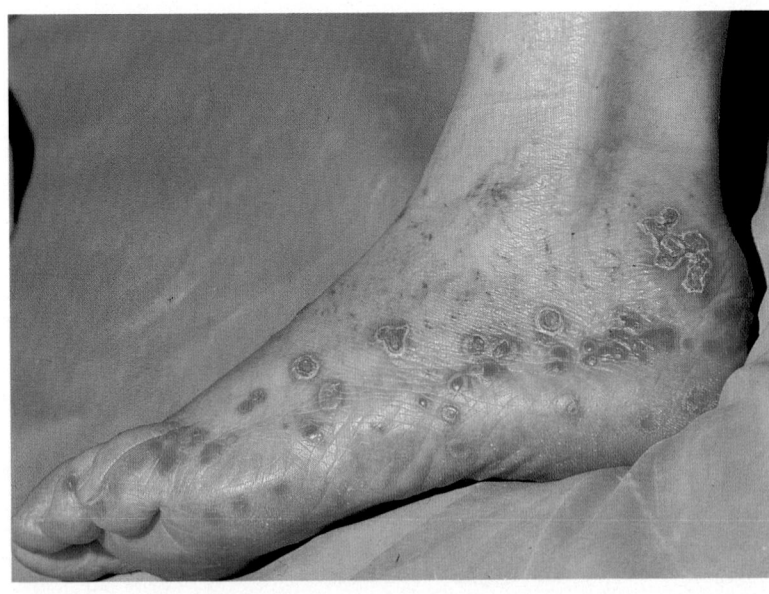

FIGURE 180-4 Reiter's syndrome, keratoderma blennorrhagicum. Red-to-brown papules, vesicles, pustules, with central erosion and confluence of lesions on the foot.

times slowly cumulative and ultimately results in an extensive poly-arthritis involving the small and large joints of the arms and legs in a pattern more similar to that of psoriatic arthritis. This cumulative pattern is usually accompanied by sustained joint disease that leads to erosions and marked periarticular osteoporosis (Fig. 180-6).

Inflammation at the sites of insertion of ligaments and tendons is a striking feature of Reiter's syndrome. In addition to the plantar fasciitis and Achilles and posterior tibial tendinitis, the enthesopathy results in chest wall and lower back pain, tenderness over ischial tuberosities and iliac crests, and dactylitis or "sausage digits." In addition to the back pain directly attributable to enthesopathy that is usually manifest as transient pain or stiffness, approximately one-quarter of patients with chronic Reiter's syndrome develop chronic sacroiliitis or a characteristic asymmetric spondylosis that limits back mobility.[84,85] The characteristic symptoms include stiffness and pain after periods of rest, such as in the early morning, with improvement upon exercise.[86]

Nail Disease

Involvement of the nail may begin as erythema of the nail fold, or more insidiously as subungual hyperkeratosis, a finding in psoriasis and Reiter's syndrome but not in rheumatoid arthritis. Small pustules develop below the nail, which then becomes thickened, yellowed, and brittle. Frank onycholysis with shedding of the nail often occurs. The acral portion of the digit may be hyperkeratotic with erythema and scaling and may exhibit a pseudoparonychia appearance. The tendency to extensive acral disease is pronounced in HIV-associated cases. In some cases of HIV-associated Reiter's syndrome, yellowing of the nails was the first manifestation of the syndrome. Pitting of the nails, characteristic of psoriasis, is not seen in Reiter's syndrome.

Other Manifestations

Urethritis and prostatitis are frequently associated findings. They may present only as sterile pyuria in the first voided specimen or range up to moderately severe dysuria with frank mucopurulent discharge. The dominant ocular lesion in Reiter's syndrome is conjunctivitis of varying intensity that usually quickly resolves. A smaller proportion of patients also exhibits uveitis, initially manifest as acute anterior iritis, which may progress to chronic iridocyclitis and visual impairment.[62,87–89] The uveitis resembles that of ankylosing spondylitis in that it is acute in onset, frequently unilateral, and spares the choroid and retina.[90] There is some controversy over whether the uveitis is an intrinsic manifestation of Reiter's syndrome or a problem stemming directly from the HLA-B27 status of the individual. Uveitis is a potentially serious problem that must be carefully evaluated and treated.

The cardiac symptoms in Reiter's syndrome include palpitations, pericardial type chest pain, and, relatively rarely, symptoms of aortic valve incompetence. Findings present in 5 percent of the patients include first-, second-, and third-degree heart block, ST segment, T- and Q-wave changes on electrocardiography, pericardial rubs, and varying degrees of aortic and occasionally mitral valve incompetence from granulomatous involvement at the aortic root.[6,19,91–93] Atrioventricular conduction disturbances may appear early in the course.[94] HLA-B27 itself, in either Reiter's syndrome or ankylosing spondylitis, is a strong risk factor for isolated aortic valve lesions, especially if associated with conduction abnormal-

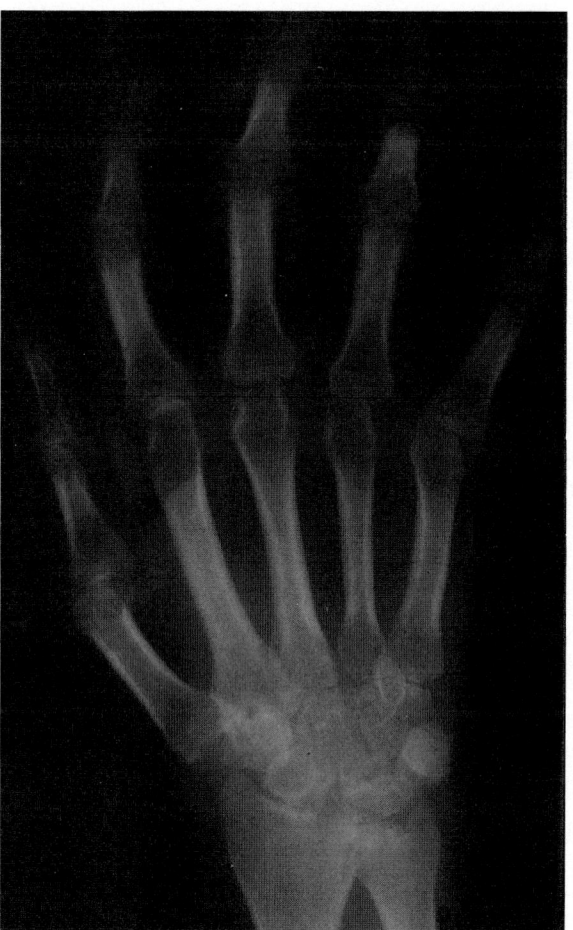

FIGURE 180-6 Juxtaarticular osteoporosis in an HIV-positive person who presented with typical Reiter's syndrome, but who exhibited a cumulative pattern of joint involvement indistinguishable from psoriatic arthritis. The involvement of the small joints in the hands is also more typical of psoriatic arthritis.

ities.[95] Relatively rare manifestations include peripheral neuropathy and other neurologic findings,[89,92,96] pleuritic and pulmonary parenchymal inflammation,[97] thrombophlebitis,[98] erythema nodosum,[99] and amyloidosis.[100]

Laboratory Findings

High levels of cytokines associated with the inflammation of Reiter's syndrome are reflected by the elevation in acute-phase reactants, a variably elevated erythrocyte sedimentation rate, hypochromic or normochromic anemia, and mild hypoalbuminemia. There are no diagnostically specific antimicrobial antibodies, although elevated antibody titers to specific enteric pathogenic agents or *Chlamydia* often help with differential diagnosis.[42–44] The reports of antibodies to chlamydial heat-shock proteins appear to be a promising new direction, but further study is required to document diagnostic usefulness[41,101] (Y. Molad, personal communication). Serum IgA levels are elevated without the formation of immune complexes, perhaps reflecting the transmucosal acquisition of infection.[102] Rheumatoid factor and classic autoantibodies are absent. Urine and stool cultures are usually nonrevealing, although the persistence of *Salmonella* carriage would be important to determine. The demonstration of persistent microorganismal components in tissue biopsies is still an experimental technique. Testing for HIV should be considered in view of the fact that HIV infection is also a sexually acquired disease, and that the clinical outlook and therapy for HIV-associated Reiter's syndrome is significantly different from that for Reiter's syndrome not associated with HIV. The assessment of the persistence of specific microorganisms related to Reiter's syndrome in the HIV-positive person assumes great importance.

Much has been written about whether or not to perform HLA typing for diagnostic reasons.[103,104] The sensitivity and specificity of determinations of the presence of HLA-B27 are approximately those of tests for antinuclear antibodies in lupus erythematosus. It is this author's view that in a classic but mild case, where Reiter's syndrome is an obvious clinical diagnosis, the only justification for HLA typing would be to assist in making a prognosis. HLA-B27 positivity is associated with more severe and protracted disease, including the occurrence of uveitis, carditis, and sacroiliitis; the presence of CREG specificities alone is associated with milder disease.[105–107] However, in the considerable proportion of more atypical cases that present problems in differential diagnosis, knowledge of an individual's HLA type can often be important in providing a correct approach. This is particularly so in the HIV-associated disorders. In the diagnosis of ankylosing spondylitis, HLA-B27 typing alone is sufficient, but in the case of Reiter's syndrome, assessment of all class I alleles is advisable to determine whether HLA-B27 CREG specificities are present and perhaps to exclude the presence of specificities associated with susceptibility to psoriasis.

The joint fluid cell count varies from occasional to over 50,000 neutrophils per μL, a level that in conjunction with the intense inflammation might otherwise suggest a septic joint and is designated *pseudosepsis*. Occasionally ''Reiter's cells'' are observed, which are macrophages that have ingested a neutrophilic leukocyte. Total joint fluid protein levels are elevated in proportion to the degree of inflammation, and because there is little or no intraarticular consumption of complement, the joint fluid complement component levels are about two-thirds of their levels in serum when normalized on a per gram of serum protein basis.[108] Glucose levels are normal, and bacteriologic cultures are uniformly negative. Much current work is directed towards identification of persisting antigenic fragments of candidate microorganisms. The presence of distinctly elevated levels of cartilage proteoglycans in Reiter's syndrome compared to rheumatoid arthritis or psoriatic arthritis has been described.[109]

Radiographic Features

Frank arthritis may initially only show signs of an effusion. Periarticular osteoporosis develops after several weeks of inflammation, and in some instances where the arthritis becomes chronic, erosions and loss of the cartilaginous joint space are seen. Enthesopathy is characterized by a combination of erosions about tendon and ligament insertions, bone lucency, and new bone formation, often in the form of spurs extending into the tendon or fascia. Widespread periosteal new bone formation can be found, especially on the bones of the pelvis and feet. Calcaneal enthesopathy is also found in psoriatic arthritis and certain metabolic arthropathies, whereas erosions of the calcaneus can be seen in rheumatoid arthritis.[110]

Sacroiliitis is typical in appearance but may be only asymmetric, distinguishing it from that found in ankylosing spondylitis. Similarly, the frank spondyloarthropathy, when present, is often asymmetric without the uniformity in extension from the lower lumbar vertebrae that occurs in psoriatic arthritis.[85] Indeed, neck involvement is rather more common in Reiter's syndrome.

Diagnosis

The diagnosis of Reiter's syndrome can be simple or exceedingly challenging. The classic presentation is a young male with an antecedent nonspecific urethritis or one of many individuals with an epidemic enteric infection. After a few days to weeks, fever, conjunctivitis, characteristic mucocutaneous disease, urethritis, florid arthritis of the knees, ankles, and feet, and extensive enthesopathy develop. However, in the majority of patients a variable number of these features are absent, and a careful differential diagnosis must be made among entities such as other spondyloarthropathies (including especially ankylosing spondylitis and psoriatic arthritis), infectious arthritis (notably that due to the gonococcus), the crystal-induced arthropathies (primarily gout), and other rheumatic diseases such as rheumatoid arthritis, Behçet's syndrome, and rheumatic fever. Difficulties may arise because elements of the early history are ignored or suppressed. The history of a sexual contact or risk factors leading to the acquisition of HIV infection may be concealed, or an episode of dysentery may be disregarded unless the patient is specifically questioned. Similarly, many of the features of the illness may be mild so that mouth ulcers, if noticed at all, are passed off as ''cold sores,'' and transient dysuria is dismissed. The remaining signs and symptoms may add up to a relatively perplexing entity.

The rapid increase in the prevalence of Lyme disease makes this diease an important differential consideration. Typically, Lyme disease is preceded by the characteristic rash of erythema migrans associated with fever, malaise, and meningitic symptoms. Conjunctivitis, nail involvement, and urethritis are absent. The joints typically involved include the knees and the temperomandibular joints; the latter are an extremely uncommon site of involvement in Reiter's syndrome. Rising titers of antibodies to *Borrelia burgdorferi* and especially the conversion of IgM to IgG antibodies are dignostic of Lyme disease. In endemic areas where seroprevalence is high, a positive test would not exclude the diagnosis of otherwise classic Reiter's syndrome.

Although gonococcal arthritis and Reiter's syndrome may superficially resemble one another in that urethritis, skin rash, oligoarthritis, and tenosynovitis occur in both, the character and natural history of the two illnesses are usually readily distinguishable. Gonococcal arthritis is more common in females, and upper limb joint involvement predominates. The arthritis is not florid and is usually preceded by insidiously developing migratory arthralgias. Enthesopathy, keratodermia blennorrhagicum, balanitis, and back pain are absent. Culture may be helpful but can be negative. That both entities can coexist should be emphasized.

The differential diagnosis between ankylosing spondylitis and Reiter's syndrome can sometimes be difficult in the early phases of the illness. When mucocutaneous disease or urethritis is present, ankylosing spondylitis can be excluded. Similarly, the abrupt onset and remittent course of Reiter's syndrome can be useful diagnostic points. Other differences require more time to be evident. Foot involvement and florid enthesopathy suggest Reiter's syndrome, but lesser degrees of hind foot involvement are seen in ankylosing spondylitis. Uveitis, isolated hip involvement, and symmetric spine and sacroiliac disease favor ankylosing spondylitis.

The differential diagnosis between psoriatic arthritis and Reiter's syndrome is discussed in detail in the chapter on psoriatic arthritis (Chap. 40). The presence of mouth ulcers, urethritis, predominant foot or lower extremity disease, and antecedent infection favor Reiter's syndrome; an insidious onset, extensive skin disease, primary upper limb arthritis, and especially distal interphalangeal joint involvement are characteristic of psoriatic arthritis. Examination of the nails, especially those of the fingers, can be of great importance in the diagnosis of either entity. Nail involvement is prevalent but distinctive in both diseases.[11] HLA typing can often be useful. In HIV infection the differential diagnosis between pustular psoriatic arthritis and Reiter's syndrome may in principle be impossible because the entities appear to be interrelated if not identical, as discussed in detail in Chap. 40.

In any florid arthritis the fluid should be studied for the presence of microorganisms by culture and staining and examined for urate crystals by polarized light microscopy. Rheumatic fever remains a rare but strong simulator of Reiter's syndrome. The antecedent pharyngitis and characteristic rash of streptococcal infection are points of differentiation, but similar cardiac and joint findings can prove problematic. Behçet's syndrome is another rare entity in North America, but the combination of mucocutaneous disease and arthritic disease in this syndrome can cause diagnostic difficulties. Neurologic findings and the pustulonecrotic pathergic lesions at injury sites, as well as extensive, painful genital and oral ulcers, suggest the diagnosis of Behçet's syndrome.

The complications of the effusive inflammatory arthritis include ruptured popliteal cysts and thrombophlebitis. The rupture of popliteal cysts with the syndrome of pseudothrombophlebitis should be differentiated from true thrombophlebitis, which can also be found in this setting due to pressure on the popliteal vein by the joint effusion and the contiguous inflammation.

Treatment

Therapy of Reiter's syndrome is difficult when the illness is sustained or severe because there are no agents capable of definitively and safely eliminating the inflammatory host response. The cutaneous manifestations and the systemic concomitants of intense inflammation (fever, mild anemia) are often the most obvious features of the illness; but despite their significant psychological impact, they are usually in themselves not the cause of significant morbidity. In contrast, arthritis, uveitis, and the more uncommon visceral manifestations, especially those of the heart, while often less overt to the patient, require therapy to prevent serious complications or disability. Physical therapy is very important to maintain range of motion and prevent joint fibrosis.

Antibiotic therapy is still controversial; newer data about microbial persistence support the viewpoint of its advocates. Clearly, Reiter's syndrome following chlamydial urethritis is a situation where short-term antibiotics are appropriate.[39] While comprehensive controlled trials are awaited, we take the interim position that in the absence of a specific known pathogen, well-tolerated doxytetracycline or tetracycline preparations are appropriate in severe, recent-onset Reiter's syndrome in HLA-B27-positive persons. Because advanced HIV infection is associated with microbial persistence, we feel that therapy of documented inciting infectious

agents in an HIV-positive individual with Reiter's syndrome is appropriate.

Because many HIV-positive patients develop Reiter's syndrome within a year of the onset of opportunistic infections, the inflammatory response of Reiter's syndrome may transactivate the otherwise predominantly latent virus. The expression of MHC class II (DR) molecules and interleukin 2 receptors on the CD4 lineage T cells are associated with this inflammatory state. For this reason and because of the generally lower level of CD4 lymphocytes in HIV-positive patients with Reiter's syndrome, therapy with zidovudine is warranted.

All patients with Reiter's syndrome must be informed about the sometimes difficult nature of the illness and its variable outcome. It is important to engender both an optimistic mentality on the ultimate outcome and a sense of realism about the potential problems. Psychological support is particularly important for this type of arthrocutaneous syndrome because of anxiety associated with sexually transmitted routes of infection and the fact that these younger patients often have not had a prior major and potentially chronic illness. Moreover, public health aspects involve other individuals in the identification of enteric or sexually transmitted routes. Available evidence suggests that reinfection may induce a recrudescence that is sometimes more severe than the original episode. Therefore, counseling must be offered on prevention by avoidance of reexposure to microorganisms, including the avoidance of travel in areas of the world with unreliable hygiene and attention to measures that reduce the likelihood of acquiring a sexually transmitted disease.

Skin Disease

The management of the acute mucocutaneous lesions of uncomplicated Reiter's syndrome is usually limited to the general measures discussed above because the lesions are rarely severe enough to mandate specific therapeutic attention. The severe, extensive, and chronic cutaneous reactions that are more common in the form of Reiter's syndrome associated with HIV infection present a much more difficult challenge. Moderate success has been obtained by treating these lesions in the same manner as pustular psoriasis. UVB irradiation, coal tar and etrinate administration, combined with very judicious use of topical steroids, form the center of the therapy.[90] When HIV infection is excluded, extremely severe skin lesions can be treated with immunosuppressive agents including methotrexate, PUVA therapy, or cyclosporine. These latter drugs are to be used in the HIV-positive person with Reiter's syndrome only under the most exceptional circumstances, because they appear to be associated with the induction of opportunistic infections and Kaposi's sarcoma.[11] Corticosteroid therapy is often not effective and may cause dermal atrophy. In HIV-positive persons, systemic corticosteroid therapy often results in the appearance of oral or esophageal candidiasis and has little or no efficacy.

Eye Disease

Conjunctivitis is a common short-lived occurrence and can be adequately managed by nonspecific local therapy. Topical antibiotics have no established efficacy. In marked contrast the development, actual or suspected, of uveitis is a threatening complication. Eye pain, ciliary flush, and other symptoms of early iritis should prompt immediate referral to an ophthalmologist for definitive evaluation and therapy. Treatment includes the use of agents that diminish intraocular tension, and intraocular or occasionally systemic steroid therapy.

Visceral Disease

The development of cardiac involvement is a potentially life-threatening complication that can either appear as a part of the initial presentation or develop in otherwise clinically stable individuals. Conduction disturbances and aortic or mitral valvular involvement mandate immediate medical evaluation. Systemic corticosteroid therapy is useful in this specialized situation.

Musculoskeletal Disease

Arthritis and enthesopathy are the symptoms that necessitate treatment in most patients. Exercise and physical therapy are important.[112] Nonsteroidal anti-inflammatory drug (NSAID) therapy is the first line of treatment. Three NSAIDs, indomethacin, naproxen, and phenylbutazone, are generally considered to be the most efficacious of this large class of agents for the therapy of Reiter's syndrome. Because of idiosyncratic reactions including cytopenias, phenylbutazone, the most effective of the agents, has fallen out of use with the major exception of treating HIV-associated cases of Reiter's syndrome. Therapy with indomethacin or naproxen is begun at the lowest dose and increased. Naproxen, 200 to 375 mg, is administered two to three times a day and is increased to the maximum recommended dose of 1500 mg over a 1- to 2-week period. Indomethacin, 25 mg, is administered two to three times a day and increased to a total of 225 mg daily. Three weeks or more should be allowed before an agent is deemed ineffective. Change to the other drug should include at least a 1-week taper of the initial drug to prevent "rebound" activation, while the alternative drug is concomitantly begun. Occasional patients may respond to other anti-inflammatory agents. In the often severe enthesopathy of HIV infection not responsive to naproxen, phenylbutazone is especially effective in doses of 100 to 200 mg two to three times a day. The untoward effects of the NSAIDs include erosive and irritative gastrointestinal effects, central asthma, headache, depression, nephropathy, antihemostatic action on platelets, salt retention with attendant congestive heart failure and hypertension, and idiosyncratic allergic responses such as cytopenias and rash.[113]

Sulfasalazine is reported to be effective in the therapy of Reiter's syndrome unresponsive to NSAIDs when given at 2 g daily in divided doses, but 21 percent of patients had to discontinue the agent because of side effects.[114] The drug is initially given at 250 to 500 mg one to two times a day to minimize the prominent untoward gastrointestinal effects of nausea and vomiting. The maintenance dose of 2 g is approached slowly over 1 to 2 months by weekly increments in dosage. Because it is slow-acting, its therapeutic effect may not be seen until after 5 months of maintenance therapy, although most patients respond by 2 months. Our unit has used this agent in open studies in HIV-infected patients with Reiter's syndrome; approximately one-third of the patients improved, one-third remained unchanged, and one-third failed to tolerate the drug. Most untoward effects resemble those of aspirin and sulfonamides, including gastrointestinal irritation, hematologic and central nervous system disturbances, nephrotoxicity, oligospermia, and hypersensitivity responses.

Immunosuppressive agents such as methotrexate or azathioprine remain choices of last resort for intractable, severe disease not associated with HIV infection. Although effective, they are contraindicated in the setting of HIV infection because most patients are very sensitive to their immunosuppressive effects.[11] Oral or parenteral methotrexate is given in weekly doses beginning at 2.5 mg and increasing in weekly or biweekly steps of 2.5 mg to a maximum of 20 mg, if necessary. The weekly dosage is divided into two or three units and given every 12 h. Methotrexate appears to be free of the mutagenic effects that characterize, for example, alkylating agents; but both immunosuppression that can be fatal even on low-dose therapy[115] and a set of idiosyncratic parenchymal disorders, including liver injury and fibrosis and lung disease, are recognized untoward effects.[116–118] Cirrhosis and lesser degrees of hepatic fibrosis primarily occur when the cumulative dose exceeds 1.5 g. Although initial and repeat liver biopsies upon reaching a total dose of 1.5 g have previously been commonly performed on patients receiving long-term methotrexate therapy,[117] and are still recommended by some,[119] it is now evident that individuals with diabetes mellitus and antecedent liver disease or injury account for most of those patients developing these complications.[120] Accordingly, greater effort is warranted in evaluating the status of the liver if therapy with methotrexate is contemplated; and it should be used only with great caution in those with liver abnormalities, diabetes mellitus, and obesity, and then only when the abnormalities are minimal.[121] Collagen deposition in the space of Disse was documented in all those taking the drug, even though frank hepatic fibrosis was not detected with light microscopy.[122] One authority has recommended liver biopsy after each 2 to 2.5 g of the drug.[120]

Particularly in the evaluation of lung disease occurring in the course of methotrexate therapy, in addition to the primary drug reaction of fibrosis,[123] the possibility of infection by agents such as *Pneumocystis carinii* and *Cryptococcus* should be considered.[124,125] Attention should be given to prior history of infection with organisms such as *Mycobacterium tuberculosis* or parasites such as *Strongyloides stercoralis,* which may become rampant upon administration of methotrexate. More recently, a syndrome of central nervous system toxicity to methotrexate has been described, consisting of headaches, dizziness, mood alteration, and memory impairment.[126]

Course and Prognosis

Increasingly, Reiter's syndrome is being recognized as an illness that may result in a relatively unfavorable outcome. Sixty-three percent of patients with Reiter's syndrome in a rural midwest setting had a prolonged or relapsing course.[27] Often, the mucocutaneous aspect of the illness remits while the arthritic manifestations persist. However, in a smaller proportion of patients, persistent dermal lesions such as balanitis can be troublesome. Patients with chronic or recrudescent illness require progressive escalation of therapy to agents that have more harmful side effects. Meticulous reexamination of the immunologic infections and epidemiologic features of these patients may provide insight into effective therapeutic interventions. A few patients with chronic disease progress into other forms of spondyloarthropathy. The HIV-associated forms of Reiter's syndrome usually illustrate the worst features of this illness. The tendency of these patients to develop chronic arthritis and skin disease indistinguishable from pustular psoriasis is a most troublesome feature.

References

1. Stoll M: (1776) Cited by Huette, in De l'arthrite dysenterique. *Arch Gen Med* **14**:29, 1869

2. Brodie BC: *Pathologic and Surgical Observations on Diseases and Joints*. London, Longman, 1818

3. Benedek TG, Rodman GP: A brief history of the rheumatic diseases. *Bull Rheum Dis* **32**:59, 1982

4. Fiessinger N, Leroy E: Contribution a l'étude d'une epidemie de dysenterie dans le Somme. *Bull Soc Med Hop Paris* **40**:2030, 1916

5. Hawkes JG: Clinical and diagnostic features of Reiter's disease: A follow-up study of 39 patients. *NZ Med J* **78**:347, 1973

6. Good AE: Reiter's disease: A review with special attention to cardiovascular and neurologic sequelae. *Semin Arthritis Rheum* **3**:253, 1974

7. Calin A: Reiter's syndrome, in *The Spondyloarthropathies,* edited by A Calin. Orlando, FL, Grune & Stratton, 1984, p 119

8. Ball J: Enthesopathy of rheumatoid and ankylosing spondylitis. *Ann Rheum Dis* **30**:213, 1971

9. Brewerton DA et al: Reiter's disease and HLA 27. *Lancet* **2**:996, 1973

10. Morrison RP et al: Chlamydial disease pathogenesis. The 57-kD chlamydial hypersensitivity antigen is a stress response protein. *J Exp Med* **170**:1271, 1989

11. Winchester R et al: The co-occurrence of Reiter's syndrome and acquired immunodeficiency. *Ann Intern Med* **106**:19, 1987

12. Duvic M et al: Acquired immunodeficiency syndrome associated psoriasis and Reiter's syndrome. *Arch Dermatol* **123**:1622, 1987

13. Iveson JMI et al: Reiter's disease in three boys. *Ann Rheum Dis* **34**:364, 1975

14. Csonka GW: Recurrent attacks in Reiter's disease. *Arthritis Rheum* **3**:164, 1960

15. Csonka GW: The course of Reiter's syndrome. *Br Med J* **1**:1088, 1958

16. Keat AC et al: Role of *Chlamydia trachomatis* and HLA-B27 in sexually acquired reactive arthritis. *Br Med J* **1**:605, 1978

17. Arnett FC: Incomplete Reiter's syndrome: Clinical comparisons with classical triad. *Ann Rheum Dis* **38**(suppl 1):73, 1979

18. Fox R et al: The chronicity of symptoms and disability in Reiter's syndrome: An analysis of 131 consecutive patients. *Ann Intern Med* **91**:190, 1979

19. Paronen I: Reiter's disease: A study of 344 cases observed in Finland. *Acta Med Scand* **131**(suppl 212):1, 1948

20. Tiwari JL, Terasaki PI: *HLA and Disease Associations*. New York, Springer Verlag, 1985

21. Hochberg MC et al: Family studies in HLA-B27-associated arthritis. *Medicine* **57**:463, 1978

22. Calin A et al: The nature and prevalence of spondylarthritis among relatives of probands with ankylosing spondylitis and Reiter's syndrome. *Arthritis Rheum* **24**:S78, 1981

23. Gofton JP et al: HLA B27 and ankylosing spondylitis in British Columbia Indians. *J Rheumatol* **2**:314, 1975

24. Lisse JR et al: High risk of sacroiliitis in HLA-B27 positive Pima Indian men. *Arthritis Rheum* **25**:236, 1982

25. Morse HG et al: High frequency of HLA-B27 and Reiter's syndrome in Navajo Indians. *J Rheumatol* **7**:900, 1980

26. Boyer GS et al: Prevalence rates of spondylarthropathies. Rheumatoid arthritis and other rheumatic disorders in an Alaskan Inupiat Eskimo population. *J Rheumatol* **15**:678, 1988

27. Michet CJ et al: Epidemiology of Reiter's syndrome in Rochester, Minnesota: 1950–1980. *Arthritis Rheum* **31**:428, 1988

28. Arnett FC et al: Incomplete Reiter's syndrome: Discriminating features and HLA-W27 in diagnosis. *Ann Intern Med* **84**:8, 1976

29. West SG, Lawless OJ: The chronic disability of Reiter's syndrome in the US Army. *Arthritis Rheum* **24**:S78, 1981

30. Paronen I: Reiter's disease. Study of 344 cases observed in Finland. *Acta Med Scand* **212**(suppl):1, 1948

31. Noer HR: An "experimental" epidemic of Reiter's syndrome. *JAMA* **198**:693, 1966

32. Aho K et al: HL-A27 in reactive arthritis. A study of *Yersinia* arthritis and Reiter's disease. *Arthritis Rheum* **17**:521, 1974

33. Hakansson U et al: HL-A27 and reactive arthritis in an outbreak of salmonellosis. *Tissue Antigens* **6**:366, 1975

34. Kaslow RA et al: Search for Reiter's syndrome after an outbreak of *Shigella sonnei* dysentery. *J Rheumatol* **6**:562, 1979

35. Manson Bahr PH: *The Dysenteric Disorders*. London, Cassel, 1991, p 71

36. Lindley RI et al: *Yersinia pseudotuberculosis* infection as a cause of reactive arthritis as seen in a genitourinary clinic: Case report. *Genitourin Med* **65**:255, 1989

37. Hayward RS et al: Relapsing *Clostridium difficile* colitis and Reiter's syndrome. *Am J Gastroenterol* **85**:752, 1990

38. Stieglitz H et al: Identification of a 2-Md plasmid from *Shigella flexneri* associated with reactive arthritis. *Arthritis Rheum* **32**:937, 1989

39. Wollenhaupt J et al: Clamydia-induced arthritis: Diagnosis— follow-up—therapy. *Wien Med Wochenschr* **140**:302, 1990

40. Schumacher HR Jr et al: Light and electron microscopic studies on the synovial membrane in Reiter's syndrome. Immunocytochemical identification of chlamydial antigen in patients with early disease. *Arthritis Rheum* **31**:937, 1988

41. Inman RD, Morrison RP: Immunoblot analysis of reactivity to chlamydial 57kD heat shock protein in Reiter's syndrome (RS) (abstract). *Arthritis Rheum* **33**:S26, 1990

42. Granfors K: Measurement of immunoglobulin M (IgM), IgG and IgA antibodies against *Yersinia enterocolitica* by enzyme-linked immunosorbent assay: Persistence of serum antibodies during disease. *J Clin Microbiol* **9**:336, 1979

43. Granfors K et al: Analysis of IgA anti-lipolysaccharide antibodies in *Yersinia*-triggered reactive arthritis. *J Infect Dis* **159**:1142, 1989

44. van Bohemen CG et al: HLA-B27M1M2 and high immune responsiveness to *Shigella flexneri* in post-dysenteric arthritis. *Immunol Lett* **13**:71, 1986

45. Gaston JS et al: In vitro responses to a 65-kilodalton mycobacterial protein by synovial T cells from inflammatory arthritis patients. *J Immunol* **143**:2494, 1989

46. Inman RD et al: HLA class I-related impairment in IL-2 production and lymphocyte response to microbial antigens in reactive arthritis. *J Immunol* **142**:4256, 1989

47. Hill JL, Lu DTY: Development of an experimental animal model for reactive arthritis induced by *Yersinia enterocolitica*. *Infect Immun* **55**:721, 1987

48. Keat A et al: *Chlamydia trachomatis* and reactive arthritis: The missing link. *Lancet* **1**:72, 1987

49. Granfors K et al: *Yersinia* antigens in synovial fluid cells from patients with reactive arthritis. *N Engl J Med* **320**:216, 1989

50. Granfors K et al: *Salmonella* lipopolysaccharide in synovial cells from patients with reactive arthritis. *Lancet* **335**:685, 1990

51. Schumacher HR Jr et al: Light and electron microscopic studies on the synovial membrane in Reiter's syndrome. Immunocytochemical identification of Chlamydial antigens in patients with early disease. *Arthritis Rheum* **31**:937, 1988

52. Hochberg MD et al: Family studies in HLA-B27 associated arthritis. *Medicine (Baltimore)* **57**:463, 1978

53. Yunus M et al: Family studies with HLA typing in Reiter's syndrome. *Am J Med* **70**:1210, 1981

54. Calin A et al: Familial aggregation of Reiter's syndrome and ankylosing spondylitis: A comparative study. *J Rheumatol* **11**:672, 1984

55. Kaslow R et al: Reiter's disease following epidemic shigellosis. *J Rheumatol* **8**:969, 1981

56. Inman RD: Postdysenteric reactive arthritis. A clinical and immunogenetic study following an outbreak of Salmonellosis. *Arthritis Rheum* **31**:1377, 1988

57. Khan MA et al: Low association of HLA-B27 with Reiter's syndrome in blacks. *Ann Intern Med* **90**:202, 1979

58. Winchester R et al: Implications from the occurrence of Reiter's syndrome and related disorders in association with advanced HIV infection. *Scand J Rheumatol* **74**:89, 1988

59. Lopez de Castro JA: HLA-B27 and HLA-A2 subtypes: Structure, evolution and function. *Immunol Today* **10**:239, 1989

60. van Seventer GA et al: Public determinants of the HLA-B7 CREG defined by antibodies and T-cell clones, in *Immunobiology of HLA*, edited by B DuPont. New York, Springer-Verlag, 1989, p 204

61. Hill AVS et al: HLA class I typing by PCR: HLA-B27 and an African B27 subtype. *Lancet* **337**:640, 1991

62. Calin A, Fries JF: An "experimental" epidemic of Reiter's syndrome revisited: Follow-up evidence on genetic and environmental factors. *Ann Intern Med* **84**:564, 1976

63. Battisto JR et al: Susceptibility to adjuvant arthritis in DA and F344 rats: A dominant trait controlled by an autosomal gene locus linked to the MHC. *Arthritis Rheum* **25**:1194, 1982

64. Nickerson CL et al: Role of enterobacteria and HLA-B27 in spondyloarthropathies: Studies with transgenic mice. *Ann Rheum Dis* **49**:426, 1990

65. Hammer RE et al: Spontaneous inflammatory disease in transgenic rats expressing HLA-B27 and human β_2m: An animal model of HLA-B27-associated human disorders. *Cell* **63**:1099, 1990

66. Inman RD: Immunogenetic aspects of host immune response. *Can J Microbiol* **34**:319, 1988

67. Winchester R et al: Immune recognition events in rheumatic disease mediated by polymorphic MHC molecules, in *The Second Swiss Seminar in Advanced Rheumatology, Bad Ragaz, 1989*, edited by F Hasler. Bad Ragaz, CIBA-GEIGY, p 29

68. Kappler J et al: Vβ-specific stimulation of human T cells by staphylococcal toxins. *Science* **244**:813, 1989

69. Schwimmbeck PL et al: Autoantibodies to HLA-B27 in the sera of HLA-B27 patients with ankylosing spondylitis and Reiter's syndrome: Molecular mimicry with *Klebsiella pneumoniae* nitrogenase reductase as potential mechanisms of autoimmune disease. *J Exp Med* **166**:173, 1987

70. Raybourne RB et al: Reaction of anti-HLA-B monoclonal antibodies with envelope proteins of *Shigella* species. Evidence for molecular mimicry in the spondyloarthropathies. *J Immunol* **140**:3489, 1988

71. Tsuchiya N et al: Autoantibodies to the HLA-B27 sequence cross-reactive with the hypothetical peptide from the arthritis-associated *Shigella* plasmid. *J Clin Invest* **86**:1193, 1990

72. Ewing C et al: Antibody activity in ankylosing spondylitis sera to two sites on HLA-B27.1 at the MHC groove region (within sequence 65–85), and to a *Klebsiella pneumoniae* nitrogenase reductase peptide (within sequence 181–199). *J Exp Med* **171**:1635, 1990

73. Cavender DE, Ziff M: Absence of Antienterobacteriaceae and anti-HLA-B27 antibodies in mitogen stimulated cultures of lymphocytes from patients with Reiter's syndrome and ankylosing spondylitis. *J Rheumatol* **15**:315, 1988

74. Calin A, Fries JF: The striking prevalence of ankylosing spondylitis in "healthy" W27 positive males and females. A controlled study. *N Engl J Med* **293**:835, 1975

75. Cuvelier C et al: Histopathology of intestinal inflammation related to reactive arthritis. *Gut* **28**:394, 1987

76. Miller LD et al: Amyloidosis in Reiter's syndrome. *J Rheumatol* **6**:225, 1979

77. Anderson CJ et al: Amyloidosis and Reiter's syndrome: Report of a case and review of the literature. *Am J Kidney Dis* **14**:319, 1989

78. Omdal R, Husby G: Renal affection in patients with ankylosing spondylitis and psoriatic arthritis. *Clin Rheumatol* **6**:74, 1987

79. Harkness AH: Reiter's disease. *Br Med J* **1**:72, 1947

80. Aho K et al: HLA B27 in reactive arthritis following infection. *Ann Rheum Dis* **34**(suppl 1):29, 1975

81. Grumet FC et al: Monoclonal antibody (B27M2) subdividing HLA-B27. *Hum Immunol* **5**:61, 1982

82. Xing-hua C, Gui-ying S: Reiter's syndrome: Clinical analysis of 22 cases. *Chinese Med J* **95**:533, 1982

83. Hancock JAH: Surface manifestations of Reiter's disease in the male. *Br J Venereol Dis* **36**:36, 1960

84. Oates JK, Young AC: Sacroiliitis in Reiter's disease. *Br Med J* **1**:1013, 1959

85. McEwen C et al: Ankylosing spondylitis and spondylitis accompanying ulcerative colitis, regional enteritis, psoriasis, and Reiter's disease. *Arthritis Rheum* **14**:291, 1971

86. Calin A et al: The clinical history as a screening test for ankylosing spondylitis. *JAMA* **237**:2613, 1977

87. Sairanen D et al: Reiter's syndrome: A follow-up study. *Acta Med Scand* **185**:57, 1969

88. Ford DK: Arthritis and venereal disease. *Br J Venereol Dis* **29**:123, 1953

89. Oates JK, Hancock JAH: Neurological symptoms and lesions occurring in the course of Reiter's disease. *Am J Med Sci* **238**:79, 1959

90. Belz J et al: Characterization of uveitis associated with spondyloarthritis. *J Am Acad Dermatol* **20**:898, 1989

91. Hall WH, Finegold S: A study of 23 cases of Reiter's syndrome. *Ann Intern Med* **38**:533, 1953

92. Csonka GW, Oates JK: Pericarditis and electrocardiographic changes in Reiter's syndrome. *Br Med J* **1**:866, 1957

93. Tucker CR et al: Aortitis in ankylosing spondylitis: Early detection of aortic root abnormalities with two-dimensional echocardiography. *Am J Cardiol* **9**:680, 1982

94. Haverman JF et al: Atrioventricular conduction disturbance as an early feature of Reiter's syndrome. *Ann Rheum Dis* **47**:1017, 1988

95. Bergfeldt L et al: HLA-B27: An important genetic risk factor for lone aortic regurgitation and severe conduction system abnormalities. *Am J Med* **85**:12, 1988

96. Hancock JAH: In *Recent Advances in Venerology*, edited by A King. London, Churchill, 1964, p 395

97. Thiers H, Pinet A: Syndrome de Reiter avec uretrite a inclusions, infiltrat pulmonaire labile et keratodermie. *Lyons Med* **184**:51, 1950

98. Csonka GW: Involvement of the nervous system in Reiter's syndrome. *Ann Rheum Dis* **17**:334, 1958

99. McMillan A: Reiter's disease in a female, presenting as erythema nodosum. *Br J Venereol Dis* **51**:345, 1975

100. Bleehen SS et al: Amyloidosis complicating Reiter's syndrome. *Br J Venereol Dis* **42**:88, 1966

101. Inman RD et al: Immunochemical analysis of immune response to *Chlamydia trachomatis* in Reiter's syndrome and nonspecific urethritis. *Clin Exp Immunol* **69**:246, 1987

102. Inman RD et al: Analysis of serum and synovial fluid IgA in Reiter's syndrome and reactive arthritis. *Clin Immunol Immunopathol* **43**(2):195, 1987

103. Calin A: HLA-B27: To type or not to type? *Ann Rheum Dis* **34**:468, 1975

104. Calin A: HLA-B27 in 1982. Reappraisal of a clinical test. *Ann Intern Med* **96**:114, 1982

105. Brewerton DA et al: HL-A 27 and arthropathies associated with ulcerative colitis and psoriasis. *Lancet* **1**:956, 1974

106. McClusky OE et al: HLA-B27 in Reiter's syndrome and psoriatic arthritis. A genetic factor in disease susceptibility and expression. *J Rheumatol* **1**:263, 1974

107. Leirisalo-Repo M et al: Follow-up study of Reiter's disease and reactive arthritis. Factors influencing the natural course and the prognosis. *Clin Rheumatol* **6**(suppl 2):73, 1987

108. Fostiropoulos G et al: Total hemolytic complement (CH50) and second component of complement (C2 hu) activity in serum and synovial fluid. *Arthritis Rheum* **8**:219, 1965

109. Saxne T et al: Cartilage proteoglycans in synovial fluid and serum in patients with inflammatory joint disease. Relation to systemic treatment. *Arthritis Rheum* **30**:972, 1987

110. Moll JM: Seronegative arthropathies in the foot. *Baillieres Clin Rheumatol* **1**:289, 1987

111. Gilkes JJ: Skin and nail changes in the arthritic foot. *Baillieres Clin Rheumatol* **1**:335, 1987

112. Yunus MB: Current therapeutic practices in spondyloarthropathies. *Compr Ther* **14**:54, 1988

113. Katz P: Reiter's syndrome, in *Current Therapy in Allergy, Immunology and Rheumatology* 3d ed, edited by LM Lichtenstein, AS Fauci. Toronto, BC Decker, 1988, p 121

114. Stroehmann I et al: Therapy of seronegative oligoarthritis with salazopyrine. *Z Rheumatol* **46**:79, 1987

115. Kohler S et al: Pancytopenia during low-dose oral methotrexate therapy of psoriatic arthritis. *Dtsch Med Wochenschr* **114**:1286, 1989

116. Black RL et al: Methotrexate therapy in psoriatic arthritis. *JAMA* **189**:743, 1964

117. Nyfors A: Benefits and adverse drug experiences during long-term methotrexate treatment of 248 psoriatics. *Dan Med Bull* **25**:208, 1978

118. Szanto E et al: Hepatotoxicity associated with low-dose, long-term methotrexate treatment of rheumatoid arthritis. *Scand J Rheumatol* **16**:229, 1987

119. Kevat S et al: Hepatotoxicity of methotrexate in rheumatic diseases. *Med Toxicol Adverse Drug Exp* **3**:197, 1988

120. Brick JE et al: Prospective analysis of liver biopsies before and after methotrexate therapy in rheumatoid patients. *Semin Arthritis Rheum* **19**:31, 1989

121. Shergy WJ et al: Methotrexate-associated hepatotoxicity: Retrospective analysis of 210 patients with rheumatoid arthritis. *Am J Med* **85**:771, 1988

122. Bjorkman DJ et al: Hepatic ultrastructure after methotrexate therapy for rheumatoid arthritis. *Arthritis Rheum* **31**:1465, 1988

123. Hand SH et al: Methotrexate pneumonitis: A case report and summary of the literature. *J Med Assoc Ga* **78**:625, 1989

124. Altz-Smith M et al: Cryptococcosis associated with low-dose methotrexate for arthritis. *Am J Med* **83**:179, 1987

125. Wallis PJ et al: *Pneumocystis carinii* pneumonia complicating low dose methotrexate treatment for psoriatic arthropathy. *Ann Rheum Dis* **48**:247, 1989

126. Wernick R, Smith DL: Central nervous system toxicity associated with weekly low-dose methotrexate treatment. *Arthritis Rheum* **32**:770, 1989

127. Bjorkman PJ et al: Structure of the human class I histocompatibility antigen, HLA-A2. *Nature* **329**:506, 1987

CHAPTER 181

Elaine Alexander

Skin Manifestations of Sjögren's Syndrome

Since the publication in 1933 of Henrik Sjögren's monograph[1] describing the sicca complex—the triad of keratoconjunctivitis sicca, xerostomia, and arthritis—there has been an ever-expanding appreciation of the multifaceted complexities of Sjögren's syndrome (SS). SS is an autoimmune glandular exocrinopathy[2] associated with lymphocytic inflammatory infiltrates and varying degrees of exocrine gland dysfunction and destruction. Although ocular and oral exocrine glands are affected most commonly, giving rise to sicca (dryness) symptoms, mucous glands in multiple other organs including the skin are also involved frequently. The mechanisms of glandular dysfunction are unknown but are not simply related to inflammation and destruction. SS may be accompanied by extraglandular manifestations that include organ-specific autoimmune disorders and a spectrum of lymphoproliferative disorders including lymphoma. Recently, nervous system complications, both peripheral and central,[3] and inflammatory vascular disease (IVD) (vasculitis)[4] have been recognized as additional extraglandular complications of SS.

SS is a common autoimmune connective tissue disease, which has been estimated conservatively to affect at least 2 percent of the adult population (>4 million Americans). SS is at least as common as rheumatoid arthritis (RA) and approximately 1000-fold more common than systemic lupus erythematosus (SLE). Although comprehensive epidemiologic studies have not been performed, a study[5] of 103 elderly women in a retirement community demonstrated definite SS in 2, probable SS in 12, and anti-Ro(SS-A) antibodies in 7. One resident had RA, and none had SLE or another rheumatic disorder. A recent Scandinavian study[6] documented definite SS in 2.7 percent of a reportedly normal elderly population. Definite primary SS was documented in 4.8 percent of a Greek geriatric population with no evidence of connective tissue disease.[7] These studies suggest that the frequency of SS may be higher than currently estimated.

SS has been defined as primary (occurring alone) or secondary (occurring in association with another connective tissue disease or lymphoproliferative disorder). There are no established American College of Rheumatology criteria for the diagnosis of SS. Several groups, however, have proposed criteria.[8] In general, ocular involvement in SS is confirmed by the presence of an abnormal Schirmer's test (≤5-mm filter paper moistening within 5 min) and positive rose bengal dye staining or abnormal slit-lamp examination. The oral manifestations of SS are diagnosed by abnormal baseline and stimulated salivary flow studies, sialography, salivary scintigraphy, or, most commonly, minor salivary gland biopsy showing focal lymphocytic inflammatory infiltrates.[9]

An abnormal ocular examination and salivary gland biopsy are considered 95 percent sensitive and 82 percent specific in the diagnosis of SS.[10] However, these criteria have been designed for research purposes. In clinical settings, the criteria are useful if they are diagnostic. Early in the course of disease or with mild disease, these diagnostic studies may be equivocally abnormal but not diagnostic. Ocular and oral symptoms and, therefore, abnormal diagnostic studies do not necessarily evolve at the same rate. Because SS is a chronic progressive disease, its manifestations may evolve slowly and insidiously, and so evaluation and establishment of diagnosis is an ongoing process, rather than a static one. Some investigators have proposed the presence of anti-Ro(SS-A)/La(SS-B) antibodies as an additional diagnostic criterion for SS.[11] Autoantibodies to Ro(SS-A)/La(SS-B) are primarily associated with SS, SLE, and presumed lupus variants (see below).[12] They are uncommon in other connective tissue diseases.[12] Approximately 40 to 50 percent of patients with SS have significant titers of precipitating autoantibodies to Ro(SS-A) [and less commonly La(SS-B)], IgG (rheumatoid factor), and nuclear antigen (ANA); and a smaller proportion may have hyperglobulinemia with polyclonal gammopathy, and/or cryoglobulinemia.[12,13] The presence of anti-Ro(SS-A)/La(SS-B) antibodies in a patient with sicca symptoms suggests primary SS or the Sjögren's/lupus (SS/LE) overlap syndrome. However, more than half of patients with primary SS are seronegative for anti-Ro(SS-A)/La(SS-B) as well as for other autoantibodies. Patients with SS who are seronegative by standard techniques for anti-Ro(SS-A)/La(SS-B) antibodies are usually also seronegative for autoantibodies to other specificities.[13] Thus, the absence of serum autoantibodies does not exclude the diagnosis of SS.

SS, despite its relatively high prevalence, is often underrecognized and underdiagnosed. There are a number of explanations for why SS has been relegated to the position of an "orphan disease":

1. There is a general lack of physician awareness of disease existence, manifestations, diagnosis, evaluation, and therapy. SS predominantly affects middle-aged women (9 women:1 man). However, it is not generally recognized that SS can affect children, adolescents, young women, and men.

2. Symptoms and external stigmata of this chronic progressive disorder may be subtle and insidious and, therefore, unrecognized by both patient and physician. Unlike SLE, SS seldom has acute protean disease flares. The arthritis of SS, in contrast to RA, is nondeforming and nonerosive.

3. Signs and symptoms of the sicca (dryness) syndrome may be attributed incorrectly to the normal aging process.

4. Multiple, often complex, complaints are often dismissed as being functional, hypochondriacal, or neurotic.

5. Multisystem complaints may make patients multi-doctor shoppers, often inadvertently precluding accurate diagnosis and effective doctor-patient relationships.

6. Cognitive and/or psychiatric impairment may modify patient perception of disease and ability to relate complaints and may impair meaningful and reliable interactions with physicians.

7. Sicca complaints and associated nonspecific musculoskeletal complaints are often considered nonconsequential annoyances rather than significant medical problems. The ubiquitous and often disabling general musculoskeletal complaints of SS (i.e., fatigue, malaise, myalgia, arthralgias, low-grade fever, recurrent lymphadenopathy, depression, attention/concentration deficits) are often attributed to "chronic fatigue syndrome" or fibromyalgia/fibrositis.

8. One or more of the many potential extraglandular manifestations of SS may not be appreciated or linked to underlying SS.

9. SS is the great mimicker. SS can mimic or coexist with many other autoimmune organ-specific, hematologic, or neurologic disorders. Thus, patients with SS are "tucked away" in general/family practice, multiple internal medicine subspecialties, ophthalmology, otolaryngology, neurology, psychiatry, dermatology, obstetrics, gynecology, and the like.

10. Patients with SS may be seronegative for autoantibodies. Not all patients with definite SS have one or more autoantibodies [i.e., anti-Ro(SS-A)/La(SS-B) antibodies, rheumatoid factor, ANA]. Approximately 40 to 60 percent of patients with SS are seronegative for these autoantibodies.

11. Patients with SS who meet only four nonspecific criteria for SLE (i.e., ANA, arthritis, cytopenia, central nervous system disease) are often misdiagnosed as having SLE. Such patients are seldom evaluated for SS.

12. Until recently, lack of patient advocacy programs has limited awareness of this disease. More efforts are needed to educate physicians and patients.

Glandular Cutaneous Manifestations of SS

The cutaneous manifestations of SS can be considered as *glandular* and *extraglandular*. The glandular cutaneous involvement in SS shares clinical features with the autoimmune glandular exocrinopathy (Table 181-1). Patients with SS commonly complain of skin dryness (23 to 67 percent).[14] Cutaneous sicca is characterized by xerosis or xeroderma (dry skin), often associated with pruritus and scaling, and, less commonly, pigmentation abnormalities and hypohydrosis (decreased sweating). The mechanisms that cause skin dryness and potential hypohydrosis have not been established. The cutaneous glands moisturize and lubricate the skin (sebaceous), produce sweat (eccrine), and secrete odiforous substances (apocrine). It is therefore reasonable to conclude that SS patients with xerosis and hypohydrosis have cutaneous glands that do not function normally or are destroyed. However, there is very little documentation of this postulate in the literature. The results of pilocarpine stimulation tests have been variable.[15] Biopsy documentation of periappendigeal lymphocytic infiltration and sebaceous gland atrophy has been reported in only a small number of SS cases with severe xerosis or hypohydrosis.[15-18] In contrast, dermal lymphocytic perivascular infiltrates have been observed more commonly.[16]

These observations suggest that other mechanisms may contribute to cutaneous glandular dysfunction in SS. Central and peripheral nervous system disease (sensory and autonomic neuropathy) can influence glandular secretion. SS patients can develop central nervous system disease[3] and commonly have peripheral neuropathy (particularly sensory and autonomic).[3,19,20] The neuropathies may be caused by IVD of the vaso nervorem.[3,19,20] Therefore, hypohydrosis in SS, at least in part, may have a neurogenic etiology that in some way impairs postglanglionic sympathetic fiber function.

Although alopecia is generally associated with SLE or systemic sclerosis, it may also develop in patients with SS. Decreased head, body, and pubic hair have been observed in patients with SS.

TABLE 181-1
Glandular Cutaneous Disease in Sjögren's Syndrome

	Cutaneous glands	
	Sebaceous	Eccrine
Cutaneous features		
Dry skin (xerosis)	+	−
Decreased sweating (hypohydrosis)	−	+
Gland dysfunction		
Pilocarpine stimulation test	−	Variable
Histopathology		
Gland destruction	Rare	Rare
Lymphocytic infiltrate		
Periappendigeal	Unusual	Unusual
Perivascular	More common	More common

All these cutaneous manifestations tend to result in the insidious development of the appearance of premature aging.

Although xerosis is the most common cutaneous manifestation of SS, involvement of contiguous mucocutaneous organs both externally and internally (''the internal skin'') gives rise to other sicca symptoms. In addition to the classic ocular symptoms associated with keratoconjunctivitis sicca (dry eyes), i.e., burning, itching, grittiness, foreign-body sensation, photophobia, matting, dryness, and decreased lacrimation, SS patients may develop palpebral and bulbar conjunctival injection, blepharitis (scaling and redness of the eyelids), blepharospasm, and ocular infections. Oral symptoms associated with xerostomia (dry mouth) include oral dryness, burning, dysphagia, stomatitis, dental caries, receding gums, pyorrhea, and halitosis. The lips are dry, the perioral skin is wrinkled and pursed, and there is angular cheilosis. There are abnormalities of taste and smell.

Mucous gland-containing structures adjacent to the oral cavity are also involved (i.e., nasopharynx, oropharnyx, sinuses, and ears). There is dryness and crusting of the nasal passages and posterior oropharynx. Mucous membrane dryness in the sinuses may result in edema, inspissated secretions, and obstruction. The external auditory canal has eczematous changes (pruritus, scaling, and crusting) with dry, potentially impacted cerumen. The eustachian tubes are also dry and may be obstructed. The dryness of the mucous membranes and the attendant breakdown of the normal, local protective mechanisms of the nasopharynx, sinuses, and ears predispose to recurrent or chronic infections such as pharyngitis, tonsillitis, sinusitis, otitis externa/media, and epistaxis. Each of these conditions is worsened or exacerbated by environmental conditions with low humidity, forced-air heating or cooling, high altitude, pollution, or environmental toxins. Dryness of the mucous membranes of the upper respiratory tract results in laryngitis sicca (hoarseness) and tracheobronchitis sicca (chronic dry nonproductive cough).

Episodic or recurrent major (parotid, submandibular, sublingual) salivary gland enlargement may occur, and the etiologies may be multifactorial. Lymph node enlargement, salivary gland duct stones with partial or complete obstruction, inspissated gravel or salivary secretions, or infection may occur. Fixed or enlarging masses may represent a developing salivary gland tumor or lymphoma (see below).

Vaginitis sicca is caused by the involvement of the glands within the vulva, cervix, and vagina and is accompanied by complaints of vaginal dryness, burning, pruritus, dyspareunia, and recurrent vaginal infections (e.g., yeast). Chronic interstitial cystitis is also secondary to SS.

Extraglandular Cutaneous Manifestations of SS

Inflammatory Vascular Disease

Clinical Features   Most of the extraglandular cutaneous manifestations of SS are secondary to vascular involvement of one type or another (Table 181-2). IVD is an extraglandular complication of SS[4,13,21-23] and occurs in approximately 20 to 30 percent of patients with SS.[7,13,14,21-23] Cutaneous IVD has a protracted course with exacerbation and remission and may become chronic. IVD

TABLE 181-2
Extraglandular Cutaneous Disease in Sjögren's Syndrome

Prominent inflammatory vascular involvement
  Inflammatory vascular disease
    Vasculopathy
    Vasculitis
  Lymphoproliferative disorders (lymphoma)
    Non-Hodgkin's B-cell
    T-cell
  Waldenström's benign hyperglobulinemia purpura
  Mixed cryoglobulinemia
  Idiopathic thrombocytopenic purpura
  Thrombotic thrombocytopenic purpura
  Chronic graft-versus-host disease
  Sweet's syndrome
Perivascular inflammation
  Subacute cutaneous lupus erythematosus
  Neonatal lupus erythematosus
  SS/LE overlap syndrome
Noninflammatory vascular disease
  Raynaud's phenomenon
  Livedo reticularis
Other
  Dermatitis herpetiformis

may be peripheral (skin, nerve, and muscle),[2] systemic (involving one or more organs),[4] or may involve the central nervous system (brain and/or spinal cord).[3,4] Cutaneous IVD mirrors IVD in other organs temporally and histopathologically and may be a marker for concomitant systemic or nervous system IVD.[24] Cutaneous lesions in SS are commonly overlooked by clinicians as a potential manifestation of vascular inflammation. The spectrum of cutaneous manifestations of IVD in SS are presented in Table 181-3.

The most common cutaneous manifestations of IVD in SS are palpable purpura and petechiae (predominantly, but not exclusively, involving the lower extremities)[4] (Fig. 181-1) These lesions are indistinguishable from those described as benign hypergammaglobulinemic purpura by Waldenström.[25,26] The latter lesions have been observed in a minority of SS patients.[16,27,28] It has been estimated that 20 to 30 percent of patients with benign hypergammaglobulinema purpura will develop SS.[2] Purpuric lesions in SS may occur in the setting of mixed essential cryoglobulinemia. SS has been observed in a significant proportion of patients described as having mixed essential cryoglobulinemia.[29,30]

The second most common cutaneous manifestation of IVD in SS is urticaria, usually chronic (persisting more than 6 weeks) (Table 181-3; Fig. 181-2).[4] These lesions are indistinguishable from those observed in hypocomplementemic urticarial vasculitis.[31] Other cutaneous presentations of IVD in SS include subcutaneous nodules (erythema nodosum lesions), erythema multiforme,

TABLE 181-3
Cutaneous Manifestations of Inflammatory Vascular Disease in Sjögren's Syndrome

Palpable purpura
Petechiae
Chronic urticaria
Nodules (erythema nodosum)
Erythema multiforme
Necrotizing panniculitis
Infarcts
Ulcers
Gangrene

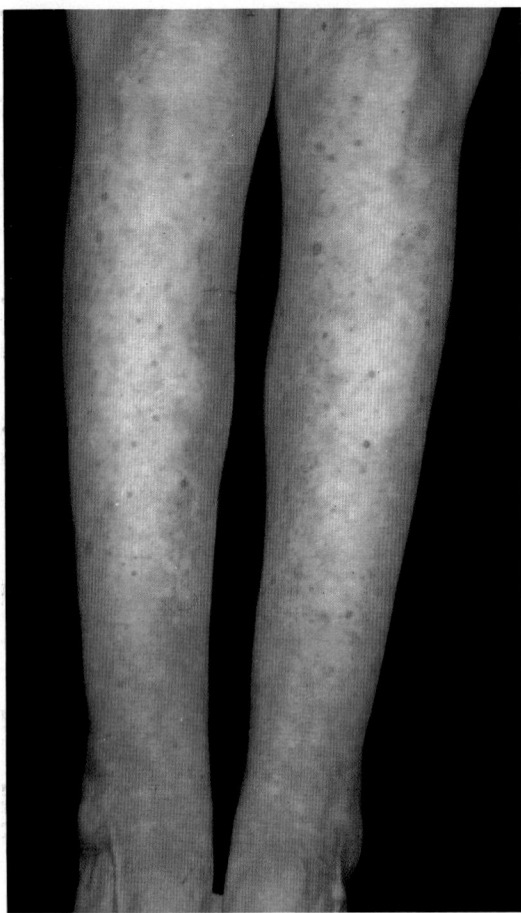

FIGURE 181-1 Lower extremity palpable purpura in an anti-Ro(SS-A) antibody-positive woman with neutrophilic inflammatory vascular disease and central nervous system disease. Patients with mononuclear inflammatory vascular disease may also have palpable purpura.

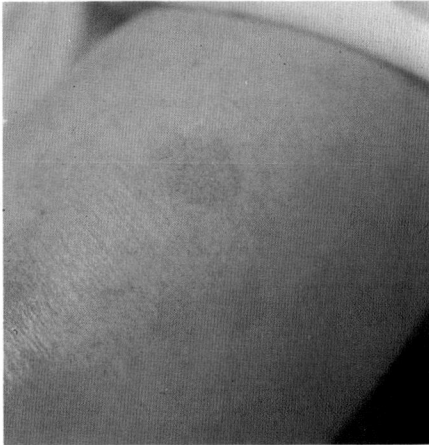

FIGURE 181-2 Chronic urticarial lesions in an anti-Ro(SS-A) antibody-negative patient with mononuclear inflammatory vascular disease and central nervous system disease. Patients with neutrophilic inflammatory vascular disease may also have chronic urticaria.

trophilic) to chronic (lymphocytic) types of IVD. First, individual patients have recurrent episodes of the same histopathologic type of IVD over time. Neutrophilic, as well as lymphocytic, IVD may be chronic and recurrent and persist for years (>40). Although it is possible that lymphocytic IVD is preceded by a brief transient influx of neutrophils, some patients have chronic neutrophilic IVD throughout the course of their illness, irrespective of the age of evolution of the cutaneous lesions. Second, lesions biopsied early in their evolution also show a similar histopathologic dichotomy. Third, both histopathologic types of IVD are associated with similar clinical cutaneous lesions. Fourth, systemic, as well as peripheral, IVD is also of two histopathologic types. Fifth, there are consistent differences in the serologic profile and complement proteins between these two types of peripheral and systemic IVD (see below). These observations strongly suggest that chronic persistent or recurrent IVD in SS may be of either histopathologic type and, within a given patient, tends to remain consistent over time.

necrotizing panniculitis, nonspecific erythematosus lesions, and, less commonly, ulcers, infarcts, or gangrene.[4]

Histopathology There are several important histopathologic features of cutaneous vascular lesions in SS.[4] We have described two distinct histopathologic types of IVD in SS: neutrophilic (leukocytoclastic) inflammatory vascular disease (Figs. 181-3, 181-4) and mononuclear (lymphocytic) inflammatory vascular disease[4,32] (Figs. 181-5, 181-6). These two histopathologic forms of necrotizing IVD in SS were first observed by Soter et al.[33] A subsequent study by Tsokos et al. confirmed these observations.[34]

Patients with recurrent episodes of cutaneous IVD generally have the same histopathologic type of disease recur over time. We have not observed a transition from neutrophilic to mononuclear IVD in individual patients, but we have observed the converse in a small subset of patients with SS. Both histopathologic forms of IVD are associated with the same clinical spectrum of cutaneous manifestations. It is not possible to predict the histopathologic type of IVD by the clinical appearance of the lesions. Both histopathologic types can induce significant vascular injury.

Several compelling observations support the hypothesis that there are two distinct histopathologic types of IVD in SS, rather than the traditionally conceived classic transition from acute (neu-

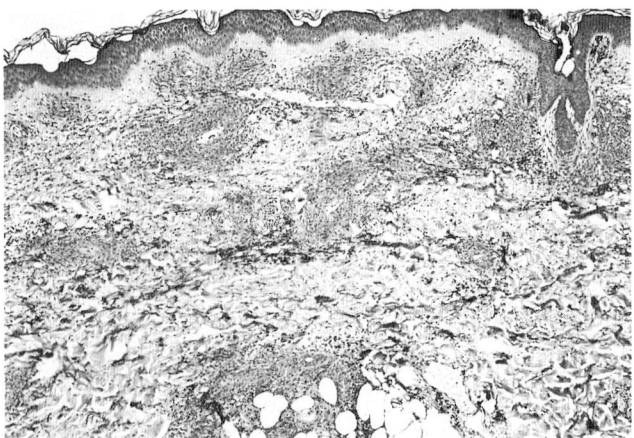

FIGURE 181-3 Neutrophilic inflammatory vascular disease involving vessels of superficial and deep dermis. Venules and arterioles are affected, and there is extensive necrosis of vessel walls with fibrin deposition and extravasation of erythrocytes. H&E, original magnification ×180.

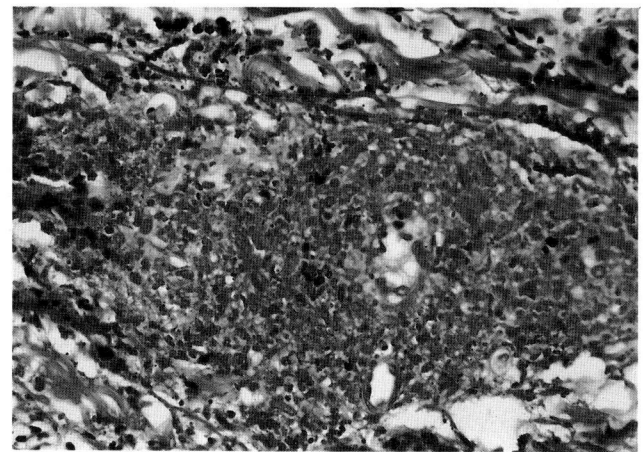

FIGURE 181-4 Early neutrophilic inflammatory vascular disease in a dermal arteriole. Endothelial cells are swollen and distorted, with lumen compromise. The integrity of the vessel wall architecture is disrupted with inflammatory infiltrates containing mononuclear cells and neutrophils. Nuclear dust is present. H&E, original magnification ×57.

IVD in SS has a predilection for certain types of blood vessels. Vessels within the upper dermis are affected most frequently, but deeper dermal vessels and vessels within subcutaneous adipose tissue also may be involved. Small vessels are preferentially affected, venules and postcapillary venules more commonly than arterioles and arteries. Finally, the cutaneous histopathologic changes mirror the IVD observed in other organs (see below).

Serologic Associations The two histopathologic types of IVD in SS have distinct serologic associations.[32] Neutrophilic IVD is characterized by a striking association with autoantibodies to Ro(SS-A) and La(SS-B) peptides, rheumatoid factor, and antinuclear antibodies. Cryoglobulins, if present, are seen in these patients. In contrast, mononuclear IVD occurs in the setting of seronegativity with respect to these autoantibodies.

The data described here are obtained from studies in which gel double-diffusion techniques were used to detect anti-Ro(SS-A) and La(SS-B) antibodies. More recent quantitative studies performed with a sensitive enzyme-linked immunosorbent assay (ELISA) using purified antigens indicate that almost all patients with SS possess Ro(SS-A) and La(SS-B) antibodies.[35] However, this ELISA technique also detects anti-Ro(SS-A) antibodies in up to 25 percent of normal controls.[12] These observations suggest that differences exist in the sensitivity and specificity of these assays. In general, Ro(SS-A) and La(SS-B) antibody detection by gel double-diffusion assay correlates with high titer antibody levels detected by ELISA, whereas a negative gel double-diffusion assay for Ro(SS-A) and La(SS-B) antibodies correlates with low titers of Ro(SS-A) and La(SS-B) antibodies.

Immune Complexes and Complement The two histopathologic types of IVD in SS are different in the quantity of circulating immune complexes.[36] IgG immune complexes, as measured by a solid-phase anti-C3 assay, are present at higher mean serum concentrations in patients with neutrophilic IVD than in patients with mononuclear IVD. There is no significant difference between the two groups with respect to immune complexes detected by a solid-phase anti-Clq binding assay. There are also differences in serum complement levels between these two groups of patients.[36] Patients with neutrophilic IVD have significantly lower mean total hemolytic complement levels than do patients with mononuclear IVD. Although there are no differences between the two groups in the mean concentrations of C3 or C4, decreased CH_{50} levels are associated with decreased concentrations of C4 and, to a lesser extent, C3. Other investigators have also found a difference in serum complement levels in the two histopathologic types of IVD. Soter et al.[33,37,38] have found that hypocomplementemia is more common in neutrophilic IVD. This form of SS vasculitis is indistinguishable from hypocomplementemia with an urticaria-like leukocytoclastic vasculitis.[39]

Serum SC5b-9 neoantigen has been observed in both histopathologic types of IVD in SS.[39] These observations indicate that the complement pathway is activated in both types of IVD, but to a greater extent in the neutrophilic form. Despite the evidence for activation of the complement pathway in IVD in SS, standard direct and indirect immunofluorescence techniques, performed on frozen

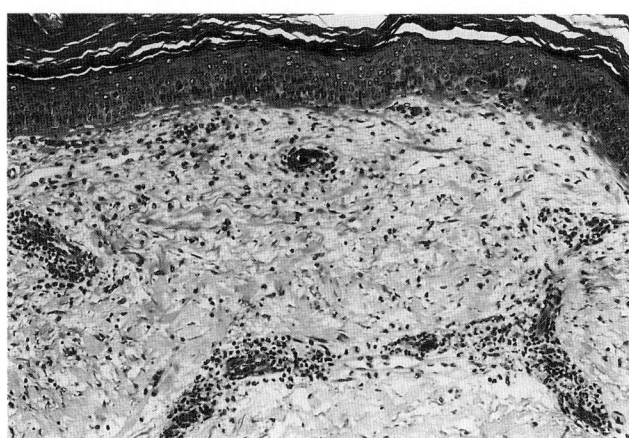

FIGURE 181-5 Mononuclear inflammatory vascular disease affecting venules and arterioles within superficial and deep dermis. H&E, original magnification ×800.

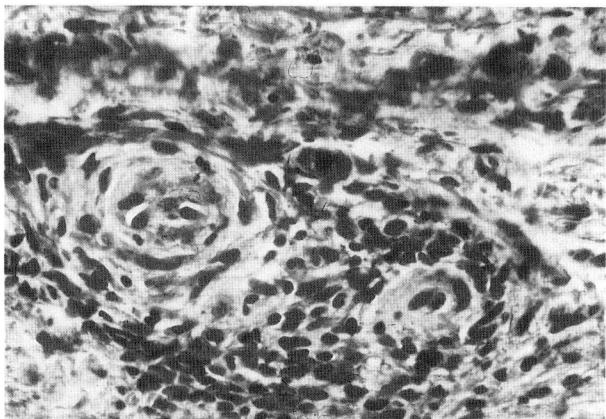

FIGURE 181-6 Mononuclear inflammatory vascular disease involving a small arteriole. Mononuclear cells surround and invade vessels, which show lumen clusion and erythrocyte extravasation. Lymphocytes and plasma cells are the predominant cell type. H&E, original magnification ×730.

sections of fresh involved vasculitic skin lesions, have demonstrated the vascular deposition of immunoglobulin or complement in only a minority of cases (Alexander, unpublished observation).

Relationship between Cutaneous IVD and Systemic or Central Nervous System IVD

Although central nervous system disease usually occurs in the absence of cutaneous IVD (particularly in early disease or young patients), the presence of recurrent or chronic peripheral (predominantly cutaneous) IVD in SS is often associated with concomitant, often subclinical systemic or neurologic disease.[3,4,24] Cutaneous IVD in SS should alert the physician to the potential presence of more extensive, systemic IVD or nervous system disease.

Both histopathologic types of cutaneous IVD can be associated with potentially serious central nervous system disease.[3,4,24] In one study, approximately two-thirds of patients with SS with biopsy-documented peripheral IVD had neurologic complications.[4] Subsequently, more than three-quarters of these patients have developed neurologic disease. Most commonly, the development of cutaneous lesions occurs concomitantly with the development of neurologic abnormalities, or may antedate the development of central nervous system disease by several years. Not uncommonly, chronic recurrent episodes of vasculitis may result in cutaneous hyperpigmentation (often diagnosed as chronic venous stasis or Schamberg's disease), which is not appreciated as a sequela of chronic IVD. Rarely, central nervous system disease antedates the development of manifestations of cutaneous IVD.

Central nervous system disease may be focal, nonfocal (psychiatric and/or cognitive dysfunction), or both.[3,40] It may mimic other neurologic disorders including multiple sclerosis, ALS, Guillain-Barré syndrome, Mollaret's meningitis, and Alzheimer's disease.[3,41] Brain magnetic resonance imaging (MRI) scans show multiple areas of increased signal intensity on T2 and proton density weighted images.[42] Analysis of cerebrospinal fluid indicates breach of the blood-brain barrier by lymphocytes with a mild mononuclear pleocytosis, intrathecal synthesis of IgG, and one or more (up to seven) clonal bands in one-half to two-thirds of patients with SS and active, progressive neurologic disease.[43,44] Histopathology demonstrates mononuclear (lymphocytic) meningeal and perivascular/vascular infiltrates (cerebral vasculopathy) with microinfarcts or hemorrhages.[3,45–47] A subset of individuals who are anti-Ro(SS-A) antibody positive, in contrast to those who are negative, may have larger (>10 mm) brain lesions on MRI, cerebral angiograms consistent with small vessel angiitis, and frank central nervous system vasculitis on histopathologic examination.[48,49] Anti-Ro(SS-A) antibody-positive patients may have catastrophic central nervous system complications (i.e., major subarachnoid or intracerebral hemorrhage).

There are similarities between the cerebral vasculopathy and cutaneous mononuclear IVD.[3,4] Mononuclear cells (predominantly lymphocytes) surround and, in some cases, invade cerebral/meningeal and cutaneous blood vessels. Small vessels are more commonly affected than large vessels. Venules and postcapillary venules are predominantly affected. Arteries and arterioles are less commonly involved and, if so, more prominently in anti-Ro(SS-A) antibody-positive individuals. Affected venules in both skin and brain show abnormal endothelial cells. At one end of the spectrum, endothelial cells are hypertrophied with the morphology of high endothelial venules. At the other extreme, varying degrees of endothelial cell damage are observed in association with micro/macro-

infarcts and/or -hemorrhages. We have not observed neutrophilic IVD within the brain, in contrast to the skin, even in the presence of concomitant systemic neutrophilic IVD and anti-Ro(SS-A) antibodies.

Cutaneous Manifestations of Lymphoproliferative Disorders Associated with SS

Patients with SS and lymphoproliferative disorders may have cutaneous lesions that are primarily a manifestation of coexistent vasculitis. Patients with SS have a 44-fold risk of developing lymphoma,[50] usually of the non-Hodgkin's B-cell type. Lymphoma is usually extraglandular, involving major parenchymal organs or lymph nodes, but lymphomatous involvement of the major salivary glands does occur. Patients with SS who develop lymphoma usually have several features of systemic extraglandular disease, including lymphadenopathy, splenomegaly, and pulmonary and/or renal infiltrates.[51] Cutaneous vasculitis (purpura) is frequent. Cutaneous lymphoma has been described in SS, particularly of the T-cell phenotype.[52] SS patients with hypergammaglobulemia, anti-Ro(SS-A) antibodies, and/or cryoglobulinemia may develop pseudolymphoma. If these patients develop frank malignancy (lymphoma), they may become hypogammaglobulinemic and lose serum autoantibodies.[51]

Cutaneous Features of Hematologic Disorders Associated with SS

Patients with SS develop autoantibodies against membrane constituents of hematopoietic cells, including lymphocytes, neutrophils, platelets, and erythrocytes. In the latter two cases, antiplatelet and antierythrocyte antibodies may give rise to idiopathic thrombocytopenic purpura (ITP) and autoimmune hemolytic anemia. ITP is associated with purpura and petechiae. Mothers with SS may passively transfer IgG antiplatelet antibodies to their neonates and induce ITP. Another hematologic disorder, thrombotic thrombocytopenic purpura, a clinical triad consisting of thrombocytopenic purpura, hemolytic anemia, and neurologic manifestations,[53] can occur in SS.[54] Since the reported cases were atypical for this disorder,[54] it may represent central nervous system SS with thrombosis.

Relationship between SS and the Presumed Lupus Variants

Primary SS is defined as an autoimmune exocrinopathy.[2] Classic SLE is characterized in its fulminant form as a disorder with prominent cutaneous manifestations, polyarthritis, polyserositis, glomerulonephritis, and central nervous system disease (particularly seizures and psychosis).[55] Antibodies to native-DNA and Sm are considered specific, but relatively insensitive, serologic markers for SLE.[55] Over the past 10 to 15 years, several disorders have been described that appear to be closely related to SLE; namely, subacute cutaneous lupus erythematosus (SCLE),[56] the Sjögren's syndrome/lupus erythematosus (SS/LE) overlap syndrome,[56–60] and the neonatal lupus erythematosus (NLE) syndrome.[61] Patients defined as having SS/LE overlap syndrome have definite SS and cutaneous manifestations of LE (SCLE skin lesions and/or photosensitivity).[57–60] Patients with SS and annular erythematosus lesions have been described.[62]

TABLE 181-4
Clinical, Serologic, and Immunogenetic Relationships between Primary SS,
Presumed Lupus Variants, and Classical SLE

	Disease category		
	Primary SS	Presumed lupus variants	Classical SLE
Clinical features			
Photosensitive dermatitis	−	+	+
SCLE-like skin lesions	−	+	−
Glomerulonephritis	−	−	+
Autoantibodies			
Ro(SS-A)/La(SS-B)	+ (often)	+ (almost always)	
nDNA	−	−	+
Sm	−	−	+
HLA class II alloantigens			
DR2	−	−	+
DR3	+	+/−	
DR3, DR5, or DRw6	+	+	−
DQw1	−	−	+
DQw2	+	+	−
DRw52	+	+	−

We have proposed that the presumed lupus variants are closely linked to each other clinically, serologically, and immunogenetically and are more closely linked to primary SS than to classical SLE (Table 181-4).[47] Clinically, each of the presumed lupus variants has prominent cutaneous features (SCLE skin lesions or photosensitivity) but few of the clinical features, such as glomerulonephritis, associated with classic SLE. SCLE is characterized by nonscarring, papulosquamous/psoriasiform or annular/polycyclic (or both) cutaneous lesions that occur in a characteristic photoexposed distribution.[63] The histopathology shows hyperkeratosis, follicular plugging, vacuolar degeneration of the basal cell layer, dermal atrophy, and perivascular inflammation. Some investigators have suggested that follicular plugging, hyperkeratosis, and density and depth of cellular infiltrates are considerably less severe than those in discoid LE lesions.[60] The mononuclear cell infiltrates are usually restricted to the perivascular and periappendageal regions of the upper one-third of the dermis. Patients with the SS/LE overlap syndrome and NLE syndrome infants develop skin lesions identical to SCLE clinically and histopathologically.[64]

Serologically, each of the presumed lupus variants has a high frequency of anti-Ro(SS-A) antibodies [a smaller proportion also has anti-La(SS-B) antibodies] but a virtual absence of autoantibodies (nDNA or Sm) associated with classic SLE.[47]

Immunogenetically, patients with the presumed lupus variants share HLA-class II alloantigen associations observed in primary SS.[47] Almost all patients are either HLA-DR3, -DR5, or -DRw6, three DR alloantigens that share amino acid sequences in the first hypervariable region of the DRβI peptide. Almost all patients are also HLA-DRw52, with which each of these three alloantigens is in linkage disequilibrium. In contrast, patients with classic SLE, glomerulonephritis, and anti-nDNA antibodies have an increased frequency of HLA-DR2, -DQw1, and specific DQB1 genes.[65]

The interrelationship among SS and the presumed lupus variants are depicted in Fig. 181-7. Patients with established SS may (often over a period of 20 to 40 years) develop clinical features of the presumed lupus variants or vice versa.[59] Likewise, most mothers who give birth to infants with NLE ultimately develop SS, cutaneous manifestations of LE, or both (SS/LE overlap syndrome). Thus, we propose that the presumed lupus variants are more closely linked nosologically to SS than to classic SLE. The classification of

patients with connective tissue disease into subcategories based on clinical, serologic, and immunogenetic features may be useful in clinical diagnosis and assessment.

Cutaneous Features of SS Occurring in Immunocompromised Hosts

An SS-like illness can develop in patients who are immunocompromised, particularly in chronic graft-versus-host disease (CGVHD) after allogenic bone marrow transplantation[66] and in retroviral illnesses (HIV and HTLV-1 infections). Patients with CGVHD develop cutaneous lesions that may be secondary to vasculitis.[67,68] Aplastic bone marrow transplant recipients treated with antithymocyte globulin have developed a serum sickness-like illness, including mononuclear cutaneous vasculitis.[69] When the granulocytes of these patients were reconstituted, the inflammatory vascular lesions changed from mononuclear to neutrophilic.[69]

HIV-associated salivary gland disease has been described in AIDS patients with parotid gland enlargement and sicca symptoms.[67] AIDS patients may develop a clinical syndrome clinically indistinguishable from SS, called diffuse infiltrative lymphocytosis syndrome, accompanied by bilateral parotid gland enlargement, xerophthalmia, and xerostomia.[68] In contrast to idiopathic primary

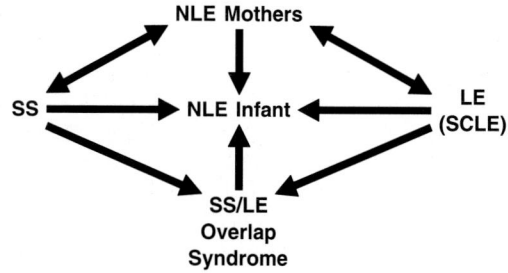

FIGURE 181-7 Interrelationship between primary Sjögren's syndrome (SS) and presumed lupus variants. LE, lupus erythematosus; NLE, neonatal LE; SCLE, systemic cutaneous LE.

SS, however, there are a peripheral CD8 (CD29) lymphocytosis and CD8+, in contrast to CD4+, lymphocytic infiltrates in the salivary glands and lungs. Patients with diffuse infiltrative lymphocytosis syndrome are usually HLA-DR5 (JVM variant) or HLA-DRw6, two alloantigens in almost all patients with primary SS and presumed lupus variants who are not HLA-DR3. Patients presenting with a SS-like illness should be tested for antibodies to HIV (HTLV-III) and HTLV-I.

Two other skin disorders of unknown etiology, dermatitis herpetiformis[70] and Sweet's syndrome,[71] have been observed in association with SS. Dermatitis herpetiformis is a chronic bullous dermatosis characterized by pruritic grouped papulovesicles distributed primarily over the extensor surfaces of the extremities, lower back, and buttocks.[70] Histopathology shows subepidermal vesicles that result from the coalescence of many neutrophilic microabscesses in the tips of dermal papillae. Patients with dermatitis herpetiformis may develop a gluten-sensitive enteropathy similar to those with adult celiac disease. Patients with primary SS and dermatitis herpetiformis both have a higher frequency of certain HLA phenotypes (HLA-B8, -DR3). Sweet's syndrome is a dermatologic disorder characterized by the presence of dull erythematous macules over the trunk and limbs.[71] Histologically, there is perivascular polymorphonuclear leukocyte infiltration and leukocytoclasis in the papillary and upper reticular dermis.

Noninflammatory Cutaneous Vascular Phenomena

Raynaud's phenomenon, triphasic peripheral digital vasospasm, occurs in approximately 20 percent of patients with SS.[14] It is also seen in a number of other rheumatic disorders such as systemic sclerosis and SLE. Livedo reticularis, cold-induced cyanotic mottling of the skin that has a characteristic "fish net" appearance, may involve the trunk as well as the extremities. These phenomena may occur alone or in association with vasculitis, cryoglobulinemia, and dysproteinemia associated with SS.

Treatment

SS is a chronic autoimmune disorder for which there is presently no cure. The treatment of glandular and extraglandular manifestations of SS is covered in detail elsewhere.[72] Briefly, treatment of the glandular exocrinopathy is symptomatic. Immunosuppressive intervention with such agents as corticosteroids, cyclophosphamide, cyclosporine, chlorambucil, and azathioprine is reserved for patients with severe progressive systemic complications, central nervous system disease, or lymphoproliferative disorders (lymphoma). Recently hydroxychloroquine has been proposed to treat patients with systemic SS, but controlled trials have not been performed.[73]

The cutaneous and mucocutaneous complications of SS are treated with modalities that preserve and restore moisture to the skin and mucous membranes. In general, the environment should prevent desiccation by enhancing humidity and should be free of pollutants and toxins. Hot baths and showers should be avoided, and the duration of exposure to water limited. Soaps containing a moisturizing cream are preferred. Moisturizing creams, particularly those that trap the body's natural moisture, should be applied while the skin is still wet. Newly available emollients contain lactic acid and alphahydroxy fatty acids and are good rehydrating agents. Ex-

cessive sun exposure should be avoided, and sun blocks should be used routinely to prevent premature aging of the skin and the predisposition for cutaneous malignancy. Hypoallergenic and nonscented cosmetics are preferred by some patients.

Vaginitis sicca is a serious symptom that may result in dyspareunia and impaired sexual performance and enjoyment. Standard lubricants are often effective in alleviating symptoms. Patients whose symptoms are not controlled by this method should be evaluated by a gynecologist to assess the need for topical or systemic hormonal supplementation and to insure that there are no attendant infections such as candidiasis.

All patients with SS syndrome and cutaneous vasculitis should be carefully evaluated for systemic or nervous system disease. Cutaneous vasculitis alone can be treated successfully with one or more drugs: hydroxychloroquine, colchicine, dapsone, or low doses of corticosteroids. Patients should be monitored serially for the reemergence of cutaneous lesions, the development of systemic complications, and drug toxicity.

References

1. Sjögren H: Zur Kenntnis der Keratoconjunctivitis sicca. *Acta Ophthalmol* 11 (suppl 2):1, 1933
2. Talal N: Sjögren's syndrome. *Bull Rheum Dis* **16**:404, 1966
3. Alexander EL: Neuromuscular complications of primary Sjögren's syndrome, in *Sjögren's Syndrome: Clinical and Immunological Aspects,* edited by N Talal et al. Heidelberg, Springer-Verlag, 1987, p 61
4. Alexander EL: Inflammatory vascular disease in Sjögren's syndrome, in *Sjögren's Syndrome: Clinical and Immunological Aspects,* edited by N Talal et al. Heidelberg, Springer-Verlag, 1987, p 102
5. Strickland RW et al: The frequency of sicca syndrome in an elderly female population. *J Rheumatol* **14**:766, 1985
6. Jacobson TH et al: Dry eyes or mouth—an epidemiological study in Swedish adults, with special reference to primary Sjögren's syndrome, in *Sjögren's Syndrome: A Model for Understanding Autoimmunity, 2nd International Symposium,* edited by N Talal. Academic, San Diego, California, 1988, p 213
7. Drosos AA et al: Prevalence of primary Sjögren's syndrome in an elderly population. *Br J Rheumatol* **27**:123, 1988
8. Prause JU et al: Definition and criteria for Sjögren's syndrome used by the contributors to the First International Seminar on Sjögren's syndrome, in *Proceedings of 1st International Seminar on Sjögren's Syndrome, 1986,* edited by R Manthorpe and JU Prause. The Almquist and Wiksell Periodical Co., Stockholm, 1986, p 17
9. Daniels TE et al: Labial salivary gland biopsy in Sjögren's syndrome: Assessment as a diagnostic criterion in 364 suspected cases. *Arthritis Rheum* **27**:147, 1984
10. Skopouli FN: Preliminary diagnostic criteria for Sjögren's syndrome, in *Proceedings of 1st International Seminar on Sjögren's Syndrome,* edited by R Manthorpe and JU Prause. The Almquist & Wiksell Periodical Company, Stockholm, 1986, p 22
11. Fox RI et al: Sjögren's syndrome: Proposed criteria for classification. *Arthritis Rheum* **29**:577, 1986
12. Harley JB: Autoantibodies in Sjögren's syndrome, in *Sjögren's Syndrome: A Model for Understanding Autoimmunity, 2nd International Symposium,* edited by N Talal. Academic, San Diego, California, 1988, p 75
13. Alexander EL et al: Sjögren's syndrome: Association of anti-Ro(SS-A) antibodies with vasculitis, hematologic abnormalities, and serologic hyperreactivity. *Ann Intern Med* **98**:155, 1983
14. Fye HK, Talal N: Skin manifestations of Sjögren's syndrome, in *Dermatology in General Medicine,* 3d ed, edited by TB Fitzpatrick et al. New York, McGraw-Hill, 1987, p 1883

15. Ellman P et al: A contribution to the pathology of Sjögren's disease. *QJ Med* **20**:33, 1951

16. Whaley K et al: Sjögren's syndrome sicca components. *QJ Med* **166**:279, 1973

17. Feuerman EJ et al: Sjögren's syndrome presenting as recalcitrant generalized pruritus. Some remarks about its relation to collagen diseases and the connection of rheumatoid arthritis with the sicca syndrome. *Dermatologica* **137**:74, 1968

18. Mitchell J et al: Anhidrosis (hypohidrosis) in Sjögren's syndrome. *J Am Acad Dermtol* **16**:233, 1987

19. Griffin JW et al: Sensory neuropathy in women with Sjögren's syndrome. *Ann Neurol* **27**:304, 1990

20. Mellgren SI et al: Peripheral neuropathy in primary Sjögren's syndrome. *Neurology* **39**:390, 1989

21. Alexander EL et al: Cutaneous manifestations of primary Sjögren's syndrome: A reflection of vasculitis and association with anti-Ro(SS-A) antibodies. *J Invest Dermatol* **80**:386, 1983

22. Alexander EL: Immunopathologic mechanisms of inflammatory vascular disease in primary Sjögren's syndrome. *Scand J Rheumatol* **61**:280, 1986

23. Alexander EL et al: Sjögren's syndrome: Association of cutaneous vasculitis with nervous system disease. *Arch Dermatol* **123**:801, 1987

24. Molina R et al: Peripheral inflammatory vascular disease (IVD) in Sjögren's syndrome: Association with nervous system complications. *Arthritis Rheum* **28**:1341, 1985

25. Waldenström J: Klinisnski metooler for pavisande av hyperproteinami och deras praktiska varde for diagnostiken. *Nord Med* **20**:2288, 1943

26. Waldenström J: Abnormal proteins in myeloma. *Adv Intern Med* **5**:398, 1952

27. Kyle RA et al: Benign hypergammaglobulinemic purpura of Waldenström. *Medicine (Baltimore)* **50**:113, 1971

28. Strauss WG: Purpura hyperglobulinemia of Waldenström. *N Engl J Med* **260**:857, 1959

29. Meltzer M et al: Cryoglobulinemia. A study of twenty-nine patients; IgG and IgM cryoglobulins and factors affecting cryoprecipitability. *Am J Med* **40**:828, 1986

30. Meltzer M et al: Cryoglobulinemia. A clinical and laboratory study. II. Cryoglobulins with rheumatoid factor activity. *Am J Med* **40**:837, 1966

31. McDuffie FC et al: Hypocomplementemia with cutaneous vasculitis and arthritis: Possible immune complex syndrome. *Mayo Clin Proc* **48**:340, 1973

32. Molina R et al: Two types of inflammatory vascular disease (IVD) in Sjögren's syndrome (SS): Differential association with seroreactivity to rheumatoid factor (RF) and antibodies to Ro(SS-A). *Arthritis Rheum* **28**:1251, 1985

33. Soter NA et al: Two distinct cellular patterns in cutaneous necrotizing angiitis. *J Invest Dermatol* **66**:344, 1976

34. Tsokos M et al: Vasculitis in primary Sjögren's syndrome. *Am J Clin Pathol* **88**:26, 1987

35. Harley JB et al: Anti-Ro(SS-A) and anti-La(SS-B) in patients with Sjögren's syndrome. *Arthritis Rheum* **29**:196, 1986

36. Alexander EL, Provost TT: Cutaneous manifestations of Sjögren's syndrome, in *Immunologic Diseases of the Skin*, edited by RE Jordan. East Norwalk, CT, Appleton/Lange, 1991, p 401

37. Soter NA et al: The complement system in necrotizing angiitis of the skin: Analysis of complement component activities in serum of patients with concomitant collagen-vascular disease. *J Invest Dermatol* **63**:219, 1974

38. Soter NA et al: Urticaria and arthralgias as manifestations of necrotizing angiitis (vasculitis). *J Invest Dermatol* **63**:485, 1974

39. Sanders ME et al: Serum SC5b-9 detects complement activation in vasculitis [inflammatory vascular disease (IVD)] in Sjögren's syndrome. *Arthritis Rheum* **32S**:R31, 1989

40. Malinow KL et al: Neuropsychiatric dysfunction in primary Sjögren's syndrome. *Ann Intern Med* **103**:344, 1985

41. Alexander EL et al: Primary Sjögren's syndrome with central nervous system dysfunction mimicking multiple sclerosis. *Ann Intern Med* **104**:323, 1986

42. Alexander EL et al: Magnetic resonance imaging of cerebral lesions in patients with Sjögren's syndrome. *Ann Intern Med* **108**:815, 1988

43. Alexander EL et al: Evidence of an immunopathogenic basis for central nervous system disease in Sjögren's syndrome. *Arthritis Rheum* **29**:1223, 1986

44. De La Monte SM et al: Polymorphous meningitis with atypical mononuclear cells in Sjögren's syndrome. *Ann Neurol* **14**:455, 1983

45. De La Monte SM et al: Polymorphous exudates and atypical mononuclear cells in the cerebrospinal fluid of patients with Sjögren's syndrome. *Acta Cytologica* **29**:634, 1985

46. Casselli RJ et al: The treatable dementia of Sjögren's syndrome. *Ann Neurol* **30**:98, 1991

47. Sato K et al: Primary Sjögren's syndrome associated with systemic necrotizing vasculitis: A fatal case (letter). *Arthritis Rheum* **30(6)**:717, 1987

48. Alexander EL et al: Immunogenetic relationship between primary SS and the lupus variants (SCLE, SS/LE overlap syndrome, and NLE). *Arthritis Rheum* **34**:R23, 1991

49. Alexander EL et al: CNS disease in Sjögren's syndrome (CNS-SS): Role of anti-Ro(SS-A) antibodies. *Arthritis Rheum* **34**:R17, 1991

50. Kassan S et al: Increased risk of lymphoma in sicca syndrome. *Ann Intern Med* **89**:888, 1978

51. Talal N, Bunin JJ: Development of malignant lymphoma in the course of Sjögren's syndrome. *Am J Med* **36**:529, 1964

52. Van der Valk PGM et al: Sjögren's syndrome with specific cutaneous manifestations and multifocal clonal T-cell populations progressing to a cutaneous pleomorphic T-cell lymphoma. *Am J Clin Pathol* **92**:357, 1989

53. Amarosi EL et al: Thrombotic thrombocytopenic purpura: Report of 16 cases and review of the literature. *Medicine (Baltimore)* **45**:139, 1966

54. Steinberg AD et al: Thrombotic thrombocytopenic purpura complicating Sjögren's syndrome. *JAMA* **215**:757, 1971

55. Tan EM et al: The revised criteria for the classification of systemic lupus erythematosus (SLE). *Arthritis Rheum* **25**:1271, 1982

56. Sontheimer RD et al: Subacute cutaneous lupus erythematosus: A cutaneous marker for a distinct lupus erythematosus subset. *Arch Dermatol* **115**:1409, 1979

57. Provost TT et al: The relationship between anti-Ro(SS-A) antibody positive Sjögren's syndrome and anti-Ro(SS-A) antibody positive lupus erythematosus. *Arch Dermatol* **124**:63, 1988

58. Provost TT et al: Ro(SS-A) positive Sjögren's lupus erythematosus (SS/LE) overlap patients are associated with the HLA Dr3 and/or DRw6 phenotypes. *J Invest Dermatol* **91**:369, 1988

59. Alexander EL et al: The immunogenetic relationship between Ro(SS-A)/La(SS-B) erythematosus overlap syndrome and the neonatal lupus syndrome. *J Invest Dermatol* **93**:751, 1989

60. Alexander EL et al: Immunogenetic relationship between primary SS and the lupus variants (SCLE, SS/LE overlap syndrome, and NLE). *Arthritis Rheum* **34**:R23, 1991

61. Watson RM et al: Neonatal lupus erythematosus. *Medicine (Baltimore)* **63**:362, 1984

62. Katayama I et al: Annular erythema associated with primary Sjögren's syndrome: Analysis of T cell subsets in cutaneous infiltrates. *J Am Acad Dermatol* **21**:1218, 1989

63. Sontheimer R et al: Lupus erythematosus, in *Dermatology in General Medicine*, 3d ed, edited by TB Fitzpatrick et al. New York, McGraw-Hill, 1987, p 1816

64. Provost TT et al: The neonatal lupus erythematosus syndrome. *J Rheumatol* **14**:199, 1988

65. Fronek Z et al: Major histocompatibility complex genes and susceptibility to systemic lupus erythematosus. *Arthritis Rheum* **33**:1542, 1990

66. Lawley TJ et al: Scleroderma, Sjögren-like syndrome, and chronic graft-versus-host disease. *Ann Intern Med* **87**:707, 1977

67. Schioat et al: Parotid gland enlargement and xerostomia associated with labial sialadenitis in HIV-infected patients, in *Sjögren's Syn-*

drome: A Model for Understanding Autoimmunity, 2d International Symposium, edited by N Talal. Academic, San Diego, CA, 1988, p 107

68. Itescu S et al: A diffuse infiltrative CD8 lymphocytosis syndrome in human immunodeficiency infection: A host immune response associated with HLA-DR5. *Ann Intern Med* **112**:3, 1990

69. Lawley T et al: A prospective clinical and immunologic analysis of serum sickness in men. *N Engl J Med* **311**:1407, 1984

70. Fraser NG et al: Dermatitis herpetiformis and Sjögren's syndrome. *Br*

J Dermatol **100**:213, 1979

71. Prystowski SD et al: Acute febrile neutrophilic dermatosis associated with Sjögren's syndrome. *Arch Dermatol* **114**:1234, 1978

72. Alexander EL: Sjögren's syndrome, in *Current Therapy in Allergy, Immunology, and Rheumatology,* edited by L Lichtenstein and AS Fauci. BC Decker, Burlington, Ontario, Canada, 1988, p 125

73. Fox RI et al: Treatment of primary Sjögren's syndrome with hydroxychloroquine. *Am J Med* **85**:62, 1988

Cutaneous Manifestations of Disease in Other Organ Systems

CHAPTER 182

Om P. Sharma

Sarcoidosis of the Skin

More than a century ago, Jonathan Hutchinson, a surgeon-dermatologist, described the first case of sarcoidosis at King's College Hospital in London. Jonathan Hutchinson's intellectual discourses, discussions, and lectures greatly impressed his contemporaries, including Sir Arthur Conan Doyle. Thus, it is not surprising that a skin disease, very much like cutaneous sarcoidosis, became a basic ingredient of the plot of *Adventures of the Blanched Soldier,* one of the Sherlock Holmes mysteries.

During most of the twentieth century, sarcoidosis remained confined to the domain of the chest physician, but its multisystem nature is now universally recognized.[1] The clinical and radiologic features of the disease are relatively clear-cut, but the diagnosis is often delayed or completely missed because of the resemblance of sarcoidosis to tuberculosis, leprosy, blastomycosis, coccidioidomycosis, berylliosis, brucellosis, and other granulomas.[2] In this chapter are described the clinical features, pathogenesis, biochemical changes, and immunologic advances in the understanding of the disease, its diagnostic criteria, and the effective management of patients suffering from cutaneous as well as multisystem sarcoidosis.

Sarcoid Granuloma

The lesion of sarcoidosis is a well-defined round or oval granuloma made up of compact, radially arranged epithelioid cells with pale nuclei. The typical giant cell of the sarcoid granuloma is of the Langhans' type in which the nuclei are arranged in an arc or a circular pattern around a central granular zone. Lymphocytes are usually seen at the periphery. Caseation is absent; fibrinoid necrosis may occasionally be seen in areas where several granulomas have coalesced (Fig. 182-1).

Monoclonal antibody techniques and indirect immunofluorescence methods have uncovered the dynamic relationship between the various components of the granuloma. The center of the granuloma is composed of macrophage-derived cells and OKT4 helper lymphocytes, whereas the periphery of the granuloma has a large number of interdigitating macrophages and OKT8 suppressor lymphocytes. The lymphokines from the inflammatory cells recruit blood-borne monocytes, prevent macrophage migration, and keep the chronic inflammatory reaction alive and efficient. It is probable

that this arrangement of interdigitating OKT8 cells on the periphery and the epithelioid cell-OKT4 pattern in the center provides an efficient perimeter defense to a persistent, poorly degradable "antigen" of low potency. This architectural arrangement is also found in cases of tuberculoid leprosy in which an efficient immune system keeps the bacillary load to a minimum; in lepromatous leprosy, in contrast, the arrangement of the immune cells is disorganized and haphazard, and bacteria abound.

The mechanisms regulating the formation and course of granulomas are not well understood. It appears that a T cell-mediated response to an antigen that has been processed and presented by macrophages to antigen-specific T lymphocytes is a fundamental step. Activated T cells orchestrate the accumulation and differentiation of mononuclear phagocytes by releasing a number of cytokines. The important cytokines released by lung T cells include interleukin 2 (IL-2), interferon-γ (IFN-γ), monocyte chemotactic factor, and migration inhibitory factor. Activated T cells also express surface markers, including IL-2 and HLA-DR class II major histocompatibility complex molecules.[3] The macrophage not only processes the antigen but also influences the granuloma formation and fibrosis by releasing a number of mediators, including IL-1, macrophage-derived fibroblast growth factor (which activates fibroblasts), fibronectin, and biologically active factor VII. Neutrophils recruited from blood by a macrophage-derived factor may participate in the development of fibrosis either by producing superoxide anion or by influencing the local concentration of immune complexes.[4]

Cutaneous Sarcoidosis

Skin lesions occur in about a quarter of patients with sarcoidosis. However, the incidence varies considerably. The lesions may be specific or nonspecific. The important specific lesions are lupus pernio, plaques, and maculopapular eruptions. The important nonspecific lesion is erythema nodosum. Other skin changes include alopecia, erythrodermas, subcutaneous nodules, erythema multiforme, itching, icthyosis, dystrophic calcifications, and verrucous outgrowths. Nail involvement is rare in sarcoidosis.[1,5]

Lupus pernio, the most characteristic of all sarcoid skin lesions, is a chronic, violaceous, indurated skin lesion with a predi-

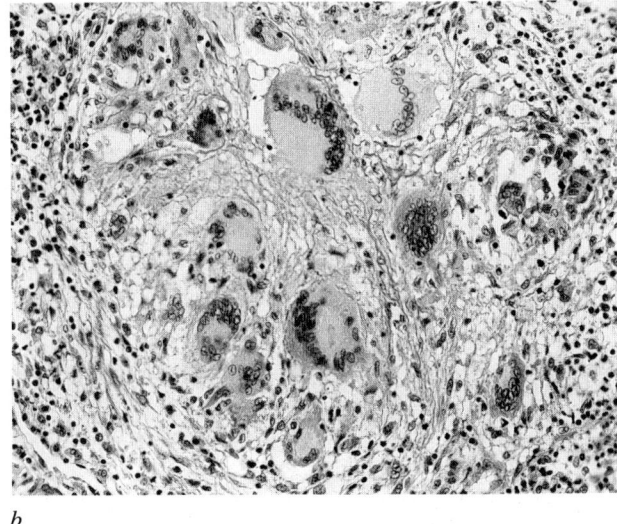

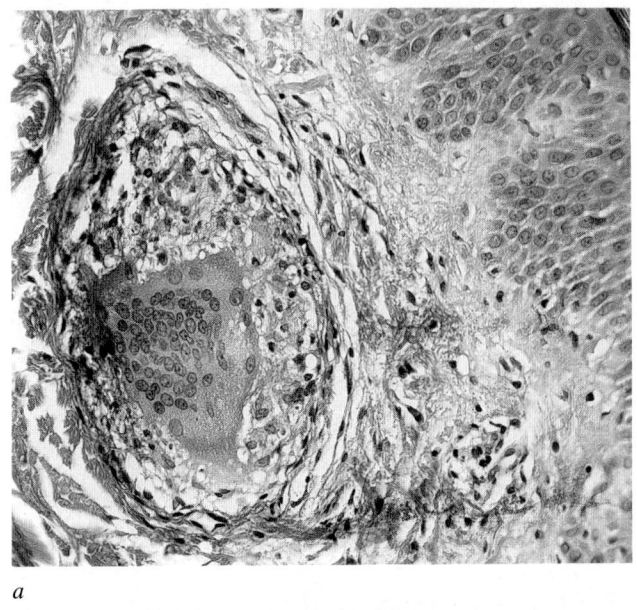

a

b

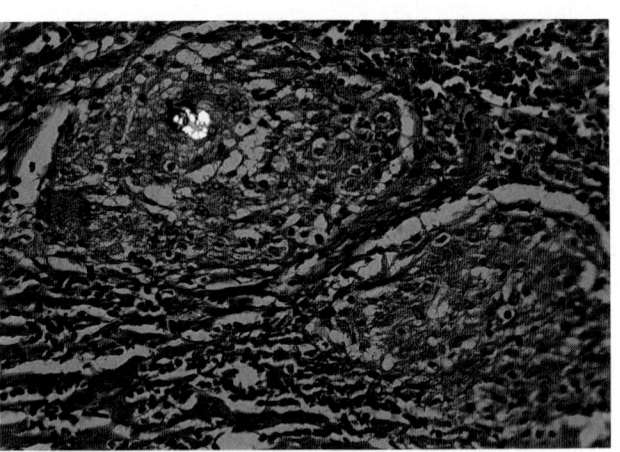

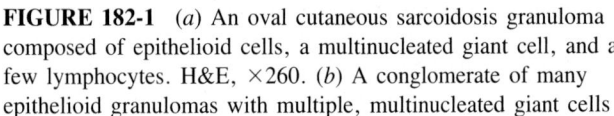

c

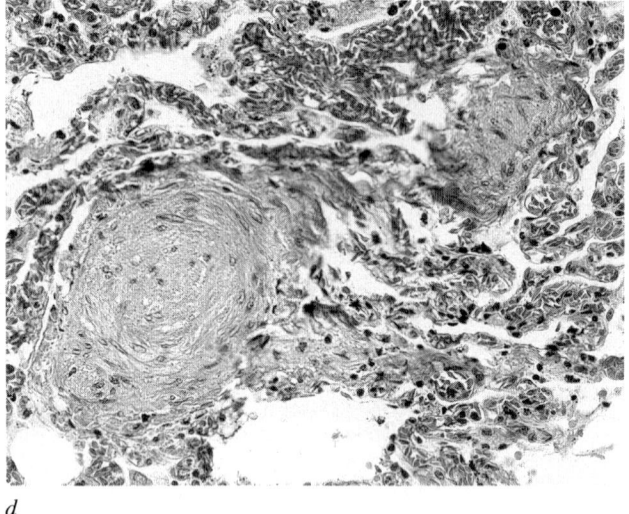

d

FIGURE 182-1 (*a*) An oval cutaneous sarcoidosis granuloma composed of epithelioid cells, a multinucleated giant cell, and a few lymphocytes. H&E, ×260. (*b*) A conglomerate of many epithelioid granulomas with multiple, multinucleated giant cells in a lymph node biopsy in sarcoidosis. H&E, ×195. (*c*) Crystalline inclusions in a sarcoid granuloma. H&E, ×169. (*d*) Late stage sarcoidosis granuloma showing hyalinization. H&E, ×75.

lection for the nose, ears, lips, and face (Fig. 182-2). It occurs commonly in women with persistent sarcoidosis with extensive pulmonary infiltration and fibrosis, chronic uveitis, and bone lesions. Occasionally, only a few tiny button-like papules or nodules may be seen involving the nasal rim. The nose lesion is often associated with granulomatous infiltration of the nasal mucosa and the upper respiratory tract.[6] Occasionally, the bony nasal septum may be destroyed. A bulbous or sausage-shaped finger in a patient with lupus pernio indicates the presence of an underlying bone lesion. Rarely, the nails may become dystrophic and brittle.

Skin plaques, like lupus pernio, are purplish, elevated, indurated patches commonly located on the limbs, face, back, and buttocks (Fig. 182-3). The distribution is usually symmetric. The center of the plaque is pale and atrophic; the periphery indurated, elevated, and dark. In the presence of large telangiectatic vessels, the lesions are called *angiolupoid*. Occasionally, the plaques, particularly in black patients, have a hypopigmented appearance—"hypomelanotic umbrella." The plaques are often associated with

chronic features of sarcoidosis including pulmonary fibrosis, bone cysts, peripheral lymphadenopathy, and uveitis. Rarely, sarcoidosis plaques may present a crusty, scaly appearance indistinguishable from psoriasis. These benignly deceptive lesions may be diagnosed in time if a biopsy specimen is obtained early.

The *maculopapular eruptions* are the most common skin manifestation of sarcoidosis in black patients. The waxy translucent lesions with a distinct flat top vary from 2 to 6 mm in diameter. They characteristically occur on the face, lids, around the orbits, in the nasolabial folds, and on the nape and upper back (Fig. 182-4).

Subcutaneous nodules, also called *Darier-Roussy sarcoidosis,* are oval, firm, painless structures that arise deep in the dermis and subcutaneous tissue of the trunk and extremities. On biopsy they show noncaseating granulomas. Rarely, these lesions may ulcerate.

Scars from atrophy, trauma, surgery, or venipuncture may become purple, swollen, and tender either at the time the patient presents or during reactivation of the disease. Biopsies of these areas show noncaseating granulomas. Ulcerative sarcoidosis is

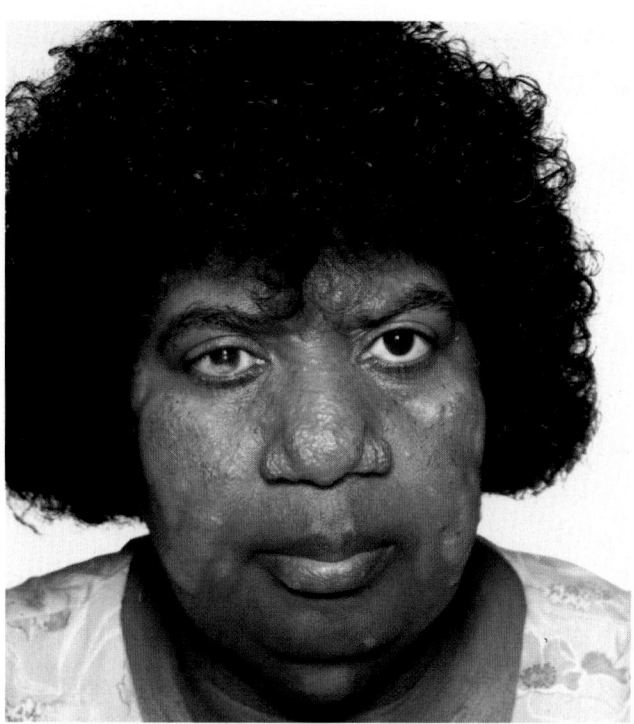

FIGURE 182-2 Lupus pernio in a black patient with chronic sarcoidosis of more than 25 years.

rare. Occurring most frequently in black women, the lesions usually involve the legs.[7] The biopsy may show typical noncaseating granulomas as well as necrotic changes (Fig. 182-5).

Erythema nodosum is a hypersensitivity reaction that results from exposure to many bacterial, fungal, and chemical antigens. It is the most common nonspecific cutaneous manifestation of sarcoidosis. Erythema nodosum is the hallmark of acute sarcoidosis, predominantly in women of childbearing age. Systemic manifestations such as fever, malaise, and polyarthralgia occur in about 50 percent of patients with erythema nodosum. Patients with erythema nodosum seldom require corticosteroid therapy because of the high rate of spontaneous resolution.

Cutaneous Sarcoidosis in Children

Although infrequent, sarcoidosis is not rare among children. In a recent review of literature, James and Kendig[8] have constructed a picture of childhood sarcoidosis from the data collected from Yugoslavia, France, Great Britain, Scandinavia, Hungary, Japan, and many areas in the United States. Intrathoracic involvement appears to be consistently present. Bilateral hilar adenopathy with and without paratracheal adenopathy is a common finding. Peripheral lymphoadenopathy occurs in about two-thirds and eye involvement in about one-third to one-fourth of children in the United States. Cutaneous lesions are frequently found, but erythema nodosum is unusual. The clinical picture in children below 4 years of age who develop sarcoidosis is different from the presentation in older children. Skin rash, uveitis, and arthritis are more common in children under 4 years of age. The rash, usually maculopapular, starts peripherally and may precede the other manifestations by several months. Intrathoracic involvement is absent in this group. The disease should be distinguished from the more common polyarticular juvenile rheumatoid arthritis (JRA), which has a later age of onset of 5 to 15 years. Thus, the diagnosis of sarcoidosis should be entertained in a child with skin rash, uveitis, lymphadenopathy, and pulmonary involvement. A rise in serum angiotensin-converting enzyme (ACE) level, although not specific for sarcoidosis, may be helpful in supplying the diagnosis and monitoring the granuloma-

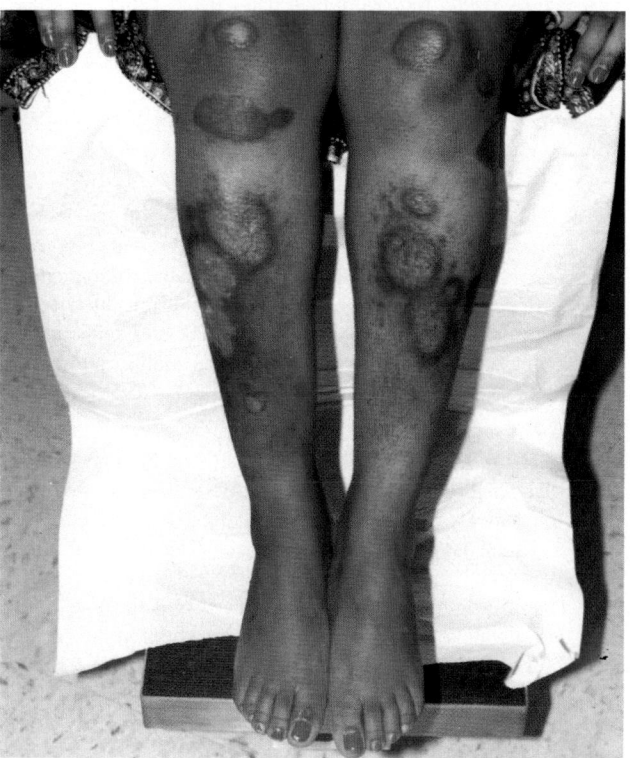

a

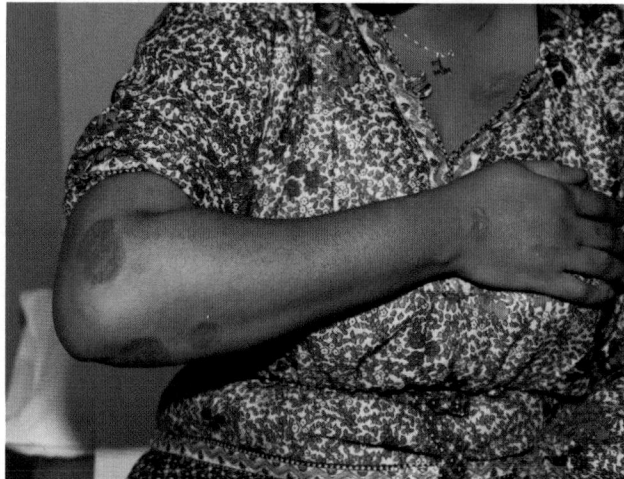

b

FIGURE 182-3 Chronic sarcoidosis skin plaques on the legs (*a*) and the arm (*b*). Occasionally, these lesions may ulcerate.

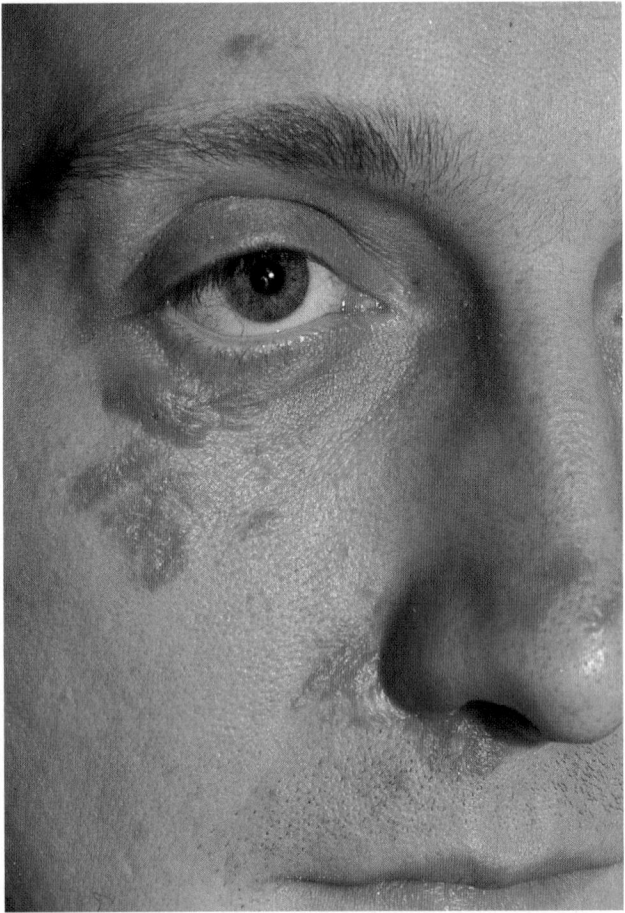

FIGURE 182-4 Sarcoidosis. Yellowish-brown plaques and papules on the face. On diascopy these lesions exhibit a pale brownish-red color.

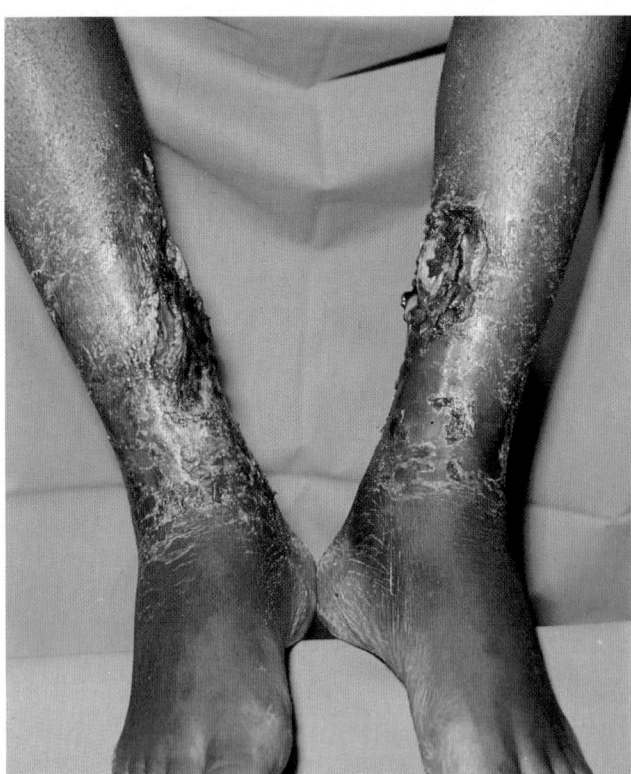

FIGURE 182-5 Chronic skin ulcers in a young black woman with sarcoidosis.

tous activity. The prognosis in children is more favorable than in adults, but for very young children with symptomatic multisystem involvement the outlook is less favorable.

The Multisystem Nature of Sarcoidosis

Because of its diverse manifestations, patients with sarcoidosis present not only to dermatologists but also to clinicians of many different specialties. Clinical manifestations depend on race, duration of the illness, site and extent of tissue involvement, and activity of the granulomatous process.

Nonspecific Constitutional Manifestations

About a third of patients with sarcoidosis complain of such nonspecific symptoms as fever, fatigue, and weight loss. Fever is generally mild, but temperatures are occasionally elevated to 39.5 or 40°C (103 to 104°F). Weight loss is generally limited to 2 to 7 kg (5 to 15 lb) during the 10 to 12 weeks before presentation. Night sweats sometimes occur. Constitutional symptoms are present more frequently in blacks and Asians from the Indian subcontinent than in Caucasians.

Lungs

Respiratory Symptoms More than one-third of patients with sarcoidosis complain of dyspnea, cough, chest pain, and tightness of the chest. The cough is usually dry. Chest pain, generally confined to the retrosternal area, may be severe and indistinguishable from cardiac pain. Occasionally, the pain may become intensified after drinking alcohol.

Chest Radiographic Abnormalities The following radiographic staging system is useful in sarcoidosis: stage 0, normal chest roentgenogram; stage I, bilateral hilar lymphadenopathy without pulmonary infiltrates; stage II, bilateral hilar lymphadenopathy with pulmonary infiltrates; stage III, pulmonary infiltrates without hilar adenopathy; and stage IV, end-stage fibrosis, bullae, and honeycombing.

Lung Function Abnormalities Extensive physiologic studies emphasize functional changes characteristic of ''restrictive impairment'' in patients with sarcoidosis. Vital capacity, residual volume, and total lung capacity are reduced. The loss of diffusing capacity remains perhaps the most common abnormality in sarcoidosis. The diffusing capacity is reduced even in patients with hilar adenopathy without any associated parenchymal infiltrates on chest x-ray film (stage I). Severe abnormalities of gas exchange are also more frequent than is generally realized. The obstruction of airways, large and small, is quite common, particularly in African American patients.[9]

Eyes

Any structure of the eye may be involved in sarcoidosis, but granulomatous uveitis is the most common eye lesion. Uveitis may be acute, subacute, or chronic.

Acute uveitis presents suddenly with redness of the eyes, watering, cloudy vision, and photophobia. Circumcorneal ciliary congestion is present, pupils are irregular, and ''mutton fat'' keratotic precipitates may be prominent in the anterior chamber. The patient may have other manifestations of early sarcoidosis, including erythema nodosum and bilateral hilar lymphadenopathy and arthralgias.

Chronic uveitis, in contrast, develops slowly and may lead to adhesions between the iris and the lens, glaucoma, cataracts, and blindness. Ciliary congestion is absent, but keratotic precipitates are present. The patient complains of pain and blurred vision. Other manifestations of chronic sarcoidosis, including lupus pernio, plaques, bone and joint lesions (Fig. 182-6), and interstitial pulmonary fibrosis may be present.

Other ocular lesions include conjunctival follicles, retinal periphlebitis, retinal hemorrhages, retinitis proliferans, cataracts, band keratopathy, proptosis, and exophthalmos.

Peripheral Lymph Nodes

The most frequently involved nodes are cervical, axillary, epitrochlear, and inguinal. In the neck, the nodes in the posterior triangle are more commonly affected than those in the anterior triangle. Enlarged nodes are discrete, shotty, mobile, painless, and free from the surrounding structures.

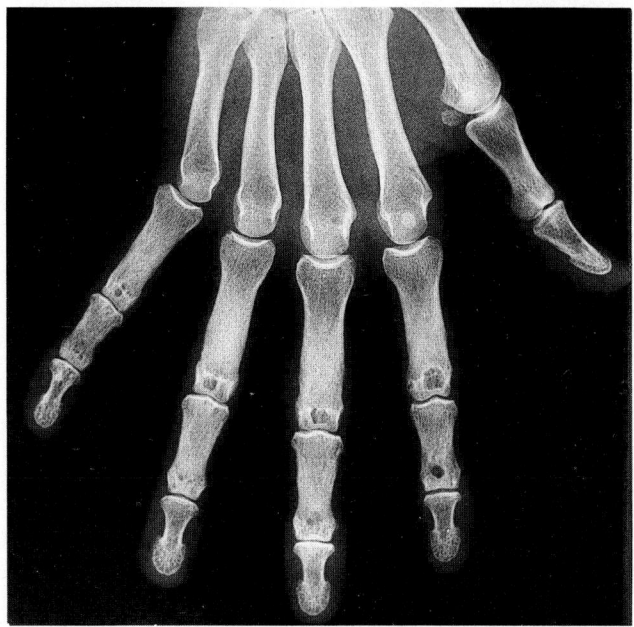

FIGURE 182-6 ''Bone cysts'' involving the small bones of a hand. These cysts, which typically involve the small bones of the feet as well as the hands, almost always are associated with chronic skin lesions.

Spleen

Although the spleen is infiltrated by sarcoid granulomas in more than 50 percent of patients, the incidence of a clinically palpable spleen is only about 15 percent. Splenic enlargement is usually silent, but, as the disease progresses, pressure symptoms, anemia, leukopenia, and thrombocytopenia are likely to occur.

Gastrointestinal Tract

The esophagus is least frequently involved by sarcoidosis. Asymptomatic granulomas occur in the gastric mucosa in 10 percent of patients. Hematemesis may occur. Intestinal involvement is rare, and there are only a few documented cases. Two patients with sarcoidosis and regional ileitis have been reported.[10] It should be emphasized, however, that the distinction between sarcoidosis confined to the intestinal tract and Crohn's or Whipple's disease may be difficult. Joints may be involved in all three conditions. Maher et al.[11] found four cases of pancreatic sarcoidosis in the literature and added one more with histologic evidence of noncaseating granulomas in the pancreas. Unexplained abdominal pain in a patient with sarcoidosis may be due to pancreatic involvement. The liver is palpable in about 20 percent of patients with sarcoidosis, and granulomas are found in 63 to 87 percent, depending on the stage and activity of the disease. Alkaline phosphatase and serum bilirubin levels may be mildly elevated in as many as 80 percent of patients. Portal hypertension is rare.

Heart

Heart involvement is clinically recognizable in about 5 percent of the patients with sarcoidosis; however, at autopsy granulomas are found in as many as 27 percent. Myocardial involvement may be present clinically in many ways, including conduction disturbances, disturbances of rhythm, sudden death, congestive heart failure, valvular involvement, pericardial disease, and myocardial infarction. Endomyocardial biopsy is of limited value because of the patchy distribution of the disease.[12]

Musculoskeletal System

The incidence of joint involvement ranges from 25 to 39 percent in various series. The onset of articular symptoms has occurred as early as 4 months and as late as 59 years of age. Joint disease was an initial manifestation of sarcoidosis in 74 (90 percent) of 83 patients in one study. Joint involvement may precede other manifestations of sarcoidosis by many years. In one of ten patients described by Patterson et al.,[13] acute arthritis preceded the established diagnosis by 16 years.

The joints most commonly affected by sarcoidosis are the knees, ankles, elbows, wrists, and small joints of the hands. The affected joints are usually swollen, warm, tender, and painful; effusions are common, particularly in patients with chronic disease. Sarcoid arthritis may be indistinguishable from that observed in rheumatic fever, rheumatoid disease, and JRA.

Kidneys

Renal involvement in sarcoidosis may result from one or more of the following mechanisms: hypercalcemia/hypercalciuria, granulomatous infiltration of the renal parenchyma, glomerular disease, or renal arteritis secondary to granulomas. The incidence of renal granulomas in sarcoid patients varies from 4 to 40 percent.

Salivary Glands

Although the parotid gland is palpable in only about 6 percent of patients, subclinical involvement is more common and may be detected by technetium 99m scan and by measuring salivary volume and amylase. Granulomas in minor salivary glands occur in as many as 50 percent of patients with mediastinal sarcoidosis but seldom occur without hilar adenopathy or other evidence of multisystem involvement.

Upper Respiratory Tract

Nasal involvement is an indicator of chronic disease, and the presence of nasal granulomas even in the early stage of the disease constitutes an indication for corticosteroid therapy. Intralesional corticosteroid injections may be beneficial for polypoidal growths. Laryngeal involvement occurs in about 5 percent of patients with sarcoidosis. The granulomatous lesions most commonly affect the epiglottis, aryepiglottic folds, arytenoids, and false cords. Ulceration is rare. A large exophytic lesion may produce severe airway obstruction.

Endocrine Glands

The pituitary and hypothalamus are the most commonly affected endocrine glands in sarcoidosis. An elevated prolactin level may be a sensitive marker of hypothalamic sarcoidosis. The thyroid, parathyroid, and adrenal glands are rarely involved.

Nervous System

Sarcoidosis may involve the nervous system in 1 to 29 percent of patients with an average of about 5 percent. The clinical diagnosis of neurosarcoidosis depends on the finding of neurologic involvement in a patient with histologically proven multisystem disease. The cranial nerves, meninges, hypothalamus, and pituitary gland are the most frequently involved sites in the central nervous system. Peripheral neuropathy, spinal cord involvement, and psychiatric manifestations are infrequent.

Laboratory Investigations

The true incidence of anemia (hemoglobin of less than 11 g) in sarcoidosis is about 5 percent. Hemolytic anemia is rare. Although corticosteroid therapy is useful in some cases, spontaneous correction of hemolytic anemia may occur. Leukopenia is a frequent finding. It may occur in the absence of splenomegaly and reflect bone marrow involvement. Leukemoid reactions and polycythemia are rare. The mean incidence of eosinophilia is about 24 percent. In

many patients, thrombocytopenia is associated with an enlarged spleen but there is some evidence that it may be an expression of a generalized immune reaction. The erythrocyte sedimentation rate is high in about two-thirds of patients, but this finding does not carry any diagnostic or prognostic complications.

Hypercalcemia

Hypercalcemia may occur in any stage of sarcoidosis. The available evidence indicates that it is due to increased intestinal calcium absorption. In normal individuals, vitamin D is converted by the liver to 25-hydroxyvitamin D, which in turn undergoes 1-hydroxylation in the kidney to form 1-25-dihydroxyvitamin D $[1,25(OH)_2 D]$, the most potent metabolite of vitamin D. In sarcoidosis, endogenous overproduction of $(3H)1,25(OH)_2 D_3$ by activated pulmonary macrophages seems to be the cause of increased intestinal absorption of calcium. Corticosteroids lower the raised calcium level to normal by inhibiting the peripheral action of $1,25(OH)_2 D_3$ and by metabolizing the compound to an inactive metabolite.[14]

Serum Angiotensin-Converting Enzyme

In sarcoidosis, the serum ACE level is raised in about 60 percent of patients. ACE activity is higher in patients with hilar adenopathy and pulmonary infiltration (stage II) than in those with either hilar adenopathy alone (stage I) or pulmonary infiltrate/fibrosis (stages III/IV). The test is positive in patients with extrathoracic sarcoidosis. Because ACE is derived from the epithelioid cells of the granulomas, it reflects the granuloma load in the body.

The diagnostic value of the serum ACE level is limited because the test has a false-negative incidence of 40 percent and a false-positive incidence of 10 percent. The test is most useful in monitoring the clinical course of the disease.[15]

Immunology

Cutaneous Anergy

The depression of cutaneous delayed-type hypersensitivity reactions is a cardinal immunologic feature of sarcoidosis. Approximately two-thirds of patients do not respond to the tuberculin test in any of the conventional strengths. However, this cutaneous anergy does not correlate with the activity of the disease, and the immunologic defect persists in most patients despite clinical and radiographic recovery.

Lymphopenia and Helper/Suppressor T Lymphocyte Ratio

Cutaneous anergy in sarcoidosis appears to be due to the unavailability of immune effector lymphocytes. Lymphopenia is a prominent feature of the disease. Monoclonal antibody techniques have enabled us to assess the helper/suppressor cell ratio of human T lymphocytes. In normal subjects this ratio in the peripheral blood is 1.8:1. In patients with low-activity sarcoidosis, the ratio is somewhat lower (1.4:1), and in patients with high-intensity alveolitis, it is significantly lower (0.8:1). The relatively high number of suppressor cells in the peripheral blood may explain in part the cutaneous and in vitro anergy in sarcoidosis.

The helper/suppressor cell ratio is significantly higher (10.5:1) at the site of tissue granulomas. The cells bearing the suppressor-cytotoxic antigen are located in a mantle surrounding the granuloma, whereas the helper-inducer cells are distributed throughout the granuloma among the aggregated epithelioid cells.

Humoral Responses and Immune Complexes

Circulating antibody production is exaggerated in sarcoidosis. Hypergammaglobulinemia occurs in perhaps half the patients and is more frequent among blacks. The prevalence of immune complexes also varies. Circulating immune complexes are present in about half the patients with acute sarcoidosis, particularly in those with erythema nodosum. In chronic disease, immune complexes are less frequent. Direct immunofluorescence techniques have demonstrated the complexes in cutaneous granulomas. It has been suggested that they alter the distribution and function of the helper and suppressor cells and macrophages.

Kveim Test

Although the Kveim test is considered specific for sarcoidosis, the potent validated antigen is not widely available. It requires 4 to 6 weeks for the Kveim nodule to mature.

Bronchoalveolar Lavage

In normal nonsmokers, the effector population of the alveolar cells consists of 93 ± 3 percent alveolar macrophages, 7 to 3 percent lymphocytes, and less than 1 percent polymorphonuclear leukocytes. In normal smokers, the proportion of polymorphonuclear leukocytes increases from less than 1 percent to 2 to 8 percent.

In patients with active sarcoidosis there is a significant increase in the number of T lymphocytes. The T cell/B cell ratio in the lung approaches 18:1, whereas the T cell/B cell ratio in the blood is only about 3:1. T lymphocytes in bronchoalveolar lavage fluid are also increased in other conditions, including hypersensitivity pneumonitis, pulmonary lymphoma, and miliary tuberculosis.[16] The expansion of the T lymphocyte population in sarcoidosis is due to an increase in CD4 (helper) T cells, whereas in hypersensitivity the expansion is due to the preferential increase of CD8 (suppressor) subsets. Other cell types, including $\gamma\delta$ + T cells, are also found in larger proportion in bronchoalveolar lavage fluids, suggesting the presence of a persistent yet unknown antigenic stimulus. B-cell activation in sarcoidosis is reflected by the increased concentration of immunoglobulins in blood and bronchoalveolar lavage fluid.

Diagnosis

The criteria for establishing the diagnosis of sarcoidosis include (1) a compatible clinical or radiologic picture, or both; (2) histologic evidence of noncaseating granulomata; and (3) negative special stains and cultures for other entities (e.g., acid fast bacilli or fungi in sputum or tissue biopsy specimens).

Recently developed tests, including serum ACE levels, lysozyme, the gallium 67 lung scan, and the bronchoalveolar lavage fluid lymphocyte count, have provided us with a better understanding of biochemical and immunologic changes of sarcoidosis but are of little help in establishing the specific diagnosis. The definitive diagnosis of sarcoidosis still requires the demonstration of noncaseating granulomas in the involved tissue.

Treatment

Corticosteroids

At present, corticosteroids are the most effective agents for influencing the course of cutaneous sarcoidosis. The skin lesions in sarcoidosis are not dangerous to life, and the patients should be treated on the basis of the severity and progression of the involvement. Oral prednisone, 20 to 40 mg daily in divided doses, is the treatment of choice. The total daily dose is then gradually reduced to maintenance levels, usually to about 10 mg daily. In many cases, after the initial 4 to 6 weeks of daily treatment, the dose may be reduced to 10 to 20 mg every other day. The alternate-day use of prednisone seems to be at least as effective as daily administration.

Disfiguring skin lesions can also be treated by intralesional injection of triamcinolone acetonide. Intralesional injection of triamcinolone acetonide diluted with 1 percent procaine to a final concentration of 2 to 5 mg/mL may be repeated at weekly intervals. On occasion, corticosteroid cream or lotions applied three to four times daily and massaged in well, are helpful.

Chloroquine

This agent is particularly useful in the management of chronic skin lesions.[17,18] The drug is administered in dosages of 250 mg twice a day for 6 months. Chloroquine may also be used together with corticosteroids to reduce the dosage of the latter. Refer to clinical precautions concerning this drug.

Immunosuppressive Drugs

Of all the immunosuppressive drugs, methotrexate seems, so far, to have the best track record in the treatment of cutaneous as well as disseminated sarcoidosis. Symptomatic and objective improvement occurred in 13 of 14 patients with refractory sarcoidosis treated with low-dose methotrexate. Four patients experienced a greater than 50 percent reduction in skin lesions. Azathioprine and chlorambucil also have been tried but with limited success.[19–21]

Other Drugs

Oxyphenbutazone, colchicine, allopurinol, levamisole, and radiation[22] have also been tried in the management of sarcoidosis.

Cosmetic Surgery

Surgical treatment may involve excision of small lesions or skin grafting of extensive sarcoid ulcers. In either case caution should be exercised because of the risk of keloid formation, particularly in black patients.[23,24]

Miscellaneous

The creative use of available cosmetic preparations in patients with disfiguring skin plaques and refractory lupus pernio can improve the quality of life both socially and psychologically.

Clinical Caution

Chloroquine administration can involve the eye and may lead to irreversible retinopathy and blindness. Therefore, regular ophthalmologic examinations are mandatory. Methotrexate may cause liver damage, and liver biopsies may be needed if the therapy is long term.

Antituberculosis therapy is not indicated routinely in patients with sarcoidosis. However, those patients who show a positive tuberculin test, if given corticosteroids, immunosuppressive drugs, or radiation, should receive prophylactic isoniazid.

ACKNOWLEDGMENT

Ms. Maggie Sharma's excellent secretarial assistance is gratefully acknowledged.

References

1. Sharma OP: Cutaneous sarcoidosis. *Chest* **61**:320, 1972
2. Williams WJ, Wallach ER: Laser microprobe mass spectrometry (LAMMS) analysis of beryllium, sarcoidosis and other granulomatous diseases. *Sarcoidosis* **6**:111, 1989
3. du Bois RM et al: Granulomatous processes, in *The Lung: Scientific Foundations,* edited by RG Crystal et al. New York, Raven, 1991, p 1925
4. Semenzato G: The immunology of sarcoidosis. *Semin Respir Med* **8**:17, 1986
5. Olumide YM et al: Cutaneous sarcoidosis in Nigeria. *J Am Acad Dermatol* **6**:1222, 1989
6. Jorizzo JL et al: Sarcoidosis of the upper respiratory tract in patients with nasal rim lesions: A pilot study. *J Am Acad Dermatol* **22**:439, 1990
7. Verdegem T, Sharma OP: Cutaneous ulcers in sarcoidosis. *Arch Dermatol* **123**:1531, 1987
8. James DG, Kendig EL Jr: Childhood sarcoidosis. *Sarcoidosis* **5**:57, 1988
9. Sharma OP, Johnson R: Airway obstruction in sarcoidosis: A study of 123 nonsmoking black American patients with sarcoidosis. *Chest* **94**:343, 1988
10. Dines DE et al: Sarcoidosis associated with regional enteritis (Crohn's disease). *Minn Med* **54**:617, 1971
11. Maher L et al: Noncaseating granuloma of the pancreas. *Am J Gastroentrol* **75**:222, 1981
12. Fleming H: Sarcoid heart disease. *Sarcoidosis* **2**:20, 1985
13. Patterson JR et al: The musculoskeletal manifestations of sarcoidosis, in *Proceedings of the Fifth International Conference on Sarcoidosis,* edited by L Levinsky, F Machoda. Prague, Charles University, 1971, p 590
14. Adams J et al: Metabolism of 25-hydroxyvitamin D₃ by cultured pulmonary alveolar macrophages in sarcoidosis. *J Clin Invest* **72**:1856, 1983
15. Romer FK: Angiotensin converting enzyme activity in sarcoidosis and other disorders. *Sarcoidosis* **2**:25, 1985
16. Hunninghake GW, Crystal RG: Pulmonary sarcoidosis: A disorder mediated by excess of helper T-lymphocytic activity at sites of disease activity. *N Engl J Med* **305**:329, 1981
17. Siltzbach LE, Teirstein AS: Chloroquine therapy in 43 patients with intrathoracic and cutaneous sarcoidosis. *Acta Med Scand* **176** (supplement 425):302, 1984
18. Adams J et al: Effective reduction in the serum 1-25-dihydroxyvitamin D and calcium concentration in sarcoidosis-associated hypercalcemia with short chloroquine therapy. *Ann Intern Med* **111**:437, 1989
19. Lower EE, Baughman RP: The use of low dose methotrexate in refractory sarcoidosis. *Am J Med Sci* **299**:153, 1990
20. Veien NK, Brodthagen H: Cutaneous sarcoidosis treated with methotrexate. *Br J Dermatol* **97**:213, 1977
21. Soriano FG et al: Neurosarcoidosis: Therapeutic success with methotrexate. *Postgrad Med J* **66**:142, 1990
22. Whittaker M et al: Sarcoidosis of penis treated by radiotherapy. *Br J Urol* **47**:325, 1975
23. Shaw M et al: Disfiguring lupus pernio successfully treated with plastic surgery. *Clin Exp Dermatol* **9**:614, 1984
24. Collison DW et al: Split-thickness skin grafting in extensive ulcerative sarcoidosis. *J Dermatol Surg Oncol* **15**:679, 1989

CHAPTER 183

David I. McLean and Harley A. Haynes

Cutaneous Manifestations of Internal Malignant Disease

Changes in the skin can be a marker for an internal malignant neoplasm. The specific relationship of the cancer with the marker can be variable. For instance, hypertrichosis lanuginosa acquisita can be a marker for many different malignant neoplasms whereas necrolytic migratory erythema is quite specific for a glucagon-producing tumor of the pancreas.

An attempt has been made to group these manifestations in a useful manner (Table 183-1). Where possible, these groupings have been made by the major clinical manifestation and will be discussed in this order. Unfortunately our lack of knowledge does not allow us to classify these diseases by a pathophysiologic approach in all cases. Indeed, there is a very large group where the biochemical relationship to the neoplasia is not yet understood.

There must be a proven association of the cutaneous eruption with a tumor. This is not difficult when the supposed manifestation is very rare and the tumor is also very uncommon. It becomes a

major problem, however, when the manifestation is very common, such as the seborrheic keratoses in the sign of Leser-Trélat, and the presumed association is with a wide spectrum of commonly occurring neoplasms. In this situation the literature becomes replete with anecdotal reports, which may or may not be an indication of whether there is a true association with the malignant neoplasm.

An attempt has been made to clarify what constitutes a true paraneoplastic syndrome.[1] There are two essential criteria: (1) the dermatosis must develop only after the development of the malignant tumor, and (2) both the dermatosis and the malignant tumor should follow a parallel course. The second criteria means that removal of the cancer results in clearing of the dermatosis, and recurrence of the cancer can cause relapse of the dermatosis (certainly relapse of the dermatosis cannot occur in the absence of the cancer). These criteria are amplified more fully in a recent discussion.[1]

TABLE 183-1
Cutaneous Manifestations of Internal Malignant Disease

I Lesions secondary to the deposition of substances in the skin	*VI* Collagen-vascular disease
A Icterus	*A* Dermatomyositis
B Melanosis	*B* Lupus erythematosus
C Hemochromatosis	*C* Progressive systemic sclerosis
D Xanthomas	*VII* Skin tumors and internal malignant disease
E Systemic amyloidosis	*A* Muir-Torre syndrome
II Vascular and blood abnormalities	*B* Gardner syndrome
A Flushing	*C* Cowden disease
B Palmar erythema	*D* Mucosal neuroma syndrome
C Telangiectasia	*E* Neurofibromatosis
D Purpura	*VIII* Hormone-related conditions
E Vasculitis	*IX* Disorders associated with primary skin cancer
F Cutaneous ischemia	*A* Nevoid basal cell carcinoma syndrome
G Thrombophlebitis	*B* Arsenical manifestations
III Bullous disorders	*X* Other disorders associated with internal malignant disease
A Bullous pemphigoid	*A* Pruritus
B Pemphigus vulgaris	*B* Erythema gyratum repens
C Dermatitis herpetiformis	*C* Subcutaneous fat necrosis
D Herpes gestationis	*D* Sweet syndrome
E Erythema multiforme	*E* Hypertrichosis lanuginosa acquisita
F Epidermyolysis bullosa acquisita	*F* Necrolytic migratory erythema
G Linear IgA dermatosis	*G* Clubbing
IV Infections and infestations	*H* Leukoderma
A Herpes zoster	*I* Peutz-Jeghers syndrome
B Herpes simplex	*J* Tuberous sclerosis
C Bacterial infections	*K* Multiple eruptive seborrheic keratoses
D Fungi and yeast infections	*L* Porphyria cutanea tarda
E Scabies	*XI* Direct tumor involvement in the skin
V Disorders of keratinization	
A Acanthosis nigricans	
B Acquired ichthyosis	
C Palmar hyperkeratosis	
D Erythroderma	
E Paraneoplastic acrokeratosis of Bazex	

Color Changes Secondary to the Deposition of Substances in the Skin

Icterus

Icterus as a manifestation of internal malignancy is generally a late sign. It is usually secondary to obstruction of the bile duct or gross intrahepatic obstruction. Extrahepatic obstruction can be secondary to malignant disease of the gall bladder, pancreas, bile duct, or adjacent bowel.

Icterus must be distinguished from other causes of yellow skin such as carotenemia and lycopenemia. Carotenemia, which can produce a carotenoderma, differs from icterus in that it is often uneven in its coloration. It is usually darkest in areas of hyperkeratotic skin such as the palms and soles. Deposition is also quite prominent on the face. The sclerae are not stained by carotene. Lycopenemia also produces a yellow color. This yellow color is also produced by carotenoids, but these are generally derived from tomatoes and tomato juice.

Melanosis

Melanosis is a condition caused by the abnormal deposition of melanin pigments in tissue. It is externally manifested by a diffuse gray-brown pigmentation of the skin, but the pigment can be deposited in most of the organs of the body (Fig. 183-1). A mild darkening of the skin may be seen with adrenal insufficiency, with ACTH-producing tumors such as primary tumors of the pituitary gland, or with other malignant tumors metastatic to the pituitary gland.[2,3]

Diffuse melanosis can also be secondary to malignant melanoma. Usually occurring late in the disease course, melanosis can, however, be the presenting sign. The pigment of the skin has been attributed to the presence of melanin granules in both the circulation and tissue macrophages[4,5] or to the presence of single-cell metastases from the primary melanoma.[6] Diffuse micrometastases can also appear in the nail matrix, leading to pigment streaks in the nail plate. Circulating tumor cells have also been found in patients with melanosis.[6] Melanuria is frequently associated with melanosis of

the skin. Urine from patients who have melanuria is usually not black when voided, but gradually darkens to a deep brown and later a black color when exposed to the air for several hours. It would appear that intermediary metabolites of tyrosine are oxidized spontaneously to melanin. Highly increased amounts of 5-S-cysteinyldopa have been reported in the urine of such patients.[7]

Andreev and Petkov noted a melasma (chloasma) type of hyperpigmentation on the face of five patients with "brain tumors."[8] In three patients the hyperpigmentation resolved after the surgical removal of the tumor.

A diffuse gray-brown pigmentation of the skin can also be produced by hemochromatosis.

Hemochromatosis

Hemochromatosis is an iron-storage disorder resulting predominantly from increased iron absorption from the gut. There is deposition of iron in the form of hemosiderin in many tissues. A third of untreated patients with hemochromatosis will develop hepatocellular carcinoma.[9] The pigment seen in hemochromatosis does not appear to be predominantly caused by iron; there is increased melanin production in these patients. Vitiligo causes a complete loss of pigment, indicating that the iron per se is a negligible contributory factor in the skin color.[10] The iron may be acting as a direct stimulant somewhere in the melanin production system or indirectly through increased melanization secondary to mild tissue injury.

Xanthomas (See also Chap. 152)

The predominant type of xanthoma associated with internal malignant disease is the plane xanthoma. The most common association of diffuse plane xanthoma is with multiple myeloma. Patients have been described with xanthomas and multiple myeloma of many types, including IgG L type,[11] IgG K type[12] and IgA type multiple myeloma.[13] Xanthomas, as well as atypical eruptive histiocytosis with lipid deposition, have also been associated with myelocytic leukemia, myelomonocytic leukemia, leukemic lymphocytic reticuloendotheliosis, diffuse histiocytic lymphoma, and in the cutaneous T-cell lymphoma.[14-20] Juvenile xanthogranuloma can be associated with juvenile chronic myeloid leukemia.[21]

Patients with xanthomas associated with cancer may be normolipemic[22] or they may, more commonly, have a hyperlipoproteinemia. Type 2A hyperlipoproteinemia has been described in association with IgG L type myeloma,[11] as has type 4 or type 5 hyperlipoproteinemia. Type 3 (broad beta) and pre-beta hyperlipoproteinemia have been described in association with IgA myeloma.[13]

Purpura may be a feature of diffuse plane xanthomas associated with malignant disease. Pinch purpura has been noted in a normolipemic patient with myeloma. Hemorrhagic bullae have been associated with xanthoma disseminatum and IgG K type multiple myeloma.[23] This patient was normolipemic. Disseminated xanthosiderohistiocytosis, a variant of xanthoma disseminatum, has been reported in association with a plasma cell dyscrasia.[24]

Systemic Amyloidosis (See also Chap. 149)

Systemic amyloidosis of both the primary type and that associated with multiple myeloma commonly have skin lesions. It is important to differentiate skin lesions of systemic amyloidosis from the far more commonly seen purely cutaneous variants of amyloidosis.

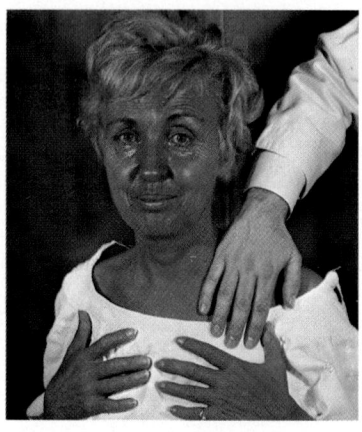
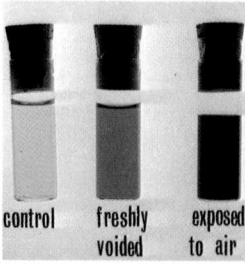

control   freshly   exposed
           voided   to air

a   *b*

FIGURE 183-1 Slate gray dermal pigmentation with metastatic melanoma and melanogenuria. (*a*) Diffuse blue argyria-like hypermelanosis. This patient died 1 month after this photograph was taken, illustrating that this bizarre argyria-like blue pigmentation is a terminal complication. (*b*) Dark urine from a patient with melanogenuria, compared with normal urine.

The typical lesions of systemic amyloidosis consist of raised waxy papules and plaques commonly involving eyelids, eyebrows, and paranasal skin, as well as lesions that can be diffusely present over the body surface. Purpura is generally seen mixed with these waxy papules but can also be seen on clinically apparently normal skin. Other changes include alopecia, macroglossia, and pallor.[25] All patients with skin lesions of systemic amyloidosis should be thoroughly investigated for multiple myeloma. Acute nonlymphocytic leukemia has also been reported in association with systemic amyloidosis treated with melphalan.[26]

Intradermal bullae have been associated with myeloma-related amyloidosis. These bullae are the result of extensive dermal infiltration with amyloid, resulting in cleavage of the uppermost dermis from the lower dermis.

Macular amyloidosis is a form of amyloidosis most commonly seen limited to the skin of the upper trunk and characterized by pruritic macular pigmented patches. Although it generally has no association with internal malignant disease, it has been reported in a patient with myelofibrosis and myeloid metaplasia.[27]

Familial cutaneous lichen amyloidosis has been reported in a large kindred in association with multiple endocrine neoplasia type 2A.[28]

Vascular and Blood Abnormalities

Flushing (See also Chap. 170)

Acquired pronounced flushing, usually of the central face and upper trunk, may be a manifestation of carcinoid syndrome, caused by carcinoid tumors.[29] These tumors may arise from the bronchus, stomach, pancreas, and thyroid, and less often from teratomas. Metastatic tumors from the small bowel are the most likely to produce flushing, but flushing can also be produced from tumors of the stomach, often immediately after food intake. Bronchus carcinoid can be associated with a particularly prolonged flushing, often with an associated periorbital edema.

When fading, the flushing of carcinoid syndrome can become gyrate. After many episodes, telangiectasia and chronic diffuse erythema can develop. Uncommonly skin sclerosis can occur. A pellagra-like dermatosis, secondary to tryptophan diversion from niacin to serotonin production, can also occur.

Although the diarrhea seen in carcinoid appears to be secondary to serotonin release, the flushing of carcinoid syndrome is secondary to the release of other vasoactive substances, such as substance P, from the tumor.[30] A somatostatin analogue (octreotide) can block at least some of the flushing.[31]

One study compared the symptomatology of patients with idiopathic flushing with that of patients with carcinoid syndrome.[32] That study showed that palpitations, syncope, and hypotension occurred only in patients with idiopathic flushing, whereas wheezing and abdominal pain occured only in patients with carcinoid. Diarrhea occurred in both.

Vasoactive substances can also be released in patients with extensive localized or systemic mastocytosis (see Chap. 161) and in patients with pheochromocytoma.

Palmar Erythema (See also Chap. 163)

Palmar erythema can be associated with advanced liver failure. Such liver failure may be secondary to either a primary or a meta-static tumor in the liver. The palmar erythema in these patients may be secondary to a high-output cardiac state. Palmar erythema, the "palmoplantar erythrodysesthesia syndrome," is common after the chemotherapy of many cancers. In that situation, it appears to be directly related to the chemotherapy, rather than the tumor.

Telangiectasia

Localized, grouped telangiectatic vessels on the anterior chest wall may be a marker for breast cancer. There is often a clinically palpable, indurated, warm, subcutaneous plaque immediately beneath the telangiectatic area. Telangiectatic vessels may also be the first evidence of dermal or subcutaneous metastases of breast cancer, as well as other malignant tumors.

Generalized telangiectasia can be a presenting factor of malignant angioendotheliomatosis (see Chap. 106). Biopsy of the telangiectatic vessels will confirm the diagnosis.

Progressive telangiectases have been associated with carcinoid tumors (see "Flushing") and with adenocarcinoma of the hepatic bile duct.[33]

Telangiectasia may also be a manifestation of a genodermatosis, which in turn can be associated with systemic malignant disease such as lymphoma. These genodermatoses include ataxia-telangiectasia (see Chap. 184), Bloom's disease, and xeroderma pigmentosum and its variant de Sanctis-Cacchione syndrome (see Chap. 158). In addition to the well-known association of lymphocytic leukemia and non-Hodgkin's lymphoma in patients with ataxia-telangiectasia, there appears to be an increased incidence of solid tumors of the oral cavity, breast, stomach, pancreas, ovary, and bladder, as well as others.[34] Female heterozygotes of ataxia-telangiectasia have a significantly increased risk of breast cancer.[35]

Purpura

Lymphoma is the most common cause of idiopathic thrombocytopenic purpura (ITP) associated with malignant disease. Hodgkin's disease is the most common associated lymphoma, and the diagnosis of ITP may precede other evidence of lymphoma.

Purpura related to cancer can occur from a wide variety of mechanisms: thrombocytopenia, consumption coagulopathy, hyper- or dysglobulinemia, vascular fragility, and vasculitis.

Disseminated intravascular coagulation (DIC) as a cause of purpura in malignant disease is most commonly associated with acute lymphocytic or myelomonocytic leukemia, in particular T-cell acute lymphocytic leukemia.[36] Many patients may not have full-blown DIC, having only biochemical or mild clinical manifestations of the process.

Thrombotic thrombocytopenic purpura, when associated with cancer, is usually a late sign.

Purpura can also be associated with the hyperglobulinemia seen in multiple myeloma or lymphoma. When purpura is secondary to the presence of cryoglobulins, lesions are often found in acral areas and may be associated with Raynaud's phenomenon. Benign hyperglobulinemic purpura can be associated with Sjögren's syndrome, which in turn can be associated with malignant disease.

Purpura, usually palpable, can also be associated with vasculitis (see Chap. 116), which in turn can be associated with cancer. It is important not to forget that a bacterial septicemia can present as a palpable purpuric eruption in patients with cancer.

Vasculitis (See also Chap. 116)

Leukocytoclastic vasculitis, such as can be seen in Henoch-Schön-lein purpura, can be very rarely associated with malignant neoplasms. The vasculitis seen in patients with malignant neoplasms does not differ clinically from that which occurs much more commonly secondary to nonneoplastic causes. It can be a presenting sign in squamous cell carcinoma, particularly of the bronchus.[37] Leukocytoclastic vasculitis can also be associated with leukemia and leukemic lymphoma.[38,39]

A periarteritis nodosa-like syndrome has also been reported in association with hairy cell leukemia, acute lymphocytic leukemia, and multiple myeloma.[40,41]

Vasculitic skin lesions can also be caused by a bacterial septicemia.

Cutaneous Ischemia

Evidence of compromised peripheral circulation can be a marker for many malignant neoplasms. It is frequently manifested by evidence of digital ischemia, either as Raynaud's phenomenon or frank gangrene.

Peripheral ischemia has been associated with many malignant neoplasms, including carcinoma of the pancreas, stomach, small bowel, ovary, and kidney, as well as lymphoma and leukemia.[42,43]

There may be associated splinter hemorrhages of the nail bed, suggestive of an underlying vasculitic process. The etiology, though, is rarely apparent.

The peripheral cutaneous ischemia of polycythemia rubra vera appears to be secondary to the increased viscosity of the peripheral circulation associated with this disease.[44] This increased viscosity may lead to frank venous thrombosis. Similarly, some patients with leukemia can develop leukostasis secondary to very high white blood cell concentrations.

The ischemia seen in cryoglobulinemia appears also to be secondary to increased blood viscosity. Cryoglobulinemia may be associated with multiple myeloma or with lymphoma.

Thrombophlebitis

Isolated vein thrombophlebitis is uncommonly associated with internal malignant disease. Multiple-lesion "migratory" superficial thrombophlebitis is much more often seen in association with cancer, and when this syndrome is present the patient should be examined carefully for occult malignant disease. The association of peripheral thrombophlebitis (phlebothrombosis) with gastric carcinoma was noted by Trousseau in the nineteenth century. Migratory superficial thrombophlebitis as a marker for cancer has been confirmed, and the association has been extended to include tumors of the pancreas, prostate, lung, liver, bowel, gallbladder, and ovary, as well as to lymphoma and leukemia. The migratory nature of the thrombophlebitis probably relates to a generalized hypercoagulable state.

Mondor's disease is thrombophlebitis of the anterior chest wall presenting as a tender or nontender cord. Usually benign, it may be associated with primary[45] or recurrent breast cancer.

Patients with deep venous thrombosis who are younger than 50 years of age appear to have a very significant risk of occult cancer (relative risk 19.0)[46] and thus should have an appropriately thorough examination and laboratory investigation. Those at greatest risk for cancer had a low hemoglobin and an eosinophilia.[47]

Bullous Disorders

Bullous Pemphigoid (See also Chap. 53)

There is probably no significantly increased risk of a malignant tumor in patients with bullous pemphigoid, other than that associated with the age of the patient.[48] However, there have been anecdotal reports showing that some patients with bullous pemphigoid clear when the concomitant tumor is treated, indicating a possible causal relationship in the rare patient.[49,50] In a patient with bullous pemphigoid and chronic lymphocytic leukemia, studies have failed to show the production of specific bullous pemphigoid antibody by the neoplastic lymphocytes,[51] suggesting that the bullous pemphigoid in that patient was not caused directly by the malignant lymphocytes.

It has not yet been shown that the immunosuppressive treatment of bullous pemphigoid has led to any increased risk of neoplasia.

Pemphigus Vulgaris (See also Chap. 52)

Pemphigus vulgaris can be associated with Hodgkin's disease, in which case the two diseases can run a parallel course.[52] A patient with lymphoma and pemphigus vulgaris had a high titer of pemphigus antibody in a tumor homogenate.[53] Pemphigus vulgaris has also been associated with Kaposi's sarcoma.[54]

The relationship of solid tumors to pemphigus vulgaris is less well defined. Pemphigus vulgaris has been reported in association with many solid tumors, but these associations have been in small series or isolated case reports. It has not been possible from these studies to decide whether there is a greater than expected incidence of pemphigus in these patients.

There is a well-defined association of pemphigus vulgaris with thymoma, with or without clinical myasthenia gravis.[55-58] Pemphigus foliaceus has been reported in association with thymoma and myasthenia gravis[59] and with hepatocellular carcinoma.[60]

Pemphigus erythematosus may be associated with bronchial carcinoma.[61]

Dermatitis Herpetiformis (See also Chap. 56)

Dermatitis herpetiformis is occasionally associated with intestinal lymphoma.[62] Patients with dermatitis herpetiformis have gluten sensitivity, and the presumed etiology of the lymphoma is the resulting chronic antigenic stimulation. The lymphoma, when it occurs, is usually a diffuse histiocytic lymphoma.[63]

Many solid tumors have also been described in association with dermatitis herpetiformis, but these reports have been isolated cases or small series. There is no indication that there are a greater than expected number of patients with dermatitis herpetiformis developing tumors other than intestinal lymphoma.

Herpes Gestationis (See also Chap. 54)

Herpes gestationis has been described in association with a hydatidiform mole[64] and germ cell tumor.[65]

Erythema Multiforme (See also Chap. 50)

Erythema multiforme does not appear to be a specific marker for any internal neoplasm. It has been reported in association with many tumors, but no studies have shown an incidence of erythema multiforme to be higher than expected. Erythema multiforme appears to occur more frequently in patients with acute leukemia, but whether this relates to the leukemia or to its treatment has not been well defined. Occurrence with monocytic and lymphocytic leukemia is more common than with granulocytic leukemia.

Erythema multiforme can occur in cancer patients secondary to drug or radiation therapy.

Epidermolysis Bullosa Acquisita (See Chap. 55)

Epidermolysis bullosa acquisita (EBA) is a very rare disorder that has been described rarely in association with carcinoma of the bronchus and with amyloidosis and multiple myeloma.[66] Most cases of EBA are not associated with cancer.

Linear IgA Dermatosis (See also Chap. 53)

Linear IgA dermatosis has been reported in association with lymphoma, chronic lymphocytic leukemia, myeloma, carcinoma of the bladder and esophagus, and with hydatidiform mole.[67,68]

Infections and Infestations

Herpes Zoster (See also Chap. 204)

Only a small percentage of patients with localized herpes zoster have a concurrent malignant disease, and investigation for malignant disease in otherwise healthy patients is not indicated. Patients with leukemia or lymphoma do have an increased risk of herpes zoster, but the herpes zoster usually occurs late in the course of their disease. The incidence of herpes zoster in patients with lymphoma is approximately 10 percent, possibly even higher in patients with Hodgkin's disease.[69] There may be an increased risk of herpes zoster in splenectomized lymphoma patients.[70] Localized herpes zoster can also occur in association with solid tumors such as breast cancer. In the case of breast cancer, the dermatomal distribution of the herpes zoster may indicate involvement of the nerve root area with metastatic tumor. The site of the primary tumor correlates with the site of herpes zoster in patients with breast cancer, cancer of the respiratory tract, and gynecologic cancer. Segmental herpes zoster can also occur after radiation therapy, presumably secondary to nerve damage with subsequent viral activation.

Disseminated herpes zoster is commonly associated with underlying malignant disease. Any patient with disseminated herpes zoster that is otherwise unexplained should be carefully examined for evidence of cancer. The most commonly associated malignant diseases are lymphoma and leukemia. Chemotherapy for cancer has also increased the risk of disseminated herpes zoster appearing in a cancer patient, presumably through suppression of the patient's immune response to the virus.

The development of herpes zoster in a previously treated lymphoma patient can be evidence of the recurrence of a lymphoma. Other evidence of the recurrence of Hodgkin's disease after remis-

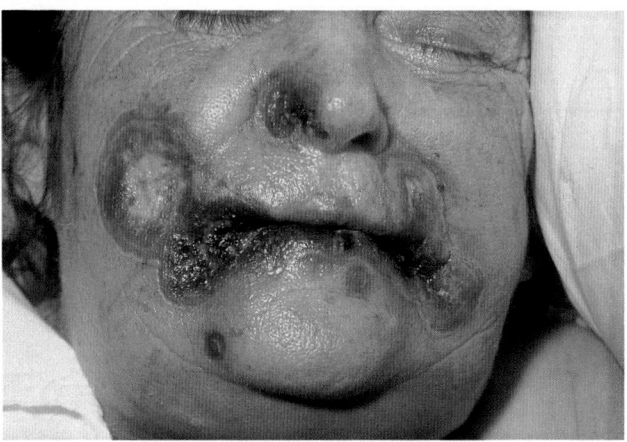

FIGURE 183-2   Female with advanced non-Hodgkin's lymphoma and chronic, ulcerative herpes simplex involving lips, cheek, and nose. (*Courtesy of Klaus Wolff, M.D.*)

sion has been preceded by herpes zoster. This sign is of particular value in patients who develop the herpes zoster more than 6 months after clinical remission.[69] The dermatome of the herpes zoster has also been found to be associated with Hodgkin's disease recurrence in that or an adjacent dermatome.[69]

Herpes Simplex

Typical localized herpes simplex is rarely a marker for cancer. Extensive, often chronic, local herpes simplex with massive ulceration and destruction of tissue (Fig. 183-2), generalized cutaneous herpes simplex, and disseminated systemic herpes simplex are indeed associated with malignant disease, which is often far advanced. Lymphoma and leukemia are most often the associated cancers, but any advanced malignant tumor can produce the compromised host immune response associated with these conditions.[71]

Generalized cutaneous herpes simplex can also be associated with extensive skin involvement, even in the presence of a reasonably intact immune system. Such generalization, called Kaposi's varicelliform eruption and most commonly seen in patients with eczema and atopic dermatitis, has been reported in association with cutaneous T-cell lymphoma.

Bacterial Infections

Bacterial infection of the skin as a marker for the presence of internal malignancy is very uncommon, and when it is associated with malignancy it is usually associated with very advanced disease. Skin lesions of a septicemia, often gram-negative, occur in cancer patients, but again generally late in the disease, as a manifestation of reduced host immunity. These skin lesions are nonspecific for the malignant disease and include pustules, nodules, vasculitic lesions, and, in *Pseudomonas* septicemia, ecthyma gangrenosum.

Fungi and Yeast

Dermatophyte infections of the skin are not associated with internal malignant disease. Deep fungal infections, with their associated skin lesions, can be associated with malignant disease. Similarly, mucosal candidiasis usually indicates a severely compromised host immune response, which can be secondary to advanced malignant disease or to chemotherapy.

Scabies

Norwegian scabies, a severe generalized form of scabies, is associated with the leukemia-lymphoma group of neoplasms, but it can be seen in any severely immunocompromised host. The scabies is frequently manifested by a minimal inflammatory response and should always be considered in patients who have advanced malignant disease associated with pruritus.

Disorders of Keratinization

Acanthosis Nigricans

Acanthosis nigricans can be classified into two major groups: benign and malignant. The benign group embraces idiopathic (including obesity-associated acanthosis nigricans), endocrine [including insulin-resistant diabetes, Stein-Leventhal syndrome, Addison's disease, pituitary tumors, and pinealoma (see Chap. 169)], and drug-related (including nicotinic acid, glucocorticoids, and diethylstilbestrol) disease. The acanthosis nigricans malignant group includes those cases associated with a malignant tumor.[72]

Polycystic ovaries, hirsutism, and acanthosis nigricans are a well-defined triad associated with hyperinsulinemia. Insulin resistance may be due to a reduced number of insulin receptors, plus, perhaps, a postbinding defect.[73–75] The elevated androgens are likely related to the hyperinsulinemia.[73] Patients with an associated acanthosis nigricans have higher testosterone levels and more intense insulin resistance.[73] In addition to defective or possibly a reduced number of receptors, endogenous beta-endorphins, high in patients with acanthosis nigricans and polycystic ovaries, may contribute to the hyperinsulinemia.[76]

Similar mechanisms may be involved in the development of paraneoplastic acanthosis nigricans in at least some patients. Very high levels of antibodies against insulin receptors in a patient with metastatic pheochromocytoma, insulin-resistant diabetes, and acanthosis nigricans have been identified. Other mechanisms that have been invoked relate to the observation that most tumors associated with acanthosis nigricans are members of the APUDoma family[77] suggesting that peptide production by the tumor may be a factor.[78]

Acanthosis nigricans, as the name implies, is a gray-brown thickening of the skin. It is manifested as symmetric, velvety, papillomatous plaques of gray-brown to black color, with increased skin-fold markings, papillomas, and skin tags (Fig. 183-3). The most common sites of involvement are the axilla, base of the neck, groin, and antecubital fossa, but the dorsum of the hand, elbow, periumbilical skin, mucous membranes, vermilion border of lips (Fig. 183-3a), and eyelids can also be involved. There may be an associated pruritus, particularly with malignant acanthosis nigricans. Malignant acanthosis nigricans is usually of sudden onset and is rapidly progressive, but it is otherwise clinically indistinguishable from benign acanthosis nigricans. Diffuse keratoderma involving the palms, soles, and flexor surfaces of the fingers

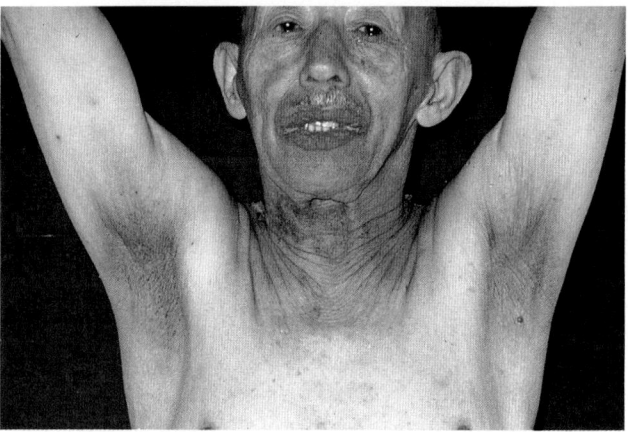

a

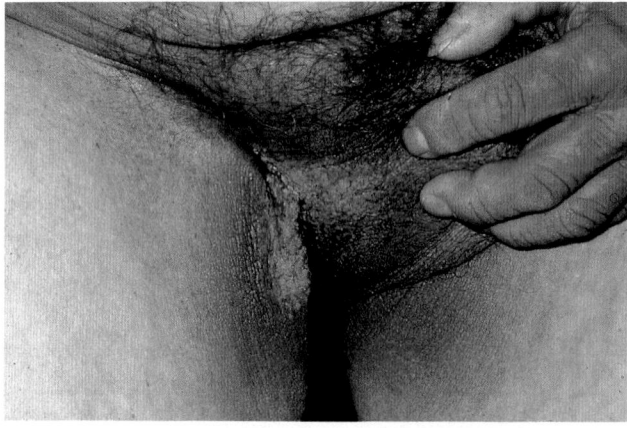

b

FIGURE 183-3 (*a*) Malignant acanthosis nigricans with pigmented, velvety, papillomatous lesions in both axillae and the neck, and papillomatous, verrucous lesions on the vermilion border of the lips. (*b*) Acanthosis nigricans in the groin and scrotal area. (*Courtesy of Fritz Gschnait, M.D.*)

and toes may be more common in malignant acanthosis nigricans than in the benign form. Such changes can be early. Acanthosis nigricans is rare in childhood and appears to have no gender predisposition.

Malignant acanthosis nigricans is usually secondary to an adenocarcinoma. The adenocarcinoma is usually intraabdominal (70 to 90 percent) and gastric (55 to 61 percent).[78,79]

Acanthosis nigricans associated with cancers at other sites is uncommon.[78] However, it has been described in association with a plethora of other malignant diseases, including carcinoma of the gallbladder, hepatocellular carcinoma, and carcinoma of the lung. Clinical changes typical of acanthosis nigricans can also be seen in non-Hodgkin's lymphoma and mycosis fungoides. The appearance of acanthosis nigricans may precede other evidence of the internal malignant disease.

Malignant acanthosis nigricans will frequently remit following extirpation of the tumor; but in general, patients with malignant acanthosis nigricans have a poor prognosis, as the tumor is commonly very advanced and extirpation is not possible.

Transient acanthosis nigricans has been reported 3 months after bone marrow transplantation for lymphoblastic lymphoma, in the absence of clinical evidence of recurrence of the lymphoma.[80]

Acquired Ichthyosis

The sudden onset of ichthyosis in an adult may indicate an occult malignant tumor, most often lymphoma. The ichthyosis is a true hyperkeratosis and can be differentiated clinically and histologically from simple dry skin (xerosis). Although the ichthyosis usually occurs as a late manifestation of a lymphoma, it may precede the diagnosis by several years. In addition to its association with Hodgkin's disease, ichthyosis has been reported in association with mycosis fungoides, other lymphomas, and multiple myeloma. Other tumors reported in association with acquired ichthyosis have included cancer of the breast, cervix, and lung, as well as Kaposi's sarcoma (with and without AIDS) and leiomyosarcoma.[81–85] In one report, a child developed a generalized icthyosis 3 weeks before presenting with a paravertebral rhabdomyosarcoma.

Follicular hyperkeratosis has been reported in association with multiple myeloma.[86] Horny follicular spicules stud the forehead, cheeks, nose, and chin and can extend to invade the upper back and arms. Microscopically, one sees a hyperkeratotic mass in the follicle mouth.

Palmar Hyperkeratosis

There are two groups of patients with palmar hyperkeratosis and associated malignant tumors: those patients with diffuse palmar hyperkeratosis and those with punctate palmar hyperkeratosis.

In 1958, diffuse hyperkeratosis, or tylosis, was reported by Howel-Evans et al.[87] to be associated in two families with an almost certain development of esophageal carcinoma by age 65. The tylosis in these patients can be separated clinically from the benign form of tylosis, which occurs at an earlier age (early childhood), has sharply delimited edges, and is of uniform thickness. In addition to the Howel-Evans families, there would appear to be a greater than expected incidence of esophageal carcinoma in other families with a pedigree of tylosis.[88]

A large kindred has been described with palmoplantar keratoderma in association with breast or ovarian carcinoma or both.[89] The clinical lesions cover the entire surface of the palms and soles and show a yellowish uniform hyperkeratosis surrounded by a red border. Histologically, the lesions show features of epidermolytic hyperkeratosis.

Direct involvement with the malignant process can also produce a hyperkeratotic state. Palmoplantar hyperkeratosis in patients with mycosis fungoides show skin infiltrates typical of the malignant disease. The picture is seen routinely in the Sézary syndrome (see Chap. 105).

The second type of palmar hyperkeratosis that may be associated with neoplasia consists of discreet hyperkeratotic papules on the palms. These patients have been reported to have a greater than expected risk of cancer of the breast and uterus, among other tumors.[90–92] While some kindreds have been described, arsenic, known to be associated with punctate palmar hyperkeratosis and an increased risk of cancer, may be responsible for other cases,[93] although studies have failed to show increased arsenic exposure on history. Other authors question the existence of the relationship of punctate palmar hyperkeratosis and internal cancer. It appears that the association, if present, is not very strong.

Palmar hyperkeratosis is also seen in paraneoplastic acrokeratosis of Bazex (see below).

Erythroderma

Erythroderma, a diffuse erythema of the skin surface usually associated with induration and scaling, is not uncommonly associated with malignancy. When associated with malignancy, it is most commonly associated with hematologic malignancies, in particular leukemia and lymphoma, where there is direct infiltration of the skin by the malignant cells. The cells are most frequently lymphocytes of T-cell type. These malignancies include Sézary syndrome and mycosis fungoides (see Chap. 105).

Among solid tumors, erythroderma has been associated with carcinoma of the lung, liver, prostate, thyroid, colon, pancreas, and stomach. The erythroderma associated with solid tumors usually occurs at a relatively late stage of the disease and may resolve after resection of the tumor. The etiology of the erythroderma associated with solid tumors is not known.

Paraneoplastic Acrokeratosis of Bazex

Paraneoplastic acrokeratosis of Bazex is a symmetric dermatosis that most commonly affects the hands, feet, ears, and nose with an erythematous psoriasiform eruption. The eruption is of a bluer hue than in psoriasis.[94] Later changes involve the cheeks, elbows, and knees, with still later changes often involving the central trunk, where bullae may be seen. Acanthosis nigricans may be an associated finding. In acrokeratosis of Bazex, the nails are involved early and severely. There is subungual hyperkeratosis, as well as a flaky white surface to the nail. The nails may be shed. The distal digits show an erythematous scaling eruption, often fissured, and often with suppuration.[95,96] Biopsy of the skin lesions of one patient showed diffuse deposition of IgA, IgM, and IgG along the basement membrane.[97] Nails appeared to have an abnormal amino acid composition.[98]

Bazex syndrome is usually associated with neoplasia of the upper respiratory system, which includes the pharynx, esophagus, tongue, and lungs, although a case associated with prostate carcinoma has been described. Lung tumors have included carcinoid. Patients with this syndrome have a virtual certainty of a tumor being present. Frequently the eruption predates evidence of the cancer, which is not diagnosed until the later stages of the syndrome.[94,99] Bazex syndrome has been reported to respond to etretinate, even though the primary lesion was left untreated.[100]

This syndrome should not be confused with follicular atrophoderma associated with basal cell carcinoma, hypotrichosis, and localized or generalized hypohidrosis, also described by Bazex.[101]

Collagen-Vascular Disease

Dermatomyositis (See also Chap. 172)

Dermatomyositis can be a marker for internal neoplasia, and the development of the dermatomyositis can predate the diagnosis of the cancer. In reviewing the world literature, Andreev reported that bronchogenic carcinoma is the most common tumor seen in association with dermatomyositis, with breast, ovary, cervix, and gastrointestinal tract tumors also being reported in a large percentage of patients.[102] In addition to these neoplasms, almost all other malignant tumors have been reported at least once in association with dermatomyositis. In spite of the multiplicity of reports, the true incidence of malignant tumors in association with dermatomyositis is quite difficult to define. In many studies, patients with polymyositis were lumped with those with dermatomyositis. Bohan et al.[103] assessed 153 patients with polymyositis-dermatomyositis and found an associated malignant tumor in 8.5 percent of the total and in 19.2 percent of men over the age of 50 years. More recent studies combining polymyositis patients with those with dermatomyositis show a similarly tenuous relationship with cancer.[104,105] Approximately 37 percent of the 650 patients with dermatomyositis alone had an underlying malignancy.[102] Bonnetblanc et al. noted that 28 percent of 118 cases of dermatomyositis had an associated malignancy.[106] Callen et al. noted a 26 percent incidence of malignancy in their patients with dermatomyositis.[107] They found that while there appeared to be a significantly increased risk of cancer in older patients with dermatomyositis, they did not feel that there was a significant relationship of polymyositis to cancer.[107] The cancers are usually identifiable by history and physical examination.[108] It would appear that adults with dermatomyositis, but not polymyositis, should be examined thoroughly for evidence of an associated malignant tumor. In children, dermatomyositis is not statistically linked to malignancy.

The clinical manifestations of dermatomyositis appear to be the same with and without a malignant tumor, although Basset-Sequin et al. noted that cutaneous necrosis and an elevated erythrocyte sedimentation rate appeared to be markers for those with cancer and, also, a reduced survival.[109] There is a suggestion that there is a male preponderance of patients with dermatomyositis associated with malignant tumors, but this has not been verified. Previous reports that biopsied muscle from patients with malignancy-associated dermatomyositis lacks an inflammatory infiltrate have recently been called into question.[103]

The cancers are usually observed with standard investigations, with extensive laboratory workup adding little.

A patient with dermatomyositis and metastatic melanoma cleared with extirpation of known tumor, but the dermatomyositis recurred simultaneously with evidence of further metastases. The relationship of the dermatomyositis to the cancer is not known, although presumably a circulating, possibly immune, factor is involved. Plasmapheresis has produced rapid clinical improvement.[110]

Lupus Erythematosus (See also Chap. 171)

Systemic lupus erythematosus (SLE) is only rarely associated with malignant neoplasia.

There is, however, a clearly recognized association between SLE and thymoma[111,112] (see also Chap. 171). A feature of many cases is erythroid aplasia.[113,114] Pemphigus erythematosus has been noted in association with malignant thymoma and myasthenia gravis, as has a pemphigus vulgaris-like eruption and positive LE cell test (see Chap. 52).

There is also an association of SLE and lymphoma.[115,116] The exact incidence and types of lymphoma associated with SLE have not been defined, but the association is probably real. In these lymphoma patients, the SLE may precede, coincide with, or follow first evidence of the lymphoma.[116]

In the large majority of reported cases, such an association with cancer is probably fortuitous. In one series, only 4 percent of SLE patients had neoplasia versus 26 percent of patients from the same institution with dermatomyositis.[117] In a single case report, SLE associated with ovarian dysgerminoma cleared after extirpation of the tumor. In another two patients, SLE developed during the course of melanoma. Despite reports such as these, it would appear that with the exception of thymoma and lymphoma, SLE is not commonly associated with internal neoplasia.

Progressive Systemic Sclerosis (See also Chap. 173)

Progressive systemic sclerosis (PSS) is not commonly associated with internal malignancy. In 727 cases of systemic scleroderma only 2.6 percent had an internal malignant lesion.[118] The only tumor that has been found to be consistently associated with PSS is carcinoma of the lung.[119–121] Almost all patients with associated lung tumors have very advanced progressive systemic sclerosis. The association is most likely one of a lung tumor developing secondary to the chronic pulmonary fibrosis.

Sclerodermatous skin changes have been reported in association with the carcinoid syndrome. Presumably, the sclerotic changes are secondary to the effect of an increased level of serotonin-like substances. These skin changes can be indistinguishable from the skin changes associated with progressive systemic sclerosis. Similar scleroderma-like changes have also been reported in a patient with myeloma.

The Werner syndrome of accelerated aging with sclerodermatous skin changes is associated with a broad range of malignant neoplasms.[122]

Skin Tumors and Internal Malignant Disease

Muir-Torre Syndrome

First described by Muir et al. in 1967 and by Torre in 1968, the essential features of the Muir-Torre syndrome are sebaceous tumors of the skin (Fig. 183-4), with or without keratoacanthomas, in association with visceral neoplasms, which are often multiple.[123,124] The sebaceous tumors are usually on the face or trunk and are usually multiple; and whereas most are sebaceous adenomas, they can include sebaceous hyperplasia, sebaceous epithelioma, and sebaceous carcinoma. Often the same patient will have the complete histologic spectrum of sebaceous tumors. Some skin lesions have histologic features of both keratoacanthoma and sebaceous proliferation.[125] Keratoacanthomas, if present, can be very large.

The visceral neoplasms are often multiple and include a wide variety of tissues. Colon cancers are particularly common and they may be associated with colonic polyposis.[123–129] Other neoplasms include other tumors of the gastrointestinal tract and tumors of the larynx and endometrium. There has been one report of an associated lymphoma. Patients with Muir-Torre syndrome appear to have a reasonably good survival, despite the profusion of neoplasms.[130] It has been suggested that a solitary benign sebaceous gland tumor of the eyelid is a good marker for the Muir-Torre syndrome and that its presence warrants review for systemic cancer.[131]

Inheritance patterns have not been well defined, but the Muir-Torre syndrome appears to be autosomal dominant.[132] There is an

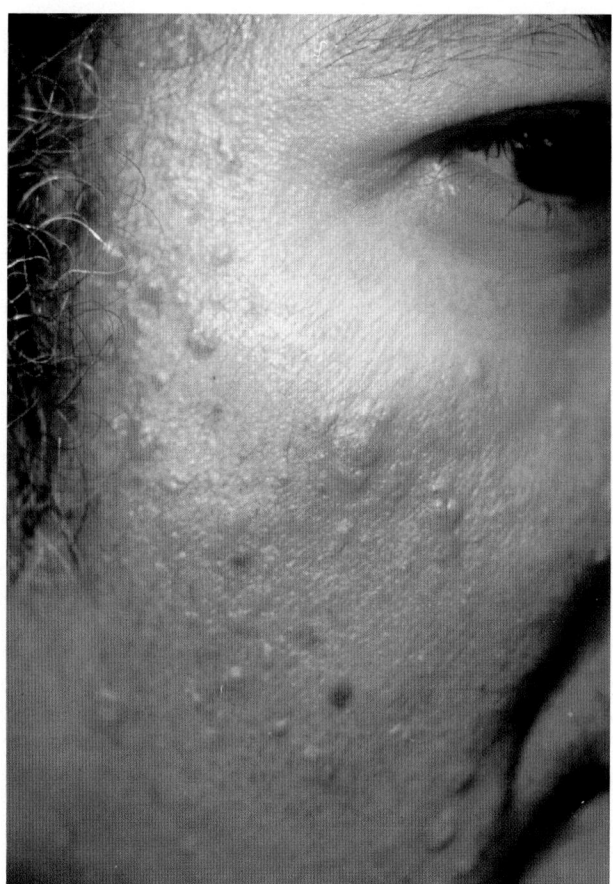

FIGURE 183-4 Muir-Torre syndrome showing typical sebaceous adenomas, in association with colonic polyposis and carcinoma in situ. (*Courtesy of T. Christensen, M.D., and R. Wilkinson, M.D.*)

association of the Muir-Torre syndrome with cancer family syndrome.[133,134]

Long-term treatment with isotretinoin appears to be useful in some patients,[135] and immunosuppression apparently exacerbates the cutaneous manifestations.[136]

Gardner Syndrome

The essential features of Gardner syndrome are intestinal polyposis (usually colonic), with a high rate of malignant transformation; epidermoid cysts, particularly of the face, scalp, and trunk; osteomatosis of the maxilla, mandible, and cranial bones; fibromas, desmoids, and other fibrous tumors of the skin and subcutaneous tissue.[137,138] Histologically, the epidermoid cysts may show areas of pilomatrixoma or a hybrid cyst with epidermal keratinization and inner root sheath keratinization. The desmoids often occur in the wounds and can be deeply invasive. At times, erroneously called sebaceous cysts, the epithelioid cysts of Gardner syndrome often precede the development of bowel cancer.

There is a virtual certainty of malignant transformation of the gastrointestinal tract polyps. Some of the polyps are almost always visible by proctoscope examination, but they can be found up to the stomach.[139] There is an association of hepatoblastoma, a rare neoplasm of infants and children with the Gardner syndrome, and there

may be some overlap of the features of Gardner syndrome and nevoid basal cell carcinoma syndrome.[140] Gardner syndrome is inherited as an autosomal dominant condition.

Cowden Disease

Cowden disease, or multiple hamartoma syndrome, was first described in 1963 by Lloyd and Dennis and was named after the propositus.[141] Inherited as an autosomal dominant trait, the distinctive cutaneous lesions are multiple tricholemmomas (Fig. 183-5a). These lesions are grouped around the mouth, nose, and ears and clinically resemble warts. Some patients also show closely set papules with a cobblestone pattern that have a fibromatous histology and also occur on the oral mucosa (Fig. 183-5b). Small keratotic lesions resembling plane warts occur on the acral skin. Patients may have an adenoid facies and high arched palate. Other cutaneous lesions can include lipomas, hemangiomas, neuromas, vitiligo, café au lait lesions, and acromelanosis.[142] Angioid streaks may be present in the retina.

Patients with Cowden disease have a greatly increased risk of breast and thyroid carcinoma. The breast changes seen in women with this syndrome range from fibrocystic disease to adenocarcinoma and can occur at a young age. Prophylactic mastectomy may be indicated.[143] Thyroid adenoma is the most common thyroid tumor in this group, but thyroid carcinoma can develop. Gastrointestinal tract polyposis is common.[144] There may also be an increased risk of gastrointestinal malignancy. One patient has been reported with a T-lymphocyte defect who eventually developed acute myelogenous leukemia. Female reproductive tract hamartomas and benign tumors are common. Squamous carcinoma of the tongue and basal cell carcinoma of the perianal skin have been reported.

The facial tricholemmomas respond well to carbon dioxide laser vaporization.

Mucosal Neuroma Syndrome

Mucosal neuroma syndrome is probably a variant of multiple endocrine neoplasia, type II (MEN II or IIA, Sipple syndrome). Also designated multiple endocrine neoplasia, type III (MEN III or IIB), the typical features include oral, nasal, upper gastrointestinal tract, and conjunctival neuromas, associated with medullary thyroid carcinoma (MTC) and pheochromocytoma. The lesions are typically soft to firm intradermal nodules. Corneal nerves may be highly visible.[145] The appearance of the neuromas usually precedes the development of cancer, but the MTC can appear in early childhood. The major cause of death in patients with MEN III is MTC, as metastases are common. The pheochromocytomas are often bilateral. Unlike MEN II, parathyroid hyperplasia is rare.

In addition to the mucosal neuromas, other abnormalities can include "blubbery" lips, a marfanoid habitus, lax joints, kyphoscoliosis, lentigines, café au lait lesions, medullated corneal nerve fibers, diverticulosis, and megacolon.[146] Localized intense itching may be a feature in some patients.

Neurofibromatosis (See Chap. 184)

Von Recklinghausen's neurofibromatosis has many associated malignant tumors.[147] Malignant schwannoma is the most common,

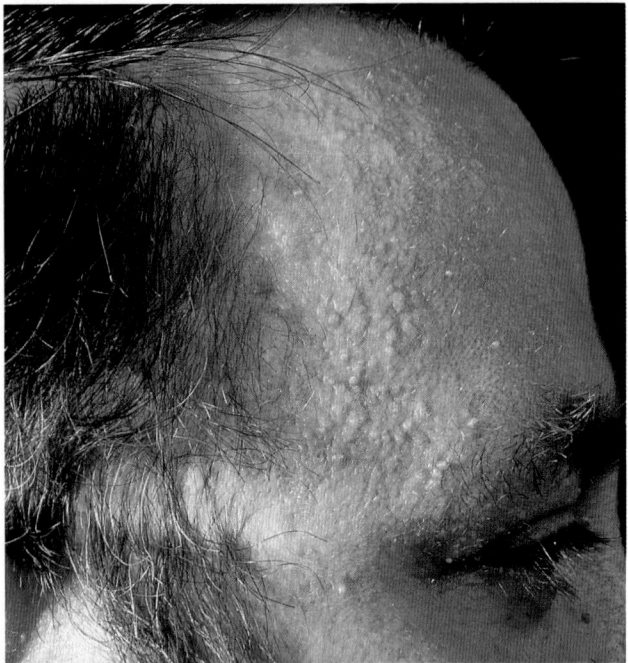

a

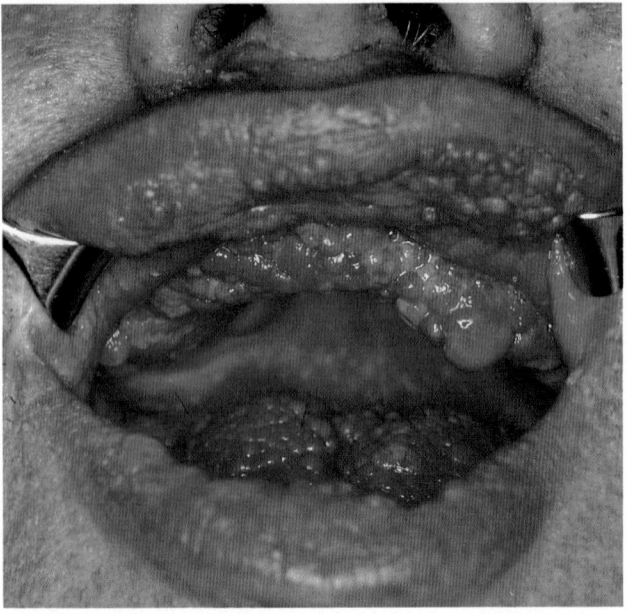

b

FIGURE 183-5 (*a*) Cowden disease with papular lesions on the forehead that histologically proved to be tricholemmomas. (*b*) Oral mucosa of same patient with multiple fibropapillomas. (*Courtesy of Peter Fritsch, M.D.*)

occurring in one series in 29 percent of patients.[148] These patients were usually over the age of 30. Other tumors include fibrosarcoma, rhabdomyosarcoma, nephroblastoma (Wilms' tumor), and acute and chronic myelogenous leukemia. There is an increased incidence of ocular melanoma, although probably not an increased incidence of cutaneous melanoma. Benign neural tumors, peripheral and intracranial, are common.

Hormone-Related Conditions

Malignant tumors may release hormones into the circulation, and such hormones can produce skin manifestations. The manifestation of such hormone excess is not specific to the tumor and can occur secondarily from an excess of that hormone from any cause.

Hirsutism may be a manifestation of an increase in circulating androgens. Such androgen excess is most typically seen with testicular or ovarian tumors. Non-androgen-regulated hair increase, hypertrichosis, may result from porphyria cutanea tarda, which may be associated with internal malignancy, or may appear as hypertrichosis lanuginosa acquisita, also secondary to internal malignant disease.

Gynecomastia in the male can be produced by an excess of estrogens. Such estrogens may be produced by a tumor of the testis. Lung tumors can also produce gynecomastia.[149]

Cushing syndrome is generally secondary to excessive ACTH production. Tumors from widely diverse sites can produce excessive ACTH. Many of these are derived from APUD tissue. The most common site is the lung, with the pancreas being the next most common.

Acne can be caused by the same tumors that produce hirsutism. Acne may also be a marker for internal malignancy in another way. Female patients with severe acne show an apparent increase in the incidence of breast cancer. Patients with breast cancer have increased sebum production.[150,151] It may well be that the stimulus for breast cancer and for increased sebum production is similar.

Other Disorders Associated with Primary Skin Cancers

Nevoid Basal Cell Carcinoma Syndrome (See also Chap. 75)

Nevoid basal cell carcinoma syndrome, or Gorlin-Goltz syndrome, is a syndrome consisting of multiple basal cell carcinomas, jaw cysts, skin pitting, skeletal abnormalities, and a tendency to malignant disease[152] (Fig. 183-6).

Both benign and malignant systemic tumors have been described in association with nevoid basal cell carcinoma syndrome. Benign tumors have included leiomyomas and fibromas of the ovary. The most common malignant tumor is medulloblastoma.[153] These tumors can occur in patients without any cutaneous basal cell carcinomas but with a family history of nevoid basal cell carcinoma syndrome. Other tumors include astrocytomas, meningiomas, and craniopharygiomas. The central nervous system tumors can occur at a very early age, sometimes in the first year of life.[154] Hodgkin's disease may be associated. Fibrosarcoma has also been reported in association with nevoid basal cell carcinoma syndrome, as has carcinoma of the maxillary antrum.

Patients with nevoid basal cell carcinoma syndrome are more sensitive to x-ray damage than normal.[155,156]

Systemic retinoids have been shown to be useful in causing the regression of some skin cancers and preventing the development of others.[157,158] The role of retinoids in preventing systemic cancers has not yet been defined.

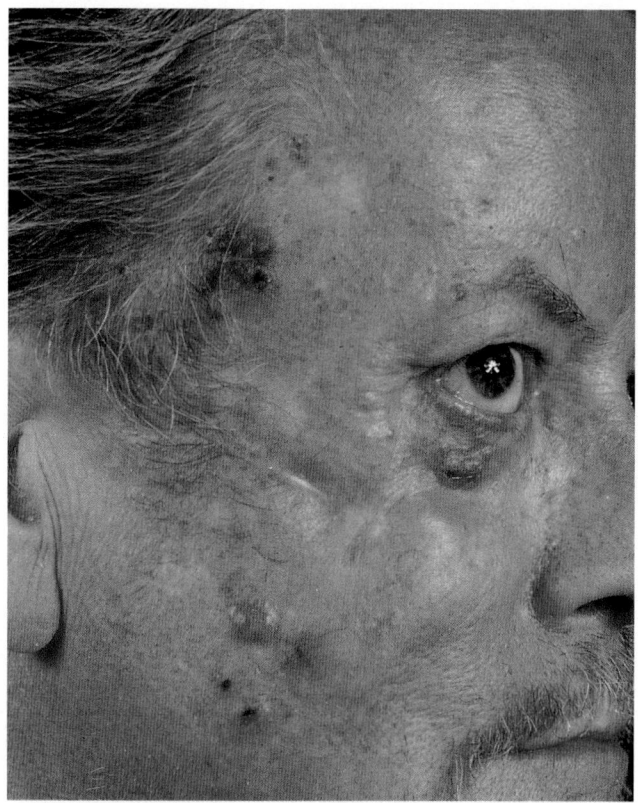

FIGURE 183-6 Patient with nevoid basal cell carcinoma syndrome with multiple basal cell carcinomas. The scarring is a result of surgery for maxillary cysts. (*Courtesy of Klaus Wolff, M.D.*)

Arsenical Manifestations

Chronic arsenic toxicity can be manifested by arsenical melanosis, plantar and palmar keratoses (Fig. 183-7), and Bowen's disease. There would also appear to be an increased risk of internal neoplasia. The risk of internal neoplasia is apparently increased if the

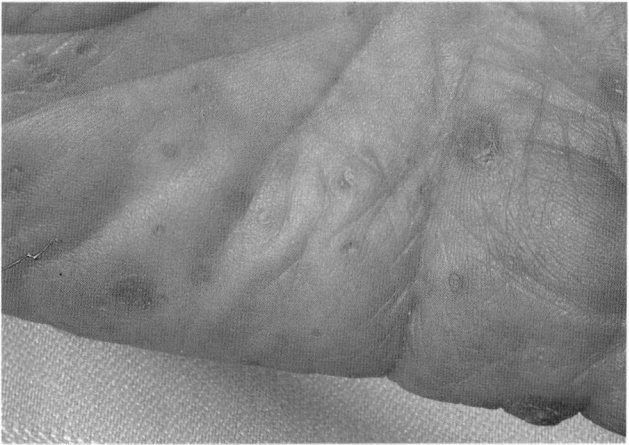

FIGURE 183-7 Punctate palmar keratoderma in a patient with previous arsenic exposure.

Bowen's disease is on non-sun-exposed skin.[159] These patients probably have their Bowen's disease secondary to previous arsenic intake. The increased cancer risk may be up to nine times the expected incidence. It has been estimated that approximately one-third of patients with Bowen's disease develop an internal malignancy 6 to 10 years after the initial diagnosis of the Bowen's disease.[160] Malignancies have included tumors of the urogenital region, mouth, esophagus, and lung. Airborne arsenic pollutants may account for an increased lung cancer rate in an industrial setting. Against the many small series that have been reported showing an increased rate of internal malignancy, there is evidence that not all patients with Bowen's disease, including both on sun-exposed and non-sun-exposed sites, have an increased risk of internal malignancy. When this large series of general Bowen's disease was compared to controls, no significant difference in systemic malignancy was found.[161] Arsenical keratoses on the palms (Fig. 183-7) and soles, a more specific finding, did correlate with an apparent increase in internal malignancy.[162]

Other Disorders Associated with Internal Malignant Disease

Pruritus

Pruritus, often accompanied by excoriations, can be a nonspecific marker of internal malignant disease. Although often associated with xerosis, the pruritus of malignant disease can occur in apparently normal skin. It can be continuous or paroxysmal. It is usually generalized.

When occurring with malignant diseases, pruritus is most commonly associated with leukemia and lymphoma, including drug-induced lymphoma.[163] The pruritus of Hodgkin's disease will often start on the legs, is usually continuous, and may be associated with a burning feeling. Pruritus is one of the most common cutaneous manifestations of leukemia, probably exceeded only by purpura. The pruritus of leukemia is usually less severe than that associated with lymphoma and is more often generalized. Although the pruritus of both leukemia and lymphoma can precede the diagnosis, it is usually a sign of late disease. The severity of the pruritus tends to parallel the course of the disease, with severe pruritus heralding a poor prognosis.[164]

Pruritus associated with bathing is a marker for polycythemia rubra vera (PRV) and is present in half of patients.[165] This itch can be severe and paroxysmal. Patients with polycythemia rubra vera can also have chronic continuous pruritus unrelated to bathing.

Severe pruritus can be a feature of Fanconi's anemia and myeloma.

Pruritus associated with visceral neoplasia is most commonly associated with pancreatic and stomach tumors[166] but may also be associated with most other solid tumors. The appearance of severe pruritus after treatment of the primary tumor may herald a tumor recurrence. Renal and liver involvement with primary or metastatic cancer can also produce pruritus secondary to the accumulation in the skin of pruritogenic metabolites. Severe pruritus of the nostrils is evidence for a central nervous system tumor,[167] with paroxysmal facial itch being associated with brainstem glioma.

Itch can also be a feature of specific tumor infiltrates in the skin. In this instance, the skin does not usually appear normal.

Erythema Gyratum Repens

Erythema gyratum repens is a cutaneous eruption consisting of concentric raised erythematous bands moving in waves over the body surface in a "wood-grain" pattern.[168] Almost all patients with this eruption have an internal malignant neoplasm. The erythematous bands in erythema gyratum repens may be flat or raised. They are frequently surmounted by a fine marginal desquamation. The erythematous bands may move at a speed of approximately 1 cm/day. Removal of the malignant tumor usually results in complete resolution of erythema gyratum repens within 6 weeks.

Almost all cases of erythema gyratum repens are associated with internal malignancy. Although first described with carcinoma of the breast,[168] erythema gyratum repens has also been found in association with tumors of the lung,[169] bladder, prostate, cervix, stomach, and esophagus and with multiple myeloma. All patients with erythema gyratum repens must be thoroughly investigated for an internal malignant disease.

Subcutaneous Fat Necrosis (See also Chap. 108)

Subcutaneous fat necrosis is a cutaneous marker for acinar cell carcinoma of the pancreas. Identical lesions can also occur with pancreatitis[170] and pancreatic pseudocyst. Subcutaneous fat necrosis associated with pancreatic disease frequently has an associated polyarthralgia, which can affect most of the joints of the body. Ankle involvement is common. Intraosseus fat necrosis can also occur,[171] with the production of osteolytic lesions visible on x-ray examination. The polyarthralgia is presumably the result of fat necrosis of the periarticular tissue. There is frequently a concomitant associated fever and eosinophilia.

The skin lesions of subcutaneous fat necrosis can be painful or painless subcutaneous nodules, which can occur anywhere on the body but are most common on the legs, buttocks, and trunk. The nodules may be fluctuant and may be skin-colored to violaceous. Clinically, they resemble the lesions of panniculitis or erythema nodosum. The skin lesions are presumably secondary to the effects of increased serum levels of lipase, amylase, or trypsin on the subcutaneous fat.

Sweet Syndrome (See also Chap. 89)

In 1964, Sweet described a syndrome, which he termed *acute febrile neutrophilic dermatosis*.[172] It consists of painful, red, raised plaques and nodules that can appear anywhere on the skin surface but occur most commonly on the face and extremities. Vesicles or pustules may cover the surface of the plaques, and the plaques often expand peripherally with central clearing. Uncommonly, lesions may resemble bullous pyoderma gangrenosum (see Chap. 93). There is frequently an associated arthritis, conjunctivitis, and episcleritis, and there is often a history of preceding respiratory tract infection. Pyrexia and neutrophilia are common. Mucosal symptoms are more prominent in those cases that are associated with cancer.[173]

Sweet syndrome may be associated with leukemia. It is most commonly associated with acute myelocytic leukemia but may also be seen in acute myelomonocytic leukemia, myelodysplastic syndrome, chronic myelogenous leukemia, acute lymphoblastic leukemia, chronic lymphocytic leukemia, hairy cell leukemia, multiple myeloma, and lymphoma. Much less commonly, it is seen with solid tumors such as adenocarcinoma, embryonal carcinoma of the testes, ovarian carcinoma, gastric carcinoma, and adenocarcinoma of the prostate and rectum (see Chap. 89).

Hypertrichosis Lanuginosa Acquisita

Hypertrichosis lanuginosa acquisita (HLA) is an acquired excessive growth of lanugo (vellus) hairs. Soft downy hairs initially cover the face and ears, but eventually all hair-bearing skin may be involved (Fig. 183-8). Associated abnormalities include a glossitis that is often painful. The tongue is studded with red papules.[174] Fully expressed HLA is usually secondary to malignant tumors, but excessive lanugo hair growth can also be caused by drugs such as exogenous steroids, phenytoin, diazoxide, streptomycin, penicillamine, cyclosporine, and minoxidil or by conditions such as anorexia nervosa.

HLA secondary to malignancy is usually abrupt in its onset and is rapidly progressive. Tumors reported in association with HLA include tumors of the colon (including carcinoid tumors), rectum, bladder, lung, pancreas, gallbladder, uterus, and breast and lymphoma.[175–177] The excessive lanugo hair growth is presumably secondary to a circulating factor produced by the tumor. Most

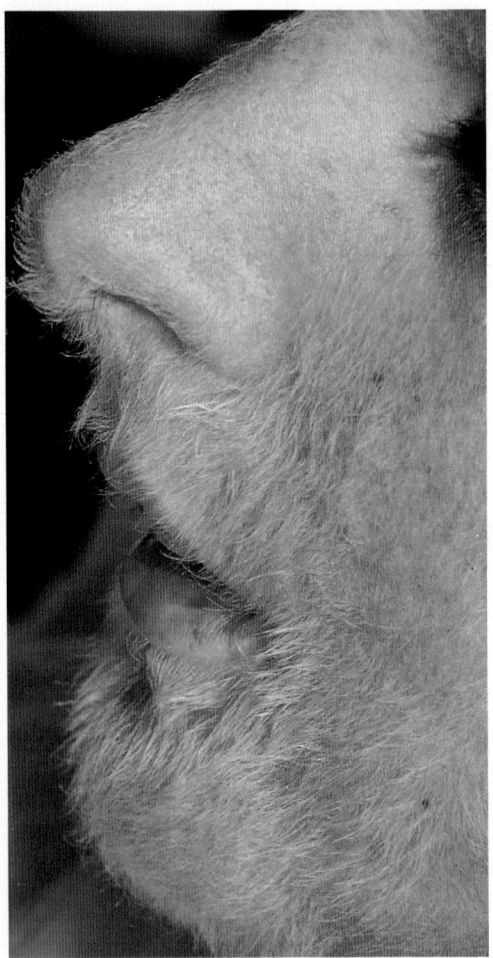

FIGURE 183-8 Hypertrichosis lanuginosa acquisita in a 19-year-old woman with pancreatic carcinoma.

of the tumors capable of producing HLA would appear to be of the APUD group.

Necrolytic Migratory Erythema (See also Chap. 164)

Necrolytic migratory erythema (NME) is a marker for an alpha-2-glucagon-producing islet cell tumor of the pancreas.[178–180] It is manifested by erythema, vesicles, pustules, bullae, and erosions, which typically involve the face, the intertriginous areas, in particular the groin, and the perigenital region (Fig. 183-9). It also involves the shins, ankles, and feet, as well as the fingertips. The vesicles are often very superficial and tend to become confluent. Patients can also have brownish-red papules scattered over much of the skin surface. Associated abnormalities include a glossitis, stomatitis, dystrophic nails, alopecia, weight loss, anemia, and diabetes.

Most patients with NME have a pancreatic tumor of the glucagon-producing type. Resection of the tumor clears the eruption, sometimes within 48 h. These patients have high blood glucagon levels. Infusion of amino acids has been reported to clear the dermatitis, as has an infusion of somatostatin or dacarbazine.[181]

The dermatitis has also occurred in patients without cancer but who have hepatitic cirrhosis and hyperglucagonemia, pancreatitis, or celiac sprue.[181]

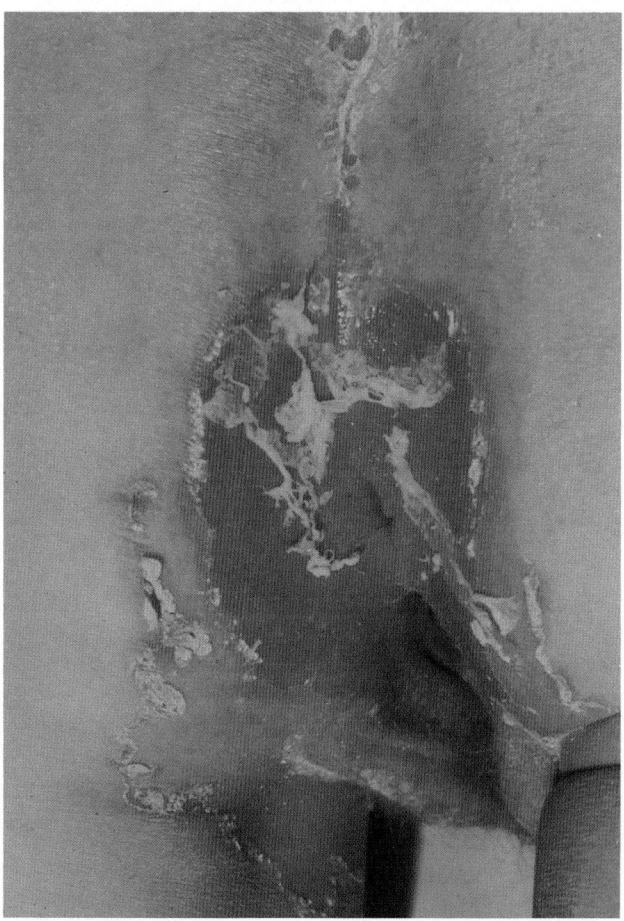

FIGURE 183-9 Glucagonoma syndrome. Flaccid vesicles and erosions in the perigenital and perianal region. (*Courtesy of Klaus Wolff, M.D.*)

Clubbing

Clubbing is the soft tissue enlargement of the tips of the fingers and toes. More typically associated with chronic lung disease, it can also be associated with neoplasms of the chest, usually of the lung. Other chest lesions include neurilemmoma of the diaphragm and cardiac tumors. It can occur secondary to chronic lung lesions such as bronchiectasis, lung abscesses, and other chronic lung disorders.

Clubbing can also be associated with intestinal polyposis of the Cronkhite-Canada types and with schistosomal colonic polyposis. Clubbing is manifested by an enlargement of the distal digits. Clubbing accompanied by subperiosteal new bone formation is called *hypertrophic osteoarthropathy*. A more florid expression of this, accompanied by acromegalic features, is called *pachydermoperiostosis*. Patients with these latter two conditions can have diffusely painful bones. Pachydermoperiostosis is usually idiopathic but can be secondary to lung cancer.[182] The clubbing and associated bone changes can be either insidious or abrupt.

The most common tumor associated with clubbing is bronchogenic carcinoma. Five to ten percent of patients with bronchogenic carcinoma develop clubbing.[183] Mesothelioma can also produce similar changes. Clubbing can also be produced by other solid tumors metastatic to the thorax and has been reported in Hodgkin's disease of the lung. Clubbing can also be seen with diffuse intestinal lymphoma.

Some patients with clubbing secondary to pulmonary disease can develop an associated thickening and yellowing of the nails, the yellow nail syndrome.

Leukoderma (See also Chap. 80)

Leukoderma is the acquired complete loss of normal skin pigment. The most common cause of leukoderma is vitiligo. Vitiligo is usually unassociated with malignant disease but has been reported rarely in association with thyroid carcinoma. Far more significant is the association of leukoderma and malignant melanoma. Depigmentation of the skin has long been known to be associated with melanocytic tumors, both benign and malignant. The halo nevus and halo melanoma are typical examples of this. Ectopic depigmentation can also occur with malignant melanoma. The appearance of leukoderma in patients after resection of their primary tumor may herald occult metastatic disease. Despite this, there is growing evidence that melanoma patients with metastic disease and leukoderma may have a relatively prolonged survival.[184] Uveitis may be an associated abnormality in patients with leukoderma and melanoma. Leukoderma may also be associated with ocular melanoma.

Peutz-Jeghers Syndrome (See also Chaps. 80 and 164)

First described by Hutchinson in 1900, the association of cutaneous and mucosal hyperpigmentation with gastrointestinal tract polyposis is now well known.[185] These gastrointestinal tract polyps can be associated with malignant tumors. The pigmentary changes involve both the skin and mucous membrane. The skin hyperpigmented macules are usually present at birth or early infancy and frequently fade at puberty. They can be typically grouped around the mouth, eyes, and nostrils, with pigmented papules also located on the fingers, palms, toes, periumbilical skin, or diffused over the skin surface. Mucosal pigmented lesions are similar but persist for life. Buccal mucosal pigmented papillomas have also been described.

The most common malignancy associated with the Peutz-Jeghers syndrome is duodenal carcinoma. These malignant tumors are frequently associated with hamartomatous polyps. The lifetime risk of a patient with Peutz-Jeghers syndrome developing an upper gastrointestinal tract malignancy is in the order of 2 to 3 percent.[186] The relative risk is 13,[187] whereas the relative risk of other non-gastrointestinal tract cancers is 9.[187] Another study showed an even greater overall cancer relative risk of 18.[188] Granulosa theca cell tumors may be present in as many as 20 percent of females with the Peutz-Jeghers syndrome and may be associated with precocious puberty. Peutz-Jeghers syndrome is inherited as an autosomal dominant condition.

Tuberous Sclerosis (See also Chap. 184)

Tuberous sclerosis can be associated with tumors within many organ systems. Most of these are hamartomatous, and some of these can become malignant. The malignant change occurring within hamartomas is usually sarcomatous, but metastatic lesions are uncommon. Malignant transformation in tuberous sclerosis is uncommon, occurring in probably no more than 5 percent of patients. Tumors of the kidney are frequently embryonal. Neural tumors are many and include glioblastoma multiforme and ependymomas. Death can result from the growth of histologically benign lesions within the central nervous system.

Multiple Eruptive Seborrheic Keratoses

Multiple eruptive seborrheic keratoses, also known as the sign of Leser-Trélat, have been mentioned in association with multiple internal malignancies.[189–191] These malignancies have included tumors of the stomach, breast, prostate, lung, and colon and malignant melanoma, as well as many references to their occurrence in lymphoma, primary lymphoma of the brain, and mycosis fungoides. They have also been mentioned in association with hyperkeratosis of the palms and soles associated with malignant disease and with acanthosis nigricans.

Evidence to support the presumed relationship of seborrheic keratoses to malignant disease is meager.[192] Most of the cancers described in association are common; seborrheic keratoses are common. Proving an uncommon causal relationship between a common cancer and a common skin sign is difficult. Reports of solitary cases abound.

A hallmark of many patients with so-called eruptive seborrheic keratoses is a cutaneous eruption that is also inflammatory. It may well be that the inflammatory dermatosis is centering around skin papillomas and seborrhoeic keratoses, making them suddenly "appear." Indeed, it is a common clinical experience to see an increase in the prominence of seborrhoeic keratoses in patients with generalized dermatitis from any cause. The sign of Leser-Trélat may or may not be a paraneoplastic syndrome.

If there is a relationship with cancer, it could be explained via growth factor or hormone effects on keratinocytes; perhaps a similar mechanism to that involved in the production of acanthosis nigricans.

The true relationship of multiple eruptive seborrheic keratoses to internal malignant disease remains to be defined.

Porphyria Cutanea Tarda (See also Chap. 150)

Porphyria cutanea tarda is clinically manifested by hypertrichosis, increased skin fragility, and bulla formation, often in sun-exposed skin. It has been associated with the development of malignant tumors, predominantly of the liver. The relative risk of hepatocellular carcinoma in patients with porphyria cutanea tarda has been estimated at 61,[193] a truly significant association. The porphyria cutanea tarda can predate or antedate the apparent development of the primary liver tumor. Porphyria has also been reported in a patient with lymphoma and an apparently normal liver.[194] Porphyria cutanea tarda can also occur secondary to chemotherapy-induced liver damage. Clinical variegate porphyria can be a marker for hepatocellular carcinoma.[195]

Direct Tumor Involvement in the Skin

Solid Tumors

Direct involvement of the skin by metastatic spread from a distant primary tumor is perhaps the most unquestioned marker for the internal malignancy. In a large review by Lookingbill et al.[196] skin involvement was the first sign of cancer in 0.8 percent of systemic cancer patients. Of this group, approximately equal numbers had direct extension to the skin, local metastases, or distant skin metastases. Direct extension was most common in patients with breast and oral cancer. Local metastases were most common in patients with breast cancer or pelvic cancer. Distant metastases were from many tumor types and sites.

Generally such a metastatic lesion is obvious, being an erythematous cutaneous or subcutaneous mass, and is frequently rapidly growing. At times, though, it can be difficult to diagnose metastatic lesions. This is especially true with metastases from breast cancer.

Most commonly breast cancer lesions metastasize to the anterior chest wall. They can typically show up as small nodules ranging from tiny 1- to 2-mm lesions to large masses of tumor. The tiny nodules can be erythematous or can be frankly hemorrhagic. The hemorrhage can be present within the nodules or in the field surrounding the nodules. Metastatic breast cancer can also present as an erysipelas-like eruption (carcinoma erysipelatodes, Fig. 183-10). A diffuse, warm, indurated plaque appears on the skin surface. Frequently, it is asymptomatic but can be painful. Even more uncommon is the leatherlike skin change of sclerosing metastatic breast cancer known as carcinoma en cuirasse, which may later develop nodules and ulcerate (Fig. 183-11). Carcinoma en cuirasse can be progressive for many years, even decades, in the absence of any apparent systemic involvement.

Metastases from malignant melanoma are usually pigmented. Often there is a bluish tint to the lesion, even if it is deep in the skin. Even if the primary tumor was pigmented, the metastases can be amelanotic. The reverse is also true.

Other tumors that commonly metastasize to skin include tumors of the lung, stomach, kidney, and ovary. The scalp is quite commonly involved by metastases from lung, kidney, and breast tumors. Alopecia may result. The face and neck may be involved by metastases from oropharyngeal carcinomas.

Metastases to the skin can appear many years after extirpation of the primary tumor. Progression, as in the case of carcinoma en

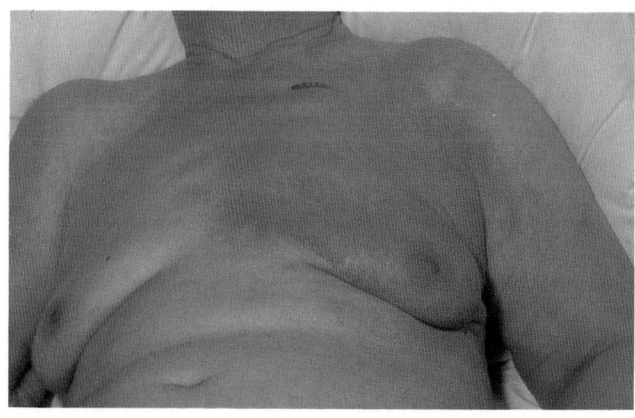

a

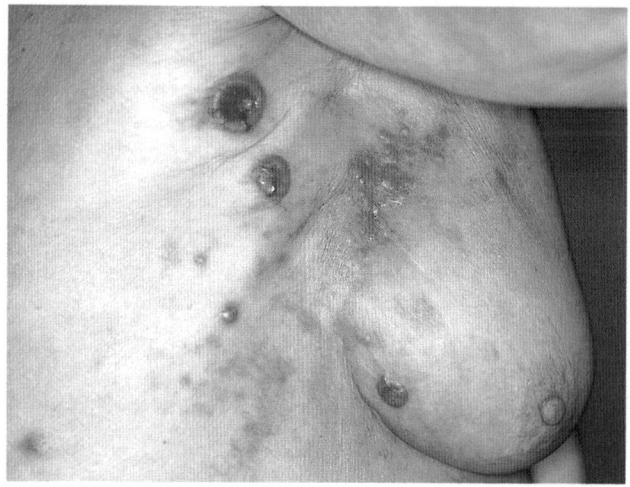

c

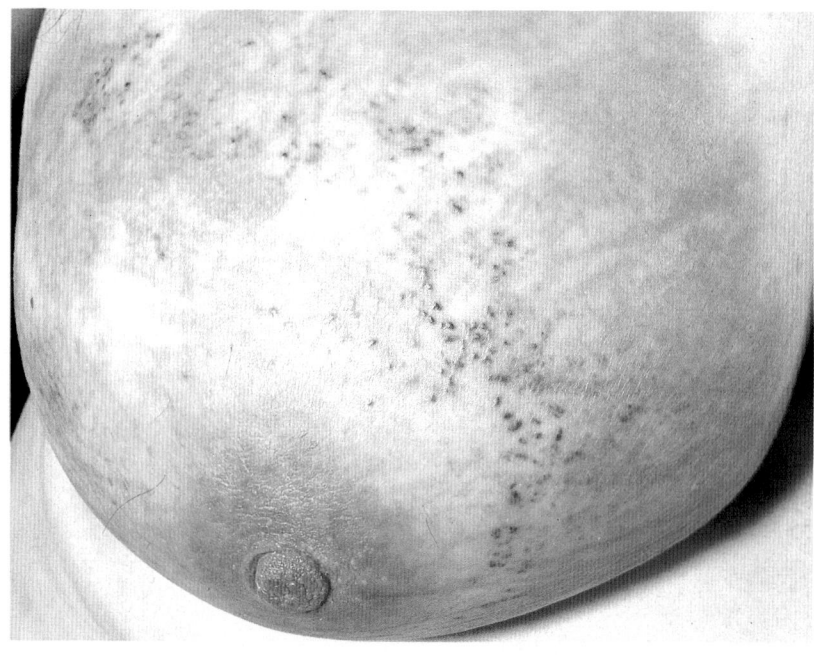

b

FIGURE 183-10 Involvement of skin by metastatic breast cancer. (*a*) Carcinoma erysipelatodes. Intralymphatic spread of mammary carcinoma that manifests as erysipelas-like erythema. (*Courtesy of Klaus Wolff, M.D.*) (*b*) In this close-up of another patient, the erysipelas-like quality of the erythema is even more evident. In addition, there are small, bright red lenticular metastases. The condition is due to an occlusion of the lympathics by cancer cells. (*c*) Metastatic breast cancer can also present as nodules. These may ulcerate and can be very painful.

cuirasse, can be very slow and may indeed not appreciably shorten life expectancy. Generally, though, cutaneous metastases herald a poor prognosis, as evidence of systemic spread to other sites is usually quickly apparent.

Metastases from renal and thyroid carcinoma may be pulsatile and may have a bruit.

Lymphoma-Leukemia

Involvement of the skin with lymphoma cells is quite common, particularly in the case of a T-cell lymphoma. Indeed, mycosis fungoides and Sézary syndrome are usually heralded by a cutaneous eruption. Like T-cell lymphomas, T-cell leukemias frequently have skin involvement. This involvement may manifest itself as a diffuse erythroderma as is seen in Sézary syndrome (see Chap. 105).

B-cell lymphomas can also involve the skin, with Hodgkin's disease being the most common. B-cell lymphoma involvement of the skin is usually manifested by the development of one or more papules or nodules. The nodules may be ulcerated or may, as they clear in the center and spread peripherally, form arcuate lesions (see Chap. 106). Alopecia can also be caused by lymphoma. Alopecia mucinosa is involvement of the hair follicles by lymphoma, with associated mucin deposition.

Aside from the erythroderma seen in T-cell leukemia, other lymphotic and myeloid leukemias can have cutaneous manifestations. The most common of these are the infiltrations of the skin produced by monocytic or myelomonocytic leukemia, which can produce a leonine facies in addition to other infiltrative plaques. The infiltrated skin frequently has a purple-colored hue. Involvement of the skin can be a presenting feature in myelomonocytic leukemia, although it generally occurs late in the course of the disease (see Chap. 160). An aleukemic leukemia cutis has also

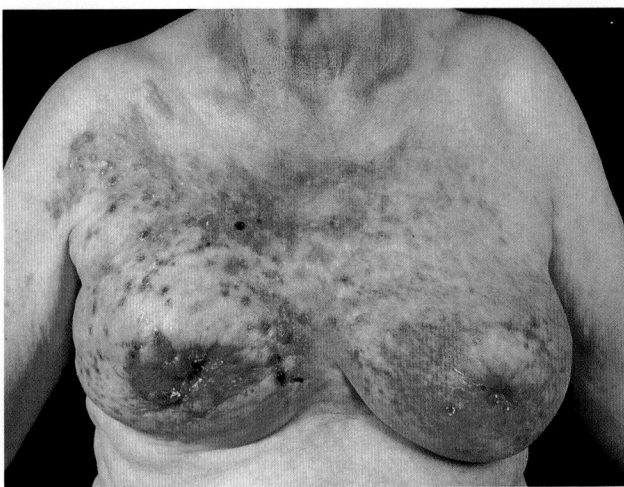

FIGURE 183-11 Cancer en cuirasse involving both breasts and thoracic wall. (*Courtesy of Klaus Wolff, M.D.*)

been described, in which an erythroderma appeared 4 months prior to the leukemia and cleared spontaneously; then typical acute myelomonocytic leukemia developed.[197] Biopsy of the precursor erythroderma showed atypical cells.

Multiple myeloma can appear as small red nodules on the skin surface with a diagnostic myeloma histology.

When assessing a solitary nodule that is histologically lymphoma but in the absence of any definable systemic disease, it is important to consider the benign cutaneous lymphoid infiltrates in the differential diagnosis.

Paget's Disease (See also Chaps. 112 and 113)

Paget's disease of the nipple is an erythematous scaling eruption that indicates ductal carcinoma of the underlying breast. Extramammary Paget's disease, which can occur in the anogenital skin, similarly may be associated with an underlying adenocarcinoma. The underlying carcinoma may be of apocrine or eccrine sweat gland origin, or can be from the rectum or urethra.

Mammary Paget's Disease This malignant neoplasm unilaterally involves the nipple, or areola, and simulates a chronic eczematous dermatitis. It usually occurs in females, with rare examples in males.[198,199] There is insidious onset over several months to years, usually in the fourth to sixth decade. Symptoms consist of itching and a feeling of discomfort, with patients reporting soiling of the bra by the exudate. Paget's disease of the nipple is usually unilateral but bilateral, symmetric involvement, either concomitantly or sequentially, has been observed as is also true for bilateral breast cancer. The lesion is a red, scaling plaque, rather sharply marginated and when scale is removed, the surface is moist and oozing (Fig. 183-12). In early stages there is no induration, but later the nipple may be flattened or depressed, indurations and infiltration develop, and a nodule or a larger lump in the underlying breast tissue may be palpated. In the initial stages regional lymph nodes are rarely found unless frank tumor or superficial ulceration is present. Differential diagnosis includes eczematous dermatitis of the nipple, which is usually bilateral and responds to topical corticosteroids. Other conditions to be considered are Bowen's disease, superficial basal cell carcinoma, and tinea. Therefore, biopsy is mandatory for verification of diagnosis. Histopathology reveals an intraepidermal, laterally spreading carcinoma consisting of large rounded cells without intercellular bridges and with large nuclei.

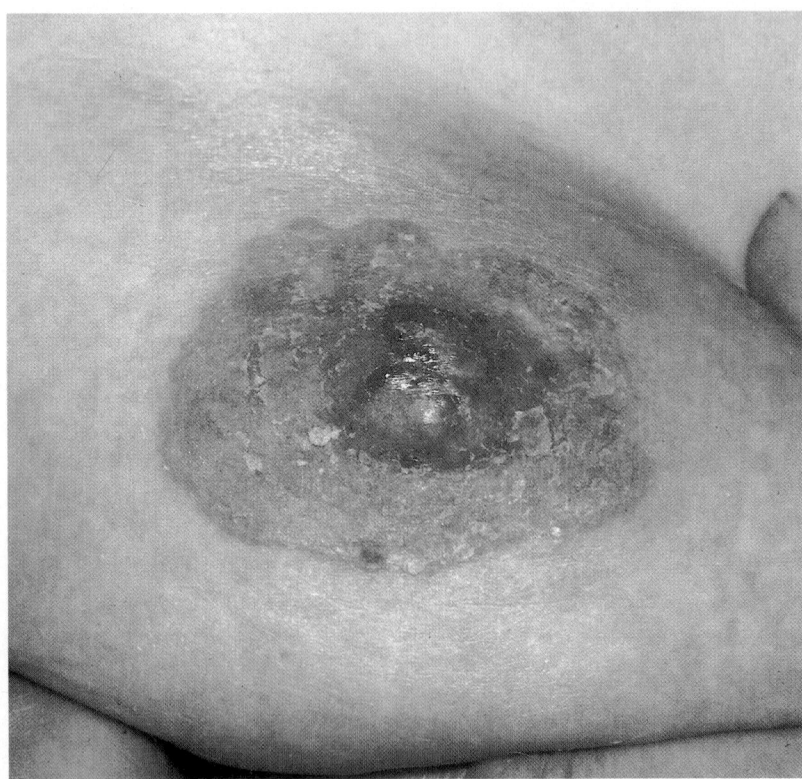

FIGURE 183-12 Paget's disease of the nipple. On the nipple and the areola mammae is a sharply demarcated erythematous area with slight scaling and an erosive and moist surface. There is a slight superficial induration. Axillary lymph nodes are not palpable.

Paget's cells are larger and stain much lighter than surrounding keratinocytes and may be PAS-positive. Subserial sections reveal that Paget's disease of the nipple extends from an intraductal mammary carcinoma.

Extramammary Paget's Disease   This is a neoplasm of the anogenital and axillary skin, histologically and clinically similar to Paget's disease of the breast, and it often represents an intraepidermal extension of a primary adenocarcinoma of underlying secretory glands. It occurs after the age of 40 and is found far more frequently in women than in men. It most commonly occurs in the genital and perigenital region and may thus involve the vulva, scrotum, penis, and the anal, perinanal and perineal skin. Other sites are the axillae, umbilicus, and presternal region. Of insidious onset the lesion spreads slowly and consists of an erythematous plaque with a velvety surface or scaling, crusting, and exudation. Borders are sharply defined with an irregular, often geographic configuration. Ulceration occurs only when the process is far advanced and at this stage lymph nodes may be palpable. Just as in Paget's disease of the nipple, the differential diagnosis includes eczematous dermatitis, intertriginous *Candida* infection, tinea corporis, erythrasma, Bowen's disease, superficial (amelanotic) spreading melanoma, and, when occurring on the vulva and penis, HPV-induced intraepithelial neoplasia (see Chaps. 112 and 113). The diagnosis must be confirmed by biopsy. Rectum, urethra, and cervix should be examined for primary adenocarcinoma. Careful examination of the anorectum must be performed by proctoscopy to search for a primary tumor.

Histopathology reveals characteristic Paget cells dispersed between keratinocytes, occurring in clusters and extending down into adnexal structures (hair follicles, eccrine ducts). Adnexal adenocarcinoma is often found when carefully searched for. Dermis shows a chronic inflammatory reaction. In later stages, the epidermis may be eroded/atrophic. The cytoplasm of Paget cells is PAS-positive and diastase-resistant, supporting a glandular origin.

The histogenesis of extramammary Paget's disease is uncertain. Paget cells in the epidermis may occur as an in situ upward extension of an in situ adenocarcinoma within deeper glands. Alternatively, extramammary Paget's disease may have a multifocal primary origin within the epidermis and its related appendages and does not represent an epidermotropic spread or metastasis from an underlying sweat gland carcinoma. Approximately 25 percent of extramammary Paget's disease can be shown to arise from a primary adenocarcinoma of underlying secretory glands. The primary tumor and Paget cells are usually mucus-secreting. Primary tumors in the anorectum can arise within the rectal mucosa or intramuscular glands.

Particularly in vulvar Paget's disease many cases have not had a documented associated underlying malignancy. There are well-documented cases where there is clearly an associated carcinoma and there are equally well-documented cases where no underlying carcinoma was found despite wide excision and extensive surgery. Studies have demonstrated the presence of carcinoembryonic antigen in each of 7 cases of mammary Paget's disease and 16 cases of extramammary Paget's disease.[200] This antigen was present in all Paget cells as well as in normal eccrine and apocrine gland cells. This additional evidence suggests that Paget cells have a glandular origin. However, it does not satisfactorily resolve the question of whether or not there is a local environmental change leading to the development of Paget's disease or, alternatively, whether there is always an underlying neoplasm.

The prognosis in both mammary and extramammary Paget's disease is related to the existence of underlying carcinoma. Treatment of choice is therefore surgery: limited or radical mastectomy or local excision for extramammary Paget's. When no underlying neoplasm is present, there is a high recurrence rate even after apparently adequate excision; this may be due to the multifocal origin within epidermis and adnexal structures and also because the intraepidermal malignancy may extend into areas where it is clinically nonapparent. Additionally, excised tissue must be carefully examined for evidence of an underlying malignancy and with regard to the lateral extension of the neoplasm. Recurrences are best managed by further excision. In situations where this is, for some reason, not possible, deep liquid nitrogen cryotherapy is an alternative.

Histiocytosis X (Langerhans Cell Histiocytosis)
(See also Chap. 160)

The classic skin lesions of Letterer-Siwe disease are fine erythematous papules surmounted by a scale. These small papules are frequently on the scalp but can be generalized. On cursory examination, the diagnosis of seborrheic dermatitis is suggested, but unlike seborrheic dermatitis, the eruption of histiocytosis X is papular and can be hemorrhagic. The red-brown papules can tend to become confluent, forming a greasy scale. Frequently, there are erosions, particularly in the flexures. Frank ulcers may occur behind the ears and in the groin. While virtually all patients with Letterer-Siwe disease have these papular skin lesions, only 30 to 50 percent of those with Hand-Schueller-Christian disease have skin lesions.

Skin lesions of eosinophilic granuloma are uncommon, but when they occur, they are usually identical to that seen in Letterer-Siwe disease. Larger papules and nodules may also occur.

Xanthomas of the skin can also be a manifestation of histiocytosis X.

References

1. McLean D: Cutaneous paraneoplastic syndromes. *Arch Dermatol* **122**:765, 1986
2. Nelson DH et al: ACTH-producing pituitary tumors following adrenalectomy for Cushing's syndrome. *Ann Intern Med* **52**:560, 1960
3. Haugen HN, Koken AC: Carcinoma of the hypophysis associated with Cushing's syndrome and Addisonian pigmentation. *J Clin Endocrinol Metab* **20**:173, 1960
4. Adrian RM et al: Diffuse melanosis secondary to metastatic malignant melanoma. *J Am Acad Dermatol* **5**:308, 1981
5. Silberberg I et al: Diffuse melanosis in malignant melanoma. *Arch Dermatol* **97**:671, 1968
6. Konrad K, Wolff K: Pathogenesis of diffuse melanosis secondary to malignant melanoma. *Br J Dermatol* **91**:635, 1974
7. Rorsman H et al: Trichochromuria in melanosis of melanoma. *Acta Derm Venereol (Stockh)* **66**:468, 1986
8. Andreev VC, Petkov I: Skin manifestations associated with tumours of the brain. *Br J Dermatol* **92**:675, 1975
9. Powell LW, Isselbacher KJ: Hemochromatosis, in *Harrison's Principles of Internal Medicine*, 12th ed, edited by JD Wilson et al. New York, McGraw-Hill, 1991, p 1825
10. Perdrup A, Poulsen H: Hemochromatosis and vitiligo. *Arch Dermatol* **90**:34, 1964
11. Marien KJC, Smeenk G: Plane xanthomata associated with multiple myeloma and hyperlipoproteinaemia. *Br J Dermatol* **93**:407, 1975

12. Wilson DE et al: Multiple myeloma, cryoglobulemia and xanthomatosis. *Am J Med* **59**:721, 1975

13. Roberts-Thomson PJ et al: Polymeric IgA myeloma, hyperlipidaemia and xanthomatosis: A further case and review. *Postgrad Med J* **51**:44, 1975

14. Lynch PJ, Winkelmann RK: Generalized plane xanthoma and systemic disease. *Arch Dermatol* **93**:639, 1966

15. Haggani MT, Hunter RD: Normolipemic plane xanthoma and histiocytic lymphoma. *Arch Dermatol* **112**:1470, 1976

16. Mays JA et al: Juvenile chronic granulocytic leukemia. *Am J Dis Child* **134**:654, 1980

17. O'Donnell J et al: Acute myelomonocytic leukemia presenting as a xanthomatous skin eruption. *J Clin Pathol* **35**:1200, 1982

18. Statham B et al: Atypical eruptive histiocytosis—a marker of underlying malignancy? *Br J Dermatol* **110**:103, 1982

19. McCadden ME et al: Mycosis fungoides associated with dystrophic xanthomatosis. *Arch Dermatol* **123**:91, 1987

20. Vail JT Jr et al: Cutaneous xanthomas associated with chronic myelomonocytic leukemia. *Arch Dermatol* **121**:1318, 1985

21. Cooper PH et al: Association of juvenile xanthogranuloma with juvenile myeloid leukemia. *Arch Dermatol* **120**:371, 1984

22. Feingold KR et al: Cutaneous xanthoma in association with paraproteinemia in the absence of hyperlipidemia. *J Clin Invest* **83**:796, 1989

23. Maize JC et al: Xanthoma disseminatum and multiple myeloma. *Arch Dermatol* **110**:758, 1974

24. Battaglini J, Olsen TG: Disseminated xanthosiderohistiocytosis, a variant of xanthoma disseminatum, in a patient with a plasma cell dyscrasia. *J Am Acad Dermatol* **11**:750, 1984

25. Brownstein MH, Helwig EB: The cutaneous amyloidoses. *Arch Dermatol* **102**:20, 1970

26. Gertz MA, Kyle RA: Acute leukemia and cytogenetic abnormalities complicating melphalan treatment of primary systemic amyloidosis. *Arch Intern Med* **150**:629, 1990

27. Coskey RJ: Macular amyloidosis. *Arch Dermatol* **111**:929, 1975

28. Gagel RF et al: Multiple endocrine neoplasia type 2A associated with cutaneous lichen amyloidosis. *Ann Intern Med* **111**:802, 1989

29. Kaplan LM: Endocrine tumors of the gastrointestinal tract and pancreas, in *Harrison's Principles of Internal Medicine,* 12th ed, edited by JD Wilson et al. New York, McGraw-Hill, 1991, p 1386

30. Vinik AI et al: Plasma substance-P in neuroendocrine tumors and idiopathic flushing. *J Clin Endocrinol Metab* **70**:1702, 1990

31. Balks HJ et al: Effect of a long-acting somatostatin analogue (octreotide) on circulating tachykinins and the pentastrin-induced carcinoid flush. *Eur J Clin Pharmacol* **36**:133, 1989

32. Aldrich LB et al: Distinguishing features of idiopathic flushing and carcinoid syndrome. *Arch Intern Med* **148**:2614, 1988

33. Rosenbaum FF et al: Essential telangiectasia, pulmonic and tricuspid stenosis, and neoplastic liver disease: A possible new clinical syndrome. *J Lab Clin Med* **42**:941, 1953

34. Morrell D et al: Mortality and cancer incidence in 263 patients with ataxia-telangiectasia. *J Natl Cancer Inst* **77**:89, 1986

35. Swift M et al: Breast and other cancers in families with ataxia-telangiectasia. *N Engl J Med* **316**:1289, 1987

36. French AJ, Lilleyman JS: Bleeding tendency of T-cell lymphoblastic leukemia. *Lancet* **2**:469, 1979

37. Cairns SA et al: Squamous cell carcinoma of bronchus presenting with Henoch-Schönlein purpura. *Br Med J* **2**:474, 1978

38. Sams WM et al: Necrotising vasculitis associated with lethal reticuloendothelial diseases. *Br J Dermatol* **80**:555, 1968

39. Greer JM et al: Vasculitis associated with malignancy. *Medicine (Baltimore)* **67**:220, 1988

40. Hughes GRV et al: Polyarteritis nodosa and hairy-cell leukemia. *Lancet* **1**:678, 1979

41. Gerber MA et al: Periarteritis nodosa, Australia antigen and lymphatic leukemia. *Nw Engl J Med* **286**:14, 1972

42. Hawley PR et al: Association between digital ischaemia and malignant disease. *Br Med J* **3**:208, 1967

43. Palmer HM: Digital vascular disease and malignant disease. *Br J Dermatol* **91**:476, 1974

44. Fagrell B, Mellstedt H: Polycythemia vera as a cause of ischemic digital necrosis. *Acta Chir Scand* **144**:129, 1978

45. Vieta JO, Heymann AD: Mondor's disease. *N Y State J Med* **77**:120, 1977

46. Goldberg RJ et al: Occult malignant neoplasm in patients with deep venous thrombosis. *Arch Intern Med* **147**:251, 1987

47. Aderka D et al: Idiopathic deep vein thrombosis in an apparently healthy patient as a premonitory sign of occult cancer. *Cancer* **57**:1846, 1986

48. Lindelöf B et al: Pemphigoid and cancer. *Arch Dermatol* **126**:66, 1990

49. Rook AJ: A pemphigoid eruption associated with carcinoma of the bronchus. *Trans St John's Hosp Dermatol Soc* **54**:152, 1968

50. Goodnough LT, Muir A: Bullous pemphigoid as a manifestation of chronic lymphocytic leukemia. *Arch Intern Med* **140**:1526, 1980

51. Cuni L: Bullous pemphigoid in chronic lymphocytic leukemia with the demonstration of antibasement membrane antibodies. *Am J Med* **57**:987, 1974

52. Sood VD, Pasricha JS: Pemphigus and Hodgkin's disease. *Br J Dermatol* **90**:575, 1974

53. Saikia NK: Extraction of pemphigus antibodies from a lymphoid neoplasm and its possible relationship to pemphigus vulgaris. *Br J Dermatol* **86**:411, 1972

54. Rosenmann E: Kaposi's disease in a patient with pemphigus vulgaris. *Israel J Med Sci* **2**:269, 1966

55. Peck SM et al: Studies in bullous disease. *Nw Engl J Med* **279**:951, 1968

56. Stillman MA, Baer RL: Pemphigus and thymoma. *Acta Derm Venereol (Stockh)* **52**:393, 1972

57. Vetters JM et al: Pemphigus vulgaris and myasthenia gravis. *Br J Dermatol* **88**:437, 1973

58. Safai B et al: Pemphigus vulgaris associated with a syndrome of immunodeficiency and thymoma: A case report. *Clin Exp Dermatol* **3**:129, 1978

59. Imamura S et al: Pemphigus foliaceus, myasthenia gravis, thymoma and red cell aplasia. *Clin Exp Dermatol* **3**:285, 1978

60. Muramatsu T et al: Pemphigus foliaceus associated with acanthosis nigricans-like lesions and hepatocellular carcinoma. *Int J Dermatol* **28**:462, 1989

61. Saikia NK, MacConnell LES: Senear-Usher syndrome and internal malignancy. *Br J Dermatol* **87**:1, 1972

62. Andersson H et al: Malignant mesenteric lymphoma in a patient with dermatitis herpetiformis, hypochlorhydria and small bowel abnormalities. *Scand J Gastroenterol* **6**:397, 1971

63. Reunala T et al: Lymphoma in dermatitis herpetiformis: Report on four cases. *Acta Derm Venereol (Stockh)* **62**:343, 1982

64. Dupont C: Herpes gestationis with hydatidiform mole. *Trans St John's Hosp Dermatol Soc* **60**:103, 1974

65. Halkier-Sorensen L et al: Herpes gestationis in association with neoplasma malignum generalisatum. *Acta Derm Venereol (Stockh)* **120**(suppl):96, 1985

66. Trump DL et al: Epidermolysis bullosa acquisita. *JAMA* **243**:1461, 1980

67. Green ST, Natarajan S: Linear IgA disease and oesophageal carcinoma. *J R Soc Med* **80**:48, 1987

68. McEvoy MT, Connolly SM: Linear IgA dermatosis: Association with malignancy. *J Am Acad Dermatol* **22**:59, 1990

69. Wilson JF et al: Herpes zoster in Hodgkin's disease. *Cancer* **29**:461, 1972

70. Monfardini S et al: Herpes zoster-varicella infection in malignant lymphoma. Influence of splenectomy and intensive treatment. *Eur J Cancer* **11**:51, 1975

71. Shneidman DW et al: Chronic cutaneous herpes simplex. *JAMA* **241**:592, 1979

72. Brown J, Winkelmann RK: Acanthosis nigricans: A study of 90 cases. *Medicine (Baltimore)* **47**:33, 1968

73. Wajchenberg BL et al: Role of obesity and hyperinsulinemia in the insulin resistance of obese subjects with the clinical triad of polycystic ovaries, hirsutism and acanthosis nigricans. *Hormone Res* **29**:7, 1988

74. Moller DE, Flier JS: Detection of an alteration in the insulin receptor gene in a patient with insulin resistance, acanthosis nigricans, and the polycystic ovary syndrome (type A insulin resistance). *N Engl J Med* **319**:1526, 1988

75. Harrison LC et al: Insulin resistance, acanthosis nigricans and polycystic ovaries, hirsutism and acanthosis nigricans. *Hormone Res* **29**:7, 1988

76. Givens JR et al: Reduction of hyperinsulinemia and insulin resistance by opiate receptor blockade in the polycystic ovary syndrome with acanthosis nigricans. *J Clin Endocrinol Metab* **64**:377, 1987

77. Hage E, Hage J: Malignant acanthosis nigricans—a paraendocrine syndrome? *Acta Derm Venereol (Stockh)* **57**:196, 1977

78. Rigel DS, Jacobs MI: Malignant acanthosis nigricans: A review. *J Dermatol Surg Oncol* **6**:923, 1980

79. Ollendorff-Curth H: Significance of acanthosis nigricans. *Arch Dermatol* **66**:80, 1952

80. Ifrah N et al: Transient acanthosis nigricans following bone marrow transplantation. *Bone Marrow Transplant* **5**(4):281, 1990

81. Krakowski A et al: Acquired ichthyosis in Kaposi's sarcoma. *Dermatologica* **147**:348, 1973

82. Majekodunmi AE, Femi-Pearse D: Icthyosis: Early manifestations of intestinal leiomyosarcoma. *Br Med J* **3**:734, 1974

83. Flint GL et al: Acquired ichthyosis. *Arch Dermatol* **111**:1446, 1975

84. Young L, Steinman HK: Acquired ichthyosis in a patient with acquired immunodeficiency syndrome and Kaposi's sarcoma. *J Am Acad Dermatol* **16**:395, 1987

85. Bechtel MA, Callen JP: Disseminated Kaposi's sarcoma in a patient with acquired ichthyosis. *J Surg Oncol* **26**:22, 1984

86. Braverman IM: *Skin Signs of Systemic Disease,* 2d ed. Philadelphia, Saunders, 1981

87. Howel-Evans W et al: Carcinoma of the oesophagus with keratosis palmaris et plantaris (tylosis). *Q J Med* **27**:413, 1958

88. Harper PS et al: Carcinoma of the oesophagus with tylosis. *Q J Med* **30**:317, 1970

89. Blanchet-Bardon C et al: Hereditary epidermolytic palmoplantar keratoderma associated with breast and ovarian cancer in a large kindred. *Br J Dermatol* **117**:363, 1987

90. Dobson RL et al: Palmar keratoses and cancer. *Arch Dermatol* **92**:553, 1965

91. Millard L, Gould D: Hyperkeratosis of the palms and soles associated with internal malignancy and elevated levels of immunoreactive human growth hormone. *Clin Exp Dermatol* **1**:363, 1976

92. Mortimer P et al: Palmar keratoses and internal malignancy. *Br J Dermatol* **109**:21, 1983

93. Andreev VC: Skin manifestations in visceral cancer, in *Current Problems in Dermatology,* series editor, H Mali. Basel, Karger, 1978

94. Jacobsen F et al: Acrokeratosis paraneoplastica (Bazex syndrome). *Arch Dermatol* **120**:502, 1984

95. Bazex A, Griffiths A: Acrokeratosis paraneoplastica—a new cutaneous marker of malignancy. *Br J Dermatol* **102**:301, 1980

96. Baran R: Paraneoplastic acrokeratosis of Bazex. *Arch Dermatol* **113**:1613, 1977

97. Pecora A et al: Acrokeratotis paraneoplastica (Bazex syndrome). *Arch Dermatol* **119**:820, 1983

98. Juhlin L, Baran R: Abnormal amino acid composition of nails in Bazex's paraneoplastic acrokeratotis. *Acta Derm Venereol (Stockh)* **64**:31, 1984

99. Richard M, Giroux JM: Acrokeratotis paraneoplastica (Bazex syndrome). *J Am Acad Dermatol* **16**:178, 1987

100. Wishart JM: Bazex paraneoplastic acrokeratosis: A case report and response to Tigason. *Br J Dermatol* **115**:595, 1986

101. Bazex A et al: Génodermatose complexe de type indéterminé associant une hypotrichose, un état atrophodermique généralisé et des dégénérescence cutanées multiples (épithéliomas basocellulaires). *Bull Soc Fr Dermatol Syphiligr* **71**:206, 1964

102. Andreev VC: Skin manifestations in visceral cancer, in *Current Problems in Dermatology,* series editor, H Mali. Basel, Karger 1978

103. Bohan A et al: A computer assisted analysis of 153 patients with polymyositis and dermatomyositis. *Medicine (Baltimore)* **56**:255, 1977

104. Manchul LA et al: The frequency of malignant neoplasms in patients with polymyositis-dermatomyositis. A controlled study. *Arch Intern Med* **145**(10):1835, 1985

105. Lakhanpal S et al: Polymyositis dermatomyositis and malignant lesions: Does an association exist? *Mayo Clin Proc* **61**:645, 1986

106. Bonnetblanc JM et al: Dermatomyositis and malignancy. *Dermatologica* **180**:212, 1990

107. Callen JP et al: The relationship of dermatomyositis and polymyositis to internal malignancy. *Arch Dermatol* **116**:295, 1980

108. Richardson JB, Callen JP: Dermatomyositis and malignancy. *Med Clin North Am* **73**:1211, 1989

109. Basset-Sequin N et al: Prognostic factors and predictive signs of malignancy in adult dermatomyositis. *Arch Dermatol* **126**:633, 1990

110. Macpherson A et al: Carcinoma associated dermatomyositis responding to plasmapheresis. *Clin Exp Dermatol* **14**:304, 1989

111. Singh BN: Thymoma presenting with polyserositis and the lupus erythematosus syndrome. *Aust Ann Med* **18**:55, 1969

112. Larsson O: Thymoma and systemic lupus erythematosus in the same patient. *Lancet* **2**:665, 1963

113. Kough RH, Barnes WT: Thymoma associated with erythroid aplasia, bullous skin eruption and the lupus erythematosus cell phenomenon. *Ann Intern Med* **61**:308, 1964

114. Takigawa M, Hayakawa M: Thymoma with systemic lupus erythematosus, red blood cell aplasia, and herpes virus infection. *Arch Dermatol* **110**:99, 1974

115. Green JA et al: Systemic lupus erythematosus and lymphoma. *Lancet* **2**:753, 1973

116. Wyburn-Mason R: SLE and lymphoma. *Lancet* **1**:156, 1979

117. Manchul LA et al: The frequency of malignant neoplasms in patients with polymyositis-dermatomyositis. A controlled study. *Arch Intern Med* **145**(10):1835, 1985

118. Tuffanelli DL, Winkelmann RK: Systemic scleroderma. *Arch Dermatol* **84**:359, 1961

119. Montgomery RD et al: Bronchiolar carcinoma in progressive systemic sclerosis. *Lancet* **1**:586, 1964

120. Romkin GH: Systemic sclerosis associated with carcinoma of the lung. *Br J Dermatol* **81**:213, 1969

121. Haggani MT, Holti G: Systemic sclerosis with pulmonary fibrosis and oat cell carcinoma. *Acta Derm Venereol (Stockh)* **53**:369, 1973

122. Hrabko RP et al: Werner's syndrome with associated malignant neoplasms. *Arch Dermatol* **118**:106, 1982

123. Muir EG et al: Multiple primary carcinomata of the colon, duodenum and larynx associated with kerato-acanthomata of the face. *Br J Surg* **54**:191, 1967

124. Torre D: Multiple sebaceous tumours. *Arch Dermatol* **98**:549, 1968

125. Burgdorf WH et al: Muir-Torre syndrome. Histologic spectrum of sebaceous proliferations. *Am J Dermatopathol* **8**:202, 1986

126. Housholder MS, Zeligman I: Sebaceous neoplasms associated with visceral carcinomas. *Arch Dermatol* **116**:61, 1980

127. Schwartz RA et al: The Torre syndrome with gastrointestinal polyposis. *Arch Dermatol* **116**:312, 1980

128. Fahmy A et al: Muir-Torre syndrome: Report of a case and re-evaluation of the dermatopathologic features. *Cancer* **49**:1898, 1982

129. Finan MC, Connolly SM: Sebaceous gland tumors and systemic disease: A clinicopathologic analysis. *Medicine (Baltimore)* **63**:232, 1984

130. Bitran J, Pellettiere EV: Multiple sebaceous gland tumors and internal carcinoma: Torre's syndrome. *Cancer* **33**:835, 1974

131. Tillawi I et al: Solitary tumors of meibomian gland origin and Torre's syndrome. *Am J Ophthalmol* **104**:179, 1987

132. Reiffers J et al: Hyperplasies sebacées, kérato-acanthomes, épithéliomas du visage et cancer du colon. *Dermatologica* **153**:23, 1976

133. Fusaro RM et al: Torre's syndrome as phenotypic expression of cancer family syndrome. *Arch Dermatol* **116**:986, 1980

134. Lynch HT et al: Muir-Torre syndrome in several members of a family with a variant of the Cancer Family Syndrome. *Am J Ophthalmol* **104**:179, 1987

135. Spielvogel RL et al: Oral isotretinoin therapy for familial Muir-Torre syndrome. *J Am Acad Dermatol* **12**:475, 1985

136. Stone MD et al: Torre's syndrome: Exacerbation of cutaneous manifestations with immunosuppression. *J Am Acad Dermatol* **15**:1101, 1986

137. Fitzgerald GM: Multiple composite odontomes coincidental with other tumorous conditions: Report of a case. *J Am Dental Assoc* **30**:1408, 1943

138. Gardner EJ: A genetic and clinical study of intestinal polyposis, a predisposing factor for carcinoma of the colon and rectum. *Am J Hum Genet* **3**:167, 1951

139. Golitz LE: Heritable cutaneous disorders which affect the gastrointestinal tract. *Med Clin North Am* **64**:829, 1980

140. Lynch PJ: Nevoid basal cell carcinoma syndrome with features of Gardner's syndrome. *Cutis* **16**:905, 1975

141. Lloyd KM, Dennis M: Cowden's disease. *Ann Intern Med* **58**:136, 1963

142. Gentry WC et al: Multiple hamartoma syndrome (Cowden's disease). *Arch Dermatol* **109**:521, 1974

143. Brownstein MH et al: Cowden's disease. *Cancer* **41**:2393, 1978

144. Taylor AJ et al: Alimentary tract lesions in Cowden's disease. *Br J Radiol* **62**:890, 1989

145. Aine E et al: Visible corneal nerve fibers and neuromas of the conjunctiva—a syndrome of type-3 multiple endocrine adenomatosis in two generations. *Graefes Arch Clin Exp Ophthalmol* **225**:213, 1987

146. Gorlin RJ et al: Multiple mucosal neuroma, pheochromocytoma and medullary carcinoma of the thyroid—a syndrome. *Cancer* **22**:293, 1968

147. Bader JL: Neurofibromatosis and cancer. *Ann N Y Acad Sci* **486**:57, 1986

148. Das Gupta TK, Brasfield RD: von Recklinghausen's disease. *Cancer* **21**:174, 1971

149. Omenn GS: Ectopic polypeptide hormone production by tumors. *Ann Intern Med* **72**:136, 1970

150. Krant MJ et al: Sebaceous gland activity in breast cancer. *Nature* **217**:463, 1968

151. Burton JL et al: Increased sebum excretion in patients with breast cancer. *Br Med J* **1**:665, 1970

152. Gorlin RJ: Nevoid basal cell carcinoma syndrome. *Medicine (Baltimore)* **66**(2):98, 1987

153. Gorlin RJ et al: The multiple basal cell nevi syndrome. *Cancer* **18**:89, 1965

154. Moynahan EJ: Basal cell nevus syndrome. *Trans St John's Hosp Dermatol Soc* **50**:187, 1964

155. Chan GL, Little JB: Cultured diploid fibroblasts from patients with the nevoid basal cell carcinoma syndrome are hypersensitive to killing by ionizing radiation. *Am J Pathol* **111**:50, 1983

156. Frentz G et al: The nevoid basal cell carcinoma syndrome: Sensitivity to ultraviolet and x-ray irradiation. *J Am Acad Dermatol* **17**:637, 1987

157. Hodak E et al: Etretinate treatment of the nevoid basal cell carcinoma syndrome. *Int J Dermatol* **26**:606, 1987

158. Cristofolini M et al: Aromatic retinoid in the chemoprevention of the progression of nevoid basal cell carcinoma syndrome. *J Dermatol Surg Oncol* **10**:778, 1984

159. Peterka ES et al: An association between Bowen's disease and internal cancer. *Arch Dermatol* **84**:623, 1961

160. Graham JH, Helwig EB: Bowen's disease and its relationship to systemic cancer. *Arch Dermatol* **80**:133, 1959

161. Andersen SLC et al: Relationship between Bowen's disease and internal malignant tumors. *Arch Dermatol* **108**:367, 1973

162. Reymann F et al: Relationship between arsenic intake and internal malignant neoplasms. *Arch Dermatol* **114**:378, 1978

163. Rubinstein N et al: Generalized pruritus as a presenting symptom of phenytoin-induced Hodgkin's disease. *Int J Dermatol* **24**(1):54, 1985

164. Feiner AS et al: Prognostic importance of pruritus in Hodgkin's disease. *JAMA* **240**:2738, 1978

165. Wasserman LR: The treatment of polycythemia vera. *Semin Hematol* **13**:57, 1976

166. Newbold PCH: Skin markers of malignancy. *Arch Dermatol* **102**:680, 1970

167. Andreev VC, Petkov I: Skin manifestations associated with tumors of the brain. *Br J Dermatol* **92**:675, 1975

168. Gammel JA: Erythema gyratum repens. *Arch Dermatol Syphilol* **66**:494, 1952

169. Appell ML et al: Erythema gyratum repens. *Cancer* **62**(3):548, 1988

170. Hughes PSH et al: Subcutaneous fat necrosis associated with pancreatic disease. *Arch Dermatol* **111**:506, 1975

171. Radin DR et al; Pancreatic acinar cell carcinoma with subcutaneous and intraosseous fat necrosis. *Radiology* **158**:67, 1986

172. Sweet RD: An acute febrile neutrophilic dermatosis. *Br J Dermatol* **76**:349, 1964

173. Clemmensen OJ et al: Acute febrile neutrophilic dermatosis—a marker of malignancy? *Acta Derm Venereol (Stockh)* **69**:52, 1989

174. Hegedus SI, Schorr WF: Acquired hypertrichosis lanuginosa and malignancy. *Arch Dermatol* **106**:84, 1972

175. Hensley GT, Glynn KP: Hypertrichosis lanuginosa as a sign of internal malignancy. *Cancer* **24**:1051, 1969

176. McLean DI, Macaulay JC: Hypertrichosis lanuginosa acquisita associated with pancreatic carcinoma. *Br J Dermatol* **96**:313, 1977

177. Jemec GBE: Hypertrichosis lanuginosa acquisita. *Arch Dermatol* **122**:805, 1986

178. McGavran MH et al: A glucagon-secreting alpha-cell carcinoma of the pancreas. *New Engl J Med* **274**:1408, 1966

179. Wilkinson DS: Necrolytic migratory erythema with carcinoma of the pancreas. *Trans St John's Dermatol Soc* **59**:244, 1973

180. Mallinson CN et al: A glucagonoma syndrome. *Lancet* **2**:1, 1974

181. Rappersberger K et al: Das Glukagonom—Syndrom. *Hautarzt* **38**:589, 1987

182. Braverman IM: *Skin Signs of Systemic Disease*, 2d ed. Philadelphia, Saunders, 1981

183. Minna JD: Neoplasms of the lung, in *Harrison's Principles of Internal Medicine*, 12th ed, edited by JD Wilson et al. New York, McGraw-Hill, 1991, p 1102

184. Nordlund JJ et al: Vitiligo in patients with metastatic melanoma: A good prognostic sign. *J Am Acad Dermatol* **9**:689, 1983

185. Jeghers H et al: Generalized intestinal polyposis and melanin spots of the oral mucosa, lips and digits. *N Engl J Med* **241**:993, 1949

186. Reid JD: Intestinal carcinoma in the Peutz-Jeghers syndrome. *JAMA* **229**:833, 1974

187. Spigelman AD et al: Cancer and the Peutz-Jeghers syndrome. *Gut* **30**:1588, 1989

188. Giardiello FM et al: Increased risk of cancer in the Peutz-Jeghers syndrome. *N Engl J Med* **316**:1511, 1987

189. Venencie PY, Perry HO: Sign of Leser-Trélat: Report of two cases and review of the literature. *J Am Acad Dermatol* **10**:83, 1984

190. Heng MC et al: Linear seborrheic keratoses associated with underlying malignancy. *J Am Acad Dermatol* **18**:1316, 1988

191. Safai B et al: Cutaneous manifestation of internal malignancies (11). The sign of Leser-Trélat. *Int J Dermatol* **17**:494, 1978

192. Rampen HJ, Schwengle LE: The sign of Leser-Trélat, does it exist? *J Am Acad Dermatol* **21**:50, 1989

193. Kauppinen R, Mustajoki P: Acute hepatic porphyria and hepatocellular carcinoma. *Br J Cancer* **57**:117, 1988

194. Maughan WZ et al: Porphyria cutanea tarda associated with lymphoma. *Acta Derm Venereol (Stockh)* **59**:55, 1979

195. Tidman MJ et al: Variegate porphyria associated with hepatocellular carcinoma. *Br J Dermatol* **121**:503, 1989

196. Lookingbill DP et al: Skin involvement as the presenting sign of internal carcinoma—a retrospective study of 7616 cancer patients. *J Am Acad Dermatol* **22**:19, 1990

197. De Coinck A et al: Aleukemic leukemia cutis. An unusual presentation of acute myelomonocytic leukemia. *Dermatologica* **172**:272, 1986

198. Jaiyesimi A et al: Carcinoma of the male breast. *Ann Intern Med* **117**:771, 1992

199. Satiani B et al: Paget disease of the male breast. *Arch Surg* **112**:587, 1977

200. Nadji M et al: Paget's disease of the skin. A unifying concept of histogenesis. *Cancer* **50**:2203, 1982

CHAPTER 184

M. Priscilla Short and Raymond D. Adams

Neurocutaneous Diseases

General Considerations

A search for a conceptual framework for the neurocutaneous diseases brings to light several logical possibilities, the most appealing of which is one based on histologic and pathogenic relationships. In pursuit of this idea, of first order of importance would be a grouping of diseases the common feature of which would be an underlying developmental fault, originating in the embryonic period and affecting cells of both skin and nervous system. The abnormalities in the two organ systems, once developed, would coexist and progress in parallel without having any direct interaction. Bourneville's tuberous sclerosis, von Recklinghausen's neurofibromatosis, and Sturge-Weber cranial hemangioma exemplify this principle.

A second category might include all the diseases in which some property common to the cells of skin and nervous system has rendered them simultaneously vulnerable to a given pathogenic agent. The latter might be a microbe (such as a virus, bacterium, or spirochete), a bacterial toxin, an exogenous poison, a deficiency state, or a metabolic (biochemical or endocrine) abnormality. Each of these agents might be taken as a subdivision of this class of disease.

Next, one might consider as a separate group all the disorders of skin consequent on a real or hypothetical abnormality of the nervous system. To take the most familiar examples, syringomyelia, congenital analgesia, polyneuropathy, and tabes dorsalis, by depriving the skin of sensory fibers which serve to protect it from injury, could result in inadvertent traumatism and chronic ulceration or unhygienic condition. And, once the skin is injured, a loss of the autonomic control of cutaneous vessels might interfere with natural healing processes, as happens in decubitus ulcerations secondary to diseases of the spinal chord.

Finally, there would be a logical position in such a classification scheme for cutaneous diseases in which the primary abnormality resides in the skin, the nervous system being secondarily affected. Reference is made here to the cutaneous furuncle that gives rise to an epidural spinal abscess; a viral exanthem that induces a postinfectious encephalomyelitis; an infected wound through which is introduced a toxin that acts by disinhibiting the motor neurons in the spinal cord, giving rise to tetanus; a cutaneous melanoma that may seed neoplastic cells through the brain without itself appearing to be in an active phase of growth.

In whatever way one might conceive of them, from a practical standpoint the neurocutaneous diseases serve to emphasize the importance of expert examination of the skin in obtaining clues as to the origin of obscure neurologic diseases and of knowing something about the way the nervous system may affect the skin and give rise to cutaneous diseases. The neurologic cases secondary to a dermatologic abnormality have no special characteristics and, being known to every student of dermatology, will not be considered further in this chapter.

This, then, is the basis of the following classification, which it is hoped will have the heuristic value of facilitating critical thinking and of putting into logical order the horde of maladies that implicate skin and nervous system either simultaneously or successively (Table 184-1).

Pathogenic Mechanisms

A general consideration of the probable causes and mechanisms of neurocutaneous diseases seems a useful theoretical introduction to our subject.

Pathologic Derangements in the Embryogenesis of the Cellular Elements of the Neural Crest

It has been shown that the symmetrically placed cells of the neural crest which, during embryonic life, lie dorsolateral to the neural tube are the common anlage of the dorsal or posterior root ganglion cells, sympathetic ganglion cells, Schwann cells, chromaffin cells, and melanocytes. Less certain is the neural crest origin of meningeal fibroblasts, endoneurial fibroblasts, and chondrocytes. Most probably they arise from mesoderm. The neural crest is said also to be involved in the formation of dental enamel.

Theoretically, then, a developmental failure or retardation of the growth and differentiation of the neural crest could result in a corresponding deficiency in all the cellular elements derived from this structure. That such a state exists has been postulated by a number of writers[1] who cite cases in which an infant or child is observed to lack sensation over the entire body, to have blond or nonpigmented hair, blue-green irides, aplasia of dental enamel, and autonomic dysfunction (manifested by pupillary and eye abnormalities ranging from a partial to complete Horner's syndrome, neurogenic anhidrosis with normal sweat glands, vasomotor instability, and urinary excretion of abnormal quantities of homovanillic and vanillylmandelic acids). This constellation of effects in the infant has been called *the syndrome of the neural crest*.

Lesser degrees of impairment of these functions, variably affecting the somatic sensory as well as the autonomic systems, have also been observed. The congenital sensory (analgesic) neuropathy with selective absence of small dorsal root ganglion cells and myelinated fibers is one example and the Riley-Day disease, a type of partial congenital dysautonomia, is another. These partial syndromes might relate to some extent to the timing of the action of the pathogenic agency, since not all the derivatives of the neural crest form and migrate at the same time during embryonic life.

Disturbances of Schwann Cell–Endoneurial Fibroblast Relationships

The Schwann cell proves to be one of the most interesting of the neural crest derivatives. Its nucleus resembles that of the fibroblast but is shorter and more oval, and its cytoplasm encloses segments of the myelin of peripheral nerves, or enfolds groups of nonmyelinated axons (Remak fibers). Thus, an intimate relationship to the axon of nerve cells stands as one of its most distinctive characteristics. The laminated myelin sheath, formed by circular infoldings of the Schwann cell cytoplasmic membrane (the molecules of lipid and protein of which the myelin sheath is constructed lie in relation to this membrane), probably is necessary for the rapid transmission of nerve impulses. Destruction of the axon results in degeneration of the myelin segments and leads to a proliferation of Schwann cells; and destruction of Schwann cells leaving the axon intact results in demyelination and interferes with axonal transmission.

Schwann cells are important in another respect—that of influencing the orientation of endoneurial fibroblasts (sheath of Henle) that surround each medullated axon. Crude lesions that interrupt the tubes of Schwann cells (bands of Bungner) disturb the spatial orientation of endoneurial fibroblasts. Similarly, fibrosis and scarring block the regeneration of injured nerve by interfering with the linear growth of Schwann cells.

Thus, there is normally a fixed relationship between axons, Schwann cells, and fibroblasts, not only in number but in spatial arrangement. Together with the axons of nerves they form an efficient neural pathway from skin to central nervous system and back. They also provide a channel along which infective agents and toxins may pass. The quantitative aspects of Schwann cells are also interesting. Because of the repeated branching and rich plexuses of nerves in the skin, the latter harbors more Schwann cells and endoneurial fibroblasts than any other organ in the human body. Any fundamental disorder of these cells might be expected to reflect itself maximally in the nerves of the skin.

The dermatologist's interest in Schwann cells and endoneurial fibroblasts emanates from the large variety of dermal lesions to which these cells give rise in neurofibromatosis. In this disease, endoneurial fibroblasts and Schwann cells undergo a limited multifocal hyperplasia (most active around puberty) in cutaneous nerve twigs and form the large number and variety of tumors to be described later in this chapter. Pigmentary changes are also induced, causing either café au lait spots or freckle-like macules. The pathogenesis of these curious focal hyperplasias of fibroblasts, Schwann cells, and melanocytes in neurofibromatosis has never been elucidated. Of course, their genetic basis is known, but what is the mechanism? One might speculate that some locally acting biochemical agent, necessary for the inhibition of the natural processes of proliferation and migration of Schwann cells and fibroblasts, is lacking during a certain period in embryonic life. Embryologists only recently have become aware of the timed sequences of natural

biochemical inhibitors of cell proliferation. Probably something has gone awry with this process. This pathogenic mechanism is not without implications in brain development as well, because there is a high incidence of cerebral dysgenesis and also of mental retardation in patients with neurofibromatosis. And in oncology it assumes importance because these benign overgrowths of tissue in nerves and brain, after years of quiescence, have a small but significant potential for malignant neoplastic transformation.

Disturbances of Melanocytes

The precursor of this cell, the melanoblast, is believed to migrate from the neural crest to the skin, to the cerebrospinal meninges, to the choroid of the eye, and to the inner ear (see Chap. 18). Melanin formation occurs also in certain neurons of the brainstem (substantia nigra, locus ceruleus, and other nuclei), but these cells are of different embryonal origin and the pigment also differs from that of epidermal melanocytes. The nerve cells retain their pigment in the human albino, whereas the melanosomes of melanocytes in the skin, hair, and meninges are deficient in melanin.

Disorders of pigmentation are discussed fully in Chap. 80. Further on in this chapter will be cited a few diseases in which pigmentary disturbances are associated with a neurologic disorder. The most familiar examples are tuberous sclerosis, neurofibromatosis, giant pigmented nevus, Waardenberg-Klein syndrome, and Chédiak-Higashi disease (see Table 184-5).

In several of these varieties of disease the melanoblasts are deficient, the melanocytes are reduced in number, melanosome formation is abnormal, or the transfer of melanosomes from melanocyte to malpighian cell (keratinocyte) is blocked. The number and variety of these disorders and their frequent conjunction with neurologic lesions strongly support the neurogenic derivation of melanocytes.

Developmental Derangements of Vascular Structures in Skin and Nervous System

The development of blood vessels in the brain and spinal cord during embryonic life occurs in a series of steps, as outlined by Streeter in the *American Embryologist.* Beginning with a complex network (rete mirabile), arteries and veins emerge and form the familiar patterns in each organ. This involves a series of regressive steps and tends to follow a metameric pattern. It is not surprising, therefore, that abnormalities of blood vessels and vascular malformations (hemangiomas), which abound in the skin and brain, might coexist if certain of these embryonic regressions failed to occur in particular regions.

Probably the most dramatic form of neurocutaneous hemangioma is exemplified by *Sturge-Weber-Dimitri disease,* a port-wine stain or nevus flammeus (feuermal, tache de feu) that occurs in association with cerebral meningeal hemangioma, cortical calcification, and glaucoma. Other examples are: the segmental *cutaneous hemangioma of the thorax,* which may be combined with a *hemangioma of the spinal meninges* in corresponding segments (Cobb's syndrome); the brachial hemangioma and hypertrophy with a cervical spinal vascular malformation (Trénauney-Weber syndrome); and the cirsoid retinal aneurysm, which is conjoined to vascular malformation of the brainstem (Bonnet-Dechaume syndrome).

TABLE 184-1

Classification of Neurocutaneous Diseases*

I Congenital and developmental neurocutaneous diseases
  A The congenital benign neoplasms and vascular formations
    † *1* Tuberous sclerosis (Bourneville's disease) (19110)
    † *2* Neurofibromatosis of von Recklinghausen (type I, 16220; type II, 10100)
    † *3* Cutaneous angiomatosis with abnormalities of the central nervous system
        †*a* Craniofacial or trigeminocranial angiomatosis with cerebral calcification (Sturge-Weber-Dimitri disease) (18530)
        ‡*b* Dermatomal hemangiomas with spinal vascular malformations (sometimes with limb hypertrophy as in Klippel-Trénauney-Weber syndrome) (14900)
    ‡ *4* Hemangioblastoma of cerebellum and retina (Lindau-von Hippel syndrome) (19330)
    ‡ *5* Familial telangiectasia (Osler-Rendu-Weber disease)
    ‡ *6* Ataxia-telangiectasia (Louis-Bar disease) (20890)
  B Developmental neurocutaneous diseases (developmental anomalies of skin and nervous system)
    ‡ *1* Congenital skin defects with gross anomalies of the nervous system (spina bifida, cranium bifidum)
        a Focal congenital skin defects and dermal hypoplasias
        ‡ (*1*) Goltz's syndrome (30560)
        ‡ (*2*) Johanson-Blizzard syndrome (24380)
        § (*3*) Wolf-Hirshhorn syndrome (4p-)
  C Congenital somatic abnormalities, including those of the nervous system and skin
    § *1* Somatic abnormalities with chromosomal changes (mongolism, or Down's syndrome; Patau's syndrome; Edward's syndrome; cri-du-chat syndrome; Turner's syndrome; Kleinfelter's syndrome)
    § *2* Somatic abnormalities with normal chromosome pattern [Papillon-Psaume syndrome, Rubenstein-Taybi syndrome, Hallerman-Streiff syndrome (23420), de Lange's Amsterdam dwarf syndrome (12247), Russell-Silver dwarf state (27005)]
  D Congenital eruptive diseases with nervous disorders
    † *1* Incontinentia pigmenti (Bloch-Sulzberger syndrome) (30830)
    ‡ *2* Hypomelanosis of Ito (incontinentia pigmenti achromians) (14615)
    § *3* Epidermolysis bullosa (22645, 13160)
    ‡ *4* Poikiloderma congenitale of Rothmund and Thomson
    ‡ *5* Anhidrotic ectodermal dysplasia (22500, 30510)
    ‡ *6* Hydrotic ectodermal dysplasia (12950)
  E Pigmentary changes of skin with neurologic disorders (see Table 184-5)
    ‡ *1* Linear sebaceous nevi (16820)
    ‡ *2* Basal cell nevus syndrome (10940)
    ‡ *3* Neurocutaneous melanosis (24940)
    ‡ *4* Moynahan's (LEOPARD) syndrome (15110)
    ‡ *5* Familial generalized melanoderma (leukomelanoderma)
    ‡ *6* Waardenburg-Klein and related syndromes (19350)
    ‡ *7* Vogt-Koyanagi-Harada syndrome
    ‡ *8* Chédiak-Higashi disease (21450)
    ‡ *9* Piebald trait (17280)
    §*10* Vitiligo, achalasia, congenital deafness (22135)
    ‡*11* Phenylketonuria (26160, 26163, 26164, 23391)
    §*12* Adrenoleukodystrophy (sex-linked, 30027, 30010; autosomal recessive, 20237)
  F The ichthyosiform dermatoses (see Table 184-3)
    ‡ *1* Ichthyosis vulgaris (14670)
    ‡ *2* Sex-linked ichthyosis (31277)
    ‡ *3* Congenital ichthyosiform erythroderma—bullous type
    ‡ *4* Sjögren-Larsson syndrome (27020)
    § *5* Conradi's syndrome (chondrodystrophia calcifans congenita) (11865)
    § *6* Rhizomelic chondroplasia punctata (21510)
    § *7* Netherton's disease (25650)
    § *8* Erythrokeratodermia variabilis (13320)
    § *9* Lamellar ichthyosis (autosomal dominant, 14675; autosomal recessive, 24210)
    §*10* Ichthyosis hystrix gravior (porcupine man)
    §*11* Unilateral congenital ichthyosiform erythroderma
    ‡*12* Refsum's syndrome (26650, 26651)

  G Looseness, redundancy, and loss of elasticity of skin (dermatochalasis, generalized elastolysis)
    § *1* Cutis laxa (autosomal dominant, 12370; autosomal recessive, 21910)
    § *2* Pterygium colli in Turner-Bonnevie-Ullrich syndrome
    ‡ *3* Noonan's syndrome (16395)
    § *4* Cutis verticis gyrata (21930)
    § *5* Melkersson-Rosenthal syndrome (15590)
  H Neurologic disorders resulting in premature aging of skin and hair
    † *1* Ataxia-telangiectasia (20890)
    † *2* Xeroderma pigmentosum (19440, 17870/ -1/ -2/ -3)
    § *3* Werner's syndrome (27770)
    § *4* Hallerman-Streiff syndrome (23420)
    ‡ *5* Cockayne's syndrome (21640)
    ‡ *6* Bloom's syndrome (21090)
    ‡ *7* Rothmund-Thomsom syndrome (26840)
    ‡ *8* Berardinelli's syndrome (26970)
    § *9* De Barsey's syndrome (21915)
    §*10* Neonatal progeroid syndrome (26409)
    ‡*11* Down's syndrome (trisomy 21)
II Diseases that simultaneously affect the cells of skin and nervous system
  A Metabolic abnormalities (including those of vitamin deficiency and endocrine diseases)
    ‡ *1* Cretinism
    ‡ *2* Pellagra (26065)
    ‡ *3* Phenylketonuria (PKU) (Følling's disease) (26160/-64, 23391)
    ‡ *4* Homocystinuria (23260)
    ‡ *5* Argininosuccinic aminoaciduria (20790)
    ‡ *6* Hartnup disease (23450)
    § *7* Hydroxykynureninuria (23680)
    § *8* Monilethrix (trichorrhexis nodosa) (autosomal dominant, 15800; autosomal recessive, 25220)
    ‡ *9* Kinky hair disease (30940)
    ‡*10* Gargoylism (Hunter-Hurler syndrome) and other mucopolysaccharidoses (MPS I—Hurler, 25280; MPS II—Hunter, 30990)
    ‡*11* Xerodermic idiocy of de Sanctis and Cacchione
    §*12* Myoclonic epilepsy of Unverricht and Lundborg
    ‡*13* Albinism and the oculocerebral syndrome of Cross and McKusick (24890)
    ‡*14* Leprechaunism (24620)
    ‡*15* Van Bogaert-Epstein-Scherer syndrome (cerebrotendinous xanthomatosis) (21730)
    ‡*16* Refsum's syndrome (26650), acanthocytosis, and Tangier disease (20540)
    ‡*17* Lipoid proteinosis (Urbach-Wiethe disease)
    §*18* Cryoglobulinemia polyneuropathy (12355)
    ‡*19* Angiokeratoma corporis diffusum (Fabry disease) (30150)
    ‡*20* Variegate porphyria (17620)
    ‡*21* Familial hyperuricemia with self-destructive biting, mental retardation, cerebral palsy, and choreoathetosis (Lesch-Nyhan syndrome)
    ‡*22* Hypoparathyroidism with superficial moniliasis, keratoconjunctivitis, and hypoadrenalism (polyglandular autoimmune syndrome) (24030)
    ‡*23* Familial dysautonomia (Riley-Day syndrome)
    ‡*24* Cockayne's syndrome (21640)
    25 Genetic myotonia syndromes
  B Toxic disorders
    § *1* Arsenic intoxication
    ‡ *2* Mercury acrodynia
    § *3* Thallium poisoning
  C Infective states, proved or suspected types
    ‡ *1* Meningococcemia, rickettsial infections, viral infections, and mycotic infections
    ‡ *2* Vogt-Koyanagi-Harada syndrome
    § *3* Behçet's syndrome (10965)
III Dermatologic disorders secondary to diseases of the nervous system
  ‡*A* Trophic changes in skin due to sensory denervation (see Table 184-7)
    § *1* Decubitus ulcerations, i.e., due to spinal cord trauma

TABLE 184-1 *(continued)*

‡ *2* Syringomyelia	*IV* Primary dermatologic diseases leading to abnormalities of nervous system
‡ *3* Chronic sensory polyneuropathies	‡*A* Tetanus
‡ *4* Congenital insensitivity to pain	‡*B* Rabies
a Familial porphyria (17600)	‡*C* Diphtheritic wound infections
b Familial amyloidosis (10480)	‡*D* Tick bites
c Hereditary radicular neuropathy	‡*E* Herpes simplex
B Factitious ulcers in hysteria and malingering	‡*F* Cutaneous melanomas
C Infections spreading from nervous system to skin	*G* Kaposi's sarcoma
‡ *1* Herpes zoster	

*Numbers in parentheses refer to entries in McKusick V: *On Line Mendelian Inheritance in Man (Machine-Readable Data File)*. Baltimore, The Johns Hopkins University (Producer); Baltimore, The William H. Welch Medical Library (Distributor).
†Major
‡Mention, but not in detail.
§Optional, mention only.

Another pathogenic mechanism must account for the *familial telangiectasia of Osler-Rendu-Weber,* where minute capillary angiomas of skin and mucous membranes evolve and (rarely) implicate parts of the cerebrum and spinal cord. In *ataxia-telangiectasia,* clusters of finely traced vessels in conjunctivae, skin of ears, and anterior thorax follow at some interval of time after degenerative changes in cerebellum and basal ganglia. The vessels appear to form as part of an inflammatory reaction or skin sensitivity. In *Fabry's disease,* a defect in alpha-galactosidase A results in skin lesions and abnormalities in endothelial and perithelial cells of vessels in the peripheral nervous system. A fault in connective tissue in skin and blood vessels appears to underlie the diseases known as *elastosis perforans serpiginosa* and *pseudoxanthoma elasticum.*

The hereditary nature of several of these neurovascular disorders is revealed in the genealogies of large families. However, chromosomal studies have yielded little information. Local factors must account for interference with the natural vascular regression of the embryonal rete mirabile. The concurrence of lesions in the nervous system and corresponding skin segments indicates an involvement of the anlage of both tissues.

It should be emphasized that neurocutaneous vascular diseases need not be based on a developmental fault. The vessels of the two organ systems may be the seat of an inflammatory process (in viremia, bacteremia, or septicemia) or an allergic vasculitis. The latter group of diseases assumes different forms, depending in part on the size of vessels involved. Such diseases demonstrate both similarities and differences between the vasculature of the brain and spinal cord and of nerves and skin. For example, in disseminated lupus erythematosus small cerebral vessels are often affected in the more advanced stages of the disease, whereas those of the spinal cord and nerves tend to be spared. However, there are many exceptions to this rule. In polyarteritis nodosa, which affects larger arteries, the vessels of the skin and cerebrospinal structures usually escape although the vessels of peripheral nerves are regularly damaged. In the disease known as granulomatous or giant-cell arteritis of the brain, cerebral vessels alone are usually involved. Of the several types of cutaneous angiitis, represented by erythema nodosum, the vessels of peripheral nerves, spinal cord, and brain are usually left untouched. In Degos' malignant necrotizing papulosis, skin lesions predominate, with frequent involvement of the intestinal tract (see Chap. 96), but there may be lesions in the vessels of the spinal cord, brain, and peripheral nerves.

Disturbed Lipocyte–Nerve Relationships

Nerve fibers exert trophic effects on fat cells—a fact long suspected from the remarkable segmental distribution of the lipodystrophic syndromes. In these, all the fat cells may vanish from part of the body, for example, one side of the face (Romberg's hemiatrophy), leaving the skin wrinkled and aged in appearance. Or all the fat cells may disappear in a band that encircles the torso in a neurodermatomal distribution. That peripheral nerve does affect fat cells was established years ago by Sidman and Fawcett,[2] who showed alteration in the appearance and chemical properties of the brown fat of animals following denervation. The relevance of these observations to humans has not been further clarified. Interruption of human nerves in the mature organism does not cause a loss of cutaneous fat, nor have nerve, root, or spinal lesions been demonstrated in human lipodystrophy. Yet, failure of grafts of fat tissue to survive in areas of lipoatrophy (in cases of segmental lipoatrophy) has led certain writers to postulate a defect in autonomic innervation, an idea that receives some support from the occasional finding of Horner's syndrome and blue or variegated iris coloration (attributed to a defect in autonomic innervation) in cases of Romberg's hemiatrophy of the face. Usually subdermal structures are not affected. The cases of atrophy of fat cells in the skin with scleroderma and localized myopathy are exceptions to this statement. Their cause is unknown. Similarly, the basis of excessive deposits of fat in hips and thighs, so striking in some women, also remains obscure. This whole question of precisely what nerve contributes to the metabolism of fat cells awaits further study.

Universal Derangements of Biochemistry of Cells, Including Those of Skin and Nervous System

Modern biochemical research has brought to light more than two hundred genetically determined metabolic diseases of the human nervous system. Some of these lead to progressive degeneration of particular systems of neurons. The enzymatic defects that account for the changes in neurons usually affect the cells of skin, blood, and other tissues, though not to a degree that alters their function. The changes in the latter structures, nevertheless, may be demonstrated by delicate biochemical tests and are visible under the electron microscope. Other diseases such as pellagra, Hartnup's disease, and variegate porphyria express themselves by syndromes comprising both cutaneous and neurologic abnormalities. Another example is phenylketonuria, in which a measurable increase in phenylalanine interferes in some unexplained way with the natural myelination of the brain in the first years of postnatal life, and, by competitively inhibiting tyrosinase, prevents normal pigmentation of skin and hair. An example of a purely exogenous neurocutaneous toxin is organic arsenic; its ingestion leads to an exfoliative dermatitis that is accompanied by polyneuropathy and hemorrhagic encephalopathy. Here the neurocutaneous link is probably the affinity between As and sulfhydryl (S–H) radicals in skin, axons of nerves, and the capillary endothelium of the cerebral white matter. All the involved structures are known to be unusually rich in mercaptans (S–H-containing proteins).

Further research will surely reveal other common chemical attributes of epithelial cells and neurons. From such data it will be possible, ultimately, to construct a more complete conceptual framework for all neurocutaneous diseases. These few examples should suffice at present to persuade the student of dermatology of the promising rewards of research in this field.

Effects of Denervating the Skin

In the context of neurocutaneous diseases, it is well to have clearly in mind the skin changes consequent on interruption of somatic motor, sensory, and autonomic nerves. Since the effects of autonomic or visceromotor and somatic sensorimotor nerves differ, they should be considered separately, even though in many diseases of the peripheral nervous system both types of fibers are affected.

Somatic Sensorimotor Denervation

Most peripheral nerves are of mixed type, i.e., they contain both sensory and motor as well as postganglionic autonomic fibers (Figs. 184-1 and 184-2). Interruption of only motor fibers may result from lesions that destroy anterior horn cells, anterior roots, and motor axons in nerves, and sensory denervation can be produced by the destruction of posterior roots, sensory ganglia, and sensory axons in nerves. Because the postganglionic sympathetic fibers arise from the sympathetic ganglia, they too can be selectively paralyzed by diseases that strike the lateral horn cells of the spinal cord, the sympathetic ganglion cells, or rami communicantes. The pathogenic agents in certain of the peripheral nerve diseases tend more or less to selectively affect one or another of these systems of motor, sensory, or autonomic nerve cells or their axons.

In complete somatic motor denervation of a limb from loss of anterior horn cells (as in poliomyelitis), there results a flaccid paralysis of muscles that then proceed to undergo severe atrophy (75 to 80 percent of their normal bulk is lost in the first 3 months). The skin is usually cool, pale, and moist, indicating preserved auto-

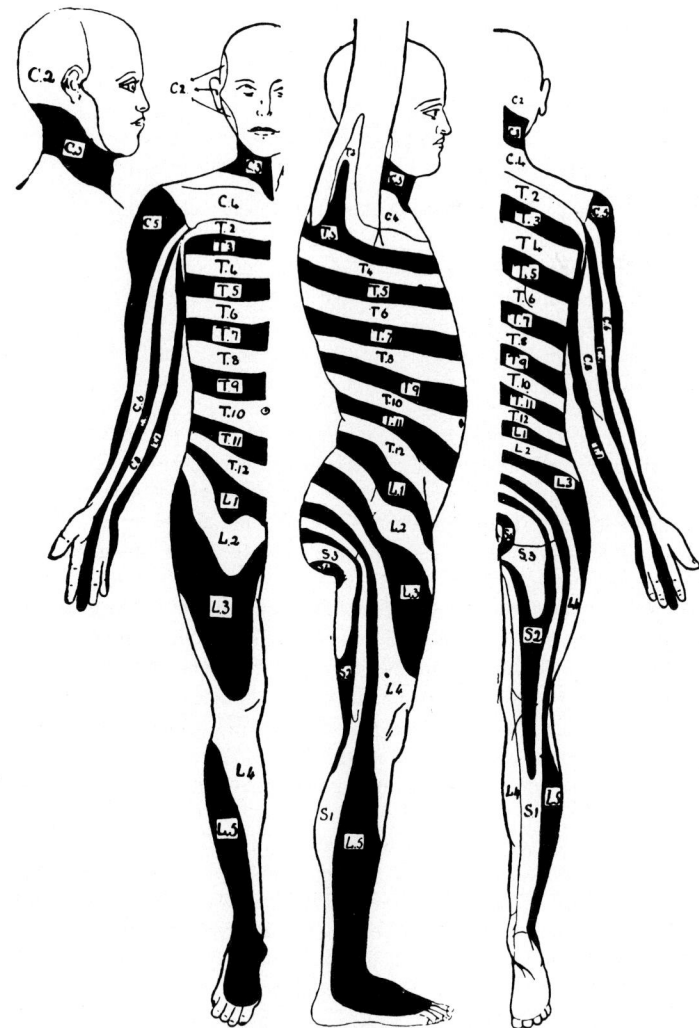

FIGURE 184-1 Distribution of the sensory spinal roots on the surface of the body. *(From Holmes G: Introduction to Clinical Neurology. Edinburgh, Livingstone, 1946.)*

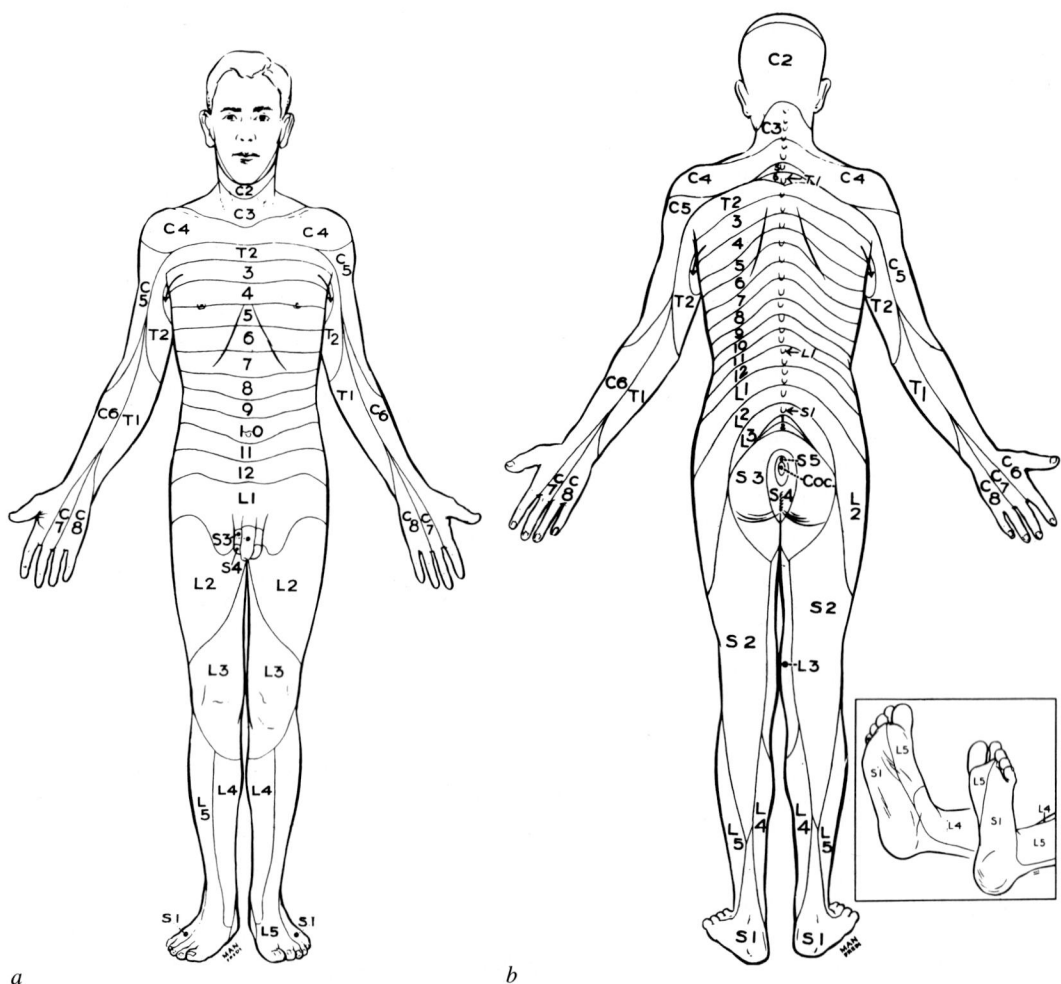

a   b

FIGURE 184-2 The cutaneous fields of peripheral nerves. (*a*) The segmental innervation of the skin from the anterior aspect. The uppermost dermatome adjoins the cutaneous field of the mandibular division of the trigeminal nerve. The arrows indicate the lateral extensions of dermatome T3. (*b*) The dermatomes from the posterior view. Note the absence of cutaneous innervation by the first cervical segment. Arrows in the axillary regions indicate the lateral extent of dermatome T3; those in the region of the vertebral column point to the first thoracic, the first lumbar, and the first sacral spinous processes. (*From Haymaker W, Woodhall B: Peripheral Nerve Injuries. Philadelphia, Saunders, 1945.*)

nomic activity. Dependency and poor venous return due to paralysis may lead to a complaint of coldness and to edema of dermal structures; but the change is nonspecific, for hysterical paralysis has the same effect. There is no change in sudomotor, pilomotor, or sebaceous activity, and responses to skin stroking and histamine injection are normal.

With sensory denervation there is a disappearance within a few days of the free nerve endings in skin and of the plexuses of cells around the hair shafts. However, the specialized endings such as Krause's end bulbs, Ruffinian plumes, and Meissner's and Pacinian corpuscles remain in a recognizable form for a long time. Denervation leads to no definite morphologic changes in sweat glands, hairs, blood vessels, or malpighian and other cutaneous cells.

Complete sensory denervation abolishes all forms of sensation (touch, pain, pressure, thermal, postural, kinesthetic). Sensory stimuli also fail to evoke spinal segmental reflex effects. After Wallerian degeneration of the sensory nerves has occurred throughout their length, a vigorous stroke of the skin still elicits immediate pallor followed by a red line of dilated capillaries in the center of the pale band. But the two changes are not followed by spreading peripheral rubor, i.e., only part of the normal *triple response* occurs. This latter response depends on the integrity of vasodilator fibers in the sensory nerves and is said to persist as long as the peripheral sensory axons are intact, even though no afferent impulses reach the spinal cord. This is called the *axonal reflex*.

Partial sensory denervation leaves the skin paresthetic and sometimes painful. The equilibrium between patterns of sensory impulses as they act on the posterior horn cells of the spinal cord is disturbed. Impulses no longer arrive in proper temporal sequence to elicit natural common sensations. Slight forms of skin stimulation induce perverted sensory experiences. For example, activation of touch fibers leads to tingling; of pressure fibers to a sense of tightness; of superficial pain and thermal fibers to prickling, smarting, or burning. In these, and more particularly in the *causalgic* syndrome of burning pain and tactile hyperpathia, the area supplied by the injured nerve may be cool and may sweat profusely or be dry, warm, and glossy, depending on whether structures under autonomic control are hyperactive or paralyzed. The sensitivity may be so severe that simple care of skin and nails is intolerable. Yellowish brown crusts then form in the territory of the nerve due to the accumulation of sebum, sweat, and dirt. The nails grow long and convex and show vertical ridging. Hair growth may increase (possibly because of the effects of vasodilatation). Since the painful limb is held motionless for long periods of time, the bones lose calcium and become osteoporotic, and the muscles undergo disuse atrophy. This combination is sometimes called *Sudeck's atrophy* or *reflex sympathetic dystrophy.*[3]

Ulceration of the denervated skin may occur as a consequence of repeated inadvertent injury, and once an ulcer is formed, the healing seems to be retarded. In the face, ulceration may extend deep into the cartilaginous structure of the nose, and infection of the cornea or entire eye may result from interruption of the first division of the trigeminal nerve. These trophic changes are initiated by trauma but may be self-induced when the patient abrades tissue because of itching and unpleasant paresthesias.

Lesions of the autonomic nervous system interrupt the innervation of smooth muscles of blood vessels, sweat glands, and pilo-erector muscles. Diseases affecting preganglionic neurons may leave the postganglionic ones untouched and vice versa. Interruption of either the pre- or postganglionic neurons of the sympathetic system cause vasomotor paralysis (rubor and orthostatic hypotension) and anhidrosis (warm and dry skin), but after a time (weeks to months) the effector organs on which postganglionic neurons terminate become hypersensitive to circulating noradrenaline (Cannon-Rosenbleuth phenomenon). As a result, Raynaud's phenomenon and excessive sweating occur. The tendency for this to happen is less with preganglionic lesions. Even after postganglionic fibers degenerate, the sweat glands and smooth muscles are relatively little changed, though the possibility of atrophy has not been well studied. Sebaceous glands are not influenced by autonomic innervation and any diseases involving them, e.g., seborrheic dermatitis and the greasy skin of Parkinson's disease, are only indirectly related to the nervous system. Probably the neurologic abnormality interferes with proper skin hygiene. Diseases affecting the parasympathetic nervous system paralyze the pupil and accommodative mechanism of the eye, reduce tearing and salivation, paralyze the bladder and bowel, and cause impotence in the male. Denervation hypersensitivity occurs here as well, at least in structures such as the pupil.

Descriptions of the Neurocutaneous Diseases

In order to facilitate exposition of the many maladies that possess in common the property of implicating the skin and the nervous system and to offer practical guidance in their recognition, the authors have chosen, perhaps out of ignorance of underlying cause and pathogenesis, to present them as four major groups (Table 184-1), according to whether the lesions of skin and nervous system appear to be relatively independent of one another and related to some indefinable common property or whether the lesions of one organ (either skin or nervous system) are dependent upon diseases in the other. This obviously leaves the largest proportion of the diseases in the first category, and these have had to be subdivided further in accordance with current concepts of probable cause and pathogenesis. The authors have yielded to tradition on another point as well—that of presenting tuberous sclerosis, neurofibromatosis, and craniocerebral hemangioma, the most familiar examples of neurocutaneous diseases, at the beginning of the ensuing discussion.

Diseases with Independent Lesions in the Skin and the Nervous System

Congenital and Developmental Neurocutaneous Diseases

Under this heading two major classes of disease have been placed: one in which a dermal abnormality of relatively stationary type is present at, or soon after, birth; the other in which it is inconspicuous at birth but continues to evolve as a series of quasi-neoplastic lesions during the early years of life. The latter, to which the term *phakomatoses* has been inappropriately applied (a term originally given the retinal lesions by Van der Hoeve in 1920[4]—from the Greek word *phakos,* meaning mother spot, mole, or freckle), includes tuberous sclerosis, neurofibromatosis, craniocerebral angiomatosis, and retinocerebellar hemangiomatosis. These diseases have been shown to possess many common features such as hereditary causation, tendency toward the formation of benign tumors or hamartomas, slow evolution of lesions in childhood and adolescence, and, in some instances, a disposition to fatal malignant transformation. Since the diseases of the second group are the most familiar of all the neurocutaneous diseases, a discussion of them will be given more space than all the others.

The Congenital Benign Neoplasms and Vascular Malformations
TUBEROUS SCLEROSIS COMPLEX (BOURNEVILLE'S DISEASE). Tuberous sclerosis is a complex congenital disease of manifestly hereditary type in which a variety of lesions arise in the skin, nervous system, heart, kidney, and other organs due to a limited hyperplasia of ectodermal and mesodermal cells. The most commonly recognized clinical manifestations comprise ash-leaf hypopigmented areas, adenoma sebaceum, epilepsy, and mental retardation.[5]

History It is stated that Virchow had recognized scleromas of the cerebrum in the 1860s and that von Recklinghausen had reported a similar case combined with multiple myomata of the heart in 1862, but Bourneville's articles, appearing between 1880 and 1900, presented the first systematic account of the disease and related the cerebral lesions to those of the skin of the face. These latter were first described in detail by Balzer and Ménétrier in 1885, and by Pringle in 1890. Vogt, in 1908, fully appreciated the significance of the neurocutaneous relationship and formally delineated the classic triad of adenoma sebaceum, epilepsy, and mental retardation.[6,7] *Epiloia,* a term introduced by Sherlock in 1911, specifies the ensemble of convulsions, mental retardation, adenoma sebaceum, and tumors of the brain and other organs, but has never gained acceptance.

Epidemiology The incidence of the disease is estimated to be approximately 3 to 10 per 100,000. The prevalence at birth is 1 in 12,000.[8,9] Reports of cases have been forthcoming from all over the world, and there seems to be no difference in frequency among Caucasians, blacks, and Asians; the two sexes are affected alike. Heredity is evident in approximately one-third of reported cases. The remaining cases are attributed to a gene mutation, the frequency of which is calculated at 1 in 12,250 to 1 in 60,000.[10] The disease involves many organs aside from skin and brain and may assume a diversity of forms, the least severe of which, viz., a forme fruste, is difficult to diagnose; hence, the true incidence of the disease cannot be fully ascertained from observations of the usual clinical syndrome. Among the feebleminded in institutions, the frequency ranges from 1 to 2.5 percent.[11] Increasing numbers of patients whose mentality is preserved and who have never had convulsions are being reported in recent medical writings. Probably incidence data drawn from surveys of mental hospital populations have tended to magnify the overall incidence of mental retardation in this disorder.[6,12]

Etiology and Pathogenesis   The cause of tuberous sclerosis is genetic; only its pathogenesis remains unknown. The chromosomes are morphologically unchanged. As was said earlier, the lesions involve cells derived from ectoderm as well as mesoderm. The cellular elements within the lesions are abnormal with respect to number and size. The tumor-like growths in different organs may include cells of more than one type, e.g., fibroblast and angioblast or glioblast and neuroblast, and their number is locally excessive. Something has gone awry with the proliferative process in embryologic development, yet it is usually kept under some degree of control, and only rarely does the growth undergo malignant transformation and metastasize. Highly specialized cells within the lesions may attain giant size; neurons three to four times normal size may be observed in the cerebral scleroses. These facts emphasize the hamartomatous character of the process and suggest that some inhibitory growth factor must be lacking at crucial moments in embryonic life and later, to account for both the hyperplasia and the hypertrophy of well-differentiated cells; Moolton[13] conceives the abnormality as a disturbance, at an embryologic level, of cellular differentiation, dependent, so he believes, on the relationship between cell competence for specialization and the amount of an organizer substance that normally provides the inductive stimulus for differentiation. The focal character of the pathologic process would argue against a systemic metabolic abnormality and would be consistent with a "two-hit" hypothesis.[14]

Genetics   Tuberous sclerosis is transmitted as an autosomal dominant disorder with variable expression and nearly complete penetrance. Approximately two-thirds of all cases are manifestations of new mutations. Of those that are familial, about one-third appear to be linked to a locus on 9q34, near the locus for ABO blood group.[15] The remainder are as yet unlinked, though in a few pedigrees there may be a connection on the 11q near the locus for the neural cell adhesion molecule (N-CAM). Unlike neurofibromatosis, which is a relatively homogeneous disease, in tuberous sclerosis there are at least three different genetic loci. This makes analysis of DNA for diagnostic purposes unavailable.

Clinical Manifestations   The disease may be present at the time of birth (the diagnosis has been made pathologically in neonatal fatalities), but more often the infant is judged at first to be normal. Attention is initially drawn to the disease by the occurrence of disordered nervous function in the form of focal or generalized seizures or by retarded psychomotor development. As with any condition leading to mental retardation, the first suspicion is raised by evidence of delay in reaching the successive milestones of natural maturation. But whatever the initial symptom, within 2 to 3 years the convulsive disorder and mental retardation become more evident and are combined. The facial cutaneous abnormality, the so-called adenoma sebaceum, appears later in childhood, usually between the fourth and tenth years, and progresses thereafter.

As the years pass, the seizures, which may at first have been focal, change pattern. In the first year or two they take the form of typical flexor (salaam) spasms or flexion myoclonus with hypsarrhythmia (irregular dysrhythmic bursts of high-voltage spikes and slow waves in the EEG); later the seizures convert to more typical generalized motor, psychomotor, and at times brief attacks, occasionally petit mal. Mental function continues to deteriorate slowly. Seizures are always the most reliable index of the cerebral lesions, and focal neurologic abnormalities (paraplegia, quadriplegia, hemi-

plegia, extrapyramidal disorders, or visual field, sensory, and speech defects), such as might be expected from the number and size of the cerebral lesions, are distinctly uncommon. Exceptionally, a spastic weakness or mild choreoathetosis of the limbs becomes manifest, and in a few cases there is associated obstructive hydrocephalus. Caron[16] and Van Bogaert et al.[17] described cases with cerebellar incoordination, but they are rare in our experience. In the Buschs' series of 12 cases,[18] only one had a spastic hemiparesis. Donegani et al.[19] comment on the rarity of cerebral diplegia and quadriplegia. Speech development is often delayed but not more so than with other forms of mental retardation.

As in any state of imbecility or idiocy, a variety of nonspecific motor peculiarities and behavioral deviations, such as crying, muttering, rocking and swaying movements, and digital mannerisms, may be noted. Characterologic and affective derangements may be added to intellectual deficiency and result in a primary type of psychosis.

The lack of parallelism between the epilepsy, mental deficit, and dermal abnormality has been noted by all experienced clinicians who have access to neurologic patients in general hospitals. Only about a third of the patients exhibit all parts of the Vogt triad. Not a few patients are subject to recurrent seizures while retaining relatively normal mental function, but of those with mental retardation nearly all have epilepsy. In other cases, only a few trivial skin lesions or a retinal phakoma may suggest the diagnosis. In these incomplete forms of disease, diagnosis may elude competent neurologists and dermatologists.

Limitations of space do not allow more than a mere catalog of other visceral abnormalities. Gray or yellow plaques (single or multiple) may be found in the retina, in or near the optic disc or at a distance from it in about 50 percent of cases. It is from this lesion, called *phakoma*, that van der Hoeve derived the term, sometimes applied to all neurocutaneous diseases of this class. Benign rhabdomyomas of the heart have a linkage with tuberous sclerosis (50 percent of all recorded cases are associated with this disease), and other benign tumors have been found in the kidneys (hamartomas of mixed cell type), liver, thyroid, testes, and gastrointestinal tract. Cysts of pleura and lungs, bone cysts in digits, and zones of marbling or densification in bones complete the picture.

In approximately 87 percent of the patients with tuberous sclerosis, congenital white skin lesions are present (Fig. 184-3). These are hypomelanotic macules (formerly referred to as partial albinism or vitiligo), appear before any of the other skin lesions, and have unique clinical and histologic features.[20] They are located in the skin over the trunk or limbs and range in size from a few millimeters to several centimeters; their orientation is often linear, the configuration being oval with one end round and the other pointed in the shape of an ash leaf. They vary in number from a few to 75 or more.

A Wood's lamp, which emits light waves of 360 nm, facilitates the demonstration of these lesions; the visualization is improved because the melanin absorbs most of the light waves of this frequency, thereby exposing areas deficient in melanin. Close examination of the skin shows no alteration of skin markings; the vascular responses to stroking appear to be normal, and there is no change in sensation or sweating over them. Unlike vitiligo macules they are seldom completely devoid of pigment, and the presence of a vascular response to cold distinguishes them from nevus anemicus, the two lesions with which they may be confused. Poliosis of scalp hair and eyelashes may also be noted. Although recognized long ago, Gold and Freeman[21] and Fitzpatrick et al.[20] have more recently emphasized their frequency and their value in the diagnosis

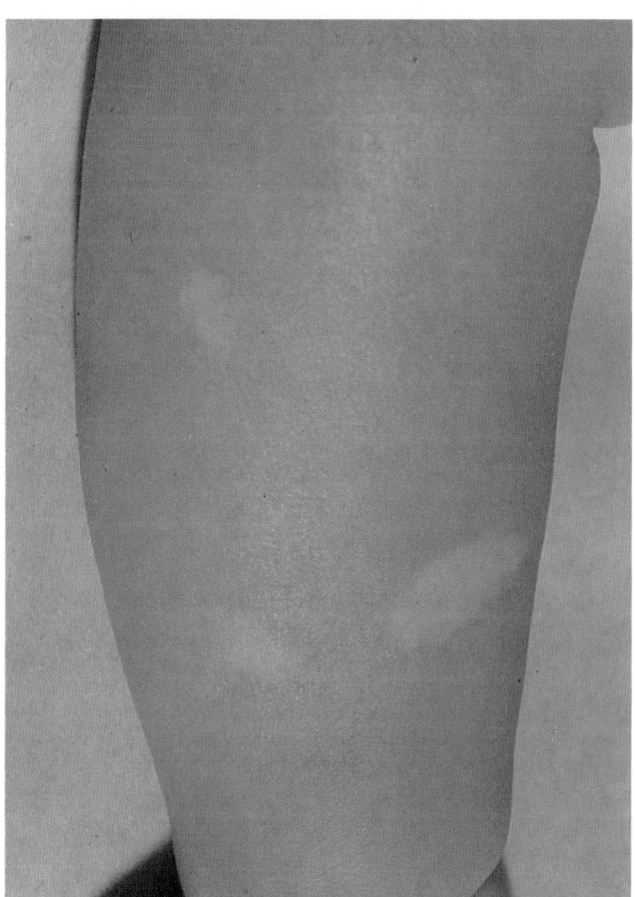

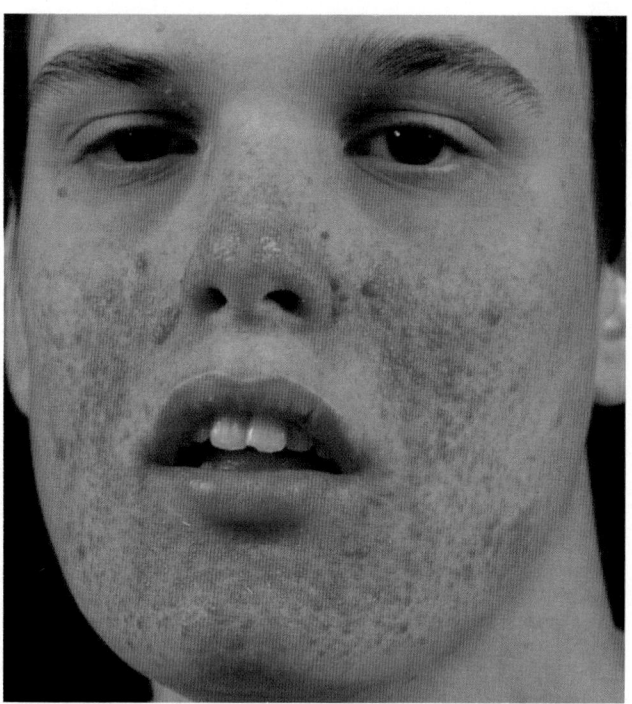

FIGURE 184-4   Adenoma sebaceum, the classic facial lesions in the tuberous sclerosis complex. These angiofibromas are typically localized on the cheeks and the nasolabial folds; they are pink or red and have a smooth surface. *(Courtesy of Klaus Wolff, M.D.)*

FIGURE 184-3   Hypomelanotic (''ash-leaf'') macules on the lower leg in a child with the tuberous sclerosis complex. *(Courtesy of Klaus Wolff, M.D.)*

of tuberous sclerosis during infancy before the other cutaneous lesions of this disease appear (see Chap. 80).

The well-developed facial lesions, diagnostic of tuberous sclerosis, are present in 50 percent of patients over 4 years of age.[6,7,22,23] Although called *adenoma sebaceum,* these tumors are actually angiofibromas (see Chap. 97); the sebaceous glands are only passively involved. Typically they are red to pink nodules with a smooth, glistening surface, localized to the nasolabial folds, cheeks, chin, and sometimes the forehead and scalp (see Fig. 184-4). The earliest manifestation of facial angiofibromatosis may be a mild erythema over cheeks and forehead, which is intensified by crying. The differential diagnosis for angiofibroma includes acne vulgaris, acne rosacea, and multiple trichoepithelioma. The latter disorder is transmitted as an autosomal dominant trait and is characterized by a similar centrofacial distribution of papules and nodules that lack the pink vascular aspect of angiofibromas. Biopsy may be necessary to distinguish these other lesions. The occurrence of large plaques of connective tissue on the forehead represents another diagnostic feature and these are similar to adenoma sebaceum except for the absence of vascular elements.

A characteristic lesion that appears on the trunk is the shagreen patch, which constitutes a presumptive diagnostic criteria (described first by Hallspean and Leredde in 1895), and is found most often in the lumbosacral region (Fig. 184-5). It appears most often as a flat, slightly elevated area of skin with a ''pigskin,'' ''elephant hide,'' or ''orange peel'' appearance. Such areas, which are in

FIGURE 184-5   Shagreen patch in tuberous sclerosis. This is a flat, elevated lesion with an ''orange-peel'' appearance. It corresponds to circumscribed subepidermal fibrosis. *(Courtesy of Klaus Wolff, M.D.)*

reality plaques of subepidermal fibrosis, usually retain a flesh color; they vary from less than 1 cm in diameter to the size of the palm.

Another common site of fibromatous involvement is the nail bed (Koenen tumors). In some patients extensive subungual fibromas disrupt the entire nail bed (Fig. 184-6). They usually appear at

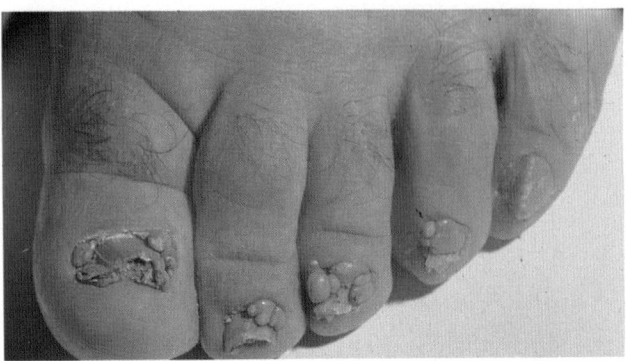

FIGURE 184-6 Koenen tumors in the tuberous sclerosis complex. These peri- and subungual fibromas are characteristic. (*Courtesy of Klaus Wolff, M.D.*)

puberty and continue to develop with age. Gingival fibromas also occur.

Other skin changes seen not infrequently, but not in themselves diagnostic, include fibroepithelial tags (soft fibromas), café au lait spots, and port-wine hemangiomas.

Pathology Brain: Grossly, the brain exhibits a number of anomalies of structure that are at once diagnostic. Broadening, unnatural whiteness, and firmness of parts of some of the cerebral convolutions are simulated by no other disease. These are the "tubers" after which the disease is named. They range from 5 mm up to 2 or 3 cm in surface diameter, and their cut surface reveals a lack of demarcation of gray cortex from white matter and the presence of white flecks of calcium salts, the latter often visible in x-rays of skull and called *brain stones*. The floors of the lateral ventricles may be encrusted with white or pinkish-white masses resembling the gutterings of a candle. When calcified, they appear in radiographs as curvilinear opacities that follow the outline of the ventricle and on noncontrast head CT scans as encroaching on the lateral ventricles and near the caudate nucleus, cerebellum, and the cortex. Nodules of abnormal tissue are observed but rarely in the basal ganglia, thalamus, cerebellum, brainstem, and spinal cord.

Under the microscope the whitish tubers are most often seen to be composed of interlacing rows of plump fibrous astrocytes (much like an astrocytoma). Derangements of cortical architecture result from abnormal-appearing glial cells. Monstrous neurons and glial cells, often difficult to distinguish from one another, and displaced normal-sized neurons contribute to the chaotic histologic appearance of cerebral cortex and ganglionic structures. There is a paucity of neurons in the cortical tubers. Some of the normal-sized or enlarged neurons are disoriented, having also lost their laminar organization. Their dendrites may lack spines and display varicosities, reminiscent of embryonic nerve cells. On ultrastructural examination, the enlarged astrocytes have multipolar processes and their cytoplasm contains glycogen filaments, membrane-bound dense bodies, and giant mitochondria. These changes reflect the dysplastic nature of the lesion, suggesting its embryonic origin.[24] Gliomatous deposits may block the aqueduct or floor of the fourth ventricle, causing the obstructive hydrocephalus. Neoplastic transformation of abnormal glial cells is a not infrequent occurrence and usually takes the form of a large cell astrocytoma, but glioblastomas and even meningiomas may develop. The phakomas of the retina are composed mainly of neuronal and glial components, but occasionally there is an admixture of fibrous tissue.

Pathology Skin: The microscopic changes of the various skin lesions are essentially of interlacing strands of fibroblasts and col-

lagen with numerous blood vessels, to which the name hamartoma has been given. A better name for the facial lesion would be angiofibroma (see Chap. 97). The ungual lesions also present the characteristics of an angiofibroma. The shagreen plaque is composed of a relatively avascular, dense, sclerotic mass of bundles of collagen fibers. In the white macules, there appears to be a reduction in the tyrosinase activity of the melanocytes compared to the normal pigmented skin surrounding the white macules. Electron microscopic studies have confirmed the findings of light microscopy, that melanocytes are present in the usual number but contain few melanosomes. This is in direct contrast to vitiligo, in which there is an absence of identifiable melanocytes. Thus it is not correct to speak of the white macules present in tuberous sclerosis as "vitiligo."

Diagnosis and Differential Diagnosis When the full combination of mental, convulsive, and dermal abnormalities are conjoined, the diagnosis is self-evident. It is the early stages of the disease and the more common forme fruste that give trouble, and here the experienced dermatologist can be of the greatest help to the neurologist. Epilepsy, i.e., flexion spasms in infancy, and delay in psychomotor development are by no means diagnostic of tuberous sclerosis, as they occur in many diseases. It is in these cases and also in every sizable population of the epileptic or mentally retarded, especially when the family history is unrevealing, that a search for the dermal equivalents of the disease—hypomelanotic ash-leaf macule, the adenoma sebaceum, the collagenous patch, the phakoma of retina, or subungual or gingival fibroma—is so rewarding. The finding of any one of these lesions provides confirmation of the forme fruste case. Adenoma sebaceum is easily confused with acne vulgaris in the adolescent and may occasionally occur alone. The elicitation of a history of epilepsy and/or the demonstration of a dull mentality is helpful but not necessary for the diagnosis of tuberous sclerosis.[12] X-ray of the skull, a search for multiple calcific densities within the brain and localized patches of hyperosteosis on the inner surface of skull, computed tomography (CT) and magnetic resonance imaging (MRI) scans to show ventricular deformity and tumor deposits along the striothalamic borders, and electroencephalography (EEG) are useful laboratory measures for corroborating the neurologic features of the disease.

Treatment Nothing can be offered in the way of prevention other than counseling as to inheritance risk by affected individuals whose children may be more severely affected than they. The medical profession does not possess the means of halting the slow march of the disease once it has begun. Anticonvulsant therapy of the standard types (phenobarbital, phenytoin, etc.) suppresses the convulsive tendency more or less effectively in many patients and should be applied assiduously. ACTH is recommended for infantile spasms and hypsarrhythmia (mountainous slow waves in the EEG). It is rather pointless to attempt to excise tumors, especially in individuals who are severely affected. The main indications for neurosurgery are intracranial hypertension and hydrocephalus. In a few instances excision of an epileptogenic focus has been beneficial. Radiotherapy is indicated for malignant neoplasms. However, there are many patients not mentally deficient who can be helped by dermabrasion, electrodesiccation, or CO_2 laser surgery of their facial lesions, with the knowledge that they will slowly regrow.[25]

Course and Prognosis In general, the disease progresses so slowly that years must elapse before one is sure of the advancing course. Of the severe cases, approximately 30 percent die before the fifth year and 50 to 75 percent before attaining adult age. Cardiac rhabdomyomas may cause hemodynamic disturbance from obstruction to blood flow or dysrhythmias, mainly in the child-age group. Status epilepticus accounted for many deaths in the past, but improved anticonvulsant therapy has reduced this hazard. Neoplasias take their toll, and several of our patients died of renal carcinomas or of malignant gliomas arising in striothalamic zones.[12]

NEUROFIBROMATOSIS. *Neurofibromatosis* is the term now given to two disorders with somewhat overlapping features. They are designated as NF1 and NF2. NF1 is von Recklinghausen's neurofibromatosis, familiar to all experienced physicians, and comprises the characteristic skin lesions (café au lait spots, intertriginous freckles, and neurofibromas) and other congenital and hamartomatous lesions of bone, endocrine glands, and the central nervous system. NF2 is delineated by the presence of bilateral acoustic neurofibromas, other cranial nerve tumors and meningiomas, and only a few, if any, skin and other visceral and skeletal abnormalities.

History The condition known as multiple idiopathic neuroma was the subject of a monograph by R. W. Smith in 1849, and even at that time he mentioned examples of the same disease having been previously recorded by other writers. But it was von Recklinghausen who, in 1882, gave the definitive account of its clinical and pathologic features and who deserves the credit for its complete identification as a nosologic entity. The monograph of Alexis Thomsen, which appeared in 1900, contains useful statistical data on a large series of cases and a full bibliography. The early monographs of Crowe et al.[26] and Canale and Bebin[27] and three more recent monographs by Riccardi and Mulvihill,[28] Riccardi and Eichner,[29] and Rubenstein and Korf[30] provide the most complete analysis of the genetic data.

NF2 had also been recognized as a distinct variety of neurofibromatosis as early as 1822, when Wishart[31] recorded a case of bilateral acoustic neuromas and multiple meningiomas. It was only recently,[32,33] however, that the new methods of molecular genetics made it possible to show that NF1 and NF2 have different chromosomal loci: NF1 on chromosome 17 and NF2 on chromosome 22. Various mutations within the NF1 gene locus were then discovered.[34,35]

Incidence and Epidemiology Crowe and Neel and their associates at the Institute of Human Biology at the University of Michigan[26] calculated that the frequency of the von Recklinghausen form of neurofibromatosis (NF1 in today's nomenclature) is 30 to 40 per 100,000. A case would be expected in one of every 2500 to 3300 births. The figures of Littler and Morton[36] confirm those of Crowe et al.[26] The carrier incidence at birth is 0.0004, and the gene frequency 0.0002. The proportion of cases arising as a new mutation is 0.56 according to Littler and Morton.[36] All ethnic groups are affected to the same degree.[29] This mutation rate of 10^{-4}, which is relatively high, is judged to be consistent with the large size of the NF1 gene—about 100 kb.[34]

The incidence of NF2 is about one-twentieth that of NF1, i.e., 1 in 50,000 to 1 in 120,000 population.[37]

Genetics Both forms of neurofibromatosis are inherited as autosomal dominant disorders. Nevertheless, there are a considerable number of new mutations. The use of markers that are tightly linked to the DNA of the cloned gene of NF1 makes prenatal diagnosis possible. DNA analysis will also permit the characterization of the mutations of NF1. Although the gene of NF2 has been sought, there have not been enough families studied to rule out genetic heterogeneity. By linkage analysis, using close-flanking DNA markers, prenatal diagnosis is now possible in some families.

Cause and Pathogenesis The function of the NF1 gene is currently being investigated. Since the gene was cloned it has been discovered that it is not transcribed in hybrids of somatic cells from two rare NF1 patients containing balanced chromosomal transloca-

tions. This finding is consistent with the hypothesis that the gene acts as a tumor suppressor, a mechanism that is known to be recessive at the cellular level. Sequence analysis of the gene has shown it to encode a protein with homology to the catalytic region of the *ras* GTPase-activating protein (GAP).[38] The expression of the NF1 gene is presently being investigated in the various lesions of neurofibromatosis by the use of antibodies against this protein.

The gene for NF2 has not been cloned. In the tumors associated with this gene, there is a loss of one copy of chromosome 22, suggesting that it too acts by inactivating another tumor-suppressor gene.[39]

Both forms of NF are believed to implicate several of the cellular derivatives of the neural crest, but why they express themselves differently in the several tissue elements affected by the disease awaits further exploration.

Clinical Manifestations At a National Institutes of Health Consensus Conference it was agreed that two or more of the following findings strongly support the diagnosis of NF1:

1. The presence of six or more café au lait macules with a diameter ≥5.0 mm in children less than 6 years of age and >15 mm in older individuals
2. Two or more neurofibromas of any type or one plexiform neuroma
3. Freckling in the axillary or inguinal regions
4. An optic nerve glioma
5. Two or more Lisch nodules (iris hamartomas)
6. Dysplasia of the sphenoid bone or thinning of the cortex of long bones, with or without pseudoarthrosis
7. A first-degree relative exhibiting these changes

For NF2 it was proposed that the diagnosis was tenable if the following criteria were satisfied:

1. The presence of acoustic neuromas bilaterally
2. A first-degree relative with NF2 and either an acoustic neuroma or any two of the following findings:
   a. a neurofibroma, meningioma, glioma, schwannoma, or
   b. juvenile posterior cataracts

In NF2 it was noted that Lisch nodules are rarely seen and that café au lait macules are less frequent than in NF1. Nevertheless, there is an obvious overlap of the two syndromes and some patients do not fit easily into either category.

In the majority of patients, as pointed out earlier by Crowe et al.,[26] spots of skin pigmentation and cutaneous or subcutaneous tumors are the basis of clinical diagnosis. These appear in increasing numbers during late childhood and adolescence. Exceptionally, a neurofibroma of a spinal or cranial nerve root, exposed during a neurosurgical procedure, may be the initial manifestation of the disease. In the large clinical survey of Crowe et al., done before the distinction between NF1 and NF2 was drawn but including mostly NF1 cases, approximately one-third were diagnosed during a medical examination for some other disease. That is to say, the disease was asymptomatic and incidental. Of the remainder, many consulted a physician because of a cosmetic problem produced by the skin lesions and the others because some of the neurofibromas or the central nervous system lesions were producing symptoms. Canale and Bebin[27] noted that in a series of 92 patients admitted to the hospital with this disease, a third presented with neurologic symptoms, the main cause of which was an offending tumor, mainly central. Typical syndromes were traced to VIII cranial nerve tumors (nerve deafness, dizziness, facial numbness, facial weakness, ataxia, and headache). Less frequent manifestations were: trigeminal neuromas (facial pain and numbness), jugular foramen syndrome (IX, X, XI cranial nerves with paralysis of vocal cords, dysphagia, paralysis of sternomastoid and trapezius muscles), hypoglossal nerve (weakness and hemiatrophy of the tongue), optic gliomas (progressive blindness and sometimes proptosis), other cranial nerve involvement, spinal root tumors with or without compression of the spinal cord, and multiple spinal or cranial meningiomas. Obviously some of Canale and Bebin's cases were examples of NF2.

Concerning the dermatologic features of NF1, patches of cutaneous pigmentation, appearing shortly after birth and occurring any place on the body, constitute the most arresting findings (Fig. 184-7a). They vary in size from 1 to 2 mm to many centimeters and range in color from light to dark brown (café au lait); seldom are they associated with any other pathologic condition at this age. Crowe et al.[26] found that 10 percent of the normal population have one or more lesions of this type, but that any patient with six or more spots exceeding 1.5 cm nearly always proved to have von Recklinghausen's disease. Of their 223 patients with this disease, 95 percent had at least one spot and 78 percent more than six spots. Freckle-like or diffuse pigmentation of the axillae is another frequent and almost pathognomonic skin lesion (Fig. 184-7b).

Multiple cutaneous tumors stand as the other principal dermatologic manifestation of the disease. These appear in late childhood or early adolescence and are cutaneous and subcutaneous. The cutaneous tumor is situated in the dermis or just beneath it and forms a discrete, soft or firm papule (called a molluscum fibrosum because of its texture) (Latin, *molluscus*, meaning soft). It varies in size from a few millimeters to 1 cm or more (Fig. 184-8a). In shape it assumes many forms: flattened, sessile, conical, pedunculated, lobulate, etc. (Fig. 184-8b). It tends to be flesh-colored or violaceous and often has a comedo at its top. When pressed, the soft tumors tend to invaginate through a small opening in the subcutaneous tissue, giving the feeling of a seedless raisin or a scrotum without a testicle. Crowe et al.[26] speak of this phenomenon as "buttonholing" and find it a most useful sign in distinguishing the lesions of this disease from other surface tumors, e.g., multiple lipomas. The number of dermal tumors in any given patient may range from a few to as many as 9000 (Fig. 184-8b). Probably every patient with von Recklinghausen's disease has at least a few of them. The subcutaneous tumors, which are also multiple, take two forms: (1) firm, discrete nodules, often attached to a nerve but not to the skin, or (2) a great overgrowth of connective tissue, sometimes reaching enormous size (*tumeur royale*). The latter occurs most often on the face, cranium, neck, and chest and may cause hideous disfigurement. When palpated these growths, which are called *plexiform neuromas* (also *pachydermatocele* or *elephantiasis neurofibromatosa*), feel like a bag of worms or strings. The underlying bone may thicken. Nerve tumors range from a few millimeters to 3 to 4 cm and occur most frequently on ulnar and radial nerves and may cause pain, muscle weakness, atrophy, and slight sensory loss. In our experience they are less frequent than cranial or spinal nerve root tumors.

Other skin lesions such as multiple pigmented nevi and cutis laxa, similar to the skin in Ehlers-Danlos disease, have been reported but it is doubtful if they bear any meaningful relationship to neurofibromatosis.

Bony skeletal abnormalities are associated only with NF1. Scoliosis is a common problem. In the general population the incidence is approximately 2 percent; in neurofibromatosis (in a series

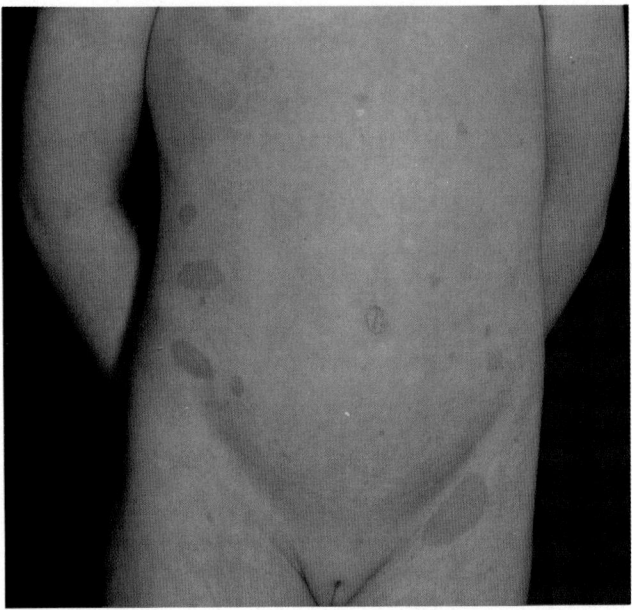

a

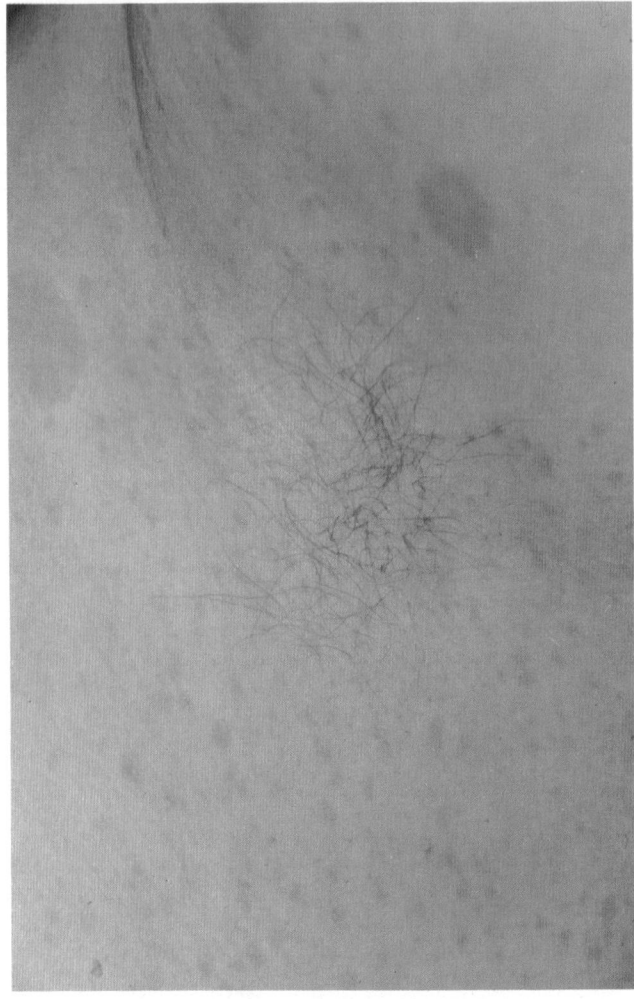

b

FIGURE 184-7 Neurofibromatosis I. (*a*) Multiple café au lait macules in a 6-year-old girl. (*b*) Axillary freckling and café au lait spots in an adult. (*Courtesy of Klaus Wolff, M.D.*)

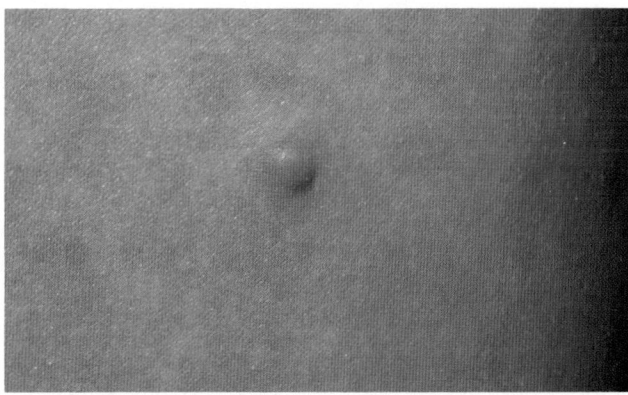

a

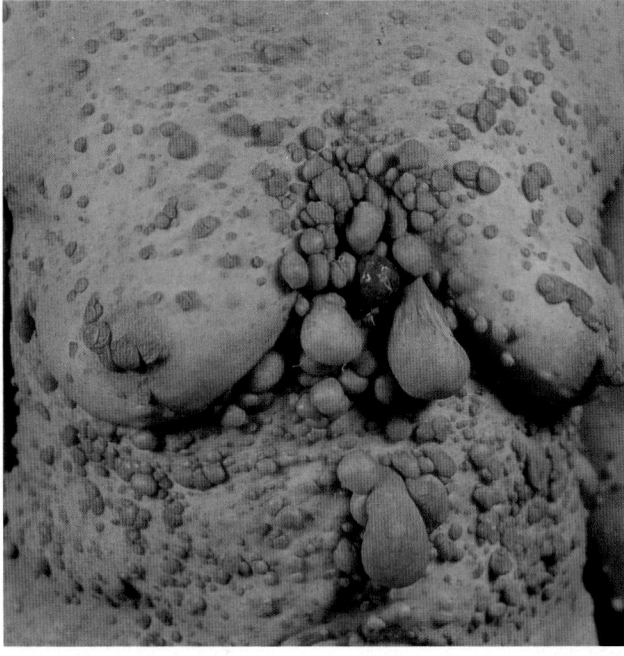

b

FIGURE 184-8 Neurofibromatosis I. (*a*) Close-up of a singular, small neurofibroma. This is a soft little nodule, which, upon pressure, will invaginate through a small hole in the dermis into the subcutaneous fat. (*b*) Hundreds of small and large, sessile and pedunculated neurofibromas cover the entire trunk of this patient. (*Courtesy of Klaus Wolff, M.D.*)

of 206 cases reported from the Philadelphia Children's Hospital[40]) the incidence was 20 percent. There are two forms of scoliosis in the NF group. In the first the deformity of spine describes a long C-shaped curve that includes eight to ten vertebrae, much like that in non-NF scoliotics. In the second, less frequent form, the curve is sharp and involves fewer vertebrae and a kyphotic element may be added. The curvature of the spine in most cases of either type is not due to neurofibromas of roots or nerves. In only a few have neurofibromas been observed in the region of scalloping of vertebral bodies, causing an imbalance of paravertebral musculature. Short stature (<5 percent in the normal population) is another frequent

skeletal finding (10 percent in one series). Pseudoarthrosis or congenital bowing of a long bone, usually the tibia, has been reported in about 8 percent. Macrocephaly (head circumference >98 percentile for age) has been recorded in 16 percent of NF1 patients, and a pulsating exophthalmos due to a defect in the sphenoid bone in 5 percent.

Mental deficiency, learning difficulties, seizures, and precocious puberty all appear to be significantly increased in NF1. In a recent survey of NF1 patients in Wales, the frequency of moderate to severe mental retardation was 3.2 percent and the figure for slight backwardness and special learning difficulties reached 30 percent.[41] Among the special developmental delays were dyslexia, motor clumsiness, and the hyperactivity syndrome. In many instances these impairments had prompted medical consultation and had for the first time called attention to the café au lait macules. Convulsions also occur but far less frequently than in tuberous sclerosis. Presumably they are related to heterotopias of glial and neural elements in the cerebrum. In a study by Duffner et al.[42] attempting to correlate these seizure states with MRI images, CT images, and EEG changes, a significant correlation was not found. Although the EEG was abnormal in 25 percent and imaging abnormalities were seen in 28 percent, they were not associated with mental deficiency. Of course the seizure group did have more EEG abnormalities. Evidently the central glial abnormality and the heterotopias found by Rosman and Pearce[43] are not attended by reliable MRI changes.

Precocious puberty has in a few instances been traced to a heterotopia of the hypothalamus. Some of these patients also have had an optic nerve glioma. The precocious puberty resulted from an activation of cells in the hypothalamus-pituitary axis. Therapy that suppresses gonadotropins and sex steroids stabilizes or causes regression of the secondary sexual characteristics and rate of skeletal maturation (bone age).

The other clinical features of neurofibromatosis are bone cysts, bone hypertrophy, pheochromocytoma, ependymomas of the spinal cord, obstructive hydrocephalus, and rarely malignant gliomas.

A separate but closely related syndrome in which multiple large zones of cutaneous pigmentation are combined with bone cysts and precocious puberty was described by Albright (see Chap. 80).

The Lisch nodules (hamartomas of iris) present as grayish-white spots, visible by direct examination; they are seen in about 10 percent of children under 6 years of age but by the sixtieth year they can be found in nearly 100 percent of patients. Of the optic nerve gliomas observed in about 15 percent of patients, only about a third are associated with loss of vision. They may be unilateral or bilateral and if not removed may extend posteriorly into the optic chiasma and hypothalamus. Malignant transformation of the NF1 lesions occurs in approximately 5 percent of patients, the most common tumor being a neurofibrosarcoma. A tendency to develop a Wilms' tumor, a rhabdomyosarcoma, or leukemia has also been noted.

The most common clinical feature of NF2 is hearing loss due to the presence of an acoustic neurofibroma, which at first may be unilateral but later may involve the other side. With increasing size of the tumor, the adjacent fifth and seventh cranial nerves are implicated as well as the lateral part of the brainstem (pons and medulla junction); the cerebellum becomes indented (cerebellopontine angle tumor) with clinical findings of facial weakness and ataxia. Cutaneous lesions are infrequent or altogether lacking. In nearly 50 percent of the patients with NF2, ophthalmologic examination reveals a posterior subcapsular cataract that may eventually become symptomatic. The other symptoms are referrable to the associated tumors that may or may not be present (meningiomas, gliomas, ependymomas, and schwannomas).[44]

Pathology The cutaneous tumors that correspond to the violaceous papule have notable features. Beneath a rather thin epidermis whose basal layer may or may not be pigmented, the natural collagen and elastin of the dermis are replaced by a bluish-gray gelatinous-appearing connective tissue. Under the microscope the cutaneous tumor is seen to be composed of loosely arranged fibroblasts. They lack the support of the normal dermal collagen, which accounts for the palpable opening in the skin.

The endoneurial fibroblasts of the schwannoma are distinguished from the fibroblasts of a typical fibroblastoma only by a tendency to form palisades and by the presence among them of Schwann cells, myelin, and axis cylinders.

The nerve tumors contain both endoneurial fibroblasts and Schwann cells, except for the optic nerve gliomas, which are combinations of astrocytes and fibroblasts. Occasionally one may find a tumor made up of partially or completely differentiated nerve cells (a typical ganglioneuroma). Special arrangements of cells, the aforementioned palisading of nuclei, tightly arranged whorls (Verocay bodies), and loose networks of vacuolated cells more fully differentiate the schwannoma from a fibroblastoma.

There has been an endless dispute as to whether the neurofibroma is a schwannoma or a fibroblastoma. We believe both elements to be present, but the Schwann cells and the axons are the identifying features. Probably the fibroblasts are the supporting interstitial elements. By cholinesterase stain one can substantiate this interpretation of their neural origin. Within such tumors there is also an increase in mast cells.

The acoustic neuroma of NF2 is more correctly a vestibular schwannoma, consisting of predominantly neoplastic Schwann cells.

The café au lait macules, on histologic examination, reveal an increase in dopa-positive melanocytes. This accounts for their darker color, in contrast to normal skin. Melanocytes contain large melanin granules that have been interpreted as giant melanosomes (on the basis of tyrosinase activity)[45] or fused lysosomes containing autophaged melanosomes.[46] Some of these giant melanosomes are transferred to keratinocytes, Langerhans cells, or dermal macrophages. They are not specific for neurofibromatosis, being found in the multiple lentigines syndrome, xeroderma pigmentosum, and the Becker hairy nevus. They are not seen in the McCune-Albright syndrome (café au lait macules, precocious puberty, bone cyst complex), which is included in the differential diagnosis.[47]

The hamartomas of the brain are amorphous clusters of glial cells, deranging the normal cellular or white matter architecture. They were thought to form a link between neurofibromatosis and tuberous sclerosis. Clinically (and now biologically), however, it is now clear that they are separate diseases.

Diagnosis and Differential Diagnosis The diagnostic features of NF1 have been reviewed previously. Often the diagnosis is suggested by the presence of café au lait spots and one of the other diagnostic criteria, such as cutaneous neurofibromas, short stature, megencephaly, learning disability, etc. Difficulty in diagnosis arises with the finding of a solitary neurofibroma or a plexiform neurofibroma without a family history. In such cases it can only be recommended that further investigation be undertaken to confirm the presence or absence of Lisch nodules by slit-lamp examination, or the presence of asymptomatic optic nerve involvement or heterotopias of the central nervous system by MRI examination of the brain. In children, café au lait spots may be missed and the Lisch nodules may not yet be present. Without other substantiating diagnostic criteria, the diagnosis must await the passage of time.

The diagnosis of NF2 is more straightforward as it is defined by the presence of bilateral acoustic neuromas. In a family at risk, the occurrence of acoustic neuromas may be as early as the teens or later in the third decade. Repeated testing of hearing, including routine audiogram plus brainstem auditory-evoked responses, is recommended along with serial MRI studies with gadolinium enhancement. The question of NF2 is difficult to answer in a person who presents with a unilateral acoustic neuroma, as there can be a delay in the occurrence of contralateral tumors. These patients need to be followed. Unilateral acoustic neuromas occurring in the general population as a rule appear in older individuals without a family history. Pathologically the tumors are different, the NF2 acoustic neuroma often being multilobed. Unilateral acoustic neuromas do occur in NF1, though rarely. The distinction of NF2 from NF1 is improved by the absence of Lisch nodules and the requisite six café au lait spots >15 mm in diameter. A detailed neurophthalmologic examination to evaluate known, suspected, or at-risk individuals is also useful in NF2, to confirm the presence of a posterior subcapsular cataract.

There are two clinical syndromes that should be mentioned in the differential diagnosis of NF1: multiple lentigines syndrome (LEOPARD syndrome), and McCune-Albright syndrome (see later). There are forms of apparent neurofibromatosis that do not fit either NF1 or NF2 diagnostic criteria: segmental NF in which neurofibromas are isolated to a single segment or side; abdominal NF in which neurofibromas are found within the gastrointestinal system without any cutaneous findings consistent with either NF1 or NF2; and persons with plexiform neurofibromas exclusively, who may represent a forme fruste of one or the other form of neurofibromatosis. NF1 in conjunction with Noonan's syndrome has been described repeatedly in both sporadic and familial cases, such that it is a recognized variant (NFNS).[48] The other syndrome that is frequently mentioned in association with NF1 is the Proteus syndrome, the disease Joseph Merrick, the "Elephant Man," had and which for many years was thought to reflect a florid example of NF1.[49,50]

Treatment For patients with NF1, routine follow-up is necessary every year or two, depending on ongoing clinical problems or for issues pertaining to genetic counseling. Baseline MRI of the brain and cervical spine are recommended, in view of the lack of clinical findings with optic gliomas. Slit-lamp examination for confirmation of Lisch nodules is recommended in children older than 6 years of age. For individuals at risk for NF2, MRI of the head in the early teens is recommended, along with audiology and brainstem auditory-evoked responses. If the initial study is negative, repeated examinations are recommended at 2-year intervals. Surgery is the mainstay of treatment of the various tumors associated with NF1. A sudden change in size or new-onset pain in a neurofibroma, particularly a plexiform lesion, should suggest the possibility of malignant transformation. There is no MRI finding that correlates with malignant change, hence biopsy is required. Radiation therapy is the mainstay, particularly for optic gliomas, and as an adjunct to surgery for astrocytomas and neurofibrosarcomas. Plastic surgery for removal of troublesome neurofibromas or for improvement of cosmetic appearance by removal of excessive soft tissue overgrowth, such as is seen with plexiform neurofibromas, is quite successful. Skeletal overgrowth such as mandibular prognathism and overgrowth of fingers is equally amenable to surgery. Orthopedic correction of pseudoarthrosis still represents a challenge, given the poor bone healing. Management of the scoliosis depends on the type and degree; the generic C-type curve responds to conservative therapy, but the more angular curve may require surgical realignment and insertion of metal rods to protect the cord from compression.

CUTANEOUS ANGIOMATOSIS WITH ABNORMALITIES OF THE CENTRAL NERVOUS SYSTEM. There are six diseases in which a cutaneous vascular anomaly is associated with an abnormality of the nervous system: (1) craniofacial, or trigeminocranial, angiomatosis with cerebral calcification (Sturge-Weber-Dimitri syndrome); (2) dermatomal hemangiomas with spinal vascular malformations (sometimes with limb hypertrophy as in Klippel-Trénauney-Weber syndrome); (3) hemangioblastoma of cerebellum and retina (Lindau-von Hippel disease); (4) familial telangiectasia (Osler-Rendu-Weber disease); (5) ataxia-telangiectasia (Louis-Bar disease); (6) angiokeratosis corporis diffusum (Fabry disease) (see Chap. 153).

Craniofacial, or Trigeminocranial, Angiomatosis with Cerebral Calcification (Sturge-Weber-Dimitri Disease) In this condition an extensive vascular nevus (port-wine stain, nevus flammeus) is observed at birth to cover a large part of the face and cranium on one side (in the territory of the ophthalmic division of the trigeminal nerve). The extent of it varies from a lesion involving only the upper eyelid to one covering the entire head and even other parts of the body (Fig. 184-9). The nevus is deep red, and its margins may be raised or flat; soft or firm papules, evidently composed of vessels, cause surface elevations and irregularities. The orbital tissue may be involved (choroidal angioma), and buphthalmos may develop later in the eye on that side, causing glaucoma and blindness. The increased cutaneous vascularity may result in overgrowth of connective tissue and underlying bone, giving rise to a deformity similar to that of the Klippel-Trénauney-Weber syndrome. Indications of cerebral involvement appear later in childhood; the most

frequent clinical manifestations are spastic hemiparesis with smallness of arm and leg, focal or unilateral seizures, hemisensory defects, and homonymous hemianopia, all on the side contralateral to the trigeminal nevus. The incidence of mental retardation is high, 55 to 92 percent of cases in one series,[51] and ranges from mild to moderately severe, depending on either unihemispheric or bihemispheric involvement. X-rays of the skull, usually negative soon after birth, will, some years later, reveal a characteristic "tram-line calcification," which outlines the convolutions of the parietooccipital cortex, and brain atrophy.

Parkes Weber was one of the first to show the association of cerebral lesion with the facial angioma, and Krabbe demonstrated that the calcification lay in the second and third layers of the cortex, which were gliotic, and not in the large numbers of surface veins and arteries in the meninges. The cortical lesion appears to be progressive and is thought to be caused by hypoxia and ischemia from the meningeal vascular malformation.

It must not be thought, however, that all cranial hemangiomas affect the cerebrum. Facial vascular nevi may occur without brain involvement, and, rarely, a cerebral meningeal angiomatosis of this type may be present without skin lesions (forme fruste of Sturge-Weber-Dimitri syndrome). When the nevus lies entirely below the ophthalmic division, i.e., below the upper eyelid and nose, the cerebral lesions are usually absent, although in a few instances a hemangioma at the base of the skull and lower face has been associated with a vascular malformation of meninges overlying the brainstem and cerebellum. Although of congenital origin, the cause and pathogenesis are unknown. Alexander and Norman[52] postulate a persistence of the primordial vascular plexus of the embryonal period of life. Familial coincidence has been observed but is exceptional (in one pair of identical twins). The chromosomes appear to be normal. The magnitude of the lesion usually contraindicates a neurosurgical approach, even when the epilepsy is recalcitrant to anticonvulsant therapy. The meningeal vascular malformation is mainly venous and in angiograms appears as a blush. However, Alexander and Norman[52] report favorable results from surgical resection of the pathologic lobe of the brain early in the course of the disease. Corpus callosotomy has also been successful in control of intractable seizures.[53]

Newer forms of laser therapy offer hope of reducing the unsightly facial nevi.

Dermatomal Hemangiomas with Spinal Vascular Malformations (Sometimes with Limb Hypertrophy as in Klippel-Trénauney-Weber Syndrome) Hemangiomas of the spinal cord may rarely be accompanied by vascular nevi in the corresponding dermatome of skin, as was pointed out by Cobb.[54] These lesions differ in no important way from the cranial hemangiomas and, like them, tend to conform to a dermatomal pattern. They are, as a rule, unilateral and are most frequent in the arm and trunk. When the cutaneous lesion involves an arm or leg, there may be enlargement of the entire limb or of fingers in combination with underdevelopment of other parts (Klippel-Trénauney-Weber syndrome). Among the dermatomal malformations should also be included that described by Van Bogaert.[55] The clinical and pathologic features of this syndrome are angiomatosis of the skin in association with diffuse meningocortical angiomatosis. The neurologic expression is mental defect, hemianopia, epilepsy, and both pyramidal and extrapyramidal disorders. The congenital poikiloderma of the skin is attributed to the cutaneous vascular abnormality. Also Brégeat[56] has described a cutaneous angioma with oculoorbital angiomatosis and thalamoencephalic involvement. It is manifested clinically by a nonpulsatile exophthalmos, photophobia, headaches, and mental

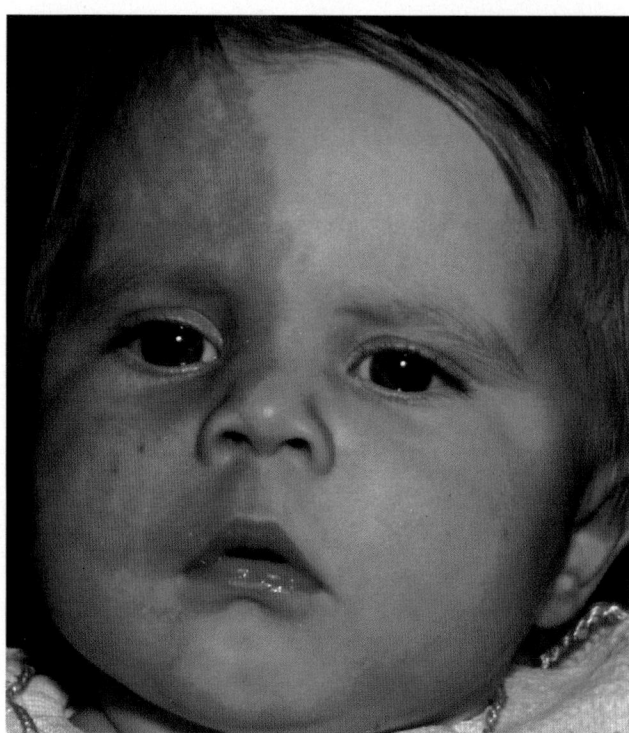

FIGURE 184-9 Vascular nevus of craniofacial angiomatosis. *(Courtesy of Klaus Wolff, M.D.)*

retardation. Ulman's name is attached to a syndrome of cutaneous angiomatosis with similar lesions in the central nervous system and viscera.[57]

A congenital angiomatous malformation, affecting the eye and upper brainstem (diencephalon), has also been described by Bonnet et al.[58] The retinal lesion, a cirsoid aneurysm, is conjoined to an arteriovenous malformation of the thalamus. There may be a cutaneous facial telangiectasia, sometimes extending to the mucous membranes. Hemianopia, oculomotor palsy with contralateral pyramidal signs, and other cranial nerve palsies occur when the vascular malformation bleeds. The condition is thought to be related to Sturge-Weber and von Hippel-Lindau diseases.

Hemangioblastoma of Cerebellum and Retina (Lindau-von Hippel Syndrome) This condition, often affecting two or more successive generations of a family, consists of a benign cerebellar tumor composed of a mass of capillaries surrounded by a cyst. The vascular nodule and its cyst slowly increase in size during childhood and adolescence and produce a cerebellar syndrome with increased intracranial pressure. One or both retinas may be the site of a tangle of small vessels, visible some distance from the optic disc, as was first pointed out by von Hippel. These retinal angiomas may lead to blindness through retinal detachment or proliferation and hemorrhage; later they may calcify. Familial incidence has been recorded many times, the transmission being that of an autosomal dominant trait.[59] Lindau, who studied the pathology of all benign cerebellar cysts, noted the frequent association of the cerebellar tumor with cysts of pancreas and kidney, angiomas of liver, and hypernephromas. The cerebellar tumor was later shown to sometimes elaborate an erythropoietin-like substance, which accounts for an accompanying polycythemia.

The majority of cases of Lindau's disease have no retinal lesions (retinal angiomas are found in only about 20 percent of cases) and are without cutaneous vascular nevi. The latter may be present, however, as was pointed out by Hall,[60] and tend to be localized to the occipitocervical region. These cases appear to provide the link between this disease and the Sturge-Weber-Dimitri syndrome.

Recent genetic studies have mapped the gene of this disease to chromosome 3p25.[61] It is linked to the locus encoding the raf-1 oncogene. Cytogenetic analysis of renal tumors associated with hemangioblastomas and of some of those which are not reveals a loss of the short arm of chromosome 3 (3p).[62] It has been suggested that the hemangioblastoma gene acts as a tumor-suppressor gene.

The treatment of the cerebellar cyst and its mural nodule is surgical excision. If the cerebellar brainstem or spinal lesions are inoperable, ionizing radiation should be employed. Obliteration of the retinal lesion by laser beam therapy at an incipient stage will save vision; hence, the family members of patients with Lindau-von Hippel disease should be followed carefully by ophthalmologists and neurologists. CT or MRI scans should be repeated every year or two after puberty.

Familial Telangiectasia (Osler-Rendu-Weber Disease) This, a vascular anomaly transmitted as a simple dominant trait, affects the skin, the mucous membranes, the gastrointestinal and genitourinary tracts, and occasionally the nervous system (see Chap. 164). The basic lesion is probably a defect in the vessel walls, analogous in some respects to Fabry's angiokeratoma corporis diffusum, in which a hereditary defect in ceramide metabolism has been found. In familial telangiectasia, the lesions range from the size of a pinhead to 3 mm or more, are of bright red or violaceous color, and blanch under pressure. Some of them form small vascular papules 2 to 3 mm in diameter. Located sparsely in the skin of any part of the body, they first appear during childhood, enlarge

during adolescence, and may assume spidery forms resembling, in late adult life, the cutaneous telangiectases of cirrhosis. The lesions cause trouble only because of their hemorrhagic tendency. During adult years they may give rise to severe and repeated epistaxis (present in 96 percent in a series of 324 patients[63]) or gastric, intestinal, or urinary tract hemorrhages. Chronic blood loss may result in an iron-deficiency anemia.[64]

The angiomas of this disease form in either the spinal cord or brain and here can produce apoplectic syndromes; or an intermittently progressive cerebral syndrome may result from a succession of small hemorrhages. Diagnosis of an unexplained gastrointestinal, genitourinary, intracranial, or intraspinal hemorrhage warrants a search for these small cutaneous lesions, which are easily overlooked. Pulmonary fistulas constitute another important feature of the generalized vascular dysplasia. Such patients are subject to brain abscesses, like the patient with congenital heart disease. The treatment may require the application of oxidized cellulose (Oxycel or Gelfoam). Although cautery eradicates a bleeding lesion, satellite ones tend to re-form. Prophylaxis has proved to be unsatisfactory. The pulmonary arteriovenous malformation can be excised, if not too large, and the common hepatic vascular malformation as well. The condition must be distinguished from the CREST syndrome (see Chap. 173).

Ataxia-Telangiectasia (Louis-Bar Disease) This hereditary disease, first described by Syllaba and Henner in 1926,[65] takes the form of oculocutaneous telangiectases combined with cerebellar ataxia, choreoathetosis, and recurrent pulmonary infections with bronchiectasis. The recurrent respiratory infections are presumably related to an associated hypoglobulinemia (immune globulin A and possibly others) resulting from hypoplasia of the thymus. The pattern of inheritance is autosomal recessive. Ataxia of voluntary movements, often with choreoathetosis, is the initial symptom, recognizable as a rule during early childhood long before the skin and conjunctival abnormalities become evident. Once fully developed, the syndrome includes slow, dysarthric speech, nystagmus, occasionally myoclonic jerks of the limbs, difficulty in initiating lateral ocular deviation from the central position, and poor voluntary control of eye movements (apraxia of gaze). Tendon reflexes are diminished or absent; intelligence may deteriorate as the disease advances; growth is retarded.

The telangiectases of conjunctivae consist of numerous tortuous vessels that issue from the canthal regions and fan out over the eyeball (Fig. 184-10*a*); the lower tarsal conjunctiva is also involved. Similar traceries of fine vessels are observed inside the helix (Fig. 184-10*b*) and over the backs of the ears, on the sides of the neck, sometimes in a butterfly area over the face, in the cubital and popliteal fossae, and on the dorsa of hands and feet. The pattern of telangiectasia appears in some patients to conform to the areas of greatest exposure to sunlight. In time the skin becomes tight and inelastic (hidebound), like that of scleroderma. The hair and skin tend to be dry and coarse with gray hair appearing in some patients.

In a study of 22 patients, café au lait spots were also observed in four and areas of hypopigmentation in eight. Several examples of cutaneous malignancy developed after the age of 21. Also, resistance to skin and pulmonary infections (bacterial, viral, fungal) is reduced. Typical atopic dermatitis was noted in two patients and nummular eczema in another.

Autopsy findings indicate that about half the patients die from pulmonary disease and most of the remainder succumb to lymphoreticular or other malignant tumors; the thymus is absent or hypoplastic, and the spleen may be reduced in size. The significant

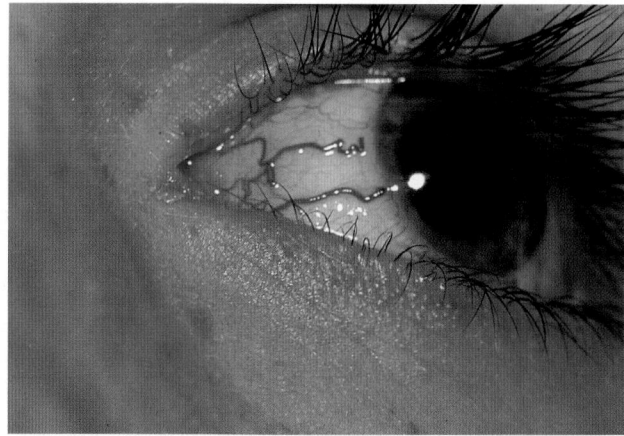

a

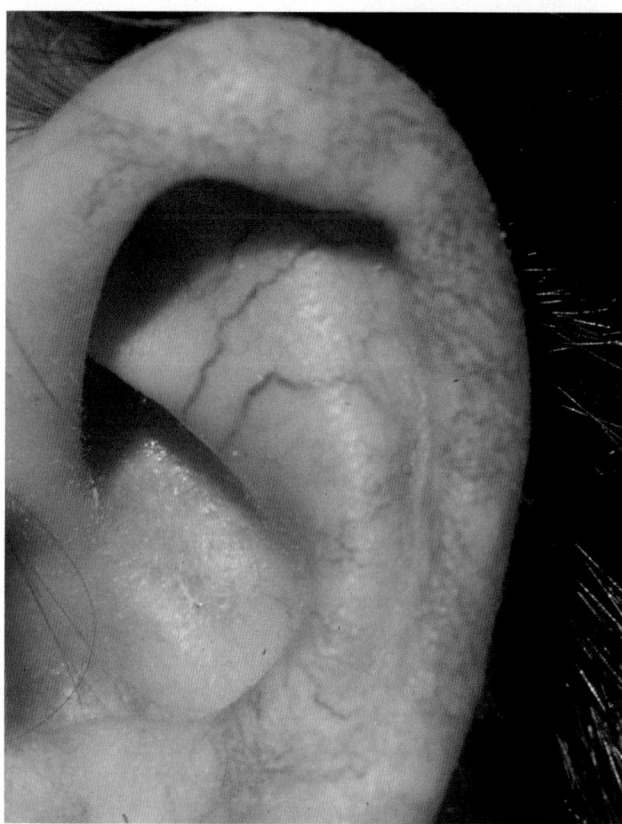

b

FIGURE 184-10 Ataxia telangiectasia. (*a*) Conjunctival telangiectasia fanning out over the eyeball. (*b*) Telangiectases inside and on the helix. *(Courtesy of Klaus Wolff, M.D.)*

pathologic abnormalities in the central nervous system are severe degeneration in the cerebellar cortex, loss of myelinated fibers in the posterior columns, and degenerative cell changes in the posterior root and sympathetic ganglia.[66]

The diagnosis is substantiated by the finding of elevated levels of alpha fetoprotein and carcinoembryonic antigen in the blood. In addition, by in vitro studies of lymphocytes, there is an increase in the number of spontaneous chromosomal breaks and rearrangements (mainly in chromosomes 2, 7, and 14). The finding of a 14:14 translocation is a predictor of leukemia.[67]

Ataxia telangiectasia is one of a group of diseases characterized by defects in the repair process of DNA damage. The others are xeroderma pigmentosum, Bloom's syndrome, and Cockayne's syndrome. In fibroblast cultures from ataxia telangiectasia, several complementation groups have been found, suggesting clinical heterogeneity. For example, one pattern of malignancy associated with ataxia telangiectasia involves solid tumors (breast, stomach, pancreas) occurring particularly in heterozygotes; and another pattern is with non-Hodgkin's lymphoma and leukemia.[68,69] A gene for ataxia telangiectasia phenotype has recently been located on chromosome 11q22-23, a site involved in the chromosome translocations in some nonlymphoid leukemias.[70] This finding may be applied to prenatal diagnosis of ataxia telangiectasia. The frequency of heterozygous carrier of the ataxia telangiectasia allele is 1 percent.[68]

Cutaneous Neurolipomatosis As a general rule, one or a few subcutaneous lipomas have no neurologic significance. However, lipomas of the brain do occasionally occur and there are instances in which they are conjoined to facial, axial, visceral, and skull lipomatosis, as described by Scherrer et al.[71] and Van Bogaert.[72] Also Krabbe and Bartels[73] have written a monograph on the subject of multiple cutaneous painless lipomas associated with pigmented skin nevi, cutaneous fibromas, mental retardation, neuropathy, and cerebellar atrophy. We have never observed such cases. Not to be confused with lipomas are the nodules of subcutaneous fat that may be extremely sensitive, as in Dercum's so-called lipodystrophy.

PATHOGENESIS OF THE PHAKOMATOSES. Common to all the diseases described above is a genetic etiology. They appear to be caused by an abnormal gene with pleiotropic potentialities, i.e., capable of affecting the development of several tissues and organs simultaneously. The hereditary patterns are usually autosomal dominant with complete or variable penetrance. The abnormal gene either acts directly on embryonic germinal layers or interferes with induction of the primary organization centers or multiple secondary ones. The variable manifestations of the phakomatoses appear to be determined by three factors: (1) specific affinity of the abnormal gene for a particular germinal layer and its derivatives; (2) the period of embryonic development when the gene intervenes; (3) the period of teratogenic sensitivity of multiple embryonic derivatives that are simultaneously damaged.[57]

Developmental Neurocutaneous Diseases (Developmental Anomalies of Skin and Nervous System) Of the various so-called classic neurocutaneous diseases thus far discussed, only the Sturge-Weber-Dimitri craniofacial angioma and possibly the hypomelanotic nevus of tuberous sclerosis are present at birth or during the first days of infancy. In contrast, many of the other congenital neurocutaneous diseases in this group are apparent at, or soon after, birth and, like the neurologic disorders with which they are associated, tend to remain more or less stationary through life.

Because the dermal abnormality attracts notice at birth or soon thereafter in this category of neurocutaneous diseases, the dermatologist may be called to the nursery to assist in its interpretation long before the symptoms and signs of nervous disease become evident. Dermatologic diagnosis, if accurate, may serve, therefore, to warn the pediatrician and neurologist of impending neurologic abnormality and encourage a search for the earliest signs of cerebral disease. Of course, recognition of these early skin anomalies requires a familiarity with the skin of the newborn.

A diffuse erythema lasting a few days is an almost universal finding in Caucasian infants and should not be confused with erythroderma. Extreme mottling of skin (livedo reticularis) is also

TABLE 184-2
Special Developmental Syndromes with Somatic, Neurologic, and Cutaneous Abnormalities

	Down's	13 Trisomy	18 Trisomy	Turner's (XO)	Kleinfelter's (XXY)	Treacher-Collins
Intelligence	Reduced	Reduced	Reduced	Normal or reduced	Reduced	Normal, reduced (5%)
Eyes	Epicanthal folds, Brushfield spots	Epicanthus variable, microophthalmia	Epicanthus variable	Normal, ptosis, epicanthus	Normal	Anti–Down syndrome slant, lower lid coloboma, absent lower eyelashes
Nose	Broad low bridge	Normal	Normal	Normal	Normal	Normal, choanal atresia
Ears	Small, deformed	Abnormal	Normal	Normal, prominent	Normal	Grossly malformed external ear canal defect
Lips and palate	Tendency to keep mouth open and tongue out	Cleft lip and palate	Cleft lip and palate	Normal	Normal	Soft palate cleft, micro-, macrostomia
Jaws	Normal	Micrognathia	Micrognathia	Micrognathia, small maxilla	Normal	Malar, mandibular hypoplasia
Cranium	Small brachy-cephalic	Small	Small	Normal	Normal	Normal
Body growth	Stunted	Underdeveloped	Underdeveloped	Short stature, absent adolescent growth spurt	Tall, with low upper to lower segment ratio	Normal
Psychomotor development	Delayed	Delayed	Delayed	Average	Slow	Normal or delayed
Dermatoglyphics	Simian line, distal axial triradius, loop patterns	Abnormal	Low arched dermal ridges	Normal, distal palmar axial triradii	Normal	Normal
Other skin abnormalities	Down syndrome spots, cutis marmorata, cutis laxa	Hemangioma, cutis laxa	Cutis marmorata, redundant skin, hirsuitism	Pytergium, pigmented nevi	None	Congenital dermal sinus, skin tags between auricle and mouth
Heredity	Trisomy 21 sporadic, maternal age	Trisomy 13 sporadic, maternal age	Trisomy 18 sporadic, maternal age	45, XO sporadic	47, XXY sporadic	Autosomal dominant
Miscellaneous	Clumsy, clinodactyly, cardiac anomalies	Holoprosencephaly, high early infant mortality	Rocker-bottom feet, clenched fist	Shield-like chest, cubitus valgus, short 4th metacarpal	Tendency to obesity with age and without testosterone therapy	Conductive hearing loss

common and must not be mistaken for scleredema or some other congenital lesion. Unnatural dryness, cracking, and flaking of skin, so typical of the postmature state (infants born beyond term), may be misleading and suggest xeroderma or ichthyosis. Indentations, hemorrhagic areas, linear erythema, or superficial erosions in the skin over the head due to pressure of a foot against the head in utero or to injury from the application of forceps may be mistaken for congenital anomalies of skin.

CONGENITAL SKIN DEFECTS WITH GROSS ANOMALIES OF THE NERVOUS SYSTEM (SPINA BIFIDA, CRANIUM BIFIDUM). Areas of the body may fail to be completely covered by skin, leaving underlying structures exposed. This dermal deficiency may be associated with other developmental defects or malformations involving bones, teeth, nails, and hair.

The most frequent examples are to be found in association with the various forms of rachischisis (spina bifida with meningocele or meningomyelocele or cranium bifidum with encephalocele). The skin may be missing or hypoplastic. Such lesions are usually midline and posterior or dorsal, and so obviously involve all tissues that they are not regarded as dermatologic problems. The least severe of them, associated with an occult defect of vertebra or cranial bone, may be revealed only by an abnormal tuft of hair or a dimple in the lumbosacral region, where there is also an absence of subcutaneous fat or dermal collagen.

Focal Congenital Skin Defects and Dermal Hypoplasias Campbell, in 1826, described focal skin defects of congenital origin in parent and child, and numerous confirmations of this finding

are to be found in the medical literature since that time. The defect may involve epidermis alone or in combination with dermis and it may extend into the subcutaneous tissue, even to underlying bone. The defect may be smooth, dry or moist, pale or red, or granular. Its borders are sharply circumscribed. The defect tends gradually to repair itself by ingrowth from adjacent tissues. Its appearance varies with age of lesion, viz., its stage of healing. Some are already cicatricized at birth. Most often they are located over the scalp, especially the occiput, but they may also occur over the trunk and limbs. Theories as to origin are speculative. The notion of inflammation of amnion with the formation of adhesions between amnion and skin (Simonart's bands), once favored, is rejected by most pathologists.

Closely related is *hypoplasia* of skin where the congenital anomaly is also circumscript and confined to the dermis. The overlying skin is extremely thin and delicate. The subcutaneous fat may herniate out through the dermal defect because of the lack of connective tissue in the dermis. The mucous membranes show a similar tendency, with papilloma formation, and the teeth and fingernails are often defective. Telangiectases and linear streaks of pigmentation appear later in the thin epidermis.

These subcutaneous abnormalities are often associated with syndactyly, spina bifida, scoliosis, microcephaly, microphthalmia, strabismus, and colobomas of iris and choroid. Some of the affected children are later found to be mentally enfeebled. Familial coincidence due to a hereditary factor has been substantiated in only a few instances.

Papillon-Psaume (oro-facial-digital) (types I, II)	Pierre-Robin sequence	Rubenstein-Taybi	Russell-Silver	Cornelia deLange	Hallerman-Streiff or François	Fanconi's
Normal (II) or reduced (I)	Normal	Reduced	Normal or reduced	Reduced	Normal or reduced	Reduced
Lateral placement of inner canthi	Normal	Anti–Down syndrome slant, epicanthal folds, strabismus	Normal	Microcornea, optic atrophy	Congenital cataracts, microphthalmia	Normal, strabismus, ptosis
Hypoplasia of alar cartilage (I), broad low nasal bridge (II), broad nasal (bifid) tip (II)	Normal	Long, beaked nose	Normal	Small, anteverted nostrils	Beaked	Normal
Normal	Normal	Low set or/malformed	Normal	Normal, lowset	Normal	Abnormal, deafness
Partial clefts (I,II), partial lip cleft and midline tongue cleft (II)	Cleft soft palate, glossoptosis	Normal, narrow palate	Inverted U-shaped mouth	Beaked upper lip, notched lower lip, high arched palate	Microstomia, narrow high arched palate	Normal
Hypoplasia	Micrognathia, early mandibular hypoplasia	Hypoplastic maxilla	Normal	Micrognathia	Micrognatia, malar hypoplasia	Normal
Normal or small	Normal or small	Microcephaly	Normal	Microcephaly	Brachycephaly, microcephaly	Microcephaly
Normal or dwarfism	Normal or small	Dwarfed	Small stature prenatal in onset	Dwarfed	Dwarfed	Dwarfed
Delayed	Normal	Delayed	Normal or slowed major motor milestones	Delayed	Delayed	Delayed
Normal	Normal	Normal	Normal	Normal, simian crease	Normal	Normal
Frontal alopecia (I), granular seborrheic skin (I)	Normal	Hirsutism, nevus flammeus	Café au lait spots	Synophrys, hirsutism, cutis marmorata	Atrophy over the nose and scalp, hypotrichosis	Brownish pigmentation over the trunk, grain, and axillae
Dominant, lethal in male (I), autosomal recessive (II)	?	Sporadic	Sporadic, X-linked	Sporadic	Recessive, dominant, and new mutations	Autosomal recessive
Brain malformation in 20% (I)	Occasional in combination with peromelia	Broad thumbs and toes, cryptorchidism, unsteady gait	Small triangular face, syndactyly of toes, clinodactyly, fasting hypoglycemia, limb asymmetry	Hands and feet small and imperfect, genitalia imperfect, hypoplastic nipples and umbilicus	Anodontia, cryptorchism	Abnormality of thumbs, absence of radial bones, renal malformations, hypoplastic bone marrow, pancytopenia

Congenital Somatic Abnormalities, Including Those of the Nervous System and Skin Unlike the first group of congenital diseases, in which defects of nervous system and skin present themselves at the moment of birth as obvious and arresting anomalies, in the following category of diseases it is a constellation of nonnervous somatic abnormalities that predominates. The skin, if altered at all, is usually not deranged in any characteristic fashion, except as part of a more general morphologic change of nose, eye, ear, lips, neck, and digits, and always the disorder is more than a purely dermal affection. The nervous system abnormality is even more elusive, ordinarily not being manifest until months or years after birth when the child fails to attain developmental milestones at the expected times. That the involvement of the nervous system should be one of the most consistent abnormalities in these many diverse syndromes, in conditions both with and without demonstrable chromosomal aberrations, probably relates to the span of time required and the complexity of cerebral development. These factors render it vulnerable at many different stages of maturation.

Occurring with monotonous frequency as common denominators in the dozen or more identifiable syndromes are microcephaly and deformities of cranium, eyes, ears, bridge of nose, jaws, lips, and digits of extremities. Certain of these regions of the body, such as inner canthus of eyes, root of nose, and maxilla, are known to be sites of intense and complex embryologic organization, which probably explains their unusual susceptibility to genetic and teratogenous influences.

The skin, if it is to be affected in any particular way, nearly always exhibits eccentricities of ridges and other markings in the palms and soles, which are also determined by genetic factors. The recognition of this fact has led to the study of anomalies of fingernails and palmar and plantar lines and creases, the scientific study of which is called *dermatoglyphics*. Students of dermatology who seek a thorough grasp of developmental disorders of the skin must acquaint themselves with the basic principles of this field. This group of diseases provides evidence, once again, of the manner in which the developmental plan of both the brain and the skin may relate to fundamental issues in embryogenesis.

The list of special syndromes in which there occurs a major abnormal deviation in somatic structure has become so lengthy that even pediatricians and pediatric neurologists concerned with developmental medicine have trouble keeping them in mind, and the number increases each year. In this discussion of them, instead of presenting a kind of catalogue, the authors have chosen to call attention to only two; the main characteristics of some of the others are listed in Table 184-2.

JOHANSON-BLIZZARD SYNDROME. This unique syndrome, in which a focal posterior scalp defect occurs, is an autosomal recessive disorder. It is characterized, in addition to the ectodermal dysplasia, by microcephaly, variable sparse hair with frontal upsweep, hypoplastic alai nasi, hypoplastic deciduous teeth and absent permanent teeth, imperforate anus, cryptorchidism, primary hypothyroidism, and malabsorption secondary to pancreatic insufficiency. Although some cases are reported with mental retardation, it is not a consistent finding.[74] Treatment with thyroid and pancreatic supplement improves growth rate, though in some cases there is no "catch-up" growth.

GOLTZ'S SYNDROME. Goltz's syndrome, or focal dermal hypoplasia, is a sex-linked dominant disorder characterized as a mesoectodermal disorder with atrophy and linear pigmentation of the skin, herniation of fat through dermal defect, and multiple papillomas of the mucous membranes or skin. Associated features include dystrophic nails, hypoplastic teeth, dental enamel abnormalities, digital syndactyly, and various ocular abnormalities (coloboma, microphthalmos, and/or aniridia). Mental retardation and microcephaly have been noted in a number of the reported cases. The absence of affected males suggests male lethality in early embryonic stage, although the evidence is not as clear as in incontinentia pigmenti. It is not known whether or not genetic heterogeneity exists for Goltz's syndrome.[75]

Congenital Eruptive Diseases with Nervous Disorders This motley group of disorders is characterized by a striking variety of skin lesions that declare their existence soon after birth or within the first weeks of life. Unlike the preceding category of diseases, in which a congenital defect is all too obvious at birth, here the skin becomes, after an interval of time, the site of a disease process. It may mimic any one of a broad spectrum of eczematoid and vesicular eruptions and, through repeated exacerbations, inevitably raises questions of infection, allergy, photosensitivity, etc. Scarring, hyperkeratosis, anhidrosis, pigmentation, inflammation, and ulceration are often present, and it is not always easy to decide whether they are primary or secondary. Only when the condition is viewed in longitudinal profile against a background of abnormalities of hair, teeth, eyes, ears, and other tissues does the pediatrician begin to think in terms of the syndromes outlined below. Familial incidence may shed light on the diagnostic puzzle, and, as months and years pass, mental retardation and other disorders of nervous function provide additional clues. Early diagnosis is nonetheless advantageous, even though it does not lead to effective therapy, because the physician and parents are then alerted to the possibility of involvement of the nervous system and defects of certain senses due to a heritable condition.

Presented below are the main features of the best known of these congenital dermal eruptions. The list is not complete; rare ones are omitted and new ones will probably be discovered and eventually find their place in the group.

INCONTINENTIA PIGMENTI (BLOCH-SULZBERGER SYNDROME). This is a sex-linked dominant disorder characterized by a disturbance of skin pigmentation combined with malformations in other systems. The skin lesions appear in the first weeks of postnatal life and evolve in three phases. In the first acute eruptive phase, there is an appearance of erythematous, vesicular, or bullous lesions over the trunk and limbs. The latter are linearly arranged (Fig. 184-11a). After several weeks to months, in the second phase, the lesions assume a verrucous, keratotic, or lichenoid aspect and persist in this form for several months (Fig. 184-11b). They may then resolve completely or leave zones of skin atrophy and hypopigmentation. The third phase is marked by hyperpigmentation, sometimes in parts not previously involved by the eruption. The zones of hyperpigmentation are curiously streaked—swirls of tan and brown like a "marble cake." Later the hyperpigmentation disappears, leaving hypopigmentation and atrophy. On histologic examination there is a decrease or absence of melanin in the basal cells of the epidermis. There is an accompanying increase in melanin in the cells of the dermis. From this presumed incontinence of epidermal cells for

melanin comes the curious name for the disease, *incontinentia pigmenti.*

Alopecia is an associated finding in nearly a third of the patients. Ocular abnormalities are present also in a third, taking the form of retrolental fibrodysplasia or pseudoglioma. Short stature, skull deformities, and cleft palate are frequent, as also are dental abnormalities (delayed dentition, partial to complete anodentia), microcephaly, psychomotor developmental delay, and mental retardation.

The gene locus for incontinentia pigmenti is thought to be an autosomal-X translocation. The breakpoint in the X chromosome in four reported cases has been in band Xp11.[76]

The differential diagnosis includes the Naegeli variant in which the cutaneous lesions are seen with equal frequency in males and females. When ocular and neurologic abnormalities are lacking, it is known as the *Franceschetti-Jadassohn syndrome.*[77] Additionally, incontinentia pigmenti must be distinguished from the autosomal dominant syndrome known as the hypomelanosis of Ito, described below.

ANHIDROTIC ECTODERMAL DYSPLASIA. This disorder is genetically heterogeneous, mainly autosomal dominant. The inheritance pattern is also recessive and sex-linked recessive in some instances. From birth the serious nature of it is suspected from the altered cranial physiognomy, with abnormalities about the eyes and, later, near-absence of teeth in both dentitions. The sex-linked form was exhibited by the "toothless men of Sind" described by Darwin in 1875.[78] The skin is dry, thin, and shiny, with prominence of the subcutaneous vessels. There is absence of the eccrine sweat glands but not the apocrine sweat glands. Later, hair over the head may be scanty and, at puberty, axillary and genital hair does not appear. A considerable proportion of the affected children are mentally retarded, though some have been able to attain upright stature and locomotion. The neuropathology has not been studied.

HIDROTIC ECTODERMAL DYSPLASIA. An autosomal dominant disorder, hidrotic ectodermal dysplasia is characterized by subtotal alopecia and dystropic nails. The sweat glands are normal. There may be hyperkeratosis of the palms and soles. Mental deficiency, epilepsy, and neural deafness have occurred in several of these patients.

LINEAR SEBACEOUS NEVI (EPIDERMAL NEVUS SYNDROME). This sporadic and, in a few cases, autosomal dominant disorder is characterized by linear sebaceous nevi of the midline of the face, which can be present at birth; it is occasionally associated with mental retardation, hemiplegia, and seizures. Seizures usually appear within the first 8 months. The mental retardation is of moderate to severe degree in the majority. Focal neurologic defects, e.g., hemiparesis or cranial nerve palsies, occur in a minority. The majority of nevi occur near the midline and involve the scalp with absence of hair. It is rarely bilateral. There are three recognized stages of evolution of lesions: infantile with yellow-orange smooth plaques; adolescent when the plaques become verrucous; and late adolescent and early adult when the lesions can progress in 20 to 30 percent of patients to more advanced lesions such as sebaceous adenomas, epitheliomas, trichilemmomas, apocrine tumors, and, rarely, basal cell carcinomas.[79] In addition there are ophthalmologic abnormalities: dermoid and lipodermoid lesions of the conjunctiva, cornea, and colombomas. The abnormalities are consistent with disordered growth and migration of cells. Mesodermal involvement is similar to that seen in other phakomatoses. The pathology is relatively specific with the finding of sebaceous glands in the second clinical stage, which distinguishes it from other phak-

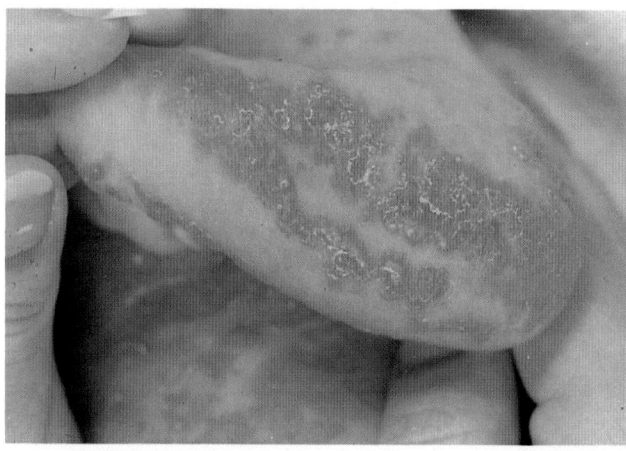

a

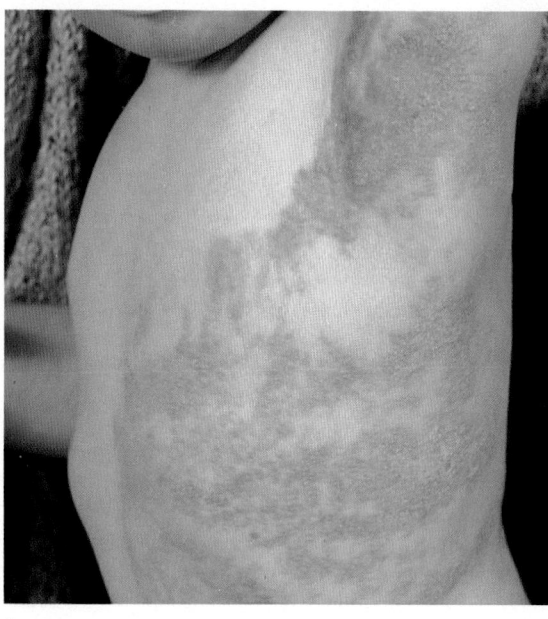

b

FIGURE 184-11 Incontinentia pigmenti. (*a*) Early lesions are erythematous papular and vesicular and are linearly arranged as on the lower arm of this baby. (*b*) Later, these lesions assume a verrucous, keratotic surface and become pigmented. *(Courtesy of Klaus Wolff, M.D.)*

omatoses. The brain lesions are variable. Unilateral hemimegalencephaly with anomalies of cortical development has been described. More frequent are ischemic and hemorrhagic vascular lesions with encephalomalacia.

BASAL CELL NEVUS SYNDROME. This syndrome, described by Gorlin and Goltz, comprises nevoid basal cell hyperplasia leading to carcinoma, palmar dyskeratoses, cysts of the jaw, lateral displacement of the inner canthi (hypertelorism), and other skeletal abnormalities (spina bifida, spade-shaped and bifid ribs). Concurrence of a variety of neurologic disorders (mental deficiency, medulloblastoma, and hydrocephalus) has been documented in several articles, and these several disorders have been incorporated into a syndrome.[80–82] Some writers refer to the familial basal cell nevus–medulloblastoma syndrome as the "fifth phakomatosis."

The basal cell carcinomas in this syndrome usually appear between puberty and age 35, mainly in the region of the face, neck, and upper trunk. The tumors are flesh-colored or reddish-brown. Only about 50 percent of patients acquire such tumors. The cysts of the jaw are mainly in the premolar region and are present in 85 percent of patients by the age of 40 years. Mental retardation is infrequent (approximately 3 percent), and in some there is an associated medulloblastoma of the cerebellum. Other skin anomalies are pits of plantar and palmar surfaces and lips and palatal clefts. A characteristic facial dysmorphism (frontal bossing, prominent supraorbital ridges, broad nasal bridge, and hypertelorism) completes the syndrome (see Chap. 75).

In 60 percent of the studied cases, basal cell nevus syndrome has arisen as a new mutation.

In the differential diagnosis one must consider Cowden's disease (see Chap. 183), which is another autosomal dominant disorder with multiple hamartomatous lesions of skin, mucous membranes, breast, and thyroid.

HYPOMELANOSIS OF ITO. Incontinentia pigmenti achromians is an autosomal dominant disorder characterized by the whorls and streaks of abnormal skin pigmentation like those seen in incontinentia pigmenti. Linear or irregular areas of hypopigmentation involving any part of the body appear within the first months of life. A Wood's lamp may be necessary to see the lesions in the fair-skinned. On histologic examination, hypopigmented whorls and streaks show normal melanocytes with decreased content of melanosomes. The hypopigmentation may also involve the hair, which is white or gray-white and often delayed in appearing. Other skin lesions are present: café au lait spots, angiomatous nevi, Mongolian blue spots, and heterochromia of the iris. In a majority of patients there are additional abnormalities, particularly neurologic. Mental retardation and seizures are frequent.[83] Neuropathologic examination has revealed many gray matter heterotopias, characterized by altered neurons and giant cells reminiscent of the other phakomatoses.[84] Ocular findings are also frequent; strabismus, microphthalmus, and nystagmus are among the abnormalities reported. Dental abnormalities similar to those seen in incontinentia pigmenti are seen. Ectrodactyly and hemihypertrophy have been reported in a number of patients. Hypomelanosis of Ito could represent chromosomal mosaicism from a postzygotic mutation, resulting in the presence of two genetically different cell lines. The risk of recurrence is low if the proband is a male, whereas if the proband is a female the risk is impossible to predict.[85]

POIKILODERMA CONGENITALE OF ROTHMUND AND THOMSON. This is an autosomal recessive disorder appearing between the third and sixth month of age and featured by diffuse erythematous skin changes, usually sparing the trunk. With time the skin becomes swollen and tense, particularly in areas exposed to the sun. Eventually the erythema fades and a network of linear telangiectases and areas of hyper- or hypopigmentation become visible (Fig. 184-12). Atrophy occurs without any scarring. The chronic poikilodermatous stage is usually present by the third to fifth year of age and persists. Photosensitivity can produce bullous lesions, although this sensitivity tends to decrease with age. Further ectodermal abnormalities include loss of scalp hair, eyebrows, and eyelashes; hypoplastic and rudimentary nails; and dental abnormalities.[86] Short stature secondary to growth hormone deficiency[87] has been observed. Cataracts appear in 75 percent of reported cases, as early as the first year of life. Intelligence is generally normal, though there have been cases with mental retardation.[88] Hypogonadism is alleged, although there is a recorded case of an affected woman who

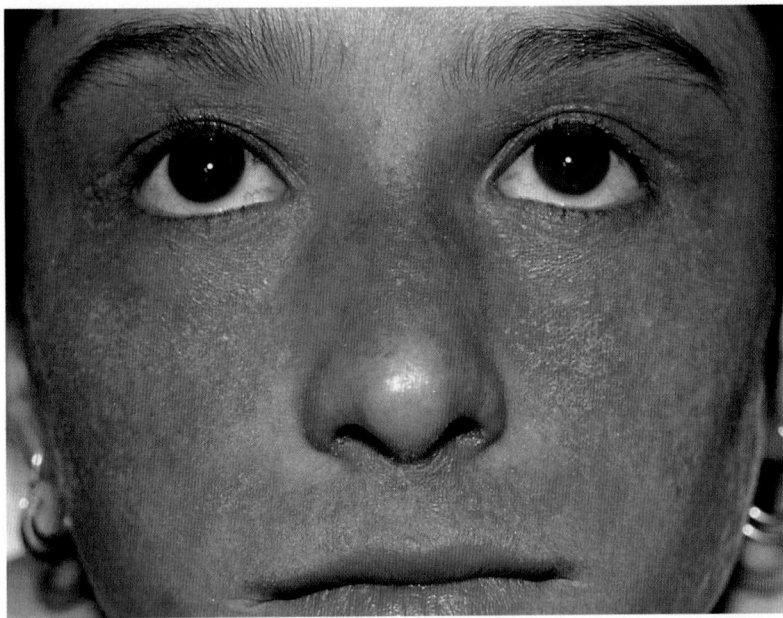

FIGURE 184-12   Poikiloderma congenitale of Rothmund and Thomson. *(Courtesy of Klaus Wolff, M.D.)*

went on to have 13 children. There have been multiple reports of the coincidental occurrence of osteosarcoma and Rothmund-Thomson syndrome.[89]

Congenital Pigmentary Disorders with Anomalous Development of the Nervous System   GIANT PIGMENTED NEVUS WITH CONCURRENT INVOLVEMENT OF MENINGES AND MALIGNANT MELANOMA (NEUROCUTANEOUS MELANOSIS) (SEE ALSO CHAPS. 81, 82).   This congenital disorder presents with one, a few, or many circumscribed, flat or raised, cutaneous pigmented nevi (color varies from light yellow to chocolate brown or black). The skin lesions tend to be oval or circular in contour, and sometimes their borders are irregular, bearing some resemblance to the outline of an animal; hence the popular belief that they are caused by a distressing maternal experience during pregnancy that has left its mark on the fetus. Lesions may be so large that they cover up to 30 percent of the body surface (Fig. 184-13). They may be present at birth, but some appear during the first year of life. The face, neck, trunk, thighs, buttocks, and external genitalia are common sites. The lesions may become less pigmented by the time of puberty, and age has another effect—to make them more elevated and corrugated or verrucous. Most of the lesions are covered with hair and a few contain cartilage. In one study of 55 patients, the dermatomal distribution of the lesions was noteworthy. They tended to originate in the posterior part of the body, near the midline; the vortex of the nevus was near the center of the spine.

Some of the more extensive elevated pigmented nevi are associated with such an exuberant growth of tissue as to resemble the elephantiasic form of neurofibromatosis, and, like the lesions in this latter condition, the tissue of the nevus reacts positively to cholinesterase stains.[90] Likewise, anomalies of skeleton (spina bifida and clubfeet), atrophy or hypertrophy of the underlying musculature of bony structures, and a tendency toward malignant degeneration are common to both the giant pigmented nevus and the elephantiasic form of neurofibromatosis. The giant nevus differs, however, in that it is not hereditary and benign tumors of the nerves are conspicuously absent.

Among the recorded examples of this disease it is to be remarked that in one series of 39 cases of pigmented nevi, 18 were in males and 29 in females. The tumors were present at birth in 8 and appeared between the ages of 1 and 5 years in 12, from 6 to 10 years in 4, from 11 to 20 years in 3, and over 20 years in 12. In the 13 autopsied cases (of the 23 that died), no fewer than 9 had metastatic melanotic carcinoma in the brain, and 2 had a diffuse melanocytosis of the leptomeninges. This last state is of particular interest insofar as many of the fully documented examples in the medical literature have been associated with extensive cutaneous nevi. The melanocytes are usually found to have proliferated abundantly. Death is usually due to communicating hydrocephalus, which is caused by obliteration of the basal subarachnoid space, interfering with the circulation of cerebrospinal fluid from over the cerebral hemispheres.[91-94] Hypo- and hyperpigmentation of the skin have been observed in conjunction with familial, spastic paraplegia and in Van Bogaert's hereditary melanosis.

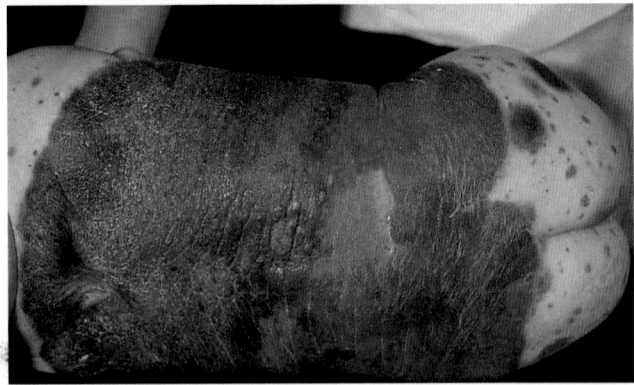

FIGURE 184-13   Giant pigmented nevus in neurocutaneous melanosis. This nevus covers the entire back and extends to the abdomen. *(Courtesy of Klaus Wolff, M.D.)*

FAMILIAL GENERALIZED MELANODERMA (LEUKOMELANO-DERMA). This is another closely related condition that appears soon after birth. The skin, according to Berlin,[95] who has described the condition in four siblings, is dry, thin, and mottled with brown or gray spots. Dwarfism and mental retardation are conjoined. Thin legs, flat nose, and defective dentition add to the grotesque appearance. In males, the penis and testicles are underdeveloped; in females, sexual development is normal. Retardation in mental development occurs in all cases. It is an autosomal recessive disorder.

WAARDENBURG-KLEIN AND RELATED SYNDROMES OF DEAFNESS (SEE ALSO CHAP. 80). Waardenburg[96] and Klein[97] have described a syndrome (now known as type I), inherited in an autosomal dominant pattern, in which developmental anomalies of eyelids, eyebrows, and root of nose are associated with a neural type of deafness.[98] The inner canthi of the eyes are displaced laterally, the eyebrows are excessively heavy, the irides are heterochromic or isochromic (pale blue). The iris may be hypoplastic, and the fundi are sometimes lacking in pigment. About half the patients have a white forelock, and a few have white areas elsewhere on the body.[99] The hair may turn gray prematurely. Piebaldness with deafness may be a closely related disorder; another is partial albinism and deafness (see Chap. 80). Other variations include type II Waardenberg with similar characteristics as type I, except for absence of dystopia canthorum,[100] and Klein-Waardenberg's syndrome, similar to type I, with skeletal muscle and bone hypoplasia[101] and can be associated with Hirschsprung disease.[102]

CHÉDIAK-HIGASHI DISEASE (SEE ALSO CHAP. 80). This syndrome is a rare autosomal recessive disorder with the cardinal features of partial albinism, photophobia, repeated pyogenic infections, terminal hepatosplenomegaly, peripheral neuropathy, seizures, and inclusions in the peripheral blood and bone marrow leukocytes. The inclusions are composed of glycolipids and have been seen in lysosomes.[103] There are giant melanosomes in melanocytes of the skin. Terminally, there may be associated cerebral lesions. Page et al.[104] found cytoplasmic lipid inclusions in the histocytic infiltrations of the brain at autopsy. Stegmaier and Schneider[105] suggest that blood smears taken from albino infants should be examined for these peculiar granulations. The giant melanosomes are demonstrable by electron microscopy and are the probable cause of the pigmentary changes seen in these patients (see Chap. 80).

MOYNAHAN'S SYNDROME (LEOPARD SYNDROME). Moynahan reported a condition of autosomal dominant inheritance in which there are multiple lentigines, genital hypoplasia, dwarfism, congenital mitral stenosis and cardiac hypertrophy, psychic infantilism, neural deafness, and mental deficiency. Moynahan believes that the disorder relates to maldevelopment of the cellular derivatives of the neural crest[106–109] (see Chap. 80).

The Congenital Ichthyotic Forms of Nervous Disease (Congenital Ichthyosis, Xeroderma, Hyperkeratosis) (See also Chap. 42)

Ichthyosis of the common variety (ichthyosis vulgaris) does not usually appear until the second year of life, but there are a number of closely related states variously designated as congenital ichthyosis, xeroderma, ichthyosiform erythroderma, etc., which are apparent at birth or during the neonatal period. The time of onset of these conditions proves not to be well documented in the literature, and, indeed, some of the neurologic syndromes with which ichthyosis is associated have been observed only in the adult, the exact beginning of the skin lesion not being known (Table 184-3). The most completely described variety was presented in 1957 by Sjögren and Larsson,[110] but prior to that time, Rud,[111] de Sanctis and Cac-chione,[112] and others had called attention to clinical cases in which ichthyosis or xerosis had been variously combined with dwarfism, endocrine abnormalities, poor muscular development, convulsions, idiocy, psychosis, and retinal lesions. Xerodermic idiocy of de Sanctis and Cacchione, despite its name, is associated with xeroderma pigmentosum, a malignant cutaneous disorder (see Chap. 158). The more important disorders associated with neurologic disease are summarized in Table 184-4.

SEX-LINKED ICHTHYOSIS (RUD'S SYNDROME). Congenital ichthyosis with infantilism, dwarfism, genital atrophy, diabetes mellitus, tetany, epilepsy, oligophrenia, polyneuropathy, retinitis pigmentosa, and macrocytic anemia make up this syndrome. For a number of years little information was available as to the nature and time of onset of ichthyosis. The ichthyosis, inherited in a sex-linked pattern, has been present at birth.[113–115]

XERODERMIC IDIOCY AND ATAXIA (LAUBENTHAL'S SYNDROME). This syndrome comprises ichthyosis, small stature, delayed dentition, mental retardation with tremor, cerebellar ataxia, and, in one instance, athetotic movements of the fingers. (The first cases were monozygotic twins.)

ICHTHYOTIC IDIOCY WITH RETINITIS PIGMENTOSA AND MUSCULAR ATROPHY (STEWART'S SYNDROME). This is a syndrome whose elements are congenital ichthyosis, idiocy, infantilism, epilepsy, arachnodactyly, muscular atrophy or hypoplasia, and atypical retinitis pigmentosa.

ICHTHYOTIC IDIOCY WITH SPASTIC PARAPLEGIA (SJÖGREN-LARSSON SYNDROME). In this disease, a congenital ichthyosis indistinguishable from ichthyosiform erythroderma, there occur, after an interval of a year or more, a spastic weakness of legs, retinal glistening, and, in 50 percent of patients, epilepsy. Dentition may be abnormal—a true dysplasia of dental enamel. The disease is inherited in an autosomal recessive pattern. Sjögren and Larsson[110] calculate that all the cases in their series from northern Sweden could be explained by the single mutation of a gene that occurred in a heterozygote about 600 years ago. The neuropathology has never been studied completely. In one case a developmental abnormality of the globus pallidus and frontal lobes was reported. Skin biopsies have revealed a picture consistent with congenital ichthyosiform erythroderma of the nonbullous type. A dermatologic study of 11 patients was made by Heijer and Reed.[116] These patients showed generalized ichthyosis but had normal scalp hair and nails. There was scaling, but no keratoderma of the palms and soles. The severity of the skin involvement appears to be unrelated to the severity of the neurologic signs.[117]

The pathogenesis of this disorder has been traced to impaired hexadecanol oxidation due to FAO (fatty alcohol oxidation—NAD^+ oxidoreductase) activity.[118] Prenatal diagnosis has been made by skin biopsy.[119]

Looseness, Redundancy, and Loss of Elasticity of Skin (Dermatochalasia, Generalized Elastolysis) (See Chap. 157)

CUTIS LAXA. In this category of developmental abnormalities the natural turgor of the skin and its tight attachments to subcutaneous tissue are lacking. As a consequence, redundancy and laxity of dermis permit extreme wrinkling, and folds of skin may be lifted from the underlying tissues. The skin is inelastic and when released does not at once return to its normal position. In some respects it resembles the skin of an aged person. The whole cutaneous surface may be involved, or only restricted regions such as neck (pterygium colli), scalp, or tongue. The condition has various clinical accompaniments such as pulmonary artery stenosis or ovarian agenesis. Hypothyroidism (cretinism) should be suspected when general laxity

TABLE 184-3
Classification of Ichthyosiform Dermatoses

Disorder	Presence at birth	Inheritance	Associated features
Ichthyosis vulgaris	No	Autosomal dominant	Atopy sometimes
Sex-linked ichthyosis	Yes	Sex-linked recessive	Corneal changes, steroid sulfatase deficiency (Xp223)
Congenital ichthyosiform erythroderma—bullous type	Yes	Autosomal dominant	Notable perinatal and childhood mortality from epidermal erosions and infections
Congenital ichthyosiform erythroderma—nonbullous type	Yes	Autosomal recessive	Growth retardation, oligophrenia, spastic paralysis, genital hypoplasia, shortened life expectancy
Sjögren-Larsson syndrome	Yes	Autosomal recessive	Severe mental retardation, spasticity, retinal glistenings
Conradi's syndrome (chondrodystrophia calcificans congenita)	Yes	Autosomal dominant	Epiphyseal calcifications and dysplastic skeletal changes, cataracts
Rhizomelic chondrodysplasia punctata (RCDP)	Yes	Autosomal recessive	Erythrodermic hyperkeratosis
Netherton's disease	Yes	Autosomal recessive	Trichorrhexis nodosa, atopy, mental deficiency, ichthyosis linearis circumflexa
Erythrokeratoderma variabilis	Sometimes	Autosomal dominant	Geographical areas of erythrokeratodermia
Sex-linked ichthyosis with mental retardation and hypogonadism (Rud's)	Yes	Sex-linked recessive	Mental retardation, hypogonadism, retinitis pigmentosa
Lamellar ichthyosis	Yes	Autosomal dominant, autosomal recessive	No
Unilateral congenital ichthyosiform erythroderma	Yes	Sex-linked dominant with male lethality	Cutaneous findings ipsilateral to malformations (hypoplastic organs and limbs); acronym CHILD syndrome given for congenital hemicysplasia with ichthyosiform erythroderma and limb defects
Ichthyosis with Down's syndrome	No	Autosomal dominant	Cataracts, mental deficiency, hypoplastic hair and nails
Mucopolysaccharidoses	No	Autosomal recessive, except for MPS II, Hunter's syndrome	Short stature, dysostosis multiplex, contractures
Tay's syndrome	Yes	Autosomal recessive	Growth retardation, mental retardation, progeroid, pili torti

of skin is present in the first days of life, for it may be one of the few indications of this disease. It is important to recognize the latter condition, for a delay in treatment results in irreparable impairment of the nervous system. The cause of cutis laxa is unknown in most instances; both familial (autosomal dominant) and nonfamilial examples have been recorded.

PTERYGIUM COLLI IN TURNER-BONNEVIE-ULLRICH SYNDROME. In the Turner-Bonnevie-Ullrich syndrome of ovarian dysgenesis in

the female, redundancy of the skin of the sides of the neck (pterygium colli) is accompanied by short stature, infantile sexual development, and multiple congenital defects, including low posterior hair line, short fourth metacarpal and metatarsal bones, and cardiac defects (bicuspid aortic valve, coarctation of the aorta, and valvular aortic stenosis). The cells contain only 45 chromosomes, one of the X pair being absent. Although the majority of the patients have had no neurologic abnormalities, the authors have observed an unusu-

TABLE 184-4
Ichthyotic Disorders with Neurologic Disease

Sjögren-Larsson syndrome	Seizures
	Spasticity
	Mental retardation
	Retinal glistenings
Conradi's syndrome	Mental retardation
Rud's syndrome	Mental retardation
	Retinitis pigmentosa
Refsum's syndrome	Peripheral neuropathy
	Retinitis pigmentosa
	Cerebellar ataxia
	Neurosensory deafness
BIDS syndrome*	Mental retardation
	Cataracts
	Microcephaly
	Dwarfism
Tay's syndrome	Mental retardation

*BIDS, *b*rittle hair, *i*ntellectual impairment, *d*ecreased fertility, *s*hort stature.

ally high incidence of slightly subnormal mentality. Because this may not be evident during infancy and early childhood and the short stature may occur only after puberty, the webbing of the skin of the neck may provide the earliest clue to the syndrome and prompt the clinician to undertake confirmatory chromosomal studies. Closely related are Noonan's syndrome and the Turner phenotype with normal karyotype.[120] See references also for other pterygium syndromes.[121–125]

LEPRECHAUNISM. A notable example of cutis laxa is observed in the syndrome known as *leprechaunism*. This is a term given to a condition in which infants of low birth weight and deficient nutrition are observed to suffer an anomaly consisting of looseness of skin including cutis gyrata, muscular wasting, retarded bone age, acanthosis nigricans, broad nose, and facial hair. The hands and feet are too large for the body. Subcutaneous fat is deficient. The male sexual organs are excessively large, and signs of precocious puberty may appear. The primary defect is a defect in the insulin receptor.[126] Death usually occurs within the first year. The hereditary pattern is autosomal recessive. A related syndrome is Seip's syndrome (lipodystrophic diabetes).

CUTIS VERTICUS GYRATA. This disorder of the scalp is characterized by the presence of folds and furrows, giving a corrugated appearance to the skin. It looks as though the head were not large enough to fill out the scalp. No satisfactory pathologic studies of the dermal condition have been forthcoming. Approximately one-fourth of the patients later exhibit mental retardation and epilepsy. Deformities of cranium, eye defects, and acromegaly may coexist. The pattern of inheritance is autosomal recessive.

MELKERSSON-ROSENTHAL SYNDROME. This condition, which rarely may have a genetic predisposition and then is inherited as an autosomal dominant trait, is featured by plication of the tongue (lingua plicata), paresis or paralysis of the muscles of facial expression on one side (like Bell's palsy), and a curious brawny edema of the lips or face on that side. The condition has usually been observed during adolescence or adult life, and its pathogenesis is unknown; therefore, unlike the other congenital and developmental neurocutaneous conditions discussed, it raises no problems during infancy.[127]

Diseases that Simultaneously Affect the Cells of Skin and Nervous System

Metabolic Abnormalities (Including Those of Vitamin Deficiency and Endocrine Diseases)

No single unifying characteristic embraces the following diseases other than the fact that some metabolic, biochemical, or endocrine abnormality has, in each instance, affected both the skin and the nervous system. The reader's attention is drawn to the most important ones, but admittedly the list is not complete, and new diseases or syndromes are being reported every month or two. Doubtless some of the diseases already described under "Congenital and Developmental Neurocutaneous Diseases" will be brought into this group as new biochemical data are obtained. A reference on this subject is the monograph by Adams and Lyon.[128] The metabolic or endocrine abnormality in each instance has been present since birth or even before, but an interval of time usually elapses before the full clinical syndrome, especially that part relative to disorders of the nervous system, becomes manifest.

Cretinism (See also Chap. 169)   This was the first neurocutaneous metabolic disease to be identified. Three types of thyroid abnormality have been delineated: first, an inherited agenesis or hypoplasia of the thyroid gland; second, a defect in thyroid metabolism[129]; and third, an acquired iodine deficiency in individuals living in regions deficient in this element. The typical physical features of cretinism are large fontanelles, facial immaturity with short nose, statural underdevelopment, large tongue, and hoarse voice.[130] Not all of these changes may be present at birth or in the first weeks of life, and the diagnosis may be delayed unless the condition is suspected because the mother is known to be hypothyroid or has had previous cretinoid children. Prolonged jaundice, an unusual degree of inactivity, and, as was mentioned above, dryness and laxity of skin and coarseness of hair are the early indications. Only as weeks and months pass do the thickness of lips, large tongue and open mouth, low-bridged nose, narrow brow, broad hands and stubby fingers, hoarse low-pitched cry, constipation, and delay in psychomotor development become manifest. Thus the dermatologist is in a particularly favorable position to assist the pediatrician in reaching an early diagnosis.

Pellagra (See also Chap. 145)   Formerly one of the most universal afflictions, this condition, now known to be due to a deficiency in nicotinic acid and other B vitamins (tryptophan deficiency may also be a factor), has been virtually eradicated in the Western world. This great advance in public health has been achieved by the fortification of the wheat flour in bread by nicotinic acid. It is still endemic in remote underdeveloped areas where green vegetables and red meat are unobtainable for parts of each year, and in chronic alcoholics and food faddists.

The skin lesions are evoked by exposure to sunlight, which leads to erythema, vesiculation, often with bullous formation, and then crusting and desquamation. The lesions appear mainly on the exposed parts of the body—backs of hands, forehead, cheeks, bridge of nose, and shins. Sebaceous plugging of skin over the nose, cheeks, and brow, and rhagades, or cracks, at the corners of the mouth are often found, but some research workers ascribe them to an associated riboflavin deficiency. The tongue and oral mucous membranes become red and smooth (lingual filiform papillae are effaced) and stomatitis and vaginitis, with fusospirochetal infections, are frequent. Later the skin becomes lichenified and pigmented.

With the skin lesions there is often a moderately severe diarrhea. Macrocytic anemia and hypochlorhydria coexist. The earliest signs of involvement of the central nervous system are general weakness and fatigability (called neurasthenia), irritability, and suspiciousness, followed within days or weeks by a confusional psychosis [incorrectly termed *dementia,* to give an alliterative term to the symptom triad of the three Ds (dermatitis, diarrhea, and dementia)]. There may also be an associated polyneuropathy. Babinski signs, sucking and grasping reflexes, and fluctuating rigidity of the limbs appear late, almost terminally. Nicotinic acid, given by injection or orally, will prevent and cure the disease. Because parts of the syndrome may be due to lack of other B vitamins (pyridoxine, riboflavin, thiamine, pantothenic acid, folic acid, and B_{12}), it is best to prescribe a balanced diet supplemented by the whole B complex. Pellagra should not be confused with Hartnup disease, in which the skin lesions are identical, or with another familial disorder with similar skin lesions but without any evidence of the tryptophan malabsorption that distinguishes it from Hartnup's disorder.[131]

Phenylketonuria (PKU) (Følling's Disease)

This, the most common of the metabolic disorders found among patients in mental institutions, is characterized by mental deficiency, epilepsy, and minor skin changes. The latter consist of decreased pigmentation of hair and skin, particularly noticeable among members of dark-skinned races, whose hair may then be brown instead of black (see Chap. 80), and a tendency in infants toward atopic dermatitis. Partington[132] noted that six of his patients developed a generalized eczema between the first and fourth month of life, and five others had dry skin and persistent nondescript rashes. Sensitivity to sunlight may prove a problem and so can lead to recognition of patients in a mental retardation hospital. It is said that Følling, who first described the disease, would find PKU patients by asking for all the patients who had an unusual degree of sensitivity to sunlight. Some patients also exhibit abnormal reactions to phenothiazine compounds.

The mental deficiency varies in degree; many children are profoundly retarded, eking out an existence in homes for the mentally enfeebled. They sit in idleness, manifesting digital mannerisms and rocking movements, making no effort to communicate by sign or word. Exceptionally, they exhibit flexion (salaam spasms) in infancy, and their limbs may be mildly spastic with increased tendon reflexes and Babinski signs. The majority show no other major neurologic abnormalities. Considering the disease in toto, the skin alterations are of relatively little importance and are seldom of value in diagnosis with one exception—in the Asian races there is a dilution of hair color; the scalp hair is normally *black,* whereas in PKU the hair is dark brown and is easily recognized as abnormal (see Chap. 80). Patients have been reported with sclerodermoid changes in the skin associated with myositis. Lowering the phenylalanine level by diet in early life prevents mental retardation and leads to improvement in skin and behavior. Some of the more recent studies of the enzymatic defect of this disease and the related clinical states are to be found in the references.[133–137]

Homocystinuria

First recognized by Carson and her collaborators in 1965,[138] this syndrome has become widely recognized among pediatricians and neurologists. It is characterized by an excessive urinary excretion of homocystine, in association with ectopia len-

tis, marfanoid habitus, fine sparse hair, malar flush, livedo reticularis, prominent joints, bilateral inguinal hernias, slight mental retardation, rare convulsions, and, later, spastic weakness of the legs or strokes (see Chap. 157).

Argininosuccinic Aminoaciduria

In this autosomal recessive disease, in which mental dullness, epilepsy, and intermittent cerebellar ataxia are related to excesses of arginine and ammonia due to a deficiency of arginosuccinate lyase activity in the urea cycle, the hair tends to be dry and brittle. When the hair is examined with a hand lens, nodose swellings and constrictions are seen along the shaft (trichorrhexis nodosa) (see Chap. 147).

Hartnup Disease

This condition is named after the family in which four of eight children had a hereditary pellagra-like skin rash aggravated by sunlight, a fluctuant cerebellar ataxia, and slight to moderate mental deficiency. These children were the result of a first-cousin marriage. One of the patients reported by the Halvorsens had premature graying of the hair.[139] The disease is extremely rare, having been identified only a few times in the United States.

From other reports it has been determined that the disease is autosomal recessive. There is an impairment of neutral amino acid transport involving and limited to the kidneys and intestines. The hyperaminoaciduria is an increased excretion of indoxyl sulfate. Tryptophan loss in the urine is excessive. The tryptophan in the small intestine is not absorbed and by bacterial action is degraded to indoles. Niacin cannot be synthesized and is deficient.[139–141]

Hydroxykynureninuria

This is an autosomal recessive disease due presumably to a deficiency of kynureninase; the nervous symptoms are much like those of Hartnup disease and congenital tryptophanuria. Sensitivity to sunlight and skin rash are associated with mental dullness and episodic ataxia.

Monilethrix (Trichorrhexis Nodosa)

(See also Chap. 61) These patients are born without hair or lose it in early infancy. The remaining hair is dry, coarse, and fragile. Alopecia is usually not complete, whether in the scalp or elsewhere.[142] Some patients exhibit defective dentition, cataracts, koilonychia, ichthyosis simplex, and mental deficiency. Monilethrix differs from pili torti, another inherited abnormality of the hair in which the shafts are flattened and twisted. (See Chap. 147 for a discussion of the metabolic disorder and its relation to argininosuccinic acid.) Both autosomal recessive and dominant forms have been reported.

Kinky Hair Disease

This disease was described in 1962 by Menkes et al.[143] as a sex-linked hereditary disorder occurring only in females (probably lethal in males). Born normally from an unaffected mother after a normal gestation, the sparse kinky hair first attracts notice. Soon thereafter, developmental delay of maturing nervous functions becomes apparent. The retardation and failure to thrive are of such severity that most of the patients have died in the first year of life, but a few live on for a few years. In 1966, Aguilar et al.[144] presented a more complete account of the disease, and details of the pathology have been amplified by Hirano et al.[145] and others[146,147] (see Chap. 61).

The abnormality of hair is not fully differentiated from monilethrix and pili torti (twisted hair), and from diseases such as were described by Robinson and Miller,[148] in which kinky hair was associated with dysplasia of dental enamel, and by Bjornstad with nerve deafness (Bjornstad's syndrome). The underlying biochemical mechanism is a failure of absorption of copper (Cu) from the intestinal tract, due to a missing enzyme. Presumably lack of Cu in the neonatal and infantile tissues (probably interfering with the action of enzymes in which Cu is a trace element) is responsible for the severe nutritional and growth defect. The defective gene has been localized to chromosome Xp13 by linkage analysis.[146]

Neuronal loss and gliosis, myelin degeneration, and deformities of Purkinje cells in the cerebellum with lack of development of proper somatic synapses underlie the neurologic abnormalities.

Tightly curled scalp hair is also an early feature of congenital lipodystrophic diabetes.

The Mucopolysaccharidoses: Gargoylism (Hunter-Hurler) and Other Syndromes

The distinctive, grotesque appearance of patients with gargoylism reflects changes in nearly every part of the body due to the abnormal deposition of a mucopolysaccharide and a glycolipid. Recently, several new variants of the disease have been described, but most of them look alike.

The most familiar types of mucopolysaccharidosis are Hunter-Hurler syndrome, Sanfilippo's syndrome, Morquio's syndrome, and Maroteaux-Lamy syndrome. In all, the clouding of corneas is diagnostic when combined with evident developmental delay, coarse facial features, short stature, stiff joints, enlarged head with hydrocephalus, hepatosplenomegaly, and retarded mentation. Characteristically the disease evolves in the first years of life and is progressive. Many succumb in late childhood. As in all the inherited metabolic forms of brain disease, there are milder variants in some, in which survival to adult years is possible, sometimes with retained intelligence.

The biochemistry of this group of diseases is described in greater detail in Chap. 21. Here it need only be pointed out that they are autosomal or sex-linked recessive defects of lysosomal enzymes involved in the degradation of glycosaminoglycans (mucopolysaccharides). The enzyme defects differ in each of the several types, which accounts for phenotypic variations.[149]

Of dermatologic interest is the common finding of hirsutism over the body, papules and nodules, and often a peculiar orange-peel appearance of the skin. Especially in the Hunter syndrome, a characteristic pebbly, waxy-appearing skin lesion covers the upper arms, back, and lateral aspects of the thighs. A second type of skin lesion occurs in the hands where the fingers may be semiflexed due to skin thickening and pseudocontractures. The skin over the hands may be thickened, lardaceous, and inelastic. Mucopolysaccharide deposition in the cytoplasm of the epidermal cells and in the fibroblasts of the dermis has been reported. Persistent tinea capitis infections, resistant to therapy, may occur, suggesting perhaps a reduced defense against infection.

Xeroderma Pigmentosum

(See also Chap. 158) Xeroderma pigmentosum (XP) represents a group of autosomal recessive disorders that can be divided into two basic forms: one associated with progressive degeneration of skin and eye, and a second with the same involvement plus progressive neurologic degeneration. Within these two forms there are nine groups characterized by defective repair of DNA following ultraviolet irradiation (shown in complementation analysis). All the diseases are deficient in gene products required for excision of damaged DNA. Groups C, E, and F have had no neurologic abnormalities. The remainder are associated with various neurologic problems. The cutaneous manifestations of XP are many: erythema, freckles, xerosis and scaling, areas of hypo-

and hyperpigmentation, telangiectasia, atrophy of the skin, actinokeratoses, and a 2000-fold increase in sunlight-induced skin cancers. The latter include basal cell and squamous cell types and malignant melanomas. The ocular manifestations of XP are conjunctivitis, ectropion, exposure keratitis, and photophobia. On neuropathologic examination there is primary neuronal degeneration of pyramidal cells of cerebral cortex, Purkinje cells of the cerebellum, deep nuclei of basal ganglia and locus ceruleus, and zona compacta of the substantia nigra, all of which are the basis of the progressive neurologic accompaniments of this skin disease. They are similar to those of Cacchione-de Sanctis disease and Cockayne's disease.[150–152]

Xerodermic Idiocy of de Sanctis and Cacchione

(See also Chap. 158) This is an autosomal recessive disorder characterized by microcephaly, progressive mental deterioration, dwarfism, choreoathetosis, ataxia, immature sexual development, and xeroderma pigmentosum (complementation group D). There is an increased incidence of leukemia in addition to skin cancer.

Cockayne's Syndrome

(See also Chap. 158) This is an autosomal recessive disorder with features of dwarfism, precociously senile appearance secondary to lipodystrophy of the face, pigmentary retinal degeneration, optic atrophy, deafness, marble epiphyses, sun sensitivity, and mental retardation. By complementation studies of RNA synthesis during cell fusion after UV exposure, three groups have been identified. There is a defect in DNA repair after incision (exonuclease reaction during DNA synthesis). A defect in DNA ligase has been postulated. Hence the disease is related to xeroderma pigmentosum. There is a reported case of a child with both xeroderma pigmentosum and Cockayne's syndrome.[153] The differential diagnosis of a child presenting with a "butterfly" rash after sun exposure would include xeroderma pigmentosum, Cockayne's syndrome, and lupus erythematosus.

Bloom's Syndrome

(See also Chap. 158) This is an autosomal recessive disorder characterized by short stature, malar hypoplasia, and telangiectatic erythema in a butterfly distribution on the face, which appears in the first year, and occasionally similar erythematous changes are seen on the dorsa of the hands and forearms.[154] Photosensitivity is present and may cause excoriation. Hypoimmunoglobulinemia is frequently present, particularly of IgA and IgM. Increased chromosomal breakage is present in culture and may be related to the increased incidence of leukemia and other malignancies. Malignancy is the cause of early mortality. There is an increased incidence in the Ashkenazim with a carrier rate of 1 in 100. Purportedly there is a defect in the DNA ligase I in Bloom's syndrome.

Albinism

(See also Chap. 80) Universal albinism, another autosomal recessive disorder, classically shows absence of marked dilution of pigment in the skin, hair, and eye. Nystagmus is frequent. There is a tendency toward early cutaneous malignant tumors. These "moon children," as they have been called, may be found even among American Indians and the aborigines of western Australia. Albinism is the result of a genetically determined deficiency of tyrosinase in melanocytes.

Albinism includes a group of disorders that have in common reduced amounts of melanin in skin, hair, and iris. In only one form of oculocerebral albinism, type IA, is there total absence of melanin. There are ten types of oculocerebral albinism (OCA) and four types of ocular albinism (OA), all of which are autosomal recessively inherited, with the exception of two forms of OA that are sex-linked and one form that is an autosomal dominant. The ocular symptoms include nystagmus, strabismus, photophobia secondary to iris translucency, and decreased visual acuity secondary to foveal hypoplasia. The cutaneous symptoms include snow-white hair and milky-white skin at birth, which is true for all ethnic backgrounds for type IA OCA. In other forms of OCA, depending on the ethnic group, the hair color may vary from light yellow to light brown at birth and darkens with age. Iris color is blue at birth for all forms, darkening to hazel and brown in most forms except for type IA. The skin color is milky- or creamy-white at birth due to lack of generalized pigment in most forms except for type IV. The skin is sensitive to UV radiation and sunlight exposure results in burns. With continued exposure, the skin becomes chronically irritated and may then develop some pigmentation. Pigmented nevi and freckles may appear within sun-exposed areas. Tyrosinase activity is variable, ranging from absent in type IA to low levels in other forms (as shown by testing by incubation of hair bulbs in tyrosine).

Two particular forms of OCA should be noted: *Hermansky-Pudlak syndrome,* type VIA, and the *Mast syndrome.* The former is an autosomal recessive disorder characterized by variable hypopigmentation, typical ocular manifestations, albinism, and hair color varying from white to red and brown. There is an increased prevalence in Puerto Rico for this type, where it is estimated to be 1 in 2000 in the general population. In addition to the features of albinism, there is an associated platelet storage deficiency with easy bruisability and prolonged bleeding after dental extraction and surgery. Drugs such as aspirin or antiprostaglandins must be avoided as they exacerbate the bleeding diathesis. In patients with Hermansky-Pudlak syndrome, there is an accumulation of ceroid-like material in the reticuloendothelial system, the lungs, heart, kidneys, oral mucosa, and gastrointestinal tract. As a result, diffuse interstitial pulmonary fibrosis and granulomatous colitis and renal insufficiency may develop, depending on the degree of accumulation. Because of increased accumulation of ceroids, patients excrete elevated levels of dolichols, which are components of lysosomal membranes, suggesting that there is a defect in the processing of lysosomal membranes. The albinism appears to be secondary to an as yet unknown metabolic defect that blocks tyrosinase activity. The lack of platelet dense bodies are a diagnostic feature, and carriers can be detected by a low level of thioredoxin reductase in skin biopsies.[155,156]

The second form of OCA, the Mast syndrome, was named after the Amish family described by Cross et al.[157] Three albino siblings were mentally retarded and had spastic diplegia, multiple ocular abnormalities, and coarse nystagmus. The inheritance was autosomal recessive.

Seip's Syndrome (Berardinelli's Syndrome) Seip's syndrome is an autosomal recessive disorder characterized by general lipodystrophy, hyperlipidemia, hepatomegaly, acanthosis nigricans, elevated basal metabolic rate, and nonketotic insulin-resistant diabetes mellitus. Occasionally it is associated with polycystic ovaries, muscular hypertrophy, and mental retardation.[158,159] In the differential diagnosis is included leprechaunism in which insulin-antagonizing and fat-mobilizing substances have been found in the urine, as in this syndrome. An autopsy case reviewed by Berge et al.[160] revealed a hypothalamic lesion of hamartomatous type. A related syndrome with partial involvement was reported by McLean and Hoefnagel,[161] in which a 16-year-old girl had involvement limited to the face, upper extremities, and upper torso. A co-occurrence of

Seip's syndrome and systemic cystic angiomatosis suggests that the same gene may be responsible for the two syndromes.[162]

Prader-Willi Syndrome This disorder represents the converse, clinically, of Seip's syndrome. It is characterized by marked hypotonia, hyporeflexia, poor feeding, cryptorchidism, and hypoplastic penis and scrotum in boys or hypoplastic labia in girls. Cytogenetically visible and submicroscopic deletions of the 15q11-12 region have been reported. Later the children are characteristically obese with small hands and feet (acromicria), short stature, gonadal atrophy, and mental retardation.

Laurence-Moon Syndrome This is an autosomal recessive disorder with the following features: mental retardation, pigmentary retinopathy, hypogenitalism, and spastic paraplegia. It differs from the *Bardet-Biedl syndrome,* which is characterized by mental retardation, pigmentary retinopathy, polydactyly, obesity, and hypogenitalism.[163]

Hypercholesterolemia with Tendon Xanthomatosis and Neurologic Abnormality (Van Bogaert-Epstein-Scherer Syndrome, Cerebrotendinous Xanthomatosis) While familial hypercholesterolemia is seldom associated with nervous disorder, there has now been described a series of cases marked by prominent xanthelasma, tendon xanthomas and progressive spastic weakness, and cerebellar ataxia of the limbs. Intellectual deterioration may be added. First described in a monograph by Van Bogaert et al.,[164] in recent years the discovery of other cases has established its existence as a clinicopathologic entity. Heavy deposits of crystalline cholesterol in the cerebellum, brainstem, and basal ganglia variably destroy parenchymal elements and excite an intense gliotic reaction. The underlying biochemical defect is a lack of the hepatic mitochondrial 26-hydroxylase involved in the normal biosynthesis of bile acids. The deficiency is inherited in an autosomal recessive pattern. Treatment with agents that decrease the level of cholestanol has improved the neurologic symptoms and reduced the xanthomas. For similar syndromes see references.[165,166]

Refsum's Syndrome and Tangier Disease Heredopathic atactica polyneuritiformis (Refsum's syndrome)[167] is an autosomal recessive disorder in which retinitis pigmentosa, deafness, and sensorimotor polyneuropathy are combined and may be accompanied occasionally by exceptional dryness and scaling of skin or frank ichthyosis. The skin disease, like that of the nervous system, is probably linked to the inability of alpha-hydroxylase to degrade phytanic acid, an exogenous fatty acid that accumulates throughout the body.[168] For the dermatologist, the diagnosis is clarified by the discovery of sensorimotor paralysis and areflexia of the limbs in patients presenting with dry, scaling skin. For the neurologist, the skin changes in a patient with chronic progressive polyneuropathy should always suggest Refsum's syndrome.[169,170]

An alpha-lipoproteinemia (Tangier disease) has been found among the inhabitants of Tangier Island in the Chesapeake Bay.[171,172] The characteristics are very large tonsils, which are covered with orange-yellow deposits, and enlarged liver, spleen, and lymph nodes. Patients with this autosomal recessive disorder have the lowest amounts of plasma alpha-lipoproteins found in any disease and profound deficiency of high-density lipoproteins (HDL) (see Chap. 152).

Tangier disease resembles Refsum's disease in its clinical neurologic manifestations.[173] Dermal deposition of cholesterol esters was found in cutaneous papules (xanthomas) or more diffusely in the skin in one case, but the skin has been clinically normal in four or five of the known living patients with Tangier disease.

Lipoid Proteinosis (Urbach-Wiethe Disease) (See also Chap. 154) Lipoid proteinosis is a rare autosomal recessive disease, typified by widespread papules, nodules, indurated plaques, and ulcerated lesions involving the skin and mucous membranes. Hoarseness is a prominent symptom, due to involvement of vocal cords and the upper respiratory tract. Lipid, protein, and carbohydrate have been demonstrated in the extracellular deposits and walls of blood vessels; hence, the designation of the disease as a *lipoglycoproteinosis*. Epilepsy, mental impairment, and indifference to pain are the reported neurologic features of this metabolic defect.

Angiokeratoma Corporis Diffusum (Fabry Disease)   This disease (see Chap. 153) was first described by Anderson and Fabry in 1898. It comprises a rash (small vascular lesions), inexplicable pains in the extremities (often lancinating and with paresthesias) indicative of a polyneuropathy, irregular fever, superficial corneal opacities, tortuosity of retinal vessels, a high incidence of cerebrovascular accidents at an early age, and cardiac and renal failure. The skin lesions may be present from childhood but usually appear later, evolving slowly but antedating the other symptoms. Typically the lesions are more or less symmetric, being most marked over bony prominences, particularly below the waist. They tend to cluster. In size they vary from a pinpoint to 3 to 4 mm; the smaller lesions are red, the larger black. Keratinized macules and papules also occur. The mucous membranes of the lips and the skin of the genitalia are involved in some cases. The vascular lesions consist of dilated vessels, but only the smaller ones blanch on pressure. Capillary dilatations cause a peculiar mottling of the palms. Angiokeratomas can be seen in other lysosomal storage diseases, fucosidosis, sialidosis, adult-type β-galactosidase deficiency, and aspartylglucosaminuria. In some patients, the general physique is poor, with slender limbs, stooped posture, and some degree of fixation of joints and even the spine. The muscles in some cases are thin and weak, possibly from atrophy of disuse occasioned by the limitation of movement and pain. The pattern of inheritance is usually that of a mendelian sex-linked trait.[174]

Studies by Sweeley and Klionsky[175] suggest there may be a defect in glycolipid synthesis resulting in an accumulation of an unidentified substance, principally in the walls of blood vessels and glomeruli. The major part of the stored material is thought to be ceramide dihexoside and trihexoside. Exceptionally, small deposits of a storage material appear in the neurons of the brain, particularly in patients whose mental capacities have declined. In this respect, the disease falls into the class of lipidoses.

The pain, acroparesthesias, and burning (chiefly of the hands), the hypersensitivity to temperature, and the anhidrosis may be due to lipid infiltration of the nerve cells, of the peripheral and autonomic nervous systems, and of vessels.[176,177] Dependent edema is part of the picture of cardiac decompensation. The vascular lesions in the brain, which may begin in adolescence or early adult life, are either embolic from heart or thrombotic. The female carrier may show only corneal opacities. Diagnosis is facilitated by the demonstration of the glycolipids (by polaroscopy) in the urinary sediment. Most patients die of uremia or heart failure in mid-adult life. The only known treatment is symptomatic. Prenatal diagnosis is available either by enzyme assay or DNA analysis. The locus for α-galactosidase A is assigned to Xq21,33-q22 and the gene for it has been cloned.[174,178] Neurologically, the disease is best listed with familial polyneuropathies, probably of vascular pathogenesis.

Variegate Porphyria (See also Chap. 150)   In this autosomal dominant disorder, the cutaneous changes of porphyria cutanea tarda are combined with the severe neurologic crises of acute intermittent porphyria.[179] This type of porphyria is very common among the Boers of South Africa.[180] These patients exhibit easy abrasion, bullae, hypertrichosis, scarring (scleroderma-like), and hyperpigmentation on the sun-exposed areas of the body. Intolerance to barbiturates and the sulfonamides has been demonstrated. Fecal and urinary coproporphyrin and porphobilinogen are increased. Goldberg[181] points out that the most striking clinical features are neurologic.

Familial Hyperuricemia with Self-Destructive Biting, Mental Retardation, Cerebral Palsy, and Choreoathetosis (Lesch-Nyhan Syndrome)   This sex-linked recessive syndrome occurs in young males who have a persistent hyperuricemia without other signs of clinical gout. The neurologic disorder takes the form of extensor spasms of the trunk, dysarthria, choreoathetosis, brisk tendon reflexes, and Babinski signs. These have appeared during the first months of life. Mental deficiency and retarded growth have been noted in all reported cases. The blood uric acid ranges from 5 to 15 mg/dL due to a deficient activity of hypoxanthine-guanine phosphoribosyltransferase. Lowering uric acid by the use of allopurinol does not alter the course of the illness. Picking and rubbing of the skin results in mutilation of the face, particularly the lower lip, and of the hands unless the patient is restrained. Sometimes it is necessary to extract the teeth to prevent biting. Tophi and gouty arthritis occur later in some cases.

The severe self-mutilation, which may result in a child literally devouring the whole lower lip, has not been explained. It is more pronounced and consistent than the self-injury of some low-grade mental defectives in whom biting of the back of the hand may be provoked during a moment of frustration or a temper tantrum. There seems to be no loss of sensation as in congenital familial sensory neuropathy with anhidrosis. At the time when the self-destructive behavior begins (usually about the age of 2 years), the uric acid content of the saliva is not greater than at other times. Prenatal diagnosis is possible by enzyme assay or by DNA analysis of amniocytes of chorionic villi.[182]

Hypoparathyroidism with Superficial Moniliasis, Keratoconjunctivitis, and Hypoadrenalism   Most of the patients with this autosomal recessive disorder follow a definite clinical sequence. The idiopathic hypoparathyroidism, with tetany and calcification of the basal ganglia and, finally, adrenal and sometimes thyroid insufficiency, develops after an infantile moniliasis of buccal mucosa and nails that continues into adult life. Chronic keratoconjunctivitis, usually not monilial, is another important feature. At autopsy the parathyroid glands are usually absent, and the adrenal glands atrophied. The disorder is included in the spectrum of Finnish inherited diseases and is also known as *polyglandular autoimmune syndrome, type I*[183,184] (see Chap. 156).

Familial Dysautonomia (Riley-Day Syndrome)   The essential features of familial autonomic dysautonomia are defective lacrimation leading to corneal ulceration, blotching of the skin, excessive sweating, and excessive drooling. Less constant findings are emotional instability, blood pressure lability, pain indifference, and faulty speech. This is an autosomal recessive disorder in which there is an enzyme defect in the metabolism and function of the catecholamines. The gene locus has been identified for this disease on 9q (personal communication, A. Blumenfeld). Nearly all the patients have been of Ashkenazi Jewish descent.[185]

Toxic Disorders

Arsenic Intoxication   Lead arsenate is the source of most of the trouble, being used in certain rural areas worldwide as an insecticide in sprays or as a powder for the extermination of boll weevils. Exposure leads to a syndrome that indicates involvement of many organs including skin (rain-drop hypo- and hyperpigmentation and keratosis as late sequelae after long-term exposure), hair, nails, gastrointestinal tract (nausea and vomiting), bone marrow (anemia and leukopenia), liver (jaundice), and peripheral and central nervous system (subacute sensorimotor polyneuropathy and convulsions and coma). Prevention of further ingestion and chelation with British antilewisite (BAL) have been the most effective treatment in the majority of patients.

Mercury and Acrodynia   Mercury intoxication causes a variety of symptoms. In Minimata disease (resulting from ingestion of an organic methylated mercurial), cerebellar ataxia and sometimes blindness develop acutely. There is no skin lesion. In young children, a syndrome known as *acrodynia* (erythrodermic neuralgia, or pink disease) has been ascribed to poisoning by this element. Irritability, photophobia, confusion, and drowsiness, the initial symptoms, are followed by a fairly typical skin eruption in 2 to 4 weeks. The hands and feet become cold, cyanotic, erythematous, and swollen. The limbs are weak. The patient constantly rubs the hands and feet, and self-mutilation may occur, as in juvenile gout, perhaps from intense pain. Stomatitis has been observed, with loss of teeth. In most of the recently reported cases, mercury has been found in the urine. The source is said to be paint or exposure to the metallic form of the element.

Thallium Poisoning   The use of thallium, formerly used as a depilatory, may result in a painful acute polyneuropathy, sometimes fatal. Loss of hair precedes or accompanies the peripheral nerve involvement.

Infective States, Proved or Suspected Types

Meningococcemia and Rickettsial, Viral, Mycotic, and Spirochetal Infections   In a variety of infections of the nervous system, the skin lesions may be among the earliest signs of a neurocutaneous syndrome. In meningococcemia, rickettsemia (Rocky Mountain spotted fever, or typhus), and some of the coxsackie- and echoviruses, the skin of the trunk and limbs may be flecked with petechiae or involved in a macular and papular rash, and only later will an infective meningitis develop. In such cases a systemic infection appears to underlie a generalized disease that may affect the skin and other organs, including the cerebrospinal meninges. The skin disease seems not to be primary.

The postexanthematous encephalomyelitides (after rubeola, variola, vaccinia, etc.) are better regarded as systemic rather than primary dermatologic diseases. However, it seems probable that affection of cutaneous structures and skin lesions might be the conditioning stimulus to an autoallergic reaction in the central nervous system. Probably antirabies treatment provides the best example, for here cutaneous or subcutaneous inoculation seems to be the most effective means of sensitizing the patient to the essential anti-

gen. Fungal infections that may attack the nervous system with regularity are rarely primary in the skin; the only examples the authors have encountered are exceptional cases of torulosis (cryptococcosis), coccidioidomycosis, actinomycosis, moniliasis, and North American blastomycosis.

Vogt-Koyanagi-Harada (Uveomeningoencephalitic) Syndrome (See also Chap. 80)   In this strange disease, presumably viral, the skin around the eyes, including the eyelashes (poliosis) and eyebrows, becomes depigmented (vitiligo).[186] There may also be scattered depigmented macules on the trunk. The uveal tracts are affected. In some cases there are also retinal detachment, papilledema, night blindness, and visual loss. Headache and mild stiffness of neck call attention to intracranial extension, and lumbar puncture reveals a pleocytosis (lymphocytic) and an elevated protein level in cerebrospinal fluid. There may be dysacousia or deafness. The course is subacute or chronic, and the process finally subsides. No treatment is known to be effective. An autoimmune process similar to Behçet's disease is suspected, i.e., a reaction against melanocytes of skin, uveal tract, and inner ear.[187] Steroid therapy, cyclosporine, and other immunosuppressive therapy has been used with success for this disorder.

Behçet's Syndrome (See also Chap. 185)   This is another presumed viral infection that affects mucous membranes (oral or genital), lungs, and cerebrum. The condition should be considered when ulcerations of mucous membranes are followed by systemic symptoms. Approximately one-quarter of the patients will have neurologic signs, such as seizures, and a variety of other focal cerebral disturbances (mild hemiparesis, hemianesthesia, aphasia, ataxia, etc.). The neurologic signs are of a type that indicate involvement of the gray and white matter of the brain (i.e., tracts and nuclear structure), and the cerebrospinal fluid usually gives evidence of the inflammatory nature of the illness in that it contains lymphocytes and protein exudate. The disease is rarely fatal, and no treatment is known to be effective. Corticosteroid and immunosuppressant therapy may be beneficial.[188]

Dermatologic Disorders Secondary to Diseases of the Nervous System

Trophic Changes in Skin due to Insensitivity

Decubitus Ulcerations   Here the disease of the nervous system obviously dominates the clinical picture, and the skin lesion represents essentially a complication of it. It would be a mistake to assume the nervous system disorder to be essential, for decubiti may develop in infirm, debilitated patients at any age. Usually some combination of immobility with prolonged pressure of skin against bony prominences must occur, but insensitivity to pain and hypotension are also important factors in the pathogenesis.

Syringomyelia   In this disease, in which cavitation of the cervical spinal cord forms during adult life, often in relation to congenital malformations of the cervical spine, skull, and cerebellum, two types of dermal abnormalities may be identified: (1) dysplasia of cutaneous and osseous structures of skull and neck; (2) trophic changes in skin and subcutaneous tissues of hands and arms. The former precedes the typical neurologic syndrome, which consists of segmental loss of pain and temperature sensation over shoulders and arms and also amyotrophy with loss of reflexes. In some cases there are skeletal abnormalities; these take the form of low hairline of scalp, short neck, asymmetric or otherwise misshapen face, and kyphoscoliosis. They indicate the existence of a congenital disturbance of cerebrocranial relationships. Less often, other structural abnormalities have been recorded, hypertrophy being the best known.

The patient may first become aware of the syringomyelic state when a burn or cut of the hand is sustained without causing pain. The odor of the burned flesh may attract attention before the patient notices that the object being grasped is scalding hot and has already seared or blistered the skin. Repeated injuries of this type may result in thickenings and callosities of skin, especially over the fingers and knuckles, and painless sores (formerly called whitlows). The nails may become deformed. Repeated injuries may cause the terminal phalanges to be absorbed or digits may drop off. More often, hands are merely edematous and swollen (*la main succulente*, of French writers), and the skin may be cold or warm, red or pale, and scaly. Many of these changes correspond to the syndrome of Morvan, in which an analgesic panaris with dermal changes of these types affects the upper extremities. The idea is now prevalent among neurologists that its basis is, in most instances, either syringomyelia or, more likely, a bibrachial sensory polyneuropathy. The resemblance to leprosy is so close that the latter must always be considered.

Tabes Dorsalis (Syphilitic Radiculitis)   This disease and also chronic polyneuropathies and congenital insensitivity to pain are other causes of painless ulcerations of skin.

Factitious Ulcers in Hysteria and Malingering

Before concluding this section on dermatologic disorders secondary to nervous system diseases, it is necessary to comment on the patient whose skin inexplicably breaks down repeatedly or persistently ulcerates in places where the circulation is ample. This may happen in the legs over the tibia in middle and late adult life consequent to stasis and a marginally reduced circulation, the latter being difficult to evaluate. But when it occurs over the volar surface of forearms or hands, especially in adolescent or adult women or after a compensable injury in either a man or a woman, it should always raise suspicion of self-inflicted injury. Usually a careful history will disclose other equally dubious past illnesses and operations—the classic form of hysteria. To make the problem more difficult, a physician who has already examined cutaneous sensation in the involved part of the body may have induced an anesthesia by suggestion, even though sensory loss is rarely found in naive hysterical individuals when first seen. Characteristically the patient states rather blandly that upon awakening he or she finds an area of redness and swelling of the skin and that an ulcer forms later. All signs of injection of a corrosive chemical or of picking at the skin with a sharp object may be obscured by the time of examination, and questions as to whether such an injury was accidentally or deliberately inflicted are denied vehemently.

The diagnosis can be difficult and depends on the establishment of a hysterical pattern of behavior with multiple bizarre illnesses in the past and the finding of a lesion in an accessible part of the body that looks as though it had been produced by the fingernail or some sharp instrument. If the physician is uncertain as to the nature of the lesion, the application of a large cast, so that the patient cannot reach the area in question, may show that healing proceeds normally.

Infections Spreading from Nervous System to Skin

Herpes Zoster   This is the classic example of a viral infection lying dormant in the nervous system and upon reactivation spreading to the skin along the branches of one or more peripheral nerves. The proof of this sequence of events is to be obtained from the clinical condition itself, where pain in one region of the body (nearly always unilateral) precedes by several days the appearance of groups of vesicles (with an erythematous base) in that region (see Chap. 204).

Primary Dermatologic Diseases Leading to Abnormalities of the Nervous System

Infections and Infestations

Tetanus   The wound that induces tetanus is nearly always located in the skin or subcutaneous tissues; only exceptionally has an operative site or an infection developing from the intestinal tract been the source. The inoculation of tetanus bacilli or their spores into abraded skin or beneath the skin by a puncture wound (rusty nail, infected hypodermic needle) seldom excites much inflammatory reaction. In fact, the skin lesion may appear so innocent as to be entirely forgotten by the patient and, even if remembered, it may appear to be quite trivial by the time the first symptoms of the nervous disorder develop—usually 5 to 15 days later. In such circumstances only the trained eye of the dermatologist may succeed in finding the primary site of dermal invasion. To locate it, however, is not without importance, for its excision and the neutralization of the residual bacilli it harbors by local injection of antitoxin is necessary if the source of toxin is to be eradicated.

The nervous disease, which consists of involuntary spasms of striated muscle, is entirely the result of the toxin elaborated by the organism.

Rabies   This disease is usually contracted from the bite of an infected carnivore (usually a dog), though scratches and abrasions and even the penetration of a mucous membrane by infected saliva from rabid animals may be the means of transmitting the viral infection. The disease is usually fatal. It can be prevented by human diploid vaccine.

Diphtheritic Wound Infections   Although diphtheritic infections seldom need to be considered in the Western world (since most children have been vaccinated against diphtheria), a chronic wound covered by a shaggy gray exudate should always be searched for Klebs-Loeffler (K-L) bacilli. Contamination of the skin lesion by these organisms may cause the ulcer and its surrounding skin to become insensitive to touch and pinprick. The adjacent muscles may become palsied. The ulcer more often occurs on the pharyngeal wall rather than the skin, though in one case seen by one of the authors it was on the buccal surface and was followed by numbness of the cheek and palsy of facial and pharyngeal muscles (Bell's palsy and dysphagia). Only after several weeks have passed (4 to 8) does a symmetric, diffuse sensorimotor polyneuropathy develop over a week or two. The protein level in the cerebrospinal fluid is elevated. Death is usually due to myocardiopathy. Treatment with intravenous penicillin or erythromycin for the infection and administration of equine diphtheria antitoxin offers some protection against the development of neuropathy (see Chap. 190).

Tick Bites (Chronic Atrophic Acrodermatitis) The bite of a certain tick (*Dermacentor andersoni*), especially in the area of the head and neck, may be followed within a few hours by rapid pulse, hyperpnea, and later, flaccid paralysis of the legs, trunk, and arms. The paralysis is believed to be due to a toxin, for removal of the tick results in recovery within a few hours. However, the tick bite may be followed by an erythematous rash, erythema chronicum migrans, which lasts for months and spreads.

Lyme Disease (See also Chap. 193) This is a multisystem disease caused by a tick-borne spirochete, *Borrelia burgdorferi,* which has three stages. In the first stage there is a characteristic skin lesion, erythema chronicum migrans, associated with headache, neck stiffness, and cerebrospinal fluid pleocytosis. The second stage may begin while the cutaneous lesion is still present or may occur months later after it has disappeared. This stage is characterized by more serious neurologic abnormalities: lymphocytic meningitis, encephalitis, myelitis, cranial neuritis, or Guillain-Barré polyneuritic syndrome. Other systemic findings in the second stage include carditis and cutaneous lesions, borrelial lymphocytoma. The third stage, which can begin months to even years later, is characterized by arthritis, a skin lesion (acrodermatitis chronica atrophicans), and progressive encephalomyelitis or latent central nervous system borreliosis, which may respond negligibly to long-term intravenous ceftriaxone. The earlier stages are successfully treated by oral and intravenous antibiotic therapy with more consistency.[189]

Herpes Simplex Herpes simplex virus, the cause of ubiquitous low-grade, recurrent lesions in the oral and genital regions, may be induced to flare up upon exposure of lips to wind and sun, trauma, and fever (particularly that accompanying certain infections such as meningococcus meningitis). Occasionally the virus passes along nerve fibers (perhaps olfactory) to reach the central nervous system, where it induces an encephalitis. Viremia is another and more likely mode of spread, especially in infants where lesions in lungs, liver, and other viscera indicate hematogenous dissemination (see Chap. 203).

Primary Neoplasms of the Skin

Cutaneous Melanomas The patient with a metastatic melanoma may present himself or herself at a medical or neurologic service with symptoms and signs of increased intracranial pressure or a focal cerebral lesion. Melanoma is one of the most frequent metastatic lesions in the brain (following lung, breast, and gastrointestinal tract in frequency), and should always be suspected in an adult with a brain tumor. Often the patient will have forgotten about the cutaneous melanoma that was removed years before, and only by inquiring about each dermal scar may the cause be ascertained. Examination of the urine for melanin by-products may confirm the diagnosis, but only if metastatic lesions in the liver are numerous[190] (see Chap. 82).

A Clinical Approach to Neurocutaneous Disease

From this lengthy survey one cannot but be impressed with the number and variety of neurocutaneous diseases. Indeed, it would seem that the nervous system is more often implicated in dermatologic disease than is any other organ in the human body. The reasons why this might be so were brought out in the discussion of pathogenic mechanisms.

It occurs to the authors that if this large compilation of data is to be useful, it must be systematized. For the novice as well as the seasoned clinician, only some type of reordering of these facts could make them immediately applicable to the common problems likely to be encountered in the clinic. This the authors have attempted to do in the following pages, considering in succession the clinical situations where a systematic knowledge of the dermatologic or neurologic aspects of these diseases might clarify the most frequently encountered medical problems.

An Infant Born with, or Developing in the First Weeks of Life, a Visible Abnormality of Skin

Here is a situation where accurate dermatologic diagnosis might serve in predicting whether the nervous system is, or will later prove to be, abnormal. One must keep in mind that clinical methods for assessing the immature nervous system at, or shortly after, birth are not wholly dependable. Since the human cerebrum is underdeveloped and functioning imperfectly, the neurologic examination perforce must be limited to the testing of muscular tone reflexes and the demonstration of certain segmental and postural automatisms, which serve only to establish the integrity of spinal cord and brainstem and peripheral sensorimotor structures. Warned through the dermatologic manifestations of an impending neurocutaneous disease, the clinician searches for evidence of a neurologic disorder more carefully.

Congenital Defects of Skin and Other Structures Of course the gross defects of spine and/or cerebrum, such as meningomyeloceles, meningoencephaloceles, or anencephalic states, which are always associated with some abnormality of the skin and subcutaneous structures, pose no diagnostic problem. It is the minor blemishes, i.e., malformations of skin and hair or subcutaneous cystlike structures, that give trouble. Many of these are of no significance and may disappear soon. Others, seemingly innocent, are of more dire significance. The observant mother who wants to know about every imperfection in her newborn infant may press for their removal. Excision without the guidance of x-ray has been a common mistake. If the defect is in the midline posteriorly, one must always consider the possibility of a small meningocele with a fistulous connection between the subcutaneous cyst and meninges. An x-ray will show the opening in the skull through which it connects with interior structures or a defect in the pedicles and spine of vertebrae. Later, such lesions may call attention to a cerebellar defect if occipital in location, or to a radicular or spinal cord abnormality of delayed onset if spinal in location. Since they may also serve as a pathway for the entrance of bacterial pathogens that give rise to brain abscess or recurrent meningitis, they should be sought in all children with intraspinal or intracranial suppuration.

Peculiarities of Skin in Conjunction with Malformations of Cranium, Eyes, Nose, Lips, Jaws, and Ears Malformations may take many forms, which deserve study and differentiation. One group in which the eyes, nose, and lips fail to form is so striking that the configuration at once reveals the nature of the associated brain anomaly, i.e., cyclopia, or arrhinencephaly. The low, beetling brow, heavy eyebrows that fuse in midline, the upturned nose, and small head betray the cerebral abnormality of de Lange's dwarf state with almost certain development of mental retardation. One group of these disorders is associated with a demonstrable chromosomal abnormality: in Down syndrome, the epicanthic folds are observable at birth and, if combined with large tongue, open mouth, round head, transverse palmar creases, displaced triradii (dermatoglyphic abnormality), short curved fifth fingers, etc., should seldom leave doubt as to diagnosis. It can be confirmed by chromosomal studies, which reveal 21 trisomy. Other somatic abnormalities point to the 13,15 and 17,18 trisomies; 4,5 deletion syndrome; mosaicism of 18; and other derangements. In these and all the other craniofacial anomalies, cerebral development tends also to be curtailed, and mental retardation can be predicted. Caution is advised in the interpretation of single abnormalities, such as epicanthic folds, for they may occur in individuals who later turn out to have normal intelligence. Table 184-2 summarizes some of the principal syndromes.

Vascular Malformations of Skin   Cutaneous hemangiomas are to be numbered among the most frequent of all somatic abnormalities. Most of the small midline hemangiomas bear no relationship to abnormalities of the nervous system, nor does the spreading nevus flammeus, which develops a few days or weeks after birth. Many of them disappear after a few months or years. Only the cranial hemangioma or truncal-brachial or crural ones are of important significance. Those of the ophthalmic-trigeminal area indicate the possibility of an ipsilateral meningeal angioma as seen in Sturge-Weber syndrome. Either focal or generalized seizures can develop, along with hemiparesis and glaucoma from an associated choroidal angioma. Incomplete forms of Sturge-Weber syndrome can occur in which eye and meningeal angiomas are present without the facial hemangioma, or a combination of only the face and eye hemangiomas without meningeal findings. A congenital brachial-cervical hemangioma with hypertrophy of the arm suggests the syndrome of Klippel-Trénaunay. It is further characterized by such vascular anomalies as lymphangiectasia, lymphedema, varicose veins, angiomas of the gut and bladder, and occasionally by limb malformations. A hemodynamically active arteriovenous malformation may be conjoined to the features of Klippel-Trénaunay-Weber syndrome. As to other neurologic disorders associated with vascular anomalies of skin, such as Osler's hemorrhagic telangiectasia syndrome with its characteristic multiple telangiectases and epistaxes, ataxia-telangiectasia, and Fabry disease, the dermal vascular lesions, as a rule, appear much later in life (late childhood or adolescence) and, in the case of ataxia-telangiectasia, long after the development of neurologic symptoms.

The Ichthyoses and Related Disorders   The group of ichthyotic states must not be confused with the simple scaling of the skin (so often seen in the postmature infant), the desquamation that follows an intrauterine rash (as in syphilis), or the dermal abnormalities of cretinism. Some of the xerodermic and ichthyotic states do not appear until weeks or months after birth. Nevertheless, they are usually noted earlier than the common variety of a hereditary ichthyosis vulgaris, the onset of which is 1 to 2 years of age. Unlike the latter they portend various neurologic abnormalities such as dwarfism, mental retardation, and a variety of generalized spastic, ataxic, and choreoathetotic states, listed under the eponyms of Rud's, Laubenthal's, Stewart's, and Sjögren-Larsson syndromes. Refsum's syndrome has also developed later in some patients with hereditary dryness of skin. The diseases listed in Table 184-4 should be considered in the differential diagnosis of ichthyotic idiocy.

Pigment Disorders of Skin   These conditions may herald the nevoid basal cell carcinoma syndrome in which there is increased risk of the development of basal cell cancers, which rarely undergo malignant transformation. There is an increased incidence of mental retardation and increased incidence of medulloblastoma. Large hyperpigmented nevi present at birth can be associated with neuromelanosis, in which the cutaneous lesions remain benign but are associated with infiltration of meninges and central nervous system with micromelanocytes that have malignant potential. Neurologic complications include intellectual deterioration, seizures, and progressive hydrocephalus. Scattered hyperpigmentation of the skin may result from chronic inflammatory states, such as incontinentia pigmenti, and occurs also in congenital melanoderma and neurofibromatosis, type I. Impairment of pigmentation may be observed in some patients with phenylketonuria. Hypomelanotic nevi may also appear in the first weeks of life and should warn the pediatrician of tuberous sclerosis, a diagnosis which may be confirmed early by the concatenation of other abnormalities (see Table 184-5).

Laxity of Skin   This too may be detected early, and a number of disorders present with the loose neck skin in infancy. It is seen commonly in Turner's syndrome (45,XO) and Noonan's syndrome (Turner-like syndrome with normal karyotype). In both the Turner and Noonan syndromes there may be mild mental retardation without other neurologic abnormality. In Ehlers-Danlos syndrome (cutis elastica syndrome), of which there are at least ten different types, hyperextensible skin can be noted early but is not appreciated until the child starts to crawl and walk. Some delay in walking can occur because of hypermobility of joints. Cutis verticis gyrata, in which the redundant skin is limited to the scalp, forewarns of mental retardation.

Excessive Hairiness of Skin   Many congenital nevi are tufted with a growth of hair, and in lumbosacral dysraphism a tuft of hair may cover an underlying neural abnormality. Early hirsutism of face and trunk could suggest a number of disorders such as Cornelia de Lange's syndrome, mucopolysaccharidoses (MPS 1, MPS I-S, MPS I-H/S, and MPS II), gangliosidosis type I, leprechaunism, trisomy 18 syndrome, Berardinelli's lipodystrophy, and Coffin-Siris syndrome. Some of the other mucopolysaccharidoses are associated with hirsutism of lesser degree and later onset. The most typical hair changes in neurologic disorders are listed in Table 184-6.

Abnormalities of Sweating, Lacrimation, Salivation, etc.   These are common to all the extensive hypoplastic or dysplastic congenital diseases of the skin. Anhidrotic ectodermal dysplasia, Fabry's disease, and incontinentia pigmenti are examples. If the skin is otherwise normal, the most likely possibility in the child is the Riley-Day dysautonomia syndrome or one of several familial or acquired polyneuropathies, including one type of congenital analgesia. The majority of the children will later be shown to have abnormalities of the peripheral nervous system, and not a few will prove to be mentally backward. In the adult, diseases of the peripheral nervous system (Shy-Drager syndrome), diabetic polyneuropathy, or one of the other familial polyneuropathies may produce a similar syndrome by affecting fibers of the autonomic nervous system.

Table 184-7 contains a listing of principal anhidrotic syndromes and their differential characteristics.

TABLE 184-5

Differential Diagnosis of Pigmentary Changes of Skin with Neurologic Disorders

	Skin criteria	Neurologic disorders
Tuberous sclerosis	Hypomelanotic patches, adenoma sebaceum, subungual fibromas, shagreen patches	Epilepsy, mental retardation
Neurofibromatosis, type I	Café au lait patches, cutaneous neurofibromas, Lisch nodules	Cranial nerve, spinal cord, spinal roots, peripheral nerve involvement
Ataxia-telangiectasia	Telangiectasia of conjunctiva, ears, neck; hypo- and hyperpigmentation	Ataxia, myoclonus, choreoathetosis, slowed voluntary eye movements, dysarthria
Chédiak-Higashi disease	Oculocutaneous hypomelanosis, hyperhidrosis, atrophic skin	Peripheral neuropathy, ataxia, seizures, behavioral abnormalities
Waardenburg-Klein syndrome	White forelock, heterochromic iridum, white eyelashes, leukoderma	Deafness, cerebellar ataxia, mental retardation
Vogt-Koyanagi-Harada syndrome	Hypomelanotic macules, poliosis	Signs of lymphocytic meningitis
Vitiligo, achalasia, congenital deafness	Vitiligo	Neuropathic muscle wasting, congenital sensorineural deafness
LEOPARD syndrome	Multiple lentigines	Sensorineural deafness
Piebald trait	Piebaldness (white forelock), hypomelanotic patches	Sensorineural deafness, ataxia, mental retardation
Neurocutaneous melanosis	Multiple nevi, giant hairy nevi in swimming trunk distribution	Macrocephaly, hydrocephalus, intellectual deterioration, seizures
Nevoid basal cell carcinoma syndrome	Basal cell carcinoma, palmar/plantar pits	Medulloblastoma, mental retardation
Phenylketonuria	Pigment dilution, eczema, scleroderma-like lesions	Seizures, mental retardation
Adrenoleukodystrophy	Bronzing	Signs secondary to leukodystrophy, dementia, optic atrophy in childhood and adolescent onset; sex-linked recessive

TABLE 184-6

Hair Changes with Neurologic Disorder

Argininosuccinic aciduria	Fragile hair, trichorrhexis nodosa
Homocystinuria	Fragile, lighter than normal siblings
Methioninuria or methionine absorption syndrome	White hair, fragile hair
Phenylketonuria	Blond hair, or usually lighter hair than in normal siblings
Bjornstad's syndrome of deafness	Pili torti
Kinky hair syndrome	Pili torti, easily broken hair
Ectodermal dysplasias: Anhidrotic Hidrotic	Sparsity and fragility of hair, lighter than in normal siblings
Lipodystrophic diabetes	Kinky hair, hirsutism
Phenytoin ingestion	Hirsutism
Gargoylism (Hunter-Hurler syndrome)	Hirsutism
	Body hair, bushy eyebrows
Cornelia de Lange's syndrome	Hirsutism, bushy eyebrows
Thallium poisoning	Total loss of hair

Light Sensitivity with or without Bulla Formation This phenomenon ordinarily does not become manifest until months have passed, as small babies are usually protected from sunlight. When present, this should always suggest one of the following diseases: xeroderma pigmentosum, Cockayne's syndrome, Chédiak-Higashi syndrome, ataxia-telangiectasia, Hartnup disease, pellagra, tryptophanuria, porphyria, Rothman-Thomson syndrome, and erythropoietic protoporphyria. In some cases the reaction to drugs such as phenothiazine or carbemazepine may produce sunlight sensitivity that needs to be distinguished from the underlying neurocutaneous syndrome.

Miscellaneous Disorders The disorders listed earlier as focal dermal hypoplasia, incontinentia pigmenti, epidermolysis bullosa, congenital melanoderma, congenital poikiloderma, basal cell nevus syndrome, orofaciodigital syndrome, and anhidrotic ectodermal dysplasia become manifest early in life and must be distinguished one from another, for they each have slightly different neurologic implications. In focal dermal hypoplasia (Goltz's syndrome), anomalies of other organs and nervous system (syndactyly, spina bifida, microcephaly, coloboma, etc.) are frequently conjoined. However, the impairment of brain development may not declare itself until later, by lesions of the nervous system that are of the acquired type also leading to microcephaly and mental retardation.

TABLE 184-7
Sensory Syndromes with Anhidrosis and Often Analgesia

	Congenital sensory neuropathy	Hereditary radicular neuropathy (HSAN-I, II) normal	Congenital indifference to pain	Syringomyelia, syringobulbia	Familial dysautonomia (HSAN-III)	Diabetic multiple neuropathy
Intelligence	Normal	Normal	Normal, mild retardation	Normal	Normal	Normal
Heredity	Recessive, dominant	Recessive, dominant	Recessive, dominant	Sporadic, dominant	Recessive	Sporadic, dominant recessive
Age of onset	Birth	Childhood	Birth	Adulthood	Birth	Associated with length of diabetes
Distribution of sensory loss	Universal	Distal extremities, mainly legs	Universal	Cervical	Spares hands, soles, neck, genital areas	Distal extremities, legs, arms
Pain and temperature perception	Absent	Absent	Absent	Absent	Absent	Reduced
Touch	Present or diminished	Absent	Normal	Normal	Normal	Reduced
Axon reflex	None	None	Present	Present	None	Reduced
Tendon reflexes	Normal or diminished	Diminished or absent	Normal	Diminished, or reduced in affected segments, with increased reflexes in lower extremities	Diminished	Diminished or absent
Motor function	Normal, delayed	Normal, diminished	Normal	Normal or reduced	Diminished	Diminished
Lesion	Small myelinated fibers reduced or absent	Loss of dorsal root ganglion cells	Normal	Nerve biopsy normal	Myelinated axons are spared, and unmyelinated axons are depleted. Marked reduction of sensory neurons, sympathetic ganglia	Segmental demyelination, loss of myelinated and unmyelinated fibers

In the closely related syndromes of incontinentia pigmenti, epidermolysis bullosa, and congenital poikiloderma, the microcephaly, mental retardation, epilepsy, and spastic paralysis of the legs may also be delayed in their appearance, but awareness of skin lesions will have alerted the pediatrician to these possibilities.

Some of the congenital neurocutaneous diseases result in a premature aging of the skin and tumor formation. These are listed in Table 184-8. In the experience of one of the authors the most difficult problem in the diagnosis of these diffuse skin lesions, some of which have vesicular, bullous, or erythematous features, has been to differentiate them from the skin lesions of congenital

TABLE 184-8
Neurologic Disorders Resulting in Premature Aging of the Skin and Hair

Ataxia-telangiectasia	Rothmund-Thomson syndrome
Xeroderma pigmentosum	Berardinelli's syndrome
Werner's syndrome	De Barsey's syndrome
Hallerman-Streiff syndrome	Neonatal progeroid syndrome
Cockayne's syndrome	Down's syndrome
Bloom's syndrome	

SOURCE: Modified from Wiedemann H: Progeria, in *Neurocutaneous Diseases. A Practical Approach,* edited by MR Gomez. Boston, Butterworths, 1987, p 250.

syphilis, rubella, cytomegalic inclusion disease, herpes simplex, and HIV-associated infections. In the latter, the affection of the nervous system is almost always accompanied by signs of disease of the liver (hepatomegaly and jaundice) and other organs, and the cerebrospinal fluid contains cells, increased protein, and sometimes the infective agent. Later, during early infancy, these congenital skin lesions must be distinguished from eczematous dermatitis.

A Child or Adult with a Disorder of the Nervous System in Which Dermatologic Study May Clarify Diagnosis

An Infant or Child, Previously Regarded as Normal, in Whom Seizures Have Developed (Massive Flexion Spasms in Infancy, Grand Mal in Childhood) As has been pointed out, during the first 2 years of life the onset of flexion, or salaam, spasms may be due to a variety of pathologic processes, some identifiable during life, others only at autopsy. In this respect this type of epilepsy differs in no important way from that which begins at a more advanced age; it merely signifies a cerebral pathologic condition of an immature nervous system without indicating the specific causative disease. Here, finding three or more white macules over the trunk or limbs or focal hypomelanosis of eyelashes is highly suggestive of tuberous sclerosis, a diagnosis which, if once considered, may then be confirmed by x-rays of the skull, CT scans, studies of the heart, kidneys, etc., even at this early age. Here the Wood's lamp is indispensable. (Occasionally such a lesion may presage ataxia-telangiectasia. Vitiligo and nevus anemicus must be distinguished.) Multiple café au lait spots will suggest neurofibromatosis. Here the point also to be noted is that pigmented patches in the skin may precede any recognizable neurologic disorder and should forewarn the dermatologist that an observed seizure or a slight backwardness may be the first and only neurologic expression of these diseases, easily missed if not sought.

Psychomotor retardation or seizures without other neurologic abnormality should suggest the possibility of an underlying phenylketonuria, histidinuria, or homocystinuria. Since all these diseases interfere to some degree with tyrosinase activity, any change in pigmentation of skin or hair must be accorded special notice. Also, the presence of a stubborn eczematous dermatitis, a notable accompaniment of some cases of phenylketonuria in infancy or childhood, should raise suspicion. Epilepsy and sensitivity to sunlight suggest the possibility of Hartnup disease.

Later in life, generalized seizures, especially when accompanied by retarded mental development, should prompt a careful search for the other skin manifestations of tuberous sclerosis as well as a variety of other metabolic derangements, such as argininosuccinic aminoaciduria, Hartnup disease, or phenylketonuria, any one of which may cause seizures.

A Child Brought to the Clinic with Retarded Psychomotor Development This, one of the most frequent of all problems in the pediatric age group, has again multiple causation, the most common being developmental faults, obstetric accidents, and a wide variety of acquired infective, traumatic, and metabolic states. Once again the dermatologist must keep in mind the portent of the group of idiopathic, vesicular, ulcerating, and fibrosing skin lesions arising in early life and leading to scaling, pigmentation, atrophy, and keratosis of the skin, and of the xerodermic, ichthyotic lesions and giant pigmented nevi. Down syndrome and the other trisomic chromosomal abnormalities form another large group (some 10 percent of patients admitted to institutions for the feebleminded) in which dermatologic clues have singular prominence. Epicanthic folds, abnormal palmar markings, and fingerprint patterns stand as the identifiable characteristics of Down syndrome. Other abnormalities of the cranium, nose, eyes, jaw, and palate should indicate the possibility of one of the other chromosomal abnormalities or of cerebral developmental anomalies without chromosomal defect (arrhinencephalia, cyclops abnormality, etc.).

The metabolic disorders constitute another small but important group of diseases, several of which can be suspected by examination of skin and hair. In cretinism the skin is cool and dry, and the hair is sparse and coarse. An erythematous scaling rash on exposed surfaces should suggest ichthyosiform erythroedema in the neonate, and later, if persistent and recurrent, Hartnup disease, hydroxykynurenuria, Cockayne's disease, or pellagra. Sensitivity to sunlight is a prominent feature of these diseases, but this trait also occurs in some cases of phenylketonuria, lipid proteinosis, and variegate porphyria. Pale papules or nodules of skin are also seen in tuberous sclerosis, as well as in Hunter's mucopolysaccharidosis, lipoid proteinosis, Farber's disease, mannosidosis, fucosidosis, and mucolipidosis.

An aspect of dermatology, recently brought to medical attention, is the use of skin biopsy in the diagnosis of hereditary metabolic diseases of the nervous system. In an easily accessible specimen of skin, prepared for electron microscopic study, one may discover subcellular particles characteristic of a disease whose only or principal manifestations are neurologic. Martin et al.[191,192] have reported their successes in the diagnosis of the following diseases: infantile and tardive forms of ceroid lipofuscinosis, mucopolysaccharidosis (Hurler, Sanfilippo A), mucolipidosis (I cell disease), acid maltase deficiency (Pompe's disease), infantile metachromatic leukodystrophy, mucolipidosis IV, infantile neuroaxonal dystrophy, galactosialidosis, and Lafora's disease.

The examination of hair, a relatively neglected part of dermatologic study, may give important leads, for a number of important metabolic neurocutaneous diseases express themselves through this appendage of skin. There may be abnormalities in growth of hair. Hirsutism is a feature of lipodystrophic diabetes, Marshall-Smith syndrome (long cranium, shallow orbits, tapered fingers, and respiratory difficulty), mucopolysaccharidoses, trisomy 18 syndrome, and the de Lange dwarf syndrome. A beaked nose, anti-mongoloid slant of eyes, and small head open the possibility of the Rubenstein-Taybi syndrome. Sparse, coarse hair is found in hypothyroidism and in anhydrotic ectodermal dysplasia. Dilution of hair color favors the diagnosis of phenylketonuria, histidinuria, and homocystinuria; the virtual absence of pigmentation favors albinism.

A white forelock should alert the clinician to the possibility of Waardenburg-Klein syndrome (with associated deafness), but it is sometimes a solitary abnormality. Depigmentation around the eyes and tufts of hair raise the question of tuberous sclerosis or Chédiak-Higashi disease, and in later life it suggests Vogt-Koyanagi-Harada disease. In argininosuccinic aminoaciduria a vertical splitting occurs between nodosities of the hair shaft (trichorrhexis nodosa); in the kinky hair syndrome the shaft is also of uneven caliber and twisted; and in monilethrix it is flattened and twisted. A hand lens permits distinctions to be drawn among these three abnormalities of hair.

Dwarfism with Mental Retardation and Other Slowly Evolving Major Neurologic Abnormalities such as Athetosis, Dystonia, Ataxia, and Spastic Diplegia Here the neurologic disorder tends to dominate the clinical picture. The child is obviously stunted, and both head circumference and body weight are down to the first percentile or below. Failure to attain the usual milestones of development in motor control, locomotion, speech, and perception can be noted even on cursory examination. Stiffness and hyperreflexia or, in the older child, tremor, ataxia, or rigidity and athetosis point to extensive involvement of motor cortices, basal ganglia, or cerebellum. Oddly enough, patients with such florid neurologic abnormalities are seldom found to have chromosomal abnormalities or biochemical disturbances. Developmental fault, a cerebral dysgenesis, or destruction of the cerebral hemispheres by hypoxia, kernicterus, or an antenatal or natal infection are the more frequent associated disease states and they seldom have dermatologic accompaniments. When there is a skin anomaly, it most often takes the form of ichthyosis or poikiloderma, which should not be difficult to recognize.

Dwarfism should raise suspicion of ataxia-telangiectasia, Lesch-Nyhan syndrome, Mast syndrome, Cockayne's syndrome, xerodermic idiocy, generalized lentigines, and poikiloderma congenitale. Of these diseases, poikilodermatous changes in the skin (hyper- and hypopigmentation with atrophy and telangiectasia) are the most common.

Familial hyperuricemia, the syndrome of Cross et al.[157] of mental deficiency, spasticity, athetosis and hypopigmentation of the skin, Hallervorden-Spatz progressive athetosis or dystonia, and Wilson's disease must also be included in the differential diagnosis. Self-mutilation suggests familial hyperuricemia (Lesch-Nyhan syndrome), whereas hypermelanosis may indicate some of the other diseases.

A Child or Adult with Cerebellar Ataxia Episodic ataxia, incoordination of limbs, and unsteadiness of gait, lasting usually for a few days after the occurrence of one or more convulsions, represents one of the more puzzling syndromes in pediatric neurology. Its differentiation taxes clinical acumen. In the very young child any convulsive illness that confines the patient to bed for days or weeks results in weakness and unsteadiness, which may be difficult to distinguish from true cerebellar ataxia. Close inspection of the limbs will show none of the usual features of cerebellar ataxia, i.e., dysmetria, lack of synergism of component muscle groups involved in skilled acts, hypotonia, or intention tremor.

Sensory ataxia can be excluded by lack of sensory deficit (particularly vibratory and position senses) and retention of tendon reflexes, which are nearly always abolished in diseases of the peripheral nervous system. Also finger ataxia (pseudoathetosis of outstretched fingers with eyes closed) and positive Romberg's sign are present. Ataxia from an overdose of phenytoin or phenobarbital given for control of the seizures, often accompanied by a pruritic macular and papular eruption, may also produce an episodic ataxia of cerebellar type. This diagnosis can be confirmed by measuring the blood levels of these drugs and observing the recession of the ataxia as the dose is reduced. Recurrent episodic ataxia should always raise suspicion of Hartnup disease or hydroxykynurenuria and other of the hyperammonemias (e.g., argininosuccinic aminoaciduria and citrullinemia). Here the dermatologic findings of skin erythema and blistering on exposure to sunlight and infrared rays are helpful to the neurologist, for they indicate Hartnup syndrome or hydroxykynurenuria. Blond coloration of hair, not concordant with race and parentage, and brittleness of hair point to argininosuccinic aminoaciduria. Urine analyses for these amino acids will confirm the clinical impression. A single attack of an acute cerebellar ataxia appearing in the wake of an infectious exanthematous disease such

as chickenpox, vaccinia, or measles is most compatible with postinfectious encephalomyelitis.

The gradual development of a persistent ataxia of cerebellar type, appearing in the first few years of life, should alert the clinician to ataxia-telangiectasia. As mentioned previously, oculomotor apraxia and a movement disorder like choreoathetosis are other components of the syndrome. The characteristic tracery of small vessels over conjunctivae, ears, neck, etc., provides the obvious clue to diagnosis. This skin change may not appear for some years, but an expectant attitude facilitates its early recognition. Tremulous ataxia combined with xeroderma, small stature, and mental retardation, sometimes with athetotic movements of the fingers, comprise the Laubenthal syndrome of xerodermic idiocy. Cerebellar ataxia with tendon xanthomatoses occurs in the van Bogaert-Epstein-Scherer form of cholesterinosis. Cerebellar ataxia with dwarfism, mental deficiency, partial deafness, and retinitis pigmentosa comprise Cockayne's syndrome.

In Cockayne's syndrome (dwarfism with kyphosis and ankylosis, mental deficiency, deafness, and retinitis pigmentosa) a cerebellar ataxia may appear early in the illness. Suspicion should be raised by the finding of a dermatitis in the "butterfly" area of the face (suggestive of lupus erythematosus). Lipodystrophy of the face is another frequent finding. The onset is at about 2 years of age, and the disease is slowly progressive, ending in blindness, deafness, idiocy, and paralysis.

Cerebellar ataxia in combination with symptoms of intracranial tumor (headaches, papilledema, vomiting) developing in childhood may, rarely, be clarified by the finding of a basal cell nevus. Additional clues are provided by the presence of hypertelorism, other skeletal anomalies, and cysts of the jaw. The cerebellar tumor usually proves to be a medulloblastoma. Giant pigmented nevi may produce a similar syndrome by metastasis of melanotic melanoma to the cerebellum or by a basal meningeal melanomatosis with hydrocephalus and a cerebral type of ataxia. In the adolescent or young adult, a cerebellar tumor, especially if familial and with coincident polycythemia, should lead to a search for von Hippel's retinal angioma. Such findings corroborate the clinical impression of Lindau's cerebellar hemangioblastoma. Ataxia is also present in some cases of cretinism, manifested early in life by excessive livedo reticularis and later by dry, cool, lax, coarse skin and thick, sparse hair.

Progressive ataxia during childhood, adolescence, or adult life with areflexia of the limbs and other signs of peripheral nerve disease receives clarification by the finding of dryness and scaling of the skin, a combination typical of Refsum's heredopathia atactica polyneuritiformis. The presence of xanthomas of the skin suggests at once the diagnosis of congenital lipodystrophic diabetes, Tangier disease, and Urbach-Wiethe lipid proteinosis.

A Child or Adult with Spastic Paraparesis Spastic weakness of the legs, out of proportion to affection of arms or cranial and trunk musculature, often presents as a relatively discrete syndrome. It may be combined with mental retardation. In its nonprogressive form the reader will recognize its identity with cerebral palsy or cerebral spastic diplegia. Not infrequently the condition becomes manifest toward the end of the first year of life, remaining thereafter rather stable. Presumably, development to the stage of standing and stepping have exposed a preexistent congenital defect.

The finding of congenital ichthyosis in conjunction with mental retardation and spastic paraparesis establishes, in most instances, the diagnosis of Sjögren-Larsson syndrome. In a case of one of the authors, however, autopsy disclosed a "globoid body" form of leukodystrophy (a hereditary disease of the cerebral white matter developing in the early years of life). Spastic weakness of the legs has been associated in some instances with homocystinuria.

Spastic paraparesis presenting in childhood or adolescence, if combined with cutaneous hypopigmentation (albinism) and multiple ocular anomalies, conforms to the Mast syndrome described by Cross et al.[157]

Chronic pigmentation of the skin with adrenal insufficiency and spastic weakness as well as other signs of progressive leukodystrophy (dementia, blindness, etc.) in boys and male adults are indicative of adrenoleukodystrophy.

An Infant, Child, or Adult with an Acute Illness Consisting of Disorder of Cerebral Function or Meningeal Irritation in Association with a Rash This clinical problem, a frequent source of perplexity to the medical staff of every large hospital, requires consideration of a variety of disease states. For one thing, there are a number of idiosyncratic reactions to a drug such as phenytoin or phenobarbital, where a pruritic macular and papular eruption on the trunk and limbs may be combined with drowsiness, confusion, ataxia, or coma (the effects produced by the direct action of the drug on the nervous system). The macular and papular rash with a lymphocytic ("aseptic") meningitis may provide the clue to one of the coxsackie- or echovirus infections and, in certain parts of the world, to a rickettsial disease.

A fading macular and papular or a vesicular eruption may be the residue of rubeola, rubella, or varicella infection that has been complicated by a postinfectious encephalomyelitis. Here history of exposure during an epidemic, details of the clinical state, and the lymphocytic pleocytosis of the cerebrospinal fluid are the main diagnostic features. The hemorrhagic rash of meningococcemia aids in the recognition or anticipation of meningococcus meningitis, and the salmon-colored mottling of the limbs, of the Waterhouse-Friderichsen syndrome.

Specific Sensory Defects in which the Diagnosis Is Aided by Dermatologic Study

Deafness One of the first responsibilities of the pediatrician or pediatric neurologist in examining a child whose psychomotor development appears to be lagging is to make sure that the whole trouble is not a lack of hearing. It is obvious enough that the auditory and visual senses are the main avenues for receiving information about the world and also that early speech development is dependent upon hearing. Deaf children show disinterest in sounds and music, do not babble in an elaborate way or imitate their mothers, and do not acquire words. They may develop their own language (idioglossia), but usually grow up as deaf-mutes.

The dermatologist may be helpful in the diagnosis of such cases. Congenital deafness, which may be either of two types, conductive or neural, may be associated with a number of disorders of keratinization and pigmentation of skin and of craniofacial development. In the Waardenburg-Klein syndrome, attention will be called to the condition by the lateral displacement of the inner canthi, hypertrichosis of the eyebrows, heterochromia of irides, and white forelock. Also, the retinal pigment of the affected eye is decreased. Albinism and deafness constitute another syndrome, the inheritance tending to follow an autosomal recessive or sex-linked

pattern. Some deaf children are piebald (autosomal dominant). In some patients with sensory nerve deafness there is pili torti, onychodystrophic nerve deafness, keratosis palmaris et plantaris, acanthosis nigricans, and ainhum. Pili torti, in which hair grows in a twisted configuration, and a cochlear type of deafness are part of Bjornstad's syndrome.

Neural deafness constitutes an element also in Refsum's syndrome, Fabry disease, Cockayne's syndrome, xeroderma pigmentosum, Laurence-Moon syndrome, Werner's syndrome, and Hunter-Hurler syndrome. Also, the conduction type of deafness appears conjoined with a number of craniofacial deformities such as the mandibulofacial dysostosis (Treacher-Collins syndrome); maldevelopment of ears (only ear pits appearing); Hallerman-Streiff, Cornelia de Lange's, and Turner's syndromes; and E trisomy, dysacousia, and deafness of nerve type may also complicate the Vogt-Koyanagi-Harada syndrome and congenital syphilis.

Blindness Obvious visual defects occasioned by microphthalmia, coloboma, retrolental fibrodysplasia, and chorioretinitis are usually unattended by dermatologic abnormalities. Ophthalmic diagnosis in other very young patients proves most difficult. There may be uncertainty as to whether disinclination to follow moving objects, a failure to peer at the mother's face, or failure to recognize her represents an inadequacy of the peripheral visual mechanism or a cerebral disease (cortical blindness). As the months pass, however, repeated examinations usually leave little doubt as to the existence of visual impairment. In these cases a clue as to an oncoming gargoylism, the osseous features of which become evident in the second and third years, may be a mistiness or cloudiness of cornea or hirsutism and an "orange-peel" quality of the skin. Similarly Refsum's syndrome and the Laurence-Moon syndrome may be suspected by the expert dermatologist before the retinal pigmentation is certain. Optic atrophy as a cause of blindness will at once be recognized as the Stewart syndrome if a congenital ichthyosis is noted. Blindness from glaucoma receives clarification when there is recognition of a craniofacial hemangioma—Sturge-Weber-Dimitri syndrome. Also, a certain number of cases of glioma of the optic nerve and chiasm will become obvious once the dermatologist confirms the presence of the skin lesions of neurofibromatosis.

References

1. Brown JW, Podosin R: A syndrome of the neural crest. *Arch Neurol* **15**:294, 1966
2. Sidman RS, Fawcett D: Effect of peripheral nerve section on brown fat. *Anat Rec* **118**:487, 1954
3. Schwartzman RJ, McLellan TL: Reflex sympathetic dystrophy. *Arch Neurol* **44**:555, 1987
4. Van der Hoeve I: Eye symptoms of tuberous sclerosis of the brain. *Trans Ophthalmol Soc UK* **40**:329, 1920
5. Gomez MR (ed): *Tuberous Sclerosis,* 2d ed. New York, Raven, 1988, p 14
6. Reed WB et al: Internal manifestations of tuberous sclerosis. *Arch Dermatol* **87**:715, 1963
7. Nickel WR, Reed WB: Tuberous sclerosis. *Arch Dermatol* **85**:209, 1962
8. Hunt A, Lindenbaum RH: Tuberous sclerosis: A new estimate of prevalence within the Oxford region. *J Med Genet* **23**:272, 1984
9. Sampson JR et al: Genetic aspects of tuberous sclerosis in the west of Scotland. *J Med Genet* **26**:28, 1989

10. Wiederholt WC et al: Incidence and prevalence of tuberous sclerosis in Rochester, Minnesota, 1950 through 1982. *Neurology* **35**:600, 1985

11. Zaremba J: Tuberous sclerosis: A clinical and genetical investigation. *J Ment Defic Res* **12**:63, 1968

12. Lagos JE, Gomez MR: Tuberous sclerosis: Reappraisal of a clinical entity. *Mayo Clin Proc* **42**:26, 1967

13. Moolton SE: Hamartial nature of the tuberous sclerosis complex and its bearing on the tumor problem. *Arch Intern Med* **69**:589, 1942

14. Caviness VS: Epilogue and unsolved questions, in *Tuberous Sclerosis,* 2d ed, edited by MR Gomez. New York, Raven, 1988, p 251

15. Haines JL et al: Genetic heterogeneity in tuberous sclerosis, study of a large collaborative dataset. *NY Acad Sci* **615**:256, 1991

16. Caron P: *Contribution à l'étude clinique de la sclérose tubéreuse,* thesis. Paris, 1939

17. Van Bogaert L et al: Étude sur la sclérose tubéreuse de Bourneville à forme cérébelleuse. *Rev Neurol (Paris)* **98**:673, 1958

18. Busch KT, Busch G: Neuro-opthalmologische Befunde bei der tuberösen Sklerose. *Klin Monatsch Augenheilkd* **141**:388, 1962

19. Donegani G et al: Contribution à l'étude de la maladie de Bourneville. *Bull Int Serv Sante Arm* **1**:359, 1963

20. Fitzpatrick TB et al: White leaf-shaped macules, earliest visible sign of tuberous sclerosis. *Arch Dermatol* **98**:1, 1968

21. Gold AP, Freeman JM: Depigmented nevi, the earliest sign of tuberous sclerosis. *Pediatrics* **35**:1003, 1965

22. Butterworth T, Wilson M Jr: Dermatologic aspects of tuberous sclerosis. *Arch Dermatol Syphilol* **43**:1, 1941

23. Gomez MR: Neurologic and psychiatric features, in *Tuberous Sclerosis,* 2d ed, edited by MR Gomez. New York, Raven, 1988, p 9

24. Trombley IK, Mirra SS: Ultrastructure of tuberous sclerosis: Cortical tuber and subependymal tumor. *Ann Neurol* **9**:174, 1981

25. Bellack GS, Shapshay SM: Management of facial angiofibromas in tuberous sclerosis: Use of the carbon dioxide laser. *Otolaryngol Head Neck Surg* **94**:37, 1986

26. Crowe FT et al: *A Clinical, Pathological and Genetic Study of Multiple Neurofibromatoses.* Springfield, IL, Charles C Thomas, 1956

27. Canale D, Bebin J: von Recklinghausen's neurofibromatosis, in *Handbook of Clinical Neurology,* edited by PJ Vinken, GW Bruyn. Amsterdam, North-Holland, 1972, p 132

28. Riccardi VM, Mulvihill JJ (eds): *Neurofibromatosis.* New York, Raven, 1981

29. Riccardi V, Eichner J: *Neurofibromatosis: Phenotype, Natural History, and Pathogenesis.* Baltimore, Johns Hopkins Univ Press, 1986

30. Rubenstein AE, Korf BR (eds): *Neurofibromatosis.* New York, Thieme, 1990

31. Wishart JH: Case of tumors in the skull, dura mater, and brain. *Edinburgh Med Surg J* **18**:393, 1822

32. Seizinger RR et al: Genetic linkage of von Recklinghausen neurofibromatosis to the nerve growth factor receptor gene. *Cell* **49**:589, 1987

33. Rouleau GA et al: Genetic linkage of bilateral acoustic neurofibromatosis to a DNA marker on chromosome 22. *Nature* **329**:246, 1987

34. Viskochil D et al: Deletions and a translocation interrupt a cloned gene at the neurofibromatosis type 1 locus. *Cell* **62**:187, 1990

35. Cawthon RM et al: A major segment of the neurofibromatosis type 1 gene: cDNA sequence, genomic structure, and point mutations. *Cell* **62**:193, 1990

36. Littler M, Morton NE: Segregation analysis of peripheral neurofibromatosis (NF1). *J Med Genet* **27**:307, 1990

37. Constantino PD et al: Neurofibromatosis type II of the head and neck. *Arch Otolaryngol Head Neck Surg* **115**:380, 1989

38. Ballester R et al: The NF1 locus encodes a protein functionally related to mammalian GAP and yeast IRA proteins. *Cell* **63**:851, 1990

39. Rouleau GA et al: Flanking markers bracket the neurofibromatosis type 2 (NF2) gene on chromosome 22. *Am J Hum Genet* **46**:323, 1990

40. Obringer AC et al: The child with neurofibromatosis, in *Neurofibro-*

matosis, edited by AE Rubenstein, BR Korf. New York, Thieme, 1990, p 150

41. Huson SM et al: A genetic study of von Recklinghausen neurofibromatosis in south east Wales. II. Guidelines for genetic counseling. *J Med Genet* **26**:712, 1989

42. Duffner PK et al: The significance of MRI abnormalities in children with neurofibromatosis. *Neurology* **39**:373, 1989

43. Rosman NP, Pearce J: The brain in neurofibromatosis. *Brain* **90**:829, 1967

44. Martuza R, Eldridge R: Neurofibromatosis 2 (bilateral acoustic neurofibromatosis). *N Engl J Med* **318**:684, 1988

45. Konrad K et al: The giant melanosome: A model of deranged melanosome morphogenesis. *J Ultrastr Res* **48**:102, 1974

46. Nakagawa H et al: The nature and origin of the melanin macroglobule. *J Invest Dermatol* **83**:134, 1984

47. Martuza RL et al: Melanin macroglobules as a cellular marker of neurofibromatosis: A quantitative study. *J Invest Dermatol* **85**:347, 1985

48. Meinecke P: Evidence that the "neurofibromatosis-Noonan syndrome" is a variant of von Recklinghausen neurofibromatosis. *Am J Med Genet* **26**:741, 1987

49. Cohen MM Jr: Further diagnostic thoughts about the Elephant Man. *Am J Med Genet* **29**:777, 1988

50. Hotamisligil GS: Proteus syndrome and hamartoses with overgrowth. *Dysmorph Clin Genet* **4**:87, 1990

51. Bebin EM, Gomez MR: The intelligence and social achievement of patients with unilateral and bihemispheric Sturge-Weber syndrome. *J Child Neurol* **3**:181, 1988

52. Alexander GL, Norman RM: *The Sturge-Weber Syndrome.* Bristol, John Wright & Son, 1960

53. Rappaport ZH: Corpus callosum section in the treatment of intractable seizures in the Sturge-Weber syndrome. *Childs Nerv Syst* **4**(4):231, 1988

54. Cobb S: Haemangioma of the spinal cord associated with skin naevi of the same metamere. *Ann Surg* **62**:641, 1915

55. Van Bogaert L: Pathologie des angiomatoses. *Acta Neurol Psych Belg* **50**:525, 1950

56. Brégeat P: Brégeat syndrome, in *Handbook of Clinical Neurology,* vol 14, *The Phakomatoses,* edited by PJ Vinken, GW Bruyn. Amsterdam, North-Holland, 1972, p 474

57. Haberland C: *Handbook of Clinical Neurology,* vol 31, *The Phakomatoses,* edited by PJ Vinken, GW Bruyn. Amsterdam, North Holland, 1977, chap 1

58. Bonnet BA et al: L'aneurysme cirsoide de la retine. *J Med Lyon* **18**:165, 1937

59. Lamiell JM et al: von Hippel-Lindau disease affecting 43 members of a single kindred. *Medicine (Baltimore)* **68**:1, 1989

60. Hall GS: Blood vessel tumors of brain with particular reference to the Lindau syndrome. *J Neurol Psychopathol* **15**:305, 1935

61. Seizinger BR et al: von Hippel-Lindau maps to the region of chromosome 3 associated with renal cell carcinoma. *Nature* **332**:268, 1988

62. Goodman MD et al: Cytogenetic characterization of renal cell carcinoma in von Hippel-Lindau syndrome. *Cancer* **65**:1150, 1990

63. Plauchu H et al: Age-related clinical profile of hereditary hemorrhagic telangiectasia in an epidemiologically recruited population. *Am J Med Genet* **32**:291, 1989

64. Peery WH: Clinical spectrum of hereditary hemorrhagic telangiectasia (Osler-Weber-Rendu disease). *Am J Med* **82**:989, 1987

65. Syllaba L, Henner K: Contribution à l'indépendance de l'athétose double idiopathique et congénital. *Rev Neurol (Paris)* **1**:541, 1926

66. Aguilar MJ et al: Pathological observations in ataxia-telangiectasia: Report of 5 cases. *J Neuropathol Exp Neurol* **27**:659, 1968

67. Boder E: Ataxia-telangiectasia, in *Neurocutaneous Diseases. A Practical Approach,* edited by MR Gomez. Boston, Butterworth, 1987, p 95

68. Swift M et al: Cancer predisposition of ataxia-telangiectasia heterozygotes. *Cancer Genet Cytogenet* **46**:21, 1990

69. Hecht F, Hecht BK: Cancer in ataxia-telangiectasia patients. *Cancer Genet Cytogenet* **46**:9, 1990

70. Swift M: Genetic aspects of ataxia-telangiectasia. *Immunodefic Rev* **2**:67, 1990

71. Scherrer JR et al: Thrombocytopenie associée à un hemangioblastome cérébelleux. *Schweiz Med Wochenschr* **95**:1456, 1965

72. Van Bogaert L: Les dysplasies à tendance blastomaleuse, in *Traité de Médicine,* vol XVI. Paris, Masson, 1949

73. Krabbe H, Bartels ED: *La Lipomatose Circonscrite Multiple.* Copenhagen, Munksgaard, 1944

74. Johanson A, Blizzard R: A syndrome of congenital aplasia of the alae nasi, deafness, hypothyroidism, dwarfism, absent permanent teeth, and malabsorption. *J Pediatr* **79**:982, 1971

75. Zuffardi O et al: Regional assignment of the loci for adenylate kinase to 9q32 and for alpha 1-acid glycoprotein to 9q31-q32. A locus for Goltz syndrome in region 9q32-qter? *Hum Genet* **82**(1):17, 1989

76. Cannizzaro LA, Hecht F: Gene for incontinentia pigmenti maps to band Xp11 with an (X:10)(p11:q22) translocation. *Clin Genet* **32**:66, 1987

77. Wettke-Schafer R, Kantner G: X-linked dominant inherited diseases with lethality in hemizygous males. *Hum Genet* **64**:1, 1983

78. Darwin C: *The Variation of Animals and Plants under Domestication,* 2d ed. London, John Murray, 1875, p 319

79. Prensky AL: Linear sebaceous nevus, in *Neurocutaneous Diseases. A Practical Approach,* edited by MR Gomez. Boston, Butterworth, 1987, p 335

80. Gorlin RJ et al: Multiple nevoid basal cell carcinoma, odontogenic keratocytes and skeletal anomalies. *Acta Derm Venereol (Stockh)* **43**:39, 1963

81. Herzberg JJ, Wiskemann A: Die fünfte Phakomatose: Basalzellnaevus mit familiärer Belastung und Medulloblastom. *Dermatologica* **126**:106, 1963

82. Hermans EH et al: Naevus epitheliomatoides multiplex een vijfde facomatose. *Ned Tijdschr Geneeskd* **103**:1795, 1959

83. Pascual-Castroveijo I: Hypomelanosis of Ito, in *Neurocutaneous Diseases. A Practical Approach,* edited by MR Gomez. Boston, Butterworth, 1987, p 85

84. Ross DL et al: Hypomelanosis of Ito (incontinentia pigmenti achromians)—a clinicopathologic study: Macrocephaly and gray matter heterotopias. *Neurology* **32**:1013, 1982

85. Donnai D et al: Hypomelanosis of Ito: A manifestation of mosaicism or chimerism. *J Med Genet* **25**:809, 1988

86. Pagon RA: Rothmund-Thomson syndrome, in *Neurocutaneous Diseases. A Practical Approach,* edited by MR Gomez. Boston, Butterworth, 1987, p 136

87. Kaufmann S et al: Growth hormone deficiency in the Rothmund-Thomson syndrome. *Am J Med Genet* **23**:861, 1986

88. Berg E et al: Rothmund-Thomson syndrome. A case report, phototesting and literature review. *J Am Acad Dermatol* **17**(pt 2):332, 1987

89. Starr DG et al: Non-dermatological complications and genetic aspects of the Rothmund-Thomson syndrome, in *Neurocutaneous Diseases. A Practical Approach,* edited by MR Gomez. Boston, Butterworth, 1987, p 136

90. Winklemann RK, Johnson LA: Cholinesterases in neurofibromas. *Arch Dermatol* **85**:106, 1962

91. Reed WB et al: Giant pigmented nevi, melanoma and leptomeningeal melanocytosis: A clinical and histopathological study. *Arch Dermatol* **91**:100, 1965

92. Henschen F: Tumoren des Zentralnervensystems und seiner Hüllen, in *Handbüch der speziellen pathologischen Anatomie und Histologie: Ekrankungen des zentralen Nervensystems,* vol XIII, edited by O Lubarsch et al. Berlin, Springer-Verlag, 1955

93. Fanconi A: Neurocutane Melanoblastose mit Hydrocephalus communicans bei zwei Säuglingen. *Helv Paediat Acta* **11**:376, 1956

94. Kaplan AM et al: Neurocutaneous melanosis with malignant leptomeningeal melanoma. *Arch Neurol* **32**:669, 1975

95. Berlin C: Congenital generalized melanoleucoderma associated with hypodontia, hypotrichosis, stunted growth and mental retardation occurring in two brothers and two sisters. *Dermatologica* **123**:227, 1961

96. Waardenberg PJ: A new syndrome combining developmental anomalies of the eyelids, eyebrows and nose root with pigmentary defects of the iris and head hair and with congenital deafness. *Am J Hum Genet* **3**:195, 1951

97. Klein D: Albinisme partiel (leucisone) accompagné de surdité d'osteomyodysplasie de l'autres malformations congénitales. *Arch Klaus Stift Vererbrungsforsch* **22**:336, 1947

98. Yoshino M et al: Incidences of dystopia canthorum and some other signs in a family with Waardenburg syndrome, type I. *Jpn J Hum Genet* **31**:373, 1986

99. Reed WB et al: Pigmentary disorders in association with congenital deafness. *Arch Dermatol* **95**:176, 1967

100. Arias S: Waardenburg syndrome—two distinct types (letter). *Am J Hum Genet* **6**:99, 1980

101. Klein D: Historical background and evidence for dominant inheritance of the Klein-Waardenburg syndrome (type III). *Am J Med Genet* **14**:231, 1983

102. Badner JA, Chakravarti A: Waardenburg syndrome and Hirschsprung disease: Evidence for pleiotropic effects of a single dominant gene. *Am J Med Genet* **35**:100, 1990

103. White JG, Clawson D: Chédiak-Higashi syndrome: Ring-shaped lysosomes in circulating monocytes. *Am J Pathol* **96**:781, 1979

104. Page AR et al: The Chédiak-Higashi syndrome. *Blood* **20**:330, 1962

105. Stegmaier OC, Schneider LA: Chédiak-Higashi syndrome. *Arch Dermatol* **91**:1, 1965

106. Moynahan E: Multiple symmetrical moles with psychic and somatic infantilism and genital hypoplasia: First male case of a new syndrome. *Proc R Soc Med* **55**:959, 1963

107. Walther RJ et al: Electrocardiographic abnormalities in a family with generalized lentigo. *N Engl J Med* **275**:1220, 1966

108. Mathews NL: Lentigo and electrocardiographic changes. *N Engl J Med* **278**:780, 1968

109. Hagler DL: Lentiginosis-deafness-cardiopathy syndrome, in *Neurocutaneous Diseases. A Practical Approach,* edited by MR Gomez. Boston, Butterworth, 1987, p 80

110. Sjögren J, Larsson T: Oligophrenia in combination with congenital ichthyosis and spastic disorders. *Acta Psychiatr Scand Suppl* **113**:9, 1957

111. Rud E: Et tilfaelde af infantilisme med tetani, epilepsi, polyneuritis ichtyosis og anaemi af perniciøs type. *Hospitalstid* **70**:525, 1927

112. de Sanctis C, Cacchione A: L'idiozia xerodermica. *Riv Sper Freniatr* **56**:269, 1932

113. Ruiz-Maldonado R: Neuroichtyosis, in *Neurocutaneous Diseases. A Practical Approach,* edited by MR Gomez. Boston, Butterworth, 1987, p 214

114. Wisiewski K et al: X-linked inheritance of the Rud syndrome (abstract). *Am J Hum Genet* **37**:A83, 1985

115. Munke M et al: Genetic heterogeneity of the ichthyosis, hypogonadism, mental retardation, and epilepsy syndrome: Clinical and biochemical investigations on two patients with Rud syndrome and review of the literature. *Eur J Pediatr* **141**:8, 1983

116. Heijer A, Reed WB: Sjögren-Larsson syndrome. *Arch Dermatol* **92**:545, 1965

117. Gedde-Dahl T et al: Autosomal recessive ichthyosis in Norway. II. Sjögren ichthyosis without CNS or eye involvement. *Clin Genet* **25**:242, 1984

118. Risso WB et al: Sjögren-Larsson syndrome: Deficient fatty alcohol: NAD$^+$ oxidoreductase (FAO) activity in mixed leukocytes (abstract). *Am J Hum Genet* **41**:A16, 1987

119. Kousseff BG et al: Prenatal diagnosis of Sjögren-Larsson syndrome. *J Pediatr* **101**:998, 1982

120. Noonan JA: Hypertelorism with Turner phenotype. A new syndrome with associated congenital heart disease. *Am J Dis Child* **116**:373, 1968

121. Tolmie JL et al: A lethal multiple pterygium syndrome with apparent X-linked recessive inheritance. *Am J Med Genet* **27**:913, 1987

122. Hall JG: Editorial comment: The lethal multiple pterygium syndromes. *Am J Med Genet* **17**:803, 1984

123. Thompson EM et al: Multiple pterygium syndrome: Evolution of the phenotype. *J Med Genet* **25**:733, 1987

124. Hall JG et al: Limb pterygium syndromes: A review and report of eleven patients. *Am J Med Genet* **12**:377, 1982

125. Graham JM, Smith DW: Dominantly inherited pterygium colli (letter). *J Pediatr* **98**:664, 1981

126. Elsas LJ et al: Leprechaunism: An inherited defect in a high-affinity insulin receptor. *Am J Hum Genet* **7**:73, 1985

127. Lygidakis C et al: Rosenthal's syndrome in four generations. *Clin Genet* **15**:189, 1979

128. Adams RD, Lyon G: *Neurology of Hereditary Diseases of Children.* New York, McGraw-Hill, 1982

129. Murray P et al: Absent and defective iodotyrosine deiodination in a family some of whose members are goitrous cretins. *Lancet* **1**:183, 1965

130. Lyons K, Jones MD (eds): *Smith's Recognizable Patterns of Human Malformations,* 4th ed. Philadelphia, Saunders, 1988, p 554

131. Freundlich E et al: Familial pellagra-like skin rash with neurological manifestations. *Arch Dis Child* **56**:146, 1981

132. Partington MV: The early symptoms of phenylketonuria. *Pediatrics* **27**:465, 1961

133. Holtzman NA et al: Effect of age at loss of dietary control on intellectual performance and behavior of children with phenylketonuria. *N Engl J Med* **314**:593, 1986

134. Woo SLC et al: Regional mapping of the human phenylalanine hydroxylase gene and PKU locus to 12q21-qter (abstract). *Am J Hum Genet* **36**:210S, 1984

135. Irons M, Levy HL: Metabolic syndromes with dermatologic manifestations. *Clin Rev Allergy* **4**:101, 1986

136. Smith I et al: New variant of phenylketonuria with progressive neurological illness unresponsive to phenylalanine restriction. *Lancet* **1**:1108, 1975

137. MacDonald ME et al: Physical and genetic localization of quinonoid dihydropteridine reductase gene on short arm of chromosome 4. *Somat Cell Molec Genet* **13**:549, 1987

138. Carson NAJ et al: Homocystinuria: Clinical and pathological review of 10 cases. *J Pediatr* **66**:565, 1965

139. Halvorsen K, Halvorsen S: Hartnup disease. *Pediatrics* **31**:29, 1963

140. Haim S et al: Cutaneous manifestations associated with aminoaciduria. Report of two cases. *Dermatologica* **156**:244, 1978

141. Levy H: Hartnup disorders, in *The Metabolic Basis of Inherited Disease,* 6th ed, edited by CR Scriver et al. New York, McGraw-Hill, 1989, p 2515

142. Schaap T et al: The genetic analysis of monilethrix in a large inbred kindred. *Am J Med Genet* **11**:469, 1982

143. Menkes JH et al: A sex-linked recessive disorder with retardation of growth, peculiar hair and focal cerebral and cerebellar degeneration. *Pediatrics* **29**:764, 1962

144. Aguilar MJ et al: Kinky hair disease. *J Neuropathol Exp Neurol* **25**:507, 1966

145. Hirano A et al: Fine structure of the cerebellar cortex in Menkes kinky-hair disease. *Arch Neurol* **34**:52, 1977

146. Danks DM: Disorders of copper transport, in *The Metabolic Basis of Inherited Disease,* 6th ed, edited by CR Scriver et al. New York, McGraw-Hill, 1989, p 1411

147. Procopis P et al: A mild form of Menkes syndrome. *J Pediatr* **98**:97, 1981

148. Robinson GC, Miller JR: Hereditary enamel hypoplasia: Its association with characteristic hair structure. *Pediatrics* **37**:498, 1966

149. Neufeld EF, Muenzer J: The mucopolysaccharidoses, in *The Metabolic Basis of Inherited Disease,* 6th ed, edited by CR Scriver et al. New York, McGraw-Hill, 1989, p 1565

150. Cleaver JE, Kraemer KH: Xeroderma pigmentosum, in *The Metabolic Basis of Inherited Disease,* 6th ed, edited by CR Scriver et al. New York, McGraw-Hill, 1989, p 2949

151. Kraemer KH et al: Xeroderma pigmentosum: Cutaneous, ocular, and neurologic abnormalities in 830 published cases. *Arch Dermatol* **123**:241, 1987

152. Robbins JH: Xeroderma pigmentosum, in *Neurocutaneous Diseases. A Practical Approach,* edited by MR Gomez. Boston, Butterworth, 1987, p 110

153. Moshell AN et al: A new patient with both xeroderma pigmentosum and Cockayne syndrome establishes the xeroderma pigmentosum complementation group H, in *Cellular Response to DNA Damage,* edited by EC Friedberg, BA Bridges. New York, Alan R Liss, 1983, p 209

154. Bloom D: The syndrome of congenital telangiectatic erythema and stunted growth. *J Pediatr* **68**:103, 1966

155. King RA: Albinism, in *Neurocutaneous Diseases. A Practical Approach,* edited by MR Gomez. Boston, Butterworth, 1987, p 311

156. Witkop CJ Jr et al: Albinism, in *The Metabolic Basis of Inherited Disease,* 6th ed, edited by CR Scriver et al. New York, McGraw-Hill, 1989, p 2905

157. Cross HE et al: A new oculocerebral syndrome with hypopigmentation. *J Pediatr* **70**:398, 1967

158. Lyons K, Jones MD (eds): *Smith's Recognizable Patterns of Human Malformations,* 4th ed. Philadelphia, Saunders, 1988, p 538

159. Berardinelli W: An undiagnosed endocrino-metabolic syndrome: Report of two cases. *J Clin Endocrinol* **14**:193, 1954

160. Berge T et al: Congenital generalized lipodystrophy: Report on one case with special reference to postmortem findings. *Acta Pathol Microbiol Scand* **84**(1): 47, 1976

161. McLean RH, Hoefnagel D: Partial lipodystrophy and familial C3 deficiency. *Hum Hered* **30**:149, 1980

162. Brunzell JD et al: Congenital generalized lipodystrophy and systemic cystic angiomatosis: The simultaneous occurrence of two unusual syndromes in a single family. *Ann Intern Med* **69**:501, 1968

163. Farag TI, Teebi AS: Bardet-Biedl and Laurence-Moon syndromes in a mixed Arab population. *Clin Genet* **33**:78, 1988

164. Van Bogaert L et al: *Une Forme Célèbre de la Cholesterinose Généralisée.* Paris, Masson, 1937

165. Menkes JH et al: Cerebrotendinous xanthomatosis. *Arch Neurol* **19**:47, 1968

166. Vjorkhem I, Skrede S: Familial diseases with storage of sterols other than cholesterol: Cerebrotendinous xanthomatosis and phytosterolemia, in *The Metabolic Basis of Inherited Disease,* 6th ed, edited by CR Scriver et al. New York, McGraw-Hill, 1989, p 1283

167. Steinberg D et al: Refsum's disease: A recently characterized lipidosis involving the nervous system. *Ann Intern Med* **66**:365, 1967

168. Mize CE et al: Phytanic acid storage in Refsum's disease due to defective alpha-hydroxylation. *Clin Res* **16**:346, 1968

169. Refsum S, Stokke O: Refsum's disease, in *Neurocutaneous Diseases. A Practical Approach,* edited by MR Gomez. Boston, Butterworth, 1987, p 225

170. Steinberg D: Refsum disease, in *The Metabolic Basis of Inherited Disease,* 6th ed, edited by CR Scriver et al. New York, McGraw-Hill, 1989, p 1533

171. Waldorf DS et al: Cutaneous cholesterol ester disposition in Tangier disease. *Arch Dermatol* **95**:161, 1967

172. Fredrickson DS: The inheritance of high-density lipoprotein deficiency (Tangier disease). *J Clin Invest* **43**:228, 1964

173. Gibbels E et al: Severe polyneuropathy in Tangier disease mimicking syringomyelia or leprosy. Clinical, biochemical, electrophysiological, and morphological evaluation, including electron microscopy of nerve, muscle, and skin biopsies. *J Neurol* **232**:283, 1985

174. Opitz J et al: The genetics of angiokeratoma corporis diffusum (Fabry's disease) and its linkage with the Xg(a) locus. *Am J Hum Genet* **17**:325, 1965

175. Sweeley CC, Klionsky B: Fabry's disease: Classification as a sphingolipidosis and partial characterization of a novel glycolipid. *J Biol Chem* **238**:3148, 1963

176. Rahman AN et al: Angiokeratoma corporis diffusum universale. *Trans Assoc Am Physicians* **74**:366, 1961

177. Cable WJL et al: Fabry disease: Impaired autonomic function. *Neurology* **32**:498, 1982

178. Desnick RJ, Bishop DF: Fabry disease: Alpha galactosidase deficiency, in *The Metabolic Basis of Inherited Disease,* 6th ed, edited by CR Scriver et al. New York, McGraw-Hill, 1989, p 1751

179. Kappas A et al: The porphyrias, in *The Metabolic Basis of Inherited Disease,* 6th ed, edited by CR Scriver et al. New York, McGraw-Hill, 1989, p 1305

180. Dean G: *The Porphyrias: A Story of Inheritance and Environment.* Philadelphia, Lippincott, 1963

181. Goldberg A: Acute intermittent porphyria: A study of 50 cases. *Q J Med* **28**:183, 1959

182. Stout JT, Caskey CT: Hypoxanthine phosphoribosyltransferase deficiency: The Lesch-Nyhan syndrome and gouty arthritis, in *The Metabolic Basis of Inherited Disease,* 6th ed, edited by CR Scriver et al. New York, McGraw-Hill, 1989, p 1007

183. Ahonen P: Autoimmune polyendocrinopathy-candidosis-ectodermal dystrophy (APECED): Autosomal recessive inheritance. *Clin Genet* **27**:535, 1985

184. Gass JDM: The syndrome of keratoconjunctivitis, superficial moniliasis, idiopathic hypoparathyroidism and Addison's disease. *Am J Ophthalmol* **54**:660, 1962

185. Axelrod FB, Pearson J: Familial dysautonomia, in *Neurocutaneous Diseases. A Practical Approach,* edited by MR Gomez. Boston, Butterworth, 1987, p 200

186. Barnes L: Vitiligo and the Vogt-Koyanagi-Harada syndrome. *Dermatol Clin* **6**:229, 1988

187. Norose K et al: Immunologic analysis of cerebrospinal fluid lymphocytes in Vogt-Koyanagi-Harada disease. *Invest Ophthalmol Vis Sci* **31**:1210, 1990

188. Wong KC et al: Behçet's disease. *Int J Dermatol* **23**:25, 1984

189. Reik L: Lyme disease, in *Current Therapy in Neurologic Disease,* edited by RT Johnson. Philadelphia, BC Dekker, 1990, p 148

190. Scott RE, Wilson DM: Role of the clinical laboratory in the diagnosis and management of malignant melanoma. *Mayo Clin Proc* **64**:837, 1989

191. Martin JJ et al: Contributions de la biopsie cutanée au diagnostic des encéphalopathies métaboliques. *Rev Neurol (Paris)* **132**:639, 1976

192. Centerick C, Martin JJ: Diagnostic role of skin or conjunctival biopsies in neurological disorders. An update. *J Neurol Sci* **65**:179, 1984

CHAPTER 185

Joseph L. Jorizzo

Behçet's Disease

Behçet's disease is a complex multisystem disease characterized clinically by the presence of oral aphthae and at least two of the following: genital aphthae, synovitis, cutaneous pustular vasculitis, posterior uveitis, or meningoencephalitis. The absence of inflammatory bowel disease and collagen vascular diseases must be documented.

Behçet's disease most often affects patients in their twenties and thirties, and men are more frequently affected than women. Pediatric cases are reported.[7]

Etiology and Pathogenesis

Genetics

Several large series in Britain, Japan, Korea, and the Middle East have shown a significant association between Behçet's disease and HLA-B51.[4,8] Familial clustering of Behçet's disease is not common but is reported.[9]

Infectious Precipitants

Early theories of the pathogenesis of Behçet's disease proposed a viral or other infectious etiology.[2,3] Extensive investigation has failed to substantiate a primary infectious etiology. The possibility that infectious agents might trigger an immunoregulatory defect in genetically predisposed individuals has been investigated by several research groups. Hybridization studies have demonstrated homology between the deoxyribonucleic acid (DNA) of herpes simplex virus type 1 and the ribonucleic acid of peripheral blood lymphocytes from patients with Behçet's disease.[10] Recent investigations, especially in Japan, have focused on immunologic alteration related to exposure to streptococcal strains such as *Streptococcus sanguis* and *S. pyogenes*.[3,11]

Historical Aspects

About 2400 years ago Hippocrates used the designation *aphthai* to refer to common oral aphthae (canker sores), and he may have described the first patient with Behçet's disease.[1] Hulusi Behçet, a Turkish dermatologist, described his patients with recurrent orogenital ulcerations and uveitis in 1937, and in 1940 he added four patients with the "triple symptom complex."[2,3] The first international multidisciplinary conference on Behçet's disease was organized by two dermatologists, Drs. Monacelli and Nazarro, in Rome in 1964. The most recent conference was held at the Mayo Clinic in 1989.[4]

Epidemiology

The prevalence of Behçet's disease is highest in Japan and Southeast Asia and in the Middle East and southern Europe.[5,6] The disease is not common in northern Europe and the United States.

Immunologic Aspects

Important early studies demonstrated autoantibodies reactive to oral mucosal antigens in patients with Behçet's disease.[12] Rogers and associates demonstrated lymphocytoxicity to oral epithelial cells.[13] Various studies have suggested that nonspecific abnormalities of cellular immunity are relevant in the pathogenesis of Behçet's disease.[14–16]

Studies have also focused on a role for circulating immune complexes and neutrophils in the pathogenesis of mucocutaneous lesions in Behçet's disease. Nazzaro[17] demonstrated that the earliest histology from aphthae, pustular vasculitic lesions, and erythema nodosum-like lesions is what we would now call a neutrophilic vascular reaction or even fully developed leukocytoclastic vasculitis, and these findings have been confirmed.[18,19] Antigen nonspecific assays for circulating immune complexes are reported to be positive in about half of patients, and they seem to correlate with disease activity.[18,20] Light, immunofluorescence, and electron microscopic studies support a neutrophilic vascular reaction or even fully developed leukocytoclastic vasculitis as the earliest finding in mucocutaneous lesions.[17–19,21] Pathergy lesions (cutaneous pustular vasculitis lesions induced by intradermal trauma) have been studied with a modification of Braverman's histamine trap test.[18,19] Patients with active disease show a neutrophilic vascular reaction or leukocytoclastic vasculitis in a biopsy specimen obtained 24 h after histamine injection and on direct immunofluorescence usually show immunoreactants in biopsy specimens obtained 4 h after histamine injection.[18,19] Studies have repeatedly suggested increased migration of neutrophils to chemoattractants in Boyden chamber or subagarose assays.[22,23] This may be due to a heat-stable serum factor.[18] The therapeutic benefit of colchicine therapy, but not of thalidomide therapy, may be due to a blockade of the ability of neutrophils to hyper-respond to serum from patients with Behçet's disease.[18,22]

Lehner's group in London has presented data to support the theory that various infectious agents could trigger a defect in immunoregulation in genetically predisposed individuals.[10] Disagreement exists as to whether subsequent tissue injury might be mediated by lymphoid cells or by circulating immune complex-mediated, neutrophil-induced vessel damage.[4]

Clinical Manifestations

Mucocutaneous Lesions

The oral aphthae that occur in patients with Behçet's disease are like those that occur in simple recurrent aphthosis, although they may be more extensive and may occur more frequently (Fig. 185-1a).[5,23] Genital aphthae are similar lesions that occur in the genital area (Fig. 185-1b). Herpes simplex should be excluded with appropriate Tzanck preparation, viral culture, or even skin biopsy.

In our opinion, cutaneous lesions that should be accepted as being diagnostically relevant in Behçet's disease should be confined to cutaneous pustular vasculitis lesions (including pathergy lesions), erythema nodosum-like lesions, Sweet's-like lesions, pyoderma gangrenosum-like lesions, and palpable purpuric lesions of necrotizing venulitis (Fig. 185-2). All of these lesions are characterized by a neutrophilic vascular reaction in their early stages.[24] Acne lesions or follicle-based pustules should not be considered relevant.

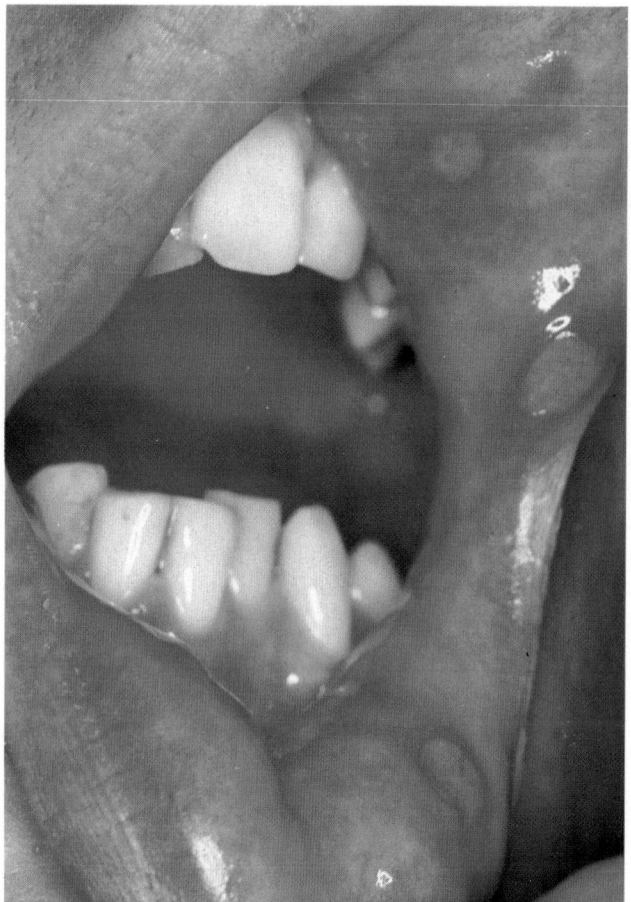

a

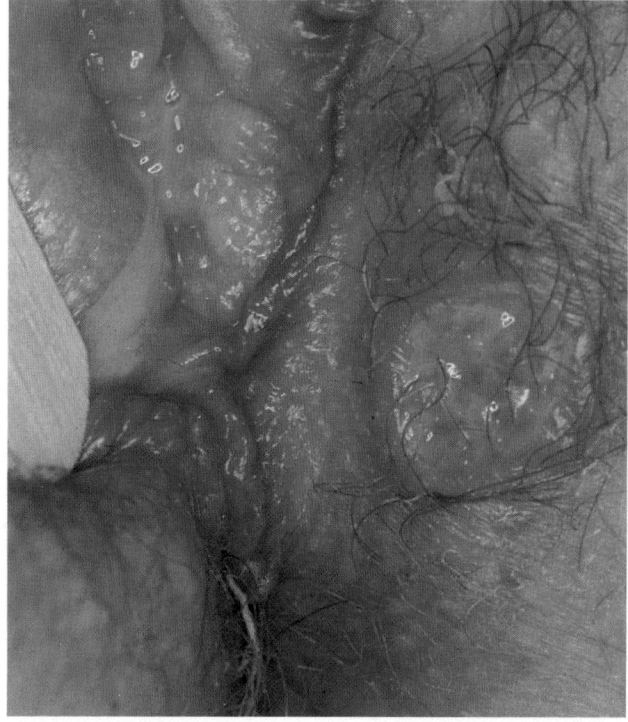

b

FIGURE 185-1 Behçet's syndrome. (*a*) On the labial mucosa there are painful aphthous-type ulcerations. (*b*) Large, painful aphthous-type ulcer on the vulva.

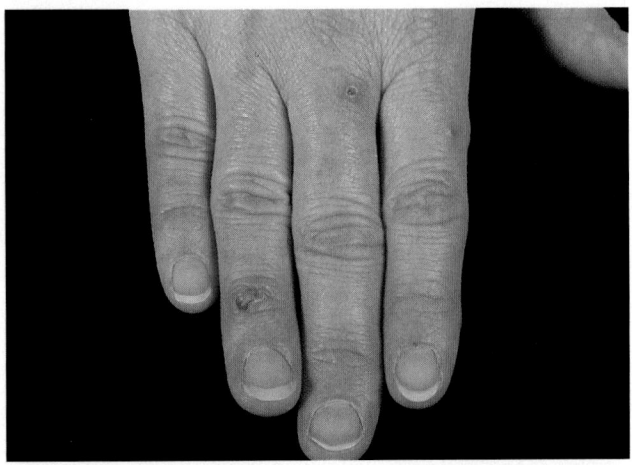

FIGURE 185-2 Pustular vasculitis lesions on the hand of a patient with Behçet's disease.

Systemic Lesions

Ocular involvement is the major cause of morbidity in patients with Behçet's disease. The most diagnostically relevant lesion is *posterior uveitis* (called *retinal vasculitis* in Great Britain). Other ocular lesions include anterior uveitis, hypopyon (now uncommon), and secondary cataracts, glaucoma, and neovascular lesions.[25,26]

The characteristic arthritis is a nonerosive, asymmetric oligoarthritis.[5,6,27] Patients with HLA-B27–positive, erosive sacroiliitis have been included in some series of patients with Behçet's disease but are more appropriately considered as a part of the Reiter's/enteropathic arthritis spectrum of disease.[4]

Significant neurologic manifestations occur in less than one-fourth of patients and may be delayed in onset. Meningoencephalitis, benign intracranial hypertension, cranial nerve palsies, brainstem lesions, and pyramidal or extrapyramidal lesions have all been described.[28,29]

Vascular involvement can be significant and includes aneurysms, arterial occlusions, venous occlusions, and varices that can be fatal.[30] Hemoptysis can occur due to vessel-based pulmonary lesions and is also potentially fatal.[31] Cardiac involvement can include myocarditis, coronary arteritis, endocarditis, and valvular disease.[32] Renal disease may be mild or asymptomatic, but in a recent series a majority of patients with active Behçet's disease had evidence of glomerular immunoreactant deposition.[33] Aphthae may occur throughout the gastrointestinal tract. Some patients with inflammatory bowel disease have been included in series of patients with Behçet's disease, but these are best excluded.[4]

Laboratory Evaluation

There are no pathognomonic laboratory abnormalities in patients with Behçet's disease. Laboratory abnormalities may occur in association with dysfunction of various organ systems, depending on clinical disease manifestations.

Histopathology

Traditional histopathologic interpretations of various types of lesions sampled in patients with Behçet's disease describe primarily a lymphocytic perivasculitis. These reports usually have focused on late lesions and on autopsy data.[34] Biopsies from the earliest mucocutaneous lesions show a neutrophilic vascular reaction with endothelial swelling, extravasation or erythrocytes, and leukocytoclasia or fully developed leukocytoclastic vasculitis with these features plus fibrinoid necrosis of blood vessel walls.[17–19,21]

Diagnosis

Behçet's disease is a complex multisystem disease that must be diagnosed by clinical criteria in the absence of a pathognomonic laboratory test. Various sets of criteria have been published; the preferred North American criteria are those of O'Duffy and associates.[35] Patients must have oral aphthae plus at least two of the following: genital aphthae, synovitis, posterior uveitis, cutaneous pustular vasculitis (our modification[18] from original pathergy) (Fig. 185-2), or meningoencephalitis in the absence of inflammatory bowel disease or collagen vascular disease.

New international criteria have been published.[36] These new criteria require the presence of oral aphthae plus two of the following: recurrent genital aphthae, eye lesions, skin lesions, or a positive pathergy test. An explanation of these criteria is given in Table 185-1. There are several problems with the new criteria. The omission of synovitis and of meningoencephalitis makes four of the five criteria variations of the same basic mucocutaneous lesion. We would require histologic confirmation that the cutaneous pustular lesions are indeed vessel-based and neutrophilic. Because 20 percent of normal young adults have oral aphthae and almost all adolescents have at least one acneiform lesion, they could practically meet the criteria if "acneiform skin lesions" are not excluded! Exclusion of inflammatory bowel disease as in the O'Duffy criteria should also be mandatory.

Reiter's disease is often confused with Behçet's disease by nondermatologists. Reiter's disease and the HLA-B27–positive spectrum of disease are characterized by an axial erosive arthritis and by psoriasiform mucocutaneous lesions and not by aphthae or pustular vasculitis. Patients with inflammatory bowel disease have an increased incidence of oral aphthae. These patients or those who have had bowel bypass or Bilroth II surgery can have a dermatosis-arthritis syndrome that mimics Behçet's disease, including an indistinguishable pustular vasculitis.[37] Eye disease is generally ab-

TABLE 185-1
Proposed International Criteria for Behçet's Disease*

Criteria	Description
Oral	Minor aphthae, major aphthae, or herpetiform ulcers observed by physicians or reported reliably by patient. Recurrent at least three times in one 12-month period.
Genital	Recurrent genital aphthae or scarring, especially scrotal in males, observed by physician or reliably reported by patient.
Eye	Anterior uveitis, posterior uveitis, cells in vitreous on slit-lamp examination or retinal vasculitis, observed by qualified physician.
Skin	Erythema nodosum-like lesions observed by physicians or papulopustular lesions consistent with Behçet's disease, observed by a physician.
Pathergy	Positive pathergy test read by a physician at 24 or 48 h, performed with oblique insertion of a 20-gauge or smaller needle under sterile conditions.

*Findings are applicable if no other clinical explanation is present.

sent in these patients. Patients with complex aphthosis have recurrent oral and genital aphthae or almost ever present, multiple (>3) oral aphthae, but no other features of Behçet's disease.[38] Patients with pustular vasculitis alone may have gonococcal or even chronic meningococcal sepsis, or the pustular vasculitis may occur as an idiopathic syndrome.[39]

Treatment

Therapy for patients with Behçet's disease can generally be divided into treatment regimens for patients with primarily mucocutaneous disease and for patients with ocular or neurologic manifestations. Palliative therapy of aphthae has included a host of agents, such as counter-irritant antipruritic agents, potent topical corticosteroids, intralesional corticosteroids, and local anesthetics. Oral colchicine, 0.6 mg orally two to three times daily as tolerated by the gastrointestinal tract, can reduce the frequency and severity of mucocutaneous lesions.[19,40] Patients should be monitored for the infrequent neutropenia that can complicate therapy. Thalidomide therapy was dramatically beneficial but is no longer available for this indication in the United States and has been replaced by dapsone therapy.[22,41] Therapeutic options available for systemic disease, particularly for severe ocular manifestations, include prednisone, prednisone plus azathioprine, cyclophosphamide (including a pulse regimen), azathioprine alone,[42] chlorambucil,[43] and cyclosporine.[44]

Course and Prognosis

The clinical course of Behçet's disease is variable. Mucocutaneous and arthritic manifestations usually occur first. Ophthalmic involvement is the leading course of morbidity. Blindness can often be prevented with early aggressive therapy of posterior uveitis. If neurologic involvement occurs at all, it is usually delayed. Death may occur from neurologic involvement, vascular disease, bowel perforation, cardiopulmonary disease, or as a complication of immunosuppressive therapy.

References

1. Feigenbaum A: Description of Behçet's syndrome in the Hippocratic third book of endemic diseases. *Br J Ophthalmol* **40**:355, 1956

2. Behçet H: Uber rezidivierende Aphthöse, durch ein Virus verusachte Geschwüre am Mund, am Auge und an den Genitale. *Dermatol Wochenschr* **105**:1152, 1937

3. Behçet H: Some observations on the clinical picture of the so-called triple symptom complex. *Dermatologica* **81**:73, 1940

4. Jorizzo JL, Rogers RS III: Behçet's disease: An update based on the International Conference held in Rochester, Minnesota, September 14 and 15, 1989. *J Am Acad Dermatol* **23**:738, 1990

5. Shimuzu T et al: Behçet's disease (Behçet's syndrome). *Semin Arthritis Rheum* **8**:223, 1979

6. Chajek T, Fainaru M: Behçet's disease: Report of 41 cases and review of the literature. *Medicine* (*Baltimore*) **54**:179, 1975

7. Ammann AJ et al: Behçet syndrome. *J Pediatrics* **107**:41, 1985

8. Yazici H et al: HLA antigens in Behçet's disease: A reappraisal by a comparative study of Turkish and British patients. *Ann Rheum Dis* **39**:344, 1980

9. Dundar SV et al: Familial cases of Behçet's disease. *Br J Dermatol* **113**:319, 1985

10. Lehner T: The role of a disorder in immunoregulation associated with herpes simplex virus type I in Behçet's disease, in *Recent Advances in Behçet's Disease,* edited by T Lehner, CG Barnes. London, Royal Society of Medicine Services, 1986, p 31

11. Niwa Y, Mizushima Y: Neutrophil-potentiating factors released from stimulated lymphocytes: Special reference to the increase in neutrophil-potentiating factors from streptococcus-stimulated lymphocytes of patients with Behçet's disease. *Clin Exp Immunol* **79**:353, 1990

12. Oshima Y et al: Clinical studies on Behçet's syndrome. *Ann Rheum Dis* **22**:36, 1963

13. Rogers RS III et al: Lymphocytotoxicity for oral epithelial cells in recurrent aphthous stomatitis and Behçet's syndrome. *Arch Dermatol* **109**:361, 1974

14. Victorino RMM et al: Cell mediated immune functions and immunoregulatory cells in Behçet's syndrome. *Clin Exp Immunol* **48**:121, 1982

15. Sakane T et al: Functional aberration of T-cell subsets in patients with Behçet's disease. *Arthritis Rheum* **25**:1343, 1982

16. Valesini G et al: Evaluation of T-cell subsets in Behçet's syndrome using anti-T–cell monoclonal antibodies. *Clin Exp Immunol* **60**:55, 1985

17. Nazzaro P: Cutaneous manifestations of Behçet's disease, in *International Symposium on Behçet's Disease in Rome,* edited by M Monacelli, P Nazzaro. Basel, Karger, 1966, p 15

18. Jorizzo JL et al: Behçet's syndrome: Immune regulation, circulating immune complexes, neutrophil migration and colchicine therapy. *J Am Acad Dermatol* **10**:205, 1984

19. Jorizzo JL et al: Behçet's syndrome: Immunopathologic and histopathologic assessment of pathergy lesions is useful in diagnosis and follow up. *Arch Pathol Lab Med* **109**:747, 1985

20. Valesini G et al: Circulating immune complexes in Behçet's syndrome: Purification, characterization and cross reactivity studies. *Clin Exp Immunol* **44**:522, 1981

21. Muller W, Lehner T: Quantitative electron microscopic analysis of leukocyte infiltration in oral ulcers of Behçet's syndrome. *Br J Dermatol* **106**:535, 1982

22. Jorizzo JL et al: Thalidomide effects in Behçet's syndrome and pustular vasculitis. *Arch Intern Med* **146**:878, 1986

23. Rogers RS: Recurrent aphthous stomatitis: Clinical characteristics and evidence for an immunopathogenesis. *J Invest Dermatol* **69**:499, 1977

24. Jorizzo JL et al: Neutrophilic vascular reactions. *J Am Acad Dermatol* **19**:983, 1988

25. Colvard DM et al: The ocular manifestations of Behçet's disease. *Arch Ophthalmol* **95**:1813, 1977

26. Dinning WJ: An overview of ocular manifestations, in *Recent Advances in Behçet's Disease,* edited by T Lehner, CG Barnes. London, Royal Society of Medicine Services, 1986, p 227

27. Yurdakul S et al: The arthritis of Behçet's disease: A prospective study. *Ann Rheum Dis* **42**:505, 1983

28. O'Duffy JD, Goldstein NP: Neurologic involvement in seven patients with Behçet's disease. *Am J Med* **61**:170, 1976

29. Inaba G: Clinical features of neuro-Behçet syndrome, in *Recent Advances in Behçet's Disease,* edited by T Lehner, CG Barnes. London, Royal Society of Medicine Services, 1986, p 235

30. Shimizu T: Vascular lesions of Behçet's disease. *Cardioangiology* **1**:124, 1977

31. Efthimiou J et al: Pulmonary disease in Behçet's syndrome. *Q J Med* **58**:259, 1986

32. James DG, Thomson A: Recognition of the diverse cardiovascular manifestations of Behçet's disease. *Am Heart J* **30**:457, 1982

33. Herreman G et al: Behçet's syndrome and renal involvement: A histological and immunofluorescence study of eleven renal biopsies. *Am J Med Sci* **284**:10, 1982

34. Lakanpal S et al: Pathologic features of Behçet's syndrome: A review of Japanese autopsy registry data. *Hum Pathol* **16**:790, 1985

35. O'Duffy JD et al: Behçet's disease: Report of 10 cases, 3 with new manifestations. *Am J Intern Med* **75**:561, 1971

36. International study group for Behçet's disease: Criteria for diagnosis of Behçet's disease. *Lancet* **335**:1078, 1990

38. Jorizzo JL et al: Complex aphthosis: A forme fruste of Behçet's syndrome? *J Am Acad Dermatol* **13**:80, 1985

39. McNeely MC et al: Primary idiopathic cutaneous pustular vasculitis. *J Am Acad Dermatol* **14**:939, 1986

40. Miyachi Y et al: Colchicine in the treatment of cutaneous manifestations of Behçet's disease. *Br J Dermatol* **104**:67, 1981

41. Sharquie K: Suppression of Behçet's disease with dapsone. *Br J Dermatol* **110**:493, 1984

42. Yazici H et al: A controlled trial of azathioprine in Behçet's syndrome. *N Engl J Med* **322**:281, 1990

43. O'Duffy JD et al: Chlorambucil in the treatment of uveitis and meningoencephalitis of Behçet's disease. *Am J Med* **76**:75, 1984

44. Nussenblatt RB et al: Effectiveness of cyclosporin therapy for Behçet's disease. *Arthritis Rheum* **28**:671, 1985

PART FIVE

Diseases due to Microbial Agents

Bacterial Diseases with Cutaneous Involvement

CHAPTER 186

Arnold N. Weinberg and Morton N. Swartz

The patient with a fever and cutaneous lesions presents one of the most challenging and frequently rewarding problems in medicine. The question of a treatable etiology (bacterial, fungal, herpes virus) should always be raised initially. The physician must actively and thoughtfully consider these possibilities and seek confirmation by appropriate studies to insure early optimal antimicrobial therapy.

Bacterial infection involving the skin may manifest itself in either of two major forms: (1) as a primarily cutaneous process, or (2) as a secondary manifestation in the skin of infection in some other organ. The cutaneous changes associated with infection are not always suppurative but may present as a vasculitis or a hypersensitivity response (e.g., lesions in subacute bacterial endocarditis or erythema nodosum).

The importance of the skin as a mirror of systemic infection cannot be overemphasized, especially when classic clinical findings are distorted as in immunocompromised patients. The timely recognition of the cutaneous clues of bacteremia may provide the early warning to consider life-threatening infections due to organisms such as *Pseudomonas aeruginosa, Salmonella typhi, Staphylococcus aureus,* and *Neisseria meningitidis.*

Natural Resistance of the Skin

The normal skin of healthy individuals is highly resistant to invasion by the wide variety of bacteria to which it is constantly exposed. It is difficult to produce localized infections such as impetigo, furunculosis, or cellulitis in laboratory animals[1] or human volunteers[2] if the integument is intact. Pathogenic organisms such as *Streptococcus pyogenes* (group A streptococcus) and *Staph. aureus* produce characteristic lesions of cellulitis and furunculosis in the absence of any obvious impairment of host defenses via disruption of the intact integument, i.e., by alcohol sponging, insect bites, an abrasion, or the introduction of a foreign body. For example, Elek[3] demonstrated that the presence of a silk suture reduces by a factor of 10,000, in the case of *Staph. aureus,* the number of organisms needed to produce an abscess in the human skin. Treatment with immunosuppressive agents can predispose patients to infections by the same organisms or by others of much lower intrinsic pathogenicity. The basis for this enhanced susceptibility of the compromised host is not understood but undoubtedly involves spe-

General Considerations of Bacterial Diseases

cific and nonspecific factors such as immunocompetence, nutritional state, and integrity of the cutaneous barrier.[4]

Bacteria are unable to penetrate the keratinized layers of normal skin and, when applied to the surface, rapidly decrease in number.[2] The nature and the relative importance of the factors thought to be involved in this local resistance to bacterial multiplication and to infection are not clear.[5] *The low pH* (approximately 5.5) *of the skin environment* has been suggested as one of these properties, but it does not appear to have an important role. Many virulent bacteria are capable of growing at pHs below that of normal skin. The presence of *natural antibacterial substances* in the sebaceous secretions may be a factor in bacterial elimination from the skin. Streptococci appear to be particularly sensitive, in vitro, to the unsaturated long-chain fatty acids of the skin lipids, but in controlled studies in humans. *S. pyogenes* (gpA) grows equally well in high- or low-lipid-containing regions.[2] Areas such as the palms and soles, lacking in sebaceous glands, remain relatively free of streptococci as well. The role of *circulating immunoglobulins, cellular immunity,* and *delayed hypersensitivity* in the defense of the skin against certain organisms is under intense investigation, especially the relationship of the thymus to Langerhans and epidermal cells and their contribution to stimulation and function of T lymphocytes.[6] IgM has not been found in normal sweat, and IgA, IgG, and IgD have been found only in minute amounts (0.01 percent of the level in serum). However, the greater frequency with which a specific cutaneous and mucous membrane mycotic infection, moniliasis, occurs in patients with severe combined immunodeficiency (e.g., Swiss type of congenital lymphopenic agammaglobulinemia) suggests a relationship. Experimental and clinical observations, summarized by Kligman et al.,[5] consistently support the importance of moisture content and the indigenous cutaneous microflora (see Chap. 17) in limiting colonization of the skin by potential pathogens. The *relative dryness* of normal skin contributes to the marked limitation of growth of bacteria, especially gram-negative bacilli with their higher moisture requirements (*Escherichia coli, Pseudomonas, Proteus*). *Bacterial interference* (the suppressive effect of one bacterial strain or species on colonization by another) exerts a major influence on the overall complexion of the skin flora. Although this effect is somewhat difficult to define, its relevance, at least in the case of colonization of the nose and skin by *Staph. aureus,* appears clear.[7] Profound changes in these bacterial interactions may be effected by the use of antibiotics.

The summation of these factors allows certain bacterial species to colonize the skin surface successfully while others are rapidly excluded. The organisms that characteristically survive and multiply in various ecologic niches of the skin constitute the ''normal cutaneous flora.'' An appreciation of the composition of this flora and the attributes of its major elements is important in understanding and treating many bacterial infections of the skin (see Chap. 17).

Pathogenesis of Bacterial Infection of the Skin

The host-bacteria relationship in infections of the skin, as in infectious disease in general, involves three major elements: (1) the pathogenic properties of the organism, (2) the portal of entry, and (3) the host defense and inflammatory response to microbial invasion of the anatomic region.

Pathogenicity of the Microorganism

The disease-producing capacity of bacteria is determined to a large measure by (1) the invasive potential (often based on antiphagocytic surface components), and (2) the toxigenic properties of the organism. A few species of bacteria (e.g., pneumococcus) appear to owe their pathogenicity solely to their ability to multiply extensively and invade tissues while resisting phagocytosis. No definable extracellular products or toxins that might contribute to their invasiveness have been discovered. Conversely, a few species have toxigenic properties that account for the local lesion (*Corynebacterium diphtheriae, Bacillus anthracis*) or systemic manifestations (*Clostridium tetani*) of a local infection. In the case of *Clostridium perfringens,* elaboration of a variety of extracellular toxins and enzymes (alpha toxin or lecithinase, proteases, collagenases) appears to play an important role in the rapidly spreading histotoxic lesions and systemic manifestations of clostridial myonecrosis. Though it is useful to distinguish between these two major pathogenic mechanisms whenever possible, most bacterial infections result from invasive and toxigenic properties of the organism. Local invasiveness (dependent to a considerable extent on the antiphagocytic M protein of the bacterial cell envelope) is an important element in streptococcal pharyngitis, but the clinical features of scarlet fever result from the elaboration of the erythrogenic toxin. For most disease-producing bacteria, including *Staph. aureus* suppurative lesions, understanding of the basis for pathogenicity is lacking. The increasing prevalence of serious infections in compromised hosts, due to ''traditionally'' nonpathogenic bacteria that include the resident skin flora, supports the concept that pathogenicity is the resultant of microorganism and host interactions.

Gram-negative bacteria (*E. coli, S. typhi, N. meningitidis, N. gonorrhoeae, Brucella melitensis,* and others) contain endotoxin, complex phospholipid-polysaccharide macromolecules (LPS), as an integral part of the bacterial cell envelope. Endotoxins, unlike exotoxins, are released only upon breakdown of the bacterial cell. Their toxicity appears to be linked principally to the lipid fraction, whereas their antigenic determinants reside with the polysaccharide component.[8] Although the biologic effects of LPS in experimental animals are numerous (shock, fever, gastrointestinal hemorrhages, leukopenia, abortion) and well studied, their role in invasiveness and the pathogenesis of localized bacterial diseases

until recently remained ill defined.[9] In the past decade this has changed considerably. Much is now known of the mechanisms by which LPS exerts its biologic effects, in systemic infections due to gram-negative bacteria or in major localized infections that may also be capable of producing the sepsis syndrome.[10] The effects are both toxic (lethality, shock, fever, anorexia and cachexia, somnolence, complement activation, disseminated intravascular coagulation, and capillary thrombosis) and immunologic (adjuvant function, polyclonal B-cell stimulation, macrophage activation, cytokine production). The two cytokines most relevant to the toxic and proinflammatory effects of LPS are produced by LPS-activated macrophages: tumor necrosis factor (TNF) and interleukin 1 (IL-1), the latter formerly known as leukocytic pyrogen.[11,12]

After it enters the circulation, TNF, among its many biologic effects, acts as an endogenous pyrogen on hypothalamic centers to induce fever.[13,14] It also acts on mononuclear phagocytes to stimulate production of IL-1 (another endogenous pyrogen), IL-6 (an inducer of production of serum amyloid A and other proteins of the ''acute phase response''), and IL-8 (an inflammatory cytokine stimulating leukocyte chemotaxis and activation). Thus, TNF initiates a proinflammatory cytokine cascade. TNF itself acts on the liver to increase synthesis of acute phase reactants, including fibrinogen. It also activates the coagulation system through its effects on vascular endothelium and it decreases blood pressure and tissue perfusion by reducing myocardial contractility and relaxing smooth muscle.

High circulating levels of TNF are demonstrable in patients with meningococcemia and other forms of severe sepsis.[15,16] Its direct role as a mediator of circulatory collapse in gram-negative bacillary bacteremia is supported by the fact that pretreatment with antibody to TNF can prevent mortality in animals (associated with hypotension and cardiac and renal failure) from experimental *E. coli* bacteremia.[17] In addition, infusion of high concentrations of purified TNF alone can produce shock and death.

LPS can directly trigger release of IL-1 from activated macrophages as well as act indirectly through initial induction of TNF. Like TNF, IL-1 acts on endothelial cells as a procoagulant and as a stimulator of leukocyte adhesion. It can cause fever, stimulate production of acute phase proteins, and initiate (in combination with TNF) muscle wasting and cachexia. IL-1 also acts in an immunomodulatory role to enhance proliferation of CD4+ T cells and to stimulate B-cell growth and differentiation.

The Shwartzman reaction is an intensified response in experimental animals to bacteria containing LPS or to purified LSP itself. LPS injected intravenously twice, 24 h apart, causes disseminated intravascular coagulation (DIC) in rabbits (systemic Shwartzman reaction); LPS injected intradermally, followed by a second (intravenous) injection, produces hemorrhagic necrosis of the skin (localized Shwartzman reaction) at the site of intradermal introduction. The necrosis stems from poor tissue perfusion as a consequence of capillary blockage by neutrophils and platelets and by local fibrin formation. TNF is the major mediator of the Shwartzman reaction; unlike TNF, IL-1 cannot directly mediate this reaction. The ability of LPS, through TNF production, to induce leukocyte adherence to capillary endothelium and to induce fibrin deposition has been suggested to be the basis for development of the hemorrhagic necrotic skin lesions (with or without direct bacterial invasion) that sometimes occur during the course of gram-negative bacillary bacteremias and meningococcemia.

Changing Patterns of Bacterial Infections of the Skin   In addition to the usual pathogens, a variety of ''nonpathogenic'' members of the cutaneous, intestinal, or respiratory tract flora are capable of producing acute disease in debilitated patients and in individuals with altered humoral or cellular defenses and with a variety of skin defects. A patient receiving immunosuppressive therapy, for example, may have an atypical streptococcal or staphylococcal lesion due to impairment of the normal inflammatory response, or an unusual organism may be causal. Pain can be the most prominent feature, and etiologic considerations should include, in addition to streptococci and staphylococci, members of the Enterobacteriaceae (*E. coli, Klebsiella-Enterobacter-Serratia, Proteus* spp.); a variety of nonfermentative gram-negative bacilli (*Pseudomonas, Aeromonas, Acinetobacter* spp., etc.); and the indigenous anaerobic flora (peptostreptococci, *Bacteroides* spp., *C. perfringens,* etc.)[4,18,19]

Portal of Entry

In laboratory animal models the pathogenic potential of many microorganisms depends, to a considerable extent, on the route of administration. Similarly, the character of the cutaneous inflammatory response to certain bacteria will be influenced by how the organisms reached the involved area. Thus, the vascular wall is often the primary site of skin involvement during bacteremic infection; hemorrhage or thrombosis with infarction is the initial manifestation. This is followed somewhat later by the cellular reaction expected from direct inoculation of the bacteria into the skin. Local inflammation and suppuration commonly accompany direct bacterial invasion of the skin, and these may, in turn, give rise to systemic spread via the rich cutaneous vascular network. Certain bacteria can produce bacteremia or distant lesions without evoking an obvious inflammatory response at the portal of entry [e.g., *Yersinia pestis, Streptobacillus moniliformis* (rat-bite fever)] even in a nonimmunosuppressed host. Occasionally a devastating *S. pyogenes* septicemia has followed closely upon an innocuous pinprick or abrasion that has not induced a significant local lesion. Table 186-1 lists those bacterial species most frequently involved in pyogenic infections of the skin.

Specific Features of Host Inflammatory Response to Cutaneous Infection

Morphologic Aspects   In view of the relatively few cell types present in the skin, it is surprising that such a variety of rather distinctive clinical responses to various bacterial infections has been catalogued. In most instances it is the anatomic site of the infection and the attendant inflammatory response pattern, rather than the specific pathogen, that provides the characteristic clinical picture. The following brief examples are expanded upon in Chapter 187.

IMPETIGO.   The very superficial location of the infection, with vesicopustule formation just beneath the stratum corneum, is the specific clinical feature.

FOLLICULITIS.   This represents a circumscribed infectious process that originates in the hair follicle and is defined by its anatomic features. It may be located superficially in the follicle or may extend more deeply to produce perifollicular inflammation.

FURUNCLE (BOIL).   This infection either complicates an antecedent folliculitis or develops as a deep-seated nodule about a hair follicle. The distinctive pathologic change results from its relation to the hair follicle; thus it does not occur in glabrous areas such as the palms. The deep location and its containment by the relatively

TABLE 186-1
Bacteria Involved in Cutaneous Infection*

I. Primary cutaneous inflammation
  A. Gram-positive bacteria
    1. *Staphylococcus aureus*
    2. Streptococci
      a. Group A
      b. Other than group A (groups B, C, D, G, particularly)
      c. Anaerobic streptococci (peptostreptococci) alone or mixed infection
    3. *Bacillus anthracis*
    4. *Corynebacterium diphtheriae*
    5. Anaerobic diphtheroids (*Propionibacterium acnes*)
    6. Aerobic diphtheroids (*Corynebacterium minutissimum*)
    7. *Clostridium perfringens*
    8. *Erysipelothrix rhusiopathiae* (erysipeloid)
    9. *Borrelia burgdorferi* (Lyme disease)
  B. Gram-negative bacteria
    1. *Francisella tularensis* (tularemia)
    2. *Pasteurella multocida* (infected animal bites)
    3. Enterobacteriaceae (*Escherichia coli, Klebsiella-Enterobacter*)
    4. Nonfermentative gram-negative bacilli (*Pseudomonas, Acinetobacter, Aeromonas*)
    5. *Malleomyces mallei* (glanders)
    6. *Pseudomonas pseudomallei*
    7. *Bacteroides* spp.
    8. *Haemophilus influenzae*
    9. Halophyllic vibrios (*Vibrio parahemolyticus, V. vulnificus,* etc.)
II. Bacteremic spread to skin
  A. Gram-positive bacteria
    1. *Staphylococcus aureus*
    2. Group A streptococci
    3. In bacterial endocarditis (acute)
      a. *Staphylococcus aureus*
      b. Streptococci (group A, group D especially)
    4. *Listeria monocytogenes*
    5. Histotoxic clostridia, primarily *Clostridium septicum*
  B. Gram-negative bacteria
    1. *Neisseria meningitidis*
    2. *Neisseria gonorrhoeae*
    3. *Pseudomonas aeruginosa*
    4. *Salmonella typhi*
    5. *Brucella* spp.
    6. *Haemophilus influenzae*
    7. *Streptobacillus moniliformis*
    8. *Pseudomonas pseudomallei* (melioidosis)
    9. *Bartonella bacilliformis*
III. Bacteremia or systemic manifestation from innocuous skin portal
  A. Gram-positive bacteria
    1. Group A streptococci
    2. *Staphylococcus aureus*
    3. *Bacillus anthracis* (rarely)
    4. *Clostridium tetani*
    5. *Leptospira interrogans* serotypes
  B. Gram-negative bacteria
    1. *Yersinia pestis* (plague)
    2. *Francisella tularensis*
    3. *Streptobacillus moniliformis* (rat-bite fever)
    4. *Brucella* spp.
    5. *Pseudomonas pseudomallei*

*Exclusive of mycobacterial and treponemal infections.

thick dermis prevent spontaneous early drainage to the surface and contribute to the hard, nodular, painful character of the lesion.

CARBUNCLE.   This is a larger, more deep-seated extension of a furuncle with infection spreading under and between fibrous tissue septums, forming a whole series of interconnected abscesses. Drainage occurs through a number of projecting necrotic points in the skin.

CELLULITIS.   This is an acute, inflammatory process in the skin, particularly in the deeper subcutaneous tissues. Because of the subcutaneous location, the borders of the lesion are usually indistinct, in contrast to the sharply defined margin of erysipelas (see below).

Interplay of Morphology and Specific Bacterial Properties

Erysipelas   This is a superficial inflammatory process of the skin and subjacent lymphatics, characterized by marked edema of the dermis and extensive invasion of connective tissue usually, but not exclusively, caused by *S. pyogenes* (gpA). The rapid progression of the process and the prominence of edema of the affected skin relate to the involvement of superficial lymphatics and the biologic properties of the microorganisms.

Influence of Hypersensitivity to Bacterial Antigens on Inflammatory Reaction in Skin

Although the introduction of certain bacteria in large numbers into the skin will elicit a local inflammatory reaction, the character and extent of this response may be modified by various host factors (e.g., leukopenia). In the case of skin infections due to *Staph. aureus,* the tendency to recur is often quite striking. Initial lesions are usually suppurative and localized, whereas subsequent infections, when due to the same antigenic strain, may have more prominent surrounding cellulitis. The immunologic response to *Staph. aureus* has been suggested as a factor in this altered inflammatory response.[20]

Vasculitis as a Cutaneous Response to Systemic Infection

Inflammatory changes in and about small blood vessels in the skin may occur in a variety of bacteremic infections in the absence of obvious localization of bacteria at these sites. The macular, papular, nodular, and petechial lesions of chronic meningococcemia show such histologic changes. The lesions of erythema nodosum have a prominent element of vasculitis even though the initiating infection (e.g., streptococcal pharyngitis) is distant and has a suppurative character. The Osler nodes and petechiae of subacute bacterial endocarditis (SBE), due to viridans streptococci, probably provide the best examples of this association of small-vessel vasculitis with bacteremia. Histologically, these lesions are more suggestive of vasculitis than of emboli. The occasional development of such lesions in profusion, localized to the lower extremities, supports the concept of cutaneous vascular inflammation rather than embolization.

Shwartzman Phenomenon in Bacteremia due to Gram-Negative Bacteria

The experimental production of a characteristic hemorrhagic necrotic reaction in the skin and in certain other organs (e.g., kidney) of the rabbit has been a subject of considerable interest for many years.[21-23] This interest has been heightened because of the gross similarity of these lesions to those that occur during the course of

meningococcemia. The Shwartzman reaction is divided into two types: local and generalized (see "Pathogenicity of the Microorganism," above). In the former, the initial ("preparatory") skin injection and the second ("eliciting" or "provocative") intravenous injection may consist of LPS from different bacterial sources. It has even been possible to elicit the reaction when the second injection has consisted of certain nonbacterial materials such as washed antigen-antibody precipitates. Following the preparatory injection, there is polymorphonuclear leukocyte "cuffing" about the small veins locally. The intravenous eliciting reaction produces peripheral vasoconstriction, particularly in the veins at the prepared skin site. Leukocyte-rich thrombi form, with ensuing occlusion of capillaries and small veins, producing necrosis of vessel walls and resulting hemorrhage. This form of response probably represents a type of hyperreactivity to LPS that can be neutralized by homologous antiserum.[24] Results of treatment of gram-negative bacteremia with human antiserum to LPS core have been encouraging in a limited clinical study.[25] Recently, treatment of patients with gram-negative bacillary bacteremia and septic shock with a human IgM monoclonal antibody (HA-1A) against the lipid A moiety of LPS has been reported, in one study, to improve survival.[26]

The typical histologic lesion of the generalized Shwartzman reaction consists of fibrin deposition within capillaries. This is particularly striking in the kidney, where characteristic bilateral renal cortical necrosis occurs. Alterations in levels of fibrinogen and other clotting factors have been found, and it appears that intravascular coagulation is the initiating event in this generalized phenomenon. Polymorphonuclear leukocytes appear to have a central role in the pathogenesis of this process, as prior induction of leukopenia with nitrogen mustard will prevent both the local and generalized reaction. Circulating fibrin monomers and inhibition of fibrinolysis appear to be essential as their absence will obviate the reaction.[22] It is possible to substitute cortisone for the preparatory injection of endotoxin in the production of the generalized Shwartzman reaction. This role of corticosteroids in the experimental Shwartzman reaction has raised questions regarding the use of these agents as adjuncts in the treatment of shock in acute meningococcemia and other gram-negative bacteremias.

It is tempting to attribute the hemorrhagic necrotic lesions that occur in meningococcemia (and gram-negative bacillary bacteremias) to this phenomenon.

Classification of Bacterial Infections of the Skin

The introduction, over the past three decades, of a variety of specific antibiotic and chemotherapeutic agents has effected rather striking changes in the management of bacterial infections. Indeed, with the availability of these drugs, the focus of attention has been on the determination of the specific bacterial cause so that the proper choice of antibacterial agent can be made. This has rendered unnecessary, and even obsolete, descriptions of some of the dermatologic entities whose status depended on imprecise morphologic criteria rather than on etiologic considerations. Consequently, from the pragmatic (therapeutic) viewpoint, the approach has been to consider and classify these infections by bacterial causation, e.g., infections due to gram-positive organisms and infections due to gram-negative organisms. Although the foregoing classification is helpful from the therapeutic point of view, there is still need for a system of categorizing bacterial infections of the skin so that the dermatologic picture will provide the basis for consideration of the most likely bacterial etiologies. To this end, the classification of skin infections as (1) primary infections (pyodermas), (2) secondary infections, and (3) cutaneous manifestations of systemic bacterial disease seems warranted. Primary bacterial infections are produced by the invasion of ostensibly normal skin by a *single* species of pathogenic bacteria. In such infections there is usually no doubt as to the primary etiologic role of the specific agent in the pathogenesis of the lesion. Treatment aimed at the bacterial pathogen almost universally results in cure of the lesion. Impetigo, erysipelas, and furunculosis are familiar examples of primary cutaneous infections. Contrastingly, secondary infections develop in areas of already damaged skin. Although the bacteria present did not produce the underlying skin disorder, their proliferation and subsequent invasion of surrounding areas may aggravate and prolong the disease. Such secondary infection may occur when the skin has been broken or bruised, primarily involved with mycotic or viral infections, or altered by sensitivity reactions or medications. In contrast to the primary infections, the secondary infections often show a *mixture* of organisms on culture, and not infrequently it is impossible to determine which plays the major role. Pathogenic organisms such as *Staph. aureus* and *S. pyogenes* (gpA), generally considered transients on the skin, can colonize such lesions and sometimes produce active secondary infection. The appearance of these lesions is not characteristic, in comparison to the primary pyodermas, but is largely dependent on the nature of the underlying skin condition. The result of antibacterial treatment is much less clear-cut, as it has no effect on the underlying process.

Table 186-2 presents an outline of infections involving the skin in a classification based upon the appearance of the lesions. In this outline, specific entities that will be discussed elsewhere in detail are described only by the appropriate chapter reference, and the more common bacterial etiologic agents are noted. This table refers exclusively to bacterial infections. Two of the categories identified in Table 186-2 present a broad differential diagnosis and warrant special consideration. These consist of infectious gangrene/gangrenous cellulitis (Table 186-3) and crepitant soft tissue wounds and cellulitis (Table 186-4). In addition, an uncommon group of infections present as chronic nodular, and sometimes ulcerative, granulomatous lymphangitis (with or without an evident initiating chancriform lesion) of a distinctive character. Because definition of the specific microbial etiology may be difficult without careful epidemiologic history, biopsy with culture, and special stains of histologic sections, and an awareness of the broad variety of microorganisms (fungi, bacteria, mycobacteria, protozoa) that may be involved, a listing of the possible causes is presented separately (Table 186-5).

Diagnostic Strategies

Direct Examination of Aspirates and Biopsies

Identification of bacteria from skin lesions may provide important information as to the cause of cutaneous infections, whether primary or secondary to systemic processes. The presence of "normal skin flora" can confuse interpretation of these cultures. All too often, the finding of a potential pathogen such as *Staph. aureus* or *P. aeruginosa* is equated with the presence of disease. It is important to recall that damaged skin (operative incisions, exudative dermatoses, etc.) provides a medium for proliferation of certain bacte-

ria. Only by correlating the clinical appearance of the lesion (local suppuration, cellulitis, etc.) with the bacteriologic data can one reach the proper decision concerning the presence of a bacterial disease. Examination of a Gram-stained smear of material from a suspected skin infection can guide decisions on early antibiotic therapy before a cultural diagnosis is made. For these reasons, bacteriologic investigation is an important part of the initial evaluation of patients with skin lesions and includes: (1) appropriate sampling, (2) interpretation of Gram-stained smears, and (3) use of selective growth media for culturing.

Gram's stain provides a very rapid method for examining a sample for number and type of bacteria, as well as for the character of the inflammatory exudate. Skin contaminants are usually recognized by being present in low concentration, often clumped in characteristic microcolonies (growth in skin crypts) and usually not associated with polymorphonuclear leukocytes. Obtaining an appropriate specimen for microscopic study and culture requires care to avoid contamination. Results of needle aspiration of superficial erysipelas lesions have been generally unrewarding. Slightly better, but still limited, results have been obtained on aspiration culture of lesions of cellulitis. Aspirates from the advancing edge of cellulitis yielded positive cultures in only 10 percent of patients, and culture of skin punch biopsy specimens taken from the leading edge were positive in only 20 percent of patients in the study by Hook et al.[27] Positive cultures (beta-hemolytic streptococci and coagulase-positive *Staph. aureus*) were more likely in patients with apparent primary sites of infection associated with the cellulitis. In another study of needle aspiration cultures of the leading edge of erythema in patients with cellulitis, the yield of pathogenic bacteria was low (15 percent) as well.[28] Others have suggested a greater yield on needle aspiration of the leading edge of cellulitis when performed in patients with underlying conditions such as diabetes mellitus and neoplastic disease.[29] A higher yield (about 50 percent) for positive cultures has been reported in aspirates obtained from the point of maximal inflammation than that (5 percent) obtained from the leading edge of cellulitis in children.[30] Our personal experience is in accord with published results for sampling *deeper* cellulitic lesions and bullae associated with acute infections. Findings on needle aspiration when positive can provide an immediate useful guide to therapy. If sterile saline is injected into a lesion that initially yields no aspirate, bacteriostatic agent-free solutions should be employed. In circumstances where no data are available from needle aspiration, a surgical biopsy may yield information that is life-saving. Local lesions of the skin and subcutaneous tissues in immunocompromised patients should always be biopsied if aspiration fails to define a pathogen.[4] Encouraging results have been reported in a series of patients with suspected necrotizing fasciitis who had biopsies done to confirm the diagnosis early in the course of this devastating infection.[31]

Methods of Culture of Skin Material

All samples for culture should be planted routinely on blood agar and inoculated into a tube of thioglycollate (anaerobic) broth. Additional media should be used as indicated by clinical findings and evaluation of the Gram-stained smear and frozen sections if a biopsy is done. If cutaneous diphtheria is a consideration, Loeffler or tellurite agar should be inoculated. When gram-negative rod infection is suspected, an EMB or MacConkey plate is used; a chocolate agar or Thayer-Martin plate incubated in a CO_2 atmosphere is indicated for suspected meningococcal or gonococcal lesions; a blood

TABLE 186-2
Bacterial Infections Involving the Skin*

I. Primary pyodermas
 A. Impetigo—group A streptococci and *Staphylococcus aureus* (see Chap. 187)
  1. Impetigo contagiosa—primarily due to group A streptococci
  2. Impetigo bullosa—primarily due to *Staph. aureus* of phage group II
 B. Folliculitis (see Chap. 187)
  1. Superficial
   a. Follicular impetigo (Bockhart's impetigo)—usually due to *Staph. aureus* but in conditions of lowered host resistance (corticosteroid and antibiotic therapy, etc.) may be due to a variety of opportunistic organisms (gram-negative coliform bacilli, particularly). The lesions consist of small globular pustules, each located about a hair.
   b. *Pseudomas aeruginosa*—associated with water exposure (see Chap. 188)
  2. Deep
   a. Sycosis barbae (usually *Staph. aureus*)
   b. Pyoderma faciale (usually *Staph. aureus*)
   c. Folliculitis decalvans—rare condition, producing a scarring type of alopecia of the scalp, attributed to chronic infection with *Staph. aureus,* but this etiologic role is not clearly established
 C. Furuncles and carbuncles (*Staph. aureus*) (see Chap. 187)
 D. Paronychia—usually of bacterial origin due to *Staph. aureus* or group A streptococci; rarely, a chronic form of the disease is due to *Pseudomonas aeruginosa*
 E. Ecthyma—group A streptococci initially (see Chap. 187); may also be due to *Pseudomonas* (see Chap. 188)
 F. Erysipelas—group A streptococci (see Chap. 187)
 G. Cellulitis—group A streptococci, *Staph. aureus,* and, less commonly, a variety of other organisms, especially in compromised hosts (see Chap. 187)
 H. Lymphangitis—usually group A streptococci, but occasionally *Staph. aureus* and other organisms (see Chap. 187)
 I. Erythrasma—*Corynebacterium minutissimum* (see Chap. 187)
II. Secondary bacterial infections
 A. Complicating preexisting skin lesions, such as:
  1. Burns (see information in Chap. 126)
  2. Eczematous dermatitis, including exfoliative erythrodermas—*Staph. aureus* or group A streptococci (see Chap. 121)
  3. Chronic ulcers (varicose, traumatic—these are particularly liable to invasion by gram-negative organisms [*Escherichia coli, Proteus, Pseudomonas*] as well as by anaerobic streptococci, *Bacteroides* or *Clostridium perfringens* [either alone or as a "synergistic" infection])
  4. Dermatophytoses—usually a *Staph. aureus* or groups A, B, C, G streptococcal infection
  5. Traumatic lesions (abrasions, infestations, insect bites, etc.)—*Pasteurella multocida, Corynebacterium diphtheriae, Staph. aureus,* gpA streptococcus
  6. Vesicular or bullous eruptions (varicella, pemphigus, etc.)—*Staph. aureus,* gpA streptococcus
 B. Distinctive dermatologic clinical entities
  1. Secondary folliculitis
   a. Acne conglobata—*Propionibacterium acnes, Staph. aureus, Proteus,* and other coliforms (particularly after antibiotic therapy)
   b. Hidradenitis suppurativa—*Staph. aureus, Proteus* and other coliforms, peptostreptotocci, *Bacteroides*
   c. Perifolliculitis capitis abscedens et suffodiens (dissecting cellulitis of the scalp)—essentially the same process as acne conglobata or hibradenitis suppurativa pathogenetically, but occurring on the scalp; secondary infection occurs with similar varieties of bacteria to the other two entities
  2. Infectious eczematous dermatitis (usually *Staph. aureus;* occasionally group A streptococci)
  3. Intertrigo (*Staph. aureus;* occasionally group A streptococci)
  4. Pilonidal and sebaceous cysts—in addition to coliform organisms; particularly in infected pilonidal cysts, there is a high incidence of anaerobic streptococci and *Bacteroides* spp.
  5. Infectious gangrene
   a. Clostridial gas gangrene (see Chap. 187)
   b. Streptococcal gangrene (see Chap. 187)
   c. Fusospirochetal gangrene—a synergistic necrotizing infection due to anaerobic organisms such as *Fusobacteria, Bacteroides, Peptostreptococcus,* and usually associated with malnutrition, agranulocytosis, and other debilitating diseases or local injury
   d. Gangrenous balanitis and perineal phlegmon—an acute cellulitis with gangrene located in the area of the genitalia, usually due to group A streptococci, enteric bacteria (*E. coli, Klebsiella, Proteus*) or anaerobes, and most commonly seen in diabetic patients
  6. Necrotizing ulcers
   a. Pyoderma gangrenosum (see Chap. 93)—many organisms (*Staph. aureus,* microaerophilic streptococci, *Proteus, E. coli,* and *Pseudomonas*) may be found secondarily in such lesions, which complicate ulcerative colitis. Proof of a primary bacterial cause of the lesions of pyoderma gangrenosum is lacking. In fact, cultures of early lesions are usually sterile.
    (1) Pyoderma vegetans—a variant of pyoderma gangrenosum with hypertrophic lesions.
   b. Progressive bacterial synergistic gangrene (Meleney) (See Chap. 187)—peptostreptococci or microaerophilic streptococci plus a second organism (*Staph. aureus, Proteus*)
   c. Synergistic necrotizing cellulitis—mixed anaerobic and facultative infection often involving skin and muscle in addition to fascia, seen in diabetic and debilitated elderly patients.
   d. Decubitus ulcer (*Staph. aureus,* coliforms, *Pseudomonas, Bacteroides, Clostridium perfringens*)
   e. Tropical ulcer
   f. Phagedenic ulcers—small, circumscribed ulcers with black necrotic centers and erythematous areolas complicating preexisting lesions (e.g., varicella); lesions look like end stage of ecthyma; usually *Staph. aureus* or *Pseudomonas* cultured from lesions
  7. Necrotizing fasciitis due to group A streptococci or to mixed anaerobic and facultative bacteria (*Bacteroides,* peptostreptococci, coliforms, etc. (See Chap. 187)

TABLE 186-2 *(Continued)*

III. Cutaneous involvement in systemic bacterial infections (exclusive of venereal diseases and mycobacterial infections)
   A. Bacteremia (see II in Table 186-1)
   B. Cutaneous lesions without direct microbial involvement of the skin
      1. Bacterial endocarditis (see Chap. 187)
         a. Subacute (usually viridans streptococci or other non-group A streptococci): petechiae; Osler's nodes; Janeway lesions, uncommonly
         b. Acute (most commonly *Staph. aureus*): petechiae; purulent purpura; Janeway lesions
      2. Streptococcosis (group A)
         a. Scarlet fever (see Chap. 187)
         b. Purpura fulminans (see Chap. 187)
      3. Chronic meningococcemia—a variety of sterile macular, papular, nodular, and hemorrhagic lesions occurring intermittently (see Chap. 188)
      4. *S. aureus* including toxin-mediated syndromes—"scalded skin" (see Chap. 187) and "toxic shock" (see Chap. 187)
      5. Erythema nodosum (see Chap. 108) associated with a variety of drugs and infections; among the latter are those due to group A
        streptococci, *Mycobacterium tuberculosis*, *M. leprae*, *Yersinia enterocolitica*, *Legionella pneumophila*
      6. Bacterids
      7. Purpura
IV. Infections due to unusual organisms (see Chap. 190)
   A. Cutaneous diphtheria
   B. Listeriosis (*Listeria monocytogenes*)
   C. Animal-borne or associated diseases
      1. *Bacillus anthracis*—cutaneous anthrax (malignant pustule)
      2. Pasteurelloses and related organisms
         a. *Francisella tularensis* (tularemia)
         b. *Pasteurella multocida*—produces infection at site of animal (usually cat) bite
         c. *Yersinia pestis* (plague)
      3. *Brucella* (*abortus, suis,* or *melitensis*)—skin lesions are rare in this systemic disease
      4. Rat-bit fever
         a. *Streptobacillus moniliformis* (Haverhill fever)
         b. *Spirillum minus* (sodoku)—exanthem with primarily erythematous macules, some papules, and nodules
      5. Erysipeloid (*Erysipelothrix rhusiopathiae*)
      6. Leptospirosis, including Weil's disease—*Leptospira interrogans* serotypes
      7. Glanders (*Pseudomonas mallei*)
   D. Diseases associated with particular geographic locations
      1. Bartonellosis (Carrion's disease)—due to *Bartonella bacilliformis*
      2. Melioidosis (*Pseudomonas pseudomallei*)
      3. Infections due to *Vibrio* spp. (*V. vulnificus, V. parahaemolyticus*)
      4. Rhinoscleroma (*Klebsiella rhinoscleromatis*)

*The localization and morphologic changes seen often constitute the initial clue in arriving at a specific etiologic cause of the skin lesion(s).

agar plate incubated in an oxygen-free atmosphere should be used if anaerobic streptococci, clostridia, or *Bacteroides* is suspected. When the skin lesions are thought to be part of a generalized infection, blood cultures should also be obtained prior to institution of antibiotic therapy.

Other Diagnostic Procedures

Fluorescent Antibody The practical use of this procedure in bacterial diseases of the skin is of limited availability at this time. Spirochetes can be demonstrated (by the direct or indirect techniques) in chancres. *N. gonorrhoeae, Actinomyces israelii, Legionella* spp., and mycobacterial isolates have been identified by this rapid method. At the present time these techniques are still in the stage of experimental development for identifying the etiologic agent in most infections of the skin.[32]

Other Immunologic Methods A variety of serologic tests may be helpful in the diagnosis of bacterial infections of the skin, particularly in those where the cutaneous manifestations are secondary to systemic disease (e.g., "rose spots" of typhoid fever). In general, these tests have proved of value in confirming a diagnosis that has already been made by direct bacteriologic identification of the offending organism (e.g., *Salmonella* agglutination, *Brucella* agglu-tination, agglutination reaction for tularemia, leptospirosis complement fixation or agglutination tests). As in any serologic test, a fourfold or greater rise in titer during the course of the illness is considered significant.

Antibiotic Therapy

The selection of the appropriate antibiotic should be made initially on the basis of the appearance of the skin lesion, the characteristics of any systemic illness, and a Gram-stained smear of material from a lesion if available to sample. Culture results and susceptibility testing of the isolated pathogen(s) are usually available within 48 h (Table 186-6).

Dosage: Methods of Administration—Excretion

Primary cutaneous infections of mild to moderate severity can be treated with local measures, topical drugs, oral antibiotics, or by a combination of these methods. Extensive infections of the skin, with or without systemic manifestations, should be vigorously treated with parenteral antibiotics in adequate dosage.

TABLE 186-3
Differential Diagnosis of Infectious Gangrene and Gangrenous Cellulitis

	Progressive bacterial synergistic gangrene	Synergistic necrotizing cellulitis	Streptococcal gangrene	Gas gangrene	Necrotizing cutaneous mucormycosis	Bacteremic pseudomonas gangrenous cellulitis	Pyoderma gangrenosum
Predisposing conditions	Surgery; draining sinus	Diabetes common	Occasionally diabetes or myxedema; after abdominal surgery	Local trauma	Diabetes; corticosteroid therapy	Burns, immunosuppression	Ulcerative colitis; rheumatoid arthritis
Pain	Prominent	Prominent	Prominent	Prominent	Minimal	Mild	Moderate
Systemic toxicity	Minimal	Marked	Marked	Very marked	Variable	Marked	Minimal
Course	Slow	Rapid	Very rapid	Extremely rapid	Rapid	Rapid	Slow
Fever	Minimal or absent	Moderate	High	Moderate or high	Low grade	High	Low grade
Anesthesia of lesion	−	−	±	−	+	±	−
Crepitus	−	Often present	−	+	−	−	−
Appearance of the involved area	Central shaggy, necrotic ulcer surrounded by dusky margin and erythematous periphery	Crepitant cellulitis; thick, copious, foul-smelling "dishwater" drainage from scattered areas of skin necrosis	Necrosis of subcutaneous tissue and fascia; black necrotic "burned" appearance of overlying skin	Marked swelling; yellow-bronzed discoloration of skin; brown bullae; green-black patches of necrosis; serosanguinous discharge	Usually a central black necrotic area with purple raised margin; also may be present as just a black ulcer	A sharply demarcated necrotic area with black eschar and surrounding erythema, resembling a decubitus ulcer; may evolve from initial hemorrhagic bulla	Begin as bullae, pustules, or erythematous nodules that ulcerate deeply; often multiple, large and coalesce; usually on lower extremities or abdomen
Etiology	Microaerophilic streptoccus plus *Staph. aureus* (or *Proteus* sometimes)	Usually a mixture or organisms (e.g., *Bacteroides*, peptostreptococci, *E. coli*, etc.)	Primarily group A streptococci; when develops secondary to abdominal surgery, enteric bacteria also involved	*C. perfringens* (occasionally other clostridia)	*Rhizopus, Mucor, Absidia*	*P. aeruginosa*	Not an infection; may be confused with such due to secondary colonization by Enterobacteriaceae, microaerophilic streptococci, *P. aeruginosa*, *Staph. aureus*

SOURCE: GL Mandell et al (eds): *Principles and Practice of Infectious Diseases*, 3d ed. New York, Churchill Livingstone, 1990, chap 74, with permission.

A number of factors must be considered in administering antibiotics: oral treatment may be limited by absorption and gastrointestinal disturbances; hypotension, severe thrombopenia, and extensive skin disease can prohibit the intramuscular route; the proper drug selected may be suitable for administration only by a specific route. Caution must be exercised in administering intramuscular medications to avoid sterile or infected abscesses. When the intravenous route is used, a needle or "heparin-lock" is preferred. Percutaneous catheters should be changed frequently (every 2 to 3 days) and all line-skin sites kept clean with a topical antibiotic ointment and sterile dressing that is changed daily.

The excretory pattern of a given antibiotic should always be considered in order to avoid toxic accumulation in the face of specific organ malfunction (e.g., use of aminoglycosides or vancomycin in the presence of renal impairment).

Toxicity

The toxicity of antibiotics should be considered on an individual basis, but some problems are applicable to all antibiotics. Hypersensitivity reactions are relatively common and may include skin rashes, fever, or more severe manifestations such as acute anaphy-

laxis or exfoliative erythrodermas. The penicillins and sulfonamides are particularly likely to produce these problems. Questions regarding previous drug allergy should be asked whenever any antibiotic is to be administered. All antibiotics alter the relative kinds and absolute numbers of the indigenous flora, and superinfection may result from their use, especially with broad-spectrum agents like the cephalosporins. Gastrointestinal disturbances and oral mucous membrane lesions are the major nonspecific types of problems encountered with alteration of the flora, although changes also occur on burn surfaces and other lesions. There are numerous other untoward reactions (renal, hematologic, hepatic, nervous system) to antibiotics that may represent acceptable risks if the reasons for use of these drugs are compelling (see footnotes, Table 186-6). The responsibility is the physician's, however, to be aware of the usual and unusual manifestations of toxicity to any of the antibiotics used and to be alert to possible novel effects in individual patients.

Antibiotic Resistance due to "R" Factors

Transferable resistance to multiple antibiotics has emerged as a widespread problem. Extrachromosomal genetic elements (R plasmids) in bacteria are the basis for such resistance.[33] Prolonged anti-

TABLE 186-4
Differential Diagnosis of Crepitant Soft Tissue Wounds*

	Clostridial cellulitis	Nonclostridial anaerobic cellulitis	Gas gangrene	Streptococcal myositis	Necrotizing fasciitis†	Infected vascular gangrene	Synergistic necrotizing cellulitis‡	Noninfectious causes of gas in tissues
Predisposing conditions	Local trauma or surgery	Diabetes mellitus; preexisting localized infection	Local trauma or surgery	Local trauma	Diabetes mellitus; abdominal surgery; perineal infection	Peripheral arterial insufficiency	Diabetes mellitus; cardiorenal disease; obesity; perirectal infection	Mechanical effects of penetrating trauma; injuries involving use of compressed air; entrapment of air under loosely sutured wounds or under ulcers; irrigation of wounds with hydrogen peroxide; intravenous catheter placement
Incubation period	Usually over 3 days	Several days	1–2 days	3–4 days	1–4 days	>5 days	3–14 days	Less than an hour
Onset	Gradual	Gradual or rapid	Acute	Not as rapid as gas gangrene	Acute	Gradual	Acute	Usually present immediately after trauma or manipulation; may not be recognized until examined several hours later
Pain	Mild	Mild	Marked	Occurs late; marked	Moderate or severe	Variable	Severe	Mild
Swelling	Moderate	Moderate	Marked	Moderate	Marked	Moderate or marked	Moderate or marked	Slight or absent
Skin appearance	Minimal discoloration	Minimal discoloration	Yellow-bronze; dark bullae; green-black patches of necrosis	Erythema	Erythematous cellulitis; areas of skin necrosis	Discolored or black	Scattered areas of skin necrosis	Only those due to initiating trauma
Exudate	Thin, dark	Dark pus	Serosanguinous	Abundant seropurulent	Seropurulent	0	"Dishwater" pus	0
Gas	++++	++++	++	±	++	+++	++	Variable but present; does not extend
Odor	Sometimes foul	Foul	Variable; slighty foul or peculiar sweet	Slight; "sour"	Foul	Foul	Foul	0
Systemic toxicity	Minimal	Moderate	Marked	Only late in course	Moderate or marked	Minimal	Marked	0
Muscle involvement	0	0	++++	+++	0	Dead	++	0

*In addition to the causes of crepitant infections in this table, *Aeromonas hydrophila* myositis may be associated with gas in soft tissues.
†The term *necrotizing fascitis* is employed here to designate forms of this syndrome of streptococcal gangrene.
‡Synergistic necrotizing cellulitis is essentially the same process as Type I necrotizing fasciitis. Since the former occasionally extends to involve muscle it is given a separate designation here; however, the two processes are clinically indistinguishable in most instances.
NOTE: ±, rarely present: ++, present to mild extent; +++, present to moderate extent; ++++, extensive.
SOURCE: GL Mandell et al (eds): *Principles and Practice of Infectious Diseases,* 3d ed. New York, Churchill Livingstone, 1990, chap 74, with permission.

biotic therapy, especially in a closed environment like a hospital, may select R-factor-carrying members of the indigenous flora (e.g., in the gastrointestinal tract), which may subsequently transfer this property to a recently acquired organism. In this way, antibiotic resistance to chloramphenicol, tetracycline, and kanamycin conferred by a plasmid in *E. coli* can be transferred during mating to a *Klebsiella* or *Salmonella* strain. As a consequence, organisms with greater intrinsic pathogenicity can become antibiotic-resistant as well. This phenomenon and its practical consequences have been verified in a number of studies.[34]

R plasmids (R factors) have been found in most pathogenic gram-negative bacteria, including *E. coli, Klebsiella, Proteus,* *Pseudomonas, Salmonella,* and *Shigella.* They are responsible also for high-level resistance to the penicillins (penicillinase plasmids) and cephalosporins.

In recent years R-factor-associated antibiotic resistance has been identified in group A and group D streptococci as well as in *Haemophilus influenzae* and *N. gonorrhoeae,* all important pathogens in skin as well as systemic infection.

Topical Antibacterial Agents

Topical antibacterial agents have frequently been used to prevent, as well as to suppress, bacterial growth in burns and other open

TABLE 186-5
Causes of Chronic Nodular (Granulomatous) Sporotrichoid Lymphangitis

Principal considerations	Relative frequency as etiology
Fungi	
Sporothrix schenkii (causative agent of sporotrichosis) (see Chap. 196)	Occasional
Mycobacteria	
Mycobacterium marinum (causative agent of "swimming pool granuloma" (see Chap 191)	Occasional
Mycobacterium kansasii	Rare
Bacteria	
Nocardia brasiliensis	Rare
Nocardia asteroides	Very rare
Francisella tularensis	Very rare
Staphylococcus aureus	Very rare
Botryomycosis (*Staph. aureus*)	Very rare
Protozoa	
Leishmania brasiliensis and *Leishmania mexicana* (causative agents of new world cutaneous leishmaniasis (see Chap. 225)	Occasional

lesions. Their greatest usefulness has been when employed along with strict aseptic techniques in preventing percutaneous line sepsis. These agents are capable of inhibiting the local flora, but, as is true of all antibiotics, they have a relatively limited spectrum of activity, which favors the emergence of bacterial resistance during treatment. In addition, topical drugs may precipitate contact dermatitis and can be absorbed to toxic levels. Furthermore, there has been very little evidence that they add a great deal therapeutically.[35] An exception to this is the result, in burn patients, of the use of sulfamylon (mafenide) acetate cream or of 0.5% silver nitrate solution. However, even with these broad-spectrum agents, resistant species, such as *Clostridium perfringens, Klebsiella,* and *Enterobacter,* may emerge as the dominant potential pathogen of the local flora.

Among the most useful topical antibacterial agents are acetic acid (1 to 5%) for *Pseudomonas* nail and toe web infections and bacitracin (500 units per milliliter or gram) for selected superficial *Staph. aureus* and streptococcal lesions. Neomycin (0.5% ointment) and gentamicin (0.17% cream) may be useful in selected patients when mixed gram-negative bacteria require local suppression. Mupirocin (2%) ointment has antibacterial activity against various streptococci and *Staph. aureus*. It is a safe and effective

TABLE 186-6
Selection of Antibiotics

Infecting agent	Drug of choice[a,b] First	Alternatives
Gram-positive cocci:		
Staphylococcus aureus or *epidermidis*		
Non-penicillinase-producing	Penicillin G or V[c]	Cephalosporin,[d] erythromycin,[e] vancomycin,[f] clindamycin[g]
Penicillinase-producing	Penicillinase-resistant penicillin[h]	Same as above for non-penicillinase-producing strains
Methicillin-resistant[i]	Vancomycin(± rifampin or gentamicin)[j]	Ciprofloxacin, trimethoprim-sulfamethoxazole[k] + rifampin
Streptococci		
Groupable (e.g., group A)	Penicillin G or V	Erythromycin, clindamycin, cephalosporin, vancomycin
Group D (enterococcus)[l] (systemic infection)	Penicillin G (or ampicillin) + gentamicin	Vancomycin + gentamicin
Nongroupable (viridans streptococci, etc.)	Penicillin G	Cephalosporin, erythromycin, vancomycin
Anaerobic	Penicillin G	Clindamycin, erythromycin, chloramphenicol,[m] cephalosporin
Gram-positive bacilli:		
Bacillus anthracis (anthrax)	Penicillin G	A tetracycline,[n] erythromycin
Borrelia burgdorferi (Lyme disease spirochete)	Tetracycline	Penicillin G, ceftriaxone, erythromycin, doxycycline
Clostridium perfringens (gas gangrene)	Penicillin G	Chloramphenicol, metronidazole,[o] clindamycin
Corynebacterium, including *C. diphtheriae*	Erythromycin	Penicillin G
Erysipelothrix rhusiopathiae	Penicillin G	Erythromycin
Leptospira spp.	A tetracycline	Penicillin G
Listeria monocytogenes	Ampicillin (or penicillin G) ± gentamicin	Trimethoprim-sulfamethoxazole, chloramphenicol, tetracycline, erythromycin
Gram-negative cocci:		
Neisseria gonorrhoeae:		
Non-beta-lactamase producing	Penicillin G	Ampicillin, amoxicillin, cefoxitin,[p] ceftriaxone, cefotaxime, ciprofloxacin
Beta-lactamase producing	Ceftriaxone	Cefoxitin,[p] cefotaxime, ciprofloxacin, chloramphenicol

TABLE 186-6 *(Continued)*

Neisseria meningitidis (meningococcus)	Penicillin G	Chloramphenicol, a sulfonamide (only if sulfonamide susceptibility of organisms is proved by appropriate quantitative methods), cefuroxime, cefotaxime, ceftriaxone
Gram-negative bacilli:		
Aeromonas hydrophilia	Gentamicin	Chloramphenicol, ciprofloxacin, trimethoprim-sulfamethoxazole
Escherichia coli (systemic infection)	Ampicillin (amoxicillin); for severe infections, ceftriaxone or cefotaxime	Ampicillin-sulbactam, broad-spectrum penicillin,[q] trimethoprim-sulfamethoxazole, chloramphenicol, aminoglycosides,[r] ciprofloxacin
Francisella tularensis (tularemia)	Streptomycin[s]	Chloramphenicol, a tetracycline
Haemophilus influenzae	Cefotaxime or ceftriaxone	Ampicillin (if beta-lactamase negative), cefuroxime, trimethoprim-sulfamethoxazole, chloramphenicol, amoxicillin-clavulanate
Klebsiella pneumoniae	Cephalosporin (1st or 2d generation); 3d generation cephalosporin for serious infections	Aminoglycosides (gentamicin, tobramycin, amikacin), chloramphenicol, ciprofloxacin, aztreonam, imipenem
Klebsiella rhinoscleromatis	Tetracycline followed by trimethoprim-sulfamethoxazole	Streptomycin
Legionella pneumophila	Erythromycin	Add rifampin; ciprofloxacin
Pasteurella multocida	Penicillin G (ampicillin)	A tetracycline, chloramphenicol, 3d generation cephalosporin, ciprofloxacin
Proteus mirabilis	Ampicillin	Cephalosporin, gentamicin, imipenem, aztreonam
Proteus—other species	Gentamicin	Cefotaxime, broad-spectrum penicillin, chloramphenicol, ciprofloxacin, trimethoprim-sulfamethoxazole, imipenem, aztreonam
Pseudomonas aeruginosa (systemic infection)	Tobramycin[t] + broad-spectrum penicillin[r]	Ceftazidime, amikacin, imipenem, aztreonam, ciprofloxacin
Pseudomonas pseudomallei	Ceftazidime + trimethoprim-sulfamethoxazole	Doxycycline, imipenem, chloramphenicol
Salmonella typhi	Chloramphenicol	Ampicillin, trimethoprim-sulfamethoxazole, ciprofloxacin
Salmonella spp.	Ampicillin (amoxicillin)	Chloramphenicol, trimethoprim-sulfamethoxazole, ciprofloxacin
Streptobacillus moniliformis (rat-bite fever)	Penicillin G ± streptomycin	Cephalosporin, a tetracycline
Yersinia pestis	Streptomycin	Chloramphenicol, a tetracycline, gentamicin

[a] Drug susceptibility testing of bacterial isolates should be performed coincident with the initial choice of an antibacterial agent. Dosages of drugs of choice are given in Chaps. 187, 189, and 190.

[b] Not all drugs are approved by the Food and Drug Administration for treatment of that infection.

[c] When used in low doses, hypersensitivity reactions (5 to 8 percent) are the major problem. Massive therapy (10 to 50 million units daily) for life-threatening gram-positive coccal infections may produce toxicity from hyperkalemia, central nervous system irritation (seizures), and Coombs-positive hemolytic anemia.

[d] A first-generation cephalosporin is preferred. Gram-negative organisms resistant to first-generation cephalosporins *may* be susceptible to second- or third-generation agents. Hypersensitivity reactions, reversible neutropenia, and, very rarely, nephrotoxicity at high doses are chief toxic problems.

[e] Side effects are uncommon except for gastrointestinal disturbances. Rarely, hypersensitivity reactions (fever or rash) and hepatotoxicity occur (with the oral erythromycin estolate preparation). Administered orally or intravenously.

[f] Causes phlebitis and fever, hypersensitivity reactions; and in the presence of renal failure or excessive dosage, ototoxicity. Should be given slowly (~1 h) i.v. to avoid histamine-like systemic effects.

[g] Gastrointestinal irritation (diarrhea) is common; rare pseudomembranous colitis and granulocytopenia.

[h] The semisynthetic penicillins (oxacillin, nafcillin, cloxacillin, dicloxacillin) cross-react with penicillin G in evoking hypersensitivity reactions.

[i] Methicillin-resistant strains are *always* cephalosporin-resistant too.

[j] Nephrotoxic and ototoxic, especially in the aged and in the presence of preexisting renal disease. Administered under the closest medical supervision with monitoring of renal (blood levels), auditory, and vestibular function.

[k] Trimethoprim-sulfamethoxazole may cause bone marrow toxicity due to either, or to combined drug effects. Hypersensitivity reactions, gastrointestinal upset, hepatitis, and anemias (megaloblastic and hemolytic) are occasionally encountered.

[l] For endocarditis or other serious infection.

[m] Chloramphenicol may depress bone marrow function, one or all elements being affected. This drug should be given only under close medical surveillance; check differential smear and white blood count;

look for a rise in serum iron levels as an indication of toxicity. Associated with the "gray syndrome" when administered without appropriate reduction in dosage to premature infants or neonates.

[n] All the tetracyclines are potent antianabolic drugs, gastrointestinal irritants; potentially hepatotoxic when doses exceed 2.0 g daily parenterally; discolor and alter organogenesis of primary and secondary teeth; photosensitizing. Outdated preparations may be nephrotoxic. All tetracyclines stimulate changes in the indigenous microflora favoring emergence of infections due to yeast and resistant staphylococci and gram-negative bacilli.

[o] Bactericidal for *Bacteroides* and *Clostridia* but variably effective in anaerobic and microaerophilic streptococcal infections.

[p] Second- (cefoxitin, cefamandol) and third- (cefotaxime, ceftazidime, cefoperazone) generation cephalosporins are occasionally drugs of choice, guided by susceptibility testing, for selected infections. In addition to cross-hypersensitivity with first-generation agents, they may cause superinfections due to their broad-spectrum activity and some may cause bleeding complications.

[q] Includes carbenicillin, ticarcillin, piperacillin, azlocillin, mezlocillin, which have similar toxic and hypersensitivity effects to penicillin. In addition they may cause bleeding, due to platelet dysfunction, as well as add a significant sodium load.

[r] Gentamicin has been used as a prototype aminoglycoside. In many situations tobramycin (or amikacin) may be selected, depending on the in vitro susceptibility of the organism involved or on known nosocomial patterns of aminoglycoside resistance.

[s] Vestibular toxicity, especially in the aged and those with renal failure, as well as hypersensitivity reactions.

[t] Tobramycin (or gentamicin) and broad-spectrum penicillins should not be mixed in the same intravenous infusion. Tobramycin has toxicity identical to gentamicin.

treatment of impetigo.[36] A number of broad-spectrum antiseptics are also available for topical use, combining antibacterial with non-irritating properties. Povidone-iodine (Betadine) is effective against most gram-positive and gram-negative bacteria but does not persist in the skin to provide a residual action. Chlorhexidine gluconate (4% solution) is an antiseptic that combines broad antibacterial properties with prolonged action due to local accumulation. An alcoholic preparation is especially effective, is not appreciably absorbed into the blood, and generally is not irritating to the skin.[37,38] These broad-spectrum antiseptics can be used prophylactically or to treat local wounds and superficially infected dermatoses.

The topical therapy of burns is discussed in Chap. 126.

References

1. Johnson JE II et al: Studies on the pathogenesis of staphylococcal infection. I. The effect of repeated skin infection. *J Exp Med* **113**:235, 1961

2. Leyden JJ et al: Experimental infections with group A streptococci in humans. *J Invest Dermatol* **75**:196, 1980

3. Elek SD: Experimental staphylococcal infections in the skin of man. *Ann NY Acad Sci* **65**:85, 1956

4. Wolfson JS et al: Dermatologic manifestations of infection in the compromised host. *Annu Rev Med* **34**:205, 1983

5. Kligman AM et al: Bacteriology. *J Invest Dermatol* **67**:160, 1976

6. Sauder DN: Immunology of the epidermis: Changing perspectives (editorial). *J Invest Dermatol* **81**:185, 1983

7. Shinefield HR et al: Bacterial interference, in *Skin Bacteria and Their Role in Infection*, edited by HI Maibach, G Hildick-Smith, New York, McGraw-Hill, 1965, chap 17

8. Elin RJ et al: Biology of endotoxin. *Annu Rev Med* **27**:127, 1976

9. Wolff SM: Biological effects of bacterial endotoxins in man. *J Infect Dis* **128**:S259, 1973

10. Young LS et al: University of California/Davis interdepartmental conferences on gram-negative septicemia. *Rev Infect Dis* **13**:666, 1991

11. Tracey KJ et al: Cachectin/tumor necrosis factor. *Lancet* **1**:1122, 1989

12. Dinarello CA et al: New concepts on the pathogenesis of fever. *Rev Infect Dis* **10**:168, 1988

13. Michie HR et al: Detection of circulating tumor necrosis factor after endotoxin administration. *N Engl J Med* **318**:1481, 1988

14. Cannon JG et al: Circulating interleukin-1 and tumor necrosis factor in septic shock and experimental endotoxin fever. *J Infect Dis* **161**:79, 1990

15. Waage A et al: Association between tumor necrosis factor in serum and fatal outcome in patients with meningococcal disease. *Lancet* **1**:355, 1987

16. Girardin E et al: Tumor necrosis factor and interleukin-1 in the serum of children with severe infectious purpura. *N Engl J Med* **319**:397, 1988

17. Tracey KJ et al: Anti-cachectin/TNF monoclonal antibodies prevent septic shock during lethal bacteraemia. *Nature* **330**:662, 1987

18. Bornstein DL et al: Anaerobic infections—review of current experience. *Medicine (Baltimore)* **43**:207, 1964

19. Fields BN et al: The so-called "paracolon" bacteria: A bacteriologic and clinical reappraisal. *Am J Med* **42**:89, 1967

20. Cluff LE: The inflammatory response of skin to bacterial invasion, in *Skin Bacteria and Their Role in Infection*, edited by HI Maibach, G Hildick-Smith, New York, McGraw-Hill, 1965, p 95

21. Thomas L: The effects of cortisone on bacterial infection and intoxication, in *Effects of ACTH and Cortisone upon Infection and Resistance*, edited by G Shwartzman, New York, Columbia Univ Press, 1953, chap 12

22. Lipinski B et al: The organ distribution of ^{125}I-fibrin in the generalized Shwartzman reaction and its relation to leukocytes. *Br J Haematol* **28**:221, 1974

23. Horn RG: Evidence for participation of granulocytes in the pathogenesis of the generalized Shwartzman reaction: A review. *J Infect Dis* **128**:S134, 1973

24. Braude AI et al: Treatment and prevention of intravascular coagulation with antiserum to endotoxin. *J Infect Dis* **128**:S157, 1973

25. Ziegler EJ et al: Treatment of gram-negative bacteremia and shock with human antiserum to a mutant *Escherichia coli*. *N Engl J Med* **307**:1225, 1982

26. Ziegler EJ et al: Treatment of gram-negative bacteremia and septic shock with HA-1A human monoclonal antibody against endotoxin. *N Engl J Med* **324**:431, 1991

27. Hook EW III et al: Microbial evaluation of cutaneous cellulitis in adults. *Arch Intern Med* **146**:295, 1986

28. Sachs MK: The optimum use of needle aspiration in the bacteriologic diagnosis of cellulitis in adults. *Arch Intern Med* **150**:1907, 1990

29. Kielhofner MA et al: Influence of underlying disease process on the utility of cellulitis needle aspirates. *Arch Intern Med* **148**:2451, 1988

30. Howe PM et al: Etiologic diagnosis of cellulitis: Comparison of aspirates obtained from the leading edge and the point of maximal inflammation. *Pediatr Infect Dis J* **6**:685, 1987

31. Stamenkovic I et al: Early recognition of potentially fatal necrotizing fasciitis. The use of frozen-section biopsy. *N Engl J Med* **310**:1689, 1984

32. Bernard P et al: Streptococcal cause of erysipelas and cellulitis in adults. A microbiologic study using a direct immunofluorescence technique. *Arch Dermatol* **125**:779, 1989

33. Elwell LP et al: Plasmid-mediated factors associated with virulence of bacteria to animals. *Annu Rev Microbiol* **34**:465, 1980

34. Falkow S: *Infectious Multiple Drug Resistance*. London, Pion, 1975

35. Editorial: Topical antibiotics. *Br Med J* **1**:1494, 1977

36. Goldfarb J et al: Randomized clinical trial of topical mucopirocin versus oral erythromycin for impetigo. *Antimicrob Agents Chemother* **32**:1780, 1988

37. Editorial: Chlorhexidine and other antiseptics. *Med Lett Drug Ther* **18**:85, 1976

38. Lilly HA et al: Detergents compared with each other and with antiseptics as skin "degerming" agents. *J Hyg (Lond)* **82**:89, 1979

Bibliography

Abramowicz M (ed): The choice of antimicrobial drugs. *Med Letter* **34**:871, 1992

Arai K et al: Cytokines: Coordinators of immune and inflammatory responses. *Annu Rev Biochem* **59**:783, 1990

Davis BD et al (eds): *Microbiology,* 4th ed. New York, JB Lippincott, 1990

Goodman LS, Gilman A: *The Pharmacologic Basis of Therapeutics,* 8th ed. New York, Macmillan, 1990

Mandell GL et al (eds): *Principles and Practice of Infectious Diseases,* 3d ed. New York, Wiley, 1990

Rosebury T: *Microorganisms Indigenous to Man.* New York, McGraw-Hill, 1962

CHAPTER 187

Morton N. Swartz and Arnold N. Weinberg

Infections due to Gram-Positive Bacteria

The majority of the primary pyodermas are due to infection with either group A streptococci or *Staphylococcus aureus*. A variety of clinical pictures may be presented by infections due to these organisms, depending on local anatomic considerations and on host factors.

Streptococcal Skin Infections

General Features

Bacteriology and Pathogenic Aspects   In view of the association of specific groups of streptococci with certain types of infections and postinfectious sequelae,[1] an understanding of the various categories of streptococci has practical value. The presence of many varieties of streptococci as commensals on mucous membranes, in the intestinal tract, and occasionally on the skin makes difficult the assessment of the significance of their isolation from the skin. Although essentially all group A streptococcal strains are beta hemolytic, not all streptococci producing beta hemolysis belong to group A. The Lancefield classification of streptococcal groups (A–T) is based on the C carbohydrate antigens of the cell wall. Because serologic grouping of streptococci is not generally available, a reasonably accurate presumptive test for group A streptococci is necessary. Bacitracin disk ("Taxos S") sensitivity has been widely used; group A organisms are, almost without exception, susceptible to the low concentration of bacitracin contained in the disk, whereas streptococci of other groups are often resistant.

The primary invasive streptococcal pyodermas are due almost exclusively to group A streptococci. The invasive potential of group A streptococci is usually considerably greater than that of other streptococci. Nonsuppurative postinfectious complications have been limited to those produced by group A organisms. Thus, group A streptococcal infections merit antibiotic treatment and eradication.

The presence of streptococci of other groups than A in skin lesions may represent either surface colonization or actual secondary infection in preexisting dermatoses. Group C and group G streptococci have occasionally been implicated in impetiginous lesions, secondarily infected dermatitis, wound infections with lymphangitis, and even in erysipelas and cellulitis. Streptococci of groups B and D have been isolated from infections of skin lesions secondary to ischemia or venous stasis and have particularly involved the perineal area and operative wound sites. As with most secondary infections, those due to group B and group D streptococci are frequently mixed infections with enteric bacteria or *Staph. aureus*. Group B streptococci may cause cellulitis in neonates and occasionally in adults. Group L streptococci (often carried by pigs, cattle, and poultry) have been responsible for impetigo, secondarily infected wounds, and paronychias in meat handlers.[2]

The hallmarks of invasive group A streptococcal infection are profuse edema, rapid spread through tissue planes, and the relatively thin character of the exudative response. Infection may spread via the lymphatic or hematogenous routes and result in a fulminant clinical course.

Epidemiology of Group A Streptococcal Infections   Group A streptococci are usually spread by transfer of organisms from an infected person or carrier through close personal contact. The major source of such spread is from patients with infections in the upper respiratory tract. A variety of skin lesions and puerperal sepsis may also be the source of intrahospital spread of infection. Group A streptococci introduced into the operating room in the form of a minor skin infection, or even through perianal carriage by a surgeon or anesthetist, may be responsible for an epidemic of streptococcal wound infections. In the past, milk- and food-borne epidemics occurred but they no longer represent a major problem.

Although viable streptococci are found on a variety of articles in the immediate surroundings of a carrier or infected individual, the major factor in spread is not the articles in the contaminated environment but rather proximity to an individual disseminating the organisms. Because many patients with group A streptococcal skin infections harbor the same organism in their pharynxes, they are, for both reasons, potential sources for spread of infection in a hospital. Particular care must be taken to prevent spread of infection by isolating such patients until antibiotic therapy has rendered them noncontagious.

Despite the salutary effects of penicillin on morbidity and mortality, the overall incidence of streptococcal disease has probably not decreased. Localized epidemics have continued to appear periodically. During such outbreaks, the carrier and infection rates in the community increase. Carriers may then enter the hospital environment. In this way, streptococci can be introduced into surgical incisions and lacerations and initiate infection. Operative infections, because of the rapidity with which they progress, may be more severe and dramatic than those caused by staphylococci.

After recovery (without antibiotic treatment) from streptococcal pharyngitis, some individuals may carry the organism for prolonged periods. The carrier state may also occur in the absence of overt antecedent infection. Ten to forty percent of school children carry group A streptococci in the throat.

Delayed Nonsuppurative Sequelae The incidence of invasive complications (lymphangitis, suppurative lymphadenitis, bacteremia) of streptococcal infections of the skin has decreased in the antibiotic era. Besides these pyogenic complications, a variety of nonsuppurative complications (acute rheumatic fever, acute glomerulonephritis, erythema nodosum) may follow group A streptococcal infections. Distinct differences exist between acute rheumatic fever and acute glomerulonephritis in the site of the antecedent infection, the length of the latent period, and the streptococcal serotypes involved.[3,4] Acute rheumatic fever may be a complication of group A streptococcal pharyngitis or tonsillitis, but it does not occur following streptococcal skin infections. In contrast, acute nephritis may follow infection of either the skin or the upper respiratory tract. The latent period between streptococcal pharyngitis and the onset of rheumatic fever is 2 to 3 weeks; whereas the latent period for pharyngitis-associated nephritis is about 10 days. A longer latent period, about 3 weeks, is characteristic of acute nephritis associated with streptococcal pyoderma. Group A streptococci are subclassified into over 80 subtypes based on antigenicity of their M proteins (fibrillar structures extending out from the cell surface). While there is as yet no strong evidence of an association between infection with any specific group A serotypes and the subsequent development of rheumatic fever, several serotypes (particularly mucoid strains of types 1, 3, 18) have been implicated in a few outbreaks of streptococcal sore throat complicated by this sequela.[5] However, there is a clear relationship between infection with certain serotypes and the subsequent occurrence of nephritis—the so-called nephritogenic serotypes. Type 12 is the classic serotype responsible for pharyngitis-associated acute nephritis, but other serotypes such as 1, 4, 25, and 49 have been implicated. The pyoderma-associated nephritogenic strains gener-

ally belong to different serotypes: types 2, 49, 55, 57, and 60.[4,6] The skin rather than the pharynx is the principal site of antecedent streptococcal infection causing nephritis, and impetigo is now the most common form of such predisposing skin infections. Major epidemics of pyoderma-associated nephritis have been observed in communities, and multiple cases of overt and subclinical nephritis have occurred within families. The frequency of acute glomerulonephritis following infection with a known nephritogenic strain is 10 to 15 percent; the frequency of rheumatic fever following an unrecognized or inadequately treated pharyngeal infection by any serotype of group A streptococcus is 2 to 3 percent or less. The distinction between nephritogenic strains of streptococci and other strains of streptococci that might be associated with rheumatic fever can be seen in studies from Trinidad, a hyperendemic area for pyoderma-associated nephritis. There, the streptococcal serotypes causing outbreaks of nephritis differed from the serotypes associated with sporadically occurring cases of acute rheumatic fever in the same population.[5]

Recent work suggests that several biologic properties are associated with broad categories of Group A streptococci. Most M proteins fall into one of two antigenic classes based on the presence (class I) or absence (class II) of a highly conserved antigenic domain. Almost all rheumatic fever outbreak-associated strains belong to serotypes of class I and require a precursor nasopharyngeal infection. However, because many class I serotypes are associated with impetigo as well and because class II serotypes are responsible for both upper respiratory and skin infections, the class of M protein alone is not a determinant of tissue tropism. Current evidence indicates differences among class I organisms that may relate to their capacities to induce rheumatic fever: class I nasopharyngeal isolates appear to lack human IgG-binding activity, whereas nearly all impetigo isolates of the same class bear human IgG receptors.[7]

Antibody Response and Immunity The immune response to group A streptococcal infection depends to a large measure on site of infection. Following streptococcal pharyngitis, specific antibodies develop to many of the extracellular enzymes of the streptococci. Eighty-five percent of patients with acute rheumatic fever and a proven preceding streptococcal infection will have an elevated or increasing antistreptolysin O (ASO) titer. The serologic demonstration of an antecedent streptococcal infection in this situation can be increased to virtually 100 percent by the simultaneous testing for several other antibodies (antihyaluronidase, anti-DNase B). Antibodies to extracellular products, with the exception of antibody to the erythrogenic toxin of scarlet fever, appear to have no effect on the manifestations of illness. Streptococcal immunity is type-specific (but not group-specific), long-lasting, and depends on the production of bactericidal antibodies to the specific M proteins of the over 80 different serotypes of group A organisms. Although recurrent pharyngeal infections due to the same serotype are most unusual, repeated clinical infections due to different types are not uncommon. Early treatment of streptococcal upper respiratory tract disease with antibiotics may suppress the appearance of type-specific antibody (and immunity) as well as the development of antibody to the extracellular products of the organism.

In contrast to pharyngeal infections, the ASO response with streptococcal skin infections or pyoderma-associated nephritis is feeble. To define the latter serologically, anti-DNase B (or antihyaluronidase) titers are much more reliable. Although pyoderma strains of streptococci produce M proteins and although type-specific antibody may develop in patients with pyoderma-associated nephritis, the frequency of production of such antibodies and their role in protection against reinfection are unclear. While pharyngeal reinfection with the same streptococcal serotype is probably unusual, some evidence suggests that the same serotype can be associated with repeated episodes of pyoderma.

Specific Diseases due to Group A (and Other) Streptococci

Superficial Pyoderma   Streptococcal pyodermas include all types of superficial streptococcal skin infections except erysipelas, i.e., impetigo, ecthyma, and secondary infections of preexisting skin lesions (e.g., insect bites, abrasions, eczema).

Impetigo (Contagiosa)   DEFINITION.   Impetigo is a primary, initially vesicular, later crusted superficial infection of the skin. It is commonly due to group A streptococci. *Staph. aureus* is the etiology of bullous impetigo (see "Staphylococcal Skin Infections" below).

EPIDEMIOLOGY AND BACTERIOLOGY.   Impetigo is a highly communicable infection predominantly of preschool-age children. Its peak seasonal incidence is in the later summer and early fall. Group A streptococcus has been the single most common isolate from impetigo in the United States.[8] Mixtures of streptococci and *Staph. aureus* have been isolated from about half the patients with nonbullous impetigo, but the role of *Staph. aureus* here appears to have been a subsidiary one. In nonbullous impetigo, *Staph. aureus* alone has been isolated from fewer than 10 percent of cases. In other parts of the world staphylococcal impetigo has been reported as more frequent.[9] Recently, the bacteriology of impetigo has been reported to be changing in the United States, with an increasing role suggested for *Staph. aureus*.[10] The relative roles for these two species in any analysis will probably vary, depending on the presence or absence of hyperendemic or epidemic streptococcal disease in the locality and on the nature of the cases selected for study. Nongroup A (groups B, C, and G) streptococci may be responsible for rare cases of impetigo; group B streptococci are associated with impetigo in the newborn. Whereas many different serotypes of group A streptococci may cause pharyngitis, a limited number of newly described types predominates in impetigo (types 49, 52, 53, 55–57, 59, and 61).

PATHOGENESIS AND PATHOLOGY.   Group A streptococci appear on normal skin of children about 10 days prior to the development of impetigo and they are not recovered from the nose and throat of the same patients until 14 to 20 days after skin acquisition of the organism. Streptococci are recovered from the respiratory tract of about 30 percent of children with skin lesions, but there is no clinical evidence of streptococcal pharyngitis. Thus, the sequence of spread in a given patient is from normal skin to lesions and eventually to respiratory tract.[11] In contrast, the sequence of spread of *Staph. aureus* (in cases of impetigo in which it is the only organism isolated) is from nose to normal skin (about 11 days later) and to skin lesions (after another 11 days).

Following acquisition of a streptococcal strain on normal skin from another family member or close contact (whose skin was already colonized or contained a pyoderma), minor traumas (insect bites, abrasions) predispose to the appearance of infected lesions.

The inflammatory process of impetigo is superficial, with a unilocular vesicopustule located between the stratum corneum above and the stratum granulosum below. This is usually situated near the opening of a hair follicle. Organisms, as well as leukocytes and epithelial cell debris, fill the vesicle.

CLINICAL MANIFESTATIONS.   *History*   Crowding, poor hygiene, and neglected minor skin trauma contribute to the spread of streptococcal impetigo in families. Minor outbreaks have also occurred among athletes involved in contact sports. Although the majority of cases occur in children, particularly of preschool age, young adults are also affected. Impetigo may complicate preexisting skin lesions such as scabies, varicella, or eczema. Systemic response is minimal unless complications occur.

Cutaneous Lesions   Streptococcal impetigo begins as transient, thin-roofed, small vesicles, sometimes with a small inflammatory halo. Pustulation rapidly occurs. Vesicles and pustules easily rupture. The purulent discharge subsequently dries, forming a thick, soft, golden-yellow "stuck-on" crust (Figs. 187-1, 187-2), the hallmark of impetigo. Removal reveals a red, weeping surface that rapidly becomes encrusted again. Exposed areas of the skin such as the face and the extremities are most commonly involved, but, in infants particularly, the lesions may occur anywhere. Satellite lesions appear, spread by autoinoculation. The individual lesions rarely exceed 1 to 2 cm, but occasionally the crusted lesions may be large through coalescence of lesions. As the process progresses peripherally, central healing occurs, producing an appearance that sometimes mimics that of a superficial fungal infection. The lesions are superficially located, do not ordinarily produce ulcerations or deep infiltration, and heal without scarring or atrophy. Regional lymphadenopathy is present in the majority of cases. Pruritus and burning may occur, but the lesions are usually painless.

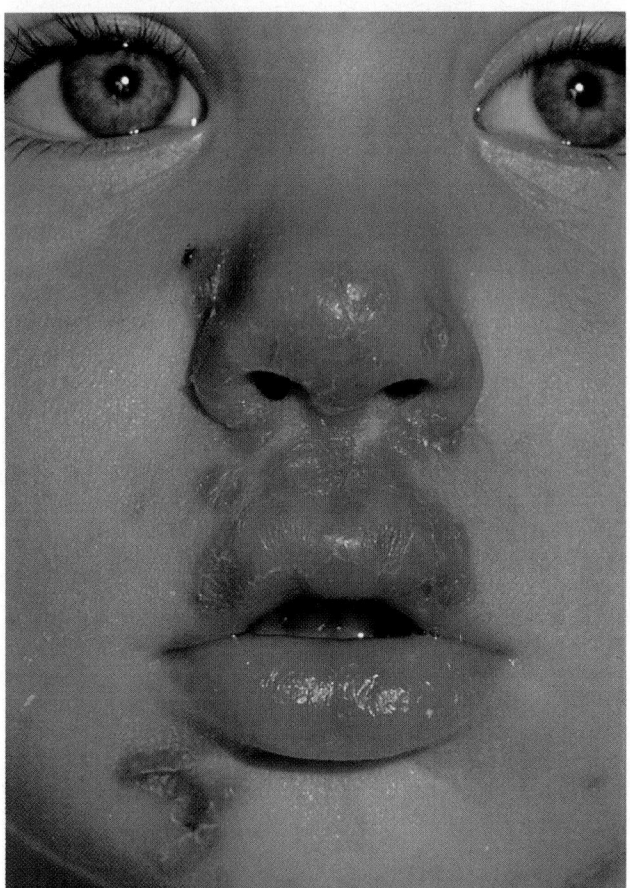

FIGURE 187-1   Impetigo. Some intact vesicles can still be recognized but most have dried to form yellowish crusts. (*Courtesy of K. Wolff, M.D.*)

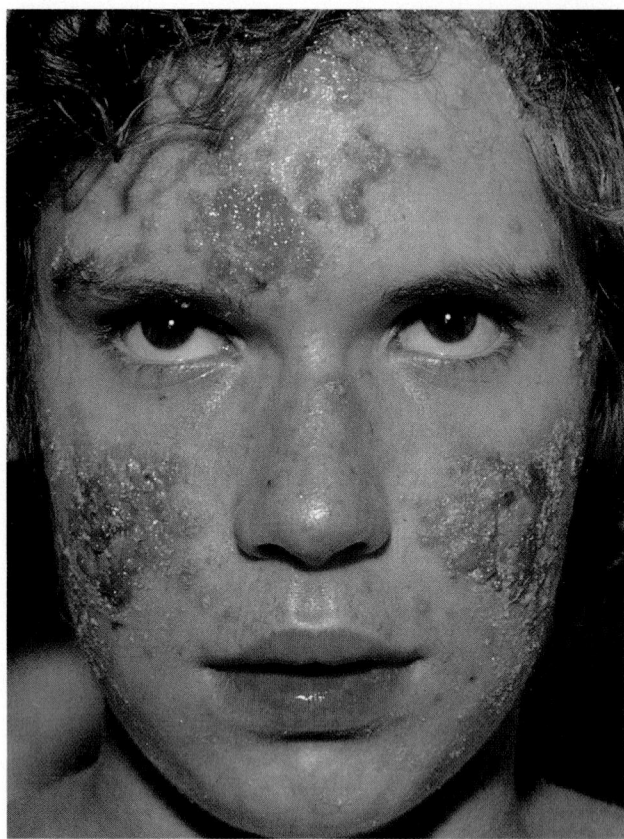

FIGURE 187-2 Impetigo. Yellowish-greyish, stuck-on crusts with inflammatory halo in the face of a young girl. (*Courtesy of K. Wolff, M.D.*)

Classical staphylococcal impetigo (see below) is characterized by intact bullae that lack a surrounding zone of erythema or by ruptured bullae with thin, "varnishlike," light brown crusts.

LABORATORY FINDINGS. A slight leukocytosis is sometimes present, more commonly in those cases due to streptococci. A Gram-stained smear of early vesicle fluid reveals gram-positive cocci. Culture of the weeping area or of the area beneath an unroofed crust reveals group A streptococci or a mixture of streptococci and *Staph. aureus* (particularly from older crusted lesions). The lesions of bullous impetigo are usually caused by *Staph. aureus* of phage group II.

DIAGNOSIS AND DIFFERENTIAL DIAGNOSIS. The diagnosis usually presents no difficulties when the lesions are seen at the stage of crusting. The initial vesicular lesion may resemble varicella, but the later crusted stage of varicella is readily distinguished by its hard, dark brown character. Occasionally, a fungal infection is suggested by the central clearing of a cluster of lesions. However, the vesicles in tinea circinata are usually very small and peripheral, and thick crusts are not formed. Herpes simplex may mimic impetigo, particularly as the contents of the vesicles become turbid. A drug eruption due to iodides and bromides may mimic a pyoderma, but it is usually not as superficial a process as impetigo and resembles a folliculitis.

COURSE AND PROGNOSIS. Untreated, the process may persist and new lesions may develop over a course of several weeks; thereafter the infection tends to resolve spontaneously unless there is some underlying cutaneous disorder such as eczema. Complicating deep cellulitis or bacteremia are most unusual. The major serious sequela is nephritis.

TREATMENT. Penicillin is the drug of choice in the treatment of streptococcal pyoderma, administered either as a single injection of long-acting benzathine penicillin (300,000 to 600,000 units for children; 1,200,000 for adults) or orally (25,000 to 100,000 units/ kg per day in divided doses every 6 h for 10 days). Erythromycin (30 to 50 mg/kg per day by mouth in divided doses every 6 h for children; 250 to 500 mg by mouth every 6 h for adults administered for 10 days) is a suitable alternative drug in patients allergic to penicillin. However, it should be noted that over 25 percent of group A streptococcal strains have become resistant to erythromycin in areas (Japan, Finland) where this antibiotic has been extensively used (or overused) for a variety of indications. Whether administration of penicillin is effective in reducing the incidence of pyoderma-associated nephritis remains a moot point. Although the latent period following impetigo is longer than that following pharyngeal infection, the mildness of the illness delays or negates the seeking of medical attention. Topical treatment (removal of dirt, crusts, and debris, by soaking with soap and water) is a valuable adjunct. Although penicillin treatment will clear the lesions of impetigo and prevent recurrence for a short time, streptococci can persist on or newly colonize normal skin in spite of this therapy.

Although topical agents (bacitracin, neomycin-bacitracin, polymyxin B-neomycin) have been used as primary treatment for streptococcal impetigo, parenteral or oral penicillin has been the most uniformly effective form of therapy.[12] However, prophylactic application of bacitracin-polysporin-neomycin ointment to insect bites and abrasions in children in an endemic area during the peak season for skin infections may be useful in preventing superficial streptococcal pyodermas.[13] Another topical antibiotic, mupirocin, in ointment form, active against *Staph. aureus* and streptococci and capable of reaching superficial skin layers, has recently been shown to be as effective as erythromycin in the treatment of impetigo that does not involve extensive areas or the scalp.[14,15]

Ecthyma DEFINITION. This disease is very similar to the superficial vesiculopurulent pyoderma, impetigo. It begins in the same fashion, but the process extends more deeply, penetrating through the epidermis to produce a shallow ulcer. Group A streptococci often initiate the disease or complicate preexisting superficial ulcers. However, lesions having the same ultimate appearance may be produced in the course of *Pseudomonas* septicemia (see Chap. 188).

CLINICAL MANIFESTATIONS. The lesions tend to occur most commonly on the lower extremities of children or neglected elderly patients following minor trauma such as insect bites or excoriations. Poor hygiene is an element in pathogenesis. Multiple ecthymatous ulcers on the ankle and dorsum of the foot were the most common pyodermas seen in the army in the rice paddies of Vietnam.[16] The initial lesion is a vesicle or vesicopustule with an erythematous base and surrounding halo. This enlarges over several days to a diameter of 0.5 to 3 cm and then crusts over. The ulcer has a "punched out" appearance when the dirty grayish-yellow crust and purulent material are removed. The margin of the ulcer is indurated, raised, and violaceous (Fig. 187-3), and the granulating base extends deeply into the dermis. The lesions are slow to heal, requiring several weeks of antibiotic treatment for resolution. Problems of spread by autoinoculation or by insect vectors and of poststreptococcal sequela (glomerulonephritis) are the same as with impetigo.

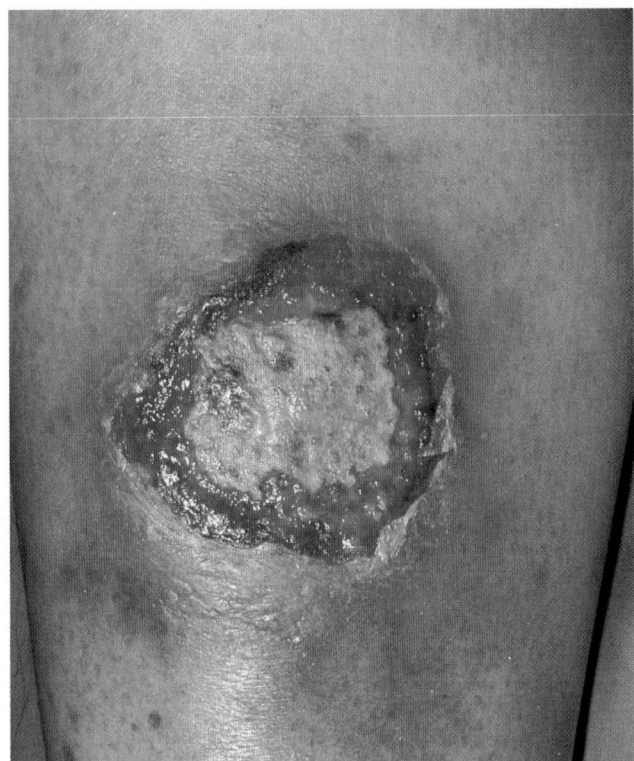

FIGURE 187-3 Ecthyma. Ulcer with a necrotic base and an inflammatory margin. (*Courtesy of K. Wolff, M.D.*)

Erysipelas DEFINITION. Erysipelas is a characteristic type of superficial cellulitis of the skin with marked lymphatic-vessel involvement due to group A (or very uncommonly group C or G) streptococci. Group B streptococci may cause erysipelas in the newborn. Rarely, a similar clinical picture may be produced by infection with *Staph. aureus*.

CLINICAL MANIFESTATIONS. *History* Erysipelas occurs most commonly in infants, very young children, and older adults; thus, not in the age groups most frequently involved in streptococcal respiratory tract infections. Predisposing circumstances include ethanol abuse, diabetes mellitus, immunosuppression, and venous or lymphatic obstruction. The process often begins in a small break in the skin, which is usually no longer evident by the time the infection has developed. The source of streptococci is commonly the upper respiratory tract, and a history of such an antecedent infection is obtained in one-third of patients. However, when the skin lesion is present, nose and throat cultures may no longer reveal streptococci. In cases of erysipelas developing after surgery or in wounds, organisms may have been transmitted from the nose, throat, or hands of attendants, the patient, or other patients. In the past, the skin of the face and head was the most common site of localization, but currently the extremities, particularly the legs, are involved most frequently.[17] In the neonate the lesion may take origin in an infection of the umbilical stump, spread rapidly over the anterior abdominal wall, and eventuate in bacteremia. In some neonates the omphalitis may be a more localized process persisting for weeks as an indolent infection at the umbilical stump. In adults, the portal of entry may be at the margin of an ulcer, at a site of chronic edema, in an area of devitalized skin, or about a dermatophytic lesion. Patients with nephrotic syndrome appear to be particularly

susceptible to erysipelas. The initial lesion begins as a small area of redness that may be easily overlooked. The febrile onset of the disease may occur quite abruptly (even before the skin lesion is recognized) and may be associated with a frank rigor. The process evolves rapidly, and the patient appears quite ill with high fever.

Cutaneous Lesions The lesion has a characteristic brawny, edematous, indurated (peau d'orange) appearance and spreads peripherally. It is hot, shiny, and bright red and has an advancing elevated margin that is sharply demarcated from the surrounding skin (Fig. 187-4). The involved area becomes painful only at this stage. The periphery of the lesion may appear irregular because of projections of the inflammatory process (Fig 187-5). As the lesion advances, no islands of normal skin are left behind. Small vesicles and occasionally large bullae may develop in the lesion, particularly in more severe infections. Petechiae and even ecchymoses may appear during the active stage. With healing, local superficial desquamation of the skin occurs.

A common form of erysipelas involves the bridge of the nose and one or both cheeks ("butterfly" distribution). The process usually halts at the hairline of the scalp or beard.

LABORATORY FINDINGS. A leukocytosis of 15,000 or greater occurs. Bacteriologic study is frequently of little help. Group A streptococci may be isolated from the throats of a few patients. Culture of the surface of the involved skin usually does not yield

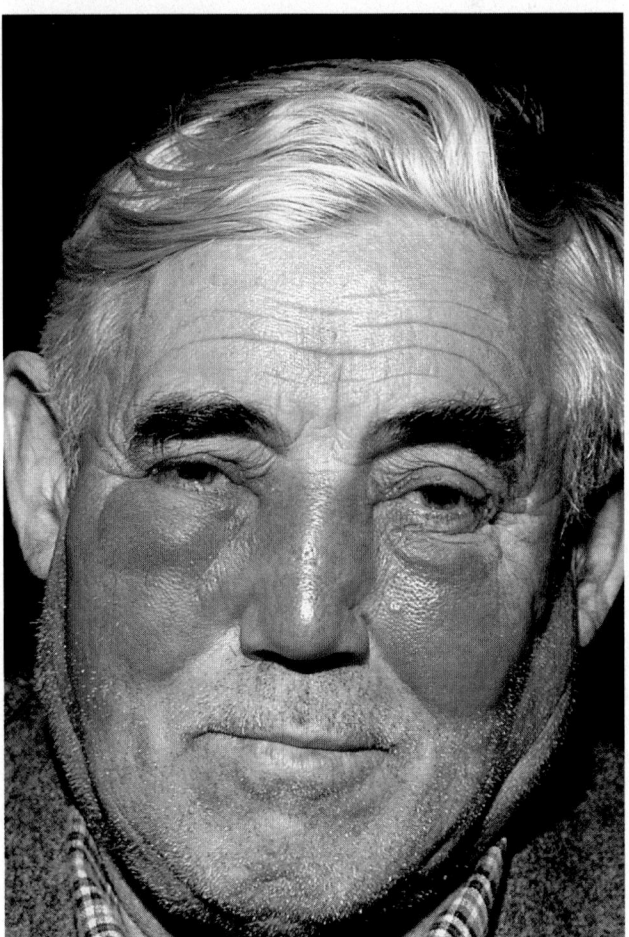

FIGURE 187-4 Erysipelas. Painful, edematous erythema with sharp margination on both cheeks and the nose. (*Courtesy of K. Wolff, M.D.*)

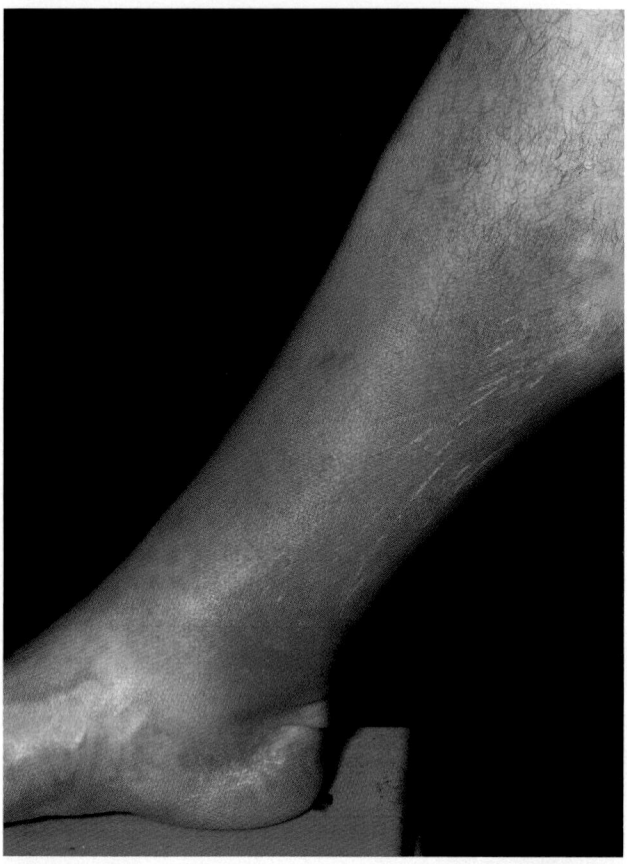

FIGURE 187-5 Erysipelas. Fiery-red, brawny, edematous erythema that is sharply and irregularly marginated. There is tenderness, and the patient has fever and chills.

group A streptococci. Streptococci are only rarely cultured from aspirated tissue fluid from the advancing edge of the lesion.

PATHOLOGY. The histologic hallmarks of this disease are intense edema, marked vascular dilatation, and a profuse infiltration of tissue spaces and lymphatic channels with streptococci. The streptococci are not found in the blood vessels themselves, but their presence in the lymphatics produces an inflammatory reaction about these vessels. The dermis is markedly edematous, and there is infiltration with neutrophils and mononuclear cells. The epidermis is only secondarily involved.

DIAGNOSIS AND DIFFERENTIAL DIAGNOSIS. The diagnosis is made on clinical grounds. Unilateral facial erysipelas may be distinguished from early herpes zoster involving the maxillary division of the fifth cranial nerve by the presence of hyperesthesia and pain prior to the appearance of lesions in the latter. Osteomyelitis of the maxillary or frontal bones (secondary to paranasal sinusitis) producing erythema and edema of overlying tissues may suggest erysipelas. The lack of sharply defined borders and evidence of sinus disease on history and transillumination serve to differentiate between these processes.

Occasionally contact dermatitis or angioneurotic edema may be mistaken for erysipelas, but the absence of fever is helpful in distinguishing these from erysipelas. An erysipelas-like skin lesion, apparently not due to infection, may occur recurrently in patients with familial Mediterranean fever.[18] Diffuse inflammatory carcinoma of the breast may present a picture mimicking low-grade erysipelas (see Chap. 183).

Erysipelas should be differentiated from erysipeloid (see Chap. 190), which commonly occurs on the hand or finger of a person in contact with fish, shellfish, or animal products and which is not associated with high fever or evidence of toxicity. Rarely, in immunosuppressed patients, skin lesions morphologically very similar to erysipelas have been produced by other organisms (e.g., coliform bacilli).

COURSE AND PROGNOSIS. Uncomplicated erysipelas remains confined primarily to the lymphatics and subcutaneous tissues. Even in the days prior to antibiotic therapy, it was often a self-limited process subsiding over 7 to 10 days. Occasionally, the organisms spread beyond the lymphatics, producing cellulitis with hemorrhagic bullae, necrosis, and subcutaneous abscesses. This sequence may then be followed by bacteremia with metastatic infection in various organs. Antibiotic therapy produces improvement in the general condition of the patient in 24 to 48 h, but it takes several more days for subsidence of the local lesion to be clearly evident. Prompt treatment prevents both suppurative and nonsuppurative complications. However, in young infants and elderly debilitated patients and in individuals receiving corticosteroids, the disease may progress with devastating rapidity to a fatal outcome.

Erysipelas has a tendency to recur in the same area, perhaps due to the predisposing effects of chronic lymphatic obstruction, edema, and even elephantiasis caused by earlier infections. Such recurrent infections may produce persistent swelling of the lips (macrocheilia), cheeks (particularly the lax tissues beneath the eyes), or lower extremities. A bizarre, irregular, cutaneous overgrowth, designated *elephantiasis nostras verrucosa,* may be produced by chronic lymphedema secondary to recurrent erysipelas. Areas of lymphatic obstruction are predisposed to recurrent infections; for example, following radical mastectomy some patients are liable to recurrent episodes of what appears to be erysipelas in the area of lymphedema.

Acute Cellulitis DEFINITION. This is an acute, spreading inflammation of the skin involving particularly the deeper subcutaneous tissues. Group A streptococci and *Staph. aureus* are by far the most common etiologic agents, but occasionally other bacteria are implicated (e.g., group B streptococci in the newborn; rarely pneumococci; in patients with underlying diabetes mellitus or an immunosuppressive illness, a variety of atypical organisms such as gram-negative bacilli and even cryptococci can be the etiology as a result of local injury or blood-borne dissemination).

CLINICAL MANIFESTATIONS. *History* Usually there is a history of an antecedent lesion (stasis ulcer, puncture wound), followed within a day or two by local erythema and tenderness. Systemic symptoms (malaise, fever, and chills) may then develop rapidly. Erythema at the site of infection rapidly intensifies and spreads. Local pain is often marked.

Cutaneous Lesions The involved area may be extensive with a markedly red, hot, infiltrated edematous appearance (Fig. 187-6). The borders of the lesion are not elevated or sharply defined. Tender regional lymphadenopathy is common, often with lymphangitis extending proximally. Superficial vesicles may form and rupture. Local abscesses may develop with necrosis of overlying skin (Fig. 187-6).

Dissecting cellulitis of the scalp (perifolliculitis capitis abscedens et suffodiens) is largely a misnomer. It represents an unusual, chronic inflammatory process of the scalp characterized by multiple, painful nodules, draining and burrowing sinuses, keloid formation, and alopecia; at some stages the process may

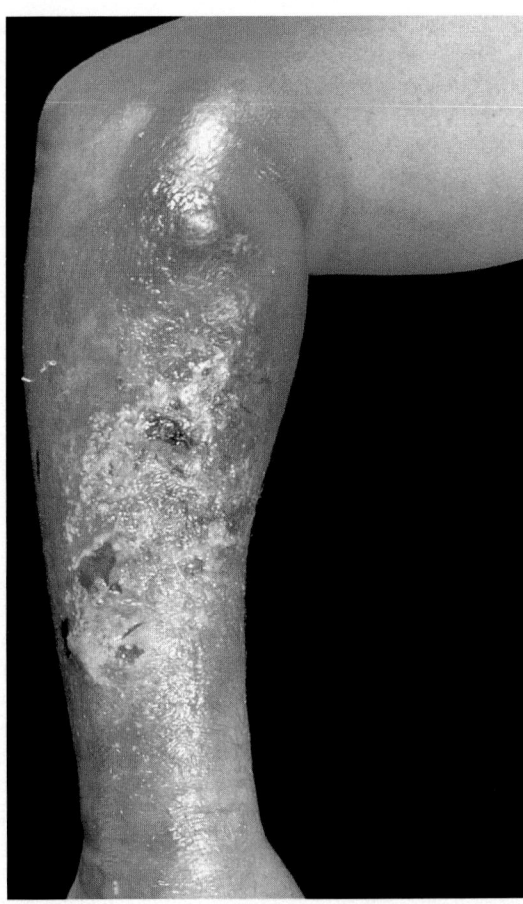

FIGURE 187-6 Cellulitis following puncture trauma. The lower arm is swollen, erythematous, and tender, and there is abscess formation, blistering, and crusting. (*Courtesy of K. Wolff, M.D.*)

resemble cellulitis. This disease usually occurs in young adults; and, in many respects, it is similar to, and may occur with, the other follicular occlusion syndromes (acne conglobata and hydradenitis suppurativa). Secondary infection may develop, requiring antimicrobial therapy. Treatment of the underlying process has included incision and drainage, x-ray epilation, and surgical excision[19]; successful short-term responses to isotretinoin have recently been noted.[20]

Streptococcal cellulitis may occur in unusual locations. Perianal cellulitis in children is a painful process with striking erythema about the anus. Perianal pruritus and blood-streaked stools are common features.[21] The involved tissues have a boggy consistency. Group A streptococci can be readily isolated from the erythematous area. Antecedent or associated streptococcal pharyngitis or impetigo is often noted.

Streptococcal cellulitis as an operative wound infection is uncommon today, in contrast to several decades ago. However, in the presence of streptococcal epidemics in the community, these organisms may be carried into the operating room and result in a particularly fulminating type of postoperative wound infection. Such sepsis may be manifest within 6 to 48 h of the surgery, more rapidly than that due to *Staph. aureus.* Hypotension (often due to bacteremia) may be the initial manifestation even before local erythema is evident. A thin serous discharge can be expressed from the

wound area, and on Gram's stain shows myriads of gram-positive cocci in chains.

An unusual form of cellulitis may occur at the saphenous vein donor site of patients who have recently undergone coronary artery bypass.[22] Erythema and edema extend along the incision; tenderness is marked. In some patients the illness is quite acute with high fever, prostration, and tachycardia. In a few patients lymphangitic streaks are evident. The localized area of tenderness and erythema may suggest thrombophlebitis. Group A streptococci have been isolated from the skin lesions or blood of a few patients. The appearance of the lesions, the occasional associated lymphangitis, and the response to treatment with penicillin G suggest that this is most often a streptococcal process. The infection probably takes origin in a minor break in the skin in the interdigital web areas, usually secondary to tinea pedis. The lymphedema resulting from lymphatic interruption accompanying saphenous vein removal predisposes to development of cellulitis once organisms reach that area. Because streptococcal infection in an area of lymphedema begets further lymphedema, episodes of infection tend to recur. Topical treatment of the interdigital dermatophytosis with miconazole or clotrimazole cream is an important element in management and prophylaxis. Although the cellulitis responds well to penicillin, the response may be slower in patients with peripheral arterial disease. Also, it is important to recognize that the *rubor* of dependency in such a patient may exaggerate the appearance of cellulitis about the saphenous incision. Thus, it is advisable to examine the leg from day to day in the same (horizontal) position.

Another unusual form of recurrent cellulitis of the lower extremities in women results from impaired lymphatic drainage due to neoplasia, radical vulvectomy or pelvic surgery, or radiation therapy. Such episodes of cellulitis have sometimes occurred temporally in relation to coitus and have been caused by group B or group G streptococci, both colonizers of the perineum and genital tract.[23]

LABORATORY FINDINGS.   There is almost always a brisk polymorphonuclear leukocytosis (15,000 to 40,000) with a marked shift to the left. Blood cultures should be performed, as the local process may be complicated by bacteremia.

DIAGNOSIS AND DIFFERENTIAL DIAGNOSIS.   Like erysipelas, the diagnosis is based almost solely on the physical appearance of the lesion. The main point of differentiation between the two lesions centers on the nature of the margin of the lesion: raised, sharply demarcated from the uninvolved skin in erysipelas; indistinct and gradually blending with uninvolved adjacent areas in cellulitis.

COURSE AND PROGNOSIS.   This process, because of its tendency to spread through lymphatics and bloodstream, is a serious disease if not treated early. In older patients, involvement of the lower extremities may be complicated by thrombophlebitis. In patients with chronic edema, the process may spread extremely rapidly and recovery may be slow, despite sterilization of the lesions by antibiotics. Occasionally, superinfection of necrotic areas, principally with gram-negative organisms, complicates recovery.

Acute Lymphangitis DEFINITION.   Acute lymphangitis is an inflammatory process involving the subcutaneous lymphatic channels. It is due most often to group A streptococci but occasionally may be caused by *Staph. aureus;* rarely, soft tissue infections with other organisms, such as *Pasteurella multocida,* may be associated with acute lymphangitis.

CLINICAL MANIFESTATIONS.   *History* The portal of entry is commonly a wound on an extremity, an infected blister, or a paronychia. The systemic manifestations of infection may occur either before any evidences of infection are present at the site of inoculation, or after the initial lesion has subsided. The patient may notice pain over an area of redness proximal to the original break in the skin. Systemic symptoms are often more prominent than one might expect from the degree of local pain and erythema.

An unusual spread of streptococcal infection of the thumb (paronychia) or of the interdigital webs between the thumb and index finger may occur occasionally.[24] Lymphatic drainage from this area can bypass the lymph nodes at the elbow and drain into the axillary nodes, which in turn communicate with the subpectoral nodes and the pleural lymphatics. As a consequence, subpectoral abscesses and pleural effusion develop. The subpectoral infection may dissect downward and appear over the lower chest and upper abdomen as an area of cellulitis. This is a very serious illness. The clinical clues to the development of this sequence of events are provided by the location of the original infection on the thumb or medial surface of the index finger and the early occurrence of axillary pain.

Cutaneous Lesions   Red linear streaks, which may be a few millimeters to several centimeters in width, extend from the local lesion toward the regional lymph nodes, which are usually enlarged and tender. The lymphangitic streaks are characteristically irregular and tender and may be mistaken for linear excoriations. Occasionally, breakdown of overlying skin and ulceration will occur in the course of bacterial lymphangitis, but this is rare in the antibiotic era.

LABORATORY FINDINGS.   The peripheral white blood cell count is elevated with a marked increase in polymorphonuclear cells. The offending organism cannot be cultured from the skin, as the infection is restricted to the lymphatic channels. However, the primary portal of entry or a suppurative lymph node, if overt infection is present, may reveal the etiologic agent.

DIAGNOSIS AND DIFFERENTIAL DIAGNOSIS.   The combination of a peripheral lesion with proximal red linear streaks leading toward regional lymph nodes is diagnostic of lymphangitis. In the lower extremities, thrombophlebitis may produce somewhat similar linear areas of tender erythema. The absence of a portal of entry and of tender regional adenopathy is helpful in distinguishing this process from lymphangitis.

COURSE AND PROGNOSIS.   The frequent development of bacteremia with metastatic infection in various organs makes this a potentially serious disease. The infection responds readily to penicillin therapy if instituted promptly.

Streptococcal Gangrene   DEFINITION.   Gangrene due to group A (occasionally C or G) streptococci is a rare entity, with a high mortality rate, usually developing at the site of a laceration, needle puncture, or surgical wound but sometimes occurring without any obvious portal of entry. Group B streptococci have caused a similar process post partum secondary to infected episiotomy incisions and in adult diabetics unrelated to obstetric complications.[25] It represents a cellulitis that has progressed rapidly to gangrene of the subcutaneous tissue, followed by necrosis of the overlying skin.[26] It is also known as *necrotizing fasciitis*. This nomenclature is confusing, because it is now recognized that the term necrotizing fasciitis includes not only group A streptococcal gangrene but also a similar-appearing entity due to other bacterial species (usually a mixture of anaerobic and facultative organisms). The latter process will be considered separately (see ''Necrotizing Fasciitis,'' below).

CLINICAL MANIFESTATIONS.   *History*   Although cases have been reported in patients with underlying diseases (diabetes, myx-

edema), the majority of cases have occurred in otherwise healthy persons, often elderly. Initially there are local redness, edema, heat, and pain in the involved area, typically on an extremity. Fever and other constitutional symptoms are prominent as the inflammatory process extends rapidly over the next 1 to 3 days.

Cutaneous Lesions   From 36 to 72 h after onset of the cellulitis, the characteristic findings of streptococcal gangrene appear: the involved area becomes dusky blue in color; vesicles or bullae containing initially yellowish, then red-black fluid appear. The bullae rupture, and extensive, sharply demarcated cutaneous gangrene develops. At this point the area may be numb, and the black necrotic eschar with surrounding irregular border of erythema resembles a third-degree burn (Fig. 187-7*a*, -7*b*). This sloughs off by the end of a week or 10 days. Peripheral areas of involvement develop about the principal lesion. Metastatic lesions may occur as a consequence of bacteremia; they may resemble purpura fulminans but rapidly go on to develop central dark-colored blebs containing streptococci. Secondary thrombophlebitis is common, but lymphangitis and lymphadenitis are not.

LABORATORY FINDINGS.   Organisms can usually be cultured from the yellow fluid in the bullous lesions. However, after these lesions rupture and undergo necrosis, a variety of other organisms not directly responsible for the lesion may be cultured from the area. Blood cultures usually contain streptococci.

PATHOLOGY.   The prominent angiitis and focal dermal necrosis with spread along fascial planes suggest that the disease is fundamentally a gangrene of the subcutaneous tissues followed by necrosis of the overlying skin. Microscopically, fibrinoid necrosis is present in the media of many arteries and veins passing through the destroyed fascia.[27] Fibrin thrombi are present. The epidermis, dermis, and skin appendages in the area of gangrene undergo coagulation necrosis. Numerous polymorphonuclear leukocytes and mononuclear cells infiltrate the lesion, and the upper layers of the dermis contain large numbers of gram-positive cocci.

DIAGNOSIS AND DIFFERENTIAL DIAGNOSIS.   The gross appearance may suggest a third-degree burn or violent trauma, particularly if the patient is not able to provide a history and if the lesions have already reached the gangrenous phase.

COURSE AND PROGNOSIS.   Prior to the availability of antibiotic therapy, the lesions commonly progressed and patients developed increasing toxemia and died from metastatic infection or shock. In rare cases, the process became sharply demarcated and self-limited. Even since the advent of antibiotics the mortality rate remains high.

TREATMENT.   Surgical debridement and decompression with removal of the gray necrotic fascia is crucial in management, along with appropriate antibiotic therapy of the streptococcal infection. Because extensive undermining is often present, thorough exploration and filleting of involved tissues is necessary to control the spreading infection. Reexploration and debridement should be performed as necessary to ensure that all necrotic tissue has been removed.

Necrotizing Fasciitis   Necrotizing fasciitis other than that due to group A streptococci will be considered here. This is a mixed infection in which one or more anaerobes (e.g., *Peptostreptococcus*, *Bacteroides*) are involved along with at least one facultative species (non-group A streptococci; members of the Enterobacteriaceae such as *Enterobacter*, *Proteus*, etc.)[28]

CLINICAL MANIFESTATIONS.   *History*   Antecedent injury to soft tissues, abdominal surgery, perirectal abscess, decubitus ulcer, and intestinal perforation are common predisposing events. Diabe-

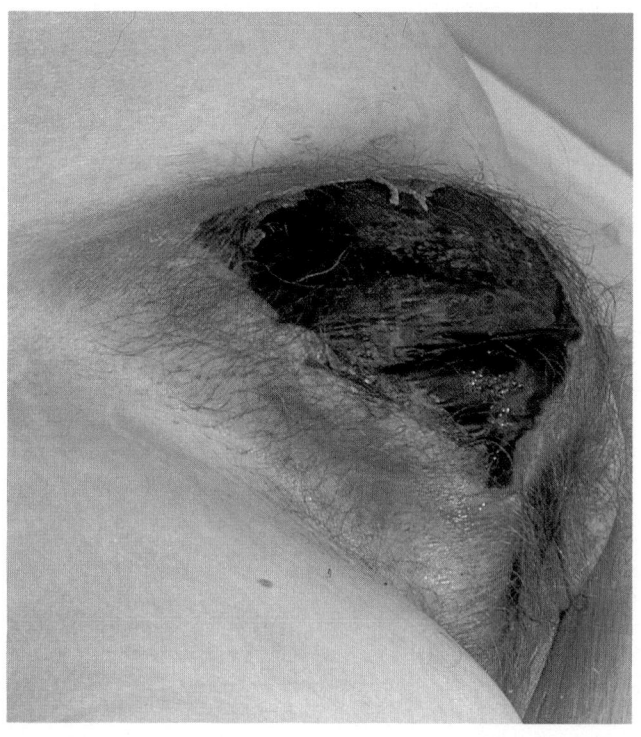

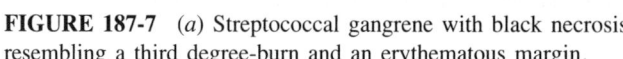

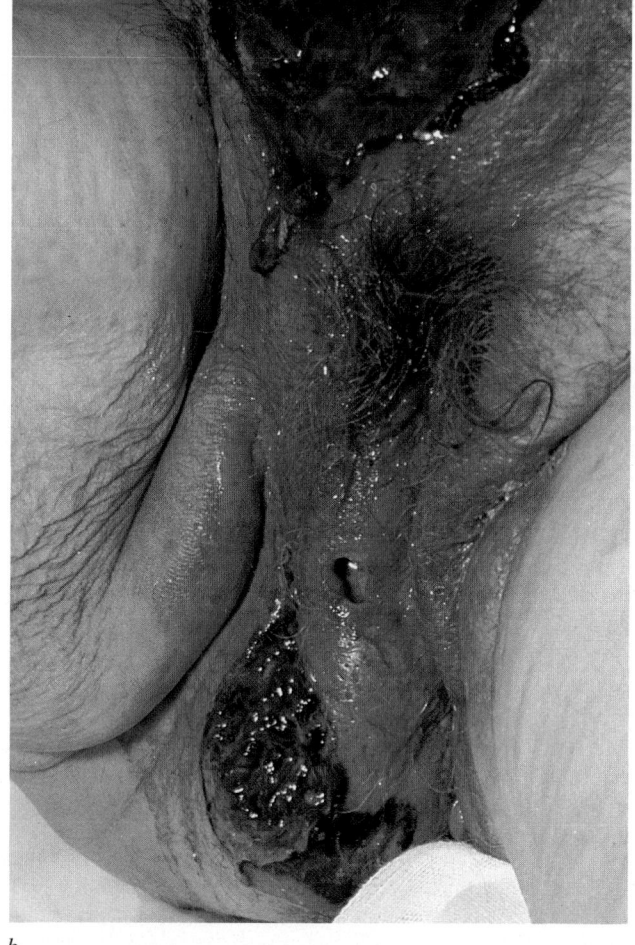

FIGURE 187-7 (*a*) Streptococcal gangrene with black necrosis resembling a third degree-burn and an erythematous margin.

(*b*) 48 h later, there is progressive gangrene of the pubic, perigenital, and perianal tissue. (*Courtesy of K. Wolff, M.D.*)

tes mellitus, alcoholism, or parenteral drug abuse are additional contributing factors. The onset is usually acute, and the course is rapidly progressive with high fever and prominent toxicity.

Cutaneous Lesions This infection most commonly occurs on the lower extremities, abdominal wall, perineum, and about operative wounds.[29] It is important to recognize that this infection may present in the thigh (dissection along the psoas muscle) or abdominal wall from an intestinal source (occult diverticulitis, rectosigmoid neoplasm). The involved area is swollen, red, warm, painful, and tender. The process is more extensive than the extent of the overlying skin changes would suggest. Within several days the skin color becomes purple, bullae develop, and frank cutaneous gangrene ensues. At this stage the involved area is no longer tender; it has become anesthetic due to occlusion of small blood vessels and destruction of superficial nerves in the subcutaneous tissues. Crepitus is often present, particularly in patients with diabetes mellitus.

A special form of necrotizing fasciitis that occurs about the male genitalia is known as *Fournier's gangrene* (streptococcal scrotal gangrene, perineal phlegmon).[30] It is caused by the same mixture of facultative and anaerobic organisms described above. In rare cases group A streptococci have been implicated. The process may be limited to the scrotum or spread to the penis, perineum, and abdominal wall. Pain, swelling, and crepitus in the scrotum are marked. Foul-smelling drainage occurs, and purplish discoloration of the scrotum progresses to frank gangrene. If the process invades the abdominal panniculus of an obese patient, especially one with diabetes mellitus, progression can be extraordinarily rapid.

Another variant of necrotizing fasciitis is known as *synergistic necrotizing cellulitis* (necrotizing cutaneous myositis, synergistic nonclostridial anaerobic myonecrosis). This process involves skin and muscle as well as fascia and subcutaneous tissue. The lower extremities, perineum, and abdominal wall are common sites.[31] The initial skin lesions may appear as skin sinuses (with surrounding areas of gangrene) draining foul-smelling brownish ("dishwater") pus. Between the draining tracks the skin appears uninvolved, even though extensive necrosis of underlying fascia, muscle, and subcutaneous tissues has occurred. Crepitus is present in about 25 percent of cases.

LABORATORY FINDINGS.   A leukocytosis is almost always present. Gram-stained smears of the exudate show a mixture of organisms (both gram-positive cocci and gram-negative bacilli of various sizes; occasionally, gram-positive bacilli consistent with *Clostridium* species are also present). Blood cultures are frequently positive for one or more bacterial species.

COURSE AND PROGNOSIS. This can be a rapidly progressive life-threatening infection if the diagnosis is not made promptly and appropriate surgical debridement is not carried out. This applies particularly when the process is secondary to a bowel perforation. Even with treatment, the mortality rate is about 35 percent.

TREATMENT. The major cause of delay in instituting appropriate therapy is the failure to appreciate involvement of fascia and deep subcutaneous tissue, leading to the misdiagnosis of this infection as cellulitis. Prompt exploration of the involved area is of paramount importance. Easy passage of a hemostat along a plane just superficial to the deep fascia (not expected with early cellulitis) should make the diagnosis. A frozen-section soft tissue biopsy performed deep enough and early in the course of the illness may provide a definitive diagnosis and expedite appropriate treatment.[32] Debridement should be carried out beyond the area of involvement until completely normal fascia is reached. All necrotic fascia and fat should be removed, and the wound should be left open. If there is any question as to the adequacy of the initial debridement, a "second-look" procedure is indicated 24 to 48 h later. Prior to obtaining results from cultures, initial antimicrobial therapy should be based on knowledge of a prominent role of anaerobic bacteria in this infection and on the specific findings on Gram-stained smear of the exudate.

Progressive Bacterial Synergistic Gangrene

DEFINITION. Progressive synergistic gangrene is a gangrenous ulceration of the skin due to a mixed bacterial infection in which microaerophilic streptococci together with *Staph. aureus* (or sometimes a gram-negative bacillus such as *Proteus*) are implicated. The lesion was designated synergistic gangrene because Brewer and Meleney[33] and Meleney[34] were able to reproduce the same type of lesion in dogs by injecting microaerophilic streptococci and *Staph. aureus* into the skin. Neither organism alone would produce such a lesion. A recent retrospective comparison of earlier reports of Meleney's progressive bacterial synergistic gangrene following abdominal surgery with reports of postoperative amebic abdominal wall gangrene suggested that the two entities were clinically indistinguishable.[35,36] The variable bacteriology of Meleney's gangrene and its nonspecific histology, coupled with the fact that amebic trophozoites might easily be missed in routine histologic sections, raised the possibility of an amebic etiology for this process. Although conceivably such may have been the case in occasional past instances following abdominal surgery in patients with unsuspected amebic colitis, it does not seem likely to apply to current cases, particularly in geographic areas where amebic disease is very rare.

CLINICAL MANIFESTATIONS. *History* This characteristic infection usually follows abdominal or thoracic infection (empyema) or trauma and is frequently associated with the use of through-and-through stay sutures in surgery. It is sometimes seen in the area of a colostomy or ileostomy opening or in proximity to a chronic ulceration on an extremity.

Cutaneous Lesions The infection usually starts in the first or second postoperative week with local redness, tenderness, and swelling. A small, painful, superficial ulcer develops and gradually enlarges. The central shaggy ulcer is characteristically surrounded by a rim of gangrenous skin. The latter, in turn, is encircled by a zone of purple erythema that blends into a peripheral pink edematous area.

LABORATORY FINDINGS. Anaerobic cultures from the advancing edematous margin of the lesion usually show microaerophilic or anaerobic streptococci, whereas *Staph. aureus* (rarely *Proteus* or

several other gram-negative bacilli) is found in the central ulcerated area.

COURSE AND PROGNOSIS. If untreated, the process extends slowly but progressively, ultimately resulting in enormous ulcerations.

TREATMENT. This is usually a very difficult lesion to treat. Local bacitracin irrigations (about 50 units/mL) and systemic antibiotic therapy with large doses of penicillin or other antibiotic (based on antibiotic susceptibility tests) are sometimes helpful. However, most often the lesion can be controlled only by wide surgical excision combined with antibiotic therapy.

Scarlet fever

DEFINITION. Scarlet fever is a diffuse erythematous eruption resulting from the production and subsequent circulation of erythrogenic toxin produced by group A streptococci usually located in a pharyngeal infection. The only difference between streptococcal tonsillopharyngitis and scarlet fever is the greater toxicity and the eruption in the latter.

BACTERIOLOGY AND PATHOGENESIS. Erythrogenic toxin is produced by most, but not all, strains of group A streptococci and is related to the presence of a lysogenic bacteriophage in the streptococcus. This relationship is very similar to that involving bacteriophage infection and toxin production in *Corynebacterium diphtheriae*. There appear to be three immunologically distinct erythrogenic toxins (types A, B, C) produced by approximately 90 percent of group A isolates. In the first half of this century, when scarlet fever was very prevalent and often severe, most scarlet fever strains of group A streptococci produced type A toxin; but in the past three to four decades strains producing either type B or combinations of type B and C toxins have predominated, perhaps related to the milder course of scarlet fever during this period. It is possible to have repeated group A streptococcal infections, but an individual usually has scarlet fever only once because of the development of protective specific antitoxic antibody. The few patients with documented recurrent attacks of scarlet fever may represent cases in which the episodes have been due to either of the other two immunologically distinct toxins. The immune status of a patient will determine the response to exposure to a given erythrogenic toxin-producing strain of group A streptococcus; it consists of two parts—type-specific antibacterial immunity and antitoxic immunity. The responses fall into three patterns: (1) Patients with type-specific antibacterial immunity (± antitoxic immunity) to a given streptococcal type (e.g., type 12) will develop no clinical disease when exposed to that type. (2) Patients with no type-specific antibacterial immunity (but with antitoxic immunity) will develop streptococcal pharyngitis. (3) Patients with neither antibacterial nor antitoxic immunity will develop pharyngitis plus scarlet fever (unless treated early with appropriate antibiotics).

It has been suggested that the rash of scarlet fever requires both the presence of erythrogenic toxin and the existence of delayed-type skin reactivity to streptococcal products, the latter stemming from prior exposure to the organism. In support of this is the observation that although streptococcal infections are not uncommon in infants and very young children, scarlet fever is rarely seen in this age group, and these infants fail to react to intradermal injection of erythrogenic toxin (Dick test). This failure to react does not appear to be correlated with transfer of antibody from the mother. Similarly, infant guinea pigs are not susceptible to intradermal injection of erythrogenic toxin. Following immunization with the toxin in Freund's adjuvant, they become sensitized and the Dick test becomes positive.

CLINICAL MANIFESTATIONS. *History* The disease usually occurs in children (the maximal incidence being in the 2- to 10-year age group) but only rarely in adults.

The clinical onset of the disease with the appearance of pharyngitis and fever is often abrupt after a 2- to 4-day incubation period. The temperature may be only slightly elevated in mild cases but it often rises rapidly to 38.9 to 40°C. Nausea and vomiting, headache, malaise, diffuse abdominal pain, and chilly sensations are prominent initial constitutional manifestations. The fever reaches its peak by the second day, and the temperature gradually returns to normal in the average case in 5 to 6 days. The rash appears 24 to 48 h after the onset of pharyngeal symptoms. Although the streptococcal focus of most patients with scarlet fever is in the pharynx, occasional patients develop a form of the disease, surgical scarlet fever, as a consequence of operative or other wound (burn, etc.) infection.

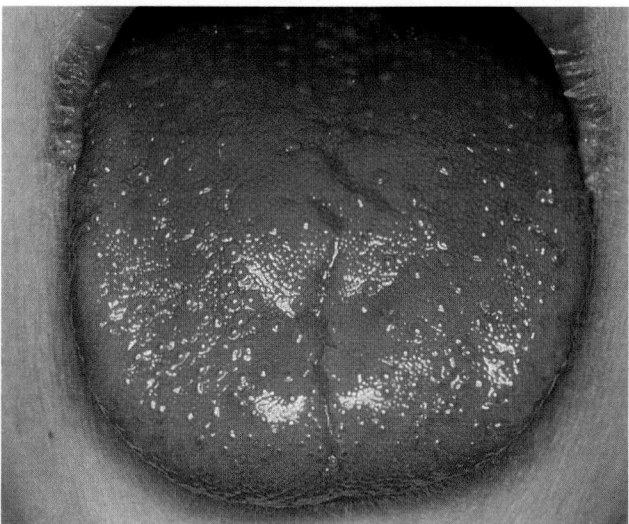

a

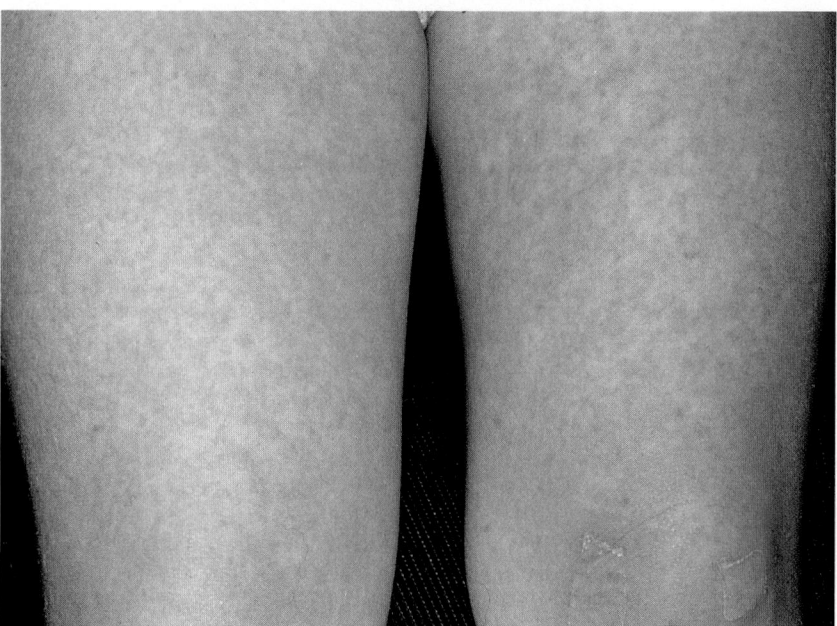

b

The acute manifestations of scarlet fever consist of those symptoms and signs related to the invasive streptococcal process at the portal of entry and those findings produced by erythrogenic toxin (malaise, nausea, vomiting, headache, fever, generalized lymphadenopathy, rash).

The severity of scarlet fever has declined over the past four decades: this trend even antedates the advent of effective antimicrobial therapy.

Cutaneous Lesions The major physical findings relate to the enanthem and exanthem.

1. *Enanthem.* The pharynx is beefy red in color, with edema involving the tonsillar area and extending anteriorly to include the soft palate and uvula. The tonsils are enlarged, reddened, and often covered with discrete patches of white or yellow exudate filling the tonsillar crypts. Occasionally, the exudate becomes confluent. Bilateral tender submandibular lymphadenopathy is present.

   During the first several days of the illness, the tongue is white and furred, but the edges and tip remain reddened. The papillae soon become reddened and hypertrophied and project through the white coating, producing what has been called the "white-strawberry" tongue. By the fourth or fifth day, the white coating has disappeared and the tongue assumes a bright red color punctuated with very prominent papillae, the so-called red-strawberry tongue (Fig. 187-8). Punctate erythema and scattered petechiae are often present over the soft palate.

2. *Exanthem.* The rash usually appears first on the neck, then rapidly encompasses the trunk, and finally spreads to the extremities (Fig. 187-8). The involvement of the body is usually complete within 36 h, but the palms and soles are spared. The rash is a diffuse erythema, blanching on pressure, with numerous 1- to 2-mm punctate papular elevations, giving a rough sandpaper quality to the skin. There are usually no discrete lesions on the face but only a marked flushing of the cheeks and forehead, contrasting quite sharply with the circumoral

FIGURE 187-8 Scarlet fever. (*a*) "Red-strawberry" tongue. (*b*) Perifollicular erythema. (*Courtesy of M. Meurer, M.D.*)

pallor. On the body the rash is most marked in the skin folds of the inguinal, auxillary, antecubital, and abdominal areas and about sites of pressure such as the buttocks and sacrum. The eruption often exhibits a linear petechial character in the antecubital fossae and axillary folds (Pastia's lines). In those cases in which the eruption is intense, pinhead vesicular lesions (miliary sudamina), seen in a variety of prolonged febrile illnesses, may appear on the abdomen and chest. In mild cases the rash may be localized to the trunk and be seen as only a faint erythema. In the black patient the rash is often difficult to recognize but may be felt as punctate papular lesions resembling "gooseflesh" or sandpaper. At its peak the rash has a diffuse, bright scarlet appearance. Capillary fragility is increased in the severer cases, and the tourniquet test result is positive. Occasional patients may develop frank purpura, with or without thrombocytopenia.

The exanthem usually persists for 4 or 5 days but in mild cases may be very transient. One of the most characteristic features of the illness is the desquamation that begins as the rash starts to fade. It commences on the face, usually about the ears, and spreads to the trunk and extremities, involving the hands and feet last (between the second and third weeks of illness). The desquamation on the face and trunk has a brawny character, and frequently a punched-out appearance of the abdomen results from the peeling off of circular areas of skin. Skin on the hands and feet is frequently shed in large sheets. The desquamation is so prominent a feature that it may be helpful in making a retrospective diagnosis in a case in which the eruption was minimal. Similar changes in the nail bed produce a transverse groove in the nails.

Other Physical Findings   Generalized lymphadenopathy is a common finding, and splenomegaly is present occasionally.

LABORATORY FINDINGS.   The blood picture in the early stages shows a polymorphonuclear leukocytosis, and later in the illness eosinophilia (5 to 10 percent) is a common finding. Throat culture reveals group A streptococci. If direct bacteriologic confirmation cannot be made during the early phases of the illness, determination of the ASO titer may provide, retrospectively, evidence of a recent streptococcal infection. Slight microscopic hematuria is found not infrequently during the peak of the exanthem and does not represent acute glomerulonephritis. It is usually transient and may be related to a generalized effect of the erythrogenic toxin on capillaries.

PATHOLOGY.   There is an outpouring of polymorphonuclear leukocytes and scattered red blood cells into the skin about small blood vessels. The punctiform lesions are represented by dilated small blood vessels and a focal accumulation of exudate. The suppurative and nonsuppurative sequelae are the same as are seen with any group A streptococcal infection.

DIAGNOSIS AND DIFFERENTIAL DIAGNOSIS.   The diagnosis is usually made on the basis of clinical features—fever, vomiting, exudative pharyngitis, and an erythematous punctiform eruption going on to desquamation. Confirmatory evidence is provided by isolation of group A streptococci from the pharynx. Two other confirmatory tests that have been employed extensively in the past are no longer necessary:

1. *Dick test:* This is a test for the presence of antitoxic immunity and is performed by an intracutaneous inoculation of 0.1 mL of a standard diluted preparation of erythrogenic toxin. The appearance of a 1-cm or greater area of local erythema at 24 h is a positive test result and indicates a lack of antitoxic immu-

nity (i.e., susceptibility to scarlet fever). A negative Dick test indicates immunity to the effects of erythrogenic toxin.

2. *Schultz-Charlton phenomenon.*   Intradermal injection of 0.1 mL of antitoxin into an area of scarlet fever rash produces "blanching" at the site of injection within 12 to 24 h. The test must be performed during the very early phase of the eruption before exudation into the lesion makes the skin changes irreversible. The blanching test is not used now because of the danger of sensitization to horse serum and because the use of antitoxin of human origin carries the risk of introducing viral hepatitis or HIV infection.

Although the total clinical picture is highly suggestive of scarlet fever (due to group A streptococci), scarlatiniform eruptions may occur in other conditions and cause confusion in diagnosis. Infection with toxin ("exfoliatin")-producing strains of *Staph. aureus* belonging to phage group II may produce a rash resembling that of scarlet fever (see section on "Staphylococcal Skin Infections" below). Strains of *Staph. aureus* producing toxic shock syndrome toxin 1 (TSST-1) are responsible for the toxic shock syndrome, an acute febrile illness that also produces a generalized scarlatiniform eruption. In infants and young children particularly, exanthem subitum and rubella may be mistaken for scarlet fever, but the lack of a pharyngeal focus is important in distinguishing these conditions. Also, neither of these processes is followed by extensive desquamation. Patients with infectious mononucleosis may develop an erythematous eruption, and this, together with lymphadenopathy and membranous pharyngitis, may mimic scarlet fever. The typical blood picture and the heterophil agglutination test are helpful points in distinguishing between these diseases. Diffuse erythroderma as part of a drug-sensitivity reaction (sulfonamides, streptomycin, penicillin) may be mistaken for scarlet fever, as may the fever and cutaneous blush associated with atropine toxicity. Sunburn in a child with pharyngitis may be a cause of confusion, but the distribution of the lesions is the crucial distinguishing point.

COURSE AND PROGNOSIS.   The acute febrile course of the untreated, uncomplicated case lasts about 4 to 5 days; desquamation may continue for several weeks thereafter. Many cases seen nowadays are mild and last only a few days. The course of the illness is dramatically altered by the administration of penicillin, which produces a prompt subsidence of fever and of constitutional symptoms. Adequate, early penicillin treatment eradicates the streptococci from the pharyngeal or other foci, interferes with the development of ASO antibodies, and prevents the development of suppurative and nonsuppurative sequelae. The prognosis is excellent, and deaths today due to scarlet fever are extremely rare.

Toxic Shock-like Syndrome due to Group A Streptococci ("Toxic Strep Syndrome")

An acute multisystem syndrome resembling that of toxic shock caused by *Staph. aureus* (see section on "Staphylococcal Skin Infections" below) has recently been attributed to infection with group A streptococci.[37,38] The initiating streptococcal infection is commonly, but not exclusively, in soft tissues (cellulitis, necrotizing fasciitis). Clinical features usually include many of the following: hypotension, chills, fever, tachycardia, myalgias, and mental changes as well as manifestations of multiorgan dysfunction (gastrointestinal abnormalities, renal failure, adult respiratory distress syndrome). Localized erythema (usually about the face) is present, but not the generalized punctate erythema of scarlet fever. Injection of bulbar and palpebral conjunctivae may be present, but not a strawberry tongue; and skin desquamation is not a later feature. Bacteremia is usually, but not invariably, absent, suggesting the toxin-associated nature of the process. It is important to recognize as well that "septic scarlet fever" may be reemerging currently, after an absence covering the postantibiotic era. Three cases of severe septic scarlet fever with the features of toxic shock were recently described in individuals with group A streptococcal cellulitis and bacteremia.[39]

A few cases of the streptococcal toxic shock syndrome have been studied microbiologically. The group A streptococcal isolates produced either type A or a mixture of types B and C pyrogenic exotoxins (also known as erythrogenic toxins). It has been postulated that the attenuated nature of scarlet fever and of nonbacteremic streptococcal infections in recent decades was associated with the virtual disappearance of group A streptococci producing pyrogenic exotoxin A and replacement with strains producing type B (or mixtures of types B and C) toxins. The resurgence of streptococcal strains producing pyrogenic exotoxin A may be responsible for the current outbreak of streptococcal toxic shock.

Cutaneous Manifestations of Subacute Bacterial Endocarditis   A variety of skin lesions have been described in subacute bacterial endocarditis (usually due to viridans streptococci). Although often ascribed to embolic phenomena, it appears that many of these lesions represent local areas of vasculitis.

PETECHIAE.   These are the most common of the skin and mucous membrane lesions in bacterial endocarditis and are found in about half of patients with this disease. These small, reddish-brown, flat lesions do not blanch on pressure. They occur particularly on the extremities and upper chest. Mucous membrane involvement (conjunctivae, palate) is common. The petechiae frequently occur in small crops. Rarely, the lesions may be extremely numerous and involve primarily the lower extremities. They usually deepen in color, last only a few days, and then fade away. It is important to distinguish capillary angiomas, which may be present on the chests of some patients, from petechiae. This can be done by applying pressure with a glass slide and demonstrating blanching of the angiomas.

The limited information on the histology of petechiae in subacute bacterial endocarditis does not suggest local bacterial multiplication or embolization as the basis for the lesions. The endothelial proliferation, hemorrhage, and round-cell infiltration found are consistent with small-vessel inflammation. Increased capillary fragility can be demonstrated in some patients.

SUBUNGUAL "SPLINTER HEMORRHAGES."   These small, dark red streaks resembling splinters beneath the nail are suggestive of the diagnosis of subacute bacterial endocarditis (Fig. 187-9). Similar lesions may occur beneath the distal portion of the nail as a result of trauma (in dishwashers, carpenters, etc.) or poor hygiene. Splinter hemorrhages may occur as part of the clinical picture in trichinosis and vasculitis. Subungual hemorrhages may occur in acute meningococcemia with extensive petechiae and purpura. "Splinters" located near the middle third of the nail are more suggestive of subacute bacterial endocarditis, as they are less likely to be of traumatic origin. True splinter lesions in subacute bacterial endocarditis will migrate distally as the nail grows out.

OSLER'S NODES.   These are split-pea-sized, erythematous, painful, nodular lesions. They appear to be in the skin and in some ways resemble an urticarial wheal, often with a whitish center. The most common location of these swellings is on the pads of the fingers and toes, on the thenar and hypothenar eminences, and over the arms. They are quite transient, lasting 12 to 24 h or perhaps several days. They are not numerous and tend to occur in crops. They may desquamate but do not ulcerate. Currently, they are seen in about 5 percent of patients with bacterial endocarditis (see Chap. 166).

Histologic examination has not confirmed the suggested embolic nature of the Osler's nodes occurring in subacute bacterial endocarditis. Endothelial swelling and a perivascular inflammatory response have been found at the center of such lesions, but no bacteria or fibrin emboli were observed. Although at first suggested as pathognomonic findings in viridans streptococcal subacute bacterial endocarditis, Osler's nodes have been observed in subacute and acute endocarditis due to a variety of organisms, including *Staph. aureus*. Histologic examination of Osler's nodes from several patients with acute endocarditis due to *Staph. aureus* and *Candida albicans* has revealed microemboli in dermal arterioles and adjacent microabscesses in the papillary dermis.[40] In these cases the responsible organism has been identified on Gram's stains or cultures of aspirates.

It appears that Osler's nodes in acute bacterial endocarditis may be caused by minute infective emboli; in subacute bacterial endocarditis they may be due to immunologic phenomena resulting in small-vessel arteritis of the skin.

JANEWAY LESIONS.   These lesions, consisting of minimally nodular hemorrhages, or occasionally erythematous macules, in the palms or soles, are seen in acute endocarditis (commonly due to *Staph. aureus*) or, infrequently, in subacute bacterial endocarditis. They may be rather numerous and, unlike Osler's nodes, are painless. Histologically, there is usually a polymorphonuclear infiltration of the walls of blood capillaries, some extravasation of red blood cells, and microabscess formation in the dermis. Gram-positive cocci in clusters have been demonstrated extracellularly in such a lesion, and *Staph. aureus* has been isolated on culture of the same lesion in a patient with *Staph. aureus* endocarditis.[41] Occasional lesions of purulent purpura (lesions with white or dark gray centers with surrounding hemorrhagic halos) may also be seen on the distal extremities in acute *Staph. aureus* endocarditis, representing progression of Janeway lesions or initial metastatic pustules (see Chap. 166).

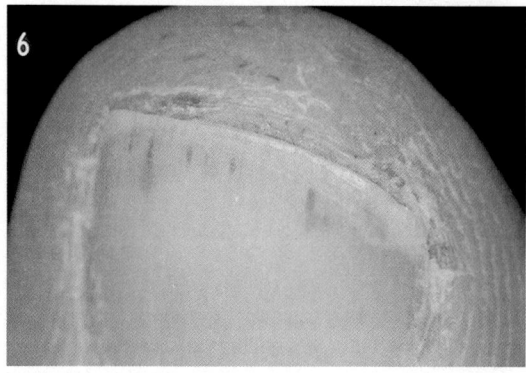

FIGURE 187-9   Splinter hemorrhages.

Poststreptococcal (Group A) Nonsuppurative Cutaneous Sequelae

Erythema Nodosum   See Chap. 108.

Erythema Marginatum (Cutaneous Lesions of Acute Rheumatic Fever)   See Chap. 178.

Purpura Fulminans (Gangrenosa) DEFINITION. Purpura fulminans is an uncommon, acute, severe, usually fatal nonspecific
hemorrhagic infarction and necrosis of the skin that occurs in the
course of, or immediately following, a variety of infections, particularly those due to group A streptococci. Marked depletion of multiple coagulation factors (disseminated intravascular coagulation)
occurs in this condition. Closely related, if not the identical process, is the symmetric peripheral gangrene that is sometimes seen
(particularly in infants) during bacteremias.

EPIDEMIOLOGY. Purpura fulminans occurs most often in children but has been seen at all ages. The antecedent or concomitant
infections with which it has been associated include those due to
bacteria (scarlet fever; group A streptococcal, staphylococcal, and
pneumococcal bacteremias; and meningococcemia) and, less commonly, those of a viral etiology (varicella). In patients with purpura
fulminans after varicella, secondary streptococcal infection may
have been an important etiologic factor.

ETIOLOGY AND PATHOGENESIS. Purpura fulminans is one of
several cutaneous syndromes whose common feature is a hemorrhagic tendency developing secondary to the acute intravascular
activation of the clotting mechanism. The exact means of initiation
of the consumption coagulopathy is not yet fully understood.
Rarely, a case appears to be associated with drug allergy. A host of
coagulation abnormalities has been noted at one time or another.
This variability probably reflects the rapid changes that occur during the evolution of the process and the effects of "secondary"
fibrinolysis. The abnormalities more commonly recorded include
thrombocytopenia; depression of prothrombin (factor II), fibrinogen (factor I), proaccelerin (factor V), and antihemophilic factor
(factor VIII); and findings of secondary fibrinolysis (i.e., increased
plasminogen levels or evidences of fibrinogen or fibrin breakdown
products). The coagulopathy and microscopic pathology in purpura
fulminans are very similar to those found in rabbits with generalized Shwartzman reaction (see Chap. 186).

CLINICAL MANIFESTATIONS. *History* The eruption develops
during, or on convalescence from, one of the infections noted earlier. Chills and fever usually herald the onset of the hemorrhagic
lesions, and the patient appears acutely ill.

Cutaneous Lesions. The lesions are localized, massive ecchymoses, often with sharp, irregular ("geographic") borders.
They are usually symmetric and on the extremities, particularly in
areas of pressure, but may involve the lips, ears, nose, and trunk.
There may be a narrow surrounding zone of erythema. Hemor-

rhagic blebs may develop in the ecchymotic areas associated with
edema of the areas. The peripheral ecchymotic lesions, especially
of the digits, may rapidly blacken and progress to gangrene
(Fig. 187-10).

Other Physical Findings. The other findings are those of a
systemically ill patient with high fever and tachycardia. The disease
often rapidly progresses over 48 to 72 h, with peripheral vasoconstriction and shock supervening.

LABORATORY FINDINGS. There is usually a leukocytosis. The
number of platelets is markedly reduced and coagulation factors V,
VII, VIII and prothrombin and fibrinogen are decreased. As a result, the prothrombin time and the partial thromboplastin time are
prolonged. Split products of fibrinogen and fibrin may be present.

PATHOLOGY. The involved areas show occlusion of arterioles
with fibrin thrombi. A dense polymorphonuclear reaction occurs in
the dermis in the areas of infarction necrosis. Bacteria are not seen
in the lesions. Similar lesions may occur in the viscera, but they are
often restricted to the skin.

DIAGNOSIS AND DIFFERENTIAL DIAGNOSIS. All the causes of
gross purpura must be considered in the differential diagnosis. The
relationship of specific infections, the striking geographic nature of
the lesions, and their location on the extremities are suggestive of
the diagnosis. Rarely, morphologically similar lesions have been
described as complications of coumarin therapy in individuals deficient in coagulation factor protein C.

TREATMENT. Treatment includes vigorous antibiotic management of any associated infection. Only if bleeding is significant
during the course of diffuse intravascular coagulation in the patient
with purpura fulminans is replacement of platelets and coagulation
factors undertaken and consideration given to the use of heparin (10
to 15 units/kg per h as a continuous intravenous infusion) to inhibit
the intravascular clotting process.

COURSE AND PROGNOSIS. The mortality rate is extremely
high. In those patients who survive, amputation of extremities or
extensive skin grafting may be necessary to deal with the gangrenous areas.

***Other Skin Lesions Accompanying or Following Group A Strep-
tococcal Infections*** ERYTHEMA MULTIFORME-LIKE LESIONS.
Round erythematous macules, up to 1.5 cm in diameter, some developing bright borders and subsequently showing clearing in the
center, may occur during bacteremia due to group A streptococci
(or *Staph. aureus*) in infants and young children (see Chap. 50).

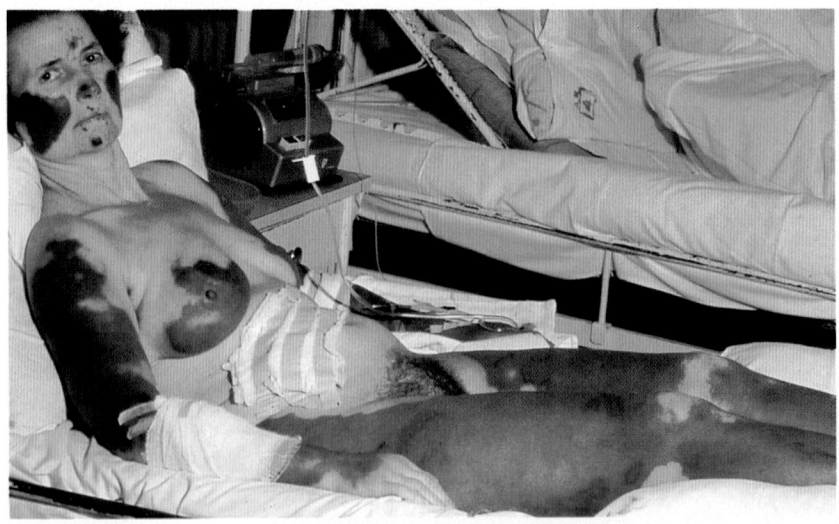

FIGURE 187-10 Purpura fulminans in
disseminated intravascular coagulation
following abdominal surgery. There are
extensive geographic areas of cutaneous
infarction involving the face, breasts, and
extremities.

ACUTE GUTTATE PSORIASIS. Rarely, erythematous, papulo-squamous, guttate psoriasiform lesions may develop during or following group A streptococcal pharyngitis or skin infections.[42] Children appear to be most commonly affected. Clearing of the lesions may occur within weeks of antimicrobial therapy of the streptococcal infection. Although the temporal relation of the two processes is striking, a direct causal connection has not been established (see Chap. 39).

Treatment of Group A Streptococcal Skin Infections

Antibiotic Management GENERAL PRINCIPLES. Penicillin G is the drug of choice in the treatment of known group A streptococcal skin infections. When the etiology is not known immediately (e.g., in cellulitis) and when *Staph. aureus* is also a distinct consideration, a semisynthetic penicillin (nafcillin or oxacillin) should be employed initially. Penicillin treatment should be continued for at least 10 days to ensure eradication of the infection. Since as many as 40 percent of isolates of group A streptococci may be resistant to the tetracyclines, this group of drugs should not be used in the treatment of known streptococcal disease. Prophylactic penicillin therapy is indicated for close family contacts (particularly children) of patients with streptococcal pharyngitis.

SPECIFIC TREATMENT. Mild infections such as impetigo, scarlet fever, or certain cases of erysipelas and cellulitis may be treated at home with intramuscular procaine penicillin (600,000 units once or twice daily), or with oral penicillin V (250 to 500 mg 4 times daily). When staphylococcal infection is suspected, oxacillin (0.5 to 1.0 g orally 4 times daily) should be substituted. In adults allergic to penicillin, erythromycin (0.25 to 0.5 g orally 4 times daily) is a reasonable alternative.

In more severe streptococcal skin infections (e.g., extensive erysipelas, cellulitis, or streptococcal gangrene), the above dosage of antibiotics is insufficient. Patients with such conditions should be hospitalized, and treatment with parenteral aqueous penicillin G (600,000 to 2,000,000 units every 4 to 6 h) should be begun. In the very ill patient in whom a staphylococcal etiology is suspected, one of the semisynthetic penicillins (e.g., nafcillin 1.0 to 1.5 g intravenously every 4 h) should be employed. In the patient with a questionable penicillin allergy, cephalothin (1.0 g intravenously every 3 to 4 h) may be substituted. If the patient has had an immediate type of reaction to penicillin (anaphylaxis or angioneurotic edema, etc.) then vancomycin (1.0 to 1.5 g intravenously daily) would be a reasonable alternative for treatment of a suspected staphylococcal infection.

LOCAL AND OTHER MEASURES. Care of the local lesion of erysipelas and cellulitis includes immobilization and elevation of the involved area to reduce local edema. Cool, sterile saline dressings decrease the local pain and are particularly indicated in the presence of bullous lesions. The use of a footboard may protect the affected area from trauma. The application of moist heat may aid in the localization of a cellulitis, but it should not be used in a patient with arterial insufficiency in the involved extremity. Subsequent drainage may be necessary for areas of abscess formation; extensive debridement and grafting may be required for the necrotic areas of streptococcal gangrene.

Superficial lesions (such as ecthyma and secondarily infected dermatoses) benefit from sterile saline dressings. Mupirocin or bacitracin ointment may be of value for softening and removing crusted lesions as well as for their antibacterial effects.

Patients hospitalized with group A streptococcal infections should be isolated until the organisms have been eradicated by antibiotic treatment.

Staphylococcal Skin Infections

General Features

Bacteriology and Pathogenic Aspects *Staph. aureus* is the causative agent in some of the primary pyodermas and cellulitides as well as a colonizer or secondary invader on diseased dermatitic skin. The organisms are readily demonstrated on smear of pus as large gram-positive cocci in small clusters.

In contrast to the relative rarity of group A streptococci, *Staph. aureus* is frequently found distributed over the skin, particularly in nasal carriers. The presence of *Staph. aureus* often represents a carrier state or its passage as a transient.[43] The biologic attributes (cellular components, extracellular products) of *Staph. aureus* bearing on the disease-producing potential of the organism are not well understood, with the exception of the role of the exfoliating toxin in the staphylococcal scalded-skin syndrome and bullous impetigo and the role of TSST in the toxic shock syndrome. The production of coagulase, leukocidin, alpha toxin, etc., may be the same in strains isolated from staphylococcal cellulitis as in those from the normal skin of the carrier. Thus, a variety of host factors (therapy with corticosteroids and immunosuppressive agents, etc.) appears to play an important, if not the major, role in the pathogenesis of staphylococcal infections. This is not to say that as yet unidentified virulence factors in certain staphylococcal isolates will not eventually explain the apparent heightened pathogenicity of particular strains. Preexisting tissue injury or inflammation (surgical wound, burn, trauma, exudative dermatitis, retained foreign body) is of major importance in the pathogenesis of staphylococcal disease. The production of coagulase, a factor capable of clotting plasma, remains, at present, the most widely employed in vitro criterion of the potential pathogenicity of a staphylococcal strain. Coagulase may play a role in the development of the staphylococcal abscess by producing local fibrin thrombi that protect organisms and concentrate toxic factors elaborated by these pathogens. The elaboration of surface slime, a substance facilitating adherence of coagulase-negative staphylococci to surfaces of foreign bodies, may contribute to the newly appreciated virulence of these organisms when they infect immunosuppressed individuals or patients with indwelling catheters or prostheses.

One of the major problems in dealing with staphylococcal infections has been the emergence of resistance to a variety of antibiotics. Although the presence of resistance, usually to penicillin G and other drugs, has been of paramount importance in the outcome of infection, there is no evidence that the intrinsic virulence of such strains is any greater than that of penicillin-sensitive organisms. The introduction of the penicillinase-resistant penicillins has altered considerably the picture for serious staphylococcal infections. *Staph. aureus* strains resistant to the semisynthetic penicillinase-resistant penicillins have emerged as a significant problem in the past 10 years in this country.

Epidemiology. The ubiquity of the staphylococcus and the difficulty in distinguishing among strains has, until recently, impeded an understanding of the epidemiology of infections due to this organism. Initially, the high frequency of staphylococcal colonization of the respiratory tract and the frequency of staphylococci in our immediate environment suggested that their spread from person to person occurred principally via respiratory transmission or fomites. Careful epidemiologic studies utilizing phage-typing techniques suggest that transfer of organisms to patients occurs predominantly via the hands of personnel rather than through the air. This appears to be particularly true in newborn nurseries, where this route is of importance in dissemination of the organisms from nasal carriers and also in transfer of staphylococci between babies. Individuals, whether infants or adults, with open staphylococcal lesions are particularly dangerous potential transmitters of infection. Good nursery technique, careful handling of patients, strict handwashing procedures, and isolation of patients with open draining staphylococcal infections are important in the reduction of transmission of staphylococci.

Immunity   The prevalence of staphylococci and staphylococcal infections is substantiated by the almost universal presence in adults of circulating antibody to one or more cell-wall antigens or extracellular toxins. The occurrence of staphylococcal infections in the presence of these antibodies suggests that they are not the primary determinants of resistance to such infections. Immunization of experimental animals with alpha toxin does not afford protection against staphylococcal disease following challenge. Hypersensitivity may play a role in recurrent staphylococcal skin infections in humans.

Superficial Staphylococcal Pyodermas

Impetigo   Two clinical types of impetigo occur. The first is a thick, yellow, crusted variety that is transiently vesicular in its early stage. Group A streptococci or a mixture of streptococci and *Staph. aureus* are usually isolated from these lesions. When both organisms are present, group A streptococci appear to be the primary pathogen and staphylococci are secondary invaders of the lesions (see earlier section on "Impetigo"). Although in the past *Staph. aureus* alone was isolated from 5 to 10 percent of cases of this type of impetigo,[6] its relative role in the United States appears to be increasing,[10] consistent with it being the etiology of a higher percentage of cases in Europe.[9] Production of bacteriocins (highly bactericidal to group A streptococci) by certain *Staph. aureus* strains (phage group 71) may be responsible for the isolation of only *Staph. aureus* from some lesions due initially to streptococci. Overall, however, it would appear that in conventional impetigo with typical crusted lesions, the group A streptococcus is etiologically most frequent; *Staph. aureus* may be responsible for a minority of cases, and these tend to heal spontaneously, faster than those due to streptococci. The second type of impetigo is bullous impetigo, characterized by large bullae that rupture and form varnishlike crusts. This infection is specifically associated with *Staph. aureus* of phage group II (usually type 71).

Bullous Impetigo   Three types of skin lesions can be produced by phage group II staphylococci: (1) bullous impetigo, (2) exfoliative disease (staphylococcal scalded-skin syndrome), (3) nonstreptococcal scarlatiniform eruption. All three represent varying cutaneous responses to an extracellular exfoliative toxin ("exfoliatin") produced by these staphylococci (for descriptions of the toxin and the latter two types of lesions see "Staphylococcal Scalded-Skin Syndrome" below and Chap. 51).

CLINICAL MANIFESTATIONS.   Bullous impetigo occurs mainly in the newborn and in older children, and is characterized by the rapid progression of vesicles to flaccid bullae (Fig. 187-11*a*, -11*b*).

The latter arise on areas of grossly normal skin, and the Nikolsky sign is not present. The bullae contain initially clear yellow fluid that subsequently becomes dark yellow and turbid. There is no erythema surrounding the bullous lesions, which are sharply demarcated. They soon rupture, collapse, and form thin, light brown crusts. *Staph. aureus* belonging to phage group II can be cultured from the contents of intact bullae. The uncommon bullous variant of varicella probably represents the occurrence of superinfection by *Staph. aureus* (phage group II) of varicella lesions. Pemphigus neonatorum (Ritter's disease) is an extensive form of bullous impetigo, often accompanied by fever, and represents the staphylococcal "scalded-skin syndrome" in the newborn (see Chap. 51). This type of infection, in the past, has spread in epidemics in infant nurseries.

Staphylococcal Scalded-Skin Syndrome (See also Chap. 51)
DEFINITION.   This is the most severe form of skin disease due to the exfoliative exotoxin produced by *Staph. aureus* of phage group II and is characterized by generalized bulla formation and exfoliation.[44] Unlike bullous impetigo, where the staphylococcal infection is in the skin at the site of the lesion, in the staphylococcal scalded-skin syndrome (SSSS) the infection is often at a distant site or not on the skin at all (bacteremia, localized abscesses, conjunctivitis).

BACTERIOLOGY AND PATHOGENESIS.   Only staphylococci belonging to phage group II (types 3A, 3B, 3C, 55, 71) appear to be responsible for the staphylococcal scalded-skin syndrome. Exfoliative toxin (ET) is produced by these organisms in vivo or in vitro on enriched media with 10% CO_2. The toxins (there are probably four molecular species) are relatively heat-stable proteins with molecular weights of about 24,000. They are antigenic and distinct from the alpha-hemolysin of *Staph. aureus*. The genes for ET production in some strains of *Staph. aureus* are extrachromosomal; in other strains they are chromosomally determined.

Staphylococcal strains isolated from the skin lesions or other sites of infection in patients with the scalded-skin syndrome, when inoculated into neonatal mice, produce generalized exfoliation. Similar changes are produced by injection of ET into mice less than 5 days of age (prior to the appearance of hair) but not in older mice. Within 1 to 2 h of injection of ET, the Nikolsky sign can be elicited. Subsequent bulla formation and exfoliation develop whether the toxin is administered intraperitoneally or subcutaneously.[45] Intradermal injection of ET in humans produces similar cutaneous changes at the site of inoculation.[46]

PATHOLOGY.   The characteristic histologic changes in SSSS are the formation of a cleavage plane high in the epidermis, in the granular cell layer, and separation of the epidermal layer by edema fluid producing typical bullae. There is little associated inflammatory reaction in the dermis or epidermis.[46]

CLINICAL MANIFESTATIONS.   Staphylococcal scalded-skin syndrome usually occurs in either newborn infants (Ritter's disease) or in young children, but it may occur in older children or rarely in adults. It begins abruptly (sometimes several days following pharyngitis, rhinorrhea, conjunctivitis, or a discrete staphylococcal infection) with diffuse erythema resembling that of scarlet fever, marked skin tenderness, and fever. Within 12 to 14 h the Nikolsky sign is present. Large flaccid bullae filled with clear fluid develop and rupture almost immediately; these are not conventional bullae but represent passive fluid accumulation beneath detached epidermis. Large sheets of skin separate, wrinkle, and exfoliate, exposing a moist, bright red surface (see Chap. 51) (Fig. 187-12). Because of the extensive exfoliation, temperature regulation and fluid balance are particular problems in the newborn. Generally,

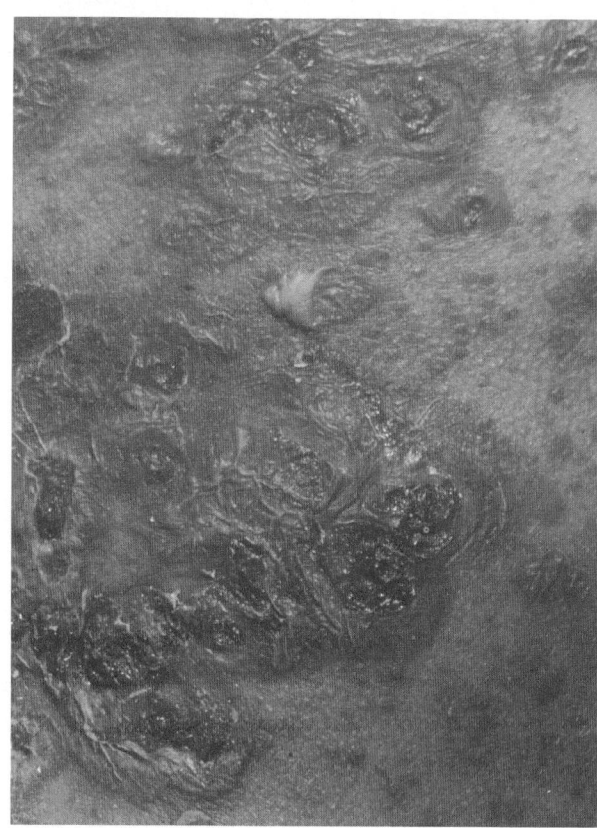

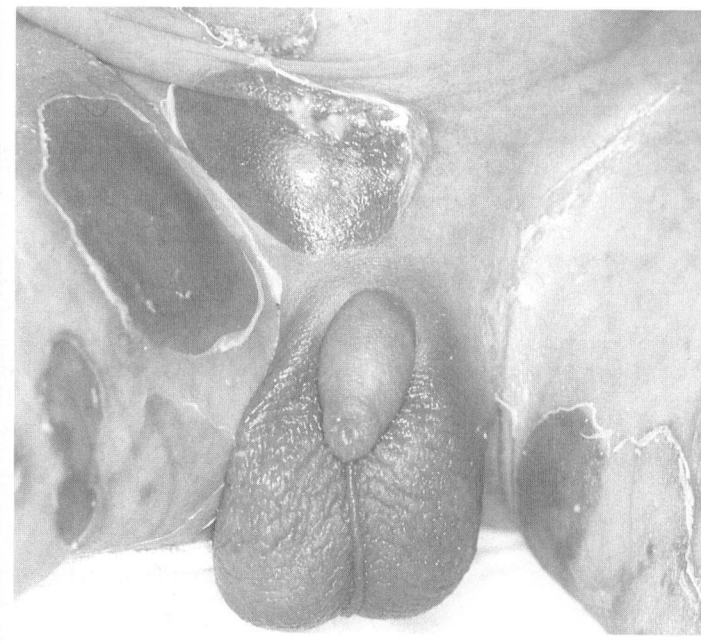

b

a

FIGURE 187-11 Bullous impetigo. (*a*) Large confluent flaccid bullae that dry to form brownish crusts. (*b*) In this infant, bullous lesions have ruptured leaving large denuded and oozing lesions. (*Courtesy of K. Wolff, M.D.*)

with appropriate antibiotic and fluid therapy, patients recover and the skin is healed within 10 to 14 days of the onset of erythema, unless secondary infection has occurred.

STAPHYLOCOCCAL SCARLET FEVER. This is identical with the generalized scarlatiniform rash with skin tenderness observed in the initial stage of SSSS. As in streptococcal scarlet fever, the skin is diffusely erythematous with a sandpaper roughness. Pastia's lines are present. Pharyngitis is not usually a feature, but patients are febrile for the first few days. The strawberry tongue and palatal enanthem are not seen. Bullae and exfoliation do not occur, although Nikolsky's sign may be present in an occasional patient. After 2 to 5 days of erythema, desquamation begins, initially on the face, and extends to involve most of the body. Healing of the skin occurs within 10 days.

Staphylococci belonging to phage group II are recovered from sites of staphylococcal infection (conjunctivitis, abscesses, bacteremia, external otitis). Staphylococcal scarlet fever can be considered a forme fruste of SSSS.

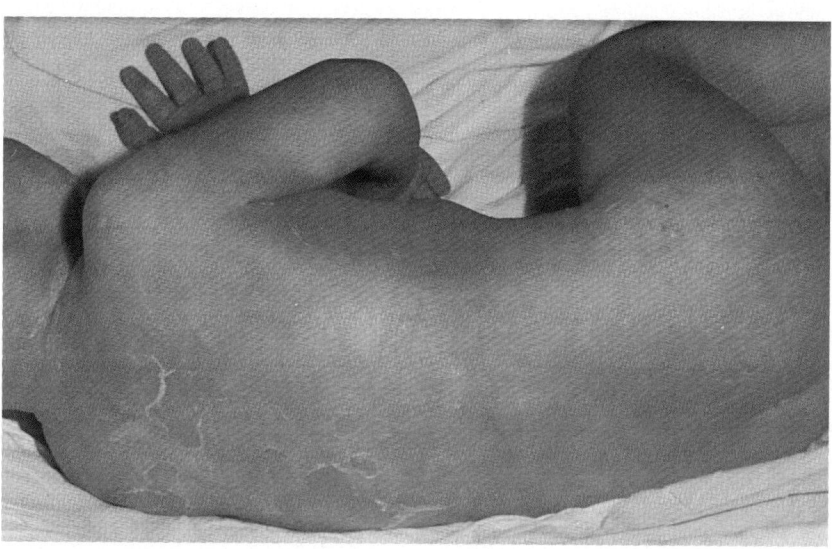

FIGURE 187-12 Staphylococcal scalded-skin syndrome. Note the large sheets of exfoliation.

Toxic Shock Syndrome DEFINITION. The toxic shock syndrome (TSS) is an acute febrile illness due to certain toxin-producing strains of *Staph. aureus* and characterized by a generalized erythematous eruption. Additional elements making up the syndrome include (1) hypotension, (2) functional abnormalities in at least three organ systems, and (3) desquamation following the scarlatiniform eruption. Over 1600 cases occurred in a nationwide outbreak between 1979 and 1982 primarily, but not exclusively, in menstruating women.[47]

BACTERIOLOGY AND PATHOGENESIS. *Staph. aureus* strains isolated from women with menstrual TSS are usually penicillin-resistant and over 93 percent of them produce TSS toxin 1 (TSST-1); 62 percent of isolates from women with nonmenstrual TSS produce this toxin, as do 20 percent of randomly tested isolates. Commonly, TSST-1 production by *Staph. aureus* is associated with tryptophane auxotrophy and with the insertion of a transposon-like segment into several sites on the chromosome.[48] Illness similar to TSS in humans can be produced in animals inoculated with either purified TSST-1 or with TSST-1–producing strains of *Staph. aureus,* and the manifestations of this illness can be prevented by TSST-1 antiserum. Many *Staph. aureus* isolates from patients with nonmenstrual TSS do not produce TSST-1; enterotoxin B is the only toxin produced by at least 38 percent of these isolates, and a few strains produce a third TSS toxin (enterotoxin C_1).[49] TSST-1 stimulates release of tumor necrosis factor (TNF), and the induction of the shock-like state appears to be related to the synergistic action of TNF with interleukin 1.[50]

In 1980, about 85 to 90 percent of cases of TSS occurred in women at the time of menstruation; almost all had been tampon (particularly superabsorbent types) users. *Staph. aureus* has been isolated from vaginal cultures of more than 90 percent of menstruating women with TSS, but from only 10 percent of healthy menstruating women. Cervicovaginal ulcerations, possibly produced or aggravated by tampon use, may have provided the initiating infection and the portal for toxin absorption in menstruating women who developed TSS. Staphylococcal infections (soft tissue, bone, lung) in children, men, and nonmenstruating women have accounted for the remaining 10 to 15 percent of cases of TSS. Between 1980 and 1990, the number of cases of menstrual TSS has declined by over 90 percent, but the number of nonmenstrual cases has remained unchanged.

CLINICAL MANIFESTATIONS. Fever, hypotension (or shock), and an erythematous rash are the initial hallmarks of TSS. The rash may be indistinguishable from that of scarlet fever or may be less striking and suggest the flush associated with fever. Desquamation of palms and soles occurs 1 to 2 weeks later. Other early clinical features may include pharyngeal redness, strawberry tongue, conjunctival injection, diarrhea, and vomiting. Evidences of multiple other organ dysfunctions are seen in TSS: (1) *muscular system—*myalgias and rhabdomyolysis, (2) *central nervous system—*toxic encephalopathy, (3) *kidney—*azotemia, (4) *liver—*elevated levels of SGOT and serum bilirubin, (5) *blood—*thrombocytopenia.

LABORATORY FINDINGS. Leukocytosis and thrombocytopenia are usually present. Microscopic hematuria may be present. Elevated BUN and creatinine levels occur in the majority of patients, and abnormal liver function tests are frequent. Increased serum creatinine kinase levels reflect muscle injury, and myoglobinuria occurs in some patients. Hypocalcemia occurs in many patients but the basis is unclear.

DIAGNOSIS AND DIFFERENTIAL DIAGNOSIS. Diagnosis is made on the basis of the clinical constellation of findings in a patient who has a *Staph. aureus* infection or in a menstruating woman, particu-larly in a tampon user. The differential diagnosis includes scarlet fever (not usually associated with hypotension or shock), streptococcal toxic shock-like syndrome, SSSS (in which bullae and a positive Nikolsky sign are expected), a febrile drug reaction (not usually associated with hypotension), Kawasaki's disease (usually in children and features prominent lymphadenopathy), and meningococcemia (in which rash is petechial rather than scarlatiniform).

TREATMENT. Staphylococcal impetigo responds quite promptly to appropriate treatment. In the adult, oxacillin (or similar penicillinase-resistant semisynthetic penicillin) 0.5 g orally 4 times daily or erythromycin (in the penicillin-allergic patient) 0.25 g orally 4 times daily should be used if the process is extensive or bullous in character. Treatment should be continued for 5 to 7 days (10 days if streptococci are isolated). Local treatment with mupirocin ointment and removal of crusts and maintenance of cleanliness, as in the management of streptococcal impetigo, is sufficient to cure many mild cases. However, the results are further improved, particularly in extensive cases, by the administration of antibiotics, as noted above. The frequency of isolation of group A streptococci makes systemic antibiotic therapy a reasonable approach in most patients with a significant degree of involvement.

Intravenous use of a penicillinase-resistant penicillin (nafcillin or oxacillin) is indicated in the initial treatment of *Staph. aureus* scalded-skin syndrome and of staphylococcal scarlet fever because of the relation of these processes to active staphylococcal infections of the skin or elsewhere and because of the rapid progression and potential seriousness of the illness. Nafcillin is administered at a dosage of 50 to 100 mg/kg per day in the newborn and at a dosage of 100 to 200 mg/kg per day (in divided doses every 4 to 6 h) for older children. The adult dose is 6 to 10 g daily, in divided doses every 4 to 6 h. Oxacillin is administered in similar dosage. A switch to oral therapy (e.g., cloxacillin 50 mg/kg per day in divided doses every 6 h) should not be made until there has been extensive clearing of the lesions or the initiating focus of staphylococcal infection has been controlled.

Systemic corticosteroids should not be used in the treatment of SSSS. Their use clinically has been associated with continued progression of the lesions, and in hydrocortisone-treated experimental animals only 1/100 to 1/1000 of the usual infecting dose of *Staph. aureus* was needed to produce exfoliation.[45] Corticosteroid therapy may be indicated in the treatment of drug-induced toxic epidermal necrolysis (TEN). In cases of TEN where it is unclear whether a staphylococcal etiology or drug sensitivity is responsible, consideration may be given to the use of combined antibiotic and corticosteroid therapy.

For topical management of the lesions of SSSS, cool saline compresses are used. Flurandrenolide ointment (0.025 to 0.05%) may be useful subsequently in selected cases where there is no direct infection of the skin.

Treatment of TSS involves (1) immediate institution of vigorous fluid replacement to combat the hypotension, (2) attention to focal staphylococcal infections (drainage of abscesses, removal of tampons), and systemic antimicrobial therapy aimed at penicillinase-producing *Staph. aureus* (nafcillin 1.0 to 1.5 g intravenously in the adult every 4 h).

Folliculitis This is a pyoderma located within the hair follicle. There are two main subdivisions: superficial and deep. Follicular impetigo (Bockhart's impetigo) is a superficial folliculitis (Fig. 187-13a). It is a form of impetigo in which a small dome-shaped pustule occurs at the opening of a hair follicle, often on the scalps of children. There are several distinctive forms of deep folliculitis.

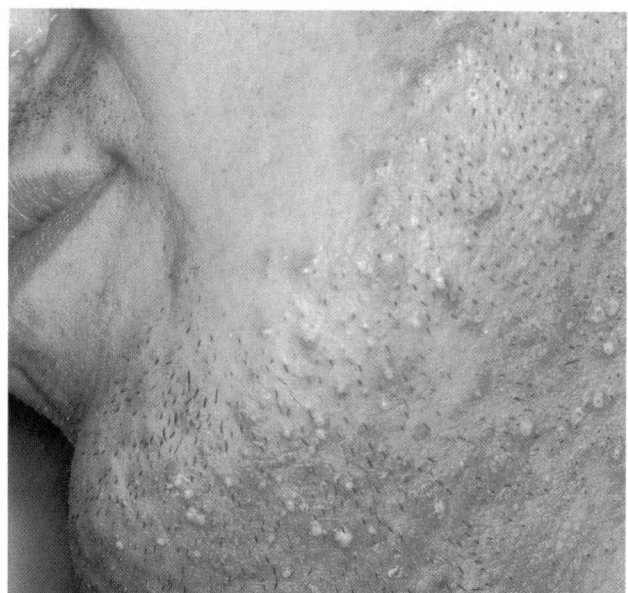

a

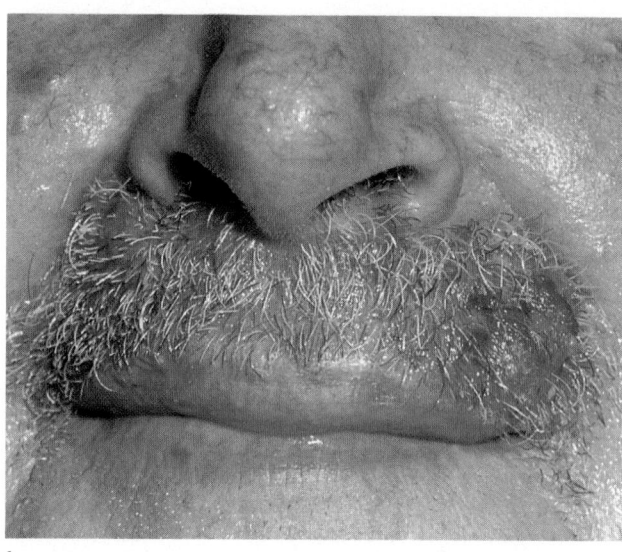

b

FIGURE 187-13 (*a*) Superficial folliculitis. Scattered, discrete pustules occurring in the ostia of the hair follicles. (*b*) Sycosis barbae. Staphylococcal folliculitis of the mustache region. (*Courtesy of K. Wolff, M.D.*)

SYCOSIS BARBAE.   This is a deep folliculitis with perifollicular inflammation occurring in the bearded areas of the face (Fig. 187-13*b*). If uncared for, the lesions become deeper seated and chronic. Local treatment with warm saline compresses and local antibiotics (mupirocin or bacitracin) is sufficient to control the infection. More extensive cases require systemic antibiotic therapy. The major condition to be considered in differential diagnosis is tinea barbae. In the latter fungal infection, the hairs are usually broken or loosened, and there are suppurative nodules rather than discrete pustules.

LUPOID SYCOSIS.   This is a deep, chronic, cicatricial form of sycosis barbae, usually occurring as a circinate lesion.

"CORAL REEF GRANULOMA."   This rare disease begins as a staphylococcal folliculitis, usually on sun-exposed areas of the upper extremities, and spreads peripherally with ulcerations, ero-

sions, and sinus tract formation.[51] There is profuse purulent drainage from multiple openings of burrowing lesions. The process continues for many months with active infection, scarring, and pseudoepitheliomatous hyperplasia progressing apace. Ultimately, the process burns itself out, leaving an irregular "coral reef" scar.

Furuncles and Carbuncles   DEFINITION.   A furuncle, or boil, is a deep-seated inflammatory nodule that develops about a hair follicle, usually from a preceding, more superficial folliculitis. A carbuncle is a more extensive, deeper, infiltrated lesion that develops when suppuration occurs in thick inelastic skin.

CLINICAL MANIFESTATIONS.   *History* Furuncles occur only in areas where there are hair follicles, particularly in regions subject to friction and perspiration: neck, face, axillae, buttocks. They may complicate preexisting lesions such as scabies, pediculosis, or abrasions, but occur more often in the absence of any local predisposing causes. In addition, a variety of systemic host factors is associated with furunculosis. These include obesity, blood dyscrasias, defects in neutrophil function (defects in chemotaxis associated with eczema and high levels of IgE; defects in intracellular killing of organisms as in chronic granulomatous disease of childhood), treatment with corticosteroids and cytotoxic agents, and immune globulin deficiency states. Whether diabetes mellitus predisposes to furunculosis is still controversial; once established, however, the process is often more extensive in patients with diabetes (Fig. 187-14). The majority of patients with problems of furunculosis appear to be otherwise healthy.

Cutaneous Lesions A furuncle starts as a hard, tender, red nodule that enlarges and becomes painful and fluctuant after several days (Figs. 187-14 and 187-15). Rupture occurs, with discharge of pus and often a core of necrotic material. The pain about the lesion then subsides, and the redness and edema diminish over several days to several weeks.

A *carbuncle* is a larger, more serious inflammatory lesion with a deeper base. It characteristically occurs as an extremely painful lesion at the nape of the neck, the back, or thighs (Fig. 187-16). Fever and malaise are often present, and the patient may appear quite ill. The involved area is red and indurated, and multiple pustules soon appear on the surface, draining externally around multiple hair follicles. The lesion soon develops a yellow-gray irregular crater at the center, which may then heal slowly by granulating, although the area may remain deeply violaceous for a prolonged period. The resulting permanent scar is often dense and readily evident.

LABORATORY FINDINGS.   Extensive furunculosis or a carbuncle may be associated with a leukocytosis, particularly when there is a large amount of unliberated pus, surrounding cellulitis, or bacteremia. *Staph. aureus* is almost always the etiology of furuncles and carbuncles.

PATHOLOGY.   A dense polymorphonuclear inflammatory process in the subcutaneous fat characterizes a carbuncle. Multiple abscesses, separated by connective tissue trabeculae, infiltrate the dermis and pass along the edges of the hair follicles, reaching the surface through openings in the undermined epidermis.

DIAGNOSIS AND DIFFERENTIAL DIAGNOSIS.   The diagnosis is made on the basis of the clinical appearance. Simple folliculitis, due to *Staph. aureus* or *Staph. epidermidis,* is easily distinguished by the absence of significant redness and induration about the hair follicle.

COURSE AND PROGNOSIS.   The major problems with furunculosis and carbuncles are bacteremic spread of infection and recurrence. Lesions about the lips and nose raise the specter of spread

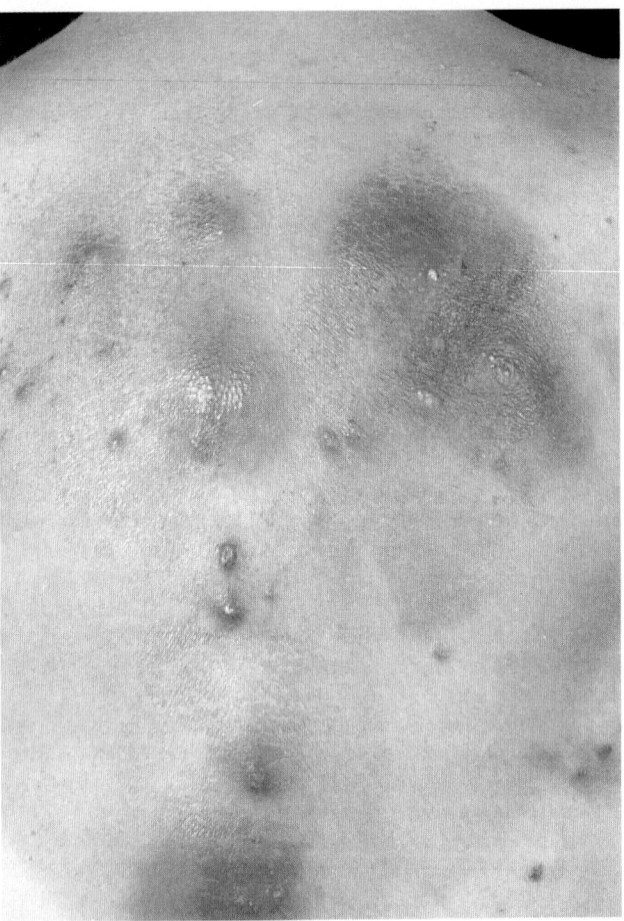

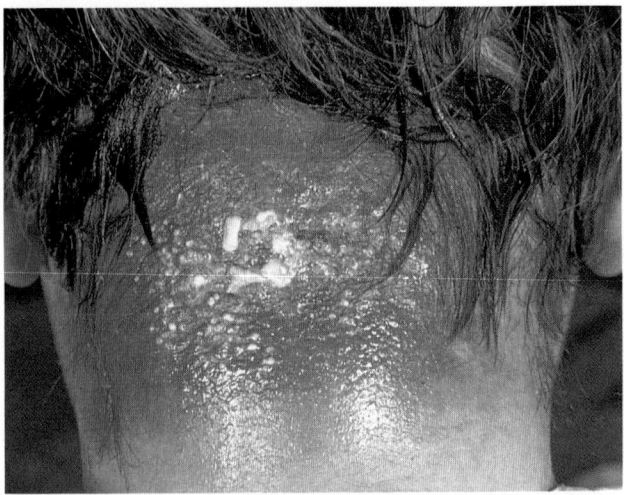

FIGURE 187-16   Carbuncle. This lesion represents multiple confluent furuncles draining pus from multiple openings. (*Courtesy of K. Wolff, M.D.*)

FIGURE 187-14   Multiple furuncles in a diabetic. (*Courtesy of K. Wolff, M.D.*)

via the facial and angular emissary veins to the cavernous sinus. Invasion of the bloodstream may occur from furuncles or carbuncles at any time, in an unpredictable fashion, producing osteomyelitis, acute endocarditis, brain abscess, or other metastatic foci. *Squeezing such lesions is particularly dangerous and frequently produces spread of infection via the bloodstream.* Fortunately, these complications are not common.

Recurrent furunculosis is a troublesome process that may recur over many years. Most often these lesions are limited to the area of the follicles, but sometimes they extend to produce surrounding cellulilitis or bacteremia. Individuals who perspire excessively or who have poor skin hygiene appear more disposed to recurrent furunculosis.

TREATMENT.   *Simple furunculosis* may be treated by local application of moist heat, which relieves discomfort, aids in the localization of the infection, and promotes drainage. Such cases do not require the use of either local or systemic antibiotics. A *carbuncle* or a *furuncle* with surrounding cellulitis, or one associated with fever, should be treated with a systemic antibiotic. In view of the high frequency of penicillin-resistant *Staph. aureus,* a semisynthetic penicillin such as oxacillin (0.50 to 0.75 g orally every 4 to 6 h in the adult) should be used. In the penicillin-allergic adult, clindamycin (150 to 300 mg orally 4 times a day) or erythromycin (0.25 to 0.5 g orally 4 times daily) may be substituted. For severe infections or infections in a dangerous area, maximal antibiotic dosage should be employed by the parenteral route, the patient should be put to bed, and the involved area should be immobilized. If methicillin-resistant *Staph aureus* is implicated or suspected in serious infections, vancomycin (1.0 to 2.0 g intravenously daily in divided doses) is indicated. Antibiotic treatment should be continued for at least 1 week.

When the lesions are large but localized, painful, and fluctuant, drainage (limited to the necrotic fluctuant area) is indicated. Antimicrobial therapy should be continued until evidences of inflammation have regressed. After adequate drainage (spontaneous or surgical) has occurred, moist dressings should not be applied because of the danger of local spread enhanced by tissue maceration. Application of a thin layer of bacitracin (500 units/g) or mupirocin (2%) ointment about the lesion protects the surrounding

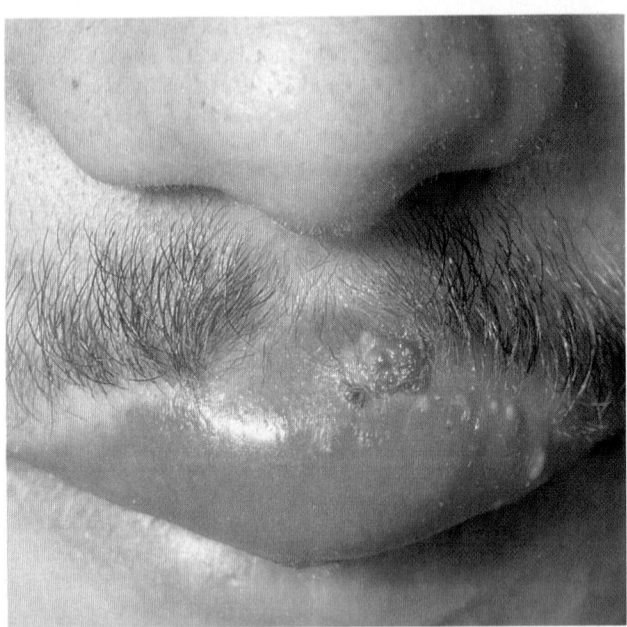

FIGURE 187-15   Furuncle of the upper lip. The lesion is nodular and the central necrotic plug is covered by purulent crust. Several small pustules are seen lateral to the center of the lesion. (*Courtesy of K. Wolff, M.D.*)

skin. Such draining lesions should be covered with a sterile dressing to prevent autoinoculation. Hands should be thoroughly washed after contact with the lesions.

The management of patients with *recurrent furunculosis* presents a special and frequently exasperating problem. There is no evidence that this disease is due to any specific staphylococcal strains with special biologic properties. In addition to the treatment of acute lesions, as above, management involves steps in the prophylaxis of recurrent episodes:

1. Careful evaluation for underlying causes.
    a. Systemic processes: previously discussed.
    b. Specific localized predisposing factors: industrial exposure to chemicals, oils; poor hygiene; obesity; hyperhidrosis; ingrown hairs; pressure from tight clothing or belts.
    c. Sources of staphylococcal contact: pyogenic infections in the family; contact sports such as wrestling; autoinoculation.
    d. Nasal carriage of *Staph. aureus:* this is the site from which dissemination of the organism may occur to other body sites. The frequency of nasal carriage varies: 10 to 15 percent in infants 1 year of age, 38 percent in college students, 50 percent in hospital physicians and military trainees.[52]
2. General skin care. The aim of these measures is to reduce the numbers of *Staph. aureus* on the skin. General skin care of both hands and body with water and soap is important (an antimicrobial soap solution, such as 4% chlorhexidine solution, may be used to decrease staphylococcal skin colonization). The patient should avoid trauma to the skin as well as potential skin irritants such as strong soaps and deodorants. A separate washcloth (and towel) should be used and carefully washed in *hot* water prior to reuse.
3. Care of clothing. Loose, lightweight, porous clothing should be worn as much as possible. Large numbers of staphylococci are frequently present on the sheets and underclothing of patients with furunculosis and may cause reinfection of the patient and infection of other members of the family. In problem cases it is not unreasonable to recommend that these items be carefully and separately washed in boiling water and changed daily.
4. Care of dressings. Dressings should be changed frequently if purulent drainage collects. They should be carefully discarded into a paper bag that can be sealed and disposed of immediately.
5. General measures. Despite the above measures, some patients continue to have recurrent cycles of lesions. Sometimes the problem can be ameliorated or abolished by removing the patient from the regular routine of work. This is particularly pertinent in individuals under considerable emotional stress and physical fatigue. A vacation for several weeks, ideally in a cool, dry climate, may help considerably by providing rest and also the time needed for carrying out the program of careful skin care.
6. Measures aimed at elimination of nasal (and skin) carriage of *Staph. aureus* (methicillin-susceptible or methicillin-resistant).
    a. Local use of antibiotic ointments in the nasal vestibule reduces nasal carriage of *Staph. aureus* and secondarily reduces the "shedding" or organisms on the skin, a process that may contribute to recurrent furunculosis. Intranasal application of a 2% mupirocin calcium ointment in a white, soft paraffin base for 5 days can eliminate *Staph.*

aureus nasal carriage in 70 percent of healthy individuals for up to 3 months.[53] (Bacitracin ointment has been used for the same purpose.) Prophylaxis with antibiotic (fusidic acid) ointment in the nares twice daily every fourth week for the patient and family members who are nasal carriers of the infecting strain (along with a peroral antistaphylococcal antibiotic for 10 to 14 days for the patient) has been employed with some success.[54]
    b. Oral antibiotics (e.g., rifampin, 600 mg orally daily for 10 days) have been effective in eradicating *Staph. aureus* from most nasal carriers for periods up to 12 weeks.[55] Such a use of rifampin for a brief period to eradicate nasal carriage of *Staph. aureus* and interrupt a continuing cycle of recurrent furunculosis might be reasonable in the patient in whom other measures have failed. However, selection of rifampin-resistant strains can occur rapidly with such therapy. The addition of a second drug (cloxacillin, if the strain is methicillin-susceptible; trimethoprim-sulfamethoxazole, ciprofloxacin, or minocycline for methicillin-resistant strains) has been employed to reduce the emergence of rifampin resistance.[56]
7. Measures of unproven worth. Staphylococcal vaccines of various types (autogenous, toxoid made from exotoxins, and bacteriophage-lysed preparations) have been used in attempts to protect against infection by inducing further humoral immunity. A controlled evaluation of the use of a staphylococcal bacteriophage-lysed vaccine showed that it had no significant effect on the course of recurrent furunculosis.[57]

Hidradenitis Suppurativa (See also Chap. 67.) DEFINITION. This is an extremely troublesome, chronic, recurrent, suppurative infection of blocked apocrine glands occurring in the axillary, perianal, and genital regions. The organisms initially found may be *Staph. aureus,* but subsequently the predominant organisms may be gram-negative bacilli such as *Proteus.*

CLINICAL MANIFESTATIONS. The initial lesions are tender, reddish purple nodules, appearing very much like furuncles. They subsequently become fluctuant, drain, and form irregular sinus tracts. Repeated crops of nodules with further burrowing constitute the usual sequence. Vegetative granular masses develop with deep boggy nodules, and there is marked hypertrophic scarring. The lesions occur in either men or women, but always after puberty. With extensive involvement, some patients exhibit constitutional symptoms such as fever and weight loss. The chronic process may eventually become quiescent after destroying most of the apocrine glands of the body.

DIFFERENTIAL DIAGNOSIS. To be considered in the differential diagnosis are acne conglobata, multiple infected sebaceous cysts, and cutaneous blastomycosis. Predominant involvement about the inguinal and perianal areas may suggest lymphogranuloma venereum.

TREATMENT. Treatment is difficult because of the multiple, deep-seated sites of inflammation and infection not accessible to antibiotics. However, guided by Gram-stained samples and cultural evidence (as well as in vitro susceptibility tests), one can employ an appropriate systemic antibiotic. This will not cure the disease but will help to quiet the active acute process. Local moist heat may help to establish drainage, but surgical drainage of the frank abscesses is usually mandatory. Unfortunately, this does not prevent recurrent infection in many residual, blind-ended sinus tracts. In the very severe cases that are marked by chronicity and scarring and have resisted the above measures, radical surgical excision of most of the involved area, followed by skin grafting, may be the only avenue remaining. This is a very extensive and difficult surgical procedure requiring considerable skill and experience. Excision of isolated, resistant, infected apocrine glands is also sometimes effective therapy.

Actinophytosis (Botryomycosis)   This a very rare pyogenic disease in humans. The lesions (usually solitary) can occur in skin, bone, liver, etc., and, on gross examination of the pus, pinhead-sized, whitish-yellow granules are evident. When examined under the microscope, as on a fresh mount or in 20% potassium hydroxide (KOH), these granules appear coarsely lobulated and are seen to contain tightly packed clublike projections (resembling the ''sulfur granules'' of actinomycosis or a mycetoma). Examination of Gram-stained preparations of crushed granules shows only masses of staphylococci, not the ray fungus appearance of actinomycosis. On histologic (hematoxylin-eosin stain) section the findings are those of a basophilic granule made up of clusters of cocci (usually within the papillary dermis) surrounded by an amorphous eosinophilic matrix (Splendore-Hoeppli phenomenon); the latter probably represents host immunoglobulin. Cultures grow out typical *Staph. aureus.*

The cases of involvement of the skin in *botryomycosis* have usually had a solitary lesion or only a few lesions, often occurring in the genital area. The lesion has the gross appearance of an infected sebaceous cyst, with mild reddening of the skin over the circumscribed, slightly tender mass. Some lesions may resemble prurigo nodularis. In the majority of reported cases, a foreign body (fish bone, broom straw, etc.) has played a role in initiating or perpetuating the lesion. Several cases have occurred in patients with the hyperimmunoglobulin E syndrome associated with recurrent staphylococcal infections and in patients with the acquired immunodeficiency syndrome (AIDS).[58] Surgical drainage will usually produce rapid resolution.

It appears that this rare lesion may be related in some way to a balance between numbers of organisms and host defenses. This condition should not be mistaken for granuloma pyogenicum (which has been given also the confusing designation botryomycosis hominis), a lesion that consists of small, pedunculated, raspberry-like vegetations of overgrowth of granulation tissue, particularly newly formed blood vessels, occurring at the site of trauma.

Skin Lesions in Staph. aureus Bacteremia and Endocarditis (See Chap. 166)   In acute bacteremia or endocarditis due to *Staph. aureus,* skin lesions can provide a clue to the nature of the infecting organism. These lesions include pustules, subcutaneous abscesses, and purulent purpura. The purulent purpura consists of an area of purpura with a white purulent center (Fig. 187-17). Gram-stained smear of the aspirated contents of the center shows gram-positive cocci in clusters and polymorphonuclear inflammatory cells.

Rarely, a patient will develop multiple, tender, 2- to 4-cm nodules in the subcutaneous tissues as part of a systemic staphylococcal infection. The overlying skin is mildly erythematous. The nodules are firm and do not suppurate. The lesions are often found on the trunk and in this location suggest those of Weber-Christian disease (relapsing febrile nonsuppurative panniculitis). Low-grade fever is associated with these lesions, but the patients do not appear acutely ill. Blood cultures have only occasionally been positive, although the lesions probably represent metastatic infection in the subcutaneous tissue. Biopsy shows a nonspecific inflammatory response, and culture of the nodule shows *Staph. aureus.* The lesions promptly regress on antibiotic treatment.

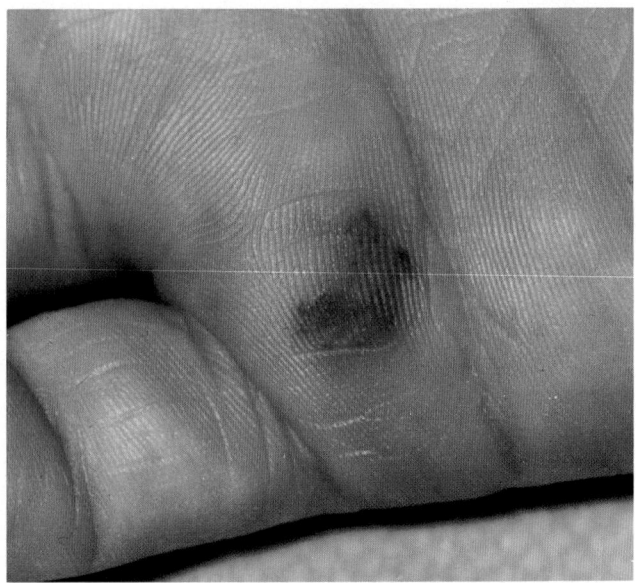

a

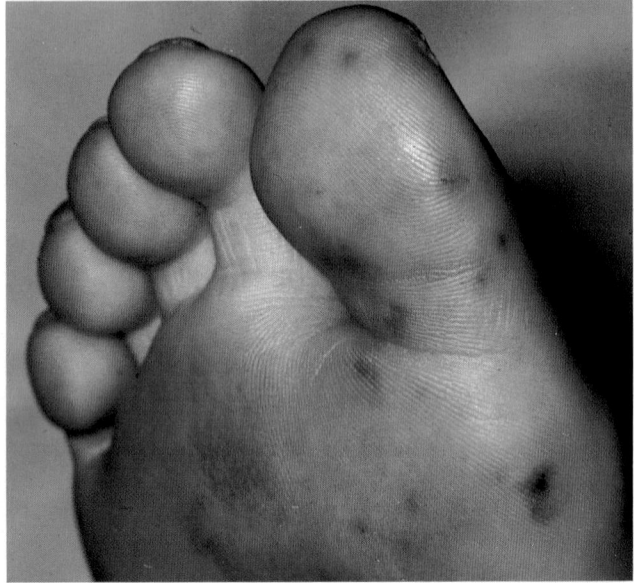

b

FIGURE 187-17   Infective endocarditis. (*a*) Janeway lesions on the hands. These are nonpainful, hemorrhagic, infarcted macules on the palms and soles. This patient had an acute *Staph. aureus* endocarditis. (*b*) Janeway lesions on the feet. (*Courtesy of David N. Silvers, M.D.*)

Staphylococcal Lymphocutaneous Syndrome   Macronodular sporotrichoid lesions on the forearm (in the distribution of nodular lymphangitis) have been reported very rarely either in the course of *Staph. aureus* bacteremia[59] or following injury to the hand or with botryomycosis.[60]

Cutaneous Manifestations of Infections due to *Clostridium perfringens (C. welchii)*

Anaerobic cellulitis and gas gangrene (myonecrosis) are two forms of *C. perfringens* infection involving subcutaneous tissues and muscles, respectively. The etiologic agent is an obligate anaerobe that is normally found in the bowel. Cutaneous manifestations are evident in each process. It should be recalled, however, that gas-forming infections may sometimes be caused by *Escherichia coli*, *Klebsiella*, *Bacteroides*, or anaerobic streptococci (see Chap. 188).

Anaerobic Cellulitis

This is a clostridial infection of devitalized tissue usually occurring in a dirty or inadequately debrided wound several days after injury. The onset is more gradual than in gas gangrene. The anaerobes are able to grow in the depths of the wound and extend rapidly through tissue planes, with attendant formation of large quantities of gas. A thin, dark gray-brown, foul, serous discharge is produced. Gram-stained smear of the drainage reveals short, plump, blunt-ended, gram-positive rods without spores and with a variable number of polymorphonuclear leukocytes. Unlike clinical gas gangrene, there is relatively little local pain or edema, change in overlying skin, toxemia, or extension of the process to involve muscle. At operation the muscles appear normal, but gas may extend diffusely and is readily evident through the exudate. This type of infection must be distinguished from clostridial myositis (gas gangrene) to avoid needless mutilating surgery and amputations. Treatment consists of opening the wound, removing necrotic debris, and administering antibiotics (penicillin preferably, or a broad-spectrum antibiotic, and metronidazole).

Anaerobic Myositis (Myonecrosis)

This is a rapidly progressing, toxemic, potentially lethal infection involving muscle but with secondary changes in the overlying skin. The infection may develop as a complication of a traumatic dirty wound with extensive muscle and soft-tissue damage. In addition, gas gangrene may also occur after surgery on the bowel or gallbladder.

The incubation period is often short (12 to 24 h) but may be delayed, and occasionally gas gangrene develops following anaerobic cellulitis. The first symptom is usually local pain, followed by edema. Gas formation is not prominent and may be completely obscured by local swelling of the subcutaneous tissues. The skin often takes on a dark yellow or bronze discoloration, with tense blebs or bullae containing dark brown fluid. A serosanguineous exudate can be expressed from the wound. Gram stain of the exudate reveals plump gram-positive rods and only a few white blood cells. Subsequently, green-black patches of necrosis of the skin at the margin of the wound may develop. Evidences of toxemia are present: high fever, tachycardia, hypotension, and oliguria. Intravascular hemolysis does not usually occur in this type of process, in contrast to septic abortion with septicemia due to this organism. The same clinical picture is produced by bacteremic *C. septicum* gas gangrene developing in the setting of occult colonic neoplasm.

Treatment consists of wide surgical debridement of all devitalized muscle and parenteral administration of penicillin (often with metronidazole) in dosage of about 10,000,000 units daily. The use of hyperbaric oxygen "drenching," particularly in patients with far-advanced disease involving the trunk in whom surgical excision would be mutilating, appears to have a place in current therapy. Polyvalent gas gangrene antitoxin (40,000 to 60,000 units every 6 h for several doses) has been administered often in the past, but there has been no clear evidence of its efficacy. This antiserum is no longer commercially available.

Cutaneous Nocardial Infections

Several types of unusual nocardial skin infections have been described: (1) cutaneous abscesses (fluctuant, nontender erythematous nodules or cold abscesses) associated with hematogenous spread from a primary infection in the lung[61]; (2) localized ulcers, abscesses, or cellulitis at sites of abrasion or thorn injuries; (3) primary lymphocutaneous *Nocardia brasiliensis* (very rarely *N. asteroides*) infection resembling the lymphocutaneous (nodular lymphangitis) syndrome,[62] more often associated with *Sporothrix schenkii* or *Mycobacterium marinum* infection; (4) mycetoma (see Chap. 196). Trimethoprim-sulfamethoxazole therapy (for several months) is the treatment of choice.

Cutaneous Infections due to Miscellaneous Gram-Positive Bacilli

Necrotizing fasciitis or isolated necrotic bullae have occurred as manifestations of localized cutaneous infections with *Bacillus cereus* in granulocytopenic patients.[63] Vancomycin intravenously is the drug of choice because this *Bacillus* species produces a beta-lactamase and is resistant to penicillin G.

Skin and soft tissue infections associated with *Corynebacterium* JK septicemia occur in granulocytopenic patients and take either of two forms: (1) primary infections (cellulitis at bone marrow biopsy sites, infection at insertion sites of intravascular catheters), and (2) secondary infections (erythematous or hemorrhagic papular rash, soft tissue abscess, or necrotic lesions) consequent on bacteremia from primary infection sites.[64] Vancomycin intravenously is the treatment of choice.

Erythrasma

Definition

Erythrasma is a common superficial bacterial infection of the skin characterized by well-defined but irregular reddish brown patches, occurring in the intertriginous areas, or by fissuring and maceration in the toe clefts.

Epidemiology

Erythrasma is widespread and has been found in about 20 percent of subjects randomly studied in a temperate climate. The generalized disease is much more common in the tropics. It is more common in men, where it may be present in an asymptomatic form in the genitocrural area. It does not appear to be significantly contagious.[65]

Etiology

The causative agent has been shown to be not a dermatophyte or *Nocardia* species, as was formerly believed, but a *Corynebacterium* species, *Corynebacterium minutissimum*. The organism is a short, gram-positive rod with subterminal granules. It is best cultivated on a medium containing 20% fetal bovine serum, 78% tissue culture medium No. 199 in 2% agar and 0.05% Tris, pH 6.8 to 7.2. Growth occurs as small, shiny, moist, whitish-gray translucent colonies, which fluoresce orange to coral-red under Wood's lamp. The organism can also be isolated on blood agar, but the colonies may not fluoresce on that medium. Related *Corynebacterium* species are associated with the lesions of trichomycosis axillaris and pitted keratolysis.

Clinical Manifestations

History The manifestations vary from a completely asymptomatic form, through a genitocrural form with considerable pruritus, to a generalized form with scaly lamellated plaques on the trunk and extremities.

Cutaneous Lesions (Fig. 187-18) The lesions are reddish-brown, rather superficial, finely scaly and finely wrinkled, and slowly spreading macular patches. Axillary and genitocrural areas are the principal sites of infection.

Pathology

Gram-stained imprints of the horny layer of the skin show rod-like, gram-positive organisms in large numbers. Bacilli have been demonstrated within cells of the horny layer on examination by electron microscope.

Diagnosis

The diagnosis is strongly suggested by the location and superficial character of the process. A characteristic ''coral-red'' fluorescence

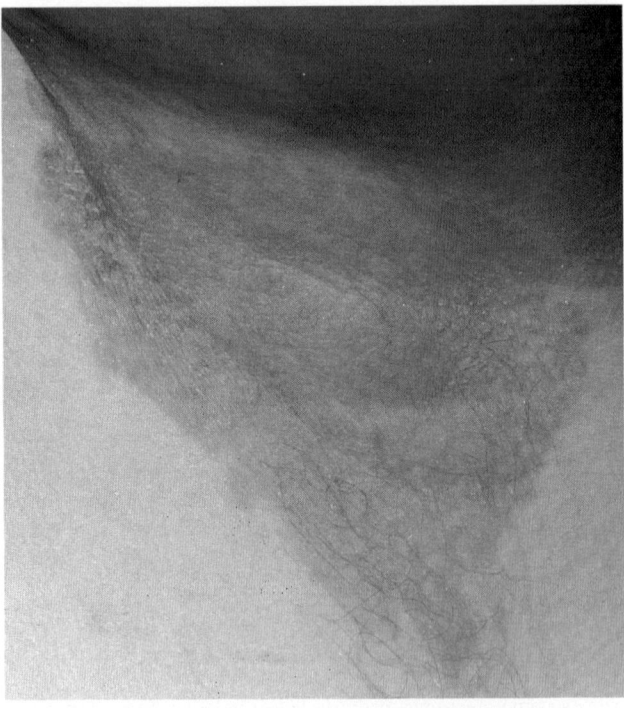

FIGURE 187-18 Erythrasma. Well-marginated brownish-reddish lesion with fine scaling at a typical site. (*Courtesy of K. Wolff, M.D.*)

seen over the involved areas under Wood's lamp confirms the diagnosis. Cultivation of the specific *Corynebacterium* in abundance from the lesion corroborates the diagnosis. Tinea versicolor is distinguished from erythrasma by the lesions on the trunk seen in the former. Tinea cruris is more rapidly progressive and has a deeper, more inflammatory character.

Treatment

A 5- to 7-day course of erythromycin, 1.0 g orally daily, usually produces clearing of the lesions within several weeks. Topical therapy is less effective, but aqueous clindamycin (2%) solution, Whitfield's ointment, or miconazole (2%) cream may be useful at times.[66]

Course and Prognosis

The disease may remain asymptomatic for years or may undergo periodic exacerbations. Relapses occasionally occur even after successful antibiotic treatment.

References

1. Duma RH et al: Streptococcal infections. A bacteriologic and clinical study of streptococcal bacteremia. *Medicine (Baltimore)* **48**:87, 1969
2. Barnham M, Neilson DJ: Group L beta-haemolytic streptococcal infection in meat handlers: Another streptococcal zoonosis? *Epidemiol Infect* **99**:257, 1987
3. Uhr JW (ed): *The Streptococcus, Rheumatic Fever, and Glomerulonephritis.* Baltimore, Williams & Wilkins, 1964
4. Wannamaker LW: Differences between streptococcal infections of the throat and of the skin. *N Engl J Med* **282**:23, 78, 1970
5. Kaplan EL et al: Group A streptococcal serotypes isolated from patients and sibling contacts during the resurgence of rheumatic fever in the United States in the mid-1980's. *J Infect Dis* **159**:101, 1989
6. Dillon HC Jr: Impetigo contagiosa: Suppurative and nonsuppurative complications. *Am J Dis Child* **115**:530, 1968
7. Bessen D, Fischetti VA: A human IgG receptor of Group A streptococci is associated with tissue site of infection and streptococcal class. *J Infect Dis* **161**:747, 1990
8. Dajani AS et al: Natural history of impetigo. II. Etiologic agents and bacterial interactions. *J Clin Invest* **51**:2863, 1972
9. Mobacken H et al: Epidemiologic aspects of impetigo contagiosa in western Sweden. *Scand J Infect Dis* **7**:39, 1975
10. Goldfarb J et al: Randomized clinical trial of topical mupirocin versus oral erythromycin for impetigo. *Antimicrob Agents Chemother* **32**:1780, 1988
11. Ferrieri P et al: Natural history of impetigo. I. Site sequence of acquisition and familial patterns of spread of cutaneous streptococci. *J Clin Invest* **51**:2851, 1972
12. Blumer JL et al: Changing therapy for skin and soft tissue infections in children: Have we come full circle? *Pediatr Infect Dis J* **6**:117, 1987
13. Maddox JS et al: The natural history of streptococcal skin infection: Prevention with topical antibiotics. *J Am Acad Dermatol* **13**:207, 1985
14. Goldfarb J et al: Randomized clinical trial of topical mupirocin versus oral erythromycin for impetigo. *Antimicrob Agents Chemother* **32**:1780, 1988
15. Britton JW et al: Comparison of mupirocin and erythromycin in the treatment of impetigo. *J Pediatr* **117**:827, 1990

16. Allen AM et al: Cutaneous streptococcal infections in Vietnam. *Arch Dermatol* **104**:271, 1971

17. Jorup-Rönström C: Epidemiologic, bacteriological and complicating features of erysipelas. *Scand J Infect Dis* **18**:519, 1986

18. Majeed HA et al: The cutaneous manifestations in children with familial mediterranean fever (recurrent hereditary polyserositis). A six-year study. *Q J Med* **75**(new series): 607, 1990

19. Williams CN et al: Dissecting cellulitis of the scalp. *Plas Reconstr Surg* **77**:378, 1986

20. Bjellerup M, Wallengren J: Familial perifolliculitis capitis abscedens et suffodiens in two brothers successfully treated with isotretinoin. *J Am Acad Dermatol* **23**:752, 1990

21. Kokx NP et al: Streptococcal perianal disease in children. *Pediatrics* **80**:659, 1987

22. Baddour LM, Bisno AL: Recurrent cellulitis after saphenous venectomy for coronary bypass surgery. *Ann Intern Med* **97**:493, 1982

23. Ellison RT, McGregor JA: Recurrent postcoital lower-extremity streptococcal erythroderma in women. Streptococcal-sex syndrome. *JAMA* **257**:3260, 1987

24. Amren DP: Unusual forms of streptococcal disease, in *Streptococci and Streptococcal Diseases,* edited by LW Wannamaker, JM Matsen. New York, Academic, 1972, p 545

25. Riefler J III et al: Necrotizing fasciitis in adults due to group B streptococcus. Report of a case and review of the literature. *Arch Intern Med* **148**:727, 1988

26. Meleney FL: Hemolytic streptococcus gangrene. *Arch Surg* **9**:317, 1924

27. Barker FG et al: Streptococcal necrotizing fasciitis: Comparison between histological and clinical features. *J Clin Pathol* **40**:335, 1987

28. Giuliano A et al: Bacteriology of necrotizing fasciitis. *Am J Surg* **134**:52, 1977

29. Casali RE et al: Postoperative necrotizing fasciitis of the abdominal wall. *Am J Surg* **140**:787, 1980

30. Finegold SM: *Anaerobic Bacteria in Human Disease.* New York, Academic, 1977, chap 13

31. Stone HH, Martin JJ Jr: Synergistic necrotizing cellulitis. *Ann Surg* **175**:702, 1972

32. Stamenkovic I, Lew PD: Early recognition of potentially fatal necrotizing faciitis. The use of frozen-section biopsy. *N Engl J Med* **310**:1689, 1984

33. Brewer GE, Meleney FL: Progressive gangrenous infection of the skin and subcutaneous tissues, following operation for acute perforative appendicitis. A study in symbiosis. *Ann Surg* **84**:438, 1926

34. Meleney FL: Bacterial synergism in disease processes with a confirmation of the synergistic bacterial etiology of a certain type of progressive gangrene of the abdominal wall. *Ann Surg* **94**:961, 1931

35. Davson J et al: Diagnosis of Meleney's synergistic gangrene. *Br J Surg* **75**:267, 1988

36. Kingston D, Seal DV: Current hypotheses on synergistic microbial gangrene. *Br J Surg* **77**:260, 1990

37. Cone LA et al: Clinical and bacteriologic observations of a toxic shock-like syndrome due to *Streptococcus pyogenes. N Engl J Med* **317**:146, 1987

38. Bartter T et al: 'Toxic strep syndrome.' A manifestation of group A streptococcal infection. *Arch Intern Med* **148**:1421, 1988

39. Shaunak S et al: Septic scarlet fever due to *Streptococcus pyogenes* cellulitis. *Q J Med* **69**(new series):921, 1988

40. Alpert JS et al: Pathogenesis of Osler's nodes, *Ann Intern Med* **85**:471, 1976

41. Cardullo AC et al: Janeway lesions and Osler's nodes: A review of histopathologic findings. *J Am Acad Dermatol* **22**:1088, 1990

42. Honig PJ: Guttate psoriasis associated with streptococcal disease. *J Pediatr* **113**:1037, 1988

43. Tuazon CU: Skin and skin structure infections in the patient at risk: Carrier state of *Staphylococcus aureus. Am J Med* **76**(5A):166, 1984

44. Dajani AS: The scalded-skin syndrome: Relation to phage-group II staphylococci. *J Infect Dis* **125**:548, 1972

45. Melish ME et al: The staphylococcal epidermolytic toxin: Its isola-

tion, characterization, and site of action. *Ann NY Acad Sci* **236**:317, 1974

46. Elias PM et al: Staphylococcal scalded skin syndrome: Clinical features, pathogenesis, and recent microbiological and biochemical developments. *Arch Dermatol* **113**:207, 1977

47. Institute of Medicine, National Academy of Science: Conference on the Toxic Shock Syndrome. *Ann Intern Med* **96**:835, 1982

48. Chu MC et al: Association of toxic shock toxin-1 determinant with a heterologous insertion at multiple loci in the *Staphylococcus aureus* chromosome. *Infect Immun* **56**:2702, 1988

49. Bohach GA et al: Analysis of toxic shock syndrome isolates producing staphylococcal enterotoxins B and C, with use of Southern hybridization and immunologic assays. *Rev Infect Dis* **11**(suppl 1):575, 1989

50. Ikejima T et al: Induction by toxic-shock-syndrome toxin-1 of a circulating tumor necrosis factor-like substance in rabbits and of immunoreactive tumor necrosis factor and interleukin-1 from human mononuclear cells. *J Infect Dis* **158**:1017, 1988

51. Greorgouras K: Coral reef granuloma. *Cutis* **3**:37, 1967

52. Berkley SF et al: A cluster of blister-associated toxic shock syndrome in male military trainees and a study of staphylococcal carriage patterns. *Milit Med* **154**:496, 1989

53. Reagan DR et al: Elimination of coincident *Staphylococcus aureus* nasal and hand carriage with intranasal application of mupirocin calcium ointment. *Ann Intern Med* **114**:101, 1991

54. Hedstrom SA: Treatment and prevention of recurrent staphylococcal furunculosis: Clinical and bacteriologic follow-up. *Scand J Infect Dis* **17**:55, 1985

55. Wheat LJ et al: Long-term studies of the effect of rifampin on nasal carriage of coagulase-positive staphylococci. *Rev Infect Dis* **5**:S459, 1983

56. Darouiche R et al: Eradication of colonization by methicillin-resistant *Staphylococcus aureus* by using oral minocycline-rifampin and topical mupirocin. *Antimicrob Agents Chemother* **35**:1612, 1991

57. Bryant RE et al: Treatment of recurrent furunculosis with staphylococcal bacteriophage-lysed vaccine. *JAMA* **194**:123, 1965

58. Patterson JW et al: Cutaneous botryomycosis in a patient with acquired immunodeficiency syndrome. *J Am Acad Dermatol* **16**:238, 1987

59. Saenz C et al: Macronodular lesions associated with *Staphylococcus aureus* bacteremia. *Arch Intern Med* **147**:793, 1987

60. Tanaka S et al: Sporotrichoid bacterial infection. *Dermatologica* **178**:228, 1989

61. Curley RK et al: Cutaneous abscesses due to systemic nocardiosis—a case report. *Clin Exp Dermatol* **15**:459, 1990

62. Tsuboi R et al: Lymphocutaneous nocardiosis caused by *Nocardia asteroides. Arch Dermatol* **122**:1183, 1986

63. Khaveri PA et al: Periodic acid-Schiff-positive organisms in primary cutaneous *Bacillus cereus* infection. *Arch Dermatol* **127**:543, 1991

64. Dan M et al: Cutaneous manifestations of infection with *Corynebacterium* group JK. *Rev Infect Dis* **10**:1204, 1988

65. Sarkany I et al: The etiology and treatment of erythrasma. *J Invest Dermatol* **37**:283, 1961

66. Sindhuphak W et al: Erythrasma. Overlooked or misdiagnosed. *Int J Dermatol* **24**:95, 1985

Bibliography

Dillon HC: Streptococcal infections of the skin and their complications: Impetigo and nephritis, in *Streptococci and Streptococcal Diseases,* edited by LW Wannamaker, JM Matsen. New York, Academic, 1972, p 571

Dillon HC et al: M-antigens common to pyoderma and acute glomerulonephritis. *J Infect Dis* **130**:257, 1974

Kapral FA, Miller MM: Product of *Staphylococcus aureus* responsible for the scalded-skin syndrome. *Infect Immun* **4**:541, 1971

Koblenzer PJ: Acute epidermal necrolysis (Ritter von Rittershain-Lyell). A clinicopathologic study. *Arch Dermatol* **95**:608, 1967

Lyell A: A review of toxic epidermal necrolysis in Britain. *Br J Dermatol* **79**:662, 1967

Rammelkamp CH Jr: Epidemiology of streptococcal infections. *Harvey Lect* **51**:113, 1957

Rudolph RI et al: Treatment of staphylococcal toxic epidermal necrolysis. *Arch Dermatol* **110**:559, 1974

Schievert PM: Staphylococcal scarlet fever: Role of pyrogenic exotoxins. *Infect Immun* **31**:732, 1981

CHAPTER 188

Arnold N. Weinberg and Morton N. Swartz

Gram-Negative Coccal and Bacillary Infections

Many of the characteristic cutaneous manifestations of infection with gram-negative organisms are due to direct microbial invasion of the skin or subcutaneous tissues. In addition, platelet depression, the dermal or generalized Shwartzman reaction, disseminated intravascular coagulation, and effects of toxic products of these bacteria may produce varied hemorrhagic cutaneous manifestations. The typical skin lesions in meningococcal or *Pseudomonas* septicemia, often among the earliest indications of generalized infection, can provide immediate and important clues to early diagnosis.

Infections due to *Neisseria meningitidis* (Meningococcus)

General Features

Three clinical syndromes associated with cutaneous involvement occur in meningococcal disease: meningitis, acute meningococcemia, and chronic meningococcemia. Skin lesions are frequently the most dramatic manifestations and graphically add to the aura of fear attached to these infections.

Bacteriology and Pathogenesis

The *Neisseria* are obligate, aerobic, gram-negative, kidney bean-shaped cocci that pair with their long axes in parallel. *N. meningitidis* grows well on blood-enriched media (chocolate agar), supplemented by an atmosphere containing 5 to 10 percent CO_2 and approximately 50 percent humidity. In potentially mixed bacterial exudates these organisms should be grown on a selective medium (e.g., Thayer-Martin); they can be distinguished from *N. gonorrhoeae* by their fermentation of both glucose and maltose rather than of glucose alone. Meningococci are separable into 13 serologic groups on the basis of capsular antigens. Agglutination and capsular swelling reactions identify groups A, B, C, Y, and W-135 as the major pathogens involved in human disease today.[1]

The presence of virulent strains colonizing the nasal mucous membranes of a nonimmune host precedes clinical disease. Initial colonization may be facilitated by pili that attach to specific receptors on nonciliated columnar mucosal epithelial cells[2,3] and by production of an IgA protease that cleaves host secretory IgA.[4] Encapsulated organisms resist phagocytosis and with the onset of a viral

respiratory infection they may multiply locally and invade the blood stream or be aspirated into the lower respiratory tract. Meningitis, meningococcemia, or pneumonitis can result. Predisposition to sporadic and occasionally recurrent meningococcal disease occurs in patients with congenital or acquired complement deficiencies, particularly late-acting components C5 to C8.[5–7]

The skin lesions associated with meningococcemia and meningococcal meningitis result from damage to small dermal blood vessels. By light and electron microscopy, bacteria are found within endothelial and polymorphonuclear cells.[8] Organisms can sometimes be seen when aspirates from involved areas of skin are Gram-stained. Local endothelial damage, thrombosis, and necrosis of the vessel walls occur. Immunoglobulins and complement are present, even in early vascular lesions.[8] Edema, infarction of overlying skin, and extravasation of red blood cells are responsible for the characteristic macular, papular, petechial, hemorrhagic, and bullous lesions. Similar vascular lesions occur in the meninges and in other tissues.

In addition to direct involvement of skin vessels by meningococci, many of the cutaneous hemorrhagic lesions may be due to the direct effects of endotoxin or via the *dermal* Shwartzman reaction. Data supporting this view have been presented showing that purified meningococcal endotoxin, in contrast to endotoxin derived from *Escherichia coli,* was uniquely potent in production of the dermal Shwartzman reaction in mice.[9] The frequency of hemorrhagic cutaneous manifestations in meningococcal infections, compared to infections with other gram-negative organisms, may be due to increased potency and/or unique properties of meningococcal endotoxins for the dermal reaction. On the other hand, lipopolysaccharide (LPS) endotoxins from meningococci and *E. coli* are equally potent producers of the *generalized* Shwartzman reaction and lethality in mice.[9]

The profound effects on small blood vessels, directly related to bacterial invasion or indirectly due to LPS endotoxin, may lead to diminished blood volume, lowered cardiac output, anoxia in vital organs, myocardial failure, hypotension, acidosis, and diffuse intravascular coagulation.[10–12]

Meningococci can be isolated from the blood in chronic meningococcemia, usually during periodic fevers, rash, and joint manifestations. The pathogenesis of this form of disease is less well understood than that of the acute process. Recent observations have linked this chronic form of meningococcal infection to absence of terminal components of complement in several patients, an association that may provide new insights into pathogenic mechanisms in this unusual host-parasite interaction.[13] The absence of bacteria, bacterial antigenic material, vascular damage, and granulocytic inflammation contrasts with the positive findings seen in acute infections. The chronic course of the disease, lack of endotoxin-like manifestations (even with demonstrated bacteremia), and the potentiality for metamorphosis to meningitis or endocarditis suggest that an unusual host-parasite relationship is central to this persistent infection.[14]

Epidemiology

Humans are the only known natural hosts, and nasopharyngeal carrier rates vary (5 to 15 percent overall) with age: ~1 percent in children 3 to 48 months of age, 5 percent in those 14 to 17 years of age, and 20 to 40 percent in young adults. In crowded conditions, such as schools or military camps, or when a carrier of a new strain develops disease in a day-care nursery or family setting, carrier rates can increase dramatically, independent of clinical disease.[15]

Asymptomatic exposure to a variety of encapsulated and non-encapsulated *N. meningitidis* strains can stimulate protective bactericidal antibody.[16] In addition, a variety of nonmeningococcal microorganisms, such as *E. coli* K1 strains and *N. lactamica*, stimulate production of cross-reacting protective antibodies to these potential pathogens.[17] Immunity to meningococci increases with age due to subclinical interactions with *N. meningitidis* or to other antigenically related bacteria. As a result, protective bactericidal antibodies, both IgG and IgM, are found in 70 to 95 percent of young adults.[18] Newborn infants are often resistant to meningococcal disease and this protection lasts until approximately 3 to 6 months of age, by which time passively acquired maternal IgG antibody levels have markedly diminished.[16–18] Some young adults with acute meningococcal disease have circulating bactericidal antibody present at the outset. This paradoxical situation may be explained by the finding that such patients can have serum IgA antibody that blocks the bactericidal reaction.[19] Even though individuals acquire group-specific antibody from subclinical exposures in youth, the presence of other immunoglobulins may interfere with this protective mechanism. Any endogenous microorganisms that stimulate IgA antibody, such as *E. coli* K1 strains, could paradoxically interfere with the protective effects of bactericidal antibody.[20]

In the past, sporadic cases (or outbreaks) often emerged in the military services in boot camp, where young, susceptible recruits are brought together in situations of overwork, stress, and crowding. This problem has been lessened considerably by the routine use in the military of quadrivalent vaccine containing polysaccharides of groups A, C, Y, and W-135. However, there is currently no effective vaccine available for group B disease due to the poor immunogenicity of group B capsular polysaccharide. Although the meningococcal polysaccharide vaccines are immunogenic in adults, they do not elicit a good antibody response in children under 2 years of age; newer generations of polysaccharide–protein conjugate vaccines appear to be more immunogenic in this age group. In civilian populations, adult family members probably introduce the organism into the household, but secondary cases are most frequently spread from children ages 1 through 14 to other family members in the same age group, especially under crowded conditions.[21] Household spread is 300 to 1000 times more frequent than secondary cases in the community at large.[22] An exception to this is the increased incidence of secondary cases in day-care centers where large numbers of susceptible children congregate.[23]

Serogroup A isolates have most often been associated with epidemic disease, but serogroups C and B are also identified in outbreaks as well as sporadic cases. Isolates belonging to groups Y and W-135 have increased in frequency in the past several decades.[24] Many of these have occurred in cases of respiratory disease in older individuals. Meningococcal disease occurs worldwide, including equatorial Africa ("meningitis belt") and Alaska. Most cases occur in early childhood (to age 4 years) and adolescence, but older individuals also become ill during epidemics. Absence of the spleen has been associated with fulminant meningococcal disease just as reported for other encapsulated organisms. *N. meningitidis* has been isolated from the genitourinary tract in individuals practicing orogenital sex and in homosexuals.[25]

Acute Meningococcemia and Meningitis

Clinical Manifestations HISTORY. The disease often follows a mild upper respiratory infection associated with headache, grippe-like complaints, nausea and vomiting, and muscle soreness. These symptoms can be so brief that fever, obtundation, and other manifestations of meningitis are the initial findings. In fulminant meningococcemia, vomiting, stupor, hemorrhagic rash, and hypotension may be evident within a few hours of onset of symptoms. Milder cases, developing at a slower pace, also occur.

CUTANEOUS LESIONS. The skin findings associated with acute meningococcal infections are characteristically petechial, but transient urticarial, macular, or papular lesions (Fig. 188-1*a*), which can resemble viral exanthems, may be noted initially.[26] The petechiae are small and irregular, have a "smudged" appearance, and are often raised with pale grayish vesicular centers. While most commonly located on the extremities and trunk, lesions can also be found on the head (Fig. 188-1*b*), palms, soles, and mucous membranes (including the conjunctivae). More extensive bullous and hemorrhagic lesions with central necrosis (suggillations) can develop. Gangrenous hemorrhagic areas (indistinguishable from purpura fulminans) (see Chap. 187) can appear in patients with severe meningococcemia, often complicated by disseminated intravascular coagulation (DIC) (Fig. 188-1*c*). Skin lesions and bacteremia are rarely seen with meningococcal pneumonia.[27]

OTHER PHYSICAL FINDINGS. Patients with meningitis display signs of meningeal irritation and altered consciousness. Occasionally, agitated or maniacal behavior predominates. Cranial nerve palsies, long-tract signs, seizures, and alterations in vital signs associated with changes in intracranial pressure may be present.

Obtundation and hypotension without meningeal signs associated with the syndrome of DIC are characteristic features of acute fulminating meningococcemia.[11] Rarely, meningococcemia may result in septic foci in other areas: (1) *septic arthritis* with a pyogenic effusion in one or several joints; (2) *purulent pericarditis* with precordial pain, enlarging cardiac silhouette, and findings of cardiac tamponade; and (3) *bacterial endocarditis*. More commonly, a delayed immune complex–mediated syndrome can result in a sterile arthritis, pericarditis, or episcleritis.

Laboratory Findings A polymorphonuclear leukocytosis is present in the peripheral blood and cerebrospinal fluid (CSF). The CSF protein level is increased, and the glucose value is commonly reduced. Characteristic organisms may be seen on Gram-stained smears of fluid, and meningococci are usually isolated from CSF. *N. meningitidis* is isolated from the blood of approximately one-third of patients with meningitis and from almost 100 percent of

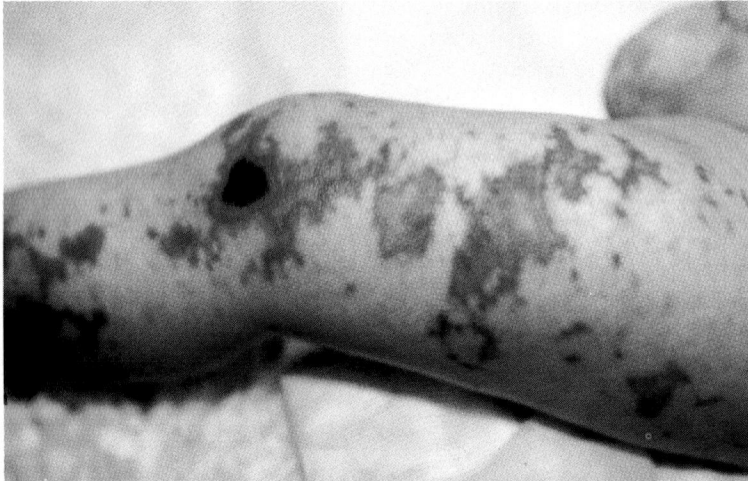

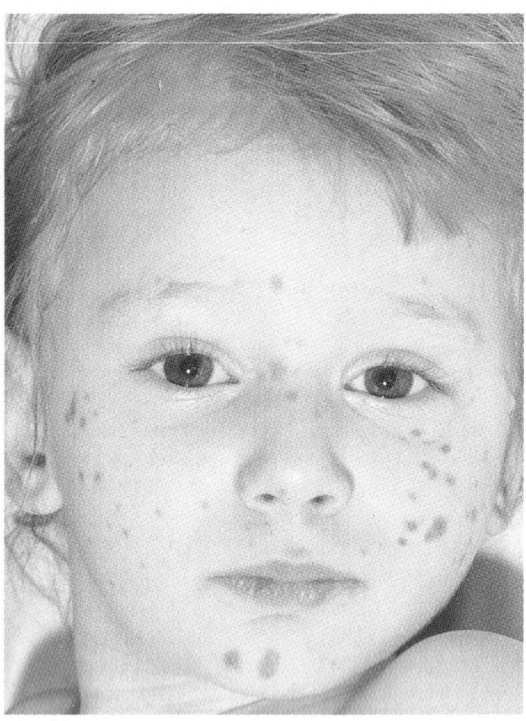

FIGURE 188-1 *Neisseria meningitidis:* Acute meningococcemia. (*a*) Transient maculopapular lesions on the upper chest. (*b*) Discrete, pink-to-purple macules and papules, as well as purpura, are seen on the face of this young child. These lesions represent early disseminated intravascular coagulation. (*c*) Maplike, gray-to-black areas of cutaneous infarction are seen in this child with disseminated intravascular coagulation.

patients with acute meningococcemia. Demonstration of organisms from cutaneous lesions has been variable. The most optimistic results include 27 positive smears and 35 cultured isolates in one series of 40 cases[28] and 70 percent positive petechial smears in another[29] but most modern reports indicate less success in finding organisms in skin lesions.

The development of rapid, accurate, and inexpensive procedures for detection of soluble antigens in CSF has been a major advance in laboratory methodology. The latex agglutination method is sensitive, and very specific, and is available as univalent or polyvalent reagents that will detect group A, B, C, Y, or W-135 antigens in CSF and possibly in concentrates of urine.[30]

Pathology See "Bacteriology and Pathogenesis," above.

Differential Diagnosis Meningococcal infection should always be considered in a patient with fever and a petechial eruption, especially if meningitis is present. The differential diagnosis should include the following conditions:

1. *Acute bacteremias and endocarditis.* Petechial eruptions may be present, with or without changes in platelet numbers. In endocarditis, mucous membrane and conjunctival lesions as well as subungual "splinter" hemorrhages occur. Very infrequently numerous petechial and purpuric lesions, almost indis-

tinguishable from those of meningococcal bacteremia, occur in patients with acute *Staphylococcus aureus* endocarditis. These patients may also have stiff neck and pleocytosis (usually without bacteria evident on Gram-stained smear of CSF) secondary to cerebral embolization or staphylococcal meningitis, completing the mimicry of systemic meningococcal disease. Usually, one or two of the skin lesions in such a patient with acute *Staph. aureus* endocarditis are those of purulent purpura; aspirate from the purulent center of the lesion usually shows gram-positive cocci in clusters (rather than gram-negative biscuit-shaped diplococci) on smear, and subsequently *Staph. aureus* is isolated on culture. This is a most important distinction to make, because treatment of *Staph. aureus* endocarditis involves a different antibiotic (nafcillin) than would be employed for the treatment of meningococcal meningitis (penicillin or ampicillin). In acute gonococcemia, the skin lesions are usually nodular, hemorrhagic, few in number, and usually located on the distal parts of the extremities (see Chap. 223).

2. *Acute "hypersensitivity" vasculitis.* The lesions are usually palpable, present in greatest profusion on the lower extremities, and are symmetric. Renal involvement and hypertension may be present. Pathologically, the major focus of inflammation is in postcapillary venules (see Chap. 116).

3. *Enteroviral infections.* Fever, petechial eruptions, and aseptic meningitis are characteristic features of enteroviral disease.

Echo (e.g., type 9) and Coxsackie viruses are most often implicated.

4. *Rocky Mountain spotted fever*. The history of exposure to ticks in an endemic area, absence of an antecedent respiratory infection, delay in appearance of the rash, and the location first on the distal parts of the extremities, including palms and soles, are helpful clues (see Chap. 197).

5. *Toxic shock syndrome* (see Chap. 187).

6. *Purpura fulminans* (see Chap. 187).

7. *Weil's disease* (*leptospirosis*) (see Chap. 190).

Course and Prognosis   Untreated, the disease usually ends fatally. The prognosis for treated meningitis or meningococcemia is excellent, with recovery in over 90 percent of patients.

In severe meningococcemia, especially with the rapid emergence of cutaneous hemorrhages, hypotension, and DIC, the entire course from onset to death can be measured in hours. These cases are often associated with massive adrenal hemorrhage (Waterhouse-Friderichsen syndrome). The mortality remains close to 100 percent, but gradations in severity of the illness make it difficult to assign an accurate prognosis in an individual case.

Chronic Meningococcemia

Clinical Manifestations   HISTORY.   Chronic meningococcemia is a rare disease, occurring much less frequently than the dermatitis-arthritis syndrome of subacute gonococcemia that it resembles. The manifestations of chronic meningococcemia are indefinite and vague at onset but tend to establish a pattern over a period of weeks or months.[31,32] Initially there may be an acute febrile illness, but this wanes and the patient is left with vague intermittent complaints of muscle aches and pains, joint soreness, mild headache, and anorexia with weight loss. The simultaneous emergence of a localized rash with several days of fever and joint soreness are characteristic symptoms. As the fever recedes, the rash usually fades too, and the patient may be totally free of overt skin manifestations for days at a time. This periodic fever and rash may recur over a period of a few weeks to as long as 6 to 8 months. The average duration of reported cases is 6 to 8 weeks. Untreated cases may eventually evolve into acute meningococcemia, meningitis, or endocarditis. Some recent case reports relate this syndrome to absence of a terminal component of complement, a finding also observed in some sporadic and recurrent acute meningococcal infections.[13]

CUTANEOUS LESIONS.   Variability is the hallmark of the eruption associated with chronic meningococcemia. Several different types of skin lesions have been noted, usually distributed about one or more painful joints or on pressure areas. They may vary in appearance and in size (1 to 20 mm) from one crop of lesions to the next and include: (1) pale to rose-colored macular and papular lesions (the most common type), occurring in about 30 percent of cases; (2) slightly indurated and tender erythema nodosum-like nodules, mainly on the lower extremities; (3) petechiae of variable size; (4) petechiae with vesicular or pustular centers; (5) hemorrhage (minute) with an areola of paler erythema (very characteristic when it occurs); (6) gross hemorrhagic areas with pale blue-gray centers; or (7) hemorrhagic tender nodules which are located deep in the dermis.

OTHER PHYSICAL FINDINGS.   Aside from the rash, the physical findings are minimal, except for occasional joint swelling and tenderness. If the disease progresses to an acute complication such as meningitis, the new findings will be those of the complicating process.

Pathology   Pathologically, the skin lesions in chronic meningococcemia differ from those in acute meningococcemia. Bacteria are absent, and meningococcal antigens cannot be recognized using fluorescent antibody techniques. In addition to the absence of bacteria or their recognized products, thrombi do not occlude capillaries and venules, endothelial cell swelling is absent, and the perivascular infiltrate consists of mixed polymorphonuclear and mononuclear cells rather than predominantly polymorphonuclear leukocytes seen in acute infections. Pathologic findings may be reported as "leukocytoclastic angiitis." An allergic basis for the skin lesions has been suggested in chronic meningococcemia, even though bacterial antigens are not identifiable.[14]

Diagnosis and Differential Diagnosis   During the febrile periods, blood cultures are frequently positive and provide the specific means of diagnosis. Serologic tests have not proved helpful, and there are no available data for the use of counterimmunoelectrophoresis (CIE) or latex agglutination in chronic meningococcemia.

A number of diseases with periodic fever, skin lesions, and joint involvement resemble chronic meningococcemia, including:

1. *Subacute bacterial endocarditis*. A prolonged febrile course with a pleomorphic petechial rash, joint symptoms, and no overt focus make this an important consideration. A prominent heart murmur, evidence of renal impairment, and positive blood cultures help to establish the diagnosis.

2. *Acute rheumatic fever*. This diagnosis may be suggested when the fever is prolonged, joint findings are prominent, and macular and papular rashes appear (see Chap. 178).

3. *Henoch-Schönlein purpura*. The petechial hemorrhagic rash in association with symptoms of arthritis and fever suggests an illness not unlike chronic meningococcemia; the eruption is more often symmetric, usually on the lower extremities only, and does not have the periodicity of the rash of meningococcemia (see Chap. 116).

4. *Rat-bite fever*. This disease may be acute (mimicking acute meningococcemia) or chronic (resembling chronic meningococcemia). Intermittent fever, rash, and joint manifestations are hallmarks of an illness that follows a rodent bite or ingestion of contaminated milk (see Chap. 190).

5. *Erythema multiforme*. This diagnosis is suggested by the symmetric distribution of the eruption and the iris-type configuration of the lesions.

6. *Gonococcemia* (chronic) (see Chap. 223). The cutaneous and joint manifestations may continue for many days or even weeks. The presence of tenosynovitis in gonococcemia, in contrast to its absence in meningococcemia, can be an important clue.

Course and Prognosis   Some patients with chronic meningococcemia spontaneously recover without specific therapy, whereas others develop serious systemic complications, such as endocarditis. The prognosis for treated infection is excellent; almost 100 percent of patients are cured with antibiotic therapy.

Primary Meningococcal Conjunctivitis

The species most commonly involved in acute bacterial conjunctivitis are *Staph. aureus, S. pneumoniae,* and *H. influenzae; N. meningitidis* is the etiology in up to 2 percent of cases, and the source of infection is most likely direct inoculation of airborne organisms from close contact with carriers or manual contact with secretions from the patient's own nasopharynx.[33] Gram-stained smear of conjunctival exudate commonly reveals gram-negative biscuit-shaped diplococci, and culture yields *N. meningitidis*. It is important to recognize that several microorganisms that can be found in infected body fluids and blood may appear morphologically similar to *N. meningitidis* on Gram stain: *N. gonorrhoeae*, *Moraxella* spp., *Acinetobacter calcoaceticus*, and *Pasteurella multocida*. Clinical features of primary meningococcal conjunctivitis include low-grade fever, conjunctival hyperemia, purulent exudate, lid edema, chemosis, photophobia, and preauricular lymphadenopathy. The majority of cases occur in children. Progression to systemic meningococcal disease occurs in about 20 percent of patients within a few hours to 4 days after the initial ocular symptoms. In view of the risk of systemic spread of infection, treatment should include not only topical antimicrobial agents (e.g., sulfonamides) but also systemically administered penicillin. Cellulitis of the cheek has complicated meningococcal conjunctivitis in one child, but meningococcal periorbital cellulitis (and bacteremia) has occurred following an upper respiratory infection in the absence of meningococcal conjunctivitis.[34]

Treatment and Prophylaxis

Chemotherapy   The therapy of meningococcal infections became complicated by the emergence of sulfonamide-resistant strains over 25 years ago. Initially, these strains belonged predominantly to serogroup B, but the majority of sulfonamide-resistant isolates in recent years have been from serogroups C or A.[1] These variations in susceptibility patterns have resulted in penicillin G supplanting the sulfonamides as the treatment of choice for acute meningococcal infections. The usual adult dosage for meningococcal meningitis is 2 million units intravenously every 2 h until approximately 7 days after the temperature has returned to normal. Treatment of chronic meningococcemia does not require "meningeal doses" of penicillin; 6 to 12 million units divided into 4 to 6 daily doses, intravenously for 10 days, should be effective therapy. In the highly penicillin-allergic patient, chloramphenicol (1.0 g intravenously every 6 h), rather than a third-generation cephalosporin, should be used. In parts of the world such as Spain where meningococci that are relatively resistant to penicillin have been isolated,[35] a third-generation cephalosporin (cefotaxime, ceftriaxone) might be considered for initial therapy. All meningococcal isolates from blood, cerebrospinal fluid, or other normally sterile body cavities should be tested for penicillin susceptibility.

Supportive Therapy   Efforts to prevent acute brain swelling are essential in patients with meningitis. These include prevention of overhydration, reduction of body temperature, and employment of agents such as mannitol or dexamethasone (if evidences of rising intracranial pressure develop).

Although it has been postulated that hypotension in acute meningococcemia may be due to adrenal failure associated with the Waterhouse-Friderichsen syndrome (adrenal hemorrhage), blood cortisol levels and corticosteroid secretion rates have been found elevated in this syndrome. The modern treatment of shock in sepsis includes appropriate use of volume expanders, beta adrenergic-stimulating drugs like dopamine or isoproterenol, sodium bicarbonate infusions for severe acidosis, and, in selected patients, peripheral vasodilators and corticosteroids.[36,37]

Severe meningococcal infections can be complicated by the syndrome of DIC. The diagnosis is usually made by a composite of associated hematologic abnormalities, including thrombopenia and hypofibrinogenemia, prolongation of the prothrombin time and partial thromboplastin time, and presence of fibrin split-products. If clinical bleeding occurs, fresh frozen plasma and heparin may be required. Each case must be individualized since therapy may be harmful and produce more problems than the DIC syndrome, especially if adult respiratory distress syndrome is also present.[38]

Prophylaxis   Reliance on sulfonamide prophylaxis has been abandoned because of the presence of sulfonamide-resistant meningococcal strains, but the need for reliable chemoprophylaxis continues to exist. In civilian experiences, especially in association with day-care nursery exposures or crowded household contacts, secondary cases can emerge rapidly, often within 24 to 48 h of an index case.[23] Currently recommended prophylactic drug regimens in the adult favor rifampin, 600 mg orally twice daily for 2 days[39]; alternatively, minocycline, 100 mg orally daily for 5 days, can be used.[40] Preliminary studies indicate that ciprofloxacin is also effective in adults in eradicating carriage.[41] The effectiveness of these agents appears to be due to their presence in effective concentrations in upper respiratory and salivary secretions.[42]

Immunization   Polysaccharide vaccines have been developed from groups A, C, Y, and W-135 *N. meningitidis* and have proved to be safe and effective in preventing meningococcal disease in adults and in children over the age of 2 years.[15,39] Group C vaccine was routinely administered to all U.S. Army inductees and has essentially eliminated group C disease from recruit camps.[15] The development of an effective group B vaccine and improved methods of stimulating protective antibody in children (less than 2 years of age) are current goals of immunization research.[43] Although chemotherapy prophylaxis provides immediate potential protection for exposure to all serogroups, immunization protection has a lag of 1 to 2 weeks and is available for serogroups A, C, Y, and W-135 only as a quadrivalent preparation.[39]

Infections due to *Pseudomonas aeruginosa*

General Features

These ubiquitous gram-negative bacilli can cause serious infections, especially in individuals with altered defenses or receiving intense antibiotic therapy, or in hospitalized patients. Cutaneous manifestations of *Pseudomonas* infections are common and characteristic. They may represent the only overt findings in septicemias or be the localizing focus in serious infections of the ear. In addition, trivial cutaneous lesions involving nails, toe webs, skin, and the external auditory canal are produced by these organisms.

Bacteriology and Pathogenesis

Pseudomonas aeruginosa is a nonfermentative, obligately aerobic, gram-negative bacillus. Some strains produce a blue pigment (pyocyanin) that is soluble in chloroform, or a yellow-green substance (fluorescein) which is water soluble. Using Wood's ultraviolet lamp, the presence of organisms in lesions of skin or nails and in the urine can be identified if fluorescein is produced by that particu-

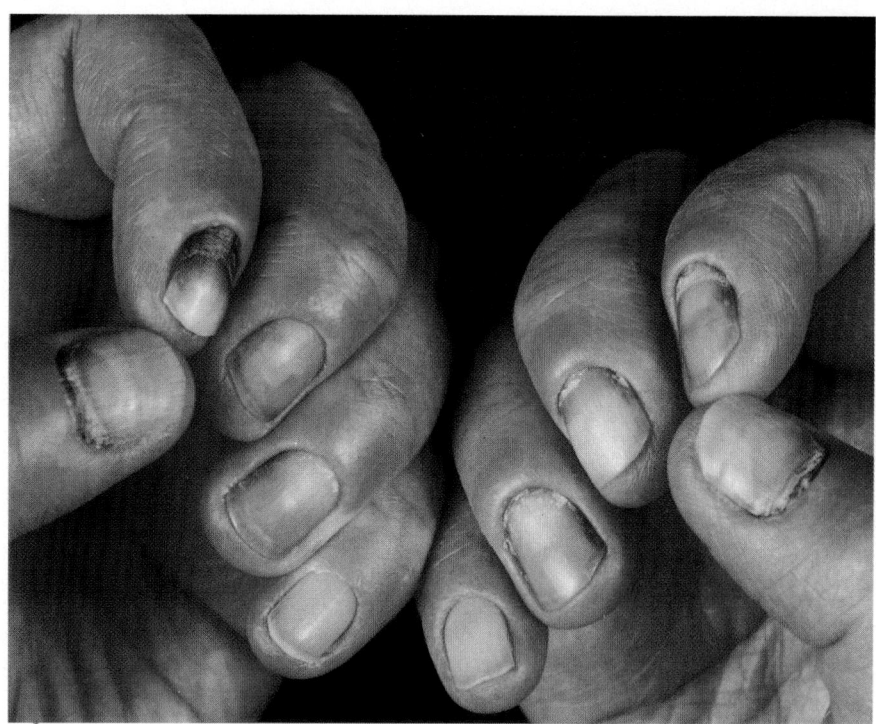

FIGURE 188-2 *Pseudomonas aeruginosa:* ''Green nails.'' This 36-year-old bartender noted a greenish discoloration of 8 of 10 fingernails during the past year. Several of the fingers show chronic candida paronychia as well.

lar strain. Either of the pigments, or their combination, impart a characteristic greenish color to the surrounding growth media or the tissue substrate involved in clinical disease (e.g., ''green nail'' syndrome, Fig. 188-2). In addition, growth of these microorganisms is often accompanied by an odor of grapes, characteristic of trimethylamine.

These organisms gain entry through breakdown of the skin or mucous membrane barriers at sites of trauma, foreign bodies (e.g., indwelling venous or urinary catheters), or via aspiration or aerosolization into the respiratory tract. Infections in otherwise healthy individuals are unusual; when they occur, the involved regions are often areas with increased moisture (toe webs, external auditory canal). Infection may begin in the base of the nail in persons having their hands in water frequently. This can progress to paronychia, followed by development of a green-blue discoloration of the nail due to local pigment production. Another example of the ability of this organism to infect healthy but moistened skin are the numerous reports of a diffuse rash on areas of skin of people immersed in public whirlpools, hot tubs (Fig. 188-3), and swimming pools.[44] These organisms can sometimes be aggressive secondary invaders in open wounds, decubitus and skin ulcerations, or in association with thermal burns. Rarely, a superficial pyoderma due solely to *Pseudomonas* is engrafted upon a generalized or localized dermatitis, such as tinea pedis or eczema, producing irregular pustular areas with macerated and eroded borders.

Serious invasive infections occur in debilitated patients; malnourished infants; individuals whose normal bacterial flora has been suppressed by antibiotics; patients with neoplastic diseases, granulocytopenias of various etiologies, or with impaired circulating or cellular immunity; and individuals requiring mechanical respiratory assistance. These organisms frequently colonize body surfaces and survive exposure to antibiotics. *Pseudomonas aeruginosa* can spread widely via the bloodstream, producing a disseminated infective vasculitis. Occasionally, features of the generalized Shwartzman reaction are found, but less frequently than in infec-

tions due to *N. meningitidis* or Enterobacterioceae. Whole dead *Pseudomonas* cells injected into experimental animals produce little if any toxicity compared to the effects of live bacteria. This suggested to Liu and his associates that the pathogenicity of this organism might reside in an exotoxin rather than in the classic endotoxin of gram-negative bacteria. Studies during the past 20 years have confirmed the relevance of a number of toxic substances to pathogenesis. Among these, collagenase and elastase may be important determinants for the development of hemorrhagic lesions. A phospholipase similar to the alpha toxin of *Clostridium perfringens* may have a major role in the pathogenesis of respiratory infections through destruction of pulmonary surfactant.[45] Studies have led to the identification and characterization of a potent protein, exotoxin A. The mechanism of action of this toxin is identical to that of diphtheria cytotoxin, but it differs in its cellular specificities, molecular properties, and clinical expression. Exotoxin A and other *Pseudomonas* toxins have been reviewed.[46] An antitoxin can neutralize the effects of the toxin in vivo. Efforts to produce a toxoid are in progress. The importance of the contribution of this exotoxin to the pathogenesis of *Pseudomonas* infections has not been definitely established. There is evidence in experimental burn sepsis that synthesis of the exotoxin occurs in local lesions, and the toxin can be identified in the serum.[47]

Epidemiology

Pseudomonas aeruginosa is found widely distributed in nature—in air, water, dust particles, and soil; thus, it is not surprising that it may contaminate plants, vegetables, and occasionally medicinal preparations such as procaine and fluorescein eye drops. In humans, the moist regions of skin folds and the external auditory canal are the most common sites of natural colonization (approximately 3 to 5 percent of individuals). *P. aeruginosa* is found in small numbers in the feces of 10 to 20 percent of the population but

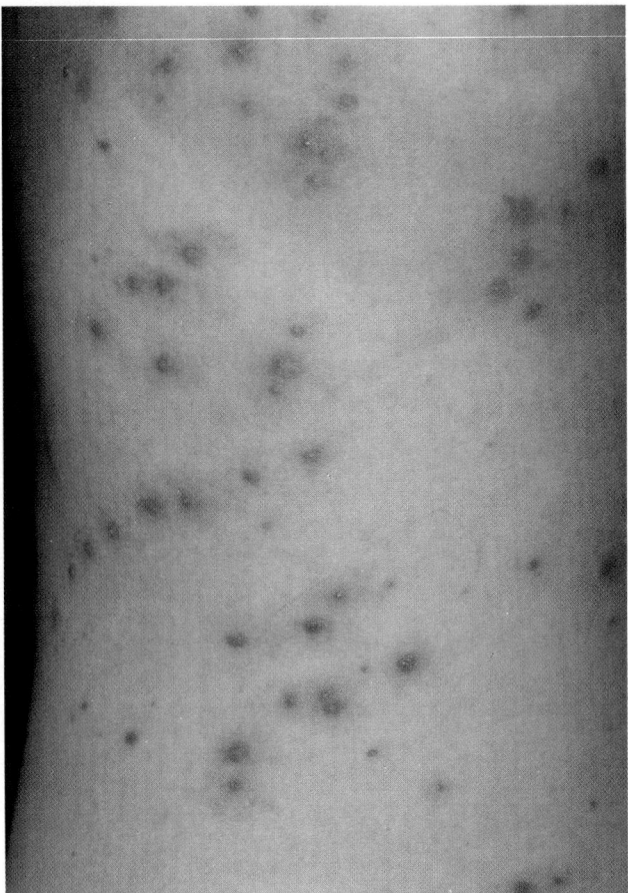

FIGURE 188-3 *Pseudomonas aeruginosa:* "Hot tub folliculitis." This 22-year-old female noted the appearance of erythematous, pruritic papules and pustules on the trunk, buttocks, and upper thighs several days after bathing in a hot tub. The eruption resolved without antibiotic therapy.

in larger numbers in as many as 35 to 50 percent of hospitalized patients. Moist or weeping cutaneous lesions (e.g., thermal burns) encourage the growth of *Pseudomonas,* as well as of other gram-negative bacteria. Procedures that increase humidity in the environment are frequently associated with overgrowth of these organisms. Systemic infection with these indigenous gram-negative bacteria depends primarily on altered susceptibility of the host rather than on spread from individual to individual or on increased pathogenicity. However, there may be exceptions to this in newborn nurseries, respiratory care units, and, occasionally, urologic wards, where dissemination from a primary source may occur. In hospitalized patients who are immunocompromised, increasing numbers become colonized and a larger number suffer disease due to this organism.

Local and Secondarily Infected Lesions

Pseudomonas produces a number of characteristic lesions. In addition, these organisms contaminate and complicate other skin diseases and open wounds.[48]

Clinical Manifestations HISTORY. Painful paronychial lesions, with or without characteristic green or blue discoloration of the

nails, occur most often in women with a history of chronic immersion of hands in water with soaps and detergents. People with toe web infection characteristically work or live in an atmosphere of high humidity and often have wet feet. Symptoms usually include slight persistent soreness and scaling of the web tissues. There are a large number of reports of therapeutic recreational whirlpool-, hot tub-, and swimming pool-associated skin rashes developing in healthy individuals within 1 to 5 days after use of public bathing facilities (Fig. 188-3). In all instances, *P. aeruginosa* was isolated in large numbers from the pool water. The skin rash was self-limited, clearing without therapy within 1 week but often accompanied by fatigue, malaise, low-grade fever, external otitis, and mastitis.[44]

CUTANEOUS LESIONS. In addition to a tender paronychial lesion, patients with "green nail" syndrome may have part or all of the associated nail colored green to blue. The color may be in horizontal bands, representing intermittent activity of the infection at the nail base (see Fig. 188-2). Individuals with toe web *Pseudomonas* infections have thick, macerated, scaling, slightly green discolored areas between the toes. External otitis due to any type of bacteria presents a characteristically swollen, macerated appearance in the local area, without any specific lesion involving the eardrum. Intense swelling and discoloration with excruciating pain on movement of the pinna are characteristic of external otitis, often referred to as "swimmer's ear." If the skin is traumatized naturally, or during a surgical procedure, local infection can spread to the pinna, producing a perichondritis and chondritis with intense tender swelling of the ear. Cartilagenous necrosis may result from pressure effects or inflammatory damage unless immediate drainage with through-and-through incisions and appropriate antibiotics are instituted. Organisms other than *P. aeruginosa* may be causal, including *Staph. aureus* and streptococci.[49]

The most severe form of this infection, malignant external otitis, has a high mortality if therapy is delayed or inadequate.[50] This serious infection usually occurs in elderly diabetics with significant small-vessel disease. The onset and early progression are insidious. Swelling, erythema, moderate discharge, and pain are present without fever or constitutional symptoms. As the surface breaks down, invasion of the soft tissues occurs at the junction of cartilage and bone, and the process then advances to involve cartilage, mastoid, and temporal bone. Inflammation at the stylomastoid and jugular foramina can lead to 7th nerve and 9th to 11th nerve palsies, the 7th being the earliest objective neurologic defect seen. Diagnosis is made clinically and early if there is adequate visibility, and granulation tissue can be seen erupting at the cartilage-bone interface in the posterior inferior canal wall. The pinna is often swollen and intense pain is present.[51]

Patients who develop folliculitis usually give a history of exposure to warm water in a whirlpool, a public bath like a hot tub, or some recreational spa for swimming or a water slide. The rash can be very local if a limb has been immersed in a whirlpool, or generalized in distribution in swim suit and intertriginous areas. The rash begins as papules, evolves to papulopustules (see Fig. 188-3), and eventually heals with fine desquamation. Pruritus and pain may accompany the lesions and localized areas of mastitis and external otitis.[44] Serotype 0-11 of *P. aeruginosa* is most commonly involved. A small outbreak of *P. aeruginosa* 0-11 folliculitis occurred in granulocytopenic patients in a cancer treatment center; but in these patients, in contrast to normal individuals with swimming pool folliculitis, the lesions rapidly became widespread and progressed to bullae, which became necrotic (ecthyma gangrenosum-like) unless systemic antibiotic treatment was initiated immediately.[52] The development of the changes of ecthyma gangrenosum represented progression of the initial folliculitis rather than the incidental occurrence of superimposed bacteremic *P. aeruginosa* lesions. Sinks and faucets in the patients' rooms were sources of *P. aeruginosa* of identical serotype.

In secondarily infected open skin areas, the presence of *Pseudomonas* is sometimes associated with a prominent greenish-blue color to the purulent exudate. Widespread, irregular, superficial pustular lesions may be superimposed on the underlying skin disease; the margins of these regions are usually sharply defined and irregular and may exhibit the characteristic grapelike odor and pigmented exudate.

Diagnosis and Differential Diagnosis   Nail and skin lesions are recognized by the characteristic pigment and "fruity" odor of the exudate. The organisms can be identified as thin gram-negative rods, or a mixed infection (e.g., with *Candida*) may be observed. Identification of the organism isolated in routine culture is based on pigment production and fermentation reactions. Fluorescence, demonstrated with a Wood's lamp, can help to support the diagnostic impression. Occasionally *Aspergillus* infection of the nails produces a greenish color, but there is usually no associated paronychia, and bacteria are not found on careful study of nail clippings. A subungual hematoma may superficially resemble *Pseudomonas* nail infection.

Course and Prognosis   Patients with minor *Pseudomonas* infections such as onychia and paronychia, toe web inflammation, whirlpool-associated skin rash, and external otitis usually improve rapidly with topical therapy and drying of the affected area. Malignant external otitis requires systemic antibiotics directed against *Pseudomonas,* utilizing an aminoglycoside and ticarcillin (or a ureido penicillin such as piperacillin) or ceftazidime. High doses and prolonged therapy are combined with surgical debridement to limit spread to bone, nervous system structures, and the meninges.[51] Ciprofloxacin may have a role in combination therapy for this infection.

Septicemia and Cutaneous Involvement

Clinical Manifestations   HISTORY.   In individuals ill with *Pseudomonas* septicemia, the history is most frequently centered around the underlying problem and antecedent therapy. A premature infant may have required resuscitation and treatment of a nonspecific pneumonitis prior to developing high fever, obtundation, and macular or hemorrhagic vesicular skin lesions. Infants may present initially with omphalitis or severe diarrhea, followed by septicemia and skin lesions. Urinary tract infections complicating congenital lesions such as exstrophy of the bladder may predispose to bacteremia. In adults, there is usually a history of antibiotic therapy, treatment with corticosteroid hormones or antitumor agents, or the use of indwelling venous catheters. Frequently, the patient is granulopenic, has already had a significant febrile illness, and may still be receiving antibiotics when one of the characteristic cutaneous manifestations develops. The local lesions are rarely painful, but in the author's experience the patient is usually too sick to focus on the local problem. Occasionally, hemorrhagic manifestations may occur secondary to involvement of small vessels supplying the skin, to platelet reduction, or to DIC.

Pseudomonas involvement of the gastrointestinal tract, particularly in the tropics, may produce the picture of an acute enteric infection with headache, high fever, diarrhea, and "rose spots"—a syndrome described as *Shanghai fever* and resembling typhoid fever.[53]

CUTANEOUS LESIONS.   The skin lesions, the most characteristic part of the physical findings in *Pseudomonas* septicemia, consist of four types[54]:

1. *Vesicles and bullae.* These occur singly or in clusters, spread in random fashion over the skin, frequently becoming hemorrhagic as they evolve (Fig. 188-4). Occasionally, in infants, they may be surrounded by large erythematous halos and may be mistaken for erythema multiforme.
2. *Ecthyma gangrenosum.* The lesion in this disorder consists of a round, indurated, ulcerated, painless area with central necrotic black or gray-black eschar and surrounding erythema (Figs. 188-4, 188-5). This lesion often evolves from a necrotic vesicle. Frequently, but not exclusively, the lesion is in the anogenital or axillary region.
3. *Gangrenous cellulitis.* This is a sharply demarcated, superficial, painless, necrotic lesion that may resemble a decubitus ulcer but is located in a nonpressure area and may complicate a prior area of injury such as a thermal burn.
4. *Macular or papular nodular lesions.* These are small, oval, and painless, located predominantly over the trunk, and resemble rose spots of typhoid fever (see above).

Another cutaneous manifestation of *Pseudomonas* septicemia, usually occurring after days or weeks, is nodular cellulitis. The lesions are red, warm, sometimes fluctuant, but often situated deeply enough to feel solid. Surgical incision reveals suppuration, and *P. aeruginosa* can be cultured from the lesions.[55] A variation of this process consists of numerous red, nonfluctant, hot, nontender, subcutaneous nodules on the trunk and extremities that may be accompanied by other characteristic lesions, such as hemorrhagic bullae and ecthyma gangrenosum.[56] Such lesions may be

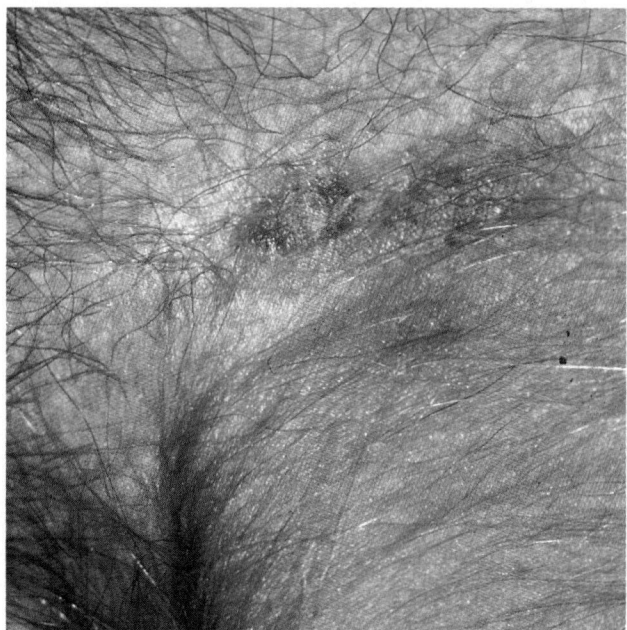

FIGURE 188-4   *Pseudomonas aeruginosa:* Ecthyma gangrenosum. Gunmetal gray, painless, infarcted lesions with surrounding erythema.

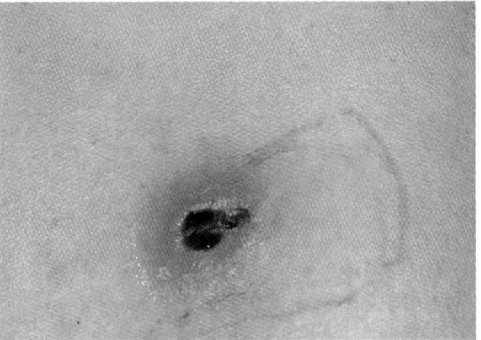

a

FIGURE 188-5 *Pseudomonas aeruginosa:* Ecthyma gangrenosum. 32-year-old male with HIV disease noted the onset of a very tender plaque on the right buttock associated with fever and malaise. (*a*) 5-day-old lesions with a central infarcted, necrotic area surrounded by erythema. (*b*) At 5-weeks, the lesions had initially improved on ciprofloxacin, which was discontinued due to an adverse drug reaction. Without antibiotic treatment, the necrotic area enlarged and was associated with bacteremia. Eventually, the lesion reepithelialized, but the patient died of pseudomonal pneumonia.

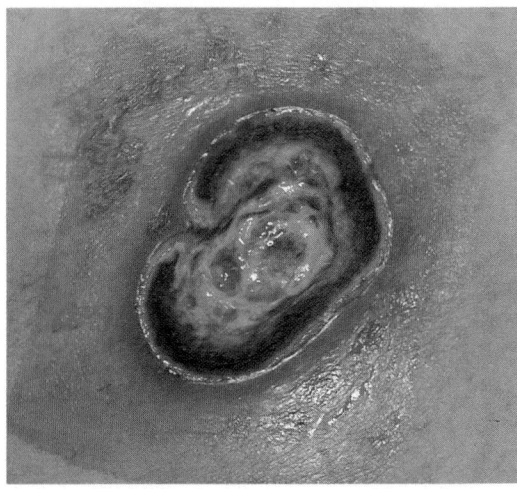

b

successfully treated by combination antipseudomonal antibiotic therapy.

Other lesions that have been described include petechiae, ecchymoses, dermal Shwartzman-like reactions, and purpura fulminans. Occasionally, the cutaneous expression of *Pseudomonas* infection may take the form of a typical erythema multiforme reaction. Patients with extensive burns may develop lesions of the above types on areas of normal skin, as well as more florid diffuse growth secondarily infecting the burn surface.

OTHER PHYSICAL FINDINGS. Patients with *Pseudomonas* septicemia frequently exhibit physical findings associated with the underlying diseases: malnutrition, mucous membrane ulcerations, glossitis and stomatitis secondary to antibiotics and granulopenia, urinary tract infections, proctitis, adenopathy, hepatosplenomegaly, and hemorrhagic bronchopneumonia.

Laboratory Findings Routine hematologic examination may reveal leukocytosis or leukopenia, with modifications based on underlying illnesses (aleukemic leukemia, leukemia, etc.). Platelets may be diminished and fibrinogen and other clotting factors reduced in association with consumption coagulopathy, liver disease, or profound malnutrition.

Characteristically, in *Pseudomonas* septicemia, aspirated material from bullae, areas of cellulitis, and papular or nodular lesions reveals numerous organisms but few leukocytes. Cultures of these lesions and of blood are almost always positive.

Pathology The distinctive finding in *Pseudomonas* lesions is a necrotizing vasculitis in which the walls of small arteries and veins are invaded by a myriad of bacteria.[57] The internal elastic lamellae may be destroyed by microbial elastase,[46] but the endothelial surface is rarely damaged and thrombosis is unusual. Extravasation occurs around the vessels, the perivascular and adventitial regions are extensively involved with edema and bland necrosis, and blood flow to the region supplied by the affected vessel is curtailed. This in turn leads to the formation of cutaneous lesions (bullae, hemorrhagic cellulitis, and gangrenous changes). Organisms tend to

spread along the exterior surfaces of vessels and invade the skin. Lungs, liver, kidneys, and brain may be similarly involved by bacterial invasion of their respective blood vessel walls, with the production of characteristic discrete nodular necrotic lesions.

Diagnosis and Differential Diagnosis The characteristic ecthyma gangrenosum skin lesions in an acutely ill patient suggests the diagnosis of *Pseudomonas* septicemia. The finding of abundant, thin, gram-negative rods with rare granulocytes in vesicle fluid or in association with gangrenous or hemorrhagic cellulitis constitutes further presumptive evidence.

The differential diagnosis of *Pseudomonas* septicemia includes other infections that can produce skin lesions through direct involvement of blood vessels (e.g., those caused by *N. meningitidis, Aeromonas hydrophilia, E. coli,* and fungi of the *Aspergillus* and *Rhyzopus* groups). In addition, other gram-negative bacteria may produce petechial, ecchymotic, and gangrenous skin lesions suggestive of the Shwartzman reaction.

Course and Prognosis *Pseudomonas* septicemia is frequently the terminal event in a complex illness involving a patient with malignant disease or altered cellular and humoral defense mechanisms. Therapy may be effective and recovery complete in some instances, especially when the septicemia occurs in patients with more favorable underlying problems like thermal burns, or in individuals with urinary tract foci of infection or in association with the use of percutaneous venous catheters.

Treatment LOCAL INFECTIONS. Superficial skin and toe web infections and onychia usually respond to acetic acid, silver nitrate, or gentian violet compresses applied 2 to 3 times daily between long periods of drying. Paronychia is best treated by surgical drainage, nail trimming, and 4% thymol in chloroform. Acetic acid in 50% alcohol, polymixin (0.1%) in acetic acid, or corticosteroids with neomycin are effective for otitis externa. When acetic acid is used topically on chronic ulcers, a 1 to 5% solution is often effective. In addition, topical silver nitrate (0.5%) or silver sulfadiazine has been used to eradicate these organisms in burn patients (see Chap. 126).

SYSTEMIC INFECTIONS. *Pseudomonas* septicemia requires early and vigorous systemic bactericidal antibiotic therapy. Effective therapeutic agents include the aminoglycosides gentamicin, tobramycin, and amikacin. One of these drugs is combined with ticarcillin, ceftazidime, or piperacillin in patients who are acutely ill. Gentamicin or tobramycin should be given every 8 h in 1.5 mg/kg doses intramuscularly or intravenously. Ticarcillin is administered in doses of 2 to 3 g every 4 h. In the presence of hypotension or of any renal impairment, the dosage of aminoglycoside antibiotics must be drastically reduced; in such circumstances, therapy should be guided by determinations of "peak" and "trough" serum levels of the aminoglycoside drug employed.

In addition to parenteral administration of antibiotics, nodular and fluctuant lesions should be drained surgically. Leukocyte transfusions have been effective in granulopenic infants, and experimental use of human immune globulins with activity against *P. aeruginosa* or specific *Pseudomonas* exotoxin A antibody preparations are under development and in early use.[39,58] A particularly difficult problem is presented by the markedly granulocytopenic patient with gangrenous cellulitis due to *P. aeruginosa* alone or in polymicrobial combination.[59] Progression of the process can be extremely rapid and thus is an indication for very prompt surgical debridement in addition to antimicrobial therapy. Complicating thrombocytopenia and DIC may supervene and add to the urgency.

PROPHYLAXIS. Infections caused by *P. aeruginosa* are difficult to treat because they often occur in altered hosts and the organisms are highly resistant to many antibiotics. There is no place for prophylactic antibiotics against *P. aeruginosa* because of drug toxicity and emergence of resistant strains. This reality has led to attempts to develop a polyvalent vaccine against the limited number of serotypes of *P. aeruginosa*. Preliminary clinical trials have been encouraging but variable in patients with thermal burns, cystic fibrosis, and in volunteers. Results are less favorable in seriously ill individuals with leukemia or other diseases with impaired host defenses. A review of the clinical aspects of *Pseudomonas* disease includes a thoughtful discussion of passive and active immunization as well as antimicrobial therapy.[60]

Skin Infections due to Other *Pseudomonas* Species

Pseudomonas putrefaciens, a psychrophilic bacterium, is a rare cause of cellulitis, particularly in the setting of chronic lower extremity infection in ulcers secondary to venous stasis.[61]

Skin Infections due to *Haemophilus influenzae*

General Features

The characteristic feature of infection of the skin with *H. influenzae* is a cellulitis that usually involves the face, neck, or upper extremities. Most cases occur in young children (6 to 24 months old), but examples in adults have been described in recent years.

Bacteriology and Pathogenesis

Haemophilus influenzae is a small, coccobacillary pleomorphic gram-negative organism. It is nonmotile and has fastidious growth requirements, including heme (X factor) and nicotinamide nucleoside (V factor). In mixed cultures the presence of organisms such as *Staph. aureus* can provide these growth factors and this allows *H. influenzae* colonies to grow well, as "satellites" of the feeding staphylococcus. There are rough and encapsulated forms, the latter divided into six serologic types (a through f) based on capsular polysaccharide antigens.

Most infections with *H. influenzae*, including meningitis, epiglottitis, and cellulitis, are caused by encapsulated type b strains (Hib). The ribosylribitol phosphate capsule inhibits phagocytosis in nonimmune individuals and allows a period of unchecked bacterial growth and invasiveness to occur. Rough, unencapsulated, nontypable, noninvasive species are commonly found in the upper part of the respiratory tract and are especially incriminated in surface infections such as exacerbations of bronchitis in older individuals with chronic lung disease and in young children with otitis media.

The mechanism involved in the development of cellulitis is uncertain, but in the majority of cases is an antecedent upper respiratory infection (URI). The characteristic localization of the cellulitis to the upper part of the body argues for the sequence of URI, fallout onto or invasion of the skin locally, and then bacteremia. This sequence is seen in adult as well as in pediatric cases. The association of otitis media with cellulitis has led to the hypothesis that the ear may serve as the primary focus in cases involving the face.[62] A primary bacteremic mechanism with secondary localization in the skin would be favored by a more random and widespread distribution of lesions than is seen. Localization of a subclinical bacteremia could follow trauma and has been suggested as a possible antecedent predisposing event.[63] The analogy to group A beta streptococcal erysipelas seems relevant, as the organisms are usually located in the upper respiratory tract, sometimes produce cellulitis locally, and bacteremia is a secondary complication, although less often seen than in Hib cellulitis.

Epidemiology

Humans are the only known natural host for *H. influenzae*. Carrier rates appear to be highest in young children between ages 1 and 5, especially in families and day-care groups with a recent case of Hib disease.[64] These potentially pathogenic bacteria are carried in the oropharynx and nasopharynx as part of the normal indigenous flora. Susceptibility to Hib disease appears to be greatest among certain ethnic groups and in socioeconomically disadvantaged populations. Genetic factors, prompt antibiotic treatment of Hib disease, congenital and acquired complement and antibody deficiency, and asplenia may also be responsible for increased susceptibility to disease and to recurrent episodes in traditional age groups as well as in adults. Spread is via droplet aerosol or close contact, and infection frequently occurs in association with a viral URI. Susceptibility to *H. influenzae* disease appears to be greatest between the ages of 3 months and 3 years. Although the early observations of Fothergill and Wright (1933) that this correlated with the absence of significant titers of bactericidal antibody have been questioned,[65] there is general agreement that complement-dependent anticapsular and bactericidal antibodies increase with age and are protective.[66] Paradoxically, Hib disease may occur in individuals endowed with adequate levels of bactericidal antibody. It has been postulated that circulating IgA antibody may block the function of specific IgG,[19] or that assay methodology provides false-positive results in vitro.[67] Although the mechanism of protection in the newborn period remains uncertain, it probably involves transplacental IgG transfer. The majority of adults beyond 15 years likewise have bactericidal and anticapsular antibody, and in this age group *H. influenzae* disease is unusual.[68]

In addition to antibody induction by clinical or subclinical *H. influenzae* disease, protective anticapsular antibody may be formed in response to cross-reacting antigens from vegetables, such as legumes, nonencapsulated *Haemophilus* species, other commensals, and enteric bacteria (e.g., *E. coli* K 100).[69]

Clinical Manifestations

History Typically, a young infant or child (under age 3) develops an area of swelling and discoloration on the face or arm following several days of coryza and abruptly rising temperature.[70] Rarely, a similar process occurs in adults as a complication of respiratory tract infection involving the upper airway.[71]

Cutaneous Lesions The typical lesion is a single, circumscribed, indurated area, usually located on the face, neck, upper chest, or upper extremity. Although described in infants as characteristically blue-red to purple-red in color and surrounded by a zone of edema, the early lesion may be an area of pale edema or erythema[63] (Fig. 188-6). The margins are indistinct, in contrast to the sharply defined borders of erysipelas. Regional adenopathy is rarely present. Occasionally, in children with Hib buccal cellulitis, erythematous buccal mucosal lesions are found on the side of the affected cheek, suggesting direct bacterial spread from the oropharynx into buccal soft tissues.[72]

When *H. influenzae* cellulitis occurs in adults, the patients are usually over 50 years of age, and the infection follows a striking sequence: marked pharyngitis at first; high fever; then rapidly progressive anterior neck swelling, tenderness, erythema, and dysphagia.[73]

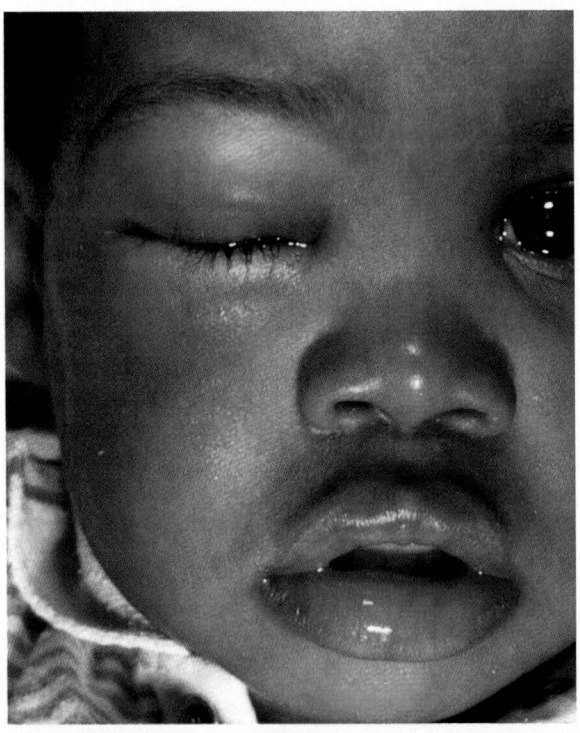

FIGURE 188-6 *Hemophilus influenzae:* Cellulitis. The right periorbital area and cheek of this febrile, 2-year-old African American child are tender, edematous, and have a violaceous-to-erythematous hue. (*Courtesy of Arthur R. Rhodes, M.D.*)

Other Physical Findings Associated infections of the upper respiratory tract including otitis media, sinusitis or epiglottitis, and pneumonia occur. The patient may appear lethargic, and, occasionally, metastatic infections such as septic arthritis or meningitis may occur. Fever, in the range of 38.9° to 40°C, is common.

Laboratory Findings

The white blood cell count is invariably elevated, usually in the 20,000 range. Blood cultures are positive in 40 to 50 percent of cases. Aspiration and culture of the margin of the cellulitis has been successful in about half the patients encountered, and Gram-stained smears should be studied.[62] Latex agglutination of soluble Hib capsule material has replaced CIE as the method of choice for antigen detection in CSF and other body fluids. It is more rapid, easier to perform, and more sensitive than CIE and can provide diagnostic information after antibiotic exposure.[30]

Pathology

No information is available about the histologic changes associated with this lesion, but the inflammatory response is doubtless an acute pyogenic reaction.

Diagnosis and Differential Diagnosis

Haemophilus influenzae cellulitis should be suspected when a child, age 3 to 24 months, develops an acute facial (buccal) cellulitis with high fever. There may be concomitant upper airway inflammation. Immediate confirmation of the diagnosis may be possible from inspection of Gram-stained smears of an aspirate of the lesion. Although cellulitis caused by other microorganisms is more common in adults, Hib disease should be considered in patients with respiratory infections and upper body cellulitis.

Streptococcal (especially group A) or pneumococcal cellulitis may produce a similar discoloration of the skin. Erysipelas, which rarely occurs in infants, is usually homogeneously erythematous and margins of the plaquelike swelling are distinct compared with the indefinite borders of *H. influenzae* cellulitis. Occasionally, *Staph. aureus* can produce a similar process, but the presence of pustules or boils is helpful in distinguishing this type of lesion.

Course and Prognosis

Most patients do well with antibiotic therapy even though the disease is usually associated with bacteremia. The patient is often brought to a physician quickly as the abrupt onset of high fever and easily observed cellulitis indicates the urgency of the situation. Constant vigil must be maintained for suppurative complications in the upper airways, meninges, lungs, bones, joints, or other organs.

Treatment and Prophylaxis

Ampicillin (150 to 250 mg/kg per day intravenously in four to six divided doses) has been effective treatment for most pediatric patients, but the emergence of plasmid-mediated (beta-lactamase-producing) ampicillin resistance in up to 45 percent of strains has led to alternative recommendations. Chloramphenicol (50 to 100 mg/kg daily in children above the age of 3 months) alone, or in combination with ampicillin, has been employed in the initial treatment of serious infections while awaiting the results of antibiotic susceptibility tests. Third-generation cephalosporins (ceftriaxone or cefotaxime) are currently the drugs of choice because of their activity against both ampicillin-susceptible and beta-lactamase-producing strains of *H. influenzae* and because of their efficacy in treating any complicating meningeal spread of infection.

Chemoprophylaxis has been studied in a variety of settings, and rifampin appears to be effective in significantly lowering carrier rates in selected populations such as households with an index case of Hib disease. At the present time rifampin is recommended for children and adults (reduced for infants) in doses of 20 mg/kg per day (up to 600 mg maximum) for 4 days, when an index case of Hib invasive disease occurs in a family where other children under age 4 reside.[74] Similar prophylaxis is recommended for nursery and day-care contacts.

Immunization with a vaccine prepared from Hib capsular polysaccharide (polyribosylribitol phosphate) has been successful in increasing circulating anticapsular antibody and protecting susceptible children over age 24 months. A newer vaccine consisting of the capsular polyribosyl ribitol phosphate conjugated to diphtheria toxoid is a better immunogen at an earlier age and is now approved for immunization of children at 18 months of age.[75] Successor conjugate vaccines (utilizing other protein components and means of conjugation) have been developed and appear to be immunogenic and effective at an even younger age, the most critical period for invasive Hib disease.

Cutaneous Manifestations of *Salmonella* Infection (Enteric Fever)

General Features

Salmonella infections are usually manifest as gastroenteritis, enteric fever (typhoidlike illness), or septicemia. "Rose spots," the classic skin lesions of systemic *Salmonella* infection, have been variably reported (10 to 60 percent) during the natural (untreated) evolution of typhoid fever, but less frequently in enteric fevers due to other *Salmonella* species.

Bacteriology and Pathogenesis

Salmonellae are not fastidious organisms, but their isolation from stool is made difficult by the fact that, when present, they represent only a small part of the abundant fecal flora. Extragastrointestinal isolates (abscesses, blood, skin lesions) are easier to identify, as they usually are pure cultures of a given *Salmonella* species. Isolation of the organisms from stool specimens is aided by the use of selective inhibiting media (e.g., MacConkey, SS agar) that decrease the growth of gram-positive organisms as well as many gram-negative species. Salmonellae are motile, gram-negative bacilli that do not ferment lactose. From a practical viewpoint, in stool bacteriology, initial selection of non-lactose-fermenting colonies is followed by biochemical and serologic (agglutination) procedures for identification and serotyping of the organism. There are three primary species: *Salmonella typhi* (1 serotype); *S. choleraesuis* (1 serotype); and *S. enteritidis* (over 1700 sero-

types). By habit, organisms are often referred to as *Salmonella* (plus serotype designation—e.g., *typhimurium*) but the correct nomenclature is *Salmonella enteritidis,* serotype *typhimurium,* etc.

There is a latent period of from 3 to as long as 50 days (usually 7 to 14) between ingestion of bacteria and the dramatic onset of clinical symptoms of enteric fever. Shorter latent periods often follow ingestion of larger numbers of organisms. When due to salmonellae other than *S. typhi,* symptoms tend to begin earlier and are milder. During the latent period, organisms multiply in the distal small bowel and invade and multiply in lymphoid tissues in the area of Peyer's patches in the terminal ileum. Invasion of the bloodstream from this focus heralds the onset of the clinical illness with chills and fever and other constitutional effects of circulating endotoxin. Manifestations of infection occur in many organs and often in a predictable sequence: respiratory and central nervous system symptoms during the first week; skin manifestations during the second week; diarrhea, usually following a period of constipation, during the second and third weeks. Bacterial invasion of the skin, liver, gallbladder, bones, and joints, as well as manifestations of endotoxemia usually occur during the bacteremic phase of the illness (first 10 days). Organisms are cleared by the reticuloendothelial system (RES), leading to hyperplasia of these elements in the liver, spleen, and lymph nodes. Persistence of organisms in the gallbladder, biliary radicals, or the RES may lead to a chronic asymptomatic carrier state.

Epidemiology

S. typhi and other *Salmonella* species causing enteric fever are acquired by ingestion of contaminated water or food. Humans are the only hosts for *S. typhi* and the chronic carrier state that may follow clinical typhoid fever is almost always asymptomatic except for manifestations of gallbladder disease if cholelithiasis and active cholecystitis are present. Other *Salmonella,* serotypes of *S. enteritidis,* e.g., *typhimurium, schottmulleri,* and *hirshfeldii,* can produce an enteric fever syndrome similar to, but usually milder than, typhoid fever. Unlike *S. typhi,* these other *Salmonella* serotypes are ubiquitous in nature (occurring in animals, birds, reptiles, poultry products) and are difficult to control as sources of human infection.

A number of factors, exclusive of inoculum size, determine whether disease will occur after ingestion of *Salmonella.* Achlorhydria and previous gastric surgery allow organisms to escape destruction by the acid barrier of the stomach. Rapid transit of a smaller inoculum in a liquid vehicle may allow adequate numbers of viable bacteria to reach the distal small bowel. Underlying illnesses such as Hodgkin's disease, which alters cellular immunity, can interfere with the host defense mechanisms that normally eradicate these pathogens; hemoglobinopathies, such as sickle cell disease, appear to predispose to systemic *Salmonella* infections and osteomyelitis by saturating the protective RES with red cell fragments and occluding small blood vessels, leading to local chronic foci; and, finally, tumor immunosuppression therapy may be factors predisposing patients to salmonellosis. Infants and young children, as well as the very elderly, appear to be especially susceptible to serious disease as well as to gastroenteritis.

Clinical Manifestations

History Symptoms begin several days to several weeks after ingestion of contaminated water or food. Headache, fever, generalized aching, bronchitis, and constipation are often present. Delirium or mental torpor are not unusual, especially when there is a high fever. The pulse rate may be slower than expected for the magnitude of the fever. Symptoms increase in intensity, and the fever often reaches 39.5° to 40.5°C by the end of the first week. During the second week, rose spots may appear on the trunk and diffuse abdominal cramping becomes prominent, sometimes accompanied by diarrhea. In areas endemic for typhoid fever, the abdominal symptoms may be present from the onset, and diarrhea can be an early manifestation too.[76]

Cutaneous Lesions   After about 7 to 10 days of high fever, the characteristic rose spots may appear. These lesions are 2 to 3 mm in size, slightly raised, pink *papules,* which blanch on pressure and are nontender. They appear in crops of approximately 10 to 20 lesions and are usually located between the nipple area and the umbilicus on the anterior trunk, rarely on the back or extremities. Without therapy, the crops of spots usually become brownish as they fade and disappear in 3 to 4 days. New lesions emerge over the ensuing 2 to 3 weeks in untreated patients. Their presence in 63 percent of a group of 62 patients in a contemporary study should encourage careful observation for this subtle rash.[77] Antibiotic therapy instituted early in the course of the illness may be responsible for the decreasing incidence of rose spots.[78] The rash is less frequently reported in blacks, but this may be because of difficulty in detecting the small, scarce lesions on dark skin.

Rose spots occur infrequently in enteric fevers caused by other *Salmonella* species, but when they do appear, they may be present in greater numbers and in a more widespread distribution.

A variety of other skin changes have been described in enteric fever during the acute phase of illness. Erythema typhosum, an erythematous rash that is confluent and widely scattered, may occur during the first week of the disease. Erythema nodosum and urticarial lesions have been noted and ascribed to hypersensitivity phenomena. Transient loss of hair and changes in nails reflect the acute catabolic stress. It is distinctly uncommon to observe herpes labialis in enteric fever.

Other Physical Findings   During the acute phase of the disease, at the time the cutaneous lesions are appearing, the patient may be disoriented and have signs of pneumonia. The abdomen is often distended, tympanitic, and diffusely tender with some localization to the right lower quadrant. The spleen is often enlarged, but may be difficult to palpate because of abdominal distension and guarding.

Laboratory Findings

Leukopenia or low normal leukocyte counts are often present, but values range from 3000 to 20,000/mm³. The percentage of mononuclear cells may be increased, and atypical lymphocytes can appear in small numbers, suggesting a viral illness. Thrombocytopenia may occur, and rarely hemolysis is observed. During the initial week of illness, blood cultures are usually positive. During the second week, or when diarrhea begins, stool cultures become positive and the white blood cell count may increase. In addition to blood and stool, the typical rose spots should be cultured, preferably using the technique of skin snips.[77] In addition to blood and fecal cultures, bone marrow and skin lesion material may be positive in approximately 65 to 95 percent of cases, even when routine blood cultures simultaneously done are negative or when antibiotics

are being administered.[78] Antibodies to somatic (''O'') antigens develop after about 2 weeks of illness and rise over the ensuing months. Unfortunately, the serologic tests (Widal agglutination) are positive in about half of patients studied, and antibodies are detected nonspecifically in a variety of other infectious diseases. A more specific and sensitive serologic test for systemic *Salmonella* infections merits development.

Pathology

The rose spot characteristically blanches on pressure, and examination of the lesion histologically reveals gross dilatation of capillaries, described by some pathologists as ''capillary atony.'' Extravasation of blood is not observed, but there is considerable edema and an abundant pericapillary infiltration with macrophages; organisms may be present within these cells.[79] Rose spots have been produced experimentally by injecting purified *S. typhi* endotoxin intradermally.[80]

Diagnosis and Differential Diagnosis

The diagnosis of *Salmonella* enteric fever may be difficult in a sporadic case, especially if the characteristic rash and gastrointestinal symptoms have not yet appeared and there is no history of travel in an endemic area. Headache, cough, and high fever are not very specific findings. However, when these symptoms are associated with delirium, relative bradycardia, and leukopenia with increased numbers of circulating mononuclear cells, the diagnosis of enteric fever should be considered. The diagnosis is usually made by obtaining blood cultures, which are positive in approximately 80 percent of untreated cases during the first week to 10 days. Serologic tests (Widal) are usually negative during the early phase of the illness and may not be diagnostic later. Likewise, enteric fever due to other *Salmonella* species can usually be diagnosed by blood cultures. Other cultured material (marrow, rose spots) may be important, especially in patients who have had prior antibiotic therapy.

The differential diagnosis includes a wide range of diseases. Prominent cough and severe headache in the early phases may suggest a viral or atypical pneumonia (caused by *Legionella pneumophila, Chlamydia pneumoniae, Mycoplasma pneumoniae;* psittacosis, or Q fever). Typhus and Rocky Mountain spotted fever can usually be excluded by geographic and epidemiologic considerations, serologic studies, the characteristic petechial component to the rash, and, in the case of spotted fever, the distribution of the rash on the distal parts of the extremities. Miliary tuberculosis may begin as an acute febrile illness with similar symptoms, leukopenia, and splenomegaly. The diagnosis may be delayed until a secondary complication such as meningitis occurs, or until biopsy material (liver, lymph node) reveals granulomas, sometimes containing acid-fast organisms.

Among the viral diseases, the diagnosis of infectious mononucleosis is suggested by headache, cough, high fever, lymphadenopathy, splenomegaly, and a blood picture with leukopenia and some atypical mononuclear cells.

Malaria and toxoplasmosis are two parasitic illnesses that deserve consideration. Epidemiologic information plus intermittency of symptoms usually suggest the diagnosis of malaria. In generalized toxoplasmosis, the symptoms may be very similar to those of early enteric fever: prominent cough, high fever, a rash that is located on the trunk, and a mononucleosis-like blood picture. The rash tends to be more florid than the crops of 10 to 20 lesions seen in enteric fever and is macular with a petechial component, rather than papular. Diagnosis usually requires identification of *Toxoplasma gondii* in biopsy material or a rising antibody titer (19S fluorescent antibody or hemagglutination inhibition).

Course and Prognosis

The response of patients with enteric fever to antibiotic therapy is usually gradual, taking 3 to 6 days for the temperature to return to normal. With prolonged treatment, the incidence of relapse has been reduced, but this will vary with the age, nutritional conditions, and general health of the patient. The major complications in the preantibiotic days were perforation and hemorrhage. Although rare, these complications still occur even with prompt, effective chemotherapy, and are responsible for approximately 75 percent of the mortality in enteric fever. Deaths have been reduced from approximately 10 percent to 1 to 2 percent with antibiotic therapy. Following typhoid fever, approximately 1 to 2 percent of patients continue to harbor organisms in the gallbladder and excrete them in the stools for an indefinite period, becoming a major potential source for infecting other individuals.

Treatment and Prophylaxis   Chloramphenicol remains the preferred drug for the treatment of the enteric fever syndrome of salmonellosis, whether it is caused by *S. typhi* or by other *Salmonella* species. It is administered intravenously, 0.75 to 1.0 g every 6 h, and should be continued for 15 to 21 days. Chloramphenicol can be given by the oral route once clinical improvement is well established, but the intramuscular route is not effective. During treatment, the synthetic functions of the bone marrow should be watched carefully with leukocyte, reticulocyte, and differential blood counts, and the patient should be under close medical supervision.

In patients for whom chloramphenicol is not the drug of choice because of allergy, toxicity, or resistance of the *Salmonella* strain, ampicillin is an alternative and may be equal to chloramphenicol in effectiveness. It should be given by the intravenous route in doses of 1.5 to 2.0 g every 4 h (in adults). The combination of trimethoprim-sulfamethoxazole (TSM) has also been extensively studied and found effective for most cases of enteric fever due to *S. typhi* or other *Salmonella* species. The dose of TSM is 160 mg trimethoprim plus 800 mg of sulfamethoxazole three times per day for 15 to 21 days. It is mandatory to carry out susceptibility tests on all isolates from cases of enteric fever as some strains are resistant to chloramphenicol, ampicillin, trimethoprim-sulfamethoxazole, or to all three agents. The fluoroquinolones (ciprofloxacin, ofloxacin) are active against drug-susceptible and multidrug-resistant (chloramphenicol, TSM, or ampicillin) *S. typhi* or other salmonellae causing enteric fever. Results of clinical trials, involving over 100 patients, indicate that blood cultures become sterile promptly on treatment with ciprofloxacin and that this drug appears to be a safe and effective alternative for chloramphenicol in the treatment of typhoid fever.[81] Ciprofloxacin is administered in 500 to 750 mg dosage orally every 12 h (or 400 mg intravenously every 12 h) in adults, for 14 to 21 days. Third-generation cephalosporins (cefotaxime, ceftriaxone, cefoperazone) are acceptable alternatives for the treatment of typhoid fever if the previously noted antimicrobials cannot be used because of resistance of the infecting strain or because of drug hypersensitivity.[82]

Corticosteroid therapy for a period of several days has been advocated in addition to antimicrobial treatment for severely toxic and febrile patients, but its efficacy is unproved. A recent report found that high doses of dexamethasone reduced mortality significantly.[83] Among the major complications, hemorrhage usually responds to conservative management, but perforation, often in the ileocecal region, requires immediate surgery.

Identification and eradication of the biliary carrier of *S. typhi* is an important preventive measure for controlling enteric fever. In the presence of stones, antibiotic therapy should be combined with cholecystectomy. In the absence of stones, a prolonged course of treatment with ampicillin or amoxicillin may eradicate the carrier site.[84] Ciprofloxacin has also been reported to be successful.[81]

Individuals traveling to areas of the world endemic for *S. typhi* or *S. paratyphi A* should be instructed in commonsense methods of eating and drinking to avoid potentially contaminated materials. Immunization is available for *S. typhi* and is probably effective for all but massive exposures, but careful personal hygiene and avoidance of suspicious water or foods (e.g., leafy greens) will eliminate most encounters with *S. typhi* and other Salmonellae capable of causing enteric fever.

Cutaneous Manifestations of Infection with Other Gram-Negative Bacilli

General Features

An acute cellulitis, with or without production of gas, may be caused by *E. coli*, *Proteus* spp., *Klebsiella* spp., *Enterobacter* spp., *Serratia marcescens*, a variety of other facultative and nonfermenting bacilli, and members of the obligate anaerobic group of *Bacteroides*. These infections have often, but not exclusively, been described in the very elderly and in diabetic patients following trauma, surgery, or bowel or perineal inflammation. Drug addicts may develop mixed infections with these organisms when "skin popping," resulting in lesions such as necrotizing fasciitis.[85] Prior exposure to broad-spectrum antibiotics and altered host defenses can predispose to this type of infection which is often nosocomial in origin. The finding of gas in the tissues frequently leads to an erroneous provisional diagnosis of clostridial cellulitis or gas gangrene.

Bacteriology and Pathogenesis

The family Enterobacteriaceae is composed of a number of bacilli that grow readily on blood agar and selective media. By means of a number of biochemical reactions and growth characteristics, seven tribes of Enterobacteriaceae have been recognized.[86] *E. coli* is closely related to *Shigella*; *Salmonella* spp. to *Citrobacter*; *Klebsiella-Enterobacter-Serratia* make up a third tribe; *Proteus-Providence* comprise a fourth main division. There are a variety of facultative gram-negative bacilli that do not belong to this family, metabolize sugars variably, and can be recognized by utilizing other specialized biochemical tests. In addition, the obligate anaerobic *Bacteroides* spp. reside in the oral cavity, colon, and female vaginal region, and are identified by their anaerobic growth requirements as well as a variety of other characteristics.[87]

Infection can result from contamination of skin or subcutaneous tissues in an area of injury, surgery, or ischemia. Bacteria can also invade the subcutaneous tissues via the circulation from a distinct source or by direct spread from contiguous structures such as the colon. By dissection along fascial planes, cellulitis can erupt in areas removed from the initial focus. The process is often necrotizing, containing a mixture of facultative and anaerobic bacteria and, especially in diabetic individuals, can be associated with gas formation (mainly hydrogen). Edema, bleb formation, ischemia, and gangrene result from thrombosis of nutrient blood vessels. The underlying muscle is almost always spared.[88] Polymorphonuclear leukocytes are abundantly present compared to the relative scarcity of acute inflammatory cells in clostridial infections.

Epidemiology

Cellulitis usually follows contamination of adjacent tissues by bowel contents or a breakdown of skin. The conditions predisposing patients to this type of infection include: (1) bowel perforation (appendicitis, neoplasm, diverticulitis, rectal mucosal tear), (2) colon surgery, (3) chronic edema, (4) vascular insufficiency, (5) decubitus ulcers, (6) percutaneous lines, and (7) superficial perineal dermatitis, including diaper rash. The health of these patients is often further impaired by poorly controlled diabetes, alterations in host defense mechanisms (granulopenia, etc.), and poor nutrition. Crepitant (gas-containing) cellulitis results from infection with gas-forming strains of bacteria (*E. coli, Klebsiella, Aeromonas hydrophila*), especially in patients with poorly controlled diabetes or when *Bacteroides* spp. or anaerobic streptococci are present too.[89] Water-related lacerations may cause soft tissue infection with *Edwardsiella tarda*.[90] Similarly, cellulitis or rapidly progressive myonecrosis due to *Aeromonas hydrophila* may follow penetrating trauma in either a freshwater environment or associated with fish or other aquatic animals.[91] Injuries on farms, particularly from corn-harvesting machinery, have been associated with gram-negative bacilli (*Enterobacter* spp. and *Xanthomonas maltophilia*).[92] Gram-negative bacillary cellulitis (due to *E. coli, Proteus* spp., or *Citrobacter freundii*) may occur in immunocompromised patients or patients with the nephrotic syndrome.[93,94] The appearance of the lesions grossly resembles those due to the more common gram-positive pathogens.

Clinical Manifestations

History Diabetes mellitus, malnutrition, chronic illness (e.g., paraplegia with decubitus ulcers), or several other conditions described under "Epidemiology" are usually present. The onset may be insidious over 4 to 5 days or abrupt, with high fever, shaking chills, hypotension, and pain in the area of cellulitis. Symptoms of gastrointestinal inflammation such as appendicitis or diverticulitis may precede the cellulitis illness. Rectal or perineal pain can indicate a local process that may be especially devastating in a patient deficient in granulocytes.

Cutaneous Lesions The areas of involvement have the typical findings of cellulitis with warmth and brawny edema. In the early stages, the skin is rarely discolored beyond a pink hue, and vesicles and blebs or bullae are almost never present. At this juncture, the process may easily be overlooked, especially if the infection is located in a less obvious area or the patient is obtunded. As the cellulitis progresses, edema and redness increase and areas of gangrene may appear. Palpable tenderness and crepitus, if present, can help define the anatomic extent of the process.

Cellulitis due to *Aeromonas hydrophila* may progress rapidly with the development, occasionally, of myonecrosis accompanied by gas spreading extensively in soft tissue planes. This process can mimic clostridial gas gangrene in its rapid onset (24 to 48 h after the initiating wound) and swift progression with pain, marked swelling, serosanguineous bullae, crepitation, and systemic toxicity. Treatment requires extensive surgical debridement and prompt initiation of antimicrobial therapy. Most isolates are susceptible to aminoglycosides, chloramphenicol, tetracycline, trimethoprim-sulfamethoxazole, and cefotaxime.

In addition to cellulitis, with or without gas formation, macular, papular, and ecthymatous lesions indistinguishable from those caused by *P. aeruginosa* occasionally occur.

SUPERFICIAL NASAL LESIONS.   Several species of *Klebsiella* that infect the upper respiratory tract can produce unique superficial diseases. Ozena is a chronic productive rhinitis caused by infection with *Klebsiella ozaenae*. The process remains internal without any cutaneous manifestations except a profuse mucopurulent foul-smelling discharge.[95] *Klebsiella rhinoscleromatis* is the etiologic agent of a hypertrophic, granulomatous infection of the external nares, which is known as rhinoscleroma. This disease often produces changes in the overlying nasal skin (Fig. 188-7) and the contiguous surfaces of the respiratory and posterior pharyngeal regions. Most cases have been described from very local areas of Eastern and Central Europe (where the disease is known as "Slavic leprosy"), from Africa, the Near East, and parts of Central and South America.[96] Dissemination of the organism is by prolonged close contact, often in family settings of crowding and poor sanitation. Infected individuals can shed organisms for years, with the result that hyperendemic areas are recognized. As seen in leprosy, the disease rarely becomes clinically apparent in children. Patients complain of chronic nasal and cutaneous discharge, obstructive symptoms, or cutaneous nasal masses. Diagnosis depends upon biopsy identification of characteristic vacuolated Mikulicz cells and isolation of the organism on routine cultures, with biochemical and serologic confirmation.[97] Both *K. ozaenae* and *K. rhinoscleromatis* are susceptible to streptomycin and the newer aminoglycosides, trimethoprim-sulfamethoxazole, tetracycline, and chlorampheni-

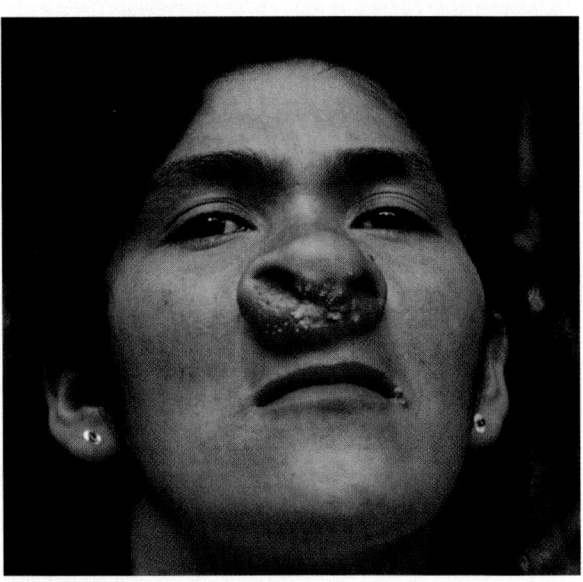

FIGURE 188-7 *Klebsiella rhinoscleromatis:* Rhinoscleroma. The nasal passages and nose are infected resulting from obstructed respiration.

col. Prolonged (6 to 8 weeks) treatment of scleroma is important, and results are favorable except for residual fibrotic and destructive changes.

Other Physical Findings   The clinical course is often dominated by systemic manifestations such as decreased mental alertness, hypotension, and dehydration. Abdominal distension and other manifestations of localized or generalized peritonitis may be present. Extreme tenderness of the rectum, with or without a mass, can indicate the local source of a perineal process.

Laboratory Findings

The leukocyte count is usually elevated, in the range of 20,000 to 30,000/mm³, but may be markedly diminished in the presence of gram-negative septicemia. Elevated blood glucose values and findings of ketoacidosis are not unusual. In the presence of crepitant cellulitis, roentgenograms of the soft tissue may show the depth and extent of the gas-forming process.[89] In the absence of palpable gas a soft tissue x-ray may indicate gas formation as part of the inflammatory process.

Pathology

Edema, necrosis, gangrene of overlying skin, and a thin exudate containing visible fat droplets and polymorphonuclear leukocytes is usually present. Gas may be seen in the subcutaneous tissues. Blood vessels are often involved in a necrotic, thrombotic inflammatory reaction. The underlying muscle is usually not involved unless there is septicemia associated with major vascular thrombosis or there is myonecrosis with *A. hydrophila* infection.

Diagnosis and Differential Diagnosis

A specific etiologic diagnosis can be made by needle aspiration of the cellulitis or an overlying bleb. Several morphologic forms of gram-positive as well as gram-negative organisms may be present, and when gas is present, anaerobic cocci and clostridia must also be considered. The presence of anaerobes in the exudate may be accompanied by a foul, fetid odor.

Course and Prognosis

The process may be indolent and quickly respond to effective antibiotic therapy. Unfortunately, especially in obese diabetic patients with perineal lesions, progression of necrotizing fasciitis may be astonishingly rapid, even with vigorous antibiotic and surgical therapy. When the process is located centrally, in the perineal-gluteal area, the mortality is often as high as 50 percent. Infection of an extremity is often treated by antibiotics and drainage and debridement, or amputation, with more favorable results. The course is often prolonged and complex due to metabolic and nutritional complications.

Treatment

Immediate antibiotic therapy and surgical drainage are essential, guided by Gram-stained smears of the exudate and the extent of the process. Extensive debridement is usually unnecessary and hyperbaric oxygen is not indicated. Judgment and experience are vital in surgical decisions that include the question of amputation. The existence of a ''feeding'' source of contamination should be sought (e.g., from a ruptured appendix, diverticulum, or rectal tear). If a lower-bowel leak is found, a diverting colostomy should be performed in addition to a local drainage procedure. Decubitus ulcers must be carefully evaluated for undermining necrosis, abscess formation, and cellulitis.[98]

Recent antibiotic usage, status of renal and hepatic function, and prior hospital exposure are factors that will help determine the choice of antibiotics. Single or multiple agents are used, depending on the above information and the results of Gram-stained smears of exudate. Hospitalized patients already exposed to antibiotics and acutely ill should be given an aminoglycoside, such as gentamicin (1.5 mg/kg every 8 h parenterally). If the cellulitis is crepitant, it may indicate coinfection with *Bacteroides fragilis,* and chloramphenicol (750 mg intravenously every 6 h) should be added. Metronidazole (2 g daily in four divided doses), clindamycin (2.4 g in four divided doses intravenously), and selected second- and third-generation cephalosporins can substitute for chloramphenicol. Tobramycin or amikacin may be preferred to gentamicin for certain hospital-acquired infections with *Pseudomonas, Klebsiella,* or *Serratia.* If gram-positive cocci are present on initial stained smears, penicillin or nafcillin should be added.

References

1. Band JD et al: Trends in meningococcal disease in the United States, 1975–1980. *J Infect Dis* **148**:754, 1983
2. Gibbons RJ, Van Houte J: Adherence in oral microbial ecology. *Annu Rev Microbiol* **29**:19, 1975
3. DeVoe IW, Gilchrist JE: Piliation and colonial morphology among laboratory strains of meningococci. *J Clin Microbiol* **7**:379, 1978
4. Kornfeld SF, Plaut AG: Secretory immunity and the bacterial IgA proteases. *Rev Infect Dis* **3**:521, 1981
5. Ross SC, Densen P: Complement deficiency states and infection: Epidemiology, pathogenesis and consequences of neisserial and other infections in an immune deficiency. *Medicine* (Baltimore) **63**:243, 1984
6. Densen P et al: Familial properdin deficiency and fatal bacteremia. Correction of the bactericidal defect by vaccination. *N Engl J Med* **316**:922, 1987
7. Ellison RT et al: Prevalence of congenital or acquired complement deficiency in patients with sporadic meningococcal disease. *N Engl J Med* **308**:913, 1983
8. Sotto MN et al: Pathogenesis of cutaneous lesions in acute meningococcemia in humans: light, immunofluorescent, and electron microscopic studies of skin biopsy specimens. *J Infect Dis* **133**:506, 1976
9. Davis CE, Arnold K: Role of meningococcal endotoxin in meningococcal purpura. *J Exp Med* **140**:159, 1974
10. DeVoe IW, Gilka F: Disseminated intravascular coagulation in rabbits: Synergistic activity of meningoccal endotoxin and materials egested from leukocytes containing meningococci. *J Med Microbiol* **9**:451, 1976
11. McGehee WG et al: Intravascular coagulation in fulminant meningococcemia. *Ann Intern Med* **67**:250, 1967
12. DeVoe IW: The meningococcus and mechanisms of pathogenicity. *Microbiol Rev* **46**:162, 1982
13. Adams EM et al: Absence of the seventh component of complement in a patient with chronic meningococcemia presenting as vasculitis. *Ann Intern Med* **99**:35, 1983
14. Fass RJ, Saslaw S: Chronic meningococcemia: Possible pathogenic role of IgM deficiency. *Arch Intern Med* **130**:943, 1972

15. Artenstein MC et al: Immunoprophylaxis of meningococcal infection. *Milit Med* **139**:91, 1974

16. Goldschneider I et al: Human immunity to the meningococcus. II. Development of natural immunity. *J Exp Med* **129**:1327, 1969

17. Robbins JB et al: Enteric bacteria cross-reactive with *Neisseria meningitidis* groups A and C and *Diplococcus pneumoniae* types I and III. *Infect Immun* **6**:651, 1972

18. Goldschneider I et al: Human immunity to the meningococcus. I. The role of humoral antibodies. *J Exp Med* **129**:1307, 1969

19. Griffiss JM, Bertram MA: Immunoepidemiology of meningococcal disease in military recruits. II. Blocking of serum bactericidal antibody by circulating IgA early in the course of invasive disease. *J Infect Dis* **136**:733, 1977

20. Griffiss JM: Epidemic meningococcal disease: Synthesis of a hypothetical immunoepidemiologic model. *Rev Infect Dis* **4**:159, 1982

21. Munford RS et al: Spread of meningococcal infection within households. *Lancet* **2**:1275, 1974

22. Meningococcal Disease Surveillance Group: Meningococcal disease. *JAMA* **235**:261, 1976

23. Jacobson JA, Holloway JT: Meningococcal disease in day-care centers. *Pediatrics* **59**:299, 1977

24. Gallaid EI et al: Meningococcal disease in New York City 1973–1978: Recognition of groups Y and W135 as frequent pathogens. *JAMA* **244**:2167, 1980

25. Salet IE et al: Seroepidemiologic aspects of *Neisseria meningitidis* in homosexual men. *Can Med Assoc J* **126**:38, 1982

26. Feldman HA: Meningoccal infections. *Adv Intern Med* **18**:177, 1972

27. Koppes GM et al: Group Y meningococcal disease in United States air force recruits. *Am J Med* **62**:661, 1977

28. Bernhard WG, Jordan AC: Purpuric lesions in meningococci infections: Diagnosis from smears and cultures of the purpuric lesions. *J Lab Clin Med* **29**:273, 1944

29. Hoyne AL, Brown RH: Meningococcic cases, an analysis. *Ann Intern Med* **28**:248, 1948

30. Tilton RC et al: Comparative evaluation of three commercial products and counterimmunoelectrophoresis for the detection of antigens in cerebrospinal fluid. *J Clin Microbiol* **20**:231, 1984

31. Benoit FL: Chronic meningococcemia. *Am J Med* **35**:103, 1963

32. Leibel RL et al: Chronic meningococcemia in childhood. *Am J Dis Child* **127**:94, 1974

33. Barquet N et al: Primary meningococcal conjunctivitis: Report of 21 patients and review. *Rev Infect Dis* **12**:838, 1990

34. Ferson M, Shi E: Periorbital cellulitis with meningococcal bacteremia. *Pediatr Infect Dis J* **7**:600, 1988

35. Mendelman PM et al: Relative penicillin G resistance in *Neisseria meningitidis* and reduced affinity of penicillin binding protein 3. *Antimicrob Agents Chemother* **32**:706, 1988

36. Winslow EJ et al: Hemodynamic studies and results of therapy in 50 patients with bacteremic shock. *Am J Med* **54**:421, 1973

37. Sprung CL et al: The effects of high-dose corticosteroids in patients with septic shock. *N Engl J Med* **311**:1138, 1984

38. Corrigan JJ Jr: Heparin therapy in bacterial septicemia. *J Pediatr* **91**:695, 1977

39. Meningococcal vaccines. *MMWR* **34**:255, 1985

40. Devine LF et al: Selective minocycline and rifampin treatment of group C meningococcal carriers in a new naval recruit camp. *Am J Med Sci* **263**:79, 1972

41. Pugsley MF et al: Efficacy of ciprofloxacin in treatment of nasopharyngeal carriers of *Neisseria meningitidis*. *J Infect Dis* **156**:211, 1987

42. Hoeprich PD: Prediction of anti-meningococcal chemoprophylactic efficacy. *J Infect Dis* **123**:125, 1971

43. Peltola H: Meningococcal disease: Still with us. *Rev Infect Dis* **5**:71, 1983

44. Gustafson TL et al: Pseudomonas folliculitis: An outbreak and review. *Rev Infect Dis* **5**:1, 1983

45. Liu PV: Extracellular toxins of *Pseudomonas aeruginosa*. *J Infect Dis* **130** (suppl):S94, 1974

46. Woods DE, Iglewski BH: Toxins of *Pseudomonas aeruginosa:* New perspectives. *Rev Infect Dis* **5**:S715, 1983

47. Saelinger CB et al: Experimental studies on the pathogenesis of infections due to *Pseudomonas aeruginosa:* Direct evidence for toxin production during pseudomonas infection of burned skin tissues. *J Infect Dis* **136**:555, 1957

48. Hall JH et al: *Pseudomonas aeruginosa* in dermatology. *Arch Dermatol* **97**:312, 1968

49. Bassiouny A: Perichondritis of the auricle. *Laryngoscope* **91**:422, 1981

50. Zaky DA et al: Malignant external otitis: A severe form of otitis in diabetic patients. *Am J Med* **61**:298, 1976

51. Doroghazi RM et al: Invasive external otitis. Report of 21 cases and review of the literature. *Am J Med* **71**:603, 1981

52. El Baz P et al: *Pseudomonas aeruginosa* 0-11 folliculitis. Development into ecthyma gangrenosum in immunosuppressed patients. *Arch Dermatol* **121**:873, 1985

53. Stanley MM: *Bacillus pyrocyaneus* infections (2 parts). *Am J Med* **2**:253, 1947

54. Forkner CE et al: Pseudomonas septicemia. *Am J Med* **25**:877, 1958

55. Reed RK et al: Peripheral nodular lesions in *Pseudomonas* sepsis: The importance of incision and drainage. *J Pediatr* **88**:977, 1976

56. Bagel J, Grossman ME: Subcutaneous nodules in *Pseudomonas* sepsis. *Am J Med* **80**:528, 1986

57. Teplitz C: Pathogenesis of *Pseudomonas* vasculitis and septic lesions. *Arch Pathol* **80**:297, 1965

58. Cryz S et al: Production and characterization of a human hyperimmune intravenous immunoglobulin against *Pseudomonas aeruginosa* and *Klebsiella* species. *J Infect Dis* **163**:1055, 1991

59. Kusne S et al: Gangrenous cellulitis associated with gram-negative bacilli in pancytopenic patients: Dilemma with respect to effective therapy. *Am J Med* **85**:490, 1988

60. Bodey GP et al: Infection caused by *Pseudomonas aeruginosa*. *Rev Infect Dis* **5**:279, 1983

61. Chen S et al: Cellulitis due to *Pseudomonas putrefaciens:* Possible production of exotoxins. *Rev Infect Dis* **13**:642, 1991

62. Nelson JD, Ginsburg CM: An hypothesis on the pathogenesis of *Haemophilus influenzae* buccal cellulitis. *J Pediatr* **88**:709, 1976

63. Dajani AS et al: Systemic *Haemophilus influenzae* disease: An overview. *J Pediatr* **94**:355, 1979

64. Granoff DM, Ward JI: Current status of prophylaxis for *Haemophilus influenzae* infections. *Curr Top Infect Dis* **5**:290, 1984

65. Shaw S et al: The paradox of *Haemophilus influenzae* type B bacteremia in the presence of serum bactericidal activity. *J Clin Invest* **58**:1019, 1976

66. Robbins JB et al: *Haemophilus influenzae* type b: Disease and immunity in humans. *Ann Intern Med* **78**:259, 1973

67. O'Reilly RJ et al: Circulating polyribophosphate in *Haemophilus influenzae* type b meningitis. *J Clin Invest* **56**:1012, 1975

68. Smith DH et al: Studies on the prevalence of antibodies to *Haemophilus influenzae*, type B, in *Haemophilus influenzae*, edited by S Sell. Nashville, Vanderbilt Univ Press, 1973

69. Schneerson R, Robbins JB: Induction of serum *Haemophilus influenzae* type b capsular antibodies in adult volunteers fed cross-reacting *Escherichia coli* 075:K100:H5. *N Engl J Med* **292**:1093, 1975

70. Granoff DM, Nankervis GA: Cellulitis due to *Haemophilus influenzae* type b antigenemia and antibody responses. *Am J Dis Child* **130**:1211, 1976

71. Drapkin MS et al: Bacteremic *Haemophilus influenzae* type b cellulitis in the adult. *Am J Med* **63**:449, 1977

72. Chartrand S, Harrison C: Buccal cellulitis reevaluated. *Am J Dis Child* **140**:891, 1986

73. McDonell M et al: *Haemophilus influenzae* type B cellulitis in adults. *Am J Med* **81**:709, 1986

74. Prevention of secondary cases of *Haemophilus influenzae* type b disease. *MMWR* **31**:672, 1982

75. Eskola J et al: A randomized prospective trial of a conjugate vaccine in the protection of infants and young children against invasive *Haemophilus influenzae* type b disease. *N Engl J Med* **20**:1381, 1990

76. Wicks ACB et al: Endemic typhoid fever: A diagnostic pitfall. *Q J Med* [*New Series XL*] **159**:341, 1971

77. Gilman RH et al: Relative efficacy of blood, urine, rectal swab, bone-marrow, and rose-spot cultures for recovery of *Salmonella typhi* in typhoid fever. *Lancet* **1**:1211, 1975

78. Gulati PD et al: Changing patterns of typhoid fever. *Am J Med* **45**:544, 1968

79. Litwack KD et al: Rose spots in typhoid fever. *Arch Dermatol* **105**:252, 1972

80. Hornick RB et al: Typhoid fever: Pathogenesis and immunologic control. *N Engl J Med* **283**:739, 1970

81. Asperilla MO et al: Quinolone antibiotics in the treatment of *Salmonella* infections. *Rev Infect Dis* **12**:873, 1990

82. Soe GB, Overturf GD: Treatment of typhoid fever and other systemic salmonelloses with cefotaxime, ceftriaxone, cefoperazone, and other newer cephalosporins. *Rev Infect Dis* **9**:719, 1987

83. Hoffman SL et al: Reduction of mortality in chloramphenicol-treated severe typhoid fever by high-dose dexamethasone. *N Engl J Med* **310**:82, 1984

84. Nolan CM, White PC: Treatment of typhoid carriers with amoxicillin. *JAMA* **239**:2352, 1978

85. Giuliano A et al: Bacteriology of necrotizing fasciitis. *Am J Surg* **134**:52, 1977

86. Brenner DJ et al: *Taxomonic and Nomenclature Changes in Enterobacteriaceae.* Atlanta, Centers for Disease Control, 1977

87. Moore WEC et al: Identification of anaerobes from clinical infections, in *Anaerobic Bacteria,* edited by A Balows et al. Springfield, IL, Charles C Thomas, 1974, p 51

88. Culbertson WR: Acute non-clostridial crepitant cellulitis. *Arch Surg* **77**:462, 1958

89. Bessman AN, Wagner W: Nonclostridial gas gangrene. *JAMA* **233**:958, 1975

90. Pitlik S et al: Nonenteric infections acquired through contact with water. *Rev Infect Dis* **9**:54, 1987

91. Heckerling PS et al: *Aeromonas hydrophila* myonecrosis and gas gangrene in a nonimmunocompromised host. *Arch Intern Med* **143**:2005, 1983

92. Agger WA et al: Wounds caused by corn-harvesting machines: An unusual source of infection due to gram-negative bacilli. *Rev Infect Dis* **8**:927, 1986

93. Asmar BI et al: *Escherichia coli* cellulitis in children with idiopathic nephrotic syndrome. *Clin Pediatr* **26**:592, 1987

94. Hick CB, Chulay JD: Bacteremic *Citrobacter freundii* cellulitis associated with tub immersion in a patient with the nephrotic syndrome. *Milit Med* **153**:400, 1988

95. Goldstein EJ et al: Infections caused by *Klebsiella ozaenae:* A changing disease spectrum. *J Clin Microbiol* **8**:413, 1978

96. Altmann G et al: Rhinoscleroma. *Isr J Med Sci* **13**:62, 1977

97. Malowany MS et al: Isolation and microbiologic differentiation of *Klebsiella rhinoscleromatis* and *Klebsiella ozaenae* in cases of chronic rhinitis. *Am J Clin Pathol* **58**:550, 1972

98. Galpin JE et al: Sepsis associated with decubitus ulcers. *Am J Med* **61**:346, 1976

CHAPTER 189

Irwin M. Freedberg

Cat-Scratch Disease

Cat-scratch disease (CSD) is a benign, usually self-limited, apparently bacterial infection, characterized in most cases by a history of a cat contact; a primary papulopustular skin lesion; and enlarged, localized lymph nodes, which may suppurate. Although there were many synonyms used for this disease in the past, the only one still relevant is *benign lymphoreticulosis*. The disease was first recognized in 1931 by Debré, although it was not formally described in the literature until 1950.[1]

Epidemiology[2–7]

The disease occurs in all ages, although approximately 50 to 80 percent of patients are less than 20 years of age. It is worldwide without any sexual, racial, or geographic predilection. Although epidemic outbreaks have been reported, CSD usually occurs throughout the year in an endemic fashion, with most cases reported in the midwinter months. Most frequently, the vector animal has been an apparently healthy cat or kitten with a negative CSD skin test (see below). CSD has also been reported after contact with dogs, monkeys, and chickens. Clinical evidence of scratches is present in half the reported cases, and in 90 percent there is a history of both cat contact and scratches. Thorns or splinters may be involved in the transmission. Usually, only one household member is affected at a time, although others may have been similarly scratched. Multiple cases in the same household have been reported, usually with exposure to the same cat, but these occur months or years apart.

The etiologic agent, if there is a specific one, has not been clearly defined. Wear and his colleagues reported the presence of delicate, pleomorphic, gram-negative bacteria in the capillaries of the lymph node of patients with CSD.[5] In 1984, Margileth and his colleagues reported bacteria in the primary lesions, and the process was named *epithelioid angiomatosis* or *bacillary angiomatosis*.[6] In 1988, these same workers reported that Koch postulates had been fulfilled.[7] Subsequent investigations have raised questions regarding these observations, and at this time the etiology still remains somewhat unclear.

Clinical Manifestations[8–17]

Cat-scratch disease is most commonly benign and self-limited. The incubation period ranges from a few days to several weeks from the original skin trauma to the onset of the primary lesion. In one-third of the patients, the primary lesion is not found, and the disease presents as asymptomatic, regional lymphadenopathy. Fever, usually of low grade, occurs in 25 to 75 percent of cases. Common symptoms include malaise, headache, generalized myalgias and arthralgias, lassitude, and chills. These symptoms tend to increase as the nodes enlarge.

When it is seen, the primary lesion may be a 0.5- to 1-cm lichenoid papule, a pustule, a nodule, a cluster of tiny nodules, or a superficial ulceration (Fig. 189-1). In 50 percent of the cases in which a primary lesion occurs, it is located on the arm or hand. The lesion persists for less than a month in approximately two-thirds of

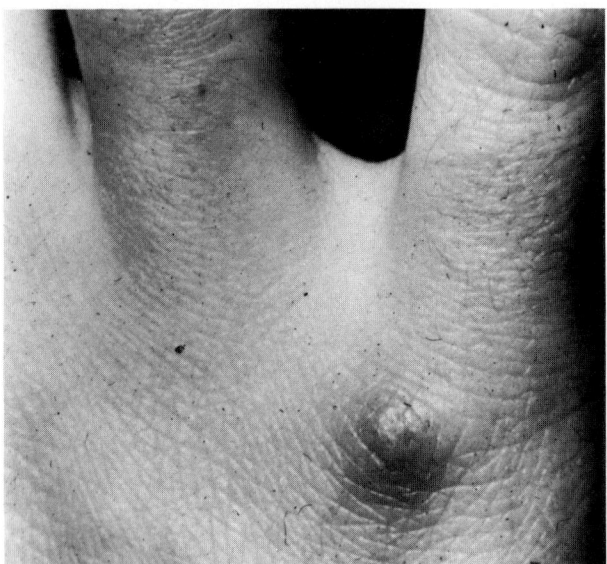

FIGURE 189-1 Cat-scratch disease. The primary lesion is a papule or nodule that has undergone necrosis with development of a central ulceration. (*Courtesy of Anne Baker, M.D.*)

cases and may last up to 2 months in the remainder. Approximately 4 percent of patients have a viral like, nonpruritic, macular and papular eruption that lasts several days. Erythema nodosum, erythema multiforme, figurate erythemas, and thrombocytopenic purpura have been reported.

The most alarming manifestation of the disease is encephalopathy, which is reported infrequently. It occurs approximately 2 weeks after the beginning of the disease and is characterized by the sudden onset of fever and coma, which may progress to convulsions. Diffuse slowing of the EEG is found associated with focal areas of low density on a computed tomography scan of the brain. The cerebrospinal fluid is usually normal, although there may be an increase in the protein or cell count. The duration of the encephalitis is usually only a few days, although deaths have been reported.

Lymphadenopathy is the hallmark of the disease. The nodes are usually unilateral, regional, and primarily cervical. However, other lymph nodes, including the axillary, epitrochlear, submandibular, inguinal, and preauricular, may be involved. The latter are seen associated with primary involvement of the eye, leading to palpebral conjunctivitis. This presentation was previously known as the *oculoglandular syndrome* or *Parinaud's syndrome,* terms also used for the oculoglandular presentation of tularemia (see Chap. 190).

Nodes are single in about half the cases and multiple in single sites in the other half. The lymphadenopathy begins within 1 to 3 weeks after the appearance of the primary lesion and is proximal to it. The nodes are initially red and tender and gradually increase in size to become fluctuant and occasionally suppurative. They usually regress within 6 weeks but may last as long as 2 years.

In 1983, a disease was described in association with human immunodeficiency virus (HIV) infection in which patients developed red, 0.1- to 0.2-cm diffuse papular lesions that were friable, tender, nonblanching, and readily bleeding. Noncutaneous involvement of bone marrow, liver, spleen, or long bones was reported, and thrombocytopenia occurred. It was initially believed that this process, which was termed *epithelioid bacillary angiomatosis*[6] and which had to be differentiated from Kaposi's sarcoma, was a manifestation of CSD occurring in immunosuppressed pa-

tients. Gram-negative, small (0.2 to 0.3 μm) pleomorphic coccobacilli were seen in the endothelium of blood vessels. As noted below, this disease responded to antibiotic therapy, in contrast to localized CSD (see Chap 215).

More recent studies, which are based upon molecular biologic investigations, indicate that the latter process is caused by an alpha purple, rickettsial-like bacterium (*Rochalimaea* p.), related but not identical to the cat-scratch bacillus. This situation still needs to be completely clarified.

Laboratory Findings

Routine laboratory tests are not helpful except to exclude other causes of lymphadenopathy. The white blood count is normal or only slightly increased with occasional eosinophilia. Sedimentation rate is commonly increased to 40 to 50 mm/h.

Cat-Scratch Skin Test[18-20]

A skin test was developed for CSD in which the source of antigen was aspirated purulent lymph node material from patients with the disease. The nature of the antigen and any other components in the skin test has not been determined. At least 6000 doses of the skin test antigens were used, and in patients with a consistent clinical picture, 98 percent of reactions were reported to be positive. In the general population, positive reactions ranged between 4 and 8 percent. For a number of reasons, including potential transmission of other diseases through the test antigen as well as lack of standardization, the test is no longer in use.

Histopathology[21-23]

The primary lesion is middermal and shows small areas of frank necrosis surrounded by necrobiosis. Surrounding the necrobiosis is a multilayered mantle of histiocytes in which the inner layer may be palisaded. Surrounding the histiocytes is a zone of lymphocytes of variable thickness and density. Multinucleated giant cells are seen in the lesion, and eosinophils can be seen in the adjacent stroma. Epidermal changes are generally varied and nonspecific, showing parakeratosis, epidermal edema, or exocytosis of inflammatory cells through the epidermis.

Microscopic changes in lymph nodes are nonspecific but may be helpful in making a diagnosis of CSD when the clinical picture is not typical. Initially, there is a reticular cell hyperplasia that progresses to an intermediate stage of caseating granulomas, simulating tuberculosis. The centers are acellular and necrotic and are surrounded by histiocytes and peripheral lymphocytes, reminiscent of the morphology found in the primary skin lesion. Late stages show multiple abscesses.

Diagnosis and Differential Diagnosis

The approach to the child or young adult with suspected CSD is the same as the approach to the patient with regional lymphadenopathy or generalized lymphadenopathy with regional accentuation.[10,11]

A diagnosis of CSD in a typical case should include (1) regional lymphadenopathy; (2) history of cat contact, cat scratch, or a consistent primary lesion; and (3) the failure to demonstrate other probable causes. When it was used, the cat-scratch skin test was considered one of the important criteria. Some investigators have stressed lymph node biopsy because of the characteristic histopathologic changes.

Treatment

Cat-scratch disease usually subsides spontaneously within a period of 1 to 2 months. Second attacks have not been reported, and sequelae from typical cases did not occur. Thus, treatment should be conservative, consisting of reassurance and analgesics. In some cases, spontaneous or therapeutic lymph node drainage is effective in relieving local pain and systemic symptoms. Antimicrobial agents have been ineffective in shortening or ameliorating the course of CSD.

In contrast, epithelioid bacillary angiomatosis, which is considered by some to be generalized CSD in an immunocompromised host, responds to antibiotics, including erythromycin, doxycycline, ciprofloxacin, isoniazid, and rifampin.[24–26]

References

1. Debré R et al: La maladie des griffes de chat. *Bull Mem Soc Med Hop Paris* **66**:76, 1950

2. Brooksaler FS, Sulkin SE: Cat-scratch disease. *Postgrad Med* **36**:366, 1964

3. Warwick WJ: The cat-scratch syndrome, many diseases or one disease? *Prog Med Virol* **9**:256, 1967

4. Emmons RW et al: Continuing search for the etiology of cat-scratch disease. *J Clin Microbiol* **4**:112, 1976

5. Wear DJ et al: Cat-scratch disease: A bacterial infection. *Science* **221**:1403, 1983

6. Margileth AW et al: Cat-scratch disease: Bacteria in skin at the primary inoculation site. *JAMA* **252**:928, 1984

7. English CK et al: Cat-scratch disease: Isolation and culture of the bacterial agent. *JAMA* **259**:1347, 1988

8. Spaulding WB, Hennessy JN: Cat-scratch disease (a study of eighty-three cases). *Am J Med* **28**:504, 1960

9. Carithers HA et al: Cat-scratch disease (its natural history). *JAMA* **207**:312, 1969

10. Moriarty RA, Margileth AM: Cat-scratch disease. *Infect Dis Clin North Am* **1**:575, 1987

11. Margileth AM et al: Systemic cat scratch disease: Report of 23 patients with prolonged or recurrent severe bacterial infection. *J Infect Dis* **155**:390, 1987

12. Carithers HA, Margileth AM: Cat-scratch disease. Acute encephalopathy and other neurologic manifestations. *Am J Ophthalmol* **145**:98, 1991

13. Milam MW et al: Epithelioid angiomatosis secondary to disseminated cat scratch disease involving the bone marrow and skin in a patient with acquired immune deficiency syndrome: A case report. *Am J Med* **88**:180, 1990

14. Koehler JE et al: Cutaneous vascular lesions and disseminated cat-scratch disease in patients with the acquired immunodeficiency syndrome (AIDS) and AIDS-related complex. *Ann Intern Med* **109**:445, 1988

15. Kemper CA et al: Visceral bacillary epithelioid angiomatosis: Possible manifestations of disseminated cat scratch disease in the immunocompromised host: A report of two cases. *Am J Med* **89**:216, 1990

16. Relman DA et al: The agent of bacillary angiomatosis. An approach to the identification of uncultured pathogens. *N Engl J Med* **323**:1573, 1990

17. Slater LN et al: *Rochalimaea henselae* causes bacillary angiomatosis and peliosis hepatis. *Arch Intern Med* **152**:602, 1992

18. Carithers HA: Cat-scratch skin test antigen: Purification by heating. *Pediatrics* **60**:928, 1977

19. Shinall EA: Cat-scratch disease: A review of the literature. *Pediatr Dermatol* **7**:11, 1990

20. Margileth AM: Cat scratch disease and nontuberculous mycobacterial disease: Diagnostic usefulness of PPD-Battey, PPD-T and cat scratch skin test antigens. *Ann Allergy* **68**:149, 1992

21. Johnson WT, Helwig EB: Cat-scratch disease (histopathologic changes in the skin). *Arch Dermatol* **100**:148, 1969

22. Czarnetzki BM et al: Cat-scratch disease skin test (studies of specificity and histopathologic features). *Arch Dermatol* **111**:736, 1975

23. Pilon VA, Echols RM: Cat-scratch disease in a patient with AIDS. *Am J Clin Pathol* **92**:236, 1989

24. Conrad SE et al: Pseudoneoplastic infection of bone in acquired immunodeficiency syndrome. A case report involving the cat-scratch disease bacillus. *J Bone Joint Surg* **73**:774, 1991

25. Holley HP Jr: Successful treatment of cat-scratch disease with ciprofloxacin. *JAMA* **265**:1563, 1991

26. Margileth AM: Antiobiotic therapy for cat-scratch disease: Clinical study of therapeutic outcome in 268 patients and a review of the literature. *Pediatr Infect Dis J* **11**:474, 1992

CHAPTER 190

Morton N. Swartz and Arnold N. Weinberg

Miscellaneous Bacterial Infections with Cutaneous Manifestations

This chapter encompasses a group of "exotic" diseases rarely seen in urban practice in the United States. The thread of continuity that can be woven among this miscellaneous group involves epidemiologic considerations. If the occupation and travel history, the possibility of animal exposure, and the duration of the incubation periods are considered, the diagnosis can often be made expeditiously. Many of the illnesses described in this chapter, e.g., anthrax and rat-bite fever, are systemic infections having a major cutaneous component that helps to suggest the proper diagnosis.

Diseases Related to Intimate Contact with Animals, Fish, Fowl, or Their Products

Anthrax

The most common form of infection with *Bacillus anthracis* is an acute cutaneous lesion called "malignant pustule."[1] Anthrax is primarily a disease of domestic and wild animals, but humans become accidentally involved through exposure to animals and their products.

Bacteriology and Pathogenic Aspects BACTERIOLOGY. *Bacillus anthracis* is a large, aerobic, gram-positive, square-ended rod that forms spores in the external environment and on culture but not in tissues. Growth occurs readily on blood agar medium without a hemolytic reaction. This characteristic, plus pathogenicity for mice and lack of motility, helps to distinguish this organism from saprophytic *Bacillus* species.

PATHOGENIC ASPECTS. *B. anthracis* has two principal virulence factors. The first is a D-glutamyl polypeptide capsule, the synthesis of which depends on the presence of a specific plasmid.[2] The second is a pair of toxins, designated *edema toxin* and *lethal toxin*. Each of the toxins consists of a pair of noncovalently linked protein components[3]: edema toxin consists of edema factor (EF) plus protective antigen (PA), the structural gene of the latter being carried on a second virulence-associated plasmid; lethal toxin consists of lethal factor (LF) plus protective antigen. Of the three proteins involved in the two toxins, one (PA) serves as the binding unit for entry of its partner into the cell by receptor-mediated endocytosis. As yet, a catalytic function is known for the toxic moiety of only one of the two toxins. EF possesses adenylate cyclase activity which, on entry into cells, is activated by cellular calmodulin, and this results in conversion of ATP to cAMP.[4] The subsequent supraphysiologic cellular levels of cAMP mediate the toxic consequences of edema toxin. Cutaneous infection usually follows introduction of spores at the site of an abrasion. Following germination, the encapsulated organisms resist phagocytosis and elaborate their toxins. Edema toxin is responsible for the characteristic gelatinous edema of the local lesion. Lethal toxin itself kills several species of experimental animals and is presumed to be the principal cause of shock and death in anthrax.

Pasteur showed in 1881 that *B. anthracis* grown at elevated temperatures were attenuated and capable of inducing immunity in animals upon subsequent challenge with virulent strains of the organism. Such vaccine strains, avirulent by virtue of their inability to produce toxins, were shown over 100 years later to have become attenuated by virtue of temperature-induced elimination of the plasmid-encoding toxin genes.[2] However, the important protective immunogen is the anthrax toxin, because vaccination with anthrax strains containing only the plasmid for capsule production, but lacking the one for toxin production, is not protective. Pasteur's vaccine was effective presumably because his attenuation procedure resulted in cultures with a relatively increased proportion of cells containing only the capsule plasmid and a *relatively decreased* proportion containing both plasmids.[5]

Epidemiology Natural infection occurs in many domestic and wild animals. Highly resistant spores persist for many years in products of these animals and in pastures where they live. Vaccination and animal control programs have essentially eliminated reservoirs of infection in the United States, but imported animal products from the Middle and Near East, Africa, India, and South America introduce spores into a selected industrial environment. Worldwide there are estimated to be from 20,000 up to 100,000 cases of human anthrax annually. Outbreaks still occur in endemic areas. In 1979 to 1980, over 6000 cases of anthrax (90 percent involving the cutaneous form, the remainder representing equally pulmonary and gastrointestinal forms) occurred in Zimbabwe.[6] Direct cutaneous contact with carcasses of infected cattle was the major means of infection; but transmission by biting flies, which had earlier fed on carcasses of animals that had died of anthrax, was also likely. Infection in the United States is almost entirely limited to persons working in animal product–associated industries, particularly individuals handling raw materials in wool factories. However, transient exposure to infected animal products (e.g., hair) from abroad through ostensibly unrelated occupations (such as one-time air-conditioning duct repairs in a wool-sorting plant) has been incriminated in acquisition of anthrax. Shaving brushes, imported bongo drums, and piano keys (ivory) have been implicated in sporadic infections in persons not related to the above industries. In recent years, as regulations to safeguard employees in these plants have been strictly enforced, cases have become extremely rare. Most often infection occurs on an exposed part (face, neck, or arms) in an area of previous scratch or abrasion, as the organisms cannot penetrate the intact epidermis. In addition to direct inoculation through abrasions, inhalation of spores may rarely result in sinus or pulmonary infection ("woolsorter's disease"). Ingestion of spores may rarely be followed by intestinal anthrax.

Clinical Manifestations HISTORY. The patient almost invariably is employed in an animal product industry, usually handling wool, goat and other animal hair, hides, bones, etc. The initial symptoms, following a 1- to 3-day incubation period, are usually low-grade fever and malaise. A painless papular lesion is usually noted on an exposed area. Itching or burning may accompany the early lesion; progressive edema, discoloration, and enlargement then occur. The initial symptoms of inhalation anthrax are insidious, with fever, fatigue, and malaise, progressing to chills, high fever, nonproductive cough, dyspnea, cyanosis, and collapse. Chest radiograph characteristically shows symmetrical mediastinal widening. In this form of the disease, as well as in septicemic anthrax (following cutaneous anthrax), meningitis may develop and dominate the clinical picture.[7] Gastrointestinal anthrax is rare in humans and, thus far, has never been reported in the United States. The disease follows ingestion of poorly cooked meat from infected animals. Although vegetative bacteria are killed by acid gastric juice, the anthrax spores are resistant and germinate in the small intestine. Clinical features consist of nausea, vomiting, abdominal pain, fever, diarrhea (sometimes bloody), dehydration, hypotension, ileus, peritoneal signs, and hemorrhagic ascites. Mortality is in the 25 to 50 percent range.[6] An uncommon but related form (oropharyngeal) of anthrax also results from ingestion of raw or undercooked meat from infected animals. Clinical features include fever, sore throat, dysphagia, ulcerative tonsillitis or tonsils (or base of tongue) covered with pseudomembrane, and cervical lymphadenopathy.[8]

CUTANEOUS LESION.   The cutaneous lesion (''malignant pustule'') is the classic primary infection in anthrax, occurring in greater than 95 percent of cases. It is most often located on an exposed area of the head, neck (Fig. 190-1), or upper extremity, beginning as a pimple or papule. The lesion enlarges and develops into a vesicle or bulla with surrounding brawny, gelatinous, nonpitting edema. During its evolution, the vesicle becomes hemorrhagic and then necrotic and may be surrounded by small satellite vesicles. The area of nonpitting edema increases, an eschar forms, and the red discoloration becomes more intense, *but without pain*. Rarely, the area of necrosis extends over most of the edematous region, or edema may be present without any detectable primary lesion or necrosis. Regional lymph nodes may be slightly enlarged and tender, but there is no lymphangitis.

OTHER PHYSICAL FINDINGS.   Systemic manifestations (high fever, tachycardia, hypotension) may accompany either extensive cutaneous involvement or dissemination from a skin site. In woolsorter's disease, tachypnea, stridor, and cyanosis may be prominent. A thick, gelatinous, hemorrhagic nasal discharge may accompany acute sinusitis due to *B. anthracis*.

Laboratory Findings   The white blood cell count is usually elevated, with a preponderance of polymorphonuclear leukocytes. If meningitis is present, the cerebrospinal fluid is characteristically hemorrhagic and gram-positive bacilli may be seen.

Pathology   The prominent features are hemorrhagic edema, dilatation of lymphatics, and necrosis of the epidermis in the area of the eschar. Bacteria may be seen in the area of cellulitis.

Diagnosis and Differential Diagnosis   The diagnosis is usually suspected on the basis of the character of the lesion and the occupational history. Demonstration of large gram-positive rods in vesicle fluid or upon aspiration beneath the eschar supports the diagnosis. Definitive diagnosis requires culture of the organism and demonstration of its susceptibility to specific bacteriophage lysis. Identification of organisms in smears of exudate or in tissue specimens is possible utilizing a direct fluorescent antibody technique. Occasionally, the organism can be isolated from the blood during the acute cutaneous illness as well as in disseminated anthrax. Retrospective serodiagnosis is possible with the demonstration of a titer rise in an indirect microhemagglutination test. Recently, electrophoretic-immunotransblots for detection of antibody to PA and enzyme-linked immunosorbent assay (ELISA) for detection of anticapsule antibodies have been shown to be helpful in the retrospective diagnosis of anthrax.

Acute staphylococcal cellulitis with a central pustular lesion or a carbuncle with necrotic eschar may be confused with early anthrax. Pyogenic staphylococcal lesions are usually very painful and tender, and the etiologic agent is usually present on Gram-stain examination.

Treatment   Parenteral crystalline penicillin G (2 million units every 6 h) is the treatment of choice. In one study, smears and cultures from vesicles or from the necrotic tissue beneath the eschar became negative within 6 h of initiation of penicillin therapy.[9] For systemic infection (inhalation, gastrointestinal, meningeal), higher doses of penicillin (2 million units every 2 h for the adult) are indicated.

Treatment of cutaneous anthrax should continue until the local edema has disappeared or the lesion has dried up, i.e., for 7 to 14 days. When the edema has almost completely resolved, penicillin therapy may be switched to the oral route to complete the treatment course. In the penicillin-allergic individual, tetracycline (1.0 to 2.0 g daily intravenously in the adult), erythromycin, or chloramphenicol are alternatives.

Incision and debridement of the cutaneous lesion should be avoided as this increases the opportunity for bacteremia. The disease does not appear to impart permanent immunity.

Two types of vaccine are available for immunization against anthrax.[5] The first vaccine is licensed for human use in the United States to protect workers in occupations that might expose them to *B. anthracis*. It is supplied by the Michigan Department of Public Health and is an aluminum hydroxide–adsorbed culture supernatant (consisting primarily of PA in a partially purified form) from a nonencapsulated, toxigenic strain. The second vaccine is for immunization of livestock against anthrax and consists of viable spores of

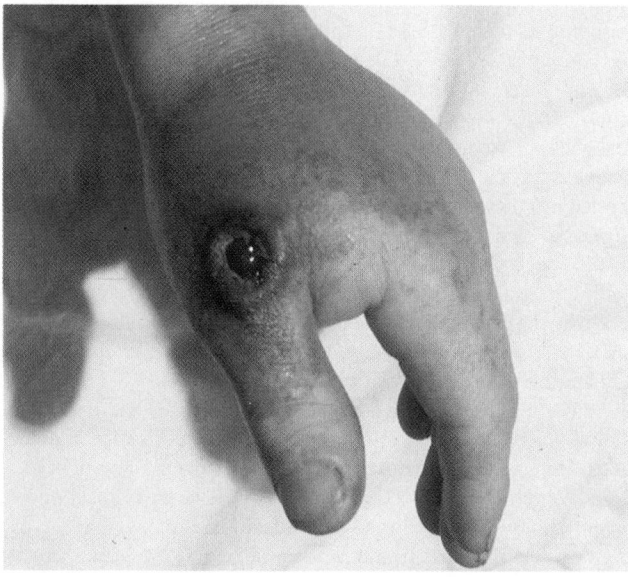

FIGURE 190-1   Anthrax. The classic cutaneous lesion of a primary infection in anthrax is a papule that evolves into a hemorrhagic bulla with surrounding brawny nonpitting edema. Note typical localization on the hand. (*Courtesy of K. Wolff, M.D.*)

an attenuated nonencapsulated, toxigenic strain. Prior to the advent of antibiotics, anthrax was treated with hyperimmune horse serum. This antitoxin preparation is no longer commercially available in the United States.

Course and Prognosis Rapid defervescence and clinical improvement follow the institution of appropriate antibiotic therapy. In pulmonary, intestinal, septicemic, and meningeal anthrax the prognosis is exceedingly grave, especially if the disease is not recognized promptly.

Brucellosis

Brucellosis is an acute or chronic infection (due to any one of four species of the genus *Brucella*) transmitted to humans from contact with animals or animal products. Such infections may be acute with bacteremia, or chronic with a variety of symptoms and signs.

Bacteriology and Pathogenic Aspects BACTERIOLOGY. The brucellae are nonmotile, coccobacillary gram-negative rods that require enriched media and an atmosphere containing 8 to 10% CO_2 for optimal growth.

PATHOGENIC ASPECTS. Contact with infected animals or contaminated excretions allows organisms to enter through small skin abrasions. Another portal for these organisms is ingestion of contaminated unpasteurized milk or cheese. The organisms can multiply intracellularly in a variety of tissues and produce acute symptoms. They may persist within cells for prolonged periods, leading to chronic brucellosis. The effects of endotoxin as well as hypersensitivity to brucella antigens appear to contribute to the clinical manifestations.

Epidemiology Domestic animals are the reservoir of brucella; humans are infected primarily by direct contact with animal material or by ingestion of raw milk or unpasteurized cheese. The majority of patients (75 percent) are males employed as abattoir workers in the meat-packing industry, engaged in livestock raising, or are veterinarians.[10] In the past, most infections in the United States were due to *B. abortus* secondary to contact with infected cattle. More recently, 70 percent of blood culture isolates from meat-processing-plant employees with brucellosis have been *B. suis*.

Another important group of patients with brucella infection are travellers who have become infected in endemic areas (countries of the Mediterranean littoral, the Middle East, Mexico) through ingestion of unpasteurized cow's or goat's milk or cheese. Unpasteurized cheese sent from abroad to friends or relatives in the United States may also be a source of infection. In recent years a brucella species, *B. canis,* that produces abortion or prostatitis and epididymitis in dogs, has been recognized as a cause of infection in individuals (pet owners, veterinarians) in contact with infected canines.

Clinical Manifestations HISTORY. In the majority of cases, contact with animals or their products is an essential feature of the history. The incubation period is usually 1 to 3 weeks, followed either by an acute febrile illness with headache (sometimes with involvement of local areas such as liver, joints, or meninges), or an indolent disease with weakness, anorexia, and low-grade fever, which may persist for weeks or months. Brucella involvement of the spine in the form of vertebral body osteomyelitis is not infrequent. Rarer forms of infection include suppurative lymphadenitis and endocarditis.

CUTANEOUS LESIONS. There are no typical cutaneous lesions, although rashes have been reported in 1 to 9 percent of cases.[11] Erythematous, papular, urticarial, and vesicular lesions may appear during the course of the illness, and burning, itching, and desquamation have also been described following contact with infected animal products.[12] Rarely, subcutaneous abscesses or cutaneous sinus tracts may develop as a result of extension of suppuration from infected lymph nodes or sites of osteomyelitis, or following introduction of organisms through a skin abrasion. A severe hypersensitivity reaction to brucella antigen may occur among veterinarians and animal handlers exposed directly to infected material. This may be manifested by an acute febrile reaction and the appearance of discrete, elevated, red papules on the hands or arms that may progress to ulceration. Dramatic reactions of this type have occurred in veterinarians who have accidentally inoculated themselves with the attenuated strain of brucella used to immunize farm animals.[13]

OTHER PHYSICAL FINDINGS. Among the characteristic findings may be lymphadenopathy, hepatosplenomegaly, suppurative arthritis, and evidence of osteomyelitis or spondylitis.

Laboratory Findings The white blood cell count is usually normal or depressed, and anemia is frequently present. Blood cultures may be positive during the acute illness.

Pathology Lesions in the liver, spleen, and other organs frequently consist of small, noncaseating granulomas. Rarely, larger areas with caseation necrosis and calcification occur in infections due to *B. suis*.

Diagnosis and Differential Diagnosis The diagnosis of brucellosis is usually based upon epidemiologic information (animal contact), cultures (blood, bone marrow, organ granulomas), and *rising* serum agglutination titer. A titer of greater than 1:160 should raise the possibility of this disease and warrant repetition of the test 7 to 14 days later. The presence of a prozone phenomenon and the development of ''blocking antibody'' may occasionally require modifications in the performance of the agglutination test. The antibody response to brucella infection is initially that of IgM followed by IgG antibodies. The IgM response may last for many months up to several years, but the IgG antibodies decrease rapidly following antimicrobial therapy. In patients with chronic symptomatology, the presence of IgG antibodies indicates continuing or recrudescent active infection.[14] Recently, use of IgM and IgG ELISA has suggested that they are very sensitive methods for detecting antibody to *Brucella,* and that a secondary increase in IgG, but not IgM, ELISA occurs in patients undergoing clinical relapse.[15] Skin testing with brucella antigen may lead to falsely positive serologic values and should not be performed. Cross reactions with *Francisella tularensis* occur uncommonly, and vaccination within the year for cholera may stimulate a brucella agglutinin titer.

The differential diagnosis includes other acute bacterial infections such as salmonellosis, listeriosis, tuberculosis, and endocarditis. Hodgkin's disease may mimic many of the findings of brucellosis. Vertebral osteomyelitis may sometimes be the primary or sole manifestation of brucellosis. Occasionally, a prolonged low-grade form of this illness is mistakenly considered as a psychoneurosis.

Treatment For the adult, tetracycline 0.5 g orally, 4 times daily for 3 to 6 weeks, is given alone or combined with streptomycin (1 g intramuscularly every 12 or 24 h for the first 7 to 14 days of treatment). Doxycycline (200 mg orally daily) has been used (in place of tetracycline) effectively in combination with streptomycin.[16] A combination of oral doxycycline plus oral rifampin (900 mg daily) for 30 to 45 days has also been effective treatment.

Course and Prognosis   Early treatment results in rapid improvement. Brucellosis relapses in approximately 3 to 10 percent of treated patients. Chronicity, often in the form of osteomyelitis or joint infection, may lead to more permanent disability.

Erysipeloid

Erysipeloid is an acute infection of traumatized skin caused by a slender, gram-positive rod, *Erysipelothrix rhusiopathiae,* occurring in fishermen, butchers, and others, such as housewives, handling raw fish, poultry, and meat products.[17]

Bacteriology   *Erysipelothrix rhusiopathiae* is a thin, gram-positive, slightly curved bacillus that tends to form filaments in culture. Growth occurs best on media fortified with serum. The bacillus is microaerophilic and nonmotile and is hardy enough to survive drying, putrefaction of tissue, and saltwater or freshwater exposure. There are certain morphologic and cultural similarities between *E. rhusiopathiae* and *Listeria monocytogenes.*

Epidemiology   *Erysipelothrix rhusiopathiae* is the cause of a cutaneous and systemic infection of swine and is present also in the slime of saltwater fish, on crabs and other shellfish, or associated with poultry (especially turkeys), meats, and by-products such as hides and bones. Occurrence of the disease is limited almost exclusively to persons handling contaminated products. Most cases occur during summer months. Usually the organisms are inoculated through a break in the skin of the hands. There have been epidemics among crab fishermen ("crab dermatitis") and bone button makers. Human infection takes one of four clinical forms: (1) localized cutaneous infection (erysipeloid of Rosenbach); (2) diffuse cutaneous form, consisting of multiple serpiginous lesions with sharply defined borders; (3) subacute bacterial endocarditis; and (4) bacteremic form without endocarditis, usually in immunocompromised patients.[18] The disease does not seem to confer lasting immunity.

Clinical Manifestations   HISTORY. Usually the patient is employed in fishing or animal product industries. Initially, there is burning pain at a site of injury. The incubation period is 2 to 7 days. A violaceous, raised area appears and enlarges. Lymphangitis and regional lymphadenopathy occasionally occur. Constitutional symptoms include low-grade fever and malaise. Occasionally, an adjacent joint is involved. Rarely, bacteremia and even endocarditis may follow.[19]

    CUTANEOUS LESION. The distinctive lesion is usually on a finger or hand, is violet or purple-red in color, warm and tender, and has well-defined, raised margins (Fig. 190-2). As the process advances peripherally, the central region clears without desquamation or ulceration.[20] The lesion may enlarge considerably. Rarely, dissemination occurs with multiple lesions distant from the original site of injury. Brownish discoloration develops as the lesion resolves.[21]

    OTHER PHYSICAL FINDINGS. Arthritis may be associated with the local lesion, and, rarely, distant joints are involved. Bronchitis may follow inhalation of organisms. Conjunctivitis also occurs. Typical peripheral stigmata as well as cardiac findings of endocarditis or septicemia have been reported.[22,23]

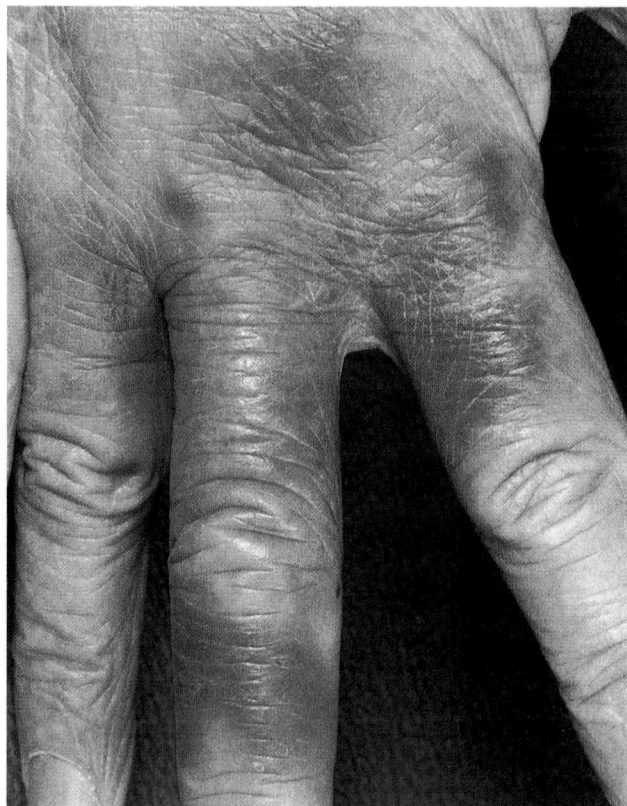

FIGURE 190-2   Erysipeloid. Characteristically, the violaceous sharply marginated lesion is composed of macules and plaques and is localized on the hand.

Laboratory Findings   There are no characteristic findings, and the organism is seldom seen on Gram stain of material from the surface of the lesion or from aspirated material. Culture of a biopsy from the advancing edge of the lesion may reveal the organism.

Pathology   Dilatation of vessels in the papillary and subpapillary areas, and perivascular cellular infiltrates deep in the dermis are present. The depth of the process may explain why organisms are rarely seen or cultured from the lesion.

Diagnosis and Differential Diagnosis   The character of the local lesion in a person handling fresh meat or fish products suggests the diagnosis. Other forms of bacterial cellulitis or erysipelas may be confused with erysipeloid. "Seal finger" may be mistaken for erysipeloid.

Treatment   Penicillin, in doses of 2 to 3 million units daily, orally or intramuscularly, for 7 to 10 days, is the treatment for erysipeloid. Erythromycin is an alternative for a penicillin-allergic patient. However, some strains are resistant to erythromycin. In vitro studies suggest that most strains are susceptible to imipenem and ciprofloxacin.[24] If arthritis, septicemia, or endocarditis is present, the dose of penicillin should be raised to 2 to 4 million units every 4 h, administered intravenously (for 4 weeks in the case of endocarditis). Vancomycin should not be used because most isolates are resistant.

Course and Prognosis   In the untreated patient, the lesion usually lasts for 2 to 3 weeks but may persist with cycles of improvement and worsening over several months. If penicillin is administered, the improvement is dramatic and recurrence is rare. In systemic infection, the course and prognosis depend on early and appropriate treatment.

Glanders

Glanders is an equine disease caused by the bacterium *Pseudomonas mallei*. This infection is rarely transmitted to humans. The clinical picture takes one of two forms: (1) an acute, febrile, disseminated, infectious process whose entire course may encompass only 10 to 30 days; (2) an indolent, relapsing, chronic infection, with multiple cutaneous and subcutaneous abscesses and draining sinuses. "Farcy," the name given to the disease in horses, refers to the nodular subcutaneous abscesses occurring along the course of lymphatics.

Bacteriology *Pseudomonas mallei* is an aerobic, nonmotile, gram-negative bacillus, with bipolar staining. It can be cultured on ordinary nutrient media. Antigenically and biochemically it is distinct from *Pseudomonas pseudomallei,* the cause of melioidosis.

Epidemiology Control measures have almost completely eradicated this previously common equine infection and essentially eliminated transmission to humans in the United States. Occasional cases still occur in Asia, Africa, and South America. Humans are infected by direct contact with horses. The organisms gain entry through abrasions in the skin, via the conjunctivae, or by inhalation or ingestion.

Clinical Manifestations HISTORY.   In the acute fulminating form, the incubation period is usually 2 to 5 days. The onset is abrupt, with headache, malaise, chills, high fever, nausea, and vomiting. In the chronic form of glanders, the onset of malaise, headache, muscle pains, arthralgias, and low-grade fever is gradual. After many weeks, typical cutaneous and subcutaneous nodules, abscesses, and draining sinuses develop.

CUTANEOUS LESIONS.   In acute glanders, a nodule or cellulitis appears at the site of inoculation. Local swelling and suppuration occur, and the lesion ulcerates. The ulcer is painful and has irregular edges with a gray-yellow base. Nodular sores rapidly develop along lymphatics draining the lesion; they become necrotic and ulcerated, and sinuses form. Regional lymphadenopathy is present. Widespread dissemination quickly follows, with multiple nodular necrotic abscesses in subcutaneous tissues and muscle. Lesions frequently coalesce into gangrenous areas. During this phase of bacteremic spread, a characteristic eruption appears, which may be generalized or localized to the face and neck. The lesions (papules, bullae, and pustules) appear in crops. Involvement of the nasal mucosa, either initially or by secondary spread, is prominent. Mucopurulent, bloody nasal discharge is commonly noted. Infection may spread to the paranasal sinuses, pharynx, and lung.

In chronic glanders, cutaneous and subcutaneous nodules appear on the extremities and occasionally on the face. The lesions ulcerate, and draining sinuses develop. Repeated cycles of healing and breakdown of nodules may continue for weeks or months. Finally, conversion to the acute form of the disease can occur.

OTHER PHYSICAL FINDINGS.   Bacteremic spread of infection may produce pneumonia, empyema, meningitis, septic arthritis, or osteomyelitis. Splenomegaly and hepatomegaly are sometimes present in both acute and chronic glanders. Pulmonary infiltrates and pneumonia occur, particularly after accidental (laboratory) inhalation.

Laboratory Findings A normal leukocyte count is usual, but a mild leukocytosis or leukopenia may occur.

Pathology In acute glanders, the pathologic picture is that of a suppurative, necrotic process, containing numerous intracellular and extracellular bacteria. In the chronic form of glanders, a granulomatous process (with few giant cells) suggesting tuberculosis is usually observed.

Diagnosis and Differential Diagnosis The diagnosis is made on the basis of the epidemiologic background, examination of Gram-stained smears of pus, isolation of the organism from abscesses or blood, and serologic tests. Acute glanders may resemble miliary tuberculosis or typhoid fever during the initial stages. The multiple subcutaneous abscesses suggest staphylococcal or mycotic infections or melioidosis. Lymphatic nodularity resembles the lesions of sporotrichosis.

Treatment Experience with modern chemotherapy is limited. Sulfonamides (sulfadiazine 100 mg/kg daily in divided doses) have been used successfully, particularly in laboratory-acquired (pulmonary) infections. A combination of intramuscular streptomycin with tetracycline has recently been recommended. Patients should be isolated.

Course and Prognosis Without antibiotic therapy, acute glanders has a mortality rate of over 90 percent. Chronic glanders has a better prognosis, especially since the advent of chemotherapy.

Streptobacillus moniliformis Infection ("Rat-Bite Fever")

Rat-bite fever is an acute infection that is usually acquired from rodents and is characterized by fever, polyarthralgias or arthritis, and a rash.[25]

Bacteriology *Streptobacillus moniliformis* is a gram-negative, pleomorphic bacillus. Growth in culture occurs as chains of bacilli and filamentous forms, interspersed with swollen bodies that look like *Candida* (*Monilia*), hence the name *moniliformis*. In blood cultures these microaerophilic organisms typically grow as small "puff balls" after prolonged incubation. On occasion, this organism may grow as an L form on initial culture.

Epidemiology *Streptobacillus moniliformis* is found in the nasopharynx of approximately 50 percent of wild and laboratory rats. In recent years, the latter have been an increasing source of infection. Sporadic cases without contact with rats have been reported. Infection may also occur following ingestion of contaminated food. One such milk-borne outbreak occurred in Haverhill, Massachusetts, in 1926, and this illness was designated "Haverhill fever" (erythema arthriticum epidemicum).[26]

Clinical Manifestations HISTORY.   The incubation period averages 1 to 5 days. The rat bite has often healed by the time the illness begins suddenly with fever, chills, headache, and myalgias.

CUTANEOUS LESIONS.   An erythematous macular or papular rash may develop within 2 to 3 days of the onset of symptoms. It is most marked on the extremities (often involving palms and soles), particularly about joints, but may become generalized, resembling measles. Sometimes the lesions are petechial.

OTHER PHYSICAL FINDINGS.   Within a week of onset arthritis can develop, involving larger joints such as the knee. This occurs in about half the patients and takes the form of either an asymmetric polyarthritis, resembling rheumatoid arthritis,[27] or a septic arthritis.[28] Regional lymphadenopathy may be present.

Laboratory Findings   Polymorphonuclear leukocytosis is common. *S. moniliformis* can usually be isolated from blood or joint fluid or sometimes from an abscess developing at the bite site. Serologic diagnosis involves use of agglutination, fluorescent antibody, or complement fixation tests.

Diagnosis and Differential Diagnosis   The skin lesions are not specific. The diagnosis should be suspected in any febrile patient with a history of a recent rat bite. Blood cultures are the best way to establish the diagnosis. The other form of rat-bite fever (*Spirillum minus*) (sodoku) may cause a similar illness, but several features are helpful in distinguishing between the two conditions[25]:

1. *Streptobacillus moniliformis* infection has a shorter incubation period (usually less than 10 days).
2. The bite site has usually healed by the time of onset of fever in *S. moniliformis* infection.
3. The incidence of arthritis is low in *S. minus* infection.

The differential diagnosis should also include meningococcemia, gonococcemia, viral exanthems, and Rocky Mountain spotted fever.

Treatment   Penicillin, 600,000 units intramuscularly every 6 h for 10 to 12 days, is the drug of choice. Tetracycline or streptomycin are alternatives in the penicillin-allergic patient.

Course and Prognosis   Untreated, the disease may last from a few days to several weeks. Rarely, it is complicated by endocarditis. Penicillin produces a prompt clinical response.

Diseases Associated Primarily with a Specific Geographic Distribution

Bartonellosis (Carrión's Disease)

Bartonella bacilliformis produces a disease exhibiting two characteristic stages: (1) a severe acute febrile illness with hemolytic anemia, known as Oroya fever; (2) a benign, nodular, cutaneous eruption, referred to as verruga peruana or Peruvian warts.[29]

Bacteriology and Pathogenic Aspects   BACTERIOLOGY.   Both phases of the disease are caused by the flagellated motile, gram-negative coccobacillus *B. bacilliformis*. This organism grows on media containing 10 percent fresh rabbit serum and hemoglobin. Growth characteristically is slow (8 to 10 days) and optimal at 25 to 27°C.

PATHOGENIC ASPECTS.   Organisms are introduced into a susceptible individual by a bite from an infected sand fly. They subsequently are found in the cells of the reticuloendothelial system and attached to red blood cells, causing them to become fragile, and leading to the profound anemia of Oroya fever.[30] Cutaneous lesions represent late bacterial invasion of the blood vessels of the dermis, resulting in proliferating vascular nodules. *B. bacilliformis* produces one or more substances capable of stimulating human endothelial cells to proliferate in vitro and to release tissue plasminogen activator, both properties characteristic of angiogenesis factors.[31] *B. bacilliformis* extracts are also able to stimulate angiogenesis in an in vivo rat model.

Epidemiology   The distribution of *B. bacilliformis* is confined to the valley regions of the Andes Mountains in South America, particularly in Colombia, Ecuador, and Peru. Humans are the only natural host, though monkeys and other animals have been experimentally infected. In an endemic area, 10 to 15 percent of patients with verruga are chronic carriers of the infection and have positive blood cultures, thus serving as a reservoir for transmission. Also, in an endemic area, over 60 percent of asymptomatic individuals have been exposed to *B. bacilliformis* and carry circulating antibodies. The nocturnal sand fly (*Lutzomyia verrucarum*) is the vector; its natural habitat is coextensive with the distribution of the disease (750 to 2800 meters elevation) in arid river valleys of the Andes.

Clinical Manifestations   HISTORY.   Characteristically, the patient lives in or has visited the endemic area but may have no recollection of having been bitten by sand flies. Since the incubation period is 19 to 30 days, there is ample time for visitors to return to distant parts of the world before the onset of symptoms. Oroya fever is characterized by intermittent fever, myalgias, malaise, headache, gastrointestinal irritability, and, finally, symptoms due to increasingly severe hemolytic anemia. During convalescence from Oroya fever, numerous discrete nodules may appear on the extremities, without recurrence of fever, malaise, or anemia. Occasionally, the cutaneous eruption occurs alone or precedes the systemic illness, and this is not accompanied by constitutional symptoms.

CUTANEOUS LESIONS.   Oroya fever is not accompanied by skin lesions. The cutaneous lesions of the second stage of the disease (verruga peruana) usually appear during convalescence from Oroya fever. The incubation period is 30 to 60 days. The most common eruption consists of miliary lesions (erythematous macules and papules) on the face and extensor surfaces of the extremities (Fig. 190-3). The lesions bleed readily and may ulcerate. The eruption heals without scarring. Involvement of the conjunctivae and nose and throat may occur. The other type of lesions are round, soft, hemangiomatous, subcutaneous nodules that may reach 1 to 2 cm in size. Sessile or pedunculated lesions also occur. They tend to occur in crops, are located on the extremities, spare the trunk, and may ulcerate and bleed.

OTHER PHYSICAL FINDINGS.   Oroya fever is accompanied by marked pallor, mild icterus, and splenomegaly.

Laboratory Findings   A profound (macrocytic) hemolytic anemia, with a reticulocytosis of up to 50 percent and erythroblasts and normoblasts in the peripheral blood, is not unusual.[32] On Giemsa-stained blood smears, numerous *B. bacilliformis* can be seen on or in red blood cells, and as many as 95 percent of cells may be parasitized. With the onset of convalescence from Oroya fever, the *Bartonella* become less numerous and change from bacillary to coccoid forms. Bilirubinemia, predominantly of the unconjugated fraction, is present. Leukocytosis may occur but is usually due to a complicating infection.

Pathology   The skin nodules show capillary and endothelial cell proliferation resembling capillary hemangiomas. They appear neo-

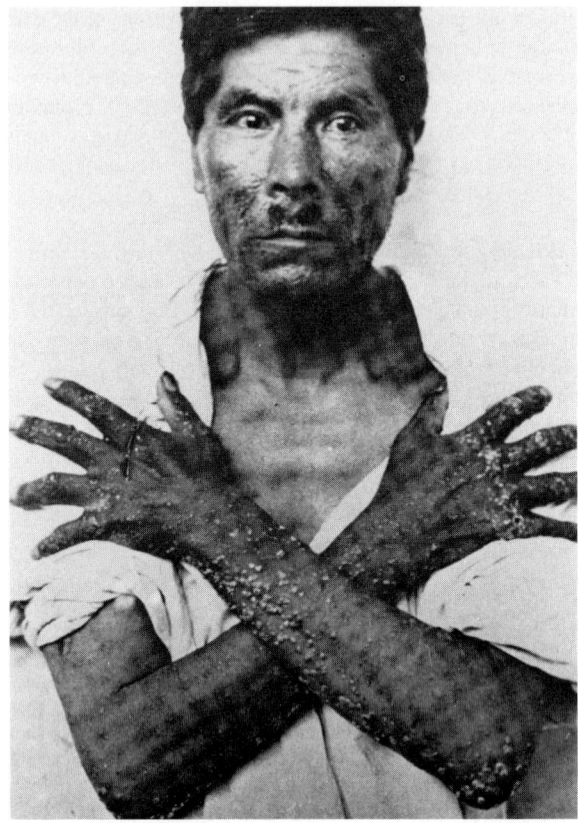

FIGURE 190-3 Bartonellosis (verruga peruana). Multiple small papules on the face and the extremities. The lesions may ulcerate. (*Courtesy of O. Canizares, M.D.*)

plastic, with many mitotic figures. Phagocytized *Bartonella* can be seen in endothelial and histiocytic cells of verrugas.[33]

Diagnosis and Differential Diagnosis The diagnosis depends primarily on an appropriate geographic history and on characterization of the etiologic agent. In Oroya fever, the organisms can be seen in red blood cells on stained smears, and blood cultures are almost always positive. In the cutaneous phase and even during convalescence, low-grade bacteremia may be present; also, organisms can be seen in and isolated from the nodular lesion.

Other rare forms of systemic (bacteremic) hemotrophic bacterial infections have been described.[34] The geographic confines of bartonellosis and the cultural characteristics of *B. bacilliformis* distinguish acute (Oroya fever) bartonellosis from these other hemotrophic infections; the distinctive skin lesions of verruga peruana are readily distinguished from the macules and petechiae that may be present in other hemotrophic bacterial infections.

Treatment Penicillin, streptomycin, tetracycline, and chloramphenicol have all been used successfully. Chloramphenicol (0.5 g orally every 4 to 6 h) is preferred if there is any suspicion of an accompanying *Salmonella* bacteremia (see Chap. 188). A therapeutic response is usually evident within 48 h. Control of sand flies with insecticides is the most important preventive measure.

Course and Prognosis The mortality rate of untreated Oroya fever is approximately 40 percent and is due to profound anemia and also to concurrent infections (malaria, amebiasis, tuberculosis, and sal-

monellosis). *Salmonella* septicemia has been reported in approximately 40 percent of affected individuals. The mechanism of this predisposition to secondary salmonella infection is unknown, but it may reflect a saturation of the reticuloendothelial system, with subsequent failure to clear these organisms.

In treated cases, the course is usually one of rapid improvement. The course and prognosis of the cutaneous syndrome are entirely favorable, in keeping with the concept that this represents a manifestation of developing immunity to the infection. Second attacks are extremely rare.

Melioidosis

Melioidosis is an infectious disease of animals and humans, endemic in Southeast Asia, but also occurring in Africa, South America, and the Middle East, between 20° north and south latitudes, and caused by the gram-negative bacillus *Pseudomonas pseudomallei*.[35] Apart from rare cases of laboratory-acquired infections, melioidosis has occurred in only those United States residents who have traveled abroad. During the war in Vietnam, extensive exposure to this organism resulted in cases of melioidosis (some fatal) among American servicemen. Melioidosis is very similar to glanders clinically and pathologically, but is entirely different epidemiologically. The clinical manifestations of this disease take one of two principal forms: (1) acute melioidosis with suppurative skin infection, pneumonia, or septicemia; (2) chronic melioidosis, the most common form of the disease, which involves the lung (unresolved pneumonia or cavitary lesions), skin (subcutaneous abscesses and draining sinuses), bones, joints, liver, spleen, etc.

Bacteriology The etiologic agent is a small, pleomorphic, gram-negative bacillus with bipolar staining that can be grown aerobically on common laboratory media.

Epidemiology The etiologic agent of melioidosis can be isolated widely from soil, vegetables, and water in the rice-growing areas of southeast Asia. Melioidosis appears to be transmitted by contamination of abraded skin with infected soil or water. The prominence of pulmonary findings in many patients, and of diarrhea in some, has suggested the possibility that it may be transmitted by inhalation or ingestion. Person-to-person transmission of melioidosis is rare.[36]

Clinical Manifestations HISTORY. The incubation period is variable. It has been as short as 3 days, and the disease has also remained latent for years. The acute pneumonic form may begin with a short prodrome (malaise, anorexia, and diarrhea), but more commonly its onset is abrupt, with chills, fever, cough, dyspnea, and chest pain. The acute septicemic form may start with an ulceration at the site of inoculation, lymphangitis, and regional lymphadenitis. In northeastern Thailand, septicemic melioidosis occurs mainly in the rainy season, primarily in rice farmers or their families. It accounts for about 20 percent of all cases of community-acquired septicemia in this region.[37] Principal predisposing factors include diabetes mellitus and renal failure but also corticosteroid therapy, leukemia, cirrhosis, and tuberculosis. In half the patients no source for the bacteremia can be identified on examination, but many have minor abrasions about the feet. Chronic melioidosis may follow the acute disease. More often it develops as an indolent pulmonary infection or as a low-grade febrile illness with multiple superficial abscesses. Recrudescence of a previous latent or clinical infection months or years (as long as 26 years) after initial exposure to the organism may be precipitated by various illnesses (e.g., thermal burns, diabetic ketoacidosis, pneumonia).[38] Recrudescent illness may take the form of localized infections such as splenic abscess, liver abscess, osteomyelitis, septic arthritis, renal abscess, subcutaneous abscesses, or lung abscess, as well as septicemia.[39] It may also take the form of persistent, unexplained fever.

CUTANEOUS LESIONS.   Cutaneous manifestations are not a specific or diagnostic feature of melioidosis. The acute septicemic form may complicate a superficial ulceration and cellulitis. Multiple superficial pustules may be present or, rarely, ecthyma gangrenosum. In chronic melioidosis, subcutaneous abscesses and draining sinuses (from bone or lymph nodes) are common features and may occur even in the absence of fever.

OTHER PHYSICAL FINDINGS.   In acute pulmonary melioidosis, the findings range from those of bronchitis to those of acute pneumonia or lung abscess. Septicemic spread of the disease leads to jaundice, hepatosplenomegaly, miliary pulmonary densities (secondary bacteremic pneumonia), myocarditis, and severe gastroenteritis. Chronic pulmonary melioidosis produces signs suggestive of fibrocavitary tuberculosis or lung abscess. The disseminated form of chronic disease may extend over many months with septic arthritis, osteomyelitis, suppurative lymphadenopathy, and visceral abscesses. In Thailand, acute suppurative parotitis constitutes 38 percent of cases of melioidosis in children.[40]

Laboratory Findings   The peripheral white blood cell count is usually normal or only moderately elevated.

Pathology   Sharply circumscribed abscesses are found in many organs and in the subcutaneous tissues. There may be a surrounding granulomatous response.

Diagnosis and Differential Diagnosis   The various forms of melioidosis and the multiplicity of organs involved characterize this disease as a great imitator. Acute melioidosis may mimic typhoid fever, staphylococcal pneumonia, mycotic infections, or septicemia. In its chronic form, it must be differentiated from pulmonary tuberculosis, nocardiosis, fungal infections, and lung abscess. Chronic skin infections and draining sinuses in individuals from endemic areas should raise the possibility of melioidosis.

The diagnosis is suspected on epidemiologic grounds and on the finding of bipolar-stained gram-negative bacilli in exudates or pus. Culture of the organism establishes the etiology. Hemagglutination, direct agglutination, and complement-fixation tests are helpful when a rise in titer is demonstrated. A positive serologic test, in the absence of a rising titer, may suggest the diagnosis but it is not definitive. The indirect hemagglutination assay (IHA) is most commonly used in southeast Asia because it is simple to perform and cheap. An IHA titer of $\geq 1:80$ is 80 to 90 percent sensitive and specific in the diagnosis of active melioidosis, but titers of $1:40$ to $1:160$ (or even above occasionally) are frequently found in healthy individuals in endemic areas.[39]

Treatment   Antibiotic susceptibility must be determined on each isolate because of variations from strain to strain. In the past, conventional treatment of melioidosis has involved tetracycline (or doxycycline), chloramphenicol, and trimethoprim-sulfamethoxazole (plus kanamycin occasionally) in combination. Due to the bacteriostatic nature of three of these drugs and due to the potentially serious toxicity of this polydrug regimen, other therapeutic programs have been sought. Most strains of *P. pseudomallei* are sus-

ceptible to some of the newer antibiotics in vitro: ceftazidime, piperacillin, imipenem, and amoxicillin-clavulanic acid. A recent multicenter clinical trial in Thailand, comparing mortality on conventional therapy with that on treatment with the combination of ceftazidime plus trimethoprim-sulfamethoxazole, significantly favored the latter, particularly in septicemic melioidosis.[41]

Surgical drainage of abscesses should be carried out, but only after initiation of appropriate antimicrobial therapy, in order to avoid a sudden septicemic episode.

Antimicrobial treatment should be continued for from 4 to 6 weeks to 4 to 6 months (the longer periods in the case of osteomyelitis or multiple suppurative foci), with initially the intravenous and then the oral route.

Course and Prognosis   The mortality rate in melioidosis depends on the clinical form of illness[41]: (1) in disseminated septicemic melioidosis (rapidly fatal bacteremia with shock and evidence of dissemination to skin and viscera), it is 87 percent; (2) in nondisseminated septicemic melioidosis (fairly rapidly progressive bacteremia with only single organ involvement), it is 17 percent; and (3) in localized melioidosis (nonbacteremic slowly progressive focal infection), it is 9 percent.

Plague

Plague is a severe, acute, febrile infection in humans caused by *Yersinia pestis*.[42] Transmission between the natural reservoir of this disease (wild and commensal rodents) and human beings is effected by fleas. Infection occurs in three forms: (1) bubonic plague; (2) bubonic-septicemic plague (a more acute and severe form of bubonic plague with bacteremia and delirium); (3) pneumonic plague (fulminant form of infection resulting from respiratory spread of *Y. pestis*).

Bacteriology   *Yersinia pestis* is an aerobic gram-negative bacillus with "safety-pin" bipolar staining. It produces an intracellular toxin (plague toxin) that is plasmid encoded and an important virulence factor.[43] Two other plasmids encode virulence factors. One plasmid mediates "the low calcium response," which occurs when *Y. pestis* is transferred from the lower temperature of the flea to the 37°C host whose intracellular (leukocytic) environment has a relatively low Ca^{2+} concentration, and which initiates selective synthesis of virulence factors.[44] The second plasmid encodes coagulase and fibrinolysin activities, which also serve as virulence factors.

Epidemiology   Endemic (sylvatic) plague is firmly established among wild rodents in the western United States. In this country, human plague is almost always fleaborne and is usually of the bubonic type. Between 1956 and 1983, 231 cases of plague were reported in the United States. Most occurred during the warmer months and were transmitted by flea bites. "Off-season" (October to February) plague occurs during rabbit-hunting season in the western states and is associated with direct contact (skinning, dressing) with animal (rabbits, bobcats) carcasses.[45] In recent years, epizootics have occurred among prairie dogs in the Southwest, and sporadic human cases have been identified on several Indian reservations.[46] The disease is also endemic in Vietnam and Africa (Tanzania, Zaire). Rarely, plague pneumonia secondary to bacteremia complicating bubonic plague may initiate respiratory spread to other persons.

Clinical Manifestations   HISTORY.   The incubation period is approximately 1 to 6 days, followed by the sudden onset of malaise, myalgias, backache, tachycardia, and high fever.

CUTANEOUS LESIONS.   In bubonic plague, the initial skin manifestation is related to the flea bite. Usually, this cannot be seen, but occasionally a small papule or vesicopustule persists. Painful, tender, enlarged lymph nodes are present in the area draining the bite site. The nodes become matted (buboes), and there is extensive surrounding subcutaneous gelatinous edema. Bacteremia may supervene and lead to overwhelming systemic illness.[47,48] In this setting petechiae and ecchymosis often occur due to the effects of plague toxin or to the development of a disseminated intravascular coagulopathy.

OTHER PHYSICAL FINDINGS.   The clinical manifestations (chills, fever, headache, nausea, vomiting, tachycardia, hypotension) of septicemic plague are similar to those of gram-negative bacillemia. Abdominal pain is a feature of almost half the cases.[49] The onset of pneumonic plague is abrupt, with high fever, tachycardia, and tachypnea. Signs of consolidation may appear, and within 24 h of onset the patient is critically ill, raising bloody sputum loaded with *Y. pestis*. Meningitis may complicate all three forms of plague.

Laboratory Findings   Leukocytosis occurs in all forms of the disease. In septicemic plague, bacilli can sometimes be seen on stained smears of venous blood (buffy coat).

Pathology   In the bubonic form, acute inflammatory changes are seen in the involved nodes.

Diagnosis and Differential Diagnosis   Bubonic plague should be distinguished from tularemia, lymphogranuloma venereum, cat-scratch disease, and suppurative lymphadenitis. Plague pneumonia must be differentiated from other acute bacterial pneumonias. Epidemiologic considerations and the tempo of the illness are major points in the differential diagnosis. Even minimal epidemiologic information provides sufficient grounds to begin treatment, for delays may be fatal in this rapidly progressive infection. The diagnosis is firmly established by examination of Gram-stained or specific fluorescent antibody–stained smears of infected material and by culture of the organism from blood, sputum, or aspirated buboes. Serologic methods can be used for retrospective diagnosis through demonstration of a fourfold of greater difference in titers between acute and convalescent sera. A convalescent passive hemagglutination titer of ≥1:16 is strongly suggestive of the diagnosis.

Treatment   Streptomycin is the drug of choice, administered intramuscularly (2 g daily in divided doses in the adult) for 10 days. Chloramphenicol or tetracycline are alternatives or may be added initially as strains resistant to streptomycin have been recovered. The dosage of chloramphenicol in the adult is 4 g daily for 2 days, followed by 3 g per day; that of tetracycline, 2.0 g daily intravenously for 1 week, then 1.5 g daily for a second week. Preliminary results suggest that gentamicin may be effective. Strict isolation of pneumonia cases is essential to prevent spread via the respiratory route. Buboes should not be drained until the lesion is well localized and the patient has been treated with antibiotics.

Course and Prognosis   Pneumonic and septicemic plague, if untreated, are almost invariably fatal. Untreated bubonic plague has a mortality rate of 30 to 70 percent. Early antibiotic therapy has reduced the mortality rate to 5 to 10 percent. Even the severest forms

of the infection respond to antibiotic treatment, if instituted promptly.

Diseases Associated with Random Animal Contact Independent of Geographic or Occupational Considerations

Francisella tularensis Infections (Tularemia)

Tularemia is a disease of humans caused by *Francisella tularensis,* an organism that normally resides in a wide range of animal species. In human beings, most cases follow direct animal contact or transmission by insect vectors. The clinical manifestations fall into six major patterns: (1) glandular, (2) ulceroglandular (most common form), (3) oculoglandular, (4) typhoidal, (5) pulmonary, and (6) oropharyngeal.[50]

Bacteriology   *Francisella tularensis* is a pleomorphic, gram-negative coccobacillus that grows best on cysteine blood agar or in thioglycollate heart infusion medium. Intracellular parasitism of the reticuloendothelial system of humans and experimental animals is characteristic.

Epidemiology   Infection in humans, particularly among hunters, most commonly follows contact with infected rabbits but may follow exposure to foxes, squirrels, skunks, and muskrats. Aquatic animals (voles, beavers) and mud and water from streams may also be a source of infection. The organisms are commonly introduced through a minimal abrasion or puncture wound. Bites of infected deerflies or ticks are also sources of infection in humans and are responsible for maintaining the disease in animals. Rarely, ingestion of meat or conjunctival contamination leads to infection.

Clinical Manifestations   HISTORY.   After an incubation period of 2 to 10 days, the onset of any of the four forms of disease is similar to that of most other acute infections: headache, malaise, myalgias, and high fever. A primary lesion then develops at the site of inoculation (usually on the hand), accompanied by regional adenopathy.

CUTANEOUS LESIONS.   In ulceroglandular tularemia, a reddish, tender papule appears at a site of trauma or insect bite, usually on a finger or hand. A small vesicular pustule may develop, and the area rapidly enlarges and becomes necrotic. The lesion then evolves to an ulcer with raised margins, often covered by a black eschar, and appears chancre-like (Fig. 190-4). Regional nodes are enlarged and tender. Systemic signs of toxicity may be marked and pneumonia may accompany dissemination of infection. A macular and papular or petechial exanthem on the trunk and extremities may occur in a minority of patients as the disease progresses. Erythema nodosum and erythema multiforme are occasional manifestations.

In oculoglandular tularemia, the organism is directly introduced via the conjunctivae. The findings are those of a purulent conjunctivitis with marked pain, edema, and congestion. Small yellow nodules may appear on the conjunctivae and ulcerate. Corneal perforation may occur. Preauricular and submaxillary adenopathy is prominent.

OTHER PHYSICAL FINDINGS.   Splenomegaly and generalized lymphadenopathy are relatively common, and hepatomegaly may occur. Elevated ALT and alkaline phosphatase levels occur in about 10 percent of patients. Ulcerative or exudative pharyngotonsillitis

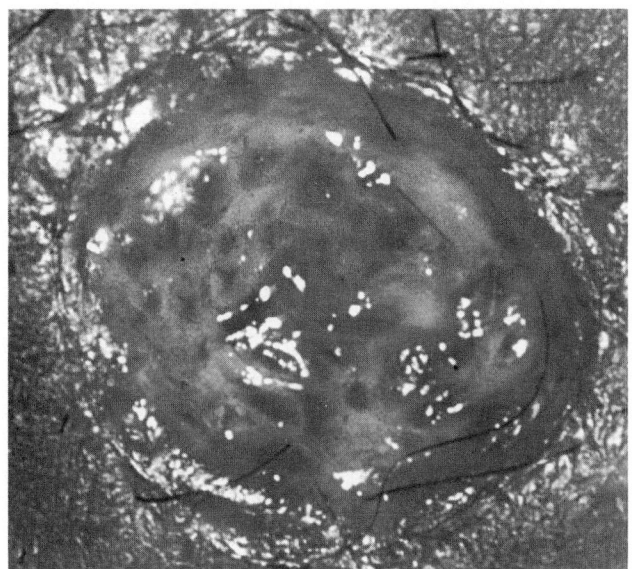

FIGURE 190-4 Tularemia. A chancre-like ulcer with raised margins on the back of the hand. There is axillary lymphadenopathy.

with cervical lymphadenopathy may follow ingestion of the organism, which may also be associated with the "typhoidal" form of the disease. Tularemic pneumonia may occur occasionally following inhalation of organisms but is more often secondary to bacteremia. Pleural effusion and mediastinal node enlargement are sometimes evident.

Laboratory Findings The white blood cell count is normal or low, but a polymorphonuclear leukocytosis may be seen. Blood cultures are only rarely positive.[51]

Pathology Following inoculation, the organism progresses through lymphatic channels and nodes to the bloodstream. The organism survives intracellularly in phagocytes, and small granulomatous lesions develop in lymph nodes, liver, and spleen. Some of the lesions may caseate or progress to frank abscess formation.

Diagnosis and Differential Diagnosis The primary lesion resembles a furuncle, paronychia, ecthyma, or the initial lesion of anthrax, *Pasteurella multocida* infection, or sporotrichosis. The prominent regional adenopathy suggests cat-scratch disease, plague, melioidosis or glanders, or lymphogranuloma venereum. Epidemiologic factors and systemic manifestations are points that suggest tularemia rather than other causes of a chancre-like lesion. A febrile illness occurring after a tick bite might suggest Rocky Mountain spotted fever, but an exanthem is usually present in that condition. The skin lesion of Lyme disease, erythema chronicum migrans, is a larger distinctive lesion that occurs after a tick bite in circumscribed geographic regions (see Chap. 193). A febrile illness with hepatomegaly and granulomas (on liver biopsy) resembles tuberculosis, brucellosis, or other causes of granulomatous hepatitis. Isolation of *F. tularensis* from ulcer, blood, or bone marrow requires special (cysteine-containing) media and is difficult to accomplish. The diagnosis is usually made by serologic (agglutination or microagglutination) tests showing a fourfold or greater rise in titer. Cross reactions occur in brucellosis. A skin test (delayed hypersensitivity), utilizing antigens from *F. tularensis,* becomes

positive during the first week of disease and may be helpful in diagnosis.[52] Unfortunately, the skin test reagent is not commercially available.

Treatment Streptomycin (1.0 to 2.0 g intramuscularly per day, in adults) is curative in all forms of tularemia if administered early. Clinical improvement is evident within 24 to 48 h, but treatment should be continued for at least 7 to 10 afebrile days. Tetracycline and chloramphenicol are alternative drugs, but clinical relapses are more frequent with these drugs, particularly if given for less than 14 days. Gentamicin has been used successfully in a small number of cases. Lymph node drainage should be avoided until late in therapy.

Course and Prognosis Untreated, the course may be weeks. Prior to the use of antibiotics, the mortality rate was about 5 percent in ulceroglandular disease and about 30 percent in typhoidal and pulmonary forms. Recovery provides immunity to systemic tularemia, but reinfection may produce a recurrent primary ulcer.

Leptospirosis

Leptospirosis is an acute febrile illness caused by any one of the serovarieties (serovars) of the species *Leptospira interrogans.* Although specific serovars have been reported with specific syndromes (canicola fever, Weil's disease, pretibial fever), any serovar may be responsible for a variety of clinical pictures, and a given clinical picture may be produced by many different serovars.[53]

Bacteriology These organisms are spirochetes that can be cultured on special (Fletcher semisolid) media. More than 170 antigenically different types have been described. They are now defined as serovarieties of the species *Leptospira interrogans.* Thus, for example, a specific antigenic serotype would bear a designation such as *L. interrogans* serovar *canicola.* The most common serovars in the United States are *canicola, icterohaemorrhagiae, pomona, autumnalis,* and *grippotyphosa.*

Epidemiology The reservoir of leptospira is in the animal population: farm animals (cattle, swine); domestic animals (dogs); wild animals (squirrels, rats). Infection in humans occurs as a result of direct contact with an animal (either a sick animal or an asymptomatic urinary "shedder"), or indirectly through contaminated water or soil. Organisms usually enter the body through a break in the skin or less often, through the mouth of conjunctiva. The disease is most prevalent among children (from playing in contaminated puddles or ponds), farmers, hunters, or abattoir workers.

Clinical Manifestations HISTORY. The incubation period is usually between 7 and 14 days, and the illness typically has a biphasic course. The onset is sudden, with headache, fever, chills, nausea, vomiting, abdominal pain, and myalgias. This initial nonspecific phase continues for about a week, when defervescence occurs. The patient is then relatively asymptomatic for several days. The second phase of illness begins with low-grade fever and often with meningeal symptoms and persists for another 2 to 4 days or even for several weeks. In the initial phase (leptospiremic), leptospiral organisms are present in the bloodstream, CSF, and other tissues. The second ("immune") phase coincides with the appearance of IgM antibodies. Clinically it is characterized by the onset of meningitis, rash, uveitis, and, in more severe cases, by hepatic and renal involvement.

CUTANEOUS LESIONS.   Scleral conjunctival injection appears on the third or fourth day of illness. Skin lesions, usually on the trunk (consisting of macules, papules, urticaria, and petechiae), occur in less than half the cases. Peripheral desquamation and infarction of portions of the hands and feet have been observed in a few children with leptospirosis.[54] Weil's disease, often but not exclusively due to serovar *icterohaemorrhagiae,* is a form of the disease with prominent hepatic (jaundice) and renal (hematuria, azotemia) involvement. Hemorrhagic manifestations occur in a variety of organs, including the skin. Pretibial ("Fort Bragg") fever is a form of leptospirosis (serovar *autumnalis*) that has a rather distinctive rash occurring on the fourth or fifth day of illness and consisting of slightly raised, 1- to 5-cm, tender, erythematous lesions on the pretibial areas.[55] The rash subsides within 4 or 7 days. Erythema nodosum has occurred in association with infection due to *L. interrogans.*[56]

OTHER PHYSICAL FINDINGS.   These depend on the particular syndrome that is presented.

1. Pyrexia of unknown origin—localizing signs lacking
2. Aseptic meningitis—nuchal rigidity
3. Weil's disease—jaundice and hepatomegaly; interstitial nephritis; generalized hemorrhagic tendency with epistaxis, hematuria, and gastrointestinal bleeding
4. Pretibial fever—splenomegaly is common

In up to 20 percent of patients with leptospirosis, generalized lymphadenopathy (particularly involving cervical nodes) may be observed. Pulmonary involvement with cough and radiologically demonstrable infiltrates occurs rarely.[57]

In children, acalculous cholecystitis has been observed occasionally as a manifestation of leptospirosis. Rarely, myocarditis is a feature of leptospirosis.

Laboratory Findings   The white blood cell count varies from a leukopenia to a mild leukocytosis. In Weil's disease, white blood cell count may reach levels of 40,000 per cubic millimeter. A cerebrospinal fluid pleocytosis, with up to several hundred mononuclear cells, may be present. Abnormalities of liver function are common, even in patients lacking overt jaundice. Azotemia and hematuria occur in patients with renal involvement, and jaundice is usually present in these.

Diagnosis and Differential Diagnosis   Skin manifestations are not specific but may suggest leptospirosis in the context of jaundice and aseptic meningitis. Conjunctival suffusion may be a helpful clue. The differential diagnosis includes viral hepatitis, all the causes of a lymphocytic meningitis, nephritis, and the causes of a fever of unknown origin. The diagnosis is established most commonly by serologic means: a fourfold or greater rise in microagglutination titer (to ≥1:100), an indirect hemagglutination test, or an IgM-specific dot-ELISA. It can also be confirmed by isolation of the organism from blood during the first 10 days of illness. In a series of cases of leptospirosis among military personnel in Panama, leptospires were isolated from blood cultures of 23 of 29 patients studied.[58]

Treatment   In the past, studies of the effectiveness of antibiotics (tetracyclines, penicillin) in the treatment of leptospirosis have been inconclusive. But in a controlled trial in anicteric leptospirosis, doxycycline therapy has proved effective, when administered early, in reducing the duration of illness and in preventing leptospiruria.[58] Doxycycline, administered orally on a once weekly basis, has been used successfully by the military as a prophylactic measure for short-term exposure in a hyperendemic area.[59]

Course and Prognosis   Recovery is the rule in anicteric cases. In the presence of jaundice, the mortality rate may be as high as 40 percent.

Pasteurella multocida Infections

Infections produced by *Pasteurella multocida* follow one of several patterns: (1) local skin infection with adenitis following animal bites (the most common form of infection); (2) septic arthritis and osteomyelitis following an animal bite (usually of the hand); (3) respiratory tract infections or colonization; (4) systemic infections such as meningitis, bacteremia, spontaneous bacterial peritonitis.[60]

Bacteriology   *Pasteurella multocida* is a small, ovoid, gram-negative rod. Its prominent bipolar staining may, from time to time, mistakenly suggest *Neisseria* or *Haemophilus influenzae.* It grows readily on nutrient blood agar, but not on MacConkey agar, and can be identified by biochemical tests and agglutination reactions.

Epidemiology   Although this organism is primarily a pathogen among animals, causing "hemorrhagic septicemia," it occasionally infects humans. *P. multocida* can be isolated from the upper respiratory tract of healthy cats, dogs, rats, and mice. Animal exposure has occurred in 70 to 80 percent of patients with *P. multocida* bacteremia, and predisposing conditions (alcoholic cirrhosis, neoplastic disease, chronic obstructive pulmonary disease) can be identified in over 75 percent.[61]

Clinical Manifestations   HISTORY.   Local pain and swelling occur within a few days of a cat or dog bite. There is little if any fever.

CUTANEOUS LESIONS.   Redness, swelling, ulceration, and a small amount of seropurulent drainage develop at the bite site. Cellulitis may progress rapidly and extensively, with associated lymphangitis. Local necrosis and abscess formation may follow.

OTHER PHYSICAL FINDINGS.   Regional adenopathy may be present. Complicating osteomyelitis may occur as a result of the introduction of organisms beneath the periosteum by the animal bite.

Laboratory Findings   Mild leukocytosis is present. After several weeks, an x-ray of underlying bone may show osteomyelitis.

Pathology   This infection produces an acute pyogenic response.

Diagnosis and Differential Diagnosis   The diagnosis is suspected when a painful infection develops at the site of an animal bite. It must be distinguished from cat-scratch disease. Local ulceration and proximal lymphadenitis mimic ulceroglandular tularemia. The diagnosis is established by isolation of the organism.

Treatment   Most strains of *P. multocida* are susceptible to penicillin, the drug of choice. In patients with simple cellulitis, oral penicillin (penicillin VK at 500 to 750 mg orally four times daily for adults) or ampicillin, or amoxicillin-clavulanate may reasonably be used, but close follow-up is mandatory. Several human isolates have been reported recently to be penicillin-resistant by virtue of plasmid-mediated beta-lactamase production.[62] If the prior animal bite is suspected to have penetrated deeply close to periosteum, parenteral penicillin (e.g., 2 to 4 million units intramuscularly daily) should be administered until the local lesion is well healed, to avert possible osteomyelitis. *P. multocida* is also susceptible to third-generation cephalosporins. For the penicillin-allergic patient, tetracycline is a suitable alternative, but susceptibility testing must always be performed. Chloramphenicol or trimethoprin-sulfamethoxazole may be effective therapy for the rare patient unable to tolerate either penicillin or tetracycline. Ciprofloxacin has activity against *P. multocida* in vitro. Abscesses should be surgically drained.

Course and Prognosis   The infection responds to local measures and antibiotic therapy.

Uncommon Diseases in Which Animal Contacts or Geographic Factors May Occasionally Be Relevant

Listeria monocytogenes Infections (Listeriosis)

Infection with *Listeria monocytogenes* produces characteristic acute disease in infants (neonatal septicemia, meningitis, and septic granulomatosis) and in both healthy and immunosuppressed adults (septicemia, meningitis, vaginal infection, pneumonitis, and oculoglandular syndrome).[63]

Bacteriology   *Listeria monocytogenes* is a small, thin, gram-positive rod that often appears coccoid in infected tissues and body fluids. It may resemble a streptococcus or pneumococcus. On the other hand, its appearance mimics that of a diphtheroid, and this pathogen has occasionally been dismissed erroneously as a "contaminant." It is non-spore-forming, beta-hemolytic, and exhibits a characteristic tumbling motility when grown in broth at room temperature. This is the classic facultative intracellular bacteria against which host resistance is mediated by thymus-derived lymphocytes (and macrophages).

Epidemiology   *L. monocytogenes* is found in the feces of many wild animals and birds and in soil and vegetation. One to four percent of humans (this is probably a minimal figure as it is difficult to isolate the organism from stool) appear to be fecal carriers of the organism. Higher rates of carriage have been observed in family contacts of patients with listeriosis. For undetermined reasons, pregnant women may acquire self-limited or asymptomatic genital infections. The highest incidence of infections is in the perinatal period, suggesting that the fetus either becomes infected in utero or on passing through the birth canal. Many but not all adult cases occur on a background of altered cellular immunity (Hodgkin's disease, immunosuppression for organ transplantation, etc.) or cirrhosis. Transfusional iron overload may also be a predisposing factor for listeriosis. *L. monocytogenes* produces a protein in culture supernatants that mobilizes iron from transferrin.[64] Because growth of this organism is stimulated by excess iron and because administration of iron compounds reduces the lethal dose of *L. monocyto-*

genes in animal models of infection, it is likely that iron overload contributes to the pathogenicity of this organism in humans. Occasionally, veterinarians handling stillborn or ill newborn animals develop cutaneous infections.

Most cases in the United States occur in urban areas without obvious animal contact. The portal of infection for most cases is unknown, but introduction through the intestinal tract seems likely. Food-borne (unpasteurized or improperly pasteurized milk or cheese; coleslaw made from cabbage grown on a farm where sheep manure had been used as fertilizer) outbreaks have been described.[64,65]

Immunocompromised and pregnant patients (neonatal infection) are at particular risk.[65,66]

Clinical Manifestations   HISTORY. Neonatal listeriosis occurs in two clinical forms—early and late onset.[67] Early-onset neonatal listeriosis develops in infants infected in utero from mothers who were undergoing a bacteremic illness with nonspecific symptoms shortly before the onset of labor. The findings of early-onset infection are evident at birth or become apparent within the first several days of life. Widespread granulomas (placenta, liver, spleen, lung, etc.) are characteristic of the syndrome known as *granulomatosis infantiseptica*. Placental, posterior pharyngeal, and multiple small cutaneous granulomas may provide clues as to the specific diagnosis. Neonatal infection, which may be due to any of a variety of agents (*Listeria*, group B streptococci, *Herpes simplex,* etc.) would be suggested in an acutely ill, moribund infant who was meconium-stained at birth and who subsequently exhibited pustular, papular, or petechial skin lesions. Late-onset neonatal listeriosis usually occurs several weeks after a normal birth, presumably resulting from postpartum acquisition. Meningitis rather than sepsis is the clinical picture. Listeriosis in the adult may present as a nonspecific acute febrile illness in which the findings of acute or subacute meningitis may predominate. Diarrhea, associated with numerous *L. monocytogenes* in the stool and blood cultures, may predate the onset of meningeal symptoms and findings by several days. *L. monocytogenes* infection in adults is not accompanied by skin lesions. Veterinarians may develop an acute febrile illness with headache, malaise, and rash 2 to 3 days after handling infected bovine fetuses.

CUTANEOUS LESIONS. In neonatal septicemia and infant granulomatosis, the skin rash consists of generalized erythematous papular or petechial lesions that may become pustular but only rarely vesicular. Veterinarians may develop tender, red papular lesions on the hands and arms, some of which evolve into pustules. Characteristic gram-positive rods can be demonstrated in these skin lesions. Tender axillary adenopathy is frequently present. In oculoglandular infection, there is acute conjunctivitis with preauricular adenitis.

OTHER PHYSICAL FINDINGS. In infants, meconium staining of the skin, hepatosplenomegaly, and lethargy are commonly present. Acute meningitis is accompanied by typical signs in infants and adults.

Laboratory Findings   A significant monocytosis occurs only rarely. In adults with meningitis, the inflammatory reaction is usually a predominantly neutrophilic pleocytosis; in infants, the response in the cerebrospinal fluid is sometimes mononuclear.

Pathology   Skin lesions show focal necrosis and infiltration by polymorphonuclear leukocytes and monocytes about blood vessels. Abscesses are found in viscera and granuloma formation may also be evident.

Diagnosis and Differential Diagnosis Listeriosis should be suspected in any newborn with meconium-stained skin who exhibits intrauterine growth retardation, fails to thrive, or develops a papular skin eruption. Gram stain of meconium shows the characteristic gram-positive rods. The skin lesions, cerebrospinal fluid, or blood cultures reveal the etiologic agent.

The differential diagnosis includes other forms of in utero neonatal infection such as toxoplasmosis, cytomegalovirus infection, rubella, disseminated *Herpes simplex* infection, and a variety of disseminated bacterial infections. The latter include those due to group B streptococci, *Escherichia coli, Salmonella,* and *Pseudomonas.*

Treatment Penicillin (or ampicillin) is the antibiotic of choice, administered by the intravenous route in neonates in 2 or 3 divided doses. Care must be exercised in adjusting the dosage of penicillin in the newborn period to 50,000 to 250,000 units/kg per day; ampicillin is administered in a dosage of 100 to 200 mg/kg per day. In adults with meningitis or bacteremia, the dosage of penicillin G should be 12 to 24 million units intravenously daily (in divided doses every 2 to 4 h) and that of ampicillin should be 12 g intravenously (in divided doses every 3 to 4 h). Gentamicin acts synergistically with ampicillin in vitro and is sometimes used in combination with the latter in treatment of *L. monocytogenes* meningitis. In nonpregnant adults who are allergic to penicillin or ampicillin, trimethoprim-sulfamethoxazole is effective therapy. Other possible, but less favored, alternatives for treatment include tetracycline and erythromycin.

Course and Prognosis In neonatal septicemia and meningitis, morbidity and mortality are high (up to 50 percent). In adult infections, treatment is effective and recovery is the rule, unless the underlying disease prevents this.

Diphtheria

Diphtheria is an acute febrile illness involving primarily the pharynx and mucous membranes of the upper respiratory tract. The major manifestations of this disease are due to (1) local membranous obstruction of the airway, and (2) the effects of a potent cytotoxin on the myocardium and peripheral nervous system. The hallmark of the local lesion is a gray, leathery membrane. Rarely, the primary lesion may be located on the skin, or the infection may complicate a preexisting wound. This is characteristically seen in tropical areas.

Bacteriology The causative organism (*Corynebacterium diphtheriae*) is a gram-positive rod that exhibits metachromatic bipolar granules on staining with methylene blue. It grows well on ordinary media, but its presence may be obscured by other bacteria in the pharynx or on the cutaneous lesion. For this reason, it is necessary to use selective media such as Loeffler's or tellurite agar to inhibit other organisms.

Identification of toxigenic strains requires either an Elek plate (agar diffusion precipitin reaction) or demonstration of protection from dermonecrosis in guinea pigs by antitoxin neutralization of a suspension of the isolate of *Corynebacterium.*

Epidemiology Humans are the only natural host for *C. diphtheriae.* The organism is carried in the pharynx of asymptomatic individuals. Infection occurs when a nonimmune person is infected by a toxigenic strain of *C. diphtheriae;* epidemics occur when such a strain becomes widespread in a population of nonimmune individuals. Most commonly, the site of primary infection is the nasopharynx or pharynx.

Cutaneous diphtheria and wound diphtheria occur in tropical areas ("jungle sore") and in association with poor hygiene. There has been an increase in skin diphtheria in the United States in the Pacific northwest and in the south.[68] The contagiousness of cutaneous diphtheria may be greater than that of respiratory infection among school children.[69]

Diphtheria is primarily a disease of young children, and in the United States most cases occur among poor, crowded, unimmunized individuals. Because of the widespread use and protective effect of toxoid immunization, the disease is rare in this country. It should be stressed, however, that this protection does not prevent the development of the carrier state and subsequent spread of organisms to susceptible individuals. In the past two decades, increasing numbers of cases have occurred in unimmunized migrant farm worker families, in older alcoholics living in "skid row" situations, and among Native Americans in the western United States and Canada. Three outbreaks, involving a total of 1100 infections (40 percent due to toxigenic strains), occurred in Seattle between 1972 and 1982. They occurred almost exclusively in indigent alcoholics, and 86 percent of these infections were cutaneous.[70] Cutaneous infections were much more common in the winter and early spring.

In underdeveloped and overcrowded parts of the world, diphtheria remains an important health problem, with many carriers and susceptible individuals. The majority of cases of cutaneous and wound diphtheria occur in this setting and are associated with poor hygiene and skin trauma.

Clinical Manifestations HISTORY. Faucial diphtheria usually presents with pharyngitis and low-grade fever. Toxicity is out of proportion to the degree of fever and local findings. As the disease progresses, swelling and pain in the neck, symptoms of airway obstruction, or unilateral nasal discharge may develop. Cutaneous diphtheria occurs in the presence or absence of pharyngeal disease. However, 20 to 40 percent of patients with cutaneous diphtheria carry the identical strain of *C. diphtheriae* in their respiratory tract. The skin lesions are usually indolent but tender and on the extremities. Symptoms of cranial or peripheral neuritis or of myocarditis may complicate the course. The latter usually occurs 5 to 14 days after the onset of the illness, whereas the former may develop any time from 2 weeks to several months after the primary lesion. Myocarditis is extremely rare as a complication of cutaneous diphtheria. Neurologic symptoms such as blurred vision, diplopia, numbness of tongue, palatal paralysis, long-tract sensory and motor findings, and the Guillain-Barré syndrome have occurred in 3 to 5 percent of patients with ulcerated diphtheritic skin lesions.

CUTANEOUS LESIONS. There are basically three types of skin involvement[71]: (1) Wound diphtheria is a secondary infection of a preexisting wound, occurs in temperate as well as tropical climates, and may involve any part of the body. This type accounts for almost all cases of cutaneous diphtheria reported in the United States. Underlying (primary) skin lesions include those due to trauma (abrasions, lacerations, burns), chronic dermatitis (eczema, scabies, etc.), and various pyodermas. A latent period of up to 3 weeks transpires between initiation of the primary lesion and evidences of superimposed diphtheritic infection (pain, erythema, tenderness, exudate). The lesion is usually partially covered with a membrane;

a purulent exudate is present, and a zone of edema and erythema surrounds the area. In the Seattle outbreak, coinfection with *Streptococcus pyogenes* occurred in 73 percent of diphtheritic skin lesions.[70] (2) Primary cutaneous diphtheria begins acutely as a tender, pustular lesion, which then breaks down and enlarges to form an oval punched-out ulcer with a gray membrane at the base. (A similar appearance may be the result of secondary infection by *C. diphtheriae* of a primary lesion of streptococcal ecthyma.) Later the membrane becomes dark brown. This ulcer does not extend below the fascia, has edematous, rolled, bluish margins, is usually located on a lower extremity, and is most often seen in the tropics. (3) Superinfection of eczematized skin lesions by *C. diphtheriae* evokes a more superficial, membranous, tender, edematous reaction.

Skin lesions with the appearance of impetigo, ecthyma, infected insect bites, etc., have been described as yielding *C. diphtheriae* on culture.[68] Whether these represent true infections with *C. diphtheriae* or are the cutaneous equivalent of the respiratory carrier state is unclear.

OTHER PHYSICAL FINDINGS.   A membranous pharyngitis may accompany cutaneous diphtheria. Cranial or peripheral nerve palsies may be present.

Laboratory Findings   The organism can be isolated on appropriate media from the skin ulcer or pharyngeal membrane.

Pathology   There is nothing characteristic about the pathologic picture of the diphtheritic lesion. The membrane is composed of coagulation necrosis and inflammatory cells.

Diagnosis and Differential Diagnosis   A presumptive diagnosis is usually based on the findings of membranous pharyngitis in faucial diphtheria and of a shallow membrane-covered ulcer in cutaneous involvement. In methylene blue–stained smears of material from the edge of the membrane, the characteristic beaded metachromatically stained rods can be seen, but proof of the diagnosis must await culture results and demonstration of toxin production. However, the presence of a pharyngeal membrane, with or without typically appearing organisms, should be presumptive evidence of infection with *C. diphtheriae,* and treatment should be started immediately. Occasionally, membranous infectious mononucleosis can mimic the picture of faucial diphtheria or be complicated by diphtheria.

Tropical ulcers may be confused with diphtheritic skin lesions, but the former usually occur in malnourished individuals and penetrate below the fascia, involving muscle and tendons. Bacterial infections in ulcerated wounds and following trauma are usually purulent and without membrane formation. Cutaneous mycotic infections are frequently more proliferative, and their margins are irregular, without surrounding reactive edema. Nonpathogenic (nontoxigenic) diphtheroids may be present in open skin lesions as superficial contaminants. Impetigo-like lesions and nondistinctive secondary pyodermas should be cultured in any contacts of a patient with diphtheria because of the contagiousness of cutaneous diphtheria.

Treatment   In faucial diphtheria, treatment consists of both specific equine antitoxin and penicillin. Treatment is initiated on the basis of clinical suspicion without awaiting cultural confirmation, as toxin elaborated in the intervening period could lead to irreversible myocardial damage.

In ulcerative cutaneous diphtheria, bed rest is essential for healing. Antitoxin in doses of 20,000 to 40,000 units is given by the intravenous route after careful testing for horse serum hypersensitivity. Injection of antitoxin as well into the subcutaneous area around the ulcer and also the surface application of antitoxin on the lesion have been suggested. Penicillin (2 to 4 million units intramuscularly daily) or erythromycin (2.0 g orally daily) is administered for 7 to 10 days. A few inducible erythromycin- and clindamycin-resistant strains of *C. diphtheriae* have been isolated recently from the lesions of cutaneous diphtheria. The lesion should be debrided and kept clean once antitoxin and antibiotics have been administered.

Close contacts of a case of cutaneous diphtheria should be examined for any skin lesions (which should be cultured for *C. diphtheriae*); the pharynx should be cultured regardless of the presence of pharyngitis or a membrane. While awaiting results of cultures, prophylactic treatment of contacts with erythromycin (or penicillin) should be initiated. In addition, if the immunization status of close contacts is unclear or incomplete, they should receive proper immunization against diphtheria. For children (7 years of age and older) and adults, the adult formulation of the combined diphtheria-tetanus toxoid (Td) preparation should be used rather than the pediatric DPT vaccine, because the latter contains a higher concentration of diphtheria toxoid as well as a pertussis component (both of which produce a higher rate of systemic reactions in older children and adults).

Course and Prognosis   If treatment is begun early, the prognosis is excellent for full recovery. In untreated, unimmunized persons with cutaneous diphtheria, ulcers may persist for as long as 6 months. Neuritic symptoms and signs may occur as late as 5 months after the onset of illness. The neurologic defects are almost always completely reversible.

Infections due to *Vibrio* Species

Infections caused by *Vibrio* species produce several different clinical syndromes: (1) gastroenteritis (the most common), (2) wound (and ear) infections, (3) septicemia (either "primary" or secondary to a wound infection).[72]

Bacteriology and Pathogenic Aspects   BACTERIOLOGY.   Nine *Vibrio* species in addition to *Vibrio cholerae* have been associated with human disease. Four species are capable of producing wound infections: *V. parahaemolyticus, V. vulnificus, V. alginolyticus,* and *V. damsela.* Of these, *V. vulnificus* is capable of causing severe wound infections and a "primary septicemia" syndrome with a mortality rate of almost 50 percent. The *Vibrio* species grow in regular blood culture media and on blood agar; they are halophilic. Selective media such as thiosulfate-citrate-bile salts-sucrose (TCBS) are necessary to isolate the organisms from stool cultures.

PATHOGENIC ASPECTS.   Markers for pathogenicity have been described for some *Vibrio* species. Almost all *V. parahaemolyticus* strains associated with disease (diarrhea, wound infections) in humans produce a hemolysin (Kanagawa phenomenon). This organism also produces a toxin capable of causing intestinal fluid accumulation in suckling mice and, as well, is capable at times of invasiveness, producing a dysentery-like syndrome. *V. vulnificus* produces extracellular collagenolytic, proteolytic, and elastolytic activities that may be important in the tissue invasiveness of this pathogen. Among the *Vibrio* species, *V. vulnificus* exhibits a striking pathogenicity when introduced into animal models by either the gastrointestinal or parenteral routes.

Epidemiology   *V. parahaemolyticus* and *V. vulnificus* are commonly found in salt water and estuarine sediments, and in fish and shellfish. The former has been implicated in 24 percent of reported cases of food-borne gastroenteritis in Japan; it also has been involved in shellfish-associated outbreaks of gastroenteritis in the United States. *V. parahaemolyticus* is responsible for occasional wound infections incurred following lacerations from shellfish or in sea water.[73] Wound infections with *V. vulnificus* typically follow cuts of the hand acquired while cleaning crabs or shrimp, or from entry of the organism through a preexisting open skin lesion exposed to seawater. *V. vulnificus* infections are endemic along the coast of the Gulf of Mexico and, to a lesser extent, along the Atlantic and Pacific coasts, particularly in the summer when seawater temperatures exceed 20°C. Primary septicemia due to *V. vulnificus* is associated with the eating of raw oysters, and particularly in the setting of hepatic cirrhosis or hemochromatosis.

Clinical Manifestations   HISTORY.   Gastroenteritis is most commonly associated with *V. parahaemolyticus,* but wound infections and septicemia also occasionally occur. After an incubation period of 4 to 96 h, abdominal cramps, nausea, and vomiting occur in the majority of patients; chills and fever occur in about 25 percent of patients. *V. vulnificus* may occasionally cause a similar gastroenteritis. More typically it is responsible for a wound infection occurring several days after a laceration sustained in sea water or brackish inland lakes. Primary septicemia with *V. vulnificus* may follow 24 to 48 h after consumption of raw oysters. This is more likely to occur in individuals with underlying chronic diseases such as cirrhosis, diabetes, leukemia, renal failure, or conditions requiring corticosteroid therapy. Fever, chills, nausea, vomiting, abdominal pain, and diarrhea are frequent symptoms in patients with primary septicemia, suggesting an initial gastrointestinal site of infection.

CUTANEOUS LESION.   Traumatic wound infections due to *V. vulnificus* may consist of pustular lesions, lymphangitis and lymphadenitis, or cellulitis. These infections may be mild or develop into rapidly progressive, painful cellulitis with myositis, extensive skin necrosis, and gangrene requiring amputation. Secondary bacteremia may ensue. Occasionally, cellulitis develops spontaneously without antecedent overt skin trauma but following exposure to sea water.

Skin lesions, in the form of large hemorrhagic bullae on the extremities or trunk, develop commonly in the course of primary *V. vulnificus* septicemia.[74] These progress to necrotic ulcers and necrotizing fasciitis and can eventuate on the lower extremity in muscle necrosis in the anterior compartment.

OTHER PHYSICAL FINDINGS.   Systemic manifestations (high fever, tachycardia, hypotension) are common in *V. vulnificus* septicemia. One-third of patients are in shock on presentation or within the first 12 h of hospitalization.

Laboratory Findings   Although *V. parahaemolyticus* usually produces a watery diarrhea, occasional patients will have a dysentery-like syndrome with leukocytes and blood present in the stool. In *V. vulnificus* primary septicemia, leukopenia is more frequent than leukocytosis. Thrombocytopenia is common and may progress rapidly to disseminated intravascular coagulation. *V. parahaemolyticus, V. vulnificus,* and other *Vibrio* species can be grown on blood agar media and isolated from routine blood cultures. TCBS media is used for isolation of *Vibrio* species from stool.

Diagnosis and Differential Diagnosis   Infection with a pathogenic *Vibrio* species should be suspected when gastroenteritis occurs in the summer months when there is a history of recent ingestion of shellfish (particularly raw oysters or crabs) or exposure to sea water, especially along the Gulf Coast. The development of unexplained fever, shock, and bullous skin lesions in a patient with cirrhosis who has recently eaten raw oysters should alert the physician to the possible diagnosis of primary vibrio septicemia.

Differential diagnosis of the gastroenteritis syndrome includes other causes of watery diarrhea (*V. cholerae,* toxigenic *Escherichia coli*). Wound infections sustained in fresh water would suggest *Aeromonas hydrophila* rather than *Vibrio* species, which are more typically involved in infected wounds sustained in a salt-water environment. Bullous lesions occurring in a hypotensive febrile patient might suggest the diagnosis of bacteremic *Pseudomonas aeruginosa* infection or even clostridial myonecrosis. The latter would be suggested by the presence of crepitus in the involved area and the presence of typical gram-positive blunt-ended bacilli in the contents of the bullae. *Pseudomonas* bacteremia would be unlikely in a nonleukopenic nonhospitalized patient without a prior history of infection and antibiotic usage.

Treatment   *V. parahaemolyticus* gastroenteritis is usually a mild to moderately severe form of diarrheal disease that requires no treatment other than oral fluid replacement (e.g., glucose-electrolyte solution). Management of *V. vulnificus* septicemia involves the treatment of hypotension with fluid replacement and treatment of systemic infection with both tetracycline (or chloramphenicol) and an aminoglycoside. There is a role for antimicrobial therapy in infected traumatic wounds due to *V. vulnificus* (or other *Vibrio* species) in view of the potential invasiveness of these organisms. Debridement of necrotic lesions is indicated.

Course and Prognosis   *V. parahaemolyticus* gastroenteritis is a self-limited disease. In contrast, the mortality rate for *V. vulnificus* primary septicemia is 50 to 60 percent, about three times as high as the mortality for wound infections due to the same organism. In view of the mortality associated with septicemic *V. vulnificus* infection, patients with cirrhosis and hemochromatosis should be advised against consuming raw shellfish or exposure of preexisting wounds to contact with warm seawater.

Rhinoscleroma

Rhinoscleroma is a chronic granulomatous disease caused by *Klebsiella rhinoscleromatis* (see Chap. 188). The principal endemic foci are in Mexico and Central and South America, but cases have also been reported from central and eastern Europe, India, North Africa, and the United States. Most cases are found in areas with primitive living conditions, and it is mildly contagious. The granulomas involve the nasal mucosa but may spread to the larynx, trachea, and bronchi. The diagnostic marker for the disease is the Mikulicz cell (a large histiocyte containing cytoplasmic bacilli). The clinical lesions consist of nodules that are painless, waxy, and red, often with ulceration (see Fig. 188-7). Treatment with streptomycin or tetracycline is often quite successful after two to three months in all but the patients with extensive disease.

References

1.   Gold H: Anthrax: A report of 117 cases. *Arch Intern Med* **96**:387, 1955

2. Green BD et al: Demonstration of a capsule plasmid in *Bacillus anthracis. Infect Immun* **49**:291, 1985

3. Singh Y et al: Internalization and processing of *Bacillus anthracis* lethal toxin by toxin-sensitive and -resistant cells. *J Biol Chem* **264**:11099, 1989

4. Gordon VM et al: Adenylate cyclase toxins from *Bacillus anthracis* and *Bordetella pertussis. J Biol Chem* **264**:14792, 1989

5. Ivins BE et al: Immunization studies with attenuated strains of *Bacillus anthracis. Infect Immun* **52**:454, 1986

6. Knudson GB: Treatment of anthrax in man: History and current concepts. *Military Med* **151**:71, 1986

7. Haight TH: Anthrax meningitis—a review of literature and report of two cases with autopsies. *Am J Med Sci* **224**:57, 1952

8. Doğanay M et al: Primary throat anthrax. A report of six cases. *Scand J Infect Dis* **18**:415, 1986

9. Ronaghy HA et al: Penicillin therapy of human anthrax. *Curr Ther Res* **14**:721, 1972

10. Buchanan TM et al: Brucellosis in the United States, 1960–1972. *Medicine (Baltimore)* **53**:413, 1974

11. Young EJ: Human brucellosis. *Rev Infect Dis* **5**:821, 1983

12. Berger TG et al: Cutaneous lesions in brucellosis. *Arch Dermatol* **117**:40, 1981

13. Spink WW: The significance of bacterial hypersensitivity in human brucellosis: Studies of infection due to strain 19 *Brucella abortus. Ann Intern Med* **47**:861, 1957

14. Young EJ: Serologic diagnosis of human brucellosis: Analysis of 214 cases by agglutination tests and review of the literature. *Rev Infect Dis* **13**:359, 1991

15. Ariza J et al: Specific antibody profile in human brucellosis. *Clin Infect Dis* **14**:131, 1992

16. Hall WH: Modern chemotherapy for brucellosis in humans. *Rev Infect Dis* **12**:1060, 1990

17. Woodbine M: *Erysipelothrix rhusiopathiae* bacteriology and chemotherapy. *Bacteriol Rev* **14**:161, 1950

18. García-Restoy E et al: Bacteremia due to *Erysipelothrix rhusiopathiae* in immunocompromised hosts without endocarditis. *Rev Infect Dis* **13**:1252, 1991

19. Grieco MH, Sheldon C: *Erysipelothrix rhusiopathiae. Ann NY Acad Sci* **174**:523, 1970

20. Nelson E: Five hundred cases of erysipeloid. *Rocky Mountain Med J* **52**:40, 1955

21. Klauder JV et al: A distinctive and severe form of erysipeloid among fish handlers. *Arch Dermatol Syphilol* **14**:622, 1926

22. Park C et al: *Erysipelothrix* endocarditis with cutaneous lesion. *South Med J* **69**:1101, 1976

23. Simberkoff MS, Rahal J: Acute and subacute endocarditis due to *Erysipelothrix rhusiopathiae. Am J Med Sci* **266**:53, 1973

24. Venditti M: Antimicrobial susceptibilities of *Erysipelothrix rhusiopathiae. Antimicrob Agents Chemother* **34**:2038, 1990

25. Brown TMcP, Nunemaker JC: Rat-bite fever. A review of the American cases with re-evaluation of etiology. *Bull Johns Hopkins Hosp* **70**:201, 1942

26. Place EH, Sutton LE: Erythema arthriticum epidemicum (Haverhill fever). *Arch Intern Med* **54**:659, 1934

27. Holroyd KJ et al: *Streptobacillus moniliformis* polyarthritis mimicking rheumatoid arthritis: An urban case of rat bite fever. *Am J Med* **85**:711, 1988

28. Anderson D, Marrie TJ: Septic arthritis due to *Streptobacillus moniliformis. Arthritis Rheum* **30**:229, 1987

29. Peters D, Wigand R: Bartonellaceae. *Bacteriol Rev* **19**:150, 1955

30. Herrer A: Bartonellosis, in *Tropical Medicine,* 5th ed, edited by GW Hunter et al. Philadelphia, Saunders, 1976, p 256

31. Garcia FU et al: *Bartonella bacilliformis* stimulates endothelial cells in vitro and is angiogenic in vivo. *Am J Pathol* **136**:1125, 1990

32. Reynafarje C, Ramos J: The hemolytic anemia of human bartonellosis. *Blood* **17**:562, 1961

33. Recavarren S, Lumbreras H: Pathogenesis of the verruga of Carrion's disease. *Am J Pathol* **66**:461, 1972

34. Archer GL et al: Human infection from an unidentified erythrocyte-associated bacterium. *N Engl J Med* **301**:897, 1979

35. Gilbert DN et al: Potential medical problems in personnel returning from Vietnam. *Ann Intern Med* **68**:662, 1968

36. McCormick JB et al: Human-to-human transmission of *Pseudomonas pseudomallei. Ann Intern Med* **83**:512, 1975

37. Chaowogul W et al: Melioidosis: A major cause of community-acquired septicemia in northeastern Thailand. *J Infect Dis* **159**:890, 1989

38. Sanford JP, Moore WL Jr: Recrudescent melioidosis: A Southeastern Asian legacy. *Am Rev Respir Dis* **104**:452, 1971

39. Leelarasamee A, Bovornkitti S: Melioidosis: Review and update. *Rev Infect Dis* **11**:413, 1989

40. Dance DA et al: Acute suppurative parotitis caused by *Pseudomonas pseudomallei* in children. *J Infect Dis* **159**:654, 1989

41. Sookpranee M et al: Multicenter prospective randomized trial comparing ceftazidine plus co-trimoxazole with chloramphenicol plus doxycyline and co-trimoxazole for treatment of severe melioidosis. *Antimicrob Agents Chemother* **36**:158, 1992

42. Davis DHS et al: Plague, in *Diseases Transmitted from Animals to Man,* 6th ed, edited by WT Hubbert et al. Springfield, IL, Charles C Thomas, 1975, p 147

43. Portnoy DA et al: Characterization of common virulence plasmids in *Yersinia* species and their role in the expression of outer membrane proteins. *Infect Immun* **43**:108, 1984

44. Mehigh RJ et al: Expression of the low calcium response in *Yersinia pestis. Microbiol Pathogenesis* **6**:203, 1989

45. Centers for Disease Control: Winter plague—Colorado, Washington, Texas 1983–1984. *MMWR* **33**:145, 1984

46. Reed WB et al: Bubonic plague in Southwestern United States. *Medicine (Baltimore)* **49**:465, 1970

47. Mengis CL: Plague. *N Engl J Med* **267**:543, 1962

48. Cantey JR: Plague in Vietnam, clinical observations and treatment with kanamycin. *Arch Intern Med* **133**:280, 1974

49. Hull HF: Septicemic plague in New Mexico. *J Infect Dis* **155**:113, 1987

50. Markowitz LE et al: Tick-borne tularemia. An outbreak of lymphadenopathy in children. *JAMA* **254**:2922, 1985

51. Evans ME et al: Tularemia: A 30-year experience with 88 cases. *Medicine (Baltimore)* **64**:251, 1985

52. Buchanan TM et al: The tularemia skin test—325 skin tests in 210 persons: Serologic correlation and review of the literature. *Ann Intern Med* **74**:336, 1971

53. Heath CW Jr et al: Leptospirosis in the United States: Analysis of 483 cases in man, 1949–1961. *N Engl J Med* **273**:857, 915, 1965

54. Wong ML et al: Leptospirosis: A childhood disease. *J Pediatr* **90**:532, 1977

55. Daniels WB, Grennan HA: Pretibial fever. *JAMA* **122**:361, 1943

56. Derham RLJ: Leptospirosis as a cause of erythema nodosum. *Br Med J* **2**:403, 1976

57. Turner JS, Willcox PA: Respiratory failure in leptospirosis. *Q J Med* **72**:841, 1989

58. McClain JBL et al: Doxycycline therapy for leptospirosis. *Ann Intern Med* **100**:696, 1984

59. Takafuji ET et al: An efficacy trial of doxycycline chemoprophylaxis against leptospirosis. *N Engl J Med* **310**:497, 1984

60. Weber DJ et al: *Pasteurella multocida* infections. Report of 34 cases and review of the literature. *Medicine (Baltimore)* **63**:133, 1984

61. Raffi R et al: *Pasteurella multocida* bacteremia: Report of thirteen cases over twelve years and review of the literature. *Scand J Infect Dis* **19**:385, 1987

62. Rosenau A et al: Plasmid-mediated ROB-1 β-lactamase in *Pasteurella multocida* from a human specimen. *Antimicrob Agents Chemother* **35**:2419, 1991

63. Gray ML, Killinger AH: *Listeria monocytogenes* and *Listeria* infections. *Bacteriol Rev* **30**:309, 1966

64. Farber JM, Peterkin PI: *Listeria monocytogenes,* a food-borne pathogen. *Microbiol Rev* **55**:476, 1991

65. Schlech WF et al: Epidemic listeriosis—evidence for transmission by food. *N Engl J Med* **308**:203, 1983

66. Stamm AM et al: Listeriosis in renal transplant recipients: Report of an outbreak and review of 102 cases. *Rev Infect Dis* **4**:665, 1982

67. Gellin BC, Broome CV: Listeriosis. *JAMA* **261**:1313, 1989

68. Belsey MA et al: *Corynebacterium diphtheriae* skin infections in Alabama and Louisiana. A factor in the epidemiology of diphtheria. *N Engl J Med* **280**:135, 1969

69. Koopman JS, Campbell J: The role of cutaneous diphtheria infections in a diphtheria epidemic. *J Infect Dis* **131**:239, 1975

70. Harnish JP et al: Diphtheria among alcoholic urban adults. A decade of experience in Seattle. *Ann Intern Med* **111**:71, 1989

71. Flor-Henry P: Cutaneous diphtheria: Brief historical review and discussion of recent literature, with presentation of two cases. *Med Serv J Canada* **17**:823, 1961

72. Morris JG, Black RE: Medical Progress. Cholera and other vibrioses in the United States. *N Engl J Med* **312**:343, 1985

73. Bonner JR et al: Spectrum of *Vibrio* infections in a Gulf Coast community. *Ann Intern Med* **99**:464, 1983

74. Tacket CO et al: Clinical features and an epidemiologic study of *Vibrio vulnificus* infections. *J Infect Dis* **149**:558, 1984

Bibliography

Berman SJ et al: Sporadic anticteric leptospirosis in South Vietnam. *Ann Intern Med* **79**:167, 1973

Gantz NM et al: Listeriosis in immunosuppressed patients. *Am J Med* **58**:637, 1975

Howe C, Miller WR: Human glanders: Report of six cases. *Ann Intern Med* **26**:93, 1947

Kerdel-Vegas F: Rhinoscleroma, in *Clinical Tropical Dermatology,* edited by O Conizares. Oxford, Blackwell, 1975

Klontz KC et al: Syndromes of *Vibrio vulnificus* infections. Clinical and epidemiologic features in Florida cases, 1981–1987. *Ann Intern Med* **109**:318, 1988

Martone WJ, Kaufmann AF: Leptospirosis in humans in the United States, 1974–1978. *J Infect Dis* **140**:1020, 1979

Riddel GS: Cutaneous diphtheria: Epidemiological and dermatological aspects of 365 cases amongst British prisoners of war in the Far East. *J R Army Med Corps* **95**:64, 1950

Roughgarden JW: Antimicrobial therapy of rat-bite fever. A review. *Arch Intern Med* **116**:39, 1965

Schmid GP et al: Clinically mild tularemia associated with tick-borne *Francisella tularensis. J Infect Dis* **148**:63, 1983

Young LS et al: Tularemia epidemic: Vermont, 1968. *N Engl J Med* **280**:1253, 1969

CHAPTER 191

Gert Tappeiner and Klaus Wolff

Tuberculosis and Other Mycobacterial Infections

It has been estimated that the genus *Mycobacterium* probably causes more suffering for humans than all the other bacterial genera combined.[1] Improved hygiene, living standards, and chemotherapy have greatly reduced the prevalence of tuberculosis in North America and Europe, but infections due to mycobacteria are still very common in the developing countries. In addition, the so-called atypical mycobacteria are increasingly recognized as human pathogens and some of them are common causes of skin disease, particularly in regions with a warm climate. The immune and tissue responses of the host play a decisive role in determining the type and extent of disease produced by mycobacterial infection. This has been studied extensively in infections with *M. tuberculosis, M. bovis,* and *M. leprae* and, to a lesser degree, with *M. ulcerans.*

In contrast to the obligate mycobacterial pathogens, which require a live host, free-living facultatively pathogenic mycobacteria in the environment only rarely cause disease by person-to-person spread.[2] Infections caused by the latter depend primarily on the occurrence and distribution of the organisms in the environment and the opportunities for contact with individuals susceptible to infection.[3–5] Previous contact with the nonpathogenic, environmental flora may be of importance in determining the nature of the immune response to subsequently encountered pathogenic species.[6] This chapter will first discuss tuberculosis of the skin—a spectrum of skin conditions due to infection with the obligatory mycobacterial pathogens, *M. tuberculosis* and *M. bovis* (including the attenuated BCG organism). Subsequently we will deal with the mycobacterioses, diseases due to infection with mycobacteria previously

designated *atypical* or *MOTT* (mycobacteria other than tuberculosis). Mycobacterial infections in AIDS are discussed in Chap. 215, and *M. leprae* infections are discussed in Chap. 192.

Classification of Mycobacteria

Mycobacteria are acid-fast, weakly gram-positive, nonsporulating, and nonmotile rods. The family Mycobacteriaceae consists of only one genus, *Mycobacteria,* which includes the obligate human pathogens, *M. tuberculosis, M. africanum, M. bovis,* and *M. leprae* as well as a number of facultatively pathogenic and nonpathogenic species, the so-called atypical mycobacteria. In the 1950s, Runyon classified atypical mycobacteria[7] into a slow-growing and a fast-growing group and subdivided the former according to pigment-forming properties in culture: group I: *photochromogens,* capable of pigment formation upon exposure to light; group II: *scotochromogens,* capable of pigment production without light exposure; and group III, *nonchromogens.* Group IV includes all *rapid growers.*

Since that time much taxonomic work has been done[3,8,9] so that the genus *Mycobacteria* stands among the best classified of bacterial genera. By 1980, 41 species of mycobacteria were recognized.[10] The main distinction, between the slow-growers and the rapid-growers, seems to have occurred early in the development of the genus.[1]

TABLE 191-1
Classification of Mycobacteria

	Runyon group
Slow-growing mycobacteria	
Obligate human pathogens	
M. tuberculosis-bovis group including bacillus	
Calmette-Guérin (BCG)	
and *M. africanum*	
Facultative human pathogens	
M. kansasii	I
M. marinum	I
M. simiae	I
M. scrofulaceum	II
M. szulgai	II
M. avium-intracellulare complex	III
M. haemophilum	III
M. ulcerans	III
M. xenopi	III
Nonpathogens	
M. gordonae	II
M. flavescens	II
M. terrae complex	III
M. triviale	III
M. gastri	III
(others)	
Rapidly growing mycobacteria	IV
Facultative human pathogens	
M. fortuitum complex including	
M. fortuitum biovar. and	
M. chelonei biovar.	
Nonpathogens	
M. smegmatis	
M. phlei	
M. vaccae	
(others)	

Note: *M. leprae* is not included in this table.

For clinical purposes, the organisms may be further subdivided into obligate and facultative pathogens and nonpathogens; a classification scheme of the genus *Mycobacteria* is presented in Table 191-1. *M. leprae* has not been included as it has not been grown in culture and thus has not been available for biochemical testing. The listing of nonpathogens or animal pathogens is not exhaustive, and some of them may still emerge as facultative pathogens.

Tuberculosis of the Skin

Definition and Classification

Tuberculosis of the skin is caused by *M. tuberculosis, M. bovis,* and, under certain conditions, the bacillus Calmette-Guérin (BCG), an attenuated strain of *M. bovis*; the clinical manifestations comprise a considerable number of skin changes, usually subclassified into more or less distinct disease forms. Morphologic classification originated at a time when the pathogenesis of tuberculosis of the skin was not well understood, and the fact that clinically similar skin manifestations may originate in different ways and may vary in their histologic appearance was not appreciated. More recent classifications are based on the mode of infection or the immunologic state of the host but they also fail to satisfy completely. The classification used in this chapter distinguishes between exogenous in-

TABLE 191-2
Classification of Cutaneous Tuberculosis

Exogenous infection
    Primary inoculation tuberculosis (infection of the nonimmune host)
    Tuberculosis verrucosa cutis (infection of the immune host)
Endogenous spread
    Lupus vulgaris
    Scrofuloderma
    Metastatic tuberculous abscess (tuberculous gumma)
    Acute miliary tuberculosis
    Orificial tuberculosis
Tuberculosis due to BCG vaccination
Tuberculids
    Tuberculids
        Lichen scrofulosorum
        Papulonecrotic tuberculid
    Facultative tuberculids
        Nodular vasculitis
        Erythema nodosum
    Non-tuberculids*

*These conditions are not related to tuberculosis but for completeness are discussed in the text.

fection and endogenous spread of *M. tuberculosis/bovis,* conditions caused by vaccination with BCG, and a group of eruptions, the tuberculids, that are nosologically and pathogenically less well understood (Table 191-2). Some entities of a nontuberculous nature, which were previously thought to be related to tuberculosis and were thus also termed *tuberculids,* will be briefly mentioned at the end of this section.

Historical Aspects

Some forms of tuberculosis of the skin, especially lupus vulgaris, were described repeatedly in the seventeenth and eighteenth centuries, and the term *lupus* was used by some of the early authors. Bayle was the first to discover that tuberculosis was not confined to the lungs but could affect the entire body. However, even after Villemin had proved that tuberculosis was infectious, tuberculous skin diseases continued to be mistaken for other dermatoses. Although tuberculosis was successfully transmitted to experimental animals and its histopathologic characteristics were described in detail by Rokitansky and by Virchow, and although the great similarity of the histologic appearance of lupus vulgaris and tuberculosis of other organs was demonstrated by Friedlaender, no absolute proof of the cause of the tuberculous skin lesions was available. Koch's[11] discovery of the tubercle bacillus and the confirmation of its role in the cause of tuberculosis of the skin finally provided this evidence.

Epidemiology and Incidence

The worldwide incidence of infectious tuberculosis is estimated to be 15 to 20 million with the highest proportion in the developing countries.[12] Tuberculosis of the skin also has a worldwide distribution; although it has been more prevalent in regions with a cold and humid climate, it is now recognized in the tropics. Reports from southeast Asia and South Africa suggest that it is not uncommon in these regions.[13-17] In European and North American countries, the incidence of skin tuberculosis has shown a steady decline over the past decades. This seems to be true for all countries and parallels the decreasing incidence of pulmonary tuberculosis. In times of crisis, e.g., after the two world wars, certain forms of skin tuberculosis occur more frequently. Malnutrition and breakdown in normal living conditions may well explain this temporary resurgence. Lower socioeconomic status seems to be associated with a higher incidence of cutaneous tuberculosis, especially of lupus vulgaris, but urban or rural residence is not. An increase in mycobacterial infection has occurred with the advent of the AIDS epidemic.

In the United States, tuberculosis of the skin has always been a rare disease. In Europe, it used to be quite common during the first quarter of this century but it now represents less than 0.5 percent of all cases seen. In Germany, only 300 to 400 new cases are estimated to occur every year.[16] In India, 0.15 percent of all outpatients at one dermatology center were recently reported to suffer from it.[18] The two most frequent forms are lupus vulgaris and scrofuloderma, but there are considerable differences in the incidence in different geographic regions[19]; in the tropics, lupus vulgaris is rare whereas scrofuloderma and verrucous lesions predominate.[12]

Lupus vulgaris is more than twice as common in women as in men, but tuberculosis verrucosa cutis is most often found in males. Generalized miliary tuberculosis is seen in infants (and in adults with severe immunosuppression or AIDS) and so is primary inoculation tuberculosis; scrofuloderma usually occurs in adolescents and the elderly, but lupus vulgaris may affect all age groups.

Etiology and Pathogenesis

M. tuberculosis, M. bovis, and, under certain conditions, the attenuated BCG organism cause all forms of skin tuberculosis. After having gained access to the host's tissues, the mycobacteria multiply intracellularly. The invasion by *M. tuberculosis* is characterized by the appearance of polymorphonuclear leukocytes, by an influx of mononuclear cells, and by the later development of epithelioid cells and necrosis. Large numbers of mycobacteria are initially found in the tissue. The mere presence of mycobacteria in the skin, however, does not necessarily lead to clinical disease, and it should be remembered that infection with *M. tuberculosis* is not necessarily synonymous with tuberculosis.

The development of a certain type of skin tuberculosis seems to depend mainly on the properties of the causative organism, the general condition and reactivity of the host, and the mode of introduction of the bacteria into the skin.

The Mycobacterium Different mammalian species vary in their susceptibility to infection with different mycobacteria. In humans, *M. tuberculosis* and *M. bovis* cause identical skin manifestations. The incidence of skin tuberculosis elicited by these two organisms varies and is determined by the probability of exposure to either human or bovine tuberculosis. On the other hand, the virulence and number of the bacteria may be subject to considerable variation.

In 50 to 90 percent of the cases of lupus vulgaris, the bacteria exhibit a low virulence[20,21] that may approach that of the attenuated BCG organism. In many forms of skin tuberculosis, the number of bacteria in the lesions is so small that it may be difficult to find them in histologic sections, whereas in the primary chancre or in acute miliary tuberculosis, large numbers of bacteria can be demonstrated in the affected tissue.

The Host The human species is quite susceptible to tuberculous infections, but differences exist among populations and individu-

als. Populations whose contact with tuberculosis spans many centuries are, in general, less susceptible than populations that have come into contact with mycobacteria recently. The decline of tuberculosis has been ascribed, in part, to a gradually enlarging population partially immunized by natural infections with a variety of mycobacteria.[21] Heredity also plays a role, for the concordance of tuberculosis is higher in monozygotic twins than in dizygotes,[22] and individuals with HLA-B15 are more susceptible to the disease.[23] Age, state of health, and somatic type of the individual are of importance, as are environmental factors. In blacks, tuberculosis frequently takes an unfavorable course, and it has been claimed that in this race tuberculin sensitivity is more pronounced than in whites.[24]

After mycobacteria have invaded the host, they may either multiply and lead to progressive disease or their multiplication is checked or completely arrested. The balance between bacterial multiplication and destruction is determined not only by the properties of the invading organisms but also by the inherent or acquired power of the host to control such an infection. The skin of an individual previously infected with tuberculosis shows an altered response upon a second exposure to the organism. This changed reactivity was first demonstrated by Koch,[25] who showed that virulent mycobacteria injected subcutaneously into a previously infected guinea pig induce a massive inflammatory response and necrosis at the site of injection. An extract containing the specific protein of the mycobacteria (tuberculin) is able to elicit the same phenomenon. I Von Pirquet[26] interpreted the different and unduly severe reaction to the second infection as altered reaction capacity of an individual ("allergic") to a repeated stimulus. Subsequently, the tuberculin reaction became a standard clinical test in tuberculosis.

The tuberculin reaction is due to delayed-type hypersensitivity mediated by sensitized T lymphocytes that, when injected into a nonsensitized individual, transfer the hypersensitivity.[27,28] Patients with sarcoidosis, whose cell-mediated immunologic capacities are compromised, will transiently support local passive transfer with living cells.[29] Conversely, patients with hypogammaglobulinemia, in whom the immunologic mechanisms mediated by circulating immunoglobulins are impaired, show no reduction in their capacity to produce hypersensitivity to tuberculin.[30]

Sensitization is induced either by the living mycobacterium (e.g., during primary infection with tuberculosis) or, under experimental conditions, with killed bacteria or with bacteria suspended in Freund's adjuvant. The substance that elicited the hypersensitivity reaction in sensitized individuals was designated *tuberculin* by Robert Koch.[25] It was obtained originally from concentrated, heat-sterilized, and filtrated cultures of mycobacteria. This "old tuberculin" (OT) was widely used for skin testing, but has now been replaced by a purified derivative (purified protein derivative, PPD). This consists of the immunologically active tuberculoproteins from which some other constituents have been removed, and is preferable to OT as its potency and composition are more consistent.[31] But even the commercial standardized PPD-tuberculins available today are subject to some variation[32] and do not eliminate cross-reactions due to sensitization by other mycobacteria.[33] The different mycobacterial species contain not only antigens unique to themselves but also antigens shared by other mycobacteria.[34] The low specificity of PPD is also due to the procedures employed in the denaturation of the antigens, and the avoidance of protein denaturation has recently yielded a class of tuberculins that are much richer in species-specific antigens than PPDs[35]; they have been given the generic name *new tuberculins*.[36]

The tuberculin reaction of a sensitized individual varies with the test dose employed and the route of administration. Local intradermal injection (the method most widely used) leads to the local tuberculin reaction, which usually reaches maximal intensity after 48 h. It consists of a sharply circumscribed area of erythema and induration and, in highly hypersensitive recipients or after large doses, may lead to a pallid central necrosis. Histologically, the earliest changes consist of an accumulation of mononuclear cells that form prominent cuffs around small veins,[37,38] and in severe reactions the small venules are plugged with leukocytes, chiefly mononuclear cells, encased in a fibrinous coagulum.[39]

Tuberculin sensitivity usually develops 2 to 10 weeks after infection with *M. tuberculosis* and tends to persist throughout life. It may diminish with age or if the infection is treated in its earliest stages. Its intensity may be reduced by conditions that diminish delayed-hypersensitivity reactions, such as acute viral infections or vaccination with live virus; immunosuppression by drugs and corticosteroids, disease, and malnutritition; and malignant disease, particularly lymphoma. About 5 percent of individuals with tuberculosis who have none of these conditions still, for unknown reasons, do not react to ordinary intermediate strength doses of tuberculin.[32]

The state of sensitivity of an individual infected with *M. tuberculosis* is of considerable significance in the pathogenesis of tuberculous skin lesions. Obviously, a primary infection of the skin (tuberculous chancre) will result in clinical manifestations that are quite different from those occurring after inoculation of mycobacteria into the skin of a previously sensitized individual (tuberculosis verrucosa cutis). Similarly, the hematogenous spread of mycobacteria in individuals with low or greatly diminished sensitivity will evolve into a skin disease (miliary tuberculosis of the skin) that is unlike that occurring in persons in whom sensitivity is high (lupus vulgaris).

The relationship between hypersensitivity and immunity in tuberculous disease is not entirely clear. At various times hypersensitivity was held responsible for immunity, and it was formerly believed that the "allergic" reaction to mycobacteria played a part in the defense mechanisms of the body. Indeed, in animals inoculated with mycobacteria there is unrestricted bacterial multiplication before the onset of hypersensitivity; bacterial destruction begins at about the time when hypersensitivity develops and is practically complete when the state of hypersensitivity has reached its maximal levels.[27] In patients with clinical tuberculosis, an increase of skin sensitivity usually indicates a rather favorable prognosis, and in tuberculous skin disease with high levels of skin sensitivity, the number of bacteria within the lesions is small. However, tuberculin sensitivity is not necessary for immunity against *M. tuberculosis,* and sensitivity and immunity do not always parallel each other.[40] There is now sufficient evidence that they are dissociable and that a high degree of tuberculin sensitivity may even be antagonistic to protection.[4] Strains of mice that become only weakly sensitive to tuberculin are relatively resistant to *M. tuberculosis* injected intravenously but are susceptible to intradermal inoculation. The opposite occurs in animals that develop high levels of tuberculin hypersensitivity.[5] Mycobacterial infection thus seems to elicit at least two cell-mediated immune responses, both of which produce positive tuberculin tests but vary in their protective efficacy, depending on the site of infection: one is the result of macrophage activation and is protective, whereas the other is a necrotizing Koch-type reaction that is usually irrelevant or antagonistic to protection.[32] It is currently believed that delayed hypersensitivity and immunity are two separate processes involving separate T-lymphocyte populations and different mediators.[4]

Any disturbance of the balance between the state of immunity on the one hand and the degree of invasion and virulence of the bacteria on the other has its bearing on the course of the disease. As in tuberculosis of other organs, this is also true for tuberculosis of the skin. Infectious diseases, particularly measles and HIV infection, as well as diabetes, lymphomas, and the systemic administration of corticosteroids or cytostatic agents may upset this balance.

Route of Infection   The mode of introduction of mycobacteria into the skin and the properties of the tissue components affected are also essential pathogenic factors. The infection may be exogenous (i.e., from an outside source), it may occur by autoinoculation, or it may be endogenous. Exogenous infection will lead to the tuberculous chancre or to tuberculosis verrucosa cutis, depending on the immunologic state of the host. Lupus vulgaris at the site of BCG vaccination represents another example of exogenous infection, in this instance by attenuated mycobacteria (see below).

Endogenous spread of mycobacteria may occur by continuous extension of a tuberculous process underlying the skin (scrofuloderma), by way of the lymphatics (lupus vulgaris), or by hematogenous dissemination (acute miliary tuberculosis of the skin or lupus vulgaris).

Finally, the structure and vascular supply of the tissue invaded by mycobacteria also has to be taken into account. Lesions developing in the upper dermis assume a clinical appearance and course quite different from those developing in the subcutaneous tissues. Impairment of local blood supply may have an important additive effect, and local injury may act as a localizing factor.[41]

Histopathology   The hallmark of tuberculosis and infections with some of the slow-growing atypical mycobacteria is the tubercle. It consists of an accumulation of epithelioid histiocytes with Langhans' giant cells among them and a varying amount of caseation necrosis in the center. This is surrounded by a rim of lymphocytes and monocytes. While this tuberculoid granuloma is highly characteristic of several forms of tuberculosis, it is not pathognomonic. Deep fungal infections, syphilis, and leprosy, among other diseases, can produce an identical picture. As in leprosy,[42] the histopathology of skin tuberculosis may be reflective of the host's immune status.[18,42]

Tuberculosis of the Skin due to *M. Tuberculosis/Bovis* Infection

Primary Inoculation Tuberculosis (Tuberculous Chancre; Tuberculous Primary Complex)

Primary inoculation tuberculosis results from the inoculation of mycobacteria into the skin of a host not previously infected with tuberculosis. The tuberculous chancre and the affected regional lymph nodes constitute the tuberculous primary complex of the skin.

Incidence   In 1930 it was estimated to constitute 0.14 percent of all primary tuberculous lesions.[43] However, it may not be quite as rare as generally believed, for in 1953 Miller[44] observed some 30 cases within a 5-year period in the northeast part of England; in some regions, particularly in Asia where the incidence of tuberculosis is still high and where living conditions and hygiene are poor, primary inoculation tuberculosis of the skin is not unusual.

Most patients are children, but the lesions may also occur in adolescents and young adults,[45–47] particularly in people working in medical care.[48–50] All parts of the body may be affected, but sites of predilection are the face and lower extremities, which are readily injured. One-third of the lesions are found on the mucous membranes of the conjunctiva and oral cavity.[44]

Pathogenesis Because tubercle bacilli cannot penetrate intact skin,[51] they are introduced into the tissue at the site of minor abrasions or wounds. Organisms from the sputum of phthisic patients are transmitted to infants by kisses; they may gain entry from contaminated dust into the skin through lacerations or at the site of pyogenic infections. Primary inoculation tuberculosis used to be a common complication of ritual circumcision when performed by tuberculous rabbis,[47,52] and a rare "venereal" inoculation tuberculosis occurred in healthy individuals after sexual contact with patients suffering from genitourinary tuberculosis.[53,54] Lesions in the mouth may be due to bovine bacilli from nonpasteurized milk and occur after mucosal trauma or tooth extraction.[44] Primary inoculation tuberculosis following mouth-to-mouth resuscitation has been reported.[55]

From 2 to 4 weeks after inoculation the skin lesion appears. Infection spreads to the regional lymph nodes, producing tuberculous lymphadenitis, and with increasing acquired immunity the process is localized to the particular region involved.

Clinical Manifestations The tuberculous chancre initially presents as a small papule, scab, or wound with little tendency to heal. A painless ulcer develops that may be quite insignificant or may enlarge to attain a diameter of over 5 cm[56] (Fig. 191-1). It is shallow with a granular or hemorrhagic base studded with miliary abscesses or covered by necrotic membranous deposits. The ragged edges are undermined and of a reddish-blue hue; as the lesions grow older they become more indurated, with thick adherent crusts.

Lacerations inoculated with tubercle bacteria may heal temporarily but break down eventually, giving rise to granulating ulcers. Lesions on the conjunctiva are characterized by shallow ulcers or fungating granulations.[44] In the mouth, painless ulcers occur on the gingiva or the palate. Primary inoculation tuberculosis of the finger may present as painless paronychia.[50] Accidental inoculations of

mycobacteria by poorly sterilized needles have resulted in subcutaneous abscesses.[57,58]

Regional lymphadenopathy develops 3 to 8 weeks after the infection (Fig. 191-1) and may rarely be the only clinical symptom. The lymph nodes enlarge slowly and harden but are usually painless. After weeks or months, cold abscesses may develop that perforate to the surface of the skin, forming sinuses. The lymph nodes draining the primary glands may also be involved.

Body temperature may be slightly raised, and occasionally lymph node enlargement, abscess formation, and perforation may take a more acute course. Fever, pain, and inflammatory swelling of the surrounding tissues, simulating a pyogenic infection,[59] are present in half the cases.

Histopathology In the early phases there is a banal acute inflammatory reaction with necrosis and ulceration, and mycobacteria are easily detected. After 3 to 6 weeks the infiltrate and the regional lymph nodes acquire a tuberculoid appearance.

Diagnosis and Differential Diagnosis Lack of awareness of the condition is probably the most common reason for a diagnostic error. Any ulcer with little or no tendency to heal and unilateral regional lymphadenopathy in a child should always arouse suspicion. Acid-fast organisms can be demonstrated in histologic sections or in smears obtained from the primary ulcer and draining glands in the initial stages of the disease but may be difficult to find in older lesions. The diagnosis is verified by bacterial culture. The reaction to intradermal PPD is negative in the initial phases, but during the course of the disease it converts to positive. A previous tuberculous infection (such as a pulmonary Ghon focus) should be reasonably well excluded.

Primary inoculation tuberculosis has to be separated, both clinically and by laboratory procedures, from the primary complexes of syphilis, tularemia, cat-scratch fever, sporotrichosis, and from ulcerative lesions of other mycobacterioses as well as from other forms of skin tuberculosis.

Course Without treatment, the condition may last up to 12 months. Skin and mucous membrane lesions heal by scarring, but in rare cases lupus vulgaris develops at the site of a healed tubercu-

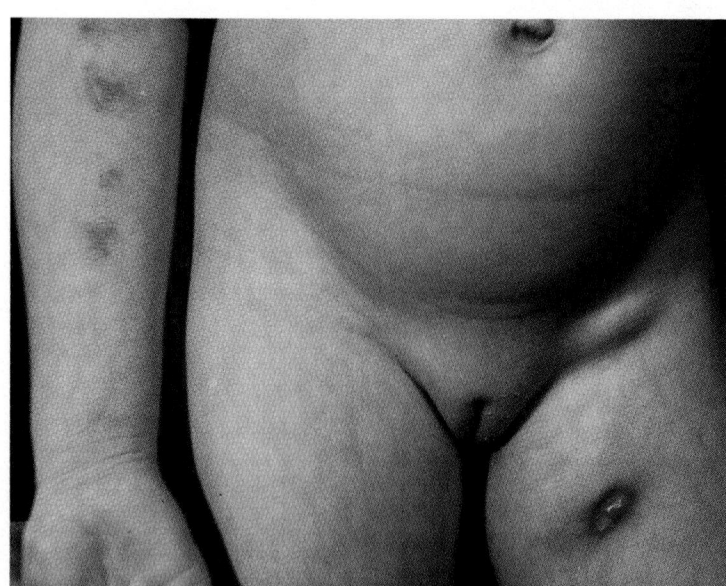

FIGURE 191-1 Primary tuberculosis of the skin. An eroded nodule arising at the site of inoculation is seen on the thigh and is associated with regional lymphadenopathy. A positive tuberculin test is noted on the arm.

lous chancre. Scars also mark the previous sites of sinuses draining liquefied lymph nodes. In more than 50 percent of the cases the regional nodes are calcified.[59]

Usually, the primary tuberculous complex procures satisfactory immunity and a state of high sensitivity, as shown by the tuberculin test. Calcification of the lymph nodes is not necessarily a sign for a favorable outcome, and reactivation of the disease may occur. Hematogenous dissemination of bacteria from such latent foci may give rise to tuberculosis of other organs, particularly of the bones and joints.[52,60] Depending on the size of the inoculum and the age and resistance of the host, primary inoculation tuberculosis may progress to acute miliary disease with fatal outcome.[47] Erythema nodosum is a feature in approximately 10 percent of the cases.[59]

Tuberculosis Verrucosa Cutis (Warty Tuberculosis)

This is a verrucous form of skin tuberculosis in previously sensitized individuals due to exogenous reinfection.

Incidence In western countries tuberculosis verrucosa cutis is one of the rare forms of skin tuberculosis, but in certain regions it may be quite common. It is the most frequently encountered form of tuberculous skin disease in Hong Kong, accounting for more than 40 percent of the cases.[15]

Pathogenesis This is an inoculation tuberculosis occurring in persons who have had previous contact with *M. tuberculosis* and who have thus acquired a certain degree of immunity and sensitivity. Tests with PPD reveal a high degree of hypersensitivity, and the regional lymph nodes are usually not involved. The inoculation of mycobacteria occurs at sites of minor wounds or abrasions, and their source is usually extraneous. Rarely, inoculation of mycobacteria may occur from the patient's own sputum. In the past, certain professional groups were most liable to develop warty tuberculosis, particularly physicians, pathologists, medical students, and laboratory attendants, who were accidentally infected by tuberculous patients or by autopsy material ("verruca necrogenica," "anatomist's wart," "postmortem wart"). Farmers, butchers, and knackers contracted the disease from tuberculous cattle and in these cases *M. bovis* was responsible. In low socioeconomic environments, children become infected by playing and sitting on ground contaminated with tuberculous sputum.[15,61]

Clinical Manifestations Tuberculosis verrucosa usually occurs on the hands, most often on the radial border of the back of the hands, and on the fingers. In children the sites of predilection are the lower extremities, which are most likely to be traumatized. The lesions are asymptomatic and start as a small papule or papulopustule with a purple inflammatory halo. The lesion becomes hyperkeratotic and warty and is often mistaken for a common wart. Slow growth and peripheral expansion lead to the development of a verrucous plaque with an irregular outline and a papillomatous horny surface (Fig. 191-2). Deep clefts and fissures extend into the underlying infiltrated base, which is brownish-red to purplish. The consistency is usually firm, but in the center it may be soft, and pus and keratinous material may be expressed from the fissures. As a rule tuberculosis verrucosa is solitary, but multiple lesions may occur. The regional lymph nodes are rarely affected.[61] Enlargement of regional lymph nodes, however, occurs after secondary bacterial infection.

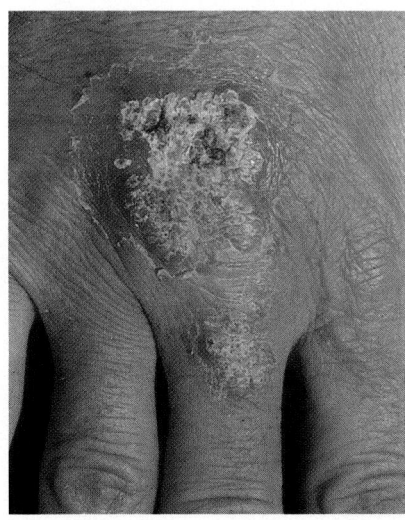

FIGURE 191-2 Tuberculosis verrucosa cutis on the back of the hand.

Histopathology (See Fig. 191-3) The most prominent features are pseudoepitheliomatous hyperplasia with marked hyperkeratosis and dense inflammatory infiltrates. Abscesses form in the superficial dermis, subepithelially, or within the pseudoepitheliomatous rete pegs. Epithelioid cells and giant cells are found in the midportions of the dermis and beneath the epidermis, but typical tubercles are uncommon. Mycobacteria can be demonstrated occasionally. At times, the dermal infiltrate may be nonspecific.[62]

Diagnosis and Differential Diagnosis Early lesions resemble warts or keratoses. Hyperkeratotic lupus vulgaris exhibits "apple-jelly" nodules at the periphery and occurs in sites where tuberculosis verrucosa is rare. Blastomycosis, chromomycosis, and bromoderma may be similar clinically and histopathologically. Negative fungal cultures and small tuberculoid foci are diagnostic aids. Chronic vegetating pyoderma and hyperkeratotic lesions due to other, atypical mycobacteria may be difficult to exclude.[63] Hypertrophic lichen planus is pruritic and more disseminated and usually other cutaneous and mucosal lesions are found. Tertiary syphilis is not quite as verrucous and is accompanied by diagnostic serologic changes.

Course The evolution of the lesions is slow, and without treatment, the course extends over many years. Secondary pyogenic infection may lead to temporary inflammatory changes of a more acute character, and lymphangitis and regional lymphadenitis ensue. Spontaneous involution does occur and usually results in sunken atrophic scars. Occasionally, ulcerative and sclerotic lesions or fungating granulomas are observed.[61]

Lupus Vulgaris

Lupus vulgaris is a chronic, progressive form of tuberculosis of the skin occurring in individuals with a high degree of tuberculin sensitivity.

Incidence Although the incidence of lupus vulgaris has steadily declined during the past decades, it was estimated in 1960 that some 50,000 new cases occur throughout the world every year.[64]

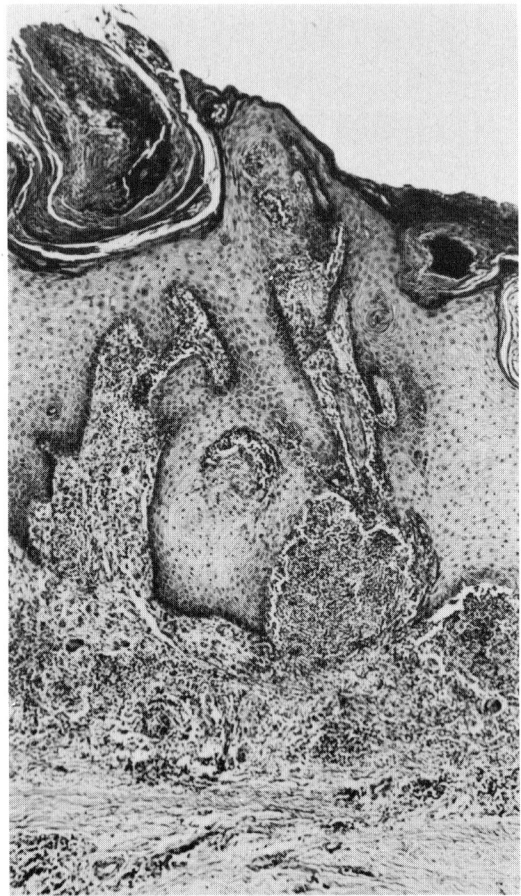

FIGURE 191-3 Tuberculosis verrucosa cutis. There is pronounced epidermal hyperplasia, with hyperkeratotic masses on the surface of the epidermis. Abscesses are seen within and below the hyperplastic epithelium, and giant cells are present in the dermal infiltrate.

Early in this century it was so common that in some European countries, special hospitals were available for the treatment of this condition alone. In 1938 the incidence in Germany was 430 per million,[65] and in the mid-1950s Denmark assessed some 775 cases per million.[64] This contrasts sharply with later figures that estimate 300 to 400 new cases of all forms of skin tuberculosis in a population of 60 million in western Germany.[16] It has always been less common in the United States than in Europe. There is a greater prevalence of the disease in regions with a cool, humid climate, but the incidence is not influenced by rural versus urban residence. Females appear to be affected about two to three times as often as males,[64,65] and all age groups are equally affected.[66]

Pathogenesis Lupus vulgaris is a postprimary form of skin tuberculosis arising in previously sensitized individuals with only moderate immunity. The lesions progress steadily, and although spontaneous involution does occur, new lesions arise within old scars. Complete healing is only rarely observed without therapy.

Lupus vulgaris originates from tuberculosis elsewhere in the body by hematogenous, lymphatic, or contiguous spread. Rarely it may follow primary inoculation tuberculosis, or BCG vaccination[67] (see below). Frequently it develops from a tuberculous condition beneath the surface of the skin, and in about 30 percent of the cases it is preceded by scrofuloderma; tuberculous involvement of the mucous membranes of the nose and throat is also a common source.[65,68]

Most often, lupus vulgaris develops after cervical adenitis or pulmonary tuberculosis. Hematogenous dissemination has also to be taken into account in those patients in whom there is no apparent tuberculosis and in whom only an old pulmonary primary complex is found. Possibly mycobacteria disseminated into the skin reside there in a latent form, to be activated by various stimuli.[69]

Clinical Manifestations The lesions are usually solitary, but two or more sites may be involved simultaneously, and in patients with active pulmonary tuberculosis, multiple foci may develop.[70,71] In about 90 percent of the patients, the head and neck are involved.[68] Lupus vulgaris usually starts on the nose or cheek and slowly extends onto adjacent areas. The earlobes are often affected, and solitary patches may be encountered on the scalp. Only a small percentage of the lesions occur on the extremities, and, except for cases with disseminated lupus vulgaris, involvement of the trunk is rare.

In general, lupus vulgaris is asymptomatic. The initial lesion is the lupus macule or papule, characterized by a brownish-red color and a soft consistency. Upon diascopy the infiltrate shows a diagnostic "apple-jelly" color, and if the lesion is probed, the instrument breaks through the overlying epidermis. Early lesions measure only a few millimeters in diameter; they are rather ill-defined, slightly raised or within the level of the skin, and may reveal a smooth surface or may be covered by a scale. Larger patches are formed by peripheral enlargement and coalescence of smaller papules, and further progression is characterized by an elevation of the lesions and a deeper brownish color (Fig. 191-4). Involution in one area and simultaneous expansion in another result in plaques with a gyrate outline. The course of this disease is marked by ulceration and scarring; thus, its clinical manifestations are diverse and a number of complications may ensue.

Plane forms manifest as flat plaques with a serpiginous or polycyclic configuration, a smooth surface (Fig. 191-5), or psoriasiform scaling. *Hypertrophic forms* may present as tumorous growths of soft consistency that exhibit a nodular surface (Fig. 191-6) or as epithelial hyperplasia with the production of hyperkeratotic masses (Fig. 191-7). Edema, lymphatic stasis, recurrent erysipelas, elephantiasic thickening, and vascular dilatation may lead

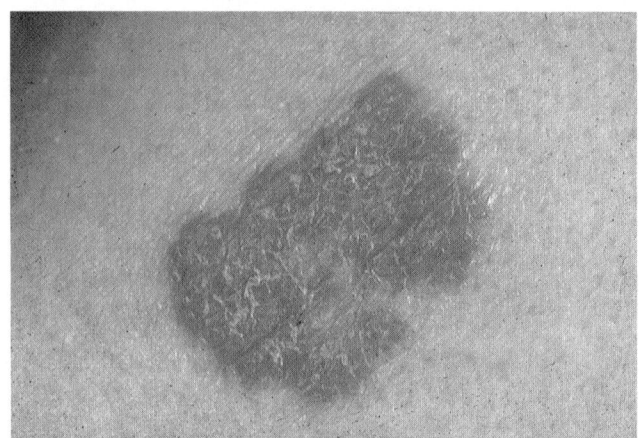

FIGURE 191-4 Slightly raised, brownish plaque of lupus vulgaris.

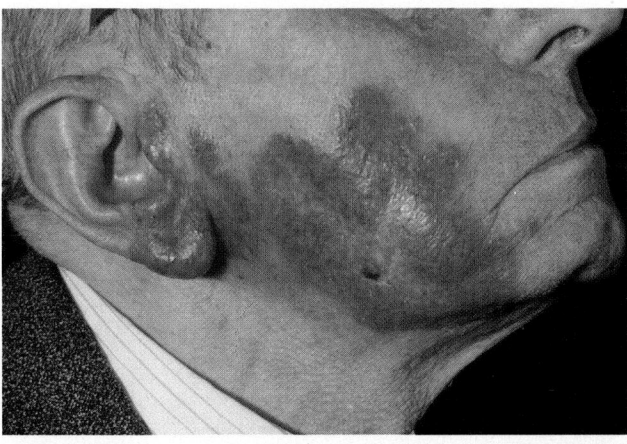

a

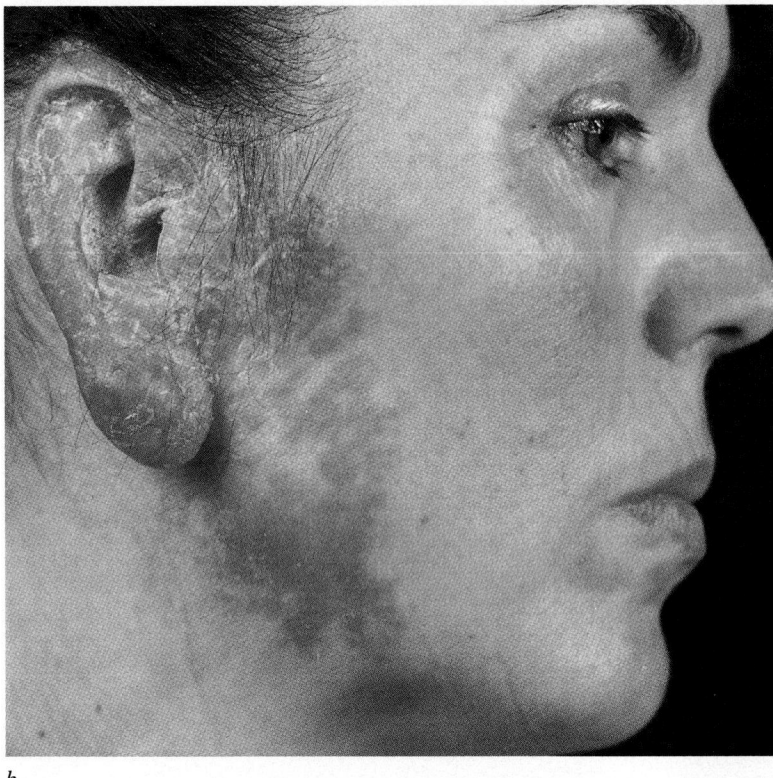

b

FIGURE 191-5 Lupus vulgaris. (*a*) Large plaque of lupus vulgaris of 10-years' duration involving the cheek, jaw, and ear. (*b*) Reddish-brown plaque which, on diascopy, exhibits the diagnostic yellow-brown color.

to gross deformity. In *ulcerative forms,* the underlying tissue may be affected by progressing necrosis, and if the nasal or auricular cartilage is involved, extensive destruction takes place (Fig. 191-8). Granulations at the floor of the ulcers lead to vegetating papillomatous lesions.

Scarring is a prominent feature of lupus vulgaris. Atrophic scars occur subsequent to or independent of ulceration, and new "apple-jelly" nodules may develop within the cicatricial areas. Sometimes scarring with excessive deformation and mutilation is very pronounced, and keloid-like fibrosis leads to contractures.

LUPUS VULGARIS OF MUCOUS MEMBRANES. The pharyngeal, oral, nasal, or conjunctival mucosae are primarily involved or are affected by extension of skin lesions. They show small, soft, gray or pink papules, ulcers, or granulating masses that bleed easily. A dry rhinitis is often the only symptom of early nasal lupus, but progressive lesions destroy the cartilage of the nasal septum; cica-

tricial deformities of the soft palate and stenosis of the larynx may also result.

LUPUS POSTEXANTHEMATICUS. Following a transient impairment of immunity, particularly after measles (thus the term *lupus postexanthematicus*), multiple disseminated lesions may arise simultaneously in different regions of the body due to hematogenous spread from a latent tuberculous focus. During and following the eruption, a previously positive tuberculin test may become negative but will usually revert to positive as the general condition of the patient improves.[72] Clinically and histopathologically, the lesions of postexanthematic lupus are typical for lupus vulgaris and this distinguishes the condition from acute miliary tuberculosis of the skin.

Histopathology (See Fig. 191-9) The most prominent feature is the formation of typical tubercles with sparse caseation necrosis.

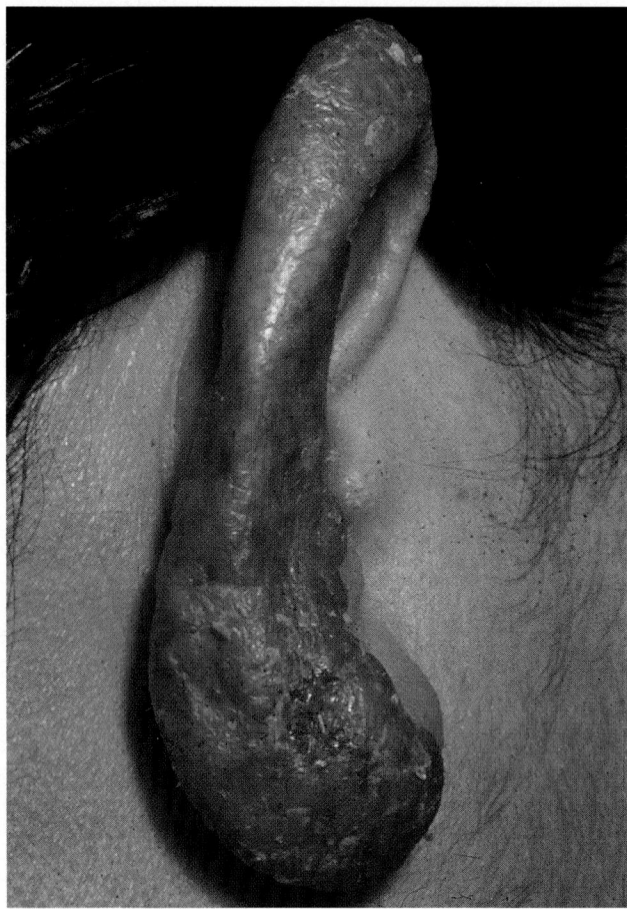

FIGURE 191-6   Hypertrophic form of lupus vulgaris involving the ear. There is a soft, brown, tumorlike thickening of the earlobe.

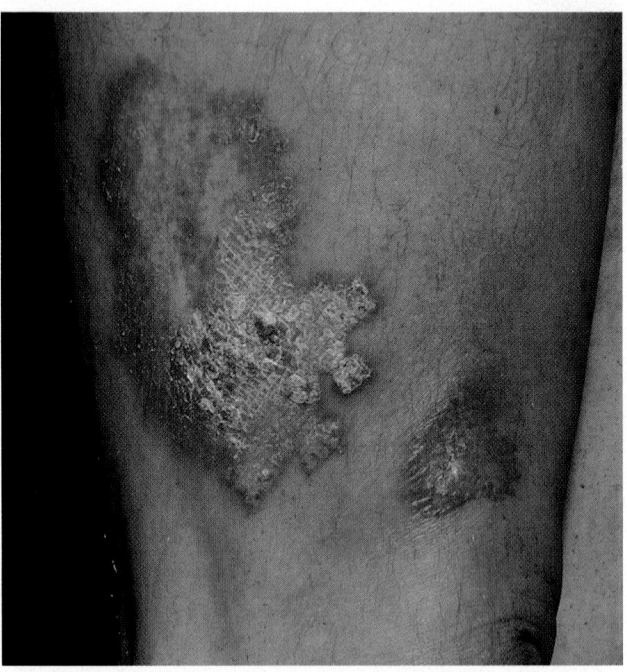

FIGURE 191-7   Hyperkeratotic lupus vulgaris on the thigh.

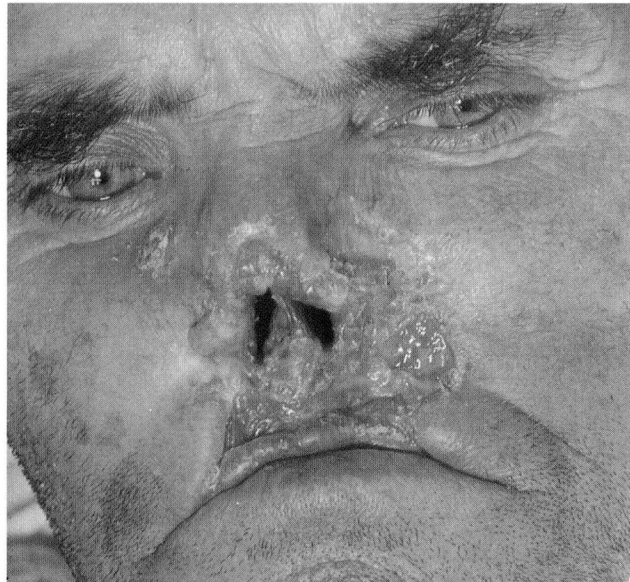

FIGURE 191-8   Lupus vulgaris of long duration, having led to the destruction of the nose. Ulcerating carcinoma has developed on the upper lip.

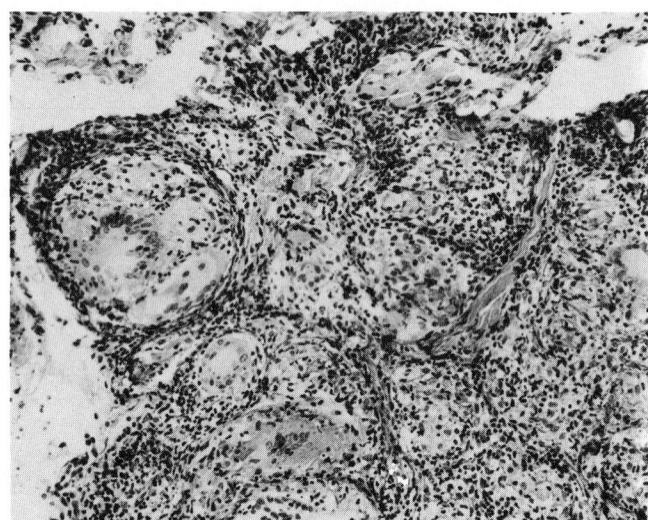

FIGURE 191-9   Lupus vulgaris. Epithelioid cell tubercles with peripheral lymphocytes but without caseation are present. Giant cells are clearly visible.

Secondary changes are often superimposed; epidermal changes include thinning and atrophy or acanthosis with excessive hyperkeratosis and, occasionally, pseudoepitheliomatous hyperplasia. Necrosis and ulceration are usually accompanied by nonspecific inflammatory reactions that may partially conceal the tuberculous structures. Granulomatous reactions of the foreign-body type may develop. Longstanding quiescent lesions are composed chiefly of epithelioid cells, and it may be impossible to distinguish them from sarcoidal infiltrates. During involution, small epithelioid foci are encased in fibrous connective tissue; they eventually disappear.

Diagnosis and Differential Diagnosis   Typical lupus vulgaris plaques do not present diagnostic problems; they have to be distinguished from lesions of sarcoidosis, lymphocytoma, discoid lupus erythematosus, tertiary syphilis, leprosy, blastomycosis or other deep mycotic infections, lupoid leishmaniasis, and chronic vegetating pyodermas. Criteria helpful in the diagnosis are the softness of the lesions, the brownish-red color, and the slow evolution. The "apple-jelly" nodules revealed by diascopy are highly characteristic; finding them may be decisive, especially in ulcerated, crusted, or hyperkeratotic lesions. Histologic examination is mandatory, and in some cases sparse acid-fast bacilli can be demonstrated. A positive culture for *M. tuberculosis/bovis* confirms the diagnosis. The tuberculin test is strongly positive except in the early phases of postexanthematic lupus.[72]

Course   Lupus vulgaris is chronic and without therapy its course usually extends over many years or even decades. Thus adults or older patients have more extensive lesions than children.[73] Although there are periods of relative inactivity, it is progressive and leads to considerable impairment of function and to disfiguration. Contractions result in a reduction of joint mobility; ulceration and destruction of the cartilaginous structures of the face, together with scarring, lead to cicatricial ectropion with its complications, microstomia with impairment of speech and food intake, and other severe mutilations.

The most serious complication of long-standing lupus vulgaris is the development of carcinoma (Fig. 191-8). Early in this century this complication was estimated to be almost 10 percent.[74] Squamous cell carcinomas outnumber basal cell carcinomas by far, and the incidence of metastases is surprisingly high.[75] There is no causal relationship between previous x-ray treatment of the tuberculous lesions and the subsequent malignancy. Sarcomas following lupus vulgaris also have been described, but some of these tumors have actually been highly dedifferentiated carcinomas.

The Relationship of Lupus Vulgaris to Tuberculosis of Other Organs   In 40 percent of patients with lupus vulgaris there is associated tuberculous lymphadenitis, and 10 to 20 percent have pulmonary tuberculosis or tuberculosis of the bones and joints.[76] The morbidity of lupus vulgaris patients from pulmonary tuberculosis is 4 to 10 times higher than in the general population, and in the majority of the cases the pulmonary disease represents postprimary phthisis.[76]

In the past it was believed that pulmonary tuberculosis associated with lupus vulgaris has a good prognosis, and a protective or immunizing effect was ascribed to the cutaneous condition.[77,78] This impression has not been substantiated. More patients with lupus vulgaris die of tuberculosis than could be predicted from the mortality ratios in the general population.[78] In some cases, lupus vulgaris may be regarded as a symptom of another tuberculous disease running a serious course.[76]

Scrofuloderma

Scrofuloderma describes a subcutaneous process originating from tuberculosis beneath the skin and leading to cold abscess formation and a secondary breakdown of the overlying skin.

Incidence   In the past, scrofuloderma was a relatively common disorder, particularly in those with tuberculosis of the lymph nodes.

It appears to be the most common form of skin tuberculosis in Mexico[79] and other tropical countries. In the United Kingdom it is more common in individuals of African or Asian origin.[80]

Pathogenesis   Scrofuloderma results from contiguous involvement of the skin overlying another tuberculous process—most commonly tuberculous lymphadenitis, tuberculosis of bones and joints, or tuberculous epididymitis. It may affect all age groups, although there is a higher prevalence among children, adolescents, and the elderly. Rarely, scrofuloderma may develop after accidental or intentional introduction of exogenous bacilli into the subcutaneous tissue by trauma or injection in those with previous latent or manifest tuberculosis.[81]

Clinical Manifestations   (See Fig. 191-10) Scrofuloderma most often occurs in the parotid, submandibular, and supraclavicular regions and on the lateral aspects of the neck[82]; owing to the involvement of lymph nodes in these areas, the lesions are often bilateral. Lesions on the extremities or on the trunk accompany tuberculous disease of the phalangeal bones, joints, the sternum, and the ribs.

The skin lesions first present as firm, subcutaneous nodules or as a well-defined, asymptomatic infiltrate, which initially is freely movable. As the infiltrate enlarges it becomes doughy, but it may take months before there is liquefaction with subsequent perforation. Ulcers and sinuses develop and discharge watery and purulent or caseous material. The ulcers are linear or serpiginous with undermined, inverted, bluish edges and uneven, soft, granulating floors. Sinusoidal tracts undermine the skin, and clefts and dissecting subcutaneous pockets alternate with soft gummatous nodules; cordlike scars develop and bridge ulcerative areas or even stretches of normal skin. Tuberculin sensitivity is usually pronounced.

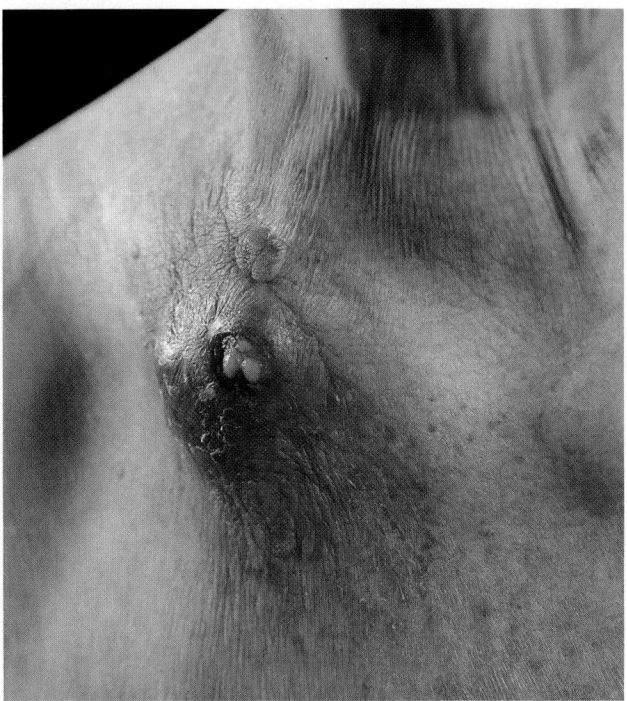

FIGURE 191-10   Scrofuloderma in the clavicular region. Note abscess formation, ulceration, and extrusion of purulent and caseous material.

Histopathology Massive necrosis and abscess formation found in the center of the lesion are nonspecific. However, the periphery of the abscesses or the margins of the sinuses contain tuberculoid granulomas and true tubercles, and *M. tuberculosis* can be found.

Diagnosis and Differential Diagnosis The more benign *M. scrofulaceum* infection must be excluded. If there is an underlying tuberculous lymphadenitis or bone and joint disease, the diagnosis usually presents no difficulty. Syphilitic gumma, deep fungal infections, particularly sporotrichosis, actinomycosis, severe forms of acne conglobata, and hidradenitis suppurativa must be excluded. Confirmation of the clinical diagnosis is by bacterial culture.

Course Spontaneous healing does occur, but the course is protracted and it may take years before the inflammatory and ulcerative lesions have been completely replaced by scar tissue. The cordlike keloidal scars are characteristic enough to permit a correct diagnosis even after the process has become quiescent. Lupus vulgaris may develop at the site of scrofuloderma or in its vicinity.

Metastatic Tuberculous Abscess (Tuberculous Gumma)

Definition and Pathogenesis The metastatic tuberculous abscess is due to hematogenous spread of mycobacteria from a primary focus during a period of lowered resistance or breakdown of immunity, resulting in single or multiple cutaneous-subcutaneous lesions. It usually occurs in undernourished children of low socioeconomic status and in immunodeficient or severely immunosuppressed patients; it may occasionally cause a carpal tunnel syndrome.[83]

Clinical Manifestations Subcutaneous abscesses, which are generally nontender and fluctuant, arise either singly or multiply on the trunk, extremities, or head (Fig. 191-11); the lesions may invade the overlying skin and break down, forming fistulas and ulcers. Metastatic tuberculous abscesses may occur not only in progressive organ tuberculosis[84] and miliary tuberculosis[85] but also without any

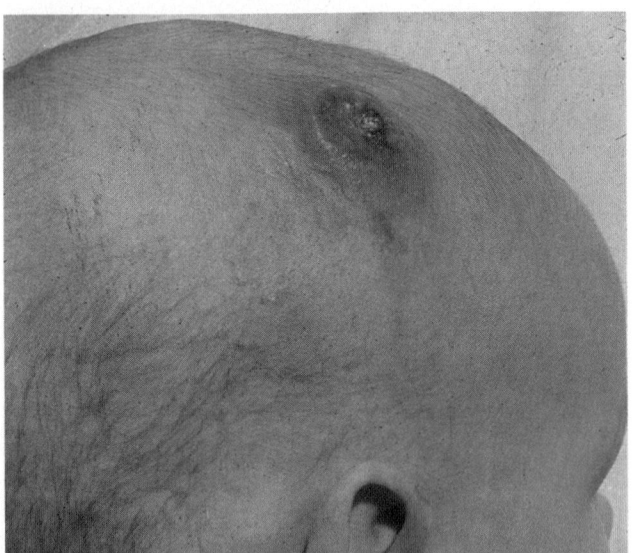

FIGURE 191-11 Metastatic tuberculous abscess on the scalp in an infant with combined immunodeficiency.

underlying tuberculous focus, suggesting silent bacteremia as the pathogenic mechanism.[70,86] Abscesses may develop at sites of previous trauma, which suggests localization of blood-borne organisms in the injured tissue.[41,86,87] Tuberculin sensitivity is usually present but is lower than in other forms of skin tuberculosis and may be absent in severely ill patients.

Histopathology As in scrofuloderma, massive necrosis and abscess formation are found. Acid-fast stains usually reveal copious numbers of mycobacteria.

Diagnosis and Differential Diagnosis All forms of panniculitis, deep fungal infections, syphilitic gumma, and hidradenitis suppurativa have to be excluded. A confirmation of the clinical diagnosis is obtained by histopathology, acid-fast stains of the tissue and smears, and bacterial culture.

Orificial Tuberculosis (Tuberculosis Ulcerosa Cutis et Mucosae)

Orificial tuberculosis occurs on the mucous membranes and the skin of the orifices due to autoinoculation of mycobacteria from progressive tuberculosis of internal organs.

Incidence The condition is rare; in one series it was found in only about 0.2 percent of patients with internal tuberculosis.[88] Males are more frequently affected than females, and although the disease may occur in practically all age groups, it is most common in middle-aged or older persons.[89]

Pathogenesis The underlying disease is far-advanced pulmonary, intestinal, or, rarely, genitourinary tuberculosis. Mycobacteria shed from these foci in large numbers are inoculated into the mucous membranes of the orifices, usually after preceding trauma. Considering the frequency of positive sputums in patients with pulmonary involvement, it is surprising that oral tuberculosis is rare. However, histologic examinations at autopsy of patients with pulmonary tuberculosis have revealed a much higher incidence of oral lesions than was expected,[90] and it may be that, clinically, many mucosal lesions go undiscovered. Most patients show a positive intradermal tuberculin reaction, but in terminal stages anergy develops.

Clinical Manifestations In orificial tuberculosis of the mouth, the tongue is most frequently affected, particularly the tip and the lateral margins, but the soft and hard palate are also common sites and lesions may develop in a tooth socket following extraction. In far-advanced cases the lips are also involved,[89,91–93] and the oral condition often represents an extension of ulcerative tuberculosis of the pharynx and larynx. In patients with intestinal tuberculosis, lesions develop on and around the anus, and in females with active genitourinary disease, the vulva is involved.

A small yellowish or reddish nodule appears on the mucosa and breaks down to form a circular or irregular ulcer with a typical "punched-out" appearance, undermined edges, and soft consistency (Fig. 191-12). Its floor is covered by pseudomembranous material and often exhibits multiple yellowish tubercles and eroded vessels. The surrounding mucosa is swollen, edematous, and inflamed. Lesions may be single or multiple and are extremely painful. The tenderness is often out of proportion to the size of the ulcers and in oral cases results in dysphagia and inability to eat.

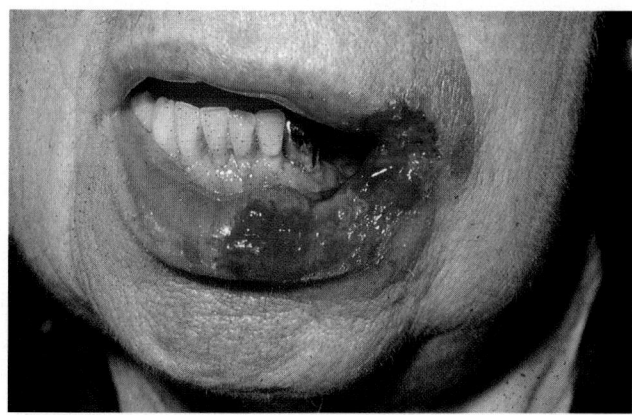

FIGURE 191-12 Orificial tuberculosis in far-advanced cavitary pulmonary tuberculosis.

Histopathology There is a massive nonspecific inflammatory infiltrate and necrosis, but tubercles with caseation may be found deep in the dermis. Mycobacteria may easily be demonstrated.

Diagnosis and Differential Diagnosis Painful ulcers of the mouth in patients with pulmonary tuberculosis should arouse suspicion. Large numbers of acid-fast organisms can be detected in smears, and bacterial culture confirms the diagnosis. Syphilitic lesions, aphthous ulcers, and carcinoma must be excluded.

Course The outcome depends on the course of the underlying disease. In general, individuals developing orificial tuberculosis run a downhill course, and as the internal condition progresses the orificial lesions enlarge and spread. Orificial tuberculosis is a symptom of advanced internal disease with a most unfavorable prognosis.

Acute Miliary Tuberculosis of the Skin

Miliary tuberculosis of the skin, which most often occurs in babies or infants, is an extremely rare skin manifestation of fulminating miliary tuberculosis due to hematogenous dissemination of mycobacteria.[94]

Pathogenesis The initial focus of infection is either meningeal or pulmonary and it may follow infections that reduce the immunologic defense mechanisms such as measles[95] and AIDS. Two babies with typical skin lesions associated with congenital miliary tuberculosis have been reported, but organisms have not been cultured from the lesions.[96] Although extremely rare, acute miliary tuberculosis does occur in adults.[97] Tuberculin sensitivity is usually absent.

Clinical Manifestations Disseminated lesions occur on all parts of the body, particularly on the trunk. They consist of minute erythematous macules or papules and of purpuric lesions. Sometimes vesicles or a central necrosis and crust develop. Removal of the crust discloses a minute umbilication.

Histopathology In the acute phases the histologic changes are nonspecific; necrosis and nonspecific inflammatory infiltrates, which sometimes form small abscesses, are prominent, and occasionally signs of vasculitis may be seen. Mycobacteria are present

both in and around blood vessels.[98] In later stages (if the patient develops immunity), lymphocytic cuffing of the vessels and even tubercles may be observed.

Diagnosis The eruption occurs in individuals already gravely ill and, because of the severity of the underlying process, often goes unnoticed. A multitude of maculopapular and purpuric rashes must be excluded, but the diagnosis is usually substantiated by the evidence of acute miliary disease of the internal organs.

Course Children usually run a downhill course, and the prognosis is poor. Cases with a favourable outcome after therapy have been described.[99,100]

Tuberculosis of the Skin due to BCG Vaccination

It is now generally accepted that vaccination with the attenuated bovine bacillus Calmette-Guérin (BCG) affords protection against tuberculosis,[101–103] but doubts about its effectiveness in developing countries have been revived.[104] However, a study from England published in 1984 has shown rather convincingly that neonatal BCG vaccination substantially reduces the incidence of childhood tuberculosis, the suggested level of protection being above 75 percent.[105] Untoward reactions are rare, but it is important to be aware of these complications, particularly as BCG vaccination in adults has come into wide use as immunotherapy for cancer. BCG is thought to have immunopotentiating effects and macrophage-activating properties and is therefore undergoing extensive clinical trials.

Approximately 2 weeks after a routine BCG vaccination,[106] an infiltrated papule develops and, after 6 to 12 weeks, attains a size of about 10 mm, ulcerates, and then slowly heals, leaving a scar.[105] Vaccination may provoke an accelerated reaction if given to a subject previously infected but with a negative tuberculin test. The regional lymph nodes may enlarge but usually heal without breaking down. Tuberculin sensitivity appears 5 to 6 weeks after vaccination.

Nonspecific complications include keloid formation, epithelial cysts, granulomas, eczema, generalized hemorrhagic rashes, erythema nodosum, and other eruptions.[106,107] Specific complications comprise tuberculous processes caused by the BCG organism.[108] The large majority of these are lymphoglandular and skin reactions that mimic cutaneous responses to ''natural'' mycobacterial infection. Their true incidence is difficult to ascertain, but it is extremely low in comparison to the great number of vaccinations performed.[101] According to Horwitz and Meyer,[108] nonfatal generalized complications occur in 1 or 2 persons per million; a perforating regional lymphadenitis was seen in 2 percent of vaccinated children in Denmark, and the incidence of postvaccinal lupus vulgaris was estimated to be from five to ten per million.[108,109] Usually the BCG reactions run a milder course than ''spontaneous'' tuberculosis of the skin and they occur more often after revaccination.[107,110]

Specific lesions originating from BCG vaccination include: (1) *Lupus vulgaris* may develop in the vicinity of the vaccination site after a latency period of several months or after 1 to 3 years. Its clinical appearance, course, and response to treatment do not differ from the usual lupus vulgaris. BCG organisms can be recovered from only one-fourth of the lesions.[108] In some cases lupus vulgaris has developed after vaccination with the Vole bacillus.[111] (2) Individuals previously sensitive to tuberculin may exhibit a type of *Koch's phenomenon*. Necrosis and ulceration occur as in normal nonsensitive individuals but with a shorter time course. Regional lymphadenitis is common, and general symptoms may be present.[108] (3) Local *subcutaneous abscesses* may form if the vaccination material has been injected too deeply into the skin, and excessive ulceration may ensue.[106] (4) Severe *regional lymphadenitis* is definitely the most common complication and occurs more often in the younger age groups. *Scrofuloderma* may develop, and suppuration may persist for 6 to 12 months. (5) Generalized *tuberculid-like eruptions* have rarely been observed.[106,107] (6) *Generalized adenitis, osteitis,* and *tuberculous foci* in *distant organs* (e.g., the joints) have occurred occasionally.[101] After repeated vaccinations *fever, chills, arthralgia,* and *malaise* may occur. *Anaphylactic* shock may be fatal[112]; *hepatic dysfunction* and noncaseous granulomas containing the organisms have been noted. *Fatal disease* due to generalized BCG tuberculosis is rare—1 per 10 million vaccinated[101]—and occurs in immunologically compromised individuals.[113] In 1980 Rosenthal[114] collected 17 fatal disseminated cases, the majority of whom had immunodeficiencies.

The Tuberculids

These were originally considered to represent recurrent disseminated or systemic skin reactions to toxins of tubercle bacilli, with a tendency to spontaneous involution, and were distinguished from "true" cutaneous tuberculosis.[115] They included lichen scrofulosorum, erythema induratum, papulonecrotic tuberculids, lupus miliaris disseminatus faciei, and some eruptions with rather exotic designations.

During the first half of this century tuberculids were eruptions quite familiar to dermatologists, but with the sharp decline in tuberculosis and its effective chemotherapy in the developed countries, the tuberculids have also become rare. This does not appear to apply to areas where tuberculosis is still not so uncommon,[17] and with the recent resurgence of tuberculosis in some western countries some tuberculids have also been observed again.[116,117]

Their pathogenesis and their relationship to tuberculosis are still poorly understood, and although there is no doubt that for some of them a relationship exists, there are good reasons to doubt it in others. Therefore it is necessary to briefly discuss the evidence for and against a relationship between tuberculids and tuberculosis. Such evidence could rest on the demonstration of mycobacteria in the lesions, on the histopathology, the patient's sensitivity to mycobacterial antigens, the presence of proven, concomitant tuberculosis elsewhere in the body, and the response to tuberculostatic therapy.

1. Mycobacteria. Early in this century several cases were described in which bacteria were recovered from skin lesions.[118–121] Some of these conditions were atypical clinically and histologically, and at that time the criteria for the identification of *M. tuberculosis* were not as stringent as today; during this period "mycobacteria" were even found in lesions of lupus erythematosus, granuloma annulare, and sarcoidosis. The results of a later study in which mycobacteria were detected in 2 out of 72 patients with erythema induratum[122] have not been confirmed,[123] and it is accepted today that mycobacteria cannot be found in tuberculids. The failure to demonstrate mycobacteria in histologic sections, by bacterial culture, or by guinea pig inoculation has been ascribed, by the supporters of the tuberculid concept, to the small number of organisms in the lesions or to their rapid destruction.[124]

2. Histology. Most tuberculids exhibit tuberculoid features histologically. However, tuberculoid granulomas are produced by a multitude of conditions, and, conversely, "tuberculids" have been described that lacked tuberculoid structures. Therefore, the histologic evidence is of questionable value.

3. Tuberculin sensitivity. The tuberculin reaction is moderate to strong in most patients and in the past was considered positive evidence for the tuberculous nature of the lesions. However, a considerable number of the patients show only a low sensitivity, and the reactions may vary within wide limits.[24] Today, it is generally agreed that a positive tuberculin reaction does not establish evidence of the pathogenesis of the tuberculids.[123–125]

4. Previous and concomitant tuberculosis of other organs. In the older literature, patients with tuberculids often presented a family or personal history of tuberculosis. Tuberculous disease was quite common in the first half of this century, and the chances of finding individuals with evidence of tuberculosis were rather high in the general population. However, in large series published in 1954[126] and in 1960,[127] active tuberculosis was found in only a small percentage of patients with tuberculids and was described to be just as common as, for instance, focal bacterial infections.[127] On the other hand, reports have been published more recently in which active tuberculosis and concomitant eruptions satisfying the clinical criteria for tuberculids are documented.[18,116,117,128] The development of lupus vulgaris from lesions of papulonecrotic tuberculid certainly appears to be a strong argument in favor of a tuberculous etiology in these cases.[17]

5. The therapeutic test. Tuberculostatics have been found beneficial in some cases, and the involution of tuberculid lesions concomitant with the improvement of underlying tuberculosis has been described.[18,117] However, it should also be kept in mind that some tuberculids tend to involute spontaneously, that some cases do not respond to antituberculous treatment,[124,129] and that many react equally well to other antibiotics or even to plain rest and nonspecific measures.[123]

In summary then, the evidence supporting the tuberculous etiology of tuberculids is largely circumstantial and not convincing in all cases. This term has obviously been used too freely in the past for conditions that are unrelated to tuberculosis; it is also clear today that some tuberculids have a multifactorial etiology and that *M. tuberculosis* or its products can, at best, be considered as one of several possible causes. On the other hand, positive evidence disproving the tuberculous nature of some of these eruptions is equally lacking, and in some an etiologic link to tuberculosis cannot be denied.

The following discussion therefore employs a restrictive classification that acknowledges as tuberculids only those conditions for which reasonable evidence supporting a tuberculous etiology exists (Table 191-3). *Tuberculids* therefore comprise only lichen scrofulosorum and papulonecrotic tuberculid. *Facultative tuber-*

TABLE 191-3
Tuberculids

Tuberculids (conditions in which *M. tuberculosis/bovis* appears to play a significant role)	1. Lichen scrofulosorum 2. Papulonecrotic tuberculid
Facultative tuberculids (conditions in which *M. tuberculosis/bovis* may be one of several etio-pathogenic factors)	1. Nodular vasculitis (erythema induratum) 2. Erythema nodosum
Non-tuberculids (conditions formerly designated tuberculids; there is no relationship to tuberculosis)	1. Lupus miliaris disseminatus faciei 2. Rosacea-like tuberculid 3. Lichenoid tuberculid

culids are conditions in which *M. tuberculosis* or its antigens can be considered as one of several possible causes: they comprise nodular vasculitis and erythema nodosum. Finally, *"non-tuberculids"* are all those conditions that were formerly regarded as tuberculids but can now be considered to be unrelated to tuberculosis.

Lichen Scrofulosorum

Lichen scrofulosorum is a lichenoid eruption of minute papules occurring in children with tuberculosis.

Incidence and Pathogenesis   The disorder was recognized by Hebra and was uncommon even in the past.[130] It usually occurred in children but also in adolescents and adults.[74] Today this diagnosis is made only rarely, but a number of well-documented cases have been described.[116,117] Lichen scrofulosorum is usually associated with chronic tuberculous disease of the lymph nodes and bones or with specific pleurisy, but is rare in phthisic patients[74]; it has been observed following BCG vaccination.[105] It is ascribed to a hematogenous spread of mycobacteria in an individual strongly sensitive to *M. tuberculosis*.[74,116,117,130]

Clinical Manifestations   The eruption is asymptomatic and is usually confined to the trunk. The lesions consist of small, firm, follicular or parafollicular papules of a yellowish or pink color; they have a flat top or bear a minute horny spine or fine scales on their surface and, rarely, there may be superficial pustulation that is barely visible. Lichenoid grouping is pronounced and results in the formation of rough, discoid plaques that tend to coalesce. The lesions persist for months, but spontaneous involution eventually ensues. Antituberculous therapy results in complete resolution within a matter of weeks.[116] An association of lichen scrofulosorum and tuberculous dactylitis has been described.[117]

Histopathology   Superficial tuberculoid granulomas develop around hair follicles but may also occur independent of the adnexae.[62] Mycobacteria are not seen in the sections and cannot be cultured from biopsy material.[116]

Diagnosis   Lichen planus, lichen nitidus, lichenoid secondary syphilis, and micropapular forms of sarcoidosis should be excluded.

Papulonecrotic Tuberculid

This is a symmetric eruption of necrotizing papules appearing in crops and healing with scar formation. The old names *folliclis* and *acnitis* probably denoted variants of this disorder.[74]

Incidence   Reports on papulonecrotic tuberculids were quite common in the older dermatologic and pediatric literature but have become rather rare. The condition still appears to be not so uncommon in populations with a high prevalence of tuberculosis—in 1974 Morrison and Fourie reported 91 cases seen in South Africa over a 17-year period.[17] It usually occurs in children or young adults.

Pathogenesis   As a rule, bacteria cannot be demonstrated in lesions, but a few authors are regularly cited who supposedly succeeded in recovering the organism.[118–121,131] However, these find-

ings do not stand up to critical analysis. In most cases a single(!) acid-fast "rod" was found histologically and, with one exception,[131] guinea pig inoculations were invariably negative. However, in a series of 91 cases published relatively recently,[17] lupus vulgaris was seen to evolve from papulonecrotic tuberculids in four patients and *M. tuberculosis* was cultured from two. This suggests that mycobacteria may have been present in the papulonecrotic lesions but does not exclude the possibility that they may have lodged in these lesions secondarily.

In most cases the tuberculin test is positive,[126] and in earlier writings the association with tuberculous lymph nodes of internal organs has been stressed.[132] In the series of Morrison and Fourie,[17] a deep focus of tuberculosis, most commonly cervical lymphadenopathy—some with scrofuloderma—was found in one-third of cases. They believe that bacilli from a tuberculous focus periodically enter the circulation, where they are opsonized and settle out, preferentially in skin capillaries, and that the papulonecrotic tuberculid represents an Arthus-like reaction followed by a delayed-hypersensitivity response to mycobacteria. Anticomplementary activity and in vivo C3 conversion observed in five patients indicate the presence of immune complexes. A prompt response to antituberculous therapy—whether a tuberculous focus was known to exist or not—has been described.[17]

An association with discoid lupus erythematosus, arthritis, or erythema nodosum has also been observed in patients with papulonecrotic tuberculid,[133] and concomitant focal bacterial infections are found frequently[127]; the antistreptolysin titer is increased in almost 65 percent of the cases,[127] and a number of them respond to antibiotics other than tuberculostatic agents.[125] Some forms of papulonecrotic tuberculid may therefore be triggered by antigens other than those of *M. tuberculosis*.

Clinical manifestations   Predilection sites are the extensor aspects of the extremities, particularly the knees and elbows, buttocks, and lower trunk (Fig. 191-13) with a symmetric distribution. Disseminated crops of dusky red, symptomless, pea-sized papules appear. They may show a central depression and an adherent crust and may develop a central necrosis that, upon removal, results in a craterlike ulcer. If the lesions are seated more deeply, they may enlarge to a diameter of 1 cm and acquire a more livid color. Localized papulonecrotic tuberculids have been reported on the penis.[134,135] There is spontaneous involution, and pitted scars result. Usually there are no systemic symptoms.

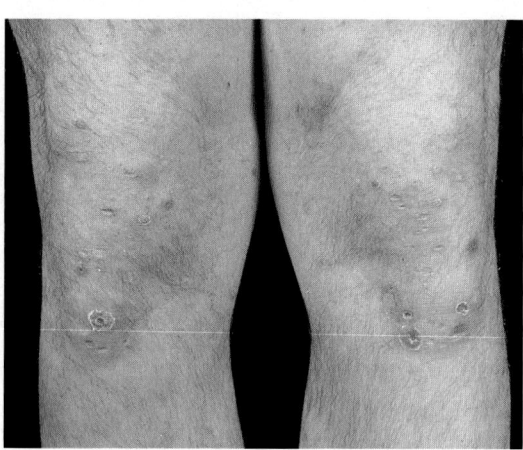

FIGURE 191-13   Papulonecrotic tuberculid on the knees.

Histopathology The most prominent feature of well-developed lesions is a wedge-shaped necrosis of the upper dermis extending to and involving the epidermis. The inflammatory infiltrate surrounding this necrotic area may be nonspecific but is usually tuberculoid. Involvement of the blood vessels is a cardinal feature and consists of an obliterative and sometimes granulomatous vasculitis leading to thrombosis and complete occlusion of the vascular channels. Recanalization of the vessels may be observed. Early lesions have been described as mimicking an Arthus-type reaction. In a reported case of papulonecrotic tuberculid, the histopathology of one lesion was considered similar to Churg-Strauss vasculitis, but an absence of eosinophils was noted.[128]

Diagnosis and Differential Diagnosis Although the clinical picture is characteristic, the diagnosis should be confirmed by histology. The exclusion of pityriasis lichenoides et varioliformis acuta may present difficulties. This condition is more widespread and also involves the trunk, palms, and soles; histologically it represents lymphocytic vasculitis.[136,137] Eruptions due to leukocytoclastic necrotizing vasculitis have also to be ruled out; the history, clinical appearance, and histology help to make the diagnosis. The distinction from lichen urticatus, prurigo, and secondary syphilis is easily established.

Nodular Vasculitis (See also Chap. 108)

This term is used to describe a chronic recurring nodular and ulcerative disorder of the lower legs. Formerly the condition was considered to be the classic example of a tuberculid and was termed *erythema induratum of Bazin*.

Incidence Nodular vasculitis is quite common, particularly in Europe. According to one report these cases comprise some 0.1 to 0.2 percent of all dermatologic patients seen at a university hospital.[123] The disease is found predominantly in women; men account only for some 5 to 10 percent of the cases.[122,123] The age of onset varies from the early teens to old age, but incidence peaks in adolescence and in menopause. There is a seasonal prevalence in winter and early spring.

Pathogenesis Most patients present with erythrocyanotic changes of the lower extremities[138] and have heavy legs, with thick and firm but not edematous skin, and follicular perniosis. Cutis marmorata is common, and the pathogenetic significance of the vasculature is clearly demonstrated by the histologic pattern, which reveals features of vasculitis. The vessels of the patients react abnormally to changes in ambient temperature. Thus the eruptions are usually associated with exposure to cold.[138]

It has long been thought that transient mycobacteremia produces a reaction that is both induced by and superimposed upon the basic circulatory disorder.[138] However, active tuberculosis is found only rarely in these patients,[123,126] and the fact that tuberculous disease has rarely developed subsequently to erythema induratum[119,123] does not establish a pathogenic link. Similarly, the tuberculin test is of no pathogenic significance; many patients exhibit high sensitivity, but up to 60 percent do not react to a 1:10,000 dilution of OT.[123]

The introductory comments on the relationship of the tuberculids to tuberculosis are particularly relevant to the problem of "erythema induratum." Nodular vasculitis[122,138] today represents a multifactorial syndrome of lobular panniculitis in which tuberculosis may or may not be one of a multitude of etiologic components. Immune complexes play a pathogenic role in this condition in which both streptococcal and (in one study) mycobacterial antigens have been found in the lesions.[139]

Today most authors accept a subdivision of the erythema induratum–nodular vasculitis complex into two groups: one with and one without tuberculous etiology.[122,123] At the same time, however, it is agreed that the term *erythema induratum* should be reserved for the first group, i.e., for those cases in which the tuberculous origin can be proven.[122,140] The demonstration of mycobacteria in culture emerges as the only reliable criterion, and because examinations of erythema induratum lesions for mycobacteria have almost invariably yielded negative results, it becomes apparent that it may be impossible to pinpoint the alleged "tuberculous" cases.

Erythema Nodosum (See Chap. 99)

Non-Tuberculids (Conditions with Nontuberculous Etiology, Previously Considered Tuberculids)

The older dermatologic literature abounds with entities that were considered tuberculous in nature. Great significance was attached to nomenclature, and the resulting confusion is still reflected in some more recent writings.[141,142] In none of these conditions has the tuberculous etiology been proved; they all exhibit tuberculoid features histologically; tuberculin sensitivity is low or inconstant; there is no associated tuberculosis; and the incidence of past tuberculous disease among patients with these conditions does not exceed that of the general population. Mycobacteria cannot be recovered from the lesions.

In order to avoid a perpetuation of the terminologic jumble, many of the older designations are not mentioned in this text. Most of them are synonymous.

Lupus Miliaris Disseminatus Faciei This is a papular eruption of the face, running a chronic course with spontaneous involution. Originally considered a variant of lupus vulgaris or a tuberculid,[141,143] there is no evidence supporting a link to tuberculosis.[144] The histology exhibits tuberculoid features; the tuberculin test is inconsistent and most often negative; the course is self-limited, leading to spontaneous involution; there is no concomitant tuberculosis[126]; mycobacteria cannot be recovered from the lesions; and there is no response to antituberculous drugs. The cause and pathogenesis of this condition are unknown and so the designation *lupus miliaris disseminatus* is not appropriate. Some cases may represent micropapular forms of sarcoidosis, but most represent a sarcoidal form of rosacea. An allergic etiology has been discussed.[144]

The eruption is not uncommon and occurs in adults and adolescents of both sexes. It consists of multiple indolent papules, 1 to 3 mm in diameter, symmetrically distributed in the centrofacial regions. The lower portions of the forehead, the bridge of the nose, the cheeks, the nasolabial folds, and the perioral areas are preferentially involved (Fig. 191-14), but occasionally more widespread dissemination occurs.[144] The papules develop quite rapidly, may be follicular or nonfollicular, and are distributed at random. Their surface is smooth, their color brownish-red; diascopy reveals an infiltrate similar to the "apple-jelly" nodules of lupus vulgaris. Their consistency is rather firm, but occasionally it may be soft, and in some cases pustulation has been observed. Histopathology reveals

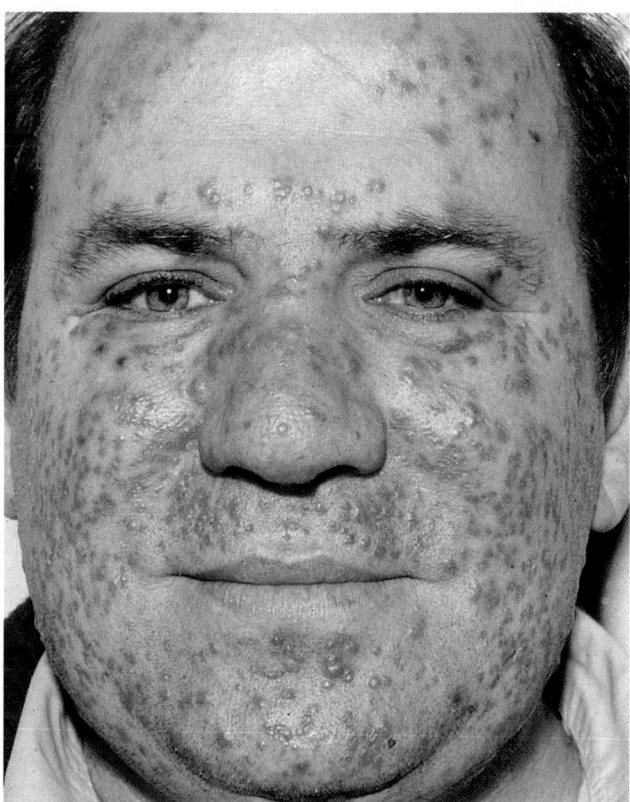

FIGURE 191-14 Condition formerly termed *lupus miliaris disseminatus faciei*, with the characteristic distribution of small follicular and nonfollicular papules. This represents a sarcoidal form of rosacea.

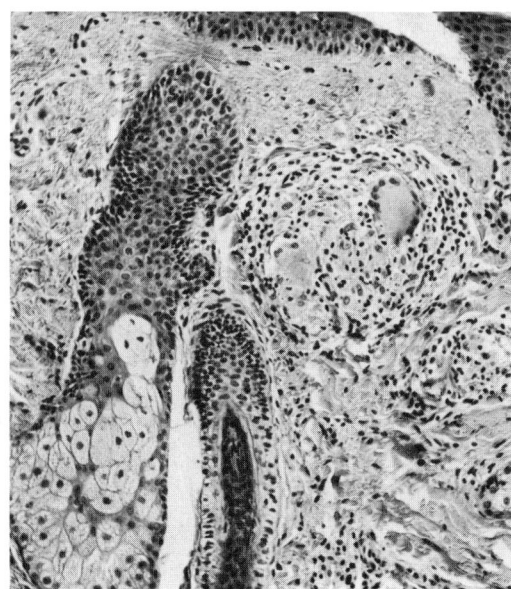

FIGURE 191-15 Histopathology of what was formerly termed *lupus miliaris disseminatus faciei*. A small tuberculoid focus consisting of epithelioid cells, Langerhans' giant cells, and peripheral lymphocytes in a perifollicular localization.

well-defined globular masses of tuberculoid structures in the upper dermis. In the center there may be frank necrosis, and thus the similarity to true tubercles may be striking (Fig. 191-15).

The condition runs a self-limited course. Individual papules regress, leaving pitted atrophic scars, and new crops of lesions arise. After a period of months or up to 2 years, the condition involutes spontaneously. Tetracyclines exert a beneficial effect.

Rosacea-like Tuberculid Originally described by Lewandowsky,[145] it is largely agreed today that rosacea-like tuberculid is simply a micropapular form of rosacea with pronounced tuberculoid features.

Lichenoid Tuberculid This condition was described by Ockuly and Montgomery[146] in a study based on 15 patients and was thought to represent a hematogenous form of skin tuberculosis. However, most cases were tuberculin-negative, epithelioid cells predominated, and only 2 out of 15 cases had evidence of tuberculosis elsewhere in the body; the eruptions were probably sarcoidal reactions. Only a few additional cases have been described.[147,148]

Clinically, there is a sudden symmetric eruption, preferentially localized on the extremities but with a tendency to generalization. The lesions are brown to violaceous papules, with a diameter of 3 to 5 mm. They may be capped by an adherent scale, and telangiectases are present. Grouping and coalescence are prominent, and annular lesions may be formed. Involution results in brownish macules but no scarring.

Histopathologically, well-demarcated "tubercles" composed chiefly of epithelioid cells, are found in the superficial and midportions of the dermis. They show a tendency for perivascular arrangement, and central necrosis is quite common.

Therapy of Skin Tuberculosis

In many respects the management of skin tuberculosis is the same as that of tuberculosis of other organs. Chemotherapy is usually the treatment of choice, but ancillary measures may be required to provide the patient with optimal care. The type of cutaneous involvement, the stage of the disease, the level of immunity, and the general condition of the patient are important factors to be considered. Cutaneous tuberculosis associated with mycobacterial disease of internal organs requires a well-coordinated, multidisciplinary plan of therapy.

Chemotherapy The aim of chemotherapy for tuberculosis is to cure the disease as rapidly as possible, to prevent the emergence of resistant strains, and to prevent relapses. Chemotherapy should consist of at least two drugs to which *M. tuberculosis* is sensitive, and it should be started as early as possible. Short-course chemotherapy (6 or 9 months) is adequate under usual circumstances, provided four or three drugs, respectively, are given.[149] Phase I of chemotherapy is directed towards the rapid destruction of large numbers of multiplying mycobacteria and therefore consists of initial, intensive chemotherapy.[32] Phase II is maintenance chemotherapy that aims at the elimination of remaining "dormant" organisms; it relies on the effect of drugs on the spurts of metabolic activity of "dormant" bacilli, which are unaffected in their nonmetabolizing state.[32]

The following drugs are currently employed in chemotherapy of tuberculosis: rifampin (rifampicin), pyrazinamide, isoniazid, streptomycin, ethambutol, and amithiozone (thioacetazone).[32,150]

In clinical practice, drug efficacy, side effects, development of resistance, and, particularly in developing countries, cost and patient compliance have to be taken into account when choosing an appropriate antituberculous treatment. First-line drugs that are highly effective and are mainly used in the initial treatment of susceptible organisms are isoniazid, rifampin, streptomycin, and ethambutol. Second-line drugs used mainly in the treatment of patients with drug-resistant mycobacteria are pyrazinamide, ethionamide, viomycin, kanamycin, capreomycin, cycloserine, and *p*-aminosalicylic acid. The quinolones,[151] and particularly their fluorinated derivates,[152] are active against *M. tuberculosis* and a number of other mycobacteria in vitro and thus may gain therapeutic importance in the future.

Isoniazid remains the mainstay of antituberculous therapy. It is both tuberculostatic and tuberculocidal in vitro. It penetrates into all body fluids and cells and also into sclerotic tissue, so that it is effective even in old fibrotic lesions. The common daily dose of the drug is 5 mg/kg with a maximum of 300 mg. Bacterial resistance to isoniazid usually develops after prolonged treatment, and because primary resistance of *M. tuberculosis* occurs (one in 10^6 tubercle bacilli), treatment with isoniazid alone will lead to selection of these bacteria.[150] Side effects seen in 5.4 percent of patients treated include fever (1.2 percent), skin eruptions (2.0 percent), peripheral neuritis (0.2 percent), and hematologic complications (agranulocytosis, eosinophilia, anemia, and thrombocytopenia).[153] Severe hepatic injury has been observed, particularly in patients older than age 35. Vasculitis, antinuclear antibodies, and arthritic symptoms may occur. Pyridoxine should be given concomitantly to prevent peripheral neuropathy, which may otherwise occur in as many as 20 percent of patients.

Ethambutol, a bacteriostatic drug given in doses of 15 to 25 mg/kg, is always used in combination with other drugs, usually rifampin and isoniazid. It accumulates in patients with impaired renal function, so the dosage must be adjusted. It should not be given to children under age 13.[150] Side effects include diminished visual acuity, rashes, and drug fever,[153] but their incidence is low.

Rifampin, a semisynthetic derivative of an antibiotic produced by *Streptomyces mediterranei*, is one of the most effective drugs for the treatment of tuberculosis. It should not be used alone, as mycobacteria rapidly develop resistance in a one-step process.[150] Although rifampin produces a number of side effects, the incidence of these is low and seldom necessitates an interruption of treatment.[150] Rifampin rapidly penetrates into tissues and cavities of the body and is rapidly bactericidal in vivo[32]; for sensitive organisms, a combination of isoniazid and rifampin is probably as effective as regimens employing three or more drugs.[154] Rifampin is administered as a single oral dose of 600 mg/day, and patients should be warned that the drug may impart an orange stain to excretions, including saliva.

Streptomycin, a time-honored antibiotic in the treatment of tuberculosis, is bactericidal for *M. tuberculosis* in vitro but its activity in vivo is essentially suppressive.[152] It does not penetrate cell membranes (and thus can not kill intracellular organisms) and has been demonstrated to be more active in an alkaline medium.[149] The toxicity of streptomycin prohibits continuous long-term therapy; nearly 75 percent of patients given 2 g of streptomycin daily for 60 to 120 days develop vestibular disturbances, including impairment of hearing.[152] Other side effects include peripheral neuropathy, dysfunction of the optic nerve, rashes, fever, exfoliative dermatitis, and blood dyscrasias, but there is less nephrotoxicity than with other aminoglycoside antibiotics.[155] Streptomycin is never used alone in the treatment of tuberculosis and since other drugs have

become available its use has been sharply reduced. It is given in doses of 1 to 2 g/day; it is usually combined with two other drugs and is employed in the more serious forms of tuberculosis.

Drug Combinations and Regimens   In the recent past clinical research on the treatment of tuberculosis has mainly been directed at identifying the best combination of drugs and the duration of treatment in phase I and phase II chemotherapy. In western countries the majority of previously untreated tuberculosis is caused by mycobacteria that are sensitive to isoniazid, rifampin, ethambutol, streptomycin, and pyrazinamide.

The following guidelines for the chemotherapy of tuberculosis in the United States have been established by a National Consensus Conference on Tuberculosis[156] and should be applied in all developed countries:

1. Extrapulmonary tuberculosis (including tuberculosis of the skin) should be treated like pulmonary tuberculosis. Drug susceptibility should always be tested; this is mandatory in cases of suspected drug resistance.
2. Adults should receive a 9-month course of isoniazid and rifampin, supplemented with ethambutol, streptomycin, or pyrazinamide in the initial phase. In infants, children, and adolescents, this initial phase therapy is only necessary when drug resistance is suspected.
3. A 6-month course of therapy is acceptable if four drugs (isoniazid, rifampin, pyrazinamide, and streptomycin or ethambutol) are given for 2 months followed by 4 months of isoniazid and rifampin.
4. Tuberculosis during pregnancy should not be treated with streptomycin and/or pyrazinamide. Immunosuppressed patients should be treated for 12 rather than 9 months.
5. Treatment schedules of less than 6-months' duration are not acceptable.

However, in circumstances in which compliance and economic problems prevail, trials of short-course chemotherapy schedules have indicated that a 6- to 9-months regimen employing rifampin and isoniazid can be sufficient if a third drug (e.g., ethambutol) is added during the initial 2 months of treatment.[149,154,157,158]

Special Considerations in the Therapy of Tuberculosis of the Skin   Essentially, the treatment of tuberculosis of the skin is that of tuberculosis in general. A full antituberculous regimen is administered even in localized forms of skin tuberculosis where a primary focus or evidence of an underlying organ tuberculosis or tuberculosis of lymph nodes exists. Special considerations may apply to tuberculosis verrucosa cutis and localized forms of lupus vulgaris without evidence of associated internal tuberculosis in which isoniazid has been given alone with a high cure rate.[159–163] Prolonged treatment, extending up to 12 months, is necessary also in these forms of lupus vulgaris, and total doses of 80 to 140 g may be required. As viable mycobacteria have been cultured from clinically healed lesions,[160] treatment should be continued for at least 2 months after complete involution of the lesions.[161] If, however, there is concomitant internal tuberculosis or if drug resistance emerges, combination therapy is mandatory in localized lupus vulgaris.

Careful observation and follow-up are essential. Surgical intervention is quite important in the treatment of scrofuloderma. It reduces morbidity and shortens the period necessary for chemotherapy. Small lesions of lupus vulgaris or tuberculosis verrucosa cutis are also best excised, but tuberculostatics should be given concomitantly. Plastic surgery is important as a corrective measure in long-standing lupus vulgaris with mutilation.

Caustics have lost their value in the treatment of localized lesions as has cryotherapy. However, in selected cases, residual lupus nodules within scarred areas may be conveniently destroyed by cryotherapy or electrocautery. Light therapy with the Finsen or the Kromayer lamp, x-ray treatment, and vitamin D_2 are obsolete.

Other Mycobacterial Diseases

For atypical mycobacterial disease in AIDS, see Chap. 215.

Historical Aspects

The pathogenic potential of slow-growing mycobacterial species other than M. leprae and M. tuberculosis has only been recognized in the past five decades. This is in part because these infections usually closely mimic infections with M. tuberculosis or, in rare instances, with other organisms, and in part because of their strict and often unusual culture requirements.

M. ulcerans was identified as the cause of an ulcerating skin condition in Australia in 1948[164] and in the Buruli district of Uganda (hence the name Buruli ulcer) in 1958.[165] M. marinum, which has been known since 1926, was isolated from patients with swimming pool granuloma in 1954.[166] Several other mycobacteria have since been identified as pathogens, and other mycobacterial species may be found to cause disease in the future.

The rapid growers have been known as human pathogens since 1938 when Da Costa isolated an organism from a postinjection skin abscess; he named it M. fortuitum.[167] It was later found to be identical with the known frog pathogen M. ranae,[168] which name has since become obsolete.[169]

The current classification of these mycobacteria is found in Table 191-1 and is discussed earlier in this chapter.

Identification of Mycobacteria

As in other infectious diseases, the diagnosis of mycobacterial infection depends on the characterization of the microorganism isolated from the host; various biologic fluids, scrapings, or biopsy specimens may be used for culture. Specimens should be sent to a special laboratory familiar with the culture requirements of mycobacteria as these vary somewhat from those of other microorganisms: correct incubation temperatures, special media, and prolonged times in culture as well as proper identification procedures are needed. It should be noted that several species of mycobacteria are sensitive to sodium, and therefore specimens should not be brought into contact with saline solutions as this may result in false-negative cultures.

Mycobacteria are identified on the basis of their rate of growth, their pigment production, and their enzymatic activities.

Antigens for intradermal skin testing (PPDs) of many of the clinically relevant mycobacterial species have been prepared in analogy to PPD from M. tuberculosis. Although a higher degree of reactivity with a particular PPD seems to correlate with that particular infection,[170] cross-reactivities are frequent, and because the

reagents are not generally available, many workers in the field feel that the use of these PPDs is limited to epidemiologic and clinical studies.[171,172]

Pathology and Pathogenesis

These infections tend to occur as sporadic cases, but certain types of exposure may lead to small community outbreaks. As in M. tuberculosis infection, any organ or organ system may be affected (Table 191-4), but there seems to be much less tendency to dissemination.

Pulmonary infections, which most frequently occur in patients with a ventilatory defect, (e.g., after long-term silica exposure), are pathologically indistinguishable from tuberculosis; however, primary complexes have usually not been identified. Skin and lymph node lesions may be granulomatous, suppurative, or mixed. They can closely mimic tuberculosis, sporotrichosis, or other conditions. Only two organisms, M. ulcerans and M. marinum, cause a disease with a distinct clinical picture.

In contrast to M. tuberculosis, atypical mycobacteria are not usually transmitted by person-to-person contact. They are acquired from environmental sources (water, soil) and their occurrence reflects their natural distribution. These mycobacteria are widely distributed in different environments and are usually commensals or saprophytes rather than pathogens.

In most instances, it is not known what allows these microorganisms to become pathogenic. However, an immunosuppressed state of the host or damage to a particular organ (e.g., in M. kansasii infection of the lung) seem to be required for the development of some types of infection. In recent years, a number of patients have developed infections with fast-growing mycobacteria after minor or major surgical procedures. Infections with atypical mycobacteria usually run a more benign and limited course than those with M. tuberculosis. They are as a rule much less responsive to antituberculous drugs but may be sensitive to other chemotherapeutic agents. The quinolones show activity against several pathogenetic mycobacterial strains in vitro.[150,151] However, adequate studies of mycobacterial drug sensitivities are still scarce.

New mycobacterial pathogens are described from time to time, suggesting that we do not yet appreciate the full pathogenic

TABLE 191-4
Mycobacterial Infections

Species	Organ involvement	
	Skin, subcutis	Lymph nodes, lungs, other
M. tuberculosis-bovis complex (including M. africanum and baciilus Calmette-Guérin)	+	+
M. marinum	+	−
M. ulcerans	+	−
M. kansasii	+	+
M. avium-intracellulare complex (including M. scrofulaceum)	+	+
M. szulgai	+	−
M. simiae	−	−
M. xenopi	−	−
M. haemophilum	+	−
M. fortuitum complex (including M. chelonei)	+	−

potential of this genus. It seems desirable to develop a unifying concept of mycobacterial disease and its treatment, but at the present time our knowledge in this area is not advanced enough to allow us to do so. Thus, skin infections with atypical mycobacteria are discussed here according to their causative organisms.

Skin Infections with Atypical Mycobacteria

Mycobacterium marinum

This mycobacterium occurs in fresh and salt water including swimming pools and fish tanks. It has been identified as the causative organism of a granulomatous eruption in swimmers since the early 1950s.[166] Depending on the source of infection, the disease occurs sporadically[173–175] or in small community outbreaks.[166,176]

Clinical Manifestations The disease begins as a violaceous papule at the site of a trauma about 2 to 3 weeks after inoculation. Patients may present with an ulcerated plaque or a psoriasiform or verrucous lesion at the site of inoculation, usually the hands, feet, elbows, or knees (Fig. 191-16). As a rule, lesions are solitary but occasionally a centripetal spread reminiscent of sporotrichosis develops.[71,176] These lesions frequently heal spontaneously within 1 to 2 years with residual scarring. Sometimes penetration to underlying structures (bursae, joints) may occur,[177] and in endemic areas, skin lesions resembling those of cutaneous leishmaniasis may develop.[178] Regional lymph nodes are usually not involved, but one patient with widespread skin and lymph node disease has been described. Occasionally the lesions are suppurative rather than granulomatous and may be multiple in normal[179] or immunosuppressed hosts.[180] Probably many of the cases thought to represent "inoculation lupus vulgaris" as well as "swimmer's lupus" have in fact been due to *M. marinum* infection.[181]

Histopathology There is a tuberculoid inflammatory infiltrate in the dermis, sometimes with abscess formation.[179,180,182,183]

Diagnosis and Differential Diagnosis As in all mycobacterial diseases, the diagnosis requires a high index of suspicion. An appropriate history (handling of fish, use of swimming pools) and the presence of a tuberculoid granuloma in histopathology are suggestive. Proof of the diagnosis can only be obtained by the demonstration of *M. marinum* in culture from a biopsy specimen. Skin testing with PPD is generally not found to be helpful. Many other granulomatous infectious processes of the skin have to be considered in the differential diagnosis; depending on the geographical area, other mycobacterial infections, blastomycosis, coccidioidomycosis, histoplasmosis, sporotrichosis, as well as nocardiosis, tertiary syphilis, and yaws have to be ruled out. The most common entities in the differential diagnoses are verruca vulgaris and tuberculosis verrucosa cutis and certain cutaneous neoplasms.

Treatment Like most atypical mycobacteria, *M. marinum* is poorly susceptible to antituberculous drugs. Therefore, past treatment usually consisted of surgical excision of skin lesions or in destruction by cryosurgery or electrodesiccation with or without adjuvant antituberculous therapy. Recently, tetracycline, minocycline, and trimethoprim-sulfamethoxazole (TMPS) have been reported to be effective;[184,185] as spontaneous healing commonly occurs, this is somewhat difficult to evaluate in the absence of

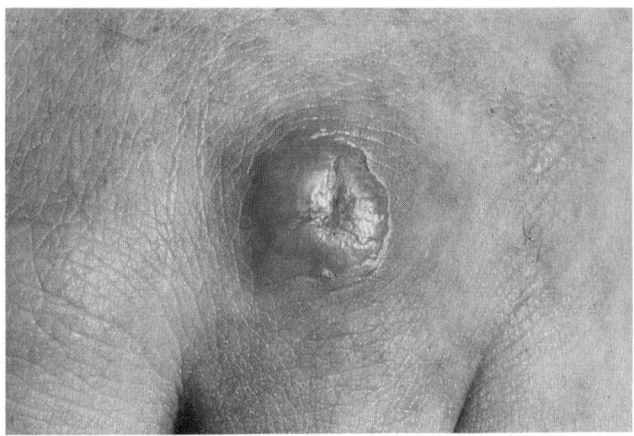

a

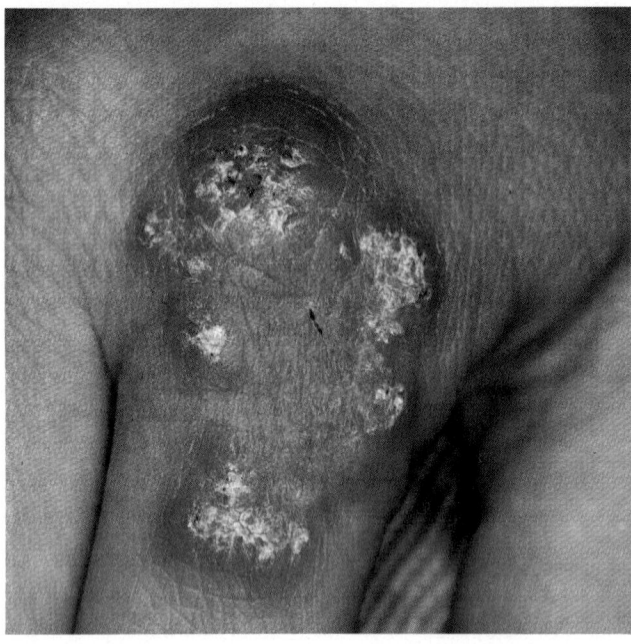

b

FIGURE 191-16 (*a*) *M. marinum* infection on the back of the hand. Granulomatous nodular lesion with central ulceration at the site of inoculation. (*Courtesy of A. Kuhlwein, M.D.*) (*b*) Verrucous, violaceous plaque with central spontaneous clearing occurring at the site of an abrasion sustained within a fish tank. Lesion was caused by M. marinum.

controlled studies. It has been recommended to begin treatment with tetracycline, 2 g per day, or minocycline, 200 mg per day, for 1 to 2 months. If there is no regression of lesions, then rifampin, 600 mg, and ethambutol, 15 mg per kg body weight daily, should be given for 18 months.[2,184]

Mycobacterium ulcerans

The natural habitat of *M. ulcerans* is still not known. It has never been found outside the human body, but the disease is most common in wet, marshy, or swampy areas.[186] It is possibly introduced into skin by microtrauma, probably by pricks or cuts from certain plants.[187] Person-to-person transmission does not seem to occur.

Clinical Manifestations   The disease is found most often in children and young adults; there is a female prevalence. After an incubation period of about 3 months, a painless subcutaneous swelling develops.[188] The nodule gradually enlarges and eventually ulcerates; a blister may develop before ulceration. The ulcer is deeply undermined, and necrotic fat is discharged (Fig. 191-17). Both the nodule and ulcer are painless, and the patient continues to feel well. The lesions may occur anywhere on the body but in adults tend to be limited to the extremities; they may be large, involving a whole limb. The ulceration may persist for months and years and then heal spontaneously. However, this may lead to an appreciable and sometimes disabling degree of scarring and to lymphedema. No lymphadenopathy or constitutional signs appear if the disease is not complicated by bacterial superinfection.

Histopathology   Central necrosis, originating in the interlobular septa of the subcutaneous fat, is surrounded by granulation tissue with giant cells but no typical caseation necrosis or tubercles. Acid-fast organisms can always be demonstrated in tissue sections of the lesions.

Diagnosis and Differential Diagnosis   Diagnosis is confirmed on the basis of histopathology and microbial culture from a subcutane-

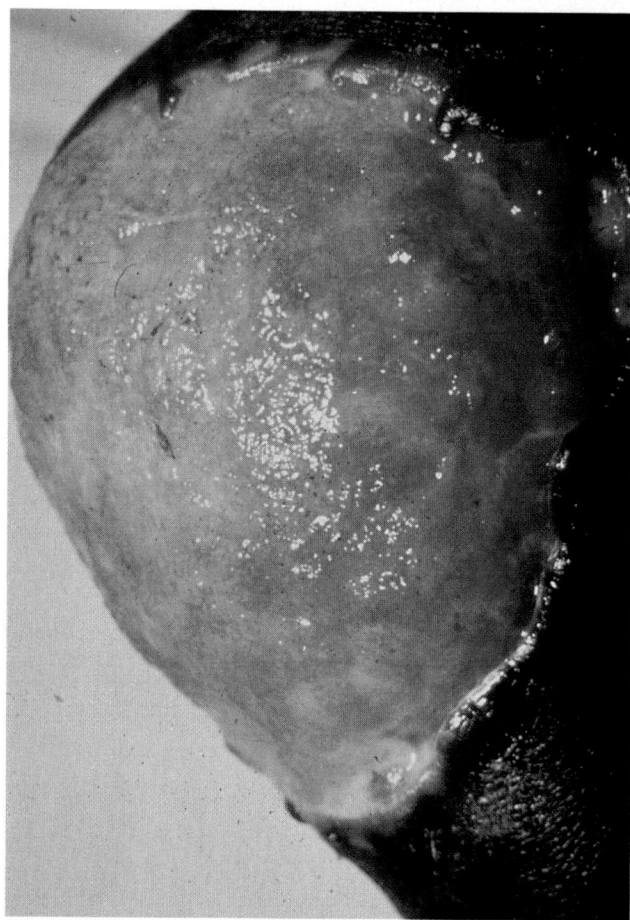

FIGURE 191-17   *M. ulcerans* infection in a child in Uganda. The knee bears an ulcer with an infiltrated undermined margin and a base of necrotic adipose and connective tissue. (*Courtesy of M. Dietrich, M.D.*)

ous node or an ulcer in an individual with a proper history. *M. ulcerans* can be isolated from diseased human tissue; its temperature requirements in culture are quite narrow (32° to 33°C). In culture, *M. ulcerans* produces a toxin that, when injected into the skin of guinea pigs, produces necrosis and ulceration that heals with scar formation after several weeks.[189] Skin testing with mycobacterial antigens is of no diagnostic value. While the lesions progress the patient is always nonreactive to an antigen prepared from *M. ulcerans*.[190] Healing of the lesions is always preceded by reversal of this anergic state. It is not yet known how this reversal is brought about; healing and progression of the ulceration may be seen in the same patient.[1]

The differential diagnosis of *M. ulcerans* infection depends on the stage of the disease. The subcutaneous nodule or node must be distinguished from a variety of processes, such as foreign body granuloma, phycomycosis, nodular fasciitis, panniculitis, nodular vasculitis, sebaceous cysts, or appendageal tumors. When the ulcerative stage is reached, necrotizing cellulitis, blastomycosis and other deep fungus infections, pyoderma grangrenosum, and suppurative panniculitis have to be considered.

Treatment   The treatment of choice is simple excision of the early lesion; when ulceration has developed, wide excision and skin grafting is necessary. Local heat therapy,[191] hyperbaric oxygen,[192] and chemotherapy with rifampin[193] and TMPS have been shown to be of some value. BCG vaccination of exposed populations seems to provide about the same amount of protection as to tuberculosis and to tuberculoid lepra.[194] Clofazimine has been shown to be ineffective.[195]

Mycobacterium kansasii

By lipid analysis this is the atypical mycobacterium most closely related to *M. tuberculosis*.[196] The organism is usually acquired from the environment; it has been found in tap water and in wild and domestic animals. Its natural habitat remains obscure but it may have a source in the urban environment. The disease is endemic in Texas, Louisiana, the Chicago area, California, and Japan. Skin disease due to *M. kansasii* usually occurs in adults with or without an underlying condition, such as Hodgkin's disease, immunosuppression for renal transplantation,[71,197] or AIDS. The route of entry is usually through minor trauma such as a puncture wound.[71]

Clinical Manifestations   *M. kansasii* infection may present in several forms: most frequently, a sporotrichoid condition develops;[198,199] sometimes, the subcutaneous tissues and deep structures are affected and this has resulted in a carpal tunnel syndrome[200] or in joint disease;[71,201,202] an ulcerated plaque may also develop as a metastatic lesion;[203] disseminated disease due to *M. kansasii* infection occurs in immunosuppressed patients[71,201] and such patients have cellulitis and abscesses rather than granulomatous lesions.[204] The most commonly affected organ is the lung, usually in patients with other pulmonary conditions (silicosis, emphysema).[205,206] It may also cause cervical lymphadenopathy. As with *M. tuberculosis*, *M. kansasii* present in nasopharyngeal secretions can lead to periorificial cutaneous infection.[206] These infections usually progress slowly,[207] although a chronic persistent lesion or even spontaneous regression may sometimes occur. Therefore drug therapy should be initiated as soon as the diagnosis is made.

Histopathology *M. kansasii* infection is histopathologically indistinguishable from tuberculosis.

Diagnosis and Differential Diagnosis The diagnosis can only be confirmed by the demonstration of *M. kansasii* in bacterial culture. Histopathology is not useful in ruling out tuberculosis, and skin testing is usually noncontributory. The differential diagnosis includes sporotrichosis, tuberculosis, *M. marinum*, *M. chelonei*, and other granulomatous infections of the skin.

Treatment *M. kansasii* is more susceptible to antituberculous drugs than other atypical mycobacteria, particularly to streptomycin, rifampin, and ethambutol. Multidrug regimens have been of value, and the in vivo response does not always parallel in vitro sensitivities.[2] As in *M. marinum* infection, treatment with minocycline hydrochloride, 200 mg daily, has resulted in complete resolution of sporotrichoid *M. kansasii* infection in one case,[208] but more extensive studies of this regimen are not yet available. In localized skin disease or in cervical lymphadenitis, surgical excision should be performed.

Mycobacterium scrofulaceum

This organism is widely distributed and has been isolated from tap water, soil, and other environmental sources. Infection probably occurs in children by accidental infestation or inhalation while playing.

Clinical Manifestations The usual manifestation of *M. scrofulaceum* infection is cervical lymphadenitis in young children, mainly between the ages of 1 to 3 years. Submandibular and submaxillary nodes are usually involved rather than the tonsillar and anterior cervical nodes characteristic for *M. tuberculosis* infection. The disease is frequently unilateral. There are no constitutional symptoms except mild pain in the neck, but nodes enlarging slowly over several weeks, eventually ulcerating and draining, are seen. There is generally no evidence of lung or other organ involvement[209]; however, in older individuals with preexisting lung disease pulmonary infection may rarely occur, and, very rarely, various internal organs may be affected, usually in patients with underlying malignant disease. Usually, however, the disease is benign and self-limited.

Histopathology *M. scrofulaceum* lymphadenitis is histopathologically indistinguishable from tuberculous disease.

Diagnosis and Differential Diagnosis Unilateral cervical lymphadenitis in a young child with a normal chest roentgenogram should suggest this diagnosis. Skin testing with PPDs is usually negative. The diagnosis needs confirmation by bacterial culture from a biopsy specimen. Differential diagnoses include all causes of cervical lymphadenopathy, both infectious and neoplastic, which must be ruled out by proper serologic, hematologic, and histopathologic investigations.

Treatment *M. scrofulaceum* is not very sensitive to antituberculous drugs; the treatment of choice for cutaneous lymph node disease is surgical excision. For more widespread disease, combinations of antituberculous drugs have to be tried until results from bacterial sensitivity testing are available.

Mycobacterium avium-intracellulare

This species complex encompasses organisms with a wide variety of microbiologic and pathogenic properties. Well over 20 subtypes can be separated by immunologic techniques,[210] although this is not necessary for clinical purposes.

They are usually grouped together with *M. scrofulaceum* in the so-called MAIS (*M. avium-intracellulare-scrofulaceum*) complex but are separated here for clinical reasons. Whereas *M. scrofulaceum* produces only a benign, self-limited lymphadenopathy with no organ involvement, *M. avium-intracellulare* usually causes lung disease or, less frequently, osteomyelitis. It may also cause a cervical lymphadenitis with sinus formation that is clinically indistinguishable from tuberculous scrofuloderma.

Clinical Manifestations Primary skin disease due to *M. avium-intracellulare* has been reported in rare instances. A chronic, slowly progressive skin condition of many years' duration has been described. In one culture-proven case, multiple lesions consisting of erythematous borders surrounding ulcers with yellow crusted bases had spread to involve 20 percent of the body surface.[211] A patient on steroid therapy developed a painless, scaling, yellow plaque on his right forearm that histopathologically resembled lepromatous leprosy but yielded *M. avium* on culture[212]; a third patient merely had a small ulcer with an erythematous border and a yellow "shaggy" base on the dorsum of his left foot.[213] Sometimes, skin involvement occurs secondary to disseminated infection with *M. avium-intracellulare*.[5] Skin lesions have included generalized cutaneous ulcerations, multiple cutaneous granulomas, infiltrated erythematous lesions on the extremities, pustular lesions, or soft-tissue swelling. *M. avium-intracellulare* infections are important in AIDS patients.[214]

Histopathology This shows noncaseating tuberculoid granulomas. Acid-fast bacilli can be found within giant cells and extracellularly.

Diagnosis and Differential Diagnosis Demonstration of *M. avium-intracellulare* in bacterial culture is necessary to establish the diagnosis. The differential diagnosis includes all chronic granulomatous conditions of the skin.

Treatment Where feasible, surgical treatment of *M. avium-intracellulare* infection is advisable as the organism seems to be poorly susceptible to chemotherapeutic agents. If dissemination of the disease does not allow curative surgery, combination therapy with multiple antituberculous drugs should be given according to the guidelines of the National Consensus Conference.[156] A synergistic effect of several antituberculous drug combinations against *M. avium-intracellulare* in vitro has been shown.[215] Experience with AIDS patients suggests that drug regimens including rifamycin (ansamycin) and clofazimine may be effective,[216,217] and ciprofloxacin has been shown to be active against some strains.[150]

Mycobacterium szulgai

The development of cervical lymphadenitis as well as cellulitis and draining nodules and plaques has been associated with *M. szulgai*.[218] The organism has also been found to cause bursitis and pneumonia; it is more susceptible to antituberculous drugs than most other atypical mycobacteria.

Mycobacterium haemophilum

This is an organism requiring media supplemented with hemin or ferric ammonium citrate in culture.[219] Not much is known about its natural habitat. It was identified as the causative organism of a subcutaneous granulomatous eruption in several immunosuppressed patients in Sydney, Australia.[219–221] Histopathologically, there was a mixed polymorphonuclear and granulomatous inflammation, the so-called dimorphic inflammatory response, with no caseation necrosis, similar to that seen in the *M. fortuitum* complex infection. The organism may be sensitive to rifampin and *p*-aminosalicylic acid, but further observations of such infections are required.

Mycobacterium fortuitum Complex

This is the only species of rapid-growing mycobacteria that has so far been found to cause human disease. The species complex includes *M. chelonei,* which is the more common pathogen, and *M. fortuitum. M. chelonei* can be divided into two subspecies, *M. chelonei chelonei,* found predominantly in Europe, and *M. chelonei abscessus,* the more common variant in Africa and the United States. *M. fortuitum* occurs in the three biotypes A, B, and C, of which type A is the most important pathogen. These organisms seem to be widely distributed and can commonly be found in soil and in water supplies. Contamination of various materials, including surgical supplies, occurs and does not always result in clinical disease.[222]

Clinical Manifestations   Infection usually follows a puncture wound or a surgical procedure. In a large series it was found that cutaneous disease accounted for 59 percent of 125 cases; of these, 54 percent were due to surgery and 46 percent to accidental inoculation.[223] When the skin and subcutaneous tissues are affected, the disease manifests itself as a painful red, infiltrated area at the site of inoculation; there are no signs of dissemination and no constitutional symptoms. This type of infection has followed augmentation mammoplasty,[224] median sternotomy,[225,226] and a variety of other procedures usually involving percutaneous catheterization. Cold postinjection abscesses, especially when occurring in the tropics, may also be due to fast-growing mycobacteria. The source seems to be contaminated injection solutions. It has been suggested that so-called fixation abscesses, found in tuberculosis patients after intramuscular injections, have frequently also been due to inoculation of *M. fortuitum* complex organisms.[227]

Primary cutaneous inoculation through skin injuries is found in all age groups and in persons without immunosuppression. The lesion presents as a dark red, infiltrated node, often with abscess formation and draining a clear liquid. Disseminated disease involving the skin also occurs, usually in immunologically compromised patients. The skin lesions consist of multiple recurring abscesses on the extremities or in a generalized maculopapular eruption. Other manifestations of *M. fortuitum* complex infection include pneumonitis or osteomyelitis, lymphadenitis, and postsurgical endocarditis.

Histopathology   The lesions are characterized by the simultaneous occurrence of polymorphonuclear microabscesses and granuloma formation with foreign body–type giant cells, the so-called dimorphic inflammatory response. There is usually necrosis but no casea-tion. Acid-fast bacilli may occasionally be demonstrated within microabscesses.

Diagnosis and Treatment   Organisms of the *M. fortuitum* complex, including *M. fortuitum* and *M. chelonei* with their subspecies, may be identified by special laboratories. This is not only of epidemiologic interest: *M. fortuitum* is more susceptible to amikacin, doxycycline, and sulfonamides than *M. chelonei,* whereas subspecies of the latter have markedly different susceptibilities to cefoxitin, erythromycin, and tobramycin. Thus, a rational treatment has to await the results of identification of the organism and in vitro susceptibility testing.

References

1. Grange JM: Mycobacteria and the skin. *Int J Dermatol:* **21**:497, 1982
2. Yeager H Jr: Other mycobacterium species, in *Principles and Practice of Infectious Diseases.* 2d ed, edited by GL Mandell et al. New York, Wiley, 1985, Chap. 207
3. Wolinsky E: Nontuberculous mycobacteria and associated disease. *Am Rev Respir Dis* **119**:107, 1979
4. Youmans GP: Relation between delayed hypersensitivity and immunity in tuberculosis. *Am Rev Respir Dis* **111**:109, 1975
5. Rook GAW, Stanford JL: The relevance to protection of three forms of delayed skin-test response evoked by *M. leprae* and other mycobacteria in mice. Correlation with the classical work in the guinea pig. *Parasite Immunol* **1**:111, 1979
6. Kardjito T, Grange JM: Immunological and clinical features of smear-positive pulmonary tuberculosis in East Java. *Tubercle* **61**:231, 1980
7. Runyon EH: Pathogenic mycobacteria. *Adv Tuberc Res* **14**:235, 1965
8. Runyon EH: Ten mycobacterial pathogens. *Tubercle* **55**:235, 1974
9. American Lung Association: *Diagnostic Standards and Classification of Tuberculosis and other Mycobacterial Diseases.* New York, American Lung Association/American Thoracic Society, 1974
10. Approved lists of bacterial names: Mycobacteria. *Int J System Bacteriol* **30**:324, 1980
11. Koch R: Die Ätiologie der Tuberculose. *Klin Wochenschr* **19**:221, 1882
12. Moschella SL: Mycobacterial infections of the skin, in *Dermatology Update, Reviews for Physicians,* edited by SL Moschella. New York, Elsevier, 1979, p 45
13. Pandhi RK et al: Cutaneous tuberculosis—a clinical and investigative study. *Indian J Dermatol* **22**:99, 1977
14. Sharma RC et al: Microbiology of cutaneous tuberculosis. *Tubercle* **56**:324, 1975
15. Wong KO et al: Tuberculosis of the skin in Hong Kong. (A review of 160 cases). *Br J Dermatol* **80**:424, 1968
16. Jung HD, Holzegel K: Klinik der Hauttuberkulose heute. *Dtsch Dermatol* **30**:365, 1982
17. Morrison JGL, Fourie ED: The papulonecrotic tuberculide. From Arthus reaction to lupus vulgaris. *Br J Dermatol* **91**:263, 1974
18. Sehgal VN et al: An appraisal of epidemiologic, clinical-bacteriologic, histopathologic and immunologic parameters in cutaneous tuberculosis. *Int J Dermatol* **26**:521, 1987
19. Spitzer R: Geographische Verteilung der Hautkrankheiten, in *Handbuch der Haut- und Geschlechtskrankheiten,* Ergänzungswerk, vol VIII, edited by J Jadassohn. Berlin, Springer-Verlag, 1967, p 1
20. Jensen KA, Frimodt-Möller J: Studies on the types of tubercle bacilli isolated from man. II. Strains with attenuated virulence. *Acta Tuberc Scand* **10**:83, 1936

21. Youmans GP et al: The biologic and clinical basis of infectious diseases, in *Tuberculosis,* edited by GP Youmans. Philadelphia, Saunders, 1975, p 371

22. Simonds B: *Tuberculosis in Twins.* London, Pitman, 1963

23. Drutz OJ, Graybill JR: Infectious diseases—tuberculosis, in *Basic and Clinical Immunology,* 6th ed, edited by DP Stites, JD Stobo, JV Wells. Norwalk, CT, Appleton/Lange, 1987, p 557

24. Rich AR: *The Pathogenesis of Tuberculosis,* 2d ed. Springfield, IL, Thomas, 1951

25. Koch R: Weitere Mitteilung über das Tuberculin. *Dtsch Med Wochenschr* 17:1189, 1891

26. von Pirquet C: Allergie. *Münch Med Wochenschr* 53:1457, 1906

27. Arnason BG, Waksman BH: Tuberculin sensitivity: Immunologic considerations. *Adv Tuberc Res* 13:1, 1964

28. Turk JL: *Frontiers of Biology,* vol IV, *Delayed Hypersensitivity.* North-Holland Research Monographs, edited by A Neuberger, EL Tatum. Amsterdam, North-Holland, 1967

29. Urbach F et al: Passive transfer of tuberculin sensitivity to patients with sarcoidosis. *N Engl J Med* 247:794, 1952

30. Good RA et al: Immunological deficiency diseases. Agammaglobulinemia, hypogammaglobulinemia, Hodgkin's disease, and sarcoidosis. *Prog Allergy* 6:187, 1962

31. Seibert FB: Progress in the chemistry of tuberculin. *Adv Tuberc Res* 3:1, 1950

32. Sbarbaro JA: Tuberculosis. *Med Clin North Am* 64:417, 1980

33. Edwards LB, Palmer CE: Epidemiological studies of tuberculin sensitivity. I. Preliminary results with purified derivatives prepared from atypical acid-fast organisms. *Am J Hyg* 68:213, 1958

34. Stanford JL, Grange JM: The nature and structure of species as applied to mycobacteria. *Tubercle* 55:143, 1974

35. Stanford JL, Rook GAW: Environmental mycobacteria and immunization with BCG, in *Medical Microbiology,* vol 2, edited by CS Easmon, J Jelsaszewicz. London, New York, Academic, 1983, p 43

36. Editorial: New tuberculosis. *Lancet* 1:199, 1984

37. Dienes L, Mallory TB: Histological studies of hypersensitive reactions. I. The contrast between the histological responses in the tuberculin (allergic) type and the anaphylactic type of skin reactions. *Am J Pathol* 8:689, 1932

38. Laporte R: Contribution à l'étude des bacilles paratuberculeux. II. Histo-cytologic des lésions paratuberculeuses. *Ann Inst Pasteur (Paris)* 65:415, 1940

39. Gell PGH, Hinde IT: The histology of the tuberculin reaction and its modification by cortisone. *Br J Exp Pathol* 32:516, 1951

40. Raffel S: The mechanism involved in acquired immunity to tuberculosis, in *Symposium on Experimental Tuberculosis: Bacillus and Host,* Ciba Foundation Symposium, edited by GEW Wolstenholme, MP Cameron. London, Churchill, 1955, p 261

41. Blacklock JWS, Williana JR: The localization of tuberculosis infection at the site of injury. *J Pathol Bacteriol* 74:119, 1957

42. Lucas SB: Histopathology of leprosy and tuberculosis—an overview. *Br Med Bull* 44:584, 1988

43. Ghon A, Kudlich H: Die Eintrittspforten der Infektion vom Standpunkte der pathologischen Anatomie, in *Handbuch der Kindertuberkulose,* edited by S Engel, CV Pirquet. Leipzig, Thieme Verlag, 1930, p 20

44. Miller FJW: Recognition of primary tuberculous infection of skin and mucosae. *Lancet* 1:5, 1953

45. Fischer I, Orkin M: Primary tuberculosis of the skin. Primary complex. *JAMA* 195:314, 1966

46. O'Leary PA, Harrison MW: Inoculation tuberculosis. *Arch Dermatol Syphilol* 44:371, 1941

47. Holt LE: Tuberculosis acquired through ritual circumcision. *JAMA* 61:99, 1913

48. Rytel MW et al: Primary cutaneous inoculation tuberculosis. *Am Rev Respir Dis* 102:264, 1970

49. Sahn SA, Pierson DJ: Primary cutaneous inoculation drug-resistant tuberculosis. *Am J Med* 57:676, 1974

50. Goette DK et al: Primary inoculation tuberculosis of the skin. Prosector's paronychia. *Arch Dermatol* 114:567, 1978

51. Koch H: Die Tuberculose des Säuglingsalters. *Ergeb Inn Med Kinderheilkd* 14:99, 1915

52. Wolff E: Über Zirkumzisionstuberkulose. *Berlin Klin Wochenschr* 58:1531, 1921

53. Strad S: Tubercular primary lesion on penis—cancer of penis. Venereal tuberculosis. *Acta Derm Venereol (Stockh)* 26:461, 1946

54. Bjørnstadt R: Tuberculosis primary infection of genitalia. *Acta Derm Venereol (Stockh)* 27:106, 1947

55. Heilman KM, Muschenheim C: Primary cutaneous tuberculosis resulting from mouth to mouth respirations. *N Engl J Med* 273:1035, 1965

56. Michelson HE: The primary complex of tuberculosis of the skin. *Arch Dermatol Syphilol* 32:589, 1935

57. Heykock JB, Noble TC: Four cases of syringe transmitted tuberculosis. *Tubercle* 42:25, 1961

58. Valledor T et al: Tuberculosis primaria de la piel en la infancia. *Rev Cutan Pediatria* 26:147, 1954

59. Miller FJW, Cashman JM: The natural history of peripheral tuberculosis lymphadenitis associated with a visible primary focus. *Lancet* 1:1286, 1955

60. Duken J: Über Verlaufsarten der extrapulmonalen Primärtuberkulose. *Z Kinderheilkd* 55:687, 1933

61. Mitchell PC: Tuberculosis verrucosa cutis among Chinese in Hong Kong. *Br J Dermatol* 66:444, 1954

62. Montgomery H: Histopathology of various types of cutaneous tuberculosis. *Arch Dermatol Syphilol* 35:698, 1937

63. Getzler NA et al: Atypical cutaneous tuberculosis. *Arch Dermatol* 84:439, 1961

64. Horwitz O: Lupus vulgaris cutis in Denmark 1895–1954. Its relation to the epidemiology of other forms of tuberculosis. *Acta Tuberc Scand* (suppl) 49:1, 1960

65. Kalkoff KW: *Die Tuberkulose der Haut.* Stuttgart, Thieme Verlag, 1950

66. Proppe A, Wagner G: Die Altersdisposition bei Lupus vulgaris. *Z Hautkr Geschlechtskr* 14:376, 1953

67. Marcussen PV: Lupus vulgaris following BCG vaccination. *Br J Dermatol* 66:121, 1954

68. Horwitz O: The localization of lupus vulgaris of the skin. *Acta Tuberc Scand* (suppl) 47:175, 1959

69. Ustvedt HJ, Ostensen IW: The relation between tuberculosis of the skin and primary infection. *Tubercle* 32:36, 1951

70. Brown FS et al: Cutaneous tuberculosis. *J Am Acad Dermatol* 6:101, 1982

71. Beyt BE et al: Cutaneous mycobacteriosis: Analysis of 34 cases with a new classification of the disease. *Medicine (Baltimore)* 60:95, 1980

72. Sundt H: A case of lupus disseminatus (postexanthematic miliary tuberculosis cutis). *Br J Dermatol* 37:316, 1925

73. Horwitz O, Christensen S: Numerical estimates of the extent of the lesion in lupus vulgaris cutis and their significance for epidemiologic and clinical research. *Am Rev Respir Dis* 82:862, 1960

74. Volk R: Tuberculose der Haut, in *Handbuch der Haut- und Geschlechtskrankheiten,* vol x/1, edited by J Jadassohn. Berlin, Springer, 1931, p 1

75. Hekele K, Seyss R: Die malignen Tumoren in Lupo vulgari. *Hautarzt* 2:349, 1951

76. Clasen K, Horwitz O: The morbidity from pulmonary tuberculosis in patients suffering from extrapulmonary tuberculosis disease, lupus vulgaris cutis. *Adv Tuberc Res* 10:237, 1960

77. Kutschera-Aichbergen H: Die Bekämpfung schwerer Lungentuberculose durch künstlich erzeugte Hauttuberculose. *Wien Klin Wochenschr* 50:1544, 1937

78. Kalkoff KW: Die Lungentuberkulosesterblichkeit bei Lupuskranken im Vergleich zu Hautgesunden. Gleichzeitig ein Beitrag zum Altersaufbau und zum Durchschnittslebensalter der westfälischen Lupuskranken. *Arch Dermatol Syphilol* 186:144, 1948

79. Amezquita R: Tuberculosis cutanea. Aspectos clinicos y epidémiológicos en Mexico. *Acta Leprologica* **16**:1, 1963

80. Editorial: Scrofula today. *Lancet* **1**:335, 1983

81. Chien JTT, Wiggins, ML: Self-inoculation with *M. tuberculosis* and *P. aeruginosa* by a diabetic woman. *Am Rev Tuberc* **69**:818, 1954

82. Michelson HE: Scrofuloderma gummosa (tuberculosis colliquativa). *Arch Syphilol* **10**:565, 1924

83. Sola Casa MA et al: Carpal tunnel syndrome as the first manifestation of subcutaneous tuberculosis. *J Am Acad Dermatol* (in press)

84. Kleid JJ, Rosenberg RF: Pulmonary tuberculosis with noncommunicating chest wall abscess. *N Y State J Med* **70**:2993, 1970

85. Munt PW: Miliary tuberculosis in the chemotherapy era: With a clinical review of 69 American adults. *Medicine (Baltimore)* **51**:139, 1971

86. Stead WW, Bates JH: Evidence of a "silent" bacillemia in primary tuberculosis. *Ann Intern Med* **74**:559, 1971

87. Glynn KP: Isolated subcutaneous abscesses caused by *Mycobacterium tuberculosis*. *Am Rev Respir Dis* **99**:86, 1969

88. Bryant JC: Oral tuberculosis. *Am Rev Tuberc* **39**:738, 1939

89. Sheingold MA, Sheingold H: Oral tuberculosis. *Oral Surg* **4**:239, 1951

90. Katz HL: Tuberculosis of the tongue. *Q Bull Seaview Hosp* **6**:239, 1941

91. Engleman WR, Putney FJ: Tuberculosis of the tongue. *Trans Am Acad Ophthalmol Otolaryngol* **76**:1384, 1972

92. McAndrew PG et al: Miliary tuberculosis presenting with multifocal oral lesions. *Br Med J* **1**:1320, 1976

93. Weaver RA: Tuberculosis of the tongue. *JAMA* **235**:2418, 1978

94. Fisher JR: Miliary tuberculosis with unusual cutaneous manifestation. *JAMA* **238**:241, 1977

95. Platou RV, Lennox RH: Tuberculous cutaneous complexes in children. *Am Rev Tuberc* **74**(2, part 11): 160, 1956

96. McCray MK, Esterly NB: Cutaneous eruptions in congenital tuberculosis. *Arch Dermatol* **117**:460, 1981

97. Schermer DR et al: Tuberculosis cutis miliaris acuta generalisata. *Arch Dermatol* **99**:64, 1969

98. Leiner C, Spieler F: Über disseminierte Hauttuberbulosen im Kindesalter. *Erg Inn Med Kinderheilkd* **7**:59, 1911

99. Lees AW, Munro ID: Skin lesions and deafness in disseminated tuberculosis. *Br Med J* **1**:496, 1954

100. Kurnedy C, Knowles GK: Miliary tuberculosis presenting with skin lesions. *Br Med J* **3**:356, 1975

101. Rouillon A, Waaler H: BCG vaccination and epidemiological situation. A decision making approach to the use of BCG. *Adv Tuberc Res:* **19**:65, 1976

102. Ten Dam HG, Hitze KL: Does BCG vaccination protect the newborn and young infant? *Bull World Health Organ* **58**:37, 1980

103. Anonymous: BCG vaccination in the newborn. *Br Med J* **281**:1445, 1980

104. Tuberculosis Prevention Trial. Trial of BCG vaccines in South India for tuberculosis prevention: First report. *Bull World Health Organ* **57**:819, 1979

105. Curtis HM et al: Incidence of childhood tuberculosis after neonatal BCG vaccination. *Lancet* **1**:145, 1984

106. Dostrovsky A, Sagher F: Dermatological complications of BCG vaccination. *Br J Dermatol* **75**:181, 1963

107. Jörgensen BB, Horwitz O: Dermatological complications of BCG vaccination. *Acta Tuberc Scand* **32**:179, 1956

108. Horwitz O, Meyer J: The safety record of BCG vaccination and untoward reactions observed after vaccination. *Adv Tuberc Res* **8**:245, 1957

109. Waaler H, Rouillon A: BCG vaccination policies according to the epidemiological situation. *Bull Int Union Tuberc* **29**:166, 1974

110. Izumi AK, Matsunaga J: BCG vaccine-induced lupus vulgaris. *Arch Dermatol* **118**:171, 1982

111. Maguire A: Lupus murinus. The discovery, diagnosis and treatment of seventeen cases of lupus murinus. *Br J Dermatol* **80**:419, 1968

112. Aungst CW et al: Complications of BCG vaccination in neoplastic disease. *Ann Intern Med* **82**:666, 1975

113. Passwell J et al: Fatal disseminated BCG infection. An investigation of the immunodeficiency. *Am J Dis Child* **130**:433, 1976

114. Rosenthal SR: *BCG Vaccine: Tuberculosis-Cancer*. Littleton, CO, PSG Publishing, 1980

115. Darier MJ: Les "tuberculides" cutanées. *Ann Dermatol Syphiligr (Paris)* **7**:1431, 1896

116. Smith NP et al: Lichen scrofulosorum. A report of four cases. *Br J Dermatol* **94**:319, 1976

117. Graham Brown RAC, Sarkany I: Lichen scrofulosorum with tuberculous dactylitis. *Br J Dermatol* **103**:561, 1980

118. Philippson L: Über Phlebitis nodularis necrotisans. *Arch Dermatol Syphilol* **55**:215, 1901

119. Whitfield A: A case of unusual papulonecrotic tuberculide. *Br J Dermatol* **25**:168, 1913

120. Tanimura C: Über papulonekrotische Tuberkulide und über den positiven Befund von Tuberkelbacillen. *Arch Dermatol Syphilol* **146**:335, 1924

121. Dittrich O: Über den Tuberkelbazillennachweis bei Tuberkuliden. *Dermatol Wochenschr* **84**:734, 1927

122. Montgomery H et al: Nodular vascular diseases of the legs. *JAMA* **128**:335, 1945

123. Eberhartinger C: Das Problem des Erythema induratum Bazin. Ein Beitrag zur Kenntnis der rezidivierenden subakuten nodösen Gefässprozesse am Unterschenkel. *Arch Klin Exp Dermatol* **217**:196, 1963

124. Miescher G: Über katamnestische Untersuchungen bei Fällen mit Tuberkulid. *Dermatologica* **110**:23, 1955

125. Flegel H: Die Stellung des Tuberculids im Rahmen der Tuberkulose. *Dermatol Wochenschr* **145**:609, 1962

126. Strauss H: Katamnestische Untersuchungen von Fällen mit Tuberkulid. *Arch Dermatol Syphilol* **198**:417, 1954

127. Sonck CE: Focal infections and tuberculids. *Acta Derm Venerol (Stockh)* **2**:195, 1960

128. Iden DL et al: Papulonecrotic tuberculid secondary to mycobacterium bovis. *Arch Dermatol* **114**:564, 1978

129. Formia FE et al: Isoniazid (nydrazid) in the treatment of cutaneous diseases: Cutaneous tuberculosis, leprosy, sarcoidosis and miscellaneous dermatoses. *Arch Dermatol Syphilol* **68**:536, 1953

130. Rauschkolb JW: Tuberculosis of the skin. *Arch Dermatol Syphilol* **29**:398, 1934

131. Leiner C, Spieler F: Zum Nachweis der bazillären Ätiologie der Folliklis. *Arch Dermatol Syphilol* **81**:221, 1906

132. Hempelmann TC: Frequency of tuberculides in infancy and childhood and their relation to prognosis. *Arch Pediatr* **34**:362, 1917

133. Irgang S: Superficial papulonecrotic tuberculid in the Negro. *Arch Dermatol Syphilol* **47**:627, 1943

134. Hellerström S: Papulo-nekrotische Tuberkulide mit Lokalisation an der Glans Penis. *Acta Derm Venereol (Stockh)* **23**:170, 1942

135. Stevanovic DV: Papulonecrotic tuberculids of glans penis. *Arch Dermatol* **78**:760, 1958

136. Szymanski FJ: Pityriasis lichenoides et varioliformis acuta: Histopathological evidence that it is an entity distinct from parapsoriasis. *Arch Dermatol* **79**:7, 1959

137. Montgomery H: *Dermatopathology*. New York, Harper & Row, 1967

138. Wilkinson DS: The vascular basis of some nodular eruptions of the legs. *Br J Dermatol* **66**:201, 1954

139. Parish WE: Microbial antigens in vasculitis, in *Vasculitis*, edited by K Wolff and RK Winkelmann. London, Lloyd Luke, 1980, p 129

140. Michelson HE: Inflammatory nodose lesions of the lower leg. *Arch Dermatol Syphilol* **66**:327, 1952

141. Laymon CW, Michelson HE: The micropapular tuberculid. *Arch Dermatol Syphilol* **42**:625, 1940

142. Bologa EI: Betrachungen zur Nosologie, Pathogenese und Erkennung der rosacea-ähnlichen Tuberculide von Lewandowsky sowie deren Beziehungen zur Rosacea. *Hautarzt* **12**:508, 1961

143. Peck SM: Beitrag zur Lehre vom Lupus miliaris disseminatus faciei. *Arch Dermatol Syphilol* **158**:545, 1929

144. Simon N: Ist der Lupus miliaris disseminatus tuberkulöser Ätiologie? *Hautarzt* **26**:625, 1975

145. Lewandowsky F: Über rosacea-ähnliche Tuberkulide des Gesichtes. *Korresp-Bl Schweiz Ärz* **47**:1280, 1917

146. Ockuly OE, Montgomery H: Lichenoid tuberculid. A clinical and histopathologic study. *J Invest Dermatol* **14**:415, 1950

147. Kowalenko W: Über ein lichenoides Exanthem unklarer Pathogenese. (Zur Kenntnis des "Lichenoid Tuberculid" von Montgomery). *Dermatol Wochenschr* **147**:13, 1963

148. Schuhmachers R: 2 Fälle eines lichenoiden Tuberculids (= Lichen scrophulosorum). *Hautarzt* **18**:81, 1967

149. Fox W, Mitchinson DA: Short course chemotherapy for pulmonary tuberculosis. *Am Rev Respir Dis* **111**:845, 1975

150. Mandell GL, Sande MA: Antimicrobial agents. Drugs used in the chemotherapy of tuberculosis and leprosy, in *The Pharmacological Basis of Therapeutics,* 8th ed, edited by A Goodman Gilman et al. New York, Pergamon, 1990, p 1146

151. Leysen DC et al: Mycobacteria and the quinolones. *Antimicrob Agents Chemother* **33**:1, 1989

152. Van Caekenberghe D: Comparative in vitro activities of ten fluoroquinolones and fusidic acid against *Mycobacterium* spp. *J Antimicrob Chemother* **26**:381, 1990

153. Pitt FW: Tuberculosis prevention and therapy, in *Current Concepts of Infectious Diseases,* edited by EW Hook et al. New York, Wiley, 1977, p 181

154. British Thoracic and Tuberculosis Association: Short-course chemotherapy in pulmonary tuberculosis. *Lancet* **1**:119, 1975

155. Sande MA, Mandell GL: Antimicrobial agents. The aminoglycosides, in *The Pharmacological Basis of Therapeutics,* 6th ed, edited by A Goodman, LS Goodman, A Gilman. New York, MacMillan, 1980, p 1162

156. Iseman MD, Sbarbaro UA: Consensus statements. *Arch Intern Med* **145**:630, 1985

157. East African/British Medical Research Councils: Controlled Clinical trial of four short-course (6 months) regimens of chemotherapy for treatment of pulmonary tuberculosis. *Lancet* **2**:237, 1974

158. East African/British Medical Research Councils: Controlled clinical trial of four short-course (6 months) regimens of chemotherapy for treatment of pulmonary tuberculosis. *Lancet* **2**:1100, 1974

159. Hentschel V: Vorschläge für eine Standardtherapie der Hauttuberculose. *Derm Monatsschr* **160**:1009, 1974

160. Meyer-Rohn J, Schulz KH: Experimentelle und klinishe Erfahrungen bei der Isonicotinsäurehydrazid-Therapie der Hauttuberkulose. *Arch Dermatol Syphilol* **197**:160, 1954

161. Krakauer R: Die Behandlung der Hauttuberkulose mit INH (Rimifon) in den Jahren 1952–1959 an der Züricher Dermatologischen Klinik. *Dermatologica* **120**:323, 1960

162. Brück D, Westbeck-Carlsson AM: Treatment of lupus vulgaris with INH exclusively. *Acta Derm Venereol (Stockh)* **44**:223, 1964

163. Ehring F: Die gegenwärtige Epidemiologie und Bakteriologie der Hauttuberkulose in der Bundesrepublik Deutschland, in *Proceedings of the 13th International Congress of Dermatology,* vol. II, edited by W Jadassohn, CG Schirren. New York, Springer, 1968, p 1308

164. MacCullum P et al: New mycobacterial infection in man: Clinical aspects. *J Pathol Bacteriol* **60**:93, 1948

165. Clancey JK et al: Mycobacterial skin ulcers in Uganda. *Lancet* **2**:951, 1961

166. Linell F, Norden A: *Mycobacterium balnei.* A new acid-fast bacillus occurring in swimming pools and capable of producing skin lesions in humans. *Acta Tuberc Scand* (suppl): **33**:1, 1954

167. Da Costa Cruz J: "*Mycobacterium fortuitum,*" un novo bacilo acido resistente patogenico par o homem. *Acta Medica Rio de Janeiro* **1**:297, 1938

168. Kuster E: Über Kaltblütentuberkulose. *Münch Med Wochenschr* **52**:57, 1905

169. Runyon EH: Conservation of the specific epithet fortuitum in the name of the organism known as *Mycobacterium fortuitum* da Costa Cruz. *Int J System Bacteriol* **22**:50, 1972

170. Marmorstein BL, Scheinhorn DJ: The role of nontuberculous mycobacterial skin test antigens in the diagnosis of mycobacterial infections. *Chest* **67**:320, 1975

171. Fogan L: Atypical mycobacteria: Their clinical, laboratory, and epidemiologic significance. *Medicine (Baltimore)* **49**:243, 1970

172. Hsu KHK: Diagnostic skin test for mycobacterial infections in man. *Chest* **64**:1, 1973

173. Brown J et al: Infection of the skin by *Mycobacterium marinum:* Report of five cases. *Can Med Assoc J* **117**:912, 1977

174. Heineman HS et al: Fish tank granuloma: A hobby hazard. *Arch Intern Med* **130**:121, 1972

175. Jänner M et al: Infektion mit *Mycobacterium marinum* aus einem Aquarium. *Hautarzt* **34**:635, 1983

176. Philpott JA et al: Swimming pool granuloma. *Arch Dermatol* **88**:158, 1963

177. Jolly HW Jr, Seabury JK: Infections with *Mycobacterium marinum. Arch Dermatol* **106**:32, 1972

178. Even-Paz Z et al: *Mycobacterium marinum* skin infections mimicking cutaneous leishmaniasis. *Br J Dermatol* **94**:435, 1976

179. King AJ et al: Disseminated cutaneous *Mycobacterium marinum* infection. *Arch Dermatol* **119**:268, 1983

180. Gombert ME et al: Disseminated *Mycobacterium marinum* infection after renal transplantation. *Ann Intern Med* **94**:486, 1981

181. Hellerstrom S: Collected cases of inoculation lupus vulgaris. *Acta Derm Venereol (Stockh)* **31**:194, 1951

182. Schaefer WB, Bavis CL: A bacteriologic and histopathologic study of skin granulomas due to *Mycobacterium balnei. Am Rev Respir Dis* **84**:837, 1961

183. Marsch WC et al: The ultrastructure of *Mycobacterium marinum* granuloma in man. *Arch Dermatol Res* **262**:205, 1978

184. Wolinsky E et al: Sporotrichoid *M. marinum* infection treated with rifampin-ethambutol. *Am Rev Respir Dis* **105**:964, 1972

185. Izumi AK et al: *M. marinum* infections treated with tetracycline. *Arch Dermatol* **113**:1067, 1977

186. Barker DJ: Epidemiology of *Mycobacterium ulcerans* infection. *Trans R Soc Trop Med Hyg* **67**:43, 1972

187. Feldman RA: Primary mycobacterial skin infection: A summary. *Int J Dermatol* **13**:353, 1974

188. Uganda Buruli Group: Clinical features and treatment of pre-ulcerative Buruli lesions (*Mycobacterium ulcerans* infection). *Br Med J* **2**:390, 1970

189. Krieg RE et al: Toxin of *Mycobacterium ulcerans.* Production and effects in guinea pig skin. *Arch Dermatol* **110**:783, 1974

190. Stanford JL et al: The production and preliminary investigation of Burulin, a new skin test reagent for *Mycobacterium ulcerans* infection. *J Hyg (Camb)* **74**:7, 1975

191. Meyers WM et al: Heat treatment of *Mycobacterium ulcerans* infections without surgical excision. *Am J Trop Med Hyg* **23**:924, 1974

192. Krieg RE et al: Treatment of *Mycobacterium ulcerans* infection by hyperbaric oxygenation. *Aviat Space Environ Med* **46**:1241, 1975

193. Stanford JL, Philipps I: Rifampicin in experimental *Mycobacterium ulcerans* infection. *J Med Microbiol* **5**:39, 1972

194. Uganda Buruli Group: BCG vaccination against *Mycobacterium ulcerans* infection (Buruli ulcer). *Lancet* **1**:111, 1969

195. Revill WD et al: A controlled trial of the treatment of *Mycobacterium ulcerans* infection with clofazimine. *Lancet* **2**:873, 1973

196. Chapman JS: *The Atypical Mycobacteria and Human Mycobacteriosis.* New York, Plenum, 1977

197. Hagmar B et al: Disseminated infection caused by *M. kansasii.* Report of a case and brief review of the literature. *Acta Med Scand* **186**:93, 1969

198. Duncan WC: Cutaneous mycobacterial infections. *Tex Med* **64**:66, 1968

199. Owens DW, McBride ME: Sporotrichoid cutaneous infection with *Mycobacterium kansasii. Arch Dermatol* **100**:54, 1969

200. Kaplan H, Clayton M: Carpal tunnel syndrome secondary to *M. kansasii* infection. *JAMA* **208**:1186, 1969

201. Owen DS, Toone E: Soft tissue infection by group I atypical mycobacteria. *South Med J* **63**:116, 1970

202. Gunther SF, Elliot RC: *Mycobacterium kansasii* infection in the deep structures of the hand. *J Bone Joint Surg* **58A**:140, 1976

203. Hirsh FS, Saffold OE: *Mycobacterium kansasii* infection with dermatologic manifestations. *Arch Dermatol* **112**:706, 1976

204. Fraser DW et al: Disseminated *Mycobacterium kansasii* infection presenting as cellulitis in a recipient of a renal homograft. *Am Rev Respir Dis* **112**:125, 1975

205. Bailey WC et al: Silico-mycobacterial disease in sandblasters. *Am Rev Respir Dis* **110**:115, 1974

206. Ahn CH et al: Ventilatory defects in atypical mycobacteriosis. *Am Rev Respir Dis* **113**:273, 1976

207. Francis PB et al: The course of untreated *M. kansasii* disease. *Am Rev Respir Dis* **111**:477, 1975

208. Dore N et al: A sporotrichoid-like *Mycobacterium kansasii* infection of the skin treated with minocycline hydrochloride. *Br J Dermatol* **101**:75, 1979

209. Lincoln EM, Gilbert LA: Disease in children due to mycobacteria other than *M. tuberculosis*. *Am Rev Respir Dis* **105**:683, 1972

210. Schaefer WB: Incidence of serotypes of *M. avium* and atypical mycobacteria in human and animal diseases. *Am Rev Respir Dis:* **97**:18, 1968

211. Cox SK, Stransbough LJ: Chronic cutaneous infection caused by *Mycobacterium intracellulare*. *Arch Dermatol* **117**:794, 1981

212. Cole GW, Gebhard J: *Mycobacterium avium* infection of the skin resembling lepromatous leprosy. *Br J Dermatol* **101**:71, 1979

213. Schmidt JD et al: Cutaneous infection due to a Runyon Group III atypical mycobacterium. *Ann Rev Respir Dis* **106**:469, 1972

214. Fainstein V et al: Disseminated infection due to *Mycobacterium avium-intracellulare* in a homosexual man with Kaposi's sarcoma. *J Infect Dis* **145**:586, 1982

215. Heifets LB: Synergistic effect of rifampin, streptomycin, ethionamide and ethambutol on *Mycobacterium intracelluare*. *Am Rev Respir Dis* **125**:43, 1982

216. Masur H et al: Effect of combined clofazimine and ansamycin therapy on *Mycobacterium avium–Mycobacterium intracellulare* bacteremia in patients with AIDS. *J Infect Dis* **155**:127, 1987

217. Agins BA et al: Effect of combined therapy with ansamycin, clofazimine, ethambutol and isomiazid for *Mycobacterium avium* infections in patients with AIDS. *J Infect Dis* **159**:784, 1989

218. Sybert A et al: Cutaneous infection due to *Mycobacterium szulgai*. *Am Rev Respir Dis* **115**:695, 1977

219. Dawson DJ, Jennis F: Mycobacteria with a growth requirement for ferric ammonium citrate, identified as *Mycobacterium haemophilum*. *J Clin Microbiol* **11**:190, 1980

220. Mezo A et al: Unusual mycobacteria in 5 cases of opportunistic infection. *Pathology* **11**:277, 1979

221. Walder BK et al: The skin and immunosuppression. *Aust J Dermatol* **17**:94, 1976

222. Centers for Disease Control: Follow-up on mycobacterial contamination of porcine heart valve prothesis—United States. *MMWR* **27**:92, 1978

223. Wallace RJ et al: Spectrum of disease due to rapidly growing mycobacteria. *Rev Infect Dis* **5**:657, 1983

224. Centers for Disease Control: Mycobacterial infections associated with augmentation mammoplasty—Florida, North Carolina, Texas. *MMWR* **27**:513, 1978

225. Robicsek F et al: *Mycobacterium fortuitum* epidemic after open heart surgery. *J Thorac Cardiovasc Surg* **75**:91, 1978

226. Hoffman PC et al: Two outbreaks of sternal wound infections due to organisms of the *Mycobacterium fortuitum* complex. *J Infect Dis* **143**:533, 1981

227. Borghans JG, Stanford JR: *Mycobacterium chelonei* in abscesses after injection of diphtheria-tetanus-polio vaccine. *Am Rev Respir Dis* **107**:1, 1973

CHAPTER 192

A. Colin McDougall and Marian I. Ulrich

Mycobacterial Disease: Leprosy

Leprosy (Hansen's disease) is often defined merely as "a chronic communicable disease caused by *Mycobacterium leprae,* mainly attacking the nerves and skin. However, a complete definition should call attention not only to bacterial etiology and the main target organs, but also to the variable immunologic response in individuals; the frequent occurrence of nerve damage that leads to loss of sensation and paralysis; and to the range of social, psychological, and economic factors that have far-reaching implications for both the patient with leprosy and the operation of control programs. A succinct definition of leprosy is liable to be misleading; it cannot describe either the remarkable range of clinical manifestations in skin, nerve, and other tissues, which depends on the cell-mediated immune capacity in different individuals, or the frequent occurrence of adverse immunologic reactions, based on either cell-mediated or immune-complex mechanisms, that are seen in most types of leprosy. These immunologic reactions account for a high percentage of the damage to nerves, eyes, and other tissues and lead, all too often, to permanent disability and deformity. The latter, in turn, is a major cause of the stigma, prejudice, social malad-

justment, and economic loss that, at least in the past, have characterized this disease.

Historical Aspects

Perhaps because of its biblical associations, it is not uncommonly asserted that leprosy is one of the oldest diseases known to humans, but in masterly reviews of its history, Cochrane and Davey[1] and Browne[2] have examined the archeological and written sources in detail, drawing attention to the fact that this assertion is by no means always supported by the available evidence and that considerable caution has to be exercised in the matter of terminology and translation from ancient languages. The earliest evidence of leprosy in skeletal remains is from the oasis of Dakhleh in Egypt, in four skulls buried in the second century B.C. Changes indicating leprosy in the bones of the hands and feet have been found in skeletons of Coptic Christians in upper Egypt, dating from the sixth century

A.D. With regard to written accounts, the earliest appear to come from India in the form of revised texts, brought together about 600 B.C. Whether leprosy arose in India or Africa, or elsewhere, and then spread, or whether it has been a disease of multifocal origin is unclear, but there is evidence to suggest that it spread from India to China in about 500 B.C. and then to Japan. The disease may have spread to the west from Greece in the third century B.C. The leprosy endemic in western Europe reached a peak between the thirteenth and fourteenth centuries, and although no estimate of the number of cases is possible, the number of leper houses and hospices (there were about 400 in the United Kingdom alone) suggests that the total must have been considerable. Although doubts have been expressed about the accuracy of diagnosis of those committed to such centers, the findings of Møller-Christensen in his excavations of the burial ground of a lazar hospital in Naestved, Denmark, revealed classic changes of leprosy in many of the skulls and bones examined.[3] From about the fifteenth century onwards, there has been a steady decline in the number of cases in Europe and particularly in Scandinavia, while the disease has spread in what are now referred to as the major endemic areas—South and Central America (including Mexico), Africa, southeast Asia, and the Far East. Significant changes have taken place in recent years with the increasing development of national leprosy control programs, the use of dapsone for treatment, and, more recently, the implementation of multidrug therapy (MDT).[4,5]

Epidemiology

More than 1.6 billion people live in countries with an estimated prevalence of leprosy of more than one case per thousand of the population; in 1988 the World Health Organization (WHO) estimated the total world prevalence to be between 10 and 12 million cases,[6] but this has recently been reduced to a total of 5.5 million requiring or receiving chemotherapy, together with 2 to 3 million with significant disabilities. With regard to the number of cases registered, there have been changes in recent years: 2.85 million in 1966, 3.6 million in 1976, and 5.4 million in 1985. The total of registered cases came down to under 4 million in 1989 and is continuing to fall, in association with the wider implementation of multiple-drug therapy (MDT) as advised by WHO. Leprosy is not confined to the four major endemic areas mentioned above but is widespread; 152 countries report cases to WHO, of which 53 are endemic for the disease. In terms of total numbers of estimated and registered cases, southeast Asia is exceptional. India has an estimated 4 million cases with approximately 2.8 million registered. There are difficulties in the collection of accurate information from leprosy-endemic countries, but in general the figures for registered (known, diagnosed) cases are considerably more reliable, than estimates of total numbers of cases. It bears emphasizing that figures of the kind mentioned above only partially describe the full extent of the leprosy problem, which frequently involves disability due to motor and sensory neuropathy, together with much social, psychological, and economic suffering. It is possible that the total number of patients requiring care because of significant levels of disability will soon outnumber those requiring, or receiving, chemotherapy.

Transmission

Despite the possibility of reservoirs of infection in certain animals and in the environment[7] (see below), leprosy is essentially a disease that is transmitted from one human being to another, and mul-

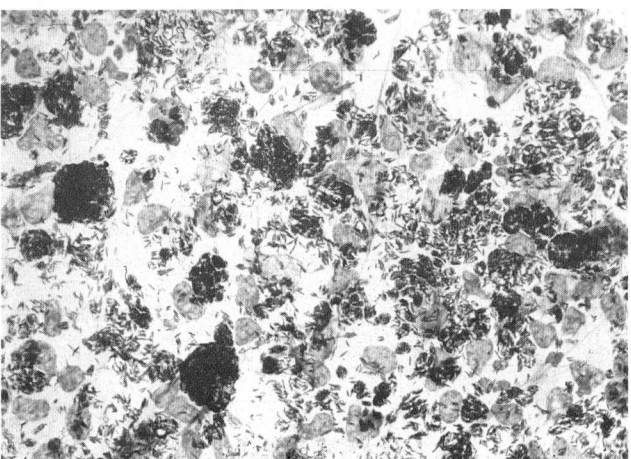

FIGURE 192-1 Smear of nasal mucus from a patient with active, untreated lepromatous leprosy. Ziehl-Neelsen stain. Bacilli: red. Nuclei of macrophages: blue. Organisms can be seen lying singly, in small groups, and also in large round or oval masses ("globi") that are characteristic of lepromatous leprosy. Original magnification ×1000.

tibacillary patients (mainly of lepromatous classification) are the main source of organisms. Such patients are capable of shedding several millions of bacilli per day from nasal and upper respiratory tract secretions (Fig. 192-1), but it is important to note that such excretion stops very soon after the initiation of effective chemotherapy. Broken skin, including lesions in untreated lepromatous leprosy that are ulcerating, may shed bacilli into the environment, but this is a relatively uncommon portal of exit. Modes of entry of bacilli into a susceptible host are unknown; they could include ingestion in food or drink, inoculation into or through the skin (bites, scratches, small wounds, tattoos, etc.), or inhalation, with deposit and entry of bacilli either in the nasal passages or in the lungs. Although nasal involvement is characteristic of lepromatous leprosy, probably at an early stage of the disease, it is not a characteristic feature of nonlepromatous leprosy, and studies of the lungs (in any form of the disease) have failed to reveal bacilli or lesions. There is no evidence for a "primary complex" either in the lungs or elsewhere, as there is in tuberculosis.

Environmental Factors

A study of the world map and the present-day distribution of leprosy suggests that socioeconomic and environmental factors may be of importance in maintaining the endemic, but it is difficult to pinpoint one factor, or even a group of factors, that may be particularly relevant. Housing, diet, water supplies, illiteracy, overcrowding, and climate have been discussed and reviewed in the literature, without any definite conclusion. Considerable gains in leprosy control, with reduction in prevalence, have been achieved in various parts of the world, using chemotherapy, in the face of adverse (and unchanged) environmental conditions. Climate is unlikely to be relevant; in the past, the disease was prevalent in Scandinavia, Siberia, and other cold regions.

Reservoirs of Infection

There is no doubt that humans with untreated lepromatous (bacilliferous) leprosy are the most important source of infection, but recent publications on naturally occurring disease in animals, indistinguishable from human leprosy, show that humans can no longer be considered the only host. Armadillos in the central and southern parts of the United States have now been shown to be naturally infected with an organism that is apparently identical to *M. leprae*.[8] Naturally occurring *M. leprae*-like infections have also been reported in mangabey monkeys[9] and a chimpanzee.[10] Furthermore, the possibility that *M. leprae* may persist in soil or vegetation has been reported and recently confirmed.[11] These reports are clearly of considerable interest, but it has to be emphasized that humans remain the most important source of infection. Untreated bacilliferous (lepromatous) cases are outstandingly important in this context, but as transmission continues to occur in many parts of the world where nonlepromatous cases predominate, the possible role of the latter in transmission should not be disregarded.[12]

Age and Sex

Leprosy is uncommon in infancy. Incidence rates attain a peak between the ages of 10 and 20 years, and prevalence rates usually rise to a peak between the ages of 30 and 50 years. There has been a gradual increase in the mean age of onset of disease, observed over the years, and the proportion of lepromatous leprosy in new cases has increased. In most parts of the world and judged by new cases and the total of those registered, leprosy is more common, often much more common, in males than in females. This difference is more marked in adults than in children and also in lepromatous leprosy as opposed to other classifications. It is unknown if this sex difference is due to social, religious, or cultural factors, or if it could possibly be an inherent characteristic of the disease. The fact that male/female ratios tend to equalize or even favor women in some areas where the lepromatous rate is low, for instance in some parts of Africa, suggests that classification is important.

Genetics

There is no clear evidence that genetic factors influence susceptibility to infection or the development of clinical leprosy, but there is good evidence that genetics greatly influence the type of disease that develops. HLA-linked genes influence the development of both tuberculoid and lepromatous leprosy; evidence to date suggests that the same HLA-DR and non-DR antigens are involved in the cellular immune response to *M. leprae* and to other mycobacterial antigens. Differences in HLA type, the cell-mediated immune response, and disease type appear to be interrelated.[13]

Etiology and Pathogenesis

Evidence indicating that leprosy is caused by infection with *M. leprae* is overwhelming and includes the establishment of disease resembling human leprosy in a number of experimental animals, including armadillos and certain primates, using inoculae obtained from patients with untreated lepromatous leprosy. As mentioned above, the concept that leprosy is confined to humans now needs revision.

Following inoculation, the vast majority of individuals appear to have complete resistance and do not proceed from the stage of infection to clinical disease. Although it has been assumed that the organisms are completely destroyed at the site of inoculation or perhaps by the immune system after circulating in the blood, this has never been proved. The possibility that some viable organisms may persist, perhaps in some form of ''primary complex'' as in tuberculosis, warrants consideration, although the site of such a complex has never been identified.

Following successful inoculation in a susceptible subject, it is thought that organisms spread by the bloodstream to invade the skin and nerves via the endothelial cells of small vessels. If bacilli survive and multiply in these sites, it is suggested that the patient may go on to develop one of the ''determined'' forms of leprosy, ranging from tuberculoid to lepromatous (see ''Classification'' below). If detected and examined at an earlier stage, changes of indeterminate leprosy may be seen in the skin; such lesions may either persist indefinitely, resolve with or without treatment, or eventually develop into one of the determined forms of the disease. Based on case histories of patients exposed to leprosy (sometimes very briefly) and then removed from the endemic area to a nonendemic area, the incubation period from exposure to the development of clinical disease is believed to be 2 to 5 years, but longer periods have been described.

Once they have developed, the ''polar'' forms of leprosy, namely tuberculoid and lepromatous, tend to be stable in the sense that patients with these forms do not change classification either as a result of treatment or adverse immunologic reaction or spontaneously. By contrast, borderline forms are unstable, particularly midborderline (BB) in both the clinical and immunologic sense, with a tendency to ''move'' in the spectrum due to reaction, or under treatment. Although BB leprosy is commonly described as the most unstable, this is not a common form of the disease to encounter in clinical practice. From the point of view of management and the prevention of damage due to reactions, borderline-tuberculoid (BT) and borderline-lepromatous (BL) forms are usually of greater practical importance.

It is a characteristic of leprosy that the nerves are affected early and constantly. It is not at all uncommon for a neurologic manifestation, such as sensory loss or muscle weakness, to develop months or even a year or so before any cutaneous lesion, although in practice, particularly in endemic areas in third-world countries, it is usual to find both dermatologic and neurologic lesions at the time of presentation for diagnosis. Pure neural leprosy is not uncommon in India (though seen only rarely in other parts of the world); as the name implies, there are no skin lesions. No good explanation has ever been offered for this unusual form of the disease.

Immunologic and Immunopathologic Aspects of Leprosy

Importance of the Host's Immune Response in Disease Manifestations

The clinical manifestations of leprosy reflect an extraordinarily complex host-parasite interaction, in which the host's immune response plays the fundamental role in determining the pathologic characteristics of the disease. Most individuals in areas in which the disease is endemic appear to be fully resistant to the development of clinical disease. Epidemiologic studies have shown that a high percentage of household and nonhousehold contacts give positive skin tests of delayed-type hypersensitivity (DTH) to crude extracts of *M. leprae*; DTH is presumably associated with at least some degree of resistance to clinical disease. The remainder of the population may develop leprosy in any of its clinical forms after exposure under appropriate conditions. The clinical spectrum of disease appears to depend exclusively on variable limitations in the host's capacity to develop effective cell-mediated immune responses to *M. leprae*.[14]

The immunologic compromise or defect whose maximum expression occurs in lepromatous leprosy is extraordinarily specific; this specificity is demonstrated by the fact that many patients with leprosy give positive skin tests to numerous other antigens that provoke DTH in vivo or in vitro. They do not show increased susceptibility to cancer, viral or mycotic infections, or other conditions that might be associated with nonspecific cell-mediated immunodeficiency.

Characteristics of *M. leprae* Associated with Pathogenicity and Virulence

The leprosy bacillus is remarkably devoid of any characteristics that are frequently associated with virulence in other microorganisms. No known exotoxins nor endotoxins are produced. Differences in epidemiologic patterns and in disease manifestations cannot at present be ascribed to different strains of *M. leprae*.[15] The pathologic consequences of infection with *M. leprae* reflect two fundamental characteristics of the bacilli: their capacity to invade and multiply within peripheral nerves and their capacity to infect and survive within endothelial and phagocytic cells in many organs of the body. Constituents of the mycobacterial cell wall, such as phenolic glycolipid I[16] and lipoarabinomannan B,[17] might be considered virulence factors, because these constituents have been reported to scavenge metabolites of the oxidative burst of phagocytic cells and to induce nonspecific inhibition of T-cell reactions through as yet undefined mechanisms.

Characteristics of the Immunologic Response

The Humoral or Antibody-Mediated Response   The presence of specific and cross-reacting antimycobacterial antibodies has been demonstrated throughout the clinical spectrum of disease. In general terms, the humoral response to *M. leprae* is most vigorous in multibacillary disease, reflecting the high bacillary load, and decreases toward the tuberculoid pole of the clinical spectrum. At present no role in protective immunologic mechanisms can be ascribed to circulating antimycobacterial antibodies; they do appear to play a role in the pathogenesis of type 2 reactional phenomena (see below), including erythema nodosum leprosum and immune-complex glomerulonephritis. Serologic tests are of particular interest in the study of leprosy in the following areas: detection of subclinical infection, monitoring of therapy, early detection of relapse or reinfection as indicated by rising antibody levels, and immunoepidemiologic studies. Undoubtedly the most widely studied specific antigen of *M. leprae* is the cell wall component phenolic glycolipid I (PGL-I), described by Brennan and Barrow.[16] This antigen, which is also present in large amounts in tissue containing viable bacilli, is highly specific and is suitable for use in enzymatic immunoassays that are easily carried out in countries where leprosy is endemic. Unfortunately, the sensitivity of these tests is quite low. Another cell membrane component, lipoarabinomannan B, appears to be a much stronger immunogen than PGL-I, but cross-reactivity with other mycobacteria complicates the interpretation of tests using this antigen. Antigenic determinants or epitopes that are specific for *M. leprae* have been reported on at least six bacillary

proteins, with molecular masses ranging from 12 to 70 kDa, but widely applicable serologic tests have not yet been developed using these proteins.

Low levels of antibodies associated with autoimmunity have been demonstrated in patients with multibacillary leprosy with some frequency, but there is little or no evidence that these antibodies contribute significantly to the pathology of leprosy; nor are they associated with autoimmune phenomena in these patients.

The Cell-Mediated Immune Response   The protective immunologic mechanisms associated with infections produced by obligatory intracellular microorganisms such as *M. leprae* appear to be mediated by specifically sensitized T lymphocytes and their soluble products. Macrophage activation by gamma-interferon and possibly by other lymphokines produced by stimulated T cells probably represents the principal immunologic defense mechanism against *M. leprae*, but other soluble cytokines such as tumor necrosis factor may play some role in protection. Cytotoxic reactions by the CD8+ class T cells, killer cells, or other leukocytes might be active in the lysis of phagocytic cells infected with *M. leprae*, but such mechanisms have not been studied in detail.

The development of T cell-mediated protective immunity is usually accompanied by the development of DTH reactions during the course of natural infections, and this relationship is very clear in leprosy. DTH reactions are clearly responsible for the pathology in the high-resistance, tuberculoid portion of the spectrum of clinical leprosy.

Undoubtedly the most widely used test for evaluating cell-mediated immunity in leprosy is the Mitsuda or lepromin skin test, performed by the intradermal injection of heat-killed *M. leprae*. These preparations act as microvaccinations and induce the formation of immune granulomatous reactions in all persons who are able to develop competent cell-mediated immune reactions to *M. leprae*. Positivity does not depend upon previous exposure to the microorganism and in no way constitutes a diagnostic test. Mitsuda positivity is clearly associated with a significant degree of resistance in patients, as it occurs toward the tuberculoid pole of the spectrum; Mitsuda-positive patients with indeterminate leprosy and positive contacts of leprosy patients are also presumed to have a significant level of resistance.

Several preparations of crude soluble extracts of purified *M. leprae*, disrupted by sonication or pressure, have been rather widely used in recent years to evaluate preexisting cell-mediated immunity to the leprosy bacillus in both patients and healthy individuals in endemic areas. These reactions are neither diagnostic nor specific for leprosy; as is the case with the classic Mitsuda reaction, positivity appears to be associated with a significant degree of resistance.

It is generally accepted that most lepromatous patients, who invariably give negative skin tests during the clinical course of their disease, do not develop or recover cell-mediated immune reactivity to *M. leprae* after they apparently have been successfully treated with chemotherapy. They remain susceptible to reinfection or to relapse from viable bacilli that may persist without dividing in the tissues for many years. Enormous effort has been devoted to try to characterize the antigen-specific immunologic defect that is observed in leprosy, particularly in the borderline and lepromatous forms of the disease. Defects have been reported in macrophages, lymphocytes, their respective cytokines, and immunoregulatory systems. Active suppressor mechanisms mediated by both macrophages and lymphocytes offer one of the more attractive possibilities to explain antigen-specific T-cell deficiency and have been described in leprosy,[18] but these studies appear to be very sensitive to variations in experimental design.

Immunopathologic Characteristics within the Clinical Spectrum

Immunologic phenomena play such a prominent role in the pathology of leprosy that some description of these features seems appropriate in any discussion of the disease.

Tuberculoid Leprosy   The relatively effective cell-mediated immune response in tuberculoid leprosy is reflected in the clinical characteristics. The characteristic immune granuloma of tuberculoid leprosy is formed by differentiated macrophages (epithelioid cells, Langhans' giant cells) surrounded by a mantle of lymphocytes. Immunocytochemical studies demonstrate the predominance of CD4+ helper-inducer T cells in these lesions and show significant numbers of cells producing interleukin 2 (IL-2) as well as cells with IL-2 receptors.[19] CD8+ cytotoxic or suppressor T cells are largely found in the lymphocytic mantle of the granuloma; it is not clear at present which of the two major activities of these cells is more important.

NERVE DAMAGE IN TUBERCULOID LEPROSY.   Cell-mediated hypersensitivity reactions are responsible for the severe nerve damage of relatively early onset that is observed in tuberculoid leprosy. This damage appears to be disproportionate to the number of microorganisms present and undoubtedly reflects both a considerable amplification of localized antigen–T cell interaction and the sensitivity of peripheral nerves to immunologic hypersensitivity mechanisms. These mechanisms may include accumulations of mononuclear cells, causing mechanical damage, and liberation of cytotoxic substances from inflammatory leukocytes. Although neural autoantibodies are present in leprosy, their role, if any, in the pathogenesis of nerve damage has not been elucidated.

Borderline Leprosy   Perhaps one of the most striking immunologic features of borderline leprosy is the lack of clinical and immunologic stability that is observed; both upgrading reactions, characterized by an increase in cell-mediated immune response, and downgrading reactions, reflecting a shift toward the lepromatous end of the spectrum, are not uncommon. Abrupt increases in cell-mediated immunity in the borderline forms of leprosy are often accompanied by relatively acute inflammatory reactions affecting skin and nerves. These inflammatory reactions are known as reversal, or type 1, reactions. Cutaneous manifestations are characterized by erythema, edema, and tenderness; sheathed nerves may suffer permanent damage if not treated appropriately. Recent studies have demonstrated the accumulation of lymphocytes with gamma/delta receptors in the reversal reactions of leprosy and suggest that this subpopulation may play a role in granuloma formation.[20] The pathogenesis of type 1 reactions is incompletely understood. They may apparently be "triggered" or precipitated by intercurrent illness, vaccination, pregnancy, absorption, or physical or psychological trauma, but many patients develop reactions suddenly and inexplicably, without any of these factors being present. Adverse immunologic reactions of the type described above are by far the most frequent and important cause of the damage that occurs in sensory, motor, and autonomic nerves.

Lepromatous Leprosy   The lesions of lepromatous leprosy are characterized by the presence of disorganized granulomas formed by nondifferentiated macrophages containing massive numbers of bacilli. In vivo and in vitro manifestations of cell-mediated protective immunity and DTH cannot be demonstrated. Immunocytochemical studies of lepromatous lesions show a CD4+/CD8+ ratio <1, with suppressor-cytotoxic cells scattered throughout the granuloma; suppressor T-cell clones have been isolated from these lesions. Cells producing IL-2 are rare in lepromatous lesions, although the number of cells with IL-2 receptors is normal.

Nerve damage occurs relatively late in lepromatous leprosy and appears to be due largely to the mechanical effects of extensive bacillary multiplication. Anesthesia or hypesthesia is a prominent feature of nerve damage, leading to the traumatic injuries that eventually cause the mutilations associated with untreated lepromatous disease.

Erythema Nodosum Leprosum   As previously mentioned, type 1, or reversal, reactions in borderline leprosy reflect an increase in the cell-mediated immune response. Erythema nodosum leprosum (ENL), which occurs in lepromatous leprosy, represents the other "reactional phenomenon" in leprosy and is known as a type 2 reaction. In addition to the erythematous inflammatory reactions of ENL, type 2 reactions can affect the kidney, eyes, bones, and joints. The presence of abundant polymorphonuclear leukocytes in ENL lesions, as well as the demonstration of immunoglobulins and complement,[21] clearly suggest that these are classic Arthus' or immune-complex type reactions. More recent studies have demonstrated a transitory increase in cell-mediated immunity during ENL reactions.[22] The initiation of the pathogenic process by an increase in cell-mediated immunity, which leads to release of mycobacterial antigen in situ in the presence of high levels of antimycobacterial antibody, rather easily reconciles the importance of both cellular and humoral mechanisms in the pathogenesis of these reactions. It remains perplexing that some patients, even with florid disease, suffer not a single episode, whereas others have repeated and debilitating reactions over a period of many years. It is also now known why the target organs for reaction and tissue damage vary so widely between patients; some experience a "full-blown" syndrome with erythema nodosum on the skin, iritis, arthritis, neuritis, and kidney complications, accompanied by fever, debility, and weight loss; others have only a relatively mild involvement of one body system. Thalidomide is extraordinarily effective in controling ENL, although it is not effective against type 1 reactions.

Modification of the Immune Response in Leprosy— Immunotherapy and Immunoprophylaxis

Convit et al.[23] demonstrated that the repeated injection of a mixture of heat-killed *M. leprae* and live BCG induced important immunologic changes in patients with multibacillary leprosy and in Mitsuda-negative indeterminate leprosy. These changes included positive DTH skin reactions, positive tests for cell-mediated immunity in vitro to *M. leprae* soluble antigen and lepromin, histologic changes in biopsy specimens compatible with a shift toward more resistant forms of disease, and a loss of suppressor cell activity. Reversal type 1 reactions were frequent during the course of immunotherapy in lepromatous patients. These patients also received chemotherapy for ethical reasons, but the phenomena described above are exceptionally rare in patients treated with chemotherapy alone and clearly suggest the activation of immunologic mechanism by the combined vaccine.

The immunologic mechanism activated by immunotherapy may include the accumulation of an active population of antigen-presenting cells and the synthesis of lymphokines, including gamma-interferon and IL-2, at the site of the immune granuloma induced by the BCG component of the mixture. Liberation of appropriate immunogens of *M. leprae* from activated macrophages as well as common cross-reactive antigens of BCG may contribute to the response. Local synthesis of IL-1 and enhanced expression of class II MHC antigens in response to BCG have also been reported.

Patients with Mitsuda-negative indeterminate leprosy usually develop cell-mediated immunity to *M. leprae* after one to three injections, and Mitsuda-negative contacts after a single dose of the combined vaccine. These observations have provided the basis for immunoprophylaxis trials in Venezuela, Malawi, India, and other countries. Several approaches to second-generation vaccines have been conceived, based on the identification of specific epitopes of *M. leprae* and their incorporation into synthetic molecules or vectors that would include adjuvant components. If one or more of these approaches to active vaccination gives promising results, leprosy control programs in the future would ideally include early action and multidrug treatment of active cases, together with vaccination of high-risk groups.

Clinical Manifestations and Classification

In 1966, Ridley and Jopling published their classification of leprosy, suggesting that the disease could be divided into five groups according to a spectrum, based on the patient's cell-mediated immune capacity: tuberculoid (TT), borderline-tuberculoid (BT), midborderline (BB), borderline-lepromatous (BL), and lepromatous (LL).[24] A summary of the main characteristics of these forms of leprosy is given in Table 192-1 and Figs. 192-2 to 192-6 illustrate some of the commonly occurring skin lesions. This system has proved extremely useful in clinical practice, and although initially considered too complicated and detailed for field work, it has been found increasingly useful in control programs.

Tuberculoid Leprosy

Tuberculoid (TT) leprosy manifests on the skin as either macules or plaques (Fig. 192-2), commonly single or few in number. The edges are well defined, and there is a tendency to central healing. The surface is typically nonsweating (dry), irregular in texture, and either hypopigmented, erythematous, or coppery in color. Hair growth is impaired, and there is reduction in or even complete loss of sensation to light touch, temperature, and pain. In clinical practice, plaques are more commonly seen than macules. A thickened peripheral nerve is often palpable in the vicinity, or a thickened cutaneous nerve may be felt entering or leaving the skin lesion. The low number of skin or skin/nerve lesions is an important characteristic of this form of leprosy. Skin smears are negative, and the lepromin test strongly positive.

Histopathology   Skin biopsy shows epithelioid cell granuloma with many peripheral lymphocytes and Langhans' giant cells. A biopsy of adequate depth will reveal nerves that are almost invariably infiltrated (often replaced) by the granuloma, occasionally showing caseation. With rare exceptions (and after a long search of many sections), bacilli are absent.

Borderline-Tuberculoid Leprosy

Borderline-tuberculoid (BT) leprosy (Fig. 192-3) has skin lesions that resemble those of TT leprosy as described above, but they are (1) more numerous—usually at least 5, commonly 10 to 20 and occasionally more; (2) less well defined at the edges; (3) often larger, occasionally involving a whole limb or other body area; and (4) more likely to vary in size, shape, and texture within the same patient. The distribution, whether macule or plaque, is asymmetric. Many peripheral nerves may be involved, again asymmetrically, and damage may be severe; patients with this classification are particularly likely to develop type 1 (cell-mediated) reactions. Sensation is moderately or markedly reduced. Skin smears are either

TABLE 192-1
Clinical Aspects of the Ridley-Jopling Classification

Observation or test	Type of leprosy				
	TT	BT	BB	BL	LL
Number of lesions	Single usually	Single or few	Several	Many	Very many
Size of lesions	Variable	Variable	Variable	Variable	Small
Surface of lesions	Very dry, sometimes scaly	Dry	Slightly shiny	Shiny	Shiny
Sensation in lesions (not face)	Absent	Moderately–markedly diminished	Slightly–moderately diminished	Slightly diminished	Not affected
Hair growth in lesions	Absent	Markedly diminished	Moderately diminished	Slightly diminished	Not affected
AFB in lesions	Nil	Nil or scanty	Moderate numbers	Many	Very many (plus globi)
AFB in nasal scrapings or in nose-blows	Nil	Nil	Nil	Usually nil	Very many (plus globi)
Lepromin test	Strongly positive (+ + +)	Weakly positive (+ or + +)	Negative	Negative	Negative

NOTE: AFB, acid-fast bacilli; TT, tuberculoid; BT, borderline-tuberculoid; BB, midborderline; BL, borderline-lepromatous; LL, lepromatous.
SOURCE: From Jopling, WH, McDougall, AC: *Handbook of Leprosy*, Heinemann, 1988, reproduced with permission.[25]

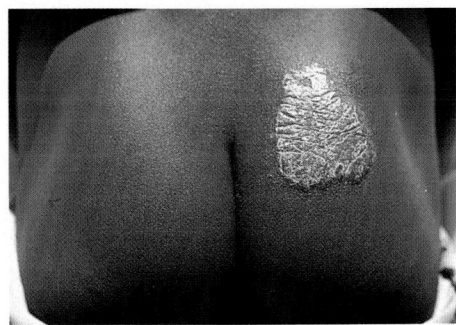

FIGURE 192-2 Single lesion of tuberculoid (TT) leprosy on the buttock; infiltrated, firm, well defined, nonsweating (dry), and completely anesthetic. Smears from the lesions: negative.

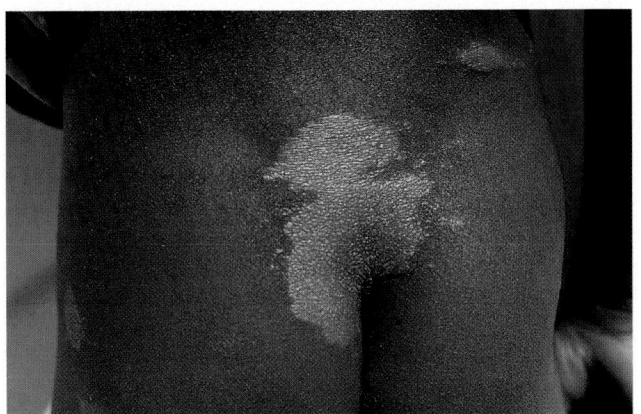

FIGURE 192-3 Multiple lesions of tuberculoid type (see Fig. 192-2), but affecting many body areas and with small "daughter" or "satellite" lesions adjacent to the main lesions. There was enlargement of greater auricular, ulnar, and lateral popliteal nerves. Borderline-tuberculoid (BT) classification. Bacteriologic index (BI) of smears from the lesions averaged 1.

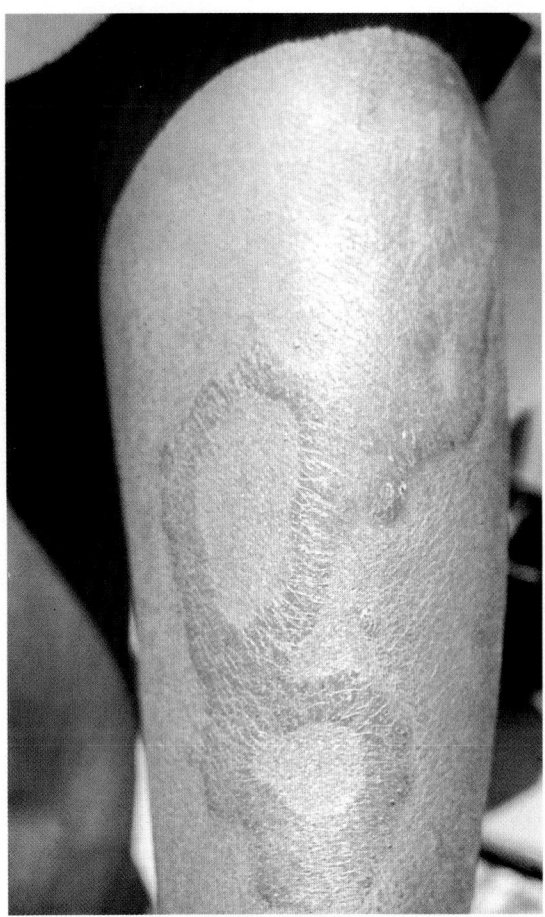

FIGURE 192-4 Fairly extensive lesions of midborderline (BB) leprosy on the right thigh; there were similar lesions with "punched-out" centers on both arms and the trunk, with involvement of both ulnar and one lateral popliteal nerve. BI, 3.

negative or only weakly positive, and the lepromin reaction is invariably positive.

Histopathology Skin biopsy shows an epithelioid cell granuloma with moderate numbers of lymphocytes scattered throughout. Giant cells tend to be foreign-body rather than Langhans' in type. Lower dermal nerves show moderate swelling and infiltration, and there is often lymphocytic infiltration of the perineurium, causing lamination.

Midborderline Leprosy

Midborderline (BB) leprosy (Fig. 192-4) typically shows a considerable number of polymorphic skin lesions, with a tendency to bilateral symmetry; in number they are more than BT and fewer than BL (see below). Macules or plaques occur and the latter exhibit curious "geographic" appearances, with poorly defined outer edges and "punched-out" or "hole in cheese" centers. Sensation in skin lesions may be slightly or moderately diminished. Damage to peripheral nerves is variable, as BB leprosy is intrinsically an unstable form of the disease (much less commonly seen in practice

than the other borderline forms) that may represent a "transition state" from either a BT or BL classification. If the patient has deteriorated (downgraded clinically and immunologically) from BT, there will be fairly widespread, asymmetric involvement of peripheral nerves as described above. If the patient has improved (upgraded) from BL (see below), perhaps under the influence of successful chemotherapy, more peripheral nerves may be affected, symmetrically, but there will be little evidence of sensory or motor damage, unless the situation is, or has been, complicated by type 1 (cell-mediated) reaction. Skin smears show moderate numbers of acid-fast bacilli, and the lepromin test is negative.

Histopathology Skin biopsy shows a diffuse epithelioid cell granuloma with scanty lymphocytes and no giant cells. The epithelioid cell areas may be edematous. Lower dermal nerves may be virtually normal or slightly swollen; the perineurium may be laminated and invaded by epithelioid cells. Bacilli are present in moderate numbers; the bacterial index (BI) (see below) is commonly 3 to 4.

Borderline-Lepromatous Leprosy

Borderline-lepromatous (BL) leprosy (Fig. 192-5) has many skin lesions, widely distributed. These are macular in the early stages

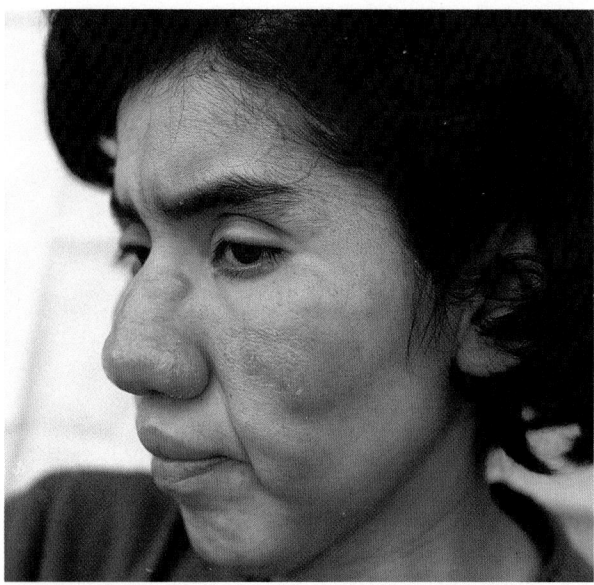

FIGURE 192-5   Active, untreated borderline-lepromatous (BL) leprosy; numerous large fleshy lesions on the face, trunk, and limbs, raised at the center and sloping towards the periphery. Moderate enlargement of one ulnar and both terminal nerves at the wrist. BI, 4.

but later develop into papules, nodules, and plaques, with a tendency to symmetry. Again, the clinical appearance and number of lesions may be influenced by the previous sequence of events: patients who have downgraded from BT may show skin lesions that are large and have some evidence of central healing. Generally, however, most patients with BL leprosy have a large number of small lesions with central, rather than peripheral, infiltration. Skin smears are markedly positive (BI, 4 to 5), and the lepromin test is invariably negative. Peripheral nerve involvement may be widespread, with a tendency to symmetry; sensory and motor damage may be marked, especially in those patients who have suffered from type 1 reactions. Patients of this classification may also experience episodes of type 2 (ENL) reaction.

Histopathology   Skin biopsy shows a macrophage granuloma with many lymphocytes. The latter may be densely packed over at least one segment of the granuloma or encompass nerve bundles and infiltrate the perineurium. Occasionally, a solitary clump of epithelioid cells is found amongst macrophages, with or without lymphocytes. Nerves often show "onion-skin" changes in the perineurium. Bacilli are numerous (BI, 4 to 5).

Lepromatous Leprosy

Lepromatous (LL) leprosy (Fig. 192-6) is a generalized, systemic disease with a continuous bacteremia, so that bacilli, often accompanied by a macrophage response, may be found in a very wide range of body tissues. In the early stages the skin shows widespread, numerous, symmetrically distributed macules that are poorly defined and often difficult to see, unless the patient is examined with care, in a good light. As the disease progresses, these tend to coalesce and involve the entire body surface, with the exception of the so-called immune areas—scalp, axillae, groin, perineum, and midline of the back. Early macules have minimal altera-

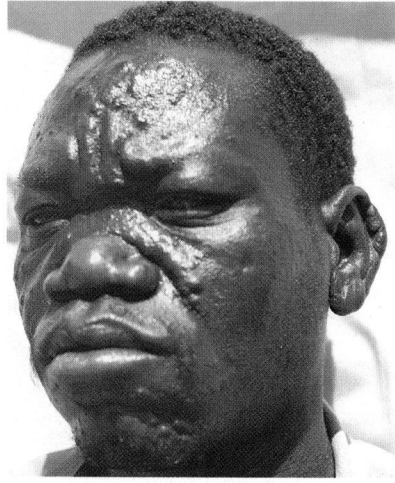

FIGURE 192-6   Active, nodular lepromatous leprosy with heavy involvement of both ears, depression of the nasal bridge, loss of eyebrows (madarosis), gynecomastia, and testicular atrophy. Slit-skin smears from all areas were highly positive. BI, 6.

tion in color but may be shiny. Characteristically, they show no alteration in sensation. If untreated at this stage, skin lesions progress to infiltration and then to the formation of nodules, especially on the forehead, ears, and face. Skin smears from early macules and from the more advanced lesions are, in the untreated patient, invariably positive (BI, 6), and similar concentrations of bacilli will be found on scraping apparently normal-looking skin between lesions. Over the cooler parts of the skin, for instance the back of the hands and the outer areas of the arms, there is a characteristic temperature-dependent sensory and autonomic loss, not recorded in other diseases. Although peripheral nerves harbor bacilli, clinical evidence of damage may not be apparent in the early stages of LL leprosy. In the later stages, there may be symmetric, firm enlargement of many nerves, with the slow onset of sensory and motor changes in their area of supply. Important changes occur in LL leprosy in the eyes, nose, testicles, kidneys, and other systems, and it is important to remember that some patients may present with ocular, renal, or other clinical features long before the diagnosis of leprosy is suspected by examination of the skin, peripheral nerves, or by the taking of skin smears or a biopsy. The lepromin test is invariably negative.

Histopathology   Skin biopsy shows an infiltrate of foamy macrophages, a variable number of which have intracytoplasmic vacuoles, some of striking size. Foamy change in macrophages is almost invariable, especially in treated cases. Lymphocytes are either scanty or absent. Multinucleate giant cells may be seen, often with large vacuoles, but Langhans' giant cells and epithelioid cells do not occur. The BI in untreated cases is invariably high (BI, 6).

Indeterminate Leprosy

It may be noticed that the Ridley-Jopling classification refers only to "determined" forms of leprosy and does not include indeterminate leprosy. This is a form of the disease with one or a few macules, hypopigmented or pink in color. If multiple, the lesions are usually asymmetrically distributed. Lesions may occur on virtually any area of the body, but as with other forms of leprosy, there is a tendency to avoid the axillae, groin, perineum, and scalp. Some loss of sensation is usually found but in areas that are very well supplied with nerve endings, such as the face, sensory testing may be of limited value, particularly in children, who have difficulty in giving meaningful replies to the stimulus. Skin smears are almost invariably negative. A skin biopsy more often than not shows non-specific changes but, occasionally, in a biopsy of sufficient depth, an acid-fast bacillus may be seen within a dermal nerve. A thickened cutaneous nerve may be seen or palpated adjacent to the lesions, or there may be enlargement of a nearby named peripheral nerve. It can thus be seen that the diagnosis of indeterminate leprosy may be difficult, particularly in differentiating it from a long list of other dermatologic conditions, especially in the tropics. However, everything possible should be done to confirm the diagnosis before the patient is registered as a case of leprosy, if only because of the sociologic implications in many communities.

Pure Neural Leprosy (Primary Neuritic Leprosy)

A form of leprosy only affecting one or more peripheral nerves seems to be well recognized, especially by leprologists in India, but it is uncommon in Africa and other endemic areas. Such cases require expert advice before diagnosis and classification. It is important to examine the entire body surface in a good light to confirm that there are in fact no subtle changes in skin pigmentation (indicating skin lesions) and also to be sure that the patient has definitely not received previous treatment. Patients with apparently "pure" neural leprosy may in fact be partly or previously treated, so that skin lesions present at the outset have disappeared by the time of presentation to another examiner. A nerve biopsy may be necessary in order to confirm the diagnosis and establish a classification, but this should be undertaken only by a qualified doctor trained in the procedure. Only sensory nerves should be biopsied, backed by adequate processing facilities and a competent histopathologist. A lepromin test is of value in classification (but not diagnosis), being strongly positive in TT and BT cases and negative in the other forms.

Histoid Leprosy

The term *histoid leproma* was introduced by Wade[26] to describe the appearances seen in hyperactive lepromatous nodules, usually in relapsed patients, including those with dapsone resistance. The lesions, which are of considerable dermatologic interest (Fig. 192-7) and likely to give rise to difficulty if leprosy is not suspected, consist of firm, erythematous or coppery, glistening nodules in the dermis or subdermis, with a tendency to occur in such situations as the midline of the chin, the antecubital fossa, and the surface of the eye, all unusual for nodules in typical LL leprosy. A biopsy characteristically shows elongated or spindle-shaped histiocytes in a whorled arrangement with large numbers of bacilli, many of them solid-staining. Although not invariably, histoid lesions are often indicative of the development of dapsone resistance.

Lucio Leprosy

This is an unusual form of leprosy, first described by Lucio and Alvarado in Mexico (see reference 27). Typically, there is a wide-

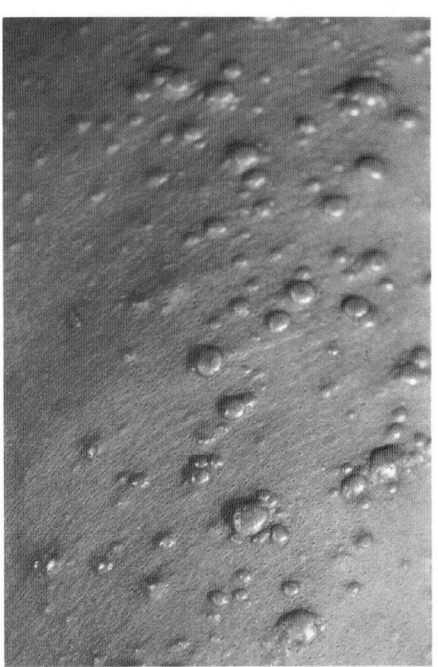

FIGURE 192-7   Numerous erythematous, round or oval, glistening nodules of histoid leprosy on the side of the chest, in a patient with dapsone resistance. Smears of the nodules were highly positive (BI, 6). (*Reproduced by permission of T. Fajardo, M.D., Eversley Childs Sanatorium, Philippines.*)

spread diffuse infiltration of the skin, without nodules, together with loss of body hair, eyebrows, and eyelashes. There is widespread sensory loss, and skin smears are heavily positive from most sites. These patients may develop a curious form of immunologic reaction, the so-called Lucio phenomenon, characterized by painful red patches, mainly on the extremities, which become necrotic and ulcerated (Fig. 192-8); the trunk and face are spared. Unlike other forms of adverse immunologic reaction in leprosy, the Lucio phenomenon occurs only in untreated patients. A further point of dif-

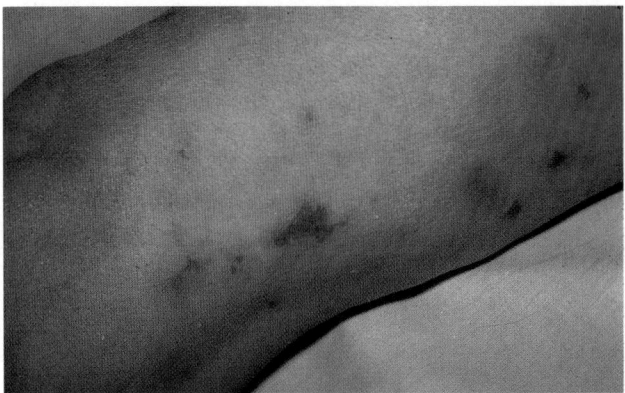

FIGURE 192-8   Serrated hemorrhagic infarcts with erythematous halos are characteristic of the Lucio phenomenon. This 50-year-old woman had recurrent eruptions of lesions for several years, complete alopecia of eyebrows and eyelashes, and nasal perforation. (*Courtesy of Thomas H. Rea, M.D.*)

ference with the immune-complex type of reaction described for lepromatous leprosy is that it responds to steroids but not to thalidomide. The histopathology has been described in detail by Rea and Ridley[28]; it includes epidermal necrosis, necrotizing vasculitis, focal endothelial proliferation of middermal vessels, and large numbers of bacilli in endothelial cells.

Adverse Immunologic Reactions

As already indicated, clinical events associated with adverse (unwelcome and potentially damaging) immunologic response are an important aspect of the whole subject. From the standpoint of the patient, they are of greater significance and often more alarming than the development of the standard, determined forms of leprosy, whether in skin or nerve. The two most important types in clinical practice are reversal reactions, also called upgrading or delayed-type hypersensitivity or type 1, and erythema nodosum leprosum (ENL), also called immune-complex or type 2. The immunologic basis of these reactions is described above.

In *reversal reactions* (type 1), there is a rapid change in some or all skin lesions; they become red, shiny, and swollen and may ulcerate. Nerves may swell, becoming painful and tender, and this may be accompanied by loss of sensation and muscular paralysis, sometimes occurring very rapidly. Abscess formation may occur, particularly in the ulnar nerve, and the extremities and/or the face may show edema. There is evidence to suggest that reversal reactions are associated with a rapid increase in cell-mediated immunity, but current immunologic research has done little to explain why this happens. Reversal reactions tend to occur after treatment has been instituted, but they are by no means uncommon in completely untreated patients. The differentiation from relapse is not always easy and may call for expert investigation, including skin biopsy.

In the *immune-complex type* of reactions (type 2), occurring typically in lepromatous (LL) and occasionally in borderline-lepromatous (BL) cases, the commonly used name erythema nodosum leprosum is understandable in view of the frequency of red nodular lesions on the skin (face, arms, and legs). However, it is misleading in that this form of reaction is usually systemic, with manifestations in many other body systems, including nerves, eyes, bones, joints, lymph nodes, kidneys, and testicles. There is commonly fever, malaise, raised sedimentation rate, and a polymorphonuclear leukocytosis. In severe cases, the skin lesions may become vesicular or bullous and ulcerate (erythema necroticans). Inexperienced observers may fail to recognize this immune-complex reaction, thinking that the skin and other lesions are manifestations of renewed activity or relapse.

Disability

A full description of deformity in leprosy is beyond the scope of this chapter, but it is a subject of prime importance in both clinical management and control programs and specialist texts should be consulted.[25,29,30] There is a good case for a policy that combines ''bacillus control'' with ''disability control,'' so that all members of the health staff are constantly aware of measures that must be taken to predict, prevent, and manage disability. Manuals outlining the steps to be taken have been fully developed by Watson in the United Kingdom.[31,32]

Social, Psychological, and Economic Aspects

No account of the clinical manifestations of leprosy would be complete without reference to the very considerable social and psychological dislocation experienced by patients with leprosy. With the possible exception of AIDS, it is doubtful if any other disease has been associated with such strong reactions of fear, revulsion, prejudice, and superstition. Although the level of ''stigma'' is low in some areas endemic for leprosy (e.g., central Africa), it remains high elsewhere. There is, however, encouraging evidence from many parts of the world that the implementation of multiple-drug therapy, exclusively on an outpatient basis, has both ''normalized'' the disease in many parts of the world and greatly lowered the level of stigma.

Diagnosis and Differential Diagnosis

The diagnosis of leprosy should be made only if one or more of the cardinal signs are present. Essentially these are (1) skin lesions of a type characteristic for leprosy, with diminution or loss of sensation; (2) enlarged peripheral nerves; and/or (3) the finding of *M. leprae*, usually in skin, less commonly in other sites. To an experienced observer, and provided the findings are reliable (notably in the case of results of slit-skin smears), any one of these cardinal signs may be sufficient for diagnosis, but it is important to realize that no one sign is absolutely dependable under all circumstances. For example, the lesions of lepromatous leprosy may be characteristic and highly positive for *M. leprae*, but they usually show little or no loss of sensation. As indicated below, enlargement of peripheral nerves may not be absolutely diagnostic of leprosy. The finding of acid-fast bacilli in skin, especially in appreciable numbers and in patients in an endemic area, is very highly in favor of leprosy, but it now has to be kept in mind that some patients in the advanced stages of AIDS may harbor vast numbers of opportunistic mycobacteria, usually *M. avium-intracellulare*, and these may be found in skin and many other tissues. The limitations and hazards of finding a few acid-fast bacilli in nasal smears or scrapings are discussed below. These reservations apply not only to the developed forms of leprosy, but also to those in which even an experienced observer has reasonable doubt. In such cases, it is better to err on the side of caution and to keep the patient under observation at regular intervals. The number of dermatologic and neurologic conditions that may cause confusion is large. They include the following: morphea, vitiligo, yaws, onchocerciasis, pityriasis alba, pityriasis versicolor, post-kala-azar dermal leishmaniasis, fungal infections, seborrheic dermatitis, nutritional dyschromia (all macular), ringworm, granuloma annulare, granuloma multiforme (Mkar disease), gyrate erythemas, Wegener's granulomatosis, tinea corporis, acquired syphilis, sarcoidosis, tuberculosis, lupus erythematosus, cutaneous leishmaniasis, neurofibromatosis, necrobiosis lipoidica, atypical necrobiosis of the face, mycosis fungoides, Kaposi's sarcoma, and infection with *M. marinum*. Neurologic conditions are less numerous and are also a less common cause of confusion: peroneal muscular atrophy (Charcot-Marie-Tooth disease), Déjerine-Sottas disease (familial hypertrophic interstitial neuritis), primary amyloidosis of peripheral nerves, syringomyelia, tabes dorsalis, hereditary sensory radicular neuropathy, congenital indifference to pain, and peripheral neuropathy of varied etiology.

Several points call for comment: (1) In the list of skin diseases, there should be little or no margin of error for anyone with dermatologic training, and for others, most mistakes should be avoidable by testing for loss of sensation, examining the peripheral nerves for enlargement or tenderness, and, in some cases, taking slit-skin smears in order to search for acid-fast bacilli. (2) The list of nerve diseases includes some that are rare or extremely rare, and in endemic areas it is important to realize that leprosy is by far the most likely diagnosis in any patient with enlargement and/or tenderness of a peripheral nerve, until proved otherwise. (3) Neither list includes a number of commonly occurring or mundane conditions that often relate to local practices and lifestyle, such as scarring of various kinds, deformity following trauma and fractures, simple postinflammatory dyschromia; these are worth study if mistakes are to be avoided.

Following inspection and palpation of skin lesions, simply testing for loss of sensation, using a wisp of cotton or something similar, is the next vital step and it is one that may establish the correct diagnosis beyond doubt. Although some loss of sensation has been described in the skin lesions of necrobiosis lipoidica,[33] psoriasis, and morphea,[34] definite loss of sensation is rare and atypical in dermatologic conditions other than leprosy, but is common and often diagnostic in leprosy. Further information may be obtained in some cases by testing for pain sensation and thermal loss. A further important step is the systematic palpation of nerves: first, in the vicinity of the lesions, especially in tuberculoid (TT) and borderline-tuberculoid (BT) cases, and second, at certain sites where named peripheral nerves run superficially. The first important point to grasp is that not all peripheral nerves that are palpable are abnormal; these include the ulnar nerve at the elbow and lateral popliteal as it curves round the neck of the fibula. The following nerves are relevant in clinical leprosy: supraorbital, zygomatic, great auricular, supraclavicular, ulnar, radial (particularly the terminal, sensory branch at the wrist), median, lateral popliteal, posterior tibial, superficial peroneal, and sural. Careful comparison of the nerves on both sides of the body is essential; with few exceptions, peripheral nerves that are palpable in the normal subject should be of the same size on both sides of the body, and a difference in size may indicate disease (the converse, namely, that a nerve is judged to be smaller than usual, is a rare finding and not relevant in this context).

Palpation of these nerves should be followed by careful sensory and motor tests for any nerves that have been found abnormal. For the assessment of motor function, a procedure of established value is the "voluntary muscle test" (VMT), which can be carried out on the eyes, hands, and feet. Essentially the VMT aims to assess muscle function in the facial, ulnar, median, and lateral popliteal nerve supply to the muscles of the eyelids, fifth finger, thumb, and foot, respectively, grading the responses as strong, weak, or paralyzed.

Laboratory Procedures and Special Examinations

Slit-Skin Smears

The slit-skin smear consists of making a small incision in the skin and of then scraping it in order to obtain tissue fluid (not blood) so that it can be examined using a modified Ziehl-Neelsen technique. It has been standard practice for the better part of this century. Ridley described the bacterial (or bacteriologic) index (BI) in which the number of bacilli in a given number of oil immersion fields (or

TABLE 192-2
The Bacterial Index (BI)—Ridley's Logarithmic Scale

0	No bacteria seen in 100 fields*
1 +	1–10 bacteria in 100 fields
2 +	1–10 bacteria in 10 fields
3 +	1–10 bacteria in an average field
4 +	10–100 bacteria in an average field
5 +	100–1000 bacteria in an average field
6 +	Many clumps of bacteria (>1000) in an average field

* "Field" means oil-immersion field in each case.

in one field) is counted. The BI ranges from 0 (no bacilli seen in 100 oil immersion fields) to 6 (1000 or more bacilli seen in an average oil immersion field)[35] (Table 192-2). In patients with active lesions, the minimum number of smears per session is three: both ear lobes and one active lesion from any part of the body. In fact, four smears is preferable and should include both ear lobes and two active lesions. Further details for the selection of sites of the taking of smears, the technique of incision and smearing, fixation, staining, interpretation, and reporting are given in standard textbooks and manuals.[36,37] Although it is often stated that the examination of skin smears is essential for the diagnosis of leprosy, the following points should be noted. (1) A very large number of cases (the majority in some situations) will be predictably negative (BI, 0), whether the smears are taken from "routine" sites, such as both ear lobes, arms, buttocks, and thighs, or from lesions, or both, because paucibacillary cases, almost by definition, are likely to be negative on skin smear examination. (2) Treated cases may become negative, in some cases quite rapidly, after the institution of treatment. (3) The value of slit-skin smear examination is entirely dependent on the accuracy and reliability of the work carried out by those who select, take, fix, despatch, stain, and interpret the slides. If this work is not consistently of high standard, inaccurate and misleading results may be produced.

Nasal Smears or Scrapings

The procedure of smearing or scraping the nose or the nasal mucosa received considerable attention in the literature in past years, but is now, justifiably, falling into disuse. As a procedure, it is somewhat difficult to perform, uncomfortable and often painful for the patient, and—most important—it rarely yields information that cannot be obtained from the proper examination of slit-skin smears. Furthermore, scanty acid-fast bacilli (usually commensals, having nothing to do with leprosy or *M. leprae*) are occasionally found, giving rise to diagnostic confusion and even alarm.

Skin Biopsy

Full technical details of the skin biopsy procedure, including the choice of site for biopsy, fixation, transport, staining, and interpretation are available in standard works and have been described in detail by Ridley.[38] Apart from the importance of choosing an active, representative part of the skin lesion, the removal of a biopsy of adequate depth is of paramount importance; it should include the lower dermis and preferably a small amount of subdermis, so that nerves that are vitally important for interpretation are included.

Nerve Biopsy

Nerve biopsy is a special procedure, to be carried out only by experienced and qualified staff, in exceptional cases in which diagnosis and classification cannot be established by other means. Only sensory nerves should be biopsied, such as the great auricular in the neck, the terminal radial at the wrist, or the sural or superficial peroneal nerves in the leg. The technique of taking the minimum number of fasciculi from a nerve trunk is described in standard works. In pure neural leprosy, a nerve biopsy may be unavoidable in order to confirm diagnosis and classification, and it may rarely be indicated in other circumstances. Experience and attention to technique are essential to ensure that there is no risk of the procedure causing deterioration of nerve function.

The Lepromin Test

This test is of value in classification and prognosis, but not in diagnosis. Thus it is not analogous (as is often mistakenly thought) with the tuberculin test in tuberculosis. Full details of the composition of lepromin solution, the technique of injection, and interpretation are available from standard texts. Once diagnosis has been established, the lepromin test may aid classification, for instance, in the Ridley-Jopling classification. However, it has little or no contribution to make to the work of a leprosy control program, in which the interval between injection and reading (3 to 4 weeks), coupled with the need to carry lepromin solution, needles, and syringes, would be deterrents.

The Pilocarpine Test

This aims to test sweating by applying a cholinergic drug to a patch suspected to be caused by leprosy, in which the parasympathetic nerve fibers controlling sweating may be damaged. An intradermal injection of 0.2 mL of a 1/1000 solution of pilocarpine is given into the patch and also into a control site. The sweat response may be assessed by inspection or by applying quinizarin powder, which changes from white to blue in the presence of sweat.

The Histamine Test

If a 1/1000 solution of histamine chlorohydrate or phosphate is injected intradermally into normal skin, it causes bright capillary dilation, known as the histamine flare, that is due to an (intact) axon reflex. If the histamine is injected into a lesion caused by leprosy, it is thought that there will be no reflex and no secondary erythema. It is our view that this test, like the pilocarpine test, is impractical under most circumstances and even likely to be misleading.

The Polymerase Chain Reaction in Leprosy

The polymerase chain reaction[39] is a powerful tool for the amplification of specific sequences of cDNA. Preliminary reports[40,41] suggest that this procedure will offer an exceptionally sensitive and specific tool for the detection of very small numbers of *M. leprae* in crude biologic samples. Future applications of this technique may be of particular importance in the diagnosis of early paucibacillary forms of leprosy, in the detection of very small numbers of persisting bacilli in treated patients, and in epidemiologic and control programs related to the study of infection rates and the detection of subclinical infections.[42]

Treatment

Treatment of the Bacillary Infection

Following the era of chaumoogra oil, dapsone was first used in the 1940s and was soon recognized to be an effective and relatively nontoxic chemotherapeutic agent. It was used extensively during the next two decades as monotherapy in most leprosy-endemic countries of the world and achieved the arrest or cure of leprosy in hundreds of thousands of cases. However, by the 1960s it became increasingly apparent that dapsone resistance was developing on a serious scale,[43] and in the 1970s various regimens of combined therapy, including isoniazid, rifampin (rifampicin), clofazimine, amithiozone (thioacetazone), thiambutosine, and the thioamides (protionamide or ethionamide), were proposed in order both to treat dapsone-resistant cases and to prevent the development of resistance in new cases. In 1981, WHO convened a meeting of experts in Geneva to discuss the formulation of regimens of short duration that could be given to all patients whatever their classification. Their prime objective was to combat the increasing problem of dapsone resistance. The resultant WHO publication, *Chemotherapy of Leprosy for Control Programmes,* has become a classic in this context.[4] It proposes that all patients, whatever their classification, should receive multidrug regimens and that for this purpose they should be divided into "pauci-" or "multibacillary" groups. Paucibacillary leprosy includes indeterminate (I), tuberculoid (TT), and borderline-tuberculoid (BT) on the Ridley-Jopling classification, whether diagnosed clinically or histopathologically, with a BI of less than 2 on the Ridley scale at any site. Multibacillary leprosy includes lepromatous (LL), borderline-lepromatous (BL), and mid-borderline (BB) in the Ridley-Jopling classification. The regimens and their duration are shown in Table 192-3. In their Sixth Report of 1988,[6] the WHO Expert Committee on Leprosy modified the

TABLE 192-3
Multidrug Regimens: Adult Doses

Multibacillary patients (LL, BL, and BB on the Ridley-Jopling scale)	
Monthly, supervised medication	Rifampin, 600 mg Clofazimine, 300 mg
Daily, unsupervised medication	Dapsone, 100 mg Clofazimine, 50 mg
Duration	A minimum of 2 years but wherever possible until slit-skin smears are negative
Follow-up after stopping treatment	A minimum of 5 years with clinical and bacteriologic examination at least every 12 months
Paucibacillary patients (TT and BT on the Ridley-Jopling scale and Indeterminate)	
Monthly, supervised mediation	Rifampin, 600 mg
Daily, unsupervised medication	Dapsone, 100 mg
Duration	6 months; all treatment then stops
Follow-up after stopping treatment	A minimum of 2 years with clinical examination at least every 12 months

SOURCE: World Health Organization Report of Study Group.[4]

above figure of a BI of "less than 2 on the Ridley scale" by advising that any case of leprosy with smear positivity, even if clinically paucibacillary, should be classified and treated as multibacillary for the purposes of multidrug therapy.

Since 1982, nearly 2 million patients have completed or are receiving treatment with these regimens, and the regimens have been shown to be widely acceptable to patients and staff, not excessively expensive, and not associated with significant toxic (drug) effects. Most important, relapse rates have been remarkably low, about 1 per 1000 for paucibacillary cases and about 0.2 per thousand for multibacillary cases. Furthermore, there is no evidence that the use of these regimens has produced (as some predicted) an increased incidence of adverse immunologic reactions, and many centers have reported a decreased incidence of erythema nodosum leprosum in lepromatous patients.

Other multidrug regimens are in use, some of them radically different, others merely modifications of the WHO pattern. Thus, a combination of isoniazid, dapsone, protionamide, and rifampin has been developed by workers in Germany and used quite extensively in Africa, South Africa,[44] and (in an eradication program) in Malta.[45] In India and some other parts of the world, rifampin, clofazimine, and dapsone are given daily for the first 14 days (intensive phase) for multibacillary patients, followed by the WHO regimen. Somewhat more complicated alternatives to those proposed by WHO are currently in use in the United States and have recently been described by Jacobson.[46]

The wide range of toxic effects that may occur during treatment with dapsone, clofazimine, or rifampin in general[47] stands in contrast to the remarkably low incidence of such effects reported in clinical practice in leprosy and in control programs. Clofazimine may cause a brownish-red pigmentation of the skin, which is unacceptable to some patients, but it is a valuable antibacillary and anti-inflammatory drug that should not be omitted from the WHO regimens (for multibacillary patients) unless it is absolutely necessary. The thioamides, originally listed by WHO in 1982 as alternatives for patients who could not accept clofazimine, have been found in several parts of the world to be hepatotoxic. Combinations that include isoniazid, rifampin, and one of the thioamides may be dangerous, especially in patients with a history or clinical evidence of liver disease, all the more so if this is associated with malnutrition and/or alcoholism.

Treatment of Adverse Immunologic Reactions

In the case of type 1, or reversal, reactions, early recognition is important because early treatment can prevent much sensory and motor damage in nerves, thus preventing deformity and disability. However, experience is still needed to decide between cases that are mild and likely to respond to chloroquine, antimonials, and even aspirin and those that are more severe, in which case the early use of steroids is essential. In the latter case, a daily dose of 60 to 80 mg may be needed to control reversal reactions, tapering off gradually over a period of weeks. Clofazimine has been found successful by some workers, but is not generally used. Thalidomide is ineffective in this type of reaction and should not be used.

Some cases of type 2, or immune-complex, reaction in lepromatous leprosy are mild and respond to general nursing, aspirin, and sedation, but steroids should be used if there is any clinical indication of neuritis, which may lead to paralysis or loss of sensation, or any other serious complications. In most cases steroids should be started at 60 mg daily, reducing after some days to a dose

that controls the reaction; 20 or 30 mg every other day may be suitable for the control of most chronic reactions. Thalidomide is generally regarded by leprologists as the drug of choice for the control of type 2 reactions, but risk of teratogenicity obviously limits its use. The usual dose is in the order of 100 mg 3 or 4 times daily, tapering down as soon as the reaction is controlled with the objective of discontinuing within about 4 weeks. More resistant and chronic cases may require a maintenance of 100 mg daily or every other day. Considering its wide use, thalidomide for this type of reaction in leprosy has proved safe; very few serious toxic reactions have been reported. The use of thalidomide in leprosy and other conditions has been extensively reviewed by Sheskin[48] and Barnhill and McDougall.[49]

In contrast to thalidomide, steroids, in the doses that are needed in order to control type 1 or type 2 reactions, carry all the usual hazards. Clofazimine is valuable not only as an antibacterial drug but also as an anti-inflammatory for the treatment and control of type 2 reactions, as first reported by Browne and Hogerzeil in 1962 from Nigeria.[50] Higher doses are needed to obtain an anti-inflammatory effect than are needed for an antibacterial effect. The starting dose should be 300 mg daily in divided doses, for a few weeks, reducing to 200 mg daily for a month or two, and then gradually to 100 mg daily. Although red-brown pigmentation of the skin is inevitable and some patients experience severe gastrointestinal side effects, most who have suffered prolonged and debilitating type 2 reactions accept this drug very well.

The Treatment and Prevention of Disability

Much can be accomplished in hospitals and special centers in the way of treatment, but the potential of patient involvement and active participation in the home is now increasingly acknowledged; it is likely to do much to prevent the occurrence of minor trauma, much of it due either to a poor perception on the part of the patient of the importance of impairment or loss of sensation, or to carelessness. The admission of patients with chronically ulcerated feet to special centers is often effective in healing ulcers (and satisfying to the staff), but is of limited long-term value once the patient has returned home. There is a case, at least in control programs, for doing as much as possible in the community. Patients with established claw hand, thenar muscle weakness, dropped foot, or paralysis of eye muscles may benefit greatly from skilled reconstructive surgery and physiotherapy, but it is important to recognize that selection of patients is of the utmost importance, as a certain level of cooperation and intelligence is essential, and that surgical techniques benefit muscle defects, not loss of sensation (Fig. 192-9).

Prevention

The spread of leprosy in a community can best be minimized by reducing or possibly even eliminating all sources of infection, with emphasis on untreated lepromatous (bacilliferous) cases. Early case detection and treatment with multidrug regimens, including rifampin, are thus of paramount importance, and there is no other measure available for prevention that is in any way comparable. There is already evidence that the systematic use of multidrug therapy for all known registered cases, and for any new cases arising, will, after a period of a few years' sustained effort, have a beneficial effect not only on prevalence (the total number of registered,

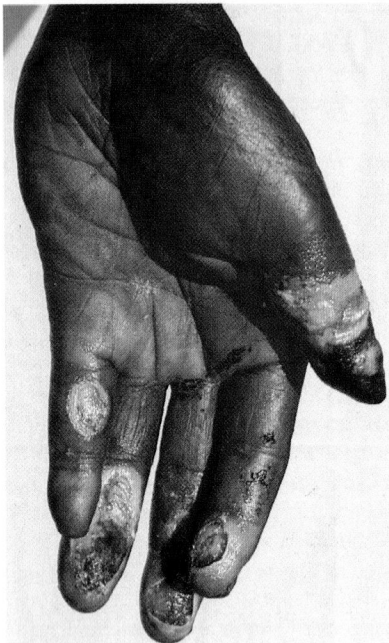

FIGURE 192-9 Severe burns and tissue destruction due to extensive loss of sensation in the hand of a patient with treated (and inactive) borderline-lepromatous (BL) leprosy. Median, ulnar, and radial nerves were all affected.

known cases) but also on incidence, suggesting that its use may be breaking the chain of infection. Chemoprophylaxis, using small doses of dapsone to prevent disease in close contacts and family members, has been used in the past. This is inadvisable and has been abandoned because it is impossible to administer and supervise systematically and also because of the risks of promoting dapsone resistance. Neither oral dapsone, nor its injectable long-acting analogue, acedapsone, are advised by the WHO Expert Committee on Leprosy for this purpose.

The subjects of immunotherapy and immunoprophylaxis have been described above. Progress is obviously being made, but from a control program point of view it is difficult to escape the comment that case detection combined with multidrug therapy is proving to be successful to a degree that was almost certainly not expected at the outset. The potential value of a vaccine, in practice, may be heavily influenced by the pace of research towards its development and availability for use, coupled with the development of a reliable skin or other test indicating which patients need vaccination.

Course and Prognosis

Following the entry of bacilli into a susceptible host (by routes that are as yet ill-defined), it is considered likely that the first lesion that can be recognized clinically and histologically is indeterminate leprosy, with the characteristics already described above. This may resolve spontaneously, or persist. If recognized and treated, it may resolve; if not treated, it may proceed to one of the developed forms of leprosy, as already described. In the case of tuberculoid (TT) leprosy, there is evidence that many, perhaps most, lesions are self-healing without treatment, but this is an unsafe assumption to

make, and all cases, whether seen individually in clinical practice or in control programs, should be treated with multidrug therapy for a minimum of 6 months. At the other end of the spectrum, lepromatous leprosy is progressive in all cases if not treated, although there is some evidence to show that if left untreated, they will eventually "subside" clinically and bacteriologically into a "burnt-out" state—usually, however, with considerable damage to skin, nerves, eyes, and other tissues. Treatment is therefore essential, and a minimum of 2 years is required. In the borderline zone, borderline-lepromatous (BL) and midborderline (BB) cases should be handled, for treatment purposes, in the same way as lepromatous (LL) cases. Borderline-tuberculoid (BT) patients, although classed as paucibacillary for the purpose of multidrug therapy, call for particular care in some instances, especially if there are many multiple macular lesions. It is vital to keep in mind the likelihood of immune-complex reactions in borderline-lepromatous (BL) and lepromatous (LL) cases and the potential damage that may take place not only in skin and peripheral nerves, but also in eyes, testicles, kidneys, and joints. Reversal reactions, if not diagnosed and treated early, may lead to tissue damage in skin, nerves, and eyes, sometimes very rapidly. The course and prognosis of indeterminate leprosy has already been discussed. Pure neural or primary neuritic leprosy, as already noted, often has a paucibacillary classification and usually responds well to treatment, without complication. For reasons that may not be entirely related to improvements in chemotherapy, the clinical profile of leprosy is changing for the better. Over the past 20 years, ulcerating nodular lesions, leonine facies, laryngeal and hard palate involvement, progressive ulcerating ENL, amyloidosis, nephrotic syndrome, and death have all become less frequent, particularly in countries operating efficient leprosy control programs.

Leprosy and AIDS

The subject of mycobacterial infections and AIDS has been reviewed in depth by Nunn and McAdam.[51] The sinister association of AIDS and tuberculosis and the threat that this poses to the management of individual cases and to control programs has been reviewed by Slutkin et al.,[52] Styblo,[53] and WHO in association with the International Union Against Tuberculosis and Lung Disease.[54]

So far, there have been only a limited number of reports describing an association of leprosy and AIDS. These have been of an essentially clinical, not epidemiologic nature,[55–58] and there is no clear evidence to date to suggest that HIV infection or frank AIDS has a significant effect on the incidence of leprosy, the clinical picture, or the response to treatment. It is not known whether immunosuppression by HIV infection will eventually be shown to hasten the development of clinical leprosy in persons who have been infected (and who may be harboring viable organisms in some, as yet, unidentified site) or bring about deterioration of disease in patients with indeterminate or tuberculoid forms of disease towards the lepromatous end of the spectrum. It has been suggested that the slow reproduction rate of *M. leprae* and the long incubation period of the disease will allow other infections to develop and become clinically significant before leprosy develops. However, a recent report by Baskin et al.[59] of dual infection by *M. leprae* and the simian immunodeficiency virus (SIV) is disquieting; an increased susceptibility to *M. leprae* was demonstrated in SIV-infected rhesus monkeys, and the authors comment, albeit by analogy, that although leprosy has so far not increased dramatically in populations where both leprosy and HIV are prevalent, such an increase may indeed by expected.

On a more practical level, it has to be remembered that leprosy control involves the use of slit-skin smear techniques; all concerned should be aware of the detailed guidelines that have been widely issued by WHO for the protection of staff against HIV infection for the proper sterilization of instruments in order to avoid transmission,[60] and in the use of vaccines, including BCG.[61] In an editorial on AIDS and leprosy,[62] Turk and Rees have included advice on the conduct of leprosy vaccine trials in areas endemic for AIDS and drawn attention to difficulties that may arise in the assessment of vaccine efficacy if subjects concerned are not tested for HIV in parallel.

References

1. Cochrane RG, Davey TF (eds): *Leprosy in Theory and Practice.* Bristol, John Wright, 1964.
2. Browne SG: The history of leprosy, in *Leprosy. Medicine in the Tropics,* edited by RC Hastings. Edinburgh, London, Melbourne and New York, Churchill Livingstone, 1985, p 1
3. Møller-Christensen V: *Bone Changes in Leprosy.* Copenhagen, Munksgaard, p 961
4. World Health Organization Report of Study Group: Chemotherapy of leprosy for control programmes. *WHO Tech Rep Ser* **675:**1, 1982
5. World Health Organisation: *Multidrug Therapy for Leprosy: An End in Sight.* World Health Organisation, Geneva, 1988
6. World Health Organisation Expert Committee on Leprosy: Sixth report, *WHO Tech Rep Ser* **768:**1, 1988
7. World Health Organisation Report of Study Group: Epidemiology of leprosy in relation to control. *WHO Tech Rep Ser* **716:**1, 1985
8. Walsh GP et al: Naturally acquired leprosy-like disease in the nine-banded armadillo (*Dasypus novemcinctus*). Recent epizootiologic findings. *J Reticulo Soc* **22:**363, 1977
9. Meyers WM et al. Naturally-acquired leprosy in a mangabey monkey (*Cerocebus* sp.). *Int J Lepr* **53:**1, 1985
10. Leininger JR et al: Leprosy in a chimpanzee. Postmortem lesions. *Int J Lepr* **48:**414, 1980
11. Kazda J et al: Acid-fast bacilli found in sphagnum vegetation of coastal Norway containing *Mycobacterium leprae*-specific phenolic glycolipid-1. *Int J Lepr* **58:**353, 1990
12. Fine PEM: Leprosy: The epidemiology of a slow bacterium. *Epidemiol Rev* **4:**161, 1982
13. Van Eden W, De Vries RRP: Occasional review—HLA and leprosy; a re-evaluation. *Lepr Rev* **55:**89, 1984
14. Convit J: Leprosy and leishmaniasis. Similar clinical-immunological-pathological models. *Ethiop Med J* **12:**187, 1974
15. Clark-Curtiss JE, Walsh GP: Conservation of genomic sequences among isolates of *Mycobacterium leprae. J Bacteriol* **171:**4844, 1989
16. Brennan PJ, Barrow WW: Evidence for species-specific lipid antigens in *Mycobacterium leprae. Int J Lepr* **48:**382, 1980
17. Brennan PJ: The carbohydrate-containing antigens of *Mycobacterium leprae. Lepr Rev* **57**(suppl 2):39, 1986
18. Mehra V et al: Lepromin-induced suppressor cells in patients with leprosy. *J Immunol* **123:**1813, 1979
19. Van Voorhis WC et al: The cutaneous infiltrates of leprosy, cellular characteristics and the predominant T-cell phenotypes. *N Engl J Med* **307:**1593, 1982
20. Modlin RL et al: Lymphocytes in human infectious disease lesions. *Nature* **339:**544, 1989
21. Wemambu SNC et al: ENL—a clinical manifestation of the Arthus phenomenon. *Lancet* **2:**933, 1969
22. Laal S et al: Natural emergence of antigen-reactive T cells in lepromatous leprosy patients during erythema nodosum leprosum. *Infect Immunol* **50:**887, 1985
23. Convit J et al: Immunotherapy with a mixture of *Mycobacterium leprae* and BCG in different forms of leprosy and in Mitsuda-negative contacts. *Int J Lepr* **50:**415, 1982
24. Ridley DS, Jopling WH: Classification according to immunity. *Int J Lepr* **34:**255, 1966
25. Jopling WH, McDougall AC: *Handbook of Leprosy,* 4th ed. Oxford, Heinemann, 1988
26. Wade HW: The histoid variety of lepromatous leprosy. *Int J Lepr* **31:**129, 1963
27. Latapi F, Zamora AC: The 'spotted' leprosy of Lucio (la lepra manchanda' de Lucio): An introduction to its clinical and histological study. *Int J Lepr* **16:**421, 1948
28. Rea TH, Ridley DS: Lucio's phenomenon: A comparative histologic study. *Int J Lepr* **47:**161, 1979
29. Hastings RC (ed): *Leprosy. Medicine in the Tropics.* Edinburgh, London, Melbourne, New York, Churchill Linvingstone, 1985
30. Bryceson A, Pfaltzgraff RE: *Leprosy. Medicine in the Tropics.* Edinburgh, London, Melbourne, New York, Churchill Livingstone, 1990
31. Watson JM: Preventing disability in leprosy patients. The Leprosy Mission International, Brentford, Middlesex, United Kingdom, 1986
32. Watson JM: Essential action to minimise disability in leprosy patients. The Leprosy Mission International, Brentford, Middlesex, United Kingdom, 1986
33. Mann RJ, Harman RRM: Cutaneous anaesthesia in necrobiosis lipoidica. *Br J Dermatol* **110:**323, 1984
34. Ghosh S, Haldar B: Quantitative evaluation of cutaneous thermal sensation in psoriasis, morphoea and vitiligo. *Indian J Dermatol Venereol Lepr* **55:**30, 1989
35. Ridley DS: Bacterial indices, in *Leprosy in Theory and Practice,* edited by RG Cochrane, TF Davey. Bristol, John Wright, 1964, p 620
36. World Health Organisation: *Manual of Basic Techniques for a Health Laboratory.* World Health Organisation, Geneva, 1980
37. Leiker DL, McDougall AC: *Technical Guide for Smear Examination for Leprosy,* 2d ed. Teaching and Learning Materials (TALMILEP). German Leprosy Relief Association, Würzburg, Germany, 1987
38. Ridley DS: *Skin Biopsy in Leprosy,* 2d ed. Documenta Geigy. Basel, 1985
39. Saiki R et al: Primer directed enzymatic amplification of DNA with a thermostable DNA polymerase. *Science* **239:**487, 1988
40. Williams PL et al: Application of polymerase chain reaction amplification technology for the detection of *Mycobacterium leprae. Int J Lepr* **58:**192, 1990
41. Plikayetes BB, Shinnick TH: Rapid, sensitive and specific detection of *mycobacteria* using gene amplification techniques. *Int J Lepr* **58:**197, 1990
42. World Health Organisation: Report of the consultation on the early diagnosis of leprosy. Geneva, May 23–25, 1990. WHO/CTD/LEP/90.2
43. Baohong J: Drug resistance in leprosy—a review. *Lepr Rev* **56:**265, 1985
44. Freerksen E: Preliminary experience with combined therapy using rifampicin and isoprodian. *Lepr Rev* **46** (suppl): 161, 1975
45. Freerksen E et al: Le Projet Malte. *Acta Leprologica* **VI:**7, 1989
46. Jacobson RR: Treatment, in *Leprosy. Medicine in the Tropics,* edited by RC Hastings. Edinburgh, London, Melbourne, New York, Churchill Livingstone, 1985
47. Jopling WH: Side effects of anti-leprosy drugs in common use. *Lepr Rev.* **54:**261, 1983
48. Sheskin J: Thalidomide in the treatment of lepra reactions. *Clin Pharmacol Ther* **6:**303, 1965
49. Barnhill RL, McDougall AC: Thalidomide: Use and possible mode of action in reactional lepromatous leprosy and various other conditions. *J Am Acad Dermatol* **7:**317, 1982
50. Browne SG, Hogerzeil LM: 'B663' in the treatment of leprosy: Preliminary report of a pilot trial. *Lepr Rev* **33:**6, 1962
51. Nunn PP, McAdam KPWJ: Mycobacterial infections and AIDS, in *Tuberculosis and Leprosy,* edited by RJW Rees. *Br Med Bull* **44:**801, 1988

52. Slutkin G et al: Tuberculosis and AIDS. The effects of the AIDS epidemic on the tuberculosis problem and tuberculosis programmes. *Bull Int Union Tuberc* **63**:21, 1988

53. Styblo K: The potential impact of AIDS on the tuberculosis situation in developed and developing countries. *Bull Int Union Tuberc* **63**:25, 1988

54. World Health Organisation: Global Programme on AIDS, Tuberculosis Unit, and the International Union Against Tuberculosis and Lung Diseases (IUATLD): Joint Working Group on HIV Infection and Tuberculosis. Geneva, January 18–19, 1988

55. Lamfers EJP et al: Leprosy in the acquired immunodeficiency syndrome. *Ann Intern Med* **107**:111, 1987

56. Kennedy C et al: Leprosy and human immunodeficiency virus infection. *Int J Dermatol* **29**:139, 1990

57. Meeran K: Prevalence of HIV infection among patients with leprosy and tuberculosis in rural Zambia. *Br Med J* **298**:364, 1989

58. Vreeburg AEM: Clinical observations on leprosy patients with HIV-1 infections in Zambia. Unpublished observations.

59. Baskin GB et al: Pathology of dual *Mycobacterium leprae* and Simian immunodeficiency virus infection in Rhesus monkeys. *Int J Lepr* **58**:358, 1990

60. World Health Organisation: Guidelines for personnel involved in collection of skin smears in leprosy control programmes for the prevention and control of possible infection with HIV. WHO/CDS/LEP/87.1

61. World Health Organisation: Special Programme on AIDS: Statement from the Consultation on Human Immunodeficiency Virus (HIV) and Routine Childhood Immunization. Geneva, August 12–13, 1987. WHO/SPA/INF/87.11

62. Turk JL, Rees RJW: AIDS and leprosy, editorial. *Lepr Rev* **59**:193, 1988

CHAPTER 193

Eva Åsbrink and Anders Hovmark

Lyme Borreliosis

Lyme borreliosis (Lyme disease, erythema migrans borreliosis, *Ixodes*-borne borreliosis) is a vector-borne infection, primarily transmitted by *Ixodes* ticks, and caused by *Borrelia burgdorferi*. The disease may affect different organs, and the clinical picture and course may be highly variable. Erythema (chronicum) migrans, borrelial lymphocytoma, and acrodermatitis chronica atrophicans (ACA) are the cutaneous hallmarks.

Historical Aspects

The three dermatologic conditions—erythema migrans, lymphadenosis benigna cutis (LABC), and ACA—have long been well known to European dermatologists. Both the atrophic and the inflammatory forms of ACA were described by different European authors more than a century ago, but the disease was first named and further characterized by Herxheimer and Hartmann in 1902. The first report of an erythema developing after a tick bite was presented by Afzelius in Sweden in 1909 and he gave it the name *erythema migrans*. A few years later the term *erythema chronicum migrans* was used in an Austrian case report by Lipschütz. The designation *lymphocytoma* was first used by Biberstein in 1923. Bäfverstedt coined the term *lymphadenosis benigna cutis* in his monograph on pseudolymphomas published in 1943.[1]

In 1941 and 1944, the German neurologist Bannwarth described a syndrome, later to be named after him, with focal and often severe radicular pain, lymphocytic meningitis, and cranial nerve paralysis. The association with tick bites and erythema migrans was later observed by Schaltenbrand.

In the United States, erythema migrans was not described until 1970. In 1977, Steere et al. reported on an epidemic form of arthritis occurring in several communities around Lyme on the Connecticut River.[2] Lyme arthritis was soon linked to a preceding erythema migrans, and manifestations from the nervous system and the heart were also found.[2]

In the beginning of the 1980s, Burgdorfer et al.[3] showed that Lyme disease was caused by tick-borne spirochetes. With use of modified Kelly medium,[4] cultivation of spirochetes from *Ixodes* ticks, from erythema migrans lesions, and from blood and cerebrospinal fluid specimens from a few patients with Lyme disease was successful. These spirochetes could be classified as a new species of *Borrelia* and were named *B. burgdorferi*.[5] Later, spirochetal cultivations and serologic tests also revealed that Bannwarth's syndrome[6] and ACA[7] were caused by *B. burgdorferi* and that these spirochetes may also cause LABC.[8] However, as all cases diagnosed as LABC probably do not have a borrelial etiology, Weber et al. introduced the term *borrelial lymphocytoma* in 1985.[9]

Epidemiology

Lyme borreliosis is a disease with a wide distribution in the northern hemisphere. Cases have been reported from Canada, 46 of the United States, most European countries, the Federal Republic of China, and Japan. In the former Soviet Union, cases have been recognized from the Baltic republics to the Pacific Ocean. It is the most common vector-borne disease of bacterial origin in the United States and Europe. There have been discussions as to whether the true incidence is rising or whether the reported increase is mainly attributable to greater recognition and awareness of this infection.

Etiology

B. burgdorferi was discovered unexpectedly in conjunction with a tick survey on Long Island, New York in 1981 and 1982.[3] The spirochete represents a new species in the genus *Borrelia* (order Spirochetales), as determined by morphologic, protein, and DNA relationship studies. Closely related species or different subtypes of

B. burgdorferi seem to exist,[6,10] but there is still no accepted system of classification.

The primary vectors of Lyme borreliosis are hard ticks belonging to the *Ixodes ricinus* complex, i.e., *I. ricinus, I. persulcatus,* and *I. ovatus* in Europe and Asia and *I. dammini, I. pacificus,* and *I. scapularis* in North America. They are three-host ticks parasitizing a wide range of animals, including humans. During feeding on a spirochetemic host, the larval or nymphal tick may become infected and it may then remain infectious throughout the rest of its life by transstadial transmission of spirochetes. The feeding activity of the different stages is often seasonal during the spring, summer, and autumn. The rate of infection in nymphs and adult ticks has been found to range from a few percent to more than 50 percent. Transovarial transmission seems to be rare. Instead the main reservoirs of *B. burgdorferi* are the hosts, mainly considered to be rodents, of the larvae and nymphs. However, many other warmblooded animals may serve as additional reservoirs. Large animals such as deer may play an important role in feeding adult ticks. In endemic areas domestic animals are frequently seropositive for antibodies to *B. burgdorferi,* and manifestations of Lyme borreliosis have been demonstrated in such animals.

Tick vectors other than those of the genus *Ixodes* may transmit *B. burgdorferi* but are less efficient vectors. Transmission of *B. burgdorferi* by nontick vectors such as deer flies, horse flies, and mosquitoes or by direct contact with fluids from infected animals has been reported. However, Lyme borreliosis obtained in other ways than through a tick bite is probably very rare.

Human Exposure to Tick Bites and B. burgdorferi Many patients with Lyme borreliosis are not aware of a preceding tick bite. The large bloodsucking adult female tick is usually easily detected. However, the small nymphal tick, which is considered to be the most important vector for transmitting *B. burgdorferi* to humans, often escapes detection. The tick drops off spontaneously, and the bites are usually painless, which may be other reasons why the tick may escape detection. In one German study of 91 humans bitten by 105 ticks known to harbor *B. burgdorferi,* only one individual developed symptomatic infection, but a seroconversion rate of 27 percent was estimated.

Clinical Manifestations

Classification of Clinical Disease By analogy with syphilis, the natural history of Lyme borreliosis can be divided into three stages based on the clinical manifestations. As the course in the individual patient does not imply a uniform temporal sequence with development of all the stages and as the infection is sometimes not manifest until stage 2 or 3, many clinicians are of the opinion that a staging system with numbers may be misleading. It has therefore been proposed that the terms *early localized infection, early disseminated infection,* and *late* or *chronic infection* should be used instead (Table 193-1). Besides the clinical picture, the duration of the disease is probably also important in therapeutic decisions. A definition of chronic or late infection as persistent infection lasting more than 12 months has been suggested. As many signs and symptoms of Lyme borreliosis are nonspecific, the cutaneous borrelial manifestations may serve as helpful and important landmarks in the identification of Lyme borreliosis.

TABLE 193-1
Classification of Lyme Borreliosis*

Early Lyme borreliosis
  Localized infection
  Erythema migrans and borrelial lymphocytoma without signs or symptoms of disseminated infection. (Regional lymphadenopathy and/or minor constitutional symptoms may be present.)
  Early disseminated infection
  Multiple erythema migrans-like skin lesions. Early manifestations of neuroborreliosis, arthritis, carditis, or other organ involvement.
Late Lyme borreliosis
  Chronic infection
  ACA. Neurologic, rheumatic, or other organ manifestations—persistent or remitting for at least 12 months.

*The classification provides a guideline for the timing of different disease manifestations.

Geographic Differences in the Clinical Picture The clinical experiences of Lyme borreliosis in Europe and in the United States have differed in some respects. Multiple erythema migrans-like lesions have been found in a higher frequency among U.S. patients (25 to 48 percent)[11,12] than among European (≤8 percent).[13,14] A higher frequency of arthritis has also been reported from the United States. In contrast, only a few U.S. cases of ACA and borrelial lymphocytoma have been described. There are historical reasons that may explain some of the different approaches to this infection; European clinicians initially focused on dermatologic and neurologic manifestations and U.S. clinicians paid special attention to joint manifestations. Thus, selection of patients from different medical specialties may at least partly explain the claims that have been made concerning geographic differences in the clinical picture. However, there may also be regional genetic differences between the spirochetes involved, which perhaps may influence the clinical picture. Other factors that may vary are genetic predispositions of the hosts and the clinical management of the infection.

Cutaneous Manifestations

Erythema Migrans

Clinical Features[11-18] Erythema migrans, the principal cutaneous hallmark of Lyme borreliosis, starts at the site of a tick bite, but it is not unusual for the bite to pass unnoticed. The incubation period may vary from a few days to 3 months but is usually 1 to 3 weeks.[11,13,14] In most endemic areas there is a peak in the occurrence during the summer or autumn months. The initial erythema is usually homogeneous (Fig. 193-1) and it sometimes remains so until it heals. However, in the majority of the lesions the center partly or totally fades, leaving an annular erythema that spreads centrifugally (Fig. 193-2). A central reddish patch, representing the site of the tick bite, may sometimes be apparent. The diameter of the erythema migrans ranges from less than one decimeter to several decimeters. The size of the lesion or the distance the erythema has migrated mostly corresponds to the duration of the infection. The peripheral reddish band may be more or less sharply demarcated and is mostly 1 to 2 cm wide. With time the erythematous border often fades; it may wax and wane and is sometimes only visible after the skin has been warmed up, for example in a hot bath. The classic lesion is round, but elliptical or irregular forms

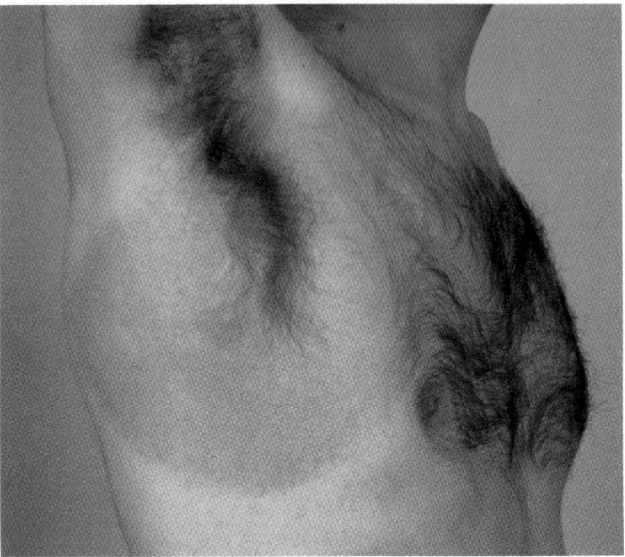

FIGURE 193-1 Homogeneous 3-week-old erythema migrans.

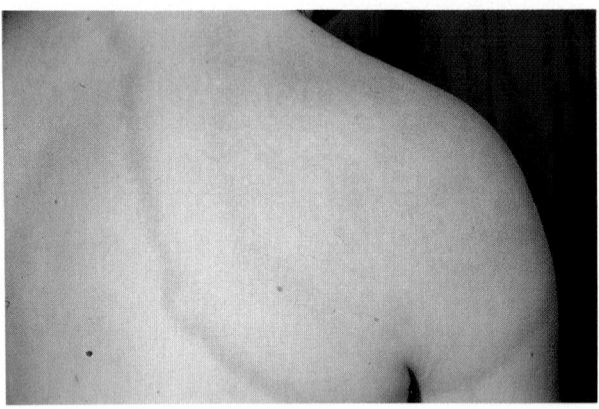

FIGURE 193-2 Annular 2-month-old erythema migrans.

may be seen. The duration of an untreated erythema migrans may vary from some days to about a year, but generally it disappears within some weeks or months.[11,16] In patients who develop extracutaneous manifestations such as meningitis, the duration of the erythema often seems to be short. Erythema migrans may appear almost anywhere on the skin surface, but the lower extremities are most usually affected.[14,17] Facial involvement is common in children.[15] The clinical spectrum of erythema migrans is wider than has previously been reported. Atypical appearances with blisters or hemorrhagic or scaling lesions may sometimes develop.[17] Other variants are small stationary erythemas or a localized swelling without any obvious erythema at the site of the tick bite.

Erythema migrans may pass unnoticed as it may be poorly visible and asymptomatic. However, many of the patients experience local itching or sensations of irritation or heat.[11–13,16] In most cases the local symptoms are mild or moderate, but in a few cases more intense dysesthesia/hyperesthesia may occur at or near the site of the eruption. Regional lymphadenopathy may be present. In at least half of the patients constitutional signs or symptoms such as headache, low-grade fever, malaise, gastrointestinal complaints, and/or myalgia/arthralgia will accompany the skin lesion or some-

times start before the erythema.[11–13,16–18] Severe fatigue or emotional disturbances such as irritability and depression may develop. Mostly the constitutional reactions are mild or moderate, of an intermittent and changing nature, and last for some days to 1 or a few weeks. If they are more pronounced or long-lasting, they may signal a disseminated infection with meningitis, and a spinal fluid examination should be performed.

Nonspecific cutaneous manifestations such as malar erythema, periorbital swelling, urticaria, maculopapular eruptions, and erythema nodosum have also been described in solitary patients with early Lyme borreliosis.[11,12,14,17]

Multiple Erythema Migrans-like Lesions   The development of secondary erythema migrans-like lesions is the cutaneous sign of hematogenous spread of spirochetes and of disseminated infection, as evidenced by successful spirochetal cultivation from secondary lesions.[12,17] The lesions may follow the initial erythema migrans or sometimes appear almost simultaneously. The multiple lesions may be homogeneous or annular; they are sometimes, but not always, smaller than a solitary erythema migrans and may be nonmigrating.

Pathology   The epidermis is usually unaffected and there is a generally sparse dermal lymphocytic infiltrate with an admixture of a few plasma cells. The infiltrate is mainly confined to the perivascular regions.

Diagnosis   The clinical picture and the characteristic evolution of the erythema are most often sufficient to make the correct diagnosis. In atypical cases the seasonal onset, the history of exposure to an area highly endemic for Lyme borreliosis, the history of a tick bite at the site of the lesion, the nonspecific histopathologic features, and/or elevated serum antibodies to *B. burgdorferi* are helpful clues. However, seronegativity does not rule out the diagnosis, as only a minority of patients with uncomplicated erythema migrans are seropositive. The diagnosis can be confirmed by cultivation of borreliae from a skin biopsy. If the lesion does not resolve after adequate antibiotic therapy, the diagnosis of erythema migrans ought to be reconsidered.

Differential Diagnosis   Important differential diagnoses are granuloma annulare, erysipelas, tinea, fixed drug eruptions, lupus erythematosus, dermatomyositis, erythema gyratum repens, and nonspecific tick or insect bite reactions. In patients with multiple lesions, erythema multiforme and Sweet's syndrome may also be differential diagnoses. Histopathologic examinations are often of help in the differentiation.

Borrelial Lymphocytoma

Clinical Features[1,8,9,19]   Borrelial lymphocytoma often, but not always, starts at the site of the tick bite. The incubation period may vary from a few weeks to several months.[8,19] Some patients have a history of a preceding erythema migrans, and others may show a concomitant erythema migrans located around or near the lymphocytoma.[1,9,19] That a lymphocytoma may start at a distance from the spirochetal inoculation is obvious in cases where it begins close to the periphery of a large migrating erythema migrans. There are also case reports of concomitant ACA or sclerotic skin lesions.[1,19]

The classic borrelial lymphocytoma presents as a solitary bluish-red nodule, 1 to 5 cm in diameter, often accompanied by

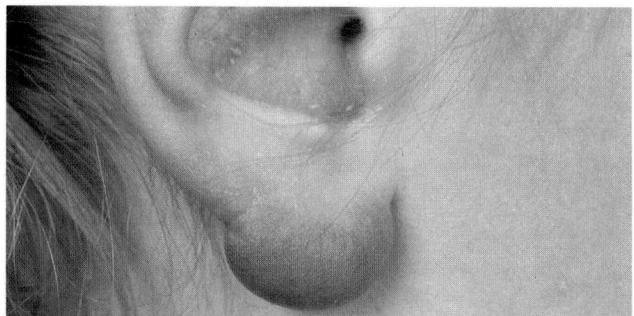

FIGURE 193-3   Borrelial lymphocytoma of 3 months' duration.

regional lymphadenopathy. Predilection sites are the ear lobe (Fig. 193-3) and the nipple/areola mammae region. Other sites of predilection are the scrotum and the nose. Ear lesions are particularly seen in children, and breast lesions in adults. The future will tell whether more unusual forms of lymphocytomas or multiple lesions can be of borrelial origin or not. In many cases there are no or only slight local symptoms, such as tenderness and itching. However, constitutional symptoms such as headache, fever, and arthralgia/myalgia may occur.

Pathology   Usually the epidermis is unaffected. There is a dense dermal lymphocytic infiltrate, mainly composed of polyclonal B cells. The presence of germinal centers (Fig. 193-4), similar to those seen in reactive lymph nodes, is a helpful clue but not an obligatory diagnostic sign.

Diagnosis   The presence of a bluish-red nodule on the ear lobe of a child suggests a borrelial lymphocytoma, as do scrotal nodules. The diagnosis should also be considered in patients with an erythematous swelling of the nipple/areola mammae region. A history of a preceding erythema migrans or a tick bite in the vicinity further supports the diagnosis. Histopathologic findings of a dense dermal lymphocytic infiltrate with germinal centers are suggestive of but not specific for borrelial lymphocytoma. Elevated serum antibody titers to *B. burgdorferi* have been found in more than half of the patients.

Differential Diagnosis   Borrelial lymphocytoma of the breast is often primarily suspected of being a malignant tumor. Conventional histopathologic examinations may be decisive in distinguishing a borrelial lymphocytoma from granuloma faciale, granuloma annulare, sarcoidosis, lupus erythematosus, polymorphous light eruptions, and arthropod bite granuloma. Lesions without germinal centers may be difficult to differentiate from malignant lymphoma. In such cases immunohistochemical characterization of the cell infiltrate is of diagnostic help.

Acrodermatitis Chronica Atrophicans

Clinical Features[7,13,15,20–27]   A connection between ACA and a preceding tick bite is very seldom suspected by patients. About 20 percent have a history of a preceding untreated erythema migrans, usually on an extremity where ACA lesions developed 6 months to 10 years later.[13,14,24] Some patients also have a history of preceding neurologic and/or rheumatic complaints. Among patients with

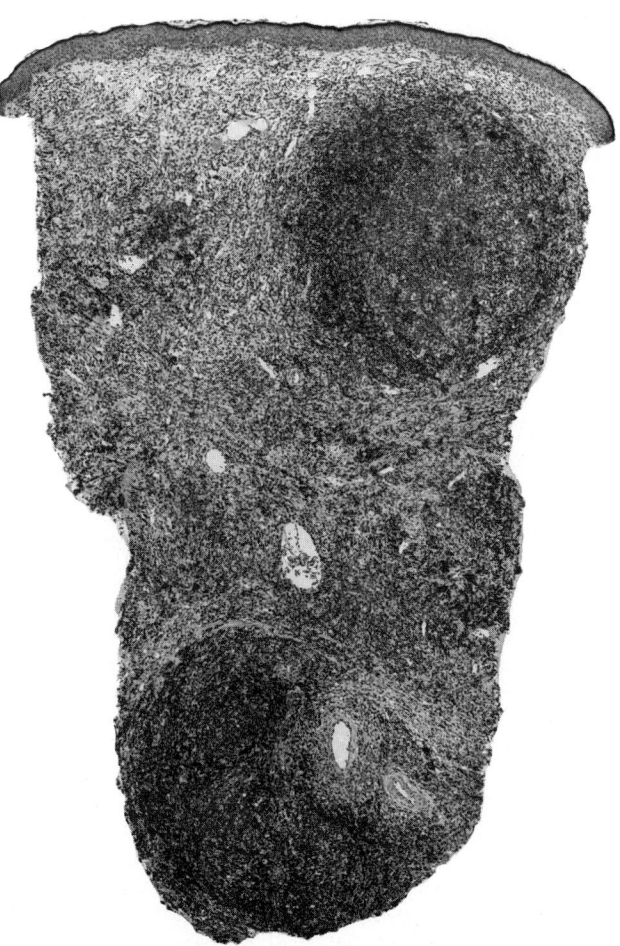

FIGURE 193-4   Borrelial lymphocytoma. Punch biopsy specimen from a scrotal lesion. In the dermis and the subcutaneous fat there is a dense lymphocytic infiltrate displaying a follicular pattern. In the uppermost follicle there is a huge germinal center. (*Micrograph by Eva Brehmer-Andersson, M.D.*)

ACA there is a preponderance of females (about 70 percent), and it is generally a disease of the middle-aged or elderly. It usually starts on the extensor aspect of one extremity. The most common site is the lower leg, with initial involvement of the foot, ankle, or knee region. The dorsal aspect of the hand or the olecranon area are other common sites. The fingers, toes, and soles may become involved. With time, more widespread involvement of the extremity may occur, and the lesions usually spread from distal to proximal sites. Additional limbs may become affected, but sometimes not until after several years. Lesions may also appear on the buttocks. More extensive involvement of the trunk or involvement of the face is uncommon. The first cutaneous sign is a bluish-red discoloration, often with edematous swelling. Sometimes the erythema may be very slight and swelling may dominate the clinical picture, suggesting venous stasis or lymphedema. A typical feature is that one of the feet or just the heel gradually increases in size.[15] ACA lesions often develop slowly and insidiously, and initially both the erythema and swelling may wax and wane.

Fibrous thickening of the skin in the form of indurated bands or nodules may develop. The most common bands are ulnar bands (Fig. 193-5a). The same area is also the most common site of single or multiple fibrotic nodules. Less often, similar bands and nodules

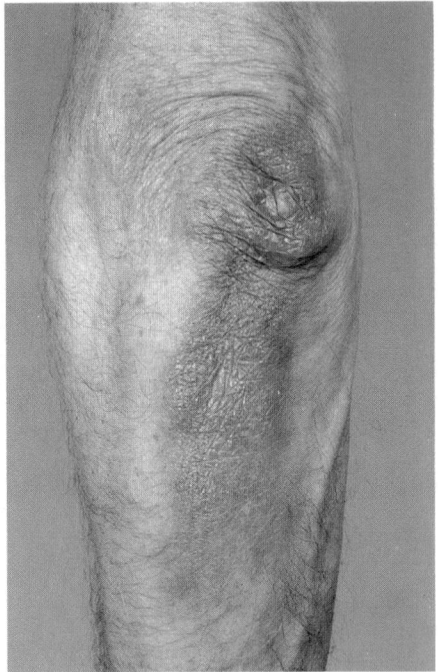

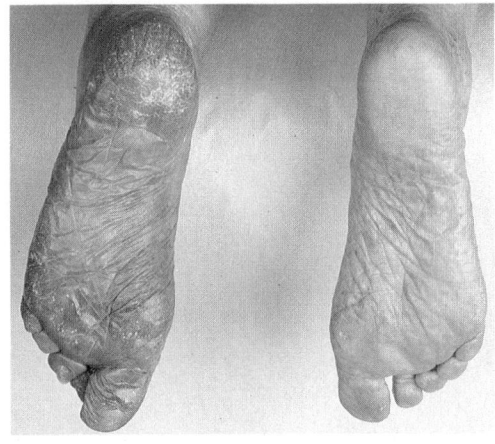

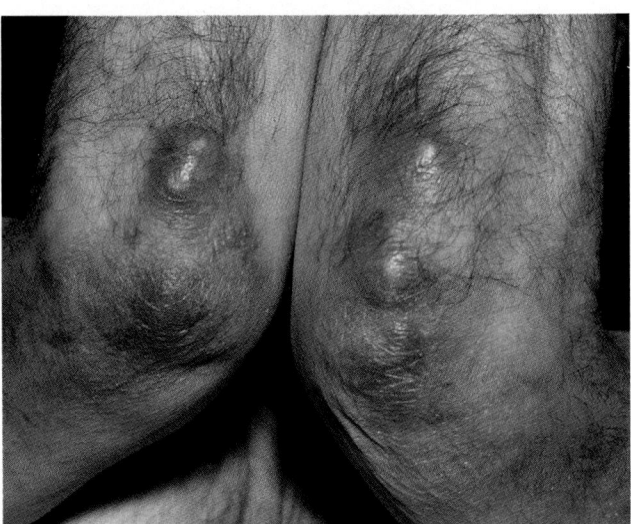

FIGURE 193-5 (a) Ulnar band in a patient with acrodermatitis chronica atrophicans that had been present for more than 10 years. *B. burgdorferi* has been cultivated from this lesion. (b) Acrodermatitis chronica atrophicans with bluish-red discoloration and advanced atrophy of the planta of one of the feet. (c) Lyme borreliosis, acrodermatitis chronica atrophicans—asymptomatic, violaceous lesions occuring on the elbows.

a

b

c

may appear in the knee region, and nodules sometimes also occur adjacent to other joints (Fig. 193-5c). The bands and nodules are generally firm, skin-colored or bluish-red, and not tender. The diameter of the nodules varies from 0.5 cm to 2 to 3 cm and the bands may be of similar width or somewhat wider.

Sclerotic skin lesions that may be clinically and histopathologically indistinguishable from localized scleroderma or lichen sclerosus et atrophicus may occur in 5 to 10 percent of patients with ACA.[24] There may be single or multiple sclerotic patches on extremities and/or the trunk. Often the sclerotic lesions develop adjacent to inflammatory or atrophic ACA lesions or there is a mixture of the different types of lesions in the same regions. The term *pseudoscleroderma* has previously been used for the sclerotic skin lesions that may occur in ACA.[26]

Inflammatory ACA lesions may persist for years or decades, with gradual conversion to atrophic skin lesions (Fig. 193-5b). The clinical picture may be one of both inflammation and atrophy in different regions in the same patient. In the advanced atrophic phase, the skin becomes cigarette paper-like and wrinkled, appendageal structures disappear, and the vessels become prominent (Fig. 193-6). Besides diffuse atrophy, macular atrophy, which has previously been described as *atrophia maculosa cutis* or *dermatitis atrophicans maculosa,* may rarely occur.

Extracutaneous Manifestations in Patients with ACA   Enlarged regional lymph nodes are common, and in rare cases a more widespread lymphadenopathy may develop. Occasionally involuntary loss of weight may occur. Migrating and/or intermittent pains are fairly frequent. A rather common and characteristic feature is pain arising from impacts against bony prominences, such as the knuckles, the olecranon, or the malleolae, underlying ACA skin lesions. As diagnosed by clinical and electroneurographic examinations, more than 50 percent of patients with ACA have peripheral neuropathy, mostly mild or moderate. This may be a sensory or motor mono- or polyneuropathy, or patchy dysesthesia, at the sites of the skin lesions. Symptoms such as hyperesthesia, muscular weakness, a feeling of heaviness, and muscle cramps are common in patients with ACA. These symptoms are mainly located in the limb(s) affected by skin lesions.

Profound fatigue, emotional disturbances, and personality changes may sometimes accompany ACA. Pathologic auditory brainstem responses, similar to those previously described in syphilis, have been found. However, there are usually no cerebrospinal fluid abnormalities in patients with ACA.

Subluxations/luxations of small joints of the fingers or toes and periosteal thickening of bones have been found underneath the skin lesions in patients with long-standing ACA.[23] Periarticular

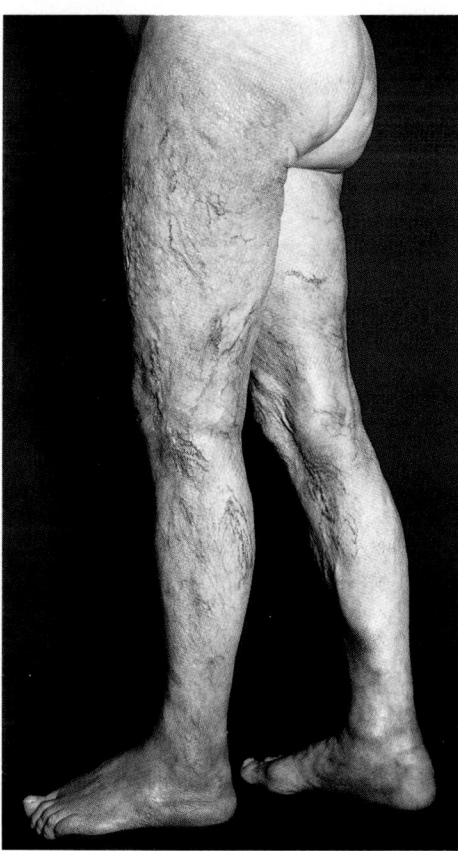

FIGURE 193-6 Acrodermatitis chronica atrophicans. Typical endstage cutaneous atrophy is seen on both legs with prominence of the veins. (*Courtesy of Klaus Wolff, M.D.*)

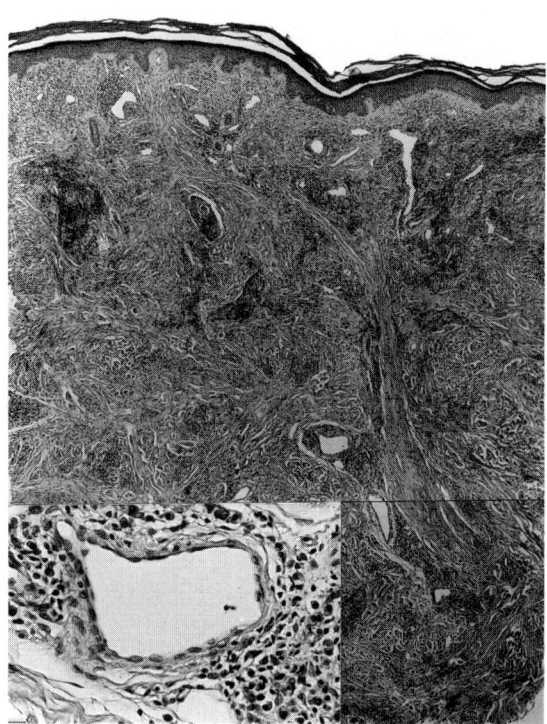

FIGURE 193-7 Acrodermatitis chronica atrophicans. Punch biopsy specimen from the elbow. Epidermis is normal. Throughout the dermis and deep in the subcutaneous fat there is a patchy cell infiltrate consisting of plasma cells and lymphocytes. Telangiectases are seen mostly in the upper dermis, but sometimes also in deeper parts. The inset exposes a telangiectatic vessel surrounded by plasma cells and lymphocytes. (*Micrograph by Eva Brehmer-Andersson, M.D.*)

manifestations such as knee or olecranon bursitis and Achilles tendinitis on the same limb as the cutaneous involvement may precede or accompany ACA. Attacks of knee-joint effusions were found to have preceded or to have occurred simultaneously with ACA in about one-fifth of investigated patients.[15]

Pathology[24,27]   There are usually no epidermal changes in the early inflammatory phase of ACA, but sometimes the epidermis is thin and shows liquefaction degeneration. The most common dermal findings are telangiectases in combination with a patchy and/or interstitial, often dense lymphocytic infiltrate with a moderate to rich admixture of plasma cells. This infiltrate may involve the whole or part of the dermis and sometimes also the subcutaneous fat (Fig. 193-7). As the disease progresses, degeneration of elastin and collagen begins. After many years or decades, advanced dermal atrophy develops, including atrophy of hair follicles and of sebaceous glands. In the advanced atrophic phase, the inflammatory cells decrease in number or almost disappear.

Sural nerve biopsies from patients with ACA and polyneuritis, as well as from some cases with early neuroborreliosis, have revealed axonal degeneration with perivascular infiltration with lymphocytes and plasma cells and obliteration of the epineural vasa nervorum.[25]

Diagnosis   The clinical recognition of ACA may be difficult. If a red-violaceous discoloration, with or without swelling, is observed on a foot or heel, the dorsal aspect of a hand, the olecranon area, or, in more advanced cases, on one or more extremities (especially in an elderly woman), a diagnosis of ACA should be considered. Cutaneous atrophy may not appear for several years and is not an obligatory clinical or histopathologic criterion for a diagnosis of ACA. Compared with the prepenicillin era, patients with advanced atrophy are seen less frequently nowadays. Instead, the diagnostic efforts should be concentrated on recognizing inflammatory ACA lesions. The clinical diagnosis should be further verified by the histopathologic pattern and by elevated serum titers of IgG antibodies to *B. burgdorferi*. The diagnosis may be confirmed by spirochetal cultivation, as borreliae may still be present in the skin even after more than 10 years of ACA. Thus, ACA is a cutaneous example of prolonged survival of *B. burgdorferi* in humans.

Differential Diagnosis   ACA lesions are frequently overlooked by the physician. Acral ACA lesions are often regarded as physiologic changes due to age or occasionally due to cold injury. A discolored, sometimes swollen and painful leg in an elderly woman is very often misdiagnosed as circulatory insufficiency, and different circulatory investigations have frequently been performed in these patients. Erythematous ACA lesions in connection with musculoskeletal pains are sometimes mistaken for connective tissue disease such as dermatomyositis. Fibrotic nodules may be confused with rheumatic nodules or gouty tophi. Patients with ACA often consult different medical specialists about signs or symptoms such as pain, joint manifestations, fatigue, or lymphadenopathy, i.e., unspecific features of Lyme borreliosis. In these cases the cutaneous ACA lesions are often neglected or misunderstood and the diagnosis of Lyme borreliosis is thus missed.

Sclerotic and other Skin Lesions

Borrelia burgdorferi may cause skin lesions that are clinically and histopathologically indistinguishable from localized scleroderma and lichen sclerosus et atrophicus, but how many sclerodermatous lesions are of borrelial origin is still controversial. A high frequency of elevated serum antibody titers to *B. burgdorferi* has been found in some studies of patients with scleroderma,[28] but this could not be confirmed by others.[29] In patients with ACA the sclerotic lesions sometimes predominate and the inflammatory ACA lesions are missed, and the patient is diagnosed as suffering from morphea or lichen sclerosus et atrophicus.[24,29]

The full clinical spectrum of dermatologic manifestations of Lyme borreliosis has probably not yet been delineated. As with syphilis, *B. burgdorferi* infection may mimic many different conditions in its clinical and histopathologic features. Granuloma annulare, eosinophilic fasciitis, benign lymphocytic infiltration (Jessner-Kanof), and anetoderma have been described in connection with Lyme borreliosis.

Extracutaneous Manifestations

Lyme borreliosis is a complex multisystem disease. Besides cutaneous involvement, manifestations from the nervous system, the joints, the heart, and the eyes may develop.

Neurologic Manifestations

Neuroborreliosis[25,30,31] may involve both the peripheral and the central nervous system (CNS).

Early Neuroborreliosis This usually begins 4 to 10 weeks after the onset of the infection. The triad of a lymphocytic meningitis, cranial neuritis, and radiculoneuritis is a typical feature of neuroborreliosis. Compared with many other bacterial meningitides, the symptoms of a borrelial meningitis may often appear mild and fluctuating. Nonspecific signs or symptoms such as fever, fatigue, malaise, vomiting, weight loss, or headache with or without neck stiffness may be the only clinical manifestations. In such cases a history of a preceding tick bite and/or a history or the presence of erythema migrans are helpful when considering the possibility of a diagnosis of neuroborreliosis. However, about one-third of the patients lack these important clues.[30]

The most common manifestations from the peripheral nervous system are radicular pains and facial palsy. In patients with a preceding erythema migrans, the skin lesion has often been located in the same part of the body as the subsequent radiculoneuritis or facial palsy. Involvement of other cranial nerves may give rise to eye muscle paresis, blindness, trigeminal neuralgia, hearing impairment, and vestibular neuritis. Paralysis of peripheral nerves in the limbs may also occur. Radicular pains may be intense and give rise to a broad spectrum of clinical features which often are initially misinterpreted. Neck pain may be misdiagnosed as cervical radiculopathy, lumbar pain as lumbago/sciatica, thoracic pain as myocar-

dial infarction, and abdominal pain as gallstones, renal calculi, or gastric ulcers. Untreated early neuroborreliosis generally heals within 3 to 6 months. However, if less than adequate therapy is given, some patients may develop manifestations from other organs or late neuroborreliosis.

Late Neuroborreliosis (Chronic or Tertiary Neuroborreliosis) This can be defined as neurologic signs and symptoms caused by *Borrelia* infection and occurring ≥ 1 year after the onset of the disease. One form of late neuroborreliosis is the chronic peripheral neuropathy that is often associated with ACA.[25] These patients usually lack spinal fluid abnormalities, in contrast to patients with severe CNS syndromes. Progressive encephalomyelitis, hemiparesis, para- and quadriparesis, ataxia, multiple sclerosis-like demyelinating disease, dementia-like deficiencies, mental changes, and incapacitating fatigue have been described, but these severe forms of late neuroborreliosis are uncommon.[31]

Rheumatic Manifestations

Reports on Lyme arthritis were first made from the United States[2,11,32] and later on from Europe.[33] Intermittent episodes of arthralgia or migrating musculoskeletal pain may occur early in the development of Lyme borreliosis. Months after the onset of the infection, a single episode or intermittent attacks of mono- or oligoarthritis may occur. In contrast to the symmetric polyarthritis seen in rheumatoid arthritis, Lyme arthritis characteristically tends to affect only one or a few large joints, most commonly the knee joint. Often the pain is not severe, and swelling of the joint usually dominates the clinical picture. Arthritic attacks can recur for months and even years. In children, Lyme arthritis may sometimes mimic juvenile rheumatoid arthritis. About 10 percent of U.S. patients with Lyme arthritis have been reported to develop chronic arthritis with erosion of cartilage and bone. According to one report, there is an association between chronic Lyme arthritis and increased frequencies of HLA-DR4, often combined with HLA-DR2.[34]

Cardiac Manifestations

The frequency of cardiac involvement in patients with Lyme borreliosis is still not well established. The most common findings have been atrioventricular conduction disturbances, the majority showing transient first-degree atrioventricular block. Occasionally complete heart block requiring a temporary pacemaker has developed. Other abnormalities have been rhythm disturbances, acute myopericarditis, pancarditis, and heart failure.[35]

Ocular Lyme Borreliosis

Early Lyme borreliosis is sometimes accompanied by conjunctivitis. Ocular motor palsies and solitary cases of iritis, iridocyclitis, choroiditis, keratitis, retinal hemorrhage, optic neuritis, ischemic optic neuropathy, and papilledema have been reported.[36]

Gestational Lyme Borreliosis

The majority of women with documented Lyme borreliosis during pregnancy appear to give birth to normal infants.[37] Solitary cases of fetal death, malformations, and prematurity have, however, been reported.

Laboratory Examination

An elevated sedimentation rate, elevated serum IgM levels, circulating immune complexes, and abnormal liver function tests are uncommon in patients with uncomplicated erythema migrans and borrelial lymphocytoma, but are somewhat more frequent in patients with multiple skin lesions or other signs or symptoms of disseminated infection and in ACA.

Detection of B. burgdorferi

Cultivation of Spirochetes   In atypical cases spirochetal cultivation, using modified Kelly medium,[4] is the most specific and reliable way of diagnosing Lyme borreliosis. *B. burgdorferi* requires microaerophilic conditions for growth and reproduces by binary fission. The optimum temperature for in vitro cultivation is 33° to 37°C. Spirochetal cultivation from human tissue or fluid has not become a routine diagnostic method in most laboratories. It is laborious and mostly a low-yielding process. One exception might be cultivation from skin specimens, as successful cultivation from more than 40 percent of skin biopsies from patients with erythema migrans has been reported from a few studies.[38,39]

In addition to cultivation from skin lesions, *B. burgdorferi* has also been cultivated from the blood, the CSF, the heart, and synovial fluid from solitary patients with Lyme borreliosis. The cultivation period has usually varied from 1 to 4 weeks.

Animals such as rabbits, Syrian hamsters, rats, and mice have been used for experimental inoculation of *B. burgdorferi* and as animal models for Lyme borreliosis.

Demonstration of Spirochetes in Tissues   Spirochetes may be demonstrated in biopsy specimens by using different silver stains. Polyclonal or monoclonal antibodies to borrelial antigens have also been used to demonstrate spirochetes in tissue specimens. These techniques for visualizing spirochetes are difficult to evaluate, however, and there may be a risk of both over- and underdiagnosis.

Polymerase Chain Reaction   In the future, amplification of borrelial DNA by the polymerase chain reaction may be of diagnostic aid.

Serology of Lyme Borreliosis

Serologic examination is at present the most important laboratory aid in diagnosing Lyme borreliosis. The serologic results must, however, be interpreted with caution, as false-negative as well as false-positive results are common with the currently used tests. In early Lyme borreliosis, particularly in patients with signs or symptoms of disseminated disease, significantly increasing IgM and/or IgG antibody titers to *B. burgdorferi* may be found in consecutive tests performed at an interval of 2 to 3 weeks. Later on, the IgG titers are often stationary and there may be difficulties in finding serologic proof of current infection. A high prevalence of seropositivity has been found among asymptomatic sports enthusiasts, outdoor workers, and other controls in endemic areas. This may limit the diagnostic value of the serologic findings, particularly in cases where only slightly elevated titers have been found. The lack of standardization also means that there may be great variations in sensitivities and specificities between different laboratories.

The tests most widely used at present for measuring antibodies to *B. burgdorferi* are the indirect immunofluorescence assay and the enzyme-linked immunosorbent assay (ELISA). Whole cells or sonicated whole cells are used as antigens. Different laboratories use different strains of *B. burgdorferi* as test antigens. In some laboratories a Reiter strain of treponemes is used in order to absorb nonspecific group antigens from the test serum.[40] The tests are of low diagnostic value in the earliest phase of Lyme borreliosis. Only 20 to 50 percent of patients with uncomplicated erythema migrans have been found to be seropositive in IgM and/or IgG ELISA.[40–43] Patients with multiple erythema migrans-like lesions and those with borrelial lymphocytoma are more often seropositive. In most cases where signs or symptoms of a disseminated infection have been present for several weeks, elevated serum titers to *B. burgdorferi* are found. Almost 100 percent of patients with ACA are seropositive and they usually show very high serum IgG titers to *B. burgdorferi.*[7,40,42,43] Serologic IgM reactivity in patients with ACA has been shown to be due to IgM rheumatoid factor activity.[40,43]

B. burgdorferi not only shares antigenic epitopes with other spirochetes but also with many common bacteria, including the normal human flora. Attempts have been made to improve ELISA by replacing the antigens used so far by fractions of spirochetes to eliminate irrelevant cross-reacting antigens. Thus, a purified *B. burgdorferi* flagellum antigen has been found to increase the sensitivity and specificity to some degree when compared with a sonicated whole-cell antigen.[43] An IgM antibody–capture ELISA with whole-cell sonic extracts as antigen has also been reported to be somewhat more sensitive than standard IgM ELISA.

With use of Western blot techniques, IgM and IgG antibodies to a number of spirochetal polypeptides have been found in sera from patients with Lyme borreliosis. Western blotting has also been used as a diagnostic tool with varying criteria for positivity in different investigations. It may be a sensitive method but has the disadvantages of being difficult to standardize, time-consuming, and nonquantitative.

False-positive serologic reactions may occur in patients with relapsing fever and syphilis. On the other hand, patients with high serum titers to *B. burgdorferi,* such as those with ACA, often have cross-reactive antibodies to treponemal antigens that are detectable in the fluorescent treponemal antibody–absorption test. However, the VDRL and Wassermann tests are negative.[7]

Cerebrospinal Fluid Examination in Neuroborreliosis   The presence of cerebrospinal fluid abnormalities with a lymphocytic pleocytosis, in combination with the finding of intrathecally synthesized antibodies to *Borrelia,* is diagnostic for neuroborreliosis with CNS involvement.[30]

Treatment

Among European dermatologists it has been the tradition since the 1940s to treat erythema migrans and ACA[27] patients with oral penicillin. Today, the opinions concerning the treatment of Lyme borreliosis are divergent,[16,44–46] some physicians preferring tetracycline or cephalosporins. There may be several explanations for the persistent controversy concerning the treatment of this infection. Few large, well-controlled treatment studies have been performed on groups of well-defined patients with similar manifestations of Lyme borreliosis. In many treatment trials, patients with uncomplicated erythema migrans have been mixed with patients who besides erythema migrans also have signs or symptoms of a disseminated infection, such as multiple erythema migrans-like skin lesions or meningitis.

Many of the minor symptoms that may occur in Lyme borreliosis, such as fatigue and musculoskeletal pain, are common and nonspecific. Thus, the evaluation of such symptoms in follow-up studies after treatment has been difficult in the absence of adequate controls.

As in syphilis, the therapeutic difficulties seem to increase with the duration of the disease. The possibility has been considered that the spirochetal division time may be longer in the late than in the early stage of syphilis and that a longer period of therapy will be needed for late cases. The same may be true for late Lyme borreliosis.

Attempts have been made to determine antibiotic sensitivities of *B. burgdorferi* in vitro and in experimental animals. As the methodology for such studies is not yet standardized, the studies should be interpreted with caution. It is not known whether the antibiotic susceptibility may differ between *B. burgdorferi* strains from different parts of the world.

The recommendations for treatment will probably be modified in the future when further treatment trials have been carried out. Current guidelines for treatment of adult patients with different manifestations of Lyme borreliosis are given below:

Treatment of Uncomplicated Erythema Migrans Phenoxymethyl penicillin (1 g orally, bid/tid) or doxycycline (100 mg orally, qd/bid) or tetracycline (500 mg orally, bid) or amoxicillin (500 mg, qid) for 10 to 14 days.

In patients with erythema migrans and concurrent manifestations from other organs, the latter may be decisive for the choice of therapy. Such manifestations are particularly common in patients with multiple erythema migrans-like lesions. Before the start of therapy in patients with erythema migrans and signs or symptoms suggestive of neuroborreliosis, a diagnostic spinal tap should be performed. Alternatively, a regimen has to be chosen that gives therapeutic CSF concentrations.

Treatment of Borrelial Lymphocytoma The same treatment regimens as for erythema migrans. In cases with a disease duration of several months, prolonged courses of antibiotics for up to 20 to 30 days may be required.

Treatment of Neuroborreliosis or Cardiac Abnormalities Penicillin G (3 g intravenously, tid/qid) or ceftriaxone (2 g intravenously, qd) for 10 to 14 days. In cases of cardiac abnormalities where only first-degree atrioventricular block is present, oral regimens have been used.

Treatment of Lyme Arthritis Doxycycline (100 mg orally, bid) or amoxicillin and probenecid (500 mg each orally, tid/qid) for 20 to 30 days or penicillin G (3 g intravenously, tid/qid) or ceftriaxone (2 g intravenously, qd) for 14 days.

Treatment of ACA Phenoxymethyl penicillin (1 g orally, tid) or doxycycline (100 mg orally, bid) for 20 to 30 days. In long-stand-

ing cases with extracutaneous complications of the joints and/or the nervous system, intravenous penicillin or ceftriaxone may be needed.

Jarisch-Herxheimer Reaction

Mild to moderate Herxheimer reactions may sometimes appear after the institution of antibiotic therapy. Intensification of the current cutaneous rash and of local symptoms or the appearance of new signs or symptoms such as fever have been reported to occur not only during the first 24 h but also later during therapy.[46,47]

Prevention

No vaccine against Lyme borreliosis is yet available. Not yet solved are whether prophylactic antibiotic therapy after a tick bite can eliminate the risk of acquiring Lyme disease and whether the value of such treatment can balance the risk of adverse reactions to antibiotics.

Protection from being bitten by ticks, by the use of protective clothing in risk areas, and body inspection and removal of any attached ticks as soon as possible, are the most important prophylactic methods. Results of animal tests have shown that it will usually take at least 24 h of attachment for an infected bloodsucking tick to transmit spirochetes to its host. The best way to remove a tick is with a pair of tweezers; the tick should be grasped as close to the skin as possible and gently pulled off.

Course and Prognosis

Natural Course (Table 193-1) On ethical grounds the natural history of untreated Lyme borreliosis cannot be studied today, and no prospective investigations on the natural course have been carried out previously on large groups of unselected patients. During the preantibiotic era and the era preceding the discovery of the etiologic agent, many of the cases of early borrelial infection probably healed spontaneously. In 1977 Steere et al. reported on 12 U.S. patients with untreated erythema migrans, six of whom had multiple skin lesions. Seven of those patients developed arthritis or arthralgia.[2] This study was later expanded to 55 untreated patients. Six patients (11 percent) developed neurologic abnormalities, two (4 percent) developed cardiac involvement, and 28 (51 percent) developed arthritis.[32] Among 16 untreated Swedish patients with solitary erythema migrans, two patients developed recurrent erythema migrans lesions, two patients developed meningitis, and one patient developed ankle arthritis during the follow-up period.[16]

Posttherapeutic Course Treatment failures have been reported with most of the different regimens. However, in the vast majority of patients antibiotic therapy results in healing of the infection. Convalescence periods of several months, especially with persisting fatigue, are not uncommon in patients treated for Lyme borreliosis.

The resolution time for erythema migrans varies.[16,44,46] In most cases the erythema starts to fade within some days after the start of therapy. In some patients the skin lesion has disappeared when the treatment is terminated, but in others it may persist for some more days. In patients with borrelial lymphocytoma, it might take more than a month after antibiotic therapy before the lesion has disappeared completely.

As a rule, the clinical improvement in ACA after antibiotic therapy occurs gradually and may continue for at least 1 year. The first sign of improvement consists in an abatement of the swelling. The cyanotic discoloration fades to varying degrees. Histologically there is a reduction in the number of infiltrating cells. Residual erythema, present several months after therapy, is generally due to hyperemia resulting from remaining dilated vessels.[20] The least satisfactory results are obtained in patients with advanced atrophy of the skin.

The therapeutic effects on borrelial sclerotic skin lesions are variable.[20,22,26,27] In some patients the lesions gradually disappear during the months after antibiotic therapy, but in others no beneficial effect is noted.

Serologic follow-up examination after therapy has shown that seroreversal tends to be slower in late than in early Lyme borreliosis. After antibiotic therapy, patients with ACA will gradually exhibit decreasing titers to *B. burgdorferi*. However, in only a minority will the titer fall to normal values within 1 year.[42,44] Serologic reactivity after therapy may perhaps persist indefinitely in patients with long-standing ACA, as in patients treated for late syphilis.

In patients with early neuroborreliosis, meningeal symptoms often improve rapidly and the effect on radicular pains is usually dramatic after initiation of therapy. Patients with hemiparesis, paraparesis, or ataxia may improve to varying extents but sometimes there will be residual sequelae.

Some patients with chronic joint involvement do not respond to antibiotic therapy, not even after repeated courses of different antibiotics. It has been speculated that *B. burgdorferi* may sometimes initiate immunologic reactions that may continue for varying lengths of time, even in the absence of live spirochetes. The value of additional treatment with corticosteroids in some cases of neuroborreliosis or Lyme arthritis is still under debate.

Reinfection in patients previously treated for erythema migrans is not unusual.[16,18]

References

1. Bäfverstedt B: *Über Lymphadenosis benigna cutis. Eine klinische und patologisch-anatomische Studie.* Stockholm, PA Norstedt, 1943

2. Steere AC et al: Erythema chronicum migrans and Lyme arthritis. The enlarging clinical spectrum. *Ann Intern Med* **86**:685, 1977

3. Burgdorfer W et al: Lyme disease—A tick-borne spirochetosis? *Science* **216**:1317, 1982

4. Barbour A: Isolation and cultivation of Lyme disease spirochetes. *Yale J Biol Med* **57**:521, 1984

5. Johnson RC et al: *Borrelia burgdorferi* sp. nov.: Etiologic agent of Lyme disease. *Int J Bacteriol* **34**:496, 1984

6. Wilske B et al: Antigenic heterogeneity of European *Borrelia burgdorferi* strains isolated from patients and ticks. *Lancet* **1**:1099, 1985

7. Åsbrink E et al: The spirochetal etiology of acrodermatitis chronica atrophicans Herxheimer. *Acta Derm Venereol (Stockh)* **64**:506, 1984

8. Hovmark A et al: The spirochetal etiology of lymphadenosis benigna cutis solitaria. *Acta Derm Venereol (Stockh)* **66**:479, 1986

9. Weber K et al: Das Lymphocytom—eine Borreliose? *Z Hautkr* **60**:1585, 1985

10. Barbour AG et al: Heterogeneity of major proteins of Lyme disease

11. Steere AC et al: The early clinical manifestations of Lyme disease. *Ann Intern Med* **99**:76, 1983

12. Berger B: Erythema chronicum migrans of Lyme disease. *Arch Dermatol* **120**:1017, 1984

13. Åsbrink E: Erythema chronicum migrans Afzelius and acrodermatitis chronica atrophicans. Early and late manifestations of *Ixodes ricinus*-borne *Borrelia* spirochetes. *Acta Derm Venereol (Stockh)* **118** (suppl):1, 1985

14. Weber K et al: Erythema-migrans-Krankheit. *Dtsch Med Wochenschr* **108**:1182, 1983

15. Åsbrink E, Hovmark A: Early and late cutaneous manifestations in *Ixodes*-borne borreliosis (erythema migrans borreliosis, Lyme borreliosis). *Ann N Y Acad Sci* **539**:4, 1988

16. Åsbrink E, Olsson I: Clinical manifestations of erythema chronicum migrans Afzelius in 161 patients. A comparison with Lyme disease. *Acta Derm Venereol (Stockh)* **65**:43, 1985

17. Åsbrink E et al: Clinical manifestations of erythema chronicum migrans Afzelius in Sweden. A study on 231 patients. *Zentralbl Bakteriol Hygiene (A)* **263**:229, 1986

18. Weber K, Neubert U: Clinical features of early erythema migrans disease and related disorders. *Zentralbl Bakteriol Hygiene (A)* **263**:209, 1986

19. Åsbrink E et al: Lymphadenosis benigna cutis solitaria—*Borrelia* lymphocytoma in Sweden. *Zentralbl Bakteriol Hygiene* **18** (suppl):156, 1989

20. Hauser W: Zur Kenntnis der Acrodermatitis chronica atrophicans. *Arch Dermatol* **199**:350, 1955

21. Hopf HCH: Acrodermatitis chronica atrophicans (Herxheimer) und Nervensystem, in *Monographien aus dem Gesamtgebiete der Neurologie und Psychiatrie.* Berlin, Springer, 1966

22. Åsbrink E et al: Clinical manifestations of acrodermatitis chronica atrophicans in 50 Swedish patients. *Zentralbl Bakteriol Hygiene (A)* **263**:253, 1986

23. Hovmark A et al: Joint and bone involvement in Swedish patients with *Ixodes-ricinus*-borne *Borrelia* infection. *Zentralbl Bakteriol Hygiene (A)* **263**:275, 1986

24. Åsbrink E et al: Acrodermatitis chronica atrophicans—A spirochetosis: Clinical and histopathological picture based on 32 patients; Course and relationship to erythema chronicum migrans Afzelius. *Am J Dermatopathol* **8**:209, 1986

25. Kristoferitsch W et al: Neuropathy associated with acrodermatitis chronica atrophicans. Clinical and morphological features. *Ann N Y Acad Sci* **539**:35, 1988

26. Jablonska S: Acrodermatitis chronica atrophicans and its sclerodermiform variety; relation to scleroderma, in *Scleroderma and Pseudoscleroderma,* edited by S Jablonska. Warsaw, Polish Medical Publishers, 1975, p 580

27. Thyresson N: The penicillin treatment of acrodermatitis chronica atrophicans. *Acta Derm Venereol (Stockh)* **29**:572, 1949

28. Aberer E et al: Evidence for spirochetal origin of circumscribed scleroderma (morphea). *Acta Derm Venereol (Stockh)* **67**:225, 1987

29. Halkier-Sörensen L et al: Antibodies to the *Borrelia burgdorferi* flagellum in patients with scleroderma, granuloma annulare and porphyria cutanea tarda. *Acta Derm Venereol (Stockh)* **69**:116, 1989

30. Stiernstedt G et al: Clinical manifestations and diagnosis of neuroborreliosis. *Ann N Y Acad Sci* **539**:46, 1988

31. Ackermann R et al: Chronic neurologic manifestations of erythema migrans borreliosis. *Ann N Y Acad Sci* **539**:16, 1988

32. Steere AC et al: The clinical evolution of Lyme arthritis. *Ann Intern Med* **107**:725, 1987

33. Herzer P et al: Lyme arthritis: Clinical features, serological, and radiographic findings of cases in Germany. *Klin Wochenschr* **64**:206, 1986

34. Steere AC et al: Association of chronic Lyme arthritis with HLA-DR4 and HLA-DR2 alleles. *N Engl J Med* **323**:1438, 1990

35. Van der Linde MR et al: Range of atrioventricular conduction disturb-

borreliae: A molecular analysis of American and European isolates. *J Infect Dis* **152**:478, 1985

ances in Lyme borreliosis: A report of four cases and review of other published reports. *Br Heart J* **63**:162, 1990

36. Winward KE et al: Ocular Lyme borreliosis. *Am J Ophthalmol* **108**:651, 1989

37. Markowitz LE et al: Lyme disease during pregnancy. *JAMA* **255**:3394, 1986

38. Åsbrink E, Hovmark A: Successful cultivation of spirochetes from skin lesions of patients with erythema chronicum migrans Afzelius and acrodermatitis chronica atrophicans. *Acta Pathol Microbiol Immunol* (sect B) **93**:161, 1985

39. Berger BW et al: Isolation and characterization of the Lyme disease spirochete from the skin of patients with erythema chronicum migrans. *J Am Acad Dermatol* **13**:444, 1985

40. Wilske B et al: Serological diagnosis of erythema migrans disease and related disorders. *Infection* **12**:331, 1984

41. Shrestha M et al: Diagnosing early Lyme disease. *Am J Med* **78**:234, 1985

42. Åsbrink E et al: Serologic studies of erythema chronicum migrans Afzelius and acrodermatitis chronica atrophicans with indirect immunofluorescence and enzyme-linked immunosorbent assays. *Acta Derm Venereol* (*Stockh*) **65**:509, 1985

43. Hansen K, Åsbrink E: Serodiagnosis of erythema migrans and acrodermatitis chronica atrophicans by the *Borrelia burgdorferi* flagellum enzyme-linked immunosorbent assay. *J Clin Microbiol* **27**:545, 1989

44. Weber K et al: Antibiotic therapy of early European Lyme borreliosis and acrodermatitis chronica atrophicans. *Ann N Y Acad Sci* **539**:324, 1988

45. Berger BW: Treating erythema chronicum migrans of Lyme disease. *J Am Acad Dermatol* **15**:459, 1986

46. Steere AC et al: Treatment of the early manifestations of Lyme disease. *Ann Intern Med* **99**:22, 1983

47. Weber K: Jarisch-Herxheimer-Reaktion bei Erythema-migrans-Krankheit. *Hautarzt* **35**:588, 1984

Fungal Diseases with Cutaneous Involvement

CHAPTER 194

Ann G. Martin and George S. Kobayashi

Superficial Fungal Infection: Dermatophytosis, Tinea, Nigra, Piedra

Mycology

Background

The dermatophytes are a group of taxonomically related fungi capable of colonizing keratinized tissues such as the stratum corneum of the epidermis, nails, hair, the horny tissues of various animals, and the feathers of birds. As a consequence of this predilection for keratin, these organisms are referred to frequently as the "keratinophilic fungi." Keratin is not an essential metabolite for these fungi, however, and the reasons for their selective colonization of tissues containing this protein are unknown.

Systematic study of dermatophytes began 150 years ago when Remak described the mycelial nature of the clinical disease favus. This observation was later supported by Schoenlein. The most significant report to follow was that of Gruby, who in 1841 isolated the organism of favus in culture and experimentally produced disease in normal skin. From a historical point of view, Gruby's studies preceded by almost four decades the work of Koch and the formulation of his criteria for assessing the etiology of infection. Despite this early start, the study of medical mycology did not witness the accelerated scientific advances seen in bacteriology and for the next 40 years the major activities were rather pedestrian. The scientific literature from this period was characterized by disorganized and incomplete descriptions of fungi found in association with skin infections. At about the turn of the century, Raymond Sabouraud began his systematic studies of the dermatophytes. Sabouraud was credited with bringing order to the chaotic situation that existed in the taxonomy of the dermatophytes. He recognized four genera of dermatophytes based on cultural and microscopic features of the fungi and clinical aspects of the diseases they produced. The culmination of this work was his classic treatise *Les Tiegnes* in 1910. Unfortunately, a period followed during which numerous species of dermatophytes were described based on their trivial morphologic differences. In 1934, Emmons critically reviewed the taxonomic status of the dermatophytes. He accepted only three genera, *Microsporum, Trichophyton,* and *Epidermophyton,* and defined each of them according to the systematic rules of nomenclature and taxonomy. Further developments occurred in 1957 when Georg reexamined the work of Emmons and supplemented it with studies on nutritional and physiologic characteristics of the dermatophytes.

Other studies have emphasized various epidemiologic and ecologic aspects of the dermatophytes. For example, of the various species of keratinophilic fungi that have been described, several have been found only in soil, and although the potential exists, most of them have not been reported to cause disease in humans or animals. From an ecologic viewpoint, these fungi are referred to as geophilic species, represented by such organisms as *M. gypseum, M. fulvum,* and *T. terrestre.* Several species are found in association with domestic and wild animals; they are called zoophilic species and include *M. canis, M. equinum, M. gallinae, M. nanum, T. verrucosum,* and *T. mentagrophytes* var. *mentagrophytes.* A third group has been found only in association with human beings. These are called the anthropophilic species and include *M. audouinii, T. rubrum, T. mentagrophytes* var. *interdigitale, T. schoenleinii, T. tonsurans, T. violaceum,* and *E. floccosum.*

A recent development in the study of these organisms has been the observation of a sexual phase of reproduction. These findings have obvious genetic implications, but there have been few studies in this regard. Of the more than 20 species in which sexual reproduction has been observed, all have been classified in the genus *Arthoderma* of the family Gymnoascaceae in the subdivision Ascomycotina. The sexual phase of *Epidermophyton* has not yet been discovered.

Mycologic Procedures

The presumptive diagnosis of dermatophyte infection should be supported by microscopy of clinical material and confirmed by culture of the specimen on suitable mycologic media. Clinical specimens must be properly collected in order to reveal fungal elements if they are present.

Microscopic Examination

1. *Hair:* When the lesions involve hairy areas of the body such as the scalp and beard, examination by ultraviolet light emitted at 365 nm (such as the Wood's lamp) will occasionally reveal hairs infected with various species of *Microsporum,* e.g., *M. audouinii, M. canis,* and *M. ferrugineum.* Scalp samples should be picked with the point of a no. 11 blade scalpel, and placed on fungal medium for culture. Suspected hairs are

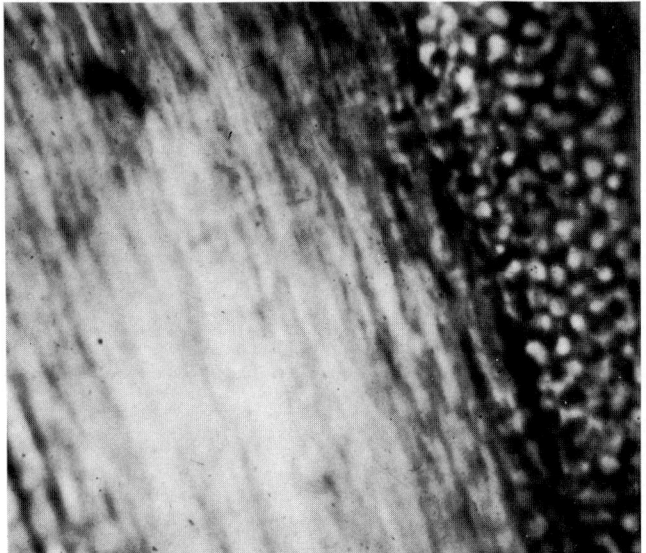

FIGURE 194-1 Microscopic examination of ectothrix type hair involvement with arthrospores outside of hair shaft.

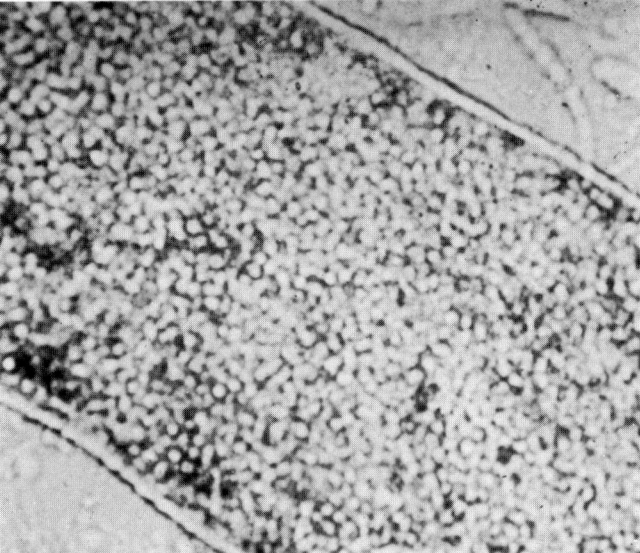

FIGURE 194-2 Microscopic examination of endothrix type hair invasion.

placed on clear microscope slides in a crop of clearing solution.* A coverslip is placed over the preparation and the specimen is examined by low-power (10× objective) microscopy. Infected hairs will appear as:

a. An ectothrix infection characterized by a mosaic of round arthrospores surrounding the hair shaft as a sheath (Fig. 194-1);

b. An endothrix infection characterized by found arthospores in a mosaic pattern contained within the hair shaft proper (Fig. 194-2); or

c. A "favic" infection that is characterized by the linear arrangement of hyphal fragments, usually vacuolated, in chains along the longitudinal axis of the hair shaft (Fig. 194-3). The type of parasitized hair caused by the various dermatophytes is summarized in Table 194-1.

2. *Skin and nails:* Skin samples are taken from the advancing margins of the lesion by scraping with the dulled edge of a scalpel and depositing onto a clear microscope slide. Nail specimens should include clippings of the entire thickness of the nail.

A coverslip is placed over the collected debris and a drop of clearing solution (10% KOH and ink) is carefully placed on the edge of the coverslip. The solution should flow evenly beneath the coverslip by surface tension. The alkaline clearing solution will digest the proteins, lipids, and most of the other epithelial debris that are present, but the fungal elements resist this treatment because of their chitinous cell wall. The clearing process can be hastened by gently heating the slide. In a positive preparation, fungi

*The clearing solution consists of 10% KOH made up in Parker Super Quink permanent Blue Black Ink. (Swartz JH, Lamkins, BE: *Arch Dermatol* **89**:149, 1964.) When KOH is added to the ink, an amorphous precipitate forms. This can be removed by centrifugation (2000 rpm/10 min). The clear supernatant fluid should be stored in a plastic bottle to prevent formation of insoluble carbonates.

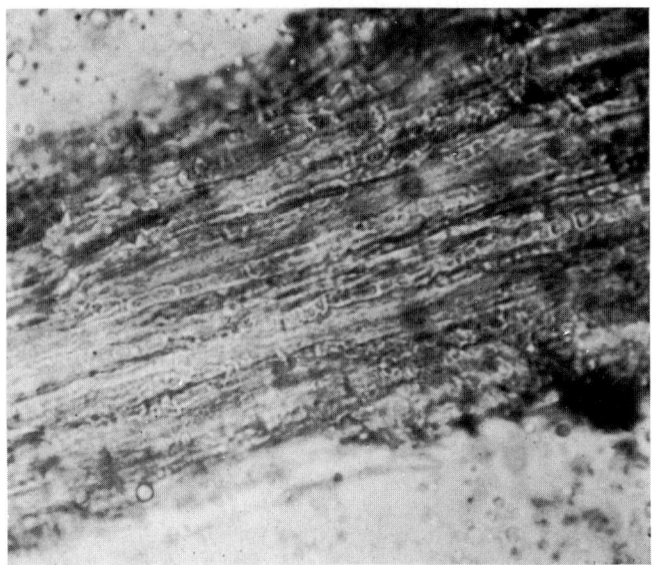

FIGURE 194-3 Favic hair invasion due to *T. schoenleinii*.

TABLE 194-1
Parasitized Hairs

Ectothrix	Endothrix	Favic
M. audouinii	*T. tonsurans*	*T. schoenleinii*
M. canis	*T. violaceum*	
M. ferrugineum		
M. gypseum		
M. nanum		
T. verrucosum		
T. mentagrophytes		

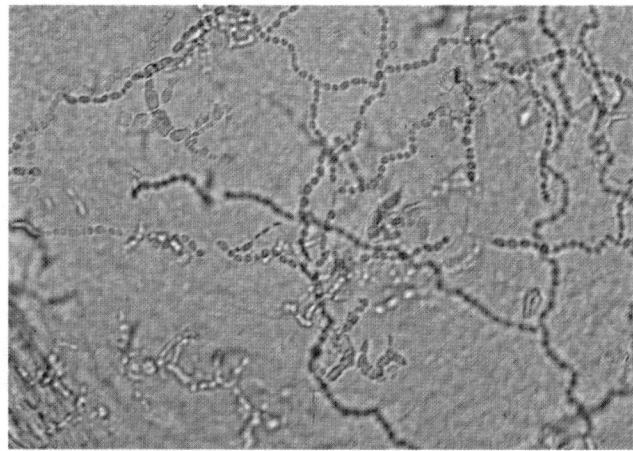

FIGURE 194-4 Skin scrapings (scales). This KOH preparation exhibits septate hyphae.

will appear as septate and branching hyphal elements (Fig. 194-4). This only denotes that fungal elements are present. In order to identify the specific agent, the organism must be cultured on suitable medium and examined accordingly.

Culture Procedures Definitive diagnosis of dermatophyte infections rests solely on the macroscopic, microscopic, and, in some cases, the physiologic characteristics of the organism. For these reasons, clinical specimens must be cultured on media suitable for growth of these fungi. Sabouraud's dextrose agar* is the most commonly used medium in medical mycology and serves as the basis for most of the morphologic descriptions of these fungi. Unfortunately, saprophytes grow rapidly and well on this medium and since they frequently contaminate body surfaces from which clinical specimens are taken, they will overgrow any pathogens that may be present, thus making it difficult to isolate and identify pathogens. To circumvent this problem, chloramphenicol (0.05 g/L) and cycloheximide (0.4 g/L) are usually incorporated into Sabouraud's dextrose agar to make the medium highly selective for the isolation of dermatophytes. The chloramphenicol inhibits bacterial growth and the cycloheximide inhibits most saprophytic fungi. It is imperative that the medium used in a given laboratory is standardized. Several good commercial variants of the standard Sabouraud medium are readily available (Mycosel, Mycobiotic medium). Cultures should be maintained at room temperature (26°C) for up to 4 weeks before they are discarded as showing no growth.

Identification and speciation of the dermatophytes require careful observation of gross colonial morphology and microscopic examination of properly prepared samples. The number of species of dermatophytes is large, and for proper identification one should rely on a suitable reference source. An excellent treatise is the manual *Dermatophytes, Their Recognition and Identification,* Revised Edition, by Gerbert Rebell and David Taplin, University of Miami Press, Coral Gables, 1979.

The remainder of this chapter is a discussion of the various clinical disorders caused by the superficial fungi and the dermatophytes.

*Sabouraud's dextrose agar, formulation: Dextrose 40 g; Peptone 10 g; Agar 20 g; distilled water adjusted to pH 5.5 1000 mL.

Dermatophytosis

Dermatophytosis represents a superficial infection of keratinized tissue caused by the dermatophytic fungi. In contrast, dermatomycosis refers to any fungal infection of the skin including the systemic or deep fungi that may have prominent cutaneous manifestations in addition to visceral disease.

History

The study of dermatophytosis has been aided by the superficial nature of its clinical manifestations. These infections were described in the earliest historic accounts. "Tinea," a name that remains today, literally refers to an insect larva (clothes moth) that was thought by the Romans to be the cause of the infection.[1]

In the 1800s, the work of a number of observers culminated in the culture of the organism responsible for favus[2] and the experimental production of diseases by cutaneous inoculation of the mold.

In 1910, Sabouraud[3] published *Les Teignes* in which he classified the dermatophytes and made other clinical and therapeutic observations that remain accurate today. For this work, Sabouraud is justly considered the father of modern medical mycology.

In the 1920s, the scientific studies of the dermatophytes by Benham and Hopkins formed the foundations of modern-day medical mycology. Subsequent work by Emmons, Conant, Geary, and others consolidated these efforts.[1] Finally, in 1959, the identification of the sexual stage of *T. ajelloi* led to taxonomic refinements that continue to assist in the scientific study of these organisms.[4]

A major therapeutic advance in dermatophytosis occurred in 1958 with the development of griseofulvin.[5] The studies of Blank and Roth solidified the role of griseofulvin in dermatologic therapeutics.[6]

Epidemiology

The dermatophytes represent 39 closely related species in three imperfect genera: *Microsporum, Trichophyton,* and *Epidermophyton.* The perfect or sexual state has now been recognized for 21 of the dermatophytes. Cleistothecia, which are fruiting bodies or ascocarps, are formed through the conjugation of two compatible mating types and sexual spores or ascospores develop within these structures. The two perfect (sexual phase, telomorphic) genera are *Nannizzia* and *Anthroderma* in the subdivision *Ascomycotina.* In general, *Nannizzia* corresponds to the *Microsporum* imperfect state, and *Arthroderma* corresponds to *Trichophyton.* No perfect state has yet been found for the genus *Epidermophyton.* The existence of a perfect state for many of the dermatophytes has allowed a more precise classification and identification of these closely related fungi.[7] For example, mating studies have been used to clarify the origin of certain isolates of *T. mentagrophytes.* The inflammatory and often incapacitation *T. mentagrophytes* infection present in many U.S. soldiers in Vietnam[8] was of a single mating strain endemic in that area and not in the United States. Hence, the infections were acquired in Vietnam—a finding that provided valuable epidemiologic data.[1] As the dermatophytes evolve toward human parasitism, their ability to form a perfect state is diminished.

Although 39 species of dermatophytes have been identified, only a few are responsible for most human infections.[1] Many of the

TABLE 194-2
Ecology of Dermatophytes

Geophilic	Zoophilic	Anthropophilic
(Microsporum boullardii)*	(M. amazonicum)	Epidermophyton floccosum
M. cookei	M. canis	M. audouinii
M. fulvum	M. distortum	M. ferrugineum
M. gypseum	M. equinum	M. praecox
(M. magellanicum)	Trichophyton equinum	T. concentricum
M. nanum	T. mentagrophytes	T. gourvilii
(M. racemosum)	var. erinacei	T. mentagrophytes
(M. ripariae)	(T. flavescens)	var. interdigitale
M. vanbreuseghemi	T. gallinae	T. megninii
T. ajelloi	T. mentagrophytes	T. rubrum
(T. georgiae)	T. mentagrophytes	T. schoenleinii
(T. gloriae)	var. quinckeanum	T. soudanense
(T. longifusum)	T. verrucosum	T. tonsurans
(T. phaseoliforme)		T. violaceum
T. simii		T. yaoundei
(T. terrestre)		
(T. vanbreuseghemii)		

*Organisms in parentheses are not known to cause human disease.
SOURCE: Modified from Otcenasek.[9]

other species are soil-inhabiting keratinophiles with little tendency to infect humans. Thus, an important concept in understanding dermatophyte infections is a knowledge of their ecology, that is, whether the particular species in question resides predominantly in the soil (geophilic), on animals (zoophilic), or on humans (anthropophilic). This concept provides a useful classification of these organisms (Table 194-2).

Geophilic organisms are adapted for soil habitation. These fungi sporadically infect humans and when they do, the resulting disease is usually inflammatory. *M. gypseum* is the most common geophile isolated in human infections. Although soil isolates of *M. gypseum* are of low virulence, strains cultured from humans are more virulent and account for epidemic spread of the infection under appropriate conditions.[10–12]

Zoophilic species primarily infect higher animals but can be transmitted to humans sporadically. The zoophiles may have specific animal hosts largely because of a special affinity for the keratin of these hosts.[9] Infections often occur in rural areas where animal contact is likely. Domestic animals and pets, however, are becoming an increasing source of these infections (i.e., *M. canis* in cats or dogs) in urban areas.[13] Transmission may occur through direct contact with a specific animal species (Table 194-3) or indirectly by infected animal hair carried on clothing or contaminated stalls, barns, or feed. Exposed areas of the body are favored sites of

infection (i.e., scalp, beard, face, arms). Although human infections with zoophiles are often suppurative, animal infection may be clinically silent. Under these conditions, animals serve as asymptomatic carriers and underscore the unique adaptation that these organisms have for their animals hosts.[9–11]

Anthropophilic species have adapted to infect humans. Unlike the sporadic geophilic and zoophilic infections, anthropophilic infections are often epidemic in nature. They are transmitted from person to person either by direct contact or indirectly through fomites. In contrast to zoophilic infections, anthropophilic organisms may produce a relatively noninflammatory infection, often located on covered areas of the body (i.e., feet, groin). The chronic *T. rubrum* infections that occur in certain individuals are examples of the tolerance that can exist for this anthropophilic equilibrium with the host.

Yet not all anthropophilic infections are noninflammatory.[1,14,15] Because of differences in susceptible hosts or strain virulence, markedly inflammatory reactions can occur. Kerion formation, suppuration, or other manifestations of inflammatory tinea can facilitate early diagnoses in these cases. Noninflammatory disease, on the other hand, fosters the existence of a clinically silent "carrier" state that serves to delay the diagnosis and propagate the infection.

Host differences play a role in the epidemiology of anthropophilic infections. Intercurrent diseases of the host are important, e.g., dermatophytosis may be more severe or recalcitrant to therapy in patients with diabetes mellitus,[16,17] lymphoid malignancies,[18] immunologic compromise,[19] or Cushing's syndrome,[20] but other factors including age, sex, race,[14] habits, geographic location,[21–23] and genetic background[24] should also be addressed.

Children are a population at risk for anthropophilic tinea capitis.[10,25–27] In one study, black male children appeared to be particularly susceptible.[14] In adults, however, tinea capitis due to anthropophilic organisms (i.e., *T. tonsurans*) is rare, and when it occurs in the United States is largely confined to blacks or Hispanics. These differences hold true even after socioeconomic factors are considered. It is clear, at least for tinea capitis, that an age-dependent incidence applies.[14] When other dermatophytoses (tinea pedis, tinea unguium, or tinea cruris) are considered, however, the reverse prevails.

TABLE 194-3
Animal Hosts for Zoophilic Dermatophytes

Organism	Animal hosts*
M. canis	Dog, cat, cattle, sheep, pigs, rodents, monkeys
M. distortum	Dog, cat, horses, monkeys
M. equinum	Horses
T. equinum	Horse, dog
T. mentagrophytes var. erinacei	Rodents (hedgehogs)
T. gallinae	Fowl, rodents, cat
T. mentagrophytes var. mentagrophytes	Cat, dog, cattle, sheep, pigs, horses, rodents, monkeys
T. verrucosum	Dog, cattle, sheep, pigs, horses

*Italics indicate the usual or preferred host.

TABLE 194-4
Geographically Limited Species

Organism	Endemic region
M. nanum	Cuba
T. concentricum	Pacific Islands, Far East, India, Ceylon; areas of North, Central, and South America
T. ferrugineum	Africa, India, eastern Europe, Asia
T. megninii	Portugal, Sardinia
T. soudanense	Central and West Africa
T. yaoundei	Central and West Africa
T. gourvilii	Central and West Africa
M. distortum	New Zealand, United States
T. equinum	Western Europe, Canada, United States
T. ajelloi	Certain areas of North and Central America, Europe, Japan, Australia

SOURCE: Adapted from Ajello.[22]

In a similar manner, sex differences play a role in susceptibility to dermatophyte infections. Overall, there appear to be fewer overt anthropophilic infections in females.[14] This may be explained partially by their less frequent exposure to an environment conducive to the spread of the organism (e.g., athletic organizations, military service). When these factors are equalized, the incidence of tinea in women approaches that in men. Yet even with this adjustment, tinea cruris remains predominantly a male dermatophytosis. *Trichophyton* tinea capitis, when occurring in adults, is far more common in women.[28]

It is well known that the type of dermatophytosis present may vary depending on geographic location.[21–23] Multiple factors are responsible for this fact. Certain strains of dermatophyte are endemic to specific geographic areas (Table 194-4). Because of patterns of travel to and from these areas, resident dermatophytes may remain restricted geographically or become more cosmopolitan. *T. yaoundei, T. gourvillii*, and *T. soudanense*, for example, are found only in Central and West Africa. *T. concentricum*—the causative organism of tinea imbricata—is found chiefly in the South Pacific.[1] With time these relationships may change. Earlier in this century, *M. audouinii* was the predominant cause of tinea capitis in the United States. In the past 10 to 15 years, *T. tonsurans* has assumed that role. The spread of this infection appears to correlate well with the ingress of Mexicans and Puerto Ricans to this country.[25,27] With the present ease of world travel, infections caused by geographically restricted dermatophytes may be seen more and more frequently in other areas of the world.[29]

Furthermore, it appears that dermatophytes indigenous to certain areas of the world have adapted themselves to their human hosts in these areas and vice versa. In Vietnam, U.S. combat personnel often acquired a disabling, inflammatory, zoophilis *T. mentagrophytes* infection. South Vietnamese soldiers under similar environmental conditions did not become infected with this organism. Presumably, adult Vietnamese had acquired a resistance to the infection.[30] Infection seen in the resident population is often chronic and noninflammatory, whereas the same infection in virgin hosts is markedly inflammatory and self-limited.

The location of the dermatophytosis is partially dependent on climatic conditions of the area and the customs of the resident population. Tinea pedis, for example, is more common in areas where occlusive footwear is used.[9] In locations where the inhabitants wear sandals or go barefoot, the infection is markedly less common. Likewise, tinea capitis is impeded in areas where the population uses hair oils.[21,22] The hair oil may inhibit initiation of the infec-

tion. In extremely hot, humid climates, tinea corporis may occur readily under occlusive garments.[10,31,32]

Finally, there is some evidence to suggest that certain human populations may be genetically more susceptible to particular dermatophyte infections. *T. concentricum* is not transmitted readily to individuals of different races living with the susceptible population.[1] One study[33] has shown convincing evidence of an autosomal recessive inheritance for the susceptibility to this infection. Likewise, *T. rubrum* infections within a household favor relatives; conjugal pairs, in contrast, are less commonly infected even though environmental exposure to the organism is equivalent.[24]

It is clear that the epidemiology of dermatophyte infections is dependent on many of the host factors discussed above. When the individual clinical infections are discussed later, these points will be expanded.

In addition to host and geographic factors, the virulence of the infecting organism must be considered. An important point is that strain-to-strain differences may exist for the same dermatophyte. The classic example is the difference between strains of *T. mentagrophytes*. *T. mentagrophytes* var. *mentagrophytes* is a zoophilic organism capable of producing a marked inflammatory infection in the human host. Its granular culture differs from the anthropophilic downy variant, *T. mentagrophytes* var. *interdigitale*. The latter variant produces a rather noninflammatory infection. The differences that exist between these two variants are alterable. Virulence may be enhanced by passage of the organism through a series of infections on guinea pigs. As the virulence is enhanced, the culture characteristics also are modified—to the granular pattern.[11,34] A similar phenomenon is postulated for different *T. rubrum* strains.[11]

Pathogenesis

How a dermatophyte infection is initiated and maintained provides information that can be useful in understanding the clinical manifestations of these infections. Much of these data have come from experimentally induced infections.[35] It takes more than just a large inoculum of fungal organisms to initiate clinical disease. Studies of experimental tinea pedis demonstrated that volunteers who immersed a foot in water teeming with *T. rubrum* or *T. mentagrophytes* failed to get an active infection unless the foot was first traumatized.[36,37] Hence, the presence of a suitable environment on host skin is of critical importance in the development of clinical dermatophytosis.[38] In addition to trauma, increased hydration of the skin with maceration is important. Occlusion with a nonporous material increases the temperature and hydration of the skin and interferes with the barrier function of the stratum corneum. Natural occlusion produced by wearing nonporous shoes definitely contributes to the development of tinea pedis.[9,10] In tropical climates, nonacclimatized subjects often develop lesions of tinea corporis, in part because of occlusive clothing.[10,31,32]

If the host skin is inoculated under suitable conditions, there follow several stages through which the infection progresses. Although initially described for tinea capitis, these stages apply to most superficial dermatophyte infections.[1,39,40] The stages include a period of incubation and then enlargement followed by a refractory period and a stage of involution.

During the incubation period, a dermatophyte grows in the stratum corneum, sometimes with minimal clinical signs of infection. A carrier state has been postulated when the presence of a dermatophyte is detected on seemingly normal skin by KOH examination or culture. There is controversy in the literature regarding the importance of the carrier state.[41-44] In tinea capitis, for example, a clinically silent carrier state has been found in 5 to 10 percent of cultured scalps in a population of school children in an endemic area.[45] In another study, dermatophytes were cultured not only from clinically apparent areas of infection but also from normal-appearing skin up to 6 cm from the margin of the lesion.[46] These findings suggest that during the early (i.e., incubation) phase of dermatophyte infections, organisms are present but are clinically silent. Only a limited number of these patients will develop clinical disease during a several-month follow-up period.[45] These individuals presumably represent true carriers.

Once infection is established in the stratum corneum, two factors are important in determining the size and duration of the lesion. These are the rate of growth of the organism and the epidermal turnover rate. The fungal growth rate must equal or exceed the epidermal turnover rate or the organism will be shed quickly.[38]

Labeling indices done from various sites in an annular dermatophytic lesion revealed a fourfold increase in epidermal turnover at the inflammatory rim of the lesion.[47] In other areas of the lesion, the labeling index was comparable to that of normal skin. It appears that the inflammatory response at the rim of the lesion stimulates an increased epidermal turnover in an effort to shed the organisms. However, there are undoubtedly lag periods between the initiation of the infection, the host inflammatory response, and the increased epidermal turnover. Therefore, probably only the organisms at the inflammatory rim are being shed, while those just ahead maintain the infection. The annular appearance of most dermatophyte infections is compatible with these findings. The center of the lesion has relatively few organisms in contrast to the "battleground" of the peripheral rim. In chronic infections (e.g., chronic *T. rubrum* infections), inflammation is often minimal. Presumably, a suppressed delayed-hypersensitivity response by the host results in less inflammation which, in turn, leads to a lowered epidermal turnover rate in the lesion. A chronic area of infection would then result.[38]

The affinity of dermatophytes for keratin is the *sine qua non* of their existence. Different species of dermatophyte are attracted to different types of keratin. *T. rubrum,* for example, seldom attacks hair but frequently involves nails and glabrous skin. *E. floccosum* rarely involves nails and never infects hair.[48] Presumably, differences in the type of keratin and/or differences in the organism's ability to metabolize this material account for these findings.

Keratinases and other proteolytic enzymes are produced by dermatophytes.[48,49] The role of these enzymes in the pathogenesis of clinical infection is not totally understood. There is evidence that actual enzymatic digestion of keratin may be occurring.[50,51] In one study, such enzymes resulted in epidermal-dermal separation.[52] In Vietnam, U.S. soldiers developed a particularly inflammatory *T. mentagrophytes* infection. Many of these organisms produced elastase, and there was a significant correlation between inflammation and elastase production.[8] The obvious conclusion of these studies is that the host immunologic response and also enzymes or toxins produced by the organism account for the clinical findings in dermatophytoses.[53]

On the other hand, there is evidence, at least from in vitro studies, that keratin is not the ideal medium for dermatophyte growth.[47] Furthermore, using a surface skin biopsy technique, certain investigators have found that dermatophytes prefer to spread between horn cells of the stratum corneum rather than through them, as might be postulated in a keratin-digestion process.[54]

So the pathogenesis of dermatophytosis is not totally understood. Other factors are probably involved that have not yet been elucidated. The host's role in these infections interacts with characteristics of the infecting organism and should be discussed separately.

Immunology

The immunology of dermatophyte infections has been studied thoroughly in recent years. Excellent reviews have been written by Emmons et al.,[55] Ahmed,[56] and Grappel et al.[57] Nevertheless, our understanding of this area is still incomplete.

Resistance to dermatophyte infections may involve nonimmunologic as well as immunologic mechanisms.[58] For example, a natural resistance to tinea capitis caused by *M. audouinii* ensues after puberty. Rothman et al.[59] have attributed this resistance to the increase in fungistatic and fungicidal long-chain, saturated fatty acids on the skin that occurs after puberty. In addition, a substance known as serum inhibitory factor (SIF) appears to limit the growth of dermatophytes, under most circumstances, to the stratum corneum.[60-62] This substance is not an antibody but is a dialyzable, heat-labile component of fresh serum.[60] Unsaturated transferrin is a likely SIF candidate.[63] Transferrin binds the iron that dermatophytes need for continued growth.[64] An alpha$_2$ macroglobin keratinase inhibitor has also been identified in serum and may modify the growth of the organisms.[65]

The importance of SIF is underscored by observations during the induction of experimental infections that skin traumatized mildly—not producing oozing or serous drainage—will support a subsequent fungal inoculation.[35] But when trauma is overly zealous and weeping of tissue fluids occurs, the experimental inoculum fails to grow.[41] Furthermore, a patient described by Blank et al.,[66] who had a low titer of SIF, developed a widespread granulomatous *T. rubrum* infection—ostensibly due to the SIF deficiency.

The consensus of most investigators is that the humoral limb of the immune system has a minor role in the development of acquired resistance to dermatophyte infections.[55-58] Infection produces precipitating, hemagglutinating, and complement-fixing IgG, IgM, IgA, and IgE antibodies.[67] However, these antibodies are not species-specific and cross-react with other dermatophytes and saprophytic fungi, including the airborne molds.[57,68] The antibodies have also been found to cross-react with the human blood group A isoantigen[69] and the intercellular substance of the epidermis.[70,71] Studies on the pathogenesis of chronic dermatophyte infections have cited these latter cross-reactions as evidence of how immunologic tolerance can occur in dermatophytosis.[56] Chronic *T. rubrum* infections and dermatophytids have been accompanied by complement-fixing and precipitating antibodies.[58] Their role in the pathogenesis of these disorders is not known. Hyperglobulinemia E is probably contributory to chronic infections, as will be discussed below.[72]

The major immunologic defense mechanism in dermatophyte infections is the type IV delayed-hypersensitivity response.[55-58,73,74] This is best illustrated during the course of human experimental infections.[75] When patients who have not been previously infected with a dermatophyte are experimentally infected with *T. mentagrophytes,* the initial response is one of slight inflammation and scaling. At this time the trichophyton skin test is negative. Between 10 and 35 days into the infection, the site abruptly becomes inflammatory and pruritic. Repeat trichophyton skin testing at this time is positive. After the development of cell-mediated immunity, the infected area becomes less inflammatory and eventually spontaneously involutes. If a second infection with the same organism is produced in the same subject at a later time, the site becomes inflammatory very early on and resolves relatively quickly. With the previous sensitization, the recall of delayed hypersensitivity to trichophyton is brisk. Organisms are less often demonstrated in these secondary reactions.[58]

A plausible mechanism by which the delayed-hypersensitivity response may cause dermatophyte inhibition has been proposed by Jones et al.[75] and others.[76,77] During the host's first exposure to the trichophyton cell wall[78,79] glycopeptide antigen,[57,58] the antigen diffuses from the stratum corneum to stimulate sensitized lymphocytes. Inflammatory mediators and lymphokines are produced by these cells and probably act on the host cells rather than on the dermatophyte. Because of this response, the epidermal barrier is abrogated, and SIF gains access to the otherwise privileged layers of the stratum corneum. SIF is fungistatic, and so the cell-mediated immune response typically leads to inhibition but not complete destruction of the dermatophyte. Hence, the organism is still identified in cultures and KOH preparations of the infected area. The greater the inflammation, however, the fewer the number of organisms that can be found. In most circumstances, therefore, the cell-mediated immunity that exists is relative rather than absolute.[75,76]

The use of the intradermal trichophyton skin test has identified two groups of patients based on the type of reaction ensuing from this test. Immediate (20 min) and delayed (48 h) reactions have been noted. The latter appears to correlate best with an active delayed-hypersensitivity response resulting from an acute infection with dermatophytes. On the other hand, patients showing immediate reactions often (75 percent) have chronic infections, most commonly with *T. rubrum*.[56,57,80-82]

The entire question of chronic dermatophyte infections deserves special consideration. Chronic infections are characterized clinically by relatively long-standing, widespread disease, often with palmar and plantar involvement, with little or no associated inflammatory response. There is often a negative delayed trichophyton skin test but a positive immediate one. The causative organism is usually *T. rubrum,* typically resistant to therapy with griseofulvin.[83,84] When other organisms are found, there may be a higher incidence of serious underlying disease (diabetes, hypercortisolism, lymphoma, etc.)[83] (Table 194-5). As many as 50 percent of patients chronically infected with *T. rubrum* have associated atopy[56,72,80,81,89]; they usually have an elevated IgE serum level.[74,90] In vitro lymphocyte transformation studies in these patients often reveal a selective failure to respond to trichophyton antigen, whereas mitogen responses remain intact.[80,84,91,92]

TABLE 194-5
Conditions Associated with Chronic Dermatophytoses

	Reference
Atopy	58,72
Cushing's disease	20
Diabetes mellitus	17
Drugs (corticosteroids)	83
Immunodeficiency diseases	58,83
Familial endocrinopathies	58
Peripheral vascular disease	83
Disorders of keratinization	58,83
Collagen vascular disease	83
Tumors (lymphoma, thymoma, Kaposi's sarcoma)	18,58,86
Chronic mucocutaneous candidiasis	83,87
AIDS	88

TABLE 194-6
Types of Dermatophytids

	Reference
Follicular papules	99
Erythema nodosum	100
Vesicular id of hands and feet	
Erysipelas-like	101
Erythema annulare centrifugum	102
Urticaria	103

There is evidence to suggest that patients with this "atopic-chronic-dermatophytosis syndrome" are capable of delayed-hypersensitivity skin test reactions, but these reactions are inhibited by the more sensitive, preceding type I response.[72] Evidence to support this conclusion comes from studies in which intradermal chlorpheniramine and trichophytin injected simultaneously are able to uncover an otherwise suppressed delayed skin test response.[90] In addition, other studies have demonstrated the antagonistic effects of histamine on the cell-mediated immune response.[93-95] This finding has important therapeutic relevance as the use of an H_2 histamine blocker (cimetidine) may prevent this antagonism and so enhance the patient's own delayed-hypersensitivity reaction.[96]

Dermatophytid reactions are an important part of the discussion of dermatophyte immunology. These are secondary inflammatory reactions of the skin at a site distant from the associated fungal infection. In contrast to material obtained from the dermatophytosis, cultures and KOH examinations of the "id" lesions are negative. Id reactions are usually accompanied by a reactive delayed trichophyton skin test. The mechanism responsible for the id response is unknown but may involve a local immunologic response to systemically absorbed fungal antigen.[55-58,97]

Clinically, id reactions may take several forms[98] (Table 194-6). These reactions tend to occur at the height of the dermatophyte infection or slightly thereafter. They also occur commonly just after initiation of systemic antifungal therapy.[100] The incidence of ids in an unselected patient population with dermatophytosis has been found to be 4 to 5 percent.[14,57] Disappearance of the dermatophytid reaction occurs when the dermatophyte infection is successfully treated. Occasionally, concomitant topical or systemic steroid therapy is warranted in addition to griseofulvin—especially if the dermatophytid is extremely widespread or inflammatory.

Clinical Types

Tinea Capitis   Tinea capitis is a dermatophytosis of the scalp and associated hair that is caused by a variety of species of the genera *Microsporum* and *Trichophyton. Epidermophyton* species have not been associated with the disease.

EPIDEMIOLOGY.   The true incidence of tinea capitis is unknown. Epidemics have occurred in the United States, but infection rates were only 5 to 20 percent of the population at risk.[104] The source of an infection depends on whether the causative organism is geophilic, zoophilic, or anthropophilic (see above). These factors also play a part in determining the degree of clinical inflammation. The anthropophilic organisms maintain their virulence in person-to-person transmission, thereby allowing epidemicity to be a prominent feature of these infections.[10] The specific organisms involved will be discussed below.

The patients most commonly affected are children between the ages of 4 and 14 years.[10] Adult infections are more unusual but do occur, especially when the causative organism is a species of *Trichophyton.*

Many studies have demonstrated a significant male predominance in infections caused by the *Microsporum* organisms. With *T. tonsurans,* the male/female infection rate is equal in childhood[104–106] but favors females in adulthood.[107–109]

In many cases, especially with inflammatory infections or in infections with *M. audouinii,* the disease is self-limited and seldom extends beyond puberty. *T. tonsurans* infections can also be self-limited[44]; however, they seem to extend into the adult population more commonly than *M. audouinii.*[110]

In some series, blacks and Hispanics have been found to have a higher incidence of tinea capitis, especially that caused by *T. tonsurans.*[104,105] Whites are affected more commonly with *Microsporum* species.[105]

Some of these differences can be explained by the fact that transmission of certain forms of tinea capitis is fostered by the existence of overcrowding or poor personal hygiene. Low socioeconomic conditions and, in one report, protein malnutrition[111] have also been implicated. It is clear that organisms responsible for tinea capitis can be cultured from brushes, combs, caps, pillow cases, theater seats, and other inanimate objects. The disease can also be transmitted from child to child through exposure at schools or daycare centers. Affected hairs can harbor infectious organisms for a year or more after they have been shed from the host.[112,113] As mentioned previously, overcrowding improves the chances for transmission. In several reports, the rate of infection appeared to vary directly with the size of the family unit.[10] On the other hand, there are cases in which individuals are spared who have had ample exposure to the disease.

The existence of an asymptomatic carrier state in tinea capitis has been repeatedly documented. The finding has important epidemiologic implications, as silent sources of infection are more difficult to detect and eradicate. In one report, school classes that had clinically affected members also had a 12 to 30 percent rate of asymptomatic carriers. In school classes without clinical disease, the rate dropped to 1 to 5 percent.[114]

ETIOLOGY AND PATHOGENESIS.   Virtually any species of *Microsporum* or *Trichophyton* can cause tinea capitis. Exceptions are *T. concentricum* and *E. floccosum.* The causative organisms can be classified according to their host preference (i.e., anthropophilic, zoophilic, geophilic) and according to whether they produce arthrospores outside or just under the cuticle of the hair (ectothrix) or within the hair (endothrix). These features are summarized in Table 194-7.

As can be seen, most of the dermatophytes causing tinea capitis have a ubiquitous geographic distribution. Others such as *M. ferrugineum* and the African species *T. yaoundei, T. gourvillii,* and *T. soudanense* cause disease in a relatively limited geographic area. It is important for the clinician to be cognizant of the prevalent organism or organisms responsible for each dermatophytosis in his or her geographic area. Although these trends are relatively stable, they are not absolutely so and may change with time. An example is the case of tinea capitis in the United States. In the 1940s the most common cause for epidemic tinea capitis in the United States was *M. audouinii.* In the late 1950s, however, *T. tonsurans* began to appear increasingly in the southwest as the primary cause of this infection. Now it is the most common cause of tinea capitis in this country.[27,105,106] *M. audouinii,* on the other hand, has inexplicably dropped from view. Similarly, changes in the frequency of certain organisms can be expected to occur elsewhere, perhaps facilitated by the ease of world travel. Rarely, tinea capitis can be caused by a mixed infection of two or more dermatophytes, and this may serve to confuse the clinical picture.[115–117]

The pathogenesis of tinea capitis has been studied by Kligman[39,40] and others. Hair appears to be susceptible to ectothrix dermatophytes during mid to late anagen. The infection usually begins in the perifollicular stratum corneum. Following a period of incubation, hyphae generally spread into and around the hair shaft. They descend into the follicle and penetrate the midportion of the hair. Subsequently, hyphae descend within the intrapilary portion of the hair until they reach the border of the keratogenous zone.

TABLE 194-7
Classification of Organisms Causing Tinea Capitis

Species	Ecology	Geographic distribution
Ectothrix		
Microsporum		
M. audouinii	Anthropophilic	Cosmopolitan
M. canis	Zoophilic	Cosmopolitan
M. gypseum	Geophilic	Cosmopolitan
M. fulvum	Geophilic	South America; rare in United States
M. ferrugineum	Anthropophilic	Africa, India, Asia, South America
Trichophyton		
T. mentagrophytes	Zoophilic, anthropophilic	Cosmopolitan
T. rubrum	Anthropophilic	Cosmopolitan
T. verrucosum	Zoophilic	Cosmopolitan
T. megninii	Anthropophilic	Europe
Endothrix		
Trichophyton		
T. tonsurans	Anthropophilic	Cosmopolitan
T. violaceum	Anthropophilic	Cosmopolitan
T. soudanense	Anthropophilic	Central and West Africa
T. gourvilli	Anthropophilic	Central and West Africa
T. yaoundei	Anthropophilic	Central and West Africa
T. schoenleinii	Anthropophilic	Europe, Near East, Mediterranean; rare in United States

TABLE 194-8
Organisms Associated with Clinical Types of Tinea Capitis*

Inflammatory	Noninflammatory	"Black dot"	Favus
M. canis	M. audouinii	T. tonsurans	T. schoenleinii
M. gypseum	T. tonsurans	T. violaceum	T. violaceum
T. mentagrophytes	M. canis		M. gypseum
T. tonsurans	M. ferrugineum		
T. verrucosum			
T. schoenleinii			
M. audouinii			
M. nanum			

*Some organisms produce more than one clinical type.

Here they continue to grow in delicate equilibrium with the keratinization process, so that they proceed no deeper than the upper limit of the keratogenous zone. The hyphae never enter the nucleated zone and, therefore, appear to discern the subtle differences between the partially keratinized and the fully keratinized hair. In this location the terminal tuft of hyphae is termed *Adamson's fringe*. Intrapilary hyphae proliferate and divide into arthrospores that reach the cortex of the hair and are transported upward on its surface. When the hair is plucked it breaks at its weakest point, just above Adamson's fringe. When the plucked hair is visualized microscopically, therefore, it is the numerous ectothrix spores that are seen, rather than the intrapilar hyphae.

With endothrix infections (e.g., *T. tonsurans*), the same process occurs until the hair is penetrated. The arthrospores are formed rapidly and in time replace much of the intrapilary keratin, while leaving the cortex intact. The hair is fragile and, with trauma, breaks at its weakest point—the surface of the scalp where it loses the supporting follicular wall. When observed clinically, the remaining hair in this infected follicle resembles a black dot, so endothrix infections are often referred to as "black dot ringworm." A final important difference between endothrix and ectothrix infections is that endothrix infections may continue past the anagen phase of the hair cycle and into telogen. Therefore, these infections tend to be more chronic than those caused by the ectothrix organisms.[15]

CLINICAL MANIFESTATIONS.   The different organisms causing tinea capitis may present with several different clinical patterns[44,104–118] (Table 194-8).

Noninflammatory, Human, or Epidemic Type   This clinical pattern is produced most commonly by *M. audouinii* or *M. ferrugineum*. The lesion begins as a small erythematous papule surrounding a hair shaft. Subsequently, the lesion spreads centrifugally, involving all hairs in its path. Typically, there is scaling with minimal inflammation. One or more well-demarcated patches are seen usually on the occiput or posterior neck. Hairs in the infected area are gray and lusterless in appearance due to their coating of arthrospores ("gray patch" ringworm) (Fig. 194-5). They frequently break off just above the level of the scalp, rather than being shed entirely.[118] Occasionally, infections with *M. audouinii* may present with just a few scattered, infected hairs that cannot be detected without a Wood's lamp examination. Kerions occur rarely (2 to 3 percent) and consist of an inflammatory, boggy mass studded with broken hairs and oozing purulent material from follicular orifices (Fig. 194-6).[119] A kerion is the clinical manifestation of the host's cellular immune response to the organism.

Inflammatory Type   In this form of tinea capitis there is significantly more inflammation present. These infections are caused most commonly by zoophilic organisms (e.g., *M. canis*) or

geophilic dermatophytes (e.g., *M. gypseum*).[120] Clinically, a spectrum of inflammatory changes may be seen, ranging from a pustular folliculitis to kerion formation. These infections usually present with more subjective symptoms of pruritus, fever, and pain. There may be associated regional lymphadenopathy. Occasionally, additional lesions are found on glabrous skin. Because of the degree of inflammation generated, scarring alopecia is often seen subsequently.

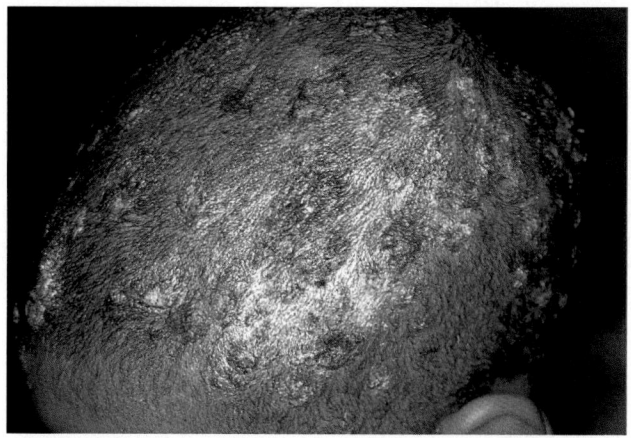

FIGURE 194-5   Tinea capitis secondary to *M. audouinii*.

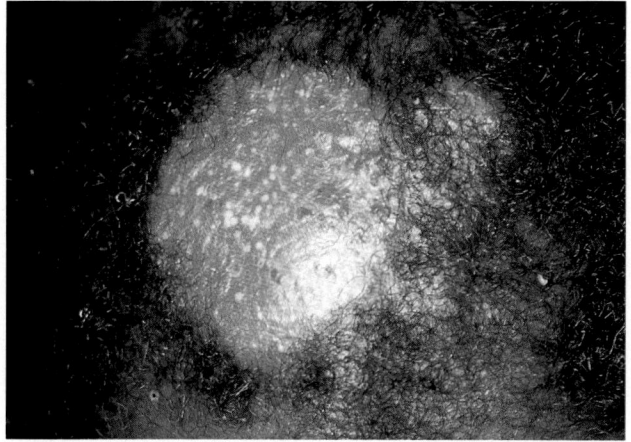

FIGURE 194-6   Kerion on scalp.

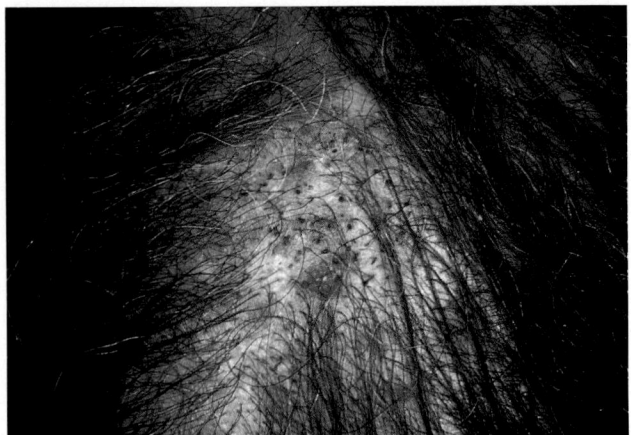

FIGURE 194-7 "Black dot" tinea capitis secondary to *T. tonsurans.*

"Black Dot" Tinea Capitis   This variety of tinea capitis is most often caused by endothrix organisms such as *T. tonsurans* or *T. violaceum.* Because of the location of the arthrospores, the hair shaft is extremely brittle and breaks at the level of the scalp. The remnant of hair left behind in the infected follicle appears as a black dot on clinical examination (Fig. 194-7). The appearance of this type of infection is variable.[110] There may be diffuse scaling with minimal hair loss and inflammation. In this circumstance, the infections can be readily confused with seborrheic dermatitis, atopic dermatitis, or psoriasis.[121] When hair loss occurs, the affected areas are characteristically multiple or polygonal in outline with indistinct, fingerlike margins.[122,123] This is in contrast to *M. audouinii infections,* which usually appear as larger, solitary, annular patches. Within the areas of involvement, "black dot" infections commonly spare some hairs so that areas of alopecia are sprinkled with a few normal hairs. "Black dot" infections may also be quite inflammatory with changes ranging from a pustular folliculitis to furuncle-like lesions or obvious kerions.[108] Finally, "black dot" tinea capitis may present without obvious black dots, making a high index of suspicion for this infection imperative.[25,121]

T. tonsurans may also infect glabrous skin or nails concurrently with scalp involvement.[119] These areas may be infected alone with complete sparing of the scalp.[124]

LABORATORY FINDINGS.   Laboratory confirmation of dermatophyte infections is imperative. Wood's lamp examination is valuable in infections caused by *M. audouinii, M. canis, M. ferrugineum,* or *M. distortum.* Here one typically sees a bright green band of fluorescence in the hair just above the level of the scalp. The examination can be positive when only a few hairs are infected. The fluorescence is thought to be produced by pteridines[125] generated as the fungus infects actively growing hairs.[1] Hairs infected in vitro do not appear to produce the substance. Rarely, Wood's lamp–negative variants of *M. audouinii* and *M. canis* are reported.[119,126] *T. tonsurans* infections typically do not fluoresce. In these instances, careful KOH examination and proper culture techniques are crucial in making the correct diagnosis.

There are several methods of obtaining material suitable for culture or examination. One may scrape the infected scaly area with a no. 15 scalpel blade or with a sterile toothbrush. In this maneuver, infected squames and portions of involved hair are recovered. The bristles of the toothbrush are then pressed directly into the appropriate culture medium. When large areas of scalp are in-

volved—as in a seborrheic dermatitis-like presentation—a sterile plastic scalp massager can be used.[27,45,127] In the case of the fluorescence-producing *Microsporum* species, the Wood's lamp may be helpful in locating individually infected hairs. These can then be plucked with epilating forceps and cultured directly. In "black dot" infections the remnant of infected hair should be extracted from the follicle, again with the use of epilating forceps or the point of a no. 11 blade, and used for KOH examination and culture.

When examining infected hairs microscopically, 10% to 15% KOH is used. The architecture of the hair is maintained if the specimen is not heated. Hence, endothrix infections can be more easily identified. An examination technique described by Shelley and Wood[128] uses xylene as the mounting medium after the plucked hair(s) is crushed. If the hairs are heavily pigmented, the melanin can be cleared partially by the use of 50% hydrogen peroxide.

Examination of the properly mounted specimen will demonstrate the type of hair parasitism involved. In ectothrix infections, arthrospores are seen outside the hair shaft (Fig. 194-1); endothrix infections have intrapilar spores (Fig. 194-2). Hyphae can be seen within the hair in both types of infection.

Specimens obtained for culture should be inoculated on Sabouraud's dextrose agar with antibiotics and incubated at room temperature. The organism can be subsequently identified by colony characteristics and microscopy.

PATHOLOGY.   In tinea capitis, hyphae are identified around and within the hair shaft. Special stains serve to emphasize their presence (i.e., PAS, methenamine silver). The dermis demonstrates a perifollicular mixed cell infiltrate with lymphocytes, histiocytes, plasma cells, and eosinophils. If follicular disruption has occurred, an adjacent foreign-body giant cell reaction is seen.[129,130]

In the more inflammatory lesion (i.e., kerions), an intense dermal infiltrate is seen with polymorphonuclear leukocytes forming abscesses in the dermis and within the follicle.[104,130] In these markedly inflammatory reactions, fungal organisms are seen with difficulty. Immunofluorescence techniques, however, have demonstrated the presence of fungal antigens.[131]

DIAGNOSIS.   The differential diagnosis of tinea capitis includes seborrheic dermatitis, atopic dermatitis,[121] and psoriasis when minimally inflammatory diffuse scaling is the major clinical presentation. When alopecia is more pronounced, diseases such as alopecia areata, trichotillomania, secondary syphilis, or pseudopelade can be entertained. Alopecia due to tinea capitis fails to produce the typical exclamation point hairs seen in alopecia areata or the artefactual-appearing areas with hairs of varying lengths seen in trichotillomania.

In inflammatory tinea capitis, bacterial pyodermas (furunculosis, impetigo) can be simulated. Folliculitis decalvans or perifolliculitis capitis abscedens et suffodiens can also enter into the differential diagnosis. After scarring has occurred, noninfectious processes such as discoid lupus erythematosus, lichen planopilaris, pseudopelade, or radiation dermatitis are often considered in the differential diagnosis.

THERAPY.   Tinea capitis may resolve spontaneously. Rothman thought that *M. audouinii* infections cleared at puberty. However, more recent data indicate that these infections, as well as many caused by *T. tonsurans,* resolve within a year without therapy and with no relation to puberty. Inflammatory zoophilic and geophilic infections tend to resolve spontaneously in a period of time that varies inversely with the inflammation. Despite the data cited above, *T. tonsurans* and *T. violaceum* infections are more prone to be persistent into adulthood than are *M. audouinii* infections.

Tinea capitis should be treated with a systemic antifungal such as griseofulvin. The usual dose is 1.0 g/day of the microcrystalline variety or 0.5 g/day of the ultramicrosized drug. For children the dose is 10 to 12 mg/kg per day. Therapy should be continued until a clinical and laboratory (culture) cure is obtained, usually 4 to 8 weeks. Although most griseofulvin therapy is conducted using daily doses, single megadose therapy has found support, particularly in economically deprived areas where access to physicians and medication is limited. In several reports, single doses of 3 to 5 g have yielded acceptable 1-year cure rates for tinea capitis caused by *M. audouinii*.[132,133] Weekly treatment protocols have also been used successfully.[134]

Occasionally, topical products are used adjunctively with systemic treatment. Topical therapy alone, however, is not advocated.

In markedly inflammatory tinea capitis, oral corticosteroids may be helpful in reducing the incidence of scarring. The therapy is particularly helpful in the treatment of kerions. The usual dose of prednisone is 1 mg/kg per day given at one time in the morning.

When anthropophilic tinea capitis is identified, it is important to examine close contacts of the patient for evidence of disease. Segregation of infected children in school is not warranted if effective therapy is provided.[104] If zoophilic organisms are cultured, examination of pets (i.e., kittens, puppies) for evidence of dermatophytes is warranted. If infection is suspected, the pets should be treated.

Tinea Favosa

Tinea favosa or favus (Latin, "honeycomb") is a chronic, mycotic infection of the scalp, glabrous skin, and/or nails characterized by the formation of yellowish crusts within the hair follicles (scutula) and eventuating in a cicatrizing alopecia.

EPIDEMIOLOGY. Favus is typically a chronic infection that begins early in life and commonly extends into adulthood.[135] The disease is seen predominantly in rural areas and often is associated with conditions of poor hygiene, malnutrition, and squalor. The infection is generally family-centered rather than school-centered as is seen commonly with other tinea capitis–producing dermatophytes. A relatively intimate and prolonged contact is probably required for transmission.[136]

Although favus is seen in families, generation after generation, attack rates within families can vary, suggesting that there may be an inherited susceptibility or resistance to the infection.[118] In addition, simple measures to improve personal hygiene in the at-risk population often result in markedly decreased transmission.[137] It is known that *T. schoenleinii* can survive for years on epilated hairs. For this reason, cleanliness with the removal of hairs or other sources of infection is an important factor in controlling the disease.[112]

Although animal favus is known to occur, there is no evidence to substantiate the existence of an animal reservoir to explain human infections.[137]

Sex differences do not seem to exist in the incidence of favus, except in those chronic infections extending into adulthood. Here, there is an increased number of females affected.[119]

ETIOLOGY. The most common dermatophyte producing favus is *T. schoenleinii*. However, other organisms can produce a favuslike clinical picture (i.e., *T. violaceum*, *M. gypseum*). A variety of different organisms are known to produce animal favus.[1]

Favus is commonly seen in certain geographic areas. In some of these locations it is the most common cause of tinea capitis.[26] The infection is endemic in the Middle East and Mediterranean basin area, southeastern Europe, France, southern Asia, and Greenland. In South Africa the disease is quite common and among the Bantu is referred to as "witkop."[1] In the Americas, endemic pockets of the disease exist. There are reports from areas of Québec, the United States (Kentucky, West Virginia, Arkansas, New York),[104] Guatemala, and Brazil.[1] In many of these areas, the infection can be traced to immigrants from endemic areas such as Russia or Poland. The disease is then passed on from generation to generation.

CLINICAL FEATURES. In the early stages of infection, hyphae invade the hair follicle and gradually distend the follicular opening. Clinically, very little is seen within the first 3 weeks of infection except a slight amount of perifollicular scaling.

Scutula are found in most cases of favus. These concentrations of hyphae and keratinous debris take root at the opening of the hair follicle. Here, they gradually expand from a yellowish-red papule to form a yellowish, cup-shaped structure that may become 1 cm or more in diameter. The center of the scutulum is often pierced by a single, lusterless, dry hair (Fig. 194-8). The color is due to the invasion of the hair by multiple intrapilar hyphae. The hair is not as brittle as with *T. tonsurans* endothrix infections, and, for that reason, hairs in favus may frequently attain a normal length. If the scutulum is removed from its attachment to the epidermis, an oozing, erythematous base is noted. Scutula may expand peripherally and, during the course of the infection, form large, adherent mats of scutula and hair. Hygienic conditions are particularly lacking in this stage of the disease, and a characteristic "mousy" odor may be appreciated.[1,7]

In the classic presentation, lesions appear in a patchy distribution on the scalp and coalesce. The borders of the infected lesions represent areas of advancing disease and are often polycyclic in shape.[137] The center of the infected area becomes extensively scarred and almost totally devoid of hair.

Besides scalp involvement, favus may involve glabrous skin and nails. The skin infections may be of various types (i.e., vesicular, papulosquamous, tinea circinata-like). Oftentimes true scutula

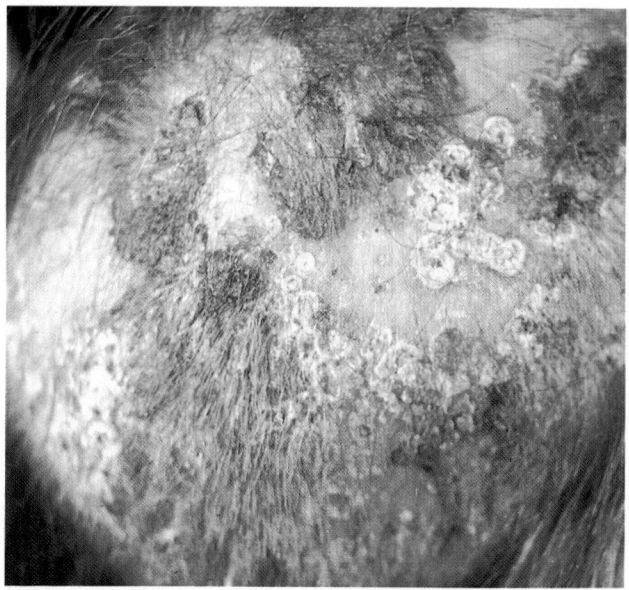

FIGURE 194-8 Tinea capitis from *Trichophyton schoenleinii* (favus). Yellowish, adherent crusts and scales, known as scutula. May be complicated by atrophy, scarring, and permanent hair loss.

are formed. Nail involvement occurs in 2 to 3 percent of infections[119] and is indistinguishable from onychomycosis due to other organisms.[55]

In some cases, especially when personal hygiene is relatively good, favus lesions may be atypical in appearance.[119,136] For example, scutula may be small or absent, and the disease may present with diffuse scaling of the scalp.[119] In these instances, the infection is difficult to distinguish from seborrheic dermatitis, psoriasis, or tinea amiantacea. In later stages of infection, a cicatricial alopecia may be present. In this end-stage presentation, the condition may be identical to that noted in cicatrizing alopecia after radiation or chemical injury or the scarring alopecia seen in some cases of pseudopelade, folliculitis decalvans, lupus erythematosus, or lichen planopilaris.

LABORATORY FINDINGS.   The laboratory diagnosis of favus requires the use of KOH examination and culture techniques discussed previously. On microscopic examination, an endothrix type of hair invasion is seen. The favus hair shows hyphae coursing lengthwise and no arthrospores.[1,7] Because of autolysis, vacant tunnels are formed within the hair and these may appear as air spaces microscopically (Fig. 194-3).[138]

With Wood's lamp examination, a pale green fluorescence is seen along the entire length of the infected hair. The fluorescence may be subtle and can be difficult to appreciate, especially in patients with gray hair.[71]

HISTOPATHOLOGY.   Using histopathologic techniques, scutula show intermingled masses of mycelia, scale, and granular debris. The degenerating hyphae and necrotic material are seen most typically in the center of the scutulum, whereas the viable organisms reside at the periphery. Under the scutulum there is an atrophic epithelium; acanthosis is noted at the lateral margins.[129] In the dermis, an extensive chronic plasma cell or granulomatous perifollicular infiltrate is commonly seen and is particularly dense subjacent to the scutulum. No fungi are noted when the dermis is examined with special stains. Fragments of hair can be seen in the dermis with polarized light. In the later stages of infection, the dermis may simply show fibrosis with a diminished inflammatory cell response.

THERAPY.   Favus is effectively treated with griseofulvin in the same dosage used in tinea capitis.[139] Nail infections require a longer course of therapy (6 to 12 months). It is important to examine and treat all affected family members simultaneously.[1] Improvement of hygienic conditions is also beneficial, as are efforts to locally debride areas of extensive crusting.

Tinea Barbae

Tinea barbae (also known as tinea sycosis, "barber's itch") is a fungal infection limited to the coarse hair-bearing beard and moustache area of men. In women and prepubertal boys, infection in the facial areas (tinea faciale) is classified with the other glabrous skin infections.[7]

EPIDEMIOLOGY.   Tinea barbae is by definition seen only in males. Usually, the infection is contracted by exposure to animals, most commonly cattle and dogs. The infection is most often seen in a rural setting,[1,7,140–144] oftentimes affecting dairy farmers or cattle ranchers. Prior to the introduction of modern-day antiseptic techniques, tinea barbae—then called barber's itch—was transmitted from person to person by contaminated barbers' razors or clippers.[1]

ETIOLOGY AND PATHOGENESIS.   Overall, the most common dermatophytes causing tinea barbae are the zoophilic organisms— *T. mentagrophytes* and *T. verrucosum*.[140,141] *M. canis* is causative in a fewer number of cases.[142] Anthropophilic organisms (*T. rubrum, T. violaceum, T. schoenleinii,* and *T. megninii*) have been implicated in urban areas[143] or in areas where these fungi are en-

demic. In general, the infection caused by the anthropophiles is less inflammatory than that caused by the zoophilic dermatophytes.

The pathogenesis of tinea barbae, while not studied as carefully as tinea capitis, is thought to be similar to that of the latter. Coarse hairs are uniquely susceptible; occasionally one may see concurrent involvement of the beard and scalp area.[118]

CLINICAL MANIFESTATIONS.   Three clinical types of tinea barbae have been recognized: (1) inflammatory or kerion-like; (2) superficial or sycosiform type[144]; and (3) the circinate, spreading type.

The inflammatory variety is analogous to kerion formation in tinea capitis (Fig. 194-9). In tinea barbae, the lesions are usually unilateral; common areas of involvement are the chin, neck, and maxillary and submaxillary areas (Fig. 194-9a). The upper lip is usually spared.[1,145] The inflammatory lesions are most often caused by *T. mentagrophytes* and *T. verrucosum*. Lesions are nodular and boggy; there is often an associated weeping of seropurulent material with subsequent crusting. Perifollicular pustulation is observed; coalescence of these inflammatory areas yields abscess-like collections of pus. The hairs within the infected areas are loose and easily epilated; commonly they are lusterless and brittle as well. Eventually, undermining and sinus tract formation can occur. Scarring and permanent alopecia are the ultimate outcome in severely affected areas.

The superficial type of tinea barbae typically resembles a bacterial folliculitis (Fig. 194-9b). There is a diffuse erythema associated with perifollicular papules and pustules.[144] The organisms causing this clinical picture are the relatively noninflammatory anthropophiles. Hairs may be affected, depending on the organism involved. For example, *T. violaceum* infections commonly result in brittle, lusterless hair due to endothrix invasion. Conversely, *T. rubrum* infections produce hair invasion less often.

The circinate tinea barbae is analogous to tinea circinata of glabrous skin. There is an active, spreading vesiculopustular border with central scaling. There may be a relative sparing of hair in this variant.[144]

Atypical tinea barbae may also be seen, especially if the course of the disease is altered by corticosteroid or other therapy.[119] Infection caused by *M. canis* may show unusual clinical patterns. For example, in children, isolated involvement of the eyebrows may occur with this organism.[1] In addition, other authors have described infected granuloma annulare-like lesions or abscess-like tumors in patients infected with *M. canis*.[146] Finally, *E. floccosum* has been found to produce verrucous, granulomatous-appearing lesions on the face and body termed *verrucous epidermophyton*.[145] One must have a high index of suspicion for these dermatophyte infections so that atypical infections can be recognized.

LABORATORY FINDINGS.   Epilated hairs or scale can be examined with 10% KOH as described for tinea capitis. Depending on the organisms involved, endothrix or ectothrix hair invasion can be seen as well as stratum corneum infections. Wood's lamp examination is useful only for infections by *M. canis*, in which a bright green fluorescence can be seen. Of course, cultures of the hair and infected squames should be done using Sabouraud's dextrose agar with antibiotics. In tinea barbae, epilated hairs may show a bulbous, white material surrounding the hair bulb; usually these hairs prove to be culture-positive.

PATHOLOGY.   Histopathologic findings are similar to those seen in tinea capitis. Fungi are seen in the hair keratin and sometimes in the stratum corneum by using special stains. No organisms are seen in the surrounding dermis. Neutrophils may be seen within the hair follicle, but a chronic, sometimes granulomatous inflam-

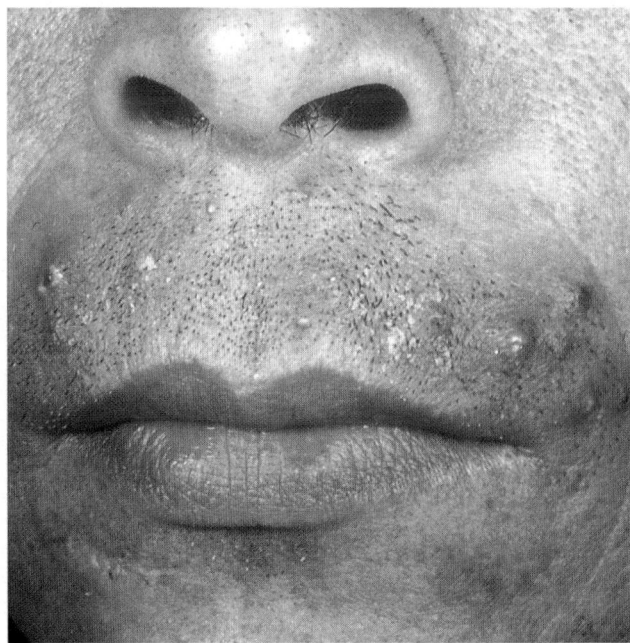

a

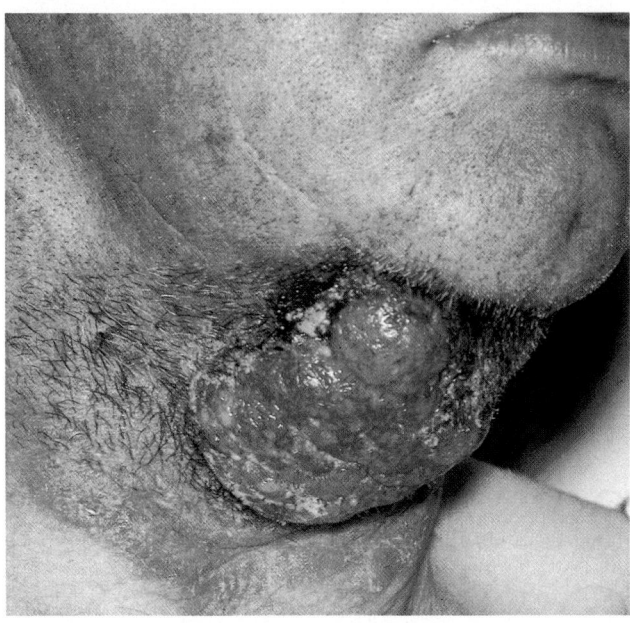

b

FIGURE 194-9 (*a*) Tinea barbae, kerion. Sharply demarcated red nodule (4.0 × 6.0 cm). The surface is moist and studded with multiple yellowish pustules. Regional lymph nodes are not enlarged. (*b*) Tinea barbae. Scattered, discrete, follicular pustules.

matory response is noted perifollicularly. In extremely inflammatory lesions, fungi may be sparse or absent.[130]

DIAGNOSIS. Tinea barbae should be differentiated from a bacterial folliculitis (sycosis vulgaris), perioral dermatitis, candidal infection, acneform dermatitis, pseudofolliculitis barbae, contact dermatitis, halogenoderma, and herpes simplex. A bacterial folliculitis is usually bilateral and may involve the upper lip. There can be more pain or fever in this instance than in tinea barbae.[145] The

other entities mentioned can be differentiated by an accurate history and the use of such diagnostic procedures as patch testing, Tzanck smears, or viral cultures.

TREATMENT. As with tinea capitis, griseofulvin in a dose of 0.5 g to 1 g per day (microsized) is used. Therapy is continued for 2 to 3 weeks after clinical resolution has occurred. Local measures such as topical antifungals, wet compresses, and debridement of crusted debris are additive. Occasionally, in severely inflammatory infections, a course of systemic corticosteroid therapy is helpful.

If no treatment is given, most inflammatory infections resolve spontaneously in a few weeks. Less inflammatory, superficial infections may, in contrast, persist for months.[1,144]

Tinea Corporis (Tinea Circinata) Tinea corporis arbitrarily includes all dermatophyte infections of glabrous skin with the exclusion of certain specific locations (i.e., palms, soles, and groin).

ETIOLOGY. All species of dermatophyte belonging to the genera *Trichophyton, Microsporum,* or *Epidermophyton* are capable of producing tinea corporis. The three most common causative organisms are *T. rubrum, M. canis,* and *T. mentagrophytes;* however, variations may occur based on the existence of endemic species in specific geographic areas.[13] Often, the prevalent organism causing tinea capitis in children in a certain geographic area is the organism producing tinea corporis in adults of the same region.[1,118] *T. concentricum* is the organism responsible for a variant of tinea corporis endemic in the Pacific Islands—tinea imbricata, which is also known as Tokelau ringworm.

EPIDEMIOLOGY. The organism responsible for tinea corporis may be transmitted by direct contact with other infected individuals or by infected animals. It may also be transmitted from inanimate fomites such as clothing and furniture. Although there is some controversy on this point, many authors feel that tinea corporis results from the transfer of infection from other involved sites on the same patient. Under appropriate environmental conditions (warmth, humidity), a reservoir of infection on the feet or elsewhere may be the source of tinea corporis.[32] Whether or not the infection originates in this manner, it is clear that a tropical or subtropical climate is associated with more frequent and severe tinea corporis.

Children appear to have an increased incidence of tinea corporis caused by zoophilic organisms. Many of these infections are with *M. canis.*[145] The organism is most likely transmitted by contact with pets (especially cats and dogs).

Tinea imbricata, caused by *T. concentricum,* has a unique epidemiology among the organisms causing tinea corporis. The organism is geographically limited to certain areas of the Far East, South Pacific, and South and Central America. Here a large proportion of the native population may be affected, but nonnatives may be spared even though they have resided in endemic areas for long periods. Like favus, tinea imbricata is probably contracted in early childhood and can persist for a lifetime.[147] There is some evidence that the susceptibility to tinea imbricata is hereditarily determined through an autosomal recessive trait.[33]

PATHOGENESIS. The organisms responsible for tinea corporis generally reside in the stratum corneum (Fig. 194-10). Presumably, serum inhibitory factor is responsible for limiting the infection.[60,61] The pathogenic sequence of events has been outlined previously. The first step involves invasion of the stratum corneum, possibly with the help of warm, moist, occlusive conditions.[148] After a 1- to 3-week incubation period, centrifugal spread occurs. The active, advancing border of infection has an increased epidermal turnover rate.[47] Presumably, the host epidermis is attempting to shed the organism by increasing epidermal turnover to exceed the fungal

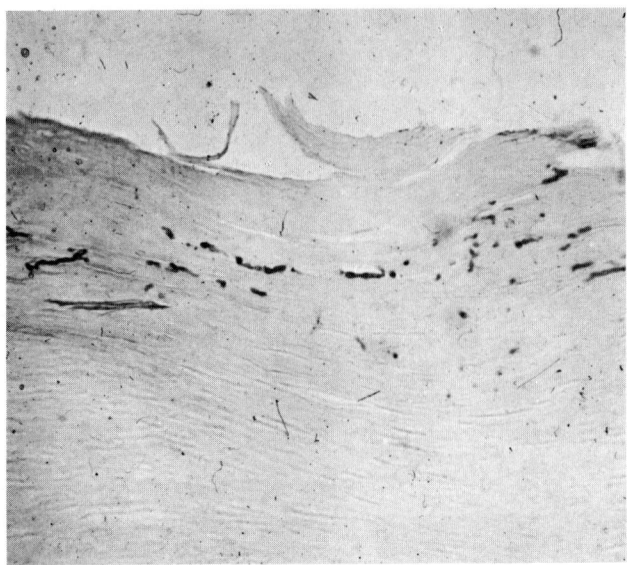

FIGURE 194-10 PAS stain of dermatophyte in stratum corneum.

growth rate. This defense mechanism is successful to a certain extent as there is relative clearing of infection in the center of the annular cutaneous lesion. Temporary resistance to reinfection occurs in this area for a variable time; however, second waves of infection are commonly seen later.[1,7]

Most organisms causing tinea corporis are located superficially in the stratum corneum. Hair follicle involvement can occur—especially with *T. rubrum* or *T. verrucosum*[130]—and seems to be associated with increased inflammation.[7] Other correlates of increased inflammation are the type of organism (zoophilic or geophilic being more inflammatory) and the nature of the host response.

CLINICAL MANIFESTATIONS. Tinea corporis may be diverse in its clinical presentation.[149–166] Table 194-9 summarizes the clinical variants that can be seen, along with distinguishing features of each. The most common presentation is the typical annular lesion with an active, erythematous and sometimes vesicular border (Fig. 194-11). Commonly, the center of the lesion shows clearing, but variations may occur. The center often shows concentric rings in tinea imbricata and *T. rubrum* infections (Fig. 194-12). With *T. rubrum* large, confluent plaques of infection may occur.[166] Polycyclic or psoriasiform lesions are also seen frequently. It is clear

TABLE 194-9
Variants of Tinea Corporis

Name	Causative organism(s)	Clinical description
Noninflammatory		
Tinea circinata	Any dermatophyte (commonly *T. rubrum*, *T. mentagrophytes*, *M. canis*)	Annular lesions with central clearing and an active, spreading border
Bullous tinea corporis[149–151]	Usually *T. rubrum*	Spongiotic or subcorneal vesicles/pustules; may be herpetiform
Tinea imbricata	*T. concentricum*	Widespread; multiple concentric, polycyclic scaly lesions with minimal inflammation; there may be an increased immediate hypersensitivity and decreased cell-mediated immunity to trichophytin antigen[147]
Inflammatory		
Kerion of glabrous skin[152]	Zoophilic organisms (usually *T. verrucosum* or *T. mentagrophytes*)	Similar to kerion of scalp
Majocchi's granuloma[153,154]	*T. rubrum*, *T. violaceum*, *T. tonsurans*, *T. mentagrophytes*	In Majocchi's original description the lesions were perifollicular, granulomatous nodules seen mostly on the scalps of children; they were often painless without pustulation, and often associated with underlying disease
Nodular granulomatous[153,154] perifolliculitis of the legs	*T. rubrum*	This variant of Majocchi's disease is characterized by lesions occurring in women on the lower two-thirds of the legs; the disease is often unilateral; *T. rubrum* is usually present elsewhere (nails, feet)
Agminate folliculitis[7]	Zoophilic organism	Well-defined, erythematous plaques studded with perifollicular pustules
Subcutaneous abscess (tinea profunda)	*T. mentagrophytes*,[155] *T. violaceum*,[156] *T. crateriforme*, (*tonsurans*),[157] *T. rubrum*,[66] *M. audouinii*[158]	Deep subcutaneous nodules are present; there is rarely lymph node involvement[158] and associated hematogenous spread[159]
Mycetoma[158]	*M. audouinii*, *T. verrucosum*, *T. mentagrophytes*, *T. violaceum*, *T. tonsurans*, *M. ferrugineum*, *M. canis*	Subcutaneous masses
Tinea faciale[159–162]	Usually *Trichophyton* species; occasionally *M. canis*	This disease represents 3 to 4% of tinea corporis; erythematous, scaly plaques with or without active borders are present; telangiectasia, atrophy, and photoexacerbation may mimic lupus erythematosus
Tinea incognito[7,163,164]	Any dermatophyte infection modified by corticosteroid treatment	Lesions are often atypical appearing; inflammation, scaling, and symptoms may be absent, or kerion-like lesions may occur; there are usually dermal nodules present
Verrucous epidermophyton[85,165]	*E. floccosum*	Verrucous-like lesions are present on the head, neck, and buttocks; cutaneous anergy may be present
Miscellaneous and wide-spread infections	*T. rubrum*[72,81–83]	There is often atrophy and a selective CMI defect to trichophytin
	M. audouinii[19]	There may be an associated depressed CMI and a deficient plasma factor needed for lymphocytic blastogenesis

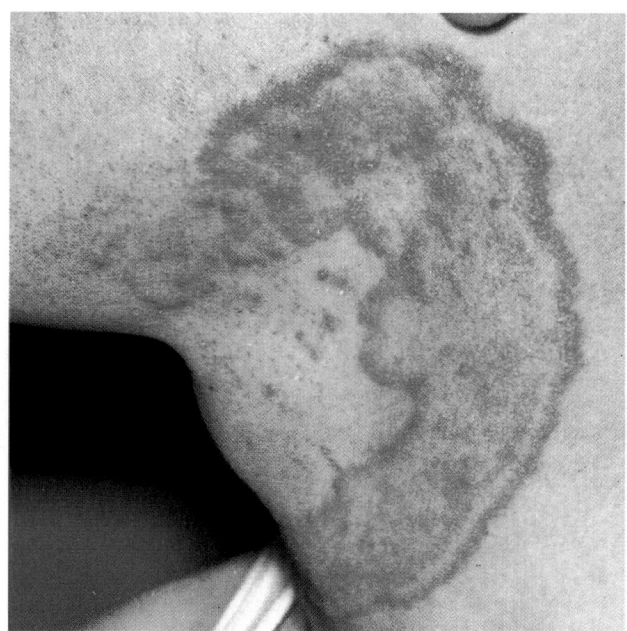

FIGURE 194-11   Tinea corporis with typical "ringworm-like" configuration.

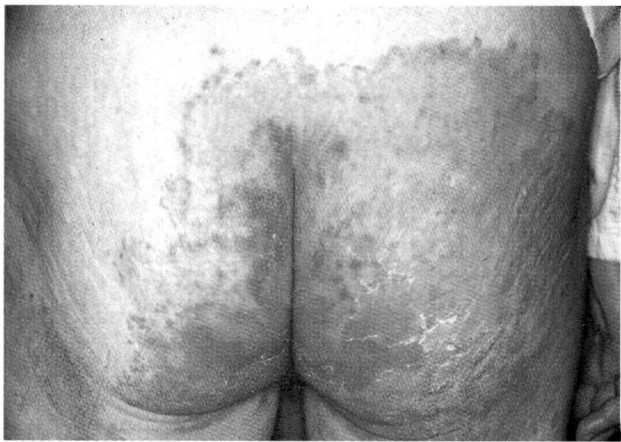

FIGURE 194-12   Polycyclic pattern of tinea corporis.

that a high index of suspicion should exist for tinea corporis. Any red, scaly rash deserves at least a thorough microscopic examination to exclude this entity.

Tinea corporis can occur on any area of the body. When the infection is due to a zoophilic organism, the lesions are commonly seen on exposed skin (head, neck, face, and arms). When such an infection occurs with *M. canis,* lesions may be unusually numerous for body ringworm. Tinea corporis due to anthropophilic organisms often occurs in occluded areas or in areas of trauma (i.e., perifolliculitis of the legs in women may be associated with leg shaving).

LABORATORY FINDINGS.   Because clinical signs are variable in many cases of tinea corporis, the clinician must often rely on laboratory findings for the correct diagnosis.

In the usual lesion of tinea corporis—the spreading ringworm with the active, erythematous border—specimens for KOH examination should be obtained from the actively spreading border of the lesion. Here organisms are more numerous, and the chances of a

positive examination are higher. One sees septate, branching hyphae in the stratum corneum (Fig. 194-4). If bullous lesions are present, the greatest numbers of organisms are found by examining the roof of the blister. Finally, if dermal granulomatous lesions occur, the greatest positivity on culture is obtained by using biopsy material as the inoculum.[152]

It is important not to rely on KOH examination alone to prove or disprove the existence of a dermatophyte infection, particularly if the index of suspicion is high. In some reports the KOH examination is positive in only one-third of patients with tinea corporis.[167] Fungal culture is imperative. Infected material should be inoculated on Sabouraud's dextrose agar with antibiotics, even when direct KOH examination is negative. Four weeks of incubation at room temperature is required before the culture plates are discarded.

PATHOLOGY.   Histopathologically, fungal organisms can be seen in the stratum corneum in the usual case of tinea circinata. With hematoxylin and eosin, they appear basophilic; with PAS, the fungal elements stain red; with silver methenamine, they stain black.[130]

If organisms are not found, the histopathology is nonspecific and may resemble an acute or chronic dermatitis. If vesiculation is present, it is often seen histologically as a spongiotic vesicle. In the nodular perifolliculitis variant caused by *T. rubrum,* there is a perifollicular granulomatous reaction, often associated with central necrosis and suppuration. Organisms are seen in the hairs as well as in the dermis. Here, spores may be large (6 μm) and located within multinucleated giant cells.[130]

DIAGNOSIS.   The differential diagnosis of tinea corporis is variable because the clinical findings are variable. In the usual annular ringworm infection, entities such as erythema annulare centrifugum (EAC), nummular eczema, and granuloma annulare (GA) should be considered. EAC generally shows scaling at the trailing edge of the advancing border, whereas tinea corporis shows scaling over the entire advancing edge. In nummular eczema, lesions show eczematous change or crusting throughout the entire lesion; no central clearing is seen. Furthermore, lesions tend to be more numerous and symmetric than in tinea corporis. In GA, intradermal papules without significant epidermal change make up the border of the lesions.

If the clinical lesion is more papulosquamous in appearance, other typically papulosquamous entities can be considered (i.e., psoriasis, lichen planus, secondary syphilis, seborrheic dermatitis, pityriasis rosea, or pityriasis rubra pilaris). Most of the above conditions are readily distinguished by their characteristic clinical features as well as by biopsy.

For the inflammatory variants of tinea corporis, bacterial, candidal, or deep fungal infections enter the differential diagnosis. Verrucous and granulomatous lesions may mimic acid-fast infections or North American blastomycosis. Deeper lesions may resemble bacterial abscesses, panniculitis, or nodular vasculitis.

Tinea faciale may resemble lupus erythematosus or dermatomyositis. The history of photoexacerbation in tinea faciale as well as the absence of a distinct raised scaly border are misleading.[160] Most tinea faciale lesions lack follicular plugging and the true poikiloderma of connective tissue diseases. Other entities to be considered include photodermatoses such as polymorphous light eruption, contact dermatitis, or acne rosacea.

TREATMENT.   For isolated lesions of tinea corporis, topical agents such as miconazole nitrate 1%, clotrimazole 2%, and other topical imidazoles or ciclopirox olamine 1% are the most effective.

For widespread or more inflammatory lesions, griseofulvin is used in a dose equivalent to 0.5 g to 1 g per day of the micronized drug. For serious infections not responding to griseofulvin, ketoconazole may be helpful (see "Therapy of Superficial Fungal Infections").

Tinea Cruris   Tinea cruris is a dermatophytosis involving the groin area and includes infections of the genitalia, pubic area, perineal and perianal skin.[168–170]

EPIDEMIOLOGY.   Tinea cruris is almost exclusively a male dermatophytosis.[28] The reasons for this preference may depend on several factors: (1) men wear more occlusive clothing than do women; (2) because of the scrotum, skin in the groin area of men may be subject to a greater area of occlusion; (3) in general, men are more physically active than women, and the groin may remain warm and moist for longer periods; (4) finally, there may be a greater incidence of other sites of dermatophyte infection in men (e.g., tinea pedis) that may function as a reservoir for new cases of tinea cruris.[1,7] Close direct or indirect physical contact does not appear to equalize the differences cited above. For example, in the examination of multiple infections within a single household, conjugal transmission is rare despite ample exposure to infectious material.[24]

The transmission of tinea cruris may occur by several mechanisms. Direct contact between infected and noninfected individuals may serve to transmit the disease in some cases. The role that trauma plays in colonization of uninvolved areas is implied but not fully appreciated. More commonly, however, indirect transmission can occur through contact with nonliving objects that carry infected scales. Cultures from items such as bed linens, towels, articles of clothing, and even bedpans and urinals have been positive for dermatophytes in situations where epidemic spread of tinea cruris is occurring.[10,171] The causative dermatophytes (especially *E. floccosum*) have been found to survive for long periods on shed squames.[1] These infected scales provide a source for future infections that is difficult to eradicate.

Environmental factors are important in the initiation and propagation of tinea cruris. It is well known that these infections occur more commonly in the summer months or in tropical climates where ambient warmth and humidity are highest. If occlusion from clothing or wet bathing apparel is added, an optimal environment for the initiation or recrudescence of this infection exists.[1,7]

A final important epidemiologic consideration is the role played by dermatophytoses elsewhere on the body in providing a reservoir for autoinfection in tinea cruris. Other sites of infection may coexist with tinea cruris. The most common association is the tinea pedis and cruris caused by *T. rubrum*.[172] Many investigators feel that the feet are a likely source of the infecting organism in nascent cases of tinea cruris.[1,168] Others have implicated the scrotum in this reservoir role. Although clinical signs of scrotal infection in tinea cruris are minimal, organisms have been detected by microscopic examination and by culture in a surprisingly high percentage of scrotal specimens.[173–175]

ETIOLOGY.   The most common organisms causing tinea cruris are *E. floccosum*, *T. rubrum*, and *T. mentagrophytes*. Differences in the number of infections caused by each organism exist and depend on the prevalence of that organism in the population being surveyed. The groin is by far the most common site for infections caused by *E. floccosum*. The epidemics of tinea cruris reported in some series are caused predominantly by this dermatophyte.[168,169] Infections with other dermatophytes, such as species of *Microsporum*, have been reported but they are extremely rare.[170]

CLINICAL MANIFESTATIONS.   Pruritus is a common symptom; pain may be present if the involved area is macerated or secondarily infected. In classic tinea cruris, one sees bilateral but often asymmetric involvement of the genitocrural area and medial upper thigh (Fig. 194-13). Often the left thigh adjacent to the scrotum is the first site involved.

The clinical lesion is characterized by a well-marginated, raised border that may be composed of multiple erythematous papulovesicles. Rarely pustules may be seen at the border, but the satellite pustules typical of candidal infections are unusual. The scrotum may appear completely normal or only minimally involved, even though microscopic examination and culture show the presence of organisms.[174] *Candida*, in contrast, often presents with obvious clinical disease on the scrotum or penis.

The two most common organisms causing tinea cruris may have differences in their clinical lesions. *E. floccosum* typically presents as described above with an active, spreading papulovesicular border and central clearing. The lesions seldom extend beyond the genitocrural crease and medial upper thigh.

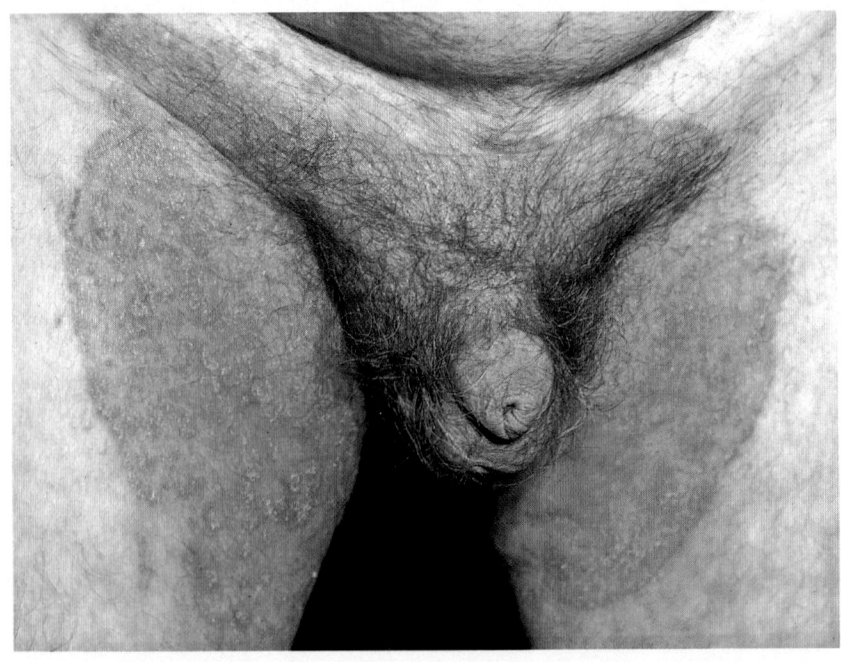

FIGURE 194-13 Tinea cruris. Scaling erythematous plaque with sharp margins.

T. rubrum lesions, however, often coalesce and spread to involve wider areas of adjacent skin in the pubic, lower abdominal, buttock, and perianal areas (Fig. 194-13).[1,7]

Secondary changes may complicate the clinical picture of tinea cruris. Chronic scratching may cause lichenification and present a lichen simplex chronicus-like picture. Secondary bacterial infection may obscure a more chronic tinea cruris. Weeping, maceration, and areas of pustulation may exist. Finally, a secondary allergic or irritant contact dermatitis may be present if sensitizing or irritating topical products have been used in treatment.

LABORATORY FINDINGS. As noted previously, infected scales examined by a 10% to 15% KOH preparation show septate hyphae coursing through infected squames. Cultures inoculated onto Sabouraud's media with antibiotics and incubated at room temperature will grow the responsible organism within 2 weeks.

PATHOLOGY. The histologic findings are identical to those described with tinea corporis.

DIAGNOSIS. The diagnosis is made by the presence of a typical clinical picture associated with positive microscopy or culture. Other dermatoses presenting a similar clinical picture in the crural area are psoriasis, seborrheic dermatitis, a therapeutic dermatitis, candidiasis, erythrasma, lichen simplex chronicus, or even Darier's disease and benign familial chronic pemphigus (Hailey-Hailey).

Candidiasis is distinguished by a greater incidence of obvious scrotal involvement and by the presence of satellite pustules peripheral to brightly erythematous plaques. Erythrasma can be distinguished by examining the suspected lesion under the Wood's lamp. The involved skin in erythrasma shows a coral red fluorescence; lesions of tinea cruris do not. Biopsy may be necessary to totally exclude some of the other diagnoses mentioned.

TREATMENT. Efforts to decrease occlusion and moisture in the involved area are helpful. This can be accomplished by lighter and better-ventilated clothing as well as by the judicious use of absorbent powder.

In most cases, tinea cruris can be managed by local topical measures. A variety of agents have been used including haloprogin, tolnaftate, and the topical imidazoles (miconazole, clotrimazole, or econazole). A powder or minimally occlusive cream base for these products is recommended.

For more widespread or inflammatory infections, treatment with griseofulvin (500 to 1000 mg/day of the microsized preparation) is indicated.

Tinea Pedis and Tinea Manuum Tinea pedis is a dermatophyte infection of the feet. Tinea manuum is a dermatophyte infection of the palmar and interdigital areas of the hand.

HISTORY. Tinea pedis represents a dermatophytosis of relatively recent onset. It probably was not common until humans began wearing occlusive footwear.[1,10] Tinea manuum was first described by Fox in 1870,[176] but tinea pedis was not reported until 1888.[177] At present both infections are common worldwide; in fact, they represent the most common forms of dermatophyte infections.

EPIDEMIOLOGY. The epidemiology of tinea pedis has been extensively studied.[10,11] The infection is common during the summer months and in tropical or semitropical climates. Footwear is an important variable, and the incidence of tinea pedis is definitely higher in any population that wears occlusive shoes.

The infection rate is increased in individuals using communal baths or pools.[178,179] The number of infections can be related to the number of people using the facilities. Cultures from swimming pool and washroom floors as well as from items of clothing in contact with infected areas[180,181] are often positive for the responsible organism. It is generally accepted, therefore, that tinea pedis is

an exogenously transmitted infection in which cross infection among susceptible individuals readily occurs.[182] Previous theories postulated that dermatophytes populate normal interdigital areas,[183–186] and that under appropriate conditions (heat, humidity, trauma), a symptomatic infection could arise from the patient's endogenous flora. In fact, these workers found that infections were difficult to produce experimentally using exogenous inocula alone.[36,37,184]

The sex and age of the host are not direct risk factors in this disease as infection rates are comparable if the nature and degree of exposure are equivalent.[10] The increasing incidence of this infection with age is probably a function of an increased opportunity for exposure. Approximately 10 percent of the total population can be expected to have a dermatophytic foot infection at any given time.[7] If only closed communities of individuals (athletic teams, military organizations, boarding schools) are considered, the rate of infection is much higher.

ETIOLOGY. Tinea pedis is caused most commonly by *T. rubrum, T. mentagrophytes,* or *E. floccosum.* In rare instances, sporadic infections with *T. violaceum, T. megninii, M. persicolor,* and *M. canis* have been described. Although slight differences may exist in relative frequency, the common causative organisms are the same worldwide. In the United Kingdom,[7] *T. rubrum* accounts for 60 percent of the cases, and *T. mentagrophytes* is seen in 25 percent. *E. floccosum* is found in 10 percent of the cases in the United Kingdom and 20 percent of the cases in the United States.[1] A 3 to 5 percent incidence of mixed infections has been noted in some series.[7]

T. rubrum commonly produces a dry, hyperkeratotic, mocassin-like involvement of the feet and/or hands (Fig. 194-14); *T. mentagrophytes* often produces a vesicular pattern; and *E. floc-*

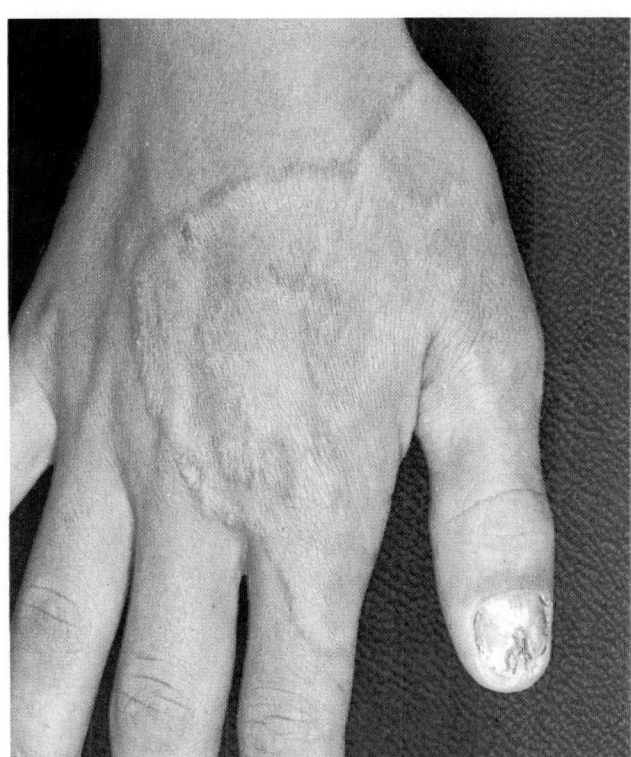

FIGURE 194-14 Tinea manus. Polycyclic pattern of an eruption composed of scaling vesicles with involvement of the thumb nail; the nail exhibits destruction of the nail plate.

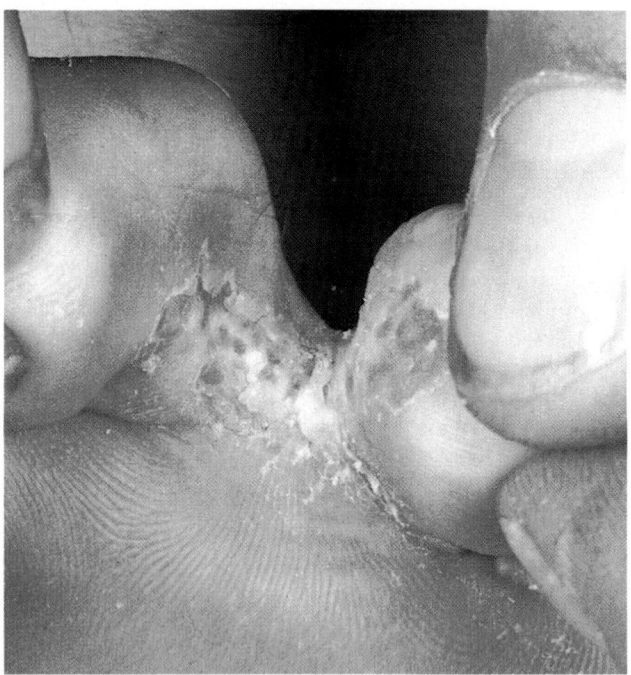

FIGURE 194-15 Tinea pedis, interdigital. The area is macerated, has opaque white scales and some erosions.

cosum may produce either of the two patterns described above. Toenail involvement, however, is less common with *E. floccosum*.

CLINICAL MANIFESTATIONS.   Tinea pedis may present as one of four clinically accepted variants or as an overlap of one or more of these types. The chronic, intertriginous type is the most common and is characterized by fissuring, scaling, and maceration in the interdigital or subdigital areas (Fig. 194-15). The lateral (i.e., 4th to 5th or 3rd to 4th) toe webs are the most common sites of infection. From here infection may spread to the sole or instep of the foot but it seldom involves the dorsum. A common aggravating feature in this type of infection is warmth and humidity. Hyperhidrosis may be an underlying problem for a number of these patients and should be treated along with the dermatophytosis.

Interesting studies on the microbial ecology of interdigital foot infections have been done by Leyden and Kligman.[185,186] It is clear that the disease we know as "athlete's foot" is not caused solely by dermatophytes. Normal-appearing toe webs have a skin flora consisting of Micrococcaceae (usually *Staphylococcus*), aerobic coryneforms, and small numbers of gram-negative organisms. Dermatophytes can also colonize normal toe webs frequently.[183,184] When toe web interspaces clinically demonstrated scaling or peeling without maceration or symptoms, the bacterial flora was unchanged from that of normal interspaces. Dermatophytes were isolated, however, in about 85 percent of these cases.

On the other hand, if an interspace showed maceration, white hyperkeratosis or erosions with increasing patient symptomatology, an overgrowth of the bacterial flora including gram-negatives was noted. Using clever manipulations of the interspace microflora in different patient groups, it was found that the clinical picture of symptomatic "athlete's foot" results from the interaction of bacteria and dermatophytes. Overgrowth of bacteria alone or the presence of dermatophytes alone produced a relatively mild clinical picture that was short-lived and relatively asymptomatic.[185,186]

Another variant of tinea pedis is the chronic, papulosquamous pattern (Fig. 194-16). This is usually bilateral and is characterized by minimal inflammation and a patchy or diffuse mocassin-like scaling over the soles. *T. rubrum* and occasionally *T. mentagrophytes* are the usual causative organisms. In addition to the feet, the hands may be involved as well as multiple toenails. A common but puzzling presentation is the "one hand, two feet" presentation observed frequently with *T. rubrum* infections (Fig. 194-17).

The third variant is the vesicular or vesiculobullous type. This is usually caused by *T. mentagrophytes* var. *interdigitale*. Small vesicles or vesicopustules are seen near the instep and on the midanterior plantar surface. Usually there is associated scaling in these areas as well as in the toe webs. Larger bullae are more unusual but can be seen. This type of infection may become clinically quiescent during the cooler months of the year only to become symptomatic again in the summer.

The fourth pattern is the acute ulcerative variant which is commonly associated with maceration, weeping denudation, and ulceration of sizable areas of the sole of the foot. Obvious white hyperkeratosis and a pungent odor are characteristically present. This infection is often complicated by a secondary bacterial (often gram-negative) overgrowth.

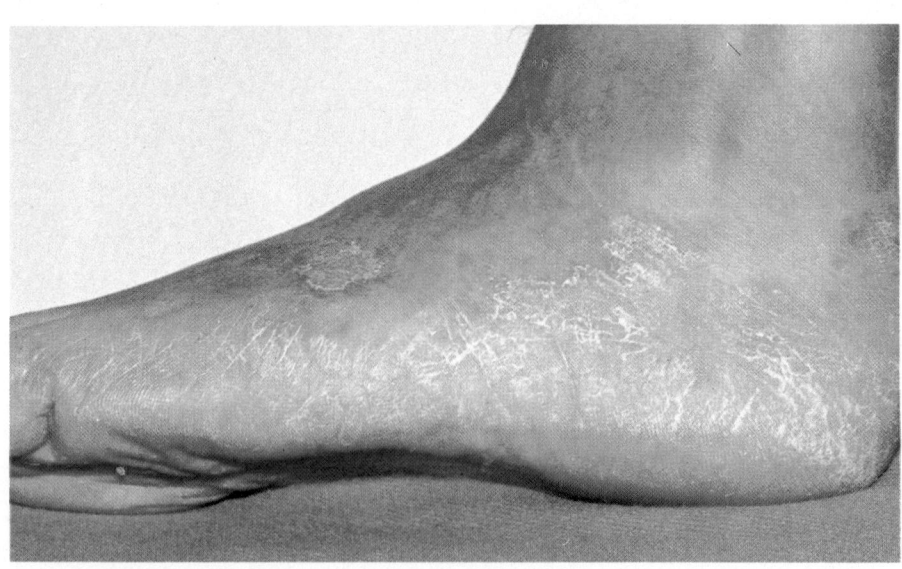

FIGURE 194-16 Tinea pedis. Superficial white scales in a moccasin-type distribution. Note arciform pattern of the scales, which is characteristic.

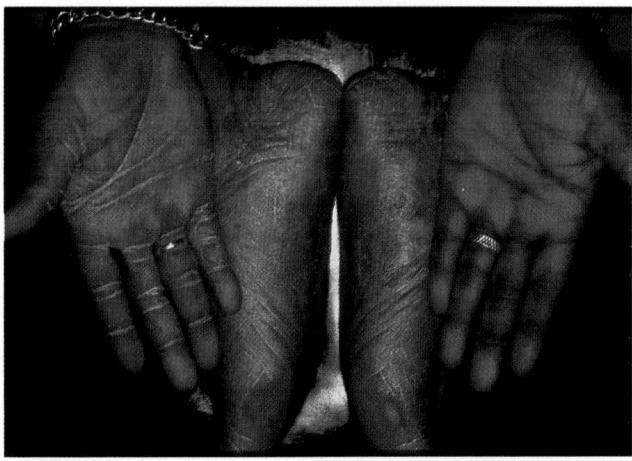

FIGURE 194-17 "One hand, two feet" presentation of *T. rubrum*.

The final two variants are commonly seen in conjunction with a vesicular "id" reaction, either as a dyshidrotic-like distribution on the hands or on the lateral foot or toe area. Cultures of these blisters are by definition sterile.

LABORATORY FINDINGS.   KOH examination of scales is positive for septate, branching hyphae in tinea pedis. If vesiculobullous lesions are present, examination of a portion of the blister roof yields the highest rate of positivity. Cultures should be done using Sabouraud's media with cycloheximide and chloramphenicol added.

PATHOLOGY.   Histologic examination reveals different patterns depending on the clinical variant involved. The hyperkeratotic, scaling variety shows acanthosis, hyperkeratosis, and a sparse, chronic superficial perivascular infiltrate in the dermis. On occasion, foci of neutrophils may be seen in the stratum corneum. In the vesicular variant, there is spongiosis, parakeratosis, and subcorneal or spongiotic intraepithelial blisters. Neutrophils are likewise seen in the stratum corneum. In both histologic patterns special stains (PAS or methenamine silver) show organisms in the horny layer.

DIAGNOSIS.   With a compatible clinical picture and a positive KOH preparation and/or culture, the diagnosis of tinea pedis can be made comfortably. If these findings are negative, however, there is a sizable differential diagnosis. Interdigital scaling, fissuring, and maceration can be seen with bacterial secondary infection. The more severe the signs and symptoms, the greater is the probability of isolating gram-negative organisms (*Pseudomonas* or *Proteus* spp. in particular). Even if dermatophytes are present, they are more difficult to isolate under these circumstances.[185,186] Other disorders to consider in evaluating an interdigital dermatosis are candidiasis, erythrasma (commonly has a coral red fluorescence with Wood's lamp examination), or soft corns.

In the scaly, hyperkeratotic variety of tinea pedis, confusion can occur with diseases such as psoriasis, hereditary or acquired keratodermas of the palms and soles, pityriasis rubra pilaris, and Reiter's syndrome. In contact dermatitis from shoes, lesions are seen on the dorsum of the foot more commonly than with tinea pedis. In children, peridigital dermatitis or atopic dermatitis is more common than tinea pedis. In the vesicular or vesiculopustular presentation, tinea pedis can be confused with pustular psoriasis, pustulosis palmaris et plantaris, and bacterial pyodermas. In many cases, careful examination of the nails can reveal convincing signs of dermatophytosis that are not seen with many of the above diagnoses.

PREVENTION AND TREATMENT.   Tinea pedis can be transmitted by contact with infected scales on bath or pool floors as well as on clothing. Laundering of clothing is not always effective in removing infectious material, and it is impossible to prevent most infected individuals from using communal baths or swimming facilities.[180] Control of concomitant hyperhidrosis is important in preventing tinea pedis. Talcum powder or antifungal powders (undecylenic acid or tolnaftate powders) can be used along with absorbent socks and nonocclusive shoes. On occasion the use of 20% to 25% aluminum chloride hexahydrate topically will help to curb excessive moisture.[187]

In overt tinea pedis, griseofulvin, ultramicrosized 0.5 g per day for 3 months is optimal. The prolonged treatment time is because of the increased turnover period of the thickened stratum corneum on the hands or feet. Cure rates with this treatment regimen are 90 percent. In intertriginous tinea pedis, griseofulvin and a topical imidazole are recommended for a 3-month course.[188]

When there is maceration, erythema, or denudation of skin associated with pain, a secondary bacterial infection must be ruled out with cultures and Gram stains. Appropriate systemic antibiotics based on sensitivity studies should be started if bacterial infection is documented. Gram-negative organisms as well as *Staphylococcus aureus* are common pathogens in this area. Adjunctive topical measures such as using antibacterial soaks (e.g., 1/4% acetic acid for *Pseudomonas* overgrowth) are helpful. Colorless Castellani's paint (phenolated resorcinol) is also used frequently.

Tinea Unguium and Onychomycosis   Tinea unguium is clinically defined as a dermatophyte infection of the nail plate. Onychomycosis, on the other hand, includes all infection of the nail caused by any fungus, including nondermatophytes and yeasts.

EPIDEMIOLOGY.   Onychomycosis is a common infection and accounts for 20 percent of all nail disease.[1] Approximately 30 percent of patients with dermatophyte infections on other parts of their body also have tinea unguium. Fungal nail infections are almost exclusively an adult malady. Children can be affected during household epidemics,[7,189] but the faster nail growth in children appears to make infection more difficult.[190] Mold infections usually affect the elderly where underlying nail diseases allow room for these secondary invaders.[191]

Although the overall susceptibility to dermatophyte nail infections is higher in men than in women, the number of cases affecting the toenails is increased in women. This may reflect differences in footwear in the female population where narrow-toed shoes allow increasing crowding of and trauma to the toenails. Paronychial infections caused by *Candida* spp. are also much more commonly seen in the fingernails of women. This most likely reflects the greater burden of wet work performed by females.[190]

The epidemiologic considerations discussed in the section on tinea pedis apply also to tinea unguium. Yet, because fungal nail infections are more chronic and recalcitrant to therapy, these infections provide an endogenous source for reinfection of the feet. This is especially true if a nidus of infection is combined with the environmental conditions of warmth and humidity provided by the climate or by occlusive footwear.[190]

ETIOLOGY AND PATHOGENESIS.   Onychomycosis can be caused not only by dermatophytes but also by certain yeasts and nondermatophytic molds.[192] The most common dermatophytes causing tinea unguium worldwide are *T. rubrum*, *T. mentagrophytes* var. *interdigitale*, and *E. floccosum*. Yet, if a dermatophyte is endemic to a certain geographic area, it is often the cause of nail

TABLE 194-10
Causative Organisms According to Anatomic Site of Infection

Tinea unguium + tinea pedis and/or tinea manuum
  T. rubrum
  T. mentagrophytes var. *interdigitale*
  E. floccosum
Tinea unguium + tinea corporis + tinea pedis
  T. rubrum
  T. mentagrophytes var. *interdigitale*
  E. floccosum
Tinea unguium + tinea capitis or favus
  T. tonsurans
  T. violaceum
  T. megninii
  T. schoenleinii
Tinea unguium + tinea imbricata
  T. concentricum

infections as well as other dermatophytoses in that area. *Microsporum* nail infections are extremely rare.[193] Table 194-10 groups the causative dermatophytes according to other anatomic areas that are often concurrently affected. Clearly *T. rubrum* is the most common cause of fingernail infections, but toenails can be infected by many of the different organisms cited.

Many nondermatophytic fungi have been associated with nail infections (Fig. 194-18).[194] Among the yeasts, *Candida albicans* is found to invade the nail only in chronic mucocutaneous candidiasis. Other species of *Candida* such as *C. parapsilosis* have been isolated from toenails.[190,192] The nondermatophytic molds have also been cultured often from nails clinically thought to be onychomycotic. Strict criteria are necessary, however, to implicate these organisms as primary pathogens as they are often considered to be contaminants when routine cultures are examined.[195] English has outlined these criteria as follows[196]: (1) if a dermatophyte is isolated on culture, it is considered to be a pathogen; (2) if a mold or yeast is cultured, it is considered significant only if hyphae, spores, or yeast cells are seen on microscopic examination; (3) confirmation of an infection by a nondermatophyte requires isolation of the organism on at least 5 out of 20 inocula without concurrent isolation of a dermatophyte. In general, it appears that nondermatophytic onychomycosis favors antecedently diseased nails or aged nails.[191] Toenails are the usual site of involvement.[197]

Zaias[192,197] has divided onychomycosis into four clinical types: (1) distal subungual onychomycosis (DSO), (2) proximal subungual onychomycosis (PSO), (3) white superficial onychomycosis (WSO), and (4) candidal onychomycosis. Characteristically, infected nails coexist with normal-appearing nails.

Distal subungual onychomycosis is the most common type and starts by invasion of the stratum corneum of the hyponychium and distal nail bed. Subsequently, the infection moves proximally in the nail bed and invades the ventral surface of the nail plate. Subungual hyperkeratosis results from a hyperproliferative reaction of the nail bed in response to the infection.[190] As the process continues, invasion of the nail plate results in a progressively dystrophic nail unit.

Proximal subungual onychomycosis is the least common variant of onychomycosis. It starts by fungal invasion of the stratum corneum of the proximal nail fold and subsequently the nail plate.

White superficial onychomycosis differs from the other variants by primarily invading the dorsal surface of the nail plate. The morphology of the fungus in WSO is typically that of a saprophyte. There are "eroding fronds" or "perforating organs" as seen with in vitro hard keratin invasion.[192,198]

Candidal onychomycosis is seen in patients with chronic mucocutaneous candidiasis. It may affect toenails and fingernails by invasion of the nail plate via the hyponychial epithelium. The entire thickness of the nail plate is commonly affected.[192] The dystrophic nails seen with candidal paronychia do not result from direct fungal invasion and should not be confused with true onychomycosis.

Table 194-11 summarizes the common causative organisms for the different variants of onychomycosis.

The mechanism and relative facility of nail invasion have been studied previously. Zaias[197] found, by using [14C]cystine-labeled keratin during in vitro invasion studies, that *T. mentagrophytes* was a more active destroyer of the nail than was *T. rubrum*. This may correlate with the clinical findings of slow, chronic infections caused by *T. rubrum*. The mechanism of nail destruction is unclear. Some authors have postulated a mechanical separation of nail laminae rather than true keratinolysis.[201] Other authors using ultramicroscopic data have seen evidence of corneocyte penetration and obvious keratinolysis.[202] Probably both mechanisms are operative, depending on the specific organisms involved.

CLINICAL MANIFESTATIONS. The different clinical types of onychomycosis have been described previously. Each type has a rather characteristic clinical picture.

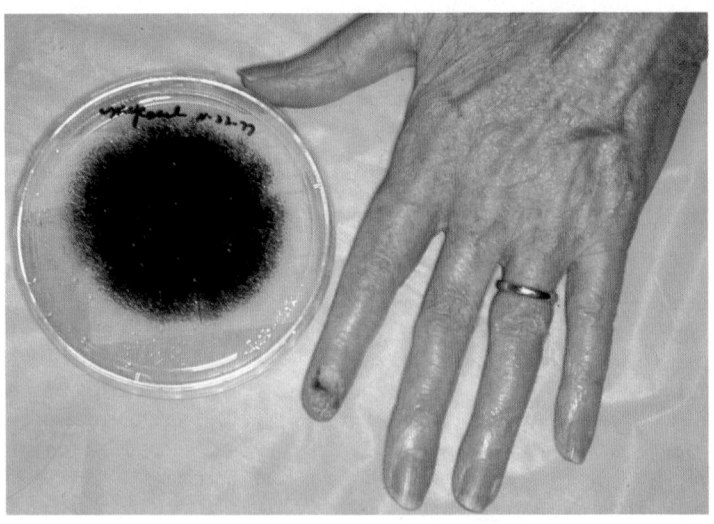

FIGURE 194-18 Onychomycosis can be due to nondermatophytic fungi including *Aspergillus niger*.

TABLE 194-11
Common Causative Organisms for Variants of Onychomycosis

Distal subungual onychomycosis (DSO)
    Toenails
        Dermatophytes: *T. rubrum, T. mentagrophytes, E. floccosum*
        Molds: *Scopulariopsis brevicaulis, Aspergillus, Fusarium, Cephalosporium*
        Yeasts: *C. albicans, C. parapsilosis, C. tropicalis, Geotrichum candidum, Hendersonula toruloidea*
    Fingernails
        Dermatophytes: *T. rubrum*
        Yeasts and molds: *C. albicans*
Proximal subungual onychomycosis (PSO)
    Toenails
        T. rubrum, T. megninii, T. schoenleinii, T. tonsurans, T. mentagrophytes
        Molds and yeasts: not documented
    Fingernails:
        Dermatophytes: *T. rubrum, T. megninii*
        Molds and yeasts: not documented
White superficial onychomycosis (WSO)
    Toenails
        Dermatophytes: *T. mentagrophytes*, rarely *T. rubrum*
        Molds: *Aspergillus, Cephalosporium, Fusarium*
    Fingernails: WSO does not occur on fingernails

SOURCE: Modified from Norton[199] and Baron.[200]

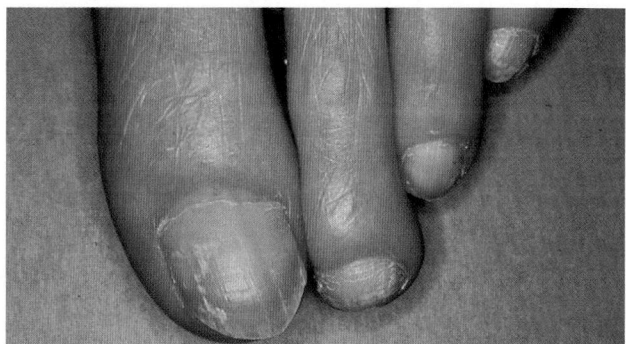

FIGURE 194-20   White superficial onychomycosis.

previously, *T. mentagrophytes* is the most common organism producing WSO. Recently, *T. rubrum* has been reported as an infrequent cause.[203]

Proximal subungual onychomycosis is the least common variant of onychomycosis. The first clinical sign of this type of infection is a whitish to whitish-brown area on the proximal part of the nail plate (Fig. 194-21). This area may gradually enlarge to affect the entire nail. As in DSO, the organisms invade the ventral surface of the nail plate from the proximal nail fold.

Candida onychomycosis is seen in patients with chronic mucocutaneous candidiasis. Both toenails and fingernails are affected. Clinically, the appearance of these nails resembles DSO with thickening of the nail bed and nail plate. In contrast to DSO, the entire nail plate is invaded by the organisms. The surface of the nail becomes opaque, rough, and furrowed. It is usually discolored and may be brownish or brownish-yellow in color. Often a surrounding paronychial inflammatory response is present, and the digit tip may become bulbous.

Distal subungual onychomycosis begins as a whitish or brownish-yellow discoloration at the free edge of the nail or near the lateral nail fold. As the infection progresses, subungual hyperkeratosis may lead to a separation of nail plate and nail bed (Fig. 194-19). Fungi invade the nail plate from the ventral surface, and in time the entire nail may become friable and discolored. The subungual debris also provides a site for opportunistic secondary infection by bacteria or other molds and yeasts. Hence, a wide spectrum of clinical changes can occur when the infection is advanced.

White superficial onychomycosis[198] appears as white, sharply outlined areas on the surface of the toenails (Fig. 194-20). The fingernails are not affected. Any area of the nail can be affected initially, and with time much of the nail surface can be involved. The surface of the nail is usually rough and friable as the "eroding fronds" of the organisms remain quite superficial. As discussed

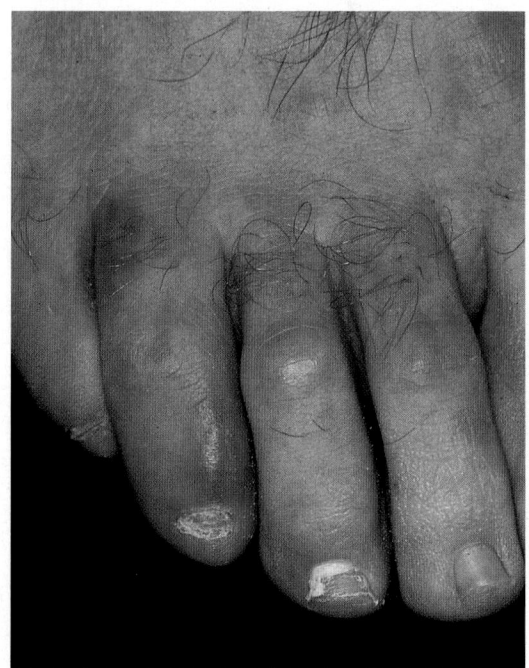

FIGURE 194-21   Proximal subungual onychomycosis in a patient with AIDS; Kaposi's sarcoma is also seen on the fourth toe.

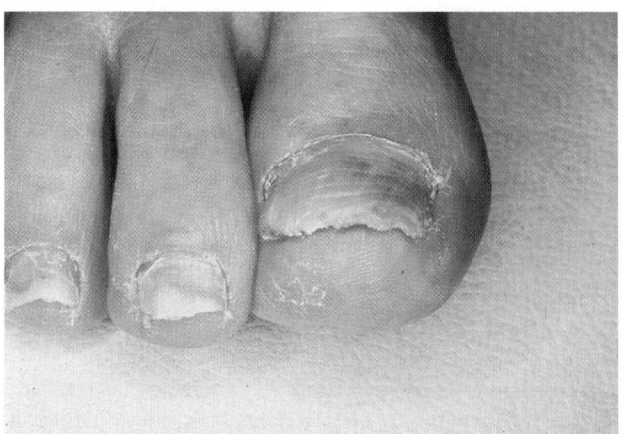

FIGURE 194-19   Distal subungual onychomycosis.

LABORATORY FINDINGS. Attempts to document fungal infections of the nail involve the use of KOH preparations and fungal cultures. Unfortunately, microscopy is often negative in nails that clinically appear to be infected. Furthermore, nails that are positive by microscopic examination often yield negative cultures.[190,194,204,205] A reason for this discrepancy is that fungi seen on KOH examination may not be viable and hence do not grow as expected. Since the most commonly sampled area of the nail is the distal tip with its associated subungual debris, we must reevaluate whether better results could be obtained by devising better sampling methods.

Samman recommends soaking full-thickness clippings of the affected nail in 5% KOH for 24 h prior to examination.[206] English[196] and others[194,207] have used a dental drill with a suction apparatus attached to obtain nail dust from affected areas. By doing this, the rate of culture positivity has been increased to 88 percent from the usual 50 to 75 percent.

Another method of sampling the nail has been described by Shelley and Wood.[208] Here one selects sites of early, active infection. These appear as whitish areas of discoloration with a normal overlying nail. A razor blade is used to trim away the normal nail and reach the powdery white area of infection. This material is then mounted with xylene and examined microscopically.

Cultures are done on Sabouraud's dextrose agar with and without added chloramphenicol and cycloheximide. Cycloheximide will suppress the growth of nondermatophytic organisms and should not be used if these fungi are suspected.

PATHOLOGY. Histologically, hyphae are seen lying between the laminae of nail parallel to the surface. The ventral nail and the stratum corneum of the nail bed are preferentially affected.[209] The epidermis may show spongiosis and focal parakeratosis. The inflammatory response in the dermis is minimal.

DIAGNOSIS. Onychomycosis can be confused with a variety of nail disorders. The diagnosis is further complicated by the high incidence of false-negative KOH examinations and cultures.

Psoriasis can closely mimic onychomycosis; however, the pitting seen in psoriasis is uncommon in fungal nail infections. The dystrophic nails seen in conjunction with hand eczema are usually transversely ridged and eczematous changes are apparent in the surrounding skin. Other disorders that can be confused with onychomycosis are the nails of Reiter's syndrome, Darier's disease, lichen planus, exfoliative dermatitis, pachyonychia congenita, and Norwegian scabies. Usually these disorders are separated from onychomycosis by history or evidence of characteristic skin lesions or biopsy findings.

White superficial onychomycosis must be distinguished from acquired or congenital leukonychias. Among these leukonychias, those due to trauma are the most common.

TREATMENT. Therapy of onychomycoses is often a challenging endeavor for the clinician. Topical agents are usually of little benefit. Systemic therapy with griseofulvin is usually effective for fingernails if given for 4 to 6 months.[210] Toenails may require 12 to 18 months to clear and are associated with a high relapse rate. Ketoconazole may be more helpful with organisms such as *T. rubrum*, but even with this drug there is a high relapse rate.

Some authors have advised chemical removal of nail using 40% urea compounds[211] or surgical avulsion of the nail combined with topical agents and oral griseofulvin.[197,206] This regimen may increase the cure rate for dermatophyte infections. Of course, avulsion or chemical destruction of the nail in nondermatophytic fungal infections is the only therapy that is effective.[197]

Tinea Nigra

Tinea nigra is a rare superficial fungal infection of the stratum corneum caused by *Exophiala werneckii*. Lesions usually appear as brownish-black, velvety macules on the palm.

History

Early reports of tinea nigra were probably erroneous descriptions of tinea versicolor.[212] The first authentic description was by Cerqueira in 1891. Horta isolated the organism and named it *Cladosporium werneckii*.[213] Subsequently, the name was changed to *Exophiala werneckii* (Horta) v. Arx.[214]

Etiology

Although the causative organism is *E. werneckii* in the vast majority of cases, there is some evidence that other species of dematiaceous fungi (*Stenella araguata*) may produce the same clinical picture.[212] The dematiaceous fungi reside in soil, sewage, decaying vegetation, and on wood or shower stalls in very humid environments.[212] Person-to-person transmission has been suspected, but occurs only rarely.[215] Yet inoculation onto the skin of volunteers has resulted in clinical disease; in one case the incubation period may have been 20 years.[216]

The disease is most commonly seen in tropical or subtropical areas (Central and South America, Africa, Asia). About 75 cases have been reported from North America since 1950.[212] Cases from Florida,[217] Texas,[218] and North Carolina[215] are well documented. With increasing awareness of the disease, more North American cases can be expected.

Clinical Manifestations

The clinical lesion appears as a slightly scaly, asymptomatic, mottled brownish or greenish-black macule on the palm or volar aspect of the fingers (Fig. 194-22). Bilateral plantar involvement[219] as well as concomitant palm and sole involvement have been reported.[217] The lesion gradually spreads centrifugally and may darken, especially at the border. The color resembles a silver nitrate stain.

Laboratory Findings

Tinea nigra is readily diagnosed by a 10% KOH examination of a scraping from the lesion. On microscopic examination, brownish or olive-colored hyphae and budding cells are seen. The hyphae are septate and freely branching, ranging from 1.5 to 5 μm in diameter. Oval to spindle-shaped yeast cells, 3 × 10 μm in size, occur singly or paired, separated by a cross wall that is centrally located.

Pathology

Skin biopsy shows hyperkeratosis without dermal inflammation. Hyphae are noted readily by H&E stain, but can be stained selectively with a Gomori methenamine silver preparation. Branched,

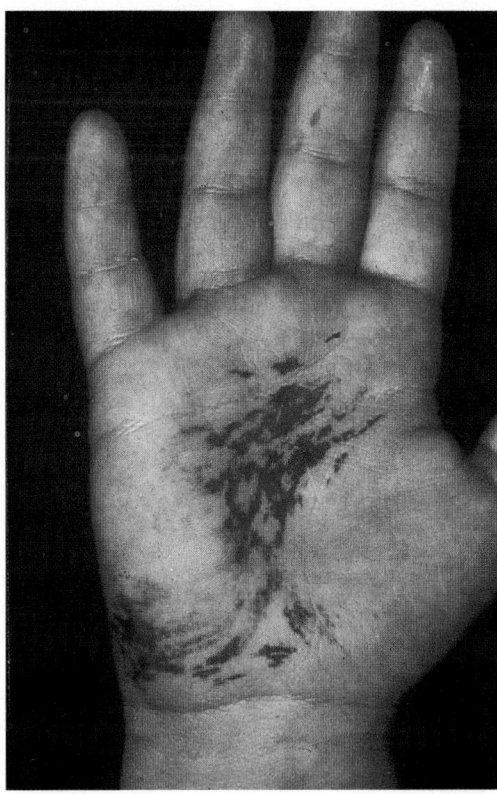

FIGURE 194-22   Tinea nigra palmaris showing an irregular, brownish-black macule on the palm. *(Courtesy of Stuart Salasche, M.D.)*

brown hyphae are seen readily in the upper layers of the stratum corneum.

Diagnosis

Tinea nigra may sometimes be confused with melanocytic lesions (i.e., junctional nevi or melanoma). The importance of recognizing this differentiation is underscored by reports of unnecessary surgical removal of lesions in misdiagnosed cases of tinea nigra.[220] Other considerations in the differential diagnosis include pigmentation from Addison's disease, syphilis, pinta, or from a variety of chemicals or dyes. All of these entities are readily excluded by KOH examination.

Treatment and Prognosis

Cure can be accomplished by the topical use of keratolytic and antifungal preparations such as Whitfield's ointment, topical 10% thiabendazole, tincture of iodine, or miconazole nitrate.[212,221] Griseofulvin is not effective. Treatment should be continued for 2 to 3 weeks to prevent recurrence.[215]

Mycology

The organism can be isolated from clinical specimens on media containing chloramphenicol and cycloheximide on which the growth is initially yeastlike and brownish to shiny black in color. Microscopic examination of these cultures reveals the typical two-celled, yeastlike morphology. As the culture ages, mycelial growth predominates. Aerial hyphae develop on the surface of the pigmented colonies, giving the appearance of a fuzzy, grayish-black growth. Microscopic examination reveals deeply pigmented thick septate hyphal cells, 7 to 10 μm in diameter.

Piedra

Piedra is an asymptomatic fungal infection of the hair shaft caused by *Piedraia hortae* (black piedra) and *Trichosporon beigelii* (white piedra).

History

The disease was reported initially by Beigel in 1865; however, he may have been describing an *Aspergillus* contaminant. The two diseases were distinguished by Horta in 1911.

Etiology

Black piedra is seen commonly in tropical areas of South America, the Far East, and the Pacific Islands. It is seen less frequently in Africa and Asia. In some cultures the infection is encouraged for social or religious reasons.[222] The scalp hair is the most commonly infected area.

White piedra is seen in temperate climates of South America, Europe, Asia, Japan, and the southern United States.[223] Beard, mustache, or pubic hair are more commonly infected than is scalp hair.[224] A recent study in Houston suggests that genital white piedra is more prevalent in Texas than previously suggested and has a variable degree of symptoms and physical findings. Transmission from person to person is felt to be rare, and travel abroad is not the source of infection.[225]

In piedra the source of infection is unknown, but related organisms can be found on animal hair, in soil, or in stagnant water.[222]

Clinical Manifestations

In black piedra, firmly attached, hard, brown-black nodules are present on the hair shaft. They vary in size from microscopic to a few millimeters and are gritty to feel. When the hair is combed, a metallic sound may be heard.[226]

In white piedra, nodules are less firmly adherent and are softer. They may vary in color from light brown to white.

Both forms of piedra may result in weakening of the hair shaft and subsequent breaks. Otherwise, the infections are asymptomatic.

There have been reports of disseminated infections with *T. beigelii* and other *Trichosporon* species.[227–231] These have occurred exclusively as opportunistic infections in an immunosuppressed host. Cutaneous manifestations of dissemination may include erythematous or purpuric papules or papulovesicles.[232] The responsible organism can be cultured from the skin lesions and seen in biopsy material.[227]

Laboratory Findings

When examined microscopically with 10% KOH, black piedra is characterized by nodules largely on the outside of the hair shaft. The periphery of the nodules shows aligned hyphae whereas the center consists of a packed, well-organized stroma of thick-walled cells (4 to 8 μm in diameter) that house the sexual (ascomycetous) phase of this organism. These are cemented together, and the resultant structure has been termed *pseudoparenchyma* because of its resemblance to organized tissue.[222,224]

The nodules of white piedra are soft in consistency, commonly intrapilar, and demonstrate less obvious external growth in comparison to black piedra. In contrast to *P. hortae*, *T. beiglii* grows in the asexual phase on infected hairs. The structure shows hyphae that are perpendicular to the hair surface and lack the organized appearance of black piedra.[222-224]

Diagnosis

Microscopic examination readily distinguishes piedra from nits, hair casts, developmental defects of the hair shaft, and trichomycosis axillaris. In the latter case, smaller nodules (<1 μm) are seen, and the hairs may fluoresce under Wood's lamp examination.

Treatment

Shaving the infected hair is curative. Treatment protocols are difficult to assess because of the high frequency of spontaneous remissions. Most authors support shaving the hair alone, or shaving the hair in conjunction with oral ketoconazole and/or topical antifungal therapy.[225]

Mycology

P. hortae grows well on most laboratory media, but *T. beiglii* is inhibited by cycloheximide-containing media. Cultures of *P. hortae* grow slowly, have a dark brown to black pigmentation, and initially have a glabrous surface upon which develop aerial mycelia. Microscopic examination reveals septate hyphae, chlamydospores, and irregularly shaped hyphal elements. The asexual phase of this fungus is most frequently cultured from clinical material. The sexual (ascomycetous) phase that occurs on infected hairs can be cultured only under various stringent culture conditions.

Clinical specimens of *T. beigelii* readily grow on Sabouraud's dextrose agar. The yeastlike growth is typically cream colored. As the colony ages, the surface growth develops furrows and convolutions that radiate out from the center. Microscopic examination reveals septate hyphae that readily fragment into arthroconidia, 3 to 7 μm in size. These cells rapidly take on an oval morphology and exhibit budding.

Antifungal Drugs

There has been a dramatic rise in the incidence of mycotic infections in recent years. This increase is due to longer life span, cancer chemotherapy, changes in antibiotic therapy, an increased use of parenteral therapy, artificial devices, organ transplantation, and new states of immunosuppression such as AIDS. Fortunately, there are many new antifungal drugs to meet our needs.[233] In the past two decades, antifungal therapy has dramatically changed. Drug selection and proper use are challenges for the practitioner.

Polyene Antibiotics

Nystatin, a polyene antibiotic, was the first specific antifungal agent.[1] Subsequently, a number of polyenes have been developed. Unfortunately, problems with solubility, stability, absorption, and toxicity have limited their use.

The polyenes are characterized by a macrolide ring of carbon atoms closed by the formation of an internal ester or lactone. A conjugated double-bond system is maintained within the lactone. The polyenes appear to act by binding to membrane sterols (i.e., ergosterol) and, in so doing, alter the permeability characteristics of the membrane. Subsequently, a loss of intracellular cations (particularly K$^+$) occurs, and cell death follows. The preferential effect of the polyenes on fungal cell membranes is explained by the more avid binding of the antibiotic to ergosterol than to cholesterol (the principal sterol in mammalian cells).[234,235]

Of the polyenes available, nystatin and amphotericin B are the only drugs used clinically. The other drugs (pimaricin, filipin, candicidin, etc.) are considered too toxic. Nystatin is insoluble in water and is not absorbed when given orally. The drug is derived from an actinomycete, *Streptomyces noursei*. Nystatin is too toxic for parenteral use but has been useful as a topical product and for oral use to clear gastrointestinal candidiasis. Topically, it is used for the therapy of cutaneous and mucous membrane candidal infections. The drug is unstable in heat, light, moisture, and air. Aqueous suspensions are stable for only 10 days under refrigeration.[236]

Amphotericin B is rarely used for superficial cutaneous fungal infections, but it is extremely effective for many systemic fungal infections. Amphotericin B is a heptaene lactone linked with mycosamine. It is the least toxic polyene for systemic use.[237] Several reviews have outlined the pharmacology of amphotericin B.[234,235,238] In addition to binding membrane sterols, amphotericin B may also act as an immunoadjuvant.[235]

Griseofulvin

Griseofulvin, 7-chloro-2',4,6-trimethoxy-6'-methylspiro-[benzofuran-2(3H),I'-(2)cyclohexene]-3,4'-dione, is a metabolic product of certain *Penicillium* species. It was discovered in 1939,[239] and its chemical structure ($C_{17}H_{17}ClO_6$) was characterized in 1947. The drug was first used medically in 1958.[5,6] Since then griseofulvin has been a safe and effective agent for cutaneous dermatophyte infections, and reports of its use in many nonfungal disease states stud the literature.

The properties of griseofulvin were described initially by Brian and his colleagues.[240] The drug was termed "curling factor" due to its ability to induce stunted and abnormal growth of certain test organisms. The precise mechanism of griseofulvin remains unclear. Griseofulvin is fungistatic and not fungicidal, even at high concentrations. It interferes with cell wall, protein, and nucleic acid synthesis of actively growing fungi. One theory holds that griseofulvin affects the microtubule system, disrupts the mitotic spindle structure, and thus arrests fungal cell growth in the M-phase.[233,241,242] In addition to the antimitotic properties of the drug, griseofulvin has also been found to be anti-inflammatory[243] and antichemotactic for polymorphonuclear leukocytes.[242]

One reason oral griseofulvin is effective lies in the ability of the drug to deposit in keratin precursor cells.[244] Griseofulvin also shows a preferential uptake in infected cells.[245] These facts together allow for the drug to disrupt fungal cells already present and provide an unfavorable environment for fungal growth.

Griseofulvin is effective in the treatment of most dermatophyte infections in a serum concentration of <1 μg/mL.[1,237] In vitro resistance to the drug can be induced by growing certain dermatophyte strains with increasing concentrations of the drug.[246] In addition, natural resistance to the drug can occur. A mean inhibitory concentration (MIC) of >3 μg/mL is considered indicative of relative griseofulvin resistance. *T. rubrum* was found to be the most common isolate in griseofulvin-resistant dermatophyte infections.[247] Griseofulvin has no activity against yeast or bacterial infections.

The absorption of griseofulvin is erratic because of low water solubility (15 μg/mL) at 37°C.[248] Absorption can be enhanced by reduction of particle size (i.e., microsized, ultramicrosized) or by administering a supersaturated solution of the drug in polyethylene glycol.[237] The absorption of griseofulvin is more rapid if taken with a fatty meal,[249] but the total absorption in 24 h is unchanged.[250] The drug has a plasma half-life of about 1 day and need only be given once daily.

After absorption from the gastrointestinal (GI) tract, the drug is detectable and selectively concentrated in the stratum corneum within 4 to 8 h. A peak plasma level of 1 μg/mL is seen at about 4 h after oral administration of 500 mg.[251] Similarly, there is a rapid disappearance of the drug from the stratum corneum within 48 to 72 h after an oral dose.[252] Griseofulvin does not fix to keratin-producing cells and moves outward with them as previous studies suggested.[253] Sweat also serves to concentrate the drug in the stratum corneum by a "wick effect."[252]

Remarkably few adverse effects have been attributed to griseofulvin. Fifty-five percent of patients complain of headaches at the onset of therapy. This is usually a transient symptom that commonly disappears with continued therapy. Other side effects include nausea, vomiting, diarrhea, and other symptoms of GI distress, and neurologic symptoms such as confusion, lethargy, and peripheral neuritis. Hypersensitivity reactions to griseofulvin include urticaria, erythema multiforme, serum sickness, and toxic epidermal necrolysis. Occasionally, a phototoxic reaction is seen. Hematologic abnormalities such as leukopenia have been reported, but fortunately are uncommon.[7,254] Finally, renal abnormalities such as proteinuria or cylinduria are described.

Griseofulvin can precipitate or aggravate systemic lupus erythematosus[254] and acute intermittent porphyria.[255] Simultaneous administration of barbiturates and griseofulvin results in lowered blood levels of griseofulvin. This is due to an interference by the barbiturate with the absorption of griseofulvin.[256] Griseofulvin diminishes the anticoagulant effect of warfarin through induction of hepatic microsomal enzymes. Finally, reduced alcohol tolerance has been reported in a few patients taking griseofulvin.[7]

The effectiveness of griseofulvin for dermatophyte infections has been well documented in the literature. Griseofulvin has been found to have the following cure rates: tinea capitis, 93.1 percent; tinea of glabrous skin, 64.8 percent; tinea of the palms and soles, 53.3 percent; tinea of the fingernails, 56.9 percent; and tinea of the toenails, 16.7 percent.[257] Reasons for failure of the drug are variable. Recently, studies demonstrating in vitro griseofulvin-resistant organisms have appeared.[247] In deciding whether or not to use

long-term griseofulvin, particularly with chronic *T. rubrum* infections, a determination of griseofulvin sensitivities may be helpful.

The dose of griseofulvin depends on the preparation used. In general, microcrystalline preparations are given in a dose of 500 to 1000 mg/day depending on body weight. In children, a dose of 10 mg/kg per day is generally used. With the ultramicronized preparations, dosages may range between one-half and two-thirds of the microsized variety.

The Imidazoles

The imidazoles are a large class of antifungals developed in the past two decades. A number of substituted imidazole derivatives are now available, including thiabendazole,[258] miconazole, clotrimazole, econazole,[259] and sulconazole. These agents are particularly useful because they are effective against a wide range of fungi, including *Candida* and dermatophytes, as well as certain bacteria.

The imidazoles, including ketoconazole, appear to function by inhibiting ergosterol synthesis in fungi by blocking C-14 demethylation. This results in a decrease in ergosterol and an accumulation of C-14 methyl sterol intermediates, such as lanosterol. This alteration in membrane sterols results in cell membrane permeability changes or structural defects that lead to growth inhibition or cell death.[260]

Applied topically in the treatment of uncomplicated dermatophytic and *Candida* infections, a representative imidazole, miconazole, has achieved a 95 percent cure rate.[237] Adverse reactions from these agents are rare, but irritant and allergic contact dermatitis have been reported.[261] The development of resistance to these agents by fungal organisms is unusual.

Ketoconazole is a dibasic piperazine imidazole that is effective orally in the treatment of several deep and superficial fungal infections. It is the first imidazole to sustain therapeutic levels after oral administration. The penetration of ketoconazole into cerebrospinal fluid and urine is not high; however, early clinical trials showed remarkable recovery rates for a range of fungal diseases. Oral ketoconazole is indicated for the treatment of the following systemic infections: candidiasis, chronic mucocutaneous candidiasis, oral thrush, candiduria, blastomycosis, coccidioidomycosis, histoplasmosis, chromomycosis, and paracoccidioidomycosis. Ketoconazole should not be used for fungal meningitis, nor is it effective against aspergillosis.

Ketoconazole is effective against dermatophytes, yeasts, and *Mallassezia furfur* and *ovale.* It is indicated for the topical treatment of tinea corporis and tinea cruris caused by *T. rubrum,* *T. mentagrophytes,* and *E. floccosum;* in the treatment of tinea versicolor caused by *M. furfur;* in the treatment of cutaneous candidiasis caused by *Candida* spp.; and in the treatment of seborrheic dermatitis. It is postulated that the therapeutic efficacy of ketoconazole in seborrheic dermatitis is due to a reduction of *M. ovale.*

The mode of action of ketoconazole is similar to that of the other imidazoles. It inhibits ergosterol synthesis in fungal cell membranes, resulting in an accumulation of lanosterol. In addition, ketoconazole may inhibit the uptake of RNA and DNA precursors by the organism and interfere with the synthesis of oxidative or peroxidative enzymes. Ketoconazole appears to have a synergistic effect with host defense mechanisms.[260] The drug, however, is fungistatic and is not able to sterilize tissues in the presence of defective cell-mediated immunity.[262]

Ketoconazole is water-soluble and well absorbed from the gastrointestinal tract. Peak serum concentrations are obtained 1 to

4 h after a 200-mg dose. Absorption may be enhanced by administering the drug with 4 mL 0.2 *N* HCl, drinking it through a plastic straw to protect the teeth, followed by a glass of water. Achlorhydria, the simultaneous administration of antacids, anticholinergics, and the H_2 blockers impair absorption. The drug is metabolized by the liver and excreted in an inactive form via the bile. The renal excretion is minimal, and alterations of drug dosage due to renal failure are unnecessary.[263]

Ketoconazole has been particularly useful in the management of chronic mucocutaneous candidiasis.[238,264] Unfortunately, resistant *C. albicans* organisms have been identified and are correlated with a poor clinical response to the drug.[265]

The drug has also been effective in dermatophyte infections and tinea versicolor. Recalcitrant griseofulvin-resistant *T. rubrum* infections usually respond to the drug but may relapse after therapy is stopped.[266–269] As expected, palmar/plantar and nail infections respond more slowly and commonly relapse after discontinuation of therapy.[266,267,270,271]

The usual dosage of ketoconazole is 200 to 400 mg/day. Side effects commonly include nausea and vomiting in 3 to 10 percent of patients. Abdominal pain, pruritus, headache, fever and chills, and photophobia are seen in fewer than 1 percent of patients.[264] Gynecomastia may occur, possibly due to an inhibition of testosterone synthesis.[272] Likewise, a block in adrenal steroid synthesis, in the absence of clinical hypoadrenalism, has been found.[273]

The most disturbing adverse effect has been the occurrence of an idiosyncratic hepatotoxic reaction to the drug.[272–275] More commonly, transient mild liver enzyme rises have been noted, which resolve with continued therapy. Symptomatic hepatic reactions have been estimated to occur in 1 in 10,000 patients treated. The reaction is usually noted early in the course of therapy and does not seem to be related to daily or cumulative dosage of the drug.[276–278] Fortunately, most of these reactions subside after the drug is discontinued.

Triazole Antifungal Drugs

Fluconazole   Fluconazole is a synthetic triazole antifungal agent approved by the Food and Drug Administration of the United States for the treatment of cryptococcal meningitis, oropharyngeal and esophageal candidiasis, and serious systemic *Candida* infections. Fluconazole is currently available in both oral and intravenous forms.[279]

The mechanism of action of fluconazole is similar to other azole antifungal agents: inhibition of the fungal cytochrome P_{450}-dependent enzymes that block the synthesis of ergosterol.[280]

Pharmacokinetic studies with fluconazole reveal high oral bioavailability with near complete absorption after a single 50-mg capsule.[281] Gastric pH does not influence the bioavailability of fluconazole, and so the drug can be taken with or without food.[282] Fluconazole exhibits low binding to plasma protein and requires adjustment of dose for patients with impaired renal function.[281] Decreased protein binding and greater polarity of the drug allows fluconazole to readily penetrate tissues and body fluids, including cerebrospinal fluid, sputum, and saliva.[283] Fluconazole is thought to be generally less toxic and more potent than imidazoles.

Investigators studying the effects of fluconazole on endocrine function found that fluconazole at doses of 200, 300, or 400 mg has no effect on testosterone plasma concentrations or on adrenocorticotropic hormone stimulation of cortisol.[284]

Side effects most commonly reported with use of fluconazole are nausea, vomiting, headache, rash, abdominal pain, and diarrhea.[280] Serious hepatic reactions are rare, but transient mild increases in SGOT, SGPT, alkaline phosphatase, and bilirubin have been reported in 5 to 7 percent of fluconazole patients.

Fluconazole has been studied for possible interactions with other commonly prescribed drugs. It was initially thought that fluconazole and its relative lack of interaction with metabolizing enzymes would allow its use with medications that presently require monitoring when used with ketoconazole. Concomitant administration of fluconazole, 100 mg, and cyclosporine is associated with minimal changes in the maximum (C_{max}) and minimum (C_{min}) concentrations of cyclosporine.[284] However, there are case reports to suggest that fluconazole interacts with cyclosporine.[285,286] This information indicates that cyclosporine levels should be monitored in patients receiving fluconazole as well. Concomitant use of fluconazole and tolbutamide results in statistically significant increases in the C_{max} and AUC (area under curve) of tolbutamide without changing the blood glucose levels.[284] This study used healthy volunteers so that extrapolation to diabetic patients is difficult. Clinical prudence suggests monitoring glucose levels when administering fluconazole and tolbutamide together.

Coadministration of rifampin and fluconazole, 200 mg, resulted in a clinically significant decrease in the half-life and AUC of fluconazole.[284] Concomitant use of warfarin and fluconazole, 200 mg, resulted in an increased prothrombin time of less than 13 percent in 12 of 13 patients. One patient, however, experienced a twofold increase in prothrombin time.[284] Therefore, careful monitoring of prothrombin time is necessary with concomitant use of fluconazole and warfarin.

Administration of fluconazole and phenytoin in the same patient resulted in a clinically significant increase in phenytoin AUC (75 percent).[284] Fluconazole levels, however, were not significantly changed. Fluconazole administration most likely inhibits metabolism of phenytoin. In any case, serum concentrations of phenytoin require close monitoring in the above situation.

While fluconazole's low MICs for *Candida* and *Cryptococcus* have been acclaimed, it has not been proven at this time to be more effective than conventional therapy for treatment of dermatophytes. The drug is very expensive and best reserved for life-threatening conditions.

Itraconazole   Itraconazole is a broad-spectrum azole dioxaline derivative that is presently under clinical investigation. The drug is highly lipophilic and can be detected in the stratum corneum up to 4 weeks after stopping treatment.[287] The drug is effective in the treatment of vaginal candidiasis, tinea versicolor, dermatophyte infections of the skin, and a variety of systemic mycoses, including aspergillosis and cryptococcal meningitis.[287]

Ciclopirox Olamine   Ciclopirox olamine (1% cream) is a substituted pyridone unrelated to azole. It has broad-spectrum activity against yeast, fungi, and various gram-positive and gram-negative bacteria.[237] It is fungicidal, accumulates inside fungal cells, and alters transmembrane transport of ions and amino acids, with loss of membrane integrity. The drug penetrates hard keratin well and may be more effective in the therapy of palmar/plantar and nail infections.[288–290]

Allylamines   The allylamines are a new class of antifungal agents with broad-spectrum action. They inhibit squalene epoxidase, an early enzyme in the pathway of ergosterol synthesis. Naftifine, the only allylamine currently available for clinical use, is effective topically. Terbinafine, a naftifine analogue under investigation, is active both topically and orally. The drug is fungicidal against dermatophytes and fungistatic against yeast organisms. The drug is extensively metabolized in the liver. Terbinafine is highly lipophilic and keratophilic, which results in a wide distribution and accumulation within stratum corneum, the hair, and sebum-rich areas of the skin.[291]

Other Topical Agents

A wide variety of older but still efficacious topical products are available for the treatment of superficial fungal infections.

Whitfield's ointment is a combination of benzoic (12%) acid and salicylic (6%) acid. It has keratolytic and antifungal properties and is used commonly for tinea nigra.

Colorless Castellani's paint has local anesthetic, antibacterial, and antifungal properties. It is particularly useful for intertriginous infections. Excessive dryness and irritation may occur, however.

Short-chain organic fatty acids and fatty acid salts have long been recognized to have antifungal properties.[292] A preparation containing 5% undecylenic acid and 20% zinc undecylenate (Desenex) is sold over-the-counter relatively inexpensively. The powder is particularly useful as a prophylactic measure for tinea pedis.

Tolnaftate (m,N-dimethylthiocarbanilic acid 0-2 naphthyl ester) is a safe, odorless, and nonstaining topical preparation that is effective against dermatophytes and tinea versicolor. It is not effective, however, against *C. albicans*. Its mode of action has not been determined.

Haloprogin (3-iodo-2-propynyl-2,4,5-trichlorphenyl ether) is effective against dermatophytes, *Candida*, and some gram-positive bacteria. The drug may work by disrupting cell membrane function. Skin irritation and contact allergy are occasional side effects.[1,237,240]

References

1. Rippon JW: Dermatophytosis and dermatomycosis, in *Medical Mycology: The Pathogenic Fungi and the Pathogenic Actinomycetes,* 3d ed. Philadelphia, Saunders, 1988, p 169
2. Gruby D: Sur les mycodermes que constituent la teigne faveuse. *C R Acad Sci (Paris)* **13**:309, 1841
3. Sabouraud R: *Les Teignes.* Paris, Masson, 1910
4. Dawson CO, Gentles JC: The perfect stage of *Keratinomyces ajelloi. Nature* **183**:1345, 1959
5. Gentles JC: Experimental ringworm in guinea pigs: Oral treatment with griseofulvin. *Nature* **182**:476, 1958
6. Blank H, Roth FJ: The treatment of dermatomycoses with orally administered griseofulvin. *Arch Dermatol* **79**:259, 1959
7. Roberts SOB, Mackenzie DWR: Mycology, in *Textbook of Dermatology,* edited by A Rook et al. London, Blackwell, 1979, p 767
8. Blank H et al: Cutaneous *Trichophyton mentagrophytes* infections in Vietnam. *Arch Dermatol* **99**:135, 1969
9. Otcenasek M: Ecology of the dermatophytes. *Mycopathologica* **65**:67, 1978
10. Philpot CM: Some aspects of the epidemiology of tinea. *Mycopathologica* **62**:3, 1977

11. Georg LK: Epidemiology of the dermatophytoses: Sources of infection, modes of transmission and epidemicity. *Ann N Y Acad Sci* **89**:69, 1960
12. Whittle CH: A small epidemic of *M. gypseum* ringworm in a plant nursery. *Br J Dermatol* **66**:353, 1954
13. Caprilli F et al: Etiology of ringworm of the scalp, beard, and body in Rome, Italy. *Sabouraudia* **18**:129, 1980
14. Blank F et al: Distribution of dermatophytosis according to age, ethnic group and sex. *Sabouraudia* **12**:352, 1974
15. Hernandez AD: An approach to the diagnosis and therapy of dermatophytosis. *Int J Dermatol* **19**:540, 1980
16. Mandel EH: Diagnosis: Tinea circinata and onychomycosis *(Trichophyton purpureum):* Resistance to griseofulvin during uncontrolled diabetes. *Arch Dermatol* **82**:1027, 1960
17. Jolly HW, Carpenter CL: Oral glucose tolerance studies in recurrent *Trichophyton rubrum* infections. *Arch Dermatol* **100**:26, 1969
18. Lewis GM et al: Generalized *Trichophyton rubrum* infection associated with systemic lymphoblastoma. *Arch Dermatol* **67**:247, 1953
19. Allen DE et al: Generalized *Microsporum audouinii* infection and depressed cellular immunity associated with a missing plasma factor required for lymphocyte blastogenesis. *Am J Med* **63**:991, 1977
20. Nelson LM, McNiece KJ: Recurrent Cushing's syndrome with *Trichophyton rubrum* infection. *Arch Dermatol* **80**:700, 1959
21. Philpot CM: Geographical distribution of the dermatophytes: A review. *J Hyg (Lond)* **80**:301, 1978
22. Ajello L: Geographic distribution and prevalence of the dermatophytes. *Ann N Y Acad Sci* **89**:30, 1960
23. Binazzi M et al: Skin mycoses—geographic distribution and present-day pathomorphosis. *Int J Dermatol* **22**:92, 1983
24. Many H et al: *Trichophyton rubrum:* Exposure and infection within household groups. *Arch Dermatol* **82**:226, 1960
25. Saferstein HL et al: Endothrix ringwork: A new public health problem in Philadelphia. *JAMA* **190**:115, 1964
26. Malhotra YK et al: A study of tinea capitis in Libya (Benghazi). *Sabouraudia* **17**:181, 1979
27. Georg LK: *Trichophyton tonsurans* ringworm—a new public health problem. *Public Health Rep* **67**:53, 1952
28. Blank F, Mann SJ: *Trichophyton rubrum* infections according to age, anatomical distribution and sex. *Br J Dermatol* **2**:171, 1975
29. Rippon JW et al: *Trichophyton simii* infection in the United States. *Arch Dermatol* **98**:615, 1968
30. Allen AM, Taplin D: Epidemic *Trichophyton mentagrophytes* infections in servicemen: Source of infection, role of environment, host factors, and susceptibility. *JAMA* **226**:864, 1973
31. Sanderson PH, Sloper JC: Skin disease in the British army in S.E. Asia III: The relationship between mycotic infections of the body and of the feet. *Br J Dermatol* **65**:362, 1953
32. Taplin D et al: Environmental influences on the microbiology of the skin. *Arch Environ Health* **11**:546, 1965
33. Ravine D et al: Genetic inheritance of susceptibility to tinea imbricata. *J Med Genet* **17**:342, 1980
34. Georg LK: The relationship between the downy and granular forms of *Trichophyton mentagrophytes. J Invest Dermatol* **23**:123, 1954
35. Knight AG: A review of experimental human fungus infections. *J Invest Dermatol* **59**:354, 1972
36. Baer RL et al: Newer studies on the epidemiology of fungus infections of the feet. *Am J Public Health* **45**:784, 1955
37. Baer RL, Rosenthal SA: The biology of fungus infections of the feet. *JAMA* **197**:1017, 1966
38. Hernandez AD: An approach to the diagnosis and therapy of dermatophytosis. *Int J Dermatol* **19**:540, 1980
39. Kligman AM: The pathogenesis of tinea capitis due to *Microsporum audouini* and *Microsporum canis:* I. Gross observations following the inoculation of humans. *J Invest Dermatol* **18**:231, 1952
40. Kligman AM: Tinea capitis due to *M. audouini* and *M. canis:* II. Dynamics of the host-parasite relationship. *Arch Dermatol* **71**:313, 1955

41. English MP, Gibson MD: Studies in the epidemiology of tinea pedis. I. Tinea pedis in school children. *Br Med J* **1**:1442, 1959

42. Davis CM et al: Dermatophytes in military recruits. *Arch Dermatol* **105**:558, 1972

43. Raubitchek F: Infectivity and family incidence of black-dot tinea capitis. *Arch Dermatol* **79**:477, 1959

44. Friedman L et al: The course of untreated tinea capitis in Negro children. *J Invest Dermatol* **42**:237, 1964

45. Ive FA: The carrier stage of tinea capitis in Nigeria. *Br J Dermatol* **78**:219, 1966

46. Knudsen FA: The areal extent of dermatophyte infection. *Br J Dermatol* **92**:413, 1975

47. Berk SH et al: Epidermal activity in annular dermatophytosis. *Arch Dermatol* **112**:485, 1976

48. Yu RJ et al: Two cell-bound keratinases of *Trichophyton mentagrophytes*. *J Invest Dermatol* **56**:27, 1971

49. Meevootisom V, Niederpruem DJ: Control of exocellular proteases in dermatophytes and especially *Trichophyton rubrum*. *Sabouraudia* **17**:91, 1979

50. Mercer EH, Verma BS: Hair digested by *Trichophyton mentagrophytes*. *Arch Dermatol* **87**:357, 1963

51. Verma BS: The use of fluorescence microscopy in the study of *in vitro* hair penetration by ringworm fungi. *Br J Dermatol* **78**:222, 1966

52. Cruickshank CND, Trotter MD: Separation of epidermis from dermis by filtrates of *Trichophyton mentagrophytes*. *Nature* **177**:1085, 1956

53. Kligman AM: Pathophysiology of ringworm infections in animals with skin cycles. *J Invest Dermatol* **27**:171, 1956

54. Marks R, Dawber RPR: *In situ* microbiology of the stratum corneum: An application of skin surface biopsy. *Arch Dermatol* **105**:216, 1972

55. Emmons CW et al (eds): Dermatophytoses, in *Medical Mycology*. Philadelphia, Lea & Febiger, 1977, p 117

56. Ahmed AR: Immunology of human dermatophyte infections. *Arch Dermatol* **118**:521, 1983

57. Grappel SF et al: Immunology of dermatophytes and dermatophytosis. *Bacteriol Rev* **38**:222, 1974

58. Dahl MV: Host defense: Fungus, in *Clinical Immunodermatology*. Chicago, Year Book, 1988, p 171

59. Rothman S et al: The spontaneous cure of tinea capitis in puberty. *J Invest Dermatol* **8**:81, 1947

60. Lorincz AL et al: Evidence for a humoral mechanism which prevents growth of dermatophytes. *J Invest Dermatol* **31**:15, 1958

61. Roth FJ et al: An evaluation of the fungistatic activity of serum. *J Invest Dermatol* **32**:549, 1959

62. Memmesheimer AR et al: Studies of fungistatic activity in normal human blood serum. *Sabouraudia* **2**:1, 1962

63. King RD et al: Transferrin, iron, and dermatophytes. I. Serum dermatophyte inhibitory component definitely identified as unsaturated transferrin. *J Lab Clin Med* **86**:204, 1975

64. Mosher WA et al: Nutritional requirements of the pathogenic mold: *T. interdigitale*. *Plant Physiol* **11**:795, 1936

65. Yu RJ et al: Inhibition of keratinases by alpha-2-macroglobulin. *Experientia* **28**:886, 1972

66. Blank HD et al: Widespread *Trichophyton rubrum* granulomas treated with griseofulvin. *Arch Dermatol* **81**:779, 1960

67. Grappel SF et al: Circulating antibodies in dermatophytosis. *Dermatologica* **144**:1, 1972

68. Jones HE et al: Apparent cross-reactivity of airborne molds and the dermatophytic fungi. *J Allergy Clin Immunol* **52**:346, 1973

69. Young E, Roth FJ: Immunological cross-reactivity between a glycoprotein isolated from *Trichophyton mentagrophytes* and human isoantigen A. *J Invest Dermatol* **72**:46, 1979

70. Peck SM et al: Intercellular antibodies: Presence in a *Trichophyton rubrum* infection. *J Invest Dermatol* **58**:133, 1972

71. Hopfer RL et al: Antibodies with affinity for epithelial tissue in chronic dermatophytosis. *Dermatologica* **151**:135, 1975

72. Jones HE: The atopic-chronic-dermatophytosis syndrome. *Acta Derm Venereol (Stockh)* **92**(suppl):81, 1980

73. Conant NF et al: Immunology of the dermatomycoses, in *Manual of Clinical Mycology,* 3d ed. Philadelphia, Saunders, 1971, p 587

74. Brahmi Z et al: Depressed cell-mediated immunity in chronic dermatophytic infections. *Ann Immunol (Paris)* **131**C:143, 1980

75. Jones HE et al: Acquired immunity to dermatophytes. *Arch Dermatol* **109**:840, 1974

76. Delamater ED, Benham RW: Experimental studies with the dermatophytes. I. Primary disease in laboratory animals. *J Invest Dermatol* **1**:451, 1938

77. Delamater ED, Benham RW: Experimental studies with the dermatophytes. II. Immunity and hypersensitivity in laboratory animals. *J Invest Dermatol* **1**:451, 1938

78. Holden CA et al: A method for identification of dermatophyte antigens *in situ* by an immunoperoxidase technique and electron microscopy. *Clin Exp Dermatol* **6**:311:1981

79. Holden CA et al: The antigenicity of *Trichophyton rubrum: In situ* studies by an immunoperoxidase technique in light and electron microscopy. *Acta Derm Venereol (Stockh)* **61**:207, 1981

80. Hanifin JM et al: Immunological reactivity in dermatophytosis. *Br J Dermatol* **90**:1, 1974

81. Hay RJ, Brostoff J: Immune responses in patients with chronic *Trichophyton rubrum* infections. *Clin Exp Dermatol* **2**:373, 1977

82. Kaaman T: The clinical significance of cutaneous reactions to *Trichophyton* in dermatophytosis. *Acta Derm Venereol (Stockh)* **58**:139, 1978

83. Hay RJ: Chronic dermatophyte infections. I. Clinical and mycological features. *Br J Dermatol* **106**:1, 1982

84. Hay RJ, Shennan G: Chronic dermatophyte infections. II. Antibody and cell-mediated immune responses. *Br J Dermatol* **106**:191, 1982

85. Marmor MF, Barrett EV: Cutaneous anergy without systemic disease: A syndrome associated with mucocutaneous fungal infection. *Am J Med* **44**:979, 1968

86. Alteras I et al: The high incidence of tinea pedis and unguium in patients with Kaposi's sarcoma. *Mycopathologica* **74**:177, 1981

87. Shama SK, Kirkpatrick CH: Dermatophytosis in patients with chronic mucocutaneous candidiasis. *J Am Acad Dermatol* **2**:285, 1980

88. Diamond RD: The growing problem of mycoses in patients infected with the human immunodeficiency virus. *Rev Infect Dis* **13**:480, 1991

89. Jones HE et al: A clinical, mycological, and immunological survey for dermatophytosis. *Arch Dermatol* **108**:61, 1973

90. Jones HE et al: Immunologic susceptibility to chronic dermatophytosis. *Arch Dermatol* **110**:213, 1974

91. Helander I: Lymphocyte transformation test in dermatophytes. *Mykosen* **21**:71, 1978

92. Hunziker N, Brun R: Lack of delayed reaction in presence of cell-mediated immunity in *Trichophyton* hypersensitivity. *Arch Dermatol* **116**:1266, 1980

93. Wang SR, Zweiman B: Histamine suppression of human lymphocyte responses to mitogens. *Cell Immunol* **36**:28, 1978

94. Rocklin RE: Modulation of cellular-immune responses *in vivo* and *in vitro* by histamine receptor-bearing lymphocytes. *J Clin Immunol* **57**:1051, 1976

95. Rocklin RE: Histamine-induced suppressor factor (HSF): Effect on migration inhibitory factor (MIF) production and proliferation. *J Immunol* **118**:1734, 1977

96. Presser SE, Blank H: Cimetidine: Adjunct in treatment of tinea capitis. *Lancet* **1**:108, 1981

97. Jillson OF: Immunology of dermatophytosis: Lack of immunity and hyperimmunity. *Cutis* **30**:159, 1982

98. Jillson OF: Dermatophytids and candidids. *Semin Dermatol* **2**:60, 1983

99. Jadassohn J: *Korblatt Schweiz Aerzte* **42**:22, 1912

100. Martinez-Roig A et al: Erythema nodosum and kerion of the scalp. *Am J Dis Child* **136**:440, 1982

101. Waisman M: Recurrent, fixed erysipelas-like dermatophytid. *Arch Dermatol* **53**:10, 1946

102. Jillson OF: Allergic confirmation that some cases of erythema annulare centrifugum are dermatophytids. *Arch Dermatol* **70**:355, 1954

103. Weary PE, Guerrant JL: Chronic urticaria in association with dermatophytosis: Response to the administration of griseofulvin. *Arch Dermatol* **95**:400, 1967

104. Rudolph AH et al: Tinea capitis, in *Clinical Dermatology,* edited by DJ Demis et al. Philadelphia, Harper & Row, 1978

105. Prevost E: Nonfluorescent tinea capitis in Charleston, SC: A diagnostic problem. *JAMA* **242**:1765, 1979

106. Laude TA et al: Tinea capitis in Brooklyn. *Am J Dis Child* **136**:1047, 1982

107. Ridley CM: Tinea capitis in an elderly woman. *Clin Exp Dermatol* **4**:247, 1979

108. Bronson DM et al: An epidemic of infection with *Trichophyton tonsurans* revealed in a 20-year survey of fungal infections in Chicago. *J Am Acad Dermatol* **8**:322, 1983

109. Seale ER, Richardson JB: *Trichophyton tonsurans:* A followup of treated and untreated cases. *Arch Dermatol* **8**:125, 1960

110. Pipkin JL: Tinea capitis in the adult and adolescent. *Arch Dermatol* **66**:9, 1952

111. Vanbreuseghem R: Tinea capitis in the Belgian Congo and Ruanda Urundi. *Trop Geogr Med* **10**:103, 1958

112. Guirges SY: Viability of *Trichophyton schoenleinii* in epilated hairs. *Sabouraudia* **19**:155, 1981

113. Rosenthal SA, Vanbreuseghem R: Viability of dermatophytes in epilated hairs. *Arch Dermatol* **85**:143, 1962

114. Clayton YM, Midgely G: New approach to the investigation of scalp ringworm in London school children. *J Clin Pathol* **21**:791, 1968

115. Crazier WJ, Searls S: "Double" or "mixed" fungal infections: Significant, or not? *Australas J Dermatol* **20**:43, 1979

116. Grigoriu D, Delacretaz J: Mixed dermatophytical infection of the scalp. *Dermatologica* **164**:407, 1982

117. Varadi DP, Rippon JW: Scalp infection of triple etiology. *Arch Dermatol* **95**:299, 1967

118. Wilson JW, Plunkett OA: Dermatophytosis, in *The Fungus Diseases of Man.* Berkeley, Univ of California Press, 1965, p 213

119. Rook A, Dawber R: Infections and infestations in *Diseases of the Hair and Scalp.* Oxford, Blackwell, 1982, p 367

120. Feuerman EJ et al: Kerion-like tinea capitis and barbae caused by *Microsporum gypseum* in Israel. *Mycopathologica* **58**:165, 1976

121. Honig PJ, Smith LR: Tinea capitis masquerading as atopic or seborrheic dermatitis. *J Pediatr* **94**:604, 1979

122. Howell JB et al: Tinea capitis caused by *Trichophyton tonsurans* (sulfureum or crateriforme). *Arch Dermatol* **65**:194, 1952

123. Rudolph AH: The clinical recognition of tinea capitis from *Trichophyton tonsurans. JAMA* **242**:1770, 1979

124. Foged EK, Sylvest B: Occurrence of *Trichophyton tonsurans* infections in the Danish island of Funen. *Acta Derm Venereol (Stockh)* **62**:159, 1982

125. Wolf FT et al: Fluorescent pigment of *Microsporum. Nature* **182**:475, 1958

126. Beare M, Walker J: Non-fluorescent *Microsporum audouinii* and *canis* infections of the scalp. *Br J Dermatol* **67**:101, 1955

127. Mackenzie DWR: "Hairbrush diagnosis" in detection and eradication of non-fluorescent scalp ringworm. *Br Med J* **2**:363, 1963

128. Shelley WB, Wood MG: New technic for instant visualization of fungi in hair. *J Am Acad Dermatol* **2**:69, 1980

129. Graham JH, Barroso-Tobila C: Dermal pathology of superficial fungus infections, in *Human Infection with Fungi, Actinomycetes, and Algae,* edited by RD Baker et al. New York, Springer-Verlag, 1971, p 211

130. Lever WF, Schaumburg-Lever G: Fungal diseases, in *Histopathology of the Skin,* 6th ed. Philadelphia, Lippincott, 1983, p 328

131. Imamura S et al: Use of immunofluorescence staining in kerion. *Arch Dermatol* **111**:906, 1975

132. Friedman L et al: The control of tinea capitis among indigent populations. *Am J Public Health* **54**:1588, 1964

133. Vanbreuseghem R et al: Mass treatment of scalp ringworm by a single dose of griseofulvin. *Int J Dermatol* **9**:59, 1970

134. Oskui J: Intermittent use of griseofulvin in tinea capitis. *Cutis* **21**:689, 1978

135. Khan KA, Anwar AA: Study of 73 cases of tinea capitis and tinea favosa in adults and adolescents. *J Invest Dermatol* **51**:474, 1968

136. Joly J et al: Favus: Twenty indigenous cases in the province of Quebec. *Arch Dermatol* **114**:1647, 1978

137. Hakendorf AJ et al: Favus. *Australas J Dermatol* **8**:22, 1965

138. Dvoretzky I et al: Favus. *Int J Dermatol* **19**:89, 1980

139. Sams WM: Favus treated with griseofulvin. *Arch Dermatol* **81**:802, 1960

140. Nierman MM, Landay ME: *Trichophyton verrucosum* in Indiana: Infection in two cases. *Cutis* **26**:591, 1980

141. Hall FR: Ringworm contracted from cattle in western New York state. *Arch Dermatol* **94**:35, 1966

142. Loewenthal K: Tinea barbae due to *Microsporum canis. Arch Dermatol* **91**:60, 1965

143. McAleer R: Fungal infection as a cause of skin disease in Western Australia. III. Tinea barbae. *Australas J Dermatol* **21**:40, 1980

144. Jansen GT et al: Tinea barbae, in *Clinical Dermatology,* edited by DJ Demis et al. Philadelphia, Harper & Row, 1978

145. Domonkos AN et al: Diseases due to fungi, in *Andrews' Diseases of the Skin,* 7th ed. Philadelphia, Saunders, 1982, p 341

146. Alteras I, Feuerman EJ: Atypical cases of *Microsporum canis* infection in the adult. *Mycopathologica* **74**:181, 1981

147. Hay RJ et al: Immune responses of patients with tinea imbricata. *Br J Dermatol* **108**:581, 1983

148. Gill KA et al: Fungus infections occurring under occlusive dressings. *Arch Dermatol* **88**:348, 1963

149. Cullen SI, Ioannides G: Bullous dermatophyte infections. *Cutis* **6**:661, 1970

150. Costello MJ: Vesicular *Trichophyton rubrum (purpureum)* infection simulating dermatitis herpetiformis. *Arch Dermatol* **66**:653, 1952

151. Tolmach JA, Schweig J: Generalized *Trichophyton purpureum* infection simulating dermatitis herpetiformis. *Arch Dermatol* **41**:732, 1940

152. Powell FC, Muller SA: Kerion of glabrous skin. *J Am Acad Dermatol* **7**:490, 1982

153. Wilson JW et al: Nodular granulomatous perifolliculitis of the legs caused by *Trichophyton rubrum. Arch Dermatol* **69**:258, 1954

154. Schreiber MM: *Trichophyton rubrum* perifollicular granuloma of legs. *Cutis* **3**:1083, 1967

155. Smith EB, Head ES: Subcutaneous abscess due to *Trichophyton mentagrophytes. Int J Dermatol* **21**:338, 1982

156. Swart E, Smit FJA: *Trichophyton violaceum* abscesses. *Br J Dermatol* **101**:177, 1979

157. Araviysky AN et al: Deep generalized trichophytosis (endothrix in tissues of different origin). *Mycopathologica* **56**:47, 1975

158. McAleer R: Fungal infection as a cause of skin disease in Western Australia. I. Tinea corporis. *Australas J Dermatol* **21**:25, 1980

159. West BC, Kwon-Chung KJ: Mycetoma caused by *Microsporum audouinii. Am J Clin Pathol* **73**:447, 1980

160. Shanon J, Raubitschek F: Tinea faciei simulating chronic discoid lupus erythematosus. *Arch Dermatol* **82**:268, 1960

161. Gilgor RS et al: Lupus-erythematosus-like tinea of the face (tinea faciale). *JAMA* **215**:2091, 1971

162. Rist TE et al: Tinea faciale: An often misdiagnosed clinical entity. *South Med J* **67**:331, 1974

163. Shapiro L, Cohen JH: Tinea faciei simulating other dermatoses. *JAMA* **215**:2106, 1971

164. Ive FA, Marks R: Tinea incognito. *Br Med J* **3**:149, 1968

165. Burkhart CG: Tinea incognito. *Arch Dermatol* **117**:606, 1981

166. Fisher BK et al: Verrucous epidermophytosis, its response and resistance to griseofulvin. *Arch Dermatol* **84**:375, 1961

167. Emtestam L, Kaaman T: The changing clinical picture of *Micro-*

sporum canis infections in Sweden. *Acta Derm Venereol (Stockh)* **62**:539, 1982

168. McAleer R: Fungal infection as a cause of skin disease in Western Australia. II. Tinea cruris. *Australas J Dermatol* **21**:33, 1980

169. Blank F, Prichard H: Epidemic ringworm of the groin. *Arch Dermatol* **85**:410, 1962

170. Gip L: Isolation of *Trichophyton gallinae* from 2 patients with tinea cruris. *Acta Derm Venereol (Stockh)* **44**:251, 1964

171. Neves H, Xavier NC: The transmission of tinea cruris. *Br J Dermatol* **76**:429, 1964

172. Rosman N: Infections with *Trichophyton rubrum*. *Br J Dermatol* **78**:208, 1966

173. Hopkins JG et al: Dermatophytosis at an infantry post. *J Invest Dermatol* **8**:291, 1947

174. LaTouche CJ: Scrotal dermatophytosis: An insufficiently documented aspect of tinea cruris. *Br J Dermatol* **79**:339, 1967

175. Davis CM et al: Dermatophytes in military recruits. *Arch Dermatol* **105**:558, 1972

176. Fox T: Tinea circinata of the hand. *Br Med J* **1**:116, 1870

177. Pellizari C: Recherche sur *Trychophyton tonsurans*. *G Ital Malattie Veneree* **29**:8, 1888

178. Gentles JC, Holmes JG: Foot ringworm in coal-miners. *Br J Ind Med* **14**:22, 1959

179. English MP et al: Studies in the epidemiology of tinea pedis. *Br Med J* **1**:1083, 1961

180. Broughton RH: Reinfection from socks and shoes in tinea pedis. *Br J Dermatol* **67**:249, 1955

181. Ajello L, Getz ME: Recovery of dermatophytes from shoes and shower stalls. *J Invest Dermatol* **22**:17, 1954

182. Munro-Ashman D, Clayton Y: Tinea pedis in adolescence. *Proc R Soc Med* **55**:551, 1962

183. Ajello L et al: Observations in the incidence of tinea pedis in a group of men entering military life. *Johns Hopkins Med Bull* **77**:440, 1945

184. Strauss JS, Kligman AM: An experimental study of tinea pedis and onychomycosis of the foot. *Arch Dermatol* **76**:70, 1957

185. Leyden JJ: Microbial ecology in interdigital "athlete's" foot infection. *Semin Dermatol* **1**:149, 1982

186. Leyden JJ, Kligman AM: Interdigital athlete's foot. *Arch Dermatol* **114**:1466, 1978

187. Leyden JJ, Kligman AM: Aluminum chloride in the treatment of symptomatic athlete's foot. *Arch Dermatol* **111**:1004, 1975

188. Arndt KA: *Manual of Dermatologic Therapeutics,* 3d ed. Boston, Little, Brown, 1983, p 82

189. Jewell EW: *Trichophyton rubrum* onychomycosis in a four month old infant. *Cutis* **6**:1121, 1970

190. Ramesh V et al: Onychomycosis. *Int J Dermatol* **22**:148, 1983

191. English MP, Atkinson R: Onychomycosis in elderly chiropody patients. *Br J Dermatol* **91**:67, 1974

192. Zaias N: Onychomycosis. *Arch Dermatol* **105**:263, 1972

193. Tuzun Y: *Microsporum* infections of the nails. *Arch Dermatol* **116**:620, 1980

194. Zaias N: Fungi in toe nails. *J Invest Dermatol* **53**:140, 1969

195. Onsberg P: The fungal flora of normal and diseased nails. *Curr Ther Res* **22**:20, 1977

196. English MP: Nails and fungi. *Br J Dermatol* **94**:697, 1976

197. Zaias N: Onychomycosis, in *The Nail: In Health and Disease.* New York, SP Medical & Scientific, 1980, p 91

198. Zaias N: Superficial white onychomycosis. *Sabouraudia* **5**:99, 1966

199. Norton LA: Nail disorders: A review. *J Am Acad Dermatol* **2**:451, 1980

200. Baron R: Onychia and paronychia of mycotic, microbial and parasitic origin, in *The Nail,* edited by M Pierre. New York, Churchill Livingstone, 1981, p 39

201. Raubitschek F, Maoz R: Invasion of nails in vitro by certain dermatophytes. *J Invest Dermatol* **28**:261, 1957

202. Meyer JC et al: Onychomycosis (*Trichophyton mentagrophytes*): A scanning electron microscopic observation. *J Clin Pathol* **8**:342, 1981

203. Reiss F: Leukonychia trichophytica caused by *Trichophyton rubrum*. *Cutis* **20**:223, 1977

204. Gentles JC: Laboratory investigations of dermatophyte infections of nails. *Sabouraudia* **9**:149, 1971

205. Davies RR: Mycological tests and onychomycosis. *J Clin Pathol* **21**:729, 1968

206. Samman PD: Fungous infection, in *The Nails in Disease,* 3d ed. London, Heinemann Medical, 1978, p 40

207. Epstein S: Examination of nails for fungi. *Arch Dermatol* **51**:209, 1945

208. Shelley WB, Wood MG: The white spot target for microscopic examination of nails for fungi. *J Am Acad Dermatol* **6**:92, 1982

209. Scher RK, Ackerman AB: Subtle clues to diagnosis from biopsies of nails. *Am J Dermatopathol* **2**:255, 1980

210. Blank H et al: Griseofulvin for systemic treatment of dermatomycoses. *JAMA* **171**:2168, 1959

211. White MI, Clayton YM: The treatment of fungus and yeast infections of nails by the method of "chemical removal." *Clin Exp Dermatol* **7**:273, 1982

212. Rippon JW: Superficial infections: Tinea nigra, in *Medical Mycology: The Pathogenic Fungi and the Pathogenic Actinomycetes,* 3d ed. Philadelphia, Saunders, 1988, p 159

213. Horta P: Sobre un caso de tinha preta e un novo cogumelo (*Cladosporium werneckii*). *Rev Med Cirug Brazil* **21**:269, 1921

214. McGinnis MR: Taxonomy of *Exophiala werneckii* and its relations to *Microsporum mansonii*. *Sabouraudia* **17**:145, 1979

215. Van Velsor H, Singletary H: Tinea nigra palmaris: A report of 15 cases from coastal North Carolina. *Arch Dermatol* **90**:59, 1964

216. Blank H: Tinea nigra: A twenty-year incubation period? *J Am Acad Dermatol* **1**:49, 1979

217. Helfman RJ: Tinea nigra palmaris et plantaris. *Cutis* **28**:81, 1981

218. Spiller WF et al: Tinea nigra. *J Invest Dermatol* **27**:187, 1956

219. Isaacs F, Reiss-Levy E: Tinea nigra plantaris: A case report. *Australas J Dermatol* **21**:13, 1980

220. Vaffee AS: Tinea nigra palmaris resembling malignant melanoma. *N Engl J Med* **283**:1112, 1970

221. Sayegh-Carreno R et al: Therapy of tinea nigra plantaris. *Int J Dermatol* **28**:46, 1989

222. Rippon JW: Superficial infections: Piedra, in *Medical Mycology: The Pathogenic Fungi and the Pathogenic Actinomycetes,* 3d ed. Philadelphia, Saunders, 1988, p 163

223. Lassus A et al: White piedra: Report of a case evaluated by scanning electron microscopy. *Arch Dermatol* **118**:208, 1982

224. Emmons EW et al (eds): Black piedra, white piedra and trichomycosis axillaris, in *Medical Mycology*. Philadelphia, Lea & Febiger, 1977, p 181

225. Kalter DC et al: Genital white piedra: Epidemiology, microbiology, and therapy. *J Am Acad Dermatol* **14**:982, 1986

226. Conant NF: Piedra, in *Manual of Clinical Mycology,* 3d ed. Philadelphia, Saunders, 1971, p 632

227. Manzella JP et al: *Trichosporon beigelii* fungemia and cutaneous dissemination. *Arch Dermatol* **118**:343, 1982

228. Winston DJ et al: Disseminated *Trichosporon capitatum* infection in an immunosuppressed host. *Arch Intern Med* **137**:1192, 1977

229. Rivera R, Cangir A: *Trichosporon* sepsis and leukemia. *Cancer* **36**:1106, 1975

230. Watson KC, Kallinchurum S: Brain abscess due to *Trichosporon cutaneum*. *J Med Microbiol* **3**:191, 1970

231. Kirmani N et al: Disseminated *Trichosporon* infection: Occurrence in an immunosuppressed patient with chronic active hepatitis. *Arch Intern Med* **140**:277, 1980

232. Evans HL et al: Systemic mycosis due to *Trichosporon cutaneum*. *Cancer* **58**:591, 1980

233. Kobayashi GS, Medoff G: Antifungal agents: Recent developments. *Annu Rev Microbiol* **31**:291, 1977

234. Medoff G, Kobayashi GS: Strategies in the treatment of systemic fungal infections. *N Engl J Med* **302**:145, 1980

235. Medoff G et al: Antifungal agents useful in therapy of systemic fungal infections. *Annu Rev Pharmacol Toxicol* **23**:303, 1983

236. Arndt KA: *Manual of Dermatologic Therapeutics,* 3d ed. Boston, Little, Brown, 1983, p 258

237. D'Arcy PF, Scott EM: Antifungal agents. *Prog Drug Res* **22**:93, 1978

238. Graybill JR, Craven PC: Antifungal agents used in systemic mycoses: Activity and therapeutic use. *Drugs* **25**:41, 1983

239. Oxford AE et al: Studies in the biochemistry of microorganisms: LX, griseofulvin, $C_{17}H_{19}O_6Cl$, a metabolic product of penicillium griseofulvum. *Biochem J* **33**:240, 1939

240. Brian PW et al: Biological assay, production and isolation of "curling factor." *Trans Br Mycol Soc* **29**:173, 1946

241. Borgers M, Van den Bossche H: The mode of action of antifungal drugs, in *Ketoconazole in the Management of Fungal Disease,* edited by HB Levine. New York, Adis Press, 1982, p 25

242. Borgers M: Mechanism of action of antifungal drugs, with special reference to the imidazole derivatives. *Rev Infect Dis* **2**:520, 1980

243. D'arcy PF et al: The anti-inflammatory action of griseofulvin in experimental animals. *J Pharm Pharmacol* **12**:659, 1960

244. McEvoy GK (ed): American Hospital Formulary Service: Drug information 88. *Am Soc Hosp Pharmacists* **76**:8, 1988

245. Anderson DW: Griseofulvin: Biology and clinical usefulness. *Ann Allergy* **23**:103, 1965

246. Lenhart K: Griseofulvin resistant mutants in dermatophytes. *Mykosen* **13**:139, 1970

247. Artis WM et al: Griseofulvin-resistant dermatophytosis correlates with *in vitro* resistance. *Arch Dermatol* **117**:16, 1981

248. Ginsburg CM et al: Effect of feeding on bioavailability of griseofulvin in children. *J Pediatr* **102**:309, 1983

249. Crounse RG: Human pharmacology of griseofulvin: The effect of fat intake on gastrointestinal absorption. *J Invest Dermatol* **37**:529, 1961

250. Epstein WL et al: Dermatopharmacology of griseofulvin. *Cutis* **15**:271, 1975

251. Sande MA, Mandell GL: Antimicrobial agents, in *The Pharmacological Basis of Therapeutics,* 6th ed, edited by AG Goodman et al. New York, Macmillan, 1980, p 1232

252. Epstein WL et al: Griseofulvin levels in stratum corneum: Study after oral administration in man. *Arch Dermatol* **106**:344, 1972

253. Scott A: Behaviour of radioactive griseofulvin in skin. *Nature (London)* **187**:705, 1960

254. Blank H: Commentary: Treatment of dermatomycoses with griseofulvin. *Arch Dermatol* **118**:835, 1982

255. Berman A, Franklin RL: Precipitation of acute intermittent porphyria by griseofulvin therapy. *JAMA* **192**:1005, 1965

256. Riegelman S et al: Griseofulvin-phenobarbital interaction in man. *JAMA* **213**:426, 1970

257. Anderson DW: Griseofulvin: Biology and clinical usefulness. A review. *Ann Allergy* **23**:103, 1965

258. Battistini F et al: Clinical antifungal activity of thiabendazole. *Arch Dermatol* **109**:695, 1974

259. MacKie RM: Topical econazole in cutaneous fungal infections. *Practitioner* **224**:1311, 1980

260. Borgers M et al: The mechanism of action of the new antimycotic ketoconazole. *Am J Med* **74**(suppl):2B, 1983

261. Samsoen M, Jelen G: Allergy to daktarin gel. *Contact Dermatitis* **3**:351, 1977

262. Graybill JR, Drutz DJ: Ketoconazole: A major innovation for treatment of fungal disease. *Ann Intern Med* **93**:921, 1980

263. Ketoconazole (Nizoral): A new antifungal agent. *Med Lett Drugs Ther* **23**:85, 1981

264. Hume AL, Kerkering TM: Ketoconazole. *Drug Intell Clin Pharm* **17**:169, 1983

265. Horsburgh CR, Kirkpatrick CH: Long-term therapy of chronic mucocutaneous candidiasis with ketoconazole: Experience with twenty-one patients. *Am J Med* **74**(suppl):23, 1983

266. Cox FW et al: Oral ketoconazole for dermatophyte infections. *J Am Acad Dermatol* **6**:455, 1982

267. Robertson MH et al: Ketoconazole in griseofulvin-resistant dermatophytosis. *J Am Acad Dermatol* **6**:224, 1982

268. Hay RJ, Clayton YM: Treatment of chronic dermatophyte infections: The use of ketoconazole in griseofulvin treatment failures. *Clin Exp Dermatol* **7**:611, 1982

269. Jones HE et al: Oral ketoconazole: An effective and safe treatment for dermatophytosis. *Arch Dermatol* **117**:129, 1981

270. Welsh O, Rodriquez M: Treatment of dermatomycoses with ketoconazole. *Rev Infect Dis* **2**:582, 1980

271. Galimberti R et al: The activity of ketoconazole in the treatment of onychomycosis. *Rev Infect Dis* **2**:596, 1980

272. Pont A et al: Ketoconazole blocks testosterone synthesis. *Arch Intern Med* **142**:2137, 1982

273. Pont A et al: Ketoconazole blocks adrenal steroid synthesis. *Ann Intern Med* **97**:370, 1982

274. Tkach JR, Rinaldi MG: Severe hepatitis associated with ketoconazole therapy for chronic mucocutaneous candidiasis. *Cutis* **29**:482, 1982

275. Heiberg JK, Svejgaard E: Toxic hepatitis during ketoconazole treatment. *Br Med J* **283**:825, 1981

276. Jones HE: Ketoconazole. *Arch Dermatol* **118**:217, 1982

277. Janssen PAJ, Symoens JE: Hepatic reactions during ketoconazole treatment. *Am J Med* **74**(suppl):80, 1983

278. Graybill JR Jr: Summary: Potential and problems with ketoconazole. *Am J Med* **74**(suppl):86, 1983

279. Fluconazole. *Med Lett Drugs Ther* **32**(818):50, 1990

280. Fluconazole: Systemic antifungal agent fluconazole receives marketing approval. *Clin Pharm* **9**:231, 1990

281. Brammer KW et al: Pharmacokinetics and tissue penetration of fluconazole in humans. *Rev Infect Dis* **12**(3):S318, 1990

282. Blum RA et al: Increased gastric pH and the bioavailability of fluconazole and ketoconazole. *Ann Intern Med* **114**:755, 1991

283. Foulds G et al: Fluconazole penetration into cerebrospinal fluid in humans. *J Clin Pharmacol* **28**:363, 1988

284. Lazar JD, Wilner KD: Drug interactions with fluconazole. *Rev Infect Dis* **12**(3):S327, 1990

285. Sugar AM et al: Interaction of fluconazole with cyclosporine. *Ann Intern Med* **110**:844, 1989

286. Collignon P et al: Interaction of fluconazole with cyclosporine. *Lancet* **1**:1262, 1989

287. Cauwenbergh G et al: Pharmacokinetic profile of orally administered itraconazole in human skin. *J Am Acad Dermatol* **18**:263, 1988

288. Sakurai K et al: Mode of action of 6-cyclohexyl-1-hydroxy4-methyl-2(1H)-pyridone ethanolamine salt (HOE 296). *Chemotherapy* **24**:68, 1978

289. Dittmar W: Penetration and antimycotic efficacy of ciclopirox olamine in keratinized body tissue. *Arzneimittelforschung* **31**:1353, 1981

290. Qadripur SA et al: On the local efficacy of ciclopirox olamine in onychomycosis. *Arzneimittelforschung* **31**:1369, 1981

291. Birnbaum JE: Pharmacology of the allylamines. *J Am Acad Dermatol* **23**(4):782, 1990

292. Lyddon FE et al: Short chain fatty acids in the treatment of dermatophytoses. *Int J Dermatol* **19**:24, 1980

CHAPTER 195

Ann G. Martin and George S. Kobayashi

Yeast Infections: Candidiasis, Pityriasis (Tinea) Versicolor

Candidiasis (or candidosis) is an infection with protean clinical manifestations, caused by *Candida albicans* or, on occasion, by other yeasts of the genus *Candida*. The infections are usually confined to the skin, nails, mucous membranes, and gastrointestinal tract but can be systemic and infect multiple internal organs.

Historical Aspects

The clinical manifestations of candidiasis have been recognized since ancient times and were discussed in the writings of Hippocrates, Galen, and Pepys. In 1839, Langenbeck discovered the organism in a lesion of thrush. Berg in 1841 and Bennett in 1844 supported this finding and demonstrated that the fungus was indeed the etiologic agent of thrush. Until the genus *Candida* was defined by Berkhout in 1923, a confusing taxonomy ensued. Initially classified as a *Sporotrichum* by Gruby, it was placed in the genus *Oidium* (*Oidium albicans*) by Robin in 1847. Later it was confused with another fungus isolated from rotting vegetation (*Monilia candida*) and was renamed *Monilia albicans* by Zopf in 1890. The name *Monilia* was stubbornly defended by Castellani and probably accounts for the term *moniliasis* being used as a synonym for candidiasis even in the relatively modern literature. Of course, the term *Monilia* is a misnomer and actually refers to the imperfect stage of certain ascomycetes; it has no relationship whatsoever to the genus *Candida*.

In 1877, further progress was made when Grawitz described the dimorphic nature of the organism. In the late 1800s and early 1900s, the protean clinical manifestations of candidiasis were recognized. In 1853 Robin first described systemic candidiasis. Cutaneous candidiasis and chronic mucocutaneous candidiasis were described relatively late, in 1907 and 1909, respectively. Diaper dermatitis was not described formally until 1911. Finally, after the genus *Candida* was established in 1923, efforts to speciate yeasts placed in this genus were forged by Martin in 1937. The importance of candidiasis as an opportunistic infection was first appreciated in the postantibiotic era of the 1940s when an increase in the number of candidal infections was noted.

Controversy over nomenclature persists, and whereas candidiasis is the accepted term for this infection in the United States, candidosis is preferred in Canada, the United Kingdom, France, and Italy.

Etiology

From a taxonomic viewpoint, the genera *Candida* and *Torulopsis* accomodate a heterogeneous collection of yeast species that do not produce ascospores or teliospores and do not possess morphologic or biochemical characteristics that would classify them in the more homogeneous genera of imperfect yeasts. At the present time, the morphologic feature that separates these two genera is based on the capacity of the yeast to form pseudomycelia (Fig. 195-1). In the genus *Candida*, pseudomycelia are well developed, whereas in the genus *Torulopsis* they are absent or poorly developed. There is presently a controversy concerning the separation of these two genera, and because the criteria for defining various genera of imperfect fungi are arbitrary, some authors have suggested they be classified in one single artificial genus (*Candida*). As this would require the renaming of a great number of species and invariably lead to confusion and disagreement among mycologists and clinicians, this chapter will recognize *Candida* and *Torulopsis* as two separate genera. Of the various species in the genus *Candida*, *C. albicans* is the most common cause of superficial and systemic candidiasis. Several of the more than 80 other species classified in this genus can also be responsible for clinical disease under certain circumstances (e.g., host immunosuppression, indwelling catheters, intravenous drug delivery). Most of these infections are systemic but can be localized (Table 195-1). Together *C. albicans* and *C. tropicalis* account for about 80 percent of the species isolated from medical specimens.[1,2] The species of *Candida* have been graded by descending degree of pathogenicity as follows: *C. albicans*, *C. stellatoidea*, *C. tropicalis*, *C. parapsilosis*, *C. kefyr*, *C. guilliermondii*, and *C. krusei*.

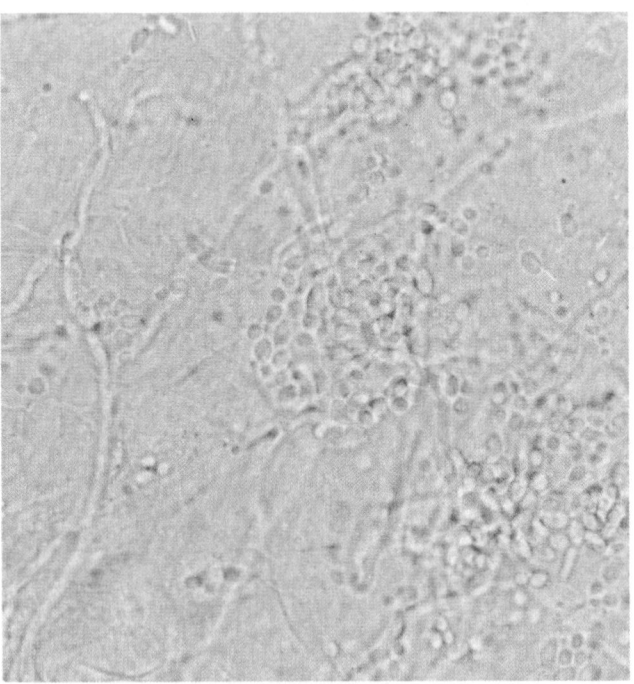

FIGURE 195-1 Candida in potassium hydroxide preparation. Pseudomycelia and clusters of grapelike yeast cells.

TABLE 195-1

Regular Isolates Other than *C. albicans* in Certain Types of Candidiasis

Causative organism	Clinical disease
C. parapsilosis	Paronychia, endocarditis, otitis externa
C. tropicalis	Vaginitis; intestinal, bronchopulmonary, and systemic infections; onychomycosis; bone and joint disease; central nervous system disease
C. stellatoidea	Vaginitis, systemic disease, bone and joint disease
C. guilliermondii	Endocarditis, cutaneous candidiasis, onychomycosis, bone and joint disease
C. kefyr	Vaginitis, urethritis
C. (Torulopsis) glabrata	Esophagitis, vaginitis, endocarditis
C. krusei	Endocarditis, vaginitis
C. zeylanoides	Onychomycosis
C. viswanathi	Central nervous system disease
C. lusitaniae	Systemic disease

TABLE 195-2

Factors Predisposing to *Candida* Infections

Mechanical factors
  Trauma (burns, abrasions, etc.)
  Local occlusion, moisture, and/or maceration (dentures, occlusive dressings or garments, obesity)
Nutritional factors
  Avitaminosis
  Iron deficiency (chronic mucocutaneous candidiasis)
  Generalized malnutrition
Physiologic alterations
  Extremes of age
  Pregnancy
  Menses
Systemic illnesses
  Down's syndrome
  Acrodermatitis enteropathica
  Diabetes mellitus and certain other endocrinopathies (Cushing's, hypoadrenalism, hypothyroidism, hypoparathyroidism)
  Uremia
  Malignancy (especially hematologic, thymoma)
  Intrinsic immunodeficiency states (DiGeorge's syndrome, Nezelof's syndrome, severe combined immunodeficiency syndrome, myeloperoxidase deficiency, Chédiak-Higashi syndrome, hyperimmunoglobulinemia E syndrome, chronic granulomatous disease, AIDS)
Iatrogenic causes
  Barrier-weak factors (indwelling catheters, intravenous drug abusers)
  X-irradiation
  Medications
  Corticosteroids and other immunosuppressive agents
  Antibiotics (especially broad-spectrum, metronidazole)
  Tranquilizers
  Oral contraceptives (especially estrogen-dominant)
  Colchicine
  Phenylbutazone

Pathogenesis

C. albicans is often found as a saprophyte and colonizes certain mucous membrane surfaces of warm-blooded animals. As many as 80 percent of normal individuals show such colonization of the oropharynx, gastrointestinal tract, and vagina.[3] In contrast, the organism is rarely isolated from normal human skin except sporadically from certain intertriginous areas. Likewise, the organism is seldom isolated from soil, vegetation, or air samples.

The development of disease due to *Candida* species is dependent on the complex interaction between the innate pathogenicity of the organism and the defense mechanisms of the host. *Candida* infections are largely opportunistic ones made possible by diminished host defenses. Certain predisposing factors have been classically associated with an increased incidence of colonization and infection by these yeasts (Table 195-2).

Various factors regarding the intrinsic pathogenicity of *Candida* species as they relate to skin and mucous membrane infections are important to consider. The species of *Candida* differ in their ability to initiate cutaneous infection in an experimental animal model.[4] Using the staphylococcal toxin epidermolysin to cleave the epidermis selectively below the granular layer, Ray et al.[5] demonstrated that only *C. albicans* and *C. stellatoidea* inoculated into this cleft were capable of invading the stratum corneum and eliciting inflammation. Other species were excluded even under occlusive experimental conditions. These findings were supported by Maibach and Kligman in experimental human cutaneous candidiasis, clearly demonstrating differences in virulence among the species of *Candida*.[6]

Other important factors in the initiation of candidal infections include adherence of the organism to epithelial cells and subsequent invasion.[3,7] The mechanism of invasion is unclear but may involve elaboration of keratinolytic enzymes, phospholipases, or strain-specific proteolytic enzymes.[8–10] Ultrastructurally, pseudohyphae can be seen penetrating intracellularly into corneocytes in clinical lesions of candidiasis. A prominent clear space is usually seen around the organisms, suggesting an ongoing process of epithelial tissue lysis.[11,12] It appears that mycelial growth predominates in invasive disease states, whereas the blastospore growth phase predominates in saprophytic states.

The induction of cutaneous candidiasis in humans under experimental conditions pointed the way to important subsequent data examining the pathogenesis of the inflammatory response in the disease. Maibach and Kligman[6] noted that the epicutaneous inoculation of *C. albicans* could produce cutaneous disease only if the site of inoculation was occluded. Within 36 to 72 h, typical erythematous, pustular lesions developed. The severity of the infection was proportional to the size of the inoculum.[13] Biopsy of these pustules showed them to be subcorneal in location. Using special stains, organisms were not seen within the pustules but were seen only in the stratum corneum. Cutaneous lesions were similarly produced using a sterile extract of disintegrated candidal cells and a sediment of killed ruptured cells. The authors postulated the existence of an endotoxin-like substance that mediated the pustular response.[6] Subsequently, Ray et al.[14] demonstrated that a purified mannan cell wall polysaccharide from *C. albicans* is capable of activating complement via the alternative pathway, thereby generating products such as C5a that induce neutrophil chemotaxis. This material also exhibits in vitro endotoxin-like activity. In this way, highly antigenic or toxic products of candidal organisms are able to induce vigorous host response mechanisms that, at the same time, both limit infection and produce the typical cutaneous manifestations of the disease. Such a mechanism may explain certain findings in systemic candidiasis. For example, circulating mannan has been demonstrated in systemic invasive candidal infections. By alternative pathway complement activation in this setting, the leukopenia and early neutrophilic tissue response associated with disseminated candidal infections may be partially explained. Furthermore, *Candida* antigen, immunoglobulin, and complement have been found in the nephritic kidney of a patient with *Candida* endocrinopathy syndrome.[15] In contrast, other cell wall "toxic" products of candidal organisms have been found to interfere with host neutrophil chemotaxis and phagocytosis.[16] Furthermore, cell wall polysaccharide products may interfere with T lymphocyte-mediated defenses.[3,17,18] The mechanisms of host defense operative during *Candida* infections are complex and still not completely understood. The broad categories include nonimmune and immune factors.[19,20]

The nonimmune factors include the following: (1) interaction with other members of the microbial flora, (2) the functional integrity of the stratum corneum, (3) the desquamation process induced by inflammation-induced epidermal proliferation, (4) opsonization and phagocytosis, and (5) other serum factors. The host microbial flora are protective in that they compete with *Candida* for nutrients and epithelial adherence sites and produce by-products toxic to the yeast. Likewise, normal intact skin with its constant sloughing and regeneration provides an effective barrier against *Candida*. Skin surface lipids are partially inhibitory as well.[3] Abrogation of this barrier by mechanical means or occlusion facilitates infection. As with cutaneous dermatophyte infections, the skin increases its turnover rate significantly during the early stages of infection, and this increased desquamation helps shed the organism.[21]

The process of phagocytosis and killing of candidal organisms is accomplished primarily by polymorphonuclear leukocytes (PMN) and macrophages. The PMN is probably the most important in this regard[22]; patients with neutropenia or diseases affecting PMN function (Table 195-2) are particularly susceptible to candidal infections. As noted previously, the PMN is the predominant early inflammatory cell seen histologically in candidal infections. It is recruited in part by mannan activation of the alternative complement pathway and the ensuing generation of potent chemotactic factors.[14] The importance of this process to host defense against *Candida* is emphasized in experimental studies on complement-depleted (using cobra venom factor) rodents or hereditary C5-deficient animals. In this setting, experimental candidal infections do not elicit a PMN response. In addition, the organism invades much more rapidly and extensively than in normal animals.[4,23] Likewise, macrophages participate in opsonization, phagocytosis, and killing of yeasts. PMN and macrophages have C3b surface receptors, and the deposition of C3b opsonins on *Candida* organisms may therefore facilitate phagocytosis.[24,25] PMN and macrophages accomplish intracellular killing by both oxidative (myeloperoxidase-hydrogen peroxide-halide system) and nonoxidative means. This mechanism is not absolute, however, and some organisms, although phagocytosed, are not killed, whereas larger hyphae may not be phagocytosed at all. However, neutrophils appear to be able to recognize these hyphae and attach to them. While not phagocytizing the yeasts, they do inflict damage by extracellular oxidative antimicrobial mechanisms.[20,26]

Serum factors that may be important in containing candidal infections include the controversial serum "clumping" factor described by Louria and Brayton.[27] Although initially thought to be important in fungistasis, this clumping phenomenon may simply reflect the entanglement of hyphal elements grown in serum.[28] Transferrin, by binding iron necessary for fungal growth, may inhibit candidal proliferation,[29] and lactoferrin, a neutrophil-derived iron-binding substance, may function similarly and also contribute to neutrophil adherence and other functions.[20,30]

The immune mechanisms responsible for protection against *Candida* infections include both humoral and cell-mediated responses. The latter are considered to be more important in this

regard. Proof for this assertion comes from experience with chronic mucocutaneous candidiasis and human immunodeficiency virus (HIV) infection, where a defect in cell-mediated immunity leads to extensive superficial candidiasis despite normal, or even exaggerated, humoral defenses. Serum antibody production to the principal cell wall glycoprotein antigens of *Candida* occurs in low titers in normal individuals. The protective role of these antibodies is controversial and may reflect a response to colonization of the gastrointestinal tract early in life. There is evidence in certain experimental situations, such as using passive transfer of serum, that a degree of protection may be provided.[31,32] Yet, in the clinical setting, it is clear that patients with primarily B-cell deficiency states are not at high risk for candidal infections.[19] There is also conflicting evidence for the role of secretory IgA in limiting mucosal infections.[19,33] It is probable that the various innate, nonimmune factors in conjunction with cell-mediated immunity and complement activation contribute more to host defense against candidal infections than does humoral immunity.[3]

Clinical Manifestations

The cutaneous and mucosal manifestations of candidiasis are varied but in most cases characteristic.

Oral Candidiasis (See also Chap. 111)

Acute pseudomembranous candidiasis or *thrush* may present early in life as candidal organisms, presumably from the maternal birth canal, colonize the mouth of the neonate. Thrush is the most common form of oral candidiasis and may affect up to 5 percent of newborns and 10 percent of debilitated, hospitalized, elderly patients.[34] Concomitant illnesses such as diabetes mellitus,[35] malignancies, and immune deficiency states may also be predisposing factors (Table 195-2). Clinically there are discrete white patches that may become confluent on the buccal mucosa, tongue, palate, and gingiva (Fig. 195-2a). This friable pseudomembrane resembles milk curds and consists of desquamated epithelial cells, fungal elements, inflammatory cells, and food debris. When scraped off, a raw, brightly erythematous surface is exposed. Microscopic examination of this material reveals masses of tangled pseudohyphae and blastospores. Severe cases may show ulcerations and necrosis of the mucosal surface.

Acute atrophic candidiasis (antibiotic candidosis) may occur de novo or after sloughing of the pseudomembrane of thrush.[34] It is commonly associated with broad-spectrum antibiotic administration but can be seen with the use of topical, inhaled, or systemic corticosteroids.[20,36] The most common location is on the dorsal surface of the tongue where there are patchy depapillated areas with minimal pseudomembrane formation.

Chronic atrophic candidiasis (denture stomatitis) (Fig. 195-2b) is a very common form of oral candidiasis among denture wearers, afflicting one in four denture wearers at some time,[37] and 60 percent of those older than 65 years of age.[38] Female patients are affected more commonly than males. The condition is characterized by chronic erythema and edema of the palatal mucosa that contacts the dentures. Angular cheilitis is commonly present as well. It is often not symptomatic or only mildly so. *C. albicans* is recovered more commonly from the surface of the denture material than from the mucosal surface.[39] Presumably, the chronic low-

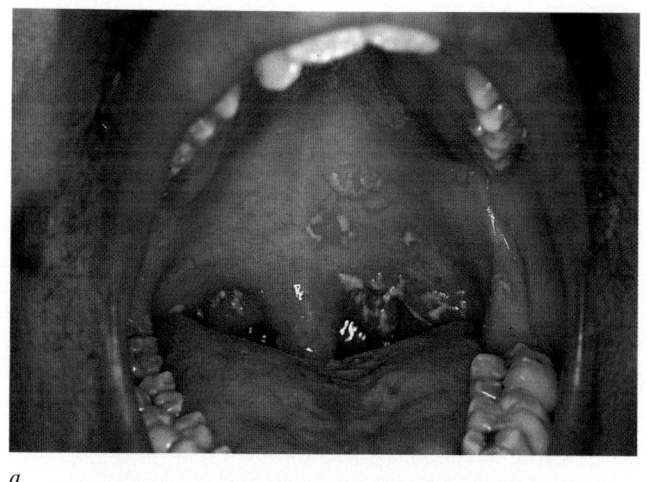

a

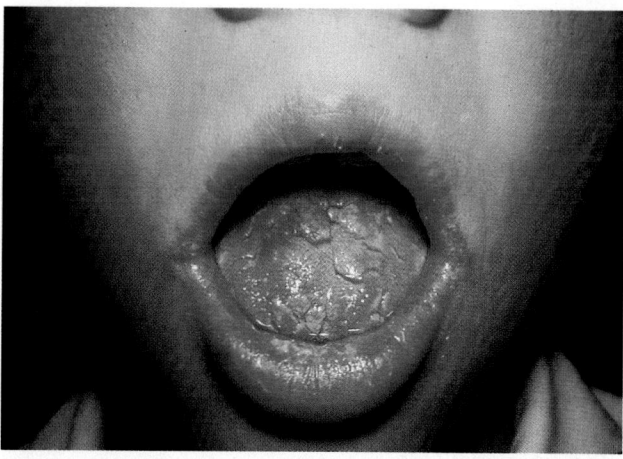

c

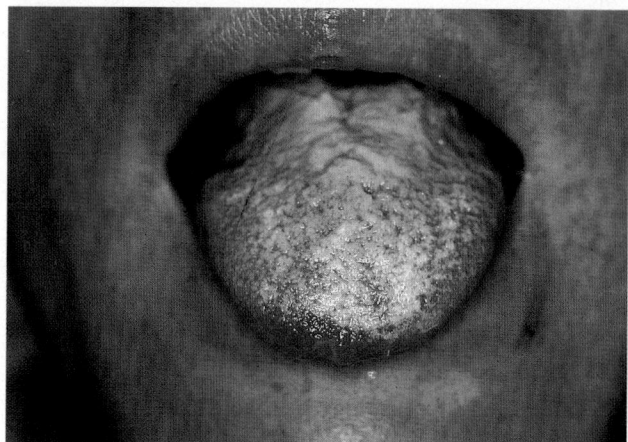

d

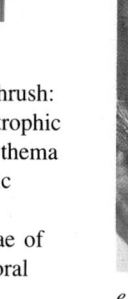

b

FIGURE 195-2 (*a*) Pseudomembranous candidiasis or thrush: note the characteristic white patches on the palate. (*b*) Atrophic candidiasis under dentures. (*c*) Candida perleche with erythema and fissuring at the corners of the mouth. (*d*) Hyperplastic candidiasis of the tongue. (*e*) Black hairy tongue is characterized by pigmented hypertrophied filliform papillae of the dorsum of the tongue and is usually associated with oral antibiotic therapy.

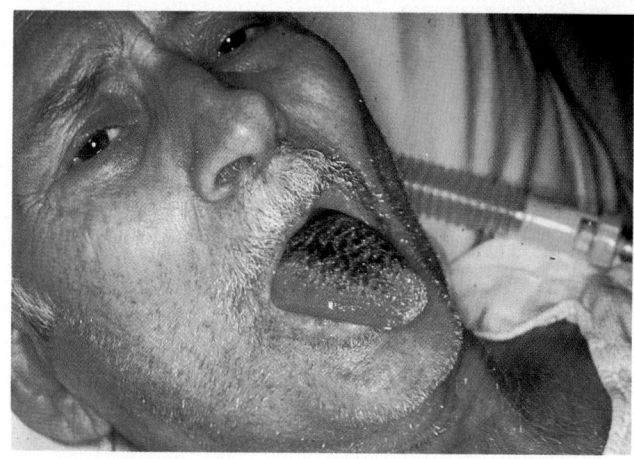

e

grade trauma and occlusion provided by dentures predisposes to candidal colonization and subsequent infection.

Candida cheilosis or *perlèche* is characterized by erythema, fissuring, maceration, and soreness at the angles of the mouth (Fig. 195-2*c*), from which the organism *C. albicans* can be isolated. It occurs in habitual lip lickers or in those elderly patients with sagging skin at the oral commissures. Loss of vertical dimension in the lower one-third of the face due to loss of dentition or poorly fitting

dentures and malocclusion may also be predisposing factors.[40] It is often associated with chronic atrophic candidiasis due to denture wear. A true candidal cheilitis has been described where chronic erosive or granular changes appear on the lower lips of compulsive lip lickers. Satellite lesions may spread beyond the vermilion in this case.[41]

Chronic hyperplastic candidiasis or candidal leukoplakia is characterized by adherent (unlike thrush), firm, raised areas on the buccal mucosa or tongue that are translucent to white in color with surrounding erythema and from which *C. albicans* can frequently be isolated (Fig. 195-2*d*).

Median rhomboid glossitis is a central papillary atrophic condition of the dorsal surface of the tongue. Some consider it to be a developmental anomaly,[42] but others point to histologic and microbiologic evidence suggesting that it represents a true candidal infection.[43]

Black hairy tongue has been associated etiologically with *C. albicans*. However, the organism probably is a secondary invader of hypertrophied filiform papillae on the dorsum of the tongue (Fig. 195-2*e*) that characterizes the condition.[1]

Oral Candidiasis in Immunocompromised and Cancer Patients

Oral candidiasis is a common complication in patients immunocompromised by irradiation, antimetabolite therapy, organ transplantation therapy, diabetes mellitus, or cell-mediated immune deficiency. An incidence of 5 percent in cancer patients and 10 percent in debilitated elderly patients has been estimated. Severe neutropenia is considered the most significant predisposing factor for life-threatening *Candida* infections. In a recent study, major *Candida* infections occurred in 84 percent of leukemic patients who had less than 1000 cells per mm^3 for 13 days.[44] In the setting of neutropenia, there is a high risk of oral candidiasis evolving to systemic infection. This may occur in several ways: (1) direct invasion of the oral mucosa through ulcerations; (2) extension of oropharyngeal infection into the esophagus, producing esophageal ulceration, fungemia, and dissemination; (3) extension into the gastrointestinal tract; and (4) aspiration of oral secretions causing *Candida* pneumonia.[45]

Oral Candidiasis and Acquired Immunodeficiency Syndrome (AIDS)

Oral candidiasis is a common, early, and often initial manifestation of infection with HIV. The disease presents as typical thrush, in association with hairy leukoplakia, or with esophageal involvement. Unexplained oral candidiasis in previously healthy adults at high risk for AIDS predicts the onset of other serious opportunistic infections or Kaposi's sarcoma over 50 percent of the time.[46] In this particular study, the diagnosis of oral candidiasis preceded the features of AIDS by a median time of 3 months. A significantly depressed T4/T8 lymphocyte ratio was present in the majority of cases.[46] In any event, the development of oral candidiasis in previously healthy adults not receiving broad-spectrum antibiotics or corticosteroids and not subject to other predisposing conditions (prolonged denture wearing, use of corticosteroid inhalers, diabetes mellitus, etc.) should strongly alert the physician to consider HIV infection.

Topical treatment of oral candidiasis is seldom effective but is worth a trial in mild cases or for prophylaxis. Generally high doses are required. Nystatin in an oral suspension, 4 to 6 million units, and clotrimazole, 10-mg troches 5 times a day, are effective. Ketoconazole (200 to 400 mg/day) may be effective in many cases; in others the results are poor. Acidifying a ketoconazole suspension and avoiding antacids aid in achieving adequate levels of drug. Newer azole derivatives, such as fluconazole and itraconazole, look promising.

Vaginal and Vulvovaginal Candidiasis

C. albicans may be isolated from vaginal cultures in roughly 8 percent of normal women. This percentage increases to 25 percent in patients with symptoms of vaginitis.[47] Factors thought to predispose to an increasing incidence of candidal vaginitis include pregnancy, diabetes mellitus, oral contraceptives, antibiotic administration, and occlusive tight-fitting garments such as pantyhose and leotards. Patients present with a thick vaginal discharge associated with burning or itching and sometimes dysuria. Examination shows whitish plaques on the vaginal wall with underlying erythema and surrounding edema. Areas of involvement may spread to the labiae and perineal area. Recurrent and chronic candidal vulvovaginitis is a particularly difficult problem for certain patients. The pathogenesis of such recurrent vaginitis is unclear and controversial but has been thought to reflect intestinal or urethral colonization or penile colonization in the male partners of affected women.[48,49] In some cases, concomitant polymicrobial infections may explain poor responses to therapy and frequent relapses.[50]

Balanitis or Balanoposthitis

Balanitis due to *C. albicans* presents as small papules or fragile papulopustules on the glans or in the coronal sulcus. These break to leave superficial erythematous erosions with a collarette of whitish scale. A thrushlike membrane may form in some cases. Infection may spread to the scrotum and inguinal areas. In diabetics or immunosuppressed patients, a severe edematous, ulcerative balanitis may occur.[51] Occasionally, patients present with a transient erythema and burning occurring shortly after intercourse with partners having candidal vaginitis. This presentation was thought to represent a hypersensitivity response to the organism.[52] Factors predisposing to balanitis include candidal vaginal infection in sexual partners, diabetes mellitus, and an uncircumcised state.

Cutaneous Candidiasis

C. albicans has a predilection for colonizing moist, macerated folds of skin. For that reason, intertrigo in its various forms is the most common clinical presentation of candidiasis on glabrous skin. Common locations for the infection include the genitocrural, subaxillary, gluteal, interdigital (Fig. 195-3*a*), and submammary (Fig. 195-3*b*) areas and between the folds of skin of the abdominal wall. Predisposing conditions include obesity, occlusive clothing, diabetes mellitus, and occupations favoring excessive exposure to moist occlusive conditions. The clinical appearance is typical and consists of pruritic, erythematous, macerated areas of skin in intertriginous areas with satellite vesicopustules. These pustules are fragile and break, leaving a red macular base with a collarette of easily detachable necrotic epidermis. Several varieties of intertrigo caused by *Candida* deserve special mention. *Diaper dermatitis* in infants can be of multiple etiologies. *Candida*, however, can colonize this area from the gastrointestinal tract of these children.[53] The chronic occlusive state provided by diaper wear propagates the infection. Lesions appear first in the perianal area and spread to the perineum and inguinal creases, with pronounced erythema in the latter area (Fig. 195-3*c*). Concomitant thrush or candidal involvement of other intertriginous areas may be present in severe cases. *Erosio interdigitalis blastomycetica* refers to interdigital candidal infection of the hands and usually affects the area between the third and fourth

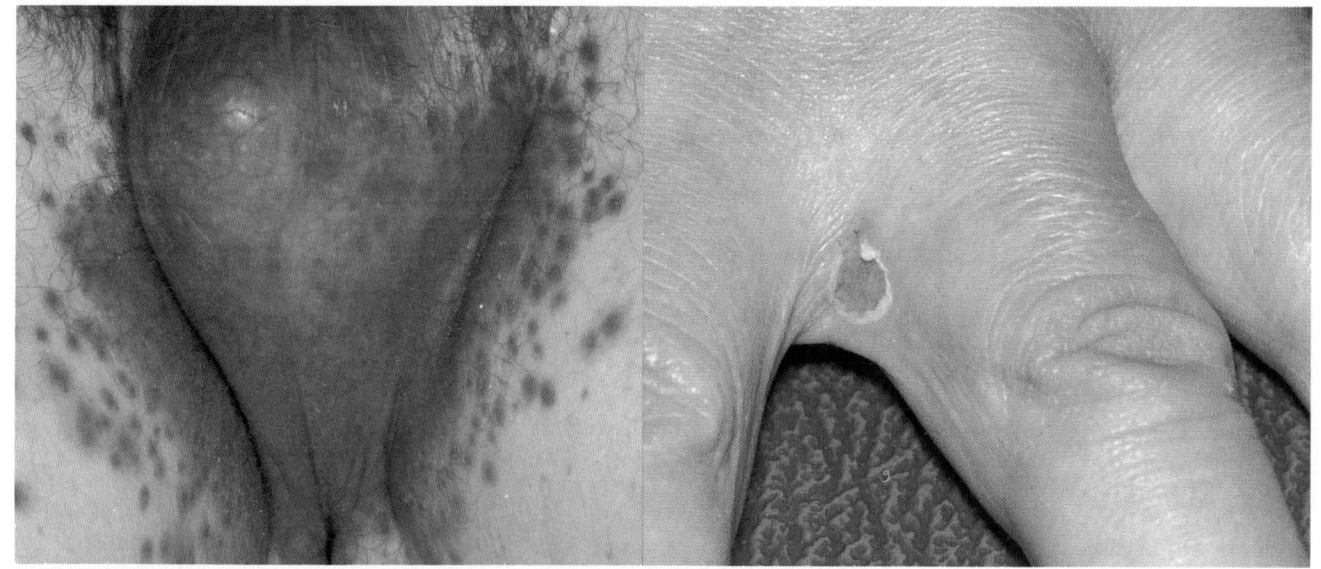

a

d

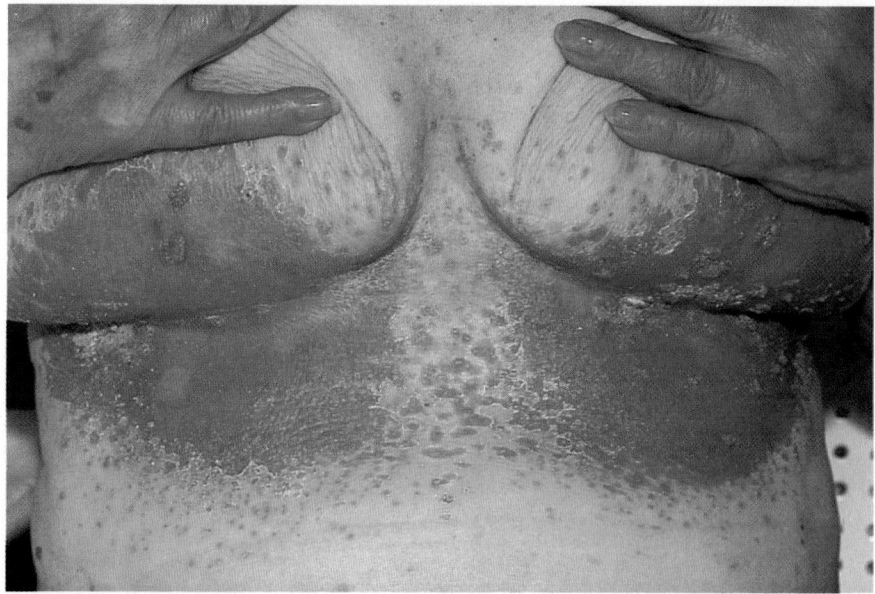

b

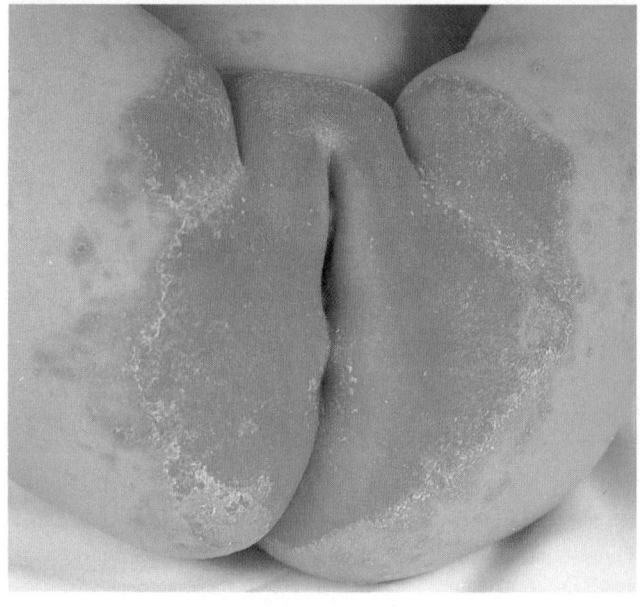

c

FIGURE 195-3 *Candida intertrigo.*
(a) Erythematous, eroded plaques
involving the scrotum and inguinal area
with satellite lesions. (*b*) Confluent and
discrete, erythematous, eroded areas with
pustular and erosive satellite lesion.
(*c*) The infant shows red macular areas
on the vulva surrounded by a delicate
collar. Outside the main lesions are a
few satellite lesions. (*d*) Erythematous
eroded area between the fingers
occurring in a waitress.

fingers (Fig. 195-3*d*). *Candida miliaria* affects the back in bedridden patients, particularly those who are febrile and sweating profusely. Lesions start as isolated vesicopustules that are positive for fungal forms. *Candida* can also colonize and infect the skin around wounds that are being dressed occlusively, especially if broad-spectrum topical antibiotics are being used.

An *erythematous pustular folliculitis* has been described due to *C. albicans.* Although the lesions are perifollicular in location, true hair shaft invasion is usually not observed.[54] A common location for these lesions is in the perioral area.[20] Typical perioral dermatitis presenting as erythematous papulopustules has been described secondary to *C. albicans,* as has a more severe pyoderma faciale-like eruption in the perioral area.[55,56]

Candida paronychia is extremely common in individuals whose hands are chronically involved in wet work (e.g., housewives, bakers, fishermen, bartenders). At times the clinical presentation may be complicated by a concomitant bacterial infection. Typically there is redness, swelling, and tenderness of the paronychial area with prominent retraction of the cuticle toward the proximal nail fold (Fig. 195-4). Occasionally, pus can be expressed from beneath this area. Secondary nail changes can occur and include onycholysis and transverse ridging of the nail plate with a brownish or green discoloration along the lateral borders. True *Candida* invasion of the nail plate occurs in chronic mucocutaneous candidiasis; in this case the entire thickness of the nail plate is involved.[57]

A more generalized cutaneous involvement can occur due to *C. albicans.* The rare syndrome of *congenital candidiasis* usually presents at birth or shortly thereafter (within 12 h of life) and is due to infection acquired in utero. The disease has been reported after amniocentesis.[58] Lesions occur diffusely over the trunk, extremities, head, and neck and spare the mouth and diaper area. They appear as red macules that progress to papulovesicles or pustules that later desquamate and resolve spontaneously. Fever and other constitutional symptoms are lacking, and patients usually have a benign course, but fatal dissemination has been described, especially in infants with low birth weights or concomitant respiratory distress.[59]

The incidence of *disseminated candidiasis* is steadily rising as more patients with serious hematologic malignancies are treated aggressively with potent immunosuppressive drugs, and more and more patients undergo bone marrow and other organ transplants.[60] Other factors that may predispose to disseminated candidal infection are listed in Table 195-2. The organisms responsible for such infections include *C. albicans, C. tropicalis, C. kefyr, C. krusei,* and *C. parapsilosis.*[61] These organisms may gain hematogenous access from the oropharynx or gastrointestinal tract, when the mucosal barrier function is compromised (e.g., mucositis secondary to chemotherapy), or through contaminated intravenous catheters. Organs most commonly involved include the lungs, spleen, kidneys, liver, heart, and brain.[62] The eye findings include an endophthalmitis that correlates well with multiple organ involvement.[63] Skin lesions occur in 10 to 13 percent of patients with disseminated infection.[64] The recognition of such lesions may be important in early diagnosis as antemortem blood cultures are negative in a high percentage of patients with autopsy-proved systemic candidiasis.[65]

The characteristic skin lesions are 0.5 to 1.0 cm erythematous papulonodules that tend to become hemorrhagic, particularly in patients with associated thrombocytopenia. They are usually located on the trunk and extremities and may be numerous or few.[66] Associated findings include fever and myalgias.[67,68] Necrotic cutaneous lesions resembling ecthyma gangrenosum (due to *Pseudomonas aeruginosa*) have also been described due to candidiasis.[69,70] A distinctive syndrome in intravenous heroin abusers has been described in which macronodular and folliculitis-like skin lesions occurred in the scalp and other terminal hair-bearing areas. Infiltration of the hair follicules with candidal organisms has been observed histologically.[71]

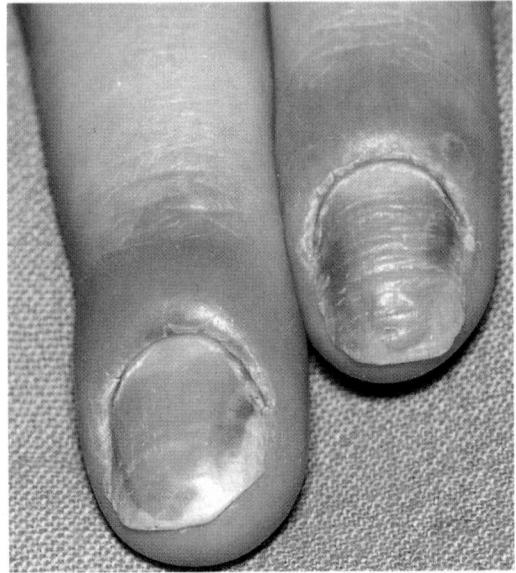
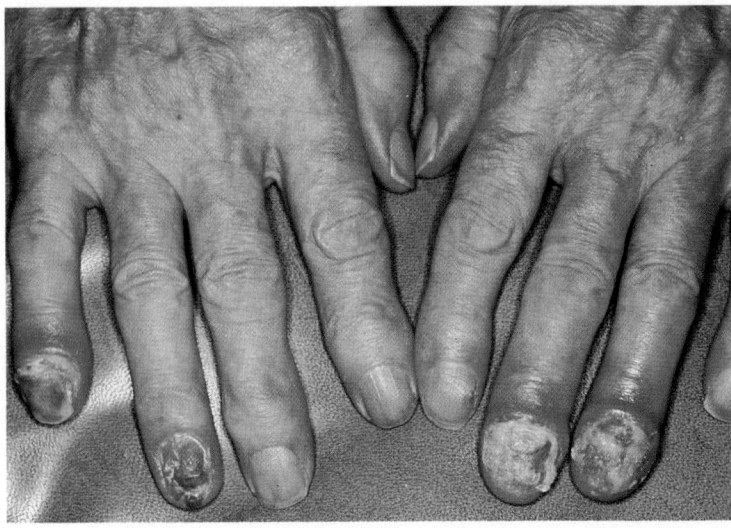

a   *b*

FIGURE 195-4 Chronic onychia and paronychia from *Candida albicans.* (*a*) Note the warm but not hot, slightly tender, edematous nail fold with some onycholysis. This is very often misdiagnosed as staphylococcal paronychia. (*b*) This is a chronic inflammatory condition of the nail fold that can also involve the nail plate.

Chronic Mucocutaneous Candidiasis

Chronic mucocutaneous candidiasis (CMC) is a term used to describe a heterogeneous group of clinical syndromes characterized by chronic, treatment-resistant, superficial candidal infections of the skin, nails, and oropharynx. There is virtually no propensity for disseminated, visceral candidiasis. In many cases there are narrow but specific abnormalities in cell-mediated immunity; in others the defects are more global. The clinical findings and immunologic defects have been extensively reviewed.[72]

Clinical Syndromes   A suitable clinical classification of the major subtypes of CMC was described by Lehner[73] and Wells et al.[74] Table 195-3 provides an updated categorization of these syndromes and a summary of their distinguishing features. In general, the various syndromes may be familial or sporadic in nature. When presenting in childhood, lesions are usually detected before the age of 3 years. Usually oral lesions or diaper dermatitis appear first, followed by angular cheilitis (perlèche), lip fissures, nail and paronychial involvement, vulvovaginitis, and cutaneous involvement. In some cases of CMC, markedly hyperkeratotic, hornlike, or granulomatous lesions may appear (*Candida* granuloma). These heavily crusted lesions may appear on the face, eyelid, scalp, lips,

or acral areas (Fig. 195-5). On the scalp they may resemble the lesions of favus and can lead to alopecia. Other cutaneous lesions may appear atypical for candidiasis and can have erythematous, serpiginous borders[75] or areas of brownish desquamation on a background of mild erythema[76] (Fig. 195-5). Concomitant dermatophyte infection of skin may commonly appear and confuse the clinical presentation.

Nail involvement is characterized by markedly thickened and dystrophic nail plates that are invaded through their entire thickness by *Candida*. The paronychial areas are red and edematous, and the digital tips are often bulbous in appearance (Fig. 195-4).

Conditions that have been associated with CMC include: *Candida* esophagitis or laryngitis,[77,78] endocrinopathies (usually hypoparathyroidism, hypoadrenalism, hypothyroidism),[79] circulating autoimmune antibodies,[80] diabetes mellitus, vitiligo with antibodies to melanocytes,[81] iron deficiency,[82] chronic active hepatitis, pernicious anemia, malabsorption, alopecia totalis, dental enamel dysplasia, keratoconjunctivitis, pulmonary fibrosis, KID syndrome (keratitis, ichthyosis, and deafness),[82] and recurrent pyogenic,[72] viral,[84] or other fungal infections.[85] When CMC first appears in adulthood, it is often associated with a thymoma and the other conditions listed in Table 195-3.[86] Some of these associations are found in only certain clinical subtypes of CMC (e.g., endocrinopa-

TABLE 195-3
Classification of Chronic Mucocutaneous Candidiasis (CMC)

Clinical syndrome	Inheritance	Age of onset	Distribution of lesions	Endocrinology	Associated findings	Notes
Chronic oral candidiasis	Sporadic	Any	Mucosa of tongue, lips, buccal cavity; perlèche; no skin or nail involvement	None	Esophagitis	Denture stomatitis is a variant
Chronic candidiasis with endocrinopathy	Autosomal recessive	Childhood	Mucous membranes, skin, and/or nails	Frequent (hypoadrenalism, hypothyroidism, hypoparathyroidism, or polyendocrinopathy)	Alopecia totalis, thyroiditis, vitiligo, chronic hepatitis, pernicious anemia, gonadal failure, malabsorption, diabetes mellitus	Endocrinopathy may be delayed in onset
Chronic candidiasis without endocrinopathy	Autosomal recessive	Childhood	Mucous membrane, perlèche, and nail involvement; less common skin involvement	None	Blepharitis, esophagitis, laryngitis	
	Autosomal dominant	Childhood		None	Dermatophytosis, loss of teeth, recurrent viral infections	
Chronic localized mucocutaneous candidiasis	Sporadic	Childhood	Mucous membrane, skin, and/or nails	Occasionally	Pulmonary infections, esophagitis	Hyperkeratotic lesions (*Candida*), granuloma
Chronic diffuse candidiasis	Autosomal recessive	Childhood	Widespread mucous membrane, skin, and nail involvement	None		Erythematous, serpiginous skin lesions
		Adolescence	Widespread mucous membrane, skin, and nail involvement	None	History of frequent courses of antibiotics	
Chronic candidiasis with thymoma	Sporadic	Adulthood (after 3rd decade)	Mucous membranes, nails, and skin	None	Thymoma, myasthenia gravis, aplastic anemia, neutropenia, hypogammaglobulinemia	CMC often precedes diagnosis of thymoma

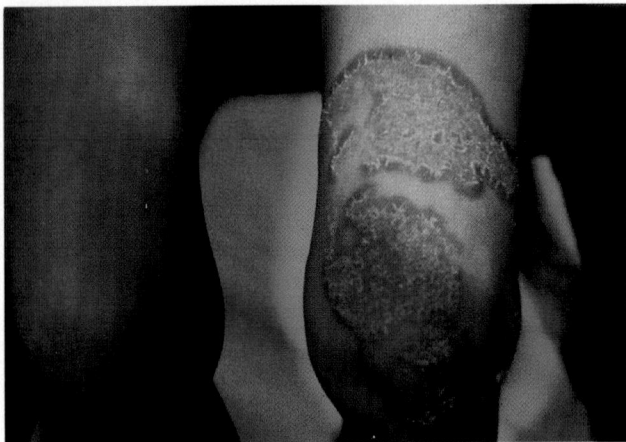

FIGURE 195-5 Mucocutaneous candidiasis. Well-demarcated serpiginous border.

thies); others are observed more broadly (e.g., esophagitis/laryngitis, dermatophytosis).

Immunology Numerous immunologic defects have been described in CMC. These usually involve abnormalities in cell-mediated immunity (CMI), whereas humoral immunity is largely intact. In up to 25 to 30 percent of patients with CMC, however, no immunologic defect can be found.[87] In many cases the CMI defects may reflect a selective deficiency in the recognition and processing of *Candida* while handling of other antigens is intact. The following is a listing of some of the commonly described immunologic abnormalities.[84,87,88]

1. There may be complete anergy to common skin test antigens or selective nonresponsiveness to *C. albicans* antigen. This group can be further divided based on in vitro lymphocyte transformation and lymphokine production studies to *Candida*. In most cases, lymphocyte response to mitogens such as phytohemagglutinin are normal in CMC.
    a. Lymphocyte transformation negative and lymphokine production positive
    b. Lymphocyte transformation positive and lymphokine production negative
    c. Both lymphocyte transformation and lymphokine production negative
2. Selective IgA deficiency
3. Plasma inhibitor to lymphocyte transformation by *C. albicans*[18]
4. Serum inhibitor of polymorphonuclear leukocyte chemotaxis[89] and killing of *C. albicans*[90]
5. Abnormal monocyte chemotactic[91] and killing responses[92]
6. Combined abnormality of monocyte mobility and phagocytosis killing[93]
7. Abnormal complement function[94]
8. Abnormal macrophage function
9. Hyperimmunoglobulinemia E and impaired granulocyte chemotaxis[95]
10. Defective suppressor T-cell function[96]
11. Defective mannan handling by monocytes[97]
12. Impaired generation of helper T cells[98]

In some cases, the observed immunologic defect is reversed after successful antifungal therapy. This suggests that a massive antigenic load (particularly mannan) may interfere with CMI—perhaps by the generation of specific T-suppressor cells.[19]

Cutaneous Candidiasis

There is controversy in the literature about the existence of allergic cutaneous reactions (id reactions) to localized infections with *C. albicans*. Certain recalcitrant cases of erythema annulare centrifugum, chronic urticaria, and groin or hand dermatitis have been attributed to this phenomenon and have cleared with successful therapy of the underlying candidal infection.

Laboratory Findings

Of the more than 80 species of yeast that have been classified in the genus *Candida,* only about 10 have been identified as capable of producing or contributing to disease of humans and animals. Because of the ubiquity of these unicellular organisms in nature and the fact that they are often found as transient colonizers of the skin and appendages of humans, the clinical diagnosis of candidiasis should be confirmed by laboratory tests for identification of the species of yeast involved. In addition to the clinical evaluation of the patient, direct microscopic examination of specimens for the presence of yeast and isolation of yeast in culture are needed for definitive proof of infection. In superficial candidal infections, the diagnosis can be made by performing an examination of skin scrapings and observing typical budding yeasts with hyphae or pseudohyphae. *C. albicans* grows readily on bacterial media, but Sabouraud's agar with added antibiotics is usually recommended for isolation. Whitish, mucoid colonies grow within 2 to 5 days. Of all superficial infections, chronic paronychiae may have the lowest yield of positive cultures.

In systemic candidiasis with skin lesions, the diagnosis can usually be made from histopathologic examination and culture of appropriate skin biopsy specimens. Blood cultures are often negative in this setting.[99] Serologic studies using immunodiffusion, counterimmunoelectrophoresis, and latex agglutination methods may be somewhat helpful in the diagnosis of systemic candidiasis. However, false-negative and false-positive reactions are common. More promising are techniques to detect circulating candidal antigens (e.g., mannan) or metabolic products (e.g., arabinitol).[100] Occasionally, muscle biopsy of symptomatic muscle groups may show organisms histologically.[68]

Microscopic Studies

Because the clinical manifestations of infections caused by species of *Candida* are protean, the type of specimen taken from patients for laboratory examination will vary from body fluids to surgical biopsy. Direct microscopic examination of these specimens for the presence of yeast forms provides rapid evidence in support of the presumptive clinical diagnosis. Body fluids such as urine and cerebrospinal fluid should be centrifuged and the sediment examined. This procedure increases the probability of finding yeasts. Sputum and other viscous secretions along with surgical biopsies and tissue scrapings must be treated with a clearing agent such as 10% potassium hydroxide (KOH) and ink before the material is examined (see Chap. 194). Yeast forms in the genus *Candida* will appear as oval budding cells, elongated filamentous cells connected in a sausage-like manner (pseudohyphae), or as truly septate hyphae (Fig. 195-1). The presence of such forms in clinical material does not permit species identification but does provide evidence that fungi consistent with the morphology of *Candida* are present. Species identification relies on isolation of the yeast in pure culture and biochemical and physiologic tests.

Culture Methods

All clinical specimens should be freshly taken and cultured onto suitable media as rapidly as possible. Sediment from centrifuged body fluids, tissue from biopsies, and scrapings should be inoculated onto Sabouraud's dextrose agar containing antibacterial antibiotics. Cultures are incubated at room temperature (25° to 27°C) and examined periodically for growth of yeast. Negative cultures are discarded after 4 weeks. All colonies of yeast must be subcultured and tested further for identifying morphologic and biochemical characteristics before they can be speciated. Several reference sources are available for speciating yeasts in the genus *Candida*. One excellent procedure is described by Warren and Shadomy in the *Manual of Clinical Microbiology*.[101]

Pathology

Superficial candidiasis is characterized by subcorneal pustules. Organisms are seldom seen within the pustule but can be visualized with the aid of a periodic acid–Schiff (PAS) stain in the stratum corneum. The histology of a candidal granuloma shows marked papillomatosis, hyperkeratosis, and a dense dermal infiltrate consisting of lymphocytes, granulocytes, plasma cells, and multinucleated giant cells. Again, organisms are usually seen only within the stratum corneum.

In systemic candidal infections with skin involvement, biopsies show focal areas in the dermis and within blood vessels where organisms can be identified using PAS or methenamine silver stains. Hematoxylin and eosin staining alone is insufficient. There may be a surrounding mononuclear cell infiltrate,[64] leukocytoclastic vasculitis, or microabscess formation. It may be necessary to do multiple sections through the biopsy material in order to identify the areas of involvement.

Diagnosis

The diagnosis of most superficial cutaneous candidal infections can be made by the typical appearance of the clinical lesions and the presence of satellite vesicopustules. This can be confirmed by KOH examination and culture of skin scrapings. Nevertheless, intertriginous candidiasis can be confused occasionally with tinea infections, eczema, seborrheic dermatitis, intertriginous psoriasis, erythrasma, bacterial intertrigo, familial benign pemphigus, Leiner's disease, glucagonoma, or flexural Darier's disease.

Candidal paronychia should be differentiated from bacterial paronychia or paronychia associated with hypoparathyroidism, celiac disease, acrodermatitis enteropathica, Reiter's syndrome, acrokeratosis paraneoplastica, or retinoid therapy.

Typical oral thrush is characteristic, but the atrophic or ulcerative forms of oral candidiasis can be confused with mucositis due to chemotherapeutic drugs, herpetic infections, erythema multiforme, pemphigus, lichen planus, histoplasmosis, leukoplakia, secondary syphilis, or an aspirin burn. Perlèche-like lesions may be seen in secondary syphilis, avitaminosis (e.g., riboflavin), glucagonoma syndrome, or iron-deficiency states.

The lesions of chronic mucocutaneous candidiasis (CMC) should be differentiated from those of tinea (e.g., favus), bacterial pyoderma, acrodermatitis enteropathica, and halogenoderma. The immunodeficiency states listed in Table 195-2 should be remembered in evaluating patients with widespread CMC.

Papular cutaneous lesions similar to those seen in systemic candidiasis can be confused with *Pityrosporum* folliculitis,[102] bacterial sepsis (e.g., gonococcal, meningococcal, pseudomonal, staphylococcal), and other disseminated fungal infections (e.g., mucormycosis, aspergillosis). Necrotic cutaneous lesions due to *Candida* may appear identical to *Pseudomonas* ecthyma or deep fungal infections (e.g., cryptococcosis, torulopsosis, or sporotrichosis).

Therapy

An important aspect of the treatment of candidiasis is the correction, if possible, of any of the predisposing factors listed in Table 195-2. For example, efforts to prevent chronic occlusion and maceration in cases of candidal intertrigo are particularly important. In systemic candidiasis, removal of potentially colonized intravenous or Foley catheters is the first step in eradication of the organism.

Fortunately, there are a number of antimicrobial agents effective against *Candida*. For oral infections, the most commonly used drugs include nystatin suspension (400,000 to 600,000 units qid) held in the mouth and then swallowed, clotrimazole troches (10 mg dissolved in the mouth five times per day), 1% to 2% gentian violet, or amphotericin B (80 mg/mL) rinses. There is some evidence that the clotrimazole troche regimen is most effective for therapy and prophylaxis of oral candidiasis.[103–105] For infants, clotrimazole 100-mg suppositories can be inserted tightly into the tip of a slit pacifier and the child allowed to suck on this qid.[106] At times, systemic therapy of strictly oral candidiasis is indicated, and ketoconazole, 200 to 400 mg per day orally, is the drug of choice.

Candidal vulvovaginitis is usually treated by one of the topical imidazole creams or tablets (e.g., miconazole, or clotrimazole). The duration of therapy is controversial, but there is evidence to suggest that high-dose, shorter courses of therapy (two 100-mg clotrimazole tablets inserted intravaginally nightly for 3 days) are as effective as the standard 7-day course.[107,108] Ketoconazole, 400 mg orally per day for 3 days, has also been used successfully.[109] For chronically recurrent vaginitis, treatment of concomitant intestinal *Candida* may be helpful (nystatin oral tablets 500,000 units qid for 10 to 14 days).[54,110] Treatment of sexual partner(s) may also be beneficial.[48,49]

Intertriginous and many of the other forms of cutaneous candidiasis (with the exception of CMC) can be treated topically with creams or ointments containing nystatin (see Chap. 194), amphotericin B, or the imidazoles (miconazole, clotrimazole, econazole, ketoconazole, or sulconazole). Powder preparations containing nystatin may be useful in moist, intertriginous areas. The long-held theory that cornstarch application exacerbates candidiasis by providing nutrient support for the organism is probably erroneous.[111]

Chronic paronychial infections due to *C. albicans* are more resistant to therapy. All wet work should be minimized. Topical therapy should be applied to the nail folds and allowed to drain under the proximal nail fold if possible. Occlusion using a finger cot may allow better drug penetration. Of the agents available, haloprogin, clotrimazole, and miconazole solutions are the most helpful. Four percent thymol in chloroform or absolute alcohol has anticandidal activity and is drying. Oral ketoconazole or even surgical marsupialization of the proximal nail fold area has been recommended in resistant cases.

Congenital cutaneous candidiasis, although it usually resolves spontaneously, can be treated with topical nystatin cream. Some authors favor treatment of all such cases in order to prevent subsequent disseminated disease.[112]

In the past, chronic mucocutaneous candidiasis has been notoriously resistant to therapy. 5-Fluorocytosine (50 to 200 mg/kg per day) has yielded excellent results but is limited due to the rapid development of resistance.[113] The mainstay of CMC therapy prior to ketoconazole was parenteral amphotericin B in low dose (15 mg/day) for 3 weeks. This low-dose protocol avoids drug side effects but it requires a 3-week hospitalization.[114]

The addition of ketoconazole to the treatment armamentarium of CMC has dramatically improved disease outcome.[115-117] The usual adult oral dose is 200 to 400 mg per day. It is essential to perform liver function tests before treatment and at monthly intervals, given the chronicity of therapy. Oral lesions usually clear early, followed by cutaneous lesions; nail infections require an average of 9 months of therapy. *C. albicans* isolates resistant to ketoconazole have been reported in CMC patients.[118,119] These isolates were resistant to all imidazole and triazole antifungals.[119]

Immune enhancers may improve the outcome of CMC or prolong clinical remission following reduction of *Candida* antigen load by antifungal therapy.[87] Transfer factor has repeatedly shown an ability to convert negative *Candida* skin tests to positive.[120,121] Other immunomodulating drugs used in the past include thymosin,[122] cimetidine,[123] and levamisole.[114] In any case, relapse is the norm when the treatment is stopped, and life-long therapy may be necessary.

The treatment of choice for systemic candidal infections continues to be parenteral amphotericin B.

"*Pityrosporum* Infections" of the Skin: Papulosquamous Tinea Versicolor, "*Pityrosporum*" Folliculitis, and Inverse Tinea Versicolor

Tinea (pityriasis) versicolor is the most common "*Pityrosporum* infection" of the skin.[124] The disease is seen as a superficial, chronically recurring fungal infection of the stratum corneum characterized by scaly, hypo- or hyperpigmented, irregular macules most often occurring on the trunk and proximal extremities. It is caused by the fungus *Malassezia furfur*, although historically the synonyms *Pityrosporum ovale*, *P. orbiculare*, and *M. ovalis* have been used interchangeably. This organism may also cause a papulopustular ("*Pityrosporum*") folliculitis that resembles the cutaneous lesions of disseminated candidiasis[125] and has been implicated

as a cause of fungal sepsis in patients receiving intravenous alimentation, particularly lipid supplementation therapy.[126] There are data that support the concept that *M. furfur* also contributes to the pathogenesis of seborrheic dermatitis.[127]

History

Tinea versicolor was first recognized as a fungal infection of the skin in 1846 by Eichstedt. For several years the disease was considered to be dermatophyte in origin, but Baillon, impressed by the yeastlike nature of the organism, coined the name *Malasezzia* in 1889 to distinguish this organism from the *Microsporum* species of dermatophytes.[128] Over the intervening years, numerous investigators claimed to have isolated the etiologic agent and suggested various epithets for their isolates, but it was not until 1951 that Gordon isolated, characterized, and authenticated the organism *M. furfur* and renamed it *P. orbiculare*.[129] A great deal of controversy has been voiced concerning the taxonomic relationship of *M. furfur*, *P. orbiculare*, *P. ovale*, and *M. ovalis* in the etiology of tinea versicolor. It is now recognized and accepted that *M. furfur* is the correct name and *P. orbiculare*, *P. ovale*, and *M. ovalis* are synonyms.[130]

Etiology and Pathogenesis

Malassezia furfur can be cultured from clinically apparent disease and normal skin and is considered part of the normal flora of skin.[131] Although *M. furfur* is common in sebum-rich areas of skin and at an age when sebum production is high, no consistent differences in surface lipid composition between patient and controls have been found.[132]

Malassezia furfur is a dimorphic, lipophilic organism that grows in vitro only with the addition of C12- to C24-sized fatty acids to the medium.[133] Under appropriate conditions it converts from the saprophytic yeast to the predominantly parasitic mycelial morphology that is associated with clinical disease. Factors responsible for mycelial transition include a warm, humid environment, an inherited predisposition, endogenous or exogenous Cushing's disease, immunosuppression, or a malnourished state.[124,134,135] There are two species in the genus *Malassezia*: *M. furfur*, which has an obligate nutritional requirement for fatty acids, and *M. pachydermatis*, which can be isolated from clinical material without addition of fatty acids to the medium. Although *M. pachydermatis* has been implicated in cutaneous infections of humans and animals and has also been associated with systemic infections,[136] in contrast to *M. furfur*, it does not have an obligate nutritional requirement for fatty acids and it does not produce hyphae.

In its true sense, tinea versicolor represents an opportunistic infection, although specific deficiencies in antibodies or complement components have not been associated with disease. Experimentally, inoculation of the organism under occlusion can cause infection. The resulting increase in humidity, temperature, and CO_2 tension appear to be important factors that make the skin susceptible to infection. When the occlusive state is terminated, self-healing occurs. The organism is not eradicated from the skin and can be cultured from clinically resolved areas.[137] It may also colonize follicular structures. For these reasons, a high clinical recurrence rate is expected.

Clinical Features

Cutaneous infections with *M. furfur* may take three forms: (1) papulosquamous lesions, (2) folliculitis, and (3) inverse tinea versicolor.

The most common presentation is scaly hypo- or hyperpigmented macules observed in characteristic areas of the body, e.g. chest, back, abdomen, and proximal extremities (Fig. 195-6). Less common areas of involvement include the face, scalp, and genitalia. The characteristic scale is described as dustlike or furfuraceous. This characteristic feature of the disease can be produced by lightly scraping the fingernail over the involved area (the "fingernail sign").[138] The color of the lesions varies from almost white to reddish-brown or fawn-colored. The presenting complaint is usually a cosmetic one as lesions often fail to tan with sun exposure. Pruritus is mild or absent.

The cause of hypopigmentation is unclear (Fig. 195-6b). Ultrastructural studies have shown an abnormality of melanosome number and packaging, with hypopigmented areas demonstrating a decreased number of individually dispersed melanosomes.[139] Extracts from *M. furfur* cultures contain C9–C11 dicarboxylic acids that may competitively inhibit tyrosinase.[140] In dark-complexioned children, a severe, rapidly spreading variant may occur (achromia parasiticus). Lesions usually begin in the diaper area and are markedly hypopigmented.[135]

Pityrosporum folliculitis is a well-recognized and often misdiagnosed clinical entity[141] (Fig. 195-7a). Lesions typically appear on the back, chest, and sometimes on the extremities. Pruritus is more common than with typical tinea versicolor. The primary lesion is a perifollicular, erythematous, 2- to 3-mm papule or pustule. Only by appropriate culture and KOH examination can it be distinguished from a bacterial folliculitis. Frequently, biopsy with special stains for fungus is necessary (Fig. 195-7b). Diabetes mellitus or prior corticosteroid or antibiotic therapy can predispose one to this disorder.[142]

Inverse tinea versicolor refers to clinical disease located predominantly in flexural areas.[143] In this location, lesions can be confused with seborrheic dermatitis, psoriasis, erythrasma, candidiasis, and dermatophyte infections.

Rarely, *M. furfur* can infect organs other than the skin. A premature infant on total parenteral nutrition with intravenous lipid supplementation has been reported who showed no skin lesions but had an extensive vasculitis of small pulmonary arteries and bronchopneumonia.[126] *Malassezia furfur* organisms were seen microscopically in areas of lipid deposition. The organism has been cultured from peritoneal dialysate, blood, and with increasing frequency in patients receiving parenteral intralipid supplementation.[144] Presumably, intravenous lipid supplementation provides an appropriate culture medium for *M. furfur*.

All of the cutaneous clinical variants have an equal sex distribution and tend to flare during warm weather. Late adolescent and early adult age groups are predominantly affected. Small children and elderly adults are infected only in unusual circumstances such as prolonged occlusion or immunosuppression.[143,145]

Immunology

Immunologic data are scarce in tinea versicolor. No specific deficiencies in antibodies or complement components have been associated with disease. Elevated specific antibody is seen in patients and also in age-matched normal controls.[146] Furthermore, Sohnle

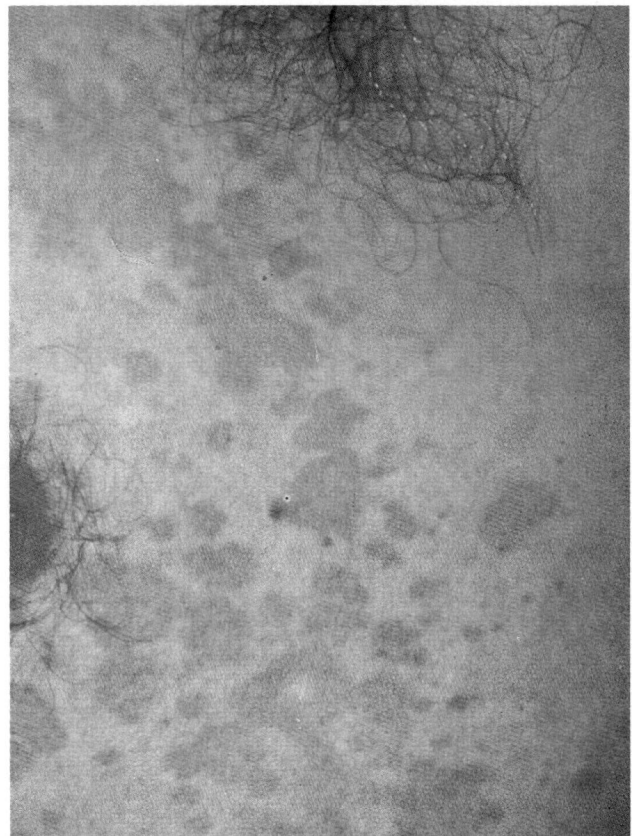

a

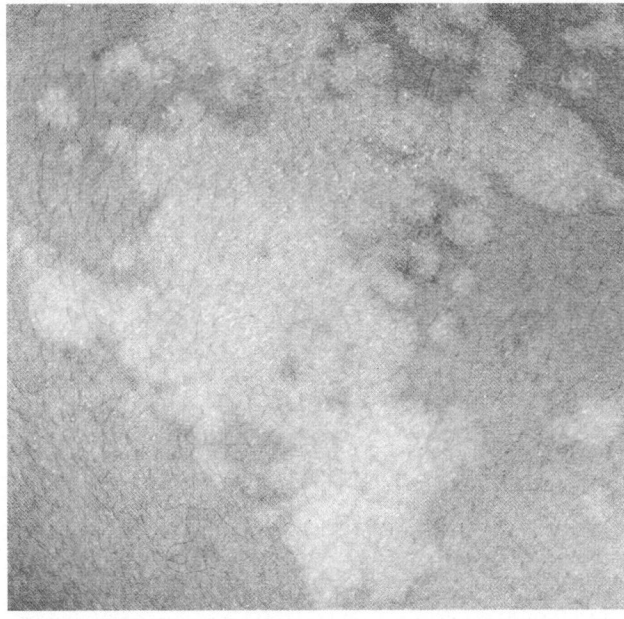

b

FIGURE 195-6 (*a*) Pityriasis versicolor. These lesions are darker because of hyperemia secondary to inflammatory response and increase in melaninization. (*b*) Tinea versicolor. There are sharply marginated uniformly hypopigmented macules with a fine, sometimes barely perceptible scale, but they are easily scraped off with a microscopic slide. When the lesions are very large, as on the left, they can be confused with vitiligo.

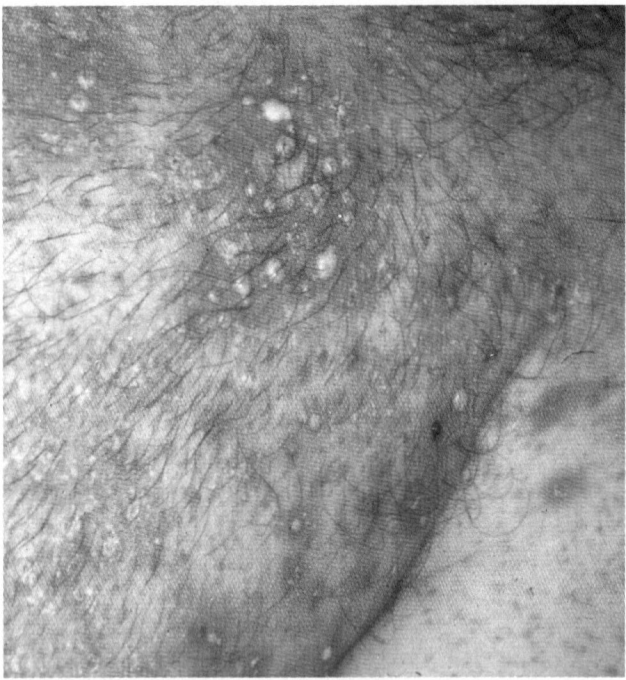

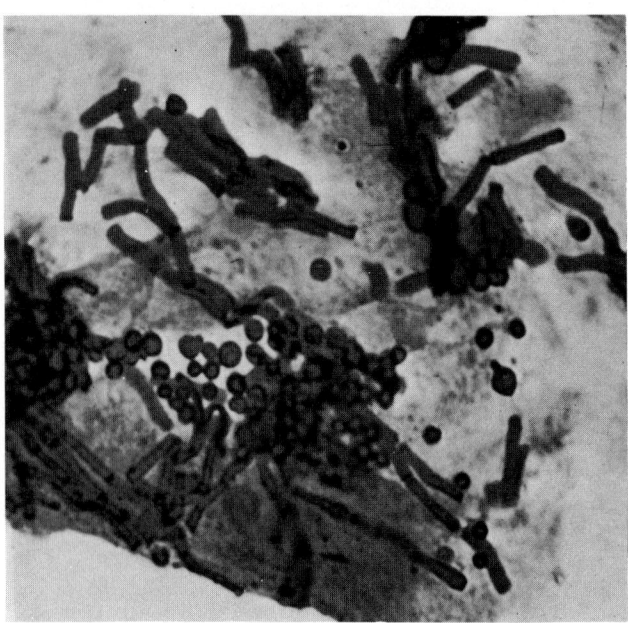

FIGURE 195-8 "Spaghetti and meatballs" appearance of tinea versicolor on KOH examination.

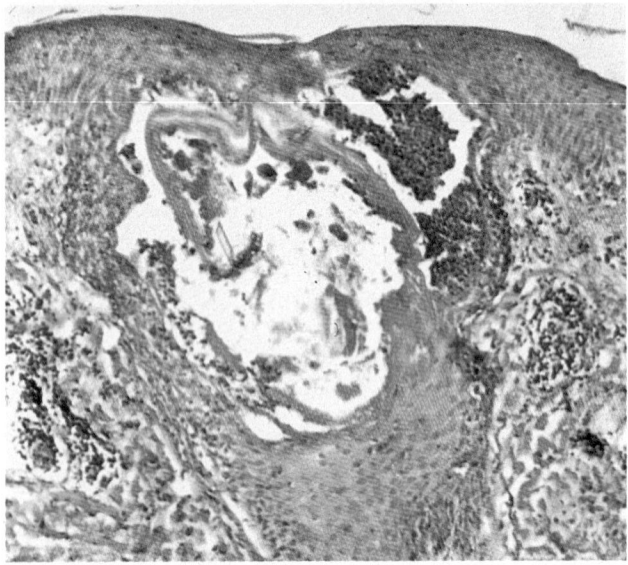

b

FIGURE 195-7 (*a* and *b*) Pityrosporum folliculitis on the anterior chest. Note the organisms in the follicular ostia on H&E.

and Collins-Lech have shown that *M. furfur* induces IgA, IgG, and IgM antibodies, and that it also activates complement through the alternative and classical pathways.[147] A defect in lymphokine production by patients with chronic tinea versicolor has been demonstrated, but the role that these and other immunologic factors play in the disease process in unknown.[148]

Laboratory Findings

The organism is readily identified in clinical material by treating specimens with 10% potassium hydroxide (KOH). Alternatively,

cellophane tape can be used to pick up skin scales from the lesion. The tape is mounted on a glass slide with methylene blue, and the organism is selectively stained.[149] Microscopically, grapelike clusters of yeasts (4 to 6 μm) and short, septate branching hyphal fragments are seen (Fig. 195-8). Cultures are not necessary for diagnosis because of the characteristic "spaghetti and meatballs" appearance of the yeast and hyphal elements seen on microscopic examination of clinical material. A Wood's lamp examination may show yellowish fluorescence of involved skin.

Pathology

In tinea versicolor, the organisms are seen in the stratum corneum. They may be observed with H&E stain alone. Periodic acid–Schiff (PAS) staining is confirmatory. There is usually no dermal infiltrate. In *Pityrosporum* folliculitis, organisms are noted in widened follicular ostia admixed with keratinous material (Fig. 195-7*b*). Rupture of the follicular wall can occur with a resulting mixed inflammatory cell and foreign-body giant cell response. Organisms can occasionally be identified in the perifollicular dermis.

Diagnosis

The clinical appearance of tinea versicolor is usually characteristic, and KOH examination is confirmatory. Occasionally, pityriasis alba, confluent and reticulated papillomatosis of Gougerot and Carteaud, pityriasis rosea, seborrheic dermatitis, vitiligo, or secondary syphilis can enter the differential diagnosis.

For the folliculitis variant, bacterial or candidal folliculitis should be considered. The skin lesions of disseminated candidiasis can sometimes be confused with *Pityrosporum* folliculitis.[125]

Treatment

There are multiple topical products that are useful in treating tinea versicolor. The most widely used has been 2.5% selenium sulfide lotion. This can be applied on a variety of schedules. We prefer to apply it liberally over and beyond the affected areas. This is left on for 5 to 10 min and then washed off. The cycle is repeated every day for 2 weeks. Subsequently, we recommend applying the drug once or twice per month to prevent recurrence. Other topical agents that have been used include miconazole 2%, clotrimazole 1%, tolnaftate, 25% sodium thiosulfate, sulfur-salicylic acid soaps or shampoos (Sebulex),[150] or keratolytic agents such as 50% propylene glycol.[151]

Griseofulvin is not helpful in this condition, but ketoconazole has been used successfully.[152] It is not necessary to give ketoconazole for the usual case of tinea versicolor. However, the drug may be useful prophylactically in a dose of 200 to 400 mg once or twice a month.[153]

Course and Prognosis

Tinea versicolor is often recurrent. Prophylactic measures, as discussed above, and fastidious cleanliness may lessen the risk of recurrence.

Mycology

Sabouraud's dextrose agar overlayed on the surface with sterile olive oil or lanolin readily supports the growth of this lipophilic, yeastlike organism. Antibiotics such as penicillin, streptomycin, and cycloheximide are incorporated into this medium when primary clinical specimens are cultured to reduce growth of contaminating organisms. Microscopic examination reveals oval budding yeast cells ~3.5 × 4.5 μm along with short, septate, and occasionally branching hyphae (Fig. 195-8). In general, cultures are not necessary for diagnosis as the organism can be demonstrated with 10% KOH.

References

1. Rippon JW: Candidiasis and the pathogenic yeasts, in *Medical Mycology: The Pathogenic Fungi and the Pathogenic Actinomycetes,* 3d ed. Philadelphia, Saunders, 1988, p 532

2. Hopfer RL: Mycology of *Candida* infections, in *Candidiasis,* edited by GP Bodey, V Fainstein. New York, Raven, 1985, p 1

3. Smith CB: Candidiasis: Pathogenesis, host resistance, and predisposing factors, in *Candidiasis,* edited by GP Bodey, V Fainstein. New York, Raven, 1985, p 53

4. Ray TL, Wuepper KD: Recent advances in cutaneous candidiasis. *Int J Dermatol* 17:683, 1978

5. Ray TL et al: Experimental cutaneous candidiasis: Role of the stratum corneum. *Clin Res* 24:495A, 1976

6. Maibach HI, Kligman AM: The biology of experimental human cutaneous moniliasis (*Candida albicans*). *Arch Dermatol* 85:233, 1962

7. King RD et al: Adherence of *Candida albicans* and other *Candida* species to mucosal epithelial cells. *Infect Immun* 27:667, 1980

8. Kapica L, Blank F: Growth of *Candida albicans* on keratin as sole source of nitrogen. *Dermatologica* 115:81, 1957

9. Pugh D, Cawson RA: The cytochemical localization of phospholipase A and lysophospholipase in *Candida albicans. Sabouraudia* 13:110, 1975

10. Staib F: Proteolysis and pathogenicity of *Candida albicans* strains. *Mycopathologia* 37:345, 1969

11. Scherwitz C: Ultrastructure of human cutaneous candidosis. *J Invest Dermatol* 78:200, 1982

12. Montes LF, Wilborn WH: Fungus-host relationship in candidiasis: A brief review. *Arch Dermatol* 121:119, 1985

13. Rebora A et al: Experimental infection with *Candida albicans. Arch Dermatol* 108:69, 1973

14. Ray TL et al: Purification of a mannan from *Candida albicans* which activates serum complement. *J Invest Dermatol* 73:269, 1979

15. Chesney RW et al: *Candida* endocrinopathy syndrome with membranoproliferative glomerulonephritis: Demonstration of glomerular *Candida* antigen. *Clin Nephrol* 5:232, 1976

16. Diamond RD et al: Properties of a product of *Candida albicans* hyphae and pseudohyphae that inhibits contact between the fungi and human neutrophils *in vitro. J Immunol* 125:2797, 1980

17. Piccolella E et al: Generation of suppressor cells in the response of human lymphocytes to a polysaccharide from *Candida albicans. J Immunol* 126:2151, 1981

18. Fischer A et al: Specific inhibition of in vitro *Candida* induced lymphocyte proliferation by polysaccharidic antigens present in the serum of patients with chronic mucocutaneous candidiasis. *J Clin Invest* 62:1005, 1978

19. Rogers TJ, Balish E: Immunity to *Candida albicans. Microbiol Rev* 44:660, 1980

20. Ray TL: Candidosis, in *Dermatologic Immunology and Allergy,* edited by J Stone. St Louis, Mosby, 1985, p 511

21. Sohnle PG, Kirkpatrick CH: Epidermal proliferation in the defense against experimental cutaneous candidiasis. *J Invest Dermatol* 70:130, 1978

22. Louria DB: *Candida* infections in experimental animals, in *Candidiasis,* edited by GP Bodey, V Fainstein. New York, Raven, 1985, p 29

23. Ray TL, Wuepper KD: Experimental cutaneous candidiasis in rodents. II. Role of the stratum corneum barrier and serum complement as a mediator of a protective inflammatory response. *Arch Dermatol* 114:539, 1978

24. Solomkin JS et al: Phagocytosis of *Candida albicans* by human leukocytes: Opsonic requirements. *J Infect Dis* 137:30, 1978

25. Wilton JMA et al: The role of F_c and $C3_b$ receptors in phagocytosis by inflammatory polymorphonuclear leukocytes in man. *Immunology* 32:955, 1977

26. Diamond RD et al: Damage to pseudohyphae forms of *Candida albicans* by neutrophils in the absence of serum in vitro. *J Clin Invest* 61:349, 1978

27. Louria DB, Brayton RG: A substance in blood lethal for *Candida albicans. Nature* 201:309, 1964

28. Lehrer RT, Cline MJ: Interaction of *Candida albicans* with human leukocytes and serum. *J Bacteriol* 98:996, 1969

29. Caroline L et al: Reversal of serum fungistasis by addition of iron. *J Invest Dermatol* 42:415, 1964

30. Boxer LA et al: Lactoferrin deficiency associated with altered granulocyte function. *N Engl J Med* 307:404, 1982

31. Pearsall N et al: Immunologic responses to *Candida albicans*. III. Effects of passive transfer of lymphoid cells or serums on murine candidiasis. *J Immunol* 120:1176, 1978

32. Mourad S, Friedman L: Passive immunization of mice against *Candida albicans. Sabouraudia* 6:103, 1968

33. Epstein JB et al: Oral candidiasis: Pathogenesis and host defense. *Rev Infect Dis* 6:96, 1984

34. Dreizen S: Oral candidiasis. *Am J Med* 77(4D):28, 1984

35. Tapper-Jones LM et al: Candidal infections and populations of *Candida albicans* in mouths of diabetics. *J Clin Pathol* 34:706, 1981

36. Pingleton WW: Oropharyngeal candidiasis in patients treated with triamcinolone acetonide aerosol. *J Allergy Clin Immunol* 60:254, 1977

37. Nyquist G: A study of denture sore mouth: An investigation of traumatic, allergic and toxic lesions of the oral mucosa arising from the use of full dentures. *Acta Odontol Scand* 10(suppl 9):II, 1952

38. Budtz-Jorgensen E et al: An epidemiologic study of yeasts in elderly denture wearers. *Community Dent Oral Epidemiol* 3:115, 1975

39. Odds FC: Candidiasis of the oropharynx, in *Candida and Candidosis.* Baltimore, University Park Press, 1979, p 83

40. Chernosky ME: Relationship between vertical facial dimension and perlèche. *Arch Dermatol* **93**:332, 1966

41. Jansen GT et al: *Candida* cheilitis. *Arch Dermatol* **88**:325, 1963

42. McCarthy PL, Shklar G: *Diseases of the Oral Mucosa.* Philadelphia, Lea & Febiger, 1980, p 88

43. Coohe BED: Median rhomboid glossitis: Candidiasis and not a developmental anomaly. *Br J Dermatol* **93**:399, 1975

44. Maksymiuk AW et al: Systemic candidiasis in cancer patients. *Am J Med* **77**(suppl):20, 1984

45. Bodey GP: Candidiasis in cancer patients. *Am J Med* **77**(suppl):13, 1984

46. Klein RS et al: Oral candidiasis in high risk patients as the initial manifestation of the acquired immune deficiency syndrome. *N Engl J Med* **311**:354, 1984

47. Odds FC: Ecology and epidemiology of *Candida*, in *Candida and Candidosis*. Baltimore, University Park Press, 1979, p 50

48. Sobel JD: Vulvovaginal candidiasis—what we do and do not know. *Ann Intern Med* **101**:390, 1984

49. Odds FC: Genital candidosis. *Clin Exp Dermatol* **7**:345, 1982

50. Meech RJ et al: Pathogenic mechanisms in recurrent genital candidosis in women. *N Z Med J* **98**:1, 1985

51. Waugh MA: Clinical presentation of candidal balanitis—its differential diagnosis and treatment. *Chemotherapy* **28**(suppl 1):56, 1982

52. Catterall RD: *Candida albicans* and the contraceptive pill. *Lancet* **2**:830, 1966

53. Rebora A, Leyden JJ: Napkin (diaper) dermatitis and gastrointestinal carriage of *Candida albicans*. *Br J Dermatol* **105**:551, 1981

54. Jorizzo JL: The spectrum of mucosal and cutaneous candidosis. *Dermatologic Clinics* **2**:19, 1984

55. Bradford LG, Montes LF: Perioral dermatitis and *Candida albicans*. *Arch Dermatol* **105**:892, 1972

56. Brandrup F et al: Perioral pustular eruption caused by *Candida albicans*. *Br J Dermatol* **105**:327, 1981

57. Zaias N: Onychomycosis. *Dermatologic Clinics* **3**:445, 1985

58. Delaplane D et al: Congenital mucocutaneous candidiasis following diagnostic amniocentesis. *Am J Obstet Gynecol* **147**:342, 1983

59. Chapel TA et al: Congenital cutaneous candidiasis. *J Am Acad Dermatol* **6**:926, 1982

60. Bodey GP: Candidiasis in cancer patients. *Am J Med* **77**(4D):13, 1984

61. Bodey GP, Fainstein V: Systemic candidiasis, in *Candidiasis,* edited by GP Bodey, V Fainstein. New York, Raven, 1985, p 135

62. Hughes WT: Systemic candidiasis: A study of 109 fatal cases. *Pediatr Infect Dis* **1**:11, 1982

63. Edwards JE et al: Ocular manifestations of *Candida* septicemia: Review of seventy-six cases of hematogenous *Candida* endophthalmitis. *Medicine* **53**:47, 1974

64. Bodey GP, Luna M: Skin lesions associated with disseminated candidiasis. *JAMA* **229**:1466, 1974

65. Bodey GP: Fungal infections complicating acute leukemia. *J Chronic Dis* **19**:667, 1966

66. Grossman ME et al: Cutaneous manifestations of disseminated candidiasis. *J Am Acad Dermatol* **2**:111, 1980

67. Jarowski Cl et al: Fever, rash, and muscle tenderness: A distinctive clinical presentation of disseminated candidiasis. *Arch Intern Med* **138**:544, 1978

68. Kressel B et al: Early clinical recognition of disseminated candidiasis by muscle and skin biopsy. *Arch Intern Med* **138**:429, 1978

69. File TM et al: Necrotic skin lesions associated with disseminated candidiasis. *Arch Dermatol* **115**:214, 1979

70. Fine JD et al: Cutaneous lesions in disseminated candidiasis mimicking ecthyma gangrenosum. *Am J Med* **70**:1133, 1981

71. Collingnon PJ, Sorrell TC: Disseminated candidiasis: Evidence of a distinctive syndrome in heroin abusers. *Br Med J* **287**:861, 1983

72. Kirkpatrick CH, Sohnle PG: Chronic mucocutaneous candidiasis, in *Immunodermatology,* edited by B Safai, RA Good. New York, Plenum, 1981, p 495

73. Lehner T: Classification and clinicopathological features of *Candida* infections of the mouth, in *Symposium on Candida Infections,* edited by HI Winner, R Hurley. Baltimore, Williams & Wilkins, 1966, p 119

74. Wells RS et al: Familial chronic mucocutaneous candidiasis. *J Med Genet* **9**:302, 1972

75. Kirkpatrick CH: Host factors in defense against fungal infections. *Am J Med* **77**(4D):1, 1984

76. Odds FC: Chronic mucocutaneous candidosis, in *Candida and Candidosis*. Baltimore, University Park Press, 1979, p 121

77. Dudley JP et al: *Candida* laryngitis in chronic mucocutaneous candidiasis: Its association with *Candida* esophagitis. *Ann Otol Rhinol Laryngol* **89**:574, 1980

78. Kobayashi RH et al: *Candida* esophagitis and laryngitis in chronic mucocutaneous candidiasis. *Pediatrics* **66**:380, 1980

79. Price ML, MacDonald DM: *Candida* endocrinopathy syndrome. *Clin Exp Dermatol* **9**:105, 1984

80. Zouali M et al: Evaluation of auto-antibodies in chronic mucocutaneous candidiasis without endocrinopathy. *Mycopathologia* **84**:87, 1983/1984

81. Howanitz N et al: Antibodies to melanocytes: Occurrence in patients with vitiligo and chronic mucocutaneous candidiasis. *Arch Dermatol* **117**:705, 1981

82. Higgs JM, Wells RS: Chronic mucocutaneous candidiasis: Associated abnormalities of iron metabolism. *Br J Dermatol* **86**(suppl 8):88, 1972

83. Harms M et al: KID syndrome (keratitis, ichthyosis, and deafness) and chronic mucocutaneous candidiasis: Case report and review of the literature. *Pediatr Dermatol* **2**:1, 1984

84. Sams WM et al: Chronic mucocutaneous candidiasis: Immunologic studies of three generations of a single family. *Am J Med* **67**:948, 1979

85. Chipps BE et al: Non-candidal infections in children with chronic mucocutaneous candidiasis. *John Hopkins Med J* **144**:179, 1979

86. Kirkpatrick CH, Windhorst DB: Mucocutaneous candidiasis and thymoma. *Am J Med* **66**:939, 1979

87. Jorizzo JL: Chronic mucocutaneous candidosis: An update. *Arch Dermatol* **118**:963, 1982

88. Valdimarsson H et al: Immune abnormalities associated with chronic mucocutaneous candidiasis. *Cell Immunol* **6**:348, 1973

89. Cates KL et al: Cell-directed inhibition of polymorphonuclear leukocyte chemotaxis in a patient with mucocutaneous candidiasis. *J Allergy Clin Immunol* **65**:431, 1980

90. Walker SM, Urbaniak SJ: A serum-dependent defect of neutrophil function in chronic mucocutaneous candidiasis. *J Clin Pathol* **33**:370, 1980

91. Synderman R et al: Defective mononuclear leukocyte chemotaxis: A previously unrecognized immune dysfunction. *Ann Intern Med* **78**:509, 1973

92. Bortolussi R et al: Phagocytosis of *Candida albicans* in chronic mucocutaneous candidiasis. *Pediatr Res* **15**:1287, 1981

93. Yamazaki M et al: A monocyte disorder in siblings with chronic candidiasis. *Am J Dis Child* **138**:192, 1984

94. Drew JH: Chronic mucocutaneous candidiasis with abnormal function of serum complement. *Med J Aust* **2**:77, 1973

95. Van Scoy RE et al: Familial neutrophil chemotaxis defect, recurrent bacterial infections, mucocutaneous candidiasis, and hyperimmunoglobulinemia E. *Ann Intern Med* **82**:766, 1975

96. Arulanantham K et al: Evidence for defective immunoregulation in the syndrome of familial candidiasis endocrinopathy. *N Engl J Med* **300**:164, 1979

97. Fischer A et al: Defective handling of mannan by monocytes in patients with chronic mucucutaneous candidiasis resulting in a specific cellular unresponsiveness. *Clin Exp Immunol* **47**:653, 1982

98. Ruiz-Arguelles A et al: Impaired generation of helper T cells in a patient with chronic mucocutaneous candidiasis and malignant thymoma. *J Clin Lab Immunol* **10**:165, 1983

99. Myerowitz RL et al: Disseminated candidiasis: Changes in inci-

dence, underlying diseases, and pathology. *Am J Clin Pathol* **68**:29, 1977

100. Penn RL et al: Invasive fungal infections: The use of serologic tests in diagnosis and management. *Arch Intern Med* **143**:1215, 1983

101. Warren NA, Shadomy HJ: Yeasts of medical importance, in *Manual of Clinical Microbiology,* 5th ed, edited by EH Lennette et al. Washington, DC, American Society for Microbiology, 1991, p 617

102. Klotz SA et al: *Pityrosporum* folliculitis: Its potential for confusion with skin lesions of systemic candidiasis. *Arch Intern Med* **142**:2126, 1982

103. DeGregorio MW et al: *Candida* infections in patients with acute leukemia: Ineffectiveness of nystatin prophylaxis and relationship between oropharyngeal and systemic candidiasis. *Cancer* **50**:2780, 1982

104. Quintiliani R et al: Treatment and prevention of oropharyngeal candidiasis. *Am J Med* **77**(40):44, 1984

105. Owens NJ et al: Prophylaxis of oral candidiasis with clotrimazole troches. *Arch Intern Med* **144**:290, 1984

106. Mansour A, Gelfand EW: A new approach to the use of antifungal agents in infants with persistent oral candidiasis. *Pediatrics* **98**:161, 1981

107. Robertson WH: A concentrated therapeutic regimen for vulvovaginal candidiasis. *JAMA* **244**:2549, 1980

108. Masterton G et al: Three-day clotrimazole treatment in candidal vulvovaginitis. *Br J Vener Dis* **53**:126, 1977

109. Fregoso-Duenas F: Ketoconazole in vulvovaginal candidosis. *Rev Infect Dis* **2**:620, 1980

110. Miles MR et al: Recurrent vaginal candidiasis: Importance of an intestinal reservoir. *JAMA* **238**:1836, 1977

111. Leyden JJ: Corn starch, *Candida albicans,* and diaper rash. *Pediatr Dermatol* **1**:322, 1984

112. Johnson DE et al: Congenital candidiasis. *Am J Dis Child* **135**:273, 1981

113. Lin C-Y: Treatment of chronic mucocutaneous candidiasis with 5-fluorocytosine. *Ann Allergy* **49**:298, 1982

114. Hay RJ: Management of chronic mucocutaneous candidosis. *Clin Exp Dermatol* **6**:515, 1981

115. Drouhet E, Dupont B: Chronic mucocutaneous candidosis and other superficial and systemic mucoses successfully treated with ketoconazole. *Rev Infect Dis* **2**:606, 1980

116. Petersen EA et al: Treatment of chronic mucocutaneous candidiasis with ketoconazole: A controlled clinical trial. *Ann Intern Med* **93**:791, 1980

117. Hay RJ et al: Treatment of chronic mucocutaneous candidosis with ketoconazole: A study of 12 cases. *Rev Infect Dis* **2**:600, 1980

118. Horsburgh CR, Kirkpatrick CH: Long-term therapy of chronic mucocutaneous candidiasis with ketoconazole: Experience with twenty-one patients. *Am J Med* **74**(suppl 1B):23, 1983

119. Smith KJ et al: Azole resistance in *Candida albicans. J Med Vet Mycol* **24**:133, 1986

120. Littman BH et al: Transfer factor treatment of chronic mucocutaneous candidiasis: Requirement for donor reactivity to *Candida* antigen. *Clin Immunol Immunopathol* **9**:97, 1978

121. Horsmanheimo M et al: Immunologic features of chronic mucocutaneous candidiasis before and after treatment with transfer factor. *Arch Dermatol* **115**:180, 1979

122. Akhter J et al: Effect of thymosin on lymphocytes from patients with chronic mucocutaneous candidiasis and endocrinopathies. *J Allergy Clin Immunol* **65**:34, 1980

123. Jorizzo JL et al: Cimetidine as an immunomodulator: Chronic mucocutaneous candidiasis as a model. *Ann Intern Med* **92**:192, 1980

124. Roberts SOB: Pityriasis versicolor: A clinical and mycological investigation. *Br J Dermatol* **81**:315, 1969

125. Klotz SA et al: *Pityrosporum* folliculitis: Its potential for confusion with skin lesions of systemic candidiasis. *Arch Intern Med* **142**:2126, 1982

126. Redline RW, Dahms BB: *Malassezia* pulmonary vasculitis in an infant on long-term intralipid therapy. *N Engl J Med* **305**:1395, 1981

127. Heng MC et al: Correlation of *Pityrosporum ovale* density with clinical severity of seborrheic dermatitis as assessed by a simplified technique. *J Am Acad Dermatol* **23**:82, 1990

128. Baillon H: *Traite de Botanique Medical Cryptoganique.* Paris, Octave Doin Editeur, 1889, p 234

129. Gordon M: Lipophilic yeast-like organisms associated with tinea versicolor. *J Invest Dermatol* **17**:267, 1951

130. Tanaka M, Imamura S: Immunological studies on *Pityrosporum* genus and *Malassezia furfur. J Invest Dermatol* **73**:321, 1979

131. Roberts SOB: *Pityrosporum orbiculare:* Incidence and distribution on clinically normal skin. *Br J Dermatol* **81**:264, 1969

132. Catterall MB: Tinea versicolor: A reappraisal. *Int J Dermatol* **19**:84, 1980

133. Porro MN et al: Growth requirements and lipid metabolism of *Pityrosporum orbiculare. J Invest Dermatol* **66**:178, 1976

134. Burke RC: Tinea versicolor: Susceptibility factors and experimental infection in human beings. *J Invest Dermatol* **36**:389, 1961

135. Rippon JW: Superficial infections: Pityriasis versicolor, in *Medical Mycology: The Pathogenic Fungi and the Pathogenic Actinomycetes,* 3d ed. Philadelphia, Saunders, 1988, p 154

136. Gueho E et al: Association of *Malassezia pachydermatis* with systemic infections of humans. *J Clin Microbiol* **25**:1789, 1987

137. Faergemann J: Experimental tinea versicolor in rabbits and humans with *Pityrosporum orbiculare. J Invest Dermatol* **72**:326, 1979

138. Dahl MV: *Common Office Dermatology.* New York, Grune & Stratton, 1983, p 35

139. Karaoui R et al: Tinea versicolor: Ultrastructural studies on hypopigmented and hyperpigmented skin. *Dermatologica* **162**:69, 1981

140. Nazzaro-Porro M, Passi S: Identification of tyrosinase inhibitors in cultures of *Pityrosporum. J Invest Dermatol* **71**:205, 1978

141. Potter BS et al: *Pityrosporum* folliculitis: Report of seven cases and review of the *Pityrosporum* organism relative to cutaneous disease. *Arch Dermatol* **107**:388, 1973

142. Berretty PJM et al: *Pityrosporum* folliculitis: Is it a real entity? *Br J Dermatol* **103**:565, 1980

143. Burkhart CG et al: An unusual case of tinea versicolor in an immunosuppressed patient. *Cutis* **27**:56, 1981

144. Wallace M et al: Isolation of lipophilic yeast in "sterile" peritonitis. *Lancet* **2**:956, 1979

145. Klotz SA: *Malassezia furfur. Infect Dis Clin North Am* **3**:53, 1989

146. DaMert GJ et al: Comparison of antibody responses in chronic mucocutaneous candidiasis and tinea versicolor. *Int Arch Allergy Appl Immunol* **63**:97, 1980

147. Sohnle RG, Collins-Lech C: Activation of complement by *Pityrosporum orbiculare. J Invest Dermatol* **80**:93, 1983

148. Sohnle RG, Collins-Lech C: Cell-mediated immunology to *Pityrosporum orbiculare* in tinea versicolor. *J Clin Invest* **62**:45, 1978

149. Popkess FG: A practical office method for the diagnosis of tinea versicolor. *Ann Allergy* **22**:42, 1964

150. Bamford JTM: Treatment of tinea versicolor with sulfur-salicylic shampoo. *J Am Acad Dermatol* **8**:211, 1983

151. Faergemann J, Fredricksson T: Propylene glycol in the treatment of tinea versicolor. *Acta Derm Venereol (Stockh)* **60**:92, 1980

152. Urcuyo FG, Zaias N: The successful treatment of pityriasis versicolor by systemic ketoconazole. *J Am Acad Dermatol* **6**:24, 1982

153. Borelli D: Treatment of pityriasis versicolor with ketoconazole. *Rev Infect Dis* **2**:592, 1980

CHAPTER 196

H. Jean Shadomy and John P. Utz

Deep Fungal Infections

With the increase in immunocompromised individuals in our population, especially those with AIDS (acquired immunodeficiency syndrome), more cases of fungal infection are being identified. Deep fungal infections are being seen to a greater extent in these patients, and skin manifestations of these infections are also on the rise.

The skin lesions seen in the systemic mycoses are, with the exception of mycetoma and perhaps sporotrichosis, acquired by the hematogenous route, rather than from direct implantation in the skin. The portal of entry is generally the respiratory tract, and a focus of infection is established in the lung. The infection may be accompanied by a spectrum of disease ranging from inapparent infection to severe, fulminant, and inexorably fatal disease. The factors responsible for the severity of disease are known in part and include the size of inoculum and predisposing factors such as immunocompetency, diabetes mellitus, Hodgkin's disease, and corticosteroid and immunosuppressive therapy. The spread of disease, characteristically hematogenous, from the focus of infection in the lung is to remote organs in patterns that are distinctive for each disease. Skin involvement is most common in blastomycosis and sporotrichosis, and these diseases are readily suspected from inspection of the lesions. Somewhat less characteristic lesions are important features in coccidioidomycosis, cryptococcosis, and in some cases of actinomycosis. Skin lesions seen in patients with AIDS may be unusual, even resembling lesions characteristic of other diseases.[1] Infection and recovery from illness are generally marked by a solid immunity. Factors responsible for this are not fully known, but circulating antibodies and cell-mediated (delayed cutaneous hypersensitivity) factors have been described for almost all infections. Contagious spread from person to person, from patient to hospital staff, or from animals to humans is not known to occur. Several systemic antimicrobial agents are useful for virtually all these diseases.

Actinomycosis

Although actinomycosis, nocardiosis, and one type of mycetoma are not caused by fungi, but rather by "higher bacteria," and treatment, therefore, is different from that of true fungi, these organisms traditionally have been placed with fungi and fungal infections, and the diseases they cause must be differentiated from fungal disease. Therefore, we have continued to place these three groups with the fungi in this chapter.

Actinomycosis is a chronic infectious disease of the cervicofacial area, thorax, or abdomen, caused by the anaerobic, grampositive bacterium *Actinomyces israelii*, a commensal of humans, characterized pathologically by a suppurative, fibrous inflammation that spreads directly to contiguous tissue. Lumpy jaw, a similar infection occurring in cattle, is caused by a related organism, *A. bovis*. Actinomycosis, usually caused by other species of *Actinomyces*, also has been reported in dogs, cats, horses, swine, goats, sheep, and other animals. It generally is caused by traumatic intrusion of the organism into tissue via plant material, broken teeth, etc. It has also been associated with intrauterine contraceptive devices.

Historical Aspects

In 1877, Bollinger[2] described the disease in cattle, and in 1878, Israel[3] reported infection in humans. In 1889, Bujwid first cultured the microorganism, and in that same year Wolf and Israel published a paper on the disease and its etiology. In 1910, Lord established that *A. israelii* is present in carious teeth and tonsils of otherwise normal persons. In an excellent review in 1938, Cope[4] summarized 1330 reported cases. Successful treatment of the disease with penicillin dates to 1943 and the report of Nichols and Harrell in 1947.[5]

Epidemiology

Actinomycosis is worldwide in distribution and is found twice as often in men as in women. Of the 13 recognized species of *Actinomyces*, all but one (*A. humiferus*, found in the soil) are normal inhabitants of the mucous membranes and oral cavities of humans and lower animals. In the United States the disease is more common in men. The incidence is difficult to determine as it is not reportable, and there is no skin test material for population surveys.

Etiology and Pathogenesis

Human disease is caused almost exclusively by *A. israelii*, infrequently by *A. bovis*, and rarely by other species. Because *A. israelii* is present in various studies in approximately 50 percent of excised tonsils and is a normal commensal of humans, the disease is regarded as being acquired endogenously by direct extension to contiguous tissues, probably as a result of minor local trauma. Even in closed lesions, however, there appears to be a synergistic relationship between *A. israelii* and a mixed flora of other bacteria. In fact, the injection of pure cultures of *A. israelii* or *A. bovis* into tissue rarely leads to disease.

Clinical Manifestations

There are three major forms of the disease: cervicofacial, thoracic, and abdominal. Literature reviews prior to 1950 indicate that 50 to 60 percent of cases were cervicofacial, 20 percent thoracic, 15 percent abdominal, and the remainder disseminate to other organs via the bloodstream, e.g., meninges or endocardium. More recent studies indicate fewer cervicofacial cases, perhaps due to rigorous regimens of antimicrobial agents.

The cervicofacial form begins as a swelling over the lower part of the face or neck with formation of an irregular, woody, indurated lesion that becomes suppurative, drains, and heals at various sites

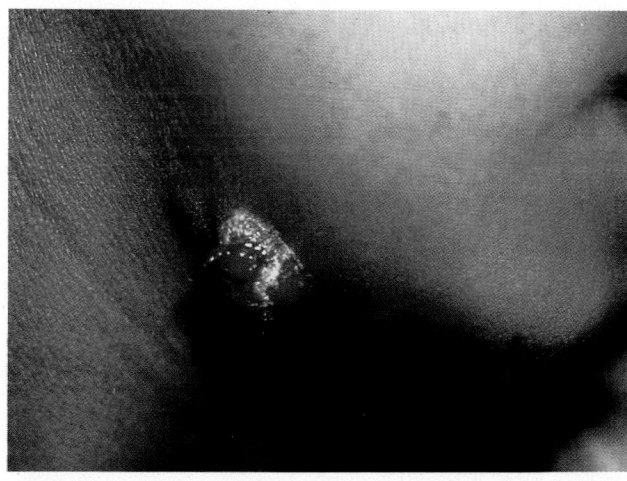

a

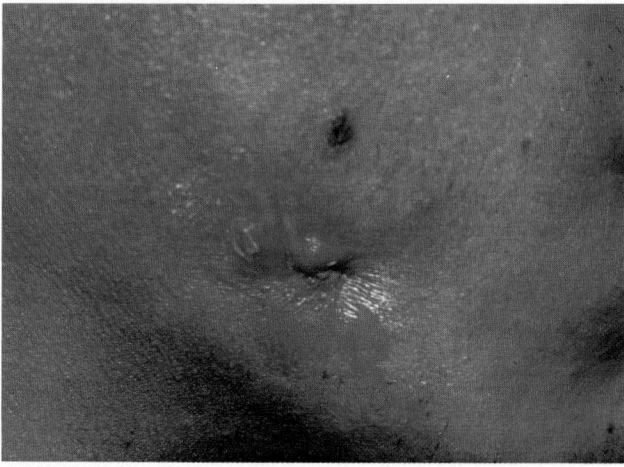

b

FIGURE 196-1 Actinomycosis, cervicofacial. (*a*) A pyogenic granuloma-like nodule is seen overlying the mandible. (*b*) A solitary lesion with a central retracted orifice of a sinus tract is seen overlying the mandible. *(Courtesy of R. Arenas, M.D.)*

(Fig. 196-1). Regional lymph node involvement is characteristically absent. Invasion and destruction of bone occur early, with periostitis and osteomyelitis.

In thoracic actinomycosis, the cutaneous lesion is generally a draining sinus tract or subcutaneous abscess, occasionally with local induration and discoloration. Productive cough and pleuritic chest pain are pulmonary symptoms. The chest x-ray characteristically shows a dense infiltrate with signs of pleural thickening and occasionally mediastinitis.

Abdominal actinomycosis presents in a cutaneous form, again as a draining sinus tract or subcutaneous abscess (Fig. 196-2). An abdominal mass is usually present, and occasionally a psoas abscess occurs. Signs of incomplete intestinal obstruction in the form of vomiting or cramping pain occasionally occur. On x-ray examination, a sinus tract sometimes can be visualized. In other instances, there is evidence of partial obstruction or an extraintestinal mass.

In all forms of the disease, there may be constitutional symptoms: fever, shaking chills, drenching night sweats, anorexia, weight loss, and marked easy fatigue.

A normocytic, normochromic anemia is frequent, but leukocytosis is mild and occasionally absent. The erythrocyte sedimentation rate is usually elevated.

Pathology

The gross pathologic picture is that of a chronic infection localized to a particular site. There are multiple, coalescent abscesses with communicating sinuses. Tissues frequently are yellow, indurated, and firm, and sandlike particles composed of tangled hyphal forms of *A. israelii* occasionally can be recognized. These are called sulfur granules. On microscopic examination, one finds chronic inflammation with granulation tissue, occasionally giant cells, and often large numbers of macrophages.

Diagnosis and Differential Diagnosis

The diagnosis is established by the isolation and identification of the causative microorganism in cultures of tissue or exudate from characteristic lesions.

A presumptive diagnosis is virtually certain if sulfur granules are seen in pus, exudate, or tissue sections.

Laboratory Diagnosis DIRECT EXAMINATION. Sputum, bronchial aspirates, pleural, joint, pericardial and other body fluids, pus, biopsy material, and intrauterine devices should be examined for sulfur granules. All granules should be studied both in a wet preparation (water, never potassium hydroxide) and by Gram stain.

Sulfur granules are irregular, hard, and usually yellowish. They vary in size from 0.1 to 5 mm, and the larger granules may be observed with the unaided eye. For examination the granules are placed in water on a microscope slide, gently crushed with a second slide, and a cover slip placed over the specimen. The granule has irregular edges; on reduction of light intensity and, preferably, with a magnification of approximately ×1000, these edges can be seen as made up of club-shaped structures. The clubs are refractile, colorless, and characteristic of *A. israelii* and *A. bovis,* as well as some other species. The tiny hyphae lying within the clubs cannot be seen without staining. Therefore, once the material has been studied as described, the cover slip is removed, and the preparation is air dried and stained by Gram stain. All of the Actinomycetales are gram-positive, with tiny (1.0 μm or less in diameter) branched and unbranched hyphal filaments. The absence of granules in a specimen does not rule out actinomycosis, nor does their presence establish the diagnosis. They may be present in other lesions (or infections) due to *Nocardia* spp. and some other bacteria, including *Staphylococcus aureus.* Even when granules are not seen, a Gram stain of the material may reveal short filaments of the actinomycetes.

In order to study tissue specimens, they generally must be fixed, sectioned, and stained with hematoxylin-eosin or other stains to ascertain the characteristic clubs with hyphae within.

CULTURE. Granules should be placed in a sterile petri dish and rinsed several times with thioglycolate broth. Upon removal from the broth they should be crushed and inoculated into tubes or on one plate each of anaerobic blood agar and phenylethyl alcohol blood agar. The actinomycetes are susceptible to antibacterial agents, and so these should not be added to culture media. Plates should be streaked for isolation of colonies. *Actinomyces* spp. are strict anaerobes and, therefore, culturing should be performed rap-

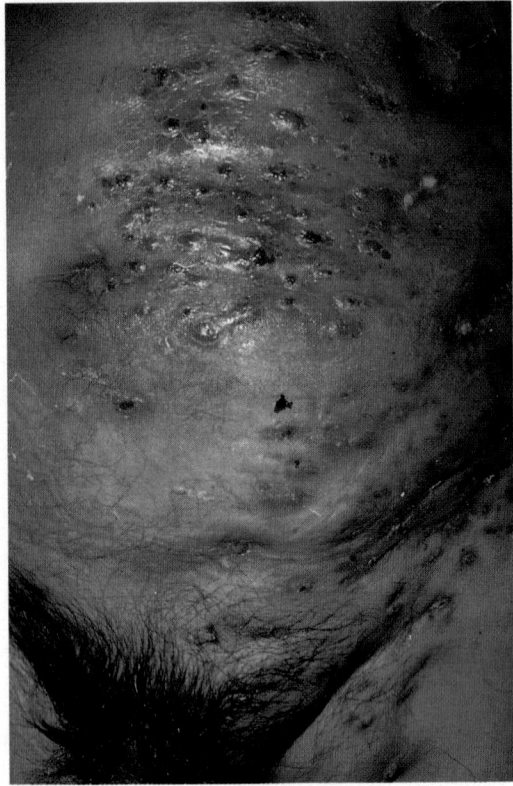

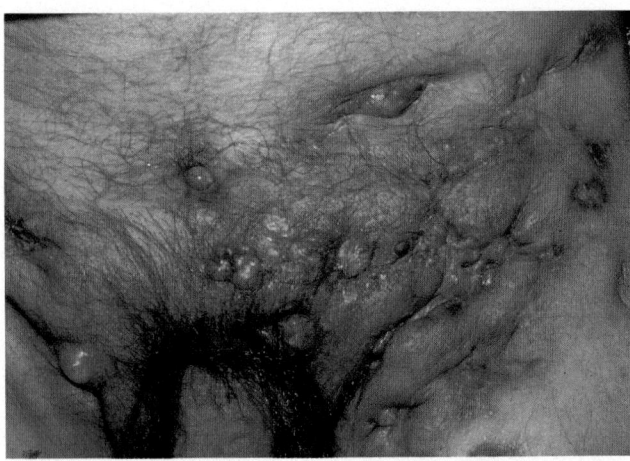

b

a

FIGURE 196-2   Actinomycosis, abdominal. (*a*) Multiple, draining sinus tracts are seen on the anterior abdominal wall. (*b*) Longstanding infection, with many scars and draining sinus tracts. (*Courtesy of R. Arenas, M.D.*)

idly, all materials placed into an anaerobic jar as soon as possible, and incubated, preferably at 35 to 37°C. Isolation of *Actinomyces* spp. from specimens with many other microorganisms may be difficult. Fluorescent antibodies from the Centers for Disease Control may be used on tissue sections and clinical specimens.

On solid agar, colonies of *A. israelii* at 48 h are long, branching, and filamentous or spider-like. After 7 to 10 days, typical colonies become white, glistening, irregular, or lobulated. They remain small and may penetrate the agar. In glucose-thioglycolate broth, *A. israelii* produces granular colonies at the bottom portion of the tube, without turbidity.

In contrast, on agar at 48 h, typical colonies of *A. bovis,* usually isolated from cattle and swine, produce pinhead size "dewdrop" colonies that enlarge by a week to 10 days, becoming similar to *A. israelii* colonies but possessing an entire border. It should be noted that cultural characteristics of the actinomycetes are variable, depending on the age and conditions of culture as well as the medium used. In glucose-thioglycolate broth, the hyphae of *A. bovis* break up early, producing turbidity and a dense sediment.

Colonies of *A. israelii* are uniformly catalase negative, differentiating this species from microorganisms previously classified as anaerobic diphtheroids. They also are urease negative and produce acid from *m*-inositol, xylose, and raffinose.

Differential Diagnosis   Cervicofacial actinomycosis must be distinguished from chronic infections due to *Mycobacterium tuberculosis, S. aureus, Nocardia asteroides,* and systemic mycoses. The abdominal form resembles other chronic infectious diseases (tuberculosis) and, occasionally, regional enteritis and malignancy. The thoracic form must be distinguished from tuberculosis, fungal infections, and malignancy.

Treatment

Treatment is twofold: surgical (incision and drainage of abscesses and excision of chronic, fibrotic, avascular tissue) and chemotherapeutic (penicillin notably).

Chemotherapy must be prolonged, usually for at least 3 months. Customary dosage early in the course is from 10 to 20 million units daily of penicillin G, administered intravenously for approximately a 4-week period. Following this, oral phenoxymethyl penicillin in daily dosage of from 4 to 6 g should be continued. Therapy should not be stopped until lesions have cleared completely or until they have been stable for 6 weeks. In patients who are allergic to penicillin, therapy may be with tetracycline, erythromycin, or chloramphenicol, each of which has been reported successful.

Course and Prognosis

The characteristic course of the disease is prolonged, indolent, and marked by the closure of one sinus tract and the opening of another.

With specific chemotherapy, most patients can be cured, although therapy is prolonged, and patients may be left with chronic residual local scarring, respiratory embarrassment from lung tissue destruction, or mild gastrointestinal obstruction.

Nocardiosis

Nocardiosis is an acute or subacute suppurative (less commonly granulomatous) infectious disease, acquired via the respiratory route, with a focus of infection in the lungs, and with frequent hematogenous dissemination, characteristically to the brain. It is caused by the aerobic actinomycete *Nocardia asteroides*, one of the "higher bacteria."

Historical Aspects

In 1888, Nocard described an illness in cattle, characterized by lymphatic swelling resembling farcy or glanders and caused by an aerobic, partially acid-fast actinomycete.[6] The first description of the disease in humans was that of Eppinger,[7] who reported a patient with brain abscess and caseous disease of the lungs and pleura. In recent years, the association with other diseases and the use of antileukemic drugs, cytotoxins, corticosteroids, and other immune depressants has been noted.

Epidemiology

Nocardiosis is worldwide in distribution and occurs most often in men 30 to 50 years of age and older.

Nocardia asteroides is found in nature in soil and in decomposing vegetation. No predilection for race or occupation has been noted.

Etiology and Pathogenesis

Nocardia asteroides is the primary agent; however, *N. brasiliensis*, *N. farcinica*, and *N. caviae* have been noted to produce the disease. These latter species are most frequently associated with mycetoma and are generally discussed as agents of that disease.

Predisposing factors are not known, and the disease is generally considered to be opportunistic. *N. asteroides* has also been reported as the cause of disease in small animals, cattle, and fish, as well as in humans.

Clinical Manifestations

Skin lesions are generally limited to sinus tracts from abscesses, although Satterwhite et al. have reported on primary cutaneous nocardiosis (Fig. 196-3).[8]

Pulmonary symptoms include cough and, occasionally, blood-tinged sputum, chest pain, and dyspnea. On x-ray examination a dense infiltrate is usually seen unilaterally, sometimes with cavitation of either the honeycomb or the large variety and frequently with markedly thickened pleurae.

It is a peculiarity of this disease that there is a strikingly increased frequency of hematogenous dissemination to the brain, with abscess formation. Findings on neurologic examination depend on the location of the lesion, but headache and signs of increased intracranial pressure are the most common. Less frequently there are abscesses in the kidney, spleen, or liver. Usually there are fever, chills, night sweats, malaise, anorexia, and weight loss. Such laboratory findings as leukocytosis, anemia, elevated sedimentation rate, and elevated serum globulin levels are also usually present.

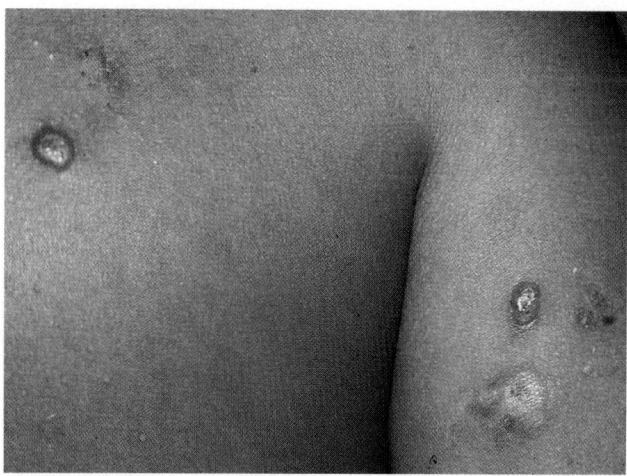

FIGURE 196-3 Nocardiosis, cutaneous. Two violaceous nodules surrounded by scars are seen on the posterior chest wall and arm.

Pathology

Tissue reaction is characteristically pyogenic, with the formation of multiple, but occasionally confluent, abscesses. There tends to be less induration, fibrotic tissue formation, and sinus tract formation than with actinomycosis, the disease it resembles.

The microorganism is seen readily on a Gram stain. Hyphae vary in size from 0.5 to 1.0 μm in diameter and up to 40 μm in length. Branching is seen frequently.

Diagnosis and Differential Diagnosis

Specific diagnosis can be established only by isolation and identification of *N. asteroides* in culture. Typical organisms seen on microscopic examination of tissues or other specimens only suggest the diagnosis, as *M. tuberculosis* is also acid-fast, and *A. israelii* branches in a similar manner.

Laboratory Diagnosis DIRECT EXAMINATION. Sputum and bronchial aspirates, pleural, joint, and pericardial fluids, pus, cerebrospinal fluid, and biopsy material should all be studied microscopically by Gram and modified acid-fast stain procedures. Small, cream- to white-colored granules may be produced, and occasionally "clubs" may be present. Granules should be studied as described for actinomycosis. When granules are not present, the microorganism is seen as freely branching filaments, which are gram-positive and partially acid-fast (destained with 0.5% aqueous sulfuric acid instead of acid alcohol).

CULTURE. Colony formation is identical at 25 to 37°C, but optimal growth is at 37°C. *N. asteroides* is sensitive to antibacterial agents, and these are not used in isolation media. The microorganism will grow on media for *Mycobacterium* spp. isolation and may be mistaken for rapidly growing members of this genus. Although *Nocardia* spp. are aerobic, they will also grow well under anaerobic cultural conditions.

Specimens are inoculated onto brain-heart infusion agar or Sabouraud agar and incubated at 25 to 30°C. Growth develops in approximately 2 weeks at 25 to 30°C and within 3 to 4 days at 37°C. Colonies vary from chalky-white to yellow and orange and are glabrous, raised, folded, and cerebriform. At maturity they may develop downy or tufted aerial hyphae. Stained smears of the hyphal growth demonstrate coccoid and bacillary forms, whereas the characteristic beaded hyphae are seen principally from broth cultures. Acid-fastness may be enhanced by growth on media containing milk (e.g., litmus milk) or on Lowenstein-Jensen media. Differentiation from other aerobic actinomycetes is based on cultural characteristics, acid-fastness, and biochemical characteristics.

Morphology Slide cultures demonstrate the ability of *N. asteroides* to produce aerial hyphae, whereas *Mycobacterium* spp. do not.

Acid-Fast Stain *N. asteroides* is acid-fast when the modified acid-fast stain is used; *Streptomyces* spp. are not.

Biochemical Reactions *N. asteroides* does not hydrolyze casein and will not grow on gelatin medium. *N. brasiliensis* hydrolyzes casein and grows well on gelatin medium. *Streptomyces* spp. hydrolyze casein but grow poorly in gelatin medium, producing a flaky or stringy type of growth. Other biochemical tests are used to differentiate the remaining *Nocardia* spp.

Differential Diagnosis It is of historical interest that the first reported patient was thought to have tuberculosis. For many years nocardiosis was not well distinguished from actinomycosis. Nocardiosis may also resemble more chronic lung and brain abscesses due to such organisms as anaerobic *Streptococcus* spp., occasionally *S. aureus*, or *Klebsiella pneumoniae*. It may mimic fungal infections such as histoplasmosis, blastomycosis, and coccidioidomycosis.

Treatment

As shown by studies in animals and experience in humans, members of the sulfonamide group, notably sulfadiazine, have been the most active chemotherapeutic agents. Chemotherapy must be combined with drainage of abscesses, but despite such therapy, treatment has been unsuccessful in so many patients that it has been customary to use another agent such as tetracycline, chloramphenicol, or large doses of penicillin (although this agent is less active in animal infections). Impressive in vitro and in vivo studies of amikacin have been confirmed by successful use in a renal transplant recipient after failure on multiple other regimens.[9]

Prognosis

Even today with newer therapy, the fatality rates approximate 50 percent. This rate appears to be due to disseminated disease and abscess formation at such vital sites as the brain when the illness is recognized and diagnosed. Furthermore, patients are usually debilitated, and host defenses are compromised either by disease or medication.

Mycetoma (Madura Foot, Maduromycosis)

Mycetoma is a localized chronic, deforming infectious disease of the subcutaneous tissues, skin, and bone, characteristically of the foot but occasionally of the hand, back, or shoulder. It follows traumatic implantation of soil organisms, at the site, of one of a variety of actinomycetes (actinomycotic) or fungi (eumycotic). Regardless of the etiologic agent, development of the disease is the same, i.e., tissues become swollen with suppurating abscesses, granulomas, and draining sinuses. Within the draining sinuses granules characteristic of the various causative organisms may be found. The actinomycetes that cause mycetoma include *Nocardia brasiliensis, N. caviae, N. farcinica, Actinomadura madurae, A. pelletieri,* and *Streptomyces somaliensis.* Eumycotic mycetoma is produced by a great number of fungi, in particular, *Pseudallescheria boydii, Madurella grisea, M. mycetomatis, Acremonium falciforme, A. recifei, Exophiala jeanselmei, Curvularia lunata, Fusarium* spp., and others. Certain lower bacteria also have been implicated, e.g., *Actinobacillus, Staphylococcus, Streptococcus, Proteus, Pseudomonas* spp., and *Escherichia coli.*

Historical Aspects

The synonym for the disease is derived from the area in India, Madura, from which the earliest cases were reported by Gill and others. In 1860, Vandyke Carter reported on a number of cases and was the first to use the term *mycetoma.*[10]

Epidemiology

In addition to India, other sites where the disease is commonly seen include the Sudan area in Africa, southern Asia, and tropical areas of Central and South America. The disease is relatively rare in the United States, although one of the causative fungi, *P. boydii*, frequently has been isolated from soil in this country. The disease is more common in blacks, a reflection of population in the geographic location of the causal microorganisms and the prevalence there of the practice of walking without shoes. The disease is more common in young adults and in workers in rural areas frequently exposed to accidental injury to the bare foot or the hand.

Etiology and Pathogenesis

Some eight species of actinomycetes and at least 16 fungi cause the disease.

Humans and animals acquire the disease through implantation by thorns, splinters, hay, and other similar materials contaminated by one of the causative fungi. The most common site for such implantation is the foot or leg, although, occasionally, the lesions are seen on the upper part of the back in individuals carrying contaminated sacks of sugar cane.[11]

Clinical Manifestations (Fig. 196-4)

The hallmark of the disease is swelling with marked distortion of the normal anatomy, draining sinus tracts, bloody or purulent drainage, and only mild impairment of mobility and relatively little pain. Development of the lesion is slow, often seen only several years after the initial implantation. The lesion is initially locally invasive and tumorlike and, as it slowly enlarges, it forms sinus tracts to the surface. Radiologic examination shows soft-tissue swelling and areas of rarefaction and fibrosis characteristic of osteomyelitis in contiguous bone.

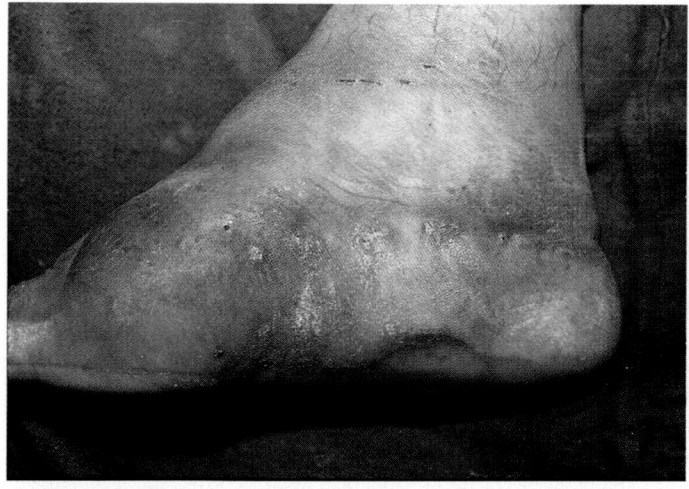

a

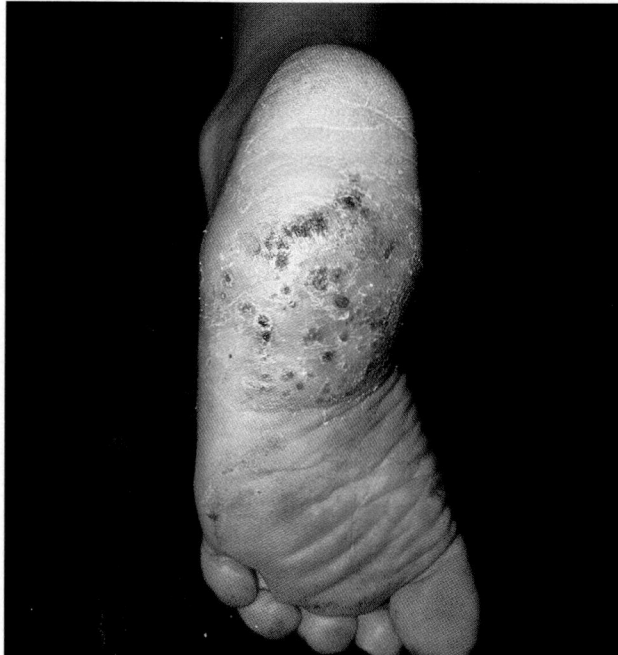

b

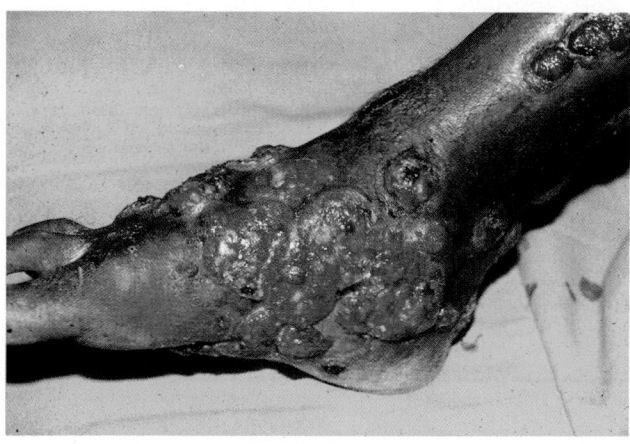

c

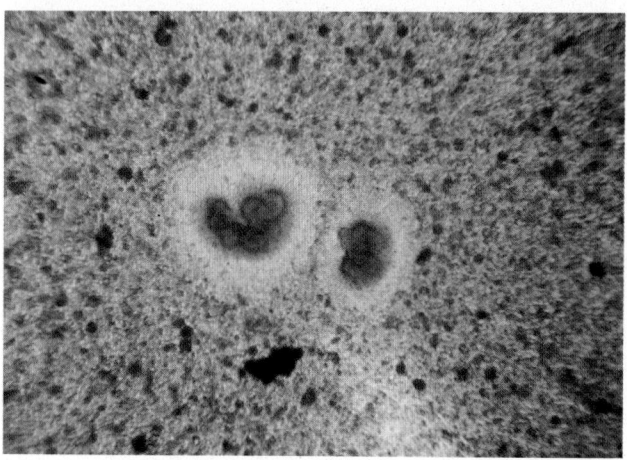

d

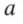

e

FIGURE 196-4   Mycetoma. (*a*) Early, with woody edema of the foot. (*b*) Brauny edema and crusted papules on the plantar foot. (*c*) Exuberant granulation tissue and edema involving the foot and leg caused by *Nocardia*. (*d*) Chronic fibrotic involvement of the foot with lymphatic spread to the popliteal fossa. (*e*) Direct examination of pus from a cutaneous lesion shows yellowish-brown granules, colonies of *Nocardia*, with a fibrin coat. *(Courtesy of R. Arenas, M.D.)*

Pathology

The gross appearance of the lesion is as described above. A characteristic finding in material draining from the sinus tracts is that of granules visible to the naked eye, which on microscopic examination are seen to be colonies of fungal hyphae with a shell or crust of fibrin derived from the host tissues (Fig. 194-4e). They vary in color from pink to yellow, white, brown, or black, and color, size, shape, and consistency tend to be characteristic for each causal microorganism. Tissue at the site of these granules characteristically shows suppuration, with epithelioid and multinucleated giant cells. Fibrosis is prominent in areas between the abscesses. Eventually, enlargement of the affected area is so dramatic that often the only method of identifying the tissue is demonstration of toes or fingers.

Diagnosis and Differential Diagnosis

Diagnosis is established by the clinical appearance of the lesion and the presence of characteristic granules; culture of pus and tissue usually shows one of the implicated fungi, but, in addition, bacteria such as *S. aureus*. Gram stain shows branching, filamentous microorganisms; aerobic and anaerobic cultures and special stains such as periodic acid–Schiff (PAS) and Gomori's methenamine silver or Gridley's may be helpful in demonstrating the causative microorganisms.

Laboratory Diagnosis   DIRECT EXAMINATION.   Biopsy material and pus from draining sinuses should be examined for granules. Processing for microscopic study and culture is as outlined under "Actinomycosis" above. If granules cannot be found in biopsy tissue, it should be teased apart and reexamined. Granules are studied for consistency, pigmentation, hyphal size and septation, morphologic characteristics, and manner of fragmentation. Direct microscopic examination is the only means of identifying whether the mycetoma is actinomycotic or eumycotic. Proper culturing of the specimen relies on this initial information.

CULTURE.   Colony production is best at 25 to 30°C or 37°C, depending upon the causative agent. Therefore, cultures should be made by cleansing the granules (see "Actinomycosis"), crushing and culturing them on Sabouraud dextrose agar, and incubating at both temperatures.

To avoid contaminated material, biopsy specimens for culture should be of deep tissue.

The microorganisms most often seen are identified in Table 196-1.

Differential Diagnosis   Mycetoma must be distinguished from osteomyelitis due to *S. aureus* (which is usually more acute and

TABLE 196-1
Microorganisms Most Often Seen in Mycetoma

Microorganism	Presentation	Culture on Sabouraud's dextrose agar	Microscopic appearance
Actinomycotic: Nocardia brasiliensis	Granules soft, irregularly spherical, white to yellow, with or without "clubs."	Small, wrinkled, heaped colony, tan to yellow or orange. May have chalky surface because of short aerial hyphae. Some strains produce browning of the medium.	Short, irregular rods, long branched hyphae in liquid culture. Partially acid-fast, often beaded hyphae. Proteolytic activity −; amylase activity −.
Actinomadura madurae	Granules large, irregular to serpiginous, white to yellow or slightly pink, "clubs" numerous, long, tapered, and sometimes branching.	Cream-colored, glabrous colony with a firm, hard surface. Some strains produce powdery, white aerial hyphae.	Delicate branched hyphae; not acid-fast; conidia in chains. Proteolytic activity +; amylase activity +.
Eumycotic: Pseudallescheria boydii	Granules soft, round or lobulated, white or yellow, no "clubs" but instead surrounded by chlamydospore-like terminal cells	Fluffy colonies, at first white but later gray to nearly black.	*Scedosporium apiospermum* stage: hyaline hyphae with pale, brown, oval to clavate conidia, on simple or branched conidiophores. Many strains also produce cleistothecia (sexual fruiting body of the *Pseudallescheria boydii* stage), particularly at the edge of the colony. Proteolytic activity +; amylase activity +.
Madurella mycetomatis	Granules hard, brittle, round or lobed, black, no "clubs," but instead chlamydospores produced at the periphery. Brown pigment particles in hyphae and chlamydospores.	Flat, membranous or fluffy colonies, tan to yellow-brown or olivaceous. Brown, diffusible pigment produced.	Chlamydoconidia. Some strains produce conidia from small phialides; black sclerotia. Proteolytic activity +; amylase activity +.
Madurella grisea	Granules soft at first, hardening with age, round or lobed, black with hyaline hyphae at the unpigmented center, dark brown hyphae at periphery. No brown pigment particles in the hyphae.	Slow-growing, tan to gray or olivaceous, velvety colony with both hyaline cylindric hyphae and chains of dark, budding cells. Chlamydospores rare.	Chlamydoconidia rare. No micro-, sclerotia, or hyphal inclusions. Proteolytic activity +; amylase activity +.
Exophiala jeanselmei	Granules soft, irregular, black, made up mostly of dark brown chlamydospores, rare brown hyphae.	Slow-growing, black colony, at first membranous, later grayish and velvety.	Begins as chains of budding cells; later hyphae develop. Conidia produced from tapering annelides. Proteolytic activity +; amylase activity +.

accompanied by more pain but less distortion of tissues) or to *M. tuberculosis.*

Treatment

Treatment of mycetomas has been notoriously unsatisfactory with a few exceptions. Those infections due to *Actinomyces* spp. have responded partially to therapy with penicillin, sulfonamides, or tetracycline. Some strains of *M. mycetomi* have been shown sensitive to levels of amphotericin B that can be achieved in the serum. However, there are no extensive data on the use of this agent in these infections.

Some attempts have been made, without notable success, to treat the disease by surgical resection of tissue. Amputation is frequently necessary.

Course and Prognosis

The course of disease is prolonged. In the areas where it occurs, it is a frequent cause of death.

Cryptococcosis (Torulosis, European Blastomycosis)

Cryptococcosis, a disease caused by the yeast *Cryptococcus neoformans* (perfect state: *Filobasidiella neoformans*), is a chronic infectious disease acquired by the respiratory route, with the primary focus of infection in the lungs; there is occasional hematogenous dissemination, characteristically to the meninges, but occasionally to the kidneys and to the skin.

Historical Aspects

Although San Felice, in 1894, reported the presence of an encapsulated yeast in peach juice, and thus probably described for the first time what is known as *C. neoformans,* it was Busse and Bushke in 1895 who first reported disease in humans. In 1905, Hansemann observed the yeast in a patient who had died of meningitis, and Verse, in 1914, recognized the disease antemortem. In 1951, an important advance occurred when Emmons reported the isolation of *C. neoformans* from soil and later from pigeon excreta, nests, and other sources associated with this bird.[12]

Epidemiology

The disease is worldwide in distribution. It is more common in males than in females by a ratio of approximately 2:1. The disease is relatively rare in children and, until the advent of AIDS, has been more common in patients over the age of 40. The important evidence of its association with pigeon excreta has been extended to show that the microorganism has been discovered in almost every area where pigeons congregate. *C. neoformans* and cryptococcosis, however, are also seen in areas of the world where pigeons are not found, and the infection must not be overlooked because of a lack of proof of association with pigeons. Disease also has been noted in patients exposed to air conditioners contaminated with pigeon excreta. Pigeon breeders have been shown to have higher levels of antibody to *C. neoformans* antigen than persons with such contact.[13] The microorganism has been isolated from other animals, including cow, cat, dog, horse, gazelle, mink, koala, and wallaby.

Etiology and Pathogenesis

The causative microorganism is *C. neoformans.* It seems highly probable that the disease is acquired by inhalation of microorganisms from dust, as the fungus is so ubiquitous. However, defective host defenses are probably equally important in disease induction. Such defects appear to be present in such diseases as diabetes mellitus, lymphoma, Hodgkin's disease, sarcoidosis, and AIDS. A focus of infection is established in the lung, and then the microorganism disseminates hematogenously.

Clinical Manifestations

Approximately 10 to 15 percent of patients have skin lesions, which usually occur as a result of hematogenous spread from the lungs. In most instances, lesions are papules or nodules with surrounding erythema (Fig. 196-5). They occasionally break down and exude a liquid, mucinous material. Other lesions less frequently noted are ulcers, acneform pustules, granulomas, and purple plaques. Although AIDS patients are particularly susceptible to

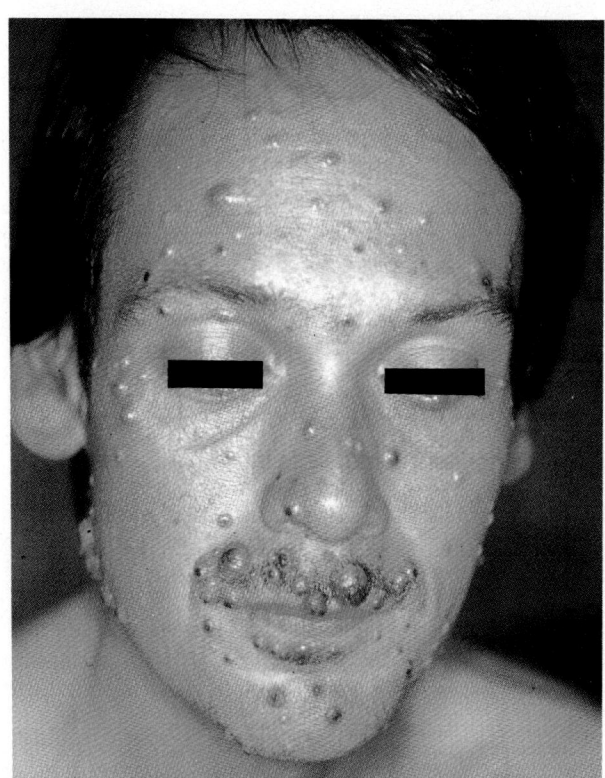

FIGURE 196-5 Cryptococcosis, disseminated. Multiple, discrete, skin-colored papules and nodules resembling molluscum contagiosum are seen on the face of a male with advanced HIV disease. *(Courtesy of Loïc Vaillant, M.D.)*

cryptococcosis (it is the second most commonly reported mycosis in AIDS), it is seen most often as a severe meningitis. Penneys and Hicks have reported unusual cutaneous cryptococcal lesions resembling molluscum contagiosum in a Haitian male with AIDS.[1]

Pulmonary disease as the sole manifestation of infection is increasing in frequency. Most patients with this condition are free of pulmonary complaints, and the lesions are discovered on a routine chest film. A few have a productive cough and, rarely, hemoptysis. The chest films show a variety of lesions, including multiple fluffy infiltrates, extensive miliary lesions, "coin" lesions, dense pneumonic infiltrates, or loculated pleural effusions. Abscesses and cavities are rare.[13] Lung lesions are often inapparent in AIDS patients.

Approximately one-third of patients have renal involvement, as attested to by the culture of *C. neoformans* from urine. Except for an occasional case of pyelonephritis or perinephric abscess, the renal form has not been well characterized.

Unlike blastomycosis, histoplasmosis, or coccidioidomycosis, cryptococcosis involves the bones and joints in less than 5 percent of cases.

The most commonly observed form of the disease is meningitis, with headache the chief complaint in approximately 80 percent of patients. Mental confusion or impaired vision is seen in about 40 percent. Onset is generally gradual, sometimes with symptoms going back to 2 or 3 months or more. In approximately 15 percent, meningitis occurs without symptoms referable to the central nervous system. Examination of cerebrospinal fluid usually reveals a leukocytosis, predominantly lymphocytic, elevated protein, and, in approximately 50 percent of patients, a depressed glucose value.[14]

Other than the above findings in the cerebrospinal fluid, consistently abnormal laboratory values are not encountered.

Pathology

A hallmark of infection is the slight or absent inflammatory response. With appropriate staining the microorganism can be seen in tissue with little round cell or polymorphonuclear response. In the brain, lytic lesions are found in which multiple, single, and budding microorganisms may be seen, again with little or no tissue response. In pulmonary lesions there may be conspicuous fibrosis.

Diagnosis and Differential Diagnosis

Diagnosis is established by isolation and identification of the causative microorganism in culture from skin lesions, pus, sputum, or urine but especially from the cerebrospinal fluid. The diagnosis is virtually established if budding yeast forms with a capsule are seen with an india ink preparation. The latex agglutination test using cerebrospinal fluid, or serum in the case of AIDS patients, has proven to be a particularly helpful, accurate, and rapid indication of disease.

In the rare instance when material for culture is not available, the diagnosis may rest on finding the characteristic fungal cells after microscopic examination of tissue sections stained with Mayer's mucicarmine stain; the capsule of the microorganism takes up the stain and is easily seen.

Laboratory Diagnosis DIRECT EXAMINATION. Cerebrospinal fluid or urine should be centrifuged and studied by india ink prepa-

ration to delineate the capsule of *C. neoformans*. Cells are surrounded by a mucopolysaccharide capsule of varying thickness. The capsule is visible in a negative fashion with reduced light intensity as a halo between the cell and the india ink particles. It may also be seen in water or cerebrospinal fluid as a slight difference in refraction of light by the experienced microscopist.

The capsule is not visibly affected by 10% KOH. When sputum or pus is mixed with this mounting agent, the microorganism and capsule may be demonstrated in outline by the cellular debris present in the specimen.

In direct examination of cerebrospinal fluid after centrifugation, care must be taken to distinguish between the microorganism and leukocytes present in the specimen.

In brain tissue crushed between a slide and coverslip to a thin layer, the microorganism and its capsule are demonstrated readily.

Other specimens generally are not studied microscopically in fresh preparations. They may be cultured, and appropriate specimens may be prepared for histopathologic procedures.

CULTURE. Culturally, *C. neoformans* is identical at 30 and 37°C and grows well on all standard mycologic media containing no cycloheximide, which inhibits it. Colonies are at first whitish-gray and pasty, with either a dull or shiny surface, and sticky and stringy due to the presence of capsular material. After about 2 weeks the color becomes tan, but the colony retains its stickiness. Occasionally other colony pigmentation may be seen, including yellow and pink.

Individual microorganisms are budding yeast cells, 5 to 20 μm in diameter, rarely producing pseudohyphae and, under standard conditions, no hyphae.

C. neoformans differs from other related organisms in having a polysaccharide capsule, a narrow pore between mother and daughter cell, in producing urease, in utilizing some sugars but fermenting none, and in growing as a yeast at both 30 and 37°C. It is differentiated from other *Cryptococcus* spp. by its sugar utilization pattern, and by the production of melanin in the presence of caffeic acid. This latter test is performed by placing material to be cultured on "birdseed agar" or "nigerseed agar," on which *C. neoformans* develops as brown colonies whereas other *Cryptococcus* spp. are cream to light tan in color.

Differential Diagnosis Cryptococcosis of the skin must be distinguished from pyoderma and other bacterial or fungal skin lesions. The pulmonary form must be distinguished from tuberculosis, malignancy, other fungal infections, and from more chronic bacterial disease. Cerebrospinal fluid findings typical of *C. neoformans* meningitis may be seen in tuberculosis, other fungal infections, sarcoidosis, meningeal carcinomatosis, and, rarely, such viral diseases as mumps and lymphocytic choriomeningitis.

Treatment

Chemotherapy is the most critical factor in the management of disease, and there are at least four options. In the rare instances in which the isolate is sensitive to it, 5-flucytosine is the first. If such data cannot be obtained or if treatment must begin immediately, amphotericin B must be used. Flucytosine is administered by the oral route in a daily dose of 150 mg/kg per day in four equally divided doses. Intervals between doses must be increased according to serum creatinine values or to creatinine clearances.

Amphotericin B is administered intravenously (see under "Blastomycosis" below). According to one schedule, optimal dose should be approximately 1 to 2 g or, by a second schedule, a 10-week course at 20 mg per day.

With meningitis both drugs must be used, in a 6-week course of therapy with a daily dose of 5-flucytosine of 150 mg/kg and of amphotericin B of 20 mg. When such therapy is unsuccessful in meningitis patients, intrathecal administration of amphotericin B is justified. The dose should not exceed 1.0 mg, at 2- to 3-day intervals. Amphotericin B should be diluted in the syringe with approximately 5.0 mL of cerebrospinal fluid.

Patients with AIDS respond poorly and relapse frequently. The best predictors of no relapse are more prolonged flucytosine during, and lower serum antigen titers at the end of, primary therapy, and continuing suppressive fluconazole therapy (200 mg/day).[16]

If other options are unsuccessful, miconazole intravenously may be useful.[17]

Course and Prognosis

Once meningitis appears, the disease is considered inexorably fatal unless treated as described above. Pulmonary forms have a more variable course, and some appear to persist for long periods without worsening or disseminating. The skin and bone forms have a chronic, slowly progressive course. Because cryptococcosis in AIDS patients is not cured, but only placed in remission, suppressive chemotherapy is required for life after the course of active treatment has ended.

Histoplasmosis

Histoplasmosis is a chronic infectious disease, acquired by the respiratory route, with a primary focus of infection in the lungs, and occasional hematogenous dissemination (characteristically to such reticuloendothelial organs as liver, bone marrow, and spleen). It is caused by the dimorphic fungus *Histoplasma capsulatum* (perfect state: *Ajellomyces capsulatus*).[18]

Historical Aspects

In 1906, Darling[19] reported his studies of a fatal illness in three patients in whom he found within macrophages microorganisms that he suspected of being protozoa. In 1934 DeMonbreum,[20] in a beautiful series of experiments, demonstrated the causative agent to be a fungus.

A second form of the disease, acute primary histoplasmosis, was delineated as a result of observations of localized outbreaks for the most part, by Christie, Peterson, Palmer, and Furcolow during the mid-1940s.

Furcolow and Brasher are also credited with the description of the third form, chronic cavitary histoplasmosis, which they identified in tuberculosis sanatorium patients who had a disease closely resembling tuberculosis, but who had negative tuberculin skin tests.[21]

Epidemiology

Although the disease has been reported from 30 widely scattered countries, it is recognized most commonly in the eastern and cen-

tral United States. In these areas up to 80 percent of the adult population demonstrate skin test evidence of prior infection. There is a marked preponderance of disease in patients above the age of 60 and (uniquely among the systemic mycoses) in infants and children below the age of 10 years. In adults the disease is more common in males. The largest recorded outbreak occurred in Indianapolis, IN, and affected some 100,000 residents.[22]

An important contribution to the knowledge of the epidemiology of histoplasmosis was the recognition by Emmons, in 1949, of the presence of the causative microorganism in soil, particularly where there has been a deposit of bird and chicken excreta. *H. capsulatum* can be recovered readily from nitrogen-rich soil, enriched with droppings of chickens, starlings, and bats. Outbreaks continue to be associated with such reservoirs.[23]

The causative fungus has been isolated from a large number of wild and domestic animals, including the dog, skunk, raccoon, woodchuck, cow, horse, and sheep. Animal-to-human or human-to-human spread does not occur.

Etiology and Pathogenesis

The causative agent is *H. capsulatum,* a dimorphic fungus. Found principally in areas of the world drained by large rivers, it is ubiquitous in nature, and because infection is widespread, as indicated by delayed-hypersensitivity skin reactions to histoplasmin, it appears certain that important factors other than exposure to the fungus are necessary for production of disease; one of these is size of the inoculum. Decreased host resistance (as seen in lymphoma and Hodgkin's disease) and impaired antibody response probably play a role, although most likely a lesser one than in other fungal infections, e.g., those due to *Candida* spp., *C. neoformans,* and the Zygomycetes. It is a defining disease in HIV-infected patients, who, thus, have AIDS.

Two varieties of the microorganism exist: *H. capsulatum* var. *capsulatum* and *H. capsulatum* var. *duboisii.* The latter variety is seen in Africa and is differentiated by the development of larger, thick-walled, oval yeast cells 10 to 15 μm in diameter in tissue, often superficially resembling the tissue phase of *Blastomyces dermatitidis.* African histoplasmosis may produce solitary lesions in cutaneous and subcutaneous tissues or bone, or multiple, disseminated lesions involving skin, subcutaneous tissues, lymph nodes, abdominal organs, or bone.[24]

Clinical Manifestations

Except in the elderly and in patients with advanced HIV disease, glabrous skin involvement in histoplasmosis is unusual, other than by the hypersensitivity phenomenon of erythema nodosum. Mucous membrane lesions due to invasion of the mouth, pharynx, and larynx by the fungus may be noted commonly in the progressive disseminated form. Reactivation of disease may lead to infection of mucocutaneous and other tissues (Fig. 196-6a).

Acute primary histoplasmosis has been characterized chiefly from observations of illness occurring in localized outbreaks in normal, immunocompetent individuals. Constitutional symptoms are commonly malaise, fever, chills, sweats, and lethargy. Pulmonary symptoms generally are those of cough, dyspnea, and, less frequently, chest pain. Chest films may demonstrate diffuse, nodular densities or, occasionally, bilateral pulmonary consolidation. Lesions may appear or heal with diffuse calcification, suggesting a miliary process.

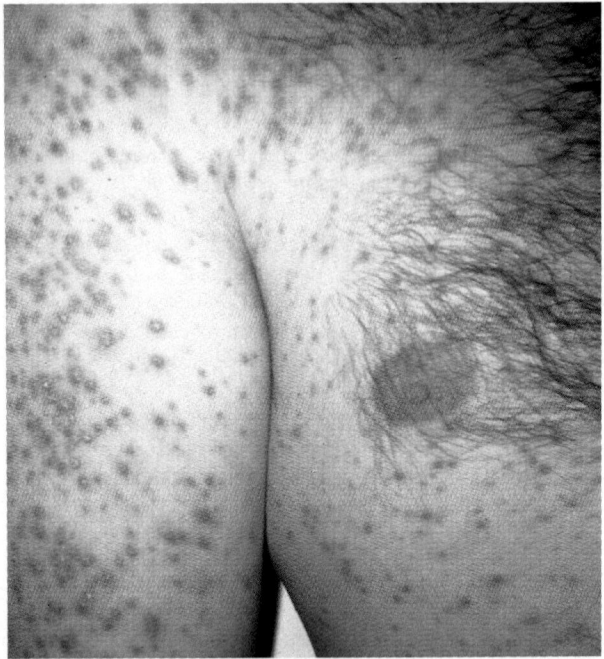

a

b

FIGURE 196-6 Histoplasmosis, disseminated. (*a*) Multiple erythematous keratotic papules and small plaques resembling guttate pattern psoriasis are seen on the chest and arm of a male with advanced HIV disease. *(Courtesy of J.D. Fallon, M.D.)* (*b*) Lesional biopsy specimen shows dermal macrophages packed with dozen of tiny yeast forms of *H. capsulatum*.

In the progressive disseminated form, the aforementioned constitutional symptoms are often present. The organ most often involved is the liver, and approximately 80 percent of patients have either abnormal function or cultural evidence of disease. An important additional lesion is ulceration of the soft palate, oropharynx, epiglottis, stomach, or intestine, resulting in pain, dysphagia, and weight loss. Overt Addison's disease or lesser manifestations of adrenal involvement may be present in the form of decreased 17-hydroxy- and 11-oxycorticoid excretion in the urine or depressed serum cortisol levels.

The chronic cavitary form is recognized from the characteristic upper-lobe pulmonary disease. A productive cough, dyspnea on exertion, and progressive respiratory embarrassment are common findings.

The usual laboratory findings in the progressive disseminated form are those of impaired liver function. Anemia and leukocytosis are present only in a minority of patients. Laboratory tests in the two other forms of disease are not especially helpful.

Pathology

Darling,[19] in his original description, reported "an intense invasion of large endothelial-like cells." The presence of *H. capsulatum* in histiocytes and macrophages is the hallmark of the histopathologic change (Fig. 196-6*b*). Lesions are seen most commonly in lymph nodes, liver, and spleen.

In nonfatal histoplasmosis, the characteristic histologic lesion is an epithelioid cell granuloma, usually with Langhans' giant cells. Such lesions may be seen in pulmonary tissue, biopsies of oral or gastrointestinal ulcers, or in the liver. Gomori's methenamine silver or the PAS stains are particularly helpful in rapid screening examinations of tissues for the presence of typically staining fungal cells.

Diagnosis and Differential Diagnosis

The diagnosis is established by the isolation and identification of the causative fungus in culture from oral lesions, bone marrow, sputum, blood, urine, lymph node, liver, or other biopsy.

H. capsulatum must be differentiated from *Coccidioides immitis, C. neoformans, Blastomyces dermatitidis, Toxoplasma gondii, Leishmania donovani, Toluropsis glabrata, Pneumocystis carinii, Penicillium mameffei,* and other microorganisms that may cause disease in immunocompromised hosts. There are various ways for these microorganisms to be differentiated. Spherules are usually seen in *C. immitis;* typical capsules of *C. neoformans* are seen with Mayer's mucicarmine stain; multinuclear fungal cells are seen in small intracellular forms of *B. dermatitidis; T. gondii* has smaller cells, which are usually not in histiocytes, and whose tachyzoites are not stained by Gomory's methenamine silver stain; and in *L. donovani* the kinetoplast can be seen easily. *T. glabrata* is rarely found within macrophages, and *P. carinii* is larger and stains intensely.

The latex agglutination test is useful for the early detection of acute histoplasmosis; the complement fixation test is a sensitive tool, but cross-reaction may occur, and the test must be performed by trained individuals; the micro-immunodiffusion test is used to detect precipitins against the H and M protein antigens of histoplasmin, even when cultures are negative from cerebrospinal fluid specimens. Used in combination, these tests can be of both diagnostic and prognostic value.[25]

Laboratory Diagnosis   DIRECT EXAMINATION.   Slide preparations may be made from specimens such as sputum, bronchial aspirates, urine, peripheral blood or bone marrow, cerebrospinal fluid, lymph nodes, and pus or material from ulcers. Preparations are fixed with methyl alcohol for 10 min and then stained with either Giemsa's or Wright's stain. Presumptive positive identification is indicated when the yeasts are found extracellularly, or intracellularly in monocytes or macrophages, as 2- to 3-μm by 3- to 4-μm microorganisms composed of deeply stained, cup-shaped protoplasm at one end of the cell, and, usually, a large clear vacuole.

Histopathologic examination of material embedded in paraffin and stained with hematoxylin and eosin or PAS stains demonstrate the microorganisms in macrophages, as above, within a granulomatous site.

CULTURE. *37°C Incubation* This temperature is not used for primary isolation, as the microorganism may not grow. Only after growth at a lower temperature is the material subcultured to an enriched medium, such as brain-heart infusion agar with cysteine, and growth at 37°C attempted to demonstrate the yeast phase.

25 to 30°C Incubation Mycosel (Difco) or Sabouraud agar is used for primary isolation. Chloramphenicol, gentamicin, streptomycin, or penicillin are added (to inhibit bacterial growth), and cycloheximide to inhibit saprophytic fungi. Colonies develop in 10 days to 4 weeks or so, producing white, cottony, aerial hyphae, which may darken to brown. Microscopically, two types of conidia are found: smooth-walled, oval or pyriform microconidia (2 to 4 μm) borne on short lateral stalks (conidiophores), and round to pyriform macroconidia (7 to 18 μm) on short or long conidiophores. These macroconidia are generally characterized by tuberculate appendages formed from condensed cell-wall material and covering the entire spore.

Macroconidia may resemble those of saprophyte *Sepedonium* spp. (inhibited by cycloheximide), and microconidia resemble those of the saprophyte *Chrysosporium* spp. However, the latter genus does not produce macroconidia and is not dimorphic.

EXOANTIGEN. As with other dimorphic fungal pathogens, if reference antisera are available, exoantigen studies may be performed on cultures. Aqueous extracts of mature mycelial cultures of the potential pathogen may be used in the exoantigen test.[26] This may be particularly useful in atypical forms of the microorganisms not readily identified in more standard methods.

Differential Diagnosis The acute primary form usually cannot be distinguished from a flu-like, acute, viral illness of the upper respiratory tract or atypical pneumonia unless microbiologic studies are performed. The progressive disseminated form most closely resembles a lymphoma, such as Hodgkin's disease, or hematogenous tuberculosis. The chronic cavitary form is distinguishable from the similar form of tuberculosis only by laboratory diagnostic tests.

Treatment

Antifungal chemotherapy is essential in those patients with more severe acute primary illness, in all patients with a progressive disseminated form of disease, and in most patients with the chronic cavitary form. Amphotericin B is presently the therapeutic agent confirmed by 30 years' experience. The details of treatment are given under "Blastomycosis" below.

Ketoconazole, in dosage of 400 to 600 mg daily, orally has been useful in preliminary studies, but amphotericin B is preferable in patients with AIDS.[27]

In some patients with chronic cavitary histoplasmosis, surgical resection of irreversibly diseased pulmonary tissue is sometimes advisable.

Course and Prognosis

The acute primary form is usually a mild disease, although fatalities have been reported in patients massively infected. In the progressive form, spontaneous recovery is rare, and 80 percent of patients die within 1 year of the diagnosis without treatment. The chronic cavitary form is less often fatal, although most patients have progressive respiratory and ventilatory impairment.

Blastomycosis

Blastomycosis is a chronic infectious disease acquired through the respiratory system, with a primary focus of infection in the lungs and with occasional hematogenous dissemination, usually to the skin, bone, and genital part of the genitourinary tract; it is caused by the dimorphic fungus, *Blastomyces dermatitidis* (perfect state: *Ajellomyces dermatitidis*).

Historical Aspects

This disease was first described in its cutaneous form by Gilchrist and Stokes at a meeting of the Baltimore and Washington Dermatologic Association in 1894.[28] In 1898, the same authors named the causative organism *Blastomyces dermatitidis*. In 1964, Emmons et al. first reported culturally authenticated cases originating outside the North American continent, in Africa.[29]

Epidemiology

Blastomycosis occurs in the Americas and Africa, principally in humans and canines. It is encountered most often in the Ohio and Mississippi River valleys. Following outbreaks, the microorganism has been isolated from river bank soil and beaver dams, but only sporadically; the natural habitat of the fungus has yet to be unequivocally demonstrated.[30,31]

Etiology and Pathogenesis

Because *B. dermatitidis* does not appear to be ubiquitous in nature and because there is no skin test survey evidence of widespread infection (as in histoplasmosis and coccidioidomycosis), disease may represent rare instances of infection. It appears to occur with increased frequency in persons who have diabetes mellitus and tuberculosis, but disease continues to be rare.

Cutaneous blastomycosis was once believed to be due to implantation into the skin. It now is known that the disease is acquired by inhalation, with a primary focus in the lungs, and that in individuals unable to contain the infection, dissemination occurs with a preponderance in skin and bone.

Clinical Manifestations (Fig. 196-7)

When infection disseminates from the lung, a number of cutaneous forms are seen. The most characteristic is an elevated, verrucous, crusted, varicolored lesion with a sharply slanting, serpiginous border and a tendency towards central healing by a thin depigmented atrophic scar. The peripheral border extends on one side only, resembling a one-half to three-quarter moon. These lesions are seen most commonly on the exposed surfaces of the body: face, hands, and arms. When one of the crusts is lifted, pus exudes. In approximately half the patients, the lesions are multiple. Another form of

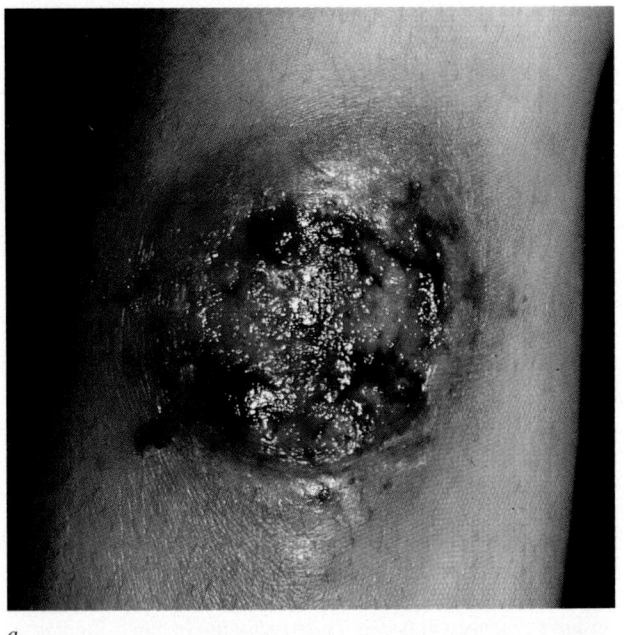

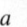
a

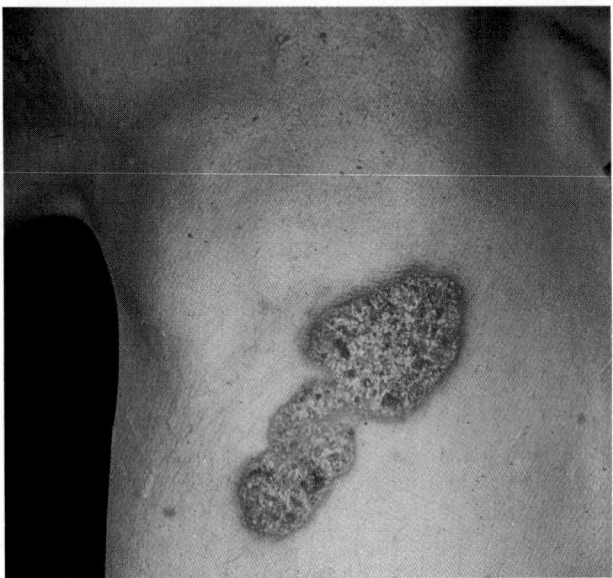
b

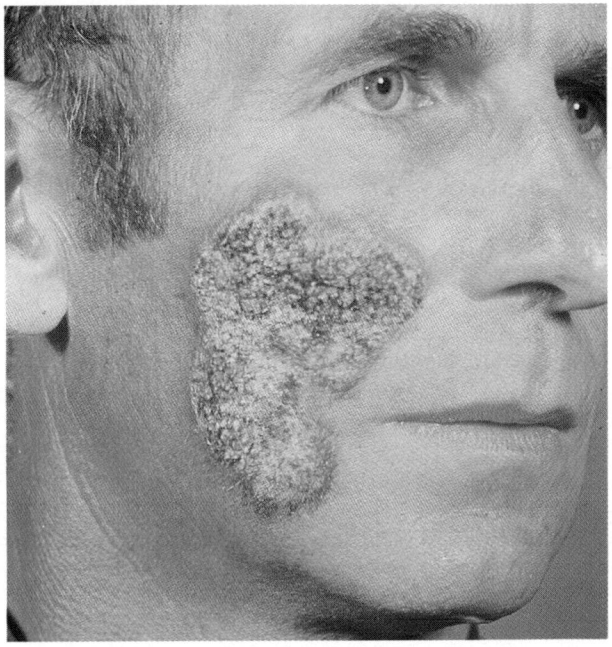
c

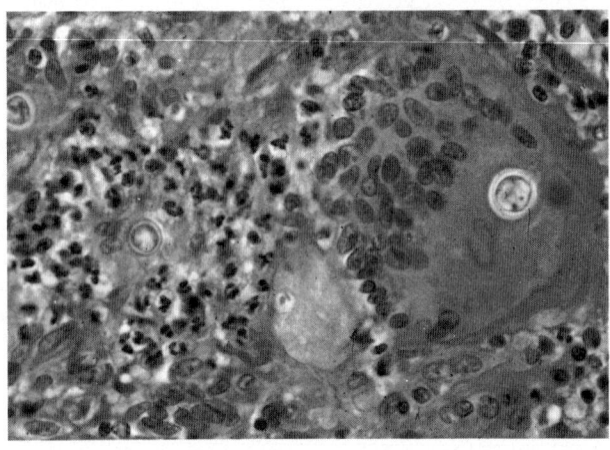
d

FIGURE 196-7   Blastomycosis. (*a*) Inflammatory plaque with ulceration resembling pyoderma gangrenosum on the calf. (*Courtesy of Elizabeth M. Spiers, M.D.*) (*b*) Older lesion, appearing as a verrucous plaque. (*c*) Chronic verrucous plaque on the cheek. (*d*) Lesional biopsy specimen shows several thick-walled budding yeast forms.

cutaneous disease is that of small superficial ulcerative lesions. A third form consists of a raised, firm, subcutaneous nodule, occasionally containing many small pustules over its surface. In extraordinarily rare instances of accidental inoculation into the skin, e.g., in a laboratory worker, the disease has been characterized by a chancre with a reddened area of induration, by lymphangitis and lymphadenopathy, and by the complete absence of hematogenous spread. Erythema nodosum may be seen, but more commonly it is a manifestation of coccidioidomycosis and histoplasmosis.

Pulmonary involvement occurs in virtually all patients but is clinically important (i.e., with lesion on chest roentgenogram or culture of the fungus from respiratory secretions) in only one-half of them. Approximately a quarter of all patients have multiple-lobe involvement. Miliary and cavitary lesions are seen occasionally. Pleural disease or pulmonary calcification is rare.

Bone lesions in the form of osteomyelitis are seen in approximately a third of the patients. The most common sites are the thoracic and lumbar vertebrae, pelvis, sacrum, skull, ribs, and long bones of the extremities. In some, extension to subcutaneous areas, with a large abscess, especially in the psoas area, may be the first manifestation. The most common symptoms are pain and tenderness at the site.

Disease of the genital tract occurs in approximately a third of the male patients. The prostate, seminal vesicles, and testes are affected: the kidney is virtually never involved. Symptoms and findings are characteristically pain, often described as "heaviness" in the perineum, or swelling of the scrotal contents.

Approximately a quarter of the patients have oral or nasal mucous membrane lesions. Of these, only one-half are from a contiguous cutaneous lesion.

Rarely, the disease may be manifest by meningoencephalitis, cerebral abscess, endocarditis, or involvement of the liver, adrenals, spleen, or gastrointestinal tract.

Constitutional symptoms such as chills, fever, night sweats, anorexia, weight loss, malaise, and lassitude are seen in only 50 percent of patients.

Leukocytosis and anemia in one-quarter of patients, increased erythrocyte sedimentation rate in two-thirds, and hyperglobulinemia in approximately three-quarters are the most common laboratory findings.

Pathology

The histologic pattern is a characteristic combination of suppurative and granulomatous change. In these inflammatory areas, especially within giant cells, the thick-walled budding fungus can be seen, even with hematoxylin and eosin stain (Fig. 196-7d). The Gridley methenamine silver stain is especially helpful in finding the fungus in screening examinations of tissue.

In skin lesions, pseudoepitheliomatous hyperplasia characteristically is seen.

Diagnosis and Differential Diagnosis

The diagnosis may be established by finding characteristic budding cells on microscopic examination of the above-mentioned specimens. Material to be examined is placed in 10% KOH or in calcofluor white (with which a fluorescence microscope must be used). This tentative diagnosis must be confirmed by culture.

In rare instances when material for culture is not available, the diagnosis rests on finding characteristic cells on microscopic examination of stained tissue sections. The cells may be confused with *H. capsulatum* var. *duboisii* (*H. duboisii* buds with a narrow attachment to the parent cell; *B. dermatitidis* buds with a wide attachment) or, more rarely, with *C. immitis* spherules (which contain endospores) or *C. neoformans* (the mucicarmine stain will differentiate the capsule of this organism from nonstaining cytoplasm of *B. dermatitidis*).

Skin and serologic tests usually are not helpful and are virtually never diagnostic in active disease.

Laboratory Diagnosis DIRECT EXAMINATION. Pus or material from the periphery of an ulcerated lesion is mixed with a drop of 10% KOH and examined microscopically. Under reduced light intensity, the fungus may be seen as 8- to 15-μm, usually single, budding cells with a thick "double-contoured" wall and wide pore of attachment. The bud often becomes as large as the parent cell before detaching. It is more difficult to differentiate the microorganism from artefacts in sputum, cerebrospinal fluid, and pleural exudates, and direct examination always should be followed by confirmatory culture. Use of calcofluor white and a fluorescence microscope circumvent the problem of artefacts, as fungi all fluoresce with this material, and most artefacts similar in appearance to the fungus are readily distinguished.

CULTURE. *37°C Incubation* Material planted on blood agar produces pseudohyphae as well as the yeastlike phase, with single and multiple budding similar to that seen in tissue. The colony is light buff to brown with a dry, wrinkled surface, sometimes described as mealy. Occasional colonies are glabrous and tan. Because this microorganism does not produce characteristic micro- or macroconidia and because it grows well at 37°C, unlike *H. capsulatum,* it should be cultured at 37°C and 25 to 30°C simultaneously.

25 to 30°C Incubation On sabouraud and Mycosel (Difco) agar, *B. dermatitidis* forms the same yeastlike growth initially as at 37°C, but then hyphae develop rapidly, and a white fluffy colony is formed. In some strains, the colony becomes brown with age and may produce a dark diffusible pigment. The hyphae are fine (2 to 3 μm in diameter) and septate. After 2 to 3 weeks, short lateral conidiophores are formed bearing single hyaline, smooth-walled conidia 2 to 10 μm in diameter. Although the conidia are usually spherical or slightly oval, in some strains of *B. dermatitidis* they may be pyriform. With development of large numbers of these conidia, the surface of the colony flattens and becomes powdery or granular.

If simultaneous culture at 37°C was not performed or was negative, the growth at 25 to 30°C should be transferred to 37°C on appropriate media to demonstrate development of the characteristic yeast colony. Likewise, transfer of a 37°C culture to 25 to 30°C will lead to development of the characteristic mold colony by which *B. dermatitidis* may be identified.

Exoantigen Exoantigen studies may be performed on cultures of *B. dermatitidis* as described for *H. capsulatum.*

Differential Diagnosis The skin lesions of blastomycosis must be distinguished from squamous cell carcinoma and chronic skin lesions due to tuberculosis, tertiary syphilis, leprosy, staphylococcal infection, and bromidism. The pulmonary lesion must be differentiated from carcinoma, atelectasis, pneumonia, tuberculosis, other fungal infections, and miscellaneous infections. The bone and genitourinary lesions resemble those of tuberculosis.

Treatment

Chemotherapy is indicated in all patients, and surgical drainage of abscesses or resection of chronically diseased tissue is occasionally essential. A number of chemotherapeutic agents have been clearly demonstrated to be efficacious.

The first chemotherapeutic agent proved effective was 2-hydroxystilbamidine. It is administered intravenously in a daily dose of 225 mg for a total dose of 8 g. This drug is well tolerated, but is relatively contraindicated in patients with hepatic disease, as it is stored in the liver.

Amphotericin B is a more effective agent. It is administered intravenously with an initial dose of 1 mg. The drug is suspended in 5% glucose solution (the drug precipitates in sodium or potassium salt solution, in a concentration not greater than 1 mg per 10 mL), and infused over a period of 2 to 4 h. The use of a smaller-gauge (no. 23 or 24) needle and heparin may be helpful in preventing phlebitis. The dosage should be increased thereafter by daily increments of 5 to 10 mg.

There are two opinions as to optimal daily dosage, total amount of drug, and duration of therapy. One recommends an optimal daily or alternate daily dose of 1 mg/kg [not to exceed 50 mg and meant to achieve a serum level approximately 10 times the minimal inhibitory concentration (MIC)], a total amount of approximately 1 to 2 g, and duration sufficient to achieve that (usually 4 to 6 weeks). A second opinion is that a lower optimal dosage of 15 to 30 mg (meant to achieve a serum level of only 2 to 3 times the MIC) is given over a duration of 10 weeks. The toxicity of the drug is usually less with the second regimen.

Amphotericin B produces fever, chills, nausea, vomiting, anorexia, headache, and, in most patients, irreversible renal damage of at least mild degree. Anemia and hypokalemia are also commonly encountered. Fifty milligrams of the succinate salt of hydrocortisone injected into the bottle or tubing at the onset of infusion is the most effective means of preventing vomiting, chills, fever, and malaise.

Preliminary data suggest that ketoconazole also may be effective in doses of 200 to 600 mg daily, orally, although it is not recommended in the rare patient with AIDS.

Course and Prognosis

It was formerly thought that the disease was inexorably fatal, but more recent studies suggest that some cases may be only mildly progressive or even self-limited. The illness should always be considered serious and deserving of treatment, because of the frequency of progressive disease and death.

Paracoccidioidal Granuloma (South American Blastomycosis, Lutz-Splendore-Almeida Disease)

Paracoccidioidal granuloma is a chronic infectious disease, characteristically beginning on the skin or mucosa about the mouth or nose, or occasionally in the lungs, with subsequent involvement of regional lymph nodes, and occasional hematogenous dissemination to the spleen, liver, lymph nodes, adrenals, and gastrointestinal tract. The causative organism is *Paracoccidioides brasiliensis*, believed to be a saprophyte of soil, associated with decaying vegetation.

Historical Aspects

In 1908 in a case report, Lutz described the fungus causing this disease.[32] A more complete description of the clinical illness and the causative microorganism was published subsequently by Splendore. Later, Almeida distinguished this illness from others with which it had been confused.[33]

Epidemiology

The causative fungus is *P. brasiliensis*. It was once believed to be introduced via traumatic implantation, but is now known to cause disease by introduction into the lungs with dissemination to other sites including the skin and mucous membranes, as is the pattern with other systemic fungal pathogens. The disease is seen in men (age 30–50) at a rate of approximately 38:1. It is believed this is due to inhibition of hypleal to yeast transformation by estrogen.[34]

Clinical Manifestations

The vast majority of patients have painful ulcerative lesions of the mouth or ulcerative or verrucous lesions of the skin. The latter most commonly are seen about the face and are usually multiple. Less frequently, a solitary pustular lesion or a subcutaneous abscess with a draining sinus tract is seen. Prior to these lesions, however, the patient may have acute or chronic pneumonia as the usual primary disease, with fever, cough, chest pain, malaise, dyspnea, and infiltrate on the chest film. Dissemination may occur to such organs as bone, adrenal glands, central nervous system, and especially, in virtually all patients, the spleen. Involvement of regional lymphatics is characteristic of the disease and, occasionally, swelling or drainage of a lymph node, especially in the cervical region, may be the first sign noted by the patient.

Pathology

The histopathologic findings characteristically are both granulomatous and suppurative. In skin lesions, there is usually pseudoepitheliomatous hyperplasia, with both the Langhans' type of granuloma and such pyogenic inflammatory cells as neutrophils, lymphocytes, plasma cells, and giant cells. In these respects, as well as in the appearance of some of the single-budding cells, the pathologic change closely resembles that of blastomycosis. However, the characteristically budding fungal cells may be seen with appropriate fungal stains.

Diagnosis and Differential Diagnosis

The diagnosis is established by demonstrating the microorganism by direct examination and by culture of the mold phase with subsequent conversion to the yeast phase. Detection of specific antigen may be necessary for definitive identification.

Laboratory Diagnosis DIRECT EXAMINATION. Sputum or other body fluids, crusts of ulcers, or pus (particularly from draining lymph nodes) may be examined microscopically in a KOH preparation. The large (10 to 60 μm in diameter) spherical to oval cells are easily visualized and appear as thick-walled cells with occasionally single or several buds, but most often with a characteristic "mariner's wheel" configuration with multiple 2- to 10-μm diameter buds with narrow points of attachment to the parent cell. Chains of multiple budding cells may be seen. It is differentiated from *B. dermatitidis* by the narrow point of bud attachment and from *C. neoformans* by the lack of a capsule.

CULTURE. *37°C Incubation* Material planted on blood agar will maintain the budding tissue form of the fungus. Growth is cream- to tan-colored, either smooth and soft in consistency or verrucose and waxy.

25 to 30°C Incubation *P. brasiliensis* is probably the slowest growing of the systemic fungi. A small, heaped colony may appear in 2 to 3 weeks, but occasionally 2 months or more may be required. On standard mycologic media (preferably neutral or alkaline in pH), the colony, usually small even at maturity, is white to beige, compact, and wrinkled or velvety. Occasionally, glabrous, irregularly folded brown colonies may develop. Primary isolation may be improved by growth on yeast extract agar. Microscopically, the colony is made up of fine septate hyphae and chlamydospores and arthroconidia. Pyriform microconidia resembling those of *B. dermatitidis* may be formed along the hyphae, although conidia may be absent or rare. Because the mold phase of *P. brasiliensis* is not characteristic, even when present, conversion to the yeast phase or detection of specific antigen may be necessary for definite identification.

EXOANTIGEN.   Exoantigen studies may be performed on cultures of *P. brasiliensis* as described for *H. capsulatum.*

Differential Diagnosis   The disease must be distinguished from blastomycosis (in which mucosal lesions are much rarer and regional lymphadenopathy is characteristically absent), tuberculosis (especially scrofula), yaws, syphilis, sporotrichosis, and leishmaniasis.

Treatment

For many years the sulfonamides have been known to suppress but not cure the infection.

Amphotericin B administered intravenously in total dosage ranging from 1 to 8 g has been shown to be effective in patients now numbering in excess of 250. In view of the known renal toxicity and the response in some patients to lower doses of drug, it would seem advisable to limit the total dose to less than 3 g. At daily doses of 1 mg/kg, approximately 4 to 8 weeks are necessary for such therapy.

Ketoconazole at doses of 200 to 600 mg daily is at least as effective as amphotericin B and has the advantage of the oral route of administration. It should not be used in patients with meningitis. Therapy needs to be given for at least a year.[35]

Course and Prognosis

Formerly, paracoccidioidal granuloma was recognized only in the advanced stage, which was invariably fatal. Earlier detection and modern antifungal drugs have altered the prognosis, and even advanced cases may be cured.

Coccidioidomycosis

Coccidioidomycosis is an acute or chronic infectious disease caused by the dimorphic fungus *Coccidioides immitis*. It is acquired by the respiratory route, primarily affecting the lungs, with occasional hematogenous dissemination to subcutaneous tissues, bone, skin or meninges.

Historical Aspects

In 1891, Posadas and Wernicke reported the first patient, a soldier in Argentina with disseminated coccidioidomycosis involving especially the skin of the face. Rixford and Gilchrist[36] reported the next case, from the San Joaquin Valley of California. They all believed that the causative microorganism was a protozoan, for which the name *C. immitis* was suggested. In 1900, Ophuls and Moffitt described an additional case and correctly identified and characterized the causative agent as a fungus.[37] In a series of papers beginning in 1915, Dickson described and identified the respiratory illness that constitutes the primary acute form of the disease. Gifford is credited with definition of the syndrome known as "San Joaquin Valley Fever," marked by fever, pleurisy, erythema nodosum, and sometimes by joint pains or rheumatism. It was Dixon and Gifford in the late 1930s who defined the mild form of the disease, rather than the rare, severe form, as the common type of coccidioidomycosis.[38]

Epidemiology

In a long series of beautifully conducted studies, Smith[39] and colleagues succeeded in defining the epidemiology of the infection in the endemic areas of southern California.

Coccidioidomycosis is sharply and dramatically limited in occurrence to southern California, Arizona, New Mexico, southwestern Texas, northern Mexico, and areas of Venezuela, Paraguay and northern Argentina. Cases reported from other areas indubitably are caused by infection by fomites or previous residence in endemic areas, e.g., cases in freight and cargo handlers in the eastern United States, and in archaeology students, and in Italians previously quartered as prisoners of war in California. It has been estimated that approximately 45,000 to 85,000 persons are newly infected with *C. immitis* annually, and of these, approximately one-half have a clinical illness. Infection appears to occur equally in both sexes and in all ages and races. However, blacks are 14 times and Filipinos 175 times more likely than Caucasians to have severe and disseminated disease. Mexicans, although darker-skinned, appear to be only about three times more susceptible to severe disease than light-skinned persons.

C. immitis is an inhabitant of soil in endemic areas, defined by dry climate (with annual rainfall of about 12 to 50 cm), alkaline soil, infrequent severe frost, and a season of several months with a mean temperature between 26 and 32°C. During the hot summer months (average temperature 38°C) the fungus remains viable in rodent burrows at depths up to 20 cm. In these burrows the rodents may become infected, and the disease also is seen in a variety of wild and domestic animals, including the dog, cat, cow, coyote, monkey, gorilla, and bat. Predators of infected wild animals usually do not become infected.

Etiology and Pathogenesis

The causative microorganism is *C. immitis* and, like other systemic pathogenic fungi, it is dimorphic. As the microorganism is so ubiquitous in certain geographic areas and, as judged by delayed-hypersensitivity skin reactions to coccidioidin, infection occurs in 80 to 90 percent of the inhabitants, it seems likely that certain factors are important in the induction and severity of the disease. Among these are race and immunosuppression. Pregnancy also predisposes towards more severe disease, even in Caucasians, and pregnant women are at least as likely as men to acquire the disseminated form of disease. However, in contrast to other systemic mycoses, diseases such as lymphoma, leukemia, and diabetes mellitus do not appear to be predisposing factors.

Clinical Manifestation

Coccidioidomycosis results from inhalation of airborne arthroconidia, causing infection in the lungs where the disease may become asymptomatic with spontaneous resolution, or symptomatic.

Erythema nodosum occurs in 5 percent of patients with a strongly reactive skin test; erythema multiforme is seen less often. In disseminated disease, there are characteristic draining sinus tracts to the skin. Granulomas and verrucous lesions, subcutaneous cellulitis, and abscesses are seen commonly; ulcerative lesions are noted less frequently.

Acute primary coccidioidomycosis, which has an incubation period of from 10 to 18 days, is usually an influenza-like illness, characterized by fever, chills, aching, malaise, pleuritic chest pain, and cough that is occasionally productive of blood-streaked sputum. Anorexia is common, and weight loss from 4.5 to 9 kg may occur during the illness.

Disseminated coccidioidomycosis (Fig. 196-8) occurs from hematogenous spread of the fungus in less than 1 percent of infections. Characteristically, there are subcutaneous cellulitis, abscess formation, and multiple draining sinus tracts, some of which heal spontaneously only to be replaced by new tracts at other sites. Cutaneous disease is seen rarely in laboratory workers and morticians. Bone is commonly involved, and osteomyelitis may be the presenting illness. The psoas area is commonly involved, with drainage posteriorly or anteriorly below the inguinal ligament. Meningitis, also a common manifestation of dissemination, is characterized by headache and stiff neck. In most patients with severe disseminated disease, such constitutional symptoms as fever and chills, weight loss, malaise, sweats, lassitude, and anorexia are present.

Chronic residual coccidioidomycosis is the term for continuing lesions in the lung such as cavities (characteristically thin-walled), pulmonary fibrosis, bronchiectasis, and calcification.

Galgiani and Ampel reportedly have the greatest experience with coccidioidomycosis in individuals infected with the human immunodeficiency virus.[40] They indicate that involvement of skin, as well as knee joint, liver, and inguinal nodes is seen in 14 percent of these patients. Additionally, illness and mortality were associated with lowered CD4 lymphocyte counts and a previous diagnosis of AIDS. Diagnosis from extrapulmonary lesions usually has been made by histologic staining of biopsy specimens.

Pathology

The early lesion of pulmonary coccidioidomycosis is a pyogenic reaction, with leukocytes around the released sporangiospores. The inflammatory response to the larger sporangia (spherules) is characteristically of granulomas surrounding the sporangia, with histiocytes, foreign-body giant cells, and lymphocytes. Although sporangia are characteristic and typical of the disease in tissue, in up to 75 percent of resected lesions, some hyphal forms and arthroconidia may be seen. When disease disseminates from the lung, characteristic lesions may be seen in skin, subcutaneous tissue, bone, meninges, lymph nodes, spleen, liver, and kidney. Suppuration or granulomatous lesions may predominate. The microorganism may be identified in tissue by the hematoxylin and eosin, Gomori's methenamine silver, and PAS stains, of which the last is preferred.

Diagnosis and Differential Diagnosis

The diagnosis is established by isolation and identification of the causative fungus in culture from sputum, sinus tract drainage, blood, urine, lymph node, or cerebrospinal fluid.

Laboratory Diagnosis　DIRECT EXAMINATION.　Because laboratory personnel working with the hyphal form of *C. immitis* are at risk, direct examination of specimen material is recommended. Specimens are best studied by microscopy in KOH or calcofluor white preparations. However, sediment from centrifuged cerebrospinal fluid may be studied directly with no mounting agent. Care

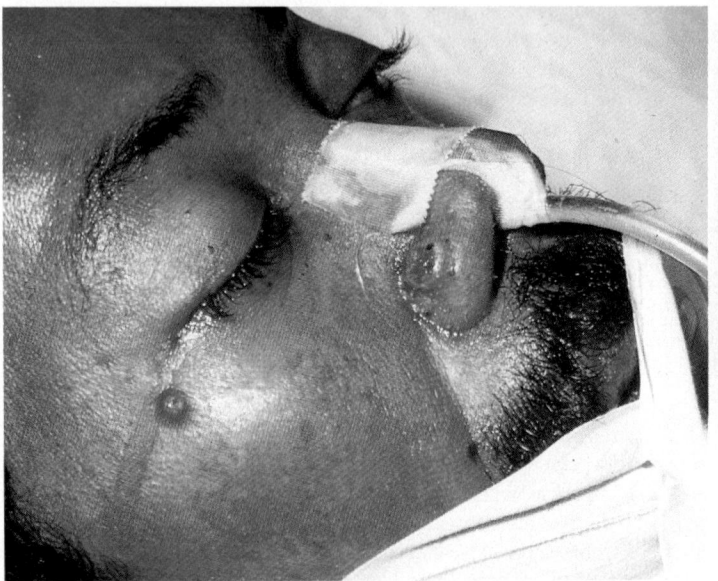

a

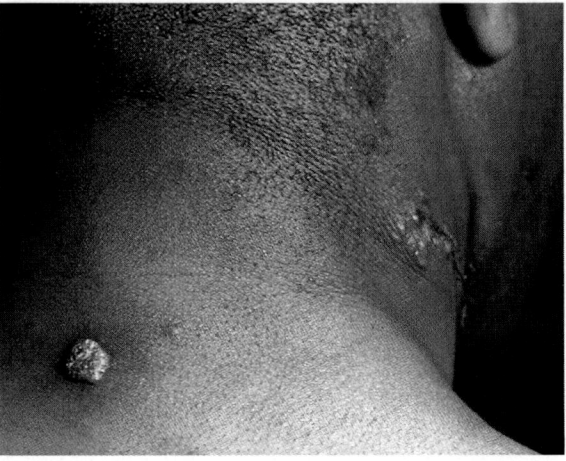

b

FIGURE 196-8　Coccidioidomycosis, disseminated. (*a*) Intact and ulcerated papules and nodules are seen on the cheek and node of this comatose patient with coccidioidomycotic meningitis. (*Courtesy of Francis Renna, M.D.*) (*b*) Several nodules are seen on the neck.

must be taken, in this latter instance, to dispose of the slide in disinfectant immediately after study, as *C. immitis* is capable of germination with production of the hyphal form under these conditions.

Because sporangia are large (30 to 60 μm), they may be visualized readily under the microscope with reduced light. However, the smaller, single sporangiospores (endospores) may be difficult to differentiate from phagocytic cells, other fungi debris, and artefacts.

CULTURE. *37°C Incubation*   Culture methods to produce the tissue phase of *C. immitis* are available but are complex and not routinely performed in the clinical laboratory. Standard media inoculated and incubated at 37°C produce the same type of growth as that seen in 30°C. When necessary, an agar medium for cultivation of spherules has been developed for the rapid in vitro conversion of hyphae to spherules.[41] In the past, intraperitoneal inoculation of laboratory animals with hyphae or spherules has been performed to convert the hyphae to spherules. Probably the most useful test for identification of colonies, not readily identifiable microscopically, is the exoantigen test (see "Histoplasmosis" above).

25 to 30°C Incubation   Specimens should always be cultured on slants rather than plates. The organism grows readily in about 2 to 4 days on conventional mycology media and produces a floccose colony, typically white, but varying in color from gray to yellow. Depending on the amount of arthroconidia formation, the colony may be floccose to powdery (the latter common in mature cultures) and cover the entire agar surface. The first characteristic thick-walled, "barrel-shaped" arthroconidia, 2 to 4 by 3 to 6 μm, appear on side branches of the vegetative hyphae in from 1 to 2 weeks after the colony is first seen. They are produced along the hyphal branches alternately with smaller thin-walled empty disjunctor cells. At maturity these empty cells rupture, freeing the infective arthroconidia. This phenomenon occurs rapidly after maturation of the culture. As with all fungal cultures, all work must be performed in a biologic safety hood. If the culture has aerial hyphae, it is advisable to flood the surface with saline solution before obtaining material either for subculture or for microscopic examination.

EXOANTIGEN.   Exoantigen studies may be performed on cultures of *C. immitis* as described previously for *H. capsulatum*.

Differential Diagnosis   The acute primary form usually cannot be distinguished from influenza or severe infection of the upper part of the respiratory tract without culture unless it has the classic hallmarks of Valley Fever. The severe disseminated form most closely resembles hematogenous tuberculosis, blastomycosis or actinomycosis, or a pyogenic infection due to *S. aureus*. Meningitis must be distinguished from that due to blastomycosis, tuberculosis, tertiary syphilis, cryptococcosis, and bacteria.

Hyphal colonies must be distinguished from other fungi, mostly contaminants, such as *Malbrachea, Arthroderma, Auxarthron, Geotrichum*, and others. These latter do not form sporangia and sporangiospores on special media although they have a varied but similar microscopic appearance.

Treatment

Antifungal chemotherapy is essential in all patients with the severe disseminated form. There is less certainty as to whether chemotherapy is necessary for patients with chronic cavities, who may need pulmonary resection, or for patients with more severe forms of acute primary disease.

Amphotericin B is not as effective in this disease as it is in cryptococcosis, histoplasmosis, or blastomycosis. More experienced workers in California believe that 3 g of drug should be the limit by the intravenous route. They also recommend for meningitis, intrathecal therapy at the cisternal site 2 to 3 times weekly for prolonged periods, e.g., at least 2 to 3 years. For greater details of the administration of amphotericin B, see the treatment sections under "Blastomycosis" and "Cryptococcosis" above.

Ketoconazole in doses (600 to 1200 mg daily) has been recommended, although recently discovered side effects have dampened enthusiasm for this drug.

Itraconazole has shown "impressive activity" in refractory coccidioidal meningitis, but controlled comparative trials have not yet been reported.[42]

Course and Prognosis

In the majority of infected residents of endemic areas, overt disease does not occur or is mild, heals spontaneously, and is not recognized to be acute primary coccidioidomycosis. This asymptomatic group of patients manifest past infection by a positive skin test with coccidioidin. Dissemination is influenced by race, pregnancy, and immunosuppression. The disseminated form must be considered serious, and patients must be studied intensely and treated as early as possible. A continuing negative delayed-hypersensitivity skin reaction to coccidioidin and a high or rising titer of serologic antibodies may serve as evidence of early or impending dissemination. Nonmeningeal disseminated coccidioidomycosis is 50 percent fatal without treatment. Meningeal disease is 100 percent fatal within 2 years without treatment.[43]

Aspergillosis

Aspergillosis comprises a group of clinical conditions unified only by sensitization to, saprophytic colonization by, or actual tissue invasion by a number of species of the genus *Aspergillus*.

Historical Aspects

Aspergillus fumigatus was first described in 1850 by Fresenius, who coined the term *aspergillosis* for this infection of the air sac of a bird. In 1856, Virchow described the human bronchial and pulmonary disease caused by the same microorganism. Renon wrote a classic review in 1897,[44] associating the microorganism with pulmonary disease in trades and occupations other than pigeon breeders. *Aspergillus* spp. have become agents of opportunistic fungal infections only relatively recently, with the advent of antibacterial chemotherapy as one of the more important predispositions to opportunistic suprainfection.

Aspergillus spp. toxins in foodstuff have also taken on importance in both animals and humans.

Epidemiology

Some 600 species of *Aspergillus* are ubiquitous saprophytes in nature and are found worldwide in soil, decaying vegetation, and other organic matter. They are thermophilic and may be found in compost heaps. Approximately 20 species have been implicated in disease.

   A. fumigatus is an important cause of severe disease and death in young birds and in penguins in zoos. However, animal-to-human spread is not considered important. In humans, it may occur as either a primary or secondary infection and is more common in men.

Etiology and Pathogenesis

Because *Aspergillus* spp. are so ubiquitous in nature, humans are exposed repeatedly and probably continuously to many species. Principally the respiratory tract, skin, cornea, external auditory canal, gastrointestinal tract, nasopharynx, vagina, and urethra have been primary sites of infections. In immunosuppressed patients, disease may be invasive, inflammatory, or granulomatous, confined to the lungs or disseminated, and is often fatal. Other modes of disease include the production of an aspergilloma or "fungus ball" in a part of the body such as the lungs. Various *Aspergillus* spp. are allergenic and produce asthma in sensitive persons. In another type of disease—of the external auditory canal in individuals with otitis externa—*A. niger* has been cultured and has been mentioned prominently as a causative factor. However, recent thinking is that the fungus is growing on the debris within the ear canal, whereas the otitis is caused by a variety of other microorganisms, particularly bacteria, growing in the cerumen and epithelial lining of the ear canal. Finally, toxicity due to ingestion of food contaminated with the mycotoxins or other metabolites of the fungus cause disease in both humans and animals.

Clinical Manifestations

Except for an occasional association with otitis externa, *Aspergillus* spp. usually are not considered factors in cutaneous disease.

   Some patients with bronchial asthma or asthmatic bronchitis show immediate-type cutaneous hypersensitivity to extracts of *Aspergillus* spp. Occasionally during attacks these species can be cultured from bronchial secretions. For these reasons, it has been customary to consider them as allergens, related to symptoms such as wheezing, shortness of breath, agitation, and cyanosis, occurring with asthma.

   One of the most characteristic and striking manifestations is the fungus ball. This is composed of colonies of *Aspergillus* spp., inflammatory exudate, cells, and fibrin in the form of a sphere measuring from 1 to 10 cm in diameter. This appears on the chest film as a ball surrounded by air within a cavity. It acts as a ball valve, trapping air during expiration and resulting in increased intracavitary pressure. This pressure tends to expand the cavity, and the fungus ball grows to fill the expanding space. Usually fungus balls are asymptomatic but they may cause hemmorhage, which can be fatal.

   In some patients, especially those with lymphoma or malignancy and those receiving corticosteroid or other immunosuppressive drugs, *A. fumigatus* is capable of invading tissue directly and of disseminating hematogenously, usually to the brain and kidney. In most such patients, the clinical picture is that of the predominating underlying disease, with general symptoms of infection, such as fever, chills, inanition, shock, altered consciousness, and anorexia. Occasionally there are pulmonary symptoms, and an infil-

trate is seen on the chest x-ray. In some instances, endocarditis with typical symptoms has been seen.

Pathology

In the characteristic pulmonary lesion, the fungus ball, there is a mass of *Aspergillus* spp. hyphae, typically without invasion or marked inflammatory response in the contiguous tissue.

   Special stains such as the Gridley, Gomori methenamine silver, or the PAS stains are necessary to demonstrate the fungi, which are seen poorly or not at all with the standard hematoxylin and eosin stain. Hyphae are branching structures at angles to each other of 45° or less, and 3 to 4 μm in diameter.

   In the invasive form of disease, the hyphae are surrounded by acute inflammatory cells and a pyogenic reaction. Rarely, there may be giant cells and granulomas.

Diagnosis and Differential Diagnosis

The ubiquitous nature of *Aspergillus* spp. complicates interpretation of the pathologic importance of any isolate from patient specimens such as sputum, skin, or pus. Furthermore, in the most common clinical form, the fungus ball, *A. fumigatus* may be cultured only with difficulty, or not at all, from the sputum. The diagnosis of disseminated disease may be made by seeing hyphae in specimens or by culturing *A. fumigatus* from tissues at autopsy or rarely at biopsy, usually too late to benefit the patient. Hyphae in tissue are often in parallel or radial formation. At times, they may appear atypically as short distorted hyphae lacking conspicuous septae. They also may be large, up to 12 μm diameter, and may be mistaken for the hyphae of a zygomycete, e.g., *Mucor* or *Rhizopus* spp. However, the branching pattern of the zygomycetes is less acute, the hyphae walls are not parallel, and the hyphae tend to be disposed in tissue in a "ribbon-like" fashion.

Laboratory Diagnosis DIRECT EXAMINATION. Potassium hydroxide preparations may be made from specimens such as bronchial washings, sputum, and biopsy material; wet mounts may be made with ear canal scrapings.

   SIGNIFICANCE OF CULTURE. As *Aspergillus* spp. are ubiquitous in nature and as a contaminant in the laboratory, a single species must be isolated repeatedly from patient specimens, and characteristic hyphal fragments must be demonstrated in tissue sections, before a disease can be called aspergillosis. When histologic specimens are not available, aspergillosis can be diagnosed by finding hyaline hyphal fragments in specimens and the culture of a single *Aspergillus* species, in the absence of any other pathogen.

   Media are usually incubated at 25 to 30°C, although *A. fumigatus* is capable of growing at temperatures of up to 45°C. Temperatures above 37°C favor development of this species and inhibit growth of many contaminants.

   Standard mycologic media (e.g., Sabouraud dextrose agar), which do not incorporate cycloheximide, may be used for patient specimens. Growth is rapid, and the characteristic structures, i.e., vesicles with phialides and phialoconidia, are produced early in colony development.

   The genus *Aspergillus* characteristically produces, along the hyphae, septate or nonseptate stalks (conidiophores) that broaden at the apex to form a vesicle. Flask-shaped projections, phialides, are produced, covering from one-third to all of the vesicle, depending upon the species. Certain *Aspergillus* species produce secondary phialides at the apex of the primary phiolides. Conidia (phialoconidia) are produced by a budding or blowing-out process, the youngest conidium being at the base of the chain. Conidia vary in color, shape, and smoothness of cell wall, and these are several of the characteristics used in their identification.

The species most often encountered as a human pathogen, *A. fumigatus,* is identified as follows: colony color, gray-green; gradual widening of the conidiophore into a vesicle; production of a single row of phialides covering the upper half to two-thirds of the vesicle; bending upwards of the lower phialides to parallel approximately the upper ones; columnar masses of gray-green conidia.

A. niger is seen frequently as a laboratory contaminant but is also associated with aspergillomas and otomycosis. The colony at first is floccose, white, becoming yellow as it matures. The surface appears to be black, but careful scrutiny indicates that the black color is made up of many vesicles covered with dark brown to black phialoconidia. Microscopically there is widening of the long, smooth conidiophores to a spherical vesicle, as well as phialides borne in a single row radially over the entire surface of the vesicle. Conidia are spherical and rough walled.

Young cultures are preferable for species identification; *The Genus Aspergillus*[45] is suggested for identification of the many *Aspergillus* species.

Differential Diagnosis   The fungus ball is generally classic in its appearance, although other fungi now have been implicated. The disseminated form must be distinguished from other severe illnesses, including bacterial sepsis, candidiasis, tuberculosis, and infection with *Pneumocystis carinii.* Otomycosis must be differentiated from chronic otitis externa from other causes, such as swimmer's ear, seborrheic dermatitis, and psoriasis.

Treatment

The otomycosis is best treated topically, not necessarily with an antifungal agent but with Burrow's solution (aluminum subacetate).

The allergic manifestations are best controlled by measures for a hypersensitivity state.

The saprophytic colonization of bronchi by *Aspergillus* spp. does not by itself warrant therapy. The fungus ball does not generally respond to chemotherapy but may need to be removed surgically if hemoptysis is severe. Intravascular (bronchial artery) coagulotherapy is in an investigative stage.

The disseminated form is generally of such short duration that chemotherapy cannot be instituted in time. Furthermore, the MIC of available antifungal drugs against most strains of *A. fumigatus* are generally greater than levels that can be obtained in the patient's serum. Despite this, however, chemotherapeutic activity of amphotericin B has been demonstrated in experimental infections in laboratory animals, and there are isolated reports of recoveries in patients who received this drug intravenously. Rather less drug is necessary than in other systemic mycoses, as the infection tends to be of shorter duration, and if the patient is living 5 to 10 days after the diagnosis is made, amphotericin B therapy can usually be discontinued. For details, see treatment section under "Blastomycosis" above.

Ketoconazole has been disappointing in preliminary studies.

Itraconazole has been successful in a few patients with amphotericin B-resistant disease, but controlled comparative trials have not yet been reported.[46]

Course and Prognosis

The otitis externa, allergic manifestations, and saprophytic colonization are virtually never disabling or fatal forms. Death by fatal exsanguination from a fungus ball rarely occurs. The invasive, systemic form is generally a fatal disease.

Mucormycosis (Zygomycosis, Phycomycosis)

Mucormycosis is an invasive fungal infection, caused by members of the order Mucorales, that manifests itself in a variety of ways. It is principally known as an acute or fulminant infectious disease, usually arising in the rhinocerebral region, with characteristic early invasion of blood vessels and with dissemination to the brain or other organs. Mucormycosis may be seen in both normal and immunocompromised individuals, although infection usually occurs in the latter. Rarely infection may be confined to the cutaneous tissues.

Another form of the disease, called entomophthoromycosis basidiobolae occurs in children (predominantly boys) and is characterized by inflammatory subcutaneous swellings, involving fat, muscle, and fascia, that spread widely over the upper part of the chest, neck, or arms and heal spontaneously. It is caused by a member of the Entomophthorales, *Basidiobolus ranarum.* Entomophthoromycosis conidiobolae, caused by *Conidiobolus coronatus,* is seen principally in adults.

Historical Aspects

The first authentic report of mucormycosis in a human was probably in 1855 when Kurchenmeister described nonseptate hyphae and a sporangium from a cancerous lung. Paltauf described the first disseminated case in 1885. However, the disease was so rarely recognized that in 1957 Baker could title a paper, "Mucormycosis: A New Disease." Indeed, the pulmonary form was rare, and the more common form was rhinocerebral mucormycosis (zygomycosis). Pulmonary mucormycosis is again being seen more often in individuals with lymphoma, leukemia, and occasionally diabetes.

In 1956, Lei-Kian-Joe and colleagues first described the characteristic subcutaneous mycosis in Indonesia caused by a strain of *B. ranarum.* Emmons, in the United States, also contributed to the knowledge of this form of disease.

Epidemiology

The pulmonary and upper respiratory forms of mucormycosis are worldwide in distribution. Infections with *B. ranarum* have been reported from Indonesia and Africa and rarely from other tropical and subtropical climates worldwide.

The causative fungi are found primarily in the genera *Mucor, Rhizopus, Absidia,* and *Rhizomucor,* although other genera have been implicated, including *Cunninghamella, Mortierella, Saksenaea, Syncephalastrum, Cokeromyces, Basidiobolus, Conidiobolus,* and others. All are ubiquitous on decaying vegetation, fruits, bread, and other vegetable material containing sugar.

Etiology and Pathogenesis

A striking feature of the pathogenesis of at least a third of the patients is concomitant diabetes mellitus. Of even greater importance, however, is the presence of diabetic ketoacidosis. In the remainder of patients, some other disease almost invariably has been present; among which have been leukemia, bone marrow hypoplasia, and malignancy. Treatment with corticosteroids, irradiation, antimetabolites, or immunosuppressive drugs also plays a role. Clark et al. recently have reported on a diabetic HIV-seropositive man with cutaneous mucormycosis.[47]

Clinical Manifestations

The orbital, nasal, sinus, or oropharyngeal form of the disease begins with pain, reddish and then gangrenous skin, or mucosal change with purulent drainage. Induration and swelling appear, so that there is often marked and disfiguring tumescence, including proptosis (Fig. 196-9). There are usually fever and leukocytosis.

Disease may begin in the lung, with pleuritic chest pain, cough, and fever. Early invasion of blood vessels is a characteristic feature, resulting in thrombosis, meningitis, and abscess formation.

The subcutaneous form usually appears over the upper part of the chest, back, neck, and arms and is marked by disfiguring swelling and boardlike induration, but entails little pain and few systemic signs and symptoms.

Primary cutaneous mucormycosis may be caused when the microorganism is injected into the cutaneous[48] or subcutaneous tissue. Reports also have noted inoculation from trauma during gardening,[48] tick implantation, automobile accidents, and use of adhesive bandages.[49] Primary cutaneous mucormycosis has mistakenly been associated with immunocompromised individuals suffering from leukemia and adenocarcinoma.[50]

Pathology

The reaction to the Mucorales is marked by early invasion of blood vessels, vascular occlusion, infarction, and ischemia or hemorrhage. Rarely there are giant cells or other manifestations of a more chronic process. In contrast to many other fungi, Zygomycetes take hematoxylin stain readily. The hyphae are characteristically large (10 to 15 μm in diameter) and rarely septate, and these distinguishing features in tissues have been the basis for diagnosis of most instances of disease.

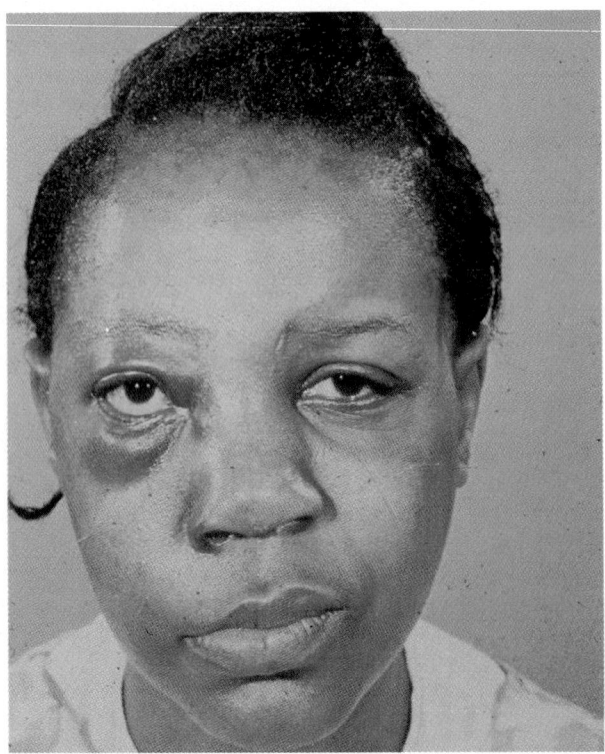

a

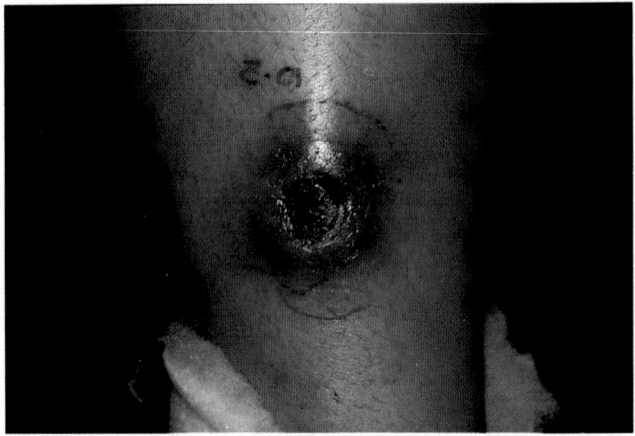

b

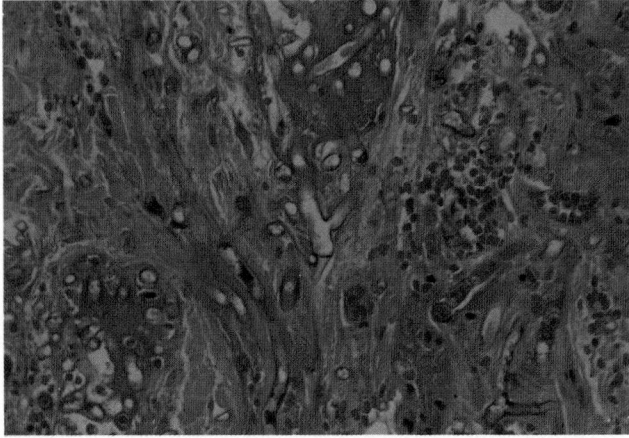

c

FIGURE 196-9 Mucormycosis. The face of this young woman with diabetes mellitus shows proptosis, unilateral facial edema, and a right-sided facial palsy associated with infection beginning in the right maxillary sinus.

Diagnosis and Differential Diagnosis

Because of the ubiquity of these fungi, care must be taken in ascribing disease to one of the Mucorales cultured. Demonstration of tissue invasion by the fungi is essential to diagnosis. Because the pulmonary and upper respiratory forms are so fulminant, the diagnosis usually must be presumptive: many patients have died before biopsy tissue sections could be studied or culture results obtained.

Laboratory Diagnosis DIRECT EXAMINATION. Because the course of most forms are so fulminant, patient specimens are not usually submitted for direct examination. However, when such material is submitted, direct laboratory examination may be useful. The causal microorganisms may be seen in pus, sputum, or biopsy specimens of nasal sinuses, by placing the tissue in a drop of KOH and teasing it apart. Calcofluor white may be added to help in finding hyphal structures. Large, broad, nonseptate, branching hyphae are characteristic of the Mucorales.

CULTURE. The significance is the same as that discussed for *Aspergillus* spp. Cultures are grown at 25 to 30°C on media that do not contain cycloheximide. In contrast to *Aspergillus* spp., zygomycetes generally do not grow above 37°C; most do not grow well above 32°C. All grow rapidly, filling the plate or tube. Differentiation is by morphologic characteristics.

EXOANTIGEN. Exoantigen studies may be performed on cultures as described for *H. capsulatum*.

Differential Diagnosis The disease of the upper respiratory tract is probably most closely mimicked by midline lethal or Wegener's granuloma. Acute orbital cellulitis, nasal sinusitis, or oral pharyngitis due to pyogenic organisms, such as *S. aureus* or *Streptococcus pyogenes,* may also resemble zygomycosis.

The subcutaneous form is so bizarre that only lymphoma or tumor, such as Burkitt's, would be suggested.

Treatment

Successful treatment of the pulmonary form has usually been with amphotericin B. For the rhinocerebral form, surgical debridement has almost always been necessary. In one summary of reported cases, overall survival increased to 70 (from 50 percent), was better when other disease was not present, was least likely when diabetes mellitus was present, and improved to 79 percent with amphotericin B and to 89 percent with accompanying surgery.

Course and Prognosis

The pulmonary and upper respiratory tract forms are usually fulminant and fatal; in the subcutaneous form, spontaneous recovery without therapy seems to occur.

Chromoblastomycosis (Chromomycosis, Verrucous Dermatitis)

Chromoblastomycosis is a chronic cutaneous and subcutaneous infection of the skin, caused by species of dematiaceous (darkly pigmented) fungi, including *Phialophora, Cladosporium,* and *Fonsecaea,* as well as a few other genera anecdotally found in the literature. All genera produce identical wartlike lesions on the skin. It is most common in the tropics and subtropics, but occasionally is seen in the United States.

Historical Aspects

Rudolph first reported a case of chromoblastomycosis from Brazil in 1914, although he did not identify a pathogenic microorganism. Lane and Medlar reported the first case from the United States in 1915, and Thaxter named the causative agent *Phialophora verrucosa.*[51] Since that time other, closely related organisms have been found to produce the same disease. The precise relationship between *P. verrucosa* and the other dematiaceous fungi, primarily causing chromoblastomycosis, *Fonsecaea pedrosoi, F. compactum,* and *Cladosporium carrionii,* is not yet known.

Etiology and Pathogenesis

The agents of chromoblastomycosis are found worldwide in soil and decaying plant material, including wood. Disease is produced by traumatic implantation, especially in individuals in the tropics and subtropics who do not wear shoes. Occasionally other parts of the body may be affected.

Clinical Manifestations (See Fig. 196-10)

Chromoblastomycosis occurs mainly in rural tropical areas and follows trauma, usually to the legs. It usually begins with a nodule that ulcerates and gradually spreads, forming a large mass on the skin surface; several nodules may coalesce. The lesions are often pedunculated and, therefore, easily traumatized and are often described as cauliflower-like because of their appearance. The infection is persistent, lasting many years, and heals with scarring and keloid formation. The disease is not systemic and is seen most frequently in males and in rural workers more often than in their urban counterparts. It is believed that this is due to environment, i.e., rural workers are less likely to wear shoes or protective clothing on their lower extremities and hence are more likely to suffer trauma on the feet and legs than are urban workers. Through such trauma the fungus is introduced into the subcutaneous tissue, where the disease begins. Lesions may also occur less frequently on the hands, arms, or trunk. Transmission does not occur from human to human or from animals to humans.

Pathology

Chromoblastomycosis is generally seen only on the body surfaces. Lesions may be pigmented in a variety of hues and range from macules to hyperkeratotic warty, pedunculated papules. Granulomas within the tissues contain foreign-body giant cells, as well as cells of chronic inflammation. Occurring alone or in clusters, which may be large, dark brown, septate cells ("copper pennies" or Medlar bodies) may be seen in the granulomas (Fig. 196-10g). At times, dematiaceous hyphae may also be found associated with these cells. Thus there is some question as to the correctness of differentiating chromoblastomycosis from pheohyphomycosis, as the latter is defined as dematiaceous hyphae within tissues. However, this question has not yet been resolved.

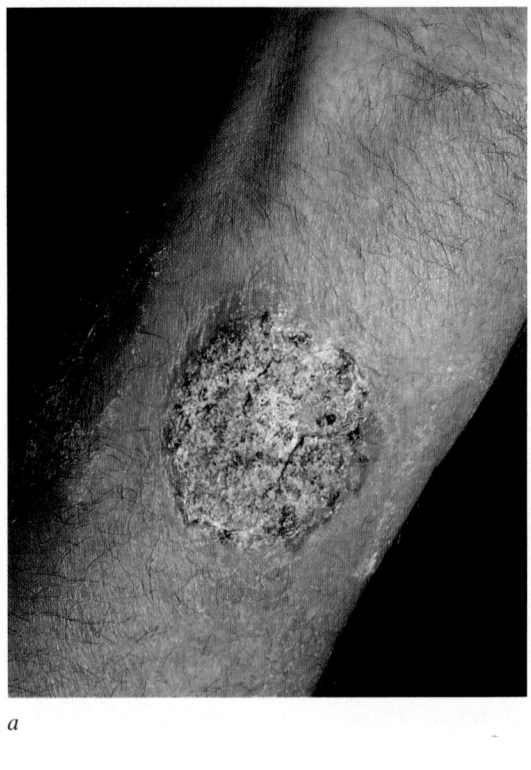

a

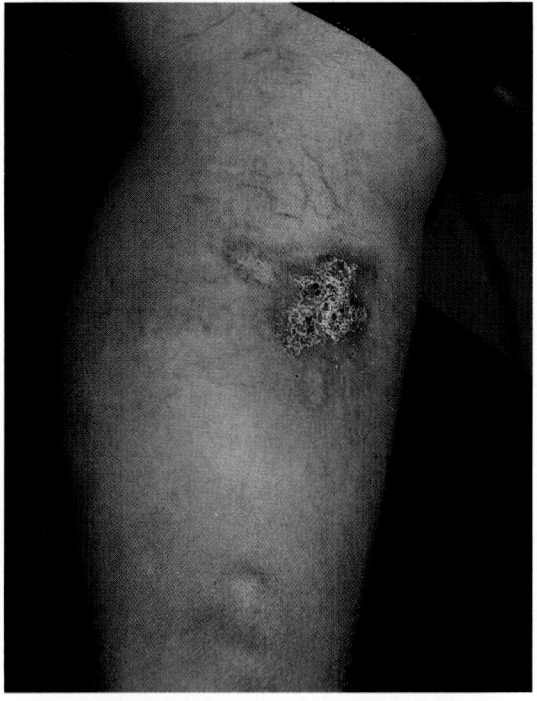

b

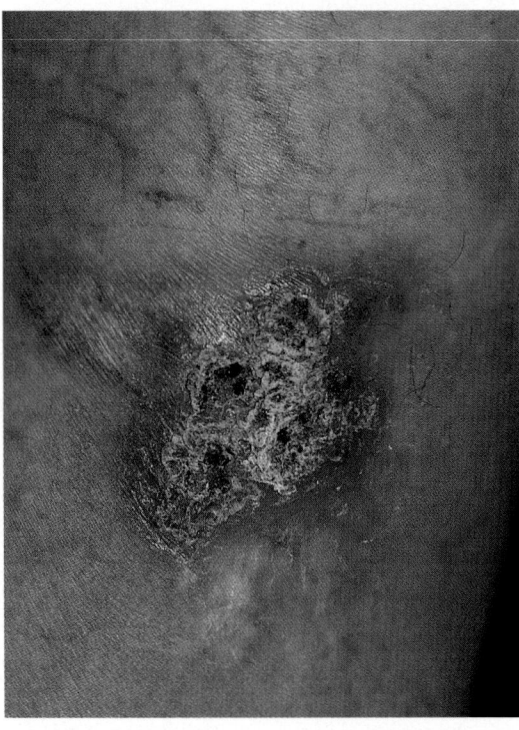

c

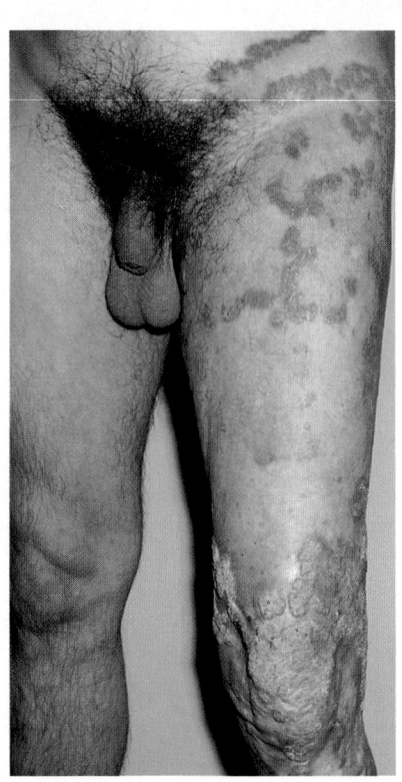

d

FIGURE 196-10 Chromoblastomycosis. (*a*) A solitary, large verrucous plaque surrounded by a halo of erythema is seen on the calf. *(Courtesy of Ted Rosen, M.D., and Howard Rubin, M.D.)* (*b*) This crusted and verrucous plaque appeared 25 years ago following a puncture wound to the area by a wooden spike. (*c*) Close-up of (*b*). (*d*) Extensive involvement of the left leg with verrucous plaques and scarring about the knee and gyrate violaceous nodules on the upper thigh and lower abdomen. *(Courtesy of Orlando Pedro, M.D.)* (*e*) Verrucous plaques with minimal edema on the medial ankle and plantar foot. *(Courtesy of Jose Francha, M.D.)* (*f*) Chronic edema of the foot and ankle with large confluent nodules. (*g*) Lesional biopsy of (*c*) shows large, dark brown, septate cells, i.e., "copper pennies" within granulomas.

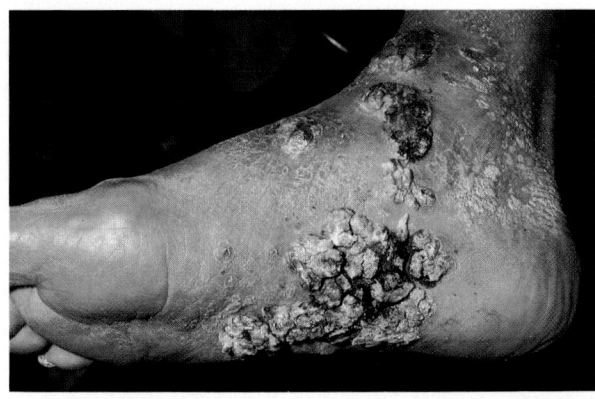

e

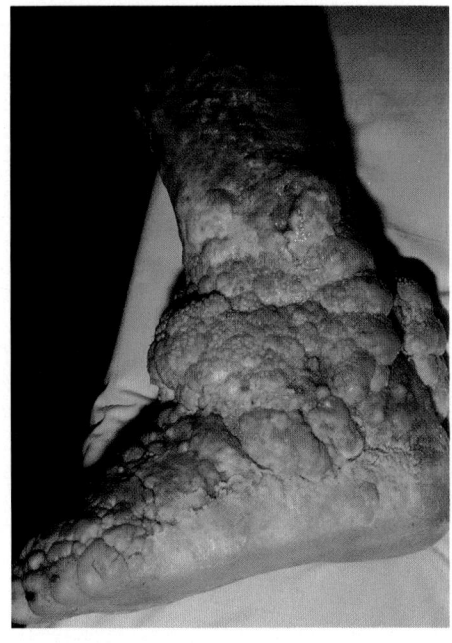

f

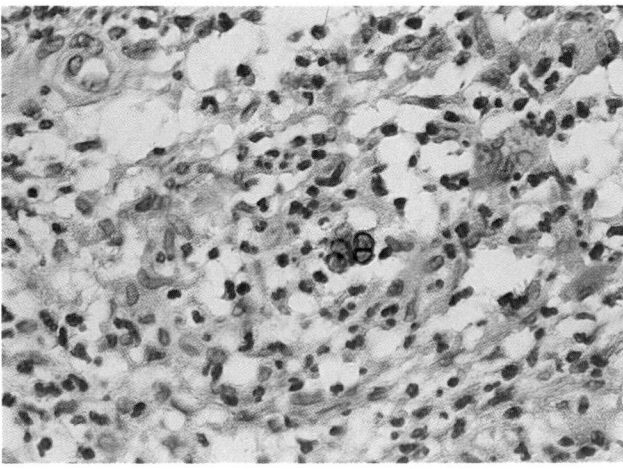

g

FIGURE 196-10 *Continued.*

Diagnosis and Differential Diagnosis

Diagnosis is generally made by examining the lesions. Occasionally the lesions must be differentiated from epidermoid tumors or carcinoma. Definitive diagnosis is made by demonstration of the dematiaceous cells within granulomas.

Laboratory Diagnosis DIRECT EXAMINATION. Skin scrapings or aspirated or biopsy material may be studied in a KOH mount, and the characteristic dematiaceous bodies and occasional hyphae may be seen readily. However, it is essential to identify the causative agent by culture, because at least one of the microorganisms occasionally producing this disease may disseminate to other organs, with a predilection for the brain.

25 to 30°C Incubation 37°C cultures of these microorganisms are not studied, as they are not diphasic. These fungi are not inhibited by cycloheximide or chloramphenicol in growth media. Therefore a medium, such as Mycosel agar (Difco), containing these antifungal and antibacterial agents may be used. Because the causal agents of chromoblastomycosis grow slowly, cultures must be kept for up to 6 weeks. The common contaminants related to these microorganisms grow more rapidly, producing larger colonies than the pathogens. Differentiation of the genera and species depends on the types of conidia produced as well as on the percentage of the various types. Identification is made primarily on microscopic characteristics, although those familiar with the genera are helped

by the size, texture, and color of the colonies produced. The species most often seen are differentiated microscopically as follows:

P. verrucosa produces phialides and phialoconidia exclusively.

F. pedrosoi produces predominantly acrogenous (conidia developing at the tip of a conidiophore or hypha) conidia. The conidia may bud, forming short, branching chains. Thick septae termed *disjunctors* are formed between conidia and between conidia and hyphae. These dark scars are seen readily and help with identification of the organism. Phialides identical to those produced by *P. verrucosa* also may be formed by this species.

F. compactum produces colonies that resemble those of *F. pedrosoi* but develop

more slowly. Conidia are borne as in *F. pedrosoi* but are rounder and formed in compact heads of short chains, which are not dissociated readily.

C. carrionii is the only etiologic agent of chromoblastomycosis in Australia. It has also been isolated in South Africa and Venezuela. Long, branching chains of small conidia resembling the saprophytic strains of *Cladosporium* are the only conidial forms seen.

Wangiella dermatitidis has been isolated a number of times from the specimens of patients with chromoblastomycosis. The culture begins as a black, slimy, moist colony. As hyphae develop, phialides and phialoconidia are produced. They differ from those of *Phialophora* by

having no collarette at the top of the phialide. This microorganism also is seen in pheohyphomycosis.

EXOANTIGEN. Exoantigen studies may be performed on cultures as described for *H. capsulatum.*

Prognosis

With early identification of the infection, surgery may be done with minimal scarring. Although the disease may progress for years with coalescence of lesions, it usually remains localized, neither producing systemic infection nor debilitating the untreated patient. There is no associated pain. However, treatment may be sought for cosmetic reasons or to allow the use of shoes.

Treatment

The treatment of choice is amphotericin B. Reports of successful treatment with potassium iodide either orally or intravenously are not convincing.

Amphotericin B may be given intravenously until a dose of 2 to 3 g is reached. It also may be injected into the skin lesions locally (for details, see "Blastomycosis" above).

Sporotrichosis

Sporotrichosis is a chronic infection that follows accidental implantation of the fungus *Sporothrix schenckii* into the skin. The disease is characterized by nodular lesions of the cutaneous and subcutaneous tissues, from which site it may spread via the lymphatics or disseminate hematogenously to the bones, joints, and other organs. Lesions in the lungs occur after inhalation or aspiration of the fungus.

Historical Aspects

The first detailed clinical description of localized sporotrichosis was made in the United States by Schenck in 1898[52]; in the same year he isolated the causative agent, *S. schenckii.*

In 1947, 3000 cases were reported from Witwatersrand, South Africa,[53] in mine workers who developed the disease within a period of approximately 2 years after contact with mine timbers on which *S. schenckii* was growing. In all cases studied, the infection was of the localized lymphatic type and none was disseminated. The epidemic was halted by use of antifungal agents on the timbers.

Epidemiology

Sporotrichosis is found worldwide and in all age groups. Although adult men are infected most often, occupation and exposure are probably more important in acquiring the disease than are race, sex, or age. The usual reservoir in nature is vegetation on which *S. schenkii* grows saprophytically, often on thorny protuberances.

Infection usually occurs after traumatic implantation of the fungus by thorns, splinters, or other sharp objects. Barberry and

rose bushes, sphagnum moss, soil, and contaminated mine timbers have most often been the source of infection in humans. Sporotrichosis is seen in animals such as the horse, dog, cat, and rat.

Etiology

The single species, *S. schenckii,* produces this disease. The fungus is diphasic with a yeastlike tissue and a hyphal phase. It is weakly pathogenic, and many strains are nonpathogenic. In most human lesions, the tissue phase is difficult to demonstrate on direct microscopic examination of exudate, skin scrapings stained with Gram's or fungal stains, or in biopsy specimens. However, asteroid bodies, (eosinophilic material surrounding the organism in tissue) may be seen. The pathology demonstrated varies with the site of inoculum, the pathogenic capabilities of the microorganism, and the response of the host to the fungus.

Clinical Manifestations (Fig. 196-11)

Cutaneous sporotrichosis presents a variety of lesions, but central lymphatic spread from a single lesion on the dorsum of the hand is most characteristic. The initial lesion begins as a papule, pustule, or nodule that ulcerates, with subsequent associated multiple cutaneous nodules spreading in linear fashion in the lymphatics to the regional lymph nodes (Fig. 196-11a). The initial lesion is indurated and ulcerative, has a ragged undetermined border, and somewhat resembles the primary lesion of syphilis. It is painless except when secondary bacterial infection is present. The disseminated form spreads from a primary lesion to lymph nodes, bone, muscle, joints, viscera, and central nervous system.

Diagnosis and Differential Diagnosis

Diagnosis is made by growing the causal agent, *S. schenckii,* from the lesion. Although lymphocutaneous lesions are typical, with an ulcer at the tip of a finger and a chain of swollen nodules along the lymphatics extending up the arm, other infections may produce similar lesions. Atypical mycobacteria producing cutaneous or lymphatic disease, tularemia, anthrax, glanders, staphylococcal lymphangitis, and some other bacterial infections may simulate the disease but are usually more acute and febrile; gummatous sporotrichosis may resemble the gumma of syphilis, and drug eruptions have been confused with this disease.

Laboratory Diagnosis DIRECT EXAMINATION. Material taken from scrapings, from a lesion or a biopsy, will rarely demonstrate the microorganism. The use of fluorescent antibody staining[54] will demonstrate the organisms when present. Microorganisms may be small, 2 to 3 μm in diameter, or typically, in secondary foci of disease, cigar shaped and 3 to 5 μm in diameter with multiple buds.

CULTURE. *S. schenckii* is one of the more rapidly growing fungal pathogens, growing on most media within 3 to 5 days. The microorganism may form a cream to dark tan, moist colony, turning nearly black and leathery with age. Colony pigment comes from the conidia, which are usually dark brown. Some cultures never produce the pigment, and others may lose the ability to form the pigment upon repeated subculture in the laboratory. Because some contaminants have similar conidia, either the yeast phase

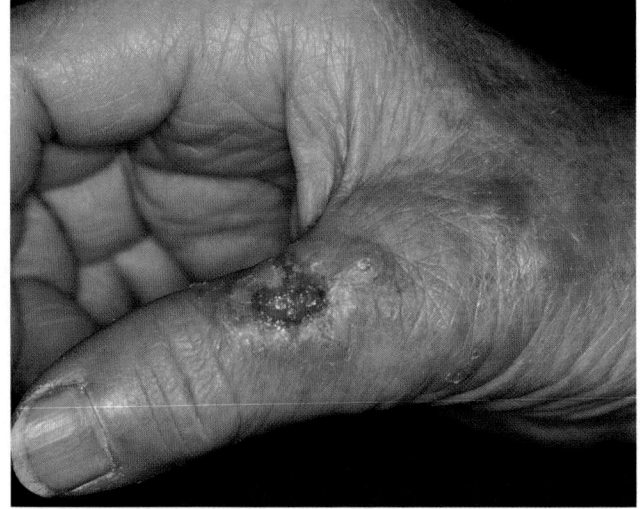

a

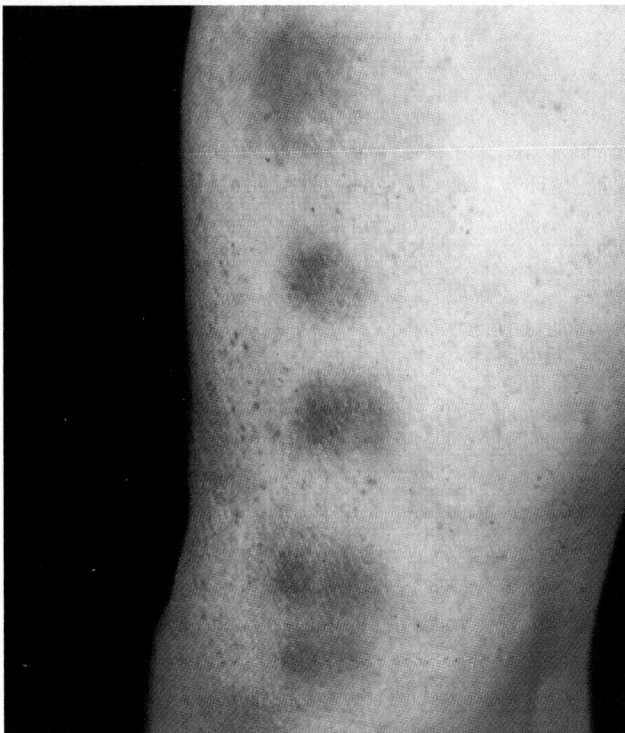

b

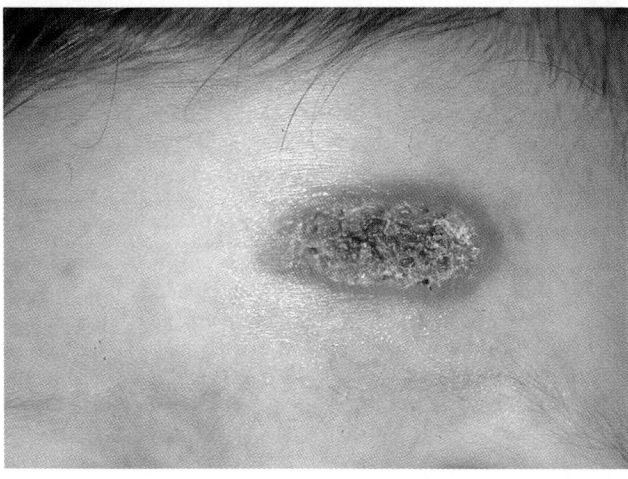

c

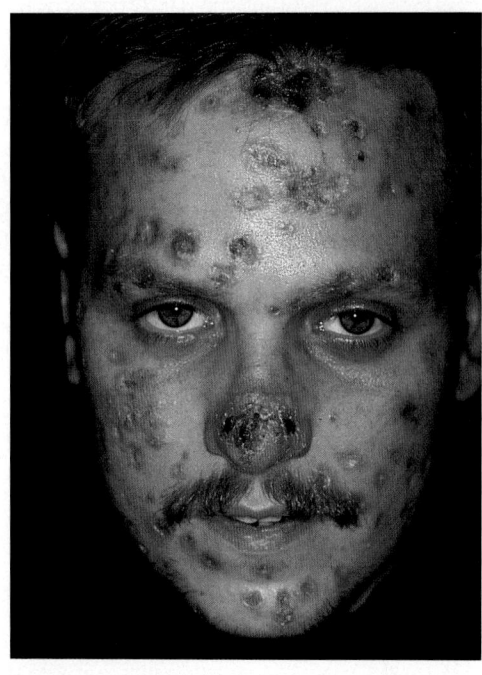

d

e

FIGURE 196-11 Sporotrichosis. (*a*) An ulcerated nodule is seen on the thumb with proximal lymphangitic spread represented by subcutaneous nodules. *(Courtesy of Takeji Nishikawa, M.D.)* (*b*) Chronic lymphangitis type, with nodule within lymphatics. (*c*) Fixed cutaneous type with a large verrucous plaque of the forehead of a child. *(Courtesy of Elyse Rafal, M.D.)* (*d*) Fixed cutaneous type with a crusted, ecthymatous, verrucous plaque on the lateral elbow.
(*e*) Disseminated (hematogenously) in a patient with advanced HIV disease with generalized crusted nodules, sparing only the palms and soles, associated with subcutaneous nodules and arthritis.

must be grown on blood agar at 37°C or the exoantigen test must be performed on the 25 to 30°C culture, if the patient history is not known.

Typical pyriform microconidia are produced along the fine hyphae and/or in arrays at the end of the lateral branches.

EXOANTIGEN. Exoantigen studies may be performed on cultures as described for *H. capsulatum*.

Treatment

The treatment is a saturated solution of potassium iodide, 10 drops three times a day after meals, until lesions have cleared; it may be necessary, in some cases, to increase the dose to maximum tolerance. When iodides are not tolerated or are ineffective, amphotericin B should be given intravenously (see "Blastomycosis" above). In preliminary studies, ketoconazole has been helpful in a few cases. Griseofulvin has been used but is not of proved value. Topical therapy is worthless.

Laboratory Techniques for Superficial and Deep Mycoses

In dealing with dermatophytic infections there is a tendency to minimize the necessity for confirmation by culture. The general impression appears to be that modern antibiotics and antifungal agents negate such requirements. However, Emmons et al.[29] state: "Clinical variations of dermatophytosis are so great and the resemblance of some other skin diseases are so close that a clinical diagnosis needs to be supported by a laboratory diagnosis." Certainly in a percentage of patients this is an accurate evaluation. Furthermore, in those instances when a dermatophytic infection is refractive to treatment, it is best to know what one is dealing with, as well as to have the culture for susceptibility testing.

Collecting the appropriate specimen, proper handling and processing, and correct culturing techniques are skills that are generally acquired through practice.

Collection and Culture of Clinical Specimens

Cultures should be examined daily. If saprophytic fungi appear, subcultures should be made of any colonies suspected of being dermatophytes or systemic fungi. All inoculated media must be held for at least 4 weeks before being considered negative.

In general, inoculated media should be incubated at room temperature (25 to 30°C) and 37°C in an attempt to isolate the tissue phase of diphasic fungi, to aid in the differentiation of *C. neoformans* from other *Cryptococcus* species, and in special instances as indicated under discussion of the various diseases.

Dermatophytes INFECTED HAIRS. Because several of the dermatophytes that infect hairs fluoresce under appropriate conditions, an ultraviolet light with a Wood's filter (3600 Å) may be used both to collect infected hairs and to separate fluorescing from nonfluorescing types of infection. It must be remembered that many other materials may also fluoresce, and the technique should be used only when the skin or scalp is clean and free from ointments. Hairs may be individually epilated with sterile forceps, or adhesive tape may be placed on the lesion surface and pulled off rapidly, removing

damaged and infected hairs. Sufficient infected hairs should be epilated for both culture and for direct KOH-mount study; at least 10 to 15 hairs should be obtained. Hairs suspected of being infected should be placed on Sabouraud dextrose agar and on a medium containing chloramphenicol and cycloheximide (Mycosel agar, Baltimore Biological Co., or Mycobiotic agar, Difco Co.). Care should be taken to ensure maximum contact of hairs with the surface of the agar. If dermatophyte test medium (DTM) is used, microscopic examination of the culture must be performed to assure that a positive (red) reaction has been produced by a dermatophyte, as certain other fungi, e.g., *Aspergillus* spp. may also give this reaction.

SKIN SCRAPINGS. The skin should be adequately cleansed, preferably with 70% alcohol. Application should be brisk, and a few minutes contact time allowed for the alcohol to control the surface contaminants. Alcohol should never be applied with cotton balls because they leave fibers that make a KOH mount difficult to interpret. The roof of unopened vesicles may be removed with sterile scissors for culture. However, suppurated or macerated areas are generally heavily contaminated with bacteria and should be avoided. One should always obtain a sample that is good both in quality and quantity. Too little material causes useless discomfort to the patient because the culture is usually negative. The best approach is to obtain sufficient material by scraping deep into the tissue, causing it to weep. *Scraping must be collected from the margins of the lesions, where the fungus is actively growing.* This area is the most productive for both culture and KOH mounts. Skin scales are placed on the surface of Sabouraud agar medium containing chloramphenicol and cycloheximide; the antibiotics are to be omitted in cases where the suspected fungus might be sensitive to either of these agents. The scales should be spread out and flattened on the surface. Scales that have excessive portions extending into the air rarely produce growth on culture media.

NAIL SCRAPINGS. The nail must be cleansed by scraping off all debris and then applying 70% alcohol, again making sure not to use cotton balls. Debris under the nail is poor material for culture. Rather, scrapings taken at the union of apparently healthy and infected nail should be used for both KOH mount and culture. All thick pieces of nail should first be sliced into smaller ones before further manipulation. After being cut into small pieces, this material should be cultured as above. If a *Candida* species rather than a dermatophyte is the suspected causal microorganism, exudate from the inflamed swollen paronychial tissue, if collected on sterile swabs, may be used for both culture and for microscopic study. However, the material from the eroded nail at the lateral fold is best for direct microscopic examination and for culture.

Specimens for Other Than Dermatophytes SPUTUM. Specimens collected prior to breakfast and after rinsing the mouth are preferable. Purulent or bloody portions of the specimen should be inoculated directly onto Sabouraud dextrose agar medium containing added chloramphenicol and cycloheximide. The latter should be incubated at both room temperature and 37°C. (If systemic infection caused by a diphasic fungus is suspected, media containing cycloheximide should be kept at room temperature only as the yeast phases of the systemic fungi are sensitive to this antibiotic at 37°C.)

URINE. A well-mixed representative sample of fresh urine should be centrifuged for 15 min at 2500 rpm. The supernatant is discarded, leaving only several milliliters, and the sediment is resuspended. Portions of this material should be inoculated onto Sabouraud dextrose agar and incubated at 37°C and at room temperature and onto one plate or tube of Sabouraud dextrose agar containing chloramphenicol and cycloheximide, at room temperature. The material should be spread to cover the entire surface.

CEREBROSPINAL FLUID. The entire specimen should be centrifuged for 15 min at 2500 rpm. The supernatant may be used for chemical evaluations or frozen and kept for serologic or other studies. Inoculation is made onto Sabouraud dextrose agar and blood agar or chocolate agar, with incubation at both room temperature and 37°C.

GRANULES. See "Actinomycosis."

BLOOD. Inoculate ≥5 mL directly into 50-mL bottles of brain-heart infusion or trypticase soy broth with sodium citrate and 5 to 8 mL Sabouraud dextrose agar added. At least two bottles should be inoculated from the same blood specimen.

BIOPSY. Inoculate pus or caseous material directly onto desired media and prepare two smears for Gram and PAS stains. *Mince the tissue with sterile scissors. Grind with sterile Sabouraud broth, and add 0.2 to 0.5 mL of the homogenate to appropriate media.*

BONE MARROW. Inoculate appropriate media by streaking the specimen across the entire surface with a loop. If the specimen is obtained in a syringe, draw up several milliliters of broth into the syringe and discharge it into 20 mL of Sabouraud broth.

Examination of Specimens in 10% to 20% Potassium Hydroxide Mounts

Dermatologic Specimens HAIR. Epilated hairs should be studied immediately. Several hairs are placed on a slide, KOH and a coverslip are added, and the slide is warmed without boiling. After sitting for 15 to 20 min, the slide may be examined for the presence of fungi. For this and most other microscopic examinations, the substage or condenser diaphragm should be closed to approximately one-half its normal opening area, and the condenser lowered until best contrast with the specimen is obtained.

All *Microsporum* spp. produce arthroconidia (usually 2 to 3 μm) around the outside of the hair shaft (ectothrix) in a mosaic fashion. *M. gypseum*, however, produces larger arthroconidia (5 to 8 μm). *Trichophyton* species produce generally larger arthroconidia, which may be either outside (ectothrix) or within (endothrix) the hair in chains. Several species produce both ectothrix and endothrix infection. Because the arthroconidia may become dislodged, particularly in heavily damaged hairs, often only the mycotic nature of the infection, and not the genus, may be determined.

T. schoenleinii is rare in the United States but may be seen in other parts of the world and in immigrants from areas where this microorganism produces disease. In such cases the yellowish scales, crusts (favic scutula), or hairs are the best material for direct microscopic examination. The microscopic field shows arthroconidia of varying size and shape. Hyphae are septate and rather coarse. In some fields the organism may be missing, but vestigial traces containing air bubbles are present, and are typical of *T. schoenleinii*.

SKIN SCRAPINGS. Several pieces of the scrapings should be placed on a glass slide without overlapping. Potassium hydroxide (10 to 20%) and a coverslip are added, and the specimen is gently heated and then allowed to stand for about 10 min. The specimen may then be studied for hyphae, arthroconidia or, occasionally, budding cells. One cannot identify specific microorganisms, only note their presence or absence.

NAIL SCRAPINGS. Several thin pieces of the specimen should be placed on a glass slide without overlapping. A few drops of KOH (10 to 20%) and a coverslip are added. The slide is *gently* heated to nearly boiling and then allowed to sit for approximately 30 min. Boiling must be avoided as it produces bubbles that both disrupt the fungus and produce artefacts. Heating is not required but hastens the action of the KOH. The specimen may then be studied for hyphae and budding cells. Several microorganisms, not dermatophytes, that cause infection in nails may occasionally be seen e.g., *Scopulariopsis brevicaulis*, *Geotrichum candidum*, various *Aspergillus* spp., *Trichosporon beigelii*, and *Candida albicans*. Therefore the presence of any type of hyphae or spore (conidia) within the scrapings must be followed by culture on media with and without cycloheximide or chloramphenicol, and if no dermatophyte is grown, microorganism usually thought to be contaminant must be considered as the actual cause of disease.

Culture of an entire nail is not recommended. However, if this is done, all of the nail should be placed in or on the surface of the agar medium. For unknown reasons, if any appreciable amount of nail is left above the agar, the microorganisms are less likely to grow.

BIOPSIED MATERIAL. This material is handled by the same general procedure as are skin scrapings. However, the tissue must first be ground or minced into minute pieces before either microscopic examination or culture.

Specimens for Other Than Dermatophytes SPUTUM. Fresh sputum, not saliva, should be collected in a sterile container. A loopful of the material is mixed with a drop of KOH (10 to 20%) on a microscope slide, a coverslip placed on top, and the specimen studied by microscope. Clearing by gentle heating may occasionally be necessary. *Candida* spp., *B. dermatitidis*, *Cryptococcus* spp., *C. immitis* spherules, and hyphal strands of either saprophytic or opportunistic fungi (e.g., *Aspergillus*, *Mucor* spp.) may be visualized in this manner. The cells of *H. capsulatum* are too small to be seen in the KOH preparation, although sputum smears dried and stained with Giemsa stain may rarely be useful for finding this microorganism under oil immersion.

URINE. Following centrifugation of the specimen, a drop of the sediment is placed on a slide and covered with a coverslip; under reduced light, hyphae and budding cells such as those produced by *B. dermatitidis* may be visualized. The Gram stain may demonstrate hyphae and yeast cells compatible with *Candida* spp.

CEREBROSPINAL FLUID. An india ink or calcofluor white preparation of the sediment is mandatory if *C. neoformans* is suspected or if yeast cells are seen in the specimen.

GRANULES. See "Actinomyces."

BONE MARROW. A small portion should be placed between two slides, smeared, and dried. Both the Gram and PAS stains are then performed.

Use of Calcofluor White M2R (Cellufluor)*

Calcofluor white is a method for rapid demonstration of fungi in specimens. It is more accurate than KOH preparations, more rapid than either PAS or other stains, may be used on a specimen even in the presence of KOH, and may be kept for months on the shelf.[55,56] The preparation of the specimen is as above, but the material must

---

*American Cyanamid.

be visualized with the use of a fluorescence microscope. Kits with the appropriate reagents may be obtained from Polysciences, Inc., Paul Valley Industrial Park, Warrington, PA, 18976-2590.

Other specimens for culture generally require special laboratory preparation or culture media. The laboratory to which the specimen will be sent should be notified first, to ensure that the most appropriate specimen will be collected and to alert the laboratory to anticipate the specimen.

Further information on culture methods may be found in references 57 and 58.

References

1. Pennys NS, Hicks B: Unusual cutaneous lesions associated with acquired immunodeficiency syndrome. *J Am Acad Dermatol* **13**:845, 1985

2. Bollinger O: Über eine neue Pilzkrankheit beim Rinde. *Zentralbl Med Wiss* **15**:481, 1877

3. Israel J: Neue Beobachtungen auf dem Gebiete der Mykosen des Menchen. *Virchows Arch [A]* **74**:15, 1878

4. Cope VZ: *Actinomycosis.* London, Oxford Univ Press, 1938, 246 pp

5. Nichols DR, Harrell WE: Penicillin in the treatment of actinomycosis (abstr). *J Lab Clin Med* **32**:1405, 1947

6. Nocard ME: Note sur la maladie des boeufs de la Guadeloupe connue sous le nom de farcin. *Ann Inst Pasteur (Paris)* **2**:293, 1888

7. Eppinger H: Über eine neue pathogene Cladothix und eine durch sie hervorgerfufene Pseudotuberculosis. *Wein Klin Wochenschr* **3**:321, 1890

8. Satterwhite TK, Wallace RJ Jr: Primary cutaneous nocardiosis. *JAMA* **242**:333, 1979

9. Yoger R et al: Successful treatment of *Nocardia asteroides* infection with amikacin. *J Pediatr* **96**:771, 1980

10. Carter HV: On mycetoma. *Trans Med Phys Soc Bomba:* vol. VI, VII, 1859, 1860

11. Mackinnon JE: Mycetomas as opportunistic wound infections. *Lab Invest* **11**:1124, 1962

12. Emmons CW: Isolation of *Cryptococcus neoformans* from soil. *J Bacteriol* **62**:685, 1951

13. Kerkering TM et al: The evolution of pulmonary cryptococcosis. Clinical implications from a study of 41 patients with and without compromising host factors. *Ann Intern Med* **94**:611, 1981

14. De Wyte CN et al: Cryptococcal meningitis: A review of 32 years' experience. *J Neurol Sci* **53**:283, 1982

15. Fink JN et al. Cryptococcal antibodies in pigeon breeder's disease. *J Allergy* **41**:297, 1968

16. Bozette SA et al: A placebo controlled trial of maintenance therapy with fluconazole after treatment of cryptococcal meningitis in the acquired immunodeficiency syndrome. *N Engl J Med* **324**:580, 1991

17. Bennett JE, Remington JS: Miconazole in cryptococcosis and systemic candidiasis: A word of caution. *Ann Intern Med* **94**:708, 1981

18. McGinnis MR, Katz B: *Ajellomyces* and its synonym *Emmonsiella. Mycotaxon* **8**:157, 1979

19. Darling ST: A protozoon general infection producing pseudotubercles in the lungs and focal necrosis in the liver, spleen, and lymph nodes. *JAMA* **46**:1283, 1906

20. DeMonbreun WA: The cultivation and cultural characteristics of Darling's *Histoplasma capsulatum. Am J Trop Med* **14**:93, 1934

21. Furcolow ML, Brasher CA: Chronic progressive (cavitary) histoplasmosis as a problem in tuberculosis sanatoriums. *Am Rev Tuberc* **73**:609, 1956

22. Wheat LJ et al: A large urban outbreak of histoplasmosis: Clinical features. *Ann Intern Med* **94**:331, 1982

23. Wheat LJ: Diagnosis and management of histoplasmosis. *Eur J Clin Microbiol Infect Dis* **8**:480, 1989

24. Drouhet E: African histoplasmosis, in *Tropical Fungal Infections,*

Bailliere's Clinical Tropical Medicine and Communicable Diseases, vol 4, *International Practice and Research,* edited by RJ Hay. Philadelphia, Bailliere Tindall, 1989

25. Lennette E et al (eds): *Manual of Clinical Microbiology,* 4th ed. Washington, DC, American Society for Microbiology, 1985

26. Kaufman L, Standard PG: Specific and rapid identification of medically important fungi by exoantigen detection. *Ann Rev Microbiol* **41**:209, 1987

27. Drugs for treatment of deep fungal infections. *Med Lett Drugs Ther* **32**:50, 1990

28. Gilchrist TC, Stokes WR: A case of pseudo-lupus vulgaris caused by blastomyces. *J Exp Med* **3**:53, 1898

29. Emmons CW et al: *Medical Mycology.* Philadelphia, Lea & Febiger, 1963

30. Klein BS et al: Two outbreaks of blastomycosis along rivers in Wisconsin. Isolation of *Blastomyces dermatitidis* from riverbank soil and evidence of its transmission along waterways. *Am Rev Respir Dis* **136**:1333, 1987

31. Klein BS et al: Isolation of *Blastomyces dermatitidis* in soil associated with a large outbreak of blastomycosis in Wisconsin. *N Engl J Med* **314**:529, 1986

32. Lutz A: Una mycose pseudococcidioidica localizado no boca e observada no Brasil. Contribucao ao conhecimento das hyfoblastomycoses americanas. *Brasil-Med* **22**:121, 1908

33. Almeida F: Consideracoes sobre a blastomicose sulamericana em sua forma queloideana. *Rev Inst Adolfo Lutz* **10**:31, 1951

34. Restrepo AM et al: Estrogen inhibition of mycelium to yeast transformation in the fungus *Paracoccidioides brasiliensis:* Implications for resistance of females to paracoccidioidomycosis. *Infect Immun* **46**:346, 1984

35. Naranjo MS et al: Treatment of paracoccidioidomycosis with itraconazole. *J Med Vet Mycol* **28**:67, 1990

36. Rixford E, Gilchrist TC: Two cases of protozoan (coccidioidal) infection of the skin and other organs. *Johns Hopkins Hosp Rep* **1**:20090, 1896

37. Ophuls W, Moffitt HC: A new pathogenic mould (formerly described as a protozoan: *Coccidioides immitis.* Preliminary report. *Phila Med J* **5**:1471, 1900

38. Dickson EC, Gifford MA: Coccidioides infection (coccidioidomycosis): The pulmonary type of infection. *Arch Intern Med* **62**:852, 1938

39. Smith CE: Epidemiology of acute coccidioidomycosis with erythema nodosum ("San Joaquin" or "Valley Fever"). *Am J Public Health* **30**:600, 1940

40. Galgiani JN, Ampel NM: Coccidioidomycosis in human immunodeficiency virus-infected patients. *J Infect Dis* **162**:1165, 1990

41. Sun SH et al: Rapid *in vitro* conversion and identification of *Coccidioides immitis. J Clin Microbiol* **3**:186, 1976

42. Tucker RM et al: Itraconazole therapy in chronic coccidioidal meningitis. *Ann Intern Med* **112**:108, 1990

43. Tomecki KJ et al: Systemic mycoses. *J Am Acad Dermatol* **21**(6):1285, 1989

44. Renon L: *Étude sur L'Aspergillose chez les Animaux et chez l'Homme.* Paris, Masson, 1897

45. Raper KB, Fennel DI: *The Genus Aspergillus.* Baltimore, Williams & Wilkins, 1965

46. Sachs MK et al: Amphotericin-resistant aspergillus osteomyelitis controlled by itraconazole. *Lancet* **335**:1475, 1990

47. Clark R et al: Cutaneous zygomycosis in a diabetic HTLV-I-seropositive man. *J Am Acad Dermatol* **22**:956, 1990

48. Costa AR et al: Subcutaneous mucormycosis caused by *Mucor hiemalis* wehmer *f. luteus* (Linnemann) Schipper, 1973. *Mycoses* **33**:241, 1990

49. Patterson JE et al: Hospital acquired gangrenous mucormycosis. *Yale J Biol Med* **59**:453, 1986

50. Umbert IJ, Daniel Su WP: Cutaneous mucormycosis. *J Am Acad Dermatol* **21**:1232, 1989

51. Lane CG: A cutaneous disease caused by a new fungus *Phialophora verruco.a. J Cutan Dis* **33**:840, 1915

52. Schenck BR: On refractory subcutaneous abscesses caused by a fungus possibly related to sporotrichia. *Bull Johns Hopkins Hosp* **9**:286, 1898

53. Helm MAF, Bermann C: Sporotrichosis infection in mines of the Witwatersrand: A symposium, in *Proceedings of the Transvaal Mine Medical Officers Association.* Johannesburg, Transvaal Chamber of Mines, 1947

54. Kaplan W, Ivens MS: Fluorescent antibody staining of *Sporotrichum schenckii* in cultures and clinical material. *J Invest Dermatol* **35**:151, 1961

55. Hageage GL, Harrington BJ: Use of calcofluor white in clinical microbiology. *Lab Med* **15**:109, 1984.

56. Monheit JE et al: Rapid detection of fungi in tissues using calcofluor white and fluorescence microscopy. *Arch Pathol Lab Med* **108**:616, 1984

57. Balows A et al: *Manual of Clinical Microbiology,* 5th ed. Washington, DC, American Society for Microbiology, 1991

58. Rippon JW: *Medical Mycology: The Pathogenic Fungi and the Pathogenic Actinomycetes,* 3d ed. Philadelphia, Saunders, 1988

Rickettsial Diseases

CHAPTER 197

William Schaffner   **The Rickettsioses**

Rickettsiae are pleomorphic coccobacillary obligate intracellular parasites. Transmitted to humans by arthropods, they produce acute systemic infections of varying severity (Table 197-1).

The most frequent rickettsial infection in the United States is Rocky Mountain spotted fever; reported cases have increased since 1960, predominantly in the southeastern states. Because the dermatologic characteristics of the rickettsioses provide the basis for clinical differential diagnosis and the initiation of proper therapy, they will be emphasized in the discussion that follows.

Historic Aspects

Classic louse-borne epidemic typhus has been one of the major scourges of civilization, particularly during periods of famine or war. As Zinsser has dramatically described, typhus—not strategy—has determined the outcome of many military campaigns, thus ex-

erting a direct influence on history. In the epidemics of typhus that swept through Russia and eastern Europe from 1918 to 1922, it is estimated that 30 million persons became ill and 3 million died.

In the 1890s, Wood and Maxcy described an unusual disease of high mortality in Idaho, which was later named Rocky Mountain spotted fever. In the early 1900s, Howard Taylor Ricketts established the tick as the vector of Rocky Mountain spotted fever. The rickettsiae were named for this investigator, who died of typhus while studying that disease in Mexico. In 1910, Brill described a series of patients in New York City who had a disease similar to, but distinct from, typhoid fever. Subsequently, Zinsser correctly postulated that this illness represented a recurrent form of epidemic typhus appearing in patients who had previously had the classic disease. In 1915, two Polish investigators, Weil and Felix, discovered that patients recovering from rickettsial infection had an agglutinin in their serums for certain otherwise unrelated *Proteus* bacteria. The Weil-Felix test is still used as a nonspecific but rapid method of screening for certain rickettsial diseases. In the 1920s

TABLE 197-1
The Rickettsial Diseases

Group	Disease	Rickettsial species	Arthropod vector	Reservoir	Weil-Felix reaction
Spotted fever	Rocky Mountain spotted fever	*R. rickettsii*	Tick	Small mammals, ticks	Positive
	Boutonneuse fever South African tick-bite fever (see Fig. 197-5) Kenya tick typhus Indian tick typhus	*R. conorii*	Tick	Dogs, rodents	Positive
	Siberian tick typhus	*R. sibirica*	Tick	Rodents	Positive
	Queensland tick typhus	*R. australis*	Tick	Marsupials, rodents	Positive
	Rickettsialpox	*R. akari*	Mite of house mouse	House mouse	Negative
Typhus	Endemic	*R. typhi*	Rat flea	Rat	Positive
	Epidemic	*R. prowazekii*	Human body louse	Humans, flying squirrel	Positive
	Brill-Zinsser disease	*R. prowazekii*		Recurrence of dormant epidemic typhus	Low or negative
	Scrub	*R. tsutsugamushi*	Mite	Rodents, mites	
Trench fever	Trench fever	*R. quintana*	Louse	Humans	Negative
Q fever	Q fever	*R. burnetii*	Inhalation of dried tick feces	Cattle, sheep, goats	Negative
Ehrlichia	Ehrlichiosis	*E. canis*	Tick	Dogs	

and 1930s, the work of Maxcy, Dyer, and others established the existence of another form of typhus transmitted not by the body louse but by the rat flea, thereby explaining the many cases of mild typhus unassociated with lousiness that had so long puzzled investigators.

Pathogenesis

Infected arthropods transmit rickettsiae to humans in two ways: ticks and mites (vectors of spotted fevers and scrub typhus) inoculate rickettsiae directly at the time of the bite, and lice and fleas (carriers of epidemic and endemic typhus) defecate feces containing rickettsiae while biting. Rickettsiae are introduced into the wound by scratching the irritated site. Rarely, epidemic typhus may be acquired via the airborne route when the garments of a patient are shaken, thus dispersing an aerosol of infected louse feces.

After inoculation it is postulated that initial rickettsial multiplication occurs at the site of introduction, and skin lesions at the site of the arthropod bite are the rule in rickettsialpox, scrub typhus, and boutonneuse fever.

Rickettsia rickettsii, the agent causing Rocky Mountain spotted fever, may be considered the rickettsial prototype. It produces the most marked pathologic changes and the most severe disease. The size of the microorganisms (0.2 by 1.0 μm) and their staining characteristics (purple with Giemsa's stain or red with Macchiavello's stain) enable them to be visualized with the light microscope if they are carefully sought in tissue sections. The members of the spotted fever group of rickettsiae multiply in both the nucleus and the cytoplasm of infected cells. Rickettsiae of the typhus group grow only in the cytoplasm.

Diffuse vasculitis is the pathologic hallmark of rickettsial disease. During the incubation period it is surmised that rickettsemia occurs, seeding the endothelial cells of capillaries, arterioles, and venules. With rickettsial multiplication the endothelial cells proliferate, swell, and degenerate, resulting in partial or complete thrombosis of the vascular lumen. In Rocky Mountain spotted fever, the rickettsiae also invade the smooth-muscle wall of arterioles, producing further vascular damage, with resultant microinfarction and extravasation. Accumulations of polymorphonuclear and mononuclear inflammatory cells surround such areas of vascular injury. These changes occur at intervals along the vessels, leaving normal vascular architecture in intervening areas. In severe cases, thrombosis involves larger vessels, and microinfarction of the affected tissue is extensive (Fig. 197-1).

The vascular lesions described account for most of the observed clinical findings, the location of the lesion determining its clinical expression. The skin most directly reflects vascular damage, the rash coinciding with the point and extent of vascular injury. In the brain the glial nodule is its counterpart; in the heart an interstitial myocarditis and microinfarctions are produced. A patchy interstitial rickettsial pneumonitis may occur.

The pathologic changes produced by the rickettsiae causing the typhus fevers closely resemble those described for Rocky Mountain spotted fever, but their extent and severity are usually more limited, there is less tendency to thrombosis, and invasion of the arteriolar smooth muscle almost never occurs (Figs. 197-2 and 197-3).

The cause of the toxic and febrile state produced by rickettsial infection remains obscure. Rickettsial toxins (lethal for mice) have been described, but their role in the pathogenesis of disease is un-

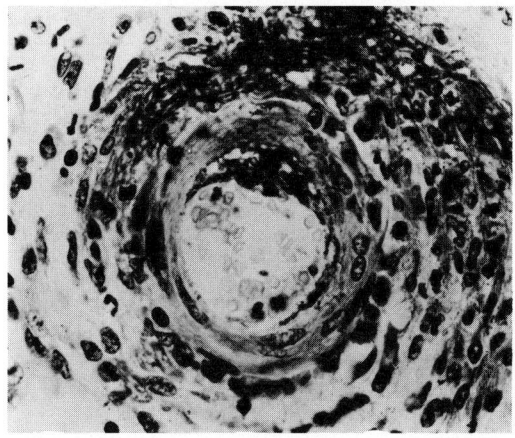

a

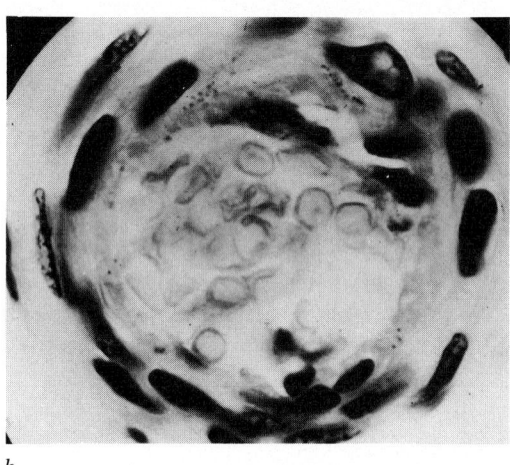

b

FIGURE 197-1 (*a*) The vascular lesion of Rocky Mountain spotted fever as seen in an arteriole in the epididymis. An early thrombus is present. (*b*) Rickettsiae are seen in endothelial cells in a biopsy from scrotal skin. (*From the collection of the late Prof. S. Burt Wolbach, with permission of Arthur T. Hertig, M.D., Dept. of Pathology, Harvard University.*)

certain. There is no explanation for the fact that the rash of Rocky Mountain spotted fever begins peripherally and spreads centrally, whereas that of typhus erupts first on the trunk and later appears on the extremities.

Rocky Mountain Spotted Fever

Rocky Mountain spotted fever, caused by *R. rickettsii* and transmitted via tick bite, is the most severe of the rickettsial infections. The illness ranges from a virtually asymptomatic form to a fulminant disease with fatality rates ranging from 20 to 80 percent in untreated cases.

The infection is seasonal, the early summer peak of the disease corresponding to the increased seasonal activity of ticks and increased human contact with them. The reservoir of the disease is thought to be in small mammals, but ticks can infect their offspring transovarially, thus also serving as a reservoir. In the western United States the wood tick, *Dermacentor andersoni,* is the vector of the disease; in the eastern United States, however, the dog tick,

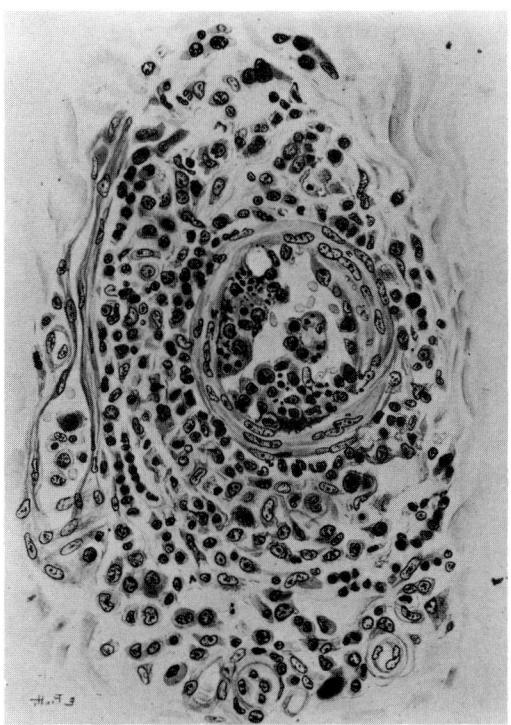

FIGURE 197-2 The vascular lesion of typhus as depicted in an artist's representation of a skin biopsy taken on the eighth day of the eruption. (*From the Wolbach collection, with permission of Arthur T. Hertig, M.D.*)

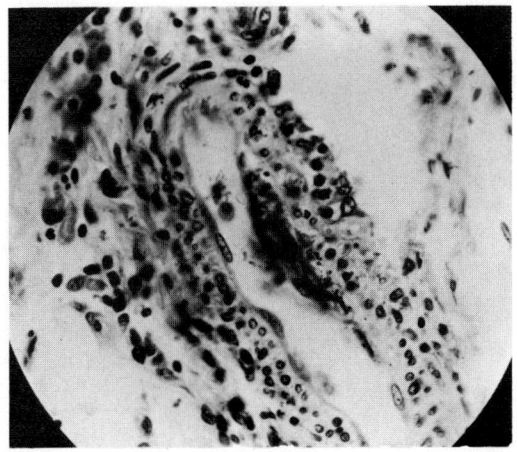

FIGURE 197-3 Thrombosis in a cutaneous arteriole from a patient with typhus. (*From the Wolbach collection, with permission of Arthur T. Hertig, M.D.*)

D. variabilis, is the principal vector. Possibly this explains the high incidence in children in the eastern United States and the high incidence in men in the mountain woods of Montana and other western states.

Clinical Manifestations

The incubation period ranges from 3 to 12 days, with a mean of 7 days. The onset is generally abrupt, with the sudden appearance of fever, chills, severe headache, myalgia, and arthralgia. The rash, the most characteristic aspect of the disease, generally appears on the fourth day of fever (range, 2 to 6 days). It goes through a very regular and unique progression, first erupting on the wrists, ankles, and forearms. It is pink and macular, fades on pressure, and is accentuated by warm compresses or a rise in the patient's temperature. After 6 to 18 h, the rash involves the palms and soles and then extends centrally to the arms, thighs, trunk, and face. After 1 to 3 days, the rash becomes macular and papular and a deeper red (Fig. 197-4). After 2 to 4 days, petechiae appear in the rash and the lesions no longer fade on pressure. Pressure from a sphygmomanometer may induce an additional shower of petechiae (Rumpel-Leede test, indicating capillary fragility), and the lesions coalesce and form ecchymoses. Small areas of gangrene may appear over the toes, fingers, earlobes, nose, scrotum, or vulva. Involvement of the scrotum or vulva often serves as a diagnostic clue. The more severe the infection, the more extensive the rash and the more rapid the progression. The rash may not be noticed in black patients. Furthermore, it now is recognized that the disease can involve many organ systems but spare the skin. Such illness without a rash has been called Rocky Mountain "spotless" fever.

The diffuse vasculitis of the severe cases results in transudation of plasma, diminishing intravascular volume, falling blood pressure, and rising pulse, and patients appear profoundly ill. These changes are accentuated by the diffuse myocarditis and by the lowered serum albumin level, thought to be a consequence of liver involvement. Such patients, especially children, may appear quite edematous. Impaired circulatory dynamics further leads to diminished renal function.

A firm spleen is palpable in half the cases. Abdominal distension and muscular tenderness may combine to mimic appendicitis or other intraabdominal disease. Severely ill patients may be comatose. Further evidence of neurologic damage, such as seizures or hemiplegia, is associated with a very poor prognosis.

On recovery, the areas involved by the rash develop secondary pigmentation, which may persist for some time.

Laboratory Diagnosis

The usual laboratory determinations do not aid in diagnosis. A normochromic, normocytic anemia may develop during the second week of the disease. The white blood cell count is generally within the normal range, although leukopenia or a mild leukocytosis may be observed. Cerebrospinal fluid examination generally reveals only a few red blood cells and lymphocytes. Thrombocytopenia and various derangements of the blood clotting mechanisms often accompany the moderate and severe forms of the disease as a consequence of diffuse intravascular coagulation. Elevated blood urea nitrogen values usually reflect a prerenal azotemia, and liver function studies show degrees of impairment, especially diminished serum albumin concentrations.

The Weil-Felix test, with OX-K, OX-19, and OX-2 strains of *Proteus vulgaris,* is used extensively to help in narrowing diagnostic possibilities to rickettsial disease. A titer of less than 1:320 is not definitely diagnostic, and demonstration of a rising titer in acute and convalescent serum specimens is desirable. The Weil-Felix test will *not* distinguish between the spotted and typhus fevers. It is thus important to have specific complement fixation or indirect fluorescent antibody studies performed with acute and convalescent serums. These tests are available through state health departments and the Centers for Disease Control in Atlanta, Georgia. Antibiotic

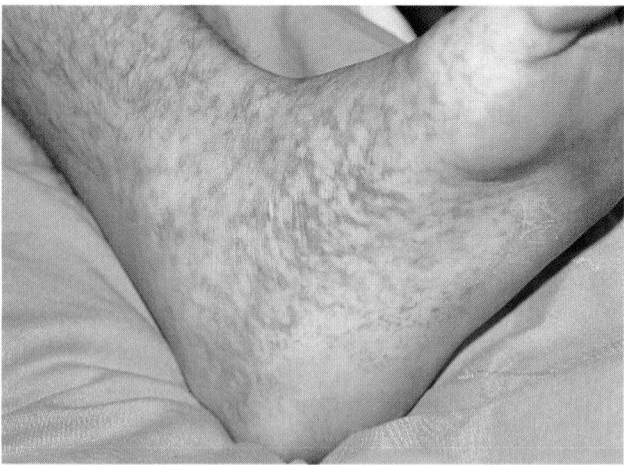

a

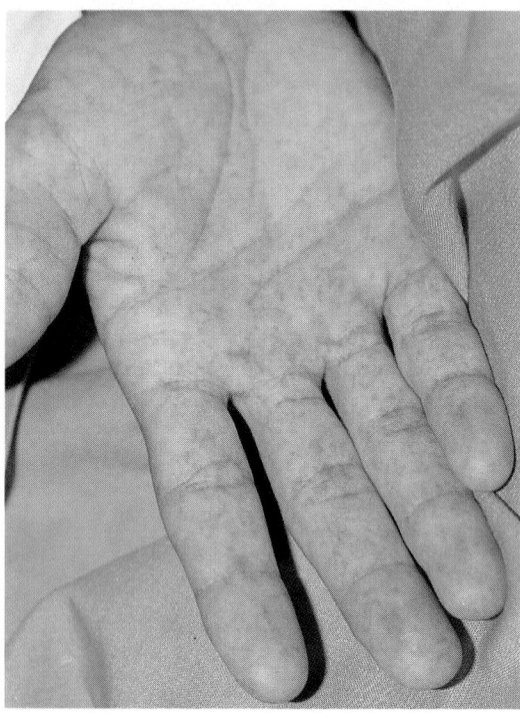

b

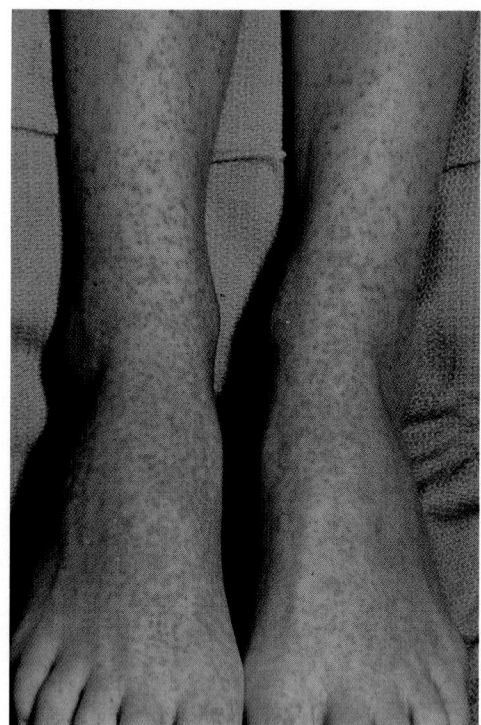

c

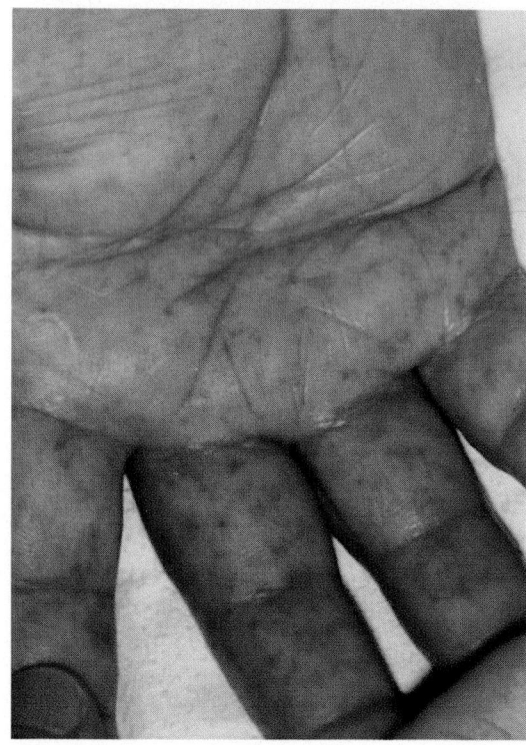

d

FIGURE 197-4 Rocky Mountain spotted fever. (*a, b*) Early macular blanchable macules and papules on the palm, soles, and ankles; no trunkal lesions were present at this time. (*c, d*) Later lesions on the ankles and palm are hemorrhagic and no long blanch with pressure; trunkal lesions were present at this time.

(*e*) Trunkal and facial hemorrhagic macules and papules 7 days after the onset of the rash. (*f*) Infarction of fingers in a patient whose course was complicated by disseminated intravascular coagulation. [(*c*), (*d*), and (*f*), *courtesy of Charles W. Stratton, M.D.*]

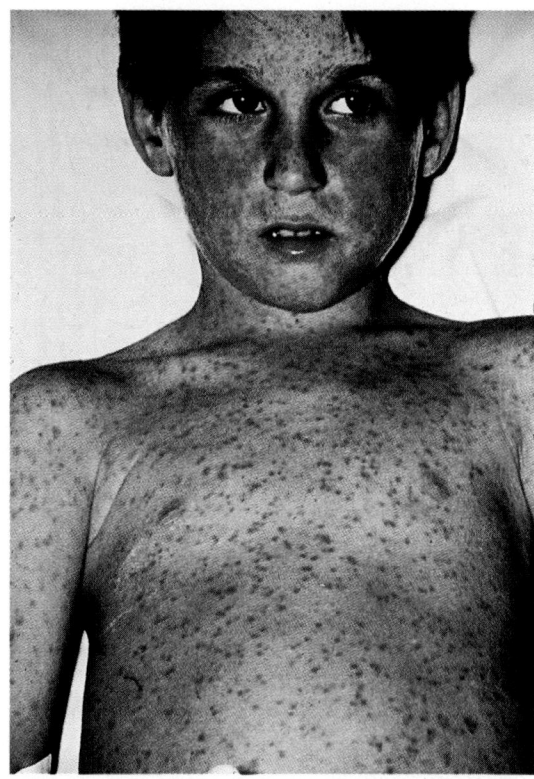

e

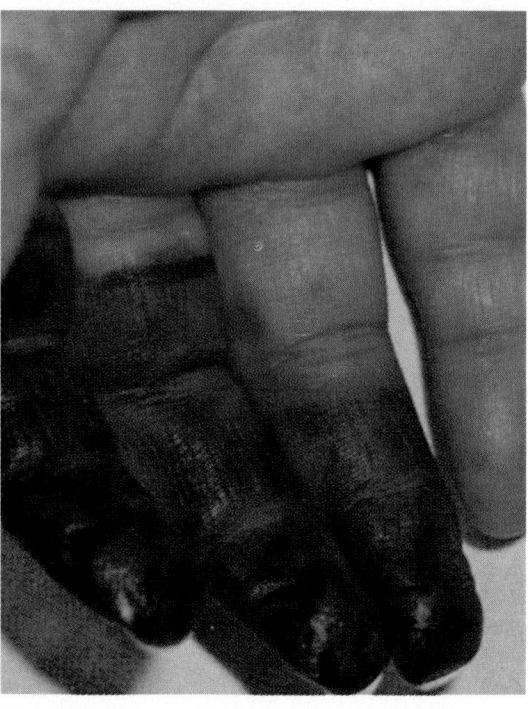

f

FIGURE 197-4 *(continued)*

therapy, if started early in illness, may delay the appearance of both Weil-Felix and more specific antibodies. Biopsy of skin lesions that can be processed within 8 h is helpful in establishing the diagnosis; the microorganisms are found by immunofluorescent staining in the walls of the small blood vessels of the skin.

Isolation of the microorganism is difficult and dangerous. Unless a laboratory specially equipped to work with rickettsiae is available, serologic methods should be relied upon to establish the diagnosis.

Differential Diagnosis

A history of tick bite in a person who has been in an endemic area is helpful but is frequently not available. The two other diseases most frequently considered are meningococcemia and measles. Meningococcemia is the most important as it, too, may kill rapidly. The rash may be entirely similar, ranging from macular to macular and papular to petechial and ecchymotic. In meningococcemia, the rash appears earlier in the course of the illness and does not have the characteristic progression of Rocky Mountain spotted fever rash. A coverslip touch preparation of a lightly scraped meningococcal lesion may reveal the microorganisms on Gram's stain. Cultures will reveal the meningococci in petechiae, blood, and cerebrospinal fluid if meningitis is present. In practice, these diseases often cannot be differentiated with certainty. Thus therapy for *both* diseases often must be instituted and subsequently modified when further information becomes available.

Coryza, conjunctivitis, cough, and Koplik's spots help to distinguish measles, in which the rash usually starts on the face and only rarely becomes petechial. The presence of edema (a parent's history of a child's puffy eyes, for example) can be very helpful in suggesting Rocky Mountain spotted fever rather than measles. So-called atypical measles (see Chap. 199) may also mimic Rocky Mountain spotted fever.

The rose spots (papules) of typhoid fever are a delicate pink, are usually few in number, and are found on the abdomen and lower part of the thorax. They do not become petechial.

Some of the enteroviruses produce summer febrile illnesses with a rash. Usually appearing in epidemics, sometimes associated with diarrhea, the illness is short and mild, and the rash only rarely becomes petechial.

Treatment

Tetracycline and chloramphenicol are extremely effective in the treatment of Rocky Mountain spotted fever when administered early in the disease. Tetracycline (10 to 20 mg/kg per 24 h given every 6 h in divided doses) can be used in persons over 9 years of age. In younger children, tetracycline produces permanent discoloration of the teeth. Chloramphenicol (50 mg/kg per 24 h every 6 h intravenously in divided doses) can be used in younger patients. Therapy is continued for about 4 days after the patient has become afebrile, to prevent relapse.

When initial therapy should also be directed against the meningococcus, 20 million units of intravenous penicillin G daily should be added to the regimen. Under *no* circumstances should the sulfonamides be employed, as they appear to *enhance* rickettsial infection.

Supportive measures, including intravenous administration of albumin, plasma, plasma expanders, or whole blood, may be of use in the severely ill patient. Corticosteroids have been employed to reduce fever and toxicity more rapidly, but whether they alter prognosis is unknown. Heparin has been administered to patients with associated disseminated intravascular coagulation, but no definite recommendation can yet be made.

Spotted Fever Groups: Boutonneuse Fever, South African Tick-Bite Fever, Siberian Tick Typhus, and Queensland Tick Typhus

The rickettsiae producing the mild diseases making up this group are closely related to one another and to *R. rickettsii,* the agent of Rocky Mountain spotted fever. The diseases are transmitted by ticks and occur in various parts of the eastern hemisphere. Boutonneuse fever, caused by *R. conorii,* is the prototype of the group.

Clinical Manifestations

After a 5- to 7-day incubation period the illness begins with fever and headache. A primary lesion, the *tache noir,* at the site of the tick bite is characteristic of all the eastern hemisphere rickettsioses. It consists of a small ulcer with a black center surrounded by a red halo. It is associated with regional lymphadenopathy. A generalized, red, macular and papular rash erupts on the fourth day (Fig. 197-5). It involves the palms and soles and rarely becomes hemorrhagic. The disease is milder than Rocky Mountain spotted fever, and those who succumb usually have underlying disease. Imported cases occurring in travelers have been described.

The Weil-Felix reaction becomes positive in convalescence and specific antibodies develop.

Treatment

Therapy with tetracycline or chloramphenicol is effective.

Rickettsialpox

Rickettsialpox, a mild disease caused by *R. akari,* was first identified in New York City in 1946. It is transmitted by the mite of the house mouse. It has been recognized in urban locations along the eastern seaboard of the United States and in Russia. It is unique among rickettsial diseases in that its eruption is vesicular.

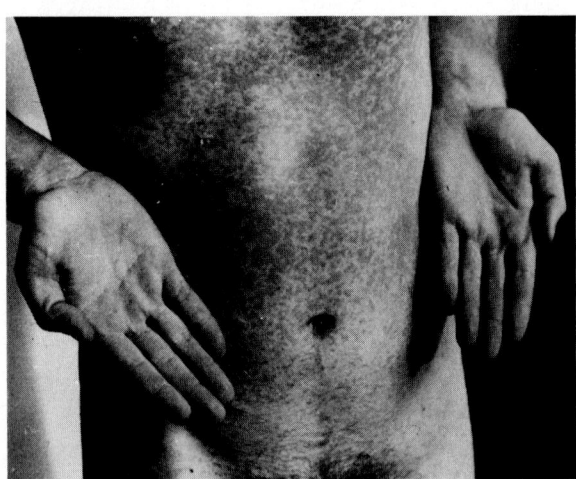

FIGURE 197-5 South African tick-bite fever. (*Courtesy of Evelyn Wallace, M.D., Monterey, California.*)

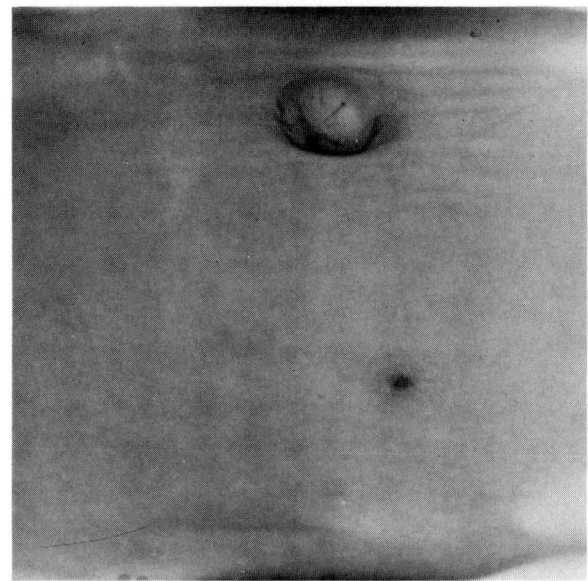

FIGURE 197-6 Rickettsialpox. Initial depicting the black eschar resulting from rupture of vesicle. (*Courtesy of F. Daniels, Jr., M.D.*)

Clinical Manifestations

A local lesion at the site of the mite bite appears 1 to 2 days after the bite and precedes the febrile illness. The lesion is a red papule that becomes quite large (1 to 1.5 cm in diameter). A vesicle forms in the center, leaving an erythematous halo. The vesicle dries and a black eschar results that is present when the patient develops systemic symptoms (Fig. 197-6). The febrile illness lasts about a week, during which period the rash appears. It is a generalized macular-papular-vesicular eruption, which is often sparse. Usually on the face, trunk, and extremities, it may involve the palms, soles, and oral mucosa. The lesions develop a scale but no permanent scars. Therapy with tetracycline or chloramphenicol shortens the course.

The Weil-Felix test remains negative after this disease, but specific complement-fixing or indirect fluorescent antibodies do develop.

Differential Diagnosis

Now that smallpox has been eradicated, the major differential diagnosis is with chickenpox. Chickenpox generally occurs in children and has no initial lesion. Its rash appears with the fever, and the whole papule is transformed into a vesicle. In rickettsialpox, fever generally precedes the rash, and the papular base is always discernible under and around the vesicle.

Typhus Group

Endemic Typhus

Endemic or murine typhus is caused by *R. typhi* (formerly *R. mooseri*), which is transmitted to humans by the rat flea. It is most prevalent about harbors and granaries where humans are likely to have contact with rats, the reservoir for the disease.

Clinical Manifestations   After an incubation period of 8 to 16 days, the onset of illness is heralded by chills, fever, severe headache, malaise, nausea, and vomiting. The rash generally appears on the fifth day. It is initially macular, becoming macular and papular. It is not petechial. The distribution of the rash helps to differentiate this disease from Rocky Mountain spotted fever. The lesions are located primarily over the trunk, with limited involvement of the face, extremities, palms, and soles, as opposed to the distal distribution of spotted fever lesions. The rash may be very evanescent and is absent in 10 percent of cases.

Typhus is generally milder than Rocky Mountain spotted fever, and it has a low mortality rate. One-fourth of patients have a palpable spleen.

The Weil-Felix test becomes positive in convalescence, and type-specific, complement-fixing and indirect fluorescent antibodies appear.

Treatment is as for the other rickettsial diseases.

Epidemic Typhus

Classical typhus is caused by *R. prowazekii* and is transmitted by the human body louse. Hence, the disease is easily spread from person to person. The reservoir for the disease is thought to be humans, lice becoming infected from patients with recrudescent typhus (Brill-Zinsser disease). Sporadic cases of classic typhus have recently been reported in this country, primarily from rural or suburban areas of the eastern United States. The majority of cases have occurred during the cold months of December, January, and February. Most of the patients have had contact with flying squirrels or their nests. This animal now has been shown to be a sylvatic reservoir of *R. prowazekii*, but the mode of transmission to humans is unknown.

Clinical Manifestations   The incubation period is about 7 days. As in other rickettsial diseases, the onset is characterized by fever, chills, headache, malaise, and weakness. On the fifth febrile day the rash appears, first in the axillae, then over the trunk, and later on the extremities. The rash initially consists of pink macules, which may become petechial and confluent (Fig. 197-7). The rash does not become papular.

Epidemic typhus is generally at an intermediate level of severity between murine typhus and Rocky Mountain spotted fever. In severe cases of louse-borne typhus, the clinical manifestations detailed for spotted fever, including widespread vascular thrombosis, are also observed (Fig. 197-8). Treatment is as for Rocky Mountain spotted fever.

In convalescence, Weil-Felix agglutinins and specific complement-fixing and indirect fluorescent antibodies develop.

Brill-Zinsser Disease

For unknown reasons, some patients who have had classic louse-borne typhus in the distant past develop a recurrence of the disease. The clinical manifestations are in all ways similar to those of a mild episode of typhus, and therapy is the same.

The Weil-Felix test is frequently negative or, at best, weakly positive, whereas specific antibodies rise rapidly to high titers in an anamnestic-like response.

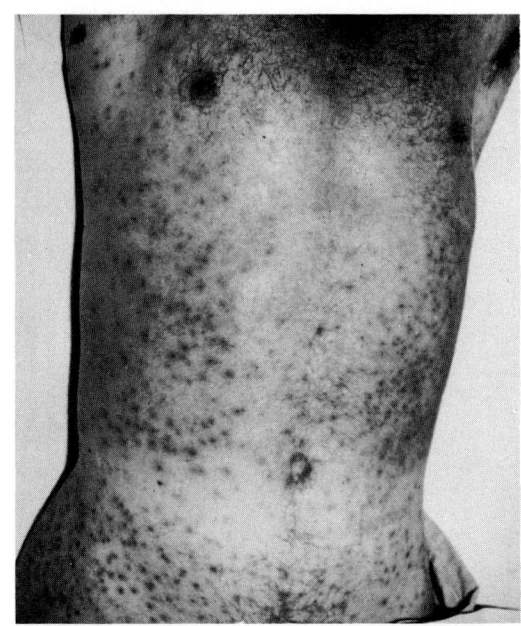

FIGURE 197-7   The diffuse macular-petechial eruption of epidemic typhus. The distribution is primarily trunkal. (*From the personal collection of Theodore E. Woodward, M.D.*)

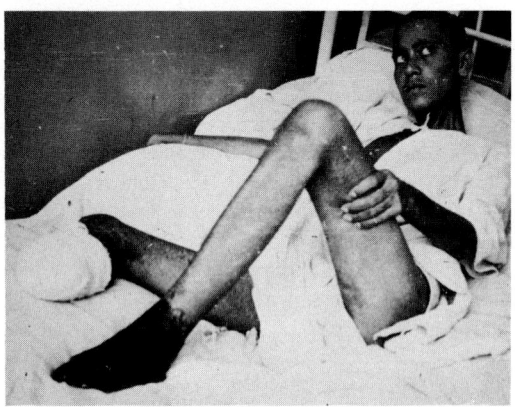

FIGURE 197-8   Epidemic typhus. Thrombosis of large vessels may result in significant gangrene. (*From the collection of Theodore E. Woodward, M.D.*)

Scrub Typhus

Rickettsia tsutsugamushi, transmitted by the bite of a mite, causes scrub typhus in India, southeast Asia, and Australia. There is marked strain variation in virulence, and mortality rates have varied from 0 to 60 percent.

Clinical Manifestations   After an incubation period of 6 to 18 days, illness begins suddenly with fever, chills, and headache. The primary lesion, a vesicle or black eschar on an erythematous papular base, can usually be found, associated with local and moderate generalized lymphadenopathy (Fig. 197-9). On the fifth day of fever the red macular and papular rash develops, primarily over the trunk. Unlike the other rickettsial eruptions, it fades within a few days.

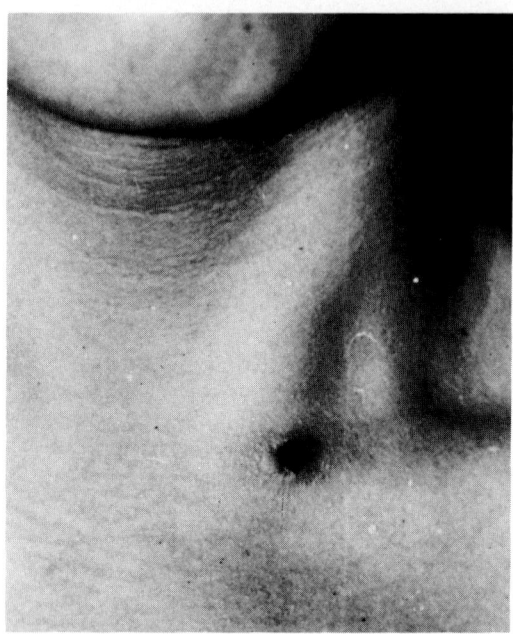

FIGURE 197-9 Scrub typhus. The primary lesion with its black eschar (''cigarette burn'') is associated with regional lymphadenopathy. (*From the collection of Theodore E. Woodward, M.D.*)

The disease resembles the other typhus fevers with two exceptions: early in the disease there is a bradycardia relative to the elevated temperature, and pneumonitis is more frequent.

Agglutinins to the OX-K strain of *Proteus* appear in convalescence. The OX-19 and OX-2 *Proteus* agglutinins remain negative. Repeated attacks of scrub typhus are not unusual, as there is considerable antigenic variation in strains.

Therapy is the same as described for the other rickettsial diseases, scrub typhus responding more rapidly than any of the other rickettsial diseases.

Trench Fever

Rickettsia quintana, a louse-transmitted microorganism, produces a mild, though sometimes prolonged, illness in humans, characterized by fever, chills, headaches, and a very characteristic myalgia, especially in the lower part of the back and in the legs. The rash consists of red macules confined to the trunk; the extremities and face are infrequently involved. The rash appears during the first day of illness and then waxes and wanes with the height of the fever. The spleen is usually palpable and quite firm. As the disease has been seen only in association with the two world wars, data on the efficacy of therapy are lacking.

Q Fever

R. burnetii, the agent of Q fever, produces an acute self-limited pneumonitis and hepatitis in humans. It does not produce cutaneous manifestations.

Ehrlichiosis

Ehrlichia canis is a rickettsial organism that has long been known to cause a febrile disease with pancytopenia in dogs. It has recently been discovered that this tick-borne organism can produce a febrile illness in humans. Over one-third of patients have a maculopapular or petechial rash that is usually limited to the trunk and proximal extremities. Serologic testing will distinguish ehrlichiosis from Rocky Mountain spotted (or ''spotless'') fever, which it most closely resembles. Tetracycline is the currently recommended therapy.

Bibliography

Barrett-Conner E, Ginsberg MM: Imported South African tick typhus. *West J Med* **138**:264, 1983

Brettman LR et al: Rickettsialpox: Report of an outbreak and a contemporary review. *Medicine (Baltimore)* **60**:363, 1981

Burnett JW: Rickettsioses: A review for the dermatologist. *J Am Acad Dermatol* **2**:359, 1980

Duma RJ et al: Epidemic typhus in the United States associated with flying squirrels. *JAMA* **245**:2318, 1981

Kirk JL et al: Rocky Mountain spotted fever: A clinical review based on 48 confirmed cases, 1943–1986. *Medicine (Baltimore)* **69**:35, 1990

Rohrbach BW et al: Epidemiologic and clinical characteristics of persons with serologic evidence of *E. canis* infection. *Am J Public Health* **80**:442, 1990

Schaffner W et al: Thrombocytopenic Rocky Mountain spotted fever: Case study of husband and wife. *Arch Intern Med* **116**:857, 1965

Torres J et al: Rocky Mountain spotted fever in the mid-south. *Arch Intern Med* **132**:340, 1973

Zinsser H: *Rats, Lice and History.* Boston, Little, Brown, 1935

Viral Diseases

Douglas R. Lowy

Skin lesions are a prominent feature of many viral diseases. In some instances, cutaneous lesions suggest a specific viral illness whose diagnosis can be quickly established by appropriate procedures. At other times, the differential diagnosis includes several viral and nonviral conditions. This situation may require costly, specialized, time-consuming, and possibly nondefinitive diagnostic procedures. However, the application of new techniques for laboratory diagnosis of viral infection will shorten the time required for diagnosis.[1] To complement advances in diagnosis, we now have several effective antiviral agents for treating at least some viral diseases with cutaneous manifestations, and other possible antiviral agents are in clinical trial.[2] Making the correct diagnosis in viral infection now has important implications for therapy as well as for prognosis. It may also contribute to the surveillance and control of infectious disease within the community.

Definition of Viruses

Viruses form a diverse group of infectious agents that share a distinctive composition and a unique mode of replication.[3,4] Viruses are not cellular organisms. Although certain viruses encode a small number of enzymes, viruses do not possess functional ribosomes or other cellular organelles. These agents therefore lack much of the machinery required for their own multiplication. They multiply only inside cells, where they make use of the cellular synthetic apparatus to produce their components. It is because of their dependence on the cell for their replication that viruses are often referred to as "obligate intracellular parasites."

The most important element of a virus is its genetic information (the viral *genome*), which may be either deoxyribonucleic acid (DNA) or ribonucleic acid (RNA), depending on the type of virus.[5] The life cycle of a virus may be divided into two parts.[6] In one part, the virus is a particle (also called a *virion*), where the viral genetic information is surrounded by a highly organized protein coat that can be seen by electron microscopy. The virus exists in this form outside of cells. The virion serves to transmit the viral genetic information, functionally intact, to a susceptible host. The second portion of the viral life cycle is that period when the viral genetic information is present inside a cell, where it is usually found in a nonparticulate form. Certain pathogenetic aspects of virus infection occur during the nonparticulate portion of the virus life cycle. The

General Considerations

duration of this intracellular phase is extremely variable, from a few hours in acute infection, to years when a virus establishes latency.

Classification of Viruses

All organisms, from bacteria to humans, are susceptible to infection by a range of viruses, but no single virus is capable of infecting all classes of cells. Each virus is broadly classified as a bacterial, plant, or animal virus on the basis of the type of cell it can infect. The animal viruses have been divided into several large groups according to the size, shape, and structure of the virion and the type of viral nucleic acid within it, as shown in Table 1. Viruses of a given group can be identified by physical methods such as the size and shape of their virions on electron microscopy, by antigenic crossreactivity, and by nucleic acid homology.[5] Although viruses have been grouped principally by virion morphology and nucleic acid composition, many functional, genetic, biochemical, and immunologic features are shared by viruses within the same group.

As noted above, the virion is composed of the viral genetic core surrounded by a protective protein coat called the *capsid*. The capsids in certain virus groups (such as herpesviruses and retroviruses) are located inside a virion *envelope* (composed of lipid, protein, and carbohydrate), which is required for infectivity (Table 1). The viral envelope is sensitive to drying, so that infectivity is lost on dry surfaces. The virions of other viruses (such as papillomaviruses) do not possess an envelope, so their capsids are called "naked." The capsid proteins are usually stable in dry environments, so viruses whose virions lack an envelope typically remain infectious for long periods after drying. In the virion, the viral genome consists of only a single type of nucleic acid, either DNA or RNA.

In most viruses, the capsid is arranged in one of two patterns: helical symmetry or icosahedral (cubic) symmetry (Table 1). Poxviruses have a more complicated structure, which is classified as "complex." In viruses with helical symmetry, the protein subunits that form the capsid are assembled in an elongated, helical form. The subunits in viruses with icosahedral symmetry are assembled into an icosahedral structure, which is a symmetric polyhedron with twenty equilateral triangular faces. Viruses within a given group may be further classified according to their relatedness at the nu-

TABLE 1
Selected Animal Virus Groups

Group	Size, nm	Symmetry	Envelope	Nucleic acid	Capsid assembly	Examples of viruses
Herpesvirus	120–200	Icosahedral	Yes	DNA	Nucleus	Herpes simplex (types 1 and 2), varicella-zoster, cytomegalo, EB
Papovavirus	45–55	Icosahedral	No	DNA	Nucleus	Papillomaviruses
Poxvirus	240 × 300	Complex	No	DNA	Cytoplasm	Molluscum contagiosum, orf, milker's nodules, variola, vaccinia, cowpox
Retrovirus	80–120	?	Yes	RNA	Cytoplasm	HIV, HTLV
Paramyxovirus	150–300	Helical	Yes	RNA	Cytoplasm	Measles, mumps
Togavirus	40–60	Icosahedral	Yes	RNA	Cytoplasm	Rubella, some arboviruses
Parvovirus	20	Icosahedral	No	DNA	Nucleus	Erythema infectiosum
Hepadnavirus	40–50	Icosahedral	No	DNA	Nucleus	Hepatitis B
Adenovirus	70–80	Icosahedral	No	DNA	Nucleus	Multiple human serotypes
Picornavirus	20–30	Icosahedral	No	RNA	Cytoplasm	Entero (coxsackie, ECHO, polio), rhino
Bunyavirus	90–100	Helical	Yes	RNA	Cytoplasm	Some arboviruses
Arenavirus	85–120	?	Yes	RNA	Cytoplasm	Lassa fever
Coronavirus	80–120	Helical	Yes	RNA	Cytoplasm	Several human serotypes
Orthomyxo-virus	80–120	Helical	Yes	RNA	Cytoplasm	Influenza types A + B + C
Rhabdovirus	70–80	Helical	Yes	RNA	Cytoplasm	Rabies
Reovirus	50–80	Icosahedral	No	RNA	Cytoplasm	Rotavirus, reovirus

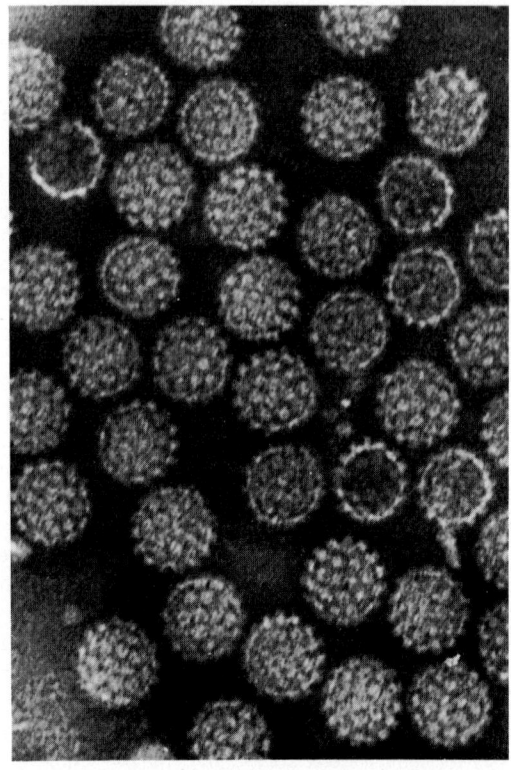

a

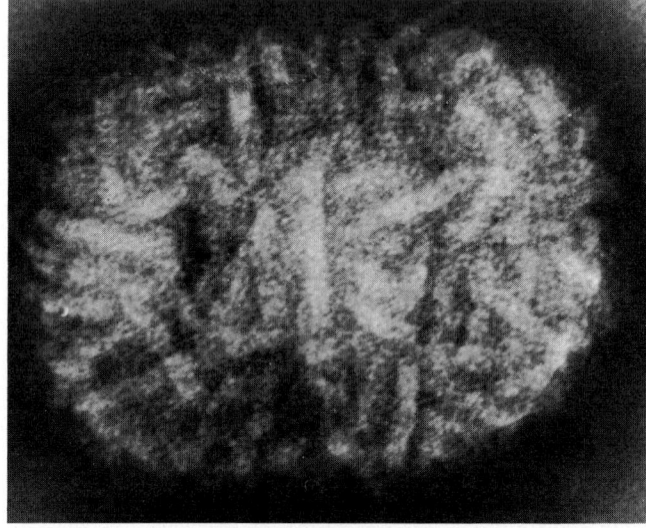

b

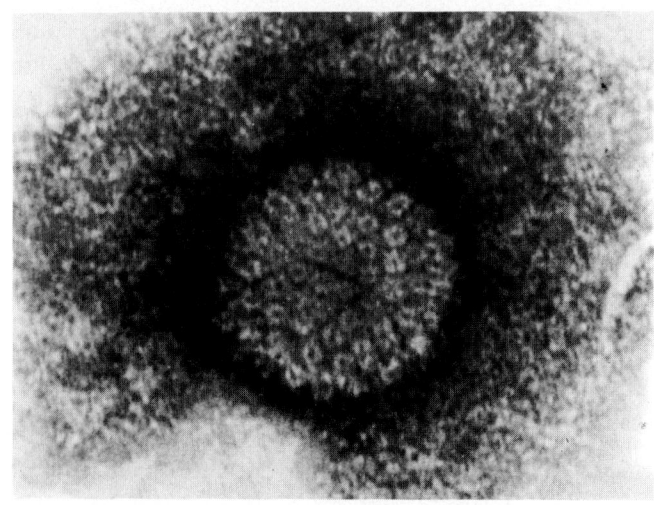

c

FIGURE 1 Electron micrographs of negatively stained virions (×200,000). (*a*) Papovavirus: multiple nonenveloped human papillomavirus (wart) virions showing capsid subunits (capsomeres). (*b*) Poxvirus: single molluscum contagiosum virus virions, showing complex tubular structures. (*c*) Herpes virus: single varicella-zoster virus virion showing capsid inside envelope. [*Parts* (a) *and* (b) *courtesy of A.F. Howartson, J.D. Almeida, and M.G. Williams. Part* (c) *by permission of Almeida JD et al, Virology 16:353, 1962.*]

cleic acid level, their antigenic crossreactivity, and the host cells that they infect.

Examples of virions from the three groups of viruses [papovaviruses (papillomaviruses), herpesviruses, and poxviruses] which multiply in the epidermis are shown in Fig. 1. The viral genomes of these three groups are composed of DNA. As noted above, papillomaviruses possess naked (nonenveloped) capsids, and herpesviruses have enveloped virions. Poxvirus virions are large, have a very complex structure, and are enveloped, but their envelope is not required for their virions to be infectious. Hence, poxviruses can remain infectious after drying.

Viral Replication

Viruses replicate inside cells by synthesizing their various structural components separately and then assembling them into multiple virions, in contrast to cells, which multiply by binary fission (the production of two progeny cells from a single parental cell).[6] As noted earlier, viruses use the host cell machinery to synthesize and assemble new virions, because these agents do not contain the apparatus required for their own replication.

It is important to recognize that viral genomes encode two different functional classes of proteins. Some virus-encoded proteins are used to form the virions; these proteins are called structural or virion proteins. Viral genomes also encode nonvirion proteins; these proteins are not incorporated into virions, although their production may be essential to the replication of the virus. Acyclovir inhibits herpesvirus replication because the drug is activated by virus-encoded nonvirion enzymes (proteins) that promote DNA synthesis.[7]

Nonvirion proteins of certain viruses may redirect the cell to synthesize the proteins required by the virus at the expense of those required for normal function of the cell. Many tumor viruses, including papillomaviruses, encode nonvirion proteins that increase cell growth and lead to inappropriate control of cell division (see Chap. 71). The intracellular pathogenicity of a virus may be due partly to effects of nonvirion proteins.[8]

The viral replication cycle, which has been studied in detail in tissue culture, involves several sequential steps: attachment (adsorption), penetration, uncoating, biosynthesis, virion assembly, and release.[6] Attachment of virions to cells involves a specific interaction between the viral capsid or envelope (for those viruses that possess enveloped virions) and receptors on the cell surface. For example, HIV enters cells via an interaction between viral envelope protein and cellular CD4 receptors.[9] Cells that lack the appropriate cell surface receptors for a particular virus will not be infected by that virus. Following penetration of the virion into the cell, cellular enzymes degrade the envelope and capsid (uncoating), which begins the nonparticulate phase of the virus life cycle.

Viruses vary in their size and complexity. The genome of poliovirus, which is a small virus with a simple virion structure, encodes a single precursor protein that is cleaved to give rise to the structural and nonstructural viral proteins. By contrast, poxviruses, whose virions are more than ten times larger than poliovirus virions and are much more complex structurally, encode dozens of structural and nonstructural proteins.

During biosynthesis, the viral genome instructs the infected cell to produce the proteins encoded by the viral genes. The virions of most viruses, including papillomaviruses, herpesviruses, and poxviruses, are assembled inside the cell and then released following cell death and lysis. However, enveloped viruses whose virions

are assembled at the cell surface (such as retroviruses and paramyxoviruses) are released by budding from intact cells; with these viruses, productive infection and release of virions may or may not be accompanied by toxic effects on the infected cell. Each virus has its characteristic site of replication within the cell. Papillomaviruses and herpesviruses are assembled in the nucleus (Figs. 2 and 3). Poxviruses, which are the only DNA viruses that replicate in the cytoplasm, synthesize their virions in organized cytoplasmic "viral factories" (Fig. 4).

Typically, hundreds or thousands of new virions are produced from each infected cell, and they in turn infect previously uninfected cells. One cycle of virus replication may last 3 to 36 h, depending on the virus and cell involved. Interruption of any step will prevent the development of new infectious virions.

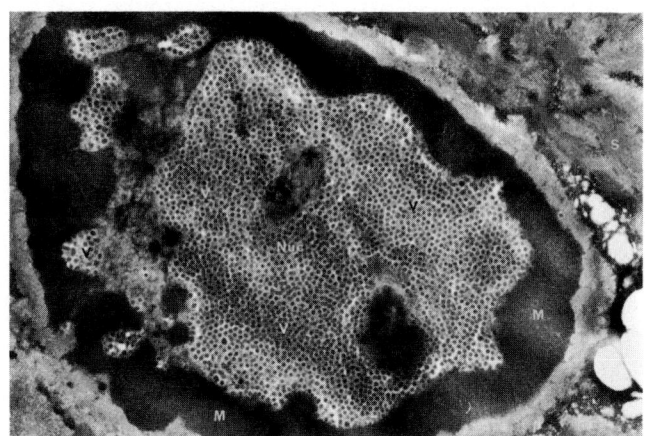

FIGURE 2 Papillomavirus (a papovavirus). Electron micrograph (×20,000). Nucleus (Nuc) of a stratum corneum cell, filled with papillomavirus virions (V); chromatin is marginated (M). Mature keratin can be seen in an adjacent cell (S).

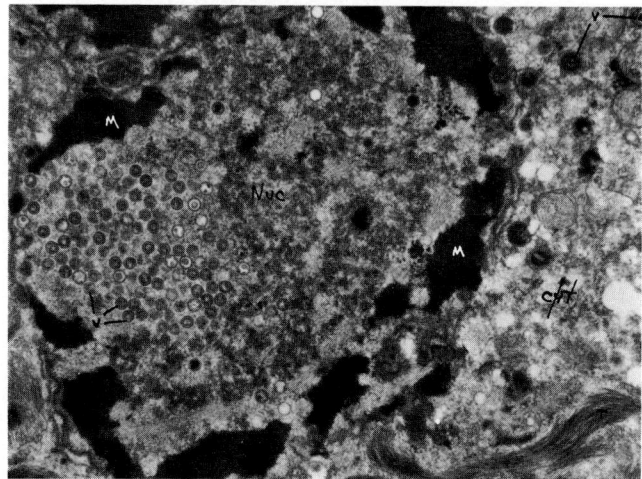

FIGURE 3 Varicella-zoster virus (a herpesvirus). Electron micrograph (×24,000). Portion of cell of the stratum spinosum. The nucleus (Nuc) contains varicella-zoster virions (V). Chromatin is marginated at (M). Virions (V) and tonofilaments (T) are shown in the cytoplasm (Cyt).

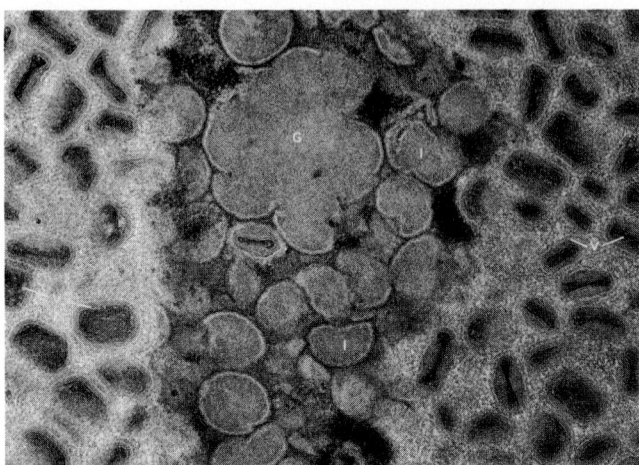

FIGURE 4 Molluscum contagiosum (a poxvirus). Electron micrograph (×45,000). Cytoplasm of a spinosum cell filled with mature molluscum contagiosum virions (V), immature virus forms (i), and viroplasm in a gyrate pattern (G).

Each virus can infect and replicate in only a limited number of cell types. The spectrum of susceptible cells depends on the virus. Human papillomaviruses (HPV) can infect a very narrow range of cells, namely certain differentiating human epidermal cells. Other viruses can infect a much broader range of cells; herpes simplex viruses can replicate in many different human and nonhuman cell types.

Even within a given tissue, a virus may be infectious only for cells with a specific degree of differentiation. The important role of the differentiated state of the cell in determining whether or not a virus will undergo replication is seen in the skin lesions of molluscum contagiosum. Since molluscum contagiosum virus (MCV) particles are sometimes found in cells of the upper dermis, the virus is capable of attachment to and penetration of these cells. MCV does not, however, replicate in dermal cells, indicating that an intracellular block to MCV synthesis exists in these dermal cells. MCV particles are also found in the basal layer of epidermal cells, but synthesis of new viral components does not begin until the cells reach the suprabasal layers. This observation implies that MCV replication can take place only in partially differentiated epidermal cells.

Cellular Consequences of Viral Infection

Typically, infected cells develop gross and often characteristic cytopathic changes and eventually die. Infections of this type are termed *cytocidal* or *lytic*. However, some viruses can replicate without causing irreversible damage to the host cell. Noncytocidal infection of this type occurs in tissue culture with measles virus and many other enveloped RNA viruses, leading to a chronically infected culture. While many retroviruses replicate without killing cells, cell lysis plays an important role in the pathogenesis of HIV infection.[10]

Two other types of noncytocidal infection are neoplastic transformation[11] and viral latency.[12] Tumor viruses, when they transform cells, alter the normal control of cellular proliferation. In gen-

eral, tumor viruses (such as the papovavirus SV-40) do not synthesize new virions in neoplastically transformed cells, although such transformation requires the continued expression of a portion of the viral genome. It is interesting to note that SV-40 is exclusively cytocidal for some cell types (permissive infection), induces transformation exclusively in other cells (nonpermissive infection), and induces both types of infection in still other cell types (semipermissive infection), again underlining the importance of the host cell in affecting the outcome of infection. Epidermal cells are semipermissive for papillomavirus infection. Virus-induced neoplasia is discussed in greater detail in Chap. 71.

Viral latency, which occurs commonly with herpes viruses, papillomaviruses, and retroviruses, represents the other type of noncytocidal infection.[12] Latently infected cells probably either produce very small numbers of new virions so that spread to uninfected cells is minimal, or they synthesize no new virus but retain an intact and potentially activatable viral genome.

Pathogenesis of Viral Infections in the Skin

Virus infections may affect the skin by three different routes: direct inoculation, systemic infection, or local spread from an internal focus. In warts, herpes simplex, chickenpox, herpes zoster, molluscum contagiosum, and smallpox, virus shedding from human skin lesions represents an important source in the transmission of virus to other people. Skin lesions may be produced by the direct effect of virus replication on infected cells, the host response to the virus, or the interaction of replication and host response. Relatively little is known about the role of the immune response in the pathogenesis of skin lesions induced by viruses.

The viruses of warts, molluscum contagiosum, vaccinia, orf, milker's nodules, and (primary) herpes simplex, all of which infect the skin by direct inoculation, replicate in the epidermis. Their viral cytopathic effects account for the appearance of early lesions. The contribution of the immune response to the evolution of these lesions remains unknown. The incubation period is generally short because the lesions develop at the site of inoculation. The incubation period for warts is longer, presumably because the virus replicates slowly or cell-to-cell spread of virus occurs to only a limited extent. Latent papillomavirus infection has been demonstrated in clinically normal laryngeal tissue of patients with a history of laryngeal papillomas, suggesting that host-specific factors may play a significant role in some papillomavirus-induced lesions.[13]

In systemic infections, the skin is infected during viremia, so that the dermis is generally infected earlier than the epidermis. It is not known how the distribution of viral exanthems is determined. In chickenpox and smallpox, the damage from cytocidal infection of the skin is a prime cause of the lesions. On the other hand, there is suggestive evidence from patients with impaired cellular immunity that the lesions of rubella and measles result in part from cell-mediated immune response to the virus. The basis of most exanthems associated with enteroviral infections remains to be established; there is significant cytocidal viral replication in the skin in hand-foot-and-mouth disease.

Recurrent herpes simplex and herpes zoster represent the local spread of virus to the skin following reactivation of the latent viral infection present in peripheral nerves. Cytocidal infection clearly plays an important role in these lesions, although lesions may contain less virus than during primary infection, presumably because of immunity.

Host Response

The severity of illness induced by a particular virus varies considerably from person to person. While the size of the viral inoculum and the portal of entry play some role, it is believed that host factors usually account for most of this variation. Both immunologic and nonimmunologic responses appear to be important.[8,14] Conversely, viral infection may have significant direct and indirect effects on the immune system,[10,15] especially those viruses that infect lymphoid cells, such as Epstein-Barr virus and HIV.

Antibody responses to viral infection represent the major host defense against reinfection by the same virus; the prophylactic administration of type-specific antibodies can prevent or modify some primary viral infections, even in patients with impaired cellular immunity. Humoral immunity is thought not, however, to contribute to the recovery from most primary viral infections, because viral infection of patients with isolated deficiencies of humoral immunity usually follows a normal course. There are several mechanisms by which antibodies may inhibit the spread of virus. These include neutralization of virus through prevention of viral attachment to target cells (which may be increased by complement), enhancement of viral uptake by phagocytic cells, which then inactivate the virus, and (complement-mediated) immune lysis of infected cells.

Specific cell-mediated immunity (CMI) is also elicited during viral infections and apparently influences the course of many viral infections. CMI is usually protective, although it may sometimes increase the degree of cellular pathology (as in the eruption of measles). Patients with impaired CMI often have difficulty handling primary or recurrent viral infection. Such patients are at risk of developing severe primary virus infections, warts, chronic herpes simplex virus infections, disseminated herpes zoster, and AIDS. The antiviral mechanisms of CMI have not yet been fully established. Sensitized T cells are known to be capable of lysing infected cells and of liberating lymphokines that attract phagocytic cells. Natural killer cells, virus-specific cytotoxic lymphocytes, and antibody-dependent cell-mediated cytotoxicity can inhibit infection under experimental conditions.

Inflammatory cells produce some of their antiviral effects via the production of interferons, a unique family of closely related cytokines that are active against viruses.[16] Interferon, which can be induced by foreign RNA or DNA (including viral nucleic acids), is secreted into the extracellular fluid. Resistance to virus infection is induced in those cells that come in contact with the interferon. Virtually all viruses induce interferon secretion and are susceptible to its action, but viruses differ greatly in their degree of interferon induction and in their sensitivity to its action. The presence of interferon correlates with the recovery phase of several viral infections. Genetic factors may also play a role in determining the outcome of viral infections. In animal models, genes can determine the susceptibility to viral infection at several levels, including virion attachment to cells, viral replication, and viral-induced immune responses.[17]

Diagnosis of Viral Infections

Four major approaches are used in the laboratory to diagnose viral infection: virus isolation, microscopy, detection of viral nucleic acids or viral antigens, and serology.[18,19] As with all laboratory tests, the results must be interpreted in the context of the clinical setting. Fortuitous infection with a virus unrelated to the illness should always be considered. For many viruses, considerable progress has been made in the development of relatively rapid assays that are sensitive and specific.[1] Most of these newer assays depend upon the ability to detect small amounts of viral nucleic acids and/or viral antigens.

Cultivation of the virus has represented the traditional "gold standard" for viral diagnosis. Virus isolation is most useful if the suspected pathogen can be readily propagated and positive results can be obtained in a short time. If necessary, more precise identification of the cultured virus can be carried out with specific tests for viral nucleic acid or viral antigen. Culture techniques for herpes simplex virus are quite sensitive, with diagnostic changes in cells often appearing within days of inoculation. The closely related varicella-zoster virus is much more difficult to grow in culture, so false-negative results are very common.

When virus isolation is attempted, specimens should be obtained as early in the disease as possible. In vesicular conditions, fluid from an early vesicle is often a good source of virus. Lesional specimens are less likely to be positive with nonvesicular exanthems. Specimens should also be obtained from other sites as indicated. Each specimen should be placed in a sterile tube with 2 to 5 mL of a buffered isotonic balanced salt solution containing penicillin and streptomycin. Preferably, it should be transported on ice immediately to the laboratory. If this is not practical, the specimen should be frozen (at $-70°C$, if possible). The suspected pathogen(s) should be indicated, as it may determine the type of cell culture or test animal to be inoculated.

The direct identification of a virus in clinical specimens can theoretically be accomplished more quickly than tests that rely on culturing the virus. This approach is especially useful for detecting those viruses that are difficult to propagate in culture and those, such as papillomaviruses, for which no reproducible culture system is available. Direct analysis may identify characteristic cells, as with Tzanck smears for herpes viruses (this test will not distinguish between herpes simplex and varicella-zoster viruses)[20] or the histologic appearance of molluscum contagiosum virus–containing lesions.

The direct identification of virus from clinical material is limited by the sensitivity of the assay. For those lesions that contain large numbers of viral particles, electron microscopy of a lesion or its extract may provide morphologic identification of the virus.[21] The positive identification of specific viral antigen in clinical material through use of immunologic techniques permits a more specific diagnosis than direct microscopy. For example, immunologic techniques can distinguish between herpes simplex virus and varicella-zoster virus.[22] Radioimmunoassay, enzyme-linked immunosorbent assay, immunoelectron microscopy, fluorescent antibody, or immunoperoxidase techniques identify viral antigen by the use of viral-specific antibody.

The use of assays based on viral nucleic acid probes is having a progressively larger impact on direct identification. The development of techniques such as the polymerase chain reaction (PCR),[23] which can specifically amplify minute quantities of viral nucleic acid, promises to revolutionize diagnostic virology.[1,24,25] Such assays are extremely sensitive, often being able to detect as few as one infected cell in 10,000, and highly specific.

Serologic studies to detect viral antibodies may be important for epidemiologic purposes, for identifying chronic infection with viruses such as HIV and hepatitis B, and for those situations where acute sera contain diagnostic antibodies, as with heterophile antibodies in infectious mononucleosis. In most acute viral illness, serologic analysis requires acute and convalescent sera, which limits its use in that setting to making a retrospective diagnosis. Paired sera are required because a positive serology during the acute phase may merely mean the individual was infected previously with a member of that virus group, but it does not have implications for the etiology of the current illness. The acute specimen should be taken as early in the illness as possible, and the convalescent specimen 2 to 4 weeks later. Serum should be separated immediately from the coagulated blood and refrigerated or preferably frozen at −20°C until antibody tests can be run simultaneously on both specimens. A fourfold or greater rise in antibody titer between first and second specimen generally indicates recent infection. A variety of assays are used to measure antibody levels, each detecting a certain type of antigen-antibody reaction. The antibody titer of a given serum is defined as the reciprocal of the highest dilution that gives a positive reaction.

Therapy and Prevention

Prophylaxis of viral infection has thus far proved more successful than the specific treatment of established infection. Vaccines have been very useful in the prevention of a variety of viral illnesses.[26] Recombinant DNA techniques are making it possible to develop effective subunit vaccines composed only of viral protein, rather than traditional vaccines, which represent either an attenuated strain of the pathogen or an inactivated preparation of the entire virus. In addition to vaccines that induce active immunity, passive immunity can be induced by administration of type-specific antibody soon after exposure, e.g., to prevent chickenpox in compromised hosts. Sensitive procedures for the detection of hepatitis B and HIV infection in potential blood donors has drastically reduced the incidence of transmission of these agents by transfusion.

Because viruses are adapted to the cells they infect and make use of cellular machinery, many chemotherapeutic agents that have been considered as potential antiviral agents affect cells to about the same extent as they affect viruses. However, this difficulty has already been overcome in several instances, and it is likely that more effective antiviral agents will be developed rapidly.[2] Most antiviral agents seek to exploit unique properties of a particular virus.[7] Azidothymidine (AZT), which is approved for use in the treatment of HIV infection, interferes with HIV replication by preferentially inhibiting synthesis of the viral genome. Acyclovir, an antimetabolite that has been approved for use in selected herpesvirus infections, is preferentially activated by herpesvirus-infected cells through its affinity for two herpesvirus enzymes involved in DNA synthesis. Interferon is a potentially potent antiviral agent that inhibits most viruses and at low dosages is relatively nontoxic to cells. Interferon has been approved for use in the treatment of certain genital papillomavirus infections and has also been helpful in the management of some children with papillomas of the larynx.

References

1. Lee PC, Hallsworth P: Rapid viral diagnosis in perspective. *Br Med J* **2**:1413, 1990

2. Galasso GJ et al (eds): *Antiviral Agents and Viral Diseases of Man*, 3d ed. New York, Raven, 1990

3. Belshe RB (ed): *Textbook of Human Virology*, 2d ed. St. Louis, Mosby Year Book, 1991

4. Fields BN, Knipe DM (eds): *Virology*, 2d ed. New York, Raven, 1990

5. Mattern CFT: Structure and classification of viruses, in *Medical Microbiology*, 3d ed, edited by S Baron. New York, Churchill Livingstone, 1991, p 559

6. Roizman B: Multiplication of viruses, an overview, in *Virology*, 2d ed, edited by BN Fields, DM Knipe. New York, Raven, 1990, p 87

7. Crumpacker CS: Molecular targets of antiviral therapy. *N Engl J Med* **321**:163, 1989

8. Nokta MA et al: Pathogenesis of viral infections, in *Antiviral Agents and Viral Diseases of Man*, 3d ed, edited by GJ Galasso et al. New York, Raven, 1990, p 49

9. Capon DJ, Ward RHR: The CD4-gp120 interaction and AIDS pathogenesis. *Annu Rev Immunol* **96**:649, 1991

10. Rosenberg ZF, Fauci AS: Immunopathogenesis of HIV infection, in *AIDS: Etiology, Diagnosis, Treatment, and Prevention*, 3d ed, edited by VT DeVita et al. Philadelphia, Lippincott, 1992, p 61

11. Bishop JM: Molecular themes in oncogenesis. *Cell* **64**:235, 1991

12. Stevens JG: Human herpesviruses: A consideration of the latent state. *Microbiol Rev* **53**:318, 1989

13. Steinberg BM et al: Laryngeal papillomavirus infection during clinical remission. *N Engl J Med* **308**:1261, 1983

14. Wittek AE, Quinan GV Jr: Immunology of viral infections, in *Textbook of Human Virology*, 2d ed, edited by RB Belshe. St. Louis, Mosby Year Book, 1991, p 116

15. McChesney MB, Oldstone MBA: Viruses perturb lymphocyte functions: Selected principles characterizing virus-induced immunosuppression. *Ann Rev Immnol* **5**:279, 1987

16. Zoon KC: Human interferons: Structure and function. *Interferon* **9**:1, 1987

17. Brinton MA, Nathanson N: Genetic determinants of virus susceptibility: Epidemiologic implications of murine models. *Epidemiol Rev* **3**:115, 1981

18. Schmidt NJ, Emmons RW (eds): *Diagnostic Procedures for Viral, Rickettsial and Chlamydial Infections*, 6th ed. Washington, American Public Health Association, 1989

19. Yolken R: Laboratory diagnosis of viral infections, in *Antiviral Agents and Viral Diseases of Man*, 3d ed, edited by GJ Galasso et al. New York, Raven, 1990, p 141

20. Solomon A et al: The Tzanck smear in the diagnosis of cutaneous herpes simplex. *JAMA* **251**:633, 1984

21. Field AM: Diagnostic virology using electron microscopic techniques. *Adv Virus Res* **27**:2, 1982

22. Goldstein LC et al: Monoclonal antibodies to herpes simplex viruses: Use in antigenic typing and rapid diagnosis. *J Infect Dis* **147**:829, 1983

23. Saiki RK et al: Primer-directed enzymatic amplification of DNA with a thermostable DNA polymerase. *Science* **239**:487, 1988

24. Wright PA, Wynford-Thomas D: The polymerase chain reaction: Miracle or mirage? A critical review of its uses and limitations in diagnosis and research. *J Pathol* **162**:99, 1990

25. Pennys NS, Leonardi C: Polymerase chain reaction: Relevance for dermatopathology. *J Cutan Pathol* **18**:3, 1991

26. Murphy BR, Chanock RM: Immunization against viruses, in *Virology*, 2d ed, edited by BN Fields, DM Kniper. New York, Raven, 1990, p 469

CHAPTER 198

Stephen E. Gellis

Rubella (German Measles)

Rubella (German measles) is a common communicable infection of children and young adults, characterized by a short prodromal period, enlargement of cervical, suboccipital, and postauricular glands, and a rash of approximately 2 to 3 days' duration. The disease has rare sequelae and, were it not for its devastating effect on the fetus, would be of relatively little significance in terms of morbidity or complications.

Epidemiology

Epidemics of rubella have been noted at 5- to 7-year intervals. The disease is worldwide in its distribution and tends to occur most frequently during the spring months in North America. It is rare in young infants and is most common in school-age children, adolescents, and young adults. It is spread via the respiratory route, and the period of infectivity extends from the end of the incubation period to the disappearance of the rash. A single attack confers lifelong immunity in most individuals, although subclinical reinfections can be demonstrated by laboratory tests in some "immune" individuals who are subsequently exposed to the wild virus. Two attacks of rubella with rash are most unlikely to be encountered; in such instances, one of the episodes is usually not rubella but is due to another viral infection.

The virus of rubella may be recovered from the pharynx as early as 7 days before and up to 14 days after the onset of the rash. Viremia is rarely demonstrated after the onset of the rash.[1]

Clinical Manifestations (Table 198-1)

The incubation period ranges between 14 and 21 days and is usually 16 to 18 days. Prodromal signs and symptoms are rare in young children, and the rash usually appears without prior complaint. In older children, adolescents, and adults, low-grade fever, headache, conjunctivitis, sore throat, rhinitis, cough, and lymphadenopathy may precede the rash by 1 to 4 days and disappear rapidly after the rash appears. In some adults, however, these symptoms and signs may persist longer and be more severe, and the infection under such circumstances may be difficult to distinguish from rubeola (measles) unless Koplik's spots characteristic of measles are observed. The rash of rubella is first noted on the face (Fig. 198-1) and rapidly spreads to the neck, arms, trunk, and legs. It consists of pink-red macules and papules which are discrete and remain so on the extremities, coalescing on the trunk to give a uniform red blush.

The rash, which usually disappears by the end of 2 or 3 days, clearing first from the face, may occasionally be followed by fine desquamation. This rapid disappearance is in contrast to measles (rubeola) in which the rash persists for longer periods. An enanthem is often seen at the end of the prodromal period or beginning of the rash, consisting of red spots, pinhead in size, scattered over the soft palate. The lymphadenopathy of rubella is striking; it involves all lymph nodes, but enlargement and tenderness are most common in the suboccipital, postauricular, and anterior and posterior cervical nodes. In older children and adults lymphadenopathy may be noted several days before the rash but in both children and adults the enlargement and tenderness are most striking on the first day of the rash. Enlargement of glands may persist for days to weeks but tenderness rapidly subsides. Splenomegaly may occasionally be detected. The fever of rubella is usually low-grade and seldom lasts beyond the first day or two of the eruption, except in individuals who have joint involvement in whom fever may persist. Arthritis due to rubella occurs much more frequently in adults than in children and is usually first noted as the rash fades. Small and large joints may become painful, with or without swelling, and may simulate rheumatic fever or rheumatoid arthritis. In one epidemic, joint involvement was seen in 25 percent of children under the age of 11 years and in 52 percent of patients 11 years of age or older.[2]

TABLE 198-1
Some Distinctive Features of the Rashes of Rubella, Measles, and Scarlet Fever

	Rubella	Rubeola (measles)	Scarlet fever
Prodromata	1–2 days of mild fever and respiratory symptoms	2–4 days of fever with moderate-to-severe respiratory symptoms	1–2 days of fever and sore throat
Duration of rash	Average 1–2 days	Average 3–5 days	Varies with treatment
Color	Pink-red	Purple-red to brown before fading	Yellow-red (may blanch on pressure)
Distribution	Scattered to generalized	Generalized (variable in modified measles) Koplik's spots (early)	Generalized (altered by treatment) Circumoral pallor "Strawberry" tongue
Nature	Macular to macular and papular Discrete with minimal coalescence about thorax	Macular to macular and papular Discrete with marked coalescence about face and thorax	Punctate lesions on erythematous skin Pinhead-sized lesions imparting sandpaper-like texture to skin Accentuation in flexor creases
Postexanthem desquamation	Occasional and branny	Common and branny	Typical and severe, often occurring on the hands and feet

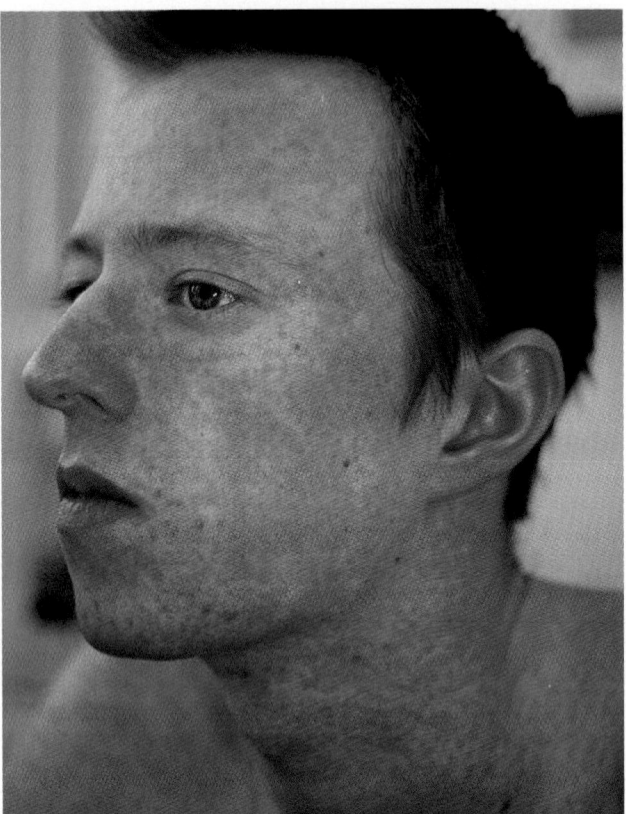

FIGURE 198-1 Rubella. Erythematous macules and papules appearing initially on the face and spreading usually within 24 h.

Striking effusions into joints have been reported. The arthritis of rubella usually lasts 1 to 2 weeks but occasionally may persist for longer periods or may be recurrent.

Complications

Rubella is essentially a benign disease. Rarely, it may produce an encephalitis which tends to be mild and is usually followed by complete recovery and no effect on intellectual function. Thrombocytopenic purpura, which may result from rubella, may be accompanied by epistaxis, petechiae, ecchymoses, intestinal hemorrhage, and hematuria. These manifestations frequently clear within a month of onset but occasionally may persist for longer periods. Rarely, a peripheral neuritis may follow rubella.

Laboratory Findings

The white blood count is usually low but may be normal. Increased numbers of atypical lymphocytes may be noted, and in some cases increased numbers of plasma cells have been reported. In cases with meningoencephalitis, varying numbers of lymphocytes may be found in the cerebrospinal fluid.

Congenital Rubella (Table 198-2)

Gregg in 1941[3] was the first to record the devastating effects of rubella infection in the fetus and to describe the congenital rubella syndrome. Approximately 50 percent of infants who acquire rubella during the first trimester of intrauterine life will show clinical signs of damage from the virus. The earlier the infection, the more severe is fetal damage. In such infants multiple congenital defects include low birth weight, microcephaly with mental retardation, cataracts, nerve deafness, and congenital heart disease (usually patent ductus arteriosus or ventricular septal defect). Following completion of organ development in the fetus, infection with rubella may produce a variable clinical picture which may include hepatitis, splenomegaly, pneumonitis, myocarditis, encephalitis, and osteomyelitis. When the bone marrow is affected, the infant may be born with thrombocytopenia and bleeding into the skin, producing a striking picture of petechiae and ecchymoses given the colorful term "blueberry muffin baby." In congenital rubella a retinopathy is commonly found, consisting of a diffuse deposit of black pigmentation.

Diagnosis

Infants with congenital rubella may be chronically infected for many months. Virus can be cultured from the nasopharynx, urine,

TABLE 198-2
Some Manifestations of the Congenital Rubella Syndrome

Teratogenic findings—congenital malformations:
1. Heart*
    a. Patent ductus arteriosus
    b. Coarctation of pulmonary vessels
    c. Ventricular septal defects
    d. Combination of above
    e. Others
2. Eye*
    a. Cataracts
    b. Microphthalmia
    c. Retinopathy
    d. Glaucoma
    e. Cloudy cornea
3. Hearing defects*
4. Central nervous system*
    a. Microcephaly
    b. Hydrocephaly
5. Bone;* disturbances of growth of skull
6. Abnormal dermatoglyphics
7. Agammaglobulinemia
8. Other organ systems
Other findings:
1. Intra- and extrauterine growth retardation*
2. Prematurity*
3. Meningoencephalitis
4. Pneumonitis
5. Hepatitis*
6. Cardiac tissue injury
7. Rarefaction bone*
8. Thrombocytopenia with or without purpura*
9. Anemia
10. Rubelliform skin rash
11. Generalized adenopathy

*More commonly encountered.
Source: Adapted from papers in Rubella Symposium, *Am J Dis Child 110*:345, 1965.

cerebrospinal fluid, and even from the lens of infants with congenital cataract. As time passes, the amount of virus shed in the nasopharynx and urine gradually declines and disappears. Approximately 85 percent of infants infected in utero will excrete virus in the first month of life; 1 to 3 percent continue to excrete virus in the second year of life. The large amounts of virus from congenitally infected infants are very hazardous to pregnant women working with such infants who may be susceptible to infection. The infant with congenital infection will usually have elevation of IgM due to antibody produced by the infant itself, together with elevated IgG caused by passive transfer of antibodies in the maternal blood. IgG traverses the placenta, in contrast to IgM, which does not. The IgG antibodies disappear over the first few months of life. Passively acquired IgG by the fetus from an immune mother may explain the rarity of acquired rubella in early infancy. The antibodies against rubella consist of neutralizing, complement-fixing, and hemagglutination-inhibition antibodies. Neutralizing and hemagglutination-inhibition antibodies usually persist for life. The hemagglutination-inhibition antibodies are easily and quickly measured and serve to determine whether a recent infection can be attributed to rubella by an increase in titer in the convalescent period over the titer in the acute stage. A fourfold increase or more is considered diagnostic of the infection. Testing for these antibodies also enables the physician to determine whether a woman of childbearing age is immune or susceptible to German measles.

Differential Diagnosis (Table 198-1)

Immunity and Immunization

Lifelong immunity usually follows an attack of rubella. Reinfection can occur but is usually not accompanied by clinical signs and symptoms. A rise in antibody level can occur; viremia from subclinical reinfection is very rare. Thus, congenital rubella is very unlikely in an infant whose mother has had an attack of rubella in the past and acquires a reinfection during pregnancy. In these instances, evaluation of fetal blood obtained by cordocentesis for specific rubella IgM antibodies or for evaluation by newer techniques using polymerase chain reaction (PCR) may help to confirm a diagnosis of fetal infection.[4,5] The availability of rubella vaccine[6,7] and its widespread use has markedly reduced the frequency of congenital infection.

In the United States, rubella vaccine is usually given together with mumps and measles vaccines in a single injection (MMR) at the age of 15 months. The ACIP recommends a second vaccination (as MMR) at age 5 to 6 years, whereas the AAP (American Academy of Pediatrics) recommends reimmunization at 11 to 12 years of age.[8,9] The child or adult to whom rubella vaccine is administered does not shed sufficient virus to infect susceptible individuals in close contact. As a result it is safe to immunize children in a family in which the mother is pregnant. If a woman of childbearing age is to be immunized, it is important to obtain her rubella hemagglutination-inhibition titer since she may be immune as a result of an unrecognized or subclinical infection in the past and will therefore not require immunization. If she is susceptible and therefore is to be immunized, she must understand that pregnancy must be avoided for the following 3 months, a period during which virus from the vaccine may persist in her tissues. If a woman shown to be susceptible to rubella because of the absence of antibody is inadvertently given vaccine when she is pregnant, abortion is no longer recommended. Although rubella vaccine virus has been demonstrated in the fetal membranes and amniotic fluid, there has been no risk of the congenital rubella syndrome. Because of the risk to the fetus from proved rubella infection in the pregnant woman, abortion is recommended if the fetus is shown to be infected.

References

1. Cooper LZ, Krugman S: Clinical manifestations of postnatal congenital rubella. *Arch Ophthalmol* **77**:434, 1967
2. Jedelsohn RG, Wyll SA: Rubella in Bermuda: Termination of an epidemic by mass vaccination. *JAMA* **223**:401, 1973
3. Gregg NM: Congenital cataract following German measles in the mother. *Trans Ophthalmol Soc Aust* **3**:35, 1941
4. Zolti M et al: Rubella-specific IgM in reinfection and risk to the fetus. *Gynecol Obstet Invest* **30**:184, 1990
5. Ho Terry L et al: Diagnosis of foetal rubella virus infection by polymerase chain reaction. *J Gen Virol* **71**:1607, 1990
6. Meyer HM, Jr et al: Attenuated rubella virus II. Production of an experimental live-virus vaccine and clinical trial. *N Engl J Med* **275**:575, 1966
7. Meyer HM, Jr, Parkman PD: Rubella vaccination: A review of practical experience. *JAMA* **215**:613, 1971
8. Anonymous: Rubella prevention. Recommendations of the immunization practices advisory committee (ACIP). *MMWR*:**39**:15,1, 1990
9. Committee of Infectious Disease of the American Academy of Pediatrics. *Red Book of the American Academy of Pediatrics* 11, 1991

Bibliography

Krugman S et al: *Infectious Diseases of Childhood*, 8th ed. St. Louis, Mosby, 1985
Feigin RD, Cherry JD: *Textbook of Pediatric Infectious Diseases*, 2d ed. Philadelphia, Saunders, 1987

CHAPTER 199

Louis Z. Cooper

Measles

Measles is a universal, highly contagious, acute viral disease of childhood. It is characterized by high fever, cough, coryza, conjunctivitis, and Koplik's spots, which precede the appearance of a florid, generalized macular and papular rash.

Historical Aspects

The term *measles* is thought to come from the Latin *misellus* or *misella,* a diminutive of the Latin *miser,* meaning miserable, which described the inmate of a medieval leper house. *Morbilli,* the diminutive of *morbus,* was introduced to distinguish minor rash disease from bubonic plague, *morbus,* the major disease. Morbilliform is a synonym for measles-like, which is still in common use.

No accurate information is available on the early history of measles. The tenth-century Arabian physician Rhazes has generally been credited with distinguishing measles from smallpox, although he cited El Yehudi, a Hebrew physician from the first century, as first describing the disease. However, it was probably not until the severe epidemics of measles during the seventeenth century that these diseases were clearly separated; e.g., the astute clinical and epidemiologic observations by Thomas Sydenham were completed at this time.[1]

In more recent times, transmission of measles to monkeys was first reported by Josias,[2] and other investigators[3,4] demonstrated that monkeys could be infected with blood or nasopharyngeal secretions obtained from patients.

The isolation of measles virus in tissue culture by Enders and Peebles[5] provided the essential techniques for definitive characterization of the virus excretion and antibody response in this disease and for its ultimate control. In 1960, Enders and his coworkers successfully attenuated measles virus,[6] and after extensive field trials, a live measles virus vaccine was licensed for general use in the United States in 1963. Since that time, the administration of approximately 200 million doses of vaccine has significantly decreased the incidence of this infection in this country.

Epidemiology

Measles is a universal illness, worldwide in distribution, that occurs primarily in children. However, the age incidence varies according to the environmental setting. In congested urban areas, the highest attack rate occurs in infancy and early childhood. In rural and less-crowded areas, the attack rate is highest in the early school years, ages 5 to 10 years. When measles has been introduced into isolated communities, the attack rate has approached 100 percent among the susceptible population of all ages. Very young infants, under 4 months of age, are usually protected by the persistence of transplacentally acquired maternal measles antibody.

Neither race nor sex affects the attack rate of measles, but the general state of health and nutrition clearly affects morbidity and mortality rates. Measles is primarily a disease of winter and spring in temperate climates, with the peak incidence of infection usually occurring in March or April.

The epidemiology of measles has changed dramatically because of the impact of massive immunization programs for eradication of the disease. A Measles Elimination Program, aided by a policy of school exclusion for those without proof of measles immunization, reduced the total number of reported cases in the United States to a low of 1497 in 1983. However, due to a combination of social factors, progressively declining immunization rates among urban poor infants and young children have led to increasing rates of measles. During the three-year period, 1989 to 1991, there were 18,000, 28,000, and almost 10,000 cases, respectively, reported nationally. Perhaps as a consequence of increased immunization efforts targeted to high-risk populations, the provisional number of cases reported in 1992 dropped to 2200. Black and Latino infants and preschool children have borne the brunt of the new epidemics. Hospitalization and death rates have been remarkably high compared to the preimmunization era (see ''Complications'' below).

Etiology and Pathogenesis

Measles virus has been classified as a paramyxovirus. Its structure and many of its biologic properties are similar to those of the larger members of the myxovirus group, i.e., mumps, Newcastle disease virus (NDV), and parainfluenza viruses. It is a heat-labile virus, with an RNA core and an outer envelope of protein and lipoprotein. The virus is stable at low temperatures (especially in the presence of protein) but is rapidly inactivated by ultraviolet radiation, ether, trypsin, acetone, and β-propiolactone. Complement fixation, hemagglutination, and hemolysis are properties of the virus that have been utilized for laboratory diagnosis (see ''Diagnosis'' below). Initial isolation in tissue culture is most readily accomplished in primary cultures of human or simian renal or human amnion cells, but the virus has been adapted by serial passage to grow well in numerous continuous cell lines.

At the time of the initial isolation of measles virus in tissue culture, certain characteristic cytopathic effects were noted that were strikingly similar to previously well-recognized pathologic changes occurring during natural infection in humans. These included formation of syncytia, or multinucleated giant cells with intranuclear and intracytoplasmic eosinophilic inclusions.

Measles virus is antigenically stable and distinct from mumps virus and the other larger myxoviruses. There is some degree of cross-reactivity with the agents of canine distemper and bovine rinderpest, but these cause no difficulty in serodiagnosis in humans.

The natural route of infection is by droplet spread of infectious secretions from an infected patient to the respiratory tract of a person who is susceptible. It is suspected that after local multiplication at this site of entry there may be an early viremia, but this has not been documented. During the prodromal period, virus can be detected in nasopharyngeal secretions, lymphatic tissue, blood, and urine,[7] and virus may persist in the urine for 4 days after onset of the rash.[8] However, viremia and pharyngeal shedding of virus cease by the second day of rash, a time when measles antibody reaches detectable levels in the serum.

The mechanism of the rash has not been established; rash may be a direct effect of viral invasion on epithelial and vascular endothelial cells, or it may result from the damaging effects of a virus-antibody complex. In support of the latter theory is the temporal relationship between onset of rash and appearance of antibody (the same is true in rubella, another exanthem) and the absence of rash in the few rare children, usually those with leukemia, who have developed chronic measles infection without rash or antibody production but with fatal giant cell pneumonia.[9] The experience of these children is in sharp contrast to that of children with classical (Bruton type) agammaglobulinemia, who respond to measles infection in a normal fashion.[10] Delayed allergy (tuberculin-type skin sensitivity) is intact in these children, and they may make small quantities of humoral antibody as well. Similarly, two complications of measles, encephalitis and thrombocytopenia purpura, are suspected of having an allergic basis, but direct evidence is not available to clarify these points.

Clinical Manifestations

The course of measles may be divided into three distinct phases: (1) an essentially asymptomatic incubation period of 10 or 11 days following exposure; (2) a prodromal phase characterized by fever, malaise, and increasing severe coryza, conjunctivitis, and cough, which persists for 3 or 4 days before (3) onset of the rash, which usually reaches its maximum within several days and rarely persists longer than 5 to 6 days. The pathognomonic Koplik's spots usually appear in the mouth 24 to 48 h before onset of the rash and may remain discrete for 2 or 3 days. A typical clinical course is illustrated in Fig. 199-1.

Prodromal Symptoms

The coryza, conjunctivitis, cough, and fever that characterize the measles prodrome increase in severity until the rash has reached its

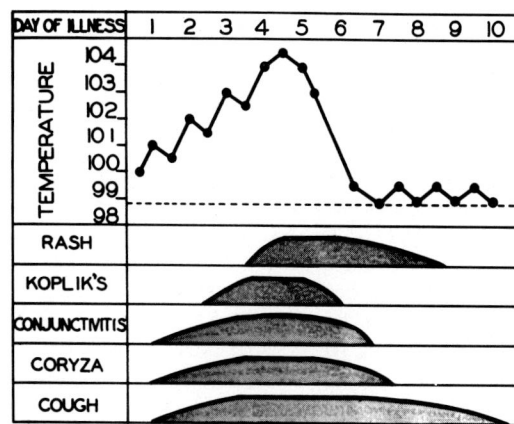

FIGURE 199-1   Schematic diagram illustrating the clinical course of typical measles. *(From Krugman S, Ward R: Infectious Diseases of Children, 3d ed. St. Louis, Mosby, 1964.)*

peak. The coryza is similar to that in a severe common cold. The conjunctivitis is most strikingly palpebral, extending to the lid margin so that the eyes appear to be red-rimmed. Lacrimation, lid edema, and photophobia accompany the conjunctivitis. A brassy or barking cough, due to the diffuse involvement of the tracheobronchial tree, may be quite severe even in the absence of a complicating pneumonia and may persist for a week after the coryza. The temperature frequently reaches 40 to 40.5°C at the peak of the rash but falls promptly to normal in the absence of complications. Generalized adenopathy is common in measles.

Rash (See Fig. 199-2b, -2c)

After a prodromal period of 1 to 7 days, an erythematous, discrete, macular and papular rash appears behind the ears and over the forehead. It spreads down over the neck and trunk and then distally over the upper and lower extremities. The hands and feet are involved. This progression is usually complete, and the rash most intense, within 3 days, which coincides with the peak of the other major clinical signs of fever, cough, and conjunctivitis. Those areas in which the rash appears first tend to be most heavily involved, and confluence of lesions on the face and upper neck is common. Lesions on the legs usually remain discrete and macular and papular. The exanthem begins to fade in the order of its appearance; sometimes clearing of the face begins on the third day while the eruption is still discrete and fresh on the legs. Although the early erythematous rash blanches on pressure, the fading rash consists of a brown staining (inflammatory melanosis with old hemorrhage) that does not blanch.[11] Variable degrees of fine, branny desquamation may be present as the rash clears. In the United States, the desquamation is never as extensive as that which may occur in severe scarlet fever, but desquamation has been described as quite marked in certain areas of the world such as Nigeria.[12]

The severe hemorrhagic measles (black measles) associated with extreme toxicity, respiratory tract and gastrointestinal bleeding, hyperpyrexia, and significant mortality rate is now rare and should not be confused with the purpuric lesions that may be seen in fair-skinned children during the course of ordinary measles.

Oral Lesions

The earliest oral lesions, according to Weinstein,[11] are a "series of pin-point elevations connected by a network of minute vessels on the soft palate." These red dots then coalesce as the entire pharynx becomes reddened. Herrman spots, bluish-gray or white areas on the tonsils, also may be present. Neither of these lesions is pathognomonic of measles. The pathognomonic lesions of measles described by Henry Koplik,[13] a New York pediatrician, begin as small, irregular, bright-red spots that usually precede onset of the rash by 24 to 48 h. In the center of each red spot is a minute bluish-white speck. These Koplik's spots are most heavily clustered on the buccal mucosa opposite the second molars (Fig. 199-2a), but occasionally are on the conjunctivae at the inner canthus, and at autopsy in the large intestine.[14] During the first day of rash, the Koplik's spots are usually easy to see as a cluster of fine grains of sand on a red background. They normally become less distinct as the rash progresses.

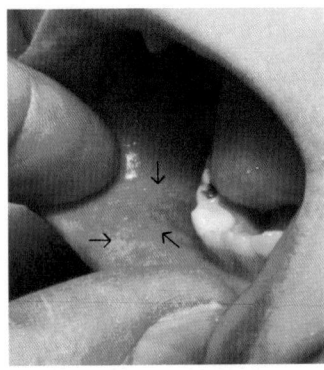

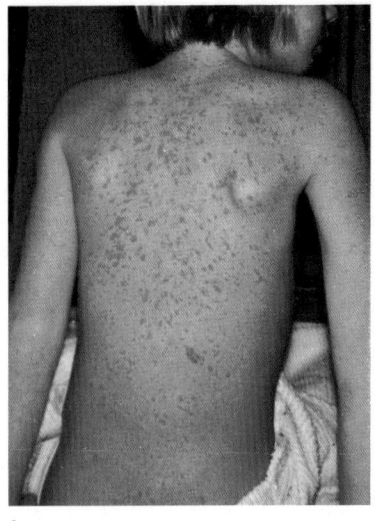

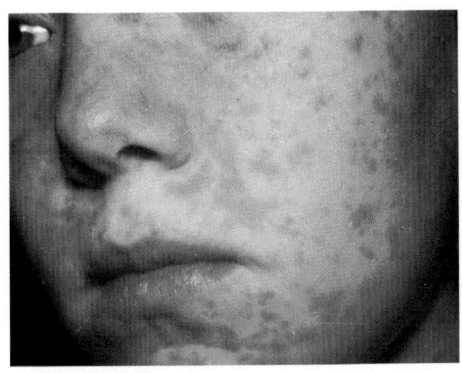

a   *b*   *c*

FIGURE 199-2 Measles (rubeola; morbilli) has a characteristic prodrome of 3 to 4 days that consists of coryza, a striking palpebral conjunctivitis with photophobia, and a "barking" cough. The first lesions appear on the soft palate as blotchy erythema, but the most pathognomonic lesions of the prodrome, if present, are the Koplik spots (*a*), which appear as tiny white lesions surrounded by an erythematous ring ("grains of sand"). Koplik's spots precede the onset of the generalized rash by 1 to 2 days, remain for 2 to 3 days, and are usually heavily clustered on the buccal mucosa opposite the second molars. The purplish red rash on the body appears first behind the ears and over the forehead and then spreads slowly to involve the entire body by the third day: the eruption extends downward over the neck and shoulders and trunk and then distally over the upper and lower extremities; the spread of this rash over the central parts of the trunk (*b*) first is in contrast with that of German measles, which spreads rapidly to involve the entire body in 1 day. The measles rash remains in its original site while it spreads to the extremities, in contrast with the rash in rubella, which disappears from each site as it spreads. The erythematous macular and papular lesions, which were discrete (*c*), become confluent on the face and upper part of the neck, whereas they may remain discrete on the legs. As the rash disappears, it becomes brownish yellow, owing to capillary hemorrhages.

Complications

The complications of measles fall into two categories: those that are due to the measles infection alone and/or the patient's response to the infection, and those due to superinfection with pathogenic bacteria. Encephalitis, which occurs in approximately 1 out of every 800 cases, is the most dreaded and unpredictable complication of measles. Although most children recover completely, death or permanent brain damage occurs in a significant minority of children who develop measles encephalitis. Purpura, usually associated with thrombocytopenia, may be severe. These complications may be due to a direct effect of measles virus on the target tissues, or there may be an immunologic component. Common bacterial complications are otitis media and pneumonia caused by the pneumococcus, group A hemolytic streptococcus, *Haemophilus influenzae,* or, occasionally, *Staphylococcus aureus*. The onset of these complications is frequently accompanied by a secondary fever spike or prolongation of fever at a time when defervescence would ordinarily be expected.

Complication rates have always been higher among the very young, the malnourished, and those with other underlying diseases. Recent outbreaks in the United States have been focused in just such inner-city populations. Approximately one-third of cases have been in children under 4 years of age. Hospitalization rates of 15 to 20 percent, usually attributed to dehydration and/or respiratory distress, have been associated with measles itself or bacterial superinfection. Although most of the deaths have occurred in young children, almost one-third of the 97 deaths in 1990 were in adults. Some of the deaths in adults were in individuals known to be immunocompromised (e.g., HIV infected). Death rates have reached almost 4 per 1000 cases, far higher than the less than 1 per 1000 experienced in the United States in the prevaccination era, but still tenfold lower than the rate seen among malnourished children in developing nations.

Measles may aggravate or exacerbate tuberculosis. The reasons for this and for the transient anergy it produces are unknown. Both measles and measles vaccine may depress the tuberculin skin test reaction for 2 or 3 weeks.

A complication, new since the "vaccine era," has been described in children who received killed measles virus vaccine and subsequently were exposed to and infected with natural measles.[15] Some of these children have developed atypical infection characterized by urticarial, vesicular, and petechial rashes, swollen hands and feet, severe pneumonia, high fever, and extreme prostration. Although children may be quite sick with this syndrome, the illness appears to be self-limited. Similarly, administration of the live attenuated measles virus vaccine after prior immunization with the killed vaccine may produce erythema, edema, and even vesiculation at the injection site, with or without fever for several days.

Another late-developing complication of measles is subacute sclerosing panencephalitis (SSPE). Patients with this progressive and usually fatal disease recover uneventfully after acute measles. Months or years later, mental and motor deterioration, often with myoclonic seizures, are associated with a characteristic spike and wave pattern of the electroencephalogram, remarkably elevated serum and cerebrospinal fluid (CSF) measles antibody titers, and elevated total CSF IgG. In brain tissue, measles virus antigen has been demonstrated by immunofluorescence, measles-like nucleocapsids have been seen on electron microscopy, and infectious virus with the characteristics of measles has been isolated in tissue culture by meticulous techniques of cocultivation and serial passage. Fortunately, this rare complication (estimated at 5 to 10 cases per million cases of measles) appears to be even less common among children protected by attenuated measles vaccines (1 case per million doses of vaccine).

Laboratory Findings

In uncomplicated measles, routine laboratory tests are unremarkable and not particularly helpful. There is a mild leukopenia, and the chest roentgenogram frequently reveals an increase in bronchovascular markings. Cytologic examination of nasal secretion and sputum may demonstrate characteristic multinucleated giant cells.

Isolation of measles virus from blood, urine, or pharyngeal secretions during the prodromal and early rash period (see "Etiology and Pathogenesis" above) requires virus laboratory facilities, which are available in only a limited number of research and reference institutions.

Serologic tests for measles include measurements of neutralizing, complement-fixing (CF), and hemagglutination-inhibiting (HI) antibodies. Paired serums taken shortly after onset of rash and 2 weeks later will show diagnostic (fourfold or greater) rises in measles antibody measured by each of these tests. Neutralizing and HI antibody persist at detectable levels for many years after natural infection (probably for life in most instances), but CF antibody persistence is not so predictable.[16] The most sensitive and convenient of these serologic tests are the HI technique[17] and the enzyme-linked immunosorbent assay (ELISA).[18] These tests, which are specific for measles, can be most helpful in clarifying the cause of the unusual case of atypical measles. Bacterial superinfections and measles encephalitis are usually associated with a polymorphonuclear leukocytosis.

Pathology

The measles exanthem begins with hyaline necrosis of epidermal cells, followed by exudation of serum around the superficial vessels in the dermis and by proliferation of endothelial cells.[19] The epithelial cells become necrotic. Intranuclear inclusions may be seen. In the later stages, there are leukocytic infiltration of the dermis and lymphocytic cuffing of vessels. In uncomplicated measles, the invariable presence of multinucleated giant cells in the respiratory tract and lymphoid tissues (Warthin-Finkeldey cells) throughout the body has been accepted as evidence of measles virus invasion of these tissues (see "Etiology and Pathogenesis" above). Tracheobronchitis is as much a part of measles as the exanthem. Rarely, a fatal pneumonia, characterized by the presence of giant cells in the lungs, occurs in children with underlying disease such as leukemia. The histopathologic characteristics of measles encephalitis are similar to those observed in other postviral encephalitides. Early lesions include lymphocytic infiltration of the walls of small veins in gray and white matter, measured cellular infiltration, degeneration of ganglion cells, and microglial proliferation. Perivascular demyelinization follows these initial changes. Adams et al.[20] described intranuclear and intracytoplasmic inclusions and small giant cells in brain tissue obtained from fatal cases of measles encephalitis. Confirmation of these observations by others would add indirect support to the concept that direct invasion of the central nervous system by measles virus is of pathogenic significance in measles encephalitis.

Diagnosis

The clinical course of full-blown measles is so characteristic that diagnosis should represent no problem. The 3- to 4-day prodrome of cough, conjunctivitis, coryza, with appearance of Koplik's spots, then a macular and papular rash, is unambiguous. Laboratory confirmation is usually not necessary. However, when measles has been modified by prophylactic administration of human immunoglobulin at the time of exposure (see "Treatment" below), the disease may be significantly attenuated; it may consist of various combinations of brief fever, cough, and rash, or it may be subclinical.

The unusual clinical picture seen in patients who develop measles despite prior immunization with inactivated (killed) measles vaccine may be diagnosed on the basis of a prior history of such immunization and recent measles exposure (see "Complications" above).

Treatment

As in other systemic viral infections, there is no specific therapy for measles. Supportive therapy, consisting of rest, diet, hydration, aspirin, a vaporizer, and mild antitussive agents appropriate for the febrile child with tracheobronchitis, is frequently helpful in management of the self-limited disease. The prophylactic administration of antibiotics is unwarranted, as it does not prevent bacterial complications and, in fact, may predispose the patient to superinfection with a treatment-resistant organism.[21] Antibiotic therapy should be instituted promptly, however, if bacterial complications develop (see "Complications" above). Therapy for measles encephalitis is also supportive.

Prevention

Measles is preventable. Guidelines for using the highly effective and safe live attenuated measles vaccine (licensed in 1963) have continued to evolve in response to the vaccine-induced changing epidemiology of the disease. A single dose of vaccine produces detectable levels of measles antibody in approximately 95 percent of recipients. Immunity from vaccine is protective against this disease, presumably for life, in most, if not all, of those who seroconvert. However, it has become clear in recent years that the 5 percent of children who fail to respond to an initial dose of measles vaccine have provided a reservoir for continued outbreaks of disease, especially in settings where large numbers of adolescents and young adults congregate (e.g., college and high school campuses).

In 1989, because of the morbidity and costs associated with the outbreaks among young people, public health authorities in the United States adopted a two-dose measles immunization schedule (a practice already in place in ten European countries). The first dose of vaccine is usually given at age 15 months, in the United States, to avoid an interfering effect from maternal measles antibody. The second dose is given prior to school entry or early in elementary school.

The major epidemics of measles experienced in 1990 and 1991 were not due to vaccine failure (i.e., the 5 percent who fail to respond to the first dose of vaccine). The failure has been in distributing vaccine to poor children. Measles vaccination rates for inner-city children age 2 years dropped to less than 50 percent, setting the stage for epidemics with an age distribution lower and complication and death rates higher than previously experienced in the United States. For control of epidemic measles, the timing and number of subsequent doses of vaccine is now adjusted by local health officials. The first dose may be given as early as 6 months of age. An "extra dose" after age 15 months, but before school entry, may be required in certain communities. It is likely that recommendations concerning the timing, number of doses, and perhaps even route of administration of measles vaccine will continue to evolve.

Immune serum globulin (ISG) may be used to modify or prevent measles if given within 6 days of exposure. The recommended dose is 0.25 mL/kg of body weight, given intramuscularly. ISG is especially valuable for infants too young for active immunization. For children and adults who are immunosuppressed, the dose is 0.5 mL/kg. The maximum dose is 15 mL. In contrast to other congenital or acquired causes of immunosuppression, HIV infection is not a contraindication for measles vaccination, but such children, when exposed, should still receive ISG.

Course and Prognosis

Uncomplicated measles runs a self-limited course, lasting about 10 days, with no sequelae. However, the prognosis varies greatly with the age of the patient, the nutritional and general health status, and, perhaps, access to early and appropriate supportive care. Prior to widespread immunization, approximately 500 deaths were attributed to measles each year in the United States. In the early 1980s, when measles cases dropped to an average of only 3000 yearly, deaths were few. In 1990, with almost 100 deaths, the rate of almost 4 per 1000 greatly exceeded the death rate of 3 per 10,000 that characterized the preimmunization era rate for infants in the United States. Morbidity and mortality in developing nations, where poverty prevents access to care, continues to reflect the general health status of children in these areas, with measles a major contributor to infant mortality. This experience offers ample justification for the World Health Organization's Expanded Program for Immunization.

References

1. Katz SL, Enders JF: Measles virus, in *Viral and Rickettsial Infections of Man*, 4th ed, edited by FL Horsfall Jr, I Tamm. Philadelphia, Lippincott, 1965, p 784
2. Josias A: Récherches expérimentales sur la transmissibilité de la rugeole aux animaux. *Med Mod* 9:158, 1898
3. Anderson JF, Goldberger J: Experimental measles in a monkey; a preliminary note. *Public Health Rep* 26:847, 1911
4. Blake FG, Trask JD Jr: Studies on measles. I. Susceptibility of monkeys to the virus of measles. *J Exp Med* 33:385, 1921
5. Enders JF, Peebles TC: Propagation in tissue cultures of cytopathogenic agents from patients with measles. *Proc Soc Exp Biol Med* 86:277, 1954
6. Enders JF et al: Studies on an attenuated measles-virus vaccine. I. Development and preparation of the vaccine: Technics for assay of effects of vaccination. *N Engl J Med* 263:153, 1960
7. Enders JF: Measles virus: Historical review, isolation and behavior in various systems. *Am J Dis Child* 103:282, 1962
8. Gresser I, Katz SL: Isolation of measles virus from urine. *N Engl J Med* 263:452, 1960
9. Mitus A et al: Persistence of measles virus and depression of antibody formation in patients with giant cell pneumonia after measles. *N Engl J Med* 261:882, 1959
10. Janeway CA, Gitlin D: The gamma globulins. *Adv Pediatr* 9:65, 1957
11. Weinstein L: *The Practice of Infectious Disease*. New York, McGraw-Hill, 1958
12. Morley DC: Measles in Nigeria. *Am J Dis Child* 103:230, 1962
13. Koplik H: The diagnosis of the invasion of measles from a study of the exanthema as it appears on the buccal mucous membrane. *Arch Pediatr* 13:918, 1896
14. Corbett EU: The visceral lesions in measles. *Am J Pathol* 21:905, 1945
15. Rauh LW, Schmidt R: Measles immunization with killed virus vaccine: Serum antibody titers and experience with exposure to measles epidemic. *Am J Dis Child* 109:232, 1965
16. Krugman S et al: Studies on immunity to measles. *J Pediatr* 66:471, 1965
17. Rosen L: Hemagglutination and hemagglutination-inhibition with measles virus. *Virology* 13:139, 1961
18. Parker JC et al: Sensitivity of enzyme-linked immunosorbent assay, complement fixation, and hemagglutination inhibition serological tests for detection of Sendai virus antibody in laboratory mice. *J Clin Microbiol* 9:444, 1979
19. Robbins FC: Measles: Clinical features. *Am J Dis Child* 103:266, 1962
20. Adams JM et al: Inclusion bodies in measles encephalitis. *JAMA* 195:290, 1966
21. Weinstein L: Failure of chemotherapy to prevent the bacterial complications of measles. *N Engl J Med* 253:679, 1955

Bibliography

Centers for Disease Control: Measles prevention: Recommendations of the Immunization Practices Advisory Committee. *MMWR* 38(suppl 9): December 1989
Markowitz LE, Orenstein WA: Measles vaccines. *Pediatr Clin North Am* 37:603, 1990
National Vaccine Advisory Committee: The measles epidemic, barriers and recommendations. *JAMA* 266:1574, 1991

CHAPTER 200

Antoinette F. Hood and Martin C. Mihm, Jr.

Hand-foot-and-mouth disease (HFMD), a distinctive clinical syndrome caused by an enterovirus, is clinically manifested by characteristic vesicular lesions in the mouth and on the extremities.

Historical Aspects

In 1957, in Canada, Robinson et al.[1] described an epidemic of vesicular stomatitis with an exanthem on the hands and feet from which coxsackievirus type A16 was isolated. A second epidemic, in England, was described by Alsop et al.[2] who coined the term *hand-foot-and-mouth disease*. Subsequently, epidemics and individual cases have been reported from around the world.

Epidemiology

The epidemic disease is usually associated with coxsackie-virus A16 or enterovirus 71.[3] Sporadic cases have been reported in association with coxsackie-virus A4–7, A9,[4] A10,[5] B2 and B5.[6] HFMD usually affects children under the age of 10, although in one series 10 of 11 patients were 15 years of age.[7]

The incubation period in HFMD is short, from 3 to 6 days. The disease is highly contagious and the spread of virus from person to person occurs by the oral–oral and fecal–oral routes.

During epidemics of HFMD, the usual spread is from child to child (horizontal spread) and then to adults (vertical spread) in various family groups. In one study 44 percent of asymptomatic family contacts had laboratory evidence of infection; 53 percent of infected asymptomatic individuals were adults.[8] A nosocomial outbreak of HFMD involving adult operating suite employees was reported in 1986.[9] In temperate climates there is usually a seasonal pattern for the occurrence of the clinical syndromes caused by enterovirus, as well as for the isolation of the virus from the sewage and fecal samples taken from populations where epidemics occur. Epidemic outbreaks of HFMD tend to occur approximately every 3 years, mainly in the warmer months.

Etiology and Pathogenesis

Infections due to an enterovirus, a member of the picornavirus group, typically develop according to a basic pathogenic mechanism.[9,10] Initial viral implantation in the buccal mucosa and ileum is followed within 24 h by extension to regional lymph nodes. At 72 h, a viremia occurs followed by the seeding of viruses to the sites of secondary infection, which, in HFMD, are the oral mucosa and the skin of the hands and feet. By the seventh day there is a rise in serum antibodies, and the virus disappears from the blood and other sites of implantation.

Hand-Foot-and-Mouth Disease

Clinical Manifestations

The typical signs and symptoms of HFMD may be preceded by a brief prodrome of 12 to 24 h characterized by low-grade fever, malaise, and abdominal pain or respiratory symptoms. The most frequent finding of the disease is ulcerative oral lesions. In one series, sore mouth and refusal to eat were the presenting complaints in over 80 percent of laboratory-confirmed cases; oral lesions were present in 100 percent.[11] The number of oral lesions averages between 5 and 10. Although the lesions may be found anywhere within the oral cavity, they appear most frequently on the hard palate, tongue, and buccal mucosa.[8] The oral lesions begin as erythematous macules and papules 2 to 8 mm in diameter, then progress to form gray, thin-walled vesicles surrounded by a zone of erythema. The vesicular stage is short and rarely seen since the vesicles progress to form shallow, yellow-to-gray ulcerations with an erythematous halo. Small lesions may coalesce to form larger ones. The tongue may become red and edematous. These lesions are usually painful and may interfere with eating; however, they usually resolve in 5 to 10 days without treatment.

The cutaneous lesions appear together with or shortly after the oral lesions. They may vary in number from a few to over 100. In general, the hands are more commonly involved than the feet; specifically, the dorsal surfaces and sides of the fingers, hands, toes, and feet are more often involved than the palms and soles. Each lesion begins as an erythematous macule or papule, 2 to 10 mm in size, in the center of which arises a gray, round to oval vesicle.[12] The lesions often run in or parallel to the skin lines (Fig. 200-1). The vesicles are often surrounded by a red areola (Fig. 200-2); they may be asymptomatic, painful, or tender. They crust after a few days and gradually disappear over the course of 7 to 10 days without scarring.

Macular and papular erythematous lesions have also been described in association with the more typical lesions of HFMD in infants. This eruption occurs principally on the buttocks but is occasionally generalized.[11–15]

Histopathology

The characteristic cutaneous lesion is an intraepidermal vesicle containing neutrophils, mononuclear cells, and proteinaceous eosinophilic material. As the lesion ages, there may be focal loss of the basal cell layer resulting in a subepidermal bulla. The roof of the blister is often necrotic with discrete eosinophilic dyskeratotic and acantholytic epidermal cells. The epidermis immediately adjacent to the vesicle exhibits intercellular and intracellular edema or so-called reticular degeneration (Fig. 200-3). Eosinophilic intranuclear inclusions have been described.[16] The dermis beneath a vesicle is edematous and contains a perivascular polymorphous infiltrate composed of lymphocytes and neutrophils.

Intracytoplasmic particles in a crystalline array characteristic of coxsackievirus have been observed with electron microscopy.[16]

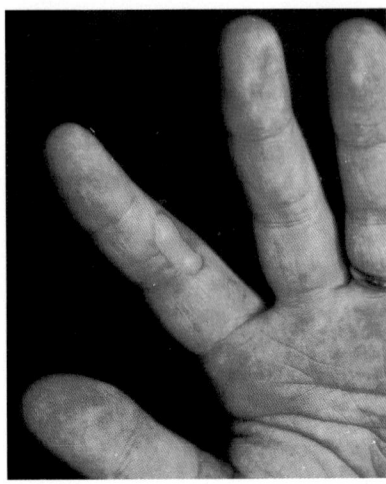
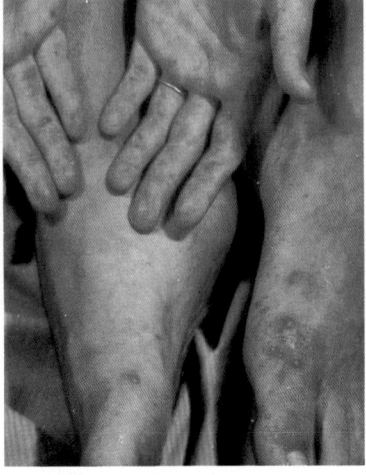

a   *b*

FIGURE 200-1 Hand-foot-and-mouth disease is manifested by vesicles, bullae, and pustules, often linear (*a*) on an erythematous base. They are often painful and are usually found on the fingers and toes (*b*). There may be an associated vesicular exanthem. The causative agent is usually coxsackievirus A16, although rarely it may be A5.

The material obtained by scraping the base of a vesicle, when smeared on a glass slide and stained with Giemsa's stain, reveals no multinucleated giant cells or inclusion bodies.[7,17]

Diagnostic Procedures

The diagnosis of HFMD is usually made on a clinical basis with the observation of ulcerative oral lesions plus an exanthem on the hands and feet occurring in association with a mild febrile illness. Leukocyte counts range from 4000 to 16,000/mm^3, occasionally with atypical lymphocytosis.

The causative viral agent may be isolated from an affected subject by inoculation of suckling mice and appropriate tissue culture with fluid from vesicles, throat washings, throat swabs, and stool specimens. More than one technique is suggested for virus isolation because the various strains of these viruses possess different characteristics and differ in their ease of isolation.

Serum-neutralizing antibody against these viruses appears early in the illness and often rapidly disappears; therefore, serologic examination performed during the course of the illness may demonstrate antibody only during the acute, and not during the convalescent, phase of the disease.

Significantly elevated titers of complement-fixing antibody may be detected in serum drawn from a patient during the convales-

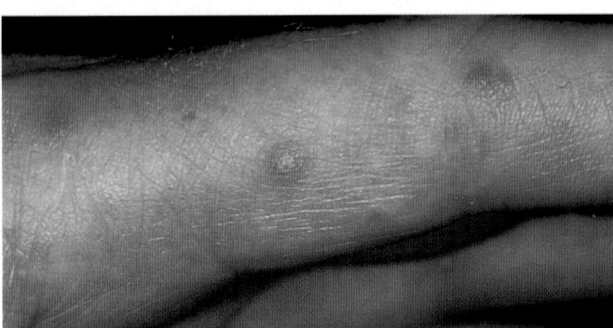

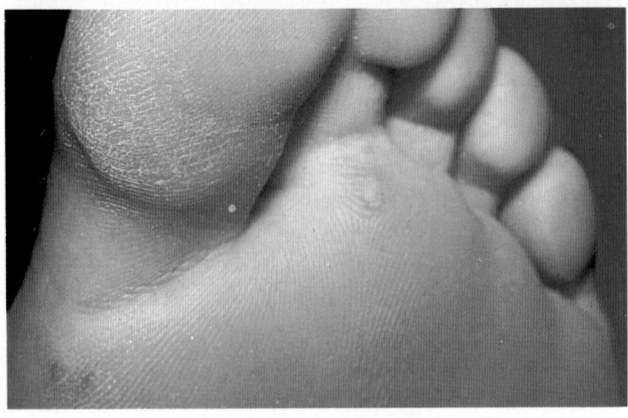

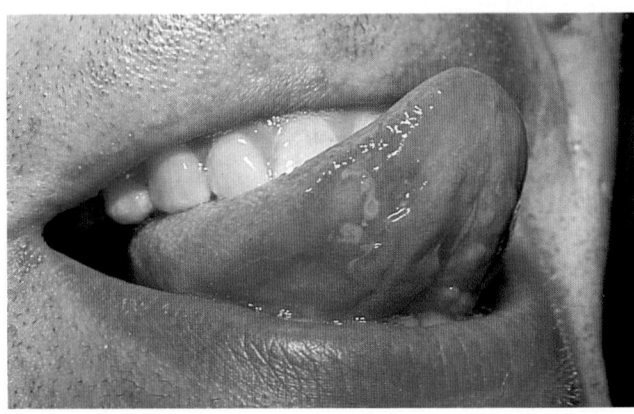

b

a

FIGURE 200-2 (*a*) Small vesicular and papular lesions distributed on the hands and feet are characteristic of hand-foot-and-mouth syndrome. (*b*) Erosions on the tongue may accompany mucosal ulcerations as part of the oral manifestation of coxsackievirus A16 infection.

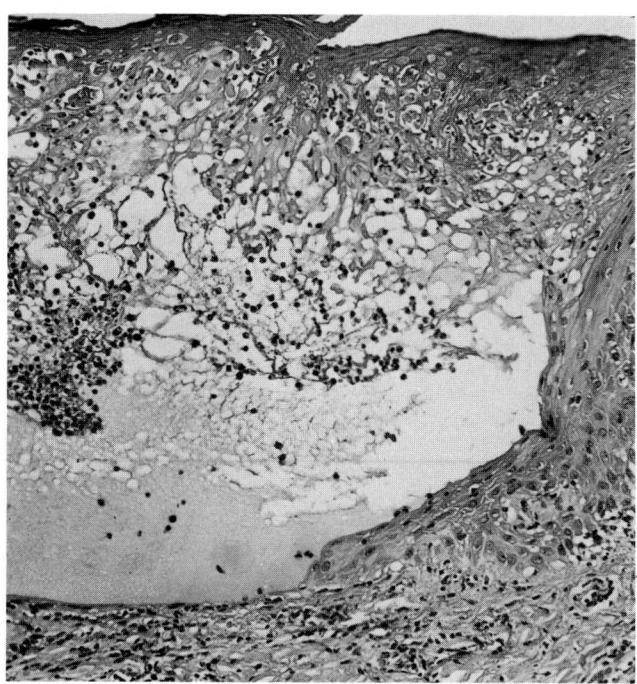

a

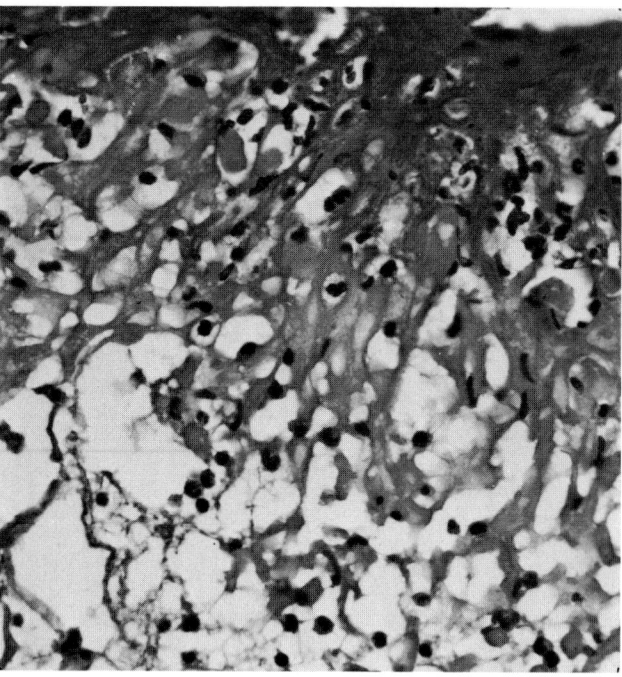

b

FIGURE 200-3 (*a*) An intraepidermal bulla with focal loss of the epidermis at the base. The blister cavity is filled with neutrophils and mononuclear cells. H&E; ×140. (*b*) Higher magnification of blister roof showing numerous dyskeratotic epidermal cells and exocytosis of mononuclear cells. H&E; ×400.

cent stage of the illness. These antibodies, however, are usually group specific, rather than type specific.

Differential Diagnosis

The occurence of oral and distal-extremity lesions in an outbreak setting is pathognomonic of HFMD. When only oral lesions are present the illness is often mistaken for aphthous stomatitis, herpes simplex virus infection, or herpangina. *Aphthae* are rarely accompanied by systemic symptoms or fever. Although fever may occur in *herpesvirus* infection, the perioral areas are often involved; cervical and submanibular adenopathy may be prominent. *Herpangina*, which usually involves the anterior fauces, tonsillar pillars, soft palate, and uvula, does not commonly involve the tongue, buccal mucosa, and gingiva.

    Erythema multiforme major may present with oral ulcerations and vesicular skin lesions; the number of cutaneous lesions present in erythema multiforme is usually greater than in HFMD, and the characteristic target lesions are frequently present. *Drug eruptions* can usually be differentiated on the basis of extensive cutaneous involvement and prominent pruritus.

Treatment

There is no specific treatment for HFMD. Topical application of dyclonine HCl solution (Dyclone) or lidocaine (Xylocaine, ointment or viscous) may reduce the discomfort accompanying the oral ulcerations.

Course and Prognosis

Patients may present with either enanthem or exanthem, but most patients manifest both aspects of the disease. In general, the disease is accompanied by minimal or mild signs and symptoms, such as low-grade fever, vague malaise, and sore mouth. Some patients, however, are afflicted with high fever, marked malaise, diarrhea, and occasionally even joint pains.[14] In Japan, epidemics of HFMD caused by enterovirus 71 have been associated with an 8 to 24 percent incidence of neurologic signs and symptoms such as headache, nuchal rigidity, hyperreflexia, tremor, ataxia, myoclonus, and CSF pleocytosis.[3] Most commonly, however, the entire disease runs its course in 7 to 10 days without the patient's awareness of debility. A few cases of prolonged or recurrent HFMD have been observed.[11,15] Serious sequelae rarely occur; however, coxsackievirus has been implicated as the etiologic agent in cases of myocarditis,[18,19] meningoencephalitis,[18] aseptic meningitis,[18,20] paralytic disease,[21] and a systemic illness resembling rubeola.[22] Infection acquired during the first trimester of pregnancy may result in spontaneous abortion.[23]

References

1. Robinson CR et al: Report on an outbreak of febrile illness with pharyngeal lesions and exanthem. Toronto, Summer 1957—isolation of group A Coxsackie virus. *Can Med Assoc J* **79**:615, 1958
2. Alsop J et al: "Hand-foot-and-mouth disease" in Birmingham in 1959. *Br Med J* **2**:1708, 1960
3. Ishimaru Y et al: Outbreaks of hand, foot, and mouth disease by enterovirus 71. *Arch Dis Child* **55**:583, 1980

4. Hughes RP, Roberts C: Hand, foot, and mouth disease associated with Coxsackie A₉ virus. *Lancet* **2**:751, 1972

5. Duff MF: Hand-foot-and-mouth syndrome in humans: Coxsackie A₁₀ infection in New Zealand. *Br Med J* **2**:661, 1968

6. Lindenbaum JE et al: Hand, foot, and mouth disease associated with Coxsackie virus group B. *Scand J Infect Dis* **7**:161, 1975

7. Miller GD, Tindall JP: Hand, foot, and mouth disease. *JAMA* **203**:827, 1968

8. Adler JL et al: Epidemiologic investigation of hand, foot, and mouth disease. Infection caused by Coxsackie A₁₆ in Baltimore, June through September 1968. *Am J Dis Child* **120**:309, 1970

9. Johnston JM, Burke JP: Nosocomial outbreak of hand-foot-and-mouth disease among operating suite personnel. *Infect Control* **7**:172, 1986

10. Cherry JD, Nelson DB: Enterovirus infections: Their epidemiology and pathogenesis. *Clin Pediatr* **5**:659, 1966

11. Evans AD, Waddington E: Hand, foot and mouth disease in South Wales, 1964. *Br J Dermatol* **79**:309, 1967

12. Higgins PG, Warin RP: Hand, foot, and mouth disease: A clinically recognizable virus infection seen mainly in children. *Clin Pediatr* **6**:373, 1967

13. Meadow SR: Hand, foot, and mouth disease. *Arch Dis Child* **40**:560, 1965

14. Fields JP et al: Hand, foot, and mouth disease. *Arch Dermatol* **99**:243, 1969

15. Mihm MC Jr et al: A clinical, epidemiologic, and virologic study of hand, foot, and mouth syndrome. *Proceedings of the Third Joint Meeting of the Clinical Society and Commissioned Officers Association of the United States Public Health Service, March 25–29, 1968, San Francisco, California*, p 64

16. Kimura A et al: Light and electron microscopic study of skin lesions of patients with the hand, foot and mouth disease. *Tohoku J Med* **122**:237, 1977

17. Cherry JD, Jahn CL: Hand, foot, and mouth syndrome. Report of six cases due to Coxsackie virus, group A, type 16. *Pediatrics* **37**:637, 1966

18. Wright HT et al: Fatal infection in an infant associated with Coxsackie virus group A, type 16. *N Engl J Med* **268**:1041, 1963

19. Baker DA, Phillips CA: Fatal hand-foot-and-mouth disease in an infant caused by Coxsackie virus A₇. *JAMA* **242**:1065, 1979

20. Froeschle JE et al: Hand, foot, and mouth disease (Coxsackie A₁₆) in Atlanta. *Am J Dis Child* **114**:278, 1967

21. Magoffin RL, Lenette EH: Nonpolioviruses and paralytic disease. *Calif Med* **97**:1, 1962

22. Gohd RS, Faigel HC: Hand-foot-and-mouth disease resembling measles. A life-threatening disease: Case report. *Pediatrics* **37**:644, 1966

23. Ogilvie MM, Tearne CF: Spontaneous abortion after hand-foot-and-mouth disease caused by Coxsackie virus A₁₆. *Br Med J* **281**:1527, 1980

CHAPTER 201

Robert H. Parrott

Herpangina

Herpangina[1-4] is a specific infectious disease in which characteristic peculiar lesions appear on the mucous membrane around the soft palate, tonsillar pillars, and fauces. In temperate climates it appears almost exclusively in the summertime and early fall, and it affects primarily children. The etiologic agent has been established as any of six or seven different group A coxsackievirus types, although some authorities have suggested that herpangina may also occur as part of a larger clinical syndrome in response to other enteroviruses.

Historical Aspects[1]

Zahorsky first described herpangina as a specific entity in 1920. Outbreaks of an illness similar to what he called herpangina were reported in summer camps and nursery schools in 1939 and 1941. Later, Huebner and his associates recovered group A coxsackieviruses from throat washings and feces of a group of patients with herpangina. This was the first suggestion that specific viruses caused the disease. The clinical association has been confirmed in many reports since that time.

Epidemiology[3]

The viruses that are responsible for herpangina may also result in subclinical infection or febrile illness without typical oropharyngeal lesions. These viruses also may be isolated from as many as 1.5 to 7.5 percent of persons who are not ill during the summer in a temperate climate. The group A coxsackieviruses may spread readily in a family or neighborhood group and from patient to patient in hospitals. Virus may persist in the feces for up to 47 days after acute infection. Fecal material is a common source of isolation of virus, although in herpangina the agent may be recovered from saliva, nasal secretions, and oropharynx, and stomach washings. Undoubtedly the major method of spread early in illness is from oropharyngeal secretions. Herpangina and the group A coxsackieviruses which cause it have been reported from many parts of the world; the disease is presumably worldwide in distribution.

Etiology and Pathogenesis[3,4]

The clinical association of group A coxsackieviruses with herpangina has occurred much more often than would be expected by chance. In most studies the virus types recovered have been the same—A2, A4, A5, A6, A8, and A10. Type 3 was found in cases of herpangina in one locale during one season. Whether the oropharyngeal lesions sometimes seen during infection with other coxsackieviruses or echoviruses should be considered herpangina is a matter of definition. The herpangina strains of group A coxsackievirus can cause febrile illness without visible oropharyngeal lesions, and this situation should be strongly suspected when one finds fever and pharyngitis in siblings of a patient who has clinically distinct herpangina.

There is no sex difference and no known difference by race or national origin in the occurrence of the disease. In Washington, D.C., 50 percent of cases occur in July, 35 percent in August, 5 percent in June, and 10 percent in September. The incubation period is approximately 4 days. Permanent immunity occurs to the type-specific agent. However, since there are several group A coxsackieviruses which can cause the disease, the clinical syndrome may recur.

Clinical Manifestations[2]

The child affected with herpangina is usually in good health until a sudden onset of fever. In Zahorsky's description: "The child feels tired and often complains of pain in the back and extremities. Headache and pains in the back of the neck are frequently marked symptoms and lead one to expect poliomyelitis at times. This impression is often accentuated by the tenderness of the extremities on movement."

In 68 cases studied at Children's Hospital in Washington, D.C., temperatures ranging from 38.3 to 40.5°C were found in 89 percent of the patients and lasted for 1 to 4 days. Five percent had convulsions with the onset of fever. Seventy percent complained of anorexia, dysphagia, or sore throat. There was vomiting in 38 percent, abdominal pain in 21 percent, and headache in 16 percent.

The characteristic feature of the disease is the presence of gray-white papulovesicular lesions, about 1 to 2 mm in diameter, which progress to slightly larger ulcers. A zone of erythema usually surrounds the lesion (Figs. 201-1, 201-2). The lesions are distributed, in order of frequency, on the anterior pillars of the tonsillar fauces, the soft palate, the uvula, and the tonsils themselves. The lesions may persist for 4 to 6 days. During the illness there is usually a diffuse pharyngeal hyperemia. Occasionally there is non-

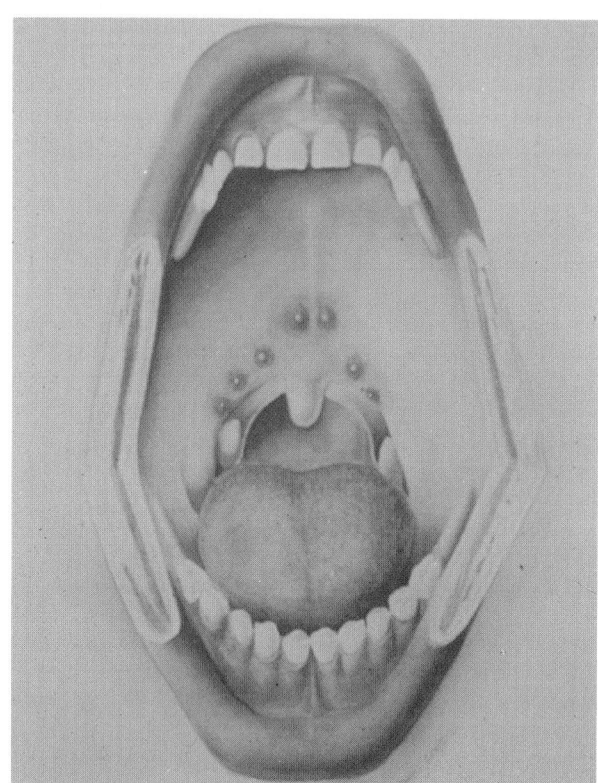

FIGURE 201-2 The typical presentation of herpangina.

purulent conjunctivitis and, rarely, a rash. Similar lesions have been reported occurring in the vagina in the course of what was otherwise typical herpangina. In the Washington, D.C., series, total peripheral white blood cell counts were under 10,000/mm³ in 53 percent of the cases, 20 percent ranged from 10,000 to 15,000, and 27 percent were over 15,000.

Pathology

The only visible lesions occurring in the course of this disease are the oropharyngeal lesions already described and the diffuse pharyngeal hyperemia. Specific histologic studies of these lesions have not been reported.

Diagnosis and Differential Diagnosis[3,5]

The diagnosis is primarily clinical. It can be confirmed in the laboratory either by obtaining material from the oropharyngeal lesions or by an anal swab for recovery of group A coxsackieviruses or by type-specific serologic study with blood specimens obtained early in the illness and during convalescence. The group A coxsackieviruses induce flaccid paralysis and marked muscle degeneration but no significant central nervous system lesions in suckling mice and cause no apparent disease in adult mice. Most of the herpangina strains of coxsackievirus can be recovered only in suckling mice and not as readily in tissue culture as most of the other coxsackieviruses.

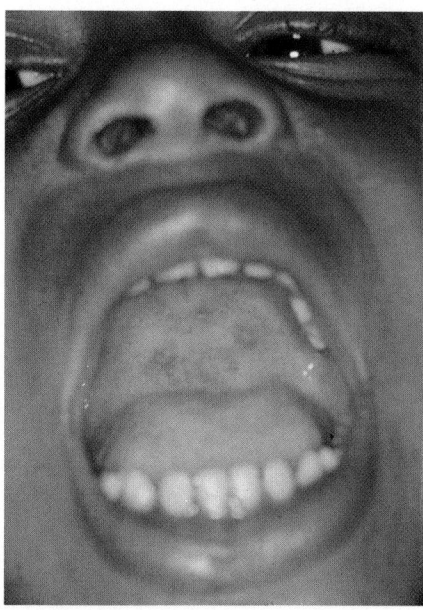

FIGURE 201-1 The typical feature of herpangina is the early presence of gray-white papulovesicular lesions on the palate. These progress to slightly larger ulcers as illustrated. A zone of erythema surrounds the lesions.

The clinical conditions which may be confused with herpangina are infectious gingivostomatitis due to herpes simplex virus, acute lymphonodular pharyngitis (also due to a group A coxsackievirus), or possibly the other oropharyngeal lesions sometimes described in the course of enteroviral infections. Infectious gingivostomatitis is also a common childhood illness. There is fever, with vesicles or ulcers in the oral cavity, occasionally in the pharynx. It occurs throughout the year. The onset is more gradual than that of herpangina. The major symptoms include fever, dysphagia, sore mouth with a very fetid odor to the breath, and bleeding gums. There are cervical lymphadenopathy and hyperemia, hypertrophy, and hemorrhage of the gums, none of which occurs in herpangina. The vesicles and ulcers are on the gums, tongue, lips, buccal mucous membrane, as well as occasionally in the location of herpangina lesions. Fever lasts longer, and the oropharyngeal lesions persist for 8 to 14 days. The child with gingivostomatitis is much more severely ill than the one with herpangina.

Acute lymphonodular pharyngitis is an illness that also primarily affects children and is due to coxsackievirus A10, as reported by Steigman et al.[5] There are headache, malaise, and anorexia with fever. Lesions located on the uvula, palate, anterior pillars, and posterior pharynx, as in herpangina, are described as raised, discrete, white-to-yellow nodules, surrounded by erythema. These lesions do not ulcerate. Symptoms and lesions persist somewhat longer than in herpangina.

Various authors have described vesicles, ulcers, and other types of lesions in the faucial and soft-palate area in the course of infection with coxsackieviruses B1 through B5, with coxsackievirus A7 and A9, and with echoviruses 9 and 16. In these cases the clinical picture is not that described by Zahorsky and others. These cases suggest that various enteroviruses may produce lesions in this particular location. Some authors have, therefore, suggested that the term *herpangina* be used as a description of oropharyngeal lesions rather than as a description of a specific disease.

In the differential diagnosis of herpangina one must also exclude occasional cases of oral candidiasis, infectious mononucleosis, the enanthems of measles, varicella, scarlatina, and diphtheria, certain heavy-metal poisonings, and deficiency diseases and hematologic disorders. Aphthae which occur as a result of trauma, allergy, or psychogenic factors are not usually accompanied by fever.

Treatment

The major importance of herpangina for the physician is that making the diagnosis relieves the fear which accompanies sudden fever in children. No specific treatment is available or necessary. Antipyretic or anticonvulsant treatment might be indicated in individual cases.

Course and Prognosis

The fever of herpangina rarely lasts more than 4 days, and the lesions rarely more than a week. With the exception of the occasional child who suffers a convulsion, the prognosis is good and the course benign.

References

1. Cole RM et al: Studies of Coxsackie viruses: Observations on epidemiological aspects of group A viruses. *Am J Public Health* **41**:1342, 1951
2. Parrott RH, Cramblett HG: Nonbacterial infections affecting nasopharynx. *Pediatr Clin North Am* **4**:115, 1957
3. Parrott RH: Clinical importance of group A Coxsackie viruses. *Ann NY Acad Sci* **67**:230, 1957
4. Cherry JD, Jahn CL: Herpangina: Etiologic spectrum. *Pediatrics* **36**:632, 1965
5. Steigman AJ et al: Acute lymphonodular pharyngitis: Newly described condition due to Coxsackie A virus. *J Pediatr* **61**:331, 1962

CHAPTER 202

Karen Wiss and Richard Allen Johnson

Erythema Infectiosum and Parvovirus B19 Infection

Erythema infectiosum (fifth disease) is an illness primarily of childhood that is characterized by a "slapped cheek" appearance of the face and an erythematous, lacy eruption on the trunk and extremities. Parvovirus B19, the etiologic agent, may also cause arthritis, aplastic crisis in patients with increased red blood cell turnover, chronic anemia in immunocompromised persons, and fetal hydrops.

Historical Aspects

The first known clinical picture of a patient with erythema infectiosum is drawn in Robert Willan's book *On Cutaneous Diseases* from 1808.[1] Throughout the 1800s, fifth disease was thought to be a mild form of rubella or measles. Tschamer described a distinct illness compatible with erythema infectiosum in 1889, although he thought it was abortive rubella.[2] It was designated fifth disease in the early 1900s, when infectious exanthems were numbered first through sixth.[3]

The first clue to the etiologic agent came in 1975 in England. During routine screening of serum from healthy blood donors for hepatitis B surface antigen, nine samples of blood had false positive results by counter immunoelectrophoresis (CIE) but were negative by the more sensitive techniques of hemagglutination and radioimmunoassay. Electron microscopy of these serum samples demonstrated viral particles that were designated B19 after a specimen label from one of the blood donors.[4] The authors postulated that this was an infectious agent because 30 percent of adults had IgG antibody to the viral antigen. It was later confirmed that B19 was a parvovirus.[5] Parvoviruses had previously been thought to infect only animals. In this manner the virus was discovered but association with a clinical illness awaited.

Parvovirus was identified as the etiologic agent of an acute febrile illness in two British soldiers in 1980[6] and was found in the serum of patients with sickle cell anemia and hypoplastic crisis in 1981.[7] The virus was suggested as a cause of aplastic crisis in sickle cell disease.

In 1983, there was an outbreak of fifth disease among London school children.[8] Serum samples from 31 schoolchildren and six exposed adults, all with clinical signs of the disease, contained parvovirus-specific IgM antibody. There was no IgM detected in exposed asymptomatic individuals. These findings suggested parvovirus B19 as the cause of erythema infectiosum.[9]

Epidemiology

Fifth disease is worldwide in distribution, can occur throughout the year, and can affect all ages. It tends to occur in epidemics, especially associated with school outbreaks in the late winter and early spring.[10] Serologic studies have shown increasing prevalence with age. Various studies indicate that from 15 to 60 percent of children ages 5 to 19 years and 30 to 60 percent of adults are seropositive.[4,11,12]

The incubation period for erythema infectiosum is from 4 to 14 days.[9,11,13,14] After intranasal inoculation of parvovirus-infected serum to healthy volunteers, low-grade fever and nonspecific complaints occurred at the time of viremia, 6 to 14 days after inoculation, and the rash appeared at day 17 or 18.[5]

Parvovirus B19 is thought to be transmitted primarily by the respiratory route via droplet aerosol[11] during the viremic phase.[15] B19 DNA has been found in respiratory secretions of viremic patients.[13,15,16] After the rash of erythema infectiosum appears, B19 is not found in respiratory secretions and is usually not present in the serum.[15] This suggests that persons with erythema infectiosum are infectious only prior to the onset of the rash.[11]

The virus seems to be effectively spread after close contact. The secondary attack rate among susceptible household contacts is approximately 50 percent.[16] Transmission may occur via blood transfusion,[4] from blood products,[17] and vertically from mother to fetus.[18]

Etiology and Pathogenesis

The B19 virus belongs to the family Parvoviridae and the genus *Parvovirus*.[19] It is small, contains single-stranded DNA, at least two capsid proteins, and one nonstructural protein that serves as a template for replication. It differs from other members of the family because it does not require coinfection with a helper virus in order to replicate.[20]

The pathogenesis of erythema infectiosum is unknown, but the mechanism may involve immune complexes.[10] The more serious manifestations of parvovirus infection relate to the fact that the virus infects and lyses erythroid precursor cells.[21] In patients with increased red blood cell destruction or loss who depend on compensatory increases in red cell production to maintain stable red cell indices, B19 infection may lead to transient aplastic crisis.[10] This includes individuals with chronic hemolytic anemias and those with anemia associated with acute or chronic blood loss. When parvovirus infects the erythroblasts in the developing fetus, the result may be hemolysis and anemia.[22] Anemia may trigger congestive heart failure, edema (hydrops), and possibly fetal death.

Clinical Manifestations

Parvovirus B19 in Children

Fifth disease usually begins with nonspecific symptoms such as headache, coryza, and low-grade fever about 2 days prior to the onset of the rash.[23] Patients may have headache, pharyngitis, fever, malaise, myalgias, coryza, diarrhea, nausea, cough, and conjunctivitis coinciding with the rash.[23] A small percentage of children develop arthralgias[23] and, rarely, children present with symptoms suggestive of juvenile rheumatoid arthritis.[24]

The characteristic rash begins with confluent, erythematous, edematous plaques on the malar eminences, the "slapped-cheeks" (Fig. 202-1). As the facial rash fades over 1 to 4 days, pink-to-erythematous macules or papules appear on the trunk, neck, and extensor surfaces of the extremities.[11] These lesions have some central fading giving them a lacy (Fig. 202-2) or reticulated appearance[23] (Fig. 202-3). The rash can be morbilliform, confluent, circinate, or annular,[11] and there have been reports of palmar and plantar involvement.[13] The eruption typically lasts 5 to 9 days but can recur for weeks or months with triggers such as sunlight, exercise,

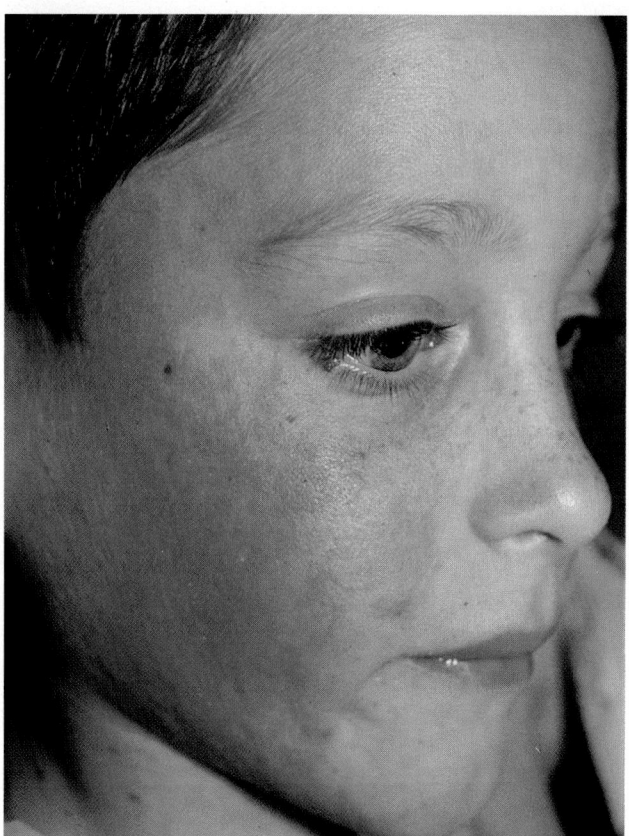

FIGURE 202-1 Child with the characteristic "slapped cheeks."

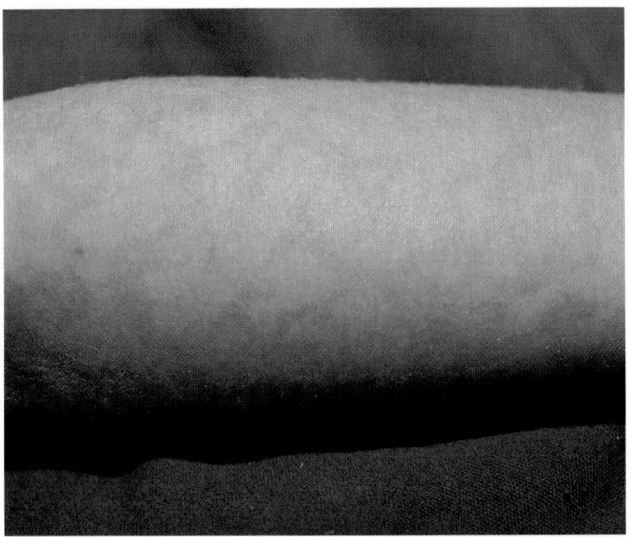

FIGURE 202-2 Lacy pink macules on the forearm.

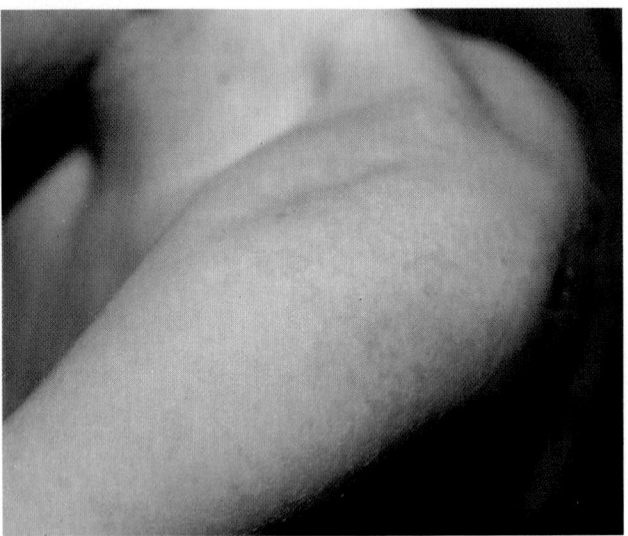

FIGURE 202-3 Reticulate erythematous macules on the trunk and upper arm.

temperature change, bathing, and emotional stress.[23] In some outbreaks, pruritus is a major feature of the rash in children.[13,14]

There have been occasional reports of parvovirus B19 associated with vascular purpura,[25] including Henoch-Schönlein purpura.[25,26] An enanthem consisting of erythema of the tongue and pharynx and red macules on the buccal mucosa and palate can occur.[27]

Parvovirus B19 in Adults

Acute arthropathy is the primary manifestation of B19 viral infection in adults.[14,28] It occurs mainly in women and affects the small joints of the hands, the knees, wrists, ankles, and feet.[29] Occasionally other joints like the spine and costochondral joints are involved.[28] This symmetric polyarthritis is usually self-limited but can be persistent or recurrent for months.[28,29] It may mimic Lyme arthritis[30] and rheumatoid arthritis.[31]

The constitutional symptoms are usually more severe in adults than in children.[32] Fever, adenopathy, and a mild arthritis without a rash is the usual course.[32] Women are more likely than men to have joint complaints and rash, while men often present only with a flulike illness.[28] Some adults may have fatigue, malaise, and depression for weeks after the infection.[32] Asymptomatic infection can certainly occur in adults as well as in children.[13,16] Twenty-six percent of adults were reported to be asymptomatic in one outbreak.[28] Parvovirus B19 has been known to cause numbness and tingling of the fingers with or without other features of fifth disease.[33] Pruritus that is sometimes severe can occur with or without a rash. It has been suggested that if pruritus is a complaint in a patient with acute-onset arthritis, parvovirus should be considered as a possible cause.[34]

The rash in adults, if present at all, is usually macular or lacy, often on the extremities, and rarely demonstrates the characteristic slapped-cheek appearance.[28] Other cutaneous manifestations associated with B19 infection in adults include purpura,[35] vesicles, pustules,[36] and palmoplantar desquamation.[37]

Complications

Transient Aplastic Crisis

Parvovirus B19 is the most common cause of transient aplastic crisis in patients with chronic hemolytic anemias.[38] This has been demonstrated in sickle cell anemia,[7,39] hereditary spherocytosis,[40] heterozygous beta-thalassemia,[41] pyruvate kinase deficiency,[42] and autoimmune hemolytic anemia.[43] The aplastic crisis may be the initial manifestation of the underlying hematologic disease.[41,43]

Patients typically have fever and constitutional complaints, followed one week later by fatigue, pallor, and worsening anemia.[44] Rarely is a rash reported with aplastic crisis. There is an absence of reticulocytes and the hemoglobin may fall below 4 g/dL.[44] Bone marrow examination shows hypoplasia or aplasia of the erythroid series. Red blood cell transfusion may be necessary and most patients recover in one week[44] although the problem can be fatal if untreated.[10] Transient red cell aplasia can occur in healthy persons without underlying hematologic abnormalities.[45] It is likely that the aplasia is missed in individuals without disorders of shortened erythrocyte survival, because the hemoglobin does not drop low enough to cause symptoms.

Chronic B19 Infection

In immunocompromised patients, B19 infection can cause a serious, prolonged anemia from persistent lysis of red cell precursors.[45] Parvovirus-related chronic anemia has been reported in HIV-infected patients,[46] in congenital immunodeficiencies,[47] with acute leukemias,[48] lupus erythematosus,[48] and during the first year of life without immunodeficiency.[49] These patients respond dramatically to intravenous gammaglobulin, which suggests that antibody is the main defense to human parvovirus infection.[50]

Fetal B19 Infection

Nonimmune fetal hydrops is the most common complication of intrauterine infection with B19.[18] Because B19 virus can infect erythroid precursors, extensive hemolysis can occur in the fetus, leading to severe anemia, tissue anoxia, and high output heart failure.[18] Brown et al., in 1984,[51] first reported a case of hydrops fetalis during an epidemic of erythema infectiosum. During another outbreak in Scotland, 2 out of 6 women infected with B19 during pregnancy had hydropic abortuses, while 4 infected women had healthy infants.[22] The overall risk of fetal death is not clearly known, but recent studies have suggested that this risk is less than 10 percent after maternal infection and is even less if the infection occurs in the second half of pregnancy.[18,52] The risk of fetal death for a woman with unknown serologic status is estimated to be less than 2.5 percent after a household exposure and less than 1.5 percent after a significant work exposure.[18] It seems that in B19-infected pregnant women, most fetuses are not infected, and, if they are infected, usually there is no adverse outcome.[45,52]

Because parvoviruses are known teratogens in animals, there has been much concern about their causing birth defects in humans.[18] In sera collected from 253 infants with a wide range of congenital abnormalities, there was no parvovirus-specific IgM detected to suggest recent infection.[53] There has been one report of a B19-infected abortus with eye abnormalities.[54] Otherwise no reports of liveborn infants with anomalies have been linked to B19 infection in utero. It has been concluded from these studies that parvovirus B19 is not a common cause of birth defects.

Laboratory Findings

In patients with erythema infectiosum, laboratory results are usually normal, including reticulocyte count, hematocrit, and tests of liver and renal function.[13,27] Patients with aplastic crisis have reticulocytopenia and anemia, the severity of which depends on the degree of the underlying anemia.[11] Reticulocytopenia, anemia, lymphopenia, neutropenia, and thrombocytopenia can occur in healthy individuals with B19 infection, although these are usually not significant enough to cause clinical symptoms.[15] The erythrocyte sedimentation rate is occasionally elevated,[24] and rheumatoid factor has been positive in some cases of parvovirus-associated arthritis.[29,31]

Pathology

Histologic examination of various tissues demonstrates homogeneous, intranuclear inclusions with peripheral condensation of chromatin in erythroid precursor cells.[22,55] Electron microscopy of these inclusions reveals parvovirus-like particles.[55] In fetal tissues, a leukoerythroblastic reaction may be seen as well.[22,51] The histologic changes in the skin of patients with erythema infectiosum have not been well characterized and are not considered diagnostic.[56]

Diagnosis

The diagnosis of erythema infectiosum is usually based on the clinical features. The differential diagnosis includes rubella, measles, scarlet fever, roseola, enteroviral infection, erysipelas on the cheek, and drug hypersensitivity. These other disorders may involve more significant systemic illness and lack the progression from the slapped cheeks to the lacy eruption on the extremities that is so characteristic of fifth disease.

Because no animal model or easy tissue culture system exists for the B19 virus, laboratory testing for the antibody or the virus is performed only in a limited number of research laboratories. The CDC currently will test the serum of patients with aplastic crisis, those with immunodeficiency and chronic anemia, pregnant women with B19 exposure, and fetal hydrops cases in which B19 infection is suspected.[10] The testing is not done on a routine basis and is arranged through state health departments.

Detection of recent infection is usually performed with assays for IgM antibody. Radioimmunoassay (RIA) or enzyme-linked immunosorbent (ELISA) techniques can detect IgM within a few days after onset of illness. IgM can be measured for up to 6 months in many cases, although there is a decline in titer in the second month after onset.[57,58] IgC can be identified with the same techniques by day 7 of the illness and lasts for years[57,58] and therefore is best used to document past infection. Parvovirus antibody is often not detectable in immunodeficient persons.[46]

B19 virus can be detected in serum during viremia by a variety of techniques, including RIA, CIE, and ELISA. The most specific tests are dot-blot hybridization[59] and the polymerase chain reaction,[60] which may allow identification of B19 DNA in serum, urine, respiratory secretions, and various tissues.

Treatment

There is no specific treatment available for parvovirus B19 infections. Erythema infectiosum is a benign condition and often no treatment is necessary. Supportive therapy for relief of fatigue, malaise, pruritus, and arthralgia may be needed. The chronic anemia is often successfully treated with commercially available intravenous gammaglobulin.[46,48,50] Aplastic crisis, which can be life threatening, may require oxygen therapy and blood transfusion.[44] Fetal hydrops has been effectively treated with intrauterine blood transfusions.[52,61]

Prevention

There is currently no vaccine to prevent parvovirus B19 infection. It is not known whether immunoglobulin given around the time of exposure will prevent infection or alter the course of the disease. Routine treatment with immunoglobulin is not recommended at the present time.[10]

Since patients with erythema infectiosum are no longer infectious by the time they develop the illness, control measures directed toward these individuals are not likely to be effective.[11] If these persons are hospitalized, no special precautions need to be taken. Because the virus is transmitted before the rash appears, the disease is easily spread in situations of close prolonged contact, such as schools, day care centers, workplaces, and homes.

Patients with aplastic crisis or immunodeficiency with chronic B19 anemia can be infectious and should be placed in respiratory and contact isolation if hospitalized. Hospital workers are at risk of contracting nosocomial infections from these patients[62] and could spread the virus to patients if adequate precautions are not taken.

Course and Prognosis

Parvovirus B19 infection in healthy individuals is self-limited. The rash of erythema infectiosum and the parvovirus arthropathy usually resolve in 1 to 2 weeks but can recur or persist for months.[23,28,29] Although, if untreated, transient aplastic crisis can be fatal, most patients recover in one week.[44] Chronic anemia from B19 usually resolves if treated with gammaglobulin.[46] Fetal hydrops can be fatal if not treated with exchange transfusion.[18]

References

1. van Elsacker-Niele AMW, Anderson MJ: First picture of erythema infectiosum (letter). *Lancet* **1**:229, 1987

2. Tschamer A: Ueber ortliche Rotheln. *Jahrbuch fur Kinderheilkunde* **29**:372, 1889

3. Shapiro L: The numbered diseases: first through sixth (letter). *JAMA* **194**:210, 1965

4. Cossart YE et al: Parvovirus-like particles in human sera. *Lancet* **1**:72, 1975

5. Summers J et al: Characterization of the genome of the agent of erythrocyte aplasia permits its classification as a human parvovirus. *J Gen Virol* **64**:2527, 1983

6. Shneerson JM et al: Febrile illness due to a parvovirus. *Br Med J* **280**:1580, 1980

7. Pattison JR et al: Parvovirus infections and hypoplastic crisis in sickle-cell anaemia (letter). *Lancet* **1**:664, 1981

8. Anderson MJ et al: Human parvovirus, the cause of erythema infectiosum (fifth disease) (letter). *Lancet* **1**:1378, 1983

9. Anderson MJ et al: An outbreak of erythema infectiosum associated with human parvovirus infection. *J Hyg (Lond)* **93**:85, 1984

10. Risks associated with human parvovirus B19 infection. *MMWR* **38**:81, 1989

11. Anderson LJ: Role of parvovirus B19 in human disease. *Pediatr Infect Dis J* **6**:711, 1987

12. Cohen BJ, Buckley MM: The prevalence of antibody to human parvovirus B19 in England and Wales. *J Med Microbiol* **25**:151, 1988

13. Plummer FA et al: An erythema infectiosum-like illness caused by human parvovirus infection. *N Engl J Med* **313**:74,1985

14. Ager EA et al: Epidemic erythema infectiosum. *N Engl J Med* **275**:1326, 1966

15. Anderson MJ et al: Experimental parvoviral infection in humans. *J Infect Dis* **152**:257, 1985

16. Chorba T et al: The role of parvovirus B19 in aplastic crisis and erythema infectiosum (fifth disease). *J Infect Dis* **154**:383, 1986

17. Mortimer PP et al: Transmission of serum parvovirus-like virus by clotting-factor concentrates. *Lancet* **2**:482, 1983

18. Torok TJ: Human parvovirus B19 infections in pregnancy. *Pediatr Infect Dis J* **9**:772, 1990

19. Siegl G et al: Characteristics and taxonomy of Parvoviridae. *Intervirology* **23**:61, 1985

20. Anderson MJ, Pattison JR: The human parvovirus. *Arch Virol* **82**:137, 1984

21. Young N et al: Direct demonstration of the human parvovirus in erythroid progenitor cells infected in vitro. *J Clin Invest* **74**:2024, 1984

22. Anand A et al: Human parvovirus infection in pregnancy and hydrops fetalis. *N Engl J Med* **316**:183, 1987

23. Feder HM, Anderson I: Fifth disease. A brief review of infections in childhood, in adulthood, and in pregnancy. *Arch Intern Med* **149**:2176, 1989

24. Reid DM et al: Human parvovirus-associated arthritis: A clinical and laboratory description. *Lancet* **1**:422, 1985

25. Lefrere JJ et al: Human parvovirus and purpura (letter). *Lancet* **2**:730, 1985

26. Lefrere JJ et al: Henoch-Schönlein purpura and human parvovirus infection (letter). *Pediatrics* **78**:183, 1986

27. Condon FJ: Erythema infectiosum—report of an area-wide outbreak. *Am J Public Health* **49**:528, 1959

28. Woolf AD et al: Clinical manifestations of human parvovirus B19 in adults. *Arch Intern Med* **149**:1153, 1989

29. White DG et al: Human parvovirus arthropathy. *Lancet* **1**:419, 1985

30. Mayo DR, Vance DW: Parvovirus B19 as the cause of a syndrome resembling Lyme arthritis in adults (letter). *N Engl J Med* **324**:419, 1991

31. Naides SJ, Field EH: Transient rheumatoid factor positivity in acute human parvovirus B19 infection. *Arch Intern Med* **148**:2587, 1988

32. Thurn J: Human parvovirus B19: Historical and clinical review. *Rev Infect Dis* **10**:1005, 1988

33. Faden H et al: Numbness and tingling of fingers associated with parvovirus B19 infection (letter). *J Infect Dis* **161**:354, 1990

34. Jacks TA: Pruritus in parvovirus infection. *J R Coll Gen Pract* **37**:210, 1987

35. Mortimer PP et al: Human parvovirus and purpura (letter). *Lancet* **2**:730, 1985

36. Naides SJ et al: Human parvovirus B19-induced vesiculopustular skin eruption. *Am J Med* **84**:968, 1988

37. Dinerman JL, Corman LC: Human parvovirus B19 arthropathy associated with desquamation. *Am J Med* **89**:826, 1990

38. Young N: Hematologic and hematopoietic consequences of B19 parvovirus infection. *Semin Hematol* **25**:159, 1988

39. Serjeant GR et al: Outbreak of aplastic crises in sickle cell anaemia associated with parvovirus-like agent. *Lancet* **2**:595, 1981

40. Tsukada T et al: Epidemic of aplastic crisis in patients with hereditary spherocytosis in Japan. *Lancet* **1**:1401, 1985

41. Lefrere JJ et al: Familial human parvovirus infection associated with anemia in siblings with heterozygous B-thalassemia. *J Infect Dis* **153**:977, 1986

42. Duncan JR et al: Aplastic crisis due to parvovirus infection in pyruvate kinase deficiency. *Lancet* **2**:14, 1983

43. Bertrand Y et al: Autoimmune haemolytic anaemia revealed by human parvovirus-linked erythroblastopenia. *Lancet* **2**:382, 1985

44. Ware R: Human parvovirus infection. *J Pediatr* **114**:343, 1989

45. Anderson LJ: Human parvoviruses. *J Infect Dis* **161**:603, 1990

46. Frickhofen N et al: Persistent B19 parvovirus infection in patients infected with human immunodeficiency virus type 1 (HIV-1): A treatable cause of anemia in AIDS. *Ann Intern Med* **113**:926, 1990

47. Kurtzman GJ et al: Chronic bone marrow failure due to persistent B19 parvovirus infection. *N Engl J Med* **317**:287, 1987

48. Koch WC et al: Manifestations and treatment of human parvovirus B19 infection in immunocompromised patients. *J Pediatr* **116**:355, 1990

49. Belloy M et al: Erythroid hypoplasia due to chronic infection with parvovirus B19 (letter). *N Engl J Med* **322**:633, 1990

50. Kurtzman G et al: Pure red-cell aplasia of 10 years' duration due to persistent parvovirus B19 infection and its cure with immunoglobulin therapy. *N Engl J Med* **321**:519, 1989

51. Brown T et al: Intrauterine parvovirus infection associated with hydrops fetalis (letter). *Lancet* **2**:1033, 1984

52. Public Health Laboratory Service Working Party on Fifth Disease. Prospective study of human parvovirus (B19) infection in pregnancy. *Br Med J* **300**:1166, 1990

53. Mortimer PP et al: Human parvovirus and the fetus. *Lancet* **2**:1012, 1985

54. Weiland HT et al: Parvovirus B19 associated with fetal abnormality (letter). *Lancet* **1**:682, 1987

55. Caul EO et al: Intrauterine infection with human parvovirus B19: A light and electron microscopy study. *J Med Virol* **24**:55, 1988

56. Ackerman AB: *Superficial Perivascular Dermatitis in Histologic Diagnosis of Inflammatory Skin Diseases.* Philadelphia, Lea & Febiger, 1978

57. Cohen BJ et al: Diagnostic assays with monoclonal antibodies for the

human serum parvovirus-like virus (SPLV). *J Hyg (Lond)* **91**:113, 1983

58. Anderson LJ et al: Detection of antibodies and antigens of human parvovirus B19 by enzyme-linked immunosorbent assay. *J Clin Microbiol* **24**:522, 1986

59. Anderson MJ et al: Diagnosis of human parvovirus infection by dot-blot hybridization using cloned viral DNA. *J Med Virol* **15**:163, 1985

60. Salimans MMM et al: Rapid detection of human parvovirus B19 DNA by dot-blot hybridization and the polymerase chain reaction. *J Virol Methods* **23**:19, 1989

61. Schwarz TF et al: Human parvovirus B19 infection in pregnancy (letter). *Lancet* **2**:566, 1988

62. Bell LM et al: Human parvovirus B19 infection among hospital staff members after contact with infected patients. *N Engl J Med* **321**:485, 1989

CHAPTER 203

Clyde S. Crumpacker and Roy M. Gulick

Herpes Simplex

The human herpes simplex virus consists of two closely related viruses designated herpes simplex virus type 1 (HSV-1) and herpes simplex virus type 2 (HSV-2) (Fig. 203-1). The viruses cause a wide variety of mucocutaneous infections and produce both primary and recurrent infections. The primary infection by herpes simplex virus is more severe and has a different natural history than recurrent disease. Following a primary infection, the virus establishes a latent or dormant state. Recurrent disease is caused by reactivation of this dormant virus which then travels down the nerve fiber to establish skin infection. The natural history and transmission of these viral infections pose a significant health problem. Effective antiviral therapy for these diseases remains an important medical goal. In this chapter, the clinical presentations, diagnosis, and treatment of herpes simplex infections will be discussed.

Epidemiology

Recurrent oral-facial herpes simplex infection, known commonly as "cold sores" or "fever blisters," afflicts between 25 and 40 percent of the United States population and is thus the most common manifestation of herpes simplex infection. Studies show that 46 percent of graduating college students have serologic evidence of HSV-1 exposure, although only 28 percent report a history of cold sores.[1] In general in adult populations from city and rural areas throughout the world, >85 percent have serologic evidence of HSV-1 exposure.[2]

Genital infection with herpes simplex virus has increased markedly during the past three decades. Patient consultations with private physicians for genital herpes increased tenfold from 1966 to 1981. Over the same period, the number of new infections increased more than sevenfold.[3]

In the United States, 16 percent of the population aged 15 to 74 has serologic evidence of previous exposure to HSV-2. Because nearly 100 percent of positive serologies are due to infections acquired sexually, it is estimated that more than 25 million Americans are infected with genital HSV-2.[4] In one study of women attending family practice clinics, 78 percent of those with serologic evidence of HSV-2 had no historical, clinical, or virologic evidence of genital herpes infection. Of these, 4 percent were asymptomatically shedding HSV.[5] Similarly, a study of college students showed only 25 percent of those exposed had a history of genital herpes.[1] From

these studies it is clear that the large majority of HSV-2 infections are clinically inapparent.

The Viruses

Herpes simplex virus types 1 and 2 contain a double-stranded linear DNA genome of molecular mass of 160×10^3 kDa surrounded by a protein coat and lipid envelope. The genomes of HSV-1 and HSV-2 have about 50 percent of the nucleotide sequence in common and 50 percent variable. The viral genomes encode for about 50 viral-specific proteins. These include five to six viral-specific glycoproteins that are present on the viral surfaces and on the surface of viral-infected cells. These glycoproteins are important for induction of neutralizing antibodies to the virus and regulate cell fusion exhibited by these viruses. Only one of these surface glycoproteins, gC for HSV-1 and gG for HSV-2, appears to be type specific. There is significant cross-reactivity of antibodies raised against the other glycoproteins between HSV-1 and HSV-2.

The major glycoproteins that induce neutralizing antibodies, the gD glycoprotein of HSV-1 and HSV-2, share 80 percent of the

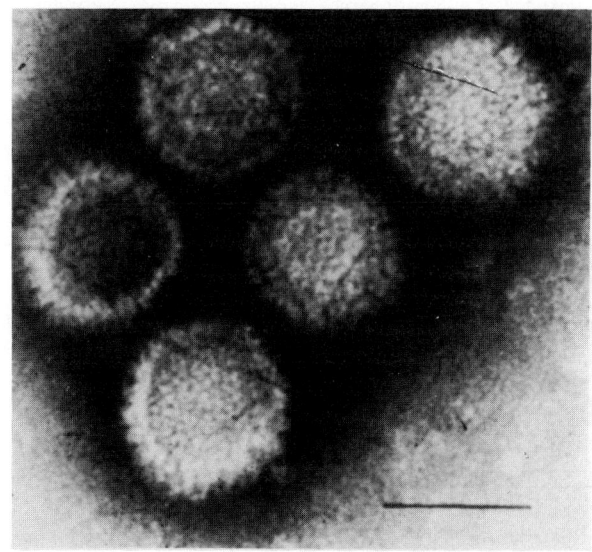

FIGURE 203-1 Herpes simplex virion.

amino acids in common, and neutralizing antibodies raised against HSV-1 readily neutralize HSV-2. The viral core proteins and structural proteins comprise 20 viral-specific proteins. The viral protein coat consists of protein arranged in 162 capsomeres around the viral nucleic acid.

The herpes simplex virus genome encodes a number of nonstructural proteins that are important for viral DNA replication. These include a viral thymidine kinase, DNA polymerase, ribonucleotide reductase, and alkaline DNAse. These enzymes have all been mapped to precise locations on the viral genome, and mutants of herpes simplex virus have been isolated that contain mutations in the genes encoding these viral enzymes. These viral enzymes, which differ in significant ways from cellular enzymes, can be selectively inhibited by antiviral drugs. The development of antiviral drugs that selectively inhibit viral-specific enzyme targets, such as viral DNA polymerase, has progressed rapidly and permitted the successful application of antiviral chemotherapy for the treatment of herpes simplex infections. The use of rapid techniques of viral diagnosis to make an early diagnosis of herpes simplex infection and begin therapy with drugs, such as acyclovir, has made it possible to treat many forms of mucocutaneous infection caused by herpes simplex virus effectively.

Primary Infection

A hallmark of infections caused by herpes simplex virus is that they occur initially in mucocutaneous locations and then remain dormant in neuronal cells located in ganglia before recurring as outbreaks of mucocutaneous infection. The natural histories of primary and recurrent infections differ, the response to treatment may differ, and they need to be considered separately. Primary infection with herpes simplex occurs primarily by direct exposure through mucocutaneous contact with another infected individual. It is estimated that 95 percent of primary genital herpes simplex infection occurs within 2 weeks of sexual contact with an infected sexual partner. In one study, in 70 percent of patients transmission appeared to result from sexual contact during periods of asymptomatic viral shedding.[6] Primary infection is defined as the first infection with herpes simplex virus in a seronegative patient. There are no reliable well-documented examples of herpes simplex virus being transmitted by the respiratory route. Even though some experimental studies have shown that the virus can persist on surfaces like towels, toilet seats, or counter tops for as long as 30 min, there is no case of a herpes simplex infection being acquired by contact with such a surface. The virus may persist in water or on a wet surface for a short period of time also, but the presence of any halogenated compound in the water inactivates the virus infectivity immediately. There is no evidence that herpes simplex infection can be acquired through water transmission.

For primary facial-oral herpes infection, exposure to herpes simplex in a mother's vaginal secretions during the process of delivery can result in a primary neonatal infection in about 50 percent of the infants exposed to the virus. This usually is first noted at day 4 to 7 of life by the development of characteristic herpetic skin lesions. The skin infection commonly occurs in areas of trauma on the body and may begin in areas where scalp electrodes were placed to facilitate fetal monitoring during labor. Neonatal infection with herpes simplex virus may also occur in the absense of skin lesions and directly involve the CNS and visceral organs such as the liver. In the absence of skin lesions, primary neonatal herpes simplex

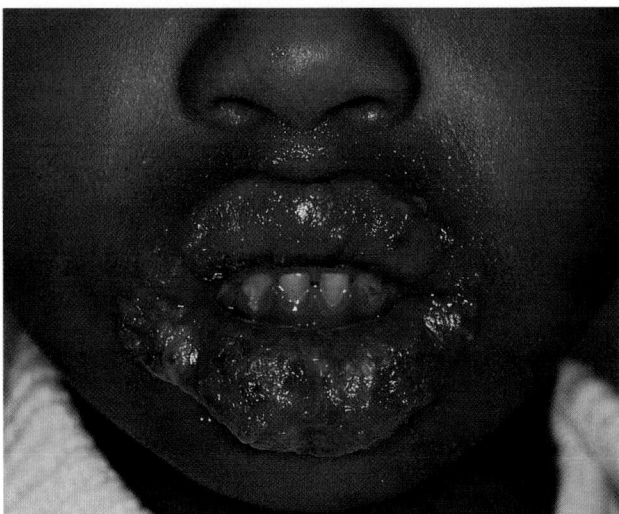

FIGURE 203-2   Primary herpetic gingivostomatitis in a child.

infection is very difficult to diagnose and remains an important challenge for the pediatric clinician. Primary herpes simplex infection in the neonate is a devastating life-threatening infection that must be diagnosed and treated promptly with antiviral drugs.

Primary facial-oral herpes infection usually occurs as an acute gingivostomatitis, and ulcers may occur throughout the buccal mucosa (Fig. 203-2). Many cases of herpes gingivostomatitis occur early in life and are probably not diagnosed. It is estimated that a great majority (>85 percent) of the worldwide population has evidence of herpes simplex facial-oral infection,[2] whereas only 37 percent of middle-class college-age American students have antibody to herpes simplex infection.[1]

Primary genital herpes infection occurs following sexual exposure in perhaps 95 percent of cases. The usual time for an outbreak of genital herpes is between 3 to 14 days following sexual relations with a person with active genital lesions.

Recurrent Infection

A characteristic feature of all the herpes viruses is that after primary infection occurs, the virus has the ability to establish latent or dormant infection and then to reactivate to produce recurrent disease (Fig. 203-3). The recurrent disease is usually milder and of shorter duration than the primary infection. In the facial-oral herpes simplex infection, the virus is almost always HSV-1 and, following the primary episode of stomatitis, the virus migrates to the trigeminal ganglion. In the ganglion of the nerve, the viral genome remains in a suppressed state primarily as a circular episome of viral DNA with very few of the viral genes being expressed. Certain triggering events such as exposure to sunlight, severe stress, or neurosurgical manipulation of the ganglia will cause the latent virus to reactivate and express its genome to make intact viral particles. The viral particles move down the nerve, probably by axonal flow, and replicate in the epithelial cells of the skin to produce an outbreak of cold sores (Fig. 203-3). Between episodes there is no evidence of viral particles, viral proteins, or viral nucleic acids in the skin at the affected site. These general principles apply to recurrent episodes of herpes infections in all common sites, especially facial-oral her-

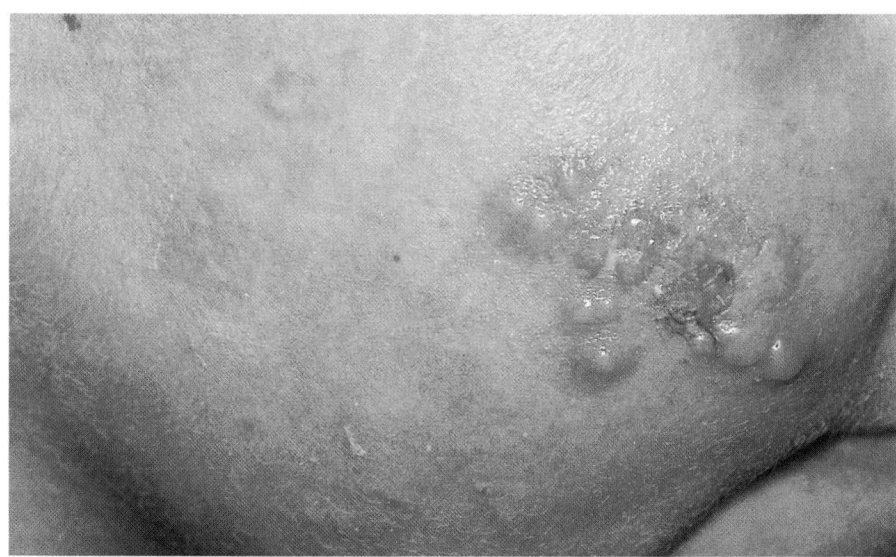

FIGURE 203-3   Recurrent facial herpes simplex with grouped vesicles and crusting.

pes, genital herpes, herpes whitlow, and herpes keratitis. In recurrent herpes infections, patients possess antibody to the virus, and immunologically active mononuclear cells and lymphocytes contribute to the pathogenesis and healing of the recurrent outbreak.

Clinical Manifestations

Primary Gingivostomatitis

Primary herpetic infection of the mouth and pharynx is a disease of children and young adults. The peak years of incidence usually occur between ages 1 and 5. A study at a large university health service estimated that primary herpes simplex virus infection was a significant cause of sore throats in college students.[7] The infection may be mild and inapparent to severe with high fever. The usual onset is with fever, sore throat and painful vesicles, and ulcerative erosions on the tongue, palate, gingiva, buccal mucosa, and lips. The vesicles on the mucous membranes coalesce to form plaques covered with a gray membrane. Severe oral lesions are associated with drooling, halitosis, enlarged lymph nodes, inability to eat, fever, and generalized complaints. The time from exposure to onset of symptoms is from 5 to 10 days. The diagnosis is suggested by the early onset of lesions in discrete clusters before they spread to extensively involve the entire buccal mucosa. Diagnosis is confirmed by culturing herpes simplex virus from the lesions, or identifying herpes simplex antigens with the use of monoclonal antibodies and immunofluorescent analysis.

The differential diagnosis of primary herpetic gingivostomatitis includes streptococcal pharyngitis, diphtheria, Coxsackie virus infection, aphthous ulcers, infectious mononucleosis, severe candidiasis, pemphigus vulgaris, Behçet's disease, erythema multiforme, and primary HIV infection.

Recurrent Facial-Oral Herpes Simplex

After a primary infection with herpes simplex virus, patients develop antibody to the virus. In one study, 27 percent of college students reported a history of cold sores.[1] It is estimated that about one-third of the population of the United States experience recurrent episodes of facial-oral infection with HSV, known as *recurrent herpes labialis* or *cold sores*. The incidence of recurrences is variable in different populations, but 15 percent of young adults surveyed had recurrences of at least one lesion per year and in a series of over 1000 young adults, 20 percent have recurrent episodes. The usual number of recurrences is 3 to 4 per year.[8,9]

The onset of a cold sore is heralded by itching and burning at the vermilion border of the lip. This may be associated with an erythematous papule that rapidly goes on to become vesicular and then to ulcerate to produce a sore. The open sore crusts over in about 4 days, the scab falls off, and complete healing occurs in 8 to 9 days. Virus can be isolated from cold sores for about 3.5 days, and the virus is HSV-1. Neutralizing antibodies do not prevent recurrent episodes, and most patients with recurrent herpes labialis have high levels of neutralizing antibody at the time of recurrence. The most common triggering events to bring on recurrent cold sores are sun exposure, trauma to the lips, emotional stress, and fatigue.[10]

Recurrent herpes labialis must be distinguished from other ulcerative lesions such as aphthous ulcers, erythema multiforme, impetigo, and vaccinia infection. The usual location for recurrent herpes labialis is at the skin-lip junction. Recurrent erosive ulcers inside the mouth are most commonly due to aphthous ulcers or erythema multiforme, rather than herpes simplex infection. An important distinguishing feature of herpes in the mouth from aphthous ulcers (canker sores) is that herpes begins as a few clustered lesions on one part of the buccal mucosa, whereas aphthous ulcers begin as sores on widely separated parts of the buccal mucosa.

Primary Genital Herpes

In industrial countries, herpes simplex virus is the most common cause of genital ulcerations and accounts for 20 to 50 percent of ulcerative lesions in patients attending sexually transmitted disease clinics. It is estimated that 95 percent of episodes of primary genital herpes occur following sexual exposure to a sexual partner with active lesions. The usual period between sexual exposure to a person with active genital herpes and development of an acute episode is from 3 to 14 days. The outbreak begins with small grouped

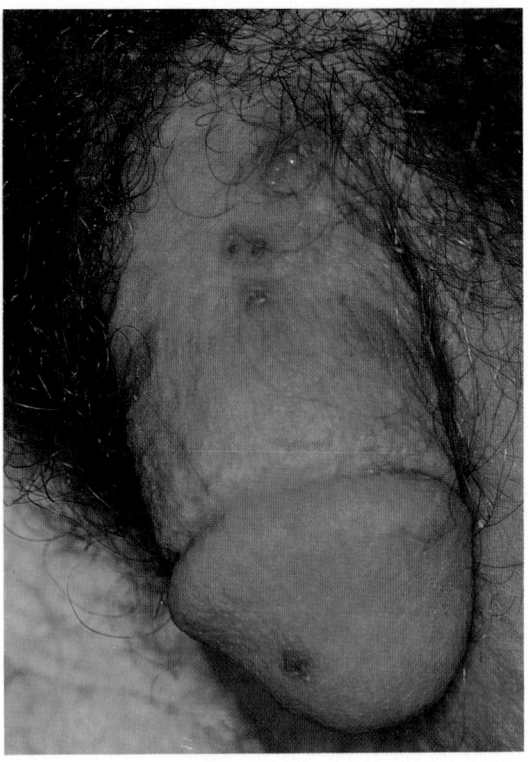

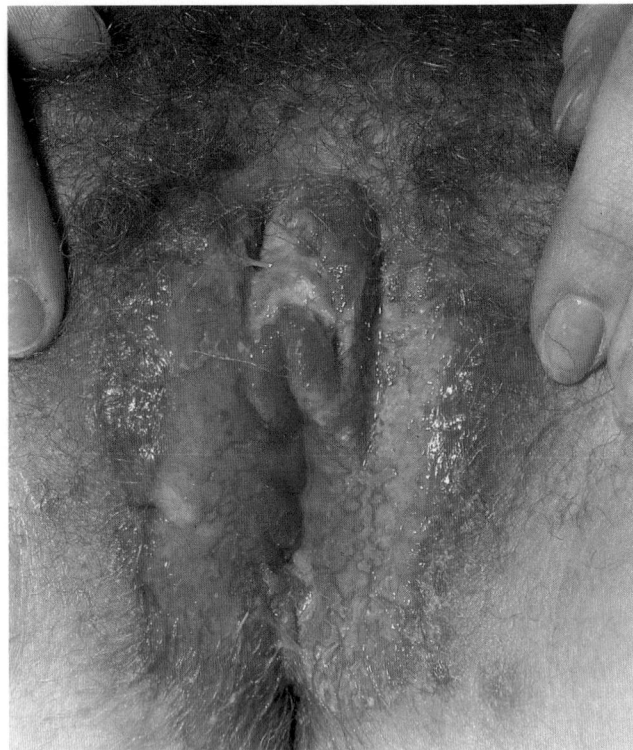

a

b

FIGURE 203-4 (*a*) Primary genital herpes simplex with vesicles. (*b*) Primary herpetic vulvitis.

vesicles (Fig. 203-4), which break and progress to ulcerative lesions in 2 to 4 days. Most patients present to the physician with ulcerative lesions. The first episode of genital herpes usually has multiple lesions, which are present bilaterally and coalesce to involve a larger surface. Recurrent genital herpes frequently presents as a single ulcer. Painful enlarged inguinal lymph nodes are common, and the nodes are usually tender on palpation, nonfixed, and slightly firm. About 35 percent of women and 13 percent of men with primary genital herpes will have an aseptic meningitis with fever, stiff neck, headache, photophobia, and pleocytosis in the spinal fluid.[11] The spinal fluid protein may be elevated to near 100 mg/dL, and the glucose may fall below 40 mg. Cells are mainly lymphocytes (200 to 1000 per mm^3). It is also clear that approximately 20 percent of patients with primary genital herpes will have painful difficulty on urination, which may require catheterization of the urinary tract for relief. This is essentially never present in recurrent genital herpes. The dominant local symptoms of primary genital herpes are pain, itching, dysuria, and vaginal and urethral discharge. The severity of these symptoms increases over the first 6 to 7 days of the illness and peaks at day 8 to 10. New lesions continue to form during the first week of illness in about 75 percent of patients. Both HSV-1 and HSV-2 cause primary genital herpes, with 80 percent being associated with isolation of HSV-2 from lesions. Both produce an identical clinical picture, but HSV-1–induced primary disease is associated with many fewer recurrences than when HSV-2 is isolated from the primary episode. Herpes simplex virus has been isolated from the pharynx of 11 percent of patients with primary genital herpes and in only 1 percent of those with recurrent disease.[11] Clinical signs of herpes simplex virus pharyngitis may be mild erythema or diffuse ulcerative and

exudative pharyngitis of the posterior pharynx. This may be associated with tender anterior cervical adenopathy and may mimic streptococcal pharyngitis.

The course of primary genital herpes may last 18 to 21 days, and virus shedding is present for about 11 days; this correlates with the time from onset of symptoms to the development of crusting. The differential diagnosis of other infections that cause genital ulcers and inguinal lymphadenopathy includes syphilis, chancroid, lymphogranuloma venereum, and granuloma inguinale.

Herpes Simplex Virus Cervicitis

Herpes simplex virus is a common etiology of cervical ulcerations. In women attending a sexually transmitted disease clinic, 88 percent of cervical ulcers were believed to be caused by HSV-2, based on culture and serologic evidence. During the first episode of HSV-2 genital infection, virus may be isolated from the cervix in 59 percent of women. In women with symptomatic recurrences, HSV-2 was isolated from the cervix in only 8 percent.[5]

Of women with cervical cultures positive for HSV-2, 50 percent showed evidence of cervical ulcers by speculum examination, whereas 65 percent had ulcerations seen by colposcopy. Cellular changes indicative of HSV infection were present on cervical cytology in 62 percent of women with positive HSV-2 cultures and in only 0.5 percent of those without positive cultures.[5]

Shedding of herpes simplex virus is found in patients both with and without symptoms of genital herpes infection. Of women with asymptomatic HSV-2 genital infections, 5 percent actively shed HSV-2, with about 40 percent of those having positive cervi-

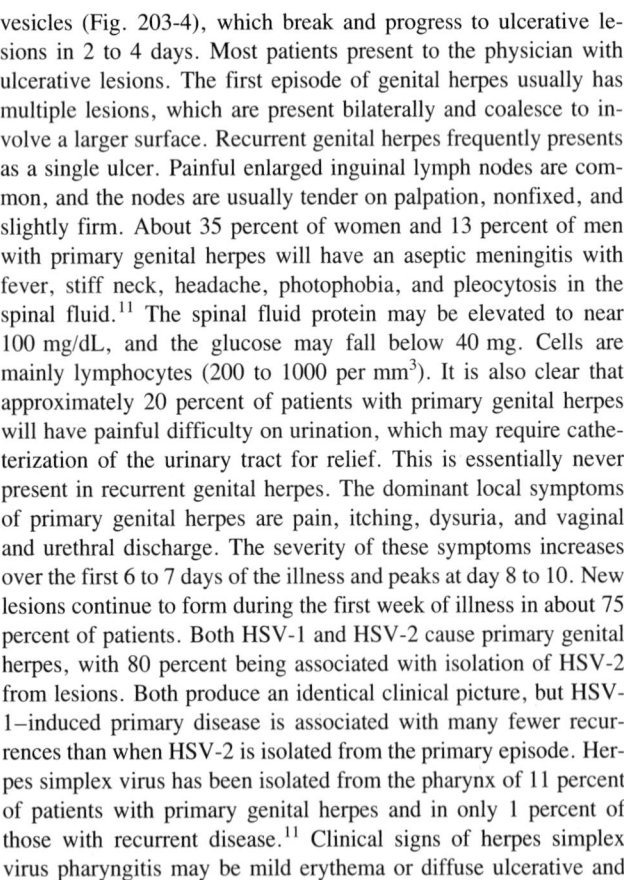

cal cultures in the absence of symptoms. Acute herpetic cervicitis may be the only manifestation of first-episode genital herpes simplex infection. In one study, 8 percent of women had mucopurulent cervicitis with positive cultures in the absence of external genital lesions.[12]

Because of the high prevalence of genital herpes infection and the amount of asymptomatic HSV-2 shedding, some authors have advocated routine screening for HSV-2 antibodies in high-risk populations to identify and counsel those with subclinical infections.[5]

Recurrent Genital Herpes

It is estimated that recurrent genital herpes infection affects about 25 million adults in the United States.[4] Following the primary infection, about 50 percent of men will have a recurrence in 4 months, whereas 50 percent of women will not have a recurrence until 8 months after the initial outbreak. Recurrent episodes may be more common in men following the initial episode, but the recurrent episodes appear to be more painful in women. The average number of recurrences is 3 or 4 per year, whereas perhaps 15 percent of patients with recurrent disease have 8 or more recurrences per year. The severity of symptoms, duration of symptoms, and duration of viral shedding are all much shorter in recurrent episodes than in primary disease. Virus can be cultured for 3 to 4 days, mean time for crusting is 4 to 5 days, and time to complete healing is 9 to 10 days in recurrent genital herpes. The mean lesion area is much smaller in recurrent disease, and new lesion formation is much less. New lesions occur for only 1 to 2 days in recurrent disease as compared to 5 to 6 days in primary disease. Symptoms of fever, aseptic meningitis, and headache are also much less frequent in recurrent disease. With recurrent disease, 40 to 50 percent of episodes have a prodrome consisting of tingling, burning, or dysesthesias that may occur 1 or 2 days to a few hours before the appearance of vesicles. This prodrome may be associated with buttock pain or pain radiating down the back of the thigh and mimicking sciatic pain. In patients with recurrent genital herpes, HSV-1 is isolated much less frequently than in primary episodes. The recurrence rate is definitely much greater with genital herpes associated with HSV-2.

A major cause of morbidity with recurrent genital herpes is the frequency of recurrences and the fear of transmission of disease to infants or to sexual partners. Patients should be instructed to avoid sexual intercourse when prodromal symptoms or lesions occur and to resume sexual activity only when lesions completely reepithelialize. Herpes can be isolated from lesions rarely at the crust stage of disease.

Herpes as a Risk Factor for HIV

Early in the AIDS epidemic, it was noted that genital ulcer disease was more common in HIV-seropositive individuals than in their HIV-negative counterparts. This was first described in East African female prostitutes[13] and men attending African sexually transmitted disease clinics,[14] where the most common etiologies of genital ulcer disease are chancroid and syphilis.

In North America and Europe, where the most common cause of genital ulcer disease is HSV-2, several studies have linked HSV-2 with exposure to HIV. In sexually transmitted disease clinics in Baltimore, HIV-positive men and women more often had a history of genital herpes and showed a higher seroprevalence rate of

HSV-2 but not HSV-1 than HIV-negative men and women.[15] In separate cohorts of gay men in San Francisco[16] and Seattle,[17] the presence of HSV-2 antibody was significantly associated with HIV seropositivity. In a Dutch cohort, a history of anogenital HSV infection was more predictive of HIV seroconversion than other sexually transmitted diseases.[18]

Sexual transmission of HIV, both homosexual and heterosexual, is facilitated by genital ulcer disease by the disruption of protective epithelial or mucosal barriers and by the presence of activated T lymphocytes at ulcer bases, which likely serve as reservoirs of virus. In fact, HIV has been cultured from the bases of genital ulcers of both men and women in Africa.[19] Because genital HSV infection is common and may have high rates of recurrence, it may serve as a major cofactor in the sexual acquisition and transmission of HIV in the developed world. This underscores the benefits of preventive ''safe sex'' measures and early antiviral treatment, which may promote ulcer healing, decrease infectivity, and prevent subsequent recurrences. Clearly, controlling genital ulcer disease, particularly herpes, is an integral part of AIDS prevention efforts.

Herpes Infection in the Immunocompromised Patient

Herpes infections are an important cause of morbidity and mortality in immunocompromised patients. Patients with defects in cellular immunity from hematologic malignancies and HIV infection and those receiving immunosuppressive agents, such as corticosteroids, or who have undergone organ transplants are particularly susceptible. Immunocompromised patients infected with herpes simplex may have self-limited, localized disease that varies little from that seen in patients with normal immunity. However, depending on the degree of immunosuppression—either the activity of the underlying disease or the length of immunosuppressive therapy—herpes infection may recur more frequently and have a more severe and prolonged course. Patients may develop deep, progressive ulcerations of mucocutaneous areas of the face, mouth, or anogenital areas (Fig. 203-5). Lesions may coalesce, becoming much larger than in patients with normal immune function. Lesions may also persist for weeks to months, with continuous shedding of isolable

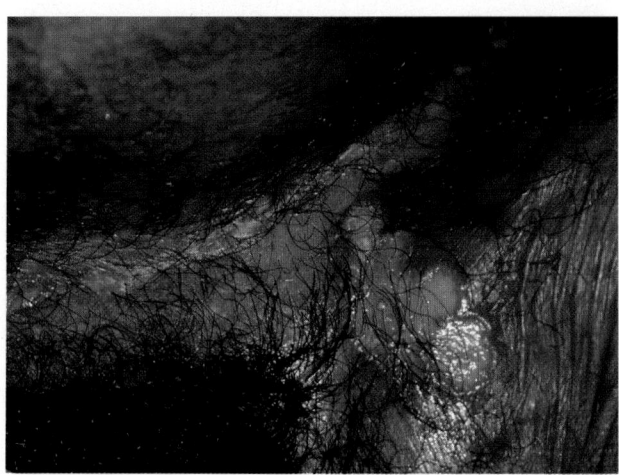

FIGURE 203-5 Chronic herpeitic ulcer. A 32-year-old male presented with these ulcers of 7-weeks duration. HIV serology was positive.

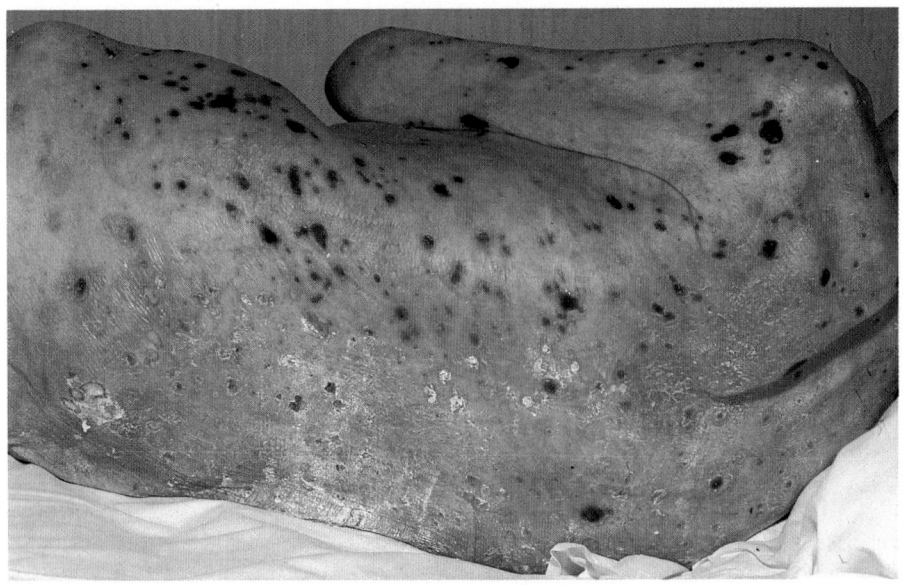

FIGURE 203-6　Disseminated herpes simplex infection. (*a*) generalized vesicles and pustules with hemorrhage and necrosis. (*b*) Generalized vesicles, pustules, erosions, and ulcerations.

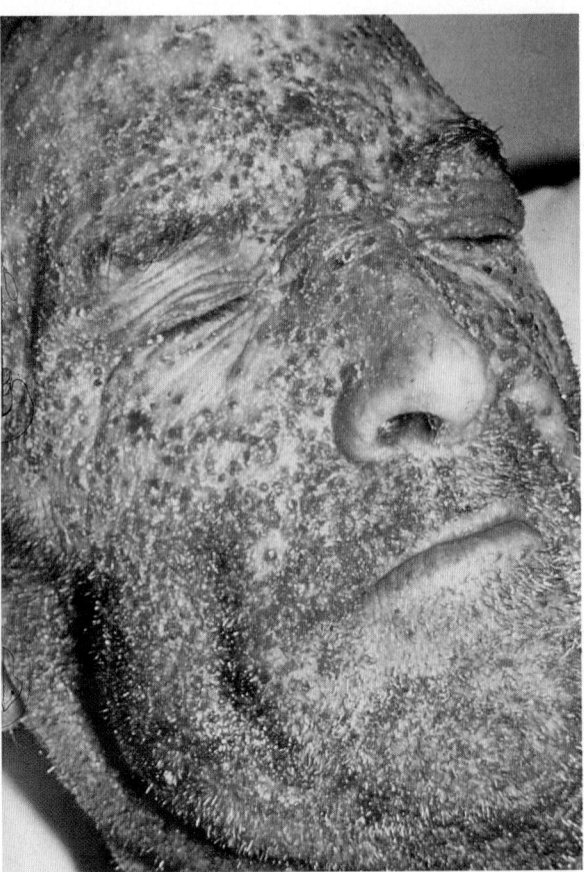

virus. The size and duration of such lesions may also predispose to bacterial or fungal superinfection. Due to the large amount of virus present, patients treated with antiviral agents may be particularly prone to develop resistant virus.

Oral mucosal lesions can produce an extensive painful stomatitis in immunocompromised patients. The differential diagnosis of oral ulcers in such patients includes herpes simplex, cytomegalovi-rus (CMV), *Candida, Histoplasma,* or primary HIV infection, and chemotherapy or allergic drug reactions. Superficial oral lesions may lead to herpes pharyngitis, esophagitis, or pneumonitis,[20] often after passage of an endotracheal or nasogastric tube. Recurrent orofacial or genital lesions may lead to viremia with subsequent seeding of viscera, including the esophagus, lungs, and liver (Fig. 203-6).

In the presence of a positive HIV serology, definitive evidence of herpes simplex infection causing a mucocutaneous ulcer that persists longer than 1 month, or bronchitis, pneumonitis, or esophagitis of any duration indicates the diagnosis of AIDS (in a patient older than 1 month).[21]

Antiviral therapy can be dramatically effective in reducing morbidity in these patients, both with early recognition and treatment of disease and in the wider use of prophylactic and suppressive therapy.

Herpes Whitlow

The term *herpetic whitlow* applies to a primary or recurrent herpes simplex infection of the fingers or hands. The disease is a common occupational hazard for medical and dental personnel, who work in and around the mouths of patients shedding the virus. Herpetic whitlow may also complicate recurrent genital herpes infections.[22]

Inoculation may occur on the fingers or hands in areas of abraded or broken skin. Following inoculation, primary infection lasts 2 to 6 weeks and is characterized by painful vesicles (Fig. 203-7), erythema, and edema, often accompanied by erythematous streaking of the forearm and tender axillary lymphadenopathy. Although the process may mimic bacterial infection, there is no evidence of pus formation.

The appearance of vesicles with subsequent progression to ulcers at the margin of the skin lesion is highly suggestive of herpetic whitlow. Confirmation by a positive Tzanck smear and viral culture will establish the diagnosis. The lesions resolve spontaneously; however, as with other sites of herpes infection, recurrences are common.

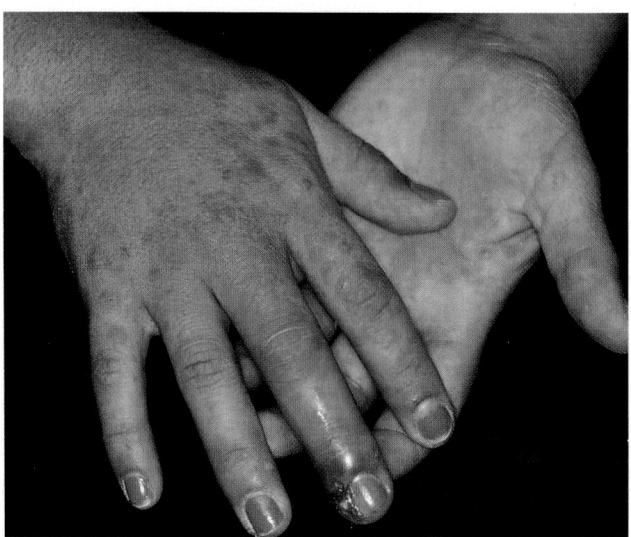

FIGURE 203-7 Herpetic whitlow of the middle finger with associated erythema multiforme in a nurse's aide.

Prevention of contact with saliva and active vesicles or ulcers is an important goal for health care workers. Routine use of latex gloves as part of universal blood and body fluid precautions will likely also reduce the risk of HSV transmission.

Although no controlled studies have been performed, there is anecdotal evidence that acyclovir is successful in the acute treatment of herpetic whitlow and may help to decrease the frequency of recurrences of disease when used prophylactically.[23,24] The latter use may be especially valuable for health care workers who otherwise might need to limit patient care responsibilities during outbreaks. A recent report described the case of a 22-year-old man with AIDS and severe herpetic whitlow of his left thumb.[25] The lesion improved during a course of ganciclovir (for presumed CMV pneumonia) then worsened despite lengthy courses of oral and intravenous acyclovir. HSV isolated from the lesion was found to be highly resistant to acyclovir and ganciclovir.

Herpes Gladiatorum

Cases of cutaneous and ocular infections with HSV-1 have occurred among wrestlers and rugby players and have been labeled *herpes gladiatorum*.[26,27] Surveys of high school and college athletic trainers suggest herpes infection among wrestlers is endemic.[28] A recent investigation of an outbreak among high school wrestlers attending a training camp supported direct skin-to-skin contact as the primary mode of transmission;[29] nearly half of the affected wrestlers reported an abrasion or break in the skin at the site of subsequent infection. The sites of skin lesions were markedly different from typical orolabial HSV-1 infections and included the head (73 percent), trunk (28 percent), and extremities (47 percent). The attack rate among wrestlers in the same practice groups was as high as 67 percent. Oropharyngeal swabs for HSV-1 culture from affected wrestlers failed to grow HSV-1 in any of those tested, suggesting that saliva was not a major source of transmission. Early identification of skin lesions and the exclusion of infected wrestlers is recommended to decrease the incidence of transmission of herpes gladiatorum.

Herpetic Keratoconjunctivitis

Herpes simplex virus infection of the eye can cause recurrent erosions of the conjunctiva and cornea. The initial phase of the ophthalmologic disease is a superficial corneal ulcer. This is usually specifically diagnosed by a slit-lamp examination. With repeated recurrences, deeper ulcers develop and stromal keratitis occurs. With each episode, stromal scarring may progress and blindness may develop. Herpes simplex keratitis is now regarded as the leading cause of infectious blindness in the United States. The differential diagnosis of herpetic keratoconjunctivitis includes herpes zoster, adenovirus infection, vaccinia, and chlamydial conjunctivitis. Early treatment with topical antiviral drugs such as vidarabine or trifluorothymidine can enhance healing and minimize stromal scarring.

Recurrent Lumbosacral Herpes Simplex

Recurrent cutaneous herpetic lesions on the low back and buttocks can occur in the absence of actual genital lesions. Recurrent outbreaks of "buttock herpes" usually occur in men and women over the age of 40 and comprise a small percentage—usually only 10 percent of herpes outbreaks in the pelvic and genital area. The lesions are frequently triggered by stress, fatigue, or the onset of the menstrual cycle. The lesions usually occur on one side of the buttocks or another, begin as clusters on an erythematous base (Fig. 203-8), and heal with hyperpigmentation and minimal scarring. Recurrences can develop on a periodic basis and go on for several years. A central feature of recurrent lumbosacral herpes simplex is the prodrome associated with deep pelvic aching for 1 to 3 days before the cutaneous lesions appear. Some patients may experience pain going down the back of the leg and mimicking "sciatic pain." Patients have even undergone myelograms in evaluation of this pain. The differential diagnosis of lumbosacral herpes simplex infection must include low back strain, herniated lumbosacral disk, impetigo, and herpes zoster.

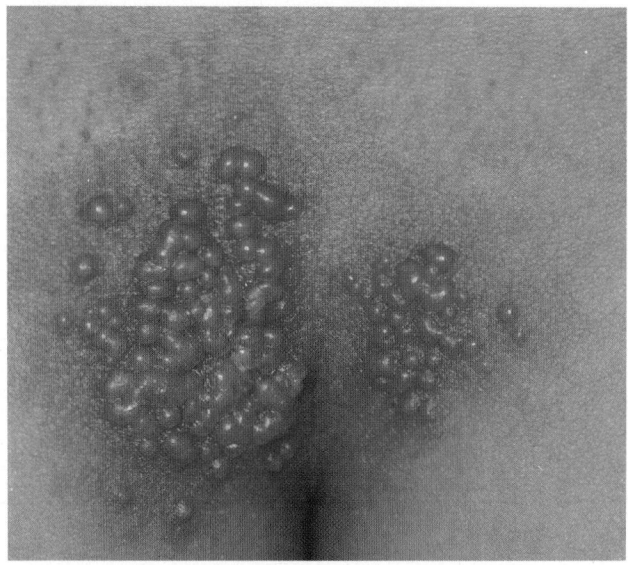

FIGURE 203-8 Recurrent lumbosacral herpes simplex.

Recurrent Herpes Simplex and Erythema Multiforme

In a subset of patients, the development of recurrent herpes simplex infection may be followed in 7 to 10 days by the development of erythema multiforme. The presentation may vary from typical erythematous papules (see Fig. 203-7) evolving into target lesions on the extremities to painful ulcerations of the oral, genital, or conjunctival mucosa. Recurrent lesions may occur as infrequently as once a year or may persist nearly continuously. Spontaneous improvement occurs over about 5 years.

Anecdotal reports suggest that acyclovir may be successful both in aborting attacks of erythema multiforme when given in the prodromal period[30] and in preventing recurrences when given continuously.[31,32] These results suggest that herpes simplex antigens are playing a crucial role in the development of erythema multiforme.

Eczema Herpeticum

Patients with preexisting skin disorders such as atopic dermatitis and Darier's disease may develop widespread cutaneous infections with herpes simplex virus. Eczema herpeticum (Fig. 203-9) begins as clusters of umbilicated vesicles in areas where the skin has been previously abnormal. The eruption spreads widely over a period of 7 to 10 days and may be associated with fever, malaise, and lymphadenopathy. The vesicular lesions coalesce into large erosions, which frequently become secondarily infected with bacteria. The primary episode of eczema herpeticum will run its usual course and heal in 2 to 6 weeks. Patients with chronic skin damage may have recurrent episodes that are milder and not associated with systemic symptoms. The differential diagnosis of eczema herpeticum includes widespread impetigo and a Kaposi's varicelliform eruption caused by vaccinia virus.

Herpes Simplex Encephalitis

Herpes simplex virus is the most common cause of sporadic encephalitis in the developed world. The virus spreads along neural pathways from sites of primary or recurrent herpes infections causing a necrotizing, hemorrhagic encephalitis, most often of the temporal lobes. It affects men and women of all ages and may occur during all seasons of the year.

A concurrent or prior diagnosis of orofacial or genital herpes simplex infection does not predict the likelihood of developing herpes encephalitis. The disease can occur in healthy adults and children without evidence of previous herpes simplex infection, although 70 percent of cases occur in patients with neutralizing antibody for herpes simplex.[33]

The onset of disease may be sudden with symptoms of fever, headache, and confusion or temporal lobe signs such as olfactory hallucinations or behavioral changes. The diagnosis is suggested by the clinical presentation, a cerebrospinal fluid (CSF) pleocytosis and elevated protein, and a temporal lobe focus of electroencephalogram signals or focal enhancement on computed tomography or magnetic resonance imaging scans.

Brain biopsy with appropriate histology and cultures remains the definitive way to make the diagnosis. The virus will grow from infected tissue in 95 percent of cases within 5 days. Spinal fluid culture is usually negative for HSV even when tissue culture is positive. Preliminary studies suggest that the use of the polymerase chain reaction for detection of herpes simplex DNA in the CSF may offer an early diagnostic advantage.[34] Untreated, herpes simplex encephalitis has greater than 70 percent mortality. Because antiviral therapy has dramatically altered the course of the disease, the institution of empiric antiviral treatment while addressing diagnostic procedure options has been recommended.[35]

Caution is advised, however, as one study demonstrated only 45 percent of patients thought to have HSV encephalitis who went

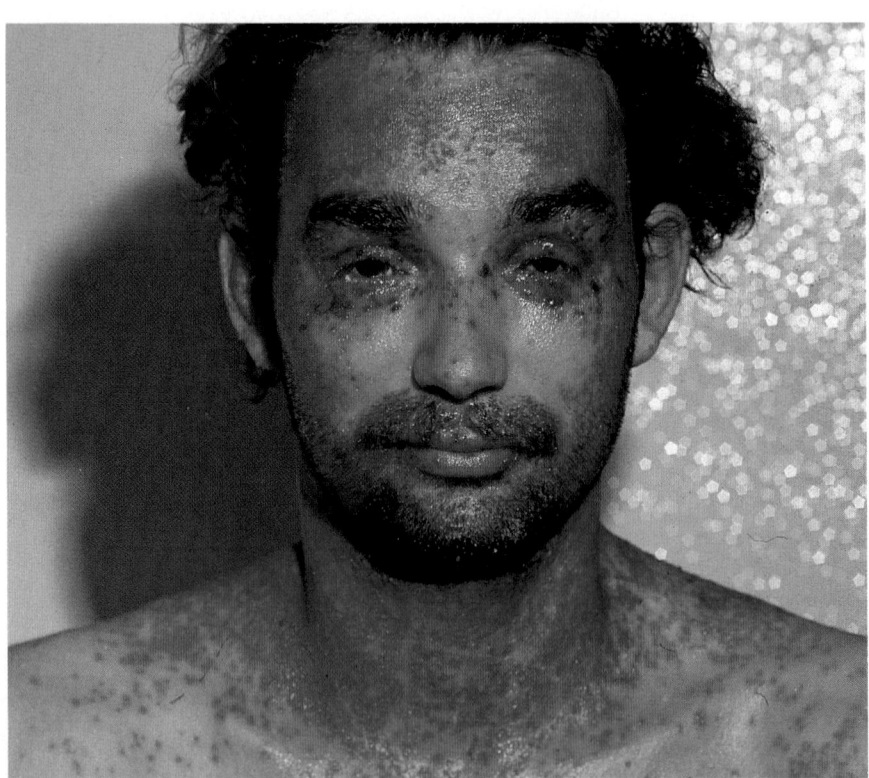

FIGURE 203-9 Eczema herpeticum in areas of atopic dermatitis.

to brain biopsy had evidence of HSV infection, whereas another 22 percent of patients had diagnoses other than HSV, including 9 percent with other treatable diseases (including bacterial, mycobacterial, rickettsial, fungal, and malignant processes).[36]

Diagnosis

Viral Culture

The most reliable way to make a precise diagnosis of herpes simplex infection is to grow the virus from skin lesions. The virus obtained from skin lesions can be quantitated by plaque titration, typed, and its sensitivity to antiviral agents determined. When compatible skin lesions are present and viral culture obtained from skin lesions yields herpes simplex virus, this essentially establishes the diagnosis. In the setting of characteristic lesions on the lip-skin junction that progress from papule to vesicle to erosion or ulcer to crusting state, the vast majority of isolates will be HSV. In our clinical trials, lesions which appear to be due to herpes will produce positive virus on culture about 85 to 90 percent of the time.[10] The percent of positive viral cultures obtained from clinical lesions is quite variable but in most large series this has varied between 60 and 90 percent. All other current methods of making a specific viral diagnosis of herpes simplex–induced skin lesions are less sensitive than viral culture.

Tzanck Preparation

A valuable clinical approach to making a rapid diagnosis of herpes virus infection relies on taking a smear of cells from the base of the skin lesion, spreading the cells on a glass slide, and staining with Wright's or Giemsa's stain to look for multinucleated giant cells in a Tzanck preparation. Both HSV and varicella zoster virus infection will result in multinucleated giant cells and a positive Tzanck smear. With experience, a clinician can reliably distinguish multinucleated giant cells from cellular debris, crushed cells, and artifacts. In the case of genital herpes, multinucleated giant cells can also be identified on cytologic examination of Papanicolaou smears. A comparison of the yield of positive cultures for HSV with the appearance of multinucleated giant cells obtained from clinical specimens of genital herpes in women revealed that about 60 percent of specimens that grew HSV also possessed multinucleated giant cells on cytologic examination. In another study of biopsy-proved HSV encephalitis, examination of brain tissue by histopathology, immunofluorescence, and electron microscopy demonstrated evidence of HSV infection in 56, 70, and 45 percent, respectively, of cases where herpes simplex virus was cultured from brain tissue.[33] This study also indicated that false-positive results were obtained in 14, 9, and 2 percent of HSV-negative specimens of brain biopsies by histopathology, immunofluorescence, and electron microscopy, respectively. Taken together, these studies document the importance of obtaining a positive culture for HSV in establishing a precise diagnosis.

Monoclonal Antibodies

The use of specific monoclonal antibodies directed against HSV-1 and HSV-2 proteins is currently established as a means of making a

rapid and precise viral diagnosis of facial-oral HSV infection and genital herpes simplex. In a study employing monoclonal antibodies to confirm HSV in tissue cultures by immunofluorescence, the monoclonal antibodies for HSV-1 and HSV-2 have proved to be sensitive and specific[37] with an 88 percent correlation with tissue culture results. The use of monoclonal antibodies has considerable utility in making rapid precise viral diagnosis of herpes infections.

Treatment of Herpes Simplex Infection

Acyclovir (9-[2-hydroxyethoxy-methyl]-guanine) is the prototype of a class of antiviral drugs that employ the viral-specific thymidine kinase (TK) enzyme to add a phosphate group to the guanosine analogue (Fig. 203-10). The guanosine analogue acyclovir, utilizes the viral TK enzyme to form the acyclovir monophosphate. Cellular guanyldylate kinase and guanosine diphosphate kinase then form acyclovir triphosphate, a potent inhibitor of viral DNA polymerase. Acyclovir triphosphate is incorporated as the terminal base in an elongating strand of DNA and functions as a chain terminator to inhibit chain elongation.[38] Acyclovir triphosphate also appears to form an irreversible bond between elongating DNA and viral DNA polymerase, leading to inactivation of the DNA polymerase.[39] This has been described as an example of how acyclovir triphosphate also acts as a competitive inhibitor of guanosine triphosphate on viral DNA polymerase function. In addition to requiring viral (TK) for activation and inhibition of viral DNA polymerase at a 30-fold less concentration of acyclovir triphosphate than is required to inhibit cellular polymerase functions, acyclovir is taken up preferentially in cells that express a viral TK activity. This third area of specificity, decreased uptake of acyclovir by uninfected cells, probably accounts for the remarkable lack of toxicity associated with high doses of acyclovir.

In carefully randomized placebo-controlled trials, acyclovir is effective in the treatment of mucocutaneous herpes simplex infections.

In addition, other drugs are being developed for treatment of HSV infections. These include foscarnet, or phosphonoformic acid, which is a direct inhibitor of the viral DNA polymerase and is effective in the treatment of acyclovir-resistant herpes simplex. Trifluorothymidine, which is phosphorylated by the cellular TK, is an approved drug for HSV keratitis and may be active as a topical

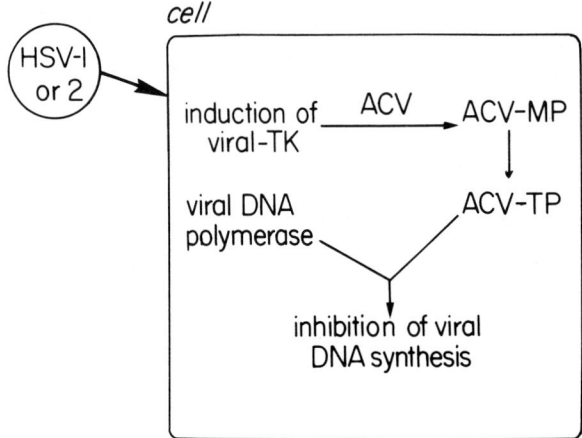

FIGURE 203-10   Acyclovir diagram.

treatment for mucocutaneous acyclovir-resistant HSV infection. Ganciclovir, primarily active against CMV infection, also has good antiviral activity against HSV. Adenine-arabinoside, which can be effective therapy against HSV encephalitis, has no activity in the treatment of mucocutaneous infections caused by HSV.

Treatment of Facial-Oral Herpes

Therapy of recurrent facial-oral herpes simplex infection with a topical 5% ointment of acyclovir polyenthylene glycol in normal patients has revealed that the early application of the ointment would result in a significant antiviral effect with the virus being eradicated more rapidly from the skin of patients treated in the first 8 h of clinical occurrence of facial-oral HSV.[40] This antiviral effect was not associated with any clinical benefit, and treated cold sores did not heal more quickly nor did pain and discomfort resolve more rapidly. Recurrence rate of facial oral herpes was not affected by acyclovir treatment. In another study in fewer patients employing acyclovir 5% ointment in modified aqueous cream, an increased rate of healing of cold sores was noted in patients treated with acyclovir.[41]

Treatment of Genital Herpes

In primary genital herpes, however, topical acyclovir or oral acyclovir therapy is associated with an antiviral effect and also more rapid healing. Topical acyclovir in a 5% ointment was applied four times a day for 7 days. Topical acyclovir reduced viral shedding from 7.0 days to 4.1 days, and time to complete crusting was reduced from 10.5 to 7.1 days.[42] Intravenous and oral acyclovir treatment of primary and initial genital herpes shortened median healing time by about 50 percent. Treatment with oral acyclovir, 200 mg, five times daily for 10 days, decreased median duration of viral shedding from 9 to 2 days, time for healing from 16 to 12 days, duration of pain from 7 to 5 days, and the number of patients forming new lesions after 48 h in therapy was decreased from 62 to 18 percent.[43] Other studies with patients having true primary disease had similar results. In nonprimary initial disease, the symptoms are intermediate in severity between primary and recurrent disease. Oral acyclovir is probably effective in treatment of nonprimary disease, but sufficient numbers of these patients have not been studied to document efficacy. In all of the studies employing oral acyclovir therapy for 10 days, there was no effect noted in the proportion of patients who developed recurrent disease episodes nor in the frequency of these episodes. When patients with severe initial cases of genital herpes have an inability to urinate and require urinary catheterization or have severe meningitis with systemic symptoms, they may require hospitalization and treatment with intravenous acyclovir. Oral acyclovir will be the therapy of choice, however, for most patients with initial disease. Oral acyclovir will replace the less effective topical acyclovir therapy for this indication.

Suppression of Recurrent Disease

In a large double-blind trial comprising 143 patients with a mean number of 1.07 recurrences of genital herpes per month, placebo was compared with oral acyclovir (200 mg) five times daily and oral acyclovir twice daily.[44] Patients received the therapy for 4 months, and 94 percent of the placebo patients experienced recur-

rences during this period compared to 29 percent of those treated with acyclovir five times daily and 35 percent of those treated with acyclovir twice daily. The recurrences while patients were taking acyclovir were less frequent and of a shorter duration than among placebo recipients, but recurrence rates returned to pretreatment rates once medication was discontinued. In another study, patients taking three or four capsules daily experienced a similar improvement.[45] In the study by Straus et al., three patients who developed recurrences while taking acyclovir had acyclovir-resistant HSV isolated from episodes that developed while they were taking the drug.[45]

These episodes were described as ''breakthrough recurrences.'' No other studies in patients with a normal immune system have been able to document the occurrence of acyclovir-resistant HSV. To date, acyclovir-resistant HSV has been detected only in patients with a compromised immune system.

Prolonged, continuous oral acyclovir treatment of normal patients with frequently recurring genital HSV infection has been successful in suppressing recurrences. A 3-year study of patients with six recurrences per year revealed that 400 mg of acyclovir orally twice per day markedly suppressed recurrent episodes.[46] The annual recurrence rate dropped from more than 12 recurrences per year at baseline to one recurrence in the third year on suppressive therapy. No significant toxic effects were observed. It was concluded that daily suppressive acyclovir therapy was effective and well tolerated. The study of long-term oral acyclovir suppression is now in the eighth year, and the medication appears to be remarkably safe. The current recommendation of the U.S. Food and Drug Administration suggests the use of oral acyclovir for 1 year in patients with six or more recurrences per year.

Treatment of Recurrent Genital Herpes

The treatment of recurrent genital herpes with acyclovir in any form has been only of limited success. Topical acyclovir treatment did not facilitate healing in women with recurrent disease, but slight beneficial effects were observed in pain reduction and healing in men. Shortened time of virus shedding was observed with topical acyclovir therapy. Due to the slight clinical benefit of acyclovir therapy in recurrent genital herpes, topical treatment of recurrent genital herpes is not justified. In a large multicenter controlled trial, oral acyclovir treatment of recurrent genital herpes was evaluated by comparing patient-initiated therapy with therapy initiated by a physician or placebo.[47] Oral acyclovir capsules (200 mg) were taken five times daily, for 5 days. When patients had acyclovir at home and initiated therapy at the onset of a prodrome or at the first sign of lesions, therapy was more effective than when it was initiated by a physician within 48 h of the onset of symptoms. The patient-initiated treatment reduced viral shedding from 3.9 days, in placebo-treated cases, to 2.1 days. Time to healing was reduced from 6.5 days, in placebo-treated cases, to 5.5 days with patient-initiated treatment. The percent of patients forming new lesions was 22 percent with placebo treatment, and this was reduced to 7 percent in the patient-initiated treatment. When patients went to a physician and initiated therapy within 48 h of the onset of lesions, new lesion formation was reduced from 22 to 16 percent. The treatment of recurrent episodes with oral acyclovir offers marginal clinical benefit, but the benefit is superior to that obtained with topical acyclovir. Patients with severe recurrent episodes who initiate therapy at the first sign of a recurrence will derive the greatest benefit. Treatment with acyclovir has no effect on subsequent recurrence rate.

Treatment of Herpes Infections in the Immunosuppressed Patient

In immunocompromised patients with severe herpes simplex infections, the need for effective antiviral therapy is greatest. In these immunocompromised patients acyclovir therapy for mucocutaneous herpes simplex infection can be lifesaving or dramatically successful. In these patients, healing of mucocutaneous herpes simplex infection occurs more quickly in those treated with acyclovir because inhibition of HSV replication reduces tissue destruction. In a randomized double-blind trial of intravenous acyclovir for culture-proved herpes simplex infection that followed bone marrow transplantation, 13 of 17 patients who received acyclovir (750 mg per square meter per day) for 7 days had a therapeutic response.[48] Only 2 of 17 placebo-treated patients improved. Intravenous acyclovir produced a shorter duration of positive cultures, shortened duration of pain, and hastened healing. These controlled trials have been performed in heart transplant patients and in other immunosuppressed patients. The accumulated data on intravenous acyclovir in immunocompromised patients with mucocutaneous herpes simplex infection indicate that acyclovir shortens the period of viral shedding, shortens the time interval to scabbing and healing, and shortens the duration of pain. On termination of acyclovir, reactivation of herpes simplex infection usually occurs. Intravenous and oral acyclovir are useful in preventing mucocutaneous herpes simplex infection in immunocompromised patients. A double-blind placebo-controlled trial of intravenous acyclovir in bone marrow transplant recipients indicated that 10 patients who were seropositive for antiherpes antibody and who received acyclovir in a dose of 250 mg per square meter every 8 h for 18 days starting at 3 days before transplantation did not develop herpes infection.[49] Virus-positive lesions developed in 7 of 10 patients who received placebo treatment. When acyclovir treatment was discontinued, however, herpes infection did develop. Oral acyclovir treatment has been found to be effective in preventing reactivation of HSV infections following bone marrow transplantation and in other immunosuppressed patients. Topical acyclovir therapy, however, has not been effective in suppressing recurrence in normal or immunosuppressed patients. In immunocompromised patients, oral acyclovir is more effective than topical acyclovir in treatment of mucocutaneous herpes infections, but severe or life-threatening infections caused by HSV should be treated with intravenous acyclovir. A comparison of the effects of vidarabine and acyclovir in the treatment of a severe mucocutaneous infection caused by HSV in the immunocompromised patient indicates that vidarabine was not very successful. Acyclovir is also much more soluble than vidarabine, and less fluid volume is required for treatment. Vidarabine is also more inhibitory for proliferating granulocytes and bone marrow cells than is acyclovir. At doses of 30 mg/kg per day, adenine-arabinoside therapy will produce a megaloblastic anemia in patients. From the standpoint of efficacy and safety, acyclovir is the preferred therapy for mucocutaneous herpes simplex infections in immunocompromised patients.

Treatment of Herpes Simplex Encephalitis

Herpes simplex virus is the most common cause of sporadic nonepidemic encephalitis. The disease commonly involves the temporoparietal lobes in a hemorrhagic necrosis, and without treatment has a mortality of greater than 70 percent. In a double-blind, placebo-controlled trial in 1977, treatment of biopsy-proved herpes encephalitis with adenine-arabinoside reduced the mortality from 70 percent in the placebo group to 44 percent survival at 6 months after treatment.[50] In a follow-up study, the mortality was reduced to 39 percent, and one-third of patients who survived had a return to normal function. The level of consciousness and age had the greatest impact on outcome. Patients under 30 years of age, and only lethargic at the beginning of therapy, had the highest recovery. Relapses after vidarabine treatment have occurred.[51]

A comparison of acyclovir at 30 mg/kg per day and vidarabine (15 mg/kg per day) for 10 days as treatment for biopsy-proved herpes encephalitis was carried out by the NIAID (National Institute of Allergy and Infectious Disease) collaborative antiviral study group of the National Institutes of Health, and acyclovir was clearly superior. The mortality of the acyclovir-treated group was 28 percent compared with 54 percent for vidarabine-treated patients. At 6 months after treatment, 38 percent of acyclovir patients were functioning normally and only 14 percent of vidarabine-treated patients were normal.[52] This study concluded that acyclovir is the preferred treatment for biopsy-proved herpes encephalitis. In another study of 53 patients where there was not uniformity of diagnosis for herpes simplex encephalitis, adenine-arabinosine therapy was associated with a mortality of 50 percent and acyclovir mortality at 6 months was 19 percent.[53]

Over two-thirds of the acyclovir survivors returned to normal function. Relapses after acyclovir therapy have also been documented.[54] Both of these studies had remarkably similar outcomes in favor of acyclovir as the preferred treatment for herpes encephalitis.

Treatment of Acyclovir-Resistant Herpes Simplex Infection

The incidence of acyclovir-resistant mucocutaneous HSV infection in immunocompromised patients, especially in AIDS patients, is being increasingly recognized. In the setting of HIV disease or severe immunosuppression, HSV is able to replicate to a high titer. The high replication role in the presence of a highly selective antiviral drug such as acyclovir permits the selection of drug-resistant mutants.[55] Acyclovir is activated by the viral TK enzyme to produce acyclovir triphosphate, a potent inhibitor of the viral DNA polymerase, and acyclovir is the prototype of effective antiviral agents employing the viral TK for activation. In AIDS patients who develop large mucocutaneous erosions due to acyclovir-resistant HSV, the mechanism of resistance is due to TK-deficient mutants of HSV. The mutant strains of HSV do not effectively phosphorylate acyclovir, and there is no inhibition of HSV replication. In bone marrow transplant recipients or leukemia patients receiving antiviral therapy, the majority of acyclovir-resistant mutants are also due to TK-deficient mutants. In this setting, however, resistance due to an altered viral DNA polymerase or an altered TK enzyme that does not phosphorylate acyclovir has also been reported.[56] In a series of 12 patients with AIDS who developed acyclovir-resistant HSV infection and large mucocutaneous lesions in spite of oral and intravenous acyclovir, all the lesions were due to TK-deficient virus.[57] Over half of the TK-deficient mutants were able to establish a latent ganglion infection, and one of the viral isolates produced cerebral infection and death in a murine model following intranasal inoculation.

An effective alternative therapy for acyclovir-resistant HSV has been developed. Foscarnet, or phosphonoformic acid, inhibits viral DNA polymerase activity directly and is an effective agent against TK-deficient HSV. In a controlled clinical trial of foscarnet compared with adenine-arabinoside in AIDS patients with acyclovir-resistant mucocutaneous HSV infection, foscarnet was associated with rapid healing and clearing of virus from infected skin lesions.[58] This trial clearly established that mucocutaneous infections with acyclovir-resistant HSV were clinically significant and could be effectively treated with alternative therapy.

Foscarnet is administered intravenously at a dose of 40 mg/kg twice a day for 14 days in patients with previous acyclovir-resistant HSV infection or large mucocutaneous lesions that fail to heal with 10 days of acyclovir. The main side effects of foscarnet are renal failure, hypocalcemia, and seizures. Renal function needs to be carefully monitored in these patients to avoid serious nephrotoxicity. Foscarnet is also effective against ganciclovir-resistant CMV and the drug will also inhibit HIV-1.

Clinical Significance of Acyclovir-Resistant Herpes Simplex Virus

The continuing emergence of HSV infection that exhibits resistance to acyclovir in immunocompromised patients is a clinically significant problem.[59] The lesions caused by these drug-resistant viruses can progress and involve a large area of skin and mucosa. The clearest evidence that these infections are clinically significant was obtained from a randomized clinical trial when acyclovir-resistant HSV infections were treated with either foscarnet or vidarabine.[58] The foscarnet-treated patients showed a dramatic healing in spite of failure of their lesions to resolve after several months of oral and intravenous acyclovir treatment. This intervention study clearly showed that acyclovir-resistant HSV caused clinically important mucocutaneous lesions that healed within 2 weeks of receiving therapy with an antiviral drug that worked by an alternative mechanism on the viral DNA polymerase. In a pediatric tertiary-care hospital, it was estimated that about 10 percent of herpes simplex viral isolates obtained during 1 year showed resistance to acyclovir, and all of these isolates were from clinically important infections.[60] In patients with AIDS, all of the acyclovir-resistant HSV mutants have been TK-deficient mutants. In bone marrow transplant recipients and in patients with leukemia, acyclovir-resistant mutant viruses have been obtained that possess an altered TK or an altered viral DNA polymerase that is not inhibited by acyclovir triphosphate. Significant clinical disease has been attributed to acyclovir-resistant TK-deficient mutants, including fatal HSV-2 meningitis, progressive HSV-1 pneumonia, and progressive HSV-1 disease in newborn infants.[59] Transmission of acyclovir-resistant HSV has not been documented. With increasing use of antiviral therapy in immunocompromised patients, it is likely that increasing cases of clinically important acyclovir-resistant infection will be observed.

References

1. Gibson JJ et al: A cross-sectional study of herpes simplex virus types 1 and 2 in college students: Occurrence and determinants of infection. *J Infect Dis* **162**:306, 1990
2. Nahmias AJ et al: Sero-epidemiological and sociological patterns of herpes simplex virus infection in the world. *Scand J Infect Dis* **69**(suppl):19, 1990
3. Becker TM et al: Genital herpes infections in private practice in the United States 1966 to 1981. *JAMA* **253**:1601, 1985
4. Johnson RE et al: A seroepidemiologic study of the prevalence of herpes simplex virus type 2 infection in the United States. *N Engl J Med* **321**:7, 1989

5. Koutsky LA et al: Underdiagnosis of genital herpes by current clinical and viral-isolation procedures. *N Engl J Med* **326**:1533, 1992
6. Mertz GJ et al: Risk factors for the sexual transmission of genital herpes. *Ann Intern Med* **116**:197, 1992
7. Glezen WP et al: Acute respiratory disease of university students with special reference to the etiologic role of *Herpes-virus hominis*. *Am J Epidemiol* **101**:111, 1975
8. Embil JA et al: Prevalence of recurrent herpes labialis and aphthous ulcers among young adults on six continents. *Can Med Assoc J* **113**:627, 1975
9. Young SK et al: A clinical study for the control of facial mucocutaneous herpes virus infections. I. Characterization of natural history in a professional school population. *Oral Surg* **41**:498, 1976
10. Bader C et al: The natural history of recurrent facial-oral infection with herpes simplex virus. *J Infect Dis* **138**:897, 1978
11. Corey L et al: Genital herpes simplex virus infections: Clinical manifestations, course and complications. *Ann Intern Med* **98**:958, 1983
12. Jeansson SS, Molin L: On the occurrence of genital herpes simplex virus infection: Clinical and virological findings and relation to gonorrhea. *Acta Derm Venereol (Stockh)* **54**:79, 1974
13. Kreiss JK et al: AIDS virus infection in Nairobi prostitutes. *N Engl J Med* **314**:414, 1986
14. Simonsen JN et al: Human immunodeficiency virus infection among men with sexually transmitted diseases. *N Engl J Med* **319**:274, 1988
15. Quinn TC et al: Human immunodeficiency virus infection among patients attending clinics for sexually transmitted diseases. *N Engl J Med* **318**:197, 1988
16. Holmberg SD et al: Prior herpes simplex virus type 2 infection as a risk factor for HIV infection. *JAMA* **259**:1048, 1988
17. Stamm WE et al: The association between genital ulcer disease and acquisition of HIV infection in homosexual men. *JAMA* **260**:1429, 1988
18. Kuiken CL et al: Risk factors and changes in sexual behavior in male homosexuals who seroconverted for human immunodeficiency virus antibodies. *Am J Epidemiol* **132**:523, 1990
19. Kreiss JK et al: Isolation of human immunodeficiency virus from genital ulcers in Nairobi prostitutes. *J Infect Dis* **160**:380, 1989
20. Ramsey PG et al: Herpes simplex virus pneumonia: Clinical, virologic and pathologic features in 20 patients. *Ann Intern Med* **97**:813, 1982
21. Centers for Disease Control and Prevention: 1993 Revised clarification system for HIV infection and expanded surveillance case definition for AIDS among adolescents and adults. *MMWR* **41**:15, 1992
22. Glogan R et al: Herpetic whitlow as part of genital virus infection. *J Infect Dis* **136**:689, 1977
23. Laskin OL et al: Acyclovir and suppression of frequently recurring herpetic whitlow. *Ann Intern Med* **102**:494, 1985
24. Gill MJ et al: Therapy for recurrent herpetic whitlow. *Ann Intern Med* **105**:631, 1986
25. Norris SA et al: Severe, progressive herpetic whitlow caused by an acyclovir-resistant virus in a patient with AIDS. *J Infect Dis* **157**:209, 1988
26. Selling B et al: An outbreak of herpes simplex among wrestlers (Herpes Gladiatorum). *N Engl J Med* **270**:979, 1964
27. White WB et al: Transmission of herpes simplex virus type 1 infection in rugby players. *JAMA* **252**:533, 1984
28. Beuler TM et al: Grappling with herpes: Herpes Gladiatorum. *Am J Sports Med* **16**:665, 1988
29. Belongia EA et al: An outbreak of herpes gladiatorum at a high school wrestling camp. *N Engl J Med* **325**:906, 1991
30. Molin L: Oral acyclovir prevents herpes simplex associated erythema multiforme. *Br J Dermatol* **116**:109, 1987
31. Lemak MA et al: Oral acyclovir for the prevention of herpes associated erythema multiforme. *J Am Acad Dermatol* **15**:50, 1986
32. Leigh IM: Management of non-genital herpes simplex virus infections in immunocompetent patients. *Am J Med* **85**(suppl 2A):34, 1988
33. Nahmias AJ et al and the Collaborative Antiviral Study Group: Herpes simplex virus encephalitis: Laboratory evaluations and their diag-

nostic significance. *J Infect Dis* **145**:829, 1982

34. Aurelius E et al: Rapid diagnosis of herpes simplex encephalitis by nested polymerase chain reaction assay of cerebrospinal fluid. *Lancet* **337**:189, 1991

35. Herpes simplex encephalitis, editorial. *Lancet* **1**:535, 1986

36. Whitley RJ et al: Diseases that mimic herpes simplex encephalitis. *JAMA* **262**:234, 1989

37. Goldstein LC et al: Monoclonal antibodies to herpes simplex viruses: Use in antigenic typing and rapid diagnosis. *J Infect Dis* **147**:829, 1983

38. Elion GB et al: Selectivity of action of an antiherpes agent 9-(2-hydroxyethoxymethyl)-guanine. *Proc Natl Acad Sci USA* **74**:5716, 1978

39. Furman PA et al: Acyclovir triphosphate is a suicide inactivator of herpes simplex virus DNA polymerase. *J Biol Chem* **259**:9575, 1984

40. Spruance SL et al: Treatment of herpes simplex labialis with topical acyclovir in polyethylene glocol. *J Infect Dis* **146**:85, 1982

41. Fiddian AP et al: Successful treatment of facial-oral herpes with topical acyclovir. *Br Med J* **286**:1699, 1983

42. Corey L et al: A trial of topical acyclovir genital herpes simplex virus infections. *N Engl J Med* **306**:1313, 1982

43. Bryson Y et al: Treatment of first episode of genital herpes simplex infection with oral acyclovir, a randomized double-blind controlled trial in normal subjects. *N Engl J Med* **308**:916, 1982

44. Douglas JM et al: A double-blind study of oral acyclovir for suppression of recurrences of genital herpes simplex virus infection. *N Engl J Med* **310**:1551, 1984

45. Straus SE et al: Suppression of frequently recurring genital herpes. *N Engl J Med* **310**:1545, 1984

46. Kaplowitz LG et al and Acyclovir Study Group: Prolonged continuous acyclovir treatment of normal adults with frequently recurring genital herpes infection. *JAMA* **265**:747, 1991

47. Reichman RC et al: Treatment of recurrent genital herpes simplex infections with oral acyclovir. *JAMA* **251**:2103, 1984

48. Wade JC et al: Intravenous acyclovir to treat mucocutaneous herpes simplex infection after marrow transplantation: A double blind trial. *Ann Intern Med* **96**:265, 1982

49. Saral R et al: Acyclovir prophylaxis of herpes-simplex virus infections. A randomized double-blind controlled trial in bone marrow transplant recipients. *N Engl J Med* **305**:63, 1981

50. Whitley RJ et al: Adenine arabinoside therapy of biopsy proved herpes simplex encephalitis. *N Engl J Med* **297**:289, 1977

51. Dix RD et al: Recurrent herpes simplex encephalitis: Recovery of virus after Ara-A treatment. *Ann Neurol* **13**:196, 1983

52. Whitley RJ et al: Vidarabine vs. acyclovir therapy in herpes simplex encephalitis. *N Engl J Med* **314**:144, 1986

53. Skoldenberg B et al: Acyclovir versus vidarabine in herpes simplex encephalitis. Randomized multicenter study in consecutive Swedish patients. *Lancet* **8405**:707, 1984

54. VanLandingham KE et al: Relapse of Herpes simplex encephalitis after conventional acyclovir therapy. *JAMA* **259**:1051, 1988

55. Schnipper LE, Crumpacker CS: Resistance of herpes simplex virus to acycloguanosine: Role of viral thymidine kinase and DNA polymerase loci. *Proc Natl Acad Sci USA* **77**:2270, 1980

56. Darby G et al: Altered substrate specificity of herpes simplex virus: Thymidine kinase confers acyclovir resistance. *Nature* **289**:81, 1981

57. Erlich KS et al: Acyclovir-resistant herpes simplex virus infections in patients with the acquired immunodeficiency syndrome. *N Engl J Med* **320**:293, 1989

58. Safrin S et al: A controlled trial comparing foscarnet with vidarabine for acyclovir-resistant mucocutaneous herpes simplex in the acquired immunodeficiency syndrome. *N Engl J Med* **325**:551, 1991

59. Chatis PA, Crumpacker CS: Resistance of herpesviruses to antiviral drugs. *Antimicrob Agents Chemother* **36**:1589, 1992

60. Englund JA et al: Herpes simplex virus resistant to acyclovir. A study in a tertiary care center. *Ann Intern Med* **112**:416, 1990

CHAPTER 204

Michael N. Oxman and Rhoda Alani

Varicella and Herpes Zoster

Varicella (chickenpox) and herpes zoster (shingles, zoster) are distinct clinical entities caused by a single member of the herpesvirus family, varicella-zoster virus (VZV). The differences between these two diseases are due to differences in the host and in the circumstances of infection, not to differences in their etiologic agent.

Varicella, an acute, highly contagious exanthem that occurs most often in childhood, is the result of primary infection of a susceptible individual. It is characterized by a short or absent prodromal period and a generalized pruritic rash consisting of successive crops of lesions that progress rapidly from macules and papules to vesicles, pustules, and crusts. In normal children, systemic symptoms are usually mild and serious complications are extremely rare. In adults and in immunologically compromised persons of any age, varicella is more likely to be associated with an extensive eruption, high fever, severe constitutional symptoms, pneumonia, and other life-threatening complications. With the increasing incidence of human immunodeficiency virus (HIV) infection over the past decade, we are now beginning to recognize more cases of complicated and atypical varicella infections.[1]

Herpes zoster is a localized disease characterized by unilateral radicular pain and a vesicular eruption that is generally limited to the dermatome innervated by a single spinal or cranial sensory ganglion. It occurs most often in elderly people. In contrast to varicella, which follows primary exogenous VZV infection, herpes zoster is the result of reactivation of an endogenous infection that has persisted in latent form within sensory ganglia following an earlier attack of varicella. As with varicella, the incidence of complicated and atypical zoster herpes has been increasing with the increasing prevalence of HIV infection in the population.[1-12]

Historical Aspects

Herpes zoster, though sometimes confused with herpes simplex and other cutaneous eruptions, has been recognized as a distinct clinical entity since ancient times. On the other hand, varicella was confused with smallpox well into the nineteenth century. Herberden

(1767) is credited with first differentiating varicella from smallpox, but more than a century later, such authorities as Osler (1892) deemed it necessary to emphasize that the two diseases were indeed etiologically distinct.[13-15] The name *chickenpox* is probably derived from the Old English *gican*, "to itch."[16] The infectious nature of varicella was demonstrated in 1875 by Steiner,[17] who transmitted the disease to volunteers by the inoculation of vesicle fluid from patients with varicella. Tyzzer described the histopathology of the skin lesions of varicella in 1906 and called attention to the characteristic multinucleated giant cells and intranuclear inclusion bodies.[18] However, it was not until 1952 that Weller and Stoddard succeeded in isolating and propagating the virus from varicella vesicle fluid in vitro.[19]

The relationship of herpes zoster to varicella was first noted by von Bokay in 1888, when he observed that susceptible children acquired varicella after contact with individuals with herpes zoster.[13,14,20] It was further supported by Lipschutz,[21] who noted that the skin lesions of herpes zoster were histologically identical to those of varicella previously described by Tyzzer.

Kundratitz (in 1922) and Bruusgaard (in 1932) inoculated children with vesicle fluid from patients with herpes zoster and demonstrated that the same agent was responsible for both diseases.[20] Some recipients developed varicella-like lesions at the site of inoculation; others developed, in addition, a generalized exanthem that resembled varicella in every respect. Uninoculated children in contact with affected recipients developed typical varicella after a normal incubation period and transmitted the disease to other contacts. Children who had previously had varicella did not develop the disease when inoculated with vesicle fluid from patients with herpes zoster or when exposed to children who had developed a varicella-like exanthem following such inoculation. Vesicles from the site of inoculation and the generalized exanthem were histologically identical to those of ordinary varicella and herpes zoster. Early serologic studies[22] demonstrated that antigens derived from vesicles and crusts of both varicella and herpes zoster reacted equally well in complement fixation tests with convalescent sera from patients with either disease. However, it was only with the isolation and propagation in vitro of the agents of varicella and herpes zoster that the common etiology of the two diseases was proved. Weller and his colleagues found that the viruses recovered from patients with varicella and herpes zoster were identical with respect to their physical, biologic, and immunologic attributes.[23,24] This identity has subsequently been confirmed in numerous studies.[14,22,25]

The neurologic implications of the segmental distribution of the lesions of herpes zoster were recognized as long ago as 1831 by Richard Bright, and the inflammatory changes in the corresponding sensory ganglion and spinal nerve were first described by von Barensprung in 1862.[26-28] The definitive work is that of Head and Campbell (1900); they published detailed postmortem examinations of 21 persons with herpes zoster, together with clinical observations on 450 individuals with the disease.[26] All the gross and microscopic pathology is described and illustrated, including the acute lymphocytic inflammation, focal hemorrhage and neuronal destruction in sensory ganglia, the degeneration of sensory nerve fibers linking the affected neurons peripherally to the involved skin and centrally to the spinal cord and brain, and the later fibrosis of severely involved ganglia and nerves. Correlation of their detailed pathologic and clinical observations enabled Head and Campbell to map the area of skin (dermatome) innervated by each of the sensory ganglia. Their findings have been confirmed repeatedly by a number of subsequent studies,[28-35] some of which employed newer techniques, such as electron microscopy and fluorescent antibody staining, to demonstrate virus particles and viral antigens within neurons and satellite cells in the sensory ganglia and within peripheral sensory nerves early in the disease. Together, these observations indicate that in herpes zoster, active infection of sensory neurons precedes involvement of the skin.

Epidemiology

Epidemiology of Varicella

Varicella is worldwide in distribution, with no evidence of differing racial or sexual susceptibility. Humans are the only known reservoir, and there is no indication that arthropod vectors play any role in transmission. In metropolitan communities in temperate climates, varicella is endemic, with a regularly recurring seasonal prevalence in winter and spring and periodic epidemics dependent upon the accumulation of susceptible persons. In urban areas of the United States, varicella is primarily a disease of childhood; 90 percent of cases occur in children less than 10 years of age and fewer than 5 percent in individuals over the age of 15.[13,14] In tropical and semitropical countries, infection is delayed and varicella is seen more often in adults. In a serologic survey of parturient women in New York City, only 4.5 percent of those born in the United States lacked antibody to VZV, whereas 16 percent of those from Latin America were seronegative.[36] The proportion of susceptible adults is even higher in Asia, Africa, and the Middle East.[14,25] This can be an important consideration in delivering health care to immigrant populations and in controlling nosocomial varicella in hospitals with patients and staff from these areas.

Military recruits from Puerto Rico and the Philippines, up to 40 percent of whom are VZV seronegative, appear to account, in part, for a recent increase in hospital admissions for varicella at United States military facilities.[36a,b] This may also reflect increasing varicella susceptibility in United States teenagers and young adults.[36a] Delayed acquisition of primary VZV infection may have serious consequences because the mortality of varicella in adults is 25 times greater than it is in children.[36c]

Despite the lability of the virus, varicella is highly contagious. Attack rates of 87 percent among susceptible siblings in households and nearly 70 percent among susceptible patients on hospital wards have been reported.[13,37] Most cases of varicella are clinically apparent, although on occasion the exanthem may be so sparse and transient that it is unnoticed. A typical patient is probably infectious for 1 to 2 days (rarely, 3 to 4 days) before the exanthem appears and for 4 or 5 days thereafter, i.e., until the last crop of vesicles has crusted. The immunocompromised patient, who may experience successive crops of lesions for a week or more, is infectious for a longer period of time. The average incubation period of varicella is 14 or 15 days, with a range of 10 to 23 days.[13,37] The incubation period is often prolonged in patients who develop varicella after passive immunization with varicella-zoster immune globulin (VZIG) or plasma (ZIP).[38-40] The major route by which varicella is acquired and transmitted is thought to be the respiratory tract. Airborne droplets constitute an important mechanism of transmission, but infection is also spread by direct contact and less often, by indirect contact. Aerosolized virus can be spread by air currents without direct contact.[41,42] Unlike the crusts of smallpox, varicella crusts are not infectious, and the duration of infectivity of droplets containing the labile VZV must be relatively limited. The mechanism by which VZV is shed is unclear. Viremia occurs during the prodromal stage, when varicella can be transmitted to the fetus in utero and by blood transfusion from a donor incubating the infection. Lesions are not confined to the skin but also occur in the respiratory, genitourinary, and gastrointestinal tracts. Though the infectiousness of patients with varicella is thought to depend largely upon virus shed from the mucous membranes of the upper respiratory tract, VZV has only rarely been cultured from pharyngeal secretions; however, the polymerase chain reaction (PCR) was used to detect VZV DNA in the oropharynx of 62 percent of infected patients.[43] In contrast, VZV can regularly be recovered from vesicle fluid.[14,25]

One attack of varicella generally confers lasting immunity to the disease. Most of the rarely reported second attacks are probably examples of cutaneous dissemination in patients with herpes zoster (see below). With the advent of new immunosuppressive agents, recurrent exogenous VZV primary infections may be seen,[44] and severely immunocompromised patients with HIV infection may become susceptible to recurrent varicella. In addition, persons who develop modified varicella (e.g., because they are infected early in infancy in the presence of maternal antibody,[44a] or have been immunized with live attenuated varicella vaccine) may develop an immune response that is more limited than that induced by unmodified natural infection. Subsequently, such individuals may respond to exogenous exposure by developing a second episode of clinical (breakthrough) varicella.[44a–c]

Epidemiology of Herpes Zoster

Herpes zoster occurs sporadically throughout the year without seasonal prevalence. It affects both sexes and all races equally. As expected with a disease that reflects the reactivation of latent endogenous infection, the occurrence of herpes zoster is independent of the prevalence of varicella, and there is no convincing evidence that herpes zoster can be acquired by contact with persons with varicella or herpes zoster.[27,45,46] Rather, the incidence of herpes zoster is determined by factors that influence the host-parasite relationship. One of these is age. The rate of occurrence is in the range of 1.3 to 5 per 1000 persons per year; although the disease may be seen in any age group, including children, more than two-thirds of reported cases occur in individuals over 50 years of age and less than 10 percent of cases occur in those under the age of 20 years.[13,27,45–51] Hope-Simpson's tabulation of data from 192 cases occurring over a 16-year period in a population of 3500 individuals showed that the annual incidence per thousand rises from 0.74 in children under 10 years of age, to a plateau of approximately 2.5 between ages 20 and 50, and thereafter increases to reach a level of over 10 in octogenarians. A population-based study of herpes zoster involving approximately 470,000 person-years of observation was carried out in Rochester, Minnesota, by Ragozzino et al. from 1945 through 1959.[51] It revealed an age-adjusted incidence rate about one-half that of Hope-Simpson's (1.3 vs. 3.0 per thousand persons per year) but otherwise yielded comparable results (Fig. 204-1); the incidence rate in both studies increased markedly with age beyond the fourth decade. The incidence of herpes zoster among those who have already had an attack appears to be at least

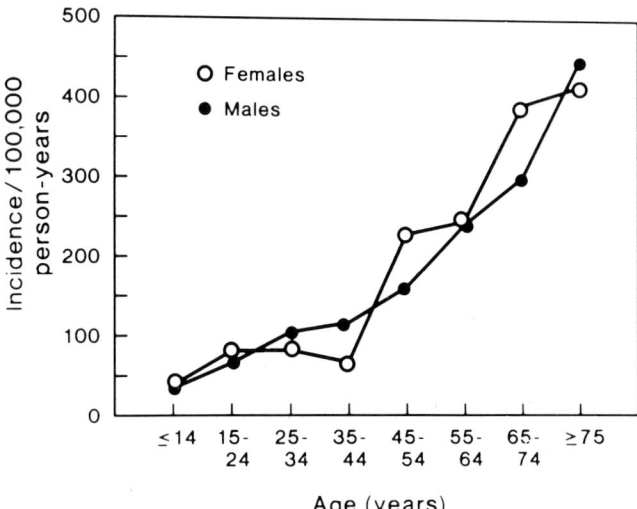

FIGURE 204-1 Incidence of herpes zoster among residents of Rochester, Minnesota, 1945–1959, by age and sex. (*Reprinted with permission from Ragozzino.*[51])

as high as that of first attacks in individuals of comparable age. Second attacks comprise 4 to 5 percent of reported series, and third attacks are not unheard of. Hope-Simpson estimated that if a cohort of 1000 people were to live to be 85 years old, half would have had an attack of herpes zoster and 10 would have had two attacks. However, patients suffering multiple episodes of zoster-like disease, especially involving the same anatomic location, are far more likely to be suffering from recurrent zosteriform herpes simplex virus infections.[52] The incidence of herpes zoster in immunosuppressed patients is increased 20 to 100 times, and the severity of the disease is also increased. The increased incidence and severity of herpes zoster in older individuals, as well as in individuals of any age who are immunosuppressed, is associated with deficient cell-mediated immune responses to VZV antigens (see below).

Herpes zoster is rare during the first few years of life. When it occurs in infants, there is usually no history of postnatal varicella, but there is almost always a history of maternal varicella during gestation.[53,54] Presumably, primary VZV infection and the establishment of neuronal latency occurred in utero.

Patients with herpes zoster are infectious. Virus can be isolated from vesicles in uncomplicated herpes zoster for up to 7 days after the appearance of the rash and for much longer periods in immunocompromised individuals. However, herpes zoster is less contagious than varicella; the infection rate in susceptible household contacts appears to be only about one-third that of varicella.[13,20,27,45]

The increased incidence of herpes zoster in immunocompromised patients with cancer had previously led many physicians to assume that the occurrence of herpes zoster in an otherwise normal individual might be an indication of underlying malignancy. A prospective study of 590 patients with herpes zoster indicated that the incidence of cancer during the first year and the first 5 years after the diagnosis of herpes zoster is the same as the incidence of cancer in the general population.[55] However, herpes zoster is sometimes an early manifestation of HIV infection. Indeed, high-risk individuals with herpes zoster should probably be evaluated for coincident HIV infection.[6,12] Herpes (zoster) in African patients was found to be a good predictor of HIV infection.[7]

Etiology

Varicella-zoster virus is a member of the herpesvirus family. Other members pathogenic for humans include herpes simplex virus type 1 (HSV-1) and type 2 (HSV-2), cytomegalovirus (CMV), the Epstein-Barr virus (EBV) of infectious mononucleosis, human herpesvirus-6 (HHV-6), the cause of roseola infantum, and the related human herpesvirus-7 (HHV-7).[56] All these herpesviruses are morphologically indistinguishable and share a number of properties, including a remarkable propensity for establishing latent infections that persist for the life of the host. VZV consists of an icosahedral capsid 100 nm in diameter that encloses the viral genome, a linear molecule of double-stranded DNA 125,000 base pairs in length. The capsid is composed of 162 protein subunits (capsomers), which resemble elongated hexagonal or pentagonal prisms with axial holes. The genome and capsid (the nucleocapsid) are surrounded by one or two additional layers of protein and, on the outside, by a loose lipoprotein envelope derived from the nuclear membrane of the host cell, containing radially oriented viral glycoproteins on its surface. The complete virion is roughly spherical, with a diameter of 150 to 200 nm.[57] Only enveloped virions are infectious, and this accounts for the lability of VZV; infectivity is rapidly destroyed by organic solvents, detergents, proteolytic enzymes, heat, and extremes of pH. More than 30 virus-specific proteins and glycoproteins have been identified in purified virions and in VZV-infected cells.[25] In addition to structural components of the virion, certain enzymes essential for virus replication, including a virus-specific DNA polymerase and a virus-specific deoxypyrimidine (thymidine) kinase, are synthesized in infected cells. Because these viral enzymes differ in substrate specificity from the corresponding host cell enzymes, they are important targets for specific antiviral chemotherapy.

The VZV genome consists of a linear molecule of double-stranded DNA 125,000 base pairs in length. It is similar in organization to the genomes of HSV-1 and HSV-2, but is approximately 17 percent shorter and has much lower guanosine plus cytosine content (46 percent vs. 68 percent and 69 percent, respectively).[57a-c] Like the genomes of HSV-1 and HSV-2, it contains covalently linked long (L) and short (S) segments, each of which consists of a unique DNA segment (U_L and U_S) flanked by internal and terminal inverted repeats (IR_L, TR_L, IR_S, TR_S) (Fig. 204-2). In the case of HSV-1 and HSV-2, both the L and S segments can invert with respect to one another to yield four isomers, which are found with equal frequency in mature virions. The genome of VZV, which is about 25,000 base pairs shorter than that of HSV-1 or HSV-2, lacks almost all of the IR_L and TR_L sequences and has a considerably shorter U_S segment (Fig. 204-2). While the S segment can invert freely, the vestigial IR_L and TR_L do not facilitate isomerization, and only two genomic isomers predominate in VZV virions.[57a,c-f] The complete sequence of the VZV genome has been determined; it contains open reading frames (ORF) corresponding to approximately 70 genes, many of which have DNA sequence and functional homology to HSV genes, and some of which can even complement their HSV homologs.[57a-e]

HSV gene expression is coordinately regulated and sequentially ordered in a cascade fashion, with three basic classes of genes: *immediate early* (IE) or *alpha, early* or *beta,* and *late* or *gamma.*[51] IE genes are the first to be expressed and generally encode regulatory proteins that downregulate further IE gene expression and induce the expression of early genes. Several of the early genes encode enzymes involved in viral DNA synthesis. Early gene

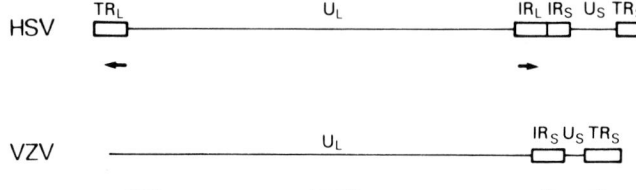

FIGURE 204-2 The genomes of HSV and VZV showing their structural relationship and the map locations of RNAs expressed during latency. Each viral genome contains long and short unique DNA segments (U_L and U_S) flanked by internal and terminal inverted repeats (IR_L, TR_L, IR_S, TR_S). The IR_L and TR_L of VSV are vestigial and not shown. Arrows show regions of the genome transcribed during latency and the direction of transcription. (*Adapted from Meier and Strauss.*[57h])

expression is followed by viral DNA replication and by the expression of late genes, most of which encode proteins and glycoproteins destined to become structural components of the virion. VZV replication has not been analyzed in such detail, but it is thought to be analogous to HSV, and VZV genes are grouped in similar classes. However, the structural differences between the HSV and VZV genomes described earlier (Fig. 204-2) result in important differences in gene representation and arrangement.[57c,d,g,h] The IR_L/TR_L of HSV contain an immediate early gene (IE 0) that encodes a protein, ICPO, implicated in the reactivation of latent virus. While there are two copies of this gene in the HSV genome, there is only one copy of the VZV homolog, ORF61, which is located in U_L. The IR_L/TR_L also encodes the HSV latency associated transcripts, (LATs), which have no counterpart in the VZV genome. Moreover, whereas the HSV genome encodes eight envelope glycoproteins, the VZV genome only encodes five. Although we do not understand the mechanisms involved, it seems likely that these genomic differences account in large part for the biological differences between HSV and VZV (Table 204-1).

There is only one VZV serotype. A number of antigens are present in the virion and produced in infected cells, but these are identical in viruses isolated from patients with varicella and herpes zoster throughout the world.[14,22,23,25,57a] However some VZV antigens cross-react with antigens of other members of the herpesvirus family and this limits the usefulness of certain serologic tests.[14,22,25,28,58]

The DNA of viruses isolated from cases of varicella and herpes zoster worldwide is basically similar, but minor variations in nucleotide sequence give the genomes of different clinical isolates of VZV slightly different restriction endonuclease cleavage patterns (i.e., each isolate has a unique pattern or "fingerprint"). More substantial differences distinguish the OKA live attenuated VZV vaccine (see below) from wild-type VZV isolates, and there is little resemblance between the restriction endonuclease cleavage pattern of VZV and those of the other human herpesviruses (HSV-1, HSV-2, CMV, and EBV).[59] These differences are useful epidemiologically, in that isolates from common source outbreaks will have identical restriction endonuclease cleavage patterns; when illness occurs in vaccinees or their contacts, the responsible agent, vaccine virus or wild-type VZV, can be determined.[25,60]

Studies of the molecular biology and pathogenesis of VZV infection have been hampered by difficulty in obtaining adequate quantities of cell-free virus and by the absence of suitable animal models. Some progress has been made in preparing cell-free virus, and the application of molecular cloning procedures has facilitated

TABLE 204-1
Comparison of Varicella Zoster Virus (VZV) and Herpes Simplex Virus (HSV)

Virus	VZV	HSV
Genome size	125,000 base pairs	150,000 base pairs
Percent G + C	46%	68%, HSV-1; 69%, HSV-2
Number of serotypes	1	2
Host range	Narrow	Broad
Cytopathic effect (CPE)	Multinucleated giant cells, eosinophilic intranuclear inclusion bodies	Multinucleated giant cells, eosinophilic intranuclear inclusion bodies
Cell free virus in tissue culture	No (Focal CPE)	Yes
Acyclovir sensitivity	++	++++
Primary Infection		
Epidemiology	Epidemic (Winter & Spring)	Sporadic
Transmission	Respiratory	Direct contact
Incubation period	Long (approx. 14 days)	Short (2–7 days)
Viremia essential	Yes	No
Disease location	Distant from portal of entry (the skin)	At portal of entry*
% Symptomatic	>95%	<25%
Recurrent Infection		
Frequency of symptomatic recurrences in lifetime	Usually once	Up to several hundred
Percent seropositives with symptomatic recurrences	10–20%	20–50%
Prodrome	Prolonged, severe pain	Short, mild dysesthesia
Distribution of lesions	Entire dermatome	Focal within dermatome
Destruction of sensory neurons during symptomatic recurrence	Yes	Probably not
Postherpetic neuralgia	Common	Very rare
Risk of recurrence	Increases with age	Decreases over time
Site of latency	Satellite cells in sensory ganglia	Sensory neurons in sensory ganglia
Asymptomatic virus shedding	No	Yes
Serologic response to recurrence	>95%	<10%
Reactivation induced by UV light	No	Yes

*Except herpes simplex encephalitis.

the physical mapping of the VZV genome. VZV has now been propagated in guinea pig cells, and a guinea pig model of VZV infection and transmission has been established.[25,61]

Pathogenesis

Pathogenesis of Varicella

Our present concept of the pathogenesis of varicella is based primarily on circumstantial evidence, analogy with experimental models of other exanthems, and postmortem examination of fatal cases. Entry of the virus is probably through the mucosa of the upper respiratory tract and oropharynx. Initial multiplication at this portal of entry results in dissemination of small amounts of virus via the blood and lymphatics (the primary viremia). This virus is removed by cells of the reticuloendothelial system, which probably constitutes the major site of virus replication during the remainder of the incubation period.

The incubating infection is partially contained by nonspecific host defenses (e.g., interferon) and by developing immune responses. In most individuals, virus replication eventually overwhelms these defenses, so that about 2 weeks after infection a much larger viremia (the secondary viremia) occurs.[42a–c,62,63] This

causes fever and malaise and disseminates virus throughout the body, especially to the skin and mucous membranes, where foci of infection are initiated by the infection of capillary endothelial cells.[18,20,64–66] The skin lesions appear in successive crops, reflecting a cyclic viremia, which in the normal host is terminated after about 3 days by VZV-specific humoral and cellular immune responses. Virus in the blood is cell-associated; it appears to circulate in mononuclear leukocytes, primarily lymphocytes.[42a–c,43,63,67,68] The frequent observations of abnormal electroencephalograms and elevated serum levels of hepatocellular enzymes in the acute stage of uncomplicated varicella[69–72] suggest the regular occurrence of asymptomatic viremic infection of many organs, including the central nervous system.

In addition to terminating the viremia, host immune responses play a critical role in limiting the progression of the focal lesions in the skin and other organs. Varicella pneumonia and most other complications of varicella reflect a failure to halt virus replication and dissemination and to limit the progression of visceral and cutaneous foci of infection.[64–67,73–75] Their common occurrence in newborns and in patients with congenital, acquired, or iatrogenic immunodeficiencies is almost certainly due in large part to depressed cellular immunity. The pathogenic basis of the greater severity of varicella in normal adults than in children, however, is unknown.

IgG, IgM, and IgA antibodies to VZV are detectable within 2 to 5 days after the onset of clinical varicella and reach maximum titers during the second or third week. Thereafter, IgG antibodies decline slowly and persist at low levels for life. IgM and IgA antibodies decline more rapidly and are generally undetectable a year after infection.[25,73,76-79] Cell-mediated immunity to VZV also develops during the course of varicella and persists for many years.[80,81] The assays usually employed measure the capacity of peripheral blood leukocytes to synthesize DNA and proliferate in vitro in response to VZV antigens, but cell-mediated immunity to VZV has also been demonstrated by other techniques, including a skin test that correlates well with the results of antibody assays and efficiently identifies susceptible individuals.[25,79a,80,82a]

Cell-mediated immunity appears to be more important than humoral immunity in recovery from varicella. The disease is not particularly severe in children with agammaglobulinemia,[83] and there is no obvious correlation between the endogenous antibody response and the severity of varicella.[73,74,76] Cellular immune responses, especially those of T lymphocytes, and perhaps interferons, are critical in limiting the extent and duration of VZV infection; it is patients with congenital, acquired, or iatrogenic defects in cell-mediated immunity who suffer severe and life-threatening varicella.[1,2,25,74,80,84-87] However, passive immunization of these immunocompromised patients with antibody to VZV can protect them from severe or fatal varicella.[38-40,88] A recent report of a 13-year-old child who lacked natural killer (NK) cells and developed severe varicella with pneumonia as well as severe infections with other herpesviruses[87] suggests that these cells may also be important in terminating primary VZV infections. Clearly, control of primary VZV infection involves a number of overlapping host defenses, and augmenting one (e.g., by administering antibody to VZV) may compensate for deficiencies in another.

Immunity to VZV is complex. In immunocompetent persons, one attack of varicella confers lasting immunity to varicella (i.e., to clinically apparent exogenous reinfection) but it does not prevent herpes zoster, a disease caused by the same virus. Serum antibody to VZV is an important factor in varicella immunity. People with detectable serum antibody do not usually become ill after exogenous exposure, whereas those devoid of serum antibody to VZV develop varicella.[89,90] Moreover, passive immunization can prevent varicella in susceptible immunocompetent individuals exposed to exogenous VZV.[37,38,91] However, the development and application of sensitive assays for humoral and cell-mediated immunity to VZV has revealed the dynamic nature of the VZV-host interaction. Subclinical reinfection, evidenced by a boost in the titer of IgG antibody to VZV, by the reappearance of IgM and IgA antibodies, and by an increase in cell-mediated immune responses to VZV antigens, is a frequent occurrence in normal immune individuals following household exposure to varicella.[76,80,92-94] This implies limited replication of VZV, at least as the portal of entry. Repeated exposures of this sort may help adults to maintain a high level of immunity to VZV.[27] Infants with transplacentally acquired maternal antibody regularly develop mild varicella after exposure,[44a] as do immunocompromised children passively immunized with varicella-zoster immune globulin (VZIG).[88] It would thus appear that the presence of antibody to VZV in a normal host, with or without VZV-specific cellular immune responses induced by previous varicella, will prevent the development of disease but not the local replication of exogenous VZV at the portal of entry. The failure of the same antibody preparations to prevent disease in immunosuppressed patients implies the need for some nonspecific, presumably cellular, component(s) that may interact with antibody—perhaps cells capable of mediating antibody-dependent cellular cytotoxicity.

It also appears that immunity in persons who develop modified varicella (e.g., because they are infected as infants in the presence of transplacentally acquired maternal antibody) is less durable than that which follows unmodified infection; such individuals may later respond to exogenous reinfection by developing mild varicella.[44a,b] Similarly, while immunologically normal recipients of live attenuated VZV vaccines (see below) have had a greatly reduced incidence of varicella after subsequent exposures, a few have developed mild varicella in spite of having vaccine-induced antibody to VZV.[44c,95-100]

Taken together, these observations suggest that antibody alone will not guarantee total immunity to varicella, unless it is the result of a previous unmodified natural infection.

Pathogenesis of Herpes Zoster

The pathogenesis of herpes zoster is not fully understood, but clinical, epidemiologic, and pathologic data as well as analogy with recurrent herpes simplex virus infections[101] support the following model.[27] During the course of varicella, VZV passes from lesions in the skin and mucosal surfaces into the contiguous endings of sensory nerves and is transported centripetally up the sensory fibers to the sensory ganglia. In the ganglia a latent infection is established and the virus then persists silently and harmlessly; it is no longer infectious and does not multiply, but it retains the capacity to revert to full infectiousness. Although VZV might also reach the sensory ganglia via the bloodstream during the course of the primary or secondary viremia of varicella, only the neural route can easily explain the coincidence of the anatomic pattern of the incidence of zoster in later life with the distribution of the rash in varicella. Herpes zoster occurs most commonly in those dermatomes in which the rash of varicella achieves the greatest density,[27,29] presumably because areas of skin with a denser rash during varicella transmit larger amounts of virus to the corresponding sensory ganglia and thus establish latent infection in a larger number of ganglionic cells. If subsequent reactivation occurs at random, zoster should occur most frequently in areas of skin innervated by ganglia with the largest number of latently infected cells.

Although the latent virus in the ganglia retains its potential for full infectivity, reversions are sporadic and infrequent. The mechanisms involved in the activation of latent VZV are unclear, but a number of conditions have been associated with the occurrence and localization of herpes zoster. These include immunosuppression in HIV infection and Hodgkin's disease and other malignancies; administration of immunosuppressive drugs and corticosteroids; irradiation of the spinal column; tumor involvement of the cord, dorsal root ganglion, or adjacent structures; local trauma; surgical manipulation of the spine; heavy metal poisoning or therapy; and frontal sinusitis, as a precipitant of ophthalmic zoster.[1,7,12,26,27,84-86,102,108,110]

Even when latent virus does revert, usually nothing perceptible happens. The minute dose of infectious virus that results is immediately neutralized by circulating antibody or destroyed by cellular immune responses before it can infect other cells and multiply enough to cause perceptible damage. The small quantity of viral antigen released into the bloodstream during such "contained reversions" stimulates host immune responses,[27,80,107,108,108a,109] and this raises the level of host resistance. A similar boost in the level of host resistance often follows contact with a patient with varicella, reflecting subclinical exogenous reinfection.[76,92-94,109] When host resistance falls below a critical level, reactivated virus can no longer be contained and the next reversion is "successful."

Virus multiplies and spreads within the ganglion, causing neuronal necrosis and intense inflammation, a process that is usually accompanied by severe neuralgia. Infectious VZV then spreads antidromically down the sensory nerve, causing intense neuritis, and is released around the sensory nerve endings in the skin where it produces the characteristic cluster of zoster vesicles. The occurrence of neuralgia several days before the rash appears and the presence of degenerative changes in cutaneous nerve fibrils on the first day of the eruption[31] provide additional evidence that infection in the sensory ganglion precedes involvement of the skin. Spread of the ganglionic infection proximally along the posterior nerve root to the meninges and cord results in local leptomeningitis, cerebrospinal fluid pleocytosis, and segmental myelitis. Infection of motor neurons in the anterior horn and inflammation of the anterior nerve root account for the local palsies that may accompany the cutaneous eruption, and extension of infection within the central nervous system may result in ascending myelitis or meningoencephalitis, rare complications of herpes zoster.[110,111]

During each successful reversion, hematogenous dissemination of virus from the affected ganglion[108,112] often produces aberrant vesicles at a distance from the primary dermatome, even in uncomplicated herpes zoster,[48] and stimulates an anamnestic immune response that terminates the infectious process. Sometimes this response is sufficiently rapid to neutralize virus released into the skin and thus prevent the development of cutaneous lesions; the result is an episode of radicular pain without eruption (zoster sine herpete) and a coincident rise in antibody to VZV. The occurrence of this syndrome has now been well documented,[27,103,107,113] as have completely asymptomatic rises in antibody to VZV that presumably reflect "contained reversions."[27,80,93,107,109] If the anamnestic host response is delayed or deficient, as it appears to be in many immunosuppressed patients, the duration and severity of the local infection is increased, and the hematogenous dissemination of VZV is more prolonged and extensive.[3–5,8–12,80,84–87,102–108,110,112,114–120] Restoration of immunity to VZV in bone marrow transplant recipients depends upon reactivation of latent VZV. Surprisingly, many of these reactivations are subclinical and result in cell-associated viremia.[80,108,123]

Hope-Simpson considered the level of antibody to be the critical determinant of the host's capacity to contain VZV reversions.[27] However, it now appears that cellular immunity is a more important factor in host resistance to these recurrent VZV infections of endogenous origin.[49,73,76,80,84–87,104–106,110,112–123]

A selective decline in cellular immune responses to VZV has been documented in elderly individuals, and this may explain the increased incidence and severity of herpes zoster observed in older people.[80,81,82a,124–126]

Clinical Manifestations

Clinical Manifestations of Varicella

Prodrome of Varicella   In young children, prodromal symptoms are uncommon, and the illness usually begins, after an incubation period of 14 to 15 days, with the onset of the rash. The rash may be accompanied by a low-grade fever and malaise. In older children and adults, the rash is often preceded by 2 to 3 days of fever, chills, malaise, headache, anorexia, severe backache, and, in some patients, sore throat and dry cough. A fleeting scarlatiniform rash is sometimes observed just before or coincident with the vesicular eruption.

Rash of Varicella   The rash begins on the face and scalp and spreads rapidly to the trunk, with relative sparing of the extremities. New lesions appear in successive crops but their distribution remains central. The rash tends to be more profuse in hollows and protected parts of the body than on prominent and exposed parts. Thus it is denser in the hollow of the small of the back and between the shoulder blades than on the scapulae and buttocks and more profuse on the medial than on the lateral aspects of the limbs. It is not uncommon to have a few lesions on the palms and soles. Vesicles often appear earlier and in larger numbers in areas of inflammation, such as diaper rash, sunburn, or eczema.

The most striking feature of the lesions of varicella is their rapid progression from rose-colored macules to papules to vesicles to pustules to crusts (Fig. 204-3a). The entire transition may take only 8 to 12 h. The typical vesicle of varicella is superficial and thin-walled, so that it looks like a drop of water lying on, rather than in, the skin. It is usually 2 to 3 mm in diameter and elliptical, with its long axis parallel to the folds of the skin. The early vesicle is surrounded by an irregular area of erythema, which gives the lesions the appearance of a "dewdrop on a rose petal."[127] The vesicle fluid soon becomes cloudy with the influx of inflammatory cells, which convert the vesicle to a pustule (Fig. 204-3b). The lesion then dries, beginning in the center, first producing an umbilicated pustule and then a crust. Crusts fall off in 1 to 3 weeks, depending on the depth of the skin involvement, leaving shallow pink depressions that gradually disappear. Scarring is rare in uncomplicated varicella.

Vesicles also develop in the mucous membranes of the mouth, occurring most commonly over the palate. Mucosal vesicles rupture so rapidly that the vesicular stage may be missed. Instead, one sees shallow ulcers 2 to 3 mm in diameter. Vesicles may also appear on other mucous membranes, including those of the nose, pharynx, larynx, trachea, gastrointestinal tract, urinary tract, and vagina, as well as on the conjunctivae.

A distinctive feature of varicella is the simultaneous presence, in any one area of the skin, of lesions in all stages of development. This is due to the rapid evolution of individual lesions and the appearance of successive crops involving the same anatomic areas. In the typical case, three crops of lesions appear over a 3-day period, but there is wide variation, ranging from a single crop of a few scattered lesions to a series of five or more crops developing over a period of a week, with innumerable lesions covering the entire body. In general, the mildest cases are seen most frequently in infants and the most severe in adults. Inapparent infections occur but are rare.[37]

Fever usually persists as long as new lesions continue to appear and its height is generally proportional to the severity of the rash. In typical cases it rarely exceeds 39°C (102°F); it may be absent in mild cases and rise to 40.5°C (105°F) in severe cases with extensive rash. Prolonged fever or recurrence of fever after defervescence may be seen with secondary bacterial infections. Headache, malaise, myalgia, and anorexia generally accompany the fever and are more severe in older children and adults. However, the most distressing symptom is usually pruritus, which is present throughout the vesicular stage.

Complications of Varicella   In the normal child, varicella is a benign disease rarely attended by serious complications. The most common complication is the secondary bacterial infection of skin lesions, usually by staphylococci or streptococci, which may produce impetigo, furuncles, cellulitis, erysipelas, and rarely gangrene. These local infections often lead to scarring and, very rarely,

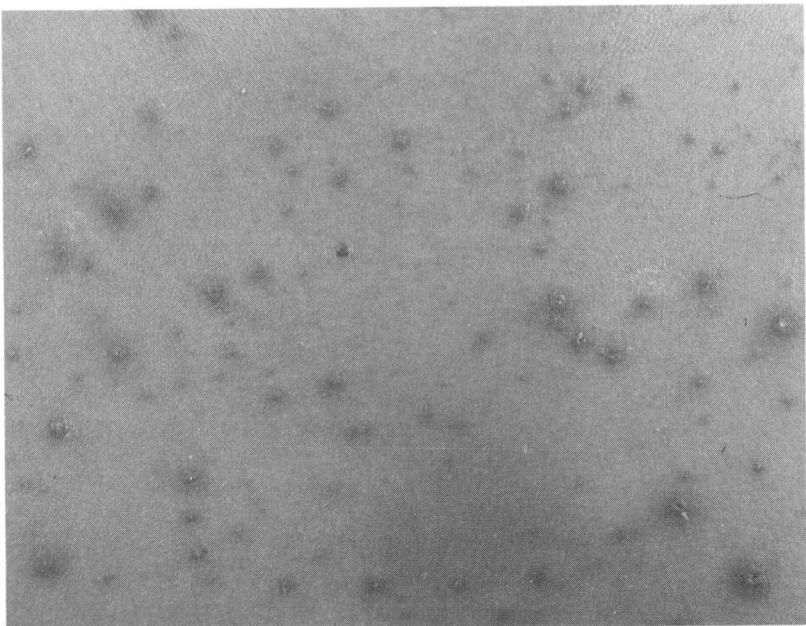

a

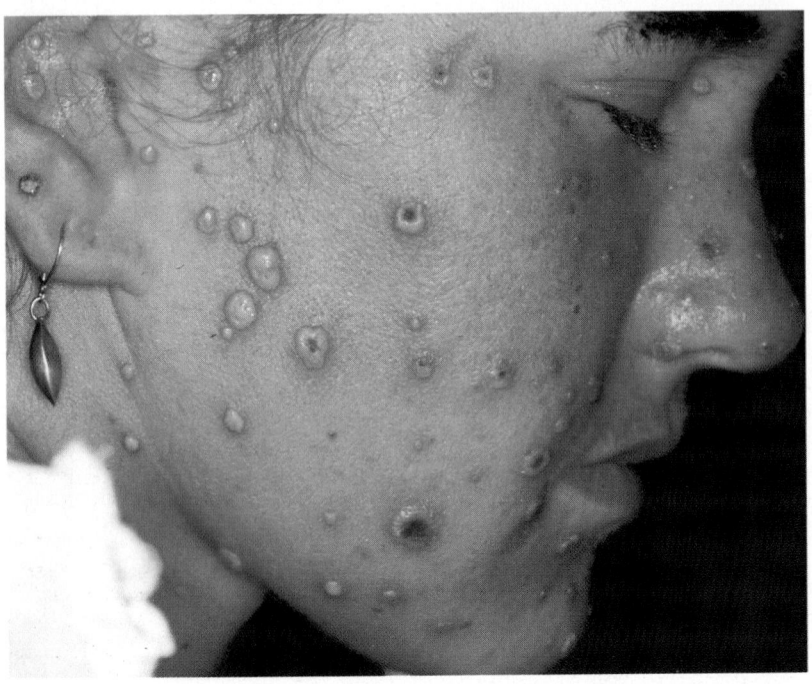

b

FIGURE 204-3 Varicella. (*a*) A full spectrum of lesions, i.e., erythematous papules, vesicles ("dewdrops on rose petals"), crusts, and erosions at sites of excoriation, is seen in a child with a typical case of varicella. (*b*) A wider range of lesions, including many large pustules, is seen in a 21-year-old female who was febrile, "toxic," and had varicella pneumonitis.

to septicemia with metastatic infection of other organs.[128–131] Bullous lesions may be produced when vesicles are infected with staphylococci that elaborate exfoliative toxin.[132] Secondary bacterial pneumonia is a rare complication that occurs mainly in children under 7 years of age and responds to appropriate antibiotic therapy, as do otitis media and suppurative meningitis.[128,133,134] In contrast to the situation in the normal host, bacterial superinfection is common and life-threatening in leukopenic patients, especially in children with leukemia who are undergoing chemotherapy.

Other complications that appear to reflect some defect in the capacity of the host to limit VZV multiplication and dissemination account for the increased morbidity and mortality of varicella in adults, in newborns, and in immunocompromised patients of any age.[1–12,54,64,74,103,129,131,133–138]

Varicella, like many other viral infections, is generally more severe in adults than in children. Fever and constitutional symptoms are more prominent and prolonged. The rash is more profuse, and complications more frequent. Primary varicella pneumonia is the major complication of adult varicella. It is rarely observed in normal children; adults account for more than 90 percent of reported cases.[1–12,36c,54,74,103,110,129,131–138]

The incidence of primary varicella pneumonia depends on the population of patients studied and on the diagnostic criteria employed. Radiographic evidence of pneumonia was found in 16 percent of healthy male military recruits with varicella, but clinical signs of pneumonia were present in only 4 percent.[139] In a more recent study, radiographic evidence of pneumonitis was found in fewer than 3 percent of healthy young military personnel with varicella.[140] The incidence and severity of varicella pneumonia are substantially higher in older patients and in the subset of adults with varicella admitted to hospitals.[133,135] Pneumonia generally appears 1 to 6 days after the onset of the rash, and the degree of pulmonary involvement correlates best with the severity of the cutaneous eruption. Some patients are virtually asymptomatic, but others develop severe respiratory embarrassment, with cough, dyspnea, tachypnea, high fever, pleuritic chest pain, cyanosis, and hemoptysis. The severity of the symptoms is usually out of proportion to the physical findings in the chest, but the roentgenogram typically reveals diffuse nodular densities throughout both lung fields, often peribronchial in distribution, with a tendency to concentrate in the perihilar regions and at the bases.[129,133,135,139,143,144] Radiographic abnormalities disappear more slowly than the symptoms of pneumonia, and occasionally the pulmonary lesions calcify and persist for years.[129,135,142] The mortality in adults with varicella pneumonia has been estimated to be between 10 and 30 percent, but it is probably less than 10 percent if immunocompromised patients are excluded.[129,135,138,141,143] It is clear from postmortem examination of fatal cases that the pneumonia is but one manifestation of widespread hematogenous dissemination, with evidence of varicella infection in virtually every organ examined.[135,143,144]

Varicella during pregnancy is a threat to both mother and fetus. Disseminated infection and varicella pneumonia may result in maternal death, but it is not clear that either the incidence or the severity of varicella pneumonia is greater when varicella occurs during pregnancy than when it occurs in the normal nonpregnant adult.[145,146] The fetus may sometimes die as a consequence of premature labor or maternal death in severe varicella pneumonia, but varicella during pregnancy has not increased the background level of fetal morbidity, mortality, or congenital malformations.[54,145,146] Nevertheless, even in uncomplicated varicella, maternal viremia may result in intrauterine (congenital) VZV infection.

When congenital VZV infection occurs early in gestation, the spectrum of disease ranges from severe congenital malformations to asymptomatic latency. A characteristic syndrome of developmental abnormalities (including hypoplasia of an extremity, cicatricial skin scarring, cortical atrophy, ocular abnormalities, and low birth weight) has been observed in infants born to women who had varicella between the seventh and twentieth weeks of gestation.[54,145–147] This is a rare occurrence, with fewer than 30 cases reported worldwide. However, maternal varicella at any stage of pregnancy can cause a fetal infection that resolves before parturition without obvious sequelae. These infants are born without visible evidence of infection, but frequently develop herpes zoster at an early age without any history of previous varicella.[53,54,145,146]

Congenital varicella (i.e., varicella occurring within 10 days of birth) appears to be more serious than varicella in infants infected postnatally, and the severity varies markedly depending on the proximity of maternal disease to delivery. When an infant acquires VZV infection in utero but is born before the transplacental passage of sufficient maternal antibody to modify the infection during its incubation period (i.e., when the rash of varicella occurs in the mother less than 5 days before or within 2 days after delivery, or begins in an infant between 5 and 10 days of age), the result is often severe disseminated varicella, with mortality as high as 30 percent. When the onset of rash in the mother is 5 days or more

before delivery (onset of rash in the infant at 0 to 4 days of age), sufficient maternal antibody has crossed the placenta to modify the infection, and all such infected infants can be expected to survive. These observations imply that immature perinatal defenses cannot, by themselves, restrain VZV replication and dissemination.[54,145,146]

The morbidity and mortality of varicella are markedly increased in immunocompromised patients, including patients with AIDS; patients with leukemia and other malignancies who are receiving corticosteroids, chemotherapeutic agents, or radiotherapy at the time of infection; patients receiving corticosteroids for diseases such as nephrotic syndrome and rheumatic fever; and patients with congenital immunologic deficiencies.[1–3,64,74,136,137,148–154] In these patients, continued virus replication and dissemination result in a prolonged high-level viremia,[67,75] a more extensive rash and a longer period of new vesicle formation, and, commonly, involvement of the lungs, liver, central nervous system, and other organs throughout the body. In one series, 19 of 60 children with leukemia who were receiving chemotherapy at the time of infection had visceral dissemination, and 4 died.[74] There was varicella pneumonia in all four fatal cases and fulminant encephalitis in two. Varicella hepatitis was also frequently present but was not fatal in the absence of pneumonia. Disseminated varicella occurred more often in children with absolute lymphopenia (less than 500 lymphocytes per cubic millimeter). Immunosuppressed and corticosteroid-treated patients may also develop hemorrhagic complications of varicella, which range in severity from mild febrile purpura to severe and often fatal purpura fulminans and malignant varicella with purpura.[103,155–159] The etiology of these hemorrhagic complications is complex and probably not the same in every case. In some, thrombocytopenia may be associated with the underlying disease, its therapy, the direct effect of VZV infection on the bone marrow, or immune-mediated platelet destruction.[103,156,160] In others, particularly those with malignant varicella and purpura fulminans, the primary factor may be infection of vascular endothelial cells, with endothelial damage initiating disseminated intravascular coagulation and thrombotic purpura.

Central nervous system (CNS) complications of varicella, which occur in fewer than 1 in 1000 cases, include several distinct syndromes[111]: (1) Reye's syndrome, (2) acute cerebellar ataxia, (3) encephalitis or meningoencephalitis, (4) acute ascending or transverse myelitis, and (5) Guillain-Barré syndrome. Varicella-associated Reye's syndrome (acute encephalopathy with fatty degeneration of the viscera), which typically occurs 2 to 7 days after the appearance of the rash, is not discernibly different from Reye's syndrome associated with influenza A, influenza B, or other viral infections. Although its pathogenesis is not understood, there is no inflammatory response in the CNS, and pathologic and virologic studies have essentially ruled out direct virus infection of the liver or brain. Instead, Reye's syndrome may be caused by some circulating toxin, perhaps a component of the virus or a substance elaborated by virus-infected cells. From 15 to 40 percent of all cases of Reye's syndrome occur in association with varicella,[161,162] and the mortality may be as high as 40 percent.[131] Reexamination of older reports of the CNS complications of varicella suggests that many of the cases described as "varicella encephalitis" in immunologically normal children were probably Reye's syndrome. Furthermore, Reye's syndrome appears to account for most of the fatalities in normal children that were attributed to varicella encephalitis. Two case series[131,163] support this conclusion. In Takashima and Becker's review of 32 fatal cases of varicella in children, all 12 that occurred in otherwise normal children had clinical and pathologic findings compatible with Reye's syndrome. Of the remaining 20, 18 occurred in children with underlying diseases (12 of whom were receiving corticosteroids) and 2 were cases of neonatal varicella. Although typical inclusions were demonstrated in the brains of only 2, all 20 of these children had evidence of widespread VZV dissemination, with inclusions in many internal organs. In a series of 96 patients hospitalized with varicella,[131] there were 17 cases of Reye's syndrome in 81 immunologically normal children, and these accounted for 7 of the 10 fatalities recorded. Another of the deaths occurred in an infant who developed varicella 7 days after delivery; CNS involvement in this case was part of a widely disseminated VZV infection.

Varicella-associated Guillain-Barré syndrome is extremely rare, and many of the cases reported are almost certainly examples of varicella myelitis. Apart from the temporal association in the few cases recorded, there is no evidence directly implicating VZV in the pathogenesis of Guillain-Barré syndrome.

In acute cerebellar ataxia, the onset of neurologic symptoms has ranged from 11 days before to 20 days after the appearance of the rash. Recovery without sequelae is the rule, and no pathologic data are available. However, its occurrence as early as 11 days before the onset of rash, i.e., during the primary viremia,[164] and the detection of VZV antigens in the cerebrospinal fluid of patients with this complication[165,166] suggest that acute cerebellar ataxia may reflect direct invasion of the CNS, presumably as a consequence of viremia and infection of vascular endothelial cells.

The pathogenesis of varicella encephalitis (meningoencephalitis) and myelitis remains obscure. Although many observers favor a postinfectious (autoimmune) demyelinating process like that observed in measles encephalomyelitis,[167] there is increasing evidence that these complications of varicella result from direct VZV infection of the CNS. The therapeutic implications of this distinction are obvious (see below). Many cases of varicella meningoencephalitis and myelitis (and most cases that have come to postmortem examination) have occurred in patients with prolonged high-grade viremia and infection of many organs in addition to the skin and mucous membranes—a setting in which direct infection of the CNS is to be expected.[67,74,110,144,163,168,169] Furthermore, whereas characteristic intranuclear inclusions in the CNS have been reported in only a few cases,[163,170] many others have shown pathologic features more consistent with direct VZV infection than with postinfectious (autoimmune) encephalomyelitis.[171] These have included perivascular infiltrates in the cortex and brainstem; scattered foci of necrosis, often hemorrhagic and often associated with swelling of endothelial cells and injury to vessel walls; and inflammatory infiltration of the leptomeninges. Moreover, because isolation of VZV from skin vesicles after more than 4 days of rash is uncommon[73] and because characteristic intranuclear inclusion bodies are not always observed in infected tissues, the failure to isolate VZV or demonstrate inclusion bodies is not compelling evidence against direct CNS infection. Finally, the infectious nature of varicella encephalitis and myelitis is further supported by the recent demonstration of antibody to VZV (presumably locally produced within the CNS) in the cerebrospinal fluid of patients with varicella encephalitis and transverse myelitis, and by the direct isolation of VZV from the cerebrospinal fluid of a patient with varicella encephalitis.[172]

Other rare complications of varicella include myocarditis, glomerulonephritis, orchitis, appendicitis, pancreatitis, gastritis and ulcerative lesions of the bowel,[173] arthritis, Henoch-Schönlein vasculitis, optic neuritis, keratitis, and iritis.[173,174] The pathogenesis of many of these complications has not been delineated, but direct

parenchymal infection or vasculitis induced by VZV infection of endothelial cells or vasculitis induced by VZV antigen-antibody complexes appear to be responsible in most cases.

Although chemical evidence of mild hepatitis is common in uncomplicated varicella,[70–72,140] clinical hepatitis is rare, except as a complication of progressive varicella.

Clinical Manifestations of Herpes Zoster

Prodrome of Herpes Zoster The first symptoms of herpes zoster are usually pain and paresthesia in the involved dermatome. This generally precedes the eruption by several days and varies from superficial itching, tingling, or burning to severe, deep boring or lancinating pain. It may be constant or intermittent and is often accompanied by tenderness and hyperesthesia of the skin in the involved dermatome. The preeruptive pain of herpes zoster may simulate pleurisy, myocardial infarction, duodenal ulcer, cholecystitis, biliary or renal colic, appendicitis, prolapsed intervertebral disk, or early glaucoma, and it may thus lead to serious misdiagnosis. Constitutional symptoms, including headache, malaise, and fever, occur in about 5 percent of patients, usually in children, and may precede the rash by 1 to 2 days.[46,50,103]

A few patients experience acute segmental neuralgia without ever developing a cutaneous eruption, a syndrome called zoster sine herpete.[103,107,113,157,175] A concurrent rise in antibodies to VZV has now been demonstrated in a number of such episodes, providing evidence that they are, indeed, manifestations of herpes zoster.[103,107,113] However, although zoster sine herpete may explain some cases of trigeminal neuralgia, most patients with this syndrome do not have serologic evidence of herpes zoster. Similarly, although facial palsy frequently complicates cephalic herpes zoster, VZV infection does not appear to be responsible for most cases of "idiopathic" facial (Bell's) palsy.[176]

Rash of Herpes Zoster The most distinctive feature of herpes zoster is the localization of the rash, which is nearly always unilateral, does not cross the midline, and is generally limited to the area of skin innervated by a single sensory ganglion (Fig. 204-4). Individual sensory ganglia are not attacked at random; herpes zoster occurs with greatest frequency in those areas in which the rash of varicella was most abundant.[27,29,51] The area supplied by the trigeminal nerve, particularly the ophthalmic division, and the trunk from T3 to L2 are most frequently affected; the thoracic region alone accounts for more than one-half of reported cases, and lesions rarely occur below the elbows or knees.[26,27,46,51,103,177] Regional lymphadenopathy occurs in the majority of cases, and the cerebrospinal fluid frequently shows a mild pleocytosis, predominantly lymphocytic, and an elevated protein content. Although the individual lesions of herpes zoster and varicella are usually indistinguishable, those of herpes zoster tend to evolve more slowly and often consist of closely grouped vesicles on an erythematous base, rather than the discrete, randomly distributed vesicles of varicella. The lesions begin as erythematous macules and papules that often first appear where superficial branches of the affected sensory nerve are given off, e.g., the posterior primary division and the lateral and anterior branches of the anterior primary division of spinal nerves.[22,26,29,157] Vesicles form within 12 to 24 h and evolve into pustules by the third day. These dry up and crust in 7 to 10

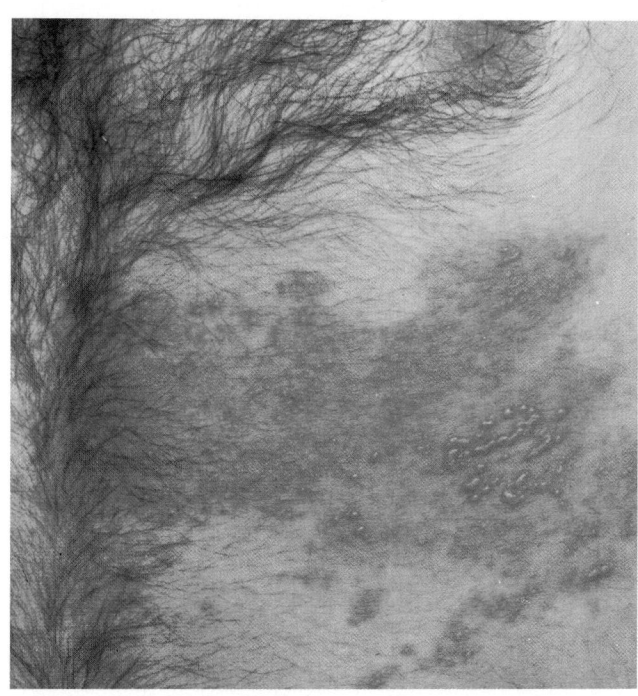

a

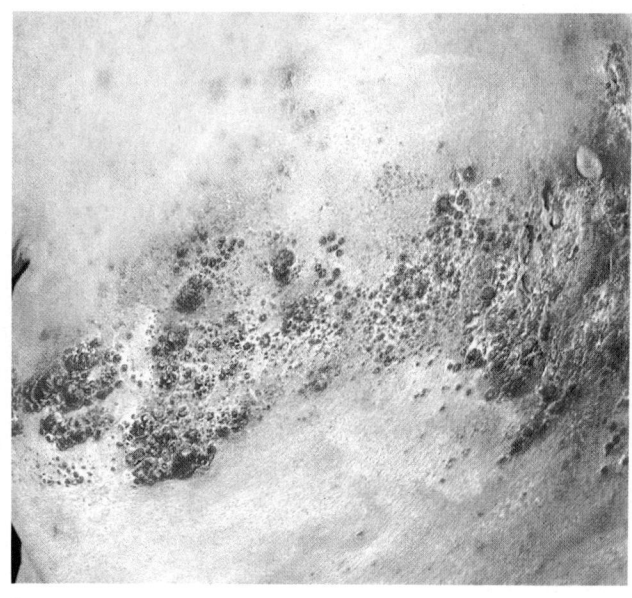

b

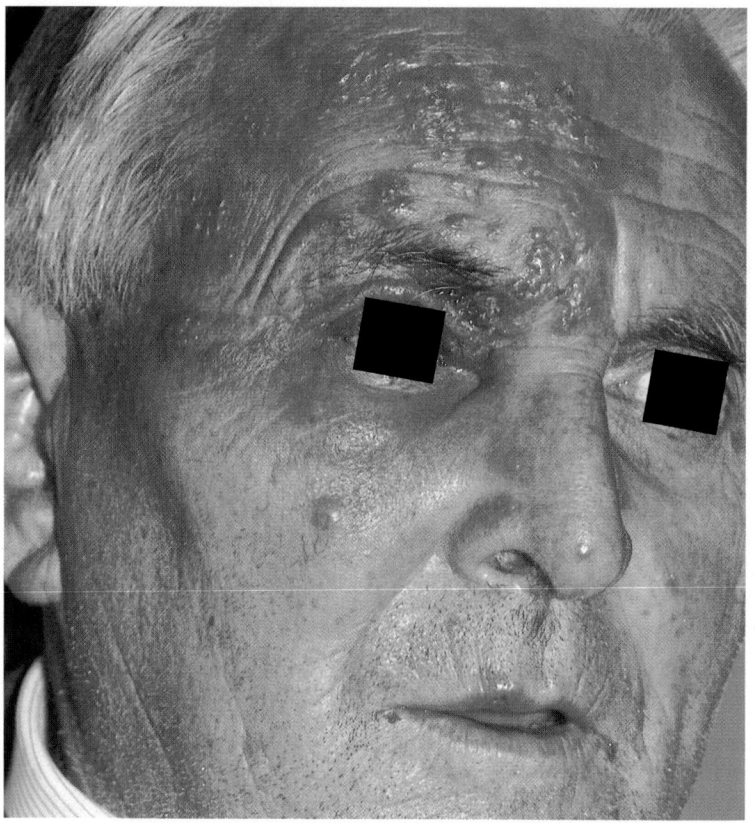

c

FIGURE 204-4   Herpes zoster. (*a*) Early involvement of a thoracic dermatome with erythema within the dermatome and areas of grouped vesicle formation. (*b*) Later involvement with crusted sites on the back where the eruption first appeared and many confluent hemorrhagic vesicles and bullae on the lateral chest wall, where the eruption appeared more recently; some vesicles are also seen outside the involved dermatome, representing hematogenous dissemination, a not uncommon occurrence. (*c*) Ophthalmic zoster: Note the involvement of the tip of the nose, which frequently signals involvement of the eye.

days. Crusts generally persist for 2 to 3 weeks (Fig. 204-4*b*). In normal individuals, new lesions continue to appear for 1 to 4 days (occasionally for as long as 7 days), and virus may be recovered from lesions for as long as a week after the appearance of the rash. The rash is most severe and lasts longest in older people and is least severe and of shortest duration in children.[46,47,103,177] Segmental

pain, a prominent feature of herpes zoster in older individuals, generally remits as the crusts fall off. Pain is seldom a significant symptom of herpes zoster in children.[178,179]

Between 10 and 15 percent of reported cases of herpes zoster involve the ophthalmic division of the trigeminal nerve (Fig. 204-4*c*). The rash of ophthalmic zoster may extend from the level

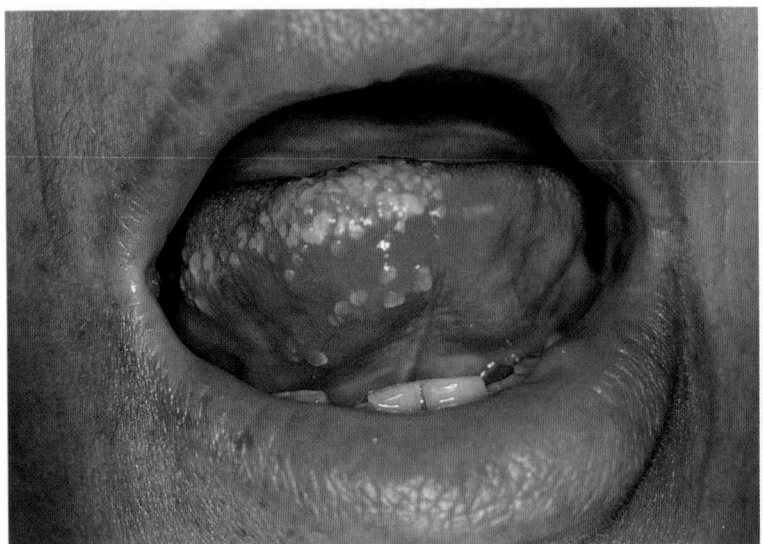

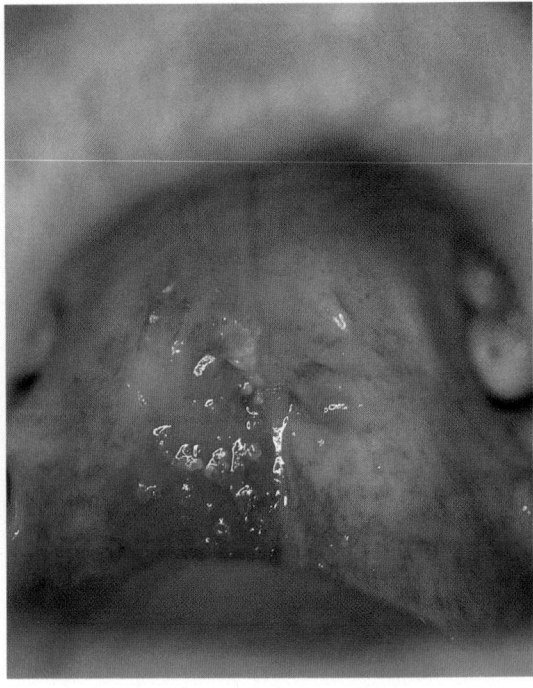

FIGURE 204-5 Cephalic herpes zoster with facial palsy (Hunt syndrome). A 60-year-old female with right-sided facial palsy and vesicles on her (*a*) tongue and (*b*) soft palate.

a

b

of the eye to the vertex of the skull, but it does not cross the midline of the forehead. When only the supratrochlear and supraorbital branches are involved, the eye is usually spared. Involvement of the vasociliary branch, as evidenced by a herpetic rash on the tip and side of the nose, occurs in 30 to 40 percent of patients and is usually accompanied by conjunctivitis and occasionally by keratitis, scleritis, iridocyclitis, extraocular-muscle palsies, ptosis, and mydriasis. Thus, when ophthalmic zoster involves the tip and the side of the nose, careful attention must be given to the condition of the eye. VZV is not, however, as pathogenic for the eye as is herpes simplex virus.

Herpes zoster affecting the second and third divisions of the trigeminal nerve and other cranial nerves is uncommon, but when it occurs it may produce symptoms and lesions in the mouth, ears, pharynx, or larynx.[28,157,180,181] The so-called Ramsay Hunt's syndrome (Figs. 204-5, 204-6), which consists of facial palsy in combination with herpes zoster of the external ear or tympanic membrane, with or without tinnitus, vertigo, and deafness, results from involvement of the facial and auditory nerves.[28] Because facial palsy is frequently associated with herpes zoster involving cranial structures other than the external ear (e.g., Fig. 204-5), the term "Ramsay-Hunt syndrome" has been replaced by "cephalic herpes zoster with facial palsy" or "Hunt's syndrome."

Complications of Herpes Zoster (Table 204-2) Postherpetic neuralgia (pain persisting after all crusts have fallen off) occurs in 10 to 15 percent of patients with herpes zoster.[51,182] It is uncommon in patients under 40 years of age but occurs in more than one-third of patients 60 years old or older, especially those with ophthalmic zoster.[46,47,51,103,182,183] Anesthesia in the involved dermatome is another common sequela and is particularly troublesome when it occurs in the area innervated by the ophthalmic nerve.[103,183,184] Postherpetic neuralgia is generally refractory to treatment but usually remits spontaneously in 1 to 6 months.

When the rash is particularly severe, as it often is in severely immunosuppressed patients, there may be superficial gangrene with delayed healing and subsequent scarring. As in varicella, secondary bacterial infection may also delay healing and cause scarring.

Ophthalmic zoster has a relatively high complication rate, especially when involvement of the nasociliary branches provides VZV with direct access to intraocular structures.[51,180,183,184] The eye is involved in 20 to 70 percent of patients with ophthalmic zoster. Complications include cicatricial lid retraction, paralytic ptosis, acute epithelial keratitis, scleritis, uveitis, secondary glaucoma, oculomotor palsies, chorioretinitis, and optic neuritis. Corneal sensation is almost always impaired, and when the impairment is severe it may lead to neurotrophic keratitis and chronic ulceration. Rarely, secondary bacterial infection may result in panophthalmitis requiring enucleation. Granulomatous cerebral angiitis with contralateral hemiplegia (see below) was observed in 4 of 86 patients with ophthalmic zoster seen at the Mayo Clinic between 1975 and 1980.[184]

Most other complications of herpes zoster appear to be associated with the spread of virus from the involved ganglion, either via the bloodstream or by direct neural extension. When patients with herpes zoster are carefully examined, 17 to 35 percent are found to have at least a few vesicles in areas remote from the involved dermatome; this is due presumably to hematogenous dissemination of virus from the affected ganglion, nerve, or skin.[22,48,103] The disseminated lesions usually appear within a week of onset of the segmental eruption and, if few in number, are easily overlooked. More extensive dissemination, producing a varicella-like eruption (generalized herpes zoster), occurs in 2 to 10 percent of unselected patients with localized zoster, most of whom have immunologic defects due to acquired immunodeficiency as seen with HIV infection,[9,12] underlying malignancy (particularly lymphomas), and immunosuppressive therapy.[9,12,45–50,80,84–87,108,110,112,114–123,154]

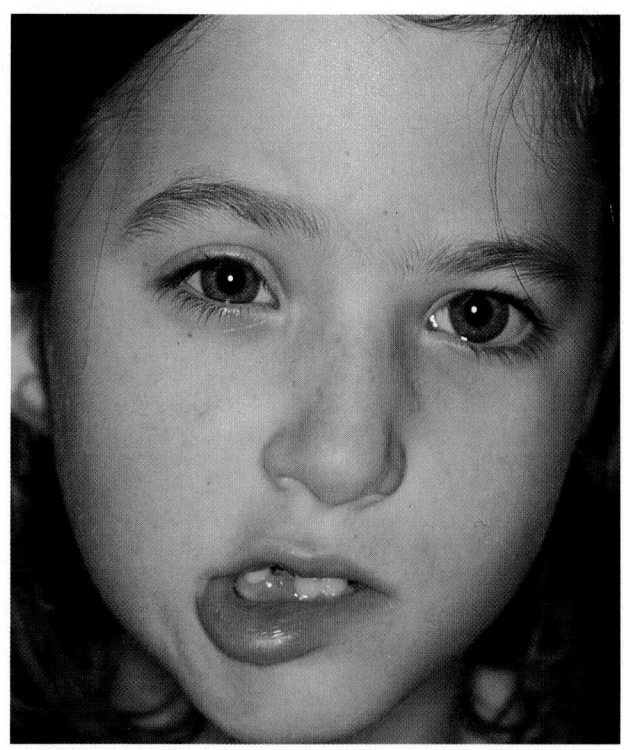

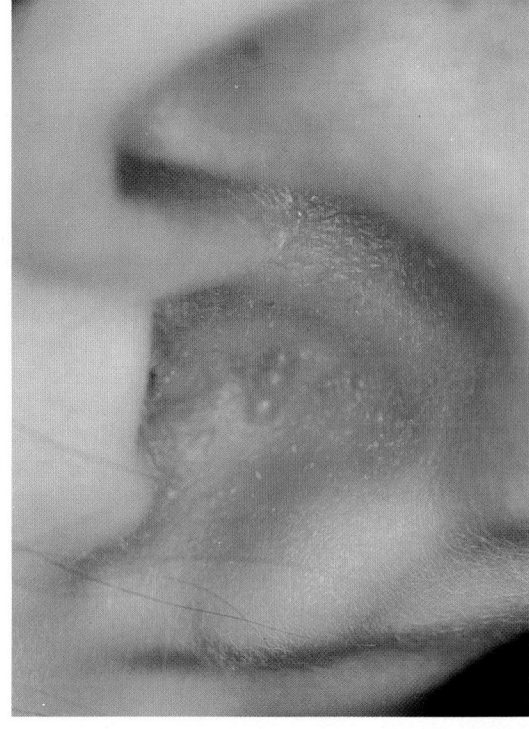

a   *b*

FIGURE 204-6 Cephalic herpes zoster: Ramsay-Hunt syndrome. An 11-year-old girl with (*a*) left-sided facial palsy and (*b*) vesicles involving only her left ear; the patient experienced no pain.

On rare occasions, most often in children, infection disseminates widely from a small, painless area of zoster.[50] In such cases, the herpes zoster may go unnoticed, and the disseminated eruption be mistaken for varicella. This probably explains some reported second attacks of varicella as well as some of the cases of "atypical generalized zoster" (a disseminated varicella-like eruption without an accompanying dermatomal rash in a person with a history of varicella) reported primarily in immunocompromised patients.[105,207] However, symptomatic reinfections do occur, espe-cially in immunocompromised patients and in people whose initial infection was modified by passively acquired antibody to VZV[14,97] (see above). These patients may have a prolonged incubation period and probably account for the majority of the cases of "atypical generalized zoster" observed in immunocompromised and apparently normal patients.[105,185]

Motor paralysis is reported in 1 to 5 percent of patients with herpes zoster. It results from the direct extension of infection from the sensory ganglion to adjacent parts of the nervous system.[26,28,103,157,166,180,183,184,186,187] Mild motor deficits are often missed in thoracolumbar zoster, but when zoster involves the cranial nerves or the extremities, the incidence of recognized motor involvement is 10 to 20 percent.[111]

Paralysis usually begins within 2 weeks of the onset of the rash and almost always involves muscle groups with innervation that is contiguous with that of the affected dermatome; oculomotor and facial palsies are seen with cephalic zoster, unilateral diaphragmatic paralysis with homolateral cervical zoster, paralysis of the trunk and limbs with zoster involving corresponding dermatomes, and dysfunction of the bladder and anus with sacral zoster.[26,28,103,157,180,183,184,186–191] Total or functional recovery occurs in most cases. Rare cases in which the involved myotome and dermatome are widely separated may be the result of more extensive myelitis.[111,187,192] Herpes zoster myelitis, with detection of VZV in the spinal cord or cerebrospinal fluid, has been reported both in typical herpes zoster and in zoster sine herpete.[192a,216]

TABLE 204-2
Complications of Herpes Zoster

Cutaneous	Visceral	Neurologic
Bacterial superinfection	Pneumonitis	Postherpetic neuralgia
Scarring	Hepatitis	Meningoencephalitis
Zoster gangrenosum	Esophagitis	Transverse myelitis
Cutaneous dissemination	Gastritis	Peripheral nerve palsies
	Pericarditis	Motor
	Cystitis	Autonomic
	Arthritis	Cranial nerve palsies
		Sensory loss
		Deafness
		Ocular complications
		Granulomatous angiitis
		(causing contralateral
		hemiparesis)

Posterior nerve roots contain sensory fibers originating in the viscera as well as the skin, which explains the occasional occurrence of visceral lesions in patients with herpes zoster. The affected viscera usually have innervation corresponding to the infected dermatome. Thus, vesicular lesions in the gastric mucosa have been observed in patients with thoracic herpes zoster,[193] and herpes zoster hemicystitis has frequently been observed in association with sacral herpes zoster.[194,195]

Although a lymphocytic pleocytosis, with or without an increase in the concentration of protein in the cerebrospinal fluid, is a regular feature of uncomplicated herpes zoster, the incidence of acute symptomatic meningoencephalitis and myelitis is low (0.2 to 0.5 percent). When these complications do occur, their onset usually follows that of herpes zoster by 7 to 10 days but may precede the rash by a week or more or follow it by up to 2 months.[111,196–200] Clinical manifestations include fever, altered sensorium (frequently with delirium and hallucinations), headache, meningismus, and cranial or extracranial nerve palsies, often at a cord level corresponding to the rash. There is a lymphocytic cerebrospinal fluid pleocytosis, with the cell count usually ranging from 10 to 500/mm^3, a moderate elevation in protein concentration, and a normal glucose concentration. However, the cell count occasionally exceeds 1000/mm^3, there may be 30 to 40 percent neutrophils, and the sugar concentration may be low. The incidence of meningoencephalitis appears to be increased in cranial zoster and in immunocompromised patients, and most cases occur in association with VZV dissemination.[110,200] Most patients recover and return to their pre-encephalitis cognitive status, but many are left with postherpetic neuralgia, chronic ophthalmologic infections, and motor palsies. Most cases probably represent actual VZV infection, with virus reaching the CNS by the hematogenous route in the course of disseminated herpes zoster or by direct extension from the involved sensory ganglion.[110,111,166,196,200]

Another complication of herpes zoster, which is being recognized with increasing frequency, is granulomatous angiitis of cerebral arteries, which is responsible for a syndrome of ophthalmic zoster and delayed contralateral hemiplegia.[201–203] It usually occurs weeks to months after the episode of ophthalmic zoster (average interval about 8 weeks) and may present as an isolated cerebral infarction, multiple cerebral infarctions, stroke-in-evolution, or transient ischemic attacks. Because the clinical manifestations are similar to hypertensive strokes and the delayed onset may obscure the relationship to herpes zoster, the syndrome is probably underdiagnosed. Cerebral arteriograms usually reveal segmental narrowing or occlusion of cerebral arteries ipsilateral to the ophthalmic zoster. Although multiple strokes may occur for several weeks, later recurrences are rare and the disease appears to be self-limited. The mortality in reported cases is about 15 percent.

Herpes Zoster in the Immunocompromised Host   Infection with the HIV, certain types of malignancy, especially Hodgkin's disease and lymphocytic leukemia, and the administration of immunosuppressive therapy (e.g., radiation, antimetabolites, antilymphocyte serum, and corticosteroids) to patients with malignant and nonmalignant diseases markedly increase the incidence and severity of herpes zoster.[1,2,8,10,12,102–106,110,114–120,204,205,207] In fact, serious complications of herpes zoster occur predominantly in such immunocompromised patients. From 20 to 50 percent of patients with Hodgkin's disease develop herpes zoster, with the highest incidence in patients with far-advanced disease and those receiving radiation and combination chemotherapy (Fig. 204-7).[102–106,115–117] In a review of 766 VZV infections in 740 cancer patients, it was noted that the greatest risk of infection was among patients with leukemia or lymphoma. The risk of dissemination of VZV was markedly increased in patients with active tumor

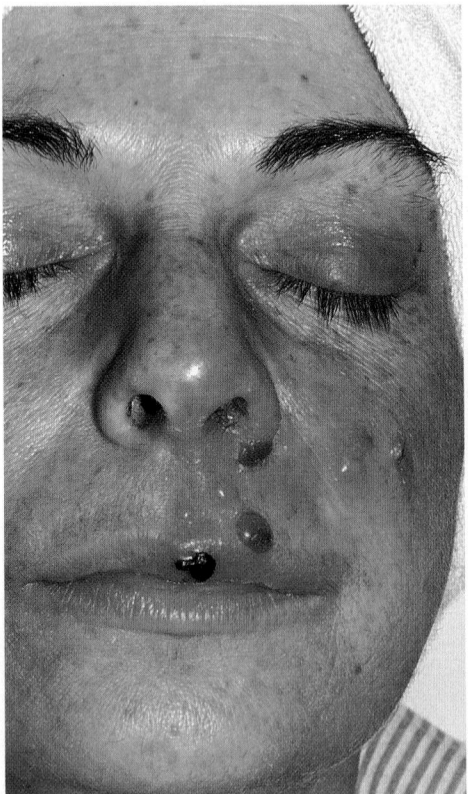
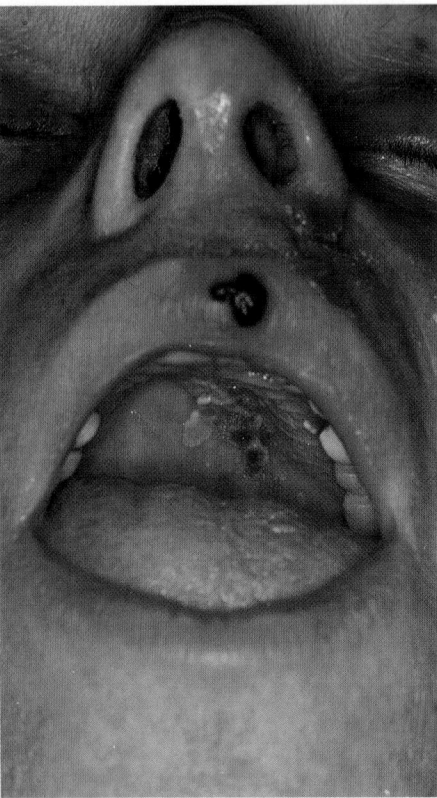

a   *b*

FIGURE 204-7   Herpes zoster, maxillary branch of cranial nerve VII. A 43-year-old female undergoing chemotherapy for lymphoma experienced extensive, painful herpes zoster of her (*a*) facial skin and (*b*) oral mucosa.

at the time of infection. When zoster occurred in these patients, it was usually within 1 month of chemotherapy or within 7 months of x-ray therapy.[204] The severity of zoster is also increased in immunocompromised patients—necrosis of skin and scarring are fairly common, as is postherpetic neuralgia, and the incidence of cutaneous dissemination is 25 to 50 percent. Approximately 10 percent of patients with disseminated cutaneous lesions develop widespread, often fatal visceral infection, particularly of the lungs, liver, and brain.[30,33,114,153,154,196,206] The incidence and severity of herpes zoster are also markedly increased in immunosuppressed recipients of solid organ and bone marrow transplants.[107,120,122,123,207] Twenty to 40 percent of bone marrow transplant recipients develop herpes zoster within 1 year of transplantation.[80,120,123,207] Disseminated infection, often without a dermatomal rash, is common, as is postherpetic neuralgia, scarring, and bacterial superinfection. Subclinical reactivation of VZV is also common in these patients and is frequently responsible for restoring their cell-mediated immunity to VZV.[80,108,120]

The incidence of herpes zoster is markedly increased in persons infected with HIV; it tends to occur early in the course and is often the first sign of their HIV infection.[6,7] Herpes zoster tends to recur in HIV-infected patients as their disease progresses, usually in another dermatome, and patients with AIDS may have severe herpes zoster with cutaneous and visceral dissemination.[1-3,9-12] Patients with AIDS and herpes zoster also tend to have chronic persistent cutaneous lesions that often have unusual morphologies. When these verrucous, hyperkeratotic, and ecthymatous lesions are biopsied, they show changes consistent with VZV infection and yield VZV when cultured.[3,5,8-12]

A syndrome resembling progressive multifocal leukoencephalopathy (PML) has been reported following herpes zoster in two immunocompromised patients.[208] Both patients exhibited steadily progressive, asymmetric, multifocal neurologic deficits, including impaired mental function and focal seizures, and died after several months. At autopsy, there were multifocal lesions, primarily at the gray-white cortical junction, with demyelination, necrosis, and eosinophilic Cowdry type A intranuclear inclusion bodies in oligodendrocytes, neurons, and astrocytes. Herpesvirus-like particles and VZV antigens were detected in these cells. A remarkable feature of these two cases was the long interval (9 to 20 months) between the episode of herpes zoster and the onset of neurologic symptoms. This, as well as the long interval between ophthalmic zoster and the onset of symptoms in patients with granulomatous angiitis, suggests that in addition to latent infections, VZV can produce prolonged "smoldering" subclinical infections, especially in patients lacking the normal defenses that eliminate virus-infected cells and prevent cell-to-cell spread of VZV infection.

The presence or absence of a normal humoral response to VZV does not appear to be a major determinant of the response of these patients to herpes zoster. Rather, cellular immunity, as measured by lymphocyte blastogenesis and interferon production following exposure to VZV antigens, appears to be a major correlate of the host's capacity to limit VZV replication and dissemination.[49,73,76,80,83–87,106,120–123,207]

Pathology

The cutaneous lesions of varicella and herpes zoster are histologically indistinguishable and are similar to those produced by herpes simplex virus. The characteristic changes in infected cells, which can be observed in tissue culture as well as in vivo, are "ballooning degeneration," with the formation of intranuclear inclusion bodies and multinucleated giant cells.[18,22] Individual infected cells become greatly enlarged with pale vacuolated cytoplasm. The nuclei exhibit margination of chromatin and contain inclusion bodies. Early in infection, the inclusion bodies may be homogeneous and moderately basophilic and they often fill the nucleus. However, they rapidly evolve into sharply demarcated acidophilic (eosinophilic) inclusion bodies that are separated from the deeply basophilic ring of marginated chromatin at the nuclear membrane by a clear zone or halo. Multinucleated giant cells are formed primarily by the fusion of adjacent infected cells.[65] Cell fusion, which is mediated by viral glycoproteins that appear on cell membranes early in the VZV replication cycle, facilitates cell-to-cell spread of infection, even in the presence of antibody capable of neutralizing extracellular virus. Neither multinucleated giant cells nor intranuclear inclusion bodies are found in the vesicular lesions caused by poxviruses (smallpox, vaccinia) or enteroviruses (echoviruses, Coxsackie viruses).

Pathology of Varicella

The initial event in the formation of the cutaneous lesions of varicella is probably infection of capillary endothelial cells in the papillary dermis, with subsequent spread of virus to epithelial cells in the epidermis, hair follicles, and sebaceous glands.[18,20–22,64,65,209] In early papular lesions, the epithelium is slightly elevated due to swelling of the infected epithelial cells and to edema and vascular congestion of the underlying dermis. In the superficial dermis, capillary endothelial cells are swollen, and their nuclei often contain intranuclear inclusion bodies. Similar inclusion bodies may be seen in the nuclei of fibroblasts in the surrounding connective tissue, which is edematous and infiltrated by small numbers of mononuclear cells. Superficial lymphatics are dilated, and cells lining these structures are also swollen and may contain intranuclear inclusion bodies. In the epidermis, the cells initially involved are those of the germinal layer and the deeper portion of the stratum spinosum. These cells show ballooning degeneration with loss of intercellular bridges and are soon separated by intercellular edema (acantholysis). A few small multinucleated giant cells, containing three to eight nuclei, are usually seen at the base and periphery of these early epithelial lesions. The papular lesions rapidly evolve into intraepidermal vesicles as a result of the infection and degeneration of increasing numbers of epithelial cells, the fusion of adjacent areas of microscopic degeneration, and the continuing influx of edema fluid which elevates the uninvolved stratum corneum to form a delicate clear vesicle (Fig. 204-8a). At this stage, the vesicle fluid contains fibrin, degenerating and "ballooned" epithelial cells, and abundant cell-free infectious VZV. Multinucleated giant cells with eosinophilic intranuclear inclusion bodies are readily found in the walls and base of the vesicle (Fig. 204-8b). As the lesions progress, polymorphonuclear leukocytes and a small number of macrophages invade from the underlying dermis, and the vesicle fluid becomes cloudy; this transforms the vesicle into a pustule. The fluid is then absorbed, with the formation of a flat adherent crust that is eventually detached by the regrowth of subjacent epithelial cells. The evolution from papule to early crusting can occur over a period of 8 to 12 h. Lesions of uncomplicated varicella usually heal without scarring. Lesions in mucous membranes develop in the same way, but the thin roof of the vesicle breaks down quickly, producing a shallow ulcer that heals rapidly.

In fatal varicella, focal lesions have been found in the mucous membranes of the respiratory, gastrointestinal, and genitourinary tracts; in the serosa of the pleural and peritoneal cavities; and in the

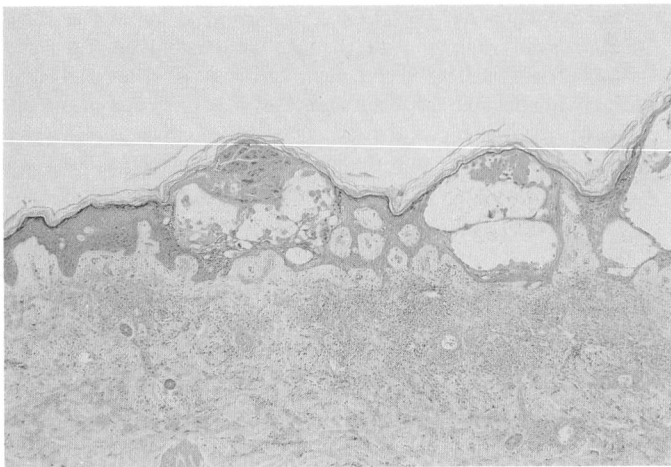

a

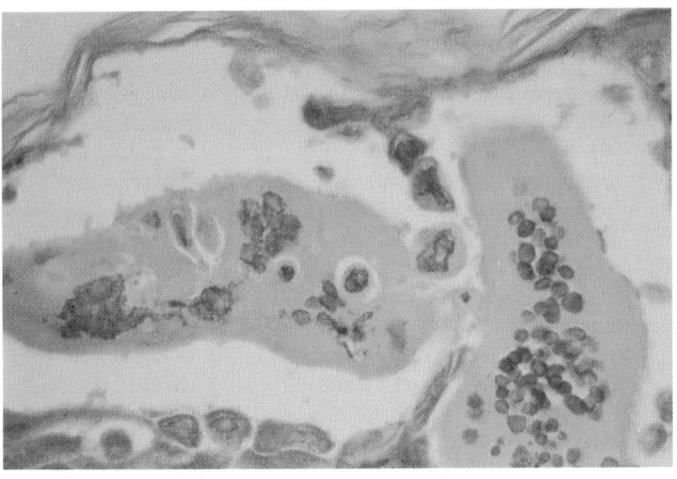

b

FIGURE 204-8 Herpes zoster, histopathology.
(*a*) intraepidermal vesicle, acantholysis, reticular
degeneration; underlying dermis shows edema and
vasculitis. (*b*) Multinucleated giant cells with characteristic
nuclear changes. (*Courtesy of Dr. Danielle Bouffard.*)

parenchyma of virtually every organ, the lungs being the most
common site of severe involvement.[22,64–66,129,143,144,157,210–212]
There is widespread vascular damage, with characteristic acidophilic intranuclear inclusion bodies in the endothelial cells lining
small blood vessels and lymphatics; capillaries within individual
lesions are often destroyed, resulting in thrombosis and hemorrhage. In varicella pneumonia, the pleura are studded with hemorrhagic nodules, and the lungs show widely disseminated interstitial
pneumonia with numerous foci of hemorrhagic necrosis. Alveoli
are filled with red blood cells, fibrin, inclusion-bearing mononuclear cells, and occasional multinucleated giant cells. Hyalin membranes are frequently seen. Typical acidophilic inclusion bodies are
also seen within hyperplastic alveolar septal cells, swollen capillary
endothelial cells, fibroblasts, and bronchiolar and tracheobronchial
epithelial cells. Similar areas of vascular damage and focal necrosis
are found in the parenchyma of the liver, spleen, and other organs
throughout the body. In some cases, characteristic intranuclear inclusion bodies may be nearly or totally absent, in spite of unmistakable clinical and pathologic evidence of extensive VZV infection
and the isolation of VZV from the liver, lungs, brain, and other
tissues.[144,211,212]

There is now compelling evidence that (except for Reye's syndrome) the central nervous system complications of varicella and
herpes zoster (see below) are the direct result of VZV infection,
rather than autoimmune demyelination, as previously thought by
many observers.[111,171]

Pathology of Herpes Zoster

Although the histopathology of the skin lesions of herpes zoster and
varicella is the same, herpes zoster is accompanied by acute inflammation of the corresponding sensory nerve and ganglion. The ganglion shows intense lymphocyte infiltration, necrosis of nerve cells
and fibers, endothelial cell proliferation and lymphocytic cuffing of
small vessels, focal hemorrhage, and inflammation of the ganglion
sheath.[26,28] Satellite cells and neurons contain characteristic acidophilic intranuclear inclusion bodies, virus particles visible by electron microscopy, and VZV antigens demonstrable by immunofluorescence.[22,30,32–35,103] Some degree of neuronal degeneration and
lymphocytic infiltration is also generally present in adjacent ganglia
on the same side. The peripheral nerve shows diffuse lymphocytic
infiltration and focal hemorrhage, with axonal degeneration and
demyelination of sensory fibers. Virus particles and VZV antigens
are present in Schwann and perineural cells. These inflammatory
and degenerative changes can be traced distally to branches inner-
vating the affected skin.[31] The inflammatory reaction in the ganglion also extends proximally to the posterior nerve root and into

adjacent regions of the cord or brainstem, producing a segmental myelitis that is predominantly unilateral and involves the posterior more than the anterior horns. There is degeneration of nerve fibers in the posterior columns and inflammatory changes in the gray matter of the posterior and anterior horns, with perivenous lymphocytic infiltration, scattered neuronal necrosis, and neuronophagia. These changes may extend two or more segments from the one corresponding to the cutaneous eruption. A mild lymphocytic leptomeningitis is generally present and is most intense over the involved segments and nerve roots. Marked inflammation and degeneration of the anterior nerve root within the meninges and in the portion contiguous to the involved sensory ganglion may also be present, producing a true motor radiculitis.[28] When extensive, the acute inflammatory response is followed by fibrosis of the ganglion and nerve.[26] These observations, as well as the isolation of VZV from sensory ganglion,[34,35,213] cerebrospinal fluid,[106,192a,197,214,215] and CNS tissue[196,208,216] indicate that the pathologic changes in herpes zoster are the direct result of VZV infection.

Herpes zoster is occasionally complicated by meningoencephalitis or myelitis, in which CNS involvement is not restricted to segments corresponding to the involved dermatome.[111] The pathologic findings in herpes zoster meningoencephalitis vary from focal mononuclear cell infiltration of the leptomeninges[103,199] to acute necrotizing encephalitis with perivenous encephalomalacia, myelin and axonal degeneration, macrophage infiltration, and typical intranuclear inclusion bodies and virus particles in oligodendrocytes, neurons, and astrocytes.[196] The presence of VZV in the involved brain tissue has been documented by virus isolation and immunoperoxidase staining in several of these patients.[196,208] Herpes zoster myelitis is rarely fatal, but in two patients who died of pulmonary embolism 12 days and 12 weeks, respectively, after the onset of herpes zoster, autopsy revealed extensive inflammatory necrosis of the spinal cord, which was maximal at the level of the dermatomal rash and extended above and below in a continuous but irregular pattern that did not correspond to any vascular topography.[192,216] In areas of most recent extension where necrosis was less complete, intranuclear inclusion bodies were present in glial nuclei.[216] VZV has also been identified in the cerebrospinal fluid of a number of patients with herpes zoster meningoencephalitis and myelitis.[106,172,197,200,208,214,215] In herpes zoster myelitis, it seems clear that VZV reaches the spinal cord by direct extension from the infected dorsal root ganglion. The pathogenesis of herpes zoster encephalitis (or meningoencephalitis) is more obscure. The presence of perivascular mononuclear cell infiltrates and demyelination, and the lack of direct evidence of VZV infection in autopsied cases, has led many observers to favor a postinfectious (autoimmune) encephalomyelitis[111] like that observed in measles encephalomyelitis.[167] However, there is now much evidence that most or all of the CNS complications of herpes zoster are the direct result of VZV infection of the tissues involved, and that the demyelination observed in herpes zoster encephalitis can be accounted for by VZV infection of oligodendrocytes.[208] The common occurrence of herpes zoster encephalitis or meningoencephalitis in association with disseminated herpes zoster suggests that virus often reaches the brain as a result of viremia.[110,111,200] However, it may also reach the brain along neural routes, especially when meningoencephalitis occurs in association with herpes zoster of cranial dermatomes.[200,208,216]

The contralateral hemiplegia that sometimes develops in patients with ophthalmic herpes zoster appears to be caused by segmental granulomatous angiitis involving ipsilateral cerebral arteries.[201–203,217,218] The temporal association with herpes zoster and the electron microscopic observation of herpesvirus-like particles in the walls of involved vessels and in adjacent glial cells[183,217,219,220] suggest that the angiitis is due to VZV infection of arterial walls. The virus may reach the vessels by direct spread from the trigeminal ganglion or along branches of the ophthalmic nerve that supply the meninges and most of the intracranial arteries that have been involved.[221]

Lesions of the skin, lungs, and other organs in fatal cases of disseminated herpes zoster are identical to those observed in fatal cases of varicella.[30,64–66,114,129,143,144,206,210,212] They result from the viremic spread of VZV in both diseases.[62,67,73,75,112]

Clinical and Laboratory Diagnoses

Clinical Diagnosis of Varicella

Varicella can usually be diagnosed clinically on the basis of the character and evolution of the rash, particularly when there is a history of exposure within the preceding 2 to 3 weeks.[127,129,157] Characteristic diagnostic features include (1) the development, after a brief and mild (or absent) prodrome, of a papulovesicular eruption accompanied by fever and mild constitutional symptoms; (2) the appearance of lesions in crops, with a predominantly central distribution including the scalp; (3) the rapid evolution of individual lesions from macules to papules to delicate thin-walled vesicles to pustules and, finally, to crusts; (4) the presence of lesions in all stages of development in any one anatomic area throughout the acute disease; and (5) the presence of lesions in the mucous membranes of the mouth.

Severe varicella, especially in immunosuppressed patients, may resemble smallpox or generalized vaccinia. Conversely, generalized vaccinia may be confused with varicella, especially in patients with immunologic defects or eczema. Since the distinction between varicella and these poxvirus infections cannot be made with certainty on clinical grounds, prompt laboratory diagnosis is required. However, the eradication of smallpox and the consequent cessation of smallpox vaccination has virtually eliminated this diagnostic problem.

Disseminated herpes simplex may occasionally resemble varicella, especially in the neonate, in immunosuppressed patients, and in patients with eczema. However, the distribution of lesions is rarely typical of varicella, and there is often an obvious concentration of lesions at the site of the primary or recurrent infection (e.g., the mouth or external genitalia). Marked toxicity and encephalitis are more common in neonatal herpes simplex than in neonatal varicella. The histopathology of lesions caused by herpes simplex virus (HSV) and VZV is indistinguishable. Thus differentiation of the two requires virus isolation or the detection and identification of viral antigens or nucleic acids in the lesions.

Other diseases that may be confused with varicella include impetigo, the vesicular exanthems of Coxsackie virus and echovirus infections (e.g., hand-foot-and-mouth disease syndrome), rickettsialpox, insect bites, papular urticaria, scabies, contact dermatitis, dermatitis herpetiformis, drug eruptions, secondary syphilis, and erythema multiforme. The character, distribution, and evolution of the lesions, together with a careful epidemiologic history, usually differentiate these diseases from varicella.[129,157] When any doubt exists, the clinical impression should receive laboratory confirmation.

Clinical Diagnosis of Herpes Zoster

In the preeruptive stage, herpes zoster is easily confused with other causes of pain such as pleurisy, myocardial infarction, cholecystitis, appendicitis, renal colic, or collapsed intervertebral disk. Sometimes the early appearance of regional lymphadenopathy and localized cutaneous sensory abnormalities (e.g., hyperesthesia, dysesthesia) provide a clue to the diagnosis. When the eruption appears, the diagnosis is almost always obvious.

Zosteriform herpes simplex is often impossible to distinguish from herpes zoster on clinical grounds. A history of multiple recurrences at the same site is common in herpes simplex but exceedingly rare in herpes zoster. Virus isolation or the identification of VZV (or HSV) antigens or nucleic acids in material obtained from the lesions is the only reliable means of differentiating these entities.

Contact dermatitis, burns, vaccinia autoinoculation, and localized bacterial skin infections may occasionally resemble herpes zoster, but a careful history and examination of the lesions (including a Tzanck smear with the identification of multinucleated giant cells and intranuclear inclusion bodies) will eliminate any confusion.

Disseminated herpes zoster may be mistaken for varicella when there is widespread dissemination of VZV from a small painless area of zoster or from the affected sensory ganglion in the absence of an obvious dermatomal eruption.[50,105,108,207] This is not infrequent in profoundly immunosuppressed peropositive persons, such as bone marrow transplant recipients.[105,108,207]

Laboratory Diagnosis

Routine laboratory determinations are not helpful in the diagnosis of either varicella or herpes zoster. Asymptomatic elevations in serum levels of alanine aminotransferase (ALT) and aspartate aminotransferase (AST) occur in the majority of children and adults with uncomplicated varicella.[70–72,140] They are highest during the first week of illness, rarely exceed 5 times the upper limit of normal, and resolve in 1 to 4 weeks.

The lesions of varicella and herpes zoster are indistinguishable by histopathology and both contain VZV virions, VZV antigens, and VZV nucleic acids. The presence of multinucleated giant cells and epithelial cells containing acidophilic intranuclear inclusion bodies distinguishes the cutaneous lesions produced by VZV from all other vesicular skin lesions except those produced by HSV. These cells can be demonstrated in Tzanck smears prepared at the bedside; material is scraped from the base of an early vesicle and stained with hematoxylin-eosin, Giemsa's, Papanicolaou's, or Paragon Multiple stain.[222,223] Every physician should become familiar with this simple diagnostic procedure and employ it in the initial evaluation of any patient with a vesicular eruption. Punch biopsies provide more reliable material for histologic examination than Tzanck smears and facilitate diagnosis in the prevesicular stage.[209] Sputum from patients with varicella pneumonia may contain desquamated respiratory epithelial cells with acidophilic intranuclear inclusion bodies, but such cells are also found in patients with pneumonia caused by measles virus and in patients with respiratory tract infections caused by HSV. The identification of herpesvirus particles in vesicle fluid or biopsy material by electron microscopy provides another means of diagnosis.[224] However, neither electron microscopy nor Tzanck smears can distinguish VZV from HSV infections.

The definitive diagnosis of VZV infection, as well as the differentiation of VZV from HSV, is accomplished by the isolation of virus in cell cultures inoculated with vesicle fluid, blood, cerebrospinal fluid or infected tissue, or by the direct identification of VZV antigens or nucleic acids in these specimens.[43,58,108,209,225,226] Virus isolation is the only technique that yields infectious VZV for further analysis, e.g., determination of its sensitivity to antiviral drugs. However, VZV is extremely labile and, except in vesicle fluid, is highly cell-associated, and this adversely affects the sensitivity of virus isolation procedures. Specimens should be inoculated into cell culture immediately. Vesicle fluid is inoculated directly and tissue specimens are minced or trypsinized, rather than homogenized, to ensure inoculation of viable cells. It is important to select new vesicles containing clear fluid for aspiration because the probability of isolating VZV diminishes rapidly as lesions become pustular. VZV is almost never isolated from crusts. In immunocompetent persons, lesions are usually virus-positive for the first 3 days in varicella and for up to a week in herpes zoster. Virus is readily isolated for longer periods in immunocompromised patients.

VZV can be isolated and propagated in vitro in monolayer cultures of a variety of human (and certain simian) cells.[22,58,229] The cytopathic effect in such cell cultures is characterized by the formation of acidophilic intranuclear inclusion bodies and multinucleated giant cells similar to those seen in the cutaneous lesions of the disease. These changes are indistinguishable from those produced by HSV, but whereas HSV is released into the medium by initially infected cells and rapidly spreads to infect the remaining cells in the culture, the cytopathic effect of VZV remains focal. This is because infectious VZV remains cell-associated and is not released into the medium by the initially infected cells; infection proceeds from cell to cell only by direct contact, and the initial foci of infection gradually enlarge. Serial passage of VZV in tissue culture requires the transfer of infected cells. Cytopathic effects of VZV are generally not apparent until several days after specimen inoculation.

A rapid and specific diagnosis can be achieved by identifying VZV antigens or nucleic acids in vesicle fluid, in cells scraped or swabbed from the base of vesicles or ulcers, in crusts, or in tissue obtained by biopsy. Viral antigens can be demonstrated in vesicle fluid or extracts of crusts by countercurrent immunoelectrophoresis (CIE) using antiserum to VZV.[230] Immunofluorescence or immunoperoxidase staining of cellular material from fresh vesicles or prevesicular lesions is a useful diagnostic technique in experienced hands; it can identify individual infected cells and structures and can detect VZV antigens relatively late in the disease when cultures are no longer positive.[32,35,58,209,227,231] Enzyme immunoassays provide another rapid and sensitive method for antigen detection.[226,232] Monoclonal antibodies have improved the specificity of these techniques, but it is always important to examine aliquots of each specimen with antisera to VZV, HSV-1, HSV-2, and control antigen in parallel, together with positive and negative virus-infected tissue controls.

Serologic tests can provide a retrospective diagnosis of varicella and herpes zoster when acute and convalescent sera are available for comparison and can also identify susceptible individuals who may be candidates for isolation or prophylaxis. The widely available complement fixation (CF) test suffers from two disadvantages: (1) a rise in CF titer to VZV or HSV is not diagnostic if antibody to both viruses increases, because infection by either virus can induce a heterologous anamnestic response; and (2) the CF antibody titer drops within months after varicella infection and may reach undetectable levels. Thus, many adults who are immune to varicella may be CF antibody-negative. Consequently, the CF test is not useful for distinguishing between immune and susceptible adults.[14,25,58,225] Indirect fluorescent antibody tests have problems of specificity similar to those of the CF test.[58,225] VZV neutralization tests are both sensitive and specific but are time consuming and technically demanding and are available only in research laboratories. A number of more sensitive techniques have been developed to measure humoral responses to VZV.[25,58,225] These include an immunofluorescence assay for antibody to VZV-induced membrane antigens (FAMA)[89,90,233] that distinguishes immune from susceptible adults; an immune adherence hemagglutination assay (IAHA), which is slightly less sensitive than the FAMA assay[234]; a rapid ^{125}I-labeled staphylococcal protein A radioimmunoassay, which is more sensitive and easier to perform than the FAMA assay[235]; enzyme-linked immunosorbent assays (ELISA), which are slightly less sensitive and specific than the FAMA assay in their ability to distinguish immune from susceptible adults, but which are simpler to perform[52,92,236,237]; and a solid-phase radioimmunoassay (RIA) for measuring VZV-specific IgG, IgM, and IgA responses.[77,93] In addition, measurement of the in vitro proliferative response of peripheral blood lymphocytes to VZV antigens[80,81,93] correlates well with immunity as measured by FAMA, RIA, and ELISA, and a VZV skin test has been widely and successfully used in Japan to distinguish between immune and susceptible individuals.[80,82,94,239] With all these assays, adequate controls are required to deal with the problem of heterotypic responses to infections by other herpesviruses.[14,25,58,79,225]

Seroconversion to VZV is indicative of varicella. However, if the "acute" serum is obtained late, it may already contain detectable antibody to VZV, and it may then only be possible to demonstate an increase (≥fourfold) in antibody titer.

Most immunocompetent patients with herpes zoster show an anamnestic increase in humoral and cell-mediated immunity to VZV,[77,93,97,107,108a,109] but this may fail to occur in immunocompromised patients. Antibody to VZV appears in the cerebrospinal fluid of most patients with herpes zoster meningoencephalitis, presumably as a result of intrathecal synthesis.[172] As in the case of herpes simplex encephalitis, this may provide a useful means for retrospective diagnosis.

The presence of VZV-specific IgM antibody is indicative of recent active infection, but it can be induced by exogenous reexposure or by asymptomatic "contained reversions" of latent VZV (Fig. 204-2), as well as by symptomatic varicella and herpes zoster.[77,79,93,109]

Treatment

Treatment of Varicella

Three antiviral chemotherapeutic agents, acyclovir [9-(2-hydroxyethoxymethyl)guanine, acycloguanosine], vidarabine (9-β-D-arabinofuranosyladenine, adenine arabinoside), and foscarnet (phosphonoformic acid), as well as human interferon-α, have shown efficacy in VZV infections.[239–242] Acyclovir, a guanosine analogue, is selectively phosphorylated by HSV and VZV thymidine kinases (it is a poor substrate for cellular thymidine kinase) and is thus concentrated in infected cells. Cellular enzymes then convert acyclovir monophosphate to acyclovir triphosphate, which

interferes with viral DNA synthesis by inhibiting viral DNA polymerase.[243] At therapeutic concentrations, acyclovir is remarkably nontoxic, with no observed effects on hematopoietic precursor cells or the immune system.[239–242] Vidarabine, a purine nucleoside analogue, is phosphorylated by cellular kinases to vidarabine triphosphate, which appears to inhibit herpesvirus DNA polymerases to a greater extent than cellular DNA polymerases.[239–242,244] Despite its clinical efficacy, vidarabine has drawbacks. It is not a selective inhibitor of virus replication (vidarabine triphosphate also inhibits cellular DNA polymerases) and thus is potentially cytotoxic. Its low solubility requires that it be administered in large volumes of fluid.[239–242] Foscarnet is an organic analogue of inorganic pyrophosphate that inhibits replication of all known herpesviruses in vitro. It exerts its antiviral activity through selective inhibition at the pyrophosphate binding site on virus-specific DNA polymerases and reverse transcriptases at concentrations that do not affect cellular DNA polymerases. Foscarnet does not require phosphorylation by thymidine kinase in order to be activated and therefore is active against VZV mutants that lack thymidine kinase activity and are resistant to acyclovir therapy.[245] Several reports have demonstrated altered or deficient thymidine kinase activity of VZV isolates in patients with HIV disease on long-term suppressive doses of acyclovir.[2–5,10] It appears that long-term low-dose acyclovir treatment selects for resistant strains of VZV in these patients who have shown good response to intravenous foscarnet therapy at 40 mg/kg every 8 h.[4]

In normal children, varicella is generally benign and self-limited. Cool compresses or calamine lotion locally, and antihistamines orally, may help control the intense pruritus of the rash. Tepid baths with baking soda (1/4 cup per tub of water) may also relieve itching. Creams and lotions containing corticosteroids and occlusive ointments should not be used. Antipyretics are rarely indicated, and it has been recommended that salicylates be avoided because of their possible association with Reye's syndrome.[162,246] Fingernails should be kept short and clean to minimize secondary skin infections and the scarring that may result from scratching. Recent studies of acyclovir treatment of healthy children 2 to 12 years of age have found that early treatment (within 24 h of the appearance of rash) with oral acyclovir (20 mg/kg four times a day for 5 days) reduced the duration and severity of chickenpox and led to early defervescence.[247–249] Recently, the Antiviral Advisory Committee of the United States Food and Drug Administration (FDA) recommended licensure of oral acyclovir for the treatment of chickenpox in the normal child and adolescent; however, to date this indication for use of acyclovir has not been approved.[250]

Normal adults frequently experience severe primary infections with VZV and have a relatively high incidence of visceral involvement and varicella pneumonia. It is reasonable to think that this subset of patients may also benefit from acyclovir therapy. A recent randomized, placebo-controlled trial of oral acyclovir in healthy adults with primary varicella infections showed that early treatment (within 24 h of onset of cutaneous lesions) with oral acyclovir (800 mg five times a day for 7 days) significantly reduced time to crusting of lesions, extent of disease, duration of symptoms, and fever.[251] Another subset of adults who might benefit from treatment of primary varicella infections is pregnant women, particularly those with exposure to varicella during the perinatal period; however, data concerning treatment of primary varicella infections in pregnant women is currently unavailable, and treatment guidelines for VZV infections in these patients have not been established.[248]

Complications are most often due to bacterial superinfection. Bacterial infections of local lesions are treated with warm soaks. Systemic antimicrobial drugs are indicated for bacterial cellulitis, otitis media, sepsis, bacterial meningitis, osteomyelitis, septic arthritis, and bacterial pneumonia. The prominence of *Staphylococcus aureus* and group A beta-hemolytic *Streptococcus* as causes of these complications should be recognized, but therapy should be guided by the results of Gram-stained smears and cultures. Antibiotics are useless in varicella pneumonia unless there is bacterial superinfection.

Varicella pneumonia is rare in normal children but more common in adults. Although it usually responds to supportive measures, including positive-pressure ventilation, antiviral chemotherapy should be used early to inhibit VZV replication. Recent studies of immunocompetent adults with primary VZV infections and VZV pneumonia demonstrated that early treatment (within 36 h of hospitalization) with intravenous acyclovir (5 mg/kg every 8 h) was useful in reducing fever and tachypnea and improved oxygenation in treated patients versus untreated ones.[139,140] Antibiotics are indicated only when bacterial superinfection develops. There is no evidence that corticosteroids are beneficial in this setting and their use is not recommended.

Reye's syndrome must be considered when a child with otherwise uncomplicated varicella develops lethargy, persistent vomiting, and confusion. Early diagnosis with supportive care and aggressive control of increased intracranial pressure and hypoglycemia should reduce the mortality and morbidity of this mysterious complication.

The most common neurologic complication of varicella in normal children is cerebellar ataxia, which is usually self-limited. However, recent evidence that it may be associated with VZV infection of the CNS (see above) suggests that the use of antiviral chemotherapy is warranted. Varicella encephalitis, meningoencephalitis, and myelitis are very rare complications in normal children. However, the evidence that they are the result of CNS VZV infection, rather than of some postinfectious autoimmune mechanism (see above) makes it reasonable to treat them with an antiviral agent. An interesting report in the literature describes a previously healthy woman who became encephalopathic secondary to disseminated VZV a few days after the onset of thoracic zoster and subsequently returned to her baseline neurologic status after 72 h of intravenous acyclovir (30 mg/kg per day). This suggests that encephalitis in VZV infections is related to direct viral infection of the CNS and that early intravenous acyclovir therapy is warranted in this setting.

Hemorrhagic complications should be treated on the basis of the results of coagulation studies and bone marrow examination. It is always important to rule out bacterial sepsis. Because of the possible involvement of VZV-induced endothelial damage in purpura fulminans, especially if this complication occurs when new vesicles are continuing to appear, these patients should receive antiviral chemotherapy.

In contrast to varicella in normal children, varicella in immunocompromised children and adults may be severe and life-threatening. Thus every effort should be made to prevent its occurrence (see "Prevention and Control" below). When this fails, antiviral therapy should be initiated as early in the illness as possible and certainly before there is any clinical evidence of disseminated disease. Patients at risk include those with HIV disease, leukemia, lymphoproliferative disorders, metastatic malignancies, and congenital and acquired immunodeficiency diseases; others at risk are newborns and patients receiving cytotoxic drugs, corticosteroids or other immunosuppressant agents, radiotherapy, or antithymocyte globulin because of organ allografts, nephrotic syndrome, collagen-vascular diseases, etc. The risk is low in patients receiving low-dose alternative-day steroid therapy but is substantial in those receiving higher doses (e.g., 1 to 2 mg/kg per day of prednisone). If possible, cancer chemotherapy should be temporarily interrupted; however, treatment of malignancy should take precedence during induction therapy or therapy for disease in relapse. When treatment is stopped, it should be resumed 21 days after exposure or 7 days after complete crusting of all lesions. Steroids should be tapered during the incubation period, and cytotoxic or other immunosuppressive therapy stopped if possible. However, patients who have received prolonged courses of corticosteroids should continue to receive replacement therapy.

In placebo-controlled therapeutic trials, intravenous acyclovir (500 mg/m^2 each 8 h for 7 days), intravenous vidarabine (10 mg/kg per day over 12 h for 5 days), and parenteral human interferon-α (3.5×10^5 units/kg per day for 2 days, then 1.75×10^5 units/kg per day for 3 days) have all been shown to markedly decrease the incidence of life-threatening visceral complications when administered within 72 h of onset to immunosuppressed patients with varicella.[153,250,252–257] These results, as well as experience gained in open protocols,[258–260] suggest that acyclovir is at least as effective as vidarabine in patients with VZV infections but is free of vidarabine's toxicity and problems of fluid overload. To date there are no comparative trials of acyclovir versus vidarabine treatment for chickenpox,[261] but studies comparing these two agents in treating immunocompromised patients with disseminated or localized zoster have shown that early treatment (within 72 h of rash) with intravenous acyclovir was significantly more effective than vidarabine in preventing dissemination of VZV, preventing complications of VZV, decreasing viral shedding time and length of healing in localized and disseminated VZV infections, and decreasing time to resolution of dermatomal pain.[205,250,262,263] Therefore, current treatment recommendations for primary varicella infection in an immunocompromised host are for intravenous acyclovir at a dose of 500 mg/m^2 every 8 h for 7 to 10 days.[250] Treatment must be initiated early in the disease to be effective, and the dosage must be reduced in patients with renal insufficiency.[241]

A number of new selective antiviral chemotherapeutic agents are currently being evaluated in clinical trials.[240] Treatment with systemic cytosine arabinoside (ara-C) or iododeoxyuridine (IUdR) should not be considered in patients with varicella or its complications. These compounds are toxic and are likely to affect the outcome of the disease adversely, especially in immunosuppressed patients.

Treatment of Herpes Zoster

During the acute phase of herpes zoster, analgesics and the application of cool compresses, calamine lotion, cornstarch, or baking soda may help to alleviate local symptoms and hasten the drying of vesicular lesions. Occlusive ointments should be avoided, and creams and lotions containing corticosteroids should not be used. After the acute phase, a bland ointment or olive oil dressings may help to soften and separate adherent crusts. Bacterial superinfection of local lesions is uncommon and should be treated with warm soaks; bacterial cellulitis requires systemic antibiotic therapy.

The major goals of therapy in patients with herpes zoster are to: (1) limit the extent, duration, and severity of disease in the primary dermatome; (2) prevent disease elsewhere; and (3) prevent postherpetic neuralgia. Since the pathology in the primary dermatome, as well as that responsible for the visceral and CNS complications of herpes zoster, appears to be the consequence of VZV replication, the first two goals can be achieved by limiting VZV replication and spread. If immunity is intact, herpes zoster is usually self-limited and there is rarely significant spread outside of the initially involved dermatome. In contrast, immunocompromised individuals, particularly those with deficiencies in cell-mediated immunity, have more severe and prolonged local disease and a much higher incidence of visceral and CNS complications. Obviously, it is these patients who have the most to gain from effective antiviral therapy.

Acyclovir has proven effective in the early treatment of acute herpes zoster. A randomized double-blind placebo-controlled study in immunocompromised patients with acute herpes zoster showed that acyclovir (500 mg/m^2 intravenously each 8 h for 7 days) halted progression of herpes zoster, both in patients with localized disease and in patients with cutaneous dissemination before treatment.[264] Acyclovir accelerated the rate of clearance of virus from vesicles and markedly reduced the incidence of visceral and progressive cutaneous dissemination. Pain subsided faster in acyclovir recipients, and fewer reported postherpetic neuralgia, but these differences were not statistically significant. No acyclovir toxicity was observed. Studies comparing intravenous acyclovir therapy to vidarabine therapy for the treatment of herpes zoster infections in immunocompromised patients showed that acyclovir was significantly more effective than vidarabine in preventing complications of VZV infection and in decreasing the period of viral shedding, healing time, and time to resolution of acute neuritic pain.[262] Acyclovir was also found to be superior to vidarabine in the treatment of immunocompromised patients with disseminated zoster.[205,250,263] Current recommendations for treatment of zoster in immunocompromised patients is intravenous acyclovir 500 mg/m^2 every 8 h for 7 to 10 days.[250]

The efficacy of vidarabine in immunocompromised patients with acute herpes zoster was established in a double-blind placebo-controlled crossover study[265] and in a randomized double-blind placebo-controlled study.[154] When administered within 72 h of the onset of rash, vidarabine (10 mg/kg intravenously over 12 h each day for 5 days) shortened the period of new vesicle formation, accelerated healing, and reduced the spread of rash over the primary dermatome. Vidarabine also markedly reduced the incidence of cutaneous dissemination and of visceral and CNS complications. Vidarabine did not reduce the incidence of postherpetic neuralgia (45 percent in patients older than 38 years of age) but appeared to reduce its duration and to reduce the duration of acute pain. Due to the increased side effects and decreased efficacy of vidarabine versus acyclovir therapy in immunocompromised patients, current treatment recommendations favor acyclovir as the drug of choice for VZV infections in this setting.

Human interferon-α (1.7 or 5.1×10^5 units/kg per day intramuscularly for 7 days) has also been shown to reduce new vesicle formation, cutaneous and visceral dissemination, and visceral and CNS complications.[266,267] Interferon also appears to reduce the incidence of postherpetic neuralgia. Although reasonably well tolerated in these trials, interferon appears to be somewhat more toxic than vidarabine.[239–242,268]

Nucleoside analogues capable of inhibiting VZV replication have been administered parenterally in attempts to control the multiplication and dissemination of VZV in immunocompromised patients with herpes zoster. Both ara-C and IUdR have proved ineffective and toxic when administered systemically. Immunocompro

mised patients with herpes zoster who have a deficient or delayed antibody response to VZV have an increased incidence of severe disease and dissemination.[49,269,270] This led Stevens and Merigan[271] to conduct a double-blind controlled therapeutic trial of zoster immune globulin (ZIG) in immunocompromised patients with herpes zoster. Despite a much higher titer of antibody to VZV, ZIG did not appear superior to the normal immune serum globulin control in preventing dissemination or diminishing postherpetic neuralgia.

The efficacy of intravenous acyclovir in normal adults with herpes zoster has been evaluated in three small double-blind placebo-controlled trials.[272–274] Acyclovir (5 mg/kg or 500 mg/m^2 each 8 h for 5 days) shortened the period of virus shedding and of new vesicle formation, accelerated healing, and shortened the duration of pain during the acute phase of the disease. However, there was no effect on the incidence of postherpetic neuralgia. The greatest effect of acyclovir treatment was observed in patients older than 67 years of age and those with fever (i.e., patients in whom the disease is more severe and prolonged without therapy) and in patients treated early.[272] No toxicity was observed in acyclovir recipients.

There have been several studies to determine the efficacy of oral acyclovir in the treatment of healthy adults with zoster.[275–278] Studies of elderly patients treated with 800 mg orally five times a day for 10 days showed significant decreases in healing time, period of viral shedding, and acute pain versus untreated patients when therapy was initiated within 48 h of the appearance of vesicles. Variable effects on postherpetic neuralgia following oral acyclovir therapy have been observed.[275–278] It is therefore recommended that oral acyclovir therapy be given to healthy adults (over the age of 50) with zoster, within 48 h of the onset of vesicles if no contraindication to such therapy is apparent.

Topical treatment for zoster has also been attempted with limited success. Well-controlled studies of IUdR in dimethylsulfoxide (DMSO) have demonstrated that topical application of 5 to 40% IUdR in 100% DMSO, beginning early in the course of uncomplicated herpes zoster, shortens the vesicular phase and accelerates healing and may also reduce the duration of pain.[103,279] However, these effects are small, the treatment protocol is inconvenient, and IUdR is not effective in more convenient ointment formulations.

Postherpetic neuralgia, once established, is often refractory to therapy. Fortunately, it resolves spontaneously in most patients—within 3 months in about 50 percent and within a year in 75 percent or more. Nevertheless, a number of patients are left with persistent, often disabling, pain. Conventional analgesics should be tried but often fail, as do narcotics, which also carry a risk of addiction. A wide range of therapies has been advocated, including epidural injection of local anesthetic and corticosteroid, acupuncture, biofeedback, subcutaneous injections of triamcinolone, and systemic administration of a variety of compounds, but most have not been validated by controlled trials. Though of unproved benefit, an initial trial of cutaneous stimulation, either by frequent rubbing with a dry towel or with a cutaneous electrical stimulator, is advocated by many experts.[280] This should be continued for several weeks before being abandoned. The typical dull persistent aching pain of postherpetic neuralgia will often respond to tricyclic antidepressants.[280] In a controlled trial, amitriptyline provided excellent pain relief in about two-thirds of patients with postherpetic neuralgia. Amitryptyline and fluphenazine, alone or in combination, have been shown to be useful for acute neuritis and may be of some benefit in postherpetic neuralgia. Carbamazepine may also be effective, especially for the lancinating pain that develops in some patients.[280] Capsaicin (*trans*-8-methyl-*N*-vanillyl-6-nonenamide) is a chemical known to deplete substance P—an important endogenous neuropeptide that acts as a chemomediator of nociceptive impulses from the periphery to the central nervous system. Substance P is found in high levels in sensory nerves supplying sites of chronic inflammation. A small clinical trial of topical capsaicin for 4 weeks in patients with postherpetic neuralgia demonstrated significant effects of this therapy on pain, with 75 percent of patients experiencing substantial pain relief.[281] Capsaicin is currently available for use in patients with neuralgia and may be effective in patients with refractory postherpetic neuralgia.

The possibility that postherpetic neuralgia may be caused by inflammation, necrosis, and subsequent scarring of the sensory ganglion and contiguous neural structures has provided the rationale for the use of corticosteroids during the acute phase of herpes zoster in an attempt to prevent this complication. Two small controlled trials have suggested that the oral administration of 48 mg of triamcinolone or 40 mg of prednisolone per day, beginning during the early eruptive phase of the disease, may reduce the duration of postherpetic neuralgia in otherwise healthy patients over 60 years of age.[282,283] No complications of corticosteroid therapy were observed in either study. A more recent large, randomized double-blind controlled trial of prednisolone for postherpetic neuralgia demonstrated no significant effect of steroid therapy in the prevention of postherpetic neuralgia.[284]

The eye is involved in 20 to 50 percent of patients with ophthalmic zoster, and the advice of an ophthalmologist should be sought in treating these patients. Therapy of ocular VZV infections is controversial. Mydriatics are used to prevent synechiae, and topical corticosteroids are frequently recommended for keratitis and uveitis, although their efficacy is unproved.[183] Topical antiviral drugs (IUdR, vidarabine, trifluorothymidine) are also frequently recommended and should be included whenever corticosteroids are used.

In summary, herpes zoster in immunologically normal persons less than 50 years of age is generally benign and self-limited and is very rarely complicated by postherpetic neuralgia. Thus antiviral therapy is not recommended.

In immunologically normal older persons (over 50 years of age), the major complication of herpes zoster is postherpetic neuralgia, which can be expected to develop in 20 percent or more of these patients. The high incidence of ocular and CNS complications observed in patients with ophthalmic zoster, including the syndrome of delayed contralateral hemiplegia,[51,184,201–203] warrants consideration of antiviral therapy. It is therefore recommended that patients over 50 years of age with zoster be treated with oral acyclovir (800 mg five times a day for 7 days).

Immunocompetent patients of any age who develop significant cutaneous dissemination (e.g., 20 or more vesicles at a distance from the primary dermatome) should be carefully evaluated, and those with evidence of visceral or CNS involvement should receive intravenous acyclovir antiviral therapy. It might seem reasonable to use oral acyclovir to treat all patients who are able to take it, but it has been noted that oral administration of acyclovir does not allow patients to consistently attain therapeutic blood levels of acyclovir.

In immunocompromised patients of any age with herpes zoster, the major objective is to prevent local, visceral, and CNS complications, which are the direct consequence of VZV replication and spread. Accordingly, such patients are prime candidates for intravenous antiviral therapy. It is important to begin intravenous therapy early in this setting because of the close temporal proximity of the onset of cutaneous dissemination to the onset of visceral and CNS complications; one would rather not wait for the occurrence of cutaneous dissemination to initiate antiviral therapy. Current treatment recommendations for immunocompromised patients are for intravenous acyclovir, 500 mg/m^2 or 10 mg/kg each 8 h for 7 days, or until there is no longer evidence of continuing VZV replication. Untreated immunocompromised patients who develop cutaneous dissemination or evidence of visceral or CNS involvement should be treated with intravenous acyclovir at this same dosage until there is no longer evidence of VZV replication. Patients with CNS involvement should probably be treated longer, and the physician should be alert for relapse. Both acyclovir and vidarabine require dose reduction in patients with renal insufficiency.[241]

Prevention and Control

Prevention and Control of Varicella

Varicella is almost always a benign disease in normal children. Because infection results in lifelong immunity, its acquisition in childhood eliminates the problem of varicella in the adult years. Therefore, no preventive measures are recommended for a normal child who has been exposed to varicella.

On the other hand, varicella is potentially fatal in susceptible patients with HIV disease, those undergoing immunosuppressive therapy, those with an immunosuppressive malignancy such as Hodgkin's disease, susceptible newborn infants, and even normal adults. Thus it is desirable to prevent or modify varicella in these high-risk individuals. Potential approaches include passive immunization, active immunization, chemoprophylaxis, and prevention of exposure.

Passive immunization with large doses (0.6 to 1.2 mL/kg) of standard human immune serum globulin (ISG) administered within 3 days of exposure to VZV was shown to attenuate but not prevent varicella in normal children.[37] Passive immunization with zoster immune globulin (ZIG), prepared from the plasma of donors recovering from herpes zoster and containing a high titer of antibody to VZV, has been shown to prevent varicella in susceptible normal children when administered within 3 days of exposure[91] and to modify the disease in immunosuppressed children.[38,40] One-third of the immunosuppressed recipients developed subclinical infection, and the disease was mild in most of the others. Similarly, zoster immune plasma (ZIP) obtained from otherwise healthy individuals during convalescence from varicella or herpes zoster has been shown to modify or prevent varicella in susceptible high-risk children when it is administered within 5 days of exposure.[39,285] In contrast to the favorable outcome in these passively immunized, high-risk children is the 32 percent mortality reported in a group of 106 leukemic children with unmodified varicella.[151] In order to overcome the relative shortage of zoster convalescent plasma and ZIG for the growing population of immunosuppressed patients, Zaia et al.[286] screened outdated blood from blood banks and used those units with high levels of antibody to VZV to prepare batches of immune globulin (VZIG) with antibody levels equivalent to those in ZIG. In a randomized double-blind trial of their capacity to protect immunosuppressed children from severe varicella, ZIG and VZIG were comparable.[88] Clinical infection occurred in 44 percent of VZIG recipients and 37 percent of ZIG recipients, with no significant difference in severity in the two groups. Subclinical infections occurred in 16 percent of VZIG and 31 percent of ZIG recipients. The incubation period is prolonged in ZIG, ZIP, and VZIG

TABLE 204-3

Criteria for the Use of Varicella-Zoster Immune Globulin (VZIG) for the Prophylaxis of Varicella*

1. Susceptible to varicella
   a. Children <15 years of age with no or unknown history of varicella or herpes zoster
   b. Bone marrow transplant recipients regardless of pretransplantation history of varicella or herpes zoster
   c. Immunocompromised adolescents and adults (≥15 years of age) with no or unknown history of varicella or herpes zoster
   d. Normal adolescents and adults (≥15 years of age) with no or unknown history of varicella or herpes zoster who lack antibody to VZV†
2. One of the following underlying illnesses or conditions
   a. Leukemia or lymphoma
   b. Congenital or acquired immunodeficiency
   c. Bone marrow transplant recipient regardless of pretransplantation history of varicella or herpes zoster
   d. Immunosuppressive treatment (including corticosteroids)
   e. Newborn of mother who had onset of varicella within 5 days before delivery or within 48 h after delivery
   f. Premature infant (≤28 weeks gestation) whose mother lacks a history of varicella or herpes zoster
   h. Any infant ≤14 days of age whose mother lacks a history of varicella or herpes zoster
   i. Susceptible pregnant or nonpregnant adult†
3. One of the following types of exposure to person or persons with varicella or herpes zoster
   a. Continuous household contact
   b. Playmate contact (generally >1 h play indoors)
   c. Hospital contact (in same 2- to 4-bed room or adjacent beds in a large ward or prolonged face-to-face contact with an infectious staff member or patient)
   d. Intrauterine contact (newborn of mother with onset of varicella 5 days or less before delivery or within 48 h after delivery)
4. Time elapsed after exposure is such that VZIG can be administered within 96 h of exposure (but preferably sooner)

*Patients should fulfill all four criteria.
†New serologic tests that permit the rapid identification of susceptible individuals, and the increased availability of VZIG, now make it possible to passively immunize susceptible pregnant and nonpregnant adults with recognized exposure to varicella. Immunologically normal adults with no history of varicella or herpes zoster are generally considered immune unless it is demonstrated that they lack serum antibody to VZV.[287]

recipients who develop clinical disease. Recommended criteria for the use of VZIG are listed in Table 204-3. The availability of serologic tests that permit the rapid identification of susceptible individuals, and the increased availability of VZIG, now make it possible to identify and passively immunize susceptible pregnant[54,288,289] and nonpregnant adults with recognized exposure to varicella.

Unfortunately, protection afforded by VZIG is transient, whereas most susceptible people will experience repeated exposures to VZV. Furthermore, exposure to VZV is often unrecognized, and thus large numbers of immunocompromised patients will continue to develop unmodified varicella in spite of the availability of VZIG. Continuous prophylaxis by administration of VZIG on a monthly or bimonthly schedule is impractical; what is needed is a safe means of inducing long-lasting immunity to VZV in immunocompromised patients and susceptible adults.

Almost two decades ago Dr. M. Takahashi and his colleagues announced the development of a live attenuated VZV vaccine (OKA strain) prepared by serial passage in human and guinea pig cell cultures of a strain of VZV isolated from a varicella vesicle.[290] Despite concerns about its degree of attenuation, capacity to induce latent infections, and safety in immunocompromised patients, it has

been extensively evaluated in Japan and recently in the United States.[95,96,98–100,290–311] Large-scale studies of the OKA strain varicella vaccine in healthy children have shown consistent evidence for high seroconversion rates after one or two administrations of vaccine-strain virus.[98,100,305] In one study, 96 percent of healthy children who received the VZV vaccine seroconverted as evidenced by newly detectable circulating VZV antibodies, and 99 percent of these children maintained positive antibody titers 1 year after vaccination.[98] Additionally, long-term immunity of recipients of the OKA strain of vaccine has been reported to occur 7 to 10 years after vaccination.[312] Side effects of the vaccine in healthy children are that it induces a mild papular or papulovesicular rash and slight fever in a small minority. Virus is rarely isolated from the rash in normal recipients, and there is no apparent transmission to contacts. However, in contrast to natural varicella, a few of these immunized normal persons have developed very mild varicella on subsequent exposure to VZV; the virus isolated from such patients is wild-type VZV.[98,100] Herpes zoster has developed in less than 0.3 percent of normal childhood recipients of the vaccine.[309] When children with leukemia in remission and off chemotherapy are vaccinated, fewer than 10 percent develop a papular or papulovesicular rash, and most develop antibody and cell-mediated immunity to VZV. When children on chemotherapy have it stopped for 1 week before and 1 week after vaccination, up to 40 percent develop rash.[296,302,303,309] When the rash is vesicular, vaccine virus can be isolated and transmitted to susceptible normal siblings who develop mild varicella.[310] When vaccinated leukemic children are exposed to VZV, most are protected, and only 10 to 20 percent develop clinical varicella, which is generally mild. Although initially rates were thought to be similar,[306,307] long-term follow-up of leukemic patients who have received the varicella vaccine indicates that leukemic vaccinees develop herpes zoster at a lower rate than leukemic patients with a history of natural varicella.[276] It is thought that the lower incidence of zoster in vaccinees may be related to the milder form of varicella that these patients develop, and hence the fewer dermatomes affected by vaccine strain virus, or the decreased ability for latent vaccine strain-virus to reactivate.[306,308] A recent study of siblings of children with malignancies showed a 10 percent rate of transmission of vaccine-strain virus to the immunocompromised siblings. These observations indicate that the OKA VZV vaccine can be safely administered to susceptible immunosuppressed children and will help protect them from the morbidity and mortality that would otherwise result from subsequent exposures to varicella. Even in normal individuals, the immunity induced by the vaccine is not as solid as that induced by wild-type VZV infection. A study of 187 healthy adults immunized with the OKA strain of varicella vaccine showed a 94 percent seroconversion rate following two doses of vaccine; however, 12 patients developed mild breakthrough varicella after a known exposure to VZV, and 44 percent of patients with known household exposure developed varicella.[99] All patients who were vaccinated experienced a markedly attenuated course of VZV infection, with the average number of lesions in these patients being 24. Twenty-five percent of vaccinees lost antibodies to VZV over time but continued to experience modified disease and showed partial protection against severe varicella.[99]

It is expected that the attenuated OKA VZV vaccine will be available in the United States within the next year. This represents a tremendous advance in our ability to cope with the problem of varicella in immunocompromised patients and nonimmune adults. The indications for vaccination of healthy children and previously infected elderly individuals remain less obvious. Proponents of the use of this vaccine in healthy children suggest that the decrease in costs associated with childhood VZV infections (e.g., parental time off from work to care for the sick child) afforded by vaccination may justify the use of this vaccine in this subset of the population. These issues are still being debated and, with the release of the vaccine in the United States, are likely to be clarified over the next few years.

Chemoprophylaxis has not been developed for VZV. Exposure of susceptible patients to VZV warrants reduction in the dosage of corticosteroids to physiologic levels and the elimination or reduction of immunosuppressive drugs until their varicella has resolved or until it is clear that they have escaped infection. Such patients should receive VZIG immediately after exposure.

There is no need to prevent exposure of susceptible normal children to VZV; patients with varicella need only be kept at home until all vesicles have crusted.[14,129] On the other hand, rigid isolation should be enforced to prevent infection of susceptible immunocompromised patients and newborn infants. Contact with patients with varicella and herpes zoster, and with persons who may be incubating varicella, must be avoided. Hospital personnel without a clear history of varicella or herpes zoster should be tested for antibody to VZV so that appropriate leave from work can be instituted following an exposure to VZV. Hospitals should develop and implement effective procedures to prevent nosocomial varicella.[14,41,129,165] If such exposure occurs or is suspected, susceptible immunocompromised patients and newborn infants should receive prophylaxis with VZIG.

Prevention and Control of Herpes Zoster

Herpes zoster is a sporadic disease that results from reactivation of latent endogenous VZV, rather than from exogenous infection. Thus, attempts at prophylaxis must be aimed at preventing the reactivation of endogenous VZV or inhibiting its subsequent replication and spread. It appears that natural resistance to herpes zoster is maintained by periodic antigenic stimulation, which results from subclinical episodes of exogenous reinfection and endogenous reactivation. The increased incidence and severity of herpes zoster observed in elderly persons appears to be associated with depressed immunity to VZV, primarily depressed cell-mediated immunity.[124–126] Depressed cell-mediated immunity also appears to be responsible for the increased incidence and severity of herpes zoster in immunocompromised patients. Accordingly, one approach to the prevention of herpes zoster is the stimulation of immunity to VZV in elderly and other high-risk individuals. Studies have shown that healthy adults over 60 years of age who have had zoster develop higher numbers of VZV-specific T lymphocytes after infection than age-matched controls. It is presumed that this increase in cell-specific immunity to VZV affords protection against additional episodes of zoster. Studies have been done of healthy adults over 55 years of age with a history of previous primary VZV infection who received the Oka varicella vaccine to determine the effect on VZV-specific T lymphocytes and VZV immunity. An increase in VZV-specific T lymphocytes and VZV immunity was demonstrated in these patients after vaccination that was similar to the increased immunity to VZV observed after an episode of zoster.[294,295,298] These findings suggest that vaccination of this subset of patients may be useful in preventing zoster infections; however, it remains to be seen whether immunization of such individuals will result in a reduction in the incidence and severity of herpes zoster. The use of live attenuated vaccines is generally to be avoided in immunocompromised individuals, but the current VZV vaccine has proved to be relatively safe and effective in immunocompromised children with leukemia and other malignancies (see above) and may therefore be useful in stimulating VZV immunity in this subset of patients.

With the increased prevalence of HIV disease and associated increased incidence of VZV infections, the question of suppressive treatment of such patients with acyclovir has been raised. Studies in bone marrow transplant (BMT) recipients who received intravenous acyclovir for 23 days after BMT and were then randomized to receive 6 months of oral acyclovir or placebo showed a significantly decreased incidence of zoster in the patients receiving acyclovir. However, 6 months after discontinuation of therapy, the incidence of zoster in the two groups was identical. This study suggests prophylactic doses of acyclovir in BMT patients may be useful in the peritransplant period when these patients are most susceptible to VZV recrudescence.[313] The occurrence of acyclovir-resistant VZV as seen in patients with HIV disease who have been on long-term acyclovir therapy[2–5,10] raises the question of selection for resistant strains of VZV in BMT patients treated prophylactically with acyclovir. It appears that more studies of prophylactic acyclovir therapy are needed to assess the efficacy of such treatment and the risks of selection for acyclovir-resistant VZV.

Patients with herpes zoster are infectious and may transmit varicella to susceptible individuals. Thus, susceptible high-risk patients should be protected from contact with individuals with herpes zoster.

Course and Prognosis

Course and Prognosis of Varicella

In the normal child, varicella is a benign disease rarely attended by serious complications or sequelae. New skin lesions continue to appear for about 3 days and are all crusted by day 5; the rash persists for about a week. Fever is mild and persists as long as new lesions continue to appear. The disease is often trivial in young children but tends to be more severe in older children and adults. Except for Reye's syndrome (which occurs in immunocompetent children), serious complications of varicella occur almost exclusively in neonates, adults, and immunocompromised patients (see above), and these account for most of the morbidity associated with the disease. Mortality in the United States is less than 4 per 100,000, with most deaths occurring in patients with underlying diseases or Reye's syndrome.

Course and Prognosis of Herpes Zoster

In the normal host, herpes zoster is a self-limited disease with little direct mortality. The rash is usually preceded by 1 to 3 days of neuralgic pain in the involved dermatome. New lesions continue to appear for 2 to 4 days (occasionally for as long as a week) and resolve somewhat more slowly than those of varicella; lesions generally crust in 7 to 10 days and the crusts fall off after about 2 weeks. The most common complication is postherpetic neuralgia, which is uncommon in normal persons under 40 years of age but occurs in more than one-third of patients over 60 years of age. Postherpetic neuralgia is especially common in patients with ophthalmic zoster and in immunocompromised patients. Mortality in herpes zoster is associated with failure of the host to limit virus replication and dissemination; it occurs almost exclusively in immunocompromised patients.

References

1. Jura E et al: Varicella-zoster virus infections in children infected with human immunodeficiency virus. *Pediatr Infect Dis J* **8**:586, 1989

2. Pahwa S et al: Continuous varicella-zoster infection associated with acyclovir resistance in a child with AIDS. *JAMA* **260**:2879, 1988

3. Jacobson MA et al: Acyclovir-resistant varicella zoster virus infection after chronic oral acyclovir therapy in patients with the acquired immunodeficiency syndrome (AIDS). *Ann Intern Med* **112**:187, 1990

4. Safrin S et al: Foscarnet therapy in five patients with AIDS and acyclovir-resistant varicella zoster virus infection. *Ann Intern Med* **115**:19, 1991

5. Linnemann CC et al: Emergence of acyclovir-resistant varicella zoster virus in an AIDS patient on prolonged acyclovir therapy. *AIDS* **4**:577, 1990

6. Friedman-Kien AE et al: Herpes zoster: A possible early clinical sign for development of acquired immunodeficiency syndrome in high-risk individuals. *J Am Acad Dermatol* **14**:1023, 1986

7. Colebunders R et al: Herpes zoster in African patients: A clinical predictor of human immunodeficiency virus infection. *J Infect Dis* **157**:314, 1988

8. LeBoit PE et al: Chronic verrucous varicella-zoster virus infection in patients with the acquired immunodeficiency syndrome (AIDS)—histologic and molecular biologic findings. *Am J Dermatopathol* **14**:1, 1992

9. Gilson IH et al: Disseminated ecthymatous herpes varicella-zoster infection in patients with acquired immunodeficiency syndrome. *J Am Acad Dermatol* **20**:637, 1989

10. Hoppenjans WB et al: Prolonged cutaneous herpes zoster in acquired immunodeficiency syndrome. *Arch Dermatol* **126**:1048, 1990

11. Alessi E et al: Unusual varicella zoster virus infection in patients with the acquired immunodeficiency syndrome (letter). *Arch Dermatol* **124**:1011, 1988

12. Cohen PR et al: Disseminated herpes zoster in patients with human immunodeficiency virus infection. *Am J Med* **84**:1076, 1988

13. Gordon JE: Chickenpox: An epidemiological review. *Am J Med Sci* **244**:362, 1962

14. Weller TH: Varicella-herpes zoster virus, in *Viral Infections of Humans, Epidemiology and Control,* 3d ed, edited by AS Evans. New York, Plenum 1989, p 659

15. Osler W: *The Principles and Practice of Medicine.* New York, Appleton, 1892, p 65

16. Scott-Wilson JH: Why "chicken" pox? *Lancet* **1**:1152, 1978

17. Steiner: Zur Inokulation der Varicellen. *Wien Med Wochenschr* **25**:306, 1875

18. Tyzzer EE: The histology of the skin lesions in varicella. *Phillipp J Sci* **1**:349, 1906

19. Weller TH, Stoddard MB: Intranuclear inclusion bodies in cultures in human tissue inoculated with varicella vesicle fluid. *J Immunol* **68**:311, 1952

20. Bruusgaard E: The mutual relation between zoster and varicella. *Br J Dermatol Syphilol* **44**:1, 1932

21. Lipschutz B: Untersuchungen über die Atiologie der Krankheiten der Herpesgruppe (Herpes zoster, Herpes genitalis, Herpes febrilis). *Arch Dermatol Syphilol* **136**:428, 1921

22. Taylor-Robinson D, Caunt AE: *Varicella Virus.* Vienna, Springer-Verlag, 1972

23. Weller TH, Witton HM: The etiologic agents of varicella and herpes zoster: Serologic studies with the viruses as propagated in vitro. *J Exp Med* **108**:869, 1958

24. Weller TH et al: The etiologic agents of varicella and herpes zoster: Isolation, propagation, and cultural characteristics in vitro. *J Exp Med* **108**:843, 1958

25. Weller TH: Varicella and herpes zoster. Changing concepts of the natural history, control, and importance of a not-so-benign virus. *N Engl J Med* **309**:1362, 1434, 1983

26. Head H, Campbell AW: The pathology of herpes zoster and its bearing on sensory localization. *Brain* **23**:353, 1900

27. Hope-Simpson RE: The nature of herpes zoster: A long-term study and a new hypothesis. *Proc R Soc Med* **58**:9, 1965

28. Denny-Brown D et al: Pathologic features of herpes zoster: A note on "geniculate herpes." *Arch Neurol Psychiatr* **51**:216, 1944

29. Stern ES: The mechanism of herpes zoster and its relation to chicken-pox. *Br J Dermatol Syphilol* **49**:263, 1937

30. Cheatham WJ: The relation of heretofore unreported lesions to pathogenesis of herpes zoster. *Am J Pathol* **29**:401, 1953

31. Muller SA, Winkelmann RK: Cutaneous nerve changes in zoster. *J Invest Dermatol* **52**:71, 1969

32. Esiri MM, Tomlinson AH: Herpes zoster: Demonstration of virus in trigeminal nerve and ganglion by immunofluorescence and electron microscopy. *J Neurol Sci* **15**:35, 1972

33. Ghatak NR, Zimmerman HM: Spinal ganglion in herpes zoster. *Arch Pathol* **95**:411, 1973

34. Bastian FO et al: Herpesvirus varicellae: Isolated from human dorsal root ganglia. *Arch Pathol* **97**:331, 1974

35. Aoyama Y et al: Demonstration of viral antigens in herpes simplex and varicella-zoster infection. *Recent Adv RES Research* **14**:90, 1974

36. Gershon AA et al: Antibody to varicella-zoster virus in parturient women and their offspring during the first year of life. *Pediatrics* **58**:692, 1976

36a. Gray GC et al: Increasing incidence of varicella hospitalizations in United States Army and Navy personnel. Are today's teenagers more susceptible? Should recruits be vaccinated? *Pediatrics* **86**:867, 1990

36b. Longfield JN et al: Varicella outbreaks in army recruits from Puerto Rico: Varicella susceptibility in a population from the tropics. *Arch Intern Med* **150**:970, 1990

36c. Preblud SR et al: Varicella: Clinical manifestations, epidemiology and health impact in children. *Pediatr Infect Dis* **3**:505, 1984

37. Ross AH: Modification of chicken pox in family contacts by administration of gamma globulin. *N Engl J Med* **267**:369, 1962

38. Gershon AA et al: Zoster immune globulin: A further assessment. *N Engl J Med* **290**:243, 1974

39. Balfour HH Jr et al: Prevention or modification of varicella using zoster immune plasma. *Am J Dis Child* **131**:693, 1977

40. Orenstein W et al: Prophylaxis of varicella in high-risk children. Dose-response effect of zoster immune globulin. *J Pediatr* **98**:368, 1981

41. Leclair JM et al: Airborne transmission of chickenpox in a hospital. *N Engl J Med* **302**:450, 1980

42. Gustafson TL et al: An outbreak of airborne nosocomial varicella. *Pediatrics* **70**:550, 1982

42a. Asano Y et al: Viremia is present in incubation period in non-immunocompromised children with varicella. *J Pediatr* **106**:69, 1985

42b. Asano Y et al: Severity of viremia and clinical findings in children with varicella. *J Infect Dis* **161**:1095, 1990

42c. Ozaki T et al: Viremic phase in nonimmunocompromised children with varicella. *J Pediatr* **104**:85, 1984

43. Sawyer MH et al: Detection of varicella-zoster virus DNA in the oropharynx and blood of patients with varicella. *J Infect Dis* **166**:885, 1992

44. McNamara MP et al: Exogenous reinfection with varicella-zoster virus (letter). *N Engl J Med* **317**:511, 1987

44a. Baba K et al: Immunologic and epidemiologic aspects of varicella infection acquired during infancy and early childhood. *J Pediatr* **100**:881, 1982

44b. Gershon AA et al: Clinical reinfection with varicella-zoster virus. *J Infect Dis* **149**:137, 1984

44c. Gershon AA: Live attenuated varicella vaccine: Protection in healthy adults compared with leukemic children. *J Infect Dis* **161**:661, 1990

45. Seiler HE: A study of herpes zoster particularly in its relationship to chickenpox. *J Hyg (Camb)* **47**:253, 1949

46. Burgoon CF et al: The natural history of herpes zoster. *JAMA* **164**:265, 1957

47. de Moragas JM, Kierland RR: The outcome of patients with herpes zoster. *Arch Dermatol* **75**:193, 1957

48. Oberg G, Svedmyr A: Varicelliform eruptions in herpes zoster—some clinical and serological observations. *Scand J Infect Dis* **1**:47, 1969

49. Miller LH, Brunell PA: Zoster: Reinfection or activation of latent virus? *Am J Med* **49**:480, 1970

50. Rogers RS, Tindall JP: Herpes zoster in children. *Arch Dermatol* **106**:204, 1972

51. Ragozzino MW et al: Population-based study of herpes zoster and its sequelae. *Medicine (Baltimore)* **61**:310, 1982

52. Kalman CM, Laskin OL: Herpes zoster and zosteriform herpes simplex infections in immunocompetent adults. *Am J Med* **81**:775, 1986

53. Brunell PA, Kotchmar GS: Zoster in Infancy: Failure to maintain virus latency following intrauterine infection. *J Pediatr* **98**:71, 1981

54. Brunell PA: Varicella in pregnancy, the fetus, and the newborn: Problems in management. *J Infect Dis* **166**(suppl):S42, 1992

55. Ragozzino MW et al: Risk of cancer after herpes zoster. A population-based study. *N Engl J Med* **307**:393, 1982

56. Roizman B: Herpes viridae: A brief introduction in *virology,* edited by BN Fields and DM Knipe. New York, Raven, 1990, p 1787

57. Almeida JD et al: Morphology of varicella (chickenpox) virus. *Virology* **16**:353, 1962

57a. Gelb LD et al: Varicella-zoster virus, in *Virology,* edited by BN Fields and DM Knipe. New York, Raven, 1990, p 2011

57b. Davidson AJ et al: The complete DNA sequence of varicella-zoster virus. *J Gen Virol* **67**:1759, 1986

57c. Davidson AJ: Varicella-zoster virus. *J Gen Virol* **72**:475, 1991

57d. Ostrove JM: Molecular biology of varicella-zoster virus. *Adv Virus Res* **38**:45, 1990

57e. Croen KD et al: Patterns of gene expression and sites of latency in human nerve ganglia are different for varicella-zoster and herpes simplex viruses. *Proc Natl Acad Sci USA* **85**:9773, 1988

57f. Straus SE: Clinical and biological differences between recurrent herpes simplex virus and varicella-zoster virus infections. *JAMA* **262**:3455, 1989

57g. Croen KD, Straus SE: Varicella-zoster virus latency. *Annu Rev Microbiol* **45**:265, 1991

57h. Meier JL, Straus, SE: Comparative biology of latent varicella-zoster virus and herpes simplex virus infections. *J Infect Dis* **166**:S13, 1992

58. Gershon AA et al: Varicella-zoster virus, in *Manual of Clinical Microbiology,* 5th ed, edited by Balows A et al. Washington, DC, American Society for Microbiology, 1991, p. 838

59. Martin JH et al: Restriction endonuclease analysis of varicella-zoster vaccine virus and wild-type DNAs. *J Med Virol* **9**:69, 1982

60. Straus SE et al: Genome differences among varicella-zoster virus isolates. *J Gen Virol* **64**:1031, 1983

61. Myers MG, Connelly BL: Animal models of varicella. *J Infect Dis* **166**:S48, 1992

62. Feldman S, Epp E: Detection of viremia during incubation of varicella. *J Pediatr* **94**:746, 1979

63. Asano Y et al: Viral replication and immunologic responses in children naturally infected with varicella-zoster virus and in varicella vaccine recipients. *J Infect Dis* **152**:863, 1985

64. Cheatham WJ et al: Varicella: Report of two fatal cases with necropsy, virus isolation, and serologic studies. *Am J Pathol* **32**:1015, 1956

65. Johnson HN: Visceral lesions associated with varicella. *Arch Pathol* **30**:292, 1940

66. Eisenbud M: Chickenpox with visceral involvement. *Am J Med* **12**:740, 1952

67. Myers MG: Viremia caused by varicella-zoster: Association with malignant progressive varicella. *J Infect Dis* **140**:229, 1979

68. Koropchak CM et al: Investigation of varicella-zoster virus infection by polymerase chain reaction in immunocompetent host with acute varicella, *J Infect Dis* **163**:1016, 1991

69. Gibbs FA et al: Electroencephalographic abnormality in "uncomplicated" childhood diseases. *JAMA* **171**:1050, 1959

70. Pitel BA et al: Subclinical hepatic changes in varicella infection. *Pediatrics* **65**:631, 1980

71. Myers MG: Hepatic cellular injury during varicella. *Arch Dis Child* **57**:317, 1982

72. Ey JL et al: Varicella hepatitis without neurologic symptoms or findings. *Pediatrics* **67**:285, 1981

73. Gold E: Serologic and virus-isolation studies of patients with varicella or herpes-zoster infection. *N Engl J Med* **274**:181, 1966

74. Feldman S et al: Varicella in children with cancer: Seventy-seven cases. *Pediatrics* **56**:388, 1975

75. Feldman S, Epp E: Isolation of varicella-zoster virus from blood. *J Pediatr* **88**:265, 1976

76. Brunell PA et al: Varicella-zoster immunoglobulins during varicella, latency, and zoster. *J Infect Dis* **132**:49, 1975

77. Arvin AM, Koropchak CM: Immunoglobulins M and G to varicella-zoster virus measured by solid-phase radioimmunoassay: Antibody responses to varicella and herpes zoster infections. *J Clin Microbiol* **12**:367, 1980

78. Wittek AE et al: Serum immunoglobulin A antibody to varicella-zoster virus in subjects with primary varicella and herpes zoster infections and in immune subjects. *J Clin Microbiol* **18**:1146, 1983

79. Schmidt NJ, Gallo D: Class-specific antibody responses to early and late antigens of varicella and herpes simplex viruses. *J Med Virol* **13**:1, 1984

79a. Rotbart HA et al: Immune responses to varicella-zoster virus infections in healthy children. *J Infect Dis* **167**:195, 1993

80. Arvin AM: Cell-mediated immunity to varicella-zoster virus. *J Infect Dis* **166**:S35, 1992

81. Levin MJ et al: Immune responses of elderly individuals to a live attenuated varicella vaccine. *J Infect Dis* **166**:253, 1992

82. Asano Y et al: Soluble skin test antigen of varicella-zoster virus prepared from the fluid of infected cultures. *J Infect Dis* **143**:684, 1981

82a. Takahashi M et al: Immunization of the elderly and patients with collagen vascular diseases with live varicella vaccine and use of varicella skin antigen. *J Infect Dis* **166**:S58, 1992

83. Good RA, Zak SJ: Disturbances in gamma globulin synthesis as "experiments of nature." *Pediatrics* **18**:109, 1956

84. Armstrong RW et al: Cutaneous interferon production in patients with Hodgkin's disease and other cancers infected with varicella or vaccinia. *N Engl J Med* **283**:1182, 1970

85. Ruckdeschel JC et al: Herpes zoster and impaired cell-associated immunity to the varicella-zoster virus in patients with Hodgkin's disease. *Am J Med* **62**:77, 1977

86. Patel PA et al: Cell-mediated immunity to varicella-zoster virus infection in subjects with lymphoma or leukemia. *J Pediatr* **94**:223, 1979

87. Biron CA et al: Severe herpesvirus infections in an adolescent without natural killer cells. *N Engl J Med* **320**:1731, 1989

88. Zaia JA et al: Evaluation of varicella-zoster immune globulin: Protection of immunosuppressed children after exposure to varicella. *J Infect Dis* **147**:737, 1983

89. Gershon AA, Krugman S: Seroepidemiologic survey of varicella: Value of specific fluorescent antibody test. *Pediatrics* **56**:1005, 1975

90. Zaia JA, Oxman MN: Antibody to varicella-zoster virus-induced membrane antigen: Immunofluorescence assay using monodisperse gluteraldehyde-fixed target cells. *J Infect Dis* **136**:519, 1977

91. Brunell PA et al: Prevention of varicella by zoster immune globulin. *N Engl J Med* **280**:1191, 1969

92. Iltis JP et al: Comparison of Raji cell line fluorescent antibody to membrane antigen test and the enzyme-linked immunosorbent assay

for determination of immunity to varicella-zoster virus. *J Clin Microbiol* **16**:878, 1982

93. Arvin AM et al: Immunologic evidence of reinfection with varicella-zoster virus. *J Infect Dis* **148**:200, 1983

94. Kamiya H et al: Diagnostic skin test reaction with varicella-zoster virus antigen and clinical application of the test. *J Infect Dis* **136**:784, 1977

95. Kuter BJ et al: Oka/Merck varicella vaccine in healthy children: final report of a 2-year efficacy study and 7-year follow-up studies. *Vaccine* **9**:643, 1991

96. Arbeter AM et al: Varicella vaccine trials in healthy children. *Am J Dis Child* **138**:434, 1984

97. Gershon AA et al: Varicella vaccine: The American experience. *J Infect Dis* **166**:S63, 1992

98. White CJ et al: Varicella vaccine (VARIVAX) in healthy children and adolescents: Results from clinical trials, 1987 to 1989. *Pediatrics* **87**:604, 1991

99. Gershon AA et al: Immunization of healthy adults with live attenuated varicella vaccine. *J Infect Dis* **158**:132, 1988

100. Johnson C et al: Humoral immunity and clinical reinfections following varicella vaccine in healthy children. *Pediatrics* **84**:418, 1989

101. Stevens JG: Latent herpes simplex virus and the nervous system. *Curr Top Microbiol Immunol* **70**:31, 1975

102. Shanbrom E et al: Herpes zoster in hematologic neoplasias: Some unusual manifestations. *Ann Intern Med* **53**:523, 1960

103. Juel-Hensen BE, MacCallum FO: *Herpes Simplex, Varicella and Zoster.* Philadelphia, Lippincott, 1972

104. Sokal JE, Firat D: Varicella-zoster infection in Hodgkin's disease. *Am J Med* **39**:452, 1965

105. Schimpff S et al: Varicella-zoster infection in patients with cancer. *Ann Intern Med* **76**:241, 1972

106. Feldman S et al: Herpes zoster in children with cancer. *Am J Dis Child* **126**:178, 1973

107. Lubey JP et al: A longitudinal study of varicella-zoster virus infections in renal transplant recipients. *J Infect Dis* **135**:659, 1977

108. Wilson A et al: Subclinical varicella-zoster virus viremia, herpes zoster, and T lymphocyte immunity to varicella-zoster viral antigens after bone marrow transplantation. *J Infect Dis* **165**:119, 1992

108a. Weigle KA, Grose C: Molecular dissection of the humoral immune response to individual varicella-zoster viral proteins during chickenpox, quiescence, reinfection, and reactivation. *J Infect Dis* **149**:741, 1984

109. Gershon AA et al: IgM to varicella-zoster virus: Demonstration in patients with and without clinical zoster. *Pediatr Infect Dis* **1**:164, 1982

110. Dolin R et al: Herpes zoster-varicella infections in immunosuppressed patients. *Ann Intern Med* **89**:375, 1978

111. McKendall RR, Klawans HL: Nervous system complications of varicella-zoster virus, in *Handbook of Clinical Neurology,* vol 34, edited by PJ Vinken, GW Bruyn. Amsterdam, North-Holland, 1978, p 161

112. Feldman S et al: A viremic phase for herpes zoster in children with cancer. *Pediatrics* **91**:597, 1977

113. Easton HG: Zoster sine herpete causing trigeminal neuralgia. *Lancet* **2**:1065, 1970

114. Merselis JG Jr et al: Disseminated herpes zoster. *Arch Intern Med* **113**:679, 1964

115. Goffinet DR et al: Herpes zoster-varicella infections and lymphoma. *Ann Intern Med* **76**:235, 1972

116. Goodman R et al: Herpes zoster in children with stage I–III Hodgkin's disease. *Radiology* **118**:429, 1976

117. Reboul F et al: Herpes zoster and varicella infections in children with Hodgkin's disease. *Cancer* **41**:95, 1978

118. Novelli VM et al: Herpes zoster in children with acute lymphocytic leukemia. *Am J Dis Child* **142**:71, 1988

119. Balfour HH Jr: Varicella zoster virus infection in the immunocompromised host. *Scand J Infect Dis* **78**:69, 1991

119a. Wilson A et al: *J Infect Dis* **165**:119, 1992

120. Ljungman P et al: Clinical and subclinical reactivations of varicella-zoster virus in immunocompromised patients. *J Infect Dis* **153**:840, 1986

121. Stevens DA et al: Cellular events in zoster vesicles: Relation to clinical course and immune parameters. *J Infect Dis* **131**:509, 1975

122. Pollard RB et al: Specific cell-mediated immunity and infections with herpesviruses in cardiac transplant recipients. *Am J Med* **73**:679, 1982

123. Meyers JD et al: Cell-mediated immunity to varicella-zoster virus after allogenic marrow transplant. *J Infect Dis* **141**:479, 1980

123a. Arwin AM: Cell-mediated immunity to varicella zoster virus. *J Inject Dis* **166**:S35, 1992

124. Miller AE: Selective decline in cellular immune response to varicella-zoster in the elderly. *Neurology* **30**:582, 1980

125. Berger R et al: Decrease of the lymphoproliferative response to varicella zoster virus antigen in the aged. *Infect Immun* **32**:24, 1981

126. Burke BL et al: Immune response to varicella-zoster in the aged. *Arch Intern Med* **142**:291, 1982

127. Wesselhoeft C: The differential diagnosis of chicken pox and smallpox. *N Engl J Med* **230**:15, 1944

128. Bullowa JGM et al: Complications of varicella I. Their occurrence among 2,534 patients. *Am J Dis Child* **49**:923, 1935

129. Krugman S et al: Varicella-zoster infections, in *Infectious Diseases of Children,* 8th ed. St Louis, Mosby, 1985, p 433

130. Smith EW et al: Varicella gangrenosa due to group A-hemolytic streptococcus. *Pediatrics* **57**:306, 1976

131. Fleisher G et al: Life-threatening complications of varicella. *Am J Dis Child* **135**:896, 1981

132. Melish ME: Bullous varicella: Its association with the staphylococcal scalded skin syndrome. *J Pediatr* **83**:1019, 1973

133. Weinstein L, Meade RH: Respiratory manifestations of chicken pox. *Arch Intern Med* **98**:91, 1956

134. Singer J: Postvaricella suppurative meningitis. Case reports and review of the literature. *Am J Dis Child* **133**:934, 1979

135. Triebwasser JH et al: Varicella pneumonia in adults. *Medicine* (Baltimore) **46**:409, 1967

136. Haggerty RJ, Eley RC: Varicella and cortisone. *Pediatrics* **18**:160, 1956

137. Gershon A et al: Steroid therapy and varicella. *J Pediatr* **81**:1034, 1972

138. Guess H et al: Population-based studies of varicella complications. *Pediatrics* **78**:723, 1986

139. Haake DA et al: Early treatment with acyclovir for varicella pneumonia in otherwise healthy adults: Retrospective controlled study and review. *Rev Infect Dis* **12**:788, 1990

139a. Weber DM, Pellecchia JA: Varicella pneumonia: Study of prevalence in adult men. *JAMA* **192**:527, 1965

140. Wallace MR et al: Treatment of adult varicella with oral acyclovir. A randomized, placebo-controlled study. *Ann Intern Med* **117**:358, 1992

141. Schlossberg D, Littman M: Varicella penumonia. *Arch Intern Med* **148**:1630, 1988

142. Mackay JB, Cairney P: Pulmonary calcification following varicella. *N Z Med J* **59**:453, 1960

143. Sargent EN et al: Varicella pneumonia. A report of 20 cases, with postmortem examination in six. *Calif Med* **107**:141, 1967

144. Waring JJ et al: Severe forms of chickenpox in adults. *Arch Intern Med* **69**:384, 1942

145. Oxman MN et al: Management at delivery of mother and infant when herpes simplex, varicella-zoster, hepatitis or tuberculosis have occurred during pregnancy, in *Current Topics in Infectious Diseases,* vol 4, edited by JS Remington, MN Swartz. New York, McGraw-Hill, 1983, p 224

146. Gershon AA: Chickenpox, measles, and mumps, in *Infectious Diseases of the Fetus and Newborn Infant,* 3d ed, edited by JS Remington, JO Klein. Philadelphia, Saunders, 1990

147. Williamson AP: The varicella-zoster virus in the etiology of severe congenital defects. *Clin Pediatr* **14**:553, 1975

148. Finkel KC: Mortality from varicella in children receiving adrenocorticosteroids and adrenocorticotropin. *Pediatrics* **28**:436, 1971

149. Scheinman JI, Stamler FW: Cyclophosphamide and fatal varicella. *J Pediatr* **74**:117, 1969

150. Lux SE et al: Chronic neutropenia and abnormal cellular immunity in cartilage-hair hypoplasia. *N Engl J Med* **282**:231, 1970

151. Hattori A et al: Use of live varicella vaccine in children with acute leukemia or other malignancies. *Lancet* **2**:210, 1976

152. Feldhoff CM et al: Varicella in children with renal transplants. *J Pediatr* **98**:25, 1981

153. Whitley RJ et al: Vidarabine therapy of varicella in immunosuppressed patients. *J Pediatr* **101**:125, 1982

154. Whitley RJ et al: Early vidarabine therapy to control the complications of herpes zoster in immunosuppressed patients. *N Engl J Med* **307**:971, 1982

155. Smith H: Purpura fulminans complicating varicella: Recovery with low molecular weight dextran and steroids. *Med J Aust* **54**(II):685, 1967

156. Feusner JH et al: Mechanisms of thrombocytopenia in varicella. *Am J Hematol* **7**:255, 1979

157. Christie AB: Chickenpox (varicella); herpes zoster, in *Infectious Diseases: Epidemiology and Clinical Practice,* 3d ed. Edinburgh, Churchill Livingstone, 1980, pp 262, 278

158. Charkes ND: Purpuric chickenpox: Report of a case, review of the literature, and classification by clinical features. *Ann Intern Med* **54**:745, 1961

159. Yeager AM, Zinkham WH: Varicella-associated thrombocytopenia: Clues to the etiology of childhood idiopathic thrombocytopenic purpura. *Johns Hopkins Med J* **146**:270, 1980

160. Espinoza C, Kuhn C: Viral infection of megakaryocytes in varicella with purpura. *Am J Clin Pathol* **61**:203, 1974

161. Centers for Disease Control: Reye syndrome—United States, 1984. *MMWR* **34**:13, 1985

162. Lichtenstein PK et al: Grade I Reye's syndrome. A frequent cause of vomiting and liver dysfunction after varicella and upper-respiratory-tract infection. *N Engl J Med* **309**:133, 1983

163. Takashima S, Becker LE: Neuropathology of fatal varicella. *Arch Pathol Lab Med* **103**:209, 1979

164. Goldston AS et al: Cerebellar ataxia with preeruptive varicella. *Am J Dis Child* **106**:197, 1963

165. Peters ACB et al: Varicella and acute cerebellar ataxia. *Arch Neurol* **35**:769, 1978

166. Puchhammer-Stöckl E et al: Detection of varicella-zoster DNA by polymerase chain reaction in the cerebrospinal fluid of patients suffering from neurological complications associated with chicken pox or herpes zoster. *J Clin Microbiol* **29**:1513, 1991

167. Johnson RT et al: Measles encephalomyelitis—clinical and immunological studies. *N Engl J Med* **310**:137, 1984

168. Applebaum E et al: Varicella encephalitis. *Am J Med* **15**:223, 1953

169. Boughton CR: Varicella-zoster in Sydney: II. Neurological complications of varicella. *Med J Aust* **53**(II):444, 1966

170. Nicholaides NJ: Fatal systemic varicella. A report of 3 cases. *Med J Aust* **44**(II):88, 1957

171. Griffith JF et al: The nervous system diseases associated with varicella. *Acta Neurol Scand* **46**:279, 1970

172. Gershon AA et al: Varicella-zoster-associated encephalitis: Detection of specific antibody in cerebrospinal fluid. *J Clin Microbiol* **12**:764, 1980

173. Sherman RA et al: Fatal varicella in an adult: Case report and review of the gastrointestinal complications of chickenpox. *Rev Infect Dis* **13**:424, 1991

174. Baird RE et al: Varicella arthritis diagnosed by polymerase chain reaction. *Pediatr Infect Dis J* **10**:950, 1990

175. Lewis GW: Zoster sine herpete. *Br Med J* **2**:418, 1958

176. Adour KK: Current concepts in neurology: Diagnosis and management of facial paralysis. *N Engl J Med* **307**:348, 1982

177. Brown GR: Herpes zoster: Correlation of age, sex, distribution, neuralgia, and associated disorders. *South Med J* **59**:576, 1976

178. Winkelmann RK, Perry HO: Herpes zoster in children. *JAMA* **171**:112, 1959

179. Brunell PA et al: Zoster in children. *Am J Dis Child* **115**:432, 1968

180. Harding SP et al: Natural history of herpes zoster ophthalmicus: Predictors of postherpetic neuralgia and ocular involvement. *Br J Ophthalmol* **71**:353, 1987

180a. Eisenberg E: Intraoral isolated herpes zoster. *Oral Surg* **45**:214, 1978

181. Clark J: Herpes zoster of right glossopharyngeal nerve. *Lancet* **1**:38, 1979

182. Hope-Simpson RE: Postherpetic neuralgia. *J R Coll Gen Pract* **25**:571, 1975

183. Liesegang TJ: Diagnosis and therapy of herpes zoster ophthalmicus. *Ophthalmology* **98**:1216, 1991

184. Womack LW, Liesegang TJ: Complications of herpes zoster ophthalmicus. *Arch Ophthalmol* **101**:42, 1983

185. Patterson SD et al: Atypical generalized zoster with lymphadenitis mimicking lymphoma. *N Engl J Med* **302**:848, 1980

186. Grant BD, Rowe CR: Motor paralysis of the extremities in herpes zoster. *J Bone Joint Surg* **43A**:885, 1961

187. Thomas JE, Howard FM: Segmental zoster paresis—a disease profile. *Neurology* **22**:459, 1972

188. Kendall D: Motor complications of herpes zoster. *Br Med J* **1**:616, 1957

189. Brostoff J: Diaphragmatic paralysis after herpes zoster. *Br Med J* **2**:1571, 1966

190. Jellinek EH, Tulloch WS: Herpes zoster with dysfunction of bladder and anus. *Lancet* **2**:1219, 1976

191. Izumi AK, Edwards J: Herpes zoster and neurogenic bladder dysfunction. *JAMA* **224**:1748, 1973

192. Rose FC et al: Zoster encephalomyelitis. *Arch Neurol* **11**:155, 1964

192a. Heller HM et al: Varicella-zoster virus transverse myelitis without cutaneous rash. *Am J Med* **88**:550, 1990

193. Wisloff F et al: Herpes zoster of the stomach. *Lancet* **2**:953, 1979

194. Gibbon NOK: A case of herpes zoster with involvement of the urinary bladder. *Br J Urol* **28**:417, 1956

195. Richmond W: The genitourinary manifestations of herpes zoster. *Br J Urol* **46**:193, 1974

196. McCormick WF et al: Varicella-zoster encephalomyelitis. *Arch Neurol* **21**:559, 1969

197. Gold E, Robbins FC: Isolation of herpes zoster virus from spinal fluid of a patient. *Virology* **6**:293, 1958

198. Applebaum E et al: Herpes zoster encephalitis. *Am J Med* **32**:25, 1962

199. Norris FH et al: Herpes-zoster meningoencephalitis. *J Infect Dis* **122**:335, 1970

200. Jemsek J et al: Herpes zoster-associated encephalitis: Clinicopathologic report of 12 cases and review of the literature. *Medicine (Baltimore)* **62**:81, 1983

201. Reshef E et al: Herpes zoster ophthalmicus followed by contralateral hemiparesis: Report of two cases and review of literature. *J Neurol Neurosurg Psychiatry* **48**:122, 1985

202. Bourdette DN et al: Herpes zoster ophthalmicus and delayed ipsilateral cerebral infarction. *Neurology* **33**:1428, 1983

203. Hilt DC et al: Herpes zoster ophthalmicus and delayed contralateral hemiparesis caused by cerebral angiitis: Diagnosis and management approaches. *Ann Neurol* **14**:543, 1983

204. Rusthoven JJ et al: Varicella-zoster infection in adult cancer patients—a population study. *Arch Intern Med* **148**:1561, 1988

205. Whitley RJ et al: Disseminated herpes zoster in the immunocompromised host: A comparative trial of acyclovir and vidarabine. *J Infect Dis* **165**:450, 1992

206. Pek S, Gikas PW: Pneumonia due to herpes zoster: Report of a case and review of the literature. *Ann Intern Med* **62**:350, 1965

207. Locksley RM et al: Infection with varicella-zoster virus after bone marrow transplantation. *J Infect Dis* **152**:1172, 1985

208. Horten B et al: Multifocal varicella-zoster leukoencephalitis temporally remote from herpes zoster. *Ann Neurol* **9**:251, 1981

209. Olding-Stenkvist E, Grandien M: Early diagnosis of virus-caused vesicular rashes by immunofluorescence on skin biopsies. *Scand J Infect Dis* **8**:27, 1976

210. Frank L: Varicella pneumonitis: Report of a case with autopsy observations. *Arch Pathol* **50**:450, 1950

211. Rotter R, Collins JD: Fatal disseminated varicella in adults. Report of a case and review of the literature. *Wis Med J* **60**:325, 1961

212. Sander J et al: Fatal varicella pneumonia. *Scand J Infect Dis* **2**:231, 1970

213. Shibuta H et al: Varicella virus isolation from spinal ganglion. *Arch gesamte Virusforshung* **45**:382, 1974

214. O'Donnell PP et al: Recurrent herpes zoster encephalitis. *Arch Neurol* **38**:49, 1981

215. Andiman WA et al: Zoster encephalitis. Isolation of virus and measurement of varicella-zoster-specific antibodies in cerebrospinal fluid. *Am J Med* **73**:769, 1982

216. Hogan EL, Krigman MR: Herpes zoster myelitis. *Arch Neurol* **29**:309, 1973

217. Doyle PW et al: Herpes zoster ophthalmicus with contralateral hemiplegia: Identification of cause. *Am J Clin Pathol* **14**:84, 1983

218. Rosenblum WL, Hadfield MG: Granulomatous angiitis of the nervous system in cases of herpes zoster and lymphosarcoma. *Neurology* **22**:348, 1972

219. Reyes MG et al: Viruslike particles in granulomatous angiitis of the central nervous system. *Neurology* **26**:797, 1976

220. Linnemann CC, Alvira MM: Pathogenesis of varicella-zoster angiitis in the CNS. *Arch Neurol* **37**:329, 1980

221. Mayberg MR et al: Trigeminal projections to supratentorial pial and dual blood vessels in cats demonstrated by horseradish peroxidase histochemistry. *J Comp Neurol* **223**:46, 1984

222. Blank H et al: Cytologic smears in diagnosis of herpes simplex, herpes zoster, and varicella. *JAMA* **146**:1410, 1951

223. Barr RJ et al: Rapid method for Tzanck preparations. *JAMA* **237**:1119, 1977

224. Folkers E et al: Rapid diagnosis in varicella and herpes zoster: Re-evaluation of direct smear (Tzanck test) and electron microscopy including colloidal gold immunoelectron microscopy in comparison with virus isolation. *Br J Dermatol* **121**:287, 1989

225. Weller TH: Varicella and herpes zoster, in *Diagnostic Procedures for Viral, Rickettsial and Chlamydial Infections*, 5th ed, edited by EH Lenette, NJ Schmidt. Washington, DC, American Public Health Association, 1979, p 375

226. Richman DD et al: Rapid viral diagnosis. *J Infect Dis* **149**:298, 1984

227. Sadick NS et al: Comparison of detection of varicella-zoster virus by the Tzanck smear, direct immunofluorescence with a monoclonal antibody, and virus isolation. *J Am Acad Dermatol* **17**:64, 1987

228. Schirm J et al: Rapid detection of varicella-zoster virus in clinical specimens using monoclonal antibodies on shell vials and smears. *J Med Virol* **28**:1, 1989

229. Weinberg A et al: Improved detection of varicella-zoster infection with a spin amplification shell vial technique and blind passage. [in press]

230. Frey HM, Steinberg SP: Rapid diagnosis of varicella-zoster virus infections by countercurrent immunoelectrophoresis. *J Infect Dis* **143**:274, 1981

231. Schmidt NJ et al: Direct immunofluorescence staining for detection of herpes simplex and varicella-zoster virus antigens in vesicular lesions and certain tissue specimens. *J Clin Microbiol* **12**:651, 1980

232. Cleveland PH, Richman DD: Enzyme immunofiltration staining assay for immediate diagnosis of herpes simplex virus and varicella-zoster virus directly from clinical specimens. *J Clin Microbiol* **25**:416, 1987

233. Williams V et al: Serologic response to varicella-zoster membrane antigens measured by indirect immunofluorescence. *J Infect Dis* **130**:669, 1974

234. Kalter ZG et al: Immune adherence hemagglutination: Further observations on demonstration of antibody to varicella-zoster virus. *J Infect Dis* **135**:1010, 1977

235. Richmann DD et al: A rapid radioimmunoassay using ^{125}I-staphylococcal protein A for antibody to varicella-zoster virus. *J Infect Dis* **143**:693, 1981

236. Shanley J et al: Enzyme-linked immunosorbent assay for detection of antibody to varicella-zoster virus. *J Clin Microbiol* **15**:208, 1982

237. LaRussa P et al: Comparison of five assays for antibody to varicella-zoster virus to the fluorescent antibody to membrane antigen assay. *J Clin Microbiol* **25**:2059, 1987

238. Steinberg SP, Gershon AA: Measurement of antibodies to varicella-zoster virus using a latex agglutination test, *J Clin Microbiol* **29**:1527, 1991

239. Steele RW et al: Varicella zoster in hospital personnel: Skin test reactivity to monitor susceptibility. *Pediatrics* **70**:604, 1982

240. Dolin R: Antiviral chemotherapy and chemoprophylaxis. *Science* **227**:1296, 1985

241. Savoia M, Oxman MN: Guidelines for antiviral therapy, in *Current Therapy in Infectious Disease: 1985–1986,* edited by EH Kass, R Platt. Toronto/Philadelphia, BC Dekker, 1986, p 1

242. Nicholson KG: Antiviral therapy. Varicella-zoster virus infections, herpes labialis and mucocutaneous herpes, and cytomegalovirus infections. *Lancet* **2**:677, 1984

243. Elion GB: Mechanism of action and selectivity of acyclovir. *Am J Med* **73**:7, 1982

244. Schwartz PM et al: Antiviral activity of arabinosyladenine and arabinosylhypoxanthine in herpes simplex virus-infected KB cells. Selective inhibition of viral deoxyribonucleic acid synthesis in the presence of an adenosine deaminase inhibitor. *Antimicrob Agents Chemother* **10**:64, 1976

245. *Physicians' Desk Reference,* 47th ed. Medical Economics Data, 1993, p 643

246. Fulginiti VA et al: Aspirin and Reye syndrome. *Pediatrics* **69**:810, 1982

247. Dunkle LM et al: A controlled trial of acyclovir for chickenpox in normal children. *N Engl J Med* **325**:1539, 1991

248. Rothe MJ et al: Oral acyclovir therapy for varicella and zoster infections in pediatric and pregnant patients: A brief review. *Pediatr Dermatol* **8**:236, 1991

249. Balfour HH et al: Acyclovir treatment of varicella in otherwise healthy children. *J Pediatr* **116**:633, 1990

250. Whiteley RJ: Therapeutic approaches to varicella-zoster virus infections. *J Infect Dis* **166**(suppl 1):S51, 1992

251. Wallace MR et al: Treatment of adult varicella with oral acyclovir—a randomized placebo-controlled trial. *Ann Intern Med* **117**:358, 1992

252. Prober CG et al: Acyclovir therapy of chickenpox in immunosuppressed children—a collaborative study. *J Pediatr* **101**:622, 1982

253. Arvin AM et al: Human leukocyte interferon in the treatment of varicella in children with cancer. *N Engl J Med* **306**:761, 1982

254. Whitley RJ, Gnann JW: Acyclovir: A decade later. *N Engl J Med* **327**:782, 1992

255. Nyerges G, Meszner Z: Treatment of chickenpox in immunocompromised children. *Am J Med* **85**(suppl 2A):94, 1988

256. Nyerges G et al: Acyclovir prevents dissemination of varicella in immunocompromised children. *J Infect Dis* **157**:309, 1988

257. McGregor RS et al: Varicella in pediatric orthotopic liver transplant recipients. *Pediatrics* **83**:256, 1989

258. Serota FT et al: Acyclovir treatment of herpes zoster infections. *JAMA* **247**:2132, 1982

259. Balfour HH Jr: Intravenous acyclovir therapy for varicella in immunocompromised children. *J Pediatr* **104**:134, 1984

260. Shulman ST: Acyclovir treatment of disseminated varicella in childhood malignant neoplasms. *Am J Dis Child* **139**:137, 1985

261. Shulman ST: Acyclovir treatment of disseminated varicella in childhood malignant neoplasms. *Am J Dis Child* **139**:137, 1985

262. Shepp DH et al: Current therapy of varicella zoster virus infection in immunocompromised patients. *Am J Med* **85**(suppl 2A):96, 1988

263. Vild'e JL et al: Comparative trial of acyclovir and vidarabine in disseminated varicella-zoster virus infections in immunocompromised patients. *J Med Virol* **20**:127, 1986

264. Balfour HH Jr et al: Acyclovir halts progression of herpes zoster in immunocompromised patients. *N Engl J Med* **308**:1448, 1983

265. Whitley RJ et al: Adenine arabinoside therapy of herpes zoster in the immunosuppressed. *N Engl J Med* **294**: 1193, 1976

265. Whitley RJ et al: Adenine arabinoside therapy of herpes zoster in the immunosuppressed. *N Engl J Med* **294**: 1193, 1976

266. Merigan TC et al: Human leukocyte interferon for the treatment of herpes zoster in patients with cancer. *N Engl J Med* **298**:981, 1978

267. Merigan TC et al: Short-course human leukocyte interferon in treatment of herpes zoster in patients with cancer. *Antimicrob Agents Chemother* **19**:193, 1981

268. Winston DJ et al: Recombinant interferon alpha-2a for treatment of herpes zoster in immunosuppressed patients with cancer. *Am J Med* **85**:147, 1988

269. Rifkind D: The activation of varicella-zoster virus infections by immunosuppressive therapy. *J Lab Clin Med* **68**:463, 1966

270. Mazur MH et al: Serum antibody levels as risk factors in the dissemination of herpes zoster. *Arch Intern Med* **139**:1341, 1979

271. Stevens DA, Merigan TC: Zoster immune globulin prophylaxis of disseminated zoster in compromised hosts. *Arch Intern Med* **140**:52, 1980

272. Peterslund NA et al: Acyclovir in herpes zoster. *Lancet* **2**:827, 1981

273. Bean B et al: Acyclovir therapy for acute herpes zoster. *Lancet* **2**:118, 1982

274. McGill J et al: A review of acyclovir treatment of ocular herpes zoster and skin infections. *J Antimicrob Chemother* **12**:45, 1983

275. Wood MJ et al: Efficacy of oral acyclovir treatment of acute herpes zoster. *Am J Med* **85**(suppl 2A): 79, 1988

276. Huff JC et al: Therapy of herpes zoster with oral acyclovir. *Am J Med* **85**(suppl 2A):84, 1988

277. McKendrick MW et al: Oral acyclovir in acute herpes zoster. *Br Med J* **293**:1529, 1986

278. Wassilew SW et al: Oral acyclovir for herpes zoster: A double-blind controlled trial in normal subjects. *Br J Dermatol* **117**:495, 1987

279. Wildenhoff KE et al: Treatment of herpes zoster with idoxuridine ointment, including a multivariate analysis of symptoms and signs. *Scand J Infect Dis* **11**:1, 1979

280. Price RW: Herpes zoster. An approach to systemic therapy. *Med Clin North Am* **66**:1105, 1982

281. Bernstein JE et al: Treatment of chronic postherpetic neuralgia with topical capsaicin. *J Am Acad Dermatol* **17**:93, 1987

282. Eaglstein WH et al: The effects of early corticosteroid therapy on the skin eruption and pain of herpes zoster. *JAMA* **211**:1681, 1970

283. Keczkes K, Basheer AM: Do corticosteroids prevent postherpetic neuralgia? *Br J Dermatol* **102**:551, 1980

284. Esmann V et al: Prednisolone does not prevent post-herpetic neuralgia. *Lancet* **2**:126, 1987

285. Geiser CF et al: Prophylaxis of varicella in children with neoplastic disease: Comparative results with zoster immune plasma and gamma globulin. *Cancer* **35**:1027, 1975

286. Zaia JA et al: A practical method for preparation of varicella-zoster immune globulin. *J Infect Dis* **137**:601, 1978

287. Centers for Disease Control: Varicella-zoster immune globulin for the prevention of chickenpox. *Ann Intern Med* **100**:859, 1984

288. Miller E et al: Outcome in newborn babies given anti-varicella-zoster immunoglobulin after perinatal maternal infection with varicella-zoster virus. *Lancet* **2**:371, 1989

289. *Report of Committee on Infections Diseases. Varicella-Zoster Infections,* 22d ed. Elk Grove Village, IL, American Academy of Pediatrics, 1991, p 517

290. Takahashi M et al: Live vaccine used to prevent the spread of varicella in children in hospital. *Lancet* **2**:1288, 1974

291. Brunell PA et al: Administration of live varicella vaccine to children with leukemia. *Lancet* **2**:1069, 1982

292. Asano Y et al: Five-year follow-up study of recipients of live varicella vaccine using enhanced neutralization and fluorescent antibody membrane antigen assays. *Pediatrics* **72**:291, 1983

293. Asano Y et al: Long-term protective immunity of recipients of the OKA strain of live varicella vaccine. *Pediatrics* **75**:667, 1985

294. Weibel RE et al: Live attenuated varicella virus, vaccine. Efficacy trial in healthy children. *N Engl J Med* **310**:1410, 1984

295. Hayward A et al: Varicella-zoster virus-specific immunity after herpes zoster. *J Infect Dis* **163**:873, 1991

296. Brunell PA: Chickenpox—examining our options (editorial). *N Engl J Med* **325**:1577, 1991

297. Hardy I et al: The incidence of zoster after immunization with live attenuated varicella vaccine—a study in children with leukemia. *N Engl J Med* **325**:1545, 1991

298. Hayward A et al: Varicella-zoster virus (VZV)-specific cytotoxicity after immunization of nonimmune adults with OKA strain attenuated VZV vaccine. *J Infect Dis* **166**:260, 1992

299. Levin MJ et al: Immune response of elderly individuals to a live attenuated varicella vaccine. *J Infect Dis* **166**:253, 1992

300. Arbeter AM et al: Combination measles, mumps, rubella and varicella vaccine. *Pediatrics* **78**:742, 1986

301. Brunell PA et al: Combined vaccine against measles, mumps, rubella, and varicella. *Pediatrics* **81**:779, 1988

302. Englund JA et al: Placebo-controlled trial of varicella vaccine given with or after measles-mumps-rubella vaccine. *J Pediatr* **114**:37, 1989

303. Gershon AA et al: Varicella vaccine: The American experience. *J Infect Dis* **166**(suppl 1):S63, 1992

304. Gershon AA et al: Measurement of antibodies to VZV by latex agglutination (abstr). Presented at the Society for Pediatric Research Meeting, Baltimore, MD, 1992

305. Weibel RE et al: Live Oka/Merck varicella vaccine in healthy children. *JAMA* **254**:2435, 1985

306. Lawrence R et al: The risk of zoster after varicella vaccination in children with leukemia. *N Engl J Med* **318**:543, 1988

307. Williams DL et al: Herpes zoster following varicella vaccine in a child with acute lymphocytic leukemia. *J Pediatr* **106**:259, 1985

308. Hayawaka Y et al: Biologic and biophysical markers of a live varicella vaccine strain (Oka): Identification of clinical isolates from vaccine recipients. *J Infect Dis* **149**:956, 1984

309. Plotkin SA et al: Zoster in normal children after varicella vaccine (letter). *J Infect Dis* **159**:1000, 1989

310. Gershon AA, Steinberg SP, and the Varicella Vaccine Collaborative Study Group of the National Institute of Allergy and Infectious Diseases: Persistence of immunity to varicella in children with leukemia immunized with live attenuated varicella vaccine. *N Engl J Med* **320**:892, 1989

311. Diaz PS et al: Lack of transmission of the live attenuated varicella vaccine virus to immunocompromised children after immunization of their siblings. *Pediatrics* **87**:166, 1991

312. Asano Y et al: Long-term protective immunity of recipients of the OKA strain of live varicella vaccine. *Pediatrics* **75**:667, 1985

313. Perren TJ et al: Prevention of herpes zoster in patients by long-term oral acyclovir after allogeneic bone marrow transplantation. *Am J Med* **85**(suppl 2A):99, 1988

CHAPTER 205

Kathryn E. Bowers and Richard Allen Johnson

Cytomegalovirus Infection

In the developed countries, 40 to 80 percent of young adolescents have become infected by the ubiquitous cytomegalovirus (CMV).[1] The gradual rise in the percentage of those seropositive for CMV in subsequent years is most often accounted for by sexual transmission.[2] By old age, nearly everyone has been infected by the virus.[3] After primary CMV infection, which is most often subclinical and asymptomatic, the virus persists in a lifelong latent stage with the omnipresent potential for reactivation. Symptomatic clinical infection in immunocompetent hosts is rare. Clinically apparent disease may manifest itself in neonates and the immunosuppressed or immunocompromised host. With increasing numbers of organ transplant recipients and individuals infected with the human immunodeficiency virus (HIV), the incidence of symptomatic CMV-associated morbidity and mortality has also increased. Unlike herpes simplex virus (HSV) and varicella-zoster virus (VZV) infections, CMV infection only rarely affects the skin.

CMV was first observed in kidney epithelial cells of a stillborn infant in 1881. Weller named the virus in 1960 based on its cytopathic effect.[4] The term "cytomegalic inclusion disease" was coined even before the virus was discovered, based on the large cells with intranuclear inclusions. The virus, composed of double-stranded DNA, is a member of the *Herpesviridae* family which includes HSV types 1 and 2, VZV, Epstein-Barr virus (EBV), and human herpes virus 6 (HHV-6). The CMV genome is the most complex of all the DNA viruses and is 50 percent larger than that of herpes simplex.[5] Like the other herpes viruses, CMV normally exists in certain tissues in a latent state after the primary infection. CMV can be isolated from urine, breast milk, semen, tears, feces, saliva, blood, cervical secretions, and lymphocytes in healthy persons.[6] Human CMV cannot be readily grown in any experimental animal; many other subtypes of CMV exist and are species specific.[3]

Epidemiology

Humans are believed to be the only reservoir of human CMV. Transmission occurs throughout the year via intimate contact with body fluids such as saliva, cervical secretions, semen, breast milk, feces, and blood (Table 205-1).[1] Virus excretion may be prolonged in infected individuals, leading to an increased duration of exposure of seronegative individuals to the virus.

CMV seroprevalence varies considerably in different population groups throughout the world. Groups with a poor socioeconomic status have a higher rate of seropositivity, regardless of hygiene practices.[7] In the United States, African Americans, Hispanics, and Native Americans acquire the infection at an earlier age than their Caucasian middle-class counterparts.[1,7] Healthy adults are exposed to CMV through blood transfusions and sexual contact (oral, orogenital, or genital).[1,7]

Two periods of increased risk for CMV infection occur: the perinatal period (36 to 56 percent of infants are exposed in the first year of life) and the reproductive years.[3] Infants with CMV-sero-positive mothers are exposed to the virus during passage through the birth canal and while breast feeding, and later within their family and while at day care centers.[8] Adolescents have an annual CMV seroconversion rate of 2 to 10 percent.[9]

Primary CMV infection in adults after exposure to children in day care has been well documented. The annual seroconversion rate of seronegative day care workers is >10 percent.[10] As many as 80 percent of toddlers in day care centers have asymptomatic CMV infection with prolonged viral shedding through the urine, saliva, and respiratory tract.[10,11] Seroconversion of the adults is directly related to the rates of CMV excretion of the children at these centers.[10,11] When a CMV-infected child returns home, 50 percent of the susceptible family members seroconvert within 6 months.[12] Medical care workers do not appear to be at an increased risk of seroconversion through patient contact.[13]

Sexual transmission in both heterosexual and homosexual populations is the predominant mode of transmission in adults. Outbreaks of CMV mononucleosis have been well documented in sexual partners in college communities.[3] High titers of CMV have been found in semen and cervical specimens of healthy adults attending sexually transmitted disease clinics; a history of multiple sexual partners is the strongest predictor of infection.[5] Eight to ten percent of women shed CMV from the cervix; an association exists between chronic cervicitis and CMV infection.[5]

CMV is transmissible through sexual intercourse in homosexual men; CMV antibodies are present in 94 percent of homosexual men versus 54 percent of heterosexual controls.[6,14] Using Southern blot hybridization, multiple strains of CMV may be detected in homosexual men with AIDS, a phenomenon not ordinarily observed in a healthy population.[15] Thirty percent of asymptomatic homosexual men have CMV in their semen; CMV seroprevalence increases with age, number of sexual partners, and participation in anal-receptive intercourse.[5] CMV is excreted for a more prolonged period in semen than urine.[5] Reinfection with CMV through passive anal intercourse may account for the high degree of CMV and other infectious gastrointestinal diseases seen in HIV-positive patients.[8] CMV seropositivity is common among African patients

TABLE 205-1
Transmission of Cytomegalovirus

Congenital	AIDS
Primary maternal infection	Primary infection: rare
Maternal reactivation	Reactivation
Perinatal	Superinfection
Exposure through birth canal	Transplant patients
Hospital nursery	Primary infection: donor
Breast feeding	Reactivation: host
Toddlers/young children	Superinfection: donor
Day care centers	Blood/blood product transfusion
Other children/family members	
Adolescents/young adults	
Heterosexual activity	
Homosexual activity	

with AIDS, but the incidence in hemophiliacs parallels that in the normal population.[16]

CMV was originally thought to be the etiologic agent for AIDS.[1,7] African patients with Kaposi's sarcoma have an increased incidence of anti-CMV antibodies.[3] In homosexual men with Kaposi's sarcoma, CMV RNA and early antigens have been demonstrated; however, other studies have not linked CMV and either classic or HIV-associated Kaposi's sarcoma.[6] Whether CMV has any role in the pathogenesis of Kaposi's sarcoma remains to be determined.

With an increasing number of heart, lung, kidney, and bone marrow transplantation recipients and immunocompromised HIV-infected persons, CMV-associated morbidity and mortality are rising concomitantly. These patients may become chronic carriers of CMV. The majority of CMV-related morbidity and mortality represents reactivation of the virus in the host; primary infection has been associated with more severe disease.[9] Bone marrow transplant recipients have the highest incidence of CMV-related mortality.[17]

The risk of acquiring CMV from a unit of blood is estimated to be 3 to 4 percent, is highest with fresh blood, and is reduced with leukocyte-depleted or cryopreserved blood, possibly because CMV may be associated with the polymorphonuclear leukocyte.[1,7,18] Infants, in whom primary CMV infection may cause high morbidity and mortality, require as little as 50 to 100 ml of a CMV-seropositive blood transfusion to become infected.[3,8] CMV infection associated with cardiopulmonary bypass and infusion of a large volume of blood products, the so-called postperfusion syndrome, may develop in as many as 14 percent of patients, 4 percent of whom will be symptomatic.[19] CMV-seronegative individuals in certain risk groups, i.e., pregnant women, premature infants, bone marrow recipients, and HIV-infected persons, should be identified and transfused with only CMV-seronegative or specially treated blood products.[20]

Ulcerative colitis may be related to previous CMV infection, because the virus has been found in the crypts and inflamed mucosa of the gastrointestinal tract.[21] The virus has a predilection for all portions of gastrointestinal mucosa; serious enteric CMV infections may occur in transplant recipients.

CMV may play a role in atherogenesis. CMV and HSV antigens have been found in arterial smooth muscle cells, where they may induce an inflammatory reaction, proliferation of smooth muscle cells, and accumulation of cholesterol. Heart transplant recipients who develop CMV infection are at higher risk of developing severe coronary artery disease in the transplanted organ.[22]

Nucleic acid sequences specific for CMV have been found localized to the pancreatic Langerhans cells of patients with type 2 diabetes mellitus. CMV antigens have also been detected in peripheral blood monocytes of patients with diabetes; persistent infection may be a factor in the pathogenesis of type 1 diabetes mellitus.[23,24]

Cutaneous Manifestations of CMV Infection

Cutaneous lesions associated with CMV are rare and nonspecific. Underlying disorders associated with CMV cutaneous involvement include HIV disease, malignant neoplasms, burns, and iatrogenic immunosuppression occurring with organ transplantation. Most reported patients with cutaneous CMV have evidence of disseminated infection; all patients who died have had either concurrent systemic CMV infection, other overwhelming infections, or systemic diseases.[25,26]

TABLE 205-2
Cutaneous Manifestations of Cytomegalovirus

Papules[27,28]	Ulcerations[25,36,44–49]
Verrucous plaques/nodules[29–32]	Pyoderma[31]
Vesicles[33–36]	Morbilliform rash[36,42,48,50]
Epidermolysis[37]	Urticaria[51]
Purpura[36,38–41]	Granulation tissue/burns[52]
Petechiae[2,41–43]	Dermatitis, diaper[26]

Multiple morphologic patterns from vesicles to verrucous plaques have been described in the reported cases of cutaneous CMV; these are tabulated in Table 205-2. Urticarial and morbilliform eruptions are reported more frequently in healthy patients who have a CMV mononucleosis-like syndrome and have received recent antibiotic therapy such as ampicillin.[53] The finding of CMV-induced cytopathic changes in lesional skin biopsies probably indicates widespread tissue infection and does not necessarily mean that the CMV infection is the cause of the cutaneous change (Fig. 205-1).

The most specific cutaneous manifestation of CMV is ulceration, especially in the perianal area. Ulcerations were present in 30 percent of the reported cases of cutaneous CMV.[25] One of the earliest reported cases of cutaneous CMV was an otherwise healthy elderly woman with perianal and rectal ulcerations.[6] Ulcerations on the buttocks, perineum, and thigh with visceral involvement have

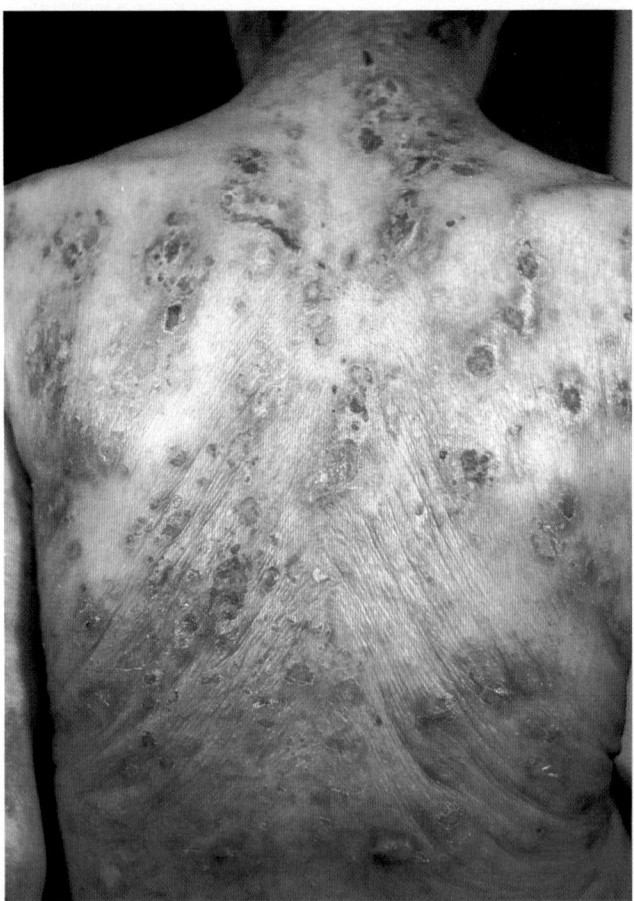

FIGURE 205-1 Papules and nodules on the back of a patient with Hodgkin's disease and disseminated CMV. (*From Sugiura,[30] with permission.*)

also been well described.[4,6,8,25] All patients with ulcerations died. Horn and Hood[54] demonstrated histologic and immunohistochemical evidence of CMV infection in five consecutive patients with immunosuppression and perineal ulcers. Clinically, these ulcers resembled a chronic herpetic infection. The authors hypothesized that CMV may be a direct cause of the ulcer or evidence of a subclinical infection, or may reflect disseminated CMV infection.[54]

Multiple organisms, including *Staphylococcus aureus* and acid-fast bacilli, as well as HSV, may be found in association with CMV in skin biopsies.[27,28,32,55] Smith et al.[32] reported two patients with concurrent epidermal involvement with both CMV and HSV, documented by both immunohistochemical and DNA hybridization studies, in two HIV-infected patients. Two reported cases have been associated with disseminated intravascular coagulation.[43,48]

In summary, cutaneous manifestations of CMV infection are usually not distinctive enough to confirm the diagnosis. Certain risk groups have distinctive patterns of primary and reactivated infection. In contrast to the healthy host, in whom the disease is usually asymptomatic, the immunocompromised host may present with mononucleosis, pneumonitis, hepatitis, encephalitis, gastroenteritis, choreoretinitis, or a cutaneous eruption.[14]

CMV Infection in Pregnancy

Approximately 2 percent of CMV-seronegative pregnant women develop an asymptomatic primary CMV infection during pregnancy. A mononucleosis-like syndrome with a rubelliform or morbilliform rash has been reported.[6] The two principal sources of CMV infection for women of child-bearing age are sexual intercourse and exposure to young children attending day care centers.[56] Intrauterine infection occurs in 55 percent of fetuses whose mothers have a primary CMV infection.[3] An adverse outcome is more likely if the virus is transmitted in the first trimester. Congenital infection is equally common in babies of mothers who are infected with CMV before the pregnancy; however, maternal immunity reduces the severity of infection in these infants.[8] Congenital CMV infection is more common in infants of young, single, primigravida mothers who also have other sexually transmitted diseases such as gonorrhea.[56,57]

Congenital CMV Infection

CMV is the major infectious cause of mental retardation and deafness in the United States.[58] CMV infection, part of the TORCH syndrome [*t*oxoplasmosis, *o*ther (syphilis/bacterial sepsis), *r*ubella, *c*ytomegalovirus, *h*erpes simplex virus], is the most common congenital viral infection.[59] One percent of infants born in the United States become infected with CMV in utero and may shed virus in saliva and urine for up to 5 years.[3] Less than 10 percent of infected infants have clinical manifestations of the virus.[6] Sixty-five percent of infants with symptomatic CMV infections experience long-term sensorineural hearing loss, mental retardation, learning disabilities, and seizures.[1] The infant mortality rate of congenital CMV infection is 20 to 30 percent; hydrocephalus and intracranial calcification are poor prognostic signs.[6] Involvement of the CNS, inner ear, and the choroid of the eye are unique to congenital CMV infection.[3] Fifteen percent of asymptomatic infants develop sequelae later in life.[6]

Primary maternal CMV infection during the first 24 weeks of gestation carries the highest risk of permanent sequelae for the

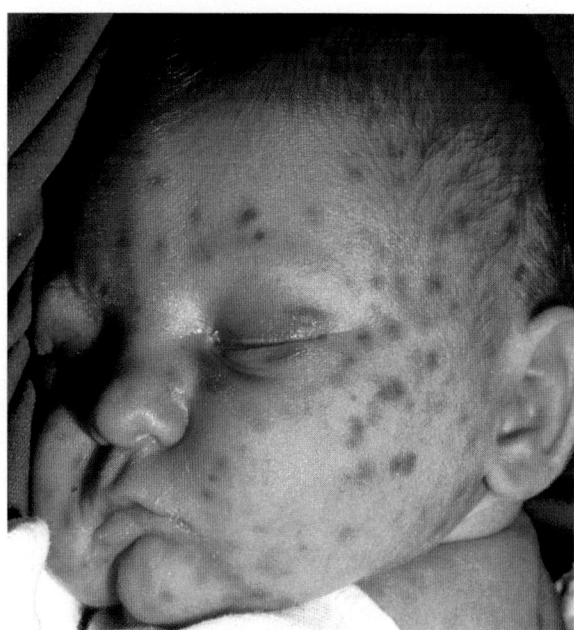

FIGURE 205-2 Infant with congenital CMV infection: "blueberry muffin baby." (*From Groark and Jampel,[60] with permission.*)

fetus.[10] Infants born of mothers who were infected in the first trimester may be small for gestational age and may have microcephaly, intracranial calcifications, retinitis, and optic nerve malformations (coloboma). Infants infected in later trimesters may have acute visceral disease with hepatitis, pneumonia, purpura, and disseminated intravascular coagulation.[13]

The diseases that comprise the TORCH syndrome may each have a similar clinical picture. The major clinical manifestations of the TORCH syndrome are hepatomegaly, splenomegaly, microcephaly, deafness, chorioretinitis, thrombocytopenia, jaundice, and purpura ("blueberry muffin baby").[6] Fulminant infection with CMV was originally termed congenital cytomegalic inclusion disease.[3]

The "blueberry muffin baby," first described in the 1960s by Brough et al., had purpuric macules and papules, manifestations (see review by Lesher[6]), of persistent dermal hematopoiesis (Fig. 205-2). During normal fetal development, erythropoiesis occurs in the dermis. The persistence of these blood-forming elements may be the result of tissue hypoxia, chronic anemia, or a direct or indirect effect of the virus on the vascular mesenchyme.[60] These dark blue to violaceous, raised or flat, purpuric lesions present within 24 to 48 h of birth, resolve with a copper color, and are present in 31 percent of infants with the TORCH syndrome.[61]

Recovery of CMV from the urine, throat, or other body fluids during the first week of life is the ideal method for diagnosis since serologic tests are inaccurate because of maternal antibodies and the small amount of IgM produced by the infant.[13,62] A positive viral culture during the first 3 weeks of life indicates congenital CMV infection.

CMV Infection in Children

Acquisition of CMV is common during the first year of life, usually from the infant's mother.[63] Ten to fifteen percent of healthy term infants may be exposed to CMV through the birth canal or from breast milk, but they rarely develop symptomatic CMV infection.[63] Infants who acquire the virus during the perinatal period begin to shed the virus at 4 to 8 weeks and for up to 2.5 years.[3] Preterm or low-birth-weight infants are at greater risk for developing signs and symptoms of infection with CMV and may develop a mononucleosis-like syndrome.[63] Outbreaks of CMV infection have occurred in neonatal intensive care units in high-risk seronegative infants.[3]

Papular acrodermatitis of childhood (Gianotti-Crosti syndrome) is associated with many viral illnesses such as enterovirus, hepatitis B, adenovirus, and CMV. CMV hepatitis may accompany this syndrome as described by Berant et al.[64]

Viral or bacterial illness may precede the development of scleredema. A preceding CMV illness may have contributed to the development of scleredema in an infant with CMV viruria and pneumonia described by Heilbron and Saxe.[65]

Helm et al.[59] described an infant with disseminated CMV in the KID syndrome (*k*eratitis, *i*chthyosis, and *d*eafness). Autopsy documented multiorgan involvement with CMV inclusions and a lower esophageal ulcer.[59] Children with KID syndrome usually have problems with recurrent bacterial and yeast infections secondary to defective T-cell immunity.

A dramatic case of ulcerative perianal diaper dermatitis heralded systemic CMV infection in an infant with AIDS described by Thiboutot et al.[26] The diaper area was covered with vesicles, pustules, and bullae on an erythematous base (Fig. 205-3). CMV was cultured from the skin biopsy and characteristic viral inclusions were conspicuous on histology. Disseminated infection involving the blood, urine, lung, and eyes was subsequently diagnosed. The infant died within 1 month of the diagnosis despite treatment with ganciclovir.

Petechiae in an infant with acute graft-versus-host disease were reported to be secondary to generalized CMV.[43] CMV has the potential to infect human natural killer cells, monocytes, and B- and T-cell lymphocytes.[43] A 7-year-old girl with CMV mononucleosis developed purpuric papules in a livedoid and annular pattern with histology demonstrating a lymphocytic vasculitis. No viral inclusion bodies were seen in the histologic sections.[66]

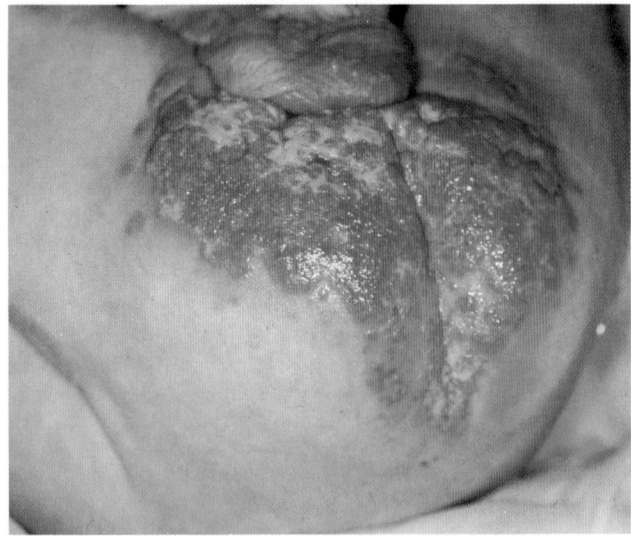

FIGURE 205-3 Infant with AIDS and diaper dermatitis secondary to disseminated CMV. (*From Thiboutot et al.,[26] with permission.*)

CMV Infection in Healthy Adults

Most individuals eventually become infected with CMV; primary infection is usually subclinical and symptomatic. A mononucleosis-like syndrome may develop in healthy adults, usually in an older group than those susceptible to EBV-associated mononucleosis. Women in the third decade are most commonly affected. CMV mononucleosis may also be caused by blood and leukocyte transfusions.[3]

CMV mononucleosis often poses an initial diagnostic problem. The most common presenting signs and symptoms are fever, abnormal liver function tests, a negative heterophile antibody test, and blood smears with an atypical lymphocytosis indistinguishable from that of EBV infectious mononucleosis.[67] These patients tend to have less severe pharyngitis, lymphadenopathy, and splenomegaly than EBV-infected patients.[6,66] A short-lived rubelliform type rash, lasting from several hours to days, occurs predominantly on the lower extremities, although it may be generalized and is seen in 31 percent of patients.[6,19] This maculopapular rash occurs in the majority of patients treated with ampicillin or amoxicillin during the initial phase of the illness; the identical phenomenon occurs in EBV mononucleosis.[19]

Immunologic abnormalities, such as the presence of mixed cryoglobulins, cold agglutinins, rheumatoid factor, and antinuclear antibodies, are observed with both CMV and EBV infection.[3] Although the prognosis is usually excellent, complications of CMV mononucleosis include thrombocytopenia, granulomatous hepatitis, pneumonitis, hemolytic anemia, meningoencephalitis, myocarditis, vasculitis, and the Guillain-Barré syndrome.[63] Spear et al.[68] reported a case of an adult patient with acute CMV mononucleosis and erythema nodosum without viral inclusions in the skin biopsy.

CMV Infection in Immunocompromised Individuals

Prolonged parenteral corticosteroid therapy alone has a minimal effect on reactivation of CMV.[69] The incidence of CMV reactivation and symptomatic infection is significantly increased in patients with neoplasia, especially lymphoma and leukemia, and in transplant recipients.[3] Patients receiving chemotherapy experience an increase of primary CMV infection, both subclinical and symptomatic.[63] Systemic manifestations of CMV infection include a mononucleosis-like syndrome, pneumonitis, hepatitis, gastroenteritis or gastrointestinal ulcerations, and chorioretinitis.[35] Neutropenia alone does not appear to be an independent risk factor for developing CMV disease.[3]

CMV Infection in HIV-Infected Individuals

Reactivated latent CMV infection is exceedingly common in HIV-infected individuals. CMV affects more organs in HIV patients than in the transplant population.[8] CMV viremia with pneumonia and necrotizing adrenalitis may be one of the leading causes of death; 77 to 90 percent of patients with AIDS also have CMV disease at the time of death.[32,70] Concurrent CMV infection may potentiate the immunosuppressive effects of HIV, enhancing HIV replication at the cellular level by transactivation.[5,16] Dissemination of CMV is associated with fever, wasting, and inanition. A catabolic state in the patient with AIDS can be reversed with therapy for CMV, suggesting that CMV may contribute significantly to the pathology of the overall disease state.[58,70]

Five percent of patients with AIDS have CMV pneumonia, characterized by increasing shortness of breath and an interstitial pattern on chest x-ray.[71] More commonly, CMV is a coinfecting agent in the lung, usually with *Pneumocystis carinii*; it is unclear whether CMV is a true pulmonary pathogen in these cases.

Subacute encephalitis may be caused by CMV, and symptoms include headaches, personality changes, and somnolence.[71] Multiple endocrinopathies have also been reported.[8] CMV may cause inflammation of the gastrointestinal mucosa with symptoms of esophagitis, colitis, pancreatitis, and cholecystitis. Other pathogens such as *Mycobacterium avium-intracellulare* and *Cryptosporidia* may be cultured as copathogens.[3] The colon is most frequently involved, followed by the esophagus, rectum, and small bowel.[1]

CMV retinitis occurs in 30 percent of patients with AIDS in the United States and may cause blindness if untreated.[72] Patients with CMV retinitis are usually viremic and have symptoms of decreased visual acuity and multiple spots interfering with vision. Viral replication occurs at a very high level; numerous virions may be detected in the retina by electron microscopy.[9] The characteristic retinal findings are yellow-white exudates and hemorrhages at the periphery of the fundus, described as resembling ''crumbled cheese with ketchup.''[73] Ganciclovir is effective in the treatment of CMV retinitis, but therapy must be continued indefinitely because lesions recur if the drug is discontinued. Despite therapy, retinal detachment may occur and is related to extensive viral-induced retinal necrosis.[73]

CMV Infection in Transplantation Recipients

Transplanted bone marrow, kidney, heart, lung, and liver are often reservoirs of CMV and may infect the host with a new strain of CMV or cause a primary infection in the seronegative host.[8] CMV infection is diagnosed by a rise in antibody titers or isolation of the virus in 85 percent of seropositive transplant recipients and 53 percent of seronegative recipients.[3] Iatrogenic immunosuppression is the most important parameter for CMV reactivation; it does not prevent development of an antibody response to the CMV, except in the presence of severe infection.[3] Cyclosporine use is a low risk factor for reactivation but, once it occurs, cyclosporine cripples the host response.[69] The use of antilymphocyte globulin greatly increases reactivation of CMV.[69]

Half of renal transplant recipients experience CMV disease, which is responsible for 25 percent of the deaths in these patients, 20 percent of graft failures, 30 percent of febrile episodes, and 35 percent of leukopenic episodes.[74] A distinct glomerulopathy may occur with renal dysfunction.[1] Fortunately, symptomatic disease occurs 3 to 4 months after transplantation, when immunosuppressive drug doses are being decreased.[58] Fever may be the only manifestation of active CMV infection, although leukopenia, thrombocytopenia, pneumonitis, hepatitis, retinitis, and encephalitis may also occur.[63]

The risk of developing significant CMV-induced disease in solid organ transplant recipients occurs between weeks 4 and 12 after transplantation.[75] In heart and lung transplant recipients, gastrointestinal disease (gastritis, esophagitis, perforation, and hemorrhage) is the most prominent manifestation of CMV; the overall frequency of severe CMV disease and CMV mycocarditis is higher in this group than in those who receive other organ transplants.[69,75] CMV hepatitis is a more common complication of liver transplants and is often difficult to distinguish from organ rejection, other than by liver biopsy, in that both are associated with fever and elevated liver function tests.[3]

CMV-seropositive bone marrow transplant recipients have a higher incidence of subsequent CMV disease related to reactivation of latent virus. Donor marrow and blood product transfusion are important sources of CMV infection in seronegative transplant patients.[76] The major morbidity from CMV disease occurs during the first 40 days after transplantation, before engraftment and resumption of immune function.[58] CMV pneumonia is the most frequent cause of CMV-related morbidity in bone marrow transplant recipients, with a mortality rate approaching 85 percent.[77] The interstitial pneumonia may be an immunopathologic process mediated by a specific T-cell response to CMV antigens, enhanced by graft-versus-host disease.[17] Combined therapy with ganciclovir and immune globulin has improved survival in these patients.[17,77] The CMV virus may also be responsible for a delay in the immunologic recovery of bone marrow transplant patients with secondary effects on the immune system including leukopenia, decreased cell-mediated immunity with increased risk of other opportunistic infections, and altered macrophage function.[63,76] The risk of superinfection is directly related to the degree of leukopenia (<3000 leukocytes/mm^3), decrease in CD4 cell counts, and increase in CD8 cell counts.[69]

Diagnosis

Prompt diagnosis of disseminated CMV is important because of the availability of specific and effective antiviral agents. CMV infection is often asymptomatic and must be distinguished from mere viral shedding. Cutaneous infection with CMV has a characteristic histopathologic morphology, with preferential involvement of endothelial and ductal cells much more commonly than of epithelium. The characteristic ''owl's eyes'' basophilic intranuclear inclusion is good evidence of CMV infection (Fig. 205-4).[78] However, there is a false-negative rate of at least 12 percent with light microscopy alone.[25]

Infection can be confirmed by viral culture techniques, traditionally from the urine, blood, and throat. Viremia, diagnosed by buffy-coat cultures, is one of the best indicators of active systemic CMV infection.[31] However, asymptomatic viremia and viruria may occur, especially in patients with advanced HIV disease. CMV grows slowly, and only in fibroblast culture, compared with other herpes viruses, which grow rapidly in both fibroblast and epithelial (amnion) cell cultures.[34] CMV-induced cytopathic effects in con-

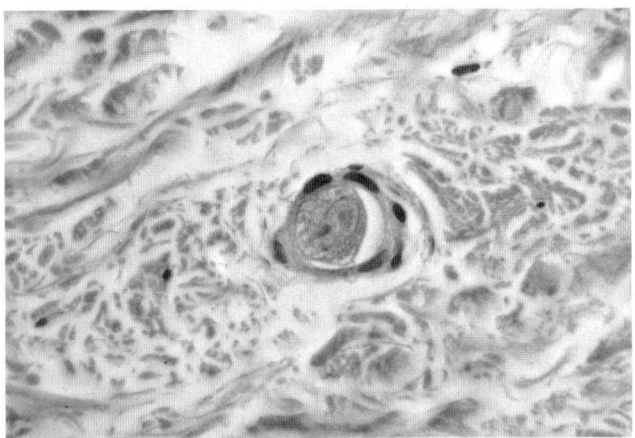

FIGURE 205-4 Intranuclear inclusions in a cell infected by CMV. (*From Konstadt et al.,*[2] *with permission.*)

ventional cultures are noted within 1 to 2 weeks, although they may be delayed for as long as 6 weeks if viral titers are low.[79] CMV cultured from a skin biopsy specimen indicates the presence of virus either in the tissue itself or in the circulating blood within it. Because acutely ill adults may have no specific symptoms or signs and may shed CMV intermittently and in small quantities, culture techniques are unreliable[13] so buffy coats should be checked for evidence of viremia, which is usually greater than viruria and correlates with active disease.[79]

Viremia is present long before an anti-CMV IgM immune response. The presence of IgM antibodies indicates infection within the last 12 to 16 weeks; IgM antibodies detected by ELISA can occur with primary infection and as a result of reactivation and exogenous reinfection.[79] CMV seroconversion or a fourfold rise in IgG antibody titers in the sera of an acutely ill patient compared with convalescent sera indicates active CMV infection.[63] Both maternal and infant sera should be evaluated in order to diagnose a congenital infection.[5] Antibody production may be decreased in the presence of overwhelming infection; the immunosuppressed patient may not be able to mount an immune response to the virus.[79]

On histology and electron microscopy, HSV and VZV have only intranuclear inclusions, whereas CMV may have both intranuclear and intracytoplasmic inclusions. Electron microscopy cannot be relied on to confirm the diagnosis of CMV because it is time consuming, expensive, and may fail to allow CMV to be distinguished from other human herpes viruses.

Immunohistochemical and immunoperoxidase testing with CMV-specific monoclonal antibodies is rapid, generally available, and may be used on tissue or fluid samples. An early, 72-kDa CMV protein is detectable within hours on flat monolayers of centrifuged samples using monoclonal antibodies. This process, the shell vial technique, works best on urine and bronchoalveolar lavage specimens and less well on buffy-coat samples.[79,80] A biotin-labeled, cloned probe of CMV, used for in situ DNA hybridization has little cross-reactivity with the other herpes viruses and may be used on formaldehyde-fixed or paraffin-embedded samples. If suitable primers, distinct sequences, and problems of cost and availability are solved, polymerase chain reaction (PCR) may become the gold standard for detecting CMV.[81] Whether PCR can differentiate between latent and active CMV infection is not known.

Differential Diagnosis

CMV infection should be included in the differential diagnosis of an immunosuppressed patient with fever and a generalized or unexplained localized rash, especially if cutaneous ulceration occurs. Because of the multiple case reports of HSV coexisting with CMV, the possibility of an associated HSV or VZV infection must be considered in chronic ulcers and diagnosed by viral culture, immunohistochemistry, or DNA in situ hybridization.

The differential diagnosis of a neonate with purpuric macules and papules should include CMV, the other TORCH infectious agents, lymphoma, leukemia, neuroblastoma with cutaneous metastases, twin transfusion syndrome, hereditary spherocytosis, neonatal systemic lupus erythematosus, and neonatal sepsis.[60]

Dermatopathology

The diagnosis of CMV infection by histologic findings alone is not always possible since the typical CMV-associated inclusions may be subtle. The typical cytomegalic cell is characterized by the following features: a diameter of 20 to 40 μm; large intranuclear inclusion(s) (8 to 10 μm); a clear halo around the nuclear inclusion; a rim of nuclear material (1 to 2 μm); cytoplasmic inclusions (2 to 4 μm).[6] The intracytoplasmic inclusions appear as granular, periodic acid-Schiff-positive, perinuclear structures.[32]

The intranuclear inclusions are identical to those seen in HSV or VZV infections, although those occurring with CMV may be larger.[32] The characteristic ''owl's eyes'' intranuclear inclusion (Fig. 205-4) indicates CMV infection and often persists for some time, in comparison with the evanescent structure in HSV-infected cells.[32]

Intraepithelial involvement by CMV occurs in the kidney, lung, salivary gland, gastrointestinal tract, and rarely skin.[31] CMV usually infects endothelial cells; involvement of the vascular endothelium is specific for disseminated CMV infection.[6] Myerson et al.[82] postulated that the commonly multifocal nature of CMV infection is due to the hematogenous dissemination with local spread via infection of the endothelial cells. CMV usually also infects ductal structures and sweat glands.[32,48]

In three patients with AIDS, CMV was unexpectedly found in biopsy specimens of clinically normal skin. Clinically occult CMV probably occurs more commonly than recognized and may be only an incidental finding in the immunocompromised patient.[6,83] Investigators do stress the importance of searching for active visceral involvement especially in the lungs and eyes if there is evidence of CMV on a skin biopsy specimen in an immunocompromised patient.

Pathogenesis

Some strains of CMV are more virulent than others in vivo.[1] Pariser[48] has hypothesized that an initial reactivation of CMV leads to viremia in the immunosuppressed host. The virus infects the vascular endothelium, resulting in an exanthem. As involvement of the vessels increases, vasculitis occurs and the destruction of blood vessels causes secondary ulceration.[6] A prominent neutrophilic perivascular infiltrate may be observed around CMV-infected vessels.[48] Endothelial cells have the ability to phagocytose the virus, and an oncogenic potential of the virus has been demonstrated in vitro.[48,73]

The polymorphonuclear leukocyte is the main source of CMV in the blood.[1] Cells that carry latent infection may be present in many organs, and circulating white blood cells or stromal cells may be the source of infection in transplant patients.[8] Rubin[69] hypothesized that the virus is present at multilple sites, in more than one cell type, and that reactivation may be caused by many stimuli.

Beta$_2$-microglobulin, present in most body fluids, has a high binding affinity for CMV and protects it against immune destruction.[1] CMV also binds nonspecifically to the Fc receptor of immunoglobulins, and that binding provides the virus with another immune protective coat.[1] The finding that lymphocyte proliferative responses to mitogens and viral antigens are decreased in the presence of CMV provides evidence for an immunosuppressive role of CMV in the host.[1]

The most potent reactivator of CMV is exogenous immunosuppressive therapy.[69] Cell-mediated immunity and the activity of cytotoxic T cells are of prime importance in determining the outcome and severity of CMV infection.[17] CMV suppresses functioning of cytotoxic T cells, with decreased CD4 cells and increased CD8 cells leading to an overall depression in cell-mediated immunity.[69] Macrophage phagocytosis and presentation are disrupted, especially in the lung, and immune mediators such as interferon alpha are decreased.[76] Natural killer cells and cytotoxic T cells are important not only for recovery from a CMV infection, but also for surveillance and prevention of viral reactivation.[69]

CMV encodes for glycoproteins that are homologous to class I MHC antigens and causes up-regulation of class II MHC antigens in transplanted grafts, which may play a role in allograft rejection.[69] In heart transplant recipients, CMV is associated with early allograft rejection and an increased incidence of graft atherosclerosis.[69] The virus may directly mediate injury to the vascular endothelium with secondary lipid deposition.[69]

Humoral immunity can modify the degree of infection, for example, in newborns who acquire a perinatal CMV infection but have circulating maternal CMV antibodies. The administration of CMV immune globulin decreases the incidence of CMV illness in seronegative transplant recipients.[17]

Course and Prognosis

Early diagnosis and treatment of disseminated CMV may lead to a successful outcome, as reported by Sugiura.[30] The treatment of CMV retinitis has been successful with ganciclovir and phosphonoformate (foscarnet), although therapy must be continued for life. The response rates of other manifestations of CMV infection are difficult to assess because of the sporadic case reports and the presence of coinfecting agents. Patients with cutaneous CMV have a very poor prognosis, with a mortality rate that approximates 85 percent within 6 months, although most of these cases were reported before the general use of improved antiviral agents.[25]

Treatment

High-dose acyclovir can be used effectively as prophylaxis against CMV infection, although it is ineffective against active viral disease.[69] Ganciclovir is a nucleoside analogue of acyclovir that differs by one hydroxyl side chain. Unlike acyclovir, ganciclovir does not require viral thymidine kinase for phosphorylation and activation.[17] Ganciclovir is 50 times more effective than acyclovir in vitro against CMV and inhibits viral DNA polymerase.[30]

Eighty-five percent of patients with CMV retinitis respond within 2 weeks of therapy with ganciclovir.[73] One-third of patients with AIDS must discontinue therapy because of drug-related adverse side effects such as neutropenia, thrombocytopenia, and central nervous system changes. Significant hematologic toxicity may occur with combination therapy with ganciclovir and zidovudine. In those individuals who tolerate the medication, therapy must be continued on a long-term basis since ganciclovir is virostatic and not virocidal. Patients with CMV retinitis will usually relapse within 1 month after discontinuation of therapy.[73] Prophylactic ganciclovir has been used successfully in bone marrow transplant patients to prevent CMV interstitial pneumonia.[77] Ganciclovir-resistant strains of CMV have been reported in as many as 7 percent of patients treated longer than 3 months.[84]

Trisodium phosphonoformate (foscarnet), the newest antiviral approved for CMV retinitis, inhibits DNA polymerase of human herpes viruses and also the reverse transcriptase of human immunodeficiency virus in vitro. This drug may also be used for acyclovir-resistant HSV and VZV because it works at a different site than

acyclovir.[85] A more prolonged long-term survival of patients with CMV retinitis has been reported with phosphonoformate treatment compared with ganciclovir treatment.[86] Phosphonoformate holds promise in the treatment of CMV infections and may be effective in bone marrow transplant patients. The dose-limiting side effects are nephrotoxicity and anemia without neutropenia.[73] A case of a bone marrow transplant patient has been reported in whom three strains of CMV were isolated, one of which was resistant to both ganciclovir and phosphonoformate.[87]

Alpha interferon may prevent serious CMV infections in seropositive renal transplant patients.[5] A trial of CMV hyperimmune globulin as an effective prophylaxis in bone marrow transplantations from seropositive donors demonstrated a decrease in viremia but no overall difference in long-term survival; other studies have shown conflicting results.[88,89] Interleukin-2 partially restores CMV-specific cell-mediated immune responses in vitro, but it has not been studied as a form of therapy.[16]

Researchers have developed several live attenuated vaccines against CMV for at-risk individuals such as young adults and transplant candidates.[90] Immunity wanes rapidly and there is a theoretical concern regarding the oncogenic potential of a live CMV vaccine. In the future, combination therapy with less toxic antiviral drugs, immunomodulators, and prevention strategies may hold promise in decreasing the morbidity and mortality of severe CMV infections in at-risk groups.

References

1. Alford CA, Britt WJ: *Cytomegalovirus in Virology,* 2d ed. New York, Raven, 1990, p 1981
2. Konstadt JW et al: Disseminated cytomegalovirus infection with cutaneous involvement in a heart transplant patient. *Clin Cases Dermatol* **2:**2, 1990
3. Ho M: Cytomegalovirus, in *Principles and Practices of Infectious Diseases,* 3d ed. New York, Churchill Livingstone, 1990, p 1159
4. Weller TH et al: Serologic differentiation of viruses responsible for cytomegalic inclusion disease. *Virology* **12:**130–2, 1960
5. Smiley L, Huang ES: Cytomegalovirus as a sexually transmitted infection, in *Sexually Transmitted Diseases,* 2d ed. New York, McGraw-Hill, 1990, p 415
6. Lesher JL: Cytomegalovirus and the skin. *J Am Acad Dermatol* **18:**1333, 1988
7. Alford CA et al: Congenital and perinatal cytomegalovirus infections. *Rev Infect Dis* **12:**S745, 1990
8. Ho M: Epidemiology of cytomegalovirus infections. *Rev Infect Dis* **12:**S701, 1990
9. Zaia JA: Epidemiology and pathogenesis of cytomegalovirus disease. *Semin Hematol* **27:**5, 1990
10. Adler SP: Cytomegalovirus and child day care: Evidence for an increased infection rate among day-care workers. *N Engl J Med* **321:**1290, 1989
11. Murph JR et al: The occupational risk of CMV infection among day care workers. *JAMA* **265:**603, 1991
12. Yow MD: Congenital cytomegalovirus disease: A NOW problem. *J Infect Dis* **159:**163, 1989
13. Yow MD: CMV infection in young women. *Hosp Practice* **25:**61, 1990
14. Jacobson MA, Mills J: Serious cytomegalovirus disease in the acquired immunodeficiency syndrome. *Ann Intern Med* **108:**585, 1988
15. Spector SA et al: Identification of multiple CMV strains in homosexual males with AIDS. *J Infect Dis* **150:**953, 1984
16. Schooley RT: Cytomegalovirus in the setting of infection with human immunodeficiency virus. *Rev Infect Dis* **12:**S811, 1990

17. Winston DJ et al: Cytomegalovirus infections after allogeneic bone marrow transplantation. *Rev Infect Dis* **12**:S776, 1990

18. Dorkin RJ et al: Survival of cytomegalovirus in viremic blood under blood bank storage conditions. *J Infect Dis* **161**:1310, 1990

19. Cohen JI, Corey GR: Cytomegalovirus infection in the normal host. *Medicine (Baltimore)* **65**:100, 1985

20. Sayers MH et al: Reducing the risk for transfusion-transmitted cytomegalovirus infection. *Ann Intern Med* **116**:55, 1992

21. Diepersloot RJA et al: Acute ulcerative proctocolitis associated with primary cytomegalovirus infection. *Arch Intern Med* **150**:1749, 1990

22. Melnick JL et al: Possible role of cytomegalovirus in atherogenesis. *JAMA* **263**:2204, 1990

23. Lohr JM, Oldstone MBA: Detection of cytomegalovirus nucleic acid sequences in pancreas in type 2 diabetes. *Lancet* **336**:644, 1990

24. Pak CY et al: Association of cytomegalovirus infection with autoimmune type 1 diabetes. *Lancet* **2**(8601):1, 1988

25. Toome BT et al: Diagnosis of cytomegalovirus infection: A review and report of a case. *J Am Acad Dermatol* **24**:857, 1991

26. Thiboutot DM et al: Cytomegalovirus diaper dermatitis. *Arch Dermatol* **127**:396, 1991

27. Kwan TH, Kaufman HW: Acid-fast bacilli with cytomegalovirus and herpes inclusions in the skin of an AIDS patient. *Am J Clinic Pathol* **85**:236, 1986

28. Boudreau S et al: Dermal abscesses with *Staphylococcus aureus*, cytomegalovirus and acid fast bacilli in a patient with AIDS. *J Cutan Pathol* **15**:53, 1988

29. Fenoglio CM et al: Kaposi's sarcoma following chemotherapy for testicular cancer in a homosexual man: Demonstration of cytomegalovirus RNA in sarcoma cells. *Hum Pathol* **15**:53, 1982

30. Sugiura H: Successful treatment of disseminated cutaneous cytomegalic inclusion disease with Hodgkin's disease. *J Am Acad Dermatol* **24**:346, 1991

31. Bournerias I et al: Unusual cutaneous cytomegalovirus involvement in patients with acquired immunodeficiency syndrome. *Arch Dermatol* **24**:346, 1989

32. Smith KJ et al: Concurrent epidermal involvement of cytomegalovirus and herpes simplex virus in two HIV-infected patients. *J Am Acad Dermatol* **25**:500, 1991

33. Blatt J et al: Cutaneous vesicles in congenital cytomegalovirus infection. *J Pediatr* **92**:509, 1978

34. Bhawan J et al: Vesiculobullous lesions caused by cytomegalovirus infection in an immunocompromised adult. *J Am Acad Dermatol* **11**:743, 1984

35. Feldman PS et al: Cutaneous lesions heralding disseminated cytomegalovirus infection. *J Am Acad Dermatol* **7**:545, 1982

36. Lee JY: Cytomegalovirus infection involving the skin in immunocompromised hosts. *Am J Clin Pathol* **92**:96, 1989

37. Muller-Stamou A et al: Epidermolysis in a case of severe cytomegalovirus infection. *Br Med J* **7**:609, 1974

38. Symers WS: Generalized cytomegalic inclusion body disease associated with *Pneumocystis* pneumonia in adults. *J Clin Pathol* **13**:1, 1960

39. Sandler A, Snedeker JD: Cytomegalovirus infection in an infant presenting with cutaneous vasculitis. *Pediatr Infect Dis J* **6**:422, 1987

40. Bamji A, Salisbury R: Cytomegalovirus and vasculitis. *Br Med J* **1**:623, 1978

41. Elenitsas R, Cohen BA: Cutaneous cytomegalovirus in a liver transplant patient. *Transplant Proc* **20**:656, 1988

42. Robson GS, Mackay IR: Generalized cytomegalovirus infection in a patient with lupoid hepatitis. *Aust Ann Med* **18**:147, 1969

43. Tawfik N, Jimbow K: Acute graft-vs-host disease in an immunodeficient newborn possibly due to cytomegalovirus infection. *Arch Dermatol* **125**:1685, 1989

44. Williams G et al: Cytomegalic inclusion disease and *Pneumocystis* infection in an adult. *Lancet* **2**:951, 1960

45. Minars N et al: Fatal cytomegalic inclusion disease. *Arch Dermatol* **113**:1569, 1977

46. Walker JD, Chesney TM: Cytomegalovirus infection of the skin. *Am J Dermatopathol* **4**:263, 1982

47. Naroneczna I, Kay S: Fatal disseminated cytomegalic inclusion disease in an adult presenting with a lesion of the gastrointestinal tract. *Am J Clin Pathol* **47**:124, 1967

48. Pariser RJ: Histologically specific skin lesions in disseminated cytomegalovirus infection. *J Am Acad Dermatol* **9**:937, 1983

49. Patterson JW et al: Cutaneous CMV infection in a liver transplant patient: Diagnosis by in situ DNA hybridization. *Am J Dermatopathol* **10**:524, 1988

50. Lin CS et al: Cytomegalic inclusion disease of the skin. *Arch Dermatol* **10**:524, 1981

51. Humphreys DM, Myers A: Cytomegalovirus mononucleosis with urticaria. *Postgrad Med J* **51**:404, 1975

52. Swanson S, Feldman PS: Cytomegalovirus infection initially diagnosed by skin biopsy. *Am J Clin Pathol* **15**:113, 1987

53. Feldman YM, Nikitas JA: Cytomegalovirus infection. *Cutis* **27**:562, 1981

54. Horn TD, Hood AF: Cytomegalovirus is predictably present in perineal ulcers from immunocompromised patients. *Arch Dermatol* **126**:642, 1990

55. Lee JY, Peel R: Concurrent cytomegalovirus and herpes simplex infection in skin biopsy specimens of two AIDS patients with fatal CMV infection. *Am J Dermatopathol* **11**:136, 1989

56. Pass RF et al: Young children as a probable source of maternal and congenital cytomegalovirus infection. *N Engl J Med* **316**:1366, 1987

57. Fowler KB, Pass RF: Sexually transmitted disease in mothers of neonates with congenital cytomegalovirus infection. *J Infect Dis* **164**:269, 1990

58. Merigan TC, Resta S: Cytomegalovirus: Where have we been and where are we going? *Rev Infect Dis* **12**:S693, 1990

59. Helm K et al: Systemic cytomegalovirus in a patient with the keratitis, ichthyosis and deafness (KID) syndrome. *Pediatr Dermatol* **7**:54, 1990

60. Groark SP, Jampel RM: Violaceous papules and macules in a newborn. *Arch Dermatol* **125**:113, 1989

61. TORCH syndrome and TORCH screening (editorial). *Lancet* **335**:1559, 1990

62. Spector SA: Diagnosis of cytomegalovirus infection. *Semin Hematol* **27**:11, 1190

63. Pomeroy C, Englund JA: Cytomegalovirus: Epidemiology and infection control. *Am J Infect Control* **15**:107, 1987

64. Berant M et al: Papular acrodermatitis with cytomegalovirus hepatitis. *Arch Dis Child* **58**:1024, 1983

65. Heilbron B, Saxe N: Scleredema in an infant. *Arch Dermatol* **122**:1417, 1986

66. Weigand DA et al: Vasculitis in cytomegalovirus infection. *Arch Dermatol* **116**:1174, 1980

67. Horwitz CA et al: Clinical and laboratory evaluation of cytomegalovirus induced mononucleosis in previously healthy individuals. *Medicine (Baltimore)* **65**:124, 1986

68. Spear JB et al: Erythema nodosum associated with acute cytomegalovirus mononucleosis in an adult. *Arch Intern Med* **148**:323, 1988

69. Rubin RH: Impact of cytomegalovirus infection on organ transplant recipients. *Rev Infect Dis* **12**:S754, 1990

70. Lerner CW, Tapper ML: Opportunistic infection complicating acquired immune deficiency syndrome. *Medicine (Baltimore)* **63**:155, 1984

71. Drew WL, Erlich KS: Herpes viruses in AIDS patients. Cytomegalovirus. *J Critical Illness* **4**:20, 1989

72. Buhles WC et al: Ganciclovir treatment of life or sight-threatening cytomegalovirus infection: Experience in 314 immunocompromised patients. *Rev Infect Dis* **10**:S495, 1988

73. Bloom JN, Palestine AG: The diagnosis of cytomegalovirus retinitis. *Ann Intern Med* **109**:963, 1988

74. Marker SC et al: Cytomegalovirus infection: A quantitative prospective study of three hundred twenty consecutive renal transplants. *Surgery* **89**:660, 1981

75. Kaplan CS et al: Gastrointestinal cytomegalovirus infection in heart and heart-lung transplant recipients. *JAMA* **149**:2095, 1989

76. Levin MJ: Current approaches to the prevention and treatment of cy-

tomegalovirus disease after bone marrow transplantation: An overview. *Semin Hematol* 27:1, 1990

77. Schmidt GM et al: A randomized, controlled trial of prophylactic ganciclovir for cytomegalovirus pulmonary infection in recipients of allogeneic bone marrow transplants. *N Engl J Med* 324:1005, 1991

78. Drew WL: Diagnosis of cytomegalovirus infection. *Rev Infect Dis* 10:S468, 1988

79. Chou S: Newer methods for diagnosis of cytomegalovirus infection. *Rev Infect Dis* 10:S468, 1990

80. Shuster EA: Monoclonal antibody for rapid laboratory detection of cytomegalovirus infections: Characterization and diagnostic application. *Mayo Clin Proc* 60:577, 1985

81. Cassol SA et al: Primer mediated enzymatic amplification of cytomegalovirus DNA. *J Clin Invest* 83:1109, 1989

82. Myerson D et al: Widespread presence of histologically occult cytomegalovirus. *Hum Pathol* 15:430, 1984

83. Horn TD, Hood AF: Clinically occult cytomegalovirus present in skin biopsy specimens in immunosuppressed hosts. *J Am Acad Dermatol* 21:781, 1989

84. Drew WL et al: Prevalence of resistance in patients receiving ganciclovir for serious cytomegalovirus infection. *J Infect Dis* 163:716, 1991

85. Balfour HH: Management of cytomegalovirus disease with antiviral drugs. *Rev Infect Dis* 12:S849, 1990

86. Jabs DA et al: Mortality in patients with AIDS treated with either foscarnet or ganciclovir for cytomegalovirus retinitis. *N Engl J Med* 326:213, 1992

87. Knox KK et al: Cytomegalovirus isolate resistant to ganciclovir and foscarnet from a bone marrow transplant patient. *Lancet* 337:1292, 1991

88. Bowden RA, Meyers JD: Prophylaxis of cytomegalovirus infection. *Semin Hematol* 27:17, 1990

89. Bowden RA et al: Cytomegalovirus (CMV)-specific intravenous immunoglobulin for the prevention of primary CMV infection and disease after marrow transplant. *J Infect Dis* 164:483, 1991

90. Plotkin SA et al: Vaccines for the prevention of human cytomegalovirus infection. *Rev Infect Dis* 12:S827, 1990

CHAPTER 206

James C. Niederman

Epstein-Barr Virus Infections

Epstein-Barr virus (EBV), a lymphotropic member of the herpes virus group, infects human populations throughout the world. EBV is the causal agent of infectious mononucleosis (IM) and is associated with African Burkitt lymphoma (BL), nasopharyngeal carcinoma (NPC), and lymphomas or lymphoproliferative syndromes in patients with either primary immunodeficiency disease or acquired immunodeficiency.

Historical Aspects

EBV was discovered by electron microscopic studies of tumor cells from biopsies of BL grown in tissue culture. This tumor, usually involving the jaw, is the most common childhood malignancy in certain parts of East Africa and was first described by Burkitt in 1958.[1] Because its geographic distribution was similar to that of certain mosquito-borne diseases in equatorial Africa, the search for a causal arbovirus was undertaken. In 1964, Epstein, Achong, Barr, and Pulvertaft established continuous lymphoblastoid cell lines from BL explants; subsequently, virus particles having structural characteristics of the herpes virus group were identified in thin sections of such cell lines.[2–4] In 1966, Henle and Henle demonstrated that cells producing the viral particles contained antigen detectable by indirect immunofluorescence when sera from BL patients were used as the source of antibody.[5]

Two years later, investigations utilizing such antibody measurements demonstrated that EBV is the cause of infectious mononucleosis.[6,7] The studies established that EBV antibodies are regularly absent before the onset of IM and develop during the disease. EBV-specific IgM antibody is present in sera collected 1 to 6 weeks after onset of symptoms and usually disappears in 3 to 6 months;[8] IgG responses are also detectable during early illness and have been demonstrated in sera collected many years after clinical disease.[9,10]

Further evidence of the causative relationship is the presence of EBV in cultures of circulating lymphocytes of patients with acute IM as well as from subjects with a past history of the disease.[11,12]

Epidemiology

Seroepidemiologic studies have demonstrated that absence of EBV antibody correlates with susceptibility to infection and conversely the presence of antibody indicates immunity.[9,10] Environmental, hygienic, and socioeconomic factors generally determine the age at which infection occurs. In populations from tropical and developing areas, infections are acquired early in life, and almost all children under 3 years of age are antibody-positive. Among individuals living in more affluent environments, exposure is delayed and usually only 50 to 60 percent of older children and young adults have demonstrable antibody responses. In general, IM emerges as an important clinical entity only when sufficient numbers of susceptibles reach the ages of 15 to 25 years before acquiring infection. Large prospective studies involving more than 2600 young adults in England and the United States demonstrated that over a period of 4 to 8 years EBV seroconversion occurred in 44 percent of susceptibles.[9,10,13] Measurements of apparent and inapparent infections indicated a clinical/subclinical ratio of 1:2 to 1:3 in adults.

Etiology and Pathogenesis

EBV is tropic for B lymphocytes, which apparently become infected in the oropharynx through salivary exchange; infected B cells then circulate in the blood and are distributed to bone marrow and the entire lymphoreticular system. When lymphoproliferation occurs, there are large numbers of atypical lymphocytes in the peripheral blood. Relatively few lymphocytes are actually infected, but the number is sufficient to initiate prompt responses by both helper and suppressor T cells and later by cytotoxic T cells. Such reactions result in production of interleukin-2 and promote proliferation of specific T8 lymphocytes and to a lesser extent other suppressor cell activity.

EBV is present in oropharyngeal secretions during acute IM, and virus excretion in low titers continues intermittently throughout life.[14–16] The virus has been detected in throat washings from approximately 20 percent of normal seropositive persons who lack a history of IM, indicating that oropharyngeal excretion is common after subclinical infection. If saliva from healthy EBV antibody-positive persons is sufficiently concentrated, up to 100 percent of such individuals may be found to be shedding virus.[17] Both parotid duct epithelium and oropharyngeal squamous epithelial cells harbor EBV-DNA and are sites of viral replication and release, suggesting that chronic epithelial replication brings about continuous reinfection of B lymphoid cells.[18–21] By means of culture and cytohybridization, EBV has also been detected in uterine cervical secretions; such findings imply that cervical epithelium may be another site of EBV replication.[22]

Clinical Manifestations

EBV infections acquired early in life are asymptomatic or associated with nonspecific symptoms suggesting an upper respiratory infection. Classic IM develops in primary infections of older children, adolescents, and young adults. In adults an incubation period of 30 to 50 days has been established on the basis of contact infections.[23] Following blood transfusion IM associated with the development of heterophile and EBV antibodies developed 5 weeks later.[24] Children appear to have a shorter incubation period, but there is relatively little information on this point.

In IM a 3- to 5-day prodromal period, associated with dissemination of EBV throughout the body, is characterized by malaise, mild headache, and fatigue. During the acute disease, clinical responses are variable in severity. Most common are fever, sore throat, and cervical adenopathy. These occur in 80 percent of cases. Diffuse hyperemia and hyperplasia of oropharyngeal lymphoid tissue are present; a gelatinous grayish-white exudative tonsillitis persisting for 7 to 10 days occurs in approximately half of the cases. During the first week, small petechiae are present at the border of the hard and soft palates in about one-third of patients. In adults, a fluctuating fever reaching 38 to 39°C or higher persists for 7 to 10 days and falls gradually over the next 10 days. Tender lymphadenopathy is the hallmark of IM; cervical nodes are most commonly enlarged, but axillary, epitrochlear, inguinal, mediastinal, and mesenteric nodes may also be involved.

Splenomegaly occurs in approximately 50 percent of patients and is usually maximal during the second and third weeks of disease. Although hepatomegaly is present in only 10 to 15 percent, serum transaminase and lactic acid dehydrogenase levels are abnormally elevated for several weeks in almost all cases. Frank jaundice develops in less than 5 percent and is usually mild. Rarely, central nervous system complications occur; they include aseptic meningitis, Bell's palsy, meningoencephalitis, transverse myelitis, cerebellar ataxia, and acute psychosis. Recovery is usually complete, although fatalities have been associated with encephalitis. Hematologic complications are also unusual, although hemolytic anemia, marked neutropenia, and mild to moderate thrombocytopenia have been reported during the early weeks of disease.[25–28] Splenic rupture is a rare complication necessitating immediate splenectomy.

Fatal mononucleosis has been reported in persons having underlying immune defects, such as the X-linked lymphoproliferative syndrome in boys,[29] and in young children with poorly defined immunologic abnormalities.[30] Rarely, fatal IM occurs in previously healthy adults without evidence of underlying pathology.[31]

Dermatologic Findings

A wide variety of skin manifestations are associated with clinical IM; the incidence of cutaneous eruptions ranges from 3 to 16 percent. The rash is usually macular or maculopapular, although erythematous, vesicular, morbilliform, petechial, and purpuric exanthems have also been described.[32–38] In most instances, skin eruptions are located on the trunk and upper arms; occasionally, the face and forearms are involved. The rash usually appears during the first week of illness and may persist for 1 to 7 days. Urticarial lesions located on the abdomen, arms, and legs with sparing of palms and soles have been described and may be associated with the presence of cold agglutinins and acrocyanosis.[39–44]

The increased frequency of skin rashes in IM patients treated with ampicillin was first reported in 1967.[45,46] Seven to 10 days after initiation of antibiotic therapy, a generalized erythematous maculopapular eruption develops (Figs. 206-1, 206-2) mainly over the trunk and extremities, including the palms and soles.[45–48] The rash becomes confluent over exposed areas and pressure points, particularly over extensor surfaces; it persists for approximately 1 week and desquamation may continue for several more days. High levels of IgM and IgG antibodies to ampicillin have been demonstrated during acute IM.[49] Hypersensitivity skin rashes may also develop with the use of ampicillin analogues, such as amoxicillin, and certain other penicillins, including methicillin; the drug-associ-

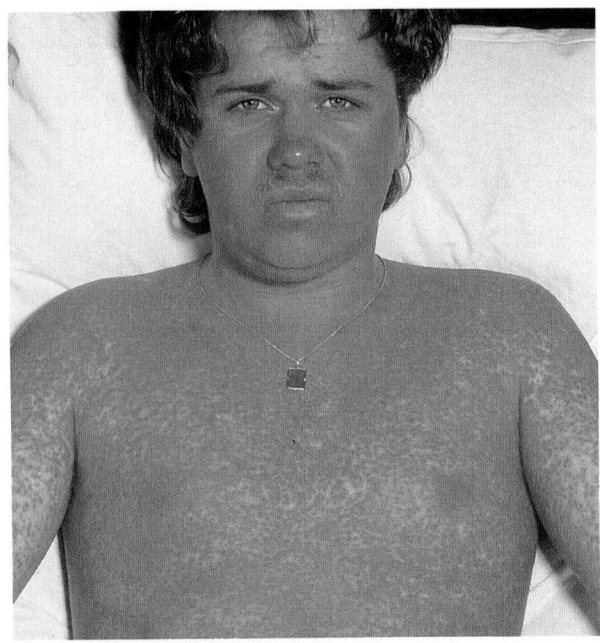

FIGURE 206-1   Generalized ampicillin exanthem in a patient with infectious mononucleosis. (*Courtesy of Helmut Hinton, M.D., University of Innsbruck.*)

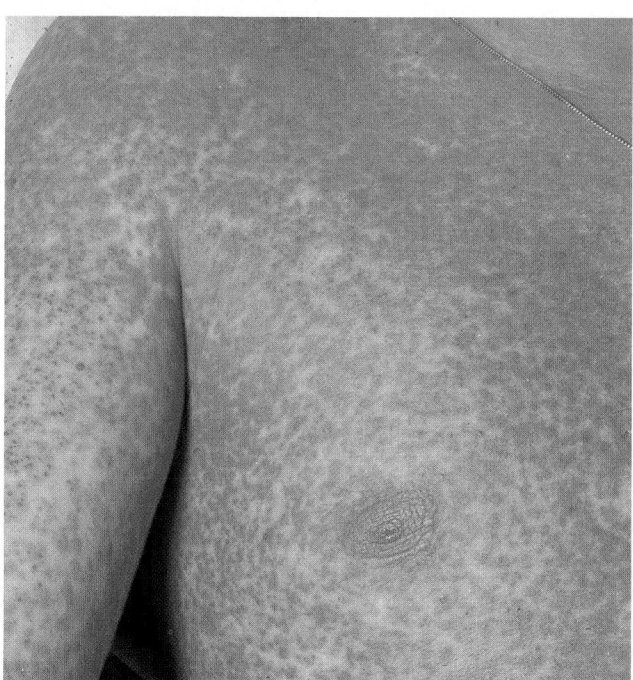

FIGURE 206-2 Close up of ampicillin eruption shown in Figure 206-1. (*Courtesy of Helmut Hinton, M.D., University of Innsbruck.*)

ated reactions are temporary, however, and do not recur when such drugs are used after acute mononucleosis has subsided.[50–53]

It is obvious that EBV can infect human epidermis and produce cutaneous disease,[20,21,54,55] but the exact mechanism is unclear; epithelial cell expression of the C3d EBV receptor has been demonstrated in several investigations[20,55] but other studies suggest actual fusion of epithelial cells with infected lymphocytes.[56,57]

EBV has been implicated in hairy leukoplakia, an oral lesion which is associated with human immunodeficiency virus (HIV) infection (Fig. 206-3) and is a predictive marker of subsequent clini-

cal progression to AIDS.[58–61] EBV-DNA has been found in superficial, intermediate, and prickle cell epithelial layers but not in the basal layer.[62]

EBV genome copies have also been detected in epidermal cells from a widespread erythematous and purpuric maculopapular eruption in a patient with chronic lymphocytic leukemia.[63] This interaction between EBV and cutaneous epithelium suggests the possibility of a role for the agent in other undiagnosed epithelial lesions.[64]

Cases of Gianotti-Crosti syndrome in children have been reported in association with primary EBV infection. A distinctive eruption characterized by symmetric, nonpruritic, lichenoid papules develops on the face, limbs, and buttocks.[65,66]

Ill-defined skin rashes have been described in rare cases of EBV-associated hemophagocytic and X-linked lymphoproliferative syndromes.[29,67] The virus has also been detected in labial ulcerations developing during clinical IM.[68]

An association between EBV and ataxia telangiectasia is suggested by the presence of elevated anti-early antigen (EA) responses in some patients with this disorder.[69,70] Oculocutaneous telangiectasias develop at about 3 years of age and usually involve bulbar conjunctivae, periorbital skin, malar eminences, ears, and antecubital fossae.

Periorbital Edema

In 30 to 40 percent of IM cases, edema of the eyelids occurs during the first week of symptoms. It lasts for only several days and has no relationship to severity of illness. Puffy swelling of the upper lids with narrowing of palpebral fissures may be as striking as that observed in patients with trichinosis or chronic renal disease.[34,37]

Oral Lesions

The palatal petechiae located at the border of the hard and soft palates consist of 5 to 20 reddish circumscribed lesions, 1 to 2 mm

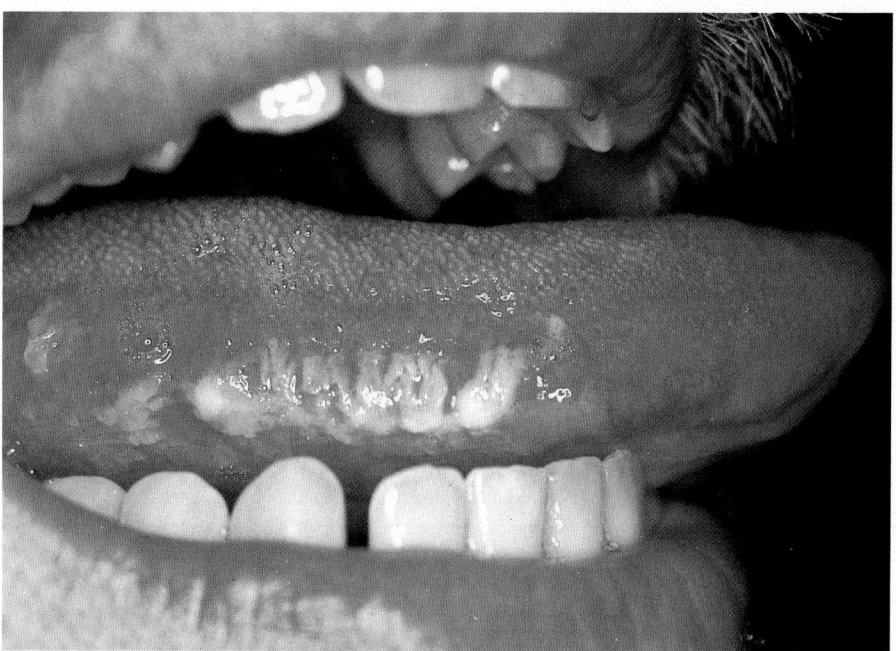

FIGURE 206-3 Oral hairy leukoplakia associated with HIV infection.

in diameter, which occur in crops and usually persist 3 to 4 days.[71] Their appearance is suggestive but not pathognomonic of IM.

Laboratory Findings

The presence of increased numbers of lymphocytes and atypical lymphocytes in peripheral blood is essential to the diagnosis of IM; total lymphocyte counts may constitute 50 to 60 percent of peripheral blood leukocytes. In the first week of illness the white blood cell count is normal or moderately decreased. By the second week leukocytosis develops with more than 10 percent atypical lymphocytes; such cells vary in size and staining characteristics, with indented, oval, or horseshoe-shaped nuclei and basophilic, vacuolated, foamy cytoplasm. During early illness, the atypical lymphocytes in which EBV has multiplied are B cells; later, the atypical cells are primarily T cells with immunoregulatory function.

Antibody Responses

Heterophile antibodies, first reported in 1932 by Paul and Bunnell as agglutinins for sheep erythrocytes,[72] are demonstrable in about 90 percent of adult IM cases. Differential absorption techniques distinguish between naturally occurring antibodies to Forssmann antigen, serum sickness antibodies and IgM heterophile responses; the latter may be present at the onset of disease or appear later in the course of illness. Heterophile antibodies usually are detectable for 3 to 6 months; in general, the higher the titer attained during acute disease, the longer such antibodies persist during convalescence.

Specific antibodies to EBV-associated antigens develop regularly. Viral capsid (VCA)-specific IgM and IgG are present early in illness; VCA-IgM responses disappear after several months, whereas VCA-IgG antibodies persist for life. Antibodies to EBV-EA complexes, associated with viral replication, are demonstrable in 70 to 80 percent of patients during the acute disease and usually disappear after 6 months. Recent studies suggest, however, that antibody to the R component of the EA complex may persist in healthy subjects for years following IM.[73]

Antibodies to the EBV nuclear antigen complex (EBNA) usually develop in the third or fourth week after onset; all late convalescent sera contain EBNA antibodies.

Pathology

Generalized lymphadenopathy, nasopharyngeal lymphoid hyperplasia, and splenomegaly develop during the course of the disease. Histopathologic studies of tissues obtained at an occasional autopsy or made available from volunteers demonstrate widespread focal and perivascular aggregates of mononuclear cells throughout the body.[74,75] Nonlymphoid organs, such as the liver, lungs, heart, kidneys, and central nervous system, are sites of focal infiltrations which may be associated with functional abnormalities. Bone marrow hyperplasia develops regularly and in some instances small granulomas are present which are nonspecific and have no prognostic significance. The pathology of CNS lesions is not clear but may be due to proliferation of EBV-infected B cells within the central nervous system; lymphocytes harboring EBV have been demon-

strated in cerebrospinal fluid from a patient with complicating meningoencephalitis.[76]

Diagnosis

Diagnosis of acute IM is made on the basis of both clinical features and specific laboratory findings; the latter include characteristic hematologic changes consisting of lymphocytosis with atypical lymphocytes and elevated titers of heterophile and EBV antibody responses. Approximately 10 percent of adult IM patients are heterophile antibody-negative; in such circumstances EBV-specific antibody determinations are necessary.

Treatment

In most cases, treatment of IM patients is largely supportive and symptomatic. Antibiotics have no influence on the course of an EBV infection unless a throat culture is positive for group A beta-hemolytic streptococci, which occurs in approximately 20 percent of cases. During the early febrile period, rest in bed is advisable. In addition to suppressing fever, salicylates and saline gargles usually relieve the sore throat and headache; in more severe cases codeine or meperidine (Demerol) may be necessary. In patients who have severe pharyngotonsillitis with oropharyngeal edema and airway encroachment, a short course of steroids should be given. Prednisone (or its equivalent) in an initial dosage of 10 to 15 mg four times daily is administered for 24 to 48 h. The daily dose is then decreased by 5 mg daily so that steroid treatment is discontinued in approximately 10 days. Corticosteroid therapy is also employed in the treatment of other major complications of IM, including hemolytic anemia, thrombocytopenic purpura, neurologic sequelae, myocarditis, pericarditis, and severe generalized dermatologic lesions. In cases with profound thrombocytopenia, refractory to corticosteroid administration, splenectomy may be necessary.[77]

The patient's physical activity is determined on an individual case basis during convalescence; participation in contact sports and excessive exertion are prohibited during acute illness and also in the presence of splenic enlargement. Rupture of the spleen associated with severe abdominal pain may be fatal if not recognized and treated with blood transfusions and splenectomy.

In most EBV infections the use of antiviral chemotherapeutic agents such as acyclovir, which acts on the lytic phase of EBV replication, is not warranted; the drug has minimal effect on IM symptoms and limits the level of oropharyngeal virus replication only during the period of drug administration.[78] Acyclovir treatment has little or no effect in limiting the number of EBV-infected B cells in the peripheral circulation.

Course and Prognosis

Most cases of IM in older age groups are mild or moderate in severity. Acute symptoms may last 2 to 3 weeks, and as a rule patients recover uneventfully during a period of 4 to 6 weeks' convalescence. Rarely, laboratory results resolve more slowly, and symptoms, including fatigue, malaise, intermittent sore throat, and cervical adenopathy, may persist for several months. However, recent studies have cast strong doubt on a proposed direct relationship between EBV and chronic fatigue syndrome, which lasts 6 months or more.[79-80]

References

1. Burkitt D: A sarcoma involving the jaws in African children. *Br J Surg* **46**:218, 1958

2. Epstein MA et al: Virus particles in cultured lymphoblasts from Burkitt's lymphoma. *Lancet* **1**:702, 1964

3. Epstein MA, Barr YM: Cultivation in vitro of human lymphoblasts from Burkitt's malignant lymphoma. *Lancet* **1**:252, 1964

4. Pulvertaft RJV: Cytology of Burkitt's tumor (African lymphoma). *Lancet* **1**:238, 1964

5. Henle G, Henle W: Immunofluorescence in cells derived from Burkitt's lymphoma. *J Bacterol* **91**:1248, 1966

6. Henle G et al: Relation of Burkitt's tumor-associated herpes-type virus to infectious mononucleosis. *Proc Natl Acad Sci (USA)* **59**:94, 1968

7. Niederman JC et al: Infectious mononucleosis: Clinical manifestations in relation to EB virus antibodies. *JAMA* **203**:205, 1968

8. Hampar B et al: Serologic evidence that a herpes-type virus is the etiologic agent of heterophile-positive infectious mononucleosis. *Proc Natl Acad Sci (USA)* **68**:1407, 1971

9. Evans AS et al: Seroepidemiologic studies of infectious mononucleosis with EB virus. *N Engl J Med* **279**:1123, 1968

10. Niederman JC et al: Prevalence, incidence and persistence of EB virus antibody. *N Engl J Med* **282**:361, 1970

11. Diehl V et al: Demonstration of a herpes group virus in cultures of peripheral leukocytes from patients with infectious mononucleosis. *J Virol* **2**:663, 1968

12. Nilsson K et al: The establishment of lymphoblastoid cell lines from adult and fetal human lymphoid tissue and its dependence on EBV. *Int J Cancer* **8**:443, 1971

13. University Health Physicians et al: Infectious mononucleosis and its relationship to EB virus antibody. *Br Med J* **4**:643, 1971

14. Miller G et al: Prolonged oropharyngeal excretion of Epstein-Barr virus following infectious mononucleosis. *N Engl J Med* **288**:229, 1973

15. Niederman JC et al: Infectious mononucleosis: EB-virus shedding in saliva and the oropharynx. *N Engl J Med* **294**:1355, 1976

16. Morgan DG et al: Site of Epstein-Barr virus replication in the oropharynx. *Lancet* **2**:1154, 1979

17. Rickinson AB et al: The Epstein-Barr virus as a model of virus-host interactions. *Br Med J* **41**:75, 1985

18. Sixbey JW et al: Epstein-Barr virus replication in oropharyngeal epithelial cells. *N Engl J Med* **310**:1225, 1984

19. Wolf H et al: Persistence of Epstein-Barr virus in the parotid gland. *J Virol* **51**:795, 1984

20. Sixbey JW et al: Replication of Epstein-Barr virus in human epithelial cells infected in vitro. *Nature* **306**:480, 1983

21. Sixbey JW et al: Human epithelial cell expression of an Epstein-Barr virus receptor. *J Gen Virol* **68**:805, 1987

22. Sixbey JW et al: A second site for Epstein-Barr virus shedding: The uterine cervix. *Lancet* **2**:1122, 1986

23. Hoagland RJ: The incubation period of infectious mononucleosis. *Am J Public Health* **54**:1699, 1964

24. Blacklow NR et al: Mononucleosis with heterophile antibodies and EB virus infection. Acquisition by an elderly patient in a hospital. *Am J Med* **51**:549, 1971

25. Carter RL: Granulocyte changes in infectious mononucleosis. *J Clin Pathol* **19**:279, 1966

26. Clarke BF, Davies SH: Severe thrombocytopenia in infectious mononucleosis. *Am J Med Sci* **248**:703, 1964

27. Cantow EK, Kostinas JE: Studies on infectious mononucleosis. IV. Changes in the granulocytic series. *Am J Clin Pathol* **46**:43, 1966

28. Penman G: Extreme neutropenia in glandular fever. *J Clin Pathol* **21**:48, 1968

29. Grierson H, Purtilo DT: Epstein-Barr virus infections in males with X-linked lymphoproliferative syndrome. *Ann Intern Med* **106**:538, 1987

30. Robinson JE et al: Diffuse polyclonal B-cell lymphoma during primary infection with Epstein-Barr virus. *N Engl J Med* **302**:1293, 1980

31. Snydman DR et al: Infectious mononucleosis in an adult progressing to fatal immunoblastic lymphoma. *Ann Intern Med* **96**:737, 1982

32. Sadusk JF: The skin eruption and false-positive Wasserman in infectious mononucleosis. *N Intern Clinics* **1**:239, 1941

33. Paul JR: Infectious mononucleosis. *Bull NY Acad Med* **15**:43, 1939

34. Bernstein A: Infectious mononucleosis. *Medicine* **XIX**:85, 1940

35. Contratto AN: Infectious mononucleosis: A study of one-hundred and ninety-six cases. *Arch Intern Med* **73**:449, 1944

36. Milne J: Infectious mononucleosis. *N Engl J Med* **233**:727, 1945

37. McCarthy JT, Hoagland RJ: Cutaneous manifestations of infectious mononucleosis. *JAMA* **187**:153, 1964

38. Petrozzi JW: Infectious mononucleosis manifesting as a palmar dermatitis. *Arch Dermatol* **104**:207, 1971

39. Africk JA, Halprin, KM: Infectious mononucleosis presenting as urticaria. *JAMA* **209**:1524, 1969

40. Cowdrey SC, Reynolds JS: Acute urticaria in infectious mononucleosis. *Ann Allergy* **27**:182, 1969

41. Tyson CJ, Czarny D: Cold-induced urticaria in infectious mononucleosis. *Med J Aust* **1**:33, 1981

42. Barth JH: Infectious mononucleosis (glandular fever) complicated by cold agglutinins, cold urticaria and leg ulceration. *Acta Derm Venereol (Stockh)* **61**:451, 1981

43. Dickerman JD et al: Infectious mononucleosis initially seen as cold-induced acrocyanosis: Association with auto-anti-M and anti-I antibodies. *Am J Dis Child* **134**:159, 1980

44. Horwitz CA et al: Cold agglutinins in infectious mononucleosis and heterophile-antibody-negative mononucleosis-like syndrome. *Blood* **50**:195, 1977

45. Patel BM: Skin rash with infectious mononucleosis and ampicillin. *Pediatrics* **40**:910, 1967

46. Pullen H et al: Hypersensitivity reactions to antibacterial drugs in infectious mononucleosis. *Lancet* **2**:1176, 1967

47. Nazareth I et al: Ampicillin sensitivity in infectious mononucleosis—temporary or permanent? *Scand J Infect Dis* **4**:229, 1972

48. Levene G, Baker H: Drug reactions: Ampicillin and infectious mononucleosis. *Br J Dermatol* **80**:417, 1968

49. McKenzie H et al: IgM and IgG antibody levels to ampicillin in patients with infectious mononucleosis. *Clin Exp Immunol* **26**:214, 1976

50. Bjorg M et al: Temporary skin reactions to penicillins during the acute stage of infectious mononucleosis. *Scand J Infect Dis* **7**:21, 1975

51. Mulroy R: Amoxicillin rash in infectious mononucleosis. *Br Med J* **1**:554, 1973

52. Morris J: Infectious-mononucleosis rash after Talampicillin (Letter). *Lancet* **1**:423, 1976

53. Fields DA: Methicillin rash in infectious mononucleosis (Letter). *West J Med* **133**:521, 1980

54. Young LS et al: Epstein-Barr virus receptors on human pharyngeal epithelia. *Lancet* **1**:240, 1986

55. Niedobitek G et al: Epstein-Barr virus complement receptor and epithelial cells. *Lancet* **2**:110, 1989

56. Niedobitek G et al: Identification of Epstein-Barr virus infected cells in tonsils of acute infectious mononucleosis by in situ hybridization. *Hum Pathol* **20**:796, 1989

57. Bayliss, CF, Wolf, H. Epstein-Barr virus induced cell fusion. *Nature* **287**:164, 1980

58. Greenspan D et al: Oral "hairy" leucoplakia in male homosexuals: Evidence of association with both papillomavirus and a herpes-group virus. *Lancet* **2**:831, 1984

59. Greenspan D et al: Oral hairy leucoplakia: Human immunodeficiency virus status and risk for development of AIDS. *J Infect Dis* **155**:475, 1987

60. Greenspan JS et al: Replication of Epstein-Barr virus within the epithelial cells of oral "hairy" leukoplakia, an AIDS-associated lesion. *N Engl J Med* **313**:1564, 1985

61. Conant MA: Hairy leukoplakia. A new disease of the oral mucosa. *Arch Dermatol* **123**:585, 1987

62. DeSouza YG et al: Localization of Epstein-Barr virus DNA in the epithelial cells of oral hairy leukoplakia by in situ hybridization on tissue sections. *N Engl J Med* (letter) **320**:1559, 1987

63. Fermand JP et al: Detection of Epstein-Barr virus in epidermal skin lesions of an immunocompromised patient. *Ann Intern Med* **112**:511, 1990

64. Allday MJ, Crawford DH: Role of epithelium in EBV persistence and pathogenesis of B-cell tumours. *Lancet* **1**:855, 1988

65. Lowe L et al: Gianotti-Crosti syndrome associated with Epstein-Barr virus infection. *J Am Acad Dermatol* **20**:336, 1989

66. Taieb A et al: Gianotti-Crosti syndrome: A study of 26 cases. *Br J Dermatol* **115**:49, 1986

67. Reisman RP, Greco MA: Virus associated hemophagocytic syndrome due to Epstein-Barr virus. *Hum Pathol* **15**:290, 1984

68. Portnoy J et al: Recovery of Epstein-Barr virus from genital ulcers. *N Engl J Med* **311**:966, 1984

69. Joncas J et al: Unusual prevalence of antibodies to Epstein-Barr virus early antigen in ataxia telangiectasia. *Lancet* (letter) **1**:1160, 1977

70. Peterson RDA et al: Ataxia telangiectasia. Its association with a defective thymus, immunological-deficiency disease and malignancy. *Lancet* **1**:1189, 1964

71. Caird F, Holt PR: The enanthem of glandular fever. *Br Med J* **1**:85, 1958

72. Paul JR, Bunnell WW: The presence of heterophile antibodies in infectious mononucleosis. *Am J Med Sci* **183**:90, 1932

73. Horwitz CA et al: Long-term serological follow-up of patients for Epstein-Barr virus after recovery from infectious mononucleosis. *J Inf Dis* **151**:1150, 1985

74. Custer R, Smith EB: The pathology of infectious mononucleosis. *Blood* **3**:830, 1948

75. Carter RL, Penman HG (eds): Histopathology of infectious mononucleosis, in *Infectious mononucleosis*. Oxford, Blackwell, 1969, p 146

76. Schiff J et al: Cell-associated Epstein-Barr virus in the cerebrospinal fluid of a patient with meningo-encephalitis complicating infectious mononucleosis. *Yale J Biol Med* **55**:59, 1982

77. Ellman L et al: Platelet autoantibody in a case of infectious mononucleosis presenting as thrombocytopenic purpura. *Am J Med* **55**:723, 1973

78. Ernberg I, Anderson J: Acyclovir efficiently inhibits oropharyngeal excretion of Epstein-Barr virus in patients with acute infectious mononucleosis. *J Gen Virol* **67**:2267, 1986

79. Straus SE: The chronic mononucleosis syndrome. *J Inf Dis* **157**:405, 1988

80. Holmes GP et al: Chronic fatigue syndrome: A working case definition. *Ann Intern Med* **108**:387, 1988

CHAPTER 207

Mihael Skerlev and *Richard Allen Johnson*

Human Herpesvirus-6 Infection and Exanthem Subitum (Roseola Infantum)

Exanthem subitum (roseola infantum) is a disease seen mostly in children 6 months to 2 years of age characterized by the sudden onset of a maculopapular rash following 3 to 5 days of high fever. The name is derived from the Greek and Latin term "exanthema subitum," which means "sudden rash." The older name, "roseola infantum" (Latin, "the pink rash of infants"), reflects some morphologic aspects of the disease.

Historical Aspects

Zahorsky, in 1913, was the first to describe this disease as "roseola infantum." Although Willan, Zahorsky,[2] and others made previous descriptions of the disease, it is obvious that many different eruptions (e.g., rubella, toxic erythema, measles) were confused with what is now referred to as exanthem subitum. The name "exanthem subitum" was introduced by Veeder and Hempelmann[3] in 1921 "as being descriptive of the most striking clinical symptom, namely, the sudden, unexpected appearance of the eruption on the fourth day."

Epidemiology

There are no consistent epidemiologic studies on the prevalence and incidence of exanthem subitum, probably (but not only) because of the character of the disease (i.e., mild course, short duration, self-limited, negligible sequelae). It is not a reportable disease and is frequently misdiagnosed,[4] which makes epidemiologic follow-up quite difficult. According to some reports, exanthem subitum occurs less frequently than other childhood exanthemas;[1,2,4] however, Barenberg et al. report it is the most common exanthem in children under 2 years of age.

On a global basis, the disease is ubiquitous. The majority of cases occur sporadically and without known exposure, although some epidemics have been reported in maternity hospitals.

Unlike other childhood infectious exanthems, there is no characteristic seasonal or monthly incidence of exanthem subitum, i.e., the results reported by different authors who followed large groups of children over a few years' period[1,4,7] showed such uncharacteristic variations that no significant difference was apparent. However, in his review of 243 cases over a 10-year period, Juretic[7] noted that May was the peak month of occurrence.

The typical age range is between 6 months and 2 years, but occasional cases have been observed in older children and young adults, as well as in infants younger than 6 months of age.[6] Maternal antibodies play an important role in immunity, in that clinical infection before 6 months of age is uncommon.

The incubation period, according to epidemic outbreaks, is estimated to be 5 to 15 days.[1,2,4,6] Exanthem subitum is contagious and some secondary cases in families have been observed.[1,2,4]

According to the results of most large studies[5,8,9] boys and girls are equally affected, although some older reports suggested that girls may be more often affected than boys.[10]

The reason that some data about exanthem subitum are contradictory might be due to the fact that many epidemiologic studies are not up-to-date and are based mostly on clinical observations. An etiologic agent of exanthem subitum has recently been identified (since 1988), but further laboratory studies might provide more precise and accurate information on the epidemiology of this disease.

Etiology and Pathogenesis

During the latter half of this century, a number of papers have been published regarding identification of the etiologic agent of exanthem subitum.[11–13] Many viruses that were believed to be the causative agent have been incriminated, such as echovirus 16,[14,15] different types of coxsackieviruses,[16,17] adenoviruses, parainfluenzae type 1 virus,[18,19] etc. In 1988 Yamamashi and associates[20] provided very convincing evidence that human herpesvirus-6 (HHV-6) is the etiologic agent of exanthem subitum. In fact, the first isolation of HHV-6 was reported by Salahuddin et al. in 1986[21] as the isolation of a previously unrecognized human herpesvirus from cultures of peripheral blood mononuclear cells derived from patients with lymphoreticular disorders. Salahuddin et al. thought, at the time of their report, that the newly discovered virus infected only B cells, and they proposed the name "human B lymphotropic virus" (HBLV). Later, the virus was isolated from T cells as well[22] and the name HBLV did not seem appropriate; the term human herpesvirus-6 is preferred. HHV-6 belongs to the *Herpesviridae* group and it differs from the other herpesviruses in its gross genome structure,[23] which is a linear, double-stranded DNA molecule. The HHV-6 virus produces a characteristic cytopathic effect in cell cultures.[23] From that point of view, exanthem subitum can be considered a "primo-infection" with HHV-6 in early infancy.[26,27] Current information suggests[28] that after the primary infection in childhood, the virus persists or remains latent in asymptomatic adults. Moreover, it seems very likely that a large number of children in the first two years of life become infected by the virus, but only a small percentage develop typical clinical features of exanthem subitum. Apart from virus isolation from blood mononuclear cells[21,28] in very high concentration during the febrile phase of the disease, the seroconversion (of anti-HHV-6 antibodies in infected individuals) provides strong additional evidence for HHV-6 as the etiologic agent of exanthem subitum.

This disease is now considered to be a consequence of primary infection with HHV-6 in early infancy, but the consequences of primary infection in adults are still unclear. There are some reports correlating HHV-6 with the chronic fatigue syndrome (a condition characterized by fatigue, fever, disability, malaise, lymphadenopathy, etc.).[29,30] It was also thought that HHV-6 infection could acti-

vate or accelerate human immunodeficiency virus infection, but recent studies have not proved such a hypothesis.[31]

Clinical Manifestations

The striking and characteristic symptoms of exanthem subitum are prodromal high fever persisting 3 to 5 days, the disappearance of the general symptoms, and the onset of rash lasting 1 to 2 days. The features of exanthem subitum have been reviewed in several papers and textbooks; excellent clinical descriptions can be found in the older literature.[1–3]

General Findings

The onset of the disease is abrupt and the only symptom in the first phase of the disease is a high fever ranging from 38.9 to 40.6°C. The fever remains consistently high, with moderate morning remission, until the fourth day, when it falls precipitously to normal, coincidentally with the appearance of the rash. In spite of a high fever, the infant usually is in no distress. Nocturnal restlessness and daytime drowsiness have sometimes been noted.

On physical examination, a number of other symptoms may be noted: inflammation of the pharynx and tonsils, a mild injection of the tympanic membrane, lesions of the soft palate, Berliner's physical sign (i.e., the characteristic facies due to the palpebral edema, which parents describe as "heavy eyelids" or a "droopy" or "sleepy" appearance of their child, bulging of the anterior fontanelle, and minor enlargement of the occipital, nuchal, and retroauricular lymph nodes. Vomiting, diarrhea, catarrhal, or any other general symptoms apart from those mentioned above are uncommon.

Dermatologic Findings

The rash appears as the fever falls (usually on the fourth day of the disease, as mentioned above) and develops very rapidly ("exanthema subitum" means "sudden rash"), lasts 1 to 2 days, and is fully evolved within 12 h. The eruption consists of small, often tender macules or maculopapules, 1 to 5 mm in diameter, that blanch on pressure and very often are surrounded by a whitish areola or halo. The lesions may be solitary or coalescent. The rash is characteristically localized on the trunk and neck, but it can also be present on the lower part of the face and extremities.

The lesions may occasionally be very sparse and limited only to areas of the trunk. Even in the papular form, the lesions are barely raised above the skin surface. The rash is usually not pruritic although the child might feel some discomfort. Desquamation and subsequent hyperpigmentation, as a rule, do not occur (this may be important for the differential diagnosis; see below).

Laboratory Findings

Classical laboratory tests are not strictly specific for exanthem subitum, so from the practical point of view, the diagnosis is based on history and physical examination. Leukopenia is usually found, ranging from 3000 to 5000 white blood cells/mm^3. A relative lymphocytosis and atypical lymphocytes are often reported.

Great progress has been made in the specific serology since 1988 when HHV-6 as the causative agent of exanthem subitum was convincingly reported. Specific serologic tests are now available for diagnostic purposes and their use is advised by some authors[27,34] for establishing the diagnosis. Immunofluorescence tests (direct and indirect) are available; the anticomplement immunofluorescence (ACIF) test is preferred by several authors.[21-23] Japanese investigators[27] obtained very specific results with neutralization tests, suggesting that the titers of specific anti-HHV-6 IgM and IgG antibodies in this test are higher than the titers of antibodies in the immunofluorescence test. In addition to specific serologic tests, the polymerase chain reaction (PCR) technique, which can detect very low concentrations of viral DNA in cell cultures, has been successful at detecting HHV-6 DNA in patients with exanthem subitum.[35] The PCR technique, although not yet available commercially as a routine diagnostic method, appears to be the preferred test because of its sensitivity, specificity, and efficiency; results can be obtained in 1 to 2 days, and a very low concentration of HHV-6 can be detected. Besides specific serologic tests and PCR technique, virus isolation can be performed from the peripheral blood mononuclear cells.[36-38]

Diagnosis and Differential Diagnosis

The diagnosis of exanthem subitum is usually made in the second or eruptive phase of the disease. The 4-day period of high fever occurring in an otherwise well infant, followed by lysis of the fever and subsequent appearance of the rash, strongly suggests the diagnosis. Most likely, the majority of cases of primary HHV-6 infection and exanthem subitum do not follow this scenario precisely. However, numerous infections of early infancy should be considered in the differential diagnosis; for practical purposes, the most relevant clinical diagnoses to be considered include rubella, measles, erythema infectiosum (fifth disease), scarlet fever, and drug eruptions.

In rubella, the prodromal fever is very short (a few hours), the fever rises with the eruption, children of all ages are susceptible, it is very contagious, and occurs mostly in spring.[1] In exanthem subitum, the prodromal fever lasts 4 days and falls to normal as the eruption appears, children in early infancy are the most susceptible, it is slightly contagious, and can appear in any season. Frequently an antibiotic or antipyretic is given to an infant with a febrile illness and the subsequent infectious exanthem may be confused with an exanthematous drug eruption. Drug eruptions tend to last longer than the exanthem of exanthem subitum and are usually very pruritic.

In measles, catarrhal prodromal symptoms, Koplik spots, the presence of measles in the community, and the slow spread of the exanthem from the head inferiorly and centrifugally help to distinguish it from exanthem subitum. Of interest is the report by Japanese authors of simultaneous infection by both HHV-6 and measles in two infants, confirmed by specific immunofluorescence assay and by electron microscopy.[39]

Erythema infectiosum (fifth disease) is characterized by the simultaneous occurrence of an exanthem and low-grade fever. In the prodromal phase, gastrointestinal symptoms are commonly present. The exanthem characteristically occurs on the face in a lacelike pattern; typically the eruption resolves and recurs on repeated occasions.

Scarlet fever is most often associated with pharyngitis or tonsillitis. The exanthem is characterized by diffuse erythema, accentuated about hair follicles are in flexural areas. Desquamation commonly occurs 1 to 2 weeks following the onset of the illness. The diagnosis can be confirmed by throat cultures and antistreptococcal antibody testing.

The differential diagnosis also includes exanthems associated with other viral agents such as adenovirus, echovirus, coxsackievirus, and rotaviruses.[40]

Treatment

Most cases of exanthem subitum do not require treatment. The disease is self-limited without associated sequelae. Symptomatic treatment might be used to treat the fever. In vitro testing of HHV-6 has indicated that ganciclovir and foscarnet antiviral agents are more effective than acyclovir.[41]

Course and Prognosis

The course of exanthem subitum is mild, the disease is self-limited, and there are usually no sequelae. The most common complications are seizures. It is still not clear whether seizures occur as a consequence of the fever, or from the HHV-6 infection. Rarely, meningoencephalitis has been reported as a complication of exanthem subitum.[42,43] Intussusception, associated with hyperplasia of intestinal lymphoid tissue, has recently been reported in three Japanese infants with HHV-6 infection.[44] Fulminant hepatitis in infants and adults has also been reported in association with primary HHV-6 infections, confirmed by isolation of the virus with positive serology.[45]

Although the etiology and pathogenesis of exanthem subitum and HHV-6 infections have been clarified during the past few years, the route of infection, the circumstances leading to latent or manifest infection, and a role of persistent infection with HHV-6 in the pathogenesis of some chronic diseases in adults are questions to be elucidated in the next few years.

References

1. Zahorsky J: Roseola infantum. *JAMA* **61**:1446, 1913
2. Zahorsky J: Roseola infantilis. *Pediatrics* **22**:60, 1910
3. Veeder BS, Hempelmann TC: A febrile exanthem occurring in childhood (exanthem subitum). *JAMA* **77**:1787, 1921
4. Clemens HH: Exanthem subitum (roseola infantum): Report of 80 cases. *J. Pediatr* **26**:66, 1945
5. Berenberg W et al: Roseola infantum (exanthem subitum). *N Engl J Med* **241**:253, 1949
6. James U, Freier A: Roseola infantum. An outbreak in a maternity hospital. *Arch Dis Child* **23–24**:54, 1948–1949
7. Jeretic M: Exanthem subitum: A review of 243 cases. *Helv Pediatr Acta* **18**:80, 1963
8. Zahorsky J: Roseola infantum: The rose rash of infants. *Arch Pediatr* **42**:410, 1925

9. Letchner A: Roseola infantum: A review of fifty cases. *Lancet* **2**:1163, 1955

10. Faber HK, Dickey LB: The symptomatology of exanthem subitum. *Arch Pediatr* **44**:491, 1927

11. Gurwith M et al: Exanthem subitum not associated with rotavirus. *N Engl J Med* **305**:174, 1981

12. Hellström B, Vahlquist B: Experimental inoculation of roseola infantum. *Acta Paediatr* **40**:189, 1951

13. Kempe CH et al: Studies on the etiology of exanthema subitum (roseola infantum). *J Pediatr* **37**:323, 1977

14. Hall CB et al: The return of Boston exanthem. Echovirus 16 infections in 1974. *Am J Dis Child* **131**:323, 1977

15. Neva FA et al: Clinical and epidemiological features of an unusual epidemic exanthem. *JAMA* **155**:544, 1954

16. Cherry JD: Newer viral exanthems. *Adv Pediatr* **16**:233, 1969

17. Cherry JD et al: Coxsackie B5 infections with exanthems. *Pediatrics* **31**:455, 1963

18. Neva FA, Enders JF: Isolation of cytopathogenic agent from an infant with a disease in certain respects resembling roseola infantum. *J Immunol* **72**:315, 1954

19. Watson GI: The roseolar reaction. *Br Med J* **4**:719, 1974

20. Yamanashi K et al: Identification of human herpesvirus-6 as a causal agent for exanthem subitum. *Lancet* **1**:1065, 1988

21. Salahuddin SZ et al: Isolation of a new virus, HBLV, in patients with lymphoproliferative disorders. *Science* **234**:596, 1986

22. Whittle H: A novel lymphotropic herpesvirus. *Lancet* **2**:390, 1987

23. Lopez C et al: Characteristics of human herpesvirus-6. *J Infect Dis* **157**:1271, 1988

24. Briggs M et al: Age prevalence of antibody to human herpesvirus-6. *Lancet* **1**:1058, 1988

25. Lusso O et al: In vitro cellular tropism of human B-lymphotrophic virus (human herpesvirus-6). *J Exp Med* **167**:1659, 1988

26. Wiersbitzky S et al: New knowledge of Zahorsky exanthema subitum (critical 3-day fever, exanthema, roseola infantum). *Kinderarztl Prax* **57**:155, 1989

27. Suga S et al: Neutralizing antibody assay for human herpesvirus-6. *J Med Virol* **30**:14, 1990

28. Takahashi K et al: Human herpesvirus-6 and exanthem subitum. *Lancet* **1**:1463, 1988

29. Kirchesch H et al: Seroconversion against human herpesvirus-6 (and other herpesviruses) and clinical illness. *Lancet* **2**:273, 1988.

30. Strauss SE: The chronic mononucleosis syndrome. *J Infect Dis* **157**:405, 1986

31. Fox J et al: Antibody to human herpesvirus-6 in HIV-1 positive and negative homosexual men. *Lancet* **2**:396, 1988

32. Berliner BC: A physical sign useful in diagnosis of roseola infantum before the rash. *Pediatrics* **25**:1034, 1960

33. Oski FA: Roseola infantum. Another case of bulging fontanel. *Am J Dis Child* **101**:376, 1961

34. Irving WL, Cunningham AL: Serological diagnosis of infection with human herpesvirus type 6. *Br Med J* **300**:156, 1990

35. Kondo K et al: Detection of polymerase chain reaction amplification of human herpesvirus-6 DNA in peripheral blood of patients with exanthem subitum. *J Clin Microbiol* **28**:970, 1990

36. Asano Y et al: Simultaneous occurrence of human herpesvirus-6 infection and intussusception in three infants. *Pediatr Infect Dis J* **10**:335, 1991

37. Asano Y et al: Viremia and neutralizing antibody response in infants with exanthem subitum. *Lancet* **114**:535, 1989

38. Suga S et al: Human herpesvirus-6 infection (exanthem subitum) without rash. *Pediatrics* **83**:1003, 1988

39. Suga S et al: Simultaneous infection with human herpesvirus-6 and measles in infants. *J Med Virol* **31**:306, 1990

40. Goodyear HM et al: Acute infectious exanthemas in children: A clinico-microbiological study. *Br J Dermatol* **124**:433, 1991

41. Burns WH, Sandford GR: Susceptibility of human herpes 6 to antiviral in vitro. *J Infect Dis* **162**:634, 1990

42. Burnstine RC, Paine RS: Residual encephalopathy following roseola infantum. *Am J Dis Child* **98**:144, 1959

43. Ishiguro N et al: Meningo-encephalitis associated with HHV-6 related exanthem subitum. *Acta Paediatr Scand* **79**:987, 1990

44. Asano Y et al: Simultaneous occurrence of human herpesvirus 6 infection and intussusception in three infants. *Pediatr Infect Dis J* **10**:335, 1991

45. Sobue R et al: Fulminant hepatitis in primary herpes-6 infection. *N Engl J Med* **324**:1290, 1991

CHAPTER 208

Meredith A. Simon, Douglas J. Ringler, and

Ronald D. Hunt

B Virus (*Herpesvirus simiae*)

B virus (*Herpesvirus simiae*, herpesvirus B, simian herpesvirus, cercopithecine herpesvirus 1) is indigenous in primates of the *Macaca* species. The virus produces primary disease in its natural hosts comparable to that associated with herpes simplex 1 in human beings, with seropositivity in clinically normal macaques ranging from 2.5 to over 90 percent, depending on the population studied.[1] Human infection with B virus has occurred, albeit rarely, in people who work with macaques or with tissues from macaques. The disease in humans frequently includes rapidly progressive neurologic symptoms.

Historical Aspects

Between 1932 and 1989, 18 human infections with B virus, confirmed by virus isolation, were reported, and at least 13 others are probable from clinical signs, exposure to macaques, and seroconversion.[1,2] Of the 31 reported cases, 21 have been fatal, and at least 5 of the nonfatal cases resulted in moderate to severe residual neurologic impairment. Human infections with B virus are of interest to dermatologists because in most cases the portal of entry for the virus is the skin, often with a vesicular eruption at the site of inocu-

TABLE 208-1
Human Infections with B Virus Confirmed by Virus Isolation

Case	Year	Mode of exposure	Species	Skin lesions	Other symptoms	Outcome	Reference
1	1932	Bite, hand	Mm	Yes	Encephalitis, ascending myelitis	Death at 17 days	11
2	1949	Saliva to wound on hand	Mm, Mf	Yes	Encephalitis, lymphadenitis	Death after a "few" days	36
3	1957	Aerosol?	Mm (?)	No	Encephalitis	Death at 7 days	37
4	1957	Handled autopsy material (cleaned skull)	Mm	No	Encephalitis	Death at 2 days	38
5	1957	Bite, finger	Mm	Yes	Encephalitis	Death at 8 days	38
6	1957	Unknown	Mm or Mf	No	Encephalitis	Death at 2 days	39
7	1958	Cuts, hand, from tissue culture	Mm or Mf	Yes	Encephalitis	Death at 15 days	38
8	1958	Needlestick	Mm or Mf	NR	Ascending myelitis	Death at 7 days	38
9	1958	Bite, hand, needlestick	Mm or Mf	No	Encephalitis	Death at 3 days	38
10	1960	Scratches, possible aerosol	Mm	No	Pneumonia, encephalitis	Death at 38 days	40
11	1963	Aerosol?	Mm, Cpa	Yes	Pneumonia, encephalitis	Severe neurologic impairment; died 3 years after acute illness	41
12	1970	Unknown, possible recurrent	Mm, possibly others	Yes (trigeminal zoster)	Ascending myelitis, encephalitis	Survived; severe neurologic impairment	42
13	1987	Bite, thumb	Mm	No	Myelitis, encephalitis	Death at 6 months	3,4
14	1987	Bite, forearm	Mm	Yes	Encephalitis	Death at 6 weeks	3,4
15	1987	Scratch	Mm?	Yes	None	Recovered	3,4
16	1987	Contaminated wound on finger	Human	Yes	None	Recovered	3,4
17	1989	Bites	Mm or Mf	Yes	Encephalitis	Death at 10 days	2
18	1989	Needlestick	Mm	No	None	Recovered	43

Note: Cpa = *Cercopithecus aethiops*, Mf = *Macaca fascicularis*, Mm = *Macaca mulatta*, NR = not reported.

lation (Tables 208-1 and 208-2). Recently, a confirmed case of human to human transmission of B virus was reported.[3,4]

Classification

B virus is a member of the alphaherpesvirus group, which comprises the epidermo/neurotropic viruses.[5-7] This group includes herpes simplex virus types 1 and 2, herpes varicella/zoster and at least seven herpesviruses of nonhuman primate origin (Table 208-3). In the natural host, alphaherpesviruses are most often associated with mild to inapparent disease, but the virus remains latent, usually in ganglia, for the life of the individual. Infection of aberrant hosts by these viruses frequently produces severe, generalized, often fatal disease.

All the alphaherpesviruses contain a linear double-stranded DNA of approximately 10^8 M_r, surrounded by a nucleocapsid consisting of an icosahedral arrangement of 162 capsomers within a

pleomorphic outer envelope (Fig. 208-1). The genome encodes approximately 50 viral proteins, including several antigenic glycoproteins expressed on both infected cells and virions. Extensive cross-reactivity of neutralizing antibodies to different alphaherpesviruses has been observed, especially those of herpes simplex, B virus, and SA8.[7-9]

In addition to these surface glycoproteins, the genome also encodes approximately 20 structural and 20 nonstructural proteins, including viral-specific enzymes required for DNA synthesis. These enzymes differ sufficiently from cellular enzymes in that they represent targets for therapeutic intervention.

B Virus in Monkeys

B virus was first isolated from tissues from a human who died of encephalomyelitis in 1932.[10,11] Onset of disease was 3 days after a bite from an apparently normal rhesus monkey (*M. mulatta*). Since

TABLE 208-2
Other Probable Human B Virus Cases

Case	Year	Mode of exposure	Species	Skin lesions	Basis for diagnosis	Outcome	Reference
19	1956	Scratch	Mm or Mf	NR	Seroconverted	Survived; moderate neurologic impairment	38
20	1957	Scratches, bite, hand	Mm, Mf	No	Increasing titer to B and herpes simplex	Death at 30 days	44
21	1957	Bites, fingers	Mm, Mf	No	Increasing titer	Survived; mild neurologic impairment	45
22	1965	Bite	Cpa	NR	Increasing titer	Death at 20 days	1
23	1973	Bites?	Mm	No	Increasing titer	Survived; mild neurologic impairment	46*
24	1989	Bite	Mm or Mf	NR	CSF antibodies	Recovered	2

*Seven additional cases mentioned.
Note: Cpa = *Cercopithecus aethiops,* CSF = cerebrospinal fluid, Mf = *Macaca fascicularis,* Mm = *Macaca mulatta,* NR = not reported.

the original description, the virus has been isolated from tissues of several species of macaques,[12–14] a finding suggesting that these animals are reservoirs; however, natural B virus infection of non-human primates was not described until 1958.[15,16]

Clinical Manifestations

The disease was seen in a group of young, newly imported rhesus monkeys. Lesions were found in 332 of 14,400 animals examined (2.3 percent). They consisted of an initial vesicular eruption on the tongue, the lips, or rarely elsewhere on the skin, similar to primary herpes simplex 1 in humans (Fig. 208-2). The vesicles occurred singly or in groups and soon ruptured to form ulcers covered by fibrinonecrotic plaques, sharply demarcated from surrounding normal tissue. These ulcers healed in 1 to 2 weeks, depending on the degree of secondary infection, and no visible scar remained. B virus was isolated from unruptured vesicles. Some animals also exhibited a mucopurulent nasal discharge or conjunctivitis.

Pathology

Histopathologic examination of the ulcers revealed two distinct zones in the epithelium: a central area of necrosis surrounded by a zone of ballooning degeneration. Typical eosinophilic intranuclear inclusions were most commonly seen at the junction of these two zones, often within multinucleated cells. The underlying dermis or mucosa was infiltrated by inflammatory cells, both mono- and polymorphonuclear. Subsequently, granulation tissue formed, followed by reepithelialization and resolution.

In 12 animals with oral lesions, additional tissues were examined. Lesions were observed in the pons and medulla (10 of 12), liver (7 of 12), and kidney (3 of 12). Generally, these lesions consisted of areas of degeneration and/or necrosis, with neutrophilic and mononuclear inflammation, and rare intranuclear inclusions. None of the affected animals were demonstrably ill.

Epidemiology

Since this original report, others have also described the disease in rhesus monkeys and similar oral lesions have been described in *M.*

fascicularis (cynomolgus monkeys),[17] *M. fuscata, M. cyclopis,*[18] and *M. arctoides.*[19] Fatal disseminated B virus infection has been reported in *M. radiata,*[20] *Erythrocebus patas,* and *Colobus abyssinicus,*[21] and rarely in rhesus[22,23] and cynomolgus monkeys.[16,24]

Serologic evidence of B virus infection in nonhuman primates indicates a high rate of exposure in wild-caught animals, with an age-related increase in incidence and a major increase at approximately the time of puberty. Crowding and group housing contribute to the spread of the virus, and the incidence increases rapidly in newly formed captive colonies.[25] Transmission is mediated by direct contact with the virus or virus-containing fomites; virus can be isolated from saliva, conjunctiva, vagina, blood, rectum, and vesicular fluid from infected animals, including those that are clinically normal.[1,23,24,26] Venereal transmission has been suggested as a principal means of spread, but overt genital lesions are rare.[26] A simian virus analogous to herpes simplex type 2 has not been identified.

No studies have specifically addressed the incidence of virus shedding among clinically normal, antibody-positive animals, but it has been estimated to be 2 to 3 percent.[27] Once infected, a macaque should be considered to be infected and potentially shedding B virus for life.

Latent herpes simplex infections in humans are known to be activated by stress and/or fatigue[28] and can become disseminated in immunocompromised individuals, including infants. Latent infections of B virus have been recognized in macaques.[13,26,29] B virus has been isolated from trigeminal and other sensory ganglia in clinically normal animals. These observations, the similarity of the lesions in the natural host, and close serologic relationships suggest that B virus is the simian counterpart to herpes simplex. Reactivation of B virus has been described rarely, possibly because the primary lesions have not been observed. However, the stress of experimental studies and confinement may be responsible for recrudescent disseminated B virus infection in some cases.

B Virus in Humans

Continued interest in B virus has been maintained because of the potential for human infection and the severity of the disease in most human infections. All human B virus cases had previously involved

TABLE 208-3
Alphaherpesviruses of Primates

Scientific name	Common name	Host(s)	Disease	Reference
Human herpesvirus 1 and 2	Herpes simplex (types 1 & 2)	Human beings	Usually self-limiting, mucocutaneous vesicles	47
		Gibbons	Self-limiting vesicles or encephalitis	48
		Owl monkeys, tamarins, marmosets	Generalized fatal infection	19, 49, 50
Saimirine herpesvirus 1	Herpes T (Herpes M, Herpes platyrrhinae)	Squirrel monkey	Usually self-limiting mucocutaneous vesicles	51
		Owl monkeys, marmosets, tamarins	Fatal generalized infection	50, 52
Cercopithecine herpesvirus 1	Herpesvirus simiae (B virus)	Macaques	Usually self-limiting, mucocutaneous vesicles	15
		Human beings, marmosets, patas monkeys, colobus monkeys	Fatal encephalomyelitis	11, 21, 34
Cercopithecine herpesvirus 2	SA8	African green monkeys	Myelitis	53, 54
		Baboons	Usually latent	55
Human herpesvirus 3	Herpes varicella/zoster	Human beings	Chickenpox, shingles	56
		Great apes	Chickenpox	57, 58
Cercopithecine herpesvirus 6, 7, and 9	Simian varicella (Delta, Medical Lake, Liverpool vervet monkey viruses)	African green monkeys, patas, monkeys, *M. nemestrina*, *M. fuscata*, *M. fascicularis*	Chickenpox-like disease	59, 60, 61
Ateline herpesvirus 1	Spider monkey herpesvirus	Spider monkeys	Usually latent, may cause generalized fatal infection	62

direct contact with monkeys or tissues from monkeys, with one notable exception (Table 208-1). Virus cannot penetrate intact skin. Human infection may occur through monkey bites or scratches, by contamination of wounds with infected fluids or cell culture materials, or possibly by aerosol inhalation of infected secretions.[27,30]

Clinical Manifestations

The first symptoms of infection are local erythema and induration at the point of inoculation, followed by vesicular lesions, recorded in 10 of the 18 cases confirmed by virus isolation (Table 208-1). Additional vesicular lesions have occurred at other cutaneous sites and in the oropharynx (case 10, Table 208-1). Early generalized symptoms of the human illness vary, but they include fever, lymphadenitis and lymphangitis, gastrointestinal symptoms, and flulike aches and pains. In all of the fatal cases and several of the others, these symptoms were followed by rapid progression (within days) to neurologic signs and symptoms, which included hyperesthesia, ataxia, and ascending, flaccid paralysis. In the fatal cases, death was due to encephalomyelitis.

Pathology

Histopathologic changes are comparable to those of fatal systemic herpes simplex in infants. Encephalomyelitis, most severe in the brain stem and spinal cord, is the most commonly described change. The lesions are comparable to those observed in several viral diseases, including perivascular cuffs and infiltration of the neuropil by mononuclear and polymorphonuclear inflammatory cells, foci of hemorrhage and necrosis, edema, and degeneration of neurons. Eosinophilic intranuclear inclusions typical of herpesviral infections are seen rarely. Involvement of other organs occurs, with focal hemorrhage and necrosis often seen in liver, spleen, lymph nodes, and adrenal glands.

Epidemiology

The possibility of reactivation of latent B virus infection in a human is raised in case 12 of Table 208-1. This individual presented with lesions compatible with herpes zoster and had a history of zoster-like disease; ascending myelitis and encephalitis followed. B virus

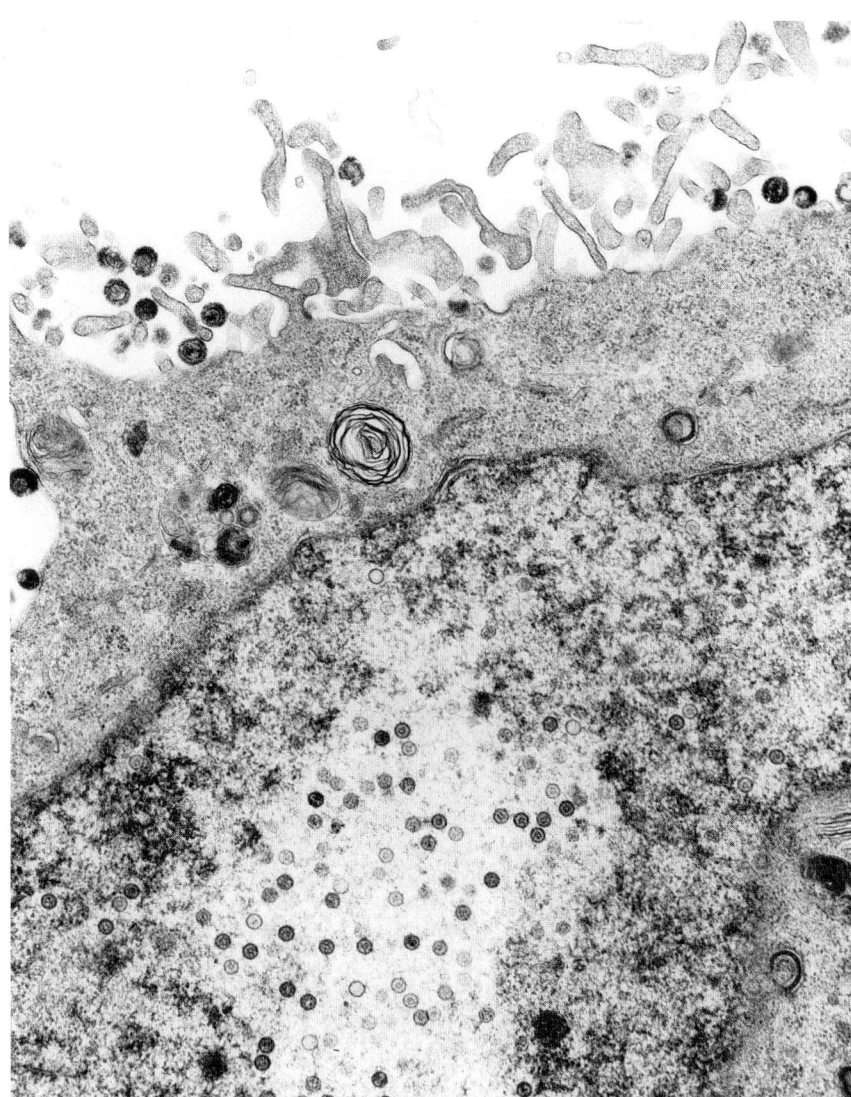

208-1 OMK cell infected with B virus isolated from a cynomolgus monkey (*M. fascicularis*). Note the nucleocapsids within the cell nucleus and enveloped virions at the cell surface and within cytoplasmic vacuoles. ×37,500.

was isolated from skin lesions. The patient's last direct exposure to macaques occurred at least 10 years before this illness, and no known contact with monkey tissue had occurred for at least 6 months preceding his illness. Neutralizing antibody titers to B virus rose from 1:8 in an early acute serum to 1:256 a month later, while the herpes simplex titer remained constant.

Person-to-person transmission of B virus has recently been documented (case 16, Table 208-1). The wife of an animal technician who subsequently died of B virus infection was directly involved with the care of her husband's herpetic skin lesions and acquired a B virus infection in a wound on her finger. She also developed asymptomatic conjunctival shedding, which lasted over 2 weeks.

Diagnosis

B virus infection should be considered when a patient has a history of exposure to macaques or tissues from macaques, especially when the history includes a bite, scratch, or possible wound con-

tamination. It also may be prudent to investigate the possibility of B virus infection in a person who handles macaques and has a history of suspected herpes zoster. The index of suspicion should be high when such a patient has vesicular lesions and lymphadenopathy. Neurologic symptoms that cannot be explained by trauma may also suggest B virus infection in a patient who has worked with macaques.

Serologic diagnosis of B virus infection is complicated by the extensive cross-reactivity with herpes simplex virus. Most adults have antibodies to herpes simplex and, although most human sera contain higher neutralizing antibodies to herpes simplex than to B virus, an unequivocal diagnosis based on serology alone is difficult. Newer serologic techniques, which minimize cross-reactivity, have been developed.[31,32] An increasing neutralizing titer to B virus, without a corresponding increase in herpes simplex titer is presumptive evidence of B virus infection. Individuals who work with macaques should have serial blood samples taken for antibody determinations, or at least saved for future reference.

Virus isolation was the basis for the original diagnosis of B virus infection and should be attempted in suspected cases. In early

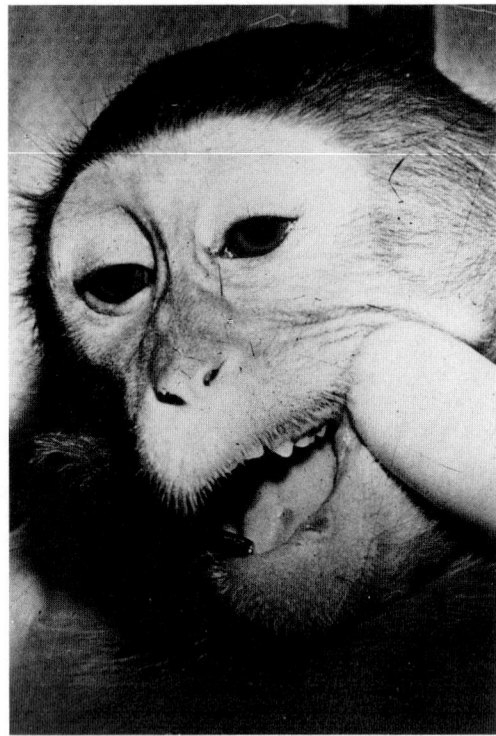

FIGURE 208-2 Labial and lingual ulcers in a rhesus monkey (*M. mulatta*) infected with B virus. (*Courtesy of William C. Cole, D.V.M. and the Journal of the American Veterinary Medical Association*).

reported fatalities, virus was isolated from the central nervous system in autopsy material; more recently B virus has been successfully isolated from vesicular fluid and skin punch biopsy specimens, allowing earlier diagnosis.

Treatment

The nucleoside analogues acyclovir, ganciclovir, and desciclovir[33,34] have been used successfully in experimental infections of rabbits and primates. Intravenous followed by oral acyclovir has been used in three cases of culture-confirmed, cutaneous B virus infection in humans. No progressive symptoms occurred in these patients and all became culture-negative (cases 15, 16, and 18, Table 208-1). Three other patients (cases 13, 14, and 17, Table 208-1) were treated unsuccessfully with intravenous acyclovir and two of them also with ganciclovir after the onset of neurologic symptoms.

Prognosis

The prognosis for encephalitic B virus infections is poor. Earlier diagnosis and institution of antiviral therapy may prevent disease progression and can render patients culture-negative. Caution must be used in interpreting these results, however, because the number of cases is limited, as is our knowledge of possible undiagnosed localized B virus infections and the possibility of reactivation of latent infections.

Prevention

The occurrence of four cases of B virus infection prompted the Centers for Disease Control (CDC) to establish guidelines for prevention of B virus infection in animal handlers.[35] These guidelines describe procedures for safe handling of monkeys and for dealing with potential exposure to B virus. Physicians managing potential cases and wishing further information may want to consult the Viral Exanthems and Herpesvirus Branch, Division of Viral Diseases, CDC, and for laboratory assistance, the Southwest Foundation for Biomedical Research (Dr. Julia Hilliard).

References

1. Palmer AE: B virus, *Herpesvirus simiae:* Historical perspective. *J Med Primatol* **16**:99, 1987
2. Centers for Disease Control: B virus infections in humans—Michigan, *MMWR* **38**:453, 1989
3. Centers for Disease Control: B-virus infection in humans—Pensacola, Florida. *MMWR* **36**:289, 1987
4. Holmes GP et al: B virus (*Herpesvirus simiae*) infection in humans: Epidemiologic investigation of a cluster. *Ann Intern Med* **112**:833, 1990
5. Matthews REF: Classification and nomenclature of viruses. *Intervirology* **17**:1, 1982
6. Wildy P: Herpesvirus. *Intervirology* **25**:117, 1986
7. Ludwig H et al: B virus (*Herpesvirus simiae*), in *The Herpesviruses,* 2d ed, edited by B Roizman. New York, Plenum, 1983, p 385
8. Eberle R et al: Relatedness of glycoproteins expressed on the surface of simian herpes-virus virions and infected cells to specific HSV glycoproteins. *Arch Virol* **109**:233, 1989
9. Hilliard JK et al: Simian alphaherpesviruses and their relation to the human herpes simplex viruses. *Arch Virol* **109**:83, 1989
10. Gay FP, Holden M: The herpes encephalitis problem, II. *J Infect Dis* **53**:287, 1933
11. Sabin AB, Wright AM: Acute ascending myelitis following a monkey bite, with the isolation of a virus capable of reproducing the disease. *J Exp Med* **59**:115, 3 plates, 1934
12. Melnick JL, Banker DD: Isolation of B virus (herpes group) from the central nervous system of a rhesus monkey. *J Exp Med* **100**:181, 1954
13. Wood W, Shimada FT: Isolation of strains of virus B from tissue cultures of cynomolgus and rhesus kidney. *Can J Public Health* **45**:509, 1954
14. Krech U, Lewis LJ: Propagation of B-virus in tissue cultures. *Proc Soc Exp Biol Med* **87**:174, 1954
15. Keeble SA et al: Natural virus-B infection in rhesus monkeys. *J Pathol Bacteriol* **86**:189, 1958
16. Keeble SA: B virus infection in monkeys. *Ann NY Acad Sci* **85**:960, 1960
17. Hartley EG: Naturally-occurring "B" virus infection in cynomolgus monkeys. *Vet Rec* **76**:555, 1964
18. Endo M et al: Etude du virus B au Japon. II. Le premier isolement du virus B au Japon. [Virus B in Japan. II. The first isolation of virus B in Japan.] *Jpn J Exp Med* **30**:385, 1960
19. Hunt RD, Melendez LV: Herpes virus infections of non-human primates: A review. *Lab Anim Care* **19**:221, 1969
20. Espana C: *Herpesvirus simiae* infection in *Macaca radiata. Am J Phys Anthrop* **38**:447, 1973
21. Loomis MR et al: Fatal herpesvirus infection in patas monkeys and a black and white colobus monkey. *J Am Vet Med Assoc* **179**:1236, 1981
22. McClure HM et al: Disseminated herpesvirus infection in a rhesus monkey (*Macaca mulatta*). *J Med Primatol* **2**:190, 1973

23. Daniel MD et al: Multiple *Herpesvirus simiae* isolation from a rhesus monkey which died of cerebral infarction. *Lab Anim Sci* **25**:303, 1975

24. Simon MA: Unpublished observations. 1990

25. Di Giacomo RF, Shah KV: Virtual absence of infection with *Herpesvirus simiae* in colony-reared rhesus monkeys (*Macaca mulatta*), with a literature review on antibody prevalence in natural and laboratory rhesus populations. *Lab Anim Sci* **22**:61, 1972

26. Zwartouw HT, Boulter EA: Excretion of B virus in monkeys and evidence of genital infection. *Lab Anim* **18**:65, 1984

27. Whitley RJ: Cercopithecine herpes virus 1 (B virus), in *Virology,* 2d ed, edited by BN Fields, DM Knipe, New York, Raven, 1990, p 2063

28. Bader C et al: The natural history of recurrent facial-oral infection with herpes simplex virus. *J Infect Dis* **138**:897, 1978

29. Vizoso AD: Recovery of herpes simiae (B virus) from both primary and latent infections in rhesus monkeys. *Br J Exp Pathol* **56**:485, 1975

30. Chappell WA: Animal infectivity of aerosols of monkey B virus. *Ann NY Acad Sci* **85**:931, 1960

31. Hilliard JK et al: Rapid identification of Herpesvirus simiae (B virus) DNA from clinical isolates in nonhuman primate colonies. *J Virol Methods* **13**:55, 1986

32. Katz D et al: ELISA for detection of group-common and virus-specific antibodies in human and simian sera induced by herpes simplex and related simian viruses. *J Virol Methods* **14**:99, 1986

33. Boulter EA et al: Successful treatment of experimental B virus (Herpesvirus simiae) infection with acyclovir. *Br Med J* **280**:681, 1980

34. Zwartouw HT et al: Oral chemotherapy of fatal B virus (herpesvirus simiae) infection. *Antiviral Res* **11**:275, 1989

35. Centers for Disease Control: Guidelines for prevention of *Herpesvirus simiae* (B virus) infection in monkey handlers. *MMWR* **36**:680, 687, 1987

36. Sabin AB: Fatal B virus encephalomyelitis in a physician working with monkeys. *J Clin Invest* **28**:808, 1949

37. Nagler FP, Klotz M: A fatal B virus infection in a person subject to recurrent herpes labialis. *Can Med Assoc J* **79**:743, 1958

38. Davidson WL, Hummeler K: B virus infection in man. *Ann NY Acad Sci* **85**:970, 1960

39. Pierce EC et al: B virus: Its current significance. Description and diagnosis of a fatal human infection. *Am J Hyg* **68**:242, 1958

40. Love FM, Jungherr E: Occupational infection with virus B of monkeys. *JAMA* **179**:160, 1962

41. Hull RN: The simian herpesviruses, in *The Herpesviruses*, edited by AS Kaplan. New York, Academic, 1973, p 389

42. Fierer J et al: Herpes B virus encephalomyelitis presenting as ophthalmic zoster. *Ann Intern Med* **79**:225, 1973

43. Benson PM et al: B virus (*Herpesvirus simiae*) and human infection. *Arch Dermatol* **125**:1247, 1989

44. Hummeler K et al: Encephalomyelitis due to infection with *Herpesvirus simiae* (herpes B virus). *N Engl J Med* **261**:64, 1959

45. Breen GE et al: Monkey-bite encephalomyelitis: Report of a case—with recovery. *Br Med J* **2**:22, 1958

46. Centers for Disease Control: Herpes B encephalitis—California. *MMWR* **22**:333, 1973

47. Corey L, Spear PG: Infections with herpes simplex viruses (parts I and II). *N Engl J Med* **314**:686, 749, 1986

48. Smith PC et al: The gibbon (*Hylobates lar*); a new primate host for Herpesvirus hominis. I. A natural epizootic in a laboratory colony. *J Infect Dis* **120**:292, 1969

49. Melendez LV et al: Natural herpes simplex infection in the owl monkey (*Aotus trivirgatus*). *Lab Anim Care* **19**:38, 1969

50. Hunt RD, Melendez LV: Clinical, epidemiologic, and pathologic features of cytocidal and oncogenic herpesviruses in South American monkeys. *J Natl Cancer Inst* **49**:261, 1972

51. King NW et al: Overt herpes-T infection in squirrel monkeys (*Saimiri sciureus*). *Lab Anim Care* **17**:413, 1967

52. Hunt RD, Melendez LV: Spontaneous herpes-T infection in the owl monkey (*Aotus trivirgatus*). *Pathol Vet* **3**:1, 1966

53. Malherbe H, Harwin R: Neurotropic virus in African monkeys. *Lancet* **2**:530, 1958

54. Malherbe H et al: The cytopathic effects of vervet monkey viruses. *S Afr Med J* **37**:407, 1963

55. Eichberg JW et al: Clinical, virological, and pathological features of herpesvirus SA8 infection in conventional and gnotobiotic baboons (*Papio cynocephalus*). *Arch Virol* **50**:255, 1976

56. Weller TH: Serial propagation *in vitro* of agents producing inclusion bodies derived from varicella and herpes zoster. *Proc Soc Exp Biol Med* **83**:340, 1953

57. Heuschele WP: Varicella (chicken pox) in three young anthropoid apes. *J Am Vet Med Assoc* **136**:256, 1960

58. Marennikova SS et al: A generalized herpetic infection simulating smallpox in a gorilla. *Intervirology* **2**:280, 1973/1974

59. Clarkson MJ et al: A virus disease of captive vervet monkeys (Cercopithecus aethiops) caused by a new herpesvirus. *Arch Ges Virusforsch* **22**:219, 1967

60. McCarthy K et al: Exanthematous disease in patas monkeys caused by a herpes virus. *Lancet* **2**:856, 1968

61. Blakely GA et al: A varicella-like disease in macaque monkeys. *J Infect Dis* **127**:617, 1973

62. Hull RN et al: Recovery and characterization of a new simian herpesvirus from a fatally infected spider monkey. *J Natl Cancer Inst* **49**:225, 1972

CHAPTER 209

Vincent A. Fulginiti

Smallpox and Complications of Smallpox Vaccination

Smallpox (Variola)

Smallpox is an acute exanthematous disease caused by infection with poxvirus variolae. The significant clinical features include a 3-day prodromal illness and a generalized centrifugal rash with rapidly successive papules, vesicles, pustules, umbilication, and crusting within 14 days. Although the worldwide eradication of smallpox was officially announced in 1979, it is too soon to give up discussion of this disease in medical texts.

Historical Aspects

The first clinical description of smallpox was by Rhazes, an Arabian physician, in the tenth century A.D. Many curious beliefs concerning the cause and pathogenesis of the disease are recorded in the writings of the early physicians. Frequently smallpox was confused with chickenpox, syphilis, and measles. It is of interest that smallpox was known in China 11 centuries before the birth of Christ, and that inoculation to prevent the disease was described in the sixth century B.C. using dried crusts introduced into the nose. It is likely that smallpox was introduced into the Western world in the early centuries after Christ by the migrations of invading armies. Subsequent spread of smallpox in Europe and England is intertwined with the history of these areas. As one reads the various accounts of epidemics of this disease in the fifteenth and sixteenth centuries, and later in the United States, it becomes apparent that smallpox represented a major force in life, often affecting dynasties, determining the outcome of military conflicts, as well as influencing daily life. Until the advent of Jennerian vaccination, its widespread application, and the ultimate eradication of smallpox, this disease continued to be a major threat, with widespread attack rates, persistent infection within a community, and a high mortality rate.

Epidemiology

In the past decade and a half, a remarkable event occurred in public health. The efforts of many countries, coordinated by the World Health Organization, resulted in intensive case finding and application of smallpox vaccination across large populations. This resulted in the eradication of smallpox, and there have been no cases since October 1977 anywhere in the world.

Etiology and Pathogenesis

Smallpox is caused by infection with poxvirus variola. It is believed that infection occurs strictly following contact with another infected human being. Evidence is accumulating that suggests a respiratory transmission, and the epidemiologic pattern supports this concept. Skin inoculation and fomite spread also may play a role in some instances.

Following contact, an asymptomatic period of 12 to 13 days follows. Despite the lack of symptoms, viral replication is massive. The pathogenic events that occur in the human being are suggested by analogy with Jenner's experimental mousepox infection. The virus, following introduction via the respiratory tract, undergoes local multiplication in the respiratory mucosa and regional lymphoid tissue. Primary viremia occurs, which spreads the virus widely throughout the reticuloendothelial system, where a massive multiplication occurs. A secondary viremia heralds the onset of the prodromal illness, resulting in spread to many organs and tissues, with primary manifestations in the skin. It has been postulated that serum antibody is not the significant factor in recovery from initial episodes of smallpox, and it appears likely that both delayed hypersensitivity and interferon production play some role in such recovery. Hemorrhagic forms of the disease are of interest in that a profound coagulation disorder is associated with a decrease in the number of serum platelets. Recent evidence indicates that depression of platelet formation occurs routinely in smallpox infection and that the hemorrhagic forms of the disease bear some similarity to disseminated intravascular coagulation, which results in reduction in coagulation factors, extensive hemorrhage, and death.

Clinical Manifestations

History   An influenzal illness shortly after contact has been described ("illness of contact"). A history of contact is essential. Prior vaccination history and interval to symptoms are important, as the disease pattern may be altered. Prior to the onset of the typical cutaneous lesions, a prodromal period of 3 days' duration occurs, characterized by apprehension, sudden prostrating fever, severe headache, back pain, and vomiting. A prodromal rash is not uncommon; it is macular and papular or petechial, and when it occurs in the characteristic "swimming-trunk" distribution, it is felt to be pathognomonic.

Cutaneous Lesions   The disease may take various courses. In the nonvaccinated, a discrete pox eruption is the most frequent form of illness. Severe forms of the disease are associated with confluent eruptions and/or cutaneous hemorrhage. Infrequently variola may occur without eruption, or with just a few pocks. A flat erythematous macular rash may precede the appearance of tense, deep-seated papules which rapidly vesiculate. These lesions are firm and more deep-seated than those of chickenpox. The rash may be very sparse, or individual vesicles may become confluent to form large patches. As the lesions mature, the classical "pustule" occurs (Fig. 209-1). These lesions do not contain bacteria, and the cloudiness represents accumulated white blood cells, debris, and protein. Central umbilication is characteristic (Figs. 209-1 and 209-2), and eventually the lesion crusts over and heals, with scar formation.

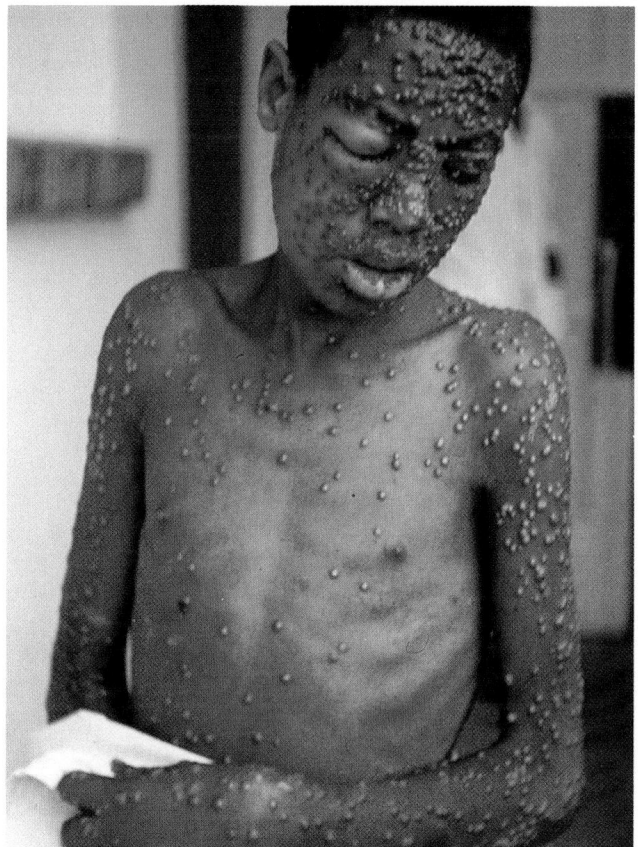

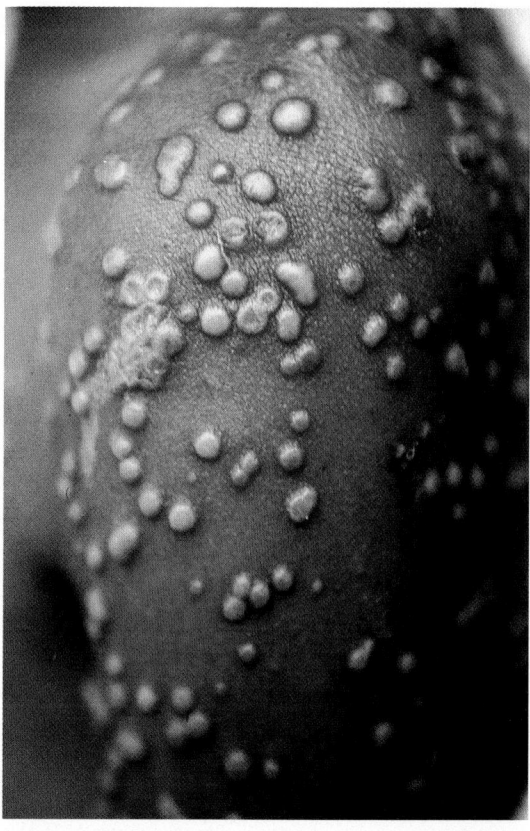

a

b

FIGURE 209-1 Pustular smallpox: tense, clouded vesicles which maintain firm feel. Note tendency to confluence and beginning central umbilication in some lesions (*b,c*).

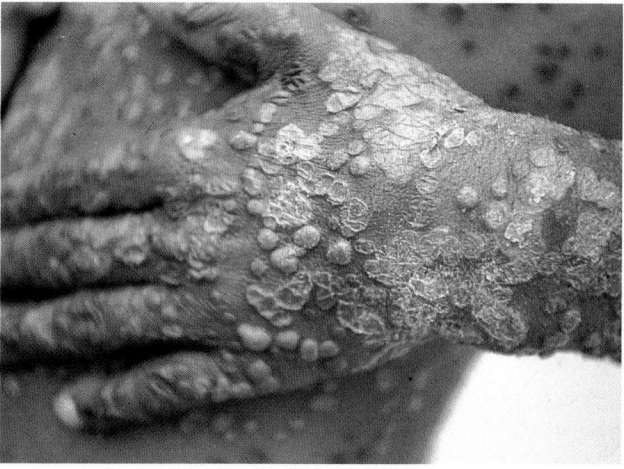

c

Although this is the classical evolution of smallpox, many variants are encountered, especially in individuals previously vaccinated. Lesions may present a flat disklike appearance or may undergo resolution without passing through the vesiculopustular stage.

There are two recognized hemorrhagic forms of the disease: one in which hemorrhage occurs in association with prodromal symptoms but death supervenes before any of the characteristic skin lesions can occur; and a second, characterized by hemorrhage into preexisting skin lesions. Both have almost universally fatal outcomes, the first within a week and the second after 8 to 12 days. Bacterial infection of smallpox lesions occurs, and localized abscesses, cellulitis, etc., may result.

Other Physical Findings Secondary viremia with spread to many organs may result in clinically apparent illness. Particularly common are ulceration of the cornea, laryngeal lesions with symptoms of obstruction in the upper part of the airway, central nervous system involvement with encephalitis or acute psychotic behavior, and, less commonly, osteomyelitis, pneumonia, and orchitis.

Laboratory Findings Usual diagnostic laboratory measurements are of little value in smallpox. The white blood cell count may be elevated early in the disease, but this is not of diagnostic significance.

Virus is present in the blood of patients during the prodrome and occasionally thereafter. Virus is uniformly found in the skin

lesions; the early papules and vesicles provide the richest source. In hemorrhagic forms of the disease, severe thrombocytopenia occurs; in addition, marked decrease in the level of accelerator globulin (factor V), moderate decreases in the amount of prothrombin and proconvertin, and a circulating antithrombin are noted in early hemorrhagic smallpox. The late hemorrhagic form of the disease is associated with a decrease in platelets without other coagulation disturbances.

Pathology

In the papular stage of the eruption, capillary dilatation and edema of the papillary layer of the dermis are observed. Perivascular in-

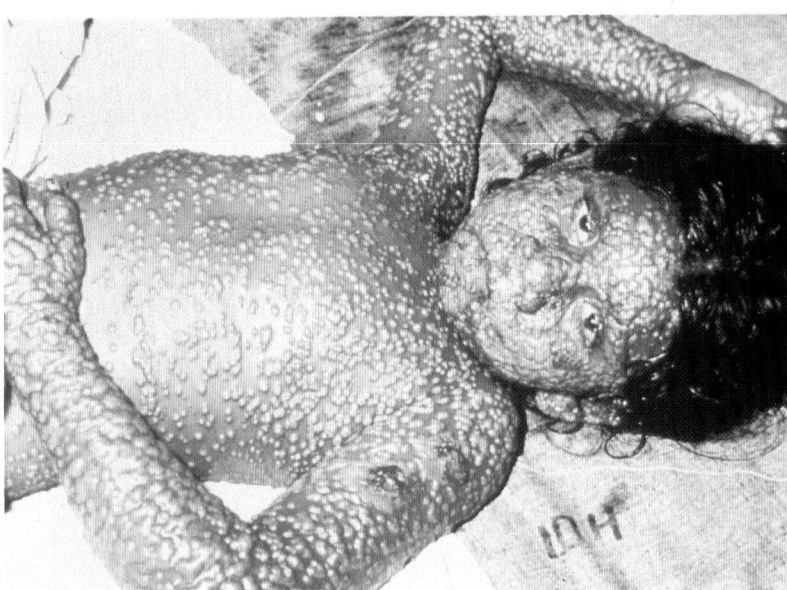

FIGURE 209-2 Confluent smallpox. Note massive numbers of lesions, all in same stage of development, and confluency of many.

flammatory changes occur, with lymphocytic and histiocytic infiltration. Thickening and vacuolization in the epithelium result in vesicle formation. The vesicle is deep and, because of the destruction of cells, becomes separate. Leukocyte infiltration results in the "pustule formation," which resolves by epithelial migration and crusting. Typical cytoplasmic eosinophilic inclusion bodies have been described (Guarnieri's bodies). Histopathologic changes in the mucosa are similar, with added ulceration.

Diagnosis and Differential Diagnosis

Typical smallpox in endemic areas usually could be diagnosed clinically, and ancillary virologic laboratory aids were usually unnecessary. However, now that smallpox has been eradicated worldwide, if a case arose, it would probably be confused with severe chickenpox or not suspected at all. For this reason virologic diagnosis would be *essential*, with confirmation of variola having global public health implications. Rapid means of laboratory diagnosis include (1) light microscopic identification of elementary bodies with appropriate stains, (2) electron microscopic identification of virus in vesicular fluid or scrapings from the base of a papule or early vesicle, and (3) fluorescent antibody staining of the virus from the same material. All these tests yield rapid, presumptive results in the hands of experienced workers, but definite diagnosis can be achieved only by isolation of the virus in the embryonated egg or in appropriate tissue culture systems and specific identification of the virus by neutralization with variola or vaccinal antiserum. Indirect but rapid methods utilize vesicular fluid as a hemagglutinin, complement-fixing, or precipitating antigen with specific variola vaccinia antiserum. Retrospective diagnosis can be afforded by evaluation of serum antibody rises in a 2- to 3-week interval, utilizing paired sera collected during the acute and convalescent phases of the illness.

In summary, the diagnosis of smallpox is primarily clinical and based upon obtaining an adequate history of exposure, the observation of an approximately 2-week incubation period followed by a severe 3-day prodrome, ultimately terminating in a typical rash with centrifugal distribution and all lesions in the same stage of development. One cannot rely on the presence of Guarnieri's bodies to establish the diagnosis, although they may be suggestive.

In the preeruptive phase of smallpox, distinction must be made from dengue, enterovirus infections, and other febrile illnesses. The prodromal rash may be confused with that of measles. History of contact and the appropriate incubation interval should serve to make one suspect smallpox.

Hemorrhagic smallpox may be confused with meningococcal septicemia, coagulation disorders, typhus, and other acute hemorrhagic exanthems. Eruptive smallpox is most frequently mistaken for chickenpox. The lack of prodromal symptoms, the successive appearance of crops of superficial vesicles, the centripetal distribution, and the varying stages of development of chickenpox lesions all serve to distinguish this disease from variola.

Treatment

This disease has now been prevented by Jennerian vaccination, but no effective specific treatment was known. Thiosemicarbazone and antivariola or antivaccinia serum and immune globulin failed in the therapy of established smallpox.

Good nursing care with attention to the prevention of secondary bacterial infection is critical in treatment. Appropriate antimicrobial therapy for bacterial complications should be employed, and attention should be paid to the nutritional, fluid, and electrolyte needs of patients.

Course and Prognosis

The overall mortality rate of smallpox approximates 25 percent, with confluent disease representing a greater risk than discrete eruptions. Fulminant smallpox is universally fatal, as are the hemorrhagic forms of the illness.

Complications of Smallpox Vaccination (Vaccinia)

Definition and Classification

Vaccination against smallpox consists of the introduction of vaccinia virus into the outer layers of the intact skin. Local multiplication of virus occurs, and in some instances regional lymphadenopathy and systemic symptoms ensue. The infection is a localized one which heals by scarring and is limited by host response. A complicated vaccination is one in which any of the above components is altered. Complications may be classified as indicated in Table 209-1.

Historical Aspects

With the eradication of smallpox in the world, the routine application of infant vaccination has been greatly diminished. As a result, complications of vaccinations are seen infrequently in most countries and not at all in many.

Epidemiology

Most complications may occur at any age, but they are usually seen among young infants and children. Primovaccination is most often administered to this age group, and almost all the significant complications occur most frequently, if not exclusively, after first vaccination. In addition, the infectious complications tend to occur in the immunologically deficient child, which also contributes to the clustering in early childhood. Bacterial superinfection in some instances is related to warm weather, with the opportunity for maceration of skin and with increased exposure of the vaccination site.

Complications are reported more commonly in the western world, despite the prevalence of vaccination in the east. This undoubtedly represents reporting differences, not a true geographic or racial relationship. The incidence of postvaccinal encephalitis appears to be higher in the Netherlands. Whether this represents a true

TABLE 209-1

Classification of Complications of Vaccination

Major category	Specific syndromes	Comment
Noninfectious rashes	Erythema multiforme	Differentiate from generalized
	Macular—toxic eruption	
	Macular and papular	
	Vesicular	
	Urticarial	
Bacterial superinfection	Streptococcal	Often hyperkeratotic
	Staphylococcal	
	Mixed	
	Tetanus	
	Syphilis	Of historical interest in U.S.
Accidental inoculation (may occur in vaccinated individual)	Normal skin	
	Abnormal skin	
	Burns	
	Pyoderma	
	Exanthem	Examples: varicella, herpes
	Eczema	
	Other dermatides:	
	Mucosal	Usually oral or conjunctival
	Corneal	Vaccinal keratitis
Congenital vaccinia		
Generalized vaccinia	Benign becoming malignant with progression	
Progressive vaccinia (vaccinia gangrenosa, vaccinia necrosum)	In immunologically normal persons	
	In hypogammaglobulinemia:	
	Congenital sex-linked	
	Thymic alymphoplasia	
	In dysgammaglobulinemia	
	With malignancies:	
	Chronic lymphatic leukemia	
	Hodgkin's disease	
	Lymphoma	
Encephalitis	Postvaccinal	
Miscellaneous	Hemolytic anemia	
	Arthritis	
	Osteomyelitis	
	Laboratory infections	
	Pericarditis and myocarditis	

racial difference or simply reflects the fact of primovaccination in the adults is not clear.

Etiology and Pathogenesis

The basic mechanisms of the complications of vaccination may be divided into three categories: (1) bacterial superinfection, (2) abnormal viral replication, and (3) altered reactivity, or ''allergy,'' to some viral component.

Bacteria can invade the vaccination site; indeed, not all vaccine is bacteriologically sterile. That superinfection is not more common is remarkable. Apparently more than contamination is necessary; those factors of greatest importance are concurrent streptococcal infection elsewhere and excessive trauma, maceration, and manipulation of the vaccination site.

Usually the virus remains localized at the site of implantation, but occasionally infection may be transposed to healthy or unhealthy skin elsewhere on the body, or even to another person. Etiologic factors include excessive manipulation, abnormal skin (burns, eczema, etc.), inflammatory lesions (blepharitis, herpes), and abnormal immune mechanisms. Any of these may contribute to spread of the virus away from the intended localized vaccination site.

Among the host factors that are responsible for limitation of viral spread and recovery from vaccination are development of serum antibody, delayed hypersensitivity, and interferon production. Serum antibody and delayed hypersensitivity are specific and are induced soon after infection; antibody would appear to be less important in recovery than delayed hypersensitivity. Interferon is nonspecific and has been found in the skin of animals recovering from vaccinia infection who have been rendered deficient in antibodies and in delayed hypersensitivity. It has also been found in human vaccination crusts. Individuals who lack antibody-synthesizing capacity may develop progressive and widespread vaccinal lesions. However, even these patients, if they retain delayed-hypersensitivity responsiveness, may undergo perfectly normal vaccinations. In addition, patients with normal antibody levels, but with absent delayed-hypersensitivity responsiveness, are susceptible to the progressive form of the disease. As indicated, interferon is also important and may account for recovery of animals in the absence of the other two functions. However, data for human beings are lacking, and the importance of this mechanism of resistance is not known.

Allergy, or presumed altered reactivity, to viral components appears to be responsible for the erythema multiforme type of skin rash observed in some individuals after primovaccination. This mechanism has also been implicated in the pathogenesis of postvaccinal encephalitis; it is assumed the virus or a virus–central nervous system complex invokes an immune response directed against brain antigens, which then results in an antigen–antibody inflammatory reaction and the clinical picture of encephalitis.

Clinical Manifestations

Erythema Multiforme-like Eruptions   An intensely erythematous macular rash may follow smallpox vaccination. This rash has the characteristics of erythema multiforme in that iris or bull's eye lesions appear and tend to coalesce. The rash is often symmetrical and florid, involving a large portion of the body. This is a totally benign manifestation representing an allergic reaction.

Bacterial Superinfection   Purulent complications of smallpox vaccination today involve principally impetiginous infection with *Staphylococcus aureus* or group A beta-hemolytic streptococci. If poultices are employed, tetanus may be introduced by the soil or dung elements incorporated in such primitive techniques.

Accidental Inoculation   Vaccinia virus can be implanted from the site of vaccination onto the skin or mucous membrane anywhere on the individual's body. They can also be transferred to another individual. Each of the lesions is characteristic of a primary smallpox vaccination with the exception that they do not tend to scar. Certain implantations may be more hazardous than the occasional single-site inoculation. These include implantation onto large areas of abnormal skin (burns or other dermatoses), into the eye (vaccinal keratitis may result), extensive mucosal lesions, and implantation around various body orifices which may impede certain bodily functions (Fig. 209-3).

Congenital Vaccinia   Vaccination of the pregnant woman may result in disseminated disease fatal to the fetus. Congenital vaccination may also occur following exposure to a vaccinated individual. The infant may be stillborn or may develop lesions shortly after birth.

Generalized Vaccinia   Generalized vaccinia as used in this classification refers to a benign generalized eruption, each lesion of which is identical to its primary smallpox vaccination. Although little is known of the immunology surrounding such a defect, it is clear that some children with isolated IgM deficiency are liable to this complication. This is not generally a lethal disease.

Progressive Vaccinia (Vaccinia Gangrenosa, Vaccinia Necrosum)   If a smallpox vaccination shows no evidence of normal resolution within 2 weeks of inoculation, a presumptive diagnosis of progressive vaccinia should be made. In this disease, the normal immunologic response to vaccination is impaired. This may occur in an

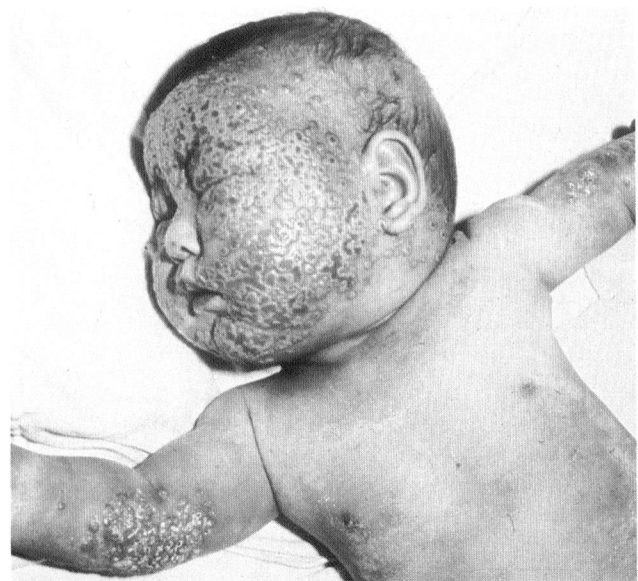

FIGURE 209-3   Eczema vaccinatum. Lesions are in areas of active eczema. Note typical vaccinal character of individual lesions.

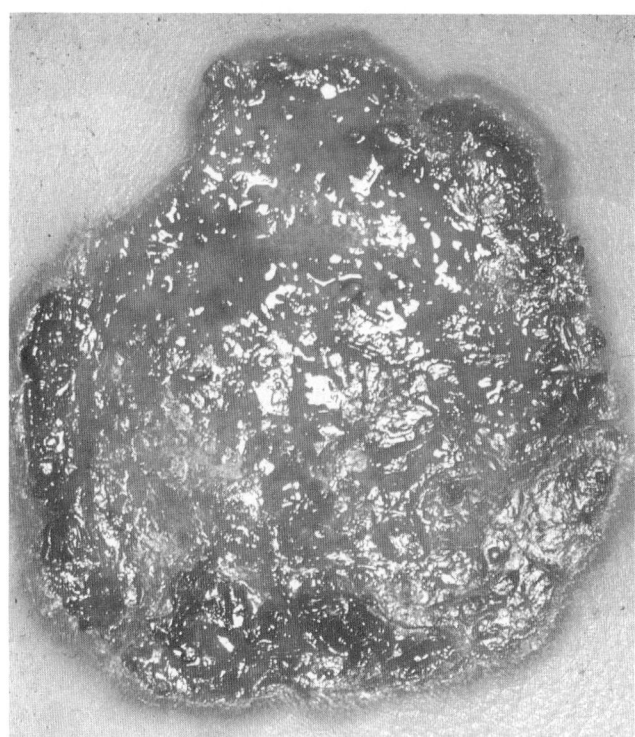

FIGURE 209-4   Progressive vaccinia: large, nonhealing vaccination site with "soft, rubbery" border, high virus content, and lack of surrounding inflammatory response; present 4 months in 10-month-old male with variant of thymic alymphoplasia.

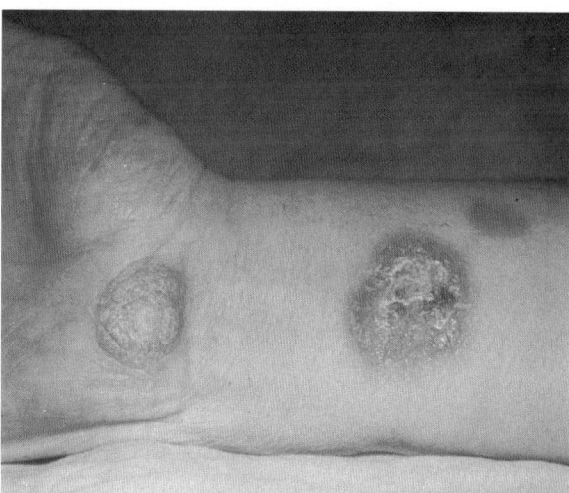

FIGURE 209-5   Secondary, viremic lesions in progressive vaccinia. Two lesions on arm, which demonstrate variability, both positive for vaccinia virus, occurred in elderly female with chronic lymphatic leukemia; complete clearing with thiosemicarbazone therapy.

otherwise normal individual or in persons with generalized defects in immunologic capacities.

In its complete form, the site of vaccination fails to heal and continues to enlarge, often for months. Usually, no systemic signs of illness are present and, in the absence of some other disease, physical findings are limited to the vaccination. These lesions differ from normal ones in that little inflammatory response is observed. The vaccination initially has a soft, rubbery appearance with little scabbing (Fig. 209-4). As the lesion progresses in size, considerable central necrosis becomes evident, and thick, dark eschars form (hence the synonym, vaccinia necrosum). The initial lesion may become huge, with the entire upper arm and shoulder involved. In many cases secondary lesions are evident; in some, satellite vaccinations occur close to the primary one, and, in addition, viremic lesions may appear at distant sites. Each of the secondary lesions progresses in the same fashion as the primary one (Fig. 209-5). Variations are observed in that the primary lesion may become ulcerative or may have a piled-up appearance, but the progression is characteristic.

Untreated disease or illness failing to respond to treatment may be of long duration, during which extensive tissue destruction, secondary bacterial infection and septicemia, mucosal lesions, pneumonia, and other complications may occur. The course is progressively downhill, although the patient may not manifest correspondingly severe constitutional symptoms until relatively late in the disease.

Encephalitis   A meningoencephalitis syndrome occurs rarely as a complication of smallpox vaccination. The sudden onset of head-

ache and vomiting in the second week after vaccination may herald this illness. Convulsions, lethargy, coma, paralysis, signs of cerebral edema, increased intracranial pressure, and focal neurologic findings may occur. In other instances the disease may resemble aseptic meningitis or myelitis.

Laboratory Findings

Virologic   Specimens from suspected vaccinal lesions can be inoculated into a variety of tissue culture systems or the embryonated hen's egg. Identification is by typical pock formation or by classical cytopathogenic effect with subsequent neutralization by antisera. Additionally, specific vaccinia antigen can be detected by a variety of antibody methods, either from the original specimen obtained from the patient or from the infected cell cultures or egg fluids.

Immunologic and Hematologic   Response to vaccinia virus may be critical in determining host susceptibility. Vaccinia-neutralizing antibody can be measured, as can a delayed-hypersensitivity reaction to inactivated vaccinia antigen.

In certain clinical states, total immunologic capacity may need to be surveyed, as the vaccinal infection is simply an indicator of a more comprehensive immunologic defect. Assays for immunoglobulin antibody capacity and for cell-mediated immune function may need to be employed.

Treatment

Complications of vaccination can be reduced by recognizing those predisposing conditions which lead to each of the separate types of complication. Thus, individuals who have eczema or other skin lesions should not be vaccinated or exposed to an individual who is vaccinated. Individuals with immunologic deficiency, receiving immunosuppressive therapy, or suffering from diseases such as lymphatic malignancies which heighten susceptibility should avoid contact with vaccinia virus and should not be vaccinated. If such individuals are exposed, use of either vaccinia immune globulin by injection or methisazone (isatin thiosemicarbazone) can be expected to reduce the risk.

In the past, administration of vaccinia immune globulin (VIG) for complications of vaccination has been facilitated by its ready availability. Currently this product is no longer produced and is in limited supply. As a result, its use should be more stringent than in the past and it should be reserved for those severe complications in which a beneficial effect has been either demonstrated or suspected. Children with erythema multiforme or simple autoinoculation disease and vaccinal encephalitis should not receive this preparation as it is of no benefit. On the other hand, those with extensive intradermal involvement such as eczema vaccinatum or burns should be treated with either VIG or methisone. VIG should be used in conjunction with methisazone and immunologic therapy in those severe complications such as progressive vaccinia.

Course and Prognosis

As indicated in the separate sections, prognosis is variable. Most complications are self-limited or respond to simple measures; a few require extraordinary forms of therapy, and even with such treatment a small group remains who are unresponsive.

Bibliography

Smallpox (Variola)

Bauer DJ et al: The chemotherapy of variola major infection. *Bull WHO* **26**:727, 1962

Bauer DJ et al: Prophylactic treatment of smallpox contacts with *N*-methylisatin β-thiosemicarbazone. *Lancet* **2**:494, 1963

Bremen JG, Arita I: The confirmation and maintenance of smallpox eradication. *N Engl J Med* **303**:1263, 1980

Dixon CW: *Smallpox.* London, Churchill, 1962

Downie AW: Smallpox, in *Medical History of the Second World War,* edited by Z Cope. London, HM Stationery Office, 1952

Downie AW, MacDonald A: Smallpox and related virus infections in man. *Br Med Bull* **9**:191, 1953

Downie AW et al: Studies on the virus content of mouth washings in the acute phase of smallpox. *Bull WHO* **25**:49, 1961

Fenner F: Global eradication of smallpox. *Rev Infect Dis* **4**:916, 1982

Kempe CH: Smallpox, in *The Biologic Basis of Pediatric Practice,* edited by R Cooke. New York, McGraw-Hill, 1965

Kempe CH, St Vincent L: Variola and vaccinia, in *Diagnostic Procedures in Viral and Rickettsial Infections,* edited by E Lennette. New York, American Public Health Association, 1964

Kempe CH et al: The use of vaccinia hyperimmune gamma globulin in the prophylaxis of smallpox. *Bull WHO* **25**:41, 1961

Rao AR et al: A study of 1,000 cases of smallpox. *J Indian Med Assoc* **35**:296, 1960

Wehrle P: A reality in our time—certification of the global eradication of smallpox. *J Infect Dis* **242**:636, 1980

WHO Expert Committee on Smallpox: *WHO Technical Report Series* **283**:1, 1964

Complications of Smallpox Vaccination (Vaccinia)

Adels BR, Oppe TE: Treatment of eczema vaccinatum with *N*-methylisatin beta-thiosemicarbazone. *Lancet* **1**:18, 1966

Barbero GT et al: Vaccinia gangrenosa treated with hyperimmune vaccinal gamma globulin. *Pediatrics* **16**:609, 1955

Daly JJ, Jackson E: Vaccinia gangrenosa treated with *N*-methylisatin β-thiosemicarbazone. *Br Med J* **2**:1300, 1962

Davidson E, Hayhoe FG: Prolonged generalized vaccinia complicating acute leukemia. *Br Med J* **2**:1298, 1962

Dimson SB: Eczema vaccinatum. *Lancet* **2**:73, 1962

Ellis PP, Wenograd L: Ocular vaccinia. *Arch Ophthalmol* **68**:600, 1962

Erichson RB, McNamara MJ: Vaccinia gangrenosa: Report of a case and review of the literature. *Ann Intern Med* **55**:491, 1961

Fekety FR Jr et al: Vaccinia gangrenosa in chronic lymphatic leukemia. *Arch Intern Med* **109**:205, 1962

Flewitt TH, Ker FL: A case of vaccinia necrosum (progressive vaccinia) with severe hypogammaglobulinemia, treated with *N*-methylisatin β-thiosemicarbazone (33T57). *J Clin Pathol* **16**:271, 1963

Fulginiti VA, Kempe CH: Poxvirus diseases, in *Brennemann's Practice of Pediatrics,* vol II, part 1, edited by V Kelley. Hagerstown, MD, Harper & Row, 1937, p 1

Fulginiti VA et al: Therapy of experimental vaccinal keratitis. *Arch Ophthalmol* **74**:539, 1965

Greenberg M: Complications of vaccination against smallpox. *Am J Dis Child* **76**:492, 1948

Kaufman H et al: A cure of vaccinia infection by 5-iodo-2'-deoxyuridine. *Virology* **18**:567, 1962

Kempe CH: Studies on smallpox and complications of smallpox vaccination. *Pediatrics* **26**:176, 1960

Kempe CH, Benenson AS: Smallpox immunization in the United States. *JAMA* **194**:161, 1965

Kempe CH et al: Hyperimmune vaccinal gamma globulin. *Pediatrics* **18**:177, 1956

Naidoo P, Hirsch H: Prenatal vaccinia. *Lancet* **1**:196, 1963

Nanning W: Prophylactic effect of antivaccinia gamma globulin against postvaccinal encephalitis. *Bull WHO* **27**:317, 1962

Neff JM: Smallpox vaccination: Minimal complication rates, United States, 1963. Presentation at Annual Epidemiologic Intelligence Service, Communicable Disease Center, April 1965

O'Connel CJ et al: Progressive vaccinia with normal antibodies: A case possibly due to deficient cellular immunity. *Ann Intern Med* **60**:282, 1964

Sathe PV et al: Prevention of postvaccinal tetanus. *Indian J Pediatr* **31**:306, 1965

Spillane JD, Wells CEC: The neurology of Jennerian vaccination: A clinical account of the neurological complications which occurred during the smallpox epidemic in South Wales in 1962. *Brain* **87**:1, 1964

Sussman S, Grossman M: Complications of smallpox vaccination. Effects of vaccinia immune globulin therapy. *J Pediatr* **67**:1168, 1965

Wielenga G et al: Prenatal infection with vaccinia virus. *Lancet* **1**:258, 1961

CHAPTER 210

Ullin W. Leavell, Jr., and Robert J. Jacob

Orf

Contagious ecthyma, or contagious pustular dermatitis, is a disease that is caused by the orf virus. The disease is endemic among sheep, goats, and musk oxen (i.e., ruminants) and can be transmitted to humans. Early authors who suggested that the disease was transmitted from animals to humans included Brandenberg, Newsom and Cross, and Peterkin. The disease usually develops in the vicinity of the mouth and nose of animals and manifests itself as nodules on exposed areas of the skin. Lesions are similar in humans and animals and heal in about 35 days. The disease is classified as a near-neoplasm, since it stimulates pseudoepitheliomatous hyperplasia and causes a finger-like downward proliferation of the epidermis.

Epidemiology and Etiology

The disease has been reported exclusively in the white race. Age is not a factor; the disease has been seen in patients as young as 10 and as old as 72 years. It is commonplace among sheepherders in all parts of the world. Not all cases are thoroughly documented because many patients do not seek medical advice. Farmers and veternarians are most likely to be exposed to the virus, and immunosuppression and skin lesions increase susceptibility in exposed persons. The disease is more prevalent in the spring when newborn lambs, lacking immunity, fall prey to the disease. Individuals feeding milk from bottles to infected, orphaned lambs frequently come in contact with the lamb's sore mouth, and may contract the disease. The virus may be acquired indirectly from knives, barbed wire, barn doors, towels, and vehicles that have contacted infected animals.

The virus is sturdy, surviving the winter months on barn doors, feeding troughs, and fences. Susceptible lambs become infected from contact with virus-containing objects. It has been found in goats, camels, bighorn sheep, mountain goats, and wild sheep. Pregnancy and fetal development have not been reported to be affected by infection with the virus.

Immunity

Previous cutaneous infection results in lesions that are less pronounced. Recurrences of the eruption have been reported in a patient 8 months after the initial lesion. Experimental inoculation of vaccine indicates that reinoculation will take place in 3 to 5 months. The best prevention in animals is vaccination every 6 to 8 months. After vaccination with the orf virus, mules, deer, musk oxen, moose, and wapiti calves have developed the disease.

Molecular Anatomy of Orf

Orf virus could be considered a prototype for the genus *Parapoxvirus*. It is an ovoid particle about 250 nm by 160 nm. The surface tubules of parapoxvirus appear as a twinelike structure 10 nm to 20 nm wide forming a long crisscross design that extends for up to 1 μm in length. This design is easily seen on negatively stained preparations by electron microscopy (Fig. 210-1). This structure helps distinguish a parapoxvirus from an orthopoxvirus in that or-

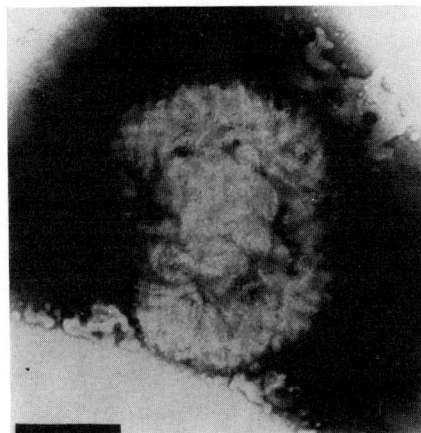

a

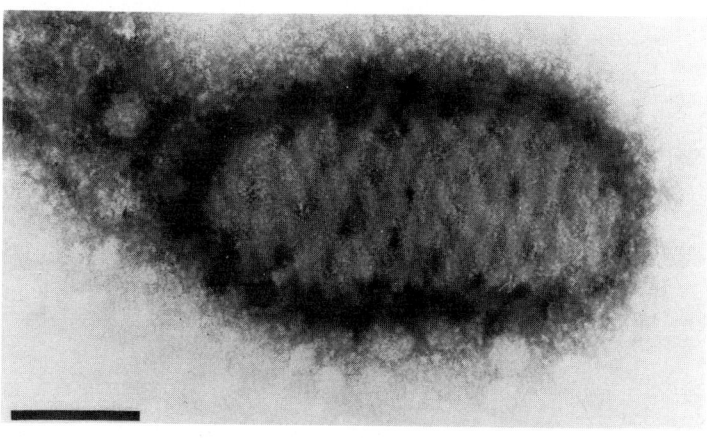

b

FIGURE 210-1 Electron micrographs of negatively stained preparations of (*a*) orthopoxvirus and (*b*) parapoxvirus (orf) isolated from vesicular fluid and representing the ''M'' forms of poxviruses. The bars represent 100 nm. (*Reprinted with permission from ''An Atlas of Mammalian Viruses,'' edited by EL Palmer, ML Martin. Copyright CRC Press, Inc., Boca Raton, FL)*

thopoxviruses have an irregular arrangement of tubules in their outer membranes. Orf virus shows serologic cross-reactivity with another parapoxvirus, milker's nodules virus. Parapoxviruses are sensitive to heating at 58°C (136°F) for 30 min and resistant to lipid solvents such as ether and chloroform. The virus's resistance to long-term drying is important for the enzootic spread of infection.

The virus will not produce pocks on the chorioallantoic membrane (CAM) of fertilized eggs. However, the virus will grow plaques in cultured cells such as bovine (BEL) and ovine (OEL) embryonic lung cells, lamb testes (LT), and bovine fetal spleen cells. The orf virus has a DNA genome that is smaller than orthopoxvirus, but contains a 64 percent G + C content that is higher than orthopoxvirus. However, the DNA contains an inverted terminal repeat (ITR), that is cross-linked and contains a sequence pattern reminiscent of orthopoxviruses.

Restriction endonuclease (RE) "fingerprint" analysis of orf DNA reveals heterogeneity in the genome structure that is consistent with reports of antigenic variation in the virus. RE analysis could not resolve orf virus into groups of ovine and human strains. Point mutations, substitutions, and deletions of base pairs, inversions and transpositions, and minor alterations of sequences throughout the DNA are probably responsible for this difference in RE fingerprints. This pattern is similar to what has been seen in other poxviruses. Although Southern blot analysis did not reveal any insertion of host DNA within the orf genome, it did reveal that several field isolates lack a large segment (i.e., 14 to 19 percent) of DNA that is found in the commonly used vaccine strain (i.e., CE).

Molecular Pathogenesis

The virus grows on primary human amnion and other cell cultures (see above), producing cells with pyknotic nuclei and vacuolated cytoplasm. Later, plaques form as holes in the monolayer, surrounded by clumps of granular cells. Cytopathic effect is seen during orf virus replication with complete virions forming at 12 to 16 h pi. Ultrastructural changes seen were a result of areas of viral production in the cytoplasm. These areas contained immature viral particles in the form of trilamina structures.

During the period of viral replication, the nuclear chromatin marginates to the nuclear membrane. Distinct morphologic changes can be seen in the nucleoplasm around 36 h pi. These changes can be seen as an accumulation of tubules and the formation of fine filaments that appear to be independent of the development of mature virus particles. Accumulation of intranuclear tubules may be a host phenomenon, and intranuclear tubules and filaments represent an indirect cellular response to viral infection, rather than viral products.

Clinical Manifestations

The cutaneous lesions average 1.6 cm in diameter. Usually only one lesion is present, although as many as 10 have been reported. The lesion is most commonly located on the dorsal aspect of the right index finger. Regional lymphadenopathy is common; lymphangitis and fever may occur. Fever disappears within 3 to 4 days, lymphangitis within 3 to 4 weeks. Toxic erythema, erythema multiforme, and a widespread papulovesicular eruption of the skin and

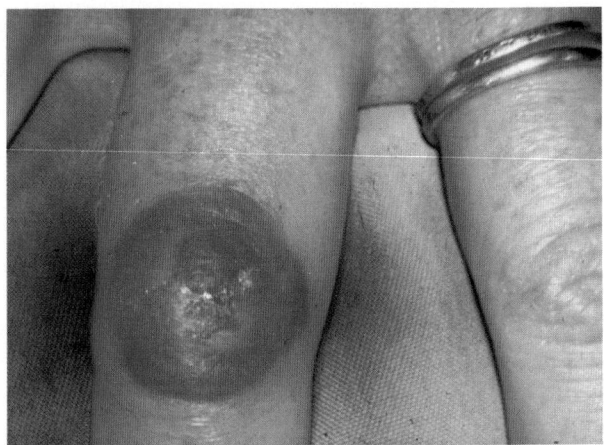

FIGURE 210-2 The target phase shows a white circle with central and peripheral erythema.

mucosae may occur. Amputation of a finger was necessary in a patient receiving immunosuppressive drugs for lymphoma.

The disease advances through six stages, healing uneventfully in about 35 days. Each stage lasts approximately 6 days. The papular phase shows a red, elevated lesion. The target stage has a nodule with a red center, a white middle ring, and a red periphery (Fig. 210-2). A red, weeping surface is present during the acute phase and the lesion may be elevated, appearing to be a rapidly growing infected tumor (Fig. 210-3). In the regenerative state, a thin, dry crust through which black dots may be seen, covers the surface of the nodule. Small papillomas appear over the surface of the lesion during the papillomatous stage. In the regressive stage, a thick crust develops over the surface of the lesion, the papillomas decrease in size, and elevation of the lesion subsides.

Pathology

The papular state of orf has not been studied in humans. In the target stage, intranuclear and intracytoplasmic inclusions are present in superficial, vacuolated epidermal cells in areas corresponding to the white ring (Fig. 210-4). Intracytoplasmic and intranuclear inclusions may also be seen. There is an infiltrate of plasma cells, macrophages, histiocytes, and lymphocytes. The acute state is distinguished by loss of epidermis over the central part of the lesion. Peripherally, there is reticular degeneration. Microvesicles

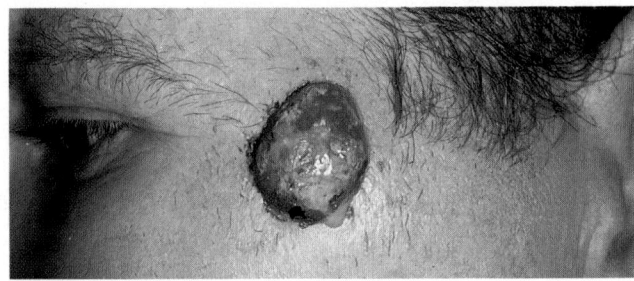

FIGURE 210-3 In the acute phase there is weeping of the surface overlying an elevated tumor.

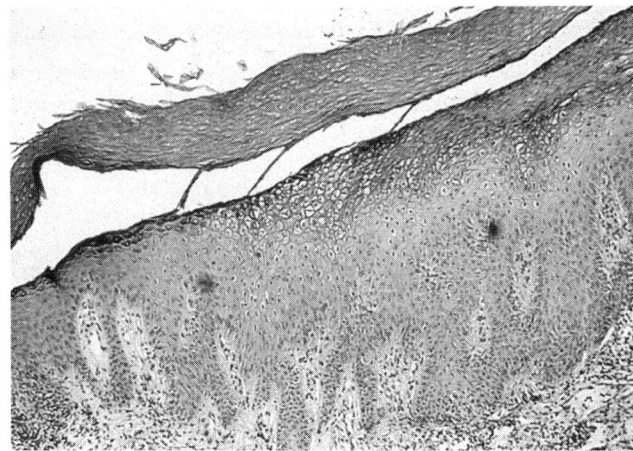

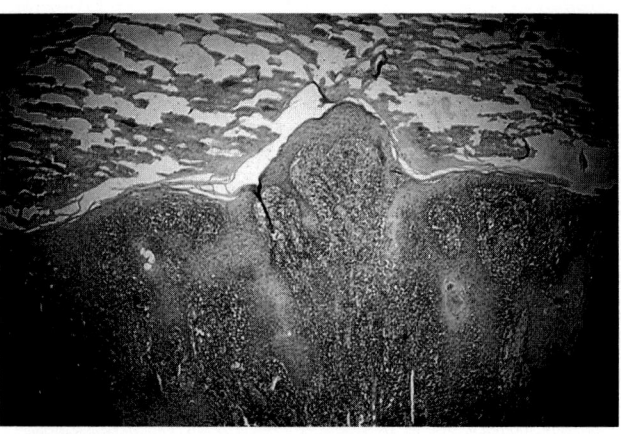

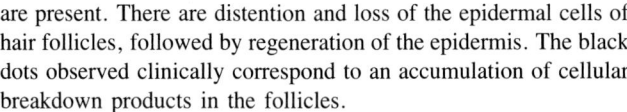

FIGURE 210-4 In the target stage vacuolated epidermal cells advance peripherally, leaving behind epidermal thickening and pyknotic epidermal cells. ×250.

FIGURE 210-5 In the papillomatous phase there is a papilloma and finger-like downward projections of the epidermis. ×250.

are present. There are distention and loss of the epidermal cells of hair follicles, followed by regeneration of the epidermis. The black dots observed clinically correspond to an accumulation of cellular breakdown products in the follicles.

Many papillary elevations and finger-like downward projections of the epidermis are seen in the papillomatous stage (Fig. 210-5). In the regressive stage, the papillomas are reduced in size, and histiocytes, macrophages, lymphocytes, and plasma cells are decreased in number.

Acanthosis within the first week, followed by a finger-like downward proliferation of the epidermis are features suggesting neoplasia. Papillomatosis and acanthosis occur within the papilloma. The infiltrate in the dermis contributes to the growing tumor.

The pathology of human regional lymph nodes has not been studied. In sheep, however, there is a progressive increase in the size of the lymph nodes and in the plasma cell infiltrate over a 14-day period.

Diagnosis

The diagnosis of orf is established by a history of contact with infected animals, the appearance of the lesions, passage of the virus to sheep cell cultures, fluorescent antibody tests, and electron microscopy (Fig. 210-6). Electron microscopy of sheep tissue reveals partially and/or totally encapsulated viroplasm and nucleoids, and mature oval particles with a riblike outer structure. Elongated virions with central narrowing and bending of the elementary bodies may be present. Structures reminiscent of the virus have been seen in the nucleus and cytoplasm of epidermal cells. A spiral form in the virus is typical for a member of the parapoxviruses. Complement-fixing antigen has been advanced as the most sensitive diagnostic technique for diagnosing contagious ecthyma. T-cell function, phytohemagglutinin reaction, and K-cell activity have been normal.

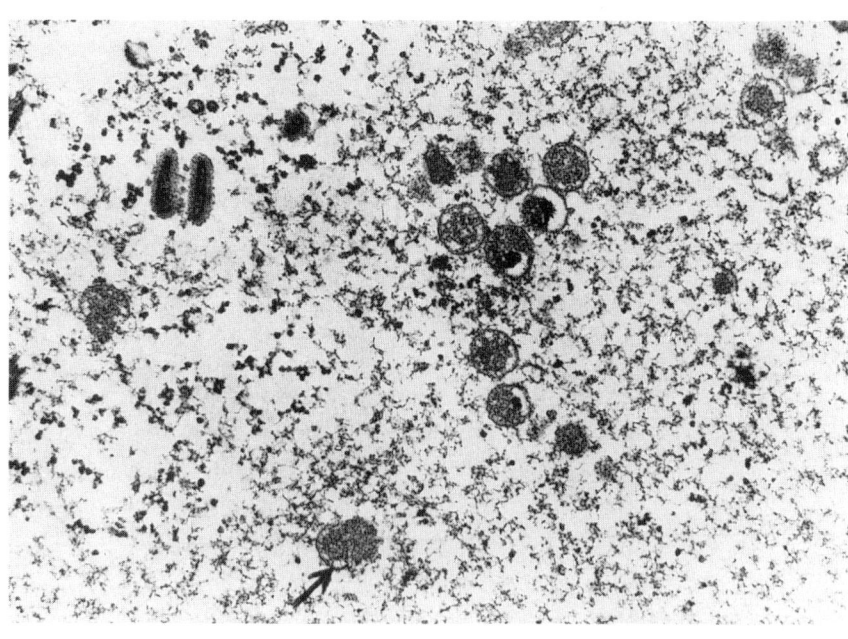

FIGURE 210-6 An electronmicrograph shows viroplasm, partially encapsulated viroplasm, and mature viral particles. ×36,750. (*Reprinted by permission of Albert J. Dalton, M.D., National Institute of Health, Bethesda, Maryland.*)

Treatment

Treatment is not specific. Compresses, culture and sensitivity testing, and appropriate antibiotics are of value for secondary bacterial infection. After excision and cautery, lesions heal uneventfully within 2 to 3 weeks. Corticosteroids and immunosuppressive drugs should be avoided, inasmuch as acanthosis and pseudoepitheliomatous hyperplasia may appear earlier and be more extensive as a result of their administration. No underlying disease has been found as a predisposition, nor has any residual pathologic change been reported. The prognosis is excellent.

BIBLIOGRAPHY

Brandenberg TO: Lip and leg ulceration in sheep with report of two cases in man. *JAMA* **8**:818, 1932

Carr RW: A case of orf contracted by a human from a wild Alaskan mountain goat. *Alaska Med* **10**:75, 1968

Cutler TP: Orf: A report of a case. *Clin Exp Dermatol* **6**:205, 1981

Dupre A et al: Orf and atopic dermatitis. *Br J Dermatol* **105**:103, 1981

Erickson GA et al: Generalized contagious ecthyma in a sheep rancher: Diagnostic considerations. *J Am Vet Med Assoc* **166**:262, 1974

Esposito JL et al: Intragenomic sequence transposition in monkeypox virus, *Virology* **109**:231, 1981

Fraser KM et al: Sequence analysis of the inverted terminal repetitions in the genome of the parapoxvirus, orf virus. *Virology* **176**:379, 1990

Garon C et al: Visualization of an inverted terminal repetition in vaccinia virus DNA. *Proc Natl Acad Sci USA* **75**:4863, 1978

Gold P et al: Localization of nucleotide phosphorylase within vaccinia virus. *Proc Natl Acad Sci USA* **60**:845, 1968

Gourreau J et al: Orf recontamination 8 months after the original infection. Review of the literature apropos of the case. (French) *Ann Dermatol Venereol* **113**:1065, 1986

Guss SB: Contagious ecthyma (sore mouth, orf). *Mod Vet Pract* **61**:335, 1980

Hessami M et al: Isolation of parapoxviruses from man and animals: Cultivation and cellular changes in bovine fetal spleen cells. *Comp Immunol Microbiol Infect Dis* **2**:1, 1974

Holowczak JA et al: Poxvirus DNA. Curr Topics Microbiol Immunol **17**:27, 1982

Leavell UW Jr: Ecthyma contagiosum. *J Ky Med Assoc* **58**:42, 1960

Leavell UW Jr et al: Ecthyma contagiosum (orf). *South Med J* **58**:238, 1965

Leavell UW Jr et al: Orf: Report of 19 human cases with clinical and pathological observations. *JAMA* **204**:657, 1968

Mayr A et al: *Virologische Arbeitsmethoden*, vol 1, *Zellkulturen-Bebrutete Huhnereier-Versuchstire.* Jena, VEB J Fischer-Verlag, 1974

Nagington J et al: The structure of the orf virus. *Virology* **23**:461, 1964

Newsome IE et al: Soremouth transmissible to man. *J Am Vet Med Assoc* **84**:799, 1934

Peterkin GAG: The occurrence on humans of contagious pustular dermatitis of sheep ("orf"). *Br J Dermatol* **49**:492, 1937

Pospischil A et al: Nuclear changes in cells infected with Parapoxvirus Stomatitis Papulosa and orf: An in vivo and in vitro ultrastructure study. *J Gen Virol* **47**:114, 1980

Rafii F et al: Comparison of contagious ecthyma virus genomes by restriction endonucleases. *Arch Virol* **84**:283, 1985

Robinson G et al: The genome of orf virus: Restriction endonuclease analysis of viral DNA isolation from lesions of orf in sheep. *Arch Virol* **71**:43, 1982

Taieb A et al: Orf and pregnancy. *Int J Dermatol* **27**:31, 1988

Wilkinson JD: Orf: A family with unusual complications. *Br J Dermatol* **97**:447, 1977

Yeh HP, Soltani K: Ultrastructural studies in human orf. *Arch Dermatol* **109**:390, 1974

CHAPTER 211

Douglas R. Lowy

Milker's Nodules and Molluscum Contagiosum

Milker's Nodules

Milker's nodule is a benign viral skin disease that generally consists of one or a few nodules on the hand or forearm. The virus is usually transmitted to cattle handlers from infected cows.

Etiology

The disease is caused by paravaccinia virus, a poxvirus that is endemic in cattle.[1] Lesions in cows, which may be chronic and recur-

rent, appear mainly on the teats, although other areas may be affected. In cows the condition is called *pseudocowpox*. There is no cross-immunity with the cowpox, vaccinia, or variola group of poxviruses. Bovine papular stomatitis is a closely related poxvirus infection of cattle characterized by lesions around the mouth[2]; because it induces lesions in humans that are identical to milker's nodules, some investigators believe that the two viruses may be identical.[3]

Paravaccinia virus can be propagated in bovine and human cells in tissue culture.[4,5] It resembles the virus of orf (ecthyma contagiosum) morphologically and serologically,[6-8] but the two viruses can be distinguished by viral DNA hybridization.[9] As is true of other poxviruses, paravaccinia is a large (150 by 300 nm) brick-shaped DNA virus that contains many enzymes and replicates in foci in the cytoplasm of infected cells.[10] Infection often induces a mild degree of hyperplasia. The disease has been transmitted experimentally from human to human and from human to cow.[11]

Epidemiology

Milker's nodule has a worldwide distribution, occurring where cattle are found. Most cases are sporadic, but small epidemics have been reported. Because the disease is usually transmitted to humans by direct contact with infected cattle, milkers are most at risk. Cases also occur among stockyard and slaughterhouse workers. Most cases arise in individuals who have recently become milkers, and infection in humans usually induces lasting immunity. Indirect transmission from virus-contaminated material to patients with burned skin has been reported.[12] The incidence of subclinical infection is not known. Although infectious virus is found in human lesions, person-to-person transmission under natural conditions has not been documented.

Clinical Manifestations

The typical case consists of a single asymptomatic or slightly painful 1-cm nodule on a finger.[13,14] There are usually no more than four lesions, and they are generally confined to the hand and forearm (Fig. 211-1). Rarely, other areas of the skin may be involved, or numerous lesions may be present. Lymphadenopathy is uncommon.

The incubation period is usually 4 to 7 days, but may be as long as 2 weeks. In the absence of secondary bacterial infection, each lesion usually heals spontaneously in 4 to 6 weeks without scar formation. Leavell and Phillips[14] have described six clinical stages, each lasting about a week. Initially, the lesion begins as an erythematous macule, which soon becomes papular. The target stage is next: the lesion, which is papulovesicular, has a red center, surrounded by a white ring and a red halo. This stage is followed by a period of weeping and erosion. The lesion then becomes a firm, crusted nodule. Next, small papillomatous elevations develop on the nodule. Finally, during the regressive stage, the lesion darkens and sloughs.

Pathology

Pathologic changes are present in both epidermis and dermis; the precise histologic appearance depends on the clinical stage.[14] Epidermal changes include hyperkeratosis, parakeratosis, acanthosis, and striking elongation of the rete ridges. These alterations increase progressively as the lesion develops. In early lesions the upper portion of the malpighian layer may contain balloon cells and cells with many intracytoplasmic and some intranuclear inclusions. Later, reticular degeneration, multilocular vesicles, spongiosis, and intracellular edema may be the prominent findings. The dermis contains a marked increase in the number of capillaries and a nonspecific inflammatory infiltrate that is most intense during the acute weeping stage. Electron micrographic examination of the superfi-

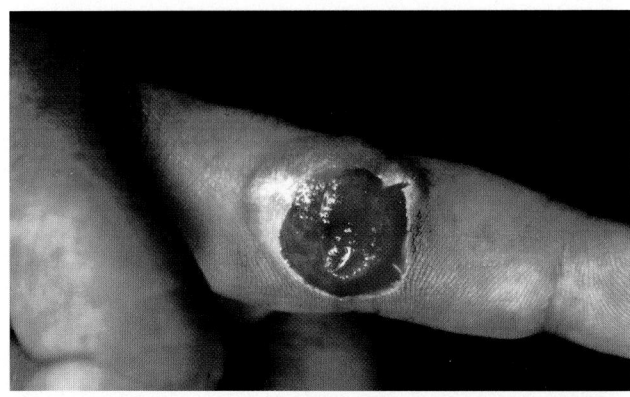

a

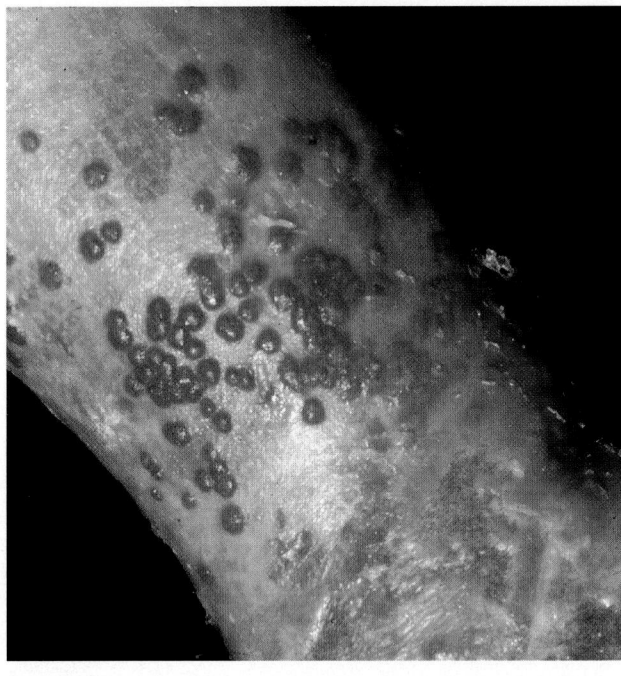

b

FIGURE 211-1   Milker's nodule. *(a)* Firm, purple, eroded nodule occurred following milking a cow. *(b)* Multiple, purple papules and nodules occurred in a second degree scalding burn sustained in a milking barn.

cial portion of a lesion usually reveals the characteristic cytoplasmic viral particles.

Diagnosis and Differential Diagnosis

The diagnosis is generally based on the history, clinical appearance, and biopsy. It can be established more definitively by the electron microscopic demonstration of viral particles or by propagation of the virus in tissue culture. Orf and bovine papular stomatitis must be excluded by history.

Milker's nodule must be differentiated from many other conditions, including true cowpox, herpetic whitlow, pyoderma, anthrax, tularemia, primary inoculation tuberculosis, atypical mycobacterial infection, syphilitic chancre, sporotrichosis, and pyogenic granuloma.

Course, Prognosis, Treatment, and Prevention

Because the disease is self-limited, only symptomatic therapy is generally indicated. Prevention is limited to the isolation of infected animals.

Molluscum Contagiosum

Molluscum contagiosum is a common, benign, viral disease of the skin and mucous membranes that generally affects children. In adults, the condition may be transmitted sexually. The fully developed lesion is an umbilicated papule, and most patients have multiple lesions.

Etiology

Molluscum contagiosum virus (MCV) is a poxvirus that is distinct morphologically, serologically, and pathologically from other poxviruses.[15,16] It is a large (200 by 300 nm) DNA virus that replicates in the cytoplasm of infected cells and induces hyperplasia, as do other poxviruses. Unlike most other poxviruses, MCV has not been reproducibly propagated in tissue culture. A report of the successful tissue culture growth of MCV[17] has not been confirmed.[18] Using viral particles extracted from lesions, minor differences are found in viral proteins[19] and in restriction endonuclease cleavage patterns of viral DNA.[20] Two different MCV strains (I and II) have been identified, based on restriction endonuclease digestion patterns.[21,22] MCVI is more prevalent than MCVII.[23,24] No clinical differences have been noted between the two strains.

Experimental transmission to humans has been achieved, with a reported incubation period of 2 to 7 weeks.[15] Attempts to induce the disease experimentally in other species have been unsuccessful. MCV infection was thought to be confined to humans, but lesions that are clinically and histologically identical to those in human disease have been reported in the chimpanzee and kangaroo in captivity.[25,26]

Epidemiology

The disease occurs throughout the world, but its frequency varies considerably.[15] On some Pacific islands, 5 percent of children under 10 years may be affected. The prevalence rate in the United States is much lower. Although the disease may develop at any age, the vast majority of cases are found in children, with boys being affected more often than girls. Multiple familial cases are uncommon.

The disease is believed to be transmitted primarily by person-to-person spread and possibly by fomites. Outbreaks have been reported among children attending swimming pools, and genital lesions in adults are probably transmitted sexually.[27,28] As with other sexually transmitted viral diseases, the incidence of genital molluscum increased between the 1960s and 1980s.[29,30] The incidence of subclinical infection is unknown. The role of humoral immunity is unclear, although experimental studies suggest that many adults are resistant to infection.[31] Individuals with impaired cellular immune function may have widespread lesions.[32,33] Patients with AIDS are at particular risk of MCV infection, with prevalence rates of 9 to 18 percent having been reported[34,35]; the lesions may be extensive and refractory to treatment.

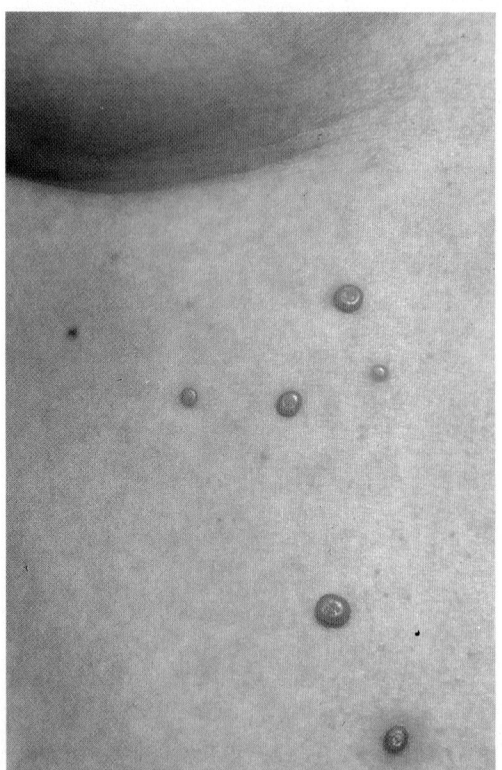

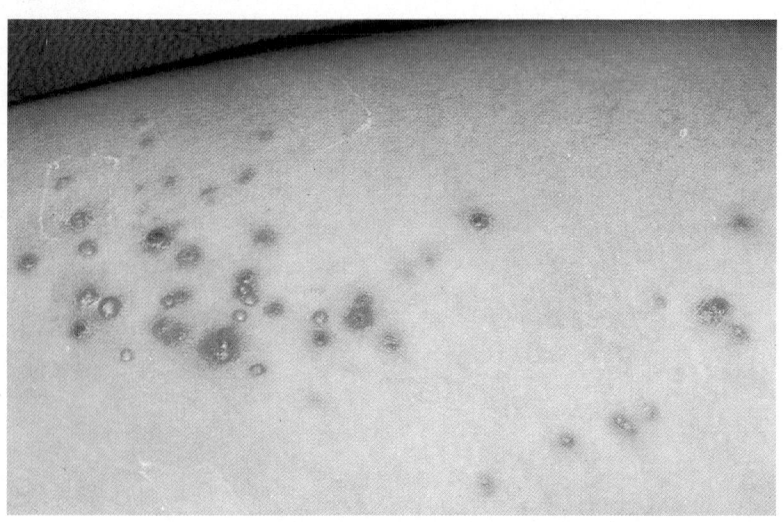

FIGURE 211-2 Molluscum contagiosum. *(a)* Discrete, solid, skin-colored papules, 1.0 to 2.0 mm in diameter with central umbilication. *(b)* Multiple, scattered, and discrete lesions, some of which are inflamed.

Clinical Manifestations

The lesions, which begin as minute papules, are usually 3 to 6 mm, although rarely they may be as large as 3 cm in diameter. The individual lesions are discrete, smooth, pearly to flesh-colored, dome-shaped papules, often with central umbilication; the white curdlike core may be easily expressed.[36]

Lesions may be located on any area of the skin and mucous membranes. They are usually grouped (Fig. 211-2) in one or two areas but may be widely disseminated. Most patients have fewer than 20 lesions, although some may have several hundred. In temperate climates, the head, eyelids, trunk, and genitalia are affected most often (Fig. 211-3). In the tropics, lesions occur most commonly on the extremities.

Although lesions are usually asymptomatic, pruritus may be present, and an eczematous reaction may develop around some lesions. Conjunctivitis and keratitis may complicate lesions around the eyelid. Patients with atopic dermatitis or other conditions with impaired immune function may develop widespread lesions, and secondary bacterial infection also occurs.

Pathogenesis and Pathology

The rate of cell division in the basal layer of lesional skin is twice that of normal skin.[37] This correlates with an apparent increase in the number of receptors for epidermal growth factor (EGF) in infected cells[38] and indirect evidence that MCV synthesizes an EGF-like growth factor, as do other poxviruses.[22] Viral growth is confined to the epidermis; virus particles are synthesized in cytoplasmic foci of cells in the malpighian and granular layers.[31,37] The infected cells, which are interspersed with uninfected cells, move more quickly than uninfected cells through the epidermis. Viral

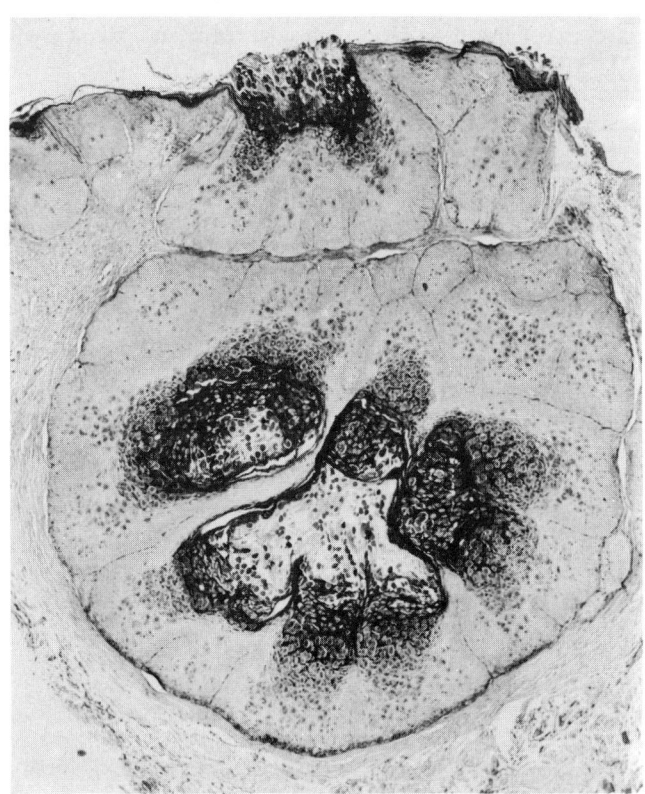

FIGURE 211-4   Molluscum contagiosum. Extensive downgrowth of infected cells bearing the large, eosinophilic cytoplasmic inclusion bodies. ×40. *(Micrograph by Wallace H. Clark, Jr., M.D.)*

antigen is present in infected cells, and 90 percent of patients possess circulating antibody to this antigen. Immunocompetent cells are absent from the infected epidermis, even when they are present in the underlying dermis.[38]

The histologic appearance of the hypertrophied and hyperplastic epidermis is characteristic (Fig. 211-4).[36,39] Above the normal-appearing basal layer are lobules of enlarged epidermal cells that contain multiple Feulgen-positive intracytoplasmic inclusion bodies (*molluscum bodies* or *Henderson-Paterson bodies*). These inclusion bodies, which contain the viral particles, increase in size as the infected cell moves toward the surface. In the horny layer, the molluscum bodies are enmeshed in a fibrous network that dissolves in the center of the lesions, forming the central core, which is composed primarily of molluscum bodies.

Diagnosis and Differential Diagnosis

The diagnosis is usually made by the distinctive clinical appearance of the lesions, by stained smears of the expressed core, and by biopsy. Molluscum contagiosum must be differentiated from warts, varicella, pyoderma, papillomas, epitheliomas, and lichen planus. Cutaneous cryptococcal infection in patients with AIDS may mimic the appearance of MCV infection.[40]

Treatment

Because the condition is usually self-limited and lesions heal without scarring in the absence of secondary bacterial infection, treat-

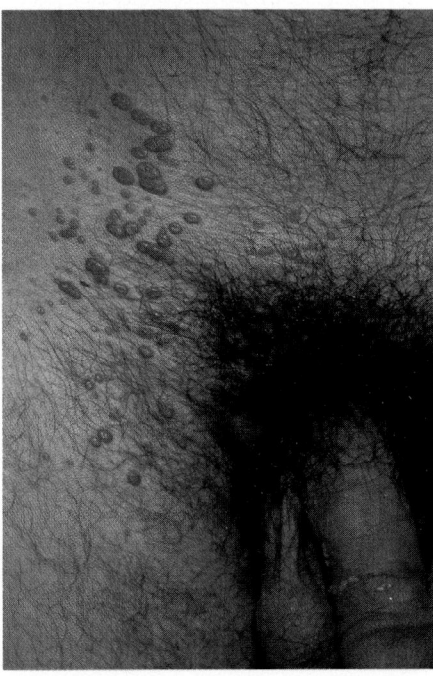

FIGURE 211-3   Molluscum contagiosum. Multiple umbilicated papules are seen on the abdomen, thigh, and penis of this 33-year-old HIV infected male.

ment is not always mandatory. Removal of lesions with a sharp curette or liquid nitrogen is simple, relatively painless, and usually effective. More than one treatment session is often necessary, because of recurrence or the development of new lesions. Treatment may be especially difficult in patients with impaired immune function.

Course and Prognosis

Individual lesions may last 2 to 4 months, but the development of new lesions by autoinoculation is common. Most cases resolve spontaneously in 6 to 9 months, but some persist for years.

References

Milker's nodules

1. Moscovici C et al: Isolation of a viral agent from pseudocowpox disease. *Science* **141**:915, 1963
2. Bowman KF et al: Cutaneous form of bovine papular stomatitis in man. *JAMA* **246**:2813, 1981
3. Rossi CR et al: A paravaccinia virus isolated from cattle. *Cornell Vet* **67**:72, 1977
4. Friedman-Kien AE et al: Milker's nodules: Isolation of a poxvirus from a human case. *Science* **140**:1335, 1963
5. Thomas V: Biochemical and electron microscopic studies of the replication and composition of milker's node virus. *J Virol* **34**:244, 1980
6. Nagington J et al: Milker's nodule virus infections and their similarity to orf. *Nature* **208**:505, 1965
7. Leavell UW et al: Orf: Report of 19 human cases with clinical and pathological observations. *JAMA* **204**:657, 1968
8. Lard SL et al: Differentiation of parapoxviruses by application of orf virus-specfic monoclonal antibodies against cell surface proteins. *Vet Immunol Immunopathol* **28**:247, 1991
9. Gassmann U et al: Analysis of parapoxvirus genomes. *Arch Virol* **83**:17, 1985
10. Caplen HS, Holowczak JA: Some enzymatic activities associated with purified parapoxvirions. *J Virol* **46**:384, 1983
11. Sonck CE, Penttinen K: Milker's nodules: Transmission from man to man. *Acta Derm Venereol (Stockh)* **34**:420, 1954
12. Schuler G et al: The syndrome of milker's nodules in burn injury: Evidence for indirect transmission. *J Am Acad Dermatol* **6**:334, 1982
13. Wheeler CE, Cawley EP: The etiology of milker's nodules. *Arch Dermatol* **75**:249, 1967
14. Leavell UW Jr, Phillips IA: Milker's nodules: Pathogenesis, tissue culture, electron microscopy, and calf inoculation. *Arch Dermatol* **111**:1307, 1975

Molluscum Contagiosum

15. Postlethwaite R: Molluscum contagiosum: A review. *Arch Environ Health* **21**:432, 1970
16. Brown ST et al: Molluscum contagiosum. *Sex Trans Dis* **8**:227, 1981

17. Francis RD, Bradford HB Jr: Some biological and physical properties of molluscum contagiosum virus propagated in tissue culture. *J Virol* **19**:382, 1976
18. McFadden G et al: Biogenesis of poxviruses: Transitory expression of molluscum contagiosum early functions. *Virology* **94**:297, 1979
19. Oda H et al: Structural polypeptides of molluscum contagiosum virus: Their variability in various isolates and location within the virion. *J Med Virol* **9**:19, 1982
20. Parr RP et al: Structural characterization of the molluscum contagiosum virus genome. *Virology* **81**:247, 1977
21. Darai G et al: Analysis of the genome of molluscum contagiosum virus by restriction endonuclease analysis and molecular cloning. *J Med Virol* **18**:29, 1986
22. Porter CD, Archard LC: Characterization and physical mapping of molluscum contagiosum virus DNA and location of a sequence capable of encoding a conserved domain of epidermal growth factor. *J Gen Virol* **68**:673, 1987
23. Porter CD et al: Molluscum contagiosum virus types in genital and non-genital lesions. *Br J Dermatol* **120**:37, 1989
24. Scholz J et al: Epidemiology of molluscum contagiosum using genetic analysis of the viral DNA. *J Med Virol* **27**:87, 1989
25. Dagnall BG, Witson GR: Molluscum contagiosum in a red kangaroo. *Austr J Dermatol* **15**:115, 1974
26. Douglas JD et al: Molluscum contagiosum in the chimpanzee. *J Am Vet Med Assoc* **151**:901, 1967
27. Brown ST et al: Molluscum contagiosum: Sexually transmitted disease in 17 cases. *J Am Vener Dis Assoc* **1**:35, 1974
28. Wilkin JK: Molluscum contagiosum venereum in a women's outpatient clinic: A venereally transmitted disease. *Am J Obstet Gynecol* **128**:531, 1977
29. Becker TM et al: Trends in molluscum contagiosum in the United States, 1966–1983. *Sex Transm Dis* **13**:88, 1986
30. Oriel JD: The increase in molluscum contagiosum. *Br Med J* **294**:74, 1987
31. Shirodaria PV, Matthews RS: Observations on the antibody responses in molluscum contagiosum. *Br J Dermatol* **96**:29, 1977
32. Solomon LM, Telner P: Eruptive molluscum contagiosum in atopic dermatitis. *Can Med Assoc J* **95**:978, 1966
33. Peachy RDG: Severe molluscum contagiosum infection with T-cell deficiency. *Br J Dermatol* **97**(suppl):49, 1977
34. Goodman DS et al: Prevalence of cutaneous disease in patients with acquired immunodeficiency syndrome (AIDS) or AIDS-related complex. *J Am Acad Dermatol* **17**:210, 1987
35. Matis WL et al: Dermatologic findings associated with human immunodeficiency virus infection. *J Am Acad Dermatol* **17**:746, 1987
36. Uehara M, Danno K: Central pitting of molluscum contagiosum. *J Cutan Pathol* **7**:149, 1980
37. Epstein WL, Fukuyama K: Maturation of molluscum contagiosum virus (MCV) in vivo: Quantitative electron microscopic autoradiography. *J Invest Dermatol* **60**:73, 1973
38. Viac J, Chardonnet Y: Immunocompetent cells and epithelial cell modifications in molluscum contagiosum. *J Cutan Pathol* **17**:202, 1990
39. Kwittken J: Molluscum contagiosum: Some new histologic observations. *Mt Sinai J Med* **47**:583, 1980
40. Rico MJ, Penneys NS: Cutaneous cryptococcosis resembling molluscum contagiosum in a patient with AIDS. *Arch Dermatol* **121**:901, 1985

Douglas R. Lowy and Elliot J. Androphy

Warts

Warts, or verrucae, are benign epithelial proliferations of the skin and mucosa caused by infection with *papillomaviruses*.[1] These viruses do not produce acute signs or symptoms but induce slow-growing lesions that can remain subclinical for long periods of time. A subset of the human papillomaviruses has been associated with the development of epithelial malignancies.

Historical Aspects

Cutaneous warts were known to the ancient Greeks and Romans, and, until the nineteenth century, genital warts were believed to be a form of syphilis or gonorrhea. The viral etiology of warts was inferred from the observation that inoculation of wart filtrates from which cellular and bacterial products were removed could induce papillomas at the site of injection. All warts were considered to be derived from a single virus, because isolates from cutaneous, genital, or laryngeal warts could induce papillomas at other sites. However, recent advances in recombinant DNA technology have identified at least 65 different human papillomavirus (HPV) genotypes, many of which are associated with distinct regional predilection, histopathology, and biology.[2]

Etiologic Agent

The papillomaviruses (PVs) form a family of double-stranded DNA viruses that are distantly related to the other members of the Papovavirus class (which includes simian virus 40, polyomavirus, BK virus, and JC virus).[3] Detergent-disrupted PV particles expose common structural antigens shared by all PVs but not by other viruses.[4] Antibodies to such shared antigens can be used to detect structural (or capsid, see below) PV antigens in clinical materials, including formalin-fixed tissue (Fig. 212-1).

Recombinant DNA technology has enabled the viral genomes (the complete viral DNA) to be molecularly cloned from clinical lesions, and the complete nucleotide sequence has been determined for the genomes of several human and animal PVs.[2,3] Comparison of these PV DNAs reveals that they share a similar genetic organization (Fig. 212-2) and are predicted to encode related protein products.[5]

The PV genome is present within the viral particle as a covalently closed, supercoiled circle of double-stranded DNA. The genome is composed of about 8000 nucleotide base pairs, which is about one-twentieth the size of a herpesvirus genome, and encodes approximately 9 proteins, which are historically divided into two groups. The genes required for replication of the viral DNA are labeled "E" (for "early," being expressed before the "L" or "late" genes, see below). These "E" genes do not encode a DNA polymerase or thymidine kinase, and therefore PVs are not suscep-

tible to inhibition by acyclovir. PVs contain two "L" genes, which encode the structural proteins that form the capsid (outer protein shell) of the viral particle (virion).

The spherically shaped virion measures 55 nm in diameter and surrounds the viral DNA. Unlike many other viruses (e.g., herpesviruses, human immunodeficiency virus, and measles virus), the PV capsid is not surrounded by a lipoprotein envelope. This lack of a lipid envelope is associated with greater stability of the virus, as manifested by its resistance to freezing or desiccation. Exposure of virions to formalin, detergents, or high temperature can reduce viral infectivity, but PV virions can remain infectious for years when warts are stored in glycerol at room temperature.

All PVs are highly host specific, which means that PVs from one species do not induce papillomas in heterologous species. HPVs do not infect laboratory animals, rodent models for laboratory investigation are not available, and it is not yet possible to propagate the PVs in tissue culture. These obstacles stand in the way of determining the mechanism and biologic consequences of PV infection. However, recent applications of recombinant DNA technology have partially circumvented these problems and have provided new insights into the molecular mechanisms of PV pathogenesis (see below).

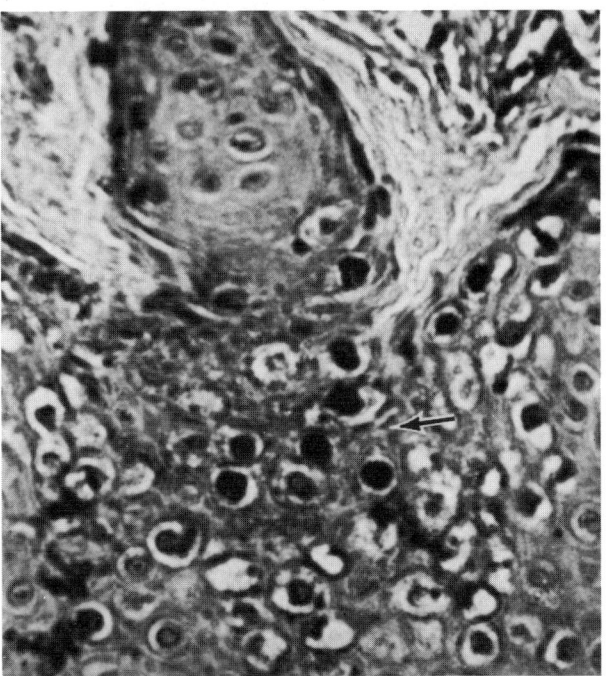

FIGURE 212-1 Immunoperoxidase assay of a verruca in which the darkly stained nuclei (arrow) represent cells that contain PV virion structural antigens. The positive nuclei are found in some, but are not limited to, koilocytotic cells.

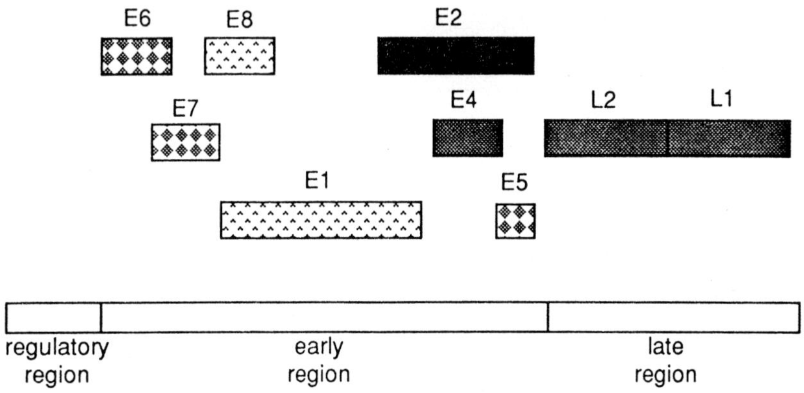

FIGURE 212-2 Genetic organization of papillomaviruses. All papillomavirus genomes are composed of approximately 8000 nucleotide base pairs, represented as a linear sequence but actually a closed circle of double-stranded DNA. The boxes depict the viral genes, each of which encodes a protein. The regulatory region is a DNA segment that does not encode proteins but has been shown to be involved in expression of the viral genes and replication of the viral DNA. In general, E6, E7, and E5 represent transforming genes; E1 and E2 coordinate replication and expression of the viral genome; and the L1 and L2 proteins form the viral capsid. E4 encodes a protein that may be involved in the release of the virus from the cell's keratin framework. For details, see text.

Human Papillomavirus Types

It is now recognized that there are many different HPV types.[1-3] In principle, HPVs can be classified by the ability of antisera to distinguish their capsid antigens, and antisera made by immunization with intact PV virions can generate type-specific antibodies.[4] Because serologic typing would require the generation of specific antisera to each HPV type, the lack of in vitro methods to culture HPVs makes it cumbersome to use this approach. HPV typing by serologic methods is therefore used only rarely. Furthermore, antibodies to structural viral proteins cannot be used to confirm the presence of HPV in cells that do not synthesize large numbers of virions and are therefore negative in many genital warts, bowenoid papulosis, dysplasias, and HPV-associated malignancies.

The various HPV types are currently discriminated according to the relatedness of their DNA, using molecularly cloned HPV DNAs of known type as standards. Typing of HPV is therefore according to genotype, rather than serotype. The relatedness of different HPV DNAs is usually determined by molecular hybridization techniques. In this approach, an HPV type is determined by measuring the efficiency with which an HPV DNA whose type is known specifically binds (hybridizes) to an unknown HPV DNA. Because the complementarity of double-stranded DNA permits specific high-affinity binding, DNA of HPVs of the same type will bind to each other with high efficiency, whereas HPV form a different type will bind poorly or not at all. These hybridization techniques are much more sensitive than serologic methods and do not require HPV protein synthesis in the infected cell for detection.

Two HPVs are said to be different types when their DNAs hybridize less than 50 percent as efficiently to each other as to themselves. Therefore a new HPV type is defined when it hybridizes by less than 50 percent to all other HPV types. However, 50 percent hybridization in this context implies close to 90 percent identity at the DNA sequence level.

Using the above definition, 65 different HPV genotypes have been identified over the past two decades (see Table 212-1).[2] Most

TABLE 212-1
Clinical Associations of HPV Types

HPV type	Most common clinical lesion	Uncommon or rare involvement	Potential oncogenicity
1	Deep plantar/palmar warts	Common warts	—
2, 4	Common warts	Plantar, palmar, mosaic, oral, and anogenital warts	—
3, 10	Flat warts	Flat warts in EV	HPV 10 rare in cervical and vulvar carcinomas
5, 8, 9, 12, 14, 15, 17, 19–24	Macular warts in EV	Immunosuppression	HPVs 5, 8, 9 isolated from SCCs
6, 11	Anogenital warts, cervical condylomata	Bowenoid papulosis, common warts	Verrucous carcinoma; rare in penile, vulvar cervical, and other urogenital tumors
7	Butcher's warts	—	—
13	Oral focal epithelial hyperplasia	—	—
16, 18, 31, 33, 35	Bowenoid papulosis, cervical condylomata	Anogenital warts	Genital and cervical dysplasias and carcinomas, rare in cutaneous SCC

NOTE: HPV, human papillomavirus; EV, epidermodysplasia verruciformis; SCC, squamous cell carcinoma. For additional HPV types and references, see reference 2.

HPV types can be placed into one of three categories: those viruses usually isolated from genital-mucosal lesions (genital-mucosal types, such as HPVs 6, 11, 16, and 18); those viruses usually isolated from nongenital lesions in the general population (nongenital types, such as HPVs 1, 2, 3, and 4); and those usually isolated from epidermodysplasia verruciformis (EV), a disease of unique susceptibility resulting in chronic HPV infection (EV-specific types, such as HPVs 5 and 8, see Chap. 213). Some HPV types are closely related to each other by molecular hybridization and tend to induce similar lesions. Examples include types 3 and 10, which induce flat warts, types 6 and 11, which induce genital-mucosal warts (condyloma acuminata), and types 5 and 8, which induce scaling lesions in EV.

Another important distinction is that a subset of HPV genotypes appear to have malignant potential. For example, almost all cutaneous squamous cell carcinomas that arise in patients with EV contain HPVs 5 or 8, whereas benign lesions, even in the same patient, may harbor many other HPV types. Similarly, the majority of cervical carcinomas contain HPVs 16 or 18, whereas HPVs 6 and 11, which are often found in benign cervical disease, are only rarely identified in cervical malignancies.

Diagnostic kits to identify certain genital-mucosal HPV types are now commercially available. The polymerase chain reaction (PCR), and related advances in molecular diagnostics, may further facilitate the routine molecular detection of HPV.[6] PCR, which can specifically amplify even a few DNA molecules to readily detectable levels, represents an extremely sensitive and specific method to identify the presence and type of HPV DNA in any lesion. PCR has been successfully applied to detect and type HPV DNA in paraffin-embedded tissue blocks that are decades old.[7]

Epidemiology

HPV infection occurs commonly in humans. Transmission of HPV probably depends on several factors, including the location of lesions, quantity of infectious virus present, degree and nature of the contact, and general and HPV-specific immunologic states of the exposed individuals. The source or reservoir for HPV is believed to be individuals with clinical or subclinical infection as well as infectious virus that may be present in the environment. Since HPVs do not replicate in other species, an animal reservoir is unlikely. Patients with impaired cell-mediated immunity (CMI) are particularly susceptible to HPV infection. Warts develop in the majority of renal transplant patients on immunosuppressive therapy.[8]

Nongenital warts occur most commonly in children and young adults, in whom the incidence may approach 10 percent.[9] Since the 1960s, there has been a sixfold increase in the number of office visits for anogenital warts, which now represent more than three times the number of visits for genital herpes.[10] The age-specific incidence of nongenital warts differs form that of anogenital warts. Anogenital warts, which are uncommon in children, are sexually transmitted. In one study, genital warts were clinically detectable in two-thirds of the sexual contacts of individuals with genital warts but were not more frequent in sexual contact of individuals with cutaneous warts.[11] Although several different HPV types may be isolated form anogenital and cervical lesions, high concordance for the same HPV type has been found among sexual partners.[12]

Although genital warts in children may be sexually transmitted, often as a consequence of sexual abuse, such warts in infants and children may also result from virus inoculation at birth or from incidental spread form cutaneous warts. In contrast to anogenital lesions in adults, a significant proportion of genital warts in children contain HPV types that are usually isolated from nongenital warts.[13,14] Respiratory (laryngeal) papillomas contain the same HPV types as are found in anogenital papillomas. About one-half of respiratory papillomas occur in infants and young children. In this age group, the condition is believed to have been transmitted from mothers with genital HPV infection when the infant aspirates infectious virus during birth.[15] The incidence of respiratory papillomas is much lower than that of genital HPV infection, and the factors that predispose to the development of clinical respiratory lesions have not been elucidated.

Pathogenesis

The roles of immunity and genetic susceptibility to PV infection are poorly understood.[16] Individuals with defective CMI are particularly susceptible to PV infection and are notoriously resistant to treatment.[17] Several phenomena suggest that the immune system plays a significant role in wart regression, namely, observations that flat warts may regress spontaneously in association with a mononuclear cell infiltrate[18] and that treatment of one or a few warts may lead to resolution of many or all warts in nonimmunosuppressed patients, although this outcome is the exception rather than the rule. Host factors may also be important in limiting PV infection, because even those with multiple verrucae rarely have widespread dissemination over the body surface. Humoral immunity could be important in protecting the individual from reinfection, and low titer antibodies have been detected to several viral proteins. In uncontrolled studies, vaccination with wart extracts has been reported effective in prevention of condyloma acuminatum recurrence.[19]

HPV infection is thought to be acquired through inoculation of virus into the viable epidermis through defects in the epithelium. Maceration of the skin is probably an important predisposing factor, as suggested by the increased incidence of plantar warts in swimmers who frequent public pools.[20] Once an individual has been infected, new warts may develop over a small area or in distant sites. Each new lesion probably results either from the initial exposure or from skin-associated virus, rather than from blood-borne infection. Autoinoculation of virus into apposed lesions is commonly seen on adjacent digits and in the anogenital region.

Following entry through the superficial epithelium, it is believed that a single viral genome becomes resident within the epithelial basal cells, where the viral DNA is maintained at one to two copies of extrachromosomal, circular double-stranded DNA per cell. It is clear that in cows with bovine papillomavirus infection, the viral genetic information is present in basal cells.[21] As the basal cells replicate, the viral genome is also duplicated and transported within the cells as they migrate upward through the differentiating epithelium. The epidermis is acanthotic due to hyperplasia of the proliferative basal cell population and retention of the upper stratifying keratinocytes.

After experimental PV inoculation, a clinically detectable verruca usually requires from 2 to 9 months to develop. This implies a relatively long period of subclinical infection, which could represent an unrecognized source of infectious virus. HPV DNA has been detected in normal-appearing mucosa of the larynx of patients with respiratory papillomatosis who were in clinical remission[22] and in normal-appearing skin adjacent to treatment sites of recurrent genital warts.[23] It is not known whether this is a subclinical state of infection or true "latency" (i.e., non-replicating and transcriptionally inactive virus).

The relative abundance of virus particles in a verruca varies with the clinical setting and the HPV type. Newer lesions tend to contain more virions than do older verrucae. Plantar warts containing HPV 1 have a high number of virions, anogenital verrucae typically have small quantities of mature virus particles, and common warts usually have intermediate numbers. Not only does the quantity of viral DNA present differ among these lesions, but also the proportion that is enclosed within the infectious virions varies among these verrucae.[24]

Viral RNA expression (transcription) occurs mostly in the upper malpighian layer, just before the granular layer, where viral DNA replication begins and may result in hundreds of copies of viral DNA per cell. The viral capsid proteins (L1 and L2, Fig. 212-2) are synthesized and assembled into virions in the nuclei of the cells at this level (Fig. 212-1). The virions encapsidate the viral DNA within the infected cell as it migrates to the stratum corneum. There is experimental evidence that a viral protein (HPV-16 E1-E4) collapses the cytoplasmic keratin filament network.[25] This is postulated to enable release of the virions so that they can be directly inoculated into another site or desquamated into the environment.

Because virions are not detected in the lower epithelial levels in warts, it is believed that viral transcription, DNA replication, and late protein production are coordinated by the state of differentiation of the infected epithelial cell. The inability to propagate PVs in cultured cells is probably a consequence of the inability to reproduce the milieu required for physiologic differentiation. Further support for the hypothesis that production of virus particles and virion antigens depends on the state of epithelial differentiation is that as benign papillomas progress toward dysplasia, virion production decreases.[26] Capsid proteins are almost never observed in frank malignancies, although PV DNA is present. It has become possible to cultivate some HPVs by exposing epithelial cells to infectious virions, then placing them under the renal capsule of an immunodeficient (nude) mouse for prolonged periods. In this system, the epithelial cells differentiate, stratify, and resemble a verruca histologically, and the full virus replication cycle occurs, producing infectious virions.[27]

Experimental evidence from cell culture systems has shown that PV genes can alter cell proliferation, a characteristic common to many tumor viruses. Several different transformation assays have been developed to examine the biologic effects of PV genes in vitro.[28] For example, cells may lose contact inhibition and continue to divide, exhibit increased DNA synthesis and replication rates, lose growth factor dependence, or become immortal instead of exhibiting a finite lifespan in vitro. Three different viral genes have been shown to confer these properties: E5, E6, and E7 (Fig. 212-2). The relative activity of these genes varies with the PV. The viral E5 genes encode proteins that appear to activate growth factor receptors.[29] In the bovine (cow) papillomavirus, which induces fibropapillomas, E5 appears to activate preferentially the receptors for platelet-derived growth factor (PDGF),[30] which are abundant in dermal fibroblasts but not epithelial cells.

These experimental systems have shown that the genital-mucosal HPVs that are highly associated with cervical carcinomas, such as HPVs 16 and 18, are significantly more active than those not commonly isolated with cervical neoplasms, such as HPVs 6 and 11.[31] In one assay, keratinocytes or cervical cells were grown on a raft that provided an air-media interface. Introduction of HPV-

16 or -18 DNA induced a disorganized pattern of differentiation with suprabasal mitotic figures resembling squamous cell carcinoma in situ, whereas the cells retained a normal pattern of stratification when HPV-6 or -11 DNA was used.[32] In other in vitro models, introduction of HPV-16 or -18 DNA into cultured human epithelial cells resulted in an increased growth rate, resistance to differentiation, and the ability to be continuously passaged; HPV-6 and -11 DNA were much less active.

In cutaneous and cervical epithelial cells, transformation is best achieved with both E6 and E7 from HPVs 16 or 18. These two HPV genes are preferentially retained and expressed in cervical cancers, implying that transformation assays measure a property that is closely related to the oncogenic potential of these viruses in cervical infection. One mechanism by which the E6 and E7 proteins exert their effects is by each binding to a different cellular protein that inhibits normal epithelial cell growth. The two proteins, p53 and the retinoblastoma susceptibility protein (Rb), are apparently inactivated by binding to E6 and E7, respectively, thereby relieving infected cells from the normal growth inhibitory activities of p53 and Rb.[31]

Clinical Manifestations

Warts are commonly classified by their clinical location or morphology and can be separated into cutaneous and extracutaneous PV infections.

Cutaneous Infections (Figs. 212-3 through 212-8)

Common warts (verruca vulgaris) are scaly rough papules or nodules that can be found on any skin surface (Table 212-1). They occur most often as single or grouped papules on the hands. Flat warts (verruca plana) are 2 to 4 mm, slightly elevated flattopped papules that have minimal scale. Verrucae may also be filiform or appear as cutaneous horns. These are most frequent on the face, hands, and lower legs. Plantar and palmar warts are thick, endophytic, and hyperkeratotic lesions that may be painful with pressure. Punctate black dots ("seeds") are seen after shaving away the outer keratinous surface and represent thrombosed capillaries in the papilloma. Mosaic warts result from the coalescence of plantar or palmar warts into large plaques. Some immunologically normal individuals develop exuberant warts of the palms or soles that are refractory to treatment. Butcher's warts are verrucous papules, usually multiple, on the dorsal, palmar, or periungual hands and fingers of meat cutters.[33] Epidermodysplasia verruciformis is discussed in Chap. 213.

Anogenital warts (also known as condylomata acuminata, genital warts, or venereal warts) consist of epidermal and dermal papules or nodules on the perineum, genitalia, crural folds, and anus. They vary in size and can form large, exophytic ("cauliflower like") masses, especially in the moist environment of the perineum. Discrete 1- to 3-mm sessile warts may occur on the penile shaft. Lesions that resemble common warts also occur in this region but are unusual. Warts may extend internally into the vagina, urethra, and rectum.

Bowenoid papulosis (see also Chap. 112) is a clinicopathologic entity in which HPVs have been identified.[34,35] These appear as 2- to 3-mm papules, often multiple, of the external male and

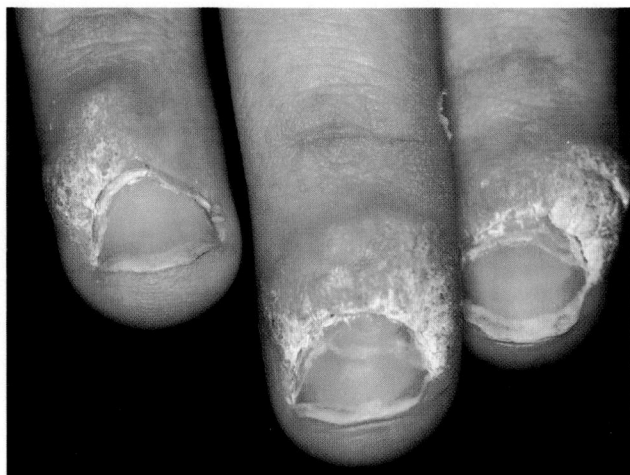

a

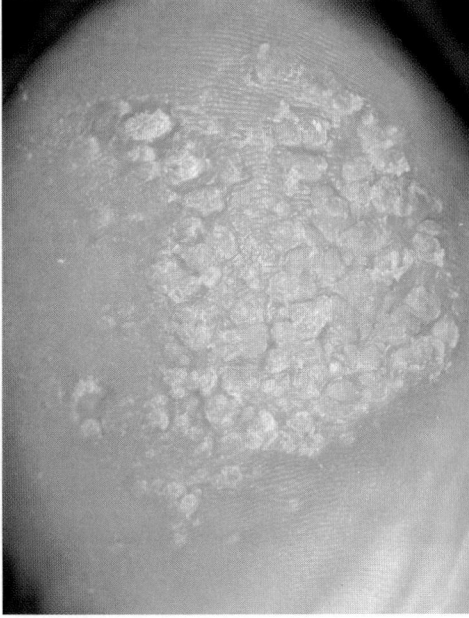

c

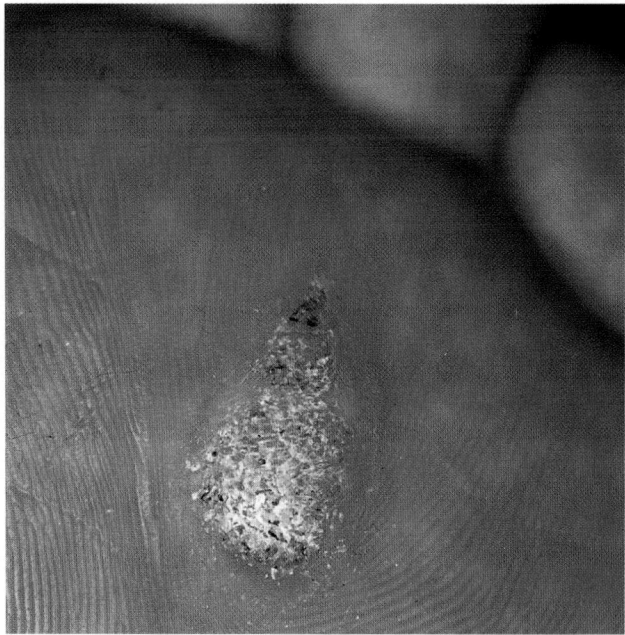

b

FIGURE 212-3 *(a)* Common wart, periungual. Multiple, confluent kerototic papules are seen around the proximal periphery of the fingernails. *(b)* Common wart, verruca plantaris. *(c)* Common wart, mosaic plantar. A large hyperkeratotic plaque is seen on the heel, made up of multiple small coalescing warts.

female genitalia. Histologically there is cellular atypia resembling Bowen's disease or squamous cell carcinoma in situ. These lesions are usually infected with HPV 16, which suggests that bowenoid papulosis may be a precursor of penile and vulvar cancer. However, the rate of transition to frank malignancy is much lower for the external genitalia than for the cervix. These small papules should be treated as they may be a reservoir for transmission of potentially oncogenic HPVs.[36] As in all genital warts, virions are difficult to detect in these lesions.[37,38]

Extracutaneous (Mucosal) Infections

Oral warts are small, slightly elevated, soft, pink or white papules that may be found on buccal, gingival, or labial mucosa or hard palate.[39] Verrucous, horny papillomas may occur on the palate. Mucosal lesions of the oropharynx, termed *focal epithelial hyperplasia,* have also been demonstrated to contain HPVs.[40] In *oral*

florid papillomatosis, which is thought to be caused by a PV, multiple large verrucae appear within the oral cavity. Progression to verrucous carcinoma (see the discussion that follows) may occur. *Oral condylomata acuminata* can result from orogenital sexual contact. Warts may also occur in the urethra, usually when meatal warts are present[41]; they may spread to the urinary bladder.

Respiratory (laryngeal) papillomatosis is characterized by multiple benign, noninvasive warts that usually involve the larynx but may extend to the oropharynx and bronchopulmonary epithelium. Presenting symptoms commonly include hoarseness and stridor. Most cases occur in infants, where the lesions may block the airway, but the condition may develop at any age. These HPV-associated papillomas may spontaneously remit, especially at puberty, but recurrences are common, perhaps because of the persistence of viral DNA despite clinical remission.[22] Because the HPVs isolated from these lesions are the same types as those of cervical warts, respiratory papillomatosis is thought to result from seeding of the larynx during parturition from virus present in maternal condyloma acuminatum or cervical papillomas. Several studies have demonstrated an epidemiologic correlation of condylomata in mothers of infants with this disease.[15] Nonetheless, cervical and external genitalia warts are common in the child-bearing years, whereas respiratory papillomatosis of infants is rare. It is controversial whether Cesarean section should be performed in mothers with condylomata, as this procedure itself has some attendant risk.

Many clinical lesions of the uterine cervix contain HPVs. These lesions are usually termed *cervical warts* or *atypical condylomata.* They are usually flat, and their visualization may require colposcopy and enhancement following acetic acid application,

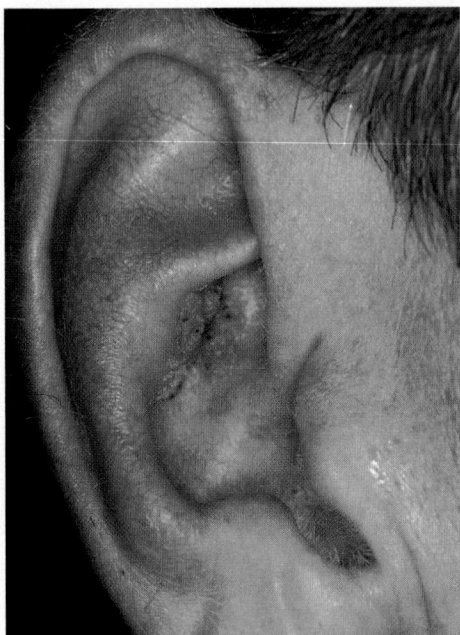

FIGURE 212-4 Common wart. A large hyperkeratotic nodule is seen on the ear.

which makes them appear as white patches (Fig. 212-9). Atypical condylomata may mimic cervical dysplasia or carcinoma in situ histologically, with nuclear atypia and disorganized differentiation. Cells with a central nucleus and a surrounding clear halo (*koilocytotic cells*) may be seen histologically in these lesions as well as in common verrucae. The natural history of cervical warts is not known, but progression to cervical dysplasia and carcinoma in situ is supported by several studies.[42,43] PV virion antigens can be detected in fixed biopsies and Papanicolaou's stains of cervical warts and dysplasias.[44]

Relation of Papillomaviruses and Malignancy

Although most PVs are associated with biologically benign lesions, epidemiologic and experimental studies suggest that certain PV genotypes have oncogenic potential. In humans, the association with infection by specific HPV types was first noted in patients with epidermodysplasia verruciformis (see Chap. 213). Squamous cell carcinoma may arise in sun-exposed warts in EV lesions, usually those with HPVs 5 or 8. Progression of the verrucae in respiratory papillomatosis to invasive squamous cell carcinoma can occur subsequent to X-irradiation. Immunosuppressed renal allograft patients have developed cutaneous squamous cell carcinoma containing HPV-5 DNA.[45] The benign epidermal hyperplasia induced in rabbits by the (Shope) cottontail rabbit PV can spontaneously convert to invasive squamous cell carcinoma.[46] Small doses of chemical carcinogens induce a high rate of malignant conversion in those lesions. In cattle, esophageal papillomas induced by BPV 4 become malignant if the infected animals graze on bracken fern, which contains a potential carcinogen. These observations and the long latency to malignant progression suggest that PVs do not induce

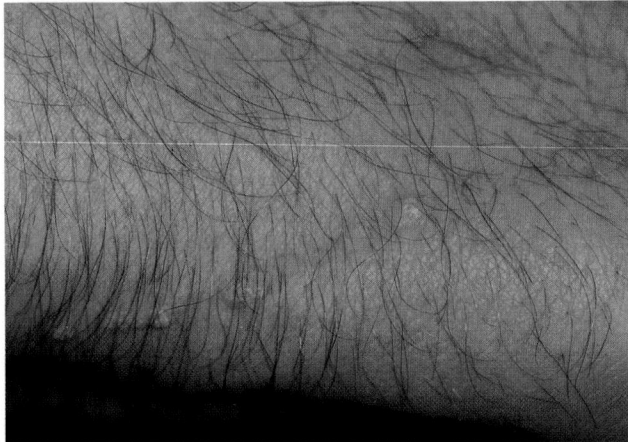

a

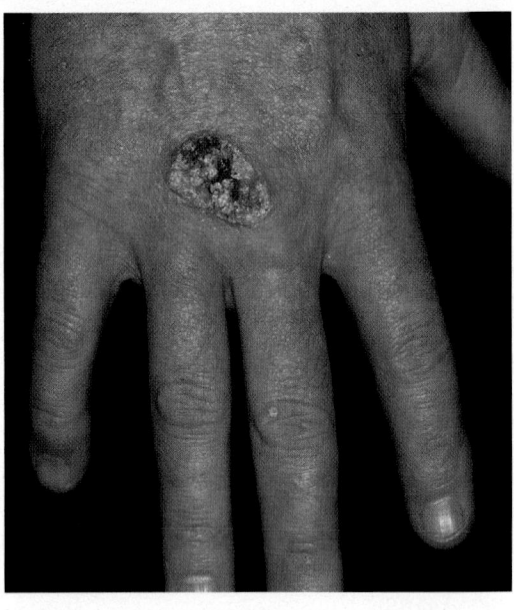

b

FIGURE 212-5 *(a)* Common wart with Koebnerization. A linear arrangement of warts is seen on the elbow, arising at the site of an abrasive injury. *(b)* Common wart. A giant wart is seen on the dorsum of the hand in a renal transplant recipient; the lesions were resistant to treatment but resolved spontaneously when immunosuppressive therapy was discontinued.

malignant tumors directly; it is more likely that potentially oncogenic PVs act by predisposing the infected cell to become malignant.

The verrucous carcinoma is a low-grade, well-differentiated squamous cell carcinoma that is locally invasive but rarely metastasizes. HPVs not usually associated with malignancy (such as HPVs 6 or 11) are usually found in these tumors. The giant condyloma acuminatum, also called the *Buschke-Lowenstein tumor,* and the squamous cell carcinoma that may arise from oral florid papillomatosis are forms of verrucous carcinoma. *Epithelioma cuniculatum,* another rare type of verrucous carcinoma, is found on the sole and is thought to arise from a plantar wart.

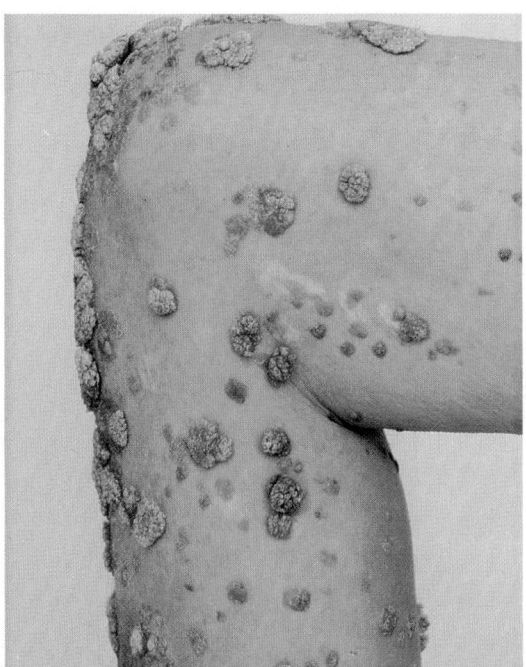

FIGURE 212-6 The large, scaly, and horny warts contain HPV 2. The smaller, flatter, less scaly papules are warts that contain HPV 3.

Epidemiologic evidence has linked condylomata acuminata, penile, vulvar, and anal carcinoma with HPV infection.[47] As discussed above, only a limited set of HPVs are isolated in cervical tumors. Although HPVs 6 and 11 are most common in cervical papillomas and early dysplasias, they are rarely identified in cervical cancers, whereas the opposite distribution is seen with HPVs 16, 18, 31, and 33. The relative risk of anogenital warts and cervical warts developing into squamous cell carcinoma, particularly for those lesions containing HPVs 16, 18, 31, and 33, is not yet known. HPV 16 has also been identified in digital cancers.[48] In summary, HPVs usually induce benign verrucae, but specific HPV genotypes can induce the development of malignant epithelial tumors. Although HPV infection may be necessary, it is not sufficient and most likely requires other cofactors to alter the cell to a malignant phenotype.[49]

Histopathology

Verrucae consist of an acanthotic epidermis with papillomatosis, hyperkeratosis, and parakeratosis (Fig. 212-10); some correlations can be made with HPV type.[50,51] The elongated rete ridges often point toward the center of the wart. The dermal capillary vessels are prominent and may be thrombosed. Mononuclear cells may be present. Large keratinocytes with an eccentric, pyknotic nucleus surrounded by a perinuclear halo, termed *koilocytotic cells* or *koilocytes,* are characteristic of HPV-associated papillomas. Koilocytes do not usually contain keratohyaline granules, although they occur in the malpighian layer. PV-infected cells may have small, eosinophilic granules and dense clumps of basophilic keratohyaline granules. These granules may be composed of or associated

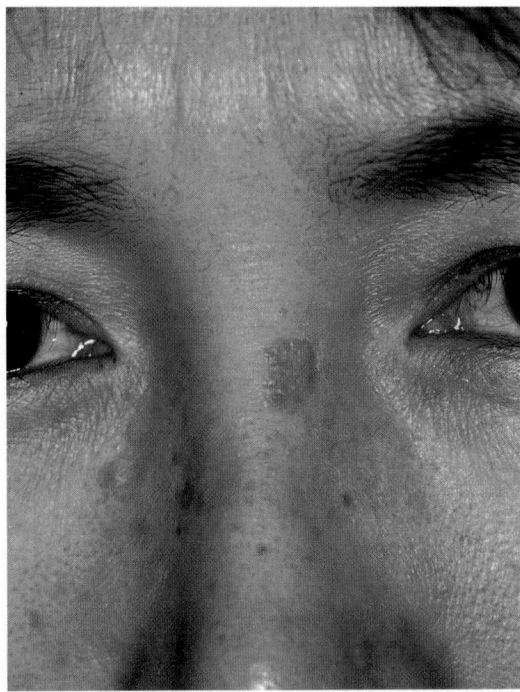

a

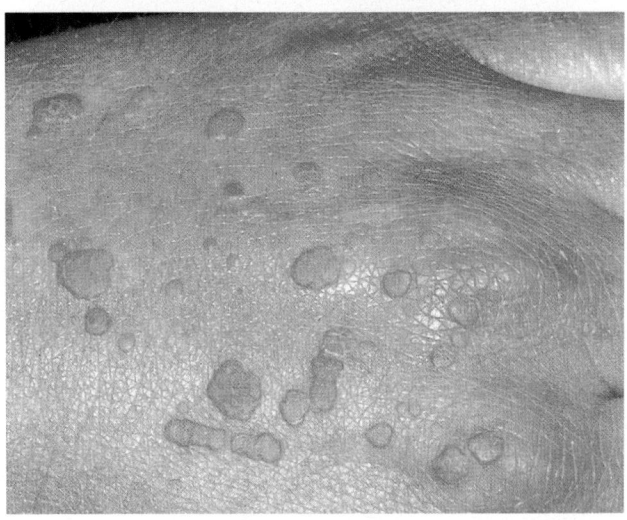

b

FIGURE 212-7 Common wart, verruca plana. *(a)* A single pink flat topped lesion is seen on the nose. *(b)* Mesalike flat topped papules. The linear configuration in the lower part of the picture is due to autoinoculation.

with the PV E4 (E1-E4) protein[52] and are not conglomerates of virus particles. Flat warts have less acanthosis and hyperkeratosis and do not have parakeratosis or papillomatosis. Koilocytotic cells are usually abundant, indicating the viral origin of the lesion. Anogenital warts may have from slight to extensive acanthosis and parakeratosis; they lack a granular layer as they are within or adjacent to a mucosal surface. The rete ridges often form thick bands extending extensively into the underlying, highly vascular dermis. Koilocytes are often observed in these viral papillomas.

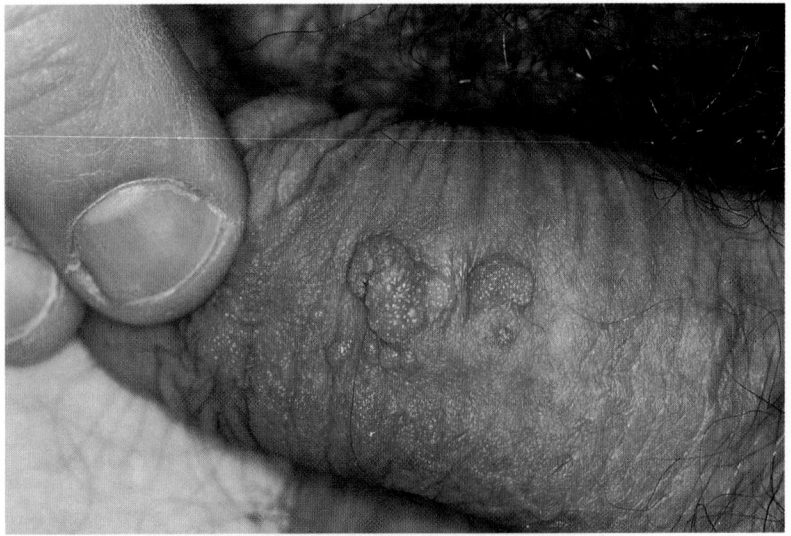

a

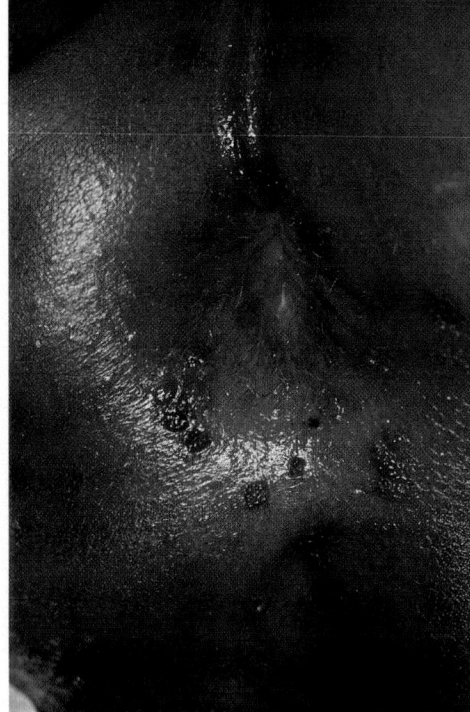

c

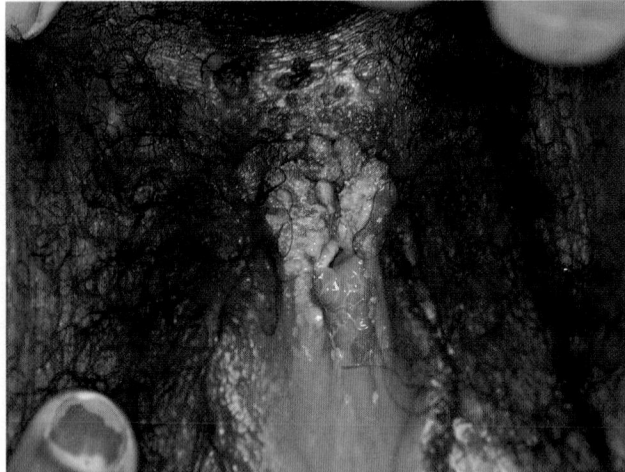

b

FIGURE 212-8 Mucosal wart. *(a)* Multiple condyloma acuminata are seen on the shaft of the penis. *(b)* Multiple confluent condylomata are seen on the labia minora. *(c)* Multiple condylomata are seen on the perineum of this 20-month-old boy, who was infected during vaginal delivery; his mother was not aware of her infection, but on examination was found to have several small condylomata.

Diagnosis

The diagnosis of viral wart is usually made by the clinical appearance but can also be suggested by histologic examination. Immuno-histochemical detection of PV structural proteins may confirm the presence of virus in a lesion. DNA hybridization techniques, which are currently limited to research laboratories, may soon be more widely available (see above). Application of 3 to 5% acetic acid to genital warts enhances detection of these lesions, particularly with colposcopic magnification,[12] although diagnosis should not rest only on the presence of white lesions, as there may be false-positives.

Cutaneous warts are common in children and young adults but also occur in patients over 40 years of age. Multiple warts that do not spontaneously resolve, always recur after treatment, persist for years, or have an unusual morphology, especially if familial, suggest epidermodysplasia verruciformis. Immunocompromised patients, such as those with lymphoproliferative disorders or on chemotherapeutic drugs, may have multiple warts.

Differential Diagnosis

Papules of lichen planus may resemble flat warts; they may be differentiated by the presence of Wickham's striae and buccal involvement. Acrokeratosis verruciformis and epidermolytic hyperkeratosis are characterized by verrucous papules on the extremities. Common lesions such as seborrheic keratoses, nevi, acrochordons, clavi, and squamous cell carcinomas may resemble verrucae. Syphilitic condylomata need to be differentiated from venereal warts.

Treatment

The approach to management of warts depends on the age of the patient, the extent and duration of lesions, the patient's immunologic status, and the patient's desire for therapy. Children with

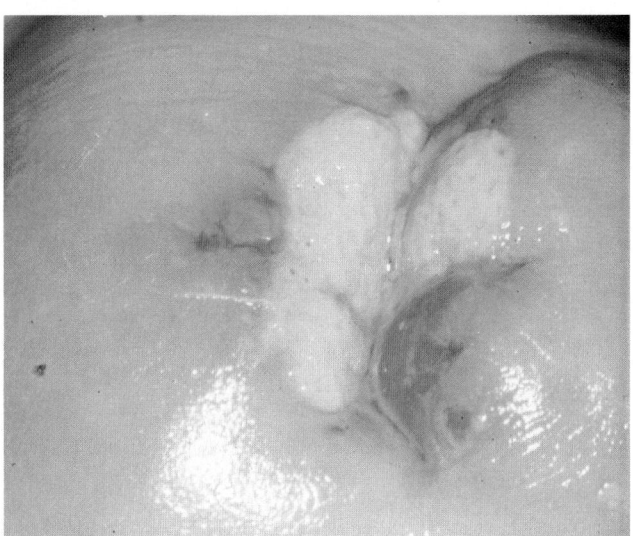

FIGURE 212-9 Colposcopic view of cervical condylomata after treatment with acetic acid for visualization as white, elevated patch.

common warts may not require therapy. Studies of spontaneous regression of warts in children suggest that two-thirds will remit within 2 years, with remaining verrucae continuing to resolve at this rate.[53] However, new warts may appear while others are regressing.

Current treatments for verrucae involve physical destruction of the infected cells. The existence of multiple treatment modalities reflects the fact that none is uniformly effective or directly antiviral. Choice of treatment depends on the location, size, number, and type of wart, as well as the age and cooperation of the patient.

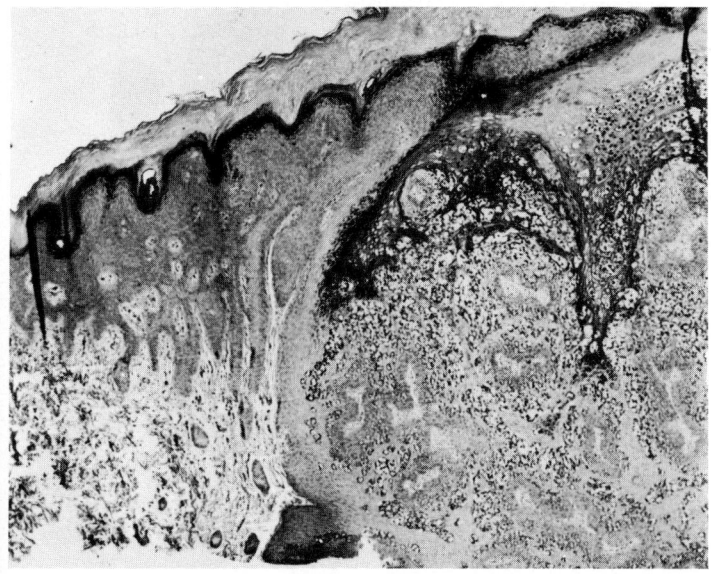

FIGURE 212-10 Verruca vulgaris. The process is one of extensive hyperplasia, and the hyperplastic cells contain both intranuclear and intracytoplasmic inclusion bodies. ×40 *(Micrograph by Wallace H. Clark, Jr., M.D.)*

Pain, inconvenience, risk of scarring, and experience of the physician are considerations to evaluate prior to treatment. In patients with anogenital warts (including bowenoid papulosis), sexual partners should be examined and treated if necessary. In females, evaluation of the uterine cervix should be performed; male contacts of women with cervical disease should also be examined.[12] Therapy for bowenoid papulosis with standard techniques such as cryotherapy, electrodesiccation, or excision is indicated, for although the papulosis may spontaneously remit, HPV 16 is frequently found.

Cryotherapy with liquid nitrogen is a common and effective treatment for most warts. Caustics and acids such as salicylic acid, lactic acid, and trichloroacetic acid destroy and peel off infected skin. Retinoic acid has been used topically for flat warts and probably has a similar mechanism of action. Cantharidin is an extract of the green blister beetle that leads to blistering and focal destruction of epidermis. Induction of allergic contact dermatitis with dinitrochlorobenzene (DNCB) allows localization of inflammation to warts on which DNCB is painted; it has been speculated that this treatment stimulates local immunity. DNCB is positive in the Ames bacterial test of mutagenicity and its use remains controversial.

A variety of chemotherapeutic agents are also widely employed. Topical podophyllin resin is a common treatment, particularly for anogenital warts, as it is more effective on mucosal surfaces. However, podophyllin is often said to be contraindicated during pregnancy,[54] and the potency of podophyllin preparations may be highly variable. Purified podophyllotoxin, whose activity is reproducible from batch to batch, has been approved for treatment of genital warts.[55] Application of 5-fluorouracil has been reported to be effective in some cases of flat warts and condylomata acuminata,[56] and direct instillation has been used for urethral warts.[57] Intralesional bleomycin may eradicate verrucae but should be used cautiously due to the possibility of extensive tissue necrosis.[58] Warts may be curetted or surgically excised, particularly large anogenital warts unresponsive to topical treatments. Electrodesiccation of condylomata acuminata requires local anesthesia but is effective. The CO$_2$ laser can be used to destroy resistant warts or those where careful control of width and depth are necessary, such as in large periungual warts. A surgical mask should be used because infectious HPV has been identified in the vapor plume with laser or with electrocoagulation of warts.[59] Microscopically controlled (Mohs) surgery has been particularly useful in the treatment of verrucous carcinoma.

Interferon has been effective in short-term studies in reducing warts in laryngeal papillomatosis and epidermodysplasia verruciformis, but lesions recur when therapy is stopped.[60–62] Recombinant interferon-α was approved for intralesional injection of refractory genital warts in 1989, and interferon derived from human leukocytes has recently become available.[63] X-irradiation of verrucae is contraindicated because of its association with development of malignancy in respiratory papillomatosis.

References

1. Jablonska S, Orth G (eds): *Warts/Human Papillomaviruses,* Clin Dermatol vol 3. Philadelphia, Lippincott, 1985
2. De Villiers E: Heterogeneity of the human papillomavirus group. *J Virol* **63**:4898, 1989
3. Salzman NP et al: *The Papovaviridae,* vol 2, *The Papillomaviruses.* New York, Plenum, 1987

4. Jenson SB et al: Immunological relatedness of papillomaviruses from different species. *J Natl Cancer Inst* **64**:495, 1980

5. Danos O et al: Comparative analysis of the human type Ia and bovine type 1 papillomavirus genomes. *J Virol* **46**:557, 1983

6. Bauer HM et al: Genital human papillomavirus infection in female University students as determined by a PCR-based method. *JAMA* **265**:472, 1991

7. Brandsma JL et al: Detection and typing of papillomavirus DNA in formaldehyde-fixed paraffin-embedded tissue. *Arch Otol Head Neck Surg* **116**:844, 1990

8. Barr BB et al: Human papilloma virus infection and skin cancer in renal allograft recipients. *Lancet* **1**:124, 1989

9. Laurent R et al: Epidemiology of HPV infection. *Clin Dermatol* **3**:64, 1985

10. Condyloma acuminatum—United States, 1966–1981. *MMWR* **32**:306, 1983

11. Oriel JD: Natural history of genital warts. *Br J Vener Dis* **47**:1, 1971

12. Barrasso R et al: High prevalence of papillomavirus-associated penile intraepithelial neoplasia in sexual partners of women with cervical intraepithelial neoplasia. *N Engl J Med* **317**:916, 1987

13. Cohen BA et al: Anogenital warts in children. Clinical and virologic evaluation for sexual abuse. *Arch Dermatol* **126**:1575, 1990

14. Obalek S et al: Condylomata acuminata in children: Frequent association with human papillomaviruses responsible for cutaneous warts. *J Am Acad Dermatol* **23**:205, 1990

15. Mounts P, Shah KV: Respiratory papillomatosis: Etiological relation to genital tract papillomaviruses. *Prog Med Virol* **29**:90, 1984

16. Kirchner H: Immunobiology of human papillomavirus infection. *Prog Med Virol* **33**:1, 1986

17. Morison WL: Viral warts, herpes simplex and herpes zoster in patients with secondary immunodeficiencies and neoplasms. *Br J Dermatol* **92**:625, 1975

18. Rogozinsk TT et al: Role of cell mediated immunity in spontaneous regression of plane warts. *Int J Dermatol* **27**:322, 1990

19. Abcarian H et al: Long-term effectiveness of the immunotherapy of anal condyloma acuminatum. *Dis Colon Rectum* **25**:648, 1982

20. Gentles JC et al: Foot infections in swimming baths. *Br Med J* **2**:260, 1973

21. Burnett S et al: Localization of bovine papillomavirus type 1 E5 protein to transformed basal keratinocytes and permissive differentiated cells in fibropapilloma tissue. *Proc Natl Acad Sci USA* **89**:5665, 1992

22. Steinberg BM et al: Laryngeal papillomavirus infection during clinical remission. *N Engl J Med* **308**:1261, 1983

23. Ferenczy A et al: Latent papillomavirus and genital warts. *N Engl J Med* **313**:784, 1985

24. Grussendorf-Cohen E-I et al: Correlation between content of viral DNA and evidence of mature virus particles in HPV-1, HPV-4, and HPV-6 induced virus acanthomata. *J Invest Dermatol* **81**:511, 1983

25. Doorbar J et al: Specific interaction between HPV-16 E1-E4 and cytokeratins results in collapse of the epithelial cell intermediate filament network. *Nature* **352**:824, 1991

26. Morin C et al: Confirmation of the papillomavirus etiology of condylomatous cervix lesions by the peroxidase-antiperoxidase technique. *J Natl Cancer Inst* **66**:831, 1981

27. Kreider JW et al: Laboratory production in vivo of infectious human papillomavirus type 11. *J Virol* **61**:590, 1987

28. DiMaio D: Transforming activity of bovine and human papillomaviruses in cultured cells. *Adv Cancer Res* **56**:133, 1991

29. Martin P et al: The bovine papillomavirus E5 transforming protein can stimulate the transforming activity of EGF and CSF-1 receptors. *Cell* **59**:21, 1989

30. Petti L et al: Activation of the platelet-derived growth factor receptor by the bovine papillomavirus E5 transforming protein. *EMBO J* **10**:845, 1991

31. Werness BA et al: Role of the human papillomavirus oncoproteins in transformation and carcinogenic progression, in *Important Advances in Oncology,* edited by JT De Vita. Philadelphia, Lippincott, 1991, p 3

32. McCance DJ et al: Human papillomavirus type 16 alters human epithelial cell differentiation in vitro. *Proc Natl Acad Sci USA* **85**:7169, 1988

33. Orth G et al: Identification of papillomaviruses in butcher's warts. *J Invest Dermatol* **76**:97, 1981

34. Zachow KR et al: Detection of human papillomavirus DNA in anogenital neoplasias. *Nature* **300**:771, 1982

35. Ikenberg H et al: Human papillomavirus type-16 related DNA in genital Bowen's disease and in bowenoid papulosis. *Int J Cancer* **32**:563, 1983

36. Obalek S et al: Bowenoid papulosis of the male and female genitalia: Risk of cervical neoplasia. *J Am Acad Dermatol* **14**:433, 1986

37. Guillet GY et al: Bowenoid papulosis: Demonstration of human papillomavirus (HPV) with anti-HPV immune serum. *Arch Dermatol* **120**:514, 1984

38. Gross G et al: Bowenoid papulosis. *Arch Dermatol* **121**:858, 1985

39. Syrjänen SM: Human papillomavirus infections in the oral cavity, in *Papillomaviruses and Human Disease,* edited by K Syrjänen et al. Berlin, Springer, 1987, p 104

40. Pfister H et al: Characterization of human papillomavirus type 13 from focal epithelial hyperplasia Heck lesions. *J Virol* **47**:363, 1983

41. Sand PK et al: Evaluation of male consorts of women with genital human papilloma virus infection. *Obstet Gynecol* **68**:679, 1986

42. Reid R et al: Genital warts and cervical cancer: I. Evidence of an association between subclinical papillomavirus infection and cervical malignancy. *Cancer* **50**:377, 1982

43. Welker PG et al: Natural history of cervical epithelial abnormalities in patients with vulvar warts. *Br J Vener Dis* **59**:327, 1983

44. Meisels A et al: Human papillomavirus infection of the cervix: The atypical condyloma. *Acta Cytol* **25**:7, 1981

45. Lutzner MA et al: Detection of human papillomavirus type 5 DNA in skin cancers of an immunosuppressed renal allograft recipient. *Lancet* **2**:422, 1983

46. Kreider JW: The Shope papilloma to carcinoma complex of rabbits: A model system of neoplastic progression and spontaneous regression. *Adv Cancer Res* **35**:81, 1981

47. Schiffman MH: Recent progress in defining the epidemiology of human papillomavirus infection and cervical neoplasia. *J Natl Cancer Inst* **84**:394, 1992

48. Moy R et al: Human papillomavirus type 16 DNA in periungual squamous cell carcinomas. *JAMA* **261**:2669, 1989

49. zur Hausen H: Human papillomaviruses in the pathogenesis of anogenital cancer. *Virology* **184**:9, 1991

50. Gross G et al: Correlation between human papillomavirus (HPV) type and histology of warts. *J Invest Dermatol* **78**:160, 1982

51. Jablonska S et al: Cutaneous warts. Clinical, histologic, and virologic correlations. *Clin Dermatol* **3**:71, 1985

52. Rogel-Gaillard D et al: Human papillomavirus type 1 E4 proteins differing by their N-terminal ends have distinct cellular localizations when transiently expressed in vitro. *J Virol* **66**:816, 1992

53. Messing AM et al: Natural history of warts: A two year study. *Arch Dermatol* **87**:306, 1963

54. Bargman H: Is podophyllin a safe drug to use and can it be used during pregnancy? *Arch Dermatol* **124**:1718, 1988

55. Beutner KR et al: Patient-applied podofilox for treatment of genital warts. *Lancet* **8**:31, 1989

56. Goette DK: Topical chemotherapy with 5-fluorouracil. *J Am Acad Dermatol* **6**:633, 1981

57. Carpiniello VL et al: Long-term followup of subclinical human papillomavirus infection treated with the carbon dioxide laser and intraurethral 5-fluorouracil: A treatment protocol. *J Urology* **143**:726, 1990

58. Shumer SM et al: Bleomycin in the treatment of recalcitrant warts. *J Am Acad Dermatol* **9**:91, 1983

59. Sawchuk WS et al: Infectious papillomavirus in the vapor of warts treated with carbon dioxide laser or electrocoagulation: Detection and protection. *J Am Acad Dermatol* **21**:41, 1989

60. Haglund S et al: Interferon therapy in juvenile laryngeal papillomatosis. *Arch Otolaryngol* **107**:327, 1981

61. Steinberg BM et al: Persistence and expression of human papillomavirus during interferon therapy. *Arch Otolaryngol Head Neck Surg* **144**:27, 1988

62. Androphy EJ et al: Response of warts in epidermodysplasia verruciformis to treatment with systemic and intralesional alpha interferon. *J Am Acad Dermatol* **11**:197, 1984

63. Reichman RC et al: Treatment of condyloma acuminatum with three different interferon-α preparations administered parenterally: A double-blind, placebo-controlled trial. *J Infect Dis* **162**:1270, 1990

CHAPTER 213

Stefania Jablonska

Human Papillomavirus: Epidermodysplasia Verruciformis

Epidermodysplasia verruciformis (EV) is a rare, lifelong, sporadic or familial, genetic autosomal recessive disease, associated with human papillomaviruses. The disseminated wartlike or pityriasis-versicolor-like lesions persist from early childhood and, in about one-third of patients, cutaneous carcinomas develop in adult life. This heritable disease is of great interest because it is the first model of cutaneous viral oncogenesis in humans.

History

EV was first described in 1922 by Lewandowsky and Lutz[1] as a genodermatosis characterized by vacuolar degeneration of epidermal cells, with a predisposition to malignant transformation.[2] A relationship to disseminated warts, based on the morphology of the lesions, was confirmed by successful auto- and heteroinoculation and detection of viral particles. Human papilloma viruses (HPVs) specific for EV (EV HPVs) were first characterized in 1978.[3] So far, there are known to be at least 17 EV-specific HPVs, but only a few of them are found in carcinomas developing from EV lesions.

Epidemiology

The disease is worldwide in distribution, and HPV types do not differ in various continents. HPV-3 and HPV-10, commonly found in patients with EV, are also found in normal individuals with flat warts. About a dozen other HPVs are found in the benign lesions of patients with EV and only rarely infect normal individuals. HPV-5 and HPV-8 are associated with malignant lesions in patients with EV. Patients with EV are often infected with more than one HPV. In some immunosuppressed patients, widespread warts appear that may be associated with EV HPVs. Also, DNA of EV HPVs has been found in developing cancers.[4–7] EV-HPV-related DNA sequences have also been detected in single carcinomas in the general population.[7] The role of these viruses in cutaneous tumors of immunologically competent hosts remains unknown, and there is no evidence that carcinomas in the general population are associated with EV HPVs, at least not those that are presently recognized and can be detected with available probes.

Etiology and Pathogenesis

EV is probably a polygenic and multifactorial disease involving genetics, infectious agents, and environmental factors.

Genetics

The role of genetic factors is suggested by the familial occurrence and parental consanguinity in many cases. There is no racial or sexual predisposition. The mode of inheritance is apparently autosomal recessive, although one family was shown to have an X-linked recessive inheritance and in another EV affected only women.[8] The main genetic defect involves an abnormal susceptibility to specific HPVs. There is some analogy to another hereditary tumor, retinoblastoma, which also appears in familial and sporadic forms and is related to absence of the suppressor gene (antioncogene) Rb-1 that prevents progression of the cell to malignancy. It is conceivable that in patients with EV there is also a defect of a suppressor gene whose presence correlates with lack of pathogenicity of EV HPVs for the normal population. The transforming proteins of some potentially oncogenic HPVs (eg., HPV-16) were shown to bind to the pRB domain, which acts as a cellular antioncogene, and to cancel its inhibitory activity. In immunocompromised patients suppression may be lost by mutation or gene rearrangement, and thus keratinocytes could become permissive for EV HPVs. However, the suppressor gene in EV remains unknown.

HPV Types Associated with Benign Lesions of EV

The presence of crystalline viral particles is easily established by electron microscopy because the lesions usually harbor a high number of HPVs. Molecular cloning of the viral genomes made it possible to characterize at least 17 EV HPVs.[8] In addition, a frequent finding is HPV-3 or the related HPV-10, responsible for flat warts in the general population, appearing in association with EV HPVs. HPV-3 and HPV-10 found in patients with EV do not differ from those responsible for plane warts not related to EV. There is almost no homology between EV HPVs and HPVs inducing plane or common warts in the general population.

The most frequently encountered EV HPVs are HPV-5, -8, -17 and -20. Most patients are infected with several EV HPVs.

EV HPVs Associated with Cancers

Although there are multiple EV-specific HPVs in lesions of EV, only some are associated with carcinomas originating from these lesions.[8,9] The fully organized viral particles are found rarely, but molecular hybridization procedures have shown DNA of HPV-5 and HPV-8 in the majority of carcinomas. Thus these two somewhat related EV HPVs have the highest oncogenic potential. In single tumors, HPV-14 and HPV-17 have been detected. In contrast to genital mucosa-specific viral sequences integrated into cellular DNA and associated with anogenital tumors (HPV-16, -18, -31, and others), EV HPVs in cutaneous tumors remain extrachromosomal (nonintegrated), even in metastatic carcinomas.[10] Malignant transformation of HPV-3-induced EV lesions is exceptional and is probably related to the action of some cocarcinogens.

Role of Immunologic Factors in the Pathogenesis of EV

Immune responses appear to play an important role in the pathogenesis of the disease[11] because EV-like syndromes have been reported in immunosuppressed populations, even in patients with AIDS.[12]

Humoral Immunity　Specific antibodies are either undetectable or present in low titer. Otherwise, humoral immunity is fully preserved. However, humoral immune responses do not play an essential role in HPV infections.

Cell-Mediated Immunity　Cellular responses are believed to be important in controlling viral infections. Most patients with EV have a decreased number of T and T-helper cells and a lowered response to mitogens, and they are unable to develop contact sensitivity to dinitrochlorobenzene (DNCB).[11] However, the defect in cell-mediated immunity is only partial, because the functions of Langerhans cells, suppressor lymphocytes, cytotoxic cells, and cells generating angiokines are preserved.[13] The defect in cellular immunity relates mainly to inhibited specific responses of T cells and natural killer cells to EV-specific HPV-encoded antigens.[14,15] This specific defect may explain why EV patients develop lesions induced by EV-specific HPVs but, in spite of immunosuppression, are usually not abnormally susceptible to other viral and bacterial infections.

Cofactors of HPV Oncogenesis

Carcinomas develop from only some benign EV lesions associated with potentially oncogenic HPVs. Oncogenesis involves a multistage, long-term process requiring the action of some cocarcinogens. The most important factor in oncogenesis appears to be UV irradiation since cancers develop primarily on sun-exposed areas, preferentially on the forehead, i.e., at sites most involved by actinic keratoses in the general population.[2,11] Since chronic

trauma is another cofactor, malignancies commonly develop, for example, in macerated anogenital areas and retroauricularly.

Clinical Manifestations

There are two main varieties of EV: the typical form associated with EV HPVs and the form associated with HPV-3.[2,3,8,11,16]

EV Associated with EV HPVs

Cutaneous lesions vary: Flat (plane), wartlike lesions; red macules; and achromic, brownish, or pityriasis-versicolor-like plaques may be present. The flat wartlike lesions are localized mostly to the extremities and the face (Figs. 213-1 to 213-3). They are usually somewhat flatter than plane warts, with uneven outlines; they are also much more abundant, not infrequently confluent, and widely

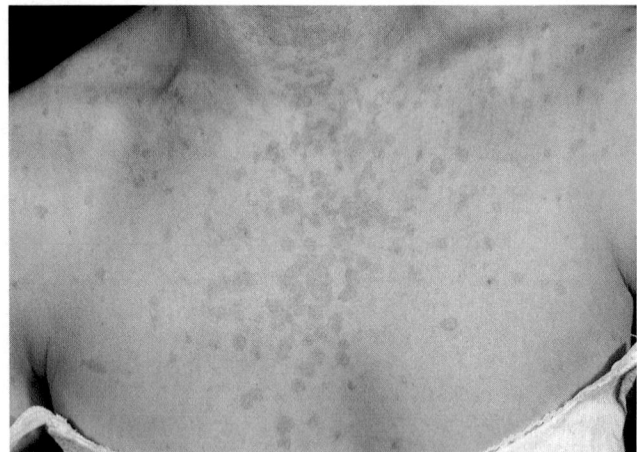

FIGURE 213-1　Red-brown, pityriasis(tinea)-versicolor-like macules in a typical location on the thorax, induced by HPV-5.

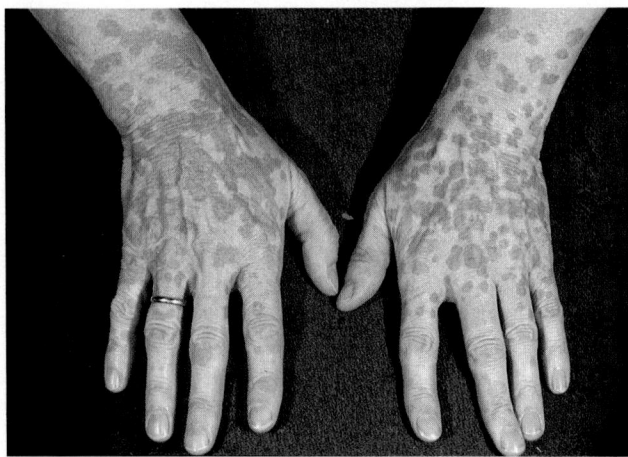

FIGURE 213-2　Plane wartlike lesions on the dorsa of the hands and forearms, associated with HPV-5 and -8. The lesions are numerous, flat, reddish, and partly confluent.

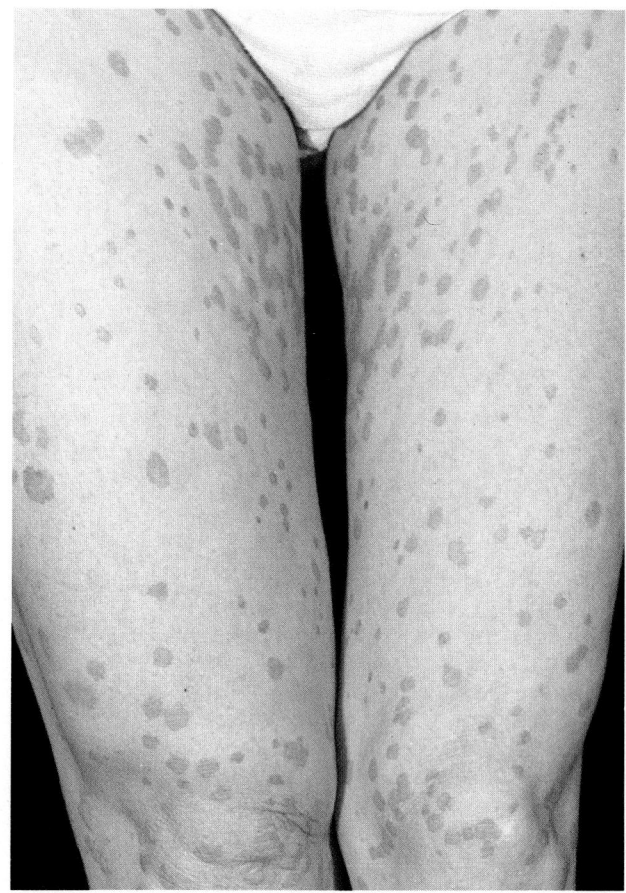

FIGURE 213-3 Red macules and plane wartlike lesions widely disseminated over the entire skin. Some form large plaques, and some appear in a linear distribution (Koebnerization). These lesions were associated with HPV-5, -21, and -23.

disseminated on the proximal and distal parts of the extremities. Actinic keratoses and malignant tumors develop from flat wartlike or seborrheic wartlike lesions on the face in the third and fourth decades of life. On the trunk, the red, brownish, or achromic lesions are macular, and if not abundant, may be overlooked. Oral and genital mucosa are, as a rule, not involved.

In some patients, the infection with EV-specific HPVs is mixed with HPV-3. In these cases flat (plane) warts are widespread, localized all over the body, but usually more pronounced in locations characteristic for plane warts in the general population, i.e., on the dorsa of the hands and feet, and on the face.

The lymph nodes are not involved. The general condition of patients is satisfactory, with no visceral involvement. However, patients with HPV-3-induced EV are susceptible to other infections. Single cases have been reported to be associated with mental retardation.[8,11]

EV Associated with HPV-3

In this variety of EV, lesions of the flat wart type are widely disseminated over the body, extremities, and face. The single lesions may be indistinguishable from typical flat warts; however, they are mostly larger, plaquelike, and more brownish, with polycyclic out-

lines. Because in this variety of EV there is a more pronounced decrease in cell-mediated immune responses than in the variety induced by EV HPVs, common or genital warts may appear at some time in the disease. Unlike EV induced by EV HPVs, EV associated with HPV-3 progresses to malignant transformation only exceptionally, e.g., after intensive sun exposure or x-ray therapy.

Tumors Associated with EV

Tumors in patients with EV may be benign (papillomas), premalignant, or malignant.

Papillomas Benign proliferation of pigmented verrucae of the seborrheic type and of papillomas is a frequent finding in both forms of EV. The preferential sites for papillomas are the forehead, periorbital region, neck, and anogenital area.

Actinic Keratoses These small, red, keratotic and scaling lesions appear mostly on the forehead, in the frontal areas, usually in great number. In contrast to the rare (approximately 5 percent) malignant conversion of actinic keratoses in the general population, in EV patients such a transformation occurs progressively in numerous lesions. Red plaques and wartlike lesions in other locations may also change into premalignant lesions: actinic keratoses or Bowen's disease.

Malignant Tumors Carcinoma in situ, microinvasive and invasive, develops preferentially on the forehead and the scalp but may occur on the hands, in traumatized areas, or elsewhere on the body. The tumors grow slowly, and if located periorbitally or on the lip, they do not destroy the eyeball or oral mucosa. Although locally destructive, these cancers do not metastasize if not treated with radiation or other cocarcinogens (Fig. 213-4). There are no internal malignancies related to HPVs. In rare instances, lymphomas have been reported, but their relationship to EV is not established.

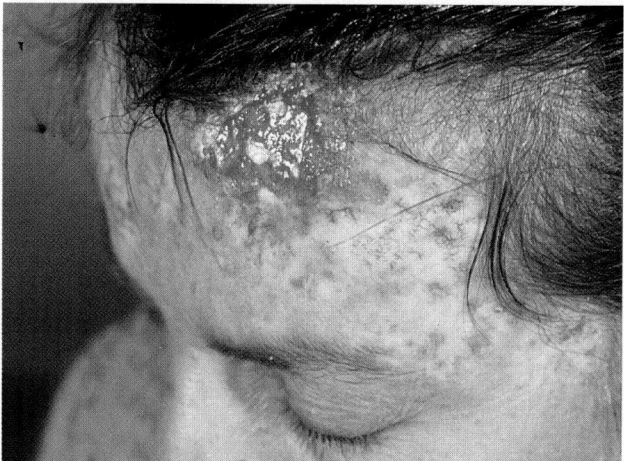

FIGURE 213-4 Invasive cancer in a patient infected with numerous EV HPV-5, -8, -9, -14, and others. In the tumor cells, DNA HPV-5 was detected in a high copy number. This large squamous-cell carcinoma did not metastasize and did not recur after surgery. There are numerous actinic keratoses on the forehead.

Laboratory and Special Examinations

Routine laboratory examinations are within normal limits.

Virologic Studies[17]

1. The presence of papillomaviruses may be established in formalin-fixed, paraffin-embedded tissue by the peroxidase-antiperoxidase technique using antibodies against disrupted viral particles. This method detects only the group-specific papillomavirus antigen.
2. Detection of type-specific viral nucleic acid is possible with various techniques:
    a. The most sensitive but time-consuming is Southern blot hybridization performed on tissue scrapings or on specimens.
    b. Dot blot hybridization with extracted DNA and filter in situ hybridization are more rapid and simple tests, but they are less sensitive and yield more false-positive results.
3. In situ hybridization makes it possible to correlate the location of viral genomes in the tissue with cellular abnormalities. The method can be applied to routinely processed, paraffin-embedded tissue. After DNA is denatured, it is hybridized to radioactively or chemically labeled viral DNA. The sensitivity of the method is much inferior to that of Southern blot.

Immunologic Studies

Of practical significance are tests for cell-mediated immune responses, number of T cells, OKT 4/OKT 8 ratio of peripheral lymphocytes, mitogenic responses, natural killer cell activity, and DNCB sensitization, as well as cutaneous bacterial tests and others.

Pathology

Pathology of EV Induced by EV HPVs

A characteristic feature of this type of EV is the presence of large, clear, dysplastic cells arranged in nests in the granular and spinous layers, not infrequently starting suprabasally and replacing almost the entire epidermis. The nucleoplasm is clear, with margination of the chromatin, and the cytoplasm is finely granular with characteristic prominent keratohyalin granules of different sizes and shapes. This cytopathic effect is related to replication of EV HPVs (Figs. 213-5 and 213-6). The histopathologic pattern is diagnostically significant and is identical in lesions induced by various EV HPV types, regardless of their clinical morphology.[2,3,7–9,11,16]

Pathology of EV Lesions Induced by HPV-3

The flat wartlike lesions have all the characteristic histologic features of HPV-3- or HPV-10-induced warts in the general population. The stratum corneum is loose, with a basket-weave appearance. The main feature is perinuclear vacuolization of the cells in the upper layers of the epidermis; the nuclei are small and pyknotic and cytoplasmic membranes are sharply defined. Such cells show some similarity to "birds' eyes"[11] (Fig. 213-7).

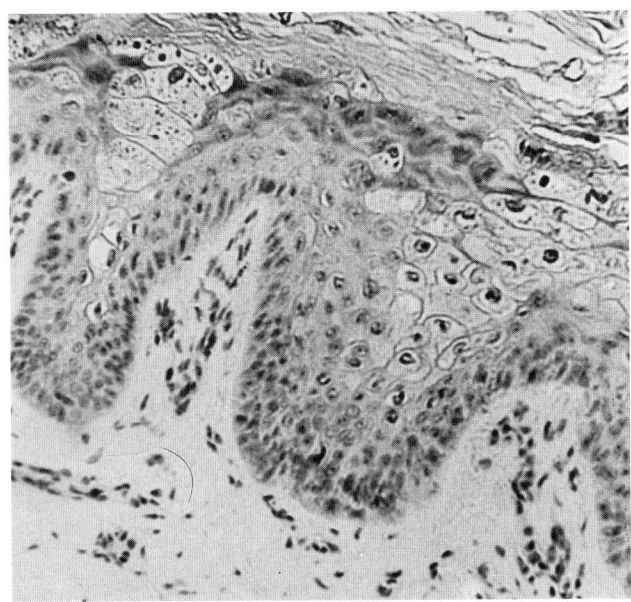

FIGURE 213-5 Histology of an HPV-5-induced wart. Loose, basket-weave-like hyperkeratosis, clear large cells arranged in nests in the granular and spinous layers. Their nuclei are shrunken and pyknotic, and the clear cytoplasm is dotted with dispersed keratohyalin granules of different sizes and shapes. Typical cytopathic effect of EV-specific HPVs. H&E, ×180.

Pathology of Tumors

Papillomas If induced by EV-specific HPVs, the characteristic cytopathic effect may be seen in the superficial layers of the epidermis. Otherwise, the structure is of the papilloma type, with no signs of malignant proliferation. Papillomas induced by HPV-3 are typical of papillomas not related to EV.

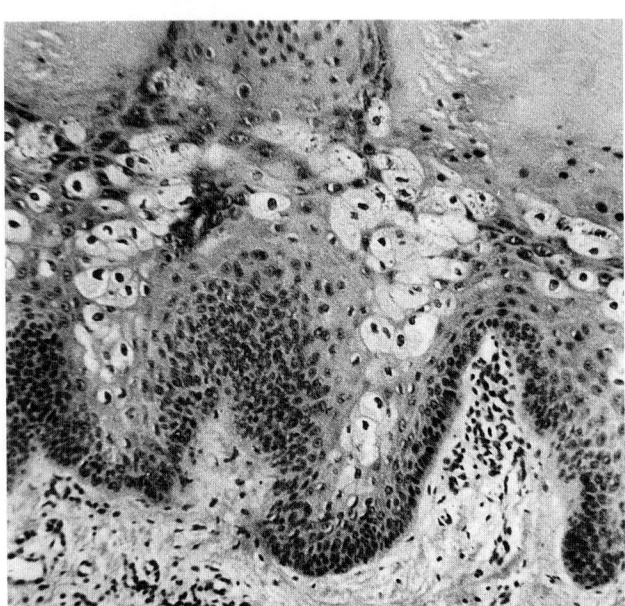

FIGURE 213-6 Characteristic cytopathic effect of EV-specific HPV in a patient found to be infected with HPV-5, -8, and -9. Very abundant clear large cells with small pyknotic nuclei replace almost the entire epidermis. H&E, ×200.

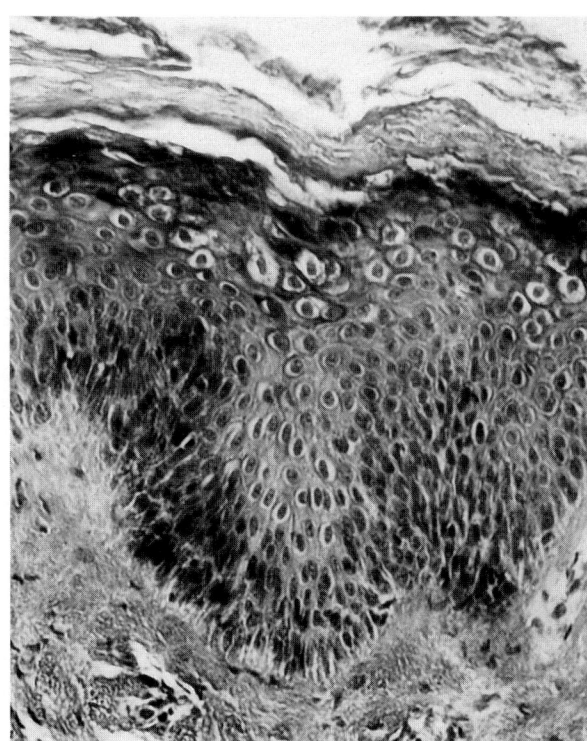

FIGURE 213-7 Histology of HPV-3-associated plane wartlike lesion in a patient with EV. The pattern is characteristic of a plane wart with numerous cells showing perinuclear vacuolization in the granular and upper spinous layers. H&E, ×200.

Actinic Keratoses The pathology of actinic keratoses originating from benign EV lesions is similar to that of actinic keratoses in the general population, with more pronounced Bowen's atypia. There are numerous pleomorphic cells with large hyperchromatic nuclei (Fig. 213-8), multinucleated and dyskeratotic cells, and abnormal mitotic figures. In very early malignancies, the characteristic cyto-

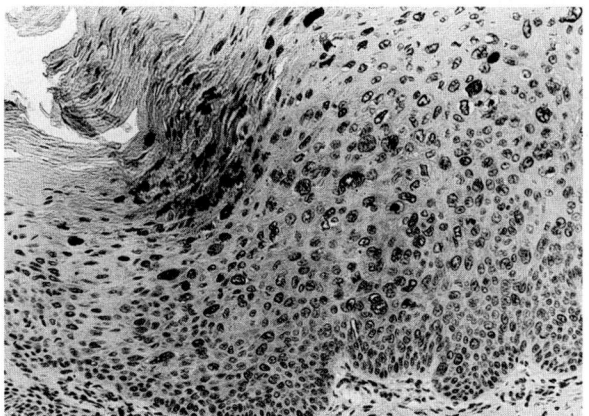

FIGURE 213-8 Histology of actinic keratosis in a patient with EV. In situ hybridization demonstrated that large, strongly basophilic, parakeratotic nuclei contained HPV-5 DNA. There are numerous atypical pleomorphic and dyskeratotic cells. H&E, ×125.

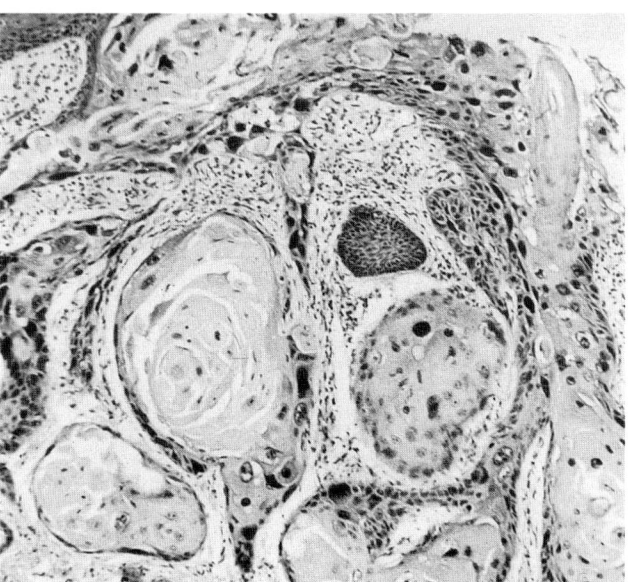

FIGURE 213-9 Squamous cell carcinoma associated with HPV-5 DNA. A characteristic feature of early EV carcinoma is pronounced keratinization. Multiple horn pearls, with fully or partly keratinized centers, contain numerous dyskeratotic cells. H&E, ×180.

pathic effect can be observed in the superficial layers of the epidermis, whereas the proliferating downward rete ridges display atypical changes. Microinvasive squamous cell carcinomas usually retain features of Bowen's atypia, with monstrous dyskeratotic and pleomorphic cells (Fig. 213-9).

Electron Microscopic Findings

EV Induced by Specific HPVs The characteristic feature of lesions induced by EV HPVs is a clear nucleus with margination of chromatin and prominent nucleoli. Numerous nuclei are filled with crystalline viral particles. The cytoplasm is devoid of all cytoplasmic organelles except for ribosomes and scattered uneven keratohyalin granules not associated with tonofilaments[7,11] (Fig. 213-10).

HPV-3-Induced EV Perinuclear vacuolization is related to the displaced cytoplasmic structures at the cell periphery. There is no clearing of nucleoplasm and margination of chromatin, as in the EV-HPV-induced variety, although the nuclei are also filled with crystalline viral particles.[7,11]

Carcinomas In addition to all the characteristics of carcinomas not related to EV, there are usually abundant apoptotic bodies and other signs of dyskeratosis. Viral particles are absent.

Diagnosis and Differential Diagnosis

Diagnosis of EV is easy if the cutaneous lesions are widespread. It rests on the characteristic distribution of wartlike, macular, and

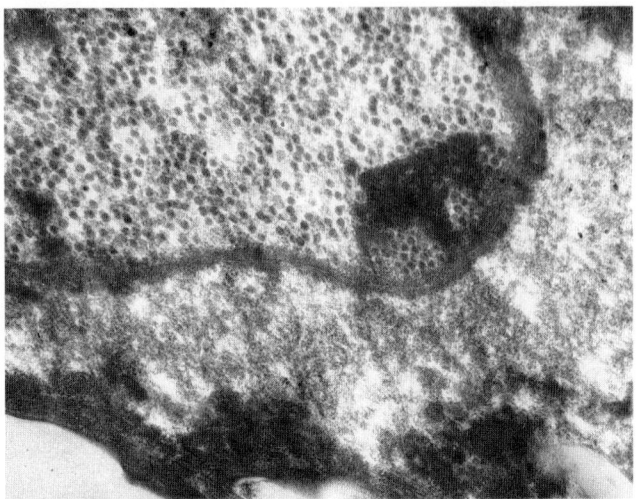

FIGURE 213-10 Electron microscope view of an EV lesion induced by HPV-5. Chromatin is marginated and the nucleus and nucleolus are filled with viral particles. The cytoplasm exclusively contains ribosomes. ×40,000.

pityriasis-versicolor-like lesions, the onset of the disease in early childhood, and otherwise good health with no visceral involvement. There may be a positive family history. Diagnosis is confirmed by the characteristic histopathology, detection of viral particles by electron microscopy, and especially by molecular hybridization procedures for characterization of EV HPVs.

Patients infected with EV HPVs should be carefully screened for premalignant lesions in sun-exposed areas, mainly on the forehead. The reported onset of EV in the fourth decade of life is probably due to recognition of multiple facial cancers as the first symptom of the disease, while macular lesions on the trunk must have been overlooked. EV induced by EV HPVs should be differentiated from generalized flat warts coexistent with pityriasis versicolor. Some cases may be somewhat similar to unusual lichen planus.

Of practical significance is differentiation of true EV from an EV-like syndrome in the immunosuppressed population. This syndrome can be distinguished by its later onset, less widespread cutaneous lesions, and presence of other symptoms of immunosuppression. EV induced by HPV-3 should be differentiated from disseminated verrucae planae, which are not lifelong, are preferentially located on the extremities and the face, and are not associated with brownish or achromic plaques. Acrokeratosis verruciformis differs in its more restricted verruca-plana-like changes, localized mainly on the hands and feet, the stationary character of the disease, the dominant mode of inheritance, and the histopathologic features (absence of cytopathic effect characteristic of HPV-3).

Treatment

There is no effective therapy for EV, and in only one case has the EV-HPV-induced variety been reported to regress spontaneously (see below). However, some new experimental therapies appear to be beneficial in inducing temporary regression or improvement of benign lesions. No local therapy has been successful.

Retinoids

The benign lesions of both forms of EV improve considerably upon systemic administration of retinoids.[18,19] Isotretinoin (13-*cis* retinoic acid) appears to be somewhat more effective than etretinate (daily dose 50 mg). The daily dose of isotretinoin is 1 mg/kg for 6 to 9 months. After some improvement is achieved, if there are no significant side effects, a maintenance dose of 10 to 25 mg twice weekly may be continued for several months, and the therapy may be repeated with the reappearance of premalignant lesions.

Although retinoids do not induce clearing of the lesions associated with EV HPVs, they appear to prevent development of new actinic keratoses and/or microinvasion and invasion of carcinomas in situ. Thus retinoids are indicated mainly for patients with numerous premalignant and early malignant changes and a progressive disease.

Treatment of Premalignant and Malignant Lesions

The local application of 5% 5-fluorouracil ointment, retinoic acid (0.05 to 0.1%), 2% isotretinoin, or some stronger new retinoid (0.5% arotinoid sulfone cream) or lotion is effective for very early malignancies and premalignant lesions. Advanced tumors should be removed either by surgery or cryosurgery. Radiotherapy is contraindicated. X-rays are one of the most potent cocarcinogens for HPV-induced lesions; after regression of irradiated tumors, there are usually recurrences displaying invasive growth and higher malignancy, and sometimes metastases.

Because there are usually numerous steadily appearing and progressive malignant lesions on the forehead, we replace the frontal skin with a lesion-free graft taken from the interior aspect of the arm. Healing is very good, probably because of the increased activity of TGF-β in EV lesions. We have not seen cancers in the grafts during 14 years of follow-up, while in the surrounding skin numerous premalignant and early malignant lesions have developed.

Interferons

Interferons-α, -β, and -γ have been tried at various doses (1, 1.5, 3, 6, 9 million U/day), but the improvement was transitional.[20] Another experimental therapy is the combined use of etretinate or isotretinoin with interferon-α_2 (1.5 to 6 million U/day). The experimental intralesional application of interferons-α or -γ appears to be a promising method of treatment for Bowen's carcinomas, both in situ and microinvasive, and for basal cell carcinomas originating from actinic keratoses. Interferon is given in injections of 3 million U two to three times weekly for 3 to 4 weeks. Some tumors regress, and histologic examination does not show any trace of malignancy. Because this heritable disease is lifelong and potentially dangerous, experimental therapies with retinoids and interferons are worth trying.

Immunologic Therapies

These therapies aimed at provoking immune responses are unsuccessful because the defect of cellular immunity is apparently specific for the HPV type and cannot be overcome by nonspecific stimulation. Sensitization with dinitrochlorobenzene (DNCB) is ineffective because, in this population; DNCB allergy cannot be evoked.

Prevention

The greatest priority is preventing premalignant and malignant lesions. Children in affected families should use sunscreens and avoid exposure to sunlight. Since the disease appears to be transmitted as an autosomal recessive trait, the children of patients with EV are usually unaffected.

X-ray therapy for any lesions of EV is strongly contraindicated. Frontal skin with numerous malignancies should be replaced by a skin graft from the non-sun-exposed areas to prevent deeply destructive tumors. Prevention by effective vaccination or other means is not yet possible.

Course and Prognosis

The course of the disease induced by EV HPVs or by mixed infection with EV HPV and HPV-3 is, in most cases, progressive. However, the rate of progression differs considerably. In some patients with widespread benign lesions, there are no carcinomas, and the tumors, if they develop, are of the papilloma type. In a large percentage of patients, actinic keratoses appear in the third and fourth decades of life, and both carcinoma in situ and invasive tumors appear initially on the forehead, then on the trunk and extremities. This malignant transformation originates from actinic keratoses. If patients are protected from carcinogens, their general health is satisfactory. In two heavily immunosuppressed patients we have seen malignancies not related to HPV (lymphoma in one case, and astrocytoma in another).

In EV associated with HPV-3, there is no danger of malignant conversion unless the patients become additionally infected with EV HPVs. However, HPV-3-induced disease is also usually unresponsive to any therapy and the lesions are lifelong. Since this population has more depressed cell-mediated immunity than patients with the variety induced by EV HPVs, they are more prone to concomitant viral, bacterial, and mycotic infections.

We have observed an unusual case of regression of HPV-3-induced familial EV after two consecutive pregnancies and deliveries. In two other patients with HPV-3-induced EV, infection with EV HPVs developed progressively and Bowen's type carcinomas appeared in sun-exposed areas. This pattern favors a close relationship between EV associated with specific HPVs and the form associated with HPV-3. The latter cannot be regarded as a harmless disease.

References

1. Lewandowsky F, Lutz W: Ein Fall einer bisher nicht beschriebenen Hauterkrankung. Epidermodysplasia verruciformis. *Arch Dermatol* **141**:193, 1922
2. Jablonska S et al: Epidermodysplasia verruciformis as a model in studies on the role of papovavirus in oncogenesis. *Cancer Res* **32**:585, 1972
3. Orth G et al: Characterization of two types of human papillomavirus in lesions of epidermodysplasia verruciformis. *Proc Natl Acad Sci USA* **75**:1537, 1978
4. Lutzner M et al: A potentially oncogenic human papillomavirus (HPV5) found in two renal allograft recipients. *J Invest Dermatol* **75**:353, 1980
5. Gassenmaier A et al: Papillomavrius DNA in warts of immunosuppressed renal allograft recipients. *Arch Dermatol Res* **278**:219, 1986
6. Barr BBB et al: Human papilloma virus infection and skin cancer in renal allograft recipients. *Lancet* **2**:124, 1989
7. Jablonska S: Human papillomaviruses in skin carcinomas, in *Papillomaviruses and Human Cancer,* edited by H Pfister. Boca Raton, FL, CRC Press, 1990, p 45
8. Orth G: Epidermodysplasia verruciformis, in *The Papovaviridae*, vol. 2, *The Papillomaviruses,* edited by HP Salzman, PM Howley. New York, Plenum, 1987, p 199
9. Orth G et al: Epidermodysplasia verruciformis: A model for the role of papillomaviruses in human cancer. *Cold Spring Harbor Conference on Cell Proliferation* **7**:259, 1980
10. Ostrow RC et al: Human papillomavirus DNA in cutaneous primary and metastasized squamous cell carcinomas from patients with epidermodysplasia verruciformis. *Proc Natl Acad Sci USA* **79**:1634, 1982
11. Jablonska S, Orth G: Epidermodysplasia verruciformis. *Clin Dermatol* **3**:83, 1985
12. Prose NS et al: Widespread flat warts associated with human papillomavirus type 5: A cutaneous manifestation of human immunodeficiency virus infection. *J Am Acad Dermatol* **23**:978, 1990
13. Majewski S et al: Partial defects of cell-mediated immunity in patients with epidermodysplasia verruciformis. *J Am Acad Dermatol* **15**:966, 1986
14. Majewski S et al: Natural cell-mediated cytotoxicity against various target cells in patients with epidermodysplasia verruciformis. *J Am Acad Dermatol* **22**:423, 1990
15. Cooper KD et al: Antigen presentation and T-cell activation in epidermodysplasia verruciformis. *J Invest Dermatol* **94**:769, 1990
16. Orth G et al: Epidermodysplasia verruciformis: Characteristics of the lesions and risk of malignant conversion as related to the type of human papillomavirus lesions. *Cancer Res* **39**:1074, 1979
17. Pfister H: Detection of human papillomavirus infection and prospects for diagnosis, in *Papillomaviruses and Human Cancer,* edited by H Pfister. Boca Raton, FL, CRC Press, 1990, p 226
18. Lutzner MA et al: Oral aromatic retinoid (Ro 10-9359) treatment of two patients suffering with the severe form of epidermodysplasia verruciformis, in *Retinoids,* edited by CE Orfanos et al. Berlin, Springer Verlag, 1981, p 407
19. Jablonska S et al: Ro-9359 in epidermodysplasia verruciformis, in *Retinoids,* edited by CE Orfanos et al. Berlin, Springer Verlag, 1981, p 401
20. Androphy EJ et al: Response of warts in epidermodysplasia verruciformis to treatment with systemic and intralesional alpha interferon. *J Am Acad Dermatol* **11**:197, 1984

CHAPTER 214

E. Tschachler, B. Hanchard, and M.S. Reitz, Jr.

Human Retroviral Disease: Human T-Lymphotropic Viruses

Viruses have attracted attention as pathogens in malignant and autoimmune diseases in animals ever since Peyton Rous discovered, at the beginning of the century, that a virus could cause solid tumors in fowls.[1] The Rous sarcoma virus, named after its discoverer, turned out to contain an RNA genome[2] but appeared to exist as a DNA provirus in infected cells.[3,4] This paradox was resolved when Baltimore[5] and Temin and Mizutani[6] independently discovered a polymerase that was able to use RNA as a template to produce DNA, i.e., the reverse transcriptase (RT). Viruses that contain an RNA genome and an RNA-dependent DNA polymerase belong to the family of Retroviridae (for an extensive review of taxonomy of retroviruses see reference 7).

Much effort was invested during the 1960s and 1970s in the search for human retroviruses in various diseases, and a plethora of reports claiming evidence for the existence of human retroviruses detected by electron microscopy,[8-12] reverse transcriptase activity,[13-15] serologic cross-reactivity,[16-18] and nucleic acid homology[19,20] has been compiled over the past decades. However, the lack of convincing evidence led many researchers to believe that human retroviruses did not exist until Poiesz and coworkers, in 1980, isolated a retrovirus from lymphocytes of a patient with cutaneous T-cell lymphoma[21] and subsequently from a patient with leukemia classified as Sézary syndrome.[22] Independently of this work, Miyoshi and coworkers isolated a retrovirus from a coculture of normal blood T lymphocytes with lymphocytes from a Japanese leukemia patient.[23,24] In the following years, the U.S. and Japanese isolates were shown to be indistinguishable by nucleic acid comparison,[25,26] and the name *human T-cell leukemia virus* type I (HTLV-I) was proposed[27] for all isolates previously called adult T-cell leukemia virus (ATLV) in Japan and HTLV in the United States. The association between the infection by HTLV-I and the occurrence of adult T-cell leukemia/lymphoma (ATL), as defined by Uchiyama and coworkers,[28] had been well established in the meantime by seroepidemiologic[29-33] and molecular[25,34-37] studies.

In 1982, a second human retrovirus, related to but distinct from HTLV-I,[38] was isolated from a cell line derived from a patient with hairy cell leukemia[39] and was named HTLV-II.[38] Although isolated from a leukemic patient, a clear association to a distinct disease has not been accomplished for HTLV-II so far.

Since the discovery of the HTLVs, other human retroviruses—human immunodeficiency virus types 1 and 2 (HIV-1 and -2)—have been isolated, and HIV-1 has been identified as the infectious agent that causes the acquired immunodeficiency syndrome (AIDS, see Chap. 215). Human retrovirology has become a very rapidly developing area of medical research during the last decade.

Virology

HTLV-I and -II are related but distinct type C human retroviruses. Many strains of HTLV-I have been isolated from different areas of the world, including the United States, the Caribbean islands, and Japan.[40] From sequencing data obtained from different laboratories, it appears that the overall sequence variation between different HTLV-I isolates is no higher than 3.5 percent.[41-45] Although the genomic organization of HTLV-I and -II is quite similar, the nucleotide sequence conservation between these two viruses is only about 55 percent.[46] Like other enveloped retroviruses, their genome consists of a dimer of identical RNA subunits. After infection of host cells the RNA genome is transcribed into DNA by the viral RT. The viral DNA is subsequently integrated into the host cell genome as a provirus. The organization of the HTLV-I provirus is depicted in Fig. 214-1; it contains dual long terminal repeats (LTR) at the 3′ and 5′ ends and *gag, pol,* and *env* genes that encode integral components of the virions. In addition to these genes, both the HTLV-I and -II genomes contain an extra sequence of about 1.6 kb between the *env* and the 3′ LTR, which was originally called "pX."[34] Whereas the full-length genomic RNA codes for *gag* and *pol* proteins, and the *env* proteins are translated from singly spliced mRNAs, the pX genes are expressed from RNA produced by double splicing mechanisms. The pX region codes for two transregulatory genes termed *tax* (*t*ransactivator in the region *x*) and *rex* (*re*gulator in the region *x*). The functions of these two genes have been elucidated in the past few years: genes in the pX region are essential for HTLV replication.[47] The 40-kDa HTLV-I *tax*-gene product acts in trans by activating the viral LTR[48,49] and increasing viral RNA synthesis, and the 27-kDa *rex* protein promotes the export of the viral structural, i.e., genomic, and envelope mRNAs to the cytoplasm,[50] where they can be translated. (For review of regulation of HTLV-I gene expression see reference 51.)

In contrast to its name, which suggests a limited host cell range, HTLV-I can productively infect a wide variety of cells of different species in vitro.[52-54] Infection of human, monkey, and rabbit T lymphocytes by HTLV-I in vitro leads to their continuous growth in tissue culture and the development of cell lines with growth characteristics of transformed cells.[24,55-58]

The exact mechanisms that lead to transformation after HTLV-I infection are not known because, unlike rapidly transforming animal retroviruses,[59] the HTLV-I genome lacks cell-derived oncogenes that could account for its capacity to immortalize cells. HTLV-I seems also not to transform cells by integrating at a specific site in the host genome. Although monoclonal integration of the virus is observed in HTLV-I–associated ATL,[37,60] no common site of integration has been found in the analysis of tumor cells from different patients.[36] Although it has not been formally proven, it is generally thought that HTLV-I regulatory genes participate in HTLV-I–mediated transformation of infected cells. It has been shown that HTLV-I *tax* not only acts on the viral promoter[48,49] but also serves to transactivate cellular genes, including genes for cytokines and cytokine receptors.[61-63] Additional lines of evidence that HTLV-I regulatory genes participate in leukemogenesis come from a report by Grassman et al.,[64] who showed that introduction of the pX region into primary human T lympho-

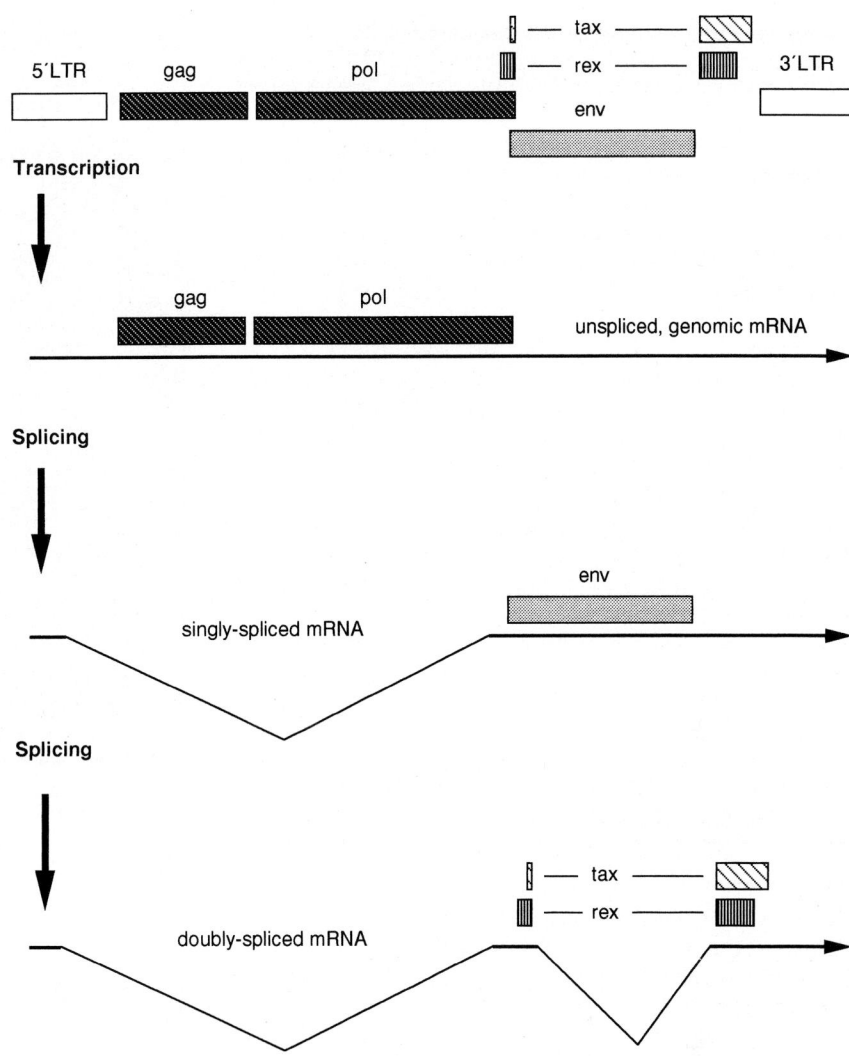

FIGURE 214-1 Genomic organization of the HTLV-I provirus and expression of viral structural and regulatory genes.

cytes is sufficient to initiate continuous growth of these cells in culture in the presence of interleukin 2 (IL-2). In this context it is also of interest that mice transgenic for the HTLV-I *tax* gene develop nerve sheath tumors in which the *tax* protein is expressed.[65]

Although HTLV-II has been less well studied than HTLV-I, most of the properties described for the latter, including the transformation of T cells in vitro and the presence and importance of transregulatory genes, are also true for the former.[47,66] To date, however, no disease has been associated with HTLV-II infection, except for two cases of a rare T-cell variant of hairy cell leukemia.[38]

Epidemiology

The regional distribution of infection with HTLV-I and -II has been determined primarily by seroepidemiologic methods using immunofluorescence assays with fixed infected cells as a substrate; by enzyme-linked immunosorbent assay (ELISA) or radioimmunoassay (RIA) employing whole disrupted virus; and by radioimmunoprecipitation assays using labeled purified viral proteins. At this level HTLV-I infection cannot be distinguished from HTLV-II infection,[67,68] and epidemiologic data obtained primarily by serol-

ogy should refer to HTLV-I/II rather than HTLV-I seroprevalence. To accomplish distinction of the two viruses, virus isolation and typing with monoclonal antibodies or nucleic acid analysis had to be performed in the past. More recently, quick distinction between infection with HTLV-I and -II has become feasible through amplification and analysis of distinct viral sequences from infected cells by the polymerase chain reaction (PCR).[67,68]

By seroepidemiologic and molecular studies, HTLV-I shows an endemic pattern in southern Japan, comprising Kyushu, Shikoku, and the Ryuku islands including Okinawa,[69] where seroprevalence ranges from 1 up to 36 percent, depending on the location and the age group investigated.[70,71] Similar endemic patterns can be found in the Caribbean islands, particularly Jamaica, Trinidad, Tobago, Martinique, Haiti, Guadeloupe, and Barbados,[69] and in equatorial Africa.[72,73]

Other clusters of HTLV-I/II seropositive populations have been reported from Panama,[74] Brazil,[75] Colombia,[76] and Venezuela.[77] In the United States the presence of HTLV-I was confirmed in certain populations for the first time in 1982.[78] A more recent seroepidemiologic survey performed by the American Red Cross showed a seroprevalence for HTLV-I/II of 0.025 percent among 39,898 U.S. blood donors in eight geographically diverse areas,[79] and clusters of HTLV-I/II seropositivity have been reported among intravenous drug users.[67,80]

The mode of transmission of HTLV-I/II appears to be quite analogous to that of HIV-1, although in contrast to HIV-1, which can be transmitted cell-free, HTLV-I/II is poorly infectious except by cell-to-cell contact, which makes it less infectious than HIV-1. Ample epidemiologic data exist primarily from longitudinal studies in Japan, and it has become well established that sexual transmission of HTLV-I from male-to-female, female-to-male, and male-to-male occurs.[69,81,82] In vertical transmission of HTLV-I, transmission from mother to child via breast feeding appears to play a more important role than perinatal or intrauterine transmission.[83,84] Programs to eradicate HTLV-I from the endemic areas in Japan by changing the habits of breast feeding are underway.

In parenteral transmission, approximately one-half of patients who received transfusions from an HTLV-I–infected donor seroconverted[85,86] whereas cell-free fresh frozen plasma appears not to be infectious.[86] Transfusion-mediated HTLV-I infection in Japan has been virtually terminated by mass screening of donated blood. In the United States, a screening program for blood units was initiated in 1989. Parenteral transmission via needle sharing very likely accounts for the clusters of HTLV-I/II seropositivity in intravenous drug users in certain areas of the United States and Europe. There is no indication that arthropod-borne transmission of HTLV-I occurs.

The Natural Course of HTLV-I Infection and Clinical Disease Spectrum

Although HTLV-I was initially isolated from leukemic patients, infection with this virus does not necessarily lead to development of leukemia. From Japanese epidemiologic studies, it appears that the annual incidence rate of ATL among HTLV-I carriers older than 40 years is approximately 0.6 to 1.7 per 1000.[87] The cumulative incidence rate of ATL in HTLV-I carriers approximates 2 to 5 percent. The latent period from infection to outbreak of leukemia is 20 years or more, as concluded from migrant studies.[88] The average age of onset of ATL[89] differs in patients from Japan (56 years) and the Caribbean (43 years).

Neurologic Disease

HTLV-I has been implicated as the causative agent in chronic progressive myelopathies, i.e., *tropical spastic paraparesis* (TSP) in the Caribbean[90] and *HTLV-I–associated myelopathy* (HAM) in Japan.[91] Because these two conditions appear to be identical, the terms *TSP* and *HAM* are now used synonymously. Patients suffering from TSP/HAM are generally younger than ATL patients, and the latency from infection to development of clinical neurologic symptoms has been described to be very short in individual cases.[92]

Concomitant Infectious Disease

Infective dermatitis (Fig. 214-2) is a severe, chronic relapsing eczema in children,[93] associated with infection by *Staphylococcus aureus* and beta-hemolytic *Streptococcus*.[94] The association of infective dermatitis with HTLV-I infection has recently been reported.[95] Bacterial infection in infective dermatitis is difficult to control and although it responds to antibiotic treatment, prolonged

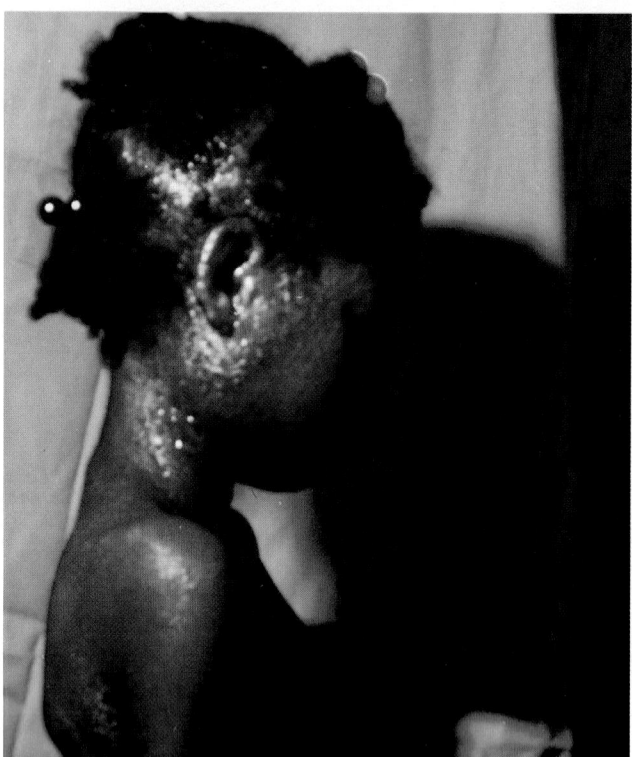

FIGURE 214-2 Infective dermatitis in a 10-year-old HTLV-I–infected Jamaican girl. (*Courtesy of L. LaGrenade, M.D., University of the West Indies, Kingston, Jamaica.*)

therapy is necessary and relapses are common after discontinuation.[95] Immunosuppression observed by other investigators in HTLV-I carriers[96] as well as in ATL patients[97–100] may play a role in the pathogenesis of infective dermatitis. Future longitudinal epidemiologic and molecular studies should help to elucidate the contribution of disturbances of the immune system to the clinical picture observed in infective dermatitis. Such studies should also help to answer the question raised by LaGrenade and coworkers[95]: whether infective dermatitis represents a "preleukemic syndrome" that ultimately leads to the development of ATL. Indeed, long-lasting (21 years) cutaneous prodromes have been described in a patient who finally developed ATL.[101] Further evidence for infective dermatitis in childhood being associated with subsequent development of ATL comes from a recent report on a patient in Jamaica who developed ATL 17 years after having been diagnosed as having infective dermatitis.[102]

Immunosuppression and development of *opportunistic infections* are complications frequently observed in ATL patients,[98–100] and Essex and colleagues have reported that HTLV-I–infected individuals are overrepresented among patients hospitalized for infectious diseases in an endemic area in southwestern Japan.[103] In this context it is interesting that lymphocytes from healthy HTLV-I carriers[104] and from TSP/HAM patients[105] proliferate spontaneously in vitro and this indicates that subtle disturbances of immunoregulation can occur without manifestations of HTLV-I–associated disease.

Besides the diseases mentioned, there are also reports of other disorders occurring in HTLV-I infected patients, such as *polymyositis*[106] *chronic inflammatory arthropathy*,[107] and *peripheral neuropathy*.[108] However, future epidemiologic and virologic studies

TABLE 214-1
Clinical Signs of ATL*

	Geographic area		
	Southeast United States[99]	Japan[110]	Caribbean[102]
Leukemia	80%[†]	90%	60%
Bone marrow involvement	30%	45%	63%
Lymphadenopathy	100%	48%	87%
Spleen involvement	NR[‡]	55%	37%[§]
Liver involvement	(2/2)[¶]	52%	37%[§]
CNS involvement	20%	NR	NR
Skin involvement	70%	52%	35%
Lytic bone lesions	(4/8)[¶]	NR	15%
Number of patients	10	29	82

*Without differentiation between acute, smoldering, chronic, or crisis type ATL.
†Percentage of patients showing involvement.
‡NR: not reported.
§Reported as hepatosplenomegaly.
¶Number of patients showing involvement/number of patients tested.

will be necessary to establish a causative role of the virus in the pathogenesis of these diseases.

Adult T-Cell Leukemia/Lymphoma

ATL was first described by Uchiyama and coworkers in 1977[28] as a distinct malignancy of mature T cells occurring primarily in patients born in southwestern Japan. In 1982, Catovsky and coworkers[109] described ATL in West Indian immigrants in London; this encouraged Blattner and colleagues[32] to investigate the West Indies as a major region where HTLV-I infection and ATL are endemic. HTLV-I was linked to ATL by virus isolation from leukemic cells[23,24,55,56] as well as by extensive seroepidemiologic[29–33] and molecular studies.[25,35–37]

Three different courses have been described: (1) *acute, prototype ATL,* (2) *chronic ATL,*[110] and (3) *smoldering ATL.*[111] Smoldering and chronic ATL may convert into acute ATL, which has led some authors to speak of *crisis-type ATL.*[111] Recently still another form, i.e., *cutaneous-type ATL,* has been proposed by Jono and colleagues[112] for patients with involvement of the skin but without leukemia and without apparent signs of involvement of other organs.

Prototype ATL is a fatal malignancy of adult onset with a clinical presentation that appears to be identical in all endemic areas.[28,98,99,109,113,114] It is characterized by the variable combination of multiorgan involvement (Table 214-1) with the presence of multilobate leukemic cells in the peripheral blood (Fig. 214-3). Organ involvement can add significantly to morbidity; central nervous system involvement may alter the mental status of the patient[99]; involvement of the liver may lead to abnormalities in liver function tests and jaundice[99]; and lung involvement may lead to tachypnea, dyspnea, and cyanosis.[99,115]

The skin involvement in ATL varies considerably among patients but is present to a variable degree in all forms of ATL.[99,110,111,113,114,116] Skin lesions may appear as uncharacteristic erythematous patches, as papular and nodular tumors (Fig. 214-4), and as erythroderma. Nonspecific skin lesions may precede the onset of acute ATL for up to 2 decades.[101] Specific skin infiltrates may occur as first manifestations of ATL,[110] and show monoclonality of skin-infiltrating cells by the criteria both of T-cell-receptor rearrangement and integration of HTLV-I DNA.

This occurs at a time when circulating T cells of these patients still appear unaffected.[116] For this latter situation, the term *cutaneous-type ATL* has been proposed.[112] However, it is questionable whether this form indeed represents an independent course of ATL or reflects improved diagnostic measures that lead to very early diagnosis of prototype or chronic ATL.

A striking feature in a high percentage of patients with acute ATL is a refractory hypercalcemia, which may represent the first sign of the disease and indicates an aggressive course.[98,99,109,110,117] Patients may present with weakness, lethargy, polyuria, and polydypsia. Lytic bone lesions resembling those of multiple myeloma are often present at diagnosis, and levels of alkaline phosphatase may be elevated.[98,99,109,110,114,118] Parathyroid hormone levels[98] and 1,25-dihydroxyvitamin D levels[119] are normal in ATL patients with hypercalcemia, and it has been postulated that factors produced by leukemic cells are involved in osteoclast activation that leads to the clinical symptoms.[98] A variety of cytokines produced by HTLV-I–infected cells or cells derived from ATL patients[120,121] have been suggested to account for hypercalcemia and bone resorption in ATL patients.

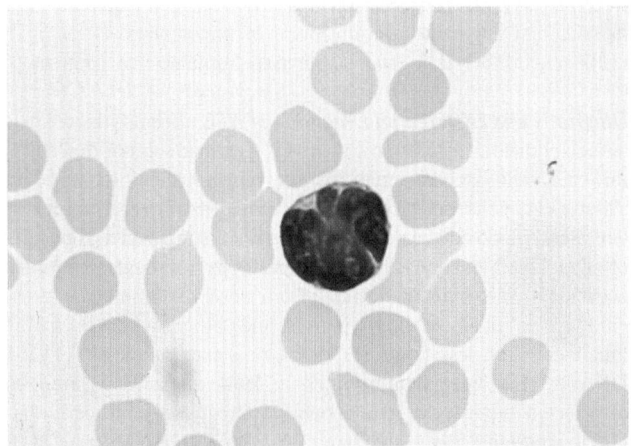

FIGURE 214-3 Abnormal lymphocyte with multilobate nucleus ("flower cell") from the peripheral blood of a patient with ATL. (*Courtesy of K. Takatsuki, M.D., Kumamoto University, Japan.*)

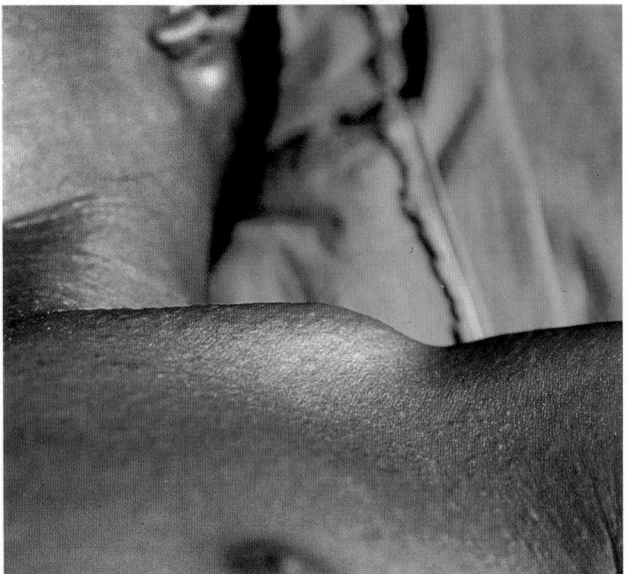

a

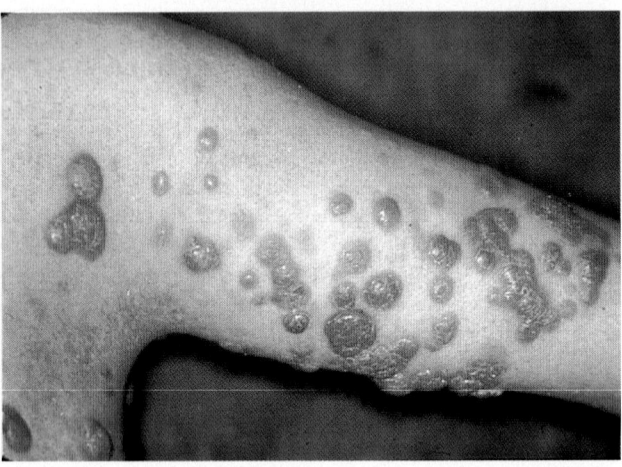

c

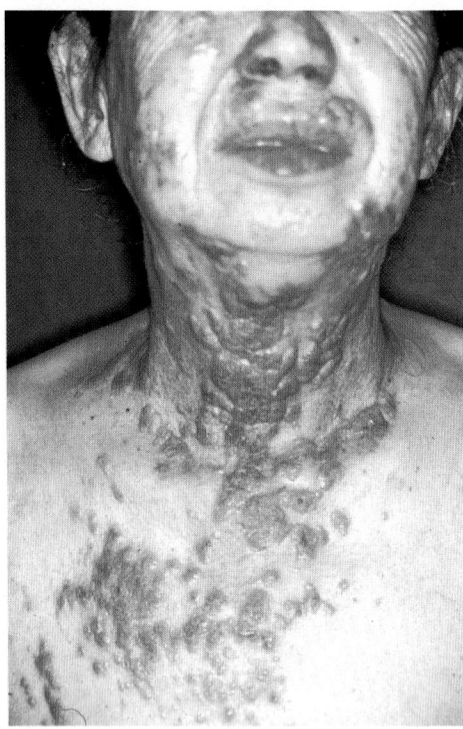

b

FIGURE 214-4 Skin manifestations of ATL. (*a*) Generalized papular infiltrates and enlarged retroauricular lymph node in a Jamaican patient with prototype ATL. (*b* and *c*) Nodular skin tumors in Japanese ATL patients. (*Courtesy of K. Takatsuki, M.D., Kumamoto University, Japan.*)

Recently, several reports established a link between hypercalcemia in ATL and augmented serum levels of tumor necrosis factor α (TNF-α),[122] TNF-β,[123] and parathyroid hormone-like peptide.[124]

Diagnosis and Differential Diagnosis of ATL Besides the characteristic clinical course of prototype ATL, examination of the leukemic cells yields a characteristic picture: numerous multilobate cells, called ATL cells or "flower" cells (Fig. 214-3), are present in peripheral blood and can usually be readily distinguished from cells of other T-cell leukemias by light microscopy, although sometimes occasional cells indistinguishable from Sézary cells may be present.[98,125–127] In smoldering-type ATL and chronic-type ATL multilobate cells are less frequent. Monoclonal integration of HTLV-I DNA[36,37] has been demonstrated in leukemic cells as well as in affected organs. By immunophenotyping, leukemic cells display predominantly a mature CD2+/CD3+/CD4+/CD8 − /CD25 + phenotype.[128–131] Although most of these T-cell markers can be found on other T-cell malignancies, the expression of CD25 can be regarded as a distinguishing marker between ATL and Sézary syndrome.[131]

The histopathologic features seen in affected organs and lymph nodes (Fig. 214-5*a*) are more variable than the picture encountered in peripheral blood, and ATL is associated with lymphomas of several histologic subtypes (Table 214-2). Distinction of ATL from other peripheral T-cell lymphomas, especially HTLV-I–positive and –negative cases, cannot be accomplished on morphologic grounds alone. Evaluation of the clinical picture, course of the disease, and the presence of multilobate lymphocytes in the peripheral blood are essential for diagnosis. Difficulties can also be encountered in differentiating skin involvement of ATL from mycosis fungoides/Sézary syndrome, since focal epidermal infiltration by T cells or Pautrier's microabscesses (Fig. 214-5*b*) can be present in skin lesions of ATL.[135,136] Indeed, the diseases of patients from whom the original U.S. HTLV-I isolates were obtained were classified as Sézary syndrome[22] and cutaneous T-cell lymphoma,[21] respectively. Seropositivity for HTLV-I and/or the presence of HTLV-I provirus in the leukemia cells and lymphomatous lesions establish the diagnosis of ATL.

Prognosis and Therapy of ATL Acute ATL is an aggressive disease with a poor prognosis. The presence of hypercalcemia, high LDH levels, and an excessively high white blood cell count indicate a 50 percent survival time of less than 6 months.[137] Controlled randomized studies comparing different therapeutic protocols have not been performed for ATL. Combination cytotoxic therapy (CHOP, COMLA, VEPA, CAP) has been reported by several groups[28,99,109,110]; however, long-term remission cannot be ob-

TABLE 214-2
Histologic Classification of ATL as Compared in Three Classification Systems for Non-Hodgkin's Lymphoma

Rappaport[132]	Working formulation[133]	Lymphoma Study Group[134]	Number of patients (%)		
			Hanchard et al.[102]	Chan et al.[135]	Broder et al.[98]
Well-differentiated lymphocytic	Small cell	Small cell	2(3)	2(2)	0
Poorly differentiated lymphocytic	Unclassifiable	Medium-sized cell	7(11)	34(36)	2(15)
Mixed cell	Mixed small and large	Mixed cell	10(16)	8(8)	5(38)
Histiocytic/ undifferentiated	Large cell	Large cell, small, noncleaved	33(52)	8(8)	1(8)
Histiocytic/ mixed cell	Large cell, immunoblastic	Pleomorphic	11(18)	40(42)	5(38)
Other	Other	Other	—	3(3)	—
Total number of patients			63	95	13

SOURCE: Modified from Broder et al.[98]

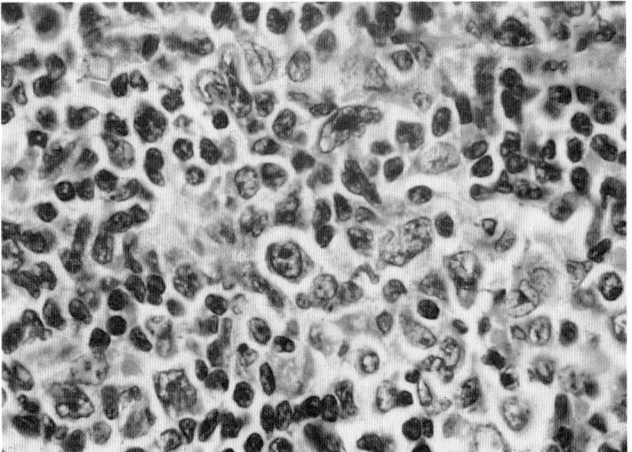

a

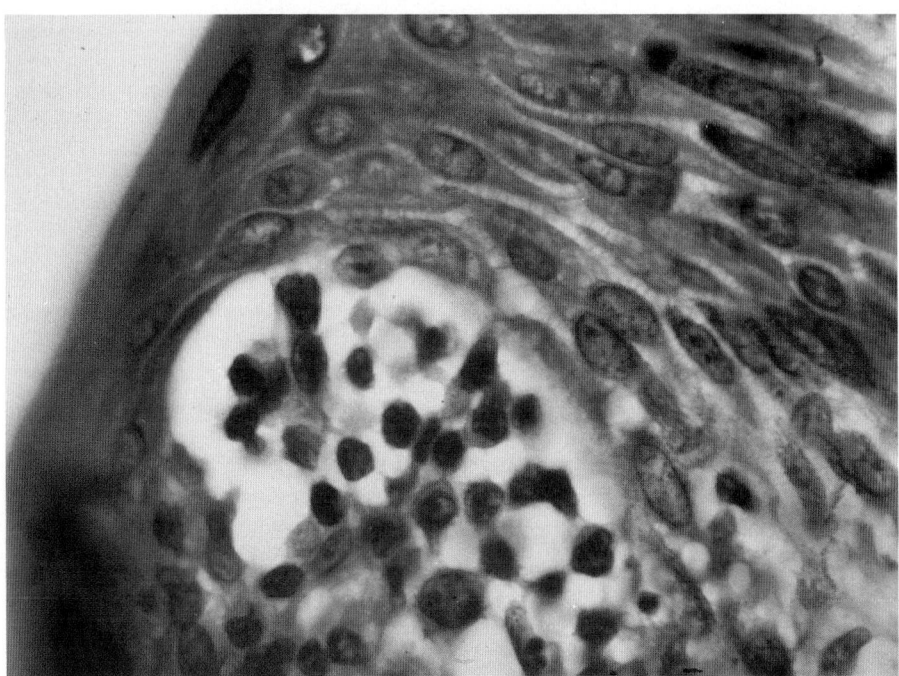

b

tained with any of the therapeutic approaches reported. Complications of chemotherapy include septicemia and opportunistic infections.[99,110,117] The course of smoldering and chronic ATL is less dramatic, and involvement of inner organs and hypercalcemia are observed less frequently.[110,111] Because patients suffering from smoldering or chronic ATL have a better prognosis than those with acute ATL, they should not be treated by chemotherapy unless they enter a more acute phase of their disease.

ATL cells express IL-2-receptor alpha chain (CD25) moieties on their surface.[129,131] This feature has led investigators to employ anti-CD25 antibodies to target leukemic cells.[98] Although antibodies alone are not effective, results obtained with antibodies coupled to Ricin A or other toxic agents might prove promising in the future. Another therapeutic approach following the same avenue is currently being followed in Japan where a fusion protein between IL-2 and diphtheria toxin is being investigated as a possible thera-

FIGURE 214-5 (*a*) Histology of a lymph node of an ATL patient showing pleomorphic large cell lymphoma. (*b*) Pautrier's microabscess in a cutaneous lesion of an ATL patient.

peutic agent.[89] Extracorporeal photochemotherapy,[138] as an alternative therapeutic protocol primarily for the treatment of chronic and smoldering ATL, is also currently being investigated in Japan.[89]

The Role of HTLV-I–Related Retroviruses in Cutaneous T-Cell Lymphoma (CTCL)

Reports about the presence of retroviral particles in the skin and lymph nodes of patients with mycosis fungoides and Sézary syndrome and in T-cell lines from a Sézary syndrome patient[139–141] have, in the past, implicated a retrovirus in the pathogenesis of these diseases. Serologic surveys for HTLV-I in CTCL patients from the United States and Europe revealed seropositivity rates of less than 1 percent[142] and up to 12 percent,[143] respectively. Recently, Manzari and coworkers demonstrated the presence of nucleic acid sequences cross-hybridizing with HTLV-I in a B-cell line derived from a patient with a CD25− CTCL.[144] Other investigators found HTLV-I–related sequences in DNA from cutaneous lesions of HTLV-I–seronegative patients with CD30+ CTCL[145] and in a cell line derived from a mycosis fungoides patient by Southern hybridization. Furthermore, sequences related to different parts of HTLV-I could be amplified from DNA of skin lesions of five HTLV-I–seronegative mycosis fungoides patients by PCR.[146] It is not established at the moment whether these HTLV-I–related sequences represent defective forms of HTLV-I or whether they represent parts of a HTLV-I–related virus. Future investigations, i.e., virus isolation and characterization, will be necessary to study the possible role of retrovirus in the pathogenesis of CTCL.

References

1. Rous P: A sarcoma of the fowl transmissible by an agent separable from the tumor cells. *J Exp Med* **13**:397, 1911
2. Crawford LV, Crawford EM: The properties of Rous sarcoma virus purified by density gradient centrifugation. *Virology* **13**:227, 1961
3. Temin H: The effects of actinomycin D on growth of Rous sarcoma virus in vitro. *Virology* **20**:577, 1963
4. Bader JP: The role of deoxyribonucleic acid in synthesis of Rous sarcoma virus. *Virology* **22**:462, 1964
5. Baltimore D: RNA-dependent DNA polymerase in virions of RNA tumor viruses. *Nature* **226**:1209, 1970
6. Temin H, Mizutani S: RNA-directed DNA polymerase in virions of Rous sarcoma virus. *Nature* **226**:1211, 1970
7. Teich N: Taxonomy of retroviruses, in *RNA Tumor Viruses*, edited by R Weiss et al. Cold Spring Harbor, NY, Cold Spring Harbor Laboratory, 1984, p 25
8. Burger CL et al: Virus-like particles in human leukemic plasma. *Proc Soc Exp Biol Med* **115**:151, 1964
9. Seman G, Seman C: Electron microscopic search for virus particles in patients with leukemia and lymphoma. *Cancer* **22**:1033, 1968
10. Parsons PG et al: Detection in human melanoma cell lines of particles with some properties in common with RNA tumour viruses. *Int J Cancer* **13**:606, 1974
11. Kalter SS et al: C-type particles in normal human placentas. *J Natl Cancer Inst* **50**:1081, 1973
12. Balda BR et al: Oncornavirus-like particles in human skin cancers. *Proc Natl Acad Sci USA* **72**:3697, 1975
13. Gallo RC et al: RNA dependent polymerase in human acute leukemic cells. *Nature* **228**:927, 1970
14. Kiessling AA et al: Deoxyribonucleic acid polymerase activity associated with a plasma particulate fraction from patients with chronic lymphocytic leukemia. *J Virol* **7**:221, 1971
15. Chandra P et al: Biochemical and immunological characterization of a reverse transcriptase from human melanoma tissue. *Cancer Lett* **5**:299, 1978
16. Stand M, August JT: Structural proteins of mammalian oncogenic RNA viruses: Multiple antigenic determinants of the major internal protein and envelope glycoprotein. *J Virol* **13**:171, 1974
17. Mellors RC, Mellors JW: Type C RNA virus-specific antibody in human systemic lupus erythematosus demonstrated by enzymeimmunoassay. *Proc Natl Acad Sci USA* **75**:2463, 1978
18. Lewis RM et al: C-type viruses in systemic lupus erythematosus. *Nature* **252**:78, 1974
19. Wong-Staal F et al: Proviral sequences of baboon endogenous type C RNA virus in DNA of human leukaemic tissues. *Nature* **262**:190, 1976
20. Reitz MS et al: Primate type-C virus nucleic acid sequences (wooly monkey and baboon types) in tissues from a patient with acute myelogenous leukemia and in viruses isolated from cultured cells of the same patient. *Proc Natl Acad Sci USA* **78**:2113, 1976
21. Poiesz BJ et al: Detection and isolation of type C retrovirus particles from fresh and cultured lymphocytes of a patient with cutaneous T-cell lymphoma. *Proc Natl Acad Sci USA* **77**:7415, 1980
22. Poiesz BJ et al: Isolation of a new type C retrovirus (HTLV) in primary uncultured cells of a patient with Sézary T-cell leukemia. *Nature* **294**:268, 1981
23. Miyoshi I et al: Type C virus particles in a cord blood T-cell line derived from cocultivating normal human cord leukocytes and human leukaemic T cells. *Nature* **294**:770, 1981
24. Miyoshi I et al: Transformation of normal human cord lymphocytes by co-cultivation with a lethally irradiated human T-cell line carrying type C virus particles. *GANN* **72**:997, 1981
25. Reitz MS et al: Relatedness by nucleic acid hybridization of new isolates of human T-cell leukemia-lymphoma virus (HTLV) and demonstration of provirus in uncultured leukemic blood cells. *Virology* **126**:688, 1983
26. Watanabe T et al: HTLV type I (U.S. isolate) and ATLV (Japanese isolate) are the same species of human retrovirus. *Virology* **133**:238, 1984
27. Watanabe T et al: Retrovirus terminology. *Science* **222**:1178, 1983
28. Uchiyama T et al: Adult T-cell leukemia in Japan: Clinical and hematologic features of 16 cases. *Blood* **50**:481, 1977
29. Hinuma Y et al: Antibodies to adult T-cell leukemia-virus-associated antigen (ATLA) in sera from patients with ATL and controls in Japan: A nation-wide sero-epidemiologic study. *Int J Cancer* **29**:631, 1982
30. Kalynaraman VS et al: Natural antibodies to the structural core protein (p24) of the human T-cell leukemia (lymphoma) retrovirus found in sera of leukemia patients in Japan. *Proc Natl Acad Sci USA* **79**:1653, 1982
31. Robert-Guroff M et al: Evidence for human T-cell lymphoma-leukemia virus infection of family members of human T-cell lymphoma-leukemia virus positive patients. *J Exp Med* **157**:248, 1983
32. Blattner WA et al: The human type-C retrovirus, HTLV in Blacks from the Caribbean region, and relationships to adult T-cell leukemia/lymphoma. *Int J Cancer* **30**:257, 1982
33. Yamamoto N et al: Adult T-cell leukemia (ATL) virus-specific antibodies in ATL patients and healthy virus carriers. *Int J Cancer* **32**:281, 1983
34. Seiki M et al: Human adult T-cell leukemia virus: Molecular cloning of the provirus DNA and the unique terminal structure. *Proc Natl Acad Sci USA* **79**:6899, 1982
35. Seiki M et al: Human adult T cell leukemia virus: Complete nucleotide sequence of the provirus genome integrated in leukemia cell DNA. *Proc Natl Acad Sci USA* **80**:3618, 1983
36. Seiki M et al: Nonspecific integration of the HTLV provirus in adult T-cell leukemia cells. *Nature* **309**:640, 1984

37. Yoshida M et al: Monoclonal integration of human T-cell leukemia provirus in all primary tumors of adult T-cell leukemia suggests causative role of human T-cell leukemia virus in the disease. *Proc Natl Acad Sci USA* **81**:2534, 1984

38. Kalyanaraman VS et al: A new subtype of human T-cell leukemia virus (HTLV-II) associated with a T-cell variant of hairy cell leukemia. *Science* **218**:571, 1982

39. Golde DW et al: Human T-lymphocyte cell line producing colony stimulating factor. *Blood* **52**:1068, 1978

40. Gallo RC: Human T-cell leukemia-lymphoma virus and T-cell malignancies in adults. *Cancer Surv* **3**:113, 1984

41. Ratner L: Molecular variation of human T-lymphotropic viruses and clinical associations, in *Human Retrovirology: HTLV*, edited by WA Blattner. New York, Raven, 1990, p 49

42. Ratner L et al: Nucleotide sequence analysis of a variant of human T-cell leukemia virus (HTLV-Ib) provirus with a deletion in pX-I. *J Virol* **54**:781, 1985

43. Malik KTA et al: Molecular cloning and complete nucleotide sequence of an adult T cell leukemia virus/human T cell leukemia virus type I (ATLV/HTLV-I) isolate of a Caribbean origin: Relationship to other members of the ATLV/HTLV-I subgroup. *J Gen Virol* **69**:1695, 1988

44. Hiramatsu K et al: Molecular cloning of the closed circular provirus of human T cell leukaemia virus type I: A new open reading frame in the *gag-pol* region. *J Gen Virol* **68**:213, 1987

45. Tsujimoto A et al: Nucleotide sequence analysis of a provirus derived from HTLV-I-associated myelopathy (HAM). *Mol Biol Med* **5**:29, 1988

46. Shimotohno K et al: Complete nucleotide sequence of an infectious clone of human T-cell leukemia virus type II: An open reading frame for the protease gene. *Proc Natl Acad Sci USA* **82**:3101, 1985

47. Chen ISY et al: The x gene is essential for HTLV replication. *Science* **229**:54, 1985

48. Sodroski JG et al: Trans-acting transcriptional activation of the long terminal repeat of human T lymphotropic viruses in infected cells. *Science* **225**:381, 1984

49. Felber BK et al: The pX protein of HTLV-I is a transcriptional activator of its long terminal repeats. *Science* **229**:675, 1985

50. Hidaka M et al: Post-transcriptional regulator (rex) of HTLV-I initiates expression of viral structural proteins but suppresses expression of regulatory proteins. *EMBO J* **7**:519, 1988

51. Smith MR, Greene WC: Molecular biology of the human T-cell leukemia virus (HTLV-I) and adult T-cell leukemia. *J Clin Invest* **87**:761, 1991

52. Clapham P et al: Productive infection and cell free transmission of human T-cell leukemia virus in a non-lymphoid cell line. *Science* **222**:1125, 1983

53. Weiss RA et al: Envelope properties of human T-cell leukemia viruses. *Curr Top Microbiol Immunol* **115**:235, 1985

54. Hoxie JA et al: Infection of human endothelial cells by human T-cell leukemia virus type 1. *Proc Natl Acad Sci USA* **81**:7591, 1984

55. Popovic M et al: Isolation and transmission of human retrovirus (human T-cell leukemia virus). *Science* **219**:856, 1983

56. Yamamoto N et al: Transformation of human leukocytes by cocultivation with an adult T-cell leukemia virus producer cell line. *Science* **217**:737, 1982

57. Miyoshi I et al: Transformation of monkey lymphocytes with adult T-cell leukemia virus. *Lancet* **1**:1016, 1982

58. Miyoshi I et al: Transformation of rabbit lymphocytes with T-cell leukemia virus. *GANN* **74**:1, 1983

59. Teich N et al: Pathogenesis of retrovirus-induced disease, in *RNA Tumor Viruses*, edited by R Weiss et al. Cold Spring Harbor, NY, Cold Spring Harbor Laboratory, 1984, p 785

60. Wong-Staal F et al: A survey of human leukemias for sequences of a human retrovirus. *Nature* **302**:626, 1983

61. Inoue J et al: Induction of interleukin-2 receptor gene expression by p40x encoded by human T-cell leukemia virus type I. *EMBO J* **5**:2883, 1986

62. Cross SL et al: Regulation of the human interleukin-2 receptor α chain promoter: Activation of a nonfunctional promoter by the trans-activator gene of HTLV-I. *Cell* **49**:47, 1987

63. Wano Y et al: Stable expression of the Tax gene of type I human T-cell leukemia virus in human T cell activates specific cellular genes involved in growth. *Proc Natl Acad Sci USA* **85**:9733, 1988

64. Grassman R et al: Transformation to continuous growth of primary human T lymphocytes by human T-cell leukemia virus type I X-region genes transduced by a Herpesvirus Saimirii vector. *Proc Natl Acad Sci USA* **86**:3351, 1989

65. Hinrichs SH et al: A transgenic mouse model for human neurofibromatosis. *Science* **237**:1340, 1987

66. Chen ISY et al: Human T-cell leukemia virus type II transforms normal human lymphocytes. *Proc Natl Acad Sci USA* **80**:7006, 1983

67. Lee H et al: High rate of HTLV-II infection in seropositive IV drug abusers in New Orleans. *Science* **244**:471, 1989

68. Kwok S et al: Enzymatic amplification of HTLV-I viral sequences from peripheral blood mononuclear cells and infected tissues. *Blood* **72**:1117, 1988

69. Blattner WA: Retroviruses, in *Viral Infections of Humans: Epidemiology and Control*, edited by AS Evans. New York, Plenum, 1989, p 545

70. Maeda Y et al: Prevalence of possible adult T-cell leukemia virus carriers among volunteer blood donors in Japan: A nation-wide study. *Int J Cancer* **33**:717, 1984

71. Kajiyama W et al: Seroepidemiologic study of antibody to adult T-cell leukemia virus in Okinawa, Japan. *Am J Epidemiol* **123**:41, 1986

72. Saxinger WC et al: Human T-cell leukemia virus (HTLV-I) antibodies in Africa. *Science* **225**:1473, 1984

73. de Thé G et al: Human retroviruses HTLV-I, HIV-1 and HIV-2 and neurological diseases in some equatorial areas of Africa. *AIDS* **2**:550, 1989

74. Reeves WC et al: Human T-cell lymphotropic virus type I (HTLV-I) seroepidemiology and risk factors in metropolitan Panama. *Am J Epidemiol* **127**:532, 1988

75. Cortes E et al: HIV-1, HIV-2 and HTLV-I in high-risk groups in Brazil. *N Engl J Med* **320**:953, 1989

76. Maloney EM et al: A survey of the human T-cell lymphotropic virus type I (HTLV-I) in southwestern Colombia. *Int J Cancer* **44**:419, 1989

77. Merino F et al: Natural antibodies to human T cell leukemia/lymphoma virus in healthy Venezuelan population. *Int J Cancer* **34**:501, 1984

78. Blayney DW et al: The human T-cell leukemia-lymphoma virus in the southeastern United States. *JAMA* **250**:1048, 1983

79. Williams AE et al: Seroprevalence and epidemiological correlates of HTLV-I infection in U.S. blood donors. *Science* **240**:643, 1988

80. Robert Guroff M et al: Prevalence of antibodies to HTLV-I, -II and -III in intravenous drug abusers from an AIDS endemic region. *JAMA* **255**:3133, 1986

81. Bartholomew C et al: Transmission of HTLV-I and HIV among homosexuals in Trinidad. *JAMA* **257**:2604, 1987

82. Tajima K et al: Epidemiological features of HTLV-I carriers and incidence of ATL in an ATL-endemic island: A report of the community-based co-operative study in Tsushima, Japan. *Int J Cancer* **40**:741, 1987

83. Hino S et al: Mother-to-child transmission of human T-cell leukemia virus type I. *Jpn J Cancer Res* **76**:474, 1985

84. Ando Y et al: Transmission of adult T-cell leukemia retrovirus (HTLV-I) from mother to child: Comparison of bottle- with breast-fed babies. *Jpn J Cancer Res* **78**:322, 1987

85. Hino S et al: Transfusion-mediated spread of the human T-cell leukemia virus in chronic hemodialysis patients in a heavily endemic area, Nagasaki. *GANN* **75**:1070, 1984

86. Okochi K et al: A retrospective study on transmission of adult T cell leukemia virus by blood transfusion: Seroconversion in recipients. *Vox Sang* **46**:245, 1985

87. Kondo T et al: Risk of adult T-cell leukemia/lymphoma in HTLV-I carriers. *Lancet* **2**:159, 1987

88. Greaves MF et al: Human T-cell leukemia virus (HTLV) in the United Kingdom. *Int J Cancer* **33**:795, 1984

89. Yamaguchi K et al: Pathogenesis of adult T-cell leukemia from clinical pathologic features, in *Human Retrovirology: HTLV*, edited by WA Blattner. New York, Raven, 1990, p 163

90. Gessain A et al: Antibodies to human T-lymphotropic virus type 1 in patients with tropical spastic paraparesis. *Lancet* **2**:407, 1985

91. Osame M et al: HTLV-I associated myelopathy, a new clinical entity. *Lancet* **1**:1031, 1986

92. Gout O et al: Rapid development of myelopathy after HTLV-I infection acquired by transfusion during cardiac transplantation. *N Engl J Med* **84**:383, 1990

93. Sweet RD: A pattern of eczema in Jamaica. *Br J Dermatol* **78**:93, 1966

94. Walshe MM: Infective dermatitis in Jamaican children. *Br J Dermatol* **79**:229, 1967

95. LaGrenade L et al: Infective dermatitis of Jamaican children: A marker for HTLV-I infection. *Lancet* **336**:1345, 1990

96. Tachibana N et al: Suppression of tuberculin skin reaction in healthy HTLV-I carriers from Japan. *Int J Cancer* **42**:829, 1988

97. Sato E et al: Autopsy findings of adult T-cell leukemia/lymphoma, in *Adult T-Leukemia and Related Diseases*, edited by M Hanaoka et al. Tokyo, Jpn J Cancer Res Monogr, 1982, p 51

98. Broder S et al: T-cell lymphoproliferative syndrome associated with human T-cell leukemia/lymphoma virus. *Ann Intern Med* **100**:543, 1984

99. Bunn PA et al: Clinical course of retrovirus-associated adult T-cell lymphoma in the United States. *N Engl J Med* **309**:257, 1983

100. Matsumoto M et al: Adult T-cell leukemia-lymphoma in Kagoshima district, southwestern Japan: Clinical and hematological characteristics. *Jpn J Clin Oncol* **9**:325, 1979

101. Bunker CB et al: Indolent cutaneous prodrome of fatal HTLV-I infection. *Lancet* **335**:426, 1990

102. Hanchard B et al: Childhood infective dermatitis evolving into adult T-cell leukemia after 17 years. *Lancet* **338**:1593, 1991

103. Essex ME et al: Seroepidemiology of human T-cell leukemia virus in relation to immunosuppression and the acquired immunodeficiency syndrome, in *Human T-Cell Leukemia/Lymphoma Virus*, edited by RC Gallo et al. Cold Spring Harbor, NY, Cold Spring Harbor Laboratory, 1984, p 355

104. Krämer A et al: Spontaneous lymphocyte proliferation in symptom-free HTLV-I positive Jamaicans. *Lancet* **2**:923, 1989

105. Jacobson S et al: Immunologic findings in neurological diseases associated with antibodies to HTLV-I:activated lymphocytes in tropical spastic paraparesis. *Ann Neurol* **23**:196, 1988

106. Morgan OSTC et al: HTLV-1 and polymyositis in Jamaica. *Lancet* **2**:1184, 1989

107. Sato K et al: Arthritis in patients infected with human T lymphotropic virus type I. Clinical and immunopathologic features. *Arthritis Rheum* **34**:714, 1991

108. Vernan JC et al: Pseudo-amyotrophic lateral sclerosis peripheral neuropathy and chronic polyradiculoneuritis in patients with HTLV-I associated paraplegias in HTLV-I and the nervous system, in *Neurology and Neurobiology*, edited by G Roman et al. New York, Alan R. Liss, 1989, p 361

109. Catovsky D et al: Adult T-cell lymphoma-leukemia in Blacks from the West Indies. *Lancet* **1**:639, 1982

110. Kawano F et al: Variation in the clinical course of adult T-cell leukemia. *Cancer* **55**:851, 1985

111. Yamaguchi K et al: A proposal for smoldering adult T-cell leukemia (smoldering ATL):A clinicopathologic study of 5 cases. *Blood* **62**:758, 1983

112. Jono M et al: ATL (adult T-cell leukemia/lymphoma) and skin eruptions. *Hihubyou-shinryou* (Jpn) **9**:206, 1987

113. Gibbs W et al: Non-Hodgkin lymphoma in Jamaica and its relationship to adult T-cell leukemia/lymphoma. *Ann Intern Med* **106**:361, 1987

114. Hanchard B et al: Adult T-cell leukemia/lymphoma (ATL) in Jamaica, in *Human Retrovirology:HTLV*, edited by WA Blattner. New York, Raven, 1990, p 173

115. Yoshioka R et al: Pulmonary complications in patients with adult T cell leukemia. *Cancer* **55**:2491, 1985

116. Dosaka N et al: Examination of HTLV-I integration in the skin lesions of various types of adult T-cell leukemia (ATL):Independence of cutaneous-type ATL confirmed by Southern blot analysis. *J Invest Dermatol* **96**:196, 1991

117. Grossmann B et al: Hypercalcemia associated with T-cell lymphoma-leukemia. *Am J Clin Pathol* **75**:149, 1981

118. Blayney DW et al: The human T-cell leukemia/lymphoma virus, lymphoma, lytic bone lesions and hypercalcemia. *Ann Intern Med* **98**:144, 1982

119. Dodd RC et al: Calcitriol levels in hypercalcemic patients with adult T-cell lymphoma. *Arch Intern Med* **146**:1971, 1986

120. Wano Y et al: Interleukin 1 gene expression in adult T cell leukemia. *J Clin Invest* **80**:911, 1987

121. Tschachler E et al: Human T-lymphotropic virus I-infected T cells constitutively express lymphotoxin in vitro. *Blood* **73**:194, 1989

122. Matsuda K et al: Hypercalcemia and serum TNF in T-cell leukemia. *Lancet* **335**:1032, 1990

123. Ishibashi K et al: Tumor necrosis factor-β in the serum of adult T-cell leukemia with hypercalcemia. *Blood* **77**:2451, 1991

124. Watanabe T et al: Constitutive expression of parathyroid hormone-related protein gene in human T cell leukemia virus type 1 (HTLV-1) carriers and adult T cell leukemia patients that can be trans-activated by HTLV-1 tax gene. *J Exp Med* **172**:759, 1990

125. Takatsuki K et al: Adult T cell leukemia: Proposal as a new disease and cytogenetic, phenotypic and functional studies of leukemic cells. *Jpn J Cancer Res* **28**:13, 1982

126. O'Brien CJ et al: The histopathology of adult T-cell lymphoma/leukemia in blacks from the Caribbean. *Histopathology* **7**:349, 1983

127. Swerdlow SH et al: Caribbean T-cell lymphoma/leukemia. *Cancer* **54**:687, 1983

128. Hattori T et al: Surface phenotype of Japanese adult T-cell leukemia cells characterized by monoclonal antibodies. *Blood* **58**:645, 1981

129. Uchiyama T et al: A monoclonal antibody (anti-Tac) reactive with activated and functionally mature human T cells. II. Expression of Tac antigen on activated cytotoxic killer cells, suppressor cells, and on one or two types of helper T cells. *J Immunol* **126**:1398, 1981

130. Yamada Y: Phenotypic and functional analysis of leukemic cells from 16 patients with adult T-cell leukemia/lymphoma. *Blood* **61**:192, 1983

131. Waldmann TA et al: Functional and phenotypic comparison of human T cell leukemia/lymphoma virus positive adult T cell leukemia with human T cell leukemia/lymphoma virus negative Sézary leukemia, and their distinction using anti-Tac. *J Clin Invest* **73**:1711, 1984

132. Rappaport H: Tumors of the hematopoietic system, in *Atlas of Tumor Pathology*, section 3, fascicle 8. Washington, DC, US Armed Forces Institute of Pathology, 1966

133. National Cancer Institute sponsored study of classifications of non-Hodgkin's lymphomas: Summary and description of a working formulation for clinical usage: The Non-Hodgkin's Lymphoma Pathologic Classification Project. *Cancer* **49**:2112, 1982

134. Suchi T et al: Some problems on the histopathological diagnosis of non-Hodgkin's malignant lymphoma—a proposal of a new type. *Acta Pathol Jpn* **29**:755, 1979

135. Chan HL et al: Cutaneous manifestations of adult T cell leukemia/lymphoma. *J Am Acad Dermatol* **13**:213, 1985

136. Maeda K, Takahashi M. Characterization of skin infiltrating cells in adult T-cell leukemia/lymphoma (ATLL) clinical, histological and immunohistochemical studies on eight cases. *Br J Dermatol* **121**:603, 1989

137. Shimoyama M et al: Major prognostic factors of adult patients with advanced T-cell lymphoma/leukemia. *J Clin Oncol* **68**:169, 1988

138. Edelson R et al: Treatment of cutaneous T-cell lymphoma by extracorporal photochemotherapy. *N Engl J Med* **316**:297, 1987

139. Van der Loo EM et al: C-type virus-like particles specifically localized in Langerhans and related cells of the skin and lymph nodes of patients with mycosis fungoides and Sézary syndrome. *Virchows Arch* **31**:193, 1979

140. Kaltoff K et al: C-type particles are inducible in SE-Ax, a continuous T-cell line from a patient with Sézary's syndrome. *Arch Dermatol Res* **280**:264, 1988

141 Unge T et al: Detection of T-lymphotropic virus-like particles in cultures of peripheral blood lymphocytes from patients with mycosis fungoides. *Proc Natl Acad Sci USA* **88**:7630, 1991

142. Gallo RC et al: Association of the human C type retrovirus with a subset of adult T-cell cancer. *Cancer Res* **43**:3892, 1983

143. Lange-Wantzin G et al: Occurrence of human T cell lymphotropic virus (type I) antibodies in cutaneous T cell lymphoma. *J Am Acad Dermatol* **15**:598, 1986

144. Manzari V et al: HTLV-V: A new human retrovirus isolated in a Tac-negative T cell lymphoma/leukemia. *Science* **238**:1581, 1987

145. Anagnostopoulos I et al: Detection of HTLV-I proviral sequences in CD30-positive large cell cutaneous T-cell lymphomas. *Am J Pathol* **137**:1317, 1990

CHAPTER 215

Richard Allen Johnson and Jeffrey S. Dover

Cutaneous Manifestations of Human Immunodeficiency Virus Disease

Human immunodeficiency virus (HIV) disease was first recognized in 1981 as an acquired immune deficiency manifested by the opportunistic infections *Pneumocystis carinii* pneumonia (PCP) and chronic herpetic ulcers and by the opportunistic neoplasia Kaposi's sarcoma. In the initial reports, the first patients with HIV disease to be recognized were homosexual men, followed later by injecting drug users (IDUs). Within a year, this acquired immune deficiency was reported in persons in these two groups in Europe and Australia. Within a few years, however, it was recognized that the majority of individuals with HIV disease, on a global basis, were in Africa and did not share the characteristics of engaging in male-male sexual intercourse or injecting drug use.

The demographics of the HIV epidemic are changing rapidly, with a near steady-state of the number of HIV-infected individuals in industrialized countries, such as the United States, but with an explosion of the number of new infections in many parts of Asia. The population of persons with HIV disease has been compared with an iceberg, those symptomatic represented by the visible portion and the larger, submerged invisible portion representing those with undetected, asymptomatic HIV disease. On a worldwide basis, accurate detection and reporting of persons with HIV infection is complex for several reasons. The majority of persons who become infected with HIV do not experience significant symptoms during primary infection and are, therefore, not identified at that time. During the greater part of the natural history of HIV disease, the individual feels relatively well, does not seek medical attention, and again goes undetected. Only those with endstage disease experience symptomatic illness, seek medical care, and are thus diagnosed serologically.

In industrialized regions such as North America and Europe, individuals at risk for HIV infection may be identified if they choose to be HIV serotested. A deterrent to HIV serotesting, however, is the absence of laws preventing discrimination against those found to be HIV infected. In developing regions of the world such as Africa, South America, and parts of Asia, the health care system is such that HIV testing is either not available or prohibitively expensive. Epidemiologic surveys in these regions are unreliable. The diagnosis of HIV disease is commonly based on clinical findings.

Etiology and Epidemiology

Etiology

The human immunodeficiency virus is a lymphotropic human retrovirus. Two types have been identified: HIV-1 is the cause of nearly all HIV infection in the United States and Europe; HIV-2 infection has been detected mainly in West Africa, with isolated cases elsewhere. Both these closely related HIV types cause nearly indistinguishable clinical HIV disease.

The first detected human retrovirus, human T-cell lymphotropic virus I (HTLV-I), was identified and reported in 1980, only 3 years prior to the detection of HIV. HTLV-I is also thought to have originated in Africa and spread to various geographic loci around the world, similar to the pattern of spread of HIV. Montagnier and colleagues[1] were the first to identify and report HIV in 1983, followed by the report of Gallo and coworkers in 1984.[2]

Origins

The origins of HIV are unclear[3]; however, the most likely scenario is that HIV was introduced into humans from another primate in sub-Saharan Africa.[4] Both HIV-1 and HIV-2 are thought to have existed in rural Africa prior to the onset of the HIV pandemic and probably entered the human population several decades ago. Urbanization is thought to have brought the virus to population centers. Greater sexual freedom in cities is associated with loss of tribal traditions, a migrant-worker system that encourages multiple partners and stimulates demand for prostitution, and poverty, which also promotes prostitution.[5,6]

Transmission

HIV is transmitted by the same three modes as hepatitis B virus: sexual contact with an infected person; significant exposures to infected blood or blood products, including needles shared among

IDUs; and perinatally from an infected mother to her child.[7] During the first decade of the HIV pandemic (1981 to 1990), the route of transmission varied greatly between industrialized and developing countries. In industrialized continents such as North America, Europe, and Australia, HIV was transmitted most commonly by male-male sexual intercourse and injecting drug use when needles were shared. In sub-Saharan Africa, HIV was transmitted mainly via male-to-female or female-to-male sexual intercourse. In spite of public education, the majority of lay population is still unsure about the modes of transmission and harbors fears that HIV can be transmitted by other, as yet, undetected modes.

In the United States beginning in the 1970s, HIV transmission occurred mainly during male-male sexual intercourse, receptive anal intercourse being the most efficient mode of transmission. Currently, the number of new cases of HIV infection is shifting from homosexual and bisexual men, who successfully reduced risky sexual practices, to IDUs who share needles, crack cocaine addicts, and their sexual partners.

HIV is present at contagious levels in blood, genital secretions, and breast milk. Transmission occurs most efficiently by injection of a large volume of HIV-infected blood. Rarely, infection has also occurred by spillage of HIV-infected blood on skin or mucosa that is either abraded or inflamed, with breaks in the integrity of the epithelium. Transmission has also occurred through organ transplantation from an HIV-infected donor. Extracellular HIV has been found in blood and in seminal fluid, raising the possibility of cell-free transmission. HIV has been demonstrated to infect, multiply, and destroy Langerhans cells of the epidermis and mucosa.[8]

Sexual Transmission   Risk factors that increase the likelihood of sexual transmission of HIV include coexistence of sexually transmitted diseases (STDs) (syphilis, chancroid, genital herpes, chlamydial infections, vaginal trichomoniasis, gonorrhea), lack of circumcision, lack of condom use, receptive anal intercourse, and advanced HIV-related immunosuppression in the index case.[9] In Africa, the presence of genital ulcers has been associated with increased risk for heterosexual transmission of HIV.[10–12] In homosexual men in the United States, a history or serologic evidence of syphilis, a history of herpes simplex virus (HSV) infection, and antibody to HSV-2 have been associated with HIV infection,[13] whereas cytomegalovirus (CMV), Epstein-Barr virus (EBV), or HSV-1 antibodies were not associated with increased risk for HIV infection.[14] HIV-1 appears to have a low rate of transmission for each sexual encounter.[15,16]

Perinatal Transmission   Associated with the increasing number of HIV-infected females of childbearing age around the world, perinatal HIV transmission from infected women to their children is occurring more frequently.[17–19] Early in the HIV epidemic, transmission of HIV to the fetus was thought to occur in the majority of pregnancies of HIV-infected women; however, more recent data suggest transmission occurs in 10 to 30 percent of pregnancies.[20] Transmission occurs most often in utero; however, it can also occur during vaginal delivery or through ingestion of breast milk.[21,22] The later the pregnancy occurs in HIV disease, the more likely the mother is to infect the fetus.

Transmission through Blood, Blood Products, or Tissue Transplantation   Prior to reliable HIV serotesting, HIV was inadvertently transmitted by the administration of blood or blood products.

Transfusion with HIV-infected blood is the most efficient mode of transmission of HIV, up to 90 percent of recipients becoming infected.[23,24] As of 1991, 1 percent of adults and 5 percent of children with HIV disease had hemophilia or other coagulation disorders.[25] Currently, the risk of transmission of HTLV-I and II and HIV-1 in the United States is very low but still present, calculated as 1 in 60,000 units, from donors who are retrovirus infected but seronegative at the time of donation.[26] HIV has also been transmitted to recipients of tissue transplantation, i.e., kidney, liver, and bone grafts.[27–29]

Transmission in Injecting Drug Users and Their Sexual Partners
In 1991 in the United States, 19 percent of men with late symptomatic and advanced HIV disease were heterosexual men with a history of injecting drug use; an additional 7 percent were men who had had sex with other men.[30] Fifty-one percent of women with late symptomatic and advanced HIV disease had a history of injecting drug use, and an additional 21 percent had a history of sexual contact with an IDU. Fifty-nine percent of children with HIV disease were born to mothers who were IDUs or sexual partners of IDUs. Persons with HIV disease who continue use of injected drugs have a more rapid progression of HIV disease than those who stop or are in methadone treatment.[31]

Transmission in Health Care Workers   Up to 30 percent of individuals who sustain a puncture wound with an instrument tainted with hepatitis B virus–contaminated blood will become infected; in contrast, when HIV is present on the instrument, transmission occurs in only 1 in 300 such injuries.[32] In late 1992, 7652 health care workers were known to be HIV-infected; 94 percent were infected through nonoccupational exposures. Most of the infections sustained by health care workers who were occupationally infected occurred following a puncture, and only four occurred following mucocutaneous exposure.[33,34]

Global Aspects of the HIV Epidemic[35]

In 1980, estimates are that 100,000 persons were infected with HIV worldwide. In mid-1992, it was estimated that a total of 13 million persons—12 million adults (7 million men and 5 million women) and 1 million children—are infected, the majority of whom were infected via heterosexual intercourse.[36–38] The majority of these persons are in sub-Saharan Africa (>8 million), with 1 million each in North America and Latin America, 1 million in Asia, and half a million in Europe. Of the 12 million HIV-infected adults, 85 percent were infected by sexual transmission, 7 percent by injecting drug use, and 5 percent by contaminated blood.

By the year 2000, an estimated 40 to 110 million individuals will have become HIV infected worldwide, with 20 million cases of advanced HIV disease in adults and 3 million in children. India, which currently has an estimated 1 million persons infected of a total population of 800 million, will have the largest number of HIV-infected individuals. By the turn of the millenium, the annual number of new HIV infections is predicted to be somewhat less than 100,000 in North America, 700,000 in Africa, and 1.3 million in Asia.

The seroprevalence of HIV-1 antibodies is highest in cities such as New York, San Francisco, and Miami in homosexual men and in IDUs. Of interest, in a retrospective study of stored sera from 585 persons attending methadone maintenance clinics between 1972 and 1976, none of the sera had HIV antibodies; however, 18 percent were reactive to HTLV-I or -II. In a study of seroprevalence of anti-HIV-1 antibodies in serum samples from 26 hospitals in 21 cities conducted over an 18-month period (January, 1988 to June, 1989), the overall seroprevalence rate was 1.3 percent, ranging from 0.1 percent to 7.8 percent.[39] In hospitals with low seroprevalence, HIV-1 infections were seven times more common in men; in those with high seroprevalence, the median ratio was 2.9. In hospitals in communities with a high prevalence of HIV infection, 1.1 to 3.8 percent of 15 to 19-year olds and 18 to 22 percent of 25 to 44-year-old men were seropositive for HIV-1.

Natural History

HIV disease is a continuum progressing from primary infection to death, with a sequence of opportunistic infections and malignancies marking the gradual destruction of the immune system. In many ways, the slowly progressive decline in immune function occurring in HIV disease is analogous to the slowly progressive vascular disease that complicates diabetes mellitus. Many lay persons as well as health care workers are not aware of the continuum of HIV disease; rather, they falsely conceptualize HIV disease as having two stages: an asymptomatic pre-AIDS period followed by AIDS. Medically, the acquired immunodeficiency syndrome is defined by precise clinical and laboratory parameters. However, ''AIDS'' always generates an emotional response of varying degrees as well as the scientific connotation, analogous to the emotional response to ''herpes,'' which was generated by lay writings about ''the incurable venereal disease'' in the early 1980s.

Following transmission of HIV, the natural history of HIV disease can be divided into stages, using clinical and/or laboratory parameters. These stages are not sharply demarcated from each other clinically; however, they are helpful conceptually in following the course of HIV disease. During each stage, certain clinical events can be anticipated, and CD4+ cell counts fall within a certain range. The terms *late symptomatic* and *advanced stage HIV disease,* which cover the stage designated as the acquired immunodeficiency syndrome, lack the emotionally charged eponym AIDS.

Knowledge of the natural history of HIV disease is of practical importance in the care of the patient by the dermatologist. For example, a febrile patient with late symptomatic stage HIV disease and a CD4 cell count of >200/mm^3 presenting with umbilicated, shiny papules on the face is much more likely to have molluscum contagiosum than cryptococcosis with hematogenous dissemination to the skin. Although a common cutaneous presentation of disseminated cryptococcosis is molluscum contagiosum-like facial lesions, cryptococcosis usually occurs in patients with CD4 cell counts of ≤50/mm^3. A chronic herpetic ulcer of ≥1-month duration is a clinical marker of advanced HIV disease and is an AIDS-defining condition in a person without other causes of immunocompromise. Oral hairy leukoplakia is a manifestation of EBV infection of the glossal mucosa and appears in patients with late symptomatic HIV disease.

Several different staging systems for HIV disease have been proposed and are in use, including the Centers for Disease Control (CDC) surveillance case definition of AIDS, the Walter Reed classification system for HIV infection, the World Health Organization (WHO) clinical case definition for AIDS where diagnostic resources are limited, and a broader staging system using the CD4+ cell count.

Centers for Disease Control Staging: Surveillance Case Definition of AIDS

The CDC defined the end stage of HIV disease as the acquired immunodeficiency syndrome, or AIDS, a decade ago. No single definition of AIDS is practical on a worldwide basis. In industrialized countries, where serologic testing is readily available, the CDC criteria are used. In developing countries, such as those in sub-Saharan Africa, serologic and other sophisticated testing procedures are not available, and clinical criteria are used to make the diagnosis of AIDS.[40,41] The term *AIDS-related complex,* or *ARC,* has been applied to less severe signs and symptoms, accompanied by a measurable depletion of immune competence.

The CDC established and updated criteria for diagnosing AIDS[42]:

1. In an individual whose HIV status is unknown or inconclusive and who has no other cause for immunodeficiency, the following mucocutaneous findings are AIDS defining:
   a. Candidiasis of the esophagus, trachea, bronchi, or lungs (however, not oropharangeal candidiasis alone)
   b. Cryptococcosis with hematogenous dissemination to skin
   c. Herpes simplex virus mucocutaneous ulcer that persists longer than 1 month
   d. Kaposi's sarcoma in a patient younger than 60 years.
2. In an individual who is HIV seropositive, the following are AIDS defining:
   a. Coccidioidomycosis or histoplasmosis with hematogenous dissemination to skin
   b. Kaposi's sarcoma at any age.

The new AIDS case definition proposed by the CDC in 1992 (see Table 215-1) includes those persons already meeting the 1986 AIDS definition and adds all adults and adolescents infected with HIV with CD4 lymphocyte counts <200/mL.[43] The 1992 revision attempts to include manifestations of HIV disease common among women and IDUs.[44] Cohort studies have shown that 80 percent of persons with CD4 lymphocyte counts <200/mL develop an AIDS-related opportunistic infection or malignancy within 3 years.[45-47]

The impact of the revision of the case definition of AIDS is predicted to change the distribution characteristics of cases (e.g., heterosexual IDUs composed 18 percent of cases meeting the old criteria, 35 percent of cases meeting only the new criteria, and 23 percent of all cases).[48]

World Health Organization Staging

In many developing nations, laboratory confirmation of HIV infection is not possible because of the cost and lack of adequate health care facilities. As such, the WHO has proposed an alternative definition for AIDS, in geographic areas where only clinical parameters can be used (see Table 215-2).

Staging by CD4+ Cell Counts

An alternative to the CDC staging of HIV disease, which essentially makes two major groupings of HIV-infected non-AIDS and AIDS, is a staging system that is based on the CD4+ cell count as a measure of the degree of destruction of the immune system (Table 215-3).[49] This staging system defines five stages rather than two:

TABLE 215-1

1992 Revised Classification System for HIV Infection and Expanded AIDS Surveillance Case Definition for Adolescents and Adults

	Clinical categories		
CD4+ cell categories	A, asymptomatic or PGL	B, symptomatic, not A or C conditions	C, AIDS-indicator conditions
1 >500/mm^3	A1	B1	C1
2 200–499/mm^3	A2	B2	C2
3 <200/mm^3 AIDS-indicator cell count	A3	B3	C3

A3, B3, C1, C2, C3 illustrate the expansion of the AIDS surveillance definition. People with AIDS-indicator conditions (category C) are currently reportable to the health department in every state and United States territory. In addition to people with clinical category C conditions (categories C1, C2, and C3), persons with CD4+ lymphocyte counts <200/mm^3 (categories A3 or B3) also will be reportable as AIDS cases.

Description of Clinical Categories

A: One or more of the conditions listed below with documented HIV infection. Conditions listed in categories B and C must have occurred.
   Asymptomatic HIV infection
   Persistent generalized lymphadenopathy (PGL)
   Acute (primary) HIV infection with accompanying illness or history of acute infection

B: Symptomatic conditions that meet at least one of the following criteria: (1) the conditions are attributed to HIV infection and/or are indicative of a defect in cell-mediated immunity; or (2) the conditions are considered by physicians to have a clinical course or management that is complicated by HIV infection.

C: Any condition listed in the 1987 Surveillance Case Definition for AIDS. The conditions in this category are strongly associated with severe immunodeficiency, occur frequently in HIV-infected individuals, and cause serious morbidity and mortality.

TABLE 215-2

Provisional World Health Organization (WHO) Clinical Case Definition for AIDS Where Diagnostic Resources Are Limited

Adults

AIDS in an adult is defined by the existence of at least two of the major signs associated with at least one minor sign, in the absence of known causes of immunosuppression such as cancer or severe malnutrition or other recognized causes.

Major signs
   Weight loss greater than 10 percent of body weight
   Chronic diarrhea for more than 1 month
   Prolonged fever for more than 1 month (intermittent or constant)

Minor signs
   Persistent cough for more than 1 month
   Generalized pruritic dermatitis
   Recurrent herpes zoster infection
   Oropharyngeal candidiasis
   Chronic progressive and disseminated herpes simplex virus infections
   Generalized lymphadenopathy

The presence of generalized Kaposi's sarcoma or cryptococcal meningitis is sufficient for the diagnosis.

Children

Pediatric AIDS is suspected in an infant or child presenting with at least two major signs associated with at least two minor signs in the absence of other known causes of immunosuppression.

Major signs
   Weight loss or abnormally slow growth
   Chronic diarrhea for more than 1 month
   Prolonged fever for more than 1 month

Minor signs
   Generalized lymphadenopathy
   Oropharyngeal candidiasis
   Repeated common infections (otitis, pharyngitis, etc.)
   Persistent cough for more than 1 month
   Generalized dermatitis
   Confirmed maternal HIV infection

acute retroviral syndrome (CD4+ cell count range of 1000 to 500 per mm^3), symptomatic (750 to 500), early symptomatic (500 to 200), late symptomatic (200 to 50), and advanced HIV disease (50 to 0). The combined stages of late symptomatic and advanced HIV disease are similar to the CDC definition of AIDS.

Acute Retroviral (Primary HIV) Infection In the majority of persons, primary HIV infection is subclinical and asymptomatic and therefore escapes diagnosis. Many persons with symptomatic primary HIV-1 infection, however, have been identified and studied, with documentation of symptoms, signs, and laboratory parameters. Presumably, primary HIV-2 infection, although less well studied, behaves in a similar manner. Estimates of the incidence of symptomatic primary HIV infection range from 1 to 50 percent.[50] When symptomatic, primary HIV infection is most commonly accompanied by fever and mild systemic symptoms, usually not severe enough to cause the patient to seek medical advice. Less commonly, the presentation is of an acute febrile illness, presenting with findings of or resembling influenza, mononucleosis, aseptic meningitis, myelopathy, encephalitis, polyneuropathy, Guillain-Barré syndrome, or brachial neuritis.[51–53] Unless the symptomatic patient presents to a physician knowledgeable about primary HIV infection, documentation of primary HIV infection may be missed. The incubation period (from presumed exposure to development of acute febrile illness) ranges from 3 to 6 weeks, varying with the route of infection and the size of the viral inoculum. Symptoms include fever, rigors, lethargy, malaise, sore throat, anorexia, myalgia, arthralgia, headache, stiff neck, photophobia, nausea, diarrhea, abdominal cramps, and pain.

Cutaneous findings in acute HIV infection are not unique but rather resemble those usually associated with many other acute viral infections. The most characteristic exanthem has much of the morphology and distribution of the papulosquamous eruption of

TABLE 215-3
Stages of HIV Disease

Stage		Clinical features	Typical duration	CD4+ cell range, cell/mm³
I	Acute retroviral syndrome	Brief mononucleosis-like illness	1–2 weeks	1000–500
II	Asymptomatic	No symptoms or signs other than lymphadenopathy	10+ years	750–500
III	Early symptomatic	Non-life threatening infections, chronic or intermittent illness	0–5 years	500–100
IVa	Late symptomatic	Increasingly severe symptoms, life-threatening infections, cancers	0–3 years	200–50
IVb	Advanced	Increasing hazard of death, less transferrable "opportunistic" infections	1–2 years	50–0

secondary syphilis, i.e., pink to red macules and papules, 5 to 10 mm in diameter, occurring on the upper trunk (Fig. 215-1) and palms and soles; an exanthem may also occur.[54,55] Lesions remain discrete and do not become confluent. Individual lesions may become keratotic or hemorrhagic. Less commonly, oropharyngeal, esophageal, and/or genital erosions or ulcerations have been reported to occur in acute symptomatic HIV infection.[56,57] Oropharyngeal and esophageal candidiasis has been reported in patients with acute immunodeficiency as part of severe, symptomatic, primary HIV infection.[58,59] These cutaneous findings are detected in up to 75 percent of symptomatic patients. Physical examination often reveals findings of aseptic meningitis and lymphadenopathy.[60] The acute illness usually lasts 1 to 2 weeks.

Diagnosis of primary HIV infection is made by documentation of HIV seroconversion using enzyme-linked immunosorbent assay (ELISA) confirmed by Western blot assay; by isolation of HIV

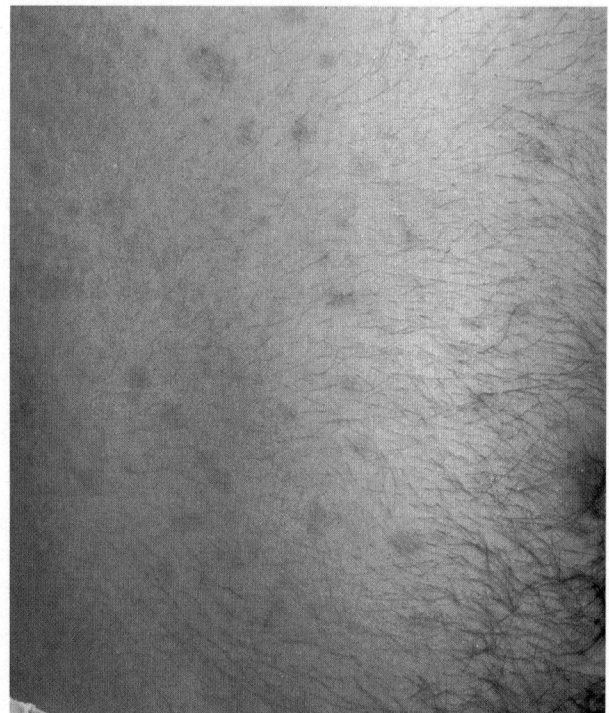

FIGURE 215-1 Primary HIV infection. Discrete erythematous macules and papules are seen on the trunk of a young male with an acute mononucleosis-like syndrome. (*Courtesy of Mark Drabkin, M.D.*)

from blood or cerebrospinal fluid (CSF); or by demonstration of the HIV p24 antigenemia.[61,62] Anti-HIV antibodies usually do not appear until 6 weeks after onset of the acute illness. The differential diagnosis of acute HIV infection presenting with acute mononucleosis or aseptic meningitis syndrome and an infectious exanthem includes viral agents, bacterial agents, rickettsial infections, and miscellaneous agents such as mycoplasma, *Strongyloides*, and *Toxoplasma*.

Laboratory findings often include leukopenia, elevated erythrocyte sedimentation rate, and lymphocytic CSF pleocytosis. HIV can be cultured from blood and CSF at this time. During the first week of symptomatic primary HIV infection, a pronounced lymphopenia with significantly depressed numbers of CD3+, CD4+, CD8+, and B cells had been documented.[63] In a small subset of homosexual men, integrated HIV-1 genome has been demonstrated in peripheral blood lymphocytes with no antibody response for almost 3 years, at which time seroconversion occurs. Lesional biopsy specimens associated with primary HIV infection are nonspecific and show a superficial perivascular and perifollicular mononuclear cell infiltrate of predominantly CD4+ cells.[64]

The role of antiretroviral therapy for acute symptomatic HIV infection or following a needlestick injury is unknown. Zidovudine therapy begun within hours following needlestick or inadvertent infusion of HIV-infected blood has failed to prevent seroconversion in reported cases.

The prognosis for patients with prolonged symptomatic primary HIV infection appears to be significantly poorer than for those patients with asymptomatic or mild primary infection. Patients with long-standing, severely symptomatic primary HIV infections (duration ≥14 days) have a much shorter period before progression to AIDS.[65] Seventy-eight percent of these patients experienced an AIDS-defining illness within 3 years, compared with 10 percent of patients with asymptomatic or mild primary infection. Extensive CD4 lymphocyte depletion is common in early HIV infection; frequent screening is indicated to identify newly infected patients who might benefit from antiretroviral therapy.[65]

After primary infection, the HIV becomes latent for a variable period of time: In the majority of patients latency is measured in years, in a minority in months or in decades. The factors that govern the persistence of HIV within the host and ultimately the transition from latent to fulminant infection are not known. Multiple variables are known to influence the rate of progression of HIV disease: size of virus inoculum, the site of infection, immune status of the host,[66] variable virulence of certain HIV strains,[67] and reactivation of herpesvirus infection contribute to induction of HIV expression and potentially modify and accelerate the course of HIV disease.[68]

The period of time from primary HIV infection to advanced HIV disease is highly variable.[69–71] In a cohort of HIV-infected homosexual males from San Francisco, approximately 50 percent developed AIDS within 11 years after becoming infected. The period of time for developing AIDS following infection by blood transfusion in adults is reported to vary from 6.5 to 11 years.[72] In a study of 89 persons infected by contaminated blood products in France, the mean incubation period was 62 months.[73]

MARKERS OF DISEASE PROGRESSION. The CD4+ (helper) lymphocyte count is used most extensively as an indirect marker of progression of HIV-induced immunodeficiency.[74] The normal CD4+ cell count ranges from 31 to 61 percent of the total lymphocyte count. The CD8+ (suppressor) lymphocyte count normally ranges from 18 to 39 percent of the total lymphocyte count. B cells make up the remainder of the blood lymphocytes, ranging from 5 to 20 percent of the total lymphocyte count. Patients with symptomatic or advanced HIV disease usually have CD4 cell counts below 20 percent of the total lymphocyte count. The absolute CD4 count is used as a guideline for several therapeutic interventions: low-dose zidovudine therapy is begun if the CD4 cell count is <500/mm³; prophylaxis for PCP is begun when the CD4 cell count is <200/mm³. Others tests used to follow the course of HIV disease include serum quantitative levels of beta₂ microglobulin,[75,76] neopterin,[77,78] and p24 antigen.[79,80]

Asymptomatic (Early) Disease

Asymptomatic HIV disease, as the name implies, is characterized by the absence of signs or symptoms of HIV infection, with the exception of diffuse reactive lymphadenopathy (persistent generalized lymphadenopathy, or PGL) and/or headache. Anxiety, fatigue, and depression may be experienced during this stage of HIV disease but may be related to awareness of impending morbidity and mortality rather than organic disease.

The duration of asymptomatic HIV infection is highly variable, dependent on unknown and known variables such as inoculum size, coexistence of other disorders, and age. In a large cohort of homosexual men with HIV disease who were studied prospectively, the median time from primary HIV infection to advanced HIV disease was 10.8 years.[81] Similar figures have been reported in other risk groups in the United States.[82–85]

The CD4 cell count in asymptomatic HIV disease ranges from 750 to 500 per mm³. Other laboratory parameters vary but may include mild abnormalities of the hemogram including anemia, neutropenia (decrease of neutrophils and/or lymphocytes), and/or thrombocytopenia and an elevated erythrocyte sedimentation rate. Serologic tests for *Toxoplasma gondii,* hepatitis B virus, and syphilis as well as tuberculin testing for tuberculosis are usually obtained in persons with newly diagnosed HIV disease, including the asymptomatic stage. Determination of CD4+ cell counts is advised more frequently as levels decline: every 6 to 12 months if >500/mm³; every 3 months if <500/mm³. Currently, antiretroviral therapy is advised if the CD4+ cell count is <500/mm³. Zidovudine has been available since 1987 and was initially used alone. Various combinations of zidovudine, ddI, and/or ddC are currently being used. Once CD4+ cell counts have fallen to <200/mm³, primary prophylaxis for PCP is begun with either trimethoprim-sulfamethoxazole, dapsone, or aerosolized pentamidine.

Early Symptomatic Disease

With progressive loss of CD4 cells and other parts of the immune system, asymptomatic disease progresses to early symptomatic HIV disease, which is defined by a CD4+ cell count in the range of 500 to 200 per mm.³ The initial nomenclature for symptomatic HIV disease was ARC. Symptoms experienced during early symptomatic disease include fever, night sweats, chronic diarrhea, fatigue, headache, and oral findings related to candidiasis and hairy leukoplakia. These symptoms may be associated with opportunistic infections and neoplasms, and their presence must be ruled out before symptoms are ascribed to HIV disease alone.

Late Symptomatic Disease

Late symptomatic HIV disease is defined as a CD4+ cell count in the range of 200 to 50 per mm³. The older CDC classification designates late symptomatic and advanced HIV disease stages as the acquired immunodeficiency syndrome (AIDS), but many clinicians caring for persons with HIV disease prefer the new staging. During the late symptomatic stage, opportunistic infections, such as chronic herpetic ulcers and esophageal candidiasis, and neoplasms such as Kaposi's sarcoma are common, as are many other disorders. Because of the risk of PCP, primary prophylaxis is begun with either trimethoprim-sulfamethoxazole, dapsone, or aerosolized pentamidine. Prophylaxis against other opportunistic infections is currently under investigation, including cryptococcal meningitis, central nervous system (CNS) toxoplasmosis, *Mycobacterium avium-intracellulare* (MAI), and cytomegalovirus (CMV) retinitis. Symptomatic illnesses and other disorders are treated as they occur.

Advanced Disease

Advanced HIV disease exists when severe immune dysfunction occurs (CD4+ cell count <50/mm³) and the patient is subject to one of many life-threatening infections or neoplasms. In a cohort of HIV-infected persons from North America, Europe, and Australia whose date of seroconversion was known, the incubation time to the development of an AIDS-defining event varied with the various risk groups, possibly because of different exposures to potential opportunistic pathogens.[86] No differences in incubation times were found among homosexual men infected in different continents or in different years (prior to and after January 1, 1985). Children with hemophilia developed AIDS more slowly than homosexual men, mainly because homosexual men had an added risk factor of Kaposi's sarcoma. Progression time to AIDS was significantly faster in older men, but not in older homosexual men.

The cause of death in HIV disease has changed due to various medical interventions and varies in populations in different geographic regions around the world. In a report of 126 patients from Providence, Rhode Island, who died after 1988, bacterial infections were the most common cause of death (30 percent).[87] Prior to 1988, PCP was the most common cause of death in HIV disease, but in this study group accounted for only 16 percent of deaths. Other causes of death included other opportunistic infections (25 percent), wasting/encephalopathy (8 percent), liver failure (7 percent), unknown (6 percent), lymphoma (5 percent), non-HIV-related causes (2 percent), and Kaposi's sarcoma (1 percent). In a report of the causes of death in 75 patients with HIV disease from the National Institutes of Health, 51 percent experienced respiratory failure due to PCP, bacterial pneumonia, CMV pneumonia, Kaposi's sarcoma, or cryptococcosis as the primary cause of death; 16 percent had neurologic disease as the primary cause.[88] All 75 patients had one or more disease processes identified in their lungs or pleurae at autopsy. In an autopsy study from the Ivory Coast, tuberculosis was the cause of death in 35 percent of adults with HIV disease, compared to 15 percent for toxoplasmosis, 11 percent for bacteremia, 6 percent for bacterial pneumonia, and only 2.5 percent for PCP.

Mucocutaneous Findings

Hundreds of disorders occurring on the skin and mucosa have been reported to occur in HIV disease. The remainder of this chapter discusses these findings in the following sequence: neoplasia, common infectious and noninfectious findings, and uncommon and rare infectious and noninfectious findings in HIV disease; there are also separate headings for oral findings and findings in HIV disease in children.

The many types of mucocutaneous lesions occurring in HIV disease and the disorders associated with them are listed in Table 215-4. The list must be continually revised. The cause of different types of lesions varies in different geographic regions of the world.

Neoplasia

Kaposi's sarcoma (KS), anorectal squamous cell carcinoma, undifferentiated non-Hodgkin's B-cell lymphoma, and primary CNS lymphoma have been shown to occur with increased incidence in HIV disease.[89] Although not proven, the incidence of nonmelanoma skin cancer, Hodgkin's lymphoma, and T-cell lymphomas may also be increased. These opportunistic neoplasias may be the consequence of opportunistic oncogenic infectious agents occurring in advanced HIV disease. In general, HIV-associated neoplasias are more aggressive, respond poorly to treatment, and are associated with a higher morbidity and mortality compared to the same tumors in non-HIV-infected individuals.

HIV-Associated Kaposi's Sarcoma (See also Chap. 99)

Classification   Kaposi's sarcoma (KS), an endothelially derived, multifocal tumor, was first reported by Moritz Kaposi in 1872 as "idiopathic pigmented sarcoma of the skin."[90] The original description, now termed *classic KS*, presents particularly in men of Mediterranean or eastern European ancestry as a rare, slowly growing tumor consisting of hyperpigmented cutaneous nodules most commonly found on the lower extremities. In the 1950s, a separate subtype, termed *endemic African KS*, was described in young, black, male adults in equatorial Africa.[91] In the 1960s, the first cases of KS associated with iatrogenic immunosuppression were described in renal transplant recipients and others treated with immunosuppressive drugs.[92]

HIV-Associated (Epidemic) KS   With the first reports of HIV disease, the 1980s brought an explosion of cases of KS,[93] the most common malignant complication of HIV disease.[94,95] In the United States, KS is at least 20,000 times more common in persons with HIV disease than in the general population and 300 times more common than in other immunosuppressed groups.[96] Ninety-five percent of HIV-associated KS occurs in homosexual and bisexual men, 9 percent of whom are also IDUs. KS has developed in only 3 percent of heterosexual IDUs in the United States, in 3.5 percent of blood transfusion recipients, in 1.5 percent of hemophiliacs, and in 1.9 percent of heterosexual contacts of known HIV-infected individuals.[94] The incidence of KS in men with HIV disease appears to have decreased since 1981, from 40 percent at the outset of the HIV epidemic to the present rate of less than 20 percent.[94,97,98]

Etiology and Pathogenesis   Several contributing factors have been implicated in the etiology and pathogenesis of AIDS-related KS: (1) a genetic predisposition; (2) infectious agents; (3) hormonal, neural, and vascular factors; (4) carcinogenic effects on vascular tissue; and (5) the status of the underlying immune system.[94,99,100] Genetic and hormonal influences are suggested by the increased incidence of HLA-DR5, both in individuals with classic KS and in those with HIV disease, and by the striking male predominance in patients with KS. Ninety-five percent of all cases of HIV-associated KS in the United States and Europe occur in homosexual and bisexual men.[94] In mice transfected with the transactivating gene of HIV, only the male animals develop KS.[101] HIV-associated KS cells have been cultured in vitro, and a growth factor produced by CD4+ T lymphocytes infected by one of the retroviruses isolated. It was demonstrated that cultured KS cells produce factors that support their own growth and that of other cells and possess angiogenic activity that induces vascular lesions histologically resembling human KS lesions when the cells are inoculated subcutaneously into mice. This information suggests that HIV itself may play a role in the induction and proliferation of KS.[102,103]

Epidemiologic information suggesting that KS may be caused by a sexually transmitted infectious agent includes: (1) the increased prevalence of KS in homosexual men compared to other risk factors; (2) the increased prevalence of KS in female partners of bisexual men compared to the partners of IDUs; and (3) the declining incidence of KS in homosexual men coinciding with the adoption of safer sexual practices since the early 1980s.[94,104] Two percent of a cohort of homosexual men with KS in New York City were not HIV infected. This suggests that another infectious agent concurrent with HIV in the male homosexual population may be causative of KS, and that HIV is likely a cofactor in the pathogenesis of KS in HIV disease.[104] Human papillomavirus (HPV) DNA sequences have been found in 11 of 69 biopsy specimens from homosexual men with HIV-associated KS, in 3 of 11 specimens from homosexual men with KS but with no evidence of HIV infection, and in 5 of 17 specimens from elderly HIV-negative men and women with KS. HPV DNA sequences were not found in 35 normal skin specimens tested.[105] In another study, HPV-related antigens have also been identified in dermal cells of KS biopsy specimens. These findings suggest that HPV may play a role in the pathogenesis of various forms of KS.

Retrovirus-like particles have been identified in the endothelial cells of cutaneous KS occurring in non-HIV-infected individuals in an endemic focus of KS in the Peloponnesus in Greece.[106] Avian hemangiomatosis, which is caused by a retrovirus, resembles human KS clinically and histopathologically, with characteristics including predilection for skin, multicentricity with organ involvement, and recurrence after excision.[107] It has been hypothesized that HIV-associated KS, like avian hemangiomatosis, may be caused by an as-yet unknown non-HIV retrovirus.

Symptoms   The most common symptom associated with mucocutaneous KS is the cosmetic disfigurement caused by nodular lesions and edema. Patients feel stigmatized as the lesions commonly appear on the face, making it apparent to friends, colleagues, and strangers that the patient has AIDS. The lesions themselves are usually initially painless, even those that enlarge to tumorous masses. Bulky lesions on the lower legs and feet, especially when associated with edema, may become eroded and ulcerated and cause significant pain. These lesions frequently become secondarily infected with *Staphylococcus aureus* or *Pseudomonas aeruginosa*, causing additional pain.

TABLE 215-4
Differential Diagnosis by Type of Cutaneous Lesions Occurring in HIV Disease

Lesion Type	Differential Diagnosis	Lesion Type	Differential Diagnosis
Papules, nodules		Folliculitis	S. aureus
Any location	Botryomycosis, staphylococcal		C. albicans
	Mycobacterial, environmental		Pityrosporum ovale
	Verruca vulgaris, verruca plana		Eosinophilic folliculitis
	Bacillary angiomatosis		Papular eruption of AIDS
	Scabies, scabetic nodules	Psoriasiform (papulosquamous)	Seborrheic dermatitis
	Disseminated deep mycotic infection		Tinea versicolor
	Cryptococcosis		Dermatophytosis
	Histoplasmosis		Psoriasis vulgaris
	Coccidioidomycosis		Psoriasis, inverse pattern
	Kaposi's sarcoma		Reiter's syndrome
	Basal cell carcinoma		Xerosis/ichthyosis
	Squamous cell carcinoma	Eczematous dermatitis	Atopic dermatitis
Facial	Molluscum contagiosum		Seborrheic dermatitis
	Verruca vulgaris, verruca plana		Scabies
	Disseminated deep mycotic infection	Urticaria	Drug eruption
	Kaposi's sarcoma		Idiopathic
	Basal cell carcinoma	Erythema multiforme	Drug eruption
	Squamous cell carcinoma		HSV-associated
Anogenital	Condylomata acuminata	Morbilliform eruption	Acute HIV exanthem
	Intraepithelial neoplasia		Infectious exanthem
	Molluscum contagiosum		Drug eruption
	Scabies, scabetic nodules	Purpura ± palpable	Thrombocytopenic purpura
	Kaposi's sarcoma		Hypersensitivity vasculitis
	Squamous cell carcinoma arising in intraepithelial neoplasia		Extrapulmonary pneumocystosis
			Infectious endocarditis
Crusted papules/nodules	Impetigo	Erosion(s), ulcer(s)	
	Ecthyma	Any site	
	Mycobacterial, environmental		HSV: primary, recurrent, chronic
	Ecthymatous VZV infection (painful)		CMV infection
	Disseminated deep mycotic infection		Ecthyma
	Kaposi's sarcoma		Nocardiosis
	Basal cell carcinoma		Mycobacterial, environmental
	HSV, chronic ulcers		Deep mycotic infection
Vesicles, bullae, pustules			Mycobacterial infection
Solitary	Bullous impetigo		Fixed drug eruption
	Ecthyma gangrenosum	Anogenital	Fixed drug eruption, including foscarnet
	Drug eruption		HSV ulcer chronic
Multiple	Grouped: HSV infection, primary or recurrent		CMV
	Zosteriform: herpes zoster, herpes simplex		Bacterial infection: ecthyma gangrenosum
	Bullous impetigo		Balanitis circinata (Reiter's syndrome)
	Ecthyma gangrenosum	Generalized pruritus, ±skin changes	Atopic dermatitis
	Disseminated zoster		Scabies
	Disseminated herpes simplex		HIV-associated eosinophilic folliculitis
	Infectious endocarditis		Papular eruption of HIV disease
	Pustular psoriasis		Adverse cutaneous drug reaction
	Reiter's syndrome/keratoderma blenorrhagica	Scars	Intravenous drug use
	Erythema multiforme		Skin "popping"
	Toxic epidermal necrolysis	Nail/paronychial changes	Dermatophytosis, proximal superficial
Acneiform	Acne vulgaris		Candida paronychia and onychomycosis
	Rosacea		S. aureus whitlow
	Perioral dermatitis		Psoriasis: pits, onycholysis, subungual hyperkeratosis
	Disseminated histoplasmosis		Beau's lines
	Eosinophilic folliculitis		Zidovudine pigmentation
	Papular eruption of AIDS		Yellow nail syndrome

NOTE: VZV, varicella-zoster virus; HSV, herpes simplex virus; CMV, cytomegalovirus.

Clinical Findings HIV-associated KS presents initially as an asymptomatic, erythematous macule or papule (Fig. 215-2*a*, -2*b*), often with a yellow-green bruiselike halo, commonly mistaken for a bruise. Lesions enlarge at varying rates, becoming violaceous nodules or plaques in months or years, and are usually oval or fusiform in shape. Older lesions may have varying degrees of hy-perkeratosis, especially on the lower legs. The surface of lesions on the upper body tends to remain shiny. Early lesions appear relatively flat and their extent is best judged by palpation. Nearly all KS lesions, even early lesions that appear to be macular, can be identified by palpation, in comparison with a bruise or ecchymosis, which is usual not palpable. The most common sites for KS to

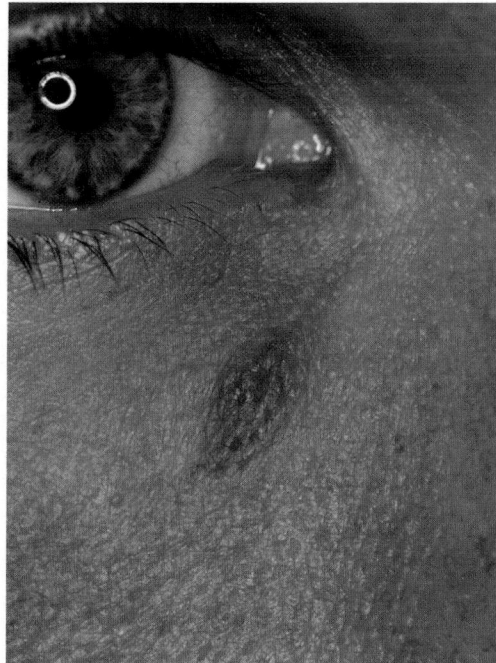

a

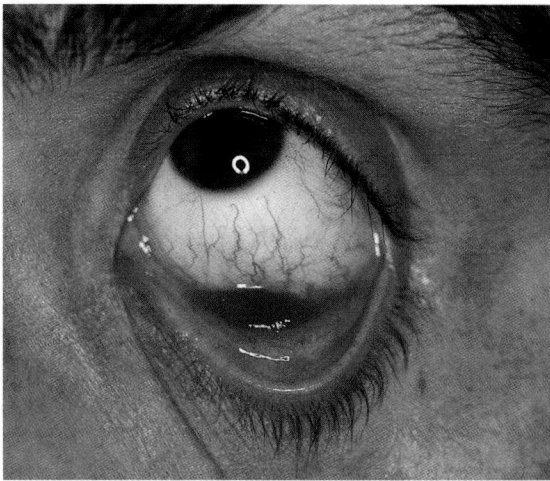

c

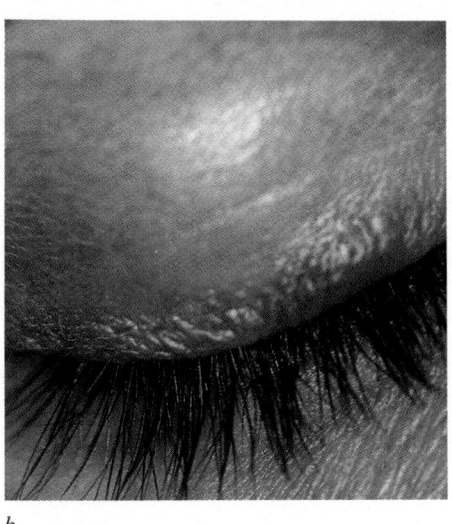

b

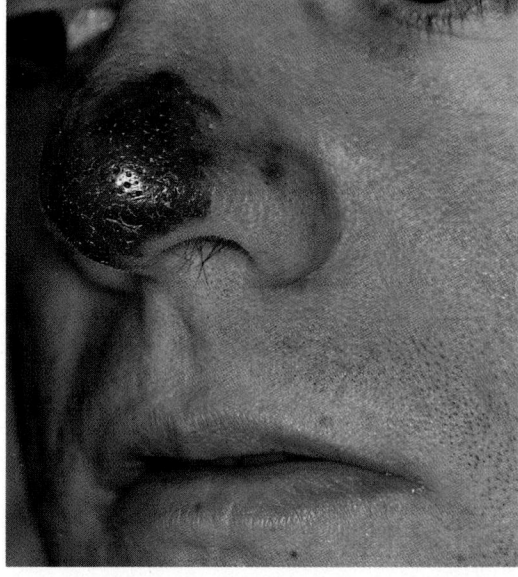

d

FIGURE 215-2 HIV-associated Kaposi's sarcoma, early lesions. *(a)* This violaceous, teardrop-shaped macule on the cheek was the first lesion detected by the patient. *(b)* This solitary nodule on the margin of the upper eyelid was not detected by the patient. *(c)* For nearly a year, this patient had only mucosal lesions on the conjunctiva and palate. *(d)* Violaceous plaque on the tip of the nose, a common site for this disfiguring lesion; the lesion is only slightly raised and could be easily masked with a cosmetic.

occur are, in decreasing order of incidence, the trunk, leg, arm, face, and oral cavity.[108]

KS lesions often have several characteristic arrangements. Individual lesions commonly arise at one site in clusters, giving a follicular pattern (Fig. 215-3*a*), although the lesions themselves do not arise at the hair follicle; this arrangement is common on the trunk and lower extremities. Another arrangement, less common than the follicular pattern, is the pityriasis rosea-like pattern (Fig. 215-3*b*) with discrete oval papules and nodules occurring along the lines of cleavage on the trunk; the lesions are usually of the same age and are similar in morphology.[109] Koebnerization of KS can

also occur at the site of various types of cutaneous injury, e.g., venipuncture or intravascular catheter sites, BCG injection, abscess formation, and contusions.[110] In the majority of patients with HIV-associated KS, the distribution of lesions lacks symmetry, with many on one side of the body but few on the corresponding opposite side.

In addition to papules, nodules, and plaques, cutaneous KS is often accompanied by varying amounts of edema. The most common site for edema is the lower leg (Fig. 215-4*a*–*c*). Edema occurs in areas that have numerous cutaneous KS lesions, from the leaky new vasculature in the mass of KS. Edema also occurs at dependent

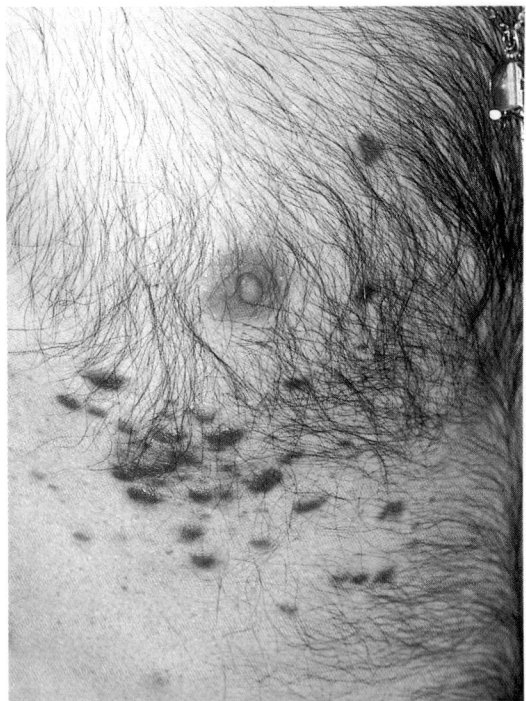

a

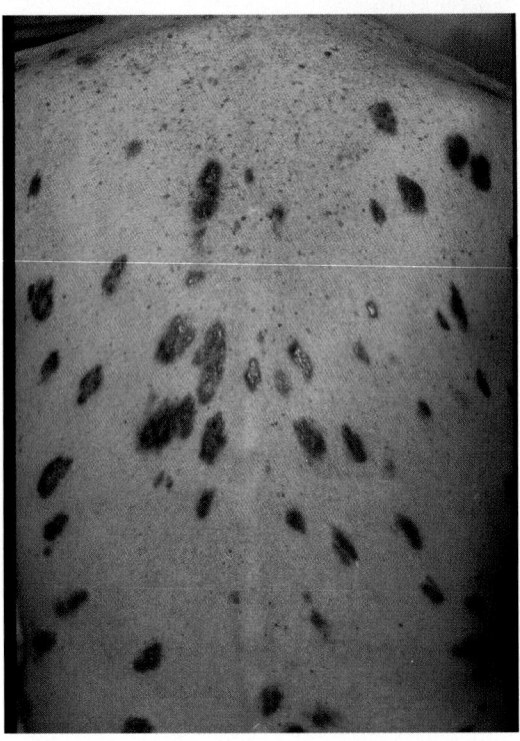

b

FIGURE 215-3 HIV-associated Kaposi's sarcoma, arrangement of lesions. *(a)* Follicular pattern: a cluster of violaceous papules and nodules of varying size are seen on the lateral chest wall; the interlesional skin has a greenish-yellow hue secondary to erythrocyte extravasation and breakdown to biliverdin. *(b)* Pityriasis rosea-like pattern: Multiple oval violaceous nodules are seen on the back; KS lesions had been present for 1 year.

sites. Leg edema can appear prior to the appearance of nodular KS lesions, secondary to obstruction of deeper lymphatic structures in the leg itself or the pelvis. Facial edema is also common, either with numerous nodular lesions or with very few, related to deeper lymphatic obstruction (Fig. 215-4*d*). In patients with involvement of several weeks' to months' duration, edema is dependent, facial edema being most pronounced in the morning and improving as the patient is upright during the daytime. Edema of the lower extremities is least in the morning when arising and worsens during the daytime if the patient is in the upright position. After many months, edema of the lower extremities is not reversible because of fibrotic changes.

Old tumorous KS lesions and sites with edema are subject to secondary bacterial infection in areas of erosion, ulceration, or hyperkeratosis. The most common bacterial pathogens causing secondary infection of KS lesions are *S. aureus* and *P. aeruginosa*. KS lesions on the lower legs and feet are most likely to become secondarily infected because of frequency of ulceration and edema formation (Fig. 215-5).

The oral cavity is commonly involved with HIV-associated KS. The palate is the most common site of involvement with early lesions appearing as a violaceous macular stain, usually on the hard palate. In time, these lesions can become more voluminous, forming papules and nodules, which occasionally become ulcerated (Fig. 215-6*a*, -6*b*). Lingual lesions most commonly appear as solitary papules or nodules and are violaceous or white because of overlying hyperkeratosis. In the majority of persons with oral involvement, KS is asymptomatic. In some patients, oral lesions may become very large, painful, and cosmetically disfiguring.

Diagnosis and Differential Diagnosis Early lesions, in the patch stage, can be easily mistaken for a bruise, insect bite, or nevomelanocytic nevus. The differential diagnosis for later lesions in the plaque stage includes psoriasis, lichen planus, secondary syphilis, insect bites, nevomelanocytic nevi, nonmelanoma skin cancer, melanoma, and metastatic visceral malignancies.

Clinical Course Epidemic KS may precede or develop concurrently with other HIV-related symptoms or it may develop late in the course of disease, months to years after the presentation of other HIV-related findings, such as opportunistic infection.[91] Infrequently, HIV-infected patients with KS may remain free of other symptoms and signs of HIV for years. Occasionally, epidemic KS lesions resolve spontaneously.[111] Epidemic KS often involves the viscera, including the gastrointestinal tract, lymph nodes, liver, lung, spleen, and kidneys; occasionally it occurs in the absence of cutaneous involvement.[112,113]

Systemic administration of pharmacologic doses of corticosteroids, such as given for treatment of acute PCP, may be associated with the appearance or acceleration of KS, which can regress or disappear when corticosteroids are withdrawn. KS may also appear or progress following a severe episode of opportunistic infection, such as PCP.

Prognosis The course of patients with HIV-associated KS is variable and appears to be related to the activity of HIV disease and the degree of underlying immunosuppression, rather than to the KS itself.[114] However, patients with HIV-associated KS uncommonly succumb to KS itself. Patients with KS, advanced immunodeficiency, and opportunistic infections do poorly and substantially worse than those individuals who develop KS early on after HIV

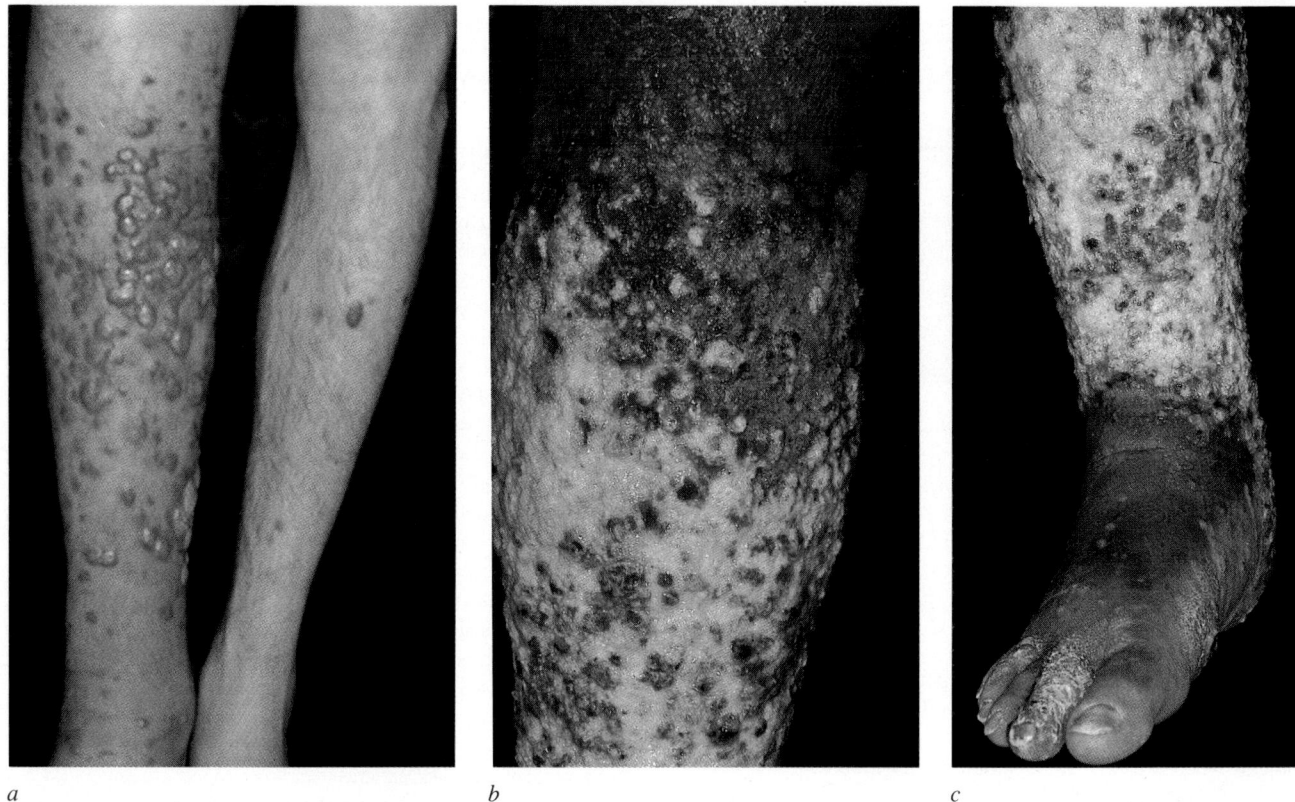

a   *b*   *c*

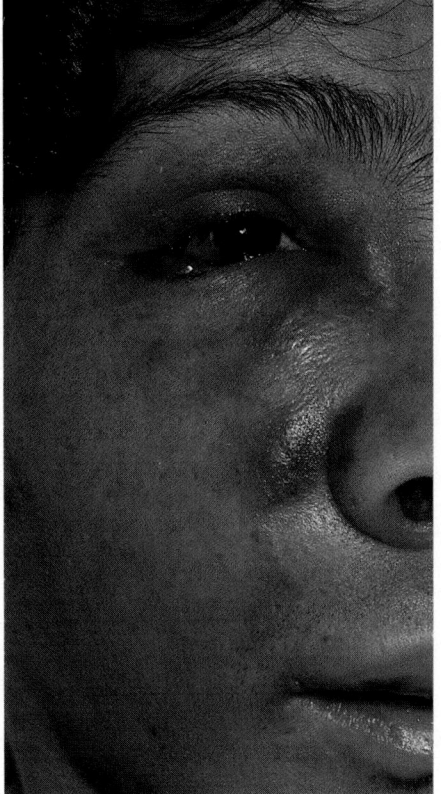

d

FIGURE 215-4 HIV-associated Kaposi's sarcoma with edema. *(a)* Confluent nodules associated with striking edema on one leg, essentially sparing the other. *(b, c)* Striking edema of the leg, with an elephantiasis nostras verrucosa; the dark pigmentation of the skin is mainly hemosiderin and not melanin. The patient had red hair and phototype II skin. *(d)* Striking unilateral facial edema associated with exuberant enlargement of KS in the ipsilateral nasal cavity, gingiva, and palate occurred over a 2-week period of time.

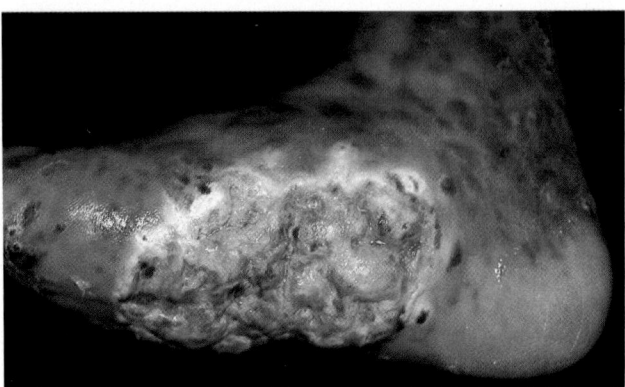

FIGURE 215-5 HIV-associated Kaposi's sarcoma with secondary infection. Massive involvement of the foot is seen with confluence of tumorous lesions, edema formation, hyperkeratosis, and erosion. The yellowish region on the plantar foot as well as the webspaces were infected with *P. aeruginosa,* very painful, and associated with fever. Marked improvement followed intravenous antibiotic and radiotherapy.

infection.[115] In a prospective study, patients who first presented with KS alone and had a peripheral blood CD4 count of >300/mm^3 had the best prognosis, with a median survival of 32 months.[116] Patients who developed an opportunistic infection within 3 months of presentation of their KS had the worst prognosis, with a median survival of 7 months.

Treatment (See Table 215-5) Initial treatment for KS should include an antiretroviral agent, such as zidovudine, even though no direct anti-KS activity has been demonstrated.[117,118] This suggestion is supported by the following: (1) KS activity is related to the degree of immunosuppression; (2) it is the immunosuppression that is the ultimate nemesis of HIV-infected patients; (3) in instances where the immunosuppression is reversed the KS clears; and (4) there is some evidence that antiretroviral drugs may have a synergistic effect with some directly anti-KS agents.[118,119]

Although mucocutaneous KS is not usually life-threatening, lesions that are cosmetically disfiguring or are large, ulcerated,

TABLE 215-5
Treatment of Kaposi's Sarcoma

Local
  Cryotherapy
  Intralesional vinblastine
  Intralesional interferon-α
  Radiotherapy
Systemic
  Interferon-α
  Interferon-α and zidovudine
  Cytotoxic chemotherapy
    Single agent
      Adriamycin
      Bleomycin
      Vinblastine
      Vincristine
      Oral etoposide
    Combination chemotherapy
      Vinblastine and vincristine
      Bleomycin and vincristine
      Bleomycin, vincristine, and adriamycin

bleeding, painful, or rapidly proliferating are indications for treatment. Localized KS is best treated by a variety of local modalities. KS is radiosensitive, and for locally aggressive or cosmetically disturbing lesions, radiotherapy is the treatment of choice.[120,121] An example of the use of localized radiotherapy is a study of the treatment of KS of the male genitalia (Fig. 215-6*d*): of 25 evaluable courses of radiation in 19 men with genital KS, in which treatment consisted of 600 to 3000 cGy in fractions of 150 to 800 cGy, 9 had a complete response and 14 a partial response. Treatment was well tolerated in all except one patient who developed local ulceration.[122] Similar responses have been obtained in larger series of patients with both localized and widespread disease, in which the overall response rates approached 90 percent, with complete response rates of 60 percent.[123,124] To limit the incidence of severe reactions, which was initially 17 percent, the authors suggest using a single fraction of 800 cGy for all KS lesions of skin regardless of site. Treatment of oral KS lesions may be followed by severe mucositis.[125] Recent data confirm that both skin and mucous membranes in AIDS patients are generally radiosensitive and that this must be considered in calculating dosimetry.[123]

Other local treatments include cryotherapy; surgical excision; and intralesional vinblastine, vincristine, bleomycin, or interferon-α. Intralesional vinblastine (0.1 to 0.2 mg/mL, 0.1 mL per 0.5 cm^2 of KS tumor) has been used to treat palatal, gingival, and lingual KS lesions. A single injection with vinblastine in ten patients resulted in mean reduction in tumor size of palatal lesions of 51 percent. In four patients receiving repeat treatments to the same lesions, the overall size reduction was 71 percent. The mean combined reduction in surface area of the palatal lesions was 63 percent. Gingival and lingual lesions showed more complete reduction in size than the palatal lesions treated. The main side effect was localized pain, which was controlled with oral analgesics.[126] In a study of cutaneous lesions using vinblastine (0.01 to 0.02 mg/mL, 0.1 mL/lesion, every 2 weeks for up to three treatments) 25 of 190 lesions cleared completely and 149 had partial improvement.[127]

Intralesional interferon has also been shown to be effective on KS lesions of the skin, conjunctiva, and oral cavity. Lesions were injected with interferon-α_{2a} (from 3 to 5 million units, depending on the volume of the lesion, three times per week for 4 weeks) with placebo controls. All lesions treated with interferon cleared, whereas those treated with placebo did not. No relapse has been observed during an average of 12 months after treatment. Histologic examination showed substitution of the interferon-treated tumor nodules with fibrotic tissue. Side effects were reported to be mild. In comparison with intralesional vinblastine, however, intralesional interferon required 12 treatments, versus only 2 with vinblastine during a 4-week period, and is 10 to 100 times more expensive.[128]

Cryotherapy with liquid nitrogen spray produces at least 50 percent cosmetic improvement, especially in deeply violaceous, 1- to 2-cm nodules occurring on the head and neck. In a study of 20 patients in whom two to four individual lesions were treated three times with 3 weeks between treatments, each treatment consisting of two freeze-thaw cycles and thaw times of 11 to 60 s, complete responses lasting at least 6 weeks were produced in 80 percent of KS lesions treated. Histopathology of treated lesions correlated poorly with cosmetic improvement. The response rate did not appear to be related to CD4 cell count, repsonse to prior chemotherapy, nor the presence of B symptoms (see Table 215-1), although patients without previous opportunistic infections were more likely to have a good response. Side effects of pain and blistering were well tolerated.[129]

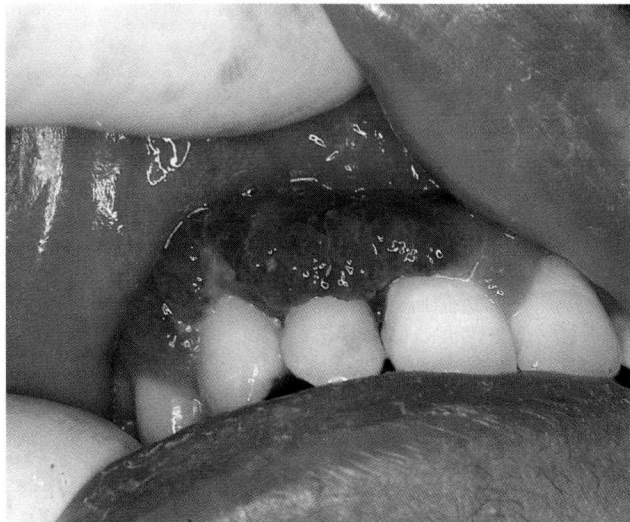

a

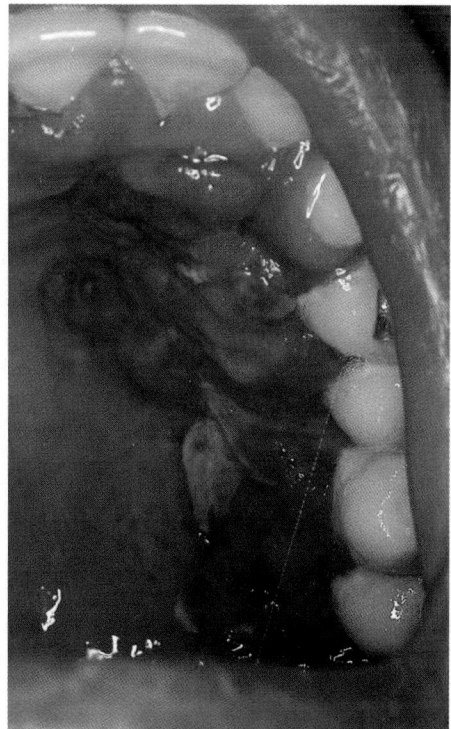

b

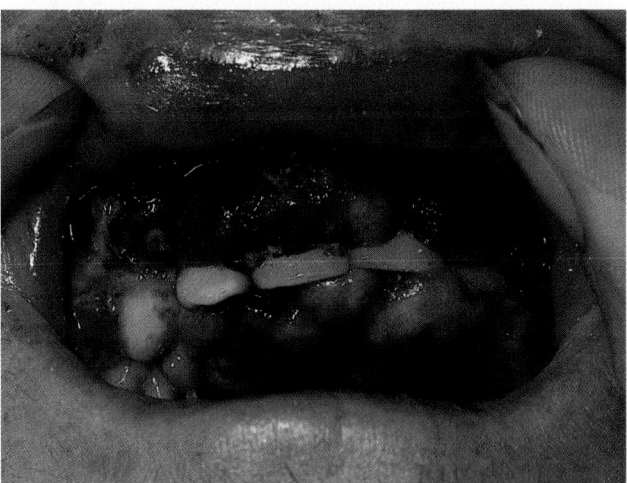

c

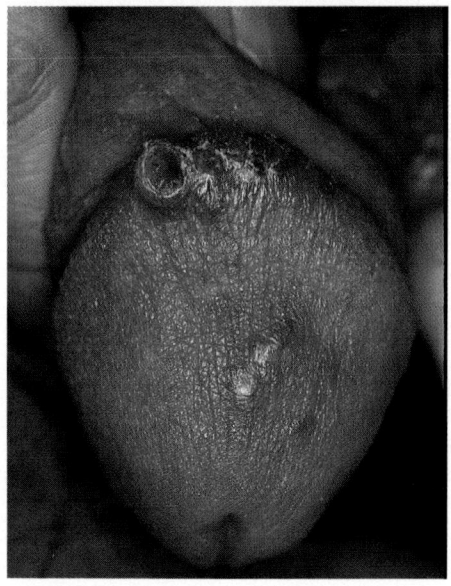

d

FIGURE 215-6 HIV-associated Kaposi's sarcoma with mucosal involvement. *(a)* (Same patient as in Fig. 215-4*d*.) Extensive infiltration of the gingiva is seen, associated with *(b)* involvement of the palate as well (note areas of ulceration); *(c)* 4 months later, the patient experienced explosive enlargement of facial KS (Fig. 215-4*d*) as well as oral KS. *(d)* Nodular lesions, some of which are hyperkeratotic, are seen on the glans penis; lesions resolved following radiotherapy.

Indolent disseminated cutaneous KS is best treated with immunotherapy or chemotherapy. Interferon-α, the most successful immune modulator so far used, is cytotoxic to T cells, increases natural killer cell activity, and has direct antiproliferative and antiviral properties.[118] Systemic interferon-α treatment (5 to 12 million units/day), usually requiring 6 to 8 weeks for an initial response, is most effective in indolent or slowly growing KS in patients with CD4 lymphocyte counts >400/mm^3 who have few systemic symptoms and no opportunistic infections. In these cases, the response rate is up to 50 percent. In unselected cases, the overall response rate is 25 to 30 percent. In an effort to reduce systemic side effects of interferon, which are frequent when doses of 20 million units or more per day are used, combined therapy of zidovudine and interferon-α have been attempted. Antitumor effect can be seen with doses as low as 4.5 million units per day when combined with zidovudine; however, the combination also produces dose-limiting side effects.[130]

Cytotoxic chemotherapy may be attempted in patients with CD4 cell counts <200/mm^3 with indolent disseminated KS where immunotherapy has failed, for asymptomatic visceral disease, and for extensive cutaneous KS (more than 50 lesions or more than 10 new lesions per month). The presence of tumor-associated edema or the presence of symptomatic visceral disease regardless of CD4 count is a strong indication for multiagent chemotherapy.[131] Traditional chemotherapeutic agents, such as vinblastine, etoposide (VP16), and adriamycin, produce high tumor-response rates but are myelosuppressive and potentially immunosuppressive. Vincristine and bleomycin, both of which are marrow-sparing agents, may be the agents of choice.[132,133] Studies have been conducted to evaluate the toxicity and efficacy of these two relatively marrow-sparing chemotherapy regimens in the treatment of advanced or progressive epidemic KS.[134] Bleomycin has been used relatively successfully as a single agent, with the disease improving or at least stabilizing in 78 percent of the 60 patients treated. Side effects were no more common in these patients than in non-HIV-infected cancer patients.[135,136] In a study of 33 patients, chemotherapy regimens consisted of bleomycin (10 mg/m^2), vincristine (1.4 mg/m^2, 2 mg maximum), and adriamycin (doxorubicin) at either 10 mg/m^2 or 20 mg/m^2 given IV, every 2 weeks, until intolerable toxicity or maximum antitumor response. Major responses (complete or partial remission) were attained in 79 percent of the cases. Bone marrow suppression consisted primarily of neutropenia, which occurred in a third of the patients. Variables significantly associated with shorter survival included low hemoglobin (<10 g/dL), low Karnofsky performance status (<70 percent), and weight loss. Opportunistic infections occurred in the majority of cases during administration of chemotherapy. A separate trial at the same institution used low-dose bleomycin, vincristine, and adriamycin.[137] The major response rate was 88 percent, although 52 percent of the patients became neutropenic. The most striking difference from the standard regimen was that the frequency of opportunistic infections was only 25 percent. Newer chemotherapeutic approaches employ hematopoietic growth factors such as erythropoietin or granulocyte or granulocyte-macrophage colony-stimulating factor with cytotoxic chemotherapy and antiviral therapy.

Although each of the treatments reported above helps to control the KS, none has been demonstrated to actually improve patient survival.[138]

Other HIV-Associated Malignancies

Lymphoma B-CELL LYMPHOMA. The incidence of primary lymphoma of the central nervous system and undifferentiated non-Hodgkin's lymphoma are increased in HIV disease.[89,139] Most lymphomas reported have been B-cell neoplasms, although peripheral nonepidermotropic T-cell lymphomas have also been described. The diagnosis of these aggressive tumors is often made at a more advanced stage of disease, and the response to therapy is usually poor. Extranodal disease occurs frequently in B-cell non-Hodgkin's lymphoma. Cutaneous extranodal involvement occurs in 8.2 percent, approximately equal to that seen in this tumor type in non-HIV-infected patients. Scalp involvement is less frequent than in non-HIV-infected individuals.[140]

T-CELL LYMPHOMA. Epidermotropic T-cell lymphoma has been described in HIV-infected individuals. Patients may present with patch-, plaque-, or tumor-stage disease indistinguishable from mycosis fungoides, with nodular lesions and focal epidermotropism, or with exfoliative erythroderma with large numbers of circulating Sézary cells. HTLV-I serology has been negative in most individuals tested.[141–144] Immunophenotyping of the lymph

nodes and skin infiltrates reveal a suppressor cell (CD8) predominance.

HTLV-I–ASSOCIATED LYMPHOMA. HTLV-I, the first detected human retrovirus, which also results in immunodeficiency, is endemic in Japan, the Caribbean, Africa, and the southeastern United States and has the same mode of transmission as HIV-1 and HIV-2. HTLV-I is the causative agent for acute T-cell leukemia/lymphoma (ATLL), which is frequently accompanied by infiltrative skin lesions. IDUs are dually infected with both HIV and HTLV-I in up to 27 percent of individuals in cities such as Queens, NY, and Newark, NJ. The natural history of HTLV-I infection is quite different from that of HIV infection; only 1 in 1500 individuals infected with HTLV-I might be expected to develop ATLL, with a mean incubation period of more than 20 years. To develop symptomatic HTLV-I and HIV infection at the same time, HTLV-I infection would have to be contracted 10 years or more prior to the HIV infection. In a study of HIV-1 and HTLV-I or -II infection in IDUs from the middle atlantic and central regions of the United States, dually infected subjects had more clinical symptoms related to immunodeficiency but a lower prevalence of HIV antigenemia.[145] One case of coinfection has been reported in a 43-year-old black homosexual male who presented with generalized lymphadenopathy but without skin lesions and was diagnosed as having ATLL.[146] Treatment with combined chemotherapy resulted in remission of the ATLL. Because of the increasing numbers of individuals infected with both HTLV-I and HIV among IDUs in the United States and other risk groups in Africa and South America, overlapping manifestations of combined infection might be anticipated.[147,148] Kaposi's sarcoma has also been reported to occur in a patient with HTLV-I–induced ATLL.[149] The KS erupted after induction of a partial remission of ATLL, but regressed when the ATLL subsequently relapsed.

Nonmelanoma Skin Cancer BASAL CELL AND SQUAMOUS CELL CARCINOMAS. Cutaneous malignancies may also be increased in this group of individuals, just as they are in other immunocompromised individuals. Multiple squamous cell carcinomas,[150] multiple warts in association with an evolving squamous cell carcinoma,[151] and metastatic basal cell carcinoma have been reported in patients with AIDS.[152] In a 4-year, retrospective, case-controlled study in San Francisco, 48 HIV infected individuals had 116 nonmelanoma skin cancers, of which 101 were basal cell carcinomas, and 15 low-grade squamous cell carcinomas. Neither the number of lesions nor type of cancer correlated with the degree of immunosuppression, while risk factors for cancers in these patients were the same as those in the general population.[153]

ANOGENITAL SQUAMOUS CELL AND CLOACOGENIC CARCINOMA. The incidence of squamous cell carcinoma of the cervix appears to be increased in women with HIV disease. This population has higher grade dysplasia, more widespread cervical involvement, and more frequent involvement of the vulva and vagina than women without HIV disease. Recurrence rate after local ablative therapy is also higher (36 versus 8 percent).[154] These findings in New York City have also been seen in Colombia, where a cohort of 300 HIV-infected women were prospectively studied and found to have a greater likelihood of developing cervical carcinoma with lower CD4+ cell counts. Cervical neoplasia was found in 15 percent with CD4+ cell counts >500/mm^3, compared to 29 percent in those with cell counts <200/mm^3.[155]

Surveillance and epidemiologic data evaluated from the Northern California Cancer Center of the surrogate population of single, never-married men in San Francisco, 28 to 49 years of age, reveals a greater than sevenfold increase in the incidence of invasive squamous cell carcinoma of the anus during the years 1987 to 1989, compared to the incidence during the period 1973 to 1978.[156] Reported anal cytology data from 28 HIV-negative and 34 HIV-infected homosexual men showed abnormal Pap smears in 28 percent of the HIV-seropositive compared with only 7 percent of the HIV-seronegative individuals. Evidence of HPV infection was present in 64 percent of the HIV-seropositive group and in only 38 percent of the HIV-seronegative group. A CD4+ cell count below 200/mm[3] was significantly associated with both abnormal Pap smears.

Cloacogeni carcinoma is increased in homosexual males at high risk for HIV infection and is specifically associated with receptive anal intercourse.[157] With increasing degrees of HIV-induced immunodeficiency, the incidence of intraepithelial neoplasia and invasive squamous cell carcinoma increases. HPV infection has been suggested in the pathogenesis of this disease because of the increased incidence of anal condylomata in this patient population and because papillomavirus antigens have been identified in anorectal carcinoma.

Dysplastic Nevi and Melanoma Seven patients with HIV disease having new eruptive nevi with clinical and histologic features of dysplastic nevi have been reported to date.[158] Seven others with coexistent malignant melanoma have also been reported.[159-161] The fact that neither dysplastic nevi nor melanoma is increased in patients with other immunosuppressive states makes the significance of these reports difficult to interpret. Nevertheless, continued surveillance of individuals at risk is warranted, considering that established data on melanoma in non-HIV-immunosuppressed individuals would suggest a poor prognosis for melanoma in HIV disease.

Common Mucocutaneous Manifestations of HIV Disease

Infectious Complications

Bacterial Infections Bacterial infections occur commonly in HIV disease as a result of multiple effects on the immune system.[162] A compromised cell-mediated immune system (loss of T-helper cells and diminished cytokine production) and abnormal macrophage function result in loss of protection against some bacterial pathogens such as *Salmonella, Listeria,* and mycobacteria. Altered B-cell function results in reduced specific antibody production against encapsulated organisms such as *Streptococcus pneumoniae* and *Haemophilus influenzae.* Significant neutrophil dysfunction (impaired chemotaxis, phagocytosis, and bacterial killing) in late HIV disease results in functional ''neutropenia,'' which may be combined with actual neutropenia associated with drug toxicity (zidovudine, ganciclovir), bone marrow dysfunction, or bone marrow infections (*M. avium-intracellulare*).[163] Loss of integrity of the skin, oral mucosa, gastrointestinal mucosa, and tracheobronchial tree provides portals of entry for organisms into tissue and the bloodstream. Sites of placement of intravascular catheters, frequently used to treat infections such as CMV retinitis, often become colonized and infected by nosocomial pathogens, such as methicillin-resistant *S. aureus* and antibiotic-resistant gram-negative rods.

In a group of 46 adult patients with HIV disease who came to autopsy in 1983 to 1987, 83 percent had documented nonmycobacterial bacterial infections some time during the course of their illness; 74 percent of the patients had parasitic infection, 67 percent had viral infections, 61 percent had fungal infections, and 26 percent had mycobacterial infections.[164] Fifty-four percent of the autopsied patients had *S. aureus* infections, 15 percent had *P. aeruginosa* infections, and 13 percent had enterococcal infections. Twenty-six percent had undiagnosed bacterial infections at time of autopsy. Nosocomial bacterial infections in HIV disease occur at the rate of 3.46 per thousand hospital days, compared with 1.49 in non-HIV-infected patients, the intravascular catheter site being the site of infection and source of bacteremia in the majority.

INFECTIONS DUE TO GRAM-POSITIVE BACTERIA. *Staphylococcus aureus Infection* *S. aureus* is the most common bacterial pathogen in HIV disease, causing cutaneous and systemic infections that are associated with significant morbidity and mortality. *S. aureus* initially colonizes the nose and other sites such as the perineum; it may subsequently cause primary infections or secondarily infect underlying dermatoses or breaks in the epidermal integrity. In asymptomatic and symptomatic HIV-infected individuals, the *S. aureus* nasal carriage rate is twice that of control groups.[165-167] *S. aureus* may also be locally invasive at the nasal carriage site, causing abscess formation.[168] Prophylaxis with agents such as trimethoprim-sulfamethoxazole for PCP is associated with a decreased nasal carrier rate as well as a reduced rate of infections; treatment of *M. avium-intracellulare* infection with agents such as rifampin or the newer macrolide antibiotics, clarithromycin or azithromycin, are also prophylactic against staphylococcal carriage and infection.

No HIV disease–specific staphylococcal infections occur in HIV disease. Rather a wide range of primary *S. aureus* cutaneous and soft tissue infections occur, the incidence increasing with the degree of immunocompromise. Primary staphylococcal infections include impetigo, bullous impetigo,[169] and ecthyma; papular and plaquelike folliculitis (Fig. 215-7*a*)[170]; furuncles and carbuncles (Fig. 215-7*b*); cellulitis; botryomycosis[171-173]; pyomyositis[174,175]; and rhabdomyolysis.[176] The staphylococcal toxin syndromes of nonmenstrual toxic shock syndrome,[177] staphylococcal scalded skin syndrome,[178] and a recalcitrant, erythematous, desquamating disorder associated with toxin-producing staphylococci[179] have been reported in HIV disease. Secondary infection of underlying dermatoses and superinfections occur commonly in persons with scabies, chronic atopic (eczematous) dermatitis that may be associated with elevated IgE levels,[180] excoriations, herpetic ulcers, KS, molluscum contagiosum, injection sites in IDUs, and intertrigo.[181] Line sites such as intravascular catheters[182] and chest tubes (Fig. 215-7*c*) are frequently infected.

Staphylococcal bacteremia may complicate either primary or secondary cutaneous infections; however, the most common site for hematogenous dissemination is the intravenous catheter, the source of 73 percent of cases of bacteremia in one report.[183] Thirty-five percent of patients with staphylococcal bacteremia who survived initial antibiotic therapy experienced late metastatic complications. Staphylococcal bacteremia associated with intravascular catheters is difficult to cure unless the catheter is removed.[184,185] Other predisposing factors for staphylococcal bacteremia include injecting drug use, lymphedema secondary to KS, and neutropenia. Staphylococcal sepsis has also been reported to complicate secondary infection of underlying dermatoses such as psoriasis[186] or scabies.

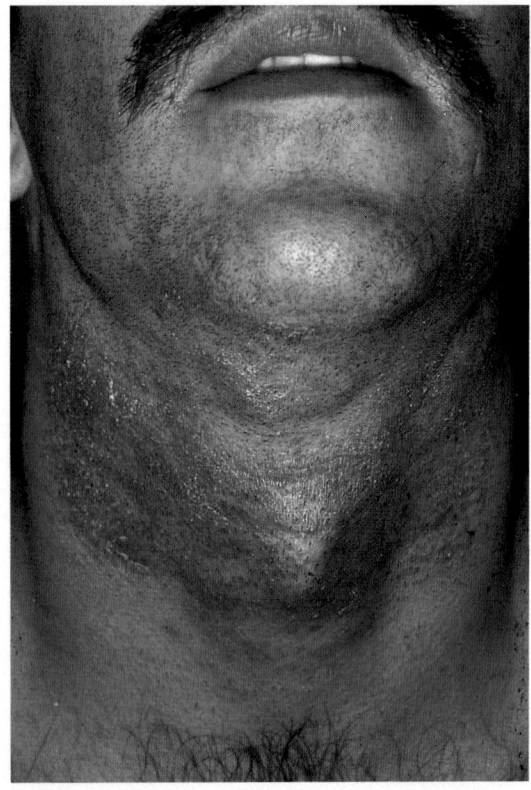

a

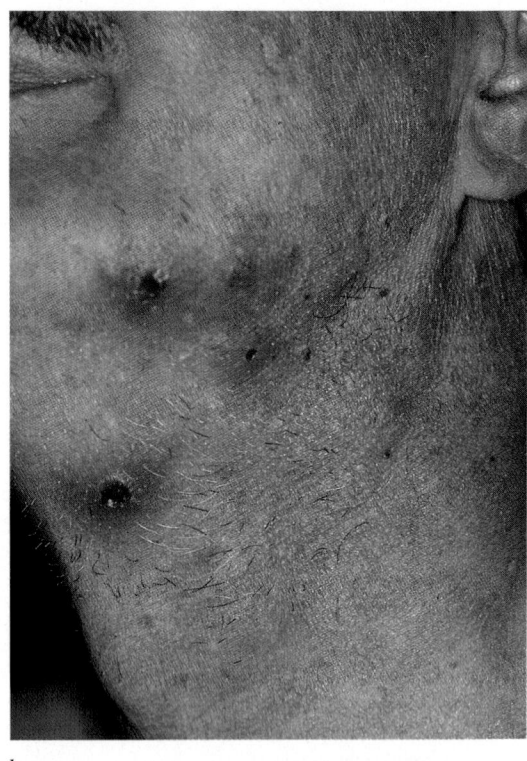

b

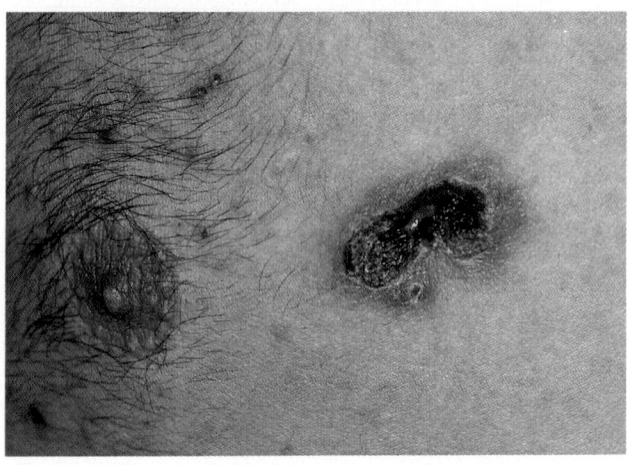

c

FIGURE 215-7 *S. aureus* infection. *(a)* A large erythematous, scaling plaque is seen on the neck, from which a heavy growth of *S. aureus* was cultured; the lesion cleared with mupirocin ointment treatment. *(b)* Multiple furuncles, seen on the neck, were also present on the scalp; continuous prophylactic dicloxacillin was required to prevent recurrence of lesions. *(c)* Ecthymatous lesions on the chest wall are seen at the site of chest tube as well as other areas of impetigo and folliculitis; the patient died 2 weeks later of staphylococcal septicemia, seeding from his multiple cutaneous infected sites.

As with the majority of infections in HIV disease, staphylococcal infections tend to be recurrent. Treatment should be directed at the acute infection and eradication of any underlying dermatoses, nasal carriage of *S. aureus,* and chronic oral prophylaxis with antistaphylococcal antibiotic. Helpful topical prophylactic regimens include the daily application of mupirocin to the nares and a benzoyl peroxide bar for bathing. Rifampin, 600 mg daily orally, is effective for eradication of nasal carriage of *S. aureus.*

Streptococcus pyogenes Infections Severe infection with group A beta-hemolytic streptococcus (GAS), resembling toxic streptococcal syndrome and the streptococcal toxic shocklike syndrome, has been reported in HIV disease,[187,188] presenting as a lymphadenitis with surrounding cellulitis, scarlatiniform rash, fever, diarrhea, and hypotension. Meningitis associated with a

scarlatiniform rash has been reported in an HIV-infected child.[189] Milder infections with lymphadenitis have also been reported.[190]

Intravascular Line-Related Infections Intravascular catheter–related infections occur commonly in HIV disease, often necessitating removal of the device. The most common etiologic agent is *S. aureus,* but a number of organisms have been reported to cause infection, including *P. aeruginosa, Candida albicans,* and *Stomatococcus mucilaginosus.*[191] Patients may present with fever, phlebitis, a new cardiac murmur, or local tenderness at the insertion site (Fig. 215-8*a,* -8*b*). The infecting agent can be isolated from the catheter and/or blood culture.

Fungal Infections SUPERFICIAL DERMATOMYCOSES. Although the frequency of dermatophyte infection in HIV disease appears to be no higher than in control groups, the severity and variability of presentation is increased in HIV disease. HIV-infected homosexual males have a 37.3 percent rate of dermatophyte colonization of the feet, compared to 31.8 percent in non-HIV-infected homosexual males and 8.6 percent in heterosexual males.[192] Tinea faciale mimicking seborrheic dermatitis (Fig. 215-9*a*),[193] and tinea manus and tinea pedis with marked hyperkeratosis, resembling keratoderma blenorrhagica, have been reported.

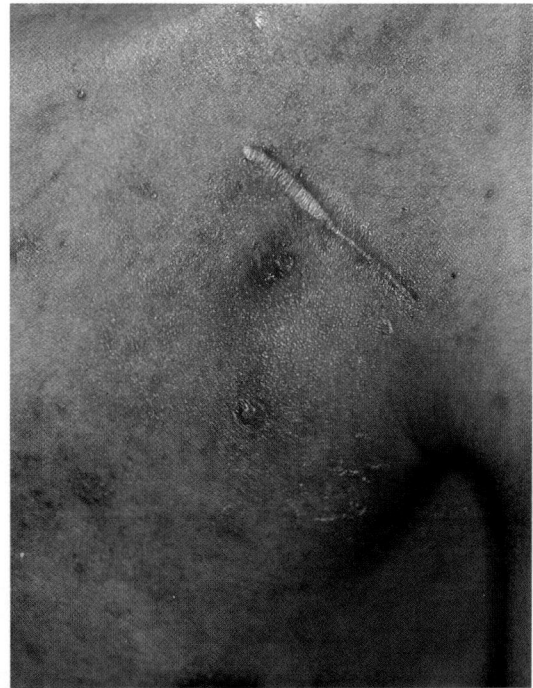

a

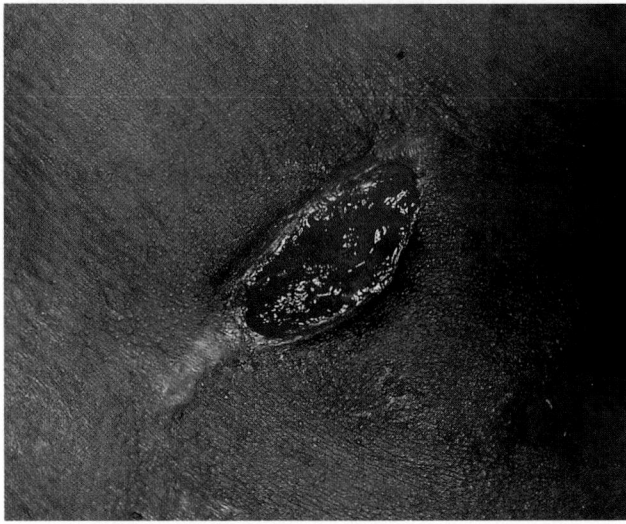

b

FIGURE 215-8 *S. aureus* infection of an intravenous catheter. *(a)* A recently placed intravascular catheter site is seen on the chest wall with several inflammatory papules, which were early lesions of staphylococcal folliculitis; *(b)* in 1 week, the catheter site had become infected and the line was removed.

Onychomycosis is common in HIV disease and differs from that in non-HIV-infected persons.[194] Proximal subungual onychomycosis (Fig. 215-9*b*), which is uncommon in the normal host, is common in HIV disease. Superficial white onychomycosis (chalky white involvement of the outer nail plate, usually caused by *Trichophyton mentagrophytes*) is common and usually caused by *T. rubrum*.[195] Both hands are often involved with mycotic kerato-

derma (compared to one hand in the normal host). Involvement of all fingernails may occur in a short time period (Fig. 215-9*c*) and this involvement is not rare.

In a study of 62 HIV-infected patients with advanced immunodeficiency referred for onychomycosis, 87.1 percent had involvement of the toenails, 8 percent of the fingernails, and 4.8 percent of both areas.[196] In 88.7 percent of this group, the nail involvement was reported to be proximal subungual onychomycosis. The classic distal subungual form was found in only 3.2 percent of patients, and white superficial onychomycosis in 4.8 percent. Dermatophytes were the most commonly isolated fungus, *T. rubrum* accounting for 58 percent; *C. albicans* was isolated alone from the nails in seven patients and *Pityrosporum ovale* was the only etiologic organism found in two.

Superficial infection of the scalp and other hair-bearing sites, caused by dermatophytes[197] and other fungi such as *Scopulariopsis brevicaulis,* may be associated with significant hair loss.

Dermatophyte infections in HIV disease are chronic and recurrent.[198] Because many patients are taking oral imidazoles such as ketoconazole, fluconazole, or itraconazole for candidiasis or cryptococcosis, dermatophytoses are inadvertently treated and kept under control.

CANDIDIASIS. In 1981, a new syndrome of mucosal candidiasis and PCP occurring in homosexual men was reported, later to be designated the acquired immunodeficiency syndrome.[199] Oropharyngeal candidiasis probably occurs in all those with HIV disease at some point during the course of illness, a consequence of defective T cell–mediated host defenses rather than of more pathogenic candidal strains.[200,201] The oropharynx is the most common site of mucosal candidiasis; the infection may extend into the esophagus and/or tracheobronchial tree. Candidal vulvovaginitis is common in HIV-infected women and is often the first clinical expression of immunodeficiency, even before oropharyngeal involvement.[202] In contrast, *Candida* intertrigo, which is more common than mucosal candidiasis in the normal host, is uncommon in adults with HIV disease. In the 1990s, a diagnosis of oropharyngeal candidiasis in the absence of predisposing local or systemic causes should always raise the issue of HIV serotesting.

Oropharyngeal and esophageal candidiasis has been reported to occur as a manifestation of primary HIV infection.[203–207] The incidence of candidiasis increases with advancing immunodeficiency. Mucosal candidiasis may develop in asymptomatic HIV-infected individuals but is more common in those with moderate reduction in the CD4 cell count. Eight percent of patients with stage II HIV disease (Table 215-3) have documented oropharyngeal candidiasis, 6.5 percent in stage III, 32 percent in stage IVa, and 81 percent in stage IVb. HIV-infected women with CD4 cell counts 200 to 500/mm³ had a 33 percent incidence of vaginal candidiasis, and 44 percent if the CD4 cell count was <200/mm³. Esophageal candidiasis, an AIDS-defining condition, occurs only with advanced CD4 cell count reduction (<100/mm³).

Oropharyngeal candidiasis is often asymptomatic. Patients may complain of a soreness or burning sensation in the mouth, sensitivity when eating spicy foods, and/or a reduced or altered sense of taste. Patients with oropharyngeal candidiasis may also have esophageal candidiasis with associated retrosternal burning or odynophagia; however, symptomatic esophageal candidiasis may occur in the absence of apparent oropharyngeal infection. In a study from Providence, RI, of 117 HIV-infected women, recurrent candidal vaginitis was the most common initial clinical manifestation of HIV disease (43 of 117 women).[208]

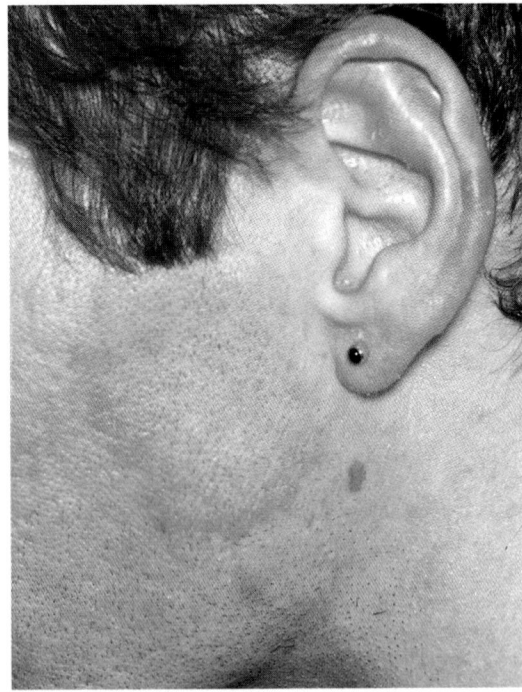

a

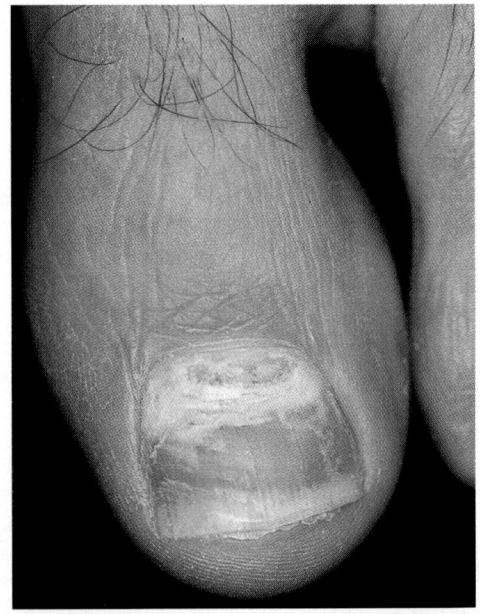

b

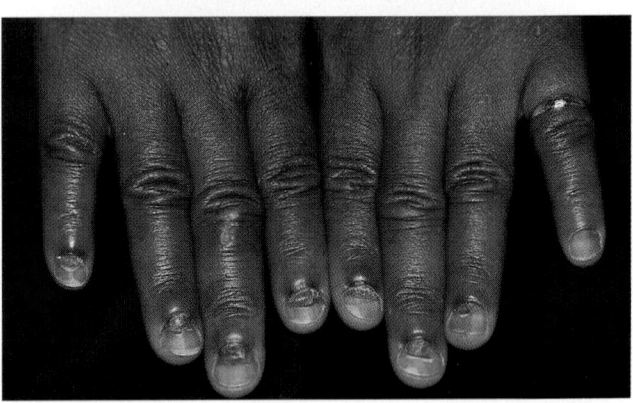

c

FIGURE 215-9   Dermatophytosis. *(a)* Tinea facialis with a well-demarcated annular plaque on the cheek that also involved much of the ear. *(b)* Tinea unguium with proximal subungual onychomycosis involving the great toenail, occurring in a 3-week period. *(c)* A very unusual involvement of all ten fingernails, involving the proximal nail plate, occurred over a 2-week period.

Oropharyngeal candidiasis presents in four different patterns: pseudomembranous (thrush), erythematous (atrophic), hyperplastic, and as an angular cheilitis. Erythematous candidiasis appears as patches of erythema, most commonly in the vault of the mouth on the hard and/or soft palate, and is easily missed on physical examination (Fig. 215-10*a*). On the dorsal surface of the tongue, erythematous candidiasis appears as depapillated areas with a smooth red glossal mucosa. Pseudomembraneous candidiasis appears as white, cottage cheeselike flecks at any site on the oropharynx and usually lacks any inflammatory response in the involved areas (Fig. 215-10*b*, -10*c*). Some patients, however, exhibit findings of both erythematous and pseudomembranous candidiasis on the oropharyngeal mucosa (Fig. 215-10*d*). Hyperplastic candidiasis occurs on the dorsum of the tongue, appearing as a white coating. Angular cheilitis is an intertrigo that occurs at the corners of the lips, usually with erythema but at times with a thrushlike membrane (Fig. 215-10*e*). Vulvovaginal candidiasis presents as erythema, often with white caseous plaques involving both the vulva and vagina or either site alone, and often associated with a burning or itching sensation. *Candida* intertrigo or paronychia is not common in the majority of HIV-infected persons. Chronic candidal paronychia and nail dystrophy are common in young children with HIV disease.[209]

Documented esophageal and/or tracheopulmonary candidiasis in a known HIV-seropositive individual is an AIDS-defining condition. Esophagoscopy is advised to document esophageal candidiasis in any patient who continues to have esophageal symptoms after adequate anticandidal therapy. In spite of a high prevalence of candidiasis in HIV-infected individuals, disseminated candidiasis is distinctly uncommon, probably because of B-cell activation and the presence of anticandidal protective antibody.

The main differential diagnosis of oropharyngeal candidiasis is oral hairy leukoplakia. Demonstration of candidal pseudohyphae by PAS stain is often seen as an incidental finding in non-candidal oral pathology in HIV-infected persons. Oropharyngeal candidiasis is diagnosed by demonstration of candidal pseudomycelial forms on potassium hydroxide preparation; however, it should be noted that, in one study, 49.1 percent of HIV-infected males had a positive smear but no clinical signs of oral candidiasis.[210] Isolation of *C. albicans* on culture is not diagnostic of candidiasis.

Treatment of mucosal candidiasis should be directed at control of symptomatic candidiasis and is usually followed by secondary prophylaxis. Topical treatments rely on high patient compliance in that they require administration 4 to 5 times daily; however, they are usually preferred over systemic drugs for initial treatment. The

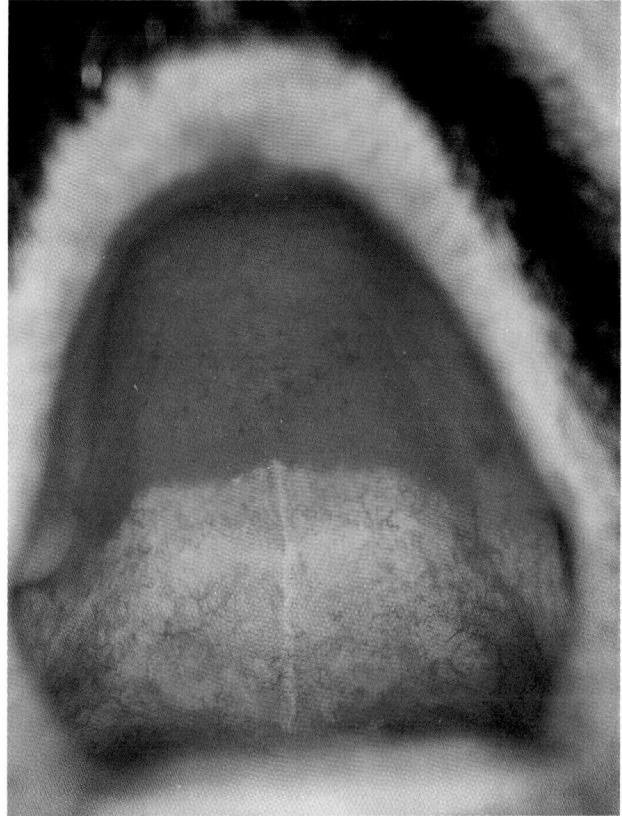

a

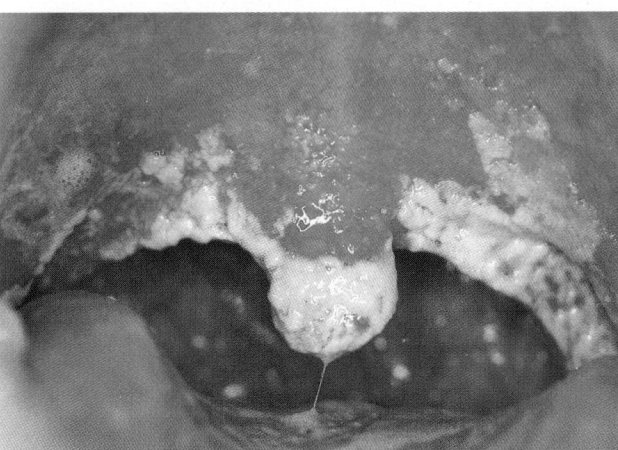

b

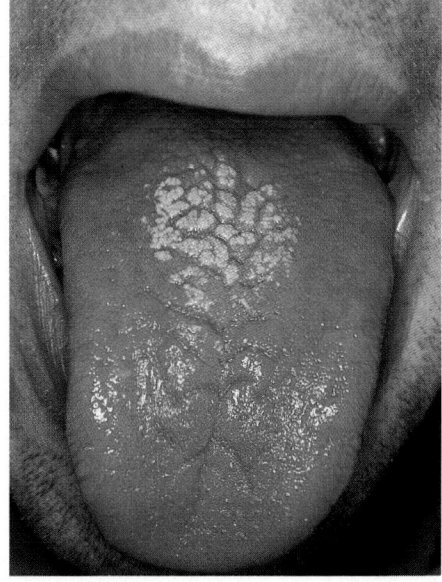

c

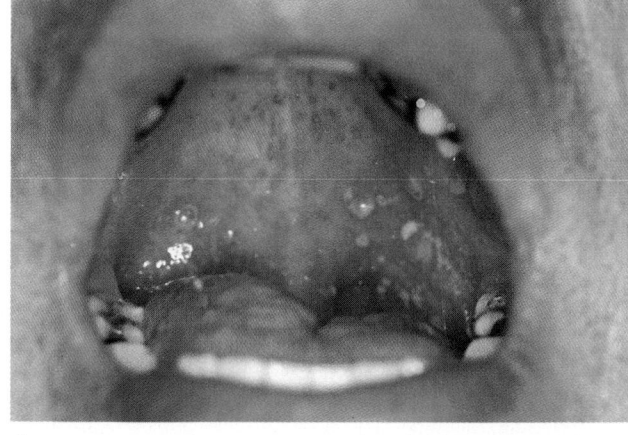

d

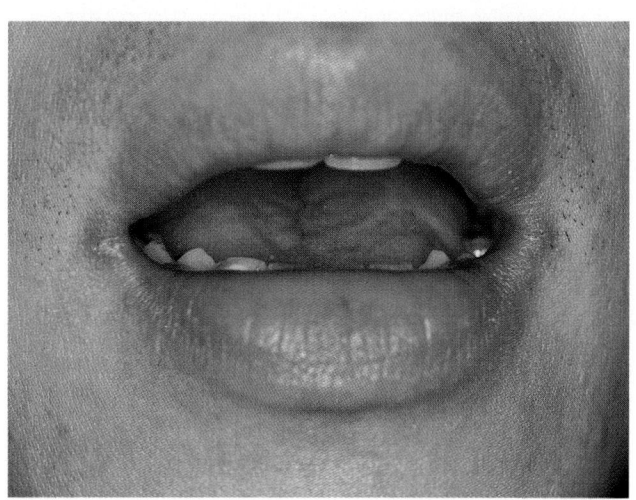

e

FIGURE 215-10 Oropharyngeal candidiasis. *(a)* Atrophic type with well-demarcated patches of erythema on the palate. *(b)* Pseudomembranous candidiasis appears as cream-colored cheesy plaques on the soft palate and uvula; and *(c)* as a dusting of powdered sugar on the dorsum of the tongue. *(d)* Erythematous and pseudomembranous candidiasis is seen on the soft palate. *(e)* Erythema is seen at the angles of the mouth, i.e., angular cheilitis, which accompanied oropharyngeal involvement as well.

imidazoles, ketoconazole, fluconazole, and itraconazole, are available for systemic therapy in the United States. Optimal absorption of ketoconazole and itraconazole occurs with an acidic gastric pH. Because many patients with advanced HIV disease are achlorhydric, absorption of ketoconazole and itraconazole is often suboptimal. Fluconazole is more effective than ketoconazole in the treatment of oropharyngeal[211,212] and esophageal candidiasis.[213,214] One added advantage of fluconazole over ketoconazole and itraconazole is the lack of effect of the gastric pH on absorption of fluconazole; however it is much more expensive than ketoconazole. As with most infections in HIV-infected individuals, secondary prophylaxis of oropharyngeal and esophageal candidiasis is required.[215,216]

PITYROSPORON INFECTION. *Pityrosporum ovale* causes *Pityrosporum* folliculitis and infection of intravascular catheters and is thought to have a significant role in the pathogenesis of seborrheic dermatitis.[217] The exact relationship *P. ovale* in the pathogenesis of seborrheic dermatitis in HIV disease is unclear. Seborrheic dermatitis, which occurs in the majority of HIV-infected patients,[218] has been associated with *P. ovale* colonization in some studies, the density of *P. ovale* on the involved skin correlating with severity of the dermatitis.[219,220] Another study concluded that *Pityrosporum* yeasts play no role in seborrheic dermatitis in HIV disease.[221]

In most patients with HIV disease and seborrheic dermatitis, the dermatosis is asymptomatic except for its cosmetic appearance. Clinically, seborrheic dermatitis appears as scaling and erythema in the hair-bearing areas such as the eyebrows, nasolabial folds, beard and mustache areas, retroauricular fold, scalp, chest, and pubic area. The main differential diagnosis is with dermatophytosis, psoriasis, and Reiter's syndrome. The histology of seborrheic dermatitis occurring in conjunction with HIV disease differs from that in non-HIV patients, with added features of spotty keratinocytic necrosis, leukoexocytosis, and superficial perivascular infiltrate of plasma cells and neutrophils with leukocytoclasis.[222] Seborrheic dermatitis in HIV disease remains relatively easy to control. Low-potency topical corticosteroids or topical antifungal preparations containing ketoconazole[223] or fluconazole are usually effective; however, relapse occurs if treatment is discontinued. The effect of oral imidazoles on seborrheic dermatitis has not been reported.

Pityrosporum folliculitis is characterized by numerous pruritic follicular papules and/or pustules occurring on the upper trunk and proximal arms. Potassium hydroxide preparation of lesional scrapings shows yeast forms only in comparison to the spores and hyphal forms seen in pityriasis versicolor. *Pityrosporum* yeasts are also seen in hair follicles in lesional skin biopsy. Tinea versicolor can be very extensive, especially in HIV-infected patients living in tropical climates. Both *Pityrosporum* folliculitis and pityriasis versicolor respond to a 10- to 14-day oral course of ketoconazole.

OTHER SUPERFICIAL MYCOSES. Other superficial mycoses have been reported in HIV-infected individuals, including invasive trichosporosis (*Cladosporium cladosporioides*) arising at the site of an intravascular catheter and appearing clinically as a 5-mm violaceous crusted nodule at the site of a tetanus skin test[224]; alternariosis presenting as an eschar on the leg; and superficial *Curvularia* phaeohyphomycosis presenting as a superficial keratotic lesion of the scrotum.

Viral Infections Viruses are major pathogens causing opportunistic infections in HIV disease (Table 215-6), many of which are manifested at mucocutaneous sites. Viral infections in HIV disease range from cosmetically disfiguring facial molluscum contagiosum to extensive common or genital warts to life-threatening or blinding cytomegaloviral disease.

TABLE 215-6
Opportunistic Viral Pathogens in HIV Disease

Virus	Disease
Herpesviruses	
HSV-1 and -2	Anogenital and oral ulcerations, encephalitis
VZV	Zoster, retinitis, disseminated infection
CMV	Retinitis, encephalitis, pneumonitis, adrenalitis, hepatitis, colitis
EBV	Oral hairy leukoplakia, Burkitt's lymphoma, CNS lymphoma
Pox virus	Molluscum contagiosum
Papovaviruses	
JC virus	Progressive multifocal leukoencephalopathy
HPV	Verruca vulgaris, gential warts, intraepithelial neoplasia, squamous cell carcinoma
Hepatitis B virus	Hepatitis, hepatic carcinoma
HTLV-I	Adult T-cell leukemia/lymphoma, tropical spastic paraparesis

NOTE: HSV, herpes simplex virus; VZV, varicella-zoster virus; CMV, cytomegalovirus; EBV, Epstein-Barr virus; JC virus (causes progressive multifocal leukoencephalopathy); HPV, human papilloma virus.

HERPES FAMILY OF VIRUSES. Herpesvirus reactivation in HIV disease is commonly associated with morbidity and, at times, mortality during the gradually emerging immunodeficient state. Of the six human herpesviruses, herpes simplex virus types 1 and 2 (HSV-1, -2), varicella-zoster virus (VZV), cytomegalovirus (CMV), Epstein-Barr virus (EBV), and human herpesvirus 6 (HHV-6), many exist in a latent phase of infection in otherwise healthy persons. Following onset of immunodeficiency, any of these viruses can become activated from the latent phase, causing various clinical patterns of infection. Reactivated herpesvirus infections may contribute to induction of HIV expression and potentially modify and accelerate the course of HIV disease.[225]

HSV-1 and HSV-2 Infections Genital herpes as well as other genital ulcerative diseases are risk factors for acquisition of HIV infection during sexual intercourse.[226–228] Reactivation of latent HSV infection is one of the most common viral complications of HIV disease. An early harbinger of the impending HIV epidemic was the observation of chronic perianal HSV infections associated with a severe, previously undetected, acquired immunodeficiency.[229,230] Chronic nonhealing perianal HSV ulcers, an opportunistic infection, associated with an acquired immunodeficiency were other early clues to the forthcoming HIV epidemic.

The majority of adults have latent HSV infection, which can be documented by detection of type-specific IgG antibody. The most common sites for these outbreaks are, in order of frequency, perianal, genital, orofacial, and digital (Fig. 215-11).[231] The majority of reactivation HSV infections in early HIV disease heal within 1 to 2 weeks without treatment.

With increasing immunodeficiency, recurrent HSV infection may become persistent and progressive. Erosions occurring at the usual sites enlarge and deepen into painful ulcers with raised margins. Multiple, large herpetic ulcers with angulated borders can be confused with neurotic exoriations.[232] Untreated, these ulcers may become confluent, forming large lesions involving large areas of the face, perineum, or genital region. Herpetic infection of one or more fingers can form severely painful, large whitlows.[233–235] Mucosal HSV infection may occur in the oropharynx, extending to the esophagus and causing severe odynophagia,[236] or may arise in the anorectum. Failure of adequate oral or intravenous treatment of herpetic lesions usually indicates the emergence of acyclovir-resistant HVS strains (Fig. 215-11f).[237] Large atrophic scars may follow healing of deep herpetic ulcers. Hematogenous dissemination with visceral infection is rare.[238,239]

Herpetic ulcers must be considered in the differential diagnosis of any ulcerative or crusted lesion occuring in HIV disease, especially at anogenital or facial sites. The differential diagnosis includes a wide category of infectious diseases. The diagnosis is made on clinical findings confirmed by a variety of laboratory tests. The most reliable method to make a precise diagnosis of HSV infection is to grow the virus from lesional samples. The isolated virus can be quantitated by plaque titration, typed, and its sensitivity to antiviral agents determined. The use of specific monoclonal antibodies directed against HSV-1 and HSV-2 proteins is an established means of making a rapid and precise viral diagnosis of HSV infection. The traditional test for dermatologists, the Tzanck test, which looks for giant epithelial or adnexal cells, preferably multinucleated, in smears of lesional exudate, is useful but is not always positive, even in frank herpetic lesions; its reliability is completely dependent on the skill of the microscopist. Lesional biopsy is helpful when giant epidermal cells are detected but cannot distinguish HSV from VZV infection.[240]

Herpetic lesions in early HIV disease usually heal without treatment. For recurrent herpes in early HIV disease, oral acyclovir 400 mg three times a day for 5 days is effective. One recommendation for prophylactic and suppressive treatment of recurrent HSV infection in HIV disease is oral acyclovir 400 mg five times a day for 5 days or until the eruption clears and then 400 mg three times a day for 1 or 2 months followed by 400 mg twice a day thereafter.[241] In more advanced HIV disease, oral acyclovir 400 mg five times a day or intravenous acyclovir 5 mg/kg every 8 h for 7 to 14 days is recommended.[242,243]

Herpetic lesions that fail to respond or that enlarge in spite of oral and intravenous acyclovir treatment should be evaluated promptly for the presence of acyclovir-resistant virus. High-dose continuous-infusion acyclovir has been reported to be effective in treatment of acyclovir-resistant chronic herpetic ulcers.[244] Intravenous foscarnet (trisodium phosphonoformate) is effective for acyclovir-resistant herpetic infections.[245–249] With continued administration of antiviral agents in the treatment of chronic HSV ulcers, HSV-2 has developed resistance to both acyclovir and foscarnet.

Varicella-Zoster Virus Infections   Primary infection with VZV is always symptomatic (varicella or chickpox) and is followed by a lifelong latent phase of infection, which can become reactivated (zoster). Immunocompromised persons who experience primary VZV infection or reactivation of latent virus are at significant risk for developing severe disease and experiencing high morbidity and mortality. Children with HIV disease represent the largest reservoir of VZV-susceptible immunodeficient children in the world, numbering several million in Africa. The nosology of varicella in HIV disease, however, is still very scanty. Primary VZV infection occurring in HIV disease may be severe, prolonged, and complicated by VZV dissemination (pneumonia, hepatitis, encephalitis, pancreatitis), bacterial superinfection, and death.[250,251] Fulminant varicella may occur relatively early in the course of HIV disease.[252]

A second episode of varicella can occur in HIV disease, presumably following infection with a different strain of VZV than that which caused primary varicella. Rather than resolving, persistent crusted lesions can occur at sites of initial vesicle formation, lasting for weeks or months.[253]

Zoster or reactivation of latent VZV infection is a major marker for faltering immunity and its occurrence should always raise the issue of the need for HIV serotesting with any patient. In the United States and in Africa, zoster in HIV disease has been reported to occur at seven times the expected incidence.[254,255] Conversely, 8 to 13 percent of those with an AIDS-defining condition have a history of prior zoster.[256] In a cohort study of 287 homosexual men with well-defined dates of HIV seroconversion and 419 HIV-seronegative homosexual men, the incidence of zoster was significantly higher among HIV-seropositive men (29.4 cases per 200 person-years) than among HIV-seronegative men (2.0 cases per 1000 person-years).[257] The overall age-adjusted relative risk was 16.9.

Zoster often occurs early in the course of HIV disease and, in children, can occur soon after varicella.[258] In the cohort study of 287 homosexual men, the risk of zoster was not associated with duration of HIV infection and was not predictive of faster progression to AIDS.[257] In a different study, reactivation of latent VZV infection correlated with moderate HIV-induced immunodeficiency, occurring earlier than oral hairy leukoplakia and oropharyngeal candidiasis.[255] Of HIV-infected individuals presenting with thoracic zoster, 7 of the 33 progressed to AIDS in a mean of 13 months (range, 1 to 28 months) following the zoster. Another study reported that 23 percent developed AIDS within 2 years after the diagnosis of zoster, 46 percent within 4 years, and 73 percent within 6 years. Extent of dermatomal involvement, severity of pain, and involvement of cranial or cervical dermatomes have been correlated with a poor outcome of HIV disease.

Because zoster often occurs early in HIV disease, the course is fairly uneventful for the majority of patients. It is most often dermatomal, but may be multidermatomal (Fig. 215-12*a*), recurrent within the same dermatome, or disseminated. The eruption may be bullous, hemorrhagic, or necrotic and be accompanied by severe pain. The majority of HIV-infected patients with zoster experience an uneventful recovery, but atypical clinical courses are not uncommon. Limited cutaneous dissemination of zoster secondary to viremia is common in some patients with zoster; however, uneventful recovery is the rule.[259,260] Ophthalmic zoster has the highest incidence of serious complications, which include corneal ulceration,[261,262] variable decrease of visual acuity,[263] and retinal necrosis.[264] Viral encephalitis can occur via entry into the brain by VZV infection of the optic nerve,[265] as well as follow hematogenous dissemination.[266] Systemic dissemination of zoster with hepatitis, encephalitis, or pneumonitis is uncommon.[267]

An uncommon, previously unreported complication of cutaneous VZV infection[268] is VZV lesions that persist for months following either primary[269] or reactivation VZV infection with a pattern of zoster[270,271] or disseminated infection.[272–274] This complication is referred to as chronic verrucous or ecthymatous VZV infection. Lesions may persist for months, either in the localized or disseminated form, and appear as hyperkeratotic, ulcerated, painful nodules, often with central crusting and/or ulceration with a border of vesicles (Fig. 215-12*b*, -12*c*).[275] A rare complication of zoster is the occurrence of a granulomatous vasculitis in the involved dermatome, without persistence of the VZV genome, possibly as a reaction to minute amounts of viral proteins.[276]

Diagnosis of primary VZV infection can usually be made on the clinical findings, but some children experience delay or absence of the typical mucocutaneous findings of varicella. Diagnosis of zoster is usually apparent on the clinical findings; however, zosteriform herpes simplex must be ruled out. The most reliable and rapid laboratory confirmation of VZV infection is detection of viral antigen on a smear of the base of a vesicle or erosion by monoclonal antibody detection. Tzanck test with detection of giant and, at times, multinucleated acanthocytes is often helpful, but does not

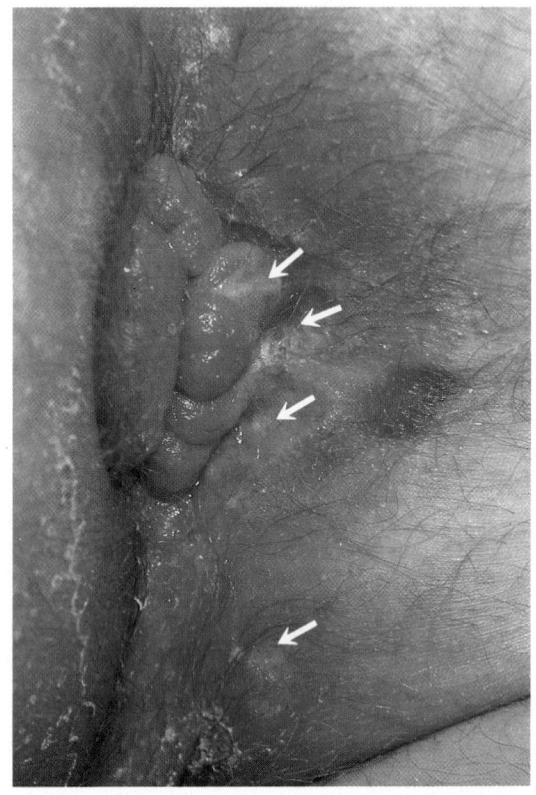

a

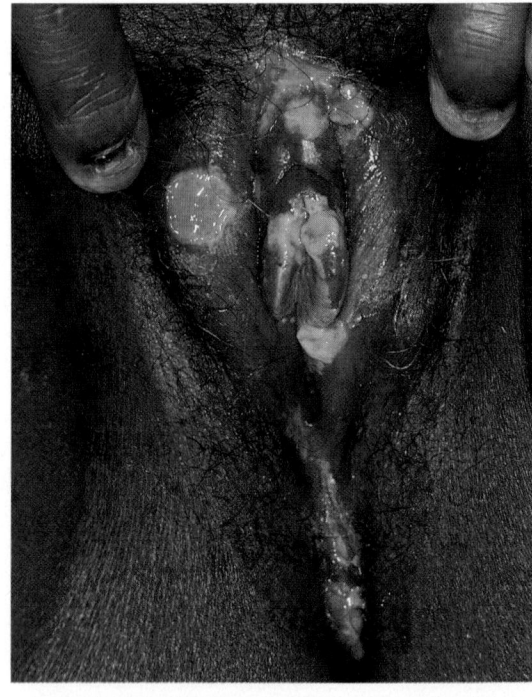

c

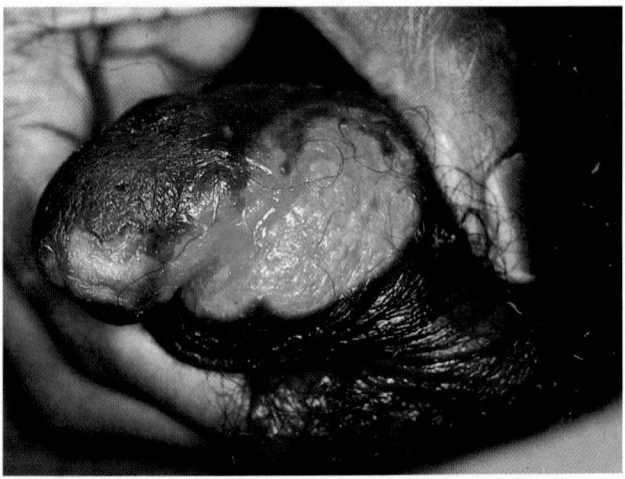

b

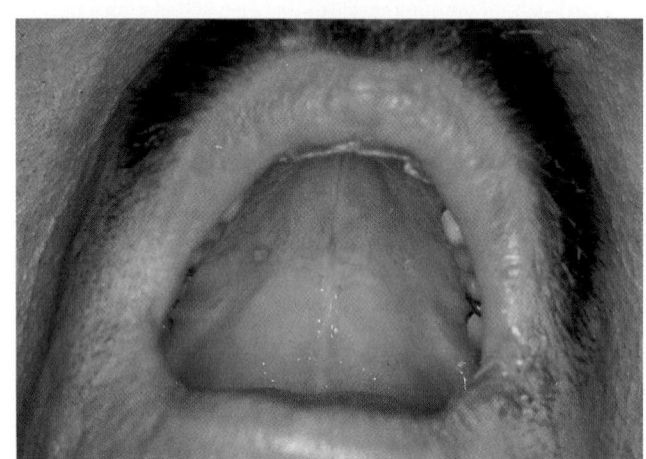

d

FIGURE 215-11 Herpes simplex virus infection. *(a)* Multiple, very painful ulcers, which had been present for 3 weeks, are seen in the perianal region, as well as a violaceous nodule of Kaposi's sarcoma. *(b)* Chronic ulcer on the shaft of the penis with signs of an older reepithelialized lesion on the glans. *(c)* Large, very painful ulcers had been present for only 2 weeks; they healed promptly on oral acyclovir. *(d)* Crusted erosion on the left angle of the lips accompanied by erosions on the palate; lesions healed promptly with oral acyclovir. *(e)* Chronic, painful, herpetic whitlow on a single digit was healing on oral acyclovir. *(f)* Extensive, erosive, painful ulcer involving the entire lower half of the face, it was unresponsive to IV acyclovir. *(Courtesy of C. Lisa Kauffman, M.D.)*

distinguish VZV from HSV. Isolation of VZV on culture is more difficult than isolation of HSV; however, it is necessary for determination of sensitivities to antiviral agents. Lesional biopsy is also helpful in establishing a diagnosis, especially in unusual manifestations of VZV infection such as ecthymatous or chronic verrucous lesions, but distinction from HSV infection is not usually possible histologically.

Treatment of VZV infection in HIV disease is not clearly defined. HIV-infected children exposed to VZV, whether varicella or zoster, should be treated prophylactically with varicella-zoster

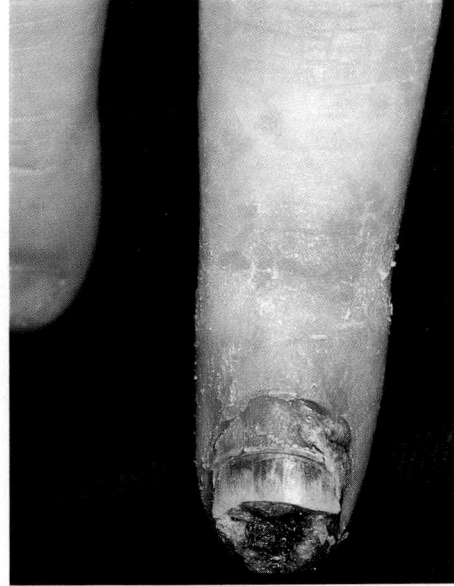

e

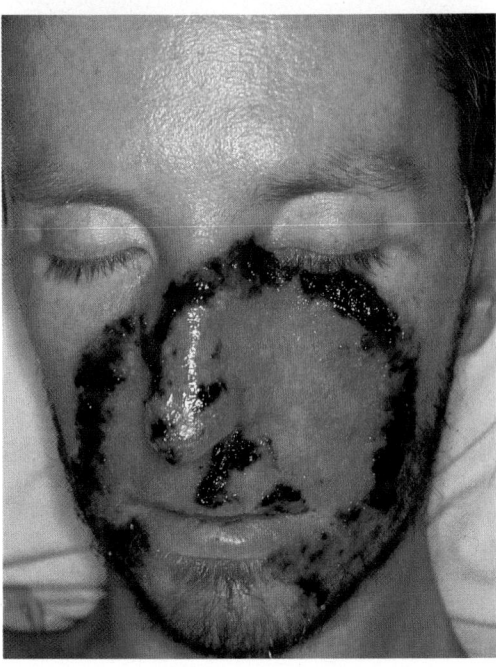

f

FIGURE 215-11   *(continued)*

immune globulin and possibly also with acyclovir. Most persons with zoster occurring in early HIV disease do well without antiviral therapy. Oral acyclovir (800 mg every 4 h for 7 to 10 days) is probably adequate for zoster occurring in adults with mild to moderate immunodeficiency. Current recommendations for treatment of primary or reactivation VZV infection is advanced HIV disease is intravenous acyclovir, 10 mg/kg every 8 h for 7 days, adjusted for renal function.[242] Because of the risk of visual impairment following ophthalmic zoster, all patients should be treated with intravenous acyclovir. Parenteral corticosteroids, often given to diminish postherpetic neuralgia, are usually contraindicated in HIV

disease. As with HSV infections, acyclovir-resistant strains emerge following prolonged acyclovir treatment; most of these resistant strains respond to foscarnet therapy.[277–279]

Epstein-Barr Virus Infection   Epstein-Barr virus selectively infects cells of the B-lymphocyte lineage and certain types of squamous epithelium. The majority of adults have been infected with EBV and harbor the latent virus. After primary replication of orally transmitted EBV in oropharyngeal epithelium, virion entry into the B-cell system provides a means of long-term viral carriage and serves to disseminate the infection to other sites.

With advancing immunodeficiency in HIV disease, EBV replication occurs with the resultant clinical manifestations: oral hairy leukoplakia (OHL), classic Burkitt's lymphoma, and EBV-positive large-cell lymphoma. EBV DNA can be detected in the oral epithelium in HIV-infected patients who have no clinical signs of OHL, and its detection may be a marker for advanced HIV disease.[280]

With the exception of a few observed cases occurring in immunosuppressed organ transplant patients,[281,282] OHL is a lesion specific to HIV-induced immunodeficiency. OHL usually occurs 5 to 10 or more years after primary HIV infection and has been noted in >50 percent of homosexual and bisexual males with HIV disease; it correlates with moderate to advanced immunodeficiency, when the CD4 count has declined to a median count of 390 cells per mm^3. In those patients who have not been diagnosed with AIDS at the time of detection of OHL, the probability of developing AIDS has been reported to be 48 percent by 16 months after detection, and 83 percent by 31 months.[283] Persons with OHL with a history of hepatitis B virus infection have a fourfold risk for early progression to AIDS; those with syphilis, have a nearly threefold risk for early AIDS diagnosis.[284]

Clinically, OHL presents as hyperplastic, verrucous, white to grayish white epithelial plaques. Although described as hairy, the most frequently noted characteristic lesion that occurs on the tongue has a corrugated appearance, with parallel white rows arranged nearly vertically (Fig. 215-13). Useful diagnostic criteria for OHL are a white lesion on the lateral margin of the tongue that does not rub off, that has the clinical appearance of hairy leukoplakia, that changes from day to day, and either has the characteristic histologic features of the lesion or does not respond to antifungal therapy. OHL may exist as a single lesion or as three to six discrete plaques separated by normal-appearing mucosa and is usually bilateral. The most common location is the lateral surface of the tongue, frequently extending onto the contiguous dorsal or ventral surfaces; the buccal mucosa and soft palate are much less commonly involved.

The diagnosis of OHL is relatively easy to make on clinical findings; however, if the diagnosis is in doubt, it should be confirmed by biopsy. The differential diagnosis includes hyperplastic oral candidiasis, condyloma acuminatum, geographic tongue, lichen planus, tobacco-associated leukoplakia, mucous patch of secondary syphilis, squamous cell carcinoma, occlusive trauma, and pseudo oral hairy leukoplakia.[285] Biopsy of OHL demonstrates acanthosis, marked parakeratosis with the formation of ridges and keratin projections, areas of ballooning cells resembling HPV-induced koilocytosis, and little or no dermal inflammatory reaction. Some studies report immunohistochemical findings suggesting HPV as well as EBV. Electron microscopy demonstrates 100-nm intranuclear virions and 240-nm encapsulated virus particles, consistent with a herpes group virus. Using in situ hybridization of tissue sections, EBV DNA is seen in the nuclei of the upper portions of the epithelium. Keratinocytes are widely infected with

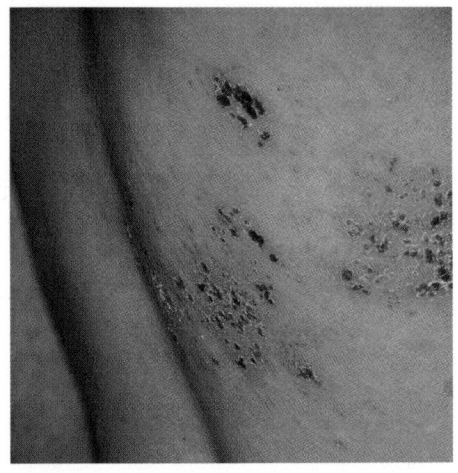

a

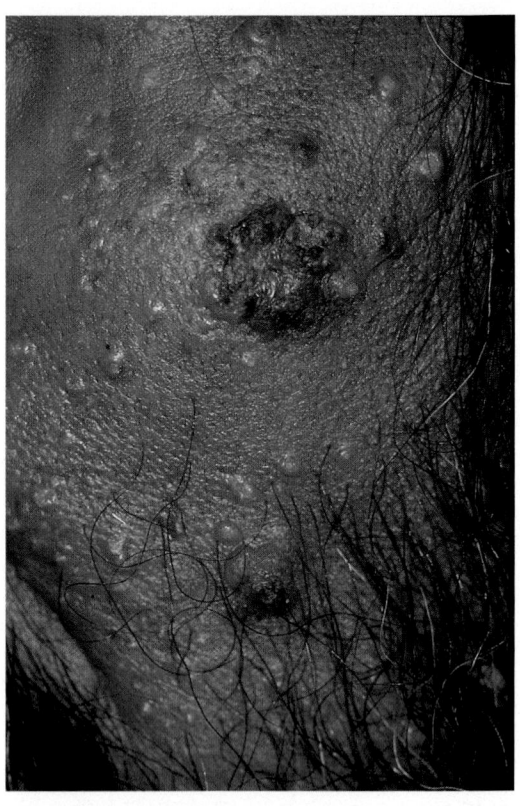

b

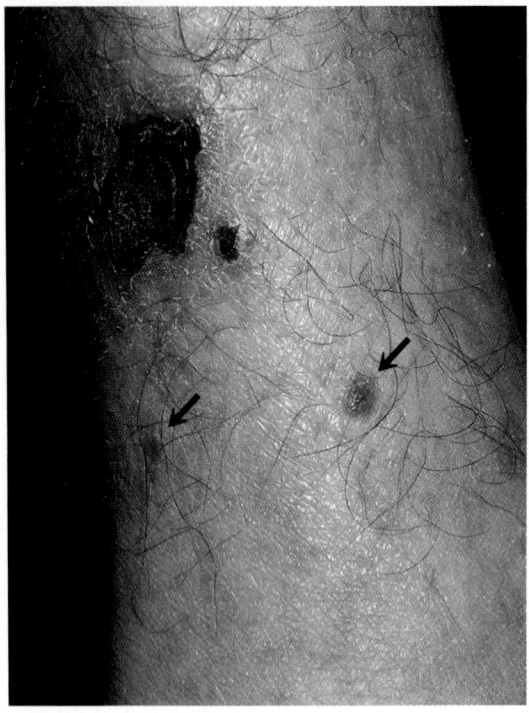

c

FIGURE 215-12 Varicella-zoster virus infection. *(a)* The crusted lesions of multidermatomal zoster are seen on the posterolateral chest wall in a young male with oral candidiasis; zoster was the presenting complication of HIV disease. *(b)* Ecthymatous VZV lesion, present for 2 months, is seen on the cheek of a male, who also had extensive facial molluscum contagiosum; 12 similar, very painful lesions were scattered in a generalized distribution. *(c)* A large painful, crusted lesion, present for 3 months, is seen on the lower calf; hemorrhagic pustules were also present in the same dermatome.

EBV; however, expression of viral antigens and replication appears dependent on some process in the epithelial cell maturation-differentiation phase.

For the most part, OHL is asymptomatic. Once OHL has been pointed out to the patient, however, its presence may be associated with some degree of anxiety. Patients should be reassured and instructed that OHL is not candidiasis. Topically applied podophyllin is effective in treating OHL, but lesions tend to recur in weeks to months.[286,287] Lesions may disappear shortly after beginning treatment with zidovudine, acyclovir, desciclovir, ganciclovir, or foscarnet but do not respond to anticandidal therapy.[288]

HUMAN PAPILLOMAVIRUS. Subclinical infection with HPV is nearly universal in humans, and clinical warts are very common in most individuals during the first few decades. It is well recognized that immunosuppressed persons such as organ transplant recipients have a higher incidence of HPV infections.[289] Likewise, in HIV

disease the prevalence of HPV infection is increased, with a higher incidence of common and genital warts, intraepithelial neoplasia, and possibly invasive squamous cell carcinoma.[290,291] In most persons with HIV disease and HPV infection, warts are not unusual in morphology, number, or response to treatment. An unusual pattern of extensive verruca plana and tinea versicolor-like warts, similar to the pattern seen in epidermodysplasia verruciformis, has also been reported in which HPV-5 was detected.[292,293] With moderate or advanced HIV-induced immunodeficiency, warts may become much more numerous and refractory to usual treatment modalities.

The presence of condylomata acuminata, occurring exclusively at anal/perianal sites in males, is associated with homosexual anogenital intercourse and with increased risk for HIV infection.[294] Condylomata acuminata in HIV-infected homosexual males are difficult to treat and are more likely to recur following CO_2 laser

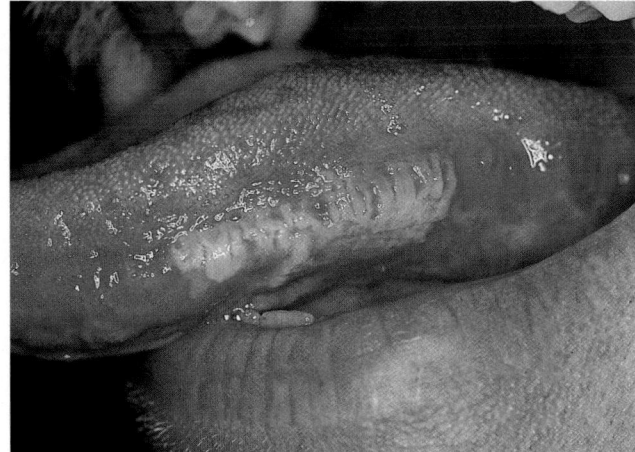

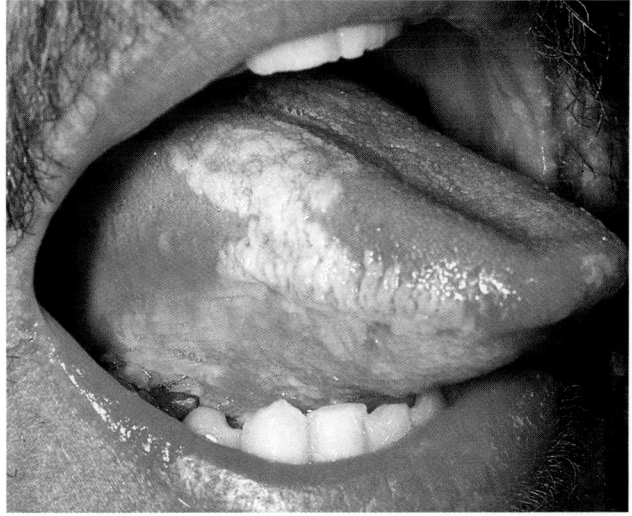

a

b

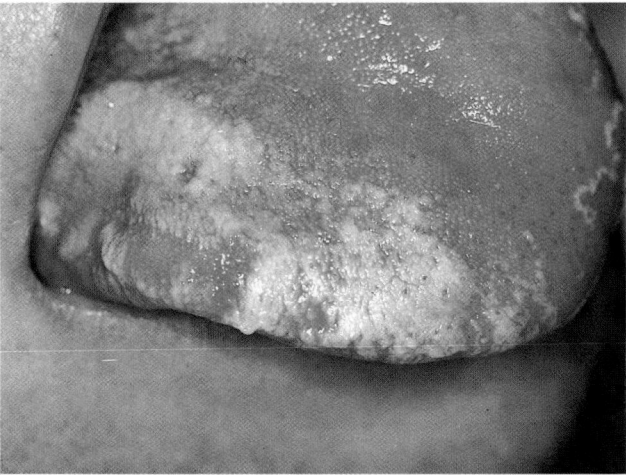

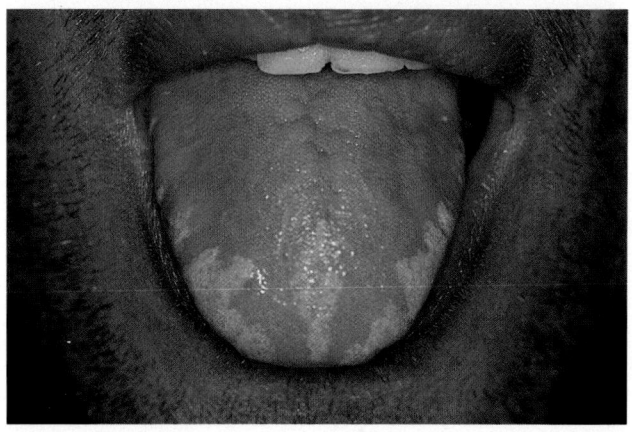

c

d

FIGURE 215-13   Epstein-Barr virus infection, oral hairy leukoplakia. *(a)* A well-demarcated, white plaque with corrugated surface is seen on the inferolateral aspect of the tongue; similar involvement, although less striking, was also present on the other side of the tongue. *(b)* White plaques are seen on three surfaces of the tongue. *(c)* Well-demarcated white plaques are seen on the dorsum of the tongue. *(d)* Well-demarcated white plaques extend from the inferolateral aspect of the tongue to the dorsum.

treatment than in non-HIV-infected subjects, independent of CD4 cell counts. Homosexual males with anal condylomata who experienced two or more recurrences following laser ablation had an 86 percent likelihood of being HIV-infected.

Of concern in HIV patients with moderate to advanced immunodeficiency is infection by potentially oncogenic types of HPV, i.e., 16, 18, 31, 33, 35. The incidence of intraepithelial neoplasia in HIV-infected patients is markedly increased both in women with cervical intraepithelial neoplasia (CIN)[295] and homosexual men with anogenital intraepithelial neoplasia (AIN).[296,297] Female prostitutes with HIV disease and CIN have been reported to be infected with multiple HPV types.[298] HPV DNA has been detected in anal swabs from 54 percent of HIV-infected male homosexuals.[299] Cytologic specimens from 39 percent of individuals demonstrated abnormalities ranging from atypia in 19 percent to AIN in 15 percent. Infection with multiple HPV types was documented in 12 percent and was associated with a high risk ratio for atypia. Median CD4 cell counts were significantly lower in individuals with cytologic abnormalities than in those with normal cytology. Similarly,

HIV-infected women had rates of cervical dysplasia five to ten times higher than non-HIV-infected women, i.e., up to 33 percent. To date, an increased incidence of invasive squamous cell carcinoma has not been documented in patients with AIN or in HIV-infected females with CIN; however, with improved antiretroviral therapy and longer survival, invasive squamous cell carcinoma arising in HPV-induced AIN or CIN may become a major clinical problem.

Clinically, the morphology of common warts, i.e., verruca vulgaris, verruca plana, and verruca plantaris, is not unusual in HIV disease (see Chap. 212). Warts, however, may be extensive, forming coalescent plaques, and be refractory to the usual treatments (Fig. 215-14*a*). The beard area is a common site of involvement, where the HPV is spread while shaving. These lesions must be distinguished from molluscum contagiosum, which occurs more commonly on the face than do warts. An unusual clinical presentation is flat warts associated with a pityriasis versicolor-like hypopigmentation, resembling the HPV-induced lesions seen in the inherited disorder epidermodysplasia verruciformis (Fig.

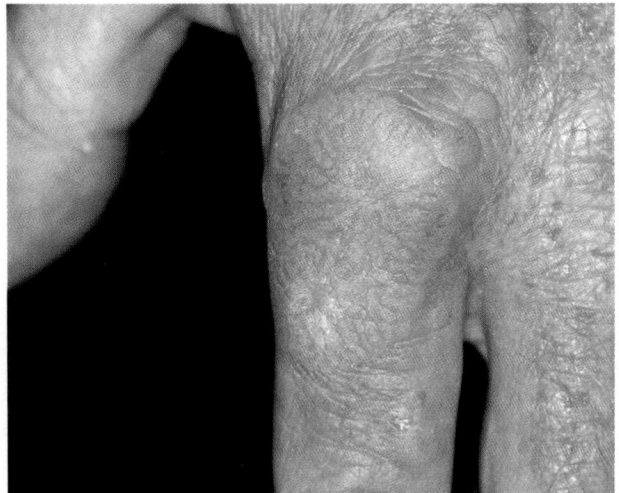

a

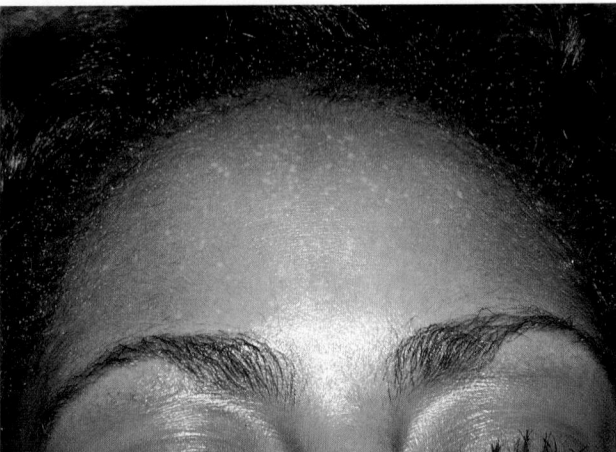

b

FIGURE 215-14 Human papillomavirus infection, common warts. *(a)* This large wart on the knuckle had been present for several years, was refactory to weekly cryosurgery, and was reduced in bulk by the patient, being frequently abraded using sandpaper. *(b)* Numerous, pityriasis versicolor-like hypopigmented flat warts are seen on the forehead.

215-14*b*).[292] In the four patients reported, HPV types 5 and 8 were identified, types usually occurring only in persons with epidermodysplasia verruciformis.[293]

The clinical morphology of mucosal warts is also not unusual in HIV disease (see Chaps. 112, 113, 212). However, as with common warts, mucosal warts may be profuse, confluent, and voluminous[300,301] and resistant to the usual modalities of therapy. Mucosal warts occur commonly on the anogenital and oral epithelia (Fig. 215-15*a*). Acetowhitening, a phenomenon in which mucosal HPV lesions turn white following a 5-min application with 5% acetic acid–soaked gauze, is helpful in detecting subclinical lesions. Lesions that have a different morphology than neighboring mucosal warts may represent bowenoid papulosis or intraepithelial neoplasia (Fig. 215-15*b*) and should be biopsied for a histologic diagnosis.[302]

The diagnosis of common and mucosal warts is usually made on clinical findings. Common warts must be differentiated most often from molluscum contagiosum, which occurs more frequently in HIV disease than do common warts. The differential diagnosis of

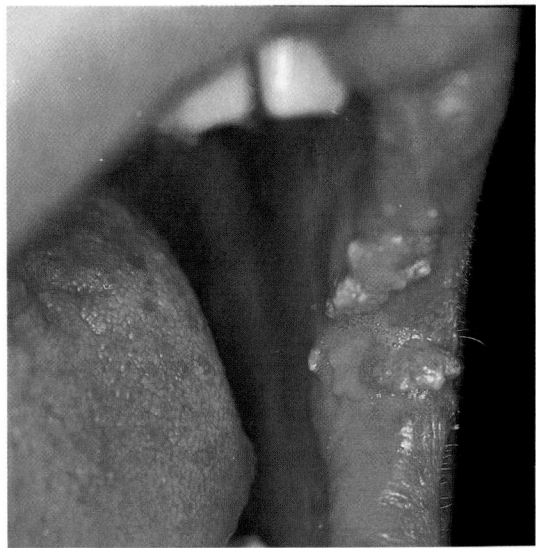

a

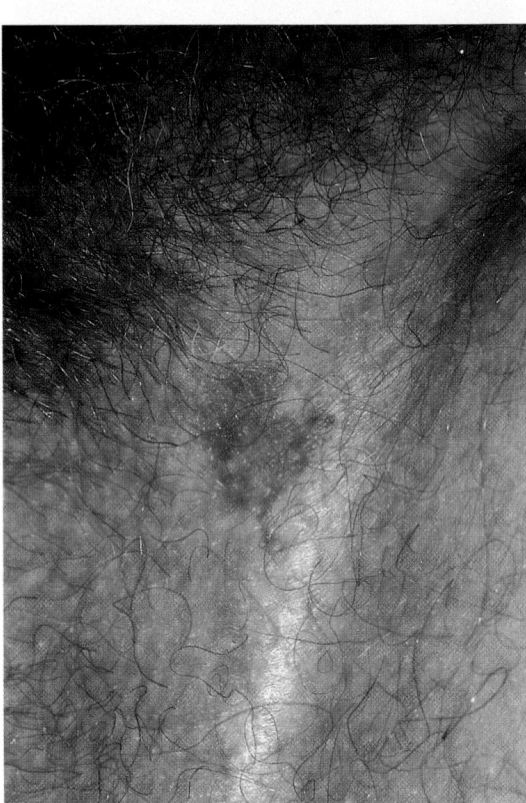

b

FIGURE 215-15 Human papillomavirus infection, mucosal. *(a)* Large condylomata acuminata are seen on the labial mucosa of this 20-year-old female, who also had vulvar and cervical condylomata. *(b)* Solitary hyperkeratotic brown plaque in the inguinal region; lesional biopsy specimen showed intraepithelial neoplasia.

mucosal warts includes condylomata lata, intraepithelial neoplasia, bowenoid papulosis, squamous cell carcinoma, molluscum contagiosum, lichen nitidus, lichen planus, normal sebaceous glands, angiokeratoma, pearly penile papules, folliculitis, moles, seborrheic keratoses, skin tags, pilar cyst, and scabetic nodules. In some cases, lesional biopsy should be obtained to rule out intraepithelial neoplasia or squamous cell carcinoma in situ (see "Neoplasia," above).

Condylomata recur after appropriate therapy in a high percentage of patients, due to persistence of latent HPV in normal-appearing perilesional skin. The major significance of HPV infection is the oncogenic potential. HPV types 16, 18, 31, and 33 are the major etiologic factors for cervical dysplasia and cervical squamous cell carcinoma, bowenoid papulosis, in situ and invasive carcinoma of the penis, and anal squamous cell carcinoma of homosexual/bisexual males.

Treatment of verruca vulgaris and condyloma acuminatum varies with the stage of HIV disease. Even in the normal host, subclinical HPV infection probably persists lifelong, and there is currently no cure. In the HIV-seropositive individual with little or no demonstrable immunodeficiency, the usual guidelines for therapy should be followed[303] (see Chap. 212). In advanced HIV-induced immunodeficiency, complete eradication of benign HPV-induced lesions is unlikely, and aggressive treatments such as CO_2 laser surgery may be contraindicated due to the high failure rate and associated morbidity. Isotretinoin and interferons may be helpful in some patients. Development of intraepithelial neoplasia should be monitored by appropriate cytologic smears and/or lesional biopsy.

MOLLUSCUM CONTAGIOSUM. Molluscum contagiosum is a common poxvirus infection of keratinized skin, which resolves spontaneously in the immunocompetent host, usually within a year, even in the absence of treatment. Transmission is usually via skin-to-skin contact, occurring commonly in children and sexual partners. The clinical course of molluscum contagiosum in HIV disease differs significantly from that in the normal host and is an excellent clinical marker of the degree of immunodeficiency. In a report on molluscum contagiosum in HIV disease, the mean CD4 cell count of patients with extensive involvement was 17/mm^3.[304]

Between 10 and 20 percent of patients with symptomatic HIV disease and AIDS are reported to have molluscum contagiosum.[305–307] Solitary papules can be quite large, up to 10 mm. More common, however, is the appearance of multiple (50 to 100) typical-appearing papules occurring most commonly on the face (Fig. 215-16a), eyelids, and neck, and in the intertriginous sites in the axillae, groins, or buttocks. In males with HIV disease, lesions are often confined to the beard area, the skin having been inoculated during the process of shaving; discontinuation of shaving does reduce the appearance of new lesions. A helpful diagnostic finding to distinguish the papules of molluscum contagiosum from other papular lesions is multiple keratotic plugs seen in a specimen frozen in liquid nitrogen (Fig. 215-16b). Beard-area lesions may be flat and confluent, best observed by sidelighting, and appear as a "cobblestoned" surface with few, if any, typical discrete umbilicated papules. In Caucasian patients, the papules are skin colored, leading to variable cosmetic disfigurement. In Latino or African-American patients, however, hyperpigmentation or postinflammatory hypopigmentation following treatment accentuates the cosmetic disfigurement (Fig. 215-16c). Occasionally, large lesions can become confluent, forming large "cluster-of-grapes" lesions.[308]

The diagnosis of molluscum contagiosum in the HIV-infected patient is usually made on clinical grounds. The differential diagnosis of a solitary lesion of molluscum contagiosum includes a common wart, basal cell carcinoma,[309] keratoacanthoma, and squamous cell carcinoma. The differential diagnosis of multiple facial lesions includes hematogenous dissemination to the skin of cryptococcosis, histoplasmosis, and coccidioidomycosis. Early biopsy of a facial lesion with a touch preparation is indicated if the papules appear at all atypical or appear suddenly in a patient with

fever, headache, confusion, or pulmonary infiltrate. In comparison to the course of molluscum contagiosum in nonimmunodeficient individuals in whom lesions resolve spontaneously, the course in HIV-infected patients is one of persistence and recurrence. Viral structures consistent with molluscum contagiosum have been demonstrated within clinically normal epidermis surrounding lesions, suggesting the mechanism by which new lesions sprout up at treatment sites.[310]

Treatment of molluscum contagiosum should be directed at controlling the numbers and bulk of cosmetically disturbing lesions rather than at eradication of all lesions. Liquid nitrogen cryosurgery is the most convenient method and usually must be repeated every 2 to 4 weeks. Electro- or CO_2 laser coagulation may be more effective but is usually more painful and has the potential for aerosolizing HIV. Curettage is also effective but is bloody. Discontinuation of shaving is helpful in camouflaging existing lesions and often reduces spread to new sites. In most cases, cure of molluscum contagiosum cannot be accomplished, and new lesions tend to occur subsequently. Initiation of zidovudine therapy has been reported to be associated with the disappearance of extensive lesions of molluscum contagiosum.

HUMAN T-CELL LYMPHOTROPIC VIRUS I. Human T-cell lymphotropic virus I, the first retrovirus identified in humans, is transmitted by the identical routes as HIV. Significant percentages of populations of areas such as Japan, Africa, the Caribbean, and the United States are infected with HTLV-I. In the United States, IDUs are dually infected with HTLV-I and HIV. The effect on the morbidity and mortality of persons with coinfection of HTLV-I and HIV is not known. In a retrospective study of a cohort of Peruvian men with HIV disease, 18 percent were also infected with HTLV-I or -II.[311,312] At the time of the study, the mortality was 63.3 percent in those infected with HIV only and was 80 percent in those dually infected. Survival time from onset of late symptomatic and advanced HIV disease to death was shorter in the dually infected group (5 months) than in those with HIV infection alone (10 months). The results of larger studies are needed before the effect of dual infection is known.

Sexually Transmitted Diseases In the majority of cases, HIV transmission occurs during sexual intercourse. Many patients with HIV disease have had other sexually transmitted diseases (STDs) in addition to HIV infection.

SYPHILIS. The incidence of acquired syphilis in the United States has reached a 40-year high. Prior to the HIV epidemic, two-thirds of syphilis cases occurred in homosexual men; currently, however, the incidence in this group has fallen by 50 percent, presumably due to safer sexual practices. In heterosexual men and women in large cities such as San Francisco and New York, the incidence of syphilis has increased by over 75 percent. In heterosexual individuals, syphilis occurs with increasing incidence in IDUs, users of crack cocaine who exchange sex for drugs, and the sexual partners of both groups, especially in Latinos and African-Americans living in large cities. The incidence of congenital syphilis in infants of mothers in these groups is also increasing. Genital ulcer disease is recognized as an important cofactor in HIV transmission; thus an epidemic of syphilis among heterosexuals increases the risk of concurrent HIV infection.

Coinfection with both *Treponema pallidum* and HIV may alter the usual course of either disease when occurring alone. Individuals with genital ulcer disease such as syphilis with a chancre are at increased risk for becoming HIV-positive if exposed to an HIV-infected sexual partner. In the reverse clinical circumstance, an individual with long-standing HIV infection with some degree of

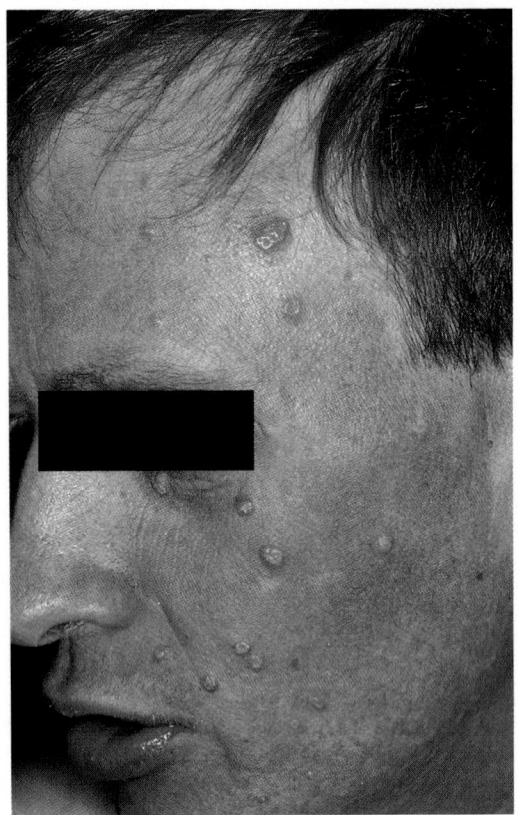

a

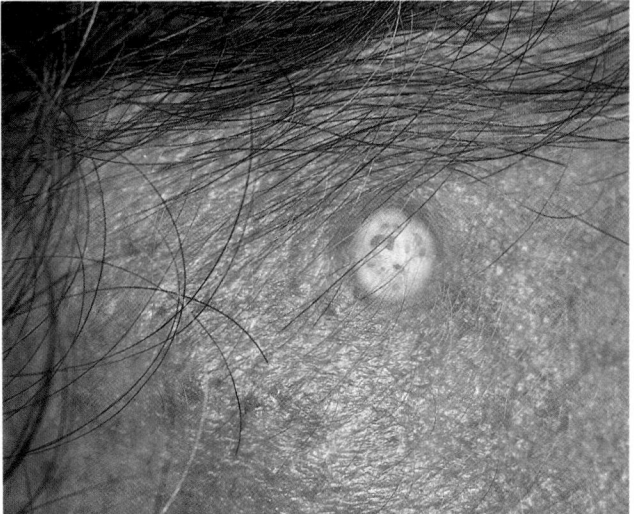

b

FIGURE 215-16 Molluscum contagiosum. *(a)* Pink
umbilicated papules are seen scattered on the face. *(b)* A papule
treated with liquid nitrogen shows multiple keratotic plugs,
typical of molluscum contagiosum in HIV disease. *(c)* The
unusual feature of molluscum contagiosum in HIV-infected
patients is the large number of lesions and their occurrence on
the face.

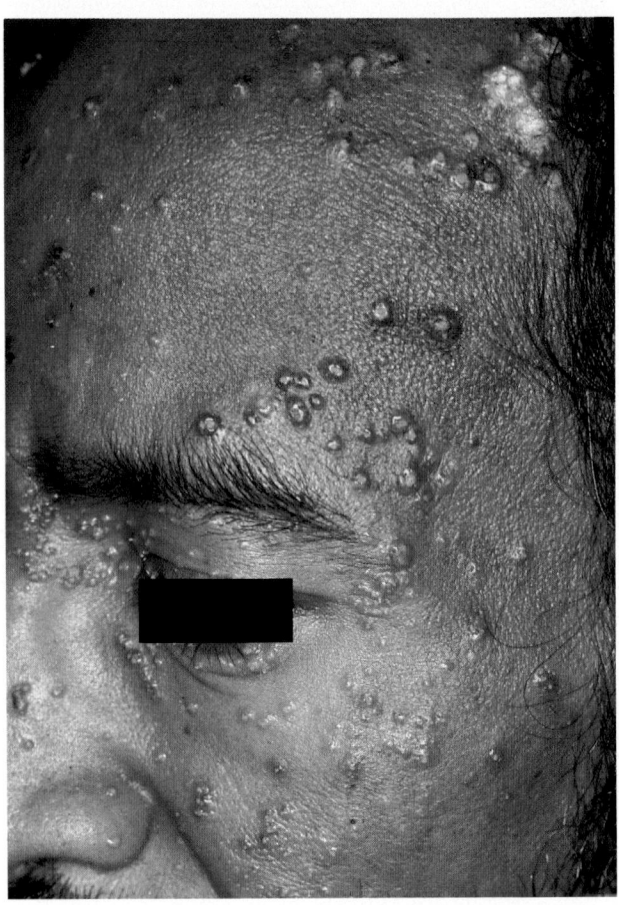

c

immunodeficiency who becomes infected with *T. pallidum* may
experience an altered course of syphilis.

The cutaneous findings of syphilis occurring in the setting of
HIV disease are not unusual in the majority of patients. In the
HIV-infected patient with moderate to advanced immunodeficiency
who becomes infected with *T. pallidum,* the following variations
from the expected course of syphilis have been noted: (1) limited or
absent antibody responses to infection with repeatedly negative reagin and treponemal antibody testing; (2) increased severity of the
clinical manifestations; (3) painful rather than the usually painless
chancre of primary syphilis due to secondary infection; (4) shorter
latency period before development of meningovascular syphilis;
(5) rapid progression to tertiary disease within the first year of infection; (6) lack of response to penicillin therapy; and (7) relapse
without reexposure despite ''adequate'' treatment.[313] Indurated,
shiny, erythematous, confluent plaques on the face and scalp with
associated alopecia and tautness of skin have been reported in secondary stage infection.[314] Lues maligna, a rare form of secondary
syphilis, has also been reported in HIV disease; it is characterized
by pleomorphic skin lesions including pustules, nodules, ulcers,
and a necrotizing vasculitis.

The majority of HIV-infected persons who acquire syphilis
have the expected clinical course of disease, expected serologic

findings in serum and CSF, and respond to the recommended therapeutic regimens. In a small percentage of persons, however, the
clinical course, serologic response, and response to antibiotic treatment are unusual. The major variations of syphilis in HIV-infected
persons are: a greater likelihood of ocular (retrobulbar optic neuritis)[315,316] and neurologic disease,[317,318] an accelerated course or
more florid clinical findings,[319–324] a greater likelihood of treatment failure,[325–328] and failure to develop the usual STS responses

in serum and CSF.[329] Because unusual clinical presentations or failures of treatment are reported as single or a few cases, the percentage of cases of syphilis with an unusual clinical course of disease in HIV-infected patients in unknown. An inadequate immune response to *T. pallidum* is considered to cause the various abnormalities in the course of syphilis in the HIV-infected patient.[330]

Nearly all HIV-infected patients with symptomatic neurosyphilis have positive syphilis serologies.[331] Although uncommon, seronegative primary and secondary syphilis have been reported.[332] Normally, treponemal tests remain positive throughout life. Seven percent of seropositive asymptomatic HIV-infected patients with a history of syphilis and 38 percent of those with symptomatic HIV infection with a history of syphilis have been reported to lose reactivity of treponemal tests.[333]

HIV testing is advised for all sexually active patients with syphilis. Neurosyphilis should be considered in the differential diagnosis of neurologic disease in HIV-infected persons. When clinical findings suggest syphilis but serologic tests are negative or confusing, alternative tests such as biopsy of lesions, dark-field examination, and direct fluorescent antibody staining of lesion material should be used.

Penicillin regimens should be used whenever possible for all stages of syphilis in HIV disease. Erythromycin has been reported to be ineffective at curing secondary syphilis in HIV disease.[334] CSF examination and/or treatment with a regimen appropriate for neurosyphilis is necessary for all patients coinfected with syphilis and HIV, regardless of the clinical stage of syphilis. Patients should be followed clinically and with quantitative nontreponemal serologic tests (VDRL, RPR) at 1, 2, 3, 6, 9, and 12 months after treatment. Patients with early syphilis whose titers increase or fail to decrease fourfold within 6 months should undergo CSF examination and be re-treated. In such patients, CSF abnormalities could be due to HIV-related infection, neurosyphilis, or both. Although the CDC does not recommend a different regimen for syphilis in HIV-infected patients, some experts feel that a second or a third dose of penicillin should be given at 1-week intervals.[22,46,335] Because *T. pallidum* may persist in the CNS of the HIV-infected patient in spite of adequate antibiotic treatment, the possibility of chronic maintenance treatment, analogous to secondary prophylaxis of cryptococcal meningitis, has been raised.[25]

Arthropod Infestations SCABIES. During early HIV infection, with the immune system relatively intact, scabies behaves as it does in non-HIV-infected individuals. Pruritus with or without rash is a very common complaint in HIV-infected persons; scabies is relatively common and should always be included in the differential diagnosis of pruritus. As immunodeficiency progresses, HIV-infected patients are more liable to experience crusted (Norwegian) scabies in which the number of infesting mites can increase into the millions.[336] Although usually a generalized process, crusted scabies has been reported to be limited to a single digit.[337] Generalized scaling to marked hyperkeratosis may resemble psoriasis vulgaris, keratoderma blenorrhagica of Reiter's syndrome, or Darier's disease.[338] Crusted scabies occurring in HIV-infected infants may be confused with seborrheic dermatitis or atopic dermatitis. Because of the number of organisms in crusted scabies, recurrences are common, and hospital epidemics may occur. Excoriations often become secondarily infected with *S. aureus,* which in some patients causes an invasive infection complicated by septicemia, and death.

Scabies must always be considered in the differential diagnosis of pruritus in HIV-infected patients, even in those who have experienced prior episodes of exanthematous drug eruptions and/or eosinophilic folliculitis. Use of potent topical corticosteroids for such previously diagnosed pruritic conditions may mask the presence of scabetic infestation. Topical treatment with lindane or permethrin lotion is effective; in crusted scabies, total-body application may be required. Keratolytic agents may be needed in crusted scabies to debride hyperkeratotic areas, in conjunction with debridement of involved nails.

Common Noninfectious Complications

Disorders of Epidermal Cell Kinetics and Differentiation
SEBORRHEIC DERMATITIS (see also *Pityrosporum* infection).   Seborrheic dermatitis is common in HIV disease, the severity varying with the stage of immunodeficiency[339]; in one report, the incidence was 4.7 percent in early disease and 26.7 percent in those with late-stage disease.[340] Clinically, seborrheic dermatitis in HIV disease is unusual only in its severity, involving the hairy regions of the scalp, face, axillae, and pubic area, and in its resistance to usual banal treatments (Fig. 215-17).

PSORIASIS VULGARIS.   In two large series, psoriasis has been reported to occur in 1.3 percent[341] and 2 percent[342] of persons with HIV disease. The prevalence of psoriasis appears to be no higher than in the general population, where it is estimated at 1.6 percent, but the prevalence of psoriatic arthritis (1.7 percent) is higher than expected (0.10 percent).[343] The presence of peripheral arthritis in 18 men with HIV-associated psoriasis was 32 percent and correlated with the presence of HLA-B27 (Fig. 215-18).[344] The presence

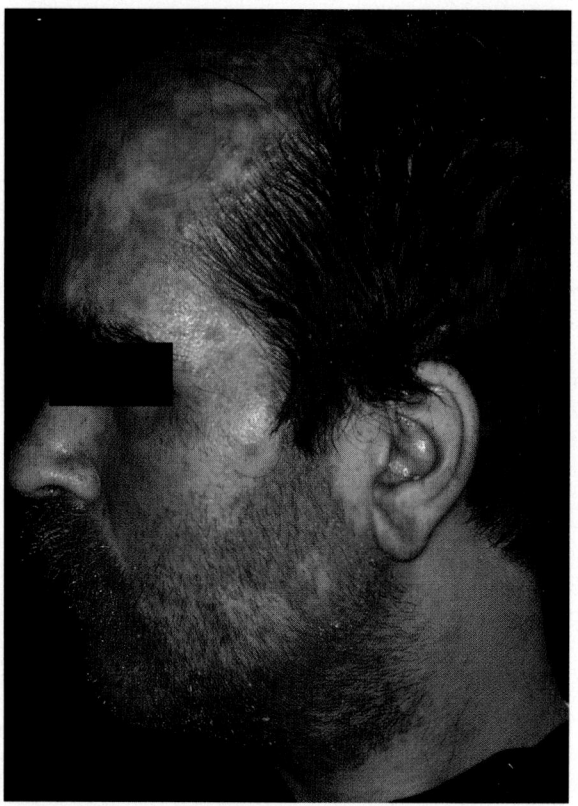

FIGURE 215-17 Seborrheic dermatitis. Striking erythema and greasy scaling is seen on the head and neck of this person with advanced HIV disease.

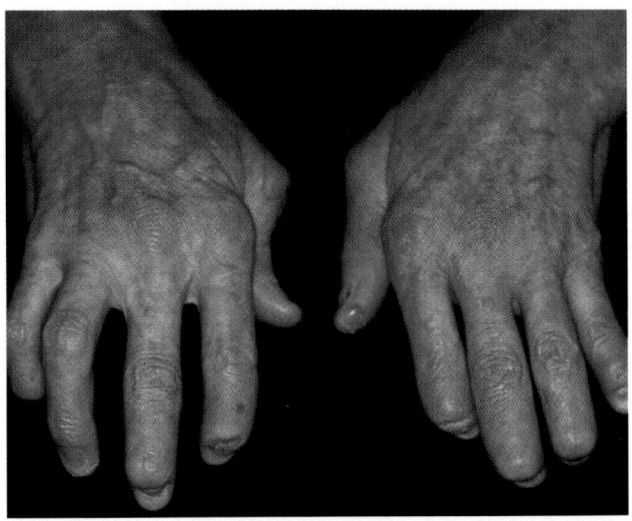

FIGURE 215-18 Psoriatic arthritis. Marked joint deformity is seen on the hands; similar changes were also present on the feet. Recalcitrant psoriasis vulgaris and psoriatic arthritis had begun 6 months previously.

of HLA-Cw6 and other HLA antigens previously found to be related to psoriasis unassociated with HIV infection is less commonly found in patients developing psoriasis after HIV infection.[342]

Mild preexisting psoriasis, in an individual with or without a family history of psoriasis, may suddenly undergo severe exacerbation in patients with advanced HIV disease. More commonly, psoriasis is first noted at some point after HIV seroconversion.[345–347] No unusual clinical lesions occur in persons in whom psoriasis and HIV disease coexist. Psoriasis does tend to become more severe as the degree of immunodeficiency increases.[348] Onset of psoriasis in any person at risk for HIV disease should promptly raise the issue of HIV serotesting.

The histology of psoriasis in persons with HIV disease differs from the histology of psoriasis in those without HIV infection. The dermal infiltrate in HIV-infected individuals has fewer T cells and significantly more plasma cells.[349] Despite early failures of in situ hybridization, HIV RNA transcripts have now been identified in 5 of 15 lesional skin biopsies using this technique, whereas RNA transcripts were absent in normal-appearing skin from HIV-infected individuals and in psoriatic skin of normal controls.[350] The transactivating *tat* gene and the HIV provirus of transgenic mice have been reported to produce epidermal hyperplasia either directly or by cytokine production, suggesting that HIV may play a direct role in the genesis of psoriasis in HIV-infected individuals. Interferon-γ stimulates monocytes/macrophages to produce and release large amounts of neopterin, a molecule that decreases upon cyclosporine-induced improvement in psoriasis. Significantly increased serum interferon-γ has been identified in HIV-infected individuals, suggesting that it may play a pathogenic role in HIV-associated psoriasis.[351].

HIV-associated psoriasis occasionally responds to antiretroviral treatment with zidovudine.[345,352] A trial of zidovudine is recommended in patients not being treated with antiretroviral drugs. Limited disease usually responds well to routine topical therapy with topical corticosteroids, anthralin, or tar. Widespread disease tends to respond less well. Although ultraviolet B and PUVA (psoralen plus UVA) have been used effectively,[351] con-

cerns remain regarding the immunosuppressive potential of phototherapy in HIV disease.[353] Five patients with psoriasis and HIV disease who were treated with PUVA for two 4-week periods 2 months apart remained well for the entire 1-year follow-up period, and markers of progression of HIV disease remained stable or improved.[354] Similar concerns about other systemic treatments also exist. Methotrexate and agents that are immunosuppressive are generally contraindicated in treatment of HIV-associated psoriasis because of the potential for further immunosuppression, leukopenia, and infection. However, cyclosporine has been used successfully in a person with HIV disease and severe psoriasis, with complete clearing of the skin for over a year as well as general improvement in the patient's well-being and no deterioration in his immune status.[355] It seems clear that drugs with immunosuppressive action, such as cyclosporine, should be used with great caution in HIV disease.[345,355] The retinoid etretinate, which does not affect the immune system, may be useful in treating some persons with psoriasis and HIV disease.[345] Psoriasis occasionally improves or disappears completely in advanced HIV disease.[355,356]

ICHTHYOSIFORM DERMATOSES. Xerosis or acquired ichthyosis (Fig. 215-19), reported to occur in 23 to 30 percent of HIV-infected individuals,[357–359] may be related to chronic illness, malnutrition, poor hygiene, or immunologic deficit. The lack of correlation of the prevalence or of the severity of either the ichthyosis or xerosis with the degree of immunosupression[289,290] suggests that the relationship is more complex and may be directly related to the HIV.[360,361]

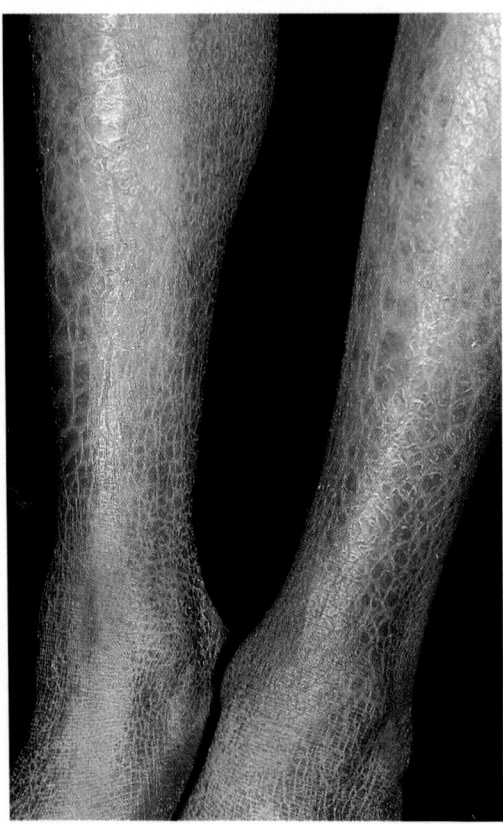

FIGURE 215-19 Acquired ichthyosis. A tesselated pattern is seen on both legs and feet in this male with advanced HIV disease; ichthyosis appeared 1 year previously and had a generalized distribution.

Papular and Pruritic Eruptions

Pruritus is a common complaint in patients with late symptomatic and advanced HIV disease. Although usually accompanied by cutaneous findings, pruritus may occur without lesions and probably occurs on a "metabolic" basis. Most patients with pruritus, however, do have associated primary and secondary cutaneous findings. Papular eruptions can occur as follicular and nonfollicular lesions, i.e., papules, pustules, or nodules[362]; commonly, although not universally, their presence and severity correlate with the severity of HIV disease. Several of these eruptions have distinctive clinical or histologic features, including HIV-associated eosinophilic folliculitis, *Pityrosporum* folliculitis, demodicidosis, heightened response to insect bites, and prurigo nodularis. In many patients, the eruption is clinically and histologically nonspecific[363] and difficult to treat effectively, although it responds somewhat to topical antipruritics and to potent topical corticosteroids.

Follicular Pruritic Eruptions STAPHYLOCOCCUS AUREUS
FOLLICULITIS. *S. aureus* commonly causes folliculitis that is often accompanied by an eczematous dermatitis secondary to scratching. The pathogenesis of the combination of pruritus plus *S. aureus* infection plus eczematous dermatitis occurring in HIV disease is not known. Diagnosis of *S. aureus* folliculitis with or without eczematous dermatitis is made by Gram's stain and culture of lesional exudate. Patients with *S. aureus* infection and eczematous dermatitis should be treated with topical steroids and antibacterial therapy with topical agents, washing with a benzoyl peroxide preparation followed by application of mupirocin (pseudomonic acid) ointment to the nares and involved skin, as well as oral antibiotics. In that staphylococcal folliculitis and eczema tend to recur, prophylactic use of benzoyl peroxide and mupirocin are often useful in preventing recurrence.

HIV-ASSOCIATED EOSINOPHILIC FOLLICULITIS.   A chronic, pruritic, culture-negative folliculitis that is unresponsive to systemic antibiotic therapy occurs in HIV disease—HIV-associated eosinophilic folliculitis.[364] It has some similarities to Ofuji's disease or eosinophilic pustular folliculitis, a rare eruption consisting of sterile, pruritic papules and pustules on the face, trunk, and extremities. Eosinophilic folliculitis may be accompanied by peripheral leukocytosis and eosinophilia and is characterized histologically by neutrophilic and eosinophilic infiltration of hair follicles.[364–366] Pruritus and advanced immunodeficiency appear to be constant features.[299–301] Clinically, eosinophilic folliculitis is characterized by multiple follicular and nonfollicular, urticarial papules, most commonly involving the upper trunk, face, and proximal extremities (Fig. 215-20).

The diagnosis of eosinophilic folliculitis is made by the histologic findings. The differential diagnosis most commonly includes acne vulgaris, rosacea, scabies, and staphylococcal folliculitis. Elevated peripheral eosinophil counts, without leukocytosis, and increased IgE levels occur in the majority of cases. Ultraviolet B phototherapy, potent topical corticosteroids, and the nonsedating antihistamines astemizole and cetirizine[367] have been reported to ameliorate the pruritus significantly and also to clear the eruption.[299,301] Despite these encouraging reports, treatment is usually extremely difficult.

Other Causes of Pruritus Other papular eruptions have been reported in HIV disease, but the lack of diagnostic criteria prevents definitive diagnosis; clinical and histologic findings are nonspecific.[368–372]

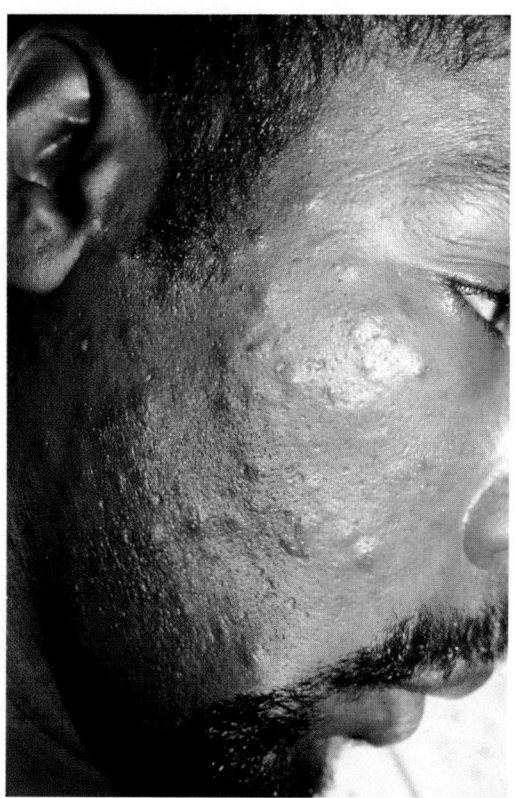

FIGURE 215-20   HIV-associated eosinophilic folliculitis. Numerous papules, follicular and nonfollicular, are seen on the face; lesions were also present on the upper trunk and neck; the diagnosis was made on lesional skin biopsy.

Follicular, inflammatory, pruritic papules may represent either an exaggerated response to insect bites[373] or a localized *S. aureus* infection.[374] Antibodies to bullous pemphigoid appear to be increased in the serum of patients with HIV disease and chronic pruritus,[375] the frequency of antibodies increasing with advancing HIV disease. Seventy-five percent of a subgroup of these individuals with a papulovesicular pruritic eruption related to HIV infection had antibodies to bullous pemphigoid.

Disorders of the Oral Mucosa

All individuals with HIV disease experience disorders of the oral mucosa during the course of their illness (Table 215-7). Some disorders occur early in the course of HIV disease and their detection on routine physical examination should raise the issue of HIV serotesting. In a study of 103 consecutive patients with late symptomatic and advanced HIV disease, oropharyngeal candidiasis was the most common oral finding, diagnosed in more than 90 percent.[376] Other orolabial findings included herpetic ulcers (10 percent), xerostomia (10 percent), exfoliative cheilitis (9 percent), hairy leukoplakia (7 percent), Kaposi's sarcoma (4 percent), patchy depapillation of the tongue (6 percent), and ulcers of uncertain cause (3 percent). Other studies have found similar oral diseases but with slightly different frequency.

Aphthous Ulcers Minor recurrent aphthous ulcerations (RAU) are common lesions in all populations but tend to occur more often and

TABLE 215-7

Differential Diagnosis by Type of Oropharyngeal Lesions in HIV Disease

Papules, nodules, plaques	Candidiasis, hyperplastic Hairy leukoplakia Condylomata acuminata Intraepithelial neoplasia Invasive squamous cell carcinoma Lymphoma
Leukoplakia	Hair leukoplakia Candidiasis, pseudomembranous (thrush) Condylomata acuminata Intraepithelial neoplasia Invasive squamous cell carcinoma
Pigmented macules	Candidiasis, atrophic Kaposi's sarcoma Zidovudine pigmentation
Erosion(s), ulcer(s)	
Solitary	Aphthous ulcer HSV Histoplasmosis Cryptococcosis Fixed drug reaction
Multiple	Aphthous ulcers HSV Candidiasis, atrophic Histoplasmosis Cryptococcosis Erythema multiforme Fixed drug reaction

NOTE: HSV, herpes simplex virus.

be larger in persons with advancing HIV-induced immunodeficiency. The minor RAU are small, self-limited, rarely progress to involve the hypopharynx or esophagus, and do not usually cause significant pain on swallowing (odynophagia). Major RAU (defined as >1.0 cm in diameter) are extremely painful ulcerations of the oral mucosa, hypopharynx, and esophagus; they can heal with scarring and are rare in immunocompetent individuals but develop more commonly in patients with AIDS.[377] Ulceration may be so extensive, often involving the tongue (Fig. 215-21), gingiva, lips, and esophagus, and pain upon swallowing may be so severe that rapid weight loss ensues.

Diagnosis of large RAU is usually made on clinical findings; however, large persistent ulcers should be biopsied to rule out squamous cell carcinoma, lymphoma (Fig. 215-22), herpetic ulcers, and deep fungal infections such as histoplasmosis or cryptococcosis. Ulceration of the gingiva must be differentiated from acute ulcerative necrotizing gingivitis. Lesional biopsy specimens of RAU show diffuse inflammation and necrosis affecting the oral mucosa, submucosa, muscle, and connective tissue.

Major RAU are usually refractory to topical treatment. Oral corticosteroids are relatively contraindicated because of the risk of activation of a latent infection. Thalidomide given orally at a dose of 100 mg once or twice daily is very effective in the treatment of severely painful major aphthous ulcers that limit nutrition.[378] Recurrence of major aphthous ulcers is common and can be treated with either another short course of thalidomide or low-dose daily or alternate day administration. Side effects include sedation, constipation, peripheral neuropathy, neutropenia, and birth defects associated with administration during early pregnancy.

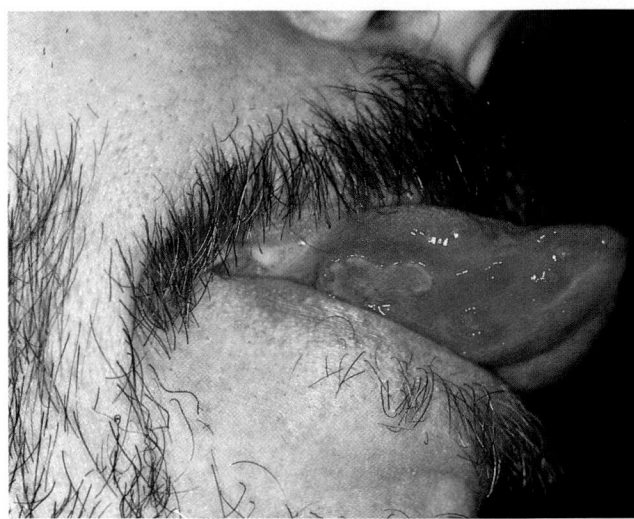

FIGURE 215-21   Major aphthous ulcer. A very large, deep ulcer is seen on the inferolateral aspect of the tongue. This painful lesion interfered with eating and was associated with significant weight loss. The ulcer healed in 10 days when the patient was treated with thalidomide, 100 mg daily by mouth.

Adverse Cutaneous Drug Reactions

The incidence of cutaneous eruptions from a variety of drugs, especially antibacterial agents, is high in HIV disease. The most common offending agents are sulfonamides and amoxicillin-clavulanate. The incidence of multiple-drug reactions is also increased.[379] Although the pathogenesis of the high rates of adverse reactions in HIV disease is unknown, underlying infections with CMV or EBV may have a role, as such reactivity to ampicillin and amoxicillin occurs in patients with primary EBV or CMV mononucleosis.[380]

Trimethoprim-sulfamethoxazole (TMP-SMZ) (Bactrim, Septra), used commonly in HIV disease for treatment of and prophy-

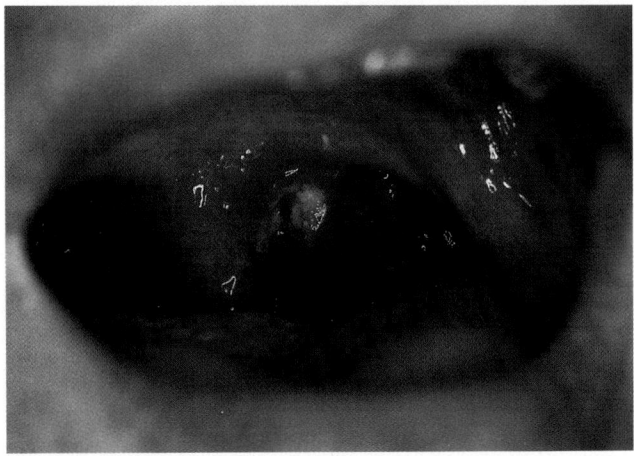

FIGURE 215-22   Lymphoma, pharyngeal. This patient with advanced HIV disease and a history of painful major aphthous ulcers presented with this painful pharyngeal ulceration. Lesional biopsy showed non-Hodgkin's lymphoma, which responded to radiotherapy.

laxis against PCP, is more effective than the alternatives, dapsone or aerosolized pentamidine. Sulfonamides are also the mainstay of therapy for prophylaxis and treatment of CNS toxoplasmosis. Between 50 and 60 percent of HIV-infected patients treated with intravenous TMP-SMZ develop an exanthematous eruption associated with fever 1 to 2 weeks after starting therapy,[381,382] ten times more often than the general population. Alternative treatments for PCP in sulfa-sensitive patients are intravenous pentamidine or desensitization to the sulfonamide. Successful desensitization has been accomplished in patients with prior exanthematous or urticarial reactions to dapsone, sulfadiazine, and TMP-SMZ.[383–387]

Pentamidine has been reported to cause severe adverse reactions in up to 20 percent of HIV-infected patients.[337] Prophylactic treatment for PCP includes low-dose daily TMP-SMZ, weekly sulfadoxine-pyrimethamine (Fansidar), and monthly aerosolized pentamidine. Although these agents have lower adverse reaction rates than high-dose intravenous TMP-SMZ, they are not without cutaneous side effects. Fansidar has been reported to cause erythema multiforme and fatal toxic epidermal necrolysis,[388] and aerosolized pentamidine to cause a widespread, erythematous, maculopapular, pruritic eruption.[389]

Severe bullous eruptions appear to be much more frequent in HIV disease. In a report of six cases of erythema multiforme major and six of toxic epidermal necrolysis (TEN), all adverse reactions were to sulfonamide: sulfadiazine in six cases, TMP-SMZ in two, and Fansidar in two.[390,391] By the end of 1992, a total of 25 cases of TEN had been reported in HIV disease. Of 80 cases of TEN reviewed in France over a 6-year period from 1984 to 1989, 14 individuals had HIV disease; sulfa drugs were the most common offending agents in this group.[392] During this study period, the number of cases of TEN was 375 times that expected. In all cases, TEN occurred in patients with advanced HIV disease and had a 21 percent mortality rate in these 14 patients. In the other 11 patients with TEN in HIV disease, the mortality rate was 55 percent. Early TEN is difficult to distinguish from an exanthematous drug reaction; TEN, however, often has early mucosal involvement.[392]

Although uncommon, adverse drug reactions have been linked to zidovudine; they include hyperpigmentation, acne, pruritus, urticaria, and leukocytoclastic vasculitis.[393] The most common cutaneous reaction is a longitudinal, brown-black streak of hyperpigmentation of the nail plate, occurring in up to 40 percent of zidovudine-treated individuals,[394] a phenomenon noted more commonly in African-Americans than in Latinos or Caucasians. Nail dyschromia is not associated with drug dose, HIV risk group, or stage of HIV disease; the pigmentary changes are usually noted within 4 to 8 weeks after initiating zidovudine treatment but may occur as late as 1 year later.[395] Pigmentation usually begins proximally and progresses distally to occasionally involve the free margin of the nail plate. Longitudinal streaks are most common, but diffuse pigmentation and transverse bands may occur. Thumbnail pigmentation develops most frequently, and the thumbnail is usually the first affected, followed by the fingernails then the toenails.[395] Zidovudine-induced nail dyschromia is caused by increased melanogenesis of the nail matrix; clippings of involved nails reveal melanin granules within the nail plate.[394] Hyperpigmentation of mucous membranes and skin also occurs, although mucosal pigmentation is much more commonly observed in more heavily melanized persons.[396] Longitudinal melanonychia has also been reported in HIV disease, independent of zidovudine.[397] Diffuse hyperpigmentation mimicking primary adrenal insufficiency has been reported in two zidovudine-treated patients with AIDS.[398]

Increased eyelash growth and other types of hypertrichosis have been reported in AIDS patients, reported both in patients on zidovudine[399,400] and in individuals never exposed to the drug.[401] Although infrequent, severe exanthematous eruptions warranting drug withdrawal occur in approximately 1 percent of zidovudine-treated patients within 8 to 12 days following initiation of therapy. Successful desensitization has been accomplished in allergic individuals (D.K. McFadden, personal communication, 1990).

Foscarnet (trisodium phosphonoformate) has been reported to cause painful, penile ulcers in almost 30 percent of patients undergoing high-dose induction therapy for CMV retinitis, within 7 to 24 days after starting treatment.[402] The ulcers, which may represent a fixed drug eruption, cleared spontaneously despite continued treatment in one-half of those affected.

Systemic treatment with methotrexate for psoriasis and with corticosteroids for vasculitis, non-Hodgkin's lymphoma, and opportunistic infections has precipitated both rapid proliferation and the sudden appearance of KS.[276,403]

Cutaneous Changes in Nutritional Disorders

Weight loss occurs commonly in HIV disease and is often secondary to malabsorptive diseases and/or enterocolitis. In some persons, no cause other than HIV disease can be found. This progressive weight loss occurs commonly in HIV disease in sub-Saharan Africa, where it is known as "slim" disease,[404] and may cause death through progressive wasting before opportunistic infections or malignancies occur. The wasting syndrome also occurs in persons with HIV disease in industrialized countries, the most apparent cutaneous findings being loss of subcutaneous fat and musculature.

Mucocutaneous Findings in Children

HIV disease in children differs somewhat from that in adults in both the natural history and clinical presentation.[405–407] Approximately 1 percent of all patients with AIDS in the United States have been children under 13 years of age. In one-half of these children, the diagnosis is made in the first year of life. Seventy-five percent of all cases of HIV disease in children is transmitted perinatally. In industrialized countries, the majority of children with HIV disease are children of IDUs or of bisexual fathers.[308] Because vertical transmission (transmission from mother to child) accounts for the overwhelming majority of HIV disease in children, a rise in the number of those cases is predicted, associated with the escalating number of young HIV-infected women. Prior to the availability of HIV serotesting of blood, children also became infected through blood and blood product administration, most often in the neonatal period.[408]

In hemophiliacs, the incubation period is longer for those infected at a younger age.[409] Young hemophiliacs with low CD4 cell counts are less likely to progress to advanced HIV disease than older hemophiliacs with similar counts.[410] In sharp contrast, children infected by vertical transmission of HIV experience a shorter incubation period and more rapid progression of HIV disease.[411,412] In children, in comparison to adults, opportunistic infections such as PCP may occur when CD4 cell counts are well above 200/mm^3. Measles and varicella in children with HIV disease are often associated with high morbidity and mortality.

In contrast to adults with HIV disease, children experience striking B-cell defects early in the disease, presenting with bacterial infections such as impetigo, cellulitis, skin abscesses, otitis media, sinusitis, pneumonia, and sepsis.[352] Polyclonal hypergammaglobulinemia with elevated IgA, IgD, IgE, and IgG are often seen very early in HIV disease.[413] Children with advanced HIV disease eventually develop immune system abnormalities similar to those seen in adults, including low CD4 lymphocyte counts and poor T-cell response to mitogens, but these occur much later in the course of the disease.

The cutaneous manifestations of HIV disease in children differ both in type and in frequency from those seen in the adult. There is no single mucocutaneous disease that is pathognomonic in children with HIV infection.[351] The characteristic opportunistic infections, such as PCP, and the unusual malignancies, such as KS, occurring in adults are less common in children.[414,415] Candidiasis of the oral mucosa, skin, and esophagus; herpetic gingivostomatitis; and staphylococcal skin infection are the most common cutaneous manifestations of pediatric HIV disease. These infections are similar to those occurring in nonimmunocompromised children, differing only in severity and frequency of recurrence.[351]

Other disorders reported associated with pediatric HIV disease include seborrheic and atopic dermatitis, hypersensitivity vasculitis, nutritional deficiencies, drug eruptions, and pyoderma gangrenosum.[351,362,416]

Uncommon and Miscellaneous Mucocutaneous Manifestations of HIV Disease

Infectious Complications

Gram-Negative Coccal and Bacillary Infections PSEUDOMONAS. *Pseudomonas aeruginosa* has been reported to cause primary cutaneous infections, such as cellulitis that may ulcerate (Fig. 215-23) (e.g., ecthyma gangrenosum), malignant otitis media, and infection at catheter sites, and secondary infection of underlying disorders such as KS.[417–419] Cutaneous *P. aeruginosa* infection occurs via local invasion, commonly gaining entry by apocrine gland infection in the anogenital or axillary regions, or by hematogenous dissemination to the skin. Cutaneous pseudomonal infection may extend into the blood stream, with resultant bacteremia and seeding of many organ systems. In a retrospective study of adults with AIDS admitted during a 16-month period, 5 percent had community-acquired bacteremia; *P. aeruginosa* was the cause of bacteremia in 7 percent of the bacteremic group.[420]

Compresses moistened with 5% acetic acid (white vinegar) are effective in treatment of superficially infected lesions such as ulcerated and/or hyperkeratotic KS on the lower legs, feet, and webspaces.[421] Oral administration of ciprofloxacin is recommended for treatment of nonbacteremic pseudomonal infection; intravenous administration of agents such as imipenem is indicated for invasive infections. As with other infections in HIV disease, pseudomonal infections tend to recur. Pseudomonal infections in HIV disease usually have a poor prognosis with high morbidity and mortality.[417,422]

SALMONELLOSIS.   Recurrent *Salmonella* bacteremia is an AIDS-defining condition. Cutaneous abscess formation has been reported occurring over the zygomatic arch in an HIV-infected patient with recurrent *S. enteritidis* gastroenteritis and bacteremia.[423] The cutaneous abscesses resulted from hematogenous seeding of the skin.

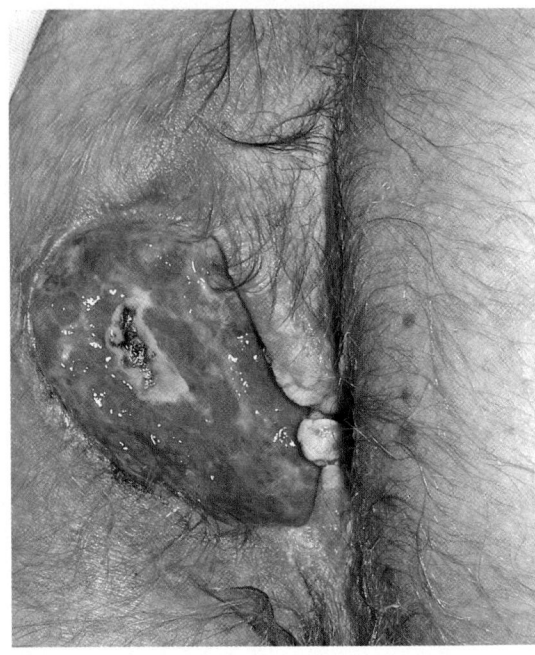

FIGURE 215-23 *P. aeruginosa* infection, ecthyma gangrenosum. A large ulcer is seen on the buttock, caused by pseudomonal cellulitis with a septic vasculitis; the primary event was the cutaneous infection, with secondary bacteremia. The patient required a diverting colostomy but was eventually reanastomosed once the ulcer healed.

NOCARDIOSIS.   Nocardiosis, caused by aerobic actinomycetes, can occur either as localized or disseminated infection. The majority of infections, caused by *Nocardia brasiliensis*, are limited to the skin and subcutaneous tissues. Systemic nocardiosis is most commonly caused by *N. asteroides* but can also be caused by *N. brasiliensis* and *N. caviae*. Nocardiosis in HIV disease is rare; prophylaxis for PCP with sulfonamides may also provide primary prophylaxis for nocardiosis. Primary cutaneous nocardiosis in HIV disease has been reported to occur at the site of heroin injection; abscesses appeared initially and evolved into large ulcerations.[424] *Nocardia asteroides* was cultured from a lesional skin biopsy. Systemic nocardiosis with lymph node or pulmonary infection can drain to the skin.[425,426]

MISCELLANEOUS.   Severe B-cell dysregulation may result in frequent and severe pyogenic infections, such as meningococcemia with fever and petechiae.[427] Infections caused by *Streptococcus pneumoniae* and *H. influenzae* have also been reported.[428]

MYCOBACTERIOSES.   *Mycobacterium tuberculosis* In developing countries, tuberculosis is the most common opportunistic infection in HIV disease; however, cutaneous tuberculosis is relatively uncommon. Whether HIV-associated tuberculosis is usually a primary, reactivated, or secondary exogenous infection is uncertain.[429] In the United States, the tallies of new cases of tuberculosis had fallen to a low until 1985; subsequently, the numbers have increased to 23,500 in 1989, with 4350 cases of extrapulmonary tuberculosis.[430,431] In large urban centers such as New York, the number increased markedly from 2000 cases in 1986 to 2800 in 1990. This increased incidence is presumably related to the HIV epidemic, homelessness, and immigration. The current epidemic of tuberculosis is occurring mainly in HIV-infected persons, IDUs, African-Americans, and Latinos. As has been true in the past, most cases of symptomatic tuberculosis represent reactivation of latent infection. Primary pulmonary tuberculosis does occur in HIV disease and may have an accelerated course.[432] Of great concern in the tuberculosis occurring in HIV disease is the appearance of multiple-drug-resistant strains of *M. tuberculosis,* resulting in mortality rates that reach 80 percent 2 to 3 months after diagnosis.[433,434]

In non-HIV-infected persons, the incidence of extrapulmonary tuberculosis is 15 percent; in HIV infection, 20 to 40 percent. As HIV disease progresses, the incidence of extrapulmonary tuberculosis increases to 70 percent. The most common routes of spread of tuberculosis to extrapulmonary sites include contiguous spread and acute hematogenous spread, in nodes or abscesses.

The etiologic agents of human tuberculosis include *M. tuberculosis, M. bovis,* and occasionally bacillus Calmette-Guérin (BCG). Although never common, cutaneous tuberculosis appears to occur more often in HIV-infected persons. Nosocomial transmission of tuberculosis can occur from patient to patient as well as from patient to health care workers.[435]

Cutaneous tuberculosis is highly variable in its clinical presentation and depends on prior infection with *M. tuberculosis* and therefore delayed hypersensitivity to the organism, the immunologic status of the patient, the route of inoculation of mycobacteria into the skin, mode of spread to the skin, number and virulence of the bacilli, age of patient, and presence or absence of an internal tuberculous focus. Cutaneous tuberculosis occurs following infection with *M. tuberculosis* from an exogenous source or by autoinoculation or endogenous spread from another site. Modes of endogenous spread to skin include: direct extension from underlying tuberculous infection, i.e., lymphadenitis[436] or tuberculosis of bones and joints, resulting in scrofuloderma[437]; lymphatic spread to the skin, resulting in lupus vulgaris; and hematogenous dissemination, resulting in either acute miliary tuberculosis,[438–440] lupus vulgaris, or metastatic tuberculosis abscess.[441]

Several patients with HIV disease who had been immunized previously with BCG developed reactivation BCG infection. One developed disseminated *M. bovis* infection after immunization; another developed BCG lymphadenitis 30 years after BCG immunization.[442–444]

Mycobacterium avium-intracellulare (MAI) Complex   Although disseminated MAI infection occurs commonly in HIV-infected patients with advanced immunodeficiency, symptomatic cutaneous MAI involvement is rare.[445] MAI is the most common cause of disseminated bacterial infection in patients with advanced HIV disease.[446] In a study of 2006 patients followed over a 3-year period from the day of diagnosis of AIDS with monthly lysis-centrifugation blood cultures, 21 percent had positive MAI cultures at 1 year and 43 percent at 2 years following diagnosis.[447] The incidence of MAI complex bacteremia was directly related to the CD4 cell counts: 39 percent of patients with CD4 cell counts of $<10/mm^3$, 30 percent with <10 to $19/mm^3$, 20 percent with <20 to $39/mm^3$, 15 percent with <40 to $59/mm^3$, 8 percent with <60 to $99/mm^3$, and 3 percent with <100 to $199/mm^3$. MAI bacteremia may eventually occur in most, if not all, HIV-positive patients who do not die from another HIV-related event. In a study of the incidence of disseminated MAI complex infection, 16 percent of patients with AIDS had disseminated MAI complex infection, characterized by fever, anemia, weight loss, diarrhea, and elevated alkaline phosphatase.[448]

It is difficult to interpret both the culture of MAI from and the demonstration of acid-fast bacilli in skin biopsy specimens of patients with HIV disease whose CD4 cell counts are $<10/mm^3$, in that approximately 40 percent have MAI bacteremia. MAI can be

detected within a biopsy of such skin lesions as KS, but in most circumstances the presence of MAI is incidental, having no part in the pathogenesis of the cutaneous lesion. MAI infection has been reported in three patients who presented with either submandibular, axillary, or inguinal lymphadenitis.[449] Following incision and drainage or spontaneous rupture, scrofuloderma occurred, with the formation of deep ulcerative lesions; resolution occurred after a short course of routine antituberculous therapy. Subcutaneous masses can also represent underlying MAI osteomyelitis.[450]

Other Environmental Mycobacterioses   *M. haemophilum* infection of the skin has been reported to induce erythema, swelling, painful nodules, and abscess formation in patients with advanced HIV disease.[451–455] Recovery of *M. haemophilum* requires a high level of clinical suspicion and special handling of mycobacterial cultures by the microbiology laboratory, including cultivation on enriched chocolate agar or heme-supplemented media and incubation at 30°C for up to 8 weeks. Response to antimycobacterial therapy has been poor, and disease tends to recur and progress.

M. fortuitum infection has been reported on the lower abdomen and extremities in an IDU with HIV disease; the infection presented as multiple subcutaneous nodules with areas of necrosis, ulceration, and abscess formation with associated erythema and edema of the legs.[456,457] The therapeutic response was poor.

M. marinum infection has been reported in a male with HIV disease, presenting as three nodules on the dorsum of the hand, associated with ipsilateral axillary lymphadenopathy. The patient did own a fish tank, the probable source of infection of this environmental mycobacterium. The only treatment at this time was surgical excision. Eighteen months later, the patient returned with new nodular skin lesions over the upper arm, associated with fever, malaise, pulmonary symptoms, and hemoptysis. Cultures of skin, blood, bone marrow, and bronchial secretions grew out *M. marinum.* In spite of treatment with clofazimine, ciprofloxacin, and ethionamide, the skin lesions enlarged; the patient died from disseminated *M. marinum* infection 3 months later.

Leprosy   The interrelationship of *M. leprae* and HIV in dually infected persons has not been adequately studied to date.[458–461] Tropical areas such as Africa and India, which have a high prevalence of leprosy, are expected to bear the brunt of the HIV epidemic during the next decade. Current estimates are that 12 million persons worldwide have leprosy and that by the end of the 1990s, up to 120 million persons will have HIV disease. It is probable that leprosy will accelerate the course of HIV disease and that HIV infection will result in a higher ratio of cases of lepromatous versus tuberculoid leprosy and resistance to antilepromatous therapy.[462,463]

The natural history of leprosy in HIV disease has been reported in 275 patients from Haiti; 6.5 percent of the entire cohort were HIV seropositive. No difference in HIV seropositivity was detected in patients with either lepromatous or tuberculoid types of leprosy. Twenty-two percent of HIV-seropositive patients developed new skin lesions and lepromin anergy during the course of dapsone/rifampin leprosy therapy, as compared to 0.8 percent of HIV-seronegative patients.

Fungal Infections   SUPERFICIAL MYCOSES OTHER THAN CANDIDIASIS AND DERMATOPHYTOSIS. Other superficial mycoses have been reported in HIV-infected individuals, including invasive trichosporonosis arising at the site of a Hickman catheter and appearing clinically as a crusted nodule; *Cladosporium cladosporioides* causing a 5-mm violaceous, pustular nodule at the site of a tetanus skin test[464]; alternariosis presenting as an eschar on the leg[465]; and superficial *Curvularia* phaeohyphomycosis presenting as a superficial keratotic lesion of the scrotum.[466]

DEEP MYCOSES. The pathogenesis of the deep mycotic infections cryptococcosis, coccidioidomycosis, and histoplasmosis resembles that of tuberculosis: primary pulmonary infection following the inhalation of air contaminated with these organisms. The initial response to this event is a polymorphonuclear leukocyte one, which serves to limit the extent of primary infection. However, the definitive host response is a cell-mediated immune response, which limits both the impact of postprimary systemic dissemination of the organisms and prevents the subsequent breakdown of sites of dormant infection. Thus, AIDS patients are at risk for three patterns of infection: (1) progressive, primary infection with systemic spread due to a failure of the normal cell-mediated immune response; (2) reactivation of dormant sites of infection, with secondary systemic dissemination of the organisms; and (3) reinfection in a patient who has lost the protective immunity engendered years previously on exposure to this same organism, with such reinfection resulting in a pattern of disease akin to that seen in patients with progressive primary infection. Whenever systemic dissemination of these organisms occurs, there is an approximately 10 percent incidence of mucocutaneous disease—often as the first recognizable manifestation of systemic infection. In a study of 980 patients with AIDS from Dallas, 4 percent had disseminated histoplasmosis and 7 percent had disseminated cryptococcal infection.[467]

The cornerstone of diagnosis of deep mycotic infection with hematogenous dissemination to the skin is lesional biopsy for culture and pathologic examination. Lesional biopsies have two purposes: diagnosis of a particular skin lesion and early recognition of disseminated infection in an immunocompromised host. Because of these dual objectives, any unexplained skin lesion in the patient with HIV infection should be considered for biopsy. The differential diagnosis of patients with skin lesions possibly due to systemic fungal infection includes molluscum contagiosum, verruca vulgaris, verruca plana, disseminated herpetic or varicella infection, bacillary angiomatosis, and furunculosis.

The diagnosis of cutaneous infection with *Cryptococcus neoformans, Coccidioides immitis,* or *Histoplasma capsulatum* is *prima facie* evidence of disseminated infection and must be treated as such. Primary infection of the skin is vanishingly rare and should be considered only in such unusual circumstances as direct inoculation in a laboratory. The traditional therapy for such infection has been prolonged courses of intravenous amphotericin B. More recently, it has been shown that lifelong therapy with drugs such as fluconazole are necessary to prevent relapse in this patient population.

Cryptococcosis C. neoformans is a ubiquitous, worldwide fungus, which often causes an asymptomatic primary pulmonary infection followed by spontaneous resolution but persistence of the fungus within the lesion. With advancing HIV-induced immunodeficiency, *C. neoformans* often reactivates, spreading hematogenously to the meninges, skin, and other organs. It is the second most common fungal opportunist in HIV-infected individuals, causing symptomatic cryptococcosis in approximately 5 percent of patients with AIDS.[468] Cryptococcosis is less common than PCP or mucosal candidiasis but is by far the most common life-threatening fungal pathogen in HIV disease.

Patients with CNS cryptococcosis may present with symptoms of malaise, fever, headache, nausea, or vomiting that may occur over a few days to several months; more specific findings include personality change, confusion, loss of memory, and symptoms of cranial nerve palsies. Hematogenous dissemination of *C. neofor-*

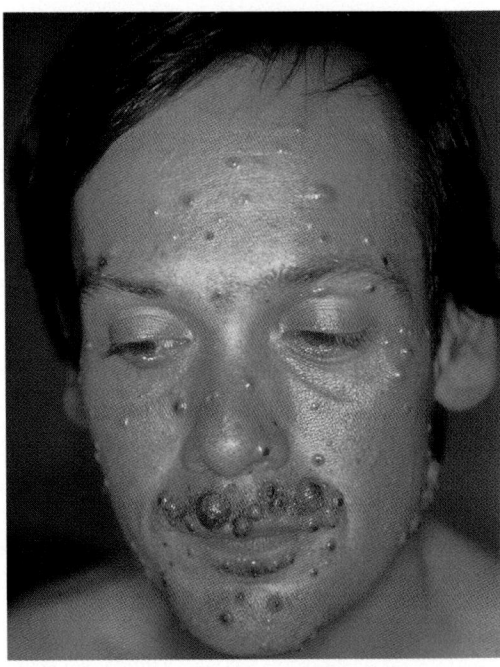

FIGURE 215-24 Cryptococcosis, disseminated. Multiple, discrete, skin-colored papules and nodules resembling molluscum contagiosum. *(Courtesy of Loïc Vaillant, M.D.)*

mans to the skin, which occurs in 5 to 10 percent of patients with disseminated infection, results in lesions of various morphologies that are, generally, asymptomatic. Skin lesions may be present for weeks or many months before presentation.[469]

The most common types of skin lesions in disseminated cryptococcosis are papules or nodules that strongly resemble molluscum contagiosum (Fig. 215-24). Other types of cutaneous lesions include pustules, cellulitis, ulceration, panniculitis, palpable purpura, subcutaneous abscesses, and vegetating plaques.[470–473] Lesions commonly occur on the face but may be widespread. Oral nodules and ulcers also occur alone or with cutaneous lesions. The papules and nodules of cryptococcosis, ranging from solitary to greater than 100 in number, are usually skin-colored, with little if any inflammatory erythema, and lack the central umbilication or keratotic plug characteristic of molluscum contagiosum. Occasionally, crusting or ulceration occurs that resembles lesions seen in herpes simplex virus infection. In black or Latino patients, they may be hypo- or hyperpigmented. Cryptococcal cellulitis presenting with a red, hot, tender plaque also occurs in immunodeficient hosts. Cutaneous cryptococcosis may occur in the absence of demonstrable fungal infection in the lung or meninges. Hematogenous dissemination of *Histoplasma capsulatum* or *Coccidioides immitis* can produce identical skin lesions on the face.

Diagnosis of hematogenous dissemination of *C. neoformans* to the skin is made by skin biopsy, the specimen showing cryptococcal yeast forms with routine stains of the biopsy or of a touch preparation.[474] Tzanck smears obtained by scraping the top of a lesion, placing the material on a glass slide, fixing the methyl alcohol, and staining with rapid Giemsa technique[475] show multiple encapsulated and budding yeast. India ink preparation of lesional skin scraping can also be used to demonstrate encapsulated and budding yeast forms. *C. neoformans* can also be isolated on culture of the skin biopsy specimen.

Therapy for cryptococcal meningitis is intravenous amphotericin B, which may be given with oral 5-flucytosine or fluconazole. The bone marrow toxicity of 5-flucytosine often precludes its use in HIV-infected patients, especially in patients receiving zidovudine. Cutaneous cryptococcal lesions resolve 2 to 4 weeks after beginning effective primary antifungal therapy but relapses occur in over 50 percent of patients once primary induction therapy is stopped. Chronic prophylaxis with fluconazole is effective.

Coccidioidomycosis   *C. immitis* is limited in geographic distribution to the western hemisphere, in arid regions of the southwestern United States, Mexico, and Central and South America. Many residents of these regions have subclinical primary pulmonary infection. With progressive HIV disease, *C. immitis* can become activated from latent infection to cause disseminated disease. It reactivates and disseminates hematogenously, with resultant chronic progressive granulomatous infection in skin, lung, bone, and meninges. Cutaneous lesions of disseminated coccidioidomycosis are usually asymptomatic, beginning as papules and evolving to pustules, plaques, or nodules with minimal surrounding erythema. Facial lesions, which are most common, resemble molluscum contagiosum. In time, lesions may enlarge and become confluent, with formation of abscesses, multiple draining sinus tracts, ulcers, subcutaneous cellulitis, verrucous plaques, granulomatous nodules, and, with healing, scars. Unlike histoplasmosis and cryptococcosis, the oral mucous membranes are spared.

Disseminated coccidioidomycosis is diagnosed culturally by isolating the fungus from infected tissues. Serum complement fixation titers are often helpful in diagnosing the disease, but may be absent in the setting of HIV disease.[476]

Histoplasmosis   *H. capsulatum* is restricted geographically, and so disseminated infection occurs less often in HIV disease than does cryptococcosis. *H. capsulatum* occurs only in certain regions of the western hemisphere (east central portion of the United States—Ohio and Mississippi River valleys, Virginia, and Maryland—as well as parts of Central America); a variant, *H. capsulatum* var. *duboisii*, occurs in Africa. In endemic geographic areas, e.g., Indiana, disseminated histoplasmosis is the leading opportunistic infection in HIV disease.[477]

Histoplasmosis presents with a variety of cutaneous findings in approximately 10 percent of disseminated cases in HIV-infected patients. Disseminated histoplasmosis presents in HIV-infected patients as an acute, subacute, or chronic illness, often accompanied by fever, weight loss, hepatosplenomegaly, and pulmonary symptoms. Cutaneous findings include erythematous macules; necrotic or keratin-plugged papules and nodules; pustules, folliculitis, acneform lesions, a rosacea-like eruption, and a guttate psoriasis-like eruption (Fig. 215-25); ulcers; vegetative plaques; or panniculitis. Several different morphologic lesions may occur on a patient. Lesions occur most commonly on the face, followed by the extremities and trunk. Oral mucosal lesions include nodules and vegetations; ulceration occurs on the soft palate, oropharynx, epiglottis, and nasal vestibule. A subtle, widespread, exanthematous or psoriasiform eruption may occasionally develop in HIV-infected patients already on systemic antifungal therapy, in whom systemic symptoms are completely lacking. Hepatosplenomegaly and/or lymphadenopathy occur commonly in patients with disseminated histoplasmosis.

Skin biopsy, touch, or crushed tissue preparation can be used to identify *C. immitis* and *H. capsulatum*. Treatment is with intravenous amphotericin B. Recurrences are common; weekly maintenance amphotericin B infusions or oral fluconazole have been used in prophylaxis.

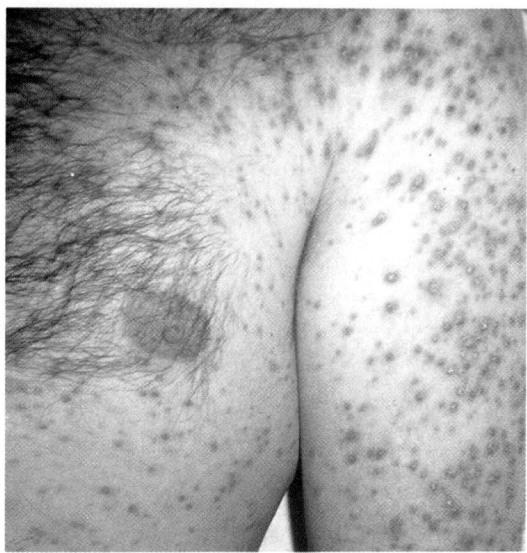

a

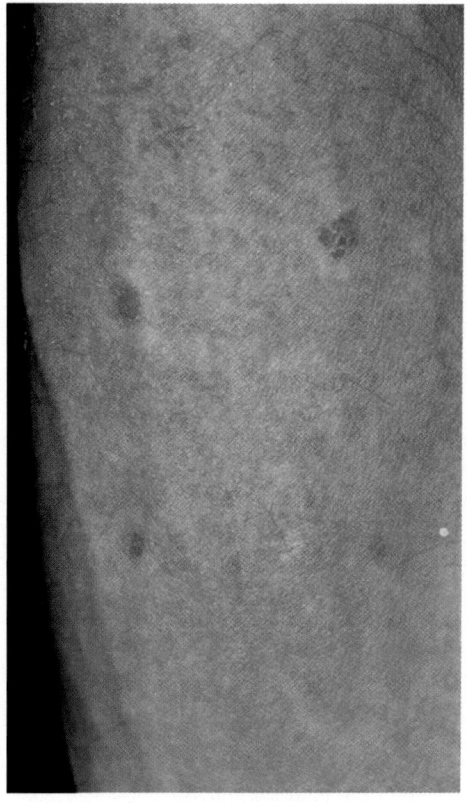

b

FIGURE 215-25   Histoplasmosis, disseminated. *(a)* A guttate psoriasis-like eruption appeared during a 1-week period, associated with fever in this patient with advanced HIV disease. *(Courtesy of J. D. Fallon, M.D.) (b)* After stopping secondary prophylaxis with fluconazole, the papulosquamous eruption recurred; lesional skin biopsy showed *H. capsulatum.*

Sporotrichosis *Sporotrix schenkii* is ubiquitous in the environment in rotting organic matter. Percutaneous inoculation results in limited forms of sporotrichosis (chancriform or sporotrichoid pattern) in the immunocompetent patient; in HIV disease, the reported cases are all of disseminated infection involving skin and other organ systems. The most likely site from which primary sporotrichosis disseminates is the lung.

The reported cutaneous findings of sporotrichosis in HIV disease are distinctly different than in nonimmunocompromised hosts, i.e., the cutaneous findings arise from hematogenous dissemination of *S. schenckii* to the skin rather than localized infection at the site of inoculation. The reported findings range from a papulosquamous eruption[478] to papulonodular lesions that may become crusted, hyperkeratotic, eroded, or ulcerated.[479–481] Individual lesions may remain discrete or become confluent. Subcutaneous nodules, 1 to 2 cm in diameter, also occur. The distribution of lesions is usually generalized, normally sparing the palms, soles, and oral mucosa. Dissemination to the eye may occur, with hypopeon, scleral perforation, and prolapse of the uvea.[482,483] Joint infection with frank arthritis is also common in the disseminated form of sporotrichosis occurring in HIV disease.[484] Other organs involved in disseminated sporotrichosis in HIV disease include lung, liver, spleen, intestine, and meninges.[485] As with other infections in HIV disease, sporotrichosis tends to relapse in spite of seemingly adequate treatment or prophylaxis.

The diagnosis of disseminated sporotrichosis is usually made more easily in patients with HIV disease. Because of immunodeficiency, *S. schenckii* are much more numerous in cutaneous lesions and can be demonstrated on Gram's stain of lesional exudate or on histology of lesional biopsy. Confirmation of the presence of *S. schenckii* is made by culturing the organism from lesional biopsy, joint aspiration, or blood culture. Although the experience of treatment of disseminated sporotrichosis in HIV disease is limited, the most effective agents are amphotericin B and itraconazole. Amphotericin B is administered intravenously. Itraconazole is given orally with a loading dose of two 800-mg doses followed by 400 mg/day. Like ketoconazole, itraconazole requires an acid gastric pH for absorption.

Blastomycosis The dimorphic fungus *Blastomyces dermatitidis* is confined to certain endemic geographic regions of the midwestern and south-central United States. To date, blastomycosis has occurred only rarely in HIV disease and is not recognized as an AIDS-defining opportunistic infection.[486–489] Blastomycosis in HIV disease occurs in two patterns: localized pulmonary infection and disseminated or extrapulmonary disease. In the largest series of blastomycosis occurring in HIV disease reported to date, with 15 patients from different tertiary hospitals in the United States, 7 patients had localized pulmonary infection and 8 had disseminated disease. CNS infection occurred in 40 percent of cases. Six patients died within 21 days of presentation with blastomycosis, four patients with disseminated disease and two with fulminant pulmonary disease. Three of eight patients with disseminated blastomycosis had cutaneous involvement with papular and crusted facial lesions.

Aspergillosis Invasive aspergillosis is a rare opportunistic infection in HIV disease. In a report of 18 patients, the most common organ infected was the lung, and less commonly the brain, heart, kidney, sinuses, and skin; half the patients had multiorgan involvement.[490] Risk factors for invasive aspergillosis in HIV disease included leukopenia and therapy with corticosteroids, broad-spectrum antibiotics, and antineoplastic agents. Primary cutaneous aspergillosis has been reported to occur under adhesive tape near intravascular catheter sites. Skin lesions appeared as skin-colored to pink umbilicated papules, resembling molluscum contagiosum.[491] Biopsy specimens showed rupture of hair follicles with foci of fungal hyphae; *A. fumigatus* was identified on culture. The majority of patients with invasive systemic aspergillosis die, despite treatment with amphotericin B.[492,493]

Penicilliosis *Penicillium marneffei* is a dimorphic fungus endemic to countries of southeast Asia and the southern part of China. As of mid-1992 in the English-language literature, 29 cases of *P. marneffei* infection had been reported to occur in HIV disease.[494–499] In the largest series of 21 patients,[500] the clinical presentation included fever, cough, and generalized papular skin lesions. The most common cutaneous presentation was a generalized papular rash, occurring most frequently on the face, pinnae, upper trunk, and arms. In some patients, papules had central necrotic umbilication, resembling molluscum contagiosum. Genital ulcers were also reported, ranging in sizes from <1 cm to 3 cm in diameter. Oral lesions included papules and ulcers.

Penicilliosis should be considered in the differential diagnosis of HIV disease of patients from endemic countries of southeast Asia and China presenting with fever, cough, and a generalized papular eruption. A presumptive diagnosis of *P. marneffei* infection can often be made by microscopic examination of Wright's-stained bone marrow aspirate and/or touch smears of skin specimens obtained by biopsy, and confirmed by culture. *P. marneffei* has a characteristic appearance on touch smears, showing septate yeast cells within macrophages. Amphotericin B and itraconazole are reported to be effective in treatment, with clinical findings resolving after about 2 weeks of treatment.

Rickettsial Infections ROCHALIMAEA HENSELAE AND BACILLARY ANGIOMATOSIS. *Rochalimaea henselae* is a newly recognized fastidious gram-negative bacillus that has been associated with four clinical syndromes: bacillary angiomatosis (BA), relapsing fever with bacteremia, peliosis hepatis, and cat-scratch disease.[501–503] Bacillary angiomatosis occurs most commonly in the setting of HIV-induced immunodeficiency and is characterized by vascular neoplasms resembling pyogenic granulomas or KS.[504] The etiologic agent of BA, *R. henselae*, is a previously undescribed rickettsia-like organism related to *R. quintana*, the etiologic agent of trench fever.[505,506] The cutaneous lesions of BA resemble verruga peruana, the chronic cutaneous manifestation of infection with *Bartonella bacilliformis*. Patients with BA usually have moderate to advanced HIV-induced immunodeficiency, but rarely, BA occurs in immunocompetent, non-HIV-infected individuals. Transmission is thought to occur via breaks in the skin, with resultant bacteremia and seeding of multiple organs.

Whether asymptomatic or latent infection occurs in humans is not known. The most common risk factor for BA is HIV infection with advanced immunodeficiency. The incubation period is unknown but is probably days to weeks. Patients with localized infection may be free of systemic symptoms, but localized skin lesions may be painful in comparison to the lesions of KS, which are usually not painful. Those with more widespread disseminated infection usually experience fever, malaise, and weight loss.

Clinically, the cutaneous lesions of BA, which was initially called a pseudo-Kaposi's sarcoma, are red to violaceous, dome-shaped papules or nodules resembling angiomas (Fig. 215-26a, -26b), ranging in size from a few millimeters up to 2 to 3 cm in diameter. Less commonly, domed subcutaneous masses occur (Fig. 215-26c).[507] Lesions are soft to firm and may be tender to palpation. These lesions are usually situated in the dermis and may show thinning or erosion of overlying epidermis; occasionally they may

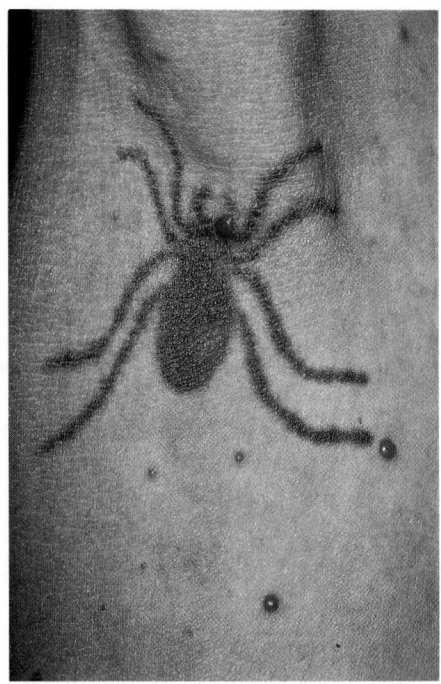

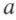

a

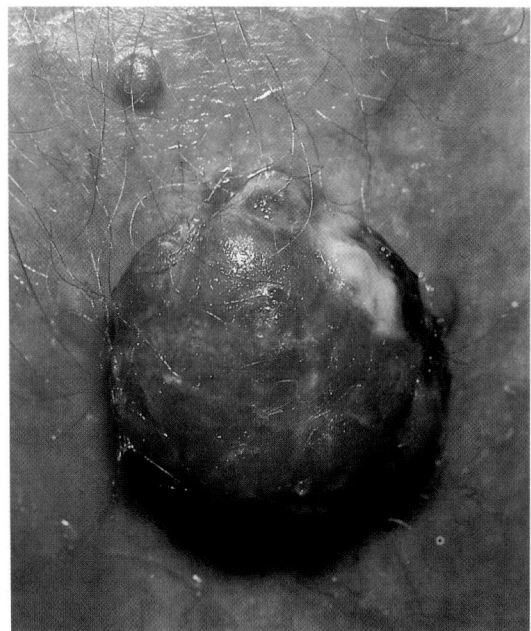

b

FIGURE 215-26 Bacillary angiomatosis. A 31-year-old male presented with the following lesions: *(a)* Cherry hemangioma-like lesions are seen on the forearm; similar lesions were also present on the arms and both thighs. Lesions erupted during a 1-week period and were associated with fever. *(b)* A solitary 2-cm pyogenic granuloma-like lesion was also present over the shin. *(c)* Several weeks earlier, ten tender, meatball-sized nodules were noted on the medial thighs. All lesions resolved following initiation of orally administered erythromycin.

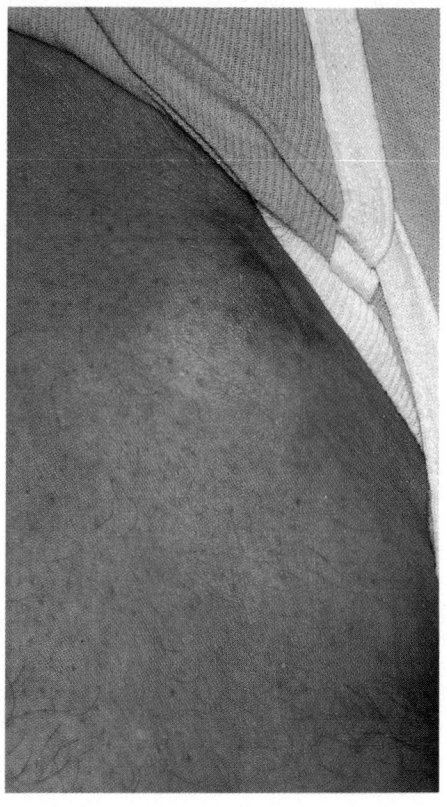

c

be located deeper in subcutaneous tissue. The number of lesions ranges from solitary to more than a 100 and, rarely, greater than 1000. Nearly any site may be involved, but the palms, soles, and oral cavity are usually spared. Following hematogenous or lymphatic dissemination, the spectrum of internal disease caused by *R. henselae* includes soft tissue masses, bone marrow involvement, lymphadenopathy, splenomegaly, and hepatomegaly; internal involvement can occur with or without cutaneous lesions.

The diagnosis of BA is made by the demonstration of pleomorphic bacilli on a Warthin-Starry or similar silver stain or by electron microscopic examination of lesional skin biopsy. Percutaneous liver biopsy in patients with peliosis hepatis is relatively contraindicated because of the vascular nature of the lesions and the risk for uncontrolled bleeding. The differential diagnosis of the cutaneous lesions of BA includes KS, pyogenic granuloma, epithelioid (histiocytoid) angioma, cherry angioma, sclerosing hemangioma, verruga peruana lesions of bartonellosis, and disseminated cryptococcosis.

The histopathology of lesional skin biopsy specimens of BA is distinctive and usually diagnostic. Two patterns of lobular proliferations of capillaries and venules are seen.[502] The first pattern, seen in pyogenic granuloma-like lesions, is characterized by proliferation of small, round blood vessels with a plump endothelial cell lining associated with cuboidal endothelial cells in the interstitium. The stroma is edematous and loose, but endothelial cells are closely grouped. The inflammatory infiltrate is composed of lymphocytes,

histiocytes, and neutrophils. The overlying epidermis may show collarette formation, thinning, or ulceration. Few if any bacteria are visualized by silver stain. The second pattern is dense and cellular, usually arising more deeply in the dermis, and is seen in plaque lesions and subcutaneous masses. Stroma is compact, composed of endothelial cells; the bulk of the lesion is made up of myriad small, round blood vessels lined by plump endothelial cells. The inflammatory infiltrate is composed of neutrophils. The interstitium shows a granular amphophilic material. Abundant clusters of bacilli, corresponding to sites of granular material, are visualized by silver stain. Histology of liver lesions shows peliosis hepatis, which is characterized by the formation of blood-filled cysts, with clusters of bacilli in the connective tissue rims of the cysts.[508] *R. henselae* can be cultured from biopsy specimens of BA; however, isolation is not possible in most microbiology laboratories.

The course of BA is variable. In some patients, lesions regress spontaneously. BA infection may spread hematogenously or via lymphatics to involve bone marrow, bone, spleen, and liver. Death may occur secondary to laryngeal obstruction, liver failure, or pulmonary infection. The antibiotics of choice are erythromycin, given at a dose of 250 to 500 mg orally four times daily until the lesions resolve, usually 3 to 4 weeks, and doxycycline, 100 mg twice daily.

Viral Infections   MEASLES.   Measles has been uncommon in the industrialized nations because of childhood immunization; in third world countries such as Africa, measles is common and is associated with significant morbidity and mortality. In the United States, focal epidemics have occurred due to failure of immunization. Measles occurring in the setting of HIV disease in unvaccinated persons has high morbidity and mortality.[509] The immunogenicity of measles vaccine in children with HIV infection is low, with only 25 percent of immunized HIV-infected children developing antibody detected by ELISA.[510] Clinically, measles occurring in HIV disease may be atypical with a prolonged period of rash or absence of exanthem or enanthem.[511,512] Diagnosis of measles is usually made on clinical findings; however, in cases when the exanthem is atypical, documentation of seroconversion is helpful. In some cases, seroconversion does not occur due to abnormal B-cell function; lesional skin biopsy is helpful, showing multinucleated keratinocytes. Children who develop measles may have severe or occasionally fatal infection.

CYTOMEGALOVIRUS.   Seroprevalence studies of cytomegalovirus (CMV) infection indicate that nearly 100 percent of homosexual and bisexual males and IDUs are infected with CMV. Most cases of primary CMV infection are asymptomatic; following primary infection, CMV enters a latent phase of infection, during which asymptomatic viral shedding in saliva, semen, and/or urine is extremely common.

CMV is the most common viral pathogen in patients with advanced HIV-induced immunodeficiency. In a study of 82 HIV-1–seropositive persons, 51.7 percent of those with either ARC or AIDS had evidence of CMV infection of circulating polymorphonuclear cells, whereas no infection was detected among the 50 asymptomatic HIV-infected persons. Manifestations of CMV infection include retinitis, esophagitis, colitis, gastritis, hepatitis, and encephalitis. In a multicenter study of 1002 persons with AIDS or ARC, median survival after diagnosis of CMV disease was 173 days, and CMV was an independent predictor of death.[513] Disseminated CMV has been demonstrated in 93 percent of patients with AIDS; at autopsy, however, association with skin lesions was not reported. CMV reactivation and dissemination are common events as immunodeficiency worsens. As an opportunistic organism, CMV commonly infects the retina, causing a sight-threatening retinitis,[514] and the large intestine, causing colitis manifested by intractable diarrhea. Widespread infection is associated with a generalized wasting syndrome, pneumonitis and encephalitis. CMV infection, although present within various organs as documented by viral culture, is not necessarily the cause of the tissue dysfunction.[515]

Specific CMV-induced skin lesions have not been identified in HIV-infected individuals. Evidence for CMV infection in a variety of mucous membrane lesions has been reported, implied by specific cytopathic changes in biopsy specimens demonstrated by light and electron microscopy, immunofluorescence, immunoperoxidase, and in situ hybridization techniques; however, the role of CMV in the pathogenesis of the lesions is not certain. Perianal ulceration caused by CMV occurs as the infection spreads from contiguous gastrointestinal sites. CMV was considered to be the cause of perianal and oral ulceration in five AIDS patients with advanced disease, based on typical histologic changes and positive fluorescent monoclonal anti-CMV antibody studies. Empirical treatment with acyclovir failed, but all ulcers healed with either foscarnet or ganciclovir treatment. Other reported presentations of CMV infection in the skin of HIV-infected individuals include macular purpura of the extremities associated with leukocytoclastic vasculitis and small, keratotic, verrucous lesions, 1 to 3 cm in diameter, scattered on the trunk, limbs, and face.

Infestations   PROTOZOAN INFESTATIONS.   Protozoan infestations are among the most common opportunistic infections in HIV disease; mucocutaneous involvement, however, is uncommon.[516]

Extrapulmonary Pneumocystosis   In late symptomatic and advanced HIV disease, an extracellular microorganism *Pneumocystis carinii,* which exists silently in our environment, becomes an opportunist, most commonly causing PCP. Currently, prophylaxis (primary) for CPC is begun when the CD4 cell counts fall below 200/mm³; secondary prophylaxis is given following episodes of symptomatic PCP. Trimethoprim-sulfamethoxazole is the most effective prophylaxis[517]; other prophylactic regimens include monthly aerosolized or parenteral pentamidine or orally administered dapsone or pyrimethamine-sulfadoxine (Fansidar).

Extrapulmonary *P. carinii* infection (pneumocystosis) is uncommon but may be the initial presentation of HIV disease.[518] Pneumocystosis of the external auditory canals presents with unilateral or bilateral polypoid masses, which may be accompanied by loss of hearing. Similar lesions may occur at the tympanic membrane, middle ear, and mastoid air cells. The infection is thought to occur by retrograde spread via the eustachian tube and not by hematogenous or lymphatic spread. Aerosolized pentamidine prophylaxis reduces the incidence of otic pneumocystosis, but because the drug is concentrated in the lung, disseminated extrapulmonary pneumocystosis may still occur in patients receiving the drug by this route. Gangrene of the foot has been reported in a patient with widespread pneumocystosis; microemboli containing *P. carinii* were present in smaller arterioles and capillaries within necrotic skin of the toes. Widespread violaceous papules and nodules arising on the torso, arms, and legs, resembling KS have also been described.[519] Extrapulmonary *P. carinii* infection is treated with trimethoprim-sulfamethoxazole, trimethoprim and dapsone, or parenteral pentamidine.

Leishmaniasis   Although not included in the CDC surveillance case definition for AIDS, visceral leishmaniasis may be an opportunistic infection of HIV disease and, as such, may be considered an AIDS-defining condition.[520] Current estimates are that more than 100 million persons are infected with *Leishmania* spp. worldwide. The course of persons with HIV disease who harbor *Leishmania* is not yet determined.[521]

Persons with HIV disease and leishmaniasis may present with typical lesions of cutaneous infection.[522] Patients with prior cutaneous leishmaniasis or asymptomatic primary infection may harbor *Leishmania* in the reticuloendothelial system.[523] As immunodeficiency progresses, the protozoans may escape confinement by immune surveillance and present with visceral leishmaniasis (kala-azar).[524] Presumed primary leishmanial infection has been reported in an HIV-infected homosexual male, presenting as a rectal mass transmitted as a venereal infection.[525]

Visceral leishmaniasis is being reported with increased frequency in HIV disease. Investigators from Spain have reported 16 patients with HIV disease who developed visceral leishmaniasis, 5 of whom had late symptomatic or advanced disease.[526] The clinical presentation of visceral leishmaniasis was typical; leishmanial serology, however, was negative in 93 percent of these patients. Forty-three percent experienced a chronic course with multiple relapses despite alternative treatment. In another series, seven of nine patients with HIV disease and visceral leishmaniasis had not experienced a previous major AIDS-defining opportunistic infection.[527]

Diagnosis of leishmaniasis may be confirmed by demonstration of *Leishmania* on lesional skin biopsy and bone marrow aspiration.[528] Serologic tests for leishmaniasis are not reliable in persons with HIV disease. The incidence of relapse of visceral leishmaniasis is high in HIV disease. Interferon-γ has been reported to be an effective adjunct in treating relapsing leishmaniasis.[529]

Cutaneous Toxoplasmosis Approximately half the population of the United States has been infected with the obligate intracellular protozoa *Toxoplasma gondii*. In the immunologically normal host, primary toxoplasmal infection is associated with no or minimal symptoms and is followed by a dormant or latent phase. In patients with HIV disease, *T. gondii* reactivation commonly presents with CNS complaints suggestive of encephalitis or of a focal lesion. Epidermotrophic cutaneous toxoplasmosis is rare.[530] In a case report, a person with HIV disease presented with a generalized eruption consisting of 5- to 10-mm, erythematous, blanching, nontender papules occurring on the face, trunk, legs, and arms, sparing the palms and soles, and accompanied by fever, hepatosplenomegaly, and weight loss. Bone marrow biopsy demonstrated tachyzoites of *T. gondii*; however, lesional skin biopsy failed to demonstrate *T. gondii*. The skin lesions cleared during the course of treatment of the toxoplasmosis with sulfadiazine and pyrimethamine.

Amebiasis Acanthamoeba has been reported to cause a dermal nodule on the leg.[531]

ARTHROPOD INFESTATIONS. *Demodicidosis Demodex folliculorum* causes a pruritic papulonodular eruption, occurring on the scalp, face, and neck, in persons with HIV disease.[532] Skin scrapings suspended in mineral oil show innumerable *Demodex* mites. Lesional skin biopsy specimens show a dense lymphoeosinophilic inflammatory infiltrate in the papillary and midreticular dermis and, at times, in a perifollicular arrangement. Demodicidosis must be differentiated from staphylococcal folliculitis, HIV-associated eosinophilic folliculitis, pityrosporum folliculitis, and the other nonspecific papular eruptions of HIV disease. Treatments with permethrin cream or topical lindane are effective.

Noninfectious Complications

Disorders of Keratinization and Epidermal Appendages Erythroderma, an uncommon event in HIV disease, may be related to atopic dermatitis, psoriasis vulgaris, photosensitivity dermatitis,[533,534] the hypereosinophilic syndrome,[535] coexistent HTLV-I infection,[536] and CD8 (cytotoxic T cell) phenotype cutaneous T-cell lymphoma.[537,538]

Pityriasis rubra pilaris (PRP) has been reported in eight persons with HIV disease since 1991.[539-543] Three of the patients also

had severe nondulocystic acne,[540,541] one of whom also had hidradenitis suppurativa. The number of reports of this relatively uncommon disorder and the rapid and prolonged clearing in two zidovudine-treated patients suggest an association between HIV disease and PRP, and that HIV may play a pathogenic role in PRP and other papulosquamous disorders occurring in HIV disease.

Hair alterations, such as thinning of scalp and body hair, occur commonly in persons with advanced HIV disease. In one large series, 5 of 33 patients with HIV disease had diffuse hair loss, compared to 0 of 204 individuals in the control group.[357] Sudden premature graying is also seen, probably as a result of malnutrition. Other reported hair alterations in HIV disease include alopecia areata; hypertrichosis of the eyelashes; and lengthening, lightening color, and softening of hair in blacks.

Nail changes are seen in as many as 32 percent of patients with symptomatic HIV infection.[544] None of the nail changes are pathognomonic of HIV disease. However, several findings should raise the possibility of HIV disease: proximal white subungual onychomycosis, or superficial white onychomycocsis, especially of the fingernail[545]; multinail candidal infection of the nail bed and/or plate; destructive psoriatic nail dystrophy; and squamous cell carcinoma of the nail bed in a young adult.[546] Yellow discoloration of the nails has been reported in several studies of persons with advanced HIV disease and PCP.[289,547] Whether the nail changes fulfill the criteria of yellow nail syndrome or simply represent discoloration of the nails is debatable.[548,549] Zidovudine-induced pigmentation is also a nail change seen in association with HIV disease.

Porphyria cutanea tarda (PCT) has been reported to have occurred in nearly 50 persons with HIV disease. Clinical lesions of PCT may occur prior to the diagnosis of HIV infection[550-553] or later in the course.[554,555] Underlying liver disease is common in persons with HIV disease and PCT; porphyrin metabolism may be affected by HIV infection or by hepatic dysfunction associated with chronic hepatitis B virus infection or alcohol ingestion.[556]

Granuloma annulare (GA) has been reported in HIV disease.[557] Lesions typical of localized and generalized GA have been observed. In several cases, the eruptions have been surprisingly transient.[288] Perforating GA[558] and reactive perforating collagenosis[559] have also been reported. An atypical generalized form of GA, which can be clinically indistinguishable from the papular eruption of AIDS and from the lichenoid granulomatous papular dermatosis associated with HIV infection, has also been described.[331,560,561] Skin biopsy may be helpful in distinguishing these entities.

Acne conglobata,[562] anetoderma,[563] papular mucinosis,[564] and calciphylaxis[565] have all been reported in HIV disease; however, the scanty number of case reports prevents drawing any conclusion of the association of these disorders with HIV disease.

Epidermotropic T-cell lymphoma has been reported in seven persons with HIV disease. Three patients had patch, plaque, or tumor stage disease indistinguishable from mycosis fungoides, two had one or more nodular lesions with focal epidermotropism, and two had exfoliative erythroderma with large numbers of circulating Sézary cells. HTLV-I serology was negative in three individuals tested.

The incidence of primary lymphoma of the CNS and undifferentiated non-Hodgkin's lymphoma is increased in patients with HIV disease.[566] Most reported lymphomas have been B-cell neoplasms, although peripheral nonepidermotropic T-cell lymphomas have also been described. The diagnosis of these aggressive tumors is often made at a more advanced stage of disease, extranodal involvement is often present, and the response to therapy is usually poor.

Lymphomatoid granulomatosis (LG) represents an angiocentric immunoproliferative disorder with a wide clinical spectrum of disease, ranging from spontaneously regressing lesions to evolution into a monomorphic T-cell lymphoma. LG has been reported in HIV disease, presenting as painful, aphthous ulcerlike lesions of the oral and esophageal mucosa.[567] The differential diagnosis of painful oral and esophageal ulcers includes recurrent aphthous ulcers and infectious etiologies such as HSV, CMV, *C. albicans,* and *H. capsulatum.* In another report of five cases of LG in HIV disease, four had CNS involvement.[568] The characteristic histologic features, best seen in ulcer margins and deeper submucosal tissues, are an angiocentric concentration of mononuclear cells, some of which are atypical. Therapy of LG, including prednisone and cyclophosphamide, is unsatisfactory in HIV-infected patients in that both agents are commonly contraindicated.

Idiopathic thrombocytopenic purpura (ITP), characterized by bruising, nonpalpable petechiae and hemorrhage, and thrombotic thrombocytopenic purpura have been reported in HIV disease. ITP is most commonly a disorder of young women, and its occurrence in young men was one the features of HIV disease recognized in the early phase of the epidemic.[569,570]

Cutaneous leukocytoclastic vasculitis has been reported in HIV disease,[393,571,572] as has polyarteritis nodosa.[284] Whether the vasculitis is caused by HIV itself is not known. In one patient with necrotizing vasculitis, HIV was cultured from peripheral nerves but not from the vasculitic infiltrate.[573] In three patients with HIV disease, CMV was implicated in the pathogenesis of their vasculitis.[284]

Vitiligo has been reported in four patients with HIV disease,[574] suggesting that vitiligo may be an autoimmune disease triggered by viral infection in a genetically predisposed host.

Sicca syndrome has been reported in HIV disease and may differ from typical Sjögren's syndrome in that most patients were male, without significant autoantibody levels, with a profound salivary gland inflammatory infiltrate, and of different HLA types.[284]

Reiter's syndrome has been reported in 1.7 to 10 percent of persons with HIV disease, compared to a 0.06 percent prevalence in healthy men 20 to 29 years old.[575–577] Onset of Reiter's syndrome occurs before or simultaneously with the onset of symptomatic HIV disease. Articular symptoms can precede onset of immunodeficiency by up to 14 months and may often be the first manifestation of HIV infection. Mucocutaneous manifestations include urethritis, conjunctivitis, keratoderma blenorrhagicum, circinate balanitis, and painless oral ulcers. Joint disease is characterized predominantly by severe, persistent oligoarticular arthritis, primarily affecting the large joints of the lower extremities, and occasionally by sacroiliitis.[575] Organisms known to trigger Reiter's syndrome are rarely found in HIV-infected patients with Reiter's syndrome. Some patients, however, do have culture-negative diarrheal illness or culture-negative urethritis at the time of onset of Reiter's syndrome.[577] In a case study of 21 patients with HIV-associated incomplete or complete Reiter's syndrome, HLA-B27 occurred in 15 (71 percent). Antecedent infection with bacteria associated with reactive arthritis was documented in 30 percent of these individuals, further emphasizing the similarity of this syndrome with non-HIV-associated Reiter's syndrome. The finding of extensive clinical overlap between psoriatic arthritis, psoriasis, and Reiter's syndrome; the absence of HLA antigens previously found to be associated with psoriasis; and the increased prevalence of HLA-B27 in HIV-infected patients with psoriatic arthritis[344] suggest a close association between psoriasis and Reiter's syndrome in this population.[285,578]

References

1. Barre-Sinoussi F et al: Isolation of a T-lymphotropic retrovirus from a patient at risk for acquired immune deficiency syndrome. *Science* **220**:868, 1983

2. Gallo RC et al: Frequent detection and isolation of cytopathic retroviruses (HTLV-III) from patients with AIDS and at risk for AIDS. *Science* **224**:500, 1984

3. Kyle WS: Simian retroviruses, poliovaccine, and origin of AIDS. *Lancet* **339**:600, 1992

4. Essex M: Origin of AIDS, in *AIDS: Etiology, Diagnosis, Treatment and Prevention,* edited by VT DeVita Jr, S Hellman, SA Rosenberg, Philadelphia, Lippincott, 1992, p 3

5. Neal K: Origins of HIV. *Lancet* **340**:58, 1992

6. Larson A: Social contact of human immunodeficiency virus transmission in Africa: Historical and cultural bases of east and central African sexual relations. *Rev Infect Dis* **2**:716, 1989

7. Lifson AR: Transmission of the human immunodeficiency virus, in *AIDS: Etiology, Diagnosis, Treatment and Prevention,* 3d ed, edited by VT DeVita Jr, S Hellman, SA Rosenberg, Philadelphia, Lippincott, 1992, p 111

8. Stingl G et al: Langerhans cells in HIV-1 infection. *J Am Acad Dermatol* **22**:1210, 1990

9. Kirby PK et al: The challenge of limiting the spread of human immunodeficiency virus by controlling other sexually transmitted disease. *Arch Dermatol* **127**:237, 1991

10. Kreiss JK et al: Isolation of human immunodeficiency virus from genital ulcers in Nairobi prostitutes. *J Infect Dis* **160**:380, 1989

11. Nsubuga P et al: The association of genital ulcer disease and HIV infection at a dermatology-STD clinic in Uganda. *J AIDS* **3**:1002, 1990

12. Latif AS et al: Genital ulcers and transmission of HIV among couples in Zimbabwe. *AIDS* **3**:519, 1989

13. Stamm WE et al: The association of genital ulcer disease and acquisition of HIV infection in homosexual men. *JAMA* **260**:1429, 1988

14. Holmberg SD et al: Prior herpes simplex virus type 2 infection as a risk factor for HIV infection. *JAMA* **259**:1048, 1988

15. Padian NS et al: The effect of number of exposures on the risk of heterosexual transmission. *J Infect Dis* **161**:883, 1990

16. European Study Group on Heterosexual Transmission of HIV: Comparison of female to male and male to female transmission of HIV in 563 stable couples. *Br Med J* **304**:908, 1992

17. Fallon J et al: Human immunodeficiency virus infection in children. *J Pediatr* **114**:1, 1989

18. Goedert JJ et al: Mother-to-infant transmission of human immunodeficiency virus type 1: Association with prematurity or low anti-gp120. *Lancet* **2**:1351, 1989

19. Cowan MJ et al: Maternally transmitted HIV infection in children. *AIDS* **2**:437, 1988

20. European Collaborative Study: Children born to women with HIV-1 infection: Natural history and risk of transmission. *Lancet* **337**:253, 1991

21. Ziegler JB et al: Postnatal transmission of AIDS-associated retrovirus from mother to infant. *Lancet* **1**:896, 1985

22. Stiehm ER, Vink P: Transmission of human immunodeficiency virus infection by breast-feeding. *J Pediatr* **118**:410, 1991

23. Donegan E et al: Transfusion Safety Study Group: Transmission of HIV-1 by component type and duration of shelf storage before transfusion. *Transfusion* **30**:851, 1990

24. Donnegan E et al: Infection with human immunodeficiency virus type 1 (HIV-1) among recipients of antibody-positive blood donations. *Ann Intern Med* **113**:733, 1990

25. Centers for Disease Control: *HIV/AIDS Surveillance Report,* October 1991, pp 1–18

26. Nelson KE et al: Transmission of retroviruses from seronegative donors by transfusion during cardiac surgery. A multicenter study of HIV-1 and HTLV-I/II infections. *Ann Intern Med* **117**:554, 1992

27. Kumar P et al: Transmission of human immunodeficiency virus by transplantation of a renal allograft, with development of the acquired immunodeficiency syndrome. *Ann Intern Med* **106**:244, 1987

28. Centers for Disease Control: Human immunodeficiency virus transmitted from an organ donor screened for HIV antibody–North Carolina. *MMWR* **36**:306, 1987

29. Centers for Disease Control: Transmission of HIV through bone transplantation: Case report and public health recommendations. *MMWR* **37**:597, 1988

30. Lifson AR: Transmission of the human immunodeficiency virus, in *AIDS: Etiology, Diagnosis, Treatment, and Prevention,* 3d ed, edited by VT DeVita Jr, S Hellman, SA Rosenberg. Philadelphia, Lippincott, p 114

31. Weber R et al: Progression of HIV infection in misusers of injected drugs who stop injecting or follow a programme of maintenance treatment with methadone. *Br Med J* **301**:362, 1990

32. Henderson DK et al: Risk for occupational transmission of human immunodeficiency virus type 1 (HIV-1) associated with clinical exposures: A prospective evaluation. *Ann Intern Med* **113**:740, 1990

33. Centers for Disease Control: Update: Human immunodeficiency virus infections in health-care workers exposed to blood of infected patients. *MMWR* **36**:285, 1987

34. Gershon RRM et al: The risk of transmission of HIV-1 through nonpercutaneous, non-sexual modes: A review. *AIDS* **4**:645, 1990

35. Mann JM, Welles SL: Global aspects of the HIV epidemic, in *AIDS: Etiology, Diagnosis, Treatment and Prevention,* 3d ed, edited by VT DeVita Jr, S Hellman Jr, SA Rosenberg. Philadelphia, Lippincott, 1992, p 89

36. Padian N et al: Male to female transmission of human immunodeficiency virus. *JAMA* **258**:788, 1987

37. Peterman TA et al: Risk for human immunodeficiency virus transmission from heterosexual adults with transfusion-associated infections. *JAMA* **259**:55, 1988

38. Johnson AM et al: Transmission of HIV to sexual partners of infected men and women. *AIDS* **3**:367, 1989

39. St. Louis ME et al: Seroprevalence rates of human immunodeficiency virus infection at sentinel hospitals in the United States. *N Engl J Med* **323**:213, 1990

40. Widy-Wirski R et al: Evaluation of the WHO clinical case definition for AIDS in Uganda. *JAMA* **260**:3286, 1988

41. Pan American Health Organization: Working group on AIDS case definition. *Epidemiol Bull* **10**:9, 1990

42. Centers for Disease Control: Classification system for human T-cell lymphotrophic virus type III/lymphadenopathy-associated virus infections. *MMWR* **35**:334, 1986

43. Centers for Disease Control: Revision of the CDC surveillance definition for acquired immunodeficiency syndrome. *MMWR* **40**:787, 1991

44. Chang SW et al: The new AIDS case definition. Implications for San Francisco. *JAMA* **267**:973, 1992

45. Phillips AN et al: Serial CD4 lymphocyte counts and development of AIDS. *Lancet* **337**:389, 1991

46. Moss AR et al: Seropositivity for HIV and the development of AIDS or AIDS-related condition: Three year follow-up of the San Francisco General Hospital cohort. *Br Med J* **296**:745, 1988

47. Lang W et al: Patterns of T lymphocyte changes with human immunodeficiency virus infection: From seroconversion to the development of AIDS. *J AIDS* **2**:63, 1989

48. Selik RM et al: Impact of the 1987 revision of the case definition of acquired immune deficiency syndrome in the United States. *J AIDS* **3**:73, 1991

49. Clinical spectrum of HIV disease, in *AIDS: Etiology, Diagnosis, Treatment and Prevention,* 3d ed, edited by VT DeVita Jr, S Hellman, SA Rosenberg, Philadelphia, Lippincott, 1992, p 123

50. Gaines H: Primary HIV infection. *Scand J Infect Dis* **61**(suppl):1, 1989

51. Ho DD et al: Primary human T-lymphotropic virus type III infection. *Ann Intern Med* **103**:880, 1985

52. Denning DW et al: Acute myelopathy associated with primary infection with human immunodeficiency virus. *Br Med J* **294**:142, 1987

53. Sinicco A et al: Acute HIV-1 infection: Clinical and biological study of 12 patients. *J AIDS* **3**:260, 1990

54. Hulsebosch HJ et al: Human immunodeficiency virus exanthem. *J Am Acad Dermatol* **23**:483, 1990

55. Hillman RJ et al: Acute seroconversion to HIV in male prostitute as a consequence of occupational exposure. *AIDS* **3**:925, 1990

56. Rabeneck L et al: Acute HIV infection presenting with painful swallowing and esophageal ulcers. *JAMA* **263**:2318, 1990

57. Peña JM et al: Esophageal candidiasis associated with acute infection due to the human immunodeficiency virus: Case report and review. *Rev Infect Dis* **13**:872, 1991

58. Peña JM et al: Esophageal candidiasis associated with acute infection due to human immunodeficiency virus: Case report and review. *Rev Infect Dis* **13**:872, 1991

59. Decker CF et al: Esophageal candidiasis associated with acute infection due to human immunodeficiency virus. *Clin Infect Dis* **14**:791, 1992

60. Gaines H et al: Clinical picture of primary HIV infection presenting as a glandular-fever-like illness. *Br Med J* **297**:1368, 1988

61. Tindall B et al: Primary human immunodeficiency virus infection: Clinical and serologic aspects. *Infect Dis Clin North Am* **2**:329, 1988

62. Fox R et al: Clinical manifestations of acute infection with human immunodeficiency virus in a cohort of gay men. *AIDS* **1**:35, 1987

63. Gaines H et al: Immunological changes in primary HIV-1 infection. *AIDS* **4**:995, 1990

64. McMillan A et al: Immunohistology of the skin rash associated with acute HIV infection. *AIDS* **3**:309, 1989

65. Weiss PJ et al: Initial low CD4 lymphocyte counts in recent human immunodeficiency virus infection and lack of association with identified coinfections. *J Infect Dis* **166**:1149, 1992

66. McCune JM: HIV-1. The infective process in vivo. *Cell* **64**:351, 1991

67. Learmont J et al: Long-term symptomless HIV-1 infection in recipients of blood products from a single donor. *Lancet* **340**:863, 1992

68. Laurence J: Molecular interactions among herpesviruses and human immunodeficiency virus. *J Infect Dis* **162**:338, 1990

69. Anderson RM, May RM: Epidemiological parameters of HIV infection. *Nature* **333**:514, 1988

70. Berkelman RL et al: Epidemiology of human immunodeficiency virus infection and acquired immunodeficiency syndrome. *Am J Med* **86**:761, 1989

71. Moss AR, Bacchetti P: Natural history of HIV infection. *AIDS* **3**:55, 1989

72. Downs AM et al: Transfusion-associated AIDS cases in Europe: Estimation of the incubation period, distribution and prediction of future cases. *J AIDS* **4**:805, 1991

73. Msellati P et al: A cohort study of 89 HIV-1-infected adult patients contaminated by blood products: Bordeaux 1981–1989. *AIDS* **4**:1105, 1990

74. Fernández-Cruz E et al: Immunological and serological markers predictive of progression to AIDS in a cohort of HIV-infected drug users. *AIDS* **4**:987, 1990

75. Anderson RE et al: Use of β_2-microglobulin level and CD4 count to predict development of acquired immunodeficiency syndrome in persons with human immunodeficiency virus infection. *Arch Intern Med* **150**:73, 1990

76. Hofmann B et al: Serum beta2-microglobulin level increase in HIV infection: Relation to seroconversion, CD4 T-cell fall and prognosis. *AIDS* **4**:207, 1990

77. Kramer A et al: Neopterin: A predictive marker of acquired immune deficiency syndrome in human immunodeficiency virus infection. *J AIDS* **2**:291, 1989

78. Melmed RN et al: Serum neopterin changes in HIV-infected subjects: Indicator of significant pathology, CD4 T cell changes, and the development of AIDS. *J AIDS* **2**:70, 1989

79. Eyster ME et al: Predictive markers for the acquired immunodeficiency syndrome (AIDS) in hemophiliacs: Persistence of p24 antigen and low T4 cell count. *Ann Intern Med* **110**:963, 1989

80. Rinaldo C et al: Association of human immunodeficiency virus (HIV) p24 antigenemia with decrease in CD4+ lymphocytes and onset of acquired immunodeficiency syndrome during the early phase of HIV infection. *J Clin Microbiol* **27**:880, 1989

81. Lemp GF et al: Projections of AIDS morbidity and mortality in San Francisco. *JAMA* **263**:1497, 1990

82. Eyster ME et al: Natural history of human immunodeficiency virus infections in hemophiliacs: Effects of T-cell subsets, platelet counts, and age. *Ann Intern Med* **107**:1, 1987

83. Ward JW et al: The natural history of transfusion-associated infection with human immunodeficiency virus. *N Engl J Med* **321**:947, 1989

84. Moss AR, Bacchetti P: Editorial review: Natural history of HIV infection. *AIDS* **3**:55, 1989

85. Schoenbaum EE et al: HIV infection and intravenous drug use. *Curr Opin Infect Dis* **3**:80, 1990

86. Biggar RJ et al: AIDS incubation in 1981 seroconverters from different exposure groups. *AIDS* **4**:1059, 1990

87. Stein M et al: Causes of death in persons with human immunodeficiency virus infection. *Am J Med* **93**:387, 1992

88. McKenzie R et al: The causes of death in patients with human immunodeficiency virus infection: A clinical and pathologic study with emphasis on the role of pulmonary disease. *Medicine (Baltimore)* **70**:326, 1991

89. Biggar RJ et al: Cancer among New York men at risk of acquired immunodeficiency syndrome. *Int J Cancer* **43**:979, 1989

90. Kaposi M et al: Idiopathiches multiples pigment Sarcom der Haut. *Dermatol Syph* **4**:265, 1872

91. Friedman-Kien AE, Saltzman BR: Clinical manifestations of classical, endemic African, and epidemic AIDS-associated Kaposi's sarcoma. *J Am Acad Dermatol* **22**:1237, 1990

92. Harwood HR et al: Kaposi's sarcoma in recipients of renal transplants. *Am J Med* **67**:759, 1979

93. Friedman-Kien AE et al: Disseminated Kaposi's sarcoma in homosexual men. *Ann Intern Med* **96**:693, 1982

94. Haverkos HW: Factors associated with the pathogenesis of AIDS. *J Infect Dis* **156**:251, 1987

95. Krigel RL, Friedman-Kien AE: Epidemic Kaposi's sarcoma. *Semin Oncol* **17**:350, 1990

96. Beral V et al: Kaposi's sarcoma among persons with AIDS: A sexually transmitted infection? *Lancet* **335**:123, 1990

97. Rutherford, GW, Kahn JO: The epidemiology of AIDS-related Kaposi's sarcoma. *J AIDS* **3**(suppl 1):54, 1990

98. Rutherford GW et al: The epidemiology of AIDS-related Kaposi's sarcoma in San Francisco. *J Infect Dis* **159**:569, 1989

99. Connor E et al: Cutaneous acquired immunodeficiency syndrome-associated Kaposi's sarcoma in pediatric patients. *Arch Dermatol* **126**:791, 1990

100. de Wit R: AIDS-associated Kaposi's sarcoma and the mechanism of interferon alphas activity. A riddle with a puzzle. *J Intern Med* **231**:321, 1992

101. Vogel J et al: The HIV *tat* gene induces dermal lesions resembling Kaposi's sarcoma in transgenic mice. *Nature* **335**:606, 1988

102. Salahudin SZ et al: Angiogenic properties of Kaposi's sarcoma-derived cells after long term culture in vitro. *Science* **242**:430, 1988

103. Ensoli B et al: AIDS-KS-derived cells express cytokines with autocrine and paracrine growth effects. *Science* **243**:223, 1989

104. Friedman-Kien AE et al: Kaposi's sarcoma in HIV-infected homosexual men. *Lancet* **335**:168, 1990

105. Huang YQ: HPV-related DNA sequences in Kaposi's sarcoma. *Lancet* **339**:515, 1992

106. Rappersberger K et al: Endemic Kaposi's sarcoma in human immunodeficiency virus type 1-seronegative persons: Demonstration of retrovirus-like particles in cutaneous lesions. *J Invest Dermatol* **95**:371, 1990

107. Dictor M, Järplid B: The cause of Kaposi's sarcoma: An avian retroviral analog. *J Am Acad Dermatol* **18**:398, 1988

108. Myskowski PL et al: AIDS-associated Kaposi's sarcoma: Variables associated with survival. *J Am Acad Dermatol* **18**:1299, 1988

109. Rendon MI et al: Linear cutaneous lesions of Kaposi's sarcoma: A clinical clue to the diagnosis of AIDS. *Arch Dermatol* **124**:327, 1988

110. Janier M et al: The Koebner phenomenon in AIDS-related Kaposi's sarcoma. *J Am Acad Dermatol* **22**:125, 1990

111. Real FX, Krown SE: Spontaneous regression of Kaposi's sarcoma in patients with AIDS (letter). *N Engl J Med* **313**:1659, 1985

112. Barrison IG et al: Upper gastrointestinal Kaposi's sarcoma in patients positive for HIV antibody without cutaneous disease. *Br Med J* **296**:92, 1988

113. Lemlich G et al: Kaposi's sarcoma and AIDS. Postmortem findings in twenty-four cases. *J Am Acad Dermatol* **16**:319, 1987

114. Safai B, Schwartz JJ: Kaposi's sarcoma and the acquired immunodeficiency syndrome, in *AIDS: Etiology, Diagnosis, Treatment, and Prevention,* 3d ed, edited by VT De Vita Jr et al. Philadelphia, Lippincott, 1992, p 209

115. Volberding PA: Clinical features and staging, in *Kaposi's Sarcoma: Pathophysiology and Clinical Management,* edited by M Ziegler, RF Dorfman. New York, Marcel Dekker, 1988, p 169

116. Chachoua A et al: Prognostic factors and staging classifications of patients with epidemic Kaposi's sarcoma. *J Clin Oncol* **7**:774, 1989

117. Lane HC et al: Zidovudine in patients with human immunodeficiency virus (HIV) infection with Kaposi's sarcoma. A phase II randomized, placebo-controlled trial. *Ann Intern Med* **111**:41, 1989

118. Groopman JE, Scadden DT: Interferon therapy for Kaposi's sarcoma associated with AIDS. *Ann Intern Med* **110**:335, 1989

119. Kovacs JA et al: Combined zidovudine and interferon-alfa therapy in patients with Kaposi's sarcoma and the acquired immunodeficiency syndrome (AIDS). *Ann Intern Med* **111**:280, 1989

120. El-Akkad et al: Kaposi's sarcoma and its management by radiotherapy. *Arch Dermatol* **122**:1396, 1986

121. Le Bourgeois JP et al: Radiotherapy of epidemic Kaposi's sarcoma in patients with AIDS. Analysis of 149 cases treated by extended and/or localized cutaneous irradiation. *Ann Dermatol Venereol* **117**:17, 1990

122. Vapnek JM et al: Acquired immunodeficiency syndrome-related Kaposi's sarcoma of the male genitalia: Management with radiation therapy. *J Urol* **146**:333, 1991

123. Berson AM et al: Radiation therapy for AIDS-related Kaposi's sarcoma. *Int J Radiat Oncol Biol Phys* **19**:569, 1990

124. Cooper JS et al: Intentions and outcomes in the radiotherapeutic management of epidemic Kaposi's sarcoma. *Int J Radiat Oncol Biol Phys* **20**:419, 1991

125. Cooper JS, Fried PR: Toxicity of oral radiotherapy with acquired immunodeficiency syndrome. *Otolaryngol Head Neck Surg* **113**:327, 1987

126. Epstein JB: Oral Kaposi's sarcoma with acquired immunodeficiency syndrome. Review of management and report of the efficacy of intralesional vinblastine. *Cancer* **64**:2424, 1989

127. Neuman SB et al: Treatment of epidemic Kaposi's sarcoma (KS) with intralesional vinblastine injection (IL-VBL). *Proc Am Soc Clin Oncol* **7**:5, 1988

128. Sulis ML et al: Interferon administered intralesionally in skin, conjunctiva and oral cavity lesions in patients with AIDS-related Kaposi's sarcoma. *Eur J Cancer Clin Oncol* **25**:759, 1989

129. Tappero JW et al: Cryotherapy for cutaneous Kaposi's sarcoma (KS) associated with acquired immunodeficiency syndrome (AIDS): A phase II trial. *J AIDS* **4**:839, 1991

130. Krown SE: Approaches to interferon combination therapy in the treatment of AIDS. *Semin Oncol* **1**(suppl):38, 1990

131. Krown SE et al: Kaposi's sarcoma, in *Medical Management of AIDS Patients*. *Med Clin North Am* **76**:235, 1992

132. Gelmann EP et al: Combination chemotherapy for disseminated Kaposi's sarcoma in patients with the acquired immunodeficiency syndrome. *Am J Med* **82**:456, 1987

133. Gill PS et al: Advanced AIDS-related Kaposi's sarcoma. Results of pilot studies using combination chemotherapy. *Cancer* **65**:1074, 1990

134. Laine L et al: The response of symptomatic gastrointestinal Kaposi's sarcoma to chemotherapy: A prospective evaluation using an endoscopic method of disease quantification. *Am J Gastroenterol* **85**:959, 1990

135. Lassoued K et al: Treatment of the acquired immune-deficiency syndrome-related Kaposi's sarcoma with bleomycin as a single agent. *Cancer* **66**:1869, 1990

136. Caumes E et al: Cutaneous side effects of bleomycin in AIDS patients with Kaposi's sarcoma. *Lancet* **336**:1593, 1990

137. Gill PS et al: Systemic treatment of AIDS-related Kaposi's sarcoma: Results of a randomized trial. *Am J Med* **90**:427, 1991

138. Gill PS et al: Clinical effect of glucocorticoids on Kaposi's sarcoma related to the acquired immunodeficiency syndrome. *Ann Intern Med* **110**:937, 1989

139. Myskowski PL et al: Lymphoma and other HIV-associated malignancies. *J Am Acad Dermatol* **22**:1253, 1990

140. Burns MK et al: Nodular cutaneous B-cell lymphoma of the scalp in the acquired immunodeficiency syndrome. *J Am Acad Dermatol* **25**:933, 1991

141. Goldstein J et al: Cutaneous T-cell lymphoma in a patient infected with human immunodeficiency virus type 1. *Cancer* **66**:1130, 1990

142. Kaplan LD et al: AIDS-associated non-Hodgkins lymphoma in San Francisco. *JAMA* **261**:719, 1989

143. Shpall SN et al: Cutaneous T cell lymphoma in patients with HIV disease. *J Cutan Pathol* **17**:317, 1990

144. Crane GA et al: Cutaneous T-cell lymphoma in patients with human immunodeficiency virus infection. *Arch Dermatol* **127**:989, 1991

145. Lee HH et al: Patterns of HIV-1 and HTLV-I/II in intravenous drug users from the middle Atlantic and central regions of the USA. *J Infect Dis* **162**:347, 1990

146. Shabita D et al: Human T-cell lymphotrophic virus type I (HTLV-I)-associated adult T-cell leukemia-lymphoma in a patient infected with human immunodeficiency virus type 1 (HIV-1). *Ann Intern Med* **111**:871, 1989

147. Cortes E et al: HIV-1, HIV-2, and HTLV-I in high-risk groups in Brazil. *N Engl J Med* **320**:953, 1989

148. Baurmann H et al: Adult T-cell leukemia associated with HTLV-I and simultaneous infection with human immunodeficiency virus type 2 and human herpesvirus 6 in an African woman: A clinical, virologic, and familial serologic study. *Am J Med* **85**:853, 1988

149. Greenberg SJ et al: Kaposi's sarcoma in human T-cell leukemia virus type 1-associated adult T-cell leukemia. *Blood* **76**:971, 1990

150. Ourcy WL, Jakubek DJ: Multiple squamous cell carcinomas and human immunodeficiency virus infection. *Ann Intern Med* **106**:33, 1987

151. Milburn PB et al: Disseminated warts and evolving squamous cell carcinoma in a patient with acquired immunodeficiency syndrome. *J Am Acad Dermatol* **19**:401, 1988

152. Sitz KV, Keppen M: Metastatic basal cell carcinoma in acquired immunodeficiency syndrome-related complex. *JAMA* **257**:340, 1987

153. Lobo DV et al: Nonmelanoma skin cancers and infection with the human immunodeficiency virus. *Arch Dermatol* **128**:623, 1992

154. Frichter R et al: Cervical intraepithelial neoplasia in HIV-infected women, abstract No. 0057. VIII International Conference on AIDS, Amsterdam, July 19–24, 1992

155. Klein RS et al: A prospective study of genital neoplasia and human papillomavirus (HPV) in HIV-infected women, abstract No. 0527. VIII International Conference on AIDS, Amsterdam, July 19–24, 1992

156. Palefsky J et al: Anal cytologic abnormalities and papilloma virus infection in men with HIV infection, abstract No. 0058. VIII International Conference on AIDS, Amsterdam, July 19–24, 1992

157. Daling JR et al: Sexual practices, sexually transmitted diseases, and the incidence of anal intercourse. *N Engl J Med* **317**:973, 1987

158. Duvic M et al: Eruptive dysplastic nevi associated with human immunodeficiency virus infection. *Arch Dermatol* **125**:397, 1989

159. Rivers JK et al: Malignant melanoma in a man seropositive for the human immunodeficiency virus. *J Am Acad Dermatol* **20**:1127, 1989

160. Tindall B et al: Malignant melanoma with human immunodeficiency virus infection in three homosexual men. *J Am Acad Dermatol* **20**:587, 1989

161. McGregor JM et al: Cutaneous malignant melanoma and human immunodeficiency virus (HIV) infection: A report of three cases. *Br J Dermatol* **126**:516, 1992

162. Zuger A: Bacterial infections in AIDS: Part I. *AIDS Clin Care* **4**:69, 1992

163. Ellis M et al: Impaired neutrophil functions in patients with AIDS or AIDS-related complex: A comprehensive evaluation. *J Infect Dis* **158**:1268, 1988

164. Nichols L et al: Bacterial infections in the acquired immune deficiency syndrome. Clinicopathologic correlations in a series of autopsy cases. *Am J Clin Pathol* **92**:787, 1989

165. Ganesh R et al: Staphylococcal carriage and HIV infection (letter). *Lancet* **2**:558, 1989

166. Raviglione MC et al: High *Staphylococcus aureus* nasal carriage in patients with acquired immunodeficiency syndrome or AIDS-related complex. *Am J Infect Control* **18**:64, 1990

167. Battan R et al: *S. aureus* nasal carriage among homosexual men with and without HIV infection. *Am J Infect Control* **19**:99, 1991

168. Henry K et al: Nasal septal abscess due to *Staphylococcal aureus* in a patient with AIDS. *Rev Infect Dis* **10**:428, 1988

169. Donovan B et al: Bullous impetigo in homosexual men—a risk marker for HIV-infection? *Genitourin Med* **68**:159, 1992

170. Becker BA et al: Atypical plaquelike staphylococcal folliculitis in human immunodeficiency virus-infected persons. *J Am Acad Dermatol* **21**:1024, 1989

171. Patterson JW et al: Cutaneous botryomycosis in a patient with acquired immunodeficiency syndrome. *J Am Acad Dermatol* **16**:238, 1987

172. Toth IR, Kazal HL: Botryomycosis in acquired immunodeficiency syndrome. *Arch Pathol Lab Med* **111**:246, 1987

173. Weitzner JM et al: Successful treatment of botryomycosis in a patient with acquired immunodeficiency syndrome. *J Am Acad Dermatol* **21**:1312, 1989

174. Schwartzman WA et al: Staphylococcal pyomyositis in patients infected by the human immunodeficiency virus. *Am J Med* **90**:595, 1991

175. Widrow C et al: Pyomyositis in patients with the human immunodeficiency virus: An unusual form of disseminated bacterial infection. *Am J Med* **91**:129, 1991

176. Sesma P et al: Rhabdomyolysis, infection due to the human immunodeficiency virus, and staphylococcal bacteremia. *Clin Infect Dis* **15**:1054, 1992

177. Kline MW, Dunkle LM: Toxic shock syndrome and the acquired immunodeficiency syndrome. *Pediatr Infect Dis J* **10**:736, 1988

178. Donohue D et al: Staphylococcal scalded skin syndrome in a women with chronic renal failure exposed to human immunodeficiency virus. *Cutis* **47**:317, 1991

179. Cone LA et al: A recalcitrant, erythematous, desquamating disorder associated with toxin-producing staphylococci in patients with AIDS. *J Infect Dis* **165**:638, 1992

180. Scully M, Berger TG: Pruritus, *Staphylococcal aureus,* and human immunodeficiency virus infection. *Arch Dermatol* **126**:684, 1990

181. Duvic M: Staphylococcal infections and the pruritus of AIDS-related complex. *Arch Dermatol* **123**:1599, 1987

182. Skoutelis AT et al: Indwelling central venous catheter infections in

patients with acquired immune deficiency syndrome. *J AIDS* **3**:335, 1990

183. Jacobson MA et al: *Staphylococcus aureus* bacteremia and recurrent staphylococcal infection in patients with acquired immunodeficiency syndrome and AIDS-related complex. *Am J Med* **85**:172, 1988

184. Dugdale D, Ramsey PG: *Staphylococcus aureus* bacteremia in patients with Hickman catheters. *Am J Med* **89**:137, 1990

185. Raviglione MC et al: Infections associated with Hickman catheters in patients with acquired immunodeficiency syndrome. *Am J Med* **86**:780, 1989

186. Jaffe D et al: Staphylococcal sepsis in HIV antibody seropositive psoriasis patients. *J Am Acad Dermatol* **24**:970, 1991

187. Hewitt WD, Farrar WE: Case report: Bacteremia and ecthyma caused by *Streptococcus pyogenes* in a patient with acquired immunodeficiency syndrome. *Am J Med Sci* **295**:52, 1988

188. Janssen F et al: Group A streptococcal cellulitis-adenitis in a patient with acquired immunodeficiency syndrome. *J Am Acad Dermatol* **24**:363, 1991

189. Marshall GS et al: Meningitis caused by toxigenic group A beta-hemolytic *Streptococcus* in a pediatric patient with acquired immunodeficiency syndrome. *Pediatr Infect Dis J* **10**:339, 1991

190. Ho DD, Murata GH: Streptococcal lymphadenitis in homosexual men with chronic lymphadenopathy. *Am J Med* **77**:151, 1984

191. Decker C et al: *Stomatococcus mucilaginosus* intravascular catheter-related infection in a patient with AIDS. *Infect Dis Clin Prac* **1**:174, 1992

192. Torssander J et al: Dermatophytosis and HIV infection. A Study in homosexual men. *Acta Derm Venereol (Stockh)* **68**:563, 1988

193. Perniciaro C, Peters MS: Tinea faciale mimicking seborrheic dermatitis in a patient with AIDS. *N Engl J Med* **314**:315, 1986

194. Daniel CR et al: The spectrum of nail disease in patients with human immunodeficiency virus infection. *J Am Acad Dermatol* **27**:93, 1992

195. Lee MM et al: Onychomycosis (letter). *Arch Dermatol* **126**:402, 1990

196. Dompmartin D et al: Onychomycosis and AIDS. Clinical and laboratory findings in 62 patients. *Int J Dermatol* **29**:337, 1990

197. Hevia O et al: Nonscalp hair infection caused by *Microsporum canis* in patient with acquired immunodeficiency syndrome. *J Am Acad Dermatol* **24**:789, 1991

198. Wright DW et al: Generalized chronic dermatophytosis in patients with human immunodeficiency virus type 1 infection and CD4 depletion. *Arch Dermatol* **127**:265, 1991

199. Gottlieb MS et al: *Pneumocystis carinii* pneumonia and mucosal candidiasis in previously healthy homosexual men. Evidence of a new acquired cellular immunodeficiency. *N Engl J Med* **305**:1425, 1981

200. Matthews R et al: Candida and AIDS: Evidence for protective antibody. *Lancet* **2**:263, 1988

201. Whelan WL et al: *Candida albicans* in patients with the acquired immunodeficiency syndrome: Absence of a novel or hypervirulent strain. *J Infect Dis* **162**:513, 1990

202. Imam N et al: Heirarchical pattern of mucosal *Candida* infections in HIV-seropositive women. *Am J Med* **89**:142, 1990

203. Pedersen C et al: *Candida* esophagitis associated with acute human immunodeficiency virus infection. *J Infect Dis* **156**:1419, 1987

204. Podzamezer D et al: Esophageal candidiasis in the diagnosis of HIV-infected patients. *JAMA* **259**:1569, 1988

205. Dull JS et al: Oral candidiasis as a marker of acute retroviral illness. *South Med J* **84**:733, 1991

206. Peña JM et al: Esophageal candidiasis associated with acute infection due to human immunodeficiency virus: Case report and review. *Rev Infect Dis* **13**:872, 1991

207. Decker CF et al: Esophageal candidiasis associated with acute infection due to human immunodeficiency virus. *Clin Infect Dis* **14**:791, 1992

208. Carpenter CCJ et al: Human immunodeficiency virus infection in North American women: Experience with 200 cases and a review of the literature. *Medicine (Baltimore)* **70**:307, 1991

209. Prose NS: HIV infection in children. *J Am Acad Dermatol* **22**:1223, 1990

210. Torssander J et al: Oral *Candida albicans* in HIV infection. *Scand J Infect Dis* **19**:1597, 1987

211. De Wit S et al: Comparison of fluconazole and ketoconazole for oropharyngeal candidiasis in AIDS. *Lancet* **1**:746, 1989

212. Thorsen S, Mathiesen LR: Fluconazole for ketoconazole-resistant oropharyngeal candidiasis in HIV-1 infected patients. *Scand J Infect Dis* **22**:375, 1990

213. Chave J-P et al: Single-dose therapy for esophageal candidiasis with fluconazole. *AIDS* **4**:1034, 1990

214. Laine L et al: Fluconazole compared with ketoconazole for the treatment of candida esophagitis in AIDS. A randomized trial. *Ann Intern Med* **117**:655, 1992

215. Esposito R et al: Maintenance therapy of oropharyngeal candidiasis in HIV-infected patients with fluconazole. *AIDS* **4**:1033, 1990

216. Stevens DA et al: Thrush can be prevented in patients with acquired immunodeficiency syndrome and the acquired immunodeficiency syndrome-related complex. *Arch Intern Med* **151**:2458, 1991

217. Eisenstat BA, Wormser GP: Seborrheic dermatitis and butterfly rash in AIDS. *N Engl J Med* **311**:189, 1984

218. Mathes BM, Douglass MC: Seborrheic dermatitis in patients with acquired immunodeficiency syndrome. *J Am Acad Dermatol* **13**:947, 1985

219. Groisser D et al: Association of *Pityrosporum orbiculare (Malassezia furfur)* with seborrheic dermatitis in patients with acquired immunodeficiency syndrome. *J Am Acad Dermatol* **20**:770, 1989

220. Heng MCY et al: Correlation of *Pityrosporum ovale* density with clinical severity of seborrheic dermatitis as assessed by a simplified technique. *J Am Acad Dermatol* **23**:82, 1990

221. Wikler JR et al: Quantitative skin cultures of *Pityrosporum* yeasts in patients seropositive for the human immunodeficiency virus with and without seborrheic dermatitis. *J Am Acad Dermatol* **27**:37, 1992

222. Soeprona FF et al: Seborrheic-like dermatitis of acquired immunodeficiency syndrome. A clinicopathologic study. *J Am Acad Dermatol* **14**:242, 1986

223. Skinner RB et al: Seborrheic dermatitis and acquired immunodeficiency syndrome. *J Am Acad Dermatol* **14**:147, 1986

224. Drabick JJ et al: Cutaneous cladosporiosis as a complication of skin testing in men positive for human immunodeficiency virus. *J Am Acad Dermatol* **22**:135, 1990

225. Laurence J: Molecular interactions among herperviruses and human immunodeficiency viruses. *J Infect Dis* **162**:338, 1990

226. Holmberg SD et al: Prior herpes simplex virus type 2 infection as a risk factor for HIV infection. *JAMA* **259**:1048, 1988

227. Stamm WE et al: The association of genital ulcer disease and acquisition of HIV infection in homosexual men. *JAMA* **260**:1429, 1988

228. Hook EW III et al: Herpes simplex virus infection as a risk factor for human immunodeficiency virus infection in heterosexuals. *J Infect Dis* **265**:251, 1992

229. Siegal FP et al: Severe acquired immunodeficiency in male homosexuals, manifested by chronic perianal ulcerative herpes simplex lesions. *N Engl J Med* **305**:1439, 1981

230. Quinnan GV et al: Herpes virus infections in the acquired immunodeficiency syndrome. *JAMA* **252**:72, 1984

231. Norris SA et al: Severe, progressive herpetic whitlow caused by acyclovir-resistant virus in a patient with AIDS. *J Infect Dis* **157**:209, 1988

232. Don PC et al: Herpetic infection mimicking chronic neurotic excoriation. *Int J Dermatol* **30**:136, 1991

233. Norris SA et al: Severe, progressive herpetic whitlow caused by an acyclovir-resistant virus in a patient with AIDS. *J Infect Dis* **157**:209, 1988

234. Baden LA et al: Off-center fold: Persistent necrotic digits in a patient with acquired immunodeficiency syndrome. *Arch Dermatol* **127**:113, 1991

235. Glickel SZ: Hand infections in patients with acquired immunodeficiency syndrome. *J Hand Surg [Am]* **13A**:770, 1988

236. Sacks SL et al: Progressive esophagitis from acyclovir-resistant herpes simplex. Clinical roles for DNA polymerase mutants and viral heterogeneity? *Ann Intern Med* **111**:893, 1989

237. Erlich KS et al: Acyclovir-resistant herpes simplex virus infections in patients with the acquired immunodeficiency syndrome. *N Engl J Med* **320**:293, 1989

238. Zimmerli W et al: Disseminated herpes simplex type 2 and systemic *Candida* infection in a patient with previous asymptomatic human immunodeficiency virus infection. *J Infect Dis* **157**:597, 1988

239. Marks GL et al: Mucocutaneous dissemination of acyclovir-resistant herpes simplex virus in a patient with AIDS. *Rev Infect Dis* **11**:474, 1989

240. Kory WP et al: Dermatopathologic findings in patients with acquired immunodeficiency syndrome. *South Med J* **80**:1529, 1987

241. Conant MA: Prophylactic and suppressive treatment with acyclovir and the management of herpes in patients with acquired immunodeficiency syndrome. *J Am Acad Dermatol* **18**:186, 1988

242. Drugs for viral infections. *Med Lett Drugs Ther* **34**:31, 1992

243. Whitley RJ, Gnann JW Jr: Acyclovir: A decade later. *N Engl J Med* **327**:782, 1992

244. Engel JP et al: Treatment of resistant herpes simplex virus with continuous-infusion acyclovir. *JAMA* **263**:1662, 1990

245. Sall RK et al: Successful treatment of progressive acyclovir-resistant herpes simplex virus using intravenous foscarnet in a patient with the acquired immunodeficiency syndrome. *Arch Dermatol* **125**:1548, 1989

246. Chatis PA et al: Successful treatment with foscarnet of an acyclovir-resistant mucocutaneous infection with herpes simplex virus in a patient with acquired immunodeficiency syndrome. *N Engl J Med* **320**:297, 1989

247. Hardy WD: Foscarnet treatment of acyclovir-resistant herpes simplex virus infection in patients with acquired immunodeficiency syndrome: Preliminary results of a controlled, randomized, regimen-comparative trial. *Am J Med* **92** (suppl 2A):30S, 1992

248. Safrin S et al: A controlled trial comparing foscarnet with vidarabine for acyclovir-resistant mucocutaneous herpes simplex in the acquired immunodeficiency syndrome. *N Engl J Med* **325**:551, 1991

249. Lietman PS et al: Clinical pharmacology: Foscarnet. *Am J Med* **92** (suppl 2A):8S, 1992

250. Jura E et al: Varicella-zoster virus infections in children infected with human immunodeficiency virus. *Pediatr Infect Dis J* **8**:586, 1989

251. Perronne C et al: Varicella in patients infected with the human immunodeficiency virus. *Arch Dermatol* **126**:1033, 1990

252. Nousbaum JB et al: Deux manifestations inhabituelles d'une par le virus LAV-HTLV III: BCGite et varicelle pulmonaire. *Rev Pneumol Clin* **42**:310, 1986

253. Pahwa S et al: Continuous varicella-zoster infection associated with resistance in a child with AIDS. *JAMA* **260**:2879, 1988

254. Friedman-Kien AE et al: Herpes zoster: A possible early clinical sign for development of acquired immunodeficiency syndrome in high-risk individuals. *J Am Acad Dermatol* **14**:1023, 1986

255. Colebunders R et al: Herpes zoster in African patients: A clinical predictor of human immunodeficiency virus infection. *J Infect Dis* **157**:314, 1988

256. Melbye M et al: Risk of AIDS after herpes zoster. *Lancet* **2**:728, 1987

257. Buchbinder SP et al: Herpes zoster and human immunodeficiency virus infection. *J Infect Dis* **166**:1153, 1992

258. Patterson L et al: Clinical herpes zoster shortly following primary varicella in two HIV-infected children. *Clin Pediatr (Phila)* **28**:354, 1989

259. Williamson BC: Disseminated herpes zoster in a human immunodeficiency virus-positive homosexual man without complications. *Cutis* **40**:485, 1987

260. Cohen PR et al: Disseminated herpes zoster in patients with human immunodeficiency virus infection. *Am J Med* **84**:1076, 1988

261. Kestelyn P et al: Severe herpes zoster ophthalmicus in young African

adults: A marker for HTLV-III seropositivity. *Br J Ophthalmol* **71**:806, 1987

262. Shuler JD et al: External ocular disease and anterior segment disorders associated with AIDS. *Int Ophthalmol Clin* **29**:98, 1989

263. Seiff SR et al: Use of intravenous acyclovir for treatment of herpes zoster ophthalmicus in patients at risk for AIDS. *Ann Ophthalmol* **20**:480, 1988

264. Chess J et al: Zoster-related bilateral acute retinal necrosis syndrome as presenting sign in AIDS. *Ann Ophthalmol* **20**:431, 1988

265. Rostad SW et al: Transsynaptic spread of varicella zoster virus through the visual system: A mechanism of viral dissemination in the central nervous system. *Hum Pathol* **20**:174, 1989

266. Ryder JW et al: Progressive encephalitis three months after resolution of cutaneous zoster in a patient with AIDS. *Ann Neurol* **19**:182, 1986

267. Cohen PR, Grossman ME: Clinical features of human immunodeficiency virus-associated disseminated herpes zoster virus infection—a review of the literature. *Clin Exp Dermatol* **14**:273, 1989

268. LeBoit PE et al: Chronic verrucous varicella-zoster virus infection in patients with the acquired immunodeficiency syndrome (AIDS). *Am J Dermatopathol* **14**:1, 1992

269. Leibovitz E et al: Chronic varicella zoster in a child infected with human immunodeficiency virus: Case report and review of the literature. *Cutis* **49**:27, 1992

270. Hoppenjans WB et al: Prolonged cutaneous herpes zoster in acquired immunodeficiency syndrome. *Arch Dermatol* **126**:1048, 1990

271. Disler RS, Dover JS: Chronic localized herpes zoster in the acquired immunodeficiency syndrome. *Arch Dermatol* **126**:1105, 1990

272. Gilson IH et al: Disseminated ecthymatous herpes varicella-zoster virus infection in patients with acquired immunodeficiency syndrome. *J Am Acad Dermatol* **20**:637, 1989

273. Alessi E et al: Unusual varicella zoster virus infection in patients with the acquired immunodeficiency syndrome. *Arch Dermatol* **124**:1011, 1988

274. Janier M et al: Chronic varicella zoster infection in acquired immunodeficiency syndrome. *J Am Acad Dermatol* **18**:584, 1988

275. Gulick RM et al: Varicella-zoster virus disease in patients with human immunodeficiency virus infection. *Arch Dermatol* **126**:1086, 1990

276. Langenberg A et al: Granulomatous vasculitis occurring after cutaneous herpes zoster despite absence of viral genome. *J Am Acad Dermatol* **24**:429, 1991

277. Linnemann CC Jr et al: Emergence of acyclovir-resistant varicella zoster virus in an AIDS patient on prolonged acyclovir therapy. *AIDS* **4**:577, 1990

278. Jacobson MA et al: Acyclovir-resistant varicella-zoster virus infection after chronic oral acyclovir therapy in patients with the acquired immunodeficiency syndrome (AIDS). *Ann Intern Med* **112**:187, 1990

279. Safrin S et al: Foscarnet therapy in five patients with AIDS and acyclovir-resistant varicella-zoster virus infection. *Ann Intern Med* **115**:19, 1991

280. Näher H et al: Detection of Epstein-Barr virus-DNA in tongue epithelium of human immunodeficiency virus-infected patients. *J Invest Dermatol* **97**:421, 1991

281. Reggiani M, Pauluzzi P: Hairy leukoplakia in liver transplant patient. *Acta Derm Venereol (Stockh)* **70**:87, 1990

282. Epstein JB et al: Hairy leukoplakia-like lesions in immunosuppressed patients following bone marrow transplantation. *Transplantation* **46**:462, 1988

283. Greenspan D et al: Relation of oral hairy leukoplakia to infection with the human immunodeficiency virus and the risk of developing AIDS. *J Infect Dis* **155**:475, 1987

284. Greenspan D et al: Risk factors for rapid progression from hairy leukoplakia to AIDS: A nested case-control study. *J AIDS* **4**:652, 1991

285. Fisher DA, Greenspan JS: Oral hairy leukoplakia unassociated with

human immunodeficiency virus: Pseudo oral hairy leukoplakia. *J Am Acad Dermatol* 27:257, 1992

286. Lozada-Nur F: Podophyllin resin 25% for the treatment of oral hairy leukoplakia: An old treatment for a new lesion. *J AIDS* 4:543, 1991

287. Sanchez M et al: Treatment of oral hairy leukoplakia with podophyllin. *Arch Dermatol* 128:1659, 1992

288. Greenspan D et al: Efficacy of desciclovir in the treatment of Epstein-Barr virus infection in oral hairy leukoplakia. *J AIDS* 3:571, 1990

289. Briggaman RA, Wheeler CE: Immunology of human warts. *J Am Acad Dermatol* 1:297, 1979

290. Palefsky J et al: Anal intraepithelial neoplasia and papillomavirus infection among homosexual males with group IV HIV disease. *JAMA* 263:2911, 1990

291. Maiman M et al: Colposcopic evaluation of human immunodeficiency virus-seropositive women. *Obstet Gynecol* 78:84, 1991

292. Prose NS et al: Widespread flat warts associated with human papillomavirus type 5: A cutaneous manifestation of human immunodeficiency virus infection. *J Am Acad Dermatol* 23:978, 1990

293. Berger TG et al: Epidermodysplasia verruciformis-associated papillomavirus infection complicating human immunodeficiency virus. *Br J Dermatol* 124:79, 1991

294. Critchlow CW et al: Association of human immunodeficiency virus and anal human papillomavirus infection among homosexual men. *Arch Intern Med* 152:1673, 1992

295. Feingold AR et al: Cervical cytologic abnormalities and papillomavirus in women infected with human immunodeficiency virus. *J AIDS* 3:896, 1990

296. Scholefield JH et al: Anal and cervical intraepithelial neoplasia. Possible parallel. *Lancet* 2:765, 1989

297. Mougin C et al: Prevalence of oncogenic human papillomavirus DNA in lesions of the anogenital region of human immunodeficiency seropositive men: Correlation between histological features and in situ hybridization signal. *Eur J Dermatol* 2:231, 1992

298. Icenogle JP et al: Genotypes and sequence variants of human papillomavirus DNAs from human immunodeficiency virus type 1-infected women with cervical intraepithelial neoplasia. *J Infect Dis* 166:1210, 1992

299. Bradshaw BR et al: Human papillomavirus type 16 in a homosexual man. *Arch Dermatol* 128:949, 1992

300. Forman AB, Prendiville JS: Association of human immunodeficiency virus seropositivity and extensive perineal condylomata acuminata in a child. *Arch Dermatol* 124:1010, 1988

301. Laraque D: Severe anogenital warts in a child with HIV infection (letter). *N Engl J Med* 320:1220, 1989

302. Ikenberg H et al: Human papillomavirus type 6-related DNA in genital Bowen's disease and Bowenoid papulosis. *Int J Cancer* 32:563, 1983

303. Beck DE: Surgical management of anal condylomata in the HIV-positive patient. *Dis Colon Rectum* 33:180, 1990

304. Schwartz JJ, Myskowski PL: Molluscum contagiosum in patients with human immunodeficiency virus infection. A review of twenty-seven patients. *J Am Acad Dermatol* 27:583, 1992

305. Sarma DP, Weilbaecher TG: Molluscum contagiosum in the acquired immune deficiency syndrome. *J Am Acad Dermatol* 13:682, 1985

306. Matis WL et al: Dermatologic findings associated with human immunodeficiency virus infection. *J Am Acad Dermatol* 17:746, 1987

307. Katzman M et al: Molluscum contagiosum and the acquired immunodeficiency syndrome: Clinical and immunological details of two cases. *Br J Dermatol* 116:131, 1987

308. Sugihara K et al: Molluscum contagiosum associated with AIDS: A case report with ultrastructural study. *J Oral Pathol Med* 19:235, 1990

309. Fivenson DP et al: Giant molluscum contagiosum presenting as a basal cell carcinoma in an acquired immunodeficiency syndrome patient. *J Am Acad Dermatol* 29:912, 1988

310. Smith KJ et al: Molluscum contagiosum. Ultrastructural evidence for its presence in skin adjacent to clinical lesions in patients infected with human immunodeficiency virus type 1. *Arch Dermatol* 128:223, 1992

311. Gotuzzo E et al: The impact of human T-lymphotrophic virus type I/II infection on the prognosis of sexually acquired cases of acquired immunodeficiency syndrome. *Arch Intern Med* 152:1429, 1992

312. Cleghorn FR, Blattner WA: Does human T-cell lymphotropic virus type I and human immunodeficiency virus type 1 coinfection accelerate acquired immunodeficiency syndrome? The jury is still out. *Arch Intern Med* 152:1372, 1992

313. Gregory N et al: The spectrum of syphilis in patients with human immunodeficiency virus infection. *J Am Acad Dermatol* 22:1061, 1990

314. Glover RA et al: An unusual presentation of secondary syphilis in a patient with human immunodeficiency virus infection. *Arch Dermatol* 128:530, 1992

315. Zaidman GW: Neurosyphilis and retrobulbar neuritis in a patient with AIDS. *Ann Ophthalmol* 18:260, 1986

316. Zambrano W et al: Acute syphilitic blindness in AIDS. *J Clin Neuro Ophthalmol* 7:1, 1987

317. Reid SE, Anzarut A: Neurosyphilis and stroke in a patient with antibodies to the human immunodeficiency virus. *Am J Med* 87:119, 1989

318. DiNubile MJ et al: Acute syphilitic meningitis in a man with seropositivity for human immunodeficiency virus infection and normal numbers of CD4 T lymphocytes. *Arch Intern Med* 152:1324, 1992

319. Radolf JD, Kaplan RP: Unusual manifestations of secondary syphilis and abnormal humoral response to *Treponema pallidum* antigens in a homosexual man with asymptomatic human immunodeficiency virus infection. *J Am Acad Dermatol* 18(suppl):423, 1988

320. Johns DR et al: Alteration in the natural history of neurosyphilis by concurrent infection with human immunodeficiency virus. *N Engl J Med* 316:1569, 1987

321. Musher DM et al: Effect of human immunodeficiency virus (HIV) infection on the course of syphilis and on the response to treatment. *Ann Intern Med* 113:872, 1990

322. Katz DA, Berger JR: Neurosyphilis in acquired immunodeficiency syndrome. *Arch Neurol* 46:895, 1989

323. Hook EW III: Syphilis and HIV infection. *J Infect Dis* 160:530, 1989

324. Berger JR: Spinal cord syphilis associated with human immunodeficiency virus infection: A treatable myelopathy. *Am J Med* 92:101, 1992

325. Matlow AG, Rachlis AR: Syphilis serology in human immunodeficiency virus-infected patients with symptomatic neurosyphilis: Case report and review. *Rev Infect Dis* 12:703, 1990

326. Hutchinson CM et al: Characteristics of patients with syphilis attending Baltimore STD clinics: Multiple, high-risk subgroups and interactions with human immunodeficiency virus infection. *Arch Intern Med* 151:511, 1991

327. Fiumara N: Human immunodeficiency virus infection and syphilis. *J Am Acad Dermatol* 21:141, 1989

328. Berry CD et al: Neurologic relapse after benzathine penicillin therapy for secondary syphilis in a patient with HIV infection. *N Engl J Med* 316:1587, 1987

329. Bowen DL et al: Immunopathogenesis of the acquired immunodeficiency syndrome. *Ann Intern Med* 103:704, 1985

330. Tramont EC: Syphilis in the AIDS era. *N Engl J Med* 316:1600, 1987

331. Matlow AG, Rachlis AR: Syphilis serology in human immunodeficiency virus-infected patients with symptomatic neurosyphilis: Case report and review. *Rev Infect Dis* 12:703, 1990

332. Hicks CB et al: Seronegative secondary syphilis in a patient infected with the human immunodeficiency virus (HIV) with Kaposi's sarcoma. *Ann Intern Med* 107:492, 1987

333. Haas JS et al: Sensitivity of treponemal tests for detecting prior

treated syphilis during human immunodeficiency virus infection. *J Infect Dis* **162**:862, 1990

334. Duncan WC: Failure of erythromycin to cure secondary syphilis in a patient infected with the human immunodeficiency virus. *Arch Dermatol* **125**:82, 1989

335. Musher DM: Syphilis, neurosyphilis, penicillin, and AIDS. *J Infect Dis* **163**:1202, 1991

336. Donabedian H, Khazan U: Norwegian scabies in a patient with AIDS. *Clin Infect Dis* **14**:162, 1992

337. Arico M et al: Localized crusted scabies in the acquired immunodeficiency syndrome. *Clin Exp Dermatol* **17**:339, 1992

338. Inserra DW, Bickley LK: Crusted scabies in acquired immunodeficiency syndrome. *Int J Dermatol* **29**:287, 1990

339. Mathes BM et al: Seborrheic dermatitis in patients with acquired immunodeficiency syndrome. *J Am Acad Dermatol* **13**:947, 1985

340. Matis WL et al: Dermatologic findings associated with human immunodeficiency virus infection. *J Am Acad Dermatol* **17**:746, 1987

341. Duvic M et al: Acquired immunodeficiency syndrome-associated psoriasis and Reiter's syndrome. *Arch Dermatol* **123**:1622, 1987

342. Kaplan MH et al: Antipsoriatic effects of zidovudine in human immunodeficiency virus-associated psoriasis. *J Am Acad Dermatol* **20**:76, 1989

343. Calabrese LH et al: Rheumatic symptoms and human immunodeficiency virus infection. The influence of clinical and laboratory variables in a longitudinal cohort study. *Arthritis Rheum* **34**:257, 1991

344. Reveille JD et al: Human immunodeficiency virus-associated psoriasis, psoriatic arthritis, and Reiter's syndrome: A disease continuum? *Arthritis Rheum* **33**:1574, 1990

345. Duvic M et al: Acquired immunodeficiency syndrome-associated psoriasis and psoriasis and Reiter's syndrome. *Arch Dermatol* **123**:1622, 1987

346. Lazar AP, Roenigk HH: AIDS and psoriasis. *Cutis* **39**:347, 1987

347. Johnson TM et al: AIDS exacerbates psoriasis (letter). *N Engl J Med* **313**:1415, 1985

348. Obuch ML et al: Psoriasis and human immunodeficiency virus infection. *J Am Acad Dermatol* **27**:667, 1992

349. Horn TD et al: Characterization of the dermal infiltrate in human immunodeficiency virus-infected patients with psoriasis. *Arch Dermatol* **126**:1462, 1990

350. Mahoney SE et al: Human immunodeficiency virus transcripts identified in HIV-related psoriasis and Kaposi's sarcoma lesions. *J Clin Invest* **88**:175, 1991

351. Fuchs D et al: Interferon-gamma concentrations are increased in sera from individuals infected with the human immunodeficiency virus. *J AIDS* **2**:158, 1989

352. Duvic M et al: Remission of AIDS-associated psoriasis. *Lancet* **2**:627, 1987

353. Stanley SK et al: Induction of expression of human immunodeficiency virus in a chronically infected promonocytic cell line by ultraviolet radiation. *AIDS Res Hum Retroviruses* **5**:375, 1989

354. Ranki A et al: Effect of PUVA on immunologic and virologic findings in HIV-infected patients. *J Am Acad Dermatol* **24**:404, 1991

355. Allen BR: Use of cyclosporin for psoriasis in HIV-positive patient. *Lancet* **339**:686, 1992

356. Colebunders R et al: Psoriasis regression in terminal AIDS. *Lancet* **339**:1110, 1992

357. Valle S-L: Dermatologic findings related to HIV infection in high-risk individuals. *J Am Acad Dermatol* **17**:951, 1987

358. Goodman DS et al: Prevalence of cutaneous disease in patients with AIDS or ARC. *J Am Acad Dermatol* **17**:210, 1987

359. Coldiron BM, Bergstesser PR: Prevalence and clinical spectrum of skin disease in patients infected with the human immunodeficiency virus. *Arch Dermatol* **125**:357, 1989

360. Brenner S: Acquired ichthyosis in AIDS. *Cutis* **39**:421, 1987

361. Young L, Steinman HK: Acquired ichthyosis in a patient with AIDS and Kaposi's sarcoma. *J Am Acad Dermatol* **16**:395, 1987

362. Liautaud B et al: Pruritic skin lesions: A common initial presentation of acquired immunodeficiency syndrome. *Arch Dermatol* **125**:629, 1989

363. Smith KJ et al: Papular eruption of human immunodeficiency virus disease. A review of the clinical, histologic, and immunohistochemical findings in 48 cases. *Am J Dermatopathol* **13**:445, 1991

364. Rosenthal D et al: HIV-associated eosinophilic folliculitis: A unique dermatosis associated with advanced HIV infection. *Arch Dermatol* **127**:206, 1991

365. Buchness MR et al: Eosinophilic pustular folliculitis in the acquired immunodeficiency syndrome. *N Engl J Med* **318**:1183, 1988

366. Soeprono FF, Schinella RA: Eosinophilic pustular folliculitis in patients with the acquired immunodeficiency syndrome. *J Am Acad Dermatol* **14**:1020, 1986

367. Harris DWS et al: Eosinophilic pustular folliculitis in an HIV-positive man: Response to cetirizine. *Br J Dermatol* **126**:392, 1992

368. James WD et al: A papular eruption associated with T-cell lymphotrophic virus type III disease. *J Am Acad Dermatol* **13**:563, 1985

369. Hevia O et al: Pruritic papular eruption of the acquired immunodeficiency syndrome: A clinicopathologic study. *J Am Acad Dermatol* **24**:231, 1991

370. Colebunders R et al: Generalized papular pruritic eruption in African patients with human immunodeficiency virus infection. *AIDS* **1**:117, 1987

371. Pardo RJ et al: UVB phototherapy of the pruritic papular eruption of the acquired immunodeficiency syndrome. *J Am Acad Dermatol* **26**:423, 1992

372. Ansary MA et al: *A Colour Atlas of AIDS in the Tropics.* London, Wolfe, 1989, p 28

373. Sundharam JA: Pruritic skin eruption in the acquired immunodeficiency syndrome: anthropod bites? *Arch Dermatol* **126**:539, 1990

374. Scully M, Berger TG: Pruritus, *Staphylococcus aureus,* and human immunodeficiency virus infection. *Arch Dermatol* **126**:684, 1990

375. Kinloch-de-Loes S et al: Bullous pemphigoid antibodies, HIV-1 infection and pruritic papular eruption. *AIDS* **5**:451, 1991

376. Phelan JA et al: Oral findings in patients with AIDS. *Oral Surg Oral Med Oral Pathol* **64**:50, 1987

377. Bach MC et al: Odynophagia from aphthous ulcers of the pharynx and esophagus in AIDS. *Ann Intern Med* **109**:338, 1988

378. Youle M et al: Treatment of resistant aphthous ulcerations in HIV seropositive patients using thalidomide, abstract, book 2, 321. IV International Conference on AIDS, Stockholm, June 12–16, 1988

379. Wignants H et al: Multiple drug reactions in a patient with AIDS. *Lancet* **2**:1455, 1989

380. Greenberger RG, Patterson R: Management of drug allergy in patients with acquired immunodeficiency syndrome. *J Allergy Clin Immunol* **79**:484, 1987

381. Gordin FM et al: Adverse reactions to trimethoprim-sulfamethoxazole in patients with the acquired immunodeficiency syndrome. *Ann Intern Med* **100**:495, 1984

382. Matsuyasu R et al: Cutaneous reaction to trimethoprim-sulfamethoxazole in patients with AIDS and Kaposi's sarcoma. *N Engl J Med* **308**:1535, 1983

383. Moreno JN et al: Oral desensitization to sulfadiazine and trimethoprim-sulfamethoxazole (TMP-SMX) in 4 patients with AIDS. *N Engl J Med* **308**:340, 1983

384. Tenant-Flowers M et al: Sulfadiazine desensitization in patients with AIDS and cerebral toxoplasmosis. *AIDS* **5**:311, 1991

385. Torgovnick J, Arsura A: Desensitization to sulfonamides in patients with HIV infection. *Am J Med* **88**:548, 1990

386. Shafer RW et al: Successful prophylaxis of *Pneumocystis* pneumonia with trimethoprim-sulfamethoxazole in AIDS patients with previous allergic reactions. *J AIDS* **2**:389, 1990

387. Metroka CE et al: Desensitization to dapsone in HIV-positive patients. *JAMA* **267**:512, 1992

388. Raviglione MC et al: Fatal toxic epidermal necrolysis during prophylaxis with pyrimethamine and sulfadoxine in a human immunodeficiency virus-infected person. *Arch Intern Med* **148**:2683, 1988

389. Berger TG et al: Aerosolized pentamidine and cutaneous findings. *Ann Intern Med* **110**:1035, 1989

390. Roujeau JC et al: Toxic epidermal necrolysis. *J Am Acad Dermatol* **23**:1039, 1990

391. Porteous DM, Berger TG: Severe cutaneous drug reactions (Stevens-Johnson syndrome and toxic epidermal necrolysis) in human immunodeficiency virus infection. *Arch Dermatol* **127**:740, 1991

392. Saiag P et al: Drug-induced toxic epidermal necrolysis (Lyell's syndrome) in patients infected with the human immunodeficiency virus. *J Am Acad Dermatol* **26**:5676, 1992

393. Torres RA et al: Zidovudine-induced leukocytoclastic vasculitis. *Arch Intern Med* **152**:850, 1992

394. Don PC et al: Nail dyschromia associated with zidovudine. *Ann Intern Med* **112**:145, 1990

395. Prose NS et al: Disorders of the nails and hair associated with human immunodeficiency virus infection. *Int J Dermatol* **31**:453, 1992

396. Greenberger RG, Berger TG: Nail and mucocutaneous hyperpigmentation with azidothymidine therapy. *J Am Acad Dermatol* **22**:237, 1990

397. Gallais V et al: Acral hyperpigmented macules and longitudinal melanonychia in AIDS patients. *Br J Dermatol* **126**:387, 1992

398. Merenich JA et al: Azidothymidine-induced hyperpigmentation mimicking primary adrenal insufficiency. *Am J Med* **86**:469, 1989

399. Klutman NE, Hinthorn DR: Excessive growth of eyelashes in a patient with AIDS being treated with zidovudine. *N Engl J Med* **324**:1896, 1991

400. Sahai J et al: Zidovudine-associated hypertrichosis and nail pigmentation in an HIV-infected patient. *AIDS* **5**:1395, 1991

401. Kaplan MH et al: Acquired trichomegaly of the eyelashes: A cutaneous marker of acquired immunodeficiency syndrome. *J Am Acad Dermatol* **25**:801, 1991

402. Van der Pijl JW et al: Foscarnet and penile ulceration. *Lancet* **335**:286, 1990

403. Gill PS et al: Clinical effects of glucocorticoids on Kaposi's sarcoma related to the acquired immunodeficiency syndrome. *Ann Intern Med* **110**:937, 1989

404. Serwadda D et al: Slim disease: A new disease in Uganda and its association with HTLV-III infection. *Lancet* **2**:1849, 1985

405. Prose NS: Human immunodeficiency virus infection in childhood: The disease and its cutaneous manifestations. *Adv Dermatol* **5**:113, 1990

406. Straka BF et al: Cutaneous manifestations of AIDS in children. *J Am Acad Dermatol* **18**:1089, 1988

407. Lim W et al: Skin diseases in children with HIV infection and their association with degree of immunosuppression. *Int J Dermatol* **29**:24, 1990

408. Wykoff RF et al: Immunologic dysfunction in infants infected through transfusion with HTLV-III. *N Engl J Med* **31**:294, 1986

409. Goedert JJ et al: A prospective study of human immunodeficiency virus type 1 infection and the development of AIDS in subjects with hemophilia. *N Engl J Med* **321**:1141, 1989

410. Becherer PR et al: Human immunodeficiency virus-I disease progression in hemophiliacs. *Am J Hematol* **34**:204, 1990

411. Scott GB et al: Survival in children with perinatally acquired immunodeficiency virus type I infection. *N Engl J Med* **321**:1791, 1989

412. Auger I et al: Incubation periods for pediatric AIDS patients. *Nature* **336**:575, 1988

413. Straka BF: Immunization of children infected with human T-lymphotrophic virus type III/lymphadenopathy associated virus. *JAMA* **256**:2477, 1986

414. Gutierrez-Ortega P et al: Kaposi's sarcoma in a 6-day-old infant with HIV. *Arch Dermatol* **125**:432, 1989

415. Connor E et al: Cutaneous acquired immunodeficiency syndrome-associated Kaposi's sarcoma in pediatric patients. *Arch Dermatol* **126**:791, 1990

416. Paller AS et al: Pyoderma gangrenosum in pediatric acquired immunodeficiency syndrome. *J Pediatr* **117**:63, 1990

417. Kielhofner M et al: Life-threatening *Pseudomonas aeruginosa* infec-

418. Sangoerzan JA et al: Cutaneous manifestations of *Pseudomonas* infection in the acquired immunodeficiency syndrome. *Arch Dermatol* **126**:832, 1990

419. Franzetti F et al: *Pseudomonas* infections in patients with AIDS and AIDS-related complex. *J Intern Med* **231**:437, 1992

420. Krumholz HM et al: Community-acquired bacteremia in patients with acquired immunodeficiency syndrome: Clinical presentation, bacteriology, and outcome. *Am J Med* **86**:776, 1989

421. Milner SM et al: Acetic acid to treat *Pseudomonas aeruginosa* in superficial wounds and burns (letter). *Lancet* **340**:61, 1992

422. Lozano F et al: Life-threatening *Pseudomonas aeruginosa* infections in patients with infection due to human immunodeficiency virus. *Clin Infect Dis* **15**:751, 1992

423. Indrisano JP, Simon GL: Facial *Salmonella* abscess. *Ann Intern Med* **110**:171, 1989

424. Boixeda P et al: Cutaneous nocardiosis and human immunodeficiency virus infection. *Int J Dermatol* **30**:804, 1991

425. Kim J et al: Nocardial infection as a complication of AIDS: Report of six cases and review. *Rev Infect Dis* **13**:624, 1991

426. Javaly K et al: Nocardiosis in patients with human immunodeficiency virus infection. Report of 2 cases and review of the literature. *Medicine (Baltimore)* **71**:128, 1992

427. Aguado JM et al: Meningococcemia: An undescribed cause of community-acquired bacteremia in patients with acquired immunodeficiency syndrome (AIDS) and AIDS-related complex. *Am J Med* **88**:314, 1990

428. Ho D et al: Pathogenesis of infection with human immunodeficiency virus. *N Engl J Med* **317**:278, 1987

429. Harries AD: Tuberculosis and human immunodeficiency virus infection in developing countries. *Lancet* **335**:387, 1990

430. Centers for Disease Control: Tuberculosis statistics in the United States, 1989. *MMWR* **38**:1, 1990

431. Barnes PF et al: Tuberculosis in patients with human immunodeficiency virus infection. *N Engl J Med* **324**:1644, 1991

432. Daley CL et al: An outbreak of tuberculosis with accelerated progression among persons infected with the human immunodeficiency virus. An analysis using restriction-fragment-length polymorphisms. *N Engl J Med* **326**:231, 1992

433. Hopewell PC et al: Impact of human immunodeficiency virus infection on the epidemiology, clinical features, management, and control of tuberculosis. *Clin Infect Dis* **15**:540, 1992

434. Edlin BR et al: An outbreak of multidrug-resistant tuberculosis among hospitalized patients with the acquired immunodeficiency syndrome. *N Engl J Med* **326**:1514, 1992

435. Dooley SW et al: Nosocomial transmission of tuberculosis in a hospital unit for HIV-infected patients. *JAMA* **267**:2632, 1992

436. Pedersen C, Nielsen JO: Tuberculosis in homosexual men with HIV disease. *Scand J Infect Dis* **19**:289, 1987

437. Hartstein M, Leaf, HL: Tuberculosis of the breast as a presenting manifestation of AIDS. *Clin Infect Dis* **15**:692, 1992

438. Stack RJ et al: Miliary tuberculosis presenting as skin lesions in a patient with acquired immunodeficiency syndrome. *J Am Acad Dermatol* **23**:1031, 1990

439. Rohatgi PK et al: Acute miliary tuberculosis of the skin in acquired immunodeficiency syndrome. *J Am Acad Dermatol* **26**:356, 1992

440. Mehlmauer MA et al: Keratotic papules and nodules and hyperkeratosis of palms and soles in a patient with tuberculosis and AIDS-related complex. *J Am Acad Dermatol* **23**:381, 1990

441. Lupatkin H et al: Tuberculous abscesses in patients with AIDS. *Clin Infect Dis* **14**:1040, 1992

442. Boudes P et al: Disseminated *Mycobacterium bovis* infection from BCG vaccination and HIV infection. *JAMA* **262**:2386, 1989

443. Armbuster C et al: Disseminated bacille Calmette-Guérin infection in an AIDS patient 30 years after BCG vaccination. *J Infect Dis* **162**:1216, 1990

444. Reynes J et al: Bacille Calmette-Guérin adenitis 30 years after im-

munization in a patient with AIDS (letter). *J Infect Dis* **160**:727, 1989

445. Friedman BR et al: *Mycobacterium avium-intracellulare:* Cutaneous presentations of disseminated disease. *Am J Med* **85**:257, 1988

446. Horsburgh CR Jr: *Mycobacterium avium* complex infection in the acquired immunodeficiency syndrome. *N Engl J Med* **324**:1332, 1991

447. Nightingale SD et al: Incidence of *Mycobacterium avium-intracellulare* complex bacteremia in human immunodeficiency virus-positive patients. *J Infect Dis* **165**:1082, 1992

448. Havlik JA et al: Disseminated *Mycobacterium avium* complex infection: Clinical identification and epidemiologic trends. *J Infect Dis* **165**:577, 1992

449. Barbaro DJ et al: *Mycobacterium avium–Mycobacterium intracellulare* infection limited to the skin and lymph nodes in patients with AIDS. *Rev Infect Dis* **11**:625, 1989

450. Cohen OJ, Squires K: *Mycobacterium avium* osteomyelitis as the presenting manifestation of AIDS. *Infect Dis Clin Prac* **1**:110, 1992

451. Males BM et al: *Mycobacterium haemophilum* infection in a patient with acquired immunodeficiency syndrome. *Am J Med* **84**:640, 1988

452. Rogers PL et al: Disseminated *Mycobacterium haemophilum* infection in two patients with the acquired immunodeficiency syndrome. *Am J Med* **84**:640, 1988

453. Kristjansson M et al: *Mycobacterium haemophilum* infection in immunocompromised patients: Case report and review of the literature. *Rev Infect Dis* **13**:906, 1991

454. Dever LL et al: Varied presentations and responses to treatment of infections caused by *Mycobacterium haemophilum* in patients with AIDS. *Clin Infect Dis* **14**:1195, 1992

455. Centers for Disease Control: *Mycobacterium haemophilum* infections—New York City Metropolitan Area, 1990–1991. *MMWR* **40**:636, 1991

456. Sack JB: Disseminated infection due to *Mycobacterium fortuitum* in a patient with AIDS. *Rev Infect Dis* **12**:961, 1990

457. Shafer RW, Sierra MF: *Mycobacterium xenopi, Mycobacterium fortuitum, Mycobacterium kansasii,* and other nontuberculous mycobacteria in an area of endemicity for AIDS. *Clin Infect Dis* **15**:161, 1992

458. Lamfers EJP et al: Leprosy in the acquired immunodeficiency syndrome. *Ann Intern Med* **107**:111, 1987

459. Meeran K: Prevalence of HIV infection among patients with leprosy and tuberculosis in rural Zambia. *Br Med J* **298**:364, 1989

460. Turk JL et al: AIDS and leprosy (editorial). *Lepr Rev* **59**:193, 1988

461. Leonard G et al: Prevalence of HIV infection among patients with leprosy in African countries and Yemen. *J AIDS* **3**:1109, 1990

462. Gormus BJ et al: Interactions between simian immunodeficiency virus and *Mycobacterium leprae* in experimentally inoculated Rhesus monkeys. *J Infect Dis* **160**:405, 1989

463. Kennedy C et al: Leprosy and human immunodeficiency virus infection. A closer look at the lesions. *Int J Dermatol* **29**:139, 1990

464. Drabick JJ et al: Cutaneous cladosporiosis as a complication of skin testing in a man positive for human immunodeficiency virus. *J Am Acad Dermatol* **22**:135, 1990

465. Kevy-Klotz B et al: Alternariose cutanée au cours d'un sida. *Ann Dermatol Venereol* **112**:739, 1985

466. Duvic M et al: Superficial phaeohyphomycosis of the scrotum in a patient with the acquired immunodeficiency syndrome. *Arch Dermatol* **123**:1597, 1987

467. Nightingale SD et al: Disseminated histoplasmosis in patients with AIDS. *South Med J* **83**:624, 1990

468. Chuck SL, Sande MA: Infections with *Cryptococcus neoformans* in AIDS. *N Engl J Med* **321**:794, 1989

469. Blauvelt A, Kerdel FA: Cutaneous cryptococcosis mimicking Kaposi's sarcoma as the initial manifestation of disseminated disease. *Int J Dermatol* **31**:279, 1992

470. Rico MJ, Pennys NS: Cutaneous cryptococcis resembling molluscum contagiosum in a patient with AIDS. *Arch Dermatol* **121**:901, 1985

471. Picon I et al: Cutaneous cryptococcis resembling molluscum contagiosum: A first manifestation of AIDS. *Acta Derm Venereol (Stockh)* **69**:365, 1989

472. Borton LK, Wintroub B: Disseminated cryptococcosis presenting as herpetiform lesions in a homosexual man with acquired immunodeficiency syndrome. *J Am Acad Dermatol* **10**:387, 1984

473. Miller SJ: Cutaneous cryptococcosis resembling molluscum contagiosum in a patient with acquired immunodeficiency syndrome. *Cutis* **41**:411, 1988

474. Porges DY, Krueger JG: A novel use of the cryptococcal latex agglutination test for rapid presumptive diagnosis of cutaneous cryptococcosis. *Arch Dermatol* **128**:461, 1992

475. O'Keefe EJ et al: Diff-Quik stain for Tzanck smears. *J Am Acad Dermatol* **13**:148, 1985

476. Antoniskis D et al: Seronegative disseminated coccidioidomycosis in patients with HIV infection. *AIDS* **4**:691, 1990

477. Wheat LJ: Histoplasmosis in Indianapolis. *Clin Infect Dis* **14**(suppl 1):S91, 1992

478. Oscherwitz SL, Rinaldi MG: Disseminated sporotrichosis in a patient infected with human immunodeficiency virus. *Clin Infect Dis* **15**:568, 1992

479. Bibler MR et al: Disseminated sporotrichosis in a patient with HIV infection after treatment of acquired factor VII inhibitor. *JAMA* **256**:3125, 1986

480. Shaw JC et al: Sporotrichosis in the acquired immunodeficiency syndrome. *J Am Acad Dermatol* **21**:1145, 1989

481. Fitzpatrick JE, Eubanks S: Acquired immunodeficiency syndrome presenting as disseminated cutaneous sporotrichosis. *Int J Dermatol* **27**:406, 1988

482. Heller HM, Fuhrer J: Disseminated sporotrichosis in patients with AIDS: Case report and review of the literature. *AIDS* **5**:1243, 1991

483. Kurosawa A et al: *Sporotrix schenckii* endophthalmitis in a patient with human immunodeficiency virus infection. *Arch Ophthalmol* **106**:376, 1988

484. Lipstein-Kresch E et al: Dissemiated *Sporotrix schenkii* infection with arthritis in a patient with acquired immunodeficiency syndrome. *J Rheumatol* **12**:805, 1984

485. Penn CC et al: *Sporotrichosis schenckii* meningitis in a patient with AIDS. *Clin Infect Dis* **15**:740, 1992

486. Chiu J et al: Disseminated blastomycosis in HIV infected patients, abstract No. 7209, IV International Conference on AIDS, Stockholm, June 12–16, 1988

487. Kitchen LW et al: Concurrent pulmonary *Blastomyces dermatitidis* and *Mycobacterium tuberculosis* infection in an HIV-1 seropositive man (letter). *J Infect Dis* **160**:160, 1989

488. Herd AM et al: Miliary blastomycosis and HIV infection. *Can Med Assoc J* **143**:1329, 1990

489. Fraser VJ et al: Two cases of blastomycosis from a common source: Use of DNA restriction analysis to identify strains. *J Infect Dis* **163**:1378, 1991

490. Minamoto GY et al: Invasive aspergillosis in patients with AIDS. *Clin Infect Dis* **14**:66, 1992

491. Hunt SJ et al: Primary cutaneous aspergillosis near central venous catheters in patients with the acquired immunodeficiency syndrome. *Arch Dermatol* **128**:1229, 1992

492. Pursell KJ et al: *Aspergillus* species colonization and invasive disease in patients with AIDS. *Clin Infect Dis* **14**:141, 1992

493. Pulmonary aspergillosis in the acquired immunodeficiency syndrome. *N Engl J Med* **324**:654, 1991

494. Peto TEA et al: Systemic mycosis due to *Penicillium marneffei* in a patient with antibody to human immunodeficiency virus. *J Infect* **16**:285, 1988

495. Piehl MR et al: Disseminated penicilliosis in a patient with acquired immunodeficiency syndrome. *Arch Pathol Lab Med* **112**:1262, 1988

496. Sathapatayavongs B et al: Disseminated penicilliosis associated with HIV infection (letter). *J Infect* **19**:84, 1988

497. Hulshof CMJ et al: *Penicillium marneffei* infection in an AIDS patient (letter). *Eur J Clin Microbiol Infect Dis* **9**:370, 1990

498. Tsang DNC et al: *Penicillium marneffei:* Another pathogen to con-

sider in patients infected with human immunodeficiency virus. *Rev Infect Dis* **13**:766, 1991

499. Jones PD, See J: *Penicillium marneffei* infection in patients infected with human immunodeficiency virus: Late presentation in an area of nonedemicity. *Clin Infect Dis* **15**:744, 1992

500. Supparatpinyo K et al: *Penicillium marneffei* infection in patients with human immunodeficiency virus. *Clin Infect Dis* **14**:871, 1992

501. Slater LN et al: *Rochalimaea henselae* causes bacillary angiomatosis and peliosis hepatis. *Arch Intern Med* **152**:602, 1992

502. Webster GF et al: The clinical spectrum of bacillary angiomatosis. *Br J Dermatol* **126**:535, 1992

503. Schwartzman WA: Infections due to *Rochalimaea:* The expanding clinical spectrum. *Clin Infect Dis* **15**:893, 1992

504. Stoler PE: The expanding spectrum of a new disease (editorial). *Arch Dermatol* **126**:808, 1990

505. Relman DA et al: The agent of bacillary angiomatosis. An approach to the identification of uncultured pathogens. *N Engl J Med* **323**:1573, 1990

506. Reed JA et al: Immunocytochemical identification of *Rochalimaea henselae* in bacillary (epithelioid) angiomatosis, parenchymal bacillary peliosis, and persistent fever with bacteremia. *Am J Surg Pathol* **16**:650, 1992

507. LeBoit PE: Bacillary angiomatosis. *West J Med* **156**:191, 1992

508. Perkocha LA et al: Clinical and pathological features of bacillary peliosis hepatis in association of human immunodeficiency virus infection. *N Engl J Med* **323**:1581, 1990

509. Kaplan LJ et al: Severe measles in immunocompromised patients. *JAMA* **267**:1237, 1992

510. Krasinski K et al: Measles and measles immunity in children infected with human immunodeficiency virus. *JAMA* **261**:2512, 1989

511. Markowitz LE et al: Fatal measles pneumonia without rash in a child with AIDS. *J Infect Dis* **158**:480, 1988

512. McNutt NS et al: Cutaneous manifestations of measles in AIDS. *J Cutan Pathol* **19**:315, 1992

513. Gallant JE et al: Incidence and natural history of cytomegalovirus disease in patients with advanced human immunodeficiency virus disease treated with zidovudine. *J Infect Dis* **166**:1223, 1992

514. Heineman M-H: Characteristics of cytomegalovirus retinitis in patients with acquired immunodeficiency syndrome. *Am J Med* **92**(suppl 2A):12S, 1992

515. Horn TD, Hood AF: Cytomegalovirus is predictably present in perineal ulcers from immunosuppressed patients. *Arch Dermatol* **126**:642, 1990

516. Curry A et al: Opportunistic protozoan infections in human immunodeficiency virus disease: Review highlighting diagnostic and therapeutic aspects. *J Clin Pathol* **44**:182, 1991

517. Kovacs JA, Masur H: Prophylaxis for *Pneumocystis carinii* pneumonia in patients infected with human immunodeficiency virus. *Clin Infect Dis* **14**:1005, 1992

518. Raviglione MC: Extrapulmonary pneumocystosis: The first 50 cases. *Rev Infect Dis* **12**:1127, 1990

519. Litwin MA, Williams CM: Cutaneous *Pneumocystis carinii* infection mimicking Kaposi's sarcoma. *Ann Intern Med* **117**:48, 1992

520. Alvar J et al: Association of visceral leishmaniasis and human immunodeficiency virus infections. *J Infect Dis* **160**:560, 1989

521. Flegg PJ, Brettle RP: Visceral leishmaniasis in HIV-infected patients. *AIDS* **4**:365, 1990

522. Pialoux G et al: Cutaneous leishmaniasis in an AIDS patient: Cure with itraconazole. *J Infect Dis* **162**:1221, 1990

523. Josep Condom M et al: Asymptomatic leishmaniasis in the acquired immunodeficiency syndrome (AIDS). *Ann Intern Med* **111**:767, 1989

524. Rodrigues Coura J et al: Disseminated American cutaneous leishmaniasis in a patient with AIDS. *Mem Inst Oswaldo Cruz* **82**:581, 1987

525. Rosenthal PJ et al: Rectal leishmaniasis in a patient with acquired immunodeficiency syndrome. *Am J Med* **84**:307, 1988

526. Montalban C et al: Visceral leishmaniasis (kala-azar) as an opportun-

istic infection in patients infected with the human immunodeficiency virus in Spain. *Rev Infect Dis* **11**:655, 1989

527. Berenguer J et al: Visceral leishmaniasis in patients infected with the human immunodeficiency virus (HIV). *Ann Intern Med* **111**:129, 1989

528. Yerba M et al: Dissemination-to-skin kala-azar and the acquired immunodeficiency syndrome. *Ann Intern Med* **108**:490, 1988

529. Lortholary O et al: Interferon-γ associated with conventional therapy for recurrent visceral leishmaniasis in a patient with AIDS. *Rev Infect Dis* **12**:370, 1990

530. Mawhorter SD et al: Cutaneous manifestations of toxoplasmosis. *Clin Infect Dis* **14**:1084, 1992

531. Gonzalez MM et al: AIDS associated with *Acanthamoeba* infection and other opportunistic organisms. *Arch Pathol Lab Med* **110**:749, 1986

532. Dominey A et al: Papulonodular demodicidosis associated with acquired immunodeficiency syndrome. *J Am Acad Dermatol* **20**:197, 1989

533. Toback AC et al: Severe chronic photosensitivity in association with acquired immunodeficiency syndrome. *J Am Acad Dermatol* **15**:2056, 1986

534. Herman LE, Kurban AK: Erythroderma as a manifestation of the AIDS-related complex. *J Am Acad Dermatol* **17**:507, 1987

535. May LP et al: Hypereosinophilic syndrome with unusual cutaneous manifestations in two men with HIV infection. *J Am Acad Dermatol* **23**:202, 1990

536. Harper ME et al: Concomitant infection with HTLV-1 and HTLV-III in a patient with T8 lymphoproliferative disease. *N Engl J Med* **315**:1073, 1986

537. Janier M et al: Pseudo-Sézary syndrome with CD8 phenotype in a patient with AIDS. *Ann Intern Med* **110**:738, 1989

538. Janniger CK et al: Erythroderma as the initial presentation of the acquired immunodeficiency syndrome. *Dermatologica* **183**:143, 1991

539. Blauvelt A et al: Pityriasis rubra pilaris and HIV infection. *J Am Acad Dermatol* **24**:703, 1991

540. Auffret N et al: Pityriasis rubra pilaris in a patient with human immunodeficiency virus. *J Am Acad Dermatol* **27**:260, 1992

541. Martin AG et al: Pityriasis rubra pilaris in the setting of HIV infection: Clinical behaviour and association with explosive cystic acne. *Br J Dermatol* **126**:617, 1991

542. Le Bozec P et al: Pityriasis rubra pilaris in a patient with acquired immunodeficiency syndrome. *Ann Dermatol Venereol* **118**:862, 1991

543. Menni S et al: Pityriasis rubra pilaris in a child seropositive for the human immunodeficiency virus. *J Am Acad Dermatol* **26**:1009, 1992

544. Valenzano L et al: Compromissione ungeale in corso di AIDS. *G Ital Dermatol Venereol* **123**:527, 1988

545. Dompmartin D et al: Onychomycosis and AIDS: Clinical and laboratory findings in 62 patients. *Int J Dermatol* **29**:337, 1990

546. Daniel CR et al: The spectrum of nail disease in patients with human immunodeficiency virus infection. *J Am Acad Dermatol* **27**:93, 1992

547. Chernosky ME, Finley VK: Yellow nail syndrome in patients with AIDS. *J Am Acad Dermatol* **13**:731, 1985

548. Sher RK: Acquired immunodeficiency syndrome and yellow nails. *J Am Acad Dermatol* **18**:758, 1988

549. Haas A, Dover JS: Yellow nail syndrome and acquired immunodeficiency disease. *J Am Acad Dermatol* **14**:845, 1986

550. Wissel PS et al: Porphyria cutanea tarda associated with the acquired immunodeficiency syndrome. *Am J Hematol* **25**:107, 1987

551. Reynaud P et al: Porphyria cutanea tarda as initial presentation of the acquired immunodeficiency syndrome in two patients. *J Infect Dis* **161**:1032, 1990

552. Lobato MN, Berger TG: Porphyria cutanea tarda associated with the acquired immunodeficiency syndrome. *Arch Dermatol* **124**:1009, 1988

553. Hogan D et al: Human immunodeficiency virus infection and porphyria cutanea tarda. *J Am Acad Dermatol* **20**:17, 1989

554. Lafeuillade A et al: Porphyria cutanea tarda associated with HIV infection. *AIDS* **4**:924, 1990

555. Blauvelt A et al: Porphyria cutanea tarda and human immunodeficiency virus infection. *Int J Dermatol* **31**:474, 1992

556. Boisseau AM et al: Porphyria cutanea tarda associated with human immunodeficiency virus infection. A study of four cases and review of the literature. *Dermatologica* **182**:155, 1991

557. Ghadially R et al: Granuloma annulare in patients with human immunodeficiency virus infection. *J Am Acad Dermatol* **20**:232, 1989

558. Huerter CJ et al: Perforating granuloma annulare in a patient with acquired immunodeficiency syndrome. *Arch Dermatol* **123**:1217, 1987

559. Bank DE et al: Reacting perforating collagenosis in a setting of double disaster: Acquired immunodeficiency syndrome and end-stage renal disease. *J Am Acad Dermatol* **21**:371, 1989

560. Jones SK, Haman RRM: Atypical granuloma annulare in patients with the acquired immunodeficiency syndrome. *J Am Acad Dermatol* **20**:299, 1989

561. Viraben R, Dupre R: Lichenoid granulomatous papular dermatosis associated with human immunodeficiency virus infection: An immunohistochemical study. *J Am Acad Dermatol* **18**:1140, 1988

562. Resnick SD et al: Acne conglobata and a generalized lichen spinulosis-like eruption in a man seropositive for human immunodeficiency virus. *J Am Acad Dermatol* **26**:1013, 1992

563. Ruiz-Rodriguez R et al: Anetoderma and human immunodeficiency virus infection. *Arch Dermatol* **128**:661, 1992

564. Ruiz-Rodriguez R et al: Papular mucinosis and human immunodeficiency virus infection. *Arch Dermatol* **128**:995, 1992

565. Cockerell CJ, Dolan ET: Widespread cutaneous and systemic calcification (calciphylaxis) in patients with the acquired immunodeficiency syndrome and renal disease. *J Am Acad Dermatol* **26**:559, 1992

566. Myskowski PL et al: Lymphoma and other HIV-associated malignancies. *J Am Acad Dermatol* **22**:1253, 1990

567. Lin-Greenberg A et al: Lymphomatoid granulomatosis presenting as ulcerodestructive gastrointestinal tract lesions in patients with human immunodeficiency virus infection. A new association. *Arch Intern Med* **150**:2581, 1990

568. Montilla P et al: Lymphomatoid granulomatosis and the acquired immunodeficiency syndrome. *Ann Intern Med* **106**:166, 1987

569. Kim HC et al: Immune thrombocytopenia in hemophiliacs infected with HIV and their response to splenectomy. *Arch Intern Med* **149**:1685, 1989

570. Plantanias LC et al: Thrombotic thrombocytopenic purpura as the first manifestation of HIV infection. *Am J Med* **87**:699, 1989

571. Velji AM: Leukocytoclastic vasculitis associated with positive HTLV III serologic findings. *JAMA* **256**:2196, 1986

572. Chren MM et al: Leukocytoclastic vasculitis in a patient infected with HIV. *J Am Acad Dermatol* **21**:1161, 1989

573. Calabrese LH et al: Systemic necrotizing vasculitis and the human immunodeficiency virus (HIV): An important etiologic relationship. *Arthritis Rheum* **31**(suppl 2):S35, 1988

574. Duvic M et al: Human immunodeficiency virus-associated vitiligo. Expression of autoimmunity with immunodeficiency. *J Am Acad Dermatol* **17**:656, 1987

575. Kaye BR: Rheumatologic manifestations of infection with human immunodeficiency virus (HIV). *Ann Intern Med* **111**:158, 1989

576. Solomon G et al: Arthritis, psoriasis and related syndromes associated with HIV infection (abstr). *Arthritis Rheum* **31**(suppl 2):S12, 1988

577. Winchester R et al: The co-occurrence of Reiter's syndrome and acquired immunodeficiency syndrome. *Ann Intern Med* **106**:19, 1987

578. Lin RY: Reiter's syndrome and human immunodeficiency virus infection. *Dermatologica* **176**:39, 1988

CHAPTER 216

Donald Y.M. Leung and Anne W. Lucky

Kawasaki Disease

Kawasaki disease (KD) is an acute vasculitis of unknown etiology that most frequently affects infants and children under 5 years of age. No objective or specific test exists for the diagnosis of this disease. The guidelines set by the Centers for Disease Control (CDC),[1] are outlined in Table 216-1. In atypical cases, patients with fever and fewer than four of the principal symptoms can be diagnosed as having KD when coronary artery disease is detected by two-dimensional echocardiography or coronary angiography. In the latter situation, every attempt should be made to exclude other diagnoses.

Historical Aspects

Kawasaki disease, originally named mucocutaneous lymph node syndrome, was first recognized and described in Japan in 1967 by Dr. Tomisaku Kawasaki.[2] He reported his experience with 50 children who had been seen during the preceding 6 years at the Tokyo Red Cross Medical Center. These children manifested a constellation of findings distinct from any previously described disease. After this description, numerous cases were reported throughout Japan. Dr. Kawasaki's first description in the English language of the disease appeared in 1974.[3] In 1976, the syndrome was first reported in the United States by Melish, Hicks, and Larson in a group of 12 children from Honolulu seen between 1971 and 1973.[4] Since then, KD has been recognized worldwide in children of every racial group.

Whether KD is truly a new disease or syndrome, or an illness that has simply become more prevalent, is still controversial. It has been reported that KD and infantile polyarteritis nodosa are pathologically indistinguishable.[5] Furthermore, an autopsy description of coronary artery aneurysms in a 7-year-old boy who died in 1871 at St. Bartholomew's Hospital in London bears striking similarity to descriptions of KD.[6]

TABLE 216-1
Diagnostic Criteria for Kawasaki Disease

Fever of 5 or more days without other explanation, and at least four of
the five following criteria:
  Bilateral nonexudative conjunctival injection
  One of the following changes in the oropharynx:
    Injected or fissured lips
    Injected pharynx
    ''Strawberry tongue''
  One of the following extremity changes:
    Erythema of the palms or soles
    Edema of the hands or feet during the acute phase
    Periungual desquamation
    Polymorphous exanthem
    Acute nonsuppurative cervical lymphadenopathy (>1.5 cm in
      diameter)

Epidemiology

Although KD occurs worldwide in children of all racial groups, it is
clearly most prevalent in Japan and in children of Japanese ancestry. According to the last nationwide survey of KD in Japan,
83,857 patients were reported to have had this illness by the end of
1986.[7] In Japan, nationwide epidemics occurred in 1979, 1982,
and again in late 1985 to early 1986. In 1982 alone, 15,519 cases
were reported and, in 1986, 12,847 cases were reported. The incidence of KD in Japan has increased from 1967 to the present.
During that period, 88.5 percent of cases involved children less
than 4 years of age. The ratio of males to females was 1.4:1. The
incidence rate was the highest for children 9 to 11 months of age.
The endemic annual incidence of KD is approximately 67 cases per
100,000 children younger than 5 years old in Japan

Both the endemic and the epidemic form of KD in Japan occur
most commonly in the late winter and spring, with another period
of slightly increased incidence during late fall. KD only rarely occurs in the same school, day care center, or household. In Japan,
the recurrence rate of KD has been reported to be 3.9 percent and
the proportion of sibling cases 1.4 percent.[7] Thus person-to-person
transmission of the disease appears to be unlikely.

In the United States, a passive surveillance system precludes
accurate estimation of the annual incidence of KD. Nevertheless,
epidemiologic findings in the United States and other countries are
strikingly similar to those in Japan.[8] Between July 1976 and December 1985, 2126 cases of KD in the United States were reported
to the CDC. An increase in the number of new cases reported to the
CDC from 1981 through 1985 suggests a rising incidence rate.[8] KD
has been reported in all 50 states and occurs sporadically or as
temporally limited community-wide epidemic outbreaks. Epidemics of KD have occurred primarily in late winter and spring at
approximately 3-year intervals. In Boston and in Rochester, New
York, outbreaks were associated with a rise in the incidence of KD
in children under 5 years of age, from 1.6 and 5.6 per 100,000 per
year, respectively, to 66 and 179 per 100,000 per year during the
epidemic period.[9] The prevalence of KD is highest among Asians,
intermediate in blacks, and lowest in Caucasians.[10] Regardless of
the racial group affected, however, the clinical picture is similar.

In the United States and Europe, the peak reported incidence
of KD occurs in children between 12 and 24 months of age, and
over 80 percent of cases occur in children younger than 5 years of
age. KD rarely occurs in adolescents or children under 6 months.
Whether KD occurs in adults at all remains controversial. Early
reports of adults with KD appear to have represented toxic shock

syndrome. Males develop KD at a rate that is approximately 1.6
times greater than females. In studies of outbreaks in the United
States, children with KD have generally belonged to families of
higher socioeconomic status.

Because of the striking racial differences in the incidence of
KD, possible genetic factors have been investigated. HLA-typing
studies have yielded conflicting data.[11,12] Recently, a ninefold increased prevalence of atopic dermatitis was reported among children who acquire KD.[13] This observation is intriguing because patients with atopic dermatitis have underlying immunoregulatory
abnormalities and because there is a very high incidence of atopic
dermatitis in Japan. In one survey of Japanese children, 31 percent
examined had atopic dermatitis[14] as opposed to a prevalence of 2 to
4 percent in American children.[15] This observation supports the
notion that host immunologic factors may play a role in the pathogenesis of KD.

Clinical Manifestations

General Features

The mucocutaneous manifestations of KD are varied and not all
children exhibit each feature. The major diagnostic criteria for KD
are listed in Table 216-1 and reviewed by Hick and Melish[16] and
Rowley et al.[17] KD is a triphasic illness beginning with an acute
phase that lasts 10 to 14 days, followed by a subacute phase of
approximately 25 days, and a convalescent phase that lasts nearly
70 days. The cardinal feature of the acute phase is a prolonged high
fever that frequently spikes to 40°C (104°F) and is associated with a
toxic appearance in virtually all patients. In the absence of anti-
inflammatory therapy, the duration of fever is usually 1 to 2 weeks.

Approximately 90 percent of children with KD develop an
exanthem in the first days of their acute febrile illness (Fig.
216-1).[18] The eruption favors the trunk and proximal extremities

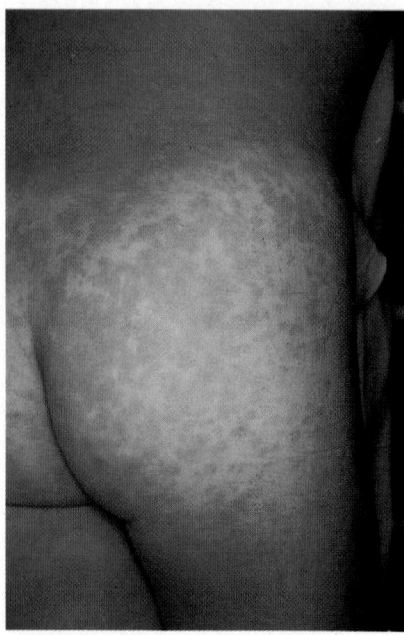

FIGURE 216-1 A generalized urticarial, morbilliform eruption
appeared early in the febrile course of this 5-year-old boy with
Kawasaki disease.

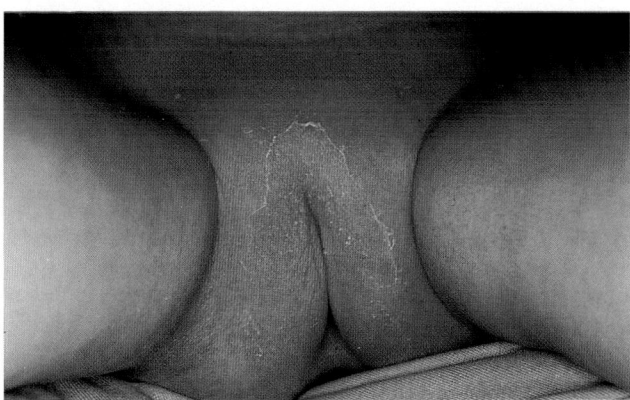

FIGURE 216-2 Generalized erythema and early desquamation in the perineal area of a 4-year-old girl with Kawasaki disease. This feature occurs early in the illness and involves 67 percent of affected children.

but can be generalized. It can be quite variable, having been described as macular, papular, morbilliform, urticarial, and even "target-like," resembling erythema multiforme. There has been very little published describing the histopathology of the exanthem. The initial rash is indistinguishable from an acute viral exanthem or adverse drug reaction. The rash of KD is rarely vesicular or bullous.

One of the earliest and most recently recognized signs of KD is a characteristic perineal eruption (Fig. 216-2).[19] In one study of 58 children, ages 2 months to 11 years, 67 percent had the perineal eruption. Onset is usually within the first 6 days of the illness; it presents as a diffuse macular or plaque-type blanching erythema involving part or all of the perineal skin. These involved areas can be warm and tender. Within 48 h, the erythematous areas begin to desquamate. This desquamation occurs earlier than that of the palms and soles.

In 90 percent of patients, a nonexudative conjunctival injection begins shortly after the onset of fever and generally involves the bulbar conjunctivae more severely than the palpebral conjunctivae. Conjunctival vessels become engorged and dilated. There is no purulent discharge, crusting, or matting of the eyelashes such as in bacterial conjunctivitis. Conjunctivitis is associated with anterior uveitis by slit-lamp examination in approximately 83 percent of patients examined within the first weeks of illness.[20]

Oral mucosal findings are very characteristic of KD and occur in almost all cases (Fig. 216-3). The lips become "cherry red," dry, and often cracked, producing small hemorrhagic fissures. In contrast to staphylococcal scalded-skin syndrome, there is no radial crusting of the perioral skin. There are no punctate ulcerations such as those seen in herpes gingivostomatitis or aphthae, and no diffuse erosions with confluent hemorrhagic crusts such as those seen in Stevens-Johnson syndrome. The tongue has been described as "strawberry" with hypertrophied papillae and hyperemia, but only about half the cases seem to have this feature.

Profound edema and erythema of the distal aspects of the hands and feet with fusiform swelling of the fingers are also noted in almost all cases (Fig. 216-4). Onset of edema and erythema is usually within a few days of the onset of illness. These hyperemic areas are subject to desquamation 10 to 18 days later. The desquamation characteristically begins at the tips of the fingers and toes and may develop either fine peeling or shredding of thick "casts" of palmar and plantar skin similar to that seen in scarlet fever.

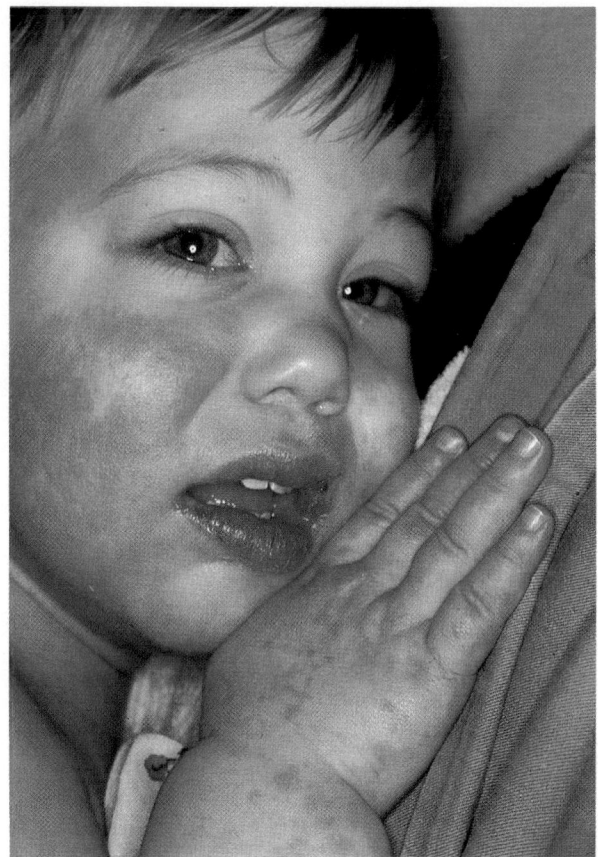

FIGURE 216-3 This boy with Kawasaki disease has "cherry red" lips with a few hemorrhagic fissures. His oral mucosa and conjunctivae are injected, and he has a generalized morbilliform eruption.

Generalized fine desquamation, especially in the areas of the skin that had previously been erythematous, is also common at this time (Fig. 216-5). Because of the severe systemic nature of the illness and the prolonged high fever, it is not surprising that some children develop telogen effluvium with significant but transient

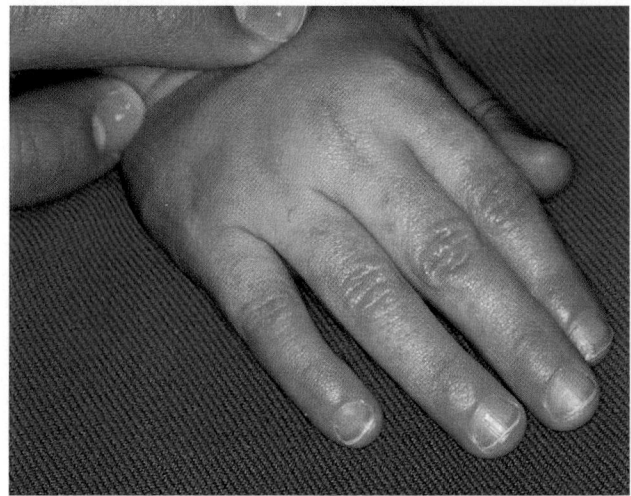

FIGURE 216-4 Erythema and edema of the distal fingertips are characteristic of the early phase of Kawasaki disease.

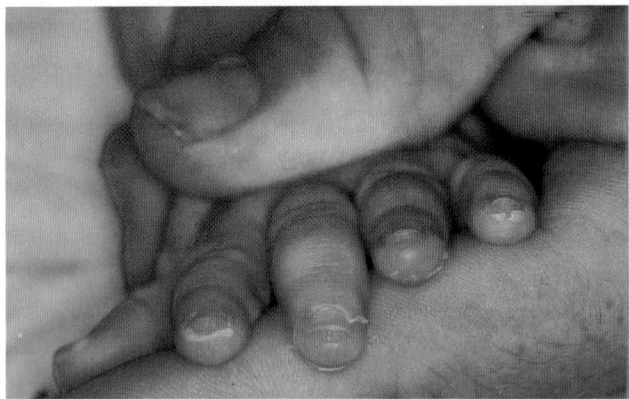

FIGURE 216-5 Desquamation starting at the tips of the fingers occurs 10 to 18 days after the onset of illness, as illustrated in this 3-month-old infant.

hair loss 6 to 12 weeks after the acute phase of the illness. Similarly, Beau's lines of the nails and/or shedding of the nails have been observed weeks to months later.

Lymphadenopathy is the least frequent finding and is seen in less than 75 percent of patients. The adenopathy generally consists of a single enlarged nonsuppurative cervical node measuring at least 1.5 cm. Arthralgia and arthritis occur in approximately one-third of patients. During the acute phase, the arthritis usually involves the small joints whereas involvement of the large weight-bearing joints usually occurs in the second and third weeks of the illness.[8,16] Urethritis associated with sterile pyuria is frequently present in acute KD (Table 216-2). Aseptic meningitis is usually associated with mild mononuclear cell pleocytosis of the cerebrospinal fluid and with normal glucose and protein. Hydrops of the gallbladder may be present with or without obstructive jaundice.[21] Diarrhea, vomiting, abdominal pain, cranial nerve palsies, otitis media, and infarction of organs whose vascular supplies are compromised by thrombosis may also be presenting symptoms. Sensorineural hearing loss has also been associated with KD.[22]

During the convalescent phase, there is generally a paucity of physical findings. Patients who suffer cardiovascular complications from this illness may have persistent cardiac abnormalities including chronic myocardial dysfunction, aortic or mitral regurgitation, and cardiac arrhythmias. Occasionally a patient may experience clinical exacerbation, with recurrence of fever and other acute clinical signs such as rash and conjunctival injection, after the exacerbation had appeared to resolve.[22,23] Such recurrences happen most

TABLE 216-2
Associated Clinical Features of Kawasaki Disease

Cardiovascular abnormalities:
  Myocarditis
  Arterial aneurysms
  Pericarditis
  Aortic or mitral regurgitation
  Ventricular arrhythmias
Arthralgia and arthritis
Urethritis with sterile pyuria
Aseptic meningitis
Hydrops of the gallbladder
Diarrhea, vomiting, or abdominal pain

often within a few weeks of the onset of illness and may be associated with an increased risk of coronary artery disease.

Cardiac Manifestations

Abnormal cardiac findings are a hallmark of KD.[24] Myocarditis is often observed during the first week after the onset of fever.[25] Pericardial effusion may develop toward the latter part of the acute phase and is secondary to myopericarditis. It is rare that these patients progress to cardiac tamponade, and the pericardial effusion generally resolves spontaneously. Congestive heart failure may be caused by myocarditis in the acute phase. During the subacute stage, congestive heart failure is usually caused by myocardial dysfunction secondary to ischemia or infarction.

Coronary artery ectasia or aneurysms occur in 15 to 25 percent of patients with KD.[26,27] Dilatation of the coronary arteries may be detected by echocardiography beginning 7 days after the onset of fever, usually peaking 3 or 4 weeks into the illness. A minority of patients, approximately 5 percent, may suffer from aortic regurgitation or mitral regurgitation due to valvulitis or transient papillary muscle dysfunction, or as a complication of myocardial infarction.

On cardiac examination, patients with acute KD often present with tachycardia and gallop rhythms that are excessive for the fever and anemia associated with the illness. In a minority of patients a pericardial friction rub, dysrhythmias, aortic and mitral regurgitation, the findings of congestive heart failure, and the appearance of peripheral arterial aneurysms appear during the latter part of the acute phase or during the subacute phase.

Laboratory Findings

During the acute phase of KD, leukocytosis develops with a left shift. A normocytic, normochromic anemia without evidence of hemolysis or reticulocytosis appears during the first week of illness and persists until the inflammatory process subsides.[28] Increased platelet turnover occurs, with marked hypercoagulability in the acute phase. Thrombocytosis peaks typically in the third to fourth week after the onset of fever.[29] Elevation of liver transaminases, usually two- to threefold, is common in the acute phase, usually with a cholestatic profile of elevated bilirubin and alkaline phosphatase. Sterile pyuria due to urethritis is observed in up to 75 percent of patients during the first week of illness. Early in the disease, acute-phase reactants such as C-reactive protein and serum α_1 antitrypsin increase with the onset of fever and persist for 6 to 10 weeks. Similarly, erythrocyte sedimentation rates are uniformly elevated in patients with acute KD. Elevation of the latter typically persists after resolution of fever, a feature that may help distinguish KD from common viral illness. Although patients with KD have a marked polyclonal B-cell activation, their sera do not contain the usual autoantibodies associated with collagen-vascular disease, i.e., no rheumatoid factor or antinuclear or anti-DNA antibodies are present. Circulating immune complexes can be detected during the second or third week of illness.[30] These immune complexes probably play no role in the pathogenesis of the vasculitis but may contribute to the arthritis that often occurs in KD 3 weeks after the onset of fever.

Electrocardiographic changes may be present in over half of patients with acute KD. These abnormalities include prolonged PR interval, left ventricular hypertrophy, abnormal Q waves, ventricular dysrhythmias, and nonspecific ST-T wave changes. Two-dimensional echocardiography has been used extensively for assessment of ventricular function, the anatomy of the proximal coronary arteries, and the presence of a pericardial effusion.[31] In general, it is preferable to obtain a baseline two-dimensional echocardiogram before the seventh day of illness (before the onset of coronary dilation) and a repeat echocardiogram 3 to 5 weeks after the onset of illness (when coronary artery abnormalities are likely to be detected). Coronary arteriography is generally reserved for the patient with persistent abnormalities on echocardiograms or any patient with symptoms of myocardial ischemia. It is especially useful for visualization of coronary artery stenoses or distal coronary artery lesions that are difficult to define by two-dimensional echocardiography.

Pathology

Extensive gross and microscopic studies have been carried out at autopsies of KD patients who died in different phases of their illness. The case-fatality ratio for KD is approximately 0.4 percent, with most deaths resulting from cardiovascular complications.[7] Fujiwara and Hamashima[32] have classified the pathology of this syndrome into four stages according to the duration of illness at death.

Stage 1 (0 to 9 days after onset) is characterized by acute vasculitis and perivasculitis of small blood vessels, including arterioles, venules, and capillaries. Microscopically, the acute vascular lesion in KD is associated with evidence of endothelial activation and endothelial cell (EC) damage.[33] These histologic changes include EC swelling, increased EC replication, the adhesion of leukocytes to the endothelial wall, and EC necrosis, with or without immunoglobulin deposition. The lesion is also associated with the infiltration of both neutrophils and mononuclear cells. The mononuclear cells consist of activated CD4+ T cells and monocyte/macrophages.

Recent studies by Terai and coworkers[34] have demonstrated the expression of major histocompatibility complex (MHC) class II antigens on the coronary arterial endothelium in a patient with KD but not in normal controls. Gamma interferon (IFN-γ) is a potent in vivo inducer of MHC class II antigens, and interleukin 1 (IL-1) as well as tumor necrosis factor (TNF-α) play an important role in the induction of leukocyte adhesion molecules.[35] Thus the induction of MHC class II antigens on EC as well as the observation of leukocyte adhesion to EC in the vascular lesion of KD suggest that cytokine-induced endothelial antigens may play an important role in the pathogenesis of this disease.

In the larger arteries, the initial inflammation involves the intima and the vasa vasorum without inflammation of the media.[32] Pericarditis, myocarditis, inflammation of the atrioventricular conduction system and endocarditis with valvulitis are also present.

Stage 2 (12 to 25 days after onset) is characterized by a thrombotic diathesis and a marked infiltration of inflammatory cells into the media of the coronary arteries and other medium-sized arteries, leading to formation of aneurysms. At this stage, it is presumed that aneurysms form as a result of the destruction of the blood vessel walls that follows release of proteolytic enzymes and inflammatory mediators into the media. In stage 3 (28 to 31 days), the acute inflammatory process regresses, and granulation in the coronary arteries is noted. In stage 4 (40 days to 4 years) scar formation and organization of thrombi occur. This process can result in severe stenosis of the coronary arteries and other medium-sized arteries.

The peak time of death is 3 to 4 weeks after onset of the acute illness. Death can occur as early as during the first week of illness and as late as 14 years after the acute illness. During stage 1 of KD, patients usually die of acute myocarditis or cardiac arrhythmia due to inflammation of the atrioventricular conduction system. In stage 2 of the disease, death can result from rupture of the coronary arteries, myocarditis that includes lesions of the atrioventricular conduction system, or myocardial insufficiency due to thrombosis of the coronary arteries. Sudden death late in the illness (stage 3), or years after recovery from acute KD (stage 4), may occur as the result of myocardial infarction in children with residual coronary artery aneurysms and stenoses.

It is worth emphasizing that although coronary arteries are invariably involved in this disease, almost any other medium-sized or large blood vessels may be involved when examined at autopsy. Aneurysm formation has been reported in the femoral, iliac, renal, axillary, and brachial arteries.[32,36] KD is a systemic vasculitis that can affect most small and medium-sized blood vessels. Cutaneous vasculitis, however, is not a prominent feature of KD.

Etiology and Pathogenesis

Etiology

The etiology of KD is currently unknown. Extensive epidemiologic studies searching for environmental toxins and laboratory culturing of body fluids for known microbial organisms have failed to uncover an etiologic agent for KD.[37] Nevertheless, it is widely believed that KD is caused by an infectious agent because of the acute self-limited nature of this disease, seasonal incidence, geographical clustering of outbreaks, the clinical symptoms of fever and exanthem mimicking other infectious diseases, and the unique susceptibility of young children suggesting that immunity to the KD agent develops early in life. Reports that *Propionibacterium acnes*,[38] *Rickettsiea*,[39] Epstein-Barr virus,[40] mercury,[41] and retroviruses[42,43] may be possible causative agents of KD have not been confirmed.

Several epidemiologic risk factors have been reported. First, in two of three outbreaks of KD in which case-control data were collected, there was a significantly higher incidence of antecedent respiratory illness in patients with KD than in controls.[44,45] This association between KD and an antecedent respiratory illness has been observed in some subsequent uncontrolled studies but not in several others.[46] Thus it is not clear whether antecedent illness is a true risk factor for KD or simply a marker for another associated event. Second, studies carried out in Denver and Los Angeles have observed a statistically significant association between exposure to freshly shampooed carpets and the subsequent onset of KD.[47] This association has not been confirmed in studies done in other geographic locations.[48] Third, several recent CDC outbreak investigations indicate that parents of KD patients reported living significantly closer to bodies of water, such as creeks or drainage ditches, than did parents of case controls.[46,49] These investigators suggested that living near water may be a marker for an arthropod vector or an animal reservoir.

The infrequent person-to-person transmission, the differences in racial incidence, and the findings of vasculitis and arthritis suggest that KD may be caused by an infectious agent that leads to an immune-mediated syndrome in certain genetically or immunologically susceptible individuals. The observation that KD is rarely seen in patients above the age of 8 years or below the age of 6 months suggests that the general population incurs asymptomatic infection and develops protective antibodies. Susceptibility to KD may thus be linked to an absence of antibody to the putative KD agent.

Immunopathogenesis

Although multiple factors are likely to be involved in the pathogenesis of KD, several observations suggest that immune activation is involved in the pathogenesis of this disease. First, the acute phase of KD is characterized by an immunoregulatory imbalance that consists of increased numbers of activated helper T cells and monocytes, a deficiency of CD8+ suppressor/cytotoxic T cells, and a marked polyclonal B-cell activation.[50–52] Recent studies by Lang et al. demonstrating elevated serum-soluble IL-2 receptor levels in acute KD provides additional evidence that this illness is associated with significant lymphocyte activation.[53] Second, the immune activation associated with acute KD is accompanied by elevated serum levels of IL-1,[54] TNF-α,[51,55] IFN-γ,[56] and IL-6.[57] Furthermore, peripheral blood mononuclear cells from KD patients during the acute phase but not in the convalescent phase of their illness spontaneously produce high levels of IL-1[58] and TNF-α.[59] Third, the histologic lesion, as discussed in the previous section, suggests a role for immune-mediated vascular injury.[32,33] Fourth, the acute phase of KD is associated with the appearance of circulating antibodies that are cytotoxic against vascular EC prestimulated with IL-1, TNF-α,[60] or IFN-γ,[61] but not against unstimulated EC. Finally, successful treatment of patients with intravenous gamma globulin (IVGG) plus aspirin reduced the immune activation associated with this disease.[62] In contrast, KD patients treated with aspirin alone have prolonged T-cell and B-cell activation.

Many of the clinical features of KD could be related to the marked immune activation associated with this disease. The high fever and increased levels of circulating acute phase reactants may be a function of increased IL-1, TNF-α, and/or IL-6 production. The lymphadenopathy may be related to the marked activation of the T- and B-cell system. The increased production of IL-1, TNF-α, and IFN-γ in this disease can predispose patients to vascular injury in several ways. IL-1 and TNF-α elicit an overlapping set of proinflammatory and prothrombotic responses in EC.[35] Both cytokines have been reported to induce expression of endothelial-leukocyte adhesion molecule 1 (ELAM-1), which is involved in the adhesion of polymorphonuclear leukocytes (PMN) to the EC surface, and increase expression of intercellular adhesion molecule 1 (ICAM-1), which is involved in the adhesion of PMN, monocytes, and lymphocytes to EC by interaction with leukocyte cell surface molecules of the CD11/CD18 complex. IL-1 and TNF-α also enhance the recruitment of leukocytes by inducing the production of chemotactic factors (IL-8, MCP-1, colony-stimulating factors) by monocytes and EC.[63] Exposure to IL-1 and/or TNF-α profoundly alters the antithrombotic properties of EC by inducing tissue-type procoagulant activity, increasing tissue-type plasminogen activator, and decreasing the thrombomodulin-protein C anticoagulation pathways. Unlike IL-1 and TNF-α, IFN-γ induces EC to act as antigen-presenting cells without inducing proinflammatory or prothrombotic activities. IFN-γ induces MHC class II antigens, increases IL-1 and IL-6 production by EC, and increases ICAM-1 expression on EC. These effects play a critical role in integrating EC into immunologic reactions.

The observation that acute KD is associated with the production of circulating antibodies directed toward cytokine-inducible endothelial antigens suggests that these patients generate an immune response directed to their abnormally stimulated vascular endothelium. This aberrant immune response, which includes the functional alteration of endothelial thrombotic properties and the induction of leukocyte adhesion molecules and chemotactic factors, contributes to the influx of inflammatory cells into the media, with consequent weakening of the vessel wall and predisposition to arterial aneurysm formation. Thus it has been hypothesized that there are two requirements for EC injury in KD: first, that increased cytokine production induces new EC antigens, and second, possibly related to the polyclonal B-cell activation in this disease, that there is the generation of antibodies directed to these induced neoantigens. This hypothesis is supported by the observation that clinical improvement of patients with acute KD is associated with a reduction in cytokine secretion, thus reversing the expression of new endothelial antigens which act as targets for immune-mediated injury.

Differential Diagnosis

KD has clinical features compatible with infection, hypersensitivity reactions, or exposure to environmental toxins. The differential diagnosis of KD should include staphylococcal and streptococcal scarlet fever, staphylococcla "scalded-skin" syndrome, toxic shock syndrome, viral exanthem, Rocky Mountain spotted fever, leptospirosis, infantile polyarteritis nodosa, mercury toxicity (acrodynia), Stevens-Johnson syndrome, erythema multiform, adverse drug reaction, and juvenile rheumatoid arthritis. KD has a variety of mucocutaneous manifestations, some of which are characteristic but many of which are shared with these other infectious and reactive disorders. The correct diagnosis of Kawasaki disease hinges on recognizing the cumulative combination of mucocutaneous, systemic, and laboratory findings.

Treatment

Specific therapy for KD awaits identification of its etiologic agent. Current management focuses on the reduction of symptoms and complications resulting from the inflammatory process associated with this illness. Therapy for the mucocutaneous manifestations of the disease is entirely symptomatic and includes emollients for desquamating skin and antihistamines for pruritus. Aspirin (ASA) remains the mainstay of therapy because of its anti-inflammatory and antithrombotic actions. ASA is administered in doses of 80 to 100 mg/kg of body weight per day (or higher in certain instances) to achieve a serum salicylate level of 20 to 25 mg/dL during the acute phase of the illness. At therapeutic doses ASA has been shown to reduce fever, toxicity, and joint symptoms within 48 h.[64] After defervescence, the ASA dose is reduced to 3 to 5 mg/kg of body weight per day to continue inhibiting platelet activity. Some investigators add dipyridamole, 1 mg/kg of body weight per day, to further inhibit platelet aggregation.[65] Platelet inhibitory therapy is continued until the platelet count, sedimentation rate, and echocardiogram are normal, and indefinitely if coronary artery aneurysms persist. Digitalis and diuretics are used as needed in patients with congestive heart failure.

At present, systemic corticosteroids are contraindicated in the treatment of KD. Several small studies in Japan have reported that patients treated with corticosteroids alone or in combination with ASA have a higher frequency of coronary aneurysms and of subsequent myocardial infarction and death.[66] Other nonsteroidal anti-inflammatory agents have not been sufficiently studied.

To date, no definitive prospective study has proved that high-dose ASA therapy prevents coronary artery abnormalities. Recently, several randomized multicenter studies in Japan and the United States have demonstrated that high-dose IVGG is safe and effective in reducing the prevalence of coronary artery abnormalities when administered early in the course of KD.[67–70]

In the only prospective, randomized, multicenter trial performed in the United States, investigators compared the efficacy of IVGG plus ASA with that of ASA alone in the treatment of acute KD.[67] Patients randomly assigned to the gamma globulin group received IVGG, 400 mg/kg of body weight per day for 4 consecutive days. Both treatment groups received ASA, 100 mg/kg per day, through the fourteenth day of illness, then 3 to 5 mg/kg per day. Two weeks after enrollment, 18 of 78 children (23 percent) treated with ASA alone had coronary artery abnormalities compared with 6 of 75 children (8 percent) treated with IVGG plus ASA ($p = .01$). Seven weeks after enrollment, abnormalities were present in 18 percent of the ASA group and in 4 percent of the IVGG group ($p = .005$). No children had serious adverse effects from receiving IVGG. In a single-center study, Rowley and co-workers [70] demonstrated that IVGG not only reduced the overall prevalence of coronary artery abnormalities, but also prevented the formation of giant aneurysms, the most serious form of coronary abnormality caused by this disease. Finally, Newburger and co-workers[71] also found that abnormalities of left ventricular systolic function and contractility improve more rapidly in children treated in the acute phase with high-dose IVGG together with ASA than in those treated with ASA alone.

The American Academy of Pediatrics recommends that all patients with acute KD should receive treatment with IVGG.[72] The optimal dose and duration of IVGG therapy is still under investigation. Indeed, recent studies suggest that the administration of IVGG at 2 g/kg as a single dose is just as effective as 400 mg/kg of body weight for 4 consecutive days.[73]

The mechanism(s) by which high-dose IVGG works to reduce the vasculitis associated with acute KD has yet to be established.[74] IVGG, however, is known to work rapidly in reducing laboratory parameters of the acute-phase response associated with KD,[67] and this finding suggests a generalized anti-inflammatory effect. In this regard, it has been reported that before therapy, peripheral blood mononuclear cells from patients with acute KD spontaneously secrete high levels of IL-1,[58] an endogenous pyrogen, and tissue vascular endothelial cells express IL-1-inducible endothelial activation antigen. IL-1 secretion remained high in IVGG-treated patients in whom coronary artery abnormalities developed. However, IL-1 secretion levels fell to normal in patients who responded to IVGG therapy and had no coronary artery abnormalities. Furthermore, following IVGG therapy there was no EC activation in patients who clinically responded to IVGG. In contrast, patients with persistent fever had evidence of persistent endothelial activation.

These data support the notion that IVGG may work in KD by reducing cytokine-inducible endothelial activation. These observations may be clinically important because duration of fever is a strong risk factor for the development of coronary artery aneurysms.[75] Furthermore, clinical trials demonstrating that IVGG decreases the prevalence of coronary artery aneurysms in KD also found that the duration of fever is significantly shortened in the IVGG-treated group.[67]

For KD patients with ischemic symptoms secondary to coronary artery disease, the options include intravenous streptokinase or urokinase when a thrombus is present,[76] balloon angioplasty, and/or coronary artery bypass grafting. Long-term patency of saphenous vein grafts has been a problem, but use of internal mammary artery grafts yielded improved results.[77]

Course and Prognosis

The major long-term morbidity in KD is related to cardiovascular complications from this disease. Most children (50 to 67 percent) with arterial aneurysms show angiographic regression within 6 months to 2 years after the onset of the disease.[78] The likelihood of resolution of the aneurysms appears to be determined by the initial size of the aneurysm; smaller aneurysms have a greater likelihood of regression.[79] Patients with giant aneurysms, i.e., those with a maximum diameter greater than 8 mm, have the worst prognosis. Nakano and colleagues[80] reported that 71 percent of patients with giant aneurysms progressed to stenosis or obstruction over an 11-month follow-up period. Tatara and Kusakawa[81] reported that 30 percent of giant aneurysms developed obstruction at a mean follow-up of 32 months. Nearly all late deaths from KD occur in this subgroup of patients.[81]

Long-term studies are needed to determine whether the intimal damage suffered during acute KD predisposes patients to late cardiovascular complications. Indeed, pathologic examination of regressed arterial aneurysms has revealed fibrous intimal thickening despite normal artery diameters.[82] The histologic abnormalities in arteries with regression of aneurysm have raised concerns that such segments may be predisposed to the premature development of other forms of cardiovascular disease such as atherosclerosis. Furthermore, studies of vascular distensibility in regressed aneurysms have demonstrated reduced vascular reactivity during pharmacologic vasodilation with intravenous nitroglycerin or dipyridamole.[83]

It is worth noting that children without known cardiac sequelae during the first month of KD appear to return to their previous state of health without signs or symptoms of cardiac impairment. It is generally recommended, however, that these children be followed every 3 to 5 years to rule out the development of myocardial dysfunction, late-onset valvular regurgitation, or premature coronary artery disease.

References

1. Rauch A, Hurwitz E: Centers for Disease Control case definition for Kawasaki syndrome. *Pediatr Infect Dis* **4**:702, 1985
2. Kawasaki T: Acute febrile mucocutaneous syndrome with lymphoid involvement with specific desquamation of the fingers and toes in children: Clinical observations of 50 cases. *Jpn J Allergol* **16**:178, 1967
3. Kawasaki T et al: A new infantile febrile mucocutaneous lymph node syndrome (MLNS) prevailing in Japan. *Pediatrics* **54**:271, 1974
4. Melish ME et al: Mucocutaneous lymph node syndrome in the United States. *Am J Dis Child* **130**:599, 1976
5. Landing BH, Larson EJ: Pathological features of Kawasaki disease (mucocutaneous lymph node syndrome). *Am J Cardiovascular Pathol* **1**:215, 1987
6. Gree SJ: Cases of morbid anatomy: Aneurysms of coronary arteries in a boy. *St Bartholomew's Hosp Rep* **7**:1871

7. Yanagawa H et al: A nationwide incidence survey of Kawasaki disease in 1985-1986 in Japan. *Pediatrics* **80**:58, 1987

8. Rauch AM: Kawasaki syndrome: Critical review of U.S. epidemiology. *Prog Clin Biol Res* **250**:33, 1987

9. Bell DM et al: Kawasaki syndrome: Description of two outbreaks in the United States. *N Engl J Med* **304**:1568, 1981

10. Shulman ST et al: Risk of coronary abnormalities due to Kawasaki disease in urban area with small Asian population. *Am J Dis Child* **141**:420, 1987

11. Kato S et al: HLA antigens in Kawasaki disease. *Pediatrics* **61**:252, 1978

12. Matsuda I et al: HLA antigens in mucocutaneous lymph node syndrome. *Am J Dis Child* **131**:1417, 1977

13. Brosius K et al: Association of Kawasaki syndrome with atopic dermatitis. *J Ped Infect Dis* **7**:863, 1988

14. Ogawa F et al: Investigation of skin diseases: An examination made together with the mass examination of three year old children in Morika City. *Pediatr Dermatol* **1**:59, 1982

15. Leung DYM et al: Atopic dermatitis, in *Dermatology in General Medicine*, 3rd ed, edited by TB Fitzpatrick et al. New York, McGraw-Hill, 1987, p 1385

16. Hicks RV, Melish ME: Kawasaki syndrome. *Pediatr Clin North Am* **33**:1151, 1986

17. Rowley AH et al: Kawasaki syndrome. *Rev Infect Dis* **10**:1, 1988

18. Bligard CA: Kawasaki disease and its diagnosis. *Pediatr Dermatol* **4**:75, 1987

19. Friter BS, Lucky AW: The perineal eruption of Kawasaki syndrome. *Arch Dermatol* **124**:1805, 1988

20. Burns JC et al: Anterior uveitis associated with Kawasaki syndrome. *Pediatr Infect Dis* **4**:258, 1985

21. Suddleson EA et al: Hydrops of the gallbladder associated with Kawasaki syndrome. *J Pediatr Surg* **22**:956, 1987

22. Sundel RP et al: Sensorineural hearing loss associated with Kawasaki disease. *J Pediatr* **117**:371, 1990

23. Vargo TA et al: Recurrent Kawasaki disease. *Pediatr Cardiol* **6**:199, 1986

24. Kato H et al: Myocardial infarction in Kawasaki disease: Clinical analyses in 195 cases. *J Pediatr* **108**:923, 1986

25. Yutani C et al: Histopathological study on right endomyocardial biopsy of Kawasaki disease. *Br Heart J* **43**:589, 1980

26. Kato H et al: Fate of coronary aneurysms in Kawasaki disease: Serial coronary angiography and long-term follow-up study. *Am J Cardiol* **49**:1758, 1982

27. Suzuki A et al: Coronary arterial lesions of Kawasaki disease: Cardiac catheterization findings of 1100 cases. *Pediatr Cardiol* **7**:3, 1986

28. Melish ME: Kawasaki syndrome: A 1986 perspective. *Rheum Dis Clin North Am* **13**:7, 1987

29. Burns JC et al: Coagulopathy and platelet activation in Kawasaki syndrome: Identification of patients at high risk for development of coronary artery aneurysms. *J Pediatr* **105**:206, 1984

30. Mason WH et al: Circulating immune complexes in Kawasaki syndrome. *Pediatr Infect Dis J* **4**:48, 1985

31. Capannari TE et al: Sensitivity, specificity and predictive value of two-dimensional echocardiography in detecting coronary artery aneurysms in patients with Kawasaki disease. *J Am Coll Cardiol* **7**:355, 1986

32. Fujiwara H, Hamashima Y: Pathology of the heart in Kawasaki's disease. *Pediatrics* **61**:100, 1978

33. Hirose S, Hamashima Y: Morphological observations on the vasculitis in the mucocutaneous lymph node syndrome. *Eur J Pediatr* **129**:17, 1978

34. Terai M et al: Class II major histocompatibility antigen expression on coronary arterial endothelium in a patient with Kawasaki disease. *Hum Pathol* **21**:231, 1990

35. Cotran RS, Pober JS: Endothelial activation: Its role in inflammatory and immune reactions, in *Endothelial Cell Biology*, edited by N Simionescu, M Simionescu. New York, Plenum, p 335

36. Fukushige J et al: Spectrum of cardiovascular lesions in mucocutaneous lymph node syndrome: Analysis of eight cases. *Am J Cardiol* **45**:98, 1980

37. Rauch AM: Kawasaki syndrome: Review of new epidemiologic and laboratoy developments. *Pediatr Infect Dis J* **6**:1016, 1987

38. Kato H et al: Variant strain of Propionibacterium acnes. A clue to the aetiology of Kawasaki disease. *Lancet* **2**:1383, 1983

39. Hamashima Y et al: Rickettsia-like bodies in infantile acute febrile mucocutaneous lymph-node syndrome. *Lancet* **2**:42, 1973

40. Kikuta H et al: Kawasaki disease and an unusual primary infection with Epstein-Barr virus. *Pediatrics* **73**:413, 1984

41. Adler R et al: Metallic mercury vapor poisoning simulating mucocutaneous lymph node syndrome. *J Pediatr* **101**:967, 1982

42. Shulman S, Rowley A: Does Kawasaki disease have a retroviral etiology? *Lancet* **2**:545, 1986

43. Burns JC et al: Polymerase activity in lymphocyte culture supernatants from patients with Kawasaki disease. *Nature* **323**:814, 1986

44. Dean A et al: An epidemic of Kawasaki syndrome in Hawaii. *J Pediatr* **100**:552, 1982

45. Bell D et al: Kawasaki syndrome: Description of two outbreaks in the United States. *N Engl J Med* **304**:1568, 1981

46. Rauch AM: Kawasaki syndrome: Issues in etiology and treatment. *Adv Pediatr Infect Dis* **4**:163, 1989

47. Patriarca P et al: Kawasaki syndrome: Association with the application of rug shampoo. *Lancet* **2**:578, 1982

48. Rogers M et al: Kawasaki syndrome: Is exposure to rug shampoo important? *Am J Dis Child* **139**:777, 1985

49. Rauch MA et al: Outbreak of Kawasaki syndrome, Denver, CO. Proceedings of the Twenty-fifth Interscience Conference on Antimicrobial Agents and Chemotherapy. Minneapolis, 1985, p 162

50. Leung DYM et al: Immunoregulatory abnormalities in mucocutaneous lymph node syndrome. *Clin Immunol Immunopathol* **23**:100, 1982

51. Furukawa S et al: Peripheral blood monocyte/macrophage and serum tumor necrosis factor in Kawasaki disease. *Clin Immunol Immunopathol* **48**:247, 1988

52. Leung DYM et al: Immunoregulatory T cell abnormalities in mucocutaneous lymph node syndrome. *J Immunol* **130**:2002, 1983

53. Lang BA et al: Serum-soluble interleukin-2 receptor levels in Kawasaki disease. *J Pediatr* **116**:592, 1990

54. Maury CPJ et al: Circulating interleukin-1 in patients with Kawasaki disease. *N Engl J Med* **319**:1670, 1988

55. Maury CPJ et al: Elevated circulating tumor necrosis factor-alpha in patients with Kawasaki disease. *J Lab Clin Med* **113**:651, 1989

56. Rowley AH et al: Serum interferon concentrations and retroviral serology in Kawasaki syndrome. *Pediatr Infect Dis J* **7**:663, 1988

57. Ueno Y et al: The acute phase nature of interleukin 6: Studied in Kawasaki disease and other febrile illness. *Clin Exp Immunol* **76**:337, 1989

58. Leung DYM et al: Endothelial cell activation and increased interleukin 1 secretion in the pathogenesis of acute Kawasaki disease. *Lancet* **2**:1298, 1989

59. Lang BA et al: Spontaneous tumor necrosis factor production in Kawasaki disease. *J Pediatr* **115**:939, 1989

60. Leung DYM et al: Two monokines, interleukin 1 and tumor necrosis factor, render cultured vascular endothelial cells susceptible to lysis by antibodies circulating during Kawasaki syndrome. *J Exp Med* **164**:1958, 1986

61. Leung DYM et al: IgM antibodies present in the acute phase of Kawasaki syndrome lyse cultured vascular endothelial cells stimulated by gamma interferon. *J Clin Invest* **77**:1428, 1986

62. Leung DYM et al: Reversal of immunoregulatory abnormalities in Kawasaki syndrome by intravenous gammaglobulin. *J Clin Invest* **79**:468, 1987

63. Mantovani A, Dejana E: Cytokines as communication signals between leukocytes and endothelial cells. *Immunol Today* **10**:370, 1989

64. Koren G et al: Probable efficacy of high-dose salicylates in reducing coronary involvement in Kawasaki disease. *JAMA* **254**:767, 1985

65. Fitzgerald GA: Dipyridamole. *N Engl J Med* **316**:1247, 1987

66. Kato H et al: Kawasaki disease: Effect of treatment on coronary artery involvement. *Pediatrics* **63**:175, 1979

67. Newburger JW et al: Treatment of Kawasaki syndrome with intravenous gammaglobulin. *N Engl J Med* **315**:341, 1986

68. Nagashima M et al: High-dose gammaglobulin therapy for Kawasaki disease. *J Pediatr* **110**:710, 1987

69. Furusho K et al: High-dose intravenous gammaglobulin for Kawasaki disease. *Lancet* **2**:1055, 1984

70. Rowley AH et al: Prevention of giant coronary artery aneurysms in Kawasaki disease by intravenous gammaglobulin therapy. *J Pediatr* **113**:290, 1988

71. Newburger J et al: Left ventricular contractility and function in Kawasaki syndrome. Effect of intravenous gammaglobulin. *Circulation* **79**:1237, 1989

72. American Academy of Pediatrics: Intravenous γ-globulin use in children with Kawasaki disease. *Pediatrics* **82**:122, 1988

73. Newburger JW and the U.S. Multicenter Kawasaki Study Group: Preliminary results of multicenter trial on IVGG treatment of Kawasaki disease with single infusion vs four-infusion regimen. *Pediatr Res* **27**:22A, 1990

74. Leung DYM: Immunomodulation by IVGG in Kawasaki disease. *J Allergy Clin Immunol* **84**(Part 2):588, 1989

75. Koren G et al: Kawasaki disease: Review of risk factors for coronary aneurysms. *J Pediatr* **108**:388, 1986

76. Terai M et al: Coronary arterial thrombi in Kawasaki disease. *J Pediatr* **106**:76, 1985

77. Kitamura S et al: Severe Kawasaki heart disease treated with an internal mammary artery graft in pediatric patients. A first successful report. *J Thorac Cardiovasc Surg* **89**:860, 1985

78. Takahashi M et al: Regression of coronary aneurysms in patients with Kawasaki syndrome. *Circulation* **75**:387, 1987

79. Fujiwara T et al: Size of coronary aneurysm as a determinant factor of the prognosis in Kawasaki disease: Clinicopathologic study of coronary aneurysms. *Prog Clin Biol Res* **250**:519, 1987

80. Nakano H et al: Repeated quantitative angiograms in coronary arterial aneurysm in Kawasaki disease. *Am J Cardiol* **56**:846, 1985

81. Tatara K, Kusakawa S: Long-term prognosis of giant coronary aneurysm in Kawasaki disease: An angiographic study. *J Pediatr* **111**:705, 1987

82. Tanaka N et al: Pathological study of sequelae of Kawasaki disease (MCLS). With special reference to the heart and coronary arterial lesions. *Acta Pathol Jpn* **36**:1513, 1986

83. Matsumura K et al: Coronary angiography of Kawasaki disease with the coronary vasodilator dipyridamole: Assessment of distensibility of affected coronary arterial wall. *Angiology* **39**:141, 1988

SECTION 35

Sexually Transmitted Diseases

CHAPTER 217

Alfred R. Eichmann

Definition and Classification

The term *venereal disease* lacks a precise medical definition because these diseases can also be acquired without sexual contact and are not limited to the genital region. It originally comprised the classical infections gonorrhea, syphilis, and chancroid. Most of the nations engaged in World War I attempted to control these diseases by legislation and the statutory regulations thus established led to a discrimination against patients with venereal diseases. In the second half of the twentieth century the term *sexually transmitted disease* (STD) has become generally accepted. The word *transmitted* implies that sexual contact is the sole mode of transmission. The more correct designation *transmissible* has not yet received general acceptance. According to the International Union against Venereal Diseases and Treponematoses (IUVDT) and the World Health Organization (WHO), three groups of diseases belong to the spectrum comprising STDs,[1] and these are listed in Table 217-1.

The STDs have the following characteristics in common: they are infectious, they are transmitted predominantly by sexual contact, their primary manifestation occurs mainly in the anogenital region, and they do not confer lasting immunity.

Incidence of Bacterial STDs

The most important bacterial STDs include: gonorrhea, syphilis, chlamydial infections, and, in most developing countries, chancroid.

Gonorrhea

The incidence curves for gonorrhea in the western world have shown a steady decline since World War I both with respect to incidence and sex ratio. Sweden has an excellent and smoothly running reporting system which is a source of reliable data. Thirty years ago the male/female ratio was 4:1, now it is close 1:1.[2] Selective culture media and improved contact-tracing may have contributed to this development. In the United States morbidity has steadily declined since the end of World War II, but since 1967 the incidence has increased by about 15 percent. The maximum was reached in 1975, with 473 cases per 100,000 inhabitants.[3] In con-

Introduction

trast to the declining incidence, the proportion of penicillinase-producing *Neisseria gonorrhoeae* strains has risen in the US in recent years.[4] This development has led to more treatment failures and to complications in the course taken by the disease.

Syphilis

Syphilis is regarded as a typical example of an STD which can be controlled by public health measures. Its incidence in the western world in recent decades shows a curve similar to that of gonorrhea. In the US the incidence of primary and secondary syphilis reached a peak of 76 cases per 100,000 during the World War II followed by

TABLE 217-1
Classification of Sexually Transmitted Diseases by Infectious Agents

I. **Bacterial Agents**
   Neisseria gonorrhoeae
   Chlamydia trachomatis
   Treponema pallidum
   Haemophilus ducreyi
   Mycoplasma hominis
   Ureaplasma urealyticum
   Calymmatobacterium granulomatis
   Shigella spp.
   Campylobacter spp.
   Group B streptococcus
   Bacterial vaginosis-associated organisms
II. **Viral Agents**
   Human (alpha) herpesvirus 1 or 2 (herpes simplex virus)
   Human (beta) herpesvirus 5 (formerly cytomegalovirus)
   Hepatitis virus B
   Human papilloma viruses
   Molluscum contagiosum virus
   HIV (human immunodeficiency virus)
III. **Protozoal Agents**
   Entamoeba histolytica
   Giardia lamblia
   Trichomonas vaginalis
IV. **Fungal Agents**
   Candida albicans
V. **Ectoparasites**
   Phthirus pubis
   Sarcoptes scabiei

a steady decline until 1958 (4 per 100,000). Subsequent peaks were registered in 1965 (12 per 100,000) and 1982 (22 per 100,000),[5] which were followed by a fall to 16.2 per 100,000 in 1987, very probably as a consequence of the anti-AIDS campaign. 1987 once again witnessed a rise in the incidence figures, particularly among blacks and Hispanic heterosexuals in urban centers.[6]

Chancroid

Chancroid is an STD which occurs predominantly in subtropical and tropical zones. Sporadic outbreaks are observed in countries with a temperate climate. These can usually be traced to highly sexually active individuals who enter a nonendemic area.

In the US between 1000 and 2000 cases have been reported annually in recent years, and in 1985 this threshold was exceeded for the first time. In the context of tourism medicine, it is important to know that chancroid is much more common than syphilis in many tropical countries.[7]

Chlamydia trachomatis

Chlamydia trachomatis (Ct) infections have become the commonest STD in the second half of the 1980s.[8,9] Why should chlamydial infections become more frequent while the incidence of gonorrhea and syphilis declines? The diagnostic methods for the detection of Ct are more complicated and intricate than those used for gonorrhea and syphilis and in many places these methods are only now becoming available. Furthermore, treatment of Ct is a long-term therapy and, because of lack of compliance, may show higher failure rates than the single dose therapies used in gonorrhea and syphilis.

Incidence of Viral Sexually Transmitted Diseases

The principal viral STDs are genital herpes and human papilloma viruses.

Genital Herpes Simplex

Since the mid-1960s an 8.8-fold increase in newly diagnosed herpes infection has been observed in the US, i.e., a rise from 18,000 cases in 1966 to 157,000 cases in 1984.[10] Most affected was the 20- to 29-year-old age group. Seroepidemiological studies have shown that less than 25 percent of seropositive individuals are clinically symptomatic.[11] This large reservoir of asymptomatic patients with herpes genitalis constitutes an essential epidemiologic problem.

Genital Human Papilloma Virus (HPV)

Once the association between HPV-infections (in particular HPV 16 and 18) and precancerous and invasive lesions of the genital mucosa became known, HPV infections attracted increased attention.[12] The epidemiology of the HPV viruses is similar to that of herpes genitalis, in that subclinical infections are more common than clinically manifest disease.[12] Kiviat estimates that of the 122

million people between the ages of 15 and 49 in the US, 1 percent have visible genital warts, 2 percent subclinical only colposcopically visible lesions, and 7 percent clinically inapparent HPV infections.[13] The natural course taken by anogenital HPV infections is largely unknown. The investigations of Grussendorf et al.[14] suggest that HPV infections can also heal spontaneously as the patient grows older. They showed that HPV-DNA could be detected in the penile epidermis of 8 percent of clinically healthy patients between 16 and 35 years of age but in only 2 percent of the 36- to 85-year-old age group. Cervical carcinoma as a possible sequela of HPV infection of the cervix adds a new and serious dimension to HPV-infections both with regard to epidemiology and prognosis.[12]

HIV Infection

The sexual transmission of the HIV infection in developing countries occurs mainly by heterosexual contact; for the Central African countries it is calculated that more than 90 percent of the infections occur heterosexually. Heterosexual infection occurs more frequently in women than in men. A study in Kinshasa showed that in the 15- to 29-year-old age group women were infected four times more frequently than men.[15] In industrialized countries the sexual transmission of HIV is very different from that in Africa. Thus, in the US the majority of HIV infections are acquired through homosexual contacts, especially by anal intercourse. In 1988 only 5 percent of new HIV infections were acquired heterosexually.[16] A significant increase of heterosexual infections has recently also been observed in the US, but so far mostly among certain minorities: the incidence in black women is twenty times more frequent and in Hispanic women four times more frequent than in white women.[17] The incidence of drug abuse in black and Hispanic women in large cities may play a role in this context.

Interaction Between HIV and Other STDs   STDs can influence the transmission of HIV. Of particular significance are STDs which destroy the integrity of the epithelium or cause an inflammatory reaction in the anogenital mucosa, because these lead to an increase, at the site of transmission, of the number of HIV-infected lymphocytes in a seropositive person and of potential target cells for HIV in seronegative individuals. Studies of homosexual and heterosexual populations have shown that STDs are more common in persons infected with HIV than in comparable control groups.[18] Genital ulcers represent an important cofactor for the heterosexual transmission of HIV[19] and have been identified as an independent risk factor for HIV-seroconversion both in prostitutes[20] and in men[21] in Nairobi. The high incidence and prevalence of genital ulcers in Africa is possibly an important factor in the more frequent heterosexual dissemination of HIV on this continent.

Risk Factors and Risk Behavior

A *risk factor* is defined as a variable of the person who has a statistically significant relationship with the disease. It is now more important to speak of risk behavior than of risk groups. Campaigns providing information on the transmission of HIV have taught homosexuals to modify their risk behavior, and, as a consequence, the incidence of new HIV infections has been reduced in this group. Important risk factors and risk behaviors for STDs are presented in Table 217-2.

TABLE 217-2
Risk Factors and Risk Behavior for STD

Risk factors	Risk behavior
Age	Sexual behavior
Smoking	More frequent partner
Alcohol	exchange
Drug abuse	Number of new partners per
Other STD	unit of time
Absence of circumcision	Sexual preference
Contraception	Sexual practices
	Health behavior
	Poor body hygiene
	Delayed medical consultation
	Lack of compliance
	Prostitution

Drug Abuse

The studies of intravenous drug abusers have concentrated mainly on "needle-sharing" and less on sexual behavior. Needle-sharing results in high incidences of HIV and hepatitis B infections. (For instance, in a treatment center for drug addicts in Brooklyn, 64.9 percent of women and 59 percent of men were HIV-positive.[22]) Drug addiction in adolescents easily leads to "drugs for sex" behavior, and many i.v. drug addicts finance their drug consumption by prostitution. At present, there are hardly any useful investigations of this serious epidemiologic problem.

Absence of Circumcision

The preputial inner membrane is not keratinized and is therefore sensitive to physical damage and microbial attack. In addition, the preputial sac forms a kind of "moist chamber" for microbes acquired during sexual intercourse which plausibly explains why genital infections more easily infect the uncircumcised man. In an Australian study it was demonstrated that for uncircumcised men the risk of acquiring gonorrhea or herpes genitalis was twice as high as for circumcised men, and in the case of candida infection and syphilis the risk was five times higher.[23]

Contraception

Contraception affects the transmission and consequences of STD in various ways. The condom has assumed a leading role in anti-AIDS campaigns worldwide. Laboratory investigations have shown that latex condoms are impermeable to all of the microbes important in STD.[24] The other barrier device, the diaphragm, has not met with a high degree of acceptance by broad sections of the population owing to difficulties in its use. Spermicides have been shown in vitro studies to damage STD agents as well as the cell wall of sperm. The most commonly used substance in the US is nonoxynol-9, which has been shown to be effective against *N. gonorrhoeae*, HSV, *Treponema pallidum*, HIV, and *Chlamydia trachomatis*.[25] Its practical use as an intravaginal sponge and its low cost permits widespread use among the low income sections of the population.

Intrauterine devices have lost their popularity since it has been established that they double the risk of pelvic inflammatory disease (PID).[26] The most widely used method of contraception in western industrialized countries is the use of oral contraceptives. Various multicenter studies in the US have shown that the use of ovulation inhibitors leads to a more than 50 percent reduction in the risk of PID.[27] The effectiveness of barrier methods and chemical prophylaxis relies on their use during intercourse and thus heavily depends on compliance and degree of instruction. Worldwide efforts thus focus on publicizing the use of condoms and simple intravaginal chemical methods (sponges).

Sexual Behavior

The AIDS epidemic in the 1980s has dramatically demonstrated how important knowledge of the sexual behavior of a given population is for the understanding of the epidemiology of STD. Various components of sexual behavior show a connection with the incidence of STD: sexual experience and activity, age, onset of sexual activity, the number of sexual partners within a fixed time period, frequency of sexual relations, mode of partner recruitment, and sexual practices. It has been shown for adolescents that in recent decades the onset of sexual activity occurs at an increasingly earlier age. Sexual relationships between teenagers tend to be somewhat intermittent and only a small group within the whole adolescent population shows high sexual activity. The number of new partners per unit time is a crucial factor in the risk of acquiring an STD. This has been established for all commonly occurring STDs.[28]

Prostitution

Prostitution is practiced by men, women, and children, and both prostitutes and their customers come from all social classes and cultural groups. Prostitution has always had a central epidemiologic significance for STDs but the relationship between prostitution and the epidemiology of STD is complex. Prostitutes represent a very heterogeneous socioeconomic group. The incidence of STD is higher in the prostitutes of the lower socioeconomic classes,[29] but it has to be admitted that scarcely any studies of "upper class" prostitutes are available. These socioeconomic differences are also reflected in HIV incidence in prostitutes of various countries and geographic regions. The percentage of prostitutes found to be HIV-positive ranges from 0 percent in Copenhagen and 6.9 percent in New York City to 56 percent in Nairobi and 80 percent in Rwanda.[30]

The proportion of prostitutes who are HIV-positive is a general marker for the spread of HIV in the general population: the higher the prevalence of the infection among prostitutes, the greater is the significance of the heterosexual dissemination of HIV. Drug abuse is widespread in practically all forms of prostitution. Among prostitutes who are drug addicts the prevalence of STD is higher, and this is particularly true for HIV-infection. For instance, in one study 31 percent of drug-addicted prostitutes in New York were HIV-positive.[30] The place of work (street, bar, club, hotel, brothel), the nature of the sexual service, the number of customers, as well as the use of preventive measures all bear on the risk to the customer and the prostitute of acquiring an STD.

Demographic and Social Factors

The highest incidence of STD is found in the large cities (inner city and slums) of both the western industrialized world and developing countries. Both population groups show similarities: a relatively higher proportion of sexually active adolescents in the total population, high rates of population increase, temporary or permanent migration of larger sections of the population (migrant workers), poverty, harsh and unstable social conditions, riots, and even wars.[31,32] All of these factors favor prostitution, drug abuse, and drug trafficking. Such an environment is conducive to a high incidence of almost all STDs. From an epidemiologic point of view the phenomenon of the migrant worker in Africa has contributed decisively to the massive heterosexual dissemination of HIV.[33]

International Travel and STD

Movements of populations have always been an important factor in the spreading of STD. History shows this to have been particularly true for times of major wars. As a consequence of air travel, travel activity has now attained colossal dimensions. In the jet age the traveller, after being infected with an STD, can return home well within the incubation period of practically every STD. STD can be both imported and exported by travellers.

Business trips are undertaken by a great variety of professional groups: business people, engineers, journalists, flight crews, etc., and tourist trips are made by the million every year. The tourist behaves differently in a foreign country than at home. Sexual contacts are made more easily, more frequently, and more casually, and there is thus a much higher risk of being infected with an STD. Many tourist trips are blatantly advertised as "sex trips." In most industrialized countries a considerable portion of the STDs are acquired abroad.[34,35] The worldwide dissemination of the penicillin-resistant gonococcal strains is a classic example of the epidemiologic consequences of international travel. The first PPNG strain (penicillinase-producing *N. gonorrhoeae*) was identified in the US in 1976,[36] and by 1980 PPNG strains had spread around the world to 43 countries.[37] The worldwide dissemination of HIV also serves as an example of the immense epidemiologic significance of international travel.

References

1. *World Health Statistics Quarterly* **41**:90, 1988
2. Danielson D: Gonorrhoea in Sweden past and present. *Scand J Infect Dis Suppl* **69**:69, 1990
3. CDC: Gonorrhea annual survey 1983. *MMWR* **32**:22, 1984
4. CDC: Antibiotic resistant strains of *N. gonorrhoeae*. *MMWR* **36** (supplement 5 S), 245, 1987
5. CDC: Syphilis: United States 1983. *MMWR* **33**:433, 1984
6. Wendel GD: Early and congenital syphilis. *Obstet Gynecol Clin North Am* **16**:479, 1989
7. Piot P, Meheus A: Epidémiologie des maladies sexuellement transmissibles dans les pays en développement. *Ann Soc Belge Med Trop* **63**:87, 1983
8. Washington AE et al: Chlamydia infections in the United States. *JAMA* **257**:2070, 1987
9. Treharne JD, Goh BT: *Chlamydia trachomatis* infections in the United Kingdom, in *Proceedings of the European Society for Chlamydia Research,* Bologna, Italy, May 30–June 1, 1988, p 33
10. Backer TM et al: Epidemiology of genital herpes infections in the United States. The current situation. *J Reprod Med* **31**:359, 1986
11. Lee R et al: New type-specific antigens for detecting antibodies to herpes simplex virus type 1 (HSV 1) and type 2 (HSV 2), presented at the *International Society for STD Research,* Brighton, England, 1985
12. Koutsky L et al: Epidemiology of genital human papillomavirus. *Epidemiol Rev* **10**:122, 1988
13. Kiviat N et al: Prevalence of genital papillomavirus infection among women attending a college student health clinic or STD clinic. *J Infect Dis* 293, Feb. 1989
14. Grussendorf-Conen ES et al: Human papillomavirus genomes in penile smears of healthy men (letter). *Lancet* **1**:1092, 1986
15. Nzila N et al: Married couples in Zaire with discordant HIV-serology, presented at *Fourth Int. Conference on AIDS,* Stockholm, June 1988
16. Shapiro CN et al: Review of human immunodeficiency virus infection in women in the United States. *Obstet Gynecol* **74**:800, 1989
17. Liberatos P et al: The measurement of social class in epidemiology. *Epidemiol Rev* **10**:87, 1988
18. Simonsen JN et al: HIV infection among men with sexually transmitted diseases: Experience from a center in Africa. *N Engl J Med* **319**:274, 1988
19. Kreiss JK et al: Isolation of human immunodeficiency virus from genital ulcers in Nairobi prostitutes. *J Infect Dis* **160**:380, 1989
20. Plummer F et al: Co-factors in male-female transmission of HIV (abstract 4554), in *Program and Abstracts IVth International Conference on AIDS,* Washington, DC, Bio-Data, 1988
21. Cameron DW et al: Incidence and risk factors for female to male transmission of HIV (abstract 4061), in *Program and Abstracts IVth International Conference on AIDS,* Washington, DC, Bio-Data 1988
22. Lange WR: Geographic distribution of human immunodeficiency virus markers in parenteral drug abusers. *Am J Public Health* **78**:443, 1988
23. Parker SW et al: Circumcision and sexually transmissible diseases. *Med J Aust* **2**:288, 1983
24. Grimes DA, Cates W: Family planning and sexually transmitted diseases, in KK Holmes et al (eds): *Sexually Transmitted Diseases,* 2d ed. McGraw Hill, New York, 1990, p 1087
25. Rosenberg JM et al: Effect of the contraceptive sponge on chlamydia, gonorrhea and candidiasis. *JAMA* **257**:2308, 1987
26. Grimes DA: Intrauterine devices and pelvic inflammatory diseases: Recent developments. *Contraception* **36**:97, 1987
27. Rubin GL et al: Oral contraceptives and pelvic inflammatory disease. *Am J Obstet Gynecol* **144**:630, 1982
28. Aral SO, Holmes KK: Epidemiology of sexual behavior and sexually transmitted diseases, in KK Holmes et al (eds): *Sexually Transmitted Diseases,* 2d ed. McGraw Hill, New York, 1990, p 29
29. Meheus A et al: Prevalence of gonorrhoea in prostitutes in a Central African town. *Br J Vener Dis* **50**:50, 1974
30. Padan NS: Prostitute women and AIDS: Epidemiology. *AIDS* **2**:413, 1988
31. Martin CJ: The agrarian question and migrant labor: The case of western Kenya. *J Afr Stud* **11**:164, 1985
32. Harris FR, Wilkins RW: *Quiet Riots: Race and Poverty in the United States.* New York, Pantheon, 1988
33. Piot P et al: AIDS: An international perspective. *Science* **239**:573, 1988
34. De Schryver A, Meheus A: International travel and sexually transmitted diseases. *World Health Statistics Quarterly* **42**:90, 1989
35. Eichmann AR, Pifaretti JC: Penicillinase producing *N. gonorrhoeae* in Zurich, Switzerland. *Br J Vener Dis* **60**:147, 1984
36. Ashford WA et al: Penicillinase producing *Neisseria gonorrhoeae*. *Lancet* **1**:657, 1976
37. WHO: Surveillance of β-Lactamase producing *N. gonorrhoeae*. *Wkly Epidem Rec* **17**:133, 1982

CHAPTER 218

Miguel Sanchez and Anton F. H. Luger

"Syphilis simulates every other disease. It is the only disease necessary to know. One then becomes an expert dermatologist, an expert laryngologist, an expert oculist, an expert internist and an expert diagnostician."

Sir William Osler

Syphilis

Syphilis is a communicable disease caused by the motile microaerophilic spirochete *Treponema pallidum,* which is a natural pathogen only for humans.[1] It is usually contracted through sexual exposure, less commonly through transplacental transmission, very rarely through blood transfusion, and, in extremely unusual circumstances, from contact with infected laboratory animals.[1] During this century, dermatologists have been recognized as experts in the diagnosis and treatment of the protean manifestations of syphilis.[2] Although the diagnosis is frequently suspected from examination of skin lesions, syphilis should be regarded from its onset as a systemic disease with an extraordinary variety of organ involvement reflected in William Osler's mock-Biblical injunction "Know syphilis in all its manifestations and relations, and all other things clinical will be added unto you." Despite significant advances, many aspects of this "great imitator" remain obscure, and the disease continues to confound and challenge the clinician, the epidemiologist, and the social scientist.

History

There are several theories regarding the spread of syphilis. The *Columbian theory,* which proposes that some of the 50 crew members who survived Christopher Columbus' first trip contracted syphilis from natives on the island of Hispaniola (Haiti), is supported by medical records of three Spanish sailors who developed unexplained "bubas" upon their return from the voyage. Some of these infected adventurers reportedly joined the multinational army of Charles VIII of France and proceeded to spread the disease through Italy in their march to conquer the kingdom of Naples.[3] The 1495 victory over Naples was brief as the French army, devastated by the disease, had to retreat, providing the disbanded missionaries a further opportunity to spread the infection throughout other European countries.[4] Reportedly, Portuguese sailors under Vasco da Gama then transported the disease to India and later to China.

However, a careful evaluation of the historic facts and a precise appraisal of clinical and epidemiologic evidence[5] oppose the reliability of the story, which, in spite of all adverse arguments, has been continuously repeated since the beginning of the sixteenth century.

Syphilitic bone changes have been found in Australian, African, and Central American pre-Columbian fossils. Also, historic writings allude to the presence of syphilis in ancient China, Greece, and Rome, often masquerading under the guise of "venereal leprosy."[6] Treponemes infect rabbits and some primates, and syphilis may originally have been a less serious infection of humans and animals that differentiated into venereal and nonvenereal diseases between 15,000 and 3000 B.C.[7]

In the fifteenth century, scientific publications referred to the new scourge as the "great pox." Elsewhere, the disease was named by different countries after rival nationalities: the Russians dubbed it the "Polish disease," the French called it the "Italian disease," and so on, with the term "French disease" (morbus gallicus), coined by the Italians, becoming particularly popular.[6] In 1530, the physician and poet Girolamo Fracastoro published the poem "Syphilis Sive Morbus Gallicus," which told the story of the wealthy and handsome mythical shepherd Syphilus afflicted with a repulsive venereal disease as punishment for blasphemy against the god Apollo. The poem included a vivid and detailed description of syphilitic manifestations, and the name of the shepherd became synonymous with the disease. The other name by which the disease is commonly referred, *lues* (from the Latin for "plague" or "pestilence"), was coined by the sixteenth century physician-poet Jean Fernel, who first differentiated between the primary and secondary stages.

By the conclusion of the sixteenth century, the communicable nature as well as the cutaneous, oral, skeletal, and visceral manifestations of the disease were well recognized. Treatment with guaiac wood, sulfur baths, mercury ("two minutes with Venus, two years with Mercury"), and inorganic arsenic had been introduced.

Attempts to elucidate the etiology of syphilis were set back by John Hunter's notorious experiment in 1767 during which he inoculated himself with urethral pus. When he developed gonorrhea and syphilis, he mistakenly concluded that these were the same disease. No further argument ensued until 1837, when Phillipe Ricord distinguished syphilis from gonorrhea and classified the primary, secondary, and tertiary stages of the disease.[8] Around 1880, Hutchinson described the triad of late congenital syphilis (keratitis, labyrinthitis, and notched teeth).

The modern era of syphilis research began in 1903 with the experimental transmission of the disease from men to apes by Metchnikoff and Roux. In 1905, the German protozoologist Fritz Schaudinn and the syphilologist Erich Hoffman collaborated to identify in chancres corkscrew-shaped organisms that appeared pale after staining; and, hence, were named *Spirochaeta pallida.* Recognized later as a treponeme, the organism was renamed *Treponema pallidum.*[9] Only 4 years later, the Nobel laureate immunologist Paul Ehrlich introduced his "magic bullet," the arsenical Salvarsan, as a cure for syphilis. This was the first time that a specific chemical agent had been demonstrated to destroy a specific microorganism.[9] Shortly thereafter, August Wassermann and his colleagues applied the complement-fixation reaction to develop a diagnostic test for syphilis.

Other notable contributions include serologic standardization by Kolmer, the codification of existing knowledge about syphilis in John Stoke's *Modern Clinical Syphilology,* intensive intravenous chemotherapy using arsenoxide in 1933, and the development of the first treponemal-specific serologic test by Nelson. These efforts, however, were completely overshadowed in 1944 with the demonstrated efficacy of penicillin in early syphilis.[10] Within 10 years the dramatic decline in the incidence of syphilis moved experts to prematurely predict the extinction of the disease. This prompted the American Board of Dermatology and Syphilology to drop the last word from its name.[3]

The pandemic of syphilis-like disease occurring at the end of the fifteenth century was associated with severe and often fatal systemic manifestations that are rarely seen in the twentieth century. Lesions of the skin, mucous membranes, and bones were frequently extensive, destructive, and disfiguring. But now, exuberant secondary lesions of skin and mucous membranes, ulcerative lesions, gummata, secondary infectious relapse, cardiovascular disease, and early prenatal syphilis are seldom seen in immunocompetent patients. On the other hand, reinfection with syphilis, once rare, is common, and multiple genital chancres, anorectal chancres, and atypical chancres, as well as the classic Hunterian chancre, are familiar presentations of modern syphilis.

Syphilologists have suggested that the disease has evolved from its original virulent presentation into a more stable and predictable course. Another possibility is that clinicians, aided by better educated patients who seek medical attention earlier, may be diagnosing the more subtle manifestations. Treatment with penicillin may also have altered the "natural course" of the disease.

Numerous political figures, composers, authors, and painters reportedly have been infected with syphilis,[4] and a great deal of speculation has been voiced about how the disease may have influenced the course of history and art.[11]

Epidemiology

Syphilis occurs in all parts of the world and respects no social class. The disease is far more common in urban than in rural communities. The exact incidence or prevalence of venereal syphilis can only be studied from areas of the world with reliable reporting systems. In developing countries trends can only be inferred. In the United States and the United Kingdom, early syphilis (primary and secondary disease) is more common in the sexually active years. The most frequent groups affected are young adults 20 to 24 years of age, followed by adults in their twenties and thirties, teenagers, and middle-aged persons between 40 and 49 years of age.[12] Men used to have from two to six times greater incidence of syphilis than women, reflecting the difficulty of diagnosing women with concealed lesions as well as greater promiscuity, both heterosexual and homosexual, in men. Recently, however, this ratio has narrowed to less than 2:1.[13]

During World War I, concern about syphilis reached unprecedented proportions after 13 percent of American military draftees were found to be infected with syphilis or gonorrhea. This led to several public health measures to contain the disease, including congressionally sponsored quarantines and compulsory premarital screening.[14] The incidence continued to climb and peaked during the years between 1935 and 1947 as efforts to combat syphilis were restrained by a "conspiracy of silence." As the leader of the social

hygiene movement, Prince Morrow, noted: "Social sentiment holds that it is a greater violation of the properties of life publicly to mention venereal disease than privately to contract it."[15] Surgeon General Thomas Parran, in his ambitious campaign to wipe out the "shadow on the land," called for a "Wassermann dragnet" to screen the population vigorously and to institute partner notification through "shoe leather epidemiology."[9] These public health interventions did not limit the spread of syphilis effectively.[16]

During World War II, efforts at public education and prostitution control were intensified. The armed forces distributed condoms and provided immediate treatment without punitive measures. In early 1943, John Mahoney of the U.S. Public Health Service found that penicillin cured syphilis in rabbits and later that year demonstrated efficacy in humans.[10] No disease has ever been more dramatically affected by antibiotics. The widespread use of penicillin reduced the number of cases 18-fold from a high of 72 cases per 100,000 in 1943 to about 4 per 100,000 in 1956.[17] This was followed by a subsequent rise, another slowdown with renewed control efforts in 1962, and then a 34 percent increase in new cases from 1969 to 1973. Although permissiveness, promiscuity, and the pill (the "three P's"), associated with relaxed sexual restraints dating from the 1960s, have been blamed for the resurgence in venereal diseases, there was actually a downward trend in new cases of syphilis in the mid-1970s.[18] This was possibly related to control efforts and to the beneficial effect on incubating syphilis of antibiotics used for other infections. Unfortunately, a decrease in syphilis tends to be accompanied by a proportional lack of concern by the medical community, government, and the public.[9] Between 1978 and 1981, the number of reported cases in the United States increased by 43 percent.[19] In 1985, the rates of early syphilis began to increase after 5 years of steady decline. As a result, from 1985 to 1990, the estimated annual rate of new cases of primary and secondary syphilis skyrocketed from 11.5 to 20.2 and the rate of cases of syphilis at any stage rose from 28.50 to 53.8 per 100,000 persons. In 1990, with a total of 50,223 reported cases of early syphilis and 134,375 cases at any stage, the incidence of syphilis surged to the highest level in 50 years.[20]

Previously, men with same-sex partners constituted a large portion of syphilis cases. Forty six percent of all males with syphilis in the United States in 1976 contracted the disease from other men,[21] and similar statistics were recorded in England.[22] However, changes in sexual practices to reduce the risk of HIV infection have dramatically reduced the proportion of syphilis among white homosexual and bisexual men from between 50 and 70 percent of all male cases in the late 1970s to between 10 and 20 percent in 1986.[23]

The present outbreak is occurring primarily among African American heterosexual men and women in cities.[24] A primary factor is the trading of sex for drugs, particularly free-basing cocaine (crack), which is being abused in epidemic proportion.[25,26] Possible but less important factors include the inefficacy on incubating syphilis of spectinomycin, recommended for most of the past decade to treat gonorrhea, and possible reactivation of syphilis in HIV-infected individuals. The high number of infected young women has resulted in an alarming increase in new cases of congenital syphilis.[27] This is a particularly challenging problem as crack addicts are less likely to seek and receive prenatal care. Prenatal syphilis had also declined from 4085 reported cases (all types) in 1962 to 287 in 1981, but then began to climb, paralleling the rising incidence of early syphilis in the population. In the second half of 1987, the rate of congenital syphilis increased to 10.5 cases per 100,000 births.[28] From 1986 through 1988, the number of cases in New York City increased by 500 percent.[29] By the end of 1991,

4352 cases had been reported throughout the country. Because only about 12 percent of all cases are reported to federal agencies, the actual number of syphilis cases is estimated to be much higher. Notably, this increase is occurring at a time when rates for gonorrhea are declining.[11] These changes have not been apparent in western European countries.[30] In Great Britain, the 1988 incidence of early syphilis was 1.5 per 100,000 in men and 0.5 per 100,000 in women.[31] Venereal syphilis appears to be increasing in most developing countries, but statistics are not reliable. High incidence rates exist in El Salvador, Chile, Johannesburg, and New Guinea.[32] Even a rich developing country such as Singapore has an estimated annual incidence rate of 72 cases per 100,000 persons. Despite therapeutic "magic bullets," syphilis has proven to be a tough enemy. Elimination or even control of the disease will require creative public health interventions, socioeconomic support, and further advances in the basic biology of the organism and the immune response of the human host.[33]

Etiology

The causative agent of syphilis, *Treponema pallidum,* is a corkscrew-shaped prokaryotic microorganism that belongs to the order Spirochaetales ("coiled hair"), a class of bacteria with flexible, helically coiled cell walls.[34] The organism, which is only pathogenic to humans, cannot be distinguished from those which cause pinta (*T. carateum*), yaws (*T. pertenue*), or endemic syphilis. *T. pallidum* belongs to the same family as *Borrelia* and *Leptospira.* This explains the confusion sometimes encountered in differentiating diseases caused by these organisms through serologic tests.[35] Other treponemes include the animal pathogens, *T. cuniculi* (rabbit syphilis), *T. Fribourg-Blanc* (monkey syphilis), and *T. hyodysenteria* (swine dysentery).[36] Some human or animal nonpathogenic saprophytic treponemes, such as *T. microdentium, T. macrodentium, T. denticola, T. orale,* and *T. vincentii,* are particularly abundant in the oral or anal cavities, making the diagnosis of lesions in these areas unreliable by dark-field microscopy but possible with special immunoperoxidase stains.[37] *T. pallidum* measures between 5 and 20 μm in length and 0.1 and 0.2 μm in width with tapered ends and 8 to 14 regular rigid spirals, which on fixation produce a wavy appearance with a wavelength of 1.1 μm and an amplitude of 0.2 to 0.3 μm.[36] Six fibrils maintain the spiral structure and may contribute to its motility. Because its narrow width renders the organism undetectable by light microscopy without silver impregnation, dark-field microscopy is needed for diagnosis.[38] The treponemes look like mobile strings of beads ambulating with a flexion and back and forth movement. This rotary motion is said to be characteristic of virulent treponemes and to facilitate penetration through tissue.

Three main elements are evident from ultramicroscopic studies: the protoplasmic cylinder (protoplast), axial filament, and outer envelope (cell wall). The protoplast is enclosed by a frail cytoplasmic membrane that functions as an osmotic barrier and is thus essential for cell metabolism, especially absorption and excretion. The axial filament consists of six to eight elastic fibrils that are twisted around the protoplast in one or two bundles and may be responsible for the helicoid form. The outer envelope is composed of three layers. Understanding the biologic and chemical properties of the outer envelope is important because antibiotics, such as penicillin, disrupt its synthesis. Also, a great deal of research is being undertaken to determine the value of cell-wall proteins in the development of a syphilis vaccine as well as to develop tests to differentiate between different pathogenic treponemes.[33] Because in comparison to most bacteria the outer envelope contains a paucity of integral transmembrane proteins to serve as targets for specific antibodies, the organism could more easily evade host humoral defenses.[39] Some of these molecules are proteolipids with structures unique to bacteria. The lipid moiety may anchor the membrane and contribute to its rigidity.

The inner layer of the outer envelope contains the heteropolymer peptidoglycan macromolecule, the mureine sacculus, which is formed by main strands of alternating sequences of *N*-acetyl muramic acid and *N*-acetyl-glucosamine. The muramic acid groups of these strands are cross-connected by tetrapeptide side chains. The peptidoglycan lattice functions as a strong skeleton for the organism, preserves its form, protects the fragile cytoplasm against physical insult, and functions as an inert filter for larger molecules.[40] During periods of cell growth, the peptidoglycan macromolecule enlarges, a process which occurs in about 30 steps and requires a number of enzymes. At first the main strings of the lattice become severed by hydrolases (*N*-acetyl − muramidase = lysozyme). Consecutively guiding molecules transport prefabricated precursors of chain components through the cytoplasmic membrane to the holes in the net. Then, 10 to 15 enzymes facilitate the incorporation of the new elements into the gaps, thus reforming the strings. One of the last steps in the biosynthesis, the cojoining of the side chains, is catalyzed by three enzymes, D-alanyl-D-alanyl-carboxypeptidase, peptidoglycan-endopeptidase, and particularly by peptidoglycan-transpeptidase.[41] An extracellular amorphous slime layer, perhaps resulting from production of mucopolysaccharides, can be demonstrated by ruthenium red staining surrounding live *T. pallidum* and may protect the organism against phagocytosis.[42]

Replication occurs via fission, with an interval of 30 to 33 h between divisions. *T. pallidum* was once considered an obligatory anaerobe, despite its ability to live in the human host where oxygen tension is quite high. Observations of *T. pallidum* in baby hamster kidney cells cultured in the presence of 7% CO_2 in air and the maintenance of the organism in aerobic fibroblast cell cultures for several weeks using special medium have challenged all traditional views.[43] In fact, *T. pallidum* requires molecular oxygen for survival in cell-free and tissue culture systems.[44] The organism possesses a cytochrome system, has superoxidase dismutase and catalase activity,[45] and metabolizes glucose and pyruvate aerobically.[46] The sole useful way of culturing virulent strains of *T. pallidum* is by inoculation of infected material into rabbit testicles. An orchitis develops, and organisms may be reliably recovered between the sixth and tenth day after inoculation. The test is cumbersome because material from the infected testicle must be injected into the testicle of another rabbit to grow sufficient numbers of treponemes.[38] The growth of treponemes in tissue culture has produced limited success. The estimated sensitivity of the rabbit infectivity test for detection of virulent *T. pallidum* is approximately ten organisms. Until the structure of this organism is better understood, the complex immunologic interactions in syphilis cannot be unraveled.

Immunology

Although the clinical course and diverse manifestations of syphilis have been recognized for centuries, wide gaps in our understanding of the immunopathogenesis of this disease remain. Although many studies on the subject have been published, investigators have needed to confront the limitation of available experimental animal models[36] and the challenge of adapting new experimental techniques.[33] In addition, the immune responses may be different depending on the time at which the infection is studied. As a result, contradictory conclusions have been reported, which confound our understanding of the complex immune interactions.

Unlike nonpathogenic treponemes, *T. pallidum* invades the mucosal surfaces and abraded skin of humans.[36] Although a receptor site has not been identified, the spirochete attaches itself to mammalian cells.[47] Recently it has been shown that *T. pallidum* not only penetrates living cells but can move through endothelial cells in vitro[48] and within 8 h can go through the epithelial, connective tissue, and muscle layers of intact murine abdominal walls.[49] Several molecules such as proteoglycans, fibronectin, lactoferrin, and transferrin become bound to the surface of the treponemes.[50] In addition to protecting the organism from immune attack, a coat of host-derived macromolecules may help to neutralize host defenses, such as proteases, and provide nutrients.[50] Fibronectin may aid treponemal adhesion to cells, proteoglycans may mediate incorporation of host lipoproteins, and cholesterol and transferrin may provide necessary iron. Following penetration into tissue, *T. pallidum* replicates and some organisms are drained by lymph nodes and spleen. The spirochete has chemotactic factors[36] that attract neutrophils to the inoculation site.[51] Phagocytosis readily occurs without need for opsonization, which indicates that immunoglobulins are present on the surface of the treponemes.[52] However, it has been speculated that the ingested organisms are not necessarily destroyed and that some treponemes are able to repel phagocytosis.[36]

Neutrophils in early skin lesions are replaced by lymphocytes,[53] over 90 percent of which are thymus-dependent (T-cell) lymphocytes.[54] Macrophages, plasma cells, and a few neutrophils constitute the remaining cells in the infiltrate.[55] Chondroitin sulfate and hyaluronic acid, which have been reported to modulate immune surveillance, are present in the center of the chancre.[56] Lymphocytes secrete lymphokines, which attract and activate macrophages.[57] Then, in the presence of exogenous antibody, the macrophages ingest and destroy the organisms.[58] It should be noted that confirmation of this role of macrophages is uncertain. Under investigational conditions, the rate of clearance of treponemes, following activation of macrophages, has been reported to be both higher[59] and unaffected.[60] However, electron microscopic and immunofluorescent studies on chancres that show degeneration of treponemes and the presence of treponemal antigens within macrophages provide evidence for an important role.[53,61] This effect may be aided by immune serum, which enhances phagocytosis, presumably by opsonization, and the antibody subclass IgG2, which enhances killing by macrophages.[61]

Treponemal-nonspecific and -specific antibodies are detectable by Western blot and radioimmunoassay techniques at the time or shortly after the chancre appears. Production of IgM precedes IgG. The subclasses of IgG1 and IgG3 are primarily expressed, whereas IgG2 and IgG4 are present at very low concentration, if at all.[62] In rabbits, the IgM response is most intense at the height of the clinical disease, whereas IgG peaks following resolution of the clinical infection.[63]

Paradoxically, soon after the combined efforts of humoral and cell-mediated immunity appear to have eliminated practically every organism and brought the infection under control, the disease becomes generalized and systemic. At this stage, called *secondary syphilis,* antibody titers reach high levels, but this peak reflects the activity of the disease and the tissue response to infection rather than the degree of humoral protection. Still, the humoral immune response clearly modifies the lesions of secondary syphilis in hu-

mans, which would otherwise look like primary chancres.[36] During this time, resistance to new infection develops, although delayed-type hypersensitivity to treponemal antigens is virtually absent.[64] The defect in cell-mediated immunity is highly specific for the spirochete, and, except for depressed blastogenic response to some fungal antigens, the response to other antigens and mitogens is normal.[65]

Investigators have attempted to explain this suppression through a number of observations. Decreased responsiveness to peripheral blood lymphocytes from humans and rabbits has been reported,[66,67] although not from rabbit spleens and lymph nodes, which provide more reliable measures. Macrophages have been implicated in the suppressed concavalin A responses of some spleen cells.[68] In part, the suppressed cell-mediated activity could be explained by defective lymphokine and monokine production, but our present knowledge of these substances in syphilis is incomplete. Although macrophage activating factors are produced by rabbit spleen cells,[69] interleukin 2 (IL-2) production by spleen cells could only be demonstrated 30 days after treponemal infection.[33] Secretion of IL-1 by rabbit spleen cells and macrophages has been found to be reduced on day 10[33] and is also decreased in hamsters. An absolute and relative lymphocytopenia has been observed in patients with primary and secondary syphilis.[70] In primary syphilis, T-helper lymphocytes appear to be reduced.[70] In contrast, in secondary syphilis, the number of lesional cytotoxic suppressor cells and N34+ (dendritic and activated) T cells is higher,[71] but the number of circulating T8 cells is decreased.[70] The natural killer cell activity decreases in early and latent syphilis as levels of nontreponemal antibodies become elevated.[72]

The suppression of cell-mediated immunity, coupled with unchecked proliferation of the organisms, leads to prolonged antigenemia in the presence of rising antibody levels. This condition is highly suitable for the formation of immune complexes.[73] Indeed, in some patients with early syphilis and most cases of secondary syphilis, immune complexes composed of immunoglobulins, complement, and treponemal outer membrane antigens can be measured.[74] Complement appears to have an important role as there is evidence that in its absence, virulent treponemes can resist antibody binding.[75] Also, complement may lyse the treponemal outer membrane exposing masked antigenic determinants.[75]

As the secondary lesions resolve, a stage called "latency" is entered. At this time delayed-type hypersensitivity, as measured by skin testing with treponemal extracts, reappears.[64] This period may last indefinitely, may end abruptly within a few months by a relapse of secondary syphilis, or may end from 1 to 20 years later as tertiary syphilis in the forms of neurologic or cardiovascular disease or gummas.[76] The granulomatous histologic nature of the gummatous infiltrate indicates that the response is primarily cell-mediated. Presumably the immune reaction is directed to invading treponemes, but organisms in tissue are scant and have been interpreted as artefacts by some investigators.[36] The spirochetes have rarely been demonstrated by immunofluorescent techniques.[77] During the early stages of infection, skin lesions show inflammation and masses of treponemes. Skin tests with inactivated treponemes are negative. In contrast, during the late stage, the pathogen elicits in the sensitized host the formation of granulomas consisting of epithelioid and giant cells. There are few if any organisms in the lesions, and skin tests are positive.

Much remains to be learned about the mechanisms leading to the appearance of "protective" immunity.[78] In humans, immunity to reinfection develops but only if the disease is untreated and allowed to persist. According to the *Finger-Landsteiner law,* patients develop a chancre, a papule, or a gumma depending on whether they are reinoculated with *T. pallidum* during the primary, secondary, or tertiary stages of syphilis, respectively. This finding was confirmed 50 years after it was proposed[79] by studying the reaction of previously infected prisoners to reinoculation with *T. pallidum*. Most patients who had been treated for early syphilis developed typical chancres containing treponemes, whereas patients with untreated latent syphilis were refractory to reinoculation. Many patients with late latent or congenital syphilis did not develop lesions or a change in nontreponemal antibody titers. A significant proportion, however, developed dark-field negative lesions associated with elevated Venereal Disease Research Laboratory (VDRL) titers, and a few developed gummas at the inoculation site.[79] This study illustrates that late syphilitic infection resists rechallenge with *T. pallidum,* whereas patients treated for early disease are susceptible to reinfection. It also argues against the impression that *T. pallidum* in human and rabbit tissue persists years after ''adequate'' antibiotic therapy for late latent disease.[80] Evidence for the importance of humoral factors in the development of syphilis immunity has been provided by a number of studies. Good correlation exists between the development of resistance to reinfection and the elevated titers of immobilizing and inactivating antibodies to *T. pallidum* present in latent and tertiary disease. In rabbits, emergence of resistance correlates with the presence of neutralizing antibody and complement in serum.[81] In this animal model, daily infusion of immune serum did not prevent reinfection but altered the appearance, severity, and duration of the lesions.[82] In addition, a factor in immune serum that prevents attachment of the treponemes to the host's cells[83] has been proposed to be an antibody, directed against treponemal mucopolysaccharidase, which presumably disrupts the organism's surface.[56]

The cell-mediated immune response is also essential.[84] Modulation of cellular immunity by immunosuppressive agents[85] affirms a crucial role for lymphocytes in resistance to syphilitic infection. In animal studies, immunity could not easily be transferred by transfusions of lymphocytes from infected rabbits,[86,87] although similar experiments in hamsters[88] and guinea pigs succeeded.[89] In fact, both helper and cytotoxic/suppressor T cells conferred some resistance to primary infection with *T. pallidum,* although to a lesser degree than whole T-cell suspensions. Immune lymphocytes injected into a site of treponemal infection also rendered some protection.[90] Immunity can also be transferred to animals with repeated infusions of irradiated treponemes but not with dead organisms.[33]

Understanding the details involved in the emergence of resistance to *T. pallidum* is integral to the development of a syphilis vaccine. The focus of current syphilis research has centered on the identification and characterization of outer membrane antigenic polypeptides.[91,92] Although antigens that can stimulate T-cell responses have been found, very little is known about their function.

A protective vaccine against syphilis will require considerably more investigation. In the only promising study so far, repeated immunization of rabbits with purified antiendoflagellar antigen over 32 weeks did not prevent reinfection, but the lesions occurred earlier, had a flatter, softer appearance, and resolved more rapidly.[93,94]

Other aspects of syphilitic infection need to be explained. Clearly, both the humoral and cell-mediated arms of the immune system play significant roles in protection against *T. pallidum* and are activated early in the disease. However, the vigorous immune response does not avert the eventual course of the infection. The means by which this slow treponeme resists the host's immune attack, which effectively clears practically every organism from early lesions, remains a mystery. As an explanation it has been reported that a partial inhibition of the cell-mediated response accounts for the failure to eradicate all live organisms from early lesions.[65] Two tests for cellular immunity, mitogen-induced blast transformation and leukocyte migration, are impaired in lymphocytes from animals and humans with early syphilis.[89–92] Furthermore, patients with syphilis have a depletion of lymphocytes in the paracortical or thymic area of lymph nodes as seen in the runting syndrome of infected neonatal rabbits.[95] However, other data suggest normal lymphocyte function in early syphilis. In syphilitic rabbits, lymphoid cells from lymph nodes and spleens extracted between the 6th and 31st day of infection proliferated when exposed to *T. pallidum* antigens after exposure.[68]

If a defect is indeed present, it could result from either suppression or dysfunction of cell-mediated immunity[33] and could be produced either by altered lymphocytes or suppressive serum factors, such as glycosaminoglycans,[96] immune complexes,[97] or other substances.[98] In support of suppressive factors in serum is the observation that levels of anti-T-lymphocyte antibodies may be reduced by incubation with syphilitic serum.[99] On the other hand, a suppressed response to antigen could merely result from an ''immunofocusing'' mechanism by the host.[100]

Others have proposed that certain anatomic sites such as the brain, eye, and aorta may not be readily accessible to immune products; that the organism remains undetected inside the host's cells; or that it is hidden or protected from the host by the slimy mucopolysaccharide coat surrounding the cell wall. Also, it has been suggested that partial tolerance develops due to antigenic competition from simultaneous exposure to a large number of antigens in the outer membrane.[101] However, there is little evidence to support these theories. A recently published study in rabbits attempts to explain the suppression that follows an initially normal immune response. According to the investigators, early on, immunity is normal and results in annihilation of most treponemes. However, treponemal products are able to induce the host macrophages to secrete twice as much prostaglandin E_2 (PGE_2). As a result, IL-2 synthesis by these cells is halved and, consequently, T-cell proliferation is inhibited, leading to suppressed immunity that enables the remaining intact organism to proliferate even in the presence of antibody. This suppression persists for at least 1 month and can be reversed by indomethacin or the combination of IL-1 and -2.[102] Investigators have reported that the outer membrane of *T. pallidum* has a paucity of polypeptides that can serve as targets for specific antibodies[91] and that as a result of molecular ''mimicry,'' these surface proteins may not be very immunogenic.[101] This structural pattern would represent a new and innovative bacterial adaptation to evade immune attack. However, over 25 different *T. pallidum* antigens have already been identified, and some of these polypeptides, perhaps due to associated lipid modifications, are very immunogenic.[102] Furthermore, proteins do not necessarily need to be surface-exposed to stimulate a protective T-cell response.[103]

Despite the close structural similarities between *T. pallidum* and other human pathogenic treponemes, there are differences in the immunopathogenesis by each of these organisms. Patients with pinta (*T. carateum*) cannot easily be infected with *T. pallidum* or *T. pertenue,* which causes yaws, but patients with yaws or syphilis readily contract pinta. Patients who have yaws are protected against developing syphilis, but the reverse is not certain. Prenatal transmission and late complications involving the cardiovascular and neurovascular systems occur rarely in nonvenereal syphilis and not at all with yaws and pinta.[104] *T. pertenue* can be inoculated into monkeys, rabbits, and hamsters, although similar attempts with *T. carateum* have succeeded only in chimpanzees. Such variations would dispute the allegation that all four diseases are caused by the same organism and represent different infection patterns based on temperature changes.[105] However, the organisms are so similar that *T. pallidum* and *T. pertenue* could not be distinguished by the sensitive polymerase chain reaction.[106] No doubt, advances in technology will provide answers to the complexity of syphilitic infection that has puzzled physicians for centuries.

Clinical Manifestations

Classification

The natural history of syphilis may be described by using a combination of an older clinical and a more recent epidemiologic terminology.

The older classification is based on clinical manifestations of disease and includes the primary stage (chancre), secondary stage (mucocutaneous lesions with lymphadenopathy and other organ system involvement), the latent stage (reactive serologic test for syphilis in the absence of signs or symptoms of disease), and the tertiary stage (cardiovascular, central nervous system, cutaneous, and visceral involvement).

The epidemiologic classification is based on the duration of infection and communicability and is divided into early and late stages. Previously, 4 years was the dividing line between early and late disease. Now, based on information that 95 percent of relapses develop by the second year following healing of secondary syphilis,[76] the generally accepted span is 2 years. However, limitations in budgets and health department personnel have influenced these classifications so that in the United States, early latent syphilis has come to mean syphilis without signs and symptoms for less than 1 year.[107] Because early symptomatic syphilis is continually infectious and early latent disease intermittently so, the yield of positive serologic tests is high among sexual contacts of these patients. Late latent syphilis, on the other hand, is only, and then rarely, infectious to the newborn, and epidemiologic investigation of sexual contacts beyond the immediate family is generally unproductive.

For treatment purposes, there is yet another classification, in which duration of disease is the determining factor. Involvement of the central nervous system tends to occur after the first year of infection, so syphilis of more than 1 year's duration as well as indeterminate syphilis are treated with the same antibiotic regimen as asymptomatic neurosyphilis.

The following is a convenient classification of acquired syphilis, combining the clinical, epidemiologic, and treatment factors (see also Table 218-1):

1. Early syphilis includes primary and secondary disease, as well as clinical relapses due to inadequate therapy, and usually lasts less than 1 year for treatment purposes.
2. Latent disease is subdivided into early (less than 2 years) and late (2 years or more) stages for contact tracing, and less than or more than 1 year for treatment purposes.
3. Late syphilis includes manifest disease: late benign (gumma), cardiovascular, and central nervous system involvement.

TABLE 218-1
Stages of Syphilis

Stage	Comment
Early	"Infectious"
Primary	
Secondary	
Latent	Infectivity decreases rapidly with time
Early	Spontaneous cure (30%)
Late	Persistent latent disease (30%)
Late (tertiary)	Disease manifestations
	CNS
	Cardiovascular
	Late benign gummata

Transmission

Syphilis can be contracted through direct contact with an infected lesion, blood transfusion, ingestion of menstrual blood or vaginal secretions, and transplacental transmission from mother to fetus. Fomites are only a hypothetical means of transfer and account for very few, if any, infections. Prosectors, blood handlers, and laboratory technicians are at risk for accidental inoculation with infected material.

Progression of Disease

Syphilis has been described as an on- and off- and on-again disease.[107] At the site of inoculation, a chancre develops after an asymptomatic incubation period that ranges from 10 to 90 days and averages 21 days. The duration of the incubation period varies with the number of inoculated spirochetes. In volunteer prisoners, chancres developed 18.6 days after experimental inoculation with 10,000 spirochetes, versus 28.1 days after inoculation with 10 organisms.[79]

Presumably, the long replication time of *T. pallidum* accounts for the variation in incubation period observed with the inoculum size.[107] Regardless of the size of the inoculum, no primary lesions develop earlier than 10 days.[79] Untreated chancres persist from 1 to 6 weeks, before healing without scar formation. The lesions of secondary syphilis erupt 6 to 12 weeks after the onset of the primary lesion but may develop months later or, in up to 15 percent of cases, before the chancre disappears. The secondary stage usually recedes in 4 to 12 weeks.

Most of our knowledge of the natural course of syphilis is derived from three studies. In *the Oslo study* conducted in Oslo, Norway, between 1891 and 1910, 2181 cases of early syphilis were untreated by Dr. Caesar Boeck who believed that the complications of the disease did not justify the danger of mercury therapy. The records of 953 patients (44 percent of the original group) were traced, analyzed, and reported in 1955[108] following a more limited, earlier publication by Gjestland. The report has been criticized for its emphasis on autopsies, death certificates, and hospital admissions, which biased the results towards a more serious prognosis.[109] However, the study, which will undoubtedly never be repeated, provides the best available account of the outcome of untreated syphilis. In the notorious *Tuskegee "experiment,"* conducted between 1936 and 1973, 800 black males with latent syphilis were untreated and compared to a normal control group. Not only are the conclusions of this study limited because of its restriction to a single race, sex, and socioeconomic class, but the reports are difficult to interpret as they follow no set protocol.[110] The *Rosahn study* is a review of autopsies and is biased because the population studied obviously had a poor outcome.[111]

According to the Oslo study, approximately 25 percent of patients experience clinical relapse of secondary syphilis, and in this group one-quarter had multiple episodes. More than two-thirds of the relapses occurred by the end of 6 months, 90 percent by the end of the first year, and 95 percent within 2 years. None occurred beyond the sixth year.[76]

The median duration of the primary and secondary stages combined is 3.1 months in males and 4.4 months in females, whereas the median duration of the secondary stage alone is 2.1 months in males and 3.5 months in females.[76] So an untreated patient usually becomes noninfectious as early as 6 months after the disease has been contracted. In 95 percent of cases, immunologic changes prevent the appearance of lesions in the skin and mucous membranes after this time, but do not prevent progression of the organisms to other tissues. Although the danger of direct transmission is low after 4 to 5 years of established infection, inoculation from gummas has occasionally been noted.[79]

Latent syphilis follows the secondary stage and may persist for life in an asymptomatic form in about two-thirds of untreated patients. The rest develop tertiary syphilis, which becomes manifest as late benign gummas (16 percent) or cardiovascular (9.6 percent) or central nervous system (6.5 percent) disease.[76] Syphilis was the cause of death of 11 percent of the patients in the Oslo study. In African American patients, the mortality may be even higher, as 50 percent of autopsies from untreated black males with syphilis of over 10 years' duration show cardiovascular disease.[112] Taken together, available studies show that syphilis causes increased mortality, and that 15 to 40 percent of untreated patients develop tertiary disease. As the eminent venereologist Rudolph Kampmeier wrote in 1943: "It would be of great value if the prognosis of untreated syphilis were accurately known (but) this is not known and probably never will be known in these days of more or less universal treatment of the disease."[113]

Primary Syphilis

The characteristic lesion of primary syphilis, the chancre (Fig. 218-1), appears at the site of treponemal penetration. A dusky red macule turns into an indolently growing, inflammatory papule. Ulceration in the center of the papule usually compels the patient to seek medical evaluation, although in 15 to 30 percent of cases the lesions go unnoticed. The chancre, which is round or oval and approximately 1 to 2 cm in size, has sharply defined, regular, raised, indurated borders. The "ham-colored" base usually has a smooth surface but may be covered with a grayish slough or hemorrhagic crust. The lesion feels firm, rubbery, and, when uncomplicated by trauma or impetiginization, is painless. If squeezed, a thin serous exudate teeming with spirochetes is expressed. Untreated, the chancre persists for 3 to 6 weeks but resolves within 1 to 2 weeks after treatment. However, deviation from the above description is common, and the classic "Hunterian" chancre is now seen in only about 60 percent of cases.[114,115] In one study of male patients, 23 percent had more than one chancre, 8 percent had multiple lesions with edema or phimosis, 4.5 percent had erosive balanitis, and 1.1 percent had lymphangitis or thrombophlebitis of the dorsal vein. In other reports, the frequency of multiple lesions was

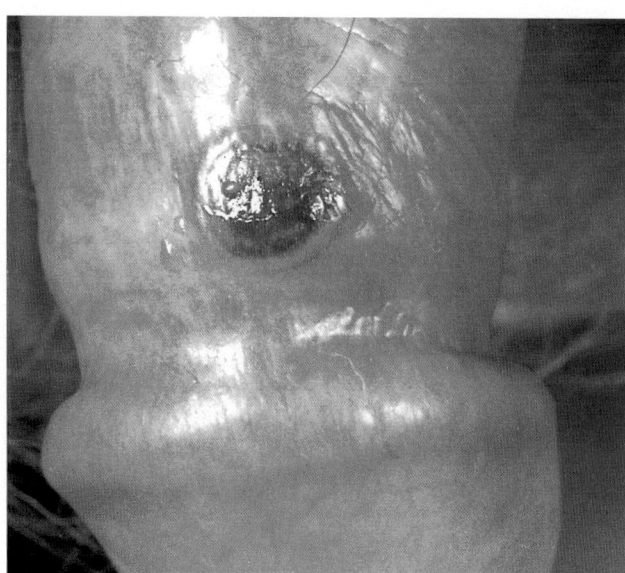

FIGURE 218-1 Primary syphilitic chancre. Painless, firm, buttonlike, eroded nodule (chancre) occurring at the site of entry of treponeme.

found to be as high as 47 percent.[114] The increased incidence of herpes genitalis, with erosions that facilitate treponemal penetration, may be the reason for the rising number of multiple chancres. In males, the regularly involved locations are the glans, the coronal sulcus, and the foreskin, but other genital areas including the urethra can be affected. Lesions at the urethral orifice may present as nongonococcal urethritis or cause an inflammatory phimosis that can eventuate in penile gangrene. When the foreskin is retracted, chancres in the mucosal surface cause it to flip briskly, a sign dubbed "the dory flop" by John Stokes. In females, the labia, fourchette, urethra, and perineum are affected in descending order of frequency. Chancres of the cervix constitute as many as 44 percent of female cases, but regularly go undetected. Lesions in females and extragenital chancres in both sexes lack "cartilaginous" firmness but, instead, are characterized by an edematous induration. Kissing chancres are particularly common in areas of skin-to-skin contact such as the vulva.

Extragenital chancres have become more common due to the increased popularity of oral and anal sex, and any evaluation of their frequency would need to consider the sexual practices of the patients. It is generally accepted that the number falls between 5 and 8 percent.[116,117] About two-thirds occur above the neck and approximately half of these are seen on or close to the lips (Fig. 218-2) or in the oral cavity.[118] The rest appear on the fingers, breasts, trunk, abdomen (Fig. 218-3), and extremities.[116] Anorectal chancres form 4 to 10 percent of cases of extragenital primary syphilis,[119] an incidence that seems unexpectedly low for the years preceding safe-sex practices. The disease is underdiagnosed and should be considered in any at-risk person with rectal pain, bloody stools, anal fissures, or a precipitously appearing mass or ulcer in the anorectal area.[121] Chancres of the fingers usually occur in medical and dental personnel and tend to be painful.

In 70 to 80 percent of primary syphilis cases, one or more firm, movable, discrete lymph nodes, or "bubos," appear around the first week of infection.[114] These are usually unilateral at first and most commonly palpated in the inguinal area, although in fe-

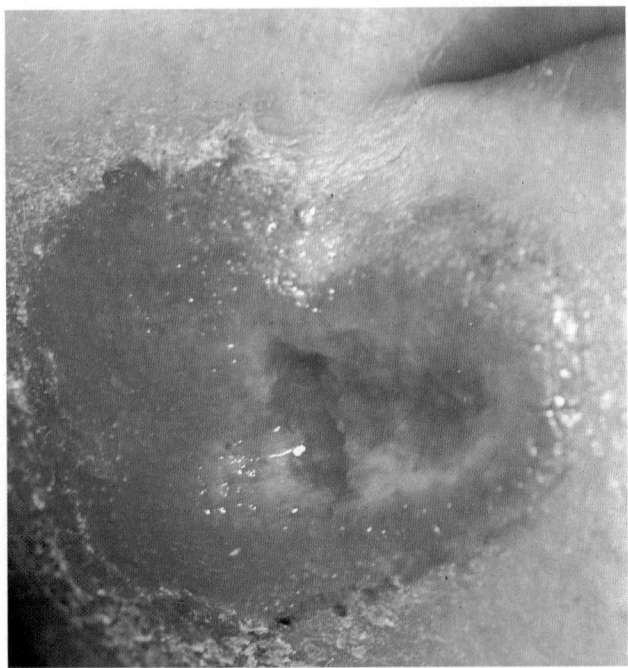

FIGURE 218-2 Primary syphilis. Extragenital chancre.

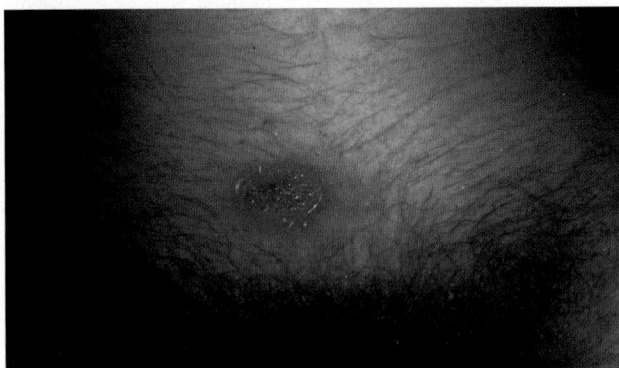

FIGURE 218-3 Primary syphilitic chancre on the lower abdomen, an unusual area.

males the femoral area is often involved. The bubos are characteristically painless, although in one study 14 percent of the nodes were tender.[114] At this stage, dark-field examination of the chancre is the investigative procedure of choice[120] and is positive unless the patient applied or ingested antibiotics or the ulcer base is dry and healing. Nontreponemal serologic tests are usually negative at the onset of the primary chancre.[120,121] The presence of other sexually transmitted infections, especially chancroid and herpes simplex, in syphilitic chancres is well documented.[122] The diseases most frequently misdiagnosed as primary syphilis are chancroid, traumatic ulcers, and herpes genitalis. The latter is particularly important in immunocompromised patients as the appearance of herpetic lesions in these patients is often one or more slowly enlarging ulcers. The differential diagnosis also includes granuloma inguinale, lymphogranuloma venereum, bacterial infections, squamous cell carcinoma,[123] Behçet's disease, fixed drug eruption, and causes of erosive balanitis or vulvitis such as candidiasis, psoriasis, Reiter's syndrome, and lichen planus.[124] All these entities can be differenti-

ated through clinical inspection coupled with cultures, smears, serology, and histopathologic examination.[125] Relapses of primary syphilis, termed *monorecidive* or *chancre redux,* are rare.[126]

Secondary Syphilis

Unfortunately, delays in diagnosis and treatment of syphilis resulting from physician failure to recognize the signs and symptoms of the secondary stage of the disease continue to be reported.[123] Not all patients present with a classic textbook picture. In fact, systemic signs, symptoms, and mucocutaneous manifestations may be subtle, transient, and easily overlooked, and the lesions can imitate other skin diseases. A wise clinician, probably once humbled by an earlier misdiagnosis, learns to include the "great imitator" when faced with clinical features that cannot be readily explained.[127] Because the clinical presentation results from propagation of spirochetes from a primary chancre, it has been suggested that *disseminated syphilis* is a better term for this stage of the disease. It is commonly stated that patients with secondary syphilis are ill with a flulike prodrome that can include malaise, appetite loss, fever, headache, stiff neck, lacrimation, myalgia,[128] arthralgia, nasal discharge, and depression. However, the majority of patients present with only an eruption.

Almost 60 percent of patients with latent or late syphilis deny a history of secondary disease, as the signs, unless severe, are easily overlooked and forgotten. One-quarter of these patients cannot recall the appearance of a chancre either.[129] The frequency of organ involvement differs somewhat among different studies.[123,130] In a series of 2269 cases of secondary syphilis, the skin was involved in 81.1 percent, the oral cavity and pharynx in 36.3 percent, the genitalia in 19.9 percent, the central nervous system in 9.9 percent, the eyes in 4 percent, and visceral organs in 0.2 percent.[123]

Cutaneous manifestations, termed *syphilids,* are observed in 80 to 95 percent of secondary syphilis cases.[131] Over 95 percent of the eruptions have one or four patterns: macular, maculopapular, papular, and annular.[131] Nodular and pustular syphilids are found less frequently, and vesiculobullous lesions are seen only in prenatal syphilis and not at all in adults. Lesions of secondary syphilis tend to have a symmetric pattern early in the disease and become polymorphic later. According to classic teachings, pruritus is generally not present, but in some reports between 8 to 42 percent of the patients experienced itching.[130,132] Pruritus appears to be more common in black and in immunocompromised patients. As a rule, the secondary lesions heal without scar formation in 2 to 10 weeks, with or without treatment. According to some reports, secondary syphilis has become less polymorphous and more predictable, but unusual cases are still being described.[133]

Macular Syphilid   Referred to in old textbooks as "roseola syphilitica," the eruption consists of nonscaling, pink, discrete, oval spots, about 1 to 2 cm in size, which predominantly involve the torso and flexor aspects of the upper extremities (Fig. 218-4). The exanthem may be confused with scarlet fever, which is macular at the start, or measles. The face is usually spared, but any area, including the palms and soles, can be involved. The macules do not tend to follow the lines of cleavage. Some lesions may progress to an annular or maculopapular morphology. The lesions, which are easily missed in blacks, usually begin 9 to 10 weeks following infection and 3 to 6 weeks after the chancre. Macular syphilids represent the earliest cutaneous manifestation of the secondary stage and have been reported to constitute about 10 percent of sec-

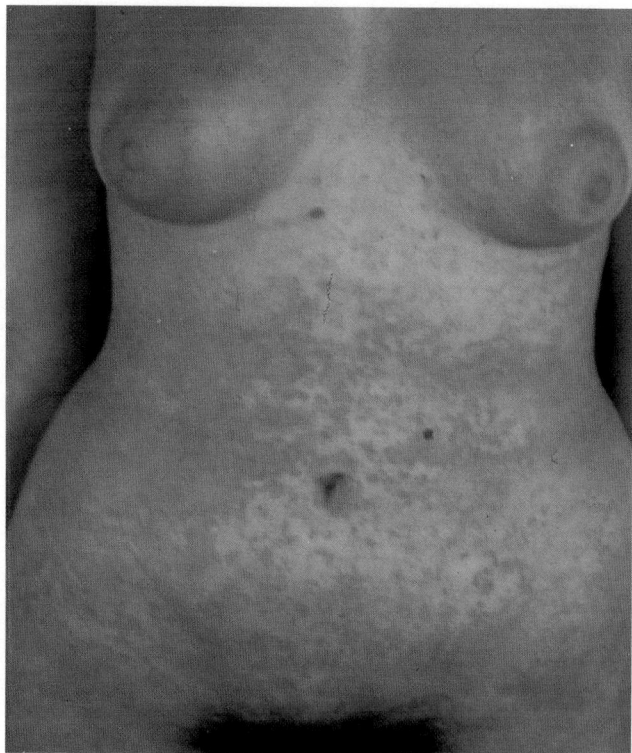

FIGURE 218-4 Macular secondary syphilis with discrete, pink, nonscaling, oval macules and small patches.

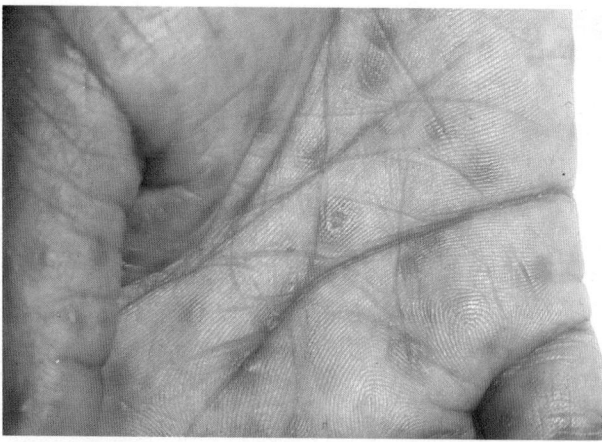

a

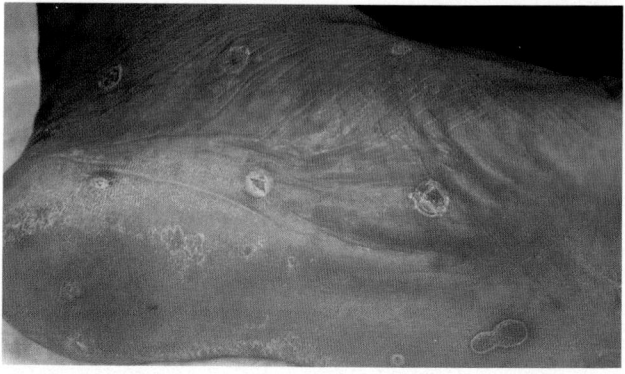

b

FIGURE 218-5 Scaly papular and macular lesions of the palms (*a*) and soles (*b*) are strongly suggestive of secondary syphilis.

ondary syphilis eruptions,[131] but in our experience, as well as others', they are rarer.[134]

Maculopapular Syphilid Reported in 22 to 70 percent of secondary syphilis cases,[131] this eruption is commonly encountered in practice. It represents an evolution of the macular syphilid as some lesions become thickened and develop a dark coppery hue. The genitalia and the face are often involved, especially the seborrheic areas and the hairline, giving a crownlike pattern known as the "corona veneris." The distinct brown-red macules and papules on the palms and soles are helpful in diagnosis (Fig. 218-5*a*, -5*b*).

Papular Syphilids This group of syphilids includes papulosquamous, follicular, lenticular, corymbose, nodular, and annular varieties.

1. *Papulosquamous syphilids* are discoid, copper-colored or erythematous, oval or circular, indurated papules or plaques with a flat, shiny, scaly surface (Fig. 218-6*a*, -6*b*). An annular, serpiginous, concentric (cockade syphilid), or arcuate configuration is often seen. When the lesions are pruritic and lichenoid, the eruption may be difficult to distinguish from lichen planus[135] and, when the scaling is thick, from psoriasis. The occasional presence of the Koebner phenomenon further contributes to this confusion. A thin, white ring of scales on the surface of the lesion, known as Biette's collarette (Fig. 218-7), is a helpful diagnostic sign, although, contrary to Dr. Biette's opinion, it is not pathognomonic. On the soles, the lesions may be hyperkeratotic and the infiltration diffuse, so that the condition may be mistaken for calluses (clavi syphilitici) or tinea.

2. *Follicular syphilids* have been called "lichen syphiliticus" or "miliary papular syphilids" and consist of pinpoint acuminate or rounded, erythematous papules that erupt in crops on the torso and extremities. This syphilid is uncommon and occurs predominantly in debilitated persons such as alcoholics.

3. *Lenticular syphilids* consist of pinhead to lentil size, brown to red papules with smooth surfaces or fine scaling. The face, especially the forehead, buccal commissures, and nasolabial folds, and the genitalia are the favored sites. Lesions do not coalesce.

4. *Corymbose ("bombshell") syphilids* are rare and seldom occur before 6 to 8 months of infection.[136] Typically a large central papule is surrounded by smaller satellite raised lesions. It has been suggested that these patients have immunologic disorders.

5. *Nodular syphilids* are being reported with increasing frequency in the modern era. The eruption is frequently misdiagnosed as lymphoma or a granulomatous process[137] (Fig. 218-8).

6. *Annular syphilids* (Fig. 218-9) consist of oval or round ringlike papules that occur predominantly in blacks and have a predilection for the face, anogenital area, body folds, palms, and soles.[131] Because the lesions in the face are approximately the size of coins, the eruption has been dubbed the "nickel and dime syphilid." Sarcoid, granuloma annulare, and tinea corporis are routinely mistaken for this syphilid.

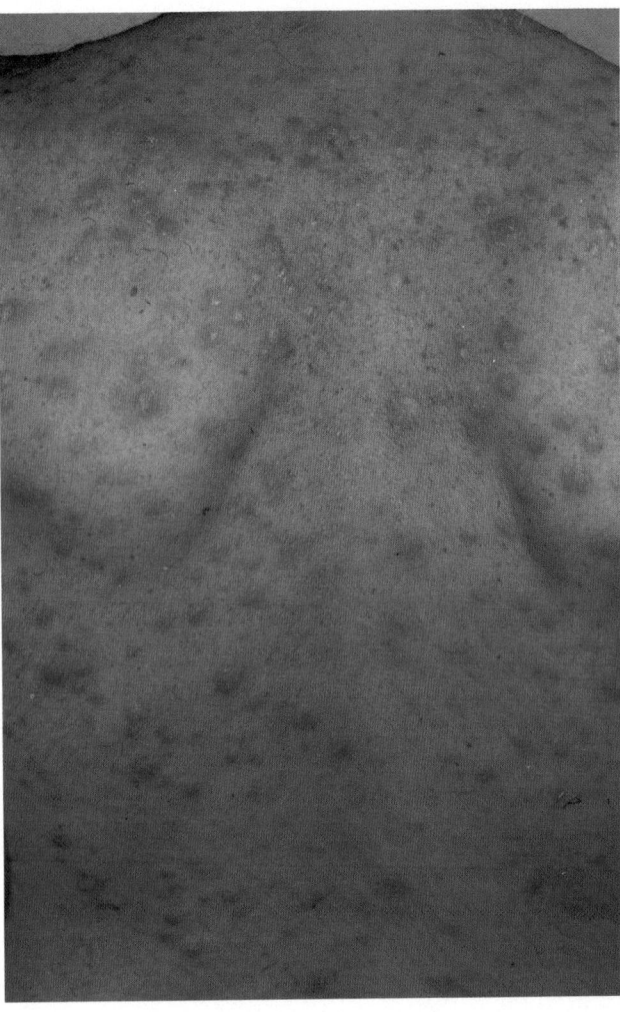

a

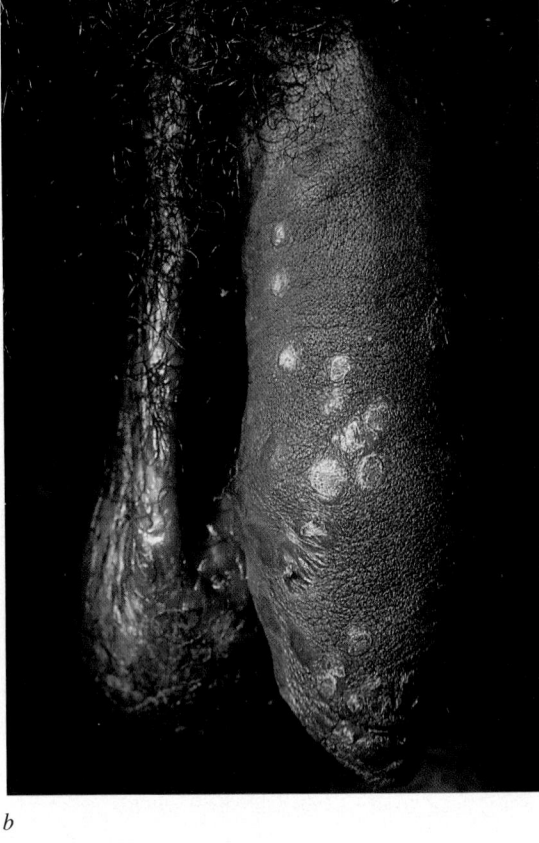

b

FIGURE 218-6 (*a*) Papulosquamous secondary eruption.
(*b*) The penile shaft is a frequently affected site.

Pustular Secondary Syphilids These eruptions encompass several morphologic variants. These include the *miliary pustular syphilid* with small, acuminate pustules and papules that resolve with depressed, pigmented scars[196]; *acneform, varioliform* (Fig. 218-10), or *obtuse syphilids* with large, acuminate perifollicular pustules,

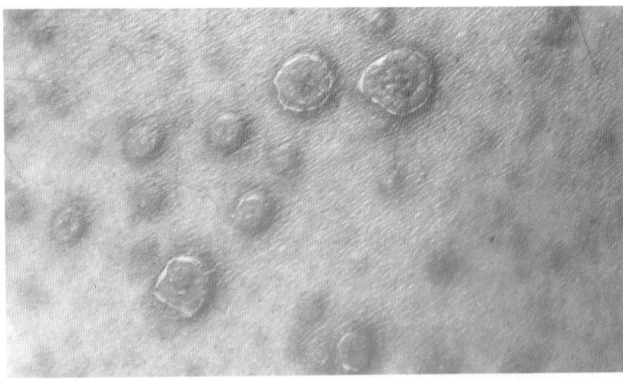

FIGURE 218-7 Secondary syphilis. Close up of pink papules of varying size with collarettes of fine scale and central crust in the larger lesions.

often with polyporphism[138]; and the *impetiginoid* or *ecthymiform syphilids* with flat pustules that become confluent and covered with a large crust called a carapace. A rare follicular papulopustular form has been associated with abnormal findings in cerebrospinal fluid.

Malignant syphilids, also known as "lues maligna," "rupial syphilid," or "pustuloulcerative syphilid," consist of widespread papulopustules. These become necrotic and break down to form ulcers covered by layers of thick, dirty crust that resemble an oyster shell ("rupioid") (Fig. 218-11).[139] The eruption, which involves predominantly the face and scalp, is associated with pain, toxicity, arthralgias, and occasionally hepatitis. In some cases, the lesions resemble chancres.[139] Oral ulcers and mucous patches are seen. Apparently this syphilid was more common in the seventeenth century, when it was known as "la grand verole." It has been reported that all patients with malignant syphilids have abnormal immune systems or preceding poor health, but recently reported cases argue against this.[140] With some exceptions, such as HIV-infected individuals,[141] most patients probably have a selective, undefined impairment in their ability to mount a normal immunologic response to *T. pallidum*.[131] Although, in one report, three cases were traced to the same source,[142] infected contacts usually have a more benign course, and no evidence supports the contention that the responsible treponeme is more virulent.

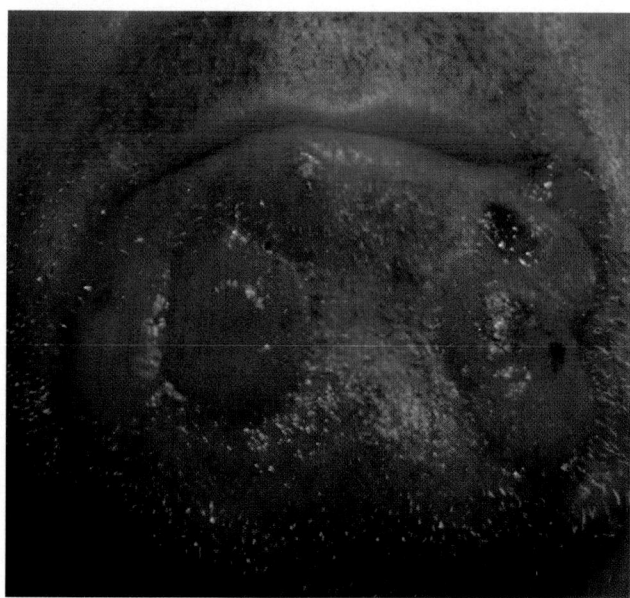

FIGURE 218-8   Nodular secondary syphilis lesions may be clinically misdiagnosed as lymphoma or granulomatous disease.

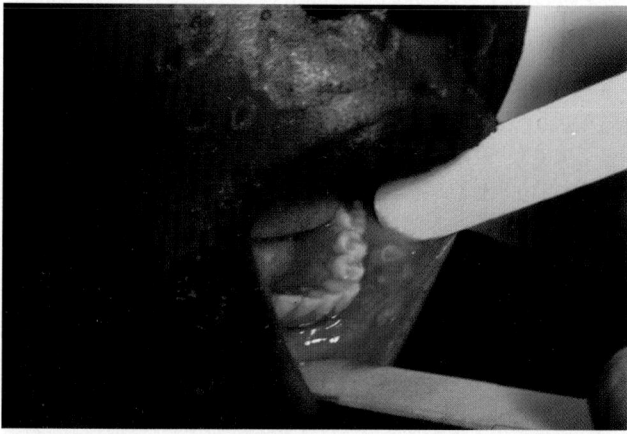

FIGURE 218-9   Annular syphilids occur predominantly in black individuals, often on the face.

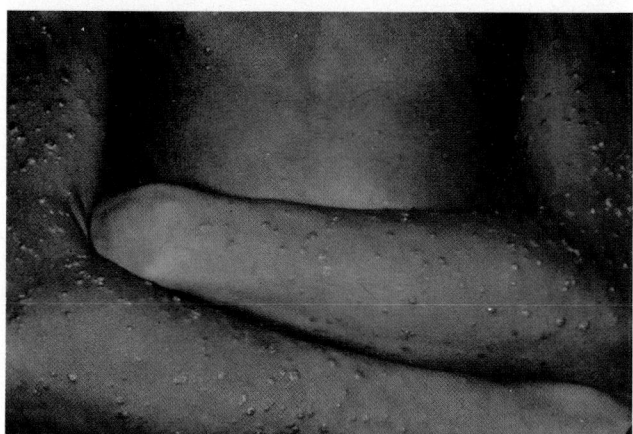

FIGURE 218-10   Varioliform type of pustular syphilid.

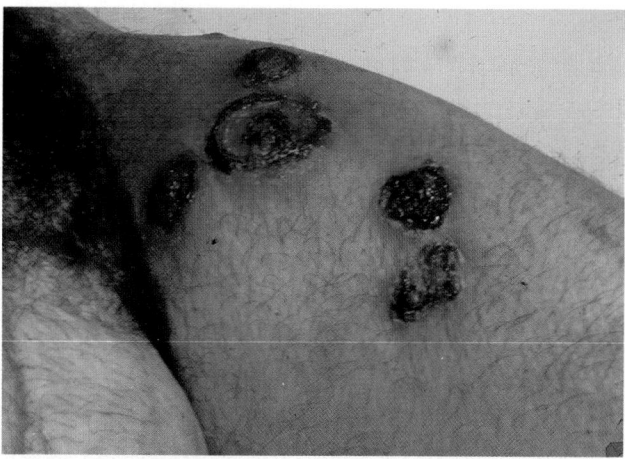

FIGURE 218-11   ''Rupioid'' or ''malignant'' syphilid with necrotic lesions that ulcerate and are covered by layers of dirty-appearing crusts.

Pigmentary Changes   Postinflammatory hyperpigmentation often follows healing. On the sides of the neck an interesting pattern consisting of hypopigmented macules superimposed on linear pigmented reticulated patches is known as ''leukoderma colli syphiliticum'' or the ''necklace of Venus.''[143] Similar lesions may occur on the penis as well as other areas.[144] In dark-skinned individuals intense loss of pigment within the affected areas may resemble vitiligo. When dermal atrophy, possibly related to inflammation-induced elastin degradation, is present, the appearance resembles anetoderma. Hypopigmentation in syphilis results from partial inhibition of melanogenesis, as the number of melanocytes is normal or only slightly reduced.[145]

Mucous Membrane Lesions   These moist lesions, which have been reported in 20 to 70 percent of patients with secondary syphilis, are full of spirochetes and extremely infectious. Three manifestations occur: condyloma lata, mucous patches, and pharyngitis. The last two heal spontaneously within 2 to 3 weeks, but condylomata persist for months.

    Condyloma lata consist of flesh-colored or hypopigmented, oozing papules that become flattened and macerated. Their surface may be smooth, papillated, or covered with cauliflower-like vegetations (Fig. 218-12). The common sites are the genital and anal areas and, less frequently, the buccal commissures, axilla, inframammary folds, and interdigital webs of toes. Lesions in intertriginous areas may erode or proliferate, forming elevated, brown, velvet-like plaques or grouped hypertrophic, nodular lesions that resemble raspberries (''frambesiform syphilid'').[146] Bacterial overgrowth produces a foul odor.

    Mucous patches are macerated, gray, rounded, flat papules present in as many as 20 percent of all cases. The epithelium sloughs off, leaving a nontender, denuded or abraded area anywhere in the mouth but especially on the tongue and lips (Fig. 218-13). The tonsils, epiglottis, and aryepiglottic folds may be affected, resulting in hoarseness. Confluence of several denuded lesions on the tongue has been termed ''plaques fauchées en prairie.'' At the labial commissures, slightly elevated mucous patches with central linear erosions, known as ''split papules,'' are sometimes seen in relapsing syphilis. Mucous patches also appear in the mucosal surface of the genitalia and anus. In these areas, papules are more likely to become eroded or ulcerated due to friction.

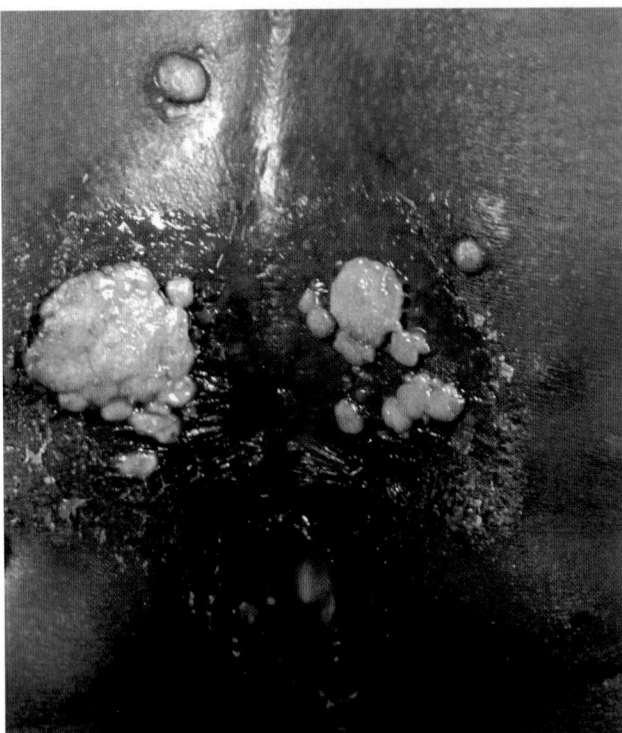

FIGURE 218-12 Condylomata lata. Cauliflower-like aggregations of hypopigmented, moist papules with smooth macerated surface.

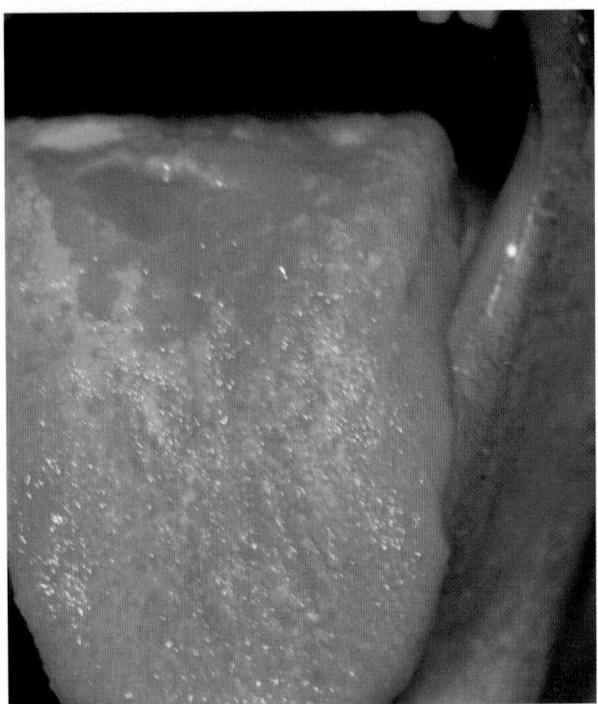

FIGURE 218-13 Mucous patch on the tongue.

Pharyngitis of variable degrees may be identified by an alert clinician in a quarter or so of cases, although sore throat is rare. Diffuse redness of the pharynx and tonsils may be very mild or severe with edema and erosions. Pseudomembranes and necrosis

have been reported, and laryngeal involvement may produce hoarseness.

Nail Changes In secondary syphilis, nail changes may be due to involvement of either the nail matrix, or the nail folds. In the nail plate, brittleness, splitting, onycholysis, pitting, lunular elkonyxis, fissuring (onyxis craquelé) and dystrophy have been described. The nail plate growing during the infectious episode may become dull, dry, and thickened or develop Beau's lines and latent onychomadesis. Amber-colored plates resembling artificial nails have been reported to be characteristic of late syphilis. Another presentation is paronychia of the lateral and proximal nail folds.[147] If prolonged, the skin can break down, leaving a horseshoe ulcer. Under the nail plate, an exudate forms that causes separation and even shedding of the nail plate, exposing an ulcerated nail bed. The new nail is deformed.

Alopecia Alopecia has been described in 3 to 7 percent of cases and includes two types. The more characteristic consists of small irregular patches of hair thinning throughout the scalp but predominantly on the occipital and parietal regions (Fig. 218-14). Because the margins are not sharp, the term *moth-eaten* is often used descriptively.[148] Occasionally the eyebrows, beard, and other hair-bearing areas are affected. Regardless of treatment, scars do not form, and the hair eventually regrows. The other type is a telogen effluvium that occurs 3 to 5 months after the infection begins.[130]

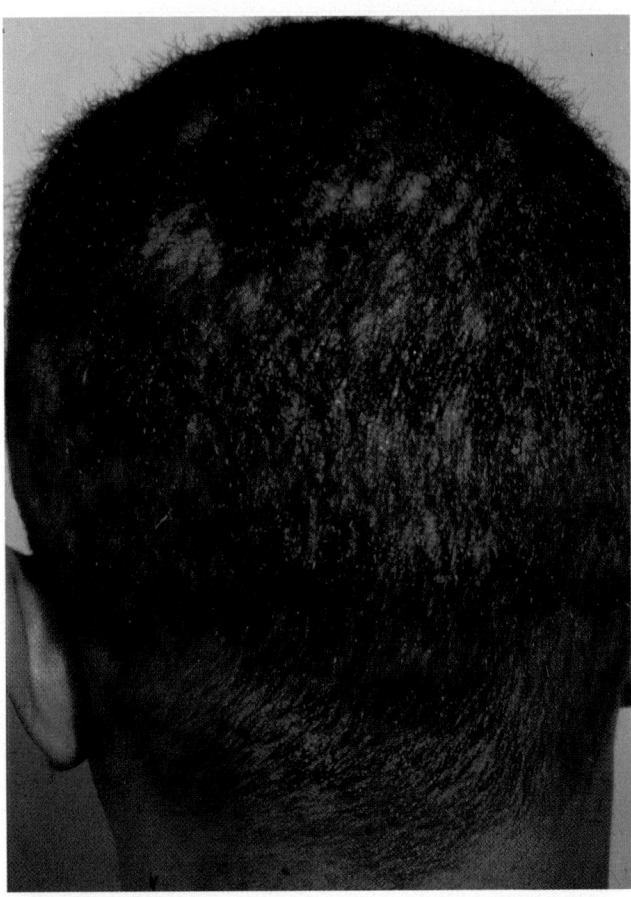

FIGURE 218-14 "Moth-eaten" alopecia with irregular patches of hair thinning.

Associated Clinical Manifestations

Lymphadenopathy   Enlarged nodes are present in over 85 percent of cases.[18] In descending order of frequency, the inguinal, axillary, cervical, epitrochlear, femoral, and supraclavicular chains are involved. Typically the nodes are movable, firm, rubbery, discrete, bilateral, symmetric, and nontender. Painful adenopathy, however, can occur[149] and in one report was associated with alcohol abuse.[150]

Mild splenomegaly is common. Other abnormalities include anemia, leukocytosis, relative lymphopenia, elevated sedimentation rate, and false-positive serologic tests.[151]

Renal   Acute membranous glomerulonephritis, usually manifested by the nephrotic syndrome, is reversible with treatment and resembles the glomerulopathy of prenatal syphilis. Deposition of C3 and treponemal antigen-antibody immune complexes has been demonstrated.[152,153]

Hepatic   Although usually subclinical, the incidence of hepatitis was 9.7 percent in one study and may be more common than has been accepted.[151,154] Jaundice is seldom detected. More typical presentations include tender hepatomegaly and an asymptomatic elevation of alkaline phosphatase or, in fewer cases, transaminases. The cause appears to be invasion of the liver by treponemes. Histopathologic examination shows a nonspecific reactive hepatitis and occasional cholestasis.[155]

Gastric   Epigastric pain and postprandial vomiting may be due to eroded, ulcerated or polypoidal stomach lesions that heal with antibiotics.[156] Erosive syphilitic gastritis usually affects the antrum of the stomach.

Ophthalmologic   Iritis, which is the most common eye complication, occurs in less than 3 percent of all cases and then, late in the disease, usually with relapsing syphilis. Condyloma lata may appear on the eyelids. Uveitis, chorioretinitis and rarely, vasculitic occlusion of the central retinal vein and artery are also observed.[157] Symptoms include photophobia; lacrimation; red, painful eyes; and blindness.[158] Topical corticosteroid administration without antibiotics is contraindicated. A number of eye manifestations have been reported in HIV infected patients with syphilis.[159]

Auditory   There are a few reports of sensorineural hearing loss in early acquired syphilis.[160] The condition worsens rapidly and tends to be bilateral.[161] Vestibular involvement with labyrinthitis is rare. The cause is usually basilar meningitis with damage to the eighth nerve. It has been estimated that, despite antibiotic therapy, 0.02 percent of early syphilis cases will develop meningitis and that 20 percent of these patients will experience eighth nerve disease.[162]

Musculoskeletal   Because bone and joint involvement is not readily apparent, the impression has been that it is rare. However, different studies have found rates ranging from 0.15 to 4 percent clinically and 9 percent radiologically.[163] The principal symptoms are local pain, erythema, doughy tumefaction, and warmth. Favored affected sites are the long bones of the extremities, especially the tibia, and the skull with resulting persistent headaches.

Radiographs and more sensitive bone scans demonstrate any combination of periostitis, osteomyelitis, bone destruction, and sclerosis.[164–166] Radiographic changes may take up to 11 months for complete resolution.[165] Back pain, arthralgias, arthritis, teno-synovitis, and bursitis, which have been reported in as many as 4 percent of all cases, may be severe and persist for several months.[163,167]

Generalized myalgias are common in the secondary stage, and muscle weakness may occasionally imitate an inflammatory myopathy.[168] Contractures of the biceps rarely occurs in early syphilis.

Cardiopulmonary   Lesions in the lungs[169] and heart conduction defects[170] have been reported but are extremely rare.

Neurologic   Abnormal findings in the cerebrospinal fluid are commonly observed in early syphilis and will be discussed in the section on neurosyphilis.

Relapsing Syphilis

After the initial secondary stage has cleared, around 25 percent of untreated patients will experience recrudescence of secondary lesions, despite the absence of reinfection. The manifestations include reappearance of typical chancres or any of the characteristic eruptions associated with secondary syphilis, including mucous patches, split papules, and condyloma lata. These lesions tend to be less extensive and are frequently confined to the genital, anal, and oral areas. Because patients may be unaware of the lesions or insufficiently concerned to seek medical help, relapsing syphilis is particularly alarming from an epidemiologic standpoint.[131] Other presentations include periostitis, usually over the tibia; iritis; and hepatitis.

Histopathology of Early Syphilis

The histologic changes in the primary stage depend on the area of the chancre examined (Fig. 218-15). In the border of the lesion the epidermis is slightly acanthotic, whereas towards the center, it becomes thinner, edematous, and penetrated by lymphocytes. As expected in an ulcer, the epidermis is missing in the center. The dermal infiltrate is composed predominantly of lymphocytes and plasma cells with only a few histiocytes and neutrophils. It is dense near the center of the lesion but in the periphery is limited to the perivascular areas. This infiltrate extends into the vessel walls. The capillaries show endothelial proliferation and swelling. Unless antibiotics have been taken, numerous spirochetes can be demonstrated with silver stains or labeled specific antibodies in the epidermal and dermal layers, particularly around the capillaries.

In secondary syphilis, the histologic findings, as expected from the diverse cutaneous manifestations, are variable.[171] Macules have no epidermal changes, whereas the epidermis of papulosquamous lesions shows psoriasiform epidermal hyperplasia, parakeratosis, and often focal spongiosis, basal vacuolar changes, and microabscesses with neutrophils.[55,171] Other common epidermal changes are epidermal pallor, keratinocyte necrosis, extravasated red blood cells, and exocytosis of mononuclear cells.[171] The diagnosis may be difficult to differentiate clinically and histologically from psoriasis[55] or lymphoma.[149] The lichenoid infiltrate, which contains many plasma cells, may involve both the superficial and deep dermis and, in one-third of the cases, surrounds adnexal, vascular, and neural structures. The infiltrate may also be T-shaped or perivascular. As the lesions become older, small epithelioid granulomas, which may have Langhans or foreign-body type giant cells, become more numerous.[171,172]

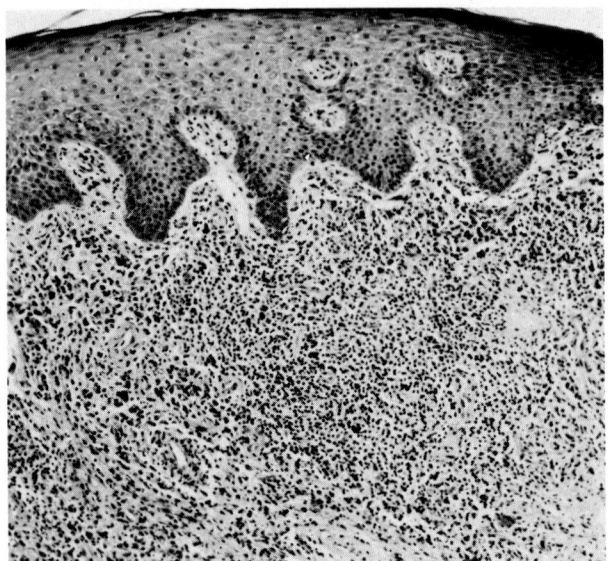

FIGURE 218-15 Primary syphilis, the chancre. The process is characterized by a dense infiltrate of inflammatory cells, including lymphocytes, histiocytes, and plasma cells. Vascular spaces are frequently difficult to identify due to endothelial swelling.

Dilatation and thickening of the blood vessels, which usually show a proliferation of swollen vacuolated endothelial cells, are the most common findings and have been reported in half to almost all of studied cases.[173] It should be noted that in up to 25 percent of the cases, the changes are not diagnostic because vascular changes are not evident and plasma cells are scant or absent. Therefore, the pathologist should be alerted when syphilis is a diagnostic consideration so that appropriate stains are done.[55] A central epidermal invagination with a hyperkeratotic plug containing parakeratotic cells is the typical finding in *syphilis cornée*. Lesions of condyloma lata are histologically similar to those of papular syphilis. The only difference is that the epithelium is more hyperplastic and edematous. The lesions of malignant syphilis ulcerate due to epidermal and dermal necrosis, which results from vascular occlusion caused by the severe endothelial changes and fibrinoid deposition in the vessel wall.[174] In some cases, the distinction between late secondary and early tertiary syphilis can be difficult because epithelioid granulomas are usually present in both.[175] Moreover, granulomas may be absent in some tertiary lesions, and the presence of numerous plasma cells and vascular changes resemble secondary syphilis.

The lymph nodes in early syphilis are infiltrated with chronic inflammation that includes abundant plasma cells. Follicular hyperplasia, endothelial proliferation, and, at times, noncaseating granulomas are also present.[3] When treponemes cannot be identified with silver stains, immunologic methods can help. Immunoperoxidase staining of the organisms with anti-T-pallidum antiserum and a goat-antirabbit IgG-horseradish peroxidase conjugate can be done in formalin-fixed, paraffin-embedded tissue.[176] Direct immunofluorescence testing with fluorescein-labeled syphilitic rabbit serum requires frozen sections.[177] These techniques are so sensitive that recently the diagnosis of tertiary syphilis was made on the exhumed mummified body of an Italian noblewoman who died in 1568 at the age of 65.[178]

Latent Syphilis

If untreated, the next stage of syphilis is an asymptomatic state in which the only manifestation is reactive serologic testing. Due to the frequency of false-positive nontreponemal tests, the reactivity is always confirmed with a more specific treponemal serologic test. This latent stage may continue as such for life or may be interrupted by relapse or tertiary disease. Being a diagnosis of exclusion, it is assumed that careful examination for mucocutaneous lesions and organ involvement has been conducted. Evaluation of the heart and aorta with radiographs or ultrasound studies is recommended. Also, neurosyphilis should be excluded by examination of the cerebrospinal fluid (CSF), although, due to concern about complications from the procedure, a spinal tap is now seldom done unless neurologic signs or symptoms are present. This is unfortunate because it allows some cases of asymptomatic neurosyphilis to pass unnoticed until irreversible damage occurs. Documentation of inadequate antibiotic levels measured in the CSF during benzathine penicillin administration and reports of rapid progression to neurosyphilis in treated HIV-infected patients reinforce the need to diagnose CNS infection before symptoms develop. The duration of infection should be determined by history and previous serologic tests, because, for therapeutic and epidemiologic purposes, the latent stage is divided into early and late periods, as previously discussed. However, this may not always be possible, and the clinician must settle for a diagnosis of ''indeterminate'' latency, which is treated in the same manner as late latent disease. Likewise, an investigation of previous treatment should be undertaken, for, in latent syphilis, nontreponemal tests may remain elevated for months or years after adequate therapy or be persistently elevated due to a ''serofast'' state. If treatment or lack of reinfection cannot be confirmed, then, from a public health standpoint, these patients should be assumed to be infected and should be treated. A record of the nontreponemal test titer and the administered therapy should be given to the patient. Too often, patients are unnecessarily re-treated over and over again because such records are not readily available.

Benign Tertiary (Late) Syphilis

This designation includes any symptomatic syphilitic manifestation, after the secondary and relapsing stages, that does not involve the cardiovascular or nervous systems. At the turn of the century, the incidence in untreated men and women was 14.4 and 16.7, respectively,[76] but now this stage is rarely seen. In the United Kingdom, the incidence varied between 1.81 to 4.56 new cases per 100,000 population from 1976 to 1980.[179] The decline may reflect inadvertent treatment of syphilis through widespread use of antibiotics for other infections rather than a change in the course of the disease. The more commonly involved organs are the skin (70 percent), mucous membranes (10.3 percent), and bones (9.6 percent), but the characteristic lesions, gummas, may appear in practically any organ system. The skin is affected in over half the patients with involvement of more than one organ. Spontaneous healing of the gumma does not usually occur.[179]

Evidence such as the development of gummas at the inoculation site in two volunteers previously treated for syphilis supported the theory that gummas develop at the site of reactivation of endogenous foci of treponemes in previously sensitized individuals who are reinfected or inadequately treated.[180]

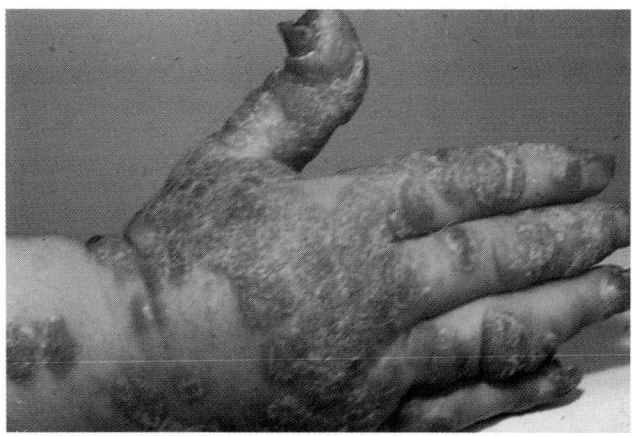
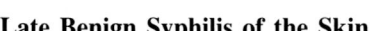

FIGURE 218-16 Late benign syphilis showing nodules and plaques with different configurations and waxy scale, which resemble psoriasis.

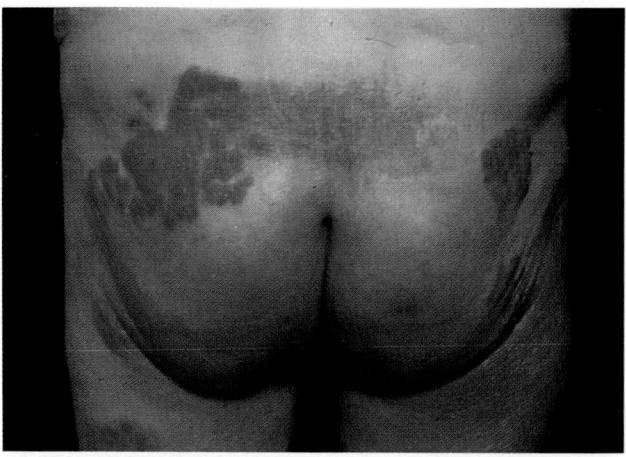

FIGURE 218-17 Sarcoid-like granulomatous plaques of late benign syphilis.

Late Benign Syphilis of the Skin

Cutaneous manifestations may develop any time after the secondary stage resolves, with "precocious" lesions noted within the first 2 years and the late syphilids between 2 to 30 years. In general, most cases occur within 3 to 7 years. Isolated examples of gummas have appeared as long as 60 years after infection. Such late-developing lesions are generally associated with neurosyphilis. The longer the interval before the appearance of the skin lesions, the more solitary and destructive the process.

Serologic tests for syphilis are usually but not always reactive with high titers. Even without therapy, there is a tendency to partial healing, but new lesions occur on the periphery, and spontaneous complete healing is unusual.[76] Scarring is notable for its noncontractile and atrophic quality. Skin lesions in benign tertiary syphilis are classified into precocious syphilids and late syphilids. Late syphilids include nodules and noduloulcerative lesions, pseudochancre redux, and gummas. The nodular tertiary syphilid differs from the gummatous syphilid in that the lesions are more superficial. All cases respond dramatically to penicillin.

Precocious tertiary syphilids were somewhat common in the preantibiotic era. The lesions usually occurred during the first 4 years of infection but occasionally appeared within weeks in a particularly aggressive precocious form. The skin manifestations have characteristics that border between secondary and late cutaneous lesions and consist of localized or generalized grouped papules with some degree of ulceration. Treponemes are rarely demonstrated, and the lesions heal with little or no scarring.

Nodular and noduloulcerative lesions (tubercular syphilids) begin as superficial, firm, pink to purple, papules or nodules that measure several millimeters to 2 cm in size. The lesions appear in a grouped configuration, rapidly extending peripherally in an irregular manner. Over weeks or months, central healing and advancing borders produce plaques with annular, arciform, serpiginous or polycyclic configurations that may reach over 30 cm. Occasionally, waxy scales may impart a psoriasiform character (Fig. 218-16), and the lesions may also closely resemble granuloma annulare, sarcoid, or lupus vulgaris (Fig. 218-17). In contrast to the latter, they are firmer. As the nodules grow, the skin appears red and eventually breaks down, resulting in ulcerations with raised borders

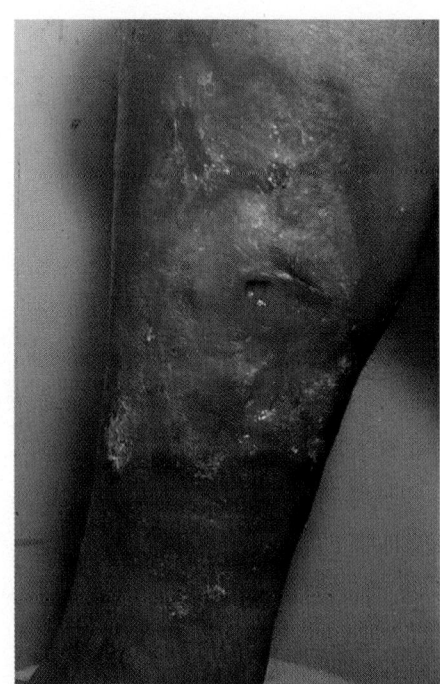

FIGURE 218-18 Noduloulcerative late syphilid.

and slightly purulent, crusted surfaces (Fig. 218-18). These are asymptomatic and have a predilection for the extensor arms, back, and face. Even if untreated, the lesions heal over the years, leaving noncontractile, atrophic scars with increased or decreased pigmentation.

Gummas are painless pink to dusky red nodules of various sizes (Fig. 218-19). The lesions, which favor sites of previous trauma, may occur anywhere in the body but are more common on the scalp, forehead, buttocks, and presternal, supraclavicular, or pretibial areas. Ulceration may occur and is typically cylindrical, punched out, and covered with adherent yellowish-white slough. The ulcer has a clean granulomatous base and may increase in size, remain unchanged, or heal spontaneously. More superficial gummas heal with noncontractile atrophic scars, whereas deeper lesions

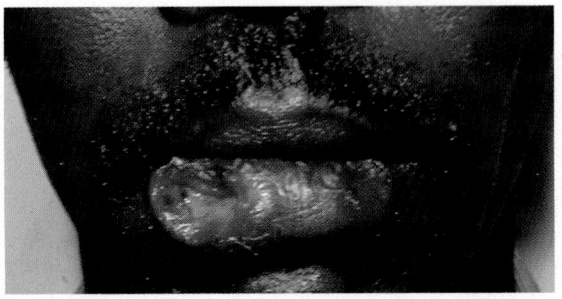

FIGURE 218-19 Ulcerated gumma on the lower lip.

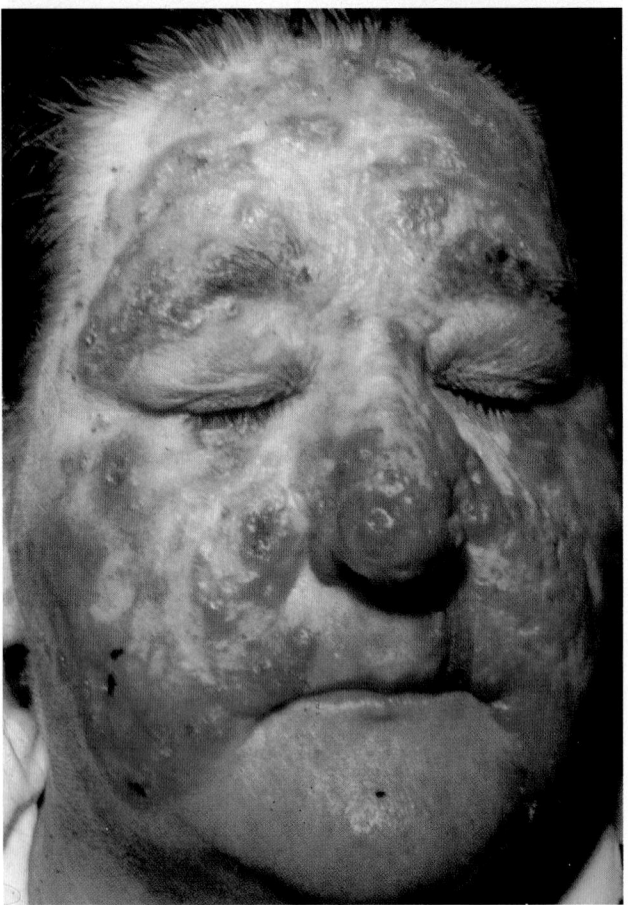

FIGURE 218-20 Large gummas on the face with central clearing and scalloped borders, which have small abscesses and ulcerations.

leave thickened, pitted, ridged scars. Characteristically, the nodule feels rubbery, but with accumulation of necrotic tissue, the lesion develops the consistency of a cold abscess. When gummas spread laterally with small ulcerations and abscesses, they may be indistinguishable from noduloulcerative syphilids (Fig. 218-20). Large gummas may have several skin perforations and undergo necrotic changes that cause destruction of the intervening bridges of skin. Various geometric configurations are assumed. As the central gumma heals, new lesions develop on the periphery, forming scalloped borders. Gummas are rarely contagious, but transfer of infection from the lesions has been reported. Histopathologic findings

include an infiltrate of lymphocytes, histiocytes, plasma cells, and fibroblasts as well as granulomas with caseation necrosis surrounded by epithelioid and giant cells. The blood vessels show endothelial swelling and, less frequently, luminal narrowing, wall thinning, and cellular infiltration. In the skin the infiltrate involves the dermis and subcutaneous tissues. Noduloulcerative lesions differ in that the granulomas are limited to the dermis, and necrosis is minimal or absent except when ulceration occurs. Demonstration of *T. pallidum* is difficult even with indirect immunofluorescence.[77]

Pseudochancre redux is a term describing a solitary gumma of the penis.

Mucous Membrane Lesions of Late Benign Syphilis

The most commonly involved mucous membranes are the palate and the bony and cartilaginous structures of the nose. Ulcers in these areas may cause destruction (saddle nose) (Fig. 218-21) or perforations that sometimes persist despite treatment. Gummas, nodules, and diffuse inflammation, with ulcers covered by a gray slough, may appear in the tonsils and pharynx. The lips and buccal membranes are rarely affected. Lesions on the tongue consist of either a single, elastic, painless tumor, which undergoes necrosis and ulceration, or a diffuse, gummatous infiltration, which often develops into a chronic interstitial glossitis with superficial, atrophic changes or deep fissuring (Fig. 218-22). These chronic interstitial or superficial changes remain precancerous even after adequate therapy for syphilis and must be periodically examined. Gummas of the larynx may produce hoarseness or aphonia, but involvement of the trachea and bronchi is rare. Late syphilis of the lung may be manifested by chronic pulmonary infection with miliary lesions, a mass, or pleural effusion and can be confused with tuberculosis.

Late Syphilis of Bone and Joints

Skeletal changes occur commonly and are classified as gummatous osteitis, periostitis, and sclerosing osteitis.[181] The bones most commonly affected are the tibia, clavicle, skull, fibula, femur, and humerus, but the disease can involve almost any osseous structure. The chief symptoms are nocturnal pain and swelling, and the most common sign is tenderness. Radiographic examinations are rarely helpful unless signs or symptoms of bone disease are present.

Gummatous osteitis is a destructive or osteomyelitic lesion associated with periosteal and/or osteal changes, with varying degrees of sclerosis occurring in neighboring bone. Swelling and sinus tract formation of surrounding soft tissues are commonly observed. A common site is the sternal end of the clavicle. Localized osteoporosis, which is frequently confused with tuberculosis or neoplasm, tends to occur at the diaphysis of long bones and rarely at the shaft.

Periostitis is characterized by periosteal thickening and a localized density that is similar to cortical bone. It often appears as a laminated periosteal reaction, but a more exuberant lacy pattern or diffuse thickening can be accompanied by destruction of bone.[182]

Sclerosing osteitis, in which a gumma may be small or obscure, represents a lesion with increased density and is usually accompanied by a periosteal reaction. Other manifestations include obliteration of the marrow cavity (ivory bone), which may be confused with tuberculosis or tumor. Lesions in the lamina externa of the skull (caries sicca) are usually a reliable sign of late benign

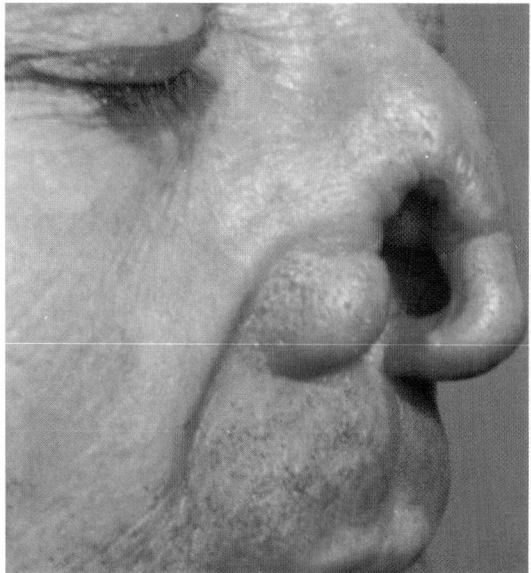
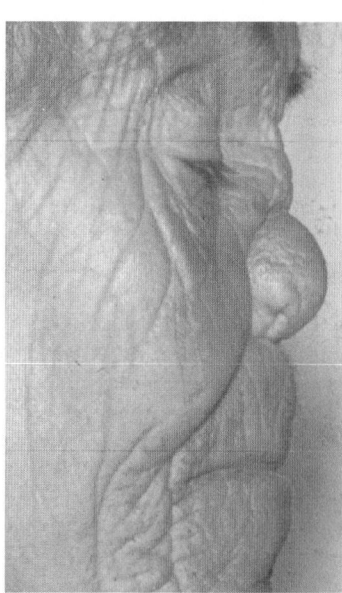

FIGURE 218-21 (*a*) Nasal perforation due to nasal gumma; (*b*) saddle nose following gummatous destruction of nasal bone. (*Courtesy of Klaus Wolff, M.D.*)

a

b

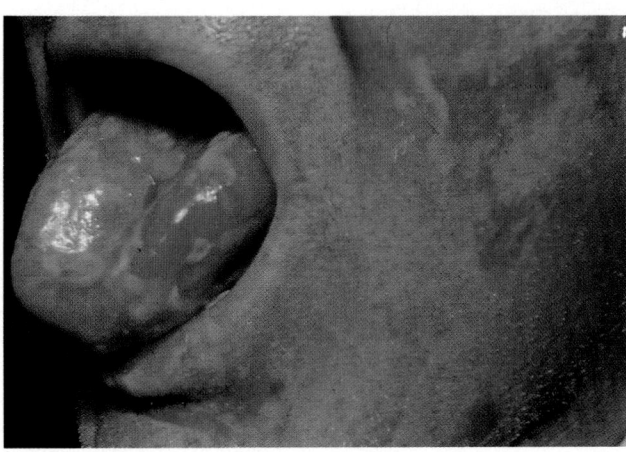

FIGURE 218-22 Syphilitic chronic interstitial glossitis with superficial, atrophic, leukoplakic changes.

syphilis. Antisyphilitic therapy decreases the symptoms and progression of disease, but bone lesions heal slowly.

Joint manifestations of late syphilis include arthralgias, synovitis, and arthritis and are caused by adjacent periostitis or gummatous infiltration from adjacent bone or skin lesions. Occasionally, bilateral syphilitic bursitis (of Verneuil) ulcerates, exposing the gelatinoid bursal contents. Juxtaarticular nodes, or "fibroid gummata," are multilobed, firm lesions occurring beneath the skin in the region of joints. The nodes enlarge slowly, sometimes ulcerate, and respond to antibiotics.

Late Benign Syphilis of Other Organ Systems

Almost any visceral organ may be affected in late tertiary syphilis. Late syphilis of the gastrointestinal tract includes involvement of the parotid glands (parotitis or gumma), esophagus (gummatous obstruction), stomach (gumma presenting as peptic ulcer or scirrhous carcinoma), and liver (hepar lobatum caused by multiple

gummas). Although seldom clinically enlarged in late syphilis, the spleen has, in rare instances, been found to contain gummas at autopsy. Gummas may also appear in the pancreas, kidneys, heart, brain, bladder, cervix, breasts, thyroid, and adrenal glands. Late syphilis of the eye is rare and appears in the form of a chronic iritis, chorioretinitis, interstitial keratitis, and atrophy of the optic nerve. Painless, fibrosing interstitial orchitis can result in atrophy. The diagnosis of benign tertiary syphilis is made through a combination of clinical findings confirmed by serologic tests and histopathologic examination.

Cardiovascular Syphilis

Presently regarded as a "medical curiosity," cardiovascular syphilis was still responsible for 1492 deaths between 1976 and 1985.[182] In the Oslo study, the disease was clinically apparent in 13.6 percent of males and 7.6 percent of females and was the primary cause of death in 15.1 percent of males and 8.2 percent of females.[76]

Although myocardial disease may be the presenting manifestation, in essence, cardiovascular syphilis is a disease of the aorta.[182,183] This fact was first recognized in the sixteenth century by Ambrose Pare, who, nevertheless, erred in attributing the cause of the aneurysm to a complication of treatment. Even in 1875, William Welch's report that syphilis was a cause of aortic aneurysms was ignored until, 30 years later, Reuter demonstrated spirochetes within the vessel walls in active aortitis.

Presumably, during the early stages of syphilis, treponemes invade the aortic wall, where they can remain dormant indefinitely. The organism's predilection for the ascending aorta is probably explained by the large number of lymphatics and vasa vasorum in this portion of the vessel. Infiltration of the vasa vasorum in the intima layer by lymphocytes and plasma cells produces an obliterative endarteritis, which, over the years, weakens the wall of the aorta. The inflammatory changes also impair the blood flow to the aortic media. This results in necrosis of the muscular and elastic tissues of this layer and consequential scarring. Fibrous thickening of the adventitia and atherosclerotic plaques in the intima impart the "tree bark" appearance that is highly suggestive of syphilis. Spotty calcification of the plaques outline the descending aorta and produce the radiologic sign termed *eggshell calcification*. The histopathologic appearance of chronic syphilitic aortitis consists of thin, uneven, serpiginous scars that are analogous to healed skin lesions. Miliary gummas are common in the adventitia.

Prior to the introduction of penicillin, syphilis accounted for 25 to 30 percent and 5 to 10 percent of all cardiac disease occurring in blacks and Caucasian patients respectively. In one study the manifestations included aortic insufficiency in 5.3 percent, saccular aneurysms in 2.5 percent, osteal stenosis in 0.5 percent, and uncomplicated aortitis, discovered at autopsy, in 0.03 percent. Men are affected three times more often than women. Cardiovascular syphilis is found predominantly in acquired syphilis and only in individuals who are infected after the age of 14. Since overt clinical cardiovascular disease occurs around 15 to 30 years following initial infection, most patients are between 40 and 55 years of age. Only 7 percent of cases with cardiovascular syphilis develop symptoms or signs within 5 years of infection.

Uncomplicated aortitis occurs predominantly in the ascending aorta, with fewer than 10 percent of the cases involving the abdominal aorta and only 2 percent affecting the portion below the renal artery. The disease comprises between 27 and 36 percent of cardiovascular syphilis cases but is asymptomatic and is usually found inadvertently at postmortem examination.[184] The diagnosis is suspected when linear calcifications of the anterolateral aortic wall are present in chest radiographs. Such symptoms as angina and congestive heart failure are not usually due to aortitis, but rather to associated atherosclerosis, hypertension, or more advanced aortic disease.

Aortic aneurysms reportedly form between 3 to 5 years following development of aortitis. Focal weakening of the wall results in a saccular aneurysm, whereas diffuse weakening produces fusiform involvement of the ascending and transverse aorta with subsequent dilation of the aortic ring. Aneurysms comprise 20 percent of cases with cardiovascular syphilis.[185] The number is actually 40 percent if patients who also have coronary, ostial, or aortic valvular disease are included.[186] Over 60 percent of aneurysms involve the ascending aorta, and 25 percent affect the transverse arch.[187] Abdominal aneurysms, which usually form above the renal arteries, occur about one-tenth as infrequently as thoracic lesions. Uncommonly, fusiform or saccular aneurysms form in the innominate artery and present with symptoms of cerebral emboli.[187] Presumably because of the thickened vessel wall and cicatricial changes in the media, aortic aneurysms rarely dissect.[188] However, the variety of symptoms and signs moved William Osler to admit that "there is no disease more conducive to clinical humility than aneurysms of the aorta."

Compression of the bronchi or trachea may cause respiratory obstruction, cough, hemoptysis, or atelectasis, and impingement on the recurrent laryngeal nerve leads to hoarseness. Flushing, distension of the superficial veins of the head and neck, edema, drowsiness, seizures, and other symptoms of the superior vena cava syndrome may occur.[189] Direct pressure on the sternum or rib cage produces chest discomfort, and erosion of the vertebrae causes back pain. About 60 percent of syphilitic abdominal aneurysms present as a palpable, pulsating mass. Less often, a mass in the chest wall, which erodes through the anterior chest wall, is the earliest sign of an ascending aortic aneurysm. One third of all cases die from spontaneous rupture.[190] The treatment of syphilitic aneurysm is surgical.

Coronary ostial stenosis, found in 25 to 30 percent of cases of cardiovascular syphilis, is believed to result from aortitis.[191] In addition, 90 percent of patients with diseased coronary ostia have aortic vascular involvement, as would be expected from the close proximity of these two structures. However, only one of 35 cases in a recent report had concommitant aortitis.[192] The condition is difficult to differentiate from atherosclerotic heart disease as angina pectoris and congestive heart failure with diffuse myocardial fibrosis are the usual findings. Clues to the cause of the angina are the relative young age of the patient, the poor response to vasodilators, and concomitant aortic regurgitation. Characteristically, the pain is most intense at night. The demonstration of coronary ostial narrowing without angiographic evidence of atherosclerosis in a patient with reactive syphilis serology strongly implies the diagnosis. Acute myocardial infarction is uncommon because ostial narrowing occurs gradually, permitting an adequate collateral circulation to form. When ostial obstruction occurs precipitously, the myocardial ischemia is so extensive that the patient usually dies instantaneously. In the absence of coronary artery bypass surgery, the prognosis is poor.[193]

Aortic valvular disease is a common manifestation of cardiovascular syphilis and is seen in about 30 percent of patients with tertiary disease. It is a very late complication caused by dilation of the aortic ring and subsequent fibrosis and shrinkage of the valvular leaflets. The resulting aortic insufficiency results in regurgitation of blood back into the left verticle, producing a volume overload and, eventually, hypertrophy and dilation of the chamber. Due to vasodilation of the peripheral circulation, a low diastolic pressure and a warm flush appear. However, the condition is usually asymptomatic until severe enough to produce congestive heart failure. The characteristic physical finding is a soft diastolic blowing murmur heard best over the second right intercostal space. If the pulse pressure is significantly wide, a ventricular diastolic gallop with a tambour-like quality of the second heart sound, or a diastolic, rumbling, "Austin Flint" murmur may be audible at the apex. Chest radiographs and electrocardiograms will be consistent with cardiomegaly, which is said to be greater in syphilitic than in other etiologies of aortic regurgitation.

Without treatment, the prognosis is so dismal that in one series more than half the patients died within 3 years after the onset of congestive heart failure.[194] Therefore, the valve should be replaced as soon as cardiac decompensation symptoms or chest pain begin. Surgical intervention is quite successful when undertaken before the left ventricle has been grossly hypertrophied and deformed.[195]

Myocardial disease occurs in only 2.4 percent of cardiovascular syphilis cases.[196] The gummas may be single or multiple, small or large, and localized or scattered. The latter results in a diffuse gummatous myocarditis. The most frequently involved locations are the left ventricle and the ventricular septum, where gummas can cause heart block and conduction defects.[197] Cases of myocardial aneurysm and rupture of the ventricle or papillary muscles as a result of gummas are exceedingly rare.

In summary, cardiovascular disease is an uncommon but life-threatening manifestation of late syphilis that is usually treatable if diagnosed early. Before casually dismissing reactive serologic tests as indicative of latent syphilis, the clinician needs to consider the possibility of cardiovascular pathology in every patient.

Neurosyphilis

Neurosyphilis has become so rare, that even neurologists familiar with the disease disagree on the diagnosis of recently reported cases.[198] In the pre-penicillin era, neurosyphilis developed in 9.4

percent of males and 5.0 percent of females with untreated syphilis and constituted about 29 percent of syphilis cases examined in an urban tertiary care hospital. Central nervous system (CNS) disease developed among those infected under the age of 15 but rarely after the age of 40. Symptoms seldom appear until 5 to 35 years after the initial infection.

In 1976, when the Centers for Disease Control last recorded statistics for neurosyphilis, there were 2903 reported cases out of a total of 71,761 syphilis patients. Now, the number of patients appears to be rising. In part, this is due to accelerated progression to neurosyphilis associated with HIV infection, but even before this epidemic, an increase in cases had been reported from several western European countries.

Essentially, neurosyphilis is a chronic meningitis that can involve the blood vessels and parenchymal tissue of the brain and spinal cord.[199] Presumably, hematogenous dissemination of spirochetes to the CNS occurs in early syphilis. Using auditory electrical analysis, subclinical brainstem lesions have been detected in 6 of 11 cases of secondary and latent syphilis.[200] Treponemes are reportedly found in the CSF of 15 to 40 percent of patients with early syphilis.[201] In one study, T. pallidum was cultured from half the patients with secondary syphilis, the only patient with primary syphilis, and none with latent syphilis. However, in other reports, around 16 percent of patients with indeterminate latent syphilis had reactive CSF serologies and pleocytosis and, of these, one-quarter were asymptomatic.

As the early syphilis stages abate, the spirochetes presumably remain dormant if the patients are untreated and, in some situations, reportedly even after treatment. In others, asymptomatic neurosyphilis either persists or, in 5 to 10 percent of cases, progresses to tabes or paresis or meningovascular disease. The protean nervous system manifestations caused by syphilis defy exact categorization, especially since the pathologic reactions and clinical syndromes often overlap, but the Merrit classification (Table 218-2) is widely used.[202] This scheme divides neurosyphilis into asymptomatic, meningeal, meningovascular, parenchymatous, and gummatous.

Asymptomatic neurosyphilis indicates the presence of CSF abnormalities due to T. pallidum in the absence of neurologic clinical signs or symptoms.[203] The diagnosis is made from clinical findings and serologic tests.[204] Nontreponemal assays may be nonreactive in as many as 39 percent of patients,[201] but treponemal tests are almost always positive in the serum as well as in the CSF. Before the introduction of penicillin, between 23 and 87 percent of the cases progressed to clinical neurologic disease. Notably, neurosyphilis does not always become symptomatic or cause obvious neurologic damage.

Meningeal and vascular syphilis may occur early or late. *Acute syphilitic meningitis,* which suggests a septic meningitis, occurs during the first 12 months of infection and is accompanied by a secondary syphilis eruption in 10 percent of the cases.[200] *Chronic meningitis* presents within the first 5 years of infection and produces signs and symptoms associated with the cerebral cortex, optic nerve area, and posterior fossa. Hydrocephalus from CSF obstruction, cranial nerve palsies, and thrombosis of small cortical vessels result in a varied constellation of symptoms. Common complaints are headache, neck stiffness, and fever. Papilledema, usually with little loss of vision, is a principal finding of hydrocephalus. The more commonly involved nerves are the third, sixth, seventh, and eighth. With acute meningitis, sensorineural deafness, which characteristically involves the higher frequencies, develops within days in 20 percent of the cases and is often preceded by tinnitus.[205] *Focal cerebral meningeal syphilis* is caused by compression and invasion of the brain by a gumma that usually arises from the pia mater. Because serologic tests can be unreactive in the serum and the CSF, a biopsy may be required for diagnosis. The gumma responds poorly to antibiotics, so that surgical resection may be necessary.

Cerebrovascular syphilis includes those cases of neurosyphilis characterized by endarteritis and, consequentially, thrombotic infarction. The name is misleading because the pathogenesis invariably stems from an underlying chronic meningitis. Because the neurologic signs are focal, the clinical picture resembles atherosclerotic thrombotic disease, but the patient is often a young adult. About half the cases experience premonitory symptoms such as dizziness, headaches, memory loss, and personality changes.[206] Depending on the artery involved, patients may present with almost any neurologic picture. The most frequent neurologic deficit is hemiparesis or hemiplegia, followed in frequency by aphasia and seizures. Therefore, this diagnosis should be considered in anyone with adult-onset epilepsy or strokes.

Spinal meningeal or vascular syphilis, even at its peak, occurred in only 3 percent of patients with untreated syphilis. The meningomyelitis usually begins over 20 years after the initial infection, with paresthesias and spastic weakness of the legs. These symptoms are followed by various combinations of sensory loss, sphincter disturbances, pain, and muscular atrophy.[206-208] *Spinal vascular syphilis* produces sudden flaccid paraplegia, sensory deficits, and urinary retention. With incomplete transection, the presentation resembles a Brown-Séquard hemisection syndrome.[202]

Pachymeningitis with inflammation and thickening of the dura mater usually involves the cervical area and causes pain, muscle atrophy, sensory loss, diminished tendon reflexes, and, ultimately, spastic paraplegia with sensory loss.[206] The symptoms of a *spinal gumma* are produced by compression like a rapidly growing intraspinal neoplasm. These diseases become symptomatic between 5 to 30 years after initial infection, and males are affected four times more frequently than females. Serologic tests are frequently reactive in the blood and CSF. The prognosis depends on the degree of irreversible neurologic damage that occurred prior to treatment.

Parenchymatous neurosyphilis is divided into two well-known syndromes. Treponemal invasion into the parenchyma of the posterior columns and posterior root of the spinal cord results in progres-

TABLE 218-2
Classification of Neurosyphilis

Type	Predominant findings
Asymptomatic	Abnormal CSF Early (0–5 years) Late (over 5 years)
Cerebromeningeal	Meningitis and cranial nerve palsies Acute Chronic
Cerebral-vascular	Hemiparesis, Aphasia, Seizures
Spinal meningovascular	Meningomyelitis
Parenchymatous	General paresis (paresis) Tabes dorsalis Optic atrophy
Focal gummatous	Cerebral or spinal compression
Atypical (forme-fruste) presentations	Tinnitus, deafness dizziness, pupillary changes, seizures, organic mental syndrome, pyramidal signs and other isolated or combined neurologic abnormalities

sive locomotor ataxia, better known as *tabes dorsalis*. This once common manifestation, which occurs in the fifth or sixth decade of the untreated patient's life, has become rare.[209] The early symptoms are ataxia, paroxysms of lightning pain, paresthesias, loss of tendon reflexes, and pupillary abnormalities. Stabbing pains in visceral organs such as the abdomen, rectum, and larynx simulate surgical emergencies. Particularly disconcerting are the periodic gastric crises with severe abdominal pain, nausea, and vomiting. As the disease progresses, the patient may develop impotence, urinary retention, loss of vision, and anesthetic plantar ulcers (mal perforans).

The ataxia, which initially consists of stumbling and difficulty in walking, is related to a loss of position sense and, therefore, worsens in the dark, but is compensated by visual orientation. The *Romberg sign* is positive, which means that the patient stumbles when the feet are held close together, with the eyes closed. Sluggish pupillary reactivity occurs early and is seen in 90 percent of cases. The distinctive *Argyll-Robertson pupils,* in which the pupils accommodate appropriately to objects but do not react to light, are seen later. Cranial nerves, such as the optic and oculomotor, may be atrophied, and eighth nerve involvement is found in approximately 25 percent of cases. *Charcot joints,* another manifestation, are enlarged, painless, uninflamed joints, with or without deformity or effusion, in the lower extremities and spine. They result from repeated traumatic fractures, dislocations, erosions, and bony repairs. Although serum and CSF serologic tests are reactive in early tabes dorsalis, they may be negative late in the disease. The disorder is rarely fatal, but the patient becomes disabled, incapacitated, and dependent.

Treponemal infection of the cerebral cortex results in *dementia paralytica,* which is better known as *general paresis of the insane.* Depending on the damaged area, the symptoms may be psychiatric, neurologic, or both. In the pre-penicillin era, this disease was diagnosed in 5 to 10 percent of psychotic patients admitted for the first time to a psychiatric institution.[210] In the Oslo study, it developed in 2.5 percent of males and 1.4 percent of females. Although now rare, it has been reported in about 10 percent of diagnosed cases of neurosyphilis in current times.[211] The disease begins about 15 years after the initial infection. The major pathology is chronic meningoencephalitis, which severely disturbs cerebrocortical function and results in gross atrophy of the frontal and temporal lobes, granulations in the ventricles, hydrocephalus, and widened cerebral sulci. The onset may be sudden but is more commonly insidious with changes in personality and behavior. These include irritability, forgetfulness, inability to concentrate, and headaches. Then, impaired judgment, emotional lability, and inappropriate social or moral behavior follow. Delusions of grandeur with marked euphoria occur in 20 percent of the cases.[212] It has been remarked, humorously but realistically, that everyone in contact with the paretic suffers but the patient. Paranoia, tantrums, and alcohol abuse may appear. Full-blown psychosis is followed by a period of neurologic decline. Tremors in the hands, lips, and tongue; seizures of any type, and incontinence of urine and feces are common.[212] Neurologic signs include monoplegias; speech or handwriting disorders; accentuated tendon reflexes; and irregular, small, unequal pupils that react poorly to light. At this point a paralytic facies devoid of facial expression is typical. Mental and neurologic deterioration progresses to death in an average of $2\frac{1}{2}$ years from pneumonia, infected pressure ulcers, or septicemia. The clever Holmes mnemonic—*p*ersonality, *a*ffect, *r*eflexes (hyperactive), *e*ye changes, *s*ensorium (delusions), *i*ntellect impairment, and *s*peech dyparthria—can help the physician consider the diagnosis in time

to help the patient.[213] The impression can then be confirmed with serum and CSF serologic tests, which are reactive in almost all cases. Adequate antibiotic therapy halts progression of the disease in 80 percent of patients. However, the clinical picture may sometimes worsen due to a "therapeutic paradox."

Optic atrophy may occur as an isolated finding. The visual loss begins in one eye but soon involves the other. Optic atrophy also results from syphilitic optic neuritis. In both conditions the CSF is usually abnormal. Differentiation may be possible through the visual evoked response (VER), as the latency is only abnormal in optic neuritis.[214] Penicillin does not restore vision but prevents further loss.

A combination of more than one form of neurosyphilis may be present in the same patient, resulting in a puzzling neurologic picture. Furthermore, perhaps as a result of partial but insufficient therapy, the classic forms of neurosyphilis are becoming less common, and the manifestations are more atypical. There are recent reports of patients with blurring of vision accompanied by Argyll-Robertson pupils or with isolated bilateral oculomotor nerve paresis or with tinnitus and variable auditory deficits. The presentation may be ophthalmic symptoms, confusion, personality changes, or persistent dizziness. The diagnosis of neurosyphilis should be strongly considered in a young adult with a stroke, new seizure disorder, confusional syndrome, or dementia.

Congenital Syphilis

As early as 1529, Paracelsus recognized that syphilis could infect the fetus, although genetically, "from father to son," rather than transplacentally. Due to another popular misconception, wet nurses were then publicly paraded and flogged, with the backing of medical authorities, for supposedly transmitting the disease to their previously healthy charges. In time, the mode of transmission became clear, but not until the nineteenth century was the disease systematically studied. In 1854, the French physician Paul Diday made significant contributions with his popular manual, "Treatise on Syphilis of the Newborn and Infants of the Breast," in which he colorfully described the syphilitic newborn as "a little wrinkled, pot bellied old man with a cold in his head." Not long after, Jonathan Hutchinson reported his famous triad of late congenital syphilis: keratitis, deafness, and notched teeth. Finally, the writings of Alfred Fournier detailed the course, management, and social implications of the disease and, among other accomplishments, influenced premarital counselling for a century. Despite the popularity of the term *congenital syphilis,* prenatal syphilis is more correct as the manifestations of the intrauterine infection may develop at any time before or after delivery rather than always being present at birth as congenital implies.

Syphilis may cause preterm delivery, stillbirth, congenital infection, or neonatal death.[215] As stated in "Kassowitz Law," the danger to the fetus varies inversely with the length of untreated syphilis in the mother.[216] Almost all infants born to mothers with untreated secondary syphilis at any time during gestation become infected, although one-half of the offspring have no clinical disease.[217] In contrast, 10 percent of the infants born of females with late latent disease have clinical manifestations, and 20 percent are stillborn or premature.[217] In general, 25 percent of infected fetuses die in utero. Almost half of infants born to mothers with active syphilis develop the disease, another quarter are seropositive without clinical manifestations, one-quarter die in utero, and one-quarter are not infected.[218] Among neonates with signs and symptoms of syphilis, 25 percent die shortly after birth unless treated.

Treatment of the mother with penicillin prevents prenatal syphilis in at least 98 percent of infants.[219] Understandably, the prevalence of prenatal syphilis closely parallels the number of syphilis cases among heterosexuals, which, as previously discussed, has been dramatically increasing. The long-held belief that syphilis does not infect the fetus before 18 weeks of gestation is incorrect, although organisms are sparsely found.[220] Furthermore, consistent with the inability of the fetus to mount an immune response before the fourth month, little inflammation is present.[221] It has been suggested that a deficiency of some biochemical treponemal requirement in the young fetus best explains the minimal damage produced by the infection in the first trimester.[222] Even later on, the inflammatory changes in the placenta are more pronounced than those of the fetus, and, at delivery, a fibrosed, large, pale placenta may provide the only evidence for a presumptive diagnosis.[215] Necrotizing funisitis, an inflammation of the matrix of the umbilical cord associated with phlebitis and thrombosis, results in stillbirths.[223] A consequence of prenatal syphilis is depressed dehydroepiandrosterone sulfate production of fetal adrenals, which causes reduced estrogen secretion.[224]

Clinical Manifestations

Prenatal syphilis is divided into early and late stages. It is important to note that prenatal syphilis is often undetected. In 80 percent of cases, the diagnosis is missed until the first year of life, and, in one series, the average age of diagnosis was 30 years. Most infants are asymptomatic, and even when manifestations develop, these are often subtle and nonspecific. For this reason, more than 80 percent of cases remain undiagnosed until after 1 year of age.[225]

In early prenatal syphilis, clinical manifestations develop within the first 2 years of life. This stage is comparable to the secondary stage of acquired syphilis as treponemes are transported through the placental circulation and disseminate throughout the fetus. Notably, the primary stage is bypassed. The disease behaves in a more "malignant" manner than the adult counterpart, resulting in perinatal death in almost half the untreated cases born with obvious signs and symptoms. However, due to improved perinatal care the mortality rate has plummetted even in underdeveloped countries.[226]

Affected infants tend to be irritable, small for dates or premature, and cry feebly.[227] However, the presentations are varied. In descending order of frequency, the manifestations found in a recent report were low birth weight, hepatosplenomegaly, anemia, jaundice, thrombocytopenia, skin lesions, respiratory distress, rhinitis, and pseudoparalysis.[226] Rhinitis, or "snuffles," usually develops in the second to third week of life and may be the earliest clinical sign (Fig. 218-23a). Initially thin, a mucoid nasal discharge, teeming with spirochetes, can become purulent or bloody. Ulceration of the nasal septum may occur.[227] If untreated, flattening of the nasal bridge results in the characteristic saddle or "fleur de lis" nose. Rhinitis has been reported in 73.4 percent of active congenital syphilis cases. Within 12 h of initiation of penicillin, the discharge becomes no longer contagious.

Bone and joint lesions, although usually asymptomatic, are the most common early findings and have been reported in 97 percent of autopsied infants younger than 6 months of age. In many of these cases, healing occurs regardless of treatment, which suggests that the nature of the lesions may be trophic rather than infectious.[216] The long bones are predominantly affected.

The most common osseous lesion, osteochondritis, is diagnosed by its characteristic radiographic "sawtooth" appearance in the metaphysis. In the medial aspect of the proximal tibial metaphysis, this defect occurs in one-fifth of early cases and has been called the *Wimberger* or *cat-bite sign.* Longitudinal lines of rarefaction, like "celery sticks," may expand into the diaphysis. Metaphyseal fractures may occur. The pain produced by osteochondritis of the long bones, or epiphysitis, is exacerbated by movement so that the child keeps the affected limb still, a sign referred to as *pseudoparalysis of Parrot.*

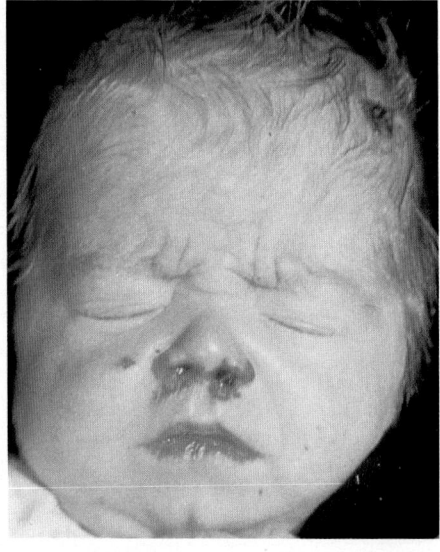
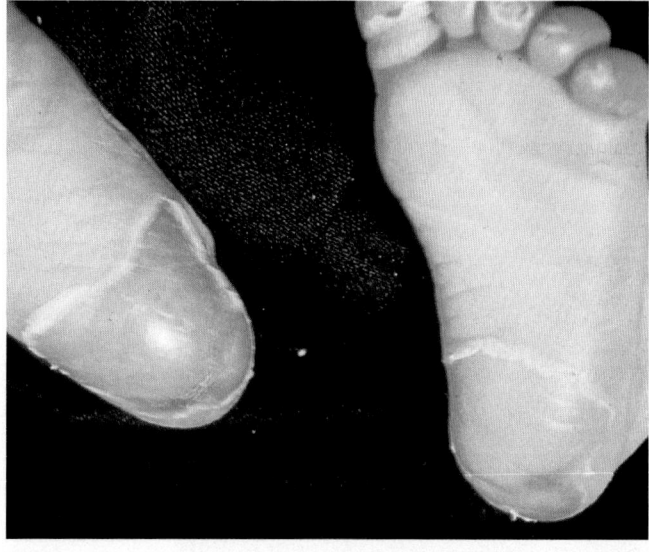

a   *b*

FIGURE 218-23   Prenatal syphilis: (*a*) Snuffles, rhagades, and an ulcerated syphilid on the forehead. (*b*) Bullous, erosive lesions on the soles ("syphilitic pemphigoid"). *(Courtesy of Klaus Wolff, M.D.)*

Painful periostitis, commonly observed in the latter half of the first year, may lead to blunting of the scapular spines and anterior tibial margins in later life. The resulting multiple layers of new bone produce the radiographic "onion-peel periosteum" sign. Osteomyelitis syphilitica, with endosteal infiltration and rarefaction of the compact substance of long bones, is rather rare. Osteitis of the fingers is uncommon but may produce dactylitis during the first 2 years of life.[216]

Even without treatment, the osteitis resolves by the end of the first year. Skull osteitis produces softening, or *craniotabes,* which indents on pressure "like stiff parchment."[216]

Mucocutaneous manifestations occur in about half of the cases under 6 months[227] and, like secondary syphilis lesions, usually consist of a maculopapular exanthem or coppery red macules and papules, with or without scale, predominantly on the palms, soles, and diaper areas.[227] In moist areas the papules become macerated and confluent, just like condylomata lata. Pustules may appear on the fingers, toes, and at the angles of the mouth.[227] Mucous patches may also be present. Ulcerations within lesions around the mouth, nose, or anus may heal with *rhagades,* (Parrot's lines) depressed linear scars that radiate from the orifice like the spokes of a wheel (Fig. 218-24). The eruptions may also be annular or corymbiform. Quite rare, but characteristic for the disease, are bullae, between 1 and 5 cm in diameter, with serous or purulent fluid. Commonly known as *syphilitic pemphigoid,* the blisters are invariably a sign of severe disease; they are highly infectious and may be generalized or, more often, limited to the extremities including the palms and soles (Fig. 218-23*b*)[227]. Other lesions such as macules, papules, and pustules may be present. Frequently, the skin of the syphilitic neonate is dry and wrinkled and, in newborns with fair skin, has a café au lait hue.[222]

Lymphadenopathy occurs in half the cases but may not be prominent. The presence of firm, movable, nontender epitrochlear nodes is especially characteristic for prenatal syphilis.

Hematologic manifestations include anemia, thrombocytopenia, and leukocytosis or leukopenia. The cause of the anemia is usually Coombs-negative hemolysis. Petechiae due to low platelets may appear. Monocytosis and neutrophilic leukocytosis are common, and leukemoid reactions have been reported.[216]

Central nervous system involvement is ten times more frequent in Caucasian than black infants. Routinely, infants are irritable. They may have bulging fontanelles, nuchal rigidity, and seizures. CSF examination shows lymphocytosis, increased protein, and reactive serology in 40 to 60 percent of all syphilitic infants. However, only 10 percent of these develop symptomatic neurosyphilis, which does not usually become clinically evident until the third to

sixth month of life. It is essentially meningovascular and can present as various neurologic syndromes.[216]

Nephropathy is due either to acute proliferative or to membranous glomerulonephritis and is rare.

Ocular disease consists of chorioretinitis, glaucoma, or uveitis. The chorioretinitis is diagnosed by its characteristic "salt and pepper" pattern at the periphery of the fundus.

Other manifestations include myocarditis, pancreatitis, peritonitis, and pneumonitis alba, which may predispose to chronic lung disease. Myocarditis is present in 10 percent of dead syphilitic infants but does not appear to be a problem in survivors.

Although students are often asked about the order of frequency of late congenital syphilis signs, a review of the literature illustrates that this information varies in different reports. In the pre-penicillin era, eye lesions constituted the most common finding, followed by keratitis, frontal bossing, saber shins, dental malformations, saddle nose, and asymptomatic neurosyphilis, in descending order. However, two more-recent studies reported contradictory findings. In one, frontal bossing was the most common finding followed, in descending order, by high arched palate, saddle nose, and tooth abnormalities; whereas in the second series, these signs were infrequently observed. Instead, eye lesions, interstitial keratitis, and scaphoid scapula occurred more often.[222]

Essentially, the stage of *late congenital syphilis* corresponds to tertiary syphilis in the adult. The salient exception is that the heart is relatively spared. Syphilis is the most common cause of nonimmune hydrops fetalis, resulting in pallor, edema, and a bloated abdomen.[215] Manifestations appear after the age of 2 years but rarely past the age of 30. The signs can be divided into two groups, consisting of permanent "stigmata" or malformations and continuously active pathologic processes (Table 218-3). Most of the manifestations are not specific, with the exception of the the notched upper central incisors or "mulberry molars" and the characteristic interstitial keratitis. The characteristic facies can be recognized in famous paintings.[228]

Interstitial keratitis (Fig. 218-25*a*) occurs in 8.8 percent of cases, and the average age of onset is 13.5 years for males and 27.1 years for females. The presenting symptoms are tearing, pain, cor-

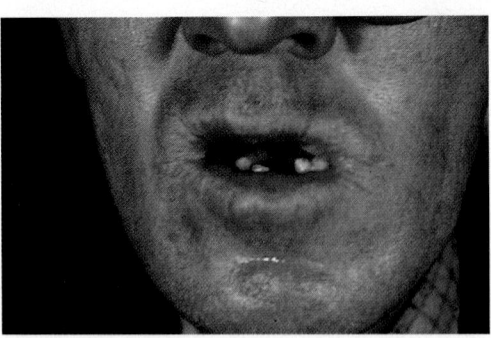

FIGURE 218-24 Parrot's lines are linear, depressed scars around the mouth.

TABLE 218-3
Signs in Late Congenital Syphilis

Stigmata	Active disease
Opthalmic	
Retinitis	Interstitial keratitis
Oral	
Hutchinson's teeth	
Mulberry molars	
High arched palate	
Ears, nose, throat	
Saddle nose	Gummas in nose or palate
Orthopedic	
Frontal bossing	Periostitis
Short maxilla	Dactylitis
Protuberant mandible	Clutton's joints
Saber shins	
Scaphoid scapula	
Thickened medial clavicle	
Neurologic	Eighth nerve deafness
	Neurosyphilis
Mucocutaneous	Gummas
	Gummatous inflammation
Gastrointestinal	Hepatomegaly
	Splenomegaly

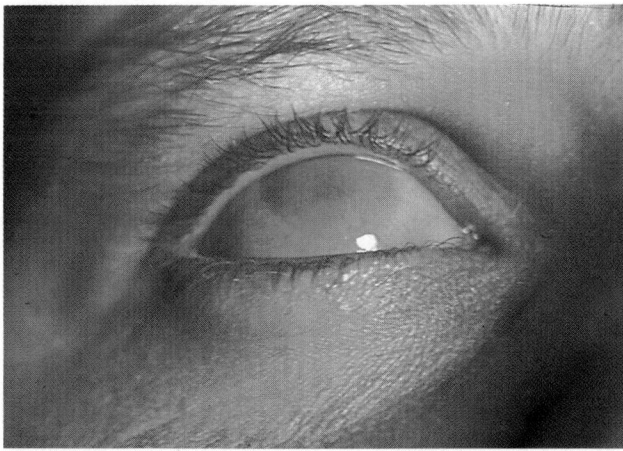

a

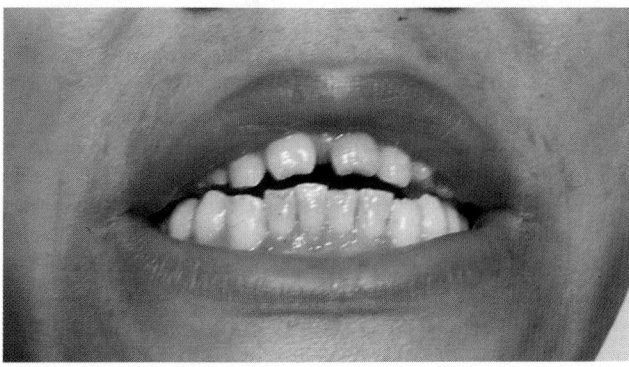

b

FIGURE 218-25 (*a*) Interstitial keratitis. *(Courtesy of Klaus Wolff, M.D.)* (*b*) Hutchinson's teeth.

neal injection, and photophobia in one eye. Within 2 months the second eye is also involved in 80 to 90 percent of patients.[229] The intermittently relapsing course eventuates in corneal clouding (syphilitic nebulae) or glaucoma. The cause appears to be an immunologic reaction in tissue invaded and sensitized by treponemes in the prenatal period. Neovascularization of the cornea may result in a "*salmon*" patch appearance. "*Ghost vessels*" may be noted by slit-lamp examination and represent residual scarring in these vessels.[216] Because corneal scarring is limited and sometimes absent, corneal transplantation often restores vision. Iritis and iridocyclitis may also be found but usually early in congenital syphilis.

Neurosyphilis without symptoms occurs in one-third to one-half of patients and is diagnosed only through abnormal CSF findings. Symptomatic disease is rare and usually delayed until puberty. Many of the clinical patterns described in acquired adult neurosyphilis are seen, and juvenile paresis, the most common, affects 1 to 5 percent of all congenital syphilis cases. The presentation often involves personality and behavior changes, such as deteriorating school performance and inappropriate emotional responses. Within a year any combination of ataxia, dysarthria, tremors, and seizures develop.[222]

Bilateral neural deafness has been reported in 3.3 to 38 percent of cases, usually in adolescence. The early symptoms are vertigo, occasionally with nausea and tinnitus. The deafness, which progresses despite antibiotics, is caused by osteochondritis of the otic capsule resulting in cochlear degeneration. At first, high fre-

quencies are lost. It is one of the few causes of a positive Hennebert's sign.[216] The response to systemic corticosteroids has been encouraging.[230]

Cutaneous manifestations consist of gummas and gummatous inflammation just as in late benign syphilis. Parrot's lines may still be visible (Fig. 218-24).

Bone manifestations, such as arthritic perisynovitis, epiphysitis, and periostitis, may also occur in late prenatal infection. Chondroosteoarthritis, which may lead to ankylosis, produces the rare *von Gies joint.* Fusiform swelling caused by periostitis produces a number of common manifestations. The *Higoumenakis sign,* which occurs occasionally but is a rather nonspecific and vague finding, is a unilateral, irregular enlargement of the sternoclavicular portion of the clavicle secondary to burned-out periostitis. Observed in only 4.1 percent of patients are *saber shins,* the anterior bowing and thickening from periostitis of the midportion of the tibia. *Frontal bossing of Parrot,* present in 86.7 percent of cases, is a thickened, prominent forehead produced by lens-shaped bony prominences that develop from localized periostitis of the frontal and parietal bones. *Scaphoid scapulae,* manifested by a concavity of the vertebral border of the scapulae, were observed in only 0.7 percent of cases. A *short maxilla,* with a shallow dish configuration, results from impaired development due to syphilitic rhinitis and was present in 83.3 percent of cases. *Mandibular protuberance,* or bulldog jaw, was found in 25.8 percent. The size is normal but appears proportionally larger in comparison to the size of the small maxilla.

Clutton joints typically refer to symmetric, nontender swelling of the knees, which often follows trauma and produces a bilateral hydroarthrosis. In some cases, however, the condition may be accompanied by fever, redness, warmth, and pain. It represents a synovitis without involvement of bone or cartilage. Systemic corticosteroids are the preferred treatment.

Paroxysmal cold hemoglobinuria may occur as the only manifestation. Muscle cramping, chills, and dark red or black urine follows cold exposure. In addition, fevers, urticaria, Raynaud's phenomenon, and jaundice may be present. Antibiotics decrease or abolish the episodes.

Dental abnormalities are caused by treponemal invasion of the tooth buds. The pathognomonic *Hutchinson's teeth* refer to widely spaced permanent upper incisors that are small, screwdriver- or peg-shaped, wide at the gingival margin, and notched at the biting edge due to defective enamel production (Fig. 218-25b).[231] These changes may also affect the upper, lower, and lateral incisors. The diagnosis can be made radiologically by the first year of life. *Mulberry* or *Moon's molars,* found in 65 percent of cases, are dome-shaped and have numerous diminutive cusps arrayed in a tight circle at the top of the dome.[231] Although all the molars may be affected, the diagnostic one is the first lower molar. Due to defective enamel, these teeth are predisposed to caries and are rarely present beyond adolescence. The dental changes can be prevented if treatment is initiated before the third month of age.

Deformities, such as painless perforation of the nasal septum or soft palate and deep ulcers of the pharynx and tongue, can occur as a result of gummas.

Diagnosis

Dark-field examination of the umbilical vein at delivery will be positive in over half the cases of early prenatal syphilis. Nasal secretions and mucocutaneous lesions should be similarly tested. In

TABLE 218-4
Congenital Syphilis Diagnostic Classification

Definite/Confirmed
Identification of *T. pallidum* by dark-field microscopy, fluorescent
  antibody, or other specific stains in specimens from lesions,
  automaterial, placenta, or umbilical cord
Compatible (Formerly ''Probable'' or ''Possible'')
A reactive serologic test for syphilis (STS) in a stillborn
                              or
A reactive STS in an infant whose mother had syphilis during
  pregnancy and was not adequately treated, regardless of symptoms in
  the infant
                              or
A reactive VDRL test in cerebrospinal fluid
                              or
A reactive STS in an infant with any of the following signs: snuffles,
  condyloma lata, osteitis, periostitis or osteochondritis, ascites, skin and
  mucous membrane lesions, hepatitis, hepatomegaly, splenomegaly,
  nephrosis, nephritis, hemolytic anemia
                              or
Fourfold or greater rise in titers* of nontreponemal tests (VDRL or
  RPR) and a confirmed treponemal test (FTA-ABS or MHA-TP) over
  a 3-month interval
                              or
A reactive treponemal test or nontreponemal test that does not revert to
  nonreactive in 6 months
Unlikely
Infants who never had a reactive STS
                              or
Asymptomatic live-born infants whose mothers were treated for syphilis
  during pregnancy and subsequently experienced a fourfold or greater
  fall in titer provided the infant's own STS is also fourfold or lower
  than the maternal titer at the time of treatment*

* ''Fourfold rise in titer,'' ''fourfold fall in titer,'' and other similar
  phrases refer to changes in serum titers of at least 2 dilutions (2
  ''tubes''), e.g., from 1:2 to 1:8 (and the reverse), or from 1:4 to
  1:16 (and the reverse), or from 1:32 to 1:8 (and the reverse).
NOTE: For explanations of serologic tests, see text.
SOURCE: Centers for Disease Control: *MMWR*, vol 37, No S-1, Jan 15,
1988

the absence of clinical disease in a suspected infant, reliance on
serologic tests becomes necessary (Table 218-4).

Syphilis and HIV Infection (See also Chap. 215)

Complex interactions between syphilis and HIV infection can alter
the clinical manifestations and natural course of both diseases. It
has been suggested that syphilis may accelerate development of
immunodeficiency in HIV-infected persons and, conversely, that
HIV infection causes reactivation of dormant syphilis. Furthermore, an unusual manifestation of syphilis may be the initial manifestations of HIV infection. It would be expected that a depressed
cellular immunity could lead to more rapid progression of syphilis
with increased complications.[232]

Concomitant infection with HIV may result in failure to respond to recommended doses of penicillin,[233] relapses despite adequate treatment,[234,235] accelerated development of neurosyphilis,[235] or progression to late benign disease in only a few
months.[236–239] The possibility that treatment failures and relapses
represent reinfection must always be considered, as initial denial

may be retracted after the patient has gained confidence and trust in
the physician. Over 40 cases of HIV-associated neurosyphilis have
been reported,[233] and in one study conducted over 42 months, 44
percent of the neurosyphilis cases were HIV infected.[234] Most
cases comprise asymptomatic or meningovascular neurosyphilis,
but focal gummata and other forms of neurosyphilis have also been
reported. Neurosyphilis may be the first clinical manifestation of
HIV infection.[233] However, large prospective studies to address the
frequency of these cases have not yet been published, and at present
most experts feel that neurosyphilis does not develop frequently.[232]

Diagnosing syphilis in HIV-seropositive patients may also be
more difficult. Secondary syphilis can present with atypical urticarial, granulomatous, or ulcerating plaques.[240] Furthermore, antibody titers may not be as accurate an indicator of disease activity.
Dysregulation of the humoral immune response may result in uncontrolled production of antibodies with extremely elevated titers.[237] A report that B-cell activation results in a high rate false-
positive nontreponemal serologic tests in these patients has not
been substantiated.[241] On the other hand, even after adequate dilutions, treponemal or nontreponemal tests may rarely be negative.[233]

Therefore, biopsy of skin lesions is recommended, but, to add
to the confusion, the classic pathologic findings may be absent. A
superficial perivascular mononuclear cell infiltrate with eosinophils
may be the only finding, leading to a misdiagnosis of HIV-associated papular dermatosis in cases eventually diagnosed with special
stains. However, with some exceptions,[242] most cases follow the
expected clinical course and serologic drop after treatment.[243]

Based on theoretical supposition, it has been repeatedly proposed that immunosuppression resulting from advanced seronegative, clinically asymptomatic syphilis predisposes to the development of AIDS.[244] Although serologic tests for syphilis are frequent
in HIV-infected patients, a popular viewpoint notes that well before
the HIV epidemic, depressed cell-mediated immunity among homosexuals exposed to chronic or recurrent viral, bacterial, and parasitic infections prevented full expression of nontreponemal serologic tests. As a consequence, syphilis has been widely undetected in
this group.[244] Recent findings of reactive IgM antibodies to treponemal proteins in HIV patients with and without a previous history
of syphilis support this theory.[233]

What appears certain is that a history of syphilis is associated
with higher risk of HIV infection,[245] perhaps because the genital
ulceration provides an easy entry to the virus into the systemic
circulation. Although the same is true for other ulcerative infections, such as herpes simplex and chancroid, numerous studies
have demonstrated that syphilis is far more common in HIV-reac-
tive individuals than in uninfected persons, even when the analysis
was limited to heterosexuals.[245]

In a small but significant study that included 15 HIV-infected
and 25 HIV-seronegative patients with primary and secondary
syphilis, *T. pallidum* was isolated from the CSF by rabbit inoculation in similar proportions from both groups. Only CSF leukocytosis was more common (67 percent vs. 25 percent) in the HIV-
seropositive group.[235] Notably, one injection of benzathine penicillin failed to eradicate CNS infection in three of the four
HIV-infected cases with positive treponeme cultures. This has led
to considerable discussion about the adequate treatment of early
syphilis with HIV infection. Surprisingly, official treatment recommendations have not been changed,[246] but a number of experts are
advocating procaine penicillin schedules for neurosyphilis or at
least three injections of benzathine penicillin 1 week apart.[239] CSF
examination is now recommended for all HIV-seropositive patients

with syphilis at any stage.[235] However, patients with CSF abnormalities including positive serologic tests should be cautiously diagnosed as having asymptomatic neurosyphilis, as CSF leukocytosis or elevated protein are present in up to 60 percent of nonsyphilitic HIV-infected patients.[247]

Serology

In 1906, August von Wassermann and his colleagues developed a complement fixation test using the treponeme-gorged livers of stillborn infants with congenital syphilis. It was discovered that the antibodies, or *reagins,* were not specific, and alcoholic extracts from beef hearts were used as substrate with excellent results. The antigenic substance from beef hearts was found to be a phospholipid called cardiolipin. In 1946, the venereal disease research laboratory (VDRL) test, a flocculation assay, used cardiolipin, lecithin, and cholesterol for antigen.[248] Only 3 years later, with the development of the *Treponema pallidum* immobilization (TPI) test, efforts toward a *T. pallidum*-specific test became successful, and the test became the yardstick of syphilis serology for a quarter of a century.[249] The method was based on the observation that serum from syphilitic patients immobilizes living *T. pallidum.*

Advances in the use of indirect immunofluorescence led to the development of the fluorescent *Treponema pallidum* antibody (FTA) test in 1957, which was subsequently improved with an additional absorption step and is now commonly used under the name of FTA-ABS test. Other advances include the introduction of the *T. pallidum* hemagglutination (TPHA) test in 1965 and the enzyme-linked immunosorbent assay (ELISA) adaptation in 1975.

New Developments

Besides these major advances, many other improvements, variants, and techniques have been reported. Some of the new methods still use nontreponemal substances (cardiolipin-lecithin-cholesterol).[250] Others employ preparations of flagellae or axial filaments of *T. phagedenis,* biotype Reiter antigens,[251] monoclonal antibodies,[252] protein fractions from *T. pallidum,* or recombinant fragments of *T. pallidum* DNA.[253] The results appear very promising; however, experience with these tests is limited.

Nonspecific antibodies (reagins) are directed against lipoidal antigens of *T. pallidum* as well as against the mitochondrial and nuclear membranes of human cells (autoantibodies). *T. pallidum* appears to contain a phospholipid that resembles the component of human mitochondrial membrane and that stimulates the production of two different types of antibodies. Antiphospholipid antibodies, which react in the VDRL, probably result from the interaction of *T. pallidum* with human tissue and can be differentiated from mitochondrial cardiolipin antibodies.[254] These antibodies are measured by nontreponemal tests[255] or serologic tests for syphilis (STS) that employ cardiolipin-lecithin antigens. Lipoidal antigens are present in normal tissue but are particularly evident in conditions associated with nuclear destruction.[255] These conditions generate autoantibodies that may produce false-positive reactions to nontreponemal tests.

Specific antitreponemal antibodies are directed against *T. pallidum* and are measured with assays which require the organism or its components. Various techniques are employed to eliminate group-specific antibodies directed against nonpathogenic spirochetes.

Classification by Chemical Structure

IgM Antibodies The earliest humoral immune response by the human host to infection with *T. pallidum* is the production of antibodies of the IgM class. These can be detected in the serum towards the end of the second week of infection.[255] Because memory cells do not synthesize IgM antibodies, generation of these immunoglobulins is terminated soon after the elimination of the antigen.[249] The determination of treponemal IgM antibodies has useful potential and may contribute to the diagnosis of syphilis in a number of difficult clinical situations. A reactive IgM test in untreated persons is proof of active disease and indicates the need for treatment.[249]

The titers of IgM antibodies drop swiftly after treatment. Reactivity ceases within 3 to 9 months after therapy of early syphilis,[256,257] but may persist for 12 to 18 months after treatment of late disease.[249,256,257] In late disease, the generation of the IgM class autoantibodies, directed against antitreponemal IgG, may cause false reactivity. On the other hand, a competitive inhibition of IgM production by high titers of IgG may cause false nonreactive results in early syphilis.[249,257] Reappearance of IgM reactivity after repeated nonreactivity strongly suggests reinfection. Persistence of reactivity after therapy indicates treatment failure, as long as false-positive results due to autoantibodies of the IgM class[249,256] can be excluded.

Due to their large size, IgM molecules cannot traverse the placenta or pass through the intact blood-CSF barrier. IgM reactivity in the serum of a newborn confirms prenatal infection, and detection of antitreponemal IgM in the CSF indicates neurosyphilis if the blood-CSF barrier function is normal.

7S IgM Antibodies IgM antibodies of low molecular weight that migrate at 7 S units rather than the usual 19 S units in the ultracentrifuge have frequently been found at high titers in the sera of patients with early syphilis and persist at low titers over a long period of time.[258] Their significance is not yet clear.

IgG Antibodies IgG antibodies become detectable by the fourth to fifth week of infection. The titers peak within the first year of the disease,[38] usually during the secondary stage, and decrease in the stage of latency. IgG synthesis is continued at low titers by memory cells for years and even throughout life, despite elimination of the antigen. Therefore, the detection of IgG antibodies does not render definitive conclusions about the activity of the disease or the efficacy of treatment. The IgG molecules are small enough to cross the placenta and the blood-CSF barrier easily, so their presence in the serum of newborns or in the CSF does not prove congenital syphilis or neurosyphilis.

IgA Antibodies The significance of IgA class antibodies has not been thoroughly investigated. It has been reported that antitreponemal IgA in the CSF may promote development of neurosyphilis by competitively inhibiting IgG and blocking the complement cascade.[259]

IgD Antibodies Antitreponemal IgD antibodies can be detected in the sera from patients in all stages of syphilis, which indicates a high specificity.[260] However, assessment of any diagnostic value requires further investigation.

Assays for the Detection of Antibodies of the IgM and IgG Class

The VDRL Test (Table 218-5) The serum is inactivated by heating at 56°C for 30 min. If lipoidal antibodies are present in the serum, flocculation occurs upon mixture with the antigen. The antigen consists of 0.03 percent cardiolipin, 0.9 percent cholesterol, and 0.21 percent lecithin.[38,255] The result is macroscopically visible within 5 to 10 min,[249] but use of a microscope facilitates the evaluation in borderline cases. The test becomes reactive 4 to 5 weeks after infection and reverts to negative in about one-fourth[261] to over one-third of cases during late latency. The results are reported as nonreactive, reactive, and weakly reactive. A ''rough'' appearance[38] is a term similar to weakly reactive. Such results should not be disregarded until more specific tests are performed, because in 36.4 percent of weakly reactive tests, the treponemal assays are positive. The sensitivity and specificity of the results during the different stages of syphilis are shown in Table 218-5. The agreement rate with the results of tests using specific *T. pallidum* antigen (TPHA, FTA-ABS) is close to 90 percent during early stages, but drops to 29 to 43 percent during late latency.[249] Nevertheless, the sensitivity and specificity of the VDRL are better than those for other assays using lipoidal antigens.

A quantitative evaluation, which consists of serial dilutions of the sample with saline in a geometric progression by a factor of 2 (1:2, 1:4, 1:8, etc.), should be performed. The highest dilution that gives a positive result is reported as the ''titer.'' A high titer (above 1:16) usually indicates active disease, whereas low titers (below 1:8) may remain unchanged for years following therapy of late disease. With treatment, the titers should decline by a factor of four within 3 months in primary or secondary syphilis or within 6 to 12 months in early latent syphilis. If an initially high titer (greater than 1:32) fails to decrease, the patient should be evaluated for neurosyphilis and retreated appropriately. A fourfold titer increase indicates reinfection or treatment failure.

Patients who are treated within 3 months of infection become nonreactive during the following 6 to 12 months, but reactivity may last for up to 60 months at low titers if therapy is administered later in the early stages. In one study, 18 percent of tests from patients treated for secondary syphilis remained reactive at low titers for 30 to 35 years. On the other hand, 56 percent of patients who were treated during the late phase, became nonreactive within 5 years.

TABLE 218-5
Current Tests in Routine Syphilis Serology

Tests for detection of IgM and IgG antibodies		
Lipoidal antigen	*T. pallidum* antigen	Tests for the selective detection of IgM antibodies
	FTA-ABS	
VDRL	TPHA	19S-IgM–FTA-ABS
RPR	MHA-TP	IgM-SPHA
TRUST	HTTS	IgM-ELISA
	Bio Enzabead	

NOTE: For explanations of serologic tests, see text.

TABLE 218-6
Causes of False-Positive Nontreponemal Tests

Acute	Chronic
Mycoplasma pneumonia	Leprosy
Enterovirus infections	Systemic lupus erythematosus
Infectious mononucleosis	Hashimoto's thyroiditis
Narcotic abuse	Rheumatoid arthritis
Advanced tuberculosis	Rheumatic heart disease
Scarlet fever	Connective tissue disease
Viral pneumonia	Hepatic cirrhosis
Brucellosis	Periarteritis nodosa
Rat-bite fever	Malignant tumors
Relapsing fever	Familial
Leptospirosis	
Measles	
Mumps	
Malaria	
Lymphogranuloma venereum	
Trypanosomiasis	
Protein deficiency	
Psittacosis	

False-negative results occur during very early infection or in latent and late syphilis. The tests of approximately 1 percent of secondary syphilis patients are falsely reported as nonreactive due to the ''prozone phenomenon,'' since, unless the serum is diluted, the high levels of antibody prevent flocculation.

Biologic false-positive results (Table 218-6) may be seen in 0.25 to 0.85 percent[262] of all sera examined and constitute 4.8 percent[263] of positive tests. Most of the false-positive results, which are predominantly caused by autoantibodies of the IgM class (rheumatoid factor), show titers between 1:1 and 1:4. Occasionally higher values are observed. Biologic false-positive results may be transient and ''acute'' (<6 months) or longer lasting and ''chronic'' (>6 months). The higher number of false-positive reports among pregnant women stems from the frequency of testing during gestation rather than a true increase. False-positive reactions occur frequently in narcotic addicts and may persist even after 14 months of drug abstinence. Patients with chronic biologic false-positive results are more likely to develop an autoimmune disorder.[264,265]

The VDRL test offers a number of advantages. The test can be performed easily in any laboratory with basic equipment. The results are reliable and can be obtained within 40 min. The reagents and the technique are standardized, and the results are comparable all over the world. Finally, the VDRL is the least expensive of all syphilis serology tests.[262] The main disadvantage is a low sensitivity during the late stages of syphilis. Furthermore, the antigen must be freshly prepared daily, and the serum must be heat-inactivated before testing. In some regards, the latter can now be considered an advantage because this procedure inactivates HIV.

Variations of the VDRL Test   *The unheated serum reagin (USR) test* uses a stabilized antigen that differs negligibly from the VDRL reagent. It does not need to be prepared daily and is only slightly more expensive. The test is performed with unheated serum. The results are comparable to the VDRL, although the sensitivity and specificity are a little lower.

The rapid plasma reagin (RPR) test is performed with unheated serum on small plastic cards. The antigen and the technique are the same as in the VDRL. Charcoal particles are added to the antigen and cause flocculation of black particles that can easily be read without a microscope. The specificity is almost identical to the VDRL test. The advantage over the VDRL test is the simplified technique. The test can be performed without laboratory equipment, and the results are available within 5 min. The disadvantages are a slightly lower sensitivity[266] and somewhat higher costs.

The automated reagin test (ART) uses the reagents of the RPR test but can be performed in autoanalyzers. The results of photometric reading are printed on record forms.

The reagin screen test (RST) uses a stabilized RPR antigen with lipid-soluble Sudan black diazodye instead of charcoal. The technique is the same as in the RPR, and the results do not differ.

The toluidine red unheated serum test (TRUST) is identical to the RPR, except that the antigen remains stable over a period of 6 months. Toluidine red pigment is substituted for charcoal and provides better visualization. A comparative evaluation of the VDRL, RPR, and TRUST results revealed differences below 2 percent in sensitivity, specificity, and reproducibility.[266]

Treponemal Tests (Table 218-5)

Tests Using T. pallidum Antigen These methods employ whole *T. pallidum* or its fragments as antigen. The assays render results that are close to optimal. The specificity and sensitivity range between 94 and 100 percent during the secondary and the late phases of the disease (Table 218-7). Therefore, the tests seem almost unsurpassable in these stages. However, the high sensitivity of these tests permits detection of very small amounts of antibodies, and so the assays cannot be used for assessment of the efficacy of treatment or evaluation of cure.

During recent years, recombinant generation of *T. pallidum* DNA and development of monoclonal antibodies directed against *T. pallidum*[33,267] have formed the basis for promising new assays.

Fluorescent Treponemal Antibody-Absorption (FTA-ABS) Test The serum of the patient is first mixed with a sorbent containing an extract from Reiter treponemes in order to absorb nonspecific treponemal antigens. The absorbed serum is then added to a glass slide on which *T. pallidum* (Nichols strain) is fixed. Antibodies to *T. pallidum,* present in the serum, bind to the surface of the organisms and are stained by incubation with fluorescent conjugated rabbit antihuman globulin. Lyophilized treponemes can be stored for a long period without loss of antigenic quality.

The FTA-ABS shows reactivity with 19S IgM, 7S IgG, and IgA antibodies directed against *T. pallidum*. The intensity of fluorescence is reported as nonreactive $(-)$, marginal or borderline $(+/-)$, or reactive $(+, ++, +++, ++++)$. A quantitative evaluation can be performed by serial dilutions in a progression by a factor of 3 (1:5, 1:15, 1:45, etc.). However, such evaluation has very little value in routine testing.[255]

Reactivity begins during the third week of infection. The test rarely becomes nonreactive in untreated patients, and reactivity continues even after successful therapy. In one study, 20 of 23 patients (87 percent) with primary syphilis and all 53 patients with secondary syphilis had reactive FTA-ABS tests 30 to 35 years after adequate treatment.[249] At present, the FTA-ABS is the most sensitive serologic test in the early stages of syphilis, rivaled only by the TPHA.[268] The automated version of the FTA-ABS test correlates well with the manual method and may be more specific. False-positive and false-negative results occur in up to 7 percent and 3 percent of samples, respectively. Failures are usually related to inefficient reagents. An evaluation of four different kits revealed considerable deviation. The ability to detect reactive serum samples varied between 83 and 95 percent, and the capability to identify nonreactive samples ranged between 81 and 16 percent. Reproducibility averaged 42 percent.[269] As demonstrated by these results, a standard in the manufacture of FTA-ABS reagents is needed.

False-negative results are very rare.[255] False-positive FTA-ABS reactions occasionally develop in healthy adults with negative lipoidal tests. Many of these revert to negative within a year.[270] False-positive FTA-ABS tests are usually related to the presence of autoantibodies, such as rheumatoid factors, but may occur due to cross-reactivity in *Borrelia* infections.[35] False-positive FTA-ABS tests usually have a beaded fluorescent appearance like a string of shining pearls and only rarely a uniform pattern. In certain patients with systemic lupus erythematosus (SLE), the anti-DNA antibodies responsible for the beading pattern are inhibited when the serum is preincubated with calf thymus DNA. In other cases, the reactivity is not related to anti-DNA antibodies and may disappear as IgM decreases with aging of the serum.

Advantages of the FTA-ABS test include detection of recent infection 1 to 2 weeks before other assays and high specificity and sensitivity, which render reliable results. However, performance of the test requires highly trained personnel. It is time-consuming, and reading the results is tiresome. Because of the expense, it should be applied as a method for confirmation when reactivity is detected in other assays.

The T. pallidum Hemagglutination Assay (TPHA) An ultrasonicate of *T. pallidum* (Nichols strain) is fixed to the surface

TABLE 218-7
Sensitivity and Specificity of Serological Tests

| | Sensitivity | | | | |
	Primary	Secondary	Latent*	Late*	Specificity
VDRL	80 (74–87)	100	80 (71–100)	71 (37–94)	98
RPR	86 (81–100)	100	80 (71–100)	73 (36–96)	98
FTA-ABS	98 (93–100)	100	80 (53–100)	96	99
MHA-TP	82 (69–90)	100	100	94 (100)	99
19S-IgM–FTA-ABS	98 (93–100)	100	100	?	99
SPHA	82 (69–90)	100	100	95	97
Captia M	82	60	53	34	?

*Widely variable results reported in the literature.
NOTE: For explanations of serologic tests, see text.
SOURCE: Adapted from references 2, 3, and 91.

of sheep erythrocytes, which are pretreated with formalin and tannin. Antibodies to *T. pallidum* in the patient serum cause agglutination that can be seen without the need of a microscope. Before the test, nonspecific group antibodies, which might cause false reactivity, are eliminated by incubation of the serum with an absorbing diluent that contains rabbit serum, rabbit testicular extract, fragments of membranes of sheep and beef erythrocytes, and Reiter treponemes. The results are reported as reactive if agglutination occurs at a dilution of 1:80 or more. Preliminary results can be read about 3 to 4 h, but final analysis is made after 18 h. Reactivity can be expected around the fourth to fifth week of infection.

Quantitative evaluation is performed by serial dilution of the serum with the absorbing diluent in a geometric progression by a factor of 2 (1:80, 1:160, 1:320, etc.). The sensitivity and specificity of the TPHA is superior to the VDRL and to the FTA-ABS, except in primary syphilis. During this stage of the disease, the reactivity depends on the IgM-binding capacity of the reagents, which may vary in different kits. The margin of error is very small and ranges between 0.008 percent false-negative and 0.07 percent false-positive findings.

False-positive results may originate from heteroagglutination or from group-specific antibodies.[249] Cross-reactivity may accompany infections with *Borrelia burgdorferi*.[35] Even after treatment, reactivity continues at high titers indefinitely. The test can easily be performed in laboratories with basic equipment, with simple training of technicians. The TPHA test renders the most reliable results in syphilis serology among presently available tests. However, the reagents are rather expensive, and quality may vary in products from the same manufacturer. Internal quality control and proficiency testing are very important, due to lack of standardization.

VARIANTS. The *microhemagglutination assay with T. pallidum antigen* (MHA-TP) is performed on microtiter plates and requires less serum and reagents. The results are ready after 4 h and can be read in a magnifying mirror. The specificity and sensitivity are the same as in the TPHA. The great advantage of the MHA-TP over the TPHA is that costs are reduced to almost one-tenth.

The *automated microhemagglutination assay with T. pallidum antigen* (AMHA-TP) involves the automated filling of the wells of the microtiter plate and serial dilutions, which saves personnel time and minimizes technical error. The machines are expensive and their use is cost effective only if the number of daily examinations exceeds 200.

The *hemagglutination treponemal test for syphilis* (HTTS) is performed in the same manner as the MHA-TP, employs the same sorbent as the FTA-ABS, but uses glutaraldehyde-stabilized turkey erythrocytes as carriers of the *T. pallidum* antigen.

The *microcapsule agglutination test for T. pallidum antibodies* (MCA-TP) is another variant that uses chemically stabile plastic capsules coated with *T. pallidum* antigen, instead of erythrocytes. The IgM reactivity and, consequentially, the sensitivity during the primary stage are superior to the MHA-TP.[271]

The *fingerprick MHA-TP* is practical in children. Two or three drops of blood from the pierced finger tip are soaked into filter paper and transported to the laboratory. Concordance with the standard MHA-TP is 99.5 percent.[249]

Enzyme-Linked Immunosorbent Assay

ELISA has been heralded as the model test system in currently used immunologic procedures.[38] The antigen is fixed to the walls of the wells in microtiter plates. Then serum is added and rinsed off after an incubation period of 30 to 60 min. Antibodies to *T. pallidum* bind to the antigen and react in a second incubation with an enzyme-labeled antihuman globulin. Usually horseradish peroxidase or alkaline phosphatase is used for marking. After rinsing, a substrate (e.g., *o*-phenylendiamine for peroxidase or *p*-nitrophenyl phosphate for alkaline phosphatase) is added and the color of the solution turns yellow. The result is available within 3 to 4 h. The test can be automated and performed in a processor.

Many variations using nonspecific VDRL-antigen[250,255] axial filaments,[272] the flagella of *T. phagedenis*, protein fractions of *T. pallidum*,[273] or recombinant DNA–derived *T. pallidum* membrane proteins[274] have been developed. However, standardized reagents are not yet available, and evaluation is limited.

VARIANTS. The *Bio Enzabead test* uses *T. pallidum* antigen fixed to ferrous metal beads. Control beads are coated with normal rabbit testicular extract and are used to determine nonspecific reactions. The reagents are commercially available. Correlation with treponemal and nontreponemal tests is about 95 percent.

The *enzyme-linked immunofiltration assay* uses *T. pallidum* antigen fixed on nitrocellulose filter sheets. Antigen-antibody binding is accelerated by passing the serum through the antigen-coated filter. The indicator system is the same as in the ELISA technique. Results are available within 15 min and are comparable to those of standard treponemal tests.[275]

The *enzyme immunoassay for detecting IgG antibodies to T. pallidum* (EIA Captia Syphilis G) is a variant of the Captia M test. The sensitivity and specificity appear to be comparable to the FTA-ABS and the MHA-TP,[276] but further evaluation is required.

Assays for the Selective Detection of IgM Antibodies to T. pallidum

IgM molecules are rather labile and may degrade under the influence of enzymes or at elevated temperatures or during prolonged storage. The serum should be frozen, but conveyance in plastic tubes with styropore boxes and storage in a refrigerator between periods of transportation keeps the loss within reasonable limits.[249]

The *IgM–FTA-ABS test* is performed and read in the same manner as the FTA-ABS test, but an anti-IgM conjugate labeled with fluorescein isothiocyanate is used instead of antihuman globulin. False-positive results due to autoantibodies occur, even after rheumatoid factor is absorbed. Furthermore, false-negative results arise from competitive binding of anti-treponemal IgG. This test can no longer be recommended.

The *19S-IgM–FTA-ABS test* requires filtration of the IgM fraction from the serum.[255] The FTA-ABS test is then performed with the pure IgM fraction. The specificity and sensitivity is very high. Reactivity usually sets in around the end of the second week of infection and ceases within 3 to 6 months after effective treatment of early syphilis and within 12 months in patients with late disease.[249] Unfortunately, false-reactive results may occur in up to 3.4 percent of all positive sera, and false-nonreactive findings may be observed in 3.6 percent of all samples,[256,257] particularly in late disease. This test, which is expensive, requires specially equipped laboratories and properly trained personnel. The introduction of a high-performance liquid chromatography technique for isolation of the IgM fraction[249] may permit more widespread use.

The *IgM-solid phase hemadsorption assay* (IgM-SPHA) is a simple and inexpensive method for the detection of *T. pallidum*-specific IgM.[277] Wells of microtiter plates are coated with μ-chain-specific anti-IgM serum. Patient serum is added, incubated, and rinsed off. IgM antibodies bind to the walls and react in a second step with TPHA antigen as used in the MHA-TP. Agglutination at 1:4 is considered borderline and at or above 1:8 is positive. After effective treatment, the titers drop, and absence of reactivity can be expected within 3 to 6 months in early syphilis and within 3 to 12 months in late disease. Compared to other IgM tests, the sensitivity is around 96 percent and the specificity is about 97.4 percent. False-negative results occur in about 8 percent of reactive samples, predominantly during the primary and late stages. False-positive findings may be observed in up to 1 percent.[256] The advantages are its simple technique and low cost, and the test is superior to the VDRL in the assessment of treatment and the diagnosis of reinfection.[249] In untreated persons, a reactive result indicates almost with certainty the need for therapy, but a nonreactive result does not exclude infection. In cases of doubt, nonreactive SPHA results should be checked by the 19S-IgM–FTA-ABS test, especially if evidence such as a high VDRL titer suggests active disease.

The *T. pallidum-specific IgM hemagglutination test* (TP-IgM-HA) uses human erythrocytes to bind IgM antibodies from the serum of the patient. In a second step, *T. pallidum*-specific IgM reacts with erythrocytes covered with *T. pallidum* antigen. The overall sensitivity of the test was 99.7 percent and the sensitivity 97.6 percent when compared to the 19S-IgM–FTA-ABS test.[278]

The *IgM-ELISA test* is much less expensive compared to the 19S-IgM–FTA-ABS test and offers comparable sensitivity and specificity.[249] In this technique, the walls of the wells of microtiter plates are coated with *T. pallidum* antigen and incubated with serum in serial dilutions. After rinsing, enzyme-labeled antihuman IgM is added and the test then continues as in the ELISA procedure. Another version uses polystyrol beads as carriers for the antigen.

The Captia M Test   Diluted serum is dispensed into microtiter plate wells coated with μ-chain-specific rabbit antibodies against human IgM and incubated. IgM antibodies bind to the wall with the C terminal of the Fc fragment, then a tracer complex consisting of purified *T. pallidum* antigen, biotinylated monoclonal antibody to *T. pallidum*, and horseradish peroxidase streptavidin is added. The antigen of the tracer complex binds to the *N* terminal of the Fab fragment of the *T. pallidum*-specific IgM antibodies on the walls. It is detected there by the biotinylated monoclonal antibodies, which in turn link with the streptavidin conjugate horseradish peroxidase. After rinsing, tetramethylbenzidine is added as a substrate, producing a blue color in positive samples. The reagents are commercially available. A comprehensive evaluation has not yet been published, but preliminary results are very promising. Rheumatoid factors and competitive inhibition by antitreponemal IgG apparently do not interfere with the method.[249] The test offers a high sensitivity and specificity, particularly during the first weeks of infection, but seems to be less sensitive during late disease.[249] In an evaluation of Captia M-tested samples from 180 persons, the sensitivity was 100 percent in congenital syphilis, 82 percent in the primary stage, 60 percent in the secondary period, 53 percent during latency, and 34 percent in neurosyphilis.[279] With the resurgence of early syphilis and congenital syphilis, the interest in IgM tests has considerably increased.[280,281] The sensitivity and specificity of current tests for syphilis serology in the different stages of the disease are presented in Table 218-7. A brief review of selected aspects in the interpretation of serologic test results is presented in Table 218-8.

Unexpected Reactive Results

In all persons with unexpectedly reactive findings in serologic syphilis tests, the examination should be repeated in order to exclude technical errors. Discrepant results in the FTA-ABS and in the MHA-TP should be reevaluated on new blood samples and supplemented by IgM tests. In uncertain cases, the patient should be carefully examined for symptoms of congenital syphilis or active disease. Cardiovascular syphilis, neurosyphilis, and congenital syphilis should be considered. If late disease cannot be excluded, the patient should be treated with a regimen appropriate for neurosyphilis.

Signs of Activity   *Activity of the disease* is indicated by VDRL titers above 1:16 and by positive IgM-SPHA titers of 1:8 or more. In 1 to 2 weeks, both VDRL and IgM-SPHA titers should rise further or, at least, remain at the same values. However, a reactive result in the VDRL at a titer below 1:16 does not necessarily exclude active disease.

Treatment failure is indicated when the VDRL titer remains unchanged at a high dilution (1:32 or more), and/or if the IgM-SPHA titer does not change, and/or if the reactivity in the IgM tests does not cease within 6 to 12 months after adequate therapy (Table 218-8).

Reinfection   A fourfold increase of the VDRL titer or newly reactive IgM tests with rising IgM-SPHA test titers signals reinfection. Treponemal-specific tests are generally not valuable in evaluating reinfection or relapse (Table 218-8). However, active disease is

TABLE 218-8
Diagnostic Interpretation of Results in Syphilis Serology

Test			
VDRL	MHA-TP	FTA-ABS	Interpretation
−	−	−	No syphilis (or incubating syphilis)
+	+	+	Syphilis (except in infants whose mothers have these antibodies)
+	+	ND	Syphilis
+	−	−	BFP, late syphilis, residual seroreactivity after treatment
+	−	+	Early infection?
+	+	−	Latent infection?
−	+	−	Late infection?
−	+	+	BFP or late infection?

NOTE: For explanation of serologic tests, see text; +, positive; −, negative; ND, not done; BFP, biologic false-positive result.

improbable if the MHA-TP titer is 320 or below[282] and remains the same at reexamination 2 or 3 weeks later.

Congenital Syphilis IgG antibodies of adequately treated mothers can pass the placenta and appear in the sera of healthy newborns. In such infants, the titers decrease spontaneously, and reactivity ceases within 3 to 6 months in the VDRL and within 6 to 12 months in the MHA-TP and the FTA-ABS. Reactivity in the 19S-IgM–FTA-ABS, the IgM-SPHA test, or in the Captia M test of the serum of newborns is proof of prenatal syphilis. The benefits of examining all pregnant women with syphilis[283] has been conclusively demonstrated to be cost effective. The benefits of testing hospitalized patients outweigh the arguments and objections against it.[284,285]

Limitations of financial resources affect screening recommendations to a large degree. The World Health Organization has recommended prenatal screening with nontreponemal tests of all females at risk of infection in industrialized countries and, particularly, in areas of endemic treponematoses, because in these groups the focus of interest is detection of early syphilis. However, in high-standard hospitals where the late manifestations of syphilis must not be overlooked, the simultaneous use of nontreponemal as well as treponemal tests is quite justified.

Diagnosis of Neurosyphilis

There is not a single clinical sign that is exclusively specific for neurosyphilis, and so reliable diagnostic criteria by laboratory examinations are of paramount importance (Table 218-9).

The classic laboratory investigation of the cerebrospinal fluid by the Dattner-Thomas formula cannot provide much diagnostic support. Increased cell count above 5 cells/mm³ (500 cells/mL,

TABLE 218-9

Impact of Laboratory Findings on the Diagnosis of Neurosyphilis

---

Neurosyphilis can practically be ruled out by
  Nonreactive CSF TPHA
                     and/or
  Nonreactive CSF FTA-ABS
                    and by
  TPHA index results below 70.
Neurosyphilis is most improbable at
  Serum TPHA (MHA-TP) titers of 320 or below
                   and
  CSF TPHA titers of 320 or below
                  and at
  Nonreactive CSF IgM-SPHA results.
Suspicion of neurosyphilis is justified by appropriate clinical symptoms
  plus CSF cell count above 5×10^6/L (5 cells/mm³)
                   and
  Total protein values above 400 mg/L
                   and
  IgG index above 0.7
                   and
  Positive CSF VDRL result.
Neurosyphilis is most probable at
  TPHA index between 70 and 500.
The diagnosis of neurosyphilis can be made at
  TPHA index results above 500 at intact blood-CSF barrier function
                   and at
  Reactivity in the CSF IgM-SPHA test at titers of 1:1 and above.

NOTE: For explanation of serologic tests, see text.

5×10^6 cells/L) and total protein above 400 mg/L indicate inflammation (specific as well as nonspecific) in the presence of normal blood-CSF barrier function. Both might be normal or slightly elevated in asymptomatic disease as well as in tabes dorsalis, and pathologic findings may be encountered in nonsyphilitic CNS diseases.

Syphilis serology of the CSF has limited diagnostic value. The CSF VDRL result may be nonreactive in up to 73 percent of patients with active disease, particularly in asymptomatic forms and in tabes dorsalis.[286] Two HIV-infected patients with active neurosyphilis (meningitis and radiculopathy) had negative CSF VDRL, which converted to positive 12 days and 3 months, respectively, after initiation of parenteral penicillin.[241] The FTA-ABS and the TPHA test may render reactive results in patients with adequately treated syphilis by transudation of *T. pallidum*-specific IgG from the serum. False-positive CSF FTA-ABS results have been reported in HIV-infected persons without syphilis.[287] On the other hand, *nonreactive CSF FTA-ABS and/or CSF TPHA results practically exclude neurosyphilis*. A patient with adequately treated syphilis without involvement of the CNS but with neurologic disease from nonsyphilitic meningitis or encephalitis, neoplasms, hemorrhage, or cerebral malaria may have false-positive serology results with abnormal CNS cell counts and chemistries that would indicate an incorrect diagnosis of neurosyphilis.

Methods for the Detection of Intrathecal Production of *T. pallidum*-specific Immunoglobulins

The detection of intrathecal synthesis of *T. pallidum*-specific antibodies of the IgM and/or the IgG class would indicate active neurosyphilis. However, it is difficult to determine whether the antibodies are produced intrathecally or are derived from the serum. At normal blood-brain filter conditions, the total IgG values are 200 to 500 times higher in the serum than in the CSF.[288] Therefore, all calculations of intrathecal IgG production should consider the blood-CSF barrier function as indicated below:

$$\text{Albumin quotient} = \frac{\text{CSF albumin (mg/dL)}}{\text{serum albumin (mg/dL)}}$$

Normal values range between 0.0018 and 0.0074. The IgG index (formerly called protein quotient) is calculated as follows:

$$\text{IgG index} = \frac{\text{Total CSF IgG/Total serum IgG}}{\text{CSF albumin/Serum albumin}}$$
$$= \frac{\text{total CSF IgG} \times \text{serum albumin}}{\text{total serum IgG} \times \text{CSF albumin}}$$

Values above 0.7 indicate intrathecal IgG production. Some authors use the CSF antibody titer against adenovirus group antigen by an ELISA assay for the assessment of the blood-CSF barrier function.[289] About 89 percent of normal Americans living in Atlanta have detectable adenovirus antibodies in the serum but not in the CSF. Therefore, identification of these antibodies in the CSF indicates a damaged blood-CSF barrier function, provided that contamination of CSF with blood can be excluded. The detection of antitreponemal IgM in the CSF and nonreactive CSF adenovirus antibody test is consequently indicative of neurosyphilis.[289] The first formula suggested for the calculation of intrathecal production of *T. pallidum*-specific IgG was reported in 1980.[290]

$$\text{TPHA index} = \frac{\text{liquor TPHA titer}}{\text{albumin quotient}} \times 10^3$$

Normal values are below 70, results of 70 to 500 strongly suggest neurosyphilis, and findings above 500 can be considered indicative of intrathecal production of *T. pallidum*-specific IgG and thus of active neurosyphilis.[291] The formula has been modified in the following way:

$$\text{``Modified'' TPHA index} = \frac{\text{CSF TPHA titer/serum TPHA titer}}{\text{albumin quotient}}$$

Values below 0.8 are considered normal. Results between 0.8 and 2 may suggest intrathecal production of *T. pallidum*-specific IgG and an outcome above 2 indicate neurosyphilis. Further investigations led to the description of the ITPA index[292]:

$$\text{ITPA index} = \frac{\text{CSF TPHA titer} \times \text{normal serum IgG}}{\text{serum TPHA titer} \times \text{total CSF IgG}}$$

Normal values range between 0.5 and 2. Results above 2 are considered indicative of active neurosyphilis. The three parameters were compared on the basis of serum and CSF findings of 45 patients with active neurosyphilis and of 67 patients with adequately treated syphilis in whom neurosyphilis was excluded (control group).[291] The modified TPHA index and the ITPA index rendered a considerable number of false-negative (2.2 percent and 13.3 percent) and false-positive (52.2 percent and 44.7 percent) results. On the other hand, the outcome of the TPHA index did not fail to indicate a case of active neurosyphilis and did not reveal pathologic findings in the control group. The diagnosis of neurosyphilis can now effectively be supported by the results of laboratory examinations as indicated in Table 218-9.

Therapy

The use of mercury, iodides, bismuth, organic arsenicals, and fever therapy constituted pharmacologic weapons that sometimes harmed the patient more than the spirochete. The organic arsenicals, which were the most effective among the lot, were widely used in the treatment of early syphilis until the introduction of penicillin. Many interesting reviews have been written about these therapies.[293–295]

Penicillin

Penicillin remains the mainstay of treatment and the standard by which other modes of therapy are judged. Although, on rare occasions, organisms have been found to persist after adequate therapy in humans and animals, there is no indication that *T. pallidum* has acquired resistance to the drug. Beta-lactam antibiotics work by irreversible binding to the transpeptidase enzymes required for biosynthesis of the outer envelope. Consequentially, the holes in the envelope lattice, which occur during phases of growth, do not close, and the net becomes fragile. The resulting high osmotic pressure within the protoplasmic cylinder causes bulging of the inner membrane and bursting of the treponeme.

Beta-lactam antibiotics are bactericidal. The bactericidal effect depends entirely on uninterrupted maintenance of effective concentrations. Because penicillin does not interfere with the synthesis of transpeptidases, the intact bacteria can resume growth and generate new organisms within 20 min of inadequate penicillin levels.

The concentrations of penicillin must be in the range of 0.0025 units/mL in order to kill 50 percent of *T. pallidum* within 16 h.

More than 10 times this concentration, or 0.03 units/mL, is recommended for a minimum duration of 7 to 10 days in early syphilis and longer in late syphilis.

The amount of penicillin required to prevent disease increases with the interval between inoculation and therapy, as well as with the number of organisms in the inoculum. Approximately 3 percent of males with gonococcal urethritis also have incubating syphilis, and treatment with short-acting procaine penicillin is sufficient to abort syphilitic infection as so few treponemes are present. Because *T. pallidum* divides every 33 h in early lesions, treatment requires effective antibiotic levels in serum and tissue for an uninterrupted and prolonged period of time.

Experimental latent syphilis requires penicillin therapy of even longer duration. This is, perhaps, due to the slower replication of organisms in late compared to early disease, rather than to the number of spirochetes present. According to reports, a very high concentration of penicillin in blood and tissue is attained by intravenous infusion of 4 million units of water-soluble penicillin G at 4-h intervals.[296] Although oral penicillin can achieve adequate serum and tissue levels, it is not recommended because effectiveness is reduced as patients often forget to take one or more doses. In addition, irregular absorption of the antibiotic can result in inadequate serum levels.

Other Drugs

Other antibiotics, such as tetracycline, erythromycin, and nonpenicillin beta-lactam compounds (particularly third-generation cephalosporins such as ceftriaxone), have strong antitreponemal activity in experimental and clinical trials. Chloramphenicol has been studied in only a small number of patients. It probably has some benefit in primary syphilis, but its bone marrow toxicity makes it a poor choice. Spectinomycin is ineffective, and rifampin, clindamycin, kanamycin, and trimethoprim-sulfamethoxazole may actually enhance the growth of *T. pallidum* in vitro. Streptomycin, polymyxin, bacitracin, novobiocin, griseofulvin, and metronidazole may suppress the development of clinical lesions and extend the period of latency but may not, ultimately, prevent late disease.

Microbial Persistence

Even after "adequate" penicillin therapy, the spirochete may persist in tissue. Treponemes have been found in the CSF,[297,298] anterior chamber of the eye,[299] lymph nodes, temporal arteries, bone,[300] and perilymph of the middle ear.[301] Although the methodology of these observations has been questioned and treponemal forms have been observed in tissue of patients with no evidence of syphilis, a large body of evidence suggests that *T. pallidum* may persist in some patients despite adequate treatment of early or late syphilis.[302] Electron micrographic studies of early lesions have shown treponemes inside the cytoplasm and even the nuclei of cells. Although the organisms are destroyed with macrophages and neutrophils, they may remain intact within plasma cells, fibroblasts, and even spermatocytes. Within 3 to 6 h after the administration of penicillin, extracellular spirochetes are destroyed, although intracellular organisms may remain intact. Whether these intracellular organisms retain their virulence is unknown. In fact, the persistence of treponemes after treatment may not appreciably influence therapeutic results. If benzathine penicillin, which has been prescribed for early syphilis since 1954, were an inadequate therapy, a dramatic increase in late manifestations would be expected. Instead, the morbidity due to late manifestations decreased by 88 percent from 1943 to 1971. Certainly, no antibacterial therapy is infallible, but treatment failures are very rare and regularly respond to a second course of penicillin at the same, or somewhat higher, doses.

The significance of treponemes in the spinal fluid continues to be debated.[302] The concentration of penicillin in the CSF ranges between 1 and 10 percent of the serum level, but even a single injection of benzathine penicillin produces effective levels in the perivascular areas where the treponemes are found and the syphilitic tissue damage is located. However, because the greatest reasonable margin of safety is indispensable and benzathine penicillin produces relatively low serum levels, it is not recommended for patients with CNS involvement.

Treatment Guidelines

The treatment schedules recommended by the Centers for Disease Control (CDC)[303] and by the World Health Organization (WHO)[291] were updated in 1989 and represent the culmination of available information and clinical experience (Table 218-10).

Penicillin remains the only therapy that has been widely used for neurosyphilis, congenital syphilis, or syphilis during pregnancy. Therefore, allergy skin testing and desensitization is recommended for any of these patients who also has a history of penicillin allergy, although the minor determinant mixture for penicillin is not currently available commercially.

Early Syphilis—Primary, Secondary, Latent Syphilis of Less Than One (CDC) or Two Years' (WHO) Duration Benzathine penicillin remains the drug of choice for primary and secondary syphilis, as it provides effective treatment in a single visit.[291,303] Therapeutic results collected from multiple studies show that 97 percent of 1381 persons with seronegative primary syphilis were clinically well with serologically unreactive tests 2 to 10 years after therapy. The 3 percent failure rate was attributed to reinfections.[304–306] In penicillin-allergic patients, doxycycline or erythromycin can be prescribed. The efficacy of erythromycin in all stages of syphilis and its ability to prevent the stigmata of congenital syphilis are questionable and many failures have been reported.

Latent Syphilis of Indeterminate or More Than One (CDC) or Two (WHO) Years' Duration, Cardiovascular, and Late Benign Syphilis (Gummas) All patients should have a thorough clinical

---

TABLE 218-10
Treatment Guidelines for Syphilis

Centers for Disease Control[303]	World Health Organization[291]
Primary, secondary, or early latent syphilis (< 1 year)	
Benzathine penicillin G 2.4 million U IM × 1 dose	(Early latent syphilis is defined as latent disease for <2 years.)
Alternative regimen:	Same
Doxycycline 100 mg bid × 2 weeks	Alternative regimen:
or	Procaine penicillin G 1.2 million U IM × 10 days
Tetracycline 500 mg qid × 2 weeks	
or	
Erythromycin 500 mg qid × 2 weeks	
Late latent (>1 year) syphilis gummas, and cardiovascular syphilis	
Benzathine penicillin G 2.4 million U IM 1 week apart × 3 consecutive weeks	(Late latent syphilis is defined as latent disease for >2 years.)
Alternative regimen:	Procaine penicillin 1.2 million U IM daily × 20 days
Doxycycline 100 mg bid × 4 weeks	Alternative regimen:
or	Benzathine penicillin G 2.4 million U IM 1 week apart × 3 consecutive doses
Tetracycline 500 mg qid × 4 weeks	
Neurosyphilis	
Aqueous penicillin G 2–4 million U q 4 h IV × 10–14 days	Same
Alternative regimen:	Alternative regimen:
Procaine penicillin G 1.2 million U IM daily with probenecid 500 mg qid orally × 10–14 days followed by benzathine penicillin G 2.4 million U IM weekly × 3 consecutive weeks	Procaine penicillin G 1.2 million U IM daily with probenecid 500 mg qid orally × 10–14 days
Patient should be desensitized if allergic to penicillin. Ceftriaxone, 1 g daily × 14 days, may be effective.	or
	Doxycycline 100 mg bid orally × 30 days
	or
	Tetracycline 500 mg qid orally × 30 days
Syphilis in pregnancy	
Penicillin regimen appropriate for stage of disease. Desensitize for penicillin allergy. Ceftriaxone is potentially valuable but not yet recommended.	Same
Prenatal syphilis	
Newborns:	Birth to 2 years:
Aqueous penicillin G 50,000 U/kg q 8–12 h IV × 10–14 days	Benzathine penicillin G 50,000 U/kg IM if neurosyphilis has been ruled out.
or	Aqueous penicillin G 50,000 U/kg IM or IV bid × 10 days
Procaine penicillin G 50,000 U/kg IM daily × 10–14 days	Aqueous procaine penicillin G 50,000 U/kg IM qid × 10 days
After newborn period:	Over 2 years of age:
Benzathine penicillin G 50,000 U/kg IM up to 2.4 million U	Aqueous penicillin G 200,000–300,000 U/kg per day up to 12–24 million U/day IV in 4–6 doses × 10–14 days
Neurosyphilis or no CSF examination:	
Penicillin G 50,000 U/kg q 4–6 h IV × 10–14 days	

examination. Preferably, any patient with syphilis of more than 1 year's duration should have a CSF examination, but, to an extent, performance of lumbar puncture can be individualized. In asymptomatic individuals, the yield of positive lumbar punctures is low. However, CSF examination is clearly indicated in certain situations, such as presence of neurologic signs or symptoms, treatment failure, therapy other than penicillin, serum nontreponemal antibody titer greater than 1:32, evidence of active syphilis (aortitis, gumma, iritis), and reactive HIV serology. If the CSF examination demonstrates abnormal, unexplainable findings, patients should be treated for neurosyphilis.

The outcome of treatment of late latent syphilis has not been conclusively studied, but in 469 patients followed for up to 12 years after treatment, the spinal fluid remained normal, and no evidence of cardiovascular syphilis was reported.[306]

Cardiovascular Syphilis   Cardiovascular syphilis is usually not diagnosed until the patient has become symptomatic. Because advanced symptomatic disease is associated with poor prognosis regardless of treatment,[307] some experts prefer to treat cardiovascular disease with the same regimens as neurosyphilis. The evidence suggests that penicillin has a beneficial effect in the majority of patients, although efficacy is difficult to evaluate as most symptomatic patients received additional therapies such as digitalis and diuretics.[308] Subjective improvement and reduction in diastolic murmur were the most impressive findings. Another study with follow-up from 6 months to 5 years found that, with penicillin treatment, asymptomatic patients remained well, with no deterioration of aortic insufficiency. In patients with aortic insufficiency, aneurysms, or both, who were treated with penicillin and followed for 6 to 72 months, 62.6 percent had symptomatic improvement, whereas the disease progressed in 4 percent of asymptomatic and 4.5 percent of symptomatic patients.

Late Benign Syphilis   Because up to 25 percent of patients with gummas will also have cardiovascular syphilis or neurosyphilis, careful evaluation of the patient and CSF examination are obligatory for determination of optimal therapy. The gummas heal slowly over several months, depending on the extent of tissue destruction.[306] Gummas of the brain or spinal cord may need surgical excision.

Quantitative nontreponemal serologic tests should be repeated at 6 and 12 months. If titers increase fourfold, if an initially high titer fails to decrease, or if the patient develops signs or symptoms attributable to syphilis, the patient should be reevaluated for neurosyphilis and re-treated appropriately.

Neurosyphilis   Evaluation of regimens with oral tetracyclines in neurosyphilis is not yet available.[291] Third-generation cephalosporins, especially ceftriaxone (1 g daily for 14 days), appear promising. In most of 8706 cases of neurosyphilis treated with penicillin with doses varying from 2 to 20 million units daily, a favorable clinical outcome was recorded. Penicillin cured, improved, or stabilized the disease in 75 percent of patients with general paresis and taboparesis (48 percent cured); in 72 percent with tabes dorsalis (47 percent cured); in 78 percent with meningovascular disease or meningitis (81 percent cured); in 88 percent with miscellaneous conditions (18 percent cured); and in 91 percent of cases with asymptomatic disease.[309]

In one study, when symptoms worsened, about half of those patients re-treated subsequently improved with larger doses of penicillin.[310] Optic atrophy, alone or in conjunction with tabes dorsa-

lis, and eighth nerve-related deafness are notoriously resistant to treatment. No case of blindness due to optic atrophy was reversible with penicillin, although lack of progression or improvement occurred in 3 to 60 percent. Eighth nerve deafness appears to benefit from the combination of penicillin and prednisone, but controlled studies are not available for substantiation.[11] If CSF pleocytosis is present, CSF examination should be repeated every 6 months until the cell count is normal. If it has not decreased at 6 months, or is not normal by 2 years, re-treatment should be strongly considered.[303]

Pregnancy   Pregnant women should be screened early, and those with seropositive results should be considered infected unless treatment can be verified and sequential serologic antibody titers convincingly demonstrate an appropriate response. In populations with suboptimal utilization of prenatal care, patients should be screened and, if necessary, treated as soon as the pregnancy is detected. In areas of high syphilis prevalence or in patients at high risk, screening should be repeated in the third trimester and again at delivery.[303]

In case of doubt, re-treatment is warranted as the potential benefits outweigh the possible risks. The WHO recommends repeat serology tests 4 weeks after the ones obtained during the first antenatal visit and, if the tests are negative, at the beginning of the third trimester. The inclination to treat syphilis during pregnancy must be tempered with the knowledge that false-positive serologic tests are not uncommon. Therefore, all positive serologic tests should be confirmed by specific assays for antitreponemal antibody.

Treatment with penicillin is strongly recommended in pregnancy. The only potential serious side effect is the Jarisch-Herxheimer reaction, which may precipitate labor ("placental shock"). However, the association of spontaneous abortion with this phenomenon is debatable and should not delay treatment of maternal syphilis with anything less than full doses of penicillin.

The antibiotic readily crosses the placenta. Aqueous penicillin G and procaine penicillin G produce high fetal blood levels 60 to 90 min after injection and reach a peak concentration of 20 to 30 percent (rarely 75 percent) of the maternal serum level. Therefore, 2.4 million units of benzathine penicillin would not consistently provide effective levels in the fetus. Monthly evaluations are mandatory, and re-treatment given if needed. The antibody response should be the same as for nonpregnant patients.

The prognosis of infants born to syphilitic mothers treated during pregnancy is encouraging. In a study of 414 pregnant women with early syphilis treated with varying amounts of penicillin (600,000 to 10 million units), only 5.3 percent of the neonates had syphilis and a "normal" rate of stillbirths was reported. The failures were observed in females treated late in pregnancy and during relapses or reinfection.[311]

Infected pregnant women with penicillin allergy should be desensitized and treated. Erythromycin is prescribed only when penicillin desensitization is impossible. Erythromycin is not an adequate drug for the pregnant patient because its ability to cross the placenta is fair to poor.[312] Infants born to mothers who received erythromycin for syphilis during pregnancy should be thoroughly evaluated for active disease, treated with penicillin, and closely followed.[313] Tetracycline is avoided because of deposition in bone and enamel with resulting staining of the teeth.[291] Although the permanent teeth are normal, the child may experience considerable psychologic and social adjustment problems from this disfigurement. Third-generation cephalosporins are potentially valuable in the treatment of syphilis during pregnancy because adequate treponemecidal fetal blood levels are achieved. These agents appear to be safe in the pregnant patient and they have been reported to be effective, in anecdotal cases. Despite insufficient data, treatment with ceftriaxone can be considered in pregnant women with penicillin allergy that is not manifested by anaphylaxis.[291]

It is essential that infants born to seropositive mothers who remained untreated or received treatment less than 1 month before delivery or at any time during pregnancy with a non-penicillin regimen be evaluated. Also, the offspring of mothers who did not have the expected decrease in serologic titers after treatment need to be carefully observed. The neonate's evaluation should include a thorough physical examination, nontreponemal antibody titer, CSF analysis, long bone x-rays, other tests as clinically indicated (e.g., chest x-ray), and, if possible, FTA-ABS on the purified 19S-IgM fraction of serum. These infants should be treated if they have any evidence of active disease by physical examination or radiographs, a reactive CSF VDRL, abnormal unexplained CSF findings, quantitative nontreponemal serologic titers that are fourfold or higher than their mother's, or reactive FTA-ABS 19S-IgM antibody. Even with a normal evaluation, infants should be treated if their mothers have untreated syphilis or evidence of relapse or reinfection after therapy.

Seropositive untreated infants must be reexamined at 1, 2, 3, 6, and 12 months of age. In the absence of infection, nontreponemal antibody titers should be decreasing by 3 months of age and should have disappeared by 6 months of age. Unless this is the case, the child should be treated. If treponemal antibodies persist beyond the first year of life, the infant should also be treated for congenital syphilis.[303] Treated infants should be followed with nontreponemal antibody titers, which should disappear by 6 months of age. Treponemal tests, however, may remain positive despite effective therapy. Infants with documented CSF pleocytosis should be tapped every 6 months until the cell count is normal. If the cell count is still abnormal after 2 years or if a downward trend is not present at each examination, the infant should be re-treated. The CSF VDRL should also be checked at 6 months, and re-treatment is administered if it is still reactive.

There are no adequate data to advocate the treatment of prenatal syphilis with antibiotics other than penicillin. Oral erythromycin may be effective in a dose of 7.5 to 12.5 mg/kg 4 times daily for 30 days.[291] For children who are allergic to penicillin and older than 8 years, a dose of 30 mg/kg daily of oral tetracycline, up to 2 g per day, for 15 days in early disease and 30 days in late disease may be effective.[291]

Persons Exposed to Syphilis (Epidemiologic Treatment) Persons sexually exposed to a patient with early syphilis should be evaluated clinically and serologically.[303] In this situation, the risk of contracting infection is around 10 to 62 percent after a single contact. It may be advisable to treat prophylactically persons exposed more than 90 days previously if serologic test results are not immediately available or compliance appears uncertain. Patients who have other sexually transmitted diseases should have a serologic test for syphilis.[303] Even though syphilis is usually not sexually transmitted 2 years after the initial infection, contact investigation of the family members is indicated to exclude syphilis in a spouse or children. Patients suspected of syphilis contact should be examined, and an STS checked every month for a maximum of 3 months from the last exposure with the contact. Alternatively, treatment for incubating syphilis with the same regimens used for primary syphilis should be considered if compliance with testing cannot be guaranteed.

HIV-Associated Syphilis Penicillin is recommended for all stages of syphilis in HIV-infected patients. Skin testing to confirm penicillin allergy may be used, although data in these patients are inadequate. No change in therapy of early syphilis for HIV-coinfected patients has been recommended; however, CSF examination is advocated or treatment with higher doses of penicillin. Although CSF abnormalities may be due to HIV-related infection, if neurosyphilis cannot be excluded, the patient should be treated for this problem. Evaluation with quantitative nontreponemal serologic tests at 1, 2, 3, 6, 9, and 12 months after treatment is essential. Patients with early syphilis whose titers increase or fail to decrease fourfold within 6 months should undergo CSF examination and re-treatment.

Penicillin Allergy Testing Ninety percent of patients with histories of ''penicillin allergy'' have negative skin tests and can be given penicillin safely. The other 10 percent with positive skin tests have an increased risk of penicillin allergy and should undergo desensitization (Table 218-11). Radioallergosorbent test (RAST) results are not determinative as penicillin-specific IgE antibodies may be detected in persons without penicillin allergy, and a negative outcome does not definitely exclude penicillin allergy.[314] Patients with a history of penicillin allergy but with no reaction to penicillin skin tests, who are not on antihistamines, and who had a positive histamine control on skin testing should be given 250 mg of penicillin orally and observed for 1 h. Patients who tolerate this dose well may be treated with penicillin as needed.

Desensitization The procedure described is not actually a desensitization but an immunotolerance induced by administration of very small doses of antigen. Hypersensitivity to penicillin still persists, but antibodies of the IgE class bind to scanty amounts of antigen. Therefore, the reaction is faint and remains subclinical. Because serious IgE-mediated allergic reaction can occur, the procedure should be done in a hospital. The antigens (Table 218-12) should be diluted 100-fold for preliminary testing if there has been an immediate generalized reaction within the past year. The test is unreliable if antihistamines have been administered within the last 48 h.

EPICUTANEOUS SCRATCH OR PRICK TEST. Apply one drop of material to the volar forearm, pierce the epidermis without drawing blood, and observe for 20 min. If there is no wheal greater than 4 mm, proceed to the intradermal test.

INTRADERMAL TEST. Inject 0.02 mL intradermally with a 27-gauge short-bevelled needle and observe for 20 min.

INTERPRETATION. For the test to be interpretable, the negative (saline) control must elicit no reaction and the positive (histamine) control must elicit a positive reaction. A positive test is a wheal greater than 4 mm in diameter to any penicillin reagent. In a negative test, the wheals at the site of the penicillin reagents are equivalent to the negative control. All other results are indeterminate.

Complications of Therapy

The Jarisch-Herxheimer reaction is a clinical syndrome consisting of fever, headache, flare of mucocutaneous lesions, tender lymphadenopathy, pharyngitis, malaise, myalgias, and leukocytosis with lymphopenia within 12 h of therapy for syphilis.[315] The fever peaks in 6 to 8 h, usually around 39°C (102.2°F), but can be as high as 42°C (107.6°F). It occurs in 55 percent of seronegative and 95 percent of seropositive primary and secondary syphilis cases. Focal

TABLE 218-11
Oral Desensitization Protocol

Penicillin V dose	Suspension (units/mL)	mL	Amount	
			Cumulative	
			Units	Dose (units)
1	1,000	0.1	100	100
2	1,000	0.2	200	300
3	1,000	0.4	400	700
4	1,000	0.8	800	1,500
5	1,000	1.6	1,600	3,100
6	1,000	3.2	3,200	6,300
7	1,000	6.4	6,400	12,700
8	10,000	1.2	12,000	24,700
9	10,000	2.4	24,000	48,700
10	10,000	4.8	48,000	96,700
11	80,000	1.0	80,000	176,000
12	80,000	2.0	160,000	336,700
13	80,000	4.0	320,000	656,700
14	80,000	8.0	640,000	1,296,700

NOTE: Observation period: 30 min before parenteral administration of penicillin.

TABLE 218-12
Reagents for Desensitization

Major Determinants
Benzylpenicilloyl polylysine (major, Pre-Pen,* 6×10^{-5} M)
Benzylpenicillin (10^{-2} M or 6000 U/mL)
Minor Determinants
Benzylpenicilloic acid (10^{-2} M)
Benzylpenilloic acid (10^{-2} M)
Positive control (histamine, 1 mg/mL)
Negative control (buffered saline solution)

*Taylor Pharmacl Co., Decator, Illinois.

or cutaneous manifestations are noted in 11 percent of treated early syphilis and in almost half of those with febrile reaction. The Jarisch-Herxheimer reaction in early syphilis is of no consequence. Patient education about the reaction and simple analgesics for symptoms are the only precautions and treatment required.

The frequency decreases in late secondary syphilis and is usually absent in latent syphilis. However, 53 to 95 percent with paresis, 9 to 23 percent with tabes, and 12 to 36 percent with other types of neurosyphilis have developed fever after treatment with penicillin. Febrile reactions are more common when the CSF contains high numbers of cells and protein. Convulsions, worsened dementia, psychosis, and meningismus have occurred in about 2 percent of neurosyphilis cases treated with penicillin. Death is rare, occurring only once among 1086 paretic patients.[310] The occurrence of Jarisch-Herxheimer reactions in cardiovascular syphilis is difficult to document. About half of infants with early and 39 percent of those with late disease develop febrile reactions. Rare cases of elevated liver function tests and the nephrotic syndrome have been reported.

Acute inflammatory changes, which occur within 4 to 6 h after treatment, consist of dilatation of the small dermal vessels, followed by endothelial swelling and migration of leukocytes through the vessel walls into the surrounding edematous tissue. It has been proposed that death of spirochetes is followed by massive phagocytosis with release of a leukocyte pyrogen that cause the reaction. Also, treponemal endotoxin and cell-mediated phenomena have been implicated,[316] but the pathogenesis remains unknown. It seems probable that plasma kinins may influence the course, but the complement system does not appear to play a role.[317] Systemic corticosteroids modify the febrile reaction without affecting the skin lesions or the leukocytosis and, if administered 12 h prior to or at the time of treatment, suppress or mitigate the reaction.

Therapeutic paradox, or deterioration of tertiary syphilis after therapy, results from rapid decomposition of gummatous tissue. The deterioration may extend to the surrounding tissue that is histologically but not yet clinically involved. Scarring worsens the appearance of the lesions. Separating these changes, which are by no means limited to the skin, from syphilitic disease becomes a dilemma. For instance, worsening of the aortic insufficiency murmur has been reported from this complication.

Another penicillin-associated adverse effect, *the pseudoanaphylactic reaction (Hoigne syndrome)* is associated with intramuscular procaine penicillin.[318] It occurs in approximately 1 case per 1000 treatments and is more common in males. The reaction is characterized by auditory or visual disturbances, unusual taste sensation, fear of imminent death, violent combativeness, neuromuscular twitching, occasional grand mal seizures, loss of consciousness, elevated blood pressure, and tachycardia and rarely lasts longer than 30 min. Treatment consists of observation and sedatives or anticonvulsants. Inadvertent intracapillary infusion of procaine or, less likely, penicillin during intramuscular injection resulting in microembolization has been proposed as the mechanism.[319]

References

1. Musher DM: Syphilis (Review). *Infect Dis Clin North Am* **1**:83, 1987
2. Dover JS, Arndt KA: Dermatology. *JAMA* **261**:2838, 1989
3. Felman YM: Syphilis from 1495 Naples to 1989 AIDS. *Arch Dermatol* **125**:1698, 1989
4. Ober WB: To cast a pox: The iconography of syphilis. *Am J Dermatopathol* **11**:74, 1987

5. Luger A: Standort und Ausblick der deutschsprachigen Dermatologie, in *Zum 100jahrigen Bestehen der Deutschen Dermatologischen Gesellschaft,* edited by G Stüttgen. Berlin, Grosse Verlag, 1989

6. Sparling FP: Natural history of syphilis, in *Sexually Transmitted Diseases,* edited by RD Caterall, CS Nichol. London, Academic, 1990, p 213

7. Rothschild BM: On the antiquity of treponemal infection. *Med Hypotheses* **28**:181, 1989

8. Ricord P: *Traite Practique des Maladies Vénériennes.* Paris, De Just Bouvier et Eike Bouvier, 1838

9. Brandt AM: The syphilis epidemic and its relation to AIDS. *Science* **239**:375, 1988

10. Mahoney JF et al: Penicillin treatment of early syphilis. A primary report. *Vener Dis Inform* **24**:355, 1943

11. Morton RS: Syphilis in art: An entertainment in four parts. *Genitourin Med* **66**:112, 1990

12. Department of Health and Social Security Annual Report: Sexually transmitted diseases. *Br J Vener Dis* **59**:206, 1983

13. Melvin SY: Syphilis: Resurgence of an old disease. *Prim Care* **17**:47, 1990

14. Brandt AM: Sexually transmitted disease: Shadow on the land, revisited (comment). *Ann Intern Med* **112**:481, 1990

15. Morrow PA: Publicity as a factor in venereal prophylaxis. *JAMA* **47**:1244, 1906

16. Andrus JK et al: Partner notification: Can it control syphilis? *Ann Intern Med* **112**:539, 1990

17. Tramont EC: Syphilis in the AIDS era. *N Engl J Med* **316**:1600, 1987

18. Centers for Disease Control: Reported morbidity and mortality in the United States, 1976: Annual summary of morbidity and mortality. *MMWR* **25**:2, 1977

19. Centers for Disease Control: Syphilis trends in the United States. *MMWR* **35**:441, 1981

20. Summary of Notifiable Diseases, United States, 1989. *MMWR* **53**:1, 1989

21. Rolfs RT, Cates W Jr: The perpetual lessons of syphilis. *Arch Dermatol* **125**:107, 1989

22. Willcox PR: Changing patterns of treponemal disease. *Br J Vener Dis* **50**:169, 1974

23. Increases in primary and secondary syphilis—United States. *MMWR* **36**:393, 1987

24. Rolfs RT, Nakashima AK: Epidemiology of primary syphilis in the United States, 1981–1989. *JAMA* **264**:1432, 1990

25. Rolfs RT et al: Risk factors for syphilis: Cocaine use and prostitution. *Am J Public Health* **80**:853, 1990

26. Leads from the MMWR. Relationship of syphilis to drug use and prostitution—Connecticut and Philadelphia, Pennsylvania. *JAMA* **261**:353, 1989

27. Petrone ME et al: Epidemiology of congenital syphilis. *N J Med* **86**:965, 1989

28. Cohen DA et al: The effects of case definition in maternal screening and reporting criteria on rates of congenital syphilis. *Am J Public Health* **80**:316, 1990

29. Congenital syphilis—New York City, 1986–1988. *MMWR* **38**:825, 1989

30. Adler M: The epidemiology of sexually transmitted diseases in the West. *Semin Dermatol* **9**:96, 1990

31. Tang A, Barlow D: Resurgence of heterosexually acquired early syphilis in London (letter). *Lancet* **2**:166, 1989

32. Goeman J, Piot P: The epidemiology of sexually transmitted diseases in Africa and Latin America. *Semin Dermatol* **9**:105, 1990

33. Development of a treponemal vaccine. Current status and recommendation for further research. Report of a World Health Organization Consultative Group, Birmingham, UK, April 1989

34. Baseman JB: The spirochetes, in *Microbiology,* edited by BD Davis et al. Philadelphia, Lippincott, 1990, p 673

35. Magnarelli LA et al: Cross-reactivity of nonspecific treponemal antibody in serologic tests for Lyme disease. *J Clin Microbiol* **28**:1276, 1990

36. Musher DM: Biology of *Treponema pallidum,* in *Sexually Transmitted Diseases,* edited by RD Caterall, CS Nichol. London, Academic, 1990, p 205

37. Fohn MJ et al: Specificity of antibodies from patients with pinta for antigens of *Treponema pallidum* subspecies *pallidum. J Infect Dis* **157**:32, 1988

38. Larsen SA, Hunter EF: Syphilis, in *Sexually Transmitted Diseases,* edited by RD Caterall, CS Nichol. London, Academic, 1990, p 927

39. Rudolf JD et al: Outer membrane ultrastructure explains the limited antigenicity of virulent *Treponema pallidum. Proc Natl Acad Sci USA* **86**:2051, 1989

40. *Syphilis, a Synopsis,* US Dept of Health, Education, and Welfare publication No. 1660. Washington, DC, Government Printing Office, 1968

41. Martin HH: Wirkungsmechanismus einiger antibakterieller Antibiotika und ihre Bedeutung fur die Chemotherapie von Treponemainfektiohen. *Hautarzt* (suppl)**1**:227, 1976

42. Zeigler JA et al: Demonstration of extracellular material at the surface of pathogenic *T. pallidum* cells. *Br J Vener Dis* **52**:1, 1976

43. Rathlev T: Investigations on in vitro survival and virulence of *T. pallidum* under aerobiosis. *Br J Vener Dis* **51**:296, 1976

44. Fitzgerald TJ et al: Interaction of *Treponema pallidum* with cultured mammalian cells: Effects of oxygen, reducing agents, serum supplements, and different cell types. *Infect Immun* **15**:444, 1977

45. Baseman JB et al: Virulent *Treponema pallidum:* Aerobe or anaerobe? *Infect Immun* **13**:704, 1976

46. Austin FE et al: Distribution of superoxide dismutase, catalase, and peroxidase activities among *Treponema pallidum* and other spirochetes. *Infect Immun* **33**:372, 1981

47. Fitzgerald FT et al: *Treponema pallidum* (Nichols strain) in tissue cultures: Cellular attachment, entry, and survival. *Infect Immun* **11**:1141, 1975

48. Thomas DD et al: *Treponema pallidum* invades intercellular junctions in endothelial cell monolayers. *Proc Natl Acad Sci USA* **85**:3608, 1988

49. Riviere GR et al: In vitro model of *Treponema pallidum* invasiveness. *Infect Immun* **57**:2267, 1989

50. Alderete JF, Baseman JB: Serum lipoprotein binding of *Treponema pallidum:* Possible role for proteoglycan. *Genitourin Med* **65**:177, 1989

51. Musher DM et al: The interaction between *Treponema pallidum* and human polymorphonuclear leukocytes. *J Infect Dis* **147**:77, 1983

52. Alderete JF, Baseman JB: Surface-associated host proteins on virulent *Treponema pallidum. Infect Immun* **26**:1048, 1989

53. Baker-Zander SA, Sell S: A histopathologic and immunopathologic study of the course of syphilis in the experimentally infected rabbit. *Am J Pathol* **101**:387, 1980

54. Bjerke JR et al: In situ identification of mononuclear cells in cutaneous infiltrates in discoid lupus erythematosus, sarcoidosis and secondary syphilis. *Acta Derm Venereol* (Stockholm) **61**:371, 1980

55. Jeerapaet P, Ackerman AB: Histologic patterns of secondary syphilis. *Arch Dermatol* **107**:373, 1973

56. Fitzgerald TJ, Johnson RC: Mucopolyssaccharides of *Treponema pallidum. Infect Immun* **24**:261, 1979

57. Lukehart SA: Activation of macrophages by products of lymphocytes from normal and syphilitic rabbits. *Infect Immun* **37**:64, 1982

58. Alder JD et al: Phagocytosis of *Treponema pallidum* subsp. *pertenue* by hamster macrophages on membrane filters. *J Infect Dis* **160**:289, 1989

59. Hardy PH et al: Macrophages in immunity to syphilis: Suppressive effect of concurrent infection with *Mycobacterium bovis* BCG on the development of syphilitic lesions and growth of *Treponema pallidum* in tuberculin-positive rabbits. *Infect Immun* **26**:751, 1979

60. Graves S: Susceptibility of rabbits to *Treponema pallidum* after infection with *Mycobacterium bovis. Br J Vener Dis* **44**:394, 1979

61. Azadegan AA et al: Synergistic effect of macrophage activation and

immune serum, especially IgG2, on resistance to infection with *Treponema pallidum* subsp. *endemicum* in hamsters. *Reg Immunol* **1**:3, 1988

62. Baughn RE et al: Ig class and IgG subclass responses to *Treponema pallidum* in patients with syphilis. *J Clin Immunol* **8**:129, 1988

63. Lukehart SA et al: Characterization of the humoral immune response of the rabbit antigens of *Treponema pallidum* after experimental infection and therapy. *Sex Transm Dis* **13**:9, 1986

64. Wright DJM, Grimble AGS: Why is the infectious stage of syphilis so prolonged? *Br J Vener Dis* **50**:45, 1974

65. Pavia CS et al: Cell mediated immunity during syphilis (review). *Br J Vener Dis* **54**:144, 1978

66. From E et al: Reactivity of lymphocytes from patients with syphilis towards *Treponema pallidum* antigen in the lymphocyte migration and lymphocyte transformation tests. *Br J Vener Dis* **56**:224, 1976

67. Musher DM et al: Lymphocyte transformation in syphilis: An in vitro correlate of immune suppression in vivo? *Infect Immun* **11**:1261, 1975

68. Lukehart SA et al: Characterization of lymphocyte response in early experimental syphilis. In vitro response to mitogens and *Treponema pallidum* antigens. *J Immunol* **124**:454, 1980

69. Schell RF et al: Induction of acquired cellular resistance following transfer of thymus-dependent lymphocytes from syphilitic rabbits. *J Immunol* **114**:550, 1975

70. Jensen JR, From E: Alterations in T lymphocytes and T-lymphocyte subpopulations in patients with syphilis. *Br J Vener Dis* **58**:18, 1982

71. Tosca A et al: Infiltrate of syphilitic lesions before and after treatment. *Genitourin Med* **64**:289, 1988

72. Jensen JR et al: Fluctuations in natural killer cell activity in early syphilis. *Br J Vener Dis* **59**:30, 1983

73. Jorizzo JL et al: Role of circulating immune complexes in human secondary syphilis. *J Infect Dis* **153**:1014, 1986

74. Folds JD et al: Lymphocyte transformation and the effect of circulating immune complexes in humans with syphilis. *Sex Transm Dis* **9**:109, 1982

75. Radolf JD et al: The surface of virulent *Treponema pallidum:* Resistance to antibody binding in the absence of complement and surface association of recombinant antigen 4D. *Infect Immun* **52**:579, 1986

76. Clark EG, Danbolt N: The Oslo study of the natural course of untreated syphilis: An epidemiologic investigation based on a re-study of the Boeck-Bruusgaard material. *J Chronic Dis* **2**:311, 1955

77. Handsfield HH et al: Demonstration of *Treponema pallidum* in a cutaneous gumma by indirect immunofluorescence. *Arch Dermatol* **119**:677, 1983

78. Sell S, Norris SJ: The biology, pathology and immunology of syphilis. *Int Rev Exp Pathol* **24**:203, 1983

79. Magnuson HG et al: Inoculation syphilis in human volunteers. *Medicine (Baltimore)* **35**:33, 1956

80. Dunlop EMC: Persistence of treponemes after treatment. *Br Med J* **2**:577, 1972

81. Riviere GR et al: In vitro model of *Treponema pallidum* invasiveness. *Infect Immun* **57**:2267, 1989

82. Bishop NH, Miller JN: Humoral immunity in experimental syphilis. I. The demonstration of resistance conferred by passive immunization. *J Immunol* **117**:191, 1976

83. Hayer NS et al: Parasitism by virulent *Treponema pallidum* of host cell surfaces. *Infect Immun* **17**:174, 1977

84. Gschnait F et al: Laboratory evidence of impaired cellular immunity in different states of syphilis. *J Invest Dermatol* **79**:40, 1982

85. Lukehart SA et al: Effect of cortisone administration on host-parasite relationships in experimental syphilis. *J Immunol* **127**:1361, 1981

86. Sell S et al: Experimental syphilitic orchitis in rabbits. Ultrastructural appearance of *Treponema pallidum* during phagocytosis and dissolution by macrophages in vivo. *Lab Invest* **46**:355, 1982

87. Smogor W, Metzger M: Enriched immune T cell suspension protects rabbits against infection with *Treponema pallidum*. *Arch Immunol Ther Exp* **32**:685, 1984

88. Schell RF et al: Endemic syphilis: Transfer of resistance to *Treponema pallidum* strain Bosnia A in hamsters with a cell suspension enriched in thymus-derived cells. *J Infect Dis* **141**:752, 1980

89. Wicher V et al: Adoptive transfer of immunity to *Treponema pallidum* Nichols infection in inbred strain 2 and C4D guinea pigs. *Infect Immun* **55**:2502, 1987

90. Metzger M: The role of immunologic responses in protection against syphilis, in *The Biology of Parasitic Spirochetes,* edited by RC Johnson. New York, Academic, 1976, p 327

91. Radolf JD et al: Outer membrane ultra-structure explains the limited antigenicity of virulent *Treponema pallidum. Proc Natl Acad Sci USA* **86**:2051, 1989

92. Walker EM et al: Demonstration of rare protein in the outer membrane of *Treponema pallidum* subsp. *pallidum* by freeze-fracture analysis. *J Bacteriol* **171**:5005, 1989

93. Borenstein LA et al: Immunization of rabbits with recombinant *Treponema pallidum* antigen 4D alters the course of experimental syphilis. *J Immunol* **140**:2415, 1988

94. Champion CI et al: Immunization with *Treponema pallidum* endoflagella alters the course of experimental rabbit syphilis. *Infect Immun* **58**:3158, 1990

95. Festenstein HC et al: Runting syndrome in neonatal rabbits infected with *Treponema pallidum*. *Clin Exp Immunol* **2**:311, 1967

96. Strugnell RA et al: Experimental syphilitic orchitis. Relationship between *Treponema pallidum* infection and testis synthesis of proteoglycans. *Am J Pathol* **133**:110, 1988

97. Baughn RE et al: Detection of circulating immune complexes in the sera of rabbits with experimental syphilis: Possible role in immunoregulation. *Infect Immun* **29**:575, 1980

98. Baker-Zander SA et al: Serum regulation of in vitro lymphocyte responses in early experimental syphilis. *Infect Immun* **37**:568, 1982

99. Thompson JJ et al: Immunoregulatory properties of serum from patients with different stages of syphilis. *Br J Vener Dis* **56**:210, 1980

100. Roberts NJ: The concept of immunofocussing illustrated by influenza virus infection. *Rev Infect Dis* **10**:1071, 1988

101. Marchitto KS et al: Monoclonal antibodies directed against major histocompatibility complex antigens bind to the surface of virulent *Treponema pallidum* isolated from infected rabbits or humans. *Cell Immunol* **101**:633, 1986

102. Chamberlain NR et al: Major integral membrane protein immunogens of *Treponema pallidum* are proteolipids. *Infect Immun* **57**:2872, 1989

103. Baker-Zander SA et al: Development of cellular immunity to individual soluble antigens of *Treponema pallidum*. *J Immunol* **141**:4363, 1988

104. Kerdel-Vegas F: Yaws, pinta, in *Textbook of Dermatology,* 3d ed, edited by A Rook et al. Oxford, Blackwell, 1979, p 736

105. Hollander DH: Treponematosis from pinta to venereal syphilis revisited: Hypothesis for temperature determination of disease patterns. *Sex Transm Dis* **8**:34, 1981

106. Noordhoek GT et al: Polymerase chain reaction and synthetic DNA probes: A means of distinguishing the causative agents of syphilis and yaws? *Infect Immun* **58**:2011, 1990

107. Crissey JT, Denenholtz DA: Natural course of syphilis. *Clin Dermatol* **2**:34, 1984

108. Bruusgaard E: Ueber das Schicksal der nicht spezifisch behandelten Leutiker. *Arch Dermatol Syphilol* **157**:309, 1929

109. Sowder WT: An interpretation of Bruusgaard's paper on the fate of untreated syphilitics. *Am J Syphil Gonor Vener Dis* **24**:684, 1940

110. McDonald CJ: The contribution of the Tuskegee study to medical knowledge. *J Natl Med Assoc* **66**:1, 1974

111. Rosahn PD: Autopsy studies in syphilis. *J Vener Dis Inform* (suppl 2021), US Public Health Service, Venereal Disease Division, 1947

112. Peters JJ et al: Untreated syphilis in the male negro: Pathologic findings in syphilitic and nonsyphilitic patients. *J Chronic Dis* **1**:127, 1955

113. Kampmeier RH: *Essentials of Syphilology*. Philadelphia, Lippincott, 1943, p 215

114. Chapel TA: The variability of syphilitic chancres. *Sex Transm Dis* **5**:68, 1978

115. Notowicz A, Menke HE: Atypical primary syphilitic lesions on the penis. *Dermatologica* **147**:328, 1973

116. Tucker HA, Mulhern JL: Extragenital chancres, a review of 219 cases. *Am J Syph Gonor Vener Dis* **32**:364, 1948

117. Allison SD: Extragenital syphilitic chancres. *J Am Acad Dermatol* **14**:1094, 1986

118. Fiumara NJ, Berg M: Primary syphilis in the oral cavity. *Br J Vener Dis* **50**:463, 1974

119. Berger TG: Rectal disease in infectious syphilis. *J Assoc Milit Dermatol* **8**:3, 1982

120. Hart G: Syphilis tests in diagnostic and therapeutic decision making. *Ann Intern Med* **104**:368, 1986

121. Wendl RB et al: The VDRL slide test in 3222 cases of darkfield positive primary syphilis. *South Med J* **64**:5, 1971

122. Lundquist CD: A mixed infection of syphilis and chancroid. *J Am Acad Dermatol* **10**:354, 1984

123. Chapel TA: Physician recognition of the signs and symptoms of secondary syphilis. *JAMA* **246**:250, 1981

124. Kraus SJ: Diagnosis and management of acute genital ulcers in sexually active patients. *Semin Dermatol* **9**:160, 1990

125. Dangor Y et al: Accuracy of clinical diagnosis of genital ulcer disease. *Sex Transm Dis* **17**:184, 1990

126. Mehta SP: A case of monorecidive syphilitic chancre. *Sex Transm Dis* **8**:222, 1981

127. Jackson R: Jonathan Hutchinson on Syphilis. *Sex Transm Dis* **7**:90, 1980

128. Anderson J et al: Primary and secondary syphilis, 20 years experience. Diagnosis, treatment, and follow up. *Genitourin Med* **65**:239, 1989

129. Pariser H: Studies on the transmobility of syphilis. *Am J Syph Gonor Vener Dis* **25**:239, 1941

130. Chapel TA: The signs and symptoms of secondary syphilis. *Sex Transm Dis* **7**:161, 1980

131. Crissey JT, Denenholz DA: Clinical picture of infectious syphilis. *Clin Dermatol* **2**:39, 1984

132. Allyn B: Pruritus in syphilis. *Arch Dermatol* **113**:1295, 1977

133. Willcox JR: An atypical case of secondary syphilis. *Br J Vener Dis* **57**:30, 1981

134. Musher DM: Syphilis. *Infect Dis Clin North Am* **1**:83, 1987

135. Lochner JC, Pomeranz JR: Lichenoid secondary syphilis. *Arch Dermatol* **109**:81, 1974

136. Kennedy CTC, Sanderson KV: Corymbose secondary syphilis. *Arch Dermatol* **116**:111, 1980

137. Graham WR, Duvic M: Nodular secondary syphilis. *Arch Dermatol* **118**:205, 1982

138. Mikhail GR, Chapel TA: Follicular papulopustular syphilid. *Arch Dermatol* **100**:471, 1969

139. Petrozzi JW et al: Malignant syphilis—severe variant of secondary syphilis. *Arch Dermatol* **109**:387, 1974

140. Held JL et al: Noduloulcerative or "malignant" syphilis occurring in an otherwise healthy woman: Report and review of a dramatic dermatosis. *Cutis* **45**:119, 1990

141. Shulkin D et al: Lues maligna in a patient with human immunodeficiency virus infection. *Am J Med* **85**:425, 1988

142. French CH: Malignant syphilis. *J R Army Med Corp* **4**:477, 1905

143. Fiumara NJ, Cahn T: Leukoderma of secondary syphilis: Two case reports. *Sex Transm Dis* **9**:140, 1982

144. Pattman RS: Reversible penile leukoderma in a man with secondary syphilis: A case report. *Sex Transm Dis* **9**:96, 1982

145. Frithz A et al: Leukoderma syphiliticum: Ultrastructural observations of melanocyte function. *Acta Derm Venereol (Stockh)* **62**:521, 1982

146. Beck MH et al: Secondary syphilis with framboesiform facial lesions. *Br J Vener Dis* **57**:103, 1981

147. Kingsbury DH et al: Syphilitic paronychia: An unusual complaint. *Arch Dermatol* **105**:458, 1972

148. Shiv SP: Unusual location of syphilitic alopecia. *Sex Transm Dis* **9**:41, 1982

149. Hartsock RJ et al: Luetic lymphadenitis—a clinical and histologic study of 20 cases. *Am J Clin Pathol* **53**:304, 1970

150. Wright DJM: Alcoholic lymphalgia in early syphilis. *Postgrad Med J* **45**:191, 1969

151. Kopf RS: Case records of the Massachusetts General Hospital. *N Engl J Med* **309**:35, 1983

152. Gamble CN, Reardan JB: Immunopathogenesis of syphilitic glomerulonephritis. *N Engl J Med* **292**:449, 1975

153. O'Regan S et al: Treponemal antigens in congenital and acquired syphilitic nephritis. *Ann Intern Med* **85**:325, 1976

154. Terry SI et al: Prevalence of liver abnormality in early syphilis. *Br J Vener Dis* **60**:83, 1984

155. Schlossberg D: Syphilitic hepatitis: A case report and review of the literature. *Am J Gastroenterol* **82**:552, 1987

156. Chung KY et al: Syphilitic gastritis: Demonstration of *Treponema pallidum* with the use of fluorescent treponemal antibody absorption complement and immunoperoxidase stains. *J Am Acad Dermatol* **21**:183, 1989

157. MacFaul PA, Catterall RD: Acute choroido-retinitis in secondary syphilis: Presence of spiral organisms in the aqueous humor. *Br J Vener Dis* **47**:159, 1971

158. Smith JL: Acute blindness in early syphilis. *Arch Ophthalmol* **90**:256, 1973

159. McLeish WM et al: The ocular manifestations of syphilis in the human immunodeficiency virus type 1-infected host. *Ophthalmology* **97**:196, 1990

160. Darmstadt GL, Harris JP: Luetic hearing loss: Clinical presentation, diagnosis, and treatment (review). *Am J Otolaryngol* **10**:410, 1989

161. Balkany TJ, Dans PE: Reversible sudden deafness in early acquired syphilis. *Arch Otolaryngol* **104**:66, 1978

162. Guttenplan M, Hendrix RA: Otosyphilis: A practical guide to diagnosis and treatment (review). *Trans PA Acad Ophthalmol Otolaryngol* **41**:834, 1989

163. Waugh MA: Bony symptoms in secondary syphilis. *Br J Vener Dis* **52**:204, 1976

164. Dismukes WE et al: Destructive bone disease in early syphilis. *JAMA* **236**:2646, 1976

165. Hansen K et al: Bone lesions in early syphilis detected by bone scintigraphy. *Br J Vener Dis* **60**:265, 1984

166. Olle-Goig JE et al: Bone invasion in secondary syphilis: Case reports. *Genitourin Med* **64**:198, 1988

167. Kazlow PG et al: Polyarthritis as the initial symptom of secondary syphilis: Case report and review. *Mt Sinai J Med* **56**:65, 1989

168. Durston JHJ, Jefferiss FJG: Syphilitic myositis. *Br J Vener Dis* **51**:141, 1975

169. Biro L et al: Secondary syphilis with unusual clinical and laboratory findings. *JAMA* **206**:889, 1969

170. Ince WE, Mahabir BS: Wenckebach phenomenon occurring in secondary syphilis. *Br J Vener Dis* **50**:97, 1974

171. Tosca A et al: Infiltrate of syphilitic lesions before and after treatment. *Genitourin Med* **64**:289, 1988

172. Kahn LB, Gordon W: Sarcoid-like granulomas in secondary syphilis. *Arch Pathol* **92**:334, 1971

173. Abell E et al: Secondary syphilis: A clinicopathological review. *Br J Dermatol* **93**:53, 1975

174. Fisher DA et al: Lues maligna. *Arch Dermatol* **99**:70, 1979

175. Lantis LR et al: Sarcoid granuloma in secondary syphilis. *Arch Dermatol* **99**:748, 1969

176. Beckett JH, Bigbee JW: Immunoperoxidase localization of *Treponema pallidum*. *Arch Pathol* **103**:135, 1979

177. Yobs AR et al: Fluorescent antibody technique in early syphilis. *Arch Pathol* **77**:220, 1964

178. Fornaciari G et al: Syphilis in a renaissance Italian mummy. *Lancet* **2**:614, 1989

179. Clark EG, Danbolt N: The Oslo study of the natural course of un-

treated syphilis: An epidemiologic investigation based on a re-study of the Boeck-Bruusgaard material. *Med Clin North Am* **48**:613, 1964
180. Olansky S: Late benign syphilis. *Med Clin North Am* **48**:653, 1964
181. Kampmeier RH: The late manifestations of syphilis: Skeletal, visceral, and cardiovascular. *Med Clin North Am* **48**:667, 1964
182. Webster B et al: Studies in cardiovascular syphilis: III. The natural history of syphilitic aortic insufficiency. *Am Heart J* **46**:117, 1953
183. Jackman JD Jr, Radolf JD: Cardiovascular syphilis (review). *Am J Med* **87**:425, 1989
184. Heggtveit HA: Syphilitic aortitis. *Circulation* **29**:346, 1964
185. Kampmeier RH: Saccular aneurysm of the thoracic aorta: A clinical study of 633 cases. *Ann Intern Med* **12**:624, 1938
186. Crissey JT, Denenholtz DA: Cardiovascular syphilis. *Clin Dermatol* **2**:117, 1984
187. Tadavarthy SM et al: Syphilitic aneurysms of the innominate artery. *Radiology* **139**:31, 1981
188. Humphries JO, Bulkey BH: Syphilitic cardiovascular disease, in *The Heart, Arteries and Veins,* 5th ed, edited by JW Hurst et al. New York, McGraw-Hill, 1982, p 1425
189. Phillips PL et al: Syphilitic aortic aneurysms presenting with the superior vena cava syndrome. *Am J Med* **71**:171, 1981
190. Farooki MA: Aneurysms in the United States and the United Kingdom. *Int Surg* **58**:475, 1973
191. Holt S: Syphilitic ostial occlusion. *Br Heart J* **39**:469, 1977
192. Miller GAH et al: Isolated coronary ostial stenosis. *Cath Cardiovasc Diagn* **12**:30, 1986
193. Weinstein G, Killen DA: Innominate artery-coronary artery bypass graft in a patient with calcific aortitis. *J Thorac Cardiovasc Surg* **79**:312, 1980
194. Kampmeier RH, Combs SR: The prognosis in syphilitic aortic insufficiency. *Am J Syph Gonor Vener Dis* **24**:578, 1940
195. Grabau W et al: Syphilitic aortic regurgitation—an appraisal of surgical treatment. *Br J Vener Dis* **52**:366, 1976
196. Clawson BJ, Bell ET: The heart in syphilitic aortitis. *Arch Pathol Lab Med* **4**:922, 1927
197. Lev M, Bharati S: Atrioventricular and intraventricular conduction disease. *Arch Intern Med* **135**:405, 1975
198. Beck-Sague CM et al: Neurosyphilis and HIV infection. *N Engl J Med* **317**:1473, 1987
199. Swartz MN: Neurosyphilis, in *Sexually Transmitted Diseases,* 2d ed, edited by KK Holmes et al. New York, McGraw-Hill, 1990, p 231
200. Melvin ET, Mildvan D: Acute syphilitic meningitis: A case report. *Mt Sinai J Med* **46**:201, 1979
201. Luger A et al: Diagnosis of neurosyphilis by examination of the cerebrospinal fluid. *Br J Vener Dis* **57**:232, 1981
202. Merritt HH: *Textbook of Neurology,* 6th ed. Philadelphia: Lea & Febiger, 1979, p 135
203. Wolters EC et al: Central nervous system involvement in early and late syphilis: The problem of asymptomatic neurosyphilis. *J Neurol Sci* **88**:229, 1988
204. Davis LE, Schmitt JW: Clinical significance of cerebrospinal fluid tests for neurosyphilis. *Ann Neurol* **25**:50, 1989
205. Steckelberg JM, McDonald TJ: Otologic involvement in late syphilis. *Laryngoscope* **94**:753, 1984
206. Agdal N et al: Pachymeningitis cervicalis hypertrophica syphilitica. *Acta Derm Venereol (Stockh)* **60**:184, 1980
207. Holmes MD et al: Clinical features of meningovascular syphilis. *Neurology* **34**:553, 1984
208. Fisher M, Poser CM: Syphilitic meningomyelitis. *Arch Neurol* **34**:785, 1977
209. Towpik J, Nowakowska E: Changing patterns of late syphilis. *Br J Vener Dis* **46**:132, 1970
210. Catterall RD: Neurosyphilis. *Br J Hosp Med* **17**:585, 1977
211. Hooshmand H et al: Neurosyphilis: A study of 241 patients. *JAMA* **219**:726, 1972
212. Dawson-Butterworth K, Heathcote PEM: Review of hospitalized cases of general paralysis of the insane. *Br J Vener Dis* **46**:295, 1970
213. Lukehart SA, Holmes KK: Syphilis, in *Harrison's Principles of In-*
ternal Medicine, 12th ed, edited by JD Wilson et al. New York, McGraw-Hill, 1991, p 651
214. Kerty E et al: Visual evoked response in syphilitic optic atrophy. *Acta Ophthalmol* **64**:553, 1986
215. Wendel GD: Gestational and congenital syphilis (review). *Clin Perinatol* **15**:287, 1988
216. Shulz KF et al: Congenital syphilis, in *Sexually Transmitted Diseases,* 2d ed, edited by KK Holmes et al. New York, McGraw-Hill, 1990, p 821
217. Fiumara N et al: The incidence of prenatal syphilis at the Boston City Hospital. *N Engl J Med* **247**:48, 1952
218. Danholt N et al: The Oslo study of untreated syphilis: A restudy of the Boeck-Brunsgaard material concerning the fate of syphilitics who receive no specific treatment. *Acta Derm Venereol (Stockh)* **34**:34, 1954
219. Ingraham NR, Beerman H: The present status of penicillin in the treatment of syphilis in pregnancy and infantile congenital syphilis. *Am J Med Sci* **219**:433, 1950
220. Harter CA, Benirschke K: Fetal syphilis in the first trimester. *Am J Obstet Gynecol* **124**:705, 1976
221. Silverstein AM: Fetal immune responses in congenital infection *N Engl J Med* **286**:1413, 1972
222. Crissey JT, Denenholz DA: Congenital syphilis. *Clin Dermatol* **143**:161, 1984
223. Fojaco RM et al: Congenital syphilis and necrotizing funisitis. *JAMA* **261**:1788, 1989
224. Parker CR Jr, Wendel GD: The effects of syphilis on endocrine function of the fetoplacental unit. *Am J Obstet Gynecol* **159**:1327, 1988
225. Kaufman RE et al: Questionnaire survey of reported early congenital syphilis. *Sex Transm Dis* **4**:135, 1977
226. Chawla V et al: Congenital syphilis in the newborn. *Arch Dis Child* **63**:1293, 1988
227. Fiumara NJ: Syphilis among mothers and children. *Ann N Y Acad Sci* **549**:187, 1988
228. Borroni G: A case of late congenital syphilis at the Metropolitan Museum of Art, New York. *Am J Dermatopathol* **10**:448, 1988
229. Fiumara NJ, Lessell S: Manifestations of late congenital syphilis. *Arch Dermatol* **102**:78, 1970
230. Hahn RD et al: Treatment of neural deafness with prednisone. *J Chronic Dis* **15**:395, 1962
231. Curtis AC, Philpott OS: Prenatal syphilis. *Med Clin North Am* **48**:707, 1984
232. Hook EW III: Syphilis and HIV infection. *J Infect Dis* **160**:530, 1989
233. Musher DM et al: Effect of human immunodeficiency virus (HIV) infection on the course of syphilis and on the response to treatment. *Ann Intern Med* **113**:872, 1990
234. Johns DR et al: Alteration in the natural history of neurosyphilis by concurrent infection with the human immunodeficiency virus. *N Engl J Med* **316**:1569, 1987
235. Lukehart SA et al: Invasion of the central nervous system by *Treponema pallidum:* Implications for diagnoses and therapy. *Ann Intern Med* **109**:855, 1988
236. Dawson S et al: Benign tertiary syphilis and HIV infection. *AIDS* **2**:315, 1988
237. Gregory N et al: The spectrum of syphilis in patients with human immunodeficiency virus infection. *J Am Acad Dermatol* **22**:1061, 1990
238. Bari MM et al: Ulcerative syphilis in acquired immunodeficiency syndrome: A case of immunodeficiency virus. *J Am Acad Dermatol* **21**:1310, 1989
239. Felman YM: Recent developments in the diagnosis and treatment of sexually transmitted diseases: Infectious syphilis and acquired immunodeficiency syndrome (review). *Cutis* **44**:288, 1989
240. Breneman DL et al: Granulomatous secondary syphilis in a patient with human immunodeficiency virus infection. *Cutis* **44**:377, 1989
241. Kvinesdal B, Pedersen NS: False positive HIV antibody tests in RPR reactive patients. *JAMA* **260**:923, 1988

242. Frederick WR et al: Secondary syphilis and HIV infection, abstract No. 1175. Abstracts of the 28th Interscience Conference on Antimicrobial Agents and Chemotherapy, Washington, DC, 1988

243. Haas JS et al: Sensitivity of treponemal tests for detecting prior treated syphilis during human immunodeficiency virus infection. *J Infect Dis* **162**:862, 1990

244. McKenna JJ et al: Unmasking AIDS: Clinical immunosuppression and seronegative syphilis. *Med Hypothesis* **21**:421, 1986

245. Quinn TC et al: Human immunodeficiency virus infection among patients attending clinics for sexually transmitted diseases. *N Engl J Med* **318**:197, 1988

246. Centers for Disease Control: Recommendations for diagnosing and treating syphilis in HIV-infected patients. *MMWR* **37**:601, 1988

247. Hollander H: Cerebrospinal fluid normalities and abnormalities in individuals infected with human immunodefiency virus. *J Infect Dis* **158**:855, 1988

248. Harris A et al: A microflocculation test for syphilis using cardiolipin antigen. *J Vener Dis Inform* **27**:169, 1946

249. Luger A: Serological diagnosis of syphilis: Current methods, in *Immunological Diagnosis of Sexually Transmitted Diseases*, edited by H Young and A McMillan. New York, Marcel Dekker, 1988, p 249

250. White TJ, Fuller SA: Visuwell Reagin, a non-treponemal enzyme-linked immunosorbent assay for the serodiagnosis of syphilis. *J Clin Microbiol* **27**:2300, 1989

251. Pedersen NS et al: Enzyme-linked immunosorbent assays for detection of immunoglobulin M to nontreponemal and treponemal antigens for the diagnosis of congenital syphilis. *J Clin Microbiol* **27**:1835, 1989

252. Ijsselmuiden OE et al: Development and evaluation of a monoclonal antibody inhibition enzyme-linked immunosorbent assay to diagnose syphilis. *Genitourin Med* **65**:308, 1989

253. Ijsselmuiden OE et al: Sensitivity and specificity of an enzyme-linked immunosorbent assay using the recombinant DNA-derived *Treponema pallidum* protein TmpA for serodiagnosis of syphilis and the potential use of TmpA for assessing the effect of antibiotic therapy. *J Clin Microbiol* **27**:152, 1989

254. Bernard C et al: Biological true and false serological tests for syphilis and their relationships with antiphospholipid antibodies. *Dermatologica* **180**:151, 1990

255. VanDyck E et al: Bench level laboratory manual for sexually transmitted diseases. WHO/VDT/89:443, WHO, Geneva 32–42, 1989

256. Luger A: Die IgM-Diagnostik in der syphilis-serologic. *Wienr Klin Wochenschr* **95**:843, 1983

257. Muller F, Wollemann G: Analysis of specific immunoglobulin M. Immune response to *Treponema pallidum* before and after penicillin treatment of human syphilis. *Eur J Sex Transm Dis* **2**:67, 1985

258. Tanaka S et al: Low molecular weight-IgM antibody in syphilis detected by *Treponema pallidum* immune adherents (TPTA) test. *Med Microbiol Immunol* **173**:155, 1984

259. Gschnait F et al: Cerebrospinal fluid immunoglobulins in neurosyphilis. *Br J Vener Dis* **57**:238, 1981

260. Tonescu AD et al: Quantitative profile of cardiolipin and group treponemal IgD antibodies in syphilis estimated by single radial immunodiffusion techniques. *Arch Roum Pathol Exp Microbiol* **48**:19, 1989

261. Hart G: Syphilis test in diagnostic and therapeutic decision making. *Ann Intern Med* **104**:368, 1986

262. Larsen SA et al: Syphilis serology and darkfield microscopy, in *Sexually Transmitted Diseases*, 2d ed, edited by KK Holmes et al. New York, McGraw-Hill, 1990, p 927

263. Luger A et al: Screening for syphilis with the AMHA-TP-test. *Eur J Sex Transm Dis* **1**:25, 1983

264. Harvey AM, Shulman LE: Connective tissue disease and the chronic biologic false positive test for syphilis (BFP reaction). *Med Clin North Am* **50**:1271, 1966

265. Catterall RD: Systemic disease and the biologic false positive reaction. *Br J Vener Dis* **48**:1, 1972

266. Phaosvasdi S et al: Rapid plasma reagin test (PRP) compared to venereal diseases research laboratory test (VDRL) for the diagnosis of syphilis in pregnancy. *J Med Assoc Thai* **72**:202, 1989

267. Wicher K, Wicher V: Immunopathology of syphilis, in *Pathogenesis and Immunology of Treponemal Infection,* edited by RF Schell, DM Musher. New York, Marcel Dekker, 1983, p 139

268. Luger A et al: Specificity of the *Treponema pallidum* haemagglutination test. *Br J Vener Dis* **57**:178, 1981

269. Beebe JL, Nouri NJ: Comparative evaluation of commercial fluorescent treponemal antibody absorbed test kits. *J Clin Microbiol* **19**:789, 1984

270. Burns RE: Spontaneous revision of FTA-ABS test reactions. *JAMA* **234**:617, 1975

271. Kobayashi S et al: Microcapsule agglutination test for *T. pallidum* antibodies. A new serodiagnostic test for syphilis. *Br J Vener Dis* **59**:1, 1983

272. Ijsselmuiden OE et al: Line immunoassay and enzyme-linked line immunofiltration assay for simultaneous detection of antibody to two treponemal antigens. *Eur J Clin Microbiol Infect Dis* **8**:716, 1989

273. Farshy CE et al: Fourstep enzyme-linked immunosorbent assay for detection of *Treponema pallidum* antibody. *J Clin Microbiol* **21**:387, 1985

274. Schouls LM et al: Overproduction and purification of *Treponema pallidum* recombinant-DNA-derived proteins TmpA and TmpB and their potential use in serodiagnosis of syphilis. *Infect Immun* **57**:2612, 1989

275. Ijsselmuiden OE et al: Enzyme-linked immunofiltration assay for rapid serodiagnosis of syphilis. *Eur J Clin Microbiol Infect Dis* **6**:281, 1987

276. Young H et al: Screening for treponemal infection by a new enzyme immunoassay. *Genitourin Med* **65**:72, 1989

277. Schmidt BL: Solid phase hemadsorption: A method for rapid detection of *Treponema pallidum* specific IgM. *Sex Transm Dis* **7**:53, 1980

278. Sato T et al: *T. pallidum* specific IgM haemagglutination test for serodiagnosis of syphilis. *Br J Vener Dis* **60**:364, 1984

279. Ijsselmuiden OE et al: An IgM capture enzyme linked immunosorbent assay to detect IgM antibodies to treponemes in patients with syphilis. *Genitourin Med* **65**:79, 1989

280. Sanchez PJ et al: Molecular analysis of the fetal IgM response to *Treponema pallidum* antigens: Implications for improved serodiagnosis of congenital syphilis. *J Infect Dis* **159**:508, 1989

281. Wendel GD: Early and congenital syphilis. *Obstet Gynecol Clin North Am* **16**:479, 1989

282. Luger A et al: Laboratory support in the diagnosis of neurosyphilis. WHO/VDT/RES **88**:379, WHO, Geneva 1988

283. Garland SM, Kelly VN: Is antenaial screening for syphilis worth while? *Med J Aust* **151**:370, 1989

284. Klaus MV et al: Routine screening for syphilis is justified in patients admitted to psychiatric, alcohol, and drug rehabilitation wards of the Veterans Administration Medical Center. *Arch Dermatol* **125**:1644, 1989

285. Luger A: Syphilisserologic. *Schrifttum Praxis* **2**:89, 1987

286. Davis LE, Schmitt JW: Clinical significance of cerebrospinal fluid tests for neurosyphilis. *Ann Neurol* **25**:50, 1989

287. Breustedt W et al: Positive fluorescent treponemal antibody absorption test in cerebrospinal fluid of neurosyphilitic persons infected with human immunodeficiency virus. *Arch Dermatol* **125**:1712, 1989

288. Delpech B, Lichtblau E: Etude quantitative des immunoglobulines G et de l'albumine du liquide cephalorachidien. *Clin Chim Acta* **37**:15, 1972

289. Cerny EH et al: Adenovirus ELISA for the evaluation of cerebrospinal fluid in patients with suspected neurosyphilis. *Am J Clin Pathol* **84**:505, 1985

290. Luger A et al: Diagnosis of neurosyphilis by examination of the cerebrospinal fluid. *Br J Vener Dis* **57**:232, 1981

291. World Health Organization: STD treatment strategies. WHO consultation on development of sexually transmitted diseases treatment strategies. Geneva 4–6, Sept, 1989. WHO/VDT/89–447

292. Muller F: Specific immunoglobulin M and G antibodies in the rapid diagnosis of human treponemal infection. *Diagn Immunol* **4**:1, 1986

293. Kampmeier RH: Syphilis therapy: An historical perspective. *J Am Vener Dis Assoc* **3**:99, 1976

294. Luger A: Geschichte der Venerologie, in *Standort und Aublick der Deutschen Dermatologie,* edited by G Stuttgen (Herausgeber). Berlin, Grosse, 1989, p 150

295. Waugh MA: History of clinical developements in sexually transmitted diseases, in *Sexually Transmitted Diseases,* 2d ed, edited by KK Holmes et al. New York, McGraw Hill, 1990, p 1

296. Wecke J et al: *Treponema pallidum* in early syphilitic lesions in humans during high dose penicillin therapy. *Arch Dermatol* **257**:1, 1976

297. Polnikorn N et al: Penicillin concentrations in cerebrospinal fluid after different treatment regimens for syphilis. *Br J Vener Dis* **56**:363, 1980

298. Tramont EC: Persistence of *Treponema pallidum* following penicillin G therapy. Report of 2 cases. *JAMA* **236**:2206, 1976

299. Hardy JB et al: Failure of penicillin in a newborn with congenital syphilis. *JAMA* **212**:1345, 1970

300. Dunlop EMC: Persistence of treponemes after treatment. *Br Med J* **2**:577, 1972

301. Weit RJ, Milko DA: Isolation of spirochetes in perilymph despite prior anti-syphilitic treatment. *Arch Otolaryngol* **101**:104, 1975

302. Luger A: The problem of persisting treponemes. *Hautartz* **31**:237, 1980

303. Centers for Disease Control: 1989 Sexually Transmitted Diseases Treatment Guidelines. *MMWR:* **suppl vol 38**, September 1989

304. Fiumara NJ: Treatment of seropositive primary syphilis: An evaluation of 196 patients. *Sex Transm Dis* **4**:92, 1977

305. Fiumara NJ: Treatment of secondary syphilis: An evaluation of 204 patients. *Sex Transm Dis* **4**:96, 1977

306. Idsoe O et al: Penicillin in the treatment of syphilis. *Bull WHO* (suppl) **1**:1, 1972

307. St John RK: Treatment of cardiovascular syphilis. *J Am Vener Dis Assoc* **3**:148, 1976

308. Edeiken J et al: Further observations on penicillin-treated cardiovascular syphilis. *Circ Res* **6**:267, 1952

309. Rothenberg R: Treatment of neurosyphilis. *J Am Vener Dis Assoc* **3**:153, 1976

310. Hahn RD et al: Penicillin treatment of general paresis (dementia paralytica). *Arch Neurol Psychol* **81**:557, 1959

311. Cole HN et al: Penicillin in the treatment of syphilis in pregnancy. *J Vener Dis Inform* **30**:95, 1949

312. Philipson A et al: Transplacental passage of erythromycin and clindamycin. *N Engl J Med* **288**:1219, 1973

313. Hashisaki P et al: Erythromycin failure in the treatment of syphilis in a pregnant woman. *Sex Transm Dis* **10**:36, 1983

314. Simon C, Stille W: *Antibiotikatherapie in Klinik und Praxis.* Stuttgart, Aufiage, Schattauer, 1989

315. Brown ST: Adverse reactions in syphilis therapy. *J Am Vener Dis Assoc* **3**:172, 1976

316. Sheldon WH et al: The production of Herxheimer reactions by injection of immune serum in rabbits with experimental syphilis. *Am J Syphilol* **35**:405, 1951

317. Aronson IK et al: Jarisch-Herxheimer reaction in complement depleted rabbits. *Br J Vener Dis* **57**:226, 1981

318. Galpin JE et al: ''Pseudoanaphylactic'' reactions from inadvertent infusions of procaine penicillin G. *Ann Intern Med* **81**:358, 1974

319. Downtham TF et al: Systemic toxic reactions to procaine penicillin G. *Sex Transm Dis* **5**:4, 1978

CHAPTER 219

Miguel Sanchez and Anton F. H. Luger

Endemic (Nonvenereal) Treponematoses

The endemic treponematoses, endemic syphilis, yaws, and pinta, are a group of chronic bacterial infections caused by treponemes.[1] The use of the term *endemic* may not be appropriate to distinguish these diseases from sexually transmitted *T. pallidum* infection, when one considers that venereal syphilis has been endemic in many parts of the world for as long as accurate epidemiologic records have been available. Other terms, such as ''nonvenereal'' and ''tropical'' have been proposed but *endemic* better describes the continued occurrence within circumscribed areas.[1–5]

The endemic treponematoses are transmitted by direct, and only rarely through indirect, contact between children and adolescents living under social, economic, and hygienic deprivation. The clinical course usually progresses from primary lesions, to secondary eruptions, to late manifestations. Cardiovascular, central nervous system, and prenatal involvement are usually not observed in endemic treponemal infections, but rare exceptions have been reported.[6] The causative organisms of the endemic treponematoses and venereal syphilis are morphologically identical. Dissimilarities

in clinical expression have been attributed to minor mutations in treponemes, to variation in host immunity, or to the environment, but supporting experimental evidence is scanty. There are minor differences in DNA sequence[7] and in some antigens, but the common determinants prevail by far.[8,9] *T. pallidum* and *T. pertenue* produce lesions with slightly different morphologic appearance and *T. carateum* causes disease only in humans and higher primates.[10] Furthermore, incomplete cross-immunity studies in rabbits confirm the differences among these organisms.[11] The epidemiologic characteristics of endemic treponematoses versus venereal syphilis are summarized in Table 219-1.

Yaws and pinta are diseases of hot, humid tropical climates. Because these diseases spread by direct contact with infected skin lesions, trauma and lack of protective clothing are probably important factors in their transmission. Endemic syphilis, which occurs in dry desert regions where the affected populations wear clothing, is transmitted mostly through saliva and less by skin-to-skin contact.[12] Due to mass treatment of endemic treponematoses in many

TABLE 219-1
Epidemiological Characteristics of Treponemal Diseases*

Epidemiological characteristics	Treponemal disease			
	Venereal syphilis	Endemic syphilis	Yaws	Pinta
Occurrence	Sporadic urban	Endemic rural	Endemic rural	Endemic, rural
Geographical distribution	World wide	Southwest Asia, sub-Saharan regions of Africa	Africa, southeast Asia, Western Pacific, South America, Caribbean	Central and South America, Mexico
Climate in which the disease mostly occurs	All types	Arid, warm	Humid, warm	Semi-arid, warm
Age group with peak incidence (years)	18–30	2–10	2–10	15–30
Transmissibility	High	High	High	Low
Mode of transmission:				
Direct (person to person)				
Sexual	Usual	No	No	No
Nonsexual	Rare	Yes	Usual	Probable
Indirect				
Utensils	Rare	Rare	Rare	Unknown
Contaminated fingers	Unknown	Probable	Probable	Unknown
Congenital	Occasional	Exceptional	No	No
Reservoir	Adults	Children 2–15 years old: contacts in home, school and village; latent cases are capable of becoming active.	Children 2–15 years old: contacts in home, school and village; latent cases are capable of becoming active.	Cases with long-standing skin lesions

*Reprinted from Ref. 1 with permission from WHO.

countries over the past three decades, the younger generations are no longer immune to venereal syphilis. As a result, the incidence of venereal syphilis is rising in urban and rural areas of developing countries where the disease was practically unknown 35 years ago.[2] However, in some areas of central and west Africa, the Pacific islands, and Latin America, where the levels of poverty and hygiene have not improved, the number of cases of endemic treponematoses has dramatically increased.[3] In 1988, 2.5 million persons, 80 percent of whom were children, suffered from early communicable disease, and 100 million children were exposed to infection.

The diagnosis of endemic syphilis, yaws, and pinta can be made from the typical clinical manifestations but should be confirmed by dark-field examination and serologic tests. Lipoidal antigen tests, like the VDRL and RPR, suffice in the field. Treponemal tests, such as the FTA-ABS, and MHATP should be used to confirm difficult cases and to differentiate biologic false-positive reactions (see Chap. 218). Screening in children is facilitated by the fingerprick method.

Endemic "Nonvenereal" Syphilis (Bejel, Novjeva, Dichiwa, Skerljevo, Frenjak, Sibbens, Button Scurvy, Radesyge)[1,13]

The multitude of local names for this disease indicates that a common origin was not recognized until the beginning of the twentieth century. At present, the disease occurs mainly among nomads and semi-nomads in western Asia, Pakistan, Saudi Arabia, Sudan, the sub-Saharan regions, Mali, Nigeria, Upper Volta, Burkina-Faso, Mauritania, and Australia.[13] Foci of endemic syphilis with a prevalence rate as high as 4 percent were found in certain European countries such as Yugoslavia after World War II but have been eradicated through WHO-UNICEF-sponsored mass-treatment campaigns.[12] Small foci of endemic syphilis in large cities of Europe and the United States after World War II and during the 1960s resulted from crowded conditions. The source of infection in such outbreaks was usually communicable lesions in venereally infected adults. Under the right conditions endemic syphilis can cause a venereal form of the disease, although strains isolated from nonvenereal syphilis may behave somewhat differently in rabbits and hamsters than treponemes of venereal syphilis.[11]

Clinical Manifestations

Infection occurs when a child comes in contact with contagious lesions. The mode of transmission is presumed to be infected saliva, and the portal of entry can be the mucous membranes of the mouth, tonsils, or larynx. Primary chancres are rarely noted because the inoculum is usually small and invasion is not confined to a circumscribed area. Occasionally, an infected child may infect a previously uninfected mother, producing a primary "throwback" infection, such as a nipple chancre during nursing.

The presentation of endemic syphilis is similar to secondary syphilis. Mucous patches (Fig. 219-1), condylomata lata, angular cheilitis and cutaneous papular eruptions comparable to those seen

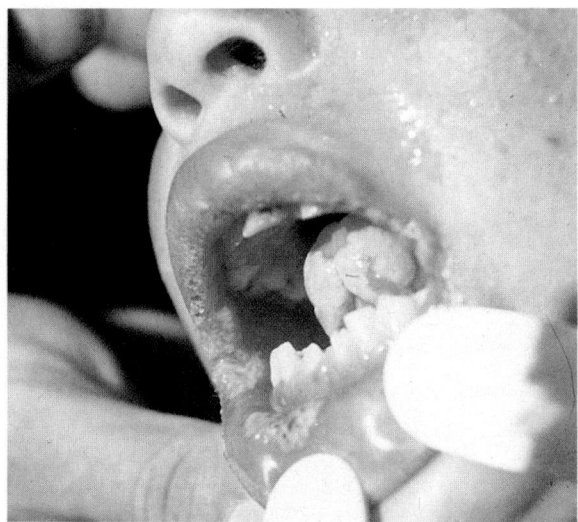

FIGURE 219-1 Nonvenereal syphilis. Mucous patches of lips and tongue.

in venereal syphilis are common. By the time signs and symptoms become evident, serologic tests are invariably reactive. The histopathologic changes are identical to those in respective lesions of venereal syphilis. Compared to venereal syphilis, early lesions heal more slowly and, without treatment, persist for 6 to 9 months. Healing of the secondary lesions is followed by a latent period of variable duration. Many patients develop gummas in the skin, nasopharynx, and bones. These late lesions appear to be provoked by trauma or reinfection in individuals previously sensitized to *T. pallidum*. Saddle nose deformity, perforation of the palate, and gangosa, which refers to massive destruction of the whole nose and adjacent maxilla, including the upper lip (Fig. 219-2), are late com-

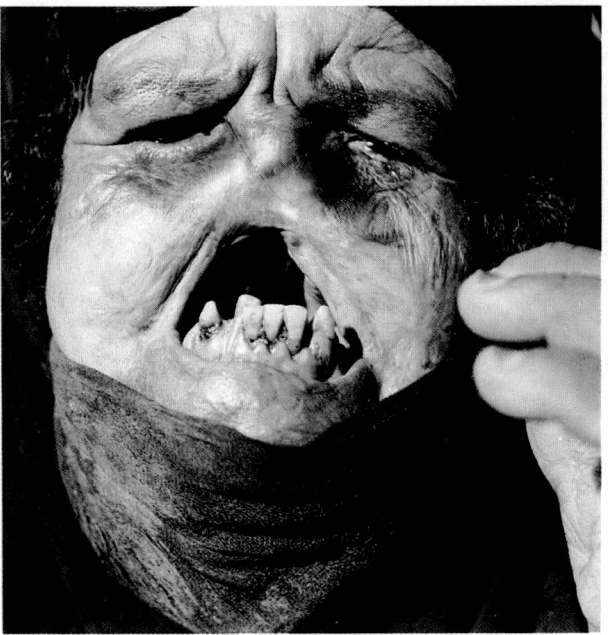

FIGURE 219-2 Gangosa may be a late manifestation of venereal and nonvenereal syphilis, as well as of yaws.

plications. The histopathology of late disease resembles that of venereal syphilis.

Cardiovascular and neurologic involvement has been infrequently reported in hypoendemic areas and has not been well studied. Also rare are the stigmata of prenatal syphilis. Most women become infected during their childhood, many years before pregnancy, and, therefore, the chance of prenatal transmission is remote.

Yaws (Framboesia, Buba, Pian)

Yaws[1,13] is caused by *Treponema pertenue* and is found in hot, humid regions around the equator, in Central and West Africa, in Latin America (Brazil, Colombia, Ecuador, Guyana, Surinam, Dominica, Haiti, Martinique) and in Asia (Indonesia, Papua New Guinea, South Pacific islands, Democratic Kampuchea, and Sri Lanka).[3,4,14] Like endemic syphilis, yaws is predominantly a disease of childhood and poverty, and about 70 percent of infections occur before the age of 10. It is not transmitted sexually but through direct contact with oozing lesions and possibly by flies.

Course of the Disease

After an incubation period, which is usually between 2 weeks and 6 months, but may be as long as 5 years, a lesion appears at the site of inoculation. Secondary lesions erupt 3 to 12 weeks after the initial lesion and, if untreated, heal in 3 to 6 months. The disease becomes latent, but relapses may occur for up to 4 years. Spontaneous cure or permanent latency may follow. Some patients develop tertiary lesions of the skin and bones after 5 to 10 years. Although yaws does not commonly involve the cardiovascular or nervous systems and does not usually affect the fetus, rare cases of prenatal transmission and cardiovascular, visceral, neurologic, and neuroophthalmologic involvement have been reported.[6] The disease is divided into early yaws and late yaws.

The primary lesion, or "mother yaw," is commonly single but may be multiple. It usually begins as a nontender papule which becomes granulomatous and ulcerates. Regional nodes are enlarged, firm, and painless. Primary lesions may persist for 2 to 6 months and heal spontaneously with an atrophic depressed scar which has an achromic center. Inoculation occurs at the site of wounds, abrasions, phagedaenic ulcers, or excoriated insect bites.

In the skin, secondary lesions, or "daughter yaws," are similar to the primary papule but smaller (Figs. 219-3, 219-4). Papillomatous, vegetating papules and small plaques covered with fibrinous exudate and resembling raspberries (framboesides) or scaly papular, corymbiform, or circinate lesions that resemble those of secondary syphilis (pianides) may appear on any part of the body. In mucocutaneous areas the lesions resemble condylomata lata and are frequently localized around orifices, usually the mouth, nose, anus, and vulva. On the palms and soles the lesions may be hyperkeratotic. In early yaws, osteitis and periostitis may develop.[15] Affected bones can be tender and may be visibly deformed due to thickening. The secondary lesions disappear spontaneously within months, and the disease progresses to a latent stage.

Late lesions are localized predominantly on the lower extremities. These include cutaneous and subcutaneous nodules, tuberoulcerative lesions and gummas, juxta-articular nodes of knees and elbows, palmoplantar keratoderma, saddle nose deformity, and

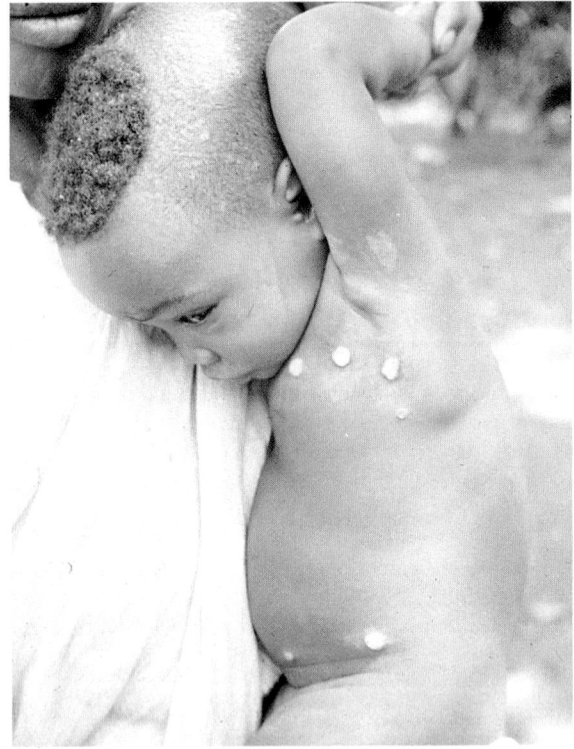

a

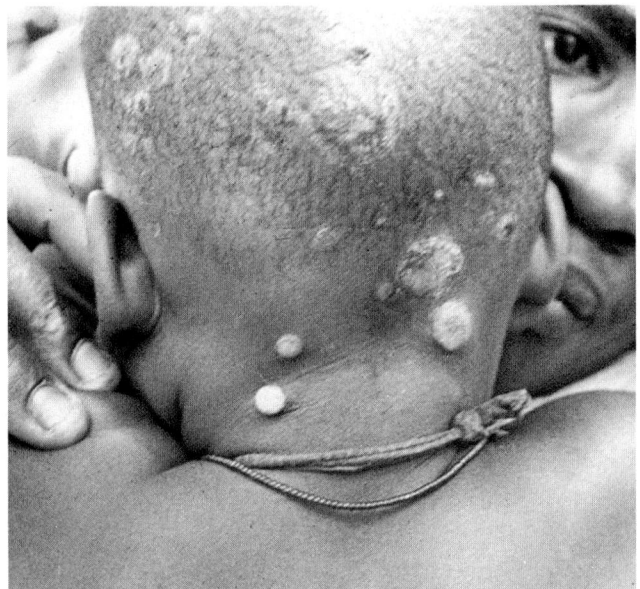

b

FIGURE 219-3 (*a,b*) Early secondary lesions of yaws (i.e., "daughter" yaws), showing crusted and ulcerated plaques and papules.

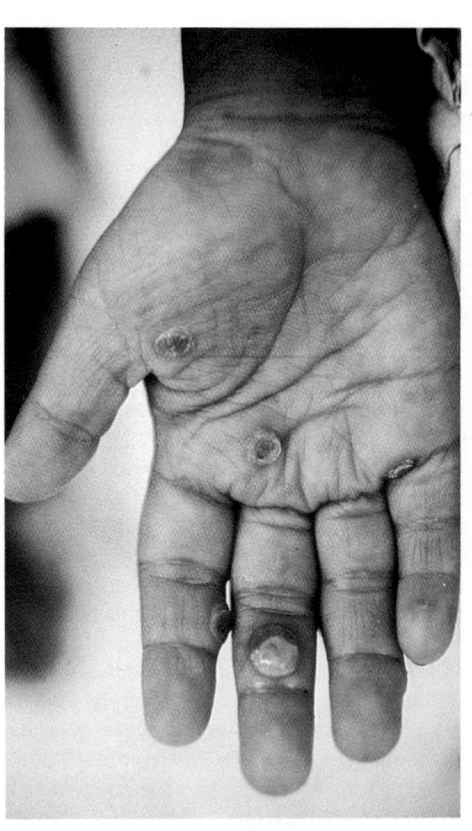

a

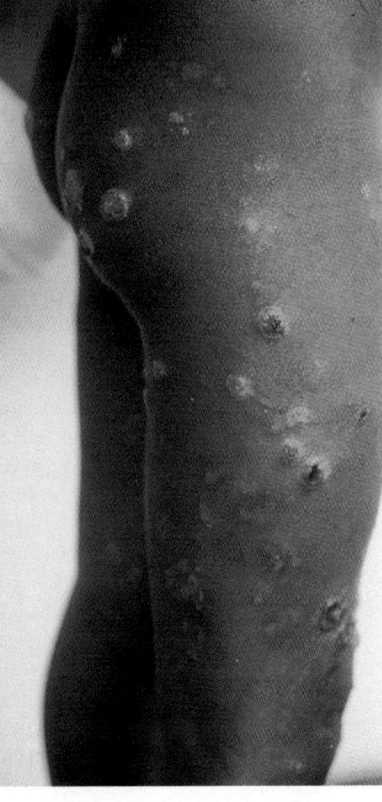

b

FIGURE 219-4 (*a*) A four-year-old girl suffering from early infectious yaws. Multiple skin lesions were present. On the hands crusted, vesiculous, papillomatous skin lesions were observed. Darkfield examination of skin lesions revealed the presence of many treponemes. Serology: VDRL ++, TPHA 2+, FTA-Abs 3+. (*b*) A three-year-old boy suffering from early infectious yaws. Multiple lenticular and nummular crusted ulcerated papulous skin lesions are present on the buttocks and lower extremities. Darkfield examination positive. Serology: VDRL +++, TPHA 2+, FTA-Abs 3+. (*Courtesy of H.J.H. Engelkens, M.D., J. van der Stek, M.D., and E. Stolz, M.D.*)

sabre tibia. Pintoid dyschromia are vitiliginous patches on the soles, palms, and wrists. Yaws is the most mutilating treponemal infection and gangosa occurs in 1 percent of patients (Fig. 219-2). Hypertrophic osteitis of the nasal process of the maxilla (Gondou) may slowly progress over 5 to 20 years and chronic obstruction of the eyes can lead to blindness.

Histopathology

In the primary lesion, there is marked acanthosis, papillomatosis and epidermal edema. Neutrophils migrate into the epidermis and form epidermal abscesses. The dermis becomes primarily infiltrated with plasma cells, but also with neutrophils, lymphocytes, histiocytes, fibroblasts, and eosinophils. Unlike in syphilis, the blood vessels in primary yaws show little or no proliferation of endothelial cells. Secondary lesions show histologic changes similar to those in primary lesions, and the epidermal changes resemble those of condylomata lata. However, the infiltrate has a diffuse arrangement rather than a perivascular localization as in condylomata lata. In late yaws, the ulcerative lesions resemble late syphilis except that vascular changes in late yaws are slight or absent. Treponemes can be easily seen between epidermal cells with silver stains or direct immunofluorescence of primary and secondary lesions.

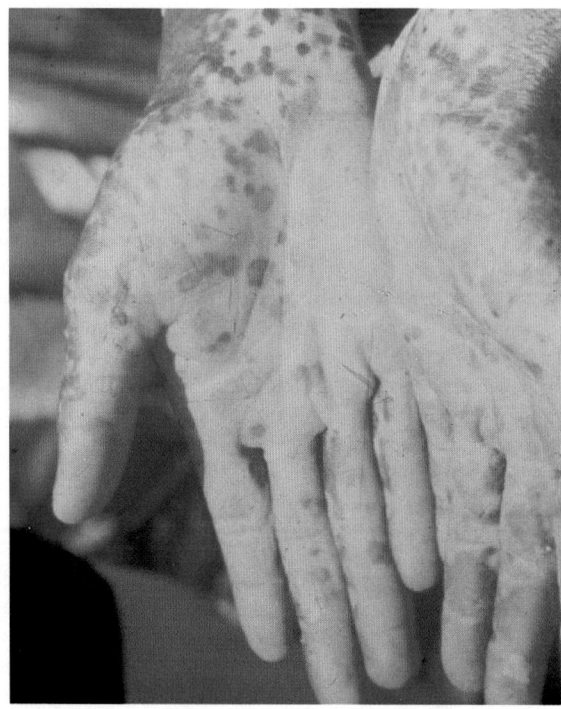

FIGURE 219-5 Late phase of pinta. Depigmentation and hyperpigmentation in healed lesions of wrists and palms.

Pinta (Carate, Purú-Purú, Mal De Pinto)

Pinta[1,13] is caused by *Treponema carateum* and was once prevalent in hot semi-arid coastal regions and in high altitudes. The disease was widespread in Cuba, southern Mexico, Colombia, Venezuela, Guyana, Ecuador, Peru, Bolivia, and Brazil. Presently, it is largely confined to Mexico, Central America, and Colombia,[4] and the incidence continues to decline.[13] It is a disease of underprivileged children and young adults and affects mostly blacks and native Indians. Transmission is by direct contact of abraded skin with an infected lesion. Long before the Spanish conquest, pinta was well known to Caribe and Aztec Indians. The disease was described by Valdez and Cortez between 1505 and 1515, and the causative microorganism was detected by Grau and Armenteros in Cuba in 1938 and confirmed by Leon in Mexico in 1942.

The clinical manifestations are confined to the skin. The primary stage consists of one or more erythematous desquamating patches on the face, arms, legs, or other uncovered areas. The lesions enlarge by peripheral extension and by fusion with satellite papules to form psoriasiform, lichenoid, or hyperkeratotic annular plaques which can grow over a period of months to years to sizes as large as 20 cm. The secondary stage is usually seen 2 to 5 months later, when new erythematous, scaly plaques encircle the primary lesion or become disseminated. Thereafter, the typical dyschromic areas of hyperpigmentation and depigmentation appear (Fig. 219-5). Originally pink or red, the lesions turn brown or copper and then slate blue or black. The pigment changes proceed irregularly. Depigmentation is characteristic of the late stage of the disease. At this stage, any variation of dyschromia, hypochromia, and achromia may be seen in the same patient. The surface of late lesions become thin, dry, and wrinkled. Generalized dermatopathic lymphadenopathy accompanies the last two stages of pinta. Demonstration of treponemes in tissue is difficult. Systemic symptoms are absent, and there is no cardiovascular or neurologic involvement.

Histopathology[16]

In early lesions, the epidermis shows slight acanthosis and intra- and extracellular edema. Lymphocytes permeate the epidermis, and there is hydropic degeneration with loss of melanin in the basal layer. Many melanophages are present in the upper dermis. Ultrastructural investigations have demonstrated that the treponemes cause irreversible damage to melanocytes. A dense infiltrate of plasma cells, lymphocytes, and, occasionally, histiocytes and neutrophils is found in the upper dermis around enlarged blood and lymph vessels. Numerous treponemes are usually visible in the epidermis.

Hyperpigmented lesions of late pinta are characterized by epidermal atrophy, absence of melanin in basal cells, accumulation of melanophages, and a scant lymphocytic dermal infiltrate. Treponemes are still seen in the epidermis. Hypochromic and achromic macules or patches of late pinta show degenerative basal layer changes, atrophy of the dermis and appendages, degeneration of elastic fibers, with accumulation of elastotic material. Melanin is completely absent, even in the dermis. Inflammation and treponemes cannot be found. Electron microscopic examination reveals the absence of basal epidermal melanocytes, but Langerhans cells are present and some of them contain a few melanosomes enclosed within lysosomes.

Immunity

Immunity from reinfection and superinfection develops during the late stages. Experiments have demonstrated the absence of cross-immunity among pinta, syphilis, and yaws in their early stages. However, a variable degree of cross-immunity is present in the late stages and is more evident in pinta and less in syphilis. Patients with pinta, "pintosos," are resistant to inoculation with *T. pallidum* during the late stage of the disease, but patients at any stage of syphilis or yaws are easily infected with pinta. Antibodies to lipoidal antigens can be found in the serum 2 to 3 months after the onset of the disease, and treponemal tests are also reactive. Nontreponemal and treponemal tests at any stage of pinta have been found unreactive in the cerebrospinal fluid.

Treatment

Endemic treponematoses are very sensitive to penicillin and other antibiotics. A single injection of benzathine penicillin at a dose of 0.6 million units for children under 10 years of age or 1.2 million units for all other cases and contacts is adequate therapy. Since these diseases rarely occur as isolated cases, they are best managed by mass campaigns.[1] In cases of penicillin allergy, oral erythromycin, 8 mg/kg four times daily, should be given for 15 days to children under 8 years of age. Older children should receive 250 mg four times daily orally for 15 days. Adults may be treated with the same regimen of tetracycline prescribed for early venereal syphilis.

Epidemiologic Treatment

The number of cases within a community largely depends on its living conditions (Table 219-2). Both treatment and clinical mani-

TABLE 219-2
WHO Recommendations[1] for Treatment of Endemic Treponematoses

1) *Total mass treatment (TMT)* in hyperendemic areas: the entire population should be treated.

2) *Juvenile mass treatment (JMT)* in mesoendemic areas: all active cases under 15 years of age and all contacts should receive treatment.

3) *Selective mass treatment (SMT)* in hypoendemic areas: treatment should be given to all active cases, all persons living in the same household, and all contacts.

Surveillance after treatment[1,13]

It is practically impossible to find all communicable cases in remote areas. These undetected cases represent future foci of infectivity unless the campaign is followed by further measures. Surveillance is the essential key element in effective control.[5] Resurveys should begin 6 months after initial treatment. Further surveys depend on the incidence of new cases but should be scheduled at least every 2 years.

festations are influenced by the disease's incidence, which epidemiologically is determined by the number of seropositive children 6 years of age. The conditions may be holoendemic (more than 90 percent of children at 6 years of age are seropositive), hyperendemic (over 50 percent), mesoendemic (between 10 and 50 percent), and hypoendemic (below 10 percent).[1,13] Despite a simple and effective therapy, persons still become disfigured and incapacitated by these diseases in epidemic proportions. Familiarity with the habits of the affected populations and an understanding of epidemiologic principles are indispensable for the future eradication of these diseases.

References

1. Perine PL et al: Handbook of endemic treponematoses. *World Health Organization*. Geneva, 1984
2. Luger A, Meheus A: Alarming spread of endemic treponematoses. *Zeitschrift fur Hautkrankheiten* **63**:463, 1988
3. Willcox RR: Mass treatment campaigns against the endemic treponematoses. *Rev Infect Dis* **7**:278, 1985
4. World Health Organization: Yaws and other endemic treponematoses. Report of a regional meeting. Brazzaville, 2–6 Feb. 1986. Regional office for Africa. Brazzaville. WHO, 1986
5. Hopkins DR: Control of yaws and other endemic treponematoses. Implementation of vertical and/or intergrated programs. *Rev Infect Dis* **7**:338, 1985
6. Roman CG, Roman LM: Occurrence of congenital, cardiovascular, visceral, neurologic and neuro-ophthalmologic complications in late yaws: A theme for future research. *Rev Infect Dis* **8**:760, 1986
7. Fieldsteel HH: Genetics of treponema, in *Pathogenesis and Immunology of Treponemal Infection,* edited by RF Shell, D Musher. New York, Marcel Dekker, 1983, p 39
8. Bakker-Zander SA, Lukehart SA: Molecular basis of immunological cross reactivity between *Treponema pallidum* and *Treponema pertenue.* *J Infect Immunol* **42**:634, 1983
9. Thornburg RW, Baseman JB: Comparison of major protein antigens and protein profiles of *Treponema pallidum* and *Treponema pertenue.* *J Infect Immunol* **42**:623, 1983
10. Turner TB, Hollander DH: Biology of treponematoses. WHO Monograph series 35, Geneva, 1957
11. Hardy PH: Pathogenic treponemes, in *The Biology of Parasitic Spirochetes,* edited by RC Johnson. New York, Academic, 1976, p 107
12. Willcox RR: The epidemiology of the spirochetoses—a worldwide view, in *The Biology of Parasitic Spirochetes,* edited by RC Johnson. New York, Academic, 1976, p 133
13. Luger A: Endemic treponematoses, in *Sexually Transmitted Diseases,* edited by LC Parish, F Gschnait. New York, Springer-Verlag, 1988, p 32
14. St. John RR: Yaws in the Americas. *Rev Infect Dis* **7**:266, 1985
15. Engelkens HJM et al: Radiological and dermatological findings in two patients suffering from early yaws in Indonesia. *Genitour Med* **66**:259, 1990
16. Lever WF and Lever GS (eds): *Histopathology of the Skin.* Philadelphia, Lippincott 1990, p 358

Alfred R. Eichmann

Chancroid

Chancroid is a sexually transmitted, acute, ulcerative disease, usually localized on the genitals or anus and often associated with an inguinal bubo. The disease is caused by *Haemophilus ducreyi*, a gram-negative, facultative anaerobic bacillus that requires hemin (x factor) for growth.

Historical Aspects

Chancroid, or soft chancre (ulcus molle), was first distinguished from syphilis by Basserau in France in 1852.[1] The causative bacillus was discovered and described in 1889 by Ducrey, a bacteriologist at the University of Naples.[2] Unna described the histology of chancroid and found the chains of gram-negative rods in the lesion.[3] It is still unclear who was the first to culture *H. ducreyi*, as a number of authors at the turn of the century claimed to have first isolated the agent. In his review, Albritton[4] has credited Himmel[5] with the first unequivocal isolation of *H. ducreyi*.

Epidemiology

Chancroid is most common in developing countries, especially in tropical and subtropical areas. It is the most common cause of genital ulcerative disease in adults in Africa and many other parts of the developing world.[6] In Nairobi, Kenya, over 5000 patients with chancroid are seen annually in only one major clinic for sexually transmitted diseases.[7] In the United States, the annual incidence of chancroid decreased markedly between 1950 and 1978,[8] but in 1985 the annual number of reported cases rose above 2000 for the first time, and in 1987 and 1990, 5000 and 4200 cases, respectively, were reported. In 1990, the annual incidence of chancroid was 1.7 cases in 100,000.[9]

Males are far more affected than females. The ratio of males to females in most nonmilitary epidemics has been 10:1.[8] The reason for this difference is not clearly understood, but it seems that the environment provided by the foreskin makes males more susceptible to *H. ducreyi*.[10]

The prevalence of chancroid is higher in lower socioeconomic groups who frequent prostitutes. Lower-class prostitutes appear to be a reservoir in all reported outbreaks of this disease.[11] Recently, several studies from Africa have shown that chancroidal ulcers are an important risk factor in the heterosexual spread of HIV-1.[12] Until now the epidemiology of chancroid has been poorly documented because of little interest and lack of accurate and simple diagnostic tools (phenotypic markers for strain typing). It is still not clear whether there is an asymptomatic reservoir of *H. ducreyi* and what the risks of transmission are.[6]

Etiology

Taxonomy

Haemophilus ducreyi is a gram-negative, facultative anaerobic bacillus that requires hemin (x factor) for growth. The organism is small, nonmotile, and non-spore-forming and typically exhibits streptobacillary chaining, especially in cultures. The exact taxonomy is still controversial. The current classifications list *H. ducreyi* as a true *Haemophilus* species. Some biochemical properties, however, put this organism close to the Pasteurellaceae.[5]

Biochemistry

Haemophilus ducreyi has few distinguishing biochemical factors. Nitrate reduction is characteristic of the genus. All reported strains are oxidase-positive and catalase-negative and have a broad range of phosphatase activity. The alkaline-phosphatase reaction is used as a differential marker of identification.[4] The differentiation from other hemin-requiring strains of *Haemophilus* rests on the non-requirement of *H. ducreyi* for nicotinamide adenine dinucleotide (NAD, V factor) and its failure to produce H_2S, catalase, or indole.[11]

Growth Requirements

Haemophilus ducreyi is a fastidious bacillus. In order to get optimal rates of positive cultures, Nszane et al.[13] recommend the use of two media simultaneously: gonococcal agar supplemented with bovine hemoglobin and Mueller-Hinton agar supplemented with chocolate horse blood, each with 5% fetal calf serum. Growth is best at 30 to 33°C in a water-saturated atmosphere.[14]

Genetics

The strains of *H. ducreyi* appear to be a serologically and biochemically homogeneous group. *H. ducreyi* shares a significant gene pool with members of the Pasteurellaceae and the Enterobacteriae. The core plasmid for the various plasmids conferring ampicillin resistance is also found in other species of *Haemophilus* and *Neisseriae*.[4] Beta-lactamase production is mediated by plasmids with a molecular mass of 5700 or 5000 kDa.[15] These plasmids are identical to the two types of *N. gonorrhoeae* beta-lactamase plasmids. A 3200-kDa plasmid, mediating beta-lactamase production has also been reported.[16] Additionally, a 3600-kDa plasmid encoding for beta-lactamase production in *H. ducreyi* was found in isolates from a chancroid outbreak in California in 1983.[17]

Pathogenesis

Very little is known about the pathogenesis of *H. ducreyi* infection. Trauma or abrasion are thought to be necessary for the penetration of the bacillus into the epidermis. No toxins or extracellular enzymes of *H. ducreyi* have been described, and virulence factors are not known. The almost complete absence of microorganisms in the bubo also remains unexplained.

Clinical Manifestations

The incubation period is between 3 and 7 days and is rarely more than 10 days. No prodromal symptoms are known. The chancre begins as a soft papule surrounded by erythema. After 24 to 48 h it becomes pustular, eroded, and ulcerated. The edges of the ulcer are often ragged and undermined, and its base is usually covered by a necrotic, yellowish-gray exudate covering a granulation tissue that bleeds readily on manipulation. In contrast to syphilis, chancroid ulcers are usually tender and quite painful and often multiple. Half of the males present with a single ulcer. The diameter varies from 1 mm to 2 cm.[18] In males, most lesions are found on the external or internal surface of the prepuce, on the frenulum, and on the glans (Fig. 220-1), and edema of the prepuce is often present. The urethral meatus and shaft of the penis and the anus are involved less frequently. Only rarely is the chancre localized in the urethra, causing purulent urethritis.[19]

In females, the lesions are usually localized on the vulva, especially on the fourchette, the small labia, and vestibule. Vaginal, cervical, and perianal ulcers have also been described.[18] Extragenital lesions of chancroid have been reported on the breasts, fingers, thighs, and within the mouth. Trauma and abrasion may be important for localization of such extragenital manifestations.

A bubo, i.e., a painful inguinal adenitis, occurs in up to 50 percent of patients and appears within a few days to 2 weeks (average 1 week) after onset of the primary lesion (Fig. 220-2). The adenitis is unilateral in most patients, and erythema of the overlying skin is typical. Buboes can become fluctuant and rupture spontaneously. Pus draining from a bubo is usually thick and creamy. Lymphadenitis is less common in females.

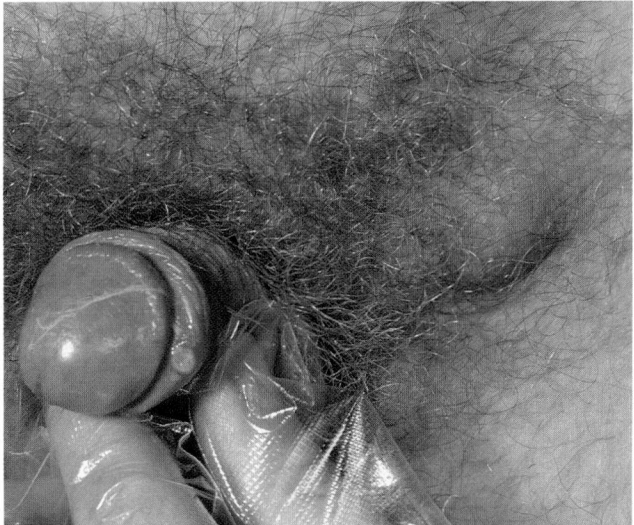

FIGURE 220-2   Small chancroid ulcer on the internal surface of the prepuce with inguinal adenitis.

Clinical Variants of the Soft Ulcer

Besides the common types of chancroid described above, a number of clinical variants have been reported.[20]

1. Giant chancroid is a single lesion that extends peripherally and shows extensive ulceration.
2. Large serpiginous ulcer is a lesion that becomes confluent, spreading by extension and autoinoculation. The groin or thigh may be involved (ulcus molle serpiginosum).
3. Phagedenic chancroid is a variant caused by superinfection by fusospirochetosis. Rapid and profound destruction of tissue can occur (ulcus molle gangrenosum).
4. Transient chancroid is a small ulcer that resolves spontaneously in a few days. It may be followed 2 to 3 weeks later by an acute regional lymphadenitis (French: *cancre mou volant*).
5. Follicular chancroid consists of multiple small ulcers in a follicular distribution.
6. Papular chancroid consists of a granulomatous ulcerated papule and may resemble donovanosis or condyloma latum (ulcus molle elevatum).

Mild systemic symptoms can accompany chancroid but are rare. Systemic infection by *H. ducreyi* has never been observed.

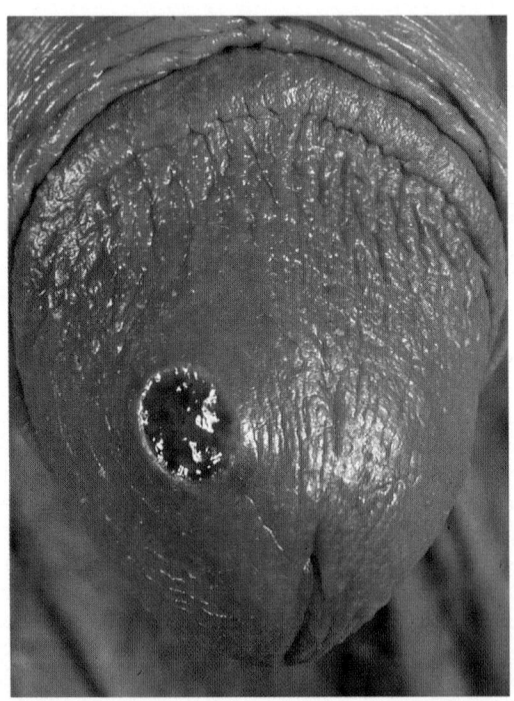

FIGURE 220-1   Sharply circumscribed ulcer on the glans.

Laboratory and Special Examination

The laboratory diagnosis of chancroid depends on the isolation of *H. ducreyi* from an anogenital ulcer. After specimens have been scraped from an ulcer, direct examination using Gram or Giemsa stain (Fig. 220-3)[21] or even electron microscopic examination[22] is recommended as a first step, but the result can be misleading because of the polymicrobial flora of most genital ulcers.[23] The bacilli are usually found in small clusters or parallel chains of two or three organisms streaming along strands of mucus (Fig. 220-3). This pattern has been described as a "school of fish" or "railroad-track" appearance. Cotton or calcium-aginate swabs are recommended for specimen collection.

The bacillus will survive only 2 to 4 h on a swab unless refrigerated. No satisfactory transport system is available. The simultaneous use of two primary isolation media supplemented with hemoglobin and serum are recommended for high culture sensitivity (see above).[13] Small, nonmucoid, yellow-gray, translucent colonies appear in 2 to 4 days after inoculation. Typically, these colonies can be pushed intact across the agar surface. The identification of *H. ducreyi* is performed following the recommendations of Lubwama[24]: demonstration of hemin requirement, oxidase- and catalase-test, beta-lactamase test, and H_2S and indole activity. Testing of antibiotic susceptibility is recommended because clinically significant antimicrobial resistance of *H. ducreyi* has become common.[25]

In the case of bubo formation, the extent of the enlarged lymph nodes can be demonstrated by computed tomography of the groin.[26] In some cases a biopsy of the ulcer can be diagnostic. The typical histologic findings are three vertically arranged zones: a superficial necrotic zone, followed by a zone of new blood vessel formation, and a deep zone consisting of a dense lymphocytic and plasma cell infiltrate. *H. ducreyi* is rarely demonstrated in tissue sections.[27]

Two previously common diagnostic procedures are obsolete: the Ito-Reenstierna skin test is only of historic interest,[28] and auto-inoculation should not be performed as a diagnostic procedure because false-positive and false-negative results may occur as other

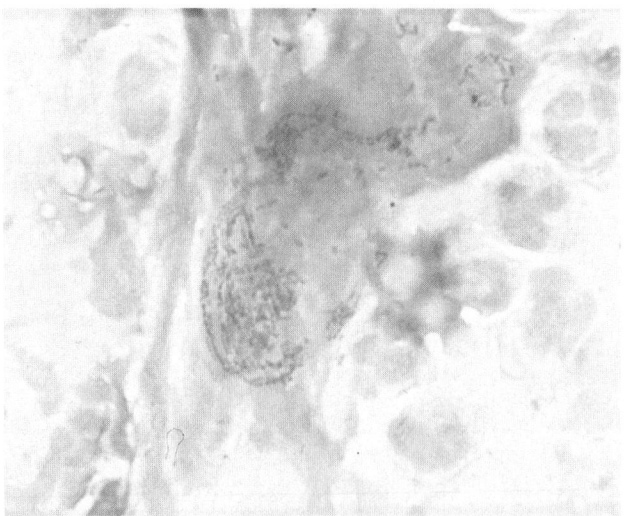

FIGURE 220-3   Smear from chancroid ulcer (Giemsa stain).

pathogens are also inoculated by this method.[29] Many attempts have been made to develop a reliable serologic test for chancroid, but such a test is still not available.

Differential Diagnosis

The three classic etiologic agents for genital ulceration are *H. ducreyi, Treponema pallidum,* and *herpes simplex.* The clinical appearance of the diseases caused by these three organisms can be extremely variable both in males and females,[30,31] and in a high percentage of genital ulcers no pathogen can be isolated.[32]

The clinical diagnosis alone is inadequate, and, according to most authors, the direct microscopic examination of smears is also insufficient for a proper diagnosis of chancroid.[24] Thus, isolation of *H. ducreyi* on appropriate media and subsequent biochemical identification is essential for a reliable diagnosis.

A syphilitic chancre must be excluded by dark-field examinations and repeated serologic tests. Herpes simplex virus can be diagnosed by culture or by routine electron microscopy using the negative-stain procedure. Lymphogranuloma venereum (LGV) can be excluded by a negative LGV complement fixation test (titer less than 1:16) and by failure to demonstrate a significant rise in the titer on repeated testing after 3 weeks.

Donovanosis (see Chap. 222) and superinfected traumatic lesions must be considered in the differential diagnosis, and it should be kept in mind that mixed infections (chancroid and syphilis, chancroid and herpes simplex) occur.

Treatment

The antibiotic susceptibility pattern of *H. ducreyi* has changed, making previously recommended treatments obsolete. A plasmid-mediated resistance in *H. ducreyi* has been described for ampicillin,[33] sulfonamides,[34] chloramphenicol,[35] tetracycline,[36] and kanamycin.[37]

The Centers for Disease Control currently recommends as treatment for chancroid ceftriaxone, 250 mg intramuscularly in a single dose, or erythromycin base, 500 mg orally 4 times a day for 7 days.[38]

Based on in vitro susceptibility, the most active drugs against *H. ducreyi* are ceftriaxone,[39] ciprofloxacin (500 mg intramuscularly),[40] and roxithromycin.[41] The first two of these agents are effective in single-dose regimens, whereas the optimal dosage and duration of treatment of roxithromycin remain to be established. A 3-day combination of amoxicillin with clavulanic acid is also effective,[42] and effectiveness has also been shown for the quinolones rosoxacin, ciprofloxacin, enoxocin, norfloxacin, and fleroxacin.[25] On the other hand, single-dose treatment with trimethoprim-sulfamethoxazole (640/3200 mg) is inferior to the other regimens.[39]

Local treatment consists of antiseptic dressings (i.e., povidone-iodine). Suppurative nodes should not be incised. If necessary, they can be punctured to prevent spontaneous rupture and sinus tract formation. A large syringe should be used and the fluctuant buboes entered laterally through normal skin. In patients with phimosis, a circumcision may be necessary when all active lesions have healed. Relapses occur in about 5 percent of the patients even after correct treatment has been performed. In such cases, treatment with the original regimen is recommended. Failure to treat the sexual partner is usually the cause of the relapse.

Prevention

Patients should be advised to abstain from sexual activity until all lesions have cleared. Sexual contacts should be examined and treated. Epidemiologic treatment of contacts has been recommended, and many authors feel that these persons should be treated even in the absence of clinical disease, as asymptomatic carriage of *H. ducreyi* is possible.[43]

Epidemiologic Association with Human Immunodeficiency Virus Type 1

Many studies, mainly in Africa, have consistently found that genital ulcers increase the risk of sexual transmission of HIV.[44] In a prospective study, HIV-infected males were three times more likely to have had a recent history of genital ulcers.[45] In another prospective study of seronegative males, those presenting with chancroid had a fivefold risk of seroconversion during follow-up compared to males with urethritis.[46] Genital ulcers are also a major risk factor for HIV infection among prostitutes. There is a tenfold increased risk among prostitutes with ulcers, compared to a cohort without ulcerations.[47]

The histologic structure of chancroid ulcer supports the hypothesis that these lesions may facilitate entrance and egress of HIV-1. Other studies have shown that HIV-1 can readily be recovered from the exudate of genital ulcers in HIV-1-infected patients.[12] It has also been shown that failure of a single-dose therapy for chancroid in males was associated with HIV-1 seropositivity.[12] It is likely that HIV-1 and *H. ducreyi* can interact in several ways to mutually increase transmission.

The epidemiologic control of chancroid may be a very important strategy to interrupt the heterosexual spread of HIV in some parts of the world. Accordingly, patients with chancroid should be tested for HIV seropositivity. HIV-seropositive patients with culture-proven chancroid should be treated with a multiple-day regimen.

Course and Prognosis

The disease is self-limited, and systemic spread does not occur. Without treatment, genital ulcers and inguinal abscesses have occasionally been reported to persist for years. Local pain is the most frequent complaint.

Infections do not confer immunity, and reinfections are possible. Patients have to be instructed to use condoms properly to avoid reinfections.

ACKNOWLEDGMENT

I am grateful to René Rüdlinger, M.D., for reading the manuscript.

References

1. Basserau L: *Traité des Affections de la Peau Symptomatiques de la Syphilis*. Paris, Ballière, 1852
2. Ducrey A: Experimentelle Untersuchungen über den Ansteckungsstoff des weichen Schankers und über die Bubonen. *Monatsschr Prakt Dermatol* **9**:387, 1889
3. Unna PG: Der Streptobacillus des weichen Schankers. *Monatsschr Prakt Dermatol* **14**:485, 1892
4. Albritton WL: Biology of *Haemophilus ducreyi*. *Microbiol Rev* **53**:377, 1989
5. Himmel J: Contributions à l'étude de l'immunité des animaux vis-à-vis du Bacille du chancre mou. *Ann Inst Pasteur (Paris)* **15**:928, 1901
6. Piot P, Meheus A: Epidémiologie des maladies sexuellement transmissibles dans les pays en développement. *Ann Soc Belg Med Trop* **63**:87, 1983
7. Kibukamusoke JW: Venereal disease in East Africa. *Trans R Soc Trop Med Hyg* **59**:642, 1965
8. Schmid GP et al: Chancroid in the United States, reestablishment of an old disease. *JAMA* **258**:3265, 1987
9. Centers for Disease Control: *Sexually Transmitted Disease. Surveillance: 1990*. Atlanta, U.S. Dept. of Health and Human Services, Public Health Service, 1991
10. Hart G: Venereal disease in a war environment: Incidence and management. *Med J Aust* **1**:808, 1975
11. Ronald AR, Albritton W: Chancroid and *Haemophilus ducreyi*, in *Sexually Transmitted Diseases*, 2d ed., edited by KK Holmes et al, New York, McGraw-Hill, 1990
12. Jessamine PG et al: HIV, genital ulcers and the male foreskin: Synergism in HIV-1 transmission. *Scand J Infect Dis* **69** (suppl): 181, 1990
13. Nszane H et al: Comparison of media for the primary isolation of *H. ducreyi*. *Sex Transm Dis* **11**:6, 1984
14. Sottnek FO et al: Isolation and identification of *H. ducreyi* in a clinical study. *J Clin Microbiol* **12**:170, 1980
15. Brunton J et al: Molecular epidemiology of beta-lactamase-specifying plasmids of *H. ducreyi*. *Antimicrob Agents Chemother* **21**:857, 1982
16. Handsfield HH et al: Molecular epidemiology of *H. ducreyi* infections. *Ann Intern Med* **95**:315, 1981
17. Anderson B et al: Common β-lactamase specifying plasmid in *H. ducreyi* and *N. gonorrhoeae*. *Antimicrob Agents Chemother* **25**:296, 1984
18. Hammond GW et al: Clinical, epidemiological, laboratory and therapeutic features of an urban outbreak of chancroid in North America. *Rev Infect Dis* **2**:867, 1980
19. Kunimoto DY et al: Urethral infection with *H. ducreyi* in men. *Sex Transm Dis* **15**:37, 1988
20. Gaisin A, Heaton CL: Chancroid: Alias the soft chancre. *Int J Dermatol* **13**:188, 1975
21. Borchardt KA, Hake AW: Simplified technique for diagnosis of chancroid. *Arch Dermatol* **102**:190, 1970
22. Marsch WC et al: Ultrastructural detection of *H. ducreyi* in biopsies of chancroid. *Arch Dermatol Res* **263**:153, 1978
23. Chapel T et al: The microbiological flora of penile ulcerations. *J Infect Dis* **137**:50, 1978
24. Lubwama SW et al: Isolation and identification of *H. ducreyi* in a clinical laboratory. *J Med Microbiol* **22**:175, 1986
25. Dangor Y et al: Treatment of chancroid. *Antimicrob Agents Chemother* **34**:1308, 1990
26. Hartmann AA et al: Intravenous single-dose certriaxone treatment of chancroid. *Dermatologica* **183**:132, 1991
27. Sheldon WH, Heyman A: Studies on chancroid: Observations on the histology with an evaluation of biopsy as a diagnostic procedure. *Am J Pathol* **22**:415, 1946
28. Ito T: Klinische und bakteriologische Studien über Ulcus molle und Ducrey'sche Streptobazillen. *Arch Dermatol Syphilol* **116**:341, 1913
29. Stüttgen G: *Ulcus molle*. Berlin, Grosse Verlag, 1981

30. Fast MV et al: The clinical diagnosis of genital ulcer disease in men in the tropics. *Sex Transm Dis* **11**:72, 1984

31. Plummer FA et al: Clinical and microbiologic studies of genital ulcers in Kenyan women. *Sex Transm Dis* **12**:193, 1985

32. Taylor DN et al: The role of *H. ducreyi* in penile ulcers in Bangkok, Thailand. *Sex Transm Dis* **11**:148, 1984

33. Brunton JL et al: Plasmid mediated ampicillin resistance in *H. ducreyi. Antimicrob Agents Chemother* **15**:294, 1979

34. Albritton WL et al: Plasmid mediated sulfonamid resistance in *H. ducreyi. Antimicrob Agents Chemother* **21**:159, 1982

35. Roberts MC et al: Molecular characterization of chloramphenicol resistant *H. parainfluenza* and *H. ducreyi. Antimicrob Agents Chemother* **28**:176, 1985

36. Albritton WL: Plasmid mediated tetracycline resistance in *H. ducreyi. Antimicrob Agents Chemother* **25**:187, 1984

37. Sanson-Le Pors MJ et al: Plasmid mediated aminoglycoside phosphotransferases in *H. ducreyi. Antimicrob Agents Chemother* **28**:315, 1958

38. Centers for Disease Control: *Sexually Transmitted Diseases. Summary: 1990.* Atlanta, U.S. Dept. of Health and Human Services, Public Health Services, 1990

39. Schmid GP: Treatment of chancroid 1989. *Rev Infect Dis* **12**(suppl):6, 1990

40. Ballard RC et al: Treating chancroid: Summary of studies in southern Africa. *Genitourin Med* **65**:54, 1989

41. Haase DA et al: Clinical evaluation of rosoxacin for the treatment of chancroid. *Antimicrob Agents Chemother* **30**:39, 1986

42. Ndimya-Achoha JO et al: Augmentin in the treatment of chancroid. Three day oral course. *Genitourin Med* **62**:202, 1986

43. Kinghorn GR: Genital colonisation with *Haemophilus ducreyi* in the absence of ulceration. *Eur J Sex Transm Dis* **1**:89, 1983

44. Kreiss JK et al: AIDS-virus infection in Nairobi prostitutes; spread of epidemic to East Africa. *N Engl J Med* **314**:414, 1986

45. Simonsen JN et al: Human immunodeficiency virus infection among men with STD. *N Engl J Med* **319**:274, 1988

46. Cameron DW et al: Female to male transmission of HIV in Nairobi. *Lancet* **1**:403, 1989

47. Plummer FA et al: Cofactors in male to female transmission of HIV, abstract no. 4554. IVth International Conference on AIDS, Stockholm, June 12–16, 1988

CHAPTER 221

Richard B. Rothenberg

Lymphogranuloma Venereum

Lymphogranuloma venereum (LGV) is a sexually transmitted disease of chlamydial etiology with protean clinical manifestations involving the lymphatic system.[1] It should be considered in the differential diagnosis of benign and malignant lymphadenopathy, genital lesions, proctocolitis, and rectal stricture. LGV, along with other causes of genital ulcer disease, is increasingly important as a potential facilitator of human immunodeficiency virus (HIV) transmission.[2,3]

History

The disease has a colorful nosologic history including such designations as tropical or climatic bubo, third, fourth, fifth, or sixth venereal disease, lymphopathia venerea, and Nicolas-Favre disease—but the current name is now universally accepted. The first major clinical description appeared in 1913, and inclusion bodies in material from lesions were demonstrated 10 years later. In 1930, the disease was produced experimentally by intracerebral inoculation of monkeys with pus from a bubo of LGV.[4] In 1940 Rake et al.[5] grew the organism, then thought to be a filterable virus, in the yolk sac of embryonated eggs. Development of several techniques in the past 20 years, including the use of cycloheximide-treated McCoy cells for tissue culture[6] and the microimmunofluorescence test,[7] has greatly enhanced the study of the chlamydial diseases.

Epidemiology

LGV probably occurs all over the world, with endemic foci in tropical and subtropical countries, but few, if any, systematic data describe incidence or prevalence. In the United States, the number of cases reported yearly declined from 2526 in 1947 to a stable level of 200 to 300 during the 1980s (Fig. 221-1). The chief foci of activity have been the District of Columbia and the southeastern United States, affecting predominantly blacks of low socioeconomic status. Age-specific attack rates are highest in the 20- to 40-year-old group. The disease is spread by direct inoculation from genital fluids, but transmission efficiency is not known. Women may be asymptomatic and culture positive and may serve as a reservoir for infection,[8] as they do for gonorrhea and other genital chlamydial infections.

Etiology

The disease is caused by members of the genus *Chlamydia* (previously known as *Bedsonia*) whose structure, metabolism, DNA and RNA content, and method of reproduction make them similar to *Rickettsia*.[9,10] The species, *Chlamydia trachomatis,* has two major biologic varieties (*biovars*): trachoma, or TRIC organisms, and LGV organisms. The latter, in turn, are characterized by three major serologic varieties (or *serovars*)—L1, L2, and L3. The LGV serovars are distinguished by their preferential infectivity for lymph nodes, intracerebral lethality for mice, and different behavior in cell culture.[1] Experimentally, the LGV serovars produce severe hemorrhagic proctitis in monkeys, and TRIC serovars do not.[11] The two biovars, however, share a major cross-reacting antigen which complicates serologic distinction between them. In recent years, however, the development of monoclonal antibody and DNA probes has materially enhanced the specificity of laboratory diagnosis.[12]

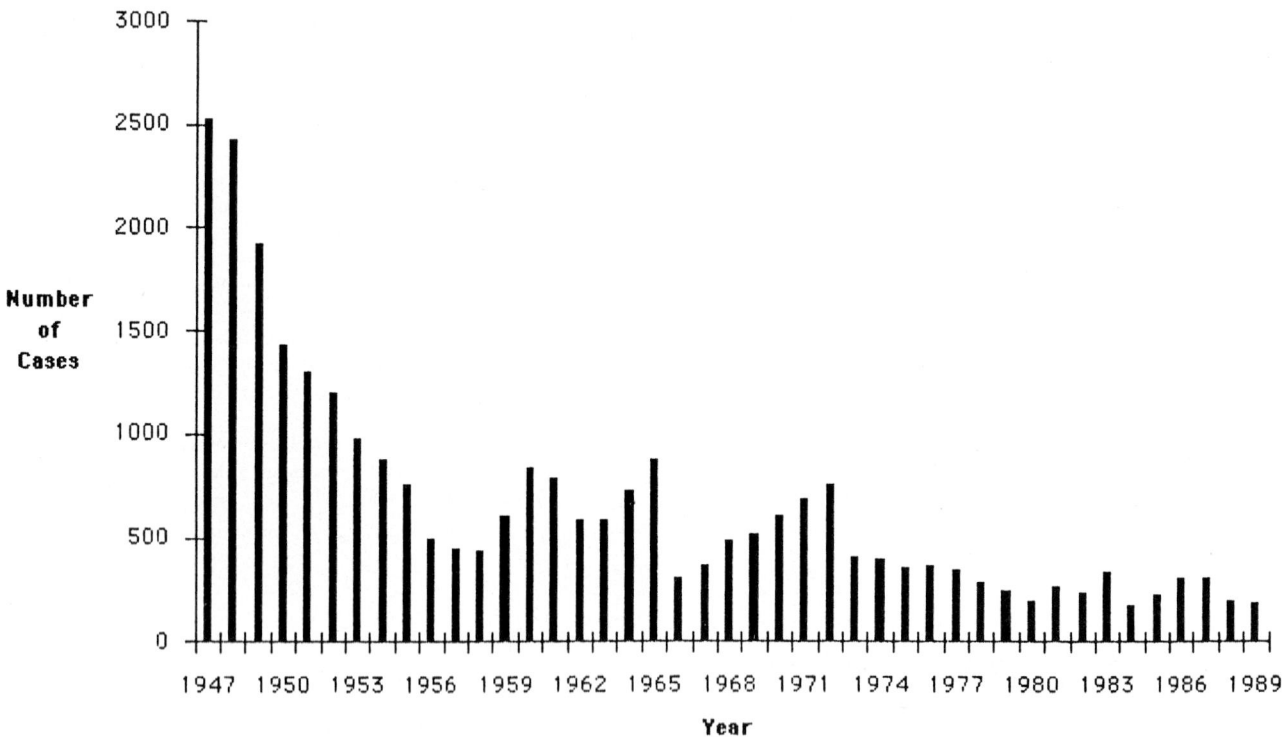

FIGURE 221-1 Yearly cases of lymphogranuloma venereum, United States, 1947–1989.

Clinical Manifestations

LGV is contracted by direct contact with infectious secretions, almost exclusively through sexual activity. The portal of entry and the initial symptoms are determined by the nature of the sex act; inoculation is usually genital, but it may be rectal or pharyngeal.[13] The incubation period varies from 3 to 30 days if primary lesions occur, but it may be longer if adenopathy is the only manifestation.[14] The period of infectiousness and transmission rates are not clearly defined.

Acute and chronic manifestations characterize both the genital (or inguinal) and rectal syndromes. The primary lesion is a 5- to 8-mm soft, erythematous, painless erosion (Fig. 221-2) that heals spontaneously in a few days. Occasionally, a button-like papule may appear which is also transient. Such lesions are reported by a fourth to a third of patients. Secondary inguinal adenopathy begins 1 to 2 weeks after the primary lesion as discrete, movable, tender nodes which later coalesce to form a firm, fist-sized, elongated, immovable mass. These may occur above and below Poupart's ligament, giving rise to the "groove" sign (Fig. 221-3). Nodes are bilateral in one-third of cases.[14] Rupture of fluctuant nodes may lead to chronic sinus formation. Initially, the overlying skin is often slightly reddened and edematous, but it later may become thickened and develop a characteristic purplish hue. Generalized systemic symptoms such as fever, chills, and malaise may be prominent. Meningoencephalitis, hepatosplenomegaly, arthralgia, stiff neck, and headache may also occur.[8] In untreated cases, the lymphadenopathy usually subsides spontaneously in 8 to 12 weeks.[14]

Late complications of the male inguinal syndrome are rare. Elephantiasis of the penis and scrotum characterized by infiltrative, ulcerative, and fistular lesions occur in approximately 4 percent of

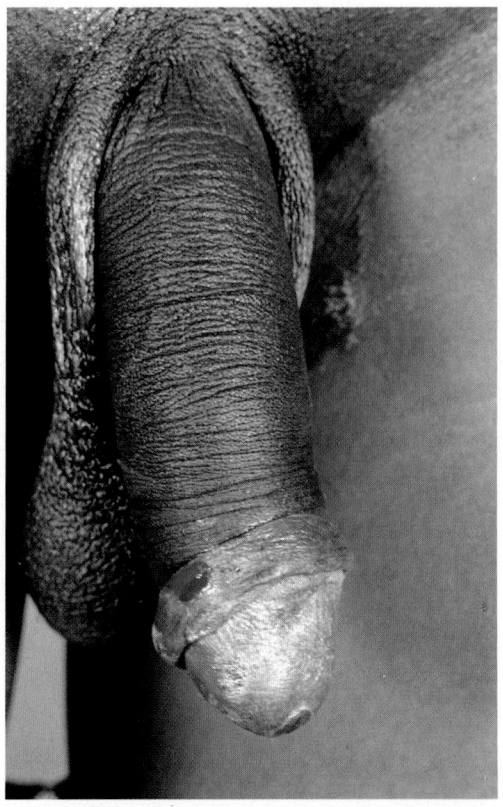

FIGURE 221-2 Lymphogranuloma venereum. Soft painless erosion on the prepuce. (Courtesy of I.M. Freedberg, M.D.)

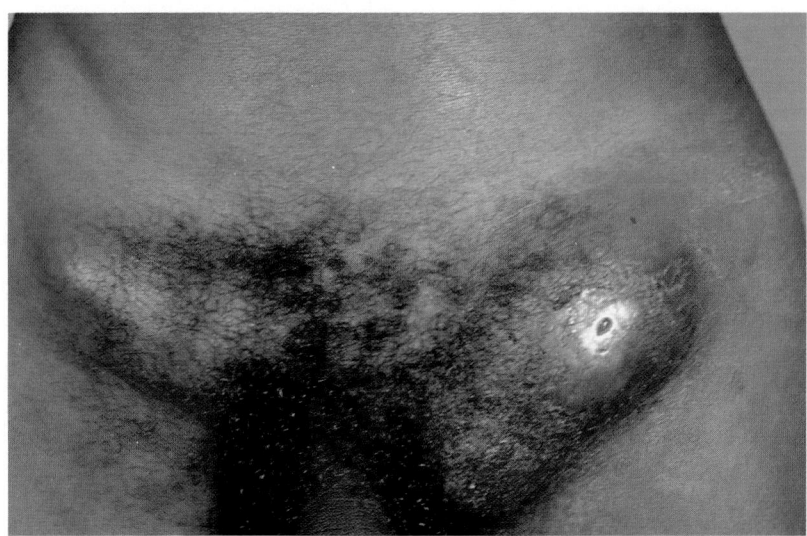

FIGURE 221-3 Lymphogranuloma venereum. Bilateral, firm, immovable masses above Poupart's ligament. (Courtesy of I.M. Freedberg, M.D.)

cases.[15] Recent reports of LGV mimicking cervical lymphoma in a homosexual male practicing fellatio[16] and a heterosexual male engaging in cunnilingus[17] emphasize the need for a detailed history. The physician must be alert, as well, to the potential for local community outbreaks.[18]

The acute rectal syndrome occurs more frequently in women than men. In men, direct inoculation of the anal canal is believed to be the mode of entry, whereas the internal lymphatic drainage of the proximal two-thirds of the vagina has been invoked as the source for women. In both sexes, acute manifestations include rectal pain, tenesmus, and mucosanguineous rectal discharge, with typical findings of proctocolitis on sigmoidoscopy. It is important to distinguish LGV from other forms of inflammatory bowel disease, particularly in homosexual men.[19,20] The major late manifestation is rectal stricture. In women, late scarring, fistulas, ulceration, and elephantiasis of the perineum, called *esthiomene,* may require radical surgical intervention.[21]

Various dermatologic conditions have been reported in association with acute manifestations, including erythema nodosum, erythema multiforme, scarlatiniform exanthem, and urticaria.[4] In addition, photosensitivity has been reported in as many as 35 percent of patients, occasionally associated with conjunctivitis, joint involvement, and erythema nodosum.[4] Sonck[22] observed a photosensitivity reaction in 140 of 400 LGV cases studied. This reaction was manifest 1 to 2 months after onset of bubo formation and occurred in 60 percent of the chronic and about 20 percent of subacute cases. Punctiform, red papules appeared on the skin 30 min to 3 h after exposure to sunlight. Accompanying this reaction was conjunctivitis in 19 percent, joint involvement in 33 percent, and erythema nodosum in 16 percent of persons with the photosensitivity reaction. The possible allergic or autoimmune nature of these phenomena is supported by the frequent appearance of biologic false-positive tests for syphilis (estimated at 20 percent of cases), the high incidence of cryoprecipitins and rheumatoid factor, and the high serum levels of IgA and IgG in both acute and chronic syndromes.[23]

As noted, as a cause of genital ulceration, LGV may play a role in facilitating transmission of HIV. Because of its lymphatic manifestations and potential effects on the immune system, it may play a role in the differential diagnosis of acquired immunodeficiency syndrome (AIDS) as well. In one reported case, for example, disseminated Kaposi's sarcoma mimicked LGV in its initial presentation.[24] The syndrome of angioimmunoblastic lymphadenopathy has been reported in association with LGV[25] and may, as occurred in one case, lead to progressive immunologic deterioration and rapidly fatal immunoblastic lymphoma.

Pathology

In general, histopathologic changes of LGV are nonspecific. Primary ulcers are characterized by an exudate of fibrin, polymorphonuclear leukocytes, and cellular debris.[26] Skin test sites or rectal lesions may contain epithelioid nodules, plasma cells, and occasional giant cells, but these changes are not diagnostic. Stellate triangular abscesses may be observed in biopsy specimens of lymph nodes and are characteristic, but not pathognomonic, of LGV.[27] The pathology of LGV-induced proctocolitis is characterized by crypt distortion, submucosal fibrosis, neuromatous hypertrophy, follicular inflammation, and occasional granuloma formation. It may be difficult to distinguish these changes from those associated with Crohn's disease, although localization of lesions is of considerable help (proximal in Crohn's disease, distal in LGV).[28] It is likely that LGV is not etiologically associated with Crohn's disease.[1]

Diagnosis

Clinical diagnosis of LGV is greatly enhanced by laboratory confirmation. Definitive diagnosis is possible through isolation of the organism from tissue or body fluids,[6] and distinction among the three serovars can be made using microimmunofluorescence techniques.[1] Since tissue culture may not be readily available, the clinician must often rely on serologic methods. First developed in the 1930s, the complement fixation test has long been the mainstay of diagnosis of LGV. It suffers from lack of specificity: virtually all members of the genus *Chlamydia* share the target antigen.[29] Although less than 3 percent of the general population has a titer as high as 1:16,[30] 40 to 50 percent of women with uncomplicated TRIC-agent cervical infection had titers of 1:16 to 1:32; similar titers occurred in 15 to 20 percent of men with TRIC-associated urethritis.[3] A titer of 1:64 or greater is, however, highly suggestive of LGV. Coupled with a fourfold change in titer (which is not uniformly detected), a high titer greatly increases diagnostic assurance. The microimmunofluorescence test, originally developed as a guide to identification of organisms, has been successfully adapted as a serologic test. It responds, similar to the complement fixation test, to the broadly reactive range of antibodies produced by patients with LGV. Again, very high titers of IgG antibody are usual in patients with acute infection. Other tests, including ELISA and radioimmunoassay methods, are also available but appear to offer little advantage.[32]

The Frei test, an intradermal inoculation of killed LGV organisms, was important to diagnosis for many years. Its sensitivity and specificity are in serious doubt, however,[30] and the test is now of historic interest only, since the antigen is no longer commercially available.

Differential Diagnosis

In view of the nonspecific nature of signs and symptoms, acute LGV should be considered in the differential diagnosis of syphilis, herpes progenitalis, granuloma inguinale, and chancroid, as well as bacterial, fungal, and tuberculous skin infection. Adenopathy may require consideration of benign and malignant lymphoproliferative disorders (e.g., infectious mononucleosis, Hodgkin's disease), particularly in the presence of oral and cervical infection. Late manifestations must be distinguished from neoplastic skin disease, filariasis, rectal cancer, inflammatory bowel disease, and hidradenitis suppurativa.

Treatment

Antibiotics are effective in the acute illness but may have little or no effect on late lymphatic pathology. Standard regimens include sulfisoxazole 1 g 4 times a day for 3 weeks, or tetracycline 500 mg 4 times a day for at least 2 weeks.[33] Other tetracycline derivatives such as minocycline have also been demonstrated to be effective. Buboes should be aspirated, rather than incised and drained, to avoid formation of fistulous tracts. With treatment, prognosis for avoidance of late complications is excellent.

References

1. Schachter J, Osoba AO: Lymphogranuloma venereum. *Br Med Bull* **39**:151, 1983
2. Piot P, Plummer FA, Rey MA, et al: Retrospective seroepidemiology of AIDS virus infection in Nairobi populations. *J Infect Dis* **155**:1108, 1987
3. Cameron DW, Plummer FA, Simonsen JN, et al: Female to male heterosexual transmission of HIV infection, Nairobi (abstract), in *Proceedings of the Third International Conference on AIDS,* Washington, DC, June 1–5, 1987
4. Koteen H: Lymphogranuloma venereum. *Medicine* (Baltimore) **24**:2, 1945
5. Rake G et al: Agent of lymphogranuloma venereum in the yolk sac of the developing chick embryo. *Proc Soc Biol Med* **43**:332, 1940
6. Evans RT, Woodland RM: Detection of chlamydiae by isolation and direct examination. *Br Med Bull* **39**:181, 1983
7. Wang SP: A microimmunofluorescence method. Study of antibody response to TRIC organisms, in *Trachoma and Related Disorders Caused by Chlamydia Agents,* edited by RL Nichols. Amsterdam, Excerpta Medica, 1971, p 273
8. Becker LE: Lymphogranuloma venereum. *Int J Dermatol* **15**:26, 1976
9. Schachter J: Chlamydial infection. *N Engl J Med* **298**:428, 490, 540, 1978
10. Moulder JW: The relationship of the psittacosis group (*Chlamydia*) to bacteria and viruses. *Annu Rev Microbiol* **20**:107, 1966
11. Quinn TC, Taylor HR, Schachter J: Experimental proctitis due to rectal infection with *Chlamydia trachomatis* in nonhuman primates. *J Infect Dis* **154**:833, 1986
12. Tompkins LS: Recombinant DNA and other direct specimen identification techniques. *Clin Lab Med* **5**: 99, 1985
13. Terho P: *Chlamydia trachomatis* and clinical genital infections: A general review. *Infection* **10** (suppl 1):S5, 1982
14. Conizares O: *Modern Diagnosis and Treatment of the Minor Venereal Diseases.* Springfield, IL, Charles C Thomas, 1954
15. Hopsu-Havu VK, Sonck CE: Infiltrative, ulcerative, and fistular lesions of the penis due to lymphogranuloma venereum. *Br J Vener Dis* **49**:193, 1973
16. Thorsteinsson SB et al: Lymphogranuloma venereum. A cause of cervical lymphadenopathy. *JAMA* **235**:1882, 1976
17. Andrada MT et al: Oral lymphogranuloma venereum and cervical lymphadenopathy: Case report. *Milit Med* **139**:99, 1974
18. McLelland BA, Anderson PC: Lymphogranuloma venereum. Outbreak in a university community. *JAMA* **235**:56, 1976
19. Geller SA et al: Rectal biopsy in early lymphogranuloma venereum proctitis. *Am J Gastroenterol* **74**:433, 1980
20. Klotz SA, Drutz DJ, Tam MR, et al: Hemorrhagic proctitis due to lymphogranuloma venereum serogroup L2; diagnosis by fluorescent monoclonal antibody. *N Engl J Med* **308**:1563, 1983
21. Hirschberg SM, Horton CE: Radical perineal resection for far-advanced lymphogranuloma venereum. *Plast Reconstr Surg* **51**:217, 1973
22. Sonck CE: On the occurrence of solar dermatitis in lymphogranuloma inguinale. *Acta Derm Venereol* (*Stockh*) **20**:529, 1939
23. Sonck CE et al: Autoimmune serum factors in active and inactive lymphogranuloma venereum. *Br J Vener Dis* **49**:67, 1973
24. Aghadiuno PU, Jankey N, Barton EN, et al: Kaposi's sarcoma in the acquired immune deficiency syndrome (AIDS), presenting as lymphogranuloma venereum (LGV) in a promiscuous Trinidadian male. *Trop Geo Med* **39**:88, 1987
25. Senitzer D, Gibbons J, Gohara A et al: Infectious antecedent of immunoblastic lymphoma; progressive immunosuppression in a patient with lymphogranuloma venereum. *Am J Med* **8**:163, 1985
26. Smith EB, Custer RP: The histopathology of lymphogranuloma venereum. *J Urol* **63**:546, 1950
27. Robbins SL (ed): *Pathology.* Philadelphia, Saunders, 1967, p 366
28. de la Monte SM, Hutchins GM: Follicular proctocolitis and neuromatous hyperplasia with lymphogranuloma venereum. *Hum Pathol* **16**:1025, 1985
29. Treharne JD, Forsey T, Thomas BJ: Chlamydial serology. *Br Med Bull* **39**:194, 1983
30. Schachter J et al: Lymphogranuloma venereum. I. Comparison of the Frei test, complement-fixation test and isolation of the agent. *J Infect Dis* **120**:372, 1969
31. Schachter J, Dawson C: Lymphogranuloma venereum. *JAMA* **236**:915, 1976
32. Darougar S: The humoral immune response to chlamydial infection in humans. *Rev Infect Dis* **7**:726, 1985
33. Centers for Disease Control: 1985 STD treatment guidelines. *MMWR* **34**(4s):1, 1985

CHAPTER 222

Richard B. Rothenberg

Granuloma Inguinale

Granuloma inguinale is an indolent, progressive, ulcerative, and granulomatous skin disease caused by *Calymmatobacterium granulomatis*. It is probably spread by both homosexual and heterosexual venereal contact and by nonvenereal means as well.[1] Untreated, it exhibits no tendency to go into spontaneous remission and in later stages may be severely debilitating.

History

The first description is credited to McLeod in 1882, who termed the illness *serpiginous ulcer*.[2] Many other names have been suggested, but aside from granuloma inguinale, only the term *donovanosis* persists. Donovan, in 1905, first described the bipolar-staining, intracellular inclusions in macrophages from lesion exudate (termed *Donovan bodies*). These organisms were grown in embryonated eggs in 1943[3]; requirements for growth on artificial media were established in 1959.[4]

Epidemiology

Sporadic cases of granuloma inguinale occur worldwide, but endemic foci are usually seen only in tropical and subtropical environments, such as New Guinea, central Australia, the Caribbean, and parts of India.[5] Recently, a focus was recognized in South Africa, after an apparent eclipse of 50 years.[6] Since 1970, fewer than 100 cases per year have been reported in the United States; in 1989, there were only 7. Certain marked racial and ethnic predispositions have been noted—higher incidence in blacks than in whites in the United States; in natives than in Europeans in Papua, New Guinea; in Hindus than in Moslems in India—but there is no evidence for specific racial susceptibility. Rather, socioeconomic status and living conditions may be a major risk factor.

The venereal nature of transmission has been debated for many years and is supported by the genital site of early lesions, the prominence of perirectal disease in male homosexuals, and the predominant occurrence of infection in the sexually active age group.[7] The possibility of nonvenereal transmission is suggested by the occurrence of disease in sexually inactive children, the infrequency of infection in partners repeatedly exposed to open lesions, and the infrequency of infection in sexually active people (e.g., prostitutes) in some endemic areas.[1,8] It seems clear, however, that granuloma inguinale is one of a class of diseases causing genital ulceration that may predispose persons to the transmission of HIV.[9]

Etiology and Pathogenesis

The causative agent (formerly termed *Donovania granulomatis*) is a gram-negative rod with some antigenic properties in common with the *Klebsiella* group. It has been demonstrated in fecal flora,[10] and there is evidence by electron microscopy that it may share bacteriophage with Enterobacteriaceae.[11,12] Studies by light microscopy of plastic-embedded material with polychromatic staining demonstrate bacteria within vacuoles of cells and thereby fail to corroborate the presence of bacteriophage-like entities.[13] These data support the hypothesis that disease transmission may occur through fecal contamination in environments with lower levels of hygiene and may also explain the occurrence of disease in males practicing rectal intercourse.

Antibody against the organism may be detected by complement-fixation test, though the test has little diagnostic value. Circulating antibody, which does not affect the relentless course of untreated disease, has raised the possibility that a defect in cell-mediated immunity may predispose the patient to clinical illness, as is the case in the other diseases caused by intracellular organisms (e.g., leprosy and tuberculosis.)[14]

Clinical Manifestations

The primary lesion may be a buttonlike papule, a subcutaneous nodule, or an ulcer. The incubation period is poorly defined and may range from 2 weeks to 3 months. Experimental human inoculation has produced lesions after latency of 21 days.[7] Papules or nodules are quickly denuded and ulcerate within several days. The subcutaneous nodule, if large enough, may be mistaken for a lymph node, giving rise to the term *pseudobubo*. True adenopathy is rare. In men, the penis, scrotum, and glans are the most common sites of primary lesions; in females, the labia minora, mons veneris, and fourchette. Lesions of the cervix may occur in as many as 10 percent of infected women, and the disease may involve the uterus and adnexa as well.[15] Typically, the disease spreads, either by direct extension or autoinoculation, to the inguinal and perineal skin.

Four major clinical varieties are described[16]: the *nodular* variety is characterized by soft, red nodules which eventually ulcerate and present a bright-red granulating surface (Fig. 222-1); the *ulcerovegetative* variety (most common) (Fig. 222-2) develops from the nodular type and consists of large, spreading, exuberant ulcers; the *hypertropic* form (relatively rare) exhibits a proliferative reaction and formation of large vegetating masses; and the *cicatricial* type produces spreading scar tissue formation which is a direct consequence of disease spread per se, rather than of healing. Superinfection with fusospirochetal organisms may give rise to necrotic lesions with massive tissue destruction, similar to the situation in so-called phagedenic chancroid. The disease may rarely progress to destroy genital and inguinal tissue.[17] Elephantiasis of the penis, scrotum, or vulva may follow involvement with granuloma inguinale.

Extragenital lesions are reported in 6 percent of cases, with occasional systemic involvement, notably in the gastrointestinal tract and bone,[18] including the bony orbit and orbital skin.[19]

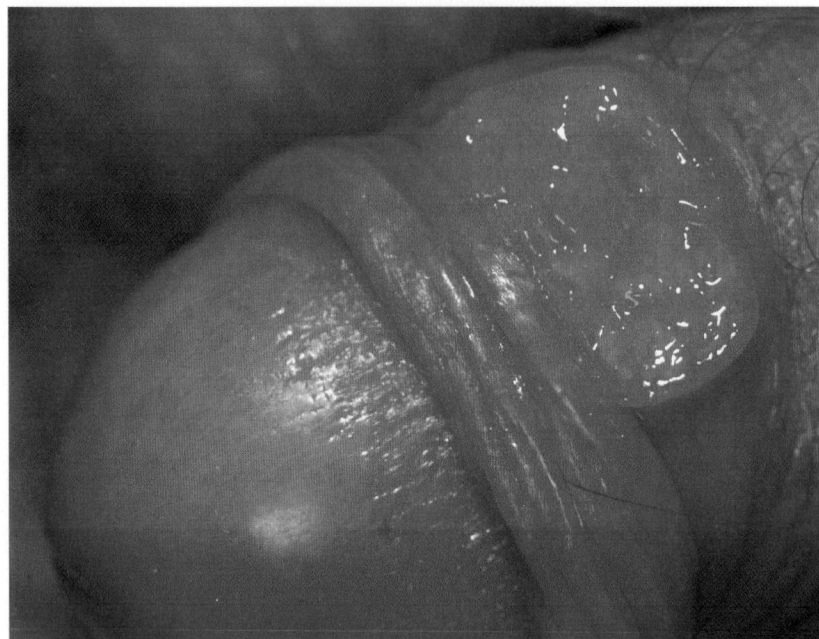

FIGURE 222-1 Granuloma inguinale: nodular variety evolving into large exuberant ulcer. *(Courtesy of A. Eichmann, M.D.)*

Chronic ulcerating oral mucosa lesions may occur with or without associated genital lesions[20,21] and may resemble actinomycosis.[22] Rarely, granuloma inguinale may affect cervical lymph nodes and resemble tuberculous lymphadenitis.[23] A single case report documented a primary extragenital occurrence of granuloma inguinale in the axilla.[24] The disease shows no tendency toward spontaneous healing, though lesions may be stable for long periods of time. There is believed to be an increased incidence of squamous cell carcinoma of the genital skin in granuloma inguinale.[25]

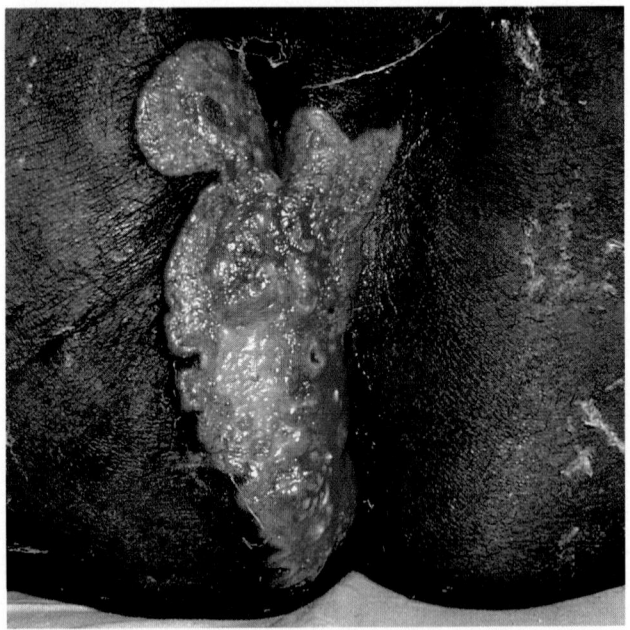

FIGURE 222-2 Granuloma inguinale: large ulcerovegetative type.

Pathology

Histologically, the skin exhibits a massive cellular reaction, predominantly polymorphonuclear, with occasional plasma cells and, rarely, lymphocytes.[5] The marginal epithelium demonstrates acanthosis, elongation of rete pegs, and pseudoepitheliomatous hyperplasia.[13] These latter changes are highly suggestive of early malignancy and squamous cell carcinoma. Hypertropic and cicatricial forms demonstrate the appropriate increase in fibrous tissue. Typically, large mononuclear cells containing numerous cytoplasmic inclusions (the Donovan bodies) are scattered throughout the lesions. These are considered to be diagnostic of granuloma inguinale and are often best demonstrated with special stains, such as Giemsa's stain, Delafield's hematoxylin, Dieterle's silver stain, and the Warthin-Starry stain.[5]

Diagnosis

The diagnosis of granuloma inguinale is usually made by history, clinical appearance, and a crush or touch preparation stained with Wright's or Giemsa's stain from a punch biopsy specimen. Superficial curettings are usually inadequate because of bacterial contamination. Donovan bodies are seen as deeply staining, bipolar, safety pin-shaped rods in the cytoplasm of macrophages (Fig. 222-3). Diagnosis may require multiple specimens since clinical varieties differ in the quantity of organisms present. Rapid-staining techniques [such as the RapiDiff stain (Clinical Science Diagnostics Ltd.)] are now readily available and suitable for use under a variety of field conditions.[26] Serologic tests, such as the use of complement fixation, have evoked some research interest, but have little practical application.

In its typical form, granuloma inguinale is easily differentiated from other ulcerative and granulomatous skin diseases, but atypical

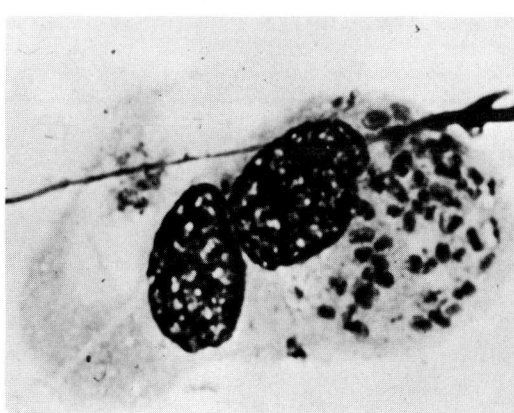

FIGURE 222-3 Granuloma inguinale: tissue smear showing Donovan bodies, which are gram-negative and readily stained with Giemsa's stain.

forms may be difficult to distinguish from syphilis, chancroid, lymphogranuloma venereum, tuberculosis of skin, cutaneous amebiasis, and filariasis. Squamous cell carcinoma with metastases may be closely mimicked by granuloma inguinale and its associated osteolytic bone lesions.

Treatment

Numerous drugs have been found useful in treating granuloma inguinale, including streptomycin, chloramphenicol, tetracycline, ampicillin, and gentamicin. Case series, usually assembled over a decade or more, offer a variety of regimens[27-29]; controlled trials are not available. Tetracycline, 500 mg 4 times a day for 3 to 4 weeks, appeared to be a good initial choice, but resistance to this therapy, alone or in combination with sulfisoxazole, was observed in U.S. military personnel in Vietnam. Ampicillin was successful in all but 2 of 31 cases of granuloma inguinale acquired in Vietnam, with complete healing of local lesions which occurred primarily on the penis or in the groin. In the same series, lincomycin was successfully used in penicillin-allergic individuals.[30] A preliminary report suggests that the 4-fluoroquinolone antibiotics (norfloxacin) may be effective.[31] Response may be monitored by clinical appearance and serial biopsy specimens examined for persistent presence of Donovan bodies. In early cases, prognosis for complete healing is good. In late cases, irreparable tissue destruction may have supervened, and radical surgery may be required.[32]

References

1. Goldberg J: Studies on granuloma inguinale. VII. Some considerations of the disease. *Br J Vener Dis* **40**:140, 1964
2. McLeod K: Précis of operations performed in the wards of the first surgeon, Medical College Hospital, during the year 1881. *Indian Med Gazette* **11**:113, 1882
3. Anderson K, DeMonbreun WA, Goodpasture EW: An etiologic consideration of *Donovania granulomatis* cultivated from granuloma inguinale (three cases) in embryonic yolk. *J Exp Med* **81**:25, 1943
4. Goldberg J: Studies on granuloma inguinale: IV. Growth requirements of *Donovania granulomatis* and its relationship to the natural habitat of the organism. *Br J Vener Dis* **35**:266, 1959
5. Sehgal VN, Shyam Prasad AL: Donovanosis: Current concepts. *Int J Dermatol* **25**:8, 1986
6. Freinkel AL: The enigma of granuloma inguinale in South Africa. *S Afr Med J* **77**:301, 1990
7. Rajam RV, Rangiah PN: Donovanosis (granuloma inguinale, granuloma venereum). WHO Monogr Ser, no. 24, 1954
8. Kuberski T: Granuloma inguinale (donovanosis). *Sex Transm Dis* **7**:29, 1980
9. Piot P, Laga M: Genital ulcers, other sexually transmitted diseases, and the sexual transmission of HIV. *Br Med J* **298**:623, 1989
10. Goldberg J: Studies on granuloma inguinale. V. Isolation of bacterium resembling *Donovania granulomatis* from the faeces of a patient with granuloma inguinale. *Br J Vener Dis* **38**:99, 1959
11. Kuberski T et al: Ultrastructure of *Calymmatobacterium granulomatis* in lesions of granuloma inguinale. *J Infect Dis* **142**:744, 1980
12. Davis CM: Granuloma inguinale: A clinical, histological, and ultrastructural study. *JAMA* **211**:632, 1970
13. Dodson RF et al: Donovanosis: A morphologic study. *J Invest Dermatol* **62**:611, 1974
14. Maddock I et al: Donovanosis in Papua New Guinea. *Br J Vener Dis* **52**:190, 1976.
15. Sengupta SK, Das N: Donovanosis affecting cervix, uterus and adnexae. *Am J Trop Med Hyg* **33**:632, 1984
16. D'Aunoy R, Von Haam E: Granuloma inguinale. *Am J Trop Med Hyg* **17**:747, 1967
17. Fritz GS et al: Mutilating granuloma inguinale. *Arch Dermatol* **111**:1464, 1975
18. Kirkpatrick DJ: Donovanosis (granuloma inguinale): A rare cause of osteolytic bone lesions. *Clin Radiol* **21**:101, 1970
19. Endicott JN et al: Granuloma inguinale of the orbit with bony involvement. *Arch Otolaryngol* **96**:457, 1972
20. Rao M et al: Oral lesions of granuloma inguinale. *J Oral Surg* **34**:1112, 1976
21. Garg BR et al: Donovanosis (granuloma inguinale) of the oral cavity. *Br J Vener Dis* **51**:136, 1975
22. Coovadia YM, Steinberg JL, Kharsany A: Granuloma inguinale (donovanosis) of the oral cavity: A case report. *S Afr Med J* **68**:815, 1985
23. Freinkel AL: Granuloma inguinale of cervical lymph nodes simulating tuberculous lymphadenitis: Two case reports and review of published reports. *Genitourin Med* **64**:339, 1988
24. Spagnolo DV, Coburn PR, Cream JJ, et al: Extragenital granuloma inguinale (donovanosis) diagnosed in the United Kingdom: A clinical, histological, and electron microscopical study. *J Clin Pathol* **37**:945, 1984
25. Stewart DB: Ulcerative and hypertrophic lesions of the vulva. *Proc R Soc Med* **61**:363, 1968
26. O'Farrell N, Hoosen AA, Coetzee K, et al: A rapid stain for the diagnosis of granuloma inguinale. *Genitourin Med* **66**:200, 1990
27. Rosen T, Tschen JA, Ramsdell W, et al: Granuloma inguinale. *J Am Acad Dermatol* **11**:433, 1984
28. Wysoki RS, Majmudar B, Willis D: Granuloma inguinale (donovanosis) in women. *J Reprod Med* **33**:709, 1988
29. Latif AS, Mason PR, Paraiwa E: The treatment of donovanosis (granuloma inguinale). *Sex Transm Dis* **15**:27, 1988
30. Breschi LC et al: Granuloma inguinale in Vietnam: Successful therapy with ampicillin and lincomycin. *J Am Vener Dis Assoc* **11**:118, 1975
31. Ramanan C, Sarma PSA, Ghorpade A, et al: Treatment of donovanosis with norfloxacin. *Int J Dermatol* **29**:298, 1990
32. Parkash S, Radhakrishna K: Problematic ulcerative lesions in sexually transmitted diseases: Surgical management. *Sex Transm Dis* **13**:127, 1986

CHAPTER 223

David S. Feingold and Monica Peacocke

Gonorrhea

Gonorrhea is a bacterial infection caused by *Neisseria gonorrhoeae,* a gram-negative diplococcus whose only natural reservoir is humans. The infection is almost always contracted during sexual activity.

The usual presentation in males is acute urethritis and, in females, cervicitis, which may be asymptomatic. Other parts of the genitourinary apparatus, and as well as the rectum, pharynx, and eye may be infected. Occasionally bacteremia occurs, which is regularly associated with arthralgia and skin lesions; metastatic infection in joints or other foci may ensue. Although good treatment is available, the disease remains an important public health problem causing a large percentage of female sterility and considerable morbidity in both sexes.

Historical Aspects

The name *gonorrhea* is attributed to Galen who thought the urethritis represented abnormal flow of semen, hence the combination of *gonos,* "seed" and *rhoea,* "flow." The slang name for gonorrhea, *clap,* likely derives from a French word for brothel, *clapoir.*

Early confusion among the venereal diseases was augmented by the unfortunate experiment of John Hunter in 1767. He inoculated himself with a presumed gonococcal urethral exudate, only to develop syphilis. With isolation of the causative organism of gonorrhea by Neisser in 1879, positive identification of the disease became possible.

Treatment for gonorrhea has progressed from sandalwood oil to urethral irrigations with potassium permanganate to sulfonamides in the 1930s. Resistance to sulfonamides developed rapidly, but, fortunately, in the 1940s the exquisite sensitivity of gonococcal strains to penicillin was discovered. The emerging problem of penicillin resistance of the organism will be discussed later in this chapter.

Epidemiology

The incidence of gonorrhea in the United States increased dramatically in the 1960s and early 1970s to over 1 million reported cases annually. It is estimated that less than one-third of the new cases are reported. In the 1980s there was a slow decline in reported cases to about 800,000 per year. Why was there an explosive increase in gonorrhea, a disease for which effective therapy is available, followed by a gradual decline? An analysis of this two-phase trend ascribes the changes to several factors.[1] The epidemic was intensified first by behavioral factors, including increased sexual activity, changes in birth control methods, high population mobility, and an increase in repeated infections, and second by increased reporting when the federal gonorrhea screening effort was introduced in 1972. The subsequent decrease in incidence in the United States resulted from the herculean efforts of the U.S. Public Health Ser-

vice through the national control program to detect and treat asymptomatic gonococcal infections.

The disease is spread almost exclusively by sexual activity, although newborns may be infected by exposure during parturition. While all age groups are susceptible, infection is more prevalent in the 15- to 35-year-old age group. The disease is concentrated in high-density population centers, with a core group of active transmitters.[2] However, the mobility of individuals results in the occurrence of gonorrhea everywhere.

A signal event which has affected the epidemiology of gonorrhea is the dramatic increase in resistance of *N. gonorrhoeae* to antibiotics. Since the availability of sulfonamides and penicillin in the 1940s, antimicrobial resistance in *N. gonorrhoeae* has been evolving. The appearance of penicillinase-producing strains of *N. gonorrhoeae* in the United States in 1975 accelerated the trend toward greater antibiotic resistance. Penicillinase (beta-lactamase) synthesis in these organisms depends on the presence of plasmids, extrachromosomal packets of DNA, which can be transferred among organisms. At least five beta-lactamase plasmids of *N. gonorrhoeae* have been reported. Chromosomal resistance to penicillin and tetracycline is also occasionally at levels sufficient to result in treatment failure.[3] The explosive epidemic of antibiotic-resistant cases of gonorrhea in the late 1980s is graphically shown in Fig. 223-1. For all practical purposes in most areas penicillin is no longer the treatment of choice for gonorrhea.

Etiologic Agent and Pathogenesis

N. gonorrhoeae is a gram-negative diplococcus with distinctive morphology; the cocci are flattened and the long axes of the bean-shaped organisms are parallel. Gonococci tolerate oxygen but usually require 2 to 10 percent of CO_2 in the growth atmosphere. The organisms have narrow temperature (35 to 37°C) and pH (7.2 to 7.6) optima for growth. Although fragile, they have relatively simple growth requirements. Defined media are now available on which the organisms will grow readily. Different strains have somewhat different growth requirements. Careful study of these requirements has led to a system of typing gonococcal isolates called *auxotyping.*[4] Auxotyping was an important advance, since the ability to tell one *N. gonorrhoeae* isolate from another made epidemiologic studies feasible. Several other efforts to type gonococci are in the developmental stage. These include sensitivity to bacteriocins, the presence of specific lipopolysaccharide antigens, the presence of specific pili or outer membrane proteins, and the use of monoclonal antibodies.[5]

Kellogg and coworkers recognized four colony types of *N. gonorrhoeae.*[6] Only types 1 and 2 were pathogenic for humans. These types were also found to possess surface hairlike structures termed *pili.* The nature of pili as virulence factors has not been clarified; pili may foster adherence of gonococci to mucosal surfaces or resistance to phagocytosis. Other virulence factors are being identified. These may include capsular production in vivo,

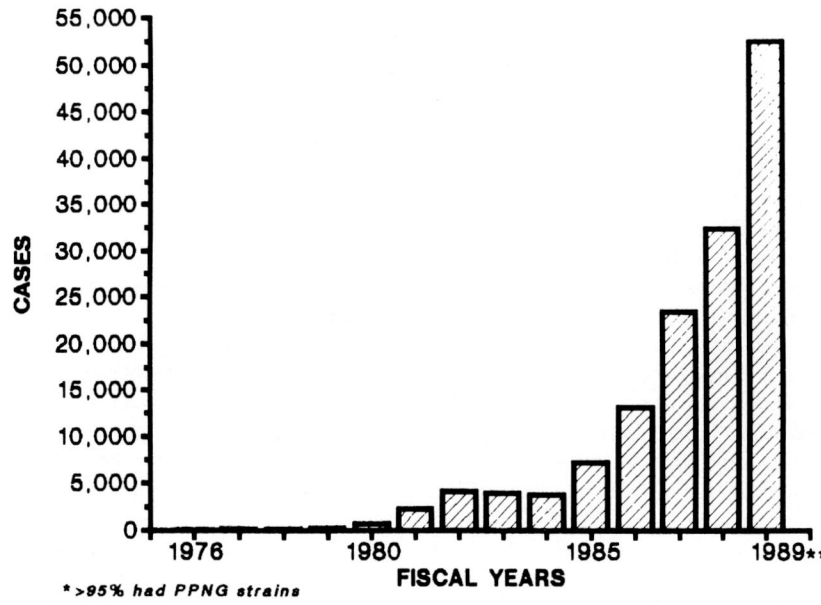

FIGURE 223-1 Reported antibiotic-resistant cases of gonorrhea in the United States, fiscal years 1976–1989. (*From Toomey KE: Sex Transm Dis 17:218, 1990, with permission.*)

resistance to the immune bactericidal action of serum, and the ability of gonococci to survive in the presence of various competing commensal organisms. Griffiss and Artenstein[7] point out that all *Neisseria* are organisms adapted to moist mucous membranes. Of them, the meningococcus and the gonococcus are the ones capable of escaping from host restraints, proliferating rapidly, and even invading the bloodstream. The reason why certain organisms occupy particular ecological niches and the factors conferring virulence are only beginning to be understood.

Clinical Manifestations

Signs, symptoms, complications, and the natural history of gonorrhea differ dramatically between males and females. However, careful studies have exposed the myth that males with gonorrhea are symptomatic and females asymptomatic.

Males

After a single exposure to an infected contact, about 25 percent of males will develop gonorrhea. It has been estimated that 85 percent of men with gonococcal urethritis develop an acute process with discomfort, dysuria, and purulent discharge usually ensuing from 2 to 10 days after exposure. Figure 223-2 shows a typical purulent discharge. Fifteen percent of urethritis in the male is minimally symptomatic or asymptomatic. Since these patients may not receive treatment, they tend to accumulate in the population. The resultant point prevalence of minimally symptomatic or asymptomatic male gonorrhea may be as high as 40 percent.[8] Clearly these men are capable of spreading disease. Untreated symptomatic urethritis subsides over several days to weeks but occasionally local complications such as epididymitis, seminal vesiculitis, and prostatitis occur. Anorectal[9] and pharyngeal[10] gonococcal colonizations are not common. The incidence of positive cultures correlates with the practices of passive rectal intercourse and fellatio, respectively. Since symptoms of proctitis and pharyngitis correlate poorly with

positive cultures, colonization of these areas rather than overt infection is likely to be what occurs.

Females

When an uninfected woman is exposed to an infected man, gonorrhea ensues over half the time. Once infected, the specific symptoms and signs of acute salpingitis may occur (20 to 40 percent) or the less specific symptoms of dysuria, increased discharge, or abnormal bleeding (20 to 30 percent) may be seen within a few days to a few weeks. Thirty to sixty percent of infected women will be minimally affected or asymptomatic yet remain long-term carriers capable of transferring the infection.[11,12] As described for men,

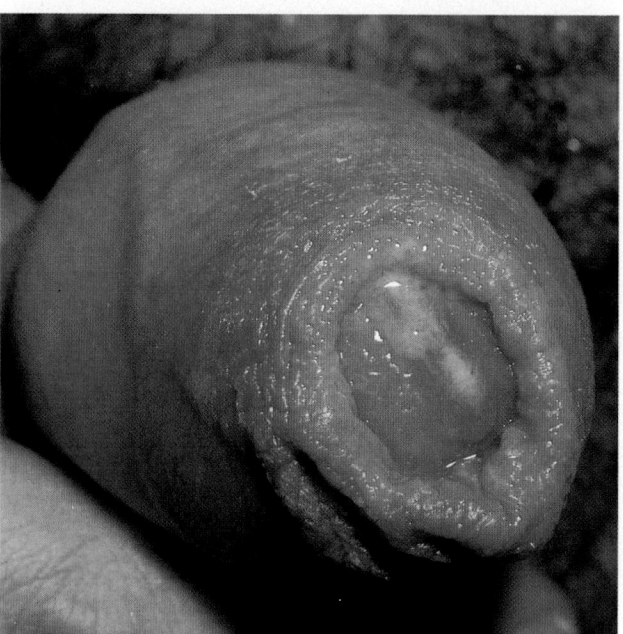

FIGURE 223-2 Purulent urethral discharge.

these cases will accumulate since symptomatic gonorrhea is treated preferentially. Since none of the symptoms or signs is diagnostic of gonorrhea, cultures of endocervix, urethra, rectum, and pharynx should be carried out if the disease is suspected or the patient is reported as a contact of gonorrhea.

Pelvic inflammatory disease (PID) is the most important complication of gonococcal infection. PID is the result of ascending infection from the endocervix, causing endometritis and/or salpingitis and/or pelvic peritonitis. Clinical findings can vary from crampy abdominal pain with minimal tenderness in mild cases to fever, severe abdominal pain, and exquisite tenderness with adnexal masses in florid cases. Prompt diagnosis and aggressive treatment are mandatory since infertility, ectopic pregnancy, and chronic pelvic pain are frequent complications. Several organisms other than *N. gonorrhoeae* may cause PID. The etiologic diagnosis, which will be discussed subsequently, may be difficult. Tragically, the role of "silent" or asymptomatic PID in causing adverse reproductive sequelae is becoming increasingly appreciated.

Disseminated Gonococcal Infection (DGI)

Spread of *N. gonorrhoeae* to the bloodstream has been estimated to occur in 1 to 3 percent of patients with gonorrhea,[13] with the majority of cases in females. Although endocarditis and meningitis have been reported, they are rare complications. Arthritis and skin lesions, on the other hand, are regularly associated with DGI. The syndrome is so characteristic that a presumptive diagnosis can usually be made on clinical grounds alone; the syndrome has been labeled the arthritis-dermatitis syndrome. The onset of gonococcal bacteremia usually occurs with menstruation or pregnancy in females. In males, DGI is most often seen in association with asymptomatic infection. Fever, chills, polyarthralgias, arthritis, and tenosynovitis are common. In the early stages of the disease, skin manifestations occur that are quite characteristic (Fig. 223-3). The

skin lesions typically are few in number (often less than a dozen) and concentrated on the extremities, usually acral and often around the joints. The lesions may be petechial or papular; however, they usually evolve into vesicles or pustules on an erythematous base which may become hemorrhagic. Sometimes they present as hemorrhagic bullae. Prompt diagnosis and therapy are mandatory since delay may result in frank pyogenic arthritis with potential for joint destruction.

It has been recognized that organisms causing DGI often differ from those causing urethritis. Most strains of gonococci are susceptible to the complement-mediated bactericidal action of normal serum; the strains causing DGI are resistant.[13] This important observation may explain why some gonococci are capable of causing bacteremia while others are restricted to mucous membranes. In support of the necessity for serum resistance in strains causing DGI are the reports that patients deficient in the late complement components, which are required for serum killing, are peculiarly susceptible to recurrent neisserial sepsis.[14]

The pathogenesis of the arthritis-dermatitis syndrome is unclear. Bacteremia regularly occurs early in the course of DGI, but it has been suggested that most signs and symptoms of DGI are manifestations of immune-complex formation. (See also Chap. 188.)

Miscellaneous Clinical Manifestations

In rare cases, an ulcer or abscess may appear on the raphe of the penis. Gonococcal perihepatitis is a complication of gonococcal peritonitis with hepatic capsular fibrosis and adhesions (Fitz-Hugh–Curtis syndrome).[15] Adhesions such as those between the hepatic capsule and the anterior abdominal wall can cause discomfort which may be persistent and difficult to diagnose.

Gonococcal ophthalmia neonatorum is neonatal purulent conjunctivitis contracted by the newborn in passage through an infected birth canal. Reappearance of this in greater numbers in the 1970s was probably a reflection of the higher incidence of gonorrhea combined with a more casual enforcement or execution of silver nitrate prophylaxis of newborns.[16]

Cornified squamous epithelium is quite resistant to infection with *N. gonorrhoeae*, hence vulvovaginitis is infrequent in adult women. However, in children, the vagina is lined with columnar epithelium; acute vulvovaginitis is the usual manifestation of genital gonococcal infection in the prepubescent female.

Pathology

The picture of active gonococcal infection is usually that of an acute or subacute inflammatory response with polymorphonuclear leukocytes predominating. The histopathology of the vesiculopustular lesions of DGI consists of infiltrates of neutrophils admixed with some mononuclear cells and red blood cells. Fibrinoid necrosis of vessel walls may be seen. The bullae are subepidermal in location.[17] Bacteria are rarely seen in or grown from the skin lesions.

Diagnosis

Definitive diagnosis of gonorrhea depends upon identification of the organisms by Gram stain and/or culture. A positive Gram stain

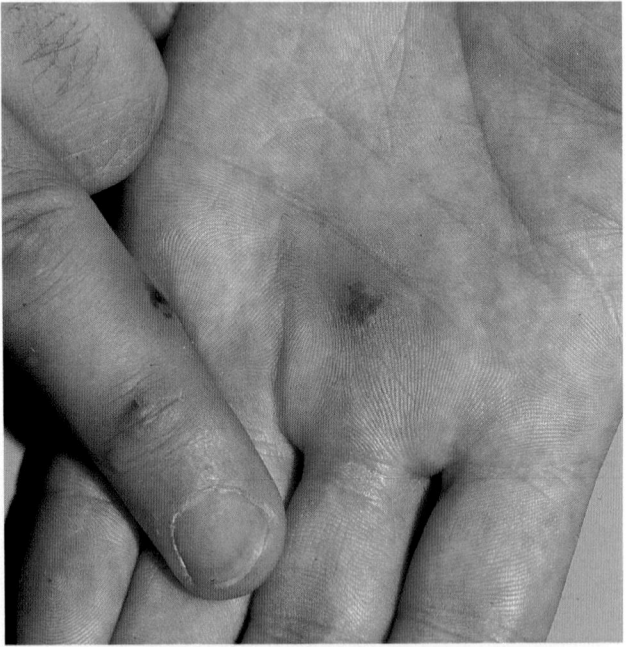

FIGURE 223-3 Disseminated gonococcal infection. Lesions on the fingers and palm consisting of pustules and hemorrhagic, necrotic pustules, which are slightly tender.

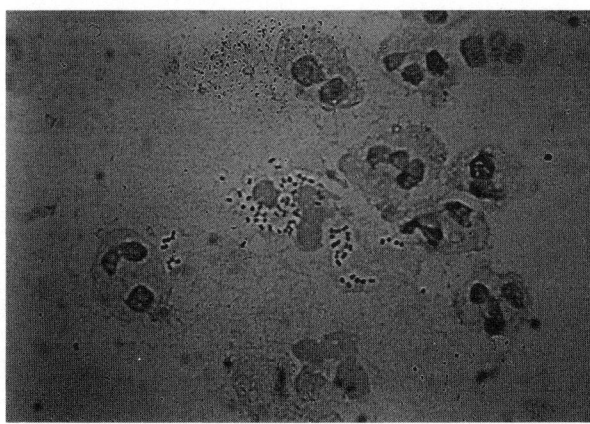

FIGURE 223-4 Diagnostic Gram-stained smear of urethral exudate of man with gonococcal urethritis.

consists of characteristic gram-negative diplococci in the cytoplasm of neutrophils (Fig. 223-4). A positive Gram stain from the male urethra is considered diagnostic. Gram stain of endocervical discharge is not usually done since even a positive smear is not considered diagnostic; culture confirmation is required. In women, endocervical cultures give a higher yield of positives than vaginal cultures. In males without exudate, swabs for culture should be inserted several centimeters into the urethra. In women with gonorrhea, not only endocervical cultures, but rectal, urethral, and pharyngeal cultures should be obtained. In DGI, blood, skin lesions, and joint effusions should be cultured. Skin lesions are regularly negative; joint fluid is usually negative until acute purulent arthritis occurs. Blood cultures are positive only early in the disease. Thus, the diagnosis of DGI frequently must be made on clinical grounds only. This rarely presents a problem since the clinical picture, especially the skin lesions and the tenosynovitis, is quite characteristic.

When culturing an area in which a mixed bacterial flora is unusual, e.g., synovial fluid or male urethra, chocolate agar may be used for isolation. When culturing an area which has an exuberant flora such as the throat, rectum, or endocervix, one should use selective media containing antimicrobials which inhibit organisms other than *Neisseria*. Modified Thayer-Martin is the medium usually employed. Transgrow is a similar medium but it also contains CO_2 and is a good transport medium for gonococci.

In addition to *N. gonorrhoeae,* several other organisms cause PID, including *Chlamydia trachomatis,* endogenous anaerobic and aerobic bacteria, and, probably, genital mycoplasmas. It is clearly advantageous for proper therapy to know the causative organism. Endocervical cultures are the only practical way to distinguish between gonococcal and nongonococcal PID; patients in whom gonococci are grown from the cervix are assumed to have gonococcal PID.[18] Several serologic tests for gonorrhea are in the developmental stage. As yet, none shows the requisite sensitivity or specificity. Possibly the greatest value of these tests, if perfected, will be in confirming the etiology of PID and establishing the diagnosis of DGI. No one advocates that they replace culture techniques for the diagnosis of routine gonorrhea, but a possible role for serologic tests for screening or case finding has not been ruled out.[19]

Differential Diagnosis

The differential diagnosis of genitourinary gonococcal disease in the female includes the following:

1. *Trichomonas vaginalis* infection. This usually presents as a profuse, frothy, foul, vaginal exudate, at times with urethritis. A positive saline preparation for the protozoa is diagnostic.
2. *Candida albicans* infection. Often this presents as a pruritic infection with creamy or curdy exudate, and diagnosis depends on identification of the organism by smear and/or culture.
3. *Gardnerella vaginalis* or bacterial vaginosis. There is still dispute about the role of various organisms in bacterial vaginosis. However, the syndrome is well defined, with malodorous, gray, acidic discharge that shows "clue" cells on smear and yields a "fishy" amine odor on alkalinization with potassium hydroxide. All patients with vaginal discharge should be cultured for gonococci. Even though inflammatory vaginitis is rarely seen with gonorrhea alone, mixed infections do occur rather commonly.

In men, urethritis can also be caused by multiple organisms. *T. vaginalis* and *C. albicans* can infect the male and be asymptomatic or cause urethritis or balanitis. Some urethritis has been attributed to *Herpesvirus hominis.* However, even more common than gonorrhea as a cause of urethritis in many populations is so-called nongonococcal or nonspecific or postgonococcal urethritis.

Nongonococcal urethritis (NGU) may be the most common sexually transmitted disease in humans in most industrialized countries, although reporting is not required in the United States. It is characterized by dysuria, often by urethral discharge or urinary frequency, and by the absence of *N. gonorrhoeae.* In contrast to classic gonococcal urethritis, NGU usually has a longer incubation period, a less acute onset, and scanty urethral discharge; at times, no discharge is evident, only urethral discomfort or tenderness. Occasionally, co-infection with *N. gonorrhoeae* occurs and urethritis remains following effective antibiotic therapy for gonorrhea; this has been labeled *postgonococcal urethritis.*

Until the mid-1970s, causative agents of NGU were not identified; however, it was clear that symptoms usually yielded to therapy with tetracyclines. Now there is good evidence that at least two organisms are responsible for NGU. *Chlamydia trachomatis* has been demonstrated convincingly to cause most of the cases of NGU. *Ureaplasma urealyticum* and possibly a few other organisms may be responsible for some of the remaining cases of NGU.

Because NGU has been the subject of such intensive study recently and is so common, it is also discussed separately in the following chapter (Chap. 224).

Treatment and Control

Ideal therapy for gonococcal urethritis would have the following attributes in addition to curing urethritis. It should be given as a single dose; it should abort co-incubating syphilis; it should cure coexisting chlamydial infections. No single drug regimen achieves these ideals. The staff and consultants of the Centers for Disease Control offered their most recent guidelines for treatment of gonorrhea in 1989.[20]

At the time of the last edition of this text three antibiotic regimens were recommended: (1) Aqueous penicillin IM plus probenecid; (2) tetracycline four times daily for 7 days; (3) amoxicillin or ampicillin plus probenecid in a single oral dose. Five years later none of these are considered good choices. Choices (1) and (3) were obviated by the high incidence of penicillinase-producing strains of *N. gonorrhoeae.* Choice (2) fails too frequently because of the increasing incidence of chromosomal-mediated tetracycline resistance.

In 1989 no single recommendation was made for treating gonorrhea in all patients, at all sites of infection, and in all geographic locations. The standard therapy recommended in uncomplicated infections of the urethra, cervix, rectum, or pharynx in nonpregnant adults is a single IM dose of 250 mg of ceftriaxone plus doxycycline 100 mg orally twice daily for 7 days (for coincubating chlamydial infection).

Alternatives to the standard therapy include: (1) Patients unable to tolerate ceftriaxone should be given spectinomycin (2 g IM in one dose); (2) patients with pharyngeal infection who can't tolerate ceftriaxone should receive nine tablets of trimethoprim-sulfamethoxazole (720 mg/3600 mg) in one daily dose for 5 days; (3) other options are ciprofloxacin (500 mg orally in one dose), norfloxacin (800 mg orally in one dose), cefuroxime axetil (1 g orally in one dose with 1 g probenecid), ceftizoxime (500 mg IM in one dose), and cefotaxime (1 g in one dose). To all these treatments doxycycline 100 mg twice daily for 7 days should be added.

Posttreatment test-of-cure is no longer considered mandatory with ceftriaxone or spectinomycin regimens. It is still recommended for the other regimens which have been less well studied.

Control of the gonorrhea epidemic probably depends more on other factors than the details of therapy of acute disease. It is essential to educate the public about venereal disease, including signs and symptoms, methods of prevention, and resources available. Medical personnel must also be made aware of the most effective case-finding techniques, including screening of at-risk populations and aggressive search for contacts of patients with gonorrhea. More controlled sexual activity in the wake of the AIDS epidemic, including widespread use of condoms, will probably help ameliorate the epidemic of gonorrhea.

References

1. Schnell D et al: A time series analysis of gonorrhea surveillance data. *Stat Med* **8**:343, 1989
2. Rothenberg RB, Potterat JJ: Temporal and social aspects of gonorrhea transmission: The force infectivity. *Sex Transm Dis* **15**:88, 1988
3. Johnson SR, Morse SA: Antibiotic resistance in *Neisseria gonorrhoeae*: Genetic mechanisms of resistance. *Sex Transm Dis* **15**:217, 1988
4. Carifo K, Catlin BW: *Neisseria gonorrhoeae* auxotyping: Differentiation of clinical isolates based on growth responses on chemically defined media. *Appl Microbiol* **26**:223, 1973
5. Tam MR et al: Serological classification of *Neisseria gonorrhoeae* with monoclonal antibodies. *Infect Immun* **36**:1042, 1982
6. Kellogg DS et al: *Neisseria gonorrhoeae*. II. Colonial variation and pathogenicity during 35 months in vitro. *J Bacteriol* **96**:596, 1968
7. Griffiss JM, Artenstein MS: The ecology of the genus *Neisseria*. *Mt Sinai J (NY)* **43**:746, 1976
8. Handsfield HH et al: Asymptomatic gonorrhea in men—diagnosis, natural course, prevalence and significance. *N Engl J Med* **290**:117, 1974
9. Klein EJ et al: Anorectal gonococcal infection. *Ann Intern Med* **86**:340, 1977
10. Wiesner PJ et al: Clinical spectrum of pharyngeal gonococcal infection. *N Engl J Med* **288**:181, 1973
11. McCormack WM et al: Clinical spectrum of gonococcal infection in women. *Lancet* **1**:1182, 1977
12. Wiesner PJ, Thompson SE III: Gonococcal diseases. *Disease-a-Month* **XXVI**:2, 1980
13. Schoolnik GK et al: Gonococci causing disseminated gonococcal infection are resistant to the bactericidal action of normal human sera. *J Clin Invest* **58**:1163, 1976
14. Petersen BH et al: Human deficiency of the eighth component of complement. *J Clin Invest* **57**:283, 1976
15. Reichert JA, Valle RF: Fitz-Hugh–Curtis syndrome. *JAMA* **236**:266, 1976
16. Snowe RJ, Wilfert CM: Epidemic reappearance of gonococcal ophthalmia neonatorum. *Pediatrics* **51**:110, 1973
17. Lever WF, Schaumburg-Lever G: *Histopathology of the Skin,* 6th ed. Philadelphia, Lippincott, 1983
18. Eschenback DA et al: Polymicrobial etiology of acute pelvic inflammatory disease. *N Engl J Med* **293**:166, 1975
19. Dans PE et al: Gonococcal serology: How soon, how useful and how much. *J Infect Dis* **135**:330, 1977
20. Centers for Disease Control. 1989 sexually transmitted diseases treatment guidelines. *MMWR* **38**(suppl 5–8), 1989

CHAPTER 224

Alfred R. Eichmann

Other Venereal Diseases

Urethritis with an identified pathogen (except gonococci) is referred to as a nongonococcal urethritis (NGU). The term nonspecific urethritis describes a urethritis caused by an unidentified organism.

Genital Chlamydia Infections

Fifteen different serotypes of *Chlamydia trachomatis* are presently known: A, B, Ba, and C are considered to be the causative agents of trachoma, D–K the infectious agents of urogenital and other diseases, and L1–L3 the causative pathogens of lymphogranuloma venereum.

Epidemiology

In the United States about 4 to 6 million adults per year contract the disease, as do 5 percent of all newborn babies.[1] In England the prevalence of NGU was 447 per 100,000 in 1986, and among nongonococcal genital infections in women it was 205 per 100,000.[2] In screening investigations of asymptomatic women, the prevalence was found to be between 3 and 5 percent[3] and in female college students, 8 to 10 percent.[4] The prevalence is similar in men: 3 to 5 percent in asymptomatic men in the total population and 15 to 20 percent of all men in STD clinics.[5]

Etiology and Pathogenesis

Chlamydiae have a cell wall and contain DNA and RNA in the cytoplasm; they are endowed with a characteristic metabolism and are bacteria. However, they are energy-requiring parasites which can only multiply within other cells. The chlamydiae form inclusions in the cytoplasm. Reproduction occurs by binary fission. In cell culture, this cycle of development takes 48 to 72 h.[6] The chlamydial infection leads to an immune response in the form of circulating antibodies and cellular immunity.[6]

Clinical Manifestations

Infections of the Female Genital Tract   The most important clinical manifestations in women of chlamydial infections include: mucopurulent cervicitis, acute urethral syndrome, pelvic inflammatory disease (PID) and postpartum endometritis. Sequelae include extrauterine pregnancy, tubal infertility, and cellular atypia of the cervix.

CERVICITIS.   *Chlamydia trachomatis* (Ct) attacks the cylindrical epithelium of the cervix. This cervicitis cannot be distinguished clinically from an inflammation of the cervix of different etiology. About 30 to 50 percent of the women with proven chlamydial cervicitis show no clinical symptoms. In women who do, the principal symptom is mucopurulent discharge, followed by hypertrophic ectopia, post-coital bleeding and spotting.[7] Cervical ectopia is often associated with the identification of Ct.[8]

ENDOMETRITIS.   A chlamydial endometritis results from the ascension of chlamydial cervicitis. Histologic signs of endometritis are found in about half of the patients with mucopurulent chlamydial cervicitis.[9]

PELVIC INFLAMMATORY DISEASE (PID).   PID is the most severe complication of the lower genital tract. The frequency of laparoscopically identified PID caused by Ct is about 50 percent.[10] Women with PID have a four- to sevenfold increase in risk of infertility (from tubal obliteration), and each new infection approximately doubles the infertility risk.[10] The identification of the pathogen in the case of chlamydial salpingitis requires laparoscopy.

PERIHEPATITIS (Fitz-Hugh–Curtis syndrome).   Ct can pass from the cervix via the endometrium and the uterine tubes and reach the region of the right diaphragm. There it causes a perihepatitis which does not involve the liver parenchyme. Clinically it is characterized by piercing pain below the right costal arch. Symptoms are reminiscent of those seen in acute cholecystitis or pleuritis. Perihepatitis appears to be more common in chlamydial infections than in gonorrhea.[11]

Infections in Men   The genital manifestations of Ct infection are very similar to those of gonococcal infection. Mucous membranes are infected first, and later more invasive infection occurs. Infection by the serotypes D–K can result in the following syndromes in men: nongonococcal urethritis (NGU), postgonococcal urethritis, prostatitis, deferentitis, epidydimitis, and proctitis. The most frequent clinical symptom in the male is urethritis. In 30 to 50 percent of the patients with NGU Ct can be found. The incubation period ranges from 7 to 21 days. The symptoms are in general the same as in gonococcal urethral infection, but they start later and are milder.

Urethritis caused by Ct is more often asymptomatic than urethritis caused by *Neisseria gonorrheae*. Coinfection with *N. gonorrheae* and Ct in the male is found in about 15 to 35 percent of patients with gonorrhea. Ct causes postgonococcal urethritis in 70 to 80 percent of patients[12] and is the cause of acute deferentitis and epidydimitis in young men (< 35 years of age) in more than 50 percent of cases. Untreated deferentitis/epidydimitis produces an obliteration of the vas deferens, and sterility can result if both sides are affected. Identification of the causative pathogen in an aspirate and increased levels of IgG and IgM antibodies in the serum provide verification of the diagnosis.[13] The role of Ct in prostatitis is still controversial. In one study only 13 percent of the patients with nonbacterial prostatitis had antibodies to Ct in the serum and prostatic secretions, and none of the patients had positive cultures of Ct in prostatic fluid.[14] Taylor-Robinson et al. were unable to detect either chlamydiae in culture or Ct antibodies in aspirated prostatic secretions from 50 patients with abacterial prostatitis.[16] Other authors[15] were able to find Ct in the prostatic secretions of 26 men with urethritis.

Ct proctitis is frequently seen in homosexual men, caused by the serotypes D–K. About 50 percent of the men with proctitis present clinical symptoms: anorectal pain and bleeding, mucous discharge and diarrhea. Crohn's disease has to be excluded in these patients.[17] Ct is present in about 80 percent of patients with Reiter's syndrome,[18] where it is considered to have a trigger function.

Infections in Newborn Children   These infections are a direct consequence of a genital chlamydial infection of the mother.

CHLAMYDIAL PNEUMONIA IN THE NEWBORN.   Chlamydial pneumonia is often afebrile and is accompanied by a pertussis-like cough and mucous sputum. X-ray reveals symetrical interstitial infiltrates. Laboratory findings include marked eosinophilia, hypergammaglobulinemia, and IgM antibodies to *chlamydia*.[19]

INCLUSION PARTICLE-CONJUNCTIVITIS.   Ct can be isolated from 15 to 20 percent of all children with postnatal blennorrhea. The conjunctivitis appears between days 5 to 15 and is often unilateral. The eyelids are edematous and inflamed and a suppurative secretion is observed. For confirmation of the diagnosis, material is taken from the conjunctiva of the lower eyelid.[19]

Laboratory Examinations

Specimen Isolation   The correct method of specimen isolation is the basis of a successful identification. The identification of chlamydiae is made from a specimen taken from the superficial epithelial cells and not from the exudate. Therefore, mucus and exudate are first removed, and the specimen is obtained from the urethra, cervix, rectum, or tubes (by laparoscopy) using a cotton-wooltipped wire swab which is vigorously rubbed against the mucosal surface.

Direct Identification of the Pathogen   For the direct identification of the pathogen monoclonal antibodies labelled with fluorescein are used (Fig. 224-1). The ELISA (enzyme linked immunosorbent assay) technique enables the identification of Ct to be made directly from the swab specimen. Recently, direct identification has also been made with luminescence-labelled DNA probes.[20]

Culture Methods.   Cultural identification in McCoy cells has proved to be reliable. After 48 to 72 h of culture inclusion bodies can be detected directly in the cells.

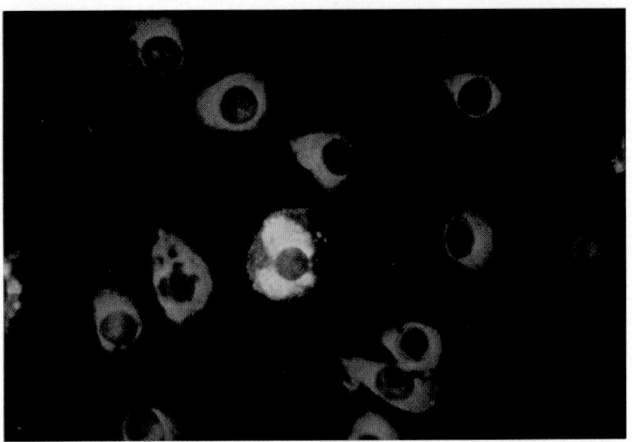

FIGURE 224-1 Detection of *Chlamydia trachomatis* by direct immunofluorescence with monoclonal antibodies.

Serology. All organisms of the genus *Chlamydia* possess a common group-specific antigen which stimulates the formation of IgM, IgA, and IgG antibodies in infected patients. The antibodies can be detected using a micro-immunofluorescence test or the ELISA technique in the case of invasive forms of the infection. Serologic methods are without significance in localized chlamydial infections.

Diagnosis

The definitive diagnosis results from the direct or indirect (serologic) identification of the causative pathogen.

Treatment

Tetracyclines and the macrolides are the antibiotics of choice. Oral doses of 500 mg four times daily are recommended for oxytetracycline, 100 mg twice daily for doxycycline, and 500 mg four times daily for erythromycin. The duration of treatment varies from 7 to 21 days.[21] The same doses are applicable in the case of invasive chlamydial infections except that treatment should be extended to at least 2 to 3 weeks. Sexual partners and the mothers of infected newborns must be examined and treated. In cases of PID and perihepatitis antibiotic therapy should last 4 weeks and be combined with metronidazole (400 mg twice daily).

Prevention

Effective prevention consists in the careful examination and treatment of all sexual partners. If techniques for appropriate diagnosis are not available it is recommended that patients with NGU and nongonococcal mucopurulent cervicitis undergo tetracycline therapy just as for proven chlamydial infections. Patients at risk during pregnancy must be examined and treated prophylactically when indicated.

Genital Mycoplasmas

Mycoplasmas are the smallest self-replicating microorganisms. In the genital region the three species *Mycoplasma hominis, Ureaplasma urealyticum,* and *M. genitalium* have been detected and correlated with genital disease. Whether these mycoplasmas have definite pathogenic properties is still a matter of controversy. Mycoplasmas are found relatively frequently on the genital mucosa in sexually active people, without giving rise to any manifest disease. The frequency of the colonization of the genital mucosa increases with sexual experience and the number of partners.[22]

Pathogenesis

It has still not been determined whether *M. hominis* and *U. urealyticum* cause NGU. Many investigations have implicated *Ureaplasma* as a cause of NGU, since clinical improvement of urethritis occurs when therapy is administered.[23] Arguments against the etiologic role of the mycoplasmas were provided by identical isolation rates from NGU patients and healthy controls.[24] Intraurethral self-inoculation, on the other hand, leads to NGU and pyuria.[22]

Detection and Treatment

Mycoplasma can be detected by culture from swabs. To date 7 serotypes of *M. hominis* and 14 serotypes of *U. urealyticum* are known. Whether a relationship exists between individual serotypes and particular diseases is unknown. In addition to NGU, mycoplasmas have been considered as possible etiologic agents in other diseases: adnexitis, puerperal fever, fever after abortion, natural miscarriage, prostatitis, and bartholinitis.[22] Mycoplasmas are quite sensitive to tetracyclines, and erythromycin. Dosage and duration of treatment are equivalent to those used against chlamydial infections.

Trichomonas Vaginalis

Since the reporting of STD is not obligatory in most countries, reliable figures are hard to find. In most western countries, however, trichomonal infections seem to be declining.[25] Transmission results from sexual contact. Perinatal infection is the most frequent nonvenereal form of transmission.[26] The causative pathogen can survive for several hours on moist objects and in body fluids.[27]

Clinical Manifestations

The most common clinical symptoms in women are a yellow vaginal discharge, abnormal vaginal odor, pruritus, reddening and swelling of the vulva, and punctate petechiae of the cervix ("strawberry cervix") (Fig. 224-2). More than half of all infected women show symptoms.[28] The majority of infected men are asymptomatic. In males the most common symptoms are milky discharge and dysuria.[29] Serious complications are unknown.

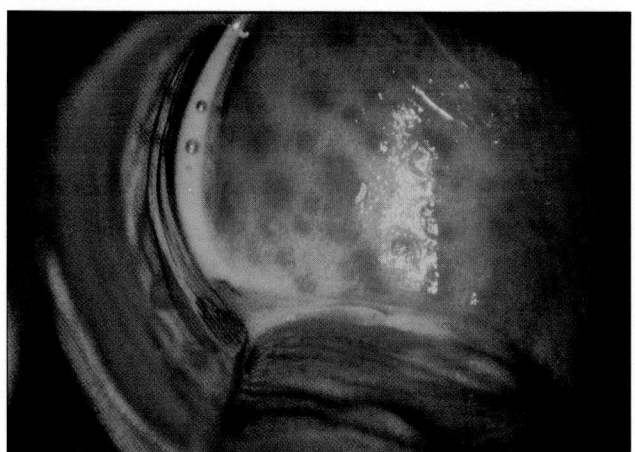

FIGURE 224-2   Trichomonas vaginalis infection: "Strawberry" appearance of cervix with punctate bleeding erosions. (*Courtesy of U. Lauper, M.D., Zürich, Switzerland.*)

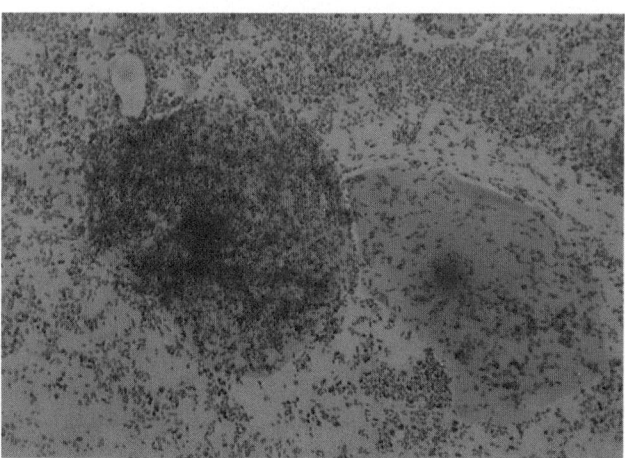

FIGURE 224-4   Colpitis due to *Haemophilus vaginalis.* Clue cells, Gram-staining. (*Courtesy of U. Lauper, M.D., Zürich, Switzerland.*)

Diagnosis

The 10 to 20 μm protozoan with 4 to 5 flagellae can be directly detected on a "wet-mount". Phase contrast or dark-field microscopy is helpful (Fig. 224-3). In women, the specimen must be taken from the vagina since the causative pathogen only attacks the multilayered squamous epithelium. Attempts to demonstrate the causative organism in men are not always successful, but trichomonas vaginalis can be detected in the urinary sediment. Various culture media are available from industrial sources.

Therapy

The therapy of choice is nitroimidazoles such as metronidazole. This can be given orally as a 2 g single dose (in one day) or 250 mg three times daily for 7 days.[30]

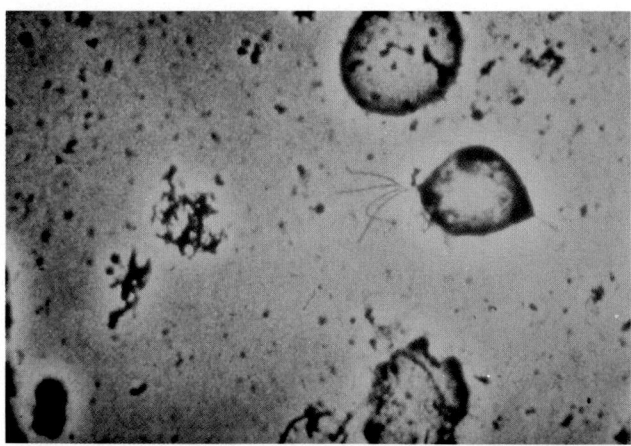

FIGURE 224-3   Trichomonas vaginalis, phase-contrast microscopy. (*Courtesy of U. Lauper, M.D., Zürich, Switzerland.*)

Bacterial Vaginosis (BV)

Bacterial vaginosis is the most common cause of vaginal symptoms in women of childbearing age.[31] Clear proof of a sexual mode of transmission is lacking, but there are indications for it. Symptoms alone are not sufficiently reliable for a diagnosis, and, in order to establish the diagnosis of BV, three of the following four criteria must be met: (1) vaginal pH higher than 4.5; (2) homogeneous milky vaginal discharge; (3) development of fishlike amine odor if 10% KOH is added to the vaginal secretion; (4) detection of clue cells in smears.[32] Four etiologically different microbes can be isolated: *Gardnerella vaginalis, Bacteroides* spp., *Mobiluncus,* and *Mycoplasma hominis.* These bacteria are present in a 100,000-fold higher concentration in women with BV than in healthy women.[33] Clue cells are desquamated vaginal epithelial cells which are covered with vaginal bacteria (Fig. 224-4). This gives them a granular appearance. The most effective therapy is 500 mg metronidazole orally twice daily for 7 days.

Cytomegalovirus (CMV) as a Sexually Transmitted Disease

CMV belongs to the herpes group of viruses and is ubiquitous. The transmission of the virus can occur in a maternal-fetal or sexual manner or as a result of blood transfusion, particularly in the developing countries. CMV has been detected in saliva, sperm, and cervix[34] and is particularly common in homosexual men. In homosexuals infected with AIDS, CMV is detected in all body fluids. In the normal host, CMV infections usually develop asymptomatically, though they can elicit a mononucleosis-like syndrome. In immunocompromised patients, CMV infection manifests as esophagitis, pneumonia, retinitis, meningoencephalitis, and colitis. The diagnosis of CMV infection can be made serologically, electron microscopically, or immunohistochemically by direct detection of the virus. Gangciclovir (DHPG) is used as treatment in immunocompromised patients.[35]

Pediculosis Pubis (the Crab Louse)

Crab lice are mainly transmitted as a result of close body contact. A few days after transmission itching develops in the pubic hair (later also in the armpits, beard, and eyelashes). Clinical findings include nits on the hairs, adult lice which adhere to the skin, and taches bleues, which are bluish spots on the skin at the site of feeding. Treatment consists of topical application of γ-hexachlorocyclohexane (lindane), primethrin, or malathion in various galenical forms. (See also Chap. 227.)

Viral Hepatitis

Among the types of viral hepatitis, hepatitis B, in particular, can be transmitted sexually. The HBs-antigen has been detected in the blood, saliva, tears, vaginal secretions, and sperm of infected patients. Multicenter studies have shown that 6.1 percent of male homosexuals are HBs-antigen carriers and 52 percent are seropositive for anti-HBs.[36] Hepatitis B can also be transmitted heterosexually as a result of vaginal intercourse. It is estimated that every fifth case of hepatitis B is transmitted heterosexually in the US.[37]

References

1. Washington AE, Hohnson RE: Chlamydia trachomatis infections in the United States. What are they costing us? JAMA 257:2070, 1987
2. Treharne JD, Goh BT: Chlamydia trachomatis infections in the United Kingdom. Proc of the European Soc. Chlamydia Research. University of Bologna, p. 33, 1988
3. Meijer CJ et al: Prevalence of Chlamydia trachomatis infection in a population of asymptomatic women. Eur J Clin Microbiol Infect Dis 8:127, 1989
4. Swinher ML et al: Prevalence of Chlamydia trachomatis cervical infection in a college gynecology clinic. Sex Trans Dis 15:136, 1988
5. Stamm WE et al: Chlamydia trachomatis urethral infections in men. Prevalence, risk factors, and clinical manifestations. Ann Intern Med 100:47, 1984
6. Schachter J: Biology of Chlamydia trachomatis, in Sexually Transmitted Diseases, 2d ed, edited by KK Holmes et al. New York, McGraw Hill, 1990, p 167
7. Harrison HR et al: Cervical Chlamydia trachomatis infection in university women. Relationship to history, contraception, ectopy and cervicitis. Am J Obstet Gynecol 153:244, 1985
8. Paavonen J et al: Genital Chlamydia trachomatis infections in patients with cervical atypia. Obstet Gynecol 54:291, 1978
9. Paavonen J et al: Prevalence and manifestations of endometritis among women with cervicitis. Am J Obstet Gynecol 152:280, 1985
10. Paavonen J: Clinical manifestations and therapy of genital chlamydia infections in women, in: Proceedings of the European Society for Chlamydia Research: Bologna-Italy May 30–June 1, p 153
11. Wølner-Hansen P: Perihepatitis in chlamydial salpingitis. Lancet 1:901, 1980
12. Oriel JD, Ridgway GL: Genital infection by Chlamydia trachomatis. London, Edwards Arnold 1982, p 144
13. Doble A et al: Acute epididymitis: A microbiological and ultrasonographic study. Br J Urol 63:90, 1989
14. Mårdh PA et al: Role of Chlamydia trachomatis in non-acute prostatitis. Br J Vener Dis 54:330, 1978
15. Nilsson S et al: Isolation of C.t. from the urethra and prostatic fluid in men with signs and symptoms of acute urethritis, in Studies on C.t. as a Cause of Lower Urogenital Tract Infections. Thesis Acta Dermatovener suppl. 93, 1981
16. Doble A et al: The role of Chlamydia trachomatis in chronic abacterial prostatitis. J Urol 141:323, 1989
17. Quinn TC et al: Chlamydia trachomatis proctitis. N Engl J Med 305:195, 1981
18. Kousa et al: Frequent association of chlamydial infection with Reiter's syndrome. Sex Transm Dis 5:57, 1978
19. Beem MO, Saxon OM: Chlamydia trachomatis infections in infants, in Chlamydial Infections, edited by PA Mårdh. Amsterdam, Elsevier Biomedical, 1982, p 199
20. Le Bar W et al: Comparison of DNA-probe, monoclonal antibody enzyme immunoassay and cell culture for detection of Chlamydia trachomatis. J Clin Microbiol 27:826, 1989
21. Stamm WE, Holmes KK: Chlamydia trachomatis infections of the adult, in Sexually Transmitted Diseases, edited by KK Holmes et al. McGraw Hill, New York, 1990, p 189
22. Taylor-Robinson D: Genital mycoplasma infection. Clin Lab Med 9:501, 1989
23. Ford DK, Smith JR: Non-specific urethritis associated with a tetracycline-resistant T-mycoplasma. Br J Vener Dis 50:373, 1974
24. McCormack et al: The genital mycoplasmas. N Engl J Med 288:78, 1973
25. Schon M et al: Trichomonas vaginalis is now a very rare disease in Sweden. Scandinavian Society for Genitourinary Medicine, Vth meeting, 1988, p 37
26. Bramley M: Study of female babies of women entering confinement with vaginal trichomoniasis. Br J Vener Dis 52:58, 1976
27. Lossick JS: Epidemiology of urogenital trichomoniasis, in Trichomonads Parasitic in Humans, edited by BM Honigberg, New York, Springer, 1989, p 313
28. Wølner-Hansen P et al: Clinical manifestations of vaginal trichomoniasis. JAMA 261:571, 1989
29. Latif AS et al: Urethral trichomoniasis in men. Sex Transm Dis 14:9, 1987
30. U.S. Departement of Health and Human Services: STD Treatment Guidelines, 1985. Washington, D.C.: U.S. Government Printing Office, 1985
31. Amsel R et al: Nonspecific vaginitis: Diagnostic criteria and microbiological and epidemiologic associations. Am J Med 74:14, 1983
32. Holst E et al: Bacterial vaginosis: Microbiological and clinical findings. Eur J Clin Microbiol 6:536, 1987
33. Martins J et al: Relationship of vaginal Lactobacillus species cervical Chlamydia trachomatis and bacterial vaginosis to preterm birth. Obstet Gynecol 71:89, 1988
34. Ho M: Cytomegalovirus, Biology and Infection. Plenum, New York, 1982
35. Chachoua A et al: Ganciclovir in the treatment of cytomegalovirus gastrointestinal disease with the acquired immunodeficiency syndrome. Ann Intern Med 107:133, 1987
36. Schredder MT et al: Hepatitis B in homosexual males: Prevalence of HBV infection and factors related for transmission. J Infect Dis 146:7, 1982
37. Centers for Disease Control: Changing patterns of groups at high risk for hepatitis B in the United States. MMWR 37:429, 1988

Infestations

CHAPTER 225

Fuad S. Farah, Sidney N. Klaus, Shoshana

Frankenburg, Amy D. Klion,

and Thomas B. Nutman

Protozoan and Helminth Infections*

Parasitic diseases are attracting more medical and public health attention than hitherto, in both endemic areas and the technologically advanced countries. The World Health Organization (WHO) has taken the lead in the effort to bring researchers and technologists to the endemic areas. The WHO program is aimed at comprehensive research of six tropical diseases and at training local personnel in the endemic areas who will ultimately carry on and continue the various programs concerned with these issues.

Although endemic, many of the parasitic diseases are being seen in nonendemic areas with greater frequency. The ease and speed of travel have decreased the importance of geographic limitations. It is therefore increasingly important for physicians to familiarize themselves with diseases that are not so common in their own environments.

The parasites that cause diseases with cutaneous manifestations belong for the most part to the protozoa and the helminth worms, including the Nematodes (round worms), Trematodes (flukes), and Cestodes (tapeworms) of the phylum Platyhelminthes.

Protozoa

The protozoa are single-cell organisms capable of performing all necessary functions of life. Those of dermatologic interest include members of the superclass Sarcodasica, family Endamoebidae, represented by *Entamoeba histolytica,* which infests the human intestine and may occasionally invade the skin. Among the Flagellata (superclass Mastigophrasaica) there are two groups of major medical interest: those that inhabit the gastrointestinal and genitourinary tracts and are transmitted from person to person, e.g., *Giardia* and *Trichomonas,* and those that live in the bloodstream and tissue and require an invertebrate vector, e.g., *Leishmania* and *Trypanosoma,* and constitute some of the most serious parasites of humans.

The diagnosis of most protozoan and helminth parasitic infections depends primarily upon the recognition of the morphologic features of the parasite. Microscopy remains the most used and useful tool, although not the only method available.

Helminths

The nematodes are round worms; some are completely parasitic, whereas others live freely in water or soil. *Ancylostoma, Nectar,* and *Strongyloides* are free-living parasites whose ova hatch in the soil. *Strongyloides stercorales* is capable of completing its life cycle either in the soil or by the larvae infecting animals (ingested by dogs or cats) or humans through the skin, producing ground itch. The larvae reach the bronchi and lung through the bloodstream and are swallowed to reach the intestine; there they develop into adults. This type of life cycle also applies to *Ancylostoma duodenale* and *Nectar americanus.* Larvae of other species that do not infect the human intestines may penetrate the human skin and produce irritation (creeping eruptions).

Ascaris, which does not affect the skin directly although it may be responsible for urticaria in endemic areas, has a similar life cycle to *Strongyloides.* The ova hatch in the human intestine and the larvae migrate to the lung via the bloodstream. They then reach the buccal cavity and are swallowed, eventually reaching the intestine and maturing into adults. The female lays her eggs, which are excreted and await ingestion by the host for continuation of the life cycle. This life cycle differs from that of *Enterobius vermicularis,* another parasite infecting humans, in which the female migrates to the anal region to lay her eggs, the larvae not migrating in the body but causing itching in allergic individuals.

The adult *Dracunculus* (guinea worm) lives in the connective tissue of humans and other vertebrates, usually just under the skin. The female discharges large numbers of larval forms through a craterlike ulcer when in contact with water. These infect *Cyclops* (water fleas), which upon ingestion by the host repeat the cycle.

Trichinella spiralis is an intestinal parasite of humans and other mammals. Young larvae bore through host tissue (intestinal mucosa) to reach the blood vessels through which they disseminate throughout the body. The majority of the larvae encyst in striated muscles. Ingestion of the cysts found in the muscle by another host will continue the life cycle.

Wuchereria bancrofti live in lymphatics, whereas *Onchocerca volvulus* and *Loa loa* live in connective tissue; infection of the host

*The chapter was a combined effort. Specific authorship is as follows: "Leishmaniasis" was written by SN Klaus and S Frankenburg; a portion of "Helminth Infections" (lymphatic filariasis, loiasis, and onchocerciasis) was written by AD Klion and TB Nutman; FS Farah wrote the balance of the chapter.

is by blood-sucking (*Brugia malayi* and *B. timori*) and tissue-feeding insects, respectively.

The trematodes (flukes) parasitize various cavities of the body (intestines, ducts associated with the gastrointestinal tract, the bladder, or lungs). The discharged eggs require water and a mollusk for further development. The egg is ingested by the snail or hatches into a free-swimming larva, the miracidium, and finds its way to the snail. In the snail it develops into a spherocyst, divides asexually, and produces many larvae (rediae) that develop into cercariae. These cercariae enter the host either by ingestion (*Fasciola hepatica*) or by penetrating the skin of fish (*Clonorchis sinensis*), the latter being ingested by humans. In *Schistosoma,* the cercariae enter the host through the skin. Cercariae of species not infective to humans may enter the skin of humans and produce cutaneous symptoms known as ''swimmer's itch,'' cercarial dermatitis, or schistosome dermatitis.

The cestodes parasitize an intermediate host. *Taenia solium* infects humans in the tapeworm stage and pigs in the bladder worm. *Echinococcus* infects the dog in the tapeworm stage and the human in the hydatid cyst form. Cysticerci may parasitize humans and affect the skin, causing the condition known as sparganosis.

Protozoan Infections

Amebiasis

Amebae are unicellular spherical organisms composed of an ectoplasm and an endoplasm. In the trophozoite stage, amebae reproduce by binary fission. When conditions become unfavorable, the amebae encyst, becoming capable of survival for prolonged periods and of transfer to other hosts. The cyst encysts in the colon, divides, and forms new trophozoites. Nonpathogenic forms of amebae may be differentiated from the pathogenic forms morphologically.

In the intestine, *Entamoeba histolytica* usually lives harmlessly in the human bowel (asymptomatic amebiasis). Occasionally, it becomes pathogenic for reasons not presently known, resulting in invasive amebiasis. Colonization occurs by repeated, rapid binary division. Invasion is accomplished by lytic digestion of the intestinal epithelium. Invasion is not accompanied by a host inflammatory response. However, amebic lesions, especially extraintestinal ones, are more prone to secondary infection. Overall case fatality in amebic dysentery is around 2 percent but is much higher in infants and children (27 percent).

Cutaneous amebiasis occurs less frequently than intestinal amebiasis, except for a group with cutaneous infection of the genitalia. The skin is involved by direct extension from the involved colon, an amebic liver abscess, following surgical intervention in colonic or hepatic amebiasis, or, less commonly, through direct inoculation by contact with infectious material. Common sites of involvement are the anus and the buttocks, the penis, and the face. Penile amebiasis may appear as the only lesion, acquired by heterosexual or homosexual intercourse with persons who suffer from amebic dysentery.

Characteristically, the skin lesions spread quickly. The course is faster in younger patients. Early diagnosis is important; however, the skin lesion itself is not diagnostic and consists of an invading ulcer or an ulcerated granuloma (ameboma). The ulcer has raised, thickened borders and often undermined edges with an erythematous surrounding zone. It is often covered by a purulent exudate with necrotic slough. It is very painful and is usually associated with regional lymphadenopathy.

Other skin conditions associated with amebiasis include urticaria and pruritus, which are said to improve with treatment of the amebiasis.

Cutaneous amebiasis should be distinguished from epithelioma, other granulomas, and syphilis. Finding trophozoites at the base of the ulcer on biopsy or in the fresh material from the edge of the ulcer confirms the diagnosis. Repeated stool examinations should also be made, despite a negative history of dysentery. Gel diffusion and latex agglutination test may be helpful.

The prognosis is good if the diagnosis is made early and treatment initiated immediately. It is, however, serious or fatal in untreated and neglected cases. Patients with acquired immunodeficiency syndrome (AIDS) are more likely to have amebiasis and are less equipped to resolve the infection as cell-mediated immunity plays a major role in limiting the infection and preventing reinfection. This group of patients is more likely to have more invasive disease, and one expects more cutaneous involvement.

The treatment of the skin lesions should include treatment of the luminal and colonic amebiasis as well as the extraintestinal infection. Metronidazole serves well to treat both manifestations; usually 750 mg given orally three times daily for 10 days is an effective amebicide. Intravenous use of the same dose may at times be necessary. A follow-up treatment for the luminal disease is recommended. Such agents as di-iodohydroxyquinoline (Iodoquin), 650 mg three times daily for 20 days, paromomycin (Humatin), 25 to 30 mg/kg body weight per day in 3 divided doses for 1 week, or diloxanide furoate (Furamide), 500 mg three times daily for 10 days, are now available through the Centers for Disease Control. Emetine (dehydroemetine; Mebadin) remains effective in a dosage of 1 mg/kg body weight per day for 5 days, not to exceed 60 mg per day; patients should be monitored closely for cardiac toxicity with repeated electrocardiograms. Chloroquine phosphate may also be used. Local irrigation and cleaning of the skin ulcer may be helpful.

Flagellate Protozoa of the Blood and Tissues

Flagellate protozoa that inhabit the human bloodstream and tissues are *Trypanosoma* (*T. rhodesiense, T. gambiense, T. cruzi,* and *T. rougeti*) and *Leishmania* (*L. tropica, L. braziliensis,* and *L. donovani*). These organisms require two hosts, a human and an insect or other mammal. *Leishmania, T. gambiense,* and *T. rhodesiense* multiply as flagellates in the midgut of the insect and migrate anteriorly to the proboscis. *T. cruzi* moves posteriorly in the vector's gut and is evacuated with the feces.

Trypanosomiasis

Protozoa of the genus *Trypanosoma* are widely distributed around the equator (15° N–S) in Africa (African trypanosomiasis) and between 40° N in the United States and 43° S in Argentina (American trypanosomiasis).

The trypanosomes are flagellated protozoa. The flagellum arises from near the posterior kinetoplast and emerges anteriorly. It has an undulating membrane. It circulates in the bloodstream as a trypomastigote, usually about 15 to 30 μm in length. When taken up by the vector, it lodges in the midgut, multiplies by binary fission, migrates to the salivary gland, and becomes infective in 2 weeks (*T. rhodesiense*) or 3 weeks (*T. gambiense*).

T. cruzi, the cause of American trypanosomiasis (Chagas' disease), invades the reticuloendothelial system, myocardium, endocrine glands, and glial cells. Here the parasite is in the amastigote (leishmanial) form, measures 1 to 5 μm, and is characterized by a larger nucleus. It transforms to the trypomastigote form when outside the cell, is ingested by the vector, is passed through the vector's liquid feces while the vector is feeding, and is introduced into the skin wound. In this respect, it differs from African trypanosomiasis and from leishmaniasis.

African Trypanosomiasis   Humans are the natural host of *T. gambiense* transmitted by tsetse flies of the genus *Glossina palpalis*. *T. rhodesiense* (morphologically similar to *T. gambiense*) is transmitted by *G. moristans* and primarily infects animals, most notably antelopes. *T. rhodesiense* is primarily a zoonotic, but infections in humans are acute and fulminant. Age, sex, and occupation do not influence the incidence of infection, except through the degree of exposure to the tsetse fly. *T. gambiense* is more prominent in central and west Africa, and *T. rhodesiense* is more common in east Africa. There are about 200 endemic foci and about 20,000 cases of trypanosomiasis reported each year.

Following the infected bite of the fly, dissemination occurs through the lymphatics, with spread to the central nervous system in *T. gambiense* infections. Often there are no cutaneous lesions, but, at times, the fly bite is followed by the formation of a red nodule, 1 to 3 cm in diameter, surrounded by a waxy white halo (trypanosome chancre), seen mostly in Europeans, not in Africans. It is accompanied by lymphangitis and lymphadenopathy without suppuration and subsides within a few days. By the second week, fever and constitutional symptoms develop, followed by a generalized pruritic exanthem similar in appearance to erythema multiforme. Lymph node enlargement is prominent, particularly the posterior cervical chain (Winterbottom's sign). Cardiac involvement may occur, as well as debility and central nervous system symptoms including lethargy, irresponsibility, headaches, seizures, ataxia, and paresis; death almost invariably follows.

Edema of the eyelids is transient and painful; the hands and feet are also involved. Large erythematous, often annular, eruptions appear on the trunk. Erythema nodosum sometimes occurs. Disseminated intravascular coagulation occurs in only a few patients, but cold hemagglutinins are regularly found. Low serum complement levels are detected. Pruritus is prominent.

The trypanosome survives the host defenses by its ability to vary the antigenic type on the surface coat, resulting in recurrent waves of parasitemia.

Diagnosis may be difficult in nonendemic areas, but a history of recent travel to an endemic area should raise suspicion. Immunologic tests may be helpful, including immunofluorescent antibody tests, enzyme-linked immunosorbent assay (ELISA), and indirect hemagglutination tests. Finding the parasite in the blood smear should be attempted and is diagnostic. Circulating complexes are found and may serve to monitor the effectiveness of treatment.

American Trypanosomiasis   Also known as Chagas' disease, American trypanosomiasis is a parasitic disease caused by *T. cruzi* and is transmitted by blood-sucking insects of the family Triatomidae (order Hemiptera; "kissing bugs"). The insect vectors are widely distributed in the western hemisphere, including Texas and the southwestern United States through Central and South America. However, no definite cases have occurred in the United

States in spite of the presence of the vector, and the area of distribution of the disease is more limited (42° N to 43° S) than the range of the insect distribution. *T. cruzi* exists in many animal reservoirs, such as dogs, cats, monkeys, and pigs, and in rodents such as squirrels. About 20 to 30 percent of an estimated population of 15 million are infected. It is the leading cause of death (Chagas' heart disease) among young and middle-aged adults in many areas of South America.

In the tissue, *T. cruzi* invades the cells of the reticuloendothelial system, transforms to the Leishman-Donovan forms, and incites an immediate reaction with edema and cellular infiltration manifested as subcutaneous swelling. Some 4 to 5 days later, the infection spreads through the lymphatics, and the draining lymph nodes become enlarged, edematous, and infiltrated with lymphocytes and plasma cells. There is hepatosplenomegaly. At a later stage, the parasite escapes into the bloodstream, becomes flagellated, and again penetrates a cell and repeats the cycle. Various tissues and organs are involved, particularly the spleen and liver. In the myocardium, the resultant scarring leads to serious effects. In the brain, localization of the parasites leads to neurologic symptoms. Tissue damage results from the rupture of the parasitized host cells and the accompanying mononuclear inflammatory response. As mentioned above, the most susceptible cells are those of cardiac, striated, and smooth muscle cells; mononuclear phagocytes; and glial cells. The cycles of parasitism are thought to be associated with variations in the trypanosomal antigens. There may be immune hemolysis based on antigen-antibody reactions.

Clinically, the lesions appear at the site of inoculation within 5 days in the majority of patients. The portal of entry is the conjunctiva (in 80 percent of the cases), evidenced by periocular edema and inflammation of the lacrimal glands known as the "eye sign," "Romana's sign," or "oculoglandular complex." If the inoculation is in the skin, then a "cutaneous adenopathy complex" or "chagoma" develops, which is characterized by a tumorlike lesion on the chest, back, or legs. In children, it is often followed by myocarditis or encephalitis and may end fatally. Hepatosplenomegaly, edema, and various forms of cutaneous exanthems appear, some resembling erythema multiforme. Recurrence of the skin lesions is frequent. Subacute or chronic forms of the disease are almost always associated with myocarditis and some possibly with gastrointestinal manifestations such as megacolon or megaesophagus. Chronic heart failure is frequent in advanced cases. Cardiac inflammation has been seen even in asymptomatic patients dying from other causes.

The pathogenesis of the disease has not been clarified. It may be related to toxins released by the parasite or to the deposition of immune complexes with complement (low C3 and C4 have been demonstrated in some patients). It has also been shown that the immune response, both antibody-mediated and cell-mediated, is suppressed in these infections, possibly through the generation of specific suppressor cells. Cell-mediated cytotoxicity is effective against bloodstream trypomastigotes in in vitro studies.

The diagnosis is suspected by the history and the physical findings, especially in individuals living in endemic areas, and is established in early cases by demonstrating the parasite in the bloodstream by smear or culture and in lymph node biopsy material. In subacute and chronic cases, demonstration of antibody by complement fixation, hemagglutination, or immunofluorescence tests is helpful. A highly sensitive ELISA detects circulating *T. cruzi* antigens.

Treatment is difficult because of the toxicity associated with the drugs used and the difficulty of eradicating intracellular parasites. Nifurtimox (a nitrofuran) and benznidazole (a nitroimidazole) are available. Nifurtimox is given orally, 6 to 8 mg/kg body weight for adults and 15 mg/kg for children in equally divided doses, for 2 to 4 months. Benznidazole is given orally, 5 to 7 mg/kg body weight per day in three divided doses. Skin rashes, photosensitivity, bone marrow suppression, and peripheral neuropathy must be looked for.

Early treatment in acute cases results in rapid clearing of the parasite along with clinical improvement and a better chance of survival. Treatment in chronic stages suppresses the parasitemia but does not eradicate the disease nor influence the clinical course appreciably. Therefore the beneficial effects of the treatment do not outweigh the serious side effects, and one may resort to supportive and symptomatic treatment.

Preventive measures should be aimed at reducing the risk of infection by control of the vector with the use of insecticides, by improving housing conditions, and by screening blood donors effectively.

Leishmaniasis

Leishmaniasis is the result of infection with intracellular protozoan parasites belonging to the genus *Leishmania*. The infections cause a wide spectrum of clinical changes that divide leishmaniasis into four broad divisions based on the extent and severity of involvement in the human host: cutaneous leishmaniasis (CL), diffuse cutaneous leishmaniasis (DCL), mucocutaneous leishmaniasis (MCL), and visceral leishmaniasis (VL).

The prevalence of all forms of leishmaniasis worldwide is in excess of 12 million cases. Movement of new immigrants into endemic areas, an increase in tourism to "exotic" areas of the globe, a decrease in the use of insecticides, and improvement in diagnostic methods have all contributed to raising the incidence of leishmaniasis, which the WHO estimates will soon exceed 400,000 new cases annually. The more serious forms of the disease, such as MCL and VL, cause the death of more than 75,000 persons annually.

Characterization of Leishmania Parasites The protozoan parasites that cause leishmaniasis are members of the order Kinetoplastida, family Trypanosomatidae. The organisms are found in two morphologic forms during their life cycle. In humans

and other mammalian hosts, they exist within macrophages as round to oval nonflagellated amastigotes, 2 to 3 μm in diameter. In the arthropod vectors (sandflies belonging to the genus *Phlebotomus* or *Lutzomyia*), the parasites exist as elongated flagellated promastigotes, 10 to 15 μm in length and 2 to 3 μm in width. Both forms of the parasite have a nucleus and a smaller DNA-containing kinetoplast. Although promastigotes of different *Leishmania* species vary slightly in the width-to-length ratio, amastigotes show no significant differences, and it is not possible to distinguish species of *Leishmania* by their morphology in tissue smears.

Until the past decade, different species of *Leishmania* were identified largely by the pattern of their clinical involvement. The old world forms of CL were thought to be caused by *L. tropica*, new world MCL was attributed to *L. braziliensis*, new world CL to *L. mexicana*, and VL to *L. donovani*. Recently, more precise techniques for identifying *Leishmania* species have been developed, such as monoclonal antibodies, isoenzyme characterization, and DNA hybridization. Based on findings using these techniques, the older clinical categories have been subdivided and now include the recently identified species. A practical, somewhat simplified classification scheme is found in Table 225-1.

VECTORS. *Leishmania* parasites are transmitted by phlebotomine sandflies of the genus *Phlebotomus* in the old world and *Lutzomyia* in the new world. Sandflies are small mosquito-like insects 1.5 to 4 mm in length. Their small size allows them to pass through ordinary mesh screens and mosquito netting. Sandflies are widely distributed throughout the tropics and subtropics in a variety of habitats, including deserts, rain forests, and highlands. Only the females are hematophagous (blood-sucking).

LIFE CYCLE. Parasites, in the form of amastigotes from infected tissue or blood, are taken up from the mammalian host during feeding by female sandflies. Within the midgut of the sandflies, the parasites undergo a change to the promastigote form and multiply. Once the promastigotes are fully developed, they migrate from the gut to the pharynx and proboscis, where they remain until they are injected into a new mammalian host during a subsequent blood meal (Walters, 1989).

Between 10 and 200 promastigotes enter the dermis during each feeding by an infected sandfly. Once in the dermis the promastigotes activate complement and bind C3. Many of the "free" promastigotes are thought to be destroyed by polymorphonuclear leukocytes and eosinophils, but the exact details of the early stages

TABLE 225-1
Classification of Leishmaniasis

Clinical form	Species	Major localities
Cutaneous leishmaniasis (CL):		
Old world	*L. major*	Near East, Africa
	L. tropica	Near East, former U.S.S.R.
	L. aethiopica	Ethiopia, Kenya
	L. infantum	Mediterranean rim
New world	*L. mexicana* complex	Mexico, Central America
	L. braziliensis complex	Brazil, Bolivia
	L. amazonensis	Brazil
Mucocutaneous leishmaniasis (MCL)		
Diffuse (anergic) cutaneous leishmaniasis (DCL):		
Old world	*L. aethiopica*	Ethiopia
New world	*L. braziliensis* complex	South America
Visceral leishmaniasis (VL)	*L. donovani*	India, Kenya
	L. infantum	Mediterranean rim
Uncommon forms of leishmaniasis:		
Leishmaniasis recidivans (LR)	*L. tropica*	Middle East, former U.S.S.R.
Post-kala-azar dermal leishmaniasis (PKADL)	*L. donovani*	India, Nepal, China

of infection are unknown. Some of the promastigotes become attached to receptors on the surface of dermal macrophages and are phagocytosed. Within the macrophage, the promastigotes transform into amastigotes (also called Leishman-Donovan bodies) and are incorporated into the cells' phagolysosomes (parasitophorous vacuoles). Within the phagolysosome, the parasites are able to resist destruction and multiply readily by binary fission. When a macrophage becomes filled with amastigotes, the macrophage is disrupted. The amastigotes reenter the extracellular space and are taken up again by other macrophages. The duration of the extracellular stage is unknown (Manuel, 1990).

Dissemination of the parasites from the inoculation site depends in large measure on the species of the parasite (Muller et al., 1989). Some species, such as *L. donovani* and *L. infantum,* can spread to macrophages elsewhere in the reticuloendothelial system early in the course of the illness. Other species, such as members of the *L. braziliensis* complex, travel to specific locations in the host, such as the mucosal surfaces of the nose, pharynx, and upper respiratory tract. Amastigotes of dermatotropic species, such as *L. major* and *L. tropica,* generally remain confined to the skin. The cycle of infection continues when an infected mammal is again bitten, and amastigotes are taken up by a female sandfly.

RESERVOIRS.   Each species of *Leishmania* favors one or more animal reservoirs, except *L. donovani* and *L. tropica,* which are thought to be mainly, if not exclusively, anthropomorphic. Identification and control of the reservoir may have a profound influence on the epidemiology of the disease. For example, in southern France and Spain, where dogs serve as the main reservoir for VL (caused by *L. infantum*), destruction of infected animals has led to a marked decrease in the frequency of the disease in humans. In an area of Turkmenistan, elimination of rodents harboring *L. tropica* led to a reduction from 70 percent to less than 1 percent in the incidence of CL.

Immunobiology   Leishmaniasis can be pictured as an immunologic spectrum that in many aspects parallels leprosy (Bryceson, 1972). At one pole lies CL, in which the host usually develops a protective immune response; at the other pole is VL, in which the host shows little evidence of resistance and immunosuppresion. In the middle are MCL, which provokes an intense inflammatory reaction, and DCL, in which there is extensive and widespread proliferation of the organisms of the skin, but without much inflammation or tendency for visceralization. Unlike leprosy, the extent and pattern of leishmaniasis that develops is strongly influenced by the specific species of *Leishmania* involved.

Additional factors that affect the clinical picture include the number of parasites inoculated, the site of inoculation, the nutritional status of the host, and even the nature of the last non-blood meal of the vector. Recently, a component of saliva of some new world sandfly species has been described that causes local vasodilatation and appears to enhance parasite infectivity (Titus and Ribeiro, 1988; Ribeiro, 1989). In some cases the sandfly is heavily infected, and a large load of parasites may partially block the insect's pharynx, requiring the sandfly to make multiple probes to obtain an adequate blood meal. This results in a localized cluster of cutaneous lesions in the host. Rather broad differences in the disease pattern may develop from apparently similar or identical strains of *Leishmania.* It is known that some patients who are infected by *L. major* develop inapparent infections, whereas others infected by identical *Leishmania* species show deep or widespread lesions that involve subcutaneous tissue and lymph nodes. Although CL caused by *L. aethiopica* will result in a spontaneous cure

in 80 percent of patients, widespread diffuse cutaneous lesions will develop in the remaining 20 percent.

Immunologic Response   Considerable data have been collected concerning the immunologic response by the host. Most studies point to a central role for cellular immunity in control of leishmanial infection. Although antileishmanial antibodies are produced during infection, their presence does not correlate with resolution of the disease. Important insights into the immunobiology of leishmaniasis and basic principles of cellular immunology have emerged from studies of lymphocyte-macrophage interactions in leishmaniasis. Susceptibility to disease appears to depend on both macrophage susceptibility and T-cell responses. Cultured macrophages from susceptible strains of mice allow extensive intracellular amastigote growth. Macrophages from some resistant mouse strains permit replication of the parasite in vitro, whereas macrophages from other strains do not. In addition, development of protective immunity also appears to depend on complex interactions between protective and disease-enhancing T-cell populations. The spontaneous resolution of cutaneous leishmaniasis is mediated by one or more subsets of T-helper cells, but their proliferation and expression seem to be affected by multiple factors. The protective T-helper cells appear to belong to the subpopulation known as Th1, and the disease-enhancing helper cells are known as Th2. Th1 cells are characterized by their secretion of interferon-γ and interleukin 2 (IL-2), and Th2 cells by IL-4 and IL-5. Although these studies have been performed in mice, similar mechanisms may be operative in human disease (Liew, 1989; Scott, 1989). For example, patients with active CL have circulating lymphocytes that produce interferon-γ in response to leishmanial antigen.

In general, infection and recovery are followed by lifelong immunity to reinfection by the same species of *Leishmania.* In some cases, interspecific immunology has also been reported. Currently, work is progressing toward an effective vaccine for the prevention of leishmaniasis (Modabber, 1989).

Clinical Patterns   OLD WORLD CL.   *CL Caused by L. major*   CL is found in widely scattered parts of Asia, Africa, and Europe, largely in tropical and subtropical zones, and in much of the Middle East, especially Iran, Iraq, eastern Saudi Arabia, the Jordan Valley of Israel, and the Sinai Peninsula.

The disease begins as a small erythematous papule, which may appear immediately after the bite of the sandfly or 2 to 4 weeks later. The papule slowly enlarges in size (to 2 cm or more) over a period of several weeks and assumes a more dusky violaceous hue (Fig. 225-1). Eventually the lesion becomes crusted in the center. When the crust is removed, a shallow ulcer is found, often with raised and somewhat indurated borders. In some cases the central part of the nodule becomes hyperkeratotic, and a firmly adherent horn develops over the lesion. Small satellite papules (Fig. 225-2) may also be found at the periphery of the lesion, and occasionally subcutaneous nodules develop along the course of the proximal lymphatics. Rarely, lesions become locally invasive and extend to subcutaneous tissue and even muscle. This latter occurrence may be related to specific deficiencies in the host's immune response.

After the lesion has been present for 2 months or more, peripheral spread stops, and the ulcerated nodule remains approximately the same size for another 3 to 6 months, or even longer (Fig. 225-3). The lesion then heals, usually leaving a slightly depressed scar. In some cases CL has been found to remain ''active,'' i.e., with positive smears, for 24 months or even longer. Such cases have been designated *nonhealing chronic cutaneous leishmaniasis.*

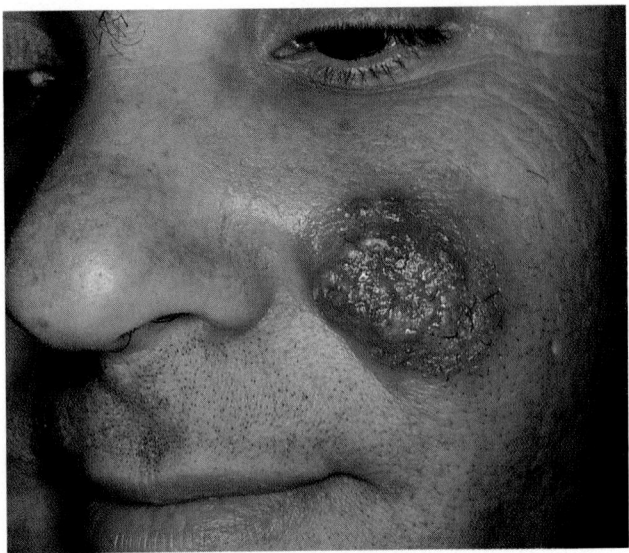

FIGURE 225-1 Cutaneous leishmaniasis. Large moist plaque on the cheek caused by *L. major*.

The number of lesions that develop in *L. major* CL depends largely on the circumstances of exposure and the extent of the infection within the sandfly. Infection with *L. major* may result in multiple lesions (Fig. 225-4); up to 100 or more have been reported in a single individual. The reservoir for *L. major* is desert rodents, and the incidence of the disease is highest in areas close to the burrows of the infected animals.

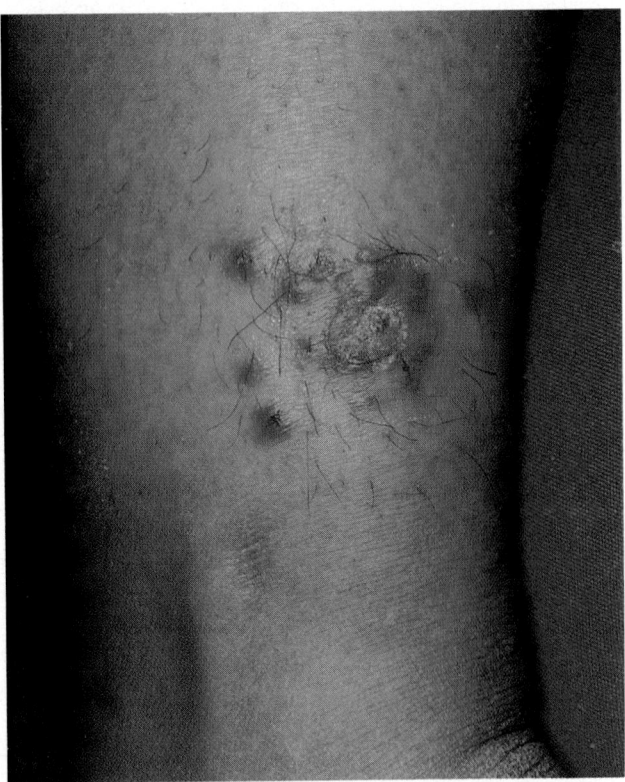

FIGURE 225-2 Cutaneous leishmaniasis, late plaque-stage cutaneous. Central plaque with peripheral satellite papules (*L. major*) is seen near the ankle.

CL Caused by L. tropica CL caused by *L. tropica* is found in Iran, Iraq, and the southern republics of the former U.S.S.R. The disease is more common in urban areas than is CL from *L. major*. *L. tropica* is largely a disease of humans, although there is recent evidence suggesting that rats also serve as reservoirs. The clinical pattern of *L. tropica* infection is similar to that of *L. major*, although lesions caused by *L. tropica* are more apt to be solitary and tend to be somewhat more inflammatory.

CL Caused by L. infantum CL caused by *L. infantum* is found in countries bordering the Mediterranean, including Spain, France, Italy, and Greece. The skin lesions are similar to those in the *L. major* form of the disease but their duration is usually shorter. Dogs serve as the reservoir for *L. infantum*. Reports from endemic areas in Spain have shown that more than 20 percent of dogs tested for the presence of *L. infantum* were harboring parasites.

CL Caused by L. aethiopica CL caused by *L. aethiopica* is found in Kenya, the Sudan, and Ethiopia. The common form of the disease seen in these areas is similar to CL caused by *L. major*; however, in a significant number of patients a widespread skin involvement develops that resembles lepromatous leprosy, known as *diffuse cutaneous leishmaniasis* (DCL) (see below).

NEW WORLD CL. *CL Caused by L. mexicana Complex* In the new world the skin lesions of CL are caused by parasites of the *L. mexicana* complex. The disease is found in Mexico, Central America, as far north as Texas, and as far south as Brazil. The vectors for this form of CL are *Lutzomyia* sandflies. The lesions develop in a similar fashion to those caused by *L. major* in the old world. Generally, a small erythematous papule develops at the site of the bite of an infected sandfly and gradually develops into an ulcerated nodule. Eventually the lesion heals, leaving a depressed scar. Although lesions can develop on any part of the body, in Mexico and Central America sores characteristically involve the pinna of the ears, so-called chiclero ulcers.

CL Caused by L. braziliensis Most cases of CL caused by *L. braziliensis* are due to transmission from forest rodent to sandfly to human, with the latter serving as a sporadic host when entering into the habitat of the forest rodent reservoirs. The clinical symp-

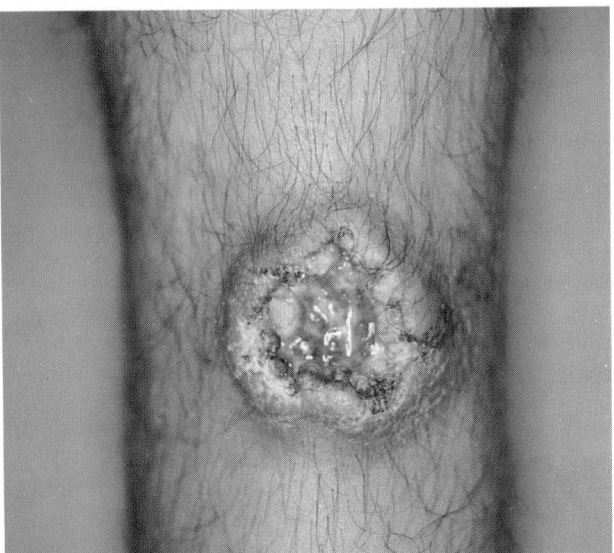

FIGURE 225-3 Cutaneous leishmaniasis, old world. A deep ulcerated lesion on the leg, caused by *L. major*, in a man with specific deficit in cell-mediated response to the parasite.

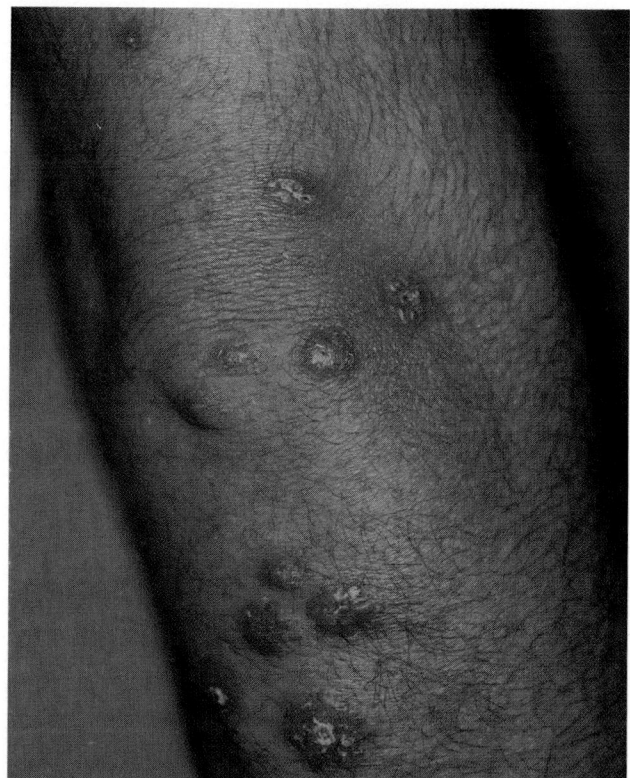

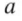

a

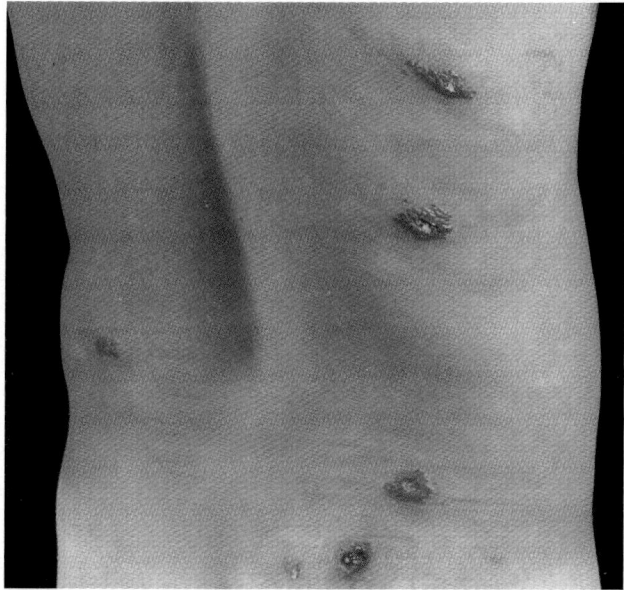

b

FIGURE 225-4 Cutaneous leishmaniasis, multiple lesions.
(a) Multiple nodules on the legs caused by *L. major*.
(b) Multiple, nodular, ulcerated lesions on the trunk at the sites
of sandfly bites.

toms of the cutaneous lesions are similar to those caused by the old
world species of *Leishmania,* except that some of the strains of the
L. braziliensis complex can invade the mucous membranes of the
mouth, nose, pharynx, and larynx, giving rise to MCL (see below)
(Fig. 225-5).

Histopathology (See Kurban, 1966) ACUTE CL. The epidermal
changes are highly variable and can range from atrophy or ulceration to hyperplasia, which may be pseudoepitheliomatous. The
most constant feature is a diffuse dermal inflammatory cell infiltrate composed of varying proportions of histiocytes, lymphocytes,
plasma cells, and neutrophils. Specific diagnosis requires identifying the amastigotes, so-called Leishman-Donovan bodies, within
the cytoplasm of dermal macrophages. In general, the number of
parasites present is inversely proportional to the duration of the
lesion. The amastigotes measure from 2 to 4 μm and are a dull
blue-gray color with hematoxylin and eosin (H&E) staining. They
are usually present in clusters. Although with Giemsa's stain the
parasites are red, in this author's experience if they are not visible
with H&E, it is rare to find them with the Giemsa's stain. In some
laboratories an immunoperoxidase monoclonal antibody stain can
be performed on paraffin sections and is sometimes more helpful
than either H&E or Giemsa staining in locating Leishman-Donovan
bodies. The histology of a longstanding lesion of acute CL may
resemble that of the chronic type, which is described below.

CHRONIC CL. In this stage the dermal infiltrate is nodular and
is characterized by tuberculoid-type histiocytic granulomas with
lymphocytes and plasma cells surrounding them. Amastigotes are
usually not detectable. Necrosis rarely occurs. This histology generates a differential diagnosis that includes other causes of tuberculoid type granulomas such as lupus vulgaris, tuberculoid leprosy,
and granulomatous rosacea. A specific diagnosis at this stage requires clinicopathologic correlation.

Diagnosis PARASITOLOGIC DIAGNOSIS (See Schnur and Jacobson,
1987). The diagnosis of CL rests on finding parasites in the skin.
The most direct method of detecting parasites is by direct smear
from a lesion. A tissue smear is obtained from the edge of an ulcer
or from the edges of a skin slit made in a papule or nodule with a
no. 11 blade. After staining with Giemsa, the amastigotes are seen
as pale-blue oval bodies with a dark-blue nucleus and a small point-
shaped kinetoplast within the cytoplasm of tissue macrophages.

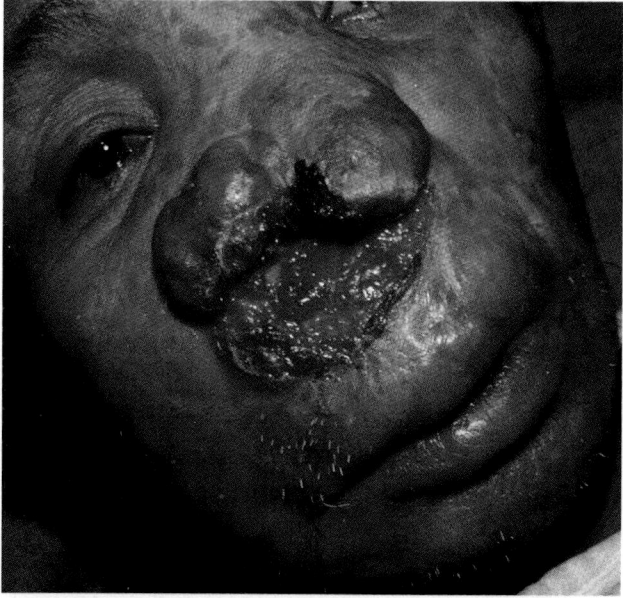

FIGURE 225-5 Mucocutaneous leishmaniasis, South
American. Painful, mutilating ulceration with destruction of
portions of the nose. (*Courtesy of Eric Kraus, M.D.*)

The organisms are enveloped by an external capsule, which may be difficult to see within the histiocyte. Occasionally, abundant organisms can be identified in an extracellular location. These bodies are generally somewhat larger than the intracellular forms, and their capsule is readily visible.

Parasites can also be cultured from tissue fluid obtained from a lesion. The material is cultured in a biphasic medium, such as Novy-MacNeal-Nicolle (NNN), or a liquid medium, such as Schneider's insect culture medium, in the presence of fetal calf serum. Promastigote forms appear after several days and can be detected in the culture medium. Cultures should not be discarded as negative before 4 weeks. Strains that do not grow in culture media may be inoculated into susceptible animals, but this method is not very practical for routine diagnosis.

IMMUNOLOGIC DIAGNOSIS.   Although both circulating and cellular responses can be demonstrated during the course of the illness, animal studies have shown that protective immunologic reaction is based solely on cell-mediated immunity. Generally, tests of immune function are of more value in following the course of the disease than they are for diagnosis.

ELISA tests for circulating antibodies are available that use purified leishmanial products as the test antigen. Antibody levels are often elevated in the early stages of CL, but they are not considered a useful diagnostic sign.

The cell-mediated immune response can be measured by the leishmanin (Montenegro) skin test, in which phenol-killed preparations of promastigotes are injected into the dermis; the extent of the inflammatory response is measured at the end of 48 and 72 h. Biopsy of a positive Montenegro test at 72 h shows a diffuse cellular infiltrate in the upper dermis, with occasional histiocytes and eosinophils.

An in vitro lymphocyte proliferation assay for cell-mediated immunity is also available. In this test proliferation of peripheral blood lymphocytes in response to a crude extract of promastigotes is measured after 6 days of incubation. This test reflects both present and past infection, so it is less useful in diagnosis than is the direct identification of the parasites (Frankenburg, 1988). Recently an assay has been developed that gives some measure of the "effector capacity" of the host. In this test peripheral blood mononuclear cells are incubated with live promastigotes, and the number of organisms ingested by monocytes is measured after a short incubation period.

Other Types of Leishmaniasis   DIFFUSE CUTANEOUS LEISHMANIASIS.   In both the old and new worlds, a form of CL is found in which large areas of the dermis become invaded by macrophage-containing organisms, without a tendency to visceralization. In the old world, this disease is caused by *L. aethiopica;* DCL is found in 20 percent of leishmaniasis patients in Ethiopia and the Sudan. In South America, DCL is attributed to a poorly characterized member of the *L. braziliensis* complex. DCL usually presents as a single nodule, which then spreads locally, often through extension from satellite lesions, and eventually by metastasis. In time, the process becomes widespread, with nonulcerating nodules appearing diffusely over the face and trunk; these lesions show a close clinical resemblance to lepromatous leprosy (Fig. 225-6a). DCL usually runs a protracted course but does not visceralize. It responds poorly to treatment.

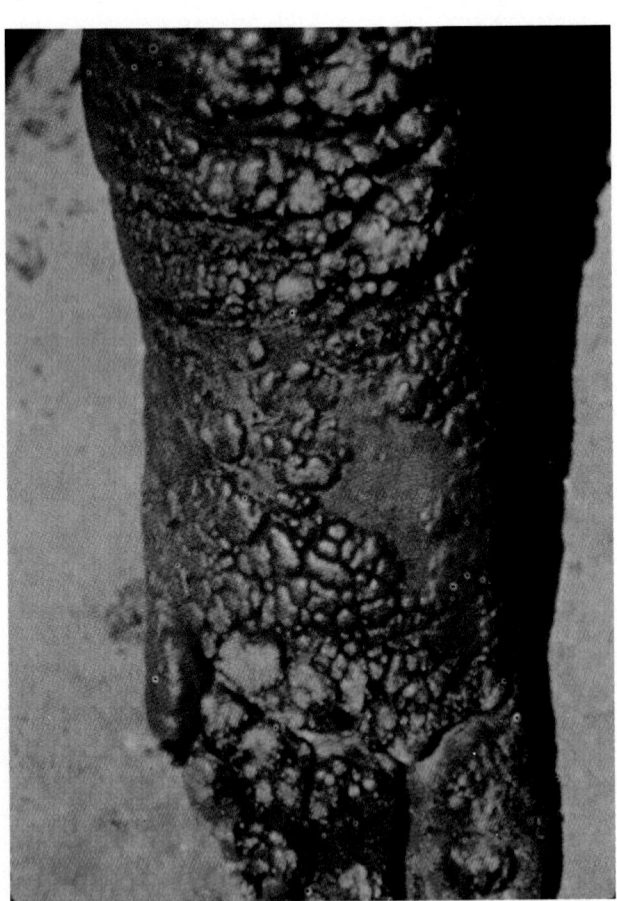

a

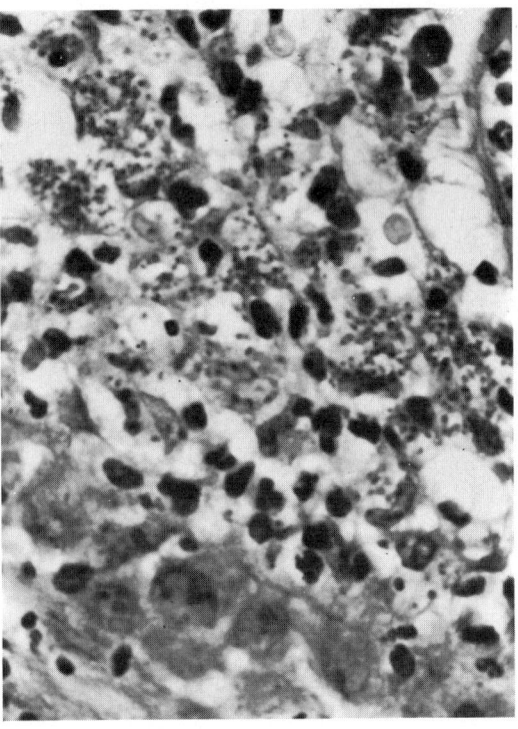

b

FIGURE 225-6 Disseminated anergic cutaneous leishmaniasis. (*a*) Confluent nodules on the foot resembling lepromatous leprosy; there was generalized cutaneous involvement as well. (*Courtesy of David Wyler, M.D.*) (*b*) Section of a nodule showing abundant leishmanial forms.

Parasites are abundant in skin smears and skin biopsies from DCL (Fig. 225-6b) and circulating antibodies are present, but tests for cell-mediated immune response, such as the Montenegro skin test and lymphocyte proliferation assay, are negative. There is still some question about the pathogenesis of this form of leishmaniasis, but most workers attribute it to deficiencies in the host's immune response, rather than to an especially virulent strain of leishmaniasis.

MUCOCUTANEOUS LEISHMANIASIS. MCL is a serious and occasionally life-threatening form of leishmaniasis, found mainly in the new world. MCL is characterized by involvement of both skin and the upper respiratory tract. The disease is caused by parasites of the *L. braziliensis* complex in South America and by *L. aethiopica* in Africa. In the form of the disease caused by *L. braziliensis*, mucosal lesions develop from cutaneous lesions in more than 75 percent of those infected. However, in infections caused by less virulent species, such as *L. braziliensis guyanensis*, nasal involvement is found in 5 percent of infected cases. In the old world, MCL can be found infrequently in patients infected by *L. aethiopica*. MCL begins with a cutaneous lesion that is identical to that of CL: a small red papule develops at the site of a sandfly bite and gradually enlarges, ulcerates, and finally heals. However, rather than showing eventual resolution, as in CL, the infection extends to the mucosa and eventually to the cartilages of the upper respiratory tract, especially the nose, oral pharynx, and, rarely, the larynx (see Fig. 225-5). Edema and inflammatory changes occur that lead to epistaxis and coryzal symptoms. Eventually there is destruction of the cartilaginous structures in the area, including the nasal septum, the floor of the mouth, and the tonsilar areas. Bony structures are usually spared. The disease leads to marked disfigurement, known as *espundia* in South America. If this form of the disease is not arrested, death usually results from superimposed bacterial infection or pharyngeal obstruction leading to acute respiratory failure or malnutrition.

The diagnosis of MCL rests largely on clinical grounds. The parasites are often difficult to demonstrate or isolate from the mucosa of the respiratory tract.

VISCERAL LEISHMANIASIS. In VL—also called kala-azar—the parasite establishes itself mainly in the bone marrow, spleen, and liver. The disease, if untreated, is often fatal, but in some areas many subclinical cases have been reported. It is a disease of all age groups. The disease is present in China, India, the former U.S.S.R., the Middle East, from east Africa through Sudan to west Africa, and across South America. The main *Leishmania* species involved are *L. donovani* in India and Africa, *L. infantum* in the Mediterranean countries, and *L. chagasi* in South America. In India the disease is transmitted directly from person to person; post-kala-azar dermal leishmaniasis (see below) may represent the human reservoir of the parasite. In other types of VL, foxes, jackals, and dogs are naturally infected, and humans are regarded as accidental hosts. The disease in this case is not believed to be transmitted directly from person to person. In India kala-azar is mostly an urban disease, but otherwise it is mostly rural. As in CL, the incubation period may last from weeks to months; then there is often a subacute febrile onset that may be so severe as to be fatal or so slight that it may be little remarked upon. The next symptom to appear is usually splenomegaly, then pancytopenia, fever, wasting, and serious imbalance of serum proteins. There is a high rate of death among untreated cases.

Definite diagnosis of VL requires the demonstration of parasites; they can be detected in smears or cultures prepared from bone marrow biopsies or in histologic sections from the spleen. Specific serologic tests are often positive in the acute stage of the disease, but cell-mediated immunity, both specific and nonspecific, are suppressed. This suppression is reversed after treatment and cure. Treatment with pentavalent antimonials (Pentostam) is usually effective against kala-azar.

LESS COMMON FORMS OF LEISHMANIASIS. *Leishmaniasis Recidivans (LR)* LR is a distinctive form of chronic cutaneous leishmaniasis that is usually a complication of an *L. tropica* infection. The lesions of LR are characterized by dusky-red plaques, with active, spreading borders and healing centers, giving rise to gyrate and annular forms. LR most commonly affects the face and can cause tissue destruction and severe deformity. Generally, the smear and culture are negative, but the patients have a strongly positive leishmanin test and tests for cell-mediated immunity are positive.

LR is difficult to treat, although intralesional injections of Pentostam have been reported to give good results in some cases.

Post-Kala-Azar Dermal Leishmaniasis (PKADL) PKADL is a rare sequel to VL that has been apparently cured following adequate treatment. The skin lesions appear a year or so after a course of therapy and consist of macular, papular, and nodular lesions on the face, trunk, and extremities. Many of the lesions take the form of hypopigmented macules and plaques. The nodules rarely ulcerate. When the lesions are numerous, the clinical picture resembles lepromatous leprosy. *L. donovani* can be recovered from the skin lesions by culture, and smears are usually positive. PKADL develops in almost 20 percent of Indian patients treated for VL and to a lesser proportion among Ethiopian patients treated for VL caused by *L. aethiopica*.

Because there is no known animal reservoir for VL in India, it is thought that patients with PKADL serve as an important human reservoir for this disease.

Treatment The treatment of leishmaniasis depends on the clinical form of the disease (Chong, 1986). CL in the old world is usually self-limited and in most cases does not require specific treatment. Treatment in this form of the disease should be given for extensive lesions, especially involving the face, or for those lesions that invade deeper tissues. The most successful therapy consists of intralesional injections of Pentostam, usually administered at weekly intervals. Up to 1 mg/kg body weight of the drug may be injected in the borders of the lesions. For very extensive lesions, Pentostam is administered intravenously. Other measures that have been advocated for the treatment of CL include freezing, local heat, oral ketoconazole, and rifampicin. Trials using these modalities have not been properly controlled, however, and their efficacy is unconfirmed.

Recently, a topically applied aminoglycoside antibiotic, paromomycin, has shown promising results in clinical trials and may develop into an alternative to the pentavalent antimonials for CL.

Treatment of DCL usually requires parenteral pentamidine.

Helminth Infections

Helminth is the Greek word for "worm" and in the more restricted sense it refers to parasitic worms. Two large phyla are mostly implicated, the Platyhelminthes (flatworms) and Nematoda (true roundworms). The two classes of Platyhelminthes, the Trematoda (flukes) and Cestoda (tapeworms), are exclusively parasitic throughout their life cycle. Many of the species of Nematoda are free-living, and some are parasitic during part or all of their lives.

Platyhelminthes (Flatworms)

Cysticercosis   Pork tapeworm infections are caused by *Taenia solium*. The human intestinal infestation is acquired by the ingestion of inadequately cooked pork containing *T. solium* cysticerci. The adult worm attaches to the intestinal mucosa and grows to a length of about 7 m. However, eggs either ingested or transferred to the mouth by poor hygiene are likely to develop into larval stages; they enter the bloodstream through penetration of the intestinal mucosa and are disseminated to various tissues, primarily the subcutaneous layer. In this case, it is a tissue cestode, and the human is its intermediate host. This is in contrast to *T. saginata* (beef tapeworm) which lives only in the intestinal tract and grows to a much longer length.

There are usually no symptoms referrable to the intestinal infestation, but cysticercosis may be associated with muscle pain, weakness, fever, and central nervous system and other organ-specific symptoms, depending on the organ involved. The diagnosis is established by finding eggs in the stool or the perianal area or by finding proglottides in the stool and by x-ray findings, complement fixation, indirect hemagglutination determination of specific IgE levels, and skin tests. Biopsy is confirmative.

Treatment is surgical removal of the cysticerci when feasible. Mebendazole deserves serious consideration, alone or in combination with surgery. It may act by preventing growth rather than by killing the parasite. For the intestinal infestation, niclosamide is effective treatment but must be used with caution because it causes digestion of the worm; eggs may be released, and cysticercosis may follow. Quinacrine is therefore a better treatment, and the dosage is 200 mg orally every 10 min for four doses. A purgative must be used the night before and again 2 h after the last dose of the medication.

Echinococcus   Echinococcus, or hydatid disease, results from tissue invasion by the tapeworms *Echinococcus granulosus* (of dogs) and *E. multilocularis* (of wild animals). Both parasitize humans in the larval stage. *E. granulosus* produces a single larval cyst (the unicellular hydatid cyst), and *E. multilocularis* produces the multilocular type (alveolar hydatid cyst). *E. granulosus* is more common and widespread. Sheep are common intermediate hosts, as are humans; cattle and pigs are less frequently affected. Humans generally are infected by ingestion of larvae in contaminated water or food. The larvae penetrate the intestinal wall and are disseminated to various parts of the body, mainly the liver, lung, and bones. The life cycle is completed when the predator eats the organs containing the hydatid cyst. The skin is occasionally involved with development of soft, flocculent, subcutaneous cysts of various sizes. These are not painful. Eventually the cysts calcify or are resorbed after several years. Urticaria may be a common and prominent complication of echinococcus due to sensitization by the products of the cyst fluid absorbed systemically. It can present a serious complication during surgery if the cyst ruptures. Severe anaphylaxis may result.

The diagnosis is established with x-ray studies, scans, skin tests, hemagglutination, and determination of specific IgE levels.

Treatment is surgical if the unilocular cysts are in an operable location. Mebendazole (Vermox) produces complete regression of intrahepatic cysts. Immunotherapeutic manipulations are under investigation.

Sparganosis   This condition, a rare zoonotic disease, has a worldwide distribution but is more common in the Orient. It is caused by the procercoid larva (sparganum) of *Spirometra mansonoides* and *S. mansoni*. The various species do not have characteristics that allow their differentiation; speciation must depend on study of the tapeworm in its definitive host (dogs, cats, or wild animals).

Infection occurs after the ingestion of the procercoid found in copepod cyclops in drinking water or from the ingestion of raw or lightly cooked muscle of the second intermediate host, namely snakes, birds, frogs, or other mammals. Application of raw flesh in the form of poultices to open lesions or to the eye or the vagina serves as a source of infection.

The larvae penetrate the intestine and develop into spargana in subcutaneous tissue or muscle. The areas affected are edematous and may be painful. The worm may migrate from one area to another, including the central nervous system, and the condition may last indefinitely.

S. mansoni has been known to acquire a gene for growth hormone from humans and has caused mice and rats to grow abnormally. This is an interesting observation that may suggest other approaches to the study of the biology of these parasites.

Treatment is by surgical removal and drainage whenever feasible. Arsenicals (neoarsphenamine) have been advised and are said to produce a good response. High doses of metronidazole and praziquantel may be attempted.

Schistosomiasis   Schistosomiasis is also known as bilharziasis, in honor of its discoverer who identified the causative agent in Cairo in 1851. The disease was known there much earlier, probably around 1100 B.C. The worms typically live in pairs in the portal system or in the vesical venules of the caval system. They can be dislodged and carried in the bloodstream to various organs at distant sites. The worms may live for up to 30 years or more in the human host.

The life cycle of these worms is complex and involves freshwater snails in which the cercariae develop and are released. The free-swimming cercariae penetrate into the skin and reach the bloodstream. The larvae mature in the portal veins and lay their eggs mostly in the pelvic veins. *Schistosoma mansoni*, common in Africa and South America, and *S. japonicum*, in the Far East, localize around the rectum and colon and pass their eggs in the feces.

S. haematobium, common in Africa, India, and the Middle East, especially the Nile delta in Egypt, localize around the bladder and pass their eggs in the urine. On contact with water the eggs develop into miracidia which seek the snail and therein develop into free-swimming cercariae. The cercariae penetrate the human skin or mucous membranes, their proteolytic secretions aiding in rapid penetration. They lose their tails and become schistosomules. The larvae are trapped in the skin of previously immunized individuals and a papular pruritic eruption appears. In the nonimmunized individual, the schistosomules move rapidly to the lymphatics and venules and thence to the lungs. Young adult schistosomes acquire antigens from the host onto their surface and become immunologically camouflaged.

The ova may work their way into the tissues where they produce a granulomatous inflammation with a tuberculoid formation and with eosinophils, histiocytes, and occasional giant cells surrounding the ovum. This reaction is probably dependent on immune mechanisms. These lesions can occur at distant ectopic sites.

There are several cutaneous lesions associated with *Schistosoma*:

Schistosomal Dermatitis   The cercariae may cause a pruritic, papular eruption indistinguishable from cercarial dermatitis due to nonhuman schistosomes.

Urticarial Reactions   Urticarial reactions appear about 4 to 8 weeks after the cercariae of *S. japonicum* and, less frequently, other human schistosomes penetrate the skin. The urticaria is mostly on the trunk and is associated with fever, malaise, abdominal pain, diarrhea, arthralgia, and hepatosplenomegaly. It is referred to as urticarial fever or Katayama disease.

Paragenital Granulomas   These occur frequently in the endemic areas of *S. haematobium* infections in the Middle East. Granulomatous lesions involve the vaginal area, perineum, and buttocks and are associated with extensive and communicating sinuses and fistulas.

Ectopic Cutaneous Schistosomiasis   Ova or dislodged flukes in pairs may become deposited in the skin as well as in other areas such as the lung, conjunctivae, and central nervous system. The trunk is most often involved with a granulomatous reaction that is flesh colored, firm, and papular, varying in size but usually in the 2- to 3-mm range. Plaques result from coalescence of the lesions. They may ulcerate or desquamate and ultimately become deeply pigmented. Skin or rectal biopsy reveals the presence of ova.

Treatment is that of the systemic bilharziasis with stibophen and other trivalent antimonials such as Astiban and niridazole (Ambilhar). Praziquantel (Biltricide) is the drug of choice and is effective against all schistosomes. It is given as 20 mg/kg body weight every 4 h for three doses and may effect a cure in 70 to 100 percent of cases. Oxamniquine (Vansil) is effective against *S. mansoni*, and netrifonate (Bilracil) is effective against *S. haematobium*.

Cercarial Dermatitis (Swimmer's Itch, Collector's Itch)   Cercarial dermatitis describes a pruritic eruption caused by the inflammatory reaction induced by the entry of cercariae into the skin. The human blood flukes (schistosomes) produce a reaction indistinguishable from the dermatitis induced by the nonpathogenic avian or mammalian flukes. Both freshwater and marine forms are responsible for the dermatitis. However, like the pathogenic forms, they require an intermediate host (a snail), and the endemicity is determined by the availability of the snail.

Collector's itch most likely results from infection with *Trichobilharzia ocellata* and *T. physellae;* these are common in swamps and in the presence of vegetation. Swimmer's itch is due to *T. stagnicolae,* whose habitat is shallow waters. The condition is found in temperate and tropical regions.

Clinically, itching is manifest at the time of exposure. The cercariae penetrate the skin by means of their spines and through the effects of proteolytic enzymes. The itching results from the acute inflammatory urticarial (edema and erythema) reaction. The

urticarial reaction subsides and is followed by a papular pruritic lesion similar to delayed-hypersensitivity reactions. The eruption appears on exposed parts and spares the areas covered by clothing. It begins to regress after about 3 days and subsides in 1 to 2 weeks. Scratching may lead to ulceration and prolongation of the dermatitis.

Treatment is symptomatic. Antipruritic preparations are used to control the itching. The cercariae do not live in the human skin, and the lesions subside spontaneously.

Nematodes (Roundworms)

Nematodes are elongated, nonsegmented animals. Their life cycle goes through an egg, four larval stages, and an adult stage. Each larval stage ends with development of a new cuticle, the older one being molted. Parasites that produce cutaneous manifestations are listed in Table 225-2.

Larva Migrans (Creeping Eruption)   Larva migrans is a characteristic cutaneous eruption caused by larvae of various nematode parasites for which the human is an abnormal final host. When the larvae migrate into and involve the viscera, the condition is referred to as visceral larva migrans, in contrast to cutaneous larva migrans. For example, *Ancylostoma braziliensis*, in central and southeastern United States, *A. canium, Uncinaria stenocephala* (hookworm of dogs), and *Bunostmum phlebotomum* (hookworm of cattle) are the common species responsible for ground itch or uncinarial dermatitis. Transient creeping eruptions result from larvae of the human hookworms, *A. duodenale* and *Necator americanus*.

The ova of these hookworms are deposited in the soil and hatch into infective larvae, which then penetrate the human skin. Sandy, warm, and shady areas are favorable. Children, farmers, gardeners, and sea bathers are likely to be exposed to the infection.

The various larvae produce a similar reaction in the skin; it begins within a few hours of exposure as a nonspecific pruritic dermatitis at the site of penetration. The skin areas involved are those in contact with the soil, usually the feet (Fig. 225-7) and buttocks. Shortly thereafter the larvae begin to migrate in the skin or remain stationary for a few weeks or months. Migration is manifested by a wandering, thin, linear, raised, tunnel-like lesion, 2 to 3 mm wide, containing serous fluid; the old lesions become dry and crusted. Many larvae may be active at one time, producing bizarre patterns. Migration may stop after a few weeks or months. The larvae move a few millimeters to a few centimeters each day, usu-

TABLE 225-2
Parasites that Produce Cutaneous Manifestations

Order	Parasite	Manifestation
Strongyloidea	*Necator americanus* } *Ancylostoma duodenale* }	Uncinarial dermatitis (ground itch)
	Ancylostoma capillaria	Larva migrans
Rhabdiasoidea	*Strongyloides stercoralis*	Larva currens
		Strongyloidiasis/ground itch
Oxyuroidea	*Enterovius vermicularis*	Oxyuriasis
Spiruroidea	*Gnathostoma spinigerum*	Gnathostomiasis
Trichuroidea	*Trichinella spiralis*	Trichinosis
Dracunculoidea	*Dracunculus medinensis*	Dracunculosis
Filarioidea	*Onchocerca volvulus*	Onchocerciasis
	Loa loa	Loiasis
	Wuchereria bancrofti } *Burgia malayi* }	Filariasis

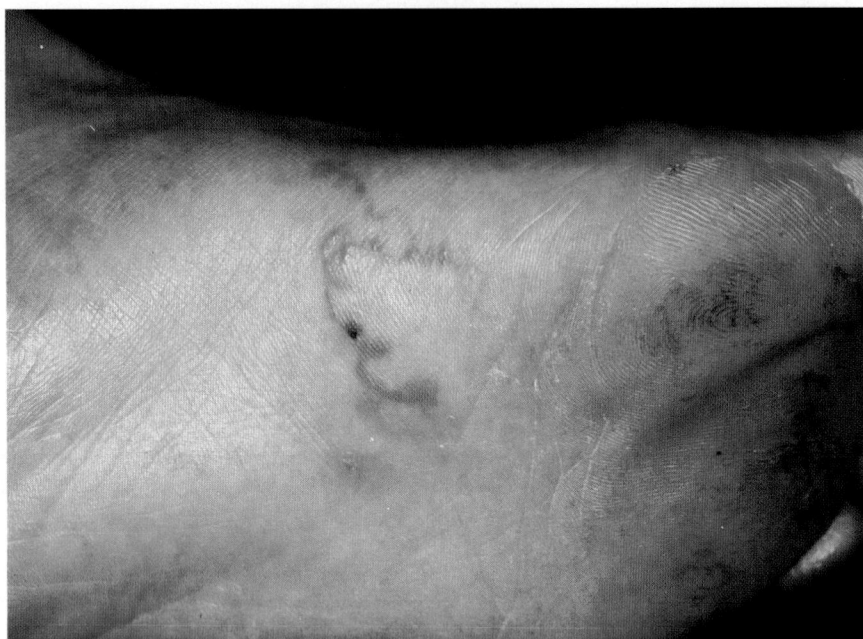

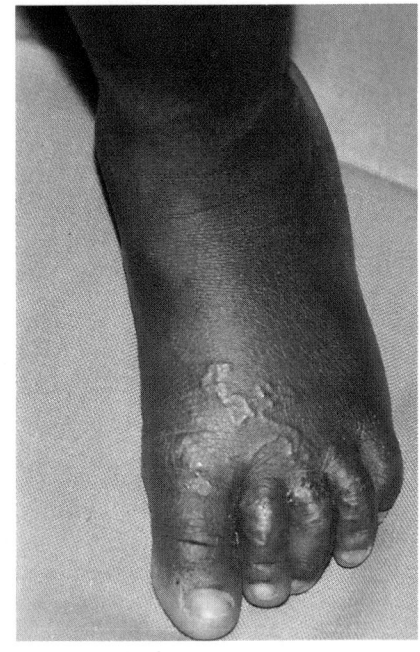

a   *b*

FIGURE 225-7 Larva migrans (creeping eruption). (*a*) Thin, erythematous, serpiginous (snakelike), papular eruption. (*b*) This eruption was effectively treated by freezing with ethyl chloride, a simple treatment widely used in endemic areas.

ally limited to a small area. They rarely travel far. The fast migration is referred to as larva currens (due to *Strongyloides stercorales*). The disease should be self-limited as humans are "dead-end" hosts. However, the natural duration of the disease is variable. Within 4 weeks, 25 to 81 percent of the larvae disappear.

Larva migrans may be associated with eosinophilia (10 to 30 percent) and Loeffler's syndrome. Visceral larva migrans due to dog or cat ascarides (*Toxocara canis*) or to other nematode larvae (*Ancyclostoma lumbridordis*) may lead to patchy, erythematous urticaria or papular eruptions accompanied by systemic illness, granulomas of the liver with hepatomegaly, pneumonitis, eosinophilia, and hyperglobulinemia.

Larva currens is a special form of cutaneous larva migrans caused by *S. stercoralis*. An intense papular eruption develops at the site of penetration, often accompanied by urticaria and a papulovesicular, edematous, or nonspecific eruption (see "Strongyloidiasis" below).

Treatment of larva migrans is best with thiabendazole (Mintezol) given in doses of 25 to 50 mg/kg body weight for 2 to 4 days and rarely longer. Pruritus subsides by the first day, and the lesions clear in 1 to 2 weeks. Topical thiabendazole as 15% cream is also effective, especially early. Freezing the affected area with dry ice or ethyl chloride may be effective if sloughing of the epidermis and the parasite is achieved. The freezing must include the advancing burrow where the parasite might be expected to be.

Strongyloidiasis Strongyloidiasis, or strongyloidal ground itch, is caused by *Strongyloides stercorales* for the most part and rarely by other *Strongyloides* species. *S. stercorales* has a life cycle similar to other hookworms, namely, larval penetration of the skin, migration to the lung, and residence in the intestine.

The infection is common in warm areas and is mostly seen in Africa, South and Central America, and the Gulf states of the United States. It is not common in colder climates.

Upon reaching the duodenum and jejunum, the larvae penetrate the mucosa and develop into 2- to 3-mm-long adults. The female starts laying eggs within a few days. The larvae develop within the egg, hatch quickly, and make their way through the feces. In the soil, when conditions are favorable, the larvae develop into free-living adults. They mate, and the resultant larvae develop into infective larvae and free-living ones. Reinfection may occur from the larvae that become infective before leaving the body. These also pass through the venous system into the lungs and continue the cycle. This form of reinfection (autoinfection) is more common in patients with immune deficiency or malnourished states and may be fatal in these patients. External reinfection may occur if the infective larvae penetrate the perineal skin.

The initial penetration of the larvae is almost always symptomless and may pass unnoticed. However, subsequent penetration may cause a macular, reddish eruption at the site. Itching may be intense. Urticaria may develop and may be generalized or localized to the involved area. In cases of external autoinfection, the larvae may migrate in the skin, usually rapidly (5 to 10 cm/h). This form of larva migrans is known as larva currens, and *S. stercorales* is virtually the only cause in humans. Systemic symptoms may occur. When in the lung, symptoms of bronchitis or pneumonitis may be observed. In severe cases, bronchopneumonia may develop. Heavy infestation may cause abdominal pain, alternating diarrhea and constipation, nausea and vomiting, anorexia, and weight loss. Mid epigastric pain may occur. In autoinfection, the larvae may be deposited in other tissues and may cause myocarditis, hepatitis, pneumonia, colitis, paralytic ileus, cholecystitis, and ascites.

The diagnosis is confirmed by demonstrating larvae in the stools. Culture methods or the Baermana larva extraction technique should be used when suspicion persists and routine stool examination fails to find the cause.

Strongyloidiasis must be differentiated from hookworm disease, ascariasis, and amebiasis, and must be considered in the differential diagnosis of atypical pneumonia. Creeping eruption (hookworm) usually occurs in exposed areas of the skin, in contrast to the covered areas involved in *S. stercorales* infections.

Treatment with thiabendazole, 50 mg/kg body weight per day for 2 days, given in one or two doses each day, effects a cure in almost all patients. Side effects are transitory and mild. Diazamine is also effective but is toxic and therefore not generally recommended.

Ground Itch (Uncinarial Dermatitis)   *Ancylostoma duodenale* and *Necatur americanus* are the two important hookworms producing similar clinical pictures. These infections are found throughout tropical and subtropical areas of the world. Both have a similar life cycle beginning with skin penetration when the skin is in contact with contaminated soil. They enter the circulatory system and the lungs, undergo considerable larval growth, and, after the fourth stage, enter the larynx and are swallowed. They attach to the mucosa of the small intestine and develop into the adult worm. *A. duodenale* infections are acquired through penetration of the skin and also through ingestion of the larvae. The worms may live for more than 10 years. Eggs are passed in the feces and, if the conditions are favorable, develop rapidly into infective larvae.

A dermatitis results from the penetration of the larvae into the skin. The feet are most commonly affected, being the part of the skin most likely to be in contact with contaminated soil. Edema and intense pruritus and a burning sensation follow. A papular eruption appears and becomes vesicular. The lesions disappear in about 2 weeks unless secondarily infected. Penetration of the larvae into an already infected individual leads to linear trails in the skin rather than the pruritic papule of the primary exposure. An urticarial rash may also develop.

Pulmonary reaction to the migration through the lung is usually mild but is significant in heavy infestations. Bronchial pneumonitis is the main manifestation. Intestinal symptoms are mild in light infections or may be absent. Heavy infections produce abdominal pain simulating peptic ulcer or cholecystitis, weakness, nausea, diarrhea, edema, and pallor. Persistent heavy infections lead to iron-deficiency anemia. This is due to blood loss caused by the laceration of the intestinal mucosa, which is produced by the attachment of the worm and by its feeding activities.

Diagnosis is made by the finding of eggs in the stools; these are detected easily by routine microscopic examination. The diagnosis should be suspected in individuals with unexplained iron-deficiency anemia, especially in endemic areas. It should be considered in the differential diagnoses of other helminth infections such as ascariasis and strongyloidiasis. The linear lesions of ground itch are more transient than those of creeping eruptions.

Treatment with tetrachloroethylene is the choice for *N. americanus* infections. A dose of 0.12 mL/kg body weight (up to 5 mL) is given on an empty stomach. It is often necessary to repeat the treatment 8 to 10 days later. The drug should not be used in pregnancy or liver and kidney disease. If ascariasis is also present, it should be treated first with piperazine. Bephenium hydroxynaphthoate is more effective for *A. duodenale* infections; it could be used for the treatment of *N. americanus* infections but is less effective. Iron-deficiency anemia should also be treated.

Enterobiasis (Threadworm)   Infection with *Enterobius vermicularis* follows the ingestion of eggs containing the infective larvae. The eggs hatch in the small intestine and migrate to the cecal area where they mature within 2 to 4 weeks. The adult female is larger than the male, being 8 to 13 mm long compared to 2 to 5 mm for

the male. When gravid, the female deposits her eggs in the perianal and perineal areas. The eggs become infective within a few hours (4 to 6) and exposed individuals become infected. The original host is subject to reinfection. Direct or indirect contamination of hands, fomites, and air form the route of spread, hence the whole household may become infected.

Pruritus ani is common in infected individuals due to mechanical irritation or allergic reactions caused by the migrating female. Intense itching may lead to lichenification, secondary infection, and scarring. Urticaria has been reported in some cases.

Systemic symptoms are, as a rule, absent. However, abdominal pain, nervousness, anorexia, loss of weight, and loss of sleep may occur. Vaginitis results from migration of the parasite to the area. Migration to the uterus and the fallopian tubes may or may not be associated with symptoms.

The diagnosis is established by having a high index of suspicion and looking for and finding the worm or the eggs in the perineal and perianal regions. The adhesive-tape technique is best suited for recovering eggs from the perineum. At times the adult worm may be seen on the surface of the stools. Routine stool examination may also be helpful.

E. vermicularis infection should be suspected in cases of salpingitis, menorrhagia, and metrorrhagia. These are due to the ectopic migration of the worm. At times the tissue reaction to the parasite incites tumors that require surgical removal.

Treatment is with pyrvinium pamoate (Povan) given as a single dose of 5 mg/kg body weight, not to exceed 250 mg. It is repeated in 1 or 2 weeks. Piperazine, 65 mg/kg body weight up to 2.5 g in a single dose, is also effective, though not always successful. Stringent hygienic measures are needed to prevent recurrences and to reduce exposure of family members. It has been suggested that treatment be given whenever symptoms appear or periodically to eliminate the infection. At times it may be desirable to treat all family members and to repeat the treatment in 2 weeks to eliminate the infection from the household.

Trichinosis   Trichinosis, also referred to as trichinelliasis or trichinellosis, is an infection by the tissue nematode *Trichinella spiralis*. It is most common in temperate climates and is rare in the tropics; the highest incidence is in Europe and North America. The infection is acquired following the ingestion of inadequately cooked, infected meat of pig, wild pig, bear, and polar bear. Of all the animals that may be infected, the pig remains the major source of the organism. Those with a particular fondness for raw pork are very susceptible to infection.

The larvae are liberated upon ingestion and penetrate the intestinal mucosa where they mature to the adult reproductive stage in about 1 week. The female measures about 4 mm, and the adult male 2 mm or less. The female larvae begin to deposit embryos in the tissue in 2 to 3 weeks. The embryos enter the circulation and are distributed to all parts of the body. In striated muscles, the embryos develop into larvae that incite an inflammatory reaction, leading to encystment of the larvae in fibrous tissue cysts. The larvae may remain infective for several years or may become calcified during the first year. Passage of the embryos through other tissues leads to intense local inflammation, but encystment occurs only in striated muscle.

Clinical manifestations begin with the stage of muscle invasion (about 1 week following infection) and last for several days or several weeks. An acute illness develops with fever, generalized muscle pain and tenderness, difficulty in respiration and in using the tongue muscles, sweating, periorbital edema, and conjunctivitis. The skin is pruritic, and urticarial, papular, macular, or petechial rashes may occur. Splinter hemorrhages may be seen, and the parasite can be readily demonstrated in biopsy specimens of the nail bed. The severity of the disease depends on the parasite load and can be fatal in severe infections. Moderate infection improves by the fifth or sixth week, at which time desquamation may be seen. Cardiovascular, neurologic, and respiratory disturbances may occur.

The condition is associated with eosinophilia in up to 90 percent of patients. Immunologic evidence of the presence of infection develops by the third week. Skin tests are not very reliable.

Treatment with thiabendazole, 50 mg/kg body weight per day for 7 days, has been found useful against the worms in the intestine and against the larval stages. Treatment is effective in early stages, but older infections do not respond. Corticosteroids may be useful in controlling the symptoms because of their anti-inflammatory effects.

Prevention of infection is important and is achieved by the proper cooking of meat. Pork cooked at outdoor barbecues is often adequately cooked on the outside but the center may be insufficiently heated to kill the parasite. Refrigeration at −18°C for 24 h is also an effective means of killing the parasite.

Dracunculosis (Guinea Worm)   Guinea or Medina worm (*Dracuncula medinensis*) is the cause of this infection in humans. It is common in the Middle East (Arabia, Iran, Pakistan), New Guinea, and Indonesia. About 40 million people are infected annually; 6 million cases occur in India alone. It is more common in drier areas than in areas with abundant rainfall.

D. medinensis is a large nematode about 1 to 2 mm wide and the female is 50 to 120 cm long; the male is shorter, measuring 4 to 8 cm and rarely up to 12 cm. The adult worm lives in subcutaneous tissues of the human.

The life cycle starts with the young worms in the body of the gravid female. The female travels to the skin, usually of the lower extremities (82 percent of the time) and elsewhere. The parasite produces a blister in the skin of the host through which the uterus is projected. Upon contact with water, as when bathing, the blister bursts, releasing the young worms into the water. The larvae (about 600 µm) are ingested by copopeds (water fleas) of the genus *Cyclops,* where they undergo one or two molts and become infective in 10 to 20 days. Definitive hosts (humans and dogs) acquire the infections by ingesting cyclops in the drinking water. The larvae are liberated in the gastrointestinal tract of the host and migrate to the connective tissue where they mature in about 8 to 12 months

from the time of entry. After fertilization, the male dies and the female travels to the skin and repeats the cycle.

There are no symptoms of infection until the skin ulcer is formed. Before the skin is broken, severe systemic symptoms develop including urticaria, erythematous rashes, malaise, and fever. Asthma may occur. There follows an intense inflammatory reaction around the anterior end of the worm, probably produced by the products of the worm or its metabolites (Fig. 225-8). The symptoms subside with the development of the ulcer. The ulcer is small, usually not larger than 5 mm, but may enlarge with secondary infection. It is possible to have more than one worm in the same individual.

After several weeks, when the process of larval discharge is completed, the worm dies and may calcify without further symptoms. Secondary bacterial infections, chronic pruritus, arthritis, synovitis, ankylosis, and contracture may develop later.

Traditional treatment is surgical removal. The worm can be removed by gently and slowly winding it on a small stick. Breakage of the worm in the process may lead to severe inflammation. Diethylcarbamazine (Banocide, Hetrazan) is effective in the early stages only. Thiabendazole has been reportedly effective in killing the worm and reducing the inflammation.

Lymphatic Filariasis   (See Fig. 225-9)   Lymphatic filariasis, chronic infection with the filarial nematodes *Wuchereria bancrofti, Brugia malayi,* and *Brugia timori,* is the most widespread of the filarial diseases, affecting up to 90 million people worldwide. While *W. bancrofti* is found throughout the tropics and subtropics, the geographic distribution of *Brugia* species is limited to areas of south and southeast Asia (for *B. malayi*) and to the Indonesian islands of Timor and Flores (for *B. timori*). The mosquito vector (*Culex, Mansonia, Aedes,* or *Anopheles*) and periodicity of blood microfilaremia (nocturnal, subperiodic, or nonperiodic) vary depending on filarial species and geographic region. Despite these differences, the life cycles and clinical manifestations of infection are quite similar for these three filarial pathogens (Partono, 1987).

Infective larvae, released by the mosquito vector while feeding, slowly mature in the human host to the 8- to 10-cm-long, threadlike, adult parasites that reside and mate in the lymph nodes and lymphatic vessels. From 3 months to 2 years after infection, sheathed microfilariae, released by the adult female, may be de-

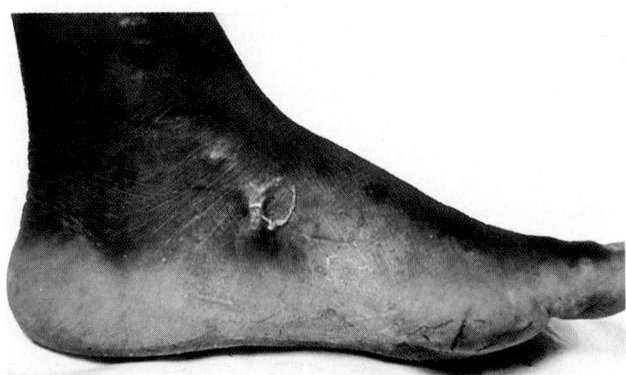

FIGURE 225-8   Dracunuclosis (Guinea worm). The worm is seen emerging from the skin on the medial side of the foot.

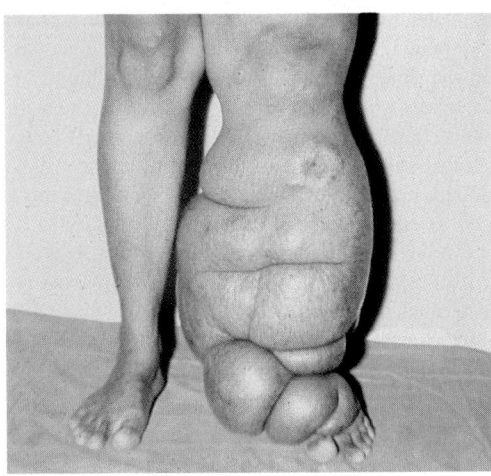

FIGURE 225-9   Lymphatic filariasis. Severe elephantiasis of the lower extremity. (*Courtesy of the Armed Forces Institute of Pathology, Washington, D.C.*)

tected in the peripheral blood and occasionally in hydrocele fluid and urine. Taken up during a blood meal by the mosquito, the microfilariae develop into infective larvae in 10 to 14 days to complete the life cycle. The three most common manifestations of lymphatic filariasis are asymptomatic microfilaremia (microfilariae in the blood), "filarial fevers," and lymphatic obstruction. "Filarial fevers" are recurrent episodes of acute adenitis and lymphangitis, accompanied by high fevers and chills. Occurring as often as ten times per year, the episodes generally last 3 to 7 days before resolving spontaneously. The characteristic "retrograde" lymphangitis extends distally from the affected lymph node. Transient lymphedema may develop during the acute attack and, in *Brugia* infections, lymphatic inflammation may lead to ulceration and draining sterile abscess formation. Microfilaremia is usually absent. With passage of time, some patients in endemic areas develop lymphatic stasis and obstruction leading to irreversible elephantiasis of the extremities (Fig. 225-9). Frequent superinfection of involved skin may contribute to this process. In *W. bancrofti* infection, genital involvement is common and includes funiculitis, epididymitis, and scrotal lymphedema or hydrocele. Obstruction and rupture of renal lymphatics may lead to intermittent chyluria.

Diagnosis may be made by morphologic identification of the microfilariae in the blood, hydrocele fluid, or urine or, rarely, by identification of an adult worm in tissue biopsy. In patients with detectable microfilariae in the blood, the characteristic clinical findings, positive antifilarial serology, and an adequate exposure history are sufficient for presumptive diagnosis.

Until recently, the only effective chemotherapy for lymphatic filariasis was diethylcarbamazine (DEC). At doses of 6 mg/kg body weight per day for 12 to 14 days, DEC is a potent microfilaricide with some activity against adult worms. Single-dose ivermectin shows similar microfilaricidal activity and posttreatment reactions and may soon replace DEC in the treatment of lymphatic filariasis because of the ease of administration (Ottesen, 1990). Although chemotherapy and conservative measures (i.e., leg elevation, elastic stockings, local foot care) may reverse early lymphedematous changes, chemotherapy is generally ineffective in cases of advanced elephantiasis. Surgical bypass of lymphatic blockages may greatly improve symptomatology in these patients.

Tropical pulmonary eosinophilia is an uncommon syndrome of filarial etiology seen primarily in young men (Uwadia, 1967). It is characterized by nocturnal asthma, fever, and adenopathy with marked peripheral blood eosinophilia ($>3000/\mu$L) in the absence of microfilaremia. Antifilarial antibody titers and IgE levels are extremely high. Chest x-rays may be abnormal, and pulmonary function tests characteristically show a restrictive defect. Treatment with DEC causes a rapid clinical improvement, although some individuals continue to have active pulmonary inflammation. Untreated, this condition leads to severely debilitating, chronic interstitial lung disease.

Loiasis *Loa loa* is a filarial parasite that causes chronic infection in humans, characterized by Calabar swellings (migratory angioedema) and subconjunctival migration of adult parasites (Fig. 225-10a). Although *Loa loa* is endemic only in central and west Africa, and a small focus in the Sudan, as many as 13 million people are estimated to be infected; in hyperendemic areas, exposure, as defined by seropositivity, approaches 100 percent.

Human infection results from the bite of an infected deerfly of the genus *Chrysops*. In the host, the infective larvae mature into adult worms that migrate through the subcutaneous tissues. After several months, adult females help to produce microfilariae, which

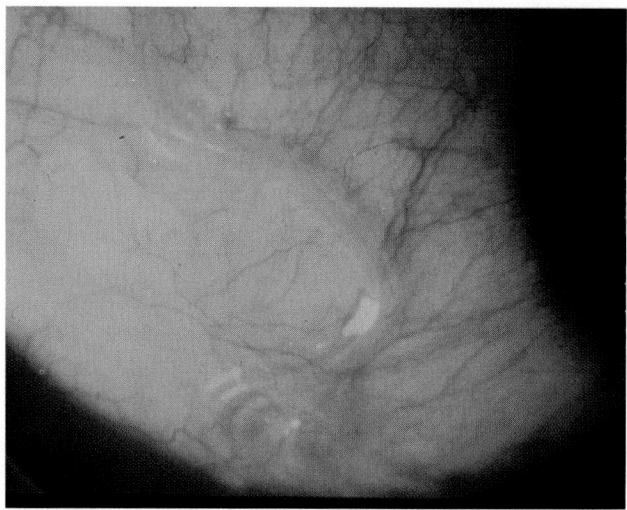

a

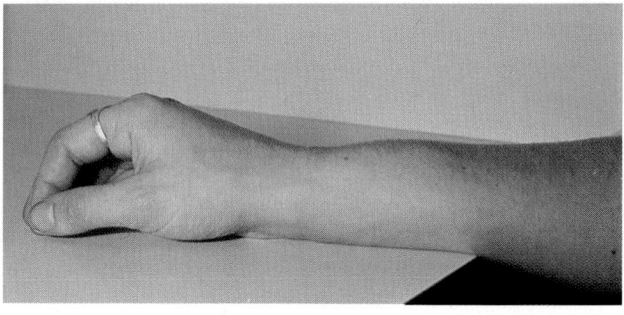

b

FIGURE 225-10 Loiasis. (*a*) Subconjunctival migration of an adult parasite. (*b*) Calabar swelling of the forearm. (*Courtesy of the Armed Forces Institute of Pathology, Washington, D.C.*)

are usually blood-borne. These may be taken up by the vector in a blood meal. Adult parasites have been reported to live up to 16 years in an untreated host.

The clinical presentation of loiasis in individuals from endemic regions differs significantly from that of long-term visitors to these regions. Endemic patients with *Loa loa* infection are often asymptomatic despite microfilaremia (detectable microfilariae in the blood) (Noireau et al., 1990). In contrast, loiasis in long-term visitors to endemic areas is characterized by Calabar swellings, areas of localized angioedema, and an absence of detectable microfilariae in the blood (Nutman et al., 1986). Often heralded by pruritus and erythema, Calabar swellings (Fig. 225-10b) may last from a few hours to several days. They often involve the extremities but may occur on the face or trunk. Nonspecific symptoms, such as generalized pruritus, arthralgia, myalgia, and fatigue, are also reported by a majority of patients. Subconjunctival migration of the adult worm ("eyeworm") is seen in a minority of endemic and nonendemic patients. Clinical complications, although rare, include cardiomyopathy, nephropathy, peripheral neuropathy, and encephalopathy.

Parasitologic diagnosis is made by morphologic identification of sheathed microfilariae in a daytime blood sample or, rarely, by surgical extraction of an adult parasite. In patients without detectable microfilaremia, the diagnosis is based on clinical presentation, laboratory tests (hypereosinophilia, elevated antifilarial antibody levels), and exclusion of other filarial infections.

Diethylcarbamazine (DEC), at a dose of 8 to 10 mg/kg body weight for 21 days, is effective against both microfilariae and adult worms, although several courses of therapy may be necessary for complete cure. Posttreatment swellings and subcutaneous nodules are common and may contain dying adult parasites. In patients with high levels of microfilaremia, concurrent administration of corticosteroids and antihistamines, as well as apheresis to reduce the parasite load, may be necessary to prevent complications of therapy (including encephalitis). DEC prophylaxis (300 mg once a week) has been shown to prevent loiasis in temporary residents of endemic areas (Nutman et al., 1988).

Onchocerciasis (River Blindness) The filarial nematode *Onchocerca vulvulus* has been estimated to infect 18 million people in equatorial Africa, Central and South America, Saudi Arabia, and Yemen and is the second leading infectious cause of blindness worldwide. Spread by the blackflies of *Simulium* spp., onchocerciasis is found primarily in hilly or mountainous areas near rapidly flowing streams or rivers where blackfly larvae breed. Humans are the only reservoir of infection in nature, although related *Onchocerca* species infect a variety of other mammals.

Infective larvae, deposited on the skin by the blackfly during a blood meal, enter the host and develop over a period of 10 to 20 months into adult parasites that are commonly found coiled in subcutaneous nodules. The adult females produce millions of sheathless microfilariae that migrate throughout the skin and subcutaneous tissues and only rarely invade the blood or internal organs. Skin microfilariae, ingested by biting blackflies, molt twice and are again ready to infect the human host in 7 to 10 days.

The clinical manifestations of onchocerciasis most commonly involve the skin, subcutaneous tissues, lymph nodes, and eye (Taylor, 1985). The characteristic "onchocercomata" are firm, mobile, nontender subcutaneous nodules (Fig. 225-11*a*), which contain adult parasites coiled within relatively acellular fibrous tissue. These nodules are characteristically located over bony prominences, most commonly over the iliac crest and buttocks in African patients and the head and shoulders in Central American patients. Early onchocercal dermatitis (Fig. 225-11*b*) may present as pruritus alone or as a generalized pruritic maculopapular eruption, with asymmetric distribution. Hyperpigmentation of affected areas is also common. With passage of time, the skin loses elasticity, becomes abnormally wrinkled and, ultimately, lichenifies and atrophies (Fig. 225-11*c*). Mottled depigmentation may be seen, especially over the shins. Enlarged inguinal and femoral nodes are common in African patients and, in extreme cases, may lead to local dependent edema ("hanging groin"). A clinical variant, "sowda," initially described in natives of Yemen, is characterized by a hypertrophic, hyperpigmented dermatitis of the lower extremities without detectable skin microfilariae.

Eye involvement occurs in patients with moderate-to-heavy infection and is most common in the savanna regions of Africa. Punctate keratitis, a result of acute inflammation around dying microfilariae in the anterior chamber, is seen early in disease. Later, chronic inflammation can lead to sclerosing keratitis and blindness. Anterior uveitis, chorioretinitis, and iridocyclitis are also seen.

Parasitologic diagnosis may be made by identification of adult parasites on nodulectomy or, more commonly, by the demonstration of microfilariae in superficial skin snips taken from the scapular, iliac, and thigh areas and incubated overnight in physiologic saline. The Mazzotti test, administration of a small test dose of diethylcarbamazine to elicit symptoms in patients with occult infec-

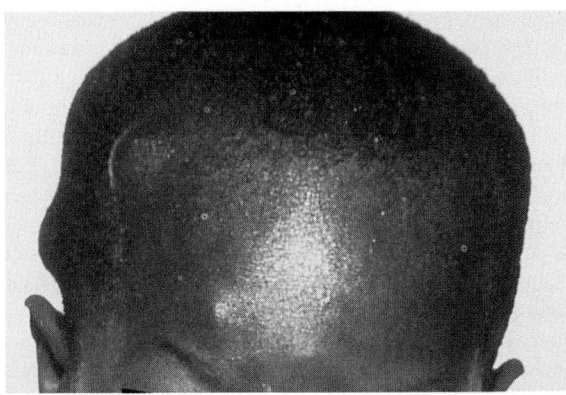

a

b

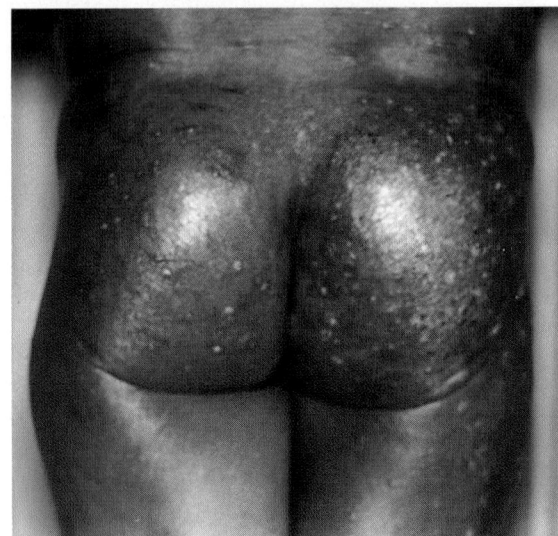

c

FIGURE 225-11 Onchocerciasis. (*a*) Subcutaneous nodules on the head of a patient with onchocerciasis. (*Courtesy of Brian O.L. Duke, M.D.*) (*b*) Early onchocercal dermatitis. (*c*) Severe lichenification of the buttocks with papular lesions caused by microfilariae. Nodular lesions with adult worms are not seen. They are mainly localized over bony prominences of the hips, ribs, knees, and elbows.

tion, is no longer recommended in routine diagnosis, as it can lead to exacerbation of ocular disease. Newer diagnostic techniques, including the use of ultrasonography to identify occult nodules and serodiagnostic tests using recombinant antigens, should prove useful in detecting patients with early infection or low levels of skin microfilariae.

The recommended treatment for onchocerciasis is ivermectin, 200 μg/kg body weight, in a single oral dose (Greene et al., 1985). As ivermectin is active only against microfilarial forms of the parasite, repeated treatment at 6- to 12-month intervals is necessary. Although a transient increase in dermatologic symptoms may occur after the initial dose of ivermectin, treatment has not been associated with an increase in ocular disease. Suramin (100 to 200 mg intravenously, followed by 1 g intravenously weekly for 5 weeks) is the only drug available that is active against the adult *Onchocerca volvulus* parasite. Because of the risk of dose-related hematologic and renal toxicity, this drug should be reserved for highly symptomatic patients unlikely to return to an endemic area.

Chemoprophylaxis has not been demonstrated to prevent onchocercal infection. Consequently, the mainstay of prevention is avoidance of blackfly bites through the use of insect repellants and proper clothing.

Bibliography

GENERAL
Botero DL: Epidemiology and public health importance of intestinal infections in Latin America. *Prog Drug Res* **19**:28, 1975
Burke JA: Round worm infections of the gastrointestinal tract—current concepts. *J Ky Med Assoc* **74**:279, 1976
Noble ER et al: *Parasitology: The Biology of Animal Parasites,* 6th ed. Philadelphia, Lea & Febiger, 1989

AMEBIASIS
Abdus-Sattar AB: An unusual case of cutaneous amebic ulcer. *J Trop Med Hyg* **82**:201, 1979
Adams AB, MacLeod IN: Invasive amebiasis 1. Amebic dysentery and its complications. *Medicine (Baltimore)* **56**:315, 1977
Biagi F, Martuschelli QA: Cutaneous amebiasis in Mexico. *Dermatol Trop* **2**:129, 1963
Faust EC: The multiple facets of *Entamoeba histolytica* infections. *Int Rev Trop Med* **1**:43, 1961
Fujita WH et al: Cutaneous amebiasis. *Arch Dermatol* **117**:309, 1981
Ganor S: *Entamoeba histolytica:* A possible cause of pruritus. *Int J Dermatol* **20**:26, 1981
Guerrant RL: The global problem of amebiasis: Current status, research needs and opportunities for progress. *Rev Infect Dis* **8**:218, 1986
Patterson M et al: Serologic testing for amebiasis. *Gastroenterology* **78**:136, 1980
Sunarwan E: A case of cutaneous amoebiasis. *Dermatologica* **151**:253, 1975
World Health Organization: Amebiasis. Report of WHO Expert Committee. *WHO Tech Rep Ser* **42**:1, 1969

TRYPANOSOMIASIS
Apted FIC: Sleeping sickness in Tanganykia—past, present and future. *Trans R Soc Trop Med Hyg* **56**:15, 1962
Apted FIC: Trypanosomiasis. *Trop Dis Bull* **61**:457, 1964
Carbonetto CH et al: Isolation of a *Trypanosoma cruzi* antigen by affinity chromatography with a monoclonal antibody. Preliminary evaluation of its possible application in serological tests. *Clin Exp Immunol* **82**:936, 1990

Chattas A et al: Chagas' disease in children (American trypanosomiasis). *Ann Pediatr* **201**:37, 1963
Davey DG: Human and animal trypanosomiasis in Africa. *Am J Trop Med Hyg* **7**:546, 1958
Greenwood BM, White HC: Complement activation in patients with Gambian sleeping sickness. *Clin Exp Immunol* **24**:133, 1976
Iayawardena AN, Waksman BH: Suppressor cells in experimental trypanosomiasis. *Nature* **265**:539, 1977
Jones IG et al: Electrocardiographic changes in African trypanosomiasis caused by *Trypanosoma rhodeniensis. Trans R Soc Trop Med Hyg* **69**:388, 1975
Kellersberger ER: African sleeping sickness. Review of 9000 cases from central Africa. *Am J Trop Med* **13**:211, 1933
Kierszenbaum F, Budzko DB: Immunization against experimental Chagas' disease by using culture forms of *Trypanosoma cruzi* killed with a solution of sodium perchlorate. *Infect Immun* **12**:461, 1975
Lambert PH, Whittle HC: The pathogenesis of sleeping sickness. *Trans R Soc Trop Med Hyg* **74**:716, 1980
Toledo-Banos HA et al: In vitro cellular immunity in Chagas' disease. *Clin Exp Immunol* **38**:376, 1979
World Health Organization: Comparative studies of American and African trypanosomiasis. *WHO Tech Rep Ser* **411**:1, 1969
World Health Organization: African trypanosomiasis. *WHO Tech Rep Ser* **63**:1, 1979

LEISHMANIASIS
Bryceson ADM; Immunological aspects of cutaneous leishmaniasis, in *Essays on Tropical Dermatology,* edited by J Marshall. Amsterdam, Excerpta Medica, 1972, p 230
Chong H: A look at trends in and approaches to the treatment of leishmaniasis. *Int J Dermatol* **25**:615, 1986
Frankenburg S: A simplified microtechnique for measuring human lymphocyte proliferation after stimulation with mitogen and specific antigen. *J Immunol Methods* **112**:177, 1988
Kurban AK et al: Histopathology of cutaneous leishmaniasis. *Arch Dermatol* **93**:396, 1966
Liew FY: Functional heterogeneity of CD4+ T cells in leishmaniasis. *Immunology Today* **10**:40, 1989
Manuel J: Macrophage-parasite interactions in *Leishmania* infections. *J Leuk Biol* **47**:187, 1990
Modabber F: Experiences with vaccines against cutaneous leishmaniasis: Of mice and men. *Parasitology* **98**:549, 1989
Muller I et al: Analysis of the cellular parameters of the immune responses contributing to resistance and susceptibility of mice to infection with the intracellular parasite, *Leishmania major. Immunol Rev* **112**:95, 1989
Ribiero JMC et al: A novel vasodilatory peptide from the salivary glands of the sand fly *Lutzomyia longipalpis. Science* **243**:212, 1989
Schnur LF, Jacobson RL: *Parasitological Techniques in the Leishmaniases.* London, Academic, 1987, vol 1, p 499
Scott P: The role of Th1 and Th2 cells in experimental cutaneous leishmaniasis. *Exp Parasitol* **68**:369, 1989
Titus RG, Ribeiro JMC: Salivary gland lysates from the sand fly *Lutzomyia longipalpis* enhance leishmania infectivity. *Science* **239**:1306, 1988
Walters LL et al: Ultrastructural biology of *Leishmania (Viannia) panamensis* (= *Leishmania braziliensis panamensis*) in *Lutzomyia gomezi* (Diptera: Psychodidae): A natural host-parasite association. *Am J Trop Med Hyg* **40**:19, 1989

CYSTICERCOSIS
Boveja UK et al: Enzyme linked immunoabsorbent assay for the diagnosis of human neurocysticercosis. *J Commun Dis* **22**:55, 1990
Faust EC et al (eds): *Clinical Parasitology,* 8th ed. Philadelphia, Lea & Febiger, 1970
Flisser A et al: Praziquantel treatment of brain and muscle porcine *Taenia solium* cysticerciasis. *Parasitol Res* **76**:640, 1990

Mahajan RC et al: Comparative evaluation of indirect hemagglutination and complement fixation tests in serodiagnosis of cysticercosis. *Indian J Med Res* **63**:121, 1975

Raimer S, Wolf JE Jr: Subcutaneous cysticercosis. *Arch Dermatol* **114**:107, 1978

Sotelo J et al: Praziquantel in the treatment of neurocysticercosis: Long-term followup. *Neurology* **35**:752, 1985

Tsang VCW et al: An enzyme linked immunotransfer blot assay and glycoprotein antigens for diagnosing human cysticercosis (*Taenia solium*). *J Infect Dis* **159**:752, 1985

ECHINOCOCCUS (HYDATID CYST)

Amman RW et al: Recurrence rate after discontinuation of long-term mebendazole therapy in alveolar echinococcosis (preliminary results). *Am J Trop Med Hyg* **43**:506, 1990

Baraka A et al: Anaphylactic reaction during hydatid surgery. An immunologic hazard. *Middle East J Anesthesiol* **5**:505, 1980

De Rosa F et al: Treatment of *E. granulosa* hydatid disease with albendazole. *Am J Trop Med Parasitol* **84**:467, 1990

Dressaint JP et al: Quantitative determination of specific IgE antibodies to *Echinococcus granulosa* and IgE levels in sera from patients with hydatid disease. *Immunology* **29**:813, 1975

Kannereo WS, Miller KL: *Echinococcus granulosa*—permeability of hydatid cyst to mebendazole in man. *Int J Parasitol* **11**:183, 1981

Kassis A, Tanner CE: Novel approach to the treatment of hydatid disease. *Nature* **262**:588, 1976

Kein P et al: Chemotherapy of echinococcus with mebendazole. Clinical observation in seven patients. *Trop Med Parasitol* **30**:65, 1979

Lightwoler MW: Immunology and molecular biology of *Echinococcus* infection. *Int J Parasitol* **20**:471, 1990

Majdaudzic J et al: Echinococcus multiloculare. *Med Welt* **32**:1060, 1981

Schanta PM et al: Chemotherapy for larval echinococcus in animals and humans. Report of workshop 2. *Parasitenka* **67**:5, 1982

Schwabe CW: *Veterinary Medicine and Human Health*. Baltimore, Williams & Wilkins, 1969

Thompson RC et al: Echinococcus: Biology and strain variation. *Int J Parasitol* **20**:457, 1990

SPARGANOSIS

Klinelles JF: The biology of spirometra. *J Parasitol* **60**:3, 1969

Kron MA et al: Abdominal sparganosis in Ecuador. A case report. *Am J Trop Med Hyg* **44**:146, 1991

Mueller JF et al: Human sparganosis in the United States. *J Parasitol* **49**:294, 1963

Phares CK, Cox GS: Molecular hybridization and immunologic data support the hypothesis that tape worm *Spirometra mansonides* has acquired a human growth hormone, in *Molecular Paradigm for Eradicating Helminth Parasites*, UCLA Symposia Series 60, edited by AJ MacInnes. New York, Alan Liss, 1987, p 391

Swartzwelde JC et al: Sparganosis in southern United States. *Am J Trop Med* **13**:43, 1964

Taylor RL: Sparganosis in the United States. Report of a case. *Am J Clin Pathol* **66**:560, 1976

SCHISTOSOMIASIS

Abdu-Aziz AH: Cutaneous bilharzial granuloma—a histologic study. *Cutis* **18**:516, 1976

Boros DL: Schistosomiasis mansoni: A granulomatous disease of cell mediated immune etiology. *Ann N Y Acad Sci* **278**:36, 1976

El-Mofty AM: Extragenital forms of cutaneous bilharziasis. *Br J Dermatol* **68**:252, 1956

El-Mofty AG et al: Evaluation of dot ELISA technique in the serodiagnosis of schistosomiasis in Egypt. *J Egypt Soc Parasitol* **20**:639, 1990

El-Zawahry M: Schistosomal granuloma of the skin. *Br J Dermatol* **77**:344, 1965

Faust EC et al: *Animal Agents and Vectors in Human Disease*. Philadelphia, Lea & Febiger, 1978, p 159

Kagan IG: Recent advances in the diagnosis of schistosomiasis. *Egypt J Bilharzia* **3**:121, 1976

Leishout LV et al: Assessment of cure in schistosomiasis with praziquantel by quantitation of circulating anodic antigen (CAA) in the urine. *Am J Trop Med Hyg* **44**:223, 1991

Watt G et al: Praziquantel in the treatment of cerebral schistosomiasis. *Lancet* **2**:529, 1986

CERCARIAL DERMATITIS (SWIMMER'S ITCH)

Cart WW: Studies on schistosome dermatitis: Status of knowledge after more than twenty years. *Am J Hyg* **52**:251, 1950

Hoeffer DF: "Swimmer's itch" (cercarial dermatitis). *Cutis* **19**:461, 1977

Mulvihill CA et al: Swimmers itch: A cercarial dermatitis. *Cutis* **46**:211, 1990

LARVA MIGRANS (CREEPING ERUPTION) AND STRONGYLOIDIASIS

Bank DE et al: The thumbprint sign; rapid diagnosis of disseminated strongyloidiasis. *J Am Acad Dermatol* **23**:324, 1990

Battistini F: Treatment of creeping eruption with topical thiabendazole. *Tex Rep Biol Med* **27**(suppl 2):645, 1969

Beaver PC: Zoonosis with particular reference to parasites of veterinary importance, in *Biology of Parasites. Emphasis on Veterinary Parasites*, edited by EJ Soulsby. New York, Academic, 1966

Campbell WC, Cuckler AC: Thiabendazole in the treatment and control of parasitic infections in man. *Tex Rep Biol Med* **27**(suppl 2):665, 1969

Davis CM, Israel RM: Treatment of creeping eruption with topical thiabendazole. *Arch Dermatol* **97**:325, 1968

Kramer MR et al: Disseminated strongyloidiasis in AIDS and non-AIDS immunocompromised hosts: Diagnosis by sputum and bronchioalveolar lavage. *South Med J* **83**:1226, 1990

Smith JD et al: Larva migrans, cutaneous strongyloidiasis. *Arch Dermatol* **112**:1161, 1976

Stone OJ et al: Cutaneous strongyloidiasis. Larva currens. *Arch Dermatol* **106**:734, 1972

GROUND ITCH (UNCINARIAL DERMATITIS)

Jung RC, McCroan JE: Efficiency of bephenium and tetrachloroethylene in mass treatment of hookworm infections. *Am J Trop Med* **9**:492, 1960

Miller TA: Hookworm infections in man. *Adv Parasitol* **17**:315, 1979

Most H: Treatment of more common worm infections. *JAMA* **185**:874, 1963

ENTEROBIASIS (THREADWORM)

Clark RF: Localized urticaria due to *Enterobius vermicularis*. *Arch Dermatol Syph* **84**:1026, 1961

Symers W St C: Pathology of oxyuriasis with special reference to granulomas due to presence of *Oxyuris vermicularis* (*E. vermicularis*) and its ova in tissues. *Arch Pathol* **50**:475, 1960

TRICHINOSIS

Barriga OO: Reactivity and specificity of *Trichinella spiralis* fractions in cutaneous and serological tests. *J Clin Microbiol* **6**:274, 1977

Gould SE: *Trichinosis in Man and Animals*. Springfield, IL, Charles C Thomas, 1970

Stone OJ et al: Thiabendazole. A probable cure for trichinosis. *JAMA* **187**:536, 1964

DRACUNCULOSIS

Faust EC et al: *Animal Agents and Vectors in Human Disease*. Philadelphia, Lea & Febiger, 1975

Hopkins DR et al: Dracunculosis eradication: Target 1995. *Am J Trop Med Hyg* **43**:296, 1990

Muller R: Dracunculosus and dracunculosis. *Adv Parasitol* **9**:73, 1971

Muller R: Guineaworm eradication. The end of another old disease. *Parasitol Today* **2**:39, 1986

Raffer G: Efficacy of thiabendazole in the treatment of dracunculiasis. *Tex Rep Biol Med* **27**(suppl 2):601, 1969

LYMPHATIC FILARIASIS

Ottesen EA et al: A controlled trial of ivermectin and diethylcarbamazine in lymphatic filariasis. *N Engl J Med* **232**:1113, 1990

Partono F: The spectrum of disease in lymphatic filariasis. *Ciba Found Symp* **127**:15, 1987

Uwadia FE: Tropical eosinophilia: A correlation of clinical, histopathologic and lung function studies. *Dis Chest* **52**:531, 1967

LOIASIS

Noireau F et al: Clinical manifestations of loiasis in an endemic area in the Congo. *Trop Med Parasitol* **41**:37, 1990

Nutman TB et al: *Loa loa* infection in temporary residents of endemic regions: Recognition of a hyperresponsive syndrome with characteristic clinical manifestations. *J Infect Dis* **154**:10, 1986

Nutman TB et al: Diethylcarbamazine prophylaxis for human loiasis. Results of a double-blind study. *N Engl J Med* **319**:752, 1988

ONCHOCERCIASIS

Greene BM et al: Comparison of ivermectin and diethylcarbamazine in the treatment of onchocerciasis. *N Engl J Med* **313**:133, 1985

Taylor HR: Infectious causes of blindness II. Onchocerciasis. *Rev Infect Dis* **7**:787, 1985

SECTION 37

Bites and Stings

CHAPTER 226

Mark Jordan Scharf and Ann Sullivan Baker

Bites and Stings of Terrestrial and Aquatic Life

The Book of Genesis promised man dominion over the fish of the sea and every living thing that moved upon the face of the earth. Unfortunately, it did not guarantee that every encounter between man and beast would be free from harm. The first two sections of this chapter consider the harmful effects of landborne animal bites as well as the bacterial and viral infections they may transmit. The remaining section reviews bites and stings and other forms of injury that may be inflicted by marine life.

Animal Bites

More than 500,000 animal bites are reported yearly in the United States; dog bites constitute the largest group. The human victim is usually a 7- to 9-year old boy, often teasing or playing with the dog. The biting dog is usually 6 to 12 months old, is often female, and is usually a working dog, such as a boxer, collie, German shepherd, Great Dane, or Saint Bernard, or a sporting dog, such as a pointer, setter, or retriever. Hounds, for some reason, are relatively safe.

The evaluation and treatment of all bite wounds should include a careful history of the incident, the type of animal, the site of the bite, and the geographic setting. Hand wounds and puncture wounds most often become infected. Most bites should be cultured and a Gram-stained smear prepared; the wound should then be washed, well irrigated, and left open. Selection of an antibiotic depends on the bite history and Gram's stain results. Most patients with deep cat bites, deep cat scratches, and sutured wounds should be treated with penicillin, amoxicillin-clavulinic acid, cefuroxime, or tetracycline because of the increased incidence of *Pasteurella multocida* infection. Tetanus immune status should be evaluated and rabies immunization considered.

Human bites and monkey bites deserve special mention as 30 percent become infected with aerobic or anaerobic mouth organisms. Anaerobic infection may spread through the metacarpal-phalangeal space and cause severe damage. The same procedure as for other animal bites should be followed, that is, culture and Gram's stain, thorough washing, and wide dissection. Wounds should be left open if possible, especially hand wounds. Patients with human bites should be treated with penicillin for 7 to 10 days. Clenched fist injuries should be evaluated by a hand surgeon.

Specific Bacterial Infections Caused by Animal Bites

Pasteurella multocida   A common organism infecting bite wounds is *P. multocida*. Disease due to this organism is now diagnosed more frequently; thus, its presence in the nasopharynx in 50 percent of dogs and 75 percent of cats is of public health importance.

Most infections in humans fall into one of three clinical patterns:

1. The most common pattern is that of *local infection with adenitis* after a dog or cat bite or scratch. In patients with a cat bite, this may then progress to tenosynovitis or osteomyelitis due to inoculation of the organism into the periosteum by the long, sharp tooth of the animal. Canine teeth are more blunt and less likely to penetrate the periosteum.
2. The second pattern is *chronic pulmonary infection,* in which *P. multocida* may occur as the primary pathogen or in association with other organisms. Bacteria may enter through the respiratory tract by inhalation of barn dust or infectious droplets sprayed by the sneeze of an animal. In such cases, the bacteria probably colonize the respiratory tract and lie dormant in the patient with chronic lung disease. Acute infection occurs only after trauma to the bronchial tree. Bronchiectasis, emphysema, peritonsillar abscess, and sinusitis have all been described with this organism.
3. Finally, *systemic infection with bacteremia or meningitis* may occur.

P. multocida is a small, gram-negative, ovoid bacillus that grows well on blood agar but does not grow on gram-negative media, such as MacConkey agar. Because of its superficial resemblance to *Haemophilus influenzae* and *Neisseria* organisms, respiratory tract and central nervous system infection with *P. multocida* may be misdiagnosed initially. Failure of growth on routine gram-negative media is an important clue.

Treatment of the patient with presumptive *P. multocida* infection (i.e., any patient with a deep cat bite or scratch or a deep dog bite) should consist of careful washing and an attempt to leave the wound open. The antibiotic of choice is penicillin, orally for 7 to 10 days, with careful follow-up of the wound. Ampicillin, amoxicillin-clavulinic acid, and tetracycline as well as ciprofloxacin and trimethoprim-sulfamethoxazole are alternatives.

Staphylococcus intermedius *S. intermedius* is an organism associated with dogs weighing more than 40 pounds.

Capnocytophaga canimorsus A fastidious, slow-growing, gram-negative rod associated with dog bites. Most infections occur in the splenectomized or immunocompromised host and present as overwhelming sepsis.

Afipia gelis and Rochalimaea Species These organisms have been described as the etiology of cat-scratch disease (see also Chap. 189).

Plague (See Chap. 190)

Tularemia (See Chap. 190)

Rat-Bite Fever (See Chap. 190)

Viral Infections Caused by Animal Bites

Rabies (See also Chap. 184) The most notorious viral disease caused by an animal bite is rabies. The epidemiology has changed in the past few years. Now, nonimmune dogs account for only 16 percent of cases, whereas sylvatic animals, such as skunks, raccoons, red and gray foxes, bats, and domestic dogs represent the greatest potential danger; rodents, such as squirrels and hamsters, are probably inconsequential as sources of rabies.

Live virus is introduced into nerve tissue at the time of the bite. The virus persists 96 h at the site and then spreads to the central nervous system. It replicates in gray matter and then spreads along autonomic nerves to the salivary glands, adrenal glands, and heart. The incubation period varies with the site of the bite, from 10 days to as long as 1 year.

Clinical features include a prodromal period of 1 to 4 days, followed by high fever, headache, and malaise. Paresthesia at the site of inoculation occurs in 80 percent of patients. The next sequence of events is familiar: agitation, hyperesthesia, dysphagia, paralysis, and death.

DIAGNOSIS. The fluorescent antibody method for the viral antigen is the most rapid and sensitive means of making the diagnosis. Brain biopsy of the animal is also useful.

PREVENTION AND TREATMENT. The most effective prevention for rabies is to avoid contact with any wild animal or any unfamiliar domestic animal. Persons at risk of unavoidable contact with rabies, such as spelunkers, veterinarians, virologists, and travelers spending time in countries where rabies is enzootic, should receive preexposure prophylaxis. Human diploid cell vaccine should be given in these cases. The neutralizing antibody titer should be followed to assure immunity in high-risk or exposed persons.

The need for postexposure prophylaxis can be determined by the answers to the following questions: What is the status of animal rabies in the locale where the exposure took place? Was the attack provoked or unprovoked? Of what species was the animal? What was the state of health of the animal?

Most animals transmit rabies virus in saliva only a few days before becoming ill themselves (dog and skunk, 5 days; fox, 3 days; cat, 1 day; bats, however, may harbor the virus for many months).

Bites by Household Pets If the dog or cat is healthy and available for observation for 10 days, do not treat the patient unless the animal develops rabies. At the first sign of rabies in the animal, treat the patient with rabies immune globulin (RIG) and human

diploid cell rabies vaccine (HDRV). The symptomatic animal should be killed and tested as soon as possible.

If the pet is rabid, or suspected of being rabid, or if it is a pet from outside of the United States (especially Latin America, Africa, and most of Asia), treat the patient with RIG and HDRV.

Bites by Wild Animals All skunks, bats, foxes, coyotes, raccoons, bobcats, and other carnivores should be regarded as rabid unless laboratory tests prove negative. Treat the patient with RIG and HDRV.

Bites by Other Animals Consider other animals (livestock, rodents, lagomorphs, e.g., rabbits, hares) individually. Local and state public health officials should be consulted about the need for prophylaxis. Bites by the following almost never call for antirabies prophylaxis: squirrels, hamsters, guinea pigs, gerbils, chipmunks, rats, mice and other rodents, rabbits, and hares.

Specifics of Treatment The most important step is to cleanse the wound immediately with a brush and soap to remove as much virus as possible. Rinse well, then perform a second scrub with green soap or alcohol, which is rabicidal.

If vaccine treatment is indicated, both RIG and HDRV should be given as soon as possible, regardless of the interval after exposure.

The administration of RIG is the more urgent procedure. If HDRV is not immediately available, start RIG and give HDRV as soon as it is obtained. RIG should be given to the patient immediately—50 percent around the site of the bite and 50 percent in the thigh or the arm. The dosage is 20 IU/kg. This passive immunization will result in the early appearance of antibody but will also inhibit development of the active antibody from the human diploid vaccine; thus, the reason for prolonged dosage of the vaccines.

Active immunization is accomplished with the human diploid cell vaccine. HDRV is given intramuscularly for a total of five doses. The doses are given on days 0, 3, 7, 14, and 28. Serum for rabies antibody testing should be collected 2 weeks after the fifth dose. If there is no antibody response, an additional booster should be given.

Management of the Patient with Clinical Rabies When the rare patient is admitted with the clinical diagnosis of rabies, several steps should be taken immediately. First the diagnosis must be made rapidly by fluorescent antibody staining of various tissues, as well as mouse inoculation with the animal's brain tissue. Elevated antibody titers in the absence of immunization are clear evidence of infection. The first signs of clinical rabies are usually nonspecific, such as malaise, anorexia, fatigue, headache, and fever. The acute neurologic illness that follows is most commonly characterized by intermittent episodes of hyperactivity. In some cases, however, a progressive paralysis is most common. The usual period from onset of symptoms to onset of coma is 10 days.

The basic clinical management consists of anticipating and preventing all treatable complications of the rabies infection. Pulmonary hypoxia should be prevented by tracheostomy at the first sign of respiratory difficulty, monitoring of actual P_{O_2}, and use of supplemental oxygen.

Anticonvulsant therapy should also be instituted. Extreme increases in intracranial pressure may be prevented by insertion of a cerebrospinal fluid reservoir connected to the lateral ventricle, allowing withdrawal of the intraventricular fluid and measurement of intracranial pressure.

Cardiac arrhythmias may be anticipated with careful monitoring.

Unfortunately there are no specific antiviral treatments for rabies at the present time.

Risk of exposure for hospital staff includes contamination of open wounds or mucous membranes with saliva or other potentially infectious material such as neurologic tissue, spinal fluid, or urine. Blood, serum, and stool are not considered infectious.

Rabies has been regarded as uniformly fatal. There have now been several cases that have survived with prolonged cardiorespiratory support. An aggressive approach in the patient with known rabies infection is certainly worthwhile.

Lymphocytic Choriomeningitis Lymphocytic choriomeningitis (LCM) virus is an infectious agent common to the house mouse but rarely transmitted to humans. More recently, outbreaks of LCM virus infection in the United States have been traced to pet hamsters. Hamsters, like mice, may excrete LCM virus for several months and may become lifelong carriers.

When humans are infected, there may be three major manifestations: a grippe-like illness, meningitis, or encephalitis. The cerebrospinal fluid formula usually reveals an increased mononuclear leukocyte count and hypoglycorrhachia. Symptomatic therapy is all that is available.

Simian Herpes B Virus Simian herpes B virus is found in old world monkeys, especially rhesus and cynomolgus species. Infection is usually caused by a bite and less commonly after inhalation of monkey saliva or contact with infected monkey cell cultures. A vesicular lesion develops at the wound site, with progressive lymphangitis and fever. Confusion, reduced tendon reflexes in lower extremities, and respiratory paralysis may follow.

Diagnosis depends on viral isolation or intranuclear inclusion bodies in lymph nodes, on a brain biopsy from patient or animal, or on a rise in neutralizing antibody titer to simian herpes B virus. Treatment is supportive.

Snake Bites

The two major poisonous snakes in the Americas are the pit viper and the coral snake. The coral snake belongs to the family Elapidae. All other poisonous snakes in this hemisphere belong to the family Viperidae. The subfamily of pit vipers includes the rattlesnake, water moccasin, and copperhead. There are about 7000 poisonous snake bites reported in the United States annually; the largest number occur in the southwestern and Gulf states.

Two poisonous snakes are native to New England. The northern copperhead, also called the highland moccasin, is pink or reddish brown and is marked with large chestnut-brown barrels resembling dumbbells or hourglasses (Fig. 226-1). The bite is painful but rarely fatal. The timber rattler is dark brown with chevrons of black and brown (Fig. 226-2).

The degree of toxicity of a snake bite depends on the potency of the venom, the amount injected, the size and condition of the snake, and the size of the person bitten. There are immediate clinical manifestations of the pit viper bite. Pain occurs at the site of the bite, as well as a wheal with local edema, numbness, and, within moments, ecchymosis and painful lymphadenopathy (Fig. 226-3). Nausea, vomiting, sweating, fever, drowsiness, and slurred speech may then develop. Bleeding of the gums and hematemesis are common hemorrhagic manifestations. For proper treatment, it is extremely important to establish that the bite is from a poisonous snake. The patient should have distinct fang punctures and immediate local pain, followed by edema and discoloration within 30 min. It is helpful to inspect the snake, since those that are poisonous may be differentiated from those that are not by the presence of fangs and the shape of the pupils (Fig. 226-4).

The limb should be immobilized and a ligature applied proximal to the wound. The ligature should be released for 90 s every 15 min. The physician should make two longitudinal incisions through the fang marks and apply suction intermittently for the first hour. An attempt should be made to neutralize the venom with immune serum. Emergency information and specific immune serum can be obtained from the Oklahoma City Poison Control Center (1-405-271-5454, 24 h a day). A photograph of snakes common to a specific geographic area is important for all hospital emergency wards.

Polyvalent pit viper antivenin should be used for all severe American snake bites except those of the coral snake. If possible, it

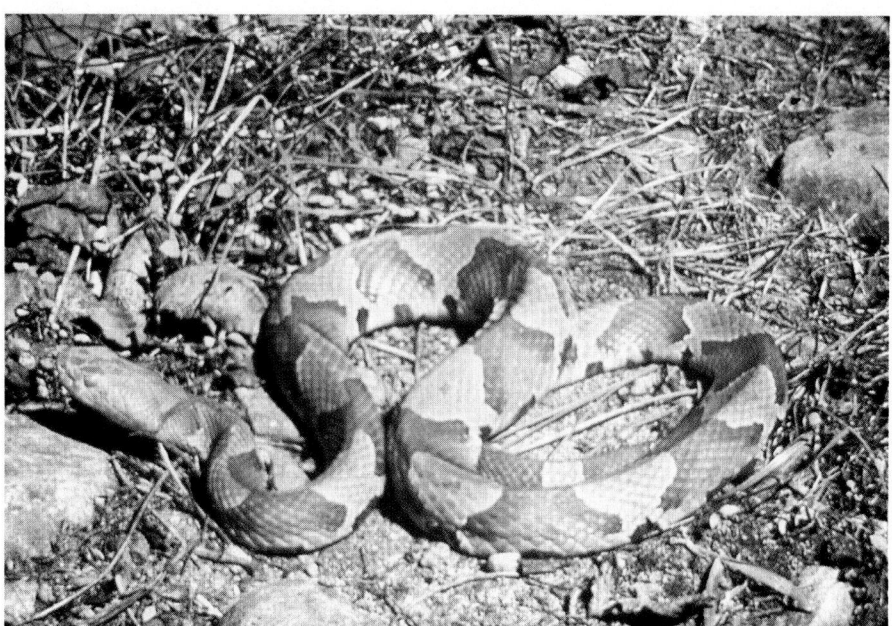

FIGURE 226-1 Northern copperhead.

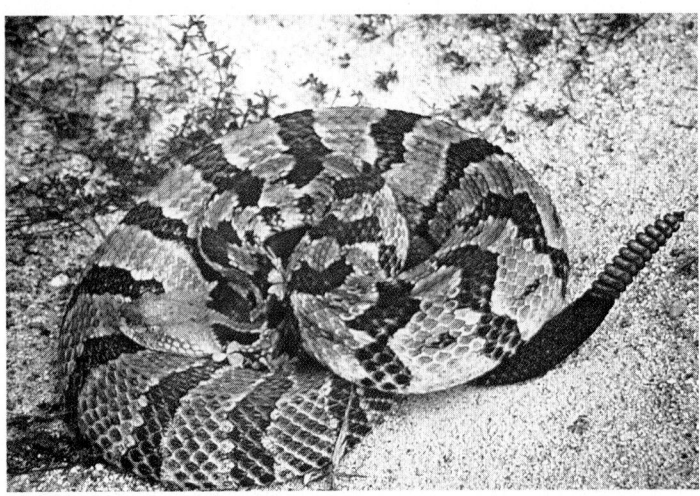

FIGURE 226-2 Timber rattler.

should be administered within 1 h of the bite, and the patient should first undergo skin testing for hypersensitivity to horse serum.

The dosage of antivenin for a moderate rattlesnake bite requires 4 to 7 vials (10 mL)—severe cases may require 15 to 20 vials; water moccasin bite requires 1 to 4 vials; for copperhead bites, antivenin is usually necessary only for a child or elderly patient. The vials should be diluted in 500 mL of normal saline and given intravenously over 30 min. Antitetanus therapy and antibiotic prophylaxis with penicillin, 2 g per day, or tetracycline, 2 g per day, should be initiated for severe bites.

Supportive treatment is important, that is, hospitalization, careful evaluation of baseline hematocrit, platelet count, and prothrombin time. The wound should be cleansed and covered. Surgical debridement of superficial necrosis should be performed between the third and tenth days.

Aquatic Bites and Stings

Seal Bite

Normally, a seal bite occurs on the finger of a trainer or a seal hunter, thus the term seal finger or Spaek finger. The etiologic

agent is unclear; *Mycoplasma phocedae* has been isolated in one case.

The incubation period of 4 to 8 days is followed by throbbing pain, erythema at the site, and swelling of the joint proximal to the bite. Untreated, Spaek finger progresses to cellulitis, tenosynovitis, and arthritis. The treatment before antibiotics were available was amputation of the affected finger to relieve the severe pain and deformity. Tetracycline, 500 mg orally four times a day for 10 days, is now the antibiotic of choice. It is also helpful to immobilize and elevate the finger as well as soak it several times a day.

Injuries Caused by Jellyfish, Portuguese Man-of-War, Sea Anemones, and Corals

Stings due to jellyfish, Portuguese man-of-war, sea anemones, and corals are the most common envenomations encountered by humans in marine environments. All these creatures are members of the phylum Cnidaria, formerly known as Coelenterata. Cnidarians are radially symmetric animals with body walls formed by an inner and outer layer of cells enclosing a jelly-like substance.[1,2] They are divided into three major classes: the first class, Hydrozoa, includes the Portuguese man-of-war, fire corals, and hydroids; jellyfish belong to the second class, called Scyphozoa; sea anemones and true corals are members of the third class, known as Anthozoa.

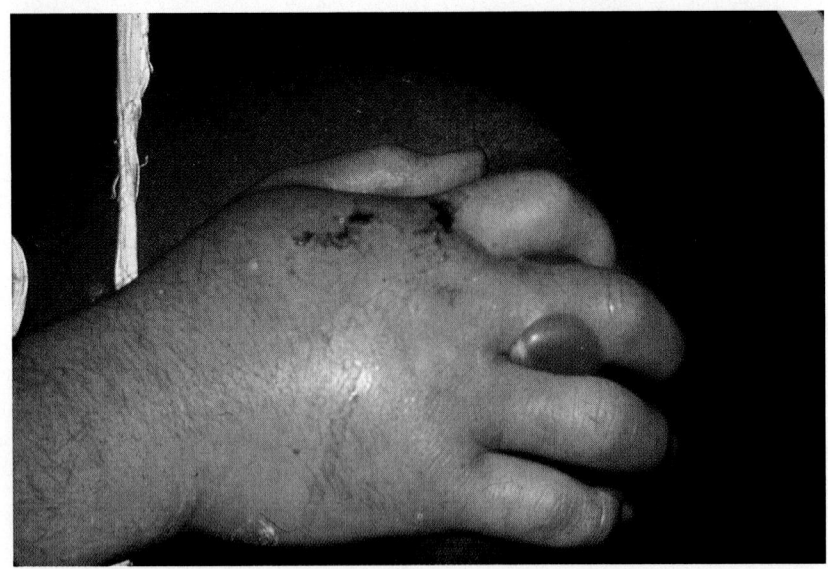

FIGURE 226-3 Copperhead snake bite.

Ways to Differentiate Poisonous From Harmless Snakes

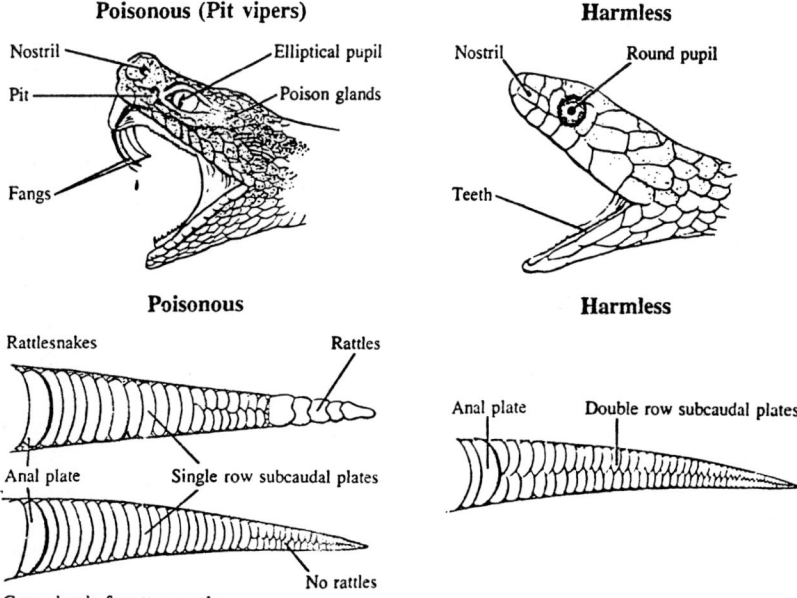

FIGURE 226-4 Identification of poisonous and nonpoisonous snakes. (*From Wingert WA, Wainschel W: A quick handbook on snake bites. Resident & Staff Physician, p 56, 1977. Reprinted with permission.*)

Almost all cnidarians possess nematocysts, or stinging capsules, which are usually concentrated on some form of tentacle. Each nematocyst contains a toxin or group of toxins and a coiled threadlike apparatus with a barbed end that functions like a flexible hypodermic syringe (Fig. 226-5). When the nematocyst comes into contact with an unwary victim, the barbed end is discharged and the toxin is injected into the skin.

Cnidarian stings may range from mild, self-limited irritations to extremely painful and serious injuries, depending on the toxin of the species involved and the magnitude of the envenomation. In certain species such as the cubomedusae, or box jellyfish, stings can be fatal.

In most cases, jellyfish stings elicit toxic rather than allergic types of reactions. These toxic reactions may be localized and/or systemic in nature and will be discussed in the following sections.

Although they occur less frequently, immediate-type hypersensitivity reactions including urticaria, angioedema, and anaphylaxis require prompt medical intervention as shock and death may ensue in highly sensitized individuals. Allergic contact dermatitis, delayed and persistent hypersensitivity reactions,[3] granuloma annulare,[4] and erythema nodosum[5] are several of the possible cutaneous reactions that can occur after jellyfish stings. A summary and classification of reactions to jellyfish stings appears in Table 226-1.

Injuries Caused by Jellyfish SEA NETTLES. Among the most common causes of jellyfish stings are the sea nettles which comprise two different species, both of which inhabit Atlantic as well as Indo-Pacific waters. *Cyanea capillata,* and its relatives, is the larger of the two species, with a bell measuring up to 1 m and numerous tentacles reaching 30 m in length[6] (Fig. 226-6).

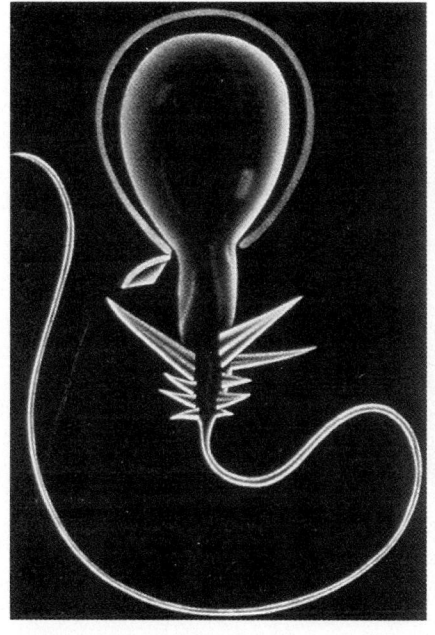
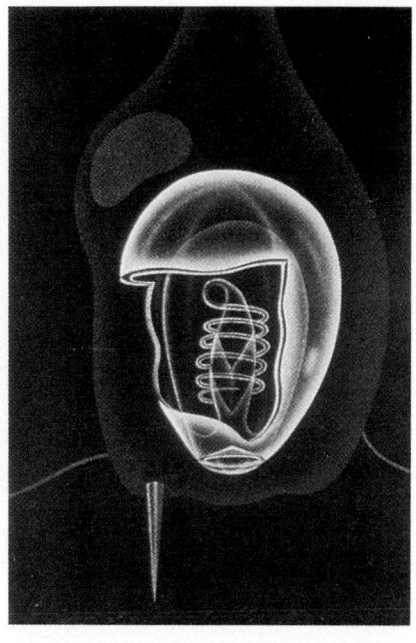

FIGURE 226-5 From left to right, a diagrammatic view of an intact and discharged coelenterate nematocyst. (*R. Kreuzinger, courtesy of World Life Research Institute.*)

TABLE 226-1
Local and Systemic Reactions to Jellyfish Stings

Reaction	Symptoms
Local reactions	
Immediate onset	Toxin-induced skin changes (wheals, papulovesicles, bullae), allergic reactions (exaggerated local reactions/angioedema)
Delayed onset	Delayed persistent reactions, recurrent reactions, persistent reactions, distant site reactions, contact dermatitis, papular urticaria, granuloma annulare, erythema nodosum
Complications and long-term sequelae	Postinflammatory pigmentary changes, scars (pruritic macular and papular), keloids, fat atrophy, neuropathy, limb necrosis due to gangrene secondary to arterial spasm, joint contractions
Systemic reactions	
Mild to moderate	Nausea, vomiting, diarrhea, headache, malaise, fever, chills, muscle aches, vertigo, ataxia, muscle weakness, delirium, Irukandji reaction
Severe or life-threatening	Immediate cardiac arrest, rapid respiratory arrest, intravascular hemolysis, delayed renal failure, allergic reactions, anaphylaxis

SOURCE: Adapted from Burnett.[6]

Chrysaora quinquecirrha is smaller, with a white or rusty bell that may reach 30 cm with four digestive tentacles hanging from it.[6]

Although sea nettle stings have not been reported to be lethal, they can be quite painful. Initially the victim experiences a sharp burning pain in the area contacted by the tentacles. Within minutes, the sting area develops a zig-zag shaped, whiplike pattern of raised red welts 2 to 3 mm wide (Fig. 226-7). The duration of acute pain may vary, but it often begins to subside in 30 min. The wheals usually subside by 1 h, but purplish-brown petechial and postinflammatory pigmentation may persist for several days in the sites of tentacle contact.

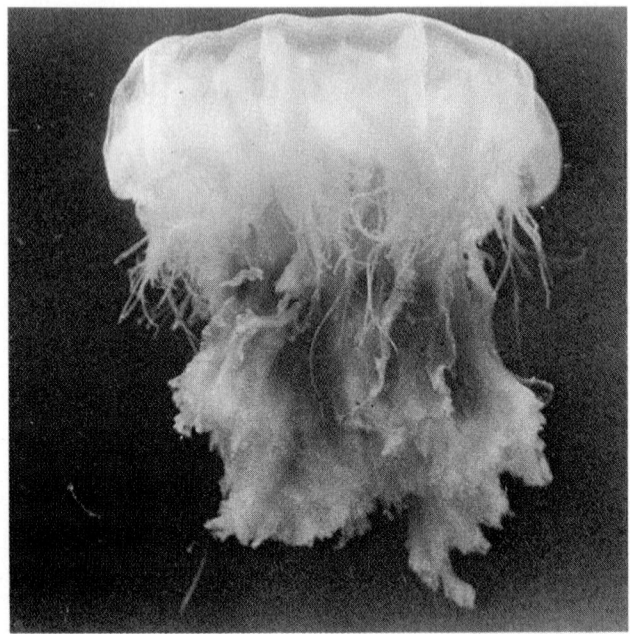

FIGURE 226-6 *Cyanea capillata*, also known as the sea nettle or lion's mane, is a common cause of jellyfish stings. *(B.W. Halstead, courtesy of World Life Research Institute.)*

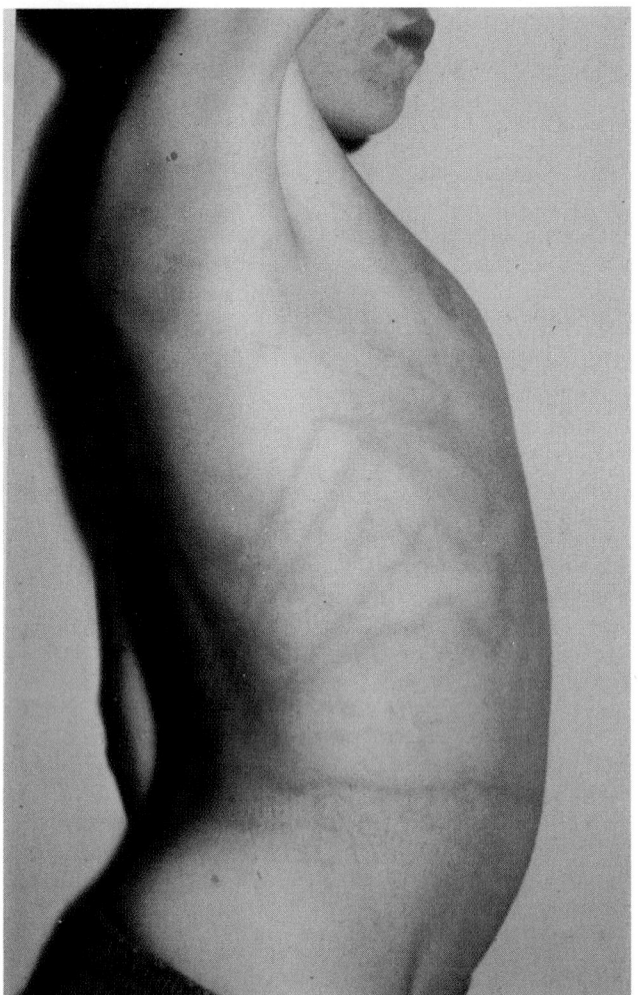

FIGURE 226-7 Whiplike sting pattern due to *Cyanea capillata* in a young boy. *(J.H. Barnes, courtesy of World Life Research Institute.)*

PORTUGUESE MAN-OF-WAR.   *Physalia physalis* is the species name for the Portuguese man-of-war, which is a member of the class Hydrozoa and is therefore not a true jellyfish. *P. physalis* is encountered in both Atlantic and Mediterranean waters and is easily recognized by its translucent blue to pink or purple, bladder-like float with multiple tentacles suspended from it (Fig. 226-8). Both the floating bell and the tentacles are composed of large colonies of hydroids. *P. physalis* is distinguished from its Pacific ocean relative *P. utriculus,* commonly known as the blue bottle, in that *P. physalis* has a larger bell ranging in size from 10 to 30 cm with multiple fishing tentacles extending up to 30 m, whereas *P. utriculus* has only a single tentacle that rarely exceeds 5 m.[6] These tentacles are armed along their entire length with hundreds of thousands of nematocysts arranged in stinging batteries, with each battery containing hundreds of nematocysts. The nematocysts remain active even after portions of the tentacles are broken off in storms or when these animals are stranded on the shoreline by high winds or waves. Beached Portuguese man-of-war can cause a severe sting when stepped on or touched. Children who are stung after handling these animals inadvertently cry and rub their eyes and may develop an acute conjunctivitis.[7]

Stings from *P. physalis* are more painful and severe than those caused by sea nettles and are more extensive and serious than those

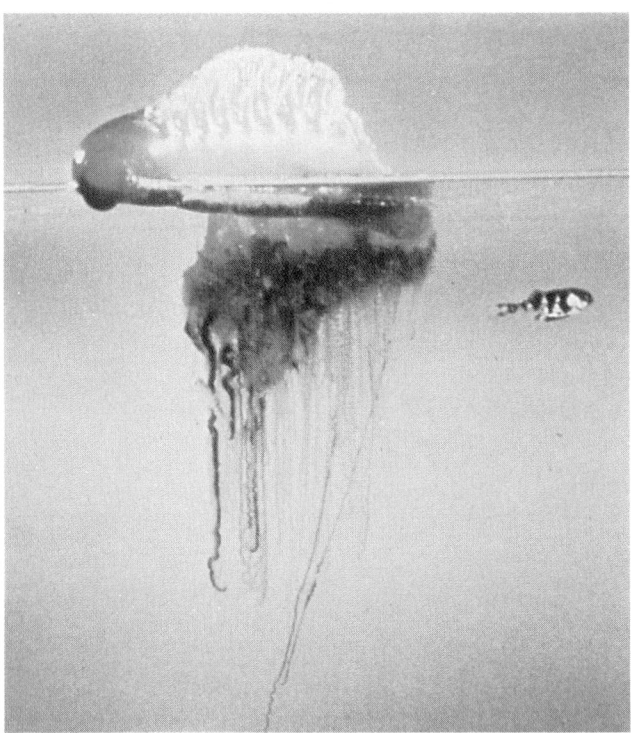

FIGURE 226-8 *Physalia physalis,* the Portuguese man-of-war, is distinguished by its bladder-like float and numerous trailing tentacles. (*B.W. Halstead, courtesy of World Life Research Institute.*)

caused by *P. utriculus.* At the moment of contact with the tentacles of *P. physalis,* the unfortunate victim experiences a sharp, shock-like, burning pain. There may be painful paresthesias or numbness in the sting area.

Initially the sting area appears as an irregular single line or multiple lines composed of red papules, beaded streaks, or erythematous welts that correspond to the areas of tentacle contact. The wheals resolve in several hours but may progress to vesicular,

hemorrhagic, necrotic, or ulcerative stages before healing[2] (Fig. 226-9). Postinflammatory striae may persist for weeks to months. Permanent scarring may occur in some instances.[7] Severe localized complications of *P. physalis* stings may also include arterial spasm in the sting site, which can result in distal digital gangrene of the affected limb.[8,9]

Within 10 to 15 min of a *Physalia* sting, the victim may develop symptoms of an envenomation reaction characterized by nausea, abdominal cramps, muscular pains, backache, irritability, dyspnea, and chest tightness. Intravascular hemolysis and acute renal failure have been reported following a severe sting by *P. physalis* in a 4-year-old girl.[10,11] Until recently, reports of fatal stingings due to *P. physalis* were not well documented; however, in 1989 there were two separate well-substantiated case reports of human fatalities caused by *P. physalis* envenomation.[12,13]

CUBOMEDUSAE (BOX JELLYFISH OR SEA WASPS). Of all the species of jellyfish that cause painful stings and distress to swimmers, the species with the most established record of lethality is the box jellyfish, *Chironex fleckeri.*[14] Since 1884 it has been responsible for at least 55 confirmed deaths throughout the Indo-Pacific region, with 40 deaths occurring along the shores of Northern Australia.[15] At least one death occurs each year in Australia.[14] The fatality is usually a child, presumably because the size of the victim and the total area of the sting determine the likelihood of mortality.

C. fleckeri (commonly known as the sea wasp) is an advanced species of jellyfish, with a semitransparent cubic bell that may grow to a volume of 9 L and weigh more than 6 kg[14] (Fig. 226-10). Trailing from the bell are up to 60 stinging tentacles, which may reach 2 to 3 m in length.[14] When a human comes into contact with a box jellyfish, some of the tentacles are torn off and adhere to the skin. Rescuers of *C. fleckeri* sting victims must exercise extreme caution, as they too are at risk of envenomation until the tentacles have been neutralized and removed.

The stings appear initially as linear welts that give the patient the appearance of having been whipped.[14] Fresh stings of *C. fleckeri* are easily recognized because they display a diagnostic frosted cross-hatched or ladder-like appearance[15] (Fig. 226-11). Conscious victims who suffer sublethal stings describe the pain as instantaneous and excruciating.[16] The pain may persist for many hours.

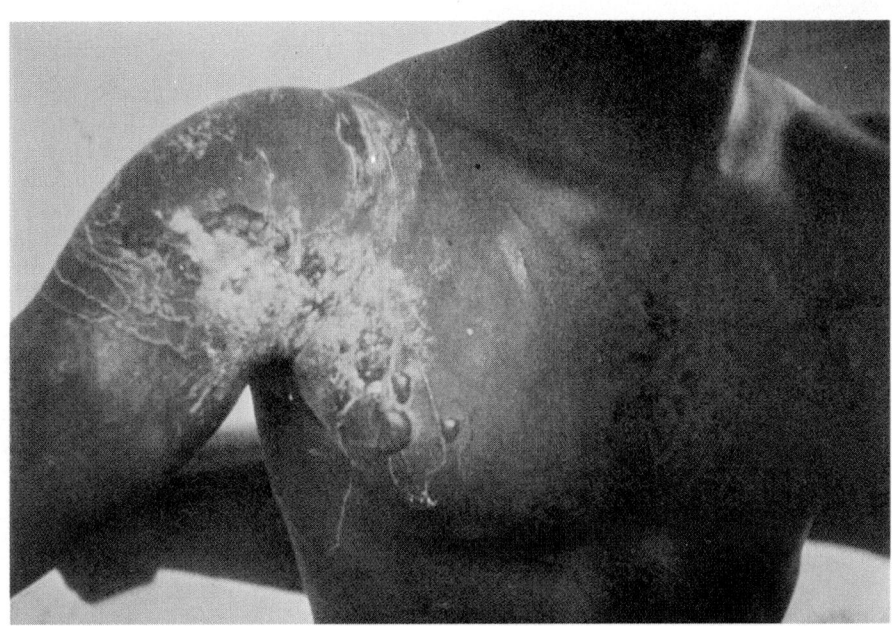

FIGURE 226-9 This unfortunate diver surfaced directly under a large Portuguese man-of-war and suffered a severe sting with bulla formation and tissue necrosis. (*S. Anderson, courtesy of World Life Research Institute.*)

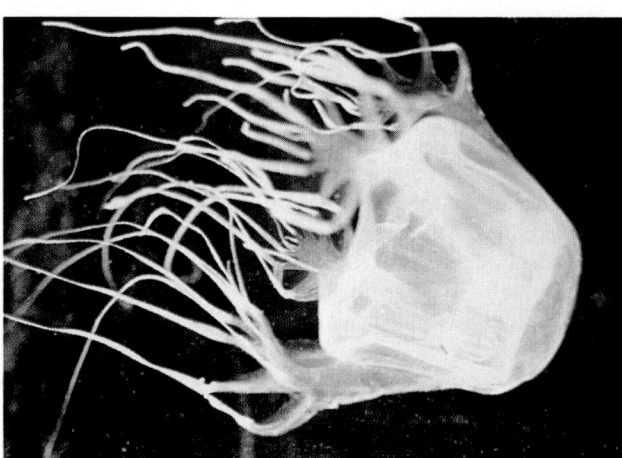

FIGURE 226-10 The deadly box jellyfish, *Chironex fleckeri*, is found in Indo-Pacific waters off the coast of Northern Australia. (*Courtesy of R. Hartwick.*[21])

Severely stung areas of skin take on a dusky cyanotic appearance and may go on to blister formation and necrosis.[16] The healing process is slow and may be complicated by bacterial superinfection.[16] Permanent scarring is often seen.

Death may ensue within minutes if ≥6 m of tentacles have made contact with the victim. Pharmacologic analysis of the venom of *C. fleckeri* has resulted in the isolation of dermatonecrotic, hemolytic, and lethal fractions.[15,17] The lethal fractions contain cardiotoxic and neurotoxic agents.[15,17] Intravascular hemolysis due to hemolytic fractions in the toxin can precipitate acute renal failure. The potent cardiotoxins can produce ventricular arrhythmias and cardiac arrest, and the neurotoxins lead to respiratory failure. First aid for these victims frequently requires cardiopulmonary resuscitation. Intravenous verapamil has been proposed for both treatment and prophylaxis of ventricular arrhythmias in sting victims.[18,19] Antivenin is available for *C. fleckeri* stings and its early use in severe envenomations may be lifesaving. In addition to blocking or reversing the systemic effects of the toxins, the antivenin has also been shown to significantly reduce the pain and inflammation at the sting site.[14,20]

Prevention and Treatment of Jellyfish Stings PREVENTION.[15,18]

1. Swim only at patrolled beaches with properly trained lifeguards and adequate treatment facilities.
2. Close bathing beaches during periods of high jellyfish infestation.
3. Avoid swimming in infested waters, especially after a storm, as stings may result from remnants of floating damaged tentacles.
4. Beware of apparently dead or beached jellyfish.
5. Wear protective clothing when snorkeling or scuba diving, such as wet suits, long-sleeved shirts, pants or long woolen underwear, and gloves.

TREATMENT. *First Aid Treatment*[1,2,6,20–23]

1. Remove or rescue the victim from the water.
2. Stabilize vital functions: airway, breathing, circulation.
3. Immobilize the affected part to prevent further envenomation by adherent tentacles.

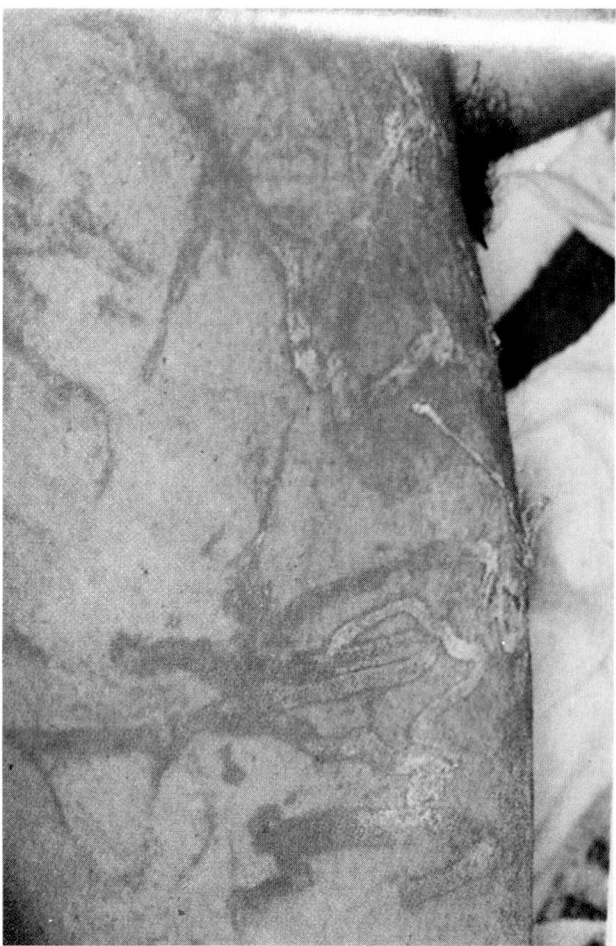

FIGURE 226-11 Characteristic frosted cross-hatched tentacle marks are diagnostic of a sting due to *Chironex fleckeri*. (*Courtesy of Townsville General Hospital, Department of Medical Illustration, Townsville, Queensland.*[21])

4. Identify the type of jellyfish sting by considering locale, time of year, and indigenous species and by observing the sting pattern. Preserve a portion of the tentacle for future identification.
5. To prevent further envenomation of the victim and to reduce the chance of a sting to the rescuer, disarm the nematocysts before removing the adherent tentacles.
   a. If *C. fleckeri* or *Physalia* species are suspected, douse or spray dilute acetic acid (3 to 10%) or household vinegar over all areas of tentacle contact for at least 30 s.[21,22]
   b. For sea nettles, mix sodium bicarbonate (baking soda) with water to form a slurry and pour over the affected area or apply the powder directly to the tentacles.[22]
   c. If vinegar or baking soda is unavailable, papain, available as a powdered meat tenderizer, may be applied directly as a powder or mixed in water as a slurry to sting areas and tentacles of both sea nettles and Portuguese man-of-war.[1,21]
   d. If nothing else is available, the tentacles can be rinsed off with seawater.
   e. Do not use fresh water, methylated spirits, or alcohol in any form to deactivate tentacles as these all may cause a rapid massive discharge of nematocysts.[1,2,21]

6. Once the tentacles have been disarmed, they may be carefully removed with a forceps or gently scraped away from the skin with a plastic card, shell, or knife.[2,23]

Treatment of Systemic Reactions

1. Support vital functions with cardiopulmonary resuscitation, oxygen, and intravenous fluids as required.[20]
2. Treat symptoms of anaphylaxis or shock with systemic epinephrine, corticosteroids, and antihistamines.[6]
3. A proximal venous-lymphatic constriction bandage should be considered in the case of severe stings where systemic reactions are present or likely to occur, where topical deactivation of tentacles is not possible, and transport to an acute care facility will be delayed.[6,23]
4. Specific antivenin is available for *C. fleckeri* stings. It is prepared by Commonwealth Serum Laboratories, Parkville, Victoria, Australia.[6] The antivenin is prepared from sheep serum and may therefore pose a risk of allergic reaction in sensitive individuals.[6] The preferred route of administration is intravenous, but it may be given intramuscularly. In severe stingings it has proved lifesaving. It is also the only treatment that can alleviate the intense pain (often within minutes of administration).[16] It may also reduce the cutaneous inflammation at the sting site and decrease the chance of scarring.[15]
5. Intravenous verapamil has been advocated both for treatment and prophylaxis of arrhythmias.[18,19]
6. For pain in severe stingings consider parenteral narcotic analgesics,[24] ice packs,[24] and antivenin in cases involving *C. fleckeri*.

Treatment of Local Reactions

1. Apply topical anesthetic ointments, creams, lotions, or sprays to relieve itching or burning pain. (Benzocaine preparations should be avoided because of the risk of contact dermatitis.)[1]
2. Cleanse ulcerated or open wounds three times daily, apply an antiseptic or antibiotic cream or ointment, and cover as needed with a light dressing.
3. Treat secondary infections with the appropriate parenteral antibiotics.
4. For delayed-type hypersensitivity reactions, use topical corticosteroids, antihistamines, and systemic corticosteroids if necessary.[6]
5. Antitetanus therapy should be considered, if indicated.
6. Ice or cold packs can relieve the pain of mild to moderate stings from many types of jellyfish.[24]
7. Aspirin or acetaminophen, alone or in combination with codeine, can be used to relieve persistent pain.[2]

Sea Anemone Dermatitis   Sea anemones are members of the phylum Cnidaria, class Anthozoa. They are sessile creatures with graceful flowery tentacles armed with nematocysts (Fig. 226-12). Although stings due to sea anemones are not as common as those due to fire corals and jellyfish, they are a frequent cause of dermatitis in sponge fishermen, sponge divers, and beachcombers who gather snails and crabs from rocky hollows along the shore.[25] Their toxicity to humans depends on the species.

The genus *Sagartia* is worth noting because it is the cause of "sponge fisherman's disease."[1] This anemone lives at the base of sponges sought by commercial fishermen. When they harvest or sort the sponges with their bare hands or forearms, they are likely to

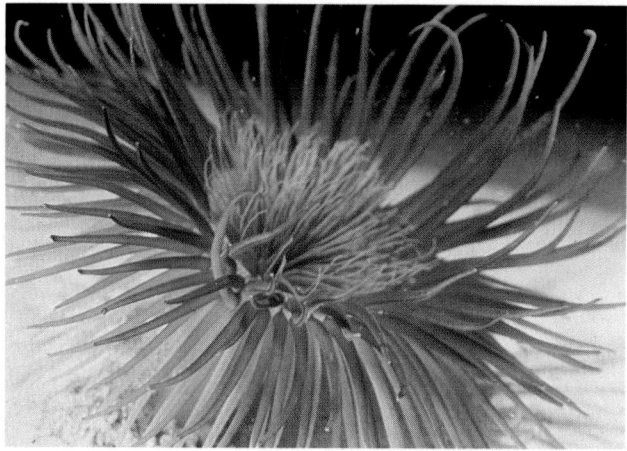

FIGURE 226-12   The flowery tentacles of the sea anemone can cause envenomations similar to jellyfish stings. (*Courtesy of Marty Gilman, Worcester, MA.*)

come into contact with the tentacles of *Sagartia*. Symptoms of itching and burning occur at the sting site within minutes of the exposure and are accompanied by erythema, edema, and vesicles.[1]

Other species of sea anemones with especially venomous stings include *Actinodendron*, *Anemonia sulcata*, and *Triactis producta*. Severe stingings may progress to vesiculation, ulceration, necrosis, and occasionally abscess formation.[2] Systemic symptoms may follow the exposure and can include headache, nausea, vomiting, fever, chills, muscle spasms, abdominal pain, malaise, thirst, and prostration.[1,2]

Treatment of sea anemone stings is similar to that of jellyfish envenomations (see above). The tentacles, if still adherent, should be removed carefully with a gloved hand and the sting area rinsed with sea water.[1] Sea anemone sting sites often heal slowly and may require treatment with antibiotics.

Injuries Caused by Fire Coral and Coral Cuts   Corals are colonial organisms belonging to the phylum Cnidaria. They form calcified structures of various sizes and shapes by cementing together their limestone exoskeletons or polyps.[25] True corals are members of the class Anthozoa. Fire corals are members of the class Hydrozoa and are not true corals, although they are similar in many ways.

Coral injuries may be divided into two major types, superficial injuries due to nematocyst stings and lacerations. It is entirely possible for both injuries to occur at the same time. Coral injuries may be complicated by foreign-body reactions, bacterial infections, and localized eczematous reactions.

Nematocyst envenomation in most true corals is a relatively innocuous experience, resulting in mild pruritic erythema that requires little if any treatment.[26] Calamine lotion or antipruritic lotions may bring relief.[27]

In contrast to true corals, the sting from the fire coral, *Millepora alcicornis*, is quite painful, as many scuba divers and snorkelers from the Florida Keys to the Caribbean will attest (Fig. 226-13). The wet mucous membrane surrounding the organism contains numerous nematocysts that readily discharge on contact with the skin, resulting in an immediate burning and stinging pain. Within one to several hours a pruritic erythematous papular eruption appears, which in severe cases may become pustular. Lesions heal in 1 to 2 weeks, often with postinflammatory hyperpigmentation.

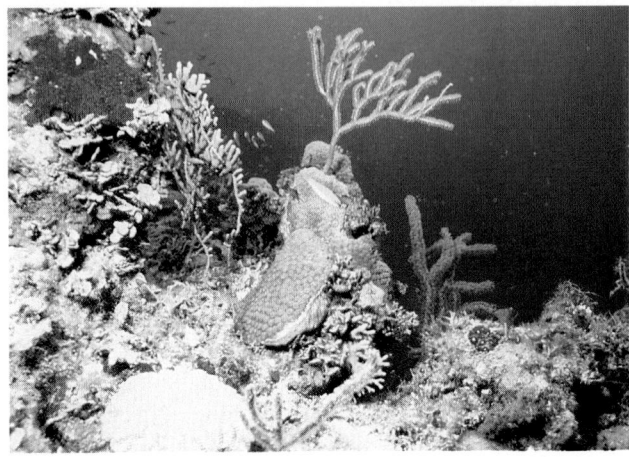

FIGURE 226-13 The mustard-colored fingerlike outcropping in the upper right quadrant of this formation of coral and hydroids is a typical example of fire coral.

The sting may be prevented by wearing protective clothing. Fire coral stings should be rinsed with sea water to remove undischarged nematocysts. Both sea water compresses, hot to the point of tolerance, and alcohol compresses are reported to inactivate the toxin. A topical steroid cream or ointment may relieve pruritus and promote healing.

Lacerations from the razor-sharp exoskeletons of coral are known collectively as coral cuts. They may be suffered by beach walkers, waders, fishermen, swimmers, surfers, and scuba and skin divers. Coral cuts can be prevented by avoiding dangerous shorelines and by wearing protective clothing such as reef boots, gloves, long pants made of a thick cut-resistant material, or a wet suit.

Coral cuts are notorious for their slow healing and their propensity for secondary infection. Factors that complicate healing in coral cuts include:

1. Wounds often involve the lower extremities and these generally heal more slowly due to decreased tissue blood supply.
2. Wound edges are often irregular, contused, crushed, and abraded.
3. Contamination of wounds is likely, due to pathogenic bacteria found in shore waters.
4. Foreign bodies, including marine algae growing on the coral or portions of the coral itself, may be implanted into the wound.
5. Victims of coral cuts are often actively engaged in water sports and may not comply with optimal wound care.[28]

Treatment of coral cuts[29] should begin with vigorous cleansing of the wound with soap and water with a soft brush or rough towel, followed by copious irrigation with saline to remove foreign bodies. If the wound is extensive, local anesthesia may be required in order to adequately cleanse, explore, debride, and achieve good hemostasis.[28] Hydrogen peroxide washing of the wound before dressing it is recommended.[25]

The decision to close a coral cut wound primarily or allow it to heal by secondary intention depends on the location of the wound, the degree of tissue trauma at the wound margins, and the likelihood of subsequent infection.[28] Facial and scalp wounds can often be converted to surgically clean wounds by debridement and closed

primarily.[28] Trunk and arm wounds may be closed primarily but require more surgical judgement. Lower extremity wounds in most cases will heal slowly by secondary intention. Tape stripping is preferable to suturing of leg wounds because sutured leg wounds have a high chance of abscess formation.[28]

Once the wound has been closed, an antibiotic ointment covered with a nonstick dressing, with an outer dressing applying light pressure for 24 to 48 h, is advisable.[28] Rest and elevation will promote healing. It should also be remembered that coral cuts are tetanus prone and require tetanus prophylaxis, depending on the patient's immunization history.[28]

Failure to remove foreign debris following a coral injury may result in foreign-body reactions. Localized episodes of dermatitis have been reported following contact with coral (Fig. 226-14). The lesions may appear within several hours and begin as erythematous papules; these coalesce to form plaques, which may become vesicular. Biopsy of these lesions reveals a superficial and middermal perivascular infiltrate of lymphocytes, eosinophils, and plasma cells resembling an arthropod bite reaction.[26] In some patients these eruptions have been recurrent. Topical steroids may be helpful in treating these eczematous reactions.

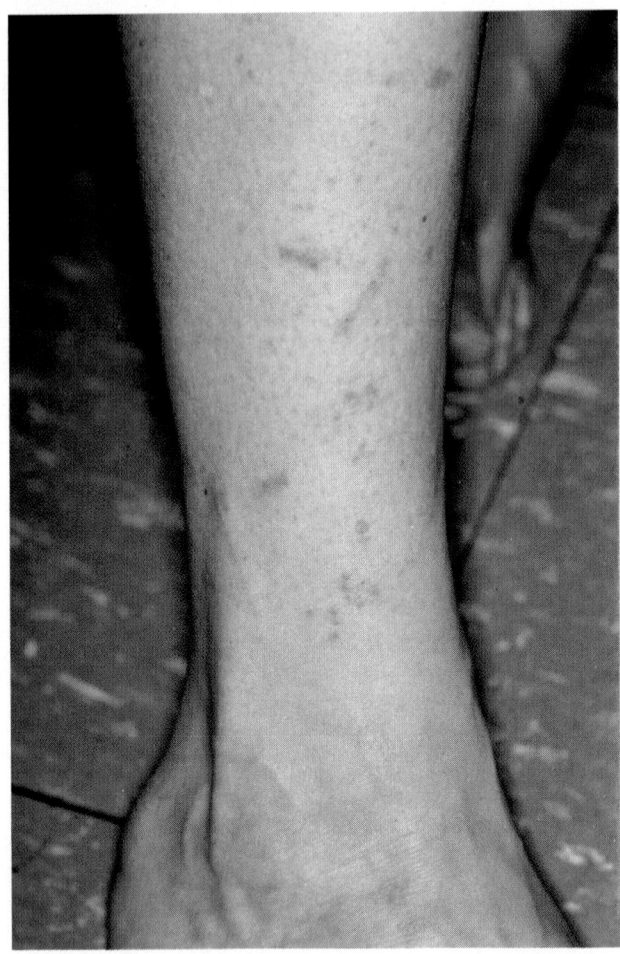

FIGURE 226-14 A contact dermatitis-like eruption resembling poison ivy occurred on the unprotected leg of this scuba diver 24 to 48 h after contact with an unknown type of coral. The eruption persisted for several weeks and cleared after treatment with topical steroid creams.

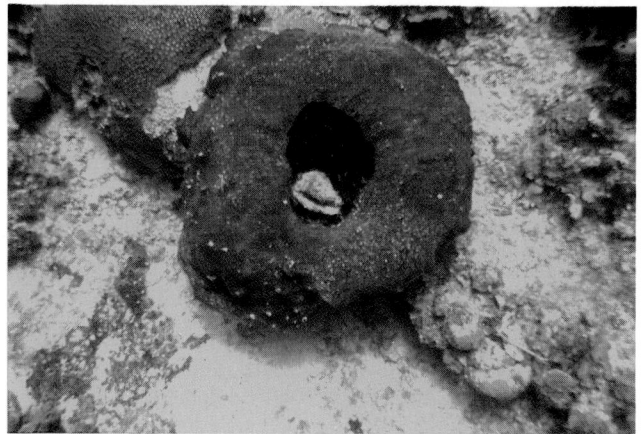

FIGURE 226-15 The poison bun sponge, *Fibula nolitangere,* can cause a severe irritant or toxin-induced contact dermatitis.

Dermatitis from Sponges

Sponges are members of the phylum Porifera, class Desmospongiae. They are simple multicellular animals that live attached to the sea bottom. Sponges grow by forming a series of hollow-centered branching tubes composed of a fibrous material called spongin, which contains spicules of calcium carbonate or silica.[1,30] Spicules from certain species of sponges are capable of penetrating the skin, causing a localized irritant or foreign-body reaction. Treatment of sponge spicule dermatitis involves tape stripping of the affected area.

There are at least 13 species of sponges that can cause a toxic dermatitis.[31] Of these the most commonly encountered are the West Indian and Hawaiian fire sponge, *Tedania ignis;* the poison bun sponge, *Fibula nolitangere* (Fig. 226-15); and the red sponge, *Microciona prolifera,* found in the northeastern United States.[31] These creatures are covered by a surface liquid, or slime, that produces an irritant or toxin-induced dermatitis when contacted by bare skin.[30]

Symptoms of itching, prickling, stinging, or burning appear within minutes of exposure and are followed within a few hours by pain, swelling, and stiffness.[1,30,31] If the fingers are involved, they often become immovable within 24 h.[1] The first cutaneous sign of sponge poisoning is local erythema, which progresses to a papular, vesicular, or bullous eruption with weeping of a serous or purulent fluid.[30,31] Desquamation of the site occurs within several days. Erythema multiforme and anaphylactoid reactions have been reported to occur in highly sensitized individuals.[32]

Treatment of sponge dermatitis is similar to that of severe poison ivy. The acute dermatitis can be treated with cool dilute vinegar soaks [30 mL of vinegar per liter of water (2 tbsp/qt water)] several times a day.[31] Soothing lotions, topical steroids, and antihistamines may improve symptoms, which usually begin to subside in several days.

Injuries due to Echinoderms: Sea Urchins, Starfish, and Sea Cucumbers

Sea Urchins Sea urchins are spiny creatures that belong to the phylum Echinodermata, class Echinoidea. They are encased in a fragile, roughly spherical, calcareous shell, which is protected by a formidable array of mobile spines and pincer-like organs known as *pedicellariae*[33] (Fig. 226-16).

Bathers, surfers, divers, and fishermen are all at risk for sea urchin injuries. These may occur when the unlucky victim steps on an urchin, driving the spines into an unprotected foot, or as a result of loss of balance or wave action, in which case the hands or other body parts may be impaled.[34] Injuries from sea urchins may be inflicted either by penetrating wounds from the animal's spines, which often break off and become imbedded in the wound, or by bites from the pedicellariae. In certain species the spines or pedicellariae are venomous. This may explain why the pain of some sea urchin wounds is so excruciating and out of proportion to the apparent injury.

Encounters with sea urchins can result in two types of reactions, immediate and delayed. Immediate reactions are usually localized and are initially manifested by a severe burning pain in the wound site, which quickly becomes red and swollen and may bleed

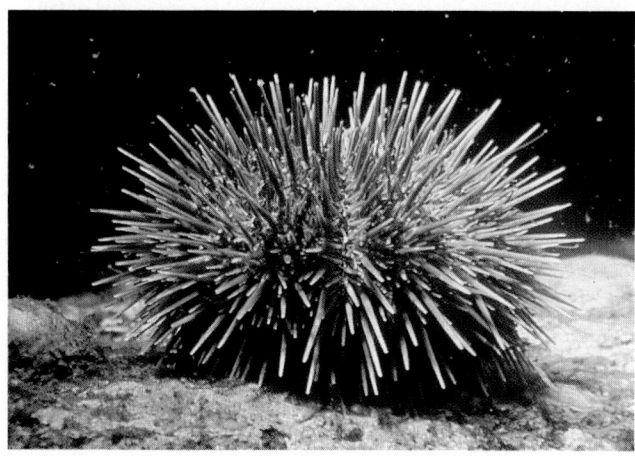

a

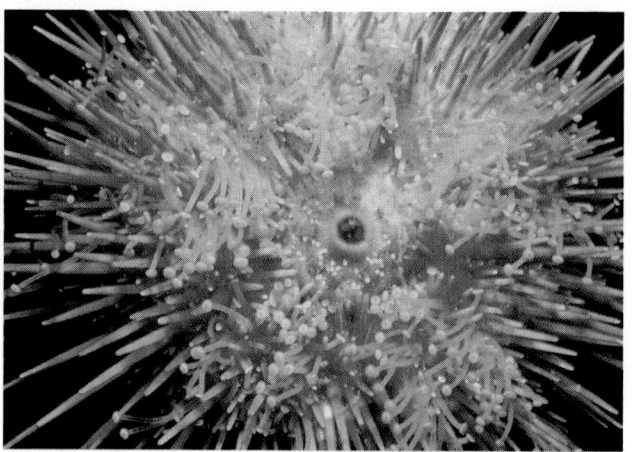

b

FIGURE 226-16 Lateral (*a*) and ventral (*b*) views of a sea urchin demonstrate this animal's protective spines and venomous pedicellaria underneath. (*Courtesy of Marty Gilman, Worcester, MA.*)

profusely.[31] There may be a black or purple discoloration at the site of the spine penetration, which can represent either retained spines in the wound or a tattoo-like effect from dye released by the spines that have exited intact. Paresthesias may develop in the wound area. Systemic symptoms are not common but can be seen in injuries due to particularly venomous species. Symptoms may include nausea, syncope, paresthesias, ataxia, muscle cramps, paralysis, and respiratory distress.[31,34]

Delayed reactions to sea urchin wounds may be nodular or diffuse; they result from a foreign-body reaction to the retained spine fragments. A granulomatous response results, which in some cases can resemble sarcoid.[33]

Nodular reactions are not usually painful and are localized to the area of spine penetration. They consist of small firm nodules, which may be flesh colored, pink, or cyanotic or may take on colors from the dye in the spines.[1,35] Nodules may have a central umbilication or a keratotic surface[35] (Fig. 226-17).

The diffuse form more commonly involves the fingers or toes and is manifested by a fusiform swelling of the affected digit with accompanying pain and loss of function.[31,33] There may be an associated tenosynovitis and destruction of the underlying bone. Sea urchin spine wounds may also cause direct mechanical injuries to nerves or joints and may be complicated by secondary infection.[31,34]

Initial first aid for the pain from immediate reactions calls for soaking the affected area in hot water [43 to 46°C (110 to 115°F)] for 30 to 90 min until maximal relief is obtained.[23,31] Infiltration of the wound site with 1 to 2% lidocaine without epinephrine may be required in some cases to produce significant pain relief.[23] Spines that are protruding from the wound may be carefully removed. They are very fragile, however, and it is very difficult to extract the entire spine intact, as it is likely to break off at the surface of the skin. More invasive attempts at spine removal should not be per-

formed without the benefit of aseptic surgical facilities and radiographs to confirm their location. Removal of the spines may be aided by the use of an operating microscope.[31]

There are anecdotal reports of pounding the wound site with a stone for the purpose of breaking up the spines into smaller fragments, which are more easily absorbed.[36] This practice has been criticized by some authors.[31] The application of ammonia compresses or freshly voided urine has also been recommended, but again these remedies are anecdotal and their value has not been proved.[33,36] Antibiotics are indicated for secondary infections, and tetanus prophylaxis should be given if indicated.

The majority of sea urchin wounds resolve without complications; however, those involving the digits, joint spaces, or nerves will require surgical intervention. Delayed nodular reactions may resolve slowly with time. Topical and intralesional corticosteroids may be efficacious for nodular reactions, and systemic corticosteroids have been recommended for diffuse reactions, but their benefit has not been clearly substantiated.[1,31,37,38] Symptomatic nodular or diffuse reactions may not resolve until the spines and granulomatous tissue have been surgically removed.[28]

Starfish   Certain species of starfish may produce puncture wound injuries similar to those caused by sea urchins. The crown-of-thorns starfish, *Acanthaster planci*, accounts for the majority of severe starfish envenomations.[31] The ice pick-like spines of *A. planci*, which may reach 4 to 6 cm in length, are covered with a thin skin and glandular tissue that produce a poisonous slime.[23,38] The resulting wound is quite painful and may be accompanied by numbness and paresthesias.[31] Systemic symptoms including nausea, vomiting, and muscle weakness are infrequent and short lived.[31] Fragments of spines and their surrounding integument may become imbedded in the wounded area, resulting in granulomatous reactions.

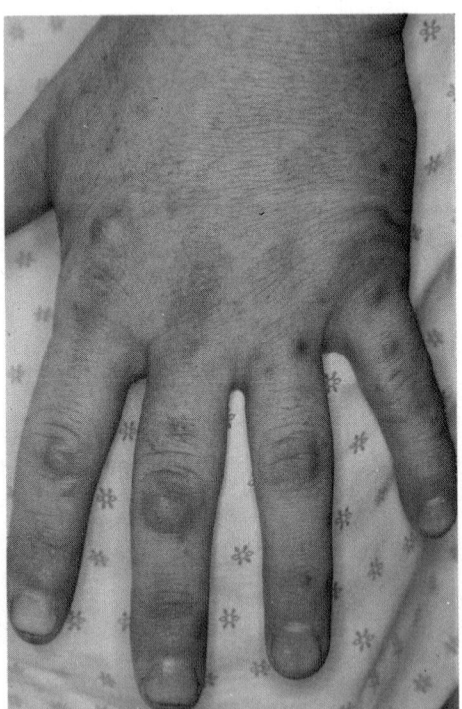

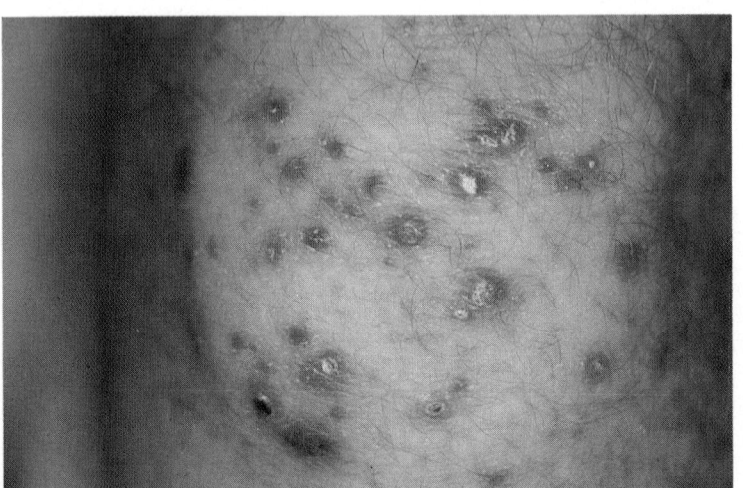

b

a

FIGURE 226-17 (*a* and *b*) Nodular reactions to imbedded sea urchin spines. (*Courtesy of Karen Rothman, M.D.*)

Treatment is similar to that of sea urchin wounds. Initial first aid should include soaking the affected area in hot water for 30 to 90 min until there is maximal pain relief.[23]

In addition to causing spinous injuries, some species of starfish may secrete a toxic substance directly into the water. When these starfish are present in large numbers, there may be sufficient amounts of this toxin to produce a pruritic papulourticarial eruption.[1,31]

Sea Cucumber Dermatitis Sea cucumbers are sausage-shaped bottom-feeding echinoderms that can produce a papular contact dermatitis by means of a toxic liquid substance, known as holothurin, which is secreted from their body walls.[1] Conjunctivitis and even blindness can result from corneal involvement if the toxin comes in contact with the eyes.[31] These animals have also been reported to ingest intact nematocysts from marine coelenterates, which they may later secrete for defensive purposes. Prevention of sea cucumber dermatitis involves protecting the skin and eyes from contact with these creatures and educating children and curious divers about the risk of handling them. Treatment consists of washing the affected area with soap and water to remove the toxin and then treating as for a mild contact dermatitis.[39]

Dermatitis and Bites from Marine Worms

Bristleworm Dermatitis Bristleworms are multisegemented marine worms of the phylum Annelida, class Polychaeta (which means "many bristles")[39] (Fig. 226-18). Each segment of the worm is armed with rows of silky or bristlelike, hollow, venom-filled setae that can easily penetrate and break off in the unprotected skin of a victim, in a fashion similar to cactus spines.[38] Contact with the bristleworm results in an erythematous papular or urticarial eruption at the site, accompanied by symptoms of paresthesias, intense itching, or burning pain.[1,38] The bristles are too small and fragile in most cases to be removed with a forceps; however, tape stripping with cellophane adhesive tape can be effective.[1,39] After the setae have been removed, the application of ammonia soaks or alcohol or water compresses may bring symptomatic relief.[1,39]

Leeches Leeches are another class of segmental worms whose bites may be encountered in fresh or salt water as well as on land. They are members of the phylum Annelida, class Hirudinea. Leeches have specialized biting jaws that allow them to attach to their host in order to feed on a meal of blood. Although freshwater leeches are capable of attaching painlessly to their human host, salt water leeches produce pain similar to a bee sting.[39] Leeches inject a powerful anticoagulant, hirudin, into the wound, as well as other antigenic substances that are capable of eliciting allergic reactions (including anaphylaxis) in sensitized individuals.[1] Local symptoms of leech bites include bleeding from the puncture marks, pain, swelling, redness, and severe pruritus; urticarial, bullous, or necrotic reactions may occur in sensitized persons.[1,39]

Severe ulcerations may result if the leech is removed forcibly and its mouth parts are left behind in the bite site. Leeches must therefore be removed carefully by inducing them to fall off by applying a noxious agent (such as alcohol, vinegar, brine, or a match flame) to their site of attachment.[1] After the leech has been removed, the wound should be carefully cleansed and minor bleeding controlled by the application of a styptic pencil.[1,39] Secondary infections may be prevented by cleansing the bite site for several days with antiseptic solutions containing alcohol or boric acid.[1]

Cercarial Dermatitis (Clam Digger's Itch) Cercarial dermatitis, also known as schistosome dermatitis or swimmer's or clam digger's itch, is an acute pruritic eruption resulting from the penetration of the skin by the cercarial forms of certain parasitic flatworms of the family Schistosomatidae.

Symptoms of cercarial dermatitis begin with urticarial-like lesions and a prickling sensation of the skin, which lasts about half an hour after exposure to cercarial-infested waters. Severe pruritus of the affected area is seen 10 to 12 h later. Within 24 h, erythematous papules appear that may progress to vesicles and later to pustules. Pain and swelling of the area accompanies the intense itching, which usually peaks in 48 to 72 h. Headache, fever, and superinfection with lymphangitis are occasionally seen.

In the Great Lakes region, several species of schistosome cercariae that cause swimmer's itch have been reported, and many other species have been discovered throughout the world in fresh as well as salt water.[40,41] The economic impact on regions with recre-

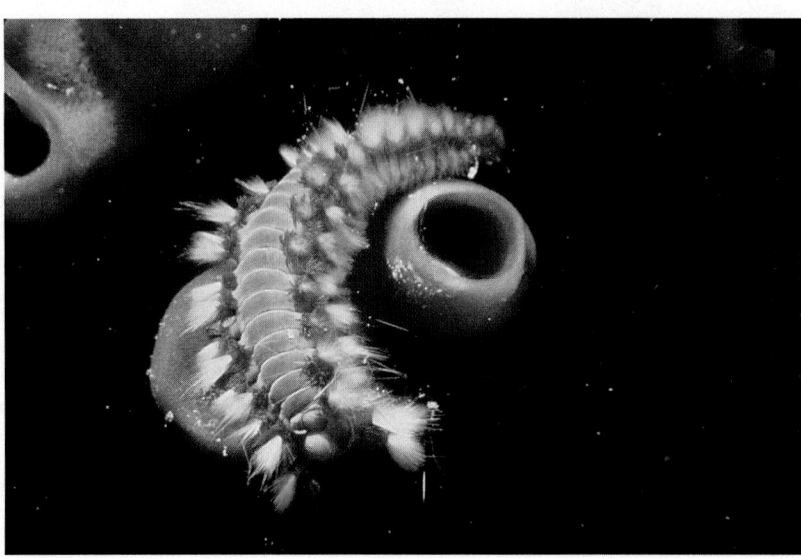

FIGURE 226-18 *Hermodice carunculata*, the West Indian bristleworm, can inflict a painful wound with its hollow, venom-filled bristlelike setae. (*Courtesy of Marty Gilman, Worcester, MA.*)

ational lakes in which the parasites are known to occur can be substantial. A severely disabling form of cercarial dermatitis affects the paddy workers and rice farmers of the Far East. Cercarial dermatitis has also been described in shallow coastal waters, notably on Long Island Sound where the condition is known to affect clam diggers, giving rise to the name, ''clam digger's itch'' (Fig. 226-19).

Humans are accidental hosts in the life cycle of dermatitis-producing schistosomes. The cycle begins when the primary host, a waterfowl, marshbird, finch, muskrat, mouse, or deer, passes schistosomal eggs in its feces into a body of water. Each egg hatches in 10 to 15 min, releasing a secondary stage miracidium. The miracidia are free-swimming and must locate and infect their definitive snail host within 12 h or they will die. The miracidia migrate to the snail's digestive gland where they develop into multiple sporocysts. In about 5 weeks the sporocysts give rise to hundreds of fork-tailed cercariae, which measure 0.75 mm in length. The cercariae are released from the snail under favorable conditions of light and heat and are carried toward the shore by prevailing winds and currents.[41] When an appropriate host is encountered, the

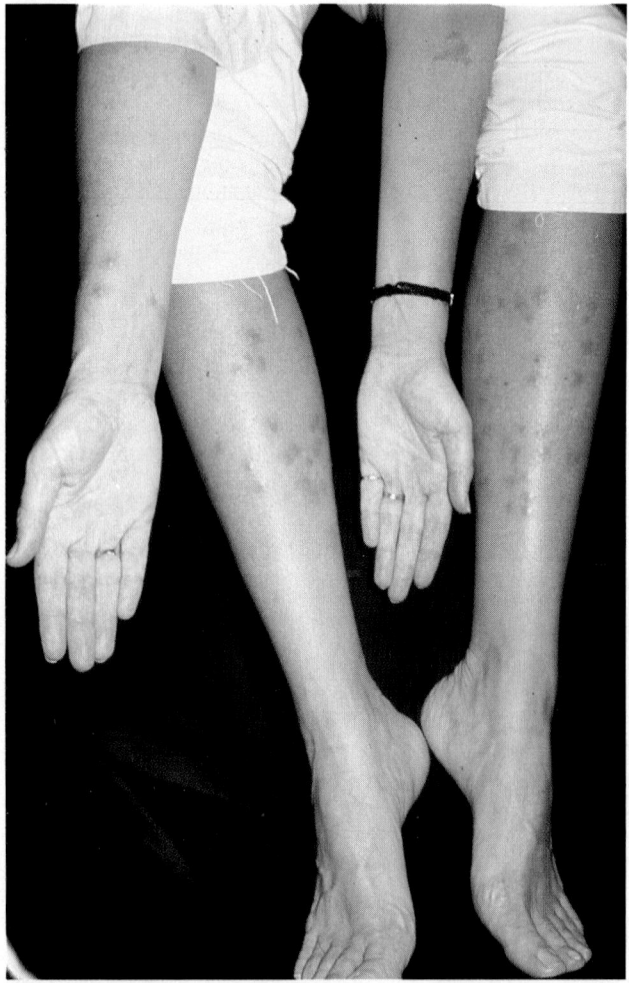

FIGURE 226-19 Intensely pruritic papulovesicles suggestive of a severe reaction to flea bites in a patient with clam digger's itch. Note that the left hand, which was not in the water and was holding the pail for collecting the clams, was spared.

cercaria attach to the skin with their oral suckers and penetrate the epidermis and dermis by means of histolytic enzymes. They lose their tails in this process and are now called schistosomulae. The schistosomulae migrate via the blood vessels through the heart and lungs to the intrahepatic veins, where they mature into adult male and female trematode flukes. When the worms mate, they pass in pairs through the mesenteric venules of the intestinal wall where the female lays hundreds of eggs.[40] The eggs then penetrate the gut wall and are discharged in the feces, and the cycle is repeated.

When cercariae that do not cause schistosomiasis in humans accidentally attach to the skin, they may penetrate the epidermis but are unable to reach the bloodstream. The organisms die in the superficial papillary dermis and undergo total histolysis within 3 to 4 days. The cercarial protein residua stimulate a delayed-type hypersensitivity response, which may increase in severity with repeated exposures.

Skin biopsies taken at 3 to 4 days reveal an amorphous eosinophilic mass at the site of the dissolved cercaria, with an intense lymphocytic infiltrate. Later, histiocytes appear in the middle and deep papillary dermis.[42]

The differential diagnosis of cercarial dermatitis includes insect bites from chiggers, mosquitoes, and fleas; contact dermatitis from poison ivy; and the stings of other marine coelenterates. In Africa, Asia, South America, and Puerto Rico, swimmer's itch must be distinguished from the dermatitis associated with human schistosomiasis, which produces an eruption with very similar but milder and more transient symptoms.[41,43] Swimmer's itch must also be distinguished from sea bather's eruption, which will be discussed in the next section.

Prevention of cercarial dermatitis in waters where swimmer's itch is known to be a problem is difficult. Avoidance of all aquatic activity is not a reasonable solution, and most swimmers or workers are not willing to apply a protective coat of petrolatum before exposure.[44] Some have advocated a brisk rubdown with a towel immediately after bathing in the belief that the cercaria can be wiped off before they can penetrate the skin, but other investigators have shown that both this and alcohol rubdowns are of little benefit. Various chemical repellents have been tried, including copper sulfate and bathing with hexachlorophene soap before exposure, but these methods remain unproved. Clothing barriers may be of some help, as cercarial dermatitis occurs more commonly on uncovered skin.

Another preventive alternative involves the elimination of the molluscan host. This can be accomplished by a variety of means, including treating the waters with various molluscicides, copper sulfate, or niclosamide. Drainage of lakes or ponds with the removal of aquatic vegetation can deprive the snails of shelter and nourishment.[41] In smaller ponds, hand removal of the snails from the banks of the water may be helpful. The most radical efforts reported involve draining the affected ponds and destroying the snails with flame throwers.[44] Under most circumstances, many of these methods are too expensive or dangerous to the environment to be practical.

Treatment of cercarial dermatitis is largely symptomatic. In mild cases antipruritic or drying lotions, oatmeal or starch baths, and antihistamines may alleviate pruritus. Aspirin may be helpful for the pain and swelling, and a bedtime sedative may be required to allow the afflicted patient much-needed sleep. Proper washing and hygiene should be maintained to prevent bacterial superinfection. In severe cases, potent topical steroids and occasionally systemic corticosteroids may be required.[44]

Sea Bather's Eruption

Sea bather's eruption, also known as marine dermatitis, is an acute dermatitis that begins shortly after bathing in sea water. It is often confused with swimmer's itch, but it is apparently not due to cercariae and can be distinguished from cercarial dermatitis by several factors (see Table 226-2). Sea bather's eruption involves areas of the body covered by bathing suits where water evaporates slowly, as opposed to the uncovered areas typical of swimmer's itch. Symptoms are not noted until the bather has left the water and may be avoided by washing and drying covered areas of skin immediately after swimming.[1,44]

The lesions begin as erythematous macules, papules, or wheals that may itch or burn (Fig. 226-20). These may progress to vesiculopapules, which crust over and heal in 7 to 10 days.[1,44] Chills and a low-grade fever may accompany the pruritus. Treatment is symptomatic with antipruritic lotions, antihistamines, and occasionally topical or systemic corticosteroids.

The etiology of seabather's eruption is unknown, although it may represent a variant of seaweed dermatitis similar to outbreaks of Lyngbya dermatitis described in Hawaii.[1] Other possibilities include coelenterate fragments, schistosomes, larval forms of marine crustaceans, dinoflagellates, and pteropods (sea butterflies).[1,44]

Injuries due to Mollusks

Cone Shell Envenomations   Cone shells are univalvular gastropods whose ornate cone-shaped shells are highly prized by shell collectors and divers. Unfortunately, a number of species have a highly developed venom apparatus that can inflict a lethal sting. Cone shells are carnivorous. They live on the ocean bottom and, depending on the species, may hunt worms, other mollusks, or fish.[45] Cone shells kill their prey by means of a spearlike venomous radular tooth that is thrust out from the animal's proboscis. Cone shell venom contains several different kinds of neurotoxins, and death may result from respiratory paralysis. There is as yet no anti-

TABLE 226-2
Comparison of Swimmer's Itch and Seabather's Eruption

Factor	Swimmer's itch	Seabather's eruption
Type of water	Fresh and salt	Salt
Part of body involved	Uncovered	Covered
Locale	Northern United States, Canada	Florida, Cuba
Cause	Cercarial forms of schistosomes	? Larval forms of crustaceans, remnants of jelly fish tentacles, others?

SOURCE: Modified from Fischer.[1]

venin for cone shell envenomations, and mortality rates for the more dangerous species (*Conus geographicus* and *C. magus*) may be as high as 15 to 20 percent.[1,45]

Injuries from cone shells are of the puncture wound variety. The degree of pain is variable, ranging from a mild stinging sensation, similar to that of an insect bite, to severe excruciating pain. Early symptoms may include edema, ischemia, numbness, and paresthesias of the wound site. Paresthesias may become widespread, with the lips and mouth commonly affected.[1,31] Localized muscular paralysis may progress to generalized weakness or paralysis with eventual respiratory distress and cardiopulmonary failure. Neurotoxic symptoms that indicate severe envenomations include diplopia, blurred vision, aphonia, dysphagia, and coma.[1,31,45]

Great care must be exercised in handling live cone shells. Thick protective gloves should be worn, and the soft underportion of the animal should be avoided. Cone shells should never be placed in pockets of clothing or swimwear as they have been known to sting through clothing.[23]

Treatment of cone shell envenomations is supportive. The victim should be kept at rest, and the sting area kept dependent and immobilized. A compression dressing should be applied to occlude lymphatic-venous, but not arterial, flow.[23] Local suction may be

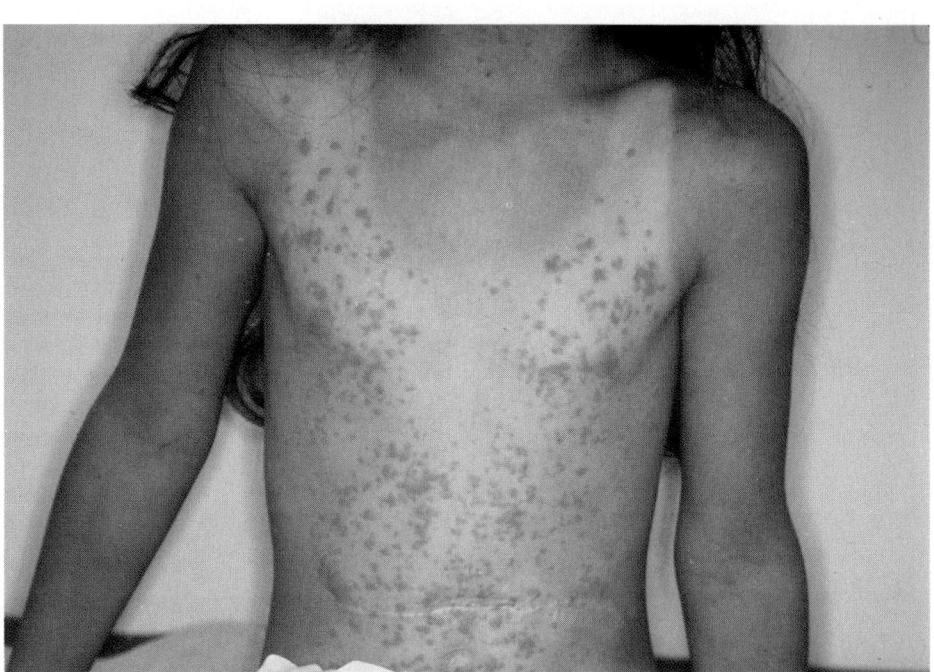

FIGURE 226-20 Sea bather's eruption in a young girl; it occurred after a swim at a Florida beach. (*Courtesy of Karen Rothman, M.D.*)

helpful if it can be applied immediately to the wound site with a plunger device, such as the Extractor (Sawyer Products, Safety Harbor, Florida).[39] No incision of the wound is required with this device.[39] Compresses or immersion of the sting area in hot water may be indicated in those cases where it is not practical to apply a lymphatic-venous compression dressing or to relieve pain in milder stings.[1,23,31] Advanced life support measures, including artificial ventilation, may be required while victims are being transported to a hospital, where they may require mechanical ventilatory support.[23]

Octopus Bites Octopuses are an advanced class of mollusks belonging to the class Cephalopoda. They are shy and reclusive creatures that tend to avoid encounters with humans; however, bites can occur when curious divers, fishermen, or beachgoers encounter these animals and handle them carelessly. The octopus bites with a parrot-like chitinous beak located on the ventral side of the head in the middle of its tentacles (Fig. 226-21).

Most octopus bites are not life threatening to humans. The bite site may be immediately painful, like a bee sting, and is recognized by the presence of two small puncture wounds, which may bleed profusely.[1] Symptoms from octopus bites are usually mild and transient and consist of redness, swelling, and itching.[46] One case of granuloma annulare has been reported to have developed around the site of an octopus bite[46] (Fig. 226-22). Paresthesias and numbness may develop at the site if the species is venomous. In more severe envenomations, these may be followed by more generalized neurologic symptoms similar to those occurring in cone shell stingings.

The most dangerous species of octopus, the Australian blue-ringed octopus, *Hapalochlaena maculosa,* is found in Australian coastal waters. Mortality rates due to bites caused by *H. maculosa* may be as high as 25 percent.[47] *H. maculosa* produces a toxin in its salivary glands, which is introduced into the bite site by the animal's powerful beak. The toxin contains a fraction identical to tetrodotoxin, which blocks peripheral nerve conduction, resulting in

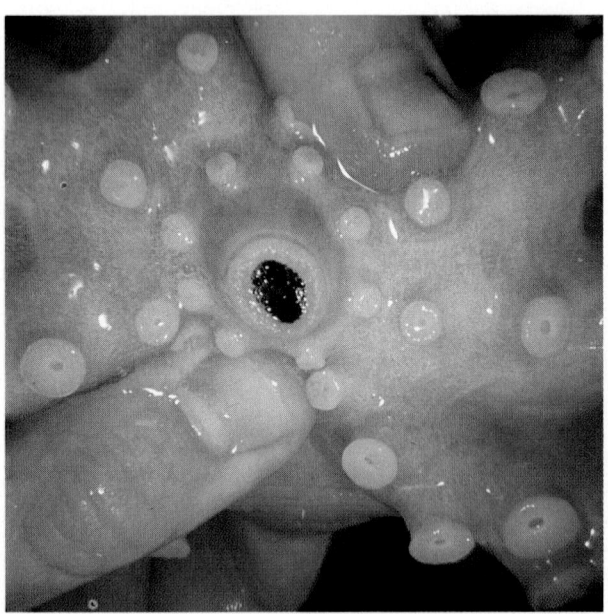

FIGURE 226-21 Ventral view of the underside of an octopus exposing the animal's centrally located mouth and parrot-like beak. (*From D. D. Fulgham.*[46])

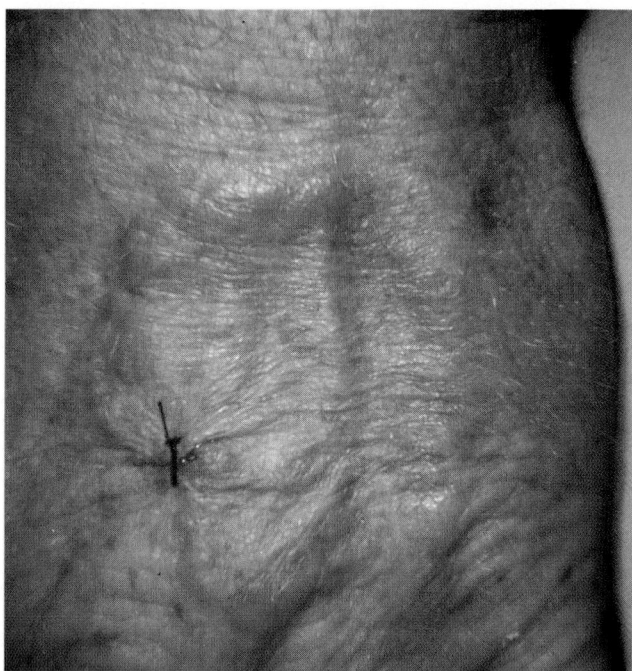

FIGURE 226-22 Granuloma annulare, which occurred on the back of the hand of a commercial fisherman several days after being bitten by a small octopus at the same site. (*From D. D. Fulgham.*[46])

paralysis of the victim with subsequent respiratory failure.[39] The bite of the blue-ringed octopus may or may not be painful, so that victims may not realize that they have been bitten until neurologic symptoms develop.[31]

Unfortunately, there is no antivenin yet for bites due to *H. maculosa*. Treatment is supportive and similar to that recommended above for severe cone shell envenomations. Immersion of the wound in hot water does not seem to be beneficial.[31] The use of the pressure-immobilization technique with a lymphatic-venous occlusive pressure dressing or the immediate application of suction to the wound site with a suction device may be of value.[23,39] Excision of the bite site down to fascia has been recommended by some authors, but is of unproved value.[1,31,47]

Injuries Due to Venomous Fish Spines

Ichthyoacanthotoxicosis is the proper term for envenomations due to puncture wounds or lacerations inflicted by the spines of venomous fish.[48] There are over 200 species of venomous fish in the world that can cause injury to humans.[31] The most notorious of these includes the stingrays, catfish, lionfish, scorpionfish, stonefish, weeverfish, toadfish, and spiny dogfish. All of these fish have in common a venom apparatus consisting of a single spine or multiple spines, in various locations, which are covered by an integumentary sheath enclosing various forms of venom glands. When the spine of the animal penetrates the victim, the sheath is torn and the venom glands release their toxins into the wound.

Stingrays Stingrays are probably the most common cause of venomous fish stings confronting humans; as many as 1500 stingray attacks are reported each year in the United States alone.[38,48] Rays are grouped into one of four categories; gymnurid (butterfly rays), urolophid (round stingrays), mylobatid (bat or eagle rays), and dasyatid (proper stingrays).[48] The groupings are based on their relative stinging ability, which depends on the size, number, and location of the caudal stinging appendages.[48,49] The most dangerous group, the dasyatid or true stingrays, have the largest spines located further out on their tails, making theirs the most potent striking weapons.[48,49] The spines have retroserrated teeth, which makes removal difficult (Fig. 226-23).

Most stingray injuries occur when bathers, waders, or fishermen accidentally step on rays as they lie partially covered with sand in shallow waters. Severe lacerations and puncture wounds are inflicted by the ray as it defensively whips its tail upward and forward when stepped on or threatened[50] (Fig. 226-24). The majority of wounds, therefore, are located on the dorsum of the foot or lower leg.[51] Penetrating wounds to other locations have occurred to fishermen stung while attempting to remove rays from their lines or nets; in a freak accident where a ray leapt from the water, striking a young boy in a small boat; and to divers engaged in feeding rays at popular dive locations.[50,51] When stingray spines penetrate the thorax or abdomen, the resulting wounds may prove fatal.[50,51]

Catfish   Both fresh and saltwater catfish are armed with stout sharp spines located immediately in front of the soft rays of their dorsal and pectoral fins.[48] Catfish defensively lock these spines into an extended position when they are handled or threatened.[51] Fishermen are commonly stung if they do not take care while attempting to remove catfish from the hooks of their fishing lines.[52] Heavy gloves, pliers, and pincer-like jaws for holding the fish afford some protection.[53] The safest approach in the absence of these devices is to maintain a safe distance from the fish and to cut the line. Fishermen and sea food processors may be stung even by dead catfish while cleaning them.[54] One author has suggested that the offending spines be removed with a pair of pliers before attempting to clean the fish, to prevent these injuries.[53]

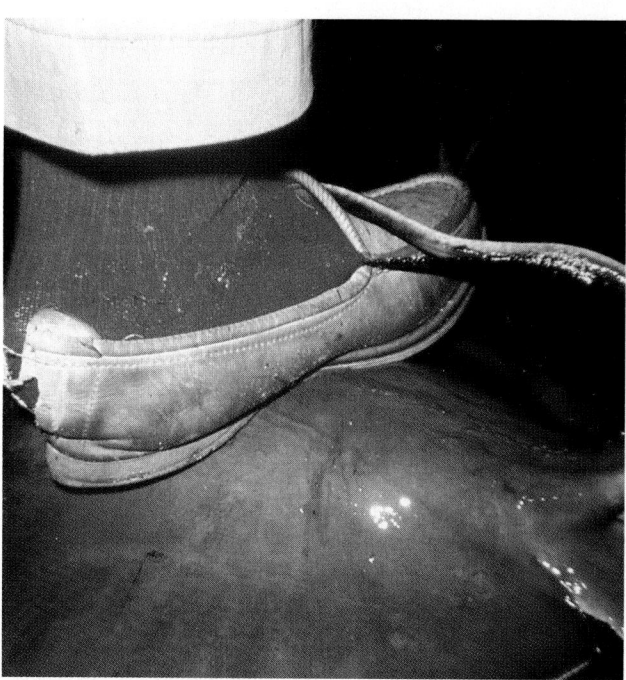

FIGURE 226-24   Stingrays reflexively swing their barbed tails up when stepped on, causing painful lacerations and puncture wounds. (The leg used for this photograph was a prosthesis; the stingray was alive.) (*Courtesy of David Fulghum, M.D.*)

Swimmers and bathers in the Amazon river are at risk for urologic injuries if they encounter a very small species of catfish called "candiru," which has the ability to enter the human urethra.[52] Barbs on the head of this fish prevent it from swimming backward out of the orifice, and surgical intervention is often required to extract the fish.[52]

Scorpionfish   Scorpionfish, family Scorpaenidae, are divided into three main groups on the basis of their stinging apparatus. All have venomous spines of varying sizes and toxicity that may be found, depending on the species, on the dorsal, pelvic, and anal locations.

Lionfish, genus *Pterois*, are found in tropical waters and are prized by fish fanciers because of their colorful and ornate fins. The spines of lionfish are long and slender with small venom glands.[31] Their stings are relatively mild and not life threatening.[38,55] Stings among amateur fish collectors are occurring more frequently because of the increasing popularity of these fish.[55]

Scorpionfish, genus *Scorpaena*, have stings that are of intermediate severity. They are bottom dwellers whose superior camouflage abilities allow them to blend in almost invisibly with their surroundings[48] (Fig. 226-25). Their spines are long and heavy and have moderate-sized venom glands.

Stonefish, genus *Synanceja*, are the most dangerous members of the scorpionfish family. They live in shallow waters, sometimes partially buried in sand or mud or in holes of rocky shoals, reef areas, or tidal pools.[38] Injuries occur when an unsuspecting wader steps on the erect venomous dorsal spine that the stonefish raises in defense. Stonefish spines are short and thick and have very large and well-developed venom glands.[31] The wounds caused by stonefish are quite severe and may be fatal.[48] Fortunately, a stonefish antivenin is available from the Commonwealth Serum Laboratories, Melbourne, Australia.[1,48]

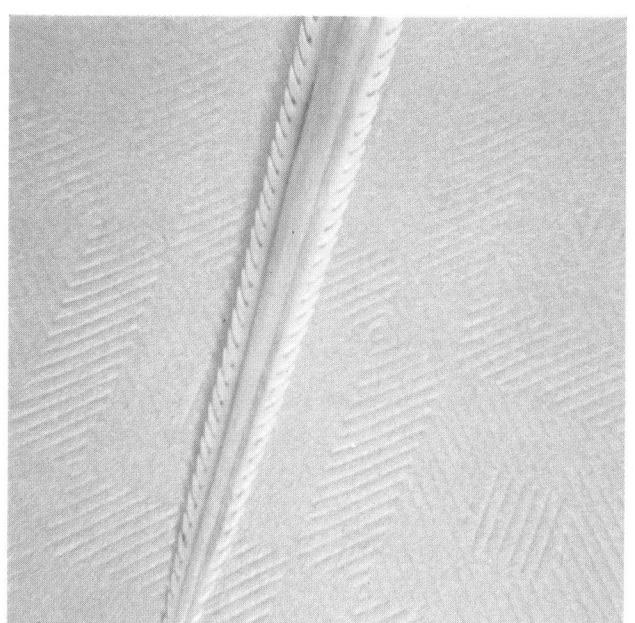

FIGURE 226-23   A close-up view of a stingray stinger devoid of its outer membrane and venom glands, demonstrating the retroserrated spine. (*Courtesy of David Fulghum, M.D.*)

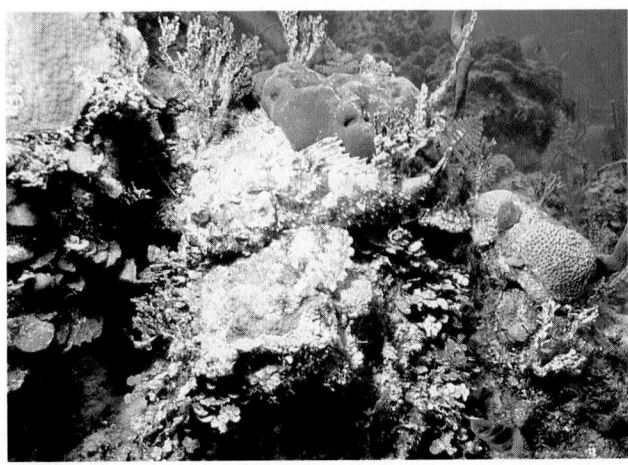

FIGURE 226-25 *Scopaena plumieri,* a species of scorpion fish, is found in the waters of the West Indies. Its camouflage abilities are exceeded only by its painful sting.

Local and Systemic Symptoms of Fish-Spine Envenomations
The toxicity of a given sting depends on a number of factors, including the species of fish involved, the location and severity of the wound, the amount of venom released, and the first aid and subsequent medical care provided to the victim. In general, these wounds produce pain out of proportion to the apparent severity of the injury. The pain is immediate and intense. In the case of scorpionfish stings, the pain may be so severe as to cause the victim to thrash about wildly, scream, and finally lose consciousness.[56]

Initially the sting site may appear pale or cyanotic. The area around the wound may be anesthetic or hyperesthetic.[31] Erythema and edema soon develop, giving the appearance of a cellulitis. Vesicles may form.[39] In severe stingings, especially those due to stonefish, the wounded area may become indurated and develop areas of ischemic necrosis with subsequent sloughing and ulcer formation.

Fish-spine wounds may be complicated by foreign-body reactions to bits of retained spines or remnants of integumentary sheath. Secondary infections must be anticipated. Healing is slow, especially in cases plagued by abscess or ulcer formation.

Systemic symptoms from toxic fish spines may range from mild to severe, depending on the species involved and the amount of venom entering the wound. They may include headache, nausea, vomiting, diarrhea, abdominal cramps and pain, fever, local lymphangitis and lymphadenitis, joint aches, muscle weakness, diaphoresis, peripheral neuropathy, limb paralysis, restlessness, delirium, seizures, cardiac arrhythmias, myocardial ischemia, hypotension, respiratory distress, and death.[31,55,56]

Prevention Prevention of toxic fish-spine wounds begins with a knowledge of and an appreciation for the various venomous species that may be encountered in a given area. Waders and bathers should shuffle their feet in order to scare away and avoid stepping on rays or scorpionfish. Fishermen must exercise care when removing rays or catfish from their fishing lines or when cleaning fish with venomous spines. Fish hobbyists and divers should wear protective clothing and avoid handling venomous species.

Treatment Puncture wounds and lacerations from venomous fish spines should be irrigated immediately with sterile saline or water, if available, and with sea water as a last resort.[23] The wounded area should then be soaked as quickly as possible in hot (not scalding) water of approximately 43 to 46°C (110 to 115°F) for 30 to 90 min

or until maximal pain relief is achieved. Hot soaks may be repeated if the pain returns. Because the wound or extremity may be partially anesthetic, it is necessary for the person administering first aid to test the water's temperature for the victim.[50] One source of hot water that is often overlooked and may be useful in an emergency is hot sea water from a boat motor's cooling system.[50]

Local infiltration of the wound with 1 to 2% lidocaine without epinephrine may bring about significant pain relief and allow for exploration of the wound after x-rays have been performed to locate retained portions of spines.[38,50] The wound should be thoroughly cleaned to remove any remnants of integumentary sheath. Cleansing with a toothbrush and a solution of hexachlorophene in 70% alcohol has been recommended.[50] Abdominal and thoracic wounds and deep wounds to the hands, feet, or fascial compartments of the legs should be explored in the operating room.[38] Debridement of necrotic tissues may be required at the time of exploration, and sequential debridement may be necessary.[38] In general, these wounds should be left open or closed loosely with tape or suture to allow for adequate drainage and to prevent abscess formation.

Tetanus prophylaxis should be administered, if indicated, and antibiotics are recommended if the wound is over 6 h old, is extensive, or involves deep puncture wounds to the hand or foot.[38,50]

Stonefish stings complicated by severe reactions may be treated with antivenin by slow intravenous infusion.[48] Antivenin is not usually required for the stings of lionfish and other species of scorpionfish other than stonefish.[38] The amount of antivenin given depends on the number of puncture wounds sustained by the victim and the response to treatment.[48] The antivenin is prepared from horse serum and its administration may be complicated by anaphylaxis in sensitized individuals.[48]

Fish Bites

There are many species of fish whose bites are dangerous to humans. Among the best known of these are the sharks, baracudas, and piraña, whose attacks may be lethal. Bluefish, which run in large schools, present a menace to swimmers and surfers and to fishers who are not wary of their vicious bites.[23] Divers must be careful of moray eels, which have powerful jaws and knifelike teeth. Although not considered venomous by most sources, they can produce deep puncture wounds and lacerations[23] (Fig. 226-26).

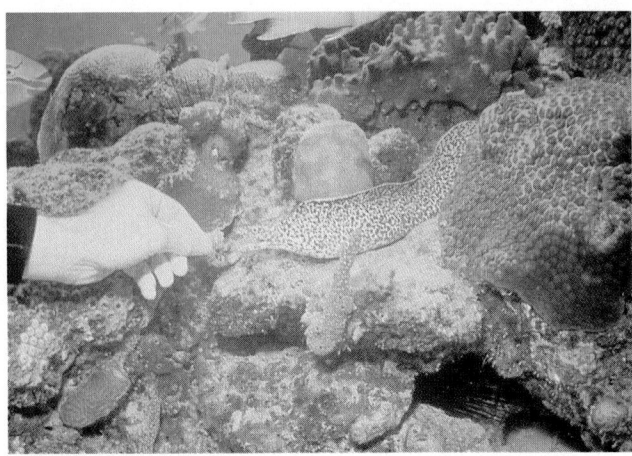

FIGURE 226-26 Moray eel bites are uncommon but have increased due to divers feeding these animals at popular dive sites. (*Courtesy of Marty Gilman, Worcester, MA.*)

Waterborne Infections (See also Section 31)

A variety of infections may result from exposures to aquatic environments. Pathogenic organisms may be actively introduced into wounds of the bites, stings, or lacerations caused by marine life; preexisting wounds may be passively infected while exposed to contaminated waters. Table 226-3 summarizes those organisms commonly associated with waterborne infections. A host of other agents, such as *Streptococcus* and *Staphylococcus* spp., *Bacter-*

TABLE 226-3
Wound Infections Associated with Waterborne Organisms

Organisms	Clinical features
Aeromonas hydrophila	Cellulitis (may be bullous) (Fig. 226-27); fasciitis; myonecrosis; bacteremia
Erysipelothrix rhusiopathiae	Slowly progressive painful cellulitis without adenopathy or lymphangitis, almost always involving the hand; septic arthritis; subacute bacterial endocarditis
Mycobacterium balnei or *marinum*	Swimming pool granuloma; fish fancier's finger (Fig. 226-28); chronic cellulitis and culture-negative ulcers
Prototothecosis	Papular or eczematoid dermatitis in immunosuppressed patients; localized infection of the olecranon bursa
Pseudomonas	Trench foot; gram-negative toe web space infections (Fig. 226-29); swimmer's ear; hot tub folliculitis
Vibrio vulnificus	Very painful cellulitis with bulla formation may progress to septicemia, especially in alcoholics, diabetics, and immunosuppressed patients. Metastatic cellulitis with bullae, meningitis, and death may result from fulminant infections

SOURCE: Adapted from Bateman JL et al: *Aeromonas hydrophila* cellulitis and wound infections caused by waterborne organisms. *Heart Lung* **17**:101, 1988.

oides fragilis, Clostridium perfringens, Escherichia coli, Salmonella enteritidis, other marine *Vibrio* species, *Chromobacterium violaceum,* and *Chlorella,* also deserve consideration when dealing with infections derived from aquatic settings.[38]

Cutaneous Manifestations of Ingesting Seafood and of Seafood Poisoning

There are several dermatologic reactions that may be seen after ingesting seafood. Urticaria, angioedema, and, rarely, leukocytoclastic vasculitis may occur in individuals sensitized to fish or shellfish (Fig. 226-30). Many seafoods, such as kelp, contain large amounts of iodine, which may cause acneform eruptions.[39]

Scombroid food poisoning involves the ingestion of spoiled fish from the Scombroidae family of fish, which includes tuna,

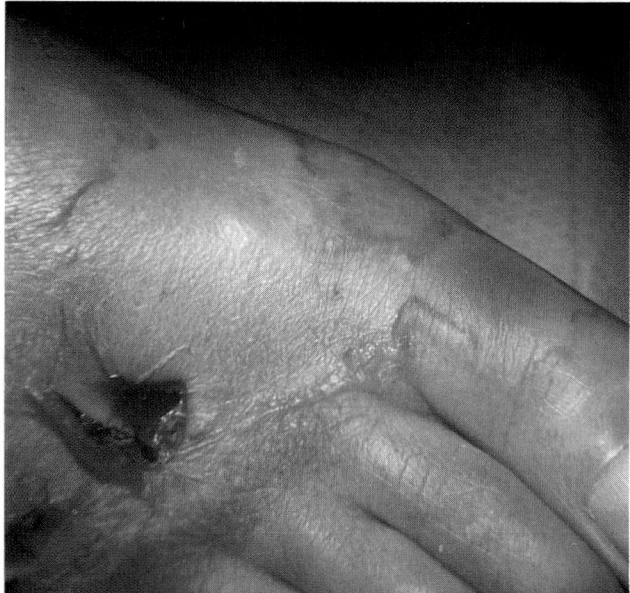

FIGURE 226-27 Bullous cellulitis due to *Aeromonas hydrophilia;* the cellulitis progressed to ischemic necrosis, requiring amputation. Unfortunately the patient succumbed to the infection. (*From Fulghum D et al: Fatal Aeromonas hydrophila infection of the skin. J South Med Assn 71:739, 1978.*)

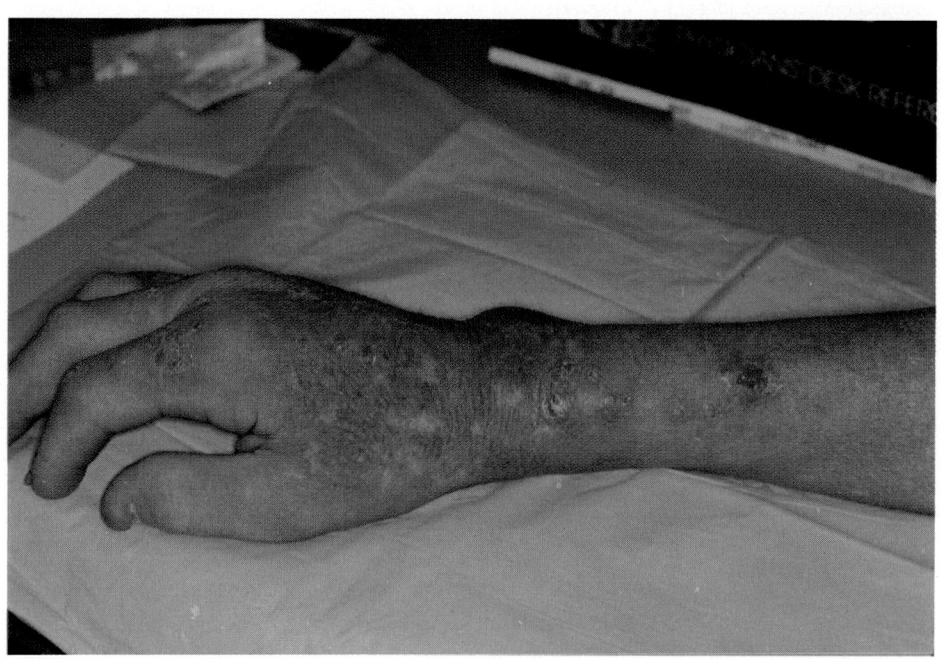

FIGURE 226-28 Fish fancier's finger with sporotrichoid spread to the wrist and arm due to a *Mycobacterium marinum* infection, which responded to minocycline. (*Courtesy of Lori Herman, M.D.*)

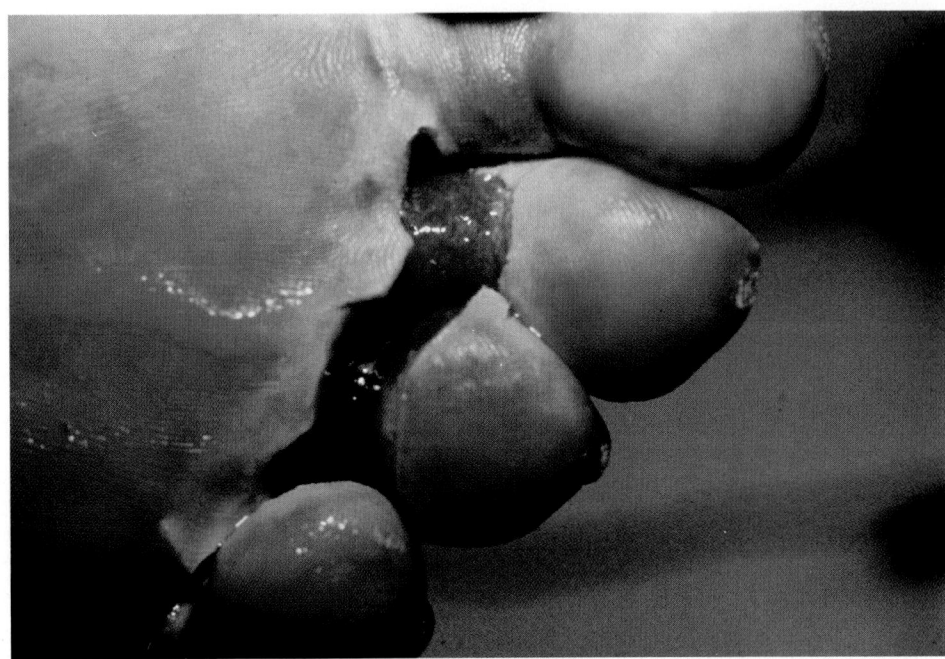

FIGURE 226-29 Gram-negative toeweb space infection due to *Pseudomonas*.

mackerel, bonita, and their relatives.[39] If these fish are not kept cold enough after being caught, their flesh develops scombrotoxins due to the bacterial breakdown of histidine into histamine, saurine, and possibly other toxic byproducts.[57] These can cause striking erythema and flushing of the face, neck, and upper trunk, as well as pruritus and urticarial and angioedematous eruptions.

Ciguatera toxin, which is produced during blooms of toxic dinoflagellates, is incorporated into the marine food chain and concentrated in the flesh of a variety of fish. Dermatologic symptoms of ingesting these fish may include generalized pruritus and diffuse erythematous macular and papular exanthems that may progress to blister formation and desquamation.[39]

ACKNOWLEDGMENT

The authors wish to thank Dr. Bruce Halstead of the World Life Research Institute, Colton, California, for allowing us to reprint the photographs from the first and second editions of *Poisonous and Venomous Marine Animals of the World*.

Bibliography

ANIMAL BITES

Berzon DR et al: Animal bites in a large city—a report on Baltimore, Maryland. *Am J Public Health* **62**:422, 1972

Goldstein EJC et al: Outpatient therapy of bite wounds: Demographic data, bacteriology and a prospective randomized trial of amoxicillin-clavulinic acid versus penicillin ± dicloxacillin. *Int J Dermatol* **26**:123, 1987

Hubbert WT et al: *Diseases Transmitted from Animal to Man*. Springfield, IL, Charles C Thomas, 1975

Kahrs RF et al: Diseases transmitted from pets to man: An evolving concern for veterinarians. *Cornell Vet* **68**:442, 1978

Strassburg MA et al: Animal bites: Patterns of treatment. *Ann Emerg Med* **10**:193, 1981

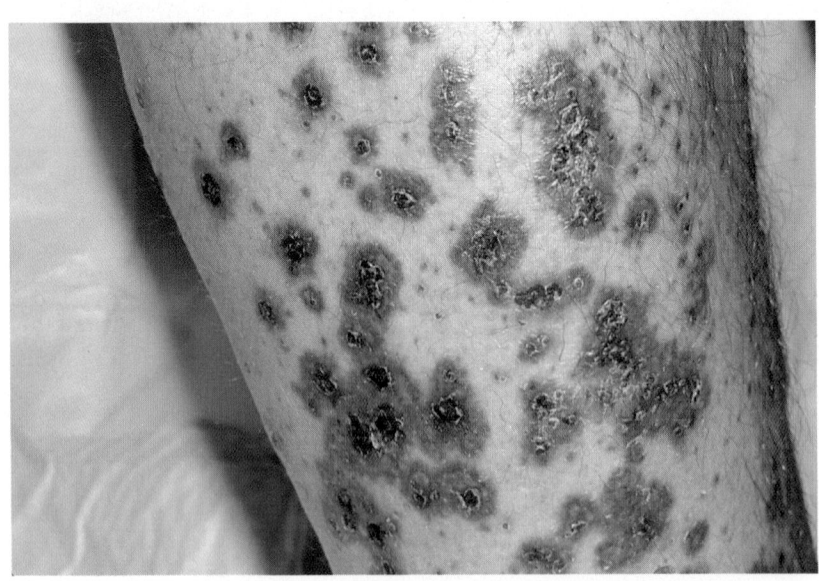

FIGURE 226-30 Leukocytoclastic vasculitis occurring in a patient, allergic to shellfish, who consumed a chowder containing quahogs, a type of clam.

Wear DJ et al: Cat scratch disease: A bacterial infection. *Science* **221**:1403, 1983

Weber DJ, Hansen AR: Infections resulting from animal bites. *Infect Dis Clin North Am* **5**:663, 1991

CAPNOCYTOPHAGA

Brenner DJ et al: *Capnocytophaga canimorsus* sp. nov. (formerly CDC Group DF-2), a cause of septicemia following dog bite and *C. cyodegmi* sp. nov., a cause of localized wound infections following dog bite. *J Clin Microbiol* **27**:231, 1989

Kullberg BJ et al: Purpura fulminans and symmetrical peripheral gangrene caused by *Capnocytophaga canimorsus* (formerly DF-2) septicemia, a complication of dog bite. *Medicine (Baltimore)* **70**:5287, 1991

DOG BITES

August JR: Dog and cat bites. *J Am Vet Med Assoc* **193**:1506, 1988

Callaham M: Prophylactic antibiotics in common dog bite wounds: A controlled study. *Ann Emerg Med* **9**:410, 1980

Klein D: Friendly dog syndrome. *N Y State J Med* **66**:2306, 1966

Parris HM et al: Epidemiology of dog bites. *Public Health Rep* **74**:891, 1959

HUMAN BITES

Mann RJ et al: Human bites of the hand: Twenty years of experience. *J Hand Surg* **2**:77, 1977

Peeples E et al: Wounds of the hand contaminated by human or animal saliva. *J Trauma* **20**:383, 1980

LYMPHOCYTIC CHORIOMENINGITIS

Biggar RJ et al: Lymphocytic choriomeningitis outbreak associated with pet hamsters. *JAMA* **232**:494, 1975

Hirsch MS et al: Lymphocytic choriomeningitis virus infection traced to a pet hamster. *N Engl J Med* **291**:610, 1974

PASTEURELLA MULTOCIDA

Gump GW, Holden RA: Endocarditis caused by a new species of *Pasteurella*. *Ann Intern Med* **76**:275, 1972

Hubbert WT et al: *Pasteurella multocida* infection due to animal bite. *Am J Public Health* **60**:1103, 1970

Jarvis WR et al: *Pasteurella multocida* osteomyelitis following dog bites. *Am J Dis Child* **135**:625, 1981

Sands M et al: Trimethoprim/sulfamethoxazole therapy of *Pasteurella multocida* infection. *J Infect Dis* **160**:353, 1989

Tindell JP, Harrison CM: *Pasteurella multocida* infections following animal injuries, especially cat bites. *Arch Dermatol* **105**:412, 1972

Weber DJ et al: ''Pasteurella multicida'' infections: Report of 34 cases and review of the literature. *Medicine (Baltimore)* **63**:133, 1984

RABIES

Anderson LJ et al: Human rabies in the United States. *Ann Intern Med* **100**:728, 1984

Bauer GM, Fishbein DB: Rabies post exposure prophylaxis. *N Engl J Med* **316**:1270, 1987

Corey L, Hattwick MA: Treatment of persons exposed to rabies. *JAMA* **232**:272, 1975

Hough SA et al: Human to human transmission of rabies virus by a corneal transplant. *N Engl J Med* **300**:603, 1979

Meyer HW: Rabies vaccine. *J Infect Dis* **2**:287, 1980

Plotkin SA: Rabies vaccination in the 1980's. *Hosp Pract* **15**:65, 1980

Porras C et al: Recovery from rabies in man. *Ann Intern Med* **85**:44, 1976

Rabies prevention: Recommendation of Immunization Practices Advisory Committee (ACIP). *MMWR* **37**:217, 1988

SEAL BITES

Beck B, Smith TG: Seal finger: An unsolved medical problem in Canada. *Technical Report of the Fisheries Research Board of Canada,* No 625. Arctic Biological Station, Ste Anne de Bellevue, Que, Fisheries and Marine Service, 1976

Eadie PA, Lee TC: Seal finger in a wildlife ranger. *Irish Med J* **83**:117, 1990

Hilenbrand FKM: Whale finger and seal finger. *Lancet* **2**:680, 1953

Madoff S et al: Isolation of a *Mycoplasma* species from a case of seal finger (abstr). American Society of Microbiology Proceedings, Dallas, TX, May 1991

Markham RB, Polk F: Seal finger. *J Infect Dis* **1**:567, 1979

SIMIAN HERPES B VIRUS

Davidson WF, Hummeier R: B virus infection in man. *Ann N Y Acad Sci* **85**:970, 1968

Hull RN: The simian herpes viruses, in *The Herpes Viruses,* edited by AS Kaplan. New York, Academic, 1973, p 390

SNAKE BITES

Garlin SR et al: Role of surgical decompression in treatment of rattlesnake bites. *Surg Forum* **30**:502, 1979

Glass TG: Early debridement in pit viper bites. *JAMA* **235**:2513, 1976

Goldstone EJC: Bacteriology of rattlesnake venom and implications for therapy. *J Infect Dis* **140**:818, 1979

Grace TG et al: The management of upper extremity pit viper wounds. *J Hand Surg* **2**:168, 1980

Johnson CA: Management of snakebite. *Am Fam Physician* **44**:174, 1991

Parrish HM et al: Poisonous snake bites in New England. *N Engl J Med* **263**:788, 1960

Russell F: Jaws that bite. *Emerg Med* **25**:40, 1978

Russell F et al: Snake venom poisoning in the United States. *JAMA* **233**:341, 1975

Snyder CC, Knowles RP: Snakebites: Guidelines for practical management. *Postgrad Med* **83**:52, 65, 71, 1988

Sutherland SK, Coulter AR: Early management of bites by the eastern diamondback rattlesnake (*Crotalus adamanteus*): Studies in monkeys (*Macaca fascicularis*). *Am J Trop Med Hyg* **30**:497, 1981

Wasserman GS: Wound care of spider and snake envenomations. *Ann Emerg Med* **17**:1331, 1988

STAPHYLOCOCCUS INTERMEDIUS

Tolan DA et al: *Staphylococcus intermedius:* Clinical presentation of a new human dog bite pathogen. *Ann Emerg Med* **18**:410, 1989

References

1. Fisher AA: *Atlas of Aquatic Dermatology.* New York, Grune & Stratton, 1978, p 10

2. Halstead BW: Coelenterate (cnidarian) stings and wounds, aquatic dermatology. *Clin Dermatol* **5**:8, 1987

3. Reed KM et al: Delayed and persistent cutaneous reactions to coelenterates. *J Am Acad Dermatol* **10**:462, 1984

4. Mandojana RM: Granuloma annulare following blue bottle jellyfish (*Physalia utriculus*) sting. *J Wilderness Med* **1**:220, 1990

5. Auerbach PS, Hays JT: Erythema nodosum following a jellyfish sting. *J Emerg Med* **5**:487, 1987

6. Burnett JW et al: Local and systemic reactions from jellyfish stings. *Clin Dermatol* **5**:14, 1987

7. Ionnides G, Davis JH: Portuguese man-of-war stinging. *Arch Dermatol* **91**:450, 1965

8. Drury JK et al: Jellyfish sting with serious hand complications. *Injury* **12**:66, 1980

9. Adiga KM: Brachial artery spasm as a result of a sting. *Med J Aust* **140**:181, 1984

10. Guess HA, Saviteer PL: Hemolysis and acute renal failure following a Portuguese man-of-war sting. *Pediatrics* **70**:979, 1982

11. Spielman FJ et al: Acute renal failure as a result of *Physalia physalis* sting. *South Med J* **75**:1425, 1982

12. Burnett JW, Gable WD: A fatal jellyfish envenomation by the Portuguese man-o'war. *Toxicon* **27**:823, 1989

13. Stein MR et al: Fatal Portuguese man-o'-war (*Physalia physalis*) envenomation. *Ann Emerg Med* **18**:312, 1989

14. Sutherland S: Lethal jellyfish. *Med J Aust* **143**:536, 1985

15. Williamson JA et al: Serious envenomation by the Northern Australian box-jellyfish (*Chironex fleckeri*). *Med J Aust* **1**:13, 1980

16. Williamson JA et al: Acute management of serious envenomation by box jellyfish (*Chironex fleckeri*). *Med J Aust* **141**:851, 1984

17. Chand RP, Selliah K: Reversible parasympathetic dysautonomia following stinging attributed to the box jellyfish (*Chironex fleckeri*). *Aust NZ J Med* **14**:673, 1984

18. Burnett JW, Calton GJ: Response of the box-jellyfish (*Chironex fleckeri*) cardiotoxin to intravenous administration of verapamil. *Med J Aust* **153**:363, 1990

19. Burnett JW: The use of verapamil to treat box-jellyfish stings. *Med J Aust* **153**:363, 1990

20. Fenner PJ et al: Successful use of *Chironex* antivenom by members of the Queensland Ambulance Transport Brigade. *Med J Aust* **151**:708, 1989

21. Hartwick R et al: Disarming the box-jellyfish: Nematocyst inhibition in *Chironex fleckeri*. *Med J Aust* **1**:15, 1980

22. Burnett JW et al: First aid for jellyfish envenomation. *South Med J* **76**:870, 1983

23. Halstead BW, Auerbach PS (eds): *Dangerous Aquatic Animals of the World: A Color Guide, with Prevention, First Aid, and Emergency Treatment Procedures.* Princeton, NJ, Darwin Press, 1990

24. Exton DR et al: Cold packs: Effective topical analgesia in the treatment of painful stings by *Physalia* and other jellyfish. *Med J Aust* **151**:625, 1989

25. Massmanian A et al: Sea anemone dermatitis. *Contact Dermatitis* **18**:169, 1988

26. Fisher AA: Water-related dermatoses. Part II: Nematocyst dermatitis. *Cutis* **25**:242, 248, 287, 314, 317, 1980

27. Weedon D et al: Coral dermatitis. *Aust J Dermatol* **22**:104, 1981

28. Cangialosi CP: Aquatic contact dermatitis. Report of two cases. *J Am Podiatry Assoc* **73**:21, 1983

29. Cooper MA: Treatment of coral cuts in Hawaii. *Hawaii Med J* **40**:73, 1981

30. Burnett JW et al: Dermatitis due to stinging sponges. *Cutis* **39**:476, 1987

31. Kizer KW: Marine envenomations. *J Toxicol Clin Toxicol* **21**:527, 1983

32. Yaffee HS, Stargardter F: Erythema multiforme from *Tedania ignis*. *Arch Dermatol* **87**:601, 1963

33. Baden HP: Injuries from sea urchins. *Clin Dermatol* **5**:112, 1987

34. Strauss MB, MacDonald RI: Hand injuries from sea urchin spines. *Clin Orthop* **114**:216, 1976

35. Baden HP, Burnett JW: Injuries from sea urchins. *South Med J* **70**:459, 1977

36. Falkenberg P: Sea urchin spines as foreign bodies—an alternative treatment. *Injury* **15**:419, 1985

37. Warin AP: Sea-urchin granuloma. *Clin Exp Dermatol* **2**:405, 1977

38. Auerbach PS: Marine envenomations. *N Engl J Med* **325**:486, 1991

39. Mandojana RM, Sims JK: Miscellaneous dermatoses associated with the aquatic environment. *Clin Dermatol* **5**:134, 1987

40. Hoeffler DF: Cercarial dermatitis. *Arch Environ Health* **29**:225, 1974

41. Hoeffler DF: "Swimmer's itch" (cercarial dermatitis). *Cutis* **19**:461, 467, 1977

42. Kirshenbaum MB: Swimmer's itch. A review and case report. *Cutis* **23**:212, 218, 1979

43. Gonzalez E: Schistosomiasis, cercarial dermatitis and marine dermatitis. *Dermatol Clin* **7**:291, 1989

44. Osment LS: Update; seabather's eruption and swimmer's itch. *Cutis* **18**:545, 1976

45. Burnett JW et al: Cone snails. *Cutis* **39**:107, 1987

46. Fulghum DD: Octopus bite resulting in granuloma annulare. *South Med J* **79**:1434, 1986

47. Rosco D: Treatment of venomous and poisonous marine animal injuries. *Int Soc Aquatic Med Newsletter* **2**(2), June 1976

48. Halstead BW, Vinci JM: Venomous fish stings (ichthyoacanthotoxicoses). *Clin Dermatol* **5**:29, 1987

49. Grainger CR: Multiple injuries due to stingrays. *J R Soc Health* **107**:100, 1987

50. Fenner PJ et al: Fatal and nonfatal stingray envenomation. *Med J Aust* **151**:621, 1989

51. Barss PL: Wound necrosis caused by the venom of stingrays: Pathological findings and surgical management. *Med J Aust* **141**:854, 1984

52. Scoggin CH: Catfish stings. *JAMA* **231**:176, 1975

53. David NF: Still more on catfish stings. *JAMA* **233**:864, 1975

54. Calton GJ, Burnett JW: Catfish (*Ictalurus catus*) fin venom. *Toxicon* **13**:339, 1975

55. Trestrail JH, Al-Mahasneh QM: Lionfish sting experiences of an inland poison center: A retrospective study of 23 cases. *Vet Hum Toxicol* **31**:173, 1989

56. Ell SR, Yates D: Marinefish stings. *Arch Emerg Med* **6**:59, 1989

57. Halstead BW: *Poisonous and Venomous Marine Animals of the World,* 2d ed. Princeton, NJ, Darwin Press, 1988

CHAPTER 227

*David C. Wilson, William H. Leyva,
and Lloyd E. King, Jr.*

Arthropod Bites and Stings

The bites and stings of arthropods cause many patients to consult physicians for relief from these vexatious creatures. Occasionally, death is caused by envenomation, particularly in infants.[1] The clinician primarily diagnoses and treats skin lesions produced by only five of the nine classes of arthropods: Arachnida, Chilopoda, Diplopoda, Crustacea, and Insecta.[2] All arthropods are invertebrates with a chitinous exoskeleton, bilateral symmetry, true segmentation, and jointed true appendages that vary from few to many (Fig. 227-1 and Table 227-1).

Histopathology

Most arthropod bites have a similar histologic reaction pattern. In the acute phase, there is variable epidermal necrosis, spongiosis, and parakeratosis with plasma exudate and a dermal inflammatory infiltrate extending upward. Dermal inflammation tends to extend into the deep dermis in a wedge-shaped pattern and surrounds vessels with some extension into dermal collagen. The infiltrate is typically of mixed composition including eosinophils, neutrophils,

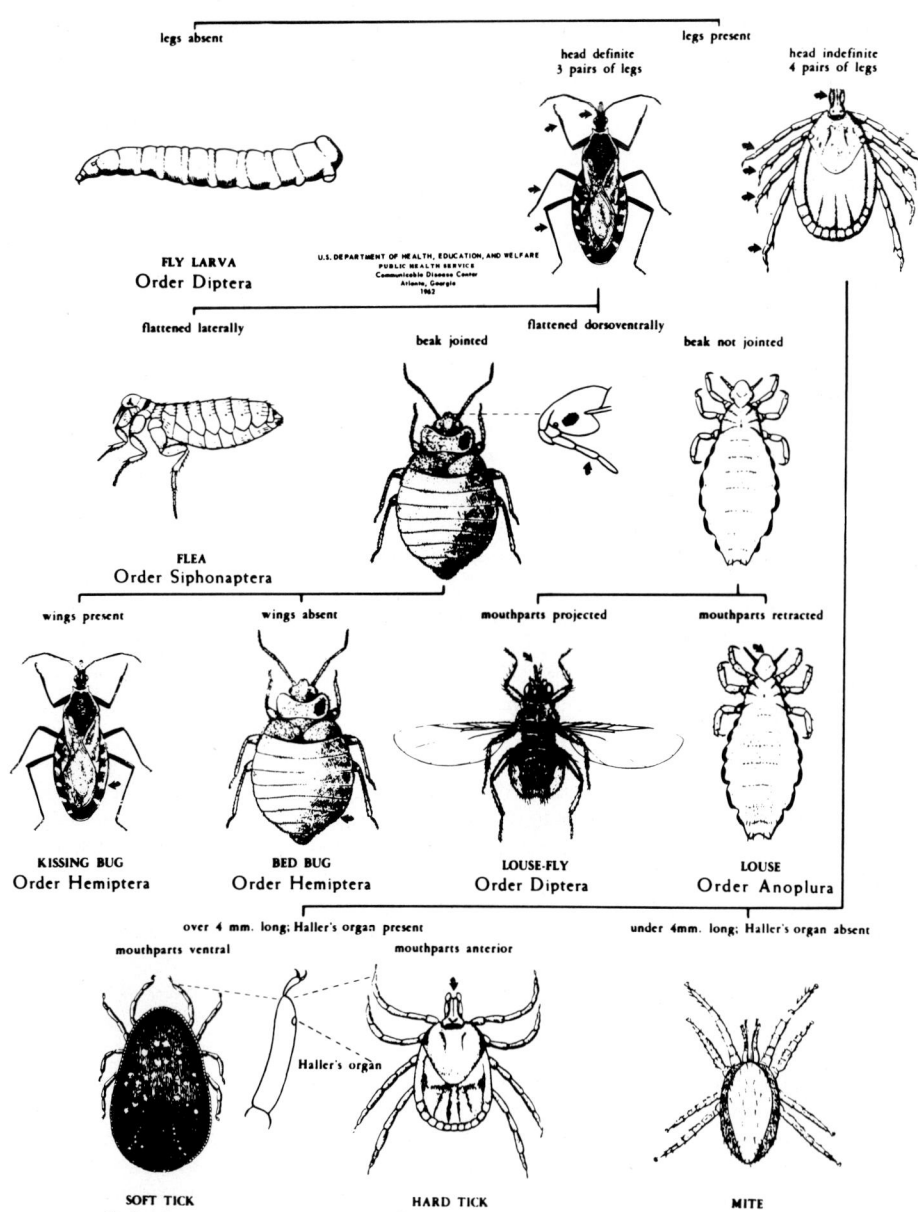

FIGURE 227-1 Pictorial key to groups of human ectoparasites. (*C. J. Stojanovich and H. G. Scott, U.S. Department of Health, Education, and Welfare, Public Health Service.*)

TABLE 227-1
Arthropods That Infest, Bite, or Sting Humans

  I. Arachnida—mites, ticks, spiders, scorpions (four pairs of legs)
    A. Acari
        1. Mites—follicle, food, fowl, grain, harvest, murine, scabies
        2. Ticks
    B. Araneae—spiders
    C. Scorpionida
 II. Chilopoda and Diplopoda—centipedes, millipedes
III. Insecta (three pairs of legs)
    A. Anoplura—lice
    B. Coleoptera—beetles
    C. Diptera—flies, mosquitoes
    D. Hemiptera—bedbugs, kissing bugs
    E. Hymenoptera—ants, bees, wasps
    F. Lepidoptera—butterflies, moths
    G. Siphonaptera—fleas

lymphocytes, and histiocytes in varying proportions. Eosinophils are usually prominent, although neutrophils may predominate in reactions to fleas, mosquitoes, fire ants, and brown recluse spiders. Bullae can form secondary to marked edema, especially in children. Insect parts are rarely seen, except for the burrowed mites of scabies within the stratum corneum and the mouthparts of ticks which may remain within the dermis after ticks are removed.

Chronic lesions most commonly result when a portion of the arthropod lodges within the skin, although hypersensitivity to the bite can be the sole cause. Chronic lesions can present diagnostic problems when they take on a pseudolymphomatous appearance.[3]

Arachnida

The Arachnida class includes three orders of medical interest: Acari (ticks and mites), Araneae (spiders), and Scorpionida (scorpions).

All adults in this class have four pairs of legs; the cephalothorax may vary, but it is typically fused. An exception to this rule is the larval stage of ticks ("seed ticks"), which have only three pairs of legs.

Acari

The mites in the order Acari of most interest to the clinician are the follicle mites, food mites, fowl mites, grain mites, harvest mites, murine mites, and scabies. With the exception of *Demodex* and scabies, these mites do not burrow and are known to drop off after feeding.[4] All mites may produce pruritus and/or allergic reactions through salivary proteins deposited during feeding. Although it is not possible to group all mites that cause human diseases into convenient categories, most of the more common mites can be grouped into three suborders:

Trombidiiformes: Harvest/chigger mites, family Trombiculidae; grain mites, family Pyemotidae; follicle mites, family Demodicidae.

Mesostigmata: Bird/rodent mites, family Dermanyssidae; straw mites, family Hemoganasidae.

Sarcoptiformes: Scabies, family Sarcoptidae; food mites, family Acaridae, family Glyciphagidae; mange, family Psoroptidae.

Follicle Mites   *Demodex* mites can be detected in sebaceous glands and hair follicles by skin biopsy of symptomatic and asymptomatic humans and other animal species.[5] Whether *Demodex* is the etiologic agent in rosacea and other dermatoses, or whether its presence reflects asymptomatic parasitosis, is not well documented. Symptoms produced by democidosis, if any, are more likely due to immunologic rather than toxicologic reactions.

Food Mites   Several species of mites that infest foodstuffs have been described. In their hypopial stage, they may be disseminated on the bodies of insects. The grain mite, *Acarus*, the cheese mite, *Glyciphagus*, and the grocery mite, *Tyrophagus*, produce papular urticaria or vesicopapular eruptions. An occupational history and skin scrapings are frequently required to separate these food mite-induced problems from scabies and other causes of papular urticaria.

Fowl Mites   Office workers, homemakers, and bird fanciers are all affected by mites that infest birds, especially pigeons that have nests or roosts near air conditioner intake ducts. *Dermanyssus gallinae* and *D. avium* are the most common fowl ectoparasites identified in the United States. These mites only temporarily infest humans. *Ornithonyssus sylviarum* is an uncommon fowl mite of the northern temperate region that can induce human skin lesions as well as transmit Western equine encephalomyelitis virus.

Grain Mites   The best studied grain mite of medical importance is the straw itch mite, *Pyemotes ventricosus*.[6] *P. ventricosus* is primarily a parasite of insect larvae that feed on grain, such as the Angoumois grain moth (*Sitotroga cerealella*) and the wheat joint worm (*Harmolita tritici*). The distribution of *P. ventricosus* is worldwide and it has been identified in over half of the United States.

P. ventricosus infests both animals and humans, occasionally producing unusual epidemics after an exposure to infested hay, grains, grasses, or straw. Affected patients often have systemic symptoms such as fever, diarrhea, anorexia, and malaise. Clinically, the lesions vary from bright red macules to varicelliform eruptions. However, identification of *P. ventricosus* in various infested grain products is often not made because of the low index of suspicion.

Harvest Mites   Perhaps the best known cause of "bites" due to mites in the United States is the chigger, mower, or harvest mite (*Trombicula alfreddugèsi* and *T. splendens*). In other parts of the world, *Trombicula* species are the vectors for *Rickettsia tsutsugamushi* in scrub typhus by *T. deliensis* and *T. akamushi*. Contact with the chigger mite usually occurs during the summer and fall when outdoor activities are maximal. Frequently, the only sign of exposure is intense pruritus on the ankles, legs, or belt line since the bright red mites ("red bugs") typically fall off after feeding or may be scratched off. In nonsensitized individuals, usually only 1- to 2-mm pruritic macules are seen, which require minimal treatment. In sensitized or allergic individuals, the reaction to the chigger infestation may be papular urticaria, vesiculation, or a granulomatous reaction with fever and lymphadenopathy. Clinically, the distribution of the lesions may be confused with other dermatoses since the type of exposure and the clothing worn greatly affect where the mites attach. Occasionally, the mites can be identified by visual inspection.

Since nonscabetic mites other than *Demodex* do not burrow into the skin, their treatment consists of a warm soapy bath to kill remaining larvae, an important step in the prevention of scrub typhus transmitted by trombiculid mites. The ultimate success of treatment in these nonscabetic cases also depends on treatment of the animal or food sources. Antipruritics are used as needed.

Animal Mites   Two species of murine mites are of medical importance throughout the world: *Ornithonyssus bacoti*, tropical rat mite, and *Allodermanyssus sanguineus*, the housemouse mite, a vector of rickettsialpox. *O. bacoti*, a vector of endemic (murine) typhus, has been noted to travel widely to obtain its blood meal if the host rats die or leave the infested nest. Persons working in areas rats commonly inhabit (groceries, granaries, restaurants, storehouses) may be affected without ever finding the mite because it drops off after each feeding.

Cheyletiellid mites are frequently harbored by dogs and cats, producing a condition sometimes referred to as "walking dandruff." Although the pet is usually asymptomatic, the person holding the pet experiences marked pruritus when the mites penetrate clothing and temporarily feed on that individual's skin. Diagnosis depends on finding the mites on the pet by microscopically examining cellophane tape applied to the pet's skin or brushings from the animal. Treatment of the pet by a qualified veterinarian resolves the symptoms.[7]

Scabies   The mite *Sarcoptes scabiei*, var. *hominis*, is the mite in the order Acari that is of most interest to physicians because of its origin in antiquity and prevalence in modern times (for reviews see Orkin et al.[8] and Burkhart[9]). The diagnosis may be easily missed and should be considered in a patient of any age with persistent generalized severe pruritus. Chronic undiagnosed scabies is the basis for the colloquial term, "the 7-year itch."

Scabies is usually spread by skin-to-skin contact, although clothing and linen may act as fomites since the mite can remain alive away from skin for 2 to 5 days.[10] The primary infestation has a 1-month incubation period before allergic sensitization occurs and itching begins. Subsequent infestations produce immediate itching.

Multiple family members are typically affected, a sign that should raise the suspicion of scabies.

Scabietic lesions are typically found on the interdigital webs, elbows, feet, genitalia, buttocks, and axillae. The head is usually spared in adults but is involved in infants. The burrow is the characteristic and diagnostic feature of the human variant of scabies. These burrows are either linear or wavy and have a small vesicle overlying the site of the female mite (Fig. 227-2). Experienced observers can detect and even remove the female mite, which appears as a small dark or gray speck below the vesicle. Occasionally, only the eggs or feces are retrieved. Excoriations and/or secondary infections may make identification of burrows very difficult. A helpful technique to detect burrows is to put on water-washable ink or topical tetracycline which fluoresces under a Wood's lamp, wash off the excess, and look for the burrows, which retain the ink or tetracycline. In animal scabies, the diagnosis is more difficult because characteristic burrows are seldom found since the mites do not persist on human skin for any length of time. Failure to identify microscopically the mites, feces, or eggs may still require a therapeutic trial when clinical suspicion is high.

Other clinical variants of human scabies are also well described.[8] Nodular lesions occur in 11 percent of patients and are most commonly seen in the groin area or axillae (Fig. 227-2c), but they may be seen elsewhere in infants. In crusted Norwegian scabies (Fig. 227-2d), literally thousands of mites instead of the usual 3 to 50 female mites may be found. These patients are highly contagious. Secondary lesions found in the typical case of acute scabies include urticarial papules, eczematous plaques, excoriations, and impetiginization of existing lesions.

The focus of treatment in scabies is directed toward the individual who harbors the burrowing mites. One of the oldest treatments for scabies is 10% sulfur in petrolatum. While this treatment is considered safe, the odor is offensive to many. Lindane (Kwell) has been a mainstay in the treatment of scabies, but concerns over potential neurotoxicity in children brought 5% permethrin cream to the forefront for these younger individuals.[11] Permethrin is now the treatment of choice for all ages. Crotamiton has also been advocated as a scabicide, though its potential toxicity is not as well characterized as that of lindane and permethrin. Resistance has been reported to both lindane and crotamiton, but these findings have been questioned.[8,12] Most problems encountered with scabies are not therapeutic but diagnostic, as clinical suspicions wax and wane with fluctuations in the prevalence of scabies in given populations.

Specific treatment instructions must be given if success is to be achieved. After a bath or shower, the entire skin surface from the neck down should be massaged with the topical medicament selected. In infants, the entire body should be treated with permethrin 5% cream. The medication is washed off 8 h after application. Reapplication in the manner described above is performed 48 h after the initial treatment.[13] Some advocate a third treatment after 7 days. All family members and close personal contacts should be treated simultaneously, and inanimate objects such as clothing should be washed or dry cleaned if they are to be used or worn within 5 days.

Posttreatment pruritus is common and may be attributed to hypersensitivity to remaining dead mites and mite products. Pruritus should be controlled with systemic antipruritics and secondary infections should be treated with appropriate antibiotics. Nodular lesions may persist for weeks and require special consideration. Intralesional corticosteroids may be helpful. PUVA photochemotherapy is effective when many lesions are present.

Ticks   Ticks are the largest members of the order Acari. They are important worldwide as vectors of systemic disease. Reactions to tick bites include foreign body reactions, reactions to salivary secretions, reactions to injected toxins, and hypersensitivity reactions.[4]

Ticks are divided into the Argasidae (soft tick) and Ixodidae (hard tick) families[2] (Fig. 227-1). The Ixodidae family is responsible for most tick-related diseases. Ticks are separated from other mites by the presence of a barbed hypostome which they use for feeding. Using their toothed chelicerae, ticks tear open the epidermis and then insert the barbed hypostome. Salivary secretions are used to soften the epidermis as well. During the insertion process, a cement-like substance is secreted which hardens and firmly anchors the hypostome to the skin. Ticks feed for about 7 days until engorged and then drop off to continue their life cycle.[4]

Tick bites occur most commonly in the spring and summer coinciding with the life cycle of the tick. Ticks have four stages of the life cycle: egg, larva, nymph, and adult. All stages require a blood meal to advance to the next stage except the egg. Eggs are deposited in early spring and develop to larvae by summer. The larvae feed once on small rodents and then are inactive over winter. The following spring larvae develop to nymphs and again find a suitable host and feed. Generally this host is a small rodent, but larger animals and humans may also become hosts. Nymphs molt to become adults in summer. After finding a suitable host for a blood meal, the adult female survives through the winter to begin the life cycle with egg laying the following spring.

Many different species of ticks are responsible for local tick bite reactions and transmission of diseases in humans. Among those most common in the United States are *Ixodes dammini, I. pacificus, I. scapularis, Amblyomma americanum* (Lone Star tick), *Dermacentor andersoni* (American wood tick), and *D. variabilis* (American dog tick). In Europe, *Ixodes ricinus* and *I. persulcatus* are important vectors of disease, especially Lyme disease.

Depending on the species of tick, the bite of the tick may or may not be painful or pruritic. Most bites are not painful. In many instances, victims are not even aware that they have been bitten and there may be only a red papule at the bite site. This papule can progress to local swelling and erythema. Blistering, severe pruritus, and ecchymosis can be seen. A cellular reaction to the bite can lead to induration and nodularity after a few days. Central necrosis and ulceration rarely occur.[4] The usual bite heals in 2 to 3 weeks, although chronic tick bite granulomas may persist for months to years. Persistent papules respond to intralesional corticosteroid injections.

TICK PARALYSIS.   Tick paralysis is thought to be caused by a toxin secreted in the saliva of the tick, although the exact nature of the toxin is unknown. Tick paralysis may be caused by 43 different species of ticks, but most human cases in the United States are attributed to *Dermacentor* species. The paralysis is an acute ascending lower motor neuron paralysis. Typically, the tick is attached from 4 to 7 days before the onset of symptoms. If the tick is found and removed, symptoms disappear rapidly in the reverse order of their appearance. Diagnosis is made by a careful search of the scalp and body for the attached tick. The diagnosis is also suggested if the patient lives in or has traveled to an area where tick paralysis is endemic. Treatment, which may require respiratory support, is merely supportive until the symptoms resolve.[14]

BABESIOSIS.   Babesiosis is a disease caused by the intracellular red blood cell parasite *Babesia microti,* which is transmitted by the larvae of *Ixodes dammini.* Eastern Long Island, Martha's Vineyard, and Nantucket are the major endemic areas. There is an in-

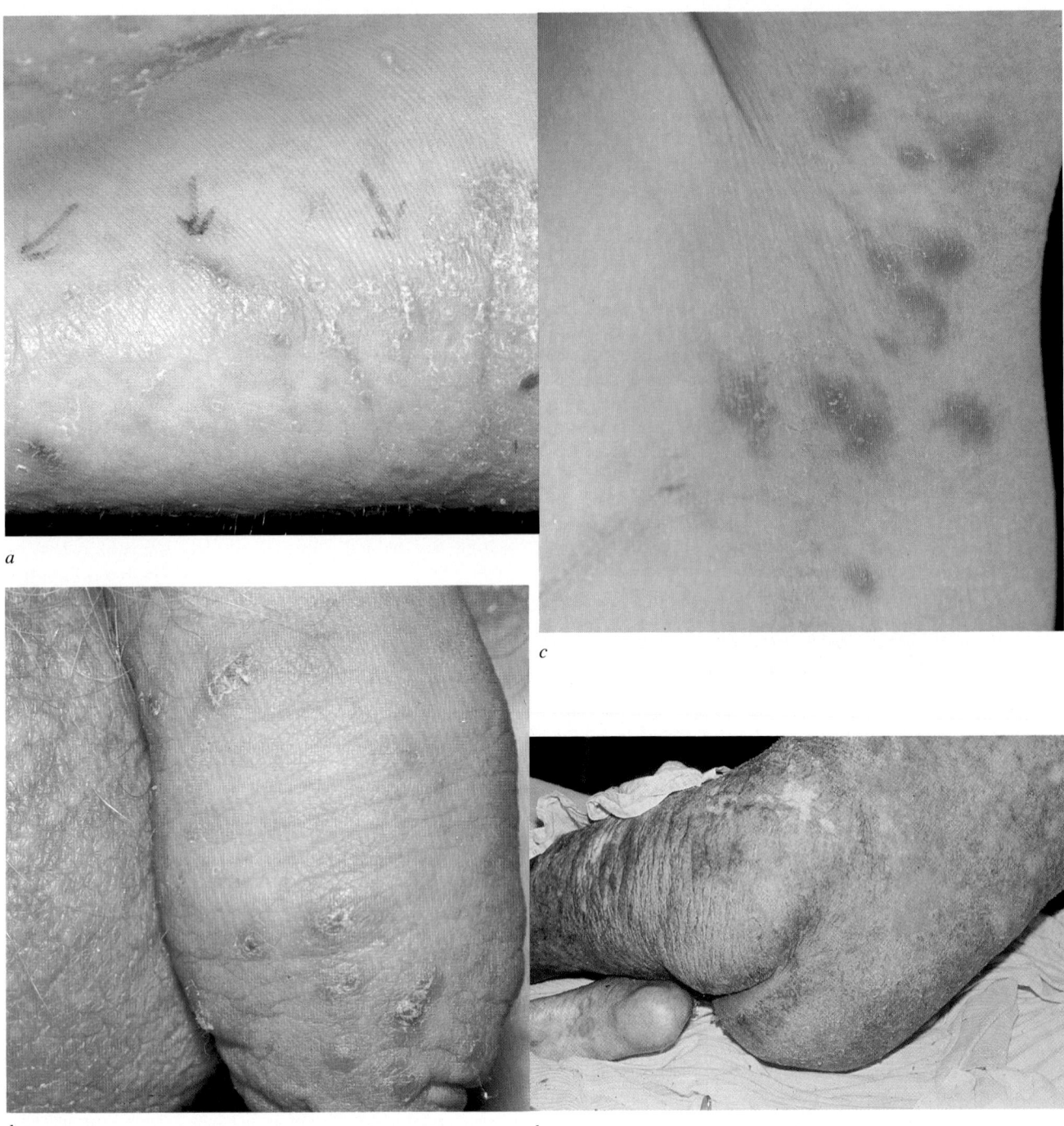

FIGURE 227-2 Scabies. (*a*) Several, slightly scaling, threadlike burrows are seen on the medial aspect of the palm, associated with a more generalized eczematous process; scrapings of a tunnel has the highest yield in detection of a scabetic mite. (*b*) The penis and scrotum are common sites for scabetic infestation; crusted, excoriated papules are seen on the prepuce and shaft. (*c*) Scabetic nodules occur in a minority of persons, especially in the axillae and genitalia, are pathognomonic, and may persist for months after successful eradication of the mite. (*d*) Crusted or Norwegian scabies in an HIV-infected person: the clinical presentation of generalized hyperkeratosis and scaling is often misdiagnosed; rather than having an infestation with a dozen mites, many thousands are present. (*Courtesy of M. Hebert, M.D.*)

creased risk in patients with T-lymphocyte depression or after splenectomy. The clinical syndrome of babesiosis includes fever, drenching sweats, myalgia, and hemolytic anemia.[15] Diagnosis is made by observation of the intracellular red blood cell parasite on a Giemsa-stained smear. The tetrad may be confused with the findings in falciparum malaria, but *Babesia*-infected red blood cells do not have pigment granules. Antibody titers are also helpful in making the diagnosis. Treatment is symptomatic in the patient with mild infection. In splenectomized patients, exchange transfusions have been helpful.[16] The combination of clindamycin and quinine has also been successful.[17]

LYME DISEASE.   (See also Chap. 193) Lyme disease (Lyme borreliosis) is now the most commonly reported tick-borne disease in the United States. It has been reported in 43 states and is most prevalent in the Northeast and upper Midwest. Lyme disease has been reported from all continents except South America and Antarctica.[18] Although not a new disease, it became well recognized in the United States in 1976 when Steere et al. investigated a cluster of arthritis in children in Lyme, Connecticut.[19] Since that time, the cause of Lyme disease was found to be a spirochete isolated from an *Ixodes dammini* tick, *Borrelia burgdorferi*. A plasmid detected in *B. burgdorferi* may explain differences in disease expression that are seen in Europe and the United States.[20] Although ticks are capable of transmitting the disease during all stages of their life cycle, the nymphal stage is the most common transmission stage. The primary vectors in the United States are *Ixodes dammini, I. pacificus,* and *I. scapularis.* Other species of ticks have also been reported as potential vectors.

The clinical manifestations of Lyme disease have been divided into three stages: erythema migrans (erythema chronicum migrans) and nonspecific constitutional symptoms (stage 1), nervous and cardiovascular system disorders (stage 2), and arthritis (stage 3). An orderly progression from one stage to another does not always occur and signs of more than one stage may coexist.

Stage 1 begins 3 to 30 days after the bite of an infected tick and is characterized by the hallmark skin finding of Lyme disease, erythema migrans. This sign is seen in 60 to 80 percent of cases of Lyme disease. Erythema migrans begins as an erythematous papule at the site of the bite and enlarges to form an annular ring. Central clearing of the ring is the usual course. Most patients describe erythema migrans as asymptomatic. Erythema migrans resolves spontaneously in weeks to months even in untreated patients. Multiple secondary annular lesions occur in 50 percent of patients as the disease progresses. These lesions may be less typical, being smaller than the primary lesion and lacking central clearing. Other cutaneous lesions seen in stage 1 include malar erythema, urticaria, periorbital swelling, and erythema nodosum.[21]

Neurologic involvement develops in 15 percent of untreated patients in stage 2. Although many manifestations are possible, meningitis and cranial (Bell's palsy) and peripheral neuropathies are common.[22] Cardiac involvement, manifested most commonly as atrioventricular block, also characterizes this stage.

The last stage of Lyme disease is characterized by arthritis. In Europe, other skin manifestations have been associated with the late stages of Lyme disease. These manifestations include acrodermatitis chronica atrophicans, lymphadenosis benigna cutis, and lesions resembling morphea or lichen sclerosus et atrophicus.[23]

Although spirochetes have been identified in some skin biopsies of patients with erythema migrans, the diagnosis of Lyme disease is accomplished with a specific enzyme-linked immunosorbent assay (ELISA) in a patient with consistent symptoms. Treatment varies with the stage of the disease but is primarily accomplished with tetracycline, 250 mg qid, or doxycycline, 100 mg bid, for 10 to 21 days. Acceptable alternatives when these agents are contraindicated include penicillin or erythromycin. More advanced disease may be treated with intravenous penicillin or ceftriaxone.

Preventing bites is the most important measure in controlling both local and systemic tick-related diseases. When exposure is anticipated, proper clothing should be worn and appropriate repellents used. Immediately after potential exposures, the skin should be carefully inspected for ticks in an attempt to remove them before they become embedded or transmit disease. Evidence suggests that the tick must remain attached for more than 24 h in most cases to transmit Lyme disease.[24] Once the tick's hypostome is secure to the skin, the tick must be forced to remove it. A colorful array of remedies has been recommended for removing the tick. These include applying noxious substances such as gasoline and chloroform or burning the tick with a match or other hot object. Suffocating the tick with petrolatum has been recommended. Physical methods such as slow steady pulling on the tick, with or without twisting, have also been advised.[25] If the hypostome is retained in the skin when the tick is extracted, it should be removed surgically. Foreign-body reactions and persistent papules are produced if tick parts remain in the wound.

Ticks are important vectors of many other diseases to humans. They play a role in transmitting viruses, rickettsia, parasites, spirochetes, and bacteria. Those of major importance are summarized in Table 227-2.[26]

Araneae

Spiders belong to the class Arachnida and are differentiated from insects by the presence of two separate body parts with five paired appendages and the absence of antennae. Spiders are carnivorous and either capture their prey in webs or attack them and inject venom through their chelicera (mandibles). In the United States, the genera *Loxosceles* and *Latrodectus* are the only species whose venom produces significant toxic effects in humans. Wolf spiders, tarantulas, jumping spiders, orb weavers, and crab spiders rarely produce cutaneous lesions by other mechanisms, such as the trauma of the bite or secondary infection.[2]

Loxosceles   There are 13 different species of *Loxosceles* in the United States and five of them, *L. reclusa, L. deserta, L. arizonica, L. laeta,* and *L. refuscens,* have been associated with cutaneous loxoscelism.[2,27] The brown recluse spider, *L. reclusa,* typifies the species and is widely distributed throughout the Southeast and the Midwest. It is often called the violin or fiddleback spider because of the violin-shaped figure on its dorsal cephalothorax (Fig. 227-3). Depending on diet and habitat, it may vary in size from 0.2 to 2.5 cm in diameter. Although its natural habitat is outdoors under dry overhanging rocks and cliffs, human environmental controls have caused it to move indoors and expand its range. Despite its usually timid nature, this spider will bite when trapped or threatened via chance encounters with humans. Since the brown recluse spider hibernates in the winter, most bites occur between March and October when humans disturb their habitat (closets, attics, outbuildings).

The venom of the brown recluse spider contains at least nine protein fractions.[28] One major fraction is a 32 kDa protein with sphingomyelinase D activity. This venom fraction aggregates

TABLE 227-2
Tick-Borne Diseases in Humans

Disease	Organism	Vector	Geographic distribution
Lyme borreliosis	*Borrelia burgdorferi*	*Ixodes dammini,* *I. pacificus, Amblyomma* *americanum, I. ricinus,* *I. persulcatus*	Northeast, Midwest, North- west United States; Europe; Asia; Australia
Relapsing fever	*Borrelia duttonii, B. hermsii,* *B. turicatae*	*Ornithodoros moubata*	Western mountains, southern Great Plains, United States
Rocky Mountain spotted fever	*Rickettsia rickettsii*	*Dermacentor andersoni,* *D. variabilis,* *Ambylomma americanum, Haema-* *physalis leporispalustris*	Western hemisphere, especially Southeast United States
Babesiosis	*Babesia microti*	*Ixodes dammini*	Coastal areas, islands off Massachusetts, Rhode Island, New York
Tularemia	*Francisella tularensis*	*Dermacentor andersoni, D. variabilis,* *Amyblomma americanum*	South, Southeast, Midwest United States
Ehrlichiosis	*Ehrlichia canis*	*Rhipicephalus sanguineus*	South, Southeast, Midwest United States
	Ehrlichia sennetsu	*R. sanguineus*	Japan
Queensland tick typhus	*Rickettsia australis*	Ixodid ticks	Eastern Australia
Spotted fever groups	*Rickettsia conorii*	Ixodid ticks	Worldwide
South African tick-bite fever	*R. conorii*	Ixodid ticks	South Africa
Asia tick fever	*Rickettsia siberica*	Ixodid ticks	Central Asia, Soviet Union
Q fever	*Coxiella burnetii*	All endemic species	Worldwide
Colorado tick fever	Orbivirus	*Dermacentor andersoni*	Rocky Mountains, northern Sierra Mountains, United States; western Canada
Tick-borne encephalitis	Flavivirus	*Ixodes persulcatus, I. ricinus*	Central Asia; Eastern Europe; Soviet Union
Tick-bite granuloma	—	All species	—
Tick paralysis	—	*Dermacentor andersoni, D. variabilis*	—

SOURCE: Adapted from Jacobs.[26]

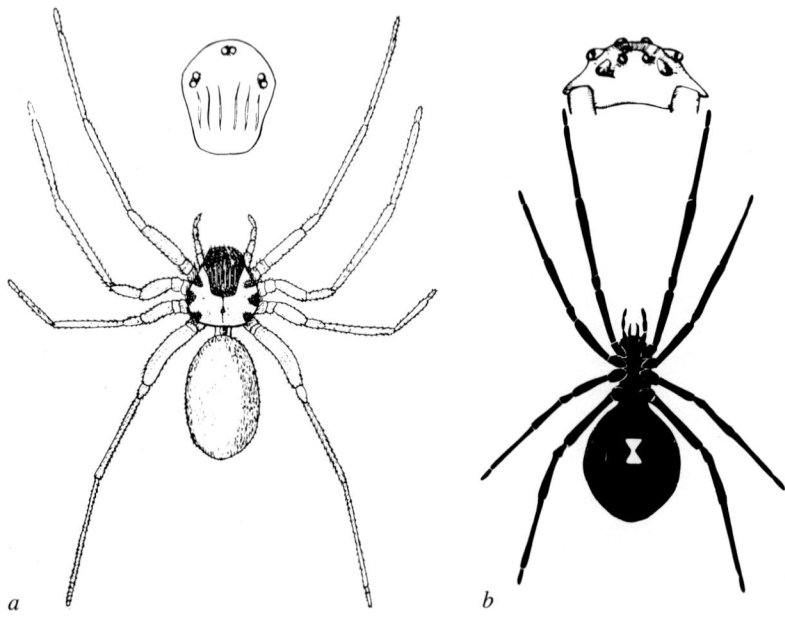

FIGURE 227-3 (*a*) Brown recluse spider. Characteristically there are six eyes in three pairs and fiddle-shaped markings on the cephalothorax. (*b*) Black widow spider, with eight eyes; it is shiny black, usually with a red hourglass marking on the underside of its abdomen. (*U.S. Department of Health, Education, and Welfare, Public Health Service.*)

platelets, generates leukocyte chemoattractants, and liberates thromboxane B_2 in vitro while producing typical skin necrosis when injected into rabbits.

Reported responses to envenomation have ranged from a mild local urticarial reaction to full-thickness skin necrosis. This re-sponse may be associated with a maculopapular exanthem, fever, headache, malaise, arthralgias, nausea, and vomiting. The bite it-self is generally painless and findings of a central papule and asso-ciated erythema may not be seen for 6 to 12 h. Few envenomations, perhaps less than 10 percent, lead to severe skin necrosis or other

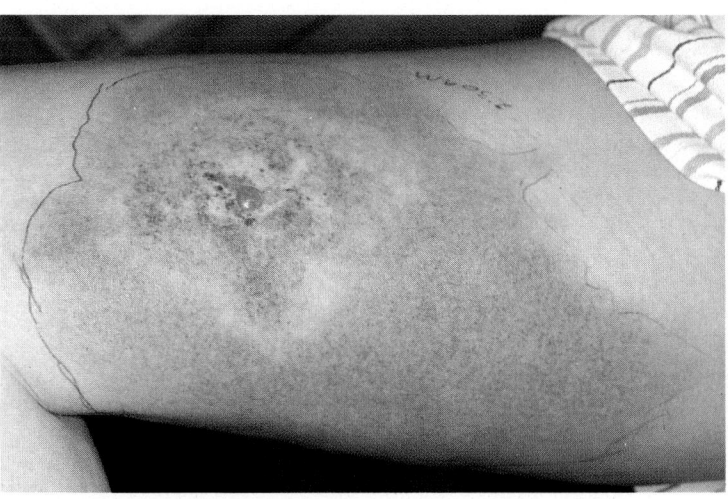

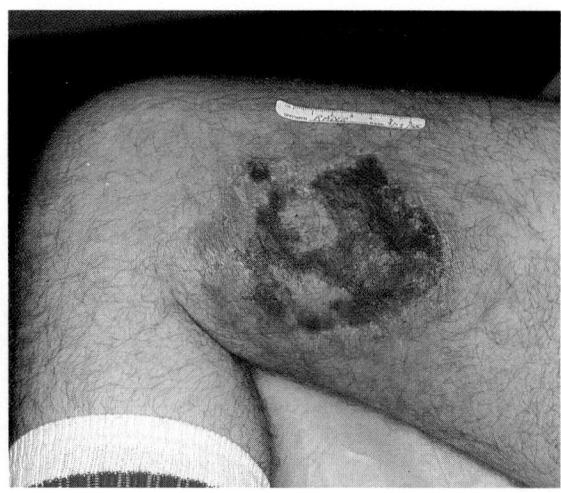

a   *b*

FIGURE 227-4 (*a*) Clinically typical brown recluse spider bite showing "red, white, and blue" sign. (*b*) Late ulcerative brown recluse spider bite with overlying eschar.

systemic manifestations. Wounds destined for necrosis generally show signs of progression within 48 to 72 h of the bite.[29] Central blistering with a surrounding gray to purple discoloration of the skin may be seen at the bite site. A surrounding ring of blanched skin is itself surrounded by a large area of asymmetric erythema leading to the typical "red, white, and blue" sign of a brown recluse bite (Fig. 227-4*a*). At this stage of evolution, these bites may be associated with significant pain related to incipient necrosis of skin and subcutaneous tissues. The resultant necrotic skin ulcer heals slowly (Fig. 227-4*b*) and may require skin grafts or flaps to reconstruct the defect. Case reports, often unconfirmed, of hemolysis, disseminated intravascular coagulopathy, convulsions, renal failure, or death have been recorded.

The histologic findings of bites are nonspecific and histologic study should not generally be pursued unless other etiologies are strongly considered. Findings include acute vasculitis, platelet thrombi, and leukocyte infiltrates.

Since the clinical appearance of a brown recluse spider bite is nonspecific, diagnosis may be difficult. The potential for exposure to *Loxosceles* spiders, identification of the arachnid, appearance of the lesion, and clinical course must all be considered. Of these, only identification of the captured spider allows for definitive diagnosis of *Loxosceles* envenomation. Laboratory tests for diagnosis are not currently available. Laboratory tests to assess for potential complications such as hemolysis are in order, particularly in children. A broad differential diagnosis must be entertained to include reactions to other biting organisms, allergic reactions, trauma, herpetic eruptions, skin abscesses, and pyoderma gangrenosum.

The treatment of brown recluse spider bites remains controversial. These authors have successfully used, both experimentally and clinically, the leukocyte inhibitor dapsone.[30] Ice and elevation are useful in reducing erythema and swelling. Corticosteroids have not proved useful for the local wound but should be considered for patients with significant systemic symptoms such as hemolysis. Antibiotics are useful in reducing the incidence of abscess formation and secondary infection in large lesions. Acute excision of the bite site should be avoided since the inflammatory reaction produced by the venom will inhibit wound healing and produce an

inferior clinical result.[28] Surgical management should be postponed until wounds have stabilized with medical management and are no longer progressing.

Latrodectus Several different species of *Latrodectus* spiders exist in the United States, but the fame and fear of *L. mactans*, the black widow, far exceed the others. *L. mactans* is the most common of the North American "widow" spiders, but *L. variolus* and *L. hesperus* can also be commonly found in a more limited distribution. All three of these spiders have the characteristic red hourglass or double triangle on the ventral surface of the abdomen; the age of the spider determines the relative amount of red on the abdomen (Fig. 227-3*b*). The red-legged widow, *L. bishopi*, is found only in southern Florida, while the brown widow, *L. geometricus*, is rarely found in the United States. Females are significantly larger than males (leg span up to 40 mm) and are the only spiders capable of envenomation. Black widows spin their large irregular webs close to the ground under debris, over hollow stumps, under woodpiles, or in front of rodent burrows. Clinging upside down to the web, they wait for prey to become entangled in the web and then quickly paralyze the prey with a bite.[31]

The venom of the black widow spider contains a neurotoxin known as alpha-latrotoxin. The envenomation produces little or no skin reaction at the bite site, but has significant systemic effects via its action at nerve terminals. Alpha-latrotoxin acts as a calcium ionophore resulting in release of massive amounts of acetylcholine from neuromuscular junctions of both sympathetic and parasympathetic nervous systems.[32]

Clinically, bites may be sensed as a pin prick or a sharp pinch. Dull aching pain or a numb sensation ensues 30 to 40 min after the bite. Skin manifestations are limited to slight erythema, local piloerection, mild edema or urtication, local perspiration, and possibly lymphangitis. Systemic symptoms peak at 1 to 8 h after the bite and may last 24 to 48 h. Severe pain in local muscle groups spreads to regional muscle groups. The characteristic crampy abdominal and chest pain may lead to confusion with acute appendicitis, renal colic, or acute myocardial infarction. Headache, restlessness, anxiety, fatigue, insomnia, salivation, lacrimation, diaphoresis, tremors, tachycardia, bradycardia, hypertension, shock, and coma have all been associated with latrodectism. Death from documented bites occurs in less than 1 percent of reported cases.[33]

Diagnosis depends on recognition of a consistent history and typical physical findings. Laboratory evaluation is not helpful, although hemoglobinuria, albuminuria, and leukocytosis may be found.

Treatment of most cases of latrodectism is supportive and generally does not require hospitalization. Exceptions to this rule include the very young and the very old, and persons with cardiovascular disease, who are at greater risk for complications. Traditional treatment with intravenous calcium gluconate (10%) and muscle relaxants has proved effective in most patients. Relief of pain with narcotics may reduce the severity of symptoms and muscle spasms.[34] Since antivenom is prepared in horses, it should be used only for severe envenomations in persons not allergic to horse serum.

Scorpions

Scorpions are of medical interest primarily in tropical and/or arid areas such as parts of the southwestern United States, Mexico, India, and the Middle East. Although capable of producing significant local wounds, the primary concern over scorpion envenomation involves the potential for serious cardiovascular complications which can be lethal. Over 600 species of scorpions have been identified worldwide with approximately 40 species identified in the United States. The family Buthidae contains almost all the dangerous species. Those of primary concern in the United States are *Centruroides sculpturatus* and *C. gertschi*.[4]

Scorpions are characterized by a body subdivided into an obvious body and tail and five obvious pairs of appendages. The second pair of appendages are quite large and terminate in a powerful pincer used to grasp prey. The tail ends in the stinger which is brought up over the body to inflict the wound (Fig. 227-5). The venom of scorpions varies from species to species. It is a neurotoxin acting through both adrenergic and cholinergic pathways.

Scorpion stings can produce both local and systemic effects. As with many other venomous arthropods, most stings occur as a result of encounters with the scorpion in a setting where it feels threatened. Most stings occur on the limbs, head, or neck. Initially, there is a sensation of sharp burning pain at the sting site which may be associated with numbness extending beyond the sting site. Re-

gional swelling can be seen. More rarely, ecchymosis and lymphangitis may occur.[35] Systemic symptoms involve primarily the neurologic, cardiopulmonary, and pancreatic systems. Neurologically, these symptoms may include convulsions, coma, hemiplegia, hyper- or hypothermia, tremor, restlessness, and irritability. Pancreatitis is a common complication of the stings of the Brazilian scorpions (*Tityus* species).[36] Deaths are most commonly related to cardiopulmonary abnormalities, particularly in children. Hypertension, arrhythmias, and pulmonary edema are seen frequently.

Therapy is aimed at inhibiting the effects of the neurotransmitters that are released by the venom. In milder cases with only local effects, therapy is largely supportive and includes local wound care, applications of ice packs, and antihistamines to control inflammation. Local injections of anesthetics may also help to control pain. Systemic effects may require a variety of medical interventions such as antihypertensive agents (hydralazine, nifedipine, or prazosin may be useful) and anticonvulsants (barbiturates).[37] Antivenin for some species is available, but its usefulness has been questioned. In the United States, antivenin is available only in Arizona.

Chilopoda and Diplopoda

Centipedes and millipedes superficially resemble each other, having one pair of legs and two pairs of legs per segment, respectively. Centipedes are nocturnal carnivores which may produce painful wounds by discharging venom through their claws as they grip the victim. In addition to severe pain, localized sweating, edema, secondary infection, and ulceration may be seen.[38] The *Scolopendra* species is found in Hawaii and the western United States and may attack and produce such lesions when its habitat is disturbed. Local injections of an anesthetic may be used to control pain. Antibiotics to control infection and corticosteroids to control inflammation may be necessary.

Millipedes are generally harmless vegetarians which neither bite nor envenomate. However, when disturbed or threatened they emit a toxic substance from repugnatorial glands on each side of each segment. This fluid may produce burning, blistering, and pigmentation of the skin. If introduced into the eye, it may cause severe inflammation.[39] For skin contact, no treatment is usually necessary other than thorough washing of the skin as soon as possible.

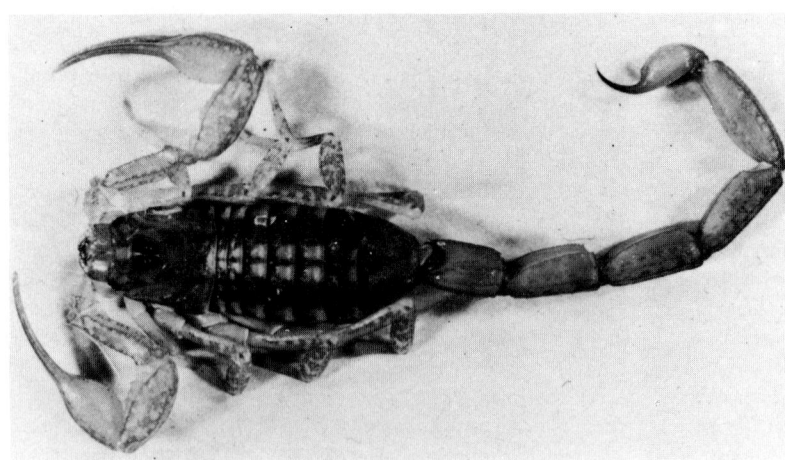

FIGURE 227-5 Scorpion. Note the pinching claws, tail, and stinger.

Insecta

Anoplura

Blood-sucking lice of the order Anoplura have long been successful obligate ectoparasites of humans. Only two species of Anoplura, *Phthirius pubis* and *Pediculus humanus,* are host-specific parasites of humans (Fig. 227-6).[2,8] Although morphologically very similar, *P. humanus* var. *capitus,* the head louse, is distinct clinically from *P. humanus* var. *corporis,* the body louse. Since interbreeding can occur, it has been speculated that the body louse evolved from the head louse after humans began to wear clothes.[6,42,43]

Pediculosis Capitis   No age or economic stratum is immune to *P. capitis.* Although the prevalence of infestation varies, crowded conditions are associated with a higher prevalence. Poor hygiene is frequently associated with pediculosis, but poor hygiene does not cause lousiness. In general, the only complaint associated with pediculosis capitis is pruritus. In long-standing or severe cases, secondary infection with cervical adenopathy may intervene. On examination, the adult *P. capitis* is frequently not observed; fewer

than 10 lice are detected in over half of the cases. In analogy to Norwegian scabies, more than 1000 head lice on a patient have been observed. On careful inspection, nits are more easily identified (Fig. 227-7). These eggs are cemented securely to the hairs and can most easily be found in the parietal and occipital areas of the scalp. By observing the distance between the scalp and the nits, one can estimate the duration of the infestation and whether the infestation remains active. Head lice may be transmitted by direct contact or via fomites such as combs, hats, and bedding.

Treatment requires the use of topical pediculocidal agents. Treatment may need to be repeated in 7 days (the time required for nits to hatch) because nits are sometimes less effectively killed than adults.[44] Lindane (gamma benzene hexachloride) (1%) has been the most widely used agent, but concerns about growing resistance and potential neurotoxicity have focused attention on other agents. Permethrin in a 1% lotion has shown high efficacy when compared with other available agents.[45] Other agents that have been used include pyrethrins, DDT, and malathion. Systemic antibiotics may be necessary if there is any secondary infection. Removal of nits after effective treatment is not necessary but may be psychologically important to the patient. All contacts should also be treated simultaneously. Fomites may be treated with hot water washing or hot air drying.

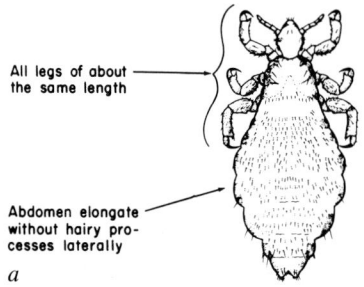
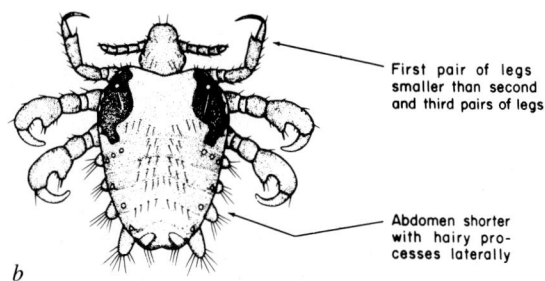

All legs of about the same length

Abdomen elongate without hairy processes laterally

a

First pair of legs smaller than second and third pairs of legs

Abdomen shorter with hairy processes laterally

b

FIGURE 227-6 Lice commonly found on humans. (*a*) Body louse or head louse, *Pediculus humanus.* (*b*) Crab louse, *Phthirius pubis.* (*U.S. Department of Health, Education, and Welfare, Public Health Service.*)

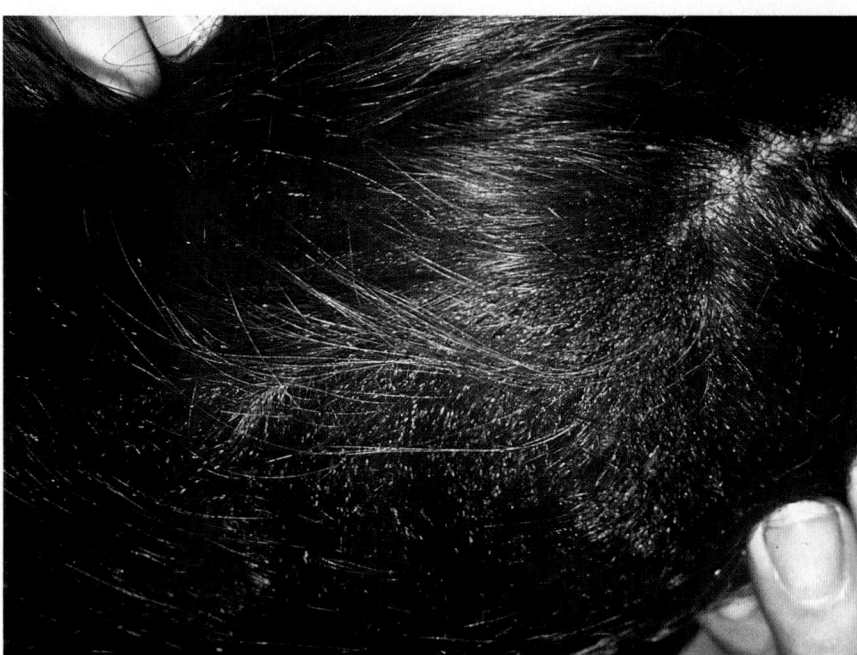

FIGURE 227-7 Pediculosis capitis. Myriads of oval, grayish-white egg capsules (nits) are firmly attached to the hair shafts.

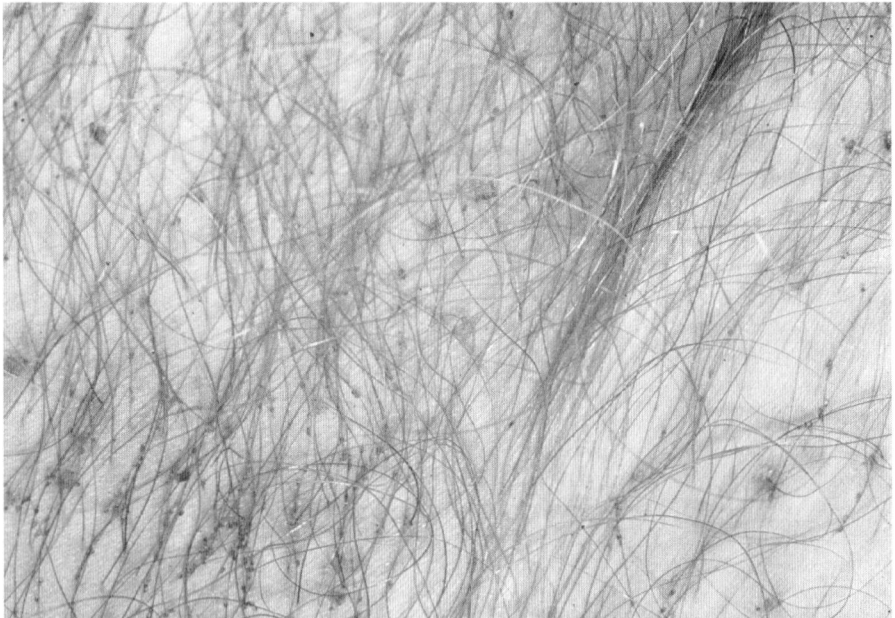

a

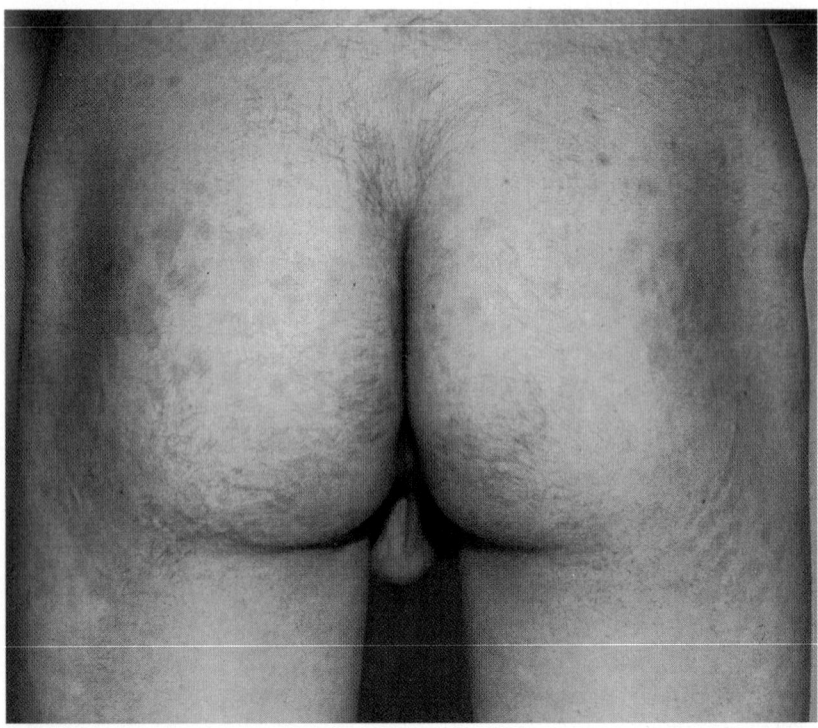

b

FIGURE 227-8 Pediculosis pubis. (*a*) Dotlike nits attached to the hair shafts can be easily seen on the pubic area of this patient, as well as several crab lice. (*b*) Maculae cerulae, slate-gray or blue-gray macules, are seen on the buttocks. (*c*) Microscopic view of an egg containing an unhatched louse, attached to a hair shaft. (*d*) Microscopic view of an adult female louse containing an egg. (*e*) Eyelash infestation with *Phthirius pubis*. Nits can be seen attached to the eyelashes. (*Courtesy of D. A. Burns.*)

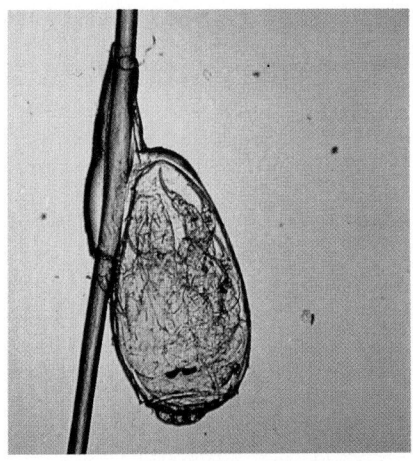

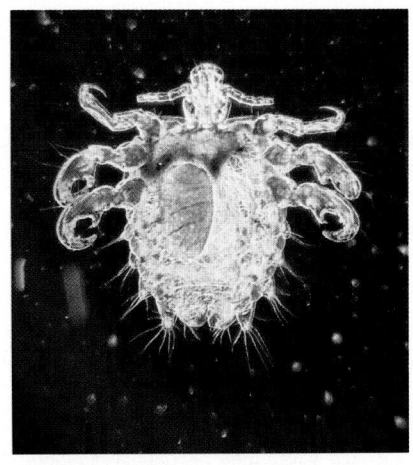

c   d

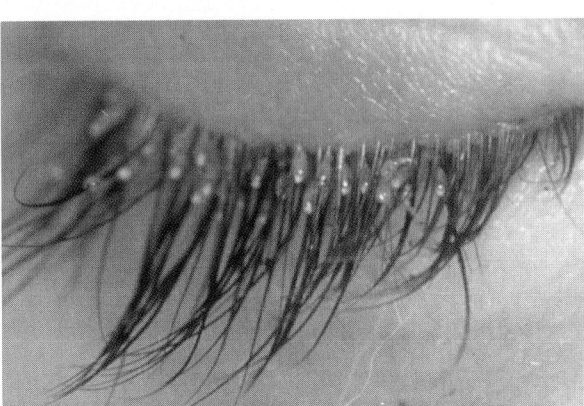

e   **FIGURE 227-8**   *(continued)*

Pediculosis Corporis   Unlike *P. capitis,* the body louse, *P. corporis,* has become relatively more rare in many affluent populations. The eggs of *P. corporis* are found predominantly on clothing and occasionally on body hairs. Since relatively few lice are found on the body, the lice and eggs should be searched for in the seams of clothing. Clinically, itch is the only symptom in most cases. Small red macules are seen in early cases, and initial lesions are often best seen on the back or under the arms. In chronic cases, excoriations, urticaria, and pigmentary changes may be seen. Pigmentation may be diffuse and can lead to confusion with other disease processes. In long-standing or severe cases, secondary infection may first appear with crusting, pus, and lymphadenopathy.[4] In uncomplicated cases, treatment requires nothing more than improved hygiene and clean clothes. In more severe cases and epidemic infestations, the ectoparasiticidal agents noted above may be necessary. Dry heat is equally effective in killing the lice and their ova in clothing.

Apart from the discomfort it may cause, the body louse is epidemiologically important as the vector of typhus, trench fever, and relapsing fever. The causative organisms are *Rickettsia prowazekii, R. quintana,* and *Borrelia recurrentis,* respectively.

Phthiriasis Pubis   The crab louse, *Phthirius pubis* (Fig. 227-8), is usually transmitted by sexual contact but may be transferred by articles of clothing or by infested hairs. In addition to pubic hair, these lice may be found on other short hairs of the body such as body hair, eyebrows, eyelashes, and hair at the edge of the scalp.

Lice may be present for up to 30 days before the symptoms of itching begin. Small blue-gray macules (maculae caeruleae) are a unique feature that may be seen. These macules are thought to be caused by the action of louse saliva on blood. A careful examination will reveal nits and the crab louse, which can frequently be seen clinging to two different hairs.

Treatment of phthiriasis pubis is the same as for pediculosis capitis with special attention paid to clothing and bedding infestation. Treatment failures can occur if other infested areas on the patient's body go untreated. Reinfestation after successful initial therapy is commonly due to reexposure to untreated sexual partners. Eyelid infestation can be treated by manual removal of nits and lice or by petrolatum occlusion. Physostigmine ophthalmic ointment and yellow oxide of mercury ointment have also been advocated.[46]

Coleoptera

Since there are over 250,000 species of beetles in the Coleoptera order, the largest order in the animal kingdom, it is not surprising that several species are of medical interest.[2] This section discusses only the beetles whose bodies contain blister-inducing irritants. Five families of Coleoptera produce chemicals that induce blistering or vesiculation upon contact with human skin: Meloidae, Staphylinidae, Paussidae, Coccinellidae, and Edemeridae. The

Spanish fly, *Lytta vesicatoria* (family Meloidae), is the most famous of the "blister beetles." Although these beetles neither bite nor sting, they produce blisters because of the chemical cantharidin which is contained in their bodies. This chemical may be emitted by the beetle, but it is most often encountered when the beetle is crushed against the skin. Several other beetle species, which contain chemicals similar to cantharidin, may be the cause of blisters in various geographic areas.[40] A characteristic clinical feature of blisters from beetles is "kissing" or touching lesions which may produce infection and ulceration. Rove beetles (genus *Paederus*), commonly noted in South America, contain the vesicant paederin. The common carpet beetle (*Anthrenus scrophulariae*) has been associated with a papulovesicular dermatitis. This condition appears to be caused by an allergic response to the larvae of the beetles and not to the beetle itself.[41] If contact with a beetle is suspected early, washing the skin with soap and water may prevent vesiculation. Symptomatic treatment with wet compresses and topical or systemic corticosteroids may be needed.

Diptera

The order Diptera consists of the two-winged or true flies, and collectively its members are responsible for the transmission of more diseases worldwide than any other arthropod order.[2] At last count, more than 100,000 species in 140 families have been described. The mosquitoes of the family Culicidae are vectors for disease throughout the world. Malaria is transmitted by the *Anopheles* mosquito while yellow fever and dengue are transmitted by the *Aedes* mosquito. Species of the genus *Culex* transmit filariasis as well as encephalitis viruses. In the continental United States, females of the genus *Aedes* are the most common cause of mosquito bites. The cutaneous reaction is produced when the female mosquito's serrated jaws disrupt the skin and she inserts her blood tube. Irritating salivary secretions are injected to anticoagulate the blood and are responsible for the edema, pruritus, and papular lesions. Mosquito bites may have an urticarial, eczematoid, or granulomatous appearance, depending on the sensitivity of the victim. Mosquitoes prefer blacks to whites, the young to the old, warm to cool skin, and scented to unscented victims. They also are attracted to bright colors and elevated carbon dioxide concentrations in the air, which make summer picnics or gatherings a favorite mosquito haunt.[47]

The black flies of the family Simulidae are also bloodsuckers. Also known as buffalo gnats, these hump-backed insects are found in tremendous swarms near fast-moving water in the late spring and early summer. Because this black fly injects an anesthetic into the wound, the initial bite is painless. However, the bite subsequently becomes extremely painful with itching, erythema, and edema, which may lead to nummular eczema, vesicles, or hard pruritic papules. A systemic reaction termed "black fly fever" producing headache, fever, nausea, and generalized lymphadenitis has been reported.[2] Black flies are vectors in the transmission of onchocerciasis (river blindness) and tularemia.

The biting midges of the genus *Culicoides,* which are also called "punkies," "no seeums," or "sand flies," are another type of bloodsucking arthropod and are known to transmit *Dipetalonema perstans.*[48] Most active in the morning and late afternoon, the female midges are vicious biters and require a blood meal to oviposit. The midge bites produce immediate pain with erythema at the bite site and 2- to 3-mm papulovesicles, followed by indurated nodules

of up to 1.0 cm which persist for many months. Unlike black flies and mosquitoes, which pupate in the water, these organisms spend their larval and pupal stages in the ground and metamorphose into adult forms at irregular intervals. Their life cycle makes mass control of this arthropod impossible.

The large family Tabandae are ferocious bloodsucking flies including horseflies, deerflies, clegs, breeze flies, greenheads, and mango flies. Species of the genus *Chrysops* are known to transmit loiasis and tularemia.[2] Because they are large flies (6 to 25 mm) with bladelike mouth parts, their bite is painful and may bleed vigorously. The cutaneous welt that is produced may be accompanied by urticaria, dizziness, weakness, wheezing, or angioedema. They are a particular problem to campers and hikers in the early spring and summer when the larval forms become adults.

Botfly larvae penetrate the skin or may be deposited onto open wounds to cause cutaneous myiasis. These larvae may be divided into three broad groups as obligatory, facultative, and accidental parasites. Larvae may be fixed to one site, or may be migratory simulating larva migrans. While many species have been described, the screw worm *Callitroga americana* is the most important in the United States. Another important species is *Dermatobia hominis,* a cause of furuncular myiasis in travelers from tropical regions. These painful lesions resemble a pyogenic furuncle but lack of response to antibiotics points to the correct diagnosis (Fig. 227-9).[49] Phlebotomid sandflies are aggressive biters that produce pruritic, inflamed, indurated lesions. More importantly, however, they are responsible for transmission of leishmanial parasites throughout the world. *Phlebotomus* species are vectors for *Leishmania donovani* and *L. tropica* while *Lutzomyia* species are vectors for *L. brasiliensis* and *Bartonella bacilliformis,* the agent of Carrión's disease.[4]

The bite of *Glossina,* the tsetse fly, produces minimal cutaneous reaction, yet among the biting flies, it ranks second only to the mosquito as a vector of human disease. Transmission occurs mainly in central Africa where *Glossina* species are vectors for the trypanosomes which cause sleeping sickness.[50]

The treatment of Diptera bites requires meticulous attention to wound care by cleansing with soap or other antiseptics to avoid secondary infection. Local application of steroid ointment and systemic treatment with antihistamines will reduce itching and redness. Although systemic allergic reactions are rare, they should be treated aggressively with epinephrine, fluids, corticosteroids, and supportive care.

Hemiptera

Most of the Hemiptera order feed on plants. Only the Cimicidae and Reduviidae families commonly feed on animals, including humans.

Cimicidae (Bedbugs)   Several genera have members that are commonly grouped as "bedbugs": *Cimex, Leptocimex, Oeciacus, Hematasiphon.* The species most common in each geographic area varies: temperate climates, *C. lectularius;* tropical climates, *C. hemipterus;* Africa and South America, *L. bonati.* Bedbugs are characteristically very flat dorsoventrally and have broad bodies. Bites by these bloodsuckers are usually not noticed immediately unless large numbers of bugs are present. Bedbugs are nocturnal feeders and can travel great distances to reach a suitable host. They may come from unusual locations: bird's nests, poultry houses, bus up-

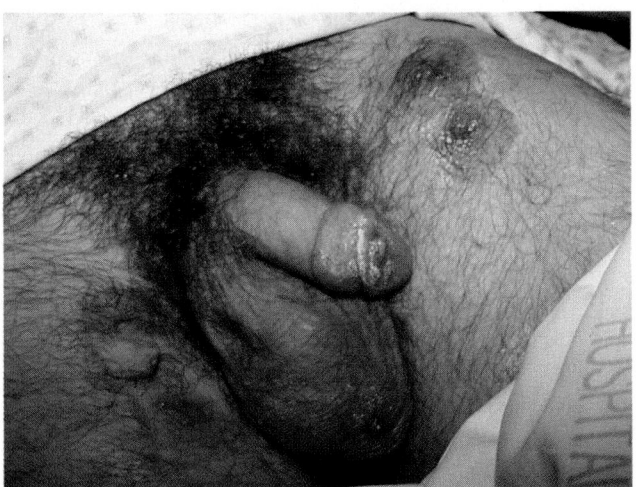

a

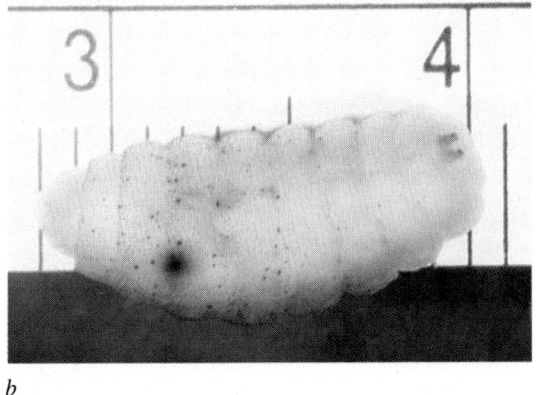

b

FIGURE 227-9 Myiasis. (*a*) Abscesses which contain the larval form of *Dermatobia hominis* are seen in the genital area and thighs. (*b*) Larva removed from the abscess.

holstery, old houses, and furniture. If only a few linear purpuric macules are present, the diagnosis may not be clinically obvious; however, allergic reactions can develop in sensitized individuals.

Reduviidae (Kissing Bugs, Assassin Bugs, Cone-Nosed Bugs)
Because several species of Reduviidae transmit *Trypanosoma cruzi*, this family is medically important. Most species are encountered in the Americas with a few in Africa, Asia, and Europe. While many predaceous reduvids produce extremely painful bites, the hematophagus reduvids, the vectors of Chagas' disease, produce painless bites. These vectors typically turn around and defecate immediately after feeding. Subsequent scratching at the bite site inoculates trypanosomes into the wound. Other reduvids defecate at a later time after feeding, reducing the possibility of disease transmission.[4] Genera involved in transmission of Chagas' disease include *Triatoma*, *Rhodnius*, and *Panstrongylus*.

Clinically, the lesions produced by Reduviidae are similar to those from other arthropods and depend on the species, type of exposure, and individual sensitivity. However, predaceous reduvid bites may produce severe local reactions, occasionally resulting in necrosis and ulceration. In some cases, they have been mistaken for spider bites.

Hymenoptera

The general family Hymenoptera includes bees (Apidae and Bombidae), wasps and hornets (Vespidae), and ants (Formicidae).[2] These insects are notorious for their painful stings which may be associated with an anaphylactic reaction and/or death.

Stings by the female bee, hornet, or wasp from the modified ovipositor (stinger apparatus) produce immediate burning and pain followed by an intense, local, erythematous reaction with swelling and urticaria. The honeybee leaves a barbed ovipositor and paired venom sacs impaled in the victim. They must be carefully removed by scraping with a fingernail or knife blade to avoid continued envenomation produced by continued action of attached musculature. The honeybee dies after stinging. Other Hymenoptera do not lose their stinging units and may use them repeatedly.

Severe systemic reactions occur in 0.4 to 0.8 percent of patients and are divided into three categories: angioedema or generalized urticaria; respiratory insufficiency from laryngeal edema or bronchospasm; and shock.[51] Case reports of acute myocardial infarction,[52] myasthenia gravis,[53] and hemolytic anemia[54] have been reported. Occasionally, major local reactions may persist at the bite site, presumably mediated by cellular immune mechanisms.[55]

Venom from the honeybee is a highly complex mixture of pharmacologically active agents. Phospholipase A, which comprises 12 percent of honeybee venom, liberates acute inflammatory mediators through the nonspecific membrane damage of its breakdown product, lysolecithin. Other venom constituents include hyaluronidase, histamine, norepinephrine, dopamine, mellitin, apamine, mast cell degranulation peptide, and minimine.[56]

The acute treatment of Hymenoptera stings is based on the severity of patient response. Cutaneous reactions may be managed by application of ice and local injection of lidocaine to relieve pain. Hypotension and respiratory failure must obviously be treated vigorously.[51] Systemic reactions require administration of subcutaneous epinephrine, while corticosteroids and antihistamines may be helpful for urticaria or edema. If a patient experiences an anaphylactic reaction and has a positive skin test, desensitization should be strongly considered. Injection of honeybee whole-body extracts has proved clinically unsatisfactory, but lyophilized venom extract injections produce blocking IgG antibodies that afford protection.[57]

Fire ants of the genus *Solenopsis* and the harvester ants of the genus *Pogonomyrmex* are aggressive and produce local skin necrosis and systemic reactions when they sting.[58,59] Imported fire ant venom contains a nonproteinaceous, hemolytic factor identified as a dialkylpiperidine derivative, solenopsin D,[56,60] which induces the lytic release of histamine and other vasoactive amines from mast cells. Clinically, the bite site starts as an intense local inflammatory reaction which becomes a sterile pustule.[56] In contrast, harvester ant venom is proteinaceous and contains histamine, kinins, hyaluronidase, hemolysins, phospholipase, smooth muscle stimulants, and other poorly defined proteins.[56]

The imported fire ants (*Solenopsis invicta*) found only in the southeastern United States are particularly vicious because they attack in groups. By securing its jaw in the victim's skin, the fire ant is able to pivot, thereby leaving a ring of pustules. Since there is no specific therapy for ant stings, therapy is symptomatic. Systemic reactions occur frequently and may require corticosteroids or anti-

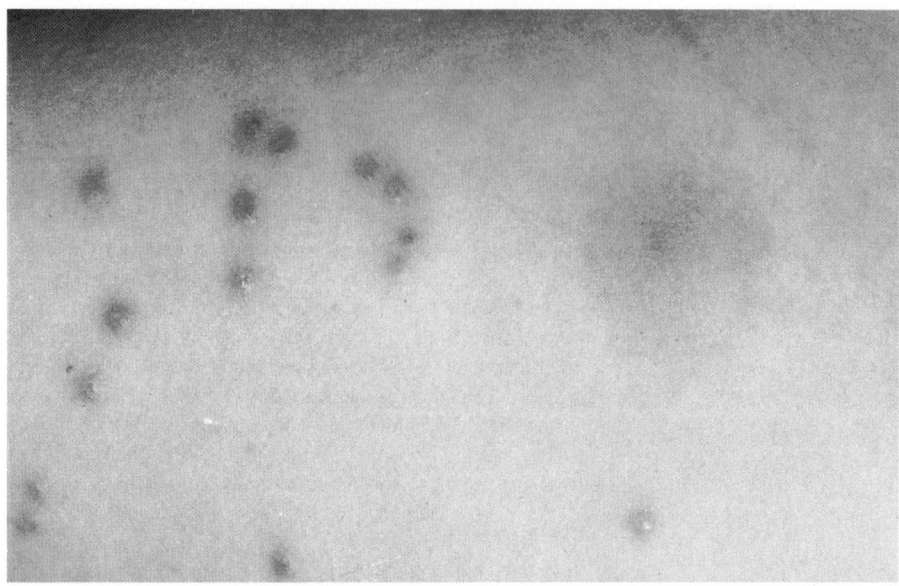

a

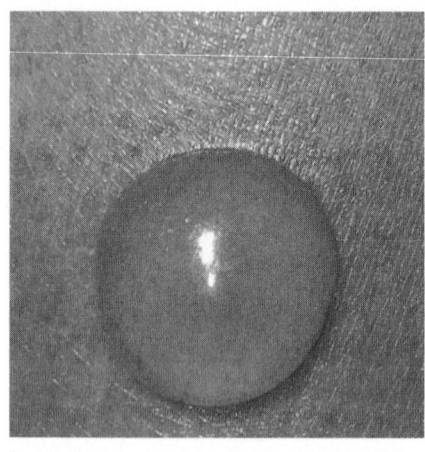

b

FIGURE 227-10   Insect bites. (*a*) Papular urticaria. Bites by fleas or bedbugs can present with the clinical picture of multiple, extremely pruritic, edematous papules. (*b*) Bullous lesions occur most commonly with flea bites, but also occur with bedbugs or contact of blister beetles on the skin.

histamines. Desensitization may be helpful to protect allergic patients.[51]

Lepidoptera

The Lepidoptera order is medically important solely because of the irritant and allergenic properties of the hairs from caterpillars and moths.[61-66] Contact with caterpillars results in burning and itching or even a stinging reaction in the case of the puss caterpillar (*Megalopyge* species), a common inhabitant in Texas. Skin lesions typically appear as papular urticaria which can become generalized in severe cases. Systemic reactions to some species have been reported. At least one caterpillar species (gypsy moth, *Lymantria dispar*) may cause irritation due to histamine contained in the lancet hairs, but the allergic potential of the same caterpillar hairs has also been demonstrated.[64] Exposure to the stinging hairs would be expected in people who spend time outdoors such as lumbermen, farmers, and even campers. However, wind-borne hairs in areas of heavy infestations have caused an epidemic in New England and even a shipboard epidemic.[63,64] Whether most "urticating" caterpillar dermatoses are due to histamine, to allergic reactions, or to both is not clear.[65,66] The caterpillars and moths most commonly

assumed to cause these problems in the United States and Latin America are the following:

Caterpillars. Brown-tailed moth (*Euproctis chrysorrhoea*); io moth (*Automeris io*); puss or flannel moth (*Megalopyge opercularis*); saddleback moth (*Sibine stimulae*).

Moths. Lymantriidae family, tussock moths; brown-tailed moth (*Euproctis chrysorrhoea*); gypsy moth (*Lymantria dispar*); Douglas fir tussock moth (*Hemorocampa pseudotsugata*); silk or peacock moth (Saturnidae family); silk moth (*Hylesia* species); io moth (*Automeris io*).

As more becomes known about the true allergenic nature of the reactions to the Lepidoptera, as well as about species specificity, some puzzling dermatoses and related mucous membrane reactions may be clarified.

Siphonaptera

Fleas have a unique body shape that is flattened laterally rather than dorsoventrally. Their ability to jump to a height of 7 in. aids in their movement from host to host.

The Pulicidae family is of interest because certain species, most notably the rat fleas (*Xenopsylla cheopis* and *X. brasiliensis*) transmit bubonic plague and endemic typhus. Other species are also capable of transmitting disease. All species bite humans since host specificity is relatively low; severe attacks may occur where the fleas that predominantly bite domestic cats (*Ctenocephalides felis*), dogs (*Ct. canus*) (Fig. 227-10), and birds (*Ceratophyllus gallinae, C. columbae*) have recently resided. Survival of adult fleas for months in the absence of host animals makes flea-borne epidemics difficult to detect and eradicate. Usually the bite of the human flea (*Pulex irritans*) causes minimal irritation in a nonsensitized person and produces typically linear or clustered urticarial papules. In allergic individuals, lesions are much more severe, and blisters and even erythema multiforme develop.

In the Tungidae family, only *Tunga penetrans*, the chigoe or sand flea, is well known to produce problems. The female sand flea burrows into the dermis of the animal host. A painful necrotic abscess forms around the site of the female sand flea and her eggs. Secondary infection and scarring are the usual major complications, although tetanus can develop in these wounds. Treatment consists of systemic antibiotics after sterile removal of early lesions, or killing the adult female with a suitable agent such as chloroform. Late lesions resolve by spontaneous ulceration.

Prevention

The biochemical bases of arthropod behavior are just now beginning to be understood.[67,68] Insect repellents such as diethyltoluamide (DEET) have been the preferred preventive agents for persons bothered by fleas, flies, mites, mosquitoes, and ticks. A variety of concentrations varying from 5 to 100% are available. Although preparations containing less than 50% DEET are almost free of side effects when applied to the skin of adults, encephalopathy in children has followed repeated and extensive application of up to 20% DEET.[69] Passive measures such as screens, nets, and clothing, especially if treated with repellents, are most effective in preventing bites. Permethrin spray, marketed as Permanone in the United States, can be applied to clothing. In contrast to DEET, permethrin is poorly absorbed and rapidly inactivated in mammals. Local reactions are uncommon and systemic effects have not been reported. Combined use of permethrin-treated clothing with DEET applied to skin gives maximum protection. A relatively new "folk medicine" mosquito repellent is "Skin-So-Soft" bath oil marketed by Avon in the United States. However, its action may be brief and the safety of repeated widespread application of the concentrated oil is unknown.[70] A number of synthetic arthropod attractants have been discovered.[68] Since pheromones have been identified for Coleoptera (beetles), Diptera (flies), Hymenoptera, and Orthoptora (cockroaches), new forms of prevention and protection from arthropod bites and stings should become available. Because no preventive measures other than killing the adult or larval forms of bees, spiders, or wasps are currently very effective, future developments are eagerly anticipated.

A variety of insecticides are available for individual or professional use. Proper use of these agents is important in the eradication of field ectoparasites inhabiting inanimate objects such as clothing, furniture, carpets, draperies, and pet bedding. Optimal results from insecticides may require consultation with a professional exterminator.

References

1. Parrish HM: Analysis of 460 fatalities from venomous animals in the United States. *Am J Med Sci* **245**:129, 1963
2. Harwood RF, James MT (eds): *Entomology in Human and Animal Health*, 7th ed. New York, Macmillan, 1979
3. Ackerman AB: *Histologic Diagnosis of Inflammatory Skin Diseases*. Philadelphia, Lea & Febiger, 1978
4. Alexander JO: *Arthropods and Human Skin*. Berlin, Springer-Verlag, 1984
5. Ayres S Jr, Ayres S III: Demodectic eruptions (democidosis) in the human. *Arch Dermatol* **83**:816, 1961
6. Betz TG et al: Occupational dermatitis associated with straw itch mites (*Pyemotes ventricosus*). *JAMA* **247**:2821, 1982
7. Rivers JK et al: Walking dandruff and Cheyletiella dermatitis. *J Am Acad Dermatol* **15**:1130, 1986
8. Orkin M et al (eds): *Scabies and Pediculosis*. Philadelphia, Lippincott, 1977
9. Burkhart CG: Scabies: An epidemiologic reassessment. *Ann Intern Med* **98**:498, 1983
10. Arlian LG et al: Prevalence of *Sarcoptes scabiei* in the homes and nursing homes of scabietic patients. *J Am Acad Dermatol* **19**:806, 1988
11. Schultz MW et al: Comparative study of 5% permethrin cream and 1% lindane lotion for the treatment of scabies. *Arch Dermatol* **126**:167, 1990
12. Rasmussen JE: The problem of lindane. *J Am Acad Dermatol* **5**:507, 1981
13. Elgart ML: Scabies. *Dermatol Clin* **8**:253, 1990
14. Abbott KH: Tick paralysis: A review. *Proc Mayo Clin* **18**:39, 1943
15. Dammin GS et al: The rising incidence of clinical *Babesia microti* infection. *Hum Pathol* **12**:398, 1981
16. Jacoby GA et al: Treatment of transfusion-transmitted babesiosis by exchange transfusion. *N Engl J Med* **303**:1098, 1980
17. Wittner M et al: Successful chemotherapy of transfusion babesiosis. *Ann Intern Med* **96**:601, 1982
18. Abele DC, Anders KH: The many faces and phases of borreliosis. I. Lyme disease. *J Am Acad Dermatol* **23**:167, 1990
19. Steere AC et al: Erythema chronicum migrans and Lyme arthritis. *Ann Intern Med* **86**:685, 1977
20. Hyde FW, Johnson RC: Characterization of a circular plasmid from *Borrelia burgdorferi*, etiologic agent of Lyme disease. *J Clin Microbiol* **26**:2203, 1988
21. Steere AC et al: The early clinical manifestations of Lyme disease. *Ann Intern Med* **99**:76, 1983
22. Pachner AR, Steere AC: The triad of neurologic manifestations of Lyme disease: Meningitis, cranial neuritis, and radiculoneuritis. *Neurology* **35**:47, 1985
23. Åsbrink E, Hovmark A: Early and late cutaneous manifestations of *Ixodes*-borne borreliosis (erythema migrans borreliosis, Lyme borreliosis). *Ann NY Acad Sci* **539**:4, 1988
24. Piesman J et al: Duration of tick attachment and *Borrelia burgdorferi* transmission. *J Clin Microbiol* **25**:557, 1987
25. Needham GR: Evaluation of five popular methods for tick removal. *Pediatrics* **75**:997, 1985
26. Jacobs RF: Tick exposure and related infections. *Pediatr Infect Dis J* **7**:612, 1988
27. Gertsch WJ: The spider genus *Loxosceles* in North America, Central America and the West Indies. *American Museum Novitates* **1907**:1, 1958
28. Rees RS et al: The pathogenesis of systemic *Loxosceles*. *J Surg Res* **35**:1, 1983
29. King LE Jr, Rees RS: Treatment of brown recluse spider bites. *J Am Acad Dermatol* **14**:691, 1986
30. King LE Jr, Rees RS: Dapsone treatment of a brown recluse bite. *JAMA* **250**:645, 1983

31. Gertsch WJ: *American Spiders*. New York, Van Nostrand Reinhold, 1979

32. Howard BD et al: Effects and mechanisms of polypeptide neurotoxins that act presynaptically. *Annu Rev Pharmacol Toxicol* **20**:307, 1980

33. Maretic Z: Latrodectism: variations in clinical manifestations provoked by *Latrodectus* species of spiders. *Toxicon* **21**:457, 1983

34. Key G: A comparison of calcium gluconate and methacarbaminol (Robaxin) in the treatment of latrodectism (black widow spider envenomation). *Am J Trop Med Hyg* **30**:273, 1981

35. Rimsza ME et al: Scorpion envenomation. *Pediatrics* **66**:298, 1980

36. Novaes G et al: Effect of purified scorpion toxin (*Tityus* toxin) on the pancreatic secretion of the rat. *Toxicon* **20**:847, 1982

37. Bawaskar HS, Bawaskar PH: Stings by red scorpions (*Buthotus tamulus*) in Maharashtra State, India: A clinical study. *Trans R Soc Trop Med Hyg* **83**:858, 1989

38. Remington CL: The bite and habits of a giant centipede (*Scolopendra subprincipes*) in the Philippines. *Am J Trop Med* **30**:435, 1950

39. Radford AJ: Millipede burns in man. *Trop Geogr Med* **27**:279, 1975

40. Nichols DSH et al: Oedermerid blister beetle dermatosis: A review. *J Am Acad Dermatol* **22**:815, 1990

41. Ahmed AR et al: Carpet beetle dermatitis. *J Am Acad Dermatol* **5**:428, 1981

42. Zinssen RH: *Rats, Lice and History*. Boston, Little, Brown, 1935

43. Buxton PA: *The Louse*, 2d ed. London, Arnold, 1947

44. Meinking TL et al: Comparative efficacy of treatments for pediculosis capitis infestations. *Arch Dermatol* **122**:267, 1986

45. Carson DS et al: Pyrethrins combined with piperonyl butoxide (RID) vs 1% permethrin (NIX) in the treatment of head lice. *Am J Dis Child* **142**:768, 1988

46. Burns DA: The treatment of *Pthirus pubis* infestation of the eyelashes. *Br J Dermatol* **117**:741, 1987

47. Frazier C: Insect reactions related to sports. *Cutis* **19**:439, 1977

48. Steffen C: Clinical and histopathological correlation of midge bites. *Arch Dermatol* **117**:785, 1981

49. File TM et al: *Dermatobia hominis* dermal myiasis: A furuncular lesion in a world traveler. *Arch Dermatol* **121**:1195, 1985

50. Taboada O: *Medical Entomology*. Washington, DC, US Government Printing Office, 1967

51. Yunginger J: Advances in the diagnosis and treatment of stinging insect allergy. *Pediatrics* **67**:325, 1981

52. Levine H: Acute myocardial infarction following wasp sting. *Am Heart J* **91**:365, 1976

53. Brumlik J: Myasthenia gravis associated with wasp sting. *JAMA* **235**:2120, 1976

54. Monzon C, Miles J: Hemolytic anemia following a wasp sting. *J Pediatr* **96**:1039, 1980

55. Case RL et al: Role of cell-mediated immunity in Hymenoptera allergy. *J Allergy Clin Immunol* **68**:399, 1981

56. Cavagnol RM: The pharmacological effects of Hymenoptera venoms. *Annu Rev Pharmacol Toxicol* **17**:479, 1977

57. Busse WW et al: Immunotherapy in bee sting anaphylaxis: Use of honeybee venom. *JAMA* **231**:1154, 1975

58. Clemmer D, Serfling RE: The imported fire ant: Dimension of the urban problem. *South Med J* **68**:1133, 1975

59. Pinnas JL et al: Harvester ant sensitivity: In vitro and in vivo studies using whole body extracts and venom. *J Allergy Clin Immunol* **59**:10, 1977

60. Lind NK: Mechanism of action of fire ant (*Solenopsis*) venoms: Lytic release of histamine from mast cells. *Toxicon* **20**:831, 1982

61. Hoover AW, Nelson E: Skin symptoms attributed to tussock moth infestation. *Cutis* **13**:597, 1974

62. Berman BA, Ross RN: Gypsy moth caterpillar dermatitis. *Cutis* **31**:251, 1983

63. Shama SK et al: Gypsy-moth-caterpillar dermatitis. *N Engl J Med* **306**:1300, 1982

64. Beaucher WN, Farnham JE: Gypsy-moth-caterpillar dermatitis. *N Engl J Med* **306**:1301, 1982

65. DeJong MCJM et al: A comparative study of the spicule venom of *Euproctis* caterpillars. *Toxicon* **20**:477, 1982

66. Bleumink E et al: Protease activities in the spicule venom of *Euproctis* caterpillars. *Toxicon* **20**:607, 1982

67. Wright RH: Why mosquito repellents repel. *Sci Am* **233**:104, 1975

68. Plimmer JR et al: Insect attractants. *Annu Rev Pharmacol Toxicol* **22**:297, 1982

69. Reeves G (ed): Are insect repellents safe? *Lancet* **2**:610, 1988

70. Abramowicz M (ed): Insect repellents. *Med Lett Drugs Ther* **31**:45, 1989

PART SIX

Therapeutics

Topical Modalities

CHAPTER 228

Jean-Claude Jamoulle and Hans Schaefer

Three factors are involved in the pharmacokinetics of topical applications of drugs: (1) *the skin,* as a target for efficacy and tolerance; (2) *the drug,* in its optimum formulation for a specific disease; (3) *the rest of the body,* which in general has to be considered from the point of view of safety. In pharmacokinetics, the role played by each of these factors is considered as a function of time.

Being a protective organ, the skin functions as a barrier to the penetration of drugs and xenobiotics into the viable tissues via the systemic circulation, and it regulates the outward migration of endogenous products. The skin barrier function has been expressed as the rate of transepidermal water loss (TEWL).[1] The TEWL measurement provides predictive information on the status of the skin and therefore on the pharmacokinetics of a drug applied topically. In vivo experiments have suggested that skin appendages could also be of significance in percutaneous absorption. If appendages are modified by a trauma, e.g., burned skin, the short-cut diffusion of drugs through those appendages might be impaired even after wound healing occurred.[2] It is also suggested that the targeting of a drug to the appendages could be beneficial in diseases such as acne.[3] In addition to its "sieving effect," the skin has a reservoir capacity and a metabolic capability; they can both influence the absorption process. Most pathologic conditions of the skin can modify the barrier function of the stratum corneum and therefore the cutaneous penetration of drugs and xenobiotics.[4] For example, it has been shown that the penetration of the antipsoriatic drug anthralin and its subsequent concentration in clinically involved psoriatic skin may increase by a factor of 10.[5] The Short Contact Therapy concept is based on this observation. It has been extended to other pharmaceutical classes such as corticosteroids.[6]

The first part of this chapter reviews the structure of the skin and how pathologic modifications of the skin structure have an effect on its barrier, reservoir, or metabolic functions. Knowledge of the skin structure and of its physiologic or pathologic modifications (by age, sex, density of hair follicles, site of application) can improve the prediction of topical pharmacokinetics in normal or diseased skin. This chapter places less emphasis on oral drugs used in dermatology because they follow the classic rules of pharmacokinetics applicable to the treatment of any other organ. One major difference, however, is the accessibility of the organ for sampling.

Two additional entities should also be taken into account in skin pharmacokinetics: the formulated product (its lipophilicity, granulometry, solubility) and the physiology of the rest of the body (temperature, blood flow, pregnancy status, liver metabolic capacity, etc.). They simultaneously influence the safety and efficacy of topical drugs (Fig. 228-1).

Pharmacokinetics and Topical Applications of Drugs

Biochemical Structure of the Skin Barrier and Pharmacokinetics

An extensive amount of information has been produced on the biochemical properties of the skin.[1,7–9] These results shed light particularly on the physicochemical structure of the stratum corneum, the main biologic system protecting the body from external aggression. Physicochemical methods of investigation are being developed to relate barrier function to stratum corneum structure.[10]

In the substructure of the stratum corneum, the lipid intercellular constituents are critical.[7] Based on published data, a hypothetical chemical structure of the skin barrier can be drawn. In theory, any perturbation of this structure will modify the barrier function of the skin and therefore the pharmacokinetics of topical drugs (Fig. 228-2).

The average composition of the stratum corneum is: 50 percent proteins, 20 percent lipids, 23 percent hydrosoluble substances, and 7 percent water. Proteins are located mainly in the intracellular space; most of the lipids are found in the intercellular space.

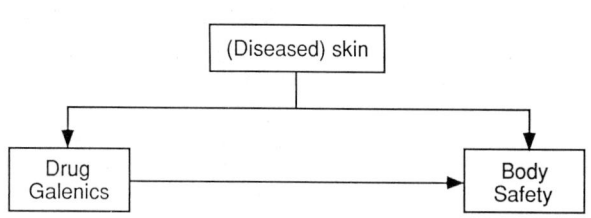

FIGURE 228-1 Relationship between the main factors in skin pharmacokinetics.

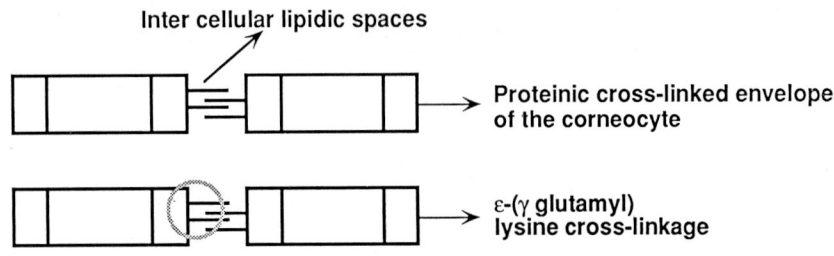

FIGURE 228-2 Hypothetical chemical structure of the skin. Covalent linkage of hydroxy-acyl sphingosines to the cross-linked envelope.[7,9] Other lipidic constituents such as cholesterol, cholesterol sulfate, and calcium ions are also involved in the structure of the intercellular constituents and could be linked to corneocytes. Other lipidic constituents can still be extracted from the stratum corneum by organic solvents.

Proteins

The inside of the corneocyte is formed by keratin filaments rich in disulfide bridges. Filaggrin, also called histidine-rich protein or stratum corneum basic protein, ensures the connection of keratin filaments. The profilaggrin (molecular mass = 300 kDa) constitutes the keratohyalin granules and is a precursor for filaggrin (molecular mass of 38 kDa). In the process of terminal differentiation of the stratum corneum, an enzymatic reaction transforms the arginine residues of filaggrin into citrulline. This process dissociates the filaggrin and the keratin filaments. A subsequent proteolysis dissociates those proteins into peptides and amino acids which are released into the uppermost layers of the stratum corneum. The amino acids produced are important for hydration of the stratum corneum, which in turn is important for its barrier and reservoir properties and therefore for controlling the penetration of drugs. The corneocyte has a cross-linked envelope that is chemically very resistant to reducing agents and surfactants. The protein framework is held together by covalent bonds. Epidermal transglutaminase links the envelope precursors by epsilon-(gamma-glutamyl)-lysine bonds. Epidermal transglutaminase is activated in the horny layer by calcium ions.[11,12]

The shape and area of the cross-linked envelope have been related to diseased status (psoriasis)[12] or to different skin sites.[13] To our knowledge, specific biochemical modifications of the protein structure have not been correlated directly with modifications of skin pharmacokinetics. The cross-linked envelope itself is coated by lipids.[9] Therefore modifications to the lipid anchorage points on the peptidic cross-linked envelope (see circle in Fig. 228-2) could alter permeability of the skin.

Enzymes and Skin Metabolism　The enzymatic activity of the skin is much reduced compared with that of the liver when expressed as weight of enzyme per weight of tissue. Nevertheless, the skin is equipped with a complete series of enzymatic systems located mainly in the epidermis and dermis.[14,15] In studies of the localization, distribution, and substrate specificity of drug-metabolizing enzymes in the skin,[16–18] significant differences have been identified between the epidermis and the dermis. Some investigators concluded that the epidermis is the principal site of drug metabolism in the skin. Nevertheless, while enzyme activity appears to be higher in the epidermis when expressed in terms of protein content, activity in terms of unit area of whole skin is higher in the dermis. For example, this pattern is reported for monoxygenase activity.[17] It should also be taken into consideration that in an area of skin the volume or weight of dermis is higher than that of the epidermis. This principle was well illustrated by Tauber and Rost[16] in a study of the rate of hydrolysis for methylprednisolone aceponate (MPA) in the epidermis and the dermis. Esterase activity for hydrolysis of 21-esters in the epidermis is approximately twentyfold higher than in the dermis, but the total contribution of the dermis and the epidermis is approximately the same because of the higher mass of the dermis. In the same study, the degradation of MPA was found to proceed more rapidly in stripped skin than in intact skin, possibly because stripping could stimulate intracellular enzyme (esterase) release or activities.

The presence and/or density of hair follicles in the skin is another factor that can influence the hydrolysis of the product applied on the skin. This factor was examined in bovine skin on adjacent regions of the snout with and without hair follicles. Viprostol had a higher hydrolysis rate in a skin specimen rich in hair follicles compared with a smooth skin specimen.[18]

The metabolic capacity of the skin can be exploited in topical therapy; for example, skin esterases have the capacity either to activate pro-drugs* or to inactivate soft drugs bearing an ester group in their pharmacophoric structure (steroid esters, benzoyl

---

*Pro-drugs are compounds that must undergo biochemical conversion before developing their pharmacologic activity.

peroxide). In the future this approach may have a beneficial effect on the therapeutic index of a topical drug family with systemic toxicity (soft drugs).

Lipids

The intercellular space in the stratum corneum is essentially composed of lipids.[19] It is produced by the excretion of membrane-coating granules. The intercellular lipids (80 percent of stratum corneum lipid content) are rich in ceramides (45 percent), cholesterol (25 percent), and free fatty acids (25 percent). Glycolipids, sterol esters, triglycerides, and cholesterol sulfate (10 percent) have also been identified. Surprisingly, the phospholipids are absent or at a very low concentration in this panel.[7] The lipid mixture plays a key role in corneocyte cohesion and in the barrier properties of the stratum corneum. Study of the molecular structure of the skin lipids has shown some degree of lipid/protein association by covalent bonds, those lipids probably being less sensitive to the extraction by solvents. Nevertheless, an important fraction of skin lipids is not linked to the proteins of the stratum corneum and therefore these lipids can be extracted by solvents such as acetone, chloroform, and ether with subsequent modification in skin permeability.

Regional variations of skin permeability[20] have been related to regional variations in the lipids of human stratum corneum.

Linoleic Acid Recent results support the hypothesis that the lipid barrier of the stratum corneum to water penetration is determined by the structural organization of the lipids and not by the exact chemical structure of the individual species of lipids. This rule may suffer one exception in the case of linoleic acid and the stereochemistry of its two double bonds. In this case, it is not only the structural organization of the lipid but also the exact chemical structure of one double bond (C_{12}-C_{13}) in a single fatty acid that can dramatically modify the barrier properties of the skin. This finding is well illustrated by the penetration-enhancing effect of oleic acid ($C_{18}H_{34}O_2$) compared with the potential barrier effect of linoleic acid ($C_{18}H_{32}O_2$).[19]

Among the different lipids found in the stratum corneum, sphingolipids have been identified as the principal mediators of the barrier function; they are enriched in linoleic acid, which plays a critical role in the formation of multilamellar sheets. Evening primrose[21] or fish oil in the diet is thought to be beneficial to the skin. In laboratory animals, arachidonic acid was shown to compensate for a linoleic acid deficiency. Physical techniques of differential scanning colorimetry (DSC) and infrared (IR) spectroscopy[22] were used to show that increases in the lipid order (or fluidity) of stratum corneum are accompanied by increases in water flux. Topical application of oleic acid has the opposite effect—it acts as a penetration enhancer.[22]

Cholesterol Sulfate In recessive X-linked ichthyosis, levels of cholesterol decrease while cholesterol sulfate content increases. The absence of the enzyme steroid sulfatase leads to the accumulation of cholesterol sulfate in intercellular bilayers in the stratum corneum.[23] These changes are expected to alter skin permeability.

Water and Mineral Constituents

The tridimensional structure of the stratum corneum is much more complex than illustrated in Fig. 228-2 because one has to take into account the presence of water (7 to 10 percent) and the association

of lipids and water creating a multilayer liposome-like structure in the intercellular space. Topical drugs have to diffuse through this structure to reach the deeper layers of the skin (epidermis or dermis).[24–26]

The water content of the stratum corneum in diseased[27] or normal[28,29] skin and its pH[28] influence its electrical characteristics (permittivity,* conductivity) and thus the diffusion of charged molecules. This influence is particularly relevant when one tries to drive molecules through the skin by application of different electrical potentials (iontophoresis).[30]

It is well known that an increased hydration of the stratum corneum, e.g., consequent to occlusion, modifies its barrier properties to certain drugs and particularly the reservoir properties of the stratum corneum (see below).[6,29]

Calcium ions have a double influence on lipids and on skin proteins.[31] A model of liposomes that mimics the intercellular lipids of the epidermal water barrier was constructed.[24] By analogy it was observed that small unilamellar liposomes prepared from stratum corneum lipids are transformed into broad multilamellar sheets in the presence of calcium. This experience demonstrates another influence of calcium ions in the skin.

The Product (Drug Substance in Its Vehicle)

The choice of a topical vehicle for a drug can serve several objectives that are sometimes conflicting: (1) to increase the penetration of a substance destined to have a systemic action; (2) to decrease permeation and hold the substance in the upper layers of the skin [i.e., antifungals (stratum corneum), retinoids (epidermis)]; and (3) to target the substance to skin appendages.

Based on the theory reported here, it is in general easy to predict how the skin structure can be modified to increase or decrease its barrier properties. The profound modifications of the skin barrier produced, e.g., by acetone, have been well documented, as have modifications by other organic solvents (DMSO, penetration enhancers). On the other hand, there is less documentation on penetration retarders such as polymers and film-forming excipients.

A very interesting study performed by Lippold and Hackemuller[32] produced evidence supporting the hypothesis that moisturizers (sodium lactate, sodium pyroglutaminate, *N*-hydroxyethylacetamide, and sorbitol) can act as penetration decelerators by increasing the resistance of intra- and intercellular penetration pathways after topical therapy. This effect was shown by a shift of the biologic activity of benzylnicotinate used as a pharmacologic indicator (Fig. 228-3).

Several decades ago, physicochemical rules governing the formulation of dermatologic products were established.[33] They showed that the physicochemical properties of drug granulometry, solubility, partition coefficient, and thermodynamic activity in the vehicle were key parameters in skin pharmacokinetics. Those general concepts can be phrased as follows referring to specific parameters.

Concentration—Solubility—Granulometry When a drug is soluble in its vehicle, a different pharmacokinetic behavior is normally noted from one vehicle to another. The quantity of drug absorbed

---

*Permittivity is the property of a material that describes the electric flux density produced when the material is excited by an electromagnetic field source.

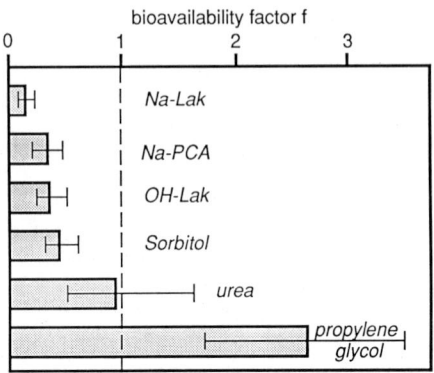

FIGURE 228-3 Influence of pretreatment with moisturizers, related substances, and propylene glycol on the bioavailability of benzyl nicotinate from soft white petrolatum: pretreatment with water (standard): f = 1; f as means (n = 10 volunteers) with 95 percent confidence limits. (By permission from B.C. Lippold and D. Hackemuller.[32])

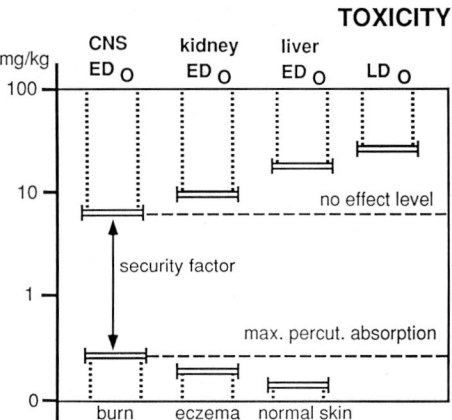

FIGURE 228-5 Hypothetical illustration of security factor as assessed by comparing dose level causing no toxic effects and maximum cutaneous absorption (ED_0 and LD_0 are "no effect level dose").

per area and time unit usually increases proportionally to the concentration of active ingredients in the vehicle. Nevertheless, when the active principle is in suspension, the drug already has its maximum thermodynamic activity and the influence of the concentration becomes less important, while all other parameters remain the same. The solubilization of the drug in suspension depends on the granulometry and eventually on the polymorphism of the active ingredient. Consequently, its diffusion in the first skin layers will also be a function of its granulometry and crystallinity.[34]

These general rules are apparently contradicted by the following application: Bioequivalence studies recently published have claimed bioequivalence for formulations of different type (e.g., ciclopirox olamine lotion and cream).[35] When two generic formulations of the same drug are compared, different pharmacokinetic profiles in the skin may lead to the same biologic efficacy if one formulation produces concentrations of drug in the skin above the saturation level of pharmacophoric receptors in the skin but below the level of toxicity (Fig. 228-4). A substantial increase of the area under the skin-vs.-time concentration curve may still give a safe product. In conclusion, when a difference in ADME (absorption, distribution, metabolism, and elimination) is observed in the skin, its clinical relevance should be established not only by determina-

tion of skin levels and pharmacokinetics, but also by correlation of pharmacotoxicologic observations with skin levels (Fig. 228-5).

The influence of vehicle, light exposure, and dose on the percutaneous absorption of retinoids was studied in vitro. The results of these studies demonstrate that retinoid absorption through monkey skin was highly vehicle dependent and followed this order: propylene glycol = isopropyl alcohol > mineral oil > diisopropyl adipate > polyethylene glycol (PEG) 400. The exposure to light does not seem to change the amount of drug that penetrates the epidermis. After application of isotretinoin to human skin in vitro, concentration in the epidermis after 24 h increases as a function of dose, but the amount of drug in the dermis and in the receptor fluid does not; these findings suggest saturation of the dermis before the epidermis, which may be due to the high lipophilicity of retinoids and to a higher affinity for lipophilic epidermal tissues than for the dermis[36] (Fig. 228-6).

Partition Coefficient of the Drug between the Vehicle and the Skin Lipids A high solubility of the active ingredient in the vehi-

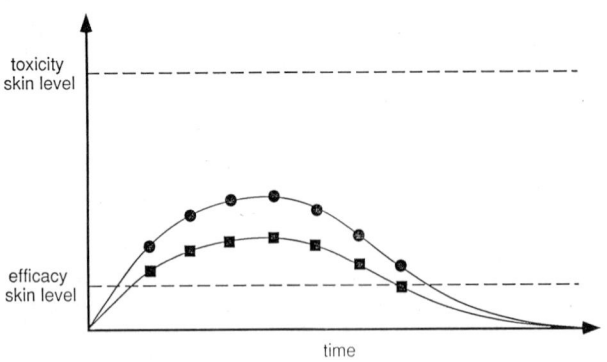

FIGURE 228-4 Possible skin levels of two topical generic formulations.

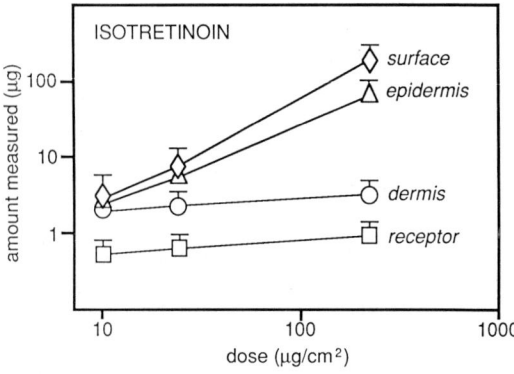

FIGURE 228-6 Amount recovered on the surface and in the epidermis, dermis, and receptor as a function of a dose of isotretinoin 24 h after application. Points represent the mean of duplicate determinations in skin from three humans. Skin from different individuals was used. The study was conducted in the light. (By permission from P.A. Lehman et al.[36])

cle and a low partition coefficient between the vehicle and the skin lipids should be unfavorable to good penetration in the skin, because the product will have a higher affinity for the vehicle and will tend to remain on the surface of the skin rather than to dissolve and diffuse in the skin lipids.[33,37]

pKa (or pKb) and Partition Coefficient   Skin penetration experiments done with simple organic acids such as benzoic acid or salicylic acid[38,39] indicated concomitantly that, in an ionized state, their penetration into the skin is lower than in a nonionized state. It has been shown also that a lipophilic counter-ion could produce a lipophilic ionic pair and increase the penetration properties of the parent ionic drug. One could hypothesize that for a highly lipophilic acid (e.g., retinoids) the ionization would improve the penetration because it would move the log P of the drug closer to the theoretical optimum value (see Fig. 228-7). Therefore, depending on the position of the drug's log P value on the axis of the graph representing log P as a function of the quantity of product penetrated through the skin (for the same alkaline counter-ion), ionization will improve or decrease the penetration properties of drugs (with equivalent molecular weight and shape).

Liposomes   Liposomes are relatively new entities in dermatology. They are usually prepared with phosphatidylcholine derivatives and cholesterol. Their exact mechanism of action in skin pharmacokinetics is not known. In theory, because of their similarity to the lipid structure of the skin, they are expected to improve the barrier properties of the skin, in particular if a liposome formulation is prepared with skin lipids. Nevertheless, phosphatidylcholine liposomes may behave differently to the skin liposome-type multilayered structure. It was proposed that a phospholipid film of liposomes applied to the skin may promote hydration of the stratum corneum and also provide an environment into which corticosteroids initially partition before a subsequent, more controlled release into the deeper layers.[40]

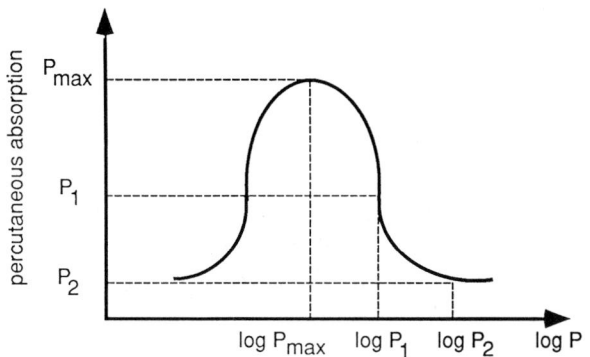

FIGURE 228-7   Cutaneous penetration. Variation of cutaneous penetration of drugs as a function of the partition coefficient. Hypothesis on the effect of counter-ions on the cutaneous penetration of highly lipophilic acid molecules.

log P_2: Partition coefficient of a very lipophilic drug (R-COOH).
log P_1: Partition coefficient of a very lipophilic drug (ionized form).
P_1: Skin penetration of the ionized form of a lipophilic drug.
P_2: Skin penetration of the nonionized form of a lipophilic drug.

Variations of the Stratum Corneum Structure

Artificial Damage to the Stratum Corneum   If the stratum corneum is nonspecifically damaged or is removed by stripping, important penetration increments can be measured.[41–43]

Age   The skin of children and particularly of newborns is more permeable than adult skin.[44]

Disease   Each dermatosis responsible for an obvious change of the skin surface is associated with a deficiency in barrier properties. This principle is observed in solar burns, eczema, mechanical irritation, infection, or conditions caused by an endogenous pathologic process.[43,45] In hyperkeratotic epidermolysis, the deficiency of the barrier function can be expressed by the TEWL. For most common dermatologic prescriptions (e.g., corticosteroids), the type and frequency of skin washing can modify the skin barrier and therefore the penetration of topical drugs.

Anatomic Site   Large differences in the stratum corneum have been identified at different anatomic sites in the same subject. For example, high postauricular skin permeability led to the development of a topical patch for an antinausea delivery system to be applied in that region. Differences of skin penetration and skin thickness are sometimes associated parameters. In vitro liberation/penetration tests on cadaver skin biopsied at different anatomic sites were used to demonstrate this statement. Rougier et al.[46] also confirmed this variation in vivo by skin stripping at different anatomic sites. Usually, the anatomic sites can be ranked in the following order of decreased permeability: postauricular, scrotum, abdomen, scalp, forearm, foot-sole.

Hydration of the Stratum Corneum   Hydration of the stratum corneum is one of the most important factors of percutaneous absorption. Under occlusion, the water content and the permeability of the stratum corneum increase, and this increases the percutaneous absorption of most compounds, e.g., corticosteroids[47] (see Fig. 228-8).

Skin Metabolism   The epidermis has its specific metabolic equipment. The activity of the esterase(s) in the skin has been well documented, probably because two major classes of skin products (corticosteroids and nitroglycerin) have ester bonds in their structure. It

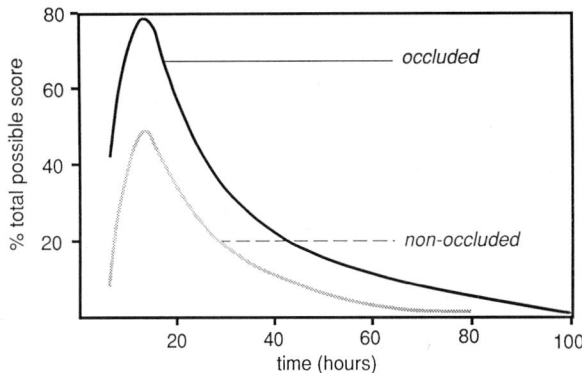

FIGURE 228-8   Blanching curves for betnovate cream. *(By permission from R. Woodford and B.W. Barry.[47])*

has been shown that the enzymatic activity of the skin can have an effect on the pharmacokinetics of nitroglycerin formulations. It can therefore be predicted that an excipient containing an esterified product as an inactive ingredient will be a competitive substrate for skin esterase(s) and in that way could increase the half-life of the active ingredient in the formulation.[48]

Systemic Exposure during Topical Therapy

A third factor in skin pharmacokinetics is the rest of the body and the physical or physiologic forces driving the drug from the deeper layers of the skin to the systemic circulation and to the other tissues or organs.[49] An increase in the dermal blood flow[50] or in the skin temperature[51] can logically increase the absorption of the product remaining in the dermis. On the other hand, vasoconstriction produced by topical application of a corticosteroid should slow down the absorption of another drug applied topically.

To study the influence of cutaneous blood flow on the transcutaneous uptake of drugs, an original in vivo model, the bipediculated dorsal flap of the hairless rat, has been developed by Auclair et al.[52] Two radiotracers were used, ^{201}Tl and ^{86}Rb. Using a different approach, Vickers[53] was able to demonstrate the prolongation of the reservoir time for radiolabeled acetylsalicylic acid by adding fluocinolone acetonide to the reservoir material.

It is particularly important to consider the entire body when one wants to prove the bioequivalence of two generic products. To assess bioequivalence, regulatory authorities seem still to give more credit to clinical studies than to topical pharmacokinetic experiments,[54] probably because of their limitations in humans[55] and because of the complexity of full ADME studies involving topical products with a low applied dose/absorption ratio.

Theory in Skin Pharmacokinetics

There is no evidence today for active transport of topical drugs within the skin. The migration of molecules from outside the body toward the bloodstream is approximately governed by diffusion laws.

Applying Fick's first law, the skin can be considered as a complex membrane and the quantity of drug J diffusing in 1 s through 1 cm^2 in the direction x equals the diffusion coefficient D times the concentration gradient ($-dc/dx$).

$$J = D \cdot dc/dx$$

During the diffusion of a substance in the stratum corneum, the concentration gradient in the distribution area is decreased. This gradient distribution is defined by Fick's second law:

$$dc/dt = D(d^2c/dx^2)$$

After mathematical transformation, one finds that the quantity of substance diffusing from the site of application to a distance d is proportional to the square root of diffusion time. This finding means that the rate of penetration decreases during the diffusion of a substance in the stratum corneum. Nevertheless, with very short distances, diffusion (and diffusion coefficient) can be considered as constant. As a first approximation, one can assume that the diffusion coefficient is constant. In addition, the relationship between the drug concentration in the formulation and at the surface of the skin is a function of K_m, the coefficient of distribution between the vehicle and the membrane.

If the difference in concentration at the top and bottom of the membrane is set as ΔC, and the thickness of the membrane set as d, the equation can be formulated as follows:

$$J = K_m \cdot D \cdot C/d = K_p \cdot \Delta C$$

$$K_p = K_m \cdot D/d$$

where J = flux of drug; K_m = distribution coefficient vehicle/membrane; D = diffusion coefficient; ΔC = difference of concentration at the top and bottom of the membrane; d = thickness of the membrane; and K_p = permeability coefficient.

There is more and more evidence today that the hair follicles (and sebaceous glands) play a role in the distribution of topical drugs. Because of these observations, skin pharmacokinetics will not be able to be considered as diffusion through a simple membrane, as stated above. For example, the effects of repeated topical applications, of occlusion, or of skin metabolism are other limitations of this theory because the skin structure can change during the treatment period. Therefore it is difficult to provide a mathematical expression for percutaneous diffusion in an anisotropic environment (e.g., in psoriatic skin). This challenge can be taken up by computer programs in the near future.

Methods Used in Pharmacokinetics

Currently, the methods used in skin pharmacokinetics have two objectives: (1) *efficacy*—methods should allow the selection of the best formulation for a given drug, and (2) *safety*—methods should give the quantity of drug delivered to the bloodstream and to different organs or tissues.

In Vitro Methods

The most popular technique used to assess percutaneous absorption is the in vitro diffusion cell.[56] The Franz diffusion cell is composed of a donor compartment and a receiver compartment, the skin being sandwiched between the donor and recipient chambers. A solution of the penetrant is applied on the stratum corneum side, and the diffusion of the drug through the skin is measured in the receiver chamber as a function of time. This method can be used to assess the influence of penetration enhancers or retarders on the stratum corneum epidermal barrier. For the application of this technique, reference is made to the above-mentioned influence of the vehicle on the penetration of retinoids in the skin (Fig. 228-6).

In Vivo Methods

Measurement of the Reservoir Properties of the Skin   The reservoir effect of the stratum corneum was described a long time ago.[57] The reservoir effect as well as the concentration gradient in the skin can easily be measured by tape stripping or slicing of skin biopsies. After cutaneous application of a radiolabeled compound, the stratum corneum can be delaminated by 15 successive tape strippings. The samples are extracted by a scintillation fluid and their radioactivity is counted. (If a sensitive "cold" assay can be developed, it is obviously not necessary to use a radiolabel.) The remaining skin layers can be sliced horizontally. Each slice can be analyzed by radiochemical detection. The amount of radioactivity found plotted as a function of time makes it possible to draw the penetration/

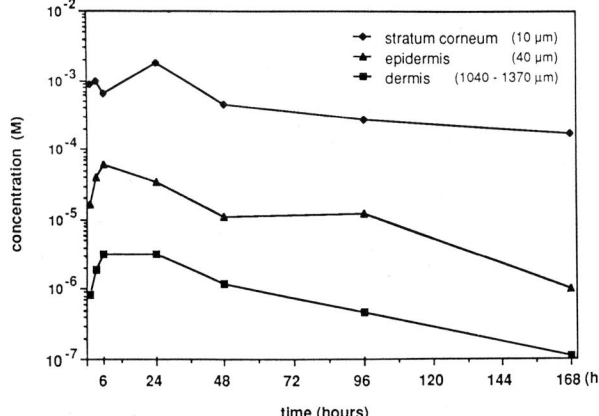

FIGURE 228-9 Molar concentration in skin layers after topical application of ^{14}C-CD 271 to rats.

distribution curve of the product in the different skin layers (Fig. 228-9).

Rougier and Lotte[58] found a relationship between the reservoir function of the stratum corneum and percutaneous absorption. The amount of product in the stratum corneum 30 min after application should predict the total absorption in the body 96 h after the application. Since its publication, the technique has been applied in various experimental conditions to characterize the different factors of skin permeability, for example, the anatomic site, application term, dose applied, and vehicle (see Rougier and Lotte[58] for a review).

Distribution of the Product in the Skin and in the Other Organs
Histoautoradiography of a biopsied skin sample is traditionally used to detect the distribution of the product remaining in the different skin layers. This technique can be applied in animals after topical or systemic administration of a radiolabeled drug.[3,18]

Skin Sandwich Flap Model Pershing, Krueger, and associates[59] developed a perfused flap model using human skin grafted to an athymic rat. Transplants from different sources can also be grafted onto the immunodepressed animal and tested in vitro or in vivo for their permeability properties.[59]

Suction Blisters When a vacuum (150 to 300 mmHg) or a vesicant (capsaicin) is applied to the skin, blisters appear on the skin surface and separate the epidermis from the dermis. The drug applied, topically or systemically, as well as its metabolites can be assayed in the blister fluid and roof of the blister. This technique recently has been applied to the study of itraconazole distribution in the skin. Surprisingly, although itraconazole is effective orally in the treatment of mycoses, the free drug concentrations measured in suction blister fluid were far lower than the minimal inhibitory concentration values for *Candida* and dermatophytes.[60] This finding must raise a question concerning the validity of the suction blister technology.

New analytic methods are being investigated to measure the skin penetration of drugs and chemicals without the need for an invasive technique. Photoacoustic spectrometry, Fourier transform infrared (spectroscopy) (FTIR)*, electron paramagnetic resonance

---

*The basis for FTIR is the conversion of the information from IR frequencies to audio frequencies to create more sensitive, accurate, and reliable spectrometers.

(EPR), and nuclear magnetic resonance (NMR) are considered for the measurement of percutaneous absorption and/or to estimate the effect of penetration enhancers on the skin.[22]

Applications of Classic Methods

Classic techniques of pharmacokinetics involving the systemic route can be applied to the topical route, if it is remembered that low concentrations in the blood do not always reflect low concentrations in the target organ when assessing activity or toxicity (Table 228-1).[61] To define the quantity of drug delivered in the body, the blood levels, target organ levels, and excretion and distribution of the drug after therapeutic cutaneous application have to be determined. Usually the limitation is the low drug levels in the body after topical application. Sometimes even radioactivity detection levels in and on the skin can be limiting. After topical application of a drug, it is sometimes easier to follow its urinary or fecal excretion than its blood profile. Models have been proposed to correlate absorption and urinary excretion in humans. These comments do not hold for transdermal therapy (e.g., nitroglycerin) when blood levels similar to systemic therapy are expected and can be easily measured.

A proposed alternative to blood sampling measures the outward migration of drugs through the skin. Topical devices have been designed to collect, over a defined period of time, the quantity of product that migrates outward from the skin.[62] Similarly to skin penetration, the inverse penetration of drug through the skin should be easier to measure in those situations in which the barrier function is weaker (diseased or damaged skin, stripped skin, hyperhydrated skin caused by occlusion, etc.).

Models for the Differentiation of Normal and Diseased Skin

Stripping and ultraviolet irradiation provide models for psoriatic or eczematous status in human skin.[41] In these conditions, a correlation exists between the degree of stratum corneum damage, the elevation of transepidermal water loss, and the skin permeability.

An essential fatty acid deficiency induces a stable model of dermatosis in hairless rats. A magnesium deficiency produces an allergy-like syndrome.[63]

TABLE 228-1

Plasma and Skin Concentrations after Cessation of Acitretin Treatment in Rats (Two Animals per Time Point)

Time, h	Plasma, ng/mL		Skin, ng/g	
	Ro 10-1670	Ro 13-7652	Ro 10-1670	Ro 13-7652
5	117	16	99	25
	68	15	125	20
10	40	42	34	<10
	95	22	33	<10
24	<2	<2	34	<10
	<2	<2	29	<10
48	<2	<2	<10	<10
	<2	<2	19	<10
72	<2	<2	11	10
	<2	<2	10	<10
96	<2	<2	24	<10
	<2	<2	NQ	<10

NOTE: NQ = Not quantifiable because of chromatographic interference.
SOURCE: Laugier et al.[61] Used with permission.

Experimental hyperproliferative epidermal disease in hairless mice can be induced by topical application of all-*trans* retinoic acid (acanthosis), by acetic acid, and by UV irradiation.[45] In these models, despite increased epidermal thickness, the in vitro percutaneous absorption of hydrocortisone was found to be increased.

Conclusion

Permeability of the skin is closely related to its lipidic constituents and to their organization. The main protein constituent of the skin seems to play the major role of a skeleton, since its contribution to increased skin thickness may not always be correlated to increased barrier properties.

Before topical application of drugs, the anatomic site, frequency of application, dose applied, disease status of the skin, and nature of the vehicle have to be evaluated cautiously, because they can dramatically modify the efficacy and safety of the drug.

Findings on the structure of skin lipids have enlightened previous pharmacologic observations (e.g., relation between linoleic acid deficiency and cutaneous dysfunction). The evolving knowledge of skin structure progresses toward a rational prediction of the physiology of skin pharmacokinetics and toward the design of new chemical entities with safer properties (soft drugs). The conjunction of different sciences from chemistry to the clinic is the key to the progress achieved in the field during the last decade and to the discovery of noninvasive approaches for skin pharmacokinetic measurements.

The activity in the skin of drugs administered by the oral route is not always consistent with skin pharmacokinetic data, and additional research is required for better understanding of the relationship between skin pharmacokinetics and oral administration.[60]

ACKNOWLEDGMENT

The authors wish to thank Dr. Peter Hebborn for his help in preparing this manuscript.

References

NOTE: This edition of the chapter "Pharmacokinetics and Topical Applications of Drugs" has focused mainly on the illustration and the discussion of articles published after 1985. Therefore, fundamental or leading publications and reviews mentioned in the previous editions have not been systematically re-cited.

1. Grubauer G et al: Lipid content and lipid type as determinants of the epidermal permeability barrier. *J Lipid Res* **30**:89, 1989
2. Illel B, Schaefer H: Transfollicular percutaneous absorption. Skin model for quantitative studies. *Acta Derm Venereol (Stockh)* **68**:427, 1988
3. Jamoulle JC et al: Follicular penetration and distribution of topically applied CD 271, a new naphthoic acid derivative intended for topical acne treatment. *J Invest Dermatol* **94**:731, 1990
4. Scott RC, Dugard PH: A model for quantifying absorption through abnormal skin. *J Invest Dermatol* **86**:208, 1986
5. Schaefer H et al: Limited application period for dithranol in psoriasis. *Br J Dermatol* **102**:571, 1980
6. Jaeger L: Psoriasis treatment with betamethasone dipropionate using short-term application and short-term occlusion. *Acta Derm Venereol (Stockh)* **66**:84, 1986
7. Swartzendruber DC et al: Molecular models of the intercellular lipid lamellae in mammalian stratum corneum. *J Invest Dermatol* **92**:251, 1989
8. Wertz PW et al: Essential fatty acids and epidermal integrity. *Arch Dermatol* **123**:1380, 1987
9. Swartzendruber DC et al: Evidence that the corneocyte has a chemically bound lipid envelope. *J Invest Dermatol* **88**:709, 1987
10. Golden GM et al: Stratum corneum lipid phase transitions and water barrier properties. *Biochemistry* **26**:2382, 1987
11. Michel S, Demarchez M: Localization and in vivo activity of epidermal transglutaminase. *J Invest Dermatol* **90**:472, 1988
12. Michel S et al: Morphological and biochemical characterization of the cornified envelopes from human epidermal keratinocytes of different origin. *J Invest Dermatol* **91**:11, 1988
13. Rougier A et al: Relationship between skin permeability and corneocyte size according to anatomic site, age and sex in man. *J Soc Cosmet Chem* **39**:15, 1988
14. Martin RJ et al: Skin metabolism of topically applied compounds. *Int J Pharmaceutics* **39**:23, 1987
15. Guzek DB et al: Transdermal drug transport and metabolism. I. Comparison of in vitro and in vivo results. *Pharmaceutical Res* **6**:33, 1989
16. Tauber U, Rost KL: Esterase activity of the skin including species variations. *Skin Pharmacol* **1**:170, 1987
17. Finnen MJ: Skin metabolism by oxydation and conjugation. *Skin Pharmacol* **1**:163, 1987
18. Nicolau G, Yacobi A: Transdermal absorption and skin metabolism of viprostol, a synthetic prostaglandin E_2 analogue. *Drug Metab Rev* **21**(3):401, 1989–1990
19. Elias PM: The essential fatty acid deficient rodent: Evidence for a direct role for intercellular lipid in barrier function, in *Models in Dermatology,* vol 1, edited by HI Maibach, NJ Lowe. Basel, Karger, 1985, p 272
20. Lampe MA et al: Human stratum corneum lipids: Characterizations and regional variations. *J Lipid Res* **24**:120, 1983
21. Chapkin RS et al: Dietary influences of evening primrose and fish oil on the skin of essential fatty acids-deficient guinea pigs. *J Nutr* **117**:1360, 1987
22. Mak VHW et al: Oleic acid concentration and effect in human stratum corneum: Noninvasive determination by attenuated total reflectance infrared spectroscopy in vivo. *J Control Release* **12**:67, 1990
23. Rehfeld SJ et al: Interactions of cholesterol and cholesterol sulfate with free fatty acids: Possible relevance for the pathogenesis of recessive X-linked ichthyosis. *Arch Dermatol Res* **278**:259, 1986
24. Abraham W et al: Stratum corneum lipid liposomes: Calcium induced transformation into lamellar sheets. *J Invest Dermatol* **88**:212, 1987
25. Elias PM et al: Epidermal permeability barrier: Transformation of lamellar granule-disks into intercellular sheets by a membrane fusion process. *J Invest Dermatol* **89**:459, 1987
26. Landmann L: Epidermal permeability barrier: Transformation of lamellar granule-disks into intercellular sheets by a membrane fusion process: A freeze-fracture study. *J Invest Dermatol* **87**:202, 1986
27. Werner YLVA: The water content of stratum corneum in patients with atopic dermatitis. *Acta Derm Venereol (Stockh)* **66**:281, 1986
28. Thune P et al: The water barrier function of the skin in relation to the water content of stratum corneum, pH and skin lipids. *Acta Derm Venereol (Stockh)* **68**:277, 1988
29. Foreman MI: Stratum corneum hydration: Consequences for skin permeation experiments. *Drug Develop Indust Pharmacy* **12**:461, 1986
30. Singh J: Effect of pH on iontophoretic and passive transport of *p*-aminobenzoic acid through full thickness rat skin. *Pharmazie* **45**:634, 1990
31. Bisset DL et al: Role of protein and calcium in stratum corneum cell cohesion. *Arch Dermatol Res* **279**:184, 1987
32. Lippold BC, Hackemuller D: The influence of skin moisturizers on drug penetration in vivo. *Int J Pharmaceutics* **61**:205, 1990

33. Lippold BC: Selection of the vehicle for topical administration of drugs. *Pharm Acta Helv* **59**:166, 1984

34. Morita M, Hirota S: Effect of crystallinity on the percutaneous absorption of corticosteroid. II. Chemical activity and biological activity. *Chem Pharm Bull (Tokyo)* **33**:2091, 1985

35. Aly R et al: Ciclopiroxolamine lotion 1%: Bioequivalence to ciclopiroxolamine cream 1% and clinical efficacy in tinea pedis. *Clin Ther* **11**:290, 1989

36. Lehman PA et al: Percutaneous absorption of retinoids: Influence of vehicle, light exposure and dose. *J Invest Dermatol* **91**:56, 1988

37. Aungst BJ et al: Contribution of drug solubilization, partitioning, barrier disruption, and solvent permeation to the enhancement of skin permeation of various compounds with fatty acids and amines. *Pharmaceut Res* **7**:712, 1990

38. Barker N, Hadgraft J: Facilitated percutaneous absorption: A model system. *Int J Pharmaceutics* **8**:193, 1982

39. Anderson BD et al: Heterogeneity effects on permeability—partition coefficient relationships in human stratum corneum. *Pharmaceutical Res* **5**:566, 1988

40. Jacobs M et al: Effects of phosphatidylcholine on the topical bioavailability of corticosteroids assessed by the human skin blanching assay. *J Pharm Pharmacol* **40**:829, 1988

41. Lamaud E, Schalla W: Influence of UV-irradiation on penetration of hydrocortisone. In vivo study in hairless rat skin. *Br J Dermatol* **111** (suppl 27):152, 1984

42. Scott RC et al: Permeability of abnormal rat skin. *J Invest Dermatol* **86**:201, 1986

43. Bronaugh RL et al: Differential rates of percutaneous absorption through the eczematous and normal skin of a monkey. *J Invest Dermatol* **87**:451, 1987

44. Barker N et al: Skin permeability in the newborn. *J Invest Dermatol* **88**:409, 1987

45. Solomon AE, Lowe NJ: Percutaneous absorption in experimental epidermal disease. *Br J Dermatol* **100**:717, 1979

46. Rougier A et al: Regional variation in percutaneous absorption in man: Measurement by the stripping method. *Arch Dermatol Res* **278**:465, 1986

47. Woodford R, Barry BW: Activity and bioavailability of a new steroid (tinobesone acetate) in cream and ointment compared with Lidex and dermovate creams and ointments and betnovate cream. *Int J Pharmaceutics* **26**:145, 1985

48. Nicolau G et al: Skin metabolism and transdermal absorption of viprostol, a synthetic PGE$_2$ analog, in the rat: Effect of vehicle. *Skin Pharmacol* **2**:22, 1989

49. Black JG, Kamat VB: Percutaneous absorption of octopirox. *Food Chem Toxicol* **26**:53, 1988

50. Siddiqui O et al: Percutaneous absorption of steroids: Relative contribution of epidermal penetration and dermal clearance. *J Pharmacokinetics Biopharmaceutics* **17**:405, 1989

51. Sasaki H et al: Effect of skin surface temperature on transdermal absorption of flurbiprofen from a cataplasm. *Chem Pharm Bull (Tokyo)* **35**:4883, 1987

52. Auclair F et al: A new model: Bipediculated dorsal flap of hairless rat for cutaneous blood flow evaluation. *Skin Pharmacol* **2**:198, 1989

53. Vickers CFH: Reservoir effect of human skin. Pharmacological speculation, in *Percutaneous Absorption of Steroids*, edited by P Mauvais-Jarvis et al. New York, Academic, 1980, p 19

54. *Approved Drug Products with Therapeutic Equivalence Evaluations.* US Department of Health and Human Services, Food and Drug Administration, Center for Drug Evaluation and Research, Office of Management. Washington DC, US Govt Printing Office, 1989

55. Jamoulle JC, Schaefer H: Percutaneous absorption, bioavailability and bioequivalence, in *In Vivo Methods, Problems and Pitfalls*, edited by V Shah, HI Maibach. New York, Plenum, 1992

56. Gummer CL et al: The skin penetration cell: A design update. *Int J Pharmaceutics* **40**:101, 1987

57. Vickers CFH: Existence of reservoir in the stratum corneum. *Arch Dermatol* **88**:72, 1963

58. Rougier A, Lotte C: Correlations between horny layer concentration and percutaneous absorption. *Skin Pharmacol* **1**:81, 1987

59. Pershing LK, Krueger G: New animal models for bioavailability studies. *Skin Pharmacol* **1**:57, 1987

60. Schafer-Korting M et al: Levels of itraconazole in skin blister fluid after a single oral dose and during repetitive administration. *J Am Acad Dermatol* **22**:211, 1990

61. Laugier JP et al: Determination of acitretin and 13-*cis*-acitretin in skin. *Skin Pharmacol* **2**:181, 1989

62. Peck CC et al: Outward transdermal migration of Theophylline. *Skin Pharmacol* **1**:201, 1987

63. Lambrey B et al: L'absorption percutanée in vivo et in vitro d'hydrocortisone à 1% chez le rat carencé en magnésium. *Acta Derm Venereol (Stockh)* **113**:87, 1985

CHAPTER 229

Kenneth A. Arndt, Paula V. Mendenhall, Kenneth B. Sloan, and John H. Perrin

The Pharmacology of Topical Therapy

One of the most rewarding aspects of the practice of dermatology is the ability to improve or eliminate most of the diverse cutaneous conditions that cause patients to consult their physicians. Just as the skin is uniquely available for inspection and for diagnostic procedures, it is easily accessible for the delivery of a myriad of effective chemical (pharmaceutical preparations) and physical (ultraviolet, laser, and ionizing radiation; cryosurgery, electrosurgery, and cold steel surgery) therapeutic modalities. Furthermore, the outcome of most therapeutic interventions is positive, i.e., the patient's disease gets objectively better. Those learning about dermatology find not only that they can diagnose previously obscure "rashes" with relative ease, but also that it is possible to treat successfully the great

majority of cases in a field formerly reputed to be plagued by chronic and incurable ills. As in the practice of other medical specialties, it is not necessary to have an exact etiologic diagnosis to offer appropriate therapy. If the physician is adept at classifying disease by reaction patterns, e.g., eczematous, benign hyperplastic, and acneform, then useful treatment can be administered even if the specific cause of the eruption is not known.

To deliver successful dermatologic therapy it is necessary to (1) be able to assess accurately the type of eruption, (2) understand the principles of use of topical preparations, (3) know the differences between dermatologic formulations and what they can do, (4) be acquainted with the structure and presumed mode of action of the many drugs available for topical use, and (5) be skilled in the delivery of the physical modes of therapy. Types of topical preparations, the factors affecting the design of topical formulations, the ingredients in topical formulations, and the appropriate administration of topical preparations containing pharmacologically active ingredients (drugs) will be discussed in this chapter. More detailed disease-related discussion and structural formulas of drugs used in topical preparations are available in monographs.[1-3]

Types of Preparations and When to Use

Commonly used topical preparations are liquid preparations used for wet dressings, soaks and baths, lotions, solutions, tinctures, and aerosols; solid or semisolid preparations such as powders, creams, gels, ointments, fixed dressings, and pastes; and occlusive or semi-occlusive wound dressings containing hydrogels, alginates, hydrocolloids, or foams. The liquid preparations are most useful for acute exudative problems and also are easiest to apply to hairy areas. Creams and ointments are more lubricating.

Liquid Preparations

Wet dressings consist of cloths or pads soaked in solutions. They soothe, cool, and dry through evaporation of water. They are indicated in the therapy of acute inflammatory states manifested by oozing, weeping, and accumulation of superficial crusts, and in treating bullous disease, erosions, and ulcers. Application of these dressings leads to vasoconstriction and hence alleviates the erythema and warmth associated with inflammation. When dressings are changed, the skin is cleansed of exudates and crusts. If dressings are left to dry in place, accumulated debris is more efficiently, though more painfully, removed (''wet-to-dry'' dressings). The most important ingredient of solutions used for wet dressings is water. Although many additives may be used, the cleansing and drying effects of the aqueous base are paramount.

Agents used for wet dressing solutions are generally either astringents or antimicrobial agents. The astringents decrease exudation through the precipitation of protein. The most commonly used additive is aluminium acetate (Burow's solution; Domeboro); a 5% concentration is diluted 1:20 to 1:40 in water. The resultant solution is easy to use and does not stain. Potassium permanganate was formerly used extensively in the treatment of fungal infections. It was felt to act as a germicide through its oxidizing action. However, it is difficult to use. It stains skin, nails, and clothing, and undissolved crystals can cause chemical burns. Agents used as antimicrobials with compresses include solutions of 0.1% to 0.5% silver nitrate, 5.0% acetic acid (especially for wounds infected with *Pseudomonas aeruginosa*), povidone iodine, and polymyxin.

Open wet dressing solutions should be liberally applied on multiple layers of an absorbent but nonirritating dressing (old bed linen, handkerchiefs, Kerlix, gauze fluffs) to the affected area for 10 to 30 min three to four times a day. The cloth is immersed in the solution and gently squeezed to remove excess water. Optimally, the dressing should be changed every 10 to 20 min. Overenthusiastic use of open wet compresses can lead to excessive drying and cooling; this problem is particularly a consideration in children. In general, no more than one-third of the total body surface should be treated at any time.

Closed wet dressings result when an impermeable cover such as plastic wrap is placed over a compress. This technique prevents evaporation, retains heat, and causes maceration; closed wet dressings may be useful in the treatment of cellulitis or abscesses but are used much less often for dermatologic eruptions.

Baths and soaks, in which parts or all of the body are immersed, are used in treating more widespread, less exudative conditions. Baths may both cleanse the skin of scales or adherent debris and be used to deliver medication to affected skin. Less drying and cooling take place because exposure to air and, hence, evaporation are decreased, yet baths and soaks are soothing, subdue itching and other cutaneous discomfort, and tend to decrease vasodilatation. Prolonged immersion may result in maceration; therefore, the duration of bathing should be limited to 30 min. The agents used for wet dressings can also be utilized for baths. Often, however, either colloid additives such as colloidal oatmeal (Aveeno) or, less frequently, starch are used for their soothing and antipruritic effects. Bath oils may be added to prevent drying of the skin. The latter are oil emulsions that are dispersed throughout the bath and coat the skin surface as the patient leaves the tub, thereby presumably decreasing evaporative water loss and thus acting as an emollient.

Some *lotions* consist of suspensions of a powder in water. Even if suspending agents are present, it is necessary to shake these preparations before application (shake lotions, such as calamine lotion). As the aqueous phase evaporates, there is drying and cooling, and a therapeutic film of powder is left on the skin. In other lotions or *solutions,* the active ingredients are dissolved so they are clear. Solutions and emulsions can be used as vehicles for drugs such as corticosteroids, antibiotics, and antineoplastic agents. All types of lotions are particularly well suited for use in hairy and intertriginous regions, and in acute exudative dermatoses.

Aerosols and *sprays* are sophisticated (and often expensive) vehicles for delivering lotions or solutions to the skin. The drug is suspended in a propellant, which allows application without touching the skin. There are relatively few general indications for their use except when the amount of inflammation, tenderness, blistering, and oozing makes direct application difficult or painful, which may occur in acute contact dermatitis such as poison oak or poison ivy. The cooling sensation of the spray may itself be antipruritic.

Solid Preparations

Powders promote drying. They are often used in body-fold areas to increase evaporation, reduce accumulation of moisture and maceration, and decrease friction between skin surfaces. Powders may contain drugs or they may be biochemically inert. There is a tendency to presume all powders are the same, but their physiochemical properties and hence their therapeutic uses vary greatly. Talc, a common ingredient of baby powder and other dusting powders, is hydrous magnesium silicate, which is totally nonabsorbent. Starch or cellulose, conversely, absorbs water and may form potentially abrasive conglomerates unless assiduously washed off before reapplying. Other powders used include zinc oxide or stearate, magnesium stearate, and bentonite. Starch-containing powders should not be used in intertriginous eruptions when infection, especially *Candida albicans,* is present, since the glycogen can be readily metabolized by these microorganisms and so lead to exacerbation of the infection. Powders containing antibacterial antibiotics (polymyxin B and bacitracin) may be useful for erosions and ulcers, while antifungal or antimonilial antibiotics (tolnaftate, nystatin) are commonly used in intertriginous areas.

Semisolid Preparations

Creams are emulsions of oil-in-water (O/W). The term *cream* was formerly also used for water-in-oil (W/O) emulsions but now, especially in dermatology, the term is used for water-miscible products only.[4] In a cream the oil droplets of natural or semisynthetic glycerides, petroleum products, waxes, sterols, volatile oils, or silicones represent the discontinuous phase and are dispersed in water or a polar liquid as the continuous phase. Such formulations require emulsifying agents and may contain preservatives. Occasionally the preservatives can act as allergens and produce an allergic contact dermatitis. O/W creams are completely miscible with the skin oils and absorb water, but they are not necessarily water soluble because of their oil content.

Gels are transparent, colorless, semisolid, colloidal dispersions. They liquefy on contact with the warm skin or by friction when rubbed into the skin, and dry as a greaseless, nonocclusive film. Gels of solvents such as water, acetone, alcohol, or propylene glycol thickened with organic polymers such as carbopols are primarily used. As with lotions, O/W creams and gels are preferable when water-washable, nongreasy, and cosmetically elegant vehicles are needed.

Ointments may be classified into three types: water-soluble, emulsifiable, and water-repellent. *Water-soluble ointments* are usually polyethylene glycol preparations (Carbowaxes). These ointments are completely water-soluble, inert polymers whose properties range from liquids to waxlike solids depending on their molecular weight. They are used as lubricants or water-soluble vehicles. *Emulsifiable ointments* are further divided into two varieties. First, *water-in-oil* (W/O) *emulsions* can absorb water into the discontinuous phase, but since oils form the continuous phase, they are difficult to wash off. Second, *absorbent ointments* such as hydrophilic petrolatum USP and Aquaphor contain hydrocarbons and emulsifying agents but no water. They are difficult to wash off and are insoluble in water, but do absorb water to form W/O emulsions. *Water-repellent ointments* consist of hydrocarbons that are insoluble in water, are difficult to wash off, do not dry out, and change little with time. Petrolatum (Vaseline), a purified semisolid mixture of hydrocarbons obtained from petroleum, is the most commonly used ingredient in these ointments. White petrolatum is decolorized and is considered more esthetically appealing than the yellow-colored Vaseline. Liquid petrolatum (mineral oil) consists of lower molecular weight hydrocarbons also obtained from petroleum. Ointments spread easily to form a protective film over the skin, and act as lubricants for dry skin and as vehicles for drugs. Petrolatum is the optimal hydrophobic vehicle. That is, it can act as a protective barrier to prevent the drying effect of aqueous formulations on the skin. If skin is hydrated by soaking in water before the application of petrolatum, the petrolatum seals in the water and becomes one of the more effective lubricants available. Ointment vehicles generally provide better topical penetration of incorporated drugs than do creams or lotion vehicles because of their occlusive nature.

Pastes are made by incorporating large quantities of fine powders into an ointment. Powders, e.g., zinc oxide and starch, usually constitute 20 to 50 percent of paste such as Lassar's. Pastes, relatively little used in today's therapeutics, are more absorptive (i.e., drying), less greasy, and often better tolerated than ointments.

They are useful to treat ulcers, subacute and chronic dermatoses, and psoriasis when, for example, anthralin is incorporated into zinc oxide paste.

Fixed dressings include tapes and plasters. In medicated tapes, the active ingredient (e.g., corticosteroid) is incorporated into the adhesive. There are also several types of nonmedicated adhesive tapes that may aid wound healing when applied to lesions such as leg ulcers. Plasters consist of self-adhesive masses spread onto supporting materials such as cloth, elasticated cloth, or plastic films. These plastic films may be water impermeable. The adhesives consist of natural or synthetic resins into which a drug, e.g., salicylic acid, is incorporated. The supporting materials afford protection from rubbing and pressure.

Wound Dressings

A wound dressing is applied to stop bleeding, absorb exudate, ease pain, and facilitate epidermal resurfacing. Until the early 1960s the general practice was to keep a wound as dry as possible. Then a variety of occlusive and semiocclusive dressings were shown to increase the rate of epithelialization by as much as 40 percent.[5] Since the tissue under the dressing remains moist, treatment with these types of dressing has been termed *moist wound healing*. Generally the type of dressing used in a particular situation is based on its adhesiveness and transparency.

A forerunner of present-day *polysaccharide dressings* was used by the ancient Egyptians when they applied disaccharides in the form of honey to wounds sustained in battle.[6] Strong solutions of sugars have high osmotic pressures and remove water from damaged tissue. Honey has the added advantage of a low pH, thus limiting bacterial growth. Today, sugar is still in use, but insoluble cross-linked dextrans or cross-linked starches as beads are preferred because they readily remove water from the surface of the wound, carrying away bacteria and cellular debris. Iodine can be trapped in starches then released for disinfection upon hydration of the starch.

Semipermeable film dressings derived from synthetic polymers, usually acrylates dissolved in solvents such as acetone and ethyl acetate,[7] have replaced the traditional collodions. When they are sprayed onto the skin, a protective film is left and is said to be impervious to bacteria. Early films developed for occlusive and semiocclusive dressings often led to skin maceration and high bacterial counts. Polyurethane films, which are permeable to water vapor and oxygen and manufactured with suitable adhesives, overcame these problems. Antimicrobials such as iodine and chlorhexidine can be incorporated into the films. Film dressings can be used in the management of catheter sites, decubitus ulcers, burns, and donor sites as well as postoperative wounds.

Current *foam dressings* are silastic or polyurethane foams.[8] The silastic foam is formed immediately before it is poured into the wound, so that secondary dressings may not be needed. The foam absorbs exudate from the wound and may be removed from and replaced into the cavity after soaking in suitable antiseptics such as chlorhexidine, and after thorough washing and squeezing to remove traces of antiseptic and water. The polyurethane foams are permeable to gases and water vapor, and the dressing takes up liquid by capillary action. The hydrophobic nature of the back of the dressings prevents penetration of liquids. These dressings are held in position by tape or bandages. Pores in the wound contact layer gradually become occluded with proteinaceous material and cellular debris; hence frequent changes of dressing may be necessary. These foams may be used in the treatment of ulcers, pressure areas, and the final stages of wound healing.

Hydrogels are insoluble polymers with hydrophilic substituents that absorb water. The polymers may be synthetic or semisynthetic such as polyacrylamide, cross-linked polyethylene oxide polymers, and modified starches as well as natural materials such as agar. The gels are available as thin sheets of fixed macrostructure that do not change shape on absorption of water, or as amorphous structures that absorb water continually and eventually may become dispersions in water. Sheet hydrogels are difficult to keep in position, need frequent changes, and are expensive.[9] The amorphous type hydrogels, on the other hand, are much more versatile and are useful in the treatment of dry, sloughy, and low-exudate wounds.

Hydrocolloid dressings are frequently based on carboxymethyl cellulose, although they may contain other polysaccharides or proteins combined with elastomers and adhesives. The dressings have backings of polyurethane films and foams. The dressings transmit water slowly across the hydrocolloid, thus keeping the wound in a moist condition and ensuring easy removal from the underlying tissue. The occlusive nature of these dressings may enhance collagen synthesis but may not change the bacteriology of the normal skin. Some of the dressings have also been reported to have fibrinolytic activity, perhaps because of the presence of pectin.[10] The hydrocolloids are useful in the management of burns, split-thickness donor sites, and pressure areas especially on heels; they are of major importance in the treatment of leg ulcers. Other types of ulcers have also been treated successfully with hydrocolloids. The rapid rate of healing and the lack of pain upon removal make them attractive for covering postoperative wounds.

Alginate dressings are composed of sodium alginate extracted from brown seaweeds. Sodium alginate is water soluble and can be converted to the insoluble calcium salt, which is then formed into films. The calcium salt is manufactured as mats for wound dressings, ropes or balls for deeper wounds, and ribbons for packing sinuses. Other dressings include a percentage of sodium alginate to increase the rate of gel formation and are useful in treating dry or lightly exuding wounds. Their hemostatic properties make alginates, especially their calcium salts, useful in first-aid dressings.[11] The dressings are useful in the management of burns and donor sites, leg ulcers, and infected traumatic wounds. Cost, as with all newly developed dressings, is a major problem with alginate dressings.

Many infected wounds produce noxious odors, the best known being those infected with *Clostridium welchii*, which causes gas gangrene. Although drugs are the best treatment, dressings containing adsorbents such as activated charcoal provide some benefit.

Factors Affecting the Design of Topical Formulations

Pharmaceutical drug preparations are used both systemically and topically to treat dermatologic conditions. For many drugs, topical administration is the preferred route because systemic administration may have serious drawbacks. Since most drugs given orally to treat dermatologic conditions do not concentrate in the skin, they often have to be administered at high levels to reach effective therapeutic levels in the epidermis and dermis. Such large doses not uncommonly cause untoward systemic side effects. Also, some

drugs that are effective in treating dermatologic diseases are simply too toxic for systemic administration at any dose.

Topical therapy, on the other hand, has many advantages. Drugs can actually be applied directly to the diseased site. The amount of drug applied can be sufficient for a therapeutic response in the skin, yet be small enough not to cause other effects after entering the systemic circulation. Further, because of their physical characteristics, some drugs can only be applied topically, and some preparations are used topically simply for their surface effects on the outermost layers of the skin.

Percutaneous Absorption

The importance of topical therapy in dermatologic conditions makes it worthwhile to discuss some of the myriads of factors involved in designing topical preparations. For any drug to be effective topically, it must be formulated at the proper concentration and in the proper vehicle. Formulation design, therefore, must take into account the physiochemical factors affecting percutaneous absorption, which include the principles of diffusion as they apply to the diffusion of the drug in the formulation and in the skin, and the partitioning of the drug from the formulation into the skin. In addition, other factors affecting percutaneous absorption, such as interactions between the skin and drug, the vehicle and skin, and the drug and vehicle, should be considered. The stratum corneum is considered to be the rate-limiting barrier to percutaneous absorption. Thus, diseased or defective stratum corneum is much more permeable than intact skin. Also, removing the stratum corneum by successive stripping with cellophane tape significantly increases the rate of permeation by most drugs. However, this increase is marginal at best for highly lipophilic drugs, which suggests that the viable epidermis presents a significant barrier to percutaneous absorption as well.[12]

There have been many studies and much speculation on how drugs diffuse through the stratum corneum. The possible routes of penetration include the skin appendages (pilosebaceous follicles or sweat glands) and the continuous stratum corneum (either intercellular or transcellular). In a review of available information, Barry[13] concludes that penetration by drugs through the appendages (shunt routes) cannot contribute appreciably to steady-state diffusion, although it may contribute in the very early stages of diffusion or may be important for ions and large polar molecules (e.g., anti-inflammatory topical corticosteroids). Permeation through the intact stratum corneum was, until recently, thought to occur primarily through the cell membranes—transcellularly. Recent evidence, however, suggests the existence of a significant intercellular volume which can accommodate diffusion by polar drugs within the aqueous regions of the intercellular bilayer structure and diffusion by nonpolar drugs within the hydrophobic regions of the lipid chains in the same structure.[14] Thus, the intercellular route of permeation may be the predominant route of diffusion for both polar and nonpolar drugs.

Diffusion is a passive process. Since the stratum corneum is not a living tissue, there is no active transport across this membrane. Passive diffusion may be regarded as a process whereby a solute moves from a region of high activity or concentration down a gradient to a region of lower activity or concentration. In the percutaneous absorption of drugs, the solute or drug is initially in a region of high concentration in its vehicle. It partitions into a region of lower concentration, which is in the first few layers of the skin itself (stratum corneum), and ultimately diffuses down a concentration gradient into the last few layers of the skin before it is carried away by the peripheral circulation. The rate of diffusion can be determined using Fick's law, according to which flux or movement across the stratum corneum (J) is shown to be directly proportional to (1) the partition coefficient (K) of the drug between its vehicle and the stratum corneum, (2) the diffusion coefficient (D) of the drug in the skin, (3) the concentration of the drug in the vehicle (C_v), and is shown to be inversely proportional to the thickness of the stratum corneum (h). A detailed description of Fick's law for molecules in general appears in Chap. 228, but, for the convenience of the reader, the equation used to describe flux is reproduced below. The partition coefficient and the concentration of drug in the vehicle are factors that can be manipulated to some degree by dosage design and can therefore influence percutaneous absorption. We will discuss those factors here in somewhat more detail.

$$J = KDC_v/h$$

The *partition coefficient* defines the distribution of a solute in solution between two different solvents or phases. In percutaneous absorption, the drug is the solute while the two phases are the vehicle and the stratum corneum. If a drug is loosely held by its vehicle (i.e., the drug is not very soluble in the vehicle), it will exhibit a large partition coefficient and will partition readily into the stratum corneum. A drug that is tightly held (i.e., the drug is very soluble in the vehicle) will exhibit a small partition coefficient and tend to remain in its vehicle rather than partition into the skin.[15] For any drug, the partition coefficient is dependent on the composition of each phase. The composition of the stratum corneum and the solubility of the drug in the stratum corneum cannot be controlled by the formulation scientist. However, it should be recognized that the composition of the stratum corneum, and hence the solubility of the drug in that phase, will change somewhat as the various components of the vehicle or formulation partition into and diffuse through the stratum corneum. On the other hand, the composition of the vehicle phase and the solubility of the drug in this phase can be designed to optimize the percutaneous absorption of the drug.[16]

One of the more important factors in the design of vehicles or formulations to optimize percutaneous absorption is the *solubility* of the drug in its vehicle. If a drug is not completely soluble in the vehicle or formulation, dissolution of the drug in the vehicle may be so slow as to become the rate-limiting step in percutaneous absorption. On the other hand, if a drug is completely in solution at saturation, diffusion of the drug to the vehicle–skin interface may become rate limiting; and if the vehicle is capable of solubilizing much more of the drug than is present (excess solubilizing capacity), then the drug will have a tendency to remain in the vehicle and not readily partition into the stratum corneum.[17] Thus, to optimize partitioning of a drug into the skin, the formulation chemist should design a formulation with the optimum amount of solubilizing capacity: sufficient capacity to solubilize completely that concentration of the drug necessary to elicit the desired therapeutic response once it is delivered to its site of action, but not so much as to hold the drug in the formulation. This optimized formulation will be different not only for each drug but also for different therapeutic concentrations of the same drug, even in the same type of formulation and containing the same types of components[18] (Fig. 229-1).

Interactions

There are many complex factors that can affect the percutaneous absorption of drugs. They can be divided into biologic factors and

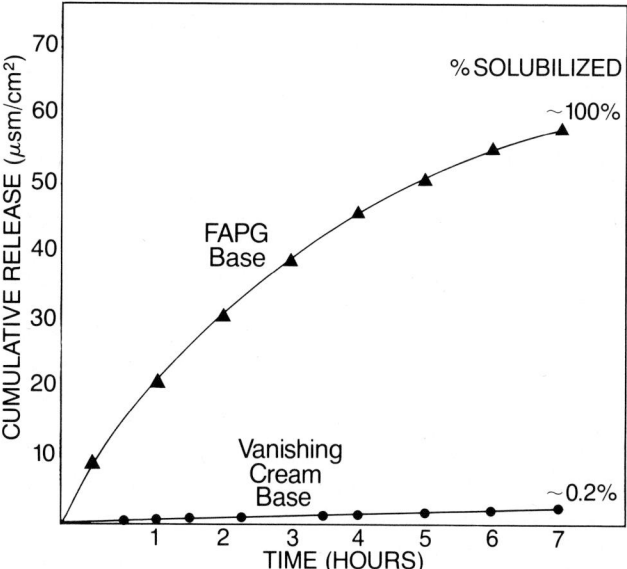

FIGURE 229-1   This figure shows the effect of the solubility of a drug vehicle on its release into skin: The more fluocinonide in the solution, the greater is the release of this corticosteroid from the vehicle.

physiochemical factors. The biologic factors are generally well known: the patient's age, the regional site of drug application, skin metabolism, changes in peripheral circulation, and the general condition of the skin.[19] The physiochemical factors that can affect percutaneous absorption may not be as well known to clinicians. These factors have been organized by Katz and Poulsen[20] and by Barry[21] into the following categories: drug–skin interactions, vehicle–skin interactions, and drug–vehicle interactions.

Drug–Skin Interactions   One type of drug–skin interaction involves skin hydration. Hydration of the stratum corneum increases its permeability to most types of drugs. It is possible that, in addition to other ways of hydrating the stratum corneum, some drugs themselves may increase hydration by exerting an osmotic effect if they permeate the skin rapidly enough to reach high concentrations in the tissue. Drugs or chemicals that have been shown to increase hydration in the stratum corneum include a complex mixture of materials called the natural moisturizing factor (NMF) of skin, urea, and even steroids such as pregnenolone and estrogens.[21]

A second type of drug–skin interaction that may affect percutaneous absorption involves the binding of drugs to the skin. If they bind strongly, it may be necessary to administer loading doses of the drug to saturate available binding sites before therapeutic activity can occur. Also, binding of a drug by the skin may affect or be affected by the application of a second drug. Complex interactions may occur, and they have not yet been studied in detail. However, one type of interaction that has been investigated is the effect of the binding of topical corticosteroids in the skin. It is known that potent fluorinated steroids form depots or reservoirs in the stratum corneum.[22] Although it is possible to elicit vasoconstrictive responses for several days after application of these steroids, whether or not the reservoirs have therapeutic significance is not clear.

Vehicle–Skin Interactions   When vehicles are applied to the skin, they may affect permeability by altering the skin's physical state. This alteration may occur as a result of the vehicle's effects on the hydration of the stratum corneum or on skin temperature, as a result of reversible effects of the vehicle on the barrier properties of the skin, or by combinations of these processes.[23,24] Different vehicles, depending on their composition, may have either positive or negative effects on stratum corneum hydration. Petrolatum-type ointments may increase hydration because of occlusive effects. Frequently, a desirable side effect of the increased hydration is an increase in the permeation of the drug. Emulsions may increase the hydration of the stratum corneum to some degree either by occlusive effects or by adding water to the tissue, depending on the type of emulsion (O/W or W/O) and the ratio of water phase to oil phase. W/O emulsions are generally more occlusive than O/W emulsions. On the other hand, glycol lotions or gels are humectants and may absorb water from the skin, thus retarding desirable drug permeation.

Temperature can also have an effect on drug permeability because the stratum corneum itself is a poor heat insulator and, under normal conditions, usually reflects the temperature of the environment. A rise in skin temperature can increase drug diffusion, because the diffusion constant is directly proportional to temperature. Generally, the use of occlusive dressings or occlusive formulations causes only a small increase in temperature, so that any increase in drug permeability due to this change is small compared with that caused by increased hydration of the stratum corneum caused by occlusion. Therefore, the effect of temperature on drug permeability is usually of minor importance.

The effectiveness of specific components of formulations to increase percutaneous absorption can be significant. Detailed lists of ideal properties of these penetration enhancers state that the ideal penetration enhancer should be pharmacologically inert, nontoxic, nonirritating, and nonallergenic.[25,26] It should be an excellent solvent for drugs and be compatible with a wide range of ingredients used in formulations. The ideal material should also be cosmetically elegant, it should be easily incorporated into all types of formulations, and its action should be reversible. While it is unlikely that the ideal penetration enhancer will be discovered, there are several available that do meet some of the criteria; among these are dimethyl sulfoxide (DMSO) and other alkyl sulfoxides such as decylmethyl sulfoxide (DCMS), dimethyl-formamide (DMF), N-methyl-2-pyrrolidone (NMP), propylene glycol (PG), azocycloalkane-2-ones such as azone, unsaturated long-chain fatty acids such as oleic acid, surfactants such as sodium lauryl sulfate (SLS), and simple alcohols such as ethanol.[27]

Barry has categorized the mechanism of action of a number of these penetration enhancers on the basis of their site of action.[28] In the proposed bilayer model of the intercellular space, it was assumed that the polar head groups of one layer of the lipid constituents (e.g., free fatty acids, triglycerides, ceramides, and cholesterol) were oriented toward an aqueous domain while their nonpolar tails were oriented toward the nonpolar tails of another layer of lipids to form a lipid domain. This orientation leads to packing of the nonpolar tails to form reasonably rigid lipid domains separated from each other by polar aqueous domains. In the proposed mechanisms, the smaller, polar penetration enhancers, such as water, ethanol, DMSO, DMF, NMP, and PG, expand the aqueous solvent shell around the polar head groups of the lipids. In this way they loosen the lipid packing to increase the fluidity of the lipid domain and hence to allow nonpolar drugs to diffuse more easily through the lipid domain. At the same time, these small polar molecules expand the volume and solubilizing capacity of the aqueous domain to make diffusion of polar drugs through the aqueous domain easier

as well. The larger penetration enhancers that were considered, such as oleic acid, azone, DCMS, and SLS, all contain a polar head group and a nonpolar hydrocarbon tail like the majority of the components of the lipid domain. In the proposed mechanism, these larger penetration enhancers insert between the constituents of the lipid domain and thus cause increased fluidity. The small polar penetration enhancers also interact with keratin to increase permeation by the intracellular route; and their accumulation in the intercellular and intracellular regions increases drug solubility in the skin and hence partitioning into the skin. However, the latter effect would occur only at high concentrations of the penetration enhancer.

Drug–Vehicle Interactions   There are certain cases in which the stratum corneum is not the rate-determining step in percutaneous absorption. The stratum corneum may be defective or even absent because of injury or disease, or there may be times when, for various reasons, diffusion of a drug within the formulation itself may be very slow. In both of these cases, the release rate of the drug from the vehicle into the skin may be the rate-limiting step in percutaneous absorption.[29] It should be recognized, however, that as the skin begins to heal, the barrier capacity of the stratum corneum may be reestablished. As this occurs, absorption of the drug from the same formulation may be slowed by the newly formed barrier.

Many factors may affect drug diffusion within the vehicle. Topical drug preparations are heterogeneous systems that contain many ingredients, some of which may interact, complex, or bind chemically to the drug in such a manner as to affect (1) the diffusion of the drug within the vehicle to the vehicle–skin interface, and (2) the partitioning of the drug into the skin. Such preparations are generally multiphase systems. Drugs in such formulations may partition into the various phases that are present. This partitioning affects the amount of drug available for absorption, because it is the external phase of a preparation that has the greatest amount of skin contact. The drug that has partitioned into the internal phase, or phases, will be less available for release into the skin. In addition, many drugs exist as polymorphs, which are different crystalline forms of the drugs, each having different physiochemical properties. The use of one particular polymorph in a formulation, or the conversion with time of one polymorph to another, affects the drug's solubility and availability.[30]

Transdermal Delivery Systems

Transdermal devices are systems that are used to deliver drugs to the systemic circulation via the skin. Although not used to treat skin disorders, transdermal devices deliver drugs through the skin to elicit systemic therapeutic effects. It is the device itself, and not necessarily the stratum corneum, that controls the rate at which the drug is delivered into the skin. In the Transdermal Therapeutic System device, a drug reservoir is separated from the skin by a polymeric membrane. This microporous membrane controls the rate at which drug is delivered to the skin and thus controls the rate of absorption. A loading or priming dose may be contained in the contact adhesive that affixes the device to the skin.

The advantages of this type of drug-delivery system include (1) eliminating the variabilities of gastrointestinal absorption and the "first-pass effect" of the liver on drug metabolism, and (2) providing constant controlled administration of a drug with a steady-state rate of delivery into the systemic circulation. Not every drug can be given by this method. To be effective in a transdermal device, the drug must be potent enough so that small doses are effective, the drug cannot irritate or sensitize the skin, and it must possess the correct physiochemical properties to partition into the stratum corneum and reach the systemic circulation.[31] Scopolamine for motion sickness is one drug that is effectively administered using a transdermal device. Drugs may also be applied topically for systemic effect without the use of specific devices, such as topical nitroglycerin creams for the treatment of angina.

Vehicle Ingredients

There are literally thousands of raw materials or supposedly inert ingredients that can be used in formulating topical preparations. As a general rule, however, those ingredients used in topical drug products tend to be less exotic than some of the newer raw materials used in some cosmetic products.

To review ingredients used in topical preparations, it is convenient to divide them into general classes and look at the most common members of each class. It should be recognized that many ingredients may serve more than one function in a particular formulation. The general classes that will be discussed are emulsifying agents, stabilizers, solvents, thickening agents, emollients, and humectants[32] (Table 229-1).

TABLE 229-1
Vehicle Ingredients—Examples of Commonly Used Agents

Emulsifying agents	**Solvents**
Cholesterol	Alcohol
Disodium monooleamido-	Diisopropyl adipate
sulfosuccinate	Glycerin
Emulsifying wax, NF	1,2,6-Hexanetriol
Polyoxyl 40 stearate	Isopropyl myristate
Polysorbates	Propylene carbonate
Sodium laureth sulfate	Propylene glycol (PG)
Sodium lauryl sulfate (SLS)	Water
Sorbitan esters	
Stearic acid	
	Thickening agents
	Beeswax
Auxiliary emulsifying agents/emulsion	Carbomer
stabilizers	Petrolatum
Carbomer	Polyethylene
Cetearyl alcohol	Xanthan gum
Cetyl alcohol	
Glyceryl monostearate	**Emollients**
Lanolin and lanolin derivatives	Caprylic/capric triglycerides
Polyethylene glycol (PG)	Cetyl alcohol
Stearyl alcohol	Glycerin
	Isopropyl myristate
	Isopropyl palmitate
Stabilizers (including preservatives,	Lanolin and lanolin derivatives
antioxidants, and chelating agents)	Mineral oil
Benzyl alcohol	Petrolatum
Butylated hydroxyanisole (BHA)	Squalene
Butylated hydroxytoluene (BHT)	Stearic acid
Chlorocresol	Stearyl alcohol
Citric acid	
Edetate disodium	**Humectants**
Glycerin	Glycerin
Parabens	Propylene glycol (PG)
Propyl gallate	Sorbitol solution
Propylene glycol (PG)	
Sodium bisulfite	
Sorbic acid/potassium sorbate	

Emulsifying Agents

Emulsions, which are dispersions of two or more immiscible liquid phases (usually an aqueous phase and an oil phase), are thermodynamically unstable. In time, they will separate into their phases because of flocculation or coalescence of the dispersed droplets. Emulsifying agents added to these systems to improve stability are surface-active agents (surfactants) which decrease surface tension. By adsorption, they form a film around each droplet of dispersed material, imparting an adequate electric potential to these droplets so that mutual repulsion will occur and thus retard coalescence.[33] There is no one ideal emulsifying agent because the properties of the two immiscible phases vary from formulation to formulation. Also, there is no ideal amount of emulsifier to use. The pharmaceutical scientist uses the minimum amount of the best emulsifying agent for a particular system necessary to impart maximum stability.

Emulsifying agents may be divided into synthetic and naturally occurring types. In practice, synthetic agents are the most widely used in pharmaceutical preparations. Synthetic emulsifying agents may be further divided into anionic, cationic, and nonionic surfactants. Soaps and sodium lauryl (dodecyl) sulfate are common examples of anionic surfactants. Alkali soaps are stable only at a high pH (>10) because the fatty acid precipitates out of solution at lower pHs. Sodium lauryl sulfate (SLS) is widely used in topical products as a detergent, wetting agent, and emulsifying agent. Unlike soaps, SLS is compatible with dilute acid, and with calcium and magnesium ions. As an emulsifying agent, SLS is usually combined with other emulsifying agents to give more stable emulsions. Sodium lauryl ether sulfate (sodium laureth sulfate) is an ethoxylated agent often used in place of SLS because it is less irritating to skin.

Cationic emulsifying agents such as quaternary ammonium salts are weak emulsifers and are generally used in combination with other emulsifying agents. They form emulsions at pHs of 4 to 6. Cationic emulsifiers are physically incompatible with anionic emulsifiers.

By far the most widely used emulsifying agents are the nonionics. The most commonly used nonionics are combinations of polysorbates and sorbitan esters (Tweens and Spans). Polysorbates are water-soluble polyoxyethylene derivatives of the fatty acid esters of sorbitol. In general, the polysorbates form O/W emulsions, which are stable and little affected by high concentrations of electrolytes or by pH changes. Sorbitans are fatty acid esters of sorbitol and its anhydrides. They are oil-soluble, water-dispersible surfactants. They form W/O emulsions, which have the same stability characteristics as the polysorbate emulsions. Because of their differing solubilities in oil and water and their tendency to form different types of emulsions (O/W vs. W/O), the polysorbates and sorbitans are commonly blended to form stable fine-textured emulsions.

In addition to the above emulsifying agents, there are also many chemicals, some of which are weak emulsifiers, that are used as auxiliary emulsifying agents or emulsion stabilizers. Glyceryl monostearate is a poor W/O emulsifying agent used by itself, but it helps stabilize emulsions when used as an auxiliary agent. Lanolin is a complex mixture of esters of alcohols and acids which has some emulsifying action because it contains cholesterol and aliphatic alcohol. Lanolin alcohol and related semisynthetic molecules impart a high gloss and creamy texture to emulsions and may help stabilize emulsions by absorption of water. Polyethylene glycols are strongly hydrophilic and useful as emulsion stabilizers. Stearyl and cetyl alcohols are weak emulsifiers of the W/O type, but, combined with water-soluble surfactant emulsifiers such as SLS, they form powerful emulsifiers of the O/W type. Emulsions formed from such mixed emulsifiers exhibit superior stability and thickening properties compared with emulsions formed with SLS alone, for instance.

Stabilizers

Included in this category is a wide variety of chemicals that are added to topical preparations to increase or help preserve their stability both initially and over time. Agents may be used to increase the stability of the drug itself or the stability of the vehicle. Preservatives, antioxidants, and chelating agents are all examples of chemical stabilizers.

Preservatives are agents that are used to prevent or inhibit microbial growth. Preservatives should be used at a level that will inhibit microbial growth throughout the life of the product, including the period of patient use. This precaution is particularly important with topical products, because every patient use is a possible source of contamination, especially if the product is dispensed in a jar. Products dispensed in tubes are less prone to contamination by bacteria on the patient's skin or in the air.

The parabens are probably the preservatives most widely used in topical preparations. Parabens are an ester of *p*-hydroxybenzoic acid. There are several esters that are used which include the methyl, ethyl, propyl, and butyl esters. As preservatives, the parabens are active against molds, fungi, and yeasts, but less effective against bacteria. They are commonly used as mixtures because of their varying activities and solubilities. In some cases they have been identified as the cause of an allergic contact reaction to vehicle contents. Also, the activity of parabens may be reduced in the presence of other formulation components such as the nonionic polysorbate surfactants. Other preservatives commonly used include benzyl alcohol, quaternary ammonium surfactants, and sorbic acid or potassium sorbate. Propylene glycol and glycerin exhibit antimicrobial activity when they are used in high concentrations (>20%).

Antioxidants are agents that inhibit oxidation and are used in products in which either the active ingredient or the vehicle may deteriorate through oxidative processes. Butylated hydroxyanisole (BHA) and butylated hydroxytoluene (BHT) are used to retard oxidative degradation in oils and fats. Propyl gallate prevents rancidity in oils and fats and also inhibits the development of peroxides in ethers and similar substances. Antioxidants used in the aqueous phase include ascorbic acid, sulfites, and amino acids containing sulfur.

Chelating agents, such as citric acid and edetate disodium (disodium EDTA), are used to complex heavy metals in aqueous phases and can be considered as synergists for the antioxidants.

Solvents

Solvents are used to increase the solubility of the active drug in the formulation or to solubilize other necessary ingredients in the product. Water, alcohol, glycerin, and propylene glycol are commonly used solvents.

Thickening Agents

Thickening agents include materials used to thicken or increase the viscosity of products or to suspend ingredients in the formulation.

They may act as emulsion stabilizers or as ointment bases. Beeswax is used to increase viscosity in ointments and enables the incorporation of water in the formulation to produce W/O emulsions. Carbomers (carbapol or carboxyvinyl polymers) are synthetic, high-molecular-weight polymers. When dispersed in water as the free acid, they form thin cloudy products. Upon neutralization with alkali hydroxides or amines, carbomers form clear gels of varying viscosities. Carbomers are also used as suspending agents. Petrolatum may be used by itself as an ointment vehicle, or in emulsions to increase viscosity and emolliency. Although petrolatum is compatible with most drugs formulated in ointments, it may not release certain drugs readily. Polyethylene, a polymer of ethylene, is resistant to oxidation and is used as a stiffening agent to replace natural waxes.

Emollients

Emollients are agents that make the skin soft and pliable by increasing hydration of the stratum corneum. They are all occlusive to some degree. The greater the occlusiveness, the greater are the decrease in water loss and resulting increase in hydration of the stratum corneum. Petrolatum is probably the most occlusive and therefore the best emollient available. Its inherent greasy feel, however, precludes its wide use alone. Petrolatum is often mixed with more cosmetically acceptable materials to produce an acceptable feeling to the skin. However, the product has been made more acceptable at the cost of decreasing its occlusiveness, so it functions less efficiently as an emollient. Compromises are made by the formulation chemist to produce products that are acceptable to the patient, yet retain emollient action. As a result, there are many emollient agents used in topical products. Cetyl alcohol and stearyl alcohol are mixtures of solid aliphatic alcohols that are used as emollients. They lubricate without being greasy and impart a smooth feeling to the skin. Isopropyl myristate and isopropyl palmitate are light mobile liquids that act as emollients without leaving a heavy, greasy feeling on the skin.

Humectants

Humectants are agents that are added to formulations on the premise that they are hygroscopic and will draw moisture into the skin. Under dry atmospheric conditions, however, humectants act in a manner opposite to that desired and actually withdraw water from the skin. Glycerin, propylene glycol, and sorbitol solutions are examples of humectants used in topical products.

Application of Topical Preparations

Amount

It is important to prescribe adequate amounts of medication for the patient. The total amount of material needed either until the patient is scheduled to return or until the eruption clears should be estimated and dispensed in one large tube, jar, or bottle. This practice ensures a higher degree of patient compliance and a greater chance of successful therapy, and it offers the possibility of cost savings to the patient. If the medication is expensive, as corticosteroids are, patients should be told the approximate cost of both generic and trade products. This information is available in the yearly editions of the American Druggist *Blue Book*,[34] the *Drug Topics Red Book*,[35] or the *Manual of Dermatologic Therapeutics*.[1] One gram of cream covers an area approximately 10 by 10 cm; an ointment spreads up to 10 percent further. The approximate amount needed for the single application of a cream or ointment to the face or hands is 2 g; to one arm or the anterior or posterior trunk, 3 g; to one leg, 4 g; and to the entire body, 30 g.

Frequency

The absorption, distribution, and excretion characteristics of parenterally administered drugs are sufficiently well known that it is usually possible to instruct the patient regarding the exact amount and frequency of use. The same type of dose-response pharmacokinetic information is much more difficult to determine for topically applied agents. Six daily treatments of a topically applied corticosteroid were found to be no more effective than three daily applications in a study of 12 patients with corticosteroid-responsive dermatoses.[36] An investigation into the percutaneous absorption of radioactive-labeled hydrocortisone applied to the shaved forearm of the rhesus monkey demonstrated no substantial difference in total absorption when a given amount was applied as a single dose or when one-third of the same amount was applied three times a day.[37] Further study is needed to determine the clinical relevance of these results for humans, but the absorption characteristics of monkey and human skin are known to be similar. One application of fluocinonide ointment was as effective as four applications a day in 52 patients with stable psoriasis,[38] while another study demonstrated that once-a-day application of betamethasone dipropionate or diflorasone diacetate ointment to 139 patients with psoriasis showed statistically significant improvement compared with subjects using vehicle alone.[39] It is likely that a single large daily application of a drug, at least of corticosteroids, could be the most efficient means of delivering it to the skin.

Acute tolerance (tachyphylaxis) to the vasoconstrictive and antimitotic effect of topically applied glucocorticoids may occur within 1 week of repeated application. After a 4-day rest period, responsiveness to the effects of the corticosteroid returns to the original level.[40] Intermittent pulse dosing of superpotent topical corticosteroids that includes 2 to 7 days without steroids[41,42] is useful for maintenance of remission of psoriasis. This regimen allows continual use of potent topical agents while minimizing the risk of both adverse effects and tachyphylaxis.

Absorption Characteristics

There is marked regional variation in the amount of drug absorbed from different body areas.[43] Approximately 1 percent of a hydrocortisone solution penetrates normal skin on the forearm, whereas it is absorbed only one-seventh as well through the plantar foot arch, but 6 times more through forehead skin and 42 times more through scrotal skin. Inflamed eczematous skin permits increased percutaneous absorption, and with conditions such as exfoliative psoriasis there seems to be little barrier to absorption at all.

When drugs such as corticosteroids are applied to the skin under an airtight occlusive plastic dressing, their efficacy and absorption are increased 10 to 100 times. Occlusion with a plastic dressing increases the skin surface area that can be treated, increases hydration and temperature, and also appears to induce a reservoir of corticosteroid in the stratum corneum that lasts for several days after application. The increased absorption of drugs applied under plastic occlusive dressings may also lead more rapidly to the appearance of undesirable side effects such as local atrophy and suppression of the HPA axis when corticosteroids are used. Also, greatly enhanced irritant or toxic side effects occur with occlusive dressings when other agents, such as tar, are used. Occlusive therapy also can promote infection, folliculitis, and miliaria and interfere with heat exchange.

A less completely occlusive dressing, the hydrocolloid patch, has recently become available for the treatment of plaques of psoriasis or other chronic recalcitrant disorders.[44] These dressings, used in combination with topical corticosteroids or other topical medications, have many potential advantages. They are flexible, self-adhesive, skin-colored, and waterproof and can therefore cover up unsightly lesions and allow patients to bathe or shower with the patch in place. The patches absorb transepidermal water, keeping the stratum corneum well hydrated, but at the same time they minimize maceration and do not cause the soggy, malodorous skin sometimes induced by plastic film occlusion. The degree of epidermal hydration is sufficient to enhance the effectiveness of topical corticosteroids to the same degree as plastic film, as measured by the blanching assay, yet because the patches are not completely occlusive, there is no significant bacterial proliferation, skin infection, or irritation. The patches are used as manufactured or cut to size, applied over a corticosteroid cream such as 0.1% triamcinolone cream, and left in place for 2 to 7 days. They may also be used to enhance the usefulness of other medications, such as anthralin. These dressings are most beneficial when treating chronic plaques of psoriasis and may also be helpful in treating disorders such as lichen planus and discoid lupus erythematosus. How well these new dressings work in association with various medications will await their widespread use and careful controlled clinical studies.[44]

Simple hydration of skin before application of topical corticosteroids may increase penetration up to fivefold. The optimal technique for applying topical medications, therefore, is first to hydrate skin by immersion in water for about 5 min and then immediately to apply the cream or ointment. If occlusion techniques are to be employed, the hydrocolloid dressing, plastic film, or body suit should be put on directly thereafter.

References

1. Arndt KA: *Manual of Dermatologic Therapeutics. With Essentials of Diagnosis,* 4th ed. Boston, Little, Brown, 1989
2. Landow RK: *Handbook of Dermatologic Treatment.* Greenbrae, CA, Jones Medical Publications, 1983, p 219
3. Madden SW (ed): *Current Dermatologic Therapy,* 3d ed. Philadelphia, Saunders, 1982
4. Barry B: *Dermatological Formulation—Percutaneous Absorption.* New York, Dekker, 1983, p 313
5. Falanga V: Occlusive wound dressings. *Arch Dermatol* **124**:872, 1988
6. Thomas S: *Wound Management and Dressings.* London, Pharmaceutical Press, 1990, p 62
7. Thomas S: *Wound Management and Dressings.* London, Pharmaceutical Press, 1990, p 25
8. Thomas S: *Wound Management and Dressings.* London, Pharmaceutical Press, 1990, p 35
9. Thomas S: *Wound Management and Dressings.* London, Pharmaceutical Press, 1990, p 52

10. Thomas S: *Wound Management and Dressings*. London, Pharmaceutical Press, 1990, p 57

11. Thomas S: *Wound Management and Dressings*. London, Pharmaceutical Press, 1990, p 46

12. Tojo K et al: Drug permeation across the skin: Effect of penetrant hydrophilicity. *J Pharm Sci* **76**:123, 1987

13. Barry B: *Dermatological Formulation—Percutaneous Absorption,* New York, Dekker, 1983, p 96

14. *Pharmacokinetics,* edited by B Shroot, H Schaefer. CIRD Symposium, Advances in Skin Pharmacology, Basel, Karger, 1987, p 121

15. Lippold BC, Schneemann H: The influence of vehicles on the local bioavailability of betamethasone-17-benzoate from solution- and suspension-type ointments. *Int J Pharmacol* **22**:31, 1984

16. Poulsen B: In *Drug Design,* vol IV, edited by E Ariens. New York, Academic, 1973, p 168

17. Poulsen BJ et al: Effect of topical vehicle composition on the *in vitro* release of fluocinolone acetonide and its acetate ester. *J Pharm Sci* **57**:928, 1968

18. Flynn G: In *Modern Pharmaceutics,* edited by G Banker, C Rhodes. New York, Dekker, 1979, p 317

19. Barry B: *Dermatological Formulation—Percutaneous Absorption.* New York, Dekker, 1983, p 129

20. Katz M, Poulsen B: In *Handbook of Experimental Pharmacology,* vol 28, part I, edited by B Brodie, J Gillette. New York, Springer-Verlag, 1971, p 117

21. Barry B: *Dermatological Formulation—Percutaneous Absorption.* New York, Dekker, 1983, p 145

22. Barry B: *Dermatological Formulation—Percutaneous Absorption.* New York, Dekker, 1983, p 116

23. Katz M, Poulsen B: In *Handbook of Experimental Pharmacology,* vol 28, part I, edited by B Brodie, J Gillette. New York, Springer-Verlag, 1971, p 121

24. Barry B: *Dermatological Formulation—Percutaneous Absorption.* New York, Dekker, 1983, p 154

25. Katz M, Poulsen B: In *Handbook of Experimental Pharmacology,* vol 28, part I, edited by B Brodie, J Gillette. New York, Springer-Verlag, 1971, p 125

26. Barry B: *Dermatological Formulation—Percutaneous Absorption.* New York, Dekker, 1983, p 160

27. Barry B: *Dermatological Formulation—Percutaneous Absorption.* New York, Dekker, 1983, p 163

28. Barry B: Mode of action of penetration enhancers in human skin. *J Controlled Release* **6**:85, 1987

29. Poulsen B: In *Drug Design,* vol IV, edited by E Ariens. New York, Academic, 1973, p 185

30. Halablain J, McCrone W: Pharmaceutical applications of polymorphism. *J Pharm Sci* **58**:911, 1969

31. Barry B: *Dermatological Formulation—Percutaneous Absorption.* New York, Dekker, 1983, p 181

32. *The Base Book*. Palo Alto, CA, Syntex Laboratories, 1982

33. Higuchi W et al: In *Remington's Pharmaceutical Sciences,* edited by A Osol. Easton, PA, Mack Publishing, 1980, p 310

34. *1991 Blue Book*. New York, American Druggist, 1991

35. *Drug Topics Red Book*. Oradell, NJ, Medical Economics, 1991

36. Eaglstein WH et al: Topical corticosteroid therapy: Efficacy of frequent application. *Arch Dermatol* **110**:955, 1974

37. Wester RC et al: Frequency of application on percutaneous absorption of hydrocortisone. *Arch Dermatol* **113**:620, 1977

38. Senter RP: Topical fluocinonide and tachyphylaxis. *Arch Dermatol* **119**:363, 1983

39. Lane AT et al: Once-daily treatment of psoriasis with topical glucocorticosteroid ointments. *J Am Acad Dermatol* **8**:523, 1983

40. du Vivier A: Acute tolerance to effects of topical glucocorticoids. *Br J Dermatol* **94**(suppl 12):25, 1976

41. Katz HI et al: Betamethasone dipropionate in optimized vehicle. Intermittent pulse dosing for extended maintenance treatment of psoriasis. *Arch Dermatol* **123**:1308, 1987

42. Hradil E et al: Intermittent treatment of psoriasis with clobetasol propionate. *Acta Derm Venereol (Stockh)* **58**:375, 1978

43. Feldman RJ, Maibach HI: Regional variation in percutaneous penetration of ^{14}C cortisol in man. *J Invest Dermatol* **48**:181, 1967

44. Ryan TJ (ed): *Beyond Occlusion: Dermatology Proceedings,* No. 137 of International Congress Symposium Series. London/New York, Royal Society of Medicine Series, 1988

CHAPTER 230

Richard B. Stoughton* and Roger C. Cornell

Corticosteroids

History

Soon after hydrocortisone became available for systemic treatment of certain inflammatory diseases, it was tried topically on some inflammatory diseases of the skin with obvious success,[1] particularly in atopic dermatitis and some other eczematous eruptions. Other analogues of hydrocortisone such as prednisone and dexamethasone followed but showed little improvement over topical hydrocortisone. In the late 1950s, triamcinolone acetonide (Kenalog) was found to be superior to hydrocortisone in clinical potency. Shortly thereafter fluocinolone acetonide (Synalar) was marketed, but it was similar to formulations of triamcinolone acetonide in potency. In 1961 a simple human bioassay that utilized the

degree of cutaneous vasoconstriction of normal human skin was found; it allowed investigators to predict clinical potency in skin diseases.[2,3] After this assay was discovered, Glaxo Laboratories used it to screen about 150 glucocorticoids rapidly and inexpensively to try to find a more potent topical glucocorticoid.[3] From these 150 steroids, betamethasone 17-valerate was selected as more potent than the others available and was soon in wide use in England as Betnovate and later in the United States as Valisone.

The inexpensive vasoconstrictor bioassay encouraged many companies to screen glucocorticoids that they already had, or to synthesize them for this purpose. Out of these programs came even more potent topical glucocorticoids such as fluocinonide (Lidex), betamethasone dipropionate (Diprosone, Diprolene), and clobetasol propionate (Temovate). The most potent glucocorticoid for topical use is clobetasol propionate which is about 1000 times more potent than hydrocortisone.

---

*Deceased.

Mechanism of Action

There are so many publications on physiologic and pharmacologic actions of glucocorticoids that it is impossible to review them in this chapter. However, a primary target for glucocorticoids that seems to be important in skin diseases is the arachidonic acid pathway for developing a cascade of inflammatory mediators. The primary initiation process of this pathway is through activity of phospholipase A. It is known that phospholipase A is inhibited by glucocorticoids, and many other steps in the arachidonic acid cascade can apparently be blocked by glucocorticoids.[4]

It is not known why some analogues are more active than others in treating skin diseases, but it is clear that the more active the glucocorticoid on skin diseases, the better it binds to the glucocorticoid receptors on the cell.[5]

A specific protein, lipocortin, has been shown to be a potent inhibitor of phospholipase A and is liberated from macrophages and other cells by glucocorticoids.[6]

In spite of all the experimental data, it is still disconcerting that we know so little about the precise molecular mechanisms by which glucocorticoids control such diseases as eczema and psoriasis.

Potency of Topical Glucocorticoids

Because of the wide range of clinical potency of topical glucocorticoid formulations, it is important to classify them into potency groups that range from those of the highest potency to those of the lowest potency (Table 230-1). Table 230-1 includes seven different groups of topical glucocorticoid formulations, all of which are distinct from the others as determined by double-blind clinical studies and vasoconstrictor assays.[7] This guide to potency is essential in selecting the most appropriate formulation for a maximum clinical response and minimum side effects.

Role of Vehicles in Release and Bioavailability

It has become very clear that the vehicle that carries the glucocorticoid can greatly influence the amount of steroid that is released in any given period of time. In turn, the amount of steroid released has been shown to increase or decrease the clinical activity and vasoconstrictive intensity of the same glucocorticoid at the same concentration. Table 230-1 shows that betamethasone dipropionate at 0.05% (Diprolene) gives the most potent response (group 1) in an optimized ointment or cream. If the same glucocorticoid at the same concentration is put into the ointment vehicle (Diprosone ointment) with less propylene glycol, it has the potency of a group 2 formulation. If the same steroid at the same concentration is put into a cream formulation with less propylene glycol (Diprosone cream), it falls into group 3. If the same betamethasone dipropionate at the same concentration is incorporated into an alcoholic lotion (Diprosone lotion), it falls into group 5. So, out of seven possible groups of potency, betamethasone dipropionate at the same concentration can be formulated to fit into four of the first five groups.

TABLE 230-1

Potency Ranking of Some Commonly Used Brand-Name Corticosteroids*

Group 1 (super-potent)	Group 4 (mid-strength)
Temovate cream 0.05%[a]	Cordran ointment 0.05%[n]
Temovate ointment 0.05%[a]	Elocon cream 0.1%[f]
Diprolene cream† 0.05%[b]	Kenalog cream 0.1%[k]
Diprolene ointment 0.05%[b]	Synalar ointment 0.025%[o]
Psorcon ointment 0.05%[c]	Westcort ointment 0.2%[p]

Group 2 (potent)	Group 5 (mid-strength)
Cyclocort ointment 0.1%[d]	Cordran cream 0.05%[n]
Diprolene cream AF 0.05%[b]	Cutivate cream 0.05%[l]
Diprosone ointment 0.05%[e]	Diprosone lotion 0.05%[e]
Elocon ointment 0.1%[f]	Kenalog lotion 0.1%[k]
Florone ointment 0.05%[g]	Locoid cream 0.1%[q]
Halog cream 0.1%[h]	Synalar cream 0.025%[o]
Lidex cream 0.05%[i]	Valisone cream 0.1%[m]
Lidex gel 0.05%[i]	Westcort cream 0.2%[p]
Lidex ointment 0.05%[i]	
Maxiflor ointment 0.05%[g]	Group 6 (mild)
Topicort cream 0.25%[j]	
Topicort gel 0.05%[j]	Aclovate cream 0.05%[r]
Topicort ointment 0.25%[j]	Aclovate ointment 0.05%[r]
	Aristocort cream 0.1%[k]
Group 3 (potent)	Desowen cream 0.05%[s]
	Synalar solution 0.01%[o]
Aristocort A ointment 0.1%[k]	Synalar cream 0.01%[o]
Cutivate ointment 0.005%[l]	Tridesilon cream 0.05%[s]
Cyclocort cream 0.1%[d]	Valisone lotion 0.1%[m]
Cyclocort lotion 0.1%[d]	
Diprosone cream 0.05%[e]	Group 7 (mild)
Florone cream 0.05%[g]	
Halog ointment 0.1%[h]	Topicals with hydrocortisone
Lidex E cream 0.05%[i]	dexamethasone, flumethasone,
Maxiflor cream 0.05%[g]	prednisolone, and methyprednisolone
Valisone ointment 0.1%[m]	

*Group 1 is the super-potent category; potency descends with each group. There is no significant difference between agents *within* groups 2 through 7; the compounds are simply arranged alphabetically. However, within group 1, Temovate cream or ointment is more potent than Diprolene cream or ointment and Psorcon ointment.

†Diprolene cream has been renamed Diprolene gel (whitener-free reformulation).

[a]Clobetasone propionate
[b]Betamethasone dipropionate (optimized vehicle)
[c]Diflorasone diacetate (optimized vehicle)
[d]Amcinonide
[e]Betamethasone dipropionate
[f]Mometasone furoate
[g]Diflorasone diacetate
[h]Halcinonide
[i]Fluocinonide
[j]Desoximetasone
[k]Triamcinolone acetonide
[l]Fluticasone propionate
[m]Betamethasone valerate
[n]Flurandrenolide
[o]Fluocinolone acetonide
[p]Hydrocortisone valerate
[q]Hydrocortisone butyrate
[r]Alclometasone dipropionate
[s]Desonide

Table 230-1 also allows one to identify other glucocorticoids that will vary in potency at the same concentration, depending on the vehicle. Among these are triamcinolone acetonide (Kenalog, Aristocort), fluocinolone acetonide (Synalar), betamethasone valerate (Valisone), mometasone furoate (Elocon) and diflorasone diacetate (Florone and Psorcon).

There is a problem with generic glucocorticoid formulations. The assumption by manufacturers of generic topical glucocorticoids that the vehicle is unimportant has led to the marketing of many generic agents that are not equivalent to the innovator product.[8] Specific examples are betamethasone valerate 0.1% cream compared with Valisone cream 0.1%, fluocinonide cream 0.05% compared with Lidex cream 0.05%, triamcinolone acetonide cream 0.1% compared with Kenalog cream 0.1%. Since over 180 generic formulations of topical glucocorticoids are now available for prescription in the United States, it is a minefield for dermatologists to negotiate. This problem has come about in part because generic manufacturers did not understand that the slight differences in vehicles could make such major differences in potency.

Role of Concentration of Steroid in Vehicles

For many years pharmaceutical companies and many physicians assumed that increasing the concentration of a given glucocorticoid in the same vehicle would result in a more potent formulation to treat skin disease. Thus there are available such formulations as Kenalog cream, lotion, and ointment, at 0.025%, 0.1%, and 0.5%, and Aristocort cream and ointment at 0.025%, 0.1%, and 0.5%. When these formulations were tested in the vasoconstriction assay, the different concentrations of steroid in the same vehicle showed no difference from one another.[9] On the other hand, others such as Synalar cream, 0.01%, 0.025%, and 0.2%, showed a stepwise increase in vasoconstrictor activity from the lowest to the highest concentration.

These unpredictable differences in the behavior of formulations in relation to differences in concentration of the same steroid again reveal the critical importance of the vehicle in determining the rate of release of the steroid to the skin surface.

Clinical Use

Responsive and Less Responsive Dermatoses

There is an almost continuous spectrum of responsiveness not only of different dermatoses but also of the same disease on different areas of the body. Rough approximations of degree of responsiveness of different dermatoses to topical application of glucocorticoids can be made by dividing them into three categories: (1) responsive, (2) less responsive, and (3) least responsive (Table 230-2). One must remember that almost all inflammatory responses in skin can be modulated if high concentrations of glucocorticoids are directly injected into the corium of such lesions, but this procedure is usually not desirable if the lesion can be controlled by topical application.

By knowing the degree of responsiveness of a given dermatosis (Table 230-2) and the degrees of potency (Table 230-1) of topical glucocorticoid formulations, one can make a reasonable estimate of the formulation group with which to begin therapy to get the maximum benefit with the minimum side effects.

Another important technique in topical therapy with glucocorticoids is to use an occlusive covering over the treated area to enhance the clinical response to the drug. All steroids elicit an enhanced clinical response when an occlusive dressing is applied. One must also remember that side effects are proportionately enhanced. One clear tape product, Cordran tape, serves well as an occlusive system for enhancing the clinical effect of the steroid it contains and is useful for treating relatively small lesions.

Regional Differences in Activity

Anyone who has attempted to treat psoriasis of the soles of the feet or the nails with the most potent topical glucocorticoid, or intertriginous psoriasis with the weakest of topical glucocorticoids, appreciates the importance of the enormous differences in penetration of steroids (or almost any other chemical) on different areas of the body. Topical steroids rarely influence psoriasis of the palms or soles or nails, but all the topical steroids including hydrocortisone (the least potent) clear most psoriatic lesions in the intertriginous areas.

Table 230-3 lists the different regions of the body and their ability to allow penetration of glucocorticoids. Table 230-3 is useful to consult when trying to make a reasonable estimate of what potency ranking (Table 230-1) to use in which area. It also may be necessary to give the patient two or more different formulations to treat properly different areas of the body involved with the same disease at the same time.

Choice of Vehicles

We have already discussed the importance of the vehicle in determining the potency (bioavailability) of the glucocorticoid in clinical

TABLE 230-2
Responsiveness of Dermatoses to Topical Application of Glucocorticoids

Most responsive	Less responsive	Least responsive
Psoriasis (intertriginous)	Psoriasis (nonplaque)	Psoriasis (hands, feet, nails)
Atopic eczema (children)	Atopic eczema (adults)	Palmoplantar psoriasis
Seborrheic dermatitis	Nummular eczema	Dyshidrotic eczema (acute and chronic)
Intertrigo	Primary irritant dermatitis	Lupus erythematosus
	Papular urticaria	Pemphigus
	Parapsoriasis	Lichen planus
	Lichen simplex chronicus	Granuloma annulare
		Necrobiosis lipoidica diabeticorum
		Sarcoidosis
		Allergic contact dermatitis
		Insect bites

TABLE 230-3
Regional Differences in Penetration of Glucocorticoids

1. Mucous membrane	6. Upper arms and legs
2. Scrotum	7. Lower arms and legs
3. Eyelids	8. Dorsa of hands and feet
4. Face	9. Palmar and plantar skin
5. Chest and back	10. Nails

Most penetration with number 1 and less penetration with increasing numbers.

use. There are many other practical aspects concerning which vehicles to use on different areas of the body, on different diseases, and in special situations.

When patients complain of "dryness," as atopic patients frequently do in cold dry weather, ointments are usually most acceptable. The main disadvantage is cosmetic. The use of glucocorticoid ointments is proportionately higher in England than in the United States, probably because of the cooler climate for most of the year in England compared with a larger population living in warm, humid climates in the United States. Ointments tend to be more occlusive than other vehicles, and that property tends to enhance penetration of the steroid.

Creams vary in their consistency and composition, but generally they are far less "greasy" than ointments and cosmetically much more acceptable. Creams also are much easier to spread on the skin. Some so-called emollient creams have more petrolatum-like derivatives, so they are more like ointments than nonemollient creams. This compromise seems to be acceptable to many patients who want the features of both creams and ointments.

Lotions usually consist of water, alcohol, and various exotic agents to make them slightly like a cream, both to help them spread on the skin and to help solubilize the steroid and enhance penetration. Glucocorticoids in only an alcohol-water base do not penetrate well when applied to human skin.

Other vehicles such as gels, aerosols, and sprays add some variety to the cosmetic aspects of these medications and occasionally to their mechanical characteristics.

Side Effects—Topical

The ability of topical glucocorticosteroids to produce side effects (Table 230-4) has become more apparent as more potent steroids have been used. Striae and atrophy may be a particular problem and are more likely in areas of sweating, occlusion, or highly penetrable areas of the skin. In general, dermal and epidermal atrophy does not occur until at least 2 to 3 weeks of steroid use. Recovery usually follows in several weeks if the steroid is promptly discontinued at the first sign of atrophic changes.[10,11]

TABLE 230-4
Topical Side Effects of Glucocorticoids

Striae and atrophy	Glaucoma
Acne	Allergic contact dermatitis
Perioral dermatitis	Hypopigmentation
Rosacea	Reduced wound healing
Purpura and telangiectasia	Hirsutism (face)
"Masking" effect	Folliculitis and miliaria

Prolonged treatment with topical steroids can result in a form of acne characterized by a wave of dense, inflamed pustules which may result in crops of comedones. In this form of acne, many lesions are in the same developmental stage; scarring is fortunately unusual.[12] Reports of perioral dermatitis have greatly increased in the past several decades because of the advent of topical steroids. Patients given topical steroids for symptoms of burning and pustulation of rosacea may initially improve, but a severe rebound consisting of edema and multiple pustules may occur[13] when treatment is discontinued, despite continued treatment, or even when a less potent agent is used. The use of mild topical steroids is appropriate for most facial dermatoses.

Purpura develops particularly when topical steroids are used on areas of already thin skin, such as the extensor arm area. The ability of steroids to "mask" recognition of many common dermatoses (e.g., fungal infections of the skin, impetigo, and scabies) by virtue of their anti-inflammatory, antiproliferative, and vasoconstrictive properties is well documented.[14] Steroids should be used around the eyes with caution. Allergic contact dermatitis associated with use of topical steroids is usually caused by vehicle and not the steroid molecule. Recently contact dermatitis to corticosteroids has apparently become a more frequent problem involving the steroid itself rather than another ingredient in the topical formulation.[15] Tixocortol pivalate, a topical glucocorticosteroid with a sulfhydryl group, has been widely used in Europe but has not been approved in the United States for topical cutaneous use. Because contact dermatitis to pure hydrocortisone still seems to be an unusual occurrence in the United States, it is possible that cross-reactivity to hydrocortisone induced by tixocortol pivalate is a possible basis for the increase in Europe.[15,16]

Side Effects—Systemic

Hypothalamic-pituitary-adrenal axis suppression has been reported with the use of virtually all topical steroids. Growth retardation in infants and children and iatrogenic Cushing's syndrome in all patients are known but rare complications of therapy.[17] Systemic side effects are related to (1) the potency of the agent; for example, as little as 2 g daily of clobetasol propionate in an erythrodermic patient can result in decreased morning plasma cortisol levels after only several days of use;[18] (2) the use of occlusion (e.g., Saran Wrap) to increase humidity around the area treated; (3) the site of application; (4) the percentage of the body covered; and (5) the status of the stratum corneum—topical steroids penetrate diseased skin far more readily than normal skin.[19]

Most topical and systemic side effects are readily reversible if recognized early by the clinician. Both topical and systemic side effects increase with increasing potency of the steroid used. Side effects may be considerably reduced if appropriate guidelines are employed.

Pediatric Use

Special considerations are needed in treating children with topical glucocorticoids. In young children with atopic dermatitis in a normal outpatient setting, routine use of even group 5 topical steroids (e.g., Valisone cream 0.1% or Synalar cream 0.025%) frequently results in adrenal-pituitary axis suppression. It is therefore highly desirable to make every effort to use only topical hydrocortisone in infants and very young children.

One must be careful not to apply topical steroids to occluded areas such as the diaper area unless caution is exercised. Children seem to be more susceptible to developing striae from the topical steroids in groups 1 to 5 (see Table 230-1).

Topical glucocorticoids have been so effective in treating many childhood dermatoses, particularly eczematous lesions, that no one would think of giving up their use, but if they are to be used it is imperative to understand their special risks and limitations in children.

Combination Products

Although a few combination products are available in the United States, development of new combination products is not encouraged by the FDA. More of these combination formulations are available in other countries. Theoretically, there should be no need for a combination when each can be obtained separately. However, practicing physicians prefer to use some agents in combination because of the simplicity of use and lower cost to the patient.

A few glucocorticoids are available in combination with antifungal and antibacterial agents. They are not widely used by dermatologists, probably because they are not available in a variety wide enough to cover a spectrum of glucocorticoid activity and to be highly effective antifungal (including antimonial and antibacterial) agents.

How Much to Apply

Most use of topical glucocorticoids is wasteful in that more is applied than is needed to give the maximum amount of penetration per unit area. Vasoconstrictor assays show that the maximum response can be derived with 4 μg of formulation per square centimeter of skin surface. This amounts to an extremely thin layer. The average patient probably applies two to four times as much. This practical point could save patients a considerable amount of money.

Dosage Schedules

Twice-a-day topical application of glucocorticoids is recommended on the labels of most formulations. No scientific evidence has ever established this twice-daily schedule as the optimum one; this dosing schedule was recommended when topical steroids were introduced and has come to be generally accepted. However, a number of investigators in many countries have reasonable evidence that the more potent formulations can be used once a day, every other day, or even less often, and that these schedules can work very well in controlling dermatitis. The simplest way to find the proper schedule is to work with the patient to find the longest elapsed time between successive applications that still controls the condition. This titration requires a motivated and intelligent patient and a person to give him or her proper instruction and follow-up.

Psoriasis in particular seems to stay well controlled with three or so applications of a group 1 (Table 230-1) formulation each week, once the disease is under good control. This persistent control may be related to the lack of the phenomenon of tachyphylaxis[20,21] to continued use of topical glucocorticoids as demon-

strated by diminished vasoconstriction, rebound of DNA synthesis, and recovery of histamine wheals. All of these biologic reactions can easily be induced by topical glucocorticoids, and they diminish with regular and continued use. The role of tachyphylaxis in treating clinical disease with topical steroids is not as obvious as is the role of tachyphylaxis in the above-described experimentally induced cutaneous reactions.

The phenomenon of a flare of psoriasis during treatment or soon after terminating treatment with a potent topical steroid may be related to an overreaction related to tachyphylaxis.

Topical glucocorticoids have been the most widely used medications in dermatologic therapy for the past 30 years. The consistent effectiveness of this class of drugs, low incidence and severity of side effects, and high patient acceptability will probably keep them in favor for years to come.

References

1. Sulzberger MD, Witten VH: The effect of topically applied compound I in selected dermatoses. *J Invest Dermatol* **19**:101, 1952
2. McKenzie AW, Stoughton RB: Method for comparing percutaneous absorption of steroids. *Arch Dermatol* **86**:608, 1962
3. McKenzie AW, Atkinson RM: Topical activities of betamethasone esters in man. *Arch Dermatol* **89**:741, 1964
4. Hammarstrom S et al: Glucocorticoid in inflammatory proliferative skin diseases reduces arachidonic and hydroxyeicosatetraenoic acids. *Science* **197**:994, 1977
5. Ponec M: Glucocorticoids and cultured human skin cells: Specific intracellular binding and structure-activity relationships. *Br J Dermatol* **107**:24, 1982
6. Blackwell GJ et al: Macrocortin: A polypeptide causing antiphospholipase effects of glucocorticosteroids. *Nature* **287**:147, 1980
7. Cornell RC, Stoughton RB: Correlation of the vasoconstrictor assay and clinical activity. *Arch Dermatol* **121**:63, 1985
8. Stoughton RB: Are generic formulations equivalent to trade name topical glucocorticoids? *Arch Dermatol* **123**:1312, 1987
9. Stoughton RB, Wullich K: Does increasing the concentration of the same glucocorticoid in brand name products result in greater topical biologic activity? *Arch Dermatol* **125**:1509, 1989
10. Lavker RM et al: Effects of topical steroids on human dermis. *Br J Dermatol* **115** (suppl 311):101, 1986
11. Katz HI et al: Betamethasone dipropionate in optimized vehicle. *Arch Dermatol* **123**:1308, 1987
12. Plewig G, Kligman AM: Induction of acne by topical steroids. *Arch Dermatol Forsch* **247**:29, 1973
13. Leyden JJ et al: Steroid rosacea. *Arch Dermatol* **110**:619, 1974
14. Ive FA, Marks R: Tinea incognito. *Br Med J* **3**:149, 1968
15. Wilkinson SM et al: Hydrocortisone: An important cutaneous allergen. *Lancet* **337**:761, 1991
16. Dooms-Goossens AE et al: Contact allergy to corticosteroids: A frequently missed diagnosis? *J Am Acad Dermatol* **21**:538, 1989
17. Fritz KA, Weston WL: Topical glucocorticosteroid, a review. *Ann Allergy* **50**:68, 1983
18. Olsen EA, Cornell RC: Topical clobetasol-17-propionate: Review of its clinical efficacy and safety. *J Am Acad Dermatol* **15**:246, 1986
19. Cornell RC, Stoughton RB: Six-month controlled study of effect of desoximetasone and betamethasone 17-valerate on the pituitary-adrenal axis. *Br J Dermatol* **105**:91, 1981
20. DuVivier A, Stoughton RB: Acute tolerance to effects of topical glucocorticoids. *Br J Dermatol* **94** (suppl 12):25, 1976
21. Singh G, Singh PK: Tachyphylaxis to topical steroids measured by histamine-induced wheal suppression. *Int J Dermatol* **25**:324, 1986

Arthur K.F. Tong and Christopher F.H. Vickers

Topical Noncorticosteroid Therapy

Topical therapy is the principal route of administration in dermatology. This is because topical treatments for the most common skin disorders, such as acne vulgaris, eczema, verrucae, localized psoriasis, are as effective or more efficacious than systemic therapy. In this chapter an attempt will be made to discuss the most commonly used noncorticosteroid agents and their mode of action, where known. The list is not exhaustive but is intended to provide an overview of the pharmacopoeia available.

Acne Therapies

Benzoyl Peroxide   Benzoyl peroxide probably owes most of its action to the fact that it is a powerful oxidizer. Its value as a comedolytic in acne[1,2] is well established and it is also effective as an antimicrobial against *Propionibacterium acnes*. Whether its action in reducing fatty acid content in sebum is secondary to its antimicrobial effect or primary is undecided.[3] Many preparations are available, but care needs to be exercised in the early stage of treatment as it is an irritant. Bleaching of skin and hair has also been reported.[4,5] Despite this, benzoyl peroxide preparations are effective in the topical therapy of acne vulgaris.

Metronidazole   Metronidazole is a synthetic agent that, when given systemically, is effective against gram-negative bacteria and protozoa. Metronidazole, 0.75% in a gel base applied topically twice daily, has been shown to be effective in the treatment of rosacea.[6]

Sulfur   Sulfur preparations are still used by some in acne. However, many studies have shown its comedogenicity.[7]

Vitamin A Acid (Tretinoin)   Vitamin A has long been known to profoundly affect the process of keratinization,[8] but topical application of vitamin A, usually in a lotion, is without significant effect. In 1962, the topical application of vitamin A acid was first reported and has since found widespread use in acne in the form of a gel or cream at 0.025% to 0.1% concentrations.[9–11] The actions of tretinoin include its effects on (1) keratinization, (2) epidermopoiesis, with the capability of restoring near-normal keratinization when that process is disorganized, (3) DNA synthesis, (4) lysosomal stabilization, and (5) prostaglandin synthesis.[12,13] By increasing the mitotic activity and the turnover of follicular epithelial cells and by regulating the maturation of epidermal cells, tretinoin effects a thickening of the granular layer and a normalization of parakeratosis. Initially, there may be redness and soreness of the skin, but the comedones then start to extrude[14,15] and do not usually re-form if therapy is continued. It is possible to minimize the initial irritation on the skin by alternate-day applications for the first 2 weeks.

Vitamin A acid, 0.1% in a simple base, is also quite effective in ichthyosis vulgaris and lamellar ichthyosis.[16] Fox-Fordyce disease (apocrine miliaria) has also been treated effectively with a 0.1% solution.[17] The use of tretinoin in the treatment of solar damage[18,19] and striae distensae[20] has been under investigation recently and has shown encouraging results.

Simplistically, it might be expected that as one of the actions of vitamin A acid is to induce a granular layer, it might benefit psoriasis, but this has not been shown in most published work.[21] Darier's disease occasionally responds dramatically, but these results again are very variable.[10] Lichen planus, plane warts, and solar keratoses have also been treated with variable success. Keratosis pilaris may also improve with tretinoin, although initial irritation is common.[22,23]

Analgesics (Topical)

Capsaicin   Capsaicin cream is derived from cayenne pepper. When applied to skin, it produces a slight burning sensation. It is believed that capsaicin works by its action on substance P, a pain-transmitter compound. It is theorized that by depleting substance P in peripheral nerve endings, pain impulses cannot be transmitted to the brain. It has been used in the treatment of postherpetic neuralgia with some success.[24]

Topical Antihistamines   Topical antihistamines, such as diphenhydramine, may have a transient antipruritic effect, but sensitization is very common and therefore they should be avoided.

Topical Anesthetics   Topical anesthetics such as benzocaine are sensitizers and should be avoided entirely. Lidocaine (USA) [or lignocaine (UK)] and other "amide"-type agents are rare sensitizers and may be used safely.[25]

Antibacterial Agents

Hydrogen Peroxide   Hydrogen peroxide, 5 to 20 volumes, has been in wide use for many years as a cleansing agent to remove purulent debris; it has a distinct antibacterial effect and the effervescent quality helps loosen crusts and debris. It may also be used to bleach hair in the treatment of hirsutism.

Silver Sulfadiazine   Silver sulfadiazine is a sulfonamide derivative and is valuable in the management of chronic ulcers and burns. It is active against a wide spectrum of gram-positive and gram-negative organisms as well as yeasts. It has a good antistaphylococcal effect both prophylactically and therapeutically.[26] Even when used over wide areas, the risk of renal damage from systemic absorption is minimal.[27] However, it should not be used in patients with glucose-6-phosphate dehydrogenase deficiency. In newborns or premature infants, the use of silver sulfadiazine may increase the risk of kernicterus. Sensitization is extremely rare, which is interesting in view of the frequent hypersensitivity to locally applied sulfonamide creams.

Antifungal Agents

Selenium Sulfide Selenium sulfide is a beneficial agent in the control of dandruff, although its use should be limited to fairly short periods, as brittleness of the hair may occur, possibly due to breakage of disulfide cross-bonds.[28] It is also commonly used as a topical application for the treatment of tinea versicolor. For this use, a 2.5% suspension of selenium sulfide is applied to the entire area from the neck down to the waist, including the upper extremities, and allowed to remain for 15 min before rinsing. This is repeated daily for 1 to 2 weeks. Thereafter, a maintenance application twice weekly may be effective for prophylaxis.

Zinc Pyrithione Zinc pyrithione is an antifungal and antibacterial agent. It is the active ingredient in several shampoos used for the treatment of seborrheic dermatitis of the scalp. It is also effective in the treatment of tinea versicolor and is used in much the same way as selenium sulfide.

Whitfield's Ointment Whitfield's ointment (12% benzoic acid and 6% salicylic acid) may be used in full or half strength in the treatment of dermatophytosis. It may, however, cause irritation to the area of application (see "Keratolytic Agents" below).

Castellani's Paint This mixture of resorcinol (10%), acetone (5%), phenol (4.5%), boric acid (1%), and fuchsin (0.3%) in water is effective in inflammatory tinea of the web spaces and acute candidal paronychia (see "Antimicrobial Agents" below).

In addition to these time-proven remedies, several very effective topical, and a few systemic, agents for the control of dermatophytoses and candidiasis became available in the past decade. These are discussed in Chaps. 194 and 195.

Anti-Hair Loss Medications

Minoxidil Minoxidil is a vasodilator used in the treatment of hypertension. For topical applications, it is formulated as a 2% solution. Its use in male-pattern alopecia is well established, with approximately 30 percent of patients obtaining good to excellent results.[29] It has also been used in alopecia areata[30] with acceptable results. Its use in female-pattern alopecia is still under investigation.[31]

Cyclosporine Cyclosporine, administered systemically, selectively inhibits T-helper cell production of interleukin 2 and increases the suppressor T-cell populations. Because one of the side effects is hypertrichosis, it has been formulated in various bases for topical use in male-pattern alopecia[32] and alopecia totalis.[33] Results so far have been mixed.

Anti-Inflammatory Agents

Bufexamac Bufexamac (*p*-butoxyphenylacethydroxine acid) is a nonsteroidal anti-inflammatory cream. Its initial promise has not been borne out; irritation and sensitization are unacceptably high and its anti-inflammatory effect is low. One interesting fact is that it appears to act as a sunscreen in the UVA range.

Coal Tar Coal tar is the product of distillation of coal during the production of gas. Very few such distilleries now exist in the western world since the discovery of natural gas deposits. The thick black viscous fluid is a combination of at least 10,000 different chemicals and only about 4 to 5 percent of them have been identified,[34] although these constitute the large majority of the crude material by weight.

One problem that exists in analyzing the active ingredients is that all coal tars are different depending on the source of the coal and the type and temperature of the distillation. The method by which crude coal tar exerts its influence is still not well understood.

Many confusing reports have appeared concerning the different fractions of tar. Phenolic constituents have been suggested as lysosomal-release agents that stimulate mitosis—hardly the desired effect in psoriasis. Other extracts appear to produce acanthosis.[35] Some studies have shown coal tars to inhibit DNA synthesis, thus acting as a cytostatic.[36] The coal tars and their actions remain one of the most intriguing and stimulating conundrums in dermatologic therapy. Many efforts have been made to produce cosmetically acceptable preparations and most have failed. The most commonly used formulations include tar gels, coal tar creams, and bath preparations. Patient compliance is always difficult, but therapeutic results in chronic eczema, especially atopic dermatitis, are gratifying. Coal tars are also formulated as shampoos and are widely used for dandruff and psoriatic and eczematous conditions of the scalp. Tars may also be prescribed in ointment or paste bases, and there are tar-impregnated bandages available that are very valuable in the management of childhood atopic eczema.

That tar is carcinogenic in animal experiments is beyond doubt.[37] Workers in the tar and pitch industry develop carcinomata, but there are very few reports of carcinomata resulting from the therapeutic use of crude coal tar, to which hundreds of thousands of patients have been exposed in all parts of the world.[38] The few reports that exist suggest that carcinomata develop when tar is applied to the flexures.

Tar is phototoxic and may induce phototoxic reactions in patients who have used it for long periods,[39] such as in the Goeckerman regime or in atopic eczema in childhood. The photosensitivity reaction is the rationale for adding UV radiation to the Goeckerman regime, but recent studies have cast doubt on its value.

Shale Tar (Ichthammol) Ichthammol is one of the time-honored therapies in dermatology. It originates from shale oil that undergoes chemical degradation with ammonia and sulfuric acid to form a sulfur-rich substance. Only certain bases, usually containing glycerin, are suitable for formulations containing ichthammol. It is believed to have anti-inflammatory and vasoactive properties and has been a standard agent in the management of eczema (especially seborrheic) and rosacea; it is used in a glycerol solution in the management of acute otitis externa where its soothing properties are legendary. There is little formal evidence of pharmacologic activity, but its continued use is testimony to its safety,[40] patient acceptance, and the symptomatic relief it gives. In contrast to coal tars, shale tars are less irritating and are not photosensitizers,[39] but they are also less effective.

Wood Tar Wood tars, of which only oil of cade (juniper tar) has any widespread use outside Scandinavia, are obtained by distilling wood under controlled conditions. Oil of cade has a strong and distinctive odor. It can be added to arachis oil or simple bases as an application to the scalp in seborrheic eczema and psoriasis. It is also a major ingredient in the so-called 20-10-5 ointment, which contains 20% oil of cade, 10% sulfur, and 5% salicylic acid. Other wood tars include oil of beech, birch, and pine. These are used in Scandinavia in a similar fashion to oil of cade. Like shale tars, wood tars do not cause photosensitivity.

Antimicrobial Agents

Chlorhexidine   Chlorhexidine is chiefly an antimicrobial and is bactericidal on contact. It is effective against a wide spectrum of gram-positive and gram-negative microorganisms, including *Pseudomonas aeruginosa*. It is also effective against common yeasts and fungi. The antimicrobial activities have a rapid onset and persist for several hours after a single application.[41] It does not lose its effectiveness in the presence of whole blood.

Dyes   Two dyes, *gentian violet* (methylrosaniline chloride) and *brilliant green* (*p*-diethylamine triphenylmethanol) in aqueous solution, retain their place in dermatology for their astringent and antimicrobial actions, especially against *Candida* and gram-negative bacterias. Hence, these dyes are effective in secondarily infected dermatophytoses.

Castellani's Paint   Castellani's paint is a magenta liquid that stains the skin red. It has bactericidal, fungicidal, as well as local anesthetic effects. It is particularly effective in inflammatory intertriginous tinea and acute *Candida* paronychia.

Iodinated Compounds   Iodine solution is bactericidal. It also kills spores when used in the proper concentration. As a 1% aqueous solution used as a hand wash, it is viricidal.[42] Iodophors are complexes of iodine with a carrier that slowly liberates inorganic iodine on contact with reducing substances. This preserves the antimicrobial activities of iodine without the irritant effects of the free tincture. However, the onset of action is slower than iodine solution (several minutes vs. less than 1 min) and they may be ineffective on contact with whole blood.

POVIDONE-IODINE.   This iodophor is commonly used for preoperative cleansing of the skin and in surgical scrubbing. It may also be used in postoperative wound care and burns. The rate of sensitization is low.

CLIOQUINOL (VIOFORM).   Clioquinol (previously called iodochlorhydroxyquin) has only mild antifungal and antibacterial actions. It may be used alone or in combination with a topical steroid such as 1% hydrocortisone cream or ointment. The latter is effective in the treatment of inflammatory dermatoses, particularly in the intertriginous areas, where the clioquinol acts to inhibit the growth of dermatophytes, *Candida,* and gram-positive cocci. Clioquinol may impart a yellowish discoloration to the skin or clothing.

Antiperspirants[43]

Aluminum Compounds   A solution of aluminum chloride in anhydrous ethyl alcohol is used in the management of hyperhidrosis.[44] The solution is applied to the axillae or the palms and soles at bedtime. Occlusion may be used to increase the effectiveness, although this may also increase the incidence of irritation. Once excessive sweating is under control, the use may be decreased to once

or twice weekly as maintenance. The mode of action is probably by inducing blockage of the sweat ducts.[45]

This preparation may also be used as a chemical cautery on the shallow wounds from curettage or shave excision procedures for hemostasis.

Aldehydes   Gluteraldehyde[46] and formaldehyde solutions applied to palms or soles may control hyperhidrosis of the palms and soles. Formaldehyde is a skin sensitizer and therefore not commonly used. Gluteraldehyde may be used on alternate days until control is achieved, then decreased to once-weekly application or used as needed. When used as a 10% solution, gluteraldehyde may leave a brown pigmentation. A 2% solution will not discolor but is less effective.

Methenamine   Methenamine is hydrolyzed to ammonia and formaldehyde when applied to the skin. A 10% solution is effective in mild to moderate hyperhidrosis and rarely produces allergic reactions.[47]

Antipruritic Agents

Camphor   Camphor is a ketone. It has two uses: first, as an additive to shake lotions for its cooling and antipruritic effect, notably in urticaria and lichen planus; second, and for a similar reason, it is added to many chilblain preparations. In concentrations of 1% to 3% it has a local anesthetic effect.

Menthol   Menthol is a cyclic alcohol. It is used interchangeably with camphor and indeed the two are often combined in one preparation. The method of action of both drugs is probably due to an induced feeling of cold that competitively inhibits itching.

Phenol   Phenol in low concentrations (0.5% to 2%) is an antipruritic through a local anesthetic effect. It is a common ingredient in many over-the-counter antipruritics. Because phenol is readily absorbed through the skin,[48] it should not be used in pregnant women or in infants less than 6 months of age. In higher concentrations phenol is widely used as a skin caustic.

Pramoxine Hydrochloride   Pramoxine hydrochloride is an antipruritic through its anesthetic actions. It is available by itself or combined with a 1% or 2.5% hydrocortisone for their anti-inflammatory properties.

Antipsoriatic Agents

Dithranol (Anthralin)   Dithranol, a mainstay of topical therapy in psoriasis, is a synthetic derivative of chrysarobin and is used widely in many different bases, paints, pastes, and wax sticks. There are also special pomades for the scalp. It stains normal skin dark brown or black and for this reason as well as its irritation of normal skin it is usual to apply it in a base that remains where it is placed and does not spread over the surface of the skin. Dithranol in white soft paraffin is used, however, in short-contact therapy,[49] in which the application is washed off after a short period of time to minimize the irritation. Salicylic acid is added to many preparations to prevent oxidative processes leading to the production of an inactive anthrone. Recently anthralin in a vanishing cream base has become available in a range of concentrations. These are cosmetically much more acceptable but are less effective therapeutically.

The mode of action of dithranol is not completely understood but it certainly inhibits glycolytic enzymes[50] and this may result from lipoid peroxidation.[51] The inhibition of enzyme activity appears to be preceded by an acanthotic effect similar to that observed with tar.[52] Dithranol acts by inhibiting mitosis,[53] although there is a contributing epidermopoietic stimulating effect. DNA uptake is inhibited.[54] Glucose-6-phosphate dehydrogenase activity in human skin is also strongly inhibited by dithranol and less so by more cosmetically acceptable derivatives such as triacetoxyanthracene.[55]

The mechanism of the staining has been extensively investigated, but no full explanation has yet been offered. Attempts to prepare a dithranol derivative that does not stain skin have so far been unsuccessful.

Chrysarobin is a derivative of the plant *Andira arobata* and a mixture of anthranols. It is still occasionally prescribed for patients who burn easily with dithranol.

5-Fluorouracil This antimetabolite has been used for limited plaque lesions of psoriasis. Although ulceration of the lesions is common, the subsequent period of remission may last several months.[56,57] Psoriasis of the nail has also been treated successfully with a 1% 5-fluorouracil solution[58] (see "Wart Therapies" below).

Oils Oils of many kinds are mainstays of dermatology mainly as bath additives (mineral oil). Coconut oil is the basis of some useful remedies for scalp psoriasis, especially in the presence of tar allergy and dithranol irritation. Sunflower seed oil has been shown to correct the results of essential fatty acid deficiency. Its clinical use in ichthyosis and atopic dermatitis has been disappointing.

Pyrogallic Acid Pyrogallic acid (1,2,3-trihydroxybenzene) has been utilized for many years in the treatment of psoriasis of the scalp, especially where scales are very thick. Patient compliance is apt to be rather low as the material tends to be very dark in color, the result of oxidative reduction.

Tars See "Anti-Inflammatory Agents" above.

Vitamin D₃ Analogue (Calcipotriol) The latest advance in the field of nonsteroidal preparations for the treatment of psoriasis is the development of the vitamin D_3 analogue calcipotriol in a cream or ointment base.[59] Vitamin D_3 inhibits proliferation of epidermal cells and at the same time induces differentiation. It also possesses anti-inflammatory actions by its potent inhibitory action on interleukin 1–induced cell proliferation. The topical analogue possesses these same properties but with a much reduced risk of producing hypercalcemia.[60,61] Its therapeutic effect on psoriasis is likely a result of all these properties. In clinical trials, the efficacy of calcipotriol is at the level of betamethasone valerate.[62,63] It is applied twice daily for up to 8 weeks. Skin atrophy is not observed. It is recommended that the serum calcium level be monitored if more than 100 g per week is used. It is also safe for use on pregnant women. Its safety on children has yet to be determined. Combined UVB phototherapy with calcipotriol may produce additional benefits.[64]

Astringents

Astringents are used to reduce weeping from acute inflammatory skin lesions or ulcers. They act by precipitating protein, thus decreasing oozing.

Aluminum Salts Aluminum acetate (Burow's solution) diluted 1:10 to 1:40 has long been used as an astringent wet dressing.[65] Over-the-counter powder packets or tablets containing aluminum sulfate and calcium acetate are available and, when dissolved in water, make a modified Burow's solution. These astringent solutions may be used as wet dressings, compresses, or soaks.

Potassium Permanganate Potassium permanganate is a strong oxidizing agent. A solution of 1:4000 to 1:16,000 dilution may be used as a wet compress on weepy areas as an astringent. Alternatively, a 1:25,000 solution may be used as a medicated bath. The oxidative property is also believed to be responsible for its germicidal and fungicidal activities. This once popular preparation is used less commonly now because of the resultant bright purple staining. This staining may be removed with a weak solution of oxalic acid or sodium thiosulfate.[66]

Silver Nitrate Silver nitrate 0.5% in aqueous solution, used as wet dressings, is valuable in the management of infected eczemas, gravitational ulcers, and indeed any weeping and/or infected skin lesions.[67] It is both an effective astringent and an antimicrobial agent, including against *Pseudomonas aeruginosa*. Its cosmetic disadvantages (staining the skin black) are outweighed by the rapid resolution of weeping and control of superficial infection, often by resistant organisms. Forty percent silver nitrate in alcohol is helpful in the management of severe folliculitis. In its solid form it may be used as a hemostat.

Normal Saline Normal saline (0.9% sodium chloride) wet-to-dry dressings are favorites of surgeons for weepy, infected wounds as a means to dry as well as debride the areas.

Lead Acetate Lead acetate was often prescribed for its astringent and antipruritic effects. It is certainly a safe and soothing preparation and is a common dermatologic preparation in developing countries.

Insecticides and Scabicides

Benzyl Benzoate Benzyl benzoate is the most commonly used scabicide in the United Kingdom. It is also effective for pediculosis capitis and pubis.

Crotamiton Crotamiton claims to be a scabicide and an antipruritic. It is, however, not particularly effective in either role.

Gamma Benzene Hexachloride Gamma benzene hexachloride as a 1% lotion is a very effective scabicide and insecticide against lice and fleas. Central nervous system toxicity from systemic absorption has been reported[68,69] and is a main concern, especially when used in infants. Aplastic anemia has also been reported.[68,70]

Malathion   Malathion is extremely effective against lice and their ova. It has a fast onset of action and is one of the least toxic organophosphorus agents. It is not available in the United States.

Permethrin   Permethrin is a synthetic pyrethroid. As a 1% cream rinse, it is effective in the treatment of head lice and the nits.[71] It acts on the cell membrane of nerve cells, causing paralysis and death. A single application, left on for 10 min, is sufficient to eliminate the infestation. Activity is still detectable at least 10 days after a single application. Permethrin 5% in a cream base is an effective scabicide.[72,73] It is safe for use in infants over 2 months of age. Animal studies have revealed no teratogenic effects on the fetus. Permethrin is also effective against ticks, mites, and fleas.

Pyrethrin   Pyrethrin in combination with piperonyl butoxide is an effective alternative to gamma benzene hexachloride in the treatment of head lice and the nits.[71] Pyrethrin is a neurotoxin, whereas piperonyl butoxide inhibits the metabolism of pyrethrin, thereby potentiating its effect. This combination has a quicker onset of action than gamma benzene hexachloride in killing head lice and is comparable in ovicidal activity. It is also effective against fleas, mosquitoes, and houseflies.

Keratolytic Agents

Alpha Hydroxy Acids   Alpha hydroxy acids (lactic acid, glycolic acid, malic acid, pyruvic acid, etc.) are extremely effective keratolytics.[74] In appropriate bases, these are effective in ichthyosis and hyperkeratotic eczema.[75] Many proprietary preparations contain these solutions as well as salicylic acid in 5% to 40% concentrations in yellow or white soft paraffin. Lactic acid 12% and glycolic acid 11% are very effective in dry skin, ichthyosis, and palmoplantar keratodermas. Other therapeutic uses are under investigation.[76]

Benzoic Acid   Whitfield's ointment (12% benzoic acid and 6% salicylic acid) is a potent keratolytic. It is used predominantly in the treatment of fungal infections. It also has a place in the management of hyperkeratotic conditions. Benzoic acid is present in smaller concentrations in many preparations designed to loosen slough.

Lactic Acid   Lactic acid 12% is very effective for dry skin, ichthyosis, and palmoplantar keratodermas.

Propylene Glycol[77]   A 40% to 60% aqueous solution of propylene glycol, under occlusion, is effective in softening the skin of patients with ichthyosis.[78] It is also available as an alcohol-cellulose gel containing 6% salicylic acid or combined with lactic acid in a lotion. These are very effective as keratolytics as well as being cosmetically acceptable.

Salicylic Acid   Salicylic acid is the oldest keratolytic known and can be used in concentrations of 0.5% to 60% in almost any base, although some emulsions are "cracked" by the addition of too high a concentration. In concentrations of 3% to 6%, it causes shedding of scales by softening the horny layers. Its widespread and prolonged use has been reported to give rise to salicylism,[79] especially in children.[48] Sensitization is unknown and irritation uncommon if care is taken to introduce low concentrations at first. It enhances

percutaneous absorption of other agents in the same base. Its action on hyperplastic keratin is probably twofold: to decrease keratinocyte adhesion[80] and thereby promote desquamation of the horny layer of the skin[81] without effect on mitotic activity[82]; and second to increase water binding, thus hydrating the keratin.[83] Some reports have suggested a direct anti-inflammatory effect, though only equivalent to 0.1% hydrocortisone.[81,84]

Urea   Urea is proteolytic at high concentrations (ca. 40%) and has been used as an aqueous solution in the management of black hairy tongue[85] and to remove nails affected by fungal infections or psoriasis. In the latter situation, the nail is isolated by occlusive collodion, and 40% urea in a lanolin base is applied as an ointment. The nail is then occluded for several days. Urea has also been added to some topical corticosteroid preparations. Five to ten percent urea in various bases is commonly recommended in the management of ichthyosis, but many patients experience burning.

Wart Therapies

Benzalkonium   This antiseptic agent is also used as a 25% solution in the treatment of plantar warts.

Cantharidin   Cantharidin is an extract from the blister beetle *Cantharis vesicatoria*. It causes an intraepidermal blister when applied to skin. For treatment of warts, it is often used in a collodion base. The efficacy may be enhanced by the addition of 30% salicylic acid.

5-Fluorouracil   5-Fluorouracil is a pyrimidine analogue that inhibits thymidylic synthetase, thereby preventing the conversion of deoxyuridylic acid to thymidylic acid and inhibiting DNA synthesis. It is available in both solution and cream forms in concentrations of 1% and 5%. It has been used successfully in the treatment of flat and mosaic warts as well as warts in the genital area.[86] It may also be very effective in some cases of periungual warts that are resistant to other commonly used modalities, such as liquid nitrogen applications. Its effectiveness may be increased by an occlusive dressing or in combination with salicylic acid.[87] Its use in actinic keratosis and other skin carcinomas is discussed in Chaps. 73 and 74.

Mono-, Di-, Trichloroacetic Acids   Monochloroacetic acid 80% penetrates the skin and may produce necrosis of the epidermis by blister formation. Saturated dichloroacetic acid or trichloroacetic acid in concentrations of 50% to 80% are less powerful but are still effective as therapies for warts. The effectiveness may be enhanced by an occlusive dressing. The application needs to be repeated at 1- to 2-week intervals until complete resolution.

Podophyllum Resin   Podophyllin is an extract from the dried roots of either *Podophyllum peltatum* or *P. emodi*. It contains several active ingredients, the most important being podophyllotoxin and β-peltatin. It acts as an antimitotic agent by preventing the formation of mitotic spindles. Thus, in treated tissues, an increase in mitotic figures in metaphase may be observed and may be confused with a squamous cell carcinoma. It is available in a range of concentrations in various vehicles such as tincture of benzoin, alcohol, or flexible collodion.

It is used most commonly in the treatment of condylomata acuminata. The resin is applied directly onto the warts, then washed off thoroughly after 2 to 4 h. The period of contact may be increased gradually in successive treatments if no ill effects are experienced. It has also been used in the treatment of black hairy tongue. For this condition, the resin is applied to the surface of the thickened tongue for 5 min, then thoroughly rinsed off (P.L. McCarthy, M.D., personal communication). It is less effective when used on keratinized skin.

Local adverse reactions include burning, pain, irritation, erosion, and itching. If applied to large areas, especially to mucosal surfaces, absorption may result in systemic side effects, which include polyneuropathy, seizure, coma, urticaria, and leukopenia. It should not be used during pregnancy.

Recently, a purified form of the resin became available as podofilox 0.5% solution.[88,89] In this form, it is applied to the warts twice daily for 3 days, followed by a rest for 4 days, and the cycle is repeated until resolution is achieved. Irritation and ulceration are the most common complaints, and the recurrence rate is high.

Salicylic Acid Salicylic acid in concentrations of greater than 6% is destructive to tissue. Hence, salicylic acid in concentrations of up to 60% in a variety of bases is available for the treatment of warts. Some formulations contain lactic acid for additional keratolytic effects (see "Keratolytic Agents" above).

References

1. Vasarinsch P: Benzoyl peroxide versus sulphur lotion. *Arch Dermatol* **98**:183, 1968

2. Kirton V, Wilkinson D: Benzoyl peroxide in acne. *Practitioner* **204**:683, 1979

3. Fulton JE, Pablo G: Topical antibacterial therapy for acne. *Arch Dermatol* **110**:83, 1974

4. Bleiberg J et al: Bleaching of hair after use of topical benzoyl peroxide acne lotion. *Arch Dermatol* **108**:583, 1973

5. Bushkell LL: Bleaching by benzoyl peroxide. *Arch Dermatol* **110**:465, 1974

6. Bleicher PA et al: Topical metronidazole therapy for rosacea. *Arch Dermatol* **23**:609, 1987

7. Mills OH, Kligman AM: Is sulphur helpful or harmful in acne? *Br J Dermatol* **86**:620, 1972

8. Kligman AM et al: Acne therapy with tretinoin in combination with antibiotics. *Acta Derm Venereol (Stockh)* **55**(suppl 74):111, 1975

9. Valle-Jones JC: Retinoic acid in the treatment of acne. *Practitioner* **213**:387, 1974

10. Günther S: Vitamin A acid in Darier's disease. *Acta Derm Venereol Suppl (Stockh)* **74**:146, 1975

11. Stutgen C: The local handling of keratin by vitamin A ointments. *Dermatologica* **124**:65, 1962

12. Logan WS: Vitamin A and keratinization. *Arch Dermatol* **105**:748, 1972

13. Rahtijarvi K: Vitamin A acid in the local treatment of congenital ichthyosiform erythroderma. Symposium. *Acta Derm Venereol Suppl (Stockh)* **74**:145, 1975

14. Kligman AM et al: Topical vitamin A acid in acne vulgaris. *Arch Dermatol* **99**:469, 1969

15. Mills OH et al: Acne vulgaris. *Arch Dermatol* **106**:200, 1972

16. Peck GL: Treatment of lamellar ichthyosis and other keratinizing disorders with oral synthetic retinoids. *Lancet* **2**:1172, 1977

17. Tkach JR: Tretinoin treatment for Fox-Fordyce disease (letter). *Arch Dermatol* **115**:1285, 1979

18. Gardner SS, Weiss JS: Clinical features of photodamage and treatment with topical tretinoin. *J Dermatol Surg Oncol* **16**:925, 1990

19. Mark R, Lever L: Studies on the effects of topical retinoic acid on photoageing. *Br J Dermatol* **122**(suppl 35):87, 1990

20. Elson ML: Treatment of striae distensae with topical tretinoin. *J Dermatol Surg Oncol* **16**:267, 1990

21. Günther S: The therapeutic value of retinoic acid in chronic discoid, acute guttate and erythrodermic psoriasis: Clinical observations in 25 patients. *Br J Dermatol* **88**:55, 1973

22. Goette DK: Keratosis pilaris clearing with topical vitamin A acid. *Acta Derm Venereol (Stockh)* **55**(suppl 74):146, 1975

23. Günther S: Use of topical retinoic acid. *Acta Derm Venereol (Stockh)* **55**(suppl 74):159, 1975

24. Bernstein JE et al: Treatment of chronic postherpetic neuralgia with topical capsaicin. *J Am Acad Dermatol* **17**:93, 1987

25. Fisher AA: *Contact Dermatitis*. Philadelphia, Lea & Febiger, 1986, p 223

26. Lowbury EJL et al: Topical chemoprophylaxis with silver sulphadiazine and silver nitrate chlorhexidine cream. Emergence of sulphadiazine resistant gram negative bacteria. *Br Med J* **1**:493, 1976

27. Cason JS et al: Antiseptic and aseptic prophylaxis for burns: Use of silver nitrate and isolators. *Br Med J* **2**:1288, 1966

28. Grover AW: Diffuse hair loss associated with selenium sulphide shampoo. *JAMA* **160**:1397, 1956

29. De Villez RL: Topical minoxidil therapy in hereditary androgenic alopecia. *Arch Dermatol* **121**:197, 1985

30. Fenton DA, Wilkinson JD: Topical minoxidil in the treatment of alopecia areata. *Br Med J* **287**:1015, 1983

31. Olsin EA: Topical minoxidil in the treatment of androgenic alopecia in women. *Cutis* **48**:243, 1991

32. Gilhar A et al: Topical cyclosporine in male pattern alopecia. *J Am Acad Dermatol* **22**:251, 1990

33. Tosti A et al: Alopecia totalis: Is treating nonresponder patients useful? *J Am Acad Dermatol* **24**:455, 1991

34. Frank HG: Coal tar constituents. *Indust Eng Chem* **55**:38, 1963

35. Wrench R, Britten AZ: Evaluation of coal tar fractions for use in psoriasiform diseases using the mouse tail test. *Br J Dermatol* **92**:569, 1975

36. Lowe NL et al: New coal tar extract and coal tar shampoos: Evaluation by epidermal cell DNA synthesis suppression assay. *Arch Dermatol* **118**:487, 1982

37. Berenblum I: Liquor picis carbonis—carcinogenic agent. *Br Med J* **2**:601, 1948

38. Rook AJ et al: Squamous epithelioma possibly induced by therapeutic application of tar. *Br J Cancer* **10**:12, 1956

39. Kaidby KH, Kligman AM: Clinical and histological study of coal tar photosensitivity in humans. *Arch Dermatol* **112**:592, 1977

40. Parfenac. *Drug Ther Bull* **12**:102, 1974

41. Peterson AF et al: Comparative evaluation of surgical scrub preparations. *Surg Gynecol Obstet* **146**:63, 1978

42. Hendley JO et al: Evaluation of virucidal compounds for inactivation of rhinovirus on hands. *Antimicrob Agents Chemother* **14**:690, 1978

43. White JW: Treatment of primary hyperhidrosis. *Mayo Clin Proc* **61**:951, 1986

44. Shelley WB, Hurley HJ: Aluminum chloride in the treatment of hyperhidrosis. *Arch Dermatol* **111**:1004, 1975

45. Holzle E, Kligman AM: The pathogenesis of miliaria rubra. Role of the resident microflora. *Br J Dermatol* **30**:279, 1979

46. Gordon HH: Hyperhidrosis: Treatment with gluteraldehyde. *Cutis* **9**:375, 1972

47. Cullen SI: Topical methenamine for hyperhidrosis. *Arch Dermatol* **111**:1158, 1975

48. Pascher F: Systemic reactions to topically applied drugs. *Int J Dermatol* **17**:768, 1978

49. Lowe NJ et al: Anthralin for psoriasis: Short-contact anthralin therapy compared with topical steroid and conventional anthralin. *J Am Acad Dermatol* **10**:69, 1984

50. Rassner G: Enzymaktivitätshemmung in vitro durch Dithrinol. *Arch Dermatol Forsch* **243**:47, 1972

51. Diezel W et al: Experiments concerning the mode of action of dithranol, increased lipid peroxidation and enzyme inhibition. *Dermatologica* **150**:154, 1975

52. Cox AJ, Watson W: Histological variations in lesions of psoriasis. *Arch Dermatol* **106**:503, 1972

53. Fisher LB, Maibach HI: The effect of anthralin and its derivatives on epidermal cell kinetics. *J Invest Dermatol* **64**:338, 1975

54. Liden S, Michaelson G: Dithranol in psoriasis. *Br J Dermatol* **91**:447, 1974

55. Raab WP: Dithranol (anthralin) versus triacetoxyanthracene. *Br J Dermatol* **95**:193, 1976

56. Ljunggren B, Moller H: Topical use of fluorouracil in the treatment of psoriasis. *Arch Dermatol* **106**:263, 1972

57. Tsuji T, Sugai T: Topically administered fluorouracil in psoriasis. *Arch Dermatol* **105**:208, 1972

58. Fredriksson T: Topically applied fluorouracil in the treatment of psoriatic nails. *Arch Dermatol* **110**:735, 1974

59. Kragballe K: Treatment of psoriasis by the topical application of the novel cholecalciferol analog calcipotriol (MC 903). *Arch Dermatol* **125**:1647, 1989

60. Kragballe K: Calcipotriol for psoriasis (letter; comment). *Lancet* **337**:1229, 1991

61. Dwyer C, Chapman RS: Calcipotriol and hypercalcaemia (letter). *Lancet* **338**:764, 1991

62. Kragballe K et al: Double blind, right/left comparison of calcipotriol and betamethasone valerate in the treatment of psoriasis vulgaris. *Lancet* **337**:193, 1991

63. Long CC, Marks R: Calcipotriol and betamethasone valerate for psoriasis (letter; comment). *Lancet* **337**:921, 1991

64. Kragballe K: Combination of topical calcipotriol (MC903) and UVB radiation for psoriasis vulgaris. *Dermatologica* **181**:211, 1990

65. Martindale W: *The Extra Pharmacopoeia.* London, Pharmaceutical Press, 1982, p 216

66. Arndt KA: *Manual of Dermatologic Therapeutics,* 4th ed. Boston, Little, Brown, 1989, p 270

67. Cason JS, Lowbury EJL: Mortality and infection in extensively burned patients treated with silver nitrate compresses. *Lancet* **1**:651, 1968

68. Rasmussen JE: The problem of lindane. *J Am Acad Dermatol* **5**:507, 1981

69. Shacter B: Treatment of scabies and pediculosis with lindane preparations: An evaluation. *J Am Acad Dermatol* **5**:517, 1981

70. Rauch AE et al: Lindane (Kwell)-induced aplastic anemia. *Arch Intern Med* **150**:2393, 1990

71. Carson D et al: Pyrethrins combined with piperonyl butoxide (Rid) vs 1% permethrin (Nix) in the treatment of head lice. *Am J Dis Child* **142**:768, 1988

72. Schultz MW et al: Comparative study of 5% permethrin cream and 1% lindane lotion for the treatment of scabies. *Arch Dermatol* **126**:167, 1990

73. Taplin D et al: Permethrin 5% dermal cream: A new treatment for scabies. *J Am Acad Dermatol* **15**:995, 1986

74. Van Scott EJ, Yu RJ: Control of keratinization with alpha-hydroxy acids and related compounds. I. Topical treatment of ichthyotic disorders. *Arch Dermatol* **110**:586, 1974

75. Swanbeck G: A new treatment of ichthyosis and other hyperkeratotic conditions. *Acta Derm Venereol (Stockh)* **48**:123, 1968

76. Van Scott EJ, Yu RY: Alpha hydroxyacids: Therapeutic potentials. *Can J Dermatol* **1**:108, 1989

77. Fine DJ, Arndt KA: *Propylene Glycol: A Review.* Princeton, Excerpta Medica, 1980

78. Goldsmith LA, Baden HP: Propylene glycol with occlusion for treatment of ichthyosis. *JAMA* **220**:579, 1972

79. Davies MG et al: Systemic toxicity from topically applied salicylic acid. *Br Med J* **1**:661, 1979

80. Baden HP: A keratolytic gel containing salicylic acid in propylene glycol. *J Invest Dermatol* **61**:330, 1974

81. Davies M, Marks R: Studies on the effect of salicylic acid on normal skin. *Br J Dermatol* **95**:187, 1976

82. Roberts DL et al: Detection of the action of salicylic acid on the normal stratum corneum. *Br J Dermatol* **103**:191, 1980

83. Huber C, Christophers E: Keratolytic effects of salicylic acid. *Arch Dermatol Res* **257**:293, 1977

84. Weirich EG et al: Dermatopharmacology of salicylic acid. *Dermatologica* **152**:87, 1976

85. Pegum J: Urea in the treatment of black hairy tongue. *Br J Dermatol* **84**:602, 1971

86. Hursthouse MW: A controlled trial on the use of topical 5-fluorouracil on viral warts. *Br J Dermatol* **92**:93, 1975

87. Goncalves JC: 5-Fluorouracil in the treatment of common warts of the hands. A double-blind study. *Br J Dermatol* **92**:89, 1975

88. Kirby P et al: Double-blind randomized clinical trial of self-administered podofilox solution versus vehicle in the treatment of genital warts. *Am J Med* **88**:465, 1990

89. Beutner KR et al: Patient-applied podofilox for treatment of genital warts. *Lancet* **1**:831, 1989

SECTION 39

Systemic Therapy

CHAPTER 232

Victoria P. Werth and Gerald S. Lazarus

Glucocorticoids are a mainstay of dermatologic therapy because of their potent immunosuppressive and anti-inflammatory properties. In 1949, Hench and coworkers[1] described the beneficial effects of cortisone in patients with rheumatoid arthritis. Since that time, glucocorticoids have been found to be useful in the treatment of numerous skin conditions. By understanding the mechanisms and properties of glucocorticoids, one can maximize their efficacy and safety as therapeutic agents.

Biology

The major naturally occurring glucocorticoid is cortisol (hydrocortisone). It is synthesized from cholesterol by the adrenal cortex. Normally, less than 5 percent of circulating cortisol is free; this portion comprises the active therapeutic molecule. The remainder is inactive because it is bound to cortisol-binding globulin (CBG, also called transcortin) (95 percent) or to albumin (5 percent). The daily secretion of cortisol ranges between 15 and 30 mg, with a diurnal peak around 8 A.M. Cortisol has a plasma half-life of 90 min. It is metabolized primarily by the liver, although it exerts hormonal effects on virtually every tissue in the body. The metabolites are excreted by the kidney and the liver.

The mechanism of glucocorticoid action involves passive diffusion of the glucocorticoids through the cell membrane, followed by binding to soluble receptor proteins in the cytoplasm.[2] This hormone-receptor complex then moves to the nucleus and regulates the transcription of a limited number of target genes.[3] Glucocorticoids decrease the synthesis of a number of proinflammatory molecules including cytokines, interleukins, and proteases.[4] In addition, glucocorticoids increase the synthesis of certain other molecules, such as lipocortin, a member of the calpactin family of molecules. The mechanism of action of lipocortin is still in dispute, but the biologic consequence is a reduction in phospholipase A_2 activity.[5] A major action of lipocortin is to reduce the release of arachidonic acid from membrane phospholipids, possibly by direct inhibition of phospholipase A_2 or by sequestration of substrate. Thus, there is less precursor available for the formation of prostaglandins and leukotrienes.[6,7] Decreasing these mediators reduces inflammation. There is usually a delay in the onset of pharmacologic activity of glucocorticoids relative to their peak blood concentrations, which is probably consequent to changes in the transcription of critical proteins.

Glucocorticoids have profound effects on the replication and movement of cells. They induce monocytopenia, eosinopenia, and lymphocytopenia and have a greater effect on T cells than B cells.[8] The lymphocytopenia appears to be due to a redistribution of cells as they migrate from the circulation to other lymphoid tissues. The increase in circulating polymorphonuclear leukocytes is related to demargination of cells from the bone marrow and a diminished rate of removal from the circulation.

Glucocorticoids affect cell activation, proliferation, and differentiation. They modulate the levels of mediators of inflammation and immune reactions. Interleukin 1 (IL-1), interleukin 2 (IL-2), and tumor necrosis factor synthesis (or release), among others, are inhibited by glucocorticoids.[9-11] Macrophage functions, including phagocytosis, antigen processing, and cell killing, are decreased by cortisol,[12,13] and this decrease affects immediate and delayed hypersensitivity.

Glucocorticoids suppress monocyte function more than polymorphonuclear leukocyte function.[14] This effect is clinically important because granulomatous infectious diseases, such as tuberculosis, are prone to exacerbation and relapse during prolonged glucocorticoid therapy. The antibody-forming cells, B lymphocytes and plasma cells, are relatively resistant to the suppressive effects of glucocorticoids. Very high doses of glucocorticoids are needed to suppress antibody production.[15]

The multiplicity of biologic effects produced by glucocorticoids emphasizes that currently there is no unifying hypothesis to explain the therapeutic efficacy of these extremely potent anti-inflammatory and immunosuppressive agents.

Pharmacology

Hydrocortisone is most often used as an anti-inflammatory drug. When it is given in moderate to high doses, its mineralocorticoid effects can be deleterious, and thus synthetic analogues of cortisol have been developed that have more anti-inflammatory properties and cause less sodium retention. Small substitutions on the basic steroid structure of three hexanes and a pentane ring (Fig. 232-1, Table 232-1) account for the differences in plasma half-life and relative anti-inflammatory and sodium-retaining potencies (Table 232-2). In general, most synthetic analogues bind less efficiently to CBG (about 70 percent binding). This property may explain, in part, their tendency to cause side effects at low dosage. The 11-betahydroxyl group in cortisol is essential for activity. Because cortisone and prednisone are 11-keto compounds, they are active only after being converted in the liver to the corresponding 11-betahydroxyl compounds (cortisol and prednisolone) (Table

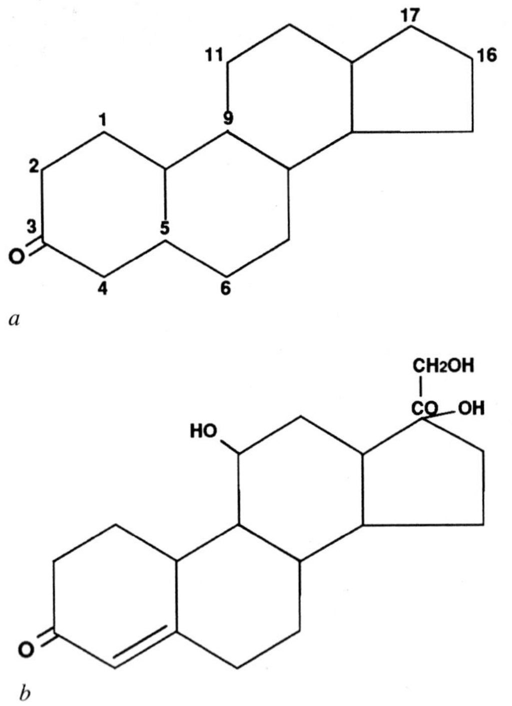

FIGURE 232-1 (*a*) Basic steroid skeleton. (*b*) The structure of hydrocortisone (cortisol).

232-1). Patients with severe liver disease generally maintain their ability to convert the 11-keto compounds; nevertheless, some authorities suggest that only the converted active compounds should be administered to these patients.[16]

Diseases Treated with Glucocorticoids

Diseases commonly treated with oral glucocorticoids include pemphigus, bullous pemphigoid, herpes gestationis, dermatomyositis, systemic lupus erythematosus (SLE), eosinophilic fasciitis, relapsing polychondritis, sarcoid, vasculitis, Sweet's syndrome, pyoderma gangrenosum, type I reactive leprosy, and capillary hemangiomas. Short courses of glucocorticoids, under appropriate conditions, are used for acute contact dermatitis and, occasionally, atopic dermatitis. Acne and hirsutism consequent to endocrinologic abnormalities can be treated with low doses of glucocorticoids at bedtime if these conditions are unresponsive to more conservative therapy. The use of glucocorticoids is controversial in the treatment of toxic epidermal necrolysis, erythema multiforme, erythema nodosum, exfoliative dermatitis, lichen planus, cutaneous T-cell lymphoma, and discoid lupus erythematosus.

Complications of Systemic Glucocorticoid Therapy

Numerous complications are associated with systemic glucocorticoid therapy (Table 232-3).[17] Complications increase with higher doses, longer duration of therapy, and more frequent dosing. However, osteoporosis and cataracts develop with alternate-day dosing, and avascular necrosis can be seen after only short courses of glucocorticoids.

Osteoporosis

Osteoporosis is seen in 40 percent of people treated with systemic glucocorticoids; it is especially prominent in children, adolescents, and postmenopausal women.[18] Corticosteroids inhibit osteoblasts,

TABLE 232-1
Comparative Structures of Glucocorticoids

	Position				
	1–2	6	9	11	16
Cortisol	—	—	—	—OH	—
Cortisone	—	—	—	=O	—
Prednisone	Double bond	—	—	=O	—
Prednisolone	Double bond	—	—	—OH	—
Methylprednisolone	Double bond	α-CH3	—	—OH	—
Triamcinolone	Double bond	—	α-F	—OH	α-OH
Dexamethasone	Double bond	—	α-F	—OH	α-CH3

TABLE 232-2
Glucocorticoids

	Equivalent glucocorticoid potency, mg	Mineralocorticoid potency	Plasma half-life, minutes
Short-acting			
Hydrocortisone (Cortisol)	20	0.8	90
Cortisone	25	1	30
Intermediate-acting			
Prednisone	5	0.25	60
Prednisolone	5	0.25	200
Methylprednisolone	4	0	180
Triamcinolone	4	0	300
Long-acting			
Dexamethasone	0.75	0	200

TABLE 232-3
Complications of Glucocorticosteroid Therapy

Central nervous system	Endocrinologic
Pseudotumor cerebri	Suppression of HPA axis
Psychiatric disorders	Growth failure
Musculoskeletal	Secondary amenorrhea
Osteoporosis with spontaneous	Metabolic
fractures	Hyperglycemia and unmasking
Aseptic necrosis of bone	genetic predisposition to
Myopathy	diabetes mellitus
Ocular	Nonketotic hyperosmolar states
Glaucoma	Hyperlipidemia
Cataracts	Alterations of fat distribution
Gastrointestinal	(typical cushingoid appearance)
Peptic ulceration	Fatty infiltration of the liver
Intestinal perforation	Drug interactions (decreased
Pancreatitis	anticoagulant effect of ethyl
Cardiovascular and fluid retention	biscoumacetate)
Hypertension	Fibroblast inhibition
Sodium and fluid retention	Inhibition of wound healing
Hypokalemic alkalosis	Subcutaneous tissue atrophy
Atherosclerosis	(striae, purpura, ecchymosis)
Hypersensitivity reactions	Suppression of host defenses
Urticaria	Immunosuppression, anergy
Anaphylaxis	Effects on phagocyte kinetics
	and function
	Increased incidence of infections

Note: HPA = hypothalamic-pituitary axis.

increase calcium excretion by the kidney, decrease intestinal calcium absorption, and concomitantly increase bone resorption by osteoclasts.[19] Serum osteocalcin, a measure of osteoblast function, decreases within a day after beginning a dosage regimen of as little as 10 mg of prednisone a day.[20] Trabecular bone is primarily affected, leading to painful vertebral fractures. A new agent, deflazacort, may have bone-sparing properties.[21]

Avascular Necrosis

Avascular necrosis is manifested by pain and limitation of motion in one or more joints. There is intraosseous hypertension, leading to bone ischemia and necrosis.[22] It is likely that intraosseous lipocyte hypertrophy causes this intraosseous hypertension in persons on glucocorticoids. Underlying diseases, such as SLE, increase the likelihood of steroid-induced avascular necrosis.[23]

Atherosclerosis

Increased risk of atherosclerosis is a concern. A number of factors that increase the risk of atherosclerosis, such as hypertension, hyperglycemia, and hyperlipidemia, are known side effects of glucocorticoids. The bimodal distribution of deaths in patients with SLE treated with glucocorticoids is documented; the early deaths are caused by active SLE whereas the late deaths are caused by myocardial infarction.[24] A similar pattern with atherosclerosis has been noted in transplant patients receiving glucocorticoids.[25]

Hypothalamic-Pituitary Axis (HPA) Suppression

The hypothalamic-pituitary axis is suppressed rapidly after the onset of glucocorticoid therapy. However, if therapy is limited to 1 to 3 weeks, the recovery of the HPA axis is rapid. Longer daily

glucocorticoid therapy is associated with suppression of the HPA axis for up to 1 year after therapy is terminated.[26] Symptoms of adrenal suppression include lethargy, weakness, nausea, anorexia, fever, orthostatic hypotension, hypoglycemia, and weight loss.

There also exists a steroid withdrawal syndrome, in which patients experience symptoms of adrenal insufficiency despite having a normal cortisol response. Symptoms most commonly include anorexia, lethargy, malaise, nausea, weight loss, desquamation of the skin, headache, and fever. Less commonly, vomiting, myalgias, and arthralgias occur. These patients have adjusted to high levels of glucocorticoids, and symptoms disappear after the glucocorticoids are restarted. This problem can be treated by slower tapering of the glucocorticoids.[27]

Drug Interactions

Glucocorticoids have a number of important drug interactions. Drugs, such as barbiturates, phenytoin, and rifampin, that induce hepatic microsomal enzymes, may accelerate the metabolism of glucocorticoids.[28] Glucocorticoids reduce the serum salicylate level and necessitate a higher dose of Coumadin for anticoagulation.

Immunologic Side Effects

Glucocorticoids impair delayed-type hypersensitivity reactions because of their inhibition of lymphocytes and monocytes. Prednisone at daily doses of 15 mg or more suppresses the response to tuberculin. It takes an average of 13.6 days for oral prednisone at 40 mg/day to inhibit the response to tuberculin.[29] Thus, even in situations requiring immediate use of prednisone, it is possible to perform simultaneously a PPD and an anergy panel. Overall, there is an increased incidence of infections attributable to both the glucocorticoids and the immunologic changes related to the underlying disease.

Concerns during Pregnancy and Lactation

Glucocorticoids cross the placenta, but they are not teratogenic. Exposed infants, as well as breast-fed infants of mothers receiving glucocorticoids, should be monitored for adrenal suppression and growth suppression.

Therapeutic Use of Glucocorticoids

Fundamental Issues

Before therapy with glucocorticoids is begun, the benefit that realistically can be expected should be weighed against the potential side effects. In dermatology, this often means assessing whether the disease is serious enough to risk exposing the patient to a toxic drug. Alternative therapies should be considered, especially if long-term treatment is contemplated. The predisposition of the patient to side effects should be included in an assessment of risk.

Rationale for Choosing among Corticosteroids

A number of considerations bear on the choice of glucocorticoids. First, a preparation with minimal mineralocorticoid effect is usually picked to decrease sodium retention. Second, the long-term oral use of prednisone or a similar drug, with an intermediate half-life and relatively weak steroid receptor affinity, may have the desired clinical effect without the greater risk of side effects observed with a drug that has a longer half-life and higher steroid receptor affinity, such as dexamethasone. Third, if a patient does not respond to cortisone or prednisone, the substitution of the biologically active form, cortisol or prednisolone, should be considered. In general, even in severe liver disease, substitution has not been proved to be very important. Fourth, methylprednisolone is used for pulse therapy because of its low sodium-retaining characteristics and high potency.

Route of Administration and Dosage Schedules

Systemic glucocorticoids can be administered orally, intralesionally, intramuscularly, and intravenously. The route and regimen are determined by the nature and extent of the disease being treated.

Oral glucocorticoids, specifically prednisone, are most commonly used. They are usually administered daily or every other day, although for acute disease multiple daily doses can be used. The initial dose must often be daily to control the disease process and can range from 2.5 mg to several hundred milligrams daily. As rapidly as possible, the dose should be tapered, as discussed under the section on adrenal suppression. If used for less than 3 to 4 weeks, glucocorticoid therapy can be stopped without tapering. The lowest possible dose of a short-acting agent every other morning minimizes side effects. Since cortisol levels peak at around 8 A.M., the HPA axis is least suppressed with this type of morning dosage. Since the drug is administered at the time of the highest level of endogenous cortisol, maximal feedback suppression of adrenocorticotropic hormone (ACTH) secretion by the pituitary is already occurring. The low levels of glucocorticoids at night allow for normal secretion of ACTH. Low doses of prednisone (2.5 to 5 mg) at bedtime have been used to maximize adrenal suppression in cases of acne or hirsutism of adrenal origin.

Intralesional glucocorticoid administration allows direct access to either a relatively few number of lesions or a particularly resistant lesion. The concentration depends on the site of injection and the nature of the lesion. Lower concentrations (2 to 3 mg/mL) are used on the face to prevent atrophy of the skin, whereas keloids may require concentrations of 40 mg/mL. In conditions requiring sustained effects, such as keloids and alopecia areata, longer-acting glucocorticoids, such as Aristospan, can be administered alone or mixed with the more typically used Kenalog. It is best to limit the total monthly dose of Kenalog to 20 mg to assure that the HPA axis will not be suppressed.

Glucocorticoids are sometimes administered intramuscularly by dermatologists. The drawbacks are erratic absorption and lack of daily control of the dose. Since Kenalog is longer acting than prednisone, there are more potential side effects, including increased HPA suppression, with serial monthly injections. We rarely, if ever, use this route of administration.

Intravenous glucocorticoids are used in two situations. One is for stress coverage for patients who are acutely ill or are undergoing surgery and who have adrenal suppression from daily glucocorticoid therapy. The other is for patients with certain diseases, such as resistant pyoderma gangrenosum, or serious SLE or dermatomyositis, to gain rapid control of the disease and thus minimize the need for long-term high-dose oral steroid therapy. Methylprednisolone is used at a dose of 500 mg to 1 g daily because of its high potency

and low sodium-retaining activity. Serious side effects associated with intravenous administration include anaphylactic reactions, seizures, arrhythmias, and sudden death. Other adverse reactions include hypotension, hypertension, hyperglycemia, electrolyte shifts, and acute psychosis. Slower administration over 2 to 3 h has minimized many of the serious side effects.

Strategies to Reduce Glucocorticoid Side Effects

Evaluation before Treatment

To minimize potential problems, the baseline evaluation should include a personal and family history, with special attention to predisposition to diabetes, hypertension, hyperlipidemia, and glaucoma. All patients should be carefully questioned for associated diseases that could be affected by steroid therapy. As an example, patients with peptic ulcer diseases could be adversely affected by steroids. Baseline blood pressure and weight should be measured. If prolonged administration is anticipated, an eye examination should be performed and a PPD and an anergy panel applied. Examination for other covert infections should be based on history and physical examination. For instance, a stool culture for *Strongyloides* should be performed for immigrants from third world countries and for Vietnam veterans. If long-term administration of glucocorticoids is anticipated, serious thought should be given to ordering a baseline spinal bone density measurement, either by quantitative CT, dual photon absorptiometry, or dual energy x-ray absorptiometry (DEXA).

Evaluation during Treatment

At follow-up visits, patients receiving chronic glucocorticoid therapy should be questioned about polyuria, polydipsia, abdominal pain, and fevers. Weight and blood pressure should be monitored. Serum electrolytes, fasting blood sugar, and cholesterol and triglyceride levels should be measured on a regular basis. Stool Hemoccults should be performed. Follow-up eye examinations should be performed with careful monitoring for the development of cataracts and glaucoma.

Preventive Measures

General   A careful initial evaluation and follow-up, as discussed in the first two sections, are mandatory. Exercise should be encouraged.

Diet   Diet should be low in calories, fat, and sodium, and high in protein, potassium, and calcium. Protein intake is important to reduce steroid-induced nitrogen wasting.[30] Alcohol, coffee, and nicotine use should be minimized.

Infections   Patients with a positive PPD should be given prophylaxis with isoniazid.[31] Anergic patients should have a baseline chest x-ray to search for evidence of previous tuberculosis. Fevers or focal findings should be evaluated with appropriate cultures and diagnostic approaches.

Gastrointestinal Complications   There is ongoing debate over whether the incidence of peptic ulcer disease is increased in otherwise normal patients receiving glucocorticoids.[32] Clearly, patients with a history of peptic ulcer disease or with a new onset of abdominal pain attributable to ulcers during glucocorticoid therapy should be carefully evaluated and treated with an anti-ulcer regimen, which can include antacids, H$_2$ receptor blockers such as ranitidine or cimetidine, or sucralfate.

Adrenal Suppression   Patients receiving daily glucocorticoid therapy for longer than 3 to 4 weeks must be assumed to have adrenal suppression that requires tapering of the glucocorticoids to allow for recovery of the HPA axis. Tapering is best performed by switching from a single daily dose to alternate-day doses, followed by a gradual reduction of the amount of the drug. The daily dose is first gradually tapered to 40 or 50 mg of prednisone. Then one of several approaches can be taken. The prednisone dose can be kept constant on one day and reduced on the alternate day by 5 mg decrements down to 5 mg a day. Alternatively, the steroid dose can be increased on one day and reduced by a similar amount on the alternate day.

After the prednisone dose is tapered to 5 mg on alternate days, the need for maintenance therapy must be assessed. The 8 A.M. plasma cortisol level is measured 4 weeks after the 5 mg dose has been reached. The morning dose of prednisone is held until the plasma cortisol level is determined. If the plasma cortisol level is greater than 10 μg/dL, the alternate day prednisone dose should be decreased by 1 mg every 1 to 2 weeks to a maintenance dose of 2 mg/day. Then the 8 A.M. plasma cortisol level should be rechecked every month until it is greater than 10 μg/dL, at which point maintenance glucocorticoids can be terminated.[33] At that point and at any point when the patient is receiving tapering doses of steroids, a stress caused, for example, by trauma, surgery, diarrhea, or fever over 38°C (101°F) can precipitate acute adrenal insufficiency related to an inadequate stress response. Patients should wear a bracelet or carry a card indicating they are receiving glucocorticoids. During such stressful situations, it is necessary to give high doses of glucocorticoids, generally 25 to 70 mg/day of prednisone or 100 to 300 mg/day of cortisol in divided doses.[34] Patients must be educated about the need for stress coverage.

In general, adrenal insufficiency resolves within 1 year of the termination of glucocorticoid therapy. An ACTH (cosyntropin) stimulation test may be performed after maintenance glucocorticoids are terminated to assess adrenal reserve. This test is performed in the office by determining a baseline cortisol level, giving an intramuscular injection of 0.25 mg of cosyntropin, and measuring the serum cortisol level again 1 h later.[33] The adrenal response is suppressed if the serum cortisol level fails to increase by at least 5 μg/dL to a stimulated value 60 min later of more than 20 μg/dL. If adequate adrenal response to stress is demonstrated, there is less concern about the endogenous cortisol response to stress. However, such a response is not a guarantee of adequate adrenal reserves if severe stress occurs, and many physicians would choose routine stress coverage with glucocorticoids without performing an ACTH stimulation test.

Osteoporosis   Attention to the prevention of osteoporosis is becoming increasingly important as newer therapies that may deter bone loss become available. Calcium and vitamin D can decrease, but not prevent, steroid-induced osteoporosis.[35] Postmenopausal women receiving estrogen supplements have markedly less osteoporosis and a 50 percent reduction in osteoporotic fractures than those not receiving supplements.[36,37] Thus, any patients receiving steroids during the first 10 to 15 years after menopause should also receive supplemental estrogen. Simultaneous cycling with Provera prevents the increased endometrial carcinoma seen in women receiving estrogen alone.[38] Glucocorticoids suppress serum testosterone in men.[39] Low serum testosterone is associated with low bone density in hypogonadal men. Bone density increases in these men when they receive supplemental testosterone.[40] Older men with low serum testosterone levels who are receiving glucocorticoids should have testosterone supplementation. Multicenter trials with newer agents such as calcitonin and bisphosphonates will likely revolutionize our approach to the prevention of osteoporosis in patients receiving chronic glucocorticoids.[41,42]

Current recommendations include baseline measurements of bone density and sequential study to identify early those who are rapidly losing bone density. These individuals can then be targeted for modification of treatment or for newer interventions with calcitonin or bisphosphonates.

Premenopausal women and men should be given elemental calcium, 500 mg, twice daily and vitamin D$_2$, 400 units, twice daily. Vitamin D at a higher dose of 50,000 units once or twice weekly has been used, but patients must be followed up very carefully in order not to precipitate hypervitaminosis D.[43] Patients with a history of renal stones should not receive supplemental calcium and vitamin D. Calcium levels should be measured in serum and in 24-h urine collections every 3 months or whenever steroid doses are substantially altered. If the urinary calcium level exceeds 250 to 350 mg/dL, the addition of 25 to 50 mg/day of thiazide will reduce the renal excretion of calcium.[44] If thiazide is not added, calcium and vitamin D supplementation should be adjusted. Older men with low serum testosterone levels may profit from testosterone supplementation.

Postmenopausal women should receive 1500 mg of elemental calcium daily in addition to the above-mentioned dose of vitamin D. Women within 10 to 15 years of menopause should also receive oral conjugated estrogen (Premarin), 0.625 mg/day. Women with a capacity to menstruate should also receive medroxyprogesterone, 10 mg daily, during the last 12 days of the month.[45] Women who are to receive hormonal therapy should not have a history of benign or malignant breast disease or other hormone-sensitive tumors, thrombophlebitis, smoking, gallstones, or a family history of breast cancer. Breast and pelvic examinations should be performed initially and at regular 6- to 12-month intervals during hormone therapy.

Calcitonin is often helpful in relieving the pain of compression fractures.[46]

Atherosclerosis   Blood pressure, serum lipids, and glucose levels should be measured serially. Abnormalities should be treated with dietary manipulation and medication as necessary. Patients who smoke should be encouraged to stop.

Avascular Necrosis   Early detection is important since early intervention may prevent progression to degenerative joint disease requiring joint replacement. Twenty percent of patients with avascular necrosis have normal x-rays. Bone scan and MRIs are more sensitive techniques for evaluating avascular necrosis. Patients should be regularly questioned about pain and limitation of motion of joints. If abnormalities develop, x-ray, bone scan, or MRI should be ordered. If imaging shows avascular necrosis, an orthopedic surgeon skilled in early intervention with core decompression may be able to halt progression of the disease. Patients with avascular necrosis have an increased risk that other joints will also be affected. The progression of avascular necrosis to destructive joint disease may require joint replacement surgery.[47]

References

1. Hench PS et al: The effect of a hormone of the adrenal cortex (17-hydroxy-11-dehydrocorticosterone (compound E)) and of pituitary adrenocorticotropic hormone on rheumatoid arthritis. *Mayo Clin Proc* **24**:181, 1949

2. Bloom E et al: Nuclear binding of glucocorticoid receptors: Relations between cytosol binding, activation in the biologic response. *J Steroid Biochem* **12**:175, 1980

3. Baxter JD et al: The adrenal cortex, in *Endocrinology and Metabolism,* edited by P Felig et al. New York, McGraw-Hill, 1988, p 511

4. Rugstad HE: Anti-inflammatory and immunoregulatory effects of glucocorticoids: Mode of action. *Scand J Rheumatol* **76** (suppl):257, 1988

5. Peers SH et al: The role of lipocortin in corticosteroid actions. *Am Rev Respir Dis* **141**:518, 1990

6. Pepinsky RB et al. Five distinct calcium and phospholipid binding proteins share homology with lipocortin 1. *J Biol Chem* **263**:10799, 1988

7. Wallner BP et al. Cloning and expression of human lipocortin 1, a phospholipase A_2 inhibitor with potential anti-inflammatory activity. *Nature* **320**:77, 1986

8. Cupps TR et al: Corticosteroid-mediated immunoregulation in man. *Immunol Rev* **65**:133, 1982

9. Stosic-Grujcic S et al: Modulation of interleukin 1 production by activated macrophages: In vitro action of hydrocortisone, colchicine and cytochalasin B. *Cell Immunol* **69**:2335, 1982

10. Smith KA: T-cell growth factor. *Immunol Rev* **51**:337, 1980

11. Beutler B et al: Cachectin and tumour necrosis factor as two sides of the same biological coin. *Nature* **320**:584, 1986

12. Balow JE et al: Glucocorticoid suppression of macrophage inhibitory factor. *J Exp Med* **137**:1031, 1973

13. Hogan MM: Inhibition of macrophage tumoricidal activity by glucocorticoids. *J Immunol* **140**:513, 1988

14. Parrillo JE, Fauci AS. Mechanisms of glucocorticoid action on immune processes. *Annu Rev Pharmacol Toxicol* **19**:179, 1979

15. Tuchinda M et al: Effect of prednisone treatment on the human immune response to keyhold limpet hemocyanin. *Int Arch Allergy* **42**:533, 1972

16. Frey FJ: Kinetics and dynamics of prednisolone. *Endocrinol Rev* **8**:453, 1987

17. Fauci AS: Glucocorticosteroid therapy, in *Cecil's Textbook of Medicine,* edited by JB Wyngaarden et al. Philadelphia, Saunders, 1988, p 133

18. Gluck OS et al: Bone loss in adults receiving alternate day glucocorticoid therapy. *Arthritis Rheum* **24**:892, 1981

19. Mitchell DR: Glucocorticoid-induced osteoporosis: Mechanisms for bone loss; evaluation of strategies for prevention. *J Gerontol* **45**:M153, 1990

20. Godschalk MF et al: Effect of short-term glucocorticoids on serum osteocalcin in healthy young men. *J Bone Mineral Res* **3**:113, 1988

21. Balsan S et al: Effects of long-term maintenance therapy with a new glucocorticoid, Deflazacort, on mineral metabolism and statural growth. *Calcif Tissue Int* **40**:303, 1987

22. Solomon L: Idiopathic necrosis of the femoral head: Pathogenesis and treatment. *Can J Surg* **24**:573, 1981

23. Zizic TM et al: Corticosteroid therapy associated with ischemic necrosis of bone in systemic lupus erythematosus. *Am J Med* **79**:596, 1985

24. Urowitz MB et al: The bimodal mortality pattern of systemic lupus erythematosus. *Am J Med* **60**:221, 1976

25. Becker DM et al: Relationship between corticosteroid exposure and plasma lipid levels in heart transplant recipients. *Am J Med* **85**:632, 1988

26. Graber AL et al: Natural history of pituitary-adrenal recovery following long-term suppression with corticosteroids. *J Clin Endocrinol Metab* **25**:11, 1965

27. Dixon RB et al: On the various forms of glucocorticoid withdrawal syndrome. *Am J Med* **68**:224, 1990

28. Gustavson LE, Benet LZ: Pharmacokinetics of natural and synthetic glucocorticoids, in *The Actual Cortex,* edited by DC Anderson, JSD Winters. Cornwall, England, Butterworth, 1985, p 235

29. Bovornkitti S et al: Reversion and reconversion rate of tuberculin skin reactions in correlation with the use of prednisone. *Dis Chest* **38**:51, 1960

30. Cogan MG et al: Prevention of prednisone-induced negative nitrogen balance: Effect of dietary modification on urea generation rate in hemodialyzed patients receiving high-dose glucocorticoids. *Ann Intern Med* **95**:158, 1981

31. American Thoracic Society. Treatment of tuberculosis and tuberculosis infection in adults and children. *Am Rev Respir Dis* **134**:355, 1986

32. Seale JP et al: Side-effects of glucocorticoid agents. *Med J Aust* **144**:139, 1986

33. Chamberlin P et al: Management of pituitary-adrenal suppression secondary to corticosteroid therapy. *Pediatrics* **67**:245, 1981

34. Baxter JD: Minimizing the side effects of glucocorticoid therapy. *Adv Intern Med* **35**:173, 1980

35. Hahn TJ et al: Altered mineral metabolism in glucocorticoid-induced osteopenia. *J Clin Invest* **64**:655, 1979

36. Christiansen C et al: Bone mass in postmenopausal women after withdrawal of oestrogen/gestagen replacement therapy. *Lancet* **1**:459, 1981

37. Kiel DP et al: Hip fracture and the use of estrogens in postmenopausal women. *N Engl J Med* **317**:1169, 1987

38. Gambrell RD: Prevention of endometrial cancer with progestogens. *Maturitas* **8**:159, 1986

39. MacAdams MR et al: Reduction of serum testosterone levels during chronic glucocorticoid therapy. *Ann Intern Med* **104**:648, 1986

40. Finkelstein JS et al: Osteoporosis in men with idiopathic hypogonadotropic hypogonadism. *Ann Intern Med* **106**:354, 1987

41. Ringe JD et al: Salmon calcitonin in the therapy of corticoid-induced osteoporosis. *Eur J Clin Pharmacol* **33**:35, 1987

42. Reid IR et al: Prevention of steroid-induced osteoporosis with (3-amino-1-hydroxypropylidene)-1,1-bisphosphonate (ADP). *Lancet* **1**:143, 1988

43. Schwartzman MS et al: Vitamin D toxicity complicating the treatment of senile, postmenopausal, and glucocorticoid-induced osteoporosis. *Am J Med* **82**:224, 1987

44. Suzuki Y et al: Importance of increased urinary calcium excretion in the development of secondary hyperparathyroidism of patients under glucocorticoid therapy. *Metabolism* **32**:151, 1983

45. Shoupe D et al: Therapeutic regimens, in *Menopause: Physiology and Pharmacology,* edited by DR Mishell. Chicago, London, Year Book 1987, p 335

46. Pun KK: Analgesic effect of intranasal salmon calcitonin in the treatment of osteoporotic vertebral fractures. *Clin Ther* **11**:205, 1989

47. Hungerford DS. Response: The role of core decompression in the treatment of ischemic necrosis of the femoral head. *Arthritis Rheum* **32**:801, 1989

Stephen I. Katz

Dapsone

In 1940, Costello[1] first described the dramatic success of sulfapyridine in treating a patient with dermatitis herpetiformis, a disease he believed to represent a form of bacterial allergy. Swartz and Lever[2] later reported the regular response of all their patients with dermatitis herpetiformis to sulfapyridine therapy. In the early 1950s, a group of drugs chemically related to sulfapyridine, the sulfones (dapsone and related compounds), were first used in treating patients with this disease.[3,4] Since dapsone is the most widely used drug among these compounds, there has been an enormous amount of research into its metabolism, mechanisms of action, and toxicity.

Pharmacology

The chemical structure of dapsone (4,4'-diaminodiphenylsulfone, DDS) is shown in Fig. 233-1. Derivatives of dapsone such as sulfoxone (no longer available in the United States) are thought to be metabolized to the parent dapsone structure. Sulfapyridine resembles dapsone in that it has an aminophenyl group attached to a sulfone (SO_2); however, on the other side of the sulfone, there is a pyridine group (Fig. 233-1). Although other sulfonamides have an aminophenyl group attached to a sulfone, they have different groups on the other side of the sulfone, and none is as effective as sulfapyridine in the treatment of inflammatory diseases. The pyridine group was thought to contribute to the beneficial effect of sulfapyridine, and other compounds such as pyribenzamine and nicotinamide were said to be useful in treating patients with dermatitis herpetiformis. Although the manufacturer of sulfapyridine has recently changed, the drug continues to be available.

After oral administration of dapsone, approximately 80 to 85 percent is absorbed, with peak levels being reached 2 to 6 h after a single dose. In patients taking 50 to 300 mg/day of dapsone, the peak levels of dapsone and its major metabolite reach 0.5 to 7 mg/L and 0.2 to 5 mg/L, respectively.[5] The half-life of dapsone in the

circulation is approximately 30 h.[6] Its retention in the body, however, is prolonged, perhaps because of its enterohepatic recirculation, since high concentrations have been detected in the bile. Dapsone and its metabolites may be transmitted through human milk[7,8] and are excreted by the kidneys.[6]

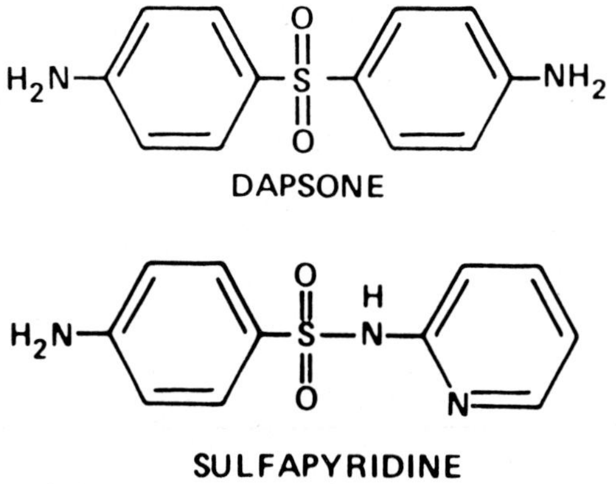

Dapsone is metabolized in the liver. The two major metabolic pathways involve acetylation and *N*-hydroxylation (Fig. 233-2). As with isoniazid and certain hydrazides and sulfonamides, dapsone and its derivatives are acetylated polymorphically, i.e., some patients rapidly acetylate dapsone to monoacetyldapsone (MADDS), the major metabolite, whereas in others this process occurs slowly. However, in humans, MADDS is rapidly deacetylated. Thus, an equilibrium is rapidly reached and sustained between MADDS and dapsone. The half-life in the body seems to be unrelated to the rate of acetylation. From a clinical standpoint, it seems that in dapsone's control of symptoms of dermatitis herpetiformis and even in its efficacy as an antileprosy drug, the dapsone dosage requirement is unrelated to acetylator phenotype.[5,9]

The other major metabolic pathway involves hydroxylation of one of the amino groups to form the aminohydroxylaminodiphenylsulfone. This compound is responsible for the methemoglobinemia, hemolysis, and Heinz-body formations, which occur regularly when dapsone is administered.[10,11] Thus, these pharmacologic side effects must be anticipated.

Drugs that interfere with the effect of dapsone include probenecid and rifampicin. Probenecid has been reported to block the renal excretion of dapsone; however, serum dapsone levels are not significantly affected.[12] When given concurrently with dapsone, rifampicin increases the rate of dapsone clearance, and this increase is most likely caused by the induction of microsomal enzymes.

Indications

Since its introduction into clinical medicine, dapsone has had therapeutic trials in a multitude of diseases. Most recently it has been introduced as adjunctive therapy (with trimethoprim) for *Pneumocystis carinii* pneumonia and has been proposed as a prophylactic agent for this infection.[13,14] A discussion of its use in leprosy, malaria chemoprophylaxis, and *Pneumocystis carinii* pneumonia is beyond the scope of this chapter. Long lists of inflammatory diseases that have responded to dapsone therapy have been generated.[15] Some of the individual reports are difficult to assess critically. Two diseases that invariably respond to dapsone therapy are dermatitis herpetiformis and erythema elevatum diutinum.[16] The dramatic dependence of patients on dapsone is best exemplified by the prompt exacerbations that follow withdrawal of the drug.

Other diseases for which dapsone therapy reportedly has been effective in some patients are rheumatoid arthritis, acne conglobata, actinomycetoma, pyoderma gangrenosum, bullous pemphigoid, scarring pemphigoid, relapsing polychondritis, the bullous eruption of systemic lupus erythematosus (SLE), granuloma faciale, subcorneal pustular dermatosis, and certain forms of leuko-

FIGURE 233-1 Chemical structure of dapsone and sulfapyridine.

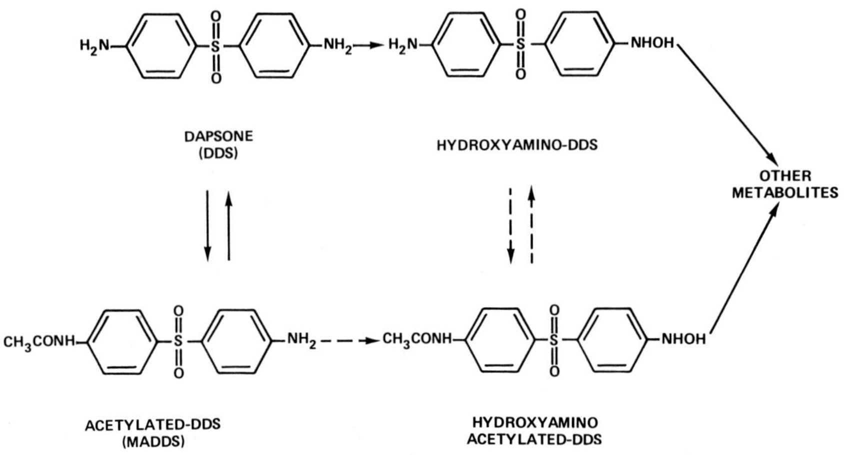

FIGURE 233-2 Dapsone metabolism in humans.

cytoclastic vasculitis. As a unifying feature, these diseases all have granulocytes (neutrophils or eosinophils) as the predominant infiltrating cell. In most diseases, the neutrophils appear early in the pathologic process. The response to dapsone therapy is not as rapid, regular, or predictable in any of these diseases as it is in dermatitis herpetiformis or erythema elevatum diutinum.

McConkey et al.[17] have provided controlled data that show dapsone therapy to be modestly effective in the treatment of some patients with rheumatoid arthritis. High dosages (up to 400 mg/day) are usually required in the treatment of otherwise unresponsive patients with cystic acne. With the advent of the new synthetic retinoids, however, a trial of dapsone therapy may no longer be necessary. A few patients with bullous pemphigoid have responded fairly dramatically to dapsone therapy.[18] Indeed, some have advocated its use as a regularly effective treatment for bullous pemphigoid.[19] Some patients with scarring pemphigoid reportedly have benefitted from dapsone therapy as well.[20]

Patients with SLE occasionally have subepidermal vesicular lesions that closely simulate dermatitis herpetiformis histologically.[21] These patients do not have an "admixture" of dermatitis herpetiformis and SLE, although the eruption is extraordinarily responsive to dapsone therapy.[22] A potentially exciting report, which was too brief and could not be evaluated, suggested the efficacy of dapsone therapy in discoid SLE.[23] Dramatic responses to dapsone have occurred in occasional patients with subacute cutaneous lupus erythematosus.[24,25] Granuloma annulare has also been reported to respond to dapsone treatment.[26,27] Some patients with subcorneal pustular dermatosis respond to and become dependent on dapsone, whereas others are unresponsive. This difference may reflect the heterogeneity of this disease, whose nosologic features have been a source of considerable debate.[28]

Although several reports suggest that dapsone therapy is remarkably effective in the treatment of relapsing polychondritis, my experiences with dapsone therapy in several patients with this condition have been uniformly unsuccessful. Occasionally, there are patients with chronic leukocytoclastic vasculitis in addition to those with erythema elevatum diutinum in whom dapsone therapy induces the prompt cessation of lesions. Since there is no uniformly successful therapy for these patients, many of whom do not seem to have associated internal problems, a short trial of dapsone therapy is warranted. In general, when a pathologic lesion is characterized by a neutrophilic infiltrate and is unassociated with an infectious agent, a trial of dapsone therapy should be considered. Even if a therapeutic trial is successful, the dose of dapsone should be de-creased to a point where lesions recur to be sure that the improvement was indeed due to dapsone and that there is a continuing need for the drug.

Adverse Effects

Dapsone therapy produces hemolysis and methemoglobinemia. The metabolite responsible for both these pharmacologic effects of sulfones has been identified as aminohydroxylaminodiphenylsulfone. Patients taking more than 50 mg/day of dapsone probably will have some degree of hemolysis that will be reflected in a lowered hemoglobin level. At 150 mg/day, dapsone may produce a decrease of as much as 2 g of hemoglobin.[29] Patients with glucose-6-dehydrogenase deficiency have a greater decrease in the hemoglobin level. Most patients tolerate a 2-g fall in the level of hemoglobin well, but the conditions of older patients or those with cardiopulmonary problems should be closely monitored or they should be given sulfapyridine. An increase in the reticulocyte count accompanies the fall in the hemoglobin level. Several months after treatment has begun, the hemoglobin level may rise almost to pretreatment levels but usually remains about 1 g below the original level.

Methemoglobinemia also regularly occurs in patients treated with sulfones but not as often as in patients treated with sulfapyridine. Methemoglobinemia is not a major problem in most patients. Even in patients taking 200 mg/day of dapsone, the level usually does not exceed 12 percent of the total hemoglobin level and is often less than 5 percent. The methemoglobin level is more pronounced at the onset of treatment and, as with hemolysis, is dose dependent. The cyanosis (which may seem more gray than blue) that results from methemoglobinemia may be seen in anyone with a methemoglobin level greater than 3 percent but may not be apparent in some patients with a level as high as 12 percent. Symptoms of methemoglobinemia include weakness, tachycardia, nausea, headache, and abdominal pains, but should not be attributed to methemoglobinemia until levels reach 20 percent or greater.

Other than these pharmacologic side effects, the adverse effects of dapsone may be idiosyncratic or allergic in nature[15,30,31] (Table 233-1). Peripheral neuropathies are one such example and usually occur at high dosage levels. Loss of motor function is the most common type of neuropathy, and it is reversible by decreasing the dose of dapsone. Sensory neuropathy is rare. Well-known side

TABLE 233-1
Adverse Reactions to Sulfones

Pharmacologic effects	Morbilliform eruptions
Hemolysis	Erythema nodosum
Methemoglobinemia	Erythema multiforme
Headache	Exfoliative dermatitis
Gastric irritation	Toxic epidermal necrolysis
Nausea	Severe hypoalbuminemia
Anorexia	Psychosis
Fatigue	Leukopenia
Hepatitis, infectious mono-	Agranulocytosis
nucleosis-like with adenopathy	Peripheral neuropathy
Cholestatic jaundice	(almost always motor)

SOURCE: Modified from Lang,[15] Alexander,[30] and Katz et al.[31]

effects include the induction of acute psychosis[32–34] and a potentially fatal mononucleosis-like syndrome that occurs during the induction of dapsone therapy in patients with leprosy.[35] Severe hypoalbuminemia with anasarca has also been reported.[36]

Agranulocytosis also may occur as a consequence of dapsone therapy. It has been estimated to occur in 0.2 to 0.4 percent of treated patients.[37] If agranulocytosis occurs, its onset is almost always during the first 3 months of therapy.[37,38] Although it is often reversible when patients stop therapy, it may be fatal. Patients should be warned to seek medical care immediately if they develop an infection during the first several months of therapy. Generally, when adverse reactions occur as a result of therapy with dapsone, dapsone derivatives and even sulfapyridine cause the same types of problems.

Information from two independent studies of carcinogenicity suggests that dapsone is a "weak carcinogen" in rats.[39,40] However, there is no similar evidence from studies in humans.

A frequently asked question is whether dapsone is safe to use during pregnancy. In one study of leprosy patients who were being treated with dapsone, 2 of 56 infants were born with congenital malformations.[41] However, there are no controlled studies in animals or people that address this point.

Monitoring of Dapsone Therapy

Before starting therapy with the sulfones or sulfapyridine, a complete blood cell (CBC) count should be done. In addition, Asians, blacks, or persons of Mediterranean descent should be tested for glucose-6-phosphate dehydrogenase deficiency, because sulfones can cause profound hemolysis in persons lacking this enzyme. After therapy is begun, a leukocyte count with a differential and hemoglobin levels should be obtained weekly for the first month and then twice a month during the next 2 months. Thereafter, CBC counts should be done periodically. Liver and renal function should also be tested before therapy starts and periodically thereafter. Once the disease being treated is under control, the dosage of dapsone should be reduced to be sure that the patient is using the minimum amount of drug required. Although in some diseases, such as dermatitis herpetiformis, the patients may alter the drug dosage according to the severity of the disease, they should be reminded not to increase the dosage by large amounts very abruptly. Because the blue-gray color of methemoglobinemia may be attributed to other causes by emergency room physicians, patients should be advised to carry a medication card in their wallets.

Mechanism of Action

The mechanisms of action of dapsone in leprosy and inflammatory diseases have been the subject of considerable study. Dapsone and its derivatives are potent oxidants with a notable influence on glutathione. Interference with the folate biosynthetic pathway of bacteria accounts for their bacteriostatic effect. Less well-known activities of dapsone involve its inhibition of choline incorporation into the lecithin of the cell membranes, thereby decreasing phospholipid synthesis.[42] Also, dapsone administered in the diet decreases visceral lesions and mortality in chickens infected with Marek's disease, in which a herpesvirus induces a lymphocytic malignant neoplasm in chickens.[43]

Numerous studies have attempted to determine how dapsone exerts its anti-inflammatory effects. Considerable evidence suggests that its anti-inflammatory effect is not related to its antibacterial effect. Dapsone inhibits lysosomal enzyme activity[44,45] and interferes with the myeloperoxidase-H_2O_2-halide-mediated cytotoxic system in polymorphonuclear leukocytes.[46,47] Although these findings may account for the effect of the drug on neutrophils or on their lysosomal enzymes at the site of injury, they probably do not account for the lack of influx of neutrophils into the dermis in treated patients. There is little evidence to support suggestions that dapsone interferes with complement activation and deposition.[48] Some in vivo studies have shown that dapsone at doses of 100 to 200 mg/kg inhibits adjuvant-induced arthritis and carrageenan-induced inflammation in rats.[49]

Several studies have suggested that dapsone and its derivatives do not affect the response of neutrophils to chemotactic stimuli. However, other studies have suggested that dapsone inhibits leukotriene B_4 binding to neutrophils,[50] and yet others have demonstrated that dapsone inhibits the neutrophil response to some chemotactic stimuli.[51,52] More extensive studies with chemotactic stimuli in varied concentrations are required to evaluate the possibility that dapsone may interfere with a specific chemotactic factor or with the response of neutrophils to such a factor.

References

1. Costello MJ: Dermatitis herpetiformis treated with sulfapyridine. *Arch Dermatol Syphilol* **41**:134, 1940.
2. Swartz JH, Lever WF: Dermatitis herpetiformis: Immunology and therapeutic considerations. *Arch Dermatol Syphilol* **47**:680, 1943
3. Cornbleet R: Sulfoxone (Diasone) sodium for dermatitis herpetiformis. *Arch Dermatol Syphilol* **64**:684, 1951
4. Kruizinga EE, Hamminga H: Treatment of dermatitis herpetiformis with diaminodiphenylsulphone (DDS). *Dermatologia* **106**:386, 1953
5. Ellard GA et al: Dapsone acetylation in dermatitis herpetiformis. *Br J Dermatol* **90**:441, 1974
6. Zuidema J et al: Clinical pharmacokinetics of dapsone. *Clin Pharmacokinetics* **11**:299, 1986
7. Sanders SW et al: Hemolytic anemia induced by dapsone transmitted through breast milk. *Ann Intern Med* **96**:465, 1982
8. Edstein S et al: Excretion of chloroquine, dapsone and pyrimethamine in human milk. *Br J Clin Pharmacol* **22**:733, 1986
9. Ellard GA et al: Dapsone acetylation and the treatment of leprosy. *Nature* **239**:159, 1972
10. Hjelm M, deVerdier CH: Biochemical effects of aromatic amines. I. Methemoglobinemia, haemolysis and Heinz-body formation induced by 4,4′-diaminodiphenylsulphone. *Biochem Pharmacol* **14**:1119, 1965

11. Grossman SJ, Jollow DJ: Role of dapsone hydroxylamine in dapsone-induced hemolytic anemia. *J Pharmacol Exp Ther* **244**:118, 1988

12. Goodwin CS, Sparell G: Inhibition of dapsone excretion by probenecid. *Lancet* **1**:884, 1969

13. Medina I et al: Oral therapy for *Pneumocystis carinii* pneumonia in the acquired immunodeficiency syndrome. *N Engl J Med* **323**:776, 1990

14. Kemper CA et al: Low-dose dapsone prophylaxis of *Pneumocystis carinii* pneumonia AIDS and AIDS-related complex. *AIDS* **4**:1145, 1990

15. Lang P: Sulfones and sulfonamides in dermatology today. *J Am Acad Dermatol* **1**:479, 1979

16. Katz SI et al: Erythema elevatum diutinum: Skin and systemic manifestations, immunologic studies, and successful treatment with dapsone. *Medicine (Baltimore)* **56**:443, 1977

17. McConkey B et al: Dapsone in rheumatoid arthritis. *J Rheumatol Rehab* **15**:230, 1976

18. Person JR, Rogers RS III: Bullous pemphigoid responding to sulfapyridine and the sulfones. *Arch Dermatol* **113**:610, 1977

19. Venning VA et al: Dapsone as first line treatment for bullous pemphigoid. *Br J Dermatol* **120**:83, 1989

20. Rogers RS et al: Treatment of cicatricial (benign mucous membrane) pemphigoid with dapsone. *J Am Acad Dermatol* **6**:215, 1982

21. Penneys NS, Wiley HE III: Herpetiformis blisters in systemic lupus erythematosus. *Arch Dermatol* **115**:1427, 1979

22. Hall RP et al: Bullous eruption of systemic lupus erythematosus: Dramatic response to dapsone therapy. *Ann Intern Med* **97**:165, 1982

23. Coburn PR, Shuster S: Dapsone and discoid lupus erythematosus. *Br J Dermatol* **106**:105, 1982

24. McCormack LS et al: Annular subacute cutaneous lupus erythematosus responsive to dapsone. *J Am Acad Dermatol* **11**:397, 1984

25. Fenton DA, Black MM: Low dose dapsone in the treatment of subacute cutaneous lupus erythematosus. *Clin Exp Dermatol* **11**:102, 1986

26. Czarnecki DB, Gin D: The response of generalized granuloma annulare to dapsone. *Acta Dermatovener* **66**:82, 1986

27. Steiner A et al: Sulfone treatment of granuloma annulare. *J Am Acad Dermatol* **13**:1004, 1985

28. Chimenti S, Ackerman AB: Is subcorneal pustular dermatitis of Sneddon and Wilkinson an entity sui generis? *Am J Dermatopathol* **3**:363, 1981

29. Cream JJ, Scott GL: Anaemia in dermatitis herpetiformis: The role of dapsone-induced haemolysis and malabsorption. *Br J Dermatol* **82**:333, 1970

30. Alexander JO: Dermatitis herpetiformis, in *Major Problems in Dermatology,* edited by A. Rook. Philadelphia, Saunders, 1975, p 291

31. Katz SI et al: Dermatitis herpetiformis: The skin and the gut. *Ann Intern Med* **93**:857, 1980

32. Sahu DM: Dapsone-induced psychosis: A case report. *Indian J Dermatol* **17**:47, 1972

33. Fine JD et al: Psychiatric reaction to dapsone and sulfapyridine. *J Am Acad Dermatol* **9**:274, 1983

34. Gawkrodger D. Manic depression induced by dapsone in patient with dermatitis herpetiformis. *Br Med J* **299**:860, 1989

35. Frey AM et al: Fatal reaction to dapsone during treatment of leprosy. *Ann Intern Med* **94**:777, 1981

36. Kingham JGC et al: Dapsone and severe hypoalbuminemia. *Lancet* **2**:662, 1979

37. Hörnsten P et al: The incidence of agranulocytosis during treatment of dermatitis herpetiformis with dapsone as reported in Sweden, 1972 through 1988. *Arch Dermatol* **126**:919, 1990

38. Liozon P et al: Agranulocytoses à la dapsone. *Am Med Interne (Paris)* **139**:469, 1988

39. *Bioassay of Dapsone for Possible Carcinogenicity.* US Department of Health, Education, and Welfare publication 77-820. National Cancer Institute Carcinogenesis Technical Reports Series, 1977

40. Griciute L, Tomatis L: Carcinogenicity of dapsone in mice and rats. *Int J Cancer* **25**:123, 1980

41. Maurus JM: Hansen's disease in pregnancy. *Obstet Gynecol* **52**:22, 1978

42. Shigeura HT et al: Metabolic studies on dapsone and sulfone derivatives in chick macrophages. *Biochem Pharmacol* **24**:687, 1975

43. Shen TY et al: Read before the American Chemical Society Abstracts Meeting. September 12–16, 1971

44. Barranco VP: Inhibition of lysosomal enzymes by dapsone. *Arch Dermatol* **110**:563, 1974

45. Mier PD, Van Den Hurk JJMA: Inhibition of lysosomal enzymes by dapsone. *Br J Dermatol* **93**:471, 1975

46. Stendahl O et al: The inhibition of polymorphonuclear leukocyte cytotoxicity by dapsone: A possible mechanism in the treatment of dermatitis herpetiformis. *J Clin Invest* **62**:214, 1978

47. Kazmierowski JA et al: Dermatitis herpetiformis: Effects of sulfones and sulfonamides on neutrophil myeloperoxidase-mediated iodinations and cytotoxicity. *J Clin Immunol* **4**:55, 1984

48. Katz SI et al: Effect of sulfones on complement deposition in dermatitis herpetiformis and on complement-mediated guinea pig reactions. *J Invest Dermatol* **67**:688, 1976

49. Williams K et al: Anti-inflammatory actions of dapsone and its related biochemistry. *J Pharm Pharmacol* **28**:555, 1976

50. Maloff BL et al: Dapsone inhibits LTB_4 binding and bioresponse at the cellular and physiologic levels. *Eur J Pharmacol* **158**:85, 1988

51. Anderson R et al: In vitro and in vivo effects of dapsone on neutrophil and lymphocyte functions in normal individuals and patients with lepromatous leprosy. *Antimicrob Agents Chemother* **19**:495, 1981

52. Harvath L et al: Selective inhibition of neutrophil chemotaxis to *N*-formyl-methionyl-leucyl-phenylalanine by sulfones. *J Immunol* **137**:1305, 1986

Gunnar Swanbeck

Aminoquinolines

The aminoquinolines are derived from quinine, a compound extracted from the bark of the cinchona tree native to South America. They have been used mainly as antimalarials. Even in dermatologic literature, these compounds are generally described under the heading of antimalarials. The antimalarials that are of dermatologic interest may all be regarded as aminoquinolines: chloroquine, hydroxychloroquine, amodiaquin, and quinacrine (Fig. 234-1). The last compound is of course more correctly classified as an acridine derivative. These four compounds are all 4-aminoquinolines. In the following discussion the word aminoquinolines designates the four compounds mentioned above.

Mode of Action

The aminoquinolines have several relatively well-defined effects on biochemical and cellular systems, the significance of which is not fully understood. Some of the more important are mentioned here.

Interactions with Nucleic Acids

Aminoquinolines bind to DNA. They also affect DNA and RNA polymerase activity and inhibit DNA replication and transcription to RNA.[1-3] This process may be directly related to DNA binding and may be involved with the antimalarial properties of these compounds and also with their inhibition of the lupus erythematosus-cell phenomenon and antinuclear antibody reactions.[4,5] This action is one possible explanation for the clinical effect of the aminoquinolines on lupus erythematosus.

Immunologic Effects

The aminoquinolines may suppress lymphocyte transformation in vitro.[6] They may also interfere with complement-dependent antigen–antibody reactions[7] and inhibit superoxide production in stimulated leukocytes.[8] No effect on the development of primary or secondary antibody response has been found.[9]

Anti-Inflammatory Activity

Chloroquine is a lysosomal stabilizer but it also inhibits hydrolytic enzymes.[10] It has also been demonstrated that chloroquine interferes with prostaglandin synthesis.[11] Another important property may be its influence on the chemotaxis of neutrophils, macrophages, and eosinophils.[12,13]

Photodermatologic Properties

There has been much work and speculation concerning the possible sun-screening effect of systemically administered chloroquine. Chloroquine absorbs in the UVA region of the spectrum and is bound in the epidermis in a relatively high concentration; however, there is no effect on the minimal erythematous dose.[14] The clinical action of chloroquine on lupus erythematosus and polymorphous light eruption may very well be explained by its effect on immunologic reactions.

Pharmacokinetics and Distribution

The aminoquinolines are all water-soluble and are readily absorbed in the gastrointestinal tract. The plasma concentration reaches a peak within about 8 h, but plasma is not cleared of the aminoquinoline within 24 h.[15] When daily doses are given, the plasma concentration increases to an equilibrium value after some weeks but remains relatively low, while the concentration in some organs may become many thousand times higher than in the plasma. The liver, spleen, lungs, and adrenal glands store chloroquine in large

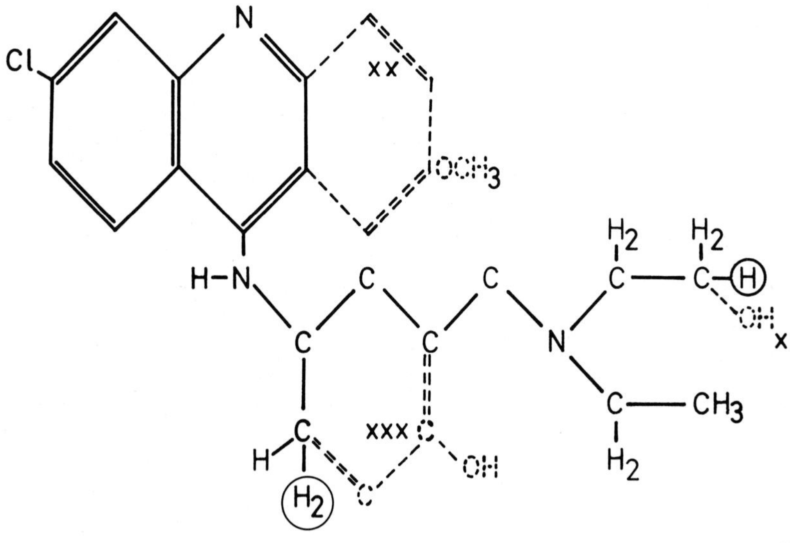

FIGURE 234-1   The aminoquinolines used in dermatology are all 4-aminoquinolines and may be regarded as derivatives of chloroquine, which is illustrated by the solid line. The other compounds are indicated by dotted lines: x = hydroxychloroquine; xx = quinacrine; xxx = amodiaquine. The two hydrogens within circles are substituted in the respective derivatives.

amounts.[16] Melanin-containing cells have a particular affinity for chloroquine,[17] and chloroquine binds to melanin in vitro.[18] The high uptake of chloroquine in the liver may be important in the use of this drug for porphyria cutanea tarda, and the melanin affinity may be the basis for the ocular side effects.

The equivalent doses of three of the aminoquinolines are 250 mg of chloroquine, 400 mg of hydroxychloroquine, and 100 mg of quinacrine.

Side Effects

Only side effects that are specific for the aminoquinolines are discussed here. The acute symptoms resulting from very large doses of chloroquine are weakness, dyspnea, hypotension, tremor, coma, convulsions, and cardiopulmonary arrest.[16] A lethal dose of chloroquine for an adult is 3 to 6 g.

All the aminoquinolines may induce leukopenia within the first few months of treatment. Aplastic anemia has been reported with the use of quinacrine, but it is a very rare side effect.

The aminoquinolines should be regarded as teratogenic. Chloroquine is capable of crossing the placenta, and congenital defects such as deafness, mental retardation, and convulsions have been described in newborn children of women who have taken chloroquine during pregnancy.[19]

Toxic psychosis, headache, and irritability have been reported as consequences of the use of both chloroquine and quinacrine.[20] However, these side effects are usually reversible and disappear when the medication is discontinued.

Among the cutaneous side effects of aminoquinolines, the exacerbation of psoriasis is well known and may lead to a generalized exfoliation. There are conflicting reports in the literature on the actual risk of using aminoquinolines in psoriasis. It is curious that antimalarials are widely used by rheumatologists for the treatment of psoriatic arthritis and they do not believe that these drugs cause flare-ups of preexisting psoriasis.

Discoloration of the skin may occur as a long-term cutaneous side effect.[16,21] A moderate dose of quinacrine rather regularly causes a yellow discoloration after a few months.

All the aminoquinolines may cause a bluish-black pigmentation of the pretibia, palate, face, and nail beds. These effects on the skin are reversible over time.

Ocular side effects are the greatest problem of the aminoquinolines, especially after long administration. Both chloroquine and hydroxychloroquine may cause deposits in the cornea that are reversible and may produce only slight symptoms in the form of halos around bright objects.[22]

Irreversible retinopathy is probably the factor that most limits use of the aminoquinolines. Most of the cases described involve chloroquine and hydroxychloroquine, although the other aminoquinolines are not safe in this respect. Hydroxychloroquine has been claimed to be safer than chloroquine with regard to induction of retinopathy.[23]

The retinopathy is certainly dose related. There are two common views about this problem. One is that the accumulated dose of chloroquine should not exceed 200 g. The other is that the daily dose of chloroquine "should not exceed 2 mg per pound of body weight" (4.4 mg/kg).[24,25] Some ophthalmologists claim that for an adult a daily dose of about 250 mg of chloroquine is safe if there is a yearly interruption of therapy for about 2 months. The patient should also be seen by an ophthalmologist at regular intervals. An interruption of the medication is, however, no guarantee against progression of the ocular problems. Systemic lupus erythematosus may itself produce ocular changes similar to those seen with aminoquinolines. However, ocular changes have also been observed in patients with rheumatoid arthritis who are taking chloroquine.[26]

Indications for Use

Malaria and rheumatoid arthritis are two of the chief indicators for aminoquinolines. They will not be discussed here because they are outside the field of dermatology. There are positive reports on the use of aminoquinolines for more than a dozen different skin diseases. Some of these findings have withstood the test of time; in other cases a single report on a rare disease has not been verified in spite of a long lapse of time since the original report was published.

Diseases for which the risk/benefit ratio seems to be favorable are lupus erythematosus, polymorphous light eruption, and porphyria cutanea tarda, and these diseases are dealt with in more detail below. Other diseases in which positive results with aminoquinolines have been reported are sarcoidosis, DNA-autosensitivity reaction, solar urticaria, scleroderma, lymphocytic infiltration of the skin, disseminated granuloma annulare, cutaneous cryptococcosis, cutaneous leishmaniasis, epidermolysis bullosa, acrodermatitis chronica atrophicans, and lichen sclerosus et atrophicus.[27]

Lupus Erythematosus (See also Chap. 171)

As early as the nineteenth century, lupus erythematosus was treated with quinine, the forerunner of the aminoquinolines. However, it was not until the 1950s that chloroquinine and its derivatives came into more general use for this disease. The first report was by Page in 1951,[28] but several more followed.

Generally the full effect of the aminoquinolines is obtained within a month. Cutaneous symptoms respond better than do systemic involvements.[29] The seriously ill patient with fever, renal damage, and hematologic abnormalities does not benefit from these compounds.

Today the aminoquinolines are mainly used in combination with corticosteroids in lupus erythematosus. The clinical effect of corticosteroids and aminoquinolines seems to be additive. However, their side effects are different and a more favorable risk/benefit ratio can be achieved by the combined use of the two types of drugs.

Although there are no convincing double-blind studies with aminoquinolines in patients with lupus erythematosus, the clinical evidence for their efficacy is overwhelming. Also the large number of studies that show a high recurrence rate after discontinuation of treatment strongly support the clinical evidence.[30,31]

Polymorphous Light Eruption (See also Chap. 135)

This disease is confined to the sun-exposed areas of the skin, and the histology of the lesions indicates that there are immunologic factors involved in the pathogenesis. Several reports indicate that chloroquine is effective in patients with this disease.[14,32] In those parts of the world where there is a season with little sun radiation, it is possible for the patient to discontinue aminoquinolines for some months and thereby decrease the risk of long-term side effects. In patients with polymorphous light eruption, aminoquinoline medication is often combined with topical sun-screening agents. PUVA therapy is definitely more effective against polymorphous light eruption than aminoquinolines. Therefore the aminoquinolines are mainly indicated when PUVA cannot be given.[33,34]

Porphyria Cutanea Tarda (See also Chap. 150)

Chloroquine is beneficial in the treatment of porphyria cutanea tarda. Its effect in this disease probably depends on mechanisms other than those in lupus erythematosus and polymorphous light eruption. It is tempting to believe that the high affinity of chloroquine for liver tissue is of primary importance.

When a daily dose of 250 mg of chloroquine is given to a patient with porphyria cutanea tarda, the following effects will be observed on the third to fourth day of medication: headache, nausea, fever, elevated transaminases, and massive excretion of uroporphyrins in the urine.[35] If the medication is stopped after a week of daily doses of 250 mg, the patient will continue to excrete porphyrins in the urine for 2 months. By the end of the third month, the patient usually has normal excretion of prophyrins, has no other symptoms of disease, and remains symptomless for 2 years or more.

The problem with this type of treatment is the acute reaction and the possible risk to the liver. Two regimens have been proposed to circumvent this problem. One is to give a small dose, 125 mg of chloroquine, twice a week over a long period.[36] The other is to perform phlebotomies three times before 250 mg chloroquine is given daily to the patient for 7 days.[37] Both methods seem to work satisfactorily.

Several theories have been proposed for the mode of action of chloroquine in porphyria cutanea tarda. It seems reasonable to assume, however, that uroporphyrins and chloroquine compete for the same binding sites in liver tissue and that chloroquine is able to displace porphyrins from the tissue. It has also been shown that chloroquine forms complexes with porphyrins.[38,39]

References

1. Kurnick NB, Radcliffe IE: Reaction between DNA and quinacrine and other anti-malarials. *J Lab Clin Med* **60**:669, 1962
2. Cohen SN, Yielding KL: Stabilization of the structure of native DNA by chloroquine and observations on the nature of the chloroquine–DNA complex. *Arthritis Rheum* **6**:767, 1963
3. Cohen SN, Yielding KL: Further studies on the mechanism of action of chloroquine: Inhibition of DNA and RNA polymerase reactions. *Arthritis Rheum* **7**:302, 1964
4. Dubois EL: Effect of quinacrine (Atabrine) upon lupus erythematosus phenomenon. *Arch Dermatol Syphilol* **71**:570, 1955
5. Bencze G, Johnson GD: Inhibition of antinuclear factor reaction by chloroquine. *Immunology* **9**:201, 1965
6. Harvitz D. Hirschorn K: Suppression of in vitro lymphocyte responses by chloroquine. *N Engl J Med* **273**:23, 1965
7. Neblett TR et al: Chloroquine: Its mechanism of action upon immune phenomena. *Arch Dermatol* **92**:720, 1965
8. Hurst NP et al: Studies on the mechanism of inhibition of chemotactic tripeptide stimulated human neutrophil polymorphonuclear leucocyte superoxide production by chloroquine and hydroxychloroquine. *Ann Rheum Dis* **46**:750, 1987
9. Kalmanson GM, Guze LB: Studies of the effects of hydroychloroquine on immune responses. *J Lab Clin Med* **65**:484, 1965
10. Weissman G: Labilization and stabilization of lysosomes. *Fed Proc* **23**:1038, 1964
11. Greaves MW, McDonald-Gibson WJ: Antiinflammatory agents and prostaglandin biosynthesis. *Br Med J* **3**:527, 1972
12. Ward PA: The chemosuppression of chemotaxis. *J Exp Med* **124**:209, 1966
13. Ganderer CA, Gleich CJ: Inhibition of eosinophilotaxis by chloroquine and corticosteroids. *Proc Soc Exp Biol Med* **157**:129, 1978
14. Cahn MM et al: Polymorphous light eruption—the effect of chloroquine phosphate in modifying reactions to ultraviolet light. *J Invest Dermatol* **26**:201, 1956
15. Rubin M, Zvaifler N: The metabolism of chloroquine. *Clin Res* **10**:22, 1962
16. Dubois EL: Anti-malarials in the management of discoid and systemic lupus erythematosus. *Semin Arthritis Rheum* **8**:33, 1978
17. Zvaifler NJ et al: Chloroquine deposition in ocular tissues. *Arthritis Rheum* **5**:667, 1962
18. Buszman E et al: Electron spin resonance studies of chloroquine–melanin complexes. *Biochem Pharmacol* **33**:7, 1984
19. Lewis R et al: Malaria associated with pregnancy. *Obstet Gynecol* **42**:696, 1973
20. Sapp OL: Toxic psychosis due to quinacrine and chloroquine. *JAMA* **187**:373, 1964
21. Tuffanelli DL et al: Pigmentation associated with anti-malarial therapy. Its possible relationship to the ocular lesions. *Arch Dermatol* **88**:419, 1963
22. Hobbs RF, Calnan CD: Visual disturbances with anti-malarial drugs with particular reference to chloroquine keratopathy. *Arch Dermatol* **80**:557, 1959
23. Finbloom DS et al: Comparison of hydroxychloroquine and chloroquine use and the development of retinal toxicity. *J Rheumatol* **12**:692, 1985
24. Bernstein HN: Chloroquine ocular toxicity. *Surv Ophthalmol* **12**:415, 1967
25. MacKenzie AH: An appraisal of chloroquine. *Arthritis Rheum* **13**:280, 1970
26. Scherbel AL et al: Ocular lesions in rheumatoid arthritis and related disorders with particular reference to retinopathy: Study of 741 patients treated with and without chloroquine. *N Engl J Med* **273**:360, 1965
27. Isacson D et al: Antimalarials in dermatology. *Int J Dermatol* **21**:379, 1982
28. Page F: Treatment of lupus erythematosus with mepacrine. *Lancet* **2**:755, 1951
29. Dubois EL: Quinacrine (Atabrine) in treatment of systemic and discoid lupus erythematosus. *Arch Intern Med* **94**:131, 1954
30. Christiansen JV, Nielsen JP: Treatment of lupus erythematosus with mepacrine. Results and relapses during a long observation. *Br J Dermatol* **68**:73, 1956
31. Merwin C, Winkelmann R: Dermatologic clinics 2. Antimalarial drugs in therapy of lupus erythematosus. *Mayo Clin Proc* **37**:253, 1962
32. Christiansen JV, Brodthagen H: The treatment of polymorphic light eruptions with chloroquine. *Br J Dermatol* **68**:204, 1956
33. Gschnait F et al: Induction of UV light tolerance by PUVA in patients with polymorphous light eruption. *Br J Dermatol* **99**:293, 1978
34. Parrish JA et al: Comparison of PUVA and beta-carotene in the treatment of polymorphous light eruption. *Br J Dermatol* **100**:187, 1979
35. Cripps DJ, Curtis AC: Toxic effect of chloroquine on porphyria hepatica. *Arch Dermatol* **86**:575, 1962
36. Kordac V et al: Chloroquine in the treatment of PCT. *N Engl J Med* **296**:949, 1977
37. Swanbeck G. Wennersten G: Treatment of porphyria cutanea tarda with chloroquine and phlebotomy. *Br J Dermatol* **97**:77, 1977
38. Moreau S et al: A nuclear magnetic resonance study of the interactions of antimalarial drugs with porphyrins. *Biochim Biophys Acta* **840**:107, 1985
39. Shanley BC et al: Evaluation of the stoichiometry and strength of chloroquine–prophyrin interactions by difference spectroscopy. *Biochem Pharmacol* **34**:141, 1985

*Jerome L. Shupack, Matthew J. Stiller,
and Guy F. Webster*

CHAPTER 235

Cytotoxic Agents and Dermatologic Therapy

The use of cytotoxic drugs is an important aspect of the treatment of skin disease. Although the list of available cytotoxic agents is lengthy, there are five drugs that have particular advantages for dermatologists: methotrexate, azathioprine, 5-fluorouracil (5-FU), cyclophosphamide, and mechlorethamine (nitrogen mustard). Cytotoxic drugs are used in some diseases to modulate the behavior of the epidermis and in others to modulate the behavior of inflammatory cells. Regardless of the target, cytotoxic drugs primarily exert their effects through inhibition of cell division, which often leads to cell death.

The concept of the cell cycle is important for understanding how cytotoxic drugs work. The cell cycle is the sequence of growth phases in which all cells of the body are involved. There are several discrete segments to the cell cycle. The G_1 phase is a period in which cell metabolism is directed toward preparing for DNA synthesis. The S phase of the cell cycle follows G_1 and is devoted to DNA synthesis. At the end of DNA synthesis, the G_2 period occurs and precedes cell division, which is termed the M phase. Cells may also enter a resting state, termed G_0, from either the G_1 or G_2 phase. The length of the G_0 phase is variable (Fig. 235-1).

Most cytotoxic drugs that are useful in dermatology fall into two broad groups, the antimetabolites and the alkylating agents. Antimetabolites mimic natural molecules and are most active while DNA is being synthesized, that is, in the S phase. Thus, these drugs require a target population that is proliferating in order to exert their effect. A corollary of this principle is that side effects of this class of drugs are most prominent in cells of the body that have an innately high proliferative index, such as visceral epithelium and bone marrow. The other group of drugs, alkylating agents, exert their effects through an actual physicochemical interaction with a preformed DNA molecule. These interactions include alkylation, cross-linking, and carbamoylation. Although drugs in this group are very effective against proliferating populations of cells, they also exert some effect on cells that are not actively synthesizing DNA. Consistent with this concept, their adverse effects are not mainly limited to proliferating cell populations, and they have a greater potential for mutagenicity.

The immunosuppressive potency of cytotoxic drugs is a double-edged sword. Infections of lethal proportion may arise quickly and quietly in immunosuppressed patients. Patients should be assessed for symptoms of infection, including fever, chills, sweats, shortness of breath, cough, headache, dysuria, and arthritis, at each visit. Patients should be instructed to report any new symptoms promptly, and physicians should be vigorous in ruling out infection by appropriate studies.

Methotrexate

Methotrexate (amethopterin) was introduced in 1948 and is the most commonly used antimetabolite in cancer treatment. It was initially used for hematologic malignancies, choriocarcinoma, and various epithelial-derived tumors. It has been used more recently in various nonmalignant diseases including rheumatoid arthritis, asthma, graft-versus-host disease, and numerous skin conditions. Because methotrexate is inherently toxic, most physicians feel uncomfortable with its use. However, the specialty of dermatology has made consistent and judicious use of this drug since the early 1960s and has generated an impressive record of safety.

Methotrexate occurs as a crystalline, yellow to brown powder that is nearly insoluble in water or alcohol. Methotrexate sodium is a yellow water-soluble powder that is used in the preparation of injectable forms of the drug.

Methotrexate is a synthetic analogue of folic acid (Fig. 235-2). It differs from folate in two regions, the substitution of an amino for a hydroxyl in the pteridine nucleus and in the methylation of the amino group between the benzoyl and pteroyl moieties. The folate vitamins function as 1-carbon carriers and are essential for the synthesis of purines and thymidylic acid. These products are required for gene synthesis and cell division.

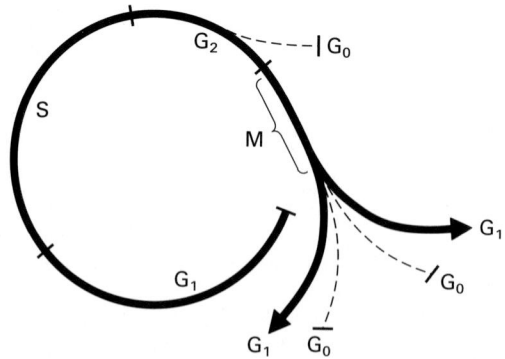

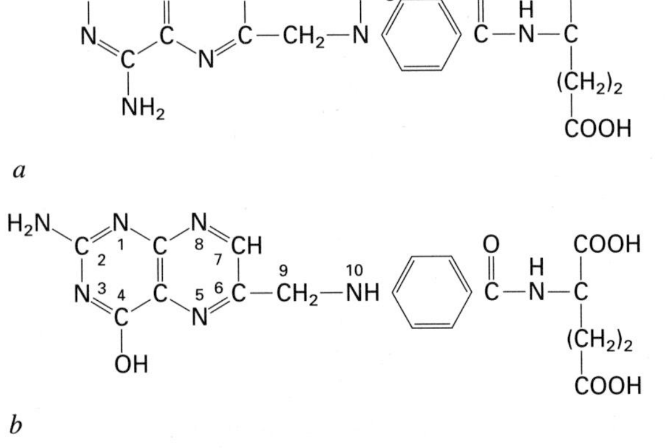

FIGURE 235-1   Diagram of the cell cycle.

FIGURE 235-2   Chemical structure of methotrexate and folic acid. (*a*) Methotrexate. (*b*) Folic acid.

TABLE 235-1
Potential Mechanisms of Methotrexate Activity in Skin Disease

Folate antagonisms/decreased cell proliferation
Suppression of inflammatory cell chemotaxis
Inhibition of monocyte/macrophage activation
Inhibition of histamine release from basophils (and mast cells?)
Inhibition of lymphocyte function

Folate exists in two forms in the body, as a monoglutamate in plasma and as a polyglutamate within cells. The polyglutamate is linked by γ-peptide bonds and is preferentially retained within cells. It is a more efficient cofactor than the monoglutamylated precursor. To be active, these folate cofactors must be reduced to tetrahydrofolate by the enzyme dihydrofolate reductase (Table 235-1). Methotrexate enters cells by two mechanisms, active transport and a carrier-independent mechanism that is active only at high methotrexate levels. Once inside the cell, methotrexate binds to dihydrofolate reductase and inactivates the enzyme. The drug is a competitive inhibitor of the natural substrate dihydrofolate. Synthesis of thymidylate is most sensitive to methotrexate-mediated folate depletion. Purine synthesis is somewhat more resistant.[1-3]

The activity of methotrexate is enhanced by polyglutamylation just as is the activity of the natural substrate. These derivatives form rapidly within cells and increase with the concentration of the drug and the duration of exposure. This form of methotrexate can persist within cells and bind more tightly to dihydrofolate reductase than does unaltered methotrexate. Glutamylation also broadens the spectrum of enzyme inhibition including thymidylate synthetase and amino imidazolecarboxamide ribonucleoside transferase. Thus, high methotrexate doses and prolonged periods of exposure produce a greater cytotoxic effect than would be predicted on the basis of drug dose alone. This fact becomes an important consideration in the design of treatment regimens, adjustment of dosages, and minimization of adverse effects.[3,4]

The mechanism of cytotoxic therapy in nonneoplastic skin disease is poorly understood, as are the diseases themselves. In skin diseases with an apparent inflammatory etiology, methotrexate may be presumed to suppress white blood cell function. In other diseases, the mechanism is less clear. For example, psoriasis is characterized by excessive growth of the epidermis and supporting vasculature and may be exacerbated by the inflammatory response. The primary defect in psoriasis may be either epidermal or inflammatory. Methotrexate may act directly to inhibit epidermal cell division or may inhibit the effect of inflammatory cells.

There are few data to prove either contention clearly. High, oncologic doses of methotrexate (for example, 100 to 250 mg/m^2 per week) have been shown to depress the antibody response to common antigens. Lower doses have been shown to suppress rheumatoid factor production. Low doses of methotrexate suppress division of mononuclear cells and inhibit their response to interleukin-2. Low-dose methotrexate suppresses neutrophil and monocyte chemotaxis both in vitro and in vivo. Langerhans cell activity is suppressed during methotrexate treatment. Leukotriene B$_4$ synthesis by neutrophils is depressed by methotrexate.[4-10] The mechanisms for most of these phenomena are not understood.

The proliferation of epidermal cells, a key issue in psoriasis, is also modulated by methotrexate. Weinstein and colleagues and others have provided strong evidence for the direct action of methotrexate on psoriatic epidermal proliferation.[11-14] Psoriatic epidermal cell division is suppressed best with systemic methotrexate. Intralesional or topical methotrexate has much less effect clinically despite evidence that local delivery of the drug suppresses the growth of normal animal skin. This discrepancy has been explained by problems in local penetration and by possible involvement of a different target for the drug. Suppression of the immune system or of systemic production of a "psoriatic factor" could be such a target.[11-14]

Pharmacokinetics

Nearly 90 percent of an oral dose of methotrexate can be recovered in the blood, but the time to peak plasma levels can vary from 1 to 5 h.[15-20] Absorption is clearly influenced by food. Pinkerton et al.[16] have shown that milk (and possibly other calcium-containing compounds) decreases bioavailability. In adults, mean bioavailability is 67 percent of the administered dose with plasma peaks between 1 and 3 h after administration of 10 mg/m^2. Divided oral doses of methotrexate (for example, three 5-mg doses separated by 12 h) result in blood levels ranging from 0.17 to 0.5 μg/ml.

The distribution of methotrexate is determined by its negative charge at neutral pH, which limits its diffusion across biologic membranes.[1] Low central nervous system penetration is a great advantage in the treatment of skin disease. However, the lower membrane transit may also result in a theoretical disadvantage. Methotrexate travels across biologic membranes very poorly. It follows that a drug that does penetrate into a third space collection, such as ascites or pleural effusion, will likewise be delayed in its exit from this area. This delay may be the mechanism for the prolonged blood levels of the drug and, to a degree, may provide the rationale for intermittent methotrexate dosing.

The mean serum half-life of methotrexate depends to a degree on the dose given. At high dosages (e.g., 30 mg/m^2), there is a triphasic elimination curve for the drug and its principal metabolite. Studies of low-dose methotrexate in rheumatoid arthritis and psoriasis show that most patients have a two-phase elimination curve. The mean serum half-life is 6 to 7 h at doses commonly used in dermatology. It should be noted that, although plasma levels fall, intracellular polyglutamylation may stabilize tissue levels of the drug, even in the absence of serum drug levels. The effect of this phenomenon on methotrexate-mediated disease suppression is not clear. Recent studies in rheumatoid arthritis suggest that its effect is negligible.[21]

Methotrexate is 50 to 60 percent bound to serum protein.[1,22] Serum protein binding is decreased in vitro and in vivo by sodium salicylate. One study noted a decrease of 50 to 70 percent. The clinical significance of such displacement is not clear.

Methotrexate is metabolized mainly in the liver. The primary metabolite is 7-OH-methotrexate, which is a weak inhibitor of dihydrofolate reductase; it is about 200 times less potent than methotrexate. Excretion of methotrexate is primarily renal; it is excreted in the renal tubules at a rate that probably exceeds inulin clearance. It is also reabsorbed by a pathway that is not well described. Various weak organic acids including aspirin, other nonsteroidal agents, and probenecid, interfere with methotrexate excretion. About 80 percent of a single dose of methotrexate eventually appears in the urine, while a smaller fraction is excreted in bile.[23-27]

Adverse Reactions

There is a large collected experience in the rheumatologic and dermatologic literature regarding the toxicity of low-dose methotrex-

TABLE 235-2
Adverse Reactions to Methotrexate

Gastrointestinal: nausea, vomiting, stomatitis, diarrhea, ulceration
Hepatic: abnormal transaminase levels, hepatitis, fibrosis, cirrhosis
Hematopoietic: anemia, thrombocytopenia, leukopenia, pancytopenia
Pulmonary: acute hypersensitivity, fibrosis

TABLE 235-3
Liver Histology Grading

Grade I:	Normal to mild fatty infiltration, portal inflammation, and nuclear variability
Grade II:	Moderate to severe fatty infiltration, nuclear variability, portal tract expansion and inflammation, and necrosis
Grade IIIA:	Mild fibrosis
Grade IIIB:	Moderate to severe fibrosis
Grade IV:	Cirrhosis

ate.[28,29] Adverse reactions may be life threatening or trivial. Table 235-2 summarizes these adverse effects.

Initially, it was suggested that the side effects of methotrexate may be lessened by administration of folinic acid. This concept is probably erroneous. Hanrahan and Russell[21] studied the effect of folinic acid on methotrexate-mediated side effects in rheumatoid arthritis and found no benefit to folinic acid "rescue."

Several principles regarding the side effects of methotrexate are generally applicable. First, higher doses cause more side effects. Second, patients who experience side effects early in therapy will probably continue to have them, and patients who are free of early complaints may be more likely to remain so during long-term treatment. Third, sicker, older, or more debilitated patients seem to experience more problems than those who are in good health. Finally, the use of divided drug dosing is often helpful in reducing side effects.

The most common complaints in methotrexate-treated patients involve the gastrointestinal tract.[28,29] Nausea and vomiting are the most frequent problems and are dose related to a great degree. They are most commonly seen with oral therapy, but they also occur with intramuscular injection; 10 to 30 percent of all patients experience some difficulty. Administration of antacids, H_2 blockers, prochlorperazine, or metoclopramide is often effective in controlling these symptoms. Diarrhea is relatively infrequent and does not limit methotrexate therapy. Gastric ulceration may rarely occur and is often exacerbated by the concurrent administration of antiarthritic drugs.

Mucocutaneous complaints are also seen fairly frequently in patients receiving this drug. Of these, oral ulcerations and soreness are most often noted. Skin ulcerations are much less frequent. When these conditions are severe enough to treat, the authors favor the use of topical anesthetics or low-potency topical corticosteroids.

A major concern in methotrexate therapy is the induction of liver fibrosis.[28-37] Methotrexate is clearly a hepatotoxic drug. Elevations in liver enzymes occur frequently in 8 to 67 percent of patients. Although disquieting, these elevations do not seem to have any value in predicting which patients will develop cirrhosis. For unknown reasons, patients with psoriasis seem to have a higher incidence of liver fibrosis than do patients with rheumatoid arthritis, who are treated with similar methotrexate regimens. Fibrosis relates to the duration of therapy, total dose, and patient age. Between 0 and 26 percent of patients receiving methotrexate have demonstrated cirrhotic changes. A somewhat larger number may show fatty infiltration and a "trivial" fibrosis.[29] Those receiving total doses of less than 1.5 g have a negligible incidence of fibrosis.[29] The course of methotrexate-induced liver disease seems to be relatively nonaggressive. In fact, several investigators have reported continuation of therapy in these patients with no adverse effects.

Since the mechanism by which methotrexate causes liver damage is not known, definitive statements cannot be made about preventing it. Experience has shown that patients with prior liver disease, diabetes, obesity, significant alcohol intake, as well as intravenous drug use are all at increased risk for hepatic fibrosis and cirrhosis.[29]

The only acceptable method for verifying methotrexate-induced cirrhosis is percutaneous needle biopsy.[30] This procedure is safe. The approximate risk of minor bleeding is 1 in 1000, while the risk of death from this diagnostic technique is 1 in 10,000.[38] Biopsy results are classified according to liver architecture, degree of inflammation and fibrosis, and presence of fat and are graded on a scale of I to IV (Table 235-3). Roenigk and colleagues[29] recommend that patients with grades I and II histology may continue therapy, grade IIIA patients may continue with a repeat liver biopsy in 6 months, and grades IIIB and IV patients should discontinue methotrexate.

There is conjecture about when a liver biopsy should first be performed. Roenigk and associates[29] recommend that liver biopsy be performed after the first 1.5 g of methotrexate have been administered. Others contend that the liver should be biopsied when it is clear that the patient is a candidate for long-term methotrexate treatment. Patients may be treated for 1 or 2 months to see if their disease is adequately suppressed and to ensure that any methotrexate side effects are tolerable. Once a commitment to long-term treatment is made by the physician and patient, the liver biopsy should be performed.

Methotrexate-induced bone-marrow suppression is not uncommon.[39-42] Because the marrow cells are rapidly proliferating, they are particularly susceptible to methotrexate. Severe bone-marrow suppression due to low-dose oral methotrexate has been reported on several occasions. The patients were anemic, neutropenic, and thrombocytopenic and showed evidence of sepsis and severe bleeding disorders. Factors that appear to put patients at increased risk for marrow toxicity include advanced age, low creatinine clearance, and concurrent administration of nonsteroidal anti-inflammatory drugs. No single cause has been identified.

Methotrexate can cause mutations in laboratory animals. However, there has been no associated increase in cancer in patients who have been treated with dermatologic doses of methotrexate. Methotrexate is teratogenic and an abortifacient. Administration during pregnancy is clearly contraindicated. The prevalence of fetal malformation during methotrexate therapy is reported at 3.4 percent. There is no apparent effect on the outcome of subsequent pregnancies. There are no reports of abnormal children fathered by men receiving methotrexate therapy, although sperm motility may be abnormal during treatment.[43-47]

Opportunistic infections have been reported in three otherwise healthy individuals receiving low-dose methotrexate (one case of *Pneumocystis* pneumonia and two cases of cyptococcosis).

Overdosage with methotrexate should be treated promptly with leucovorin (folinic acid).[29] Patients who have episodes of decreased renal function while receiving methotrexate should be

TABLE 235-4
Leucovorin Treatment of Methotrexate Overdosage

Serum methotrexate level	Leucovorin dosage*
5×10^{-7} M	20 mg q6h
1×10^{-6} M	100 mg q6h
2×10^{-6} M	200 mg q6h

*Increase proportionately for greater methotrexate levels.

TABLE 235-5
Potential Drug Interactions with Methotrexate

Nonsteroidal anti-inflammatory agents
Sulfonamides
Probenecid*
Ketotifen
Allopurinol
Ethanol*
Penicillins
Cephalosporins
Barbiturates
Phenytoin
cis-Platin and all renal-toxic drugs*

*Near absolute contraindication.

TABLE 235-6
Premethotrexate Tests

Renal	Hepatic
Urine analysis	Transaminase levels
Creatinine clearance	Alkaline phosphatase level
BUN/creatinine	Total bilirubin
Hematopoietic	Albumin
Complete blood count	
Folate level	

TABLE 235-7
Instructions for Patients Receiving Methotrexate

1. Follow instructions faithfully.
2. Take methotrexate WEEKLY (not daily).
3. Call your physician immediately if overdose is suspected.
4. Notify your physician if fever, cough, or shortness of breath develops.
5. Tell your physician about all side effects.
6. Notify all your physicians that you are taking methotrexate.
7. Drink no alcoholic beverages and take no other medications.
8. Do not take methotrexate while pregnant or trying to conceive.
9. Do not take methotrexate if you have an active infection (including cold/flu, urinary tract infection, pneumonia) without notifying your physician.
10. Allow no one else to take this medicine.

treated as they would for an overdosage. An initial dose of 10 mg of folinic acid per m^2 (about 20 mg) should be given intravenously, followed by oral doses of 20 mg every 6 h (Table 235-4). The blood level of methotrexate should be determined every 12 to 24 h. Leucovorin administration should continue until the level of serum methotrexate falls below 10^{-8} M.

There are three major groups of drug interactions: the first results from alterations in protein binding, the second from altered renal excretion, and the third from hepatotoxicity. While any drug that may enhance methotrexate toxicity should be avoided, there are several near-absolute contraindications (Table 235-5).

Treatment Recommendations

Perhaps the most effective way to reduce adverse effects from methotrexate is to exclude inappropriate patients. The ideal patient would have severe skin disease but otherwise would be healthy, young, and compliant. Patients with a history of liver disease, kidney disease, or significant risk factors for such organ impairment are not ideal candidates. The decrement in renal function that occurs as part of the aging process makes the very old patient less than ideal as well. Given the tendency to underestimate one's own alcohol intake, the admission of any drinking may constitute a relative contraindication. The use of other medications may also predispose patients to drug interactions and so may be a relative contraindication. Unfortunately, an ideal patient profile is rare, especially among patients whose disease is sufficiently severe and refractory to warrant a trial of methotrexate.

The second most effective way to reduce adverse effects is rigorous attention to detail, especially in patients who are less than ideal candidates for the drug. Such attention includes frequent follow-up, detailed reviews of systems at each visit, the monitoring of appropriate laboratory parameters (Table 235-6), and communication with the patient's general physician at appropriate intervals.

Optimal patient compliance should be promoted by detailed, clear instructions and may be reinforced by printed literature (Table 235-7). For particularly noncompliant or untrustworthy patients, the physician may elect to require an office visit for parenteral methotrexate administration.

These authors firmly believe in short-term trials of methotrexate whenever possible. Often a brief administration of methotrexate will allow a patient's disease to be controlled by less toxic therapy. Using short-term methotrexate to quiet a flare of skin disease is also particularly appropriate in patients with certain relative contraindications to prolonged therapy such as alcoholism or hepatic disease. Even when therapy is intended to be of short duration, full pretreatment tests should be performed.

Finally, it is the authors' experience that, while prudent doses of methotrexate produce great improvement, they often do not result in complete clearing of the disease. When doses of methotrexate higher than 25 mg per week are used to treat psoriasis, the side effects may outweigh any benefit. Patients' and physicians' expectations should be for effective control, not complete clearing of disease.

Specific Clinical Applications

Psoriasis   The largest and most widely accepted use for methotrexate in nonneoplastic disease is in the treatment of psoriasis. In 1987, Peckham and colleagues[48] reported that over half of the dermatologists in the United States use methotrexate for severe psoriasis. Methotrexate was second only to UV radiation as a treatment modality for severe disease. Such use dates from 1951, when it was reported that a patient's psoriasis unexpectedly cleared during treatment with methotrexate.[49]

Current use of methotrexate in psoriasis is usually limited to patients with severe disease that is refractory to conventional topical treatments. When practical, a patient with psoriasis may be allowed to fail a therapeutic trial of UVB phototherapy or PUVA photochemotherapy before methotrexate is started. The suitability of UVB therapy or photochemotherapy is limited for many individuals, and a trial of this method is often not possible for financial reasons or time considerations.

During the 1950s and 1960s, various treatment regimens were tested.[50] Weinstein and Frost[51,52] related methotrexate dosage to psoriatic cell cycle kinetics and proposed a weekly treatment regimen in which a third of the total methotrexate dose was given every 12 h over a 24-h period to achieve an effective blood level for 36 h. The intent of this regimen was to maximize the exposure of proliferating psoriatic cells to the drug. Currently, the two most common methotrexate regimens are the Weinstein-Frost regimen or a single weekly dose.

Patients who are deemed to be appropriate candidates on the basis of disease severity, general health, and personal habits and whose screening test results are acceptable are usually given a test dose of methotrexate. A dose of 2.5 mg every 12 h for three doses is given by mouth and the patient returns in 1 week for repeat laboratory tests (CBC, plus differential, BUN/creatinine, liver enzymes), a skin examination, and a review of systems. If all is in order, or if the reported side effects are minor, weekly therapy is continued after discussion with the patient. Patients with particularly severe disease often require doses of 5 mg every 12 h for maintenance. In such cases this dose is started after week 1. A period of at least 1 month at a given dose is allowed before a lack of response prompts an increased methotrexate dosage. Concomitant therapy with midpotency topical corticosteroid ointments is usually helpful.

Patients continue periodic visits until their disease is quiescent and their drug dosage is stable. At this point the authors continue therapy for several weeks to ensure that the observed improvement has stabilized and then begin a gradual methotrexate taper to the point where the disease flares. This tapering determines the dose for chronic administration.

Patients often may need methotrexate for only several months each year because their psoriasis can be well controlled by topical treatment in the interval. There are some patients whose disease does not readily respond to methotrexate. Explanations for this sort of resistance are lacking. The highest dose of methotrexate that is usually given to patients with psoriasis is a total of 22.5 mg per week, although some patients tolerate higher doses with no apparent problems. Some patients with refractory disease respond best to parenteral methotrexate, an option that may be used in selected individuals. In such resistant cases (and perhaps in all cases), the physician and patient should share the goal of effective control of disease; complete clearing may not be possible at prudent doses. In these refractory cases, combining methotrexate with PUVA photochemotherapy can enhance therapeutic efficacy without significantly increasing toxicity, as discussed in Chap. 139.

Pustular psoriasis is particularly responsive to methotrexate.[53,54] Unfortunately, no large organized studies can confirm this observation. Assuming a patient with pustular psoriasis qualifies for methotrexate therapy, the authors begin treatment with 5 mg every 12 h for three doses every 5 to 7 days until remission is achieved.

The effectiveness of methotrexate in psoriatic arthritis is less certain. Kragballe and colleagues[55] reported a retrospective study of 57 patients with psoriasis who also had seronegative arthritis. The starting dosage was 15 mg per week and the average treatment duration was 3 years. One-half of the patients reported ''modest improvement'' and one-half reported nearly complete remission. Those patients whose arthritis was of recent onset had the best response. These promising results must be tempered by the fact that

accurate grading of the initial level of joint disease may be nearly impossible in a retrospective study.

More recently, Wilkins and collaborators[56] performed a prospective double-blind, placebo-controlled study of methotrexate in patients with psoriatic arthritis. Doses were 7.5 to 15 mg per week in divided doses. An ongoing stable dose of a nonsteroidal antiinflammatory drug was permitted. Methotrexate-treated patients improved only in the area of skin involvement and in the physician's global assessment of arthritis activity. Most parameters were unchanged. It is not clear why rheumatoid arthritis appears to be more responsive to methotrexate than does psoriatic arthritis, but rheumatologists do view methotrexate as useful in psoriatic arthritis.

Reiter's Syndrome   Reiter's syndrome is a disease of skin, mucosa, and joints that is very similar to pustular psoriasis. It is often manageable with topical corticosteroids and oral nonsteroidal antiinflammatory drugs, but refractory disease may require aggressive therapy. The dermatologic and rheumatologic literature reports various treatment schedules for methotrexate in Reiter's syndrome. Lally and Ho[57] reviewed this literature and suggest treatment with 10 mg per week by mouth or intramuscular injection. Response usually occurs within weeks, although months may be required for complete clearing. Methotrexate is probably contraindicated in patients who have Reiter's syndrome associated with HIV infection. In these individuals, methotrexate may further immunosuppression. Such patients are probably best treated with etretinate.[58,59]

Sarcoidosis   Methotrexate may be quite useful in cases of refractory sarcoidosis. In 1977, Veien and Brodthagen[60] reported that refractory sarcoidosis in 12 of 16 patients was cleared by 25 mg per week of methotrexate. The authors have had experience with the use of this drug in sarcoidosis and have achieved dramatic results.[61] Methotrexate has several advantages for patients with severe sarcoidosis, most notably avoidance of the side effects of high-dose corticosteroid therapy. Since sarcoidosis is a truly chronic disease, long-term use of corticosteroids predisposes toward significant adverse affects. Disadvantages associated with methotrexate include the potential for kidney, liver, bone marrow, and pulmonary toxicity. Methotrexate may also lead to hepatic and renal involvement in patients with sarcoidosis. In patients with involvement of these organ systems who are receiving methotrexate, it may be difficult to interpret laboratory abnormalities. To date, no studies have addressed the prevalence of these side effects in patients with severe, refractory sarcoidosis.

There are many other diseases in which methotrexate is useful, including pityriasis lichenoides et varioliformis acuta,[62,63] lymphomatoid papulosis,[64,65] pityriasis rubra pilaris,[66-68] granulomatous vasculitis,[69] rheumatoid vasculitis,[69-71] polymyositis,[72-75] pemphigus vulgaris,[76,77] and lupus erythematosus.[78] In severe steroid-responsive cutaneous diseases, the concomitant use of methotrexate may allow reduction of the systemic dose of the corticosteroid.

Azathioprine

The thioprine drugs are synthetic analogues of the natural purine bases. They were first synthesized in the 1950s and many derivatives have subsequently been produced. The drug most commonly used in dermatology is azathioprine, although occasionally thioguanine or 6-mercaptopurine may be used. Allopurinol is a purine

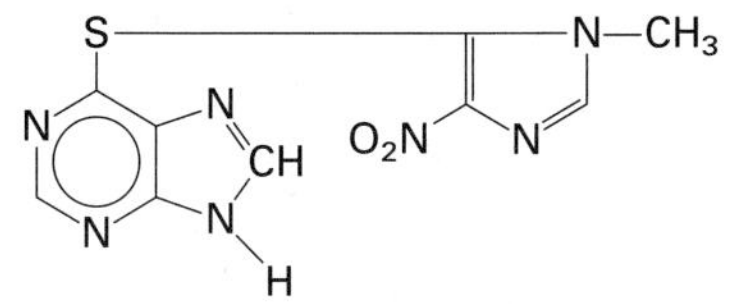

FIGURE 235-3 Chemical structure of azathioprine.

analogue that was first synthesized in a search for new cytotoxic drugs. It was later found to be useful in therapy for gout. Azathioprine was first developed as an agent to delay the metabolism of 6-mercaptopurine and is formed by attaching an imidazole ring to the sulfur at position 6 in the parent molecule[79-81] (Fig. 235-3).

The drug is a pale-yellow powder that is insoluble in water and barely soluble in alcohol. It is rendered water soluble by coadministration with sodium hydroxide. If stored in solution at alkaline pH, azathioprine degrades quickly.

The clinical activity of all the thioprine drugs is believed to stem from the inhibition of RNA and DNA synthesis and function. Azathioprine is a pro-drug that is metabolized to 6-mercaptopurine; 6-mercaptopurine is then activated by hypoxanthine-guanine phosphoribosyl transferase (HGPRT). These monophosphate nucleotide analogues then block purine synthesis at the initial step. Triphosphorylated 6-mercaptopurine is also incorporated into DNA, a process that renders the gene susceptible to strand breaks and point mutations. Cells that lack HGPRT, for example, certain tumor lines, are resistant to the cytotoxic effects of azathioprine.[82,83]

Azathioprine and 6-mercaptopurine are equivalent in potency when administered parenterally, but 6-mercaptopurine is much less effective when given by mouth.

Azathioprine is readily and fairly completely absorbed after oral administration. Plasma protein binding is about 30 percent. Azathioprine is largely dialyzable and does cross the placenta.

Only a small proportion of the thiopurines are excreted intact. Azathioprine is converted into mercaptopurine, which then undergoes oxidations to 6-thiouric acid by xanthine oxidase. Mercaptopurine may also be methylated and sulfated and then excreted in the urine.[82,84]

There is evidence that genetic polymorphism may contribute to excessive myelosuppression in some patients treated with azathioprine. An unexpected number of patients with thiopurine-induced leukopenia have no detectable levels of thiopurine methyltransferase.[85] In addition, levels of 6-thioguanine nucleotide correlate with the degree of myelosuppression in patients with pemphigus treated with azathioprine.[86] These data may be interpreted to show that any episode of leukopenia in an azathioprine-treated patient indicates abnormal sensitivity to the drug and a need for a new, lower maintenance dose.

Adverse Reactions (See Table 235-8)

Azathioprine is a generally safe drug when used carefully. A comparison of adverse reactions in patients with rheumatoid arthritis treated with methotrexate or azathioprine failed to reveal significant differences.[86]

Myelosuppression is the major toxic side effect of thioprine administration. A generalized depression of leukocytes is the most common type of myelosuppression, but any cell line may be exclusively suppressed. Since platelets have the shortest life span of all the formed elements, thrombocytopenia is the most common pre-

sentation of toxic marrow suppression. Bone marrow suppression is usually seen only at the higher dosage ranges of dermatologic azathioprine therapy.[79,86,87]

Patients receiving high doses of azathioprine may experience nausea, vomiting, and diarrhea.[79] The symptoms are usually not severe and may be minimized by using a divided dosage. A toxic hepatitis develops in about 1 percent of patients with rheumatoid arthritis who receive azathioprine. This hepatitis is characterized by extremely high alkaline phosphatase levels and is usually reversible. Hepatic venoocclusive disease has also been reported, as has pancreatitis.[88,89]

There is clearly an increased risk of infection when patients are treated with azathioprine. Since most patients treated with this drug also receive large doses of corticosteroids as part of their treatment regimen, it is difficult to assess the exact role of azathioprine in predisposing to infection. Unlike cyclophosphamide-mediated immune suppression, suppression mediated by azathioprine is not proportional to the peripheral leukocyte count. Thus, infection may occur at normal white blood cell levels.

Azathioprine infrequently causes a drug fever. The mechanism of this phenomenon is not known but clearly relates to administration of the drug. Chills, headache, and malaise often accompany the fevers.[90-92] Discontinuation of therapy is indicated.

A major concern for physicians who prescribe azathioprine is the induction of cancers. Some investigators have found no increased malignancy, while others find a significant increase. The most recent analysis of this problem suggests that hematologic malignancies, particularly non-Hodgkin's lymphoma, may be promoted. The relative risk is roughly ten- to thirteenfold, or one lymphoma per 1000 patient years of azathioprine treatment.[93]

It is not possible to interpret the relevance of these data for dermatologic diseases. It is known that there is a different incidence of azathioprine-related lymphoma in the renal transplant population, the Sjögren's syndrome population, and the rheumatoid population.[79] How patients with skin disease fare is not known. The amount of azathioprine and the duration of treatment may be important variables. In general, dermatologic doses are lower than those used in patients with renal or rheumatologic disease. Likewise, the duration of therapy for skin disease is usually much shorter than for other diseases. It is the opinion of the authors that the risk of lymphoma in patients with azathioprine-treated dermatologic disease is probably significantly less than in transplant patients or patients with arthritis. The resolution of this issue requires organized study.

Roubenoff and associates[94] reviewed the incidence of azathioprine-associated birth defects. Surprisingly, the rate of congenital malformation is only 4.3 percent. The prevalence of neonatal immunosuppression may be significant. There appears to be no adverse effect on fertility.

Azathioprine is the most commonly used thiopurine in dermatologic disease and is usually given by mouth. It is supplied as

TABLE 235-8
Adverse Reactions to Azathioprine

Myelosuppression
Infection
Drug fever
Gastrointestinal
   Nausea, vomiting, diarrhea
   Hepatitis
   Pancreatitis
Induction of malignancy

50-mg tablets and is also available in injectable form. Before therapy begins, a baseline blood count, BUN, creatinine, and liver function tests should be performed. Impaired renal function may be associated with greater toxicity even though mercaptopurine metabolites have less activity than the parent drug. During therapy, blood counts and liver function tests should be routinely performed, weekly during the first month and then every 2 or 3 weeks thereafter. Dosage increases require more frequent testing.

Some believe that patients who have previously received alkylating agents may have a greatly increased risk for subsequent malignancy after thiopurine therapy. The authors avoid the use of thiopurines in these patients when possible.

Clinical Applications

The autoimmune etiology of the pemphigus group of diseases makes them a logical choice for immunosuppressive drugs. In 1969, Wolff and Schreiner[95] reported the value of azathioprine in the treatment of pemphigus. This finding has been echoed by many other reports. Although the drug may be used as a monotherapy, it is most commonly employed as an adjunct to steroid treatment. Other steroid adjuvants such as cyclophosphamide, gold, or dapsone are in common use as well. There are no conclusive studies comparing the different agents. Steroid adjuvants are generally believed to decrease the steroid requirement in patients with pemphigus and may also speed disease resolution.

There is a suggestion that azathioprine and cyclophosphamide may also promote permanent remission of pemphigus. Because of the relative rarity and variable course of disease, there are no conclusive studies on the value of azathioprine. Bystryn[96] has reviewed the literature and finds a slightly higher rate of apparent remission in studies using azathioprine or cyclophosphamide.

It is widely held that the effect of azathioprine in pemphigus is delayed. Several weeks were said to be required for the clinical effect to be detected. Well-controlled studies have not addressed this issue.

Aberer and colleagues[97] reported a prospective long-term study of patients with pemphigus who were treated with steroids and azathioprine. The starting dose of azathioprine was 2 to 3 mg/kg per day combined with 80 to 200 mg per day of methylprednisolone. The steroid is maintained for several months and then tapered and eventually discontinued. Azathioprine was withdrawn after 4 disease-free months off steroids. Forty-five percent of patients achieved apparent remission with this drug regimen.

The authors have had favorable experience using azathioprine, 1 to 2 mg/kg per day, as therapy for pemphigus. A lower risk of neoplasia with azathioprine than with cyclophosphamide seems to be an advantage. The addition of azathioprine seems to speed steroid tapering without exacerbating the disease, and several of our patients appear to be in drug-free remission. The authors begin azathioprine therapy early in the course of the disease, usually after the first week or two, if 60 to 80 mg of prednisone has failed to control new blister formation. Azathioprine and other cytotoxic drugs have received little attention as treatment for relatively mild pemphigus. It is not known whether the potential long-term risk of azathioprine outweighs the potential benefits of inducing a long-term remission.

Other bullous diseases respond to azathioprine. There are numerous case reports endorsing use of the drug for steroid-resistant bullous pemphigoid.[98,99] Treatment regimens are similar to those used in patients with pemphigus.

The addition of cytotoxic drugs to steroid therapy has been responsible for the greatly increased survival of patients with systemic vasculitis.[100,101] Cyclophosphamide is the cytotoxic drug of choice for this application, but azathioprine is sometimes useful. Azathioprine seems more able to maintain a remission than to induce one, but it is occasionally used in patients who cannot tolerate cyclophosphamide. Since azathioprine does not induce gonadal dysfunction, it is sometimes used in patients who wish to conceive following treatment for their disease.

Various other diseases involving uncontrolled inflammation have been targets for azathioprine therapy. They include lupus erythematosus,[102] polymyositis,[103] and various photodermatoses.[104,105]

5-Fluorouracil

5-Fluorouracil (5-FU) is a frequently used cytotoxic drug in dermatology. 5-FU is an antimetabolite that mimics thymidine precursors (Fig. 235-4). Thymidylate synthetase is bound by 5-fluoro-2'-deoxyuridine, 5'-monophosphate, and this binding results in its inactivation. 5-FU may also be incorporated into RNA and thus result in inhibition of cell growth, which is not dependent on the cell cycle.

In dermatology, 5-FU use is limited to topical application. Although systemic administration is effective, the severity of side effects greatly outweighs the potential benefit in dermatologic disease. Topical 5-FU is available in 1%, 2%, and 5% strengths and is used mainly for the treatment of superficial premalignant skin disease, specifically actinic keratoses.[106] It was previously used for treatment of basal cell and squamous cell carcinomas. However, there has been a suggestion that recurrence rates are unacceptably high.[107] This high rate would be most likely with large skin tumors in which the 5-FU fails to penetrate in sufficient strength through the depth of the lesion and so destroys only its superficial portion.

Actinic keratoses are ideal targets for 5-FU. They are superficial, a therapeutic end point is easily identified, and the consequences of inadequate treatment are slight. Treatment with 5-FU is effective for a single actinic keratosis but is most advantageous when the number of lesions is great. The typical treatment regimen is twice daily application of 5-FU cream until a vigorous inflammatory response is seen in the actinic keratoses, and then to stop treatment. The time required to achieve this response varies from 2 to 4 weeks in most individuals. Emollients and, perhaps, low-potency corticosteroid preparations may then be used to soothe the irritated and uncomfortable skin. Treatment with 5-FU often reveals more actinic keratoses than were originally suspected. It is believed that these unsuspected keratoses represent incipient lesions that have yet to become clinically apparent. Thus 5-FU treatment is in a sense prophylactic and may be useful in patients who are predisposed to

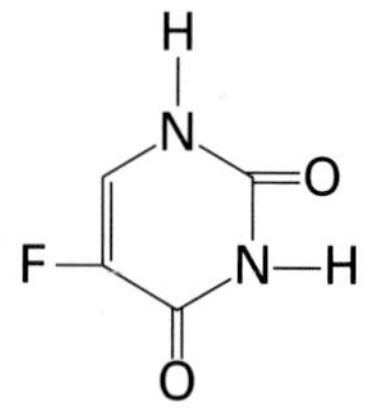

FIGURE 235-4 Chemical structure of 5-fluorouracil.

large numbers of actinic keratoses. Occasionally, the inflammatory response is inadequate and may require more frequent applications, prolonged therapy, occlusive dressings (especially on the forearms), or the use of an adjunctive agent such as tretinoin cream.

The major disadvantage of topical 5-FU is the severe irritation that results from its action. Usually the face or arms are treated. Patients experience a significant and lengthy cosmetic disfigurement which may be unacceptable. Some individuals whose jobs require public contact are often dissatisfied with 5-FU treatment.

Since systemic absorption of the drug is slight, systemic side effects are essentially nonexistent. The drug may be used in frail patients with confidence (if they can tolerate the ensuing dermatitis). Areas to be treated with 5-FU should be examined closely before treatment to ensure that there are no basal cell or squamous cell cancers whose presence may be masked by the 5-FU. Treatment with 5-FU should be withheld until any such lesions have received definitive treatment.

Hospital consultant dermatologists are familiar with the phenomonon of inflamed actinic keratoses during systemic 5-FU administration as part of cancer chemotherapy. This response is often interpreted as a ''drug reaction'' but represents the action of the systemically administered drug on actinic keratoses. Its occurrence should not be taken as a reason to discontinue systemic therapy with 5-FU.

Topical or intralesional 5-FU has also been used for keratoacanthomas, warts, and porokeratoses with varying success.[108-111] Lentigo maligna[111] also responds to 5-FU. However, more definitive therapy such as surgery should be used for this malignant lesion.

Hydroxyurea

Hydroxyurea is a low-molecular-weight drug that causes an immediate inhibition of DNA synthesis (Fig. 235-5). The drug inhibits ribonucleotide disphosphate reductase, the function of which is to convert ribonucleotides to their deoxy form. Inhibiting this enzyme limits the supply of DNA bases and thereby decreases the rate of DNA synthesis. Hydroxyurea is most active in cells with a high proliferative index.[112,113]

Hydroxyurea is well absorbed after oral administration. Serum levels peak within 2 h. Eighty percent of an oral dose can be recovered in the urine after 12 h, and at 24 h levels are negligible.

The most significant adverse effects of hydroxyurea include bone-marrow suppression and teratogenesis. Bone-marrow suppression occurs very frequently, in nearly all patients who are treated with therapeutic doses of the drug. This adverse affect reflects the susceptibility of proliferating cell populations to hydroxyurea.

The major dermatologic use of hydroxyurea is for psoriasis. Although the drug has been in existence for many years, its effect on psoriasis was not noted until the early 1970s. In a double-blind study of the treatment of psoriasis with hydroxyurea, Leavell and Yarborough[112] found that 9 of 10 cases of severe psoriasis demon-

strated clinical and histopathologic responses to hydroxyurea. Moschella and Greenwald[113] studied 60 patients whose psoriasis was treated with hydroxyurea. They found that there was a 50 to 60 percent response rate.

Because hydroxyurea has relatively little hepatic toxicity, it may be a good choice in patients who are excluded from methotrexate therapy because of liver disease. Hydroxyurea seems to be neither as effective nor as rapid in onset of action as methotrexate; however, it is clearly beneficial in some patients. To date no controlled studies have compared the effect of hydroxyurea with that of etretinate in severe psoriasis. Such studies would be valuable because the lower side-effect profile of hydroxyurea would seem to make it a superior drug in individuals who cannot tolerate methotrexate.

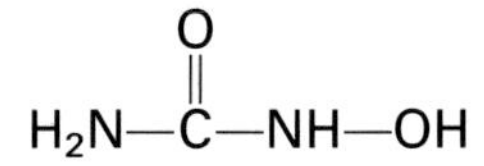

Alkylating Agents

There are two alkylating agents that are particularly useful in dermatology, cyclophosphamide and nitrogen mustard (mechlorethamine).

Cyclophosphamide

Cyclophosphamide is a derivative of nitrogen mustard (Fig. 235-6). As with other nitrogen mustards, cyclophosphamide acts primarily as a DNA cross-linker.[114]

Cyclophosphamide is a pro-drug that undergoes hepatic conversion to cytoxylamine, which is required for activity. Because the microsomal enzyme systems responsible for this activation are involved in the metabolism of other drugs, there is great potential for drug interaction during cyclophosphamide therapy. Drugs that induce these enzymes greatly alter the pharmacokinetics of cyclophosphamide.

Because cyclophosphamide interacts with preformed DNA and RNA, the drug is active against cells with a low proliferative index.

The side effects of cyclophosphamide are significant. Hematologic disturbances are frequent, especially leukopenia and thrombocytopenia.[114] The leukopenia is proportional to the degree of immune suppression and may be used as an index of the adequacy of the dosage of cyclophosphamide. Cyclophosphamide may also induce hematologic malignancy.[115]

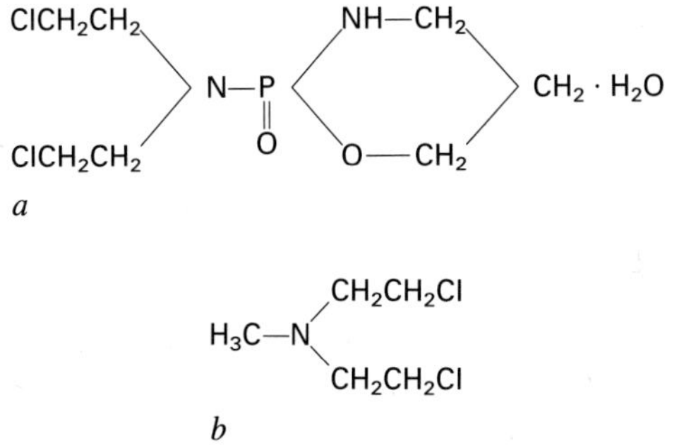

FIGURE 235-6   Chemical structure of the alkylating agents (a) cyclophosphamide and (b) mechlorethamine (nitrogen mustard).

FIGURE 235-5   Chemical structure of hydroxyurea.

Nausea and vomiting are fairly common during cyclophosphamide therapy, especially at higher doses. Alopecia often occurs, as may mucocutaneous ulcerations.[114] There is a clear increase in the incidence of low-grade squamous cell carcinoma of the skin.[115]

A hemorrhagic cystitis occurs in 5 to 10 percent of patients treated with cyclophosphamide. This cystitis is believed to be caused by the metabolite acrolein, and it occurs during therapy.[116,117] A new scavenging agent, mesna (sodium 2-mercaptoethanesulfonate), binds acrolein in the bladder and prevents severe bladder irritation. It is not known whether mesna also prevents the other common genitourinary complication of cyclophosphamide therapy, bladder cancer, which may develop in as many as 5 to 10 percent of patients.[118] No clear relationship exists between cystitis during treatment and the long-term development of cancer. Because cancers may arise many years after therapy, continued monitoring of the urinalysis is indicated.[119-123]

The use of cyclophosphamide is relatively contraindicated in patients who wish to conceive children. Although the severity of disease may demand treatment with cyclophosphamide, the patient may be rendered infertile by the drug.[94]

Infections are easily acquired during cyclophosphamide therapy, particularly after a surgical procedure.[121] Patients should be carefully watched while being treated with this drug for any evidence of infection.

The major dermatologic use of cyclophosphamide is for the treatment of autoimmune diseases. Pemphigus vulgaris in particular may be treated with cyclophosphamide in combination with prednisone.[96,122] Cyclophosphamide is usually believed to be more effective than azathioprine, although no controlled studies have been performed. Typical regimens are usually in the range of 0.5 to 1 mg/kg per day.

A major enhancement in the survival of patients with systemic vasculitis was seen with the introduction of combined steroid/cytotoxic therapy.[100,101] Diseases that were quickly lethal in the past are now controllable with such therapy. For example, the 5-year survival of patients with polyarteritis nodosa is 13 percent if the condition is untreated, 48 percent if it is treated with steroid therapy, and 90 percent if cyclophosphamide and prednisone are combined.[100,123,124] Typical doses for systemic vasculitis are 1 mg/kg per day for prednisone and 2 mg/kg per day for cyclophosphamide. Steroids are converted to an alternate-day regimen and tapered over 3 to 6 months. Cyclophosphamide is maintained for 1 year and then gradually tapered.[100,101] Resistant disease may be treated with higher doses or intravenous pulse therapy.[125]

Granulomatous vasculitis is best treated with combination therapy as well. Wegener's granulomatosis[126] and lymphomatoid granulomatosis[125,127] often require cyclophosphamide therapy for sustained remission.

Other diseases may also respond to cyclophosphamide, including Behçet's disease,[128] pyoderma gangrenosum,[129] lichen planus,[130] and lichen myxedematosus. With the availability of cyclosporine, however, cyclophosphamide may not be the drug of choice for such resistant but nonlethal inflammatory disease.

Nitrogen Mustard (Mechlorethamine)

Like cyclophosphamide, nitrogen mustard is an alkylating agent that interferes with growth in all stages of the cell cycle. The primary target of mustards is the 7-nitrogen atom of guanine, although other bases may also be alkylated.[131]

In dermatologic practice nitrogen mustard is used exclusively as a topical preparation. In high concentrations topical mustard is a vesicant and has been used in warfare. Lower concentrations are very well tolerated and of great clinical benefit in certain situations. Systemic absorption is trivial and systemic side effects are not seen.

The side effects of topical mustard are limited to the skin. Over one-half of patients on long-term treatment develop delayed hypersensitivity to the drug,[132] which is usually manifested as erythema and pruritus. If an erythematous, itchy skin disease is being treated, drug hypersensitivity may be detected through careful monitoring of new symptoms. When hypersensitivity develops, the physician has several options: discontinuation of therapy, ten- to fiftyfold dilution of the mustard preparation, or suppression of hypersensitivity with topical corticosteroids and/or UV irradiation. This last method may be particularly useful since PUVA therapy is known to deplete epidermal Langerhans cells. In support of this method is the observation that UV therapy can delay development of contact sensitization to mustard.[133] An organized study of the effects of irradiation on established sensitivity is warranted.

The other major side effect of topical nitrogen mustard is the induction of skin cancers.[134-136] These neoplasms usually occur in sun-exposed areas and are said to be due to the so-called radiomimetic effect of nitrogen mustard. This drug can act in the same manner as UV radiation in inducing usually low-grade, nonmelanoma skin cancers. The risk of squamous cell cancers and basal cell cancers increases 8.6- and 1.8-fold, respectively, after use of topical nitrogen mustard. In the opinion of the authors, the risk posed by such easily treated lesions is far outweighed by the overall benefits of the drug when used appropriately.

An important and reasonably well-resolved issue is whether the increased incidence of second hematologic malignancies and colon cancer in patients with mycosis fungoides is due to topical mechlorethamine. Since high-dose systemic mechlorethamine is not associated with these other malignancies, Vonderheid and associates have suggested that second internal malignancies reflect an underlying defect in the patients.[137,138]

The major dermatologic application of topical mustard is in the treatment of mycosis fungoides.[132,137-140] Although topical corticosteroid preparations and UV radiation, e.g., PUVA, may provide significant symptomatic relief, there is no certainty that these modalities actually alter the course of this indolent lymphoma. Topical mustard appears to be capable of inducing complete remission in at least 11 percent of patients.[137] The likelihood of complete remission is enhanced in patients in whom therapy with topical mechlorethamine begins in the early stage of mycosis fungoides.

It is usually assumed that topical nitrogen mustard is exerting cytotoxic effects in suppressing mycosis fungoides, but more may be involved. It is possible that induction of delayed hypersensitivity by the drug may call for the influx of immunoregulatory cells that limit the lymphoma by biologic means.

Topical mustard is usually dispensed either as an aqueous solution or an ointment preparation. Routinely, the contents of a 10-mg vial are rehydrated with 60 mL of tap water and promptly applied with a gauze to the entire body surface. Unused preparation may be stored in the refrigerator for up to 6 months. Extreme care must be taken to ensure that the nitrogen mustard is not inadvertantly swallowed by unknowing individuals. Aqueous preparations may prove to be more prone to sensitize patients. Definitive studies of this possibility have yet to be reported. An alternative preparation can be made by dissolving the mustard in anhydrous petrolatum. Although this method is economical, there is the potential risk of a toxic preparation being misused by individuals other than the patient.

Topical nitrogen mustard has also been used with some success in the treatment of psoriasis,[141] alopecia areata,[142] papular mucinosis (unpublished results), and histiocytosis X.[143]

References

1. Jolivet J et al: The pharmacology and clinical use of methotrexate. *N Engl J Med* **309**:1094, 1983

2. American Hospital Formulary Service: *Drug Information* **91**:584, 1991

3. Jolivet J et al: The synthesis and retention of methotrexate polyglutamates in cultured human breast cancer cells. *Ann NY Acad Sci* **397**:184, 1982

4. Anderson PA et al: Weekly pulse methotrexate in rheumatoid arthritis. *Ann Intern Med* **103**:489, 1985

5. Weinblatt ME et al: Long term prospective study of methotrexate in rheumatoid arthritis. *Arthritis Rheum* **29**(suppl):s76, 1986

6. Olsen NJ et al: Immunologic studies of rheumatoid arthritis patients treated with methotrexate. *Arthritis Rheum* **30**:481, 1987

7. O'Callaghan JW et al: The effect of low dose chronic intermittent parenteral methotrexate on delayed type hypersensitivity and acute inflammation in a mouse model. *J Rheumatol* **13**:710, 1986

8. Lammers AM et al: Reduction of LTB$_4$-induced intraepidermal accumulation of polymorphonuclear leukocytes by methotrexate in psoriasis. *Br J Dermatol* **116**:667, 1987

9. Ternowitz T, Herlin T: Neutrophil and monocyte chemotaxis in methotrexate treated psoriasis patients. *Acta Derm Venereol (Stockh)* **120**:23, 1985

10. Cream JJ, Pole DS: The effect of methotrexate and hydroxyurea on neutrophil chemotaxis. *Br J Dermatol* **102**:557, 1980

11. Gommans JM et al: Flow cytometric quantification of T6-positive cells in psoriatic epidermis after PUVA and methotrexate therapy. *Br J Dermatol* **116**:661, 1987

12. Weinstein GD, Frost P: Methotrexate for psoriasis: A new therapeutic approach. *Arch Dermatol* **103**:33, 1971

13. Newton JA et al: Study of psoriatic epidermal cell kinetics and cell death after oral methotrexate. *Dermatologica* **171**:469, 1985

14. Weinstein GD et al: Topical methotrexate therapy in psoriasis. *Arch Dermatol* **125**:227, 1989

15. Furst DE: Clinical pharmacology of very low dose methotrexate for use in rheumatoid arthritis. *J Rheumatol* **12**(suppl):11, 1985

16. Pinkerton DR et al: Can food influence absorption of methotrexate in children with acute lymphoblastic leukemia? *Lancet* **2**:944, 1980

17. Halprin KM et al: Blood levels of methotrexate in the treatment of psoriasis. *Arch Dermatol* **103**:243, 1971

18. Furst DE, Kremer JM: Methotrexate in rheumatoid arthritis. *Arthritis Rheum* **31**:305, 1988

19. Wan SH et al: Effect of route of administration and effusions on methotrexate pharmacokinetics. *Cancer Res* **34**:3487, 1974

20. Edelman J et al: Low dose methotrexate kinetics in arthritis. *Clin Pharmacol Ther* **35**:382, 1984

21. Hanrahan PS, Russell AS: Concurrent use of folinic acid and methotrexate in rheumatoid arthritis. *J Rheumatol* **15**:1078, 1988

22. Taylor JR, Halprin KM: Effect of sodium salicylate and indomethacin on methotrexate-serum albumin binding. *Arch Dermatol* **113**:558, 1977

23. Liegler DG et al: The effect of organic acids on renal clearance of methotrexate in man. *Clin Pharmacol Ther* **10**:849, 1969

24. Nierenberg DW: Competitive inhibition of methotrexate accumulation in rabbit kidney slices by non-steroidal anti-inflammatory drugs. *J Pharmacol Exp Ther* **226**:1, 1983

25. Beach BJ et al: Influence of co-trimoxizole on methotrexate pharmacokinetics in children with acute lymphoblastic leukemia. *Am J Pediatr Hematol Oncol* **2**:115, 1981

26. Evans WE, Christensen ML: Drug interactions with methotrexate. *J Rheumatol* **12**(suppl):15, 1985

27. Hendwel J, Nyfors A: Nonlinear renal elimination kinetics of methotrexate due to saturation of renal tubular reabsorption. *Eur J Clin Pharmacol* **26**:121, 1984

28. Weinblatt ME: Toxicity of low-dose methotrexate in rheumatoid arthritis. *J Rheumatol* **12**(suppl):35, 1985

29. Roenigk HH et al: Methotrexate in psoriasis: Revised guidelines. *J Am Acad Dermatol* **19**:146, 1988

30. Weinblatt ME, Kremer JE: Methotrexate in rheumatoid arthritis. *J Am Acad Dermatol* **19**:126, 1988

31. Coe RO, Bull FE: Cirrhosis associated with methotrexate treatment of psoriasis. *JAMA* **206**:1515, 1968

32. Zachariae H et al: Methotrexate-induced liver cirrhosis: Studies including serial liver biopsies during continued treatment. *Br J Dermatol* **102**:407, 1980

33. Zachariae H, Sogaard H: Methotrexate-induced liver cirrhosis: A follow-up. *Dermatologica* **175**:178, 1987

34. Roenigk HH et al: Hepatotoxicity of methotrexate in the treatment of psoriasis. *Arch Dermatol* **103**:250, 1971

35. Geronemus RG et al: Liver biopsies vs. liver scan in methotrexate-treated patients with psoriasis. *Arch Dermatol* **118**:649, 1982

36. Rademaker M et al: Magnetic resonance imaging as a screening procedure for methotrexate-induced liver damage. *Br J Dermatol* **117**:311, 1987

37. Mitchell D et al: Ultrasound and radionuclide scans poor indicators of liver damage in patients treated with methotrexate. *Clin Exp Dermatol* **12**:243, 1987

38. Tugwell P et al: Methotrexate in rheumatoid arthritis. *Ann Intern Med* **110**:581, 1989

39. Shupack JL, Webster GF: Pancytopenia following low-dose oral methotrexate therapy for psoriasis. *JAMA* **259**:3594, 1988

40. MacKinnon SK et al: Pancytopenia associated with low-dose pulse methotrexate therapy in rheumatoid arthritis. *Semin Arthritis Rheum* **15**:119, 1985

41. Maricic M et al: Megaloblastic pancytopenia in a patient receiving concurrent methotrexate and trimethoprim-sulfamethoxazole treatments. *Arthritis Rheum* **29**:133, 1986

42. Thomas DR et al: Pancytopenia induced by the interaction between methotrexate and trimethoprim-sulfamethoxazole treatments. *J Am Acad Dermatol* **17**:1055, 1987

43. Stern RS et al: Methotrexate for psoriasis and the risk of cutaneous and non-cutaneous malignancy. *Cancer* **50**:869, 1982

44. Nyfors A, Jense H: Frequency of malignant neoplasm in 248 long-term methotrexate treated psoriatics. *Dermatologica* **167**:260, 1983

45. Grunnet E et al: Studies on human semen in topical corticosteroid treated and in methotrexate treated psoriatics. *Dermatologica* **154**:78, 1977

46. Sussman A, Leonard JM: Psoriasis, methotrexate and oligospermia. *Arch Dermatol* **116**:215, 1980

47. Krough-Jensen M, Nyfors A: Cytogenic effect of methotrexate on human cells in vivo: Comparison between results obtained by chromosome studies on bone marrow cells and blood lymphocytes and by the micronucleus test. *Mutat Res* **64**:339, 1979

48. Peckham PE et al: The treatment of severe psoriasis. A national survey. *Arch Dermatol* **123**:1303, 1987

49. Gubner R: Therapeutic suppression of tissue reactivity. II. Effect of aminopterin in rheumatoid arthritis and psoriasis. *Am J Med Sci* **122**:176, 1951

50. Weinstein GD: Three decades of folic acid antagonists in dermatology. *Arch Dermatol* **119**:525, 1983

51. Weinstein GD, Frost P: Abnormal cell proliferation in psoriasis. *J Invest Dermatol* **50**:254, 1968

52. Weinstein GD, Frost P: Methotrexate for psoriasis, a new therapeutic approach. *Arch Dermatol* **103**:33, 1971

53. Ryan TJ, Baker H: Systemic corticosteroids and folic acid antagonists in the treatment of generalized pustular psoriasis: Evaluation and prognosis based on the study of 104 cases. *Br J Dermatol* **81**:134, 1969

54. Rosenbaum MM, Roenigk HH Jr: Treatment of generalized pustular psoriasis with etretinate (Ro-10-9359) and methotrexate. *J Am Acad Dermatol* **12**:357, 1984

55. Kragballe KE et al: Methotrexate in psoriatic arthritis, a retrospective study. *Acta Derm Venereol (Stockh)* **63**:165, 1983

56. Wilkins RF et al: Randomized double-blind placebo-controlled trial of methotrexate in psoriatic arthritis. *Arthritis Rheum* **27**:376, 1984

57. Lally EV, Ho GA: A review of methotrexate therapy in Reiter's syndrome. *Semin Arthritis Rheum* **15**:139, 1985

58. Winchester R et al: The co-occurrence of Reiter's syndrome and acquired immunodeficiency. *Ann Intern Med* **106**:19, 1987

59. Duvic M et al: Acquired immunodeficiency associated Reiter's syndrome and psoriasis. *Arch Dermatol* **123**:1622, 1987

60. Veien NK, Brodthagen H: Treatment of sarcoidosis with methotrexate. *Br J Dermatol* **97**:213, 1977

61. Webster GF et al: Methotrexate therapy in cutaneous sarcoidosis. *Ann Intern Med* **111**:538, 1990

62. Roenigk HH: Pityriasis lichenoides et varioliformis acuta (Mucha-Haberman). *Arch Dermatol* **104**:102, 1971

63. Lynch PJ, Saied NK: Methotrexate treatment of pityriasis lichenoides and lymphomatoid papulosis. *Cutis* **23**:634, 1979

64. Everett MA: Treatment of lymphomatoid papulosis with methotrexate. *Br J Dermatol* **111**:631, 1984

65. Wantzin GL, Thomsen K: Methotrexate in lymphomatoid papulosis. *Br J Dermatol* **111**:93, 1984

66. Brown J, Perry HO: Pityriasis rubra pilaris treatment with folic acid antagonists. *Arch Dermatol* **94**:636, 1966

67. Knowles WR, Chernosky ME: Pityriasis rubra pilaris: Prolonged treatment with methotrexate. *Arch Dermatol* **102**:603, 1970

68. Hanke CW, Steck WD: Childhood-onset pityriasis rubra pilaris treated with methotrexate administered intravenously. *Cleve Clin Q* **50**:201, 1983

69. Capizzi RL, Berlino JR: Methotrexate treatment of Wegener's granulomatosis. *Ann Intern Med* **74**:74, 1971

70. Church KS et al: Low-dose methotrexate therapy for cutaneous vasculitis of rheumatoid arthritis. *J Am Acad Dermatol* **17**:355, 1987

71. Espinoza LR et al: Oral methotrexate therapy for chronic rheumatoid arthritis ulcerations. *J Am Acad Dermatol* **15**:508, 1986

72. Fischer TJ et al: Childhood dermatomyositis and polymyositis: Treatment with methotrexate and prednisone. *Am J Dis Child* **133**:386, 1979

73. Wallace DJ et al: Combined immunosuppressive treatment of steroid resistant dermatomyositis/polymyositis. *Arthritis Rheum* **28**:590, 1985

74. Arnett FC et al: Methotrexate therapy of polymyositis. *Ann Rheum Dis* **52**:536, 1973

75. Tuffanelli DL, Lavoie PE: Prognosis and therapy of polymyositis and dermatomyositis. *Clin Dermatol* **6**:93, 1988

76. Lever WF: Methotrexate and prednisone in pemphigus vulgaris. *Arch Dermatol* **106**:491, 1972

77. Lever WF, Goldberg S: Treatment of pemphigus vulgaris with methotrexate. *Arch Dermatol* **100**:70, 1970

78. Rothenberg RJ et al: The use of methotrexate in steroid resistant systemic lupus erythematosus. *Arthritis Rheum* **31**:612, 1988

79. Nashel DJ: Mechanisms of action and clinical applications of cytotoxic drugs in rheumatic disorders. *Med Clin North Am* **69**:817, 1985

80. Bickers D et al: Cytotoxic and immunosuppressive agents, in *Clinical Pharmacology of Skin Disease*, edited by D Bickers et al. New York, Churchill Livingstone, 1984, chap 5

81. Ahmed AR, Moy R: Azathioprine. *Int J Dermatol* **20**:461, 1981

82. Chabner BA, Myers CE: Clinical pharmacology of cancer chemotherapy, in *Principles and Practices of Oncology*, 2d ed, edited by VT DeVita et al. Philadelphia, Lippincott, 1985, p 287

83. Lee MH et al: Alkaline phosphate activities of 6-thiopurine-sensitive and -resistant sublines of sarcoma 180. *Cancer Res* **38**:2413, 1978

84. Ping TL, Benet LZ: Determination of 6-mercaptopurine and azathioprine in plasma by HPLC. *J Chromatogr* **145**:237, 1978

85. Lennard L et al: Pharmacogenetics of acute azathioprine toxicity: Relationship to thiopurine methyltransferase genetic polymorphism. *Clin Pharmacol Ther* **46**:149, 1989

86. Bacon BR et al: Azathioprine induced pancytopenia: Occurrence in two patients with connective tissue diseases. *Arch Intern Med* **141**:223, 1981

87. Drugs for rheumatoid arthritis. *Med Lett Drugs Ther* **31**:61, 1989

88. Kawamski H: Azathioprine induced pancreatitis. *N Engl J Med* **289**:357, 1973

89. McKendry RJ, Cyr M: Toxicity of methotrexate compared with azathioprine in the treatment of rheumatoid arthritis. *Arch Intern Med* **149**:685, 1989

90. Singh G et al: Toxic effects of azathioprine in rheumatoid arthritis. *Arthritis Rheum* **32**:837, 1989

91. Collision DW et al: Azathioprine hypersensitivity in bullous pemphigoid. *J Clin Acad Dermatol* **23**:125, 1990

92. Lipsky BA, Hirschman JV: Drug fever, *JAMA* **245**:851, 1981

93. Silman AJ et al: Lymphoproliferative cancer and other malignancy in patients with rheumatoid arthritis treated with azathioprine. *Ann Rheum Dis* **47**:988, 1988

94. Roubenoff R et al: Effect of anti-inflammatory and immunosuppressive drugs on pregnancy and fertility. *Semin Arthritis Rheum* **18**:88, 1988

95. Wolff K, Schreiner E: Immunosuppressive therapy for pemphigus vulgaris. *Arch Klin Exp Dermatol* **235**:63, 1969

96. Bystryn JC: Adjuvant therapy for pemphigus. *Arch Dermatol* **120**:941, 1984

97. Aberer W et al: Azathioprine in the treatment of pemphigus vulgaris. *J Am Acad Dermatol* **16**:527, 1987

98. Pawlofsky C et al: Disseminated cicatricial pemphigoid. *Dermatologica* **171**:259, 1985

99. Korman N: Bullous pemphigoid. *J Am Acad Dermatol* **16**:907, 1987

100. Leavitt RY, Fauci AS: Therapeutic approach to the vasculitic syndromes. *Mt Sinai J Med* **53**:440, 1986

101. Leavitt RY, Fauci AS: Pulmonary vasculitis. *Am Rev Respir Dis* **134**:149, 1986

102. Felson DT, Anderson J: Evidence for the superiority of immunosuppressive drugs and prednisone over prednisone alone in lupus nephritis. *N Engl J Med* **311**:1528, 1984

103. Bunch TW: Prednisone and azathioprine for polymyositis. *Arthritis Rheum* **24**:45, 1981

104. Castro JL et al: Successful treatment of a musk ambrette-sensitive persistent light reactor with azathioprine. *Photodermatology* **3**:241, 1986

105. Murphy GM et al: Azathioprine treatment in chronic actinic dermatitis—a double-blind controlled trial with monitoring of exposure to ultraviolet radiation. *Br J Dermatol* **121**:639, 1989

106. Breza T et al: Noninflammatory destruction of actinic keratoses by fluorouracil. *Arch Dermatol* **112**:1258, 1976

107. Mohs FE et al: Tendency of fluorouracil to conceal deep foci of invasive basal cell carcinoma. *Arch Dermatol* **114**:1021, 1978

108. Odom RB, Goette DK: Treatment of keratoacanthomas with intralesional 5 fluorouracil. *Arch Dermatol* **114**:1779, 1978

109. Dupre A, Cvistol B: Mibelli's porokeratosis of the lips. *Arch Dermatol* **114**:1841, 1978

110. Lockshin NA: Flat facial warts treated with 5-fluorouracil. *Arch Dermatol* **115**:929, 1979

111. Gromet MA: Treatment of lentigo maligna with 5-FU. *Arch Dermatol* **113**:1128, 1977

112. Leavell VW, Yarborough JM: Hydroxyurea: A new treatment for psoriasis. *Arch Dermatol* **102**:144, 1970

113. Moschella SC, Greenwald MA: Treatment of psoriasis with hydroxyurea—an 18-month study of 60 patients. *Arch Dermatol* **107**:363, 1973

114. Fosdick WM et al: Long term cyclophosphamide therapy in rheumatoid arthritis. *Arthritis Rheum* **11**:151, 1968
115. Baker GL et al: Malignancy following treatment of rheumatoid arthritis with cyclophosphamide. *Am J Med* **83**:1, 1987
116. Cox PJ: Cyclophosphamide cystitis—identification of acrolein as the causative agent. *Biochem Pharmacol* **28**:2045, 1979
117. Townes AS et al: Controlled trial of cyclophosphamide in rheumatoid arthritis. *Arthritis Rheum* **19**:563, 1976
118. Wall RL, Clausen KP: Carcinoma of the urinary bladder in patients receiving cyclophosphamide. *N Engl J Med* **293**:771, 1975
119. Plotz PH et al: Bladder complications in patients receiving cyclophosphamide for systemic lupus erythematosus or rheumatoid arthritis. *Ann Intern Med* **91**:221, 1979
120. Pedersen-Bjergaard J et al: Carcinomas of the urinary bladder after treatment with cyclophosphamide for non-Hodgkin's lymphoma. *N Engl J Med* **318**:1028, 1988
121. Bradley JD et al: Infectious complications of cyclophosphamide treatment for vasculitis. *Arthritis Rheum* **32**:45, 1989
122. Ahmed AR, Hombal S: Use of cyclophosphamide in azathioprine failures in pemphigus. *J Am Acad Dermatol* **17**:437, 1987
123. Grohnert PP, Sheps SG: Long-term follow-up study of periarteritis nodosa. *Am J Med* **43**:8, 1967
124. Fort JG, Abruzzo JL: Reversal of progressive necrotizing vasculitis with intravenous pulse cyclophosphamide and methylprednisolone. *Arthritis Rheum* **31**:1194, 1988
125. Jenkins TR, Zaloswick AJ: Lymphomatoid granulomatosis—a case for aggressive therapy. *Cancer* **64**:1362, 1989
126. Fauci AS et al: Wegener's granulomatosis—prospective clinical and therapeutic experience with 85 patients for 21 years. *Ann Intern Med* **98**:76, 1983
127. Jambrosic J et al: Lymphomatoid granulomatosis. *J Am Acad Dermatol* **17**:621, 1987
128. Fauci AS et al: Cyclophosphamide therapy of severe systemic necrotizing vasculitis. *N Engl J Med* **301**:235, 1979
129. Newell LM, Malkinson FD: Pyoderma gangrenosum response to cyclophosphamide therapy. *Arch Dermatol* **119**:493, 1983
130. Paslin DA: Sustained remission of generalized lichen planus induced by cyclophosphamide. *Arch Dermatol* **121**:236, 1985
131. Calabresi P, Chabner BA: Chemotherapy of neoplastic disease, in *The Pharmacological Basis of Therapeutics,* 8th ed, edited by AG Gillman. New York, Pergamon, 1990, p 1209
132. Ramsay DL et al: Topical mechlorethamine therapy for early stage mycosis fungoides. *J Am Acad Dermatol* **19**:684, 1988
133. Halprin KM et al: Ultraviolet light treatment delays contact sensitization to nitrogen mustard. *Br J Dermatol* **105**:71, 1981
134. duVivier A et al: Mycosis fungoides, nitrogen mustard and skin cancer. *Br J Dermatol* **99**:61, 1978
135. Kravitz PH, McDonald CJ: Topical nitrogen mustard-induced carcinogenesis. *Acta Derm Venereol (Stockh)* **58**:421, 1978
136. Lee LA et al: Second cutaneous malignancies in patients with mycosis fungoides treated with nitrogen mustard. *J Am Acad Dermatol* **7**:590, 1982
137. Vonderheid EC et al: Long-term efficacy, curative potential and carcinogenicity of topical mechlorethamine chemotherapy in cutaneous T-cell lymphoma. *J Am Acad Dermatol* **20**:416, 1989
138. Vonderheid EC et al: Topical chemotherapy and immunotherapy of mycosis fungoides. *Arch Dermatol* **113**:454, 1977
139. Price NM et al: Topical mechlorethamine therapy for mycosis fungoides. *Br J Dermatol* **97**:547, 1977
140. Price NM et al: Ointment-based mechlorethamine treatment for mycosis fungoides. *Cancer* **52**:2214, 1983
141. Handler RM, Medansky RS: Treatment of psoriasis with topical nitrogen mustard. *Int J Dermatol* **18**:758, 1979
142. Arrazola JM et al: Treatment of alopecia areata using topical nitrogen mustard. *Int J Dermatol* **24**:608, 1985
143. Berman B et al: Histiocytosis X treated with topical nitrogen mustard. *J Am Acad Dermatol* **3**:23, 1980

CHAPTER 236

Gary L. Peck and John J. DiGiovanna*

Retinoids

Vitamin A is a necessary dietary nutrient that is important in growth, vision, reproduction, and the maintenance and differentiation of epithelial tissue for all vertebrates. The term *vitamin A* is used to characterize the biologic activity of this group of compounds rather than a particular compound. In mammals, vitamin A activity is fulfilled by three major compounds, retinol, retinal, and retinoic acid, and perhaps by some of their metabolites. The term *retinoid* refers to the entire group of compounds that includes retinol and its naturally occurring and synthetic derivatives.

The molecular mechanisms of retinoid action are undergoing intensive investigation. Two recent advances have led to a better appreciation of the scope of retinoid influence over the processes of growth and differentiation and the mechanisms through which this control might be effected. Retinoic acid is the first identified compound with the characteristics of a vertebrate morphogen. A morphogen is a substance whose concentration varies in a developing

embryo, and which the developing cells use to determine their relative position in a tissue or organ. Much of this work has been done in the chick embryo limb. In this system, retinoic acid may be a morphogen that is responsible for the three-dimensional organization of the developing vertebrate limb bud. In another significant advance, a group of high-affinity retinoic acid receptors has been discovered that act in the nucleus by binding to specific DNA regulatory sequences. These retinoic acid receptors are considered important regulatory proteins responsible for retinoid control of cell growth and differentiation.

Historical Perspective

Awareness of therapies containing vitamin A activity can be traced back to the ancient Egyptians (ca. 1500 B.C.), as evidenced by writings describing the benefits of liver as a treatment of night blindness.[1] In 1909, a fat-soluble extract from egg yolk was found to be necessary for life.[2] McCollum and Davis later used the term

*This chapter was written by John J. DiGiovanna, M.D., in his private capacity. No official support or endorsement by the National Cancer Institute is intended or should be inferred.

fat-soluble factor A for a dietary component that was important for the normal growth of animals.[3-5] The active factor "A" was associated with yellow vegetables[6] as well as with animal fats and fish oils and was subsequently named vitamin A.[7]

In 1931, vitamin A (retinol) was purified from halibut liver oil and its structural formula was determined.[8,9] In 1935, another vitamin A derivative, later identified to be retinal, was demonstrated by Wald to be important in the visual cycle.[10,11] In 1946, vitamin A acid (retinoic acid) was synthesized and shown to promote growth.[12]

Vitamin A was first used clinically during World War I in the treatment of xerophthalmia and in the prevention of night blindness. The significance of retinoids to dermatology dates back to Wolbach and Howe in 1925, when epithelial changes were identified in vitamin A-deficient animals; low levels of vitamin A were thereby related to dyskeratotic skin conditions.[13,14] Systemic vitamin A was then used clinically in the treatment of disorders such as Darier's disease and pityriasis rubra pilaris, in which follicular keratoses resemble the lesions of vitamin A deficiency.[15,16] Once the beneficial effects of vitamin A were observed in these disorders, its use spread to the treatment of other diseases of the epidermis and epidermal appendages.

Vitamin A deficiency provides a conceptual link in understanding how retinoids may be effective as therapy for a wide range of dermatologic disorders. Vitamin A deficiency is characterized by squamous metaplasia of a variety of epithelia with increased cell proliferation and hyperkeratosis, features common to many skin diseases, such as psoriasis. Vitamin A was initially related to cancer in 1926 when rats fed a vitamin A-deficient diet were found to develop carcinomas of the stomach.[17]

All-*trans* retinoic acid (tretinoin), a naturally occurring metabolite of retinol, has been used clinically in the treatment of pityriasis rubra pilaris, various ichthyoses, psoriasis, acne, and actinic keratoses.[18-20] This compound is currently accepted as standard topical therapy for acne vulgaris. Early experience with the systemic use of tretinoin was limited by its toxicity.[21]

In an effort to develop compounds that might possess a better therapeutic index than retinol or retinoic acid in the prophylaxis and treatment of cancer, a group of synthetic derivatives of retinoic acid were synthesized and developed for clinical use beginning in 1968.[22] Many chemical variations of the ring structure, the carboxylic end group, and the side chain of the retinoic acid molecule are possible.[23] More than 2000 analogues have been synthesized. Although many of them have been tested in various in vivo and in vitro models, only a few have been used in clinical trials. At present, two synthetic retinoids of appreciably different action spectra, pharmacokinetics, and side effects (Table 236-1) are commercially available: 13-*cis* retinoic acid (isotretinoin) and the trimethylmethoxyphenyl analogue of retinoic acid ethyl ester (etretinate). 13-*cis* Retinoic acid is a naturally occurring metabolite of vitamin A found in tissues in small quantities[24]; however, its usefulness in dermatology evolved before this was known. With the dramatic

response of several previously treatment-resistant dermatoses (severe cystic acne, psoriasis, and many of the disorders of keratinization) and the wide spectrum of benign and malignant conditions noted to be partially responsive, the retinoids have ushered in a new era in the therapy of skin disease.

The ability of all-*trans* retinoic acid to induce differentiation of a promyelocytic leukemia cell line (HL-60) to form granulocytic cells that are morphologically more normal and capable of phagocytosis has been known for some time,[25] but the dramatic effect on patients with acute promyelocytic leukemia has only recently received worldwide attention.[26] The profound response has recently stimulated the investigation of retinoids alone and in conjunction with other agents (e.g., interferons) for the treatment of malignancies.

Retinoid Structures and Functions

The structures and functions of the major naturally occurring retinoids are outlined in Fig. 236-1. Vitamin A is necessary for growth, differentiation, the maintenance of epithelial tissues, and reproduction. Retinol can be reversibly oxidized to retinal, the aldehyde derivative that is important in vision. Retinoic acid is an important oxidative metabolite of retinol that can substitute for some vitamin A functions. In vitamin A-deficient animals, retinoic acid can replace retinol in supporting growth promotion and in the maintenance and differentiation of epithelial tissues. Retinoic acid, however, cannot substitute for retinol in maintaining reproductive function nor for retinal in the visual cycle.

Retinoid Uptake: Dietary Intake, Serum Transport and Delivery to Target Cells

The pathway traveled by the naturally occurring retinoids from dietary precursors through absorption, serum transport, storage, and delivery to target cells is diagrammed in Fig. 236-2.[27] Retinoids are derived from retinyl esters contained in dietary animal sources (fats, fish liver oils) and from carotenoids in yellow and green leafy vegetables. Ingested retinyl esters are hydrolyzed in the intestine, leaving free retinol to be absorbed into the mucosal cells. Alternatively, a range of carotenoids can act as retinoid precursors with the most common and efficient precursor being all-*trans* beta-carotene. The dietary beta-carotene that gives rise to retinoid that the body can use is not absorbed directly, but rather as retinyl esters.[28] In the gut, carotenoids undergo oxidative cleavage of the central double bond by the action of beta-carotene-15,15'-dioxygenase to yield retinal. In the intestinal mucosa, the retinal is reduced by retinaldehyde reductase to retinol, the alcohol form.[29] The conversion of ingested carotenoid to retinoid is under physiologic control. When

TABLE 236-1
Oral Synthetic Retinoids

Generic name	Chemical name	Trade name	Principal indications	Other indications for both retinoids
Isotretinoin	13-*cis*-Retinoic acid	Accutane (USA) Roaccutane (Europe)	Cystic acne	Darier's disease Pityriasis rubra pilaris
Etretinate	Trimethylmethoxyphenyl analogue of retinoic acid ethyl ester	Tegison (USA) Tigason (other than USA)	Psoriasis	Lamellar ichthyosis, etc.

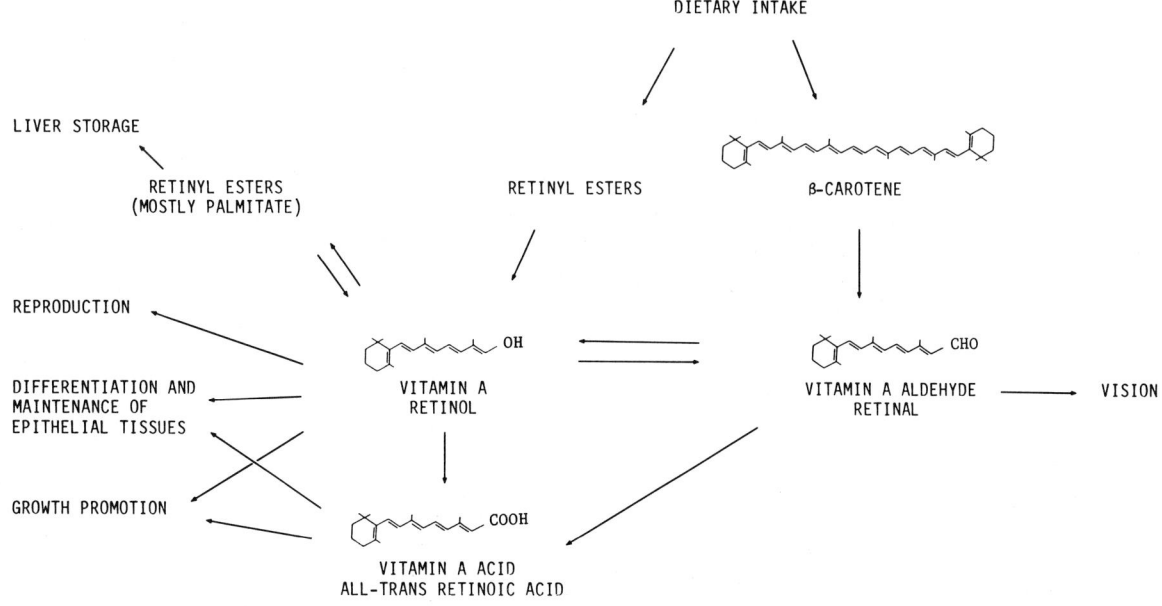

FIGURE 236-1 Structures and functions of the major naturally occurring retinoids. (*Adapted with permission from Pawson et al.*[27] *Copyright 1982, American Chemical Society.*)

large amounts of carotenoids are ingested, they are absorbed as carotenoids. Although this may lead to carotenemia and a characteristic yellow-orange skin color, it is not associated with symptoms of hypervitaminosis A.

In the intestinal cell, free retinol is then esterified (mainly as retinyl palmitate), complexed with long-chain fatty acids into chylomicrons, and transported through the lymph and then into the blood to the liver. In the liver, retinol is stored in the ester form in

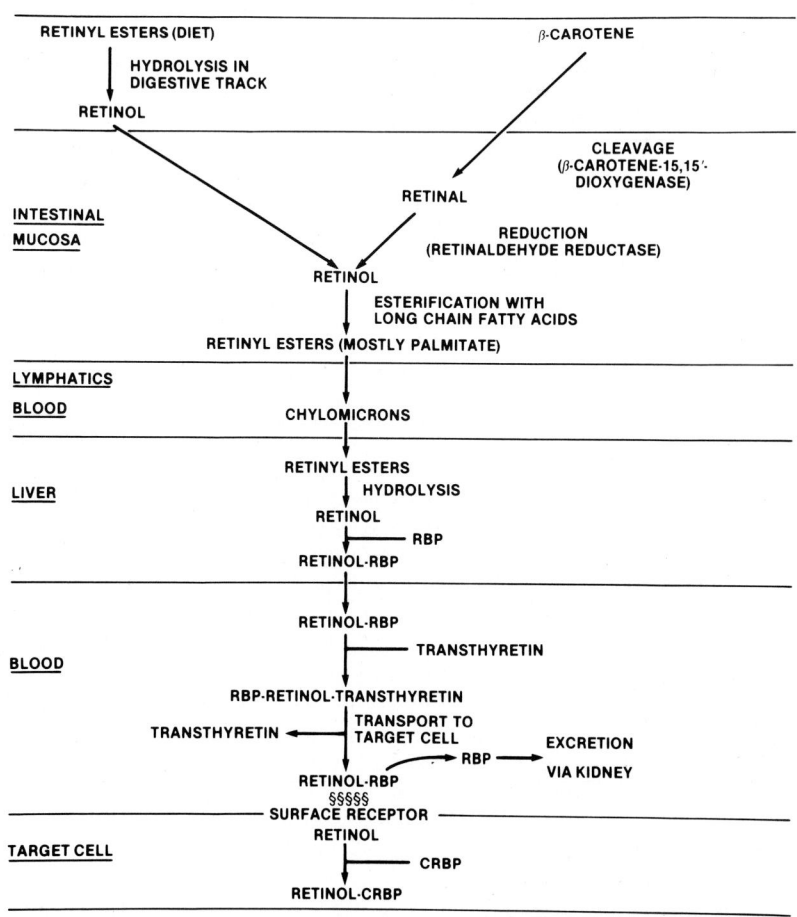

FIGURE 236-2 Retinoid uptake, storage, serum transport, and delivery to target tissues. (*Adapted with permission from Pawson et al.*[27] *Copyright 1982, American Chemical Society.*)

a small number of fat-storing, stellate cells called *vitamin A storage or Ito cells*.[30] Upon demand the ester is hydrolyzed to the free alcohol and complexed with its transport protein, the serum retinol binding protein (RBP),[31] which is synthesized in the liver.[32] Free retinol is not released from the liver unbound, but only in a 1:1 ratio with RBP.

Upon release from the liver, the RBP-retinol complex binds to prealbumin, a serum protein that has been termed *transthyretin* (TTR) to signify its role as a transport protein for both thyroxin and the RBP-retinol complex. Thyroxin is bound to TTR at a site that is independent from the RBP-retinol binding site. In the blood, retinol circulates as a complex of RBP-retinol-TTR.

On the molecular level, retinol arrives at a target cell bound to the serum RBP transport protein. The RBP-retinol complex binds to specific membrane receptors of target cells. These membrane receptors interact with the RBP-retinol complex but not to either free retinol or RBP. Retinol is then translocated into the cell. A specific cytosol binding protein [cellular retinol binding protein (CRBP)] for retinol is present within target cells. This intracellular binding protein is distinct from the serum transport protein (RBP) and binds specifically and saturably to retinol. Its exact function is not known.

All-*trans* retinoic acid is not a normal dietary constitutent. When administered, this compound is not absorbed via the lymphatics in association with lipoproteins like retinol, but is absorbed directly into the portal blood.[33] In addition, it does not bind to RBP but circulates in the serum bound to albumin.[34] Retinoic acid also has a specific intracellular binding protein, the cellular retinoic acid binding protein (CRABP). The functions of CRBP and CRABP are not known, but they may act as molecular sponges, to bind excess retinoid, thereby protecting the cell from toxic effects.

In addition to the cytosol binding proteins, a second group of retinoic acid receptors has been identified that resemble the group of steroid hormone receptors. These proteins are believed to act in the nucleus by binding to specific DNA regulatory sequences and thereby activating specific sets of genes.

Vitamin A is transported in the serum as all-*trans* retinol and that is the form that is presented to target cells. But once inside a cell, retinol must often be converted to other metabolites before it is physiologically active. For example, in the eye, retinol must be converted to retinal before it can react with opsin and function in the visual process.

Retinoid Metabolism

Although the active tissue metabolites and the mechanisms of vitamin A degradation and removal from epithelial tissues are not known, a number of retinoid metabolites have been identified. A small amount of retinoic acid is formed from retinol in tissues, and this is quickly converted to other metabolites.[35] The conversion of retinol to retinoic acid can occur in epidermis.[36] 13-*cis* Retinoic acid itself has potent biologic effects, but even further metabolic products of 13-*cis* retinoic acid have been identified. The identification of a series of nuclear receptors raises the possibility that a variety of retinoid metabolites may interact with different receptors. These interactions may vary between different tissues.

Retinol and a hydroxylated derivative of retinoic acid have been found to be phosphorylated and then glycosylated, primarily with mannose.[37–39] Retinyl phosphate and retinyl-P-sugar derivatives act as carriers of monosaccharides and may function as intermediates in cellular glycosylation reactions. The specific role of

each of these retinoid metabolites has not been elucidated. Identification of further retinoid metabolites and clarification of the biologic activity of each compound will be necessary to further clarify the exact mechanisms accounting for the various retinoid effects.

Mechanisms of Retinoid Action

Retinoids have a variety of different biologic effects. These include: (1) the regulation of growth and differentiation in epithelial and other cells, (2) inhibition of tumor promotion during experimental carcinogenesis, (3) effects on malignant cell growth, (4) effects on the immune system and inflammation, and (5) alterations in cellular cohesiveness and interaction. These effects can be understood at a cellular level by retinoid action on three parameters: proliferative capacity, differentiation state, and cell surface composition.

On a molecular level, several retinoid actions have been identified that may be responsible for modulation of these parameters. They include retinoid influences on RNA[40,41] and protein synthesis,[38,42] posttranslational glycosylation of proteins,[43] prostaglandin synthesis,[44,45] labilization of membranes, and effects on specific enzymes such as ornithine decarboxylase and collagenase. The discovery of the nuclear retinoic acid receptors was a major breakthrough in the understanding of retinoid action. The retinoic acid receptors can explain how retinoids orchestrate the regulation of diverse molecular processes. In the presence of retinoic acid, the retinoic acid receptors can bind specific DNA regulatory sequences, thereby activating specific sets of genes. By controlling the activation of sets of genes, cascades of activity can be set into motion. Retinoids may, thereby, control such diverse processes as epithelial differentiation (keratinization or cornification), embryonic morphogenesis, or carcinogenesis.

Intracellular Binding Proteins

Some retinoid actions may be mediated through intracellular receptor proteins similar to the action of several steroid hormones. A receptor protein (cytosol binding protein) may bind a hormone (or retinoid) as it enters the cytoplasm and translocate it to the nucleus. In the nucleus, another protein (nuclear receptor) could further facilitate hormone action.

Cytosol Binding Proteins Initially, a specific, soluble cellular retinol binding protein (CRBP) was identified in several tissues of the rat.[46] Subsequently, a distinct cellular retinoic acid binding protein (CRABP) was found in chick embryo skin, highlighting the physiologic role of retinoic acid in vivo and its potential importance as a separate entity from retinol.[47] CRBP and CRABP are immunologically different but have a related amino acid sequence.[48] Both have been identified in many tissues of a variety of species.[49,50] The levels of both CRBP and CRABP have been found to vary between different tissues,[51] during development,[52] and between normal and malignant tissues.[53] When adult human skin was analyzed to determine the relative contribution of epidermis and dermis to the binding found in skin, the binding from both CRBP and CRABP was confined predominantly to the epidermis, with no detectable binding in the dermis.[54]

The cytosol binding proteins also vary with development. For example, in the rat, CRBP is present in most fetal and adult tissues, but in the adult, CRABP is found only in the brain, eye, and skin.[55]

The presence of CRABP in developing tissues and its disappearance in adult tissues implicate retinoic acid and CRABP in the promotion of differentiation. This concept is supported by two facts: (1) retinoic acid is generally more effective than retinol in promoting differentiation[56] and (2) a correlation exists between the ability of some retinoids to promote differentiation and to compete for binding to CRABP.[57,58]

In some malignant tumors, the total amount of binding to these proteins is altered compared to the normal counterpart. Breast tumors often show more binding to CRABP compared to normal breast tissue.[59] The amount of CRBP binding has also been found to vary between normal and malignant tissues.[60]

Additional, distinct forms of both CRBP and CRABP have recently been identified. These include CRBP II (intestinal absorptive cells), CRBP III (fish eyes), CRABP II (chick embryo skin, muscle, and bone), and a distinct CRABP II (neonatal rats). The role of these receptors has yet to be elucidated.

Different retinoids may vary in their ability to compete for binding to the cytosol binding proteins. Both 13-*cis* retinoic acid and acitretin (trimethylmethoxyphenyl derivative of all-*trans* retinoic acid) bind to CRABP and competitively inhibit the binding of all-*trans* retinoic acid.[61,62] Although etretinate (the ethyl ester of acitretin) does not bind to CRABP, a large portion of ingested etretinate is converted to acitretin. 13-*cis* Retinoic acid was found to compete with all-*trans* retinoic acid for binding in epidermal and sebaceous follicle CRABP obtained from human facial skin, but with less affinity.[63]

The binding of these retinoids to the cytosol binding proteins may be one mechanism by which retinoids exert their clinical effects. One possible role for these binding proteins is in the translocation of retinoid from the cytosol into the nucleus, where effects on DNA, RNA, or protein synthesis may be initiated.[64] In the cytosol, retinol may be bound to CRBP until converted to retinoic acid, which then could bind to CRABP. Upon translocation to the nucleus, retinoic acid may interact with the nuclear RARs, thereby regulating retinoic acid–responsive genes.

Other hypotheses have been suggested for the function of CRABP. Retinoic acid can act as a morphogen during embryogenesis, with the concentration gradient of retinoic acid controlling the spatial pattern of limb development. Because the distribution of CRABP and retinoic acid are inversely related in the limb of the chick embryo, CRABP may be acting to control the concentration gradient of free retinoic acid.[65]

Nuclear Retinoic Acid Receptors   The recent identification of a series of nuclear retinoic acid receptors has begun to clarify and expand our understanding of not only the scope of retinoid actions but also the mechanisms capable of explaining the diversity of retinoid actions. The identification of these receptors further supports the concept that retinoids can act in a manner similar to the way steroid hormones exert their effects. That is, upon interaction with specific receptors, they can regulate the transcription of specific sets of hormone-responsive (or retinoid-responsive) genes and thereby regulate complex series of events.

Recombinant DNA technology was used to identify a family of nuclear retinoic acid receptors.[66,67] These receptors are structurally similar to those that mediate the actions of the steroid and thyroid hormones and vitamin D. All of these receptors appear to be part of a superfamily of nuclear regulatory proteins. Upon activation by their specific ligand (hormone, retinoid, etc.), they can interact with DNA to control the transcription of specific genes. It is in this way that they can control the turning on or off of complex series of events.

Three distinct retinoic acid receptor genes (α, β, and γ) have been identified in humans.[66–70] However, these three genes give rise to more than three distinct retinoic acid receptor proteins. After the transcription of these genes into RNA transcripts, these transcripts may undergo additional processing before they are translated into receptor proteins.[71] The result of this is that the three receptor genes can give rise to a large number of distinct retinoic acid receptor proteins. The possibility of a large number of distinct receptor proteins may help explain the diverse effects of retinoids on different cells and at different times (e.g., during embryonic differentiation, different phases of growth or proliferation, malignancy). That is, the effects of retinoids on different cells may be mediated by very specific RARs that are distinct from those present in other types of cells.

The three RAR genes have different patterns of expression, both between different cells and over time. Transcripts derived from the RAR-α gene are found in most embryonic and adult tissues and may be responsible for some of the general effects of retinoids on growth and differentiation. In contrast, the RAR-β gene has little expression in adult skin,[70] whereas in the mouse embryo, it is associated with areas undergoing programmed cell death.[72] These mouse embryo studies associate RAR-γ expression with cells involved in chondrogenesis and skin differentiation. In adult skin, most of the RAR receptor is derived from the RAR-γ gene. Furthermore, these RAR-γ-derived receptors are of a specific subtype (RAR-γ 1) that occurs only at low levels in other tissues.[73] Therefore, most of the direct effects of retinoic acid on skin probably occur through the RAR-γ type 1 receptors. The various subtypes of receptors seem to be expressed in a highly directed fashion, and the regulation of their expression is probably an important factor determining how retinoid effects are manifested in the skin.

Another family of nuclear receptors (RXRs) has been identified; these receptors are activated in cells exposed to retinoic acid.[74] The RXRs were initially thought to be receptors that were specific for other retinoid metabolites.[75] The RXRs do not bind all-*trans* retinoic acid, but they have recently been shown to bind and be activated by 9-*cis* retinoic acid.[76] In addition, the RXRs appear to act as coregulators necessary for the RARs (and also the thyroid and vitamin D receptors) to effectively bind their target genes.[77] A complex series of interactions between retinoid receptors and different retinoid derivatives may explain the ability of retinoids to control such a diverse series of cell and tissue behaviors.

Summary of the Mechanisms of Retinoid Action   We are beginning to understand important mechanisms that can explain many of the biologic effects of retinoids. These mechanisms involve the binding of specific RARs, activated by retinoid, to DNA. Binding of this complex to DNA initiates the transcription (turning on) of the retinoid-responsive genes. The promoters of these retinoid-responsive genes contain specific, short nucleotide sequences that act as retinoid-responsive (enhancer) elements. When an appropriately activated receptor (i.e., RAR-retinoid complex) binds to an enhancer element, there is an increase in the initiation of gene transcription by RNA polymerase of those genes controlled by that promotor. Some of the genes regulated by retinoic acid are other DNA-binding proteins, i.e., other regulatory proteins. In this manner, by increasing or suppressing the expression of other regulatory proteins, retinoids may cause changes in the expression of other genes. By changing the expression of growth factors, oncogenes, keratins, or transglutaminases, retinoids could exert widespread changes in growth or differentiation.

Retinoid Effects on Proliferative Capacity

Various retinoid effects on cellular proliferation have been described from in vitro studies. The discrepancies in observed results are probably due to differences in the systems studied, such as in cell types, culture conditions, and type and dose of retinoid. The treatment of rapidly growing cells with excess retinoid often causes growth inhibition.

Retinoid Effects on Differentiation State

Retinoids are involved in regulating cellular differentiation during embryonic development, in fully developed tissues, and in adult tissues. Recently, considerable evidence has suggested the role of retinoids as morphogens during embryonic development (see below).

The role of retinoids in maintaining the differentiated state of fully formed tissues is highlighted when retinoid is withdrawn. During retinoid deficiency, the normal growth and differentiation of a variety of adult tissues and organs (including bronchi, trachea, stomach, intestine, uterus, kidney, bladder, testis, prostate, pancreatic ducts, and skin) also do not occur.[13,78] In tissues that are normally a mucous epithelium, physiologic doses of retinoids promote differentiation in the direction of mucous secretion while inhibiting keratinization. The bladder, lung, and trachea are dependent on retinoid for maintenance of their columnar epithelia. Vitamin A deficiency in these tissues results in the development of a stratified squamous epithelium. In contrast, in the skin and other tissues that are normally stratified squamous epithelia, excess retinoids act to suppress the terminally differentiated phenotype, i.e., keratinization (cornification). For example, vitamin A in excess can inhibit keratinization and induce mucous metaplasia in chick skin[79] and hamster cheek pouch. When chick embryo skin is maintained in organ culture under the influence of retinoic acid, the epidermis transforms into a columnar mucous-secreting epithelium.[80] The ability of retinoids to alter differentiation in keratinizing epidermis probably explains the clinical benefit observed in many dermatologic disorders characterized by hyperkeratosis. This retinoid action also correlates with some of the retinoid toxicities, such as palmoplantar peeling and skin fragility, observed during systemic treatment.

Retinoids and Embryogenesis

Retinoids have recently been implicated as morphogens, molecules that have a critical role in controlling embryonic development.[81–85] Morphogens are signaling molecules that control the spatial pattern of differentiation and thereby control the shape of embryo development. Studies in the chick embryo suggest that all-*trans* retinoic acid acts as a morphogen controlling limb bud formation. A concentration gradient of all-*trans* retinoic acid seems to control the position of cells in the developing limb, and this information establishes the pattern of limb development. One proposed role for the CRABP is in the binding of retinoic acid, and the resultant steepening of the concentration gradient of free retinoic acid.[65] Retinoids may have other functions during embryogenesis, such as the control of programmed cell death. These retinoid effects may explain the mechanisms involved in retinoid teratogenicity.[86]

Retinoids, Differentiation, and Malignancy

Retinoids are involved in the relationship between differentiation and malignant transformation. For example, without retinoids the tracheal and bronchial epithelia undergo squamous metaplasia, a premalignant condition.[13] In animal studies, vitamin A deficiency yields an enhanced susceptibility to chemical carcinogenesis of the respiratory system, bladder, and colon.[87–90] Conversely, naturally occurring retinoids have been shown to protect animals against the development of carcinomas of the stomach, vagina, cervix, bronchi, trachea, and lung and against skin papillomas and carcinomas. Furthermore, some malignant cell lines can also be induced to differentiate under retinoid influence. HL-60 human promyelocytic leukemia cell lines differentiate and display characteristics of functional granulocytes. The dramatic remissions of acute promyelocytic leukemia induced by all-*trans* retinoic acid are consistent with this in vitro observation. In addition, several teratocarcinoma cell lines have been induced to differentiate on exposure to retinoic acid. The F9 teratocarcinoma cell line, for instance, differentiates into endoderm and, if subsequently exposed to dibutyryl cyclic adenosine monophosphate, into neural-like cells.[91,92] The observed effects of retinoids on differentiation, however, are not completely consistent. Retinoids can inhibit the differentiation of mesodermal tissues in chondrogenesis, osteogenesis, and in the conversion of fibroblasts to adipocytes.[93–96] Similarly, although retinoids can stimulate the differentiation of some human melanoma[97] and promyelocytic leukemia cells,[25] differentiation was suppressed in another human[98] and a hamster melanoma line[99] and in a murine leukemia line.[100]

Effects on Transformation and Carcinogenesis

Several lines of evidence support a role for retinoids as agents that suppress cancer formation. One characteristic feature of vitamin A deficiency in a variety of epithelia is a squamous metaplasia that may facilitate carcinogenesis.[56] Moreover, the addition of excess retinoid (pharmacologic doses) is associated with suppression of malignant transformation. In vitro, retinoids suppress malignant transformation caused by chemical carcinogens, ionizing radiation, growth factors, or viruses.[56,101–103] Using experimental models of carcinogenesis, retinoids interfere with tumor development in several tissues, including urinary bladder, breast, and skin.

Carcinogenesis is a multistep process. It requires an initiation step by a carcinogen and, subsequently, a promotion phase. Tumor promotors are agents that enhance carcinogenesis when administered after initiation by a carcinogen. The initiation step is irreversible, but the effect of the promoter is reversible. Retinoids can interfere with the promotion phase of carcinogenesis. After dimethylbenzanthracene (DMBA) initiation of mouse skin carcinogenesis, for example, retinoids administered during the croton-oil promotion phase can inhibit the development of skin papillomas.[104] Retinoids also have a prophylactic effect against keratoacanthomas in animal models.[105] In other animal systems, retinoids inhibit tumor formation in a variety of organs (Table 236-2).[106] In addition to the skin, chemopreventive effects of retinoids against cancer have been documented in the breast, urinary bladder, lung, prostate, cervix, and forestomach. In female Sprague-Dawley rats, the inhibition of breast tumors by retinyl acetate and retinyl methyl ether required continuous exposure to sustain the chemoprotective effect. This requirement for sustained exposure was also observed with isotretinoin, in the chemoprevention of skin cancers in high-

TABLE 236-2
Retinoids and Cancer: Laboratory Studies

Inhibit proliferation of malignant cell lines
Inhibit chemical carcinogenesis in vivo
   Bladder
   Breast
   Skin
   Lung
   Cervix
   Forestomach
Inhibition of tumor promotion and induction of ornithine decarboxylase
   by phorbol esters
Might interfere with tumor initiation
   Inhibit carcinogen-induced aryl-hydrocarbon hydroxylase
   Inhibit binding of carcinogen to DNA
Suppress malignant transformation in vivo
   Chemical carcinogenesis
   Ionizing radiation
   Sarcoma growth factor

Reprinted from Peck.[106]

risk patients with xeroderma pigmentosum. Patients who had a decrease in the rate of new tumor formation on isotretinoin had a loss of benefit within 1 to 3 months after its discontinuation.[107]

Some retinoids manifest tissue specificity. 4-Hydroxyphenyl retinamide, which is present in high levels in breast tissue, is effective in preventing breast cancer in the rat.[108] This retinoid has an antiproliferative effect on normal mammary epithelium. Eventually, it may be possible to develop retinoid molecules that can be targeted for specific organs.

Retinoids have efficacy as chemopreventive agents in animal models of other tumors such as bladder cancer.[109,110] Studies in which animals were treated with retinoids after having received full exposure to carcinogens suggest that rather than interfering with the initiation phase of carcinogenesis, retinoids were acting later, during the promotion phase. Accordingly, retinoids are considered "antipromoting" agents. Tumor promoters, such as phorbol esters, the active agents in croton oil, increase ornithine decarboxylase activity early during experimental carcinogenesis in skin.[111,112] Ornithine decarboxylase (ODC) is the rate-limiting enzyme in the synthesis of polyamines, which are involved in cell proliferation and differentiation.[113] Retinoids interfere with the ability of phorbol esters to induce ODC.[113,114] The degree of ODC inhibition was found to correlate with the ability of the retinoid to inhibit the development of skin papillomas.[115] Retinoid inhibition of proliferation of other cell types also appears to correlate with a suppression of ODC activity.[94,116]

In addition to effects on tumor promotion, there are findings to suggest that retinoids can interfere with the initiation phase of carcinogenesis. Retinoids can induce a reduction of benz[a]anthracene-induced aryl hydrocarbon hydroxylase and a decrease in binding of 7,12-dimethylbenz[a]anthracene to DNA.[117]

Although retinoids are most potent as prophylactic agents, administered before tumor development has occurred, they can interfere with the proliferation of some malignant cell lines in vitro.[56] The growth of other types of malignant cell lines can be unaffected or actually stimulated.

Retinoids have a wide variety of effects on in vitro malignant transformation, reversing or suppressing transformation caused by chemical carcinogens, ionizing radiation, and transforming peptides such as sarcoma growth factor. Retinoids also interfere with viral-induced transformation, as evidenced by the effectiveness of

etretinate in lesions of epidermodysplasia verruciformis, induced by the oncogenic human papilloma viruses.[118]

Effects on Keratinization

The process of terminal differentiation of the epidermis is called keratinization, because keratins make up the predominant protein of fully differentiated epidermal cells. Retinoids have profound effects on keratinization. Retinoic acid treatment decreases the total keratin content of keratinocytes and alters the pattern of keratin expression. Retinoids can induce fetal keratins (K 19 and K 13), which are not usually found in adult epidermis.[119,120]

During terminal differentiation, epidermal transglutaminases cross-link involucrin and other proteins to form the cornified envelope. One mechanism of retinoic acid interference with cornification is by suppressing the expression of epidermal transglutaminase.[121]

Cell Surface Alterations

Under the influence of retinoids, cell surface alterations can occur that often result in increased adhesiveness of the treated cells.[122–124] Retinoids can alter membrane microviscosity[125] and may interact directly with membranes.[126] Another direct effect on cell membranes is the production of gap junctions that allow cell-to-cell coupling and facilitate intercellular communication.[127,128]

On a molecular level, cells exposed to retinoids develop alterations in surface protein profiles,[99,124,129] increased protein glycosylation,[38] modulation of glycosaminoglycan synthesis,[122,130] and quantitative changes in surface protein receptors.[126]

Membrane Effects

Some retinoid effects may be due to direct action on cell membranes. Free retinol can have a detergent-like effect, altering membrane microviscosity, possibly through insertion directly into the membrane.[125,126] In the blood, the binding of retinol to the transport protein, RBP, minimizes this effect. One result of this detergent-like effect is the labilization of lysosomal membranes,[131,132] which may result in lysosomal enzyme release and subsequent retinoid toxicity.[133] Membrane labilization seems to be dose dependent, occurring only at high doses; at lower doses, retinoids may stabilize membranes.[134,135]

Gap Junctions

Gap junctions are communication links between cells that allow for passage of electrical signals, ions, and molecules.[136] These channels are probably important in the control of tissue organization and growth. During the development of malignancy, the number of gap junctions decreases.[137–139] In response to retinoids, gap junctions proliferate rapidly in neoplastic and embryonic keratinizing epithelia. The rapidity of the response suggests that retinoids act on these structures through a direct effect.[128,140]

Glycoconjugate Biosynthesis

During vitamin A deficiency, there is a decrease in the biosynthesis of carbohydrate-containing macromolecules in epithelial tissues.[141,142] In vitamin A-deficient animals, the synthesis of specific glycoproteins can be stimulated by the addition of vitamin A.[38,141,143] Retinoids are involved in the transfer of monosaccharides, an important step in the formation of glycoproteins. Retinoids can be phosphorylated and glycosylated, and the resulting glycosyl retinyl phosphates can serve as intermediates in glycosylation.[38,39,43] They can act as sugar carriers that donate monosaccharides to membrane proteins. Changes in cell surface glycoproteins have been related to changes in cell morphology and adhesiveness.[144-146] In addition, retinoids can also modify glycolipid biosynthesis.[147]

Glycosaminoglycan synthesis is also affected by retinoids in a manner that varies with the tissue studied. In vitro studies have described changes in heparan sulfate, chondroitin 4-sulfate, dermatan sulfate, and chondroitin 6-sulfate.[148,149] In pig and human epidermis, retinoic acid stimulates glucosamine incorporation into extracellular, surface-associated glycosaminoglycans.[150] Because glycoconjugates are involved in cellular recognition and adhesion, this may be one manner in which retinoids affect differentiation.[151]

Retinoid Effects on Proteases and Prostaglandins

Retinoids have been shown to affect proteases. Plasminogen activator cleaves plasminogen to plasmin—the enzyme that catalyzes fibrinolysis. Plasminogen activator may be important in tissue remodeling. Retinoid treatment of cell lines can cause increased secretion of plasminogen activator.[91,152-154] Another protease, collagenase, has been observed to be suppressed by retinoids.[155,156]

Inhibitory effects of retinoids on prostaglandin production in rheumatoid synovial cells has been described.[155] N-(4-hydroxyphenyl)retinamide has been shown to inhibit prostaglandins. This retinoid also inhibits breast carcinogenesis.[108,157]

Retinoid Effects on the Immune System

Retinoids are generally thought to stimulate humoral and cellular immunity, but inhibitory effects have also been observed. They can act as adjuvants in this process, enhancing antibody production in response to a variety of antigens, and have diverse effects on cell-mediated immunity. Part of the antitumor effects of retinoids may be due to these immune effects.[158-161]

Antilymphocyte serum has been found to oppose the vitamin A-induced growth inhibition of S91 melanoma in mice[158] and vitamin A-accelerated rejection of skin homographs.[161] When mice were inoculated with Lewis lung tumor cells, treatment with BCG and vitamin A was found to markedly decrease the incidence of primary tumors and lung metastases.[162]

Varied effects of retinoid have been observed on cell-mediated cytotoxicity. Low doses of retinoic acid, in vitro, stimulate cell-mediated cytotoxicity against tumors, whereas high doses abolish it.[163] Retinoic acid appeared to act as a specific adjuvant for the induction of cytotoxic (killer) T-lymphocytes.

Arginase released by activated macrophages may be responsible for the differential killing of tumor cells. Nontoxic concentrations of retinoic acid and retinol inhibit the expression of Fc receptors and enhance arginase production.[164] The retinoid effects on macrophages may occur through the inhibition of prostaglandins.[165]

Various effects of retinoids on mitogen-stimulated proliferation have also been described. Because retinoids can directly inhibit the proliferation of transformed cells in vitro in the absence of immunoregulatory cells, these immune effects are not the sole mechanism of retinoid antitumor activity. Further studies will be needed to define retinoid influence on antitumor immunity precisely.

Clinical Studies

Synthetic retinoids have profound effects on many skin diseases. Either used alone or in combination with other agents, the retinoids have been successful in clinical trials for more than a decade in the treatment of cystic acne, psoriasis, a variety of disorders of keratinization, multiple basal cell carcinomas, cutaneous T-cell lymphoma, and other skin diseases (Table 236-3). A decade of clinical and laboratory investigation into the therapeutic spectrum and the mechanisms of action of natural and synthetic retinoids preceded the clinical accomplishments observed with synthetic retinoids in dermatologic disease. For example, the chemoprevention of experimental carcinogenesis with isotretinoin provided a theoretical rationale for its use in patients with multiple basal cell carcinomas.

Cystic Acne

In 1976, patients with disorders of keratinization treated with oral isotretinoin were observed to develop drying and chapping of their facial skin similar to that seen with topical tretinoin. Because of this finding and because of the historic use of oral vitamin A and topical tretinoin in the treatment of acne, it appeared reasonable to treat acne patients with oral isotretinoin. In the first clinical trial, 14 previously treatment-resistant cystic acne patients responded dramatically to isotretinoin, at an average maximum dosage of 2.0 mg/kg body weight per day, and had an 85 percent mean reduction in lesion counts at the end of the 4-month treatment period.[166] Thirteen went on to clear completely after discontinuation of therapy, indicating that therapy need not be maintained until total improvement is observed (Figs. 236-3, 236-4, and 236-5). This continued healing was followed by prolonged remissions in all cases.

Cystic acne is unique among retinoid-responsive diseases in that most cases of even the greatest severity can be successfully treated with only one 4- or 5-month course at doses of 0.5 to 2.0 mg/kg body weight per day.[167] Only about one-third of acne patients require a second course, and only a few require additional therapy to completely clear. Because of the continued healing seen after discontinuing therapy, 2-month treatment-free evaluation periods are useful in determining which patients require additional therapy. Generally, patients with severe cystic acne located predominantly on the trunk require higher doses, up to 2.0 mg/kg per day, and longer treatment periods than do patients with facial acne.

Although isotretinoin has proved to be the most effective therapy for cystic acne, there is typically a lag period before the onset of the therapeutic effect. The usual time for a 50 percent decrease in the number of acne nodules and cysts on the face is at 8 weeks of therapy and on the trunk is at 12 weeks. Of those patients who clear completely, most remain totally free of cysts. Some patients have

TABLE 236-3
Retinoid-Responsive Diseases

Acne
   Cystic acne*
   Papular acne[†]
   Acne rosacea*
   Gram-negative folliculitis*
   Hidradenitis suppurativa[‡]
   Steroid acne[†]
   Oil acne[†]
Disorders of keratinization
   The ichthyoses*
      Ichthyosis vulgaris
      Lamellar ichthyosis
      Nonbullous congenital ichthyosiform erythroderma
      Epidermolytic hyperkeratosis
      X-linked ichthyosis
      Keratoderma palmaris et plantaris
      Mal de Meleda[†]
      Papillon-Lefevre syndrome[†]
   Darier's disease*; Hailey-Hailey disease[†]
   Pityriasis rubra pilaris*
   Erythrokeratodermia variabilis*
   Kyrle's disease[†]
   Pachyonychia congenita[†]
Skin cancer and precancer chemotherapy and chemoprophylaxis
   Basal cell carcinoma[‡]
   Squamous cell carcinoma[‡]
   Actinic keratoses[†]
   Keratoacanthoma*
   Leukoplakia[‡]
   Bowen's disease[‡]
   Mycosis fungoides[‡]
   Cutaneous metastases of malignant melanoma[‡]
Psoriasis
   Pustular psoriasis*; erythrodermic psoriasis*
   Pustular psoriasis of von Zumbusch*
   Pustular psoriasis and other pustular palmoplantar diseases*
   Psoriatic arthritis[‡]
Miscellaneous diseases[†]
   Verrucous epidermal nevi
   Subcorneal pustular dermatosis; impetigo herpetiformis
   Discoid lupus erythematosus; Reiter's syndrome
   Warts; epidermodysplasia verruciformis
   Hyperkeratotic eczema of hands and feet
   Lichen planus; lichen sclerosus et atrophicus
   Acanthosis nigricans
   Cutaneous sarcoidosis
   Scleromyxedema

* Very effective
[†] Reported
[‡] Somewhat effective

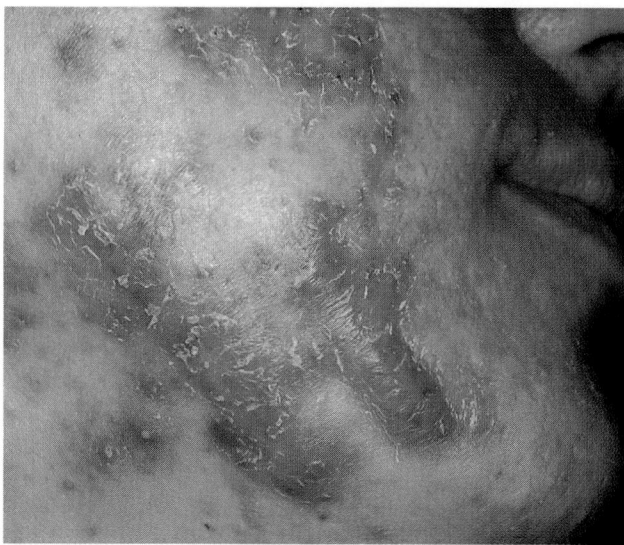

a

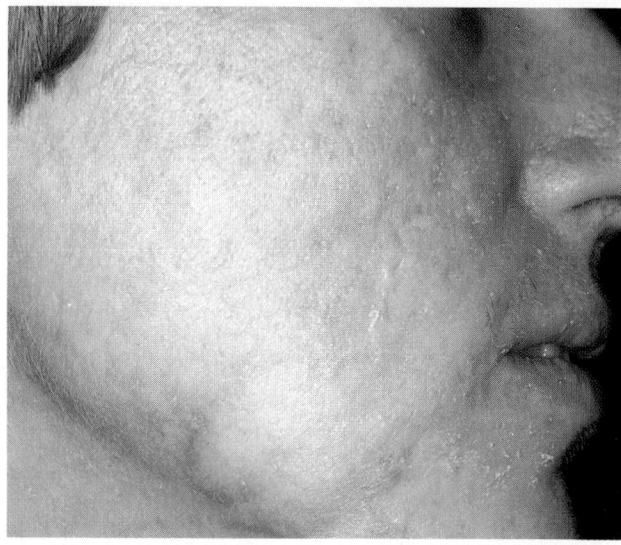

b

FIGURE 236-3 Cystic acne (note sinus tracts) before (*a*) and after (*b*) treatment with isotretinoin.

an occasional cyst or two and varying amounts of papular acne at follow-up examinations. Relapses sufficient to require further therapy with isotretinoin have been reported in about 10 to 40 percent of acne patients.[168] Tendency to relapse is dose dependent, i.e., patients treated with 0.1 mg/kg per day have a much greater tendency to relapse than those treated with 1.0 to 2.0 mg/kg per day.[169–173] Relapses are generally mild; it is unusual for the amount of acne at time of relapse to equal pretreatment severity. When mild or moderate relapses occur, a trial of conventional acne therapy is often effective. If this fails, then additional treatment with isotretinoin may be indicated.

Current dosage recommendations, based on the results of early trials treating patients with severe cystic acne, are that 1.0 mg/kg per day of isotretinoin be used for 4 or 5 months as an initial course of therapy. Although doses as low as 0.05 mg/kg per day were tested, a higher relapse rate with only a moderate reduction in incidence of side effects was reported with these doses. These data argued against the usefulness of low doses in patients with severe cystic acne. It is possible, however, that current patients with less severe forms of facial cystic acne, who are being treated earlier in order to minimize or prevent scarring and its psychosocial consequences,[174] may respond comparably and with less toxicity to a dose level of 0.5 mg/kg per day.

After observing the continuing therapeutic benefit regularly seen after the discontinuation of therapy with isotretinoin, an additional dosage schedule was designed. Comparable therapeutic results could be achieved if high initial doses (1 to 2 mg/kg per day) were given for only 2 weeks followed by lower doses (0.25 to 0.5 mg/kg per day) for the remainder of a 16-week treatment period. The higher doses (2.0 followed by 0.5 mg/kg per day) were used for patients with predominantly truncal acne, and the lower

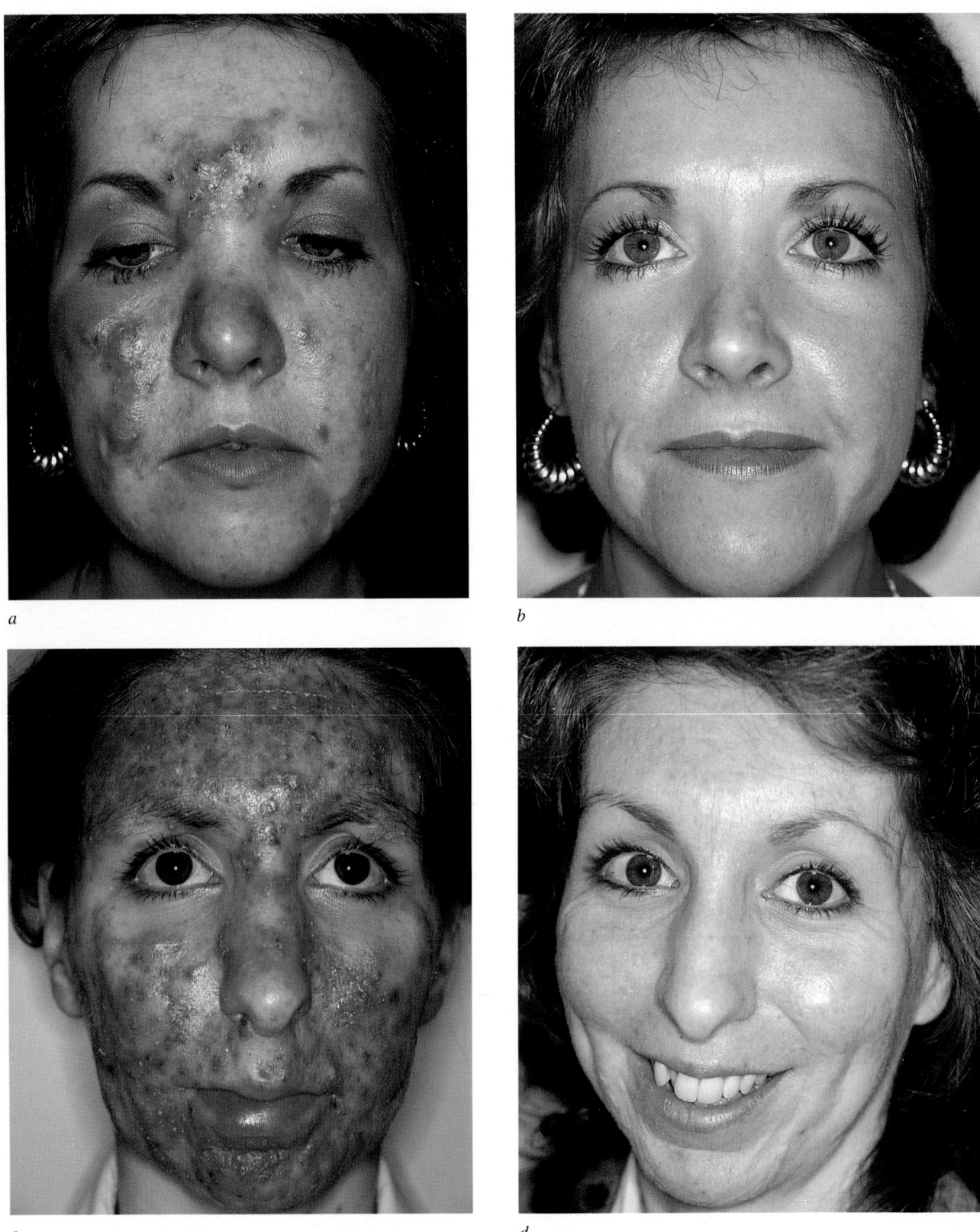

a

b

c

d

FIGURE 236-4 Severe cystic acne in females treated with oral
isotretinoin. (*a, c, e,* and *g*) Before treatment. (*b, d, f,* and *h*)
After treatment.

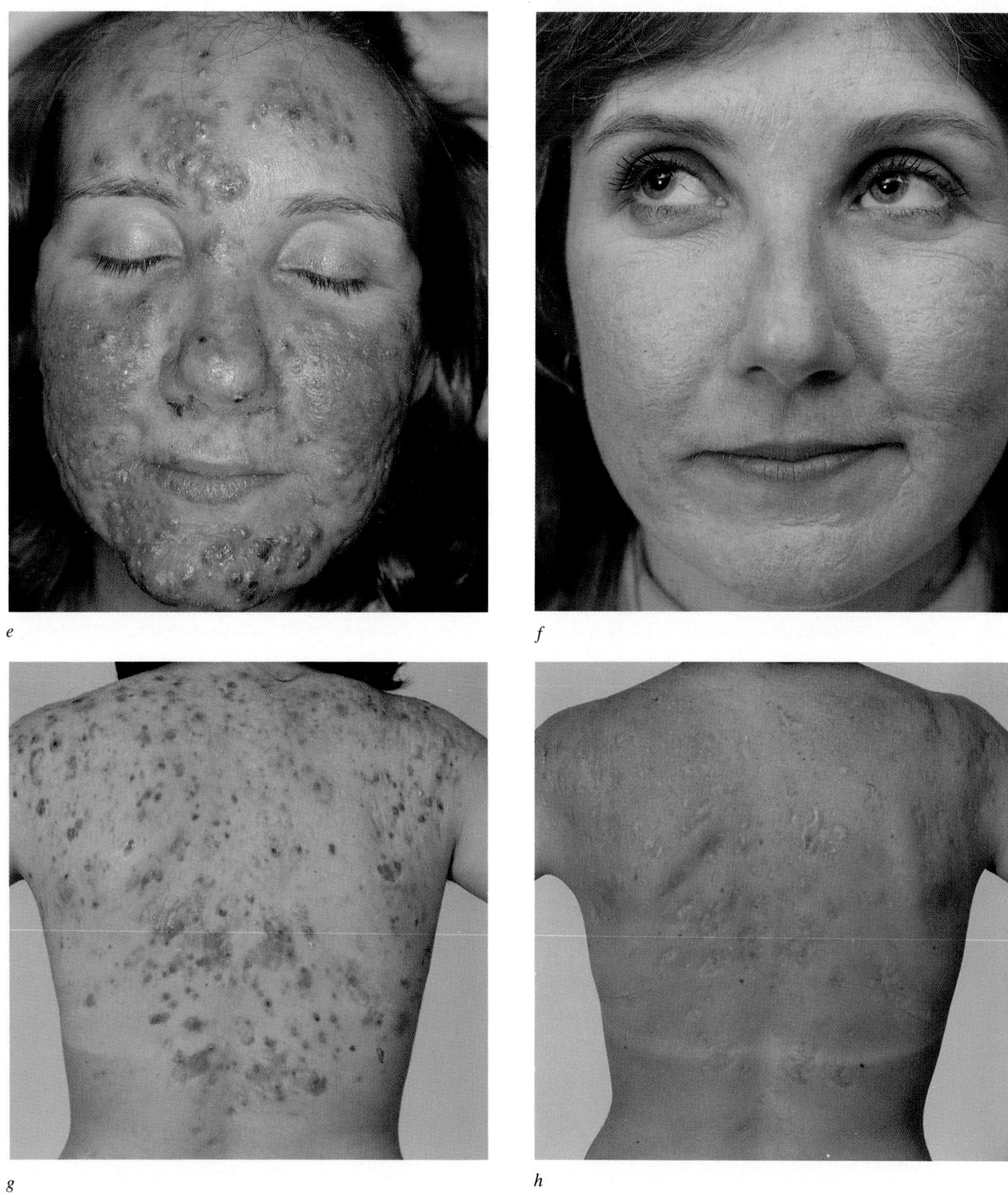

e

f

g

h

FIGURE 236-4 *(continued)*

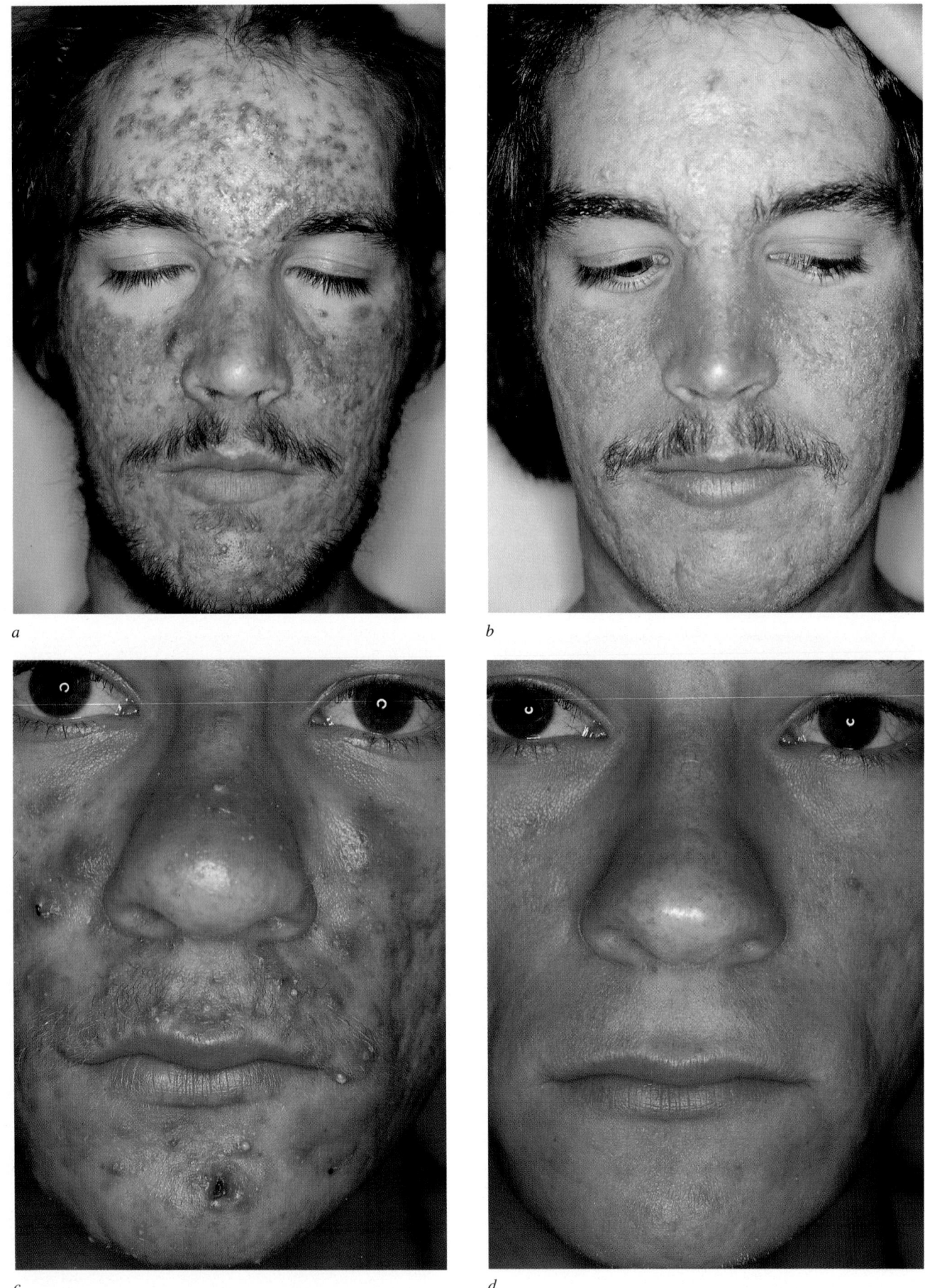

a *b*

c *d*

FIGURE 236-5 Severe cystic acne in males treated with oral isotretinoin. (*a*, *c*, and *e*) Before treatment. (*b*, *d*, and *f*) After treatment.

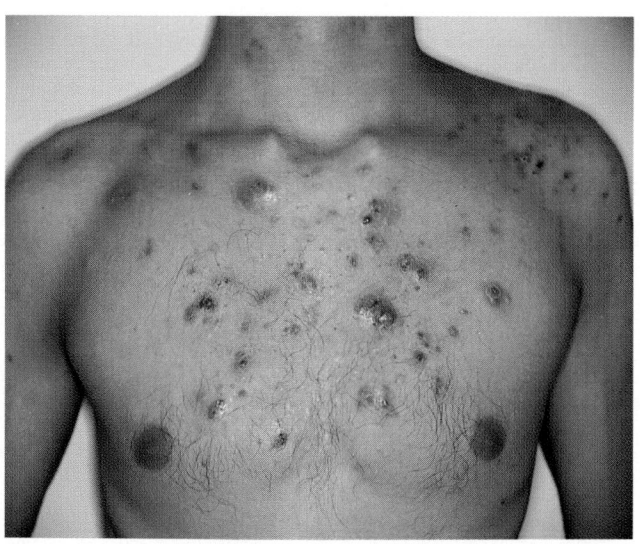
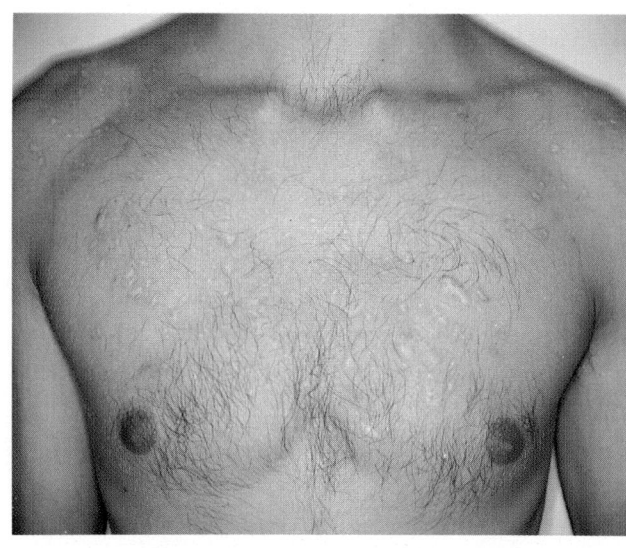

e   *f*

FIGURE 236-5 *(continued)*

doses (1.0 followed by 0.25 mg/kg per day) for facial acne patients. This high-low dosage schedule was superior to both a 2-week high-dosage schedule followed by placebo and to a constant low-dosage schedule. Specifically, the constant low-dosage schedule 0.5 mg/kg per day) led to an initial 20 percent increase in the lesion count at 2 weeks and, at the end of the 16-week treatment period, only a 50 percent reduction in lesions. In contrast, the high-low dosage schedule did not increase the mean lesion count at the 2-week observation point but did reduce acne by 75 percent at 16 weeks.

Dosage recommendations for patients who require a second course of therapy for substantial, persistent acne may require higher doses, such as 1.5 to 2.0 mg/kg per day, for an additional 4- to 6-month course of therapy. This is particularly true for acne of the nuchal region, the low back, buttocks, and thighs. Doses higher than 2.0 mg/kg per day are generally not necessary. On the other hand, when treating patients with mild to moderate acne of the face or trunk that has improved but not cleared after the initial course of therapy with isotretinoin, one may use a trial of conventional therapy prior to reinstating isotretinoin at the usual recommended dosage (1.0 mg/kg per day).

Occasionally an increased number of acne cysts was seen during the first 2 weeks of isotretinoin therapy in the initial clinical trials prior to the marketing of this agent.[175] This may have been due to isotretinoin paradoxically and temporarily increasing the number of inflammatory lesions derived from closed comedones, similar perhaps to the effect seen during initial therapy with topical tretinoin. In some reports, however, it could have been due to the abrupt discontinuation of previously used, partially effective therapy, such as oral antibiotics, 4 weeks prior to patients entering into experimental protocols with isotretinoin. Higher initial doses of isotretinoin (2.0 mg/kg per day) may minimize this initial flare. For severe flares, therapy with isotretinoin may be discontinued, and treatment with systemic corticosteroids initiated.

One other uncommon reaction in treating cystic acne with isotretinoin is the evolution of acne cysts, particularly on the trunk, into crusted pyogenic granuloma-like lesions.[176–178] These lesions may occur rarely in severe acne untreated with isotretinoin but are probably more commonly observed during isotretinoin therapy;

they readily respond to debridement of the crusts and either intralesional injection or topical application or a short course of systemic administration of corticosteroids. An additional adverse effect may be colonization of the anterior nares with *Staphylococcus aureus* during isotretinoin therapy. The use of an antibiotic ointment to the nares has been suggested for the prevention of staphylococcal folliculitis and furunculosis, which may occur late in the course of isotretinoin therapy and be confused with a relapse of acne.

In addition to cystic acne, isotretinoin therapy is effective in acne vulgaris, hidradenitis suppurativa, gram-negative folliculitis,[179] acne fulminans, acne conglobata, dissecting folliculitis of the scalp, and acne rosacea.[179] The treatment of hidradenitis with isotretinoin may be only partly effective even with prolonged therapy at 2 mg/kg per day (Fig. 236-6). However, isotretinoin can be helpful prior to surgery in reducing and delineating the extent of disease to be excised. Low-dose isotretinoin can produce a rapid therapeutic response in gram-negative folliculitis. This response is not considered to be a direct antibacterial effect but rather a secondary effect of alterations in the microenvironment.

Inhibition of sebum production with alterations in skin surface lipid film chemistry may represent a key mechanism of action of isotretinoin leading to clinical improvement in acne.[180] At peak levels of sebum suppression, the relative percentage of the skin surface lipid film composed of wax esters and squalene, which are derived from the sebaceous glands, is reduced, and the percentage of cholesterol and cholesterol esters is increased. Isotretinoin is the most effective inhibitor of sebum production known, being superior to estrogen and x-irradiation. Inhibition of quantitative sebum production (or sebum excretion rate) is almost maximal by the fourth week of treatment with isotretinoin and thus usually occurs prior to clinical improvement. Inhibition is dose dependent, and doses of 0.5 to 1.0 mg/kg per day lead to an 80 to 90 percent inhibition after 12 to 16 weeks of therapy.[181] After treatment is stopped, quantitative sebum production returns toward pretreatment levels, but long-term follow-up from 20 to 99 weeks post treatment shows an overall persistent 38 percent (range, 0 to 80 percent) inhibition.[182] Patients who received two courses of therapy with isotretinoin, for a total of 10 months, showed a persistent 60 percent decrease in quantitative sebum production when measured 1 year or more after

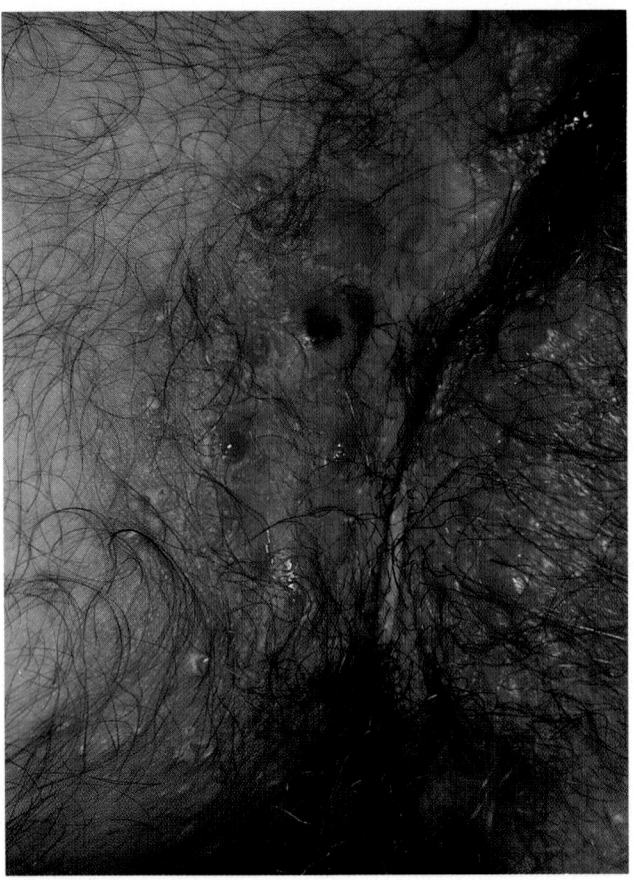

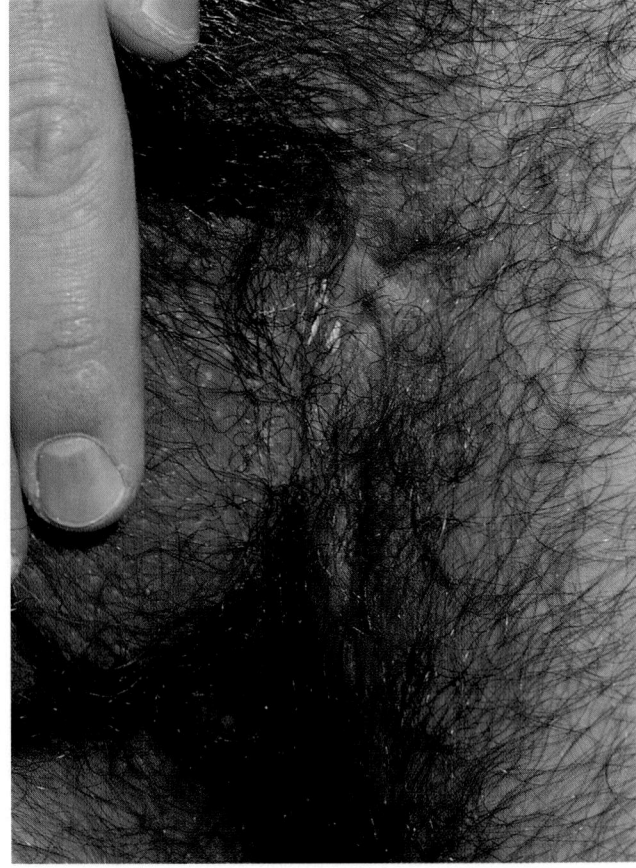

a

b

FIGURE 236-6 Hidradenitis of the groin before (*a*) and after (*b*) treatment with isotretinoin.

treatment.[183] These data suggest that prolonged remission in some patients may be related at least in part to continued partial inhibition of sebaceous glands. The histologic changes parallel and reflect the inhibition of sebum production. The sebaceous glands virtually disappear during treatment with isotretinoin and gradually recover after discontinuation of therapy.[184]

The inhibition of the wax ester secretion rate by isotretinoin was studied specifically using a bentonite clay technique.[185,186] The mean rates of wax ester secretion were greatly elevated in untreated acne patients but were suppressed below the normal range (as measured in patients without acne) during therapy. However, the post treatment secretion rates again rose above the normal range at all dose levels (0.1 to 1.0 mg/kg per day), indicating that other factors must contribute to the continued healing of acne and to the prolonged remissions observed after discontinuing therapy.

In addition to inhibition of sebum production, the mechanisms by which isotretinoin may be acting in the treatment of acne include anti-inflammatory effects, antibacterial effects, inhibitory effects of microbial enzyme activity, and desquamative effects on poral occlusion.[187–191] Isotretinoin reduces the number of *Propionibacterium acnes* on the skin surface. This probably reflects decreased follicular colonization of *P. acnes* secondary to the decrease in sebaceous secretion.

Initial studies indicated that isotretinoin does not appear to act as an antiandrogen as no change was noted in serum androgen levels[192] or gonadotropins, nor were there signs of feminization in males during therapy. Furthermore, the androgen-sensitive parts of the hamster flank organ, aside from the sebaceous component, did not involute during treatment with isotretinoin.[193] One recent report, however, documents a significant reduction in serum testosterone and urinary steroid metabolites and a change in the ratio of 5α and 5β metabolites during isotretinoin therapy, suggesting that 5α-reductase activity may be sensitive to isotretinoin.[194] In addition, isotretinoin reduced serum levels of dihydrotestosterone and 3α-androstanediol glucuronide, possibly secondary to the reduction in size of sebaceous glands, which may contribute tissue-derived androgens into the circulation.[195]

Psoriasis

Unlike acne, in which a single 4- or 5-month course of therapy with isotretinoin can lead to prolonged remissions, the treatment of psoriasis with retinoids usually requires long-term administration as relapses eventually occur in virtually all patients if therapy is discontinued (Fig. 236-7). Because of prolonged administration of retinoids, psoriasis patients are at greater potential risk of developing chronic retinoid toxicity than are acne patients. Etretinate at a dosage of 0.5 to 1.0 mg/kg per day remains the retinoid of choice in the treatment of psoriasis.[196–199] Etretinate is of particular value in the treatment of pustular psoriasis and erythrodermic psoriasis, both of which are characteristically treatment resistant, often re-

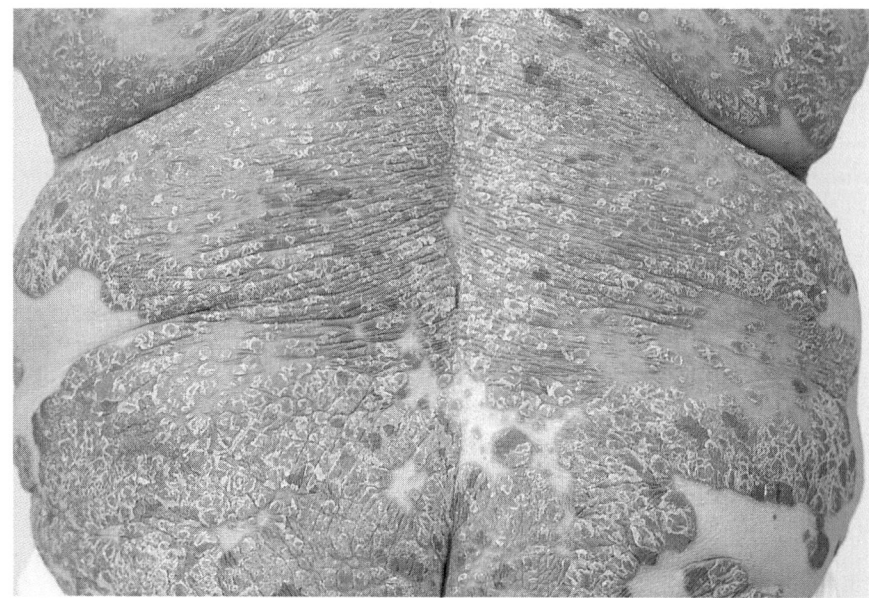

FIGURE 236-7 Generalized chronic plaque type psoriasis before (*a*) and after (*b*) treatment with etretinate.

a

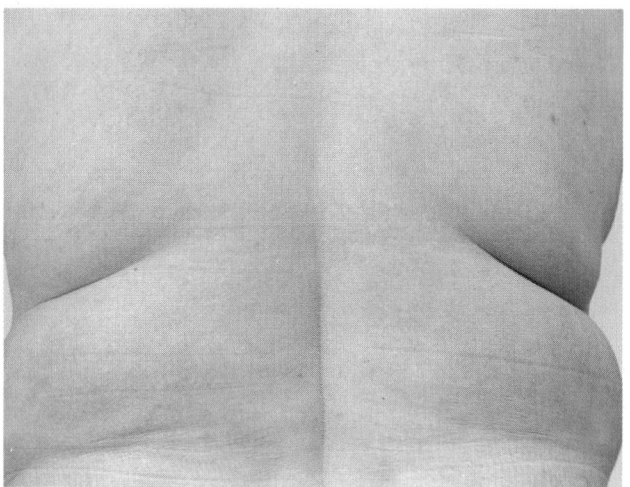

b

quiring therapy with agents such as methotrexate or cyclosporine. Isotretinoin is also effective in pustular psoriasis, providing a rapidly excreted, alternative retinoid for women of child-bearing potential.[200] Etretinate has been used both alone and in combination with other effective therapies such as anthralin, ultraviolet radiation (UVB, 280 to 320 nm), photochemotherapy (PUVA), methotrexate, and topical corticosteroids.[201–206]

Several small uncontrolled studies have indicated that most patients with psoriatic arthritis improve when treated with etretinate.[207–210] The etretinate-induced improvement allowed patients to decrease or discontinue their use of nonsteroidal anti-inflammatory agents.

Etretinate markedly augmented the response of psoriasis patients to photochemotherapy using oral methoxsalen and long-wave ultraviolet radiation (UVA, 320 to 400 nm) or PUVA.[201–203] The regimen combining a retinoid with photochemotherapy has been termed *RePUVA*. In many studies of RePUVA, etretinate has been given for 1 to 4 weeks followed by the addition of PUVA. The combined treatment considerably decreased the total amount of UVA required for clearing and accelerated the response of psoriasis to PUVA. Moreover, it was effective in patients who previously had been PUVA failures. RePUVA produced longer remissions than those induced by PUVA. Fewer side effects from etretinate were seen during RePUVA than with etretinate used alone because of the lower doses employed.

RePUVA using isotretinoin at a dose of 1 mg/kg per day was compared prospectively to RePUVA with etretinate.[211] The retinoids were given alone for 5 days prior to adding PUVA and were discontinued once psoriasis had cleared completely, at which time the patients were placed on PUVA maintenance. Even though etretinate is superior to isotretinoin when used alone in the treatment of psoriasis vulgaris, no significant difference between the two treatment regimens was observed in regard to duration of treatment required for clearing, number of UVA exposures required, and cumulative UVA dose.

Once psoriasis has cleared or markedly improved with etretinate, the subsequent posttreatment clinical course is variable. Some patients have prolonged remissions without maintenance therapy.

In other patients the therapeutic effect can often be maintained with conventional topical therapy and ultraviolet radiation, with or without low-dose etretinate (about 25 mg/day). However, relapses may occur even if etretinate therapy is maintained. Chronic maintenance therapy with etretinate may be necessary for patients with pustular psoriasis, erythrodermic psoriasis, and for those patients with severe psoriasis vulgaris who have proved to be resistent or intolerant of other treatments and who regularly demonstrate relapse on withdrawal of etretinate.

Initial dosage recommendations for the treatment of psoriasis with etretinate have been that therapy of erythrodermic psoriasis may begin at 25 to 35 mg/day and be increased to 50 to 60 mg/day within 2 to 4 weeks.[212] Pustular psoriasis may require initial doses of 75 mg/day, and chronic psoriasis vulgaris may be treated with 50 mg/day in combination with other active agents. Worsening of psoriasis may occur during the induction of etretinate therapy. This initial worsening is different from the retinoid dermatitis produced by high-dose etretinate, which can mimic psoriasis and which resolves on reduction of dosage or discontinuation of therapy.

Cutaneous Disorders of Keratinization

In 1976, isotretinoin was demonstrated effective in previously recalcitrant cases of disorders of keratinization, such as Darier's disease and pityriasis rubra pilaris.[213,214] Since then, numerous reports have indicated that these and other disorders of keratinization respond to isotretinoin, etretinate, and newer retinoids.[215] In contrast to results in acne, for which isotretinoin is more effective than etretinate, etretinate and isotretinoin gave comparable responses in Darier's disease, lamellar ichthyosis, nonbullous congenital ichthyosiform erythroderma, and pityriasis rubra pilaris.[216–218] Etretinate was superior to isotretinoin in the treatment of psoriasis, epidermolytic hyperkeratosis (Fig. 236-8), keratoderma palmaris et plantaris, X-linked ichthyosis, ichthyosis vulgaris, erythrokeratodermia variabilis, and lichen planus.

Patients with the dry, brown hyperkeratotic type of Darier's disease respond better (Fig. 236-9) and may have more prolonged remissions than those with the red, inflamed, infected variety of Darier's disease who also have marked intertriginous involvement. The latter patients are much more difficult to treat and relapse very quickly after therapy is discontinued. In one report, isomorphic reactions were noted to occur in one-third of patients with Darier's disease treated with etretinate.[217]

In a report of 45 patients with pityriasis rubra pilaris of varying duration prior to therapy, long-term remissions were noted after discontinuation of isotretinoin[218] (Fig. 236-10). Although most cases of adult-onset pityriasis rubra pilaris spontaneously clear within 3 years, this finding could indicate either that isotretinoin therapy induced or accelerated a spontaneous remission or was merely coincidental with it. In patients who did not have a complete remission after a course of therapy, new areas of involvement did not occur, and the return of disease did not reach the pretreatment degree of severity. This is in contrast to what has been observed in Darier's disease after stopping treatment with isotretinoin. Intermittent courses of therapy with prolonged treatment-free intervals may be effectively used in patients such as these. However, not all patients with pityriasis rubra pilaris respond in this manner. For instance, two patients with chronic pityriasis rubra pilaris, characterized by childhood onset, a myriad of follicular papules, and a duration longer than 10 years, responded very dramatically to treatment initially with isotretinoin and subsequently with etretinate. These patients relapsed dramatically and completely after each 4- to 6-month course of therapy over a more than 8-year period of retinoid therapy.[216]

Patients with lamellar ichthyosis treated with retinoids had a reduction in scale, increased heat tolerance and ability to sweat,

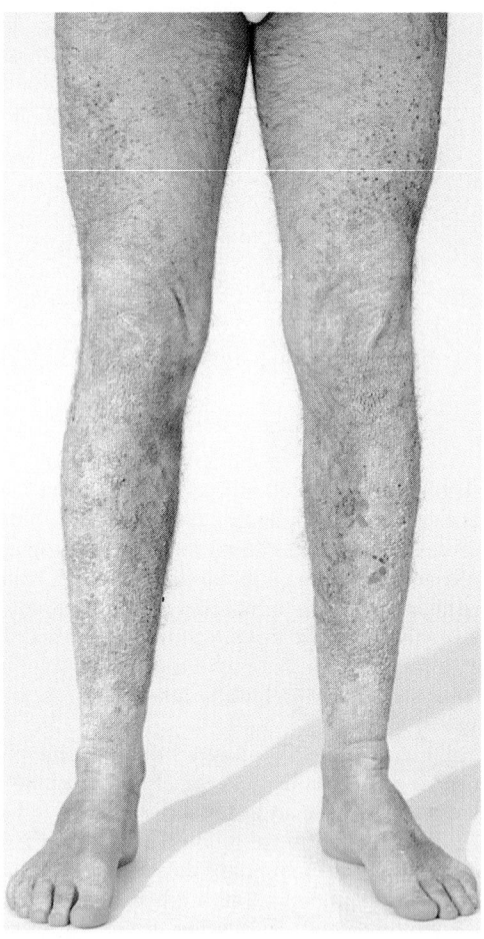

a

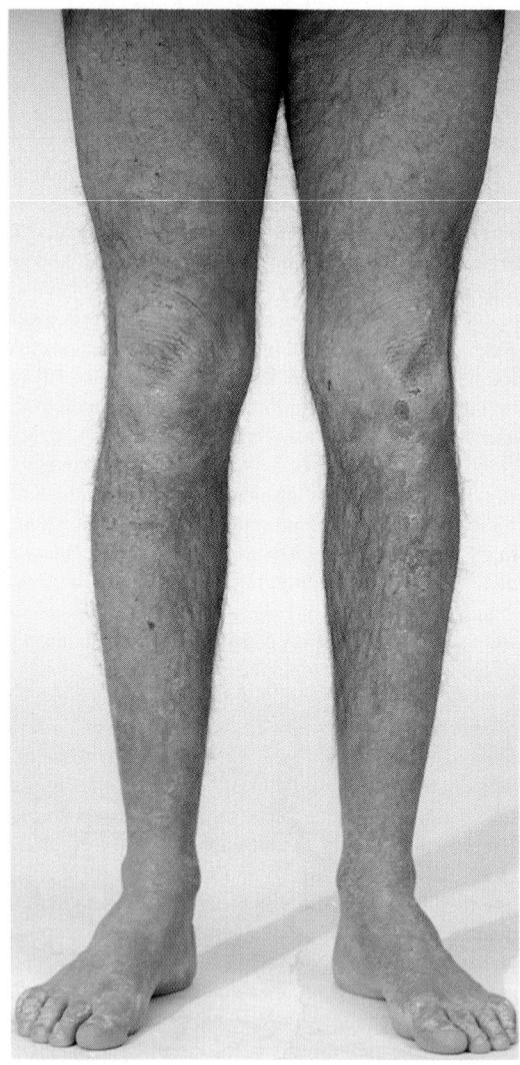

b

FIGURE 236-8 Epidermolytic hyperkeratosis before (*a*) and after (*b*) treatment with etretinate.

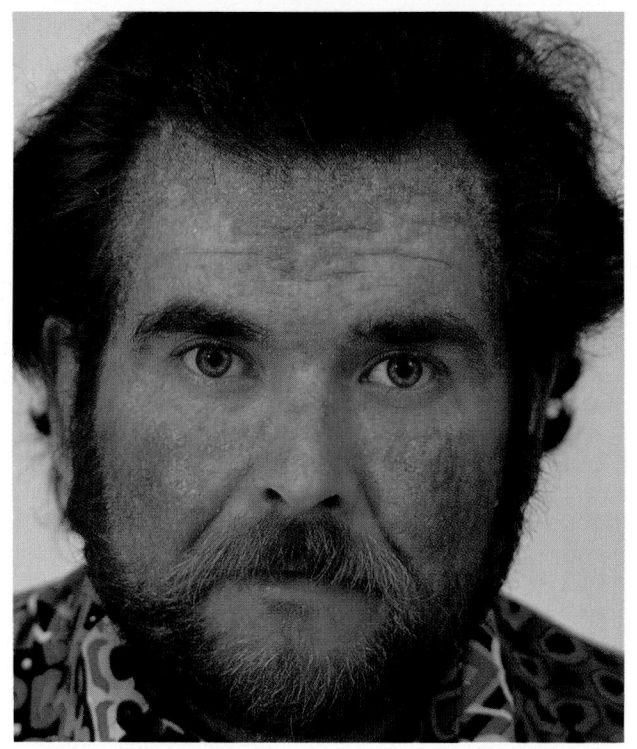
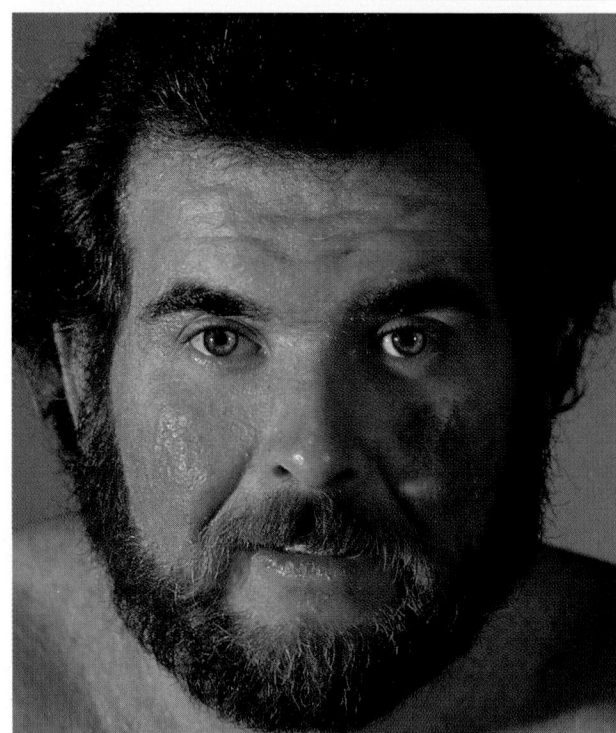

a

b

FIGURE 236-9 Darier's disease before (*a*) and after (*b*) treatment with isotretinoin.

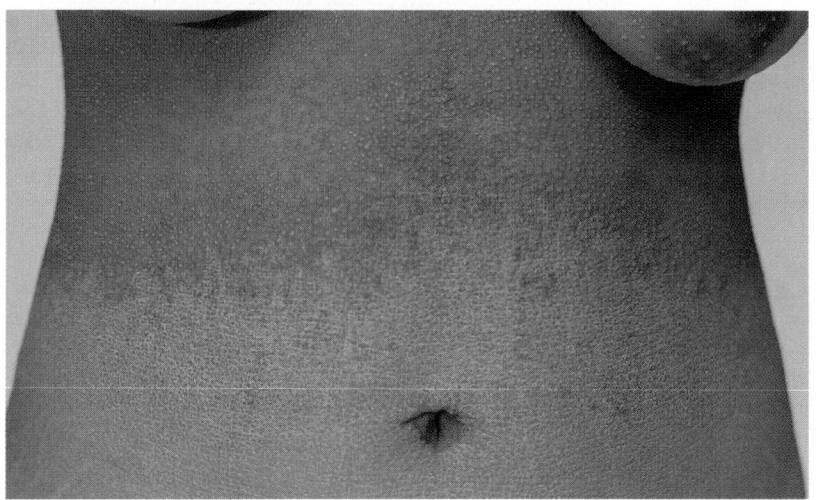

a

FIGURE 236-10 Chronic pityriasis rubra pilaris before (*a*) and after (*b*) treatment with isotretinoin.

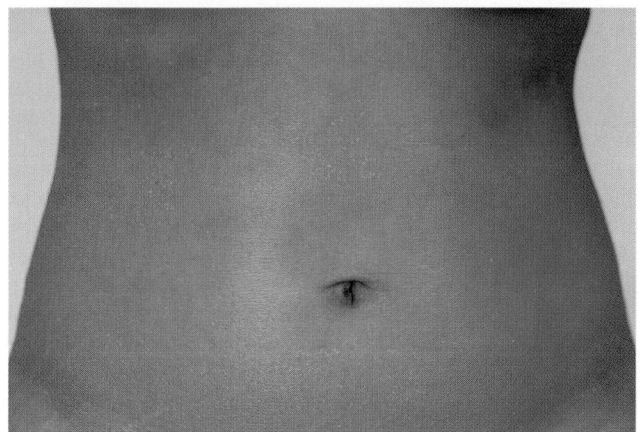

b

and improved ectropion. Clearing in these patients is usually not complete and may be greater in the summer than in the winter, when their disease is typically more severe.

Since disorders of keratinization may require long-term therapy with retinoids, the safety of chronic administration of retinoids must be addressed. Of particular concern is bone toxicity. In children, premature closure of epiphyses[219] and fractures[220] can rarely occur, as can changes in the axial skeleton resembling diffuse idiopathic skeletal hyperostosis in both children and adults.[221-223]

Unusual responses to therapy have been observed.[224] During etretinate therapy of patients with keratoderma palmaris et plantaris (epidermolytic type), epidermolytic hyperkeratosis, and pachyonychia congenita, palmoplantar blistering could be enhanced. Patients with Hailey-Hailey disease and atopic dermatitis have worsened with both retinoids, particularly at higher doses.

Cancer

The synthetic retinoids, isotretinoin and etretinate, have been used in the treatment and prevention of cutaneous malignancy in patients with a variety of conditions. These include chronic sunlight damage (basal cell carcinoma, actinic keratosis),[225] nevoid basal cell carcinoma syndrome,[214,226-228] xeroderma pigmentosum (basal cell carcinoma, squamous cell carcinoma, keratoacanthoma, actinic keratosis),[107,229] multiple keratoacanthomas (Ferguson-Smith),[230,231] porokeratosis of Mibelli with malignant degeneration (squamous cell carcinoma, Bowen's disease),[232] epidermodysplasia verruciformis,[118] oral leukoplakia,[233,234] cutaneous metastases of malignant melanoma,[235,236] and cutaneous T-cell lymphoma (mycosis fungoides and Sézary's syndrome).[237-239] Synthetic retinoids do not usually cure cutaneous tumors but do produce variable degrees of partial regression when given at high dosage (usually 1.5 mg/kg per day or more). The mechanism of action is not clear. Induction of inflammation by high-dose isotretinoin is not a necessary prerequisite for the regression of basal cell carcinoma, as both inflamed and noninflamed tumors will undergo regression.[214,226-228]

If the goal of therapy is changed from chemotherapy to chemoprevention, synthetic retinoids can have dramatic effects in preventing the formation of new skin tumors. Benefit persists only as long as therapy is maintained, particularly in patients with precancerous genodermatoses (nevoid basal cell carcinoma syndrome, xeroderma pigmentosum).[107,227,228]

In a study of five patients with xeroderma pigmentosum, high-dose oral isotretinoin (2 mg/kg per day), given for 2 years, was effective in preventing the development of new skin cancers.[107] This was the first controlled, prospective study to demonstrate cancer chemoprevention in humans. The total number of tumors in the five patients decreased from 121 (mean, 24; range, 8 to 43) in the 2 years before treatment to 25 (mean, 5; range, 3 to 9) in the 2 years of therapy, with a mean reduction in the tumor rate of 63 percent ($p = 0.019$). During the posttreatment observation period, which lasted a minimum of 9 months, a mean 8.5-fold increase in the frequency of skin cancers was observed in all five patients. These five patients and two others with xeroderma pigmentosum were enrolled in a subsequent low-dose (0.5 mg/kg per day) trial of isotretinoin.[240] The frequency of skin cancers occurring during the low-dose treatment decreased in most patients compared to their prior treatment-free interval. In some patients, there was an apparent dose response. In these patients, isotretinoin seemed to act as a switch, rapidly turning off the appearance of tumors within 2 months of the onset of therapy and quickly losing effectiveness

within 3 months of the withdrawal of treatment, findings that firmly linked isotretinoin therapy with tumor suppression.

The minimum effective dosage required to prevent the formation of basal cell carcinomas both in xeroderma pigmentosum and in the nevoid basal cell carcinoma syndrome varied between individual patients and usually ranged from 0.5 to 1.5 mg/kg per day, or 40 to 120 mg per day.

In contrast, a 3-year, placebo-controlled, multicenter trial demonstrated that very low dose isotretinoin (10 mg per day or 0.14 mg/kg per day) was not effective in reducing the incidence of new basal cell carcinomas in patients with a history of at least two prior tumors due to chronic sunlight damage.[241] In this study, treatment was associated with mucocutaneous and systemic adverse effects, including mild skeletal toxicity. For these otherwise healthy patients, it may be difficult to justify testing much higher doses of isotretinoin because of the likelihood of producing more toxicity. However, for patients with precancerous dermatoses who may develop several dozen skin cancers per year, the potential benefit of moderately higher doses of isotretinoin may outweigh the expected detriment of increased toxicity.

Isotretinoin has been reported to cause regression of squamous cell carcinoma. Complete and partial regressions occurred in four patients with large, recurrent or metastatic squamous cell carcinomas treated with oral isotretinoin, 1.0 mg/kg per day.[242] The authors suggest that retinoid activity correlates directly with the degree of differentiation of transformed cells and, therefore, the well-differentiated nature of squamous cell carcinomas may have been a factor in the excellent therapeutic responses observed. Isotretinoin, given as a chemopreventive agent, was also found to lower the rate of second primary squamous cell carcinomas among patients with previously treated head and neck cancers.[243] Although chemoprevention of potentially lethal cancer was observed, the high dose of isotretinoin used (50 to 100 mg/m^2) resulted in significant participant toxicity, with 33 percent of patients dropping out over the 12-month treatment period.

Several reports have described the beneficial responses of synthetic retinoids, either alone or in combination with other chemotherapeutic agents and with PUVA, in the treatment of cutaneous T-cell lymphoma.[237,239] When synthetic retinoids were used alone, tumors and plaques underwent marked partial regression clinically. Relapse occurred in most patients after withdrawal of therapy, indicating that treatment with synthetic retinoids is not curative. The synthetic retinoids may be active in cutaneous T-cell lymphoma by virtue of direct effects on the function of subsets of T lymphocytes.

Acute Toxicities

The acute toxicities commonly observed with the synthetic retinoids, isotretinoin and etretinate, are well tolerated, not life threatening, are dose dependent in incidence and severity, treatable with bland therapies, and reversible on discontinuation of treatment (Table 236-4). The acute toxicities of the synthetic retinoids mimic many of the findings of vitamin A intoxication but are less severe than those seen with the high doses of vitamin A required for clinical efficacy; they involve primarily the skin and mucous membranes.

The acute toxicities of the two synthetic retinoids, isotretinoin and etretinate, overlap but are not identical. Similarly, it appears that new synthetic retinoids will have unique spectra of clinical toxicity as well as efficacy. Under certain circumstances the differ-

TABLE 236-4
Retinoid Toxicity

Acute
  Mucocutaneous
    Cheilitis
    Facial dermatitis
    Xerosis with pruritus
    Conjunctivitis
    Dry nasal mucosa; minor nosebleeds
    Stratum corneum fragility (peeling from minor trauma)
    Palmoplantar peeling
    Hair loss
    Dry mouth with thirst
    Paronychia; nail plate abnormalities*
    Stickiness of skin*
    Chills*
    Inflamed urethral meatus*
    Corneal opacities[†] (reversible after discontinuation)
    Pyogenic granuloma-like lesions in acne[†]
  Systemic
    Headache*
    Arthralgias*; myalgias*
    Teratogenicity (head, ear, heart, thymus abnormalities)
    Spontaneous abortion; premature births
    Pseudotumor cerebri[†] (headache, papilledema)
    Mental depression[†]
    Inflammatory bowel disease[†]
    Urticaria; erythema nodosum[†]
    Idiopathic seizures[†]
  Laboratory
    Hyperlipidemia
      Increased triglycerides, VLDL
      Increased cholesterol, LDL*; decreased HDL*
      Eruptive xanthoma[†]
      Acute hemorrhagic pancreatitis[†]
    Elevated liver function tests (transient, minor):
      AST, ALT, alkaline phosphatase, LDH, bilirubin
    Elevated platelet counts*; leukopenia
    Hyperuricemia with gout[†]; hypercalcemia[†]
    Elevated CPK and myalgias after exercise[†]
Chronic
  Mucocutaneous—persistent, posttreatment:
    Dry eyes[†]; hair thinning[†]
  Systemic
    Vertebral abnormalities resembling diffuse idiopathic skeletal
      hyperostosis
      Osteophyte and bony bridge formation
      Anterior spinal ligament calcification
    Tendon and ligament calcification
    Premature epiphyseal closure
  Laboratory—none

* Uncommon
[†] Rare

ences in relative toxicity will influence retinoid selection in diseases in which the therapeutic effects are comparable.

As with vitamin A toxicity, the synthetic retinoids can alter tests of liver function. The tests most commonly elevated are the transaminases (AST,ALT), but occasionally other tests (alkaline phosphatase, lactic dehydrogenase, bilirubin) can also be abnormal. Elevations of transaminase occur in approximately 15 percent of patients but usually return to normal within 2 to 4 weeks and remain normal even with continued therapy with the retinoids. However, an acute hepatotoxic reaction to etretinate has occurred associated with fever and eosinophilia, possibly indicating a hypersensitivity reaction.[244] Long-term therapy with etretinate has not led to chronic liver toxicity, measured by liver function tests and by liver biopsies studied by light and electron microscopy, even in patients with preexisting liver disease.[245]

Vitamin A toxicity includes pain and tenderness in bones and joints. Arthralgias have been seen in only a minority of patients treated with synthetic retinoids, and the arthralgias disappear after discontinuation of therapy. In contrast to these retinoid-induced arthralgias, treatment of psoriatic arthritis with etretinate has led to objective improvement.

Another acute toxicity common to both vitamin A and the synthetic retinoids has been hypertriglyceridemia. The observed elevations of plasma triglycerides and very low density lipoprotein (VLDL) levels have been dose dependent and reversible on discontinuation of therapy.[246,247] Dosages of isotretinoin above 1 mg/kg per day are usually needed to elevate triglyceride levels markedly beyond the normal range. One patient, who may have had a preexisting hyperlipoproteinemia, developed eruptive xanthomas while being treated with isotretinoin at a dose of 2.5 mg/kg per day.[248] Another patient developed acute hemorrhagic pancreatitis after the plasma triglycerides exceeded 1400 mg/dL.[176] These observations have led to the recommendations to obtain fasting plasma triglyceride levels prior to initiating retinoid therapy and to discontinue therapy if triglyceride levels reach 800 mg/dL. In one report of 20 men with cystic acne of the trunk who were treated with isotretinoin at a maximum dosage of 2 mg/kg per day, the maximum increases from baseline levels were: for triglycerides, 67 percent; VLDL, 56 percent; LDL, 22 percent; and cholesterol, 16 percent. The maximum decrease in high-density lipoproteins was 10 percent.[246] Hypertriglyceridemia has also been observed with etretinate, particularly in patients with one of the following predisposing factors: obesity, high alcohol intake, diabetes, and pretreatment hypertriglyceridemia.[215] Certainly, if patients with pretreatment elevations in the level of plasma triglycerides are to be treated with retinoids, their condition must be monitored very closely. The long-term importance of this observation and the effect of dietary management of plasma triglyceride levels during therapy with retinoids remains to be determined.

Conjunctivitis, which may interfere with a patient's ability to wear contact lenses during therapy, may be a result of a decrease in the outer lipid layer of the tear film with subsequent evaporation of the aqueous phase.[249] Furthermore, *Staphylococcus aureus* has been cultured from eyelids of patients with isotretinoin-induced blepharoconjunctivitis.[250] If artificial tears and topical ophthalmologic antibiotic therapy fail to relieve the conjunctivitis, then ophthalmologic consultation should be sought. Other ophthalmologic toxicities include corneal opacities, decreased night vision, and cataracts.[251,252] Rarely, dry eyes and decreased night vision have been reported to persist after discontinuation of therapy.

Isotretinoin and etretinate are potent teratogens, and fetal deformities are the major concern in treating fertile women with oral retinoids. The birth defects characteristically induced by retinoids include central nervous system abnormalities (hydrocephalus, microcephaly), external ear abnormalities, cardiovascular abnormalities, facial dysmorphia, eye abnormalities (microphthalmia), and thymus gland abnormalities.[253,254] In some instances the above abnormalities may lead to death. Additional reported defects include premature births, parathyroid hormone deficiency, and cases of low IQ scores in the absence of obvious central nervous system abnormality. Although etretinate is a more potent teratogen in animals, more instances of fetal abnormalities have been associated with isotretinoin than with etretinate.[255] This may be due to the differences in age,[256] fertility, and compliance with birth control techniques between the groups of patients treated with these retinoids. In one report, 49 percent of 396 women, most less than 30 years old, exposed to isotretinoin during pregnancy had conceived either prior to therapy or during the first 3 weeks of therapy.[256] There is no known safe dose or duration of therapy regarding teratogenicity of retinoids. In summary, isotretinoin and etretinate are contraindicated in pregnant women and in women of childbearing potential who refuse to use or are unreliable in complying with effective contraception. Current guidelines are that contraception should be used for 1 month prior to isotretinoin therapy, during therapy, and for 1 month afterwards,[257] and that a negative pregnancy test be obtained 2 weeks prior to initiating therapy on the second or third day of a normal menstrual period. Etretinate is stored in body fat depots, has a terminal elimination half-life in plasma of about 100 days, and can be detected in serum in trace amounts for as long as 3 years after cessation of therapy.[258] Thus, it is not known when conception is safe to occur after discontinuation of etretinate.

Acitretin is the carboxylic acid metabolite of etretinate. Its spectrum of clinical efficacy and toxicity is comparable to etretinate.[259] However, it differs considerably from etretinate by having a terminal elimination half-life in plasma of only 2 days in multiple-dose pharmacoknetic studies.[260] This rapid clearance after discontinuation of acitretin therapy would create a potential major clinical advantage of reduced risk of delayed teratogenicity in comparison with etretinate. Recent studies,[260] however, have shown that etretinate has been detected in the serum after acitretin has been administered. This suggests that there may, in fact, be little clinical advantage to acitretin.

Pseudotumor cerebri has developed rarely during treatment with isotretinoin. If patients receiving isotretinoin develop persistent headache with visual changes, nausea, and vomiting, the drug should be discontinued promptly and the patient should be examined for papilledema with retinal hemorrhages. In five such cases, the patients were also being treated with tetracycline or minocycline, drugs that are known to rarely produce increased intracranial hypertension. This finding would suggest caution in combining these therapies.

Hair loss is an additional toxicologic finding that occurs both with hypervitaminosis A and also with synthetic retinoid therapy. It is more severe during treatment with etretinate. The hair loss usually occurs 3 to 8 weeks after beginning etretinate ingestion and after a minimum total dose of 2 g. It ceases 6 to 8 weeks after discontinuation of therapy, although rare instances of persistent hair loss have been reported. In the majority of cases the hair loss is a telogen effluvium; occasionally, dystrophic anagen roots are found.[261,262]

Although retinoids at high doses may inhibit spermatogenesis in animals, semen analyses from patients receiving oral retinoids have revealed no abnormalities. In fact, a return toward normal of abnormally low pretreatment sperm counts in isotretinoin-treated acne patients has been noted.[263]

Chronic Toxicity

The most common findings observed in animals and humans during chronic hypervitaminosis A intoxication have been bony changes. Demineralization, thinning of the long bones, cortical hyperostosis, periostosis, and premature closure of the epiphyses have been documented.[264-270] There are several indications that the synthetic retinoids may be capable of inducing chronic bone toxicities similar to chronic hypervitaminosis A.[271-276] Etretinate accelerated ossification of the epiphyseal line in rats given 3 mg/kg per day.[277] Radiographic evidence of partial closure of the proximal epiphysis of

the right tibia, demineralization, and altered bone remodeling occurred in a 10-year-old boy treated with high doses (3.5 mg/kg per day) of oral isotretinoin over 4½ years for epidermolytic hyperkeratosis.[219]

Children with epidermolytic hyperkeratosis, lamellar ichthyosis, psoriasis, and other disorders of keratinization have been safely and successfully treated with etretinate for over 3 years. One child treated with etretinate, however, developed two traumatic fractures during therapy.[220] Radiologically this patient's long bones were abnormally slender, but pretreatment x-rays had not been performed. It is known that in rats high-dose vitamin A and high-dose etretinate (3 mg/kg per day) may induce fractures and modeling defects of the long bones with enhanced bone resorption. The administration of etretinate did not interfere with the overall growth and development of these children as monitored by sequential height and weight measurements.

Hypervitaminosis A in adult cats causes confluent exostosis formation of the cervical spine.[278,279] Similarly, in 50 patients, 37 receiving etretinate and 13 receiving isotretinoin for periods greater than 2 years, 9 had osteophytes present at two or three vertebral levels with anterior spinal ligament calcification, but without disc space narrowing.[222] Lack of disc space narrowing eliminates degenerative joint disease as a cause of these changes. Nine patients had bone bridging, that is, the osteophytes connected two vertebrae. Patients treated with isotretinoin for longer than 2 years at a minimum dose of 1.5 mg/kg per day were considered to be at significant risk for developing vertebral osteophytes, anterior spinal ligament calcification, and bony bridging, similar to the findings of idiopathic skeletal hyperostosis and hypervitaminosis A in the adult. Furthermore, in a prospective study, vertebral osteophytes were observed to form within 12 months after the initiation of therapy with isotretinoin at 2.0 mg/kg per day.[176,223] In 84 percent of patients on long-term therapy, calcification of peripheral tendons and ligaments, especially the insertion of the Achilles tendon and the plantar ligament, may occur with both isotretinoin and etretinate.[276]

Factors in the Decision to Use Retinoids

As with other medications, a risk/benefit ratio is often useful in determining whether or not to treat a patient with synthetic retinoids. Pertinent criteria in determining a risk/benefit ratio would include:

1. *Responsiveness of the disorder to retinoids.* The complete and often prolonged benefit of isotretinoin in the treatment of severe cystic acne is optimal, in contrast to the minimal improvement and characteristic relapse after withdrawal of therapy seen in some of the disorders of keratinization.
2. *Dose of retinoid required.* Some diseases, such as nonbullous congenital ichthyosiform erythroderma and cystic acne limited to the face, respond well to lower doses of isotretinoin, whereas other diseases, such as inflammatory Darier's disease, may require higher doses. Particularly in regard to psoriasis treated with etretinate, the use of lower doses in combination with other treatments such as PUVA (RePUVA) may eliminate some toxicities that require a minimum or threshold dose.
3. *Availability of alternative treatments.* In psoriasis, acne, and certain disorders of keratinization, such as lamellar ichthyosis, alternative therapies are available. However, synthetic

retinoids may represent the only effective treatment in other diseases, such as severe cases of Darier's disease and epidermolytic hyperkeratosis.

4. *Chronicity of retinoid therapy.* Some diseases, such as inflammatory Darier's disease and epidermolytic hyperkeratosis, may relapse rapidly on withdrawal of synthetic retinoids. Other diseases, such as cystic acne, psoriasis, and hyperkeratotic Darier's disease, may have prolonged partial or complete remissions that permit retinoid-free intervals. Patients with diseases that require continuous retinoid administration may be at increased risk for developing chronic toxicity.

5. *Severity of the disease.* One is more inclined to initiate retinoid therapy in patients with severe diseases. This is especially true when educational, psychological, or physical development may be compromised. For example, early retinoid treatment of lamellar ichthyosis may prevent the development of ectropion.

6. *Age of the patient.* Children with disorders of keratinization requiring chronic, moderate- to high-dose retinoid therapy are at highest risk of developing bony toxicity. Not only would they be at risk of premature epiphyseal closure but, because of the anticipated greater lifetime exposure to the drug, they would also be at higher risk of eventually developing the vertebral changes resembling diffuse idiopathic skeletal hyperostosis.

7. *Sex of the patient.* Retinoid teratogenicity entails special risks for the female patient of childbearing age. Although isotretinoin is rapidly cleared from the body within days, etretinate can be detected in the serum for months or even years after discontinuation of therapy. Thus it is not known when it is safe to conceive after discontinuation of etretinate. Current guidelines suggest at least 12 to 18 months.

8. *Presence of other disorders that may be aggravated by retinoid usage.* Renal or hepatic compromise, preexisting hyperlipidemia, or a family history of hyperlipidemia or premature atherosclerotic cardiovascular disease should be considered in the therapeutic assessment.

9. *Concomitant use of other drugs with similar toxicities.* Estrogens and corticosteroids may elevate serum lipids. Tetracycline may rarely produce benign intracranial hypertension. In addition to retinoids, many drugs are hepatotoxic, e.g., methotrexate.

Conclusions

The synthetic retinoids, isotretinoin and etretinate, represent a fairly new class of drugs that are highly effective in the treatment of a broad spectrum of dermatologic disease. Although there is overlap in therapeutic efficacy between isotretinoin and etretinate, each agent has unique clinical indications. Isotretinoin, for example, is the drug of choice for the treatment of severe cystic acne. The use of etretinate for psoriasis, either alone or in combination with presently available therapies, has been very effective, especially for the typically treatment-resistant pustular and erythrodermic varieties. Maintenance therapy with etretinate is necessary for many psoriatic patients. Long-term safety of this treatment and the duration of teratogenic potential of this retinoid must be considered. Etretinate is stored in fat, and blood levels of etretinate have been detected for prolonged periods after discontinuation of therapy.[258,280]

Synthetic retinoids must now also be considered the most effective treatment for Darier's disease and certain other disorders of keratinization. The degree of clinical response and duration of post-treatment remission varies with the different disorders treated.

The use of synthetic retinoids in cancer prevention and therapy for both cutaneous and internal tumors is potentially the most significant clinical use of these drugs. Based on the results of preliminary studies, it appears that chronic maintenance therapy is needed for successful chemoprevention of cancer with retinoids.

Acute side effects predominantly involve the skin and mucous membranes and are reversible after discontinuation of treatment. Systemic toxicities include hypertriglyceridemia, elevations in liver function tests, arthralgias, pseudotumor cerebri, and teratogenicity. The only chronic retinoid toxicities known to date, aside from claims of persistent dry eyes or hair thinning, are radiographic changes, including calcification of the anterior spinal ligament and osteophyte and bony bridge formation of the axial skeleton, similar to the findings of diffuse idiopathic skeletal hyperostosis, and calcification of peripheral tendons and ligaments, especially the insertion of the Achilles tendon and the plantar ligament. Isotretinoin is considered to produce more radiographic toxicity in the axial skeleton than etretinate.

Based on the experience obtained with isotretinoin and etretinate, the future of the retinoids appears most promising, particularly with the expanding spectrum of retinoid-responsive diseases and with the continuing development of new synthetic compounds, such as the arotinoids,[215] that may improve still further their efficacy or tolerability.

Dr. DiGiovanna's portion of this chapter was written in his private capacity. No official support or endorsement by the National Cancer Institute is intended or should be inferred.

References

1. Mandel HG, Cohn VH: Fat-soluble vitamins, in *The Pharmacological Basis of Therapeutics,* 6th ed, edited by AG Gilman et al. New York, Macmillan, 1980, p 1583

2. Stepp W: Versuche über Fütterung mit lipoidfreier Nahrung. *Biochem Z* **22**:452, 1909

3. McCollum EV, Davis M: The necessity of certain lipids in the diet during growth. *J Biol Chem* **15**:167, 1913

4. McCollum EV, Davis M: The nature of the dietary deficiencies of rice. *J Biol Chem* **23**:181, 1915

5. McCollum EV, Kennedy C: The dietary factors operating in the production of polyneuritis. *J Biol Chem* **24**:491, 1916

6. Steenbock H: White corn vs yellow corn and a (probable) relationship between the fat soluble vitamins and yellow plant pigments. *Science* **50**:352, 1919

7. Drummond JC: The nomenclature of the so-called accessory food factors (vitamins). *Biochem J* **14**:660, 1920

8. Karrer P et al: Zur kenntnis des Vitamins-A aus Frischtranen II. *Helv Chim Acta* **14**:1431, 1931

9. Euler HV, Karrer P: The study of vitamin A concentrates. *Helv Chim Acta* **14**:1040, 1931

10. Wald GJ: Vitamin A in eye tissues. *J Gen Physiol* **18**:905, 1935

11. Wald GJ: Carotenoids and the visual cycle. *J Gen Physiol* **19**:351, 1935

12. Arens JF, van Dorp DA: A new method for the synthesis of α,β-unsaturated aldehydes. *Recl Trav Chim Pays-Bas* **67**:973, 1948

13. Wolbach SB, Howe PR: Tissue changes following deprivation of fat-soluble A vitamin. *J Exp Med* **43**:753, 1925

14. Mori SJ: Primary changes in eyes of rats which result from deficiency of fat-soluble A in diet. *JAMA* **79**:197, 1922

15. Peck SM et al: Keratosis follicularis (Darier's disease). *Arch Dermatol Syphilol* **43**:223, 1941

16. Porter AD: Vitamin A in some congenital anomalies of the skin. *Br J Dermatol* **63**:123, 1951

17. Fujimaki Y: Formation of carcinoma in albino rats fed on deficient diets. *J Cancer Res* **10**:469, 1926

18. Stuttgen G: Zur Lokalbehandlung von Keratosen mit Vitamin-A-Saure. *Dermatologica* **124**:65, 1962

19. Beer P: Studies of the effects of vitamin A acid. *Dermatologica* **124**:192, 1962

20. Kligman AM et al: Topical vitamin A acid in acne vulgaris. *Arch Dermatol* **99**:469, 1969

21. Stuttgen G: Oral vitamin A acid therapy. *Acta Derm Venereol (Stockh)* **55**(suppl 74):174, 1975

22. Bollag W: Belgian patent 752,924, July 3, 1970

23. Pawson BA: A historical introduction to the chemistry of vitamin A and its analogs (retinoids), in *Modulation of Cellular Interaction by Vitamin A and Derivatives (Retinoids)*, edited by LM DeLuca, SS Shapiro. New York, New York Academy of Sciences, 1981, p 1

24. Frolik CA: In vitro and in vivo metabolism of all-trans- and 13-cis-retinoic acid in the hamster, in *Modulation of Cellular Interaction by Vitamin A and Derivatives (Retinoids)*, edited by LM DeLuca, SS Shapiro. New York, New York Academy of Sciences, 1981, p 37

25. Breitman TR et al: Induction of differentiation of the human promyelocytic leukemia cell line (HL-60) by retinoic acid. *Proc Natl Acad Sci USA* **77**:2936, 1980

26. Huang M et al: Use of all-*trans* retinoic acid in the treatment of acute promyelocytic leukemia. *Blood* **72**:567, 1988

27. Pawson BA et al: Retinoids at the threshold: Their biological significance and therapeutic potential. *J Med Chem* **25**:1269, 1982

28. Huang H, Goodman D: Vitamin A and carotenoids. I. Intestinal absorption and metabolism of ^{14}C-labeled vitamin A alcohol and β-carotene in the rat. *J Biol Chem* **240**:2839, 1965

29. Goodman DS: Vitamin A and retinoids: Recent advances. *Fed Proc* **38**:2501, 1979

30. Hirosawa K, Yamada K: The localization of the vitamin A in the mouse liver as revealed by electron microscope radioautography. *J Elect Microsc (Tokyo)* **22**:337, 1973

31. Kanai M et al: Retinol-binding protein: The transport protein for vitamin A in human plasma. *J Clin Invest* **47**:2025, 1968

32. Muto Y et al: Regulation of retinol binding protein metabolism by vitamin A status in the rat. *J Biol Chem* **247**:2542, 1972

33. Fidge NH et al: Pathways of absorption of retinal and retinoic acid in the rat. *J Lipid Res* **9**:103, 1968

34. Smith JE et al: The plasma transport and metabolism of retinoic acid in the rat. *Biochem J* **132**:821, 1973

35. Zile M et al: Characterization of retinol β-glucuronide as a minor metabolite of retinoic acid in bile. *Proc Natl Acad Sci USA* **77**:3230, 1980

36. Connor MJ, Smit MH. Terminal-group oxidation of retinol by mouse epidermis. Inhibition in vitro and in vivo. *Biochem J* **244**:489, 1987

37. Peterson P et al: Formation and properties of retinylphosphate galactose. *J Biol Chem* **251**:4986, 1976

38. DeLuca LM: The direct involvement of vitamin A in glycol transfer reactions of mammalian membranes. *Vitam Horm* **35**:1, 1977

39. Bhat PV, DeLuca LM: The biosynthesis of a mannolipid containing a metabolite of retinoic acid by 3T12 mouse fibroblasts. *Ann N Y Acad Sci* **359**:135, 1981

40. Zachman RD: The stimulation of RNA synthesis in vivo and in vitro by retinol in the intestine of vitamin A deficient rats. *Life Sci* **6**:2207, 1967

41. Sporn MB et al: Retinyl acetate: Effect on cellular content of RNA in epidermis in cell culture in chemically defined medium. *Science* **182**:722, 1973

42. Smith KB: Early effects of vitamin A on protein synthesis in the epidermis of embryonic chick skin cultured in serum-containing medium. *Dev Biol* **30**:241, 1973

43. Wolf G et al: Recent evidence for the participation of vitamin A in glycoprotein synthesis. *Fed Proc* **38**:2540, 1979

44. Ziboh VA et al: Effects of retinoic acid on prostaglandin biosynthesis in guinea pig skin. *J Invest Dermatol* **65**:370, 1975

45. Aso K et al: The role of prostaglandin E, cyclic AMP, and cyclic GMP in the proliferation of guinea pig ear skin stimulated by topical application of vitamin A acid. *J Invest Dermatol* **67**:231, 1976

46. Bashor M et al: In vitro binding of retinol to rat tissue components. *Proc Natl Acad Sci USA* **70**:3483, 1973

47. Sani B, Hill D: Retinoic acid: A binding protein in chick embryo metatarsal skin. *Biochem Biophys Res Commun* **61**:1276, 1974

48. Eriksson U et al: The NH$_2$-terminal amino acid sequence of cellular retinoic-acid binding protein from rat testis. *FEBS Lett* **135**:70, 1981

49. Chytil F, Ong DE: Cellular-binding protein for compounds with vitamin A activity, in *Receptors and Hormone Action*, edited by BW O'Malley, L Birmbaumer. New York, Academic, 1978, p 573

50. Chytil F, Ong DE: Cellular vitamin A binding proteins, in *Vitamins and Hormones*, vol 36, edited by PL Munson et al. New York, Academic, 1978, p 1

51. Bashor M, Chytil F: Cellular retinol-binding protein. *Biochim Biophys Acta* **411**:87, 1975

52. Ong D, Chytil F: Changes in levels of cellular retinol- and retinoic acid-binding proteins of liver and lung during perinatal development of rat. *Proc Natl Acad Sci USA* **73**:3976, 1976

53. Ong D et al: Retinoic acid binding protein: Occurrence in human tumors. *Science* **190**:60, 1975

54. DiGiovanna JJ et al: Quantitative and qualitative analysis of cytosol retinoid binding proteins in human skin. *J Invest Dermatol* **80**:356, 1983

55. Chytil F, Ong DE: Cellular retinol and retinoic acid-binding proteins in vitamin A action. *Fed Proc* **38**:2510, 1979

56. Lotan R: Effects of vitamin A and its analogs (retinoids) on normal and neoplastic cells. *Biochim Biophys Acta* **605**:33, 1980

57. Jetten AM, Jetten MER: Possible role of retinoic acid binding protein in retinoid stimulation of embryonal carcinoma cell differentiation. *Nature* **278**:180, 1979

58. Trown PW et al: Relationship between binding affinities to cellular retinoic acid binding protein and in vivo and in vitro properties for 18 retinoids. *Cancer Res* **40**:212, 1980

59. Sani BP, Corbett TH: Retinoic acid-binding protein in normal tissues and experimental tumors. *Cancer Res* **37**:209, 1977

60. Ong DE et al: Cellular binding proteins for vitamin A in colorectal adenocarcinoma of rat. *Cancer Res* **38**:4422, 1978

61. Sani BP et al: Determination of binding affinities of retinoids to retinoic acid-binding protein and serum albumin. *Biochem J* **171**:711, 1978

62. Chytil F, Ong DE: Mediation of retinoic acid-induced growth and anti-tumor activity. *Nature* **260**:49, 1976

63. Puhvel SM, Sakamoto M: Cellular retinoic acid-binding proteins in human epidermis and sebaceous follicles. *J Invest Dermatol* **82**:79, 1984

64. Wiggert B et al: Differential binding to soluble nuclear receptors and effects on cell viability of retinol and retinoic acid in cultured retinoblastoma cells. *Biochem Biophys Res Commun* **79**:218, 1977

65. Maden M et al: Spatial distribution of cellular protein binding to retinoic acid in the chick limb bud. *Nature* **335**:733, 1988

66. Giguere V et al: Identification of a receptor for the morphogen retinoic acid. *Nature* **330**:624, 1987

67. Petkovich M et al: A human retinoic acid receptor which belongs to the family of nuclear receptors. *Nature* **330**:444, 1987

68. Benbrook D et al: A novel retinoic acid receptor identified from hepatocellular carcinoma. *Nature* **333**:669, 1988

69. Brand N et al: Identification of a second human retinoic acid receptor. *Nature* **332**:850, 1988

70. Krust A et al: A third human retinoic acid receptor, HRAR-γ. *Proc Natl Acad Sci USA* **86**:5310, 1989

71. Goldberg Y et al: Thyroid hormone action and the *erb* A oncogene family. *Biochimie* **71**:279, 1989

72. Dolle P et al: Differential expression of genes encoding α, β, γ retinoic acid receptors and CRABP in the developing limbs of the mouse. *Nature* **342**:702, 1989

73. Kastner P et al: Murine isoforms of retinoic acid receptor gamma with specific patterns of expression. *Proc Natl Acad Sci USA* **87**:2700, 1990

74. Manglesdorf DJ et al: Nuclear receptor that identifies a novel retinoic acid response pathway. *Nature* **345**:224, 1990

75. Mangelsdorf DJ et al: A direct repeat in the cellular retinol binding protein type II gene confers differential regulation by RXR and RAR. *Cell* **66**:555, 1991

76. Levin AA et al: 9-*Cis* retinoic acid stereoisomer binds and activates the nuclear receptor RXRα. *Nature* **355**:359, 1992

77. Yu VC et al: RXBβ: A coregulator that enhances binding of retinoic acid, thyroid hormone, and vitamin D receptors to their cognate response elements. *Cell* **67**:1251, 1991

78. Moore T: Effects of vitamin A deficiency in animals: Pharmacology and toxicology of vitamin A, in *The Vitamins*, 2d ed, vol 1, edited by WH Sebrell, RS Harris. New York, Academic, 1967, pp 245, 280

79. Fell H: The effect of excess vitamin A on cultures of embryonic chicken skin explanted at different stages of differentiation. *Proc R Soc Lond [Biol]* **146**:242, 1957

80. Peck GL et al: Effects of retinoic acid on embryonic chick skin. *J Invest Dermatol* **69**:463, 1977

81. Thaller C, Eichele G: Identification and spatial distribution of retinoids in the developing chick limb bud. *Nature* **327**:625, 1987

82. Eichele G, Thaller C: Characterization of concentration gradient of a morphogenetically active retinoid in the chick limb bud. *J Cell Biol* **105**:1917, 1987

83. Brockes JP: Retinoids, homeobox genes, and limb morphogenesis. *Neuron* **2**:1285, 1989

84. Eichele G: Retinoids and vertebrate limb pattern formation. *Trends Genet* **5**:246, 1989

85. Brickell PM, Tickle C: Morphogens in chick limb development. *Bioassays* **11**:145, 1989

86. Sulik KK et al: Teratogens and craniofacial malformations: Relationships to cell death. *Development* **103**(suppl):213, 1988

87. Nettesheim P et al: Effect of vitamin A on lung tumor induction in rats. *Proc Am Assoc Cancer Res* **16**:54, 1975

88. Cohen SM et al: Effect of hyper- and avitaminosis A on urinary bladder carcinogenicity of N-[4-(5-nitro-2-furyl)-2-thiazolyl]-formamide (FANFT). *Fed Proc* **33**:602, 1974

89. Newberne PM, Rogers AE: Rat colon carcinomas associated with aflatoxin and marginal vitamin A. *J Natl Cancer Inst* **50**:439, 1973

90. Rogers AE et al: Induction by dimethylhydrazine of intestinal carcinoma in normal rats and rats fed high or low levels of vitamin A. *Cancer Res* **33**:1003, 1973

91. Strickland S, Mahdavi V: The induction of differentiation in teratocarcinoma stem cells by retinoic acid. *Cell* **15**:393, 1978

92. Kuff EL, Fewell JW: Induction of neural-like cells and acetylcholinesterase activity in cultures of F9 teratocarcinoma treated with retinoic acid and dibutyryl cyclic adenosine monophosphate. *Dev Biol* **77**:103, 1980

93. Lewis CA et al: Inhibition of limb chondrogenesis in vitro by vitamin A: Alterations in cell surface characteristics. *Dev Biol* **64**:31, 1978

94. Takigawa M et al: Polyamine and differentiation: Induction of ornithine decarboxylase by parathyroid hormone is a good marker of differentiated chondrocytes. *Proc Natl Acad Sci USA* **77**:1481, 1980

95. DiSimone DP, Reddi AH: The influence of vitamin A (retinoic acid) on matrix induced endochondral bone differentiation. *J Cell Biol* **91**:147a, 1981

96. Murray T, Russell TR: Inhibition of adipose conversion in 3T3-L2 cells by retinoic acid. *J Supramolec Struct* **14**:255, 1980

97. Lotan R, Lotan D: Stimulation of melanogenesis in a human melanoma cell line by retinoids. *Cancer Res* **40**:3345, 1980

98. Hoal EG et al: Inhibition of pigmentation by retinoic acid in a human melanoma cell line. *Fed Proc* **41**:683, 1982

99. Avdalovic N et al: The effect of retinoic acid on the morphology and cell surface properties of a non-adhesive variant of hamster melanoma cells. *Proc Am Assoc Cancer Res* **22**:121, 1981

100. Takenaga K et al: Production of differentiation-inhibiting factor in cultured mouse myeloid leukemia cells treated with retinoic acid. *Cancer Res* **41**:1948, 1981

101. Chu EW, Malmgren RA: An inhibitory effect of vitamin A on the induction of tumors of forestomach and cervix in the Syrian hamster by carcinogenic polycyclic hydrocarbons. *Cancer Res* **25**:884, 1965

102. Davies RE: Effects of vitamin A or 7,12-dimethyl-benz(a)anthracene-induced papillomas in rhino mouse skin. *Cancer Res* **27**:237, 1967

103. Genta WM et al: Vitamin A deficiency enhances binding of benzo(a)pyrene to tracheal epithelial DNA. *Nature* **247**:48, 1974

104. Bollag W: Therapy of chemically induced skin tumors of mice with vitamin A palmitate and vitamin A acid. *Experientia* **27**:90, 1971

105. Mahrle G, Berger H: Protective effect of aromatic retinoic acid analog on skin tumor. *J Invest Dermatol* **70**:235, 1978

106. Peck GL: Retinoids in clinical dermatology, in *Progress in Diseases in the Skin,* vol 1, edited by R Fleischmajer. New York, Grune & Stratton, 1981, p 227

107. Kraemer KH et al: Prevention of skin cancer in xeroderma pigmentosum with the use of oral isotretinoin. *N Engl J Med* **318**:1633, 1988

108. Moon RC et al: N-(4-Hydroxyphenyl)-retinamide, a new retinoid for prevention of breast cancer in the rat. *Cancer Res* **39**:1339, 1979

109. Sporn MB et al: 13-*cis*-Retinoic acid: Inhibition of bladder carcinogenesis in the rat. *Science* **195**:487, 1977

110. Becci PJ et al: Inhibitory effect of 13-*cis*-retinoic acid on urinary bladder carcinogenesis induced in C57BL/6 mice by N-butyl-N-(4-hydroxybutyl)-nitrosamine. *Cancer Res* **38**:4463, 1978

111. O'Brien TG: The induction of ornithine decarboxylase as an early, possibly obligatory, event in mouse skin carcinogenesis. *Cancer Res* **36**:2644, 1976

112. O'Brien TG et al: Induction of the polyamine-biosynthetic enzymes in mouse epidermis and their specificity for tumor promotion. *Cancer Res* **35**:2426, 1975

113. Russell DH, Durie GM: *Polyamines as Biochemical Markers of Normal and Malignant Growth.* New York, Raven, 1978

114. Verma AK, Boutwell RK: Vitamin A acid (retinoic acid), a potent inhibitor of 12-O-tetradecanoyl-phorbol-13-acetate-induced ornithine decarboxylase activity in mouse epidermis. *Cancer Res* **37**:2196, 1977

115. Verma AK et al: Correlation of the inhibition by retinoids of tumor promoter-induced ornithine decarboxylase activity in mouse epidermis by vitamin A analogs (retinoids). *Cancer Res* **38**:793, 1978

116. Chapman SK: Antitumor effects of vitamin A and inhibitors of ornithine decarboxylase in cultured neuroblastoma and glioma cells. *Life Sci* **26**:1359, 1980

117. Yuspa SH et al: Retinyl acetate modulation of cell growth kinetics and carcinogen-cellular interaction in mouse epidermal cell cultures. *Chem Biol Interact* **16**:251, 1977

118. Lutzner M, Blanchet-Bardon C: Oral retinoid treatment of human papillomavirus type 5-induced epidermodysplasia verruciformis. *N Engl J Med* **302**:1091, 1980

119. Fuchs E, Green H: Regulation of terminal differentiation of cultured human keratinocytes by vitamin A. *Cell* **25**:617 1981

120. Gilfix BM, Eckert RL: Coordinate regulation by vitamin A of keratin gene expression in human keratinocytes. *J Biol Chem* **260**:14026, 1985

121. Floyd EE, Jetten AM: Regulation of type I (epidermal) transglutaminase mRNA levels during squamous differentiation: Down regulation by retinoids. *Mol Cell Biol* **9**:4846, 1989

122. Jetten AM et al: Characterization of the action of retinoids on mouse fibroblast cell lines. *Exp Cell Res* **119**:289, 1979

123. Christophers E: Growth stimulation of cultured postembryonic epidermal cells by vitamin A acid. *J Invest Dermatol* **63**:450, 1974

124. Hassell JR et al: Enhanced cellular fibronectin accumulation in chondrocytes treated with vitamin A. *Cell* **17**:821, 1979

125. Jetten AM et al: Enhancement in 'apparent' membrane microviscosity during differentiation of embryonal carcinoma cells induced by retinoids. *Exp Cell Res* **138**:494, 1982

126. Jetten AM: Modulation of cell growth by retinoids and their possible mechanisms of action. *Fed Proc* **43**:134, 1984

127. Elias PM et al: Influence of topical and systemic retinoids on basal cell carcinoma membranes. *Cancer* **48**:932, 1981

128. Prutkin L: Mucous metaplasia and gap junctions in the vitamin A acid-treated skin tumor, keratoacanthoma. *Cancer Res* **35**:364, 1975

129. Lotan R et al: Retinoic acid-induced modifications in the growth and cell surface components of a human carcinoma (HeLa) cell line. *Exp Cell Res* **130**:401, 1980

130. Shapiro SS, Poon JP: Retinoic acid-induced alterations of growth and morphology in an established epithelial line. *Exp Cell Res* **119**:349, 1979

131. Fell HG, Dingle JT: Studies on the mode of action of excess of vitamin A: VI. Lysosomal protease and the degradation of cartilage matrix. *Biochem J* **87**:403, 1963

132. Wang CC et al: Destabilization of mouse liver lysosomes by vitamin A compounds and analogues. *Biochem Pharmacol* **25**:471, 1976

133. Lazarus GS et al: Lysosomes and the skin. *J Invest Dermatol* **65**:259, 1975

134. Dingle JT: Vacuoles, vesicles, and lysosomes. *Br Med Bull* **24**:141, 1968

135. Roels OA et al: Vitamin A and membranes. *J Clin Nutr* **22**:1020, 1969

136. McNutt NS: Freeze-fracture techniques and applications to the structural analysis of the mammalian plasma membrane, in *Cell Surface Reviews,* vol 4, edited by G Poste, GL Nicholson. Amsterdam, North-Holland, 1977, p 75

137. McNutt NS, Weinstein RS: Carcinoma of the cervix: Deficiency of nexus intercellular junctions. *Science* **165**:597, 1969

138. Sheridan JD: Low-resistance junctions between cancer cells in various solid tumors. *J Cell Biol* **45**:91, 1970

139. Weinstein RS et al: The structure and function of intercellular junctions in cancer. *Adv Cancer Res* **23**:23, 1976

140. Elias PM, Friend DS: Vitamin A-induced mucous metaplasia. An in vitro system for modulating tight and gap junction differentiation. *J Cell Biol* **68**:173, 1976

141. DeLuca LM: Vitamin A, in *Handbook of Lipid Research,* vol 2, edited by LM DeLuca. New York, Plenum, 1978, p 1

142. DeLuca LM: Epithelial membranes and vitamin A, in *Mammalian Cell Membranes,* edited by GA Jamieson, DM Robinson. Boston, Butterworth, 1977, p 231

143. Wolf G: Retinal-linked sugars in glycoprotein synthesis. *Nutr Rev* **35**:97, 1977

144. DeLuca LM et al: Recent developments in studies on biological functions of vitamin A in normal and transformed tissues, in *Pure and Applied Chemistry,* vol 51. New York, Pergamon, 1979, p 581

145. Adamo S et al: Retinoid-induced adhesion in cultured transformed mouse fibroblast. *J Natl Cancer Inst* **62**:1473, 1979

146. Sasak W et al: Role of retinoids in the induction of adhesion and mannosylation of glycoconjugates of cultured spontaneously-transformed mouse fibroblasts (Balb/c 3T12-3 cells). *J Cell Biol* **79**:CS206, 1978

147. Patt LM et al: Retinol induces density-dependent growth inhibition and changes in glycolipids and LETS. *Nature* **273**:379, 1978

148. Poon JP, Shapiro SS: Retinoic acid mediated inhibition of growth in transformed epithelial cells. *Fed Proc* **37**:1392, 1978

149. Poon JP et al: Effect of vitamin A acetate on glycosaminoglycan biosynthesis in epidermal and dermal cells in vitro. *Fed Proc* **36**:748, 1977

150. King IA, Tabiowo A: Long-term effects of all-*trans*-retinoic acid on epidermal glycosaminoglycan, glycoprotein, and protein synthesis in vitro, in *Retinoids: Advances in Basic Research and Therapy,* edited by CE Orfanos et al. New York, Springer, 1981, p 473

151. Shapiro SS, Mott DJ: Modulation of glycosaminoglycan biosynthesis by retinoids, in *Modulation of Cellular Interactions by Vitamin A and Derivatives (Retinoids),* edited by LM DeLuca, SS Shapiro. New York, New York Academy of Sciences, 1981, p 306

152. Sherman MI et al: Differentiation of early mouse embryonic and teratocarcinoma cells in vitro: Plasminogen activator production. *Cancer Res* **36**:4208, 1976

153. Miskin R et al: Plasminogen activator in chick embryo muscle cells: Induction of enzyme by RSV, PMA and retinoic acid. *Cell* **15**:1301, 1978

154. Wilson EL, Reich E: Plasminogen activator in chick fibroblasts. Induction of synthesis by retinoic acid: Synergism with viral transformation and phorbol ester. *Cell* **15**:385, 1978

155. Brinckerhoff CE et al: Inhibition by retinoic acid of collagenase production in rehumatoid synovial cells. *N Engl J Med* **303**:432, 1980

156. Bauer EF et al: Inhibition of collagen degradative enzymes by retinoic acid in vitro. *J Am Acad Dermatol* **6**:603, 1982

157. Levine L: N-(4-hydroxyphenyl)retinamide: A synthetic analog of vitamin A that is a potent inhibitor of prostaglandin synthesis. *Prostaglandins Med* **4**:285, 1980

158. Felix EL et al: Inhibition of the growth and development of a transplantable murine melanoma by vitamin A. *Science* **189**:886, 1975

159. Dennert G: Retinoids and the immune system: Immunostimulation by vitamin A, in *The Retinoids,* vol 2, edited by MB Sporn et al. New York, Academic, 1984, p 373

160. Patek PQ et al: Antitumor potential of retinoic acid; stimulation of immune mediated effectors. *Int J Cancer* **24**:624, 1979

161. Medawar PB, Hunt R: Anti-cancer action of retinoids. *Immunology* **42**:349, 1981

162. Kurata T, Micksche M: Immunoprophylaxis in Lewis lung tumor with vitamin A + BCG. *IRCS J Med Sci* **5**:277, 1977

163. Dennert G, Lotan R: Effects of retinoic acid on the immune system: Stimulation of T killer cell induction. *Eur J Immunol* **8**:23, 1978

164. Rhodes J, Oliver S: Retinoids as regulators of macrophage function. *Immunology* **40**:467, 1980

165. Schultz RM et al: Regulation of macrophage tumoricidal function: A role for prostaglandins of the E series. *Science* **202**:320, 1978

166. Peck GL et al: Prolonged remissions of cystic and conglobate acne with 13-*cis*-retinoic acid. *N Engl J Med* **300**:329, 1979

167. Peck GL et al: Isotretinoin versus placebo in the treatment of cystic acne. *J Am Acad Dermatol* **6**:735, 1982

168. Cunliffe WJ, Norris JFB: Isotretinoin—an explanation for its long-term benefit. *Dermatologica* **175**(suppl 1):133, 1987

169. Jones DH et al: A dose-response study of 13-*cis*-retinoic acid in acne vulgaris. *Br J Dermatol* **108**:333, 1983

170. Strauss JS et al: Isotretinoin therapy for acne: Results of a multicenter dose-response study. *J Am Acad Dermatol* **10**:490, 1984

171. Meigel W et al: Orale Behandlung der Acne conglobata mit 13-*cis*-Retinsaure: Ergebnisse der deutschen multizentrischen Studie nach 24 wochiger Behandlung. *Hautarzt* **34**:387, 1983

172. Jones DH et al: 13-*cis*-Retinoic acid in acne (a double-blind study of dose response), in *Retinoids: Advances in Basic Research and Therapy,* edited by CE Orfanos et al. New York, Springer, 1981, p 255

173. Plewig G et al: Effects of two retinoids in animal experiments and after clinical application in acne patients: 13-*cis*-retinoic acid Ro 4-3780 and aromatic retinoid Ro 10-9359, in *Retinoids: Advances in Basic Research and Therapy,* edited by CE Orfanos et al. New York, Springer, 1981, p 219

174. Rubinow DR et al: Reduced anxiety and depression in cystic acne patients after successful treatment with oral isotretinoin. *J Am Acad Dermatol* **17**:25, 1987

175. Katz R et al: Flare of cystic acne from oral isotretinoin. *J Am Acad Dermatol* **8**:132, 1983

176. Shalita AR et al: Isotretinoin treatment of acne and related disorders: An update. *J Am Acad Dermatol* **9**:629, 1983

177. Exner JG et al: Pyogenic granuloma-like acne lesions during isotretinoin therapy. *Arch Dermatol* **119**:808, 1983

178. Holland DB et al: Inflammatory responses in acne patients treated with 13-*cis*-retinoic acid (isotretinoin). *Br J Dermatol* **110**:343, 1984

179. Plewig G et al: Action of isotretinoin in acne rosacea and gram-negative folliculitis. *J Am Acad Dermatol* **6**:766, 1982

180. Farrell LN et al: The treatment of severe cystic acne with 13-*cis*-retinoic acid. *J Am Acad Dermatol* **3**:602, 1980

181. Goldstein JA et al: Comparative effect of isotretinoin and etretinate on acne and sebaceous gland function. *J Am Acad Dermatol* **6**:760, 1982

182. Strauss JS et al: The effect of marked inhibition of sebum production with 13-*cis*-retinoic acid on skin surface lipid composition. *J Invest Dermatol* **74**:66, 1980

183. Gross EG et al: Long-term inhibition of quantitative sebum production with isotretinoin (abstr). *J Invest Dermatol* **80**:357, 1983

184. Landthaler M et al: Effects of 13-*cis*-retinoic acid on sebaceous glands in humans, in *Retinoids: Advances in Basic Research and Therapy,* edited by CE Orfanos et al. New York, Springer, 1981, p 259

185. Stewart ME et al: Effect of 13-*cis*-retinoic acid at three dose levels on sustainable rates of sebum secretion and on acne. *J Am Acad Dermatol* **8**:532, 1983

186. Stewart ME et al: Suppression of sebum secretion with 13-*cis*-retinoic acid: Effect on individual skin surface lipids and implications for their anatomic origin. *J Invest Dermatol* **82**:74, 1984

187. Camisa C et al: The effects of retinoids on neutrophil functions in vitro. *J Am Acad Dermatol* **6**:620, 1982

188. Norris DA et al: 13-*cis*-Retinoic acid has major anti-inflammatory activity in vivo. *Clin Res* **31**:593A, 1983

189. King K et al: A double-blind study of the effects of 13-*cis*-retinoic acid on acne, sebum excretion rate and microbial population. *Br J Dermatol* **107**:583, 1982

190. Leyden JJ, McGinley KJ: Effect of 13-*cis*-retinoic acid on sebum production and *Propionibacterium acnes* in severe nodulocystic acne. *Arch Dermatol Res* **272**:331, 1982

191. Jones DH et al: Effect of 13-*cis*-retinoic acid on pilosebaceous duct obstruction. *Br J Dermatol* **107**(suppl 22):35, 1982

192. Matsuoka LY et al: Effect of isotretinoin in acne is not mediated by adrenal androgens. *J Am Acad Dermatol* **20**:128, 1989

193. Gomez EC: Differential effect of 13-*cis*-retinoic acid and an aromatic retinoid (Ro 10-9359) on the sebaceous glands of the hamster flank organ. *J Invest Dermatol* **76**:68, 1981

194. Rademaker M et al: Isotretinoin treatment alters steroid metabolism in women with acne. *Br J Dermatol* **124**:361, 1991

195. Lookingbill DP et al: Effect of isotretinoin on serum levels of precursor and peripherally derived androgens in patients with acne. *Arch Dermatol* **124**:540, 1988

196. Ward A et al: Etretinate: A review of its pharmacological properties and therapeutic efficacy in psoriasis and other skin disorders. *Drugs* **26**:9, 1983

197. Ehmann CW, Voorhees JJ: International studies of the efficacy of etretinate in the treatment of psoriasis. *J Am Acad Dermatol* **6**:692, 1982

198. Mahrle G et al: Oral treatment of keratinizing disorders of skin and mucous membranes with etretinate. *Arch Dermatol* **118**:97, 1982

199. Goerz G, Orfanos CE: Systemic treatment of psoriasis with a new aromatic retinoid. *Dermatologica* **157**(suppl 1):38, 1978

200. Sofen HL et al: Treatment of generalized pustular psoriasis with isotretinoin. *Lancet* **1**:40, 1984

201. Fritsch PO et al: Augmentation of oral methoxsalen-photochemotherapy with an oral retinoic acid derivative. *J Invest Dermatol* **70**:178, 1978

202. Grupper C, Berretti B: Treatment of psoriasis by oral PUVA-therapy combined with aromatic retinoid (Re-PUVA), in *Retinoids: Advances in Basic Research and Therapy,* edited by CE Orfanos et al. New York, Springer, 1981, p 341

203. Lauharanta J et al: Aromatic retinoid (Ro 10-9359), Re-PUVA, and PUVA in the treatment of psoriasis, in *Retinoids: Advances in Basic Research and Therapy,* edited by CE Orfanos et al. New York, Springer, 1981, p 201

204. Orfanos CE et al: Oral retinoid and UVB radiation: A new alternative treatment for psoriasis on an outpatient basis. *Acta Derm Venereol (Stockh)* **59**:241, 1979

205. Van der Rhee HJ, Polano MK: Treatment of psoriasis vulgaris with a low-dosage Ro 10-9359 orally combined with corticosteroids topically, in *Retinoids: Advances in Basic Research and Therapy,* edited by CE Orfanos et al. New York, Springer, 1981, p 193

206. Orfanos CE, Runne U: Systemic use of a new retinoid with and without local dithranol treatment in generalized psoriasis. *Br J Dermatol* **95**:101, 1976

207. Brackertz D, Muller W: Die Beeinflussung der arthropathia Psoriatica und der chronischen Polyarthritis durch ein oral wirksames aromatisches Retinoid. *Verh Dtsch Ges Inn Med* **85**:1343, 1979

208. Rosenthal M: Retinoid in der Behandlung von Psoriasis-arthritis. *Schweiz Med Wochenschr* **109**:1912, 1979

209. Stollenwerk R et al: Clinical observations on oral retinoid therapy of psoriatic arthropathy (Ro 10-9359), in *Retinoids: Advances in Basic Research and Therapy,* edited by CE Orfanos et al. New York, Springer, 1981, p 205

210. Thivolet J et al: L'association retinoide aromatique PUVA-therapie dans le traitement des psoriasis arthropathiques. *Ann Dermatol Venereol* **106**:1037, 1979

211. Hönigsmann H, Wolff K: Isotretinoin-PUVA for psoriasis. *Lancet* **1**:236, 1983

212. Orfanos CE et al: Neue Aspekte und Entwicklungen der antipsoriatischen Retinoid therapie. *Hautarzt* **32**:275, 1981

213. Peck GL, Yoder FW: Treatment of lamellar ichthyosis and other keratinising dermatoses with an oral synthetic retinoid. *Lancet* **2**:1172, 1976

214. Peck GL et al: Treatment of Darier's disease, lamellar ichthyosis, pityriasis rubra pilaris, cystic acne, and basal cell carcinoma with oral 13-*cis*-retinoic acid. *Dermatologica* **157**(suppl 1):11, 1978

215. Orfanos CE et al: The retinoids—a review of their clinical pharmacology and therapeutic use. *Drugs* **34**:459, 1987

216. Peck G et al: Comparative analysis of two retinoids in the treatment of disorders of keratinization, in *Retinoids: Advances in Basic Research and Therapy,* edited by CE Orfanos et al. New York, Springer, 1981, p 279

217. Lowhagen GB et al: Effects of etretinate (Ro 10-9359) on Darier's disease. *Dermatologica* **165**:123, 1982

218. Goldsmith LA et al: Pityriasis rubra pilaris response to 13-*cis*-retinoic acid (isotretinoin). *J Am Acad Dermatol* **6**:710, 1982

219. Milstone LM et al: Premature epiphyseal closure in a child receiving oral 13-*cis*-retinoic acid. *J Am Acad Dermatol* **7**:663, 1982

220. Tamayo L, Ruiz-Maldonado R: Long-term follow-up of 30 children under oral retinoid Ro 10-9359, in *Retinoids: Advances in Basic Research and Therapy,* edited by CE Orfanos et al. New York, Springer, 1981, p 287

221. Pittsley RA, Yoder FW: Retinoid hyperostosis. *N Engl J Med* **308**:1012, 1983

222. Gerber LH et al: Vertebral abnormalities associated with synthetic retinoid use. *J Am Acad Dermatol* **10**:817, 1984

223. Ellis CN et al: Isotretinoin therapy is associated with early skeletal radiographic changes. *J Am Acad Dermatol* **10**:1024, 1984

224. Fritsch PO: Oral retinoids in dermatology. *Int J Dermatol* **20**:314, 1981

225. Moriarty M et al: Etretinate in the treatment of actinic keratosis. *Lancet* **1**:364, 1982

226. Peck GL et al: Treatment of basal cell carcinomas with 13-*cis*-retinoic acid. *Proc Am Assoc Cancer Res* **20**:56, 1979

227. Peck GL et al: Chemoprevention of basal cell carcinoma with isotretinoin. *J Am Acad Dermatol* **6**:815, 1982

228. Peck GL et al: Treatment and prevention of basal cell carcinoma with isotretinoin. *J Am Acad Dermatol* **19**:176, 1988

229. Braun-Falco O et al: Tumor prophylaxe bei Xeroderma pigmentosum mit aromatischen Retinoid (Ro 10-9359). *Hautarzt* **33**:445, 1982

230. Haydey RP et al: Treatment of keratoacanthomas with oral 13-*cis*-retinoic acid. *N Engl J Med* **303**:560, 1980

231. Berretti B et al: Aromatic retinoid in the treatment of multiple superficial basal cell carcinoma, arsenic keratosis and keratoacanthoma, in *Retinoids: Advances in Basic Research and Therapy,* edited by CE Orfanos et al. New York, Springer, 1981, p 397

232. Schnitzler L, Verret JL: Retinoid and skin cancer prevention, in *Retinoids: Advances in Basic Research and Therapy,* edited by CE Orfanos et al. New York, Springer, 1981, p 385

233. Koch HF: Effect of retinoids on precancerous lesions of oral mucosa, in *Retinoids: Advances in Basic Research and Therapy,* edited by CE Orfanos et al. New York, Springer, 1981, p 307

234. Hong WK et al: 13-*cis* Retinoic acid in the treatment of oral leukoplakia. *N Engl J Med* **315**:1501, 1986

235. Levine N, Meyskens FL Jr: Topical vitamin A acid therapy for cutaneous metastatic melanoma. *Lancet* **2**:224, 1980

236. Cassidy J et al: Phase II trial of 13-*cis*-retinoic acid in metastatic breast cancer and other malignancies. *Proc Am Soc Clin Oncol* **22**:441, 1981

237. Souteyrand P et al: Treatment of parapsoriasis en plaques and mycosis fungoides with an oral aromatic retinoid (Ro 10-9359), in *Retinoids: Advances in Basic Research and Therapy,* edited by CE Orfanos et al. New York, Springer, 1981, p 313

238. Kessler JF et al: Treatment of cutaneous T-cell lymphoma (mycosis fungoides) with 13-*cis*-retinoic acid. *Lancet* **1**:1345, 1983

239. Lippman SM, Meyskens FL Jr: Results of the use of vitamin A and retinoids in cutaneous malignancies. *Pharmacol Ther* **40**:107, 1989

240. Kraemer KH et al: Oral isotretinoin prevention of skin cancer in xeroderma pigmentosum: Individual variation in dose response (abstr). *J Invest Dermatol* **94**:544, 1990

241. Tangrea JA et al: Long-term therapy with low-dose isotretinoin for prevention of basal cell carcinoma: A multicenter clinical trial. *J Natl Cancer Inst* **84**:328, 1992

242. Lippman SM, Meyskens FL Jr: Treatment of advanced squamous cell carcinoma of the skin with isotretinoin. *Ann Intern Med* **107**:499, 1987

243. Hong WK et al: Prevention of second primary tumors with isotretinoin in squamous cell carcinoma of the head and neck. *N Engl J Med* **323**:795, 1990

244. Weiss VC et al: Hepatotoxic reactions in a patient treated with etretinate. *Arch Dermatol* **120**:104, 1984

245. Roenigk HH Jr: Liver toxicity of retinoid therapy. *Pharmacol Ther* **40**:145, 1989

246. Zech LA et al: Changes in plasma cholesterol and triglyceride levels after treatment with oral isotretinoin: A prospective study. *Arch Dermatol* **119**:987, 1983

247. Bershad S et al: Changes in plasma lipids and lipoproteins during isotretinoin therapy for acne. *N Engl J Med* **313**:981, 1985

248. Dicken CH, Connolly SM: Eruptive xanthomas associated with isotretinoin (13-*cis*-retinoic acid). *Arch Dermatol* **116**:951, 1980

249. Ensink BW, Van Voorst Vader PC: Ophthalmological side effects of 13-*cis*-retinoid therapy. *Br J Dermatol* **108**:627, 1983

250. Blackman HF et al: Blepharoconjunctivitis: A side effect of 13-*cis*-retinoic acid therapy for dermatologic diseases. *Ophthalmology* **86**:753, 1979

251. Gold JA et al: Ocular side effects of the retinoids. *Int J Dermatol* **28**:218, 1989

252. Safran AB et al: Ocular side effects of oral treatment with retinoids. A review of clinical findings and molecular mechanisms and a prospective study of the influence of acitretin on retinal function, in *Retinoids: 10 Years On,* edited by J-H Saurat. Basel, Karger, 1991, p 315

253. Lammer EJ et al: Retinoic acid embryopathy. *N Engl J Med* **313**:837, 1985

254. Stern RS et al: Isotretinoin and pregnancy. *J Am Acad Dermatol* **10**:851, 1984

255. Sulik KK, Alles AJ: Teratogenicity of the retinoids, in *Retinoids: 10 Years On,* edited by J-H Saurat. Basel, Karger, 1990, p 282

256. Dai WS et al: Epidemiology of isotretinoin exposure during pregnancy. *J Am Acad Dermatol* **26**:599, 1992

257. Dai WS et al: Safety of pregnancy after discontinuation of isotretinoin. *Arch Dermatol* **125**:362, 1989

258. DiGiovanna JJ et al: Etretinate: Persistent serum concentrations after long-term therapy. *Arch Dermatol* **125**:246, 1989

259. Gollnick H: Acitretin in psoriasis: An update, in *Retinoids: 10 Years On,* edited by J-H Saurat. Basel, Karger, 1991, p 204

260. Wiegand U-W et al: Pharmacokinetics of acitretin in humans, in *Retinoids: 10 Years On,* edited by J-H Saurat. Basel, Karger, 1991, p 192

261. Orfanos CE: Oral retinoids—present status. *Br J Dermatol* **103**:473, 1980

262. Berth-Jones J et al: A study of etretinate alopecia. *Br J Dermatol* **122**:751, 1990

263. Schill WB et al: Aromatic retinoid and 13-*cis*-retinoic acid: Spermatological investigations, in *Retinoids: Advances in Basic Research and Therapy,* edited by CE Orfanos et al. New York, Springer, 1981, p 389

264. Caffey J: Chronic poisoning due to excess of vitamin A. *Am J Roentgenol* **65**:12, 1951

265. Frame B et al: Hypercalcemia and skeletal effects in chronic hypervitaminosis A. *Ann Intern Med* **80**:44, 1974

266. Bartolozzi G, Bernini G: Chronic hypervitaminosis A. *Helv Paediatr Acta* **25**:301, 1970

267. Di Benedetto RJ: Chronic hypervitaminosis A in an adult. *JAMA* **201**:700, 1967

268. Hellriegel KP, Reuter H: Side effects of vitamins, in *Meyler's Side Effects of Drugs,* vol 8, edited by MNG Dukes. Amsterdam, Excerpta Medica, 1975, p 799

269. Pease CN: Focal retardation and arrestment of growth of bones due to vitamin A intoxication. *JAMA* **182**:980, 1962

270. Ruby LK, Mohinder AM: Skeletal deformities following chronic hypervitaminosis A. *J Bone Joint Surg* **56A**:1283, 1974

271. Lawson JP, McGuire J: The spectrum of skeletal changes associated with the long-term administration of 13-*cis*-retinoic acid. *Skeletal Radiol* **16**:91, 1987

272. Carey BM et al: Skeletal toxicity with isotretinoin therapy: A clinico-radiological evaluation. *Br J Dermatol* **119**:609, 1988

273. Ellis CN et al: Long term radiographic follow-up after isotretinoin therapy. *J Am Acad Dermatol* **18**:1252, 1988

274. Kilcoyne RF: Effects of retinoids in bone. *J Am Acad Dermatol* **19**:212, 1988

275. White SI, MacKie RM: Bone changes associated with oral retinoid therapy. *Pharmacol Ther* **40**:137, 1989

276. DiGiovanna JJ et al: Extraspinal tendon and ligament calcification associated with long-term therapy with etretinate. *N Engl J Med* **315**:1177, 1986

277. Teelmann K: Experimental toxicology of the aromatic retinoid Ro 10-9359 (etretinate), in *Retinoids: Advances in Basic Research and Therapy,* edited by CE Orfanos et al. New York, Springer, 1981, p 41

278. Seawright AA et al: Hypervitaminosis A and hyperostosis of the cat. *Nature* **206**:1171, 1965

279. Seawright AA et al: Hypervitaminosis A and deforming cervical-spondylosis of the cat. *J Comp Pathol* **77**:29, 1967

280. Rollman O, Vahlquist A: Retinoid concentration in skin, serum, and adipose tissue of patients treated with etretinate. *Br J Dermatol* **109**:439, 1983

Nicholas A. Soter

Antihistamines

The biologic effects of histamine and its release from tissues during inflammatory reactions were recognized by 1910. In 1927, Lewis suggested that a substance with biologic properties similar to those of histamine accounted for the cutaneous triple response phenomenon. Also, he showed that the intradermal injection of histamine resulted in the formation of a wheal and erythema.[1] In 1937, Bovet and Staub[2] demonstrated that some of the effects of histamine in experimental animals could be antagonized by amines containing a phenolic ether moiety. Subsequent research yielded a number of related compounds and led to the development of histamine-receptor antagonists, or antihistamines, that became available for clinical use as therapeutic agents in the 1940s.

The fact that available antihistamines were unable to block the effects of histamine on the gastric mucosa[3] suggested that histamine might exert its effects via different receptors, which were later designated H_1 and H_2.[4,5] This observation led to the synthesis of new compounds that selectively blocked histamine at the H_2-receptor site.[6] Recently, H_3 receptors[7,8] have been recognized in brain and peripheral nerve tissue in experimental animals and in the airways in humans; however, clinical therapeutic agents are not yet available to block the H_3 receptor.

All of the clinical blockers, or antagonists, of histamine are reversible competitive inhibitors of the actions of histamine at tissue receptor sites, although some of these therapeutic agents have additional actions.

Histamine

Chemistry and Metabolism

Histamine, β-imidazolylethylamine, which is present in mast cells, basophils, and platelets in association with their granules, and in the stomach, is formed by the enzymatic decarboxylation of the amino acid histidine by histidine decarboxylase. In mast cell granules, histamine is stored and bound ionically to a proteoglycan-protein complex. After its release, histamine is catabolized in one of two ways. In the more important pathway in the skin, histamine is catalyzed by histamine methyltransferase to produce methyl histamine, which is converted by monoamine oxidase to methylimidazole acetic acid. In the second pathway, histamine undergoes oxidative deamination catalyzed by diamine oxidase to form imidazole acetic acid, which is subsequently conjugated and excreted as riboxylimidazole acetic acid.

Tissue Receptors

The biologic effects of histamine result from its interactions with tissue receptors, designated H_1, H_2, and H_3. Increases in venular permeability, contraction of smooth muscle, increases in airways resistance, enhancement of chemotaxis of eosinophils and neutrophils,[9] and stimulation of nasal mucus secretion are mediated through H_1 receptors. Increases in venular permeability and in cardiac rate and force of contraction,[10] augmentation of gastric acid secretion,[11] stimulation of CD8+ T lymphocytes,[12] increases in airways mucus production, and inhibition of chemotaxis of neutrophils and eosinophils[9] are H_2-dependent actions. Inasmuch as the skin microvasculature contains both H_1 and H_2 receptors,[13] increased venular permeability depends on the interaction of histamine with both of these receptors. H_3 receptors inhibit cholinergic and noncholinergic excitatory nerves in the airways.[8] Blockade of these receptors limits the bronchoconstriction induced by histamine.

Antihistamines

Traditional, Classic, or First-Generation H_1-Type Antihistamines

The traditional, classic, or first generation H_1-type antihistamines have in common with histamine a substituted ethylamine moiety as an integral part of the molecule (Fig. 237-1). The activity of an H_1-type antihistamine is increased by the substitution of a halogen in the *para* position of the phenyl or benzyl group of R^1. For maximum activity, the terminal nitrogen of the ethylamine group should be a tertiary amine with methyl groups or a cyclic moiety in R^2 and R^3. The dextro isomer is more active than is the levo isomer. In addition, H_1-type antihistamines have a tertiary amino group linked by a two- or three-atom chain to two aromatic substituents. H_1-type antihistamines have been divided into six subgroups (Table 237-1) based on substitution at the X position with nitrogen, oxygen, or carbon.

In addition to their antihistamine actions, the H_1-type antihistamines have a number of effects that include sedation, anticholinergic activity, local anesthesia, antiemetic activity, and anti-motion sickness effects. Certain H_1-type antihistamines, such as azatadine, suppress the release of inflammatory mediators from human mast cells.[14]

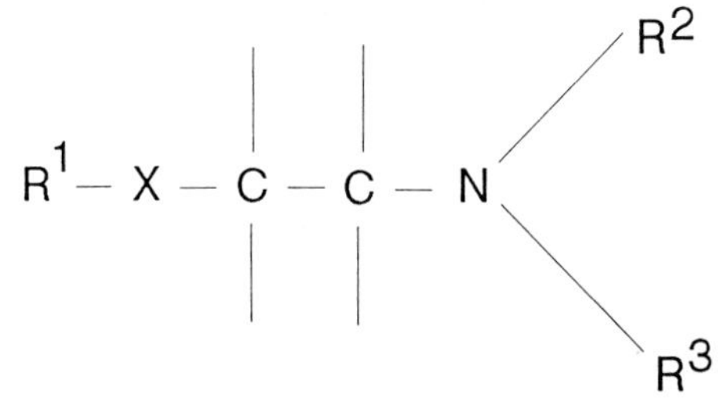

FIGURE 237-1 Ethylamine moiety present in H_1 antihistamines. R^1, aromatic and/or heterocyclic groups; X, linkage such as nitrogen, oxygen, or carbon.

TABLE 237-1

First-Generation, H_1-Type Antihistamine Drugs Available in the United States

Chemical class	Generic name
Alkylamine (propylamine)	Brompheniramine maleate Chlorpheniramine maleate Dexchlorpheniramine maleate Triprolidine hydrochloride
Aminoalkyl ether (ethanolamine)	Clemastine fumarate Diphenhydramine hydrochloride Doxylamine succinate
Ethylenediamine	Tripelennamine citrate Tripelennamine hydrochloride
Phenothiazine	Methdilazine Methdilazine hydrochloride Promethazine hydrochloride Trimeprazine tartrate
Piperidine	Azatadine maleate Cyproheptadine hydrochloride
Piperazine	Hydroxyzine hydrochloride Hydroxyzine pamoate

Pharmacokinetics H_1-type antihistamines are absorbed from the gastrointestinal tract after oral administration. Although their effects can be observed within 30 min of administration, are maximal within 1 to 2 h, and usually persist for 4 to 6 h, some of these therapeutic agents may have a longer duration of action. For example, after oral administration in single-dose studies, the serum half-lives of brompheniramine, chlorpheniramine, and hydroxyzine exceeded 20 h in adults.[15–18] The serum half-lives of chlorpheniramine and hydroxyzine are shorter in children[19,20] and longer in geriatric patients. The half-life of hydroxyzine is prolonged in patients with primary biliary cirrhosis, which suggests that its pharmacokinetics may be altered in other hepatic diseases.[21] The metabolism of H_1-type antihistamines takes place by the hepatic cytochrome P_{450} system, in which they are conjugated to form glucuronides. The H_1-type antihistamines also induce hepatic microsomal enzymes and thus may facilitate their own metabolism. Excretion of these compounds in the urine is almost complete by 24 h after administration.[18,22]

H_1-type antihistamines are conventionally administered in divided doses at intervals between 4 and 6 h. However, the observations[15–18] that one oral dose of certain of these agents is associated with longer serum half-lives suggest that some H_1-type antihistamines may not require administration so frequently as was previously indicated. The H_1-type antihistamines suppress wheal-and-erythema reactions induced by the intracutaneous injection of histamine for various time intervals depending on the agent studied.

Side Effects Approximately 25 percent of patients receiving H_1-type antihistamines experience an adverse reaction.[23] However, there are considerable variations in the responses of individual subjects. Sedation is the most common problem associated with these therapeutic agents. This sedative effect is pronounced with the aminoalkyl ether and the phenothiazine subgroups. The soporific effect of other subgroups is less marked, especially the alkylamine subgroup. The sedative effect ameliorates in most individuals within a few days of continual administration of H_1-type antihista-

mines. If tolerance to the sedative manifestations does not occur, a trial of an agent from another subgroup should be undertaken. Other central nervous system (CNS) effects include dizziness, tinnitus, incoordination, blurred vision, and diplopia. The CNS effects at times may be stimulatory, especially with the alkylamine group; these effects include nervousness, irritability, insomnia, and tremor.

Gastrointestinal complaints are the second most frequent side effects and are noted especially with the ethylenediamine group. Anorexia, nausea, vomiting, epigastric distress, diarrhea, and constipation have been reported. The administration of these agents with food may eliminate some of these manifestations.

H_1-type antihistamines have anticholinergic effects, including dry mucous membranes, difficulty in micturition, urinary retention, dysuria, urinary frequency, and impotence. These clinical manifestations have been reported with the administration of therapeutic agents from the aminoalkyl ether, the phenothiazine, and the piperazine subgroups.

Infrequent side effects of H_1-type antihistamines include headache, a sensation of tightness in the throat, tingling, and numbness. The cardiovascular effects of H_1-type antihistamines are not usually experienced after oral administration. Transient hypotension may develop after intravenous therapy, especially if the administration of the drug is rapid.

Cutaneous reactions occurring after the administration of H_1-type antihistamines are uncommon; they include eczematous dermatitis, urticaria, petechiae, fixed drug eruptions, and photosensitivity.

Acute poisoning may develop, especially in children. Hallucinations, ataxia, incoordination, athetosis, and convulsions are the major features. Anticholinergic effects include flushing, dilated pupils, and hyperthermia. Treatment for poisoning after the ingestion of H_1-type antihistamines is symptomatic and supportive.

Contraindications and Drug Interactions If patients receiving H_1-type antihistamines become sensitized to the drug, the subsequent systemic administration of the offending agent or a related compound may produce an eczematous dermatitis.[24] An important clinical example is the cutaneous eruption that occurs after the administration of drugs, such as aminophylline, that contain the ethylenediamine moiety. Allergic contact dermatitis may develop after the topical application of some H_1-type antihistamines.

When H_1-type antihistamines are consumed in combination with alcohol or other therapeutic agents with CNS depressant effects, such as diazepam, there may be an accentuation of the central depressive effects. Agents of the phenothiazine subgroup may block the vasopressor effect of epinephrine. H_1-type antihistamines are contraindicated in patients receiving monoamine oxidase inhibitors.

There are no guidelines for the use of H_1-type antihistamines in pregnant women. Their use during the last 2 weeks before delivery was associated with retrolental fibroplasia in the premature neonate.[25] A neonatal withdrawal syndrome was described in an infant born to a mother receiving 150 mg of hydroxyzine hydrochloride four times a day throughout pregnancy.[26] Teratogenic effects have been observed in experimental animals after the administration of the piperazine subgroup, but fetal abnormalities have not been reported in humans.

There is some evidence to suggest that the prolonged administration of some H_1-type antihistamines, for example chlorpheniramine for 3 weeks, may produce subsensitivity or loss of efficacy,[27] but such observations are the subject of controversy and require further study.

Low-Sedating or Second Generation H₁-Type Antihistamines

In recent years low-sedating or second-generation H_1-type antihistamines have been developed (Table 237-2). Currently terfenadine and astemizole are available in the United States. These two agents as well as cetirizine and loratadine are available in other countries. Acrivastine, azelastine, mequitazine, tazifylline, and temelastine are investigational agents being evaluated in other countries and will not be discussed further. Low-sedating H_1-type antihistamines have become popular therapeutic agents, owing to their lack of both sedative and anticholinergic side effects. These agents minimally cross the blood-brain barrier and preferentially bind to peripheral H_1 receptors. Guidelines for the use of low-sedating H_1-type antihistamines in pregnant women do not exist. The administration of low-sedating H_1-type antihistamines has not been associated with the development of subsensitivity.

Terfenadine Terfenadine,[28] the first low-sedating H_1 antihistamine approved for use in the United States, achieves peak plasma concentrations in 1 to 2 h, is metabolized in the liver, and is excreted in the urine and feces. Terfenadine suppresses cutaneous wheal-and-erythema reactions for up to 12 h. Anticholinergic and CNS effects are no greater than those that occur with placebo. Torsade de pointes, a form of ventricular tachycardia associated with prolongation of the QT interval, has been reported to occur after drug overdose[29] and in patients taking concomitant ketoconazole, macrolide antibiotics such as erythromycin, or troleandomycin.[30] Perhaps individuals with hepatic dysfunction or those susceptible to conditions associated with a prolonged QT interval may also be at risk. Rare cases of alopecia,[31] urticaria, and morbilliform eruptions[32] have been reported after the administration of terfenadine. There are no restrictions on the ability to take this drug with food.

Astemizole Astemizole[33] is a long-acting agent with a slow onset of action. Its plasma half-life is biphasic, with an initial phase of 7 to 9 days and a second phase of 19 days, owing to its metabolites. The effects of astemizole are long lasting, and it may suppress the wheal-and-erythema response after its discontinuation. The sedative effect of astemizole is no greater than that of placebo,[34] but it may cause appetite stimulation. The initial suggestion that absorption is decreased with food has not been substantiated.[35] Torsade de pointes has been reported after drug overdosage both in adults and

TABLE 237-2
Low-Sedating or Second Generation H₁-Type Antihistamines

Drug	Dosage	Onset of action	Restrictions	Side effects
Terfenadine	60 mg twice daily	Hours	Concomitant ketoconazole or macrolide antibiotics	Torsade de pointes
Astemizole	10 mg/day	Days	Empty stomach	Torsade de pointes, increased appetite
Cetirizine	10 mg/day	Hours	None	None
Loratadine	10 mg/day	Hours	None	None

in children.[36–38] The long serum half-life of astemizole may preclude its administration to women who are contemplating pregnancy and may influence the results of prick skin tests.

Cetirizine Cetirizine[39,40] is the carboxylic acid metabolite of hydroxyzine and thus is not further metabolized. Peak plasma concentrations are achieved in 1 h, and the drug is excreted unchanged in the urine. Cetirizine suppresses cutaneous wheal-and-erythema reactions for as long as 24 h. Cetirizine is less sedating than its parent compound, hydroxyzine.[41]

After the administration of cetirizine, the challenge of allergic subjects with grass pollen or 48/80 was associated with a decrease in the influx of eosinophils into the skin, as assessed by a skin-window technique.[42] In a study of pollen-sensitive persons, the oral administration of cetirizine resulted in a decrease in cutaneous wheal-and-flare reactions, in the immediate release of histamine, in the detection of platelet-activating factor, and in the influx of eosinophils, as assessed by a skin-chamber technique.[43] Moreover, cetirizine was demonstrated to have an inhibitory effect on eosinophil chemotactic responses in vitro to N-formyl-methionyl-leucyl-phenylalanine and platelet-activating factor[44] and in vivo to the influx of eosinophils induced by platelet-activating factor.[45] In subjects allergic to ragweed to whom cetirizine was administered, experimental challenge resulted in a decrease in erythema between 15 min and 4 h. In skin chambers a decrease in prostaglandin D_2 generation without an effect on histamine release was observed, with an attenuation of the migration of eosinophils, neutrophils, and basophils.[46] Such inhibition of the influx of granulocytes into skin chambers was not observed in experimental studies with terfenadine, promethazine, chlorpheniramine, and diphenhydramine.[46,47] There are no restrictions on the ability to take this drug with food or other medications.

Loratadine Loratadine[48–50] is a member of the piperidine subgroup and is related to azatadine. Peak serum concentrations are achieved in 1 to 2 h, and it is excreted in the urine and feces. Loratadine causes no greater sedative or anticholinergic side effects than does a placebo. There are no restrictions on the ability to take this agent with food or other medications. Extremely small amounts of loratadine are excreted in breast milk.[51]

H₂-Type Antihistamines

H_2-type antihistamines possess an imidazole ring and lack the aryl ring of H_1-type antihistamines. These therapeutic agents are less lipophilic, which presumably accounts for their lack of CNS effects. Although these therapeutic agents were originally developed for use in peptic ulcer disease, they have been used in dermatology because of the H_2 receptors of the cutaneous microvasculature.

Cimetidine Cimetidine was the first widely used H_2-type antihistamine, and the greatest amount of pharmacologic and clinical data has been accumulated with the use of this agent compared to other H_2 type antihistamines.

Only a small proportion of cimetidine is absorbed from the stomach; most of its absorption occurs in the small intestine. The half-life of cimetidine in plasma is approximately 2 h, with peak levels occurring 80 to 90 min after oral administration; approximately 70 percent is excreted unchanged in the urine.[6] In humans, cimetidine has been recovered from the cerebrospinal fluid of patients with high serum levels, which occurred after overdosage or impaired excretion.[52]

A side effect of cimetidine that has been reported with some frequency is mental confusion,[52] which is important in geriatric patients on regular doses and in younger individuals receiving high doses. Impairment of hepatic or renal function was found in many of the geriatric patients. Other side effects include headache, dizziness, drowsiness, malaise, muscular pain, diarrhea, and constipation.[53] Although cimetidine was initially thought to have no effect on the bone marrow, there are rare reports of granulocytopenia with a fatal outcome.[54]

Uncommon side effects of cimetidine[53,55–58] include gynecomastia with or without elevated prolactin levels in male individuals; galactorrhea with elevated prolactin levels in women; and loss of libido, impotence, and reduction of sperm counts in young men. Modest elevations in serum creatinine levels, which may decrease during therapy, are common and are reversible after withdrawal of the drug. Elevated levels of serum transaminases have been reported and are reversible. Interstitial nephritis, fever, and cutaneous eruptions that include urticaria and erythema multiforme syndrome have been observed.

Although a decrease in sebum production in patients with acne who were receiving cimetidine has been described,[59] this observation appears to be of no therapeutic value. The presence of an H_2 histamine receptor on CD8+ T lymphocytes may in part explain the augmentation of delayed-type hypersensitivity reactions with increased erythema and induration occurring after the intradermal administration of antigens.[60] In healthy volunteers, the oral administration of cimetidine was associated with an increase in the mitogen-induced proliferation of lymphocytes, a decrease in the number of CD8+ T lymphocytes, and an increase in CD4+ T lymphocytes.[61] Although cimetidine binds to nitrites in the gastrointestinal tract and may yield potential carcinogenic nitroso compounds,[62] the prolonged administration of cimetidine in high doses to rats and dogs failed to result in the development of gastric neoplasms.[63] Cimetidine, however, may mask symptoms associated with gastric carcinoma in humans.[62]

Drug interactions that have been reported with cimetidine therapy include prolonged bleeding times and prothrombin times in patients receiving concomitant oral anticoagulants and cimetidine.[64,65] Cimetidine increases the concentration of blood alcohol levels due to an inhibitory effect on gastric alcohol dehydrogenase activity.[66–69]

Ranitidine   Ranitidine[70] is absorbed with peak plasma concentrations achieved in 1 to 2 h. The oral bioavailability of ranitidine is about 50 percent and is increased in patients with liver disease. The plasma half-life is 2 to 3 h in adults and is prolonged in geriatric patients and individuals with liver or kidney diseases. Although ranitidine is metabolized in the liver, less than 10 percent of an intravenous or oral dose is excreted as metabolites. The drug and its metabolites are excreted principally in the urine; 70 to 80 percent of an intravenous dose and 30 percent of an oral dose appear in the urine as unchanged drug. Ranitidine does not bind to androgen receptors,[71] does not interfere with the hepatic metabolism of other therapeutic agents, and does not enhance cell-mediated immune responses. Ranitidine inhibits gastric alcohol dehydrogenase activity and leads to increased blood alcohol levels.[69] Ranitidine may be preferred to cimetidine in patients taking multiple drugs and in geriatric patients.

Minor adverse effects include headache, dizziness, malaise, nausea, constipation, and abdominal pain. Serum transaminase and

creatinine levels temporarily increase but return to baseline levels with continued treatment. Ranitidine appears in breast milk.

Although ranitidine interacts with other medications less frequently than does cimetidine,[72] interactions with fentanyl, metoprolol, midazolam, nifedipine, theophylline, and warfarin have been observed. Ranitidine may decrease the absorption of diazepam and reduce its plasma concentration by 25 percent.[73]

Famotidine   Famotidine differs chemically from cimetidine and ranitidine in that it contains a thiazole ring. Peak plasma concentrations occur 2 h after oral administration, and the plasma half-life is 3 to 8 h. Approximately 25 percent of the drug is excreted in the urine after a single oral dose. In patients with renal failure, the half-life of famotidine may exceed 20 h.[74] Famotidine is more potent than cimetidine and ranitidine in gastroenterologic studies of the treatment of Zollinger-Ellison syndrome.[75]

Adverse reactions are infrequent and include headache, dizziness, constipation, and diarrhea. No interference with the hepatic oxidative metabolism of diazepam, phenytoin, theophylline, or warfarin has been observed.[76] Famotidine does not inhibit gastric alcohol dehydrogenase activity[69]; it lacks antiandrogenic side effects.

Nizatidine   Like famotidine, nizatidine contains a thiazole ring. Its peak serum concentration after oral administration occurs in about 1 h, the plasma half-life is 1 to 2 h, and its duration of action is up to 10 h.[77] Nizatidine is primarily eliminated by the kidneys within 16 h.[78] The oral bioavailability of nizatidine is not affected by food.[79]

Minor gastrointestinal side effects occur; elevations of serum uric acid levels, without adverse clinical consequences, and of transaminase levels develop; and antiandrogenic effects are absent.

In healthy volunteers, drug interactions were not reported with the concomitant administration of chlordiazepoxide, diazepam, lidocaine, lorazepam, theophylline, or warfarin.[80] The administration of antacids does not decrease the absorption of nizatidine.

Other Therapeutic Agents with Antihistaminic Activity

Tricyclic Antidepressants   Tricyclic antidepressants act on both H_1 and H_2 receptors.[81,82] Doxepin, a compound related to amitriptyline, was shown to be more potent than chlorpheniramine in inhibiting experimental wheals induced by histamine.[83]

Ketotifen   Ketotifen,[84,85] a benzocycloheptathiophene derivative, prevents histamine release from mast cells induced by IgE and compound 48/80 in vitro and inhibits passive cutaneous anaphylaxis in experimental animals in vivo. Ketotifen also is an H_1-type antihistamine and a calcium channel blocker.

Antihistamines in Dermatology

General Considerations

Antihistamines have been used in dermatology primarily for the relief of pruritus and the treatment of urticaria and angioedema.[86] Although the intradermal injection of histamine consistently produces pruritus, many stimuli and other inflammatory mediators may also be responsible for pruritus. Antihistamines are effective in blocking experimental pruritus induced by histamine; however, they are of limited use in many pruritic cutaneous diseases. It has been suggested that the soporific side effect of the traditional H$_1$-type antihistamines plays a role in the treatment of pruritus.

Use in Urticaria/Angioedema

Empiric trials of traditional H$_1$-type antihistamines are used in the treatment of both acute and recurrent episodes of urticaria and angioedema.[87,88] In double-blind, placebo-controlled studies, traditional H$_1$-type antihistamines were shown to be statistically superior to placebos in the treatment of urticaria and angioedema. However, comparative studies of the subgroups of traditional H$_1$-type antihistamines have shown them to be of equal efficacy. If an agent from one therapeutic subgroup of H$_1$-type antihistamine proves ineffective, then an agent from another subgroup should be administered. At times, H$_1$-type antihistamines from different subgroups may be combined. H$_1$-type antihistamines have been reported to be of particular efficacy in some types of physical urticaria, notably hydroxyzine hydrochloride for cholinergic urticaria.[89] H$_1$-type antihistamines are used in the prevention of urticaria that occurs after the administration of radiocontrast media to patients with a history of prior reactions and in the prevention of transfusion reactions.

The low-sedating H$_1$-type antihistamines, terfenadine,[90–95] astemizole,[96–98] cetirizine,[99–101] and loratadine,[95,102] were found in double-blind, placebo-controlled studies to be statistically superior to placebo in the treatment of chronic idiopathic urticaria and angioedema.[103,104] Astemizole, however, is the only low-sedating agent currently approved for this indication in the United States. In comparative studies, in which low-sedating H$_1$-type antihistamines are compared with each other and with traditional H$_1$-type antihistamines, no single therapeutic agent commands preeminence.[92,94,105–107] Tricyclic antidepressant drugs, such as doxepin hydrochloride,[108–110] and ketotifen[111–112] have been used with therapeutic benefit in chronic idiopathic urticaria.

Traditional and low-sedating H$_1$ antihistamines may also be used in the treatment of physical urticaria. They are of value in some patients with dermographism,[113,114] cold-induced urticaria,[115] solar urticaria,[116] and delayed pressure urticaria.[117] Doxepin[118] and ketotifen[119] were used successfully in patients with various types of physical urticaria.

The combination of H$_1$- and H$_2$-type antihistamines is of benefit in a few patients with acute and chronic idiopathic urticaria and angioedema[120–125] as well as certain forms of physical urticaria.[126–133] However, one double-blind study[134] failed to show statistically significant advantage when chlorpheniramine and cimetidine were used in combination in the treatment of chronic idiopathic urticaria. The combination of H$_1$- and H$_2$-type antihistamines should be considered in patients with refractory chronic idiopathic urticaria, in whom H$_1$-type antihistamines alone or in combination are ineffective. Although an H$_2$-type antihistamine alone was claimed to control urticaria in one report,[135] their therapeutic benefit when administered as monotherapy has not been demonstrated in controlled trials.[136,137]

Use in Other Dermatologic Disorders

H$_1$-type antihistamines have been used in the treatment of pruritus of various causes and in patients with atopic dermatitis. Their effectiveness in the control of pruritus is variable, which suggests that

their efficacy may in part be related to the suppression of anxiety and their sedative effect.[138] Yet low-sedative H$_1$-type antihistamines have modified the pruritus in patients with atopic dermatitis.[139] In children with atopic dermatitis, hydroxyzine has a greater antipruritic effect than does cyproheptadine.[17]

The combination of H$_1$- and H$_2$-type antihistamines was suggested to be useful in patients with urticaria pigmentosa in anecdotal reports.[140,141] The pruritus and whealing in systemic mastocytosis and urticaria pigmentosa were modified in a double-blind trial of the administration of chlorpheniramine and cimetidine.[142] Ketotifen has also been of benefit in urticaria pigmentosa in a controlled trial.[143]

The pruritus associated with other conditions, such as allergic contact dermatitis and other forms of eczematous dermatitis, lichen planus, and infestations, and pruritus secondary to underlying medical disorders or of an idiopathic nature may benefit from the administration of H$_1$-type antihistamines. The pruritus induced by drug reactions and serum sickness may be treated with H$_1$-type antihistamines, even though these therapeutic agents will have no effect on the associated fever or arthralgias.

In anecdotal reports, cimetidine was reported to be of value in the treatment of the pruritus resulting from myelofibrosis,[144] polycythemia vera,[145] and carcinoid flush.[146] Anecdotal reports have also suggested that the combination of H$_1$- and H$_2$-type antihistamines was of value in the treatment of carcinoid flush[147] and alcohol-induced flushing.[148]

The antiandrogenic effects of cimetidine suggested its use in treating women with increased facial hair,[149] but this therapeutic regimen has not been subjected to controlled trials. Cimetidine was noted to reverse cutaneous anergy to candidin in a group of patients with chronic mucocutaneous candidiasis.[150] Other reports have noted enhanced delayed-type skin test responses in subjects treated with cimetidine.[60] This immunomodulatory effect of H$_2$-type antihistamines offers great promise and potential for therapeutic exploration.

Although ranitidine has been administered to patients with chronic urticaria,[123] studies with other H$_2$-type antihistamines in cutaneous disorders have not yet been reported.[148]

References

1. Lewis T: *The Blood Vessels of the Human Skin and Their Responses.* London, Shaw and Sons, 1927
2. Bovet D, Staub A: Action protectrice des éthers phénoliques au cours de l'intoxication histaminique. *Société de Biologie* **124**:547, 1937
3. Dale HH: The action and uses of the antihistamine drugs as applied to dermatology. *Br J Dermatol Syphilol* **62**:151, 1950
4. Ash ASF, Schild HO: Receptors mediating some actions of histamine. *Br J Pharmacol* **27**:427, 1966
5. Black JW et al: Definition and antagonism of histamine H$_2$-receptors. *Nature* **236**:385, 1972
6. Brimblecombe RW et al: Cimetidine—a non-thiourea H$_2$-receptor antagonist. *J Int Med Res* **3**:86, 1975
7. Arrang J-M et al: Highly potent and selective ligands for histamine H$_3$-receptors. *Nature* **327**:117, 1987
8. Hill SJ: Distribution, properties, and functional characteristics of three classes of histamine receptor. *Pharmacol Rev* **42**:45, 1990
9. Goetzl EJ: Regulation of the polymorphonuclear leukocyte chemotactic response by immunological reactions, in *Leukocyte Chemotaxis: Methods, Physiology, and Clinical Implications,* edited by JI Gallin, PG Quie. New York, Raven, 1978, p 161

10. McNeil JH, Verma SC: Blockade by burimamide of the effects of histamine and histamine analogues on cardiac contractility, phosphorylase activation and cyclic adenosine monophosphate. *J Pharmacol Exp Ther* **188**:180, 1974

11. Dousa TP, Code CF: Effect of histamine and its methyl derivatives on cyclic AMP metabolism in gastric mucosa and its blockade by an H$_2$ receptor antagonist. *J Clin Invest* **53**:334, 1974

12. Plaut M et al: Properties of a subpopulation of T cells bearing histamine receptors. *J Clin Invest* **55**:856, 1975

13. Robertson I, Greaves MW: Responses of human skin blood vessels to synthetic histamine analogues. *Br J Clin Pharmacol* **5**:319, 1978

14. Togias AG et al: Demonstration of inhibition of mediator release from human mast cells by azatadine base: In vivo and in vitro evaluation. *JAMA* **255**:225, 1986

15. Simons FER et al: The pharmacokinetics and antihistaminic effects of brompheniramine. *J Allergy Clin Immunol* **70**:458, 1982

16. Huang SM et al: Pharmacokinetics of chlorpheniramine after intravenous and oral administration in normal adults. *Eur J Clin Pharmacol* **22**:359, 1982

17. Simons FER et al: The pharmacokinetics and antihistaminic of the H$_1$ receptor antagonist hydroxyzine. *J Allergy Clin Immunol* **73**:69, 1984

18. Drouin MA: H$_1$ antihistamines: Perspective on the use of the conventional and new agents. *Ann Allergy* **55**:747, 1985

19. Simons FER et al: Pharmacokinetics and efficacy of chlorpheniramine in children. *J Allergy Clin Immunol* **69**:376, 1982

20. Simons FER et al: Pharmacokinetics and antipruritic effects of hydroxyzine in children with atopic dermatitis. *J Pediatr* **104**:123, 1984

21. Simons FER et al: The pharmacokinetics and pharmacodynamics of hydroxyzine in patients with primary biliary cirrhosis. *J Clin Pharmacol* **29**:809, 1989

22. Simons FER et al: Comparative pharmacokinetics of H$_1$-receptor antagonists. *Ann Allergy* **63**:20, 1987

23. Douglas WW: Histamine and 5-hydroxytryptamine (serotonin) and their antagonists, in *The Pharmacologic Basis of Therapeutics,* 7th ed, edited by LS Goodman, A Gilman. New York, MacMillan, 1985, p 590

24. Fisher AA: The antihistamines. *J Am Acad Dermatol* **3**:303, 1980

25. Zierler S, Purohit D: Prenatal antihistamine exposure and retrolental fibroplasia. *Am J Epidemiol* **123**:192, 1986

26. Prenner BM: Neonatal withdrawal syndrome associated with hydroxyzine hydrochloride. *Am J Dis Child* **131**:529, 1977

27. Bantz EW et al: Chronic chlorpheniramine therapy: Subsensitivity, drug metabolism, and compliance. *Ann Allergy* **59**:341, 1987

28. Sorkin EM, Heel RC: Terfenadine: A review of its pharmacodynamic properties and therapeutic efficacy. *Drugs* **29**:34, 1985

29. Davies AJ et al: Cardiotoxic effect with convulsions in terfenadine overdose. *Br Med J* **298**:325, 1989

30. Monahan BP et al: Torsades de pointes occurring in association with terfenadine use. *JAMA* **264**:2788, 1990

31. Jones SK, Morley WN: Terfenadine causing hair loss (unreviewed report). *Br Med J* **291**:940, 1985

32. Stricker BHCH et al: Skin reactions to terfenadine. *Br Med J* **293**:536, 1986

33. Richards DM et al: Astemizole: A review of its pharmacodynamic properties and therapeutic efficacy. *Drugs* **28**:38, 1984

34. Vanden Bussche G et al: Clinical profile of astemizole: A survey of 50 double-blind trials. *Ann Allergy* **58**:184, 1987

35. Simons FER: Recent advances in H$_1$-receptor antagonist treatment. *J Allergy Clin Immunol* **86**:995, 1990

36. Craft TM: Torsade de pointes after astemizole overdose. *Br Med J* **292**:660, 1986

37. Simons FER et al: Astemizole-induced torsade de pointes. *Lancet* **2**:624, 1988

38. Tobin JR et al: Astemizole-induced cardiac conduction disturbances in a child. *JAMA* **266**:2737, 1991

39. Wood SG et al: Metabolism and pharmacokinetics of ^{14}C-cetirizine in humans. *Ann Allergy* **59**(suppl):31, 1987

40. Sheffer AL, Samuels LL: Cetirizine: Antiallergic therapy beyond traditional H$_1$ antihistamines. *J Allergy Clin Immunol* **86**:1040, 1990

41. Seidel WF et al: Direct measurement of daytime sleepiness after administration of cetirizine and hydroxyzine with a standardized electroencephalographic assessment. *J Allergy Clin Immunol* **86**:1029, 1990

42. Fadel R et al: Inhibitory effect of cetirizine 2HCl on eosinophil migration in vivo. *Clin Allergy* **17**:373, 1987

43. Michel L et al: Inhibitory effect of oral cetirizine on in vivo antigen-induced histamine and PAF-acether release and eosinophil recruitment in human skin. *J Allergy Clin Immunol* **82**:101, 1988

44. Leprevost C et al: Inhibition of eosinophil chemotaxis by a new antiallergic compound (cetirizine). *Int Arch Allergy Appl Immunol* **87**:9, 1988

45. Fadel R: In vivo effects of cetirizine on cutaneous reactivity and eosinophil migration induced by platelet-activating factor (PAF-acether) in man. *J Allergy Clin Immunol* **86**:314, 1990

46. Charlesworth EN et al: Effect of cetirizine on mast cell-mediator release and cellular traffic during the cutaneous late-phase reaction. *J Allergy Clin Immunol* **83**:905, 1989

47. Kagey-Sobotka A et al: Terfenadine blocks both the early and late cutaneous response to antigen. *J Allergy Clin Immunol* **89**:248, 1992

48. Hilbert J et al: Pharmacokinetics and dose proportionality of loratadine. *J Clin Pharmacol* **27**:694, 1987

49. Simons FER: Loratadine, a non-sedating H$_1$-receptor antagonist (antihistamine). *Ann Allergy* **63**:266, 1988

50. Clissold SP et al: Loratadine: A preliminary review of its pharmacodynamic properties and therapeutic efficacy. *Drugs* **37**:42, 1989

51. Hilbert J et al: Excretion of loratadine in human breast milk. *J Clin Pharmacol* **28**:234, 1988

52. Schentag JJ et al: Pharmacokinetic and clinical studies in patients with cimetidine-associated mental confusion. *Lancet* **1**:177, 1979

53. McGuigan JE: A consideration of the adverse effects of cimetidine. *Gastroenterology* **80**:181, 1981

54. Chang HK, Morrison SL: Bone-marrow suppression associated with cimetidine. *Ann Intern Med* **91**:580, 1979

55. Kruss DM, Littman A: Safety of cimetidine. *Gastroenterology* **74**:478, 1978

56. Davis TG et al: Evaluation of a world wide spontaneous reporting system with cimetidine. *JAMA* **243**:1912, 1980

57. Sawyer D et al: Cimetidine: Adverse reactions and acute toxicity. *Am J Hosp Pharm* **38**:188, 1981

58. Van Thiel DH et al: Hypothalamic-pituitary-gonadal dysfunction in men using cimetidine. *N Engl J Med* **300**:1012, 1979

59. Lyons F et al: Inhibition of sebum excretion by an H$_2$ blocker. *Lancet* **1**:1376, 1979

60. Avella J et al: Effect of histamine H2-receptor antagonists on delayed hypersensitivity. *Lancet* **1**:624, 1978

61. Brockmeyer NH et al: Cimetidine and the immuno-response in healthy volunteers. *J Invest Dermatol* **93**:757, 1989

62. Elder JB et al: Cimetidine and gastric cancer. *Lancet* **1**:1005, 1979

63. Crean GP et al: Cimetidine and gastric cancer: Negative studies in dogs. *Lancet* **2**:797, 1979

64. Serlin MJ et al: Cimetidine: Interaction with oral anticoagulants in man. *Lancet* **2**:317, 1979

65. Silver BA, Bell WR: Cimetidine potentiation of the hypoprothrombinemic effect of warfarin. *Ann Intern Med* **90**:348, 1979

66. Feely J, Wood AJJ: Effects of cimetidine on elimination and actions of ethanol. *JAMA* **247**:2819, 1982

67. Seitz HK et al: *In vivo* interactions between H$_2$-receptor antagonists and ethanol metabolism in man and in rats. *Hepatology* **4**:1231, 1984

68. Caballeria J et al: Effects of cimetidine on gastric alcohol dehydrogenase activity and blood ethanol levels. *Gastroenterology* **96**:388, 1989

69. DiPadova C et al: Effects of ranitidine on blood alcohol levels after ethanol ingestion: Comparison with other H$_2$-receptor antagonists. *JAMA* **267**:83, 1992

70. Zeldis JB et al: Ranitidine: A new H$_2$-receptor antagonist. *N Engl J Med* **309**:1368, 1983

71. Jensen RT et al: Cimetidine-induced impotence and breast changes in patients with gastric hypersecretory states. *N Engl J Med* **308**:883, 1983

72. Kirch W et al: Interactions and non-interactions with ranitidine. *Clin Pharmacokinet* **9**:493, 1984

73. Hansten PD: Drug interactions of ranitidine vs cimetidine. *Drug Interact Newslett* **3**:31, 1983

74. Beradi RR et al: Comparison of famotidine with cimetidine and ranitidine. *Clin Pharmacol* **7**:271, 1988

75. Howard JM et al: Famotidine, a new, potent, long-acting histamine H$_2$-receptor antagonist: Comparison with cimetidine and ranitidine in treatment of Zollinger-Ellison syndrome. *Gastroenterology* **88**:1026, 1985

76. Friedman G: Famotidine. *Am J Gastroenterol* **82**:504, 1987

77. Stern WR: Summary of 32nd Meeting of Food and Drug Administration's Gastrointestinal Drugs Advisory Committee. *Am J Gastroenterol* **83**:417, 1988

78. Callaghan JT et al: A pharmacokinetic profile of nizatidine in man. *Scand J Gastroenterol* **22**(suppl 136):9, 1987

79. Morton DM: Pharmacology and toxicity of nizatidine. *Scand J Gastroenterol* **22**(suppl 136):1, 1987

80. Klotz U: Lack of effect of nizatidine on drug metabolism. *Scand J Gastroenterol* **22**(suppl 136):18, 1987

81. Green JP, Maayani S: Tricyclic antidepressant drugs block histamine H$_2$ receptor in brain. *Nature* **269**:163, 1977

82. Richelson E: Tricyclic antidepressants and histamine H$_1$ receptors. *Mayo Clin Proc* **54**:669, 1979

83. Sullivan TJ: Pharmacologic modulation of the whealing response to histamine in human skin: Identification of doxepin as a potent in vivo inhibitor. *J Allergy Clin Immunol* **69**:260, 1982

84. Martin U, Roemer D: The pharmacological properties of a new, orally active antianaphylactic compound: Ketotifen, a benzocycloheptathiophene. *Drug Res* **28**:770, 1978

85. Craps LP, Ney UM: Ketotifen: Current views on its mechanism of action and their therapeutic implications. *Respiration* **45**:411, 1984

86. Kerdel FA, Soter NA: Antihistamines in dermatology, in *Recent Advances in Dermatology,* vol 6, edited by AJ Rook, HI Maibach. Edinburgh, Churchill Livingstone, 1983, p 265

87. Harvey RP et al: A controlled trial of therapy in chronic urticaria. *J Allergy Clin Immunol* **68**:262, 1981

88. Coutts A, Greaves MW: Evaluation of six antihistamines *in vitro* and in patients with urticaria. *Clin Exp Dermatol* **7**:529, 1982

89. Moore-Robinson M, Warin RP: Some clinical aspects of cholinergic urticaria. *Br J Dermatol* **80**:794, 1968

90. Cerio R, Lessof MH: Treatment of chronic idiopathic urticaria with terfenadine. *Clin Allergy* **14**:139, 1984

91. Ferguson J et al: Terfenadine and placebo compared in the treatment of chronic idiopathic urticaria: A randomised double-blind study. *Br J Clin Pharmacol* **20**:639, 1985

92. Fredriksson T et al: Terfenadine in chronic urticaria: A comparison with clemastine and placebo. *Cutis* **38**:128, 1986

93. Salisbury J et al: A double-blind placebo controlled study of terfenadine in the treatment of chronic idiopathic urticaria. *Br J Clin Pract* **41**:859, 1987

94. Grant JA et al: Double-blind comparison of terfenadine, chlorpheniramine, and placebo in the treatment of chronic idiopathic urticaria. *J Allergy Clin Immunol* **81**:574, 1988

95. Belaich S et al: Comparative effects of loratadine and terfenadine in the treatment of chronic idiopathic urticaria. *Ann Allergy* **64**:191, 1990

96. Fox RW et al: The treatment of mild to severe chronic idiopathic urticaria with astemizole: Double-blind and open trials. *J Allergy Clin Immunol* **78**:1159, 1986

97. Bernstein IL, Bernstein DI: Efficacy and safety of astemizole, a long-acting and nonsedating H$_1$ antagonist for the treatment of chronic idiopathic urticaria. *J Allergy Clin Immunol* **77**:37, 1986

98. Kailasam V, Matthews, KP: Controlled clinical assessment of astemizole in the treatment of chronic idiopathic urticaria and angioedema. *J Am Acad Dermatol* **16**:797, 1987

99. Juhlin L, Arendt C: Treatment of chronic urticaria with cetirizine dihydrochloride a non-sedating antihistamine. *Br J Dermatol* **119**:67, 1988

100. Go MJT et al: Double-blind, placebo controlled comparison of cetirizine and terfenadine in chronic idiopathic urticaria. *Acta Therapeutica* **15**:77, 1989

101. Kalivas J et al: Urticaria: Clinical efficacy of cetirizine in comparison with hydroxyzine and placebo. *J Allergy Clin Immunol* **86**:1014, 1990

102. Monroe EW et al: Efficacy and safety of loratadine (10 mg once daily) in the management of idiopathic chronic urticaria. *J Am Acad Dermatol* **19**:138, 1988

103. Monroe EW: Chronic urticaria: Review of nonsedating H$_1$ antihistamines in treatment. *J Am Acad Dermatol* **19**:842, 1988

104. Soter NA: Treatment of urticaria and angioedema: Low-sedating H$_1$-type antihistamines. *J Am Acad Dermatol* **24**:1084, 1991

105. Newman Y: Antihistamine treatment of chronic urticaria: Results of a multicenter trial with azatadine and terfenadine. *Fortschr Med* **102**:967, 1984

106. Paul E, Bödeker R-H: Comparison between astemizole and terfenadine in the treatment of chronic urticaria: A randomised double blind study in 40 patients. *Z Hautkr* **60**(suppl):50, 1985

107. Cainell T et al: Double-blind comparison of astemizole and terfenadine in the treatment of chronic urticaria. *Pharmatherapeutica* **4**:679, 1986

108. Greene SL et al: Double-blind crossover study comparing doxepin with diphenhydramine for the treatment of chronic urticaria. *J Am Acad Dermatol* **12**:669, 1985

109. Harto A et al: Doxepin in the treatment of chronic urticaria. *Dermatologica* **170**:90, 1985

110. Goldsobel AB et al: Efficacy of doxepin in the treatment of chronic idiopathic urticaria. *J Allergy Clin Immunol* **78**:867, 1986

111. Saihan EM: Ketotifen and terbutaline in urticaria. *Br J Dermatol* **104**:205, 1981

112. Saihan EM, Littlewood SN: Ketotifen and terbutaline in chronic urticaria. *Br J Dermatol* **109**(suppl 24):31, 1983

113. Krause LB, Shuster S: The effect of terfenadine on dermographic whealing. *Br J Dermatol* **110**:73, 1984

114. Krause LB, Shuster S: A comparison of astemizole and chlorpheniramine in dermographic urticaria. *Br J Dermatol* **112**:447, 1985

115. Juhlin L et al: Inhibiting effect of cetirizine on histamine-induced and 48/80-induced wheals and flares, experimental dermographism, and cold-induced urticaria. *J Allergy Clin Immunol* **80**:599, 1987

116. Diffey BL, Farr PM: Treatment of solar urticaria with terfenadine. *Photodermatology* **5**:25, 1988

117. Kontou-Fili K et al: Therapeutic effects of cetirizine in delayed pressure urticaria: Clinicopathologic findings. *J Am Acad Dermatol* **24**:1090, 1991

118. Neittaanmäki H et al: Comparison of cinnarizine, cyproheptadine, doxepin, and hydroxyzine in treatment of idiopathic cold urticaria: Usefulness of doxepin. *J Am Acad Dermatol* **11**:483, 1984

119. Huston DP et al: Prevention of mast-cell degranulation by ketotifen in patients with physical urticarias. *Ann Intern Med* **104**:507, 1986

120. Phanuphak P et al: Treatment of chronic idiopathic urticaria with combined H1 and H2 blockers. *Clin Allergy* **8**:429, 1978

121. Monroe EW et al: Combined H$_1$ and H$_2$ antihistamine therapy in chronic urticaria. *Arch Dermatol* **117**:404, 1981

122. Harvey RP et al: A controlled trial of therapy in chronic urticaria. *J Allergy Clin Immunol* **68**:262, 1981

123. Paul E, Bödeker RH: Treatment of chronic urticaria with terfenadine and ranitidine: A randomized double-blind study in 45 patients. *Eur J Clin Pharmacol* **31**:277, 1986

124. Bleehen SS et al: Cimetidine and chlorpheniramine in the treatment of chronic idiopathic urticaria: A multi-centre randomized double-blind study. *Br J Dermatol* **117**:81, 1987

125. Moscati RM, Moore GP: Comparison of cimetidine and diphenhy-

dramine in the treatment of acute urticaria. *Ann Emerg Med* **19**:12, 1990

126. Matthews CNA et al: The effect of H_1 and H_2 histamine antagonists on symptomatic dermographism. *Br J Dermatol* **101**:57, 1979

127. Kaur S et al: Factitious urticaria (dermographism): Treatment by cimetidine and chlorpheniramine in a randomized double-blind study. *Br J Dermatol* **104**:185, 1981

128. Johnston WE et al: Management of cold urticaria during hypothermic cardiopulmonary bypass. *N Engl J Med* **306**:219, 1982

129. Mansfield LE et al: Greater inhibition of dermographia with a combination of H_1 and H_2 antagonists. *Ann Allergy* **50**:264, 1983

130. Breathnach SM et al: Symptomatic dermographism: Natural history, clinical features, laboratory investigations and response to therapy. *Clin Exp Dermatol* **8**:463, 1983

131. Cook J, Shuster S: The effect of H_1 and H_2 receptor antagonists on the dermographic response. *Acta Derm Venereol (Stockh)* **63**:260, 1983

132. Irwin RB et al: Mediator release in local heat urticaria: Protection with combined H_1 and H_2 antagonists. *J Allergy Clin Immunol* **76**:35, 1985

133. Duc J, Pécoud A: Successful treatment of idiopathic cold urticaria with the association of H1 and H2 antagonists: A case report. *Ann Allergy* **56**:355, 1986

134. Commens CA, Greaves MW: Cimetidine in chronic idiopathic urticaria: A randomized double-blind study. *Br J Dermatol* **99**:675, 1978

135. Farnam J et al: Successful treatment of chronic idiopathic urticaria and angioedema with cimetidine alone. *J Allergy Clin Immunol* **73**:842, 1984

136. Beauchamp C, Millares M: H_2 antagonists in hives and urticaria. *Drug Intell Clin Pharm* **19**:662, 1985

137. Theoharides TC: Histamine$_2$ (H_2)-receptor antagonists in the treatment of urticaria. *Drugs* **37**:345, 1989

138. Krause L, Shuster S: Mechanism of action of antipruritic drugs. *Br Med J* **287**:1199, 1983

139. Doherty V et al: Treatment of itching in atopic eczema with antihistamines with a low sedative profile. *Br Med J* **298**:96, 1989

140. Gerrard JW, Ko C: Urticaria pigmentosa: Treatment with cimetidine and chlorpheniramine. *J Pediatr* **94**:843, 1979

141. Fenske NA et al: Congenital bullous urticaria pigmentosa: Treatment with concomitant use of H_1- and H_2-receptor antagonists. *Arch Dermatol* **121**:115, 1985

142. Frieri M et al: Comparison of the therapeutic efficacy of cromolyn sodium with that of combined chlorpheniramine and cimetidine in systemic mastocytosis: Results of a double-blind clinical trial. *Am J Med* **78**:9, 1985

143. Czarnetzki BM: A double-blind cross-over study of the effect of ketotifen in urticaria pigmentosa. *Dermatologica* **166**:44, 1983

144. Hess CE: Cimetidine for the treatment of pruritus. *N Engl J Med* **300**:370, 1979

145. Easton P, Galbraith PR: Cimetidine treatment of pruritus in polycythemia vera. *N Engl J Med* **299**:1134, 1978

146. Wilkin JK, Rountree CB: Blockade of carcinoid flush with cimetidine and clonidine. *Arch Dermatol* **118**:109, 1982

147. Roberts LJ II et al: Blockade of the flush associated with metastatic gastric carcinoid by combined histamine H_1 and H_2 receptor antagonists: Evidence for an important role of H_2 receptors in human vasculature. *N Engl J Med* **300**:236, 1979

148. Tan OT et al: Blocking of alcohol-induced flush with a combination of H_1 and H_2 histamine antagonists. *Lancet* **2**:365, 1979

149. Vigersky RA et al: Treatment of hirsute women with cimetidine: A preliminary note. *N Engl J Med* **303**:1042, 1980

150. Jorizzo JL et al: Cimetidine as an immunomodulator: Chronic mucocutaneous candidiasis as a model. *Ann Intern Med* **92**:192, 1980

Surgery in Dermatology

CHAPTER 238

George J. Hruza and Jessica L. Fewkes

Dermatologic Surgery: Selected Aspects

During the past 20 years dermatology has evolved from a primarily medical specialty to a combined medical and surgical specialty.[1] Dermatologists have been in the forefront of the development of cutaneous laser surgery, Mohs micrographic surgery, and cosmetic surgery.[1,2] Dermatologic surgery is a required component of dermatology residency training and advanced fellowships are available at dozens of centers in the United States. Basic surgical techniques including local anesthesia, skin sterilization, surgical anatomy, wound healing, routine wound care, sutures, biopsy, basic excisional surgery, cryosurgery, electrosurgery, and curettage are described in detail in several excellent skin surgery texts.[3-9] Laser surgery of skin is discussed in Chap. 140. This chapter deals primarily with more advanced techniques including the rationale and indications for each.

Patient Selection

Before submitting a patient to any dermatologic surgery, a careful medical history, review of systems, and focused physical examination are essential. Special attention should be placed on atherosclerotic heart disease, renal disease, diabetes, immunosuppression, healing ability (poor healing, keloids, or hypertrophic scars), bleeding tendency, allergies to systemic antibiotics, local anesthetics, topical antibiotics, presence of a cardiac pacemaker, pregnancy, and history of syncope, especially from injections or phlebotomy. A detailed medication history should place special attention on platelet-inhibiting agents such as aspirin, nonsteroidal anti-inflammatory drugs, and dipyridamole; coagulation-inhibiting agents such as warfarin; β-blocking agents, tricyclic antidepressants, thyroid hormones, and monoamine oxidase inhibitors. A history of abnormal heart valves, heart murmur, or prosthetic joints or vessels should be looked for because some patients may require preoperative prophylactic antibiotics to prevent bacterial endocarditis or infection of prostheses. Smoking may interfere with survival of skin grafts or flaps because of vasoconstriction, while alcohol drinking may increase the patient's bleeding tendency by causing qualitative platelet inhibition.

Whenever possible, nonsteroidal anti-inflammatory agents, dipyridamole, warfarin, alcohol, and cigarettes should be stopped for 3 to 5 days preoperatively. Aspirin must be withheld for at least 10 days preoperatively because it causes irreversible inhibition of platelet function. Vasoconstricting agents should be used with caution in patients taking β-blocking agents, tricyclic antidepressants, thyroid hormones, and monoamine oxidase inhibitors because of the risk of severe hypertension. A detailed oral and written informed consent discussing the potential benefits, risks, and alternative treatments should be signed by the patient or, if the patient is mentally incompetent or under age 18, by the patient's legal guardian.

Mohs Micrographic Surgery

History

Frederick E. Mohs developed a technique for the in vivo fixation of rat skin tumors using a zinc chloride fixative paste with stibnite and *Sanguinaria canadensis* while he was a medical student in the 1930s. Subsequently the fixed tumor tissue was resected with serial excisions under complete microscopic control of the resection margins.[10] Mohs became a general surgeon and started to use his "chemosurgery technique" for skin cancer. He published the results from his first 440 cases in 1941.[11] In spite of high 5-year cure rates for primary basal cell carcinoma of 99 percent and 95 percent for recurrent basal cell carcinoma, the technique failed to gain widespread acceptance because it was thought to be tedious, requiring multiple stages over several days, and because early reconstruction was not possible because of an obligatory postfixation slough of remaining fixed tissue.[10,11] In the 1970s Theodore Tromovitch presented a "fresh tissue technique," in which the in vivo fixation was omitted, in a series of 75 procedures for skin cancer.[12] This modification, initially used by Mohs in 1953 for eyelid tumors, provided the highest possible cure rate with maximum tissue sparing, and made immediate reconstruction possible.[13,14] Almost all tumors can be extirpated within a few hours rather than several days, and the pain associated with in vivo fixation is eliminated.[15] With the above advantages, the fresh tissue technique has become the treatment of choice for many difficult-to-treat skin cancers.[16]

Various terms have been used over the years to describe Mohs micrographic surgery including chemosurgery (coined by Mohs),

Mohs chemosurgery, Mohs histographic surgery, microscopically controlled excision, microcontrolled surgery, and microscopically oriented histographic surgery (MOHS). In 1986 the American College of Chemosurgery named the technique *Mohs micrographic surgery, fixed tissue technique* when zinc chloride paste in vivo fixation is used, and *Mohs micrographic surgery, fresh tissue technique* when the zinc chloride fixation step is omitted.[17] Unless otherwise noted, Mohs micrographic surgery will be used to refer to the fresh tissue technique for the remainder of this chapter because almost all skin cancers treated with Mohs micrographic surgery today are treated with the fresh tissue technique.

Technique[12–15,18,19]

The diagnosis and histologic type of skin cancer are established with conventional permanent sections. After anesthesia, usually local, the lesion is debulked with a dermal curet to assess tumor extent. A saucer-shaped layer of tissue is taken around the curetted area with narrow margins beveling the incision at a 45° angle relative to the skin surface. This angle is important to facilitate proper positioning of the epidermal edge for horizontal frozen sections. The specimen is divided into conveniently sized pieces for frozen section processing, with each piece oriented relative to the defect and marked with tissue dyes. A map of the defect and specimen is drawn. The specimen pieces are turned with the deep surface facing up and mounted for horizontal frozen sections so that the epidermal, dermal, and deep margins lie in the same plane. After freezing, horizontal frozen sections are taken from the entire undersurface (margin) of the specimen. The sections are stained and examined by the Mohs micrographic surgeon, who notes any areas that contain tumor on the map, then returns to the patient and takes additional layers of tissue from the areas that still contain tumor. This process is repeated until all margins are free of tumor. At this point, the defect is ready for immediate repair or healing by secondary intention with the assurance that nearly 100 percent of the surgical margin has been examined.

The main difference between Mohs micrographic surgery and conventional excision is not in the surgical technique, but in the way that the surgical margins are examined. With conventional vertical frozen or permanent sections for examination of surgical margins, the true surgical margin is only sampled. Often, less than 0.1 percent of the true surgical margin is examined with standard vertical sections.[20] For well-confined tumors, this approach may be adequate, but for difficult skin cancers that often have an unpredictable pattern of growth with finger-like projections away from the main body of the tumor (Figs. 238-1, 238-2), total true surgical margin examination is essential to achieve a high cure rate. Also, Mohs micrographic surgery is tissue sparing because the tumor can be precisely located in the surgical defect and conservatively excised.

Indications

Locally recurrent basal cell carcinoma poses a difficult therapeutic problem. If it is re-treated by excision with conventional margin control, radiation therapy, electrodesiccation and curettage, or cryosurgery, average 5-year recurrence rates of 20 percent have been reported.[21] These high recurrence rates may occur because recurrent basal cell carcinomas grow in a very unpredictable manner throughout the scar tissue and beyond (Fig. 238-1).[22] Approxi-

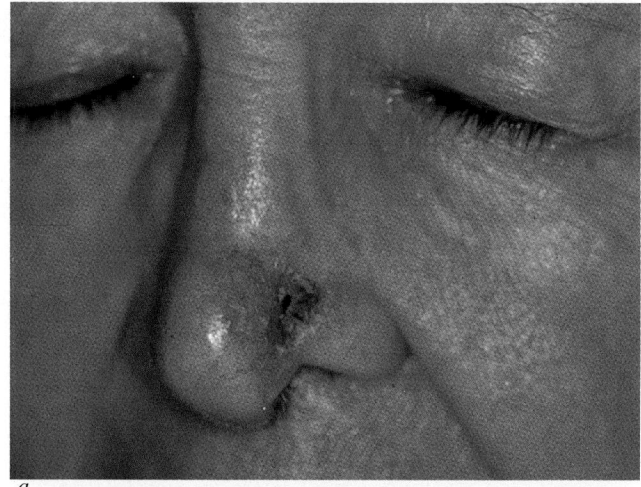

a

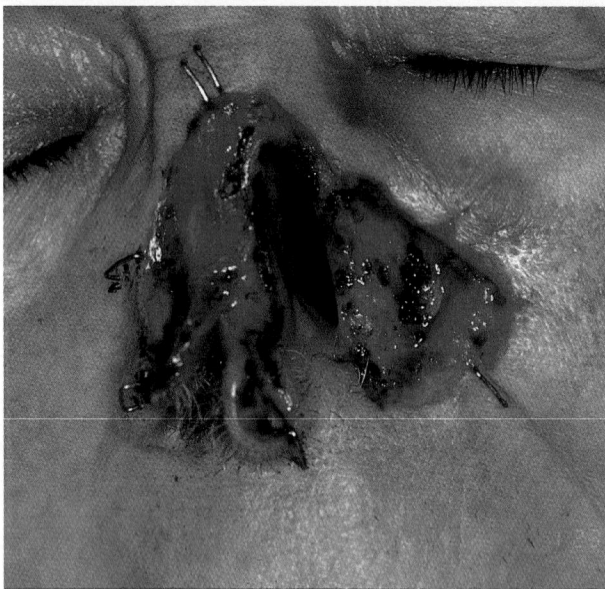

b

FIGURE 238-1 (*a*) Morpheaform basal cell carcinoma of the left nasal ala which was locally recurrent (persistent) after electrodesiccation and curettage several years previously. (*b*) Final tumor-free defect after five stages of Mohs micrographic surgery demonstrating extensive subclinical spread to involve the nasal septum, both nasal alae, medial cheek, and left nasal wall down to the maxillary bone. Staples in wound margins were used to orient tissue specimens relative to the surgical defect.

mately 50 percent of recurrences of those tumors treated by electrodesiccation and curettage reveal multiple discontiguous tumor foci.[23] Basal cell carcinoma recurrent after x-ray therapy is especially difficult to eradicate with conventional therapy.[24] With Mohs micrographic surgery, 5-year cure rates of 92 to 97 percent for recurrent basal cell carcinomas have been reported.[13,16,21]

Histologically aggressive basal cell carcinomas, including morpheaform (Fig. 238-1), sclerosing, infiltrating, and metatypical carcinomas, are significantly more invasive, aggressive, and prone to recurrence after conventional therapy.[12,25] Morpheaform basal cell carcinoma has been found to extend on average at least 7.2 mm from the clinically apparent tumor margin.[26] Metatypical (keratinizing, basosquamous) basal cell carcinoma is very aggressive with

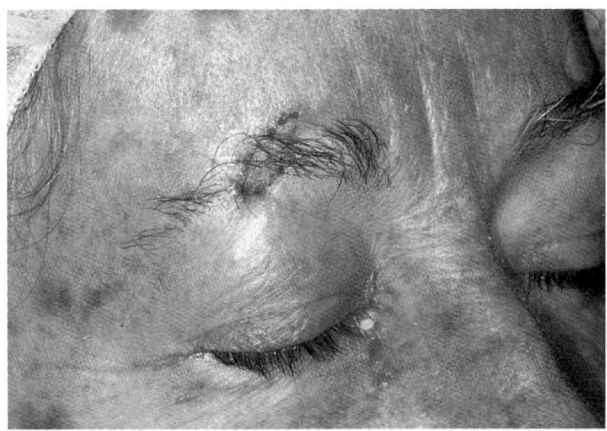

a

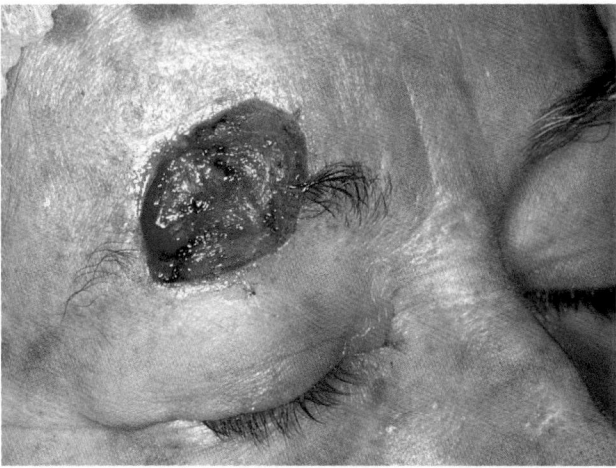

b

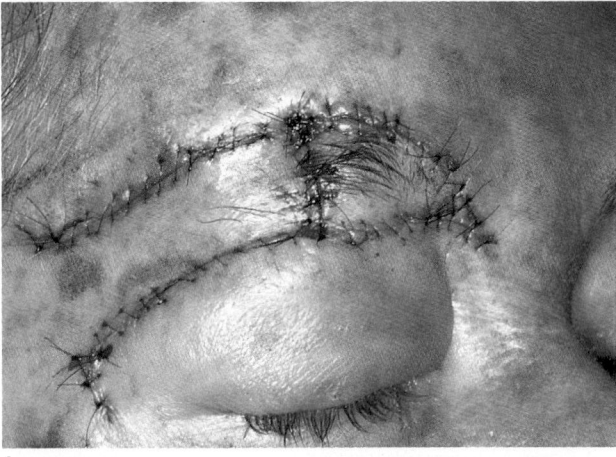

c

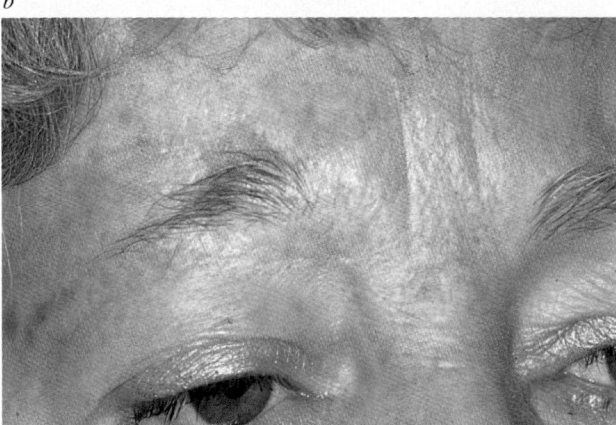

d

FIGURE 238-2 Right eyebrow primary basal cell carcinoma with ill-defined clinical margins treated with Mohs micrographic surgery followed by local flap reconstruction of the defect. (*a*) Lesion before surgery; (*b*) defect after three stages of Mohs micrographic surgery; (*c*) immediately after repair with a laterally based advancement flap and a medially based island pedicle flap; and (*d*) final result 7 months postoperatively.

a clinical behavior approaching that of squamous cell carcinoma.[25] Invasion of cartilage, bone, nerves, or blood vessels by basal cell carcinoma is a sign of an aggressive tumor with unpredictable extensions and a high recurrence rate after conventional therapy.[27] All of these aggressive tumors are most effectively treated with Mohs micrographic surgery, because all of the unpredictable extensions (Fig. 238-1), including perineural invasion, can be precisely traced.[13,14,16]

In certain anatomic locations, basal cell carcinoma may extend far beyond the clinically apparent margins. The tumor cells spread along the path of least resistance, such as fascial planes, perichondrium, periosteum, neurovascular bundles, and embryologic fusion planes.[28] This tendency of basal cell carcinoma may account for the high recurrence rate after conventional treatment reported in certain "high-risk" anatomic sites in the head and neck region.[16,25,27,29,30] In the scalp the tumor cells may spread along the galea or along hair follicles for several centimeters away from the clinically apparent tumor mass.[30] Inadequate initial treatment of periorbital basal cell carcinoma, especially of the medial canthus, may result in invasion of the lacrimal drainage system and along the periosteum deep into the orbit and ethmoidal sinuses, ultimately necessitating orbital exenteration.

Eyelid basal cell carcinoma may extend along the conjunctival surface of the tarsal plate. Eyebrow basal cell carcinoma may in-

vade along the hair follicles beyond the clinically apparent margins (Fig. 238-2). On the nose, nasal septum, ear pinna, and ear canal, the tumor cells often extend along the perichondrium and periosteum beyond the clinical margins.[14,25,29] Areas including the nasal ala groove, meilolabial fold, postauricular sulcus, and preauricular region, where embryologic fusion planes are perpendicular to the skin surface, allow unexpectedly deep invasion by tumor cells.[13,14,16,29] A recent study has shown no histologic evidence of embryologic fusion planes in adults.[31] Therefore the reason for deep tumor invasion in these sites is not clearly known. Mohs micrographic surgery is the most effective way to treat tumors in all of these high-risk locations.[13,14,16]

While most basal cell carcinomas, especially the noduloulcerative type, have grossly distinct margins that can be further delineated with curettage, there is a subset of basal cell carcinoma that has very ill-defined visible margins (Figs. 238-1, 238-2). Infiltrating and morpheaform basal cell carcinomas often present as atrophic telangiectatic macules and patches with indistinct clinical margins (Fig. 238-1) that do not become more distinct with curettage.[13] Superficial (multicentric) basal cell carcinoma may extend beyond the clinically apparent margins. A basal cell carcinoma in a field of actinic keratoses may have its clinical margins obscured by nearby lesions. Patients who have received x-ray radiation, usually for a benign condition such as acne, 30 or more years earlier, often develop basal cell and squamous cell carcinomas in the irradiation field.[32] Most of these radiation-induced basal cell carcinomas have very ill-defined clinical margins and histologically exhibit an infiltrating growth pattern. Mohs micrographic surgery can delineate the exact extent of all these ill-defined lesions with microscopic control and exact maps.[13,14]

A basal cell carcinoma that is excised with positive margins will regrow within 2 years in at least one-third of cases.[33] When tumor is present within one high-power field of the margin, the regrowth rate is 12 percent.[33] Because of these high recurrence rates, reexcision by Mohs micrographic surgery is advisable, especially if the deep margin in the head and neck area is involved by tumor, because regrowth there can result in the invasion and destruction of vital underlying structures before detection of the tumor at the skin surface.[14]

Mohs micrographic surgery is very effective in conserving tissue in cosmetic and functionally important areas, such as the nose, upper lip, ear, eyelid, eyebrow, digits, and genitalia.[14] These areas have a limited amount of excess tissue for simple, functional, and cosmetically elegant reconstructions (Fig. 238-2). Also, minimizing the risk of recurrence in these areas is important because additional surgery will make the final result even less desirable. Mohs micrographic surgery achieves a 98 to 99 percent 5-year cure rate for primary basal cell carcinoma.[34] Patients with basal cell nevus syndrome, xeroderma pigmentosum, Bazex syndrome, or Rombo's syndrome require, in addition to prophylactic measures, early treatment of their numerous basal cell carcinomas with maximal conservation of tissue.

Large and invasive squamous cell carcinomas of the skin, especially those not arising in association with actinically damaged skin, behave aggressively and are associated with a significant incidence of metastatic disease. These squamous cell carcinomas include those that are recurrent, more than 2 cm in diameter, in old scars, in areas of chronic inflammation, or present in certain high-risk anatomic locations including the lips, ears, postauricular sulcus, and nose.[13,35,36] Histologically undifferentiated squamous cell carcinomas and acantholytic squamous cell carcinomas are also prone to local recurrence and metastasis.[37] Mohs micrographic surgery is effective for the treatment of these aggressive tumors. Metastatic disease develops within 5 years in 10 to 15 percent of patients with lip squamous cell carcinoma treated by surgical excision alone.[35] With Mohs micrographic surgery, the rate of metastatic disease can be reduced to 6 percent.[13]

Dermatofibrosarcoma protuberans (DFSP) recurs in 49 percent of cases after surgical excision with negative margins.[38] Even when DFSP is resected with 3-cm margins including the underlying fascia, an 11 percent recurrence rate has been reported.[39] These high recurrence rates are due to the very extensive clinically inapparent invasion by narrow DFSP strands which can easily be missed with conventional pathologic margin checks. Mohs micrographic surgery has successfully treated DFSP in several small series (up to 10 patients each).[13,40] With follow-up periods up to 5 years, no recurrences were noted. If these results hold up over a longer period of follow-up, Mohs micrographic surgery may become the treatment of choice for DFSP. To improve the accuracy of identifying DFSP cells in frozen sections, a modification of Mohs micrographic surgery using paraffin-embedded permanent sections and immunohistochemical stains has been proposed to delineate the tumor cells better.[40,41]

The use of Mohs micrographic surgery for the treatment of malignant melanoma is controversial. Mohs has advocated the use of the fixed tissue technique to treat melanoma, reporting 5-year

cure rates comparable to, or better than, those of conventional surgical excision (Clark's level II: 100 percent; level III: 92 percent; level IV: 64 percent; level V: 33 percent).[13,42] Other surgeons who use Mohs micrographic surgery believe it does not provide any advantage over conventional surgery for melanoma because for most melanomas metastasis, rather than local recurrence, is the clinically significant problem and most frozen sections are inadequate to identify melanoma cells accurately.[14] An exception to this rule is lentigo maligna melanoma, which recurs locally in 10 percent of patients after presumably adequate excision.[43] Mohs micrographic surgery using permanent sections should be able to improve on these results.

Any tumor that is invasive locally or recurs locally and is amenable to frozen section interpretation can be treated with Mohs micrographic surgery.[14] Adnexal carcinoma, angioendothelioma, angiosarcoma, extramammary Paget's disease, leiomyosarcoma, malignant fibrous histiocytoma, Merkel's cell carcinoma, and microcystic adnexal carcinoma have been treated with Mohs micrographic surgery with mixed results.[13,14,41,44]

Wound Management

History

The oldest medical manuscript that describes wound care was written in Sumeria circa 2100 B.C. Since then, physicians have been forced to concentrate on this subject because of constant involvement in wars. Remedies for healing wounds included dousing them with wine, painting them with salves based on honey, covering them with copper-containing ointments, and wrapping them in linens soaked in beer. It was recognized fairly early that ministering to a wound, cleansing it, and providing nurturing substances to it made it heal faster and better.[45] Many experiments have been conducted recently showing that moist occluded wounds heal faster than wounds allowed to air dry. Wound healing is discussed in Chap. 9.

Second Intention Healing

Second intention healing of full-thickness skin wounds is indicated for patients who are poor surgical risks for reconstructive surgery, for patients who refuse reconstructive surgery, for infected wounds, to allow observation of a wound bed after resection of tumors at high risk for recurrence, and for selected pathologic ulcers. Wounds that are allowed to granulate are very resistant to infection and cannot form a hematoma. The locations that lend themselves best to second intention wound healing with superior cosmetic results are concave areas, such as the nose–cheek junction, medial canthus, ear concha, preauricular cheek, and retroauricular scalp. Wounds allowed to heal by second intention may decrease in size as much as 50 percent or more.[46] Superficial wounds heal with less wound contraction since there is less deposition of collagen. Therefore, a superficial wound, even on a convex surface such as the forehead or the nose, will usually heal well. Because all wounds contract to some degree, it is important that there be no "free" margin along one side of the wound that can be pulled up during wound contracture to cause distortion at the site. Such free margins may be encountered along the eyelid margins, ear margins, eyebrow, nasal ala, and lip vermilion border. These areas are better managed with appropriate reconstructive surgery.[47] Disadvantages of second intention healing include a prolonged healing time of several weeks, the need for daily wound care by the patient, and the somewhat unpredictable cosmetic results.[48]

Fusiform Excision or Closure

A fusiform (elliptical) excision is indicated for the removal of small- to moderate-sized benign or malignant neoplasms as well as for excisional biopsy. Fusiform closure can be used wherever there is sufficient skin laxity to allow direct side-to-side closure of the defect, after adequate undermining, under minimal tension, and without distortion or functional impairment of surrounding structures. For optimal cosmetic results, the long axis of the fusiform excision should be oriented along the relaxed skin tension lines, which are generally perpendicular to the muscle pull in the area, without crossing over cosmetic unit boundaries such as the nose–cheek concavity.[49] If relaxed skin tension lines are not obvious, manipulation of the skin will indicate the direction of least tension. An alternative to fusiform excision is disk excision. The lesion is excised as a circle with adequate margins, and the wound is allowed to heal by second intention or the defect is closed into a straight line with excision of the resulting bilateral standing cones of excess tissue.[8]

Local Skin Flaps

When simple primary closure cannot be done because a wound is too large, there is too much tension on the wound edges, or an unacceptable functional or cosmetic result would ensue, then a tissue movement procedure should be considered, such as a flap or a graft. A local skin flap is a portion of full-thickness skin transferred from a donor site into a surgical defect while maintaining its blood supply from the donor site via a random or axial vascular pedicle that remains attached to the donor site. The point of attachment, or pedicle, is critical for the survival of the flap because the flap receives its blood supply through this area. Therefore, for random flaps, the length-to-width ratio should not exceed 3:1 or 4:1 on the face (Fig. 238-2) and 2:1 on the trunk and extremities. The thickness of flaps also varies depending on location and should be adjusted for the site into which it will be placed.[50] Whenever possible, flap incisions should be made so that they fall into relaxed skin

tension lines (Fig. 238-2).[51] Care should be taken not to include hair in a flap that is going into an area that is not naturally hair bearing. If specifically included in the flap, the direction of hair growth should be the same as that in the area of the defect (Fig. 238-2).

Two movements occur in a flap. The action of placing the flap into the defect is the primary movement. There is also secondary movement of tissue in the donor area needed to close the secondary defect and to facilitate primary flap movement. Both movements are important in terms of distributing tension in the proper direction and over a larger area so as to minimize tension on the flap itself, which might compromise its survival.[52]

There are various kinds of flaps. In an advancement flap, the tissue movement is in a straight line from the donor area to the recipient site and it may be unilateral or bilateral (Fig. 238-2). A classic example is a bilateral advancement flap to close a moderate sized defect on the forehead with incision lines made in natural furrows of the forehead and with tissue advancement in the horizontal plane.[50] Another bilateral advancement flap is an A-to-T flap, in which incisions extend from the base of a triangular defect and the two sides are slid together along this baseline. A third similar advancement flap is a Burrow's triangle single advancement flap. Advancement flaps are commonly used for defects of hair-bearing skin in the eyebrow (Fig. 238-2) or mustache area, where orientation of the hair shafts is critical.

The rotation flap slides skin into the defect by rotating it on its axis. This flap is classically used to close relatively large defects on the cheek, forehead, or scalp. A rotation flap with a back cut can increase tissue movement in areas of limited tissue laxity, such as the nose.[53] A double rotation or an O-to-Z flap can also increase the amount of tissue rotated into the defect. Transposition flaps belong in a different category since they transpose skin from one site to another, crossing normal, nonflap skin in between. The classic transposition flap is the rhombic flap with its exact geometric design (Fig. 238-3). The defect is visualized in the shape of a rhombus with equal sides and angles opposite each other of 60° and 120°, respectively. The flap is then created by drawing a line out from and bisecting either of the 120° angles equal in length to one side. The next line creates a 60° angle with that line and is parallel to and equal to the side of the rhombus.[54] Other transposition flaps include the note flap, banner flap, nasolabial (meilolabial) flap, bilobed flap, Webster's 30° modified rhombic flap, and the Z-plasty. Transposition flaps are very versatile, being useful for the repair of various facial defects.[50]

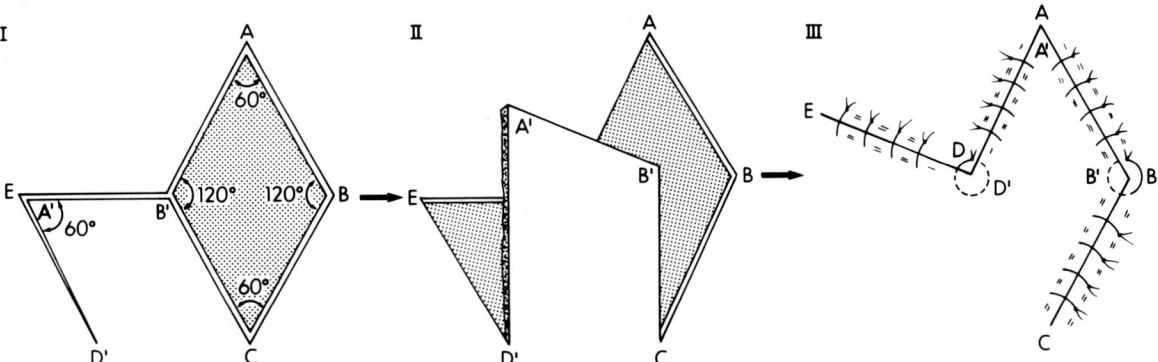

FIGURE 238-3 Rhombic transposition flap. (I) Design with shaded area representing surgical defect, (II) transposition after undermining, and (III) final suture line.

A subcutaneous island pedicle flap has had all of its connections to the epidermis and dermis severed, maintaining its blood supply only through a subcutaneous tissue pedicle (Fig. 238-2). This flap is usually slid from the defect apex into the center to close an area that would be under great tension if closed side-to-side.[55] It is often used to close defects on the side of the nose and in the meilolabial fold.[56]

The most commonly used axial vascular pedicle flap used on the face is the median forehead two-stage transposition flap. Tissue is mobilized from the forehead, based on the supratrochlear arteries, and transposed to repair large distal nasal defects with the pedicle remaining attached in the glabellar region. The pedicle is divided in approximately 2 weeks after the flap has established local blood supply from the original defect wound bed.[57]

Flaps are more delicate and therefore require more careful postoperative wound care than simple excisions. Tightly applied bandages may compromise the blood supply to the flap and cause necrosis. The area under the flap must be free of any bleeding or oozing because hemorrhage or hematoma formation may jeopardize flap survival and increase the infection rate. Patients who smoke may compromise the blood supply to the flap, and large flaps should be reconsidered in such patients.[58] The "trap door" effect occurs with some flaps when the center of the flap becomes elevated and the suture line becomes depressed. This effect is most often seen with curved transposition flaps and is probably due to centripetal contraction of the scar at the suture line and under the flap. It may resolve spontaneously over 6 to 12 months. However, if it fails to resolve spontaneously, it may respond to intralesional corticosteroids and/or flap elevation with flap thinning, possibly combined with multiple Z-plasties to break up the curved scar line.[59] The trap door effect may be prevented with wide undermining around the primary defect, proper thinning of the flap, proper size of the flap, and the use of a geometric shape for the flap.[59,60]

Skin Grafts

Grafts are totally detached from the donor site and receive all nutrients from the wound bed of the recipient site. They are named after the harvesting method (punch, pinch, dermatomal) and/or their composition (epidermis, dermis, fat, hair, cartilage, bone). Full-thickness skin grafts (FTSG) consist of epidermis with full-thickness dermis while split-thickness skin grafts (STSG) consist of epidermis with a varying thickness of dermis.

An STSG is used to cover large defects, to allow better wound bed surveillance, to line a large pedicle flap or cover the donor site of a large FTSG, or to resurface mucosa.[61] It is usually harvested from a thigh, buttock, scalp, or abdomen using a manual or power dermatome set to the desired thickness. The STSG is placed on the wound and fixed in place with absorbable sutures or staples. The main advantage of an STSG is that it will survive even in a relatively hostile environment, such as a leg ulcer. Cosmetically, this graft is suboptimal because of absent appendages, poor color match, and frequent wound contracture under the graft. For very large recipient sites, grafts may be meshed.[62] These meshed grafts are useful for coverage of lower leg ulcers because they also allow for drainage with less chance of seroma formation underneath the graft.[63] The donor site will reepithelialize rapidly and relatively painlessly with the use of biooclusive dressings.

An FTSG is generally indicated for relatively shallow full-thickness facial defects that may not be amenable to primary closure or local flap repair, or to temporarily cover a defect that needs to be observed for possible tumor recurrence. It is usually harvested from the preauricular, nasolabial, postauricular, supraclavicular, or eyelid area. An FTSG will contract less than an STSG. Appendageal structures are retained and skin color match is better than with STSG. An FTSG is harvested with a fusiform excision, often with use of a template of the defect. The graft is then trimmed to fit the defect exactly and is defatted. The donor site is closed with a primary side-to-side closure or, if it is too large, an STSG may be used to cover it. The graft is sutured onto the recipient site and a tie-over bolster dressing may be placed over the graft to keep it in place and to prevent fluid accumulation underneath the graft. Because skin grafts do not bring any blood supply with them, they are more prone to necrosis than simple closures or well-designed flaps. The color match is difficult to predict. Fairer-skinned individuals with even pigmentation and less sun damage do well with FTSG. The more darkly pigmented or mottled the surrounding skin, the less likely will there be a good color match. Uneven edges around the graft may be smoothed out with dermabrasion 6 to 8 weeks after surgery.[64]

Cultured Keratinocyte Grafts

In 1975 Howard Green and Jim Rheinwald serially cultured human keratinocytes.[65] In 1980 they were able to produce viable autologous cultured epidermal grafts suitable for placement on two burn victims.[66] By 1984 this type of graft was used to cover over 50 percent of two severely burned children.[67] Besides burn patients, these grafts can be used to cover large surgical wounds and ulcers.[68] They are very useful in patients with multiple wounds, recalcitrant large wounds, a history of skin graft failure, and limited graft donor sites, and in patients who are poor surgical risks.

There are basically two categories available today. Keratinocyte autografts are cultured from the patient's own skin and used only on that patient, while keratinocyte allografts are cultured from human newborn foreskin and used as grafts for other patients.[66,69] The success of cultured keratinocyte allografts in leg ulcers has been as high as 75 percent.[69] Because allografts appear to be as effective as autografts for wound healing, they may actually act as sophisticated biologic wound dressings that promote wound healing by producing various growth-stimulating factors. This subject is an area of intensive research at various centers.

The keratinocyte culture is started with the epidermis separated from newborn foreskin or from a 1- to 2-cm^2 biopsy specimen taken from a protected site on the patient, such as postauricular skin, axilla, or groin. The epidermis is then processed and plated, and in approximately 11 days confluent sheets of undifferentiated epithelial cells should be seen. These sheets are replated and approximately 11 days later the first grafts are ready for grafting. The undifferentiated epithelial cells are stored, and subsequent grafts take only the 10 to 11 days to prepare. Essentially, the original 2-cm^2 sample can be amplified to 100,000 times its original size.

The first graft placement is done 3 weeks after initial biopsy. Prophylactic antibiotics are given to the patient because these grafts are very susceptible to microorganisms. No preoperative topical antibiotics should be used. The grafts are pink diaphanous sheets measuring 5 × 5 cm that remain viable for 24 h in their delivery container. They are attached to petrolatum gauze to permit easier handling because they tend to float about in their medium-containing Petri dishes. They are gently placed on the wound and trimmed to fit without overlapping, and the wound is dressed. The dressing must eliminate all shearing forces to ensure graft survival, but suturing the graft to the wound bed is usually not necessary. No anesthesia is required for graft placement. These grafts contract like STSG, but cosmetically they are somewhat better because they are softer, not as stark white, and closer in appearance to the surrounding skin.[67]

Bioocclusive Wound Dressings

With the inherent difficulties of using autografts, allografts, xenografts, and cadaver skin to cover wounds, and the scientific evidence demonstrating the benefits of moist wound healing, it was natural to develop synthetic wound dressings.[70] These dressings attempt to incorporate all of the requirements for wound care and coverage. They are occlusive to encourage granulation tissue formation and to speed reepithelialization. Covered wounds are less painful and require fewer dressing changes, which is often the most uncomfortable part of wound healing for the patient.[71] They may also be able to exclude microorganisms from clean wounds. However, contaminated wounds may develop increased bacterial colonization under occlusive conditions.[72]

There are three categories of bioocclusive dressings: (1) semipermeable films, such as Op-site and Tegaderm; (2) semiocclusive hydrogels, such as Vigilon or Scherisorb; and (3) occlusive hydrocolloids, such as Duoderm or Restore. Semipermeable films allow water vapor, oxygen, and other gases to pass while preventing the passage of liquid, water, and bacteria. Because they are nonabsorbent, fluid may accumulate.[73] Aspiration of this fluid is recommended to avoid dressing changes.[74] Although these films do not adhere to the wound, they can stick to it as it reepithelializes and cause avulsion of the newly formed epidermis during dressing changes.[75] The semiocclusive hydrogels have more absorbency.[76] Because of the low P_{O_2} under these dressings, they are contraindicated in anaerobic infections. The occlusive hydrocolloids are absorbent, flexible, adhesive dressings that conform to the shape of the wound. They are impermeable to gas and moisture, and they release degradation products into the wound. The use of occlusive dressings may be slightly different for acute and chronic wounds,[75] but it is clear that covering a wound has a profound effect on all aspects of wound healing.[77] The ideal wound coverage has not been found. Future improvements may incorporate variations of the above types along with epidermal growth factors, cultured keratinocytes, and dermal components.

Nail Surgery

In addition to being cosmetically important, the nail is a functional epidermal unit used for manipulation, protection, and defense. Medical management of nail disease and nail anatomy are discussed in Chap. 62. Surgical treatment of nail diseases can offer an alternative or adjunctive therapy for many nail problems.[78]

Preoperatively, one of the important points to make to the patient is the possibility of permanent nail deformity due to the surgical procedure. Medical diseases to be looked for are Raynaud's phenomenon, peripheral vascular disease, and diabetes, all of which may increase morbidity associated with the surgery. Underlying joint or bone pathology, such as exostosis or osteomyelitis, should also be considered. The nail area is anesthetized with a digital nerve block without epinephrine to avoid vasospasm with possible ischemic injury. Small quantities of plain lidocaine are infiltrated on both sides of the proximal digit or into the surrounding web spaces. It may take as long as 15 min for the distal digit to become anesthetized. A tourniquet is placed proximal to the surgical site for intraoperative hemostasis and is left in place no longer than 15 min. Special instruments for nail surgery include either a dental spatula or Freer septum elevator to elevate the nail plate off the nail bed and a nail splitter or nail clipper to cut the nail plate.

The most frequent surgical procedure of the nail unit is biopsy for the diagnosis of inflammatory or neoplastic disease including psoriasis, lichen planus, onychomycosis, melanoma, and squamous cell carcinoma. Punch or excisional biopsy of the nail bed or matrix is preferable to shave biopsy.[79] If the disease process is in the nail bed underlying the nail plate, it is usually advisable to remove the nail plate first to gain better access to the nail bed and to be better able to achieve hemostasis. However, with a very sharp trephine, a punch biopsy can be made right through the nail plate and into the nail bed. The nail matrix (lunula) is exposed by incisions at the outer edge of the proximal nail fold, then the nail fold is everted with skin hooks. If an elliptical biopsy of the nail bed is done distal to the nail matrix, it should be oriented in a longitudinal fashion and preferably be no more than 3 mm wide to minimize scar formation.[80] If an elliptical biopsy of the nail matrix is to be done, it should be oriented transversely to prevent split-nail deformity and preferably curved slightly; care should be taken not to remove the full width of matrix because of possible resultant deformity or loss of nail growth.

Nail avulsion is indicated for temporary correction of ingrown toenails, onychogryphosis, onychomycosis, chronic paronychia, and other nail deformities as well as for access to underlying nail bed or matrix pathology. The nail plate is freed from the nail bed with a dental spatula. Further, it must be carefully loosened from the lateral and proximal nail folds. Once freed, the nail plate is grasped firmly with a hemostat and maneuvered off the nail bed.[81] The nail plate will grow back in approximately 3 months on a finger and in 6 months on a toe.[82]

Nail avulsion with matricectomy is indicated for the permanent correction and pain relief of ingrown toenails, onychogryphosis, intractable onychomycosis, and other nail deformities. After nail avulsion and exposure of the matrix, the matrix can be surgically excised, electrodesiccated, vaporized with a carbon dioxide laser, or chemically cauterized with full-strength 88% phenol.[83] If all of the matrix is not obliterated, nail spicules may grow in the area, requiring secondary procedures to eradicate them. Chemical cauterization may be more effective than excision to remove all of the nail matrix.[83] For ingrown toenails, some nail growth can often be preserved by removing only the lateral nail matrix horns while preserving the central portion of the matrix. This approach results in a narrowed nail that stays clear of the lateral nail fold. An alternative approach to ingrown toenails caused by hypertrophic or malformed lateral nail folds is to excise a wedge of the lateral nail fold down to the periosteum without removing nail matrix and thus to preserve normal nail growth. It may be necessary to excise this area to treat the problem adequately.[84]

Dermabrasion

History

The oldest recorded report of dermabrasion was in 1550 B.C. by Papyrus Ebers in Egypt, who used papyrus and pumice for smoothing the skin and removing blemishes. In 1905 Kromayer reported on the use of a burr attached to dental equipment for planing skin.[85] In 1953 modern dermabrasion was introduced by Kurtin, a dermatologist, who developed wire brush motor-driven abraders for efficient planing of the skin.[86] The technique was further refined and popularized by Orentreich, who worked with Kurtin. After a period of declining popularity during the 1960s and 1970s, dermabrasion has regained interest recently, in association with the renewed interest in dermatologic surgery.[87]

Indications

Dermabrasion exerts its therapeutic effect by removing the epidermis and superficial dermis, allowing reepithelialization primarily from the underlying adnexal structures. Therefore the technique is best used for superficial lesions on the face. The face has a large number of adnexal structures with an excellent blood supply that further improves healing. Radiodermatitis is a contraindication to dermabrasion because of a significant decrease in adnexal structures and blood supply.

Dermabrasion was developed for the treatment of postacne scars. Even though it does not totally eliminate them, a significant improvement can be expected with superficial and shallow, well-demarcated scars, as well as with saucer-shaped scars.[88] Deep icepick scars do not respond to dermabrasion alone, but they can be significantly improved with punch grafts, punch excisions, and punch elevations followed in 6 to 8 weeks by dermabrasion.[89,90] Other scars such as those caused by varicella, trauma, or surgery can be improved with dermabrasion. The best results can be achieved by dermabrading these scars 4 to 8 weeks after the injury; 8 weeks is apparently the optimal time. Earlier dermabrasion may result in scar spread due to inadequate tensile strength of the scar, whereas dermabrasion much later than 8 weeks results in less improvement.[64]

There have been at least 50 entities treated with dermabrasion.[87] Dermabrasion is especially useful for the treatment of superficial facial lesions such as adenoma sebaceum, multiple trichoepitheliomas, multiple syringomas, fine rhytids, actinic keratoses, multiple seborrheic keratoses, epidermal nevi, solar elastosis, sebaceous hyperplasia, rhinophyma, and tattoos (Fig. 238-4).[87,91] When these lesions are on the neck, trunk, or extremities, a variable amount of scarring is to be expected and has to be weighed against the benefit of removing the lesions.

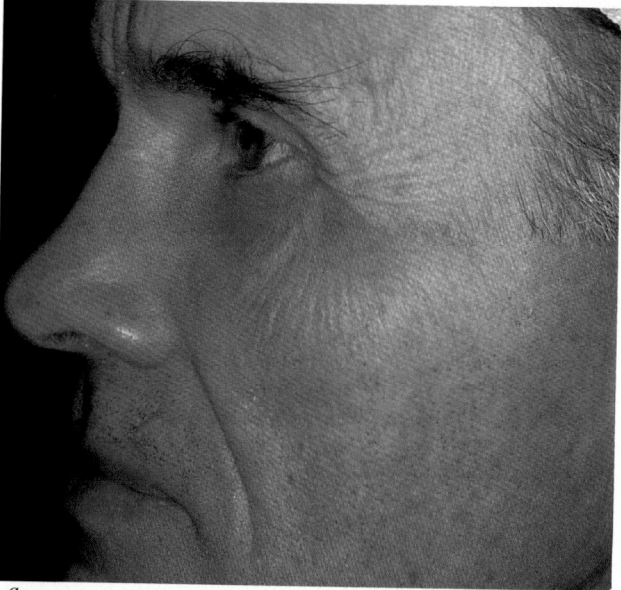

a

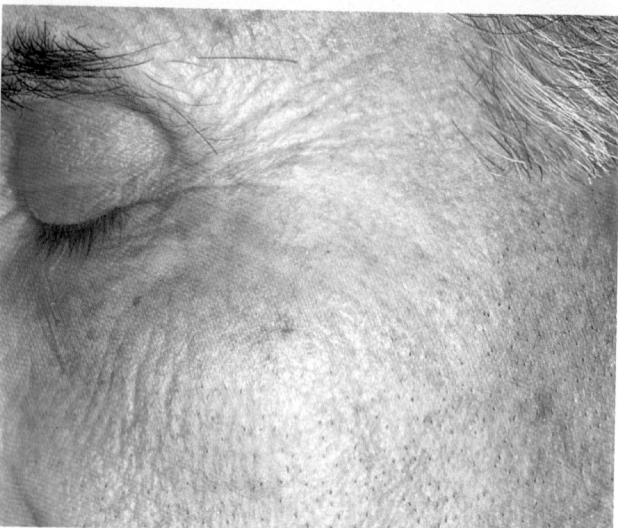

b

FIGURE 238-4 Left zygomatic cheek traumatic tattoo of many years' duration treated with spot dermabrasion.
(*a*) Preoperatively, and (*b*) 2 years postoperatively with eradication of visible tattoo pigment.

Technique

Anesthesia Full-face dermabrasion can be performed under general anesthesia, intravenous sedation with local nerve blocks, local nerve blocks alone, or in selected patients under cryoanesthesia alone. Prechilling the face enhances the effects of the hydrocarbon sprays used for cryoanesthesia.

Equipment Several motor-driven abraders are available. They are driven by either compressed gas or electricity. The gas-driven machines are capable of achieving higher revolutions per minute (40,000 to 60,000) than the electricity-driven machines (15,000 to 35,000). However, either type can generate adequate revolutions per minute for successful dermabrasion. The two main types of handpieces are the diamond fraise and the wire brush. The diamond

fraise is a stainless steel wheel on which diamond chips have been bonded. The wire brush is made of multiple wires arranged on a stainless steel wheel. The wire brush is preferred by many experienced surgeons because it cuts faster. However, the wire brush is more likely to gouge the skin than the diamond fraise. For special anatomic areas, such as the nose, the diamond fraise comes in various shapes and sizes.[88]

Careful attention has to be paid to the tissue and blood particles spread around the operating room. At the speeds used for dermabrasion, 0.6- to 0.7-μm particles, which can be deposited in lung alveoli, are produced by the centrifugal forces generated by the diamond fraise.[92] Therefore every effort must be made to minimize exposure by operating room personnel. These precautions include the use of face shields, diamond fraise guards, and 0.1-μm filter face masks, and performance of the dermabrasion with the skin frozen rigid with hydrocarbon spray cryoanesthesia.

The refrigerant sprays provide cryoanesthesia and make the skin surface rigid for efficient abrasion. Rigidity of the skin surface is especially important when using the wire brush. Freon 114 (Frigiderm, Fluoro ethyl) are used almost exclusively. The maximum cooling temperature achieved with these agents is $-40°C$ ($-40°F$).[93] Cryosthesia-30 and Cryosthesia-60 (Freon 11 and Freon 12) are used infrequently today because of concern about excessive freezing of the skin to $-66°C$ ($-87°F$) with resultant adverse sequelae of scarring and prolonged postoperative erythema.[93,94] The days of all of these refrigerants may be numbered because of mandated decreased production and a probable future ban of all chlorofluorocarbons because of atmospheric ozone depletion.

Technique[88]   Some surgeons paint the entire area to be abraded with gentian violet so that the deep color entirely fills the scars and makes identification of the scar during abrasion easier. After prechilling with ice packs, the region to be abraded is systematically divided into 3×3-cm squares that are sequentially frozen to rigidity with the refrigerant. Then the region is abraded to the desired depth, ranging from the upper papillary dermis to the midreticular dermis, depending on the requirements of each individual case. The areas are overlapped to minimize noticeable transition zones between abraded regions. The dermabrasion is carried into the hairline and over the mandibular line with feathering at the edges to minimize noticeable demarcation lines between the abraded and nonabraded areas. Hemostasis is achieved with direct pressure, or hemostatic agents such as Thrombistat may be used. Postoperatively, biooclusive dressings such as Vigilon are used to speed reepithelialization of the wound. Reepithialization is usually complete within 5 to 7 days compared with 10 to 12 days for dry wound healing with crust formation.[95]

Complications[88,96]

Properly performed dermabrasion is a safe procedure with infrequent complications. Scarring can be seen with deep abrasion, especially over bony prominences such as the mandible. Excessive freezing of the skin can increase the risk of scarring. There have been reports of atypical scarring in patients dermabraded within 6 months of completing isotretinoin treatment for acne.[97] Patients should wait at least 6 to 12 months after completing isotretinoin treatment before undergoing dermabrasion. Dermabrasion below the face and scalp and in previously x-ray-irradiated skin is associated with a high incidence of scarring because of a paucity of adnexal structures in these sites.

Pigmentary alteration is the most frequently encountered complication. A certain degree of hypopigmentation is to be expected in at least 50 percent of patients and is rarely a cosmetic problem. Irregular hyperpigmentation is more serious, but early and aggressive use of bleaching creams improves most hyperpigmentation. Black, Latino, Indian, and Asian patients are more likely to develop postinflammatory hyperpigmentation. Sun avoidance for at least 6 months after dermabrasion is essential.

Milia are routinely seen after abrasion and are usually self-limited. Pretreatment with tretinoin (Retin-A) may decrease their formation. The risk of herpes simplex and bacterial infection can be minimized with appropriate prophylactic medications.

Chemical Peel

History

The use of phenol for controlled chemical peeling of the face dates back to the early part of the twentieth century.[98] Jessner's solution for superficial skin peeling was described in 1946.[99] In the early 1960s Baker[100] and Litton[101] refined the phenol formula to the one that is still used today, while the use of trichloroacetic acid was introduced by Ayres.[102]

Definition

The success of chemical peeling of skin relies on a wounding agent, such as phenol or trichloroacetic acid, to chemically coagulate the skin to a therapeutically desired depth, followed by a slough of the damaged epidermal and dermal components and regeneration of the epidermis and upper dermis. Chemical peels are usually divided into superficial, medium, and deep peels. In general the deeper the peel the greater the therapeutic benefits as well as risks. Chemical peeling is generally restricted to the face and scalp, because peeling other regions of the body may result in a significant degree of scarring and pigmentary alteration.

Superficial Chemical Peel

Superficial peeling of the skin removes stratum corneum and variable amounts of epidermis with minimal dermal effects. Superficial peeling has been used for fine wrinkling, mild actinic damage, epidermal pigmentary changes, and as an adjunct in acne treatment.[103] However, for therapeutic effects to be noticeable, multiple weekly or monthly treatments are required. The most commonly used superficial peeling agents include 15 to 25% trichloroacetic acid, Jessner's solution (resorcinol, salicylic acid, lactic acid, ethanol), modified Unna's paste (resorcin, zinc oxide, ceyssatite, benzoin axungia), and 50 to 75% glycolic acid.[102–104] Anesthesia is generally not needed. Because the damage is so superficial, complications from light peels are rare and usually limited to postinflammatory hyperpigmentation. Long-term use of topical retinoic acid or 5 to 10% glycolic acid may achieve results similar to those of superficial chemical peels.[103–105]

Medium-Depth Chemical Peel

A medium-depth chemical peel necroses the epidermis and the papillary dermis to varying depths.[106] It is indicated for mild rhytids, mild actinic damage, irregular pigmentation, and lentigines.[106] The degree of improvement seen after a single medium-depth peel is usually more pronounced than the results seen after multiple light chemical peels. Medium-depth skin peeling can be achieved with full-strength 88% phenol and 40 to 60% trichloroacetic acid alone. However, when phenol is used, the patient has to be monitored for possible cardiac arrhythmias, and trichloracetic acid concentrations in excess of 50% are associated with an increased risk of pigmentary alteration and scarring.[107,108] To minimize these difficulties and risks, combination chemical peels have been developed.

Thirty-five percent trichloroacetic acid is combined with pretreatment of the skin with a second keratolytic agent, such as solid carbon dioxide, carbon dioxide slush, or Jessner's solution.[106] The pretreatment damages the skin barrier function, allowing the trichloroacetic acid to penetrate more deeply into the skin. Local anesthesia is often used to relieve the burning associated with the acid application. Healing with desquamation, edema, and erythema followed by reepithelialization is complete within 10 days postoperatively. Complications of medium-depth chemical peels are relatively infrequent and include pigmentary alterations, especially hyperpigmentation, herpes labialis reactivation, milia, and prolonged erythema. Significant scarring is rarely seen with combination medium-depth chemical peels.

Deep Chemical Peel

A deep chemical peel necroses the skin through the upper third of the reticular dermis and allows reepithelialization from the remaining adnexal structures.[107] It is indicated mainly for medium skin wrinkling, moderate actinic damage, and various epidermal pigmentary abnormalities.[109,110] This depth of destruction can be achieved with the Baker-Gordon phenol formula (phenol, tap water, Septisol soap, croton oil).[100] Paradoxically, the depth of phenol destruction increases with decreasing concentrations of phenol. Full-strength phenol reaches only into the papillary dermis, but the Baker-Gordon phenol formula with approximately 50% phenol penetrates into the reticular dermis.[107]

Unlike trichloroacetic acid, phenol has potentially significant side effects associated with systemic absorption from cutaneous application to intact skin. Up to 50 percent of patients having a phenol peel completed in less than 30 min demonstrated significant, mostly ventricular, cardiac arrhythmias including ventricular tachycardia.[111] To minimize the risk of cardiac arrhythmia, the phenol is applied to individual segments of the face, allowing enough time for the phenol to be metabolized and cleared from the bloodstream before continuing on to the next segment. Cardiac monitoring during, and for at least 30 min after, the procedure is essential.[108] Forced diuresis and prophylactic lidocaine may further decrease the cardiac toxicity of phenol.[108] Cardiac, hepatic, or renal disease are relative contraindications to phenol peel.

Because the application of phenol is very painful, the procedure has to be performed under heavy sedation with local anesthesia or under general anesthesia. The peel can be done either open or occluded. When phenol is occluded with waterproof tape that is left in place for 24 to 48 h, the depth of the dermal necrosis is increased, possibly because the tape causes maceration of the skin with increased phenol penetration and decreased phenol evaporation.[109]

Because of the greater depth of dermal injury with the Baker-Gordon phenol peel, the results are much more dramatic but the risk of complications is also significantly greater.[112] Hypopigmentation of any peeled area is the rule rather than the exception.[109,110,112] Therefore the ideal patient for a phenol peel is a woman with a fair complexion, blond hair, and blue eyes in whom the hypopigmentation would not be very noticeable and could be easily covered with make-up. Because men do not use make-up, they may find postpeel hypopigmentation unacceptable. Patients with a darker complexion may develop unacceptable degrees of hypopigmentation as well as postinflammatory hyperpigmentation. Sun avoidance and use of a sun screen after peeling are important indefinitely.[112] Postpeel scarring most often involves the lips, chin,

and areas of dynamic facial motion.[112] Persistent erythema, milia formation, reactivation of herpes labialis, and pyogenic infections have been reported.[112] Patients with a history of keloid formation, facial x-ray irradiation, and recent isotretinoin treatment are at an increased risk of scarring from chemical peels.[112] Very rare complications of phenol face peels, not reported with trichloroacetic acid peel, include toxic shock syndrome and laryngeal edema.

Hair Replacement Surgery

History

The idea of hair transplantation to correct baldness dates back to 1822. In the 1930s, Okuda in Japan reported the use of small hair-bearing 2- to 4-mm punch autografts to correct alopecia.[113] The Japanese were also the first to report the use of micrografts for the pubic region in 1943[114] and minigrafts for eyebrow reconstruction in 1953.[115] In the United States punch graft hair transplantation was introduced by Orentreich in 1959 when he demonstrated that androgenetic alopecia depends on the phenomenon of donor dominance.[116] Donor dominance refers to the property of hair-bearing autografts to maintain the characteristics of the donor site, including continued hair growth, when transplanted to a different recipient site.[116] The punch graft technique has been gradually refined with the addition of minigrafts and micrografts to achieve a more natural appearance of transplanted hair and to expand the indications for hair transplantation.

Various flaps and excisions have been used for reconstruction after cicatricial alopecia for many years. However, the use of scalp reduction surgery for the treatment of male pattern baldness was first introduced in the 1970s by Blanchard[117] and Unger.[118] This technique revolutionized hair replacement surgery by expanding the benefits to patients with far more extensive alopecia than would be amenable to hair transplantation alone.

Hair Transplantation

Hair transplantation has been successful only with hair-bearing autografts, except for reports of isografts between identical twins.[119] Therefore, hair transplantation involves a redistribution of existing hair; the extent and density of the area that can be covered with transplants are limited by the amount of remaining permanent fringe hair. Attempts to circumvent a paucity of donor hair by using synthetic fiber or human hair implants have uniformly resulted in severe complications including fiber/hair rejection, infection, pruritus, and cicatricial alopecia.[120] A far more successful approach has been to decrease the size of the recipient area with scalp reduction surgery (see below) in patients who have extensive androgenetic alopecia and who would otherwise not be good candidates for hair transplantation.[117,118]

Technique There are probably as many ways to perform hair transplantation as there are hair transplant surgeons. The correct placement of the frontal hairline is one of the most important aesthetic considerations. The frontal hairline should be U-shaped and the posterolateral limbs should intersect the temporal hair fringe in line with the lateral canthus. To establish a mature mildly receding hairline (Fig. 238-5a),[121] the center of the U should be approximately four finger breadths plus ¾ to 1 in. above the glabella.

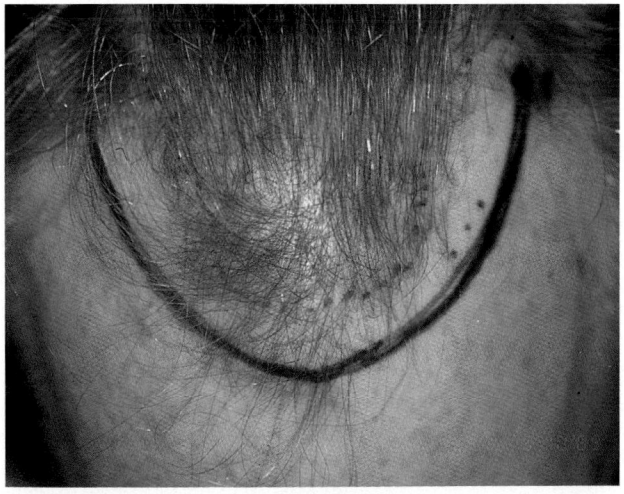

a

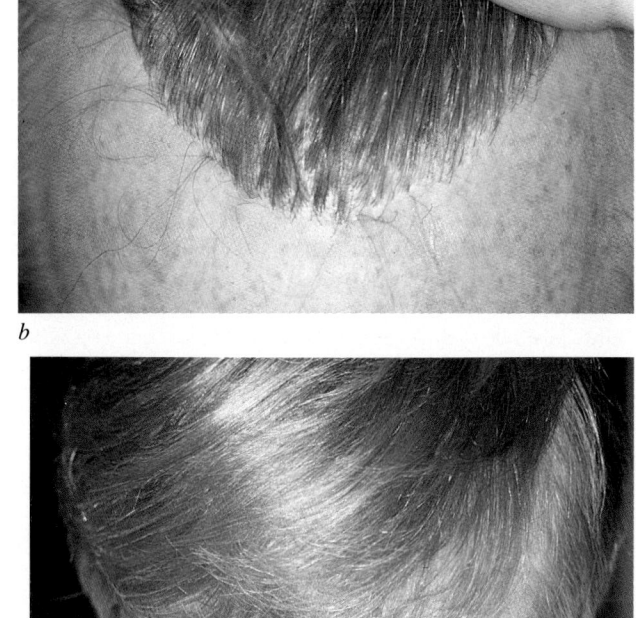

b

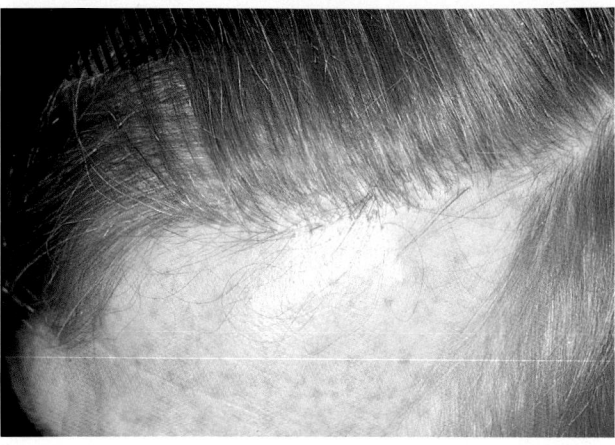

c

d

FIGURE 238-5 Hair transplantation. (*a*) Moderate frontotemporal androgenetic alopecia with proposed U-shaped hairline outlined in gentian violet; (*b*) after four punch graft sessions with hair pulled back; (*c*) close-up of transplanted hairline; and (*d*) transplanted hair in natural position.

After trimming the hairs to 3 mm and infiltrating the skin with saline to promote turgidity and straighten out the hair follicles, punch grafts are harvested with a 4-mm power punch in one or two rows from the permanent hair-bearing fringe.[122] The donor sites are closed with collapsing sutures, and the grafts are gently cleansed to remove hair spicules and excess fat. The recipient sites are prepared by a 3.5-mm power punch[123] or hand punch in alternate rows and columns, leaving a 3.5-mm space of intact skin around each recipient hole to provide adequate blood supply to the hair-bearing grafts. In the frontal area the recipient holes follow the U-shaped hairline while in the crown area the holes are placed in outward spiralling rows to recreate the occipital whorl of hair.[124] An alternative to standard round punch grafts are the square grafts proposed by Coiffman.[125] These square grafts have 25 percent more hair than round grafts of equal diameter.

The grafts are placed in the recipient holes with the appropriate hair direction, which is generally forward in the frontal region. A turban pressure dressing is placed over the grafts and removed in 24 h. To eliminate the need for a dressing and to decrease "cobblestoning" of the grafts, some surgeons advocate the use of tissue adhesive or cross-stitch suturing of the grafts in place.[126,127] The transplanted follicles experience a telogen effluvium and regrowth occurs within 2 to 4 months. The telogen effluvium may be mini-

mized by the use of topical 2% minoxidil solution in the perioperative period.[128] Complete filling of an area with punch grafts requires four hair transplantation sessions (Fig. 238-5) with the first two sessions spaced 6 weeks apart. The second, third, and fourth sessions are 4 to 6 months apart to allow the transplanted hair to grow between sessions.[129]

The standard punch graft technique achieves good hair density, but the hairline is often very abrupt and unnatural. The use of micrografts and minigrafts allows the creation of a much more natural hairline. Minigrafts are obtained by a standard round punch graft that has been divided into two "half grafts" or four "quarter grafts" with a scalpel.[130] An alternative method for obtaining minigrafts is to use small 1- to 2-mm punches to harvest from the donor sites.[131] The minigrafts are placed into slits made with a scalpel or into 1- to 2-mm round punch-graft holes in the recipient sites.[132] Micrografts are obtained by further subdivision of the standard graft to isolate only 1 or 2 hair follicles. These follicles are placed into recipient holes created with an 18-gauge needle.[133] Many have advocated the use of minigrafts and micrografts to replace standard round grafts totally in most if not all patients.[134]

Indications While standard punch graft transplantation is very effective for androgenetic alopecia in males (Fig. 238-5), micrografts and minigrafts greatly improve the aesthetic results and expand the indications for hair transplantation. Women with androgenetic alopecia are often poor candidates for standard punch grafts alone, but their alopecia can be successfully treated with minigrafts.[135] Patients with cicatricial alopecia from x-ray radiation, burns, trauma, surgery, or burned out discoid lupus erythematosus have had successful transplants.[130,136,137] Eyebrow and eyelash alopecia can be treated with micrografts if the patient trims the hair as needed.[138]

Complications Complications of properly performed hair transplantation are infrequent. Hypertrophic scars, hypopigmentation of the grafts, and a ring of scar tissue around the graft occasionally develop for poorly understood reasons.[139] Keloidal scarring can be avoided by careful patient selection. Elevation of grafts above the surrounding skin surface or ''cobblestoning'' can develop if the grafts have not been properly trimmed, the recipient area is too thin, the grafts do not fill the recipient holes correctly, there is postoperative bleeding, or inadequate pressure is applied to the grafts after placement.[139] Cobblestoning can be prevented with correct technique and corrected with light electrodesiccation of the graft surface. Inadequate cleaning of grafts may result in hair fragment implantation into the skin with a resultant granulomatous reaction. In severe cases such reactions may require removal of the involved grafts.[140] Multiple pyogenic granulomas have been reported after hair transplantation.[141] One case of osteomyelitis after hair transplantation and scalp reduction has been reported.[142] Rarely an arteriovenous fistula may develop. They usually resolve spontaneously but may require surgical dissection, ligation, and resection.[143] Intralesional corticosteroids have also been used with some success.[144]

Scalp Reduction

Scalp reduction involves the excision of alopecic scalp, relying on the patient's scalp laxity in combination with extensive subgaleal undermining of at least 10 cm on both sides of the incision.[118] The scalp excision can be repeated at 2- to 3-month intervals until the desired amount of alopecia has been excised. After the first reduction, each subsequent reduction removes less scalp.[118] There is also a degree of stretch-back after each reduction that is more evident in patients with greater scalp laxity.[145] After the final reduction the scar can be camouflaged with hair transplants.[146]

The three main scalp reduction patterns are the midline sagittal, Y-shaped, and lateral. The midline sagittal pattern removes large areas of bald scalp without altering the sensation to the scalp, but it leaves a central scar through the parietal and crown areas that may be difficult to camouflage.[146] The Y-shaped reduction eliminates the central crown region scar and removes an even greater area of alopecia while preserving sensation to the scalp.[147] The laterally based scalp reduction is excised along the existing fringe of hair in a crescent, curvilinear, or U-shape, making the resulting scars easy to hide, but there is frequent loss of sensation to the central portion of the scalp.[118,148] As an adjunct to a full scalp reduction, smaller minireductions can be performed at the time of punch grafting.[149]

To achieve greater removal of bald scalp, major scalp reductions such as the bilateral occipitoparietal flap have been proposed.[150] In these major reductions the entire occipitoparietal scalp is undermined with ligation of the occipital arteries. Very large amounts of bald scalp can be excised, but concern has been raised about the risk of scalp necrosis from this procedure.[151] An alternative modified major scalp reduction relies on undermining most of the occipitoparietal scalp while preserving the occipital arteries, thus minimizing the risk of scalp necrosis.[152]

An alternative approach to remove the maximum amount of scalp is the use of tissue expanders. The tissue expander is placed bilaterally and subgaleally under the fringe of hair and gradually inflated with weekly injections of saline. Once maximal expansion has been achieved, the expander is removed and a single scalp reduction is performed. This technique removes as much bald scalp as several serial scalp reductions.[153] For most patients the benefit of only one surgical procedure is outweighed by the significant temporary cosmetic defect experienced during the period of gradual expansion. Also, many office visits are required to fill the expander and there is an added risk of infection around the expander. Another way to stretch the scalp before a scalp reduction is to presuture the area to be excised 24 h before the actual excision of scalp.[154] Presuturing allows a larger area to be excised than would be possible otherwise. Besides being used for male pattern baldness, scalp reductions assisted with tissue expansion have been used successfully to eliminate areas of cicatricial alopecia caused by x-ray irradiation, trauma, burns, surgery, and congenital anomalies.[155]

Scalp Flaps

Frontal and central scalp alopecia can be eliminated by the temporoparieto-occipital (Juri) transposition scalp flap based on the superficial temporal artery.[156] The Juri flap requires two delays to minimize the risk of flap tip necrosis, and in skilled hands this flap is very effective. The main advantage is that the alopecic scalp can be removed and replaced with hair of normal density within a few months rather than the 18 to 24 months needed for hair transplantation. Although the hairline has excellent density and the hair continues to grow immediately after surgery, the direction of the hair is opposite the normal forward direction and so requires careful hair styling to maintain a natural appearance. The scar along the frontal hairline where the flap is inset may sometimes be quite noticeable. The risk of distal flap necrosis with attendant cicatricial alopecia is the most feared complication. However, in properly selected patients and with meticulous surgical technique, this complication appears to be quite rare. More frequent is alopecia around the donor site scar, probably due to tension on the donor site closure.[157]

A short version of the Juri flap, called a temporoparietal or Elliott flap, has been developed to decrease the potential risk of flap necrosis and patient morbidity.[158] No delays are needed. This short flap can reestablish a hairline but does not provide as much coverage as the full-length Juri flap.[159] Other flaps, such as the triple rhomboid flap and rotation flaps, have been designed to correct crown alopecia.[160,161] Microsurgical free scalp flaps have been described to correct scalp alopecia. Success with this flap depends greatly on proper technique because of the potential for extensive flap necrosis, but correctly done it can immediately reestablish a frontal hairline with correct forward hair direction.[162] One of the best uses of scalp flaps is to correct cicatricial alopecia from trauma, burns, and surgery.[162]

Filler Materials

Filler materials are used to correct various skin defects. They can be used to fill in depressed scars, age-related rhytids, and subcutaneous tissue loss. Four filler materials are currently used in the

United States and each has specific indications, advantages, disadvantages, and side effects.

Injectable Bovine Collagen

Zyderm collagen implant was approved in 1981 by the FDA to correct dermal scars and rhytids. Bovine dermal collagen consisting of 95% type I and 5% type III collagen is solubilized and purified with a combination of pepsin digestion, filtration, and ion-exchange chromatography. This material is neutralized and, after centrifugation, resuspended in solution at a concentration of 35 mg/mL for Zyderm I and 65 mg/mL for Zyderm II in phosphate-buffered saline containing 0.4% lidocaine. The collagen fibrils are cross-linked by adding glutaraldehyde during processing to form Zyplast.[88,163] This cross-linking is thought to decrease the immunogenicity of the collagen and to increase its resistance to degradation by proteolytic enzymes in the skin.[164]

Upon injection of Zyderm collagen implant into the dermis, a mild lymphohistiocytic perivascular and periadnexal infiltrate is seen during the first 3 months. The implant is found interspersed between collagen bundles, gradually travels more deeply into the dermis, and loses integrity in 6 to 9 months. Zyplast is seen in deposits that displace the host collagen. Gradually the implant is colonized by host fibroblasts that lay down new collagen by 6 months. Zyplast also gradually migrates more deeply into the dermis and is finally eliminated through the subcutaneous fat in 6 to 9 months.[163,165]

There is a 1 to 8 percent incidence of bovine collagen antibodies in patients before exposure to bovine collagen implant,[166] and only 3 to 3.5 percent of patients have a positive reaction to the first skin test.[166] Patients with high pretreatment antibody levels have a six times greater chance of developing a hypersensitivity reaction to Zyderm, and most patients with a positive skin test have bovine collagen antibodies. These antibodies do not cross-react with human collagen.[166] Most reports describe a 1 to 1.5 percent incidence of treatment site reactions in skin-test-negative patients.[167] Because most treatment site reactions occur after the first treatment, patients should have two separate skin tests before the initial treatment session.[168] Zyplast collagen appears to cause a lower level of reactivity than Zyderm.

Zyderm I and Zyderm II are implanted into the papillary dermis with a 30-gauge needle to correct fine wrinkles and superficial depressed scars, while Zyplast is injected into the middermis to correct deeper scars and furrows, such as meilolabial and glabellar folds, as well as to make lips fuller.[169] Angular cheilosis and chondrodermatitis nodularis chronica helicis have been successfully treated with Zyderm collagen implant.[88,170] Implantation of Zyplast (Keragen) under corns on the feet can provide relief.[171] Once correction has been achieved maintenance injections at 4- to 6-month intervals for wrinkles and 6- to 9-month intervals for scars are usually required to maintain correction.[172]

The most frequent complication from Zyderm/Zyplast implantation is a localized hypersensitivity reaction manifested in the skin test or treatment site by erythematous, indurated, and pruritic papules corresponding to the location of the implant. The reactions are self-limited, usually lasting 3 to 5 months, but may last as long as 18 months. All patients with localized hypersensitivity reactions develop bovine collagen antibodies.[167,173] Histologically, two-thirds of patients develop either a diffuse granulomatous reaction or a foreign body palisading granulomatous reaction, while the other third of patients have only a mild nonspecific inflammatory infiltrate.[173] Necrobiotic granulomas have also been reported.[174] The

reaction persists until the material has been digested by the host inflammatory response or eliminated from the dermis. There is no effective treatment for the hypersensitivity reaction except for symptomatic relief of pruritus with antihistamines. Corticosteroids may suppress the reaction temporarily, but they may actually prolong it by suppressing the inflammatory response needed for digestion of the implant.[164] Overcorrection with Zyderm is generally not a problem because there is significant shrinkage of the implant with resorption of the saline and lidocaine diluent. However, overcorrection with Zyplast, especially if placed too high in the dermis, results in visible beading that may persist for several months.[173]

An unusual reaction characterized by cysts and vesicles has been reported in 0.05% of cases after Zyplast implantation and in 0.002% after Zyderm implantation.[88] Eighty percent of these patients have bovine collagen antibodies. Localized tissue necrosis that heals with scarring in the area of Zyderm implantation and more often Zyplast implantation has been reported.[173] Such necrosis is usually seen in the glabellar region. The etiology of this reaction is unknown. The most serious reported adverse reaction to Zyderm implantation was one case of partial blindness, apparently caused by inadvertent intravascular injection, possibly below the dermis, with subsequent embolic occlusion of the ophthalmic vascular pathway.[88,174] To date there has been no evidence to suggest that hypersensitivity to bovine collagen implant can cause autoimmune disease in humans.[175]

Gelating Matrix Implant

Fibrel (gelatin matrix implant) was approved by the FDA in 1988 to correct depressed dermal scars. Fibrel evolved from the fibrin foam (Gelfoam) used for hemostasis since 1944.[176] Since 1957 Spangler had used fibrin foam to correct depressed scars; he treated 7000 patients by 1975 with good results.[177] Modification and refinement of this technique led to the development of Fibrel.[178] Gelatin matrix implant consists of gelatin (Gelfoam), which may provide a matrix for clotting factors and new collagen deposition, ϵ-aminocaproic acid, which inhibits fibrinolysis, and the patient's plasma, which provides fibrinogen for clot formation.[178] It is hypothesized that when Fibrel is injected under a depressed scar, localized wound healing with clot formation, fibroblast ingrowth, and new collagen deposition create new soft tissue and elevate the scar.[178]

Fibrel is reconstituted before implantation with normal saline and the patient's plasma. Most patients require local anesthesia in the area of implantation because significant burning is experienced immediately after injection. The material is implanted into the middle and upper dermis. For bound-down scars, the scar may be undermined with an undermining needle to create a pocket for the implant underneath the scar. Ecchymoses and localized edema that may take up to 1 week to resolve are frequent.[164] Even though Fibrel is being used to correct rhytids with some success, the only published large multicenter trial of Fibrel has been for the correction of depressed scars.[178,179] For depressed scars, one or two implantations achieve at least moderate correction in two-thirds of patients that lasts for at least 2 years, and in one-half of patients for at least 5 years, without significant loss of correction, measured by patient and physician evaluation as well as photogrammetric methods.[179] A maximum of only two injections were allowed as part of the study protocol. Correction of rhytids appears to have a shorter duration than correction of scars.

Fibrel appears to be less antigenic than bovine collagen implant. Before treatment all patients receive a skin test with Fibrel. The first treatment is performed 4 weeks after skin test placement.

A positive skin test reaction occurs in 1.9 percent of patients.[178] Because there appears to be no cross-reactivity with Zyderm/Zyplast, patients with bovine collagen hypersensitivity may undergo treatment with Fibrel and vice versa.[180] Localized adverse reactions other than swelling and ecchymosis have been limited to nodules persisting for 1 to several months in less than 1 percent of patients.[178] These reactions may be due to either a hypersensitivity reaction or placement of the material too superficially in the dermis.[178] No significant systemic adverse reactions have been reported with Fibrel. Patients with coagulopathies or patients receiving anticoagulants should not receive Fibrel.[178]

Silicone

The use of liquid silicone for soft tissue augmentation has been controversial, with heated debate waged in the lay press as well as in the professional literature. In most studies describing adverse reactions to silicone, the material was not pure injectable-grade silicone, or it may have been adulterated in various ways. Also, the implantation technique may have been incorrect.[181] This discussion is limited to pure injectable-grade liquid silicone (350 centistoke pure dimethylpolysiloxane).

Liquid silicone implantation is indicated for the correction of rhytids, depressed scars, and small subcutaneous contour defects.[182] Liquid silicone implantation has been used to provide relief from corns, calluses, and painful scars on soles and digits by providing a subdermal cushion under the lesion.[183] Skin testing is usually not performed before implantation. The material is implanted with a "microdroplet" technique in which individual 0.01- to 0.05-mL droplets of silicone are implanted into the superficial subcutaneous tissue or into the dermis depending on the level of the defect. Correction is primarily due to a fibroblastic capsule that forms around each droplet of silicone several weeks after implantation. Significant undercorrection at the time of implantation is desired because correction develops gradually for several weeks after implantation. Several implantation sessions at least 1 month apart are required to build up the depressed area gradually. Once achieved, the correction appears to be permanent. Successful silicone implantation depends greatly on correct technique.[182,184]

Adverse reactions to injectable-grade liquid silicone implanted with the correct microdroplet technique are very rare. The silicone may drift from the area of implantation when large amounts of silicone are injected.[185] Drifting is not seen with the microdroplet technique, which implants very small amounts of silicone. Overcorrection or lumpiness is caused by injection too superficially in the dermis or by injection of too much silicone.[184] Hyperpigmentation has been seen after superficial dermal implantation of silicone, especially in the correction of postrhinoplasty defects.[186] Superficial lymphatic obstruction with a peau d'orange appearance occurs only if very large amounts of silicone are injected or if the injection is too superficial. This problem can be avoided by correct microdroplet implantation.[182]

Most reported granulomatous reactions to silicone injections appear to be caused by adulterated forms of silicone.[184] The incidence of granulomas and "idiosyncratic" localized reactions from injectable-grade silicone has been estimated at 1 in 10,000.[184] Generally these granulomas respond to intralesional corticosteroids or antibiotics, but rarely the silicone has to be surgically removed.[184] There have been reports of systemic sclerosis associated with leaking silicone breast implants.[187] Neither systemic sclerosis nor any other collagen vascular disease has been reported after pure inject-

able-grade silicone administration by the microdroplet technique.[182,184] Silicone should never be injected into breasts because it may interfere with correct interpretation of mammograms.[184] Even though properly used injectable-grade silicone appears to be a very safe and effective filler material, it has not been approved by the FDA for any indication.

Autologous Fat Transplantation

Autologous fat transplantation was described a century ago,[188] but it was not until the 1980s, with the development of modern liposuction, that autologous fat transplantation has come into its own. Various empiric techniques have been described. Typically the fat is harvested under local anesthesia from the hips, thighs, or abdomen with a small cannula attached to a syringe. Using a syringe rather than the standard liposuction machine is thought to decrease trauma to adipocytes. The fat is allowed to separate in the syringe from blood and other debris, which are drained off. Subsequently the fat is injected into the subcutaneous tissue where augmentation is desired. Some investigators "wash" the fat with saline, Ringer's lactate, or insulin. The benefits of washing the fat, if any, are unknown. The entire procedure is performed under strict aseptic conditions. Overcorrection is necessary because only 25 to 50 percent of the fat transplant may survive. To maximize fat survival, it is harvested from areas of low vascularity, such as the thighs, and transplanted into areas of high vascularity, such as the face. Atraumatic handling of the fat is essential. The harvested fat has been used to fill in areas of age-related subcutaneous tissue loss on the face and dorsal hands, as well as for deep facial rhytids, such as meilolabial folds and glabellar furrows. Aesthetic cheek and chin augmentation can also be effective. Hemifacial atrophy and congenital soft tissue defects can be improved with fat transplants. Transplanted fat can last from a couple of weeks to several years.[189,190] Autologous fat transplantation for breast augmentation may be tempting, but the microcalcifications that often develop in the fat transplants may make mammogram interpretation difficult if not impossible.[190] Recently, Fournier described a technique for extracting autologous collagen from harvested fat; the autologous collagen can be injected into areas that require augmentation without the risk of hypersensitivity reactions that are seen with the use of exogenous materials.[191] Much clinical and basic investigation on autologous fat transplantation remains to be done before it can be considered a standard modality for soft tissue augmentation.

Liposuction

History

In the 1920s Dujarrier attempted to remove fat through a small incision, using sharp dissection to reduce the size of a famous dancer's calves.[190] The resulting injury led to complications requiring amputation of one of the dancer's legs and abandonment of the technique until the early 1970s, when Fischer, Schruddle, and Kesserling reported on sharp dissection of fat combined with the use of a suction device to remove the cut fat.[192–194] The continued reliance on sharp cutting of fat resulted in unacceptable complication rates; hematoma and seroma were the most prominent complications. Fischer in Italy and Illouz in France refined the technique by extracting fat with a blunt cannula attached to a suction device.[195,196] This technique dramatically decreased complication rates and led to the widespread popularity of liposuction among U.S. cosmetic surgeons for body sculpting. Liposuction is referred to by some surgeons as "suction-assisted lipectomy" even though lipectomy or cutting of fat is no longer part of the procedure.

Indications

Obesity results from both hypertrophy and hyperplasia of adipocytes. Liposuction removes only a relatively small number of adipocytes and is generally not useful in correcting significant obesity because resumption of excessive caloric intake by the patient can quickly reestablish the preliposuction morphology.[197] Liposuction will not improve surface skin irregularities, and if there is redundant skin preoperatively, there may be even more postoperatively that may require secondary procedures for correction. Liposuction is ideally suited for patients of normal body weight with localized fat deposits resistant to exercise and dieting, such as abdominal fat and "love handles" in men and trochanteric and gluteal regions in women. Liposuction is very effective in contouring thighs, hips, buttocks, abdomen, and knees.[198] The sculpting of calves, knees, and upper arms requires a very exacting technique but can be successful.[198] In the submental region, liposuction is often combined with rhytidectomy to remove excess skin as well as submental fat deposits.[199] Liposuction-assisted rhytidectomy has been reported to be at least as safe as standard rhytidectomy with sharp undermining.[199]

Numerous noncosmetic indications for liposuction have been proposed.[200] Large or multiple lipomas including lesions of adiposis dolorosa and of hereditary progressive nodular lipomatosis can be removed by liposuction, leaving only a very small scar at the cannula insertion point. Gynecomastia and pseudogynecomastia can be corrected by a combination of liposuction and periareolar excision of hypertrophic breast tissue, if needed. Liposuction has been used for the treatment of benign symmetric lipomatosis, hypertrophic insulin lipodystrophy, buffalo hump of Cushing's disease, lymphedema, cavernous lymphangioma circumscriptum, and axillary hyperhidrosis. Because most of these examples represent individual case reports, evaluation of therapeutic efficacy is difficult. Liposuction can facilitate flap elevation, mobilization, and defatting.[199,200]

Technique

Liposuction can be performed in most patients under local anesthesia with intravenous sedation; occasional patients require general or epidural anesthesia. When the procedure is performed under local anesthesia, a "wet" technique is used.[201] The wet or tumescent technique consists of the injection of a large volume of a very dilute mixture of lidocaine, epinephrine, sodium bicarbonate, normal saline, and hyaluronidase (optional) into the area to be treated.[201] This injection facilitates the liposuction, dramatically decreases blood loss, and minimizes postoperative discomfort. Even though very large amounts of lidocaine (as much as 35 mg/kg) are administered, lidocaine toxicity has not been encountered.[201] Even when the procedure is performed under general anesthesia, many surgeons today use the tumescent technique and omit the lidocaine from the mixture.

After the fatty deposits to be removed are marked on the standing patient, the entire procedure is performed under strictly aseptic conditions. The dilute local anesthetic is introduced into the area through a small incision into the fat compartment, and the liposuction cannula is introduced into the subcutaneous fat. Many different types of cannulae have been developed, but the most commonly used are blunt-tipped with openings to the side to minimize trauma to the fibrous septae. Also, the smaller the diameter of the cannula, the less trauma is to be expected. The fat is extracted by tunneling in various directions parallel to the skin at several levels. Often a crisscross pattern, using two entry points, is employed. The cannula opening is directed away from the skin surface so as to minimize skin irregularities postoperatively. Once the desired amount of fat has been removed, the suction is turned off and the edges of the extracted area are feathered with the cannula.[202] Fournier has proposed a syringe attached to the cannula as an alternative to the suctioning device.[203] Suction is provided by retracting the syringe plunger to create a near vacuum in the syringe and cannula. Fournier believes that better results can be achieved with this technique and that the procedure is safer. Postoperatively, the treated areas are taped and supported with pressure garments for 1 to 6 weeks. For tumescent liposuction in which less than 2000 mL of fat is removed, blood transfusion is rarely necessary, and often significantly larger volumes of fat can safely be removed without blood transfusion.[204] Large volumes removed using a "dry" technique under general anesthesia frequently require blood transfusions and significant fluid replacement.[205]

Complications

Local complications of liposuction include irregularity of the skin surface, contour deformity, hyperpigmentation, hematoma, seroma, persistent edema, loose skin, paresthesia, and skin slough.[190,206,207] Irregularity of the skin surface and loose skin, if present preoperatively, will not improve and may even worsen postoperatively. New irregularities of the skin surface can be avoided by careful technique using small-diameter cannulae, staying in the correct plane, and pointing the cannula opening away from the skin surface.[190] Contour deformity is usually due to overzealous fat aspiration. The support tape can cause hyperpigmentation in dark-skinned individuals. Patients with a history of postinflammatory hyperpigmentation should use pressure garments and bandages without tape.[190] Hematoma and seroma can be prevented by careful patient selection, gentle technique with small-diameter cannulae, pressure bandages, and, most importantly, use of the tumescent technique with epinephrine. Postoperative edema is usually self-limited and can be improved by local ultrasound therapy, massage, and perioperative corticosteroids.[190] If paresthesias develop, they almost always resolve within 1 year of surgery and are directly related to the size of the area undergoing liposuction.

Systemic complications of liposuction are extremely rare. In a review of 9478 liposuction cases performed by dermatologists, with 75 percent done under local anesthesia and 25 percent done under general anesthesia, there were five cases (0.05 percent) of excessive blood loss, two cases (0.02 percent) of infection, and no deaths.[206] Blood transfusions appear to be required with far greater frequency when the "dry" rather than the tumescent technique is used. There have been individual case reports of acute renal failure (self-limited), fat embolism syndrome (recovered), streptococcal necrotizing fasciitis (fatal), and greater saphenous vein thrombosis following liposuction. Deaths from liposuction have been associated with lack of aseptic technique and performance of other procedures concomitantly with liposuction, especially abdominoplasty. Even major liposuctions have only a 0.1 percent incidence of severe systemic complications.[207] Conservative liposuction performed by a properly trained physician using the tumescent technique appears to be a very safe procedure.

Sclerotherapy

History

Sclerotherapy of varicose veins was first attempted in 1845 with the advent of the hypodermic needle. However, because of severe to fatal complications from sepsis and emboli, the procedure was abandoned.[208] Sclerotherapy was revived in the 1930s and 1940s with the introduction of sodium morrhuate and sodium tetradecyl sulfate. At that time Biegelstein developed a method of microinjection of venules and telangiectases with 32- to 33-gauge handmade needles.[209] However, reports of anaphylactic reactions and fatalities still appeared.[208] The modern era of sclerotherapy in the United States arrived in the 1970s with reports on the safe and effective sclerotherapy of telangiectases and venules with hypertonic saline.[210]

Sclerosing Solutions

This discussion will be limited to the sclerotherapy of telangiectases and venules. For the sclerotherapy of varicose veins, the interested reader is referred to several excellent review articles.[211] Sclerosing solutions used in the United States act in one of two main ways. One depends on dehydration of endothelial cells by osmotic action with resultant injury, inflammation, and thrombus formation. The other depends on endothelial cell surface tension alteration with direct damage of the endothelial cell and resulting inflammation and thrombus formation. The only sclerosing solutions approved by the FDA for sclerotherapy are sodium morrhuate derived from cod liver oil and Sotradecol (sodium tetradecyl sulfate).[208] Sodium morrhuate is a surface-tension-acting agent that is rarely used because of the significant risk of anaphylactic reactions.[212] Sotradecol is a surface-tension-acting agent that is often used for the treatment of varicose veins, and in a dilute form, for the treatment of telangiectases. Its main disadvantages are significant pain on injection, rare anaphylactic reactions, and risk of deep ulceration at sites of extravasation.

Hypertonic 23.4% sodium chloride solution, with or without added lidocaine (Xylocaine) and heparin, is a dehydrating sclerosing agent. It is very effective and extensively used in the United States (Fig. 238-6). However, the FDA has approved it only as an abortifacient and not as a sclerosant. It causes moderate pain on injection with occasional muscle cramps and risk of ulceration at sites of extravasation. Polidocanol (Aethoxysklerol) is a surface-tension-acting agent that is very effective and painless to inject because it is a local anesthetic. There is very low risk of ulceration even with extravasation of the solution. However, Aethoxysklerol is not approved by the FDA and there is a very rare incidence of anaphylactic reactions.[212] Sclerodex (10% sodium chloride, 25% dextrose, and 1% phenethyl alcohol) is a dehydrating agent that is very effective, but it lacks FDA approval and there is risk of ulcera-

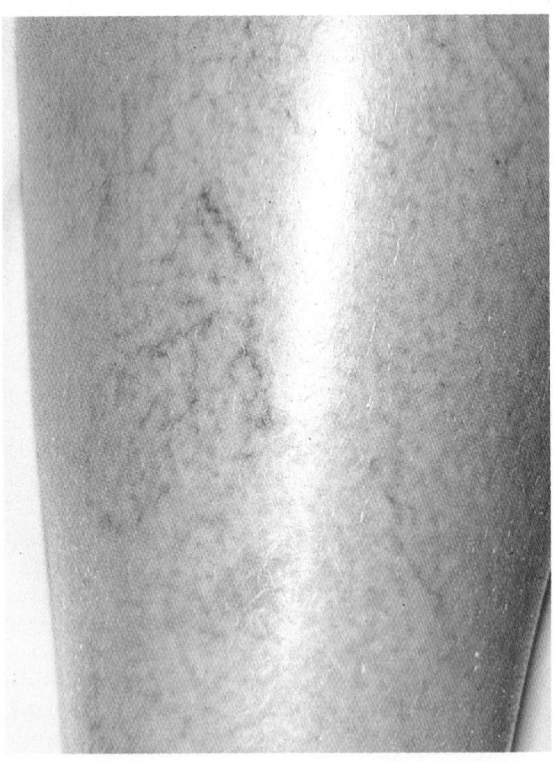

a

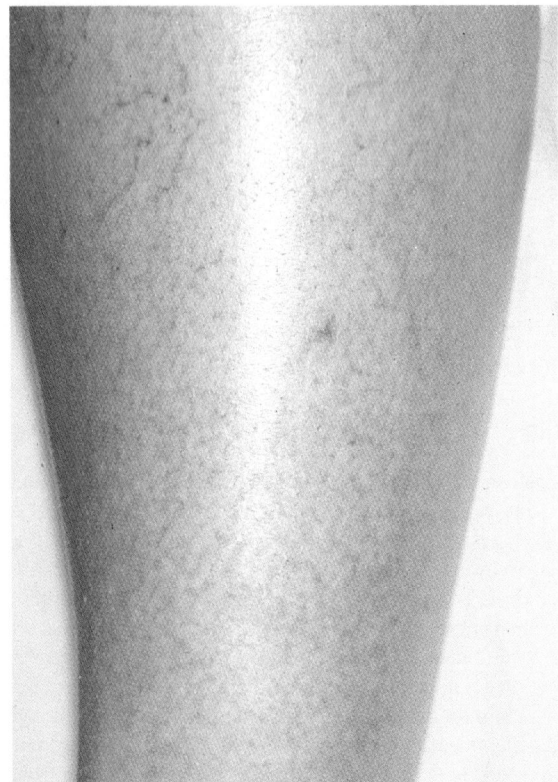

b

FIGURE 238-6 Hypertonic saline sclerotherapy of lower extremity telangiectases. (*a*) Telangiectases before sclerotherapy, and (*b*) 4 weeks after successful sclerotherapy with small resolving injection site ecchymosis.

tion at sites of extravasation.[208] The choice of sclerosing agent is usually based on physician experience. In the United States, the most popular agents are hypertonic saline and Aethoxysklerol.

Indications and Technique

Telangiectases and venules of the lower extremities from various causes can be effectively treated with sclerotherapy (Fig. 238-6). For optimal results in patients with underlying varicose veins and other venous anomalies, the underlying venous problem should be treated first with either sclerotherapy or surgery.[213] Sclerotherapy of telangiectases is generally performed for cosmetic reasons. However, some patients complain of discomfort and even pain related to their telangiectases. Successful sclerotherapy can alleviate these symptoms.[214] Postradiotherapy telangiectases can be treated with sclerotherapy.[215]

The sclerosing solution is injected into the vessel with a 30-gauge or smaller needle. The vessel is carefully cannulated under magnification and a small amount of sclerosing solution is injected until the vessel and interconnecting vessels are filled. If the material extravasates into the dermis, injection is immediately stopped, the area is massaged, and, if needed, normal saline, 1% lidocaine, or sterile water is injected into the area to dilute the sclerosant. Injecting a small amount of air before the sclerosant will help determine whether the vessel has been cannulated before injecting the sclerosing solution.[216] This step is not necessary with Aethoxysklerol because it is not significantly toxic to the dermis. Compression after sclerotherapy for varicose veins significantly improves the results.[217] However, there is controversy over whether compression after sclerotherapy of telangiectases is needed.[216,217] Fading of the treated vessels takes 3 to 4 weeks, at which time additional treatment can be performed (Fig. 238-6).

Complications

The most frequent local complication of sclerotherapy, occurring in 10 to 30 percent of cases, is linear hyperpigmentation along the course of the vessel. It is caused by hemosiderin deposition, which appears to be related to solution strength, vessel fragility, the size of the vessel treated, injection pressure, and the type of solution used. The hyperpigmentation fades in 80 percent of patients within 2 years but persists up to 5 years in the remaining 20 percent.[218] Telangiectatic matting around the area treated is seen in 5 to 35 percent of patients and represents a revascularization in the area with vessels much smaller than the original sclerosed vessel. These vessels usually resolve spontaneously or with repeated sclerotherapy, but they can rarely be permanent.[219]

Skin ulceration healing with a scar is the most feared complication, and is seen in up to 1 percent of cases.[220] However, with careful technique, avoidance of extravasation, compression of the needle entry point immediately after injection, and appropriate treatment of inadvertent extravasation, ulceration can almost always be avoided. Because Aethoxysklerol is not toxic to the dermis at concentrations of less than 1 percent, ulceration is very rare with this agent.[219]

Thrombi may be seen within 1 week of injection, especially in larger (1 to 4 mm) treated vessels. They may cause pain that can be relieved by incising the vessel and expressing the thrombus.[219] Compression may be helpful in minimizing thrombus formation.

The only systemic reactions that have been seen are allergic in nature, ranging from urticarial to anaphylactoid and anaphylactic. Sodium morrhuate and Sotradecol have a significant potential for anaphylactic reactions and fatal reactions have been reported. Aethoxysklerol has a 0.01 percent reported rate of allergic reactions, and anaphylactoid reactions are reported extremely rarely. No allergic reactions have been seen with Sclerodex or hypertonic saline.[208]

References

1. Bennett RG, Krull EA: ASDS 20th anniversary: The history of dermatologic surgery. *J Dermatol Surg Oncol* **16**:384, 1990
2. Hanke CW: The literature of dermatologic surgery 1970–present. *J Dermatol Surg Oncol* **16**:202, 1990
3. Roenigk RK, Roenigk HH Jr: *Dermatologic Surgery: Principles and Practice.* New York, Marcel Dekker, 1989
4. Kuflik EG, Gage AA: *Cryosurgical Treatment for Skin Cancer.* New York, Igaku-Shoin, 1990
5. Epstein E, Epstein E Jr: *Skin Surgery.* Philadelphia, Saunders, 1987
6. Salasche SJ et al: *Surgical Anatomy of the Skin.* Norwalk, CT, Appleton and Lange, 1988
7. Sebben JE: *Cutaneous Electrosurgery.* Chicago, Year Book, 1989
8. Swanson NA: *Atlas of Cutaneous Surgery.* Boston, Little, Brown, 1987
9. Bennett RG: *Fundamentals of Cutaneous Surgery.* St Louis, Mosby, 1988
10. Mohs FE: *Chemosurgery in Cancer, Gangrene and Infections.* Springfield, IL, Charles C Thomas, 1956
11. Mohs FE: Chemosurgery: A microscopically controlled method of cancer excision. *Arch Surg* **42**:279, 1941
12. Tromovitch TA, Stegman SJ: Microscopically controlled excision of skin tumors: Chemosurgery (Mohs), fresh tissue technique. *Arch Dermatol* **110**:23, 1974
13. Mohs FE: *Chemosurgery: Microscopically Controlled Surgery for Skin Cancer.* Springfield, IL, Charles C Thomas, 1978
14. Swanson NA: Mohs surgery: Technique, indications, applications, and the future. *Arch Dermatol* **119**:761, 1983
15. Robins P, Albom MJ: Mohs' surgery: Fresh tissue technique. *J Dermatol Surg* **1**:37, 1975
16. Robins P: Chemosurgery: My 15 years of experience. *J Dermatol Surg* **7**:779, 1981
17. Bernstein G et al: Mohs micrographic surgery. *J Dermatol Surg Oncol* **13**:13, 1987
18. Cottel WI et al: Essentials of Mohs micrographic surgery. *J Dermatol Surg Oncol* **14**:11, 1988
19. Hruza GJ: Mohs micrographic surgery. *Otolaryngol Clin North Am* **23**:845, 1989
20. Davidson TM et al: The biopsy in head and neck cancer. *Arch Otolaryngol* **11**:193, 1984
21. Rowe DE et al: Mohs surgery is the treatment of choice for recurrent (previously treated) basal cell carcinoma. *J Dermatol Surg Oncol* **15**:424, 1989
22. Menn H et al: The recurrent basal cell epithilioma. *Arch Dermatol* **103**:628, 1971
23. Wagner RF, Cottel WI: Multifocal recurrent basal cell carcinoma following primary tumor treatment by electrodesiccation and curettage. *J Am Acad Dermatol* **17**:1047, 1987
24. Smith SS, Grande DJ: Basal cell carcinoma recurring after radiotherapy: A unique, difficult treatment subclass of recurrent basal cell carcinoma. *J Dermatol Surg Oncol* **17**:26, 1991
25. Levine H, Bailin P: Basal cell carcinoma of the head and neck: Identification of the high risk patient. *Laryngoscope* **60**:955, 1980
26. Salasche SJ, Amonette RA: Morpheaform basal cell epitheliomas: A

study of subclinical extensions in a series of 51 cases. *J Dermatol Surg Oncol* **7**:387, 1981

27. Mark GJ: Basal cell carcinoma with intraneural invasion. *Cancer* **40**:2181, 1977

28. Mohs FE, Lathrop TG: Modes of spread of cancer of skin. *Arch Dermatol Syphilol* **66**:427, 1952

29. Mora CG, Robins P: Basal cell carcinomas in the center of the face: Special diagnostic, prognostic and therapeutic considerations. *J Dermatol Surg Oncol* **4**:315, 1978

30. Mohs FE, Zitelli JA: Microscopically controlled surgery in the treatment of carcinoma of the scalp. *Arch Dermatol* **117**:764, 1982

31. Wentzell JM, Robinson JK: Embryologic fusion planes and the spread of cutaneous carcinoma: A review and reassessment. *J Dermatol Surg Oncol* **16**:1000, 1990

32. Cade S: Radiation induced cancer in man. *Br J Radiol* **30**:393, 1957

33. Pascal GT et al: Prognosis of ''incompletely excised'' versus ''completely excised'' basal cell carcinoma. *Plast Reconstr Surg* **41**:328, 1968

34. Rowe DE et al: Long-term recurrence rates in previously untreated (primary) basal cell carcinoma: Implications for patient follow-up. *J Dermatol Surg Oncol* **15**:315, 1989

35. Brown RG et al: Advanced and recurrent squamous cell carcinoma of the lower lip. *Am J Surg* **132**:492, 1976

36. Dzubow LM et al: Risk factors for local recurrence of primary cutaneous squamous cell carcinomas. *Arch Dermatol* **118**:900, 1982

37. Cox FH, Becker FF: Metastatic potential of biologic variants of skin squamous cell carcinoma. *J Fla Med Assoc* **69**:516, 1982

38. Taylor HB, Helwig EB: Dermatofibrosarcoma protuberans: A study of 115 cases. *Cancer* **15**:717, 1962

39. McPeak CJ et al: Dermatofibrosarcoma protuberans: An analysis of 86 cases—five with metastasis. *Ann Surg* **166**:803, 1967

40. Robinson JK: Dermatofibrosarcoma protuberans resected by Mohs' surgery (chemosurgery). A 5-year prospective study. *J Am Acad Dermatol* **12**:1093, 1985

41. Weimar VM, Ceilley RI: Chemosurgical reports. A myxoid variant of malignant histiocytoma: Report of a case treated by Mohs' technique with a slight modification. *J Dermatol Surg Oncol* **5**:16, 1979

42. Mohs FE: Chemosurgery for melanoma. *Arch Dermatol* **113**:285, 1977

43. Coleman WP III et al: Treatment of lentigo maligna and lentigo maligna melanoma. *J Dermatol Surg Oncol* **6**:476, 1980

44. Bennett RG: Mohs' surgery. New concepts and applications. *Dermatol Clin* **5**:409, 1987

45. Majno G: *The Healing Hand.* Cambridge, MA, Harvard University Press, 1975

46. McGrath MH, Simon RH: Wound geometry and the kinetics of wound contraction. *Plast Reconstr Surg* **72**:66, 1983

47. Zitelli JA: Wound healing by secondary intention: A cosmetic appraisal. *J Am Acad Dermatol* **9**:407, 1983

48. Reed BR, Clark RA: Cutaneous tissue repair: Practical implications of current knowledge II. *J Am Acad Dermatol* **13**:919, 1985

49. Stegman SJ et al: *Basics of Dermatologic Surgery.* Chicago, Year Book Medical Publishers, 1982

50. Tromovitch TA et al: *Flaps and Grafts in Dermatologic Surgery.* Chicago, Year Book, 1989

51. Stroud MB: Design of skin flaps with a new technique using templates. *J Dermatol Surg Oncol* **13**:1171, 1987

52. Dzubow LM: Flap dynamics. *J Dermatol Surg Oncol* **17**:116, 1991

53. Wee SS et al: The frontonasal flap: Utility for distal nasal defects and technical refinements. *Br J Plast Surg* **44**:201, 1991

54. Borges AF: Choosing the correct Limberg flap. *Plast Reconstr Surg* **62**:542, 1978

55. Dzubow LM: Subcutaneous island pedicle flaps. *J Dermatol Surg Oncol* **12**:591, 1986

56. Wee SS et al: Refinements of nasalis myocutaneous flap. *Ann Plast Surg* **25**:271, 1990

57. McGregor IA: Local flaps in facial reconstruction. *Otolaryngol Clin North Am* **15**:77, 1982

58. Salasche SJ, Grabski WJ: Complications of flaps. *J Dermatol Surg Oncol* **17**:132, 1991

59. Koranda FC, Webster RC: Trapdoor effect in nasolabial flaps. *Arch Otolaryngol* **111**:421, 1985

60. Zitelli JA: The nasolabial flap as a single-stage procedure. *Arch Dermatol* **126**:1445, 1990

61. Wheeland RG: Skin grafts, in *Dermatologic Surgery: Principles and Practice,* edited by RK Roenigk, HH Roenigk, Jr. New York, Marcel Dekker, 1989, p 323

62. Davison PM et al: The properties and uses of nonexpanded machine-meshed skin grafts. *Br J Plast Surg* **39**:462, 1986

63. Berretty PJ et al: Treatment of ulcers on legs from venous hypertension by split-thickness skin grafts. *J Dermatol Surg Oncol* **5**:966, 1979

64. Katz BF, Oca MAGS: A controlled study of the effectiveness of spot dermabrasion ('scarabrasion') on the appearance of surgical scars. *J Am Acad Dermatol* **24**:462, 1991

65. Green H et al: Growth of cultured human epidermal cells into multiple epithelia suitable for grafting. *Proc Natl Acad Sci USA* **76**:5665, 1979

66. O'Connor NE et al: Grafting of burns with cultured epithelium prepared from autologous epidermal cells. *Lancet* **1**:75, 1981

67. Gallico GG et al: Permanent coverage of large burn wounds with autologous cultured human epithelium. *N Engl J Med* **311**:448, 1984

68. Hefton JM et al: Grafting of skin ulcers with cultured autologous epidermal cells. *J Am Acad Dermatol* **14**:399, 1986

69. Phillips T et al: Treatment of skin ulcers with cultured epidermal allografts. *J Am Acad Dermatol* **21**:191, 1989

70. Eaglestein WH, Mertz PM: New method for assessing epidermal wound healing: The effects of triamcinolone acetonide and polyethylene film occlusion. *J Invest Dermatol* **71**:382, 1978

71. Eaglestein WH: Experience with biosynthetic dressings. *J Am Acad Dermatol* **12**:434, 1985

72. Mertz PM, Eaglestein WH: The effects of a semiocclusive dressing on the microbial population in superficial wounds. *Arch Surg* **119**:287, 1984

73. Barnett A et al: Comparison of synthetic adhesive moisture vapor permeable and fine mesh gauze dressings for split-thickness skin graft donor sites. *Am J Surg* **145**:379, 1983

74. Alper JC et al: Use of the vapor permeable membrane for cutaneous ulcers: Details of application and side effects. *J Am Acad Dermatol* **11**:858, 1984

75. Falanga V: Occlusive wound dressings. Why, when, which? *Arch Dermatol* **124**:872, 1988

76. Mandy SH: A new primary wound dressing made of polyethylene oxide gel. *J Dermatol Surg Oncol* **9**:153, 1983

77. Alvarez OM et al: The effect of occlusive dressings on collagen synthesis and re-epithelialization in superficial wounds. *J Surg Res* **35**:142, 1983

78. Scher RK, Daniel CR: *Nails: Therapy, Diagnosis, Surgery.* Philadelphia, Saunders, 1990

79. Bennett RG: Technique of biopsy of nails. *J Dermatol Surg* **2**:325, 1976

80. Zaias N: The longitudinal nail biopsy. *J Invest Dermatol* **49**:406, 1967

81. Albom MJ: Avulsion of a nail plate. *J Dermatol Surg Oncol* **3**:34, 1977

82. Dawber R: Fingernail growth in normal and psoriatic subjects. *Br J Dermatol* **82**:454, 1970

83. Siegle RJ et al: The phenol alcohol technique for permanent matricectomy. *Arch Dermatol* **120**:348, 1984

84. Scher RK: Longitudinal resection of nails for purposes of biopsy and treatment. *J Dermatol Surg Oncol* **6**:805, 1980

85. Kromayer E: Die Heilung der Akne durch in Neves narbenlases Operations verfahren. Das Stanzen. *Illustr Monatsschr Aerztl Polytech* **27**:101, 1905

86. Kurtin A: Surgical planing of the skin. *Arch Dermatol Syphilol* **68**:389, 1953

87. Roenigk HH Jr: Dermabrasion, in *Dermatologic Surgery Principles and Practice,* edited by RK Roenigk, HH Roenigk, Jr. New York, Marcel Dekker, 1989, p 959

88. Stegman SJ et al: *Cosmetic Dermatologic Surgery.* Chicago, Year Book, 1990

89. Orentreich D, Orentreich N: Acne scar revision update. *Dermatol Clin* 5:359, 1987

90. Eiseman G: Reconstruction of the acne-scarred face. *J Dermatol Surg Oncol* 3:332, 1977

91. Roenigk HH Jr: Dermabrasion for miscellaneous cutaneous lesions (exclusive of scarring from acne). *J Dermatol Surg Oncol* 3:322, 1977

92. Wentzell JM, Robinson JK: Physical properties of aerosols produced by dermabrasion. *J Dermatol Surg Oncol* 15:233, 1989

93. Hanke CW, O'Brian JJ: A histologic evaluation of the effects of skin refrigerant in an animal model. *J Dermatol Surg Oncol* 13:664, 1987

94. Hanke CW et al: Complications of dermabrasion resulting from excessively cold skin refrigeration. *J Dermatol Surg Oncol* 11:896, 1985

95. Pinski JB: Dressings for dermabrasion: Occlusive dressings and wound healing. *Cutis* 37:471, 1986

96. Roenigk HH Jr: Dermabrasion: State of the art. *J Dermatol Surg Oncol* 11:306, 1985

97. Rubenstein R et al: Atypical keloids after dermabrasion of patients taking isotretinoin. *J Am Acad Dermatol* 15:280, 1986

98. MacKee GM, Karp FL: The treatment of postacne scars with phenol. *Br J Dermatol* 64:456, 1952

99. Urkov JC: Surface defects of skin: Treatment by controlled exfoliation. *Ill Med J* 89:75, 1946

100. Baker TJ: Chemical face peeling and rhytidectomy. *Plast Reconstr Surg* 29:199, 1962

101. Litton C: Chemical face peeling. *Plast Reconstr Surg* 29:371, 1962

102. Ayres S III: Dermal changes following application of chemical cauterants to aging skin. *Arch Dermatol* 82:578, 1960

103. Stagnone JJ: Superficial peeling. *J Dermatol Surg Oncol* 15:924, 1989

104. Van Scott EJ: Hyperkeratinization, corneocyte cohesion and alpha-hydroxy acids. *J Am Acad Dermatol* 11:867, 1984

105. Weiss J et al: Topical tretinoin improves photoaged akin: A double-blind, vehicle controlled study. *JAMA* 259:527, 1988

106. Brody HJ: Variations and comparisons in medium-depth chemical peeling. *J Dermatol Surg Oncol* 15:953, 1989

107. Stegman SJ: A comparative histologic study of the effects of three peeling agents and dermabrasion on normal and sundamaged skin. *Aesthetic Plast Surg* 6:123, 1982

108. Botta SA et al: Cardiac arrhythmias in phenol face peeling: A suggested protocol for prevention. *Aesthetic Plast Surg* 12:115, 1988

109. Alt TH: Occluded Baker-Gordon chemical peel: Review and update. *J Dermatol Surg Oncol* 15:980, 1989

110. Asken S: Unoccluded Baker-Gordon phenol peels—review and update. *J Dermatol Surg Oncol* 15:998, 1989

111. Gross BG: Cardiac arrhythmias during phenol face peeling. *Plast Reconstr Surg* 73:590, 1984

112. Brody HJ: Complications of chemical peeling. *J Dermatol Surg Oncol* 15:1010, 1989

113. Okuda S: Clinical and experimental studies of transplantation of living hairs (transl). *Jpn J Dermatol Urol* 40:537, 1939

114. Tamura H: Pubic hair transplantation (transl). *Jpn J Dermatol* 53:76, 1943

115. Fujita K: Reconstruction of eyebrow (transl). *La Lepro* 22:364, 1953

116. Orentreich N: Autografts in alopecias and other selected dermatological conditions. *Ann NY Acad Sci* 83:463, 1959

117. Blanchard G, Blanchard B: Obliteration of alopecia by hair-lifting: A new concept and technique. *J Natl Med Assoc* 69:639, 1977

118. Unger MG, Unger WP: Management of alopecia of the scalp by a combination of excisions and transplantations. *J Dermatol Surg Oncol* 4:670, 1978

119. Bertolino AP: Hair transplantation between identical twins. *J Am Acad Dermatol* 19:418, 1988

120. Lepaw MI: Therapy and histopathology of complications from synthetic fiber implants for hair replacement. A presentation of one hundred cases. *J Am Acad Dermatol* 3:195, 1980

121. Unger WP, Marritt E: General principles of recipient site organization and planning, in *Hair Transplantation,* edited by WP Unger, RAE Nordstrom. New York, Marcel Dekker, 1988, p 105

122. Alt TH: Evaluation of donor harvesting techniques in hair transplantation. *J Dermatol Surg Oncol* 10:799, 1984

123. Nusbaum BP, Lewis LA: Hair transplantation: Using a power punch in the recipient area. *J Dermatol Surg Oncol* 13:1073, 1987

124. Goldman PM: Punch grafting the crown and vertex. *J Dermatol Surg Oncol* 11:138, 1985

125. Coiffman F: Use of square scalp grafts for male pattern baldness. *Plast Reconstr Surg* 60:228, 1977

126. Morrison I: Tissue adhesives in hair transplant surgery. *Plast Reconstr Surg* 68:491, 1981

127. Orentreich N, Orentreich DS: "Cross-stitch" suture technique for hair transplantation. *J Dermatol Surg Oncol* 10:970, 1984

128. Bouhanna P: Topical minoxidil used before and after hair transplantation. *J Dermatol Surg Oncol* 15:50, 1989

129. Unger WP: Timing of sessions in hair transplantation. *Cutis* 22:214, 1978

130. Lucas MW: The use of minigrafts in hair transplantation surgery. *J Dermatol Surg Oncol* 14:1389, 1988

131. Pouteaux P: The use of small punches in hair-transplant surgery. *J Dermatol Surg Oncol* 6:1020, 1980

132. Brandy DA: Conventional grafting combined with minigrafting: A new approach. *J Dermatol Surg Oncol* 13:60, 1987

133. Marritt E: Single-hair transplantation for hairline refinement: A practical solution. *J Dermatol Surg Oncol* 10:962, 1984

134. Stough DB IV et al: Incisional slit grafting. *J Dermatol Surg Oncol* 17:53, 1991

135. Unger WP: Hair transplantation in females, in *Hair Transplantation,* edited by WP Unger, RAE Nordstrom. New York, Marcel Dekker, 1988, p 295

136. Nordstrom RE: Hair transplantation. The use of hairbearing compound grafts for correction of alopecia due to chronic discoid lupus erythematosus, traumatic alopecia, and male pattern baldness. *Scand J Plast Reconstr Surg* 14 (suppl):1, 1976

137. Stough DB III et al: Surgical improvement of cicatricial alopecia of diverse etiology. *Arch Dermatol* 97:331, 1968

138. Marritt E: Transplantation of single hairs from the scalp as eyelashes. Review of the literature and a case report. *J Dermatol Surg Oncol* 6:271, 1980

139. Tromovitch TA et al: Sequelae and complications of hair transplantation, in *Hair Transplantation,* edited by WP Unger, REA Nordstrom. New York, Marcel Dekker, 1988, p 399

140. Altchek DD, Pearlstein HH: Granulomatous reaction to autologous hairs incarcerated during hair transplantation. *J Dermatol Surg Oncol* 4:928, 1978

141. Sarnoff DS et al: Multiple pyogenic granuloma-like lesions following hair transplantation. *J Dermatol Surg Oncol* 11:32, 1985

142. Jones JW et al: Osteomyelitis of the skull following scalp reduction and hair plug transplantation. *Ann Plast Surg* 5:480, 1980

143. Semashko DC et al: Arteriovenous fistula following punch-graft hair transplantation. *J Dermatol Surg Oncol* 15:754, 1989

144. Nordstrom REA, Totterman SMS: Iatrogenic false aneurysms following punch hair grafting. *Plast Reconstr Surg* 64:563, 1979

145. Nordstrom RE: "Stretch-back" in scalp reductions for male pattern baldness. *Plast Reconstr Surg* 73:422, 1984

146. Norwood OT et al: Complications of scalp reductions. *J Dermatol Surg Oncol* 9:828, 1983

147. Unger MG: The Y-shaped pattern of alopecia reduction and its variations. *J Dermatol Surg Oncol* 10:980, 1984

148. Hitzig GS, Sadick NS: A new technique for curvilinear scalp reduction. *J Dermatol Surg Oncol* 15:1108, 1989

149. Unger WP: Concomitant mini reductions in punch hair transplant-

ing. *J Dermatol Surg Oncol* **9**:388, 1983

150. Brandy DA: The bilateral occipito-parietal flap. *J Dermatol Surg Oncol* **12**:1062, 1986

151. Unger MG: Postoperative necrosis following bilateral lateral scalp reduction. *J Dermatol Surg Oncol* **14**:541, 1988

152. Unger MG: The modified major scalp reduction. *J Dermatol Surg Oncol* **14**:80, 1988

153. Adson MH et al: Scalp expansion in the treatment of male pattern baldness. *Plast Reconstr Surg* **79**:906, 1987

154. Meirson D et al: Presuturing in alopecia reductions. *J Dermatol Surg Oncol* **16**:818, 1990

155. Roenigk RK, Wheeland RG: Tissue expansion in cicatricial alopecia. *Arch Dermatol* **123**:641, 1987

156. Juri J, Juri C: Two new methods for treating baldness: Temporo-parieto-occipito-parietal pedicled flap and temporo-parieto-occipital free flap. *Ann Plast Surg* **6**:38, 1981

157. Rabineau P: Complications of flaps in the treatment of baldness, in *Hair Transplantation,* edited by WP Unger, REA Nordstrom. New York, Marcel Dekker, 1988, p 657

158. Elliott RA Jr: Lateral scalp flaps for instant results in male pattern baldness. *Plast Reconstr Surg* **60**:699, 1977

159. Fleming RW, Mayer TG: Short vs long scalp flaps in the treatment of male pattern baldness. *Arch Otolaryngol* **107**:403, 1981

160. Juri J et al: Use of rotation scalp flaps for treatment of occipital baldness. *Plast Reconstr Surg* **61**:23, 1978

161. Stough DB, Stough DB: Triple rhomboid flap for crown alopecia correction. *J Dermatol Surg Oncol* **16**:543, 1990

162. Ohmori K: Free scalp flap. *Plast Reconstr Surg* **65**:42, 1980

163. McPherson JM et al: Development and biochemical characterization of injectable collagen. *J Dermatol Surg Oncol* **14** (suppl 1):13, 1988

164. Pollack SV: Silicone, Fibrel and collagen implantation for facial lines and wrinkles. *J Dermatol Surg Oncol* **16**:957, 1990

165. Kligman AM, Armstrong RC: Histologic response to intradermal Zyderm and Zyplast (glutaraldehyde cross-linked) collagen in humans. *J Dermatol Surg Oncol* **12**:351, 1986

166. Delustro F et al: Immunology of injectable collagen in human subjects. *J Dermatol Surg Oncol* **14** (suppl 1):49, 1988

167. Cooperman L, Michaeli D: The immunogenicity of injectable collagen. II. A retrospective review of seventy-two tested and treated patients. *J Am Acad Dermatol* **10**:647, 1984

168. Klein AW: In favor of double testing (editorial). *J Dermatol Surg Oncol* **15**:263, 1989

169. Klein AW: Indications and implantation techniques for the various formulations of injectable collagen. *J Dermatol Surg Oncol* **14** (suppl 1):27, 1988

170. Chernosky ME: Collagen implant in management of perlèche (angular cheilosis). *J Am Acad Dermatol* **12**:493, 1985

171. Croften BE et al: Report on the clinical evaluation of glutaraldehyde cross-linked collagen (Keragen) implant treatment of heloma. Durum and heloma molle. *J Foot Surg* **25**:427, 1985

172. Bailin MD, Bailin PL: Correction of surgical scars, acne scars and rhytids with Zyderm and Zyplast implants. *J Dermatol Surg Oncol* **14** (suppl 1):31, 1988

173. Stegman SJ et al: Adverse reactions to bovine collagen implant: Clinical and histologic features. *J Dermatol Surg Oncol* **14** (suppl 1): 39, 1988

174. Barr RJ et al: Necrobiotic granulomas associated with bovine collagen test site injections. *J Am Acad Dermatol* **6**:867, 1982

175. Delustro F et al: Immunity to injectable collagen and autoimmune disease: A summary of current understanding. *J Dermatol Surg Oncol* **14** (suppl 1):57, 1988

176. Bailey OT, Ingraham FD: Chemical, clinical and immunological studies on the products of human plasma fractionation. XXI. The use of fibrin foam as a hemostatic agent in neurosurgery. *J Clin Invest* **23**:591, 1944

177. Spangler AS: Treatment of depressed scars with fibrin foam: Seventeen years of experience. *J Dermatol Surg Oncol* **1**:65, 1975

178. Millikan L et al: Treatment of depressed cutaneous scars with gelatin matrix implant: A multicenter study. *J Am Acad Dermatol* **16**:1155, 1987

179. Millikan L et al: A 5-year safety and efficacy evaluation with Fibrel in the correction of cutaneous scars following one or two treatments. *J Dermatol Surg Oncol* **17**:223, 1991

180. Rosen T, Watkins HC: Use of gelatin matrix implant in patients hypersensitive to bovine collagen. *J Am Acad Dermatol* **23**:848, 1990

181. Duffy DM: Silicone: A critical review. *Adv Dermatol* **5**:93, 1990

182. Selmanowitz VJ, Orentreich N: Medical-grade fluid silicone: A monographic review. *J Dermatol Surg Oncol* **3**:597, 1977

183. Balkin SW: Treatment of painful scars on soles and digits with injections of fluid silicone. *J Dermatol Surg Oncol* **3**:612, 1977

184. Orentreich DS, Orentreich N: Injectable fluid silicone, in *Dermatologic Surgery: Principles and Practice,* edited by RK Roenigk, HH Roenigk, Jr. New York, Marcel Dekker, 1989, p 1349

185. Mason J, Apisarnthanarax P: Migratory silicone granuloma. *Arch Dermatol* **117**:366, 1981

186. Webster RC et al: Rhinoplastic revisions with injectable silicone. *Arch Otolaryngol Head Neck Surg* **112**:269, 1986

187. Varga J et al: Systemic sclerosis after augmentation mammoplasty with silicone implants. *Ann Intern Med* **111**:377, 1989

188. Neuber F: Fat transplantation (transl). *Chir Kongr Verhandl Dsch Gesellsch Chir* **22**:66, 1893

189. Glogau RG: Microlipoinjection. *Arch Dermatol* **124**:1340, 1988

190. Asken S: *Liposuction Surgery and Autologous Fat Transplantation.* Norwalk, CT, Appleton and Lange, 1988

191. Fournier PF: Facial recontouring with fat grafting. *Dermatol Clin* **8**:523, 1990

192. Fischer A, Fischer G: Revised techniques for cellulitis fat reduction in riding breeches deformity. *Bull Int Acad Cosmet Surg* **2**:40, 1977

193. Schrudde J: Lipexeresis as a new type of aesthetic plastic surgery. *Aesthetic Plast Surg* **4**:215, 1980

194. Kesserling V, Meyer R: A suction curette for removal of excessive local deposits of subcutaneous fat. *Plast Reconstr Surg* **62**:305, 1978

195. Fischer G: Liposculpture: The "correct" history of liposuction. Part I. *J Dermatol Surg Oncol* **16**:1087, 1990

196. Illouz YG: A new technique for localized lipodystrophies (transl). *Rev Chir Esth Langue Fr* **6**:3, 1980

197. Vogt T, Belluscio D: Controversies in plastic surgery: Suction-assisted lipectomy (SAL) and the HCG (human chorionic gonadotropin) protocol for obesity treatment. *Aesthetic Plast Surg* **11**:131, 1987

198. Matarasso SL: A regional approach to patient selection and evaluation for liposuction. *Dermatol Clin* **8**:401, 1990

199. Chrisman BB: Liposuction with facelift surgery. *Dermatol Clin* **8**:501, 1990

200. Coleman WP III: Noncosmetic applications of liposuction. *J Dermatol Surg Oncol* **14**:1085, 1988

201. Klein JA: Tumescent technique for regional anesthesia permits lidocaine doses of 35 mg/kg for liposuction. *J Dermatol Surg Oncol* **16**:248, 1990

202. Collins PS: The methodology of liposuction surgery. *Dermatol Clin* **8**:395, 1990

203. Fournier PF: Reduction syringe liposculpturing. *Dermatol Clin* **8**:539, 1990

204. Chrisman BB, Coleman WP III: Determining safe limits for untransfused, outpatient liposuction: Personal experience and review of the literature. *J Dermatol Surg Oncol* **14**:1095, 1988

205. Clayton DN et al: Large volume lipoplasty. *Clin Plast Surg* **16**:305, 1989

206. Bernstein G, Hanke CW: Safety of liposuction: A review of 9478 cases performed by dermatologists. *J Dermatol Surg Oncol* **14**:1112, 1988

207. Teimourian B, Rogers WB III: A national survey of complications associated with suction lipectomy: A comparative study. *Plast Reconstr Surg* **84**:628, 1989

208. Goldman PM: Sclerotherapy for superficial venules and telangiecta-

sias of the lower extremities. *Dermatol Clin* **5**:369, 1987

209. Biegelstein HI: Telangiectasia associated with varicose veins: Treatment by micro-injection technique. *JAMA* **102**:2092, 1934

210. Alderman DB: Therapy for essential cutaneous telangiectasias. *Postgrad Med* **61**:91, 1977

211. De Groot WP: Treatment of varicose veins: Modern concepts and methods. *J Dermatol Surg Oncol* **15**:191, 1989

212. Goldman MP, Bennett RG: Treatment of telangiectasias: A review. *J Am Acad Dermatol* **17**:167, 1987

213. Tretbar LL: Injection sclerotherapy for spider telangiectasias: A 20-year experience with sodium tetradecyl sulfate. *J Dermatol Surg Oncol* **15**:223, 1989

214. Weiss RA, Weiss MA: Resolution of pain associated with varicose and telangiectatic leg veins after compression sclerotherapy. *J Dermatol Surg Oncol* **16**:333, 1990

215. Gordon AB et al: Treatment of post-radiotherapy telangiectasia by injection sclerotherapy. *Clin Radiol* **38**:25, 1987

216. Bodian EL: Techniques of sclerotherapy for sunburst venous blemishes. *J Dermatol Surg Oncol* **11**:696, 1985

217. Goldman MP: Compression in the treatment of leg telangiectasia: Theoretical considerations. *J Dermatol Surg Oncol* **15**:184, 1989

218. Weiss RA, Weiss MA: Incidence of side effects in the treatment of telangiectasias by compression sclerotherapy: Hypertonic saline vs. polidocanol. *J Dermatol Surg Oncol* **16**:800, 1990

219. Goldman PM: Polidocanol (Aethoxysklerol) for sclerotherapy of superficial venules and telangiectasias. *J Dermatol Surg Oncol* **15**:204, 1989

220. Puissegur Lupo ML: Sclerotherapy: Review of results and complications in 200 patients. *J Dermatol Surg Oncol* **15**:214, 1989

PART SEVEN

Pediatric and Geriatric Dermatology

Pediatric and Geriatric Dermatology

CHAPTER 239

William L. Weston and Alfred T. Lane

The newborn period is defined as the first 30 days of life. During this period skin conditions appear abruptly and frequently frighten parents and health care givers. Neonatal skin diseases evolve much more rapidly than adult skin diseases, and some conditions that initially appear to be serious turn out to be trivial, whereas in other cases the opposite is true.[1] A thorough knowledge of the fetal skin biology and of the cutaneous lesions of newborns is expected of those providing neonatal care.

This chapter is divided into five sections: newborn skin care, transient skin disease in the newborn, birthmarks, common congenital malformations, and hereditary skin conditions with dramatic newborn presentations. Many of the disorders of the newborn are considered by their clinical features, epidemiology, etiology and pathogenesis, clinical manifestations, pathology, diagnosis, course, and prognosis only, since no treatment is required of many self-limited problems. Many of the conditions are described in detail in other portions of this textbook, and only the aspects in newborns will be considered in this chapter.

Newborn Skin Care

The full-term newborn infant's skin feels very soft and smooth. The smooth texture and softness is related to the hydration of the epidermis and the condition of the collagen and dermal matrix substances.[2] At birth the full-term infant's skin is functionally mature. The barrier portion of the epidermis, the stratum corneum, is intact and effectively protects the infant.[2–4]

Even though the infant's barrier function may be normal at birth, the infant is at increased risk for systemic toxicity of topically applied compounds.[5] The infant's surface area is great when compared with body mass. The infant's metabolism, excretion, distribution, and protein binding may be different from those of an adult.[5] The premature infant is at much greater risk than the mature newborn. The premature infant has markedly decreased epidermal barrier function and an even greater body surface area to body volume ratio.[6,7] In addition the immature organs of the premature infant may greatly change the metabolism, excretion, distribution, and protein binding of chemical agents.[5] Soaps, lotions, or other cleansing solutions can cause local or systemic toxicity in the premature infant.[5,6]

Neonatal Dermatology

The skin of the mature infant often appears dry and cracked soon after birth.[6] The stratum corneum that has accumulated in utero has not yet shed. On the ankles and wrists, fissures and bleeding may occur. During this time topical care should include moisturizing lotions or creams. The goal of therapy is to retain the soft, flexible texture of the infant's skin by hydrating and lubricating the epidermis. For infants in a dry environment, moisturizers may need to be used indefinitely. Infants in a more humid environment may need moisturizers only intermittently.

The skin care of the premature infant is much more difficult and complex that that of the full-term infant.[6,7] Not only is the barrier portion of the epidermis absent or defective, but the skin has markedly increased fragility. Because of epidermal and dermal injury, the infant may have significant cutaneous pain which is accentuated by routine handling. The infant is at risk for sepsis from skin-associated organisms. Sweating in the premature infant is functionally reduced and contributes to poor thermal regulation.[8] Heat regulation is also dysfunctional because of lack of a subcutaneous fat layer for insulation and poor autonomic control of cutaneous vessels.[9] Maintaining a humid environment decreases the infant's transepidermal water loss and assists in skin hydration. Humidity can be maintained by using a humidity-controlled isolette or by placing infants under thin plastic tents beneath infrared warmers.

Dry, flaking, fissured skin of premature infants should be treated with moisturizing creams or ointments. Petrolatum-based ointments with little or no preservatives appear to offer the greatest benefit of the lowest risk.[6,7] Ointments placed on an infant's skin under an infrared warmer will not cause cutaneous burns. Semipermeable wound dressings may offer additional cutaneous pain relief and protection, but additional studies must be done to analyze the potential for the associated risk of bacterial growth under the dressings.[7]

Transient Skin Diseases

Skin diseases encountered in newborns that begin to resolve or are completely resolved by 30 days of age are considered transient skin disease. Transient skin diseases are very common and almost expected in newborns.

Milia

Milia are multiple pinpoint papules seen over the forehead, cheeks, and nose of infants. They may be present in the oral cavity as well, where they are called *Epstein's pearls*.[10]

Milia are expected findings in the newborn. Up to 40 percent of newborns have milia on the skin and 64 percent have them on the palate.[1]

Etiology and Pathogenesis   Milia are caused by cystic retention of keratin within the superficial dermis. Trauma to the skin surface experienced during delivery may contribute.

Clinical Manifestations   Milia are 1- to 2-mm whitish, spherical papules within the outer layer of skin. They are seen prominently on the face and nose and on the cheeks as well. Usually, dozens are present. They are found also upon oral examination as 1- to 2-mm white papules on the gingiva and palate.

Pathology   On histologic examination milia appear as superficial epithelial cysts in the upper dermis, just beneath the epidermis. The cyst cavity is filled with keratin.

Diagnosis and Differential Diagnosis   Molluscum contagiosum, an acquired viral infection, may mimic milia but does not appear in the immediate neonatal period. Sebaceous gland hyperplasia also occur over the nose and cheeks of infants, but it is yellow rather than whitish.

Course and Prognosis   The cystic spheres rupture onto the skin surface and exfoliate their contents within a few weeks of birth.[1]

Sebaceous Gland Hyperplasia

Sebaceous gland hyperplasia is caused by overgrowth of sebaceous glands in skin areas where sebaceous glands are abundant. At least 50 percent of normal newborns have sebaceous gland hyperplasia. Premature infants often do not.

Etiology and Pathogenesis   Maternal androgens stimulate the overgrowth of sebaceous glands. The stimulation occurs during the last month of pregnancy, and both the number of sebaceous cells and the cell volume increases.[2]

Clinical Manifestations   Tiny (1-mm) yellow macules or papules are seen at the opening of each pilosebaceous follicle over the nose and cheeks of newborns.[1]

Pathology   Large sebaceous glands with prominent secretory cells surround the pilosebaceous follicle.

Diagnosis and Differential Diagnosis   Milia may mimic sebaceous hyperplasia but are white and cystic in appearance.

Course and Prognosis   They recede completely by 4 to 6 months of age.

Erythema Toxicum

Erythema toxicum is a transient, blotchy erythema seen in newborns. This erythema occurs in about 50 percent of term infants and less commonly in premature infants.[11]

FIGURE 239-1   Erythema toxicum. Blotchy erythematous macules with tiny central vesicles in a newborn.

Etiology and Pathogenesis   The cause of erythema toxicum is unknown.

Clinical Manifestations   Blotchy erythematous macules 2 to 3 cm in diameter, with a tiny 1- to 4-mm central vesicle or pustule, are seen in infants with erythema toxicum (Fig. 239-1). They usually begin at 24 to 48 h of age.[11] Lesions are seen on the chest, back, face, and proximal extremities, sparing the palms and soles.

Pathology   An intraepidermal vesicle is seen, filled with eosinophils.

Diagnosis and Differential Diagnosis   A smear of the central vesicle or pustule contents reveals numerous eosinophils on Wright's-stained preparations. Peripheral blood eosinophilia of up to 20 percent may accompany the accumulation of tissue eosinophils, particularly in infants with numerous lesions. Transient neonatal pustular melanosis mimics erythema toxicum, except that neutrophils rather than eosinophils are found within the pinpoint vesicles and individual lesions heal with residual pigmentation, not seen in erythema toxicum. Bacterial infections and congenital candidiasis may also mimic erythema toxicum. Bacterial and fungal culture of lesions and Gram's stain help differentiate these infections from erythema toxicum.

Course and Prognosis   The individual lesions clear in 4 to 5 days and new lesions may occur from birth to the tenth day of life. By 2 weeks of age, all lesions are resolved.

Transient Neonatal Pustular Melanosis

This blotchy erythema of the newborn heals with residual pigmentation. Transient neonatal pustular melanosis is less common than erythema toxicum and more prevalent among black newborns.

Etiology and Pathogenesis   Erythema toxicum is believed to be associated with obstruction of the pilosebaceous orifice. The cause of the condition is unknown.

Clinical Manifestations   These lesions are present at birth as vesicles, pustules, or ruptured vesicles or pustules with a collarette of surrounding scale (Fig. 239-2). Pigmented macules are also often present at birth or they develop at the sites of resolving pustules or vesicles.[12] Most lesions occur on the trunk and proximal extremities, but the palms and soles may be involved.[12]

Pathology   An intraepidermal vesicle filled with neutrophils is found.

Diagnosis and Differential Diagnosis   A smear of the vesicle or pustule contents reveals numerous neutrophils and an occasional eosinophil on Wright's-stained preparations.

Miliaria rubra is frequently confused with erythema toxicum and transient neonatal pustular melanosis. The erythema around miliaria rubra is small in area (1 to 2 mm versus 20 to 30 mm in erythema toxicum). The central vesicle or pustule may mimic the lesions of herpes simplex or bacterial folliculitis. A Gram's stain of the pustules of erythema toxicum or transient neonatal pustular melanosis will be negative. The Wright's-stained slide from a pustule of erythema toxicum shows a predominance of eosinophils, while the slide of a pustule of transient neonatal pustular melanosis usually shows a predominance of neutrophils.

Course and Prognosis   The vesicles and pustules usually disappear by 5 days of age and the pigmented macules resolve over 3 weeks to 3 months.

Mottling

Mottling is a blotchy duskiness of skin that is responsive to temperature. Virtually all babies demonstrate mottling at some time during the newborn period.

Etiology and Pathogenesis   Constriction of the deeper plexus and opening of the superficial plexus due to immaturity of the autonomic control of the skin vascular plexus is thought to be responsible for mottling.[9]

Clinical Manifestations   A lacelike pattern of dusky erythema appears over the extremities and trunk of neonates when exposed to a decrease in temperature.[1,9] This phenomenon may be sensitive to small increments of temperature change.

Diagnosis and Differential Diagnosis   The mottling disappears on rewarming.[9] Mottling that persists beyond 6 months of life may be a sign of hypothyroidism or cutis marmorata telangiectatica congenita, which can be associated with musculoskeletal or vascular abnormalities. Such mottling will not disappear with rewarming. Similarly, the livedo reticularis seen with collagen vascular disease such as neonatal lupus erythematosus will persist when the skin is warmed.

Course and Prognosis   The tendency to mottling upon exposure to cold gradually diminishes and is no longer present after 6 months of age.

Harlequin Color Change

This distinct color change of one-half of the body results from positioning. Harlequin color change is unusual in newborns and is usually seen in infants of low birth weight.

Etiology and Pathogenesis   The exact mechanism of this unusual phenomenon is not known, but immaturity of autonomic vasomotor control is thought to be responsible.

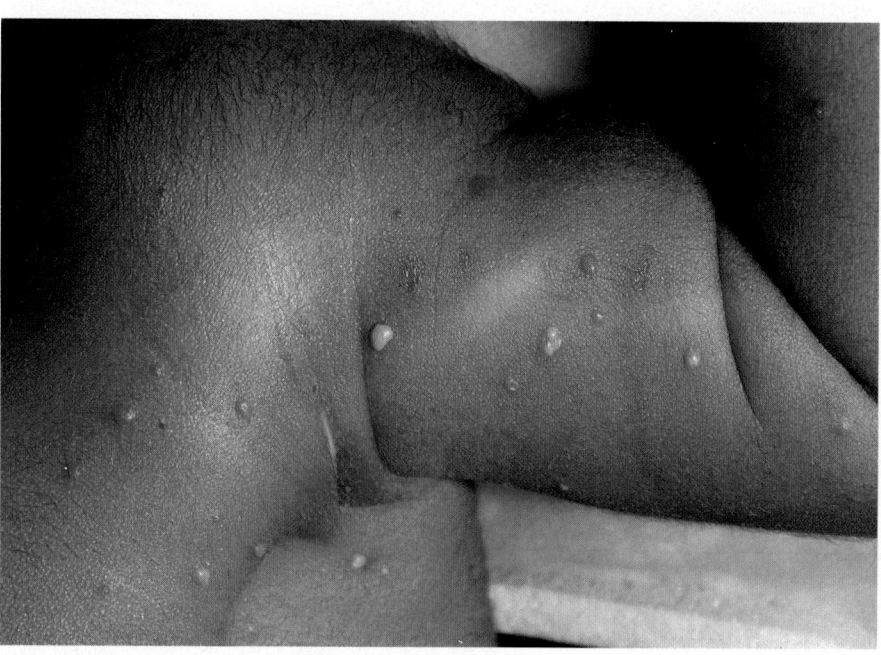

FIGURE 239-2   Transient neonatal pustular melanosis. Discrete pustules on trunk and back of a black newborn.

Clinical Manifestations When a low-birth-weight infant is placed on one side, an erythematous flush with a sharp demarcation at the midline develops on the dependent side.[1] The upper half of the body becomes pale. The color change subsides within a few seconds of placing the baby in the supine position, but it may persist for as long as 20 min.

Diagnosis and Differential Diagnosis The baby must be placed on one side for the color change to be observed. Harlequin color change is seldom confused with other vascular problems.

Course and Prognosis The color change is seldom seen after 10 days of age.

Sucking Blisters

Sucking blisters are blisters apparent at birth as the result of intrauterine sucking; however, sucking blisters are uncommon.

Etiology and Pathogenesis Vigorous sucking in utero has been postulated as the cause of these blisters.

Clinical Manifestations Sucking blisters are usually solitary intact oval blisters or erosions on noninflamed skin in the newborn.[13] They occur on the forearms, wrists, fingers, or upper lip and resolve within a few days.

Diagnosis and Differential Diagnosis Herpes virus infection or bullous impetigo are often considered when sucking blisters are encountered, but the former lesions appear on an erythematous base. Incontinentia pigmenti presents with multiple linear blisters in contrast with the solitary sucking blister. Epidermolysis bullosa usually presents with multiple new blisters that develop after birth.

Course and Prognosis Sucking blisters usually completely resolve by 14 days of age.

Subcutaneous Fat Necrosis (See also Chap. 108)

Subcutaneous fat necrosis is caused by the rupture of lipocytes resulting in a subcutaneous nodule; this is uncommon.

Etiology and Pathogenesis Cold injury is believed to be responsible for subcutaneous fat necrosis. The fat of the neonate contains more saturated fatty acids, which have a higher melting point than adult fatty acids. Once the temperature of the skin drops below the melting point of the fat, crystallization occurs within the fat of the dermal fat cells followed by a granulomatous reaction.

Clinical Manifestations In subcutaneous fat necrosis of the newborn, firm, sharply circumscribed, reddish or purple nodules appear over the cheeks, buttocks, arms, and thighs.[14,15] The lesions usually begin within the first 2 weeks of life and resolve spontaneously over several weeks. Occasionally, atrophy after the lesions heal leaves a skin depression. Infrequently, hypercalcemia can occur with or without associated irritability, vomiting, weight loss, and failure to thrive.[15,16] Serum calcium evaluations should be repeated biweekly until the lesions have totally resolved for a month or more in infants who have large plaques of involved skin or who have renal disease.[15,16]

Pathology Granulomatous inflammation with necrotic amorphous debris surround ruptured fat cells. Sometimes fat crystals are found within lipocytes.

Diagnosis and Differential Diagnosis Bacterial cellulitis or septicemic lesions may be confused with subcutaneous fat necrosis at the onset. Infants with fat necrosis appear healthy and nurse vigorously, in contrast with those with bacterial infections. The several separate lesion sites often seen in infants with subcutaneous fat necrosis would be extremely unusual in infants with cellulitis.

Course and Prognosis Lesions evolve slowly over several months. The surface discoloration changes from red to bruiselike, then fades. A hard subcutaneous mass is felt. As more subcutaneous fat is deposited in the adjacent normal skin, the lesion appears more atrophic with time. Lesions resolve by 1 year.

Sclerema (See also Chap. 108)

Sclerema is diffuse hardening of skin in a sick newborn, which is becoming rare as neonatal care improves worldwide.

Etiology and Pathogenesis Newborn exposure to low temperatures in the nursery or delivery room is believed to be responsible.

Clinical Manifestations Premature newborns who suffer hypothermia are susceptible to sclerema.[14,17] The trunk is always involved. The onset is characteristically after 24 h of age. The skin feels tight and immobile and appears yellow and shiny. Sclerema appears in severely ill newborns who have suffered sepsis, hypoglycemia, metabolic acidosis, or other severe metabolic abnormalities.

Pathology Edema of fibrous septa surrounding fat lobules, without fat necrosis, is found.

Diagnosis and Differential Diagnosis The thickening and hardening of the skin are so characteristic of sclerema that it is not confused with other disorders. The stiff-skin syndrome and other conditions characterized by contractions of extremities are present at delivery, whereas sclerema develops over several days.

Treatment Careful monitoring of the skin surface temperature of newborns who appear sick may prevent sclerema. Temperature control, nutritional replacement, correction of metabolic acidosis, and possibly repeated exchange transfusions arrest the process.[17]

Course and Prognosis Sclerema is a sign of a severely ill newborn. Mortality among infants with sclerema is high. Successful treatment reverses the thickening in several weeks.

Pustules in the Newborn

Pustules are discrete, yellow, 1- to 9-mm raised lesions that frequently have a red base. These are common in the newborn period. The incidence of bacterial sepsis is higher in preterm infants than in the full-term infants, and overall sepsis is an uncommon cause of pustules in newborns. However, the high neonatal mortality rate of unrecognized bacterial sepsis makes it imperative for clinicians to consider this possibility.

TABLE 239-1
Symptoms and Signs of Bacterial Infection in the Newborn

Symptoms	Signs
Lethargy	Pustules
Poor feeding	Jaundice
Irritability	Petechiae
Diarrhea	Pallor
	Cyanosis
	Omphalitis
	Conjunctivitis
	Enlarged liver or spleen
	Hypothermia

Etiology and Pathogenesis   Although there are many causes of pustules in the newborn, the appearance of pustules should immediately bring to mind the possibility of bacterial sepsis (Table 239-1). Pustules on the newborn skin in association with other signs or symptoms of sepsis, or when prolonged rupture of maternal membranes has occurred, should make one suspect bacterial sepsis.[18]

Clinical Manifestations   These discrete, 1- to 9-mm lesions may be observed anywhere on the skin. Pustules that appear during the first 7 days of life are a particular concern. Careful attention should be given to signs of a sick newborn such as low temperature, poor feeding, weak sucking, vomiting, irritability, and lethargy. These signs should raise the suspicion of bacterial sepsis.

Pathology   Pustules caused by bacterial infection arise as the result of accumulation of neutrophils within the skin, following dissemination of bacteria from the blood to the skin or direct bacterial invasion of the skin.

Diagnosis and Differential Diagnosis   Bacterial culture of pustules or other body fluids such as blood, urine, and cerebrospinal fluid should be performed. There is no rapid, completely reliable method of determining whether a baby has bacterial sepsis, and one should always maintain a high index of suspicion.

Other causes of pustules in the newborn may be considered after bacterial sepsis is eliminated as a possibility (Table 239-2). Erythema toxicum may occasionally be pustular, particularly if skin involvement is extensive.[11] Transient neonatal pustular melanosis mimics erythema toxicum and is characterized by pustules present at birth.[12] Herpes simplex skin infections may be pustular but are usually vesicular. Acne neonatorum is usually not present in the first 14 days of life, and evolution to the pustular stage may require several more weeks.[1,19] Candidiasis, particularly of the diaper area or of other intertriginous areas, may be pustular, and satellite pustules are characteristically found at a distance from the mar-

TABLE 239-2
Differential Diagnosis of Pustules in the Newborn

Bacterial sepsis
Erythema toxicum
Transient neonatal pustular melanosis
Herpes simplex infection
Acne neonatorum
Candidiasis
Infantile acropustulosis
Nevus comedonicus
Pustular psoriasis

gins of confluent areas of candidiasis. Congenital candidiasis, acquired in utero, may also appear as discrete pustules at birth followed by development of diffusely eczematous skin.[20] Infantile acropustulosis may appear at birth or within the newborn period as discrete pustules limited to the distal extremities, with prominent involvement of the palms and soles.[21] Nevus comedonicus is a birthmark consisting of patulous follicular openings in which pustule formation, or even deeper abscesses, may occur.[22] Psoriasis rarely occurs in the newborn period, but it also may be extensive and pustular.[23]

Course and Prognosis   Bacterial sepsis in the newborn evolves within hours and mortality is high if it remains unrecognized.

Acne Neonatorum (See also Chap. 63)

Acne that develops within the first 30 days of life is termed neonatal acne. It is estimated that 50 percent of newborns may experience neonatal acne.

Etiology and Pathogenesis   Neonatal acne may be a part of the so-called miniature puberty of the newborn. Neonatal sebaceous glands are hyperplastic, and hydroxysteroid dehydrogenase activity in these structures is high in the 2 months just before birth and at birth.[2,3] There is evidence that newborns with acne experience transient increases in circulating androgens.[19]

Clinical Manifestations   Neonatal acne is rare at birth but may appear as multiple, discrete papules at 2 to 4 weeks of age.[19] The face, chest, back, and groin are the usual areas for cutaneous lesions (Fig. 239-3). Papules evolve into pustules after a few weeks. Neonatal acne may persist up to 8 months of age.[1] There is some suggestion that infants with extensive neonatal acne may experience severe acne as adolescents.

Pathology   Sebaceous gland volume is increased and the pilosebaceous orifices are plugged with keratin. Dilated pilosebaceous structures rupture and neutrophils, or granulomatous inflammation, may occur.

Diagnosis and Differential Diagnosis   The presence of microcomedones and inflammatory papules on the facial skin is seldom confused with other conditions. The differential diagnosis of acne neonatorum is the same as for pustules in the newborn.

Course and Prognosis   Neonatal acne usually resolves spontaneously without treatment. If the involvement is severe, once daily topical therapy with 2.5% benzoyl peroxide gel can be used.[1]

Herpes Simplex Virus Infection (See also Chap. 203)

Neonatal herpes is a systemic infection in which the virus is acquired from a maternal genital herpes infection. The exact prevalence of neonatal herpes simplex is unknown, but some estimates place it at 1 per 2000 live births.[24–28]

Etiology and Pathogenesis   Herpes simplex virus is usually related to maternal infection in the birth canal.[24,26] Infected infants are likely to have had a premature birth. Infants born to mothers with a primary herpes genital infection at the time of delivery are more

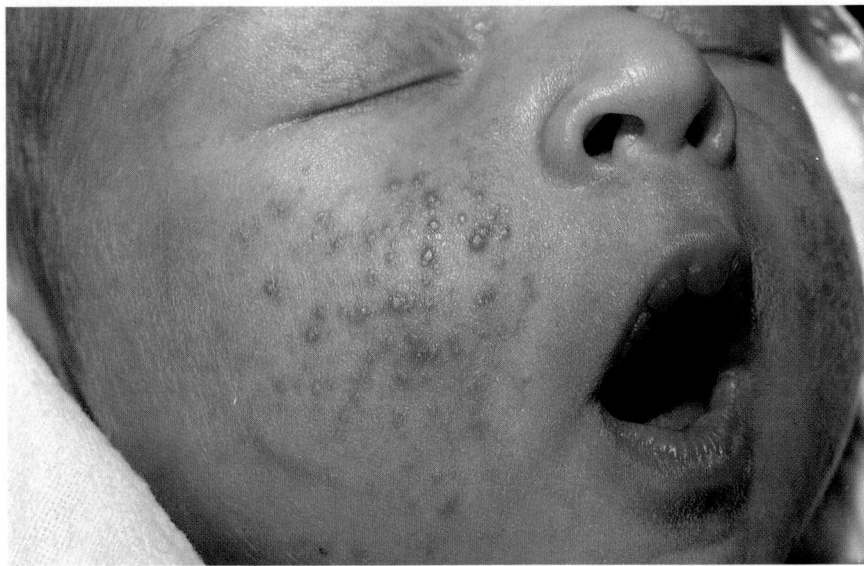

FIGURE 239-3 Neonatal acne. Microcomedones and red papules on the cheek of a 3-week-old.

likely to develop neonatal herpes simplex than infants born to mothers with recurrent genital lesions.[27] Eighty percent of neonatal infections are herpes simplex virus type 2, and 20 percent are herpes simplex virus type 1.[24]

Clinical Manifestations Grouped vesicles on an erythematous base should bring to mind neonatal herpes simplex virus infection (Fig. 239-4). Any area of skin may be involved, but vesicles on the scalp or buttocks are particularly common.[24–28] Monitoring electrodes may produce sufficient skin trauma on involved skin sites to allow invasion by the virus and to induce herpes simplex virus skin lesions. Vesicles may be present immediately at birth, but the onset after birth is more likely, with 6 days as the mean age of onset.[24–28] Some infants with neonatal herpes simplex virus will not have skin

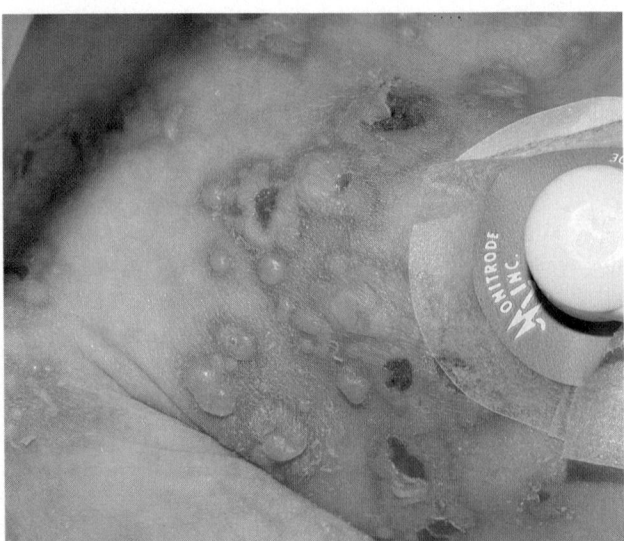

FIGURE 239-4 Herpes simplex infection. Grouped vesicles on an erythematous base. Pustules and erosions also present. (*Courtesy of Alvin H. Jacobs, M.D.*)

lesions, but 70 percent of all infants infected with herpes simplex virus display lesions.[28] Mucous membrane involvement is common.

Pathology Dermal herpes simplex infection reflects viral replication in keratinocytes. Ballooning degeneration of keratinocytes is seen in which the virus had destroyed the cells, and adjacent destruction results in an intraepidermal blister cavity. Some cells demonstrate nuclear fusion of adjacent keratinocytes, and large keratinocytes, which are mostly nuclear chromatin, form characteristic multinucleated giant cells. Inflammatory cells of all types are observed.

Diagnosis and Differential Diagnosis Other blistering diseases of the newborn such as congenital varicella, bullous impetigo, and incontinentia pigmenti may be considered in a differential diagnosis. A Wright's-stained smear of cells scraped from a vesicle base will demonstrate multinucleated giant cells and balloon cells in infants with herpes simplex virus infection. Fluorescein-tagged antiherpes simplex-virus-specific antibody may be used to examine vesicle smears or snap-frozen biopsy sections of skin to make a rapid diagnosis. Viral culture of herpes simplex virus requires 12 to 120 h to grow and, in all infected or suspected neonates, cultures of skin lesions, urine, nasopharynx, eyes, and cerebrospinal fluid are indicated.[26] Serum antibodies for herpes simplex virus are of little assistance in making the diagnosis accurately. Rapid diagnosis of herpes simplex virus is essential, and a high index of suspicion should be maintained.

Treatment Adenosine arabinoside or acyclovir, administered intravenously, are efficacious.[27] Prompt recognition and early therapeutic intervention appear to lead to an improved outcome in infected infants.[27]

Course and Prognisis Infected infants may have signs that mimic bacterial sepsis and may develop psychomotor retardation even if obvious signs of dissemination of herpes simplex virus are not evident in the newborn.

Varicella (See also Chap. 204)

Neonatal varicella is a systemic infection with varicella-zoster virus acquired during intrauterine life. Congenital varicella is rare.

Etiology and Pathogenesis   This infection is associated with maternal chickenpox 2 to 3 weeks before delivery.[24,29,30] Maternal infection with varicella-zoster virus, which may be unrecognized,[29,30] results in dissemination of the virus to the newborn. Varicella can also develop in neonates infected postnatally.

Clinical Manifestations   Lesions appear as crops of macules and papules that evolve into vesicles and then crust. The onset is within the first 10 days after birth, and mortality is as high as 20 percent in infants who develop skin lesions between 5 and 10 days of age.[24,29,31]

Pathology   Pathologic changes in skin are identical to those observed in infants with herpes simplex infection.

Diagnosis and Differential Diagnosis   Neonatal varicella may mimic herpes simplex virus in the newborn.[24,29,31] A Wright's-stained smear of cells from a blister base or a skin biopsy demonstrate the same changes seen in patients with herpes simplex virus. A maternal history of varicella and cutaneous lesions in the infant compatible with varicella are most useful in making the diagnosis. Herpes simplex virus infection and bullous impetigo are the two most important considerations in the differential diagnosis of congenital varicella. Fluorescein-tagged antiherpes-zoster-virus-specific antibody may be used to examine vesicle smears or snap-frozen biopsy sections of skin to make a rapid diagnosis. Culture identification of the virus from the vesicles may require 7 to 14 days.

Treatment   Immediate administration of zoster immune globulin to the infant is recommended if the mother is infected from 5 days before to 2 days after delivery.[31] Infected infants may require therapy with intravenous acyclovir. Passive immunization with varicella-zoster immunoglobulin should be considered when premature and term infants are exposed to varicella after birth.[31]

Course and Prognosis   Varicella may result in a severe infection, especially in premature infants. Mortality is low compared with herpes simplex infection. A few infants develop psychomotor retardation.

Impetigo (See also Chap. 187)

Impetigo is a superficial bacterial skin infection. Although uncommon, bacterial impetigo may be observed in the newborn period.

Etiology and Pathogenesis   *Staphylococcus aureus* is the predominant organism producing impetigo, including those strains capable of producing the staphylococcal scalded skin syndrome. Occasionally, group A streptococci or gram-negative bacteria can cause impetigo in the newborn period.

Clinical Manifestations   Flaccid, well-demarcated bullae may be seen and evolve into erosions.[1] Any area of skin may be involved, but the scalp, face, and diaper areas are the most common sites of infection. A collarette of scale around the erosion is characteristic of impetigo due to *S. aureus*.[32] Honey-colored crusts are less common in newborns than in older children.

Pathology   Impetigo is characterized by a subcorneal neutrophilic abscess that contains bacteria.

Diagnosis and Differential Diagnosis   Bacterial culture of skin lesions and culture of the nasopharynx will yield the organism within 24 h. A smear of vesicle contents and a Gram's stain will demonstrate the bacteria.

Treatment   The appropriate systemic antibiotic should be administered promptly to prevent sepsis and diminish spread of bacteria to other patients and hospital personnel.

Course and Prognosis   Prompt treatment results in full recovery. Undetected impetigo may result in bacterial sepsis in the newborn or premature infant with an immature immune system.

Staphylococcal Scalded Skin Syndrome (Ritter's Disease) (See also Chap. 51)

This acute bacterial infection results in red tender skin and subsequent desquamation. Ritter's disease is uncommon, although nursery epidemics have been well documented.

Etiology and Pathogenesis   Skin injury results from an intraepidermal cleavage through the granular layer of epidermis due to circulating exotoxin produced by *S. aureus*.[32] Small amounts of staphylococci, less than 10^8 organisms, may produce enough toxin to exfoliate a human. Usually, hospital personnel carry the organism into the nursery.

Clinical Manifestations   Infants 2 to 30 days old may have an abrupt onset of generalized erythema followed in 24 h by bullae with subsequent exfoliation of large sheets of skin within 48 h.[32,33] The lesions are usually around the head, neck, buttocks, groin, axilla, and periumbilical area of the abdomen.

Pathology   A subcorneal blister cavity without necrosis of the overlying stratum corneum or inflammation is seen.

Diagnosis and Differential Diagnosis   Toxic shock syndrome and toxic epidermal necrolysis should be considered in the differential diagnosis of the staphylococcal scalded skin syndrome. However, they are rarely observed in the newborn period. The flushing and blistering of diffuse cutaneous mastocytosis may be confused with scalded skin. Skin biopsy that demonstrates excessive mast cells and the recurrence of episodes will distinguish between these conditions. Cultures of the nasopharynx, rectum, and blisters are likely to yield the organism.

Treatment   Isolation of the affected newborn to prevent nursery epidemics is essential.[33] Antistaphylococcal antibiotics should be administered systemically, and aggressive fluid and electrolyte replacement should be instituted, much as it is for burn therapy.

Course and Prognosis   This is a life-threatening condition. Prompt recognition and aggressive therapy are essential.

Breast Abscess

Breast abscess is an acute bacterial infection of the breast tissue of a newborn; it is rare in the newborn period.

Etiology and Pathogenesis   *S. aureus* and gram-negative organisms are the most likely pathogens. It is believed that the bacteria enter through ductal tissue.

Clinical Manifestations   Swelling, erythema, and fluctuance in one breast of a newborn infant signify the possibility of breast abscess. Onset usually begins 5 to 20 days after birth.[34] The infant may have fever but usually is otherwise asymptomatic.

Diagnosis and Differential Diagnosis   A needle aspiration of the infection may be necessary to obtain a positive bacterial culture. Breast hyperplasia due to miniature puberty of the newborn may produce asymmetric enlargement of one breast.[34] The breast is not red or fluctuant to palpation in infants with breast hyperplasia, as it is in those with abscess.

Treatment   Systemic antibiotic therapy with the appropriate antistaphylococcal agent is usually necessary.

Course and Prognosis   With prompt antibiotic therapy, recovery is rapid. Unrecognized infection may lead to bacterial sepsis.

Omphalitis

Omphalitis is bacterial infection of the tissues around the umbilical cord, which is uncommon in the newborn period.

Etiology and Pathogenesis   Bacterial infection through the cut surface of the umbilical cord is the usual cause. It is predominantly due to *S. aureus.*

Clinical Manifestations   Redness and induration of the umbilical region are characteristic of omphalitis. Often, the redness is not well localized and spreads diffusely beyond the umbilicus.[1]

Diagnosis and Differential Diagnosis   An irritant dermatitis produced by treatment of the umbilicus with various bacteriostatic agents may sometimes mimic omphalitis.

Treatment   Prophylactic bacteriostatic agents applied to the cord in the newborn period have reduced the likelihood of this infection in many nurseries. Systemic antistaphylococcal antibiotics are the treatment of choice.

Course and Prognosis   Omphalitis usually remains localized but, if untreated, may progress to bacterial sepsis.

Caput Succedaneum and Cephalohematoma

Caput succedaneum is subcutaneous edema over the presenting part of the head[1]; cephalohematoma is a subperiosteal collection of blood.[1] Caput succedaneum is common whereas cephalohematoma is rare among newborns.

Etiology and Pathogenesis   Both lesions are due to shearing forces on the scalp skin and skull during labor.

Clinical Manifestations   Edema or hemorrhage of the scalp appears as deep swelling, with or without purpura. The swelling occurs primarily in vertex deliveries, particularly those with prolonged labor, and resolves spontaneously in 7 to 10 days. If the purpura is extensive, it can serve as a source of hyperbilirubinemia. Secondary bacterial infection of cephalohematoma may rarely occur, resulting in cellulitis.

Diagnosis and Differential Diagnosis   Caput succedaneum tends to feel soft and lacks a well-defined outline. Cephalohematoma is bounded by the suture lines of the skull and often feels fluctuant. Both lesions can mimic cellulitis or bacterial abscess. Appropriate cultures may assist in the differential diagnosis.

Petechiae and Purpura

Petechiae are nonblanching macules and purpura are bruiselike areas of skin, commonly encountered in the newborn period.

Etiology and Pathogenesis   Petechiae and purpura represent leakage of red blood cells from superficial cutaneous blood vessels into extravascular tissue. Often the results of birth trauma, these nonetheless should alert the clinician because petechiae and purpura may be presenting features of congenital infection, particularly when the newborn is small for gestational age and has hepatosplenomegaly. Petechiae and purpura are the most common cutaneous symptoms for congenital infections and may be important clues to the diagnosis.[19] Toxoplasmosis, syphilis, rubella, cytomegalovirus, and congenital herpes simplex virus infections are the usual congenital infections responsible for the production of petechiae and purpura.[18,24,25,35,36]

Clinical Manifestations   Petechiae appear as pinpoint (less than 1-mm), nonblanching, red macule whereas purpura appears as larger areas of purple macules. Newborns with congenital infection may also have other features, such as microophthalmia, congenital heart defects, cataracts, and psychomotor retardation.

Diagnosis and Differential Diagnosis   Congenital infection should be considered first as a possible cause. Serologic tests and viral cultures for the likely infections should be performed. Other causes of petechiae and purpura in the newborn include trauma: Face and scalp petechiae are common in difficult vertex deliveries or in section-assisted deliveries. Neonatal thrombocytopenia due to maternal autoantibodies, as in idiopathic thrombocytopenic purpura, or systemic lupus erythematosus, may also produce neonatal petechiae a few hours after birth. Hypoprothrombinemia may result in purpura in newborns older than 2 or 3 days as a result of vitamin K deficiency. Protein C deficiency can also cause severe purpura in neonates. Neonatal petechiae and purpura are unusual in the hemophilias, but bleeding from circumcision sites may be the first manifestation of hemophilia in the newborn period. Neonatal purpura secondary to platelet dysfunction may be observed in von Willebrand's disease or Wiskott-Aldrich syndrome.

Treatment   Treatment is guided by detection of the etiology of the petechiae or purpura.

Birthmarks

Birthmarks represent an excess of one or more of the normal components of skin per unit area: blood vessels, lymph vessels, pigment cells, hair follicles, sebaceous glands, epidermis, collagen, or elastin. Birthmarks are collections of highly differentiated cells in tissue.

Congenital malformations are most frequently observed in skin. The vascular birthmarks are the most common.[37-39] The two most common birthmarks are flat hemangiomas of a faint red color, the so-called salmon patch, and Mongolian spots.[37,39,40] Salmon patches are observed with high frequency in infants, both in white infants (703 of 1000 live births) and black infants (592 of 1000 live births).[37,39] Mongolian spots are more frequently observed in Orientals (910 of 1000 live births) and black infants (800 of 1000 live births) than in white infants (48 of 1000 live births).[39,40] Mongolian spots and salmon patches are observed at least 100 times more frequently than any other skin birthmark.

Flat Hemangiomas (See also Chap. 98)

Flat hemangiomas can be divided into those that are light red or pink in color (salmon patch, nevus flammeus) and those that are deep red or purple-red (port-wine stain). A salmon patch is present over the back of the neck in over 40 percent of infants, and over the glabella or eyelids in 20 percent. Port-wine stains occur in 0.5 percent of newborns.

Clinical Manifestations   Salmon patches appear as light red macules over the nape of the neck, the upper eyelids, and the glabella.[41,42] Port-wine stains appear as deep red or purple-red macules over the face or extremities. They are usually unilateral.[41,43-46] Occasionally, they are extensive and cover large areas of skin. Port-wine stains over the face or an extremity may be associated with soft tissue and bony hypertrophy.[41] A port-wine stain over the face may be a clue to the Sturge-Weber syndrome.[45,46] Overall, 8 percent of infants with facial port-wine stains develop Sturge-Weber syndrome, but the incidence is higher if the lesion covers the upper and lower eyelid or if the lesion is bilateral.[47] The Sturge-Weber syndrome is characterized by seizures, mental retardation, glaucoma, and hemiplegia.[43,46] Calcification of the hemangioma in the brain in patients with Sturge-Weber syndrome may be detected in childhood by skull x-ray.[46] Identification of cerebral vascular abnormalities and early calcification can be detected in infancy by computed tomography or magnetic resonance imaging. When port-wine stains are found over an extremity and are associated with soft tissue or bony hypertrophy of that extremity, the condition is called the Klippel-Trenaunay-Weber syndrome.[41,48] Elongation of an extremity can cause orthopedic deformity. Arteriovenous fistulas affect 25 percent of such patients.[48] Absence of the deep venous channels in the affected limb may be detected by venography.[48]

Pathology   Numerous dilated capillaries without endothelial change are seen on skin biopsies of lesions of adolescents or adults.[42] The capillaries are mature and represent a developmental malformation. In infants and children, the skin biopsy may be indistinguishable from normal skin.

Diagnosis and Differential Diagnosis   In an older infant, flat hemangiomas are so characteristic that they are seldom confused with other skin conditions, but in the first weeks of life raised hemangiomas may be flat and look like port-wine stains. After several weeks of life, raised hemangiomas begin to elevate the skin and become distinguished from port-wine stains. Port-wine stain lesions usually cover a larger surface area than hemangiomas and are unilateral.

Treatment   Recent data support use of a pulsed dye laser, which selectively causes thermal damage to cutaneous vasculature while sparing surrounding epidermal and dermal structures.[49,50] This therapy can commence during infancy. Therapy for the cutaneous lesion may reverse underlying soft tissue overgrowth, but bony hypertrophy or the neurologic progressions in Sturge-Weber syndrome are not affected. In addition, flat hemangiomas can be covered with make-up. If features of Sturge-Weber syndrome are present, ophthalmologic evaluation and follow-up should be done immediately.[46] The length and girth of the extremities should be carefully measured every 3 to 6 months if a port-wine stain is found over an extremity.[48] Since differences in leg length can induce scoliosis, orthopedic evaluation and assistance may be required if one leg is longer than the other.

Course and Prognosis   Flat vascular birthmarks tend to persist. Salmon patches may fade with time, but remnants may persist well into adult life.[42] Generally, eyelid lesions fade by 6 to 12 months of age, and glabellar lesions by 5 to 6 years of age. Lesions on the nape of the neck are likely to persist into adulthood.

Raised Hemangiomas (Strawberry Hemangiomas, Cavernous Hemangiomas) (See also Chap. 98)

Raised hemangiomas are red or purple-red vascular masses seen in 2 percent of newborns.

Etiology and Pathogenesis   Most raised hemangiomas are mixtures of dilated, proliferating capillaries and dilated venous channels.[51] The biologic behavior of the cavernous and mixed types is similar in children, however. Blood flow through such lesions is sluggish and platelet aggregation can occur, followed by consumption of clotting factors in the Kasabach-Merritt syndrome.[52]

Clinical Manifestations   Raised hemangiomas may not be observed at birth, but a circumscribed area of blanched skin with a few fine telangiectases may be present, representing a developing raised hemangioma. By 2 to 4 weeks of age, the skin becomes raised, with red nodules.[51,53] The lesions grow out of proportion to the baby for the first 8 to 12 months of life. Raised hemangiomas begin to show signs of involution around 15 months of age, when pale grey areas appear within the red nodule.[51,53] Soon the first sign of flattening appears. The raised lesion regresses to skin level by 5 years of age in 50 percent of patients, and by puberty in almost all patients. Most often, only redundant loose skin that was stretched during the rapid growth phase remains. In large, raised hemangiomas, ulceration of the epithelial surface often occurs when secondary bacterial superinfection results (Fig. 239-5).

There are several major complications of raised hemangiomas: (1) platelet trapping, (2) airway obstruction, (3) visual obstruction,

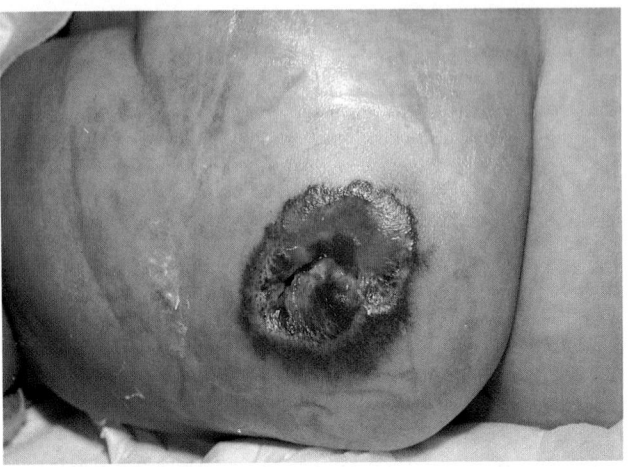

FIGURE 239-5 Ulcerated hemangioma. A 4-week-old with a large hemangioma of the buttock with central ulceration and crust.

and (4) cardiac decompensation. Platelet trapping (Kasabach-Merritt syndrome) occurs within the sluggish circulation of the raised hemangioma.[52] It usually occurs in patients with a single large hemangioma, primarily within the first 6 months of life. Platelet trapping produces easy bruising and petechiae on areas of the body not involved with hemangioma and may progress to frank hemorrhage. Often the involved hemangioma will suddenly enlarge and become very firm at the onset of the platelet trapping.[52]

Obstruction of the airway results in respiratory stridor and is usually due to subglottic hemangiomas. Infants with such hemangiomas usually have multiple hemangiomas of the skin of the head and neck.[51] Visual acuity disturbances may result either from growth of the hemangioma within the orbit, causing compression of the eyeball, or from swelling around the eyelid forcing the lid to close. Large raised hemangiomas may pool enough blood to produce high-output cardiac failure. Internal hemangioma may occur with or without cutaneous lesions.

Diagnosis and Differential Diagnosis Raised hemangiomas may be confused with pyogenic granulomas, malignant vascular tumors, and giant melanocytic birthmarks; the last may be vascular at birth and produce little pigment. Usually, these different lesions cause little confusion but occasionally, a biopsy is needed to help distinguish one from another.

Treatment The indications for treatment are obstruction of a vital orifice (airway, excretory channel), visual obstruction, platelet trapping syndrome, and cardiac decompensation. The treatment of choice is prednisone, 1 to 6 mg/kg daily.[54] Alternate-day therapy may be sufficient. Treatment for 4 to 8 weeks is often necessary. Treatment started during the growing phase of the hemangioma (1 to 8 months of age) produces the best results. The mechanism of action of prednisone is unknown, but reduction of the capillary cell division by steroids has been postulated. X-ray therapy produces poor cosmetic results, and squamous cell and basal cell carcinomas subsequently develop within the areas of radiodermatitis.[54] Surgical therapy results in significant blood loss and scarring. Newer methods to control hemangioma, such as the pulsed dye laser and the use of growth factors, are currently being tested. There is often

great pressure to treat hemangiomas for cosmetic reasons, but strict adherence to the indications for therapy is advised.[54]

Topical antibiotic or antiseptic agents will reduce secondary infection in ulcerated hemangiomas, but often oral antistaphylococcal therapy may be necessary. The rapid growth of the tumor often convinces parents that such lesions will not disappear. Careful explanation of the natural history of these lesions is necessary.[51] Photographs and measurements are useful to follow the progress of a raised hemangioma. Infants treated with prednisone should be seen every 2 weeks during therapy to monitor progress, then monthly thereafter until age 1. For other infants, a single follow-up visit in 2 weeks will reinforce the concept that treatment is not required. Monthly or bimonthly follow-up visits are advised thereafter.

Cutis Marmorata Telangiectatica Congenita

Cutis marmorata is a persistent mottling pattern due to a vascular malformation. Cutis marmorata is rare.

Etiology and Pathogenesis The disorder is considered to be a vascular ectasia of veins and, possibly, of capillaries.[55,56] Biopsy reveals tortuous, dilated veins found in the dermis and subcutaneous tissue.

Clinical Manifestations Cutis marmorata telangiectatica congenita is characterized by a mottled pattern of blue or dusky-red erythema from birth.[55,56] It is unresponsive to skin warming. Often, a single extremity is involved, but the lesions may occur bilaterally on the extremities or on the trunk.[55,56] The skin surface overlying such areas may be depressed. A gradual increase in the size of lesions is expected over the first few years of life, but most fade by adult life. There are no rigorous natural history studies of cutis marmorata telangiectatica congenita. Associations with musculoskeletal or vascular abnormalities occur.[55,56]

Diagnosis and Differential Diagnosis In contrast with cutis marmorata telangiectatica congenita, mottling of newborn skin is a transient vasodilation and is relieved by rewarming the skin. The livedo reticularis pattern of collagen vascular disease is flat, is not depressed over the discolored areas, is always bilateral, and is associated with systemic signs and symptoms.

Treatment There is no treatment. Routine evaluations should include close inspection of extremities for possible orthopedic deformity. It should be explained that cutis marmorata telangiectatica congenita is a birthmark, and that some increase is expected in the area of skin involved. It should be emphasized that it is an unusual disorder and that few data are available for predicting the course. Associated deformities should be treated as necessary.

Diffuse Neonatal Hemangiomatosis and Blue Rubber Bleb Nevus Syndrome

These are vascular syndromes consisting of multiple raised hemangiomas. Both diffuse neonatal hemangiomatosis and blue rubber bleb syndrome are rare.

Etiology and Pathogenesis In diffuse neonatal hemangiomatosis, proliferating endothelial cells and numerous capillary lumens are observed in the middermis. This syndrome has been reported in twins, but there are not enough data to determine whether it is hereditary. The lesions of blue rubber bleb nevus syndrome are more similar to cavernous hemangiomas with numerous dilated vascular channels.

Clinical Manifestations   Diffuse neonatal hemangiomatosis consists of multiple, small, raised cutaneous hemangiomas which may or may not be associated with hemangiomas in the liver, lungs, gastrointestinal tract, and central nervous system.[57,58] The raised hemangiomas may be present at birth, and more develop with time. The hemangiomas vary from 2 to 15 mm in diameter (Fig. 239-6). Spontaneous involution of the lesions has been reported.[57] Bleeding may occur into the gastrointestinal tract. The blue rubber bleb nevus syndrome is a rare disorder consisting of multiple cavernous hemangiomas of the skin and bowel.[59] The lesions are 3 to 4 cm in diameter.

Diagnosis and Differential Diagnosis   The skin hemangiomas are so characteristic that they present little difficulty in differential diagnosis. The lesions of blue rubber bleb nevus syndrome are compressible and may be painful or associated with excessive sweating. Monitoring stool samples for occult blood is helpful in identifying intestinal lesions.

Treatment   Infants with diffuse neonatal hemangiomatosis who develop complications may respond to prednisone at a dose of 2 to 6 mg/kg daily, with appropriate attention to side effects.[57] The du-

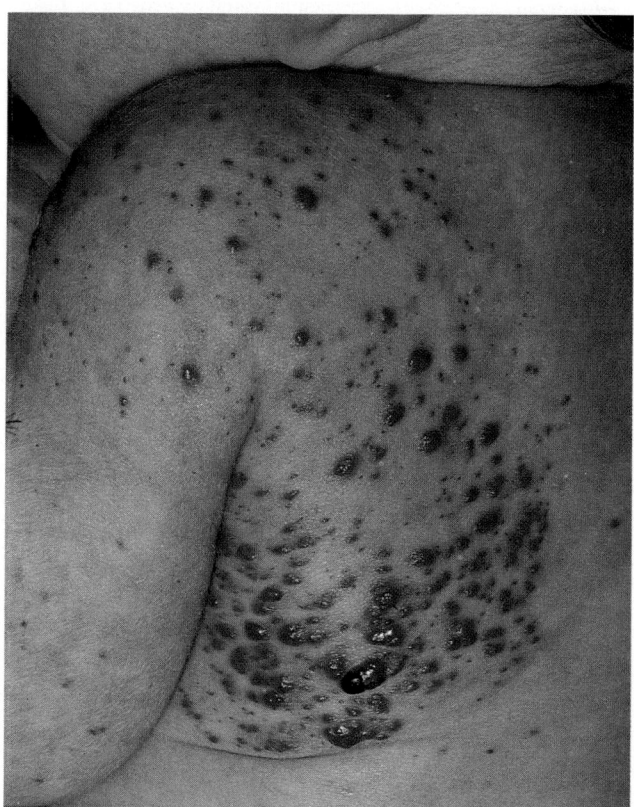

FIGURE 239-6   Diffuse neonatal hemangiomatosis. Dozens of hemangiomas grouped about the shoulder.

ration of treatment may exceed 8 to 12 weeks. The blue rubber bleb lesions are not responsive to systemic therapy and may require surgical resection.[59] Frequent stool guiac examinations will identify intestinal bleeding.

Lymph Vessel Birthmarks: Lymphangiomas (See also Chap. 98)

Lymphangiomas may be circumscribed, superficial papules or deep, cavernous nodules,[60] uncommon in the newborn period.

Etiology and Pathogenesis   Dilated, tortuous lymph vessels appear within the dermis and subcutaneous fat. Most often, many channels are found spreading from the original lesion, so that the skin surface change reflects only the tip of a triangular lesion. Cavernous lymphangiomas may involve the muscle as well.

Clinical Manifestations   Circumscribed lymphangiomas appear as a solitary group of 2- to 4-mm, gelatinous skin-colored papules limited to a skin area less than 10 cm. They are often connected to underlying venous channels, and hemorrhage into one or more papules may occur, producing sudden darkening.[60] They may be present at birth but are often not noticed until late infancy or childhood.

Cavernous lymphangiomas are rubbery, skin-colored nodules that may result in grotesque enlargement of soft tissues. They are usually solitary and involve the face, trunk, and extremities.[60] They are particularly common over the parotid area, where they are called *cystic hygromas*. They may have a rapid growth phase similar to that of raised hemangiomas.

Diagnosis and Differential Diagnosis   Circumscribed lymphangioma may be mistaken for a disorder with grouped vesicles, such as herpes simplex, herpes zoster, or dermatitis herpetiformis. However, there is no erythematous base in circumscribed lymphangioma, and the lesions appear gelatinous, not fluid-filled. As noted, hemorrhage into such lesions results in darkening, which may be confused with malignant melanoma. Cavernous lymphangiomas may be confused with lipomas, neurofibromas, and other soft subcutaneous masses.

Treatment   There is no satisfactory treatment.[60] Surgical excision can result in defects two or three times larger than the observed skin lesion, and the recurrence rate is high. Often, the lymph channels are found to surround vital subcutaneous structures, such as major arteries or nerves. The lesions are not responsive to radiotherapy or systemic steroids. Monthly or bimonthly visits in which photographs of the lesions are taken and careful measurements made are indicated initially. Eventually, semiannual or annual visits are sufficient to evaluate the lesions and commence therapy for complications.

Mongolian Spots (See also Chap. 81)

Mongolian spots are blue-black macules found on the skin of dark-skinned newborns. Infants' skin is always light at birth and becomes progressively darker with increasing age. Hyperpigmentation of the scrotum and of the linea alba is common in dark-skinned infants at birth. The most commonly observed pigmentary abnormality of infants is the Mongolian spot. Mongolian spots are found over the lumbosacral area in up to 90 percent of Oriental, black, and American Indian babies.[38-40,61]

Etiology and Pathogenesis   Mongolian spots consist of spindle-shaped pigment cells located deep within the dermis. The precise mechanism of this condition is not known.

Clinical Manifestations   Mongolian spots are blue-black macules usually found in lumbosacral skin. They are occasionally noted over the shoulders and back and may extend over the buttocks and extremities.[61]

Course and Prognosis   Mongolian spots fade somewhat with time, and the difference in pigmentation from normal skin pigment becomes less obvious as the newborn's pigment darkens. Some traces of Mongolian spots may persist into adult life.

Café au Lait Spots (See also Chap. 80)

Light brown oval macules that may appear more dark brown on black skin are found anywhere on the body and are designated café au lait spots.[38-40]

Black infants are far more likely (120 of 1000 live births) than white infants (3 of 1000 live births) to have a solitary café au lait spot. Café au lait spots persist through childhood and may increase in number with age.

Clinical Manifestations   Café au lait spots are tan macules with distinct borders. They usually are 3 to 5 mm in diameter, although huge lesions may be seen in newborns. The presence of six or more café au lait spots, greater than 5 mm at their greatest diameter, is considered by most authorities as a major clue to neurofibromatosis type 1 in prepubertal children.[62] However, newborns with neurofibromatosis type 1 may have only one or two café au lait spots and will not acquire numerous spots until 2 to 5 years of age.

Junctional Nevocellular Nevi (See also Chap. 81)

Junctional nevi are clones of pigment cells located at the junction of the epidermis and dermis, usually found in 5 of 1000 live births.

Etiology and Pathogenesis   Clones of melanocytes are present in excess at the dermal-epidermal junction. These nevi are considered to be a developmental defect.

Clinical Manifestations   Dark-brown or black macules with distinct borders are found at the junction of the epidermis and dermis.[63] As an infant ages, these nevi may become slightly raised and papular and develop intradermal melanocytes, creating a compound nevus. Often, the surface of the lesion at birth is slightly irregular.

Raised Nevocellular Nevi (See also Chap. 81)

Collections of pigment cells within the dermis produce raised nevocellular nevi. Raised nevocellular nevi occur in 10 of 1000 live births.[63,64]

Etiology and Pathogenesis   The cause of raised pigmented nevi is not known. There is no correlation with twinning, infant sex, pa-

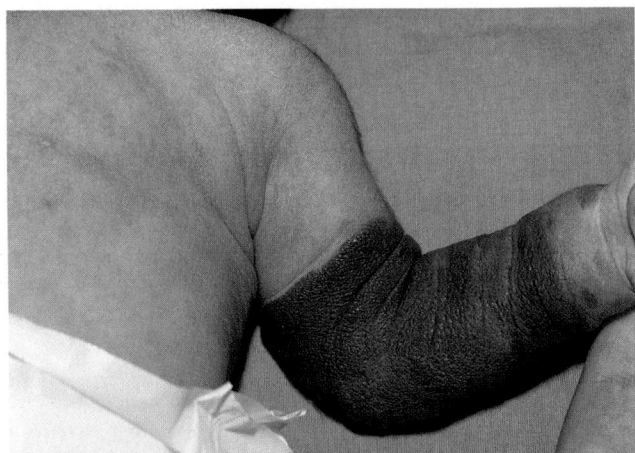

FIGURE 239-7   Giant congenital pigmented nevus. Raised pigmented lesion encircling the arm of a newborn.

rental consanguinity, parental age, birth order, radiation exposure, or drug intake.[64] They are more common in black infants than in white infants.

Clinical Manifestations   Intradermal nevi are skin-colored to tan or brown solitary papules with smooth surfaces.[63,64] Most nevi are small, measuring less than 1.5 cm at their greatest diameter. When these localized, raised pigment cell lesions are greater than 10 or 20 cm at their greatest diameter, there is a concern about their cancer potential (Fig. 239-7). Malignant melanoma may occur in such large nevi.[65] The precise estimate of cancer potential is unknown, but most authorities accept 1 percent or less.

Treatment   Prophylactic removal of large congenital nevi within the first year of life has been recommended by many authorities, although the best age for removal is unknown.[65] Equal weight should be placed on the potential for cosmetic improvement and the cosmetic deformity produced by such surgical removal. Optimal surgical results may be best when the child is older. Whether smaller lesions have any malignant potential and require removal is not known.

Hypopigmentation

Hypopigmentation is a decrease in pigment compared with normal skin. Localized areas of hypopigmented skin are uncommon in infants. A hypopigmented area of skin is found in approximately 8 of 1000 live births, and a hypopigmented tuft of hair is found in 3 of 1000 live births.[37,39,40,66,67]

Albinism (See also Chap. 80)

Albinism is the congenital inability to produce pigment; it occurs in 4 of 100,000 live births.

Etiology and Pathogenesis   All forms of albinism represent hereditary defects in the ability to produce or transfer melanin. The enzyme tyrosinase, which is pivotal in melanin production, is not functional in the most common types of albinism.

Clinical Manifestations   Ten types of oculocutaneous albinism occur. Typically, newborns with albinism have fine, white hair and pink skin at birth.[67] They may also have nevi at birth that are raised but not pigmented. Severe nystagmus and photophobia may also be present at birth.

Diagnosis and Differential Diagnosis   Fair-skinned infants and infants with phenylketonuria as well as Chédiak-Higashi syndrome may be mistakenly diagnosed as having albinism. Nystagmus is a clinical feature that often helps distinguish albinism from these other conditions.

Phenylketonuria (See also Chap. 80)

Phenylketonuria is a hereditary defect in phenylalanine metabolism. It is rare and occurs in 1 of 100,000 live births.

Etiology and Pathogenesis   Patients with phenylketonuria lack the enzymes needed to utilize phenylalanine[67] and thus develop hyperphenylalaninemia. Their hypopigmentation is thought to be related to the tight binding of phenylalanine to the receptor sites of tyrosinase so that the enzyme cannot oxidize phenylalanine to melanin.

Clinical Manifestations   Newborns with phenylketonuria have blond hair, blue eyes, and light-colored skin.[67] Routine screening tests for excessive amounts of phenylalanine in the blood will help detect this syndrome.

Diagnosis and Differential Diagnosis   Phenylketonuria should be distinguished from albinism and Chédiak-Higashi syndrome. Analysis of blood for phenylalanine is the most useful differentiating test.

Epidermal Birthmarks

Increases in mature epidermal cells, hair follicles, or sebaceous glands may appear as birthmarks.[68] Most of these lesions are present at birth, but new lesions can develop into adolescence.

Epidermal Nevi

Epidermal nevi are increases in mature epidermal cells in an area of skin; epidermal birthmarks are uncommon.

Etiology and Pathogenesis   Epidermal birthmarks are thought to be developmental.

Clinical Features   These lesions have a warty surface and appear anywhere on the body.[68] They are often linear or oval with the long axis of the lesion parallel to the long axis of the dermatome. Most lesions are present at birth, and up to 95 percent are present by 7 years of age. Initially, the lesion is barely palpable and may be a confluence of smooth-topped papules. In time the lesion becomes more wartlike and scaly. Most are 2 to 5 cm in length, but occasionally they may appear as long unilateral streaks involving an entire extremity or one side of the trunk (*nevus unius lateris*).[68] The lesions may be so extensive as to involve most of the body. The terms *ichthyosis hystrix* or *benign congenital acanthosis nigricans*

have been applied to such extensive epidermal nevi. Epidermal nevi may become erythematous and itchy during the newborn period, with episodes of redness and inflammation, and may be designated *inflammatory linear verrucous epidermal nevi* (ILVEN).[68]

Patients with epidermal nevi may have associated abnormalities.[68] They have an increased number of cutaneous lesions including café au lait spots, congenital hypopigmented macules, and congenital nevocellular nevi. They may have associated skeletal defects, seizure disorders, mental retardation, and ocular abnormalities. Patients with more extensive skin involvement have a higher association of other abnormalities than those with limited skin involvement. A birth defect clinic may be a good referral source for a multidisciplinary approach to such infants.

Pathology   Epidermal nevi show thickening of the epidermis and hyperkeratosis.[68] In some lesions, a peculiar vacuolization of the granular layer appears, and separation of the cells in that layer results in a microscopic blister cavity. This process is called epidermolytic hyperkeratosis. Inflammatory lesions are marked by dermal accumulation of inflammatory cells and alternating bands of parakeratosis. Overgrowth of sebaceous glands and apocrine glands may underlie the epidermal proliferation.

Diagnosis and Differential Diagnosis   Warts are commonly confused with epidermal nevi. Their presence from birth and linear arrangement help distinguish epidermal nevi from warts. Extensive lesions may be confused with ichthyosis, and certain features of congenital bullous ichthyosiform erythroderma may exactly mimic epidermal nevi. Some investigators feel that congenital bullous ichthyosiform erythroderma is a variant of epidermal nevi. Inflammatory linear epidermal nevi may be confused with the warty stage of incontinentia pigmenti, with lichen striatus, or with a dermatitis.

Treatment   For small lesions, surgical excision is the best treatment. Extensive lesions may be improved by mild keratolytics, such as retinoic acid cream 0.05% once daily or 12% ammonium lactate lotion several times a day, or by bland lubricant therapy. The lesions revert to their hyperkeratotic state when treatment is discontinued.

Sebaceous Nevi

Sebaceous nevi represent an excess of sebaceous glands in an area of skin. The most common of all epidermal birth marks, sebaceous nevi occurs 3 per 1000 live births.

Etiology and Pathogenesis   Like other epidermal nevi, sebaceous nevi are considered developmental.

Clinical Manifestations   Jadassohn's sebaceous nevi appear at birth as slightly raised, oval or linear areas with a yellow or orange color.[69] These nevi are common on the scalp and are devoid of hair, producing a congenital circumscribed hair loss. They may be seen on the face as well. Sebaceous nevus may be contiguous with an epidermal nevus and constitute part of the epidermal nevus syndrome.

Pathology   The sebaceous nevus is a birthmark with an increased number of mature sebaceous glands without hair follicles. Such lesions often have an increased number of apocrine glands as well.

Diagnosis and Differential Diagnosis Juvenile xanthogranulomas and xanthomas are yellow or orange lesions that may mimic sebaceous nevi. Skin biopsy will distinguish these lesions.

Treatment Surgical excision just before puberty is the treatment of choice because of the risk of basal cell carcinoma after puberty and for an improved cosmetic appearance. Lesions excised before puberty may be incompletely excised and warty growth along the surgical scar may remain.

Course and Prognosis At puberty, or with androgenic stimulation, these nevi enlarge and become warty on the surface and raised. Basal cell carcinomas will develop within the lesions after puberty on approximately 15 percent of children with sebaceous nevi.[69]

Nevus Comedonicus

Nevus comedonicus is a birthmark consisting of pilosebaceous follicles with patulous openings.[27] It is the least common epidermal birthmark. Its prevalence is not precisely known.

Etiology and Pathogenesis Nevus comedonicus is considered to be developmental.

Clinical Manifestations In nevus comedonicus, linear or oval groups of widely dilated follicular openings plugged with keratin are present at birth on the face and scalp.[27] They may become inflamed and pustular and mimic acne as the child ages. Pustules can develop within the lesions as early as 2 to 4 weeks after birth. Bilateral and widespread lesions are rare.

Diagnosis and Differential Diagnosis In contrast with nevus comedonicus, neonatal acne begins at 1 month of age and involves discrete, single lesions rather than grouped arrangements of lesions.

Treatment In small lesions, simple surgical excision is the treatment of choice. Large or extensive lesions may be controlled by applying topical retinoic acid cream once or twice daily.

Aplasia Cutis Congenita

Aplasia cutis congenita is the failure to form certain layers of skin. This condition occurs in 1 per 3000 live births. It may be seen as an autosomal dominant trait in some families or may be associated with dystrophic forms of epidermolysis bullosa.[70]

Etiology and Pathogenesis Aplasia cutis congenita is a developmental failure of skin fusion. Dermis, epidermis, and fat may all be missing, or single layers may be absent.[70]

Clinical Manifestations Aplasia cutis congenita is characterized by oval, sharply marginated, 1- to 2-cm depressed areas primarily in the midline of the posterior scalp.[70] They are hairless, may appear as an ulcer, or may be covered by a smooth, finely wrinkled epithelial membrane (Fig. 239-8). Ulcerated defects heal with scar formation. Other developmental defects, such as cleft palate or lip, syndactyly, absence of digits, and congenital heart disease may be

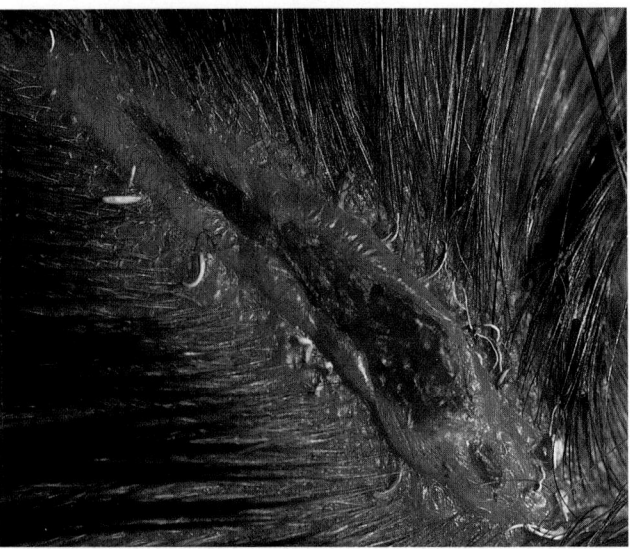

FIGURE 239-8 Aplasia cutis congenita. A newborn with a hairless crusted scalp defect.

associated.[70] Although most lesions appear on the scalp, lesions may be found on the trunk, face, or proximal extremities.

Diagnosis and Differential Diagnosis Scalp ulcers at birth may be mistaken for obstetric trauma, although a careful history will distinguish between the two. Other forms of congenital circumscribed hair loss should be considered.

Treatment If the lesion is small, surgical excision, with mobilization of the scalp and simple closure, will correct the hairless defect.[71] Hair transplantation into large defects has been successful. Convincing the parents that aplasia cutis congenita is not the result of obstetrical trauma is critical.

Connective Tissue Birthmarks (See also Chaps. 97 and 157)

Connective tissue nevi are skin lesions consisting predominantly of the elements of extracellular collagen tissue and products of fibroblasts, such as collagen, elastin, and proteoglycans.[72] All connective tissue nevi are rare, although their precise incidence is not known.

Etiology and Pathogenesis The etiology is unknown.

Clinical Manifestations Connective tissue nevi are localized areas of thickened skin appearing as multiple skin-colored papules and plaques.[72] Stretching the overlying skin will give a yellowish discoloration to these areas. They may occasionally have increased vascularity and appear red. Collagenomas are localized areas of thickened skin with multiple skin-colored papules or plaques. They may be solitary or appear in a zosteriform segmental pattern. Elastomas are solitary plaques that are present at birth and contain increases in both elastic tissue and proteoglycans.[72] Elastomas may be solitary or they may be multiple in the Buschke-Ollendorff syndrome. This autosomal dominant syndrome appears as symmetrically distributed skin-colored papules or nodules with a predilection for the lower trunk or the extremities.[72] Skin affected by these lesions may assume a thickened appearance, and the lesions may develop a lacy pattern over the trunk. X-rays may show sclerotic densities of the ends of long bones, pelvis, and hands, although such lesions are often asymptomatic. The shagreen patch of tuberous sclerosis is a connective tissue nevus. These connective tissue nevi are subtle at birth and may go unnoticed. They tend to persist throughout life.

Pathology   Connective tissue nevi are characterized by thickened, abundant collagen bundles with or without associated increases in elastic tissue.[72] Such histologic changes are difficult to appreciate unless a skin biopsy includes adjacent normal skin for comparison.

Diagnosis and Differential Diagnosis   The lesions are so characteristic that they are seldom misdiagnosed. Examination for possible associated systemic disease may be necessary.

Common Congenital Malformations of Skin

Congenital malformations are developmental defects in skin formation frequently observed in newborns. They are observed in 7 of 100 live births.[73] Ear anomalies are found in 3 of 1000 live births, and simian crease as well as lip pits are seen in 2 per 1000 live births.

Ear Anomalies

Minor abnormalities in the formation of the ear are the most common congenital malformation. Loss of the fold of the skin in the superior part of the helix is the most common type of ear anomaly.[73] Low-set ears that angle away from the eye, periauricular skin tags, auricular or preauricular pits, or auricular sinuses and/or small ears are less common. Deafness may accompany congenital malformations of the external ear or they may be associated with hemifacial microsomia (Goldenhar's syndrome).

Digital Abnormalities

A single crease on one or both upper palms is called a *simian crease*.[1,73] It is one feature of Down's syndrome but also may be observed in a variety of other syndromes, including trisomy 13, the Cornelia de Lange's syndrome, Seckel's syndrome, and the cri du chat syndrome.[73] Clinodactyly with inward curvature of a digit is often observed in the fifth finger, and overlapping of the second and third toes is also a frequently observed malformation. Partial or complete fusion (syndactyly) of the second or third toes and clubfoot also occur with relative frequency.

Genital Abnormalities

Hydrocele of one testis and hypospadias are the most common genital anomalies and malformations observed.[73] Malformations of the external genitalia may be clues to urinary tract anomalies, and investigation of the urinary tract may be indicated. They may also be clues to chromosomal abnormalities and may be associated with undescended testes.

Epicanthal Folds

Epicanthal folds of skin on the inner aspect of each eye are frequently observed. They are present in patients with chromosomal abnormalities such as Down's, Turner's, and Klinefelter's syndromes.[73]

Neural Tube Defects

Primary defects in neural tube closures, such as meningomyelocele, encephalocele, and anencephaly are relatively frequent congenital malformations.[73] In some instances, a tuft of hair that is longer and more pigmented than the adjacent scalp hair overlies the affected area of skull and is a cutaneous clue to an underlying neural tube defect.

Abnormalities of the Lip and Mouth

Pits in the lips are common. Cleft lip and cleft palate, or cleft lip alone, is less common. The finding of lip pits or cleft lips and/or cleft palate may be a clue to the so-called first arch syndrome which includes a small jaw and ocular hypertelorism.[73] A number of syndromes are associated with the first arch syndrome including Pierre Robin syndrome, orofaciodigital syndrome, and Treacher Collins syndrome.

Skin Dimpling

Infants may develop small, dimple-like, depressed scars as a result of injury during amniocentesis.[74] The skin over the lesion appears to be pulled in by absent dermis. The lesion may not be noticed until the infant is several month old and has developed additional subcutaneous fat.

Major Chromosomal Abnormalities

Chromosomal abnormalities are phenotypic expressions of an abnormal number or arrangement of chromosomes.

Epidemiology   Chromosomal abnormalities occur in 1 of 200 live births, in a higher percentage of births resulting in perinatal death, and in up to 50 percent of spontaneous abortions. Trisomy 21 is seen in 1 per 800 live births. Trisomy 18 is observed in 1 per 3000 live births, and trisomy 13-15 occurs in 1 per 5000 live births.

Trisomy 21 (Down's Syndrome)   Mothers over 40 years of age have an increased chance of giving birth to a child with Down's syndrome. Cutaneous features are most useful in recognizing this syndrome. They include prominent epicanthal folds, eyes slanting upward, small ears, simian palmar crease, excessive skin over the back of the neck, and clinodactyly of the fifth fingers.[73] These cutaneous features, plus muscular hypotonia and evidence of congenital heart disease, are the major clinical characteristics. Chromosomal analysis confirms the diagnosis. Mental retardation may be severe, and growth failure associated with congenital heart disease makes the prognosis poor.[73]

Trisomy 18 and Trisomy 13-15   In both of these chromosomal abnormalities, increased parental age has been an associated feature. Babies with trisomy 18 or trisomy 13-15 are small for gestational age, have low-set ears, simian creases, congenital heart disease, and severe mental retardation.[73] The presence of a cleft lip and palate associated with these features makes trisomy 13-15 more likely, while rocker-bottom feet and flexion contractures of the fingers make trisomy 18 more likely to be diagnosed.[73] Chromosomal analysis is required for precise diagnosis.

Turner's Syndrome   The most common sex chromosome anomaly is Turner's syndrome, in which only one X chromosome is present (XO). Newborns with Turner's syndrome exhibit webbing of the neck and marked edema of the hands and feet.[73] The neck is often quite short. Coarctation of the aorta may be an associated feature. Chromosomal analysis is necessary to confirm the diagnosis.

Klinefelter's Syndrome   Extra sex chromosomes are characteristic of Klinefelter's syndrome (XXY, XXXY, or XXXXY). A low birth weight, undescended testes, and a small penis lead to suspicion of this syndrome.[73] Hypotonia and a variety of other anomalies may also be observed. Mental deficiency is usually severe in those with this syndrome, and chromosomal analysis is required to confirm the diagnosis.

Ichthyosis (See also Chap. 42)

Ichthyosis is the term used to describe excessive scaling of the skin, which may be "fish-scale-like." It is thought to occur in 1 per 200 live births.

Etiology and Pathogenesis   All forms of ichthyosis observed in the newborn period are hereditary. Although normal infants born after 40 to 42 weeks of gestation display some scaling, as do dysmature infants, the scaling of ichthyosis is usually generalized and characterized by thick scales. Four major types of ichthyosis have been described:[75] Lamellar ichthyosis and bullous ichthyosis usually appear at birth with severe scaling. Ichthyosis vulgaris and X-linked ichthyosis may be present in the neonate or may be expressed later in childhood.

Pathology   Skin biopsy of patients with the ichthyosis syndromes often has diagnostic value. In patients with ichthyosis vulgaris, there is a thin or absent granular cell layer in addition to the hyperkeratosis. X-linked ichthyosis demonstrates hyperkeratosis with an otherwise normal-appearing epidermis.[76] Vacuolization and separation of the granular cell layer with blister cavity formation are associated with the hyperkeratosis in bullous ichthyosis. Biopsy in patients with lamellar ichthyosis may demonstrate hyperkeratosis, acanthosis, and a mild chronic inflammatory infiltrate.

Diagnosis and Differential Diagnosis   At birth, lamellar ichthyosis and bullous ichthyosis may be difficult to distinguish from one another.[76] The hereditary pattern and skin biopsy may help. As the infants age, corneal opacities and sparing of the palms and soles will distinguish X-linked ichthyosis; ectropion and eclabium will distinguish lamellar ichthyosis; and recurrent bullous episodes will distinguish epidermolytic hyperkeratosis. Measurement of steroid sulfatase activity in red blood cells may be useful in the diagnosis of X-linked ichthyosis.[76] Scaling disorders similar to lamellar ichthyosis are found in patients with many ichthyosis syndromes associated with neurologic disease.[75,76] In those with the Sjögren-Larsson syndrome, a defect in fatty alchohol dehydrogenase has been found.

Treatment   There is no satisfactory treatment for the ichthyoses. In patients with ichthyosis vulgaris and X-linked ichthyosis, hydration of the skin twice daily and the generous use of lubricants control dryness and scaling. Alpha-hydroxy acids such as lactic acid 5% ointment, citric acid 5% ointment, or 12% ammonium lactate lotion (Lac-Hydrin) applied once or more daily, may be helpful in patients with the more severe ichthyoses, although many such patients do as well with bland lubricants alone. In patients with bullous ichthyoses, systemic antistaphylococcal antibiotics are required to treat the bullous impetigo during the episodes of ichthyosis.

Great caution must be used in applying any topical agent to the skin of an infant or child. Because of their larger surface area per body weight, systemic toxicity and side effects are a risk. Topical therapy can also lead to acidosis. Recognize that both the active medication and the vehicle for the medication could cause significant toxicity in infants with significant dermatitis or even normal skin. The synthetic retinoids given orally have shown promise in the management of ichthyosis, but their use is still experimental.

Ichthyosis Vulgaris   Ichthyosis vulgaris is inherited as an autosomal dominant disease that may affect as many as 1 in 250 individuals.[75] The skin in patients with ichthyosis vulgaris usually remains normal throughout the newborn period.

X-Linked Ichthyosis   X-linked ichthyosis may appear at birth but usually appears later in infancy with scales over the posterior neck, upper trunk, and extensor surfaces of the extremities. As the child ages, the scales often become thicker and a dirty-yellow or brown color.[75] Scaling is usually mild during the first 30 days of life, and the skin is a normal color. Corneal opacities may be seen on slit-lamp examination of the eye of adults, both in patients and in carrier mothers. Palms and soles are spared, in contrast with the other forms of ichthyosis. An associated steroid sulfatase deficiency has been described in patients with X-linked ichthyoses.[75]

Lamellar Ichthyosis and Congenital Nonbullous Ichthyosiform Erythroderma   These two names are often used for the same condition. Although both conditions appear to be an autosomal-recessive trait, two separate disease entities may exist.[76] Patients with nonbullous congenital ichthyosiform erythroderma have generalized fine scales on erythematous skin.[76] Patients with lamellar ichthyosis have larger, darker, platelike scales with or without erythematosus skin. Infants with either condition can be born with a collodion membrane (Fig. 239-9). The erythroderma may fade during childhood in some patients. Ectropion and eclabium may appear shortly after birth in patients with lamellar ichthyosis.[76] The palms and soles in these patients may be greatly thickened. Skin biopsy after the collodion membrane is shed demonstrates hyperkeratosis but is otherwise not diagnostic.

Bullous Ichthyosis (Congenital Bullous Ichthyosiform Erythroderma, Epidermolytic Hyperkeratosis)   Epidermolytic hyperkeratosis, an autosomal-dominant disorder, is characterized by extensive scaling at birth, erythroderma, and recurrent episodes of bullae formation (Fig. 239-9).

ETIOLOGY AND PATHOGENESIS.   In patients with lamellar ichthyosis and bullous ichthyosis increased epidermal turnover produces excessive numbers of stratum corneum cells.[76,77] In contrast,

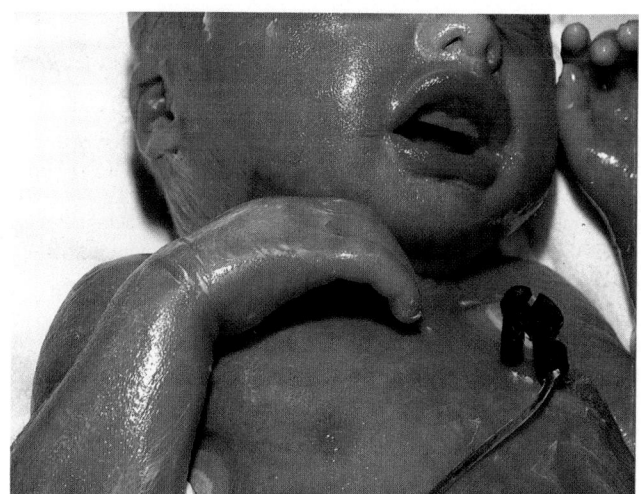

FIGURE 239-9 Collodion baby. A newborn encased in a tight membrane restricting movement.

patients with X-linked ichthyosis and ichthyosis vulgaris have normal epidermal turnover, and the accumulated scale is believed to be due to faulty shedding of the stratum corneum.[76] The role of the associated steroid sulfatase deficiency in X-linked ichthyosis is not known.[76]

CLINICAL MANIFESTATIONS.   The blisters of epidermolytic hyperkeratosis represent lysis of the epidermal granular layer, and secondary infection with *S. aureus* becomes a major difficulty in the neonatal period and during infancy.[75] As the child ages, the involvement becomes more limited. By school age, thick, warty, dirty-yellow scales with malodorous excessive bacterial colonization of the skin will have developed on the palms, soles, elbows, and knees.[75] Skin biopsy will reveal enlargement of the granular cell layer with bizarre vacuolization of the epidermal granular cells.

Pathology   Skin biopsy of the patients with the ichthyosis syndromes often has diagnostic value. In patients with ichthyosis vulgaris, there is a thin or absent granular cell layer in addition to the hyperkeratosis. X-linked ichthyosis demonstrates hyperkeratosis with an otherwise normal-appearing epidermis.[76] Vacuolization and separation of the granular cell layer with blister cavity formation are associated with the hyperkeratosis in bullous ichthyosis. Biopsy in patients with lamellar ichthyosis may demonstrate hyperkeratosis, acanthosis, and a mild chronic inflammatory infiltrate.

Diagnosis and Differential Diagnosis   At birth, lamellar ichthyosis and bullous ichthyosis may be difficult to distinguish from one another.[76] The hereditary pattern and skin biopsy may help. As the infants age, corneal opacities and sparing of the palms and soles will distinguish X-linked ichthyosis; ectropion and eclabium will distinguish lamellar ichthyosis; and recurrent bullous episodes will distinguish epidermolytic hyperkeratosis. Measurement of steroid sulfatase activity in red blood cells may be useful in the diagnosis of X-linked ichthyosis.[76] Scaling disorders similar to lamellar ichthyosis are found in patients with many ichthyosis syndromes associated with neurologic disease.[75,76] In those with the Sjögren-Larsson syndrome, a defect in fatty alcohol dehydrogenase has been found.

Treatment   There is no satisfactory treatment for the ichthyoses. In patients with ichthyosis vulgaris and X-linked ichthyosis, hydration of the skin twice daily and the generous use of lubricants control dryness and scaling. Alpha-hydroxy acids such as 5% lactic acid ointment, 5% citric acid ointment, or 12% ammonium lactate lotion (Lac-Hydrin), applied once or more daily, may be helpful in patients with the more severe ichthyoses, although many such patients do as well with bland lubricants alone. In patients with bullous ichthyoses, systemic antistaphylococcal antibiotics are required to treat the bullous impetigo during the episodes of ichthyosis.

Great caution must be used in applying any topical agent to the skin of an infant or child. Because of their larger surface area per body weight, systemic toxicity and side effects are a risk. Topical therapy can also lead to acidosis. Recognize that both the active medication and the vehicle for the medication could cause significant toxicity in infants with significant dermatitis or even normal skin. The synthetic retinoids given orally have shown promise in the management of ichthyosis, but their use is still experimental.

Hereditary Skin Diseases with Dramatic Neonatal Presentations

The Red, Scaly Newborn

Physiologic Scaling and Redness   A scaling and often red newborn may be an enigma to the inexperienced observer. A postmature baby may exhibit marked desquamation over the hands, feet, and lower trunk. If observed during the first day of life when the newborn skin is quite red, desquamation may result in an erroneous diagnosis of one of the ichthyoses.[1] Similarly, preterm infants born at 32 weeks of gestational age or earlier have red or glistening skin that similarly may be confused with ichthyosis. Such changes are transient and are often resolved within the newborn period.

Collodion Baby (See Chap. 42)   A collodion membrane is an encasement of shiny, tight, inelastic scale (Fig. 239-9). The membrane is composed of greatly thickened stratum corneum that has been saturated with water.[76,77] As the water content evaporates in extrauterine life, large fissures appear in the membrane and the membrane is shed, revealing red skin underneath. Collodion babies are quite rare.

Collodion babies appear to be tightly encased in a membrane at birth. Their appearance is frightening to health care personnel. A collodion membrane does not necessarily mean that the affected baby will develop ichthyosis, and spontaneous healing may occur. Skin biopsy of the collodion membrane is usually not diagnostic. Most collodion babies do have a form of ichthyosis, and most develop features of lamellar ichthyosis. Bullous ichthyosis, X-linked ichthyosis, and Gaucher's disease have also been reported to develop in collodion babies.[75,76]

Harlequin Fetus   A harlequin fetus is an infant born with massive plates of scales. Although this condition has been considered a more severe form of lamellar ichthyosis, most authorities now believe that it represents a distinct, rare autosomal-recessive disease. It has been associated with defects in both lipid and protein metabolism.

Harlequin fetus is usually incompatible with extrauterine life. These infants have massive, dense, platelike scales, which produce severe deformities of skeletal and soft tissues that restrict respiration.[75,76] Recently, infants treated with heroic methods have survived with residual severe ichthyosis.

Atopic Dermatitis and Seborrheic Dermatitis (See Chap. 120)

Atopic dermatitis is said to have its onset after the newborn period; the most frequently observed age of onset is 2 to 3 months.[78] If a dermatitis begins within the newborn period, many authorities designate it seborrheic dermatitis. It has now become clear, however, that infants who later develop typical atopic dermatitis may have the onset of their skin eruption within the newborn period.[1,78] In infants who have seborrheic and atopic dermatitis, there is a significant overlap both in distributions of the lesions, which involve the scalp, diaper area, and extensor area, and in the history of pruritus, feeding patterns, food intolerance, and family members with atopic disease. In newborns the dermatitis is usually acute, with extensive crusting and oozing. Physiologic overproduction of sebum occurs in the newborn period, giving any dermatitis a greasy feel to the skin surface. It is advisable to designate dermatitis seen in newborns as simply dermatitis.

Diaper Dermatitis

Diaper dermatitis occurring in the newborn period is primarily perianal and is related to the irritant substances found in stool.[79] It presents as a bright red perianal acute dermatitis. Superinfection with *Candida albicans* is frequent in neonatal perianal diaper dermatitis that lasts longer than 72 h. The role of diapers in the newborn period in preventing perianal diaper dermatitis is unclear.[80]

Scabies (See Chap. 225)

Newborns with scabies may present with a severe generalized dermatitis. They may have only a few or as many as thousands of lesions. Babies usually have involvement of the head and neck.[81] Individual burrows may be obscured and difficult to detect because of the confluence of dermatitis. The scabies mite can be recovered from papules or burrows; the hands and feet are the best sites of recovery.[81]

Histiocytosis X (See Chap. 160)

A generalized dermatitis, particularly with purpuric papules or petechiae within the dermatitis and involvement of the head and neck, is characteristic of histiocytosis X (Fig. 239-10). The skin eruption may be present at birth or may begin during the first 30 days of life. Chronic draining ears and enlargement of the liver and spleen are useful additional clues in the diagnosis.[82] Skin biopsy demonstrates the characteristic infiltration with histiocytic cells containing Langerhans-like granules.

Congenital Candidiasis

Congenital candidiasis may present at birth as generalized eczematous, scaly skin.[25] In such cases the birth canal is always infected with *Candida*. Direct microscopic examination of scales scraped from the skin's surface demonstrate yeast forms.

Epidermolysis Bullosa (See Chap. 60)

Several types of epidermolysis bullosa are evident within the first 24 h of life. Hemorrhagic blisters and bleeding erosions may be extensive. Nursery personnel may induce numerous lesions while handling the baby before the diagnosis is recognized. Other forms of epidermolysis bullosa may begin slowly, with a few lesions beginning 3 to 30 days after birth.

Diagnosis of epidermolysis bullosa in the immediate newborn period may be difficult.[83,84] There are many different types of epidermolysis bullosa that may result in mild to lethal disease.[84,85] The number of blisters in the neonate does not define the severity of the disease. The final diagnosis of the patient depends on characterization of the site of blister formation within the epidermis, basement membrane, or dermis, and on the clinical response of the patient. Diagnosis should be made through a combination of biopsies for both light and electron microscopy, and possibly by immunofluorescent mapping of antigenic sites within the basement membrane zone.[83] Extreme care must be taken in obtaining and

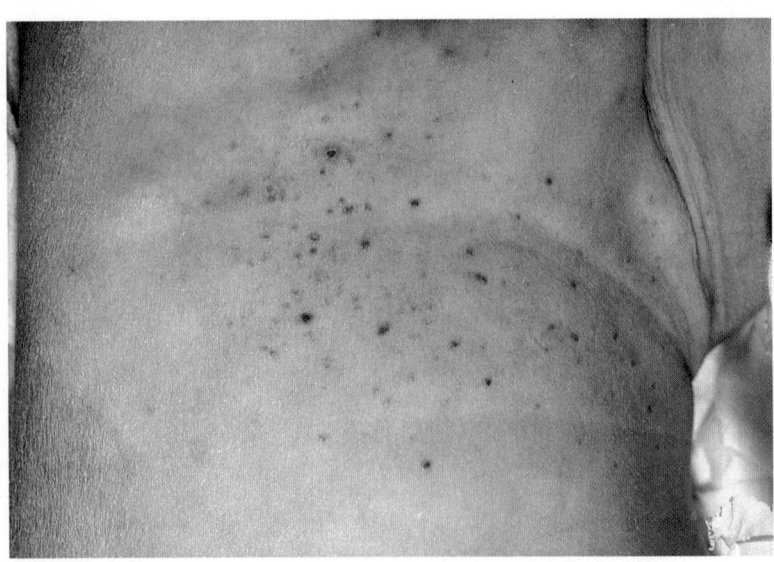

FIGURE 239-10 Histiocytosis X. A 4-week-old with enlarged inguinal lymph nodes and purpuric papules on the lower abdomen.

interpreting skin biopsies from newborns to distinguish among these mechanobullous diseases. A shave or ellipse biopsy at the edge of a blister that is less than 12 h old is preferred.

All forms of epidermolysis bullosa are related to adherence defects within the skin. Abnormalities of type VII collagen are suspected in recessive dystrophic epidermolysis bullosa, while in junctional epidermolysis bullosa, the absence of a lamina lucida protein has been noted.[87] Assistance with diagnosis and therapy can be provided by:

National Epidermolysis Bullosa Registry Headquarters[85]
The Rockefeller University
1230 York Avenue
New York, NY 10021

Acrodermatitis Enteropathica (See Chap. 146)

Acrodermatitis enteropathica is an autosomal-recessive disorder of zinc metabolism.[87]

Etiology and Pathogenesis Depletion of body zinc stores due to faulty absorption of zinc is responsible for the symptoms and signs of acrodermatitis enteropathica. It is not known whether this depletion is caused by the lack of a zinc carrier protein or by some defect of zinc absorption in the intestine. Zinc is stored in the same tissues as iron and serves as an important cofactor for a variety of enzymes such as alkaline phosphatase and carbonic anhydrase.[87] It is thought that zinc deficiency results in impairment of metalloenzyme activity, which produces the clinical features.

Clinical Manifestations Acrodermatitis enteropathica is not apparent at birth, but begins at 15 to 30 days of age, with acral skin erosions, diarrhea, and failure to thrive.[87] The erosions appear as red, moist areas over the distal extremities, including the hands and feet (Fig. 239-11), and in the perioral and perineal areas.

Often, the cutaneous features precede the diarrhea by several weeks to several months. As the disorder continues, weight loss occurs, as well as photophobia, apathy, alopecia, thrush, and paronychia due to *C. albicans*. If the child survives the infectious complications of malnutrition, the skin lesions become erythematous plaques with silvery scales that mimic psoriasis.

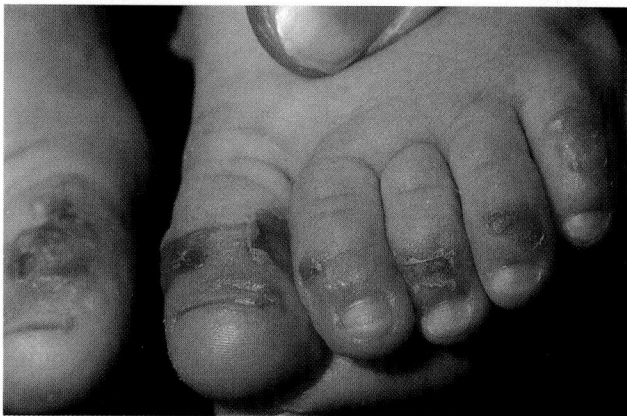

FIGURE 239-11 Acrodermatitis enteropathica. Zinc deficiency in a newborn caused erosions and crusting around the toes.

Diagnosis and Differential Diagnosis The diagnosis is made by measuring serum or plasma zinc levels.[87] There are many sources of zinc contamination in rubber stoppers and glass tubes and other blood-collecting devices that produce falsely high zinc levels. Thus the diagnosis may be obscured. Therefore blood samples should be taken with acid-washed plastic syringes and collected in acid-washed sterile plastic tubes.

Zinc deficiency also occurs in premature and term infants who are fed a diet deficient in zinc. Their clinical picture mimics that of acrodermatitis enteropathica. Occasionally, human breast milk can be low in zinc and lead to zinc deficiency in totally breast-fed infants. The lesions are often mistaken for mucocutaneous candidiasis associated with immune deficiency. Plasma or serum zinc levels distinguish between the two. Often, protein-calorie malnutrition states are considered, but lesions usually develop in such patients after 6 months of age, and the nutritional history may distinguish between the two. Histiocytosis X presents with intertriginous erosions in infancy. Acquired zinc deficiency states, such as those seen with prolonged parenteral hyperalimentation, mimic acrodermatitis enteropathica.[87]

Treatment Oral zinc sulfate, 5 mg/kg daily given in two doses, produces rapid clinical improvement.[87] Apathy disappears within 24 h, and the skin lesions and diarrhea resolve within 7 to 14 days. Photophobia, alopecia, and growth failure are reversed over the ensuing months. It is not known whether lifetime maintenance with supplemental zinc is required.

Incontinentia Pigmenti (See Chap. 80)

Incontinentia pigmenti is a hereditary condition characterized by linear rows of blisters on skin associated with ocular, CNS, and dental defects.

Etiology and Pathogenesis Incontinentia pigmenti is believed to be an X-linked trait that is lethal to males, a characteristic that explains the female predominance in this disorder.[86,88]

Clinical Manifestations Linear rows of blisters on the extremities are seen at birth (Fig. 239-12). Occasionally the trunk is also involved. These blistering episodes recur over the first 3 months of life and are replaced by warty linear areas that may last until 1 year of age.[86] Rows of brown pigmentation are then left. In addition, swirls of brown pigmentation are found on the trunk and in areas where the blisters and warty lesions did not occur. The pigmentation fades as the child ages and is usually not seen after adolescence.[88] Mental retardation, seizures, microcephaly, and other central nervous system disorders occur in 30 percent of the patients. Ocular and skeletal anomalies may also be noted.[86,88]

Pathology Skin biopsy demonstrates an inflammatory dermatitis with subcorneal vesicles filled with numerous eosinophils.[86] The warty stage is characterized merely by hyperkeratosis and chronic inflammation in the dermis. In the pigmentary stage, melanin is found free in the dermis or engulfed by dermal macrophages; this characteristic accounts for the term incontinentia pigmenti.

Diagnosis and Differential Diagnosis In the blistering stage, herpes simplex or bullous impetigo may be confused with incontinentia pigmenti, but the linear arrangement of its blisters and appropri-

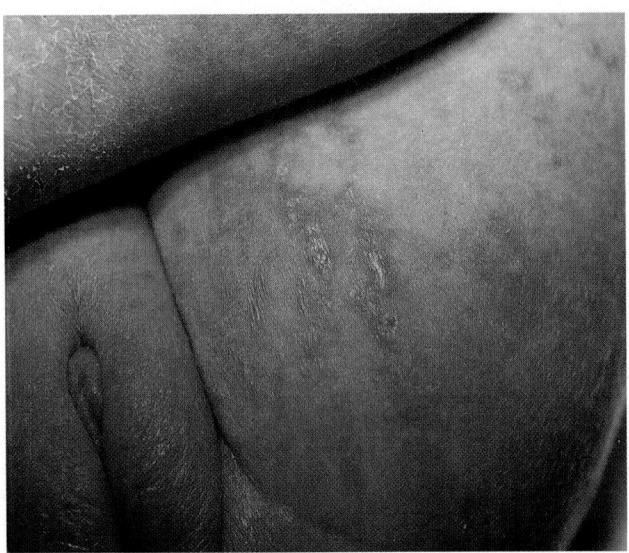

FIGURE 239-12 Incontinentia pigmenti. A newborn girl with linear rows of blisters.

ate cultures will distinguish it from these two disorders. The warty phase may mimic linear epidermal birthmarks or warts. The hyperpigmentation is uniquely arranged in whorls and is unlikely to be confused with other causes of hyperpigmentation.

Treatment There is no satisfactory treatment.

References

1. Weston WL, Lane AT. *Color Textbook of Pediatric Dermatology.* St. Louis, Mosby-Yearbook, 1991
2. Holbrook KA, Smith LT. Ultrastructural aspects of human skin during the embryonic, fetal, premature, neonatal and adult periods of life. *Birth Defects, Original Article Series XVI* 1:9, 1981
3. Lane AT. Human fetal skin development. *Pediatr Dermatol* 3:487, 1986
4. Fairley JA, Rasmussen JE. Comparison of stratum corneum thickness in children and adults. *J Am Acad Dermatol* 8:652, 1983
5. West DP, et al. Pharmacology and toxicology of infant skin. *J Invest Dermatol* 76:147, 1981
6. Lane AT. Development and care of the premature infant's skin. *Pediatr Dermatol* 4:1, 1987
7. Vernon HJ et al. The effect of a semipermeable dressing on transepidermal water loss in premature infants. *Pediatrics* 86:357, 1990
8. Harpin VA, Rutter N. Sweating in preterm babies. *J Pediatr* 100:614, 1982
9. Smales ORC, Kime R. Thermoregulation in babies immediately after birth. *Arch Dis Child* 53:58, 1978
10. Jorgenson RJ et al. Intraoral findings and anomalies in neonates. *Pediatrics* 69:577, 1982
11. Levy HL, Cothram F. Erythema toxicum neonatorum present at birth. *Am J Dis Child* 103:617, 1962
12. Ramamurthy R, Esterly NB. Transient neonatal pustular melanosis. *J Pediatr* 88:831, 1976
13. Murphy WF, Langley AL. Common bullous lesions—presumably self-inflicted—occurring in utero in the newborn infant. *Pediatrics* 32:1099, 1963

14. Fretzin DF, Arias AM. Sclerema neonatorum and subcutaneous fat necrosis of the newborn. *Pediatr Dermatol* 4:112, 1987
15. Norwood-Galloway A et al: Subcutaneous fat necrosis of the newborn with hypercalcemia. *J Am Acad Dermatol* 16:435, 1987
16. Thomsen RJ. Subcutaneous fat necrosis of the newborn and idiopathic hypercalcemia. *Arch Dermatol* 116:1155, 1980
17. Heilbron B et al. Scleredema in an infant. *Arch Dermatol* 122:1417, 1986
18. Philip AG, Hewitt JR. Early diagnosis of neonatal sepsis. *Pediatrics* 65:1036, 1980
19. Duke EMC. Infantile acne associated with transient increases in plasma concentrations of leuteinizing hormone, follicle-stimulating hormone and testosterone. *Br Med J* 282:1275, 1981
20. Kamm LA, Giacola GP. Congenital cutaneous candidiasis. *Am J Dis Child* 129:1215, 1975
21. Jarratt M, Ramsdell W. Infantile acropustulosis. *Arch Dermatol* 115:834, 1979
22. Cantu JM et al. Familial comedones. *Arch Dermatol* 114:1807, 1978
23. Farber EM, Jacobs AH. Infantile psoriasis. *Am J Dis Child* 131:1266, 1977
24. Boucher FD et al: A prospective evaluation of primary genital herpes simplex virus type 2 infections acquired during pregnancy. *Pediatr Infect Dis J* 9:499, 1990
25. Kibrick S. Herpes simplex infection at term: What to do with mother, newborn, and nursery personnel. *JAMA* 243:147, 1980
26. Prober CG et al. Use of routine viral cultures at delivery to identify neonates exposed to herpes simplex virus. *N Engl J Med* 318:887, 1988
27. Whitley R et al. A controlled trial comparing vidarabine with acyclovir in neonatal herpes simplex virus infection. *N Engl J Med* 324:494, 1991
28. Whitley RJ et al. Changing presentation of herpes simplex virus infection in neonates. *Infect Dis* 158:109, 1988
29. Rubin L et al. Disseminated varicella in a neonate: Implications for immunoprophylaxis of neonates postnatally exposed to varicella. *Pediatr Infect Dis* 5:100, 1986
30. Brice JEH. Congenital varicella resulting from infection during the second trimester of pregnancy. *Arch Dis Child* 51:474, 1976
31. Lipton SV, Brunell PA. Management of varicella exposure in a neonatal intensive care unit. *J Am Acad Dermatol* 261:1782, 1989
32. Dancer SJ et al. Outbreak of staphylococcal scalded skin syndrome among neonates. *J Infection* 16:87, 1988
33. Curran FP, Al-Salihi FL. Neonatal staphylococcal scalded skin syndrome: Massive outbreak due to an unusual phage type. *Pediatrics* 66:285, 1980
34. Rudoy RC, Nelson JD. Breast abscess during the neonatal period. A review. *Am J Dis Child* 129:1031, 1975
35. Fiumara NJ. Syphilis in newborn children. *Clin Obstet Gynecol* 18:183, 1975
36. Dudgeon JA. Congenital rubella. *J Pediatr* 87:1078, 1975
37. Jacobs AH, Walton RG. The incidence of birthmarks in the neonate. *Pediatrics* 58:218, 1976
38. Nanda A et al. Survey of cutaneous lesions in Indian newborns. *Pediatr Dermatol* 6:39, 1989
39. Alper JC, Holmes LB. The incidence and significance of birthmarks in a cohort of 4,641 newborns. *Pediatr Dermatol* 1:58, 1983
40. Hidano A et al. Statistical survey of skin changes in Japanese neonates. *Pediatr Dermatol* 3:140, 1986
41. Mulliken JB, Glowacki J. Hemangiomas and vascular malformations in infants and children: A classification based on endothelial characteristics. *Plast Reconstr Surg* 69:412, 1982
42. Leung AKC, Telmesani AMA. Salmon patches in Caucasian children. *Pediatr Dermatol* 6:185, 1989
43. Barsky SH et al. The nature and evolution of port-wine stains: A computer-assisted study. *J Invest Dermatol* 74:154, 1980
44. Shamir R et al. Nevus flammeus. *Am J Dis Child* 145:85, 1991
45. Enjolras O et al. Facial port-wine stains and Sturge-Weber syndrome. *Pediatrics* 76:48, 1985

46. Paller AS. The Sturge-Weber syndrome. *Pediatr Dermatol* **4**:300, 1987

47. Talman B et al. Location of port-wine stain and the likelihood of ophthalmologic or CNS complications. *Pediatrics* **87**:323, 1991

48. Lindenauer SM. The Klippel-Trenaunay syndrome. *Ann Surg* **162**:303, 1965

49. Tan OT, Gilchrest BA. Laser therapy for selected cutaneous vascular lesions in the pediatric population: A review. *Pediatrics* **82**:652, 1988

50. Garden JM et al. The treatment of port-wine stains by the pulsed dye laser. *Arch Dermatol* **124**:889, 1988

51. Simpson JR, Lond MB. Natural history of cavernous hemangiomata. *Lancet* **2**:1057, 1959

52. Esterly NB. Kasabach-Merritt syndrome in infants. *J Am Acad Dermatol* **8**:504, 1983

53. Amir J et al. Strawberry hemangioma in preterm infants. *Pediatr Dermatol* **3**:331, 1986

54. Sasaki GH et al. Pathogenesis and treatment of infant skin strawberry hemangiomas: Clinical and in vitro studies of hormonal effects. *Plast Reconstr Surg* **73**:359, 1984

55. Lewis-Jones MS et al. Cutis marmorata telangiectatica congenita—a report of two cases occurring in male children. *Clin Exp Dermatol* **13**:97, 1988

56. South DA, Jacobs AH. Cutis marmorata telangiectatica congenita. *J Pediatr* **93**:944, 1978

57. Esterly NB et al. Special symposia: The management of disseminated eruptive hemangiomata in infants. *Pediatr Dermatol* **1**:313, 1984

58. Golitz LE et al. Diffuse neonatal hemangiomatosis. *Pediatr Dermatol* **3**:145, 1986

59. Oranje AP. Blue rubber bleb nevus syndrome. *Pediatr Dermatol* **3**:304, 1986

60. Flanagan BP, Helwig EB. Cutaneous lymphangioma. *Arch Dermatol* **113**:24, 1977

61. Lau JTK, Ching RML. Mongolian spots in Chinese children. *Am J Dis Child* **136**:863, 1982

62. Huson S. Recent developments in the diagnosis and management of neurofibromatosis. *Arch Dis Child* **64**:745, 1989

63. Hurwitz S. Pigmented nevi. *Semin Dermatol* **7**:17, 1988

64. Castilla EE et al. Epidemiology of congenital pigmented naevi. II. Risk factors. *Br J Dermatol* **104**:307, 1981

65. Gari LM et al. Melanomas arising in large congenital nevi: A prospective study. *Pediatr Dermatol* **5**:151, 1988

66. McWilliams RC, Stephenson JBP. Depigmented hair. The earliest sign of tuberous sclerosis. *Arch Dis Child* **53**:961, 1978

67. Bolognia J, Pawlek JM. Biology of hypopigmentation. *J Am Acad Dermatol* **19**:217, 1988

68. Rogers M et al. Epidermal nevi and the epidermal nevus syndrome. *J Am Acad Dermatol* **20**:476, 1989

69. Domingo J, Helwig EB. Malignant neoplasms associated with nevus sebaceous of Jadassohn. *J Am Acad Dermatol* **1**:545, 1979

70. Frieden IJ. Aplasia cutis congenita: A clinical review and proposal for classification. *J Am Acad Dermatol* **26**:646, 1986

71. McCray MK, Roenigk HH. Scalp reduction for correction of cutis aplasia congenita. *J Dermatol Surg Oncol* **7**:655, 1981

72. Uitto J et al. Connective tissue nevi of the skin. *J Am Acad Dermatol* **3**:441, 1980

73. Holmes LB. Congenital malformations. *N Engl J Med* **295**:204, 1976

74. Bruce S et al. Skin dimpling associated with midtrimester amniocentesis. *Pediatr Dermatol* **2**:140, 1984

75. Rand RE, Baden HP. The ichthyoses—a review. *J Am Acad Dermatol* **8**:285, 1983

76. Williams ML, Elias PM. Heterogeneity in autosomal recessive ichthyosis. *Arch Dermatol* **121**:477, 1985

77. Hazell M, Marks R. Clinical, histologic, and cell kinetic discriminants between lamellar ichthyosis and nonbullous congenital ichthyosiform erythroderma. *Arch Dermatol* **121**:489, 1985

78. Yates VM et al. Early diagnosis of infantile seborrheic dermatitis and atopic dermatitis. Clinical features. *Br J Dermatol* **108**:633, 1983

79. Weston WL et al. Diaper dermatitis: Current concepts. *Pediatrics* **66**:532, 1980

80. Lane AT et al. Evaluations of diapers containing absorbent gelling material with conventional disposable diapers in newborn infants. *Am J Dis Child* **144**:315, 1990

81. Honig PJ. Bites and parasites. *Pediatr Clin North Am* **30**:563, 1983

82. Roper SS, Spraker MK. Cutaneous histiocytosis syndromes. *Pediatr Dermatol* **3**:19, 1985

83. Eady RAJ, Tidman MJ. Diagnosing epidermolysis bullosa. *Br J Dermatol* **108**:621, 1983

84. Fine JD et al. Revised clinical and laboratory criteria for subtypes of inherited epidermolysis bullosa. *J Am Acad Dermatol* **24**:119, 1991

85. Lin AN, Carter M. Epidermolysis bullosa: When the skin falls apart. *J Pediatr* **114**:349, 1989

86. Carney RG., Jr. Incontinentia pigmenti. *Arch Dermatol* **112**:535, 1976

87. Arlette JP. Zinc and the skin. *Pediatr Clin North Am* **30**:583, 1983

88. Wiklund DA, Weston WL. Incontinentia pigmenti: A four-generation study. *Arch Dermatol* **116**:477, 1980

CHAPTER 240

Nancy B. Lyon and Thomas B. Fitzpatrick

Geriatric Dermatology

Skin and Aging

Have you not a moist eye, a dry hand, a yellow cheek, a white beard, a decreasing leg, an increasing belly?
William Shakespeare, King Henry IV Part II, I, ii, 206

The aging process, unlike the specific diseases described throughout medical textbooks, inevitably affects all persons. Government and institutions arbitrarily define the geriatric population as those persons over 65 years of age. However, it is important to recognize that aging is a continuous process with a variable spectrum of manifestations. While chronologic age is a precise measurement, the physiologic age of an individual does not strictly correlate with chronologic age. Pathologic aging refers to abnormal deterioration resulting from disease. Aging, therefore is not as simplistic as it may seem.

Outward appearance loosely correlates with chronologic age and, surprisingly, correlates more strongly with physiologic age. Wrinkled and sagging skin are among the hallmarks of aging. These features are caused by an excessive laxity and loss of resiliency of the skin. In a study of 10,086 men (Longitudinal Study of the Gerontology Research Center in Baltimore, MD), Borkan and

Norris investigated the relationship between apparent age, chronologic age, and specific physiologic parameters (such as blood pressure, serum albumin and globulin, pulmonary function measurements). Individuals who appeared to be older than their chronologic age were biologically older as determined by 19 out of 24 different measurements. Kligman noted a relationship between the apparent age of a person as judged by outward appearance and the rate of chemical blistering provoked by a topical solution of 50% ammonium hydroxide. He also noted that subjects who looked older took the longest time to heal.

A confounding variable in interpreting the intrinsic changes that occur with aging in the skin is the environmental effect of prolonged sun exposure. The term *dermatoheliosis,* or *photoaging,* does not merely represent accelerated aging. Increasingly it has been appreciated that the damage resulting from chronic ultraviolet radiation exposure is distinctly separate and may compound the changes seen in intrinsic aging (refer to Table 10-4, "Features of Actinically Damaged Skin"). Several features of intrinsic aging have now been determined to contrast directly with sun-induced changes. The fine wrinkles of sun-protected aged skin contrast with the coarse furrows characteristic of cutaneous photodamage. These morphologic differences can undoubtedly be explained, at least in part, by the connective tissue of the dermis. However, dermal changes with intrinsic aging have not yet been clearly delineated. It is known that the dermis becomes thinned and less dense. Collagen fibers are coarser and less highly organized in three-dimensional array in contrast to young dermis. Elastic tissue fibers in young sun-protected skin are delicate and organized vertically to the dermal-epidermal junction. However, these are lost in aged, sun-protected skin and are tremendously increased and clumped into amorphous masses in sun-exposed skin. Truly aged skin uninfluenced by photochemistry and other extrinsic, environmentally imposed factors is most likely to be found in doubly protected areas such as the buttocks (refer to Table 10-1, "Histologic Features of Aging Human Skin").

The various diseases and disorders in geriatric dermatology are listed in Table 240-1. *This table includes two sets of numbers: the first lists cross-references to chapters in this book and the second refers to special discussions within this chapter of the features of these disorders and diseases that are unique to geriatric patients.* These discussions amplify the material presented in the various chapters of the book; for example, herpes zoster has different manifestations in elderly patients. Additionally, special reference should be made to Chap. 10, "Aging of Skin," and the tables contained therein.

1   Pruritus in Aging

Senile pruritus may be the most common disorder in elderly skin, particularly in persons over 80 years of age. It is usually associated with dry, rough, scaly skin. The pruritus is frequently worse at night and after hot baths or after the change in temperature associated with disrobing. Itch can be severe despite the lack of physical signs. It begins with xerosis, described below, frequently aggravated during winter months when the humidity is low and indoor temperatures high. Frequent bathing without the use of emollients can dry the skin further. Initially, there may be only microfissures, but the sensation of itch can be intense. Excoriations can lead to eczematous changes and eventually to infection, which can be subtle and can increase the itch sensation. Systemic causes of pruritus should be excluded. Contact dermatitis from topical medicaments may mimic xerosis. History is an important clue.

2   Connective Tissue Changes in Aging

2A   Wrinkling and Sagging Skin and Fragility   In distinct contrast to photoaged skin (see "Dermatoheliosis" below), sun-protected aged skin is uniformly pale, and the wrinkles are quite fine. Lines of facial expression are exaggerated, and there is laxity. The skin of an aged person is less resilient and is easily disrupted, with less friction and shear required to disturb its integrity. The skin may tear or even develop bullae. Blood vessels, too, are easily disrupted, leading to purpura. Some of the fragility of aged skin may be due to changes that can be seen with light microscopy.

Histologically, the stratum corneum of aged skin is unaltered, and the main change in the epidermis is a flattening of the dermal-epidermal junction. There is a slight increase in the quantity and thickness of elastic fibers in the dermis, and there is a loss of the delicate vertical elastic fibers at the dermal-epidermal junction. Collagen fibers become larger and more randomly organized, and there is a relative decrease in the proportion of soluble collagen. Glycosaminoglycans, so abundant in fetal skin, decrease rapidly early on so that adult levels are low and relatively stable. The vasculature is somewhat altered, with a relative loss of microvessels of the subepidermal capillary loops.

2B   Wound Healing   Wound healing occurs more slowly in old age. Epidermal kinetic studies demonstrate an age-related decrease in epidermal proliferation. Orentreich studied healing and epithelialization in a series of 12,000 full-face dermabrasion patients and found that healing was more efficient in younger patients, occurring in 10, 15, and 21 days, respectively, in 25-, 50-, and 75-year-old patients. It must be remembered, however, that the face is chronically sun exposed and therefore pathologic aging may be involved as well.

Wound dehiscence has been shown to increase with age following full-thickness surgical wounds. It is not known which specific factors are responsible for the delay, whether the defect lies in reepithelialization, revascularization, connective tissue synthesis, or decreased wound contraction.

3   Disorders of Altered Epidermal Kinetics

3A   Psoriasis Vulgaris   A bimodal onset of psoriasis exists with reported cases beginning from birth to 108 years. Most patients present in the third decade, with another peak (11.8 percent of 2400 patients) occurring in those over 55. With increasing age of onset there is a decrease in familial associations. Although plaque type psoriasis seems to decrease with age, flexural psoriasis tends to be more frequent in persons older than 60 years. An important therapeutic agent in psoriasis, methotrexate, may become easier to use; smaller doses may be based on a decrease in creatinine clearance, resulting in higher blood levels of methotrexate with lower doses. Psoriasis arthropathica peaks at 45 years, whereas psoriatic erythroderma peaks between 30 and 55 years. In the aged, psoriasis may lack its typical morphology, often appearing as a nonspecific eruption in unusual distributions. This blurred clinical appearance is consistent with the generalization that inflammatory reactions, regardless of course, are muted in the aged. Fewer vessels, to mention only one structural feature, reduce the inflammatory cascade.

3B   Xerosis   Rough, dry, scaling skin affects at least 75 percent of persons over the age of 64. Xerosis is esthetically unappealing, uncomfortable, pruritic, and can set the stage for eczematous erup-

TABLE 240-1
Geriatric Dermatology

	Chapter cross reference	Numbered discussions in this chapter		Chapter cross reference	Numbered discussions in this chapter
Pruritus in aging	10	1	Infections		12
Connective tissue changes in aging		2	Dermatophyte infections	194	12A
Wrinkling and sagging skin and fragility (not from sun exposure)	10	2A	Candidiasis: cutaneous, mucosal, and invasive	195	12B
Wound healing	9, 10, 238	2B	Cellulitis, including post coronary artery bypass	187	12C
Disorders of altered epidermal kinetics	11	3	Pyoderma	187	12D
Psoriasis vulgaris	39	3A	Herpes simplex: chronic herpetic ulcers, disseminated	203	
Xerosis	10, 42	3B	Herpes zoster: postzoster neuralgia, disseminated	204	12E
Vesicular and bullous diseases	53	4	Diphtheria: cutaneous, pharyngeal, and ocular	187	
Bullous pemphigoid	10,53	4A	Lyme borreliosis and acrodermatitis chronica obliterans	193	
Acneform disorders	63		Infestations		13
Rosacea	64		Scabies, including Norwegian	227	13A
Benign neoplasia	10, 77	5	Pediculosis pubis	227	
Cherry angioma	77		Pediculosis capita	227	
Skin tags (acrochordons)	77		Pediculosis corporis	227	
Colloid millium			Disorders of the feet		14
Cutaneous horns	73		Clavi, corns, calluses		14A
Fibroepithelioma			Bursitis		14B
Keratoacanthoma	76		Bunions		14C
Seborrheic keratoses	77		Intractable plantar keratoses		14D
Sebaceous adenoma (hyperplasia)	77		Neoplasia		14E
Clear cell acanthoma	77		Subungual exostosis	62	14F
Disorders of nails	62	6	Onychocryptosis	62	14G
Nail growth		6A	Onychauxis	62	14H
General aging-related nail changes	62	6B	Onycholysis	62	14I
Nail dystrophies	62	14G–K	Onychogryphosis	62	14J
Disorders of mucous membranes	111	7	Onychophosis		14K
Problems of edentulous mouth	111		Cutaneous melanoma and its precursors	81, 82	15
Cheilitis	111		Lentigo maligna	82	
Perlèche	111	7A	Lentigo maligna melanoma	82	15A
Leukoplakia	111		Superficial spreading melanoma	82	
Oral cancer	111		Desmoplastic melanoma	82	
Eczematous dermatitis		8	Nodular melanoma	82	
Nummular eczema	121	8A	Precancerous and malignant nonmelanoma cutaneous neoplasia	73–75	16
Gravitational eczema	5	8B	Angiosarcoma		16A
Asteatotic eczema	5	8C	Solar keratoses	73	
Lichen simplex chronicus	5	8D	Bowen's disease	73	
Atopic eczema	120	8E	Paget's disease of the breast	113	
Autosensitization eczema	122		Extramammary Paget's disease	113	16B
Prurigo nodularis			Basal cell carcinoma, including morpheic basal cell carcinoma	75	
Disorders due to sun exposure	133–135	9	Squamous cell carcinoma, including the lip	74	
Photoaging	240	9A	Cutaneous neuroendocrine carcinoma (Merkel cell carcinoma)	79	16C
Cutis rhomboidalis nuchae	137	9B	Cutaneous metastasis to the skin	183	
Solar lentigo	137	9C			
Favre-Racouchot disease		9D			
Solar purpura (Bateman's senile purpura)		9E			
Venous lakes		9F			
Stellate scars of the hands and forearms		9G			
Radiodermatitis, acute and chronic	127				
Photosensitivity disorders	135	10			
Actinic reticuloid	135	10A			
Drug eruptions, phototoxic	136				
Drug eruptions, photoallergic	136				
Adverse cutaneous drug reactions	142	11			
Exanthematous	142				
Fixed eruptions	142				
Warfarin necrosis	142				

TABLE 240-1 *(Continued)*

	Chapter cross reference	Numbered discussions in this chapter		Chapter cross reference	Numbered discussions in this chapter
Cutaneous manifestations of systemic malignancy, paraneoplastic syndromes	183		Dermatomyositis	172	
			Rheumatoid arthritis	178	
			Rheumatoid nodules	178	
Cowden's disease	183		Psoriatic arthritis	40	
Paraneoplastic syndromes: dermatomyositis, paraneoplastic pemphigus, acanthosis nigricans, Basex syndrome	183		Pemphigus vulgaris	52	
			Livedo reticularis	167	
			Giant cell arteritis: temporal arteritis, Takayusu's arteritis	116	
Glucagonoma and migratory necrolytic erythema	183		Hypersensitivity vasculitis, drug-induced	116	
			Wegener's granulomatosis	116	
Disorders of hair	61		Erythroderma		
Age-related changes	61		Psoriatic, pityriasis rubra pilaris, Sézary's syndrome, drug	41	
Androgenetic alopecia	61				
Graying	80				
Hair loss	61		Disorders of heat and cold		
Cutaneous lymphomas/ leukemias	105		Erythema ab igne	125	
			Chilblains	125	
Parapsoriasis en plaque	84, 105		Metabolic, endocrine		
Cutaneous T-cell lymphoma (CTCL)	105		Diabetes mellitus: diabetic dermopathy	169	
Sézary's syndrome	105		Hypothyroidism: myxedema	169	
Cutaneous B-cell lymphoma (CBCL)	106		Hyperthyroidism	169	
			Addison's disease	169	
Leukemia cutis	106		Cushing's disease	169	
Multiple myeloma	149		Gout	151	
Macroglobulinemia	152		Alkaptonuria	148	
Disorders of the anogenitalia		17	Xanthomatoses	152	
Pruritus ani and vulvae	112, 113	17A	Disorders of nutrition		
Atrophic vulvitis	113		Calorie deficiency	145	
Leukoplakic vulvitis	113		Zinc deficiency	145	
Balanitis xerotica obliterans	112		Scurvy	145	
			Pellagra	145	
Intraepithelial neoplasia	112, 113		Circulatory disorders		18
Erythroplasia of Queyrat	112		Osler's disease	184	
Squamous cell carcinoma of the penis	112		Livedo reticularis	167	18A
			Purpura, cortisone-induced	232	
Squamous cell carcinoma of the vulva	113		Ischemia and gangrene	167	
			Chronic venous insufficiency	167	
Complications of the immunocompromised host: organ transplantation, bone marrow transplantation, chemotherapy-induced			Varicose ulcers	167	
			Dependent rubor	167	18B
			Acrocyanosis	167	18C
			Sexually transmitted diseases		
Graft-versus-host disease	117		Syphilis	218	
Chronic herpetic ulcers	118		Gonorrhea	223	
Candidemia	118		Herpes simplex	203	
Neoplasia in the chronically immunosuppressed host	118		Condylomata acuminata	212	
			Intraepithelial neoplasia	212	
Immune, rheumatic disorders			Cutaneous ulcers		19
Amyloidosis	149		Leg ulcerations	5	
Lupus erythematosus syndromes	171		Pressure sores	184	19A
			Miscellaneous		20
Progressive systemic sclerosis	173		Lichen sclerosus et atrophicus	113	
Morphea	173		Skin atrophy	230	20A
Cryoglobulinemia	162		Seborrheic dermatitis	123	20B
Sarcoidosis, lupus pernio	182		Intertrigo	113	20C

tions and infection. The dryness has not been explained satisfactorily on a biochemical basis. The lipid alteration appears to be qualitative as opposed to quantitative. Although the stratum corneum compartment by some measurements has less water, aged skin as a whole appears to have more, not less, water than younger skin. The

thickness of the stratum corneum, which is the major diffusion barrier of the skin, tends to be unchanged in the aged, although the mean corneocyte area increases. The functional ability of the stratum corneum to prevent water loss increases with age unless there is gross fissuring.

The epidermis is only focally thinner, but overall is about the same in bulk. The dermal-epidermal junction flattens as a result of loss of the rete pegs. Only recently has it been appreciated that the leg skin, especially in women, who suffer more from xerosis, is not a protected area. Actinic damage, sometimes matching that of dorsal forearm skin, is common. This definitely contributes to xerosis.

Although elderly persons appear to sweat less, this is probably of little consequence in regard to dry skin. Water is not an effective therapy for xerosis, and prolonged bathing may worsen it. Sweat glands are greatly reduced in quantity and function. The eccrine secretory coil becomes architecturally distorted, appearing shrunken, dilated, and surrounded by more fibrotic tissue.

Too much emphasis has been placed on the effect of decreased sebum production as an etiologic factor. Except for the head, sebum production is quite low over the body surface owing to the sparcity of follicles. Besides, sebum is a poor "moisturizer." The skin of prepubertal children is lovely, smooth and soft despite very low levels of surface sebum. The real function of sebum is to lubricate and protect the pilage, no longer necessary for the "naked ape."

4   Vesicular and Bullous Disorders

4A   Bullous Pemphigoid   This acute, severe, self-limited blistering disease, characterized by large, tense bullae, has also been called *pemphigus of the aged* and *senile pemphigoid* as most cases occur in the seventh and eighth decades. Sixty-six percent of patients are older than 60 years at the onset. The disease is autoantibody-mediated with immune complexes, complement, and leukocytes activated at the basement membrane zone leading to cleft formation and bullae at the dermal-epidermal junction. The age-related changes probably involve both the skin and the immune system. There may be altered self-antigens or a loss of tolerance. B lymphocytes from bullous pemphigoid patients can be stimulated using mitogens to produce anti-basement membrane zone antibody, whereas lymphocytes from normal patients cannot be stimulated to produce these antibodies. Because aging is associated with a decline in T-cell function, it has been suggested that perhaps there is a loss of B-cell regulation, which normally keeps autoreactive B-cell clones in check.

5   Benign Neoplasia

The epidermis exhibits an age-related decrease in proliferative activity. Thymidine-labeling studies exhibit a 50 percent reduction in thymidine-labeling index. There is a corresponding decrease in repair rate during wound healing. However, factors governing tissue homeostasis become less well regulated. The epidermis shows a loss in architectural hierarchy and increased cell-to-cell heterogeneity. Atrophy, hyperplasia, atypia, and neoplasia can become bedfellows. Differentiation is disordered, focal proliferations of cells and tissues are commonplace in aged individuals, and increasing age strongly correlates with increased numbers of various benign neoplasms. It is rare to find persons over the age of 65 who do not exhibit proliferative growths involving keratinocytes, melanocytes, capillaries, or adnexae. Clinically, these appear as seborrheic keratoses, cherry angiomas, acrochordons, cutaneous horns, inverted follicular keratoses, clear cell acanthoma (Degos' acanthoma), lentigines, and sebaceous hyperplasia (see Table 10-3). Certain of these are more prevalent on sun-damaged skin, increasing the probability of malignant transformations.

6   Disorders of Nails   (See also "Disorders of the Feet" below)

6A   Nail Growth   Nail growth rate declines with increasing age. Bean's famous measurements of his own nail growth decreased to 0.52 mm per week in the eighth decade, as compared with 0.83 mm per week in the third decade. Orentreich correlated life expectancy with rate of decline in nail growth during aging and compared humans with beagles. The decrease in linear nail growth rate per year in humans is 0.5 percent per year from age 15 to 90 years, whereas with beagles, the decrease is 2.5 percent per year from age 1 to 14 years. He found a fivefold rate of decline in beagles, whose life expectancy is one-fifth that of humans.

6B   General Aging-Related Nail Changes   Longitudinal ridges have been reported to occur in 67 percent of persons past 70 years of age. Lamellar dystrophy, that is, brittle nails with split ends or layering is common in middle-aged women and most common in both sexes over 60 years of age. Pigmentary changes occur with age but are confounded by disease states that may contribute to apparent nail color. The lunulae become diffuse and poorly defined. There is a higher incidence of Terry's type of nails (whitish, opaque proximal nails). One study of black persons' nails showed longitudinal pigment banding in 96 percent of persons over 50 years, as compared with 2.5 percent of 0- to 3-year-olds. Onychodystrophy may be misdiagnosed as a fungal infection. Dystrophic nails due to aging are most frequent in the toenails. Contributing factors include underlying orthopedic abnormalities and trauma from ill-fitting footwear. Aged nails are frequently more convex, and the nail plate is thicker. There may be subungual hyperkeratosis. These factors may combine to produce onychogryphosis. Grotesque malformations of the nails are common in the elderly, especially in women. Unhygienic footwear is largely responsible for thickened, split, separated, rough, ridged, curved nails.

7   Disorders of Mucous Membranes

7A   Perlèche   Perlèche, derived from the French, "to lick," simply refers to inflammation and fissures of the corners of the mouth. As laxity increases with the passage of time, the redundant skin creates a fold that becomes an intertriginous zone; it is then predisposed to retention of saliva and maceration. The lateral crevices deepen and become accentuated by a combination of factors. Among these are edentulousness with partial absorption of the alveolar ridge, sagging of the skin of the cheeks, loss of elasticity from photodamage, and excessive salivation. Misdiagnosis can occur. Candidiasis is often superimposed and can be readily diagnosed by culture, responding promptly to antifungal treatment. Vitamin deficiency is often blamed but rarely proved.

8   Eczematous Dermatitis

Eczematous dermatitis represented 38 percent of the chief presenting complaints in a study involving 330 geriatric patients (average age 69.95 years). A number of disease categories are involved (see Table 240-1).

8A   Nummular Eczema   Coin-shaped eczema evolves as intensely pruritic discoid-shaped plaques. In men, the incidence rises in middle age, whereas nummular eczema may be more common in younger women. Extremities, most frequently the legs, are affected as well as the arms and hands. There may be several coinlike patches 1 to 3 cm in diameter. Relapses can be expected. Nummular eczema may sometimes be a delayed manifestation of atopic dermatitis, but most patients do not have an atopic background. Xerosis is the background for the development of nummular eczema in the elderly. Bowen's disease and superficial basal cell cancer need to be considered in persistent lesions in this age group. Colonization by *Staphylococcus aureus* is a complicating factor that is often overlooked in the choice of therapy.

8B   Gravitational Eczema   *Gravitational eczema* has replaced stasis dermatitis as a more appropriate term for the eczema that can accompany chronic venous hypertension. Actually there is an increase in blood flow within the venous circulation. The disorder is rarely seen prior to middle age. There is scaling, erythema, pigmentation, and fibrosis often associated with pruritus. Venous drainage has been compromised by a number of factors, some of which can be obesity, trauma, venous thrombosis, or multiple pregnancies. Heredity certainly plays a role by the presence of incompetent valves allowing back-flow of blood. The condition is common in the wheelchair-bound patient and in all situations where the muscle pump is not able to function in assisting blood return. Long-standing disease predisposes to ulceration with a predilection for the medial malleolus. When gravitational eczema and edema are acute in onset, an associated deep venous thrombosis must be excluded. Ischemia due to arterial impairment of blood flow is more common than is realized.

8C   Asteatotic Eczema   Asteatotic eczema, or eczema craquelatum, is a transient dermatitis related to low ambient humidity, frequent bathing, and diminished use of emollients. It is essentially a complication of xerosis, which always precedes this type of eczema. The lesions have the appearance of a cracked river bed with poorly defined borders. Pruritic and frequently tender, the dermatitis is located predominantly on extensor limbs and trunk. Asteatotic eczema usually responds readily to emollient therapy with water-in-oil emulsions.

8D   Lichen Simplex Chronicus   Lichen simplex chronicus is a circumscribed, intensely pruritic plaque of eczema that results from habitual scratching and rubbing of the skin. Lichenification is a

hallmark. The disorder is rarely seen in children and is most frequent in adults over 60 years of age. Usually there is but one lesion. Favored sites include occipital and nuchal areas in women, the perineum and scrotum in men. Wrist and leg involvement is frequent. Atopy is a predisposing factor; another is xerotic skin and its associated pruritus, which then inaugurates the itch–scratch cycle.

8E   Atopic Dermatitis   In contrast to other types of eczema, atopic dermatitis is rare in the elderly, at least in its full form. Exacerbations decrease with the passage of time, fading away to less frequent exacerbations of eczema and less extensive lesions that become more limited to the extremities. The final clinical picture may be dry, scaly skin in which pruritus is disproportionately intense. When respiratory allergy and eczema coexist, the passage of time results in clearing of the dermatitis but without a corresponding relief of asthma. This may be partially related to an attenuated inflammatory response. Aged persons exhibit a measurable decrease in irritant reactions, cutaneous blister formation, and inflammatory conditions of all kinds.

9   Disorders due to Sun Exposure

9A   Photoaging   Photoaging or dermatoheliosis is almost universal among the fair-skinned (Table 240-2). It is so commonplace that it was previously misconceived as part of the aging process itself. Photoaging is covered in detail in the second part of this chapter.

9B   Cutis Rhomboidalis Nuchae   Cutis rhomboidalis nuchae is an example of the profound textural and pigmentary changes that can occur on the neck of chronically sun-exposed persons. Coarse furrows lie in criss-cross fashion dividing thickened, leathery, ruddy-colored skin.

9C   Solar Lentigo   "Liver spots," les medallions de cimetière, sometimes called "coffin spots," are actinically induced and therefore should not be called senile lentigo. The appropriate term is *solar lentigo*; the term "liver spots" is misleading and should be discarded. The lesions may be present on ultraviolet-exposed skin in more than 90 percent of Caucasians over 70 years of age. Lesions are flat, have a uniform brown color, and are especially prominent on the dorsal hand of photodamaged older persons. The macules are usually larger than 1 cm, are multiple, and have cir-

TABLE 240-2
Dermatoheliosis ("Photoaging")

Anatomic site	Process	Clinical lesion
Keratinocyte	Variably increased	Roughness / Solar keratosis
	Reduced	Translucence
Langerhans cell	Reduced	Altered and attenuated inflammatory and immune responses
Melanocyte	Variably increased	Irregular pigmentation / Solar lentigo
	Reduced	Guttate hypomelanosis / Actinic leukoderma
Extracellular matrix	Architectural alterations / Decreased collagen / Increased glycosaminoglycans	Roughening, coarse furrowing
	Increased elastin	Solar elastosis, yellowing
Blood vessel	Proliferation, permanent dilatation	Telangiectasia
	Fragility of blood vessel and supporting tissue	Bateman's purpura

cumscribed well-defined round borders. Histologically, epidermal rete ridges are elongated with increased numbers of benign melanocytes.

9D   Favre-Racouchot Disease   Favre-Racouchot disease, also known as nodular elastosis with cysts and comedones, occurs on facial sun-exposed skin and is characterized by huge open comedones (blackheads), predominantly on the temples of some older persons. The follicular orifices are greatly dilated and contain dense impacted horn. Sebaceous glands are atrophic. Dermatoheliosis is the necessary background for the development of solar comedones. The comedones respond to topical retinoic acid.

9E   Solar Purpura (Bateman's Senile Purpura)   Purpura frequently occurs following trauma to severely sun-damaged skin of the dorsal forearm of elderly persons. Torsional stresses rapidly lead to hemorrhages that may require months for the blood pigments to be resorbed.

9F   Venous Lake   A venous lake is a venous ectasia that appears as a blue-black soft papule, typically on the lower lip and other sun-exposed areas such as the helix of the ear, the face, and the neck. Deteriorations in the three-dimensional network of connective tissue in both the vascular adventitia as well as the dermis contribute to their development. Venous lakes may be mistaken for melanomas or pigmented basal cell carcinomas. Diascopy is useful in making the diagnosis. Direct pressure created by a glass microscope slide causes a vascular lesion to blanch, thereby differentiating it from a neoplasia.

9G   Stellate Scars of the Hands and Forearms   These have been mistakenly attributed to a preexisting purpura. The latter heal without scarring. Stellate scars have been inaptly called pseudoscars (of Coulomb), but they are true scars resulting from tearing of fragile photodamaged skin.

10   Photosensitivity Disorders

10A   Actinic Reticuloid   This photosensitivity disorder occurs almost exclusively in elderly men and is associated with an exaggerated sensitivity to ultraviolet (UVA and UVB) and sometimes to visible light. Lichenified erythematous plaques occur on the forehead and the posterior nuchal area. With time the eruption becomes more deeply furrowed and intensely red, and there may be irregular areas of hyperpigmentation. There may be a gradual progression to an erythroderma. Leonine facies can develop. Itching can be intense, and there may be an associated lymphadenopathy. Due to the dense dermal lymphohistiocytic infiltrate and the hyperchromatic cells similar in appearance to Sézary cells, actinic reticuloid is classified as a pseudolymphoma. It is important to recognize that malignant lymphoma may ultimately occur. T lymphocytes are chiefly suppressor T cells (OKT8 positive, in contrast to those in cutaneous T-cell lymphoma, which are T-helper cells). Some patients have demonstrated allergic contact hypersensitivity to oleoresin extracts from *Compositae* plants or common fragrances.

11   Adverse Cutaneous Drug Reactions

It is not known whether drug reactions are intrinsically more common in the elderly, because older patients are more likely to be receiving multiple drugs, often three to five different agents. Adverse cutaneous drug effects are also undoubtedly more difficult to assess in the elderly and have variable and ambiguous expressions. Drug reactions in the elderly may be more serious than in the young. In the elderly, drugs are more likely to incite autoimmune disorders such as pemphigus, bullous pemphigoid, and lupus erythematosus-like rashes. These are reversible upon discontinuation of the drug. Photosensitivity reactions also appear to be more prevalent in older age groups. A pseudoporphyria-like presentation can occur on light-exposed areas of patients taking naproxen or furosemide. Thiazide diuretics and sulfonamide-based hypoglycemic agents can cause photosensitivity. The elderly must always be closely questioned regarding drug intake, in view of age-associated forgetfulness. Resolution of the eruption upon withdrawal of the drug is often prolonged. Anticoagulant necrosis can occur in patients taking either warfarin or heparin. Most of the nonsteroidal antirheumatoid arthritis drugs are capable of inducing photosensitivity reactions, fortunately in a minority of patients.

12   Infections

12A   Dermatophyte Infections   *Ringworm* infections, especially of the feet, are common. The usual dermatophytes prevail, often accompanied by onychomycosis. Ringworm is rarely acquired in old age. Foot ringworm is a lifelong disease, especially in men; it often worsens with age and is often misdiagnosed as dry skin. Decreased frequency of skin care, decreased epidermal turnover, and diminished immunologic function all play a role. As many as 80 percent of men over 64 years of age may have *tinea pedis*. The infection frequently exceeds the usual boundaries, with extension to beyond the fourth web space, creeping up onto the dorsum, invariably involving the nails. Sandal-type plantar involvement is common. There is often "one hand, two feet" involvement which remains an unexplained presentation. Maceration and white hyperkeratosis arise from cohabitation of dermatophyte and bacteria, frequently involving gram-negative organisms. *Tinea incognito* is a dermatophyte infection that eventuates from inappropriate, persistent use of topical corticosteroids, which allow the fungus to grow unchecked by suppressing inflammation. Diagnosis is usually delayed or missed altogether as the typical signs are missing. *Tinea cruris* may be mistakenly diagnosed in elderly men when seborrheic dermatitis is the true culprit. *Tinea capitis* is very uncommon in the elderly. Ringworm in the elderly occurs in areas with a thickened horny layer, consequently, topical therapy should be rigorous with applications two to three times daily. Effective treatment can preclude serious superinfection (see "Cellulitis" below).

12B   Candidiasis   *Candida albicans* can flourish in recesses created by redundant skin folds. Intertriginous zones are more common beneath the flabby, redundant tissues of elderly persons. For example, the inframammary creases beneath pendulous breasts, groins exposed to *Candida* from intestinal sources and kept moist with urine, and buttocks, which may rest atop plastic sheets to trap moisture, are all fertile ground for cutaneous candidiasis, which can extend onto the scrotum in men. *Candida* pustules can occur on the moist occluded back of bedridden patients, particularly those who have febrile sweats. Oral thrush may accompany severe illness. Exacerbating factors may include diabetes mellitus, systemic medications, nutritional factors, and diminished salivary function.

The oral commissures may become intertriginous zones in the elderly, predisposed to *Candida* because of redundant labial skin folds and kept warm and moist with oral secretions. Colonization by *Candida* results in a mycotic perlèche. Vulvovaginal thrush and *Candida* balanitis can be promoted by combinations of the above factors.

12C   Cellulitis   Cellulitis in the aged may lack the classic signs and often goes undiagnosed. An indolent swelling in the older patient may be the only manifestation of a soft tissue infection that would have been warm, red, and associated with fever and leukocytosis in a younger person. Predisposing factors include chronic edema, poor arterial and venous circulation, diabetes mellitus, unrecognized trauma, and portals of entry created by tinea pedis or even xerosis with erythema cracquelatum.

Cellulitis may be related to significant underlying pathology, such as cholecystitis. The process may be retroperitoneal, as in a psoas muscle abscess, which may present with cellulitis of the groin or flank. Likewise, there may be an underlying incarcerated inguinal or umbilical hernia.

Patients undergoing coronary artery bypass can develop cellulitis at the saphenous vein donor site. Cellulitis can extend along the incision and rapidly evolve into a severe febrile illness. The site of origin of the causative group A streptococci is frequently an interdigital web space fissure secondary to tinea pedis. The perisaphenous tissues are fertile soil for infection, having been deprived of their normal lymphatic drainage. The lymphotropism of streptococcal infections and the consequent lymphatic scarring create more edema and set the stage for recurrent infections. Accordingly, there needs to be meticulous search for conditions, often seemingly minor, that provide a breach of skin through which streptococci make their entrance.

Erysipelas is a special variant of cellulitis caused by beta-hemolytic streptococci and should be considered a life-threatening emergency that can evolve rapidly and dramatically. Face and scalp are favored locations, but lesions can occur anywhere, with organisms gaining entry in a web space fissure, a stasis ulcer, or from a small innocent-appearing scratch. Recurrences can occur in the same location and may warrant prophylactic antibiotic use. The sequelae of persistent livid edema on the face can produce disfiguring macrocheilia or persistent edematous periorbital tissue.

12D   Pyoderma   Pyoderma in the aged may be subtle and disguised. There may be only slight redness, tenderness, and warmth with no febrile response, even in severe infections such as carbuncles. A furuncle may simulate a cold abscess. The absence of overt clinical harbingers of infection leads to delay in recognition and treatment.

12E   Herpes Zoster   In otherwise healthy persons, herpes zoster occurs more often in the elderly and is far more serious. This is principally because of postherpetic neuralgia, which is more frequent and severe in elderly persons. The risk of postherpetic neuralgia is as high as 20 percent in patients over 60 years of age; the actual figure may approach 50 percent. In one large follow-up study, postherpetic neuralgia was present 1 month after the onset of the rash in 60 percent, by 3 months there was some pain in 24 percent, and by 6 months 13 percent still had pain. The highest prevalence is in ophthalmic zoster. A recent preliminary study of older patients (age 60) demonstrated a reduced frequency of persistent pain when intravenous acyclovir, 10 mg/kg every 8 h for 5 days, was given within 4 days of the onset of the pain or within

48 h after the onset of the rash. It is important, however, to evaluate renal function prior to high-dose acyclovir therapy in elderly patients. While this is promising, the ability to prevent neuralgia successfully is still poor. An alternative is the use of systemic corticosteroids, starting with the onset of the eruption if no contraindications exist. The dosage is 60 mg of prednisone per day, tapered to zero over a course of 4 weeks; this allegedly prevents postherpetic neuralgia in the majority of patients. The mechanisms responsible for recrudescence of the varicella zoster virus in healthy, aged persons are not known. The increased neuralgia likewise remains a mystery. In general, elderly persons have an increased tolerance to pain.

13   Infestations

13A   Scabies   The clinical presentation of scabies infestations in the elderly patient can be so varied that, although easily treated, diagnosis can be elusive. Casual skin contact can then innocently spread mites among family members or nursing home inhabitants. Three important clinical variations should be kept in mind. Cryptic cases can present with pruritus but only minimal lesions, as the hypersensitivity reaction responsible for cutaneous manifestations in younger patients may be muted in older persons. Scabies incognito can result from steroid treatment and lead to delay in diagnosis by masking signs and symptoms, which can be dramatically altered in extent and distribution. Subsequent superinfection can further confound the presentation. Nodules containing mites can persist after antiscabetic treatment. The associated histologic appearance can mimic lymphoid neoplasms. Norwegian scabies may occur in immunodepressed patients and in those who either cannot scratch effectively or who have depressed cutaneous sensation. These patients can present with extensive crusted accretions containing huge numbers of mites, creating a highly contagious situation. There may be an associated lymphadenopathy and eosinophilia. Epidemics are common in nursing homes.

14   Disorders of the Feet

The feet are frequently neglected by physicians and especially by patients who have impaired ability to care for their feet. In the elderly, the normal mechanical stresses affecting pedal anatomy, friction, compression, tension, shear, and torsion, can be exaggerated and distorted by ill-fitting footwear, abnormalities in gait, and impaired sensory input. It is not true that foot problems may be less important in the elderly who are less active than their younger counterparts. Foot health is critically important in the elderly population to maintain mobility. Decreased physical activity may be the beginning of a vicious cycle of immobility and a decreased ability for self-care. A simple foot lesion could incapacitate the elderly person and foster further musculoskeletal atrophy and decline. Podiatrist geriatricians emphasize the necessity to "keep'em walking." Toenails present a special geriatric problem, in large part associated with the impaired ability to maintain normal care; many elderly patients cannot cut their toenails.

14A   Clavi   Clavus is derived from the Latin *cornu*, a horn. Fifty percent of visits to a podiatrist are because of corns. A corn is a hyperkeratotic plaque, usually ring-shaped, sculpted into a nucleus by pressure and frictional forces from body weight, footwear, or digits pressing on each other. The differential diagnosis includes warts; however, a corn pared with a blade reveals only a central translucent core, devoid of the thrombosed capillaries characteristically seen in warts. Corns are of four types. They can be hard (heloma durum), soft, vascular, or neurovascular. Hard corns usually occur over dorsal interphalangeal joints. On the plantar surface, they are found underlying the metatarsal heads and on the great toe, beneath the interphalangeal joint or any area of increased pressure. Corns can occur subungually, between the toes, and in the nail bed sulcus. Onychoclavus is a subungual corn or heloma and usually occurs in the distal nail bed of the great toe, secondary to localized pressure on the hyponychium. The overlying nail may be distorted or split. Soft corns arise exclusively interdigitally, typically in the fourth web space. Most interdigital soft corns arise secondary to bony exostoses (usually condyles of the joints). Pressure is increased by shoes with pointed tips leading to crowding and compression of the toes. The podiatrist can supply a very effective molded plastic device that keeps the toes apart.

14B   **Bursitis**   Bursae are anatomic cushions reducing stresses on tissues. The aged person may have extreme stresses on selected sites due to impaired mobility. Bursitis can develop beneath sites of shearing stress such as corns, hallux valgus, and near the Achilles tendon. Bursitis can be traumatic or infective. As the condition may be prolonged in the aged person, fluid can form fistulous tracks towards a joint space or a sinus track to the skin, and the simultaneous occurrence of both processes can result in joint fluid leakage and the risk of serious infection.

14C   **Bunions**   A bunion is a deformity of the metatarsal phalangeal joint of the great toe. The pathophysiology is genetic and environmental. In the early stages, there is lateral deviation of the proximal phalanx over the first metatarsal head pushing medially off the underlying sesamoids. Patients usually have a history of wearing inappropriate shoes with heels too high and/or toe boxes too narrow for the feet to operate naturally. As the proximal phalanx subluxates laterally, laxity increases medially, and ligament contracture causes the deformity to become progressive. The large, often painful medial prominence of a bunion is the first metatarsal head, which is exposed to increased pressure in shoes. This prominence enlarges as the bone reacts to the increased pressure. Often a bursa can form over the head medially and this can become irritated and infected. The laterally subluxed proximal phalanx often causes an overriding second toe, which can be difficult to fit into shoes and can develop consequent painful keratoses.

14D   **Intractable Plantar Keratoses**   Callus, or tyloma, commonly develops on the plantar surface below the middle three metatarsophalangeal joints. The thickened epidermis can greatly limit mobility. The callus can vary in size, depending on its underlying cause. There are usually bony deformities that lead to increased stresses on the soft tissue of the sole of the foot, creating hyperkeratotic plaques. The keratoses can be reduced by paring, however the underlying biomechanics must be corrected in order to solve the problem. Treatment may require altering shoes, adding orthotics, and, sometimes, surgery.

14E   **Neoplasia**   The most common neoplasms are basal cell cancers and melanomas, which can be subungual. Neoplasms may be masked secondarily by traumatic hyperkeratosis. Epithelial cuniculatum is squamous cell carcinoma of the foot and looks like a wart. Because warts are uncommon in the geriatric population, verrucous

lesions mandate investigation. Epithelial cuniculatum should not be treated with radiation which can induce a more aggressive behavior pattern.

14F   **Subungual Exostosis**   This is a small bony outgrowth typically on the great toe, three times as common on the hallux relative to the fifth toe. It occurs in women more frequently than in men. The diagnosis requires x-ray. The bony growth occurs secondary to trauma.

14G   **Onychocryptosis**   Ingrown toenail occurs when a lateral portion of the nail edge, most frequently on the hallux, penetrates the neighboring soft tissue. It can be caused by improperly performed nail trimming. Other predisposing factors include ill-fitting footwear, distorted weight bearing due to abnormalities in gait, and hyperhidrosis from occlusive footwear or overuse of foot baths. It can be complicated by insidious but serious infection that may go unnoticed in this population.

14H   **Onychauxis**   Onychauxis is a condition of hypertrophied nails secondary to trauma and chronic pressure. Neglect in nail trimming leads to increased forces from footwear as the nail grows. The nail plate is typically dull and opaque and may be discolored. The condition can be misdiagnosed as a fungal infection. Complicating sequelae can include pain, subungual hemorrhage, subungual ulceration, and predisposition to tinea unguium. Treatment includes partial or total debridement of the nail plate on a regular basis, nail plate evulsion, or matricectomy.

14I   **Onycholysis**   In the elderly population onycholysis may reflect systemically impaired peripheral circulation. Dehiscence of the nail plate from the nail bed begins at the free nail margin and extends proximally. Onycholysis predisposes the nail bed to infection.

14J   **Onychogryphosis**   Synonyms for onychogryphosis include ram's horn, Osler's toe, and Hippocratic nail. The nail is club-shaped with an exaggerated, laterally extended longitudinal curvature. The greatly distorted shape results from uneven nail growth. The nail may be a dark color. Trauma, poorly fitting footwear, and failure to trim nails aggravate the problem, may result in penetration of the distal nail tip into adjacent soft tissue, and lead to infection.

14K   **Onychophosis**   Onychophosis refers to hyperkeratotic tissue occurring either on or under nail folds or subungually. The hyperkeratosis can be focal or diffuse and occurs mainly on the first and fifth toes. It is seen frequently in elderly persons and results from local mild trauma to the nail plate. The setting usually includes several predisposing factors such as xerosis and nail fold and/or nail plate deformities. Treatment includes elimination of trauma-inducing factors and debridement of the hyperkeratotic tissue. Keratolytics can be useful.

15   Cutaneous Melanoma and Its Precursors

15A   **Lentigo Maligna Melanoma**   Lentigo maligna melanoma is a large, flat, irregular, pigmented lesion that typically develops in the sixth or seventh decade of life, usually on the face. Lentigo maligna melanoma is discussed in Chap. 82.

16   Precancerous and Malignant Nonmelanoma Cutaneous Neoplasia

Nonmelanoma skin cancers are common in older persons; however, the lesions occur principally on actinically damaged skin. Skin not exposed to sun may also have an increased tendency to develop malignancies, perhaps due to a diminished cellular immune function. Genetic factors also play a role. Certainly there are elderly persons with extensive dermatoheliosis and no cutaneous malignancies.

16A   Angiosarcoma   Angiosarcoma is also known as malignant angioendothelioma and anaplastic reticulosarcoma. It is a rare tumor that, when cutaneous in origin, presents most typically on the scalp or face of elderly patients. Very rarely, angiosarcoma can arise in the setting of a chronic lymphedematous extremity. Postmastectomy lymphangiosarcoma, Stewart-Treves syndrome, occurs in the edematous upper extremity after radical mastectomy. Angiosarcoma can be mistakenly diagnosed as cellulitis or erysipelas.

16B   Extramammary Paget's Disease   Extramammary Paget's disease is a well-circumscribed erythematous plaque that can be eczematous in appearance and may have erosions or ulcerations. The location is in areas having apocrine glands, and anogenital sites predominate. Extraperineal sites include axillae and periumbilical areas. Lesions can be pruritic and painful. Underlying carcinomas are usually apocrine in origin; however, 20 percent of anogenital lesions are associated with urogenital or rectal adenocarcinomas. The treatment is surgical. Lesions can be mistakenly diagnosed as psoriasis or eczema, and the diagnosis requires a biopsy.

16C   Cutaneous Neuroendocrine Carcinoma   Cutaneous neuroendocrine carcinoma, known also as Merkel cell carcinoma, is a clinically subtle, underrecognized, highly aggressive tumor with a high rate of local recurrence following surgery. Average age at initial presentation is 68 years, with 91 percent of patients over age 50 years. The precise histogenesis is not certain. Eighty-five percent of tumors arise in areas of actinic exposure, and other ultraviolet radiation-associated neoplasias seem to be associated. The actual incidence of Merkel cell carcinoma is underrepresented in the literature because of the difficulty in making the diagnosis. The tumor has frequently been confused with other neoplasms. Prognostic variables are not known, but the majority of patients are not alive 5 years after the diagnosis is made.

17   Disorders of the Anogenitalia

17A   Pruritus Ani and Vulvae   Cutaneous perineal inflammation is common in older persons. The diagnosis must exclude underlying skin disorders, such as tinea and candidiasis. Multiple factors can work in concert in these sensitive areas. They include poor hygiene, moisture, and irritating excretions. Hemorrhoids commonly incite pruritus near the anus. Contact hypersensitivity to local preparations, residual cleansing agents, or cosmetics can play a role. There have been elderly women who responded to vulvar itching by applying a variety of household products including cleaning fluids and toothpaste. Patients are often embarrassed to talk about these problems, even though they certainly affect the quality of life.

Mild fecal incontinence can be an important cause of pruritus in persons who are scrupulous about removing feces following a bowel movement. The prevalence of fecal incontinence has been estimated at slightly over 1 percent of persons over 65 years of age. The prevalence is much higher among nursing home residents (10 to 17 percent) and hospitalized elderly persons (10 to 47 percent). Fecal incontinence related to dysfunction of the anal sphincter can cause pruritus ani without clinically apparent skin manifestations. Pruritus results from the action of pruritogenic bacterial endopeptidases contained in feces. The diagnosis of a weak anal sphincter can be made with the aid of manometry, cinedefecography, and electromyography. Treatment includes limited short-pulse therapy with a potent class I corticosteroid in severe cases having lichenification of the perianal skin. Harsh toilet paper should be replaced by cotton flannel pledgets soaked in witch hazel. Hygiene must be impeccable, and a bidet can be helpful. Topical menthol-camphor antipruritic lotions help relieve pruritus, and liberal application of talcum powder can help absorb the results of mild fecal incontinence. Dietary manipulation with high-fiber and stool-bulking supplements encourages formation of soft but solid stools as opposed to liquid stools, which are more easily leaked from a weak anal sphincter. Medical antidiarrheal agents, biofeedback training, and surgery may be indicated, depending on the etiology of the incontinence.

18   Circulatory Disorders

18A   Livedo Reticularis   In the geriatric population, livedo reticularis in a distal extremity represents atheroembolus until proved otherwise. (See Chap. 167 for discussion of multiple etiologic associations.)

18B   Dependent Rubor   Intense dependent erythema occurs due to compensatory capillary dilatation and disappears with elevation. It is often mistaken for cellulitis. There may be associated dependent edema. If ulceration exists, revascularization procedures are required. Biopsy is contraindicated.

18C   Acrocyanosis   Acrocyanosis may indicate poor cardiac output and/or insufficient environmental temperature. Incontinent, semimobile patients have additional factors associated with heat loss.

19   Cutaneous Ulcers

19A   Pressure Sores   Decubitus ulcer correctly refers to ulcers resulting from a prolonged supine, prone or lateral position (Latin *decumber,* ''to lie down''). Seventy percent of patients with pressure sores are over 70 years of age. Mortality rate is estimated at 8 percent. Risk factors other than age include neurologic deficit, malnutrition, immobilization, and debilitating medical disease. Cutaneous changes reflect only the ''tip of the iceberg.'' The skin overlying the evolving pressure sore belies the extent of tissue injury, which is cone-shaped with the apex directed toward the skin and the larger base adjacent to the bony pressure point. When combined with friction, the force required to produce ulceration can be as small as 45 mmHg. Bony prominences may receive increased force due to loss of adipose cushioning. Sedentary habits, decreased ambulatory ability, and muscle atrophy prolong the time spent in any one position. Additionally, assistance and attempts at mobilization increase the chance that shearing forces act synergistically with pressure to create tissue ischemia. With the development of the first pressure sore, the risk is compounded for the development of additional sites, in an attempt to avoid pressure on the initial site.

Decubitus ulcers are serious lesions that require prompt attention at the earliest stage of erythema. With proper turning and relief of pressure, they are completely preventable. Decubitus ulcers are more than skin deep.

20   Miscellaneous

20A   Skin Atrophy   Skin atrophy can be compounded due to a poor understanding of the correct use of medications, leading to misuse of topical steroids in the elderly patient who may have associated edema with vascular insufficiency. The geriatric dermal-epidermal interface is already compromised (see "Wrinkling and Sagging Skin and Fragility" above). The fragile skin of the poorly groomed foot is a setup for fissures, bullae, infection, and further loss of the ability to be mobile.

20B   Seborrheic Dermatitis   Although seborrheic dermatitis can affect all ages and both males and females, it becomes much more common with increasing age. The association with increasing age correlates best in men, whereas women have a peak in morbidity after puberty (maximal between 15 and 24 years), which gradually declines. There appears to be a cephalocaudad progression of the location with increasing age. Although the face and head are the predominant sites in younger age groups and certainly can be severely affected in the elderly, genitocrural and lower extremity lesions increase with age. The pubis, crural folds, gluteal cleft, and penis (seborrheic balanitis) may be involved. Lesions may be misdiagnosed as tinea infections. Striking flares of seborrheic dermatitis have been associated with confining illnesses such as coronary infarction. Exacerbations may eventuate in a diffuse erythroderma, which is often misdiagnosed. Pathogenesis may be related to changes in the cutaneous microflora. A neurophysiologic role is suggested by the association of seborrheic dermatitis with mental retardation and with Parkinson's disease. Seborrheic dermatitis may appear abruptly in the elderly, heralding the onset of Parkinson's disease. The scalp is usually involved, often giving rise to a mistaken diagnosis of dandruff. Simple dandruff declines late in adult life.

20C   Intertrigo   Intertrigo is more frequent in the elderly due to redundant skin folds and environmental factors, including temperature, moisture, friction, and inadequate hygiene. Polymicrobial secondary colonization and subsequent infection can occur. No one organism can be singled out as the main agent.

Bibliography

Balin AK, Kligman AM: *Aging and the Skin.* New York, Raven, 1989

Bean W: Nail Growth: 30 years of observation. *Arch Intern Med* **184**:497, 1974

Beauregard SA, Gilchrest BA: Survey of skin problems and skin care regimens in the elderly. *Arch Dermatol* **123**:1638, 1987

Borkan GA, Norris AH: Assessment of biological age using a profile of physical parameters. *J Gerontol* **35**:177, 1980

Braverman IM, Fonferko E: Studies in cutaneous aging. I. The elastic fiber network. *J Invest Dermatol* **78**:434, 1982

Braverman IM, Fonferko E: Studies in cutaneous aging. II. The microvasculature. *J Invest Dermatol* **78**:444, 1982

Cowdry EV: *The Care of the Geriatric Patient.* St. Louis, Mosby, 1968

Danziel K: Aspects of cutaneous aging. *Clin Exp Dermatol* **16**:315, 1991

Droller H: Dermatologic findings in a random sample of old persons. *Geriatrics* **10**:421, 1955

Everitt AV, Gal A: Age changes in the solubility of tendon collagen in the life span of the rat. *Gerontology* **16**:30, 1970

Fitzpatrick TB et al: Heritable melanin deficiency syndromes: Diagnosis and prophylactic treatment with sun-protective agents, in *Update: Dermatology in General Medicine,* edited by TB Fitzpatrick et al. New York, McGraw-Hill, 1983, p 46

Fleischmajer R, Perlish JS: Human dermal glycosaminoglycans and aging. *Biochim Biophys Acta* **279**:265, 1972

Gilchrest BA, Stoff JS: Chronologic aging alters the response to UV-induced inflammation in the skin. *J Invest Dermatol* **79**:11, 1982

Grove G et al: Use of non-intrusive tests to monitor age associated changes in human skin. *J Soc Cosmet Chem* **32**:15, 1981

Grove GL et al: Effect of aging on the blistering of human skin with ammonium hydroxide. *Br J Dermatol* **107**:393, 1982

Halasz NA: Dehiscence of laparotomy wounds. *Am J Surg* **116**:210, 1968

Holt DR, Kirk SJ: Effect of age on wound healing in healthy human beings. *Surgery* **112**:293, 1992

Holzberg M, Walker HK: Terry's nails: Reviewed definition and new correlations. *Lancet* **1**:896, 1984

Juniper J, Dykman RA: Skin resistance, sweat gland count and salivary flow. Age, race and sex differences. *Psychophysiology* **4**:216, 1967

Katlic MR (ed): *Geriatric Surgery: Comprehensive Care of the Surgical Patient.* Baltimore, Urban and Schwartzenberg, 1990

Katzberg A: The area of the dermal-epidermal junction in human skin. *Anat Rec* **131**:717, 1958

Kligman AM: Early destructive effect of sunlight in human skin. *JAMA* **210**:2377, 1969

Kligman AM: Perspectives and problems in cutaneous gerontology. *J Invest Dermatol* **73**:39, 1979

Korting GW: *Geriatric Dermatology.* Philadelphia, Saunders, 1980

Lane CG, Rockwood EM: Geriatric dermatoses. *N Engl J Med* **241**:722, 1949

Lavker RM: Structural alterations in exposed and unexposed aged skin. *J Invest Dermatol* **73**:59, 1979

Lewin K: The finger nail in general disease. A macroscopic and microscopic study of 87 consecutive autopsies. *Br J Dermatol* **77**:431, 1965

Lewis BL, Montgomery H: The senile nail. *J Invest Dermatol* **24**:11, 1955

Leyden JJ et al: Diffuse and banded melanin pigmentation in nails. *Arch Dermatol* **105**:548, 1972

Lubach D et al: Incidence of brittle nails. *Dermatologica* **172**:144, 1986

Mackinnon PCB: Variations with age in the number of palmar digital sweat glands. *J Neurol Neurosurg Psychiatry* **17**:124, 1954

Madoff RD et al: Fecal incontinence. *N Engl J Med* **326**:1002, 1992

Marks R: *Skin Disease in Old Age.* London, Martin Dunitz, 1987

Marks R: Measurement of biological ageing in human epidermis. *Br J Dermatol* **104**:627, 1981

Montagna W: Morphology of aging skin, in *Advances in Biology of the Skin,* edited by W Montagna. Oxford, Pergamon Press, 1965, p 1

Montagna W, Carlisle K: Structural changes in aging human skin. *J Invest Dermatol* **73**:47, 1979

Neale D, Adams IM: *Common Foot Disorders.* New York, Churchill Livingstone, 1985

Newcomer VD, Young EM: *Geriatric Dermatology: Clinical Diagnosis and Practical Therapy.* New York/Tokyo, Igaku-Shoin, 1989

Orentreich N, Selmanowitz VJ: Levels of biological functions with aging. *Trans N Y Acad Sci,* Series II **31**:992, 1969

Pitale M et al: An analysis of prognostic factors in cutaneous neuroendocrine carcinoma. *Laryngoscope* **102**:244, 1992

Saint-Leger D, Francois AM: Stratum corneum lipids in skin xerosis. *Dermatologica* **178**:151, 1989

Savin JA: Old skin. *Br Med J* **183**:1422, 1981

Shuster S, Black MM: The influence of age and sex on skin thickening, skin collagen and density. *Br J Dermatol* **93**:639, 1975

Silver A et al: The effect of age on human sweating, in *Advances in Biology of the Skin,* vol 6, edited by W Montagna. Oxford, Pergamon Press, 1965, p 129

Smith JG, Davidson EA: Alterations in human dermal connective tissue with age and chronic sun damage. *J Invest Dermatol* **39**:347, 1962

Tsuji T: Ultrastructure of deep wrinkles in the elderly. *J Cutan Pathol* **14**:158, 1987

Urbach E: Beitraege zur einer physiologischen und pathologischen Chemie der Haut. *Zentralbl Haut Geschlictskr* **26**:217, 1929

Young AW: Dermatologic complaints presented by 330 geriatric patients. *Geriatrics* **13**:428, 1958

Albert M. Kligman and Lorraine H. Kligman

Some authorities still believe that the striking alterations in unprotected skin, notably the face and dorsa of the hands, are merely exaggerated manifestations of normal aging.[1] However, the evidence is convincing that photoaging is not simply an acceleration of the inevitable age-dependent alterations. Photoaging denotes the gross and microscopic cutaneous changes that are a consequence of chronic solar radiation. Recent studies demonstrate that this spectrum of changes is often diametrically opposed to that which occurs in intrinsically aged skin.[2,3] Sun worshippers do look prematurely aged and this is the basis for the common misconception. Those who scrupulously avoid the sun can reach the ninth decade with smooth, unblemished skin that shows only mild thinning, loss of elasticity, and a deepening of normal expression lines. By contrast, at age 50, serious sun worshippers, especially those of skin phototype I (blue-eyed, fair skinned, Celtic ancestry who burn easily and tan poorly) have a plethora of wrinkles, with yellowed, lax, dry, leathery, knobby, blotchy skin and a variety of benign, premalignant, and malignant neoplasms.

Late nineteenth century dermatologists, notably Unna and Dubreuilh, clearly recognized the baleful influence of sunlight by comparing the integument of farmers and sailors to that of indoor workers. This was at a time when the leisured class stayed out of the sun. Today, a tan is prized by Caucasians and is ironically equated with health and beauty. Because decades of extensive sun bathing can occur before the photoaging changes become apparent to the naked eye,[4] there is a lack of urgency concerning prevention. This latent period also reinforces the impressions that actinically damaged skin differs only quantitatively from intrinsic aging. However, photoaging has distinctive and unique features that are quite different from normal aging.

Morphologic Changes in Photoaging

Elastosis, an overgrowth of abnormal elastic fibers, is a prototypical feature of actinically damaged skin[4]; it never occurs in the protected skin of even very old healthy persons. During adult life, the quantity of elastic fibers in unexposed skin increases slightly (Fig. 240-1*a*), and there is mild morphologic deteriorioration seen by electron microscopy.[5,6] However, the changes never reach the stage of coarse, tangled accretions of degraded elastic fibers that finally, in severe photoaging, degenerate into an amorphous mass (Fig. 240-1*b*). In actinically damaged skin, the glycosaminoglycans (GAGs) and proteoglycans comprising the ground substance are greatly increased, almost matching fetal skin in this regard. In protected aged skin, GAGs actually decrease.[7]

Photoaging

In the normal aging of unexposed skin, the cells of the dermis are depleted[8]; hypocellularity is the rule. Fibroblasts are scanty and shrunken and mast cells are much more scarce. This contrasts strikingly with photoaging, in which fibroblasts are numerous and hyperplastic.[9] Mast cells are abundant and partially degranulated. Histiocytes and other mononuclear cells are also increased. One might say that photoaged skin is chronically inflamed (Fig. 240-2), a process we have called *heliodermatitis*[9] and others, *dermatoheliosis* (see Chap. 137).

As elastin increases in photoaged skin, collagen proportionately decreases.[7,10] Histologically, a large portion of the dermis becomes occupied with material that was mistakenly believed to be a "basophilic degeneration" of collagen. It is now clearly recognized that this material consists of degraded elastin and microfibrillar proteins to which is bound fibronectin, a glycoprotein of the dermal matrix.[11] The massive loss of collagen and other degenerative matrix changes probably result from the proteases and lymphokines released by the perivenular inflammatory infiltrates, especially the mix of secretory products from degranulating mast cells. In normal aging, collagen, far from disappearing, becomes more stable and resistant to proteolysis.[12] The bundles become larger, forming ropelike structures.[13]

Epidermal thinning, with flattening of the dermal-epidermal junction, is characteristic of intrinsic aging. Again, the opposite holds in photoaging where the epidermis becomes thickened, a response to chronic stimulation.[14] It is only in end-stage photoaging that epidermal atrophy occurs. Acanthosis in photoaging is accompanied by cellular atypia, loss of polarity, and marked irregularities in cell size and staining properties. Melanocytes increase in size and number, whereas Langerhans cells decrease and become less functional.[15,16] In vitro, it has been shown that keratinocytes from photodamaged skin have a shorter lifespan than those from protected skin.[17] It is in this deranged milieu that various neoplasms arise, such as solar lentigines, seborrheic keratoses, keratoacanthomas, and actinic keratoses. Aside from malignant melanoma, tumors such as basal cell epitheliomas, squamous cell carcinomas, and lentigo maligna melanomas arise almost exclusively on actinically damaged skin of the face and dorsal hands and forearms. With the exception of senile (cherry) angiomas, which occur on the trunk area in nearly all aged persons, sometimes by the dozens, practically all of the important tumors that come to the attention of dermatologists originate in photoaged skin.

Finally, actinic radiation is exceedingly damaging to the microcirculation.[18] Many vessels are completely obliterated. The few that survive are variably dilated and scraggly; the normal horizontal plexuses are extinguished (Fig. 240-3*a*, -3*b*). Ultrastructurally, it has been demonstrated that vascular basement membranes are

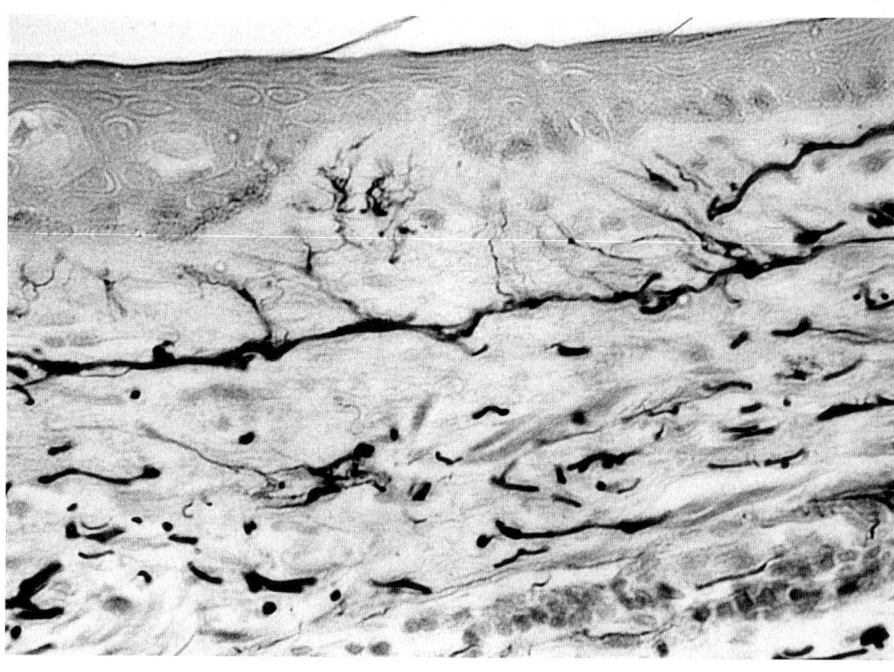

a

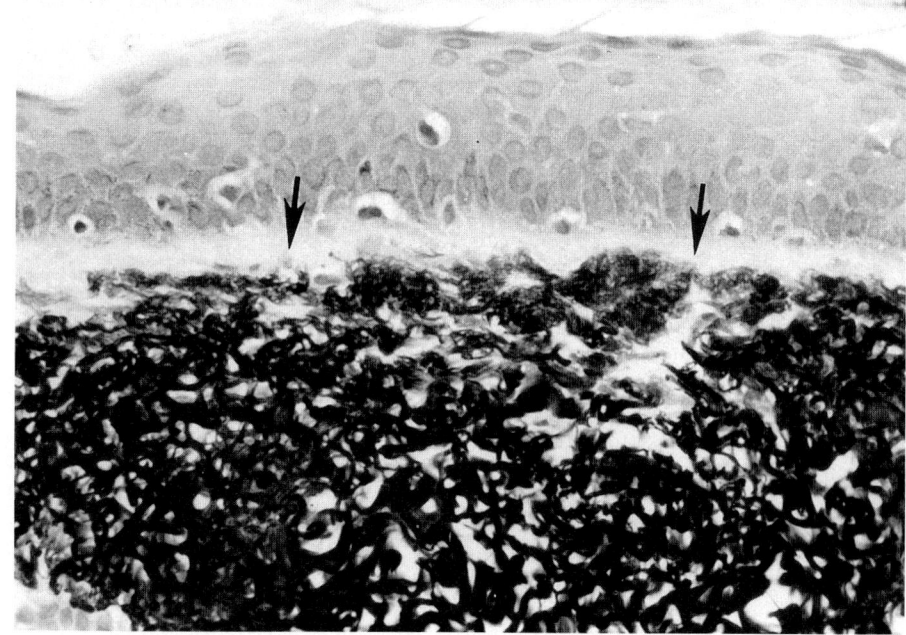

b

FIGURE 240-1 (*a*) Intrinsically aged skin. Protected abdominal skin from an 80-year-old woman shows a moderate increase and thickening of elastic fibers with resorption of most fine subepidermal fibers. The dermal-epidermal junction is flattened and dermal cells are sparse. ×270. (*b*) Photodamaged facial skin. Large masses of deranged elastic fibers characterize solar elastosis. A thin subepidermal grenz zone (arrows) is present, and the epidermis is acanthotic. ×270.

greatly duplicated.[9,19] This does not occur in healthy, intrinsically aged protected skin. In protected skin, however, as in photodamaged skin, there is a considerable deletion of small vessels, especially subepidermally where the capillary loops regress. In contrast to photodamaged skin, the vessels are not dilated or tortuous, and the overall horizontal pattern of vascular plexuses is not greatly disturbed.[20]

Pigmented skin is only partially resistant to the ravages of the sun. Even the most darkly pigmented people have only about a 10-year period of grace with regard to elastosis.[21] Gross appearance is deceiving. Still, neoplasms are rare in the skin of blacks and even Asians.

The Action Spectrum of Photoaging

Past accounts have focused on UVB (280 to 320 nm) as the portion of terrestrial solar radiation responsible for sunburning, dermal changes, and carcinogenesis. Recent experiments show that concern must be extended to UVA (320 to 400 nm). UVA can, like UVB, produce erythema, although a 500 to 1000 times greater dosage is required.[22,23] UVA also contributes, either additively or synergistically, to the sunburning effects of UVB in humans[23,24] and UVB tumorigenesis in animals.[25,26] Large single doses of UVA in humans can damage blood vessels, producing endothelial cell enlargement, vasodilatation, and extravascular infiltrates of neutro-

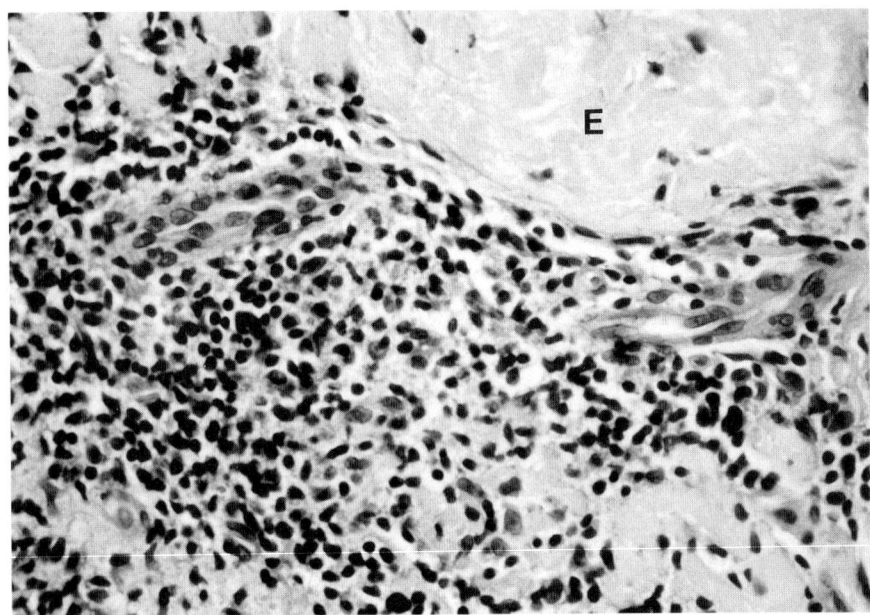

FIGURE 240-2 Marked dermal inflammatory infiltrate associated with the heliodermatitis (dermatoheliosis) that is characteristic of ongoing and chronic actinic exposure. E, epidermis. ×270.

phils.[27] Chronic exposure of hairless mice to long-wavelength UVA (>340 nm) also results in vascular damage that includes excessive duplication of basement membranes, endothelial cell cytoplasmic vacuolization, thinning, gap formation, and mitochondrial damage.[28] Exploration of the multiple effects of chronic UV exposure has been greatly aided by the hairless mouse model for photoaging.[29] It has been shown that in addition to the induction of elastosis by UVB, both the shorter (320 to 340 nm: UVA II) and longer (340 to 400 nm: UVA I) wavelength portions of UVA can produce elastosis, given a high enough dose.[30,31] The action spectrum for elastosis has been shown to be similar to that for a number of acute UV-induced damages, including erythema. As expected, UVB is the most damaging waveband because it is more energetic.[32] However, unlike clinical erythema, which requires up to a thousandfold more UVA than UVB, a 50 percent increase in elastic fibers requires only 20 times more full-spectrum UVA than UVB, but UVB is capable of producing more severe ultrastructural damage to elastic fibers than is UVA.[28,33]

As knowledge develops from experimental animal studies, it becomes increasingly evident that the UV solar spectrum does not fully account for photoaging. Sunlight is, of course, polychromatic, extending into the visible (400 to 700 nm), infrared (IR) (700 to 1,000,000 nm) and, ultimately, radiowaves. The latter can probably be ignored with regard to skin. Visible light, seemingly innocuous, has been known to cause deleterious effects ranging from phototoxic reactions[34] and solar urticaria in susceptible persons[35] to DNA cross-links[36] and UVB tumor enhancement in animals.[37]

IR radiation is inseparably linked to sunlight. Historically, heat-induced skin cancers have long been known in China, India, and Japan. In northern regions of these countries, various devices ranging from hot bricks to pots of burning coal have been used in contact with skin to maintain body warmth.[38] The peat fires of rural Ireland are also implicated in heat-induced cancers.[39] In most of these cases, hydrocarbons are a likely co-carcinogen. Long recognized as an etiologic factor in erythema ab igne, IR radiation produces a typical reticulated pattern of pigmentation of the skin's surface that is a reflection of the underlying dilated, leaking blood vessels. In addition, heat produces many changes highly reminis-

cent of actinic damage, including elastosis (Fig. 240-4), telangiectasia, marked epidermal atypia, and keratoses, some of which advance to squamous cell carcinomas. IR radiation has also been shown to enhance UVB elastosis experimentally in guinea pigs.[40] Erythema ab igne differs from photoaged skin in having deposits of hemosiderin and in not showing the final amorphous stage of elastosis.

The Biochemistry and Immunochemistry of Photoaging

Early biochemical studies on photoaged human skin demonstrated increases in GAGs with a corresponding loss of insoluble collagen and an increase in soluble collagen.[7] The availability of sufficient quantities of human skin has limited research in this area. However, in two recent studies, both acid-soluble (newly synthesized, non-cross-linked) and pepsin-soluble (partially cross-linked) collagen have been reported to be decreased in photodamaged skin.[10] Pepsin-insoluble collagen was not examined. Although it has been reported that type III collagen is increased in photodamaged skin,[41] this was not confirmed in a more recent study.[10] A similar discrepancy is seen for fibronectin in immunofluorescence studies. Chen et al.[11] have reported large amounts of fibronectin associated with elastosis, but Oikarinen and Kallioinen[10] reported no increase. Because methodologies vary and especially because the degree of chronic sun exposure is difficult to estimate in humans, much more work will be needed before these discrepancies can be resolved.

Several studies using UV-exposed hairless mice have appeared recently.[29] Unfortunately, divergent results have been reported, again largely due to different methodologies and different cumulative UV doses. However, in these cases the doses administered are known. It has become possible to begin to separate out some of the differing effects of UVA and UVB. By examining biochemical changes in collagen over time, Kligman et al.[42] found that with chronic UVB exposure total collagen increased until week 20, after which loss occurred. This result mirrored the early histo-

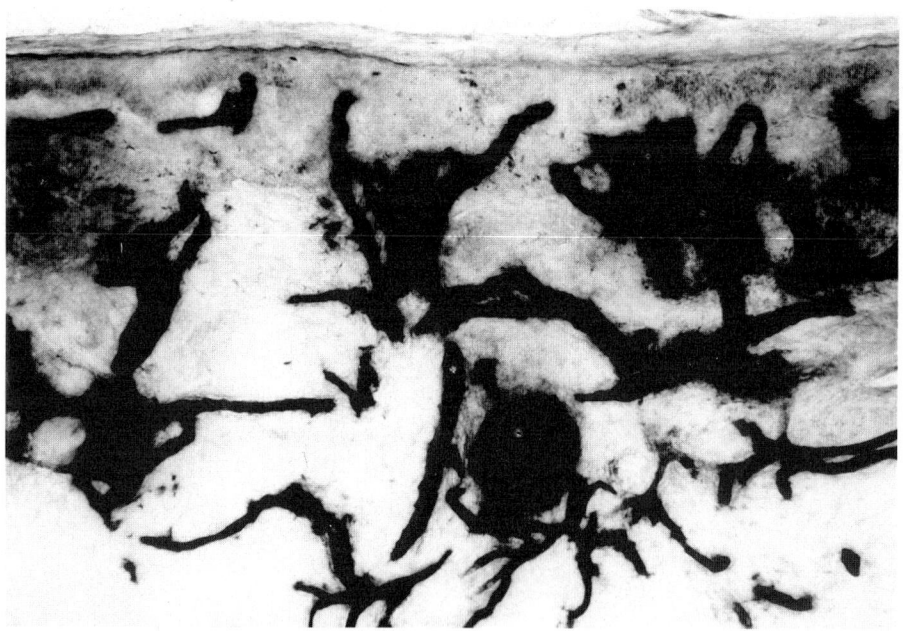

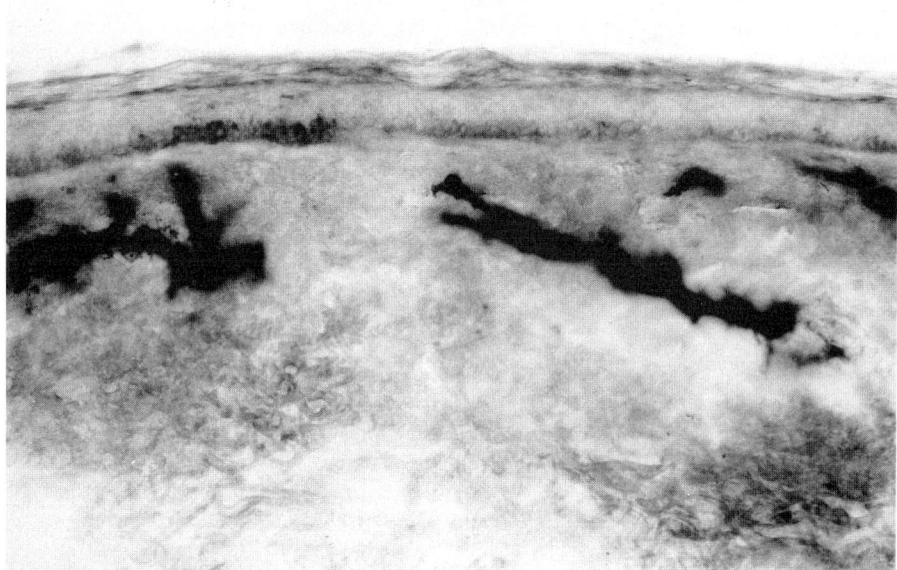

FIGURE 240-3 (*a*) Seen grossly as telangiectases, the vessels in photodamaged skin are dilated and tortuous, histologically. ×112.5. (*b*) In end-stage, severe photoaging there is massive deletion of vessels. ×112.5.

logic thickening of the upper dermis and the later loss of affinity for collagen-specific stains. Also in a time-course experiment, Plastow et al.[43] found an increase in type III collagen relative to type I. This change in ratio was not confirmed by Kligman et al.[42] or by Schwartz et al.[44] Immunochemical determination and radioimmunoassay have demonstrated that UVB radiation actually caused a loss of the aminopropeptide moiety of type III procollagen.[44] Photoaging alterations in other components of the dermal connective tissue were examined by Schwartz.[45] Immunofluorescence, biochemical, and ELISA assays showed increases in elastin, microfibrillar proteins, GAGs, and fibronectin after chronic UVB exposure of hairless mice.

The most recent biochemical studies have centered on the effects of UVA radiation on hairless mouse collagen. After only a few low-dose exposures, Johnston et al.[46] reported a reduction in prolyl hydroxylase activity. UVB had no effect on this enzyme, which is involved in posttranslational modification of nascent collagen chains. Chronic UVA radiation appears to increase significantly the resistance of collagen to digestion by pepsin.[47,48] Compared to UVB-irradiated hairless mouse skin in which 85 to 100 percent of the collagen can be digested, both full-spectrum (320 to 400 nm) and long-wavelength UVA (>340 nm) render up to 85 percent of the collagen indigestible. This phenomenon is UVA dose dependent and may be the result of increased cross-linking of the collagen.[47] Similar effects on collagen solubility have been found in intrinsically aged human skin.[49] Total collagen content of mouse skin also decreased in a UVA dose-related fashion, perhaps related to the reduced prolyl hydroxylase activity reported by Johnston et

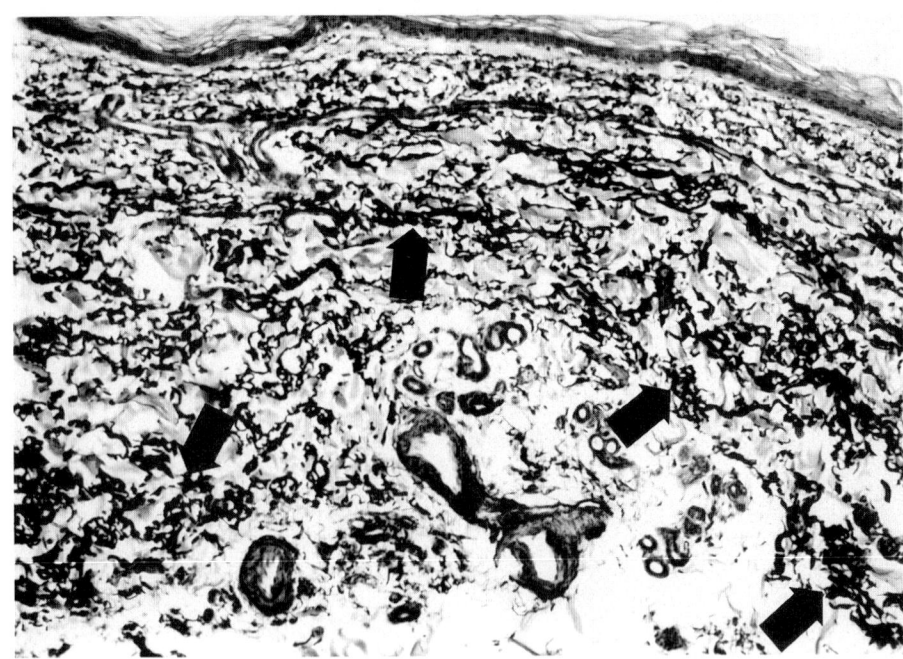

FIGURE 240-4 The deep elastosis (arrows) of infrared radiation-induced erythema ab igne. ×75.

al.[46] Fourtanier et al.[50] also found a decrease in total collagen after chronic exposure to full-spectrum UVA but not after long-wavelength UVA.

Protection Against Photoaging

Sunscreens have been demonstrated to be effective in preventing acute erythema in humans. Their efficacy against chronic UV exposure, of necessity, has to be assessed in animal models. As expected, high sun protection factors (SPFs) are more effective than low SPFs. An SPF 15 sunscreen, when applied prior to each UVB exposure, completely prevented the histologic photoaging changes induced by repeated exposure to six minimal erythema doses (MEDs).[51] Another study mimicked the human use of sunscreens in that the sunscreens were applied after varying degrees of photodamage had been produced. Sunscreens not only prevented further damage despite continued UVB radiation, but notably allowed partial reversal of the photodamage.[52] The durability of sunscreen protection was tested in a chronic study by Bissett et al.[53] The highest degree of protection was found when the sunscreen was applied 0 to 4 h prior to UVB exposure. If 6 to 8 h elapsed before exposure, protection was significantly reduced. Plastow et al.[43] found that sunscreens applied prior to each UVB exposure prevented their reported increased ratio of types III/I collagen. Broad-spectrum sunscreens (SPF 15) also prevent UVA-induced histologic photodamage in hairless mouse skin.[54] Another study[55] indicated that the addition of a UVA absorber to an SPF 2 sunscreen increased protection against chronic suberythemal doses of full-spectrum solar-simulating radiation (UVB + UVA) compared to a UVB screen alone. Histologic and collagen biochemical changes were reduced, suggesting that even short-term casual exposure, as opposed to deliberate sunbathing, may require broad-spectrum protection.

There are a number of reports that describe amelioration of photoaging damage in mouse skin by nonsunscreening agents. These protective substances include antioxidants,[56] conjugated hexadienes,[57] anti-inflammatory agents,[58] and iron chelators.[59] For

the most part, these agents were moderately effective against UVB but not against UVA damage. Physical agents such as zinc oxide or titanium dioxide added to sunscreen preparations clearly enhance UVA protection.[60] It is likely that future sunscreens will contain a "cocktail" of these various agents to reduce the effects of the small amounts of radiation that break through the UV absorbers.

Repair of Photoaged Skin

Chronically sun-exposed skin was formerly thought to be irreversibly damaged. Recent studies require a revision of this pessimistic concept. It can be stated categorically that even in the most cruelly sun-damaged skin, dermal repair goes on continuously. The famous subepidermal grenz zone, a zone of sparing from elastotic changes, affords the best evidence of ongoing repair. Long thought of as a "micro-scar" because of the parallel deposition of collagen,[61] the grenz zone is actually an area where new procollagen I is constantly being synthesized.[62] In both humans and animals, discontinuation of radiation or proper protection by sunscreens is followed by widening of the grenz zone.[51,52] As the deposition of new collagen continues, the expanding area of repair, or reconstruction zone, pushes the old elastotic dermis downward, so that a clear line of demarcation separates the newly created collagen from the degraded dermis (Fig. 240-5a, -5b). The collagen bundles in the reconstruction zone are arranged parallel to the surface but should not be regarded as a scar on this account. This zone contains many fibroblasts that are actively synthesizing collagen, as revealed by an expanded cytoplasm filled with widely dilated rough endoplasmic reticulum.[51] Our findings indicate that destruction and repair go on simultaneously under continued assault by actinic radiation. The balance is shifted toward repair when the radiation stress is relieved. Both the epidermis and dermis are capable of moderate self-restoration when exogenous injury ceases.

Thus, it is never too late to advise older persons with actinically damaged skin to protect themselves from the sun. This not only favors repair of damaged dermis but also enables some regres-

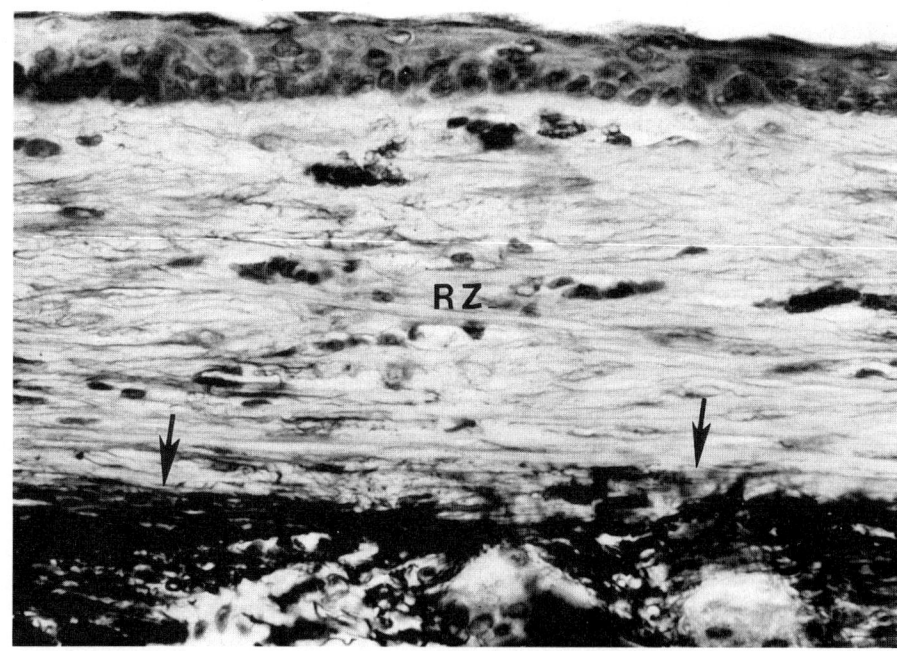

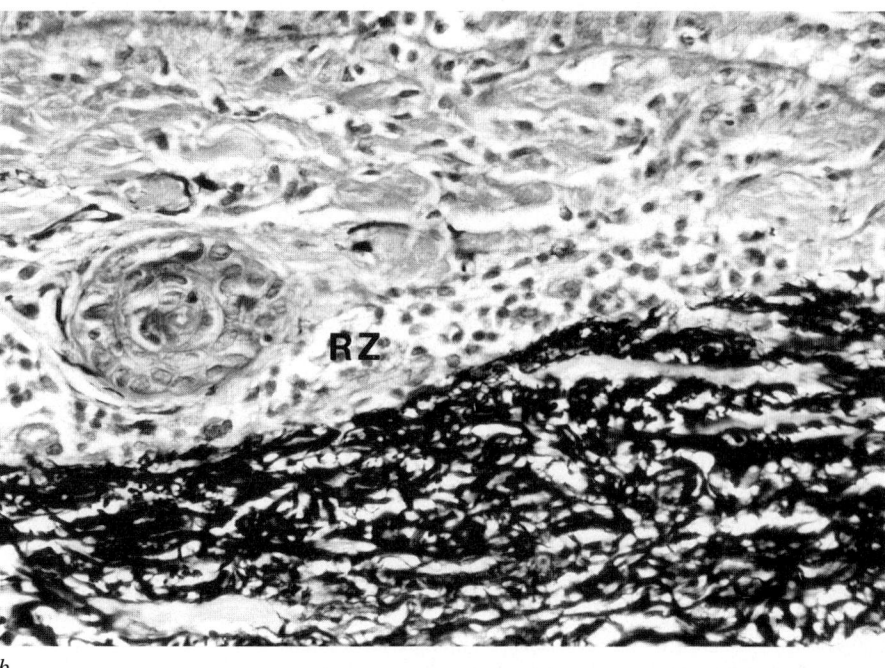

FIGURE 240-5 (*a*) Repair in hairless mouse skin. Fifteen weeks postirradiation, a reconstruction zone (RZ) of new parallel collagen compresses the elastotic fibers into a discrete band (arrows). ×270. (*b*) Repair in human skin. Biopsy from the bald scalp of retired outdoor worker after 10 years of indoor residence in a home for the aged. As in the hairless mouse, a zone (RZ) of new connective tissue has been laid down subepidermally. ×270.

sion of epithelial tumors. Clinicians in sunny areas have long realized that avoidance of sunlight may promote the disappearance of the flatter actinic keratoses.

The normal repair processes in photodamaged skin can be enhanced pharmacologically. Tretinoin (all-*trans*-retinoic acid) was the first to be assessed for this property.[63] Photodamaged hairless mice were treated topically for 10 weeks with tretinoin. In contrast to controls, the reconstruction zone of new collagen was significantly deeper in tretinoin-treated mice, with the enhanced repair being dose and time related.[63] The new collagen was histochemically, ultrastructurally, and biochemically normal.[63,64] As determined by radioimmunoassay, collagen content was increased twofold, and mRNAs for types I and III collagen were increased two-

to threefold in the tretinoin-treated skin.[64] Immunofluorescence techniques located the new collagen synthesis in the histologically defined reconstruction zone and also showed the presence of new elastin and increased fibronectin in the region.[65] Isotretinoin (13-*cis*-retinoic acid) has also been demonstrated to enhance dermal repair in mice.[66] This repair activity remains retinoid-specific.

Studies on the effects of tretinoin on human photoaging have now progressed long enough to show dermal repair in addition to the earlier reported improvement in wrinkles, roughness, epidermal atypia, and pigmented lentigines.[67,68] Angiogenesis is stimulated,[67] anchoring fibrils at the dermal-epidermal junction are increased,[69] and, after 2 to 5 years of treatment, a reconstruction zone of new collagen can be demonstrated.[70]

References

1. Montagna W, Carlisle K: Structural changes in aging human skin. *J Invest Dermatol* **73**:47, 1979

2. Balin AK, Kligman AM (eds): *Aging and the Skin.* New York, Raven, 1989, p 1

3. Gilchrest BA: *Skin and Aging Processes.* Boca Raton, FL, CRC Press, 1984, p 97

4. Kligman AM: Early destructive effects of sunlight on human skin. *JAMA* **210**:2377, 1969

5. Lavker RM: Structural alterations in exposed and unexposed aged skin. *J Invest Dermatol* **73**:59, 1979

6. Braverman IM, Fonferko E. Studies in cutaneous aging: I. The elastic fiber network. *J Invest Dermatol* **78**:434, 1982

7. Smith JG Jr et al: Alterations in human dermal connective tissue with age and chronic sun damage. *J Invest Dermatol* **39**:347, 1962

8. Andrews W et al: Changes with advancing age in the cell population of the human dermis. *Gerontologica* **10**:1, 1964

9. Lavker RM, Kligman AM: Chronic heliodermatitis: A morphologic evaluation of chronic dermal damage with emphasis on the role of mast cells. *J Invest Dermatol* **90**:325, 1988

10. Oikarinen A, Kallioinen M: A biochemical and immunohistochemical study of collagen in sunexposed and protected skin. *Photodermatology* **6**:24, 1989

11. Chen VL et al: Immunochemistry of elastotic material in sun-damaged skin. *J Invest Dermatol* **87**:334, 1986

12. Bentley JP: Aging of collagen. *J Invest Dermatol* **73**:80, 1979

13. Lavker RM et al: Aged skin: A study by light, transmission electron and scanning electron microscopy. *J Invest Dermatol* **88**:44s, 1987

14. Kligman LH: Photoaging: Manifestations, prevention and treatment, in *Dermatology Clinics,* vol 4, *The Aging Skin,* edited by BA Gilchrest. Philadelphia, Saunders, 1986, p 517

15. Gilchrest BA et al: Effect of chronologic aging and ultraviolet radiation on Langerhans cells in human epidermis. *J Invest Dermatol* **79**:85, 1982

16. Räsänen L et al: Immediate decrease in antigen-presenting function and delayed enhancement of interleukin-1 production in human epidermal cells after in vivo UVB irradiation. *Br J Dermatol* **120**:589, 1989

17. Gilchrest BA: Relationship between actinic damage and chronologic aging in keratinocyte cultures in human skin. *J Invest Dermatol* **72**:219, 1979

18. Kligman AM: Perspectives and problems in cutaneous gerontology. *J Invest Dermatol* **73**:39, 1979

19. Braverman IM, Fonferko E: Studies in cutaneous aging. II. The microvasculature. *J Invest Dermatol* **78**:444, 1982

20. Gilchrest BA et al: Chronologic aging alters the response to ultraviolet-induced inflammation in human skin. *J Invest Dermatol* **79**:11, 1982

21. Kligman AM: Solar elastosis in relation to pigmentation, in *Sunlight and Man: Normal and Abnormal Photobiological Responses,* edited by MA Pathak et al; consulting editor, TB Fitzpatrick. Tokyo, Univ of Tokyo Press, 1974, p 157

22. Kaidbey KH, Kligman AM: Acute effect of long wave ultraviolet irradiation on human skin. *J Invest Dermatol* **72**:253, 1979

23. Ying CY et al: Additive erythemogenic effects of middle (280–320 nm) and long-wave (320–400 nm) ultraviolet light. *J Invest Dermatol* **63**:273, 1974

24. Willis I et al: Effects of long ultraviolet rays on human skin: Photoprotective or photoaugmentative? *J Invest Dermatol* **59**:416, 1973

25. Willis I et al: The rapid induction of cancers in the hairless mouse utilizing the principle of photoaugmentation. *J Invest Dermatol* **76**:604, 1981

26. Kligman LH: UVA enhances low dose UVB tumorigenesis (abstr). *Photochem Photobiol* **47**:8s, 1988

27. Gilchrest BA et al: Histologic changes associated with ultraviolet-A-induced erythema in normal human skin. *J Am Acad Dermatol* **9**:213, 1983

28. Zheng P, Kligman LH: UVA radiation-induced ultrastructural changes in hairless mouse skin: A contrast to UVB-induced damage. *J Invest Dermatol* **96**:584, 1991

29. Kligman LH: The hairless mouse and photoaging: Yearly review. *Photochem Photobiol* **54**:1109, 1991

30. Kligman LH et al: The contributions of UVA and UVB to connective tissue damage in hairless mice. *J Invest Dermatol* **84**:272, 1985

31. Kligman LH et al: Long wavelength (>340 nm) ultraviolet A induced skin damage in hairless mice is dose dependent, in *Human Exposure to Ultraviolet Radiation: Risks and Regulations,* edited by WF Passchier, BFM Bosnjakovic. Amsterdam, Elsevier, 1987, p 77

32. Kligman LH, Sayre RM: An action spectrum for ultraviolet induced elastosis in hairless mice: Quantification of elastosis by image analysis. *Photochem Photobiol* **53**:237, 1991

33. Hirose R, Kligman LH: An ultrastructural study of ultraviolet-induced elastic fiber damage in hairless mouse skin. *J Invest Dermatol* **90**:697, 1988

34. Kaidbey KH, Kligman AM: Identification of topical photosensitizing agents in humans: *J Invest Dermatol* **70**:149, 1978

35. Harber LC, Bickers DR: Solar urticaria, in *Photosensitivity Diseases: Principles of Diagnosis and Treatment,* edited by LC Harber, DR Bickers. Philadelphia, Saunders, 1981, p 160

36. Gantt R et al: Visible light induces DNA crosslinks in cultured mouse and human cells. *Biochim Biophys Acta* **565**:231, 1970

37. Griffin AC et al: The effects of visible light on carcinogenicity of ultraviolet light. *Cancer Res* **10**:523, 1955

38. Kligman LH, Kligman AM: Reflections on heat. *Br J Dermatol* **110**:369, 1984

39. Cross F: On a turf (peat) fire cancer: Malignant change superimposed on erythema ab igne. *Proc R Soc Med* **60**:1307, 1967

40. Kligman LH: Intensification of ultraviolet induced dermal damage by infrared radiation. *Arch Dermatol Res* **272**:229, 1982

41. Lovell CR et al: Collagen and elastin in actinic elastosis (abstr). *J Invest Dermatol* **82**:566, 1984

42. Kligman LH et al: Collagen metabolism in ultraviolet irradiated hairless mouse skin and its correlation to histologic observations. *J Invest Dermatol* **93**:210, 1989

43. Plastow SR et al: Early changes in dermal collagen of mice exposed to chronic UVB irradiation and the effects of a UVB sunscreen. *J Invest Dermatol* **91**:590, 1988

44. Schwartz E et al: Alterations in dermal collagen in ultraviolet irradiated hairless mice. *J Invest Dermatol* **93**: 142, 1989

45. Schwartz E: Connective tissue alterations in the skin of ultraviolet irradiated hairless mice. *J Invest Dermatol* **91**:158, 1988

46. Johnston KJ et al: Ultraviolet radiation induced connective tissue changes in the skin of hairless mice. *J Invest Dermatol* **82**:587, 1984

47. Trautinger F et al: Influence of UV radiation on dermal collagen content in hairless mice (abstr). *Arch Dermatol Res* **281**:144, 1989

48. Kligman LH, Gebre M: Biochemical changes in hairless mouse skin collagen after chronic exposure to UVA radiation. *Photochem Photobiol* **54**:233, 1991

49. Schnider SL, Kohn RR: Effects of age and diabetes mellitus on the solubility of collagen from human skin, tracheal cartilage and dura mater. *Exp Gerontol* **17**:185, 1982

50. Fourtanier A et al: In vivo evaluation of photoprotection against chronic ultraviolet-A irradiation by a new sunscreen Mexoryl SX. *Photochem Photobiol* **55**:549, 1992

51. Kligman LH et al: Prevention of ultraviolet damage to the dermis of hairless mice by sunscreens. *J Invest Dermatol* **78**:181, 1982

52. Kligman LH et al: Sunscreens promote repair of ultraviolet radiation-induced dermal damage. *J Invest Dermatol* **81**:98, 1983

53. Bissett DL et al: Time-dependent decrease in sunscreen protection against chronic photodamage in UVB-irradiated hairless mouse skin. *Photochem Photobiol* **9**:323, 1991

54. Kligman LH, Dromgoole S: The effects of UVA radiation on hairless

mouse skin: Are broad spectrum sunscreens protective enough (abstr)? *Photochem Photobiol* **51**:9s, 1990

55. Harrison JA et al: Sunscreens with low sun protection factor inhibit ultraviolet A and B photoaging in the skin of hairless mice. *Photodermatol Photoimmunol Photomed* **8**:12, 1991

56. Bissett DL et al: Photoprotective effect of superoxide-scavenging antioxidants against ultraviolet-induced chronic skin damage in hairless mice. *Photodermatol Photoimmunol Photomed* **7**:56, 1990

57. Bissett DL et al: Photoprotective effect of topically applied conjugated hexadienes against ultraviolet radiation-induced chronic skin damage in the hairless mouse. *Photodermatol Photoimmunol Photomed* **7**:63, 1990

58. Bissett DL et al: Photoprotective effect of topical anti-inflammatory agents against ultraviolet radiation-induced chronic skin damage in the hairless mouse. *Photodermatol Photoimmunol Photomed* **7**:153, 1990

59. Bissett DL et al: Chronic ultraviolet radiation-induced increase in skin iron and the photoprotective effect of topically applied iron chelators. *Photochem Photobiol* **54**:215, 1991

60. Roelandts R: Which components in broad-spectrum sunscreens are most necessary for adequate UVA protection? *J Am Acad Dermatol* **25**:999, 1991

61. Serri F et al: Studies on the pathomechanics of chronic actinic dermatosis, in *Research in Photobiology,* edited by A Castellani. New York, Plenum, 1977, p 547

62. Fleischmajer R et al: Immunofluorescence analysis of collagen, fibronectin and basement membrane protein in scleroderma skin. *J Invest Dermatol* **75**:270, 1980

63. Kligman LH et al: Topical retinoic acid enhances the repair of ultraviolet damaged dermal connective tissue. *Connect Tissue Res* **12**:139, 1984

64. Schwartz E et al: Topical all-*trans* retinoic acid stimulates collagen synthesis in vivo. *J Invest Dermatol* **96**:975, 1991

65. Kligman LH et al: Quantitative assessment of elastin and fibronectin in tretinoin treated photoaged hairless mouse skin (abstr). *J Invest Dermatol* **94**:543, 1990

66. Kim et al: Effect of topical retinoic acids on the levels of collagen mRNA during the repair of UVB-induced dermal damage in the hairless mouse and the possible role of TGF-β as a mediator. *J Invest Dermatol* **98**:359, 1992

67. Kligman AM et al: Topical tretinoin for photoaged skin. *J Am Acad Dermatol* **15**:836, 1986

68. Weiss JS et al: Topical tretinoin improves photoaged skin: A double-blind, vehicle-controlled study. *JAMA* **259**:527, 1988

69. Woodley DT et al: Treatment of photoaged skin with topical tretinoin increases epidermal-dermal anchoring fibrils: A preliminary report. *JAMA* **263**:3057, 1990

70. Kligman AM, Graham GF: Histologic changes in facial skin after daily application of tretinoin for 5–6 years. *J Dermatol Treat,* in press

Note: Page numbers in **boldface** indicate major discussions; page numbers followed by the letter t or f indicate tables or figures, respectively.

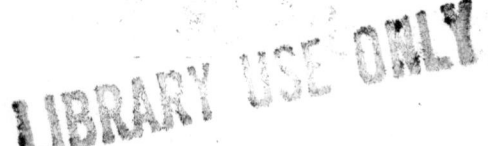

$245.00

2 vol set